The Johns Hopkins Manual of Cardiothoracic Surgery

Notice

The Johns Hopkins Manual of Cardiothoracic Surgery

David D. Yuh, MD, FACC

Associate Professor of Surgery, Division of Cardiac Surgery
Associate Professor, Center for Computer-Integrated Surgical Systems
The Johns Hopkins Hospital and Whiting School of Engineering
Johns Hopkins University
Baltimore, Maryland

Luca A. Vricella, MD, FACS

Assistant Professor of Surgery
Director, Pediatric Heart Transplantation
Division of Cardiac Surgery
The Johns Hopkins Medical Institutions
Baltimore, Maryland

William A. Baumgartner, MD

Vincent L. Gott Professor of Surgery
Chief, Division of Cardiac Surgery
Department of Surgery
The Johns Hopkins Medical Institutions
Baltimore, Maryland

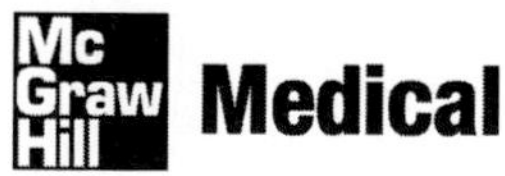

New York Chicago San Francisco Lisbon London Madrid
Mexico City Milan New Delhi San Juan Seoul Singapore Sydney Toronto

The McGraw-Hill Companies

The Johns Hopkins Manual of Cardiothoracic Surgery

1234567890 CCW/CCW 09876

ISBN-13: 978-0-07-141652-8
ISBN-10: 0-07-141652-8

This book was set in Galliard by TechBooks.
The editors were Joseph Rusko, Christie Naglieri, and Lester Sheinis.
The production supervisor was Phil Galea.
The cover was designed by Pehrsson Design.
The indexer was Alexandra Nickerson.
Courier Westford was printer and binder.

This book is printed on acid-free paper.

Library of Congress Cataloging-in-Publication Data

The Johns Hopkins manual of cardiothoracic surgery / edited by David D. Yuh, Luca A. Vricella, William Baumgartner. – 1st ed.
p., cm.
Includes bibliographical references and index.
ISBN 0-07-141652-8 (Hardcover)
1. Heart—Surgery—Handbooks, manuals, etc. 2. Chest—Surgery—Handbooks, manuals, etc. 3. Cardiovascular system—Surgery—Handbooks, manuals, etc. I. Yuh, David D. (David Daiho) II. Vricella, Luca A. III. Baumgartner, William A. IV. Title: Manual of cardiothoracic surgery.
[DNLM: 1. Cardiac Surgical Procedures—methods. 2. Thoracic Surgical Procedures—methods. WF 980 J66 2006]
RD598.J64 2006
617.89059—dc22

2006044913

DEDICATION

To my wife and best friend, Dr. Bonnie Hiatt, who allows me to forget my troubles for the day through humor, commiseration, and irreverence. A constant source of inspiration to become a better person, I will be forever indebted to her.

David D. Yuh, MD

To my wonderful Family, for the endless sacrifices, love and support.

Luca A. Vricella, MD

I wish to dedicate this book to my wife, Betsy, who has been my partner and primary support for over 40 years. She has allowed me the time to carry out many important activities such as this book.

William A. Baumgartner, MD

CONTENTS

PART III

CONGENITAL CARDIAC SURGERY

CONTRIBUTORS

Nelson Alphonso, FRCS
Consultant Paediatric Cardiac Surgeon
Alder Hey Royal Children Hospital
Liverpool, United Kingdom
Valvular Disease in Children

Robert H. Anderson, BSc, MD, FRCPath
Joseph Levy Professor of Paediatric Cardiac Morphology
Honorary Consultant
Great Ormond Street Hospital Cardiac Unit
Institute of Child Health
University College of London
London, United Kingdom
The Anatomy of Congenital Cardiac Malformations

Paolo Arciprete, MD
Department of Pediatric Cardiac Surgery
Giovanni XXIII Hospital
Bari, Italy
Atrial Septal Defects and Partial Anomalous Venous Connection

Constantine L. Athanasuleas, MD
The Norwood Clinic
Birmingham, Alabama
Myocardial Protection

Peter Attia, MD
Resident
Department of Surgery
Johns Hopkins Hospital
Baltimore, Maryland
Mediastinal Disease

Norbert Augustin, MD
Chair, Department of Cardiac Sciences
Sheihk Kalifa Medical Center
Abu Dhabi
United Arab Emirates
Ebstien's Anomaly

Anthony Azakie, MD, CM
Associate Professor of Surgery and Pediatrics
Pediatric Heart Center
University of California San Francisco
San Francisco, California
Aortopulmonary Window

Harris Baden, MD
Chief, Cardiac Intensive Care
Children's Hospital and Regional Medical Center
Assistant Professor of Pediatrics
University of Washington School of Medicine
Seattle, Washington
Extra-Corporeal Membrane Oxygenation in Pediatric Cardiac Care

Leonard L. Bailey, MD
Professor and Chair, Department of Surgery
Division of Cardiothoracic Surgery
Loma Linda University
Loma Linda, California
Pediatric Cardiac Transplant

Luigi Ballerini, MD
Consultant Pediatric Cardiologist
Department of Pediatric Cardiology and Cardiac Surgery
Ospedale Pediatrico Bambino Gesu'
Rome, Italy
Tetralogy of Fallot

Farzaneh Banki, MD
Fellow
Cardiothoracic Surgery
Division of Cardiothoracic Surgery
University of Washington
Seattle, Washington
Congenital Anomalies of the Coronary Arteries

Anshuman Bansal, BS
Research Fellow
Division of Cardiac Surgery
The Johns Hopkins Medical Institutions
Baltimore, Maryland
Reoperative Coronary Artery Bypass Surgery

John R. Barbour, MD
Resident
Department of Surgery
Medical University of South Carolina
Charleston, South Carolina
Aortic Valve Replacement, Aortic Root Replacement

Christopher J. Barreiro, MD
Resident
Johns Hopkins Hospital
Baltimore, Maryland
Reoperative Coronary Artery Bypass Surgery

Ronald D. Berger, MD, PhD
Professor of Medicine and Biomedical Engineering
Division of Cardiology
Johns Hopkins Hospital
Baltimore, Maryland
Pacemaker and Defibrillator Therapy in Cardiac Surgery Patients

Brian T. Bethea, MD
Fellow in Cardiothoracic Surgery
Division of Cardiac Surgery
Johns Hopkins Hospital
Baltimore, Maryland
Cardiac Transplantation

Kenneth C. Bilchick, MD
Fellow in Clinical Cardiac Electrophysiology
Division of Cardiology
Johns Hopkins Hospital
Baltimore, Maryland
Pacemaker and Defibrillator Therapy in Cardiac Surgery Patients

James H. Black, III, MD
Assistant Professor of Surgery
Attending Surgeon
Division of Vascular Surgery
Johns Hopkins Hospital
Baltimore, Maryland
Endovascular Repair of Thoracic Aortic Pathology

David A. Bluemke, MD, PhD
Associate Professor
Clinical Director of MRI
Departments of Radiology and Medicine
Johns Hopkins Hospital
Baltimore, Maryland
Cardiac Magnetic Resonance Imaging

Roger S. Blumenthal, MD, FACC
Associate Professor of Medicine
Director, Preventive Cardiology and the Ciccarone Center for the Prevention of Heart Disease
Division of Cardiology
Johns Hopkins Hospital
Baltimore, Maryland
Postoperative Therapies to Reduce Long-Term Cardiovascular Risk

Pramod Bonde, MD, MS, FRCSC
Research Fellow
Division of Cardiac Surgery
Johns Hopkins Hospital
Baltimore, Maryland
Surgical Management of Hypertrophic Obstructive Cardiomyopathy, Mechanical Support of the Heart

Umar S. Boston, MD
Assistant Professor of Pediatrics and Surgery
Division of Cardiothoracic Surgery
University of Tennessee/Le Bonheur Children's Hospital
Memphis, Tennessee
Double Outlet Right Ventricle

Edward L. Bove, MD
Professor of Surgery and Pediatrics
Chief, Section of Cardiac Surgery
University of Michigan
Ann Arbor, Michigan
Transposition of the Great Arteries

Christian P. Brizard, MD
Associate Professor of Pediatrics
University of Melbourne
Director, Cardiac Surgery Unit
Royal Children's Hospital
Melbourne, Australia
Valvular Disease in Children

Malcolm V. Brock, MD
Associate Professor
Division of Thoracic Surgery
Johns Hopkins Hospital
Baltimore, Maryland
Gastroesophageal Reflux and Primary Esophageal Motility Disorders

Michael M. Brook, MD
Pediatric Heart Center
University of California San Francisco
San Francisco, California
Aortopulmonary Window

Gerald D. Buckberg, MD
Professor
Department of Cardiothoracic Surgery
UCLA Medical Center
Los Angeles, California
Myocardial Protection

Anthony D. Caffarelli, MD
Resident
Department of Surgery
Stanford University Medical Center
Stanford, California
Ascending and Arch Aneurysms of the Aorta

Duke E. Cameron, MD
James T. Dresher Sr., Professor of Surgery and Pediatrics
Director, Pediatric Cardiac Surgery
Division of Cardiac Surgery
Johns Hopkins Hospital
Baltimore, Maryland
Milestones in Congenital Heart Surgery

David C. Chang, PhD
Research Associate
Department of Surgery
Johns Hopkins Hospital
Baltimore, Maryland
Thoracic Trauma

Richard E. Chinnock, MD
Director, Pediatric Heart Transplant Program
Loma Linda University Children's Hospital
Professor and Chair
Department of Pediatrics
Loma Linda University
Loma Linda, California
Pediatric Cardiac Transplantation

Michael A. Coady, MD, MPH
Assistant Professor
Director of Cardiac Transplantation
Section of Cardiothoracic Surgery
Yale University School of Medicine
New Haven, Connecticut
Chest Wall Tumors, Mechanical Complications of Myocardial Infarction

Gordon A. Cohen, MD, PhD
Chief, Pediatric Cardiac Surgery
Children's Hospital & Regional Medical Center
Associate Professor of Surgery
University of Washington
Seattle, Washington
Palliative Operations for Congenital Heart Disease, Truncus Arteriosus, Extra-Corporeal Membrane Oxygenation in Pediatric Cardiac Care, Surgery for Left Ventricular Outflow Tract Obstruction in Children, Congenital Anomalies of the Coronary Arteries

Paul M. Colombani, MD
Robert Garrett Professor of Pediatric Surgery
Children's Surgeon-in-Charge
Johns Hopkins Hospital
Baltimore, Maryland
Congenital Chest Wall Anomalies

John V. Conte, MD
Associate Director Division of Cardiac Surgery
Associate Professor of Surgery
Director of Heart and Lung Transplantation
Johns Hopkins Hospital
Baltimore, Maryland
Mechanical Support of the Heart, Surgical Ventricular Remodeling

Andrew C. Cook BSc, PhD
BHF Lecturer in Cardiac Morphology
Cardiac Unit
Institute of Child Health
University College
London, United Kingdom
The Anatomy of Congenital Cardiac Malformations

Antonio F. Corno, MD, FRCS, FACC, FETCS
Clinical Lecturer
University of Liverpool
Consultant Pediatric Cardiac Surgeon
Alder Hey Royal Children Hospital—NHS Trust
Liverpool, United Kingdom
Ebstein's Anomaly

Edward E. Cornwell, III, MD, FACS, FCCM
Professor of Surgery
Chief, Adult Trauma Service
Johns Hopkins Hospital
Baltimore, Maryland
Thoracic Trauma

Geoffrey Cousins, MD
Fellow in Cardiothoracic Surgery
Division of Cardiothoracic Surgery
Virginia Commonwealth University
Richmond, Virginia
Surgical Management of Bullous Emphysema and Spontaneous Pneumothorax

Giancarlo Crupi, MD
Attending Pediatric Cardiac Surgeon
Ospedali Riuniti
Bergamo, Italy
Cor Triatriatum

Francois Dagenais, MD
Associate Professor
Department of Cardiac Surgery
Laval Hospital
Quebec, Canada
Minimally Invasive Cardiac Surgery

Ryan R. Davies, MD
Chief Resident
Department of Surgery
Columbia University Medical Center
New York, NY
Mechanical Complications of Myocardial Infarction

Abe DeAnda Jr., MD
Associate Professor and Director
Aortic Surgery
Montefiore Medical Center
Albert Einstein College of Medicine
Bronx, New York
Pericardial Disease

Joseph A. Dearani, MD
Associate Professor of Surgery
Division of Cardiovascular Surgery
Mayo Clinic College of Medicine
Rochester, Minnesota
Double Outlet Right Ventricle

Marc R. de Leval
Professor of Cardiothoracic Surgery
Cardiac Unit
Great Ormond Street Hospital for Children—NHS Trust
London, United Kingdom
Tricuspid Atresia and the Functionally Single Ventricle

Steven R. DeMeester, MD
Associate Professor
Department of Cardiothoracic Surgery
University of Southern California
Los Angeles, California
Esophageal Perforation

Eric J. Devaney, MD
Assistant Professor of Surgery
Division of Pediatric Cardiac Surgery
University of Michigan
Ann Arbor, Michigan
Transposition of the Great Arteries

Duccio Di Carlo, MD
Staff Pediatric Cardiac Surgeon
Department of Pediatric Cardiology and Cardiac Surgery
Ospedale Pediatrico Bambino Gesu'
Rome, Italy
Tetralogy of Fallot

Maria Cristina Digilio, MD,
Medical Genetics
Ospedale Pediatrico Bambino Gesu'
Rome, Italy
Tetralogy of Fallot

Jeffrey M. Dodd-O, MD
Assistant Professor of Anesthesiology
Department of Anesthesiology
Johns Hopkins Hospital
Baltimore, Maryland
Cardiovascular Function and Physiology

John R. Doty, MD
Staff Surgeon
Division of Cardiovascular and Thoracic Surgery
LDS Hospital
Salt Lake City, Utah
Mitral Valve Disease

Yves d'Udekem d'Acoz, MD
Associate Professor of Pediatrics
University of Melbourne
Consultant Cardiac Surgeon
Cardiac Surgery Unit
Royal Children's Hospital
Melbourne, Australia
Valvular Disease in Children

Gan Dunnington, Jr. MD
Department of Cardiothoracic Surgery
Stanford University Medical Center
Stanford, California
Ventricular Assist Devices in Children

Daniel J. Durand, MD
Resident
Department of Radiology
Johns Hopkins Hospital
Baltimore, Maryland
Management of Concomitant Carotid and Coronary Artery Disease

David Efron, MD
Assistant Professor
Department of Surgery
Johns Hopkins Hospital
Baltimore, Maryland
Thoracic Trauma

John A. Elefteriades, MD
Professor and Chairman
Section of Cardiothoracic Surgery
Yale New Haven Hospital
Yale University School of Medicine
New Haven, Connecticut
Pacing of the Diaphragm

Martin J. Elliott, MD, FRCS
Professor of Cardiothoracic Surgery
Chairman, Cardiac Unit
Great Ormond Street Hospital for Sick Children—NHS Trust
London, United Kingdom
Atrioventricular Septal Defects

Nauder Faraday, MD
Associate Professor
Department of Anesthesiology & Critical Care
Medicine and Surgery
Co-Director
Cardiac Surgical
Intensive Care Unit
Johns Hopkins Hospital
Baltimore, Maryland
Coagulation and Hemostasis, Postoperative Management of the Cardiac Surgical Patient

Micah Fisher, MD
Fellow in Pulmonology
Department of Pulmonology
Johns Hopkins Hospital
Baltimore, Maryland
Benign Diffuse Pulmonary Disorders

Torin P. Fitton, MD
Fellow in Cardiothoracic Surgery
Division of Cardiac Surgery
Johns Hopkins Hospital
Baltimore, Maryland
Lung Carcinoma, Congenital Anomalies of the Sinuses of Valsalva and Aortico-Left Ventricular Tunnel

Charles D. Fraser Jr., MD
Donovan Chair and Chief
Division of Congenital Heart Surgery
Texas Children's Hospital
Professor of Surgery and Pediatrics
Baylor College of Medicine
Adjunct Professor
Department of Bioengineering
Rice University
Houston, Texas
Ventricular Septal Defects

Amy Gallo, MD
Resident, Department of Surgery
Yale University School of Medicine
New Haven, Connecticut
Chest Wall Tumors

Michael K. Gibson, MD
Assistant Professor of Oncology
The Sidney Kimmel Comprehensive Cancer Center
at Johns Hopkins
Upper Aerodigestive Group
Johns Hopkins University
Baltimore, Maryland
Neoadjuvant and Primary Chemoradiation Strategies in the Treatment of Esophageal Cancer

Ty J. Gluckman, MD
Fellow in Cardiology
Division of Cardiology
Johns Hopkins Hospital
Baltimore, Maryland
Postoperative Therapies to Reduce Long-Term Cardiovascular Risk

Allan Goldman, MD
Chief Paediatric Cardiac Intensive Care Unit
Cardiac Unit
Great Ormond Street Hospital for Children – NHS Trust
London, United Kingdom
Management of the Pediatric Cardiac Surgical Patient

Vincent L. Gott, MD
Professor of Surgery
Division of Cardiac Surgery
Johns Hopkins Hospital
Baltimore, Maryland
Milestones in Congenital Heart Surgery

Peter J. Gruber, MD, PhD
Assistant Professor of Surgery
University of Pennsylvania
Children's Hospital of Philadelphia
Philadelphia, Pennsylvania
Hypoplastic Left Heart Syndrome

Ala' Sami Haddadin, MD
Assistant Professor of Anesthesiology and Critical Care Medicine
Yale University School of Medicine
New Haven, Connecticut
Coagulation and Hemostasis, Postoperative Management of the Cardiac Surgical Patient

Dale G. Hall, MD, FACS
Staff Pediatric Cardiothoracic Surgeon
Mary Bridge/Swedish Pediatric Cardiothoracic Surgery Program
Mary Bridge Children's Hospital
Tacoma, Washington
Vascular Rings and Pulmonary Artery Sling

John W. Hammon, MD
Professor of Cardiothoracic Surgery
Wake Forest University School of Medicine
Winston-Salem, North Carolina
Cardiopulmonary Bypass

Frank L. Hanley, MD
Professor of Cardiothoracic Surgery
Director, Children's Heart Center
Department of Cardiothoracic Surgery
Stanford University School of Medicine
Stanford, California
Pulmonary Atresia With Ventricular Septal Defect and Major Aortopulmonary Collaterals

Nahidh W. Hasaniya, MD, PhD, FACS, FACC
Assistant Professor of Surgery
Division of Cardiothoracic Surgery
Loma Linda University
Loma Linda, California
Pediatric Cardiac Trasnplantation

Richard F. Heitmiller, MD
J.M.T. Finney Chairman of Surgery
Union Memorial Hospital
Baltimore, Maryland
Lung Carcinoma, Surgical Management of Esophageal Cancer

Tain-Yen Hsia, MD
Assistant Professor of Surgery
Children's Heart Program
Medical University of South Carolina
Charleston, South Carolina
Primary Coronary Artery Bypass Surgery, Patent Ductus Arteriosus

S. Adil Husain, MD
Assistant Professor of Surgery and Pediatrics
Congenital Heart Center
University of Florida School of Medicine/ Shands Hospital
Gainesville, Florida
Coarctation of the Aorta and Interrupted Aortic Arch

John S. Ikonomidis, MD, PhD, FRCS(C), FACS
Associate Professor of Surgery
Division of Cardiothoracic Surgery
Medical University of South Carolina
Charleston, South Carolina
Aortic Valve Replacement, Aortic Root Replacement

Stuart W. Jamieson, MB, FRCS
Professor and Chairman
Division of Cardiothoracic Surgery
University of California Medical Center
San Diego, California
Surgical Treatment of Chronic Pulmonary Thromboembolic Disease

Howard Jeffries, MD
Attending Physician
Cardiac Intensive Care Unit
Children's Hospital and Regional Medical Center
Assistant Professor of Pediatrics
University of Washington School of Medicine
Seattle, Washington
Extra-Corporeal Membrane Oxygenation in Pediatric Cardiac Care

Terri L. Jordan, RN, MSN, ACNP
Thoracic Surgery Coordinator
Division of Cardiothoracic Surgery
Virginia Commonwealth University
Richmond, Virginia
Surgical Management of Bullous Emphysema and Spontaneous Pneumothorax

David L. Joyce, MD
Resident
Department of Surgery
Johns Hopkins Hospital
Baltimore, Maryland
Tricuspid Valve Disease

Mazyar Kanani, PhD, FRCS
Cardiac Unit
Great Ormond Street Hospital for Children–NHS Trust
Institute of Child Health
London, United Kingdom
Atrioventricular Septal Defects

Nicholas Kang, FRACS
Consultant Cardiothoracic Surgeon
Green Lane Hospital
Auckland, New Zealand
Total Anomalus Pulmonary Venous Connection

Tom R. Karl, MD
Professor of Surgery and Pediatrics
Chief of Pediatric Cardiac Surgery
UCSF Children's Hospital
San Francisco, California
Aortopulmonary Window

Jon Kiev, MD, FACS
Chief of Thoracic Surgery
Virginia Commonwealth University
Richmond, Virginia
Surgical Management of Bullous Emphysema and Spontaneous Pneumothorax

Edward H. Kincaid, MD
Assistant Professor
Department of Cardiothoracic Surgery
Wake Forest University School of Medicine
Winston-Salem, North Carolina
Cardiopulmonary Bypass

Karen Michiko Kling, MD
Assistant Professor
Division of Pediatric Surgery
Johns Hopkins Hospital
Baltimore, Maryland
Congenital Pulmonary Anomalies

George J. Koullias, MD
Cardiothoracic Surgeon
Research Associate
Section of Cardiothoracic Surgery
Yale New Haven Hospital
Yale University School of Medicine
New Haven, Connecticut
Pacing of the Diaphragm

Hillel Laks, MD
Professor of Surgery
Division of Cardiothoracic Surgery
UCLA School of Medicine
Los Angeles, California
Pulmonary Stenosis and Pulmonary Atresia with Intact Ventricular Septum

Richard A. Lange, MD, FACC
Chief of Clinical Cardiology
E. Cowles Andrus Professor of Cardiology
Division of Cardiology
Johns Hopkins Hospital
Baltimore, Maryland
Postoperative Therapies to Reduce Long-Term Cardiovascular Risk

Rüdiger Lange, MD, PhD
Head, Department of Cardiothoracic Surgery
Deutsches Herzzentrum at the Technische Universität München
Munich, Germany
Ebstein's Anomaly

Joseph LoCicero III, MD
Professor and Chair
Department of Surgery
The University of South Alabama
Mobile, Alabama
Therapies for Benign and Malignant Pleural Diseases

Malcolm J. MacDonald, MD
Clinical Assistant Professor
Department of Cardiothoracic Surgery
Division of Pediatric Cardiac Surgery
Stanford University School of Medicine
Stanford, California
Pulmonary Atresia With Ventricular Septal Defect and Major Aortopulmonary Collaterals

Michael M. Madani, MD, FACS
Assistant Clinical Professor of Surgery
University of California Medical Center
San Diego, California
Surgical Treatment of Chronic Pulmonary Thromboembolic Disease

Carlo F. Marcelletti, MD
Director, Division of Pediatric Cardiac Surgery
ARNAS Ospedale Civico
Palermo, Italy
Congenitally Corrected Transposition

Patrick Mathieu, MD
Department of Cardiac Surgery
Laval Hospital
Quebec, Canada
Minimally Invasive Cardiac Surgery

Douglas J. Mathisen, MD
Hermes C. Grillo Professor of Thoracic Surgery
Harvard Medical School
Visiting Surgeon and Chief
General Thoracic Surgery Unit
Massachusetts General Hospital
Boston, Massachusetts
Tracheal Diseases

Susanna L. Matsen, MD
Resident
Department of Surgery
Johns Hopkins Hospital
Baltimore, Maryland
Endovascular Repair of Thoracic Aortic Pathology

D. Michael McMullan, MD
Attending Cardiac Surgeon
Children's National Medical Center
Washington, District of Columbia
Truncus Arteriosus

Avedis Meneshian, MD
Fellow in Cardiothoracic Surgery
Division of Cardiac Surgery
Johns Hopkins Hospital
Baltimore, Maryland
Surgical Management of Esophageal Cancer

R. Scott Mitchell, MD
Professor, Department of Cardiothoracic Surgery
Stanford University Medical Center
Stanford, California
Ascending and Arch Aneurysms of the Aorta

Fotios Mitropoulos, MD
Visiting Assistant Professor
Division of Cardiothoracic Surgery
UCLA School of Medicine
Los Angeles, California
Pulmonary Stenosis and Pulmonary Atresia with Intact Ventricular Septum

Susan Moffatt-Bruce, MD, PhD
Assistant Professor of Surgery
Division of Cardiothoracic Surgery
Ohio State University Medical Center
Columbus, Ohio
Lung and Heart-Lung Transplantation

Nahush A. Mokadam MD
Chief Resident
Division of Cardiothoracic Surgery
University of Washington Medical Center
Seattle, Washington
Coarctation of the Aorta and Interrupted Aortic Arch

Samia Mora, MD, MHS
Instructor in Medicine
Harvard Medical School
Associate Physician
Brigham and Women's Hospital
Boston, Massachusetts
Echocardiography in Cardiac Surgery

David L.S. Morales, MD
Congenital Heart Surgery
Texas Children's Hospital
Assistant Professor of Surgery
Baylor College of Medicine
Houston, Texas
Ventricular Septal Defects

Achintya Moulick, MD
Attending Cardiac Surgeon
Children's National Medical Center
Washington, District of Columbia
Congenital Anomalies of the Sinuses of Valsalva and Aortico-Left Ventricular Tunnel

Firas F. Mussa, MD
Fellow, Division of Vascular Surgery and Endovascular Therapy
Michael E DeBakey Department of Surgery
Baylor College of Medicine
Houston, Texas
Esophageal Perforation

Cho Ng, MD
Consultant Pediatric Intensivist
Cardiac Unit
Great Ormond Street Hospital for Children – NHS Trust
London, United Kingdom
Management of the Pediatric Cardiac Surgical Patient

Lois U. Nwakanma, MD
Research Fellow
Division of Cardiac Surgery
Johns Hopkins Hospital
Baltimore, Maryland
Thoracic Infections

Salvatore Ocello, MD
Associate Pediatric Cardiac Surgeon
Division of Cardiac Surgery
ARNAS Ospedale Civico
Palermo, Italy
Congenitally Corrected Transposition

Richard G. Ohye, MD
Assistant Professor of Surgery
Division of Pediatric Cardiovascular Surgery
University of Michigan
Ann Arbor, Michigan
Transposition of the Great Arteries

Eric A. Okum, MD
Assistant Professor
Division of Cardiothoracic Surgery
Rush-Presbyterian Medical Center
Chicago, Illinois
Pericardial Disease

Jonathan B. Orens, MD
Associate Professor of Medicine
Medical Director
Lung Transplantation Program
The Johns Hopkins Hospital
Baltimore, Maryland
Surgery and Pulmonary Physiology, Benign Diffuse Pulmonary Disorders

Nishant Patel, BA
Research Fellow
Division of Cardiac Surgery
Johns Hopkins Hospital
Baltimore, Maryland
Lung Carcinoma

Eric A. Peck, MD
Fellow in Cardiothoracic Surgery
Division of Cardiac Surgery
Johns Hopkins Hospital
Baltimore, Maryland
Off-Pump Coronary Artery Bypass

Marc Pelletier MD, MSc, FRCSC
Assistant Professor of Surgery
Department of Cardiothoracic Surgery
Stanford University School of Medicine
Stanford, California
Ventricular Assist Devices in Children

Lester C. Permut, MD
Attending, Pediatric Cardiac Surgery
Children's Hospital & Regional Medical Center
Associate Professor of Surgery
University of Washington
Seattle, Washington
Surgery for Left Ventricular Outflow Tract Obstruction in Children, Coarctation of the Aorta and Interrupted Aortic Arch

Mark D. Plunkett, MD
Pediatric Cardiac Surgeon
Mattel Children's Hospital at UCLA
Associate Professor of Surgery
Division of Cardiothoracic Surgery
UCLA School of Medicine
Los Angeles, California
Pulmonary Stenosis and Pulmonary Atresia with Intact Ventricular Septum

Zuhab A. Qamar, MD
Division of Pediatric Cardiac Surgery
University of Michigan
Ann Arbor, Michigan
Transposition of the Great Arteries

Anees J. Razzouk, MD, FACC, FACS
Chief, Division of Cardiothoracic Surgery
Professor of Surgery
Loma Linda University
Loma Linda, California
Pediatric Cardiac Transplant

Brian L. Reemsten, MD
Assistant Professor of Surgery
Division of Cardiac Surgery
University of Southern California
Los Angeles Children's Hospital
Los Angeles, California
Palliative Operations for Congenital Heart Disease

Bruce A. Reitz, MD
Norman E. Shumway Professor of Surgery
Department of Cardiothoracic Surgery
Stanford University School of Medicine
Stanford, California
Lung and Heart-Lung Transplantation, Ventricular Assist Devices in Children

Marco Ricci, MD
Associate Professor of Surgery
Division of Cardiothoracic Surgery
University of Miami Miller School of Medicine
Miami, Florida
Surgery for Left Ventricular Outflow Tract Obstruction in Children

Richard E. Ringel, MD
Associate Professor of Pediatrics
Director, Pediatric Cardiac Catheterization Laboratory
Division of Pediatric Cardiology
The Johns Hopkins Medical Institutions
Baltimore, Maryland
Patent Ductus Arteriosus, Atrial Septal Defects and Partial Anomalous Venous Connection

Mark D. Rodefeld MD
Attending Surgeon
James Whitcomb Riley Hospital for Children
Assistant Professor of Surgery
Division of Cardiothoracic Surgery
Indiana University School of Medicine
Indianapolis, Indiana
Coarctation of the Aorta and Interrupted Aortic Arch

Glen S. Roseborough, MD
Assistant Professor of Surgery
Division of Vascular Surgery
Johns Hopkins Hospital
Baltimore, Maryland
Thoracoabdominal Aneurysms

Christopher T. Salerno, MD
Corvasc MDs
Surgical Director Heart Transplant Program
St. Vincent's Hospital
Indianapolis, Indiana
Palliative Operations for Congenital Heart Disease

Nicoletta Salviato, MD
Associate Pediatric Cardiac Surgeon
Department of Pediatric Cardiac Surgery
ARNAS Ospedale Civico
Palermo, Italy
Congenitally Corrected Transposition

Christian Schreiber, MD, PhD
Deutsches Herzzentrum at the Technische Universität München
Clinic for Cardiothoracic Surgery
Munich, Germany
Ebstien's Anomaly

Dorry L. Segev, MD
Assistant Professor of Surgery
Department of Surgery
Johns Hopkins Hospital
Baltimore, Maryland
Congenital Chest Wall Anomalies

Paul Sergeant, MD, PhD
Professor of Cardiac Surgery
Gasthuisberg University Hospital
Leuven, Belgium
Off-Pump Coronary Artery Bypass

Akhil Seth, BA
Medical Student
Johns Hopkins University School of Medicine
Baltimore, Maryland
Surgical Management of Hypertrophic Obstructive Cardiomyopathy

Jay G. Shake, MD
Fellow in Cardiothoracic Surgery
Division of Cardiac Surgery
Johns Hopkins Hospital
Baltimore, Maryland
Aortic Dissection

Thomas L. Spray, MD
Chief, Division of Cardiothoracic Surgery
Alice Langdon Warner Endowed Chair
The Children's Hospital of Philadelphia
Professor of Surgery University of Pennsylvania
School of Medicine
Philadelphia, Pennsylvania
Hypoplastic Left Heart Syndrome

Denis Aleksandrovich Tereb, MD
Resident
Department of Surgery
The University of South Alabama
Mobile, Alabama
Therapies for Benign and Malignant Pleural Diseases

Tomasz Timek, MD
Resident
Department of Cardiothoracic Surgery
Stanford University Medical Center
Stanford, California
Mitral Valve Disease

Dario Troise, MD
Staff Pediatric Cardiac Surgeon
Ospedale Giovanni XXIII
Bari, Italy
Atrial Septal Defects and Partial Anomalous Venous Connection

Victor T. Tsang, MS, FRCS
Consultant Cardiothoracic Surgeon
Great Ormond Street Hospital for Sick Children – NHS Trust
London, United Kingdom
Total Anomalus Pulmonary Venous Connection

Prashanth Vallabhajosyula, MD
Resident
Department of Surgery
Johns Hopkins Hospital
Baltimore, Maryland
Primary Cardiac Tumors

Carin A. van Doorn, MD, FRCS (C/TH)
Senior Lecturer and Honorary Consultant Cardiothoracic Surgeon
Cardiac Unit
Great Ormond Street Hospital for Children – NHS Trust
London, United Kingdom
Tricuspid Atresia and the Functionally Single Ventricle

Pieter J.A. van der Starre, MD, PhD
Associate Professor
Department of Anesthesia
Stanford University Medical Center
Stanford, California
Ascending and Arch Aneurysms of the Aorta

Christina M. Vassileva, MD
Resident
Department of Surgery
Johns Hopkins Hospital
Baltimore, Maryland
Surgical Management of Endocarditis

Jens Vogel-Claussen, MD
Department of Radiology and Radiological Science
The Johns Hopkins Hospital
Baltimore, Maryland
Cardiac Magnetic Resonance Imaging

Pierre Voisine, MD
Department of Cardiac Surgery
Laval Hospital
Quebec, Canada
Minimally Invasive Cardiac Surgery

Luca A. Vricella, MD, FACS
Assistant Professor of Surgery
Director Pediatric Heart Transplantation
Division of Cardiac Surgery
The Johns Hopkins Medical Institutions
Baltimore, Maryland
Atrial Septal Defects and Partial Anomalous Venous Connection, Congenital Anomalies of the Sinuses of Valsalva and Aortico-Left Ventricular Tunnel, Milestones in Congenital Heart Surgery

Todd S. Weiser, MD
Assistant Professor of Cardiothoracic Surgery
Department of Cardiothoracic Surgery
Mount Sinai Medical Center
New York, New York
Tracheal Diseases

G. Melville Williams, MD
Professor of Surgery
Division of Vascular Surgery
Johns Hopkins Hospital
Baltimore, Maryland
Aortic Dissection

Jason A. Williams, MD
Resident
Department of Surgery
The Johns Hopkins Hospital
Baltimore, Maryland
Cardiac Transplantation

Ronald K. Woods, MD, PhD, FACS
Chief, Pediatric Cardiothoracic Surgery
Mary Bridge/Swedish Pediatric Cardiothoracic Surgery Program
Mary Bridge Children's Hospital
Tacoma, Washington
Vascular Rings and Pulmonary Artery Sling

Jeffrey J. Wu, MD
Fellow in Cardiothoracic Surgery
Division of Cardiothoracic Surgery
The George Washington University Medical Center
Washington, District of Columbia
Patent Ductus Arteriosus

Katherine C. Wu, MD, FACC
Assistant Professor of Medicine
Division of Cardiology
Johns Hopkins Hospital
Baltimore, Maryland
Echocardiography in Cardiac Surgery

David D. Yuh, MD, FACC
Associate Professor of Surgery
Division of Cardiac Surgery,
Associate Professor
Center for Computer-Integrated Surgical Systems
Johns Hopkins Hospital and Whiting School of Engineering
John Hopkins University
Baltimore, Maryland
Surgical Management of Hypertrophic Obstructive Cardiomyopathy, Congenital Esophageal Anomalies and Diaphragmatic Hernias, Primary Coronary Artery Bypass Surgery, Management of Concomitant Carotid and Coronary Artery Disease, Surgical Management of Endocarditis, Primary Cardiac Tumors, Cardiac Transplantation,

David Zaas, MD
Division of Pulmonary and Critical Care Medicine
Duke University Medical Center
Durham, North Carolina
Surgery and Pulmonary Physiology

FOREWORD

It was just a little over 100 years ago that two highly respected European surgeons basically stated that successful open heart surgery would never be achieved. Stephen Paget wrote in 1896 in his textbook *Surgery of the Chest* that "Surgery of the heart has reached the limit set by nature to all surgery; no new discovery can overcome the natural difficulties that attend a wound of the heart". A few years before Paget's statement, Theodor Billroth was reputed to have said "Anyone who operates on the heart would lose the esteem of his colleagues".

Sixty-two years ago at this institution, Drs. Alfred Blalock and Helen Taussig took an immense initial step in shattering the Paget-Billroth edict that open-heart surgery was unobtainable. These two physicians devised the Blalock-Taussig shunt procedure, primarily for children with Tetralogy of Fallot. Shortly after the first blue-baby operation in November 1944, Johns Hopkins became the world's epicenter for cardiac surgery. Day in and day out, dozens of surgeons from all over the world came to watch Alfred Blalock and his team carry out systemic-pulmonary artery shunts for complicated intracardiac defects. During the year 1947 for example, 256 patients underwent Blalock-Taussig shunt procedures at this hospital. Now, in the summer of 2006, my colleagues are preparing a manuscript that summarizes the 2000 plus patients who have undergone the Blalock-Taussig operation at this institution.

In the early 1950's, a surgical contemporary and close friend of Dr. Blalock's at the University of Minnesota was establishing a department of surgery that would be the site for the ultimate disassemblage of the Paget-Billroth pronouncement. Dr. Owen Wangensteen, Chief of Surgery at the University of Minnesota School of Medicine, encouraged three of his junior faculty to fully explore various options of open heart surgery. The first, Dr. Clarence Dennis, was unsuccessful in his attempt in 1951 to repair atrial septal defect in two children using a disc-oxygenator that he designed. Dr. John Lewis however, was successful in the performance the world's first repair of an atrial septal defect using hypothermia and inflow stasis; his first operation was in September, 1952. This technique however, imposed serious time-limits on open-heart procedures, thus ruling out repair of more complicated intraventricular defects. In May of 1953, Dr. John Gibbon at Jefferson Medical College in Philadelphia, successfully corrected an atrial septal defect in an 18 year old girl using a newly designed screen oxygenator; this obviously was a monumental achievement. Unfortunately, Dr. Gibbon's next four patients, all with a preoperative diagnosis of atral septal defect did not survive. Dr. Gibbon was so discouraged that he never again did open-heart surgery. There was a general feeling that these patients suffered from a sick heart syndrome and needed to be supported on a heart-lung machine for at least a week after surgery. This discouragement about open-heart surgery changed drastically on March 26, 1954, when Dr. C. Walton Lillehei at the University of Minnesota, closed a ventricular septal defect in a one year old boy using cross-circulation. In Dr. Lillehei's first case, the boy's father served as his oxygenator. This operation went well, but unfortunately the boy died on the 11th post-operative day of pneumonia. Dr. Lillehei was successful however with his second and third patients who underwent total correction of ventricular septal defects. Dr. Lillehei and his team proceeded to operate on 45 children over the next year; 27 had ventricular septal defects, 10 tetralogy of Fallot, 5 atrio-ventricular canal, and 3 had miscellaneous intracardiac defects. Remarkably, two-thirds of these children were discharged from the hospital with excellent long term results.

Alfred Blalock at Johns Hopkins opened up the field of closed-heart surgery in 1944 and ten years later, Lillehei established the field of open-heart surgery. Both men would be awarded the Lasker Award for their achievement. Blalock shared the Lasker award with Helen Taussig and Lillehei shared the award with his faculty colleague Richard Varco, and surgical residents Morley Cohen and Herbert Warden.

How fortunate that two young surgical house officers were able to "scrub-in" and observe Dr. Lillehei's first cross-circulation case. One was Dr. Norman Shumway and the other was myself. Dr. Shumway went on to establish the Department of Cardiac Surgery at Stanford Medical Center in 1960. His surgical contributions to our specialty have been monumental. In addition, he trained more than 100 cardiac surgeons; many would subsequently become chiefs of divisions and departments of cardiac surgery around the world.

Remarkably, all three authors of this textbook developed their cardiac surgical skills in Dr. Shumway's department at Stanford and are now faculty members in the Johns Hopkins' Division of Cardiac Surgery established by Dr. Blalock.

It's important to note that Dr. Wangensteen, a general surgeon and great admirer of Theodor Billroth, wrote in his textbook The Rise of Surgery that "The outstanding contribution in the 20th century in the advance of surgery has been intracardiac surgery".

I believe the readers of this textbook will be extremely pleased with the very comprehensive discussions presented by more than 100 authors; discussions that describe the current status of many remarkable achievements in cardiothoracic surgery during the past century.

Vincent L. Gott, MD
Professor of Cardiac Surgery

PREFACE

The Johns Hopkins Manual of Cardiothoracic Surgery was first intended as a review text for the American Board of Thoracic Surgery examinations. Although several excellent textbooks covering topics in adult cardiac, pediatric, and general thoracic surgery have been published over the years, a comprehensive single volume textbook covering all of these areas had not yet been conceived. This textbook represents a multidisciplinary effort to produce an all-inclusive core reference for all caregivers in the field of cardiothoracic surgery.

We have formatted *The Johns Hopkins Manual* to facilitate review, prefacing almost every chapter with a "Key Concepts" section highlighting the epidemiology, pathophysiology, clinical features, diagnostic and treatment strategies, and outcomes for each topic. Nevertheless, the scope of this textbook goes well beyond that of basic review, covering advanced concepts, controversial issues, and cutting edge technologies that have not yet reached widespread clinical practice. For example, we have included chapters on surgical ventricular remodeling, endovascular stent graft treatment of thoracic aortic disease, minimally-invasive cardiac operations, and the latest chemoradiation treatment strategies for lung and esophageal cancer. We have also enlisted the expertise of our cardiology colleagues who have provided excellent chapters on cardiovascular risk reduction strategies, pacemaker and defibrillator concepts, and cardiac imaging techniques.

As its title suggests, most of the contributors to the *Manual* consist of faculty, residents, fellows, and students at The Johns Hopkins Hospital. In recruiting our contributors, we were both impressed and proud of the many experts in cardiothoracic disease that call Hopkins home. Nevertheless, we also recognized that there were many topics that would be best discussed by national and international experts outside of the Hopkins community. Indeed, we are indebted to all of our contributors that have been so unselfishly generous with their time in contributing to this work.

In addition to the contributing authors, there are many other individuals to whom we owe thanks. We are indebted to our editors and production staff at McGraw-Hill. Marc Strauss, Joe Rusko, Christie Naglieri, Lester Sheinis, and Phil Galea. The painstaking permissions work provided by Jesa Wolff is also much appreciated. We would also like to thank our administrative assistants in the Division of Cardiac Surgery at Hopkins, Donna Riley, Lynn Dimarcantonio, and Genie Sessa, for providing much of the legwork on completing many of the manuscripts.

We would like to thank Vincent Gott who continues to serve as a mentor and inspiration to aspiring cardiothoracic surgeons and reminds us each day that grace and humility are amongst the most notable qualities a surgeon can hope to possess.

It is by no coincidence that each of us learned our craft in the Department of Cardiothoracic Surgery at Stanford University. We are indebted to its architect, Norman Shumway, whose technical brilliance, irreverent humor, and humility inspired many generations of leaders in our field. One of many "Normisms" espoused to his residents during operations reminds us of his enthusiasm for teaching. "Isn't this fun? Isn't this easy? What could be better? Nothing could be better!" His passing earlier this year leaves us with his amazing legacy, including the assemblage of one of the most distinguished faculties in our profession.

Finally, we give our love and appreciation to our families, who have supported and encouraged us in this endeavor.

David D. Yuh, MD
Luca A. Vricella, MD
William A. Baumgartner, MD

PART

I

GENERAL THORACIC SURGERY

CHAPTER

1 SURGERY AND PULMONARY PHYSIOLOGY

David Zaas, Jonathan B. Orens

INTRODUCTION

Pulmonary complications occur in 5 to 10 percent of all surgical patients and are a major cause of surgery-related morbidity and mortality. Approximately 25 percent of deaths within the first week after surgery are reportedly due to pulmonary complications.[1,2] Such complications after surgery have also been shown to prolong hospital stay by an average of 1 to 2 weeks.[1] Therefore, for all types of surgical procedures, it is vitally important to minimize pulmonary complications with the appropriate use of preoperative testing.

A wide range of pulmonary complications (Table 1-1) occur, most often in patients with underlying lung disease. Pneumonia occurs in 10 to 40 percent of patients after major surgical procedures and is associated with a mortality rate of 30 to 45 percent.[1,2] The incidence of postoperative pneumonia as well as other pulmonary complications is influenced by a number of variables related to both the surgery and the patient's health. Potential benefits of a thorough preoperative evaluation include the identification of patients with underlying lung disease, modification of risk factors, optimization of medical management, and avoidance of elective surgery in high-risk patients.

KEY CONCEPTS

- Epidemiology
  - Pulmonary complications occur in 5 to 10 percent of all surgical patients and have been shown to prolong hospital stay by 1 to 2 weeks. Approximately 25 percent of deaths within the first week after surgery are due to pulmonary complications.
- Pathophysiology
  - Pneumonia occurs in 10 to 40 percent of patients after major surgery and is associated with a mortality rate of 30 to 45 percent. General anesthesia can decrease lung volumes by 30 to 40 percent, and this decrease may persist for 1 to 2 weeks postoperatively.
- Clinical features
  - Cardiothoracic surgery is associated with the highest frequency of pulmonary complications. Risk factors include the type of surgery, general anesthesia, length of surgery and general anesthesia, smoking, chronic obstructive pulmonary disease, age, obesity, functional status, and a history of dyspnea.
- Diagnostics
  - Preoperative evaluation should include a directed history and physical examination to identify those patients at particular risk for pulmonary complications. Pulmonary function tests with spirometry and arterial blood gases (ABGs) should be obtained for any patient undergoing lung resection. For further risk stratification, cardiopulmonary exercise testing (CPET) is indicated in high-risk patients who do not have adequate predicted postoperative lung function. Alternatives to CPET include the shuttle-walk or stair-climb test.
- Treatment
  - Inhaled bronchodilators may successfully reverse some cases of obstructive pulmonary disease.
- Outcomes
  - Preoperative pulmonary function evaluation can stratify patients for risk, thus identifying those who can safely undergo major cardiothoracic surgery and minimizing the risk of significant morbidity and mortality.

Table 1-1 Postoperative pulmonary complications
Prolonged need for mechanical ventilation
Respiratory failure
Pneumonia
Bronchospasm
Acute respiratory distress syndrome (ARDS)
Atelectasis
Pleural effusion
Pneumothorax

Multiple risk factors for postoperative pulmonary complications have been identified; these depend on patient factors as well as the specific type of surgery and anesthesia. The location and type of surgery being performed is a major determinant of pulmonary complication risk. Cardiothoracic surgery has been repeatedly shown to have the highest frequency of pulmonary complications.[3] Upper abdominal surgery has the second highest incidence of complications, owing to the close proximity of the diaphragm. On the other hand, orthopedic and genitourinary procedures have been associated with a lower risk of postoperative pulmonary complications.[1,2,4–6] Along with the surgery itself, the type of anesthesia selected may be important in determining postoperative risks. Early literature suggests little difference between the use of regional anesthesia versus general anesthesia with regard to intraoperative and postoperative pulmonary function and complications; however, more recent studies suggest that the use of general anesthesia is associated with an increased risk of pulmonary complications.[7,8] The length of anesthesia and surgery is also associated with an increased risk of pulmonary complications.[9] In healthy patients, general anesthesia can decrease lung volumes by 10 to 30 percent; these changes may persist for 1 to 2 weeks postoperatively. The decreased lung volumes lead to a more rapid respiratory rate to maintain minute ventilation. Subsequently, the rapid shallow breathing pattern can lead to worsening oxygenation due to ventilation/perfusion mismatch or shunt through areas of atelectasis. The changes in breathing pattern can also impair the airway clearance of mucus and bacteria. These events are normally clinically silent in the host with adequate pulmonary reserve; however, they can lead to severe complications in patients with underlying lung disease.

In addition to the operation-specific risk factors described above, multiple patient-specific risk factors have been identified (Table 1-2). The identification and modification of reversible risk factors is an important component of the preoperative evaluation. One of the most important modifiable risk factors is smoking cessation several weeks prior to elective surgical procedures. This intervention significantly decreases the risk of postoperative pulmonary complications, which include atelectasis, hypoxemia, sputum production, and pneumonia.[1,2,10,11] An assessment of the surgical risk factors in combination with the clinical assessment of the patient determines which patients warrant a more thorough pulmonary evaluation of their pulmonary function prior to surgery.

Table 1-2 Patient-specific risk factors for pulmonary complications
Tobacco history
Chronic obstructive pulmonary disease
Restrictive lung disease
Age
Obesity
Functional status
Dyspnea
Impaired sensorium

INDICATIONS FOR PREOPERATIVE PULMONARY FUNCTION TESTS

A complete preoperative evaluation should include a directed history and physical to identify patients who are at increased risk of pulmonary complications. Key historical features include any history of underlying lung disease as well as an assessment of dyspnea. Unexplained dyspnea at rest or on minimal exertion should warrant a more thorough evaluation prior to any elective surgical procedure. Smoking cessation is a readily modifiable risk factor and should be recommended at least several weeks prior to surgery if possible. Any patient with a history of prior lung disease, significant tobacco use, or dyspnea with mild exertion warrants pulmonary function testing before any high-risk elective surgical procedure. The American College of Physicians recommends preoperative pulmonary function testing for the following patients[12]:

1. All patients with a history of tobacco use or dyspnea who are undergoing cardiothoracic or upper abdominal surgery
2. Any patient with unexplained dyspnea or pulmonary symptoms who is undergoing head, neck, orthopedic, or lower abdominal surgery
3. Everyone undergoing lung resection

Preoperative pulmonary function testing most often consists of spirometry and ABG analysis. However, a wide variety of tests is available through the pulmonary function lab and may be useful in selected patients. The role of these specific tests is described later in this chapter. Patients undergoing lung resection surgery are clearly at a particularly high risk of pulmonary complications and warrant a more thorough evaluation.

EVALUATION OF THE PATIENT UNDERGOING LUNG RESECTION

Several risk factors have been identified specifically for patients undergoing lung resection. Lobectomy and pneumonectomy are associated with significant morbidity in up to 30 percent of patients and death in up to 4 percent.[13] The type of surgical procedure is a major determinant of operative risks. Patients undergoing pneumonectomy have a greater operative morbidity and mortality than those who undergo only a lobectomy.[14] Older age may be an additional risk factor. Several series have reported a higher mortality in lung resection in patients above 80 years of age, especially those who undergo pneumonectomy.[14,15] Although morbidity and mortality have been shown to increase with age, there is no age cutoff beyond which lung resection is contraindicated. The increased mortality that was seen in elderly patients may simply reflect a greater number of comorbid medical conditions.

The initial evaluation of all patients considered for lung resection surgery should include ABG measurement. Hypercapnia and hypoxia may both identify patients at increased operative risk. Prior studies of surgical risk prediction have shown that baseline hypercapnia predicted an increased surgical morbidity.[16] Similarly, it has been shown that patients with hypoxia at rest or during exertion are at a higher risk of postoperative complications.[16] The assessment of oxygenation and ventilation at rest lacks adequate sensitivity and specificity in identifying high-risk surgical patients. These criteria alone should not be used to exclude patients from surgery without a more formal investigation.

Pulmonary function testing with spirometry is recommended in all patients who are scheduled to undergo a lung resection.[17] Spirometry is the most accurate and predictive pulmonary function test available. The initial use of spirometry can identify low-risk patients who can proceed directly to surgery as well as higher-risk patients who warrant further investigation. Most of these conclusions are based on patients with obstructive lung disease; they may not apply to patients with underlying restrictive lung disease. If the preoperative FEV_1 is greater than 2.0 L for a pneumonectomy or if the FEV_1 is greater than 1.5 L for a lobectomy, no further pulmonary testing is required and the patient can proceed directly to lung resection.[18] As long as these patients do not have significant interstitial lung disease or unexpected hypoxia, they have an operative mortality of less than 5 percent.[19,20] All patients who have a FEV_1 below these cutoffs require more extensive evaluation prior to lung resection (Fig. 1-1). All patients who are not clearly fit for surgery based on the above spirometry criteria warrant more extensive testing, including quantitative ventilation/perfusion scanning and complete pulmonary function testing (spirometry, lung volumes, and measurement of diffusing capacity). These additional tests are used to help predict postoperative pulmonary function. Specifically, it is recommended that patients have a postoperative FEV_1 of greater than 0.8 L and also a postoperative diffusing capacity (DLCO) of greater than 40 percent predicted.[17] Since most of the studies that determined minimum postoperative FEV_1 have involved men, an alternative cutoff of FEV_1 greater than 40 percent predicted has been proposed for women and the elderly.[17] The quantitative perfusion scan is used to estimate the percent of functional lung that is being resected.[21,22] The estimate of postoperative pulmonary function is calculated with the following equation:

$$\text{Predicted } FEV_1 = \text{preoperative } FEV_1 \times (1 - \text{percent of lung to be removed})$$

The same equation can be used to calculate the predicted postoperative DLCO. Any patient with a predicted postoperative FEV_1 and DLCO above the minimum values outlined above should have a relatively low risk of pulmonary complications and should tolerate the resection. A patient who does not have an adequate predicted postoperative lung function based on the previous tests should not be denied surgery without further evaluation if he or she otherwise appears to be an appropriate surgical candidate. These higher-risk patients may be referred for cardiopulmonary exercise testing (CPET) for further risk stratification. The measurement of the maximal oxygen consumption, $\dot{V}O_{2max}$, by CPET is the most specific predictor of postoperative pulmonary complications related to lung resection surgery.[23–26] If the measured $\dot{V}O_{2max}$ is greater than 15 mL/kg/min, the patient may be safely offered surgical resection. Any patient with $\dot{V}O_{2max}$ greater than 10 mL/kg/min is at especially high risk. Some alternatives to formal CPET that have been proposed include the shuttle-walk test or the stair-climb test.[27–29] These tests are less expensive and may be easier to obtain at some centers. Finally, in the subset of patients with emphysema and borderline pulmonary reserve based on the prior evaluation, the combination of lung resection and lung volume reduction surgery has been used in several reports and lung resection may still be considered.[30,31] Since lung resection is the only cure for many patients with localized lung cancer, the strategies of pulmonary function testing have been designed to maximize their sensitivity in identifying all patients who can safely tolerate lung resection; these strategies must be tailored to the goals of the individual patient.

INTERPRETATION OF ARTERIAL BLOOD GAS ANALYSIS

ABG analysis is relatively simple; it is readily available and provides information useful in identifying the high-risk surgical patient at an early stage. ABG measurement should be performed with the patient at rest and breathing room air if possible. Information provided by the ABG includes the partial pressure of oxygen, PO_2, partial pressure of carbon dioxide, PCO_2, and the calculated bicarbonate, HCO_3^-. The PO_2 reflects the adequacy of gas transfer from the alveoli to the blood. When measured at sea level,

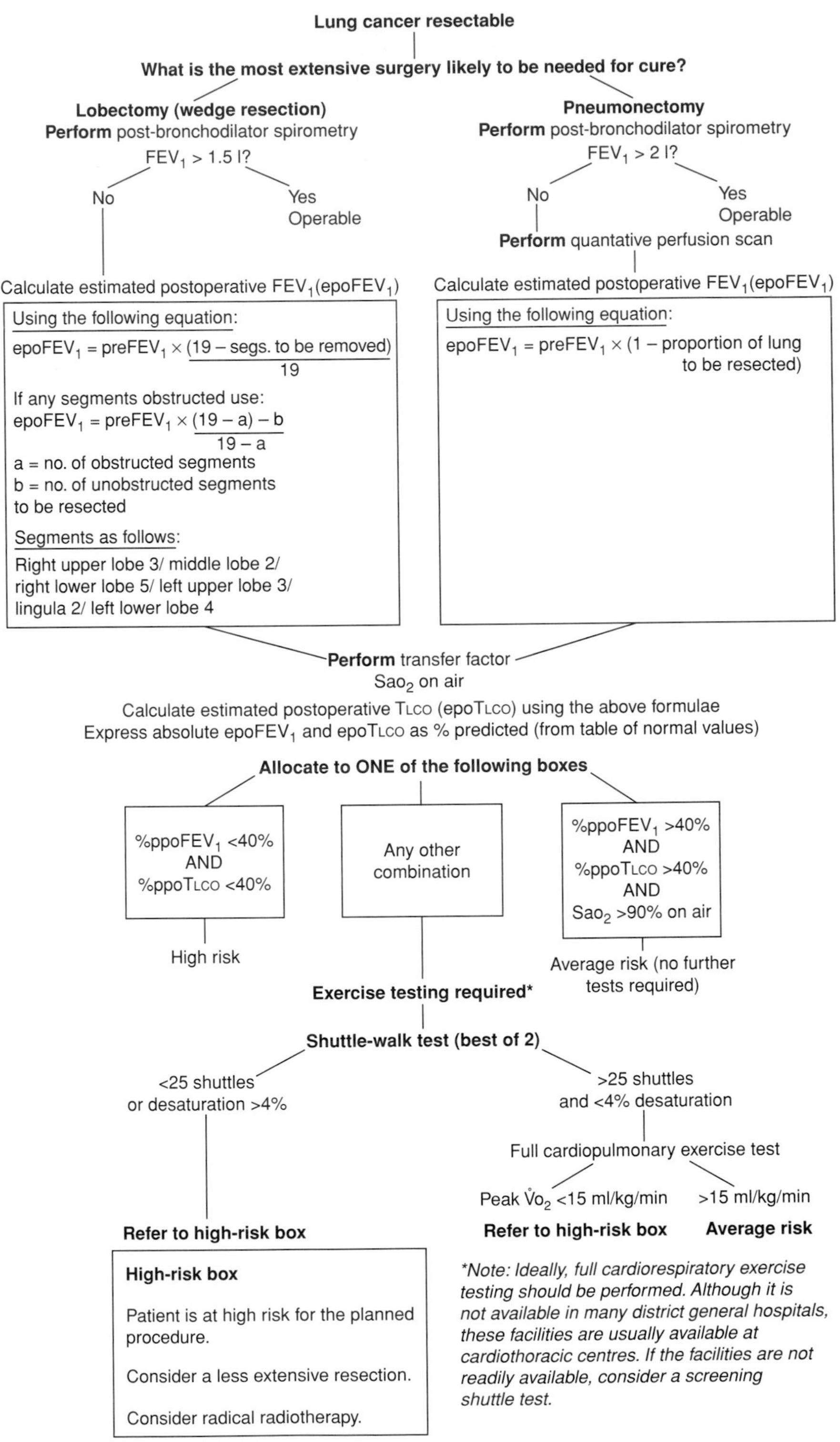

Figure 1-1 Algorithm for preoperative evaluation of candidates for lung resection. [From BTS guidelines: Guidelines on the selection of patients with lung cancer for surgery. *Thorax* 2001;56(2):89–108. With permission.]

the normal PO_2 ranges from 85 to 100 mmHg in a young, healthy adult and decreases slightly with age. PO_2 also falls with increasing altitude above sea level. The PO_2 as a measurement of oxygenation should be interpreted in terms of the oxygen dissociation curve (Fig. 1-2). Since a majority of oxygen in the blood is bound to hemoglobin, relative changes in PO_2 can reflect a wide range of changes in oxygen carrying capacity depending on the slope of the oxygen dissociation curve. Changes in PO_2 on the steep part of the oxygen dissociation curve reflect large changes

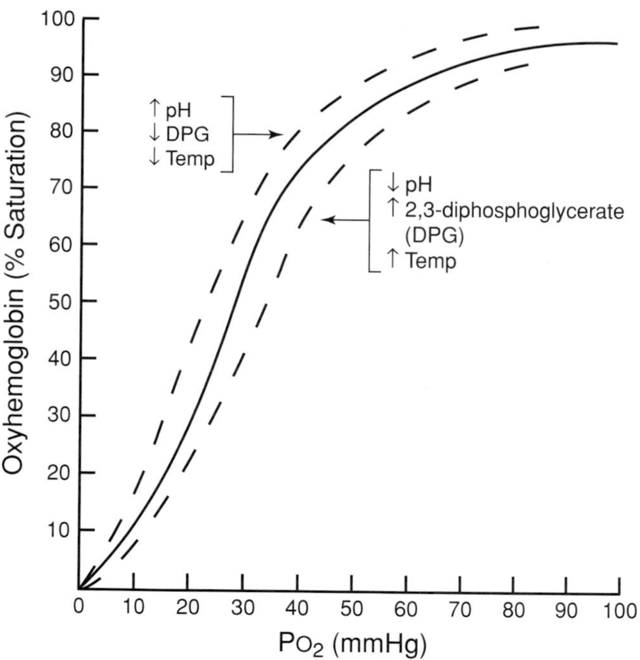

Figure 1-2 Oxygen-hemoglobin dissociation curve.

in oxygen content. In contrast, changes in Po_2 on the flat part of the oxygen dissociation curve, Po_2 greater than 70 mmHg, lead to only minor differences in oxygen content. The alveolar-arterial oxygen gradient (A–a gradient = $P_iO_2 - (PaCO_2/R) - PaO_2$) is a more sensitive measurement of gas exchange problems. Since pulmonary function normally declines with age, the normal values for A–a gradient depend on the age of the patient and can be calculated based on the following equation.

Normal A–a gradient = 2.5 + ¼ age ±2.

An elevated A–a gradient can be due to ventilation/perfusion mismatching, diffusion defects, or shunt.

The partial pressure of carbon dioxide, PCO_2, is a measurement of CO_2 production ($\dot{V}CO_2$) and alveolar ventilation ($\dot{V}_A$); that is, $PaCO_2 = \dot{V}CO_2/\dot{V}_A$. Therefore an increase in CO_2 production or a decrease in alveolar ventilation leads to an increase in PCO_2. Normally PCO_2 is tightly regulated, with normal values at rest between 38 to 42 mmHg, and they are not affected by age. Hypercapnia can be due to a wide range of causes. Total minute ventilation is composed of both $\dot{V}_A$ and dead-space ventilation ($\dot{V}_D$); that is, $\dot{V}_T = \dot{V}_A + \dot{V}_D$. Conditions such as emphysema or interstitial lung disease lead to an increase in $\dot{V}_D$ and a corresponding decrease in $\dot{V}_A$. which can result in hypercapnia with exertion or at rest. Hypoventilation can be due to a number of causes besides lung parenchymal disease, including musculoskeletal and neurologic causes. ABG analysis provides a simple measure of oxygenation and ventilation at rest. The presence of hypoxia or hypercapnia should identify a higher-risk patient who warrants a more thorough evaluation.

THE ROLE OF THE PULMONARY FUNCTION LABORATORY

Spirometry, one of the oldest clinical tests, is still utilized today. It was first used by John Hutchinson in 1848 and is the most common test performed in the pulmonary function laboratory. In undergoing spirometry, an individual first inhales to total lung capacity and then performs a forced exhalation. Spirometry measures the changes in volume during that maximal forced expiration. It is accurate and highly reproducible in patients who make a consistent effort. The results of spirometry can be depicted graphically as a flow volume loop in addition to the measurements that are traditionally reported. Flow volume loops depict both inspiration and expiration tracings, which are averaged over the multiple attempts. Recognition of flow volume loops as well as pathologic abnormalities can be a helpful addition to the other results obtained with spirometry. Fig. 1-3 shows

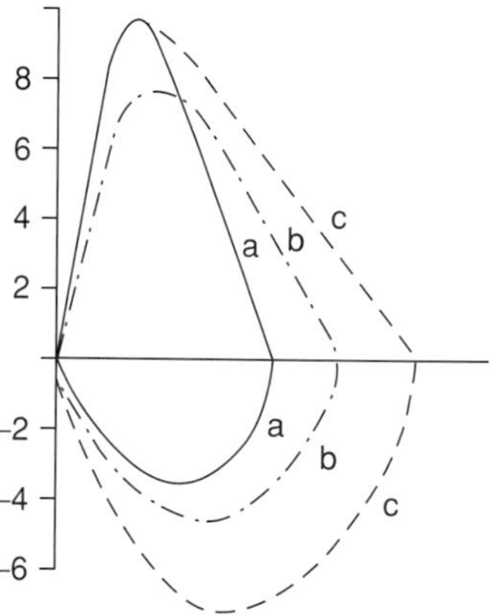

Flow volume curve in restrictive airways disease, a: early stage of restrictive type, b: late stage of restrictive type, c: normal curve

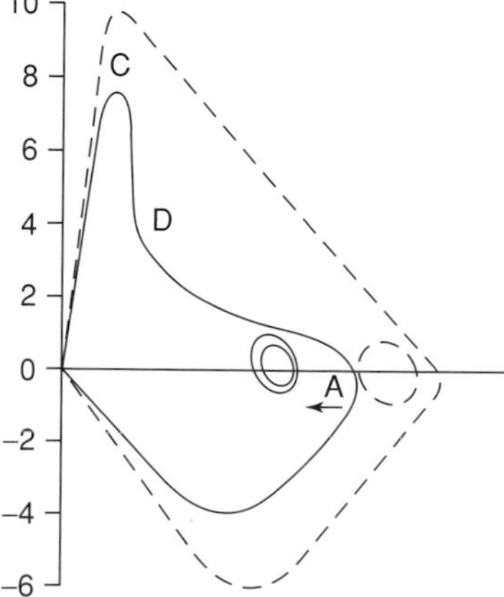

Flow volume curve in peripheral airways obstruction C; Reduced PEFR, CD : Period of high flow, CA : Curvilinear shape. Arrow : Tidal volume loop moving towards vital capacity.

Figure 1-3 Flow volume loops in restrictive and obstructive lung disease as compared to normal. [From *Lung India* 1996;14(4):169–171. With permission.]

the flow volume loops of a normal individual compared with the patterns seen in obstructive and restrictive lung disease. Obstructive lung disease is characterized by slow expiratory flow, especially at the lower lung volumes. Note the coving of the expiratory limb in the flow volume loop from a patient with obstructive lung disease. In contrast, restrictive lung disease has normal or increased expiratory flow rates but smaller volumes owing to the decreased total lung capacity. Spirometry provides several measurements that are important to understand, including the forced vital capacity (FVC), forced expiratory volume in 1 s (FEV_1), and FEV_1/FVC ratio. The FVC is a measure of the volume exhaled during the entire forced expiratory effort. The limitations to airflow reflected in the FVC are due to the dynamic compression of the airways. Three variables determine airway closure and airflow limitation: the elasticity of the lung parenchyma, the size of the airways, and the resistance to airflow. The FVC is decreased in both obstructive and restrictive lung diseases. It can also be decreased as a result of chest wall deformities, pleural disease, or neuromuscular diseases. Although the FVC measures the total volume of gas exhaled during the forced expiratory effort, the FEV_1 measures the volume of gas exhaled in the first second of exhalation (Fig. 1-4). In restrictive lung disease, the FEV_1 is decreased in similar proportion to the FVC; therefore the FEV_1/FVC ratio is normal or increased. In contrast, patients with obstructive lung disease have difficulty emptying the air within the lungs because of the collapsibility of the airways, and the FEV_1 is decreased to a greater degree than the FVC. The difficulties during exhalation seen in obstructive lung disease lead to a characteristic decrease in the FEV_1/FCV ratio. Spirometry is the only pulmonary function test needed

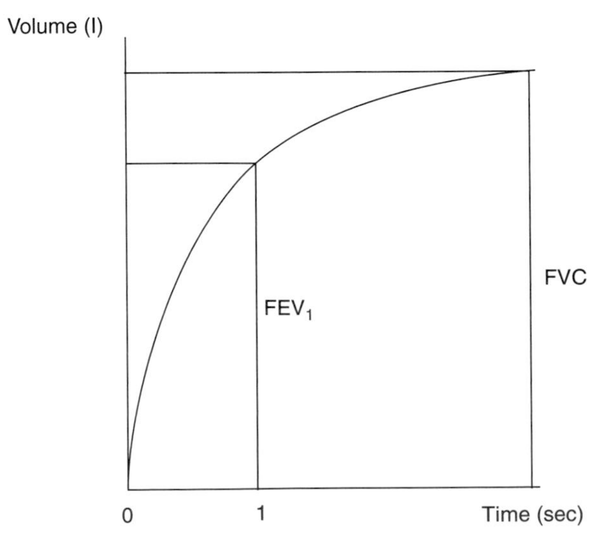

Figure 1-4 Graphic representation of forced expiratory volume at 1 s (FEV_1) as related to forced vital capacity (FVC). (From www.surgical tutor.org.)

Table 1-3 Severity of airflow obstruction based on FEV_1

FEV_1	Severity of obstruction
60–80% predicted	Mild
40–60% predicted	Moderate
Less than 40% predicted	Severe

to make the diagnosis of obstructive lung disease, and an FEV_1/FVC ratio of less than 72 percent is the diagnostic criterion of the American Thoracic Society (ATS). After a diagnosis of airway obstruction has been made, the severity of obstruction is usually determined by the percent predicted of the FEV_1, as shown in Table 1-3.

Spirometry is suggestive of restrictive lung disease when the FVC and FEV_1 are both decreased but the FEV_1/FVC ratio is normal. However, lung volumes must demonstrate a decreased total lung capacity in order to make the diagnosis. Spirometry can also be ordered with and without the use of inhaled bronchodilators to determine the amount of reversible airway obstruction. Reversible airway obstruction is defined as greater than a 12 to 15 percent improvement in the FEV_1 or FVC after treatment with an inhaled bronchodilator. The identification of patients with reversible airway obstruction can be an important component of a preoperative pulmonary evaluation, with a view to decreasing airway obstruction and minimizing surgical morbidity. Although spirometry is the most common of all the pulmonary function tests, more extensive testing of lung volumes or gas transfer is often needed.

Since spirometry measures only the volume of air exhaled, it is unable to measure the residual volume (RV) or the total lung capacity (TLC). RV is the air left in the lung after a complete exhalation. TLC equals the RV plus the vital capacity (VC) (Fig. 1-5). Several different techniques can be used to determine the TLC and RV. The three most common techniques to measure lung volume include inert gas dilution, nitrogen washout, and body plethysmography. During the inert gas dilution technique, the subject inhales a known volume and concentration of a nonabsorbable gas such as helium. After equilibration, the new concentration of the gas can be measured and the TLC calculated. The nitrogen washout technique requires the individual to breathe oxygen (without nitrogen) and inhale into a separate compartment. The volume and concentration of the exhaled nitrogen gas are measured and the TLC can be calculated. Finally, body plethysmography is based on the principle of Boyle's law ($PV = P_1V_1$). The test is performed in an airtight chamber that can measure the change in pressure and volume with respiration. This technique allows the measurement of all the gas within the lungs. A detailed discussion of each of these techniques is beyond the scope of this chapter. However, it is important to recognize that neither the inert gas technique nor the nitrogen washout technique measures the volume from poorly ventilated

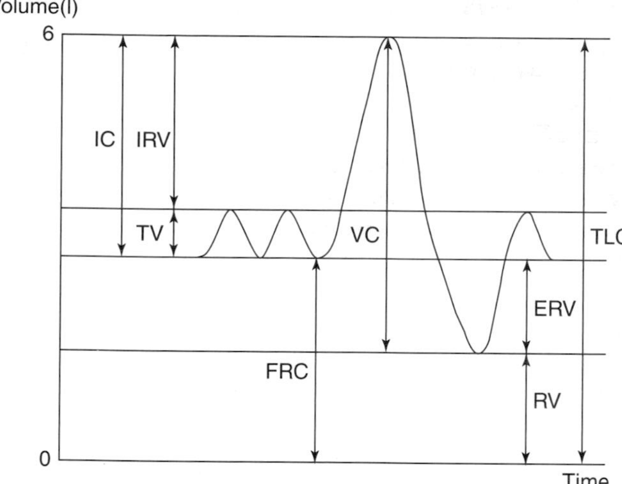

Figure 1-5 Graphic representation of spirometric relationships. (From surgical tutor.org.)
ERV = expiratory reserve volume; FRC = functional residual capacity; IC = inspiratory capacity; IRV = inspiratory reserve capacity; RV = residual volume; TLC = total lung capacity; TV = tidal volume; VC = vital capacity.

areas of the lung. Therefore both these techniques can underestimate the TLC in patients with obstructive lung disease and air trapping. Plethysmography will give an accurate measurement of lung volumes in that setting. Lung volumes are required to make the diagnosis of restrictive lung disease, which is defined by a TLC of less than 80 percent predicted and can result from a wide variety of causes, including pulmonary fibrosis, chest wall disorders, obesity, or neuromuscular disease. After confirming the presence of restriction, the VC is commonly used to quantify the severity of restriction, as shown in Table 1-4.

For patients with airway obstruction, the total lung capacity is usually normal or increased. Lung volumes are important for patients with airway obstruction and a decreased FVC in order to look for the presence of air trapping or coexistent restrictive lung disease. Air trapping is the inability to empty areas of the lung and consequent hyperinflation. Lung volumes in this setting demonstrate an elevated RV, greater than 130 percent predicted, and often an elevated TLC. A decreased TLC in the presence of airway obstruction (FEV_1/FVC lower than 72 percent) indicates a combination of obstructive

Table 1-4 Severity of restrictive ventilatory defect based on vital capacity

Vital Capacity (VC)	Severity of restriction
60–80% predicted	Mild
40–60% predicted	Moderate
Less than 40% predicted	Severe

and restrictive disease. The combination of obstruction and restriction can make the determination of pulmonary function difficult to quantify but is important to recognize. Lung volumes are not indicated in all patients who undergo spirometry, but they can be useful in patients with a decreased FVC or in patients that you suspect having restrictive lung disease of any cause.

The third most common test ordered from the pulmonary function lab is the diffusing capacity. It measures the transfer of gas from the air in the alveolar space to the hemoglobin of the red blood cells. There are four main determinants of the diffusion of gas: area of the alveolar capillary membrane, thickness of the alveolar capillary membrane, the driving pressure of the gas, and the carrying capacity of the circulating blood. Since it is not easy to measure the diffusion of oxygen, the pulmonary function lab measures the diffusion of carbon monoxide (DLCO). The DLCO closely mimics the transfer of oxygen and is used as a surrogate. In order to measure DLCO, the subject is asked to inhale to TLC and hold his or her breath for 10 s. Then the subject exhales completely and the exhaled CO is measured along with an inert gas. From this one may calculate the amount of CO that is transferred to the blood. A normal DLCO is approximately 20 to 30 mL/min/mmHg and is influenced by age, sex, and height. Since the diffusion of gas is influenced by the oxygen-carrying capacity of blood, it is important to recognize the presence of anemia, which can significantly lower the measured DLCO. There are standardized formulas that allow for the standardized correction for anemia; these should be used whenever the hemoglobin is decreased. Pathologic conditions that can lower the DLCO to less than 80 percent predicted include pulmonary fibrosis, emphysema, pulmonary hypertension, right-to-left intracardiac shunt, and anemia. A few rare conditions can elevate the DLCO (greater than 130 percent predicted); these include asthma, alveolar hemorrhage, and left-to-right intracardiac shunt. The combination of spirometry, lung volumes, and DLCO can provide a wealth of information about the pathophysiology of lung diseases. Table 1-5 depicts the expected changes seen in different lung diseases.

In summary, the measurement of pulmonary function is readily available and can provide a large amount of information that can influence the perioperative and intraoperative management of patients with lung disease. It is important to remember that borderline pulmonary function tests should not exclude a patient from surgery if he or she is otherwise a good surgical candidate. More extensive exercise testing may be useful in patients with borderline pulmonary reserve who are being considered for lung resection.

EXERCISE TESTING

Exercise testing can be used in a variety of clinical settings, including the assessment of patient suitability for

Table 1-5 Typical pulmonary function changes for specific diseases

Category	FEV_1/FVC	FVC	RV	DLCO
Asthma	Normal or ↓	↓	Normal or ↑	Normal
Emphysema	↓	Normal or ↓	↑	↓
Chronic bronchitis	↓	↓	Normal	Normal
Interstitial lung disease	Normal or ↑	↓	Normal	↓
Pulmonary hypertension	Normal	Normal	Normal	↓
Neuromuscular disease	Normal	↓	Normal or ↑	Normal

lung resection. In this setting, exercise testing has been advocated for patients at moderate to high surgical risk whose pulmonary function, based on the preliminary evaluations, does not appear to include adequate pulmonary reserve. Specifically, exercise testing may be useful in patients with obstructive lung disease and those with a postoperative predicted FEV_1 less than 1 L. It may also be informative in evaluating patients with a combination of obstructive and restrictive lung disease. Exercise testing can take several different forms. Simple tests such as the 6-min-walk or the stair-climb test have been evaluated in a small series of patients undergoing thoracotomy for lung cancer and been shown to predict operative morbidity and mortality. During the 6-min-walk test, the subject walks on level ground at a brisk pace for 6 min and the distance covered is measured in feet. A stair-climb test measures the number of steps an individual can climb at normal pace. One small study showed that a 6-min-walk distance of greater than 1000 ft was predictive of complications within 90 days, with a positive predictive value of 85 percent and a negative predictive value of 100 percent. A stair-climb test result of greater than 44 steps was also useful, with a positive predictive value of 91 percent and a negative predictive value of 80 percent.[28] For centers where formal CPET facilities are not easily accessible, these simple tests may be useful in carefully selected patients.

For most medical centers, more extensive testing can be performed with CPET, which offers the opportunity to measure the cellular, respiratory, and cardiovascular responses to exercise. CPET is underused because of a common lack of understanding of the test and the interpretation of the clinical information that it provides. There are a wide range of clinical situations in which CPET can be helpful. These include assessment of unexplained dyspnea or fatigue, disability evaluation, monitoring of response to treatment or rehabilitation programs, transplant evaluations, and preoperative risk assessment. In order to perform the test, a subject exercises on a stationary bike or treadmill, which calculates the work performed. While exercising, the individual is connected to a continuous electrocardiogram to monitor for arrhythmias or signs of myocardial ischemia. In addition, gas exchange is measured including oxygen (O_2) consumption and carbon dioxide (CO_2) production. In addition, spirometry and ABG measurements can be obtained before and after exercise. A complete discussion of the interpretation of CPET is beyond the scope of this chapter. A more comprehensive review of the details of CPET is provided elsewhere.[32]

Some of the more useful physiologic measurements provided by CPET are discussed briefly below. The most basic measurements include responses to graded exercise in terms of blood pressure, heart rate, and respiratory rate. The frequent monitoring of vital signs can provide important information regarding the cardiovascular response to stress. Blood pressure and heart rate are measured every several minutes or continuously via an arterial catheter. Normal individuals should be able to exercise to a heart rate of greater than 80 percent of the predicted maximal heart rate. In an individual who reached 80 percent of maximum heart rate without reaching other limits, physical deconditioning may be indicated. The normal blood pressure response to exercise is a moderate increase. Large increases or inappropriate decreases in blood pressure with graded exercise can help to identify cardiovascular pathology. Spirometry can also be performed as part of CPET. It is often performed before and after CPET. Decreases in FEV_1 and FEV_1/FVC can identify exercise-induced bronchospasm as a cause of dyspnea.

Most of the data provided by CPET result from measurements of exhaled gas. These measurements are interpreted in the context of the work being performed on the stationery bike or treadmill, which is recorded as well. One of the more useful measurements provided by CPET is the maximal oxygen uptake during graded exercise ($\dot{V}O_{2max}$). Oxygen consumption is determined by the cardiac output, arterial oxygen content, and extraction of oxygen by the muscles. In interpreting a CPET, $\dot{V}O_2$ is one of the first results to look at because it indicates whether the patient's physiologic responses allow him or her to reach maximal aerobic function. A subject who is unable to reach 80 percent $\dot{V}O_{2max}$ with exercise is considered to have exercise limitation. If the aerobic function is limited, reflected in a $\dot{V}O_{2max}$ less than 80 percent predicted, other measurements can be used to determine the cause of the limitation. As stated earlier, $\dot{V}O_{2max}$ is also the most studied value for predicting surgical risk, especially for patients undergoing lung resection surgery.

For patients who are identified as having exercise limitations, CPET can be helpful in determining the etiology.

Except for highly trained athletes, normal individuals are cardiac-limited in response to exercise. This limitation is indicated when the heart rate (HR) reaches more than 80 percent of the predicted maximum. Most normal subjects have a ventilatory reserve of approximately 10 L/min or 10 to 30 percent of the ventilatory capacity. The maximum ventilatory capacity is predicted by using the maximum voluntary ventilation (MVV) determined by spirometry. The percent of ventilatory capacity reached with exercise is calculated by dividing the minute ventilation ($\dot{V}_E$) by the MVV. An individual has reached his or her ventilatory limits when $\dot{V}_E$/MVV is greater than 80 percent. In addition to ventilatory limits, the respiratory system can be limiting because of problems with gas exchange or $\dot{V}/Q$ mismatching. Several different measurements can be used to identify problems with gas exchange. The arterial PO_2 normally increases with exercise owing to improved $\dot{V}/Q$ matching and increasing $\dot{V}_E$. Abnormal responses to exercise include a decrease in arterial PO_2 or an increase in the A-a gradient. The arterial PCO_2 normally decreased with exercise owing to the increased $\dot{V}_E$. An increase in the PCO_2 with the increasing $\dot{V}_E$ seen with exercise is indicative of an abnormal increase in the dead space/tidal volume ratio ($\dot{V}_D/\dot{V}_T$). Abnormalities in gas exchange can be due to pathologies within the lung parenchyma or pulmonary vascular disease.

Another value that is frequently reported is the anaerobic threshold (AT). AT is the $\dot{V}O_2$ during exercise where aerobic metabolism is supplemented with anaerobic metabolism. The level is reflected by an increase in the lactic acid within the blood. Several different methods can be used to identify the AT. For patients with arterial catheters, frequent blood sampling can be done to measure blood lactate levels. More commonly, the AT is extrapolated from measures of exhaled gas. The switch from aerobic to anaerobic metabolism leads to a cascade of physiologic events. Increasing blood lactate leads to a decrease in arterial pH, consumption of bicarbonate, and subsequent increase in CO_2 production. This is reflected in a nonlinear increase in $\dot{V}CO_2$ once the subject passes the AT. The acidosis also causes an increased ventilatory drive and increased $\dot{V}_E$. A graph of $\dot{V}CO_2$ and $\dot{V}_E$ can be used to extrapolate the AT. The AT can be used to estimate the amount of exercise or work that an individual can perform for a sustained time period.

Finally, another useful measurement provided by CPET is the O_2 pulse, which is calculated by dividing the $\dot{V}O_2$ by the HR. It also is equal to the stroke volume (SV) multiplied by the arterial to mixed venous oxygen content difference[$c(a–v)O_2$].

$$O_2 \text{ pulse} = \dot{V}O_2/HR = SV * c(a - v)O_2$$

With exercise, the O_2 pulse normally increases, mainly owing to increasing oxygen extraction by the muscles and increasing $c(a–v)O_2$. The O_2 pulse can be decreased and reaches its maximum at low levels of work in several settings, including congestive heart failure (CHF), anemia, arterial hypoxia, or elevated carboxyhemoglobin levels. These are just a few of the physiologic measurements provided by CPET. When used in the correct setting and interpreted by knowledgeable physicians, they can be extremely useful in a number of clinical settings.

SUMMARY

Cardiothoracic surgery has a high rate of pulmonary complications due to the high risk nature of the surgical procedures and also because most of the patients have underlying lung disease. The preoperative evaluation can risk stratify which patients can safely undergo these potentially life saving surgical procedures with minimal risk of significant morbidity and mortality. By understanding both the preoperative evaluation algorithm and also the different pulmonary tests, the number of patients who are offered surgery safely can be maximized and the complications limited.

References

1. Lawrence VA, Dhanda R, Hilsenbeck SG, Page CP. Risk of pulmonary complications after elective abdominal surgery. *Chest* 1996;110(3):744–750.
2. Lawrence VA, Hilsenbeck SG, Mulrow CD, et al. Incidence and hospital stay for cardiac and pulmonary complications after abdominal surgery. *J Gen Intern Med* 1995;10(12):671–678.
3. Smetana GW. Preoperative pulmonary evaluation. *N Engl J Med* 1999;340(12):937–944.
4. Arozullah AM, Daley J, Henderson WG, Khuri SF. Multifactorial risk index for predicting postoperative respiratory failure in men after major noncardiac surgery. The National Veterans Administration Surgical Quality Improvement Program. *Ann Surg* 2000;232(2): 242–253.
5. Arozullah AM, Khuri SF, Henderson WG, Daley J. Development and validation of a multifactorial risk index for predicting postoperative pneumonia after major noncardiac surgery. *Ann Intern Med* 2001;135(10):847–857.
6. Fisher BW, Majumdar SR, McAlister FA. Predicting pulmonary complications after nonthoracic surgery: A systematic review of blinded studies. *Am J Med* 2002;112(3):219–225.
7. Tarhan S, Moffitt EA, Sessler AD, et al. Risk of anesthesia and surgery in patients with chronic bronchitis and chronic obstructive pulmonary disease. *Surgery* 1973;74(5):720–726.
8. Rodgers A, Walker N, Schug S, et al. Reduction of postoperative mortality and morbidity with epidural or spinal anaesthesia: Results from overview of randomised trials. *BMJ* 2000;321(7275):1493.

9. Mitchell CK, Smoger SH, Pfeifer MP, et al. Multivariate analysis of factors associated with postoperative pulmonary complications following general elective surgery. *Arch Surg* 1998;133(2):194–198.
10. Buist AS, Sexton GJ, Nagy JM, Ross BB. The effect of smoking cessation and modification on lung function. *Am Rev Respir Dis* 1976;114(1):115–122.
11. Moller AM, Villebro N, Pedersen T, Tonnesen H. Effect of preoperative smoking intervention on postoperative complications: A randomised clinical trial. *Lancet* 2002;359(9301):114–117.
12. Zibrak JD, O'Donnell CR, Marton K. Indications for pulmonary function testing. *Ann Intern Med* 1990; 112(10):763–771.
13. Deslauriers J, Ginsberg RJ, Piantadosi S, Fournier B. Prospective assessment of 30-day operative morbidity for surgical resections in lung cancer. *Chest* 1994;106(6 Suppl):329S–330S.
14. Damhuis RA, Schutte PR. Resection rates and postoperative mortality in 7,899 patients with lung cancer. *Eur Respir J* 1996;9(1):7–10.
15. Sherman S, Guidot CE. The feasibility of thoracotomy for lung cancer in the elderly. *JAMA* 1987;258(7): 927–930.
16. Olsen GN, Block AJ, Swenson EW, et al. Pulmonary function evaluation of the lung resection candidate: A prospective study. *Am Rev Respir Dis* 1975;111(4):379–387.
17. BTS guidelines: Guidelines on the selection of patients with lung cancer for surgery. *Thorax* 2001;56(2):89–108.
18. Keagy BA, Schorlemmer GR, Murray GF, et al. Correlation of preoperative pulmonary function testing with clinical course in patients after pneumonectomy. *Ann Thorac Surg* 1983;36(3):253–257.
19. Boushy SF, Billig DM, North LB, Helgason AH. Clinical course related to preoperative and postoperative pulmonary function in patients with bronchogenic carcinoma. *Chest* 1971;59(4):383–391.
20. Miller JI Jr. Physiologic evaluation of pulmonary function in the candidate for lung resection. *J Thorac Cardiovasc Surg* 1993;105(2):347–351.
21. Schoonover GA, Olsen GN, McLain WC III, et al. Lateral position test and quantitative lung scan in the preoperative evaluation for lung resection. *Chest* 1984;86(6):854–859.
22. Wernly JA, DeMeester TR, Kirchner PT, et al. Clinical value of quantitative ventilation-perfusion lung scans in the surgical management of bronchogenic carcinoma. *J Thorac Cardiovasc Surg* 1980;80(4):535–543.
23. Bechard D, Wetstein L. Assessment of exercise oxygen consumption as preoperative criterion for lung resection. *Ann Thorac Surg* 1987;44(4):344–349.
24. Morice RC, Peters EJ, Ryan MB, et al. Exercise testing in the evaluation of patients at high risk for complications from lung resection. *Chest* 1992;101(2):356–361.
25. Smith TP, Kinasewitz GT, Tucker WY, et al. Exercise capacity as a predictor of post-thoracotomy morbidity. *Am Rev Respir Dis* 1984;129(5):730–734.
26. Walsh GL, Morice RC, Putnam JB Jr, et al. Resection of lung cancer is justified in high-risk patients selected by exercise oxygen consumption. *Ann Thorac Surg* 1994;58(3):704–710.
27. Bolton JW, Weiman DS, Haynes JL, et al. Stair climbing as an indicator of pulmonary function. *Chest* 1987;92(5): 783–788.
28. Holden DA, Rice TW, Stelmach K, Meeker DP. Exercise testing, 6-min walk, and stair climb in the evaluation of patients at high risk for pulmonary resection. *Chest* 1992;102(6):1774–1779.
29. Olsen GN, Bolton JW, Weiman DS, Hornung CA. Stair climbing as an exercise test to predict the postoperative complications of lung resection. Two years' experience. *Chest* 1991;99(3):587–590.
30. McKenna RJ Jr, Fischel RJ, Brenner M, Gelb AF. Combined operations for lung volume reduction surgery and lung cancer. *Chest* 1996;110(4):885–888.
31. Munoz JI, Pelaez MC, Alvarez MJ, et al. Lung volume reduction surgery: New expectations in the surgical treatment of lung cancer. *Chest* 1996;109(6):1664.
32. Wasserman K. *Principles of Exercise Testing and Interpretation*. 3d ed. Baltimore: Lippincott Williams & Wilkins, 1999.

CHAPTER

2 MEDIASTINAL DISEASE

Peter Attia

INTRODUCTION

The mediastinum is the region of the chest bounded superiorly by the thoracic inlet, inferiorly by the diaphragm, laterally by the pleura of the lungs, anteriorly by the sternum, and posteriorly by vertebral bodies.

EMBRYOLOGY AND ANATOMY

A firm understanding of both the embryology and anatomy of the mediastinum is essential to grasp the pathology of this body cavity. One author has referred to it as: "a topless pyramid, with a wide anteroposterior plane, a rather

KEY CONCEPTS

- Epidemiology
  - Thymoma is the most common primary neoplasm of the anterior mediastinum, with peak incidence in the third and fifth decades of life. Myasthenia occurs with a prevalence of 5–12.5 per 100,000, with women (peak incidence in 2nd to 3rd decades) affected twice as commonly as men (peak incidence in 6th to 7th decades). In most series, lymphoma is the most common neoplasm of the mediastinum. Mediastinal germ cell tumors comprise 10–15% of mediastinal neoplasms, found almost exclusively in males, usually in the third decade. Mediastinal teratomas comprise about 60% of mediastinal germ cell tumors (equal sex distribution) and mediastinal seminomas comprise approximately 40% of malignant germ cell tumors (males in 3rd to 4th decade).
- Pathophysiology
  - Pathophysiologic processes range from mass effect (e.g., superior vena cava syndrome) to antibody-mediated processes (e.g., myasthenia gravis). The most common lymphomas encountered in the mediastinum include Hodgkin's, non-Hodgkin's, and lymphoblastic lymphomas. Mediastinal teratomas generally consist of will-differentiated tissue derived from more than one of the three primitive germ cell layers. Seminomas are slow growing and slow to metastasize. Conversely, non-seminomatous germ cell tumors grow rapidly and metastasize early.
- Clinical Features
  - Although 25–50% of thymomas are asymptomatic, the most common symptoms include vague chest pain, cough, and dyspnea. Thymoma is associated with myasthenia gravis and its associated symptoms. Lymphomas typically present with "B-type" symptoms including fever, night sweats, chills, and malaise, in addition to compressive symptoms by larger lesions. Also often asymptomatic, symptoms associated with mediastinal teratomas include chest pain, fever, and dyspnea: a greater proportion of patients with mediastinal seminomas and nonseminomatous germ cell tumors are symptomatic upon presentation. About 90% of patients with seminoma have normal; α-fetoprotein (AFP) and β-human chorionic gonadotropin (β-HCG) levels; 10% have normal AFP and mildly elevated β-HCG levels. 90% of nonseminomas have elevated AFP (80%), β-HCG (30–35%), or both.
- Diagnostics
  - Diagnostic tests include plain radiography, computed tomography, magnetic resonance imaging, radionuclide studies, serum markers and tissue biopsy.

- Treatment
  - Thymoma in the absence of metastasis, is nominally treated by complete surgical resection with adjuvant/neoadjuvant therapies. Treatment for myasthenia includes immunosuppressants, cholinesterase inhibitors, plasma exchange, and surgical thymectomy. The mainstay treatments for lymphoma include chemotherapy, radiotherapy, and immune-mediate therapies. Complete surgical excision is the treatment for teratomas. Mediastinal seminomas confined to the mediastinum are treated with primary resection followed by radiation; meastatic disease in treated with cisplatin-based chemotherapy with surgical resection of residual disease. Mediastinal nonseminomatous germ cell tumors are treated primarily with chemotherapy with surgical resection reserved for residual disease.
- Outcomes
  - Most patients with myasthenia can expect normal life expectancy. Hodgkin's patients can expect a complete durable remission rate in excess of 70%. Survival for seminomatous germ cell tumors is greater than 80% at five years, whereas survival for non-seminomatous tumors is about 50%.

tight lateral plane, its base resting over the diaphragm, and its top corresponding to the base of the neck."[1] It contains vital structures of the circulatory, digestive, respiratory, and nervous systems, and its embryologic origin can be traced back to cells of ectoderm, mesoderm, and endoderm. By virtue of its proximity to vital structures, in addition to its ability to shift and compress, it plays a key role in both respiratory dynamics and hemodynamics.

Until the seventh week of development, the pericardial cavity communicates directly with the peritoneal cavity via paired pericardioperitoneal cavities. The cranial pleuropericardial membrane fuses with the mesoderm ventral to the esophagus and separates the pericardial and pleural cavities. At approximately the same time, the caudal portions of the pleuropericardial membranes fuse and, during formation of the diaphragm, separate the pleural cavity from the peritoneal cavity. The diaphragm forms from the fusion of the septum transversum, the pleuroperitoneal membranes, the dorsal mesentery of the esophagus, and the body wall. Congenital diaphragmatic hernias result from failure of these structures to fuse with the pleuropericardial membrane.[2] Germinal blastomeres migrate from one pole to the other. Failure to reach their destination may result in the development of germ cell tumors (GCTs). Similarly, intestinal and respiratory duplication cysts can occur, typically in the middle mediastinum, as a result of wayward migration patterns.

The mediastinum itself is the negative image of the organs within and surrounding it. Somewhat arbitrarily, it is divided into three (and sometimes four) regions: anterior, middle, and posterior (and superior, which, in the absence of a fourth region, is included in the anterior region). Table 2-1 shows the contents and various tumors typically found in each region. The line from the sternal angle to T4/T5 divides the mediastinum into its superior and inferior divisions. The anterior division is bounded above by the superior border of the pericardium, below by the diaphragm, anteriorly by the sternum, and posteriorly by the anterior border of the pericardium. The middle division is bounded above by the pericardial

Table 2-1 Anatomic divisions of the mediastinum with contents and tumors

Division	Contents	Tumors
Superior/anterior	**1.** Aortic arch and thoracic portions of its branches (brachiocephalic, left common carotid, left subclavian) **2.** Brachiocephalic veins, upper half of superior vena cava **3.** Vagus nerves, left recurrent laryngeal nerve, phrenic nerves **4.** Superior esophagus **5.** Upper trachea **6.** Thymus **7.** Upper portion of thoracic duct **8.** Lymph nodes	Thymoma Germ cell tumor Lymphoma Thyroid adenoma Parathyroid adenoma Lipoma Carcinoma Hemangioma
Middle	**1.** Pericardium **2.** Heart **3.** Tracheal bifurcation and mainstem bronchi **4.** Subcarinal and peribronchial nodes **5.** Ascending aorta	Bronchogenic cysts Pericardial cysts Lymphoma
Posterior	**1.** Thoracic portion of descending aorta **2.** Azygos, hemiazygos, accessory hemiazygos veins **3.** Sympathetic chains **4.** Thoracic duct **5.** Esophagus	Neurogenic tumors Enteric cysts

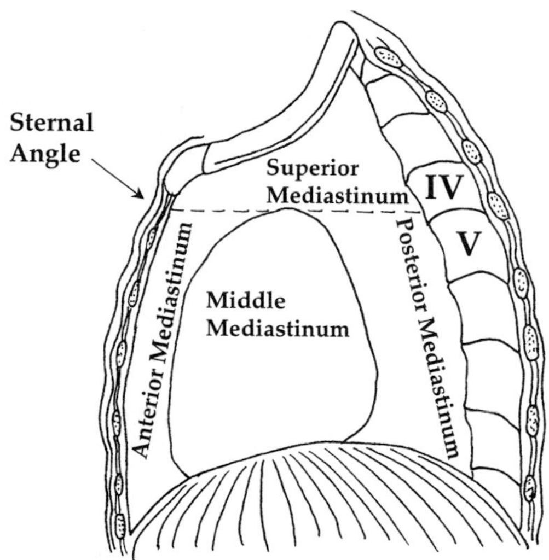

Figure 2-1 Mediastinal compartments. The plane defining the inferior border of the superior mediastinum runs from the sternal angle to the junction T4 and T5. For the purpose of discussion, the superior mediastinum is often combined with the anterior mediastinum.

reflection, below by the diaphragm, and posteriorly by the posterior border of the pericardium. The posterior division is bounded above by the superior border of the pericardium, below by the diaphragm, anteriorly by the posterior border of the pericardium, and posteri-orly by the thoracic vertebrae and mediastinal pleura (Fig. 2-1).

DIAGNOSTIC TESTS

Serum markers

Because of the diversity of pathologic conditions arising in the mediastinum, large-scale routine screening is neither warranted nor practical. However, patients with suspected GCTs should undergo serum evaluation for levels of beta human chorionic gonadotropin (β-HCG), alpha fetoprotein (AFP), and lactate dehydrogenase (LDH). Elevated levels can indicate malignancy and correlate with tumor burden, while their absence can indicate benign disease or seminoma.[3] More recently, newer markers have emerged as potential indicators of mediastinal tumors, specifically lymphoma. An elevated serum $beta_2$-microglobulin level has been demonstrated to be an independently poor prognostic factor for overall survival in patients with early-stage Hodgkin's disease.[4]

Plain radiography

In many instances, malignant and benign lesions of the mediastinum can be detected by posteroanterior and lateral radiographs.[5,6] However, with the rapid increase in and availability of other technologies, such as spiral computed tomography (CT) and magnetic resonance imagining (MRI), few if any patients will receive a diagnosis and treatment plan based solely on plain film. The likelihood that the correct diagnosis can be made from the plain film alone is significantly lower than that with CT.[7]

Computed tomography

CT of the thorax with the use of intravenous contrast has emerged as the definitive study in the workup and management of mediastinal masses. Refinement of the differential diagnosis is achieved by attention to signal intensity and degrees of tissue attenuation in addition to the presence or absence of calcification.[8] The relationship of the mass to fat and fluid further refines the differentiation of cystic, vascular, and heterogeneous masses identified by CT.[9] GCTs show roundness without distinct lobulation and frequently have calcification when they are benign, whereas malignancy is predicted by thick-walled, homogeneous images with Hounsfield units similar to water.[10] Conversely, thymoma often manifests itself as a solid mass with lobulation, occasionally with a thin rim of calcification. Additional CT findings typically found with mediastinal tumors, in addition to the presence of a mass, include pleural deposits, local infiltration of mediastinal and cardiovascular structures, and diaphragmatic deposits.[11] CT scans are most often accurate in revealing GCTs and thymolipomas.[7] CT is a useful modality for staging Hodgkin's and non-Hodgkin's lymphoma in addition to differentiating lesions of the thymus (cystic lesions versus hyperplasia versus lymphoma).[12] Currently, CT is also being used to guide needle biopsy for tissue confirmation of mediastinal masses.

Magnetic resonance imaging

MRI, which utilizes proton spin rather than an electron beam to produce an image, offers several advantages over CT. First, scans can be obtained in several planes: axial, coronal, and sagittal. Second, MRI uses gadolinium as a contrast medium, which is neither nephrotoxic nor allogeneic. MRI may be preferred for posterior mediastinal masses, while CT is still preferred for lesions that may involved lung parenchyma.[8]

Radionucleotide studies

Most radiographic studies can be broadly separated into two categories: imaging and functional. Radionucleotide studies fall into the latter category. Although the pathologies of the mediastinum are more often evaluated by techniques that focus on imaging properties, radionucleotide studies do have a small role in the workup of mediastinal masses. In particular, they are useful primarily in the evaluation of extraadrenal pheochromocytoma. A positive scan with iodine-131 metaiodobenzylguanidine (^{131}I-MIBG), an adrenergic tissue-localizing agent, is diagnostic. The addition of CT is complementary for complete anatomic detail and the facilitation of safe resection.[13]

Biopsy

Fine-needle and core-needle biopsy

Acquisition of tissue following the identification of a mediastinal mass is the next step in the workup and management of such masses. Percutaneous needle biopsy, either fine- or core-needle, is replacing the more invasive, morbid inpatient methods such as mediastinoscopy, thoracoscopy, and thoracotomy.[14] CT-guided needle biopsy (CTNB) is emerging as the procedure of choice for a number of reasons, not the least of which is the ability to perform this test in the ambulatory setting under local anesthesia. Over the past decade, CTNB has proved to be a safe, accurate, and inexpensive tool in the diagnosis of mediastinal masses from each of the mediastinal compartments.[13,15] Several large studies have found that the ability to retrieve diagnostic tissue in one attempt exceeds 70 percent for masses, including Hodgkin's and non-Hodgkin's lymphoma, in each mediastinal compartment.[14,16,17] These studies demonstrated a sensitivity in the range of 71 to 100 percent for both benign and malignant disease and a specificity in the range of 94 to 100 percent.

Mediastinoscopy, video-assisted thoracoscopic surgery (VATS), anterior mediastinotomy (Chamberlain procedure), and thoracotomy

Currently, the importance of mediastinoscopy, VATS, anterior mediastinotomy, and thoracotomy for the diagnosis of mediastinal masses has decreased. This is largely due to the proliferation of higher-quality cross-sectional imaging devices, increased accuracy of needle biopsy, and molecular methods allowing diagnoses to be made with lesser amounts of tissue than even a decade ago. The left anterior mediastinotomy is often used in conjunction with the standard cervical mediastinoscopy, in particular when access to level 5 and/or 6 nodes is warranted, whereas right anterior mediastinotomy can be used for accessing level 3, level 4, and level 10 nodes.[18] In certain suspected disease states, such as lymphoma, a greater amount of tissue may be required for diagnosis and even for therapeutic intervention than is easily obtained via needle or core biopsy. For example, immunologic treatment of lymphoma requires the isolation of antigens against which tumor vaccines are created.[19]

ANTERIOR AND SUPERIOR MEDIASTINAL MASSES

Thymoma

At birth, the thymus is a relatively large gland that is located below the superior aspect of the sternum and lies anterior to the great vessels in a roughly H-shaped configuration. Following puberty, the gland reduces in size until, by adulthood, it is merely a remnant. Its arterial blood supply most commonly arises from the inferior thyroid and internal mammary arteries, although branches may arise from the superior thyroid artery, subclavian artery, and carotid artery.[20]

Thymoma is the most common primary neoplasm of the anterior mediastinum; in some series, it is the most common primary neoplasm in the entire mediastinum.[21,22] Although thymomas can occur at any time during life, the peak incidence is between the third and fifth decades of life, and men and women are affected equally.

Clinical presentation and diagnosis

Based on the series, anywhere from 25 to 50 percent of patients with thymoma present without symptoms[23–25] and the tumor is discovered as an incidental finding on radiography. The most common symptoms are vague chest pain, cough, and dyspnea. In addition, some patients also present with constitutional symptoms such as fatigue, fever, weight loss, and limb swelling. Physical examination is often unremarkable, but patients can manifest physical signs of respiratory distress, myasthenia gravis (see below), and superior vena cava (SVC) syndrome (see below). The diagnosis of thymoma requires the acquisition of tissue. As described above, this is being done more and more frequently on an outpatient basis using CT-guided techniques and local anesthesia. The histologic classification of thymoma is an evolving and somewhat controversial issue. Traditionally, classification was based on the relative proportions of epithelial and lymphocytic cells (Table 2-2). Although not an independent predictor of survival, the epithelial cell type displays a higher rate of recurrence and tumor-related death than the other subtypes.[26,27] In the mid-1980s a second classification scheme was put forth, initially by Marino and Muller-Hermelinik and later by Kirchner and Muller-Hermelinik. This classification is based on the appearance of the tumor cells relative to thymic medullary cells and thymic cortical cells.[27,28] The six subtypes in this classification are medullary, mixed, predominantly cortical, cortical, well-differentiated carcinoma, and high-grade carcinoma, with medullary and mixed tumors demonstrating little chance of recurrence or aggressive behavior. Several reports have found this classification system to be an independent predictor of survival.[29–31]

In most series, however, clinical and pathological staging are the most important predictors of survival, in addition to ability to achieve a complete resection,[24,32,33]

Table 2-2 Traditional classification of thymic tumors based on lymphoid predominance

Subgroup	Mixture of cells
Lymphocytic	Two-thirds of cells are lymphoid
Mixed lymphoepithelial	One- to two-thirds of cells are lymphoid
Epithelial	Two-thirds of cells are epithelial
Spindle	Two-thirds of cells are epithelial and spindle

Table 2-3 Masaoka staging system for thymoma

Stage	Criteria
I	Macroscopically completely encapsulated with no microscopic extracapsular invasion
IIa	Macroscopic invasion into mediastinal fat or pleura
IIb	Microscopic invasion through the capsule
III	Invasion into adjacent structures (pericardium, great vessels, lung)
IVa	Pleural or pericardial metastases
IVb	Lymphogenous or hematogenous metastases

and many of these have demonstrated that histopathology, regardless of which system was used, had no bearing on survival.

The staging system proposed by Masaoka over 20 years ago still stands today as the most widely adapted (Table 2-3).[34] This staging system is most accurately accomplished postoperatively, with the full input from pathologic assessment.[35] Approximate 5-year survival for each the stages is as follows: stage I, 95 percent; stage II, 85 percent; stage III, 70 percent; and stage IV, 50 percent.

Treatment

Thymoma is a surgical disease provided that widespread metastases are not present at the time of diagnosis. Median sternotomy is the preferred approach, while posterolateral thoracotomy may provide some benefit in situations of bulky tumor mass necessitating control of the pulmonary vasculature. As described above, complete excision is the "gold standard" of treatment. This, in addition to the pathologic staging that accompanies it, is the most important predictor of survival. The paucity of controlled trials—randomized, prospective, or otherwise—investigating the role of neoadjuvant therapy in the management of thymoma is evident by the lack of guidelines in the literature. Several authors have discussed the role of nonsurgical (chemotherapy and/or radiotherapy) treatments in the management of malignant thymoma for patients with locally inoperable tumors or metastatic disease or as an adjunct to surgery.

A large retrospective study carried out by the Federation Nationale des Centres du Lutte Contre le Cancer (FNCLCC) across 10 French cancer centers examined the role of radiation therapy (plus or minus cisplatin-based chemotherapy) in patients with Masaoka stage III and IV disease following either partial resection or biopsy, depending on the extent of the disease. Each patient was treated with curative intent. The median dose of radiation was 50 Gy and median follow-up was 105 months. Not surprisingly, extent of resection had the largest impact on survival, with 5- and 10-year survival being 64 and 43 percent, respectively, for the resection group, and 39 and 31 percent for the biopsy group ($p < 0.02$). In addition, radiation provided a significant amount of local control, although the rate of local recurrence left the authors to conclude that doses in excess of 50 Gy were necessary to achieve sufficient local control in cases of incomplete resection.[36] A large single-institution retrospective review from Italy demonstrated that patients receiving a preoperative, or neoadjuvant, dose of 30 Gy followed by a postoperative dose of 16 to 24 Gy had a 10-year survival of 70 percent for stage III disease and 58 percent for stage IV disease. Complete resection was possible in just over half of the patients with stage III disease and none of the patients with stage IV disease.[37]

Other large reviews and single-institution retrospective studies have found that radiation in the adjuvant setting did seem to increase survival compared to historical controls in patients with stages II through IV disease[38] or at least stages III through IV.[39,40] These patients also received chemotherapy. Finally, a subset of patients' thymomas express high levels of somatostatin receptor.[41] These select patients may have thymomas sensitive to treatment with somatostatin analogues, such as octreotide, combined with prednisone.[42,43]

Clearly a prospective randomized, multicenter (given the incidence of thymoma) trial is needed to illuminate this issue. Until then, it seems that approximately 50 Gy of radiation, in addition to cisplatin-based chemotherapy, is likely to benefit patients with at least stages III and IV disease, regardless of the extent of resection, and possibly patients with stage II disease. There seems to be no role for adjuvant therapy in the management of stage I disease.

Myasthenia gravis

The first case of myasthenia gravis (MG) was described in 1672 by Thomas Willis of Oxford. However, it was not until 1934, when Mary Walker astutely noted that injection of physostigmine and neostigmine improved clinical performance in patients with this disease, that treatment became anything more than insignificant.[44] Two years later, Alfred Blalock performed the first successful thymectomy for a thymomatous patient with MG.[45] Blalock believed that one day all patients with severe MG, including nonthymomatous patients, would benefit from thymectomy[46]; in 1941, he carried out the first of such operations, publishing his series of 20 patients a few years later.[47] Today, with the many advances in the understanding of the pathophysiology of MG, similar patients still benefit from the operation performed over 60 years ago by Blalock.

Epidemiology and pathology MG occurs with a prevalence of approximately 5 to 12.5 per 100,000 population[48] or about 35,000 affected persons in the United States. Women are affected twice as commonly as men, with the peak incidence in women occurring earlier, usually during the second to third decades; in men the disease is more likely to appear between the sixth and seventh decades. MG is a condition that fits all major criteria for an autoantibody disorder[49]:

- The antibody against the acetylcholine receptor (AchR) is present in 80 to 90 percent of affected patients.

- The antibody reacts with a specific antigen (the AchR).
- The condition can be passively transferred by the antibody to an animal model, producing a similar clinical condition.
- Repeated injection of the human antigen in other species produces a model disease.
- Reduction in antibody level is associated with clinical improvement.

Despite this characterization, the interaction between the antibody and AchRs is not completely understood. For example, 10 to 20 percent of patients with MG do not have antibodies to AchR.[50] It has been proposed that these seronegative patients produce a plasma factor, distinct from the muscle-specific IgG antibodies, that bind directly to muscle membranes and activate second messengers, leading to the phosphorylation of AchRs and a reduction of AchR function.

Ultimately, the relationship between the AchR and antibody leads to a reduction in the number of AchRs at the neuromuscular junction. In addition, the neuromuscular junction (NMJ) in patients with MG has simplified, shallow postsynaptic folds, a widened synaptic space, and yet a normal nerve terminal.[49]

Clinical presentation and diagnosis In patients with MG, because of the paucity of AchRs, transmission of the action potential is decreased. This leads to decreased contraction of the target muscle fiber, clinically manifest as weakness. This usually occurs in a characteristic distribution, which Osserman has used to devise a clinical scale of disease severity.[51] Grade I disease is focal; for example, weakness of only the ocular muscles. Grade II disease is generalized and either mild (IIa) or moderate (IIb). Grade III disease is severe generalized weakness, and grade IV, or crisis, is life-threatening respiratory compromise, requiring mechanical ventilation. Approximately 15 percent of patients with MG do not progress beyond diplopia and ptosis.[52]

The diagnosis begins with a physical exam, noting weakness in ocular and bulbar muscles with progressive exercise, which resolves with rest. Following this, 2 to 8 mg of edrophonium (Tensilon), a short-acting anticholinesterase, is administered intravenously over 15 to 30 s. Within half a minute or so and lasting for 5 to 10 min, the patient experiences a marked improvement in symptoms. If the results of this test are equivocal, repetitive nerve stimulation, assay for anti-acetylcholine-receptor antibody, and single-fiber electromyography may be carried out before treatment is begun.[49]

Treatment Prior to the 1960s, approximately one-third of patients with MG died of their disease, one-third deteriorated or remained unchanged, and one-third improved.[52] Today, most patients with MG can expect to live a normal life span. The cornerstone of treatment, required by most for the duration of their lives, is immunosuppression. In addition, cholinesterase inhibitors, plasma exchange, and surgical thymectomy play a role in the acute and chronic management of MG.[53]

1. *Anticholinesterase Agents.* As an initial therapy, all patients with MG should undergo an attempt at therapy with oral anticholinesterases. The logic is simply to overcome the dearth of AchRs by providing a greater amount of acetylcholine at the neuromuscular junction. However, these medications have no role in altering either the amount of AchRs or the interaction between the AchR and antibody. As a consequence, the natural history of the disease is not altered by anticholinesterases. The usual choice of agent is pyridostigmine because it has a longer half-life than neostigmine. Its onset of action is approximately 30 min, with a peak in activity at roughly 2 h. It is usually dosed every 6 h. The side effects include abdominal pain and cramping, diarrhea, hypersalivation, bradycardia, and blurred vision. In addition, at higher doses, muscle weakness becomes a major toxicity. Low doses of atropine can alleviate some of these side effects.
2. *Short-Term Immunotherapy: Plasma Exchange and Intravenous Immune Globulin.* Plasmapheresis directly removes AchR antibodies from the circulation and produces short-term clinical improvement in patients with MG.[54–56] Its efficacy correlates roughly with the reduction of AchR-Ab titer, although antibody-negative patients have been shown to improve in the short term with plasmapheresis.[57] Treatment typically involves 2- to 4-L exchanges two to three times in a week, repeated once. The clinical improvement is usually noted quickly and lasts from several weeks to 2 months. Primary indications are for the treatment of patients in myasthenic crisis and as preoperative preparation for patients undergoing thymectomy. The major drawbacks of this therapy are the risks and complications associated with long-term use of indwelling venous catheters, including infection, venous stenosis, and thromboembolism. Like plasmapheresis, intravenous immunoglobulin (IVIG) produces a rapid clinical improvement, with an efficacy somewhere on the order of 75 percent as calculated retrospectively from eight published reports.[58] The mechanism of action is unclear, and the success of this modality does not seem to correlate with titers of AchR-Ab.[59] Side effects include headaches, fluid retention, and, rarely, renal failure.
3. *Long-Term Immunotherapy: Immunosuppressive Drugs.* Corticosteroids, primarily prednisone, are the most commonly used drugs in the treatment of MG. Their effectives in producing remission or marked improvement ranges from 30 percent for complete remission[60] to 80 percent for at least marked improvement.[61] Prednisone is initiated at 15 to 20 mg/day and increased 5 to 10 mg/day every 3 to 4 days until improvement is noted or a dose of 60 mg/day is reached. The regimen is continued for 1 to 2 years, depending on whether the patient is undergoing thymectomy, before tapering is begun. The side effects of long-term prednisone are numerous and include adrenal insufficiency, psychosis, nausea, vomiting,

anxiety, and cushingoid features. Failure to respond to prednisone or inability to tolerate the long-term side effects can prompt a trial of pulse steroids (methylprednisolone); this has been shown to result in a positive treatment response with negligible side effects in at least one double-blind trial.[62] The other commonly used medications for long-term immune suppression in patients with MG are azathioprine (Imuran) and cyclosporine (Neoral, Sandimmune). These drugs are typically used if there is a significant contraindication to the use of steroids. One randomized double-blind study found a significant advantage to oral steroids plus azathioprine versus steroids alone.[63]

4. *Thymectomy.* Thymectomy is indicated in patients with MG for two main reasons. First, the majority of patients with MG have a thymic abnormality: 60 to 70 percent have hyperplasia,[49] and anywhere from 10 to 30 percent have thymoma, depending on the series.[64,65] Second, it is generally believed that even nonthymomatous patients benefit from thymectomy.[66] As mentioned above, Blalock suggested this 60 years ago, and today most neurologists agree. In fact, current recommendations for thymectomy in nonthymomatous patients with MG are early, generalized, moderate to severe disease stabilized with medication, and resistant ocular disease.[20,67,68] There have been no randomized prospective trials examining the value and efficacy of thymectomy in nonthymomatous patients with MG, and it is unlikely that there ever will be such trials. A group at Mayo conducted a retrospective computer-assisted match of nonthymomatous patients undergoing thymectomy versus medical management of historical controls. In the surgical group, 35 percent of patients achieved a complete remission and another 33 percent had significant improvement compared to 7.6 and 17 percent, respectively, in the medically managed historical controls.[69] A 20-year review of 384 patients with MG undergoing thymectomy at a single institution in Japan revealed remission rates in the nonthymomatous patients to be 22, 37, 46, 56, 67, and 50 percent at 1, 3, 5, 10, 15, and 20 years, respectively. The remission rates for thymomatous patients were 28, 32, 23, 30, 32, and 38 percent, respectively.[70] Today, the debate is not whether nonthymomatous patients with MG should undergo thymectomy. Rather, the debate focuses on the predictors of outcome and the surgical approach and technique. Patients should not undergo thymectomy on an emergency basis—that is, if they are in crisis. Temporizing measures such as plasmapheresis should supersede surgical management in such settings. Complete removal of the thymus is essential and is associated with improved outcome, even in nonthymomatous patients.[71] As little a 3 g of residual thymus following initial operation has resulted in persistent disease and even crisis, with remission following complete resection.[72] Some authors have found the presence of a thymoma to be a poor predictor of outcome in patients with MG undergoing thymectomy,[20,65] while others have found this not to be the case in either univariate or multivariate analysis.[64,73] This disparity may be explained by the fact that MG patients with thymoma are typically older than their nonthymomatous counterparts, thereby not allowing an unbiased comparison. Nonthymomatous patients subjected to thymectomy less than 5 years after the onset of disease fare better than those with long-standing disease.[66] Despite a growing interest in minimally invasive surgery, most experts still advocate either median sternotomy or an extended cervicomediastinal approach because of the good exposure and decreased likelihood that any thymic tissue will remain,[67,71] while others have suggested a transcervical approach for nonthymomatous patients.[74,75]

Lymphomas

Incidence and epidemiology

Lymphoma is, in most series, the most common neoplasm of the mediastinum (Fig. 2-2). However, primary mediastinal lymphoma is a rare entity and accounts for only 5 to 10 percent of all lymphomas.[76] Typically, it presents as part of a systemic illness with many of the B-type symptoms (see below). Further, primary mediastinal lymphoma accounts for less than 10 percent of mediastinal lymphoma.[77] The most common types of lymphoma encountered in the mediastinum are Hodgkin's, non-Hodgkin's, and lymphoblastic lymphoma.[78] Hodgkin's lymphoma has a peak incidence in the third and fourth decades of life and females are affected more than males. The most common histologic subtype is the nodular sclerosis variant, although mixed-cellularity, lymphocyte-predominant, and lymphocyte-depleted types are also found in the mediastinum.[79] Non-Hodgkin's lymphoma presents with a more even distribution throughout the first five decades but is seen from childhood through the ninth decade. The aggressiveness of the tumor depends on the grade. Low- and intermediate-grade tumors predominate in adults, while the majority of children with

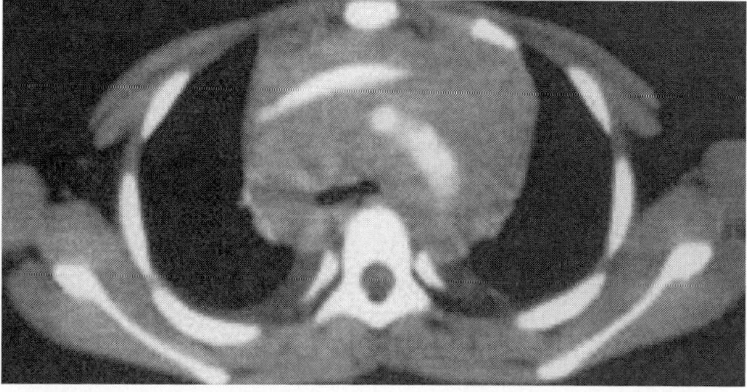

Figure 2-2 Computed tomography of lymphoma arising in anterior mediastinum.

non-Hodgkin's lymphoma have high-grade disease.[80] Lymphoblastic lymphoma is an aggressive leukemia/lymphoma seen more commonly in children and adolescents than adults and affecting males more than females. A mediastinal mass is present in 80 percent of cases.[81]

Presentation and diagnosis

The size and location of the mediastinal lymphoma dictate the symptoms associated with presentation. Larger lesions in the mediastinum cause compressive symptoms, such as chest heaviness or pain, shortness of breath, or cough. If the mass is sufficiently large, airway compression, pleural effusion, or pericardial effusion can occur.[35] Nonspecific B-type symptoms such as fever, night sweats, chills, and general malaise may also be present. Because paratracheal lymph nodes are more commonly on the right, SVC syndrome may be present in up to 60 percent of patients with mediastinal lymphoma.[82,83]

Although surgery does not often play a role in the treatment of lymphoma, it is often required for an accurate histologic diagnosis.[84,85] The surgical approach depends on the location of the mass and includes mediastinoscopy (cervical or anterior), sternotomy, thoracotomy, and VATS. In instances when airway compression makes the risks of general anesthesia too great, core or Tru-cut needle biopsy can be performed with the patient in an upright position and local anesthetic and minimal sedation.[35] However, larger amounts of lymphoid tissue are always preferred because, in addition to the specific cellularity, the architecture of the node is important for diagnosis and ultimately treatment of the lymphoma.

Treatment

Although the diagnosis of lymphoma often requires surgery, the treatment rarely does. Chemotherapy, radiation, and genetic or immune-mediated therapies play the predominant role in curing lymphoma, both mediastinal and otherwise. A thorough discussion regarding the treatment of lymphoma is beyond the scope of this chapter; however, some general principles are outlined below.

Patients with Hodgkin's lymphoma have experienced an increase in cure rate over the past several decades. Currently, patients can expect to achieve a complete durable remission greater than 70 percent of the time.[86] These cure rates are now possible because of several regimens and hybrids of regimens of chemotherapy, including mustargen, vincristine, procarbazine, and prednisone (MOPP), doxorubicin, bleomycin, vinblastine, and dacarbazine (ABVD), and bleomycin, etoposide, doxorubicin, cyclophosphamide, vincristine, procarbazine, and prednisone (BEACOPP).[87] The use of radiation therapy alone in patients with Hodgkin's disease does not appear to confer an advantage in survival,[88] while involved-field radiotherapy may benefit patients with advanced Hodgkin's disease who were partial rather than complete responders to chemotherapy.[87]

Patients with non-Hodgkin's lymphoma have not enjoyed the response rates and durable remissions that patients with Hodgkin's disease have.[89] A large multicenter trial published in 1993 confirmed that the first-line combination chemotherapy regimen consisting of cyclophosphamide, doxorubicin, vincristine, and prednisone (CHOP) is still the standard of care for patients with advanced non-Hodgkin's lymphoma.[90] Unlike Hodgkin's lymphoma, where the question remains incompletely answered, the addition of in-field radiation therapy to chemotherapy has been shown to increase survival in patients with non-Hodgkin's lymphoma.[91] Recently the development of monoclonal antibodies such has rituximab, a chimeric monoclonal antibody directed against the CD20 antigen of B cells, has significantly affected the therapy of non-Hodgkin's lymphoma.[92]

Castleman's disease

Castleman's disease, also known as angiofollicular lymphoid hyperplasia or giant lymph node hyperplasia, encompasses a heterogeneous group of lymphoproliferative disorders of unclear etiology. Histologic variants include hyaline vascular, plasma cell, and mixed histology, while clinically it exists as either a localized or mul-ticentric disease.[93] Often, the disease presents as a mediastinal mass, which may or may not cause symptoms. However, patients with this entity have also presented with diffuse adenopathy involving the inguinal, axillary, pelvic, and retroperitoneal regions.[94] Tissue diagnosis is important to avoid improper medical management. Needle biopsy is often nondiagnostic, as it is unable to preserve the architecture of the lymphoid tissue and achieve a satisfactory quantity of tissue, and thoracoscopic biopsy is potentially hazardous, as the hyperplastic tissue density is often hypervascularized and poses significant bleeding risks.[95] Complete surgical excision with appropriate follow-up is indicated for localized disease regardless of histology.[96] However, the multicentric disease, which carries a worse prognosis, requires aggressive systemic treatment.[93]

Germ cell tumors

Mediastinal germ cell tumors (GCTs) account for 10 to 15 percent of mediastinal neoplasms, making them roughly the third most common tumor of the anterior mediastinum (Fig. 2-3). There are reports, however, of GCTs arising in the posterior mediastinum with an incidence in the neighborhood of 3 to 8 percent.[97,98] The mediastinum is the most common extragonadal location for GCTs. Malignant GCTs are found almost exclusively in males, usually in the third decade, as demonstrated by a 1997 study in which 320 out of 322 mediastinal GCTs were in males.[99] Only mature teratomas affect males and females equally.[100] The earlier belief that all mediastinal GCTs arise as metastases from gonadal primary tumors was called into question by an autopsy study performed in 1976, which found that 18 out of 20 patients with mediastinal GCTs had no evidence of gonadal primary tumors.[101] However, it is imperative that patients with identified mediastinal

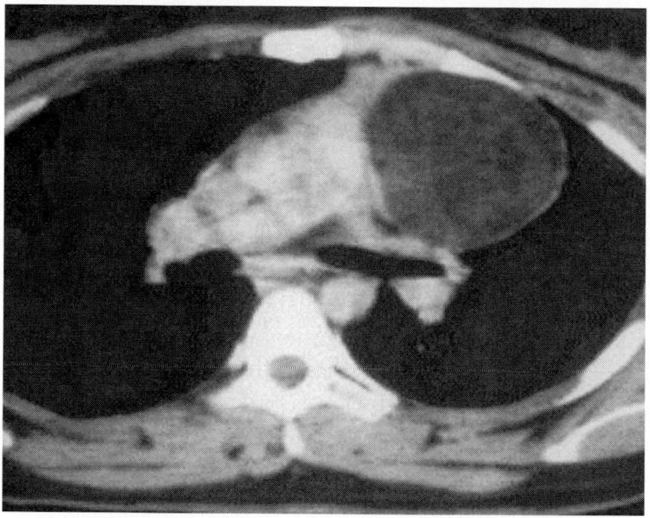

Figure 2-3 Computed tomography of mediastinal germ cell tumor.

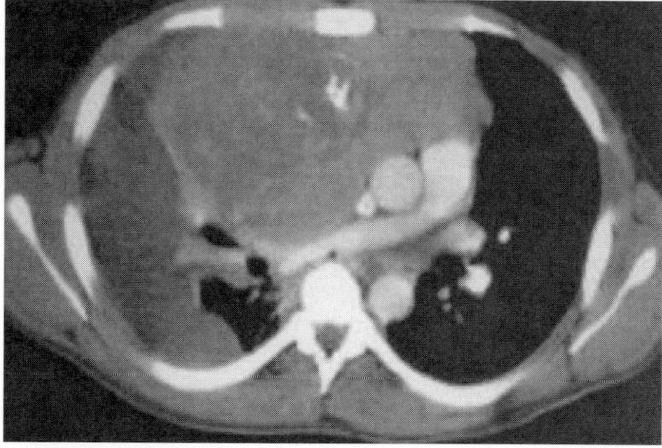

Figure 2-4 Computed tomography of mediastinal teratoma showing presence of well-differentiated structure (tooth).

GCTs undergo a thorough workup and evaluation for a primary gonadal tumor. Classification of mediastinal GCTs is divided into three broad categories: benign teratomas, malignant mediastinal seminomatous tumors, and malignant mediastinal nonseminomatous tumors.

Mediastinal teratomas

Mediastinal teratomas occur equally in men and women and represent approximately 60 percent of mediastinal GCTs.[102] The tumors are usually histologically well-differentiated and are composed of tissue from more than one of the three primitive germ cell layer. Frequently, patients are asymptomatic at the time of diagnosis. Chest pain (30 percent), fever (10 percent), and dyspnea (7 percent) were the most reported symptoms in one large series of 74 patients with mediastinal teratomas.[103] The masses are heterogeneous and up to one-quarter can display calcification on chest radiography and may demonstrate mature structures such as teeth, bone, or hair[104] (Fig. 2-4). Treatment is complete surgical excision, which is uniformly curative. There is no role for adjuvant chemotherapy or radiation.

Mediastinal seminoma

Mediastinal seminoma is a tumor primarily occurring in males in the third to fourth decades of life. These lesions represent approximately 40 percent of malignant GCTs.[105] Most patients are symptomatic at the time of presentation, but 20 to 30 percent are asymptomatic.[106] The most common symptoms include pain, dyspnea, and cough. Tumor markers play a very important role in the diagnosis of malignant GCTs. Patients with seminoma have normal alpha-fetoprotein (AFP) and beta-HCG 90 percent of the time. In 10 percent of cases, however, the AFP is normal while the beta-HCG is mildly elevated.[102] This is to be contrasted with the biochemical presentation of nonseminomatous GCTs (below). Compared with their nonseminomatous counterparts, seminomas are relatively slow-growing and slower to metastasize.[106] On CT, seminomas appear relatively homogeneous, again in contrast to nonseminomatous GCTs.[35,106] Because the histologies of mediastinal seminoma and primary gonadal seminoma are the same, all patients with a diagnosis of mediastinal seminoma should undergo meticulous evaluation for primary gonadal disease.

The mediastinal variant of seminoma shares a unique radiosensitivity with its gonadal variant.[107] For disease confined to the mediastinum at diagnosis, primary resection followed by radiation is the treatment of choice. Metastatic disease should be treated initially with cisplatin-based chemotherapy, with surgical resection of residual disease.[35,103,108] Survival at 5 years is greater than 80 percent.[107,109] The role of initial chemotherapy, instead of radiation, for disease confined to the mediastinum is unclear at this time.

Mediastinal nonseminomatous germ cell tumors

Mediastinal nonseminomatous GCTs (MNSGCTs) include embryonal cell carcinoma, endodermal sinus tumor, choriocarcinoma, and tumors of mixed germ cell histology. Like their seminomatous counterparts, they occur primarily in young men. Because these tumors grow rapidly, most patients are symptomatic at the time of diagnosis. In addition, compression and invasion of structures adjacent to the mediastinum is common; 85 to 95 percent of patients have at least one site of metastatic disease at the time of diagnosis.[110] Ninety percent of MNSGCTs are associated with elevations in AFP, beta-HCG, or both. AFP is elevated in 80 percent of patients with MNSGCTs, while beta-HCG is elevated in 30 to 35 percent of such patients.[106] An association exists between MNSGCTs and hematologic malignancies, such as leu-kemia and myelodysplastic syndrome.[111] In addition, up to 20 percent of men with MNSGCTs have Klinefelter's syndrome,[112] although the reasons for this have yet to be elucidated.

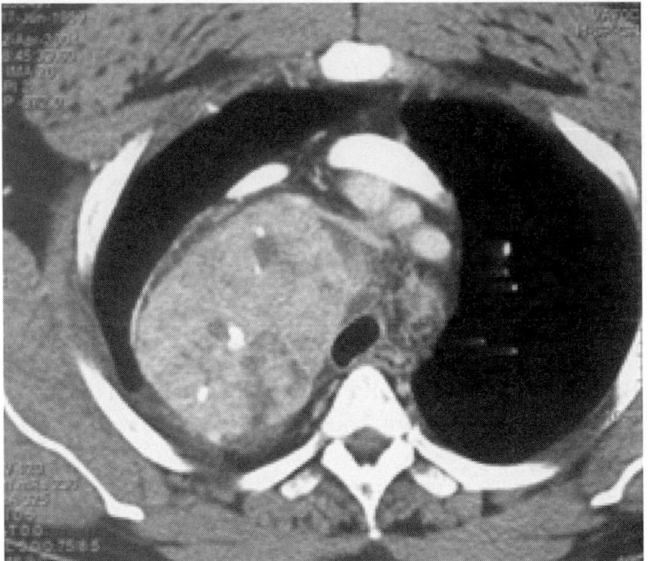

Figure 2-5 Computed tomography of mass arising in the superior mediastinum from a thyroid carcinoma.

Until the 1980s, the survival rates for patients with MNSGCTs were abysmal. Long-term survival rates were less than 10 percent.[113] However, with the advent of cisplatin-based chemotherapy regimens, survival rates have improved to greater than 50 percent.[114–116] Current regimens for MNSGCT include bleomycin, etoposide, and cisplatin. In addition, for patients who do not achieve radiographic and tumor-marker normalization, further, high-dose chemotherapy with autologous bone marrow transplantation may be indicated.[117] A recent European prospective trial found 2-year progression-free survival and overall survival rates of 64 and 68 percent, respectively, using etoposide, ifosfamide, and cisplatin, followed by autologous bone marrow transplantation.[118] Surgical resection should be reserved for residual disease, preferably in the face of normalized tumor markers.[108]

Thyroid masses

While uncommon, thyroid carcinoma can extend into the superior mediastinum (Fig. 2-5). This presentation has generally been associated with a poor prognosis.[119] However, several studies have documented long-term survival for such patients, including those with invasion into mediastinal structures including the great vessels,[120] provided that complete resection with negative margins was attainable.

MIDDLE MEDIASTINAL MASSES

Mediastinal cysts

Cystic masses comprise approximately 20 percent of all mediastinal masses[121]; while they may occur anywhere in the mediastinum, the majority are found within the middle mediastinum.

Foregut cysts

Most cystic lesions arising in the mediastinum are of congenital foregut etiology.[122] The classification of these epithelium-lined cystic structures is based on their histology rather than their anatomic location.[123] Although the reason or reasons for their formation are not known, most authors believe that foregut cysts are the result of aberrant budding or division of the primitive foregut.[103] Foregut cysts can be further subdivided into bronchogenic cysts, esophageal duplication cysts, and neuroenteric cysts. In addition, approximately 20 percent of foregut cysts are of indeterminate histology, possibly because of previous infection or hemorrhage, and cannot be further classified.[108]

Bronchogenic cysts

Bronchogenic cysts encompass approximately 60 percent of all mediastinal cystic lesions.[124] Although the majority of bronchogenic cysts arise in the mediastinum in close proximity to the trachea, main bronchi, and carina, they can also arise within the lungs,[125] inferior pulmonary ligament, pericardium, and outflow tract of the right ventricle[126] (Fig. 2-6). Histologically, they replicate the structures of the major airways. They are lined by ciliated epithelium and have focal areas of hyaline cartilage, smooth muscle, and bronchial glands within their walls.[127]

Between 60 and 80 percent of patients with mediastinal bronchogenic cysts experience symptoms.[125] Among those with intrapulmonary cysts, an even greater proportion experience symptoms.[127] Symptoms usually result from the compression of structures adjacent to the cyst. Cough and repeated infection are the most common symptoms,[128] but patients also present with complications including hemoptysis, pneumothorax, and esophageal compression.[129]

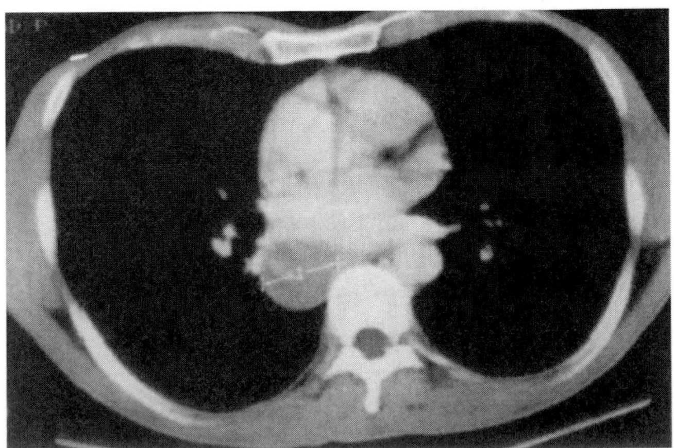

Figure 2-6 Potential anatomic locations of bronchogenic cysts. (From Cioffi et al.[130] With permission.)

Preoperative diagnosis is aided by the use of several imaging modalities including CT, MRI, and endoscopic ultrasound (EUS). Because of their heterogeneous composition, the attenuation of bronchogenic cysts varies over a range of approximately 80 Hounsfield units, from that of water to high-density fat.[130] On MRI, a T2-weighted image usually demonstrates highest signal intensity, although higher-density material within the cyst will result in increased T1 signal intensity.[131] On EUS, most bronchogenic cysts appear anechoic or hypoechoic. EUS also affords the opportunity for biopsy, usually via fine-needle aspiration (FNA). In one series of 20 patients, EUS and FNA were able to provide the diagnosis correctly in 95 percent of patients preoperatively, compared with fewer than 25 percent using CT.[132]

Definitive treatment for symptomatic cysts requires complete surgical resection whenever possible. When resection cannot be performed safely, cyst aspiration is a viable alternative, although not preferred.[133] Traditionally, resection is performed via posterolateral thoracotomy. However, video-assisted thoracoscopic surgery (VATS) has recently been demonstrated to be both safe and efficacious for the resection of mediastinal cysts.[134] In the future, a greater number of centers will likely utilize evolving technology such as robotic-assisted minimally invasive surgery, as a group at Cornell have recently reported.[135]

Some controversy exists regarding the management of asymptomatic cysts in adults. Two arguments favor resection of such cysts. First, most patients with bronchogenic cysts will eventually develop symptoms.[127,128,136] Second, operative difficulties arise in those patients who were symptomatic preoperatively compared with patients who were not. In a series of 86 patients undergoing resection of bronchogenic cysts, 35 had a complicated operation. Each of these patients was among the 62 in this series who were symptomatic.[127] Some have advocated using only the "watch and wait" approach with asymptomatic patients who have small, simple cysts. However, if an air-fluid level in the cyst is noted or the presence of malignant cells on aspiration, the development of symptoms, or cyst enlargement on follow-up, prompt surgical intervention is warranted.[137]

Esophageal duplication cysts

Esophageal or duplication cysts make up approximately 5 to 10 percent of all mediastinal cysts.[108] The majority of esophageal cysts are located on the right posterior portion of the esophagus, in the lower third.[138,139] Histologically they resemble the alimentary epithelium, and while they usually contain stratified squamous epithelium, they may contain gastric, and even pancreatic mucosa.[140] It is thought that esophageal cysts arise during early development as a result of isolated vacuoles failing to fuse into a solid, tubular esophagus and instead growing as outpouchings that can be either intramural or adjacent to the esophagus.[108,141] As with bronchogenic cysts, diagnosis is aided by CT and EUS[142]; definitive treatment is complete surgical excision. Most authors make a particular point of stressing the closure of the defect remaining following the resection, making sure to approximate exactly all muscular layers and even buttressing the repair with a nearby flap of vascularized tissue.[130] Minimally invasive techniques, most notably VATS, have been demonstrated as safe and effective ways to resect esophageal cysts as an alternative to the traditional thoracotomy.[143]

Neuroenteric cysts

By definition, a neuroenteric cyst is a hybrid of an endodermal cyst and a vertebral dysplasia.[144] Although most occur in the posterior mediastinum, on the right, usually above the carina,[145] they are discussed briefly here for the sake of completeness. Neuroenteric cysts make up approximately 2 to 5 percent of mediastinal cysts. Current evidence suggests that the notochord may play a crucial role in the development of the foregut via the sonic hedgehog–gli protein signaling pathway.[145] It is speculated that during early embryogenesis, when the notochord and primitive foregut are in close proximity, they may fuse at a certain point, whereupon a small portion of the foregut pinches off to form a cyst that retains both enteric and neural histologies[108]—the hallmark of neuroenteric cysts.

Most neuroenteric cysts become apparent during the first months of life,[144] as infants may demonstrate vertebral abnormalities such as scoliosis, hemivertebrae, and anterior spina bifida.[146] Treatment is, as in the case of the bronchogenic and esophageal cysts, compete surgical resection whenever possible.

Miscellaneous cysts (pericardial, thymic, thoracic duct)

Pericardial cysts are an uncommon, benign entity. They are most often found in the cardiophrenic angle, approximately twice as commonly on the right as on the left.[147] Other possible locations include the subcarinal site, the tracheobronchial angle, the paraauricular site above the diaphragm,[148] or in the vicinity of the aortic arch.[149] CT is most revealing in evaluating these lesions. The density of the fluid that fills the cyst is very close to that of water, approximately 0 to 20 Hounsfield units; hence the pseudonym "springwater cysts." The cysts are very thin-walled and do not enhance with intravenous contrast.[150] They are symptomatic in less than half the patients diagnosed and, more often than not, are discovered incidentally.[151] When symptomatic, they should be resected. Advocates of resecting asymptomatic pericardial cysts will argue that complications arising from ruptured cysts—including ventricular wall erosion,[152] erosion into the SVC,[153] and potential hemodynamic consequences—warrant resection in nearly all cases.[150]

Thymic cysts are very rare. However, they can be symptomatic and pose problems such as hemorrhage or tracheal/esophageal compression.[154] They usually occur in the anterior mediastinum and often demonstrate a thick, calcified capsule on imaging studies.[155] Although complete surgical resection remains the only definitive treatment, the exceedingly low risk of malignancy must be weighed against the risk of surgical intervention in asymptomatic patients whose cysts have typical radiographic findings.

Thoracic duct cysts of the mediastinum are exceedingly rare. They contain chyle and may arise as a consequence of congenital or degenerative weakness in the wall of the thoracic duct.[156] They are symptomatic in about half the cases, and the symptoms range from dysphagia and retrosternal pain to respiratory distress and SVC compression.[157] The treatment, as with other cystic lesions of the mediastinum, is surgical resection.

POSTERIOR MEDIASTINAL MASSES

Neurogenic tumors

Approximately 15 to 20 percent of adult and 30 to 40 percent of pediatric mediastinal neoplasms are neurogenic tumors.[22,77,158] Embryologically, neurogenic tumors arise from neural crest cells. They are often divided into four groups based on their cells of origin, with each group having benign and malignant variants (Table 2-4). They can originate from the nerve sheath, spinal ganglion, or parasympathetic and sympathetic components of the autonomic nervous system. Most commonly they arise in the posterior mediastinum. As a general rule, neurogenic tumors are benign and asymptomatic in adults and malignant and symptomatic in children.[159] Nerve sheath tumors arise more commonly in adults, while tumors of the autonomic nervous system arise more commonly in children.[160] Overall, 70 to 80 percent of nerve sheath tumors are benign and fewer than half produce symptoms.[77]

Tumors of the nerve sheath

Nerve sheath tumors are the most common mediastinal neurogenic tumor, representing 40 to 70 percent of all such tumors.[161–163] Ninety-five percent of these tumors are benign[164,165] and only 5 percent malignant. The benign tumors are subdivided into neurilemmomas (or schwannomas) and neurofibromas. Both are slow-growing and have

Table 2-4 Classification of neurogenic tumors

Histology	Distribution	Benign	Malignant	Demographics
Nerve sheath tumors (Peripheral nerve tumors)	40–70% of all mediastinal neurogenic tumors 95% benign (neurilemmoma and neurofibroma) 5% malignant (MTNSO)	75% neurilemmoma (schwannoma) 25% neurofibroma (30–45% associated with von Recklinghausen's neurofibromatosis)	Malignant tumor of nerve sheath origin (MTNSO), also malignant schwannoma, malignant neurofibroma, neurogenic fibrosarcoma 50–75% are associated with von Recklinghausen's neurofibromatosis	Most common neurogenic tumor in adults
Autonomic ganglion tumors	35–55% of all mediastinal neurogenic tumors	Ganglioneuroma	Ganglioneuroblastoma (composite tumor);15% of autonomic ganglion tumors	Most common neurogenic tumor in children
(Nerve cell tumors)	More than 50% are malignant		Neuroblastoma (highly malignant) 25–45% of autonomic ganglion tumors Most common extraadrenal site	60% of neuroblastomas occur before age 2
Paraganglionic tumors	Rare	Up to 30% are malignant		Present over a wide range of ages
	Active (pheochromocytoma)	Pheochromocytoma	Malignant pheochromocytoma	
	Inactive (nonchromaffin paraganglioma)	Paraganglioma	Malignant paraganglioma	Males more affected than females
Malignant small cell tumors (Askin tumor)	Rare	All malignant	Not applicable	Occur in older children and younger adults

a peak incidence in the third and fourth decades.[166] Neurilemmomas, arising from the Schwann cells, constitute 75 percent of benign nerve sheath tumors, while neurofibromas, arising from nerve sheaths, comprise the remaining 25 percent.[162] Over 90 percent of nerve sheath tumors arise in the costovertebral gutter, but they may also arise at the thoracic inlet and along the phrenic or vagus nerves.[35] Neurilemmomas are grossly encapsulated and appear grayish-tan. They appear heterogeneous on imaging studies.[167] In contrast, neurofibromas are generally homogeneous and nonencapsulated.[168] MRI is the imaging modality of choice when either of these tumors arises in the paraspinal region.[169] Most often, nerve sheath tumors do not produce symptoms and are diagnosed on routine examination. However, they can produce symptoms if they become large and compress the pulmonary parenchyma, esophagus, major airways, or major vascular structures.[170] Some 30 to 40 percent of neurofibromas arise in patients with von Recklinghausen's neurofibromatosis,[161,171] and this subset of patients tends to present earlier and have a greater predilection for malignant degeneration.[166]

The malignant nerve sheath tumors are rare, constituting approximately 5 percent of all nerve sheath tumors. They are known as malignant tumors of nerve sheath origin (MTNSO) but have also been termed malignant schwannomas, malignant neurofibromas, and neurogenic fibrosarcomas.[172,173] Between 50 and 75 percent of these malignant counterparts to neurilemmomas and neurofibromas arise in patients with von Recklinghausen's neurofibromatosis.[162,170,173] These tumors are nonencapsulated and behave aggressively, with local invasion and distant metastases being the rule rather than the exception.[159] The subset of patients with malignant schwannoma in the context of von Recklinghausen's neurofibromatosis have a very poor prognosis regardless of treatment.[160]

Tumors of the autonomic nervous system

Autonomic ganglion tumors are derived from the sympathetic or parasympathetic ganglia in the posterior mediastinum.[174] In contrast to nerve sheath tumors, they arise from the nerve cell. They constitute 20 to 50 percent of mediastinal neurogenic tumors, depending on the proportion of pediatric patients reported in the series.[162,163,165,175–177] Autonomic ganglion tumors are the most common mediastinal neurogenic tumors in children and encompass up to one-third of all pediatric mediastinal tumors.[22,158]

Histologically, these tumors exist on a continuum from ganglioneuromas, which are benign, to ganglioneuroblastomas, which are mixed, and neuroblastomas, which are malignant. Ganglioneuromas comprise 40 to 50 percent of autonomic ganglion tumors, whereas the composite ganglioneuroblastomas comprise approximately 15 percent of such tumors.[170] The remaining 35 to 45 percent of autonomic ganglion tumors are neuroblastomas, which arise in the mediastinum approximately 30 percent of the time.[178] The mediastinum is the most common extraabdominal location for this tumor. Most neuroblastomas arise in children before the age of 2[179] and symptomatic presentation is common.[159] The prognosis of children with neuroblastoma is more favorable in the group diagnosed within the first year of life compared with those diagnosed after the first year.[176]

Paraganglionic tumors

Paraganglionic tumors of the mediastinum are rare and constitute a fraction of mediastinal neurogenic tumors as compared with nerve sheath and autonomic ganglion tumors.[180] Embryologically, they arise from the neural crest and are morphologically similar to the adrenal medulla, the carotid and aortic bodies, and the organs of Zuckerkandl.[181] Within the chest, they tend to occur in one of two places: in the middle mediastinum in the vicinity of the cardiac plexus and in the posterior mediastinum along the aorticosympathetic chain in the costovertebral sulcus.[35,182,183] Paraganglionic tumors may be chemically active (functional) or chemically inactive (nonfunctional), and each of these variants may be benign or malignant. The diagnosis of a malignant variant is based on invasion and spread rather than histology. No correlation has been demonstrated between the ploidy pattern of tumors and their propensity to spread.[183] Functional tumors are histologically identical to pheochromocytomas and as such present with symptoms of catecholamine excess, including the classic triad of headache, palpitation, and episodic diaphoresis. The diagnosis is aided by the measurements of urinary catecholamines and their breakdown products in addition to ^{131}I-MIBG scans and routine radiographic imaging studies.

Malignant small cell tumors (Askin tumors)

Askin tumor, an aggressive small cell tumor of primitive neuroectodermal origin, is exceedingly rare.[184] It presents on the chest wall and primarily afflicts older children and young adults.[185] Because of its aggressive nature, the duration of symptoms is usually brief. The diagnosis is confirmed by histologic and immunohistochemical means and treatment consists of induction chemotherapy, radical resection, and postoperative chemoradiation.[186] Survival is dependent in part on the completeness of the resection.

Treatment

Surgery plays an integral role in the treatment of neurogenic tumors, both benign and malignant.[187] There is little debate about the importance of achieving a complete resection.[165,175,182,187–189] The usual approach for resection is via posterolateral thoracotomy. However, several centers are reporting successful utilization of VATS techniques for uncomplicated lesions.[190–192] Up to 10 percent of neurogenic tumors in the posterior mediastinum may exhibit intraspinal extension through an intervertebral foramen, or "dumbbell tumor."[171,193] Although the minority of dumbbell tumors are malignant, they often present with symptoms of spinal cord compression. Approximately 70 percent of dumbbell tumors are of nerve sheath origin, while the remaining 30 percent are of autonomic (sympathetic) nerve cell origin.[171] MRI has emerged as the diagnostic tool of choice for accurate preoperative evaluation of such lesions.[194] The surgical treatment of dumbbell tumors involves a combined effort of thoracic and neurosurgeons, often in a single-stage procedure,[194–196] since a laminectomy is required. Dumbbell morphology does not worsen the prognosis of these tumors.[197]

Early-stage neuroblastomas are cured by complete surgical resection.[188] For patients with stage II and III lesions, complete resection should always be attempted, followed by postoperative chemotherapy and radiation.[158,160] Three-year disease-free survival of 70 percent has been reported in patients with stage I to III disease.[158,172]

SUPERIOR VENA CAVA SYNDROME

Obstruction of blood return through the SVC results in the SVC syndrome. The characteristic signs and symptoms, described below, should alert the clinician to search for an underlying cause. Causes may be benign or malignant, and the mechanism is either external compression or internal occlusion of the SVC—sometimes both. Approximately 15,000 cases of SVC syndrome are diagnosed annually in the United States,[198] with malignancy being the underlying culprit in 80 to 95 percent of cases, depending on the patient population in the series.[93,199–201] Approximately 10 percent of patients with right-sided intrathoracic malignancies will experience SVC syndrome.[202]

The SVC is vulnerable to compression because of its position within the mediastinum and the relative position of other structures to it. Cancers of the lung and bronchus contribute most often to the extrinsic compression of the SVC. The proximity of the SVC to the bronchus, trachea, pericardium, and neighboring lymph nodes, in addition to its relatively thin wall, provides little resistance to compressive forces. The speed with which the compression occurs plays a role in the extent to which blood can travel via a collateral route. Perhaps of equal importance is the location of the occlusion—whether intrinsic or extrinsic—to the junction of the azygos vein and the SVC.[203] Obstruction above the azygocaval junction results in collateralization of the flow in the upper extremity and head through the azygos vein in an antegrade fashion to the remaining SVC and into the right atrium. Occlusion between the right atrium and the azygocaval junction results in retrograde flow of blood from the upper body through the azygos vein and ultimately to the right atrium via the inferior vena cava.

Traditionally SVC syndrome was considered an oncologic emergency.[204,205] However, it is now generally regarded that, with the exception of patients who present with airway or neurologic compromise, obtaining a diagnosis should be the first aim in treating such patients. This is the case because the slight delay in initiating treatment can be safely tolerated, since the obstruction itself will have occurred within a relatively long time frame, with only one-quarter of patients experiencing symptoms for 7 days or less.[206–209] Furthermore, "empiric" or prebiopsy radiation can significantly obscure the ability to make a definitive histologic diagnosis when tissue is biopsied.[210–212]

Signs and symptoms

The most common symptoms of SVC syndrome are a feeling of fullness in the head, edema of the face and arms, jugular venous distention, prominent venous collateral vessels on the chest wall, plethora of the face, and dyspnea.[199,205,211,213] As mentioned above, any signs of airway compromise, such as stridor or wheezing, warrant immediate intervention. Any evidence of cerebral edema or neurologic compromise should similarly invite an expeditious response of clinicians. Such symptoms portend a grave prognosis.[201]

Malignant causes

Today, neoplasm is responsible for approximately 90 percent of cases of SVC syndrome.[83,201,207] Lung cancer accounts for nearly three-quarters of this fraction,[214] with lymphoma[215,216] accounting for the majority of the remainder. Metastatic disease to the thorax from distant sites such as breast,[217] colon,[218] stomach,[219] pancreas,[220] ovary,[221] and prostate[204] make up the remaining small fraction of malignant causes of SVC syndrome.

Benign causes

Benign etiologies of SVC syndrome can be subdivided into two main groups: those resulting from infection, leading to fibrosing mediastinitis, and those resulting from iatrogenic causes. Chronic fibrosing mediastinitis arises as a complication of excessive host response to a granulomatous disease, the most common of which is due to *Histoplasma capsulatum*.[222] Other infectious agents have also been linked to fibrosing mediastinitis and SVC syndrome, including blastomycosis,[223] tuberculosis,[224] actinomycosis,[225] nocardiosis,[226] and aspergillosis.[227]

Iatrogenic causes of SVC occlusion are the most common benign etiologic factors associated with SVC syndrome and are most often related to the presence of indwelling vascular catheters.[228] The use of indwelling catheters for parenteral nutrition and antibiotics gave rise to an incidence as high as 15 percent for patients with long-term catheters at home in one large study.[229] Other iatrogenic causes of SVC syndrome include pacemaker wires[230] and chemotherapy-induced fibrosis.[231]

Diagnosis

Expeditious diagnosis and identification of the causative factor or factors is crucial in the treatment of SVC syndrome. Patients presenting with the aforementioned signs and symptoms should prompt the clinician to search for clues to the underlying cause. As many as 60 percent of patients presenting with SVC syndrome have an undiagnosed malignancy.[207] The plain radiograph is often the first study obtained, and it is abnormal in almost all instances. Widening of the mediastinum can be found between 50 and 100 percent of the time.[199,232] Additionally, hilar masses and pleural effusion are often present.[233,234] Helical CT provides excellent information about not only the patency of the SVC and the caliber of the lumen[235] but also the number and extent of collateral vessels arising as a result of the obstruction.[236] CT is highly accurate in its ability to make the diagnosis of SVC syndrome, with the additional benefit of requiring less contrast than conventional venography while being able to provide extravascular anatomic detail about the etiology of the SVC obstruction.

For patients who can tolerate contrast, it should be considered the radiographic test of choice for the diagnosis of SVC syndrome.[237] MRI also provides excellent anatomic detail and without the intravenous dye load.[238]

Obtaining a tissue diagnosis when the precipitating factor, most often a malignancy, is not known is important for initiating prompt treatment. Minimally invasive procedures such as CT-guided needle biopsy, pleural fluid sampling, and superficial lymph node biopsy can be diagnostic up to 60 percent of the time.[207] More invasive procedures such as bronchoscopy, mediastinoscopy, mediastinotomy, thoracoscopy, and thoracotomy may be reserved for situations when the former, less invasive techniques yield a diagnosis.[239] These procedures can be performed safely and accurately in more than 80 percent of cases.[240–243]

Treatment

Treatments of SVC syndrome have two aims, which are not necessarily mutually exclusive: to treat the underlying disorder and to provide symptomatic relief. The first of these aims reinforces the need for an accurate tissue diagnosis prior to treatment. As most causes of SVC syndrome are malignant, radiation and chemotherapy play an integral role in treating this condition. Short-term symptomatic relief may be provided by simple measures such as head elevation and diuretic administration. There does not appear to be any convincing evidence to support the use of corticosteroids.

A number of trials, some prospective, most retrospective, have tried to elucidate the role of radiation and/or chemotherapy in treating SVC syndrome. One large study found that initial treatment with high-dose radiation (300 to 400 cGy daily for three fractions) yielded symptomatic relief in 70 percent of patients versus 56 percent of patients receiving conventional dose (200 cGy daily for five weekly fractions), with no improvements in symptomatic relief, duration of response, or survival with the addition of chemotherapy.[244] A randomized prospective trial comparing chemotherapy with and without radiotherapy for SVC syndrome secondary to small-cell carcinoma found no additional benefit of radiotherapy following 12 weeks of chemotherapy. Eighty-four percent of patients experienced relief of symptoms (57 percent complete, 27 percent partial but significant), while 16 percent did not experience relief. There was no difference in relapse rate between patients who only received chemotherapy and those who received additional radiotherapy.[245] A large, systematic review of current treatments employed in the management of SVC syndrome found a 77 percent response rate in patients with small-cell lung cancer to chemotherapy and/or radiation with a 17 percent relapse rate. For non–small cell lung cancer, the response rate was 60 percent, with 19 percent of patients experiencing a relapse of symptoms.[246] A European study of 34 patients with an equal distribution of small and non–small cell lung cancer found a greater response rate in the patients with small-cell lung cancer than in those with non–small cell lung cancer (94 vs. 77 percent). However, the patients with non–small cell responded faster. In this study, all of the patients with small-cell lung cancer had received chemotherapy, either without response or with a relapse, demonstrating that radiation therapy can be effective for patients recalcitrant to chemotherapy.[247] Although not stated explicitly, these studies demonstrate that the response rate of the tumor to the treatment modality plays a significant role in the palliation of patients with SVC syndrome related to an underlying malignancy. Whether chemotherapy and/or radiation should be used depends on the individual tumor and the performance status of the patient.

With recent advances in the field of interventional radiology, the role for percutaneously inserted intraluminal stents to alleviate the symptoms of SVC compression or obstruction has grown. Their use has found a role in both palliating symptoms as a sole treatment modality and as an adjunct to other therapeutic interventions for patients with various etiologies of SVC syndrome.[248] Patients experience relief of symptoms within hours to days and may undergo a repeat procedure for stent occlusion.[249] Technical success rates of 100 percent are often reported, with long-term patency rates in excess of 90 percent.[250–256]

The question of whether stenting should be the first line of treatment—prior to even confirming a histologic diagnosis—has recently been examined by a group in Greece. They successfully treated 18 patients with malignancy-associated SVC syndrome with 100 percent technical success and no complications. All patients experienced relief of symptoms within hours and began radiation treatment within 24 h. The authors of this study attribute their results in part to the use long-term anticoagulation. The patients in this series were heparinized for 24 h postprocedure, as are most patients, and then started on warfarin with the goal of maintaining a prothrombin time 1.5 times the upper limit of a normal value for the remainder of their lives. At 1 year, they had achieved a clinical success rate of 89 percent.[257] Other studies have also reiterated the role for first-line stent placement with excellent results and no deleterious effect on either obtaining a diagnosis or delivering treatment for the underlying cause.[258]

Open surgical reconstruction for occlusion of the SVC is another option. Conduits have traditionally included Dacron polyester, polytetrafluoroethylene (PTFE), and autologous vein graft, most commonly saphenous. The saphenous vein is incised longitudinally and spirally wrapped around a stent. It may be sutured in the bed of the SVC or used as a bypass conduit. Initial experience with Dacron was beleaguered by reports of a high incidence of early graft thrombosis.[259] Although PTFE conduits displayed better long-term patency than Dacron, spiral saphenous vein appears to be associated with superior rates of patency on follow-up longer than 3 years.[260]

Finally, thrombolytic agents have been successfully used to treat SVC occlusion arising from indwelling catheters; however, only 20 percent of patients respond in the absence of a catheter.[200] Furthermore, the risk of pulmonary embolism from thrombi that may be attached to the catheter tip remains a potential problem.[261]

References

1. Esposito C, Romeo C. Surgical anatomy of the mediastinum. *Semin Pediatr Surg* 1999;8(2):50–53.
2. Moore KL, Persaud TV. *The Developing Human: Clinically Oriented Embryology*. William Schmitt, 1998:205–210.
3. Kollmannsberger C, Nichols C, Meisner C, et al. Identification of prognostic subgroups among patients with metastatic 'IGCCCG poor-prognosis' germ-cell cancer: An explorative analysis using cart modeling. *Ann Oncol* 2000;11(9):1115–1120.
4. Chronowski GM, Wilder RB, Tucker SL, et al. An elevated serum beta-2-microglobulin level is an adverse prognostic factor for overall survival in patients with early-stage Hodgkin disease. *Cancer* 2002;95(12):2534–2538.
5. Harris GJ, Harman PK, Trinkle JK, Grover FL. Standard biplane roentgenography is highly sensitive in documenting mediastinal masses. *Ann Thorac Surg* 1987;44(3):238–241.
6. Dewes W, Schrappe-Bacher M, Focke-Wenzel EK, Schmitz-Drager HG. [X-ray diagnosis of invasive thymoma.] *Rofo* 1986;144(4):388–394.
7. Ahn JM, Lee KS, Goo JM, et al. Predicting the histology of anterior mediastinal masses: Comparison of chest radiography and CT. *J Thorac Imaging* 1996;11(4):265–271.
8. Wyttenbach R, Vock P, Tschappeler H. Cross-sectional imaging with CT and/or MRI of pediatric chest tumors. *Eur Radiol* 1998;8(6):1040–1046.
9. Moeller KH, Rosado-de-Christenson ML, Templeton PA. Mediastinal mature teratoma: Imaging features. *AJR* 1997;169(4):985–990.
10. Mori K, Eguchi K, Moriyama H, et al. Computed tomography of anterior mediastinal tumors. Differentiation between thymoma and germ cell tumor. *Acta Radiol* 1987;28(4):395–398.
11. Yang WT, Lei KI, Metreweli C. Plain radiography and computed tomography of invasive thymomas: Clinico-radiologic-pathologic correlation. *Australas Radiol* 1997;41(2):118–124.
12. Tecce PM, Fishman EK, Kuhlman JE. CT evaluation of the anterior mediastinum: Spectrum of disease. *Radiographics* 1994;14(5):973–990.
13. Francis IR, Glazer GM, Shapiro B, et al. Complementary roles of CT and 131I-MIBG scintigraphy in diagnosing pheochromocytoma. *AJR* 1983;141(4):719–725.
14. Sklair-Levy M, Shaham D, Sherman I, et al. [Fine needle aspiration biopsy of mediastinal masses guided by computed tomography—Summary of 63 patients.] *Harefuah* 1998;134(8):599–602, 672.
15. Greif J, Staroselsky AN, Gernjac M, et al. Percutaneous core needle biopsy in the diagnosis of mediastinal tumors. *Lung Cancer* 1999;25(3):169–173.
16. Sklair-Levy M, Polliack A, Shaham D, et al. CT-guided core-needle biopsy in the diagnosis of mediastinal lymphoma. *Eur Radiol* 2000;10(5):714–718.
17. Agid R, Sklair-Levy M, Bloom AI, et al. CT-guided biopsy with cutting-edge needle for the diagnosis of malignant lymphoma: Experience of 267 biopsies. *Clin Radiol* 2003;58(2):143–147.
18. Glick RD, Pearse IA, Trippett T, et al. Diagnosis of mediastinal masses in pediatric patients using mediastinoscopy and the Chamberlain procedure. *J Pediatr Surg* 1999;34(4):559–564.
19. Fassina A, Marino F, Poletti A, et al. Follicular dendritic cell tumor of the mediastinum. *Ann Diagn Pathol* 2001;5(6):361–367.
20. Budde JM, Morris CD, Gal AA, Mansour KA, Miller JI, Jr. Predictors of outcome in thymectomy for myasthenia gravis. *Ann Thorac Surg* 2001;72(1):197–202.
21. Whooley BP, Urschel JD, Antkowiak JG, Takita H. Primary tumors of the mediastinum. *J Surg Oncol* 1999;70(2):95–99.
22. Azarow KS, Pearl RH, Zurcher R, et al. Primary mediastinal masses. A comparison of adult and pediatric populations. *J Thorac Cardiovasc Surg* 1993;106(1): 67–72.
23. Sperling B, Marschall J, Kennedy R, et al. Thymoma: A review of the clinical and pathological findings in 65 cases. *Can J Surg* 2003;46(1):37–42.
24. Moore KH, McKenzie PR, Kennedy CW, McCaughan BC. Thymoma: Trends over time. *Ann Thorac Surg* 2001;72(1):203–207.
25. Canizares MA, Arnau A, Alberola A, et al. [Thymoma. A retrospective study.] *Arch Bronconeumol* 1999;35(7): 324–328.
26. Blumberg D, Port JL, Weksler B, et al. Thymoma: A multivariate analysis of factors predicting survival. *Ann Thorac Surg* 1995;60(4):908–913.
27. Lewis JE, Wick MR, Scheithauer BW, et al. Thymoma. A clinicopathologic review. *Cancer* 1987;60(11): 2727–2743.
28. Kirchner T, Muller-Hermelink HK. New approaches to the diagnosis of thymic epithelial tumors. *Prog Surg Pathol* 1989;10:167.

29. Quintanilla-Martinez L, Wilkins EW Jr, Choi N, et al. Thymoma. Histologic subclassification is an independent prognostic factor. *Cancer* 1994;74(2):606–617.
30. Schneider PM, Fellbaum C, Fink U, et al. Prognostic importance of histomorphologic subclassification for epithelial thymic tumors. *Ann Surg Oncol* 1997;4(1): 46–56.
31. Pescarmona E, Rendina EA, Venuta F, et al. Analysis of prognostic factors and clinicopathological staging of thymoma. *Ann Thorac Surg* 1990;50(4):534–538.
32. Koga K, Matsuno Y, Noguchi M, et al. A review of 79 thymomas: Modification of staging system and reappraisal of conventional division into invasive and noninvasive thymoma. *Pathol Int* 1994;44(5):359–367.
33. Kornstein MJ, Curran WJ Jr, Turrisi AT III, Brooks JJ. Cortical versus medullary thymomas: A useful morphologic distinction? *Hum Pathol* 1988;19(11):1335–1339.
34. Masaoka A, Monden Y, Nakahara K, Tanioka T. Follow-up study of thymomas with special reference to their clinical stages. *Cancer* 1981;48(11):2485–2492.
35. Wright CD, Mathisen DJ. Mediastinal tumors: Diagnosis and treatment. *World J Surg* 2001;25(2):204–209.
36. Mornex F, Resbeut M, Richaud P, et al. Radiotherapy and chemotherapy for invasive thymomas: A multicentric retrospective review of 90 cases. The FNCLCC trialists. Federation Nationale des Centres de Lutte Contre le Cancer. *Int J Radiat Oncol Biol Phys* 1995;32(3): 651–659.
37. Urgesi A, Monetti U, Rossi G, et al. Role of radiation therapy in locally advanced thymoma. *Radiother Oncol* 1990;19(3):273–280.
38. Hejna M, Haberl I, Raderer M. Nonsurgical management of malignant thymoma. Cancer 1999;85(9): 1871–1884.
39. Latz D, Schraube P, Oppitz U, et al. Invasive thymoma: Treatment with postoperative radiation therapy. *Radiology* 1997;204(3):859–864.
40. Okada Y, Kondo T, Handa M, et al. [Surgical treatment of stage IVa thymoma.] *Kyobu Geka* 1993;46(1):35–40.
41. Lastoria S, Vergara E, Palmieri G, et al. In vivo detection of malignant thymic masses by indium-111-DTPA-D-Phe1-octreotide scintigraphy. *J Nucl Med* 1998;39(4): 634–639.
42. Palmieri G, Lastoria S, Montella L, et al. Role of somatostatin analogue-based therapy in unresponsive malignant thymomas. *Ann Med* 1999;31(Suppl 2):80–85.
43. Palmieri G, Lastoria S, Colao A, et al. Successful treatment of a patient with a thymoma and pure red-cell aplasia with octreotide and prednisone. *N Engl J Med* 1997;336(4):263–265.
44. Pascuzzi RM. The history of myasthenia gravis. *Neurol Clin* 1994;12(2):231–242.
45. Blalock A, Mason MF, Morgan HG. Myasthenia gravis and tumors of the thymic regions: Report of a case in which the tumor was removed. *Ann Surg* 1939;110, 544.
46. Kirschner PA. Thymectomy for elderly myasthenia gravis patients. *Ann Thorac Surg* 2000;69(1):313–315.
47. Blalock A. Thymectomy in the treatment of myasthenia gravis: Report of 20 cases. *J Thorac Surg* 1944;13, 316.
48. Kurtzke JF, Kurland LT. The epidemiology of neurologic disease. *Clin Neurol* 1992;4:80–88.
49. Drachman DB. Myasthenia gravis. *N Engl J Med* 1994;330(25):1797–1810.
50. Plested CP, Tang T, Spreadbury I, et al. AChR phosphorylation and indirect inhibition of AChR function in seronegative MG. *Neurology* 2002;59(11):1682–1688.
51. Osserman KE. *Myasthenia Gravis.* New York: Grune & Stratton, 1958:80.
52. Grob D, Brunner NG, Namba T. The natural course of myasthenia gravis and effect of therapeutic measures. *Ann N Y Acad Sci* 1981;377:652–669.
53. Drachman DB. *Myasthenia Gravis. Current Therapy in Neurologic Disease,* 4th ed. St. Louis: Mosby-Year Book, 1993:379–384.
54. Gogovska L, Ljapcev R, Polenakovic M, et al. Plasma exchange in the treatment of myasthenia gravis associated with thymoma. *Int J Artif Organs* 2003;26(2):170–173.
55. Qureshi AI, Choudhry MA, Akbar MS, et al. Plasma exchange versus intravenous immunoglobulin treatment in myasthenic crisis. *Neurology* 1999;52(3):629–632.
56. Clark WF, Rock GA, Buskard N, et al. Therapeutic plasma exchange: An update from the Canadian Apheresis Group. *Ann Intern Med* 1999;131(6):453–462.
57. Mossman S, Vincent A, Newsom-Davis J. Myasthenia gravis without acetylcholine-receptor antibody: A distinct disease entity. *Lancet* 1986;1(8473):116–119.
58. Arsura EL, Brunner NG, Namba T, Grob D. Adverse cardiovascular effects of anticholinesterase medications. *Am J Med Sci* 1987;293(1):18–23.
59. Dwyer JM. Manipulating the immune system with immune globulin. *N Engl J Med* 1992;326(2):107–116.
60. Mann JD, Johns TR, Campa JF. Long-term administration of corticosteroids in myasthenia gravis. *Neurology* 1976; 26(8):729–740.
61. Sanders DB, Scoppetta C. The treatment of patients with myasthenia gravis. *Neurol Clin* 1994;12(2):343–368.
62. Lindberg C, Andersen O, Lefvert AK. Treatment of myasthenia gravis with methylprednisolone pulse: A double blind study. *Acta Neurol Scand* 1998;97(6):370–373.
63. Palace J, Newsom-Davis J, Lecky B. A randomized double-blind trial of prednisolone alone or with azathioprine in myasthenia gravis. Myasthenia Gravis Study Group. *Neurology* 1998;50(6):1778–1783.
64. de Perrot M, Liu J, Bril V, et al. Prognostic significance of thymomas in patients with myasthenia gravis. *Ann Thorac Surg* 2002;74(5):1658–1662.
65. Venuta F, Rendina EA, De Giacomo T, et al. Thymectomy for myasthenia gravis: A 27-year experience. *Eur J Cardiothorac Surg* 1999;15(5):621–624.
66. De Vries SO, Oosterhuis HJ, Tolboom J, Schaafsma W. [The effect of thymectomy in patients with myasthenia gravis without thymoma: A statistical analysis.] Ned Tijdschr Geneeskd 1991;135(44):2089–2094.
67. Bulkley GB, Bass KN, Stephenson GR, et al. Extended cervicomediastinal thymectomy in the integrated management of myasthenia gravis. *Ann Surg* 1997;226(3): 324–334.
68. Wilkins KB, Bulkley GB. Thymectomy in the integrated management of myasthenia gravis. *Adv Surg* 1999;32: 105–133.
69. Buckingham JM, Howard FM Jr, Bernatz PE, et al. The value of thymectomy in myasthenia gravis: A computer-assisted matched study. Ann Surg 1976; 184(4):453–458.

70. Masaoka A, Yamakawa Y, Niwa H, et al. Extended thymectomy for myasthenia gravis patients: A 20-year review. *Ann Thorac Surg* 1996; 62(3):853–859.
71. Jaretzki A III, Penn AS, Younger DS, et al. "Maximal" thymectomy for myasthenia gravis. Results. *J Thorac Cardiovasc Surg* 1988;95(5):747–757.
72. Jaretzki A III. Thymectomy for myasthenia gravis: Analysis of controversies—patient management. *Neurology* 2003;9(2):77–92.
73. Hankins JR, Mayer RF, Satterfield JR, et al. Thymectomy for myasthenia gravis: 14-year experience. *Ann Surg* 1985;201(5):618–625.
74. Deeb ME, Brinster CJ, Kucharzuk J, et al. Expanded indications for transcervical thymectomy in the management of anterior mediastinal masses. *Ann Thorac Surg* 2001;72(1):208–211.
75. Shrager JB, Deeb ME, Mick R, et al. Transcervical thymectomy for myasthenia gravis achieves results comparable to thymectomy by sternotomy. *Ann Thorac Surg* 2002;74(2):320–326.
76. Lichtenstein AK, Levine A, Taylor CR, et al. Primary mediastinal lymphoma in adults. *Am J Med* 1980;68(4): 509–514.
77. Davis RD Jr, Oldham HN Jr, Sabiston DC Jr. Primary cysts and neoplasms of the mediastinum: Recent changes in clinical presentation, methods of diagnosis, management, and results. *Ann Thorac Surg* 1987;44(3):229–237.
78. Suster S. Primary large-cell lymphomas of the mediastinum. *Semin Diagn Pathol* 1999;16(1):51–64.
79. Keller AR, Castleman B. Hodgkin's disease of the thymus gland. *Cancer* 1974;33(6):1615–1623.
80. Jimenez-Zepeda VH, Jimenez-Zepeda RJ. [Non-Hodgkin's lymphoma: Biologic classification, diagnosis and treatment.] *Gac Med Mex* 1998;134(4):443–463.
81. Picozzi VJ Jr, Coleman CN. Lymphoblastic lymphoma. *Semin Oncol* 1990;17(1):96–103.
82. Samuels TH, Margolis M, Hamilton PA, Srigley JR. Mediastinal large-cell lymphoma. *Can Assoc Radiol J* 1992;43(2):120–126.
83. Yellin A, Rosen A, Reichert N, Lieberman Y. Superior vena cava syndrome. The myth—the facts. *Am Rev Respir Dis* 1990;141(5 Pt 1):1114–1118.
84. Glick RD, La Quaglia MP. Lymphomas of the anterior mediastinum. *Semin Pediatr Surg* 1999;8(2):69–77.
85. Petersdorf SH, Wood DE. Lymphoproliferative disorders presenting as mediastinal neoplasms. *Semin Thorac Cardiovasc Surg* 2000;12(4):290–300.
86. Canellos GP, Niedzwiecki D. Long-term follow-up of Hodgkin's disease trial. *N Engl J Med* 2002;346(18): 1417–1418.
87. Aleman BM, Raemaekers JM, Tirelli U, et al. Involved-field radiotherapy for advanced Hodgkin's lymphoma. *N Engl J Med* 2003;348(24):2396–2406.
88. Rosenberg SA, Kaplan HS. The evolution and summary results of the Stanford randomized clinical trials of the management of Hodgkin's disease: 1962–1984. *Int J Radiat Oncol Biol Phys* 1985;11(1):5–22.
89. Wilder RB, Jones D, Tucker SL, et al. Long-term results with radiotherapy for Stage I–II follicular lymphomas. *Int J Radiat Oncol Biol Phys* 2001;51(5):1219–1227.
90. Fisher RI, Gaynor ER, Dahlberg S, et al. Comparison of a standard regimen (CHOP) with three intensive chemotherapy regimens for advanced non-Hodgkin's lymphoma. *N Engl J Med* 1993;328(14):1002–1006.
91. Monfardini S, Banfi A, Bonadonna G, et al. Improved five year survival after combined radiotherapy-chemotherapy for stage I–II non-Hodgkin's lymphoma. *Int J Radiat Oncol Biol Phys* 1980;6(2):125–134.
92. Blum KA, Bartlett NL. Antibodies for the treatment of diffuse large cell lymphoma. *Semin Oncol* 2003;30(4):448–456.
93. Maslovsky I, Uriev L, Lugassy G. The heterogeneity of Castleman disease: Report of five cases and review of the literature. *Am J Med Sci* 2000;320(4):292–295.
94. Izuchukwu IS, Tourbaf K, Mahoney MC. An unusual presentation of Castleman's Disease: A case report. *BMC Infect Dis* 2003;3(1):20.
95. Rena O, Casadio C, Maggi G. Castleman's disease: Unusual intrathoracic localization. *Eur J Cardiothorac Surg* 2001;19(4):519–521.
96. Candoni A, Michelutti T, Morelli A, et al. Castleman's disease: An unusual cause of mediastinal mass and anemia. *Clin Ter* 2002;153(3):217–219.
97. Sinclair DS, Bolen MA, King MA. Mature teratoma within the posterior mediastinum. *J Thorac Imaging* 2003;18(1):53–55.
98. Smahi M, Achir A, Chafik A, et al. [Mature teratome of the mediastinum.] *Ann Chir* 2000;125(10):965–971.
99. Moran CA, Suster S. Primary germ cell tumors of the mediastinum: I. Analysis of 322 cases with special emphasis on teratomatous lesions and a proposal for histopathologic classification and clinical staging. *Cancer* 1997;80(4):681–690.
100. Weidner N. Germ-cell tumors of the mediastinum. *Semin Diagn Pathol* 1999;16(1):42–50.
101. Luna MA, Valenzuela-Tamariz J. Germ-cell tumors of the mediastinum, postmortem findings. *Am J Clin Pathol* 1976;65(4):450–454.
102. Nichols CR. Mediastinal germ cell tumors. Clinical features and biologic correlates. *Chest* 1991;99(2): 472–479.
103. Takeda S, Miyoshi S, Ohta M, et al. Primary germ cell tumors in the mediastinum: A 50-year experience at a single Japanese institution. *Cancer* 2003;97(2):367–376.
104. Lewis BD, Hurt RD, Payne WS, et al. Benign teratomas of the mediastinum. *J Thorac Cardiovasc Surg* 1983;86(5): 727–731.
105. Kilger E, Weis FC, Goetz AE, et al. Intensive care after minimally invasive and conventional coronary surgery: A prospective comparison. *Intens Care Med* 2001;27(3): 534–539.
106. Friedmann AM, Oliva E, Zietman AL, Aquino SL. Case records of the Massachusetts General Medicine. Weekly clinicopathological exercises. Case 9-2003. An 18-year-old man with back and leg pain and a nondiagnostic biopsy specimen. *N Engl J Med* 2003;348(12): 1150–1158.
107. Nichols CR. Mediastinal germ cell tumors. *Semin Thorac Cardiovasc Surg* 1992;4(1):45–50.
108. Strollo DC, Rosado de Christenson ML, Jett JR. Primary mediastinal tumors. Part 1: tumors of the anterior mediastinum. *Chest* 1997;112(2):511–522.
109. Bokemeyer C, Droz JP, Horwich A, et al. Extragonadal seminoma: An international multicenter analysis of

prognostic factors and long term treatment outcome. *Cancer* 2001;91(7):1394–1401.
110. Kesler KA, Rieger KM, Ganjoo KN, et al. Primary mediastinal nonseminomatous germ cell tumors: The influence of postchemotherapy pathology on long-term survival after surgery. *J Thorac Cardiovasc Surg* 1999; 118(4):692–700.
111. Dexeus FH, Logothetis CJ, Chong C, et al. Genetic abnormalities in men with germ cell tumors. *J Urol* 1988;140(1):80–84.
112. Nichols CR, Hoffman R, Einhorn LH, et al. Hematologic malignancies associated with primary mediastinal germ-cell tumors. *Ann Intern Med* 1985;102(5): 603–609.
113. Dulmet EM, Macchiarini P, Suc B, Verley JM. Germ cell tumors of the mediastinum. A 30-year experience. *Cancer* 1993;72(6):1894–1901.
114. Takeda S, Miyoshi S, Inoue M, et al. Clinical spectrum of congenital cystic disease of the lung in children. *Eur J Cardiothorac Surg* 1999;15(1):11–17.
115. Bukowski RM, Wolf M, Kulander BG, et al. Alternating combination chemotherapy in patients with extragonadal germ cell tumors. A Southwest Oncology Group study. *Cancer* 1993;71(8):2631–2638.
116. Nichols CR, Saxman S, Williams SD, et al. Primary mediastinal nonseminomatous germ cell tumors. A modern single institution experience. *Cancer* 1990;65(7): 1641–1646.
117. Motzer RJ, Mazumdar M, Gulati SC, et al. Phase II trial of high-dose carboplatin and etoposide with autologous bone marrow transplantation in first-line therapy for patients with poor-risk germ cell tumors. *J Natl Cancer Inst* 1993;85(22):1828–1835.
118. Bokemeyer C, Schleucher N, Metzner B, et al. First-line sequential high-dose VIP chemotherapy with autologous transplantation for patients with primary mediastinal nonseminomatous germ cell tumours: A prospective trial. *Br J Cancer* 2003;89(1):29–35.
119. Motohashi S, Sekine Y, Iizasa T, et al. Thyroid cancer with massive invasion into the neck and mediastinal great veins. *Jpn J Thorac Cardiovasc Surg* 2005;53(1): 55–57.
120. Bacha EA, Chapelier AR, Macchiarini P, et al. Surgery for invasive primary mediastinal tumors. *Ann Thorac Surg* 1998;66(1):234–239.
121. Wychulis AR, Payne WS, Clagett OT, Woolner LB. Surgical treatment of mediastinal tumors: A 40 year experience. *J Thorac Cardiovasc Surg* 1971;62(3):379–392.
122. Sirivella S, Ford WB, Zikria EA, et al. Foregut cysts of the mediastinum. Results in 20 consecutive surgically treated cases. *J Thorac Cardiovasc Surg* 1985;90(5): 776–782.
123. Ramenofsky ML, Leape LL, McCauley RG. Bronchogenic cyst. *J Pediatr Surg* 1979;14(3):219–224.
124. Petkar M, Vaideeswar P, Deshpande JR. Surgical pathology of cystic lesions of the mediastinum. *J Postgrad Med* 2001;47(4):235–239.
125. Di Lorenzo M, Collin PP, Vaillancourt R, Duranceau A. Bronchogenic cysts. *J Pediatr Surg* 1989;24(10):988–991.
126. Prates PR, Lovato L, Homsi-Neto A, et al. Right ventricular bronchogenic cyst. *Tex Heart Inst J* 2003;30(1): 71–73.
127. St Georges R, Deslauriers J, Duranceau A, et al. Clinical spectrum of bronchogenic cysts of the mediastinum and lung in the adult. *Ann Thorac Surg* 1991;52(1):6–13.
128. Patel SR, Meeker DP, Biscotti CV, et al. Presentation and management of bronchogenic cysts in the adult. *Chest* 1994;106(1):79–85.
129. Sarper A, Ayten A, Golbasi I, et al. Bronchogenic cyst. *Tex Heart Inst J* 2003;30(2):105–108.
130. Cioffi U, Bonavina L, De Simone M, et al. Presentation and surgical management of bronchogenic and esophageal duplication cysts in adults. *Chest* 1998;113(6): 1492–1496.
131. Kim Y, Lee KS, Yoo JH, et al. Middle mediastinal lesions: Imaging findings and pathologic correlation. *Eur J Radiol* 2000;35(1):30–38.
132. Wildi SM, Hoda RS, Fickling W, et al. Diagnosis of benign cysts of the mediastinum: The role and risks of EUS and FNA. *Gastrointest Endosc* 2003;58(3):362–368.
133. Whyte MK, Dollery CT, Adam A, Ind PW. Central bronchogenic cyst: Treatment by extrapleural percutaneous aspiration. *BMJ* 1989;299(6713):1457–1458.
134. Iwasaki A, Hiratsuka M, Kawahara K, Shirakusa T. New technique for the cystic mediastinal tumor by video-assisted thoracoscopy. *Ann Thorac Surg* 2001;72(2): 632–633.
135. Bacchetta MD, Korst RJ, Altorki NK, et al. Resection of a symptomatic pericardial cyst using the computer-enhanced da Vinci Surgical System. *Ann Thorac Surg* 2003;75(6):1953–1955.
136. Suen HC, Mathisen DJ, Grillo HC, et al. Surgical management and radiological characteristics of bronchogenic cysts. *Ann Thorac Surg* 1993;55(2):476–481.
137. Bolton JW, Shahian DM. Asymptomatic bronchogenic cysts: What is the best management? *Ann Thorac Surg* 1992;53(6):1134–1137.
138. Bondestam S, Salo JA, Salonen OL, Lamminen AE. Imaging of congenital esophageal cysts in adults. *Gastrointest Radiol* 1990;15(4):279–281.
139. Whitaker JA, Deffenbaugh LD, Cooke AR. Esophageal duplication cyst. Case report. *Am J Gastroenterol* 1980;73(4):329–332.
140. Reed JC, Sobonya RE. Morphologic analysis of foregut cysts in the thorax. *Am J Roentgenol Radium Ther Nucl Med* 1974;120(4):851–860.
141. Kirwan WO, Walbaum PR, McCormack RJ. Cystic intrathoracic derivatives of the foregut and their complications. *Thorax* 1973;28(4):424–428.
142. Van Dam J, Rice TW, Sivak MV Jr. Endoscopic ultrasonography and endoscopically guided needle aspiration for the diagnosis of upper gastrointestinal tract foregut cysts. *Am J Gastroenterol* 1992;87(6):762–765.
143. Lazar G, Szentpali K, Szanto I, et al. Successful thoracoscopic surgical treatment of oesophageal cyst. *Acta Chir Hung* 1999;38(2):191–192.
144. Koster B, Emons D, Kunath U, Fodisch HJ. [Neurenteric cyst of the mediastinum—case report and review of the literature.] *Klin Padiatr* 1987;199(1):1–8.
145. Azzie G, Beasley S. Diagnosis and treatment of foregut duplications. *Semin Pediatr Surg* 2003;12(1):46–54.
146. Rizalar R, Demirbilek S, Bernay F, Gurses N. A case of a mediastinal neurenteric cyst demonstrated by prenatal ultrasound. *Eur J Pediatr Surg* 1995;5(3):177–179.

147. Cangemi V, Volpino P, Gualdi G, et al. Pericardial cysts of the mediastinum. *J Cardiovasc Surg (Torino)* 1999; 40(6):909–913.
148. Volpino P, De Cesare A, Bononi M, et al. [Pericardial cysts. Report on 9 treated cases.] *G Chir* 1997;18(11–12): 811–814.
149. Stoller JK, Shaw C, Matthay RA. Enlarging, atypically located pericardial cyst. Recent experience and literature review. *Chest* 1986;89(3):402–406.
150. Kutlay H, Yavuzer I, Han S, Cangir AK. Atypically located pericardial cysts. *Ann Thorac Surg* 2001;72(6): 2137–2139.
151. Pader E, Kirschner PA. Pericardial diverticulum. *Dis Chest* 1969;55(4):344–346.
152. Chopra PS, Duke DJ, Pellett JR, Rahko PS. Pericardial cyst with partial erosion of the right ventricular wall. *Ann Thorac Surg* 1991;51(5):840–841.
153. Mastroroberto P, Chello M, Bevacqua E, Marchese AR. Pericardial cyst with partial erosion of the superior vena cava. An unusual case. *J Cardiovasc Surg (Torino)* 1996;37(3):323–324.
154. Davis JW, Florendo FT. Symptomatic mediastinal thymic cysts. *Ann Thorac Surg* 1988;46(6):693–694.
155. Rastegar H, Arger P, Harken AH. Evaluation and therapy of mediastinal thymic cyst. *Am Surg* 1980;46(4):236–238.
156. Pramesh CS, Deshpande MS, Pantvaidya GH, et al. Thoracic duct cyst of the mediastinum. *Ann Thorac Cardiovasc Surg* 2003;9(4):264–265.
157. Mattila PS, Tarkkanen J, Mattila S. Thoracic duct cyst: A case report and review of 29 cases. *Ann Otol Rhinol Laryngol* 1999;108(5):505–508.
158. Sawicz-Birkowska K, Czernik J, Chrzan R, Kolodziej J. [Mediastinal tumors in children.] *Pol Merkuriusz Lek* 2002;13(76):305–307.
159. Shields TW, Reynolds M. Neurogenic tumors of the thorax. *Surg Clin North Am* 1988;68(3):645–668.
160. Ribet ME, Cardot GR. Neurogenic tumors of the thorax. *Ann Thorac Surg* 1994;58(4):1091–1095.
161. Reed JC, Hallet KK, Feigin DS. Neural tumors of the thorax: Subject review from the AFIP. *Radiology* 1978;126(1):9–17.
162. Wain JC. Neurogenic tumors of the mediastinum. *Chest Surg Clin North Am* 1992;2:121.
163. Topcu S, Alper A, Gulhan E, et al. Neurogenic tumours of the mediastinum: A report of 60 cases. *Can Respir J* 2000;7(3):261–265.
164. Davidson KG, Walbaum PR, McCormack RJ. Intrathoracic neural tumours. *Thorax* 1978;33(3):359–367.
165. Ardissone F, Andrion A, D'Alessandro L, et al. Neurogenic intrathoracic tumors. A clinicopathological review of 92 cases. *Thorac Cardiovasc Surg* 1986;34(4): 260–264.
166. Aughenbaugh GL. Thoracic manifestations of neurocutaneous diseases. *Radiol Clin North Am* 1984;22(3): 741–756.
167. Sakai F, Sone S, Kiyono K, et al. Intrathoracic neurogenic tumors: MR-pathologic correlation. *AJR* 1992; 159(2):279–283.
168. Kumar AJ, Kuhajda FP, Martinez CR, et al. Computed tomography of extracranial nerve sheath tumors with pathological correlation. *J Comput Assist Tomogr* 1983;7(5):857–865.
169. Kiryu T, Ohashi N, Hoshi H, et al. Mediastinal schwannoma: MR imaging findings of an unusual case presenting as a lobulated mass with internal fibrous septa. *Clin Radiol* 2003;58(8):652–655.
170. Inci I, Turgut M. Neurogenic tumors of the mediastinum in children. *Childs Nerv Syst* 1999;15(8):372–376.
171. Akwari OE, Payne WS, Onofrio BM, et al. Dumbbell neurogenic tumors of the mediastinum. Diagnosis and management. *Mayo Clin Proc* 1978;53(6):353–358.
172. Strollo DC, Rosado-de-Christenson ML, Jett JR. Primary mediastinal tumors: Part II. Tumors of the middle and posterior mediastinum. *Chest* 1997;112(5): 1344–1357.
173. Ducatman BS, Scheithauer BW, Piepgras DG, et al. Malignant peripheral nerve sheath tumors. A clinicopathologic study of 120 cases. *Cancer* 1986;57(10): 2006–2021.
174. Marchevsky AM. Mediastinal tumors of peripheral nervous system origin. *Semin Diagn Pathol* 1999;16(1): 65–78.
175. Zhang H, Ping Y, Bai S. [Clinicopathological characteristics and surgical treatment of primary neurogenic tumors of the mediastinum.] *Zhonghua Zhong Liu Za Zhi* 1999;21(6):458–460.
176. Saenz NC, Schnitzer JJ, Eraklis AE, et al. Posterior mediastinal masses. *J Pediatr Surg* 1993;28(2):172–176.
177. Harjula A, Mattila S, Luosto R, et al. Mediastinal neurogenic tumours. Early and late results of surgical treatment. *Scand J Thorac Cardiovasc Surg* 1986;20(2): 115–118.
178. Swanson PE. Soft tissue neoplasma of the mediastinum. *Semin Diagn Pathol* 1991;8(1):14–34.
179. Boiko GA, Kolygin BA, Kosian VS, Belogurova MB. [Neurogenic tumors of the mediastinum in children]. *Vestn Khir Im I I Grek* 1991;146(4):75–78.
180. Olson JL, Salyer WR. Mediastinal paragangliomas (aortic body tumor): A report of four cases and a review of the literature. *Cancer* 1978;41(6):2405–2412.
181. Noorda RJ, Wuisman PI, Kummer AJ, et al. Nonfunctioning malignant paraganglioma of the posterior mediastinum with spinal cord compression. A case report. *Spine* 1996;21(14):1703–1709.
182. Lamy AL, Fradet GJ, Luoma A, Nelems B. Anterior and Middle mediastinum paraganglioma: Complete resection is the treatment of choice. *Ann Thorac Surg* 1994;57(1): 249–252.
183. Herrera MF, van Heerden JA, Puga FJ, et al. Mediastinal paraganglioma: A surgical experience. *Ann Thorac Surg* 1993;56(5):1096–1100.
184. Aggarwal M, Lakhhar B, Aggarwal BK, Anugu R. Askin tumor: A malignant small cell tumor. *Indian J Pediatr* 2000;67(11):853–855.
185. Sabate JM, Franquet T, Parellada JA, et al. Malignant neuroectodermal tumour of the chest wall (Askin tumour): CT and MR findings in eight patients. *Clin Radiol* 1994;49(9):634–638.
186. Christiansen S, Semik M, Dockhorn-Dworniczak B, et al. Diagnosis, treatment and outcome of patients with Askin-tumors. *Thorac Cardiovasc Surg* 2000;48(5):311–315.
187. Prece V, Bertagni A, Gallinaro L, et al. [Neurogenic tumors of the mediastinum.] *Ann Ital Chir* 2002;73(2): 125–127.

188. Reeder LB. Neurogenic tumors of the mediastinum. *Semin Thorac Cardiovasc Surg* 2000;12(4):261–267.
189. Luosto R, Koikkalainen K, Jyrala A, Franssila K. Mediastinal tumours. A follow-up study of 208 patients. *Scand J Thorac Cardiovasc Surg* 1978;12(3): 253–259.
190. Liu HP, Yim AP, Wan J, et al. Thoracoscopic removal of intrathoracic neurogenic tumors: A combined Chinese experience. *Ann Surg* 2000;232(2):187–190.
191. Imaizumi M, Watanabe H, Takeuchi S, et al. Video thoracoscopic resection of neurogenic tumor in a superior-posterior mediastinum: Three case reports. *Surg Laparosc Endosc* 1997;7(4):301–306.
192. Divisi D, Battaglia C, Crisci R, et al. Diagnostic and therapeutic approaches for masses in the posterior mediastinum. *Acta Biomed Ateneo Parmense* 1998;69(5–6): 123–128.
193. Heltzer JM, Krasna MJ, Aldrich F, McLaughlin JS. Thoracoscopic excision of a posterior mediastinal "dumbbell" tumor using a combined approach. *Ann Thorac Surg* 1995;60(2):431–433.
194. Ricci C, Rendina EA, Venuta F, et al. Diagnostic imaging and surgical treatment of dumbbell tumors of the mediastinum. *Ann Thorac Surg* 1990;50(4):586–589.
195. Joseph SG, Tellis CJ. Posterior mediastinal mass with intraspinous extension. *Chest* 1988;93(5):1101–1103.
196. Yuksel M, Pamir N, Ozer F, et al. The principles of surgical management in dumbbell tumors. *Eur J Cardiothorac Surg* 1996;10(7):569–573.
197. Carlsen NL, Christensen IJ, Schroeder H, et al. Prognostic factors in neuroblastomas treated in Denmark from 1943 to 1980. A statistical estimate of prognosis based on 253 cases. *Cancer* 1986;58(12):2726–2735.
198. Bilyeu JA. Superior vena cava syndrome. *J Insur Med* 2001;33(4):349–352.
199. Laguna DE, Gazapo NT, Murillas AJ, et al. [Superior vena cava syndrome: A study based on 81 cases.] *An Med Interna* 1998;15(9):470–475.
200. Dempke W, Behrmann C, Schober C, et al. [Diagnostic and therapeutic management of the superior vena cava syndrome.] *Med Klin (Munich)* 1999;94(12):681–684.
201. Parish JM, Marschke RF Jr, Dines DE, Lee RE. Etiologic considerations in superior vena cava syndrome. *Mayo Clin Proc* 1981;56(7):407–413.
202. Baker GL, Barnes HJ. Superior vena cava syndrome: Etiology, diagnosis, and treatment. *Am J Crit Care* 1992;1(1):54–64.
203. Muramatsu T, Miyamae T, Dohi Y. Collateral pathways observed by radionuclide superior cavography in 70 patients with superior vena caval obstruction. *Clin Nucl Med* 1991;16(5):332–336.
204. McGarry RC. Superior vena cava obstruction due to prostate carcinoma. *Urology* 2000;55(3):436.
205. Hsu JW, Chiang CD, Hsu WH, et al. Superior vena cava syndrome in lung cancer: An analysis of 54 cases. *Gaoxiong Yi Xue Ke Xue Za Zhi* 1995;11(10):568–573.
206. Gauden SJ. Superior vena cava syndrome induced by bronchogenic carcinoma: Is this an oncological emergency? *Australas Radiol* 1993;37(4):363–366.
207. Schraufnagel DE, Hill R, Leech JA, Pare JA. Superior vena caval obstruction. Is it a medical emergency? *Am J Med* 1981;70(6):1169–1174.
208. Wudel LJ Jr, Nesbitt JC. Superior vena cava syndrome. *Curr Treat Options Oncol* 2001;2(1):77–91.
209. Sculier JP, Evans WK, Feld R, et al. Superior vena caval obstruction syndrome in small cell lung cancer. *Cancer* 1986;57(4):847–851.
210. Loeffler JS, Leopold KA, Recht A, et al. Emergency prebiopsy radiation for mediastinal masses: Impact on subsequent pathologic diagnosis and outcome. *J Clin Oncol* 1986;4(5):716–721.
211. Markman M. Diagnosis and management of superior vena cava syndrome. *Cleve Clin J Med* 1999;66(1):59–61.
212. Escalante CP. Causes and management of superior vena cava syndrome. *Oncology (Huntingt)* 1993;7(6):61–68.
213. Bell DR, Woods RL, Levi JA. Superior vena caval obstruction: A 10-year experience. *Med J Aust* 1986; 145(11–12):566–568.
214. Fincher RM. Superior vena cava syndrome: Experience in a teaching hospital. *South Med J* 1987;80(10):1243–1245.
215. Perez-Soler R, McLaughlin P, Velasquez WS, et al. Clinical features and results of management of superior vena cava syndrome secondary to lymphoma. *J Clin Oncol* 1984;2(4):260–266.
216. Cheson BD. Hodgkin's disease, alcohol, and vena caval obstruction. *JAMA* 1978;239(1):23–24.
217. Czaykowski PM, Samuels T, Oza A. A durable response to cytarabine in advanced breast cancer. *Clin Oncol (R Coll Radiol)* 1997;9(3):181–183.
218. Dendo S, Inaba Y, Arai Y, et al. Severe obstruction of the superior vena cava caused by tumor invasion. Recanalization using a PTFE-covered Z stent. *J Cardiovasc Surg (Torino)* 2002;43(2):287–290.
219. Berrocal A, Artal A, Baron JM, Garrido P. [Superior vena cava syndrome secondary to gastric cancer.] *Rev Esp Enferm Dig* 1991;79(6):444–445.
220. Sola C, Paredes A, Villanueva C, Pallares C. [Superior vena cava syndrome as manifestation of adenocarcinoma of the pancreas.] *An Med Interna* 1989;6(5):278–279.
221. Padovani M, Tillie-Leblond I, Vennin P, et al. [Paraneoplastic superior vena cava thrombosis disclosing an ovarian tumor]. *Rev Mal Respir* 1996;13(6):598–600.
222. Urschel HC Jr, Razzuk MA, Netto GJ, et al. Sclerosing mediastinitis: Improved management with histoplasmosis titer and ketoconazole. *Ann Thorac Surg* 1990;50(2): 215–221.
223. Lagerstrom CF, Mitchell HG, Graham BS, Hammon JW Jr. Chronic fibrosing mediastinitis and superior vena caval obstruction from blastomycosis. *Ann Thorac Surg* 1992;54(4):764–765.
224. Jena RK, Patranabis N, Sarangi B. Superior vena caval syndrome due to pulmonary tuberculosis. *J Indian Med Assoc* 1996;94(9):351–352.
225. Loutsidis A, Zisis C, Rontogianni D, Bellenis I. Actinomycosis presenting as superior vena cava syndrome in a young puerperal woman. *J Thorac Cardiovasc Surg* 2000;120(5):1009–1010.
226. Abdelkafi S, Dubail D, Bosschaerts T, et al. Superior vena cava syndrome associated with *Nocardia farcinica* infection. *Thorax* 1997;52(5):492–493.
227. Takatsuka H, Wakae T, Mori A, et al. Superior vena cava syndrome after bone marrow transplantation caused by aspergillosis: A case report. *Hematology* 2002;7(3): 169–172.

228. Morales M, Comas V, Trujillo M, Dorta J. Treatment of catheter-induced thrombotic superior vena cava syndrome: A single institution's experience. *Support Care Cancer* 2000;8(4):334–338.
229. Beers TR, Burnes J, Fleming CR. Superior vena caval obstruction in patients with gut failure receiving home parenteral nutrition. *JPEN* 1990;14(5):474–479.
230. Teo N, Sabharwal T, Rowland E, et al. Treatment of superior vena cava obstruction secondary to pacemaker wires with balloon venoplasty and insertion of metallic stents. *Eur Heart J* 2002;23(18):1465–1470.
231. Turk HM, Camci C, Buyukberber S, et al. Superior vena cava syndrome caused by chemotherapy-induced fibrosis. *J Chemother* 2002;14(4):417–419.
232. Brown G, Husband JE. Mediastinal widening—a valuable radiographic sign of superior vena cava thrombosis. *Clin Radiol* 1993;47(6):415–420.
233. Lai CL, Tsai TT, Ko SC, et al. Superior vena cava syndrome caused by encapsulated pleural effusion. *Eur Respir J* 1997;10(7):1675–1677.
234. Tayade BO, Salvi SS, Agarwal IR. Study of superior vena cava syndrome—Aetiopathology, diagnosis and management. *J Assoc Physicians India* 1994;42(8):609–611.
235. Kim HJ, Kim HS, Chung SH. CT diagnosis of superior vena cava syndrome: Importance of collateral vessels. *AJR* 1993;161(3):539–542.
236. Qanadli SD, El Hajjam M, Bruckert F, et al. Helical CT phlebography of the superior vena cava: Diagnosis and evaluation of venous obstruction. *AJR* 1999;172(5): 1327–1333.
237. Raptopoulos V. Computed tomography of the superior vena cava. *Crit Rev Diagn Imaging* 1986;25(4):373–429.
238. Haddad JL, Rofsky NM, Weinreb JC, Galloway AC. SVC syndrome as a late complication of ascending aortic aneurysm repair: MR diagnosis. *J Comput Assist Tomogr* 1993;17(6):982–985.
239. Porte H, Metois D, Finzi L, et al. Superior vena cava syndrome of malignant origin. Which surgical procedure for which diagnosis? *Eur J Cardiothorac Surg* 2000;17(4): 384–388.
240. Gamez Garcia AP, Martin de Nicolas Serrahima JL, Marron FC, et al. [Surgical diagnostic procedures in superior vena cava syndrome.] *Arch Bronconeumol* 1997;33(6):284–288.
241. Jahangiri M, Goldstraw P. The role of mediastinoscopy in superior vena caval obstruction. *Ann Thorac Surg* 1995;59(2):453–455.
242. Selcuk ZT, Firat P. The diagnostic yield of transbronchial needle aspiration in superior vena cava syndrome. *Lung Cancer* 2003;42(2):183–188.
243. Bigsby R, Greengrass R, Unruh H. Diagnostic algorithm for acute superior vena caval obstruction (SVCO). *J Cardiovasc Surg (Torino)* 1993;34(4):347–350.
244. Armstrong BA, Perez CA, Simpson JR, Hederman MA. Role of irradiation in the management of superior vena cava syndrome. *Int J Radiat Oncol Biol Phys* 1987;13(4): 531–539.
245. Spiro SG, Shah S, Harper PG, et al. Treatment of obstruction of the superior vena cava by combination chemotherapy with and without irradiation in small-cell carcinoma of the bronchus. *Thorax* 1983;38(7):501–505.
246. Rowell NP, Gleeson FV. Steroids, radiotherapy, chemotherapy and stents for superior vena caval obstruction in carcinoma of the bronchus: A systematic review. *Clin Oncol (R Coll Radiol)* 2002;14(5):338–351.
247. Egelmeers A, Goor C, van Meerbeeck J, et al. Palliative effectiveness of radiation therapy in the treatment of superior vena cava syndrome. *Bull Cancer Radiother* 1996;83(3):153–157.
248. Shah R, Sabanathan S, Lowe RA, Mearns AJ. Stenting in malignant obstruction of superior vena cava. *J Thorac Cardiovasc Surg* 1996;112(2):335–340.
249. Stock KW, Jacob AL, Proske M, et al. Treatment of malignant obstruction of the superior vena cava with the self-expanding Wallstent. *Thorax* 1995;50(11): 1151–1156.
250. Solomon N, Wholey MH, Jarmolowski CR. Intravascular stents in the management of superior vena cava syndrome. *Cathet Cardiovasc Diagn* 1991;23(4): 245–252.
251. Elson JD, Becker GJ, Wholey MH, Ehrman KO. Vena caval and central venous stenoses: Management with Palmaz balloon-expandable intraluminal stents. *J Vasc Intervent Radiol* 1991;2(2):215–223.
252. Rosch J, Uchida BT, Hall LD, et al. Gianturco-Rosch expandable Z-stents in the treatment of superior vena cava syndrome. *Cardiovasc Intervent Radiol* 1992;15(5): 319–327.
253. Kishi K, Sonomura T, Mitsuzane K, et al. Self-expandable metallic stent therapy for superior vena cava syndrome: Clinical observations. *Radiology* 1993;189(2): 531–535.
254. Dyet JF, Nicholson AA, Cook AM. The use of the Wallstent endovascular prosthesis in the treatment of malignant obstruction of the superior vena cava. *Clin Radiol* 1993;48(6):381–385.
255. Rosenblum J, Leef J, Messersmith R, et al. Intravascular stents in the management of acute superior vena cava obstruction of benign etiology. *JPEN* 1994;18(4): 362–366.
256. Watkinson AF, Hansell DM. Expandable Wallstent for the treatment of obstruction of the superior vena cava. *Thorax* 1993;48(9):915–920.
257. Chatziioannou A, Alexopoulos T, Mourikis D, et al. Stent therapy for malignant superior vena cava syndrome: Should be first line therapy or simple adjunct to radiotherapy. *Eur J Radiol* 2003;47(3):247–250.
258. Lanciego C, Chacon JL, Julian A, et al. Stenting as first option for endovascular treatment of malignant superior vena cava syndrome. *AJR* 2001;177(3):585–593.
259. Avasthi RB, Moghissi K. Malignant obstruction of the superior vena cava and its palliation: Report of four cases. *J Thorac Cardiovasc Surg* 1977;74(2):244–248.
260. Kalra M, Gloviczki P, Andrews JC, et al. Open surgical and endovascular treatment of superior vena cava syndrome caused by nonmalignant disease. *J Vasc Surg* 2003;38(2):215–223.
261. Sivaram CA, Craven P, Chandrasekaran K. Transesophageal echocardiography during removal of central venous catheter associated with thrombus in superior vena cava. *Am J Card Imaging* 1996;10(4): 266–269.

CHAPTER

3 THORACIC INFECTIONS

Lois U. Nwakanma

PNEUMONIA, BRONCHIECTASIS, AND LUNG ABSCESS

Lower respiratory tract infections are important in the practice of the thoracic surgeon because their complications may require surgical intervention and they may complicate thoracic surgical procedures.

PNEUMONIA

Pneumonia is an infection of the lower respiratory tract that involves the terminal airways: respiratory bronchioles, alveolar ducts, and alveoli. There is associated inflammation of the lung parenchyma with congestion. The infection develops when the sterility of the tracheobronchial

KEY CONCEPTS

- The etiology and clinical manifestations of pneumonia depend on the environment where the disease is acquired and the host characteristics.
- Treatment of pneumonia is based on an assessment of place of therapy (outpatient, hospital ward, or ICU), the presence of coexisting cardiopulmonary disease, and the presence of modifying factors.
- Although prompt initiation of antibiotics is critical in patients with nosocomial pneumonia, all patients with suspected pneumonia should have a sampling of lower respiratory tract secretions to better guide therapy.
- Lung abscess should be managed initially with appropriate medical therapy and/or percutaneous drainage.
- Bronchiectasis is the abnormal dilatation of bronchi. It can be congenital or acquired. Surgical intervention is indicated if there is persistent recurrent infection following discontinuation of medication, massive hemoptysis, and for removal of a foreign body or tumor.
- Owing to the presence of branching hyphae, infections due to actinomycosis and nocardiosis may be mistaken for fungal infections. It is important to make the distinction because actinomycotic infections do not respond to antifungal therapy but rather to antibiotics.
- Surgical consultation is regularly requested for the diagnosis and treatment of pulmonary complications of the endemic mycoses: *Histoplasma capsulatum, Blastomyces dermatitidis* and *Coccidioidomycosis immitis,* and the yeast *Cryptococcus neoformans.* All resemble pulmonary malignancies.
- Histoplasmosis causes pericarditis, mediastinal fibrosis, and mediastinal granuloma, which can cause entrapment of vascular structures, the esophagus, and the trachea.
- Coccidioidomycosis can cause both spontaneous pneumothorax associated with effusion and thin-walled cavities that can become superinfected with tuberculosis and aspergillosis.
- Cryptococcosis can result in organ damage from tissue distortion secondary to an expanding fungal burden.
- Most patients with pulmonary aspergillosis have either impaired immunity or an underlying preexisting chronic lung disease. Aspergillomas may develop in preexisting cavities. Surgery is indicated for complications of the disease, such as massive hemoptysis.
- Surgery has largely been supplanted by multiple-regimen medical therapy for tuberculous and nontuberculous mycobacterial infections. There is still a role for pulmonary resection in multi-drug-resistant infection, cavitary lesions, and lung destruction.

tree is breached by introduction of a virulent pathogen or a defect in the host immunologic defense. Symptoms of acute lower respiratory infection may include several (in most studies, at least two) of the following: fever or hypothermia, rigors, sweats, new cough with or without sputum production or change in color of respiratory secretions in a patient with chronic cough, chest discomfort, or the onset of dyspnea. Most patients also have nonspecific symptoms, such as fatigue, myalgias, abdominal pain, anorexia, and headache.[1]

Despite advancements in the diagnosis and treatment of pneumonia in the past century, it is listed by the Centers for Disease Control and Prevention as the sixth leading cause of death in the United States and the leading cause of death from infectious diseases.[2] Contemporary management of pneumonia is based on whether the infection was acquired in the community versus in the hospital, including any care facility; the severity of illness; and the patient's comorbid conditions, including immune status.

Community-acquired pneumonia

Community-acquired pneumonia (CAP) is commonly defined as an acute infection of the pulmonary parenchyma in a patient not hospitalized or residing in a long-term-care facility for ≥ 14 days before the onset of symptoms.[1] CAP is among the leading causes of death in the United States, accounting for some 65,000 deaths in 2002[2]; it is responsible for more than 10 million physician visits a year and some 1.4 million hospital discharges.[3] The most common etiologic agent of CAP is *Streptococcus pneumoniae,* which accounts for about two-thirds of all cases of bacteremic pneumonia.[4] Other pathogens include *Haemophilus influenzae, Mycoplasma pneumoniae, Chlamydia pneumoniae, Staphylococcus aureus, Streptococcus pyogenes, Neisseria meningitidis, Moraxella catarrhalis, Klebsiella pneumoniae* and other gram-negative rods, *Legionella* species, influenza virus (depending on the season), respiratory syncytial virus, adenovirus, and parainfluenza virus. Gram-negative bacilli (Enterobacteriaceae and *Pseudomonas*) are the cause of CAP in some patients (those who have had previous antimicrobial treatment or who have pulmonary comorbidities). The frequency of other causes, such as *Mycobacterium tuberculosis, Chlamydophila psittaci* (psittacosis), *Coxiella burnetii* (Q fever), *Francisella tularensis* (tularemia), and endemic fungi (*Histoplasma, Coccidioides, Blastomyces*) vary between epidemiologic settings.[1,5,6] Certain pathogens cause pneumonia more commonly among persons with specific risk factors. For instance, pneumococcal pneumonia is especially likely to occur in the elderly and in patients with a variety of medical conditions, including alcoholism, chronic cardiovascular disease, chronic obstructive airway disease, immunoglobulin deficiency, hematologic malignancy, and human immunodeficiency virus (HIV) infection. However, outbreaks occur among young adults under conditions of crowding, as in army camps or prisons. *Legionella* is an opportunistic pathogen that is rarely recognized in healthy young children and young adults. *It is an important cause of pneumonia in organ transplant recipients* and in patients with renal failure and occurs with increased frequency in patients with chronic lung disease, smokers, and possibly those with acquired immunodeficiency syndrome (AIDS).[1] Although *M. pneumoniae* historically has been thought primarily to involve children and young adults, some evidence suggests that it causes pneumonia in healthy adults of any age.[7]

A review of published studies show that the traditional chest physical examination is not sufficiently accurate on its own to confirm or exclude the diagnosis of pneumonia.[8,9] All patients suspected to have pneumonia should undergo chest radiography[1,5,10] for the following reasons: to confirm the diagnosis, to provide information on the location and extent of disease, to explore the possibility of complications such as pleural effusion, multilobar disease, and cavitation; to detect underlying pulmonary disease or alternative diagnoses; and to monitor the progression or resolution of the disease.[11] Other appropriate tests for hospitalized patients with CAP include a complete blood cell count and differential, serum creatinine, blood urea nitrogen, glucose, electrolytes, and liver function tests. Oxygen saturation should be assessed by pulse oximetry in all admitted patients and arterial blood gas in sicker patients. There should be two pretreatment blood cultures as well as Gram's staining and culture of expectorated sputum.[1,11,12]

Other tests, which should not be performed routinely but might be useful in some patients admitted to the hospital, include the urinary antigen assays for *Legionella* species and *Strep. pneumoniae* and a direct stain (i.e., acid-fast) for the detection of mycobacterial infections in patients who are in high-risk categories for tuberculosis.[1,5,12] HIV serology with informed consent should also be considered, especially for persons aged 15 to 54 years.[1,5] Serologic testing may also include tests for viral agents, endemic fungi, and other unusual pathogens in appropriate clinical settings.[5] Invasive diagnostic techniques (transtracheal aspiration, bronchoscopy with a protected brush catheter, bronchoalveolar lavage, direct percutaneous fine-needle aspiration of the lung) are used to obtain lower airway specimens uncontaminated by oropharyngeal flora. These procedures may help to obtain early accurate diagnosis and are reserved for occasional patients who are severely ill.[1,5] Potentially infected body fluids from other anatomic sites—including pleural fluid, joint fluid, and cerebrospinal fluid (CSF)—should be obtained for chemistry, Gram's staining, and culture if warranted by the clinical presentation.[1]

Pathogen-directed antimicrobial therapy is ideal, but this is usually not feasible because no etiology can be identified in more than 50 percent of cases. Empiric

Table 3-1 Modifying factors that increase the risk of infection with specific pathogens
Penicillin-resistant and drug-resistant pneumococci
Age > 65 years
β-Lactam therapy within the past 3 months
Alcoholism
Immune-suppressive illness (including therapy with corticosteroids)
Multiple medical comorbidities
Exposure to a child in a day care center
Enteric gram-negatives
Residence in a nursing home
Underlying cardiopulmonary disease
Multiple medical comorbidities
Recent antibiotic therapy
Pseudomonas aeruginosa
Structural lung disease (bronchiectasis)
Corticosteroid therapy (> 10 mg of prednisone per day)
Broad-spectrum antibiotic therapy for > 7 d in the past month
Malnutrition

Source: From Niederman et al.[5] With permission.

antibiotic regimens should include coverage of "atypical pathogens" and changed when results of culture and in vitro sensitivity tests become available.[1,5] All admitted patients should receive their first dose of antibiotic therapy within 8 h of arrival at the hospital. This has been shown to reduce mortality at 30 days.[13] The American Thoracic Society (ATS) currently makes recommendations based on an assessment of place of therapy (outpatient, hospital ward, or ICU), the presence of coexisting cardiopulmonary disease (chronic obstructive pulmonary disease, congestive heart failure), and the presence of modifying factors (Table 3-1).[5] Most patients can be treated using monotherapy with antipneumococcal fluoroquinolone except for ICU-admitted patients who should receive beta-lactam plus either a macrolide or quinolone. Appropriate at-risk patients should receive a regimen with two antipseudomonal agents.

Hospital-acquired (nosocomial) pneumonia

Hospital-acquired pneumonia (HAP) is defined as pneumonia that occurs 48 h or more after admission and that was not incubating at the time of admission. HAP is usually caused by bacteria, is currently the second most common nosocomial infection in the United States, and is associated with high mortality and morbidity.[14] According to the report from the National Center for Infectious Diseases, nosocomial pneumonia is the most frequent hospital-acquired infection in the combined medical and surgical ICUs, which accounts for 31 percent of all infections in the ICU.[15] Risk factors for HAP include mechanical ventilation for > 48 h, residence in an ICU, duration of ICU or hospital stay, severity of underlying illness, and presence of comorbidities. Generally, loss of mechanical host defense and suppression of normal flora probably explain a major component of the increased risk of pneumonia in hospitalized patients. The most obvious compromise of normal host immunity in hospitalized patients is alteration of the mechanical components of lung defenses. For example, endotracheal intubation bypasses the mechanical barrier of the entire upper respiratory tract and compromises cough. Furthermore, even in nonintubated patients, use of sedatives, analgesics (or the pain itself), or anticholinergic agents can limit the effectiveness of cough. Many hospitalized patients are also kept in the supine position, further compromising mucociliary clearance and increasing aspiration risk. Hospitalized patients are frequently not in control of their own fluid balance, leading to decreased mucociliary clearance by dehydration or, conversely, compromise of alveolar macrophage chemotaxis and bacterial engulfment in patients with pulmonary edema.[16]

Nearly half of HAP cases are polymicrobial. Early-onset HAP (occurring in the first 4 days of hospitalization) is often caused by community-acquired pathogens such as *Haemophilus influenzae*, *Strep. pneumoniae*, or methicillin-susceptible *Staph. aureus* (MSSA). HAP developing ≥5 days after hospitalization ("late onset") is often caused by aerobic gram-negative bacilli (e.g., *Pseudomonas aeruginosa*, Enterobacteriaceae, or *Acinetobacter*) or methicillin-resistant *Staph. aureus* (MRSA).[17,18] In patients receiving mechanical ventilation, these antibiotic-resistant pathogens assume increasing importance. Other gram-negative rods, such as *Escherichia coli* and *Klebsiella* species, are also common pathogens.[17] Nosocomial viral and fungal infections are uncommon causes of HAP in immunocompetent patients. Ventilator-associated pneumonia (VAP) is a pneumonia that arises more than 48 to 72 h after endotracheal intubation.[14,17] VAP accounts for as much as 83 percent of nosocomial pneumonia and carries a particularly poor prognosis, with a reported mortality rate of up to 50 percent.[19,20]

The diagnosis of HAP is suspected if the hospitalized patient has a radiographic infiltrate that is new or progressive along with clinical findings suggesting infection, which include the new onset of fever, purulent sputum, leukocytosis, and decline in oxygenation. Most studies of nonintubated patients have involved clinical diagnosis with sputum culture.[17] Diagnosis of VAP however, based on this clinical constellation, has been challenged due to poor specificity. A recent metanalysis, showed that the most acceptable standards for the diagnosis of VAP require quantitative cultures of bronchoalveolar lavage (BAL) fluid or protected specimen brush samples.[21] BAL is also recommended if the patient is already receiving antibiotics.

The management of a patient suspected to have hospital- acquired or ventilator-associated pneumonia is summarized in Fig. 3-1. Initial inadequate antimicrobial therapy for HAP is an independent risk factor for increased

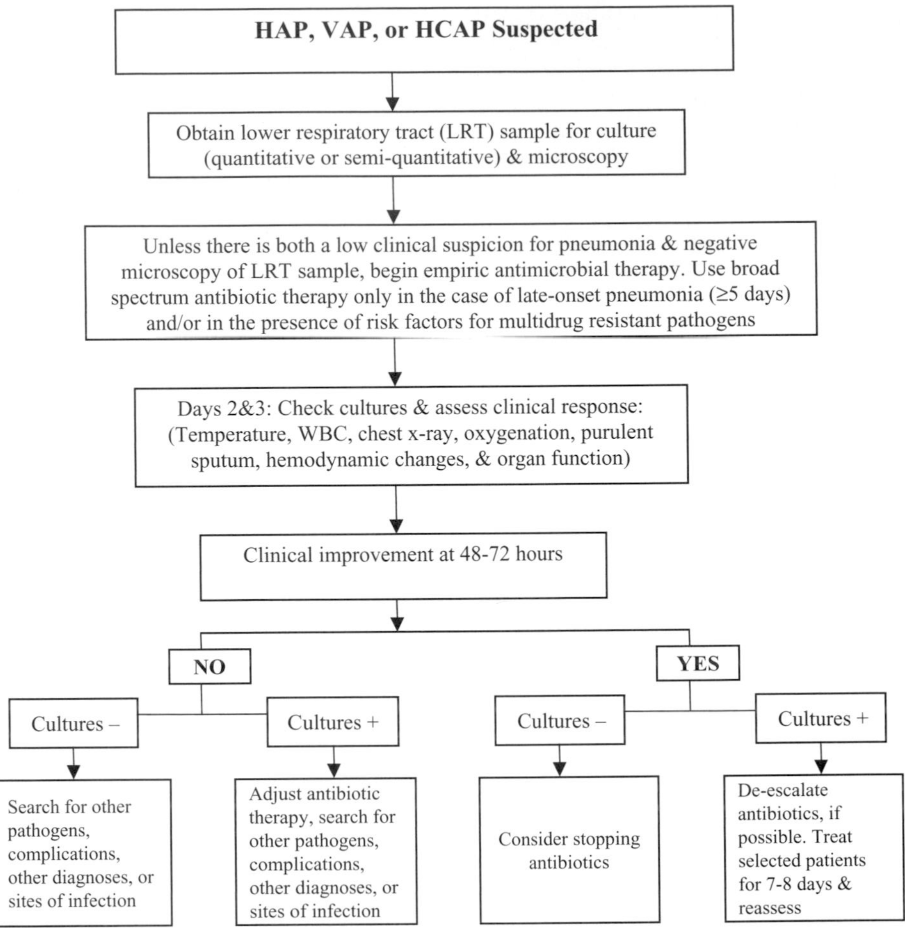

Figure 3-1 Summary of the management strategies for a patient with suspected HAP, VAP, or HCAP. (Modified from American Thoracic Society and Infectious Diseases Society of America, 2005.[17] With permission.)

mortality.[22] Initial therapy (while awaiting results of cultures) must be empiric and cover a broad spectrum of possible pathogens. Demographics, host factors (e.g., severity and acuity of illness, comorbidities), duration of hospitalization, prior antibiotic use, and antimicrobial resistance patterns within the hospital or ICU must be taken into account in selecting antibiotics for empiric treatment. Rates of resistance are influenced by type and size of hospital, ICU or non-ICU setting, anatomic site of isolation, and patterns of prior antibiotic use within individual patients or institutions. Empiric treatment for pneumonia occurring within the first 4 days of hospitalization in patients without severe comorbidities or exposure to antibiotics need not encompass *P. aeruginosa* or potentially resistant pathogens. However, broader-spectrum coverage (to include these pathogens) is advised for critically ill ICU patients requiring prolonged mechanical ventilation or those who have received prior antibiotics.[18] In this context, a combination of antipseudomonal beta-lactam (e.g., cefotetan) plus an aminoglycoside (if no contraindications to aminoglycoside use exist) can be used. Alternatively, a fluoroquinolone can be substituted for the aminoglycoside. Linezolid is an alternative to vancomycin for the treatment of MRSA. Recommended initial antibiotic therapy according to the guidelines from the American Thoracic Society and the Infectious Diseases Society of America, published in 2005, are shown in Tables 3-2 and 3-3.[17] Antibiotic therapy should be tailored appropriately when culture results become available.

Aspiration pneumonia

Aspiration is defined as the inhalation of oropharyngeal or gastric contents into the larynx and lower respiratory tract. Several pulmonary syndromes may occur after aspiration, depending on the amount and nature of the aspirated material, the frequency of aspiration, and the

Table 3-2 Initial empiric antibiotic therapy for hospital-acquired pneumonia or ventilator-associated pneumonia in patients with no known risk factors for multidrug-resistant pathogens, early onset, and any disease severity

Potential pathogen	Recommended antibiotic
Streptococcus pneumoniae[a]	Ceftriaxone
Haemophilus influenzae	*or*
Methicillin-sensitive *Staphylococcus aureus*	Levofloxacin, moxifloxacin, or ciprofloxacin
Antibiotic-sensitive enteric gram-negative bacilli	*or*
	Ampicillin/sulbactam
Escherichia coli	*or*
Klebsiella pneumoniae	ertapenem
Enterobacter species	
Proteus species	
Serratia marcescens	

[a]The frequency of penicillin-resistant *S. pneumoniae* and multidrug-resistant *S. pneumoniae* is increasing; levofloxacin or moxifloxacin is preferred to ciprofloxacin and the role of other new quinolones, such as gatifloxacin, has not been established.
Source: From the American Thoracic Society and Infectious Diseases Society of America, 2005.[17] With permission.

host's response to the aspirated material. Aspiration pneumonitis (Mendelson's syndrome) is a chemical injury caused by the inhalation of sterile gastric contents, whereas aspiration pneumonia is an infectious process caused by the inhalation of oropharyngeal secretions colonized by pathogenic bacteria. Although there is some overlap between these syndromes, they are distinct clinical entities.[23]

Aspiration of oropharyngeal or gastric contents contaminated with colonizing flora is important in the pathogenesis of ventilator-associated pneumonia. Several factors that lead to impairments in level of consciousness and/or swallowing and cough reflexes (e.g., related to cerebrovascular disease) increase the risk for the development of aspiration pneumonia. The oropharynx appears to be the most important source of microorganisms. Continuous aspiration of subglottic secretions has been associated with significant reductions in the incidence of VAP in two randomized trials.[24,25] Supine patient positioning may also facilitate aspiration, which may be decreased by a semirecumbent positioning.[26,27] Enteral nutrition has been considered a risk factor for the development of pneumonia mainly because of an increased risk of aspiration of gastric contents.[14] However, its alternative, parenteral nutrition, is associated with higher risks for infections associated with intravascular devices, complications of line insertions, higher costs, and loss of intestinal villous architecture, which may facilitate enteral microbial translocation.[17] Nasogastric intubation and gastroparesis are other known risk factors for aspiration.

Community-acquired aspiration pneumonia often is associated with anaerobic bacteria alone or aerobic species. However gram-negative bacilli such as *P. aeruginosa* and *Staph. aureus* resistant to beta-lactam and/or methicillin are the most common bacteria involved in hospital-acquired infections. Microbiology of aspiration pneumonia implicating anaerobic bacteria as major pulmonary pathogens were based on studies performed in the 1970s using transtracheal aspiration.[28,29] Some of the most common bacteria were *Bacteroides melaninogenicus, Prevotella melaninogenica, Fusobacterium nucleatum,* and anaerobic streptococci.[30] Recent studies suggest

Table 3-3 Initial empiric therapy for hospital-acquired pneumonia, ventilator-associated pneumonia, and healthcare-associated pneumonia in patients with late-onset disease or risk factors for multidrug-resistant pathogens and all disease severity

Potential pathogens	Combination antibiotic therapy
Pathogens listed in Table 3-2 and MDR pathogens	Antipseudomonal cephalosporin (cefepime, ceftazidime)
Pseudomonas aeruginosa	*or*
Klebsiella pneumoniae (ESBL[+])[a]	Antipseudomonal carbapenem (imipenem or meropenem)
Acinetobacter species[†a]	*or*
	β-Lactam/β-lactamase inhibitor (piperacillin–tazobactam)
	plus
	Antipseudomonal fluoroquinolone[a] (ciprofloxacin or levofloxacin)
	or
	Aminoglycoside (amikacin, gentamicin, or tobramycin)
	plus
Methicillin-resistant *Staphylococcus aureus* (MRSA)	Linezolid or vancomycin[b]
Legionella pneumophila[a]	

[a]If an ESBL[+] strain, such as *K. pneumoniae*, or an *Acinetobacter* species is suspected, a carbepenem is a reliable choice. If *L. pneumophila* is suspected, the combination antibiotic regimen should include a macrolide (e.g., azithromycin) or a fluoroquinolone (e.g., ciprofloxacin or levofloxacin) should be used rather than an aminoglycoside.
[b]If MRSA risk factors are present or there is a high incidence locally.
Source: From the American Thoracic Society and Infectious Diseases Society of America, 2005.[17] With permission.

that although anaerobes are quantitatively important oropharyngeal commensals, these organisms may be less important pulmonary pathogens in patients with VAP and aspiration pneumonia. The bacteriology of these syndromes reflects the fact that aerobic organisms are more likely to colonize patients at the time of aspiration. These results imply that antimicrobial agents with anaerobic coverage may not be necessarily required in the treatment of these patients.[31] The Study Group on Aspiration Pneumonia found that ampicillin plus the beta-lactamase inhibitor sulbactam, when compared to clindamycin with the optional addition of a second- or third-generation cephalosporin, was equally effective in terms of clinical response.[32]

Pneumonia in the immunocompromised host

Pulmonary infections represent the most common complication and one of the main causes of mortality in immunocompromised patients. Clinical management of these infections is complex, since virtually any microorganism may affect any immunocompromised patient at any time in the evolution, mainly depending on the net state of immunosuppression.[33] *Staph. aureus*, particularly methicillin-resistant strains, represents a serious challenge in most hospitals and is a frequent cause of pneumonia in patients receiving chronic glucocorticoid treatment.[34] Occasionally, uncommon opportunistic bacteria such as *Nocardia* may cause pneumonia. Husain et al.[35] reported an incidence of nocardial infection of 2.1 percent in lung transplant recipients. *L. pneumophila* as the causative pathogen of pneumonia is also increased in immunocompromised patients, such as organ transplant recipients or patients with HIV disease, as well as those with diabetes mellitus, underlying lung disease, or end-stage renal disease.[17,36] Pneumonia due to fungi, including *Candida* species and *A. fumigatus*, may occur in organ transplant or immunocompromised, neutropenic patients.[17,37] In fact, the incidence of invasive fungal infections has increased dramatically during the past two decades.

Although cytomegalovirus is still the most common virus affecting immunocompromised patients, recent developments in molecular-based diagnostic tools have shown that respiratory viruses (rhinovirus, adenovirus, influenza, parainfluenza, respiratory syncytial virus) also cause high rates of morbidity and mortality.[38] *Mycobacterium* infections are relatively uncommon in transplant recipients in developed countries; however, the annualized rate of infection is three- to tenfold higher than that of the general population.[39] *Pneumocystis carinii* pneumonia (PCP) is an important cause of morbidity and mortality in immunocompromised patients. PCP is frequently associated with AIDS: however, several groups of non-AIDS immunocompromised patients are also at risk for PCP. These include patients with solid tumors, those undergoing organ transplantation, or patients suffering from inflammatory conditions requiring chronic immunosuppression with corticosteroids or cytotoxic agents such as purine analogues.[40]

Overall, the high associated mortality of pneumonia in immunocompromised patients requires a rapid and sometimes invasive diagnostic approach to try to obtain an etiologic diagnosis allowing the early introduction of specific treatment.

LUNG ABSCESSES

Etiology and pathology

Lung abscess is defined as necrosis of the pulmonary tissue caused by microbial infection and the formation of cavities containing necrotic debris or fluid. The process usually begins as a localized pneumonitis. Liquefaction necrosis of the lung tissue eventually communicates with the bronchial tree. This partial internal drainage results in the classic cavity with an air-fluid level. The formation of multiple small (< 2 cm) abscesses is occasionally referred to as necrotizing pneumonia or lung gangrene. Both lung abscess and necrotizing pneumonia are manifestations of a similar pathologic process.[41]

Aspiration of infectious material is the most frequent etiologic mechanism in the development of primary lung abscess. Poor oral hygiene, dental infections, and gingival disease are common in these patients. Some of the factors that predispose to aspiration include states of compromised consciousness (e.g., cerebrovascular accident, seizure, alcoholism, anesthesia, head trauma, and coma) and esophageal disease (e.g., achalasia, reflux disease, and various causes of esophageal obstruction). Immunocompromised hosts—including patients on various chemotherapies, malnourished patients, and those with multiple trauma—are also at risk. Secondary lung abscess can occur from a hematogenous source; bronchial obstruction by tumor, stricture, or foreign body; or extension from an extrapulmonary site, such as mediastinal, subdiaphragmatic, or hepatic abscesses.[42]

The posterior segment of the right upper lobe and the superior segment of the right lower lobe are the most common locations for lung abscess. This is due to gravitation of the infectious material from the oropharynx into these dependent areas of the lung. Lung abscesses have numerous infectious causes. The dominant pathogens are *Peptostreptococcus*, *Bacteroides*, *Prevotella*, and *Fusobacterium* species.[43,44] A primary lung abscess may be caused by *Strep. pneumoniae*, *Strep. viridans*, *K. pneumoniae*, and *H. influenzae*. Selected nonbacterial pathogens that can produce lung abscess include parasites (e.g., *Entamoeba histolytica*), many fungi (e.g., *Aspergillus* species, *Histoplasma capsulatum*), and mycobacteria. A number of opportunistic infections, such as nocardiosis and aspergillosis, can dominate in lung abscess in immunocompromised hosts.

One unique mechanism for the development of lung abscesses occurs in Lemierre's syndrome, or jugular vein suppurative thrombophlebitis.[45] This infection begins in the pharynx (sometimes with an overt tonsillar or peritonsillar abscess) but spreads to involve spaces in the neck and the carotid sheath, which contains the internal jugular vein. Bacteremia, due to *Fusobacterium necrophorum*, and septic emboli to the lungs, which subsequently cavitate, are all characteristic complications of this process once the vessels are involved. Tricuspid valve endocarditis, usually due to *Staph. aureus*, also typically causes septic emboli that are widely distributed in both lungs.[46] This is a common feature of endocarditis complicating injection drug use and an infrequent complication of septic venous thrombosis in other settings.

Clinical presentation

Most of these patients present with a subacute onset of illness and do not seek medical attention for 2 weeks or more after the onset of illness. Early symptoms are often those of pneumonia—that is, malaise, anorexia, sputum-producing cough, sweats, and fever. Initially, foul sputum is not observed in the course of the infection; however, after cavitation occurs, putrid expectorations are quite prevalent. The odor of the breath and sputum of a patient with an anaerobic lung abscess is often quite pronounced and noxious and may provide a clue to the diagnosis.[41] Hemoptysis may occasionally follow the expectoration of the putrid sputum. The sputum may contain gangrenous lung tissue. Chest pain, if present, usually indicates pleural involvement.

On physical examination, a small area of dullness, indicating localized pneumonic consolidation, is found, and usually suppressed (rather than bronchial) breath sounds. Fine or medium moist crackles may be present. If the cavity is large, there may be tympany and amphoric breath sounds. Signs of pulmonary suppuration generally disappear with appropriate antibiotic therapy, but this disappearance does not necessarily denote cure. If the abscess becomes chronic, weight loss, anemia, and hypertrophic pulmonary osteoarthropathy may occur. Physical examination of the chest may be negative in the chronic phase, but rales and rhonchi are usually present.

Diagnosis

The diagnosis of a typical lung abscess can be suspected based on history and physical examination findings. Obvious oral cavity disease or predisposition to aspiration, which are the two most important factors in the development of anaerobic lung infection, should be sought. Sputum should be examined by smear and culture for bacteria, fungi, and mycobacteria. The sputum Gram's stain often shows numerous polymorphonuclear leukocytes along with a mixture of bacteria, some of which are contaminants of oral flora. When a single predominant organism is cultured, it is accepted to be the pathogen. Empyema fluid, if accessible, provides an excellent medium. Occasionally, particularly with metastatic lung abscesses, blood culture findings may be positive. Most patients never have appropriate specimens obtained for culture; they are treated empirically and do well despite the lack of exact microbiologic culture results.

Chest x-rays early in the course may show a segmental or lobar consolidation, which sometimes becomes globular as pus distends it. The distinctive characteristic of lung abscess, the air-fluid level, can be observed only on a chest x-ray film taken with the patient upright or in the lateral decubitus position (Fig. 3-2). In the presence of associated pleural thickening, atelectasis, or pneumothorax, the air-fluid level may be obscured. A computed tomography (CT) scan of the chest is valuable for better anatomic interpretation. It can demonstrate cavitation within an area of consolidation, the thickness and regularity of the abscess wall, and the exact position of the abscess with regard to the chest wall and bronchus.[47]

The indications and comparative benefits of invasive procedures such as transtracheal aspirates, transthoracic aspirates, and fiberoptic bronchoscopy are controversial and depend to a great extent on operator ability. The use of these methods to obtain appropriate culture specimens should be strongly considered in patients who do not respond to medical therapy within 2 weeks. However, dependable microbiologic data can be obtained only if these procedures are performed prior to the institution of antibiotic therapy. Most pulmonologists believe that these diagnostic procedures should not be performed routinely in all patients but should be reserved for patients with atypical presentations or unclear diagnoses. Bronchoscopy may also be used to exclude the presence of a foreign body or neoplasm and can provide drainage. These invasive procedures should be avoided in patients with coagulation disorders or bleeding tendencies and in those for whom it is difficult to provide adequate oxygenation.

Lesions that simulate bacterial lung abscess include cavitating bronchogenic carcinoma, bronchiectasis, empyema secondary to a bronchopleural fistula, tuberculosis, coccidioidomycosis and other mycotic lung infections, infected pulmonary bullae or air cysts, pulmonary sequestration, silicotic nodules with central necrosis, subphrenic or hepatic (amebic or hydatid) abscesses with perforation into a bronchus, and Wegener's granulomatosis. Detailed history, repeated clinical evaluation, and the procedures described above can usually differentiate these disorders from simple lung abscess.

Medical treatment

Appropriate use of antibiotics determines morbidity and mortality in patients with lung abscess. Clindamycin is

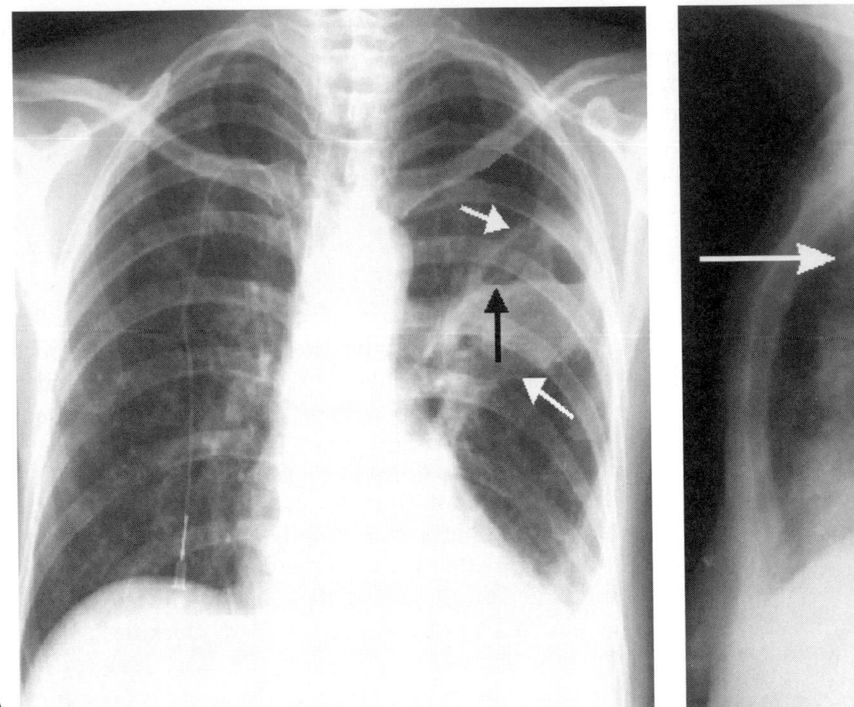

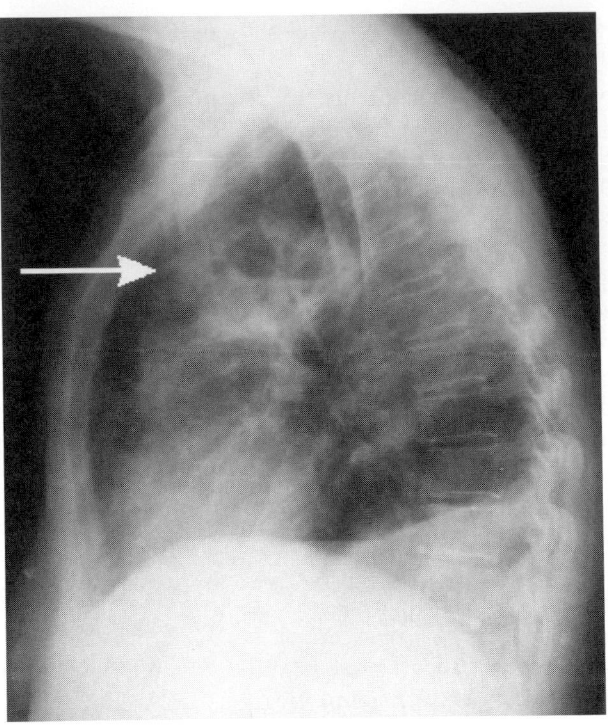

Figure 3-2 Posteroanterior and lateral chest x-ray views of a patient with lung abscess. A well-defined area of increased transparency can be seen in the left upper lobe (white arrow). More than half of the cavity is filled with fluid and air (black arrow).

currently the first choice for the treatment of anaerobic infections; penicillin is a less favored alternative.[48] The Study Group on Aspiration Pneumonia[32] also included patients with primary abscesses and found that ampicillin plus the beta-lactamase inhibitor sulbactam, as opposed to clindamycin, with the optional addition of a second- or third-generation cephalosporin, was equally effective in terms of clinical response. For gram-negative organisms as well as *Pseudomonas*, aminoglycosides and quinolones or cephalosporins can be used. Nafcillin or oxacillin or cephalexin are recommended as first-line agents for gram-positive organisms. The supportive treatment should include chest physiotherapy with postural drainage as well as nutritional support. Serial radiographs have limited use in the evaluation of response to therapy because there is often initial roentgenographic progression even in patients with a good clinical response.[49]

Surgical treatment

The availability of effective antibiotic therapy for primary lung abscess has drastically modified the natural history of the disease and diminished the role of surgery. Operative indications are less frequent in current practice, and these procedures are undertaken electively for chronic illnesses only after medical therapy has been unsuccessful. Prior to any surgical intervention, major considerations in patients with a delayed medical response include:

- An associated condition that precludes response, such as obstruction with a foreign body or neoplasm
- Erroneous microbial diagnosis with infection due to bacteria, mycobacteria, or fungi that have not have been suspected and are not being treated
- Large cavity size (usually > 6 cm in diameter) that may require prolonged therapy or empyema, which necessitates drainage
- An alternative, nonbacterial cause of cavitary lung disease, such as cavitating neoplasm, vasculitis, or pulmonary sequestration
- Other causes of persistent fever, such as drug fever or *Clostridium difficile*–associated colitis

External drainage

Indications for drainage include ongoing sepsis despite adequate antimicrobial therapy, progressively enlarging lung abscess in imminent danger of rupture, failure to wean from mechanical ventilation, and contamination of the opposite lung. These can occur when the abscess does not drain internally. In current practice, due to advances in interventional radiology, most of these lung abscesses are drained percutaneously under CT, ultrasound, or fluoroscopic guidance with acceptable success rates and morbidity.[50,51] This approach may be problematic in patients with coagulopathies if a significant amount of lung tissue must be traversed and other anatomic structures do not allow for unimpeded access to the cavity; another difficulty is posed by the presence of material within the abscess that cannot be effectively evacuated through a drainage tube. Additionally, there is always a concern for soiling the pleural space with abscess contents.[52] Direct tube drainage may be indicated in severely ill patients with large abscesses. Safe and effective pneumonostomy or cavernostomy with direct drainage (Monaldi procedure) depends on accurate topical localization of the abscess and a high degree of certainty that the underlying lung is firmly adherent to the overlying parietal pleura. But these measures have largely been replaced by percutaneous radiologic techniques.

Endoscopic drainage of lung abscesses has also been reported with acceptable outcomes.[53] The procedure is performed by placing a pigtail catheter into the abscess cavity under bronchoscopic visualization and leaving the catheter in place until the cavity has drained. It can be considered in selected patients who have an airway connection to the abscess or in whom an endobronchial obstruction that prevents drainage is present. It does not carry the risk of soiling the pleural space. Endobronchial spillage of abscess contents may be a concern in performing this intervention. The procedure should be performed only by an experienced operator. A case has also been reported using the video-assisted thoracoscopic (VATS) approach.[54]

Surgical resection

Surgical resection is now required in less than 10 percent of cases of lung abscess.[55] Indications for surgical intervention include unsuccessful medical management over a period of 8 weeks; complications such as bronchopleural fistula, empyema, massive or significant recurrent hemoptysis, and the persistence of a cavity larger than 6 cm after 8 weeks of treatment; necrotizing infection associated with multiple abscesses; and rupture into the pleural cavity with pyopneumothorax. Surgical intervention may also be indicated when there is a strong suspicion of carcinoma. Intraoperatively, the patient will require double-lumen intubation or a bronchial blocker to help prevent spillage of pus into the contralateral lung, and rigid bronchoscopy may be indicated. Careful dissection and meticulous hemostasis are very important because of the adhesions and distorted anatomy caused by the abscess. Suction decompression of large cavities prior to dissection is usually helpful. Lobectomy is typically required, as segmentectomy may be inadequate and pneumonectomy is rarely necessary. The surgeon must be skilled in resecting the abscess and in rapid clamping of the bronchus to prevent spillage into the trachea. Complete resection of involved areas as well as placement of two large-caliber tubes will help to speed recovery, prevent recurrence, and avoid the development of empyema.

BRONCHIECTASIS

Etiology and pathology

Bronchiectasis is an abnormal dilation (*ektasis* is the Greek word for dilatation) of the proximal medium-sized bronchi (> 2 mm in diameter) caused by destruction of the muscular and elastic components of the bronchial walls. It can be congenital or acquired. Acquired forms require an infectious insult, impairment of drainage, airway obstruction, and/or a defect in host defense and usually affect adults and older children. This results in damage to the muscular and elastic components of the bronchial wall both from the inciting infectious agent and from the host response. The congenital form is seen in infants and children and is due to developmental arrest of the bronchial tree. Causes include cystic fibrosis, Kartagener's syndrome, congenital deficiency of bronchial cartilage, bronchopulmonary sequestration, and various immunodeficiency disorders such as selective immunoglobulin A (IgA) and IgG deficiency, chronic granulomatous disease of childhood, and alpha$_1$-antitrypsin deficiency.[55]

Regardless of the etiology, there is abnormal bronchial dilatation with bronchial wall destruction and transmural inflammation as well as enhanced cellular and mediator responses.[56] This leads to a vicious cycle of bronchial damage, bronchial dilatation, impaired clearance of secretions, recurrent infection, and more bronchial damage. Impaired clearance of secretions causes colonization and infection with pathogenic organisms, contributing to the common purulent expectoration observed in patients with bronchiectasis. The disease typically involves the basal segments of the lower lobes and is bilateral in about 30 to 50 percent of patients. Possible offending organisms include *H. influenzae*, *Klebsiella* species, *Staph. aureus*, *M. tuberculosis*, *M. pneumoniae*, nontuberculous mycobacteria, measles, pertussis, influenza, herpes simplex, and certain types of adenovirus. Patients even with noncystic fibrotic bronchiectasis often develop chronic bronchial infection with *P. aeruginosa*. *Mycobacterium avium complex* (MAC) deserves special mention for its propensity to occur in the setting of HIV and in the host who is immunocompetent. MAC has been observed especially in women who are nonsmokers, are above 50 years of age, and have a consistent history, positive acid-fast bacilli on sputum smear, and a CT scan with small regular nodules and findings of bronchiectasis.[57]

There are three types of bronchiectasis: cylindrical (tubular, fusiform), varicose (traction), and cystic (saccular). Cylindrical bronchiectasis involves diffuse mucosal edema, with resultant bronchi that are dilated minimally but have straight, regular outlines that end squarely and abruptly. Cystic or saccular bronchiectasis has ulceration with bronchial neovascularization and a resultant ballooned appearance, which may have air-fluid levels. Varicose bronchiectasis has a bulbous appearance with a dilated bronchus and interspersed sites of relative constriction and, potentially, obstructive scarring. The latter may subsequently result in postobstructive pneumonitis and additional parenchymal damage.

Clinical presentation

Bronchiectasis can present in either of two forms: a local or focal obstructive process of a lobe or segment of a lung or a diffuse process involving much of both lungs and often accompanied by other sinopulmonary diseases, such as sinusitis and asthma.[56] Most reports of diffuse bronchiectasis and associated systemic conditions—such as inflammatory bowel disease, rheumatoid arthritis, and connective tissue diseases—are case reports.[58] Bronchiectasis is a morphologic diagnosis and may exist with relatively few symptoms. The most frequent clinical characteristics are repeated episodes of respiratory tract infections. There is usually a history of cough and daily mucopurulent, tenacious sputum production lasting months to years. Bronchiectasis should especially be suspected if the patient who presents with these complaints has no history of smoking. Other less specific symptoms include dyspnea, pleuritic chest pain, wheezing, fever, weakness, and weight loss. Hemoptysis occurs in about 50 percent of adults but is not usually severe and is rare in children. It is noteworthy that the systemic vessels, namely the bronchial arteries, are the sources of bleeding, which may pose a problem in controlling the bleeding.

Diagnosis

Diagnosis should always start with a thorough history and physical examination. Findings on physical examination are nonspecific and may include crackles, rhonchi, wheezing, and inspiratory squeaks on auscultation. General signs such as digital clubbing, cyanosis, plethora, wasting, and weight loss indicate the chronic nature of the disease. Nasal polyps and signs of chronic sinusitis may also be present. In advanced disease, the physical stigmata of cor pulmonale may be observed. Chest x-ray findings that are suggestive but not diagnostic of bronchiectasis include peribronchial thickening, volume loss and bronchial crowding, atelectasis, and persistent infiltrates. High-resolution CT scan of the chest has largely replaced bronchography for imaging diagnosis and is currently the modality of choice. The appropriate high-resolution CT study is a noncontrast study with the use of a 1.0- to 1.5-mm window every 1 cm and acquisition times of 1 s, reconstructed with the use of a high-spatial-frequency algorithm during full inspiration.[59,60] The detailed images demonstrate bronchial dilatation, peribronchial inflammation, and parenchymal disease (Fig. 3-3). In patients with abnormal, dilated bronchi, the involved airways often appear much larger than the adjacent pulmonary artery branch on cross section; this finding is referred to as the "signet-ring" sign (i.e., the internal bronchial diameter is larger than that of the adjacent pulmonary artery).[59]

Bronchoscopy can help localize the process, rule out obstructing lesions, and provide pulmonary toilet and culture samples. Some typical findings may include reddened, edematous mucosa and pitting of the mucosa due to dilatation of the ostia of the bronchus. Pus may be seen extruding from involved bronchial orifices. A ventilation/perfusion (V/Q) scan can be obtained to determine the hemodynamic features (perfused vs. nonperfused areas) of bronchiectasis, especially when surgical resection is being considered.[61]

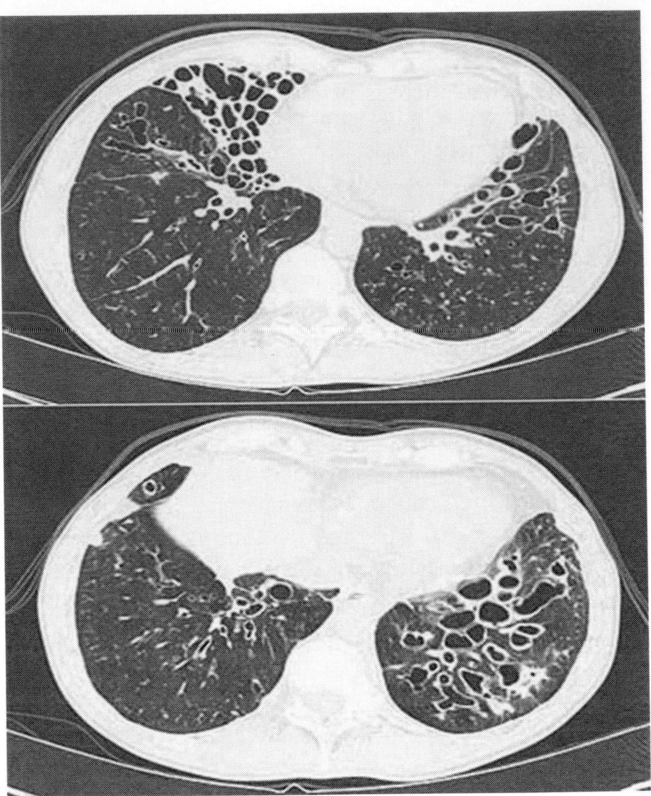

Figure 3-3 Chest CT of a patient with bronchiectasis. There are multiple dilated bronchi in the middle lobe, lingual area, and left lower lobe.

Medical treatment

Medical therapy is the primary approach and should provide appropriate antibiotic therapy, postural drainage, humidifiers, and bronchodilators as indicated, with the goal of prevention and control of exacerbations. Early antibiotic therapy for suspected exacerbations would probably limit the vicious cycle. Reasonable first choices for such therapy include a fluoroquinolone such as levofloxacin or ciprofloxacin.[62] Bronchodilators may help by presumably reversing bronchospasm associated with airway hyperreactivity and improving mucociliary clearance. Bronchoscopy with thorough suctioning of the tracheobronchial tree and irrigation with normal saline usually provides significant symptomatic relief.

Surgical treatment

The role of pulmonary resection has evolved from early curative resections for all patients to a more palliative approach limited to those with medically refractory disease or those who have complications. Surgical intervention is indicated when there is persistent recurrent infection following discontinuation of medication, in cases of massive hemoptysis, and where removal of a foreign body or tumor is indicated. Surgery may also be considered in MAC and *Aspergillus* infections. The ideal surgical candidate has unilateral, segmental, or lobar distribution of the disease and if removal of most diseased portions of the lung is feasible and will prevent recurrence. Some groups extend surgical resection to bilaterally localized bronchiectasis or complete lung destruction in the absence of other diseased areas as well as to patients with good respiratory performance.[63] The primary aim should be to perform a complete resection whenever possible for the optimal control of symptoms. This can be guided by the findings on high resolution CT scan of the chest. A V/Q scan is helpful when there are doubtful morphologic areas of bronchiectasis and there is a question regarding the need and extent of surgical resection.[63] A report of 134 patients from the Mayo clinic[64] who underwent surgical resection for bronchiectasis, showed operative mortality of 2.2 percent and the morbidity rate was 24.6 percent. About 88 percent of the patients experienced resolution or improvement of their symptoms. Similar findings were more recently reported by Balkanli et al.[65] on 238 patients who had surgery for bronchiectasis over a 10 year period. There was no operative mortality and the symptoms were resolved in 80 percent of patients. Both studies demonstrated that significantly better results were obtained in patients who had undergone a complete resection.

Preoperatively, toilet bronchoscopy should be routinely performed. For the patient with hemoptysis, one of the options to control bleeding is bronchial arterial embolization, especially if the patient is not a surgical candidate. Transplantation is indicated for diffuse cystic disease with seriously compromised pulmonary function and chronic respiratory failure.[66,67]

ACTINOMYCOTIC INFECTIONS

Owing to the presence of branching hyphae, infections due to actinomycosis and nocardiosis may be mistaken for fungal infections. It is important to make the distinction because actinomycotic infections do not respond to antifungal therapy but rather antibiotics.

ACTINOMYCOSIS

Etiology and pathology

Actinomycosis is a relatively uncommon subacute-to-chronic disease characterized by the production of suppurative abscesses or granulomas that eventually develop draining sinuses and dense scarring. These lesions discharge pus containing the organisms, which are filamentous, gram-positive, anaerobic-to-microaerophilic bacteria that are not acid fast. The branching form of the bacterium allows it to be recognized by the presence of "sulfur granules," or masses of hyphae, in the pus. In humans, actinomycosis is usually caused by *Actinomyces israelii*, which is a commensal in the normal human oropharyngeal flora that hides in the "nooks and crannies," particularly if there is poor dental hygiene. Areas of clinical manifestations of actinomycosis include cervicofacial, thoracic, and abdominal sites. Cervicofacial is the most common, comprising up to 50 percent of reported cases.[68] Infections in the soft tissues of the mouth and throat can manifest themselves as submandibular masses with chronic draining sinuses. The infection can spread by direct extension from the neck across fascial planes into the mediastinum. Interestingly, there does not seem to be any greater incidence of the disease in patients who are immunocompromised, including those with HIV, patients who have undergone organ transplantation, or those on steroids.[69] Lung infection can result from dental surgery or aspiration and after trauma, including introduction of the organism from esophageal perforation. Hematogenous spread from distant lesions is also possible and can infect preexisting cavitary disease in the lung.

Clinical presentation

Thoracic actinomycosis commonly presents as a pulmonary infiltrate or mass which, if left untreated, can spread to involve the pleura, pericardium, and chest wall with rib osteomyelitis. The patient may have any combination of the nonspecific symptoms, such as fever, dry or productive cough, blood-streaked sputum, shortness of breath, chest pain, weight loss, fatigue, and anorexia. Physical examination may reveal abnormal breath sounds. The presence of sinus tracts with drainage from the chest wall (i.e., pleurocutaneous fistula) should raise very high clinical suspicion.

Diagnosis

Definite diagnosis can be made by histopathologic examination and anaerobic culture of material from draining sinuses and abscesses. The "sulfur granules" are practically pathognomonic; they are approximately 1 mm in diameter and can be seen by the naked eye as yellowish particles. Microscopically, they are composed of branching filamentous rods that stain positive on Gram's stain (Fig. 3-4). On chest x-ray, the presence of a mass-like lesion that extends across fissures or pleura, invades into the adjacent chest wall or thoracic vertebrae, or causes local destruction of the ribs or sternum suggests thoracic actinomycosis. CT scans usually reveal an infiltrative mass with focal areas of decreased attenuation that enhance with contrast. This infiltrative mass has a tendency to invade surrounding tissues, and lymphadenopathy is uncommon.

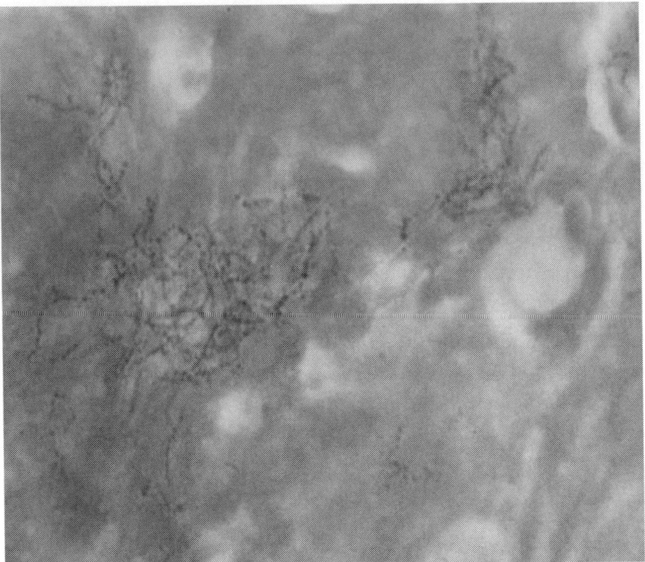

Figure 3-4 Characteristic actinomycetic granules.

Medical treatment

High-dose penicillin, administered over a prolonged period, is the cornerstone of therapy for actinomycosis. Prolonged treatment is necessary owing to the presence of surrounding dense fibrous tissues. Lack of a clinical response from a patient receiving penicillin therapy may also indicate the presence of resistant companion bacteria, which may require modification of the antibiotic regimen.

Surgical treatment

Surgical intervention may be implemented for drainage of an abscess or empyema and for radical excision of sinus tracts when feasible. Since the varieties of lung involvement are nonspecific, some of the presentations may suggest a tumor. Thus, the most common indication for surgery is exploratory thoracotomy to rule out carcinoma.[70] Rarely, actinomycosis may be complicated by an unusual but significant hemoptysis—another indication for surgery[71]—although selective bronchial artery embolization is a viable option in this setting.[72] Even if histology suggests complete resection, it must still be followed by prolonged antibiotic therapy, as surgery alone is usually not curative. Inadequate antibiotic therapy postoperatively may result in complications such as bronchopleural fistulas and empyema.[73]

NOCARDIOSIS

Etiology and pathology

Nocardiosis is an acute, subacute, or chronic suppurative infection caused by weakly gram-positive, filamentous bacteria found worldwide in soils. *Nocardia asteroides* (80 percent) and *Nocardia brasiliensis* are the principal causes of human disease. *Nocardia farcinica* is being recognized with increasing frequency. The disease has a pronounced tendency toward remission and exacerbation, and infections are localized or disseminated. Localized infection usually manifests itself as primary cutaneous or, rarely, lymphocutaneous disease. Nocardiosis is an opportunistic infection, and disseminated or fulminant disease mainly occurs in immunocompromised hosts with underlying illnesses such as chronic granulomatous disease and HIV infection as well as patients on immunosuppressive therapy.[74] Lung transplant recipients have a particularly high incidence.[35] Inhalation of the free-living organism is the likely route of infection. Introduction of *N. asteroides* via the respiratory tract results in pulmonary lesions, most often manifest as multiple abscesses. *Nocardia* abscesses are characteristically confluent, with little evidence of encapsulation, which probably accounts for the ready dissemination from the initial pulmonary focus. This organism also evades the host's bactericidal mechanisms. The primary disease, which occurs in the pulmonary system, may mimic tuberculous, staphylococcal, or mycotic infection. Hematogenous dissemination to the brain, kidneys, and liver are the most common metastatic sites.[75]

Clinical presentation

Symptoms in patients with nocardiosis are indistinguishable from those in patients with similar pulmonary infections of other microbial etiology. Cough with sputum production and fever are the dominant symptoms. Subcutaneous abscesses and draining sinuses near the chest wall that contain sulfur granules, similar to those observed in actinomycosis, are characteristic.[75] Lung examination may reveal diffuse or localized abnormal breath sounds.

Diagnosis

The diagnosis of nocardiosis is established by aerobic culture of the causative organism from the site(s) of infection. Because *Nocardia* organisms grow more slowly than common bacteria, the microbiology laboratory should always be notified when nocardiosis is clinically suspected, especially if sputum is submitted. Bronchial brushings or percutaneous transthoracic needle aspiration biopsy of the lung may help to obtain appropriate samples and avoid the need for thoracotomy. *Nocardia* organisms are not demonstrated with routine hematoxylin and eosin (H&E) stain and may be seen only by a careful search of sections stained with Gram's, *Gomori methenamine silver* (GMS) or acid-fast bacillus stain.[75]

Possible findings on chest x-ray and/or CT scan include irregular nodules (which may cavitate), reticulonodular or diffuse alveolar pulmonary infiltrates, lung abscess formation, and pleural effusion. All patients with pulmonary nocardiosis should have brain imaging by either CT scan or magnetic resonance imaging (MRI).[75]

Medical treatment

A high index of suspicion, followed by aggressive diagnosis and treatment, is necessary for optimal results; otherwise nocardiosis is associated with a high mortality rate. Sulfonamides are first-line antimicrobial therapy and sulfadiazine is generally preferred because of its central nervous system (CNS) and CSF penetration. The combination of trimethoprim/sulfamethoxazole (TMP/SMX) or minocycline in high doses are acceptable alternatives. Treatment for a minimum of 2 to 3 months is recommended; treatment for as long as 12 months may be necessary, especially for systemic disease. Prophylactic TMP/SMX should be considered in transplant centers with excess rates of nocardial infection.[76]

Surgical treatment

Surgical intervention may be required for the drainage of lung abscess or empyema or when the diagnosis of a lung lesion is unclear. Pulmonary resection for previously diagnosed *Nocardia* infection is rarely indicated.

MYCOTIC THORACIC INFECTIONS

HISTOPLASMOSIS

Etiology and pathology

Pulmonary manifestations are the hallmark of histoplasmosis, as this, also known as Darling's disease, is probably the most common of all fungal infections of the lungs. Clinical syndromes range from asymptomatic infection to diffuse alveolar disease causing respiratory difficulty and occasionally death. *H. capsulatum* is a dimorphic fungus that remains in a mycelial form at ambient temperatures and grows as yeast at body temperature in mammals. Although the fungus can be found in temperate climates throughout the world, it is endemic to the Ohio, Missouri, and Mississippi River valleys in the United States. Farmers, construction workers, and people who enjoy outdoor activities are the most at risk. The disease results from aerosolization of conidial and mycelial fragments from contaminated soil due to the excreta of chickens, pigeons, and bats, which are then deposited in the alveoli. Conversion from the mycelial to the pathogenic yeast form occurs intracellularly. The host defense includes the fungistatic properties of neutrophils and macrophages. T-lymphocytes are crucial in limiting the extent of infection. Susceptibility to dissemination is increased markedly with impaired cellular host defenses.

Clinical presentation

There is a wide spectrum of pulmonary histoplasmosis syndromes. The extent of disease and mode of presentation following initial exposure correlates with the size of the inoculum that was inhaled and the *Histoplasma*-specific immunity of the exposed subject. Thus the major clinical manifestations are asymptomatic infection, acute and subacute pulmonary histoplasmosis, chronic pulmonary histoplasmosis, and disseminated disease. Pulmonary auscultation reveals nonspecific rales, wheezes, or findings consistent with the extent of underlying pneumonitis, consolidation, or cavitation.

Asymptomatic infection

Approximately 85 to 90 percent of infected immunocompetent individuals are asymptomatic. As the cell-mediated host immunity matures, delayed-type hypersensitivity to histoplasmal antigens occurs (3 to 6 weeks after exposure). The skin antigen test for *Histoplasma* species turns positive. Over weeks to months, the inflammatory response produces calcified fibrinous granulomas with areas of caseous necrosis. Histoplasmin skin test reagents are no longer commercially available. Most asymptomatic cases are now identified by the incidental finding of enlarged mediastinal or hilar lymph nodes or pulmonary nodules seen on radiographs or CT scans obtained for the evaluation of other conditions. Perhaps the main significance of such findings is the need to differentiate them from malignancy (Fig. 3-5). The approach to the evaluation of patients with solitary pulmonary nodules has been nicely reviewed recently by Ost and colleagues.[77]

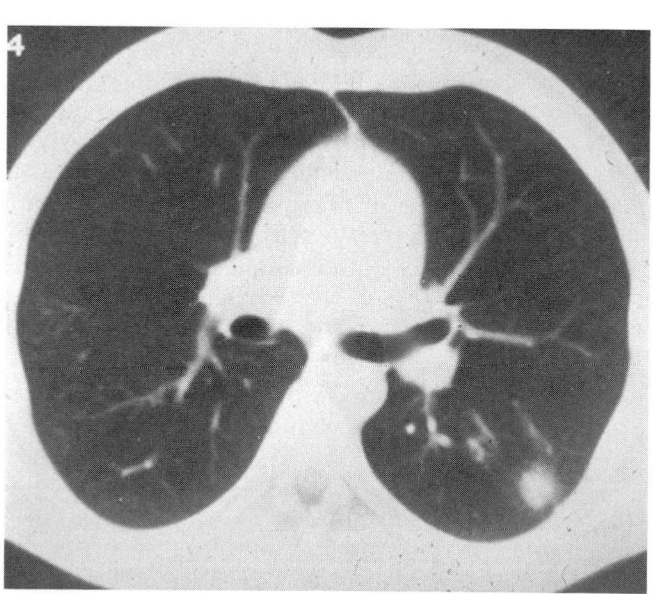

Figure 3-5 Single pulmonary nodule in a patient with histoplasmosis.

Acute and subacute pulmonary histoplasmosis

Following the more typical, low-level exposure, pulmonary illness is more commonly subacute and mild. If the host inhales a large amount of inoculum, an inflammatory response in the lung and adjacent lymph nodes results, similar to the Ghon complex of pulmonary tuberculosis.[78] This can be due to primary infection or reinfection. Nonimmune subjects usually present within 2 weeks with respiratory symptoms and diffuse pulmonary involvement radiographically. Fever, headache, malaise, myalgia, abdominal pain, and chills are common symptoms. Enlarged hilar and mediastinal lymph nodes (mediastinal lymphadenitis) are present in 5 to 10 percent of patients. Mediastinal histoplasmosis results in fibrosing mediastinitis, which can cause symptoms of compression and is the most frequent benign etiology of superior vena cava (SVC) obstruction. Significant obstruction of venous drainage may contribute to cerebral symptoms of headache, visual distortion, tinnitus, and altered consciousness. Cough, hemoptysis, dyspnea, and/or chest pain may be present; these are related to the degree of compression imposed on the pulmonary airway and circulation. Rarely, compression of the esophagus occurs, which causes dysphagia.

Chronic pulmonary histoplasmosis

This form occurs mostly in middle-aged men with underlying pulmonary disease [e.g., chronic obstructive pulmonary disease (COPD)]; it is rare in children and represents 10 percent of symptomatic cases. Chronic pulmonary histoplasmosis (CPH) resembles reactivation tuberculosis, which is a common misdiagnosis. It is associated with cough, dyspnea, chest pain, weight loss, fevers, malaise, and night sweats. The clinical course of untreated CPH is progressive, with spread to contiguous lung. Complications, such as hemoptysis and bronchopleural fistulas, may ensue. Other infections can coexist, such as mycobacterial and other fungal infections (e.g., aspergillosis). Concurrent neoplasia is not uncommon.

Radiographs typically show changes of emphysema. Airspace opacities are present and may surround preexisting bullae, producing the appearance of cavitation with air-fluid levels. In severe cases the lung disease may progress and produce diffuse confluent airspace disease. As the patient recovers, the opacities on chest x-ray become more defined and nodular in appearance. The disease is almost always in the upper lobes and may be bilateral or unilateral in distribution. The inflammatory process progressively destroys lung tissue and retracts the hilar structures upward as a consequence of the loss of lung volume. Pleural thickening adjacent to the lung disease is often present. Untreated cases may lead to progressive pulmonary fibrosis, which may result in respiratory and cardiac failure and recurrent infections. Calcified mediastinal lymph nodes or pulmonary granulomas suggest that the process had been present for several years by the time of diagnosis or that the manifestation resulted from reinfection in patients with calcifications due to prior histoplasmosis.[78]

Progressive disseminated histoplasmosis

This form occurs mostly in hosts who are immunocompromised and probably results from a failure to develop protective cellular immunity following the acute infection. Symptoms vary depending on duration of illness. The acute form may produce fever, worsening cough, weight loss, malaise, and dyspnea. The subacute form is associated with a wide spectrum of symptoms that may occur as a result of dissemination and subacute expression in the affected organs. The chronic form is associated with constitutional symptoms. Evidence for dissemination includes hepatosplenomegaly, extrapulmonary lymphadenopathy, mucosal or skin lesions, anemia, leukopenia, thrombocytopenia, or hepatic enzyme elevation. Furthermore, gastrointestinal involvement may produce diarrhea and abdominal pain. Cardiac involvement resulting in valvular disease, cardiac insufficiency, or vegetations may produce dyspnea, peripheral edema, angina, and fever. CNS involvement may produce headache, visual and gait disturbances, confusion, seizures, altered consciousness, and neck stiffness or pain. Note that subacute progressive disseminated histoplasmosis results in adrenal infection in 80 percent of patients. Radiographically, localized, cavitary, or miliary infiltrates as well as mediastinal lymphadenopathy may be present. The presence of calcified lymph nodes and lung granulomas suggests that disseminated disease has resulted from reinfection. In chronic progressive disseminated histoplasmosis, chest radiography findings usually do not reveal any active pulmonary disease. Diffuse nodular opacities can be seen on CT scan (Fig. 3-6).

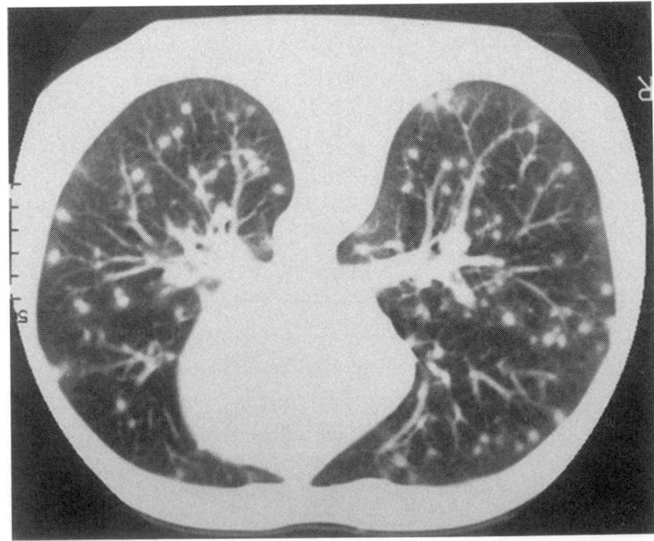

Figure 3-6 Chest CT in progressive histoplasmosis, showing diffuse pulmonary nodules.

Diagnosis

Histoplasmin skin testing is not recommended for diagnostic purposes because of the high rate of positive reactions in endemic areas and the wide variability of response. The sensitivity of laboratory tests for the diagnosis of pulmonary histoplasmosis ranges from 25 percent in patients with subacute illnesses and local manifestations following low inoculum exposure to 75 percent or more in those with acute illnesses and diffuse infiltrates who present within the first month following heavy exposure. *H. capsulatum* can be recovered from sputum, bronchoalveolar lavage (BAL) fluid, lesions, blood, or bone marrow on routine fungal cultures; but the organism grows slowly and plates must be kept up to 12 weeks. The combination of blood and bone marrow cultures increases the likelihood of positive results. In chronic or severe acute pulmonary disease, organisms can be cultured from sputum or bronchial washings. Multiple specimens increase yield. Antibody testing can be performed using immunodiffusion, complement fixation, and radioimmunoassay in increasing order of sensitivity.

Antibody levels peak 6 weeks following exposure and decline over a 2- to 5-year period. Antigen testing can also be performed with the radioimmunoassay. Antigen detection in serum and urine is useful in immunocompromised individuals, whose ability to produce antibodies may be impaired. Cross-reactivity with antigens from *Blastomyces dermatitidis* and *Coccidioides immitis* may cause a false-positive test result. Urine specimens have higher sensitivity, up to 90 percent for disseminated disease. Paired urine and serum specimens have the highest yield. A newer enzyme-linked immunosorbent assay (ELISA) using a specific monoclonal antibody has been developed; its sensitivity varies with disease presentation. Note that some patients with acute histoplasmosis may have high serum levels of angiotensin-converting enzyme. This may cause a diagnostic confusion with sarcoidosis, especially if the patient also has hilar adenopathy.

Tissue may have to be obtained from pulmonary lesions and lymph nodes by bronchoscopy, percutaneous needle biopsies, or rarely, thoracoscopy in order to make the diagnosis. Histologic findings in pulmonary histoplasmosis demonstrate a predominantly mononuclear infiltrate. Multiple caseating granulomas are characteristic, with multinucleated giant cells and possible peripheral fibrosis and central calcification. On H&E staining, the yeast form of *H. capsulatum* has a false capsule. Special stains, such as Gomori methenamine silver (GMS) or periodic acid–Schiff (PAS), may reveal budding yeast, but the organisms can be mistaken for *P. carinii* and other fungal organisms. In chronic pulmonary forms—in addition to underlying lung disease—vascular involvement, tissue necrosis, and scarring are present. Extensive fibrosis with collagen deposition is observed in fibrosing mediastinitis.[79]

The radiographic manifestations of histoplasmosis have been discussed under each form of clinical presentation. Histoplasmomas are healed pulmonary lesions that appear as residual nodules on chest radiography. These coin lesions usually are 1 to 4 cm in diameter. When yeast forms are present in the core, continued fibrosis in response to the yeast antigens adds to the fibrotic capsule, slowly enlarging the lesions. It is important to differentiate these lesions from malignancy.[78]

Pulmonary function testing can be performed to determine the extent of pulmonary involvement by evaluating the degree of restrictive defect, the presence of a small airway obstruction, the extent of diffusion impairment, and the presence of hypoxemia. It can also be used to monitor the progression of pulmonary disease in patients with chronic pulmonary histoplasmosis. Bronchoscopy with bronchial washing may be indicated to obtain diagnostic material and, if possible, transbronchial biopsy to rule out malignancy. Bronchoscopy may also be useful in hemoptysis and broncholithiasis. Echocardiography, CT scan of the abdomen, as well as CT scan and MRI of the brain should be performed when involvement of these areas is suspected. Lumbar puncture in CNS histoplasmosis demonstrates a lymphocytic pleocytosis, with elevated protein and normal or low glucose.

Medical treatment

No treatment is needed for asymptomatic immunocompetent individuals without serious underlying disease or patients with acute self-limited or mild symptoms. The antifungal therapy of choice is amphotericin B or its liposomal formulation for disseminated disease. The recommended duration of therapy is 12 weeks for acute and subacute histoplasmosis, 12 to 24 months for chronic disease, and 6 to 18 months for disseminated progressive disease. Patients with disseminated disease and HIV should be on treatment for life. Itraconazole can be used for those with moderate illness and for completion of therapy after response to amphotericin. In those who are hypoxic corticosteroids should be added.[80,81] Mediastinal and hilar lymphadenopathies usually resolve. Granulomatous inflammation causes extensive enlargement with caseating necrosis, which may fibrose with progressive healing. Occasionally, the lymph nodes may remain enlarged, compressing surrounding structures and distorting anatomic architecture.

Surgical treatment

Indications for surgery include:

- The presence of persistent or progressive cavitations with repeated relapses despite multiple courses of intensive medical treatment
- Medical therapy is insufficient to alleviate the compressive effects of progressive fibrosis, calcification, and scarring:

  - Life-threatening tracheobronchial and esophageal obstruction and bronchoesophageal fistula
  - SVC syndrome, pulmonary vascular obstruction, or middle-lobe syndrome associated with fibrosing mediastinitis
- Severe valvular insufficiency due to involvement in disseminated histoplasmosis
- Symptomatic broncholithiasis (which occurs when a calcified node erodes into a bronchus) if bronchoscopic extraction was unsuccessful

During surgery, care should be taken to avoid spilling necrotic material into the mediastinum and initiating a further fibrotic reaction.

ASPERGILLOSIS

Etiology and pathology

Pulmonary aspergillosis comprises a spectrum of mycotic diseases caused by *Aspergillus* species. Human illness is usually caused by *A. fumigatus* and *A. niger* and, less frequently, by *A. flavus* and *A. clavatus*. The transmission of fungal spores to the human host is via inhalation. *A. fumigatus* exists in two forms: (1) conidiophores, the reproductive forms that produce and release thousands of spores, and (2) hyphae, which represent mature spores characterized by a 45-degree dichotomous branching pattern. The fungus grows widely in soil, water, and decaying vegetable or animal material. The spores are readily inhaled, and the fungus is commonly found in the sputum of healthy individuals.[82] Most patients with pulmonary aspergillosis have either impaired immunity or an underlying preexisting chronic lung disease such as bronchiectasis, COPD, or tuberculosis. Impaired immunity may be secondary to alcoholism, advanced age, poorly controlled diabetes mellitus, underlying malignancy, cirrhosis, malnutrition, sepsis, AIDS, or organ transplantation.[83,84] The development of disease and its histologic, clinical, and radiologic manifestations depend on the virulence and number of spores inhaled and, more importantly, on the patient's immune status.

Clinical presentation

Pulmonary disease caused by *Aspergillus* species presents with a wide spectrum of manifestations. Pulmonary aspergillosis may present as any of three distinctive clinical syndromes: allergic bronchopulmonary aspergillosis, aspergilloma, and invasive aspergillosis.

Allergic bronchopulmonary aspergillosis

Allergic bronchopulmonary aspergillosis (ABPA) represents a hypersensitivity reaction to *A. fumigatus* in patients with poorly controlled asthma or cystic fibrosis.[85] It is associated with a type I, III, or IV allergic response to *Aspergillus* antigens. Excessive mucus production in association with impaired ciliary function leads to mucoid impaction of the airways. The plugs of inspissated mucus contain hyphal elements of *A. fumigatus* and eosinophils, but the organisms remain within the bronchial lumen; this feature differentiates ABPA from invasive aspergillosis. The inflammatory response results in damage to the bronchial wall with airway destruction and the subsequent development of bronchiectasis. ABPA was initially described as a disease characterized by episodic wheezing, pulmonary infiltrates, pyrexia, sputum and blood eosinophilia, and sputum containing brown flecks or plugs. Almost all ABPA patients have clinical asthma. The disease may progress through various stages based on clinical, serologic, and radiographic findings. These stages need not occur in order. The first four stages—which are acute, remission, recurrent exacerbation, and corticosteroid-dependent asthma—are potentially reversible with no long-term sequelae. However, the fifth stage, fibrotic lung disease in which bronchiectasis or fibrosis develops, is irreversible.[86]

Aspergilloma or saprophytic aspergillosis

Aspergilloma is the most common form of pulmonary aspergillosis. It is noninvasive, involves the colonization of a preexisting pulmonary cavity or ectatic bronchus secondary to a wide variety of underlying pulmonary conditions, and occurs most often in the upper lobe. Simple aspergilloma develops in isolated thin-walled cysts lined by ciliated epithelium while the surrounding lung is normal. Complex aspergilloma develops in cavities formed by gross disease in the surrounding lung tissue.[87] The most common underlying conditions are tuberculosis, sarcoidosis, and bronchiectasis. Histologically, the aspergilloma represents a fungal ball, or mycetoma, which consists of a mass-like conglomerate of intertwined hyphae intermingled with fibrin, cellular debris, mucus, and other blood products. This mycetoma may calcify in an amorphous or ring-like fashion. A pulmonary aspergilloma does not initiate the destructive pulmonary process, as is seen in ABPA and invasive aspergillosis. Most cases of aspergilloma are thought to arise from colonization and proliferation of the fungus in areas of devitalized lung with a poor blood supply. Most patients with pulmonary aspergilloma are asymptomatic. The most common presenting symptom, hemoptysis, has been reported in 50 to 80 percent of patients.[88] Hemoptysis is usually intermittent and scanty but may be life-threatening. When symptoms such as cough, dyspnea, malaise, and weight loss are present, they are varied and are often difficult to ascribe to the aspergilloma in the presence of underlying pulmonary disease. Fever is an unusual finding in aspergilloma and suggests an alternate cause or concurrent bacterial infection.[88] Physical examination is generally nonspecific, although localizing signs such as decreased air movement, bronchial breath sounds, and adventitial sounds are almost always heard.

Invasive pulmonary aspergillosis

Invasive pulmonary aspergillosis (IPA) is now the most common fungal pulmonary infection in severely immunocompromised patients such as hematopoietic stem cell—or organ-transplant patients with hematologic malignancies undergoing intensive chemotherapy.[89] This infectious process is characterized by the invasion of blood vessels, resulting in multifocal infiltrates. Dissemination to other organs, particularly the CNS, may occur. Invasive aspergillosis typically manifests itself with fever, cough, sputum production, dyspnea, pleuritic chest pain, and sometimes hemoptysis in patients with prolonged neutropenia or immunosuppression. Fever that persists despite the administration of broad-spectrum antibiotics is present in a majority of patients except in corticosteroid-treated patients and is often the first clinical sign. Hypoxemia is present in diffuse disease. Among patients who have undergone organ transplantation, bone marrow recipients are most at risk for *Aspergillus* infection. In patients with leukemia and lymphoma, aspergillosis may occur after chemotherapy-induced bone marrow suppression, with resultant prolonged neutropenia.[90]

Diagnosis

Several sets of diagnostic criteria incorporating the clinical, immunologic, and radiographic features of the disease have been proposed for the diagnosis of ABPA, since no single test is sufficiently discriminating. ABPA is defined by the following abnormalities: asthma, eosinophilia, a positive skin test result for *A. fumigatus*, marked elevation of the serum immunoglobulin E (IgE) level to greater than 1000 IU/dL, and positive test results for *Aspergillus* precipitins (primarily IgG, but also IgA and IgM antibodies). Chest x-ray characteristics include fleeting pulmonary infiltrates, central bronchiectasis, and mucoid impaction, which can result in lobulated masses or atelectasis. CT scanning is helpful to better define bronchiectasis; images may show that the apparent lobulated masses are mucus-filled dilated bronchi. Minor criteria for diagnosis include positive *Aspergillus* radioallergosorbent assay test results, expectoration of brown plugs, and culture findings for *Aspergillus* in sputum. Histopathology and Gomori methenamine silver staining may demonstrate degenerating eosinophils and typical fungal hyphae.

Aspergilloma does not cause many characteristic laboratory abnormalities. Although a definitive diagnosis requires lung biopsy or resection, this is rarely done. The diagnosis is usually made based on clinical and chest radiographic features coupled with serologic evidence of *Aspergillus* species. Results of the *Aspergillus* precipitin antibody test (i.e., for IgG) are usually positive. Chest radiography reveals a mass in a preexisting cavity, usually in an upper lobe, manifest by a crescent of air partially outlining a solid mass. Associated pleural thickening adjacent to the cavity is characteristic and may predate the development of an aspergilloma. CT scan images provide a better definition of the mass within a cavity and may demonstrate multiple aspergillomas in areas of extensive cavitary disease. Imaging can be performed with the patient in the supine and prone positions to demonstrate movement of the mass within the cavity.

Currently available antibody testing is not helpful for the diagnosis of invasive aspergillosis. In the appropriate clinical setting of pulmonary infiltrates in a patient who is neutropenic or immunosuppressed, visualization of the characteristic fungi, using silver stain or Calcofluor, or a positive culture result from sputum, needle biopsy, or BAL fluid should result in the prompt institution of therapy. Invasive aspergillosis demonstrates the characteristic septate hyphae, branching at acute angles, and acute inflammatory infiltrate and tissue necrosis with occasional granulomata and blood vessel invasion. Chest radiographic features are variable, including solitary or multiple nodules, cavitary lesions, or alveolar infiltrates that are localized or bilateral and more diffuse as disease progresses. A halo sign (i.e., an area of ground-glass infiltrate surrounding nodular densities on CT scan images) may be very helpful in the early diagnosis of aspergillosis. Later disease may show a crescent of air surrounding nodules, indicative of cavitation. Because *Aspergillus* is angioinvasive, infiltrates may be wedge-shaped, pleura-based, and cavitary, which is consistent with pulmonary infarction.

Medical treatment

The goals of therapy for APBA are to treat acute exacerbations of disease and prevent the development of the fibrotic stage and bronchiectasis; therefore early diagnosis is crucial. ABPA requires treatment with oral corticosteroids as a hypersensitivity reaction. Inhaled steroids are not effective. A recent double-blind, placebo-control trial has also demonstrated a potential benefit from the addition of oral itraconazole 200 mg twice daily to steroids. This may allow more rapid resolution of infiltrates and symptoms, facilitating steroid tapering or lowering the needed maintenance corticosteroid dosage.[91] Bronchodilators such as beta agonists, anticholinergics, and leukotriene antagonists are also used for the treatment of asthma symptoms in ABPA.

Medical therapy is usually not effective for the treatment of aspergilloma because amphotericin B penetrates *Aspergillus* cavities poorly. Most patients are asymptomatic and treatment is not required unless significant hemoptysis occurs, in which case surgical intervention is indicated. Invasive aspergillosis is often rapidly progressive and has a high mortality rate; therefore preventive therapy and rapid institution of therapy in patients in whom the diagnosis is suspected may be lifesaving. Prophylactic antifungal therapy with amphotericin B in high-risk patients may prevent invasive aspergillosis. The largest therapeutic experience is also with amphotericin B. Lipid formulations of amphotericin are indicated for the patient who has impaired renal function or who develops nephrotoxicity while receiving amphotericin. Oral itraconazole is an alternative for patients who can reliably take oral medication, especially those who respond to initial intravenous therapy.[92] Combination antifungal therapy sometimes may be used, or newer antifungal agents, such as caspofungin, may be instituted as monotherapy in patients in whom initial therapy with amphotericin B has failed. Voriconazole is a new broad-spectrum triazole active in vitro against various yeasts and molds including *Aspergillus* species.[93] A recent randomized trail showed that in patients with invasive aspergillosis, initial therapy with voriconazole led to better responses and improved survival and resulted in fewer severe side effects than the standard approach of initial therapy with amphotericin B.[94] For transplant patients, the level of immunosuppression should be decreased if possible.

Surgical treatment

Areas of mucoid impaction due to ABPA may have a mass-like appearance and are sometimes resected as an undiagnosed lung mass. Surgical removal of aspergilloma is definitive treatment; it has been advocated to be reserved for high-risk patients such as those with episodes of recurrent or life-threatening hemoptysis and patients who are immunocompromised.[92] This recommendation is based on earlier reports that showed significant operative morbidity and mortality, especially in patients with complex aspergilloma.[95–97] On the other hand, some recent reports demonstrate better short- and long-term outcomes and advocate early surgical resection even in patients with simple pulmonary aspergilloma and minimal symptoms.[98–101] Notably, an important factor that contributes to the high surgical risk of resection is that aspergillomas tend to develop in clinically ill individuals with poor pulmonary function. Furthermore, in complex aspergillomas, operations are often technically challenging because of the dense fibrosis around the cavity, the obliteration of pleural space and fissures, the enlarged and tortuous bronchial arteries, and the diseased pulmonary parenchyma surrounding the lesion. Inflammatory fibrosis of the pulmonary parenchyma and pleura may prevent the remaining lung from expanding fully so that it fills the pleural space after resection. For patients with life-threatening symptoms whose condition is unfit for pulmonary resection, cavernostomy and myoplasty may be considered.[102,103] Careful long-term follow-up is necessary in all patients because of the risk of recurrence. Overall, the morbidity of surgical treatment must be weighed against the clinical benefit for each patient. Bronchial artery embolization rarely produces a permanent success due to systemic collateral supply, but it may be useful as a temporizing procedure in patients with life-threatening hemoptysis.[104] Other modalities that have been used include radiation therapy and endobronchial or percutaneous intracavitary instillation of amphotericin B under fluoroscopic or CT guidance.[105,106] For invasive aspergillosis, the marginal response rates to antifungals, combined with the aggressive nature of the disease, leads to mortality rates that approach 90 percent with medical therapy alone, especially in immunocompromised patients. Aggressive surgical resection is therefore recommended for localized disease that has failed to respond to prolonged antifungal therapy.[107–109] A thoracoscopic approach has been reported that may result in a less complicated postoperative course.[110]

COCCIDIOIDOMYCOSIS

Etiology and pathology

Coccidioidomycosis is the infection caused by the dimorphic fungi of the genus *Coccidioides* (*C. immitis* and *C. posadasii*); it has been classified as a reemerging disease.[111] These fungi are endemic to certain lower deserts of the southwestern United States. Infection is acquired by inhalation of a single arthroconidium, usually dust from uncultivated soil in the endemic areas. Within the lung, an arthroconidium changes from a barrel-shaped cell to a spherical structure and then greatly enlarges. Enlarging spherules produce internal septations; within each of the resulting subcompartments, individual cells (endospores) evolve. After several days, mature spherules rupture, releasing endospores into the infected tissue. Each endospore is potentially capable of producing another spherule. If the infecting dose is huge or the person's immune status is impaired, overwhelming pulmonary disease and acute respiratory distress syndrome (ARDS) can occur. More often, localized pulmonary infection is the result. Coccidioidal pneumonia may clear, spread locally, or disseminate. Dissemination may occur during the initial illness or later with the onset of immunologic failure.

Clinical presentation

Approximately two-thirds of infected persons experience few or no symptoms. The initial, or primary, infection is called valley fever when the disease is mild. Although the symptoms of coccidioidomycosis closely resemble those of other common respiratory infections, a respiratory illness with an accompanying rash in a patient with recent exposure to an endemic area is suggestive of a coccidioidal infection.[112] Other systemic symptoms include fever, sore throat, malaise, and headache. Valley fever and acute coccidioidal pneumonia are by far the most common clinical presentations.[113] Acute coccidioidal pneumonia may be self-limited or seem to respond to treatment with antibiotics. In certain situations, acute coccidioidal pneumonia may progress to involve the pleura, the formation of a mass-like lesion, necrosis, and cavity formation (coccidioidal cavities). In approximately

5 percent of patients, pneumonia can become chronic and cavities and nodules can persist as residual pulmonary nodules and chronic fibrocavitary pneumonia. The latter is characterized by night sweats, fatigue, weight loss, chronic cough, hemoptysis, and dyspnea. If necrosis involves the pleura, rupture with contamination of the pleura and extensive bronchopleural disease can ensue. When rupture does occur, a bronchopleural fistula is formed. Dyspnea and chest pain are the most common resulting symptoms, typical of a pneumothorax. Multiple areas of the lung may be involved due to seeding of several areas or airway spread of the infection.

Diffuse pulmonary or miliary coccidioidomycosis is the pulmonary manifestation of widespread dissemination in an individual with a very poor host response or if the fungal inoculum is large. The patient may manifest ARDS with hypoxia; in some cases, hypercapnea may also occur. *Coccidioides* may invade the vasculature, and spherules can be carried hematogenously to the entire pulmonary vasculature and many organs. Extrapulmonary coccidioidomycosis can involve any organ; however, disseminated lesions are most commonly seen in the skin, lymph nodes, bones, and joints. Coccidioidal meningitis is also a manifestation of dissemination. Fortunately disseminated disease occurs in only 0.5 to 1 percent of cases.[114]

Diagnosis

The clinical presentations of coccidioidomycosis are protean, necessitating a high index of suspicion for the disease. A complete physical examination, particularly a careful exam of the skin, can provide important clues. A definitive diagnosis is established by the recovery of *Coccidioides* from respiratory secretions, tissues, or body fluids. Microscopic examination of sputum is positive in only 10 percent of cases. Bronchoscopy increases the yield dramatically, particularly if there is a lesion in the airways or parenchyma that can be biopsied. Alternatively, BAL is often useful. Respiratory samples should always be examined by cytology. Fine-needle aspiration of the lung often yields the organism, but more than one attempt is often necessary.[115] Skin tests are not helpful in making the diagnosis. If skin lesions are present, a punch biopsy is quick and often positive. Pathologic examination using a silver stain shows granulomatous inflammation with the classic double-walled spherules with endospores. Sputum samples and tissue biopsies can reveal these pathognomonic features. Serologic testing is one of the mainstays of diagnosis. The precipitin test, which measures IgM antibody, will be positive in 1 to 2 weeks and will remain positive for up to 6 months. Serology for the slower but more persistent IgG response is also tested using complement fixation or immunodiffusion assays and, more recently, enzyme immunoassay. Coccidioides will grow in nearly all laboratory media and often within the first week. The organism grows best at room temperature. A positive identification of the mold can be quickly made by a commercially available DNA probe.

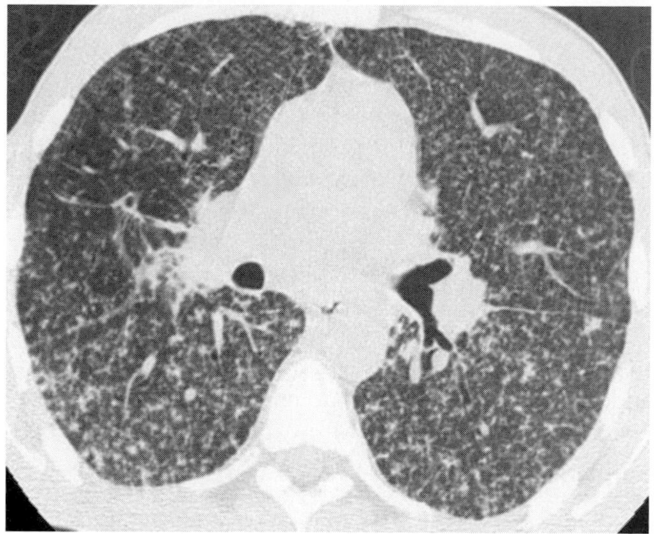

Figure 3-7 Chest CT of a patient with miliary coccidioidomycosis.

Radiographic manifestations vary depending on the clinical presentation. Residual coccidioidal cavities are commonly solitary and peripheral in location on a radiograph. Their walls are often strikingly thin with little or no discernible surrounding infiltrate. In ruptured cavities, an effusion coexists with the pneumothorax on chest x-ray, resulting in an air-fluid level. Since a spontaneous pneumothorax does not normally produce an effusion, this finding is of diagnostic significance. Chronic fibrocavitary pneumonia shows complex mixtures of infiltrate and cavitation. Hilar adenopathy is also common. A diffuse miliary or reticulonodular pattern on chest radiograph or CT scan (Fig. 3-7) is strongly associated with disseminated disease.[116] When disseminated disease is suspected, other diagnostic modalities include CT of the abdomen and pelvis and a bone scan to identify occult bony lesions. If the patient has even minimal CNS symptoms, a lumbar puncture should be performed to rule out coccidioidal meningitis.

Medical treatment

In the absence of symptoms, treatment is not recommended. Since it is possible for coccidioidal cavities to change appearance, repeat chest radiographs at intervals ranging from 6 months to 2 years, depending on their apparent stability, are helpful to determine whether the lesion is enlarging or disappearing. Treatment is recommended if symptoms such as local pleural discomfort and hemoptysis occur. Such symptoms often improve after treatment with oral antifungal agents (ketoconazole, fluconazole, or itraconazole), but they may return if treatment is discontinued. The duration of treatment is typically 1 year or longer.[117] A clinical response to treatment is usually evident by improvement in respiratory symptoms and periodic radiographs. Amphotericin B can be used for refractory infections unresponsive to oral therapy and is also the initial therapy of choice for rapidly progressive diffuse reticulonodular pneumonia and disseminated disease. As the patient's pulmonary status improves, treatment can be switched to an oral azole for at least 1 year. Patients with an underlying immunodeficiency state may have to be treated indefinitely.[115,117] A few case reports suggest that the new antifungal voriconazole is effective in disseminated disease refractory to other antifungals.[118,119]

Surgical treatment

Surgery is never the mainstay of treatment, although it may be critical for making the correct diagnosis. Cavities are considered candidates for resection if they are visible for longer than 2 to 4 years in association with symptoms, adjacent to pleura, rapidly enlarging, or thick-walled or if they contain a fungus ball. Severe or recurrent hemoptysis is a strong indication for surgery. Surgical resection has also been recommended when the cavities occur in diabetic or pregnant patients and when they coexist with pulmonary tuberculosis.[120–121]

In pyopneumothorax associated with a ruptured coccidioidal cavity, surgical resection of the cavity is the preferred approach if the condition is diagnosed promptly.[122] If the diagnosis is delayed a week or more, a conservative approach with chest tube placement and oral antifungal treatment can be attempted. Persistent bronchopleural fistulas or lungs that are restricted by residual disease are other indications for surgery. In the case of ruptured cavities, the extent of surgical resection may have to be limited because of the extensive contamination of the pleural space. Lobectomy may not necessarily be indicated, since lesser resections are associated with equally low recurrence and complications rates. [123]

BLASTOMYCOSIS

Etiology and pathology

North American blastomycosis is an endemic fungal infection predominantly seen in the south central and midwestern United States and portions of Canada. The disorder is the systemic pyogranulomatous disease caused by *B. dermatitidis*, a dimorphic organism usually acquired through inhalation of aerosolized conidia. At body temperature, these conidia transform to the yeast phase and a self-limited infection develops in the majority of persons. Rarely, blastomycosis may occur in accidental percutaneous exposure or following dog bites. Conjugal and perinatal transmissions have been reported, but person-to-person transmission is extremely rare. Most individuals who develop blastomycosis report occupations or hobbies—specifically hunting and fishing, camping, cutting timber, and operating heavy equipment—that likely enhance exposure to *B. dermatitidis*. The fungus has been identified in pigeon manure and soil. The major acquired host defense against *B. dermatitidis* is cellular immunity, which is mediated by antigen-specific T lymphocytes and lymphokine-activated macrophages. Chronic infection limited to the lungs or disseminated infection involving extrapulmonary sites develops in the minority of cases.

Clinical presentation

Blastomycosis is a systemic disease that can involve virtually any organ. Acute blastomycosis is a condition that occurs with unknown frequency among patients exposed to *B. dermatitidis* through inhalation.[124] Most of the data from outbreaks suggest that the vast majority of patients exposed to *B. dermatitidis* develop a self-limited nonspecific flu-like illness that does not progress to chronic disease.

Chronic pulmonary blastomycosis is a disease usually manifest by symptoms of chronic pneumonia, which may progress to a pyogranulomatous process. Common symptoms include weight loss, fever, night sweats, and a cough productive of purulent sputum. Hemoptysis is uncommon. The disease is difficult to distinguish clinically from other fungal pulmonary diseases, tuberculosis, nocardiosis, chronic necrotizing bacterial pneumonia, and neoplastic disease. In fewer than 10 percent of cases, pulmonary blastomycosis presents with severe clinical manifestations, ARDS, and respiratory failure. This severe and unusual manifestation occurs in both immunocompromised and otherwise normal patients and is associated with an extremely high mortality.[125] There are also several reports of so-called miliary blastomycosis associated with disseminated disease but not necessarily with frank respiratory failure.[126] Many of these patients are severely immunosuppressed, but if a diagnosis is established early, there is often a favorable outcome with appropriate systemic antifungal therapy.

Extrapulmonary involvement with *B. dermatitidis* occurs in over 50 percent of patients with chronic blastomycosis. The skin and subcutaneous tissue are the most common sites.[127] Typical lesions are verrucous (wart-like) plaques or cutaneous ulcers, frequently with a distinctive purplish hue surrounding the skin lesions. Subcutaneous disease is usually manifest as subcutaneous nodules that may suppurate and spontaneously drain, forming deep cutaneous ulcers. These lesions can easily be mistaken for pyoderma gangrenosum, squamous cell carcinoma, and other chronic cutaneous infections. Other sites that can be potentially involved include the genitourinary tract, bones, CNS, and the nasal and oral mucosa. Less common sites include the larynx, thyroid, sinuses, and eyes.

Diagnosis

The diagnosis of blastomycosis is established when *B. dermatitidis* is isolated from any clinical specimen. Transbronchial, transthoracic, or open-lung biopsy may be necessary. The organism grows well in the mycelial phase at 25 to 30°C on routine fungal media. Conversion to the yeast phase at 37°C and demonstration of morphologically typical yeast forms confirms the identity of the organism. Commercial test kits are available that allow early identification of mycelial cultures by recognition of unique deoxyribonucleic acid (DNA) sequences or fungus-specific exoantigens.[128] In culture-negative cases or before the culture becomes positive, the finding of broad-based budding yeast with a doubly refractile cell wall (Fig. 3-8) on histologic or cytologic specimens is strongly suggestive of *B. dermatitidis.* At present, there is no reliable, sensitive, and specific serologic methodology in use for routine diagnostic purposes. A new assay that measures antibody to *B. dermatitidis* by ELISA is being developed but has not been validated in humans.[127]

Radiographically, chronic pulmonary blastomycosis does not have a typical appearance. Parenchymal abnormalities may occur in the upper lobes and may appear as unilateral or bilateral lobar or segmental abnormalities. Pulmonary nodules with or without cavitation and mass-like lesions are frequently noted. The mass lesion of pulmonary blastomycosis may mimic carcinoma of the lungs. Pleural effusion and mediastinal lymphadenopathy may be seen in very few cases.

Medical treatment

There is controversy as to whether patients with acute self-limited blastomycosis should be treated with antifungal therapy. In any event, a presumptive diagnosis is not an adequate basis for therapy. Chronic blastomycosis, however, requires antifungal therapy because the disease rarely resolves spontaneously. Untreated, chronic blastomycosis can be associated with mortality rates approaching 60 percent.[129] Most experts recommend a minimum of 6 months of oral azole (typically, itraconazole) therapy for mild-to-moderate pulmonary or nonmeningeal disseminated blastomycosis. The role of the amphotericin B formulations in the treatment of blastomycosis is probably limited to patients with severe or life-threatening disease, including all patients with CNS involvement, most immunocompromised patients (including transplant recipients and HIV-infected patients), and other iatrogenically immunosuppressed patients.[130] Amphotericin B is given as "induction therapy" to gain control of the disease, and an azole is given as "consolidation therapy" to complete at least 6 months of therapy. Long-term suppressive therapy may be needed in immunocompromised patients.

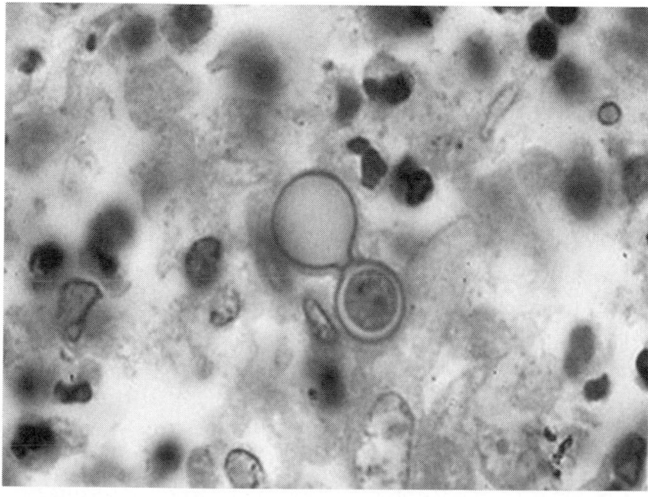

Figure 3-8 Broad-based budding yeasts typical for *Blastomyces dermatitidis.*

Surgical treatment

The main indication for surgery is usually to rule out malignancy. Surgical intervention is also necessary for drainage of large cavitary abscesses. Known blastomycotic cavitary lesions should be resected if they persist after adequate drug treatment. If the diagnosis is made only at the time of thoracotomy, drug treatment should follow operation.

CRYPTOCOCCOSIS

Cryptococcus neoformans is an encapsulated yeast. The species has four serotypes based on antigenic specificity of the capsular polysaccharide; these include serotypes A and D (*C. neoformans var neoformans*) and serotypes B and C (*C. neoformans var gattii*). The *C. neoformans var neoformans* is the most common variety in the United States and other temperate climates throughout the world; it is found in aged pigeon droppings.[131] Naturally occurring cryptococcosis occurs in both animals and humans, but animal-to-human or person-to-person transmission via the pulmonary route has not been documented. Transmission via organ transplantation has been reported when infected donor organs were used. The lungs are thought to be the initial site of almost all infections due to *C. neoformans* and, after the CNS, are the second most clinically relevant site of infection. It is postulated that humans become infected with *C. neoformans* by inhaling the basidiospore form of this fungus. Basidiospores are smaller than the yeast forms obtained from clinical samples and have much smaller polysaccharide capsules, thus facilitating deposition in the alveoli and terminal bronchioles after inhalation. The alveolar macrophages ingest the yeast.

Phagocytosis and destruction of the unencapsulated yeast cells readily occur, whereas encapsulated organisms are more resistant to phagocytosis. A cryptococcal polysaccharide capsule has antiphagocytic properties and may be immunosuppressive. Host response to cryptococcal infection includes both cellular and humoral components.

Clinical presentation

The pattern of cryptococcal pulmonary disease is extremely variable, ranging from asymptomatic saprophytic airway colonization to ARDS, which is observed in hosts who are immunocompromised (e.g., patients with AIDS, organ transplant recipients). Following inhalation, *C. neoformans* is believed to cause a small focal pneumonitis that may or may not be symptomatic. The immune status of the affected individual appears to be the most important element in determining the subsequent course of the infection (i.e., resolution of the pneumonitis vs. symptomatic dissemination). Subclinical primary infections are common and the vast majority of infected patients are asymptomatic. Symptoms may include cough with scant sputum, pleuritic chest pain, fever, weight loss, malaise, and rarely hemoptysis. Night sweats, as observed in tuberculosis, are uncommon in cryptococcal pulmonary disease but may occur with disseminated or CNS disease.[132] On occasion, cryptococcal pulmonary disease may even manifest as a slowly progressive mass that can compress thoracic structures such as the vena cava. Although chronic infection can occur, patients who are immunocompetent normally have spontaneous regression of both clinical and radiologic manifestations. Sometimes asymptomatic pulmonary infection may be followed later by the development of meningitis, which is often the first indication of disease. The presentation of pulmonary cryptococcosis in HIV-infected persons appears to be more acute and severe than in other patient groups. The severity of symptoms and extent of dissemination are inversely proportional to the CD4 lymphocyte count, with most symptomatic cases occurring in patients with counts less than 100/μL.[133]

C. neoformans infection is usually characterized by little or no necrosis or organ dysfunction until late in the disease. Organ damage may accelerate in persons with heavy infections. The lack of identifiable endotoxins or exotoxins is partly responsible for the absence of extensive necrosis early in cryptococcal infections. Organ damage stems primarily from tissue distortion secondary to the expanding fungal burden. Extensive inflammation or fibrosis is rare. The characteristic lesion consists of a cystic cluster of yeast with no well-defined inflammatory response. Well-formed granulomas generally are not present. After lung and CNS infection, the next most commonly involved organs in disseminated cryptococcosis are the skin, prostate, and medullary cavity of the bones.

Diagnosis

The diagnosis of active cryptococcal pulmonary infection can be suggested by the appearance of the characteristically encapsulated yeast forms in specimens of sputum, bronchoalveolar lavage fluid, or tissue. Culture of the organism from these same specimens can establish the diagnosis. *C. neoformans* is readily cultured in routine fungal medium that does not contain cycloheximide. In cases of clinically silent cryptococcal nodules that are sampled to rule out the possibility of malignancy, cultures of tissue can be negative despite the presence of yeast on histopathologic inspection. Cultures of associated pleural effusion should be performed, as they are usually positive.

The use of the serum cryptococcal antigen as a screening test for pulmonary cryptococcosis is less likely to be positive in the immunocompetent population than in the immunocompromised. In fact, the test is positive in virtually all patients with HIV infection and pulmonary cryptococcosis. The presence of a positive serum cryptococcal antigen titer implies deep tissue invasion and a high likelihood of disseminated disease.[134] The testing of pleural fluid for the presence of the polysaccharide antigen can be very useful in suspected cases in which cultures are negative.

Radiographic manifestation features of pulmonary cryptococcosis in patients with pulmonary cryptococcosis vary widely. Well-defined, noncalcified nodules, either solitary or a few, are the most common radiographic findings. Cavitation in cryptococcal nodules is rare. Other possible findings in the chest include lobar infiltrates, masses, hilar and mediastinal adenopathy, and pleural effusions.[135] A lumbar puncture (LP) to obtain CSF for cryptococcal antigen testing and culture is indicated if the patient has neurologic symptoms or an underlying condition that predisposes to dissemination. An LP should also be strongly considered if the patient's serum cryptococcal antigen titer is very high (> 1:250). CSF should also be tested if *Cryptococcus* is diagnosed from surgical specimen.

Medical treatment

Patients with asymptomatic pulmonary cryptococcosis with a negative serum cryptococcal antigen may not require any systemic therapy. Patients presenting with symptomatic pulmonary infection should be treated with either fluconazole or amphotericin B. Fluconazole is preferred for most patients, since it can be administered orally and is less toxic than amphotericin B. Treatment with fluconazole should be continued for 36 months in immunocompetent patients. For those individuals who are unable to tolerate fluconazole, itraconazole for 6 to 12 months is an acceptable alternative. In the presence of more severe disease, treatment with amphotericin B may be necessary for 6 to 10 weeks. In immunocompromised patients, combination therapy with the amphotericin B and flucytosine is recommended, followed by high-dose fluconazole for a total of 10 weeks. After 10 weeks of therapy, the fluconazole dosage may be reduced, depending on the patient's clinical status.[134] It is recommended that all HIV-infected individuals continue maintenance therapy for life.

Surgical treatment

Surgical excision of infected pulmonary tissue is indicated only in cases of pseudotumor-like masses that impinge on adjacent structures. However, the diagnosis is often not clear until the time of surgical resection. Once the diagnosis is established, the lesion should not be resected unless it can easily be removed by wedge resection.[136,137] Pleural effusions can be treated with systemic therapy alone and rarely require drainage.

MUCORMYCOSIS (ZYGOMYCOSIS)

Etiology and pathology

Mucormycosis refers to rare, severe infections with fungi of the order Mucorales. *Rhizopus* species are the most common causative organisms. They are saprophytic fungi that are ubiquitous in soil or decaying organic material. Spores produced by the fungi become airborne and are inhaled into the respiratory tract, which is the most common route of inoculation in a susceptible host. Humans with intact immunity are generally unaffected, but those with impairments of immunity due to cancer and its therapy, metabolic dysfunction (e.g., diabetes or ketoacidosis), or iatrogenic causes of immune suppression (e.g., steroids or cytotoxic chemotherapy) are at greatest risk for infection. Pulmonary and rhinocerebral infections predominate as a consequence of the frequency of airborne inoculation. Inhalation of spores in sawmill dust is also the source of allergic interstitial pneumonitis or alveolitis syndromes, which have been described in healthy lumber workers.[138]

Direct contamination of skin or wounds by traumatic implantation of spores from soil and other environmental sources may occur, even in the hospital setting. Ingestion of spores with subsequent invasion of the gastrointestinal tract occurs rarely. Once spores reach tissue compartments, they germinate and hyphal elements develop and proliferate. The hyphal structures of the Zygomycetes are nonseptate or have rare septa, with broad, nonparallel walls. The hyphae are highly angioinvasive. Invasion of blood vessels by hyphae characteristically results in hemorrhage, thrombosis, infarction, and tissue necrosis. Death can result from progressive tissue destruction, uncontrolled hemorrhage, or both.

Pulmonary mucormycosis is a rapidly progressive infection that occurs when the spores settle in the bronchioles and alveoli. A diffuse pneumonia with infarction and necrosis results, and the infection can spread to contiguous structures such as the mediastinum and heart. Apparent hematogenous dissemination to the brain has also been described.

Clinical presentation

Mucormycosis has a very high mortality rate of at least 50 percent. Due to the similarity in clinical features between mucormycosis and other more common filamentous fungal diseases and the difficulty in making a specific diagnosis, many cases of pulmonary mucormycosis are not suspected on the basis of clinical presentation. Neutropenic patients may present with fever refractory to broad-spectrum antibiotics, a cough that is typically nonproductive, severe or subtle pleuritic chest pain, and rapidly progressive dyspnea. Pleural rubs may also be heard on auscultation.[139] Hemoptysis is a late sign indicating fungal erosion into blood vessels. Fatal hemoptysis due to fungal invasion of the pulmonary artery or aorta has occasionally been reported. If unchecked, the infection has a propensity to invade relentlessly through multiple tissue planes and erode into the chest wall, pericardium, myocardium, superior vena cava, and diaphragm. Obstruction of major airways by endobronchial masses due to fungi has been described in diabetic patients.[140] Pulmonary involvement is often seen as a prelude to or in concert with disseminated zygomycosis. Once the disease has disseminated to other sites, including brain, skin, liver, or kidneys, the prognosis is poor. In patients with a mild degree of immune impairment, the pace of the disease is frequently less rapid. These patients may present with the slow development of cavitary lesions or pulmonary infiltrates or nodules in conjunction with fever and dry cough.

Diagnosis

The diagnosis of pulmonary mucormycosis can be difficult, since the presentation does not differ from that of diffuse pneumonias due to other microbial agents. There is a striking similarity to invasive aspergillosis. Sputum or BAL specimens can show the characteristic hyphae, which is usually the first clue to the presence of the disease.[141] However, in the case series from M.D. Anderson, only 25 percent of sputum or BAL specimens were positive premortem.[142] The hyphae can also be demonstrated on lung biopsy. A recent report of mucormycosis in cancer patients noted that about 80 percent with definite or probable pulmonary zygomycosis had a concomitant pneumonia due to another pathogen, either a mold (e.g., *Aspergillus* or *Fusarium*) or a bacterial species. Thus the presence of dual infection may obscure the diagnosis of mucormycosis. Accordingly, the detection of a Mucorales fungus in a respiratory sample should not be ignored, even if concomitant pathogens are also isolated in an immunosuppressed patient. Unfortunately, even when the correct diagnosis is made in a timely manner, the time between diagnosis and death is typically only a few days.

Radiographically, pulmonary mucormycosis may present as segmental or lobar infiltrates, isolated nodules, cavitary lesions, hemorrhage or infarction, or disseminated disease. A predilection for upper lobe involvement exists. Consolidation may be multilobar. Cavitation producing an air crescent is highly suggestive of fungal infection but does not distinguish mucormycosis from aspergillosis. Nodular lesions and pleural effusions may be present. When pulmonary mucormycosis is recognized, it should not be presumed to be isolated to that location. It is especially important to perform a CT scan of the sinuses and brain in the setting of pulmonary disease because these will be the most common sites associated with disseminated disease.[138]

Medical treatment

Early diagnosis and correction of the underlying abnormality such as control of diabetes and prompt institution of amphotericin B therapy is critical to survival. Neutropenia in association with hematologic malignancy and its treatment should be reversed, if possible, with the use of colony-stimulating factors and the withdrawal of cytotoxic chemotherapy. Attempts should be made to wean glucocorticosteroids and other immunosuppressive drugs. There is no role for flucytosine or the currently available azole antifungals in the therapy of this infection. Zaizen and coworkers detail cure of localized right-upper-lobe pulmonary mucormycosis in a poorly controlled diabetic with the combination of seven local instillations of amphotericin B via bronchoscopy, inhaled amphotericin, and intravenous amphotericin.[143]

Surgical treatment

Most patients present with multilobar involvement, which may preclude surgical resection. When feasible, extensive surgical debridement of as much involved tissue as possible is necessary. Amphotericin B is used as adjunctive therapy after aggressive surgical debridement. There are reports of patients with early pulmonary infection who were cured with lobectomies.[144-146] A case report of a cavitary rhizopus infection in a cardiac transplant recipient described a cure with the combination of surgical resection, systemic amphotericin B, and intrapleural administration of amphotericin B.[147]

CANDIDIASIS (MONILIASIS)

Etiology and pathology

Candida species are ubiquitous fungi and are the most common fungal pathogens affecting humans. They are yeast-like fungi that can form true hyphae and pseudohyphae. The genus *Candida* encompasses more than 160 species. The most common of these are *C. albicans, C. krusei, C. parapsilosis, C. tropicalis,* and *C. glabrata*. Some mycologists continue to refer to the latter species as *Torulopsis glabrata,* which is correct in terms of nomenclature.[148] For the most part, *Candida* species are confined to human and animal reservoirs; however, they are frequently recovered from the hospital environment, including on foods, countertops, air-conditioning vents, floors, respirators, and medical personnel. Although *Candida* are considered normal flora in the gastrointestinal and genitourinary tracts of humans, they have the propensity to invade and cause disease when an imbalance is created in the ecologic niche in which these organisms usually exist. The growing problem of mucosal and systemic candidiasis reflects the enormous increase in the pool of patients at risk and the increased opportunity that exists for *Candida* species to invade tissues normally resistant to invasion. *Candida* species are true opportunistic pathogens that exploit recent technologic advances to gain access to the circulation and deep tissues. Thus, needles, IV cannulas, or urinary bladder catheters are examples of the portals of infection.

Clinical presentation

The clinical manifestations of infection with *Candida* species range from local mucous membrane infections to widespread dissemination with multiorgan system failure. Pneumonia due to *Candida* is poorly defined as a clinical entity because positive cultures cannot distinguish between true infection and either colonization or contamination of samples with oropharyngeal contents.[149] In addition, the presence of clinical pneumonia may be due to coinfecting pathogens. Much more commonly, the lungs are one of many organs involved in the course of disseminated infection with *Candida* in immunosuppressed patients. In a review of a 20-year experience from the M.D. Anderson Cancer Center, there were only 55 cases of clearly documented primary candidal pneumonia in cancer patients who died.[150] The only criterion for the definitive diagnosis of candidal pneumonia was the histologic demonstration of fungus in lung tissue. In addition to the rare candidal pneumonia, other special clinical situations encountered by the thoracic surgeon in candidiasis include esophagitis and endocarditis.

Diagnosis

Species of *Candida* are present in 50 to 60 percent of respiratory secretions drawn from uninfected individuals. Studies in both cancer patients and nonneutropenic patients in an ICU setting have confirmed the lack of specificity of sputum or BAL specimens for the diagnosis of pulmonary invasion by *Candida*.[151,152] However, the presence of the fungi in bronchial or lung biopsies, in blood or deep tissue spaces is more likely due to invasive infection, especially in the immunocompromised host. This is particularly true for CSF culture, which is normally sterile. No reliable serologic test is available.

Nonspecific patchy infiltrates may be noted on radiographic imaging.

Medical treatment

If feasible, initial management should include removal of all existing portals such as central venous catheters. Management of serious and life-threatening invasive candidiasis remains severely hampered by delays in diagnosis and the lack of reliable diagnostic methods that allow for the detection of both fungemia and tissue invasion by *Candida* species.

Whenever possible, initiation of treatment for isolated candidal pneumonia should be based on histologic evidence in the nonneutropenic host. Without firm diagnostic criteria, the evaluation of antifungal therapy is difficult. Most patients with isolated candidal pneumonia have been treated with conventional amphotericin B. In contrast, patients with hematogenously disseminated infection who develop secondary candidal pneumonia should be treated for disseminated disease rather than candidal pneumonia alone. In this case, initial medical therapy should involve caspofungin, fluconazole, an amphotericin B preparation, or combination therapy with fluconazole plus amphotericin B.[149]

Surgical treatment

Surgical intervention is rarely indicated except for the occasional development of lung abscess and need for repair or replacement of valves due to candidal endocarditis.

SPOROTRICHOSIS

Etiology and pathology

Sporotrichosis is a subacute to chronic infection caused by the dimorphic fungus *Sporothrix schenckii*, which is found throughout the world in decaying vegetation, sphagnum moss, and soil. *S. cyanescens*, also found in the environment and previously thought to be nonpathogenic for humans, has been documented as a cause of infection in a heart transplant recipient.[153] *S. schenckii* exhibits thermal dimorphism. It produces hyphae in the environment at temperatures that are lower than normal human body temperatures; in comparison, it exists as a yeast form when at 37°C in human tissues. The hyphae are rather thin and septate, showing branching and stranding. The characteristic infection involves suppurating subcutaneous granulomas that progress proximally along lymphatic channels (lymphocutaneous sporotrichosis). Other tissues are involved by direct extension and, less often, by hematogenous dissemination. The most common extracutaneous sites are in the bones, joints, tendon sheaths, and bursae.

Pulmonary sporotrichosis is a rare form that appears to result from inhalation of the organism from soil. Most patients have been involved in an occupation that exposes them to aerosols from soil, but discrete point sources have rarely been identified. A chronic cavitary pneumonia, which is clinically and radiographically indistinguishable from tuberculosis and histoplasmosis, occurs in patients who usually have severe underlying COPD. Rarely, a disseminated infection occurs with disseminated cutaneous lesions and involvement of multiple visceral organs, including meningitis; this occurs most commonly in patients with AIDS.

Clinical presentation

Symptoms mimic those of tuberculosis, including constitutional complaints of fever, night sweats, weight loss, and fatigue as well as respiratory complaints including dyspnea, cough, purulent sputum, and hemoptysis. The typical patient is a Caucasian, middle-aged male who often smokes and abuses alcohol and may have underlying COPD.[154] Physical examination of patients with pulmonary sporotrichosis is dominated by the findings of the underlying COPD.

The major differential diagnoses include tuberculosis; chronic fungal infections, especially histoplasmosis; and sarcoidosis. Some patients with pulmonary involvement have evidence of dissemination to skin, osteoarticular structures, or viscera. Almost without exception, untreated pulmonary sporotrichosis progresses to death.

Diagnosis

Culture is the "gold standard" for establishing a diagnosis of sporotrichosis and is also the most sensitive method. Aspirated material from a lesion, sample from a tissue biopsy, sputum, or body fluids should be inoculated onto Sabouraud's medium or blood agar and incubated at room temperature. Incubation at this temperature facilitates growth of the mycelial phase of *S. schenckii*, with the characteristic arrangement of conidia on the hyphae. Occasionally, the organism (cigar-shaped yeast) can be visualized in biopsied tissue specimens that are stained with periodic acid–Schiff, Gomori methenamine-silver, or immunohistochemical stains. Sporotrichosis is characterized histopathologically by a mixed granulomatous and pyogenic process with occasional asteroid bodies. Asteroid bodies consist of a central basophilic yeast surrounded by eosinophilic material radiating outward like spokes on a wheel, probably representing antigen-antibody complexes. Although previously thought to be specific for sporotrichosis, this tissue reaction can be seen in other fungal infections as well.

Serology is less useful in the diagnosis of sporotrichosis than in other endemic mycoses.[155] Antibody measurement techniques demonstrate significant interlaboratory variability in sensitivity and specificity; therefore they should rarely serve as the sole basis for diagnosis. Such tests can be useful to raise diagnostic suspicion and inspire more aggressive attempts to acquire appropriate specimens

Table 3-4 Summary of actinomycotic and mycotic thoracic infections

Thoracic infection and source	Clinical presentation	Diagnosis	Medical treatment	Surgical[a] indications and treatment
Actinomycosis Oropharyngeal flora from poor dental hygiene	Pulmonary infiltrative mass. Sinus tract with drainage to the chest wall.	Sulfur granules in drainage. Anaerobic culture.	Penicillin.	Drainage of empyema. Rule out malignancy.
Nocardiosis Inhalation of organisms from soil	Pulmonary infection with subcutaneous abscess and draining sinuses.	Special stains of specimens. Aerobic culture.	Sulfonamides. Minocycline.	As above.
Histoplasmosis "Darling's disease" Inhalation of spores from bird or bat droppings	Mimics tuberculosis. Asymptomatic, acute, subacute, chronic and disseminated disease. Fibrosing mediastinitis may cause compression, such as SVC syndrome.	Caseating granulomas. Fungal culture. Antibody tests. Serum and urine antigen tests in immunocompromised patients.	Amphotericin B. Itraconazole.	Persistent or progressive cavitations. Compressive effects of progressive fibrosis.
Aspergillosis Inhalation of spores from soil, water, decaying vegetable and animal material	Allergic bronchopulmonary aspergillosis(ABPA), aspergilloma (fungus ball), invasive aspergillosis.	Asthma, eosinophilia, positive skin test and elevated serum IgE for ABPA. Serologic tests. Culture.	Itraconazole. Amphotericin B. Caspofungin. Voriconazole for invasive aspergillosis. Oral steroids for ABPA.	Resection of undiagnosed lung mass. Symptomatic or complicated aspergilloma.
Coccidioidomycosis "San Joaquin Valley fever" Inhalation of dust from uncultivated soil	Respiratory illness with rash. Acute or chronic fibrocavitary pneumonia. Spontaneous pneumothorax from rupture of thin-walled cavities associated with effusion. Coccidioidal meningitis.	Punch biopsy of skin lesions. Classic double-walled spherules with endospores. Serologic tests. Culture.	Ketoconazole, Fluconazole, Itraconazole. Amphotericin B for refractory disease.	Persistent or rapidly enlarging cavities. Pyopneumothorax.
Blastomycosis Inhalation of aerosolized spores, pigeon manure, and soil	Self-limited flu-like illness. Chronic pulmonary blastomycosis, pyogranulomatous process, rarely ARDS. Wart-like skin plaques.	Broad-based budding yeast with doubly refractile cell wall. Culture and early identification of unique DNA sequences.	Itraconazole. Amphotericin B.	Drainage of abscess. Resection of persistent cavities. Rule out malignancy.
Cryptococcosis Inhalation of basidiospores habored in aged pigeon droppings	Ranges from asymptomatic airway colonization to ARDS in immunocompromised patients. Organ damage from tissue distortion secondary to expanding fungal burden. Meningitis.	Encapsulated yeast. Culture of tissue and pleural effusions. Cryptococcal antigen testing and culture of CSF.	Fluconazole. Itraconazole. Amphotericin B with flucytosine.	Surgical excision of pseudotumor-like masses that impinge on adjacent structures.
Mucormycosis Airborne inhalation of spores from soil and decaying organic material	Rapidly progressive pulmonary and rhinocerebral infection. Propensity to invade multiple tissue planes.	Nonseptate hyphae structures. CT scan of brain and sinuses is necessary.	Amphotericin B.	Extensive surgical debridement and lung resection when feasible.

(continued)

Table 3-4 Summary of actinomycotic and mycotic thoracic infections (*continued*)

Thoracic infection and source	Clinical presentation	Diagnosis	Medical treatment	Surgical[a] indications and treatment
Candidiasis Normal GI and GU flora; access through medical invasive portals	Local mucous membrane infections can disseminate and lead to multi-organ system failure.	Definite diagnosis by demonstration of fungus in lung tissue. Positive sputum cultures cannot differentiate colonization from invasive infection.	Remove existing portals. Fluconazole. Capsofungin. Amphotericin B.	Drainage of abscess. Replacement or repair of heart valves.
Sporotrichosis Inhalation of the organism from the soil	Mimics tuberculosis. Chronic cavitary pneumonia. Dissemination to multiple visceral organs. Suppurating subcutaneous granulomas.	Culture. Cigar-shaped yeast. Thin septate hyphae. Mixed granulomatous and pyogenic process.	Amphotericin B, itraconazole.	Resection of focal lesions.

SVC = superior vena cava; ARDS = acute respiratory distress syndrome; CSF = cerebrospinal fluid; GI = gastrointestinal; GU = genitourinary.
[a]Surgical resection in most of these thoracic infections is mainly performed to rule out malignancy.

for culture. The radiographic findings are also nonspecific and are similar to those of tuberculosis: unilateral or bilateral upper lobe cavities with variable amounts of fibrosis and/or scattered nodular lesions.[155]

Medical treatment

Pulmonary sporotrichosis is difficult to treat, perhaps due to delayed diagnosis or the underlying illnesses in infected patients. If the patient is seriously ill, amphotericin B should be used initially; if not, then itraconazole can be given. Another option is to begin therapy with amphotericin B and, when the patient is stable, switch to itraconazole. The duration of azole therapy should be at least 1 year, perhaps longer in some patients.[156]

Surgical treatment

The most effective therapy for pulmonary sporotrichosis appears to be a combination of amphotericin B and subsequent surgical resection.[154] However, many patients are unable to tolerate such a procedure because of severe underlying pulmonary disease. Surgical resection is particularly useful for those patients who have focal lesions.

Thoracic *mycotic* and *actinomycotic* infections are summarized in Table 3-4.

TUBERCULOSIS AND ATYPICAL MYCOBACTERIAL DISEASES

TUBERCULOSIS

Etiology and pathology

Tuberculosis (TB) is an infectious disease that has plagued humans since the neolithic era. After decades of declining incidence in the United States, an unprecedented resurgence in TB occurred in the late 1980s and early 1990s. Deterioration of the TB program infrastructure, the HIV/AIDS epidemic, drug-resistant TB, and, less so, TB among foreign-born persons contributed to the resurgence. After its peak in 1992, the incidence has been decreasing.[157] Worldwide, TB continues to be a major health problem. There were an estimated 8.3 million new TB cases in 2000 and an estimated 1.8 million deaths from TB. TB is still on the top 10 list for all-cause, all-age worldwide mortality.[158,159]

Due to novel genetic markers, there are now five closely related mycobacteria grouped in the *M. tuberculosis* complex: *M. tuberculosis, M. bovis, M. africanum, M. microti,* and *M. canetti*.[161] *M. tuberculosis* is transmitted through the airborne route and there are no known animal reservoirs. *M. bovis* may penetrate the gastrointestinal mucosa or invade the lymphatic tissue of the oropharynx when ingested in milk containing large numbers of organisms. Human infection with *M. bovis* has decreased significantly in developed countries as a result of the pasteurization of milk and effective TB control programs for cattle. Airborne transmission of both *M. bovis* and *M. africanum* can also occur.

M. tuberculosis is a rod-shaped, slow-growing bacterium. Its cell wall has high acid content, which makes it hydrophobic, or resistant to oral fluids. The cell wall absorbs a certain dye and maintains a red color despite attempts at decolorization, hence the name acid-fast bacillus. TB is spread from person to person through the air by droplet nuclei, particles 1 to 5 μm in diameter that contain *M. tuberculosis* complex. Droplet nuclei are produced when persons with pulmonary or laryngeal TB cough, sneeze, speak, or sing. A single cough can generate 3000 infective droplets. They may also be produced by aerosol treatments, sputum induction, aerosolization during bronchoscopy, and through manipulation of lesions or processing of tissue or secretions in the hospital or laboratory. Droplet nuclei, containing two to three *M. tuberculosis* organisms, are so small that air currents normally present in any indoor space can keep them airborne for long periods of time.[161] Droplet nuclei are small enough to reach the alveoli within the lungs, where the organisms replicate. Four factors determine the likelihood of transmission of *M. tuberculosis*: (1) the number of organisms being expelled into the air, (2) the concentration of organisms in the air as determined by the volume of the space and its ventilation, (3) the length of time an exposed person breathes the contaminated air, and (4) presumably the immune status of the exposed individual.[162]

After inhalation, the droplet nucleus is carried down the bronchial tree and implants in a respiratory bronchiole or alveolus. Whether or not an inhaled tubercle bacillus establishes an infection in the lung depends on both the bacterial virulence and the inherent microbicidal ability of the alveolar macrophage that ingests it. If the bacillus is able to survive initial defenses, it can multiply within the alveolar macrophage. *M. tuberculosis* has no known endotoxins or exotoxins; therefore there is no immediate host response to infection. The organisms grow for 2 to 12 weeks, until they reach 10^3 to 10^4 in number, which is sufficient to elicit a cellular immune response that can be detected by a reaction to the tuberculin skin test.[163] Before the development of cellular immunity, tubercle bacilli spread via the lymphatics to the hilar lymph nodes and thence through the bloodstream to more distant sites.

In persons with intact cell-mediated immunity, collections of activated T cells and macrophages form granulomas that limit multiplication and spread of the organism. Antibodies against *M. tuberculosis* are formed but do not appear to be protective. The organisms tend to be localized in the center of the granuloma, which is often necrotic.[164] For the majority of individuals with normal immune function, the proliferation of *M. tuberculosis* is arrested once cell-mediated immunity develops, even though small numbers of viable bacilli may remain within the granuloma. It is estimated that approximately 10 percent of individuals who acquire TB infection and are not given preventive therapy will develop active TB. The risk is highest in the first 2 years after infection, when half the cases will occur.[165] The ability of the host to respond to the organism may be reduced by certain diseases such as silicosis, diabetes mellitus, and diseases associated with immunosuppression (e.g., HIV infection) as well as by corticosteroids and other immunosuppressive drugs.

Clinical presentation

TB inoculation can result in latent infection or active disease. Depending on the population, 10 to 30 percent of inoculated individuals progress directly to active primary disease. More commonly, however, TB inoculation results in an asymptomatic latent infection. Purified protein derivative (PPD) skin test conversion and identification of a Ghon complex (characterized by a peripheral lesion with associated hilar adenopathy) on chest radiography are the only means of identifying such cases. Patients often remain healthy for years; however, some experience reactivation of their disease due to subsequent immunologic stressors. Reactivated TB represents 90 percent of adult cases in the non-HIV-infected population and results from reactivation of a previously dormant focus seeded at the time of the primary infection. The apical posterior segments of the lung are frequently involved. Such reactivation occurs at a rate of approximately 1 percent per year in immunocompetent hosts. In immunocompromised hosts, the conversion rate increases to 10 percent. Roughly 80 percent of TB cases involve pulmonary disease, although TB can involve any organ system. In patients who are severely immunocompromised, extrapulmonary disease and atypical presentations are common.

Cough is the most common symptom of pulmonary TB. Early in the course of the illness it may be nonproductive, but subsequently, as inflammation and tissue necrosis ensue, sputum is usually produced and is key to most diagnostic methods. Fever, night sweats, anorexia, and weight loss are other classic symptoms. Hemoptysis may rarely be a presenting symptom but is usually the result of previous disease and does not necessarily indicate active TB. Hemoptysis may result from residual tuberculous bronchiectasis, caseous sloughing or endobronchial erosion, rupture of a dilated vessel in the wall of a cavity (Rasmussen's aneurysm), bacterial or fungal infection (especially *Aspergillus* in the form of a mycetoma) in a residual cavity, or from erosion of calcified lesions into the lumen of an airway (broncholithiasis). Inflammation of the lung parenchyma adjacent to a pleural surface may cause pleuritic pain. Dyspnea can occur when patients have extensive parenchymal involvement, pleural effusions, or a pneumothorax. TB may also cause severe respiratory failure, which often leads to death.[166]

Overall, the symptoms in reactivated TB typically begin insidiously and are present for weeks or months before the diagnosis is made. It is noteworthy that classic symptoms are usually absent, especially in the elderly and immunocompromised patients.

Physical findings in pulmonary TB are not generally helpful in defining the disease. Rales may be heard in the area of involvement, as well as bronchial breath sounds if there is lung consolidation. Other nonspecific findings include cachexia, hypoxia, tachycardia, and lymphadenopathy.

Diagnosis

Early identification and diagnosis of cases of active TB is key to the effectiveness of control programs. However, maintaining a high index of suspicion for TB is crucial, and diagnostic testing remains problematic. Culture of appropriate specimens for isolation of *M. tuberculosis* and susceptibility testing is the cornerstone for a diagnosis of TB, but the organism still requires weeks to grow in culture.

Pulmonary TB is diagnosed by visualization of acid-fast bacilli on a sputum smear and isolation of the organism from a culture of this sputum. Most laboratories use auramine-rhodamine or auramine O to stain the sputum, allowing scanning for fluorescence as opposed to Ziehl-Neelsen stain, which requires more time and labor to identify organisms.[162] Concentrating sputum specimens and obtaining a larger quantity of sputum (5 mL) have both been shown to increase the probability of visualizing organisms by smear. The conventional teaching is that sputum specimens should be obtained on 3 consecutive days and that first morning specimens have the highest yield. If the patient has difficulty producing sputum, inhalation of an aerosol of sterile hypertonic saline, usually produced by an ultrasonic nebulizer, can be used to stimulate the production of sputum.[170] Multiple samples increase the diagnostic yield of the test. For patients in whom a diagnosis of TB has not been established from sputum, fiberoptic bronchoscopy performed with appropriate infection control precautions may be needed with BAL. Gastric aspirates obtained in the morning can also be cultured for *M. tuberculosis* and reflect sputum swallowed over the course of the night. It is helpful in patients who cannot produce enough sputum even with induction, especially children. The disadvantage is that AFB smears cannot be done on gastric aspirates. Urine, blood, CSF, and other body fluids can also be obtained for culture. Invasive procedures to obtain specimens from the lung, pericardium, lymph nodes, and so on should be considered when noninvasive techniques do not provide a diagnosis. Many of these areas are amenable to closed techniques such as percutaneous needle biopsy or aspiration, transbronchial biopsy, or brushing, precluding a need for formal surgical procedures. In patients with hematogenous or disseminated disease, bone marrow biopsy, lung biopsy, and liver biopsy for histologic examination and culture should be considered. Appropriate measures must be taken in collecting these specimens to minimize aerosolation of *M. tuberculosis* organisms and prevent transmission of infection to personnel. Maintenance of laboratory proficiency requires continuing and frequent performance of the required tests. Adequate training in proper techniques and the availability of special containment areas are required for the safe manipulation of clinical specimens.

The tuberculin test is based on the fact that infection with *M. tuberculosis* produces a delayed-type hypersensitivity reaction to certain antigenic components of the organism that are contained in extracts of culture filtrates or "tuberculins." Tuberculin skin testing using 5 units (0.1 mL) of PPD injected intradermally (Mantoux method), usually into the volar or dorsal surface of the forearm, may be used for screening or to supplement other diagnostic testing. Induration, not erythema, is measured 48 to 72 h after injection. Tests read after 72 h tend to underestimate the true size of induration. On the basis of the sensitivity, specificity, and the prevalence of TB in different groups, three cut points have been recommended for defining a positive tuberculin reaction (Table 3-5).[162] Overall, skin testing for TB serves mainly as an epidemiologic tool to assess exposures. Patients with positive reactions may not have active TB, and 20 to 30 percent of those with a new diagnosis of active TB have negative reactions, particularly those with advanced disease.[171] Testing is also unreliable in infants, patients with immunosuppressive conditions, and those with serious illnesses.[172] There is no reliable method of distinguishing tuberculin reactions caused by vaccination with bacillus Calmette-Guérin (BCG) from those caused by natural mycobacterial infections. It is usually prudent to consider "positive" reactions to 5 tuberculin units of PPD in BCG-vaccinated persons as indicating infection with *M. tuberculosis.* Because most persons who have received BCG are from high-prevalence areas of the world, it is important that vaccinated persons who have a positive reaction to a tuberculin skin test be evaluated for TB and treated accordingly.[173]

Nucleic acid amplification tests, such as the polymerase chain reaction (PCR) and other methods for amplifying DNA and RNA, may facilitate rapid detection of microorganisms. These technologies allow for the amplification of specific target sequences of nucleic acids that can then be detected through the use of a nucleic acid probe. Both RNA and DNA amplification systems are commercially available.[174] In clinical respiratory specimens that are AFB smear–positive, the sensitivity of the amplification methods is approximately 95 percent, with a specificity of 98 percent. In specimens that contain fewer organisms and are AFB smear–negative, the nucleic acid amplification test is positive in 48 to 53 percent of patients with culture-positive TB and the specificity remains approximately 95 percent.[175] Thus, the CDC includes a positive nucleic acid amplification test in the setting of a positive smear as confirmation of the diagnosis of TB.[176]

Radiographic findings in TB depend on the stage of the infection. Primary pulmonary TB (primary exposure) is characterized by the Ghon complex and consists of (1) a subpleural (fissure) focus of inflammation and (2) infected (inflamed) lymph nodes draining the primary subpleural lesion, which manifests as ipsilateral hilar adenopathy (Fig. 3-9). Atelectasis may result from the compression of airways by enlarged lymph nodes. Overall, intrathoracic adenopathy is less common in immunocompetent adults than in children and immunosuppressed patients. Cavitation may occur in progressive primary TB if the process persists beyond the time when specific cell-mediated immunity develops.[177] Cavitation

Table 3-5 Guidelines for determining a positive tuberculin skin test reaction[a]

Induration ≥ 5 mm	Induration ≥ 10 mm	Induration ≥ 15 mm
HIV-positive persons	Recent arrivals (< 5 years) from high-prevalence countries	Persons with no risk factors for TB
Recent contacts of TB case	Injection drug users Residents and employees[a] of high-risk congregate settings: prisons and jails, nursing homes and other health-care facilities, residential facilities for AIDS patients, and homeless shelters Mycobacteriology laboratory personnel	
Fibrotic changes on chest radiograph consistent with old TB	Persons with clinical conditions that place them at high risk: silicosis diabetes mellitus, chronic renal failure, some hematologic disorders (e.g., leukemias and lymphomas), other specific malignancies (e.g., carcinoma of the head or neck and lung), weight loss of > 10% of ideal body weight, gastrectomy, jejunoileal bypass	
Patients with organ transplants and other immunosuppressed patients (receiving the equivalent of > 15 mg/day prednisone for > 1 month)	Children < 4 years of age or infants, children, and adolescents exposed to adults in high-risk categories	

[a]For persons who are otherwise at low risk and are tested at entry into employment, a reaction of > 15 mm induration is considered positive.
Source: From the American Thoracic Society and the Centers for Disease Control and Prevention, 2000.[162] With permission.

is more common in reactivation (secondary) TB. In this form, the most frequent sites of abnormalities are the apical and posterior segments of the right upper lobe and the apical-posterior segment of the left upper lobe. These lesions correspond pathologically with caseating granulomas. Miliary TB results from erosion of a parenchymal focus of TB into the blood or lymph vessel, leading to dissemination of the organism.[162] This results in evenly distributed small nodules on chest film (Fig. 3-10). Healing of the tuberculous lesions usually results in the development of fibrosis with loss of lung parenchymal volume and, often, calcification. Nodules and fibrotic lesions of old healed TB have well-demarcated, sharp margins and are often described as "hard." Old TB can also cause pleural scarring. Bronchiectasis of the upper lobes is a nonspecific finding that sometimes occurs from previous pulmonary TB.

Notably, patients with endobronchial lesions and those who are immunosuppressed may have no associated abnormalities on chest x-ray. In patients with HIV infection, the nature of the radiographic findings depends to a certain extent on the degree of immunocompromise produced by the HIV infection. TB that occurs relatively early in the course of HIV infection tends to have the typical radiographic findings described above. With more advanced HIV disease, the radiographic findings become more "atypical": cavitation is uncommon, and lower-lung-zone or diffuse infiltrates and intrathoracic adenopathy are frequent.[178]

CT scanning is more sensitive than plain chest radiography for diagnosis, particularly for smaller lesions located in the apex of the lung.[179] CT scan may show a cavity

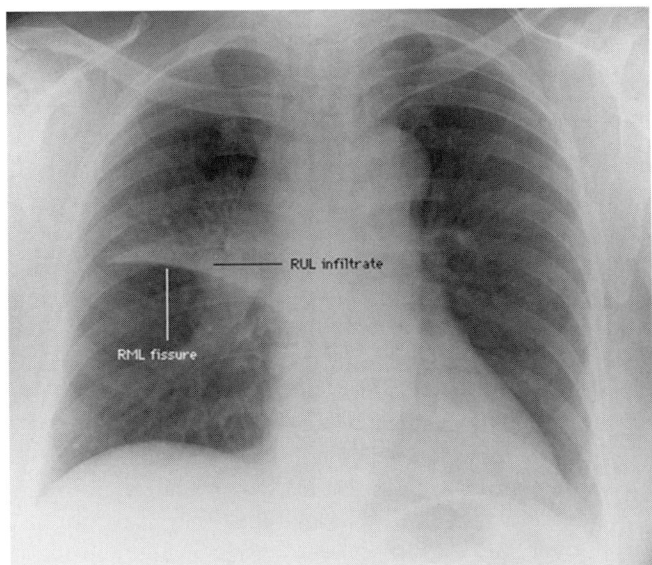

Figure 3-9 Posteroanterior chest x-ray of a patient with tuberculosis. The combination of right-upper-lobe infiltrate and hilar adenopathy should raise suspicion of tuberculosis as the potential infectious agent. RML = right middle lobe; RUL = right upper lobe.

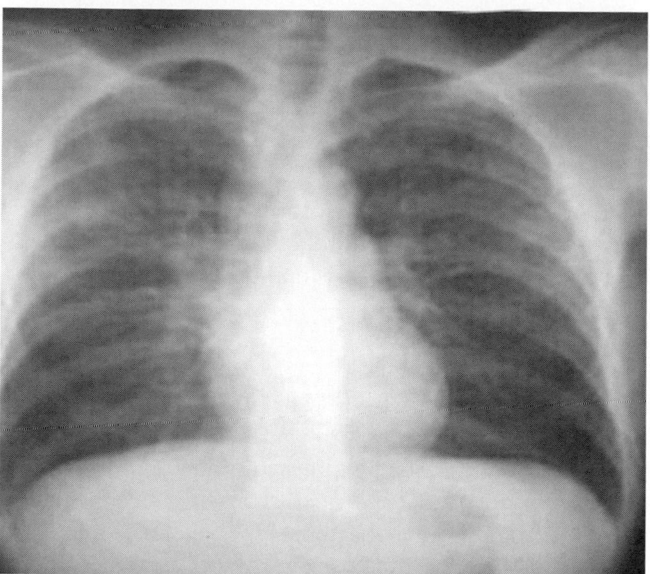

Figure 3-10 Chest x-ray of a patient with miliary tuberculosis.

(Fig. 3-11), centrilobular lesions, nodules, and branching linear densities sometimes called a "tree in bud" appearance.

Medical treatment

The overall goals for treatment of TB are (1) to cure the individual patient and (2) to minimize the transmission of *M. tuberculosis* to other persons. It is necessary to isolate any patient with suspected TB infection in a private room with negative pressure. Anyone entering should wear high-efficiency disposable masks sufficient to filter the TB bacillus. Isolation should be continued until sputum smears return negative results three consecutive times. Such sterilization usually requires 2 to 4 weeks of treatment and must be accompanied by clinical improvement.[181]

There are currently four broadly applicable recommended regimens for treating patients with TB caused by drug-susceptible organisms. Each regimen has an initial phase of 2 months followed by a choice of several options for the continuation phase of either 4 or 7 months. The initial phase is usually composed of different three- or four-drug combinations of isoniazid, rifampin, ethambutol, and pyrazinamide. The continuation phase is usually a combination of isoniazid and rifampin or rifapentin. Rifapentin is a rifampin with an increased half-life and enhanced activity against *M. tuberculosis.* Complete information can be found in the 2003 statement from the American Thoracic Society (ATS), the Centers for Disease Control and Prevention (CDC), and the Infectious Diseases Society of America (IDSA) on the treatment of TB.[182] This document contains details of specific drug therapy, including suggestions relating to monitoring for adequate response to therapy and details of monitoring for drug toxicity. Special treatment situations, including HIV infection, TB in children, extrapulmonary TB, culture-negative TB, pregnancy and breast-feeding, hepatic disease, and renal disease are discussed in detail. The use of less commonly employed antituberculous drugs for multidrug-resistant TB is also discussed.

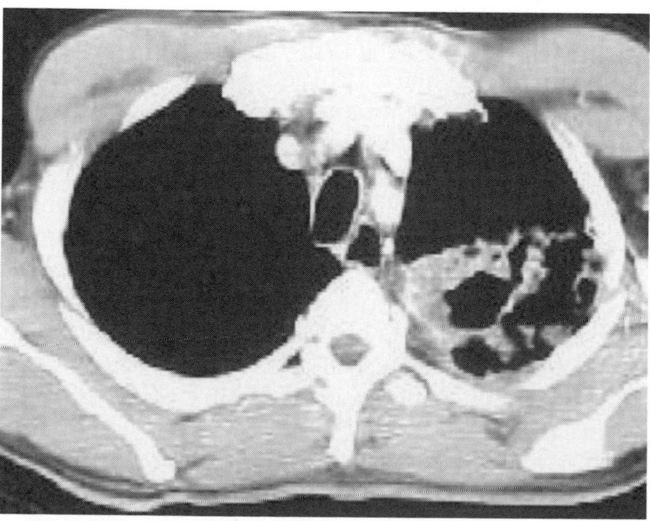

Figure 3-11 Chest CT of a patient with cavitary pulmonary tuberculosis involving the left upper lung.

Surgical treatment

Surgery has largely been supplanted by medical therapy for the treatment of pulmonary TB infection. This resulted mainly from the introduction of effective antibiotics in the 1960s. With the emergence of multidrug-resistant TB (MDR-TB), surgery is again becoming a necessary treatment modality. In destroyed lungs, cavitary disease, and patients with advanced disease, medications are often unable to penetrate the lesions. In the setting of such permanent anatomic changes, medical therapy alone has a very high failure rate; the addition of surgery with removal of the nidus of infection improves the cure rate.[183]

Contemporary indications for surgery in patients infected with *M. tuberculosis* include:

- Surgery for diagnosis of pulmonary lesions or mediastinal adenopathy of unknown etiology
- Highly resistant *M. tuberculosis* with localized disease
- Persistent cavitary disease
- Continued sputum positivity
- Destroyed lobe or lung (lung gangrene)
- Massive hemoptysis
- Bronchopleural fistula with failed tube thoracostomy
- Bronchial stenosis
- Aspergillosis complicating treatment

- Infections with mycobacteria other than tubercle bacilli
- Complications resulting from previous or insufficient surgery (e.g., delayed complications of plombage)

Excisions (segmentectomies, lobectomies, pneumonectomies) currently represent the majority of operations, followed by operations on the pleura (decortication) and rarely those on the thoracic wall (thoracoplasty, parietectomy). The basic principles remain unchanged: best available drug therapy, followed by resection of residual active foci of disease, accompanied by obliteration of abnormal pleural spaces, followed by best available drug therapy. Pomerantz et al.[184] recently reported a large series of pulmonary resection for MDR-TB. During a 17-year period, 172 patients underwent 180 pulmonary resections, which included 98 lobectomies and 82 pneumonectomies, with an acceptable operative mortality of 3.3 percent; late mortality was 6.8 percent. Significant morbidity was 12 percent. Muscle flaps were frequently used to avoid residual space and bronchial stump problems. The authors concluded that surgery remains an important adjunct to medical therapy for the treatment of MDR-TB. In the setting of localized disease, persistent sputum positivity, or patient intolerance of medical therapy, pulmonary resection should be undertaken. Other recent reports support these conclusions.[185–187]

Appropriate preoperative preparation of these patients is important. When feasible, attempts should be made to convert the patient's sputum to negative. Except in cases of emergency, such as massive hemoptysis, patients should receive at least 3 months of therapy prior to surgical consideration. Pulmonary function tests should be performed to assess the feasibility of resection, as well as CT scan of the chest to determine the extent of involvement of the lungs by the disease and to evaluate anatomic changes. Ventilation/perfusion scanning provides the important information about the amount of viable lung; if only 15 percent or less of lung tissue will remain after resection, then pneumonectomy of that lung is indicated. The nutritional status of the patient and pulmonary hygiene should also be improved prior to surgery. Bronchoscopy is essential to evaluate for tuberculous endobronchial disease and help avoid the serious postoperative complication of bronchopleural fistula. This is more likely to occur when bronchial closure encompasses an area involved by tuberculous bronchitis.

The role of surgery is to remove all gross disease, by ensuring resection of all cavitary disease as well as destroyed lung. Double-lumen endotracheal tube or bronchial blocker is essential not only to deflate the lung but also to avoid contamination of the contralateral lung. Contamination of the pleural space should be avoided when pneumonectomy is required. Complications can be minimized and an acceptable mortality rate can be achieved with an extrapleural approach supplemented by muscle flap or omentum for reinforcement of the bronchial stump.[188] Muscle flaps have been used for patients who still have positive sputum at the time of surgery, presence of bronchopleural fistula, if there is polymicrobial contamination, or if there is a need to fill space after lobectomy.[189]

Even with successful resection of pulmonary lesions due to TB, 12 to 24 additional months of chemotherapy, using drugs to which there is demonstrated susceptibility, should be given.[182]

ATYPICAL MYCOBACTERIAL INFECTIONS

There is continued growth in the number and prevalence of mycobacteria species other than the *M. tuberculosis* complex. These mycobacterial species are collectively referred to as the nontuberculous mycobacteria (NTM).[190] The most common cause of NTM pulmonary disease is *M. avium* complex (*M. avium* and *M. intracellulare*), known as MAC complex, *M. kansasii, M. abscessus, and M. fortuitum*. Other NTM (for example, *M. malmoence, M. simiae, M. szulgai, M. xenopi*) have been identified as causative agents of this disease with much lesser frequency. *M. kansasii* is the most common atypical mycobacterium in the central United States, whereas MAC is the most common in the South and Southeast.[191] NTM disease is not reportable in the United States; therefore reliable estimates of its incidence or prevalence have been limited. A CDC study from 1991 to 1992, which included results from 33 state laboratories, demonstrated that there were more isolates of *M. avium* complex than *M. tuberculosis*, with the latter representing only 26 percent of the total mycobacterial isolates. The reasons for this dramatic increase in numbers for NTM is unknown, but better clinical recognition and more culturing for both pulmonary and disseminated disease are felt to play important roles.[192] It is well documented that the reservoir for most of these infections is soil, natural waters, and aerosols created from these sources.[193] In addition, tap water, ice prepared from tap water, processed tap water for dialysis, and swimming pools can also be a source of infection with NTM. Much remains to be understood about the pathogenesis of NTM infection and disease in humans. Epidemiologic studies, skin test surveys, and, more recently, DNA fingerprinting studies suggest that person-to-person transmission of infection is rare. It is assumed that most persons are infected from environmental sources, by airborne mechanisms (especially in respiratory disease), and for some situations possibly via the gastrointestinal route.

Infections caused by NTM may take place without any obvious predisposing conditions. Coexisting medical conditions that increase the risk for developing an infection include HIV/AIDS, cystic fibrosis, diabetes mellitus, malignancy, dialysis, tissue/organ transplant, smoking,

COPD, bronchiectasis, silicosis and other pneumoconiosis, and previous TB. There is higher prevalence of NTM infections in warm climate regions, with high rates among miners. Demographically, females in the sixth decade of life or later are considered the most vulnerable to NTM infections, especially pulmonary infection with *M. avium*.

Clinical manifestations

The clinical manifestation of NTM, especially in HIV-negative patients, can be very similar to those of TB. Signs and symptoms of NTM pulmonary disease are variable and nonspecific. They include chronic cough, sputum production, and fatigue. Less commonly, malaise, dyspnea, fever, hemoptysis, and weight loss can also occur, usually with advanced NTM disease. Pulmonary disease due to *M. avium* complex in HIV-negative patients may have two types of presentations, as clarified in the recent American Thoracic Society (ATS) statement.[190] One is an apical fibrocavitary disease that has a tendency to progress within 1 to 2 years if the patient does not receive antimicrobial therapy. The other type is a bilateral or isolated right-middle-lobe/lingular nodular and interstitial/nodular disease, with a much slower progression within a period of 5 to 10 years. In addition, some authors identify "atypical manifestations" of this disease; namely, the combination of bronchiectasis and small nodules (so-called Lady Windermere syndrome) and focal mass-like opacities. In immunocompromised patients, specifically AIDS patients, MAC is the most common bacterial complication.[194] Disseminated disease is frequent, with manifestations such as hepatomegaly, diarrhea, splenomegaly, and abdominal pain.

M. kansasii causes lung disease that is clinically indistinguishable from TB. Symptoms may be less severe and more chronic compared to infection with *M. tuberculosis*. Asymptomatic infection may also occur. Rapidly growing mycobacteria include three clinically relevant species: *M. fortuitum, M. chelonae,* and *M. abscessus*. Pulmonary disease due to rapidly growing mycobacteria is predominantly due to *M. abscessus*. It has a progressive and slow course that can cause death if left untreated.

Diagnosis

As recommended in the ATS statement, the diagnosis of pulmonary NTM disease should be based on an integrated assessment of clinical manifestations, radiographic findings, and laboratory data. These organisms are commonly found in nature, and contamination of culture material or transient infection does occur. Thus a single positive culture from sputum is insufficient for diagnosis but sufficient if the organism is isolated from a transbronchial or lung biopsy specimen as well as from a bronchial wash with high bacterial contents by either or both a smear and culture. To meet the current requirements for the diagnosis, examination of three separate sputum specimens should produce at least two positive cultures, with the third being at least smear-positive, or three positive cultures even from smear-negative specimens.[190]

Radiographically, NTM tend to cause thin-walled cavities with less surrounding parenchymal infiltrate; they are associated with less bronchogenic but more contiguous spread of disease; and they produce more marked involvement of pleura over the involved areas of the lungs. Occasionally, they may produce dense pneumonic disease or a solitary pulmonary nodule without cavitation. Basal pleural disease is not often found and pleural effusion is rare. Recent studies with high-resolution computed tomography (HRCT) of the chest have shown that up to 90 percent of patients with mid- and lower-lung-field noncavitary disease with *M. avium* complex have associated multifocal bronchiectasis, with many patients having clusters of small (< 5 mm) nodules in associated areas of the lung.[195] In the case of rapidly growing mycobacteria, radiology usually shows multilobar or predominantly upper-lobe infiltrates. They can be of patchy, reticulonodular, or mixed interstitial-alveolar type. Cavitation takes place in about 15 percent of patients.[196]

Medical treatment

Medical treatment of MAC pulmonary disease has historically been frustrating and disappointing. Most first-line anti-TB drugs have 10 to 100 times less in vitro activity against *M. avium* complex isolates than against *M. tuberculosis*. This diminished activity may be due to the lipophilic cell wall of *M. avium* complex, which prevents drug penetration. Clarithromycin and azithromycin have been found to be the most effective drugs in therapy of infections caused by *M. avium* complex and some other NTM, either pulmonary or disseminated (for example in patients with AIDS).[196] The three-drug regimen of clarithromycin, ethambutol, and rifabutin appears to be the most promising in the therapy of the disseminated *M. avium* infection in AIDS patients.

The current recommendation for the treatment of pulmonary disease caused by *M. kansasii* in adults is the regimen of isoniazid, rifampin, and ethambutol given daily for 18 months with at least 12 months of negative sputum cultures. In patients who are unable to tolerate one of these three drugs, clarithromycin would seem a reasonable alternative. Pyrazinamide is unacceptable as an alternate or third drug for *M. kansasii* because all isolates are resistant.[190] The treatment of lung disease due to the rapidly growing mycobacteria is generally difficult because of their resistance to virtually all antimycobacterial drugs.[196] *M. fortuitum* is usually susceptible to other oral antimicrobial agents including the newer macrolides (clarithromycin and azithromycin) and quinolones, doxycycline and minocycline, and sulfonamides. Combination therapy of low-dose amikacin plus high-dose cefoxitin for 2 to 4 weeks almost invariably produces clinical and microbiologic improvement in *M. abscessus* infection. Imipenem appears to be a reasonable alternative to cefoxitin.

Surgical treatment

For patients with MAC, if there has been poor response to drug therapy or if the patient's isolate has become macrolide-resistant, resectional surgery should be considered, especially if the disease is localized. Recent series even in the era of macrolide therapy have shown high sputum-negative conversion rates after surgery, although with relatively high morbidity.[197,198] There is a high incidence of bronchopleural fistula even with the use of a pedicle flap closure, especially after right pneumonectomy in patients with MAC.[199] Some advocate early surgical intervention to improve outcomes.[200] Whenever possible, this surgery should be performed at centers with thoracic surgeons who have considerable experience with this type of surgery. Overall, the bilateral nature of MAC lung disease, the advanced age of the patients, and the frequency of underlying chronic lung disease have limited the number of patients who are good candidates for surgery. With the advent of rifampin containing regimens, surgery is now considered to have no role in managing routine cases of pulmonary disease due to *M. kansasii*.

For the rapidly growing mycobacteria, surgery is generally indicated with extensive disease, abscess formation, or in instances where drug therapy is difficult. Surgical resection for limited disease related to prior localized lung disease can also be curative especially in infections due to *M. abscessus*.

References

1. Bartlett JG, Dowell SF, Mandell LA, et al. Practice guidelines for the management of community-acquired pneumonia in adults. *Clin Infect Dis* 2000; 31:347–382.
2. National Vital Statistics Report. 53: Death and percentage of total deaths for the 10 leading causes of death, by race: United States, 2002. Centers for Disease Control and Prevention 2005:9.
3. DeFrances CJ, Hall MJ, Podgornik MN. 2003 National Hospital Discharge Survey. Advance data from vital and health statistics 2005;359:1–20.
4. Fine MJ, Smith MA, Carson CA, et al. Prognosis and outcomes of patients with community-acquired pneumonia. *JAMA* 1996;275:134–141.
5. Niederman MS, Mandell LA, Anzueto A, et al. American Thoracic Society. Guidelines for the management of adults with community-acquired pneumonia. Diagnosis, assessment of severity, antimicrobial therapy, and prevention. *Am J Respir Crit Care Med* 2001;163: 1730–1754.
6. Apisarnthanarak A, Mundy LM. Etiology of community-acquired pneumonia. *Clin Chest Med* 2005;26:47–55.
7. Marston BJ, Plouffe JF, File TM, et al. Incidence of community-acquired pneumonia requiring hospitalizations: Results of a population-based active surveillance study in Ohio. Community-Based Pneumonia Incidence Study Group. *Arch Intern Med* 1997;157: 1709–1718.
8. Wipf JE, Lipsky BA, Hirschmann JV, et al. Diagnosing pneumonia by physical examination: Relevant or relic? *Arch Intern Med* 1999;159:1082–1087.
9. Metlay JP, Kapoor WN, Fine MJ. Does this patient have community-acquired pneumonia? Diagnosing pneumonia by history and physical examination. *JAMA* 1997; 278:1440–1445.
10. Katz DS, Leung AN. Radiology of pneumonia. *Clin Chest Med* 1999;20:549–562.
11. Bartlett JG, Mundy LM. Community-acquired pneumonia. *N Engl J Med* 1995;333:1618–1624.
12. File TM. Community-acquired pneumonia. *Lancet* 2003; 362:1991–2001.
13. Meehan TP, Fine MJ, Krumholz HM, et al. Quality of care, process, and outcomes in elderly patients with pneumonia. *JAMA* 1997;278:2080–2084.
14. Tablan OC, Anderson LJ, Besser R, et al. Healthcare Infection Control Practices Advisory Committee, Centers for Disease Control and Prevention. Guidelines for preventing health-care–associated pneumonia, 2003: Recommendations of the CDC and the Healthcare Infection Control Practices Advisory Committee. *MMWR Recomm Rep* 2004;53:1–36.
15. Richards MJ, Edwards JR, Culver DH, et al. Nosocomial infections in combined medical-surgical intensive care units in the United States. *Infect Control Hosp Epidemiol* 2000;21:510–515.
16. Wunderink RG. Nosocomial pneumonia, including ventilator-associated pneumonia. *Proc Am Thorac Soc* 2005;2: 440–444.
17. American Thoracic Society; Infectious Diseases Society of America. Guidelines for the management of adults with hospital-acquired, ventilator-associated, and healthcare-associated pneumonia. *Am J Respir Crit Care Med* 2005; 171:388–416.
18. Lynch JP III. Hospital-acquired pneumonia: Risk factors, microbiology, and treatment. *Chest* 2001;119:373S–384S.
19. Intensive Care Antimicrobial Resistance Epidemiology (ICARE) Surveillance Report, data summary from January 1996 through December 1997: A report from the National Nosocomial Infections Surveillance (NNIS) System. *Am J Infect Control* 1999;27:279–284.
20. Chastre J, Fagon JY. Ventilator-associated pneumonia. *Am J Respir Crit Care Med* 2002;165:867–903.
21. de Jaeger A, Litalien C, Lacroix J, et al. Protected specimen brush or bronchoalveolar lavage to diagnose bacterial

nosocomial pneumonia in ventilated adults: A meta-analysis. *Crit Care Med* 1999;27:2548–2560.
22. Kollef MH, Sherman G, Ward S, et al. Inadequate antimicrobial treatment of infections: A risk factor for hospital mortality among critically ill patients. *Chest* 1999;115:462–474.
23. Marik PE. Aspiration pneumonitis and aspiration pneumonia. *N Engl J Med* 2001;344:665–671.
24. Smulders K, van der HH, Weers-Pothoff I, et al. A randomized clinical trial of intermittent subglottic secretion drainage in patients receiving mechanical ventilation. *Chest* 2002;121:858–862.
25. Mahul P, Auboyer C, Jospe R, et al. Prevention of nosocomial pneumonia in intubated patients: Respective role of mechanical subglottic secretions drainage and stress ulcer prophylaxis. *Intens Care Med* 1992;18:205.
26. Torres A, Serra-Batlles J, Ros E, et al. Pulmonary aspiration of gastric contents in patients receiving mechanical ventilation: The effect of body position. *Ann Intern Med* 1992;116:540–543.
27. Orozco-Levi M, Torres A, Ferrer M, et al. Semirecumbent position protects from pulmonary aspiration but not completely from gastroesophageal reflux in mechanically ventilated patients. *Am J Respir Crit Care Med* 1995; 152:1387–1390.
28. Gonzalez CCL, Calia FM. Bacteriologic flora of aspiration-induced pulmonary infections. *Arch Intern Med* 1975;135:711–714.
29. Bartlett JG, Gorbach SL, Finegold SM. The bacteriology of aspiration pneumonia. *Am J Med* 1974;56:202–207.
30. Bartlett JG. Anaerobic bacteria: General concepts. In: Mandell GL, Douglas RG, Bennett JE (eds). *Principles and practice of Infectious Diseases,* 3d ed. New York: Churchill Livingstone, 1990:1828–1842.
31. Marik PE, Careau P. The role of anaerobes in patients with ventilator-associated pneumonia and aspiration pneumonia: A prospective study. *Chest* 1999;115: 178–183.
32. Allewelt M, Schuler P, Bolcskei PL, et al. Ampicillin + sulbactam vs clindamycin +/− cephalosporin for the treatment of aspiration pneumonia and primary lung abscess. *Clin Microbiol Infect* 2004;10:163–170.
33. Rano A, Agusti C, Sibila O, et al. Pulmonary infections in non-HIV-immunocompromised patients. *Curr Opin Pulm Med* 2005;11:213–217.
34. Agusti C, Rano A, Filella X, et al. Pulmonary infiltrates in patients receiving long-term glucocorticoid treatment: Etiology, prognostic factors, and associated inflammatory response. *Chest* 2003;123:488–498.
35. Husain S, McCurry K, Dauber J, et al. Nocardia infection in lung transplant recipients. *J Heart Lung Transplant* 2002;21:354–359.
36. El-Ebiary M, Sarmiento X, Torres A, et al. Prognostic factors of severe *Legionella* pneumonia requiring admission to ICU. *Am J Respir Crit Care Med* 1997;156:1467–1472.
37. Shlobin OA, Dropulic LK, Orens JB, et al. Mediastinal mass due to *Aspergillus fumigatus* after lung transplantation: A case report. *J Heart Lung Transplant* 2005;24:1991–1994.
38. Garbino J, Gerbase MW, Wunderli W, et al. Lower respiratory viral illnesses: Improved diagnosis by molecular methods and clinical impact. *Am J Respir Crit Care Med* 2004;170:1197–1203.
39. Queipo JA, Broseta E, Santos M, et al. Mycobacterial infection in a series of 1261 renal transplant recipients. *Clin Microbiol Infect* 2003;9:518–525.
40. Pagano L, Fianchi L, Mele L, et al. *Pneumocystis carinii* pneumonia in patients with malignant haematological diseases: 10 years' experience of infection in GIMEMA centres. *Br J Haematol* 2002;117:379–386.
41. Bartlett JG. Lung abscess and necrotizing pneumonia. In: *Infectious Diseases.* Philadelphia: Saunders, 1992.
42. Mwandumba HC, Beeching NJ. Pyogenic lung infections: Factors for predicting clinical outcome of lung abscess and thoracic empyema. *Curr Opin Pulm Med* 2000;6:234–239.
43. Bartlett JG. Anaerobic bacterial infections of the lung and pleural space. *Clin Infect Dis* 1993;16:248–255.
44. Bartlett JG. The role of anaerobic bacteria in lung abscess. *Clin Infect Dis* 2005;40:923–925.
45. Riordan T, Wilson M. Lemierre's syndrome: More than a historical curiosa. *Postgrad Med J* 2004;80:328–334.
46. Tsao TC, Tsai YH, Lan RS, et al. Pulmonary manifestations of *Staphylococcus aureus* septicemia. *Chest* 1992;10:574–576.
47. Williford ME, Godwin JD. Computed tomography of lung abscess and empyema. *Radiol Clin North Am* 1983;21:575–583.
48. Gudiol F, Manresa F, Pallares R, et al. Clindamycin vs penicillin for anaerobic lung infections. High rate of penicillin failures associated with penicillin-resistant *Bacteroides melaninogenicus. Arch Intern Med* 1990;150:2525–2529.
49. Landay MJ, Christensen EE, Bynum LJ, et al. Anaerobic pleural and pulmonary infections. *AJR* 1980;134:233.
50. Lambiase RE, Deyoe L, Cronan JJ, et al. Percutaneous drainage of 335 consecutive abscesses: Results of primary drainage with 1-year follow-up. *Radiology* 1992;184: 167–179.
51. vanSonnenberg E, D'Agostino HB, Casola G, et al. Lung abscess: CT-guided drainage. *Radiology* 1991;178: 347–351.
52. Mueller PR, Berlin L. Complications of lung abscess aspiration and drainage. *AJR* 2002;178:1083–1086.
53. Herth F, Ernst A, Becker HD. Endoscopic drainage of lung abscesses: Technique and outcome. *Chest* 2005;127: 1378–1381.
54. Podbielski FJ, Rodriguez HE, Wiesman IM, et al. Pulmonary parenchymal abscess: VATS approach to diagnosis and treatment. *Asian Cardiovasc Thorac Ann* 2001; 9:339–341.
55. Moreschi MA, Fiel SB. An update on bronchiectasis. *Curr Opin Pulm Med* 1995;1:119–124.
56. Barker AF. Bronchiectasis. *N Engl J Med* 2002;346: 1383–1393.
57. Huang JH, Kao PN, Adi V, et al. *Mycobacterium avium-intracellulare* pulmonary infection in HIV-negative patients without preexisting lung disease: Diagnostic and management limitations. *Chest* 1999;115:1033–1040.
58. Cohen M, Sahn SA. Bronchiectasis in systemic diseases. *Chest* 1999;116:1063–1074.
59. Hansell DM. Bronchiectasis. *Radiol Clin North Am* 1998;36:107–128.

60. Munro NC, Cooke JC, Currie DC, et al. Comparison of thin section computed tomography with bronchography for identifying bronchiectatic segments in patients with chronic sputum production. *Thorax* 1990;45:135–139.
61. Ashour M. Hemodynamic alterations in bronchiectasis: A basis for a new subclassification of the disease. *J Thorac Cardiovasc Surg* 1996;112:328–334.
62. Tsang KWT, Chan W-M, Ho P-L, et al. A comparative study on the efficacy of levofloxacin and ceftazidime in acute exacerbation of bronchiectasis. *Eur Respir J* 1999; 14:1206–1209.
63. Al-Kattan KM, Essa MA, Hajjar WM, et al. Surgical results for bronchiectasis based on hemodynamic (functional and morphologic) classification. *J Thorac Cardiovasc Surg* 2005;130:1385–1390.
64. Agasthian T, Deschamps C, Trastek VF, et al. Surgical management of bronchiectasis. *Ann Thorac Surg* 1996; 62:976–978.
65. Balkanli K, Genc O, Dakak M, et al. Surgical management of bronchiectasis: Analysis and short-term results in 238 patients. *Eur J Cardiothorac Surg* 2003;24: 699–702.
66. Barlow CW, Robbins RC, Moon MR, et al. Heart-lung versus double-lung transplantation for suppurative lung disease. *J Thorac Cardiovasc Surg* 2000;119:466–476.
67. Beirne PA, Banner NR, Khaghani A, et al. Lung transplantation for non-cystic fibrosis bronchiectasis: Analysis of a 13-year experience. *J Heart Lung Transplant* 2005; 24:1530–1535.
68. Bennhoff DF. Actinomycosis: Diagnostic and therapeutic considerations and a review of 32 cases. *Laryngoscope* 1984;94:1198–1217.
69. Mabezza GF, MacFarlane J. Pulmonary actinomycosis. *Eur Respir J* 2003;21:545–551.
70. Endo S, Murayama F, Yamaguchi T, et al. Surgical considerations for pulmonary actinomycosis. *Ann Thorac Surg* 2002;74:185–190.
71. Lu MS, Liu HP, Yeh CH, et al. The role of surgery in hemoptysis caused by thoracic actinomycosis, a forgotten disease. *Eur J Cardiothorac Surg* 2003;24:694–698.
72. Hsieh MJ, Liu HP, Chang JP, et al. Thoracic actinomycosis. Chest 1993;104:366–370.
73. Mabeza GF, Macfarlane J. Pulmonary actinomycosis. *Eur Respir J* 2003;21:545–551.
74. Filice GA. Nocardiosis in persons with human immunodeficiency virus infection, transplant recipients, and large, geographically defined populations. *J Lab Clin Med* 2005;145:156–162.
75. Lerner PI. Nocardiosis. *Clin Infect Dis* 1996;22: 891–903.
76. Chapman SW, Wilson JP. Nocardiosis in transplant recipients. *Semin Respir Infect* 1990;5:74–79.
77. Ost D, Fein AM, Feinsilver SH. The solitary pulmonary nodule. *N Engl J Med* 2003;348:2535–2542.
78. Wheat LJ, Conces D, Allen SD, et al. Pulmonary histoplasmosis syndromes: Recognition, diagnosis, and management. *Semin Respir Crit Care Med* 2004;25: 129–144.
79. Goodwin RA, Owens FT, Snell JD. Chronic pulmonary histoplasmosis. *Medicine (Baltimore)* 1976;55:413–452.
80. Mocherla S, Wheat LJ. Treatment of histoplasmosis. *Semin Respir Infect* 2001;16:141–148.
81. Wheat J, Sarosi G, McKinsey D. Practice guidelines for the management of patients with histoplasmosis. *Clin Infect Dis* 2000;30:688–695.
82. Judson MA. Noninvasive *Aspergillus* pulmonary disease. *Semin Respir Crit Care Med* 2004;25:203–219.
83. Singh N, Paterson DL. *Aspergillus* infections in transplant recipients. *Clin Microbiol Rev* 2005;18:44–69.
84. Mehrad B, Paciocco G, Martinez FJ, et al. Spectrum of *Aspergillus* infection in lung transplant recipients: Case series and review of the literature. *Chest* 2001;119: 169–175.
85. Judson MA. Allergic bronchopulmonary aspergillosis. *Pulm Crit Care Update* 2003;17: lesson 17.
86. Patterson R, Greenberger PA, Halwig JM, et al. Allergic bronchopulmonary aspergillosis: Natural history and classification of early disease by serologic and roentgenographic studies. *Arch Intern Med* 1986;146: 916–918.
87. Belcher J, Plummer N. Surgery in bronchopulmonary aspergillosis. *Br J Dis Chest* 1960;54:335–341.
88. Glimp RA, Bayer AS. Pulmonary aspergilloma: Diagnostic and therapeutic considerations. *Arch Intern Med* 1983;143:303–308.
89. Cornet M, Fleury L, Maslo C. Epidemiology of IA in France: A six-year multicentric survey in the Greater Paris area. *J Hosp Infect* 2002;51:288–296.
90. Wald A, Leisenring W, van Burik JA. Epidemiology of *Aspergillus* infections in a large cohort of patients undergoing bone marrow transplantation. *J Infect Dis* 1997; 175:1459–1466.
91. Stevens DA, Schwartz HJ, Lee JY, et al. A randomized trial of itraconazole in allergic bronchopulmonary aspergillosis. *N Engl J Med* 2000;342(11):756–762.
92. Stevens DA, Kan VL, Judson MA, et al. Practice guidelines for diseases caused by *Aspergillus*. Infectious Diseases Society of America. *Clin Infect Dis* 2000;30:696–709.
93. Johnson LB, Kauffman CA. Voriconazole: A new triazole antifungal agent. *Clin Infect Dis* 2003;36:630–637.
94. Patterson TF, et al. Voriconazole versus amphotericin B for primary therapy of invasive aspergillosis. *N Engl J Med* 2002;347:408–415.
95. Faulkner SL, Vernon R, Brown PP, et al. Hemoptysis and pulmonary aspergilloma: Operative versus nonoperative treatment. *Ann Thorac Surg* 1978;25:389–392.
96. Jewkes J, Kay PH, Paneth M, et al. Pulmonary aspergilloma: Analysis of prognosis in relation to haemoptysis and survey of treatment. *Thorax* 1983;38:572–578.
97. Daly RC, Pairolero PC, Piehler JM, et al. Pulmonary aspergilloma. Results of surgical treatment. *J Thorac Cardiovasc Surg* 1986;92:981–988.
98. Babatasi G, Massetti M, Chapelier A, et al. Surgical treatment of pulmonary aspergilloma: Current outcome. *J Thorac Cardiovasc Surg* 2000;119(5):906–912.
99. Regnard JF, Icard P, Nicolosi M, et al. Aspergilloma: A series of 89 surgical cases. *Ann Thorac Surg* 2000;69: 898–903.
100. Kim YT, Kang MC, Sung SW, et al. Good long-term outcomes after surgical treatment of simple and complex pulmonary aspergilloma. *Ann Thorac Surg* 2005;79: 294–298.
101. Park CK, Jheon S. Results of surgical treatment for pulmonary aspergilloma. *Eur J Cardiothorac Surg* 2002;21: 918–923.

102. Gebitekin C, Sami Bayram A, Akin S. Complex pulmonary aspergilloma treated with single stage cavernostomy and myoplasty. *Eur J Cardiothorac Surg* 2005;27:737–740.
103. Ono N, Sato K, Yokomise H, et al. Surgical management of pulmonary aspergilloma. Role of single-stage cavernostomy with muscle transposition. *Jpn J Thorac Cardiovasc Surg* 2000;48:56–59.
104. Uflacker R, Kaemmerer A, Neves C. Management of massive hemoptysis by bronchial artery embolization. *Radiology* 1983;146:627–634.
105. Falkson C, Sur R, Pacella J. External beam radiotherapy: A treatment option for massive hemoptysis caused by mycetoma. *Clin Oncol* 2002;14:233–235.
106. Jackson M, Flower CDR, Shneerson JM. Treatment of symptomatic pulmonary aspergillomas with intracavitary instillation of amphotericin B through an indwelling catheter. *Thorax* 1993;48:928–930.
107. Robinson LA, Reed EC, Galbraith TA, et al. Pulmonary resection for invasive *Aspergillus* infections in immunocompromised patients. *J Thorac Cardiovasc Surg* 1995;109:1182–1196.
108. Pidhorecky I, Urschel J, Anderson T. Resection of invasive pulmonary aspergillosis in immunocompromised patients. *Ann Surg Oncol* 2000;7:312–317.
109. Matt P, Bernet F, Habicht J, et al. Short- and long-term outcome after lung resection for invasive pulmonary aspergillosis. *Thorac Cardiovasc Surg* 2003;51:221–225.
110. Gossot D, Validire P, Vaillancourt R, et al. Full thoracoscopic approach for surgical management of invasive pulmonary aspergillosis. *Ann Thorac Surg* 2002;73:240–244.
111. Crum NF, Lederman ER, Stafford CM, et al. Coccidioidomycosis: A descriptive survey of a reemerging disease. Clinical characteristics and current controversies. *Medicine (Baltimore)* 2004;83:149–175.
112. Yozwiak ML, Lundergan LL, Kerrick SS, et al. Symptoms and routine laboratory abnormalities associated with coccidioidomycosis. *West J Med* 1988;149:419–421.
113. Catanzaro A. Pulmonary coccidioidomycosis. *Med Clin North Am* 1980;64:461–473.
114. Stevens DA. Coccidioidomycosis. *N Engl J Med* 1995;332:1077–1082.
115. Catanzaro A. Coccidioidomycosis. *Semin Respir Crit Care Med* 2004;25:123–128.
116. Arsura EL, Kilgore WB. Miliary coccidioidomycosis in the immunocompetent. *Chest* 2000;117:404–409.
117. Galgiani JN, Ampel NM, Catanzaro A, et al. Practice guideline for the treatment of coccidioidomycosis. Infectious Diseases Society of America. *Clin Infect Dis* 2000;30:658–661.
118. Cortez KJ, Walsh TJ, Bennett JE. Successful treatment of coccidioidal meningitis with voriconazole. *Clin Infect Dis* 2003;36:1619–1622.
119. Prabhu RM, Bonnell M, Currier BL, et al. Successful treatment of disseminated nonmeningeal coccidioidomycosis with voriconazole. *Clin Infect Dis* 2004;39:e74–e77.
120. Baker EJ, Hawkins JA, Waskow EA. Surgery for coccidioidomycosis in 52 diabetic patients with special reference to related immunologic factors. *J Thorac Cardiovasc Surg* 1978;75:680–687.
121. Nelson AR. The surgical treatment of pulmonary coccidioidomycosis. *Curr Probl Surg* 1974;10:1–48.
122. Cunningham RT, Einstein H. Coccidioidal pulmonary cavities with rupture. *J Thorac Cardiovasc Surg* 1982;84:172–177.
123. Salomon NW, Osborne R, Copeland JG. Surgical manifestations and results of treatment of pulmonary coccidioidomycosis. *Ann Thorac Surg* 1980;30:433–438.
124. Pappas PG. Blastomycosis. *Semin Respir Crit Care Med* 2004;25:113–121.
125. Lemos LB, Baliga M, Guo M. Acute respiratory distress syndrome and blastomycosis: Presentation of nine cases and review of the literature. *Ann Diagn Pathol* 2001;5:1–9.
126. Isotalo PA, Ford JC, Veinot JP. Miliary blastomycosis developing in an immunocompromised host with chronic lymphocytic leukaemia. *Pathology* 2002;34:293–295.
127. Pappas PG, Dismukes WE. Blastomycosis: Gilchrist's disease revisited. *Curr Clin Top Infect Dis* 2002;22:61–77.
128. Bradsher RW, Chapman SW, Pappas PG. Blastomycosis. *Infect Dis Clin North Am* 2003;17:21–40.
129. Chapman SW. *Blastomyces dermatitidis.* In: *Principles and Practice of Infectious Diseases.* New York: Churchill Livingstone; 2000:2733–2746.
130. Chapman SE, Bradsher RW, Campbell GD, et al. Practice guidelines for the management of patients with blastomycosis. *Clin Infect Dis* 2000;30:679–683.
131. Lortholary O, Nunez H, Brauner MW, et al. Pulmonary cryptococcosis. *Semin Respir Crit Care Med* 2004;25:145–157.
132. Chu HQ, Li HP, He GJ. Analysis of 23 cases of pulmonary cryptococcosis. *Chin Med J (Engl)* 2004;117:1425.
133. Cameron ML, Bartlett JA, Gallis HA, et al. Manifestations of pulmonary cryptococcosis in patients with acquired immunodeficiency syndrome. *Rev Infect Dis* 1991;13:64.
134. Saag MS, Graybill RJ, Larsen RA, et al. Practice guidelines for the management of cryptococcal disease. Infectious Diseases Society of America. *Clin Infect Dis* 2000;30:710–718.
135. Lindell RM, Hartman TE, Nadrous HF, et al. Pulmonary cryptococcosis: CT findings in immunocompetent patients. *Radiology* 2005;236:326.
136. Johnson PC, Sarosi. The endemic mycoses: Surgical considerations. *Semin Thorac Cardiovasc Surg* 1995;7(2):95–103.
137. Wang T, Sun YE, Yu CH, et al. Surgical treatment of primary pulmonary cryptococcosis. *Zhonghua Wai Ke Za Zhi* 2005;43:1447–1449.
138. Freifeld AG, Iwen PC. Zygomycosis. *Semin Respir Crit Care Med* 2004;25:221–231.
139. Bigby TD, Serota ML, Tierney LM, et al. Clinical spectrum of pulmonary mucormycosis. *Chest* 1986;89:435–439.
140. Husari AW, Jensen WA, Kirsch CM. Pulmonary mucormycosis presenting as an endobronchial lesion. *Chest* 1994;106:1889–1891.
141. al-Abbadi MA, Russo K, Wilkinson EJ. Pulmonary mucormycosis diagnosed by bronchoalveolar lavage: A case report and review of the literature. *Pediatr Pulmonol* 1997;23:222–225.

142. Kontoyiannis DP, Wessel VC, Bodey GP, et al. Zygomycosis in the 1990s in a tertiary-care cancer center. *Clin Infect Dis* 2000;30:851–856.
143. Zaizen Y, Ohtsu T. Successful treatment of pulmonary mucormycosis, a rare pulmonary fungal infection, in a patient with diabetes mellitus. *J Thorac Cardiovasc Surg* 2002;124:838–840.
144. Brown RB, Johnson JH, Kessinger JM, et al. Bronchovascular mucormycosis in the diabetic: An urgent surgical problem. *Ann Thorac Surg* 1992;53: 854–855.
145. Murphy RA, Miller WT. Pulmonary mucormycosis. *Semin Roentgenol* 1996;31:83–87.
146. Tedder M, Spratt JA, Anstadt MP, et al. Pulmonary mucormycosis: Results of medical and surgical therapy. *Ann Thorac Surg* 1994;57:1044–1050.
147. Kfoury AG, Smith JC, Farhoud HH, et al. Adjuvant intrapleural amphotericin B therapy for pulmonary mucormycosis in a cardiac allograft recipient. *Clin Transplant* 1997;11:608–612.
148. McGinnis MR, Ajello L, Beneke ES, et al. Taxonomic and nomenclatural evaluation of the genera *Candida* and *Torulopsis*. *J Clin Microbiol* 1984;20:813.
149. Pappas PG, Rex JH, Sobel JD, et al. Guidelines for treatment of candidiasis. *Clin Infect Dis* 2004;38:161–189.
150. Haron E, Vartivarian S, Anaissie E, et al. Primary *Candida* pneumonia. Experience at a large cancer center and review of the literature. *Medicine (Baltimore)* 1993; 72:137–142.
151. Kontoyiannis DP, Reddy BT, Torres HA, et al. Pulmonary candidiasis in patients with cancer: An autopsy study. *Clin Infect Dis* 2002;34:400–403.
152. el-Ebiary M, Torres A, Fabregas N, et al. Significance of the isolation of *Candida* species from respiratory samples in critically ill, non-neutropenic patients. An immediate postmortem histologic study. *Am J Respir Crit Care Med* 1997;156:583–590.
153. Tambini R, Farina C, Fiocchi R, et al. Possible pathogenic role for *Sporothrix cyanescens* isolated from a lung lesion in a heart transplant patient. *J Med Vet Mycol* 1996;34:195–198.
154. Pluss JL, Opal SM. Pulmonary sporotrichosis: Review of treatment and outcome. *Medicine (Baltimore)* 1986;65:143–153.
155. Kwon-Chung KJ, Bennett JE. Sporotrichosis. In: *Medical Mycology*. Philadelphia: Lea & Febiger, 1992:707.
156. Kauffman CA, Hajjeh R, Chapman SW. Practice guidelines for the management of patients with sporotrichosis. For the Mycoses Study Group. Infectious Diseases Society of America. *Clin Infect Dis* 2000;30:684–687.
157. Schneider E, Moore M, Castro KG. Epidemiology of tuberculosis in the United States. *Clin Chest Med* 2005;26:183–195.
158. Corbett EL, Watt CJ, Walker N, et al. The growing burden of tuberculosis: Global trends and interactions with the HIV epidemic. *Arch Intern Med* 2003;163:1009–1021.
159. Dye C, Watt CJ, Bleed DM, Evolution of tuberculosis control and prospects for reducing tuberculosis incidence, prevalence, and deaths globally. *JAMA* 2005;293: 2767–2775.
160. van Soolingen D, Hoogenboezem T, De Haas PEW, et al. A novel pathogenic taxon of the *Mycobacterium tuberculosis* complex, *canetti:* Characterization of an exceptional isolate from Africa. *Int J Syst Bacteriol* 1997; 47:1236–1245.
161. Riley R. Transmission and environmental control of tuberculosis. In: Tuberculosis. New York: Marcel Deckker, 1993.
162. Diagnostic Standards and Classification of Tuberculosis in Adults and Children. Official statement of the American Thoracic Society and the Centers for Disease Control and Prevention. *Am J Respir Crit Care Med* 2000;161:1376–1395.
163. Dannenberg AM. Pathogenesis of pulmonary tuberculosis: Host-parasite interactions, cell-mediated immunity, and delayed-type hypersensitivity. In: Schlossberg D (ed). *Basic Principles in Tuberculosis*, 3d ed. New York: Springer-Verlag, 1992.
164. Canetti G. *The Tubercle Bacillus in the Pulmonary Lesion of Man*. New York: Springer-Verlag, 1955.
165. Styblo K. *Epidemiology of Tuberculosis.* Royal Netherlands Tuberculosis Association Selected Papers. The Hague: Royal Netherlands Tuberculosis Association, 1991.
166. Bourbonnais JM, Sirithanakul K, Guzman JA. Fulminant miliary tuberculosis with adult respiratory distress syndrome undiagnosed until autopsy: A report of 2 cases and review of the literature. *J Intens Care Med* 2005;20: 354–359.
167. Perez-Guzman C, Vargas MH, Torres-Cruz A, et al. Does aging modify pulmonary tuberculosis? A meta-analytical review. *Chest* 1999;116:961–967.
168. Peterson EM, Nakasone A, Platon-DeLeon JM, et al. Comparison of direct and concentrated acid-fast smears to identify specimens culture positive for *Mycobacterium* spp. *J Clin Microbiol* 1999;37:3564–3568.
169. Warren JR, Bhattacharya M, De Almeida KN, et al. A minimum 5.0 ml of sputum improves the sensitivity of acid-fast smear for *Mycobacterium tuberculosis. Am J Respir Crit Care Med* 2000;161:1559–1562.
170. Shinnick T, Good R. Diagnostic mycobacteriology laboratory practices. *Clin Infect Dis* 1995;21:291–299.
171. Al Zahrani K, Al Jahdali H, Poirier L, et al. Accuracy and utility of commercially available amplification and serologic tests for the diagnosis of minimal pulmonary tuberculosis. *Am J Respir Crit Care Med* 2000;162:1323–1329.
172. Canadian Thoracic Society: Essentials of tuberculosis control for the practicing physician. Tuberculosis Committee, Canadian Thoracic Society. *CMAJ* 1994; 150:1561–1571.
173. Centers for Disease Control and Prevention. The role of BCG vaccine in the prevention and control of tuberculosis in the United States. *MMWR* 1996;45:RR–4.
174. Centers for Disease Control and Prevention. Nucleic acid amplification tests for tuberculosis. *MMWR* 1996;45: 950–952.
175. American Thoracic Society. Rapid diagnostic tests for tuberculosis: What is the appropriate use? *Am J Respir Crit Care Med* 1997;155:1804–1814.
176. Catanzaro A, Perry S, Clarridge JE, et al. The role of clinical suspicion in evaluating a new diagnostic test for active tuberculosis: Results of a multicenter prospective trial. *JAMA* 2000;283:639–645.
177. Grzybowski S, Fishaut H, Rowe J, et al. Tuberculosis among patients with various radiologic abnormalities

followed by the chest clinic service. *Am Rev Respir Dis* 1971;104:605–608.

178. Chaisson RE, Schecter GF, Theuer CP, et al. Tuberculosis in patients with the acquired immunodeficiency syndrome: Clinical features, response to therapy and survival. *Am Rev Respir Dis* 1987;136:570–574.
179. Tateishi U, Kusumoto M, Akiyama Y, et al. Role of contrast-enhanced dynamic CT in the diagnosis of active tuberculoma. *Chest* 2002;122:1280.
180. Heo JN, Choi YW, Jeon SC, et al. Pulmonary tuberculosis: Another disease showing clusters of small nodules. *AJR* 2005;184:639–642.
181. Centers for Disease Control and Prevention. *Tuberculosis 2000: Fundamentals of Clinical TB and TB Control.* 1997.
182. Blumberg HM, Burman WJ, Chaisson RE, et al. American Thoracic Society/Centers for Disease Control and Prevention/Infectious Diseases Society of America: Treatment of tuberculosis. *Am J Respir Crit Care Med* 2003;167:603–662.
183. Mouroux J, Maalouf J, Padovani B, et al. Surgical management of pleuropulmonary tuberculosis. *J Thorac Cardiovasc Surg* 1996;111:662–670.
184. Pomerantz BJ, Cleveland JC Jr, Olson HK, et al. Pulmonary resection for multi-drug resistant tuberculosis. *J Thorac Cardiovasc Surg* 2001;121:448–453.
185. Shiraishi Y, Nakajima Y, Katsuragi N, et al. Resectional surgery combined with chemotherapy remains the treatment of choice for multidrug-resistant tuberculosis. *J Thorac Cardiovasc Surg* 2004;128:523–528.
186. Park SK, Lee CM, Heu JP, et al. A retrospective study for the outcome of pulmonary resection in 49 patients with multidrug-resistant tuberculosis. *Int J Tuberc Lung Dis* 2002;6:143–149.
187. Naidoo R, Reddi A. Lung resection for multidrug-resistant tuberculosis. *Asian Cardiovasc Thorac Ann* 2005;13: 172–174.
188. Brown J, Pomerantz M. Extrapleural pneumonectomy for tuberculosis.*Chest Surg Clin North Am* 1995;5: 289–296.
189. Pomerantz M, Madsen L, Goble M, et al. Surgical management of resistant mycobacterial tuberculosis and other mycobacterial pulmonary infections. *Ann Thorac Surg* 1991;52:1108–1111.
190. American Thoracic Society. Diagnosis and treatment of disease caused by nontuberculous mycobacteria. *Am J Respir Crit Care Med* 1997;156:S1–S25.
191. Nelson KG, Griffith DE, Brown BA, Wallace RJ Jr. Results of operation in *Mycobacterium avium-intracellulare* lung disease. *Ann Thorac Surg* 1998;66:325–330.
192. Ostroff S, Hutwagner L, Collin S. Mycobacterial species and drug resistance patterns reported by state laboratories– 1992. Abtract U-9. American Society for Microbiology 93rd General Meeting, Atlanta, GA, 1993: 170.
193. Falkinham JO. Epidemiology of infection by nontuberculous mycobacteria. *Clin Microbiol Rev* 1996;9: 177–215.
194. Hawkins CC, Gold JW, Whimbey E, et al. *Mycobacterium avium*-complex infections in patients with the acquired immunodeficiency syndrome. *Ann Intern Med* 1986;105:184–188.
195. Hartman TE, Swensen SJ, Williams DE. *Mycobacterium avium-intracellulare* complex: Evaluation with CT. *Radiology* 1993;187:23–26.
196. Griffith DE, Girard WM, Wallace RJ Jr. Clinical features of pulmonary disease caused by rapidly growing mycobacteria: An analysis of 154 patients. *Am Rev Respir Dis* 1993;1271–1278.
197. Shiraishi Y, Nakajima Y, Takasuna K, et al. Surgery for *Mycobacterium avium* complex lung disease in the clarithromycin era. *Eur J Cardiothorac Surg* 2002;21: 314–318.
198. Nelson KG, Griffith DE, Brown BA, Wallace RJ Jr. Results of operation in *Mycobacterium avium-intracellulare* lung disease. *Ann Thorac Surg* 1998;66:325–330.
199. Shiraishi Y, Nakajima Y, Katsuragi N, et al. Pneumonectomy for nontuberculous mycobacterial infections. *Ann Thorac Surg* 2004;78(2):399–403.
200. Shiraishi Y, Fukushima K, Komatsu H, Kurashima A. Early pulmonary resection for localized *Mycobacterium avium* complex disease. *Ann Thorac Surg* 1998;66: 183–186.

CHAPTER

4 CHEST WALL TUMORS

Amy E. Gallo, Michael A. Coady

INTRODUCTION

Chest wall tumors arise from a range of cell types including soft tissue, bone, cartilage, and metastatic disease, each with different growth potentials, presentations, diagnostic properties, and prognoses. Yet as in the case of other solid organ tumors, treatment involves multiple modalities, including chemotherapy, radiation, and the challenge of surgical resection. Although the chest wall itself is not an organ, it functions as a functional unit with complex interplay between soft tissue, bone, and cartilage. Prior to treatment, one must have a comprehensive understanding of all components involved and their integration. Soft tissue, bone, and cartilage work together to support respiration and protect underlying organs. The obligation of the thoracic surgeon is to make a diagnosis and devise a treatment plan that will offer the best chance of survival.

CLINICAL FEATURES

Chest wall tumors are rare, accounting for 1 to 2 percent of all tumors. Of these tumors, 60 percent are malignant, with 50 percent of malignancies arising from soft tissue. They account for 5 percent of all thoracic malignancies.[1]

Historically, primary chest wall tumors present as slow-growing masses, 75 percent of which are painless.[1] Painless tumors can also present as incidental findings on x-ray or computed tomography (CT) scans. Tumors that

KEY CONCEPTS

- Epidemiology
    - Chest wall tumors account for 1 to 2 percent of all tumors; 60 percent are malignant. Neoplasms can be primary soft tissue, bone, or cartilage tumors or they can be invasive or metastatic tumors. Morbidity and mortality are specific to the particular tumor.
- Clinical Features
    - 75 percent are painless and present incidentally. Metastatic tumors grow more rapidly. Patients may have constitutional symptoms.
- Diagnostics
    - Radiographic imaging is helpful to aid in diagnosis, tumor location, and evidence of metastasis. Chest radiographs, computed tomography scans, magnetic resonance imaging, and positron emission tomography scans are all diagnostic options. Biopsy assists in diagnosis and treatment planning.
- Treatment
    - Medical treatment varies with different tumors. Chemotherapy and radiation therapy are offen used; this improves survival in malignant tumors of bone and cartilage. Radiation therapy is used for soft tissue sarcomas.
    - Surgical treatment varies with different tumors. For malignant tumors, at least a 4-cm margin with the affected rib and one rib above and below the tumor is required. Chest wall reconstruction is necessary for anterior defects greater than 5 cm and posterior defects greater than 10 cm. Reconstruction can be accomplished with low morbidity and mortality in experienced hands.
- Outcome/Prognosis
    - Outcomes of treatment are tumor-dependent. Five-year survival rates for all tumors range from 14 to 86 percent.

are painful are more often malignant or originate in bone, because pain usually represents expansion into the cortex or periosteum, destruction of the cortex, or a fracture. Metastatic tumors often grow more rapidly. On physical exam, bone or cartilaginous tumors may not be palpable. If palpable, they are usually fixed to the chest wall. Soft tissue masses are more frequently mobile. Patients may also present with fever, leukocytosis, or eosinophilia.

DIAGNOSTIC MODALITIES

Following a history and physical, there are numerous radiographic modalities that contribute to the diagnosis and treatment of chest wall tumors. Chest radiographs better identify a suspected lesion's size and location. Serial radiographs are helpful in determining growth rate. CT demonstrates the relationship of a tumor to its surrounding structures. It can also delineate cystic from solid masses and bony invasion. Magnetic resonance imaging (MRI) further defines a mass by providing insight to the relationship of the mass to vascular structures, nerves, the spine, and the chest apex. CT reconstructions and MRI can also provide sagittal and coronal views. Bone scans are used to evaluate metastatic disease. Positron emission tomography (PET) is being used more frequently in oncology in general. Its use has been shown to help better differentiate benign from malignant tumors as well as delineate tumor grade. Studies are ongoing to provide parameters for analysis, but currently PET scans are a complement to biopsy and not a replacement.[2]

Biopsy has an important role in the diagnosis and management of chest wall tumors. It can provide a histologic diagnosis and grade to differentiate benign from malignant disease, which is essential for treatment planning and balancing functional preservation with the prevention of recurrence and cure of disease. For small lesions (< 2 cm) or lesions suspected to be benign, excisional biopsy is appropriate. Core biopsies and evaluations of cellular aspirates with monoclonal antibodies, immunohistochemistry, and electron microscopy are used for larger tumors. Evaluation of cellular aspirates often provides adequate diagnosis with 95 percent accuracy. Incisional biopsy is reserved for large tumors (> 5 cm), where cellular aspirates or core biopsies do not provide a diagnosis. These biopsies include 1 cm^3 of tissue with an incision that is easily excisable during subsequent tumor resection.

SOFT TISSUE TUMORS

Soft tissue tumors of the chest wall arise from both superficial and deep soft tissue, including skin, muscle, fat, lymphatics, vessels, nerves, and connective tissue. Each type has its own malignant potential and treatment (Table 4-1).

Benign soft tissue tumors

Cutaneous nevi

This is a common lesion formed by aggregates of skin melanocytes.[3] It is distinguished from melanoma pathologically and therefore excision with margins is required.

Lipomas

These are the most common soft tissue tumors of adulthood. Lipomas vary in size and present as painless, mobile, encapsulated lesions; they are most often found on proximal areas of the extremities and on the trunk. There are different subclasses of lipomas based on their morphology, but the most common subclass is the conventional lipoma, which is a well-encapsulated mass composed of mature adipocytes.[3] Treatment is excision for cosmetic reasons or for lesions where the diagnosis cannot be made clinically. Rarely, these tumors invade the underlying muscle. When they do so, a wider margin is required because recurrence is then more common.

Table 4-1 Benign soft tissue tumors of the chest wall

	Origin	Common locations	Population most often affected	Associated disorders/risk factors	Treatment
Cutaneous nevi	Melanocytes		Adults		Excision with margins
Lipoma	Adipocytes		Adults		Excision for symptoms or diagnosis
Hemangioma	Blood vessels		Children		Excision for symptoms
Lymphangioma	Lymphatics	Head/neck/axilla	Children		Complete excision
Fibroma	Fibroblasts	Near joints or pleural surfaces	Adults		Excision for symptoms
Rhabdomyoma	Skeletal muscle		Adults		Excision for symptoms
Neurofibroma	Peripheral nerve sheath		Males, ages 20–50	Von Recklinghausen's disease	Excision for symptoms or growing tumor
Desmoid tumors	Fibroblasts	Anterolateral chest wall	Teens to thirties, equally in men and women	Gardner's syndrome	Wide local excision, chemotherapy, and radiation

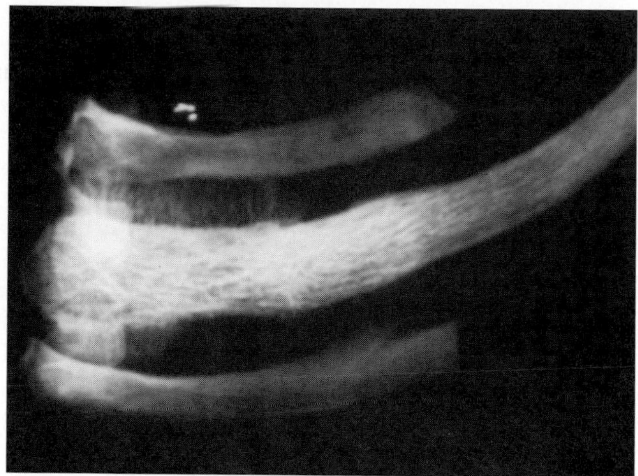
A

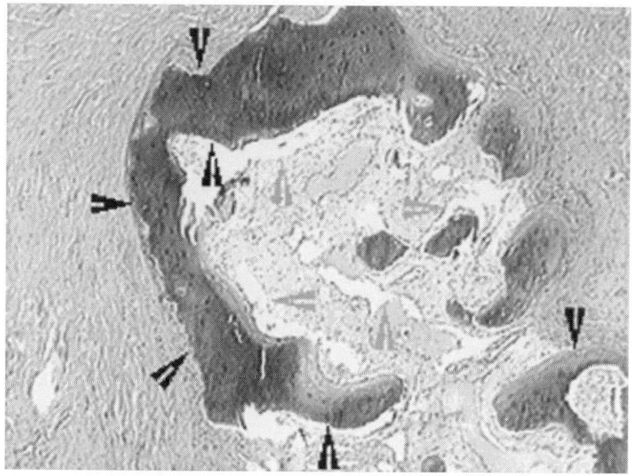
B

Figure 4-1 A. A radiograph of a resected rib in a 20-year-old female who presented with a symptomatic hemangioma. (Courtesy of the Yale Department of Radiology.) B. Cavernous hemangioma. Vascular channels (green arrows) surrounded by bone (black arrows). (From Lindquist RR, Rajan TV, Ernst L, et al: eAtlas of Pathology, uchc.edu, 1999.)

Hemangiomas

These lesions are common at birth and in young children, comprising approximately 7 percent of all benign tumors. They are composed of groups of nonencapsulated blood vessels; they may be superficial or deep, simple or cavernous. Simple hemangiomas are composed of narrow vessels and range widely in size by comparison to the dilated vessels of cavernous lesions, which are often 1 to 2 cm in diameter. Treatment on the chest wall is indicated for cosmetic reasons or with complications, including bleeding and ulceration (Fig. 4-1).

Lymphangiomas

Like hemangiomas, lymphangiomas present as both simple and cavernous types. Simple lymphangiomas are smaller, elevated lesions, 1 to 2 cm in diameter and more superficial than the cavernous type. Cavernous lymphangiomas, which tend to be larger, up to 15 cm, occur more often in children. Both types arise primarily in the head, neck, and axillary regions. Both are lined by endothelial cells on pathology and can be differentiated from hemangiomas by the lack of blood cells within their channels.[3] Treatment is complete excision to prevent recurrence. Surgery can be challenging because of the lack of a capsule and poorly defined margins.

Fibromas

These rare, slow-growing tumors arise from fibroblasts. They can present in soft tissue, near joints, or on pleural surfaces. Excision is necessary to relieve symptoms or for the sake of cosmetics.

Rhabdomyoma

This is a rare, slow-growing tumor arising from muscle. Biopsy is recommended for diagnosis. As in the case of fibromas, excision is performed to relieve symptoms and for cosmetic reasons. Symptoms may include inhibition of muscle function. Excision must be complete to prevent local recurrence.

Neurofibroma

Neurofibroma is a peripheral nerve sheath tumor most often seen in association with neurofibromatosis (von Recklinghausen disease), an autosomal dominant disorder. There are two types of neurofibromas, cutaneous and plexiform. Cutaneous neurofibromas present as nodules, sometimes with hyperpigmentation overlying their pedunculated shape; they arise only in the dermis and subcutaneous fat. Histologically they are noninvading spindle cells.[3] Their potential to transform to malignancy is low and excision is usually done only for cosmetic reasons. Plexiform lesions, on the other hand, can be associated with nerve trunks and are identified as expansions of a host nerve with a dumbbell shape on CT or MRI.[1] They have poorly differentiated margins and cannot be separated from the host nerve. Their potential to transform to malignancy is high. Treatment is excision without biopsy, and this is indicated for symptomatic lesions and those that are increasing in size. Spinal canal involvement should be investigated and documented prior to treatment (Fig. 4-2).

Desmoid tumors

Desmoid tumors arise from fibroblasts of deep fascia and muscle connective tissue. These tumors most often present in patients ranging from the teens to age 30; they occur equally in both men and women. Some 40 percent of desmoid tumors present in the shoulder and chest wall, the majority in the anterolateral chest wall (Fig. 4-3).[4] Patients often complain primarily of pain (62 percent), both from the tumor's size and local invasion

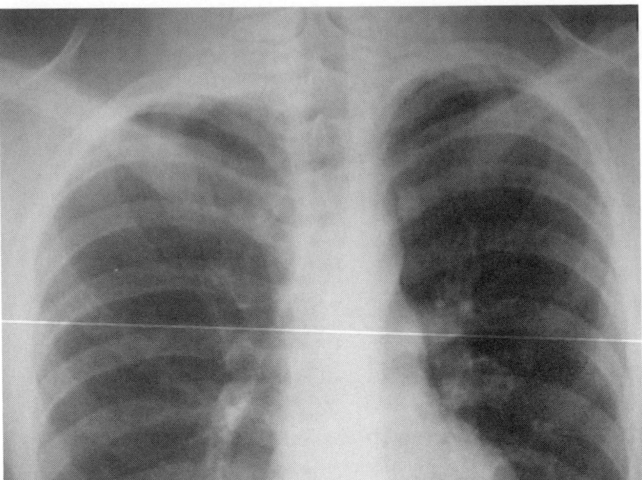

Figure 4-2 AP chest radiograph of a 25 year-old male with neurofibromatosis and several extrapleural lesions of the left neck and chest and deformities of the fourth and fifth ribs anteriorly. (Courtesy of the Yale Department of Radiology.)

into bone, nerves, vessels, and the pleural cavity.[5] This is an important feature of this benign tumor; even though the tumor itself is slow-growing along tissue planes and desmoid tumors have not been reported to have metastatic potential, they do invade local structures. Therefore local recurrence, despite excision with wide margins, is extremely common. Recurrence rates are extremely high. Surgical treatment is by wide local resection with excision of all involved structures.[5] Both chemotherapy (with doxorubicin, vinblastine, and methotrexate) and local radiation have been used to decrease local recurrence rates in patients with both negative and positive surgical margins. Radiation therapy is more commonly used.[5] Neoadjuvant treatment with doxorubicin and radiotherapy (10 × 300 cGy) has also been used to help reduce local recurrence.[6]

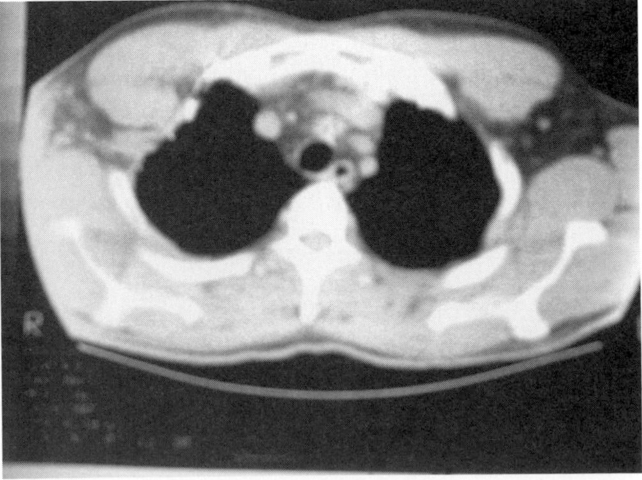

Figure 4-3 Chest CT scan of patient with a desmoid tumor of the right chest wall subsequent to radiation therapy. (Courtesy of the Yale Department of Radiology.)

Malignant soft tissue tumors

Soft tissue malignancies include skin lesions, melanoma and basal cell carcinoma, and the sarcomas. Sarcomas arise from a variety of cell types and account for 20 percent of chest wall malignancies. Prognostic factors include patient age, tumor size and grade, metastases, and surgical margins.[7] Overall, patients with low-grade sarcomas have a 90 percent 5-year survival, whereas high grade sarcomas have a 50 percent 5-year survival. Surgical treatment is excision, with a 10 to 30 percent chance of local recurrence.[8] Chemotherapy and radiation have also been used. Details regarding sarcomas from different soft tissue origins are described below (Table 4-2).

Malignant fibrous histiocytoma

This tumor is the most common sarcoma and is the most commonly evaluated neoplasm of the chest wall. Two-thirds of patients are men, and they often present late in life, from ages 50 to 70, with painless, slow-growing masses (ranging in size from 5 to 20 cm). In women, the growth rate may be accelerated during pregnancy. Malignant fibrous histiocytoma is rarely seen in childhood; when it is seen in adolescents, it is more often as the indolent angiomatoid variant. Histologically the cell of origin is not clear; the tumors are classified by cytologic pleomorphism, multinucleated cells with storiform architecture, inflamed collagen, and foamy macrophages. These tumors arise from musculature, growing along fascial planes and between muscle fibers (Fig. 4-4). Some studies have suggested that radiation therapy is a risk factor for these tumors.

Treatment is wide resection, which can often be difficult with tumor invasion. Recurrence rates are high. Neither chemotherapy nor radiation have been shown to provide statistically significant survival advantages. However at some institutions, Massachusetts General Hospital in particular, it is the policy to administer postoperative radiation, 45 Gy at 1.8 Gy per fraction over 5 weeks, in patients with marginal resection or with tumors that are diffusely infiltrating. Malignant fibrous histiocytoma metastasizes 30 to 50 percent of the time, and the 5-year survival rate is 38 percent.[3]

Rhabdomyosarcoma

This is a rare soft tissue malignancy of the thorax that arises from skeletal muscle. It most often affects children and adolescents, being rare for adults over age 45. The incidence in men is slightly greater than in women. Patients present with painless, rapidly growing masses that are intimately associated with striated muscle. Histologically, these tumors can have a variety of appearances, including different areas of cellularity, necrosis, and hemorrhage. Subclassifications of histologic variation include embryonal,

Table 4-2 **Malignant soft tissue tumors of the chest wall**

	Origin	Common locations	Population most often affected	Associated disorders/ risk factors	Treatment	5-Year survival
Malignant fibrous histiocytoma	Not well defined	Fascial planes	Males, ages 50–70	Radiation therapy	Wide resection, radiation for positive margins	38%
Rhabdomyo-sarcoma	Skeletal muscle		Male children and adolescents		Wide resection, chemotherapy, radiation	45%
Liposarcoma	Lipocytes, lipoblasts		Males, ages 40–60	Trauma	Wide resection	60%
Neurofibrosarcoma	Peripheral nerve sheath	Along intercostal nerves	Males, ages 20–50	Von Recklinghausen's disease, radiation	Wide resection	55%
Leiomyosarcoma	Smooth muscle		Female adults		Wide resection, radiation	64%

alveolar, and pleomorphic types. These subclasses may play a role in prognosis. Embryonal rhabdomyosarcoma is most common in children and carries the best prognosis, a statistically significant improvement in 5-year survival for patients with metastatic disease.[9] Treatment of rhabdomyosarcoma is wide local resection, multidrug chemotherapy, and irradiation. With these modalities, survival has been shown to be 45 percent at 5 years.[10]

Liposarcoma

Liposarcoma is another common soft tissue malignancy of the chest wall. Patients are more frequently men ranging from 40 to 60 years of age. It is a rare disease in children. An association has been made between these tumors and previous trauma. The tumors are well encapsulated and lobulated and arise from lipocytes and lipoblasts. They have a tendency to become rather large. Treatment is wide excision because local recurrence is common; chemotherapy, together or in succession, and radiation therapy have little role in treatment. Five-year survival is 60 percent.[4]

Neurofibrosarcoma

Like its benign counterpart, neurofibroma, neurofibrosarcoma is most often associated with von Recklinghausen's disease. These tumors in the chest wall grow along intercostal nerves. They are found primarily in men between the ages 20 and 50; treatment is wide local excision. Postoperative radiation and chemotherapy have been used in an attempt to improve the 55 percent 5-year survival rate[11]; however, there are currently no studies that have shown a statistically significant improvement in survival with conventional external beam radiation, brachytherapy, or chemotherapy. It is still the recommendation of some, including Neville and colleagues at the M.D. Anderson Cancer Center, to include postoperative radiation as the standard for patients less than 21 years of age regardless of surgical margins.[12]

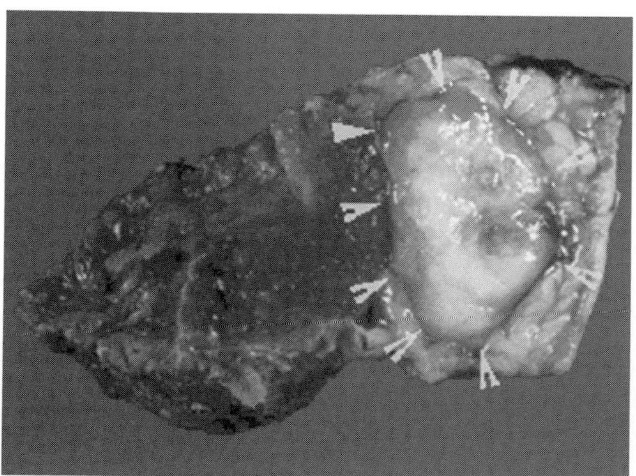
A

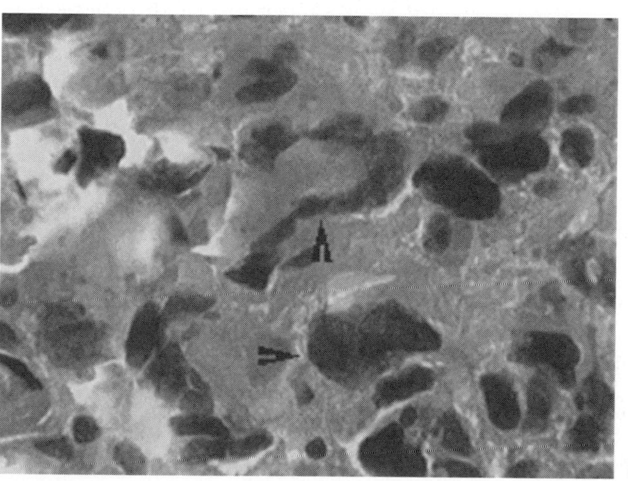
B

Figure 4-4 A. A specimen of a malignant fibrous histiocytoma. The arrow points to the tumor, which is surrounded by muscle to the left and fat to the right. B. Malignant fibrous histiocytoma. Variation in cell and nuclear size (green arrows) with typical large multinucleated giant cells (black arrows). (From Lindquist RR, Rajan TV, Ernst L, et al. eAtlas of Pathology. uchc.edu, 1999.)

Table 4-3 Benign bone and cartilage tumors of the chest wall

	Origin	Common locations in chest wall	Population most often affected	Associated disorders/risk factors	Treatment
Fibrous dysplasia	Medullary cavity of bone	Posterolateral surface of ribs	Children	Albright's syndrome	Excision
Osteochondroma	Metaphyseal cortex	Ribs	Male children		Excision for symptoms, growth, or presence in adults
Chondroma	Hyaline cartilage	Anterior rib, costochondral junction, or sternum	Ages 20–40 in both sexes		Wide resection
Langerhans cell histiocytosis	Antigen-presenting cells	Ribs	Males, infants to young adults	Letterer-Siwe disease, Hand-Schuller-Christian disease, eosinophilic granuloma	Excision or radiation for local disease, chemotherapy for systemic disease

Leiomyosarcoma

This is a less common soft tissue tumor, arising from smooth muscle and accounting for 10 to 20 percent of all sarcomas. These tumors also affect adults, but unlike other sarcomas, they are seen more commonly in women (two-thirds of cases). They present as slowly growing masses that can be painful. Histologically, the smooth muscle cells themselves contain bundles of thin filaments and vesicles; they stain with antibodies to vimentin, actin, and desmin. Treatment is wide local excision with radiation therapy. Local and metastatic recurrences are seen and 5-year survival is 64 percent.[7]

BONE AND CARTILAGE TUMORS

These tumors are also rare and account for approximately 6 percent of all primary bone tumors. However, when identified, bone and cartilage tumors of the chest wall are eight times more likely to be malignant than benign (Tables 4-3 and 4-4).

Benign bone and cartilage tumors

Fibrous dysplasia

Fibrous dysplasia accounts for 30 percent of all benign chest wall tumors. It manifests 70 percent of the time as monostotic fibrous dysplasia, or isolated lesions that affect both sexes equally. Otherwise it presents as polyostotic fibrous dysplasia, or multiple lesions that may be associated with Albright's syndrome, skin lesions, and precocious sexual maturity in girls (3 percent of cases).[3] Pathologically, these tumors are cystic lesions where fibrous material takes the place of the medullary cavity of bone (Fig. 4-5). It presents in children as a slow-growing, painless lesion on the posterolateral surface of the rib. Pain occurs with bone expansion or rib fractures due to tumor growth. Most cases are discovered incidentally on roentgenography. Findings include thinning of the cortex and a ground-glass appearance of the medulla. Symptomatic patients or those in whom the diagnosis is unclear are treated by excision, which is curative.

Osteochondroma

Osteochondroma arises from the cortical bone of the metaphyseal region, most often involving the ribs. Tumors start in childhood and are three times more common in men. They grow on a bony stalk with a cartilaginous covering over the tumor mass (Fig. 4-6). Tumors that grow on the internal side of a bone are identified on roentgenography as bone with intact cortex and stippled calcification in the area of tumor. Those that grow on the external aspect of a bone can be palpated. Treatment—which includes compete excision—is given for lesions that are symptomatic, enlarging, or those found in adults. Recurrence is rare following resection.

Chondroma

These tumors present in people (sexes equal) between 20 and 40 years of age as asymptomatic, slow-growing tumors; they represent 15 percent of all benign lesions of the ribs. The most common site is the anterior rib, costochondral junction, or sternum. The pathology of chondroma demonstrates lobules of hyaline cartilage. On

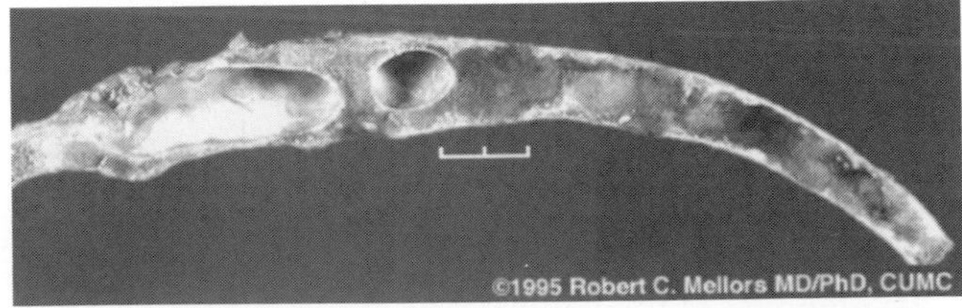

Figure 4-5 Gross specimen of the cystic lesions of fibrous dysplasia in a rib. (From Mellors RC. Bone.edcenter.med.cornell.edu, 2001.)

Table 4-4 Malignant bone and cartilage tumors of the chest wall

	Origin	Common locations in chest wall	Population most often affected	Associated disorders/risk factors	Treatment	5-Year survival
Chondrosarcoma	Cartilage	Anterior chest wall, ribs, sternum	Males, ages 30–40	Trauma	Wide resection, limited role for chemotherapy and radiation	64–86%
Osteogenic sarcoma	Bone matrix	Long bones more often than chest wall	Males, children, and teenagers	Paget's, mutations in Rb and p53, radiation therapy, bony infarcts	Chemotherapy, wide resection	14–20%
Ewing's sarcoma	Neural cell origin	Ribs	White males, ages 10–15	Gene translocations	Neoadjuvant and postoperative chemotherapy, wide resection, radiation	56–65%
Askin tumor	Neural cell origin	Ribs	Children	Gene translocations	Neoadjuvant and postoperative chemotherapy, wide resection, postoperative radiation	16%
Plasmacytoma	Plasma cells	Ribs	Males, ages 60–70	Multiple myeloma	Excision for diagnosis, otherwise radiation. Chemotherapy for multiple lesions.	20% when associated with multiple myeloma

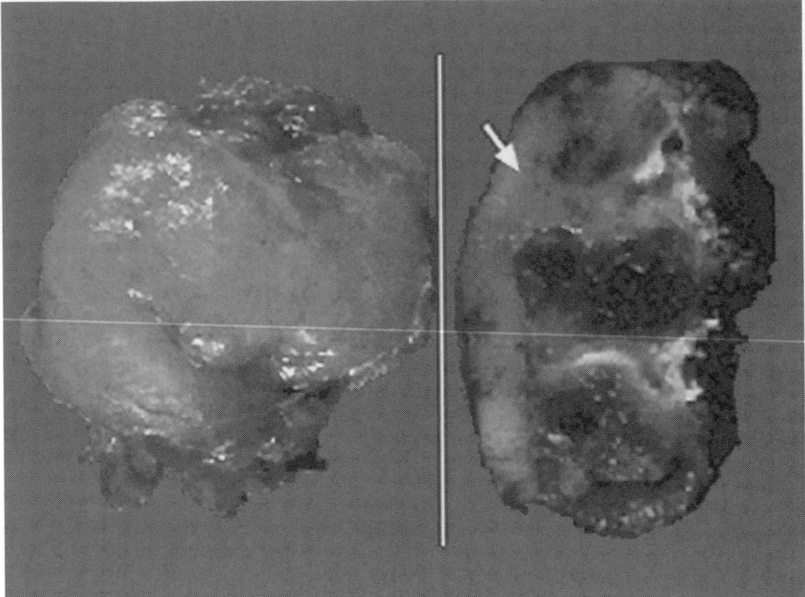

Figure 4-6 Pathologic specimen of an osteochondroma demonstrating the cartilaginous covering over the tumor mass. (From Lindquist RR, Rajan TV, Ernst L, et al. eAtlas of Pathology. uchc.edu, 1999.)

roentgenography, the tumor is a medullary or periosteal mass that is lytic in nature, with a thinning cortex and sclerotic border (Fig. 4-7). Unlike other benign tumors, chondroma is treated by complete excision with wide margins because no clear distinction can be made histologically or radiographically between chondroma and chondrosarcoma.

Langerhans cell histiocytosis

This is a disorder divided into three subtypes, Letterer-Siwe disease, Hand-Schuller-Christian disease, and eosinophilic granuloma, affecting infants, children, and young adults respectively. The three subtypes have different presentations and prognoses; however, all patients can present with destructive osteolytic bone lesions affecting almost any skeletal bone with skull being the most commonly affected. These lesions are painful when associated with fractures. On roentgenography, the cortex is disrupted and scalloped and the bone expanded. Lesions may resolve on their own or radiation or excision may cure given lesions. Patients with extensive marrow infiltrates and other symptoms of systemic diseases have been shown to benefit from chemotherapy and radiation as well.

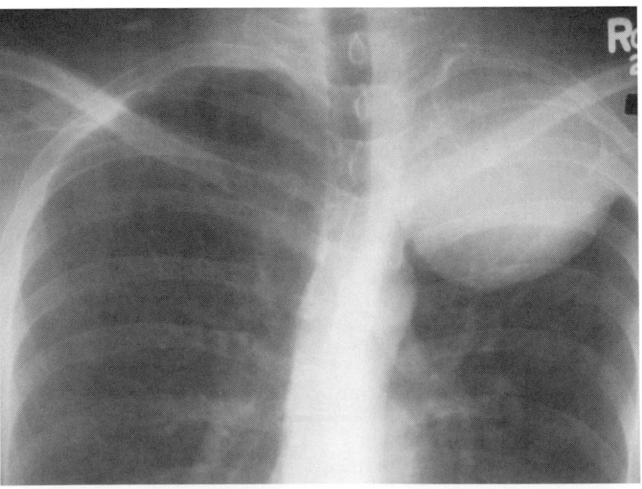

Figure 4-7 Chondroma of the first rib extending into the left hemithorax in a 30-year-old female. (Courtesy of the Yale Department of Radiology.)

Malignant bone and cartilage tumors

Chondrosarcoma

This is the most common malignancy of the anterior chest wall,[13] with approximately 20 percent of all chondrosarcomas presenting in the ribs or sternum.[14] Like chondroma, its benign counterpart, it arises 75 percent of the time from the costrochondral arches and sternum in patients 30 to 40 years of age. Unlike chondroma, it affects men twice as often as women; although it is also slow-growing, it often presents as a painful, hard, fixed mass. Trauma has been associated with these tumors. Histologically and radiographically they are difficult to distinguish from chondromas. However, there are specific prognostic indicators that help to determine prognosis.

Prognostic indicators include histologic grade, tumor size, patient's age, metastasis, and resectability. Microscopically, they are composed of malignant and

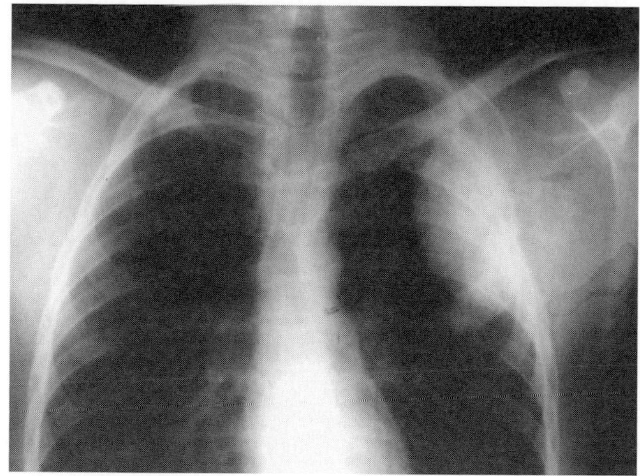

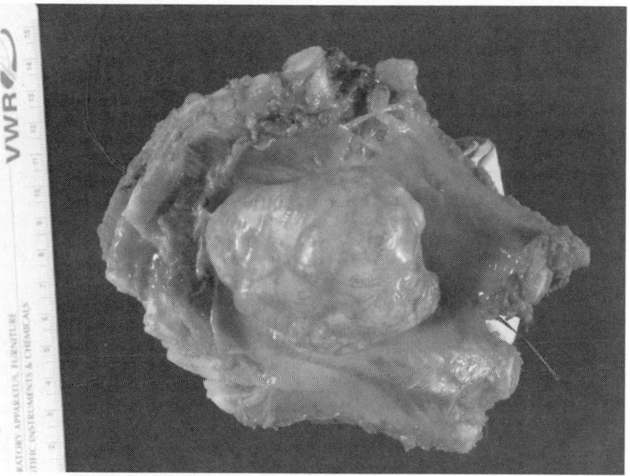

Figure 4-8 A. Radiograph of a chondrosarcoma of the third rib in a 15-year-old male who presented with a rapidly growing axillary tumor. (Courtesy of the Yale Department of Radiology.) B. Pathology specimen of a chondrosarcoma. (Courtesy of the Yale Department of Pathology.)

myxoid cartilage. X-rays demonstrate tumors that arise from the medulla, with cortical lytic lesions and some areas of thickened cortex as well as mottled or stippled calcifications on the tumor itself (Fig. 4-8). It is thought that a more radiolucent tumor represents a higher-grade lesion. Patients with low-grade tumors of mild hypercellularity have been reported to have 10-year survival rates up to 96 percent, with very few cases of metastasis. On the other hand, high-grade tumors with marked hypercellularity have demonstrated metastasis 75 percent of the time.[3] The 5-year survival rate with metastatic disease is 20 to 30 percent. Tumor size greater than 10 cm is also a poor prognostic indicator. Tumors greater than 10 cm are thought to be more aggressive. Patients who present above age 50 have also been found to have worse prognoses.[3]

Last, resectablility plays an important role in prognosis. Tumors should be treated with wide local excision, one rib above and one rib below the lesion, and with at least a 4-cm margin, including the underlying pleura, and adequate sternal margins.[4,13,14] Tumors that are widely excised have shown a 10-year survival rate of 96 percent, 65 percent with limited resection, and 14 percent with palliative resection.[1,15] Overall, 64 to 86 percent 5-year survival has been shown.[14,16–19] The local recurrence rate has also been shown to decrease significantly (up to sixfold) with adequate margins.[14] Chemotherapy and radiation therapy have had a limited role and are used primarily in patients with unresectable tumors or with positive margins.

Osteogenic sarcoma

Although this tumor is most commonly seen in long bones, it also makes up 6 percent of primary chest wall malignancies.[4] Osteogenic sarcoma is a malignant mesenchymal tumor that produces bone matrix. Patients present with a rapidly expanding, painful mass and with elevated alkaline phosphatase levels. It most commonly affects teenagers and young adults but can also be seen later in life associated with Paget's disease, with prior radiation therapy, or at regions of prior bony infarction. There is a higher incidence of osteogenic sarcoma in men. Other risk factors include mutations to the Rb gene and p53.

Osteogenic sarcoma is more virulent than chondrosarcoma, with 20 percent of patients presenting with metastasis. For this reason, workup includes a chest x-ray and CT scans of the chest and abdomen to evaluate the extent of the disease. On roentgenography, bone destruction can be evident as the tumor erodes through cortex and soft tissue. Tumors are often large. A "starburst" pattern may be visualized, which represents calcifications at right angles to the cortex (Fig. 4-9). In addition, the tumor may lift the periosteum, and the shadow between the cortex and raised periosteum forms a Codman triangle.

Treatment includes a combination of chemotherapy and surgery, with little role for radiation. In chemotherapy, the combination of vincristine, doxorubicin, and high-dose methotrexate is used for preoperative treatment of metastasis.[4] Tumors that express p-glycoprotein are thought to correlate with a better response to chemotherapeutic agents.[3] The lung is the primary location for metastasis; when possible, patients with lung metastasis will undergo resection of metastatic lesions prior to wide local excision of the primary tumor. The primary tumor is excised with the entire involved rib or bone, adjacent soft tissue and muscle, and adequate margins. The overall prognosis for osteogenic sarcoma is poor: the 5-year survival rate is 14 to 20 percent.[1,4,19,20] Poor prognosis is correlated with patients who are unresponsive to chemotherapy, have unresectable tumors, and have multifocal disease or Paget's disease.

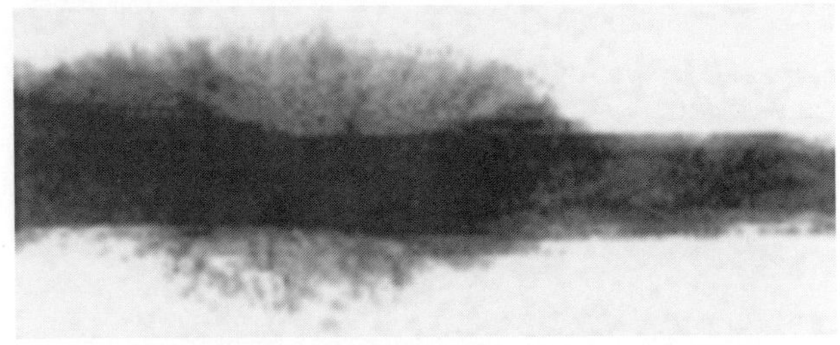

A

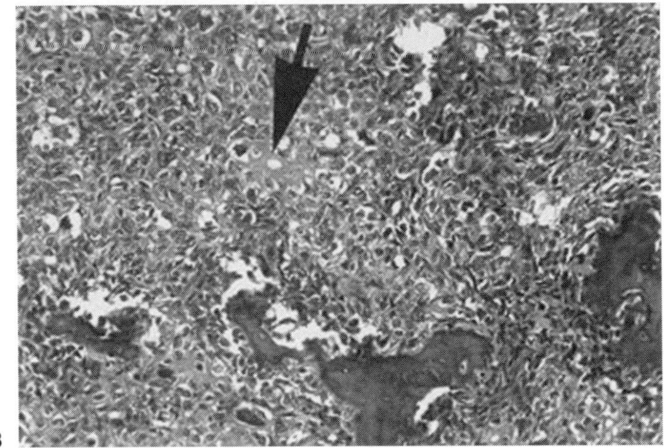

B

Figure 4-9 A. A radiograph of a rib demonstrating the "starburst" pattern visualized in osteogenic sarcoma. (Courtesy of Faxitron.) B. A microscopic look at the osteoid matrix produced by the malignant cells in osteogenic sarcoma.

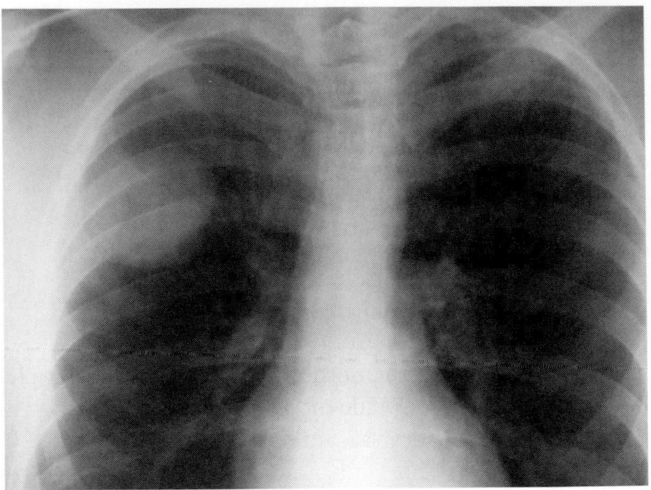

Figure 4-10 An AP chest radiograph of Ewing's sarcoma involving the right second rib in an 18-year-old male. (Courtesy of the Yale Department of Radiology.)

Primitive neuroectodermal tumors

Ewing's sarcoma is the most common chest wall malignancy in children and the third most common chest wall tumor overall. It is a tumor of neural cell origin, arising from the medullary cavity of bones and soft tissue. Microscopically, it is an abundance of small round blue cells with numerous areas of necrosis and few mitotic cells. Patients usually are between ages 10 and 15. Boys are affected twice as often as girls and whites more commonly than blacks.[21] Most patients (90 percent) have an associated gene translocation resulting in the fusion of the Ewing sarcoma gene and FLI-1 genes [t(11;22)].[22] Patients present with rapidly enlarging, painful masses, pain alone, or masses alone with or without constitutional symptoms including malaise, fever, and leukocytosis or increased erythrocyte sedimentation rates. Areas may be warm or erythematous on exam. X-rays demonstrate both lytic and blastic regions with a widened cortex and medulla. An onionskin appearance may be seen, representing elevation of the periosteum with layers of bone formation underneath (Fig. 4-10). Pathologic fractures are rare. Core or open biopsies may be more useful than cellular aspirates in helping to make a definitive diagnosis for accurate reverse-transcription polymerase chain reaction (PCR) analysis of gene translocations.[22]

Treatment is with surgery, chemotherapy (vincristine, cyclophosphamide, doxorubicin, or actinomycin D, with alternating ifosfamide and etoposide), and radiation therapy.[23] Initial adjuvant chemotherapy has been used to improve outcome and is thought to be especially important in patients who present with metastatic disease, where survival drops significantly, and where complete resection is difficult.[21,23] However, no statistically significant difference has been seen in patients treated with preoperative chemotherapy versus primary resection. Surgical treatment is wide local resection. Radiation therapy is for patients with positive margins or evidence of residual microscopic disease, but it may be avoided in patients with adequate surgical margins. Current survival rates are 56 to 65 percent in 5 years[21,23] and 43 percent in 10 years.[18]

Askin tumor is another primitive neuroectodermal tumor that was first identified in 1979 by Askin and coworkers.[24] It is a rare tumor found in the thoracopulmonary region in children. Like Ewing's sarcoma, it is diagnosed by histology and immunohistochemistry for translocations and treated with multiple modalities, including pre- and postoperative chemotherapy, radical tumor resection, and postoperative radiation therapy. Despite aggressive treatment, the survival rate is poor, with an approximately 16 percent 5-year survival.[25–27]

Plasmacytoma

Plasmacytomas are lesions of chest, ribs, sternum, scapula, and clavicle, solitary or numerous, and often associated with multiple myeloma. They arise from plasma cells and account for 20 percent of primary malignant neoplasms. Patients are older than the population that usually presents with other primary bony and cartilaginous tumors of the chest wall. Primarily men in their sixties and seventies are affected. In association with multiple myeloma, the diagnosis is made from the presence of Bence-Jones proteinuria, abnormal protein electrophoresis, bone marrow biopsies, or hypercalcemia. Approximately half of the patients who do not initially present with systemic multiple myeloma develop the disease in 10 years. Patients present with pain unaccompanied by a palpable mass. Pathologic fractures are common. X-rays demonstrate punched-out lytic lesions with cortical thinning.

Treatment is surgical excision when the lesion is isolated, and excision is also done to confirm a diagnosis. The excised bone is made up of monoclonal plasma cells. Following diagnosis, high-dose radiation therapy is the treatment of choice. Chemotherapy has a role for multiple lesions or recurrences. Wide margins have not been shown to enhance overall survival. Survival rates are as low as 20 percent in 5 years and are related to the development or presence of multiple myeloma. A survival rate of 59 percent in 10 years is seen in solitary plasmacytomas.[18]

CHEST WALL TUMORS FROM INVASION OR METASTASIS

The majority of chest wall neoplasms are tumors that spread to and extend into the chest wall. According to a 20-year study at Memorial Sloan-Kettering Cancer Center, 69 percent of chest wall tumors are due to invasion or metastasis. McCormack and coworkers have demonstrated that of 317 patients with chest wall neoplasms, 40 percent had primary lung tumors, 18 percent had mammary carcinomas, and 11 percent had metastatic sarcomas.[1] Each of these entities requires diagnostic workup and distinct clinical judgment for treatment.

Primary lung tumors

Patients with lung cancer present with chest wall invasion (T3 lesions) 5 to 8 percent of the time. They are often diagnosed with T3 lesions because they complain of pain in the chest wall. Otherwise evidence of invasion comes from diagnostic imaging, CT and MRI, and evaluation at the time of surgery. Prognostic indicators for T3 lung cancer lesions include the depth of the tumor; nodal metastasis, most importantly metastasis in the ipsilateral mediastinal and/or subcarinal lymph nodes (N2); and spinal or mediastinal involvement.[28,29] Regardless of depth and nodal metastasis, however, complete surgical resection is essential to improve survival. Numerous studies have demonstrated that an incomplete resection provides no curative benefit regardless of other prognostic indicators.[29] A study by Downey and associates showed the 3-year survival of patients with incomplete resection to be 4 percent, compared to 0 percent in patients without resection.[29]

Difficulties in surgical management arise from the intraoperative challenge of identifying tumor margins. Facciolo and colleagues studied an aggressive surgical approach to address this issue, with the following good results. They studied 104 patients with invading non–small cell carcinoma of the lung. These patients presented with either chest pain, CT or MRI evidence of invasion, or operative evidence of parietal pleural attachment without opening of the extrapleural space. Patients with Pancoast tumors or spinal invasion were excluded from the study. Each patient underwent en bloc resection of the chest wall and lung parenchyma with routine systemic dissection of all hilar and mediastinal lymph nodes for chest wall invasion. Resection of the chest wall included the involved rib or ribs and one uninvolved rib and intercostal space above and below the tumor, with the ribs divided at least 4 cm from the tumor. A radical standard lymphectomy was also done for staging and muscle flaps were used when needed for closure. Facciolo and coworkers demonstrated that all 104 patients had microscopically negative margins and 28 patients had invasion on the parietal pleura alone. These patients had a mortality of 0 percent, one case of local recurrence, and an overall 5-year survival of 61.4 percent. Patients with N0 (negative lymph nodes) versus N2 showed a 5-year survival differences of 67.3 and 17.9 percent, respectively; patients with only parietal involvement versus those with soft tissue involvement with or without bony invasion showed a 5-year survival differences of 79.1 and 54.0 percent, respectively. Also noteworthy is the fact that patients with N2 disease were given preoperative as well as postoperative chemotherapy. Patients who received postoperative radiation therapy showed an improvement in survival that was not statistically significant.[28] Currently the indications for radiation therapy are not well defined.

This aggressive surgical approach had been debated, and some would recommend resection of the pleura en bloc with the lung tumor when the parietal pleura separates easily from the intercostal structures.[1] Frozen sections have also been used intraoperatively to help evaluate the extent of invasion, but results are not always diagnostic and have underestimated the extent of disease.

Mammary carcinomas and metastatic chest wall tumors

Breast cancer remains the most common cancer among women and is know to affect approximately 200,000 women annually. Considerations for chest wall surgery in patients with breast cancer involve resection of the primary tumor, resection of local recurrences, and resection of infected tissue or tissue damaged by radiation therapy. Like other metastatic tumors from the kidney, colon, prostate, sarcomas, or salivary glands, the survival of these patients is related to the extent of their primary disease. Therefore evaluation for chest wall resection must include staging of the primary disease in addition to a needle biopsy to confirm diagnosis. Surgery is often considered appropriate for lesions that are solitary with no evidence of distant disease or for palliative reasons when patients are symptomatic.

CHEST WALL RECONSTRUCTION

Chest wall tumors vary in size, composition, growth patterns, and malignant potential. Appropriate resection is the key to improving survival in many circumstances. In an effort to allow patients the best chance of cure, wide resection guidelines consist of at least a 4-cm margin, resection of one rib above and one rib below the tumor without entering the tumor, and taking skin and parietal pleura if they are involved.[4,30] For this reason, various forms of chest wall reconstruction have been devised to maintain the structural support offered by the chest wall and assist ventilation. Reconstruction should be considered for defects greater than 5 cm (> 10 cm for posterior tumors because of scapular coverage), resection of three or more ribs, resection of two or more ribs with baseline pulmonary compromise, resection of the sternoclavicular junction, and resection of the entire sternum or upper portion with manubrium.[31] With these ideas in mind, chest wall reconstruction is a challenge for surgeons; however, with many different techniques available, this procedure has been shown to be safe and durable, providing a chance for long-term survival. In an account of 500 consecutive patients at the Mayo Clinic over 18 years and using five different muscle flaps, omental transpositions, and prosthetics, a postoperative mortality of 3 percent was shown.[32]

Prosthetic reconstruction

Prosthetic reconstruction has been established for skeletal defects that have the potential to cause respiratory compromise. Options include Prolene or polytetrafluoroethylene (Gore-Tex) soft tissue patches, polypropylene mesh, prefabricated polymethylmethacrylate ribs, methylmethacrylate "sandwiches," and iliac bone allografts.

Soft tissue patches are designed to fit a particular defect. Once a resection is complete, the defect's size is

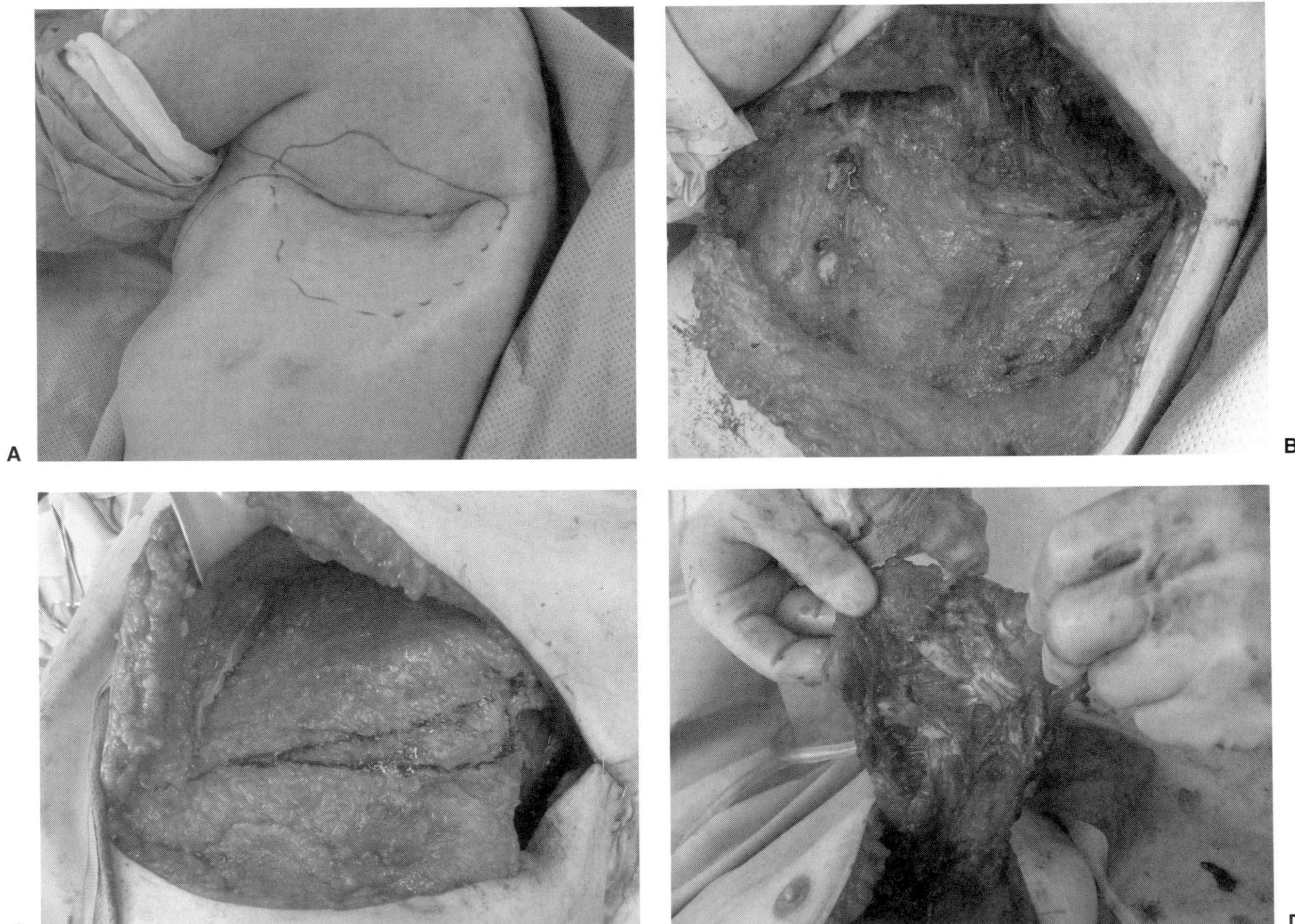

Figure 4-11 A series of pictures demonstrating the use of the pectoralis major muscle for the closure of an anterior chest wall defect. (Courtesy of Deepak Narayan, MD.)

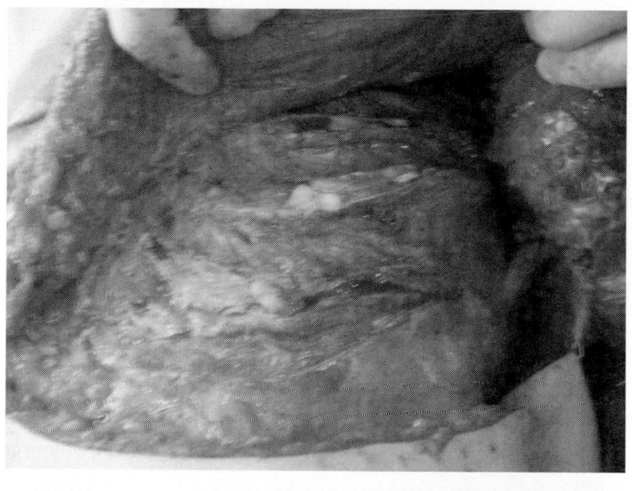
E

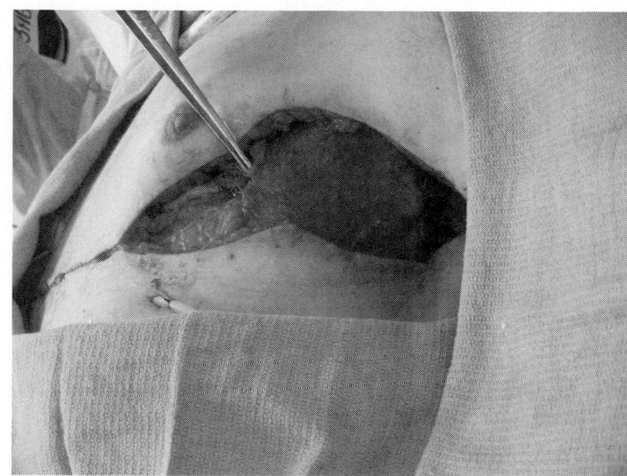
F

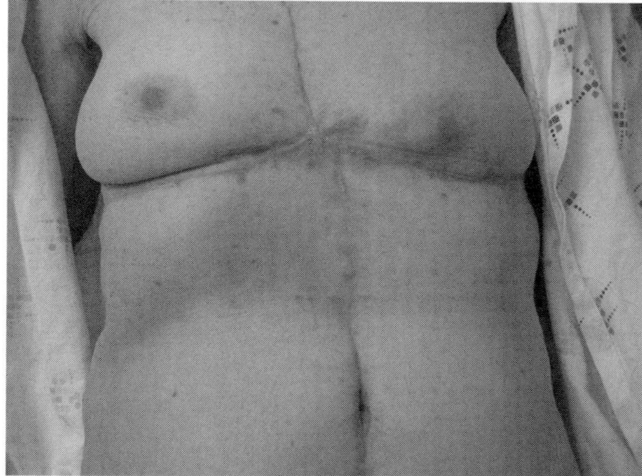
G

Figure 4-11 (*continued*)

measured and the patch created approximately 2 cm larger than the defect, allowing space to attach the patch to the chest wall. The patch is stretched over the defect to provide functional stability and a watertight seal. Mesh is fitted similarly; however, it provides slightly less mobility and is not watertight.

A methylmethacrylate "sandwich" is a rigid prosthetic that some surgeons prefer for skeletal defects, often in association with sternal or anterolateral resections. A mesh is measured to fit the defect using a gauze pattern. Then a 2- to 3-mm layer of methylmethacrylate is poured within 5 mm of the mesh edge. A second layer of mesh is then placed over the methylmethacrylate to make a sandwich. This sandwich is molded to the shape of the defect and sutured into place. Alternatively. the bottom mesh may be secured prior to forming the methylmethacrylate layer.

Iliac bone allografts have been used with muscle flap coverage to reconstruct chest walls. The allografts are tested for hepatitis B and C as well as HIV by PCR. Patients are grafted at the time of the original tumor resection. The proposed advantage is that allografts have the potential to integrate into host tissue and can be used to reconstruct larger defects than can autografts.[33] Polymethylmethacrylate ribs are used in a similar manner.[34] Stainless steel wires are used to stabilize the ribs in surgery involving large defects, where the ribs alone tend to sag. These ribs are also covered with muscle flaps.

The most important consideration in prosthetic reconstruction is infection. The use of prosthetics is contraindicated in contaminated wounds. Infected prosthetics must be removed, requiring reoperation and another method to repair persistent defects.

Soft tissue and autologous reconstruction

Soft tissue reconstructions include split-thickness skin grafts, muscle flaps, and musculocutaneous flaps, both free and with pedicles. These include flaps from the

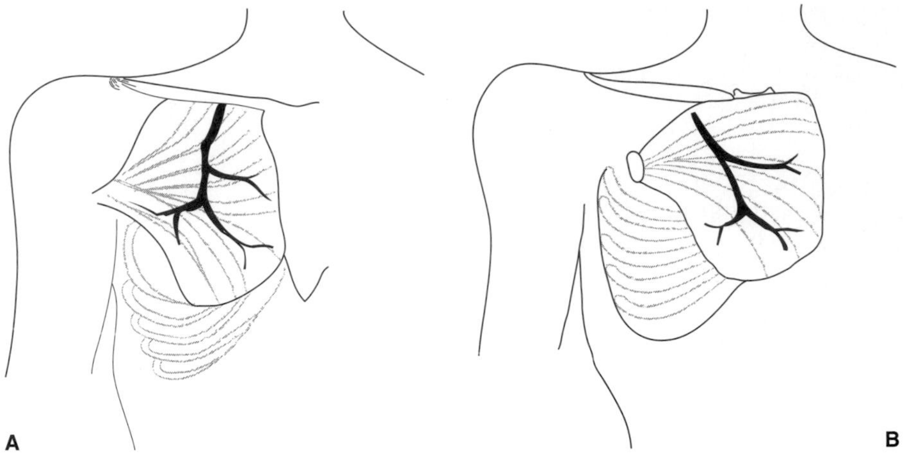

Figure 4-12 A. An illustration of the pectoralis major muscle. B. An illustration of the area covered by a pectoralis major flap. (Courtesy of Paul J. Gallo, DDS.)

pectoralis major, latissimus dorsi, rectus abdominis, trapezius, external oblique, and serratus anterior muscles. Greater omental transpositions are also used. In addition, autologous bone grafts are used for skeletal reconstruction.

Musculocutaneous flaps are frequently used following the excision of a chest wall tumor. At the Mayo Clinic, in 500 consecutive chest wall reconstructions, 470 patients underwent surgery involving 611 muscle flaps, the majority being pectoralis major flaps.[32] The advantage of these flaps is that they can cover a large surface area, and can be used in areas previously infected. Because the blood supply, or pedicle, of a flap should be axial to the incision, the choice of a particular flap depends on the location of the defect. Pectoralis major muscles are most often used for anterior central chest wall defects (Figs. 4-11 and 4-12). The latissimus dorsi muscle provides coverage for the anterior and anterolateral defects (Fig. 4-13). With the latissimus dorsi, the serratus anterior muscle can provide coverage for the intrathoracic area. The external oblique muscle is used less often, but it is helpful in closing defects at the inframammary fold (Fig. 4-14). It can also be used for closing diaphragmatic defects.

The greater omentum is used most often as a support system for skin and bone grafts. It can be used in infected sites and has the potential to cover areas often larger than can be covered by muscle flaps. It has been utilized as both a pedicle flap and as a free flap.

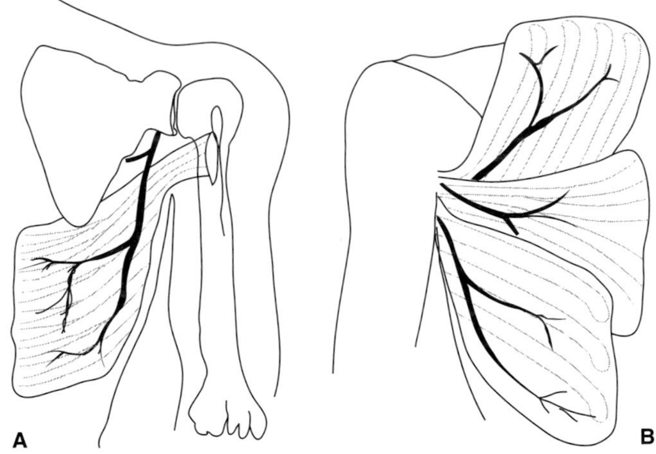

Figure 4-13 A. An illustration of the latissimus dorsi muscle. B. An illustration of the area covered by a latissimus dorsi flap. (Courtesy of Paul J. Gallo, DDS.)

SUMMARY

Chest wall tumors are rare, but they can be deadly. Their medical and surgical treatment must be well planned to give each patient the best chance for survival. Although this can be a challenge, doctors have found success and continue to learn and devise ways to improve on the diagnostic and treatment modalities already available.

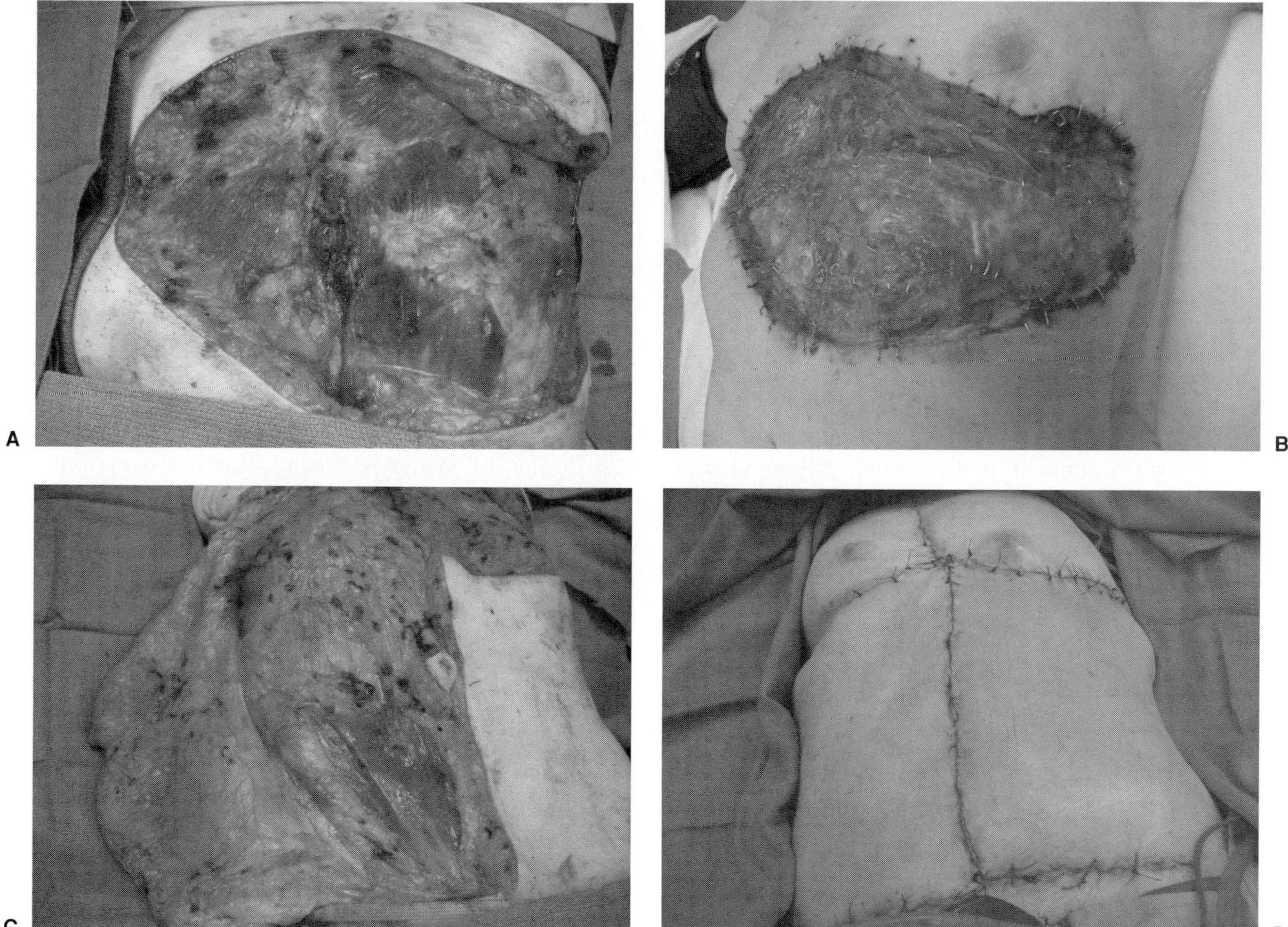

Figure 4-14 A series of pictures demonstrating the use of the external oblique muscle for an inframammary fold defect. (Courtesy of Deepak Narayan, MD.)

References

1. McCormack P. Chest wall tumors. In: Baue AE, Geha AS, Hammond GL, et al. (eds). *Glenn's Thoracic and Cardiovascular Surgery*, 5th ed. Norwalk, CT: Appleton and Lange, 1991:517–530.
2. Israel-Mardirosian N, Adler L. Positron emission tomography of soft tissue sarcomas. *Curr Opin Oncol* 2003;15(4): 327–330.
3. Cotran RS, Kumar V, Collins T. *Pathological Basis of Disease*. Philadelphia: Saunders, 1999.
4. Pairolero PC. Chest wall tumors. In: Shield TW (ed). *General Thoracic Surgery*, 4th ed. Baltimore: Williams & Wilkins, 1994:579–589.
5. Kabiri E, Al Aziz S, El Maslout A, et al. Desmoid tumors of the chest wall. *Eur J Cardio-Thorac Surg* 2001;19(5): 580–583.
6. Baliski CR, Temple WJ, Arthur K, et al. Desmoid tumors: A novel approach for local control. *J Surg Oncol* 2002;80(2):96–99.
7. Zagars GK, Ballo MT, Pisters PW, et al. Prognostic factors for patients with localized soft-tissue sarcomas treated with conservation surgery and radiation therapy: An analysis of 225 patients. *Cancer* 2003;97(10):2530–2543.
8. Chang AC, Nesbitt JC. Primary chest wall tumors. In: Cameron JL (ed). *Current Surgical Therapy*, 7th ed. St. Louis: Mosby, 2001:751–757.
9. Andrassy RJ, Wiener ES, Raney RB, et al. Thoracic sarcomas in children. *Ann Surg* 1998;227(2):170–173.
10. Maurer HM, Gehan EA, Beltangady M, et al. The intergroup rhabdomyosarcoma study I: A final report. *Cancer* 1988;61:209–220.
11. Graeger JA, Patel MK, Briele HA, et al. Soft tissue sarcomas of the adult thoracic wall. *Cancer* 1987;59:370.
12. Neville H, Corpron C, Blakely ML, et al. Pediatric Neurofibrosarcoma. *J Pediatr Surg* 2003;38(3):343–346.
13. Somers J, Faber LP. Chondroma and chondrosarcoma. *Semin Thorac Cardiovascul Surg* 1999;11(3):270–277.

14. Briccoli A, De Paolis M, Campanacci L, et al. Chondrosarcoma of the chest wall: A clinical analysis. *Surg Today* 2002;32:291–296.
15. Addis BJ. Pathology of tumors of the pleura and chest wall. In: Hoogstraten B Addis BJ, Hansen HH, et al. (eds). *Lung Tumors.* New York: Springer-Verlag, 1988:205.
16. Burt M, Fulton M, Weessner-Dunlap S, et al. Primary bony and cartilaginous sarcomas of the chest wall: Results of therapy. *Ann Thorac Surg* 1992;54:226–232.
17. King RM, Pairolero PC, Trastek VF, et al. Primary chest wall tumors: Factors affecting survival. *Ann Thorac Surg* 1986;41(6):597–601.
18. Sabanathan S, Shah R, Mearns AJ, et al. Surgical treatment of primary malignant chest wall tumors. *Eur J Cardio-Thorac Surg* 1997;11(6):1011–1016.
19. Martini N, Huvos AG, Burt ME, et al. Predictors of survival in malignant tumors of the sternum. *J Thorac Cardiol Surg* 1996;111(1):96–105.
20. Marcove R, Rosen G. En bloc resection for osteogenic sarcoma. *Cancer* 1980;45:3040.
21. Saenz NC, Hass DJ, Meyers P, et al. Pediatric chest wall Ewing's sarcoma. *J Pediatr Surg* 2000;35(4):550–555.
22. Dagher R, Pham T, Sorbara L, et al. Molecular confirmation of Ewing sarcoma. *J Pediatr Hematol Oncol* 2001;23(4):221–224.
23. Shamberger RC, LaQuaglia MP, Gebhardt MC, et al. Ewing sarcoma/primitive neuroectodermal tumor of the chest wall: Impact of initial versus delayed resection on tumor margins, survival, and use of radiation therapy. *Ann Surg* 2003;238(4):563–568.
24. Askin FB, Rosai J, Sibley RK, et al. Malignant small cell tumor of the thoracopulmonary region in childhood: A distinctive clinicopathologic entity of uncertain histogenesis. *Cancer* 1979;43:2439–2451.
25. Christiansen S, Semik M, Dockhorn-Dworniczak B, et al. Diagnosis, treatment and outcome of patients with Askin tumors. *Thorac Cardiovasc Surg* 2000;48(5):311–315.
26. Takanami I, Imamura T, Naruke M, et al. Long-term survival after repeated resections of Askin tumor recurrences. *Eur J Cardio-Thorac Surg* 1998;13(3):313–315.
27. Contesso G, Llombart-Bosch A, Terrier P, et al. Does malignant small round cell tumor of the thoracopulmonary region (Askin tumor) constitute a clinicopathologic entity? *Cancer* 1992;69(4):1012–1020.
28. Facciolo F, Cardillo G, Lopergolo M, et al. Chest wall invasion in non-small cell lung carcinoma: A rationale for en bloc resection. *J Thorac Cardiovasc Surg* 2001;121(4):649–665.
29. Downey RJ, Martini N, Rusch VW, et al. Extent of chest wall invasion and survival in patients with lung cancer. *Ann Thorac Surg* 1999;68:188–193.
30. Warzelhan J, Stoelban E, Imdahl A, et al. Results in surgery for primary and metastatic chest wall tumors. *Eur J Cardio-Thorac Surg* 2001;19(5):584–588.
31. Pairolero PC. Chest wall reconstruction. In: Shield TW (ed). *General Thoracic Surgery,* 4th ed. Baltimore: Williams & Wilkins, 1994:589–597.
32. Arnold PG, Pairolero PC. Chest-wall reconstruction: An account of 500 consecutive patients. *Plast Reconstr Surg* 1996;98(5):804–810.
33. Garcia-Tutor E, Yeste L, Murillo J, et al. Chest wall reconstruction using iliac bone allografts and muscle flaps. *Ann Plast Surg* 2004;52(1):54–60.
34. Agrawal K, Subbarao K, Nachiappan M, et al. An innovative method of reconstruction of large skeletal chest wall defects. *Plast Reconstr Surg* 1998;102(3):839–842.

CHAPTER

5 CONGENITAL ESOPHAGEAL ANOMALIES AND DIAPHRAGMATIC HERNIAS

David D. Yuh

CONGENITAL ESOPHAGEAL ANOMALIES

EPIDEMIOLOGY

Esophageal atresia

Esophageal atresia occurs in about 2.4 per 10,000 live births,[1] with a slight preponderance in males and children of older or diabetic mothers.[2] Usually sporadic, familial patterns and genomic linkages have been observed. Children born to an affected parent have a 3 to 4 percent risk, children with one affected sibling have a 0.5 to 2 percent risk, and children with two affected siblings have a risk in excess of 20 percent.[3] Associated anomalies include cardiac malformations, gastrointestinal anomalies (e.g., anal atresia), urinary tract anomalies (e.g., uni- or bilateral renal agenesis or hypoplasia, multicystic kidney, horseshoe kidney), neural tube defects, and skeletal malformations.

Esophageal duplication cysts

Esophageal duplication cysts account for 10 to 15 percent of all foregut duplication cysts and only 5 to 10 percent of all mediastinal cysts.[4]

KEY CONCEPTS

- Epidemiology
  - Esophageal atresia occurs in about 2.4 of every 10,000 live births, with a slight preponderance in males and children of older or diabetic mothers. Esophageal duplication cysts account for 10 to 15 percent of all foregut duplication cysts and only 5 to 10 percent of all mediastinal cysts. Congenital esophageal stenosis occurs in between 1:25,000 and 1:50,000 live births. Bochdalek posterolateral diaphragmatic hernias occur in 1:2000 to 1:5000 live births. Morgagni retrosternal diaphragmatic hernias comprise 1 to 5 percent of congenital diaphragmatic defects, occurring much less frequently than Bochdalek hernias.
- Pathophysiology
  - Esophageal atresia constitutes a spectrum of incomplete esophageal development, sometimes coupled with communication to the tracheobronchial tree. This can result in discontinuity between the oropharynx and stomach, leading to feeding difficulties and a predisposition for respiratory infections. Esophageal duplication cysts can occur all along the esophagus, can be intramural, partitioned completely from the esophageal true lumen, or may communicate with it. Esophageal stenosis and webs can partially or completely obstruct the esophageal lumen. Much of the morbidity associated with these esophageal malformations is derived from a spectrum of associated malformations (i.e., cardiac, renal, neurologic, skeletal). Bochdalek diaphragmatic hernias result in displacement of abdominal viscera into a pleural space (usually the left side), leading maldevelopment of the ipsilateral lung; the associated contralateral mediastinal shift can also affect contralateral lung development. The end result is hypoxia and varying degrees of pulmonary hypertension. Morgagni hernias result in herniation of abdominal viscera into the mediastinum and can cause intestinal obstructive pathophysiology.

- Clinical features
  - Esophageal atresia is suggested by polyhydramnios coupled with a small or absent stomach in utero and excessive drooling, rhonchi, aspiration, and respiratory distress during initial postnatal feedings. Esophageal duplication cysts are often asymptomatic but can cause dysphagia or respiratory compromise secondary to mass effects. Congenital esophageal stenosis and webs typically present in early infancy, leading to progressive dysphagia and vomiting with ingestion of semisolid or solid foods. In its most severe presentation, newborns with Bochdalek hernias present with severe respiratory distress with a scaphoid abdomen. Morgagni hernias usually present much later in life with more subtle gastrointestinal symptoms or discomfort.
- Diagnostics
  - Esophageal atresia is most readily diagnosed with passage and insufflation of an esophageal catheter into the blind esophageal pouch. This can be imaged with plain film radiography; abdominal air confirms a distal fistula, whereas its absence suggests pure atresia. Plain films can also suggest esophageal cysts as sharply defined, spherical or tubular masses with esophageal and/or tracheal displacement. Confirmatory studies include contrast esophagography or computed tomography. Esophageal stenosis and webs are usually adequately diagnosed with barium esophagography and endoscopy. Plain chest radiography is often diagnostic for Bochdalek and Morgagni hernias but these can be confirmed with computed tomography, magnetic resonance imaging, or ultrasound.
- Treatment
  - Operative repair of esophageal atresia nominally consists of primarily anastomosing the proximal and distal esophageal segments with ligation of associated tracheoesophageal fistulas. Esophageal cysts are generally excised. Esophageal stenosis is usually initially treated conservatively with one or several dilations. Failing conservative therapy, surgical treatment generally consists of resecting the stenotic esophageal segment with primary anastomosis. Operative repair of Bochdalek and Morgagni hernias generally consists of reducing the herniated abdominal contents to their normal intraabdominal positions, resecting of any hernia sac, and primary or patch repair of the diaphragmatic defect.
- Results/outcomes
  - Repairs of esophageal atresia and stenosis are generally associated with good results; hospital survival rates range from 85 to 95 percent. Potential complications include anastomotic leak or stricture, recurrent fistula, and gastroesophageal reflux. Surgical repair of congenital diaphragmatic hernias is associated with good results. Morbidity and mortality with Bochdalek repairs usually arise from severe pulmonary developmental compromise and/or associated malformations.

Esophageal stenosis and webs

The incidence of congenital esophageal stenosis is reported to be between 1:25,000 and 1:50,000 live births.[5] Associated anomalies include esophageal or intestinal atresia, anorectal malformations, cardiac malformations, midgut malrotation, hypospadias, chromosomal abnormalities, and malformations of the head, face, and limbs.

Embryology

Esophageal atresia

Although the embryologic basis of esophageal atresia with or without tracheoesophageal fistula is poorly understood, it is postulated that this anomaly arises from failure of early endoderm-mesoderm interactions, which normally initiate development of the tracheobronchial tree from the esophagus, leading to "trachealization" of the proximal foregut with the main bronchi branching directly from this structure and the foregut continuing caudally to the stomach.

Esophageal duplication cysts

Several theories have arisen pertaining to the embryologic origins of esophageal duplication cysts. Kirwan and colleagues have suggested that errors in epithelial cell vacuolization during esophageal luminal development in the fourth through sixth weeks of gestation may be responsible.[6] Others implicate improper tracheobronchial budding.[7] The *endoderm-ectoderm adhesion theory* proposes that discordant longitudinal growth of the neural tube and foregut creates a shear force against adhesions that normally occur between the ectodermal and endodermal layers during primitive foregut development, detaching developing enteric cells.[8] The *split-notochord theory* postulates that esophageal cysts arise when an endodermic diverticulum expands posteriorly to fill an abnormal fissure between the endodermal and ectodermal layers of the primitive foregut.

Esophageal stenosis and webs

Fibromuscular thickening is the most common cause of congenital esophageal stenosis: however, its embryologic basis remains unknown. A less common cause of stenosis is tracheobronchial remnants, which are believed to result from incomplete separation of the primitive foregut from the respiratory tract. Congenital webs are thought to occur by failure of complete vacuolization of

Table 5-1 Gross and Ladd classification schemes for esophageal atresia and tracheoesophageal fistulas

Description	EA with distal TEF	Isolated EA	"N-type" TEF	EA with proximal TEF	EA with proximal and distal TEF
Gross Classification	C	A	E	B	D
Ladd Classification	III/IV[a]	I		II	V
Frequency (%)	86.5	7.7	4.2	0.8	0.7

EA = esophageal atresia; TEF = tracheoesophageal fistula.
[a]Type III fistula enters above tracheal bifurcation; type IV fistula enters at carina.
Source: Goldstein AM, Doody DP, Donahoe PK. Esophageal atresia and tracheoesophageal fistula. In: Pearson FG, Cooper JD, Deslauriers J, et al (eds). *Esophageal Surgery.* New York: Churchill Livingstone, 2002. With permission.

the mucosa-filled primordial esophageal lumen between the sixth and tenth weeks of embryogenesis.[6]

Classification

Esophageal atresia

The anatomic variants of esophageal atresia have been classified according to several different schemes. These variants generally comprise isolated esophageal atresia, esophageal atresia with a distal tracheoesophageal fistula, esophageal atresia with a proximal tracheoesophageal fistula, esophageal atresia with proximal and distal tracheoesophageal fistulas, and a so-called N-type tracheoesophageal fistula. The most commonly used classifications are those of Ladd[9] and Gross,[10] summarized in Table 5-1.

Esophageal duplication cysts

Esophageal cysts have been observed along all points of the esophagus, including the cervical, thoracic, and abdominal segments.[11] They can be intramural, completely partitioned from the esophagus, or they may communicate with the esophagus or other abdominal viscera. The definitions and classifications of esophageal duplication cysts have varied; however, Fallon and associates[12] have classified these cysts according to histologic and embryologic features (Table 5-2).

Esophageal stenosis and webs

Like esophageal duplication cysts, esophageal stenosis and webs have been classified according to several confusing schemes. A common scheme is that described by Nihoul-Fekete and coworkers (Table 5-3).[5]

Associated congenital anomalies

Esophageal atresia

Approximately 50 percent of infants born with esophageal atresia with or without tracheoesophageal fistula have additional congenital anomalies. Associated anomalies are seen more frequently in infants with an N-type fistula and those weighing less than 2000 g. A

Table 5-2 Categories of esophageal cysts

Category	Anatomic description
Intramural esophageal cysts ("true duplication" cysts)	Exist within the esophageal wall and are lined with squamous or columnar epithelium.
Enteric cysts	Circumscribed by well-developed muscular walls and contain epithelia from different embryonic origins.
Tracheobronchial foregut duplications	Anteriorly located cysts, most likely arising from a primitive lung bud that has incompletely separated from the primitive foregut. Lined with ciliated columnar or respiratory epithelium.
Posterior cysts	Often joined to the spinal column in the posterior mediastinum.
Neurenteric cysts	A subset of dorsal enteric cysts attached to the dura through a vertebral defect, often associated with vertebral anomalies (e.g., spina bifida occulta, anterior hemivertebrae).

Table 5-3 Categories of congenital esophageal stenosis

Category	Anatomic description
Fibromuscular thickening	Diffuse fibrosis of the wall with segmental hypertrophy of the muscularis and submucosal layers. Usually located in the distal esophagus, this is the type most commonly associated with esophageal atresia.
Tracheobronchial remnants	Comprising cartilage, respiratory mucous glands, or ciliated epithelium and forming a rigid, focal stenosis; most commonly located in the distal esophagus.
Membranous web	Consists of a thin, diaphragm-like membrane lined with epithelium and with an eccentrically located opening; observed at all esophageal levels. This is the rarest type of congenital esophageal stenosis.

thorough investigation into these associated anomalies is important, as they are often responsible for the morbidity and mortality seen in these patients.

Approximately 20 to 30 percent of infants with esophageal atresia have associated cardiovascular malformations,[13] the most frequently encountered anomalies associated with esophageal atresia. The most common of these include atrial and ventricular septal defects, patent ductus arteriosus, tetralogy of Fallot, and aortic arch anomalies. Gastrointestinal anomalies occur in about 25 percent of patients with esophageal atresia; the most commonly observed anomaly is anal atresia, followed by duodenal and ileal atresia, malrotation, Meckel's diverticulum, annular pancreas, and pyloric stenosis. Fortunately, most of these anomalies are comparatively easy to repair at the time of esophageal repair. Urinary tract malformations have been observed in as many as 24 percent of patients with esophageal atresia.[14] These anomalies include uni- or bilateral renal agenesis or hypoplasia, multicystic kidney, horseshoe kidney, and vesicoureteral reflux. Permanent renal dysfunction can be avoided if such anomalies are discovered and corrected early. Neural tube defects, hydrocephalus, and vertebral or extremity anomalies comprise neurologic and skeletal anomalies associated with esophageal atresia, observed in approximately 10 percent of affected infants.[15]

Esophageal atresia is one of the components of the VACTERL syndrome (i.e., vertebral anomalies, anal atresia, cardiac anomalies, tracheoesophageal fistula with esophageal atresia, renal defects, and radial limb dysplasia).[16] VACTERL occurs in approximately 15 percent of children with esophageal atresia, resulting in heightened mortality primarily due to cardiac malformations.

Esophageal duplication cysts

Esophageal cysts are associated with esophageal atresia,[17] vertebral anomalies, and neural tube defects.

Esophageal stenosis and webs

Congenital esophageal stenosis is associated with intestinal atresia, midgut malrotation, anorectal malformations, cardiac anomalies, hypospadias, chromosomal abnormalities, and malformations of the head, face, and limbs.[5] The fibromuscular thickening and tracheobronchial remnant types of esophageal stenosis are associated with esophageal atresia.

Clinical presentation and diagnosis

Esophageal atresia and tracheoesophageal fistula

Polyhydramnios coupled with a small or absent stomach observed on prenatal ultrasound examinations suggests esophageal atresia.[18] Pure atresia nearly always results in polyhydramnios, since polyhydramnios arises from an inability of the fetus to swallow amniotic fluid through an atretic esophagus. In cases of esophageal atresia without polyhydramnios, a distal tracheoesophageal fistula often permits the amniotic fluid to pass into the stomach.

In the early postnatal period, infants with esophageal atresia suffer from excessive drooling, accumulation of saliva in the posterior pharynx, excessive salivation from the nose and mouth, and rhonchi. Left undetected, this condition often leads to aspiration, with choking, respiratory distress, and cyanosis during the initial feedings; serious aspiration may also be associated with apnea, bradycardia, and death. A distal tracheoesophageal fistula predisposes to more severe respiratory distress, since gastric secretions can reflux into the tracheobronchial tree, causing pneumonitis and pulmonary sepsis. Other signs of pure esophageal atresia include a scaphoid abdomen. Atresia associated with a distal fistula can lead to a distended abdomen as air enters the stomach from the trachea. A complete physical exam can reveal or suggest other associated anomalies. Screening tests should include an echocardiogram, renal ultrasound, voiding cystourogram, and chromosomal analysis.

The diagnosis and delineation of esophageal atresia usually begins with passage of an esophageal catheter (e.g., 10F) through the infant's mouth. With slight insufflation of the tube, plain radiography can outline the size and shape of the esophageal pouch. Infrequently, dilute barium can be used to reveal a proximal tracheoesophageal fistula. On plain films, abdominal air confirms a distal fistula, whereas its absence suggests pure atresia. Other information obtained from the plain film includes signs of pneumonitis, an abnormal cardiac silhouette suggestive of a congenital malformation or right-sided aortic arch, and skeletal malformations.

An isolated N-type tracheoesophageal fistula usually leads to coughing and choking with feeding, gastric reflux into the tracheobronchial tree, and a barking cough due to tracheomalacia. Although contrast esophagography can be used to make this diagnosis, bronchoscopy and esophagoscopy are often required.

Esophageal duplication cysts

Esophageal cysts are often detected incidentally on plain chest radiographs, since many are asymptomatic. Symptoms arising from esophageal cysts usually consist of varying degrees of dysphagia. Esophageal cysts can also lead to respiratory distress in young patients, due to reductions in ventilatory volume, tracheal compression, or extrinsic compression of large bronchi, causing emphysema from air trapping and atelectasis or consolidation from extensive alveolar collapse. Other symptoms arise from the gastric epithelial cyst lining, including esophageal perforation, hemorrhage, or ulcerative pain. Rarely, larger cysts have elicited superior vena cava syndrome and abdominal masses. Neurenteric cysts commonly cause pain. Weakness and paralysis can arise from spinal cord compression caused by intraspinal lesions.

On plain chest radiography, esophageal cysts are usually suggested by a large unilateral (propensity to the right hemithorax), sharply defined, spherical or tubular mass. Often, this mass displaces the trachea and/or esophagus. Other plain film findings may derive from associated anomalies, including vertebral anomalies (e.g., bifid vertebrae). Confirmatory studies include contrast esophagography, typically demonstrating a smooth filling defect with luminal distortion or displacement. Transthoracic ultrasonography can also be used to confirm these lesions, differentiating them by their cystic nature from solid tumors. Computed tomography is replacing ultrasonography as the imaging modality of choice. Technetium scanning can reveal cysts containing a gastric mucosal lining, particularly in patients presenting with bleeding or ulceration. Esophagoscopy cannot reliably differentiate esophageal cysts from other posterior mediastinal masses; however, this modality may be useful in identifying continuity between a cyst and the true esophageal lumen. Magnetic resonance imaging is useful in identifying any neurenteric components to esophageal cysts as well as detecting associated vertebral and intraspinal abnormalities.

Esophageal stenosis and webs

The typical presentation of congenital esophageal stenosis occurs in early infancy as progressive dysphagia and vomiting with ingestion of semisolid or solid foods. The severity of these symptoms largely depends on the degree of stenosis and its location within the esophagus; complete obstruction resembles esophageal atresia, proximal stenosis leads to an inability to swallow food, and distal lesions often result in regurgitation.

Diagnostically, barium esophagography and endoscopy are usually adequate in defining the location and severity of esophageal stenosis. Fibromuscular thickening is typically characterized by a long, tapered narrowing in the distal esophagus. Discrete, focal narrowings are more suggestive of tracheobronchial remnants. Webs or fibromuscular hypertrophy can also present as lesions in the middle or proximal third of the esophagus. Esophagoscopy usually demonstrates normal mucosa overlying a narrowed lumen; biopsy can exclude esophagitis and neoplastic lesions.

Preoperative management

Esophageal atresia and tracheoesophageal fistula

Infants with esophageal atresia and tracheoesophageal fistula should be nursed in a semiupright sitting position to reduce gastric reflux through the fistula into the tracheobronchial tree. Frequent oropharyngeal suctioning and a soft sump catheter placed into the atretic esophageal pouch can minimize aspiration events. Usually, prophylactic or therapeutic parenteral antibiotics (e.g., ampicillin and gentamicin) should be administered due to the high incidence of aspiration pneumonitis.

For infants suffering from severe aspiration pneumonitis or who are in significant respiratory distress, endotracheal intubation and mechanical ventilation is indicated. A gastrostomy should be considered to prevent continued reflux of gastric contents into the tracheobronchial tree and gastric distention. Early primary esophageal repair with division of an associated fistula can usually be performed within the first 2 days of life in stable patients without a major cardiac anomaly or respiratory compromise. Unstable patients with severe associated anomalies can be temporized with a gastrostomy until they have been optimized. In patients with congenital cardiac malformations, early primary esophageal repair can proceed in those whose circulation is not dependent on a patent ductus arteriosus.[13] In duct-dependent infants, prostaglandin E may be used to permit early repair. Otherwise, corrective cardiac surgery may have to performed first, with fistula division and gastrostomy placement sometimes performed during the cardiac operation; definitive esophageal repair should be delayed in these ill infants.

Esophageal duplication cysts

In most cases, elective surgical excision of esophageal cysts can be performed after diagnosis. In the rare cases of particularly large cysts associated with respiratory compromise, percutaneous decompression may be necessary preoperatively.[19]

Esophageal stenosis and webs

Effective treatment of congenital esophageal stenosis and webs focuses on alleviation of symptoms and preservation of normal antireflux mechanisms. Initial treatment for most children consists of esophageal dilatation by bougienage. This approach consists of a series of antegrade and retrograde dilatations with mercury-weighted tapered Maloney or Avaray bougies and is most successful in children with a thin esophageal web or mild fibromuscular thickening. This conservative, nonoperative approach is still associated with occasional complications, including esophageal leak and recurrent stenosis. Long-term results are generally good, although many patients require repeated dilatations to maintain adequate esophageal patency.[20]

Operative repair

Esophageal atresia and tracheoesophageal fistula

Bronchoscopy should be performed prior to any operative repair of esophageal atresia in order to identify all tracheoesophageal fistulas, characterize tracheomalacia, and correctly position the endotracheal tube distal to the fistula and above the carina.

The operative approach is through a right posterolateral thoracotomy running 1 cm below the scapular tip (except in the case of a right-sided aortic arch) and within the inframammary crease (Fig. 5-1). Entry is usually through the fourth intercostal space, although the third interspace may afford better access to higher proximal pouches. Approaching the esophagus along the retropleural plane can limit any postoperative leak to the retropleural space. This approach is conducted by bluntly peeling the pleura away from the chest wall from the apex of the chest to a level several interspaces below the incision and posterior to the mediastinum.

The vagus nerve is identified and carefully preserved, while the azygos vein is divided. The trachea and distal esophagus are exposed by retracting the mediastinal pleura anteriorly. The distal esophagus is then looped to control any tracheoesophageal air leak, particularly if this interferes with mechanical ventilation during the procedure. The proximal esophageal pouch is then dissected up into the neck, identifying any proximal fistula; this can be facilitated with insertion of a Bakes dilator and gentle pushing of the proximal esophagus toward the surgeon by the anesthesiologist. If the gap between the proximal pouch and distal esophagus is so large as to preclude a primary repair, circular myotomies can be made in the proximal pouch to extend its length distally. Up to three myotomies can be made safely, with each adding approximately 1 cm of length.

Any tracheoesophageal fistula is isolated and divided; the tracheal side is closed with an interrupted absorbable 5-0 suture. The distal esophagus is mobilized sufficiently to permit tension-free approximation to the upper pouch. The proximal pouch is then opened and an end-to-end single-layer anastomosis is constructed with interrupted 5-0 nonabsorbable sutures on the posterior wall, with the knots tied on the outside. A feeding tube is then passed through the nares into the stomach across the anastomosis, followed by completion of the anterior circumference of the anastomosis; the feeding tube is secured to the nares to prevent dislodgement. If the distance between the proximal pouch and the distal esophagus is particularly long or the infant is premature, a gastrostomy is placed prior to the thoracotomy and a nasogastric feeding tube is not passed.

After the anastomosis has been completed, a chest tube is placed in the immediate vicinity of the repair but is secured to the posterior chest wall to prevent direct contact with the anastomosis. The thoracotomy is then closed in standard fashion. If primary repair is not possible, the distal esophagus is oversewn and sutured to the prevertebral fascia. Delayed primary repair is then undertaken after daily dilatations of the proximal pouch for 1 to 2 months. In those rare cases where a primary repair cannot be performed, alternatives include esophageal replacement using a colon interposition graft,[21] jejunal interposition graft,[22] or gastric tube.[23] Operative results are generally good, with hospital survival rates ranging from 85 to 95 percent.[1] Morbidity and mortality usually stem from associated congenital or chromosomal defects.

Complications Complications after operative repair of esophageal atresia include anastomotic leak (15 to 20 percent), recurrent fistula (3 to 10 percent), anastomotic stricture (10 to 35), gastroesophageal reflux (55 to 82 percent), and tracheomalacia (10 to 20 percent). Anastomotic leaks are often heralded with saliva observed in the chest tube, confirmed by orally administered methylene blue dye, and localized by barium swallow. Since most leaks are small, initial conservative management with proximal esophageal suctioning, localized drainage, antibiotics, and parenteral nutrition is often successful. Larger leaks or those that do not seal after conservative management should be operatively repaired to prevent mediastinal sepsis or empyema.

Infants with recurrent tracheoesophageal fistulas usually present several months after primary repair with cyanosis, wheezing, coughing or choking with feeding; abdominal distention, and recurrent pneumonias. The initial diagnosis is generally a barium swallow to identify and localize these fistulas. Since most of them do not close with expectant management, operative repair should generally be undertaken. The operative approach is dictated by the location of the fistulas; a cervical approach is taken for proximal fistulas while more distal fistulas are accessed via the chest. The fistulas must be closed at either end, followed by interposition tissue flaps placed between the esophagus and trachea to prevent recurrence.

Esophageal anastomotic strictures are best characterized by barium swallow and usually effectively treated with balloon dilatation. Gastroesophageal reflux—accompanied by heartburn, dysphagia, chronic coughing, vomiting, and recurrent respiratory infections—is commonly encountered after esophageal atresia repair. Once confirmed with a swallow study, symptomatic patients are initially treated conservatively with antacid therapy, thickened feeds, upright feedings, and promotility

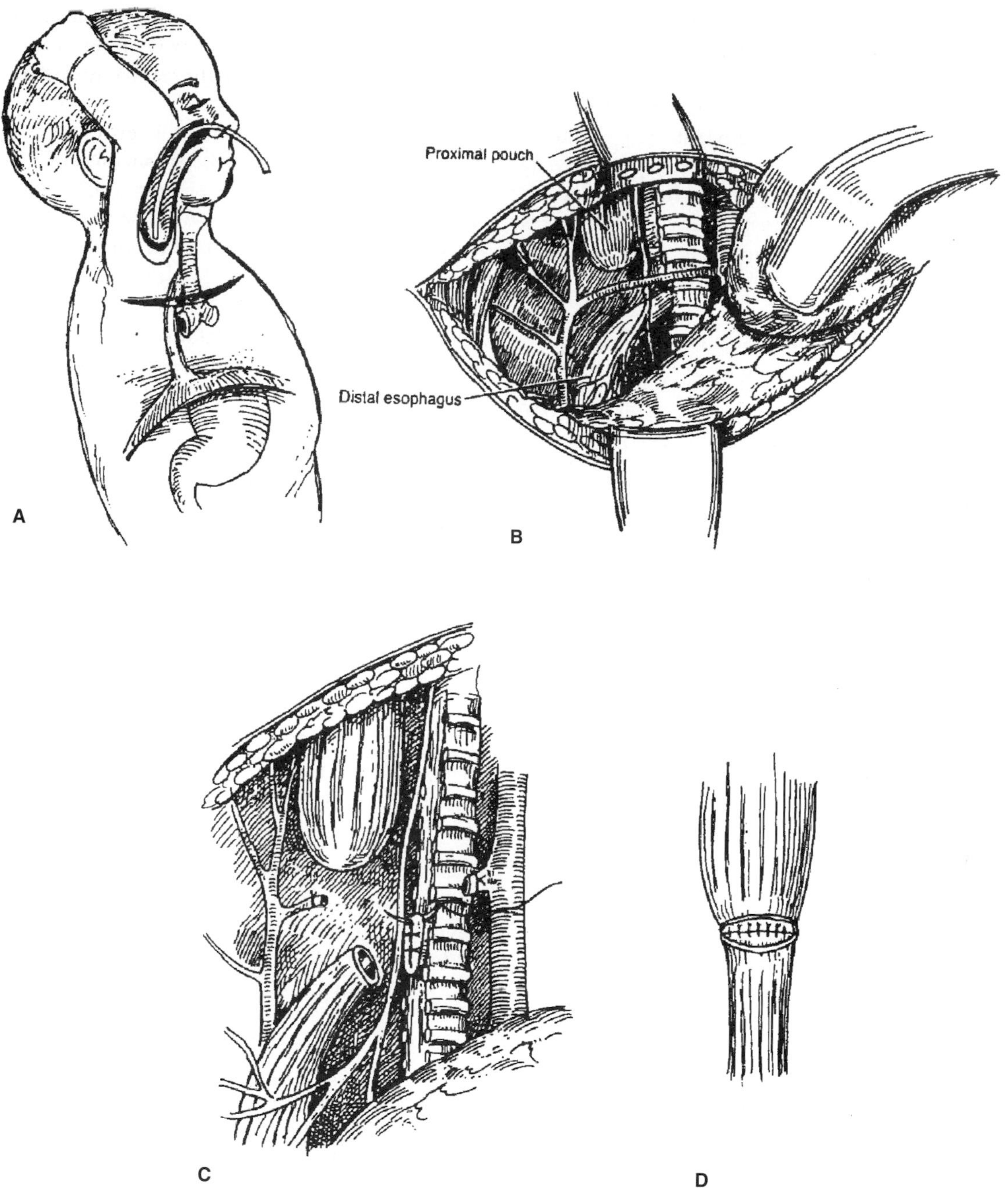

Figure 5-1 Surgical repair of type I esophageal atresia. A. A right posterolateral thoracotomy through the fourth intercostal space is a standard approach. B. The proximal esophageal pouch and distal esophagus are exposed with anterior traction of the lung and mediastinal pleura. C. Division and closure of the tracheoesophageal fistula. D. Single-layer primary anastomosis between the proximal and distal esophageal segments using interrupted absorbable sutures. (From O'Neill JA. *Operative Surgery, Principles and Techniques,* 3d ed. Philadelphia: Saunders, 1990:1072. With permission.)

agents. An antireflux procedure (e.g., partial Thal fundoplication) is considered for patients refractory to these medical measures.

Tracheomalacia, occurring in approximately 15 percent of patients after esophageal atresia repair, presents with a range of symptoms from mild expiratory stridor and barking cough to more severe cyanosis, apnea, and bradycardia. Bronchoscopy is diagnostic. Although mild symptoms often respond to expectant management, more severe symptoms require operative intervention, usually in the form of an aortopexy performed through a left thoracotomy. With this procedure, the aortic arch is sutured to the posterior sternal table to prevent its compression of the weakened tracheal wall.

Esophageal duplication cysts

Esophageal cysts are generally approached and excised through a limited posterolateral thoracotomy. Intramural cysts can be enucleated by dividing the overlying esophageal musculature, shelling out the cyst extramucosally, and maintaining esophageal wall integrity.[24] In all cases it is necessary to completely excise the cyst mucosa. Any continuity between the cyst and the esophageal lumen should be closed and the muscular esophageal wall reapproximated without creating a stricture. Operative results are generally excellent.

Esophageal stenosis and webs

If conservative management of esophageal stenosis or webs with one or more dilatations proves unsuccessful, resection with primary anastomosis should be considered. Once the stenosis has been localized, it is generally approached via a right thoracotomy for middle-third lesions or a left thoracotomy for distal esophageal lesions. Most stenoses can be resected with construction of a primary end-to-end anastomosis. Rare cases of more extensive esophageal resections may require esophageal replacement with interposition grafts. Resected stenoses near the gastroesophageal junction usually prompt a concomitant antireflux procedure to avoid significant reflux.

Complications Complications of surgical resection include anastomotic leak and gastroesophageal reflux.

An alternative to extensive resection of long fibromuscular esophageal stenoses is myotomy, although the intermediate- and long-term results are indeterminate.

CONGENITAL DIAPHRAGMATIC HERNIAS

EPIDEMIOLOGY

Posterolateral hiatal hernia (Bochdalek)

Congenital posterolateral diaphragmatic hernias occur in 1:2000 to 1:5000 live births.[25] As with congenital esophageal anomalies, associated defects are frequent, occurring in approximately 40 percent of affected patients. Associated anomalies include cardiac, renal, neural, and gastrointestinal defects (e.g., malrotation).

Retrosternal anterior diaphragmatic hernia (Morgagni)

Congenital retrosternal anterior diaphragmatic hernias comprise 1 to 5 percent of congenital diaphragmatic defects, occurring much less frequently than Bochdalek hernias. These hernias present most commonly in adulthood, with the onset of symptoms. They have a predisposition to affect obese patients and women.

Pathophysiology

Posterolateral hiatal hernia (Bochdalek)

Bochdalek hernias are caused by failure of the pleuroperitoneal canal to close during the eighth gestational week. Some 80 percent of these hernias occur on the left side. The primary pathophysiologic processes are incited by the herniation of abdominal organs into the chest through the diaphragmatic defect, compressing and impeding the growth and development of the ipsilateral lung. Mediastinal shift to the contralateral side may affect the other lung as well. A true hernial sac is encountered in only 10 percent of cases. Developmental morphologic and biochemical defects have also been observed in affected infants. These infants are susceptible to bronchopulmonary dysplasia, possibly related to defective antioxidant and surfactant mechanisms; pulmonary hypoplasia; and restrictive pulmonary physiology. Pulmonary hypoplasia and pulmonary hypertension lead to varying degrees of hypoxia and right-to-left shunting, with a heightened reactivity of these abnormal lungs to stimuli that increase pulmonary vascular resistance (i.e., hypoxia, acidosis, hypercarbia, hypothermia).

Retrosternal anterior diaphragmatic hernia (Morgagni)

Morgagni hernias are located between the xiphoid and costochondral diaphragmatic attachments and are predominantly on the right side, as the pericardium protects the left side. They are thought to arise from the failure of the transverse septum to fuse to the sternum, resulting in a triangular defect.[26] Unlike the Bochdalek hernia, a true hernial sac is usually present when abdominal viscera protrude into the mediastinum.

Diagnosis

Posterolateral hiatal hernia (Bochdalek)

Early presenting symptoms generally comprise varying degrees of respiratory compromise. The most extreme presentation is that of a newborn who is markedly dyspneic, tachycardic, and cyanotic with a scaphoid abdomen. There are signs of contralateral mediastinal and tracheal shift, with decreased breath sounds on the ipsilateral side. Plain chest radiography is often diagnostic, revealing bowel loops on the ipsilateral side, contralateral mediastinal shift, and a paucity of abdominal bowel gas patterns. The tip of any naso- or orogastric feeding tube placed may be seen above the diaphragm in the chest. Infants presenting later in life often present with feeding difficulties, colic, and growth retardation, generally depending on the size of the defect and the extent of visceral herniation into the pleural space.

Retrosternal anterior diaphragmatic hernia (Morgagni)

Symptoms vary; however, crampy abdominal pain or obstructive signs and symptoms constitute most of these. Often, plain chest radiographs display foramen of Morgagni hernias as excessively large densities in the region of the pericardial fat pad.[27] Confirmatory imaging includes computed tomography, magnetic resonance imaging, and/or ultrasonography, which show abdominal viscera within the hernial sac. In some cases, herniation of omentum only can make the diagnosis more difficult.

Preoperative management

Posterolateral hiatal hernia (Bochdalek)

Newborns presenting with respiratory distress and a clinical suspicion of a Bochdalek hernia should undergo endotracheal intubation with mechanical ventilation, paralysis/sedation, and orogastric tube decompression of the gastrointestinal tract to head off visceral distention and further respiratory embarrassment. Initial ventilatory parameters should include an inspired oxygen fraction of 100 percent, peak inspiratory pressure under 30 cmH_2O, positive end-expiratory pressure less than 5 cmH_2O, and hyperventilatory frequency; high-frequency ventilation may be useful in some settings. In order to reduce vasoreactive pulmonary hypertension, the postductal arterial oxygen tension should be maintained above 100 mmHg, carbon dioxide tension below 30 mmHg, and pH above 7.50. Tromethamine or sodium bicarbonate can be used to treat acidosis. Systolic blood pressures should be maintained above 50 mmHg, although intravenous fluids should be used sparingly. After adequate resuscitation, most of these patients should be referred for expeditious surgical repair. In patients who cannot be adequately ventilated mechanically, extracorporeal membrane oxygenation (ECMO) can be employed.

Retrosternal anterior diaphragmatic hernia (Morgagni)

Once diagnosed, patients with Morgagni diaphragmatic hernias are prepared for operative repair in a routine manner.

Operative repair

Posterolateral hiatal hernia (Bochdalek)

Most left-sided Bochdalek hernias are repaired via a transabdominal subcostal approach. Right-sided hernias are usually approached transthoracically. Herniated viscera are returned to their normal anatomic positions; any hernial sac is dissected free and resected. The lung tissue should be inspected; however, no attempt at expanding a hypoplastic lung should be made. Occasionally, extralobar pulmonary sequestration is encountered; it should be resected at this time. Once the edges of the diaphragmatic defect are defined, repair can usually be effected primarily with interrupted nonabsorbable suture material (e.g., polypropylene) in a horizontal mattress pattern. Large defects or defects whose edges are under tension should be closed with synthetic patch material (e.g., Teflon, Dacron). With these repairs, the patch is fashioned and sewn to the edges of the diaphragmatic defect with horizontal nonabsorbable sutures with or without a running buttressing suture line. Bilateral chest tubes should be placed and connected to a water seal. If the patient is stable, malrotation should be repaired at this time. In some cases, the abdominal wall fascia cannot be closed primarily. These cases are managed in similar fashion to large abdominal wall defects. Survivors of this operation generally have a good long-term prognosis, although some respiratory abnormalities have been observed in some survivors.

Retrosternal anterior diaphragmatic hernia (Morgagni)

Morgagni hernias are usually approached transperitoneally through an upper abdominal incision. The patient's habitus and size and the location of the hernial sac and its contents determine whether a subcostal, paramedian, or midline incision is used. The basic principles of hernia repair are used. Once the peritoneum is entered, the abdominal viscera are retracted from the hernial sac and returned to their normal locations. The hernial sac is then defined, taking down any associated adhesions, and resected. Small diaphragmatic defects that can be closed without tension can be repaired with nonabsorbable suture material (e.g., polypropylene), using a horizontal mattress pattern with or without a running reinforcement. Large defects or defects whose edges are under tension should be closed with synthetic patch material (e.g., Teflon, Dacron). With these repairs, the patch is fashioned and sewn to the edges of the diaphragmatic defect with horizontal nonabsorbable sutures with or without a running buttressing suture line. Morgagni repairs can be effected via a thoracic approach. In these cases the principles and techniques of repair resemble those used in the transperitoneal approach. The results with these repairs are generally excellent.

References

1. Pegoli W, Drugas G. Congenital tracheoesopheagal fistula. In: Yang SY, Cameron DE (eds). *Current Therapy in Thoracic and Cardiovascular Surgery.* Philadelphia: Mosby, 2004:94–97.
2. Skandalakis J, Gray S, Ricketts R. The esophagus. In: Skandalakis J, Gray S (eds). *Embryology for Surgeons.* Baltimore: Williams & Wilkins, 1994:65–112.
3. Pletcher BA, Friedes JS, Breg WR, Touloukian RJ. Familial occurrence of esophageal atresia with and without tracheoesophageal fistula: Report of two unusual kindreds. *Am J Med Genet* 1991;39:380–384.
4. Brock MV. Esophageal duplication cysts. In: Yang SY, Cameron DE (eds). *Current Therapy in Thoracic and Cardiovascular Surgery.* Philadelphia: Mosby, 2004:448–451.
5. Nihoul-Fekete C, De Backer A, Lortat-Jacob S, Pellerin D. Congenital esophageal stenosis: A review of 20 cases. *Pediatr Surg Int* 1987;2:86.
6. Kirwan WO, Walbaum PR, McCormack RJM. Cystic intrathoracic derivatives of the foregut and their complications. *Thorax* 1973;28:424.
7. Simpson I, Campbell PE. Mediastinal masses in childhood: A review from a paediatric pathologist's point of view. *Prog Pediatr Surg* 1991;27:92.
8. Segev DL, Donahoe PK, Doody DP. Other congenital disorders in children. In: Pearson FG, Cooper JD, Deslauriers

J, et al (eds). *Esophageal Surgery.* New York: Churchill Livingstone, 2002:207–214.

9. Ladd W. The surgical treatment of esophageal atresia and tracheoesophageal fistulas. *N Engl J Med* 1944;230:625–637.
10. Gross R. *Atresia of the Esophagus.* Philadelphia: Saunders, 1953.
11. Hocking M, Young DG. Duplications of the alimentary tract. *Br J Surg* 1981;68:92.
12. Fallon M, Gordon ARG, Lendrum AC. Mediastinal cysts of the foregut origin associated with vertebral abnormalities. *Br J Surg* 1954;41:520.
13. Mee R, Beasley S, Auldist A, Myers N. Influence of congenital heart disease on management of oesphageal atresia. *Pediatr Surg Int* 1992;7:90–93.
14. Beasley S, Phelan E, Kelly J, et al. Urinary tract abnormalities in associated with oesophageal atresia: Frequency, significance, and influence on management. *Pediatr Surg Int* 1992;7:94–96.
15. Harris J, Kallen B, Robert E. Descriptive epidemiology of alimentary tract atresia. *Teratology* 1995;52:15–29.
16. Quan L, Smith DW. The VATER association: Vertebral defects, anal atresia, t-e fistula with esophageal atresia, radial and renal dysplasia: A spectrum of associated defects. *J Pediatr* 1973;82:104–107.
17. Hemalatha V, Batcup G, Brereton RJ, et al. Esophageal atresia associated with esophageal duplication cyst. *J Pediatr Surg* 1987;22:984.
18. Beasley S, Myers N. Diagnosis of congenital tracheoesophageal fistula. *J Pediatr Surg* 1988;23:415.
19. Salo JA, Ala-Kulju KV. Congenital esophageal cysts in adults. *Ann Thorac Surg* 1987;44:135.
20. Bluestone CD, Kerry R, Sieber WK. Congenital esophageal stenosis. *Laryngoscope* 1969;79:1095.
21. Hendren WH, Hendren WG. Colon interposition for esophagus in children. *J Pediatr Surg* 1985;20: 829–839.
22. Ring WS, Varco RL, L'Heureux PR, Foker JE. Esophageal replacement with jejunum in children: An 18- to 33-year follow-up. *J Thorac Cardiovasc Surg* 1982;83:918–927.
23. Anderson KD, Randolph JG. The gastric tube for esophageal replacement in children. *J Thorac Cardiovasc Surg* 1973;66:333–342.
24. Cioffi U, Bonarina L, De Simone M, et al. Presentation and surgical management of bronchogenic and esophageal duplication cysts in adults. *Chest* 1998;113:1492.
25. Harrison MR, de Lorimier AA. Congenital diaphragmatic hernia. *Surg Clin North Am* 1981;61:1023.
26. Cordero Jr JA, Moores DWO. Morgagni and Bochdalek hernias in the adult. In: Yang SY, Cameron DE (eds). Current therapy in thoracic and cardiovascular surgery. Philadelphia: Mosby, 2004:452–453.
27. Karanikas ID, Dendrinos SS, Liakakos' TD, et al. Complications of congenital posterolateral diaphragmatic hernia in adults. *J Cardiovasc Surg* 1994;35:555.

CHAPTER

6 CONGENITAL CHEST WALL ANOMALIES

Dorry L. Segev, Paul M. Colombani

INTRODUCTION

Children with congenital chest wall anomalies present from infancy to adolescence with cosmetic, psychological, or physiologic concerns. The spectrum of major anomalies of the chest wall includes pectus excavatum, pectus carinatum, Poland's syndrome, sternal clefts, and Jeune's syndrome.[1,2] The most common anomaly, pectus excavatum, is a concave depression of the sternum that comprises at least 90 percent of referrals for chest wall defects. Genetic or chromosomal associations with chest wall deformities are rare and include connective tissue disorders such as Marfan's and Ehlers-Danlos syndromes.[3,4] A number of minor anomalies of rib and cartilage can also occur and require specific therapy. This chapter reviews the embryology of chest wall development as well as the pathophysiology, diagnosis, and treatment of the various congenital chest wall anomalies.

HISTORICAL HIGHLIGHTS

The first reported repair of the pectus excavatum deformity, by Meyer, occurred in 1911.[5] Several reviews followed, but the benchmark repair, including costal cartilage excision and sternal osteotomy, was described by

KEY CONCEPTS

- Epidemiology
  - Pectus excavatum occurs in about 1:400 live births, with a male predominance of up to 5:1. No genetic abnormalities or chromosomal aberrations have been associated with pectus excavatum, although a familial tendency has been described. Up to two-thirds of children with Marfan's syndrome and a large proportion of Ehlers-Danlos patients develop pectus excavatum deformities. The incidence of pectus carinatum is about one-tenth that of pectus excavatum, with a similar male predominance and 25 to 30 percent reported family history. Scoliosis and other spinal deformities or a family history of these are associated with pectus carinatum.
- Pathophysiology
  - Pectus excavatum is a concave depression of the sternum resulting from abnormal growth, lengthening, rotation, or increased elasticity of the costal cartilages. Reduced cardiovascular performance has been linked to this defect. Pectus carinatum results from anterior displacement of the costal cartilages due to rotation and lengthening, leading to sternal protrusion. No significant cardiopulmonary abnormalities have been demonstrated with this lesion.
- Clinical features
  - In pectus excavatum, the sternum is posteriorly retracted and differential growth of the costal cartilages often results in an asymmetric chest wall with a common right-sided rotation of the sternum and an elevated left side. Other characteristic findings include sloped ribs, rounded shoulders with a classic stooped posture, and a protuberant abdomen. It is most commonly discovered in the first few years of life. Decreased stamina and endurance during exercise and excessive tachycardia/palpitations are commonly observed with this disorder. Pain is occasionally associated with this defect. Pectus carinatum is associated with pain, respiratory symptoms, ease of injury, and psychosocial body image concerns.

- Diagnostics
  - The best radiographic imaging modality for pectus deformities is the computed tomographic scan of the chest, which provides precise information regarding cardiac displacement, lung volumes, the degree of deformity, and any associated malformations.
- Treatment
  - Surgical correction of pectus excavatum includes the modified Ravitch repair (subperichondrial resection of all abnormal costal cartilages and wedge osteotomy to correct the posterior depression of the sternum by bringing it to a more anterior and neutral position) and the Nuss repair (using a precurved substernal bar to bend the sternum and cartilages to a corrected position). Surgical correction for pectus carinatum utilizes the basic principles employed in the open Ravitch repair, namely excision of all abnormal cartilages and return of the sternum to a neutral straight position.
- Outcomes/prognosis
  - The modified Ravitch or Nuss repairs represent the "gold standard" corrective operation for pectus excavatum. Hospitalization rarely exceeds 3 days and 97 percent of patients experience a good result from the operation. Similar success rates are reported for Ravitch-type repairs of pectus carinatum. Complications include recurrence, pneumothorax, wound infection, atelectasis, and local tissue necrosis.

Ravitch in 1949 and has undergone only minor modifications in over 50 years of use.[6] Recently, experience has been growing with a minimally invasive technique for pectus excavatum repair described in 1998 by Donald Nuss.[7] Ravitch is also credited with the first repair of a pectus carinatum defect in 1952.[8] Jeune and colleagues described the syndrome of asphyxiating thoracic dystrophy in 1954,[9] and Cantrell, in 1958, described the pentalogy that includes lower sternal clefts.[10] Interestingly, Alfred Poland is eponymously associated with the syndrome that includes pectoralis muscle absence,[11] although descriptions preceded his by up to 15 years in the German and French literature.[12–14]

EMBRYOLOGY

The chest wall consists of muscles derived from myotomes and ribs, costal cartilages, and components of the sternum from the axial skeleton. Shortly after the fifth week of development, dermatomyotomes in the thoracic region split and form myotomes, from which the chest wall musculature arises. The mesenchymal costal processes of the developing thoracic vertebrae give rise to the ribs starting at week 5 postfertilization.[15,16] During the embryonic period, the costal processes become cartilaginous and finally undergo endochondral ossification to become ribs. The synovial costovertebral joints arise from the embryonic junction between the vertebrae and the costal processes. During week 6 of development, a pair of vertical mesenchymal structures, known as sternal bars, develops ventrolaterally along the body wall. These bars gradually fuse craniocaudally in the median plane as they chondrify to form precursors of the manubrium, sternebral segments of the sternal body, and xiphoid process. Ossification of the sternum also occurs in a craniocaudal fashion and is complete by 60 days postfertilization except for the xiphoid, which ossifies after birth. Incomplete sternal fusion is not uncommon and can lead to bifid xiphoid or a spectrum of sternal clefts.

PECTUS EXCAVATUM

Abnormal growth, lengthening, rotation, or increased elasticity of the costal cartilages leads to the relatively common depression of the sternum known as pectus excavatum. Clinical findings usually begin to manifest by 2 to 3 years of age, but—given the risk of acquired thoracic dystrophy or recurrence after correction in younger patients—operative intervention should occur in older children or adolescents. The physiologic benefit of pectus excavatum repair is frequently discussed but remains controversial and is based mostly on retrospective data. Two repairs are most commonly performed, an open repair, first described by Ravitch, and a less invasive bar repair, described by Nuss. The type of repair is chosen based on the surgeon's experience and the complexity of the deformity. Both techniques have demonstrated good results when the appropriate patient is selected at the appropriate age for repair.

DEVELOPMENT

There is no known cause for pectus excavatum. Cartilagenous growth appears to be abnormal, which causes either posterior depression of the sternum in the case of abnormal lengthening of the cartilages or rotation of the sternum in the case of differential cartilagenous growth. A study of the biomechanical, morphologic, and histochemical properties of cartilage from children with pectus excavatum shows decreased tension, compression, and flexure, with disrupted type II collage patterns in the deep zones of the cartilage.[17]

EPIDEMIOLOGY

Pectus excavatum is relatively common, occurring in approximately 1:400 live births, with a male predominance of up to 5:1.[18] No genetic abnormalities or chromosomal aberrations have been associated with pectus excavatum, although a familial tendency has been described.[18,19] Up to two-thirds of children with Marfan's syndrome and a high frequency of Ehlers-Danlos patients develop pectus excavatum deformities.[3,4] Children with connective tissue disorders can present later in life, have more progressive defects, and suffer from more complicated postoperative courses, but successful cosmetic and functional results can be achieved even in these patients.[4] Other associations include cardiac disorders[20] and scoliosis.[21]

PATHOPHYSIOLOGY

Pediatric surgeons performing pectus excavatum repair argue that children with pectus excavatum seem to enjoy an increase in stamina and cardiovascular performance after surgical correction. However, the magnitude of physiologic sequelae and their significance preoperatively and after surgical repair remain controversial.[22,23]

Two organ systems have been examined for physiologic differences in pectus excavatum: pulmonary and cardiovascular. Static pulmonary function tests performed at rest seem to show few abnormalities in children with pectus.[24,25] Other studies have confirmed the lack of difference in static lung volumes and baseline resting pulmonary function before and after both Ravitch and Nuss repairs,[26,27] while some even argue for a possible worsening of lung function after chest wall reconstruction.[28–31] In reviewing these studies, the majority of children are at the lower end of the "normal range" of pulmonary function, suggesting a defect. Interestingly, decreased postoperative pulmonary function testing in some studies has been found in contrast to subjective improvement in exercise stamina.[30] In some studies, including those that show no difference in resting pulmonary tests, exercise pulmonary function studies show significant differences in lung volumes in preteen and teenaged pectus patients.[24,32] A recent study by Haller and coworkers shows a lower forced vital capacity (FVC) in pectus patients before surgery, with over half complaining of exercise limitation; significant improvement was found in 66 percent of these patients after repair.[33] Patients with abnormal ventilation/perfusion scintigraphy scans have demonstrated improvement after surgical correction of pectus deformity.[34] Although vital capacities were reported as only mildly reduced or normal in pectus patients, a nonlinear increase in oxygen uptake was seen when compared with controls, possibly indicating an abnormal work of breathing during exercise.[35] In another study, all pectus patients experienced improvement in maximal voluntary ventilation and exercise tolerance.[36] Some authors believe that the improvement of pulmonary function after pectus repair can be appreciated only in children who have severe deficits preoperatively.[37]

Reduced cardiovascular performance, rather than ventilatory limitations, has been the focus of a number of studies in an effort to understand the physiologic manifestations of pectus excavatum.[38,39] Right ventricular filling seems to be diminished with this condition and somewhat alleviated after repair.[40] Kowalewski and colleagues showed increased right ventricular systolic, diastolic, and stroke volumes after surgical correction of pectus excavatum.[41] A lower heart rate and expanded cardiac stroke volume has been described after pectus repair,[30,31,36] as has a higher oxygen pulse and cardiac output.[32,33]

In addition to the apparent cardiopulmonary advantages of pectus repair, the psychological and psychosomatic aspects associated with this disease cannot be underestimated. School-aged children with pectus excavatum suffer from embarrassment, social anxiety, orientation toward failure, marked depressive reactions, feelings of stigmata, reduced tolerance of frustration, and limited capacity for work.[42] In many children, these body image issues alone merit surgical intervention; when combined with the apparent cardiopulmonary advantages of correction, these considerations should clearly urge all health care providers to be supporters and advocates of treatment of pectus excavatum.

CLINICAL FEATURES

Figure 6-1 illustrates the classic physical features of a child with pectus excavatum. Most children who present for surgical evaluation are active and healthy-appearing, with the chief complaint of a visible anatomic defect. Commonly, overgrowth of the costal cartilages cause a posterior retraction of the sternum. In addition, differential growth of the costal cartilages can result in an asymmetrical chest wall, with a common right-sided rotation of the sternum and elevation of the left side.[43] Other characteristic findings include sloped ribs, rounded shoulders with a classic stooped posture, and a protuberant abdomen. When the excavatum defect is severe, the cardiac point of maximal impact can be shifted laterally beyond the midclavicular line. Pectus excavatum is most commonly discovered in the first few years of life, although it can be apparent in the newborn period or in a delayed fashion later in development. In newborns, pectus excavatum can be associated with paradoxical chest wall movement with ventilation. Many of these anomalies can resolve spontaneously during the early years and should not be considered for surgical repair until ages 8 to 12.

Occasionally, pain can accompany the obvious visible defect as a presenting symptom. Physically active children often complain of shortness of breath during exercise or decreased exercise tolerance when compared with their peers, but they generally have no symptoms at rest. Excessive tachycardia or palpitations during mild exercise can also be seen in patients with this disorder.[18] In a 30-year review of 375 patients undergoing pectus repair, 67 percent reported preoperative decreased stamina and endurance during exercise, 32 percent had frequent respiratory

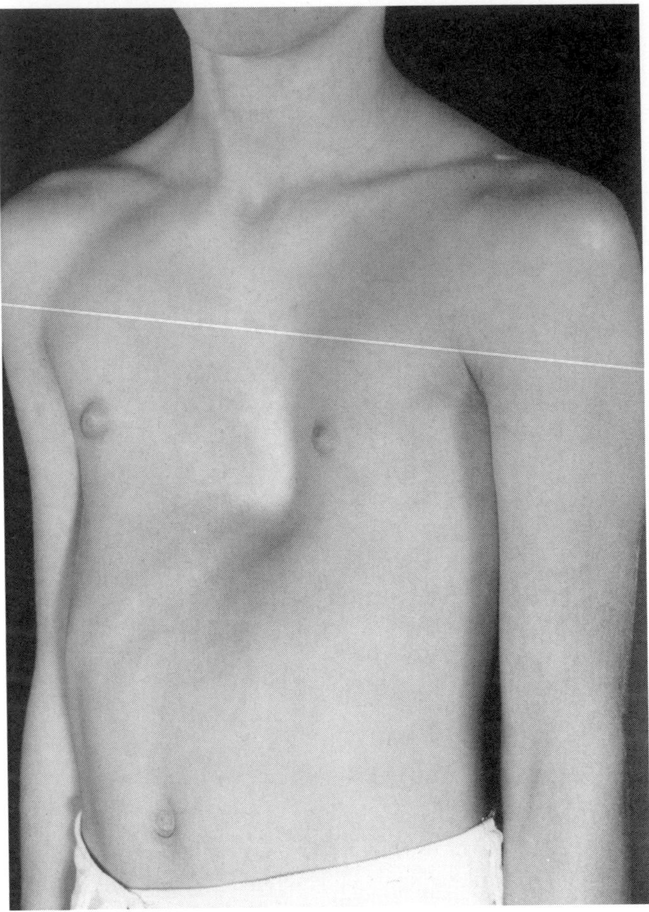

Figure 6-1 Child with pectus excavatum. Note the rounded shoulders, central defect, and "pot belly."

infections, 8 percent had chest pain, and 7 percent had asthma.[44] Another 30-year study found, at initial presentation, 56 percent of subjects with dyspnea on exertion, 29 percent with shortness of breath at rest, 10 percent with chest pain, and 10 percent with palpitations.[45] Table 6-1 summarizes the signs and symptoms of pectus excavatum.

Table 6-1 Signs and symptoms of pectus excavatum

Physical Signs
Visible depression of lower sternum
Right-sided rotation of sternum with asymmetrical chest wall
Sloped ribs
Rounded shoulders
Protuberant abdomen
Laterally displaced cardiac point of maximal impact
Associated findings of connective tissue disorders
Symptoms
Nonspecific parasternal chest pain
Decreased subjective exercise tolerance, work capacity
Frequent respiratory infections, exercise-induced asthma
Embarrassment reactions, social anxiety, depression, suicidal thoughts

IMAGING STUDIES

Regardless of the surgical approach selected, the best radiographic test for preoperative evaluation of a patient with pectus excavatum is computed tomography (CT) of the chest.[46–48] This study provides precise information regarding cardiac displacement, lung volume, and, most importantly, the most accurate measurement of the depth of the sternal defect and its relationship to the overall width of the thorax.[49] The Haller index can be obtained by measuring the ratio of the AP distance between the vertebral bodies and the sternum at its narrowest point and the transverse diameter of the chest (Fig. 6-2). This can be performed on physical exam or more reliably by CT scan. Although age and gender-related variability exists in the Haller index,[50] normal children should not have a Haller index greater than 2.5, while the severity index of those with pectus excavatum generally ranges from 3 to 6 (Fig. 6-3A and B).

INDICATIONS FOR OPERATION

Factors determining candidates for repair of pectus excavatum defects include anatomic, physiologic, psychological, considerations as well as proper timing (Table 6-2). A CT scan can accurately define the anatomic defect, including the severity index of the sternal depression as well as its effects on cardiac and pulmonary anatomy. A Haller index of 3 or greater is associated with the presence of pectus excavatum.

All candidates should undergo stress pulmonary function studies and, if indicated by stress pulmonary function or history, echocardiography. Based on patient and family history—including double joints, joint dislocations, hyperflexibility, accelerated worsening of eyesight,

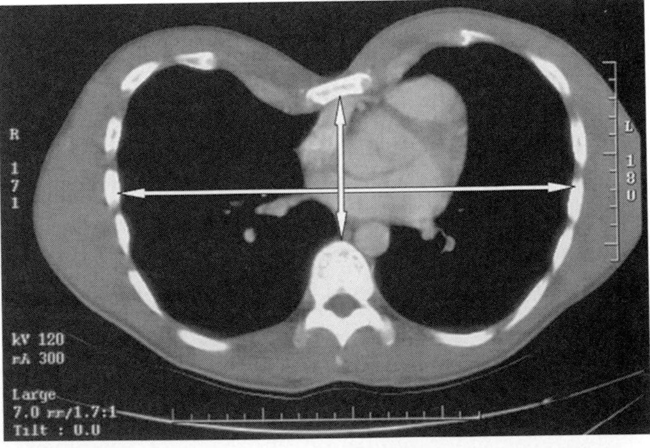

Figure 6-2 Cross-sectional CT scan to measure Haller index. CT scan taken at the deepest part of defect. Haller index is equal to the transverse diameter of the thorax divided by the anteroposterior dimension.

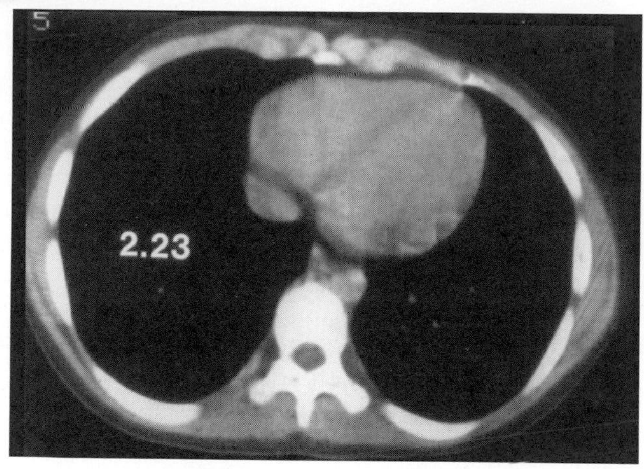

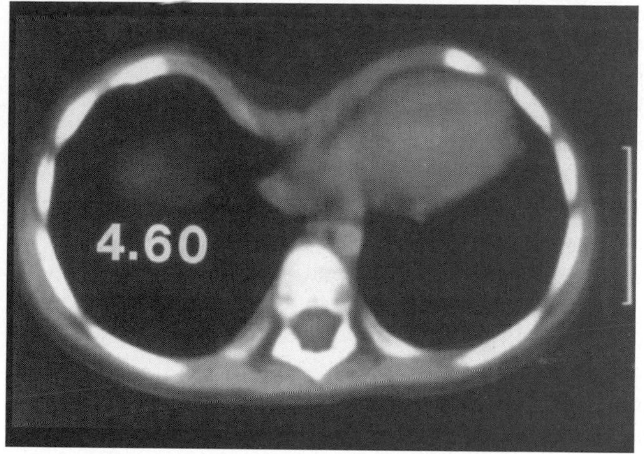

Figure 6-3 A. Chest CT scan of normal child. Haller index should be < 2.5. B. Chest CT scan of patient with severe pectus excavatum.

and mitral valve prolapse—a screen should be considered for connective tissue disease. Associated chest pain, dyspnea on exertion, decreased exercise tolerance, exercise-induced asthma, or cardiac anomalies are possible indications for operative correction.[30,31,36–39] Patients who begin with symptoms such as dyspnea on exertion or exercise-induced chest pain show significant improvement of these symptoms postoperatively.[44,51] In addition, the need for future sternotomy, as in children with Marfan's syndrome, should be considered an indication for correction in childhood.[52]

Psychological symptoms are not uncommon in these patients and include embarrassment reactions, marked depressive reactions, social anxiety, feelings of stigmata, and others.[42] These manifestations can seriously alter the mental and physical health of a child and should be strongly considered in deciding candidacy for operative repair.

Proper timing of surgical repair is essential for adequate outcome, although this is also frequently debated and based on retrospective data. In general, good results have been reported with correction in school-aged children between the ages of 8 and 16, either before or after but not during their pubertal growth spurts.[18,46,53] It remains clear that Ravitch repair in patients younger than 7 years of age should be avoided because of a higher incidence of damage to the cartilagenous growth centers, with resulting acquired Jeune's syndrome.[33,54–57] Timing should vary with indication, as with the example of lower incidence of recurrence in children with Marfan's syndrome who underwent repair after maximal growth was obtained.[58] Success has been reported with simultaneous correction of pectus excavatum and congenital cardiac defects.[59] Age should not be a barrier to repair, as excellent long-term cosmetic results and symptomatic relief approaching 90 percent have been described in adults between the ages of 16 and 68 years.[45]

Table 6-2	Indications for surgical repair of pectus excavatum deformities
Cardiorespiratory symptoms	
Exercise intolerance	
Abnormal pulmonary function testing	
Abnormal echocardiogram	
Exercise-induced asthma	
Body image issues	
Anatomic severity	
Haller index > 3.0	
External measurement > 2.5	

MODIFIED RAVITCH REPAIR

Almost 60 years ago and for several decades to follow, Ravitch described subperichondrial resection of the lower costal cartilages with wedge osteotomy of the sternum as a possible repair for pectus excavatum.[6,60–63] This has gained wide acceptance as the gold standard operation for pectus excavatum, especially for complex or recurrent cases. Extensive experience has been reported with this procedure, and outcomes are generally excellent.[46,48,64–69] One group has reported some success with a minimally invasive endoscopic Ravitch repair.[70]

Incision and exposure

A modified Ravitch repair as performed at Johns Hopkins Hospital has been described (Table 6-3). A

Table 6-3	Summary of operative steps in the modified Ravitch repair for pectus excavatum
Incision (midline or transverse) through the depth of the defect	
Skin and muscle flaps to expose sternum and costal cartilages	
Subperichondrial cartilage resections, usually four bilaterally	
Sternal mobilization and transverse osteotomy	
Sternal support; cartilage tripod and retrosternal bar	
Wound closure with retrosternal chest tube, subcutaneous drain	

transverse inframammary skin incision is utilized at the level of the deepest portion of the sternal defect. It is our experience that cosmetic outcomes from transverse incisions for this operation are more appealing than vertical ones. Upper and lower skin flaps are created in the subcutaneous layer, followed by creation of midline muscle flaps elevating the pectoralis muscles. This exposes the costal cartilages in their entire length bilaterally along the affected portion of the sternum. In most cases, this includes the fourth through seventh cartilages, but it can include as high as the second and third in severe cases of pectus excavatum. Exposure of the upper flap should extend to at least one normal cartilage cranial to the uppermost abnormal one, with the goal of excising at least four cartilages bilaterally.

Subperichondrial resection

One of the two principal goals of the operation is subperichondrial resection of all abnormal costal cartilages (Fig. 6-4A). These are resected from the lateral point of union with the rib, extending medially to the chrondrosternal junction. To keep the resection subperichondrial, the perichondrium is incised anteriorly along each cartilage, and upper and lower flaps of perichondrium are created to expose the deformed cartilage. It is imperative to keep the perichondrium entirely intact and not devascularized, as this provides the basis for new cartilage growth and subsequent bone. It is also suspected that devascularization of the perichondrium can contribute to the acquired Jeune's syndrome. During the dissection of the posterior perichondrium, care must be taken to avoid violating the pleural space.

Wedge osteotomy

The xiphoid is exposed and elevated, allowing for the creation of a substernal plane (Fig. 6-4B). This is performed mostly by blunt dissection, taking meticulous care to preserve the pleura and the pericardium as it is

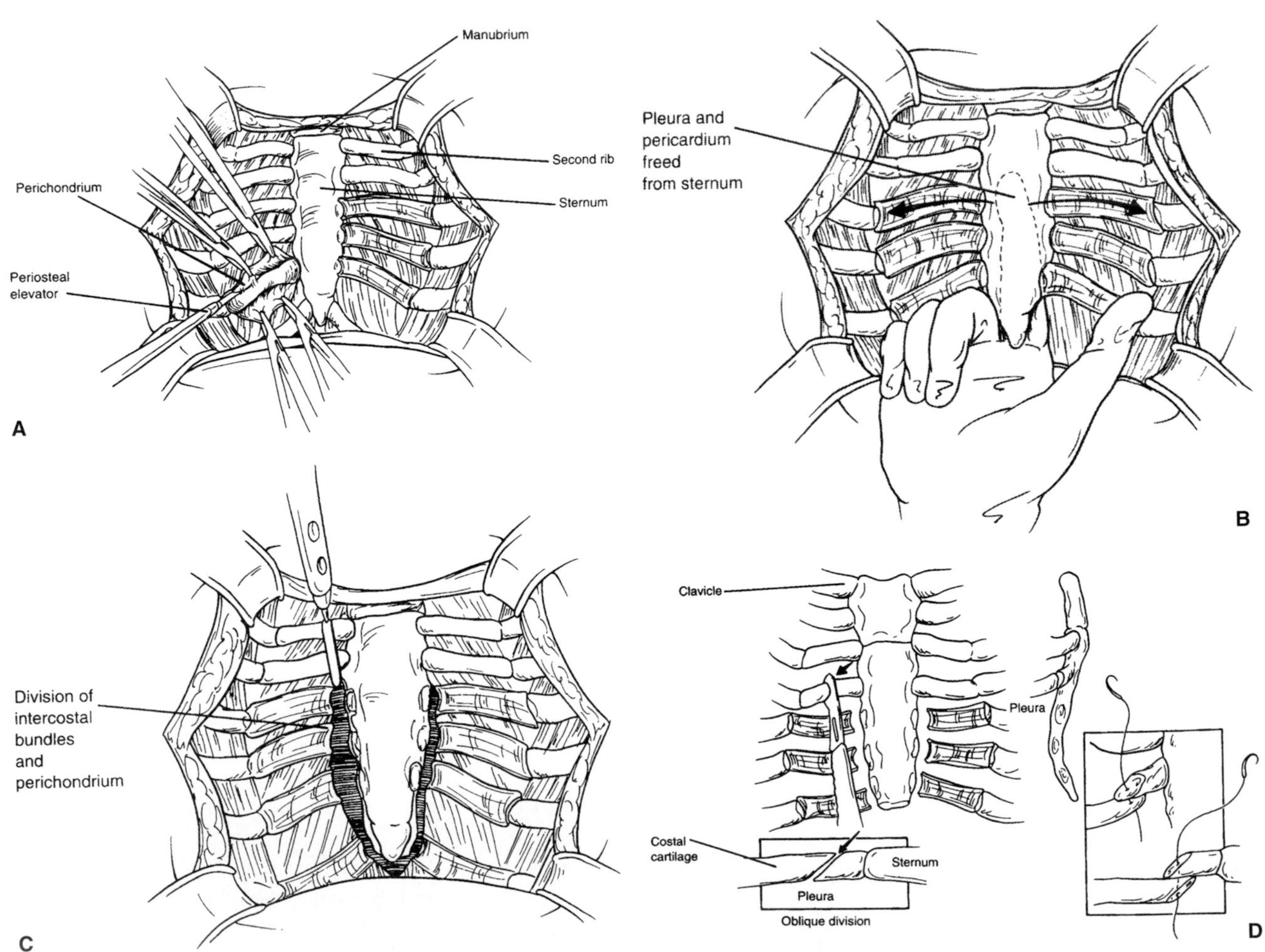

Figure 6-4 Summary of modified Ravitch procedure. A. Exposure of anterior chest wall and excision of four costal cartilages bilaterally. B. Elevation of sternum and its freeing from the underlying pleura (pericardium). C. Division of intercostal bundles. D. Oblique chondrotomy of three cartilages to form tripod. E. Transverse osteotomy. F. Placement of substernal strut.

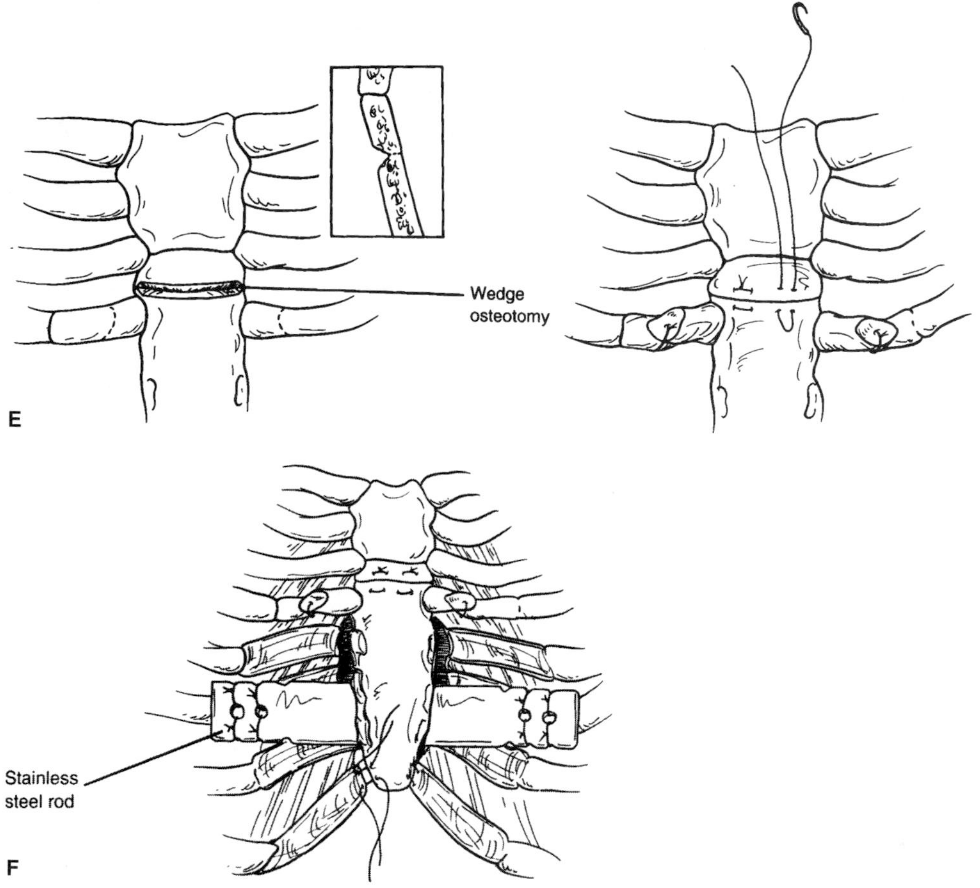

Figure 6-4 (*continued*) E. Transverse osteotomy. F. Placement of substernal strut.

swept from the posterior surface of the sternum. The perichondrial bundles at the level of all of the excised cartilages are detached from the sternum, making sure that the internal mammary artery is swept laterally with the intercostals bundle and perichondrium. Just above the resected cartilages, the wedge osteotomy is performed (Fig. 6-4C). This is an anterior, triangular incision in the anterior table of the sternum performed to correct the posterior depression of the sternum by bringing it to a more anterior and neutral position. A single osteotomy is usually performed between the second and third cartilages, although at times a second osteotomy can be performed in a more caudal location (Fig. 6-4D). Tripod supports consisting of the lowest third or fourth intact costal cartilages can be used to support the sternum as well by obliquely dividing them in a medial-to-lateral trajectory and then placing the medial portion atop the lateral. Finally, for further security, the sternal periosteum is sutured in the position fashioned during the operation (Fig. 6-4E).

Support bar

Various modalities have been described to further support the sternum after wedge osteotomy. Autologous perichondrium has been used,[71] as have various metal struts with or without synthetic envelopes.[72] We prefer selective use of stabilizing struts for patients over the age of 10 or 12 or those with connective tissue diseases such as Marfan's or Ehlers-Danlos syndrome. A substernal stainless steel bar can be placed under the distal third of the sternum and secured in place laterally to the medial aspect of surrounding ribs (Fig. 6-4F). Interrupted sutures are generally sufficient to secure the bar.

Postoperative management

It is not necessary to suture intercostal bundles that have been detached from the sternum back into place. If this defect is small, however, it can be closed by approximating nearby tissues. Retrosternal and subcutaneous chest drains are placed and can be removed 2 to 3 days postoperatively. After drains are removed, oral analgesia is sufficient and patients can be discharged within 3 to 4 postoperative days. A bladder catheter is recommended for the first day or two in the teenager and older patient, in whom urinary retention is not uncommon. Incentive spirometry is critical to prevent atelectasis. We recommend avoidance of contact sports for 6 to 8 weeks to allow cartilage regrowth and sternal fixation. A support bar, if placed, should remain for at least 6 months and can be removed in an outpatient procedure.

Outcomes and complications

For almost six decades, thousands of patients with pectus excavatum have been successfully treated with some modification of the Ravitch repair and followed for significantly long periods of time.[18,27,44–46,48,51,66,68,73–80] This is the gold standard operation to which all new techniques are compared.

The psychological benefits of the operation are clear.[42] The physiologic benefits of pectus repair remain controversial, with some groups demonstrating a measurable physiologic advantage[24,30–36,40] and others showing no difference before and after corrective operations.[26–31] It is possible that only selected patients with certain preoperative physiologic handicaps will benefit in this regard from surgical repair.

Hospitalization rarely exceeds 3 days, and 97 percent of patients experience a good result from the operation.[18] Although the operation is mostly performed in male patients, females with pectus deformities fare equally well after surgical repair.[73] Complications generally occur in fewer than 5 percent of patients undergoing a modified Ravitch repair; these are listed in Table 6-4. Early complications include pneumothorax, pleural effusion, pericarditis, seroma, wound infection, urinary retention, and atelectasis. Bar migration and pectus recurrence can occur as late complications. Acquired Jeune's syndrome is a terrible complication and is discussed later in this chapter. We find a higher incidence of urinary retention in older teenagers and adults and recommend 1 to 2 days of bladder catheterization in this population. In addition, we recommend the use of incentive spirometry to reduce atelectasis and the risk of pneumonia. We have seen recurrence in 2 percent of our patients, with a higher incidence if the operation was performed at an early age (below 7 years).

In a review of 375 patients over 30 years, Fonkalsrud and associates report 12 cases of atelectasis, 13 pleural effusions, 5 recurrences, and 3 patients with pericarditis.[44] Of 777 procedures for pectus repair in a single center, 98.5 percent were successful, with an overall complication rate of 6.7 percent, a major recurrence rate of 1.5 percent, and a minor recurrence rate of 4.5 percent.[76] Shamberger and coworkers reported 704 patients seen over a period of 30 years who were repaired by modified Ravitch technique, with 4.4 percent rate of complications including 11 cases of pneumothorax, 5 wound infections, 1 seroma, 1 hemopericardium, and 17 major recurrences (2.7 percent), of which 12 required revision.[48]

Complications may occur more commonly in adults because of the magnitude of dissection required and the anatomic difference that cartilage has developed into bone. Still, this operation is safe and successful in adults, with no statistical significance in reported complications in most studies. Of 116 patients over the age of 18 undergoing modified Ravitch repair, Fonkalsrud and colleagues report 7 pleural effusions, 2 pneumothoraces, and 2 patients with pericarditis.[51] Table 6-4 summarizes complications of the Ravitch operation.

Table 6-4 Complications following modified Ravitch repair for pectus excavatum

Early
Pneumothorax
Atelectasis
Pleural effusion
Pericarditis
Seroma
Wound infection
Urinary retention
Late
Bar migration
Recurrence
Acquired Jeune syndrome
Floating sternum

NUSS REPAIR

In 1998, Nuss reported a seminal 10-year series of 42 patients for whom he achieved adequate correction of pectus excavatum defects using a minimally invasive approach that does not involve excision of the costal cartilages.[7] Instead, through small bilateral incisions, a convex steel bar was surgically placed under the sternum to allow repositioning and remodeling of the deformed costal cartilages and sternum. After keeping the bar in place for 2 years to allow distraction and splinting of the costal cartilages as well as rotation of the sternum to a more neutral position, the bar was removed. Although a number of modifications have been described, experience with this procedure has become extensive, outcomes remain excellent, and the modified Nuss procedure has become the initial procedure of choice for many pediatric surgeons.[81–85] Success has even been reported for this procedure in the repair of patients failing modified Ravitch procedures.[86]

Incision and exposure

The patient is positioned supine on the operating table with arms abducted (Fig. 6-5A). This allows access to the lateral chest wall for bilateral 5-cm transverse incisions positioned just above the deepest portion of the sternal defect. Variations exist regarding ideal placement of the incisions and support bar. In our experience, placement of the incisions at the caudalmost portion of the defect within the costosternal region, avoiding the xiphoid, allows for optimal results in almost all types of patients. In addition, the older the patient, the more medially the bar should pass the chest wall. This provides for a shorter and thus stronger arch to elevate the sternum.

On both sides, flaps of skin and subcutaneous tissues are raised, using electrocautery to expose one intercostal space above and below the chosen incisions. This mobilization provides room for the laterally placed bar stabilizers. Using the intercostal space corresponding to the deepest portion of the sternal defect, the pleural space is entered bilaterally, protecting the lung from parenchymal injury during this maneuver. Usually the anterior axillary line is chosen as an entry point, allowing for entry where the ribs transition from the anterior to the lateral chest wall.

Retrosternal dissection

A retrosternal tunnel is next created to allow passage of the steel bar in the retrosternal space. A Crawford clamp or similar device is carefully advanced by blunt dissection from the left hemithorax to the right side. For this maneuver, bone hook elevation of the distal sternum or thoracoscopy may be helpful or necessary. We insist that the clamp pass from left to right, thus avoiding injury to the heart and pericardium. An umbilical tape is attached to the clamp and pulled retrogradely back through the retrosternal tunnel (Fig. 6-5B).

Lorenz bar

Using a series of bar templates, the appropriate size and approximate shape are selected for the stainless steel Lorenz bar (Walter Lorenz Surgical, Jacksonville, FL)

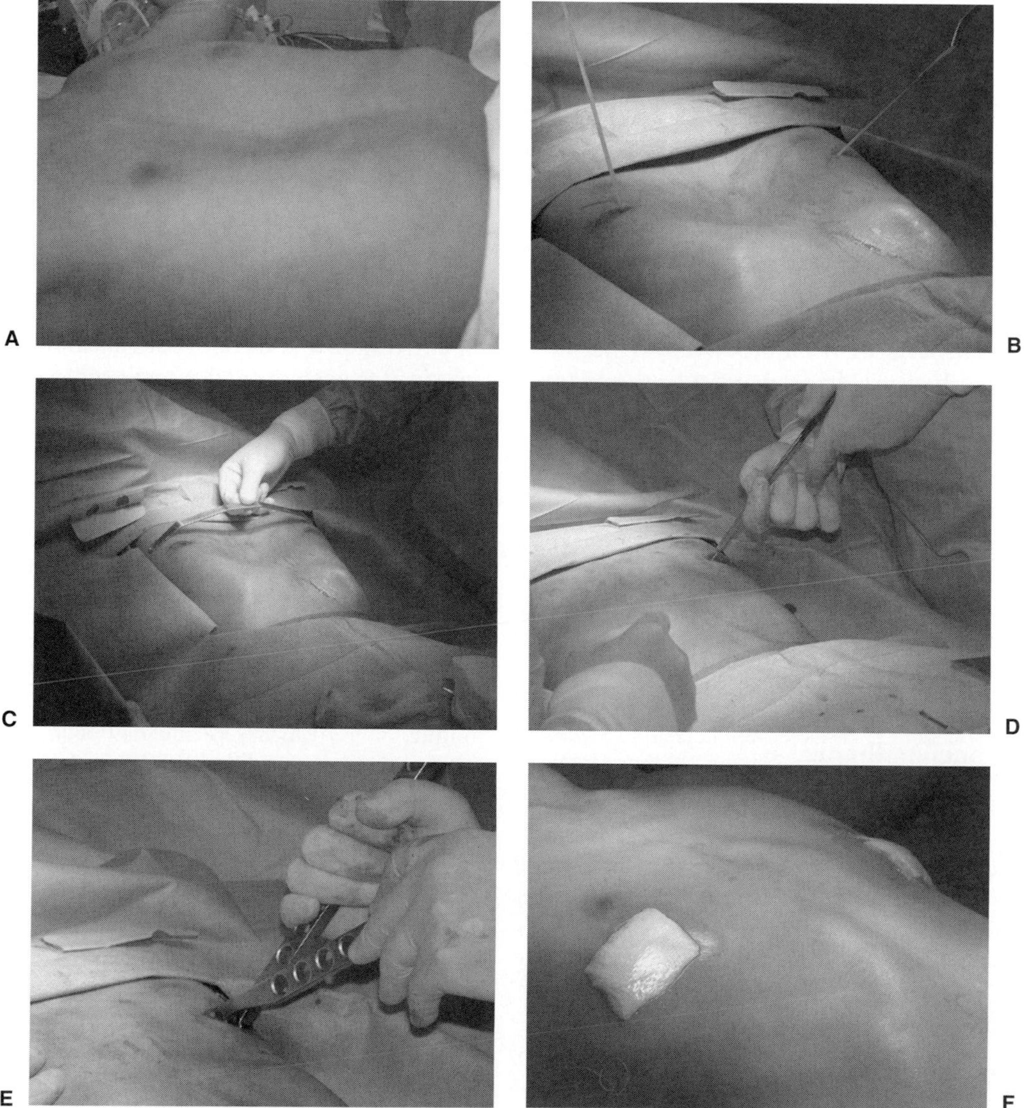

Figure 6-5 Nuss repair. A. Patient positioned for procedure with arms outstretched. B. Umbilical tape is threaded through a retrosternal tunnel. C. Lorenz bar curved to conform to patient's chest. D. After incisions are made into the pleural space bilaterally, a retrosternal tunnel is made and the bar is threaded through the tunnel, using the umbilical tape. E. Bar benders are used to bend the bar against the lateral chest wall. Stabilizing clips and stainless steel wires are used to further immobilize the bar. F. Completion of operation without chest tubes or drains.

Table 6-5	Summary of operative steps in the modified Nuss repair for pectus excavatum
1. Bilateral inframammary incisions at the deepest level of the sternum	
2. Template measurements to determine length of bar; precurve bar to chest size	
3. Development of retrostrenal plane from left to right (with or without thoracoscopy)	
4. Passage of substernal clamp/umbilical tape	
5. Insertion of pectus bar under sternum	
6. Bar rotation and application of stabilizers	
7. In situ bar bending and fixation with 5-mm or 6-mm surgical wire	
8. Wound closure	

(Fig. 6-5C). With the help of a bar-bending system, the bar is curved so that the substernal segment is as flat as possible to afford a sturdy support. One of the umbilical tapes is tied to the end of the Lorenz bar, and it is guided with the concave side up (upside down) through the retrosternal tunnel from left to right using thoracoscopy or sternal elevation (Fig. 6-5D). A steel bar turner is used to flip the bar in a craniocaudal direction and hold it in place while the correction of the pectus defect is examined (Fig. 6-5E). To remain most stable, the lateral parts of both sides of the bar arch must rest on the rib cage. Major changes to the concavity of the bar may require unflipping the bar, with or without removal, and rebending it. Minor changes can be fixed with an in situ bar-bending system, which, in our experience, allows for optimal contour and subsequent stabilization. We place bilateral stabilizing clips and bend the end of the bar to keep the stabilizer in place. The bar is also fixed to the crossing rib using no. 5 or 6 wire sutures medial to each clip. Table 6-5 outlines these steps in the operative procedure.

Evacuation of pneumothorax

In our experience, no chest tubes or drains are required (Fig. 6-5F). For closure, interrupted subcutaneous sutures are placed bilaterally but not tied. Then 40 cm of sustained inspiratory pressure is administered by the anesthesia team while the sutures are quickly pulled up and tied after the pleural air has escaped. Skin is reapproximated using a running subcuticular closure.

Postoperative management

Patients undergoing a modified Nuss procedure have a significant amount of postoperative pain; this is usually the limiting factor for discharge planning. In our experience, the analgesia requirement is even greater for this procedure than for the modified Ravitch repair. Some centers utilize a thoracic epidural for younger patients. The Lorenz substernal bar is left in place for a period of at least 2 years to allow for optimal remodeling of the costal cartilages and repositioning of the sternum. Longer bar placement may be used for patients requiring reoperation and those with elastic cartilage abnormalities. Bar removal is usually an outpatient procedure and should not be scheduled during a growth spurt.

Outcomes and complications

The original report of 42 patients by Nuss and associates in 1998[7] has been followed by two reports from his group describing a 14-year experience of repair in 329 patients, including 14 reoperations for failed Ravitch repairs and 10 for failed Nuss repairs (2 of which were performed by the Nuss group).[81,85] Perioperative antibiotics and aggressive incentive spirometry are advocated to prevent bar infection, pneumonia, and atelectasis. Epidural anesthesia is recommended for analgesia, and both thoracoscopy and sternal elevation are described for bar insertion to minimize the risk of mediastinal injury. They report no cases of cardiac perforation, thoracic chondrodystrophy, or death using these techniques. Although 52 percent of patients developed pneumothorax, most resolved spontaneously, with only 1.2 percent requiring aspiration and 1.5 percent requiring tube thoracostomy. Pericarditis responsive to either indomethacin or pericardial fluid aspiration was reported in 2.4 percent of patients in this review, pneumonia in 0.9 percent, and wound infection in 2.6 percent, responsive mostly to antibiotics but resulting in bar removal in 3 patients. Before the routine use of bar stabilizers, bar displacement occurred in 15.7 percent of patients; this was reduced to 5.4 percent with stabilizers and even further with wire sutures. In 13 percent of these patients, double stabilizing bars were used.

Several other large series have reported similarly encouraging results, with good results in over 95 percent of patients but also with a reminder that a learning curve is associated with the introduction of this new technique.[82–84,87] Quality of life has been studied objectively and, using two quality-of-life models, was found to be improved.[88] Complications of the Nuss procedure include ileus, pleural effusions, atelectasis, flipped or displaced bar, pericarditis, chronic pain, worsening of chest wall asymmetry,[87] anterior thoracic artery pseudoaneurysm, thoracic outlet obstruction,[82] sternal erosion, and liver injury.[83]

A review of three major complications following Nuss repair was reported by Moss and colleagues.[89] One patient suffered a cardiac perforation requiring urgent sternotomy and repair on cardiopulmonary bypass. A second patient required open pleural and cardiac debridement for staphylococcal sepsis, bilateral empyema, and bacterial pericarditis. Three patients suffered thoracic outlet syndrome with persistent paresthesias. Postpericardiotomy syndrome refractory to nonsteroidal anti-inflammatory treatment has also been described and treated successfully with intravenous methylprednisolone. Table 6-6 outlines the complications reported following the modified Nuss procedure.

Table 6-6	Complications of modified Nuss procedure
Early	
Pneumothorax	
Hemothorax	
Cardiac or pulmonary parenchymal injury	
Wound hematoma	
Bar movement/turning with recurrence	
Wound Infection	
Rib fracture	
Arrhythmias	
Late	
Bar movement	
Chronic pain/neuropraxia	
Erosion through sternum or rib	
Wound infection	
Recurrence	

Two reports compare the minimally invasive Nuss repair with the traditional modified Ravitch repair for surgical correction of pectus deformities.[90,91] Both provide excellent clinical and cosmetic results. Operative time is longer for the Ravitch repair, but length of stay, need for postoperative analgesia, and time to return to work are decreased. As reported in these studies, advantages of the Nuss repair include shorter operative time, smaller incisions, and less dissection at the potential expense of longer hospital stay, a high complication rate, more difficulty with success in older children and patients with connective tissue disorders, and a paucity of long-term outcome data.

ACQUIRED JEUNE'S SYNDROME

A dreaded complication of surgical correction for pectus excavatum is acquired thoracic chondrodystrophy, or acquired Jeune's syndrome (the congenital syndrome is described later in this chapter) (Fig. 6-6). In our institution we recently described 12 children referred to us for severe cardiopulmonary symptoms due to arrested chest wall growth following pectus operations.[55] These children underwent a modified Ravitch surgical repair at a very early age (< 4 years old) that involved extensive resections of five or more costal cartilages. The restriction of chest wall growth resulted in forced vital capacities (FVC) of 30 to 50 percent predicted and forced expiratory volumes (FEV_1) of 30 to 60 percent. None of the patients reviewed could perform any moderate exercise and all became symptomatic with even mild exercise.

Acquired Jeune's syndrome should not be mistaken for a recurrence of the pectus excavatum defect. The entire anterior chest wall is hypoplastic, as compared to the reversible depression of the sternum in the case of recurrent pectus. Acquired thoracic chondrodystrophy represents severe restriction of chest wall growth and movement; its natural history includes irreversible pulmonary hypertension.

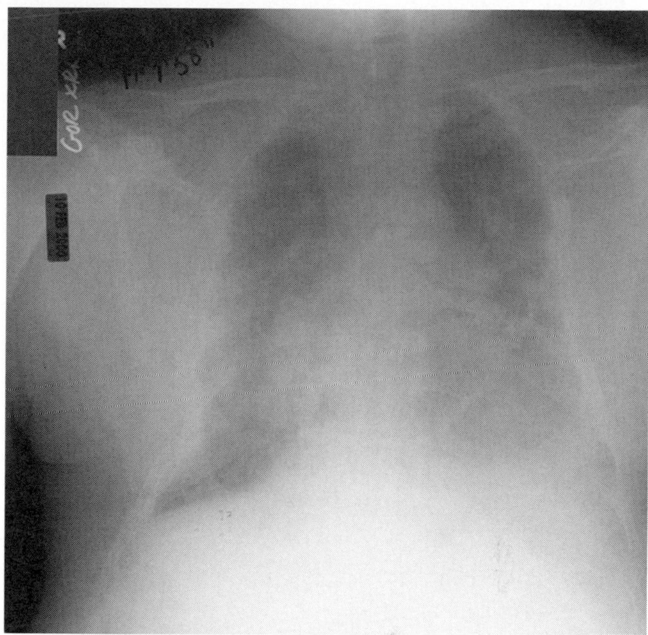

Figure 6-6 Chest x-ray of patient with acquired Jeune's syndrome. Note the small chest cavity in relation to chest wall and depressed diaphragm.

Diagnosis is best made by clinical examination and CT scanning (Fig. 6-7A and B). Pulmonary function testing reveals very severe restrictive disease, with FEVs and FVCs < 30 percent of predicted in most cases. Treatment is extensive and involves excision of all substernal cartilages, mobilization of all of the ribs to the anterior axillary line, and bar stabilization of the sternum. Rib grafts and sternal support bars may be required to stabilize the sternum after such a procedure. The use of rib grafts/compression/expansion plates and substernal support represents attempts to expand the compromised chest cavity. The best treatment for this life-threatening complication, however, is avoidance by delaying Ravitch operative repair in small children until at least the ages of 6 to 8 and minimizing chest wall resection and dissection in younger children.[55]

RECURRENT PECTUS EXCAVATUM

Up to 5 percent of patients undergoing pectus excavatum repair will have a recurrence following initial surgical correction. The incidence of this is higher in younger patients undergoing repair prior to completion of the teenage growth spurt, in patients with connective tissue disorders such as Marfan's syndrome, and in patients undergoing redo repair.[57,58] Operative repairs using modifications of the techniques of Ravitch or Nuss have been successful.[57,69,86,92]

After a Ravitch repair or one of its modifications, the incidence of recurrence in large studies with long-term

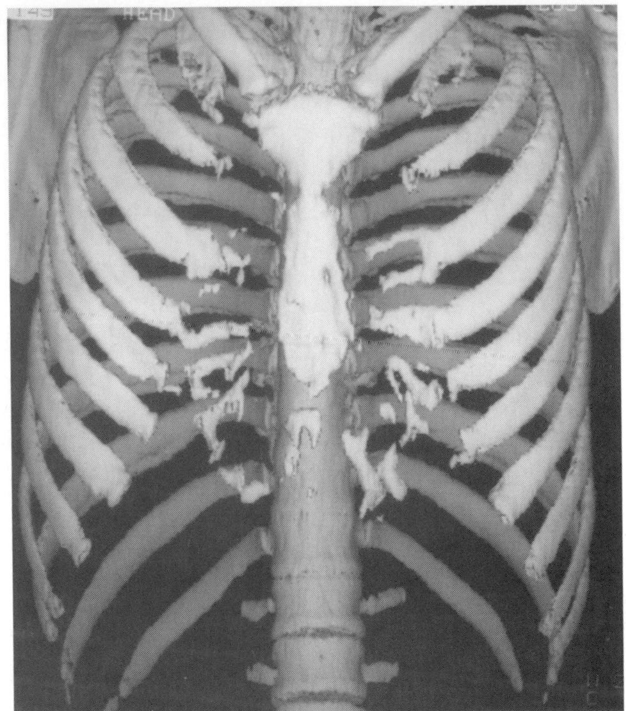

A

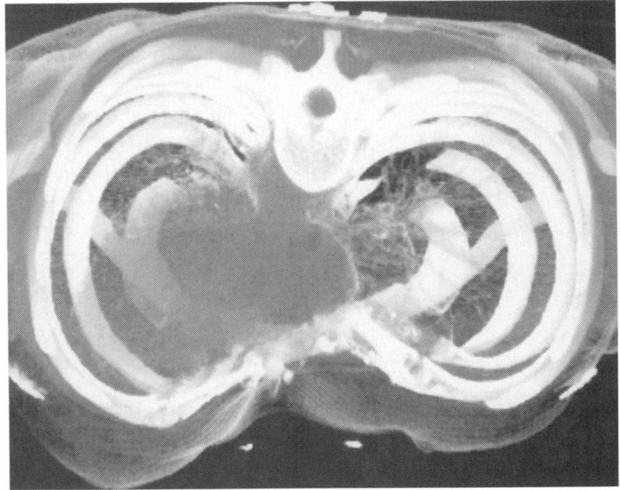

B

Figure 6-7 Recurrent pectus; three-dimensional scan reconstruction with two views (A and B) of patient with recurrent pectus excavatum.

follow-up is reported at 2 to 11 percent.[57,66,80,93] One possible cause of recurrence is fibrous nonunion of the edge of the sternum to the costal margin after cartilage resection. As the child progresses through the growth spurt of the teen years, a fibrous nonunion allowing bending of the sternum or the weight of the chest may both play a pathophysiologic role in recurrences, as most are seen in patients under the age of 12.[64] If the rib cartilages entirely fail to reattach to the edge of the sternum, an unstable anterior chest wall is created rather than a recurrence, with an easily movable or "floating" sternum.[94]

On initial evaluation of a child with chest wall abnormalities following pectus excavatum repair, a recurrence must be distinguished from a carinatum deformity, an acquired Jeune's syndrome, or a floating sternum. These last three deformities are addressed in other sections of this chapter. The severity of the recurrence should be assessed by clinical examination as well as CT scan if necessary (Fig. 6-7A and B). Pretorius and Haller studied the role of spiral CT in evaluating candidates for reoperation and found that CT could accurately define the orientation of the ribs, costal cartilages, and sternum as well as their interrelationships in both the pre- and postoperative periods. CT findings can help plan an individualized operative repair.[49,95] Pulmonary function tests as well as cardiac output measurements or echocardiography should be performed to evaluate the extent of cardiopulmonary restriction.[31,32]

Indications for reoperative correction are the same as for primary repair and include significant pain, exercise intolerance, a Haller index greater than 3.0, sternal depression greater than 2.5 cm, or significant restriction demonstrated by pulmonary function tests or cardiac evaluation. Timing is critical, and reoperation in teenagers should be postponed until growth spurts have been completed.

The choice of operation depends on the initial operation used to correct the pectus deformity, the type of recurrence, the severity of the defect, the age of the patient, and the experience of the surgical team planning the operation. Successful repairs of pectus recurrences have recently been reported in large series using both modified Ravitch procedures[69,92] and modified Nuss repairs.[86]

Important considerations in preventing recurrence after reoperative Ravitch repairs include the use of a bar placed substernally to elevate the sternum to a neutral position, wiring of the costal cartilages to the edge of the sternum, or repeat subperichondrial resections of the costal cartilages. Wedge osteotomy is usually required, as with primary Ravitch repairs.[6,57,80]

Our institutional experience with Nuss repairs as well as reports from large international series have led us to consider the following modifications to primary Nuss repairs as well as reoperations using the Nuss technique. We prefer to fix the Lorenz bar at the point where the bar exits the pleural cavity to first cross over a lateral rib. If the bar is not stable, a second wire is used at the point where the bar crosses a rib in the midaxillary line. We now use bilateral stabilizing clips much more liberally than we did in our initial experience. A second bar is used above the first if the upper sternum remains depressed or below the first if the lower costal margin remains significantly depressed. Finally, in patients with recurrences or connective tissue disorders, placement of the Lorenz bar for periods in excess of the original 2-year recommendation seems to have decreased problems in these patient populations.

PECTUS CARINATUM

INTRODUCTION

The pectus carinatum defect mirrors the excavatum defect, with anterior protrusion deformity of the chest

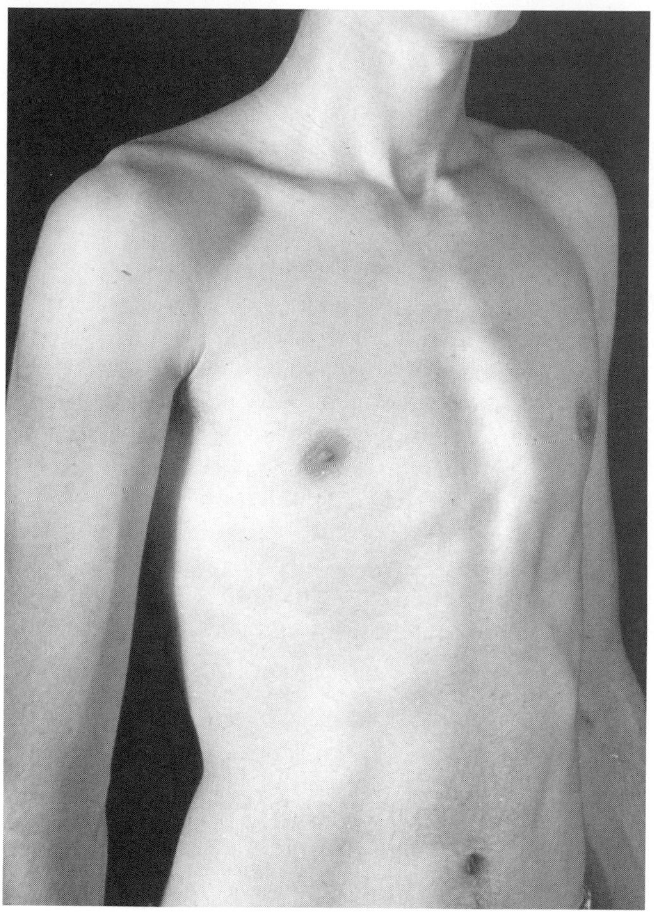

Figure 6-8 Typical pectus carinatum patient with unilateral defect.

wall. Figure 6-8 depicts the typical patient with pectus carinatum. Incidence is about one-tenth that of pectus excavatum, with a male predominance pattern like excavatum and a 25 to 30 percent reported family history.[96] Rotation and lengthening of the costal cartilages causes anterior displacement of the cartilages and resulting sternal protrusion. Carinatum can occur at any age, as early as in the toddler years, but it most commonly becomes clinically apparent in the early teenage years. A number of unusual deformities can occur, including unilateral asymmetrical patterns, mixed carinatum/excavatum lesions, and upper chondromanubrial deformities.[97] A number of large clinical reports demonstrate successful surgical correction of carinatum deformities in both male and female patients.[45,51,73,74,96,98–102]

DEVELOPMENT AND PATHOPHYSIOLOGY

As with pectus excavatum, the etiology of pectus carinatum remains unknown. Familial proclivity has been reported,[96] and dominant mutations in the type II collagen gene *COL2A1* have been associated with pectus carinatum.[103] Scoliosis and other spinal deformities or a family history of these are associated with pectus carinatum as well.

Since no significant cardiopulmonary abnormalities can be demonstrated with this lesion of the chest wall, carinatum remains a clinical diagnosis and no further diagnostic tests are required. Children with this anomaly do, however, complain on occasion of exertional dyspnea, limitations to exercise potential, frequent respiratory infections, and chest discomfort.[98,99] If necessary, CT scanning can clarify any question of differential diagnosis, better assess the anatomic defect, and help to plan the surgical correction.

Pectus carinatum can cause significant body disfigurement and pain and can have a profound effect on a growing teenager's body image (Fig. 6-9). Indications for surgical correction of pectus carinatum include pain, respiratory symptoms, ease of injury, and psychosocial concerns of body image. Because of a 20 to 30 percent chance of recurrence if this condition is corrected prior to the completion of pubertal growth spurts, repair must be deferred until the patient is fully grown, where the risk of recurrence is less than 1 percent. Table 6-7 outlines typical signs and symptoms of pectus carinatum.

Operative repair

Surgical correction for pectus carinatum utilizes the basic principles outlined earlier in this chapter for the

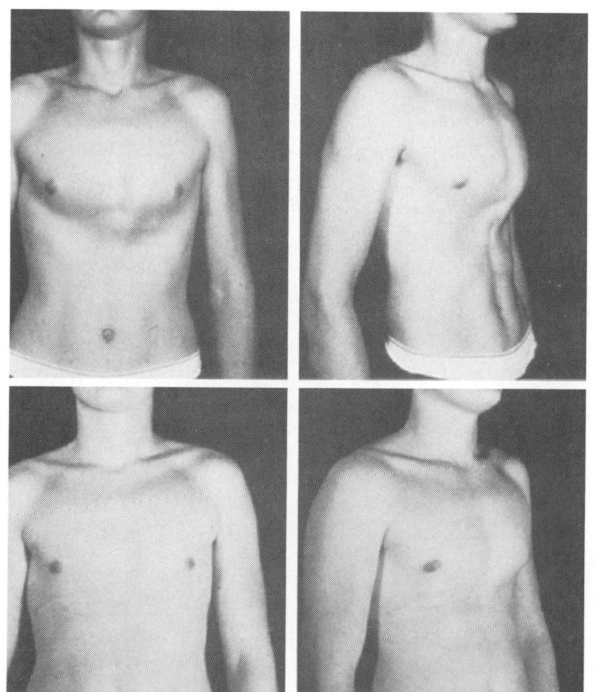

Figure 6-9 Severe pectus carinatum with bilateral involvement of costal cartilages and elevation of the sternum; pre- and postoperative views.

Table 6-7	Signs and symptoms of pectus carinatum
Physical signs	
Sternal elevation/rotation	
Unilateral or bilateral costal cartilage elevation	
Barrel chest	
Symptoms	
Parasternal pain	
Frequent injuries	
Exercise intolerance	
Decreased work capacity	

modified open Ravitch repair (Table 6-8). Surgical goals include excision of all abnormal cartilages and return of the sternum to a neutral straight position. The same incision and flaps are created as described for patients with pectus excavatum. A meticulous search should be made for abnormal cartilages, since they may be difficult to identify and those that go unrecognized are sources of recurrence. All abnormal cartilages, usually bilaterally, are resected using the subperichondrial technique of Ravitch. If the sternum remains anterior or rotated after subperichondrial resection, anterior sternal osteotomies can be performed to facilitate depression of the anterior table of the sternum to a neutral position. Oblique osteotomy corrects sternal rotation. In our institution, we use subpectoral and subcutaneous drains to avoid seromas. Hospital stay is usually 3 to 4 days, and neocartilage formation of 6 to 8 weeks' duration precludes contact sports or strenuous activity for this postoperative period.

Outcomes and complications

Fonkalsrud and Beanes have described their 30-year experience with 90 children who underwent surgical repair of pectus carinatum defects.[99] All of the children were symptomatic, including 84 with exertional dyspnea and exercise limitation, 52 with respiratory infections, 24 with asthma, and 38 with pain. Modified Ravitch-type repairs were used in all patients. Deaths were none and complications were minimal, with only 5 patients developing seroma, 3 with pleural effusions, and 2 with pneumothorax. Mean hospital stay was 2.6 days and follow-up was 12.8 years. The authors described one recurrence amenable to reoperation, and all children reported marked clinical improvement. Similar success, although with greater technical difficulty, has been reported with pectus carinatum repair in adults.[45,51,74]

Two other large series have reported success in the surgical correction of pectus carinatum defects. Saxena and Willital reviewed a 14-year experience of 111 patients using double bilateral chondrotomy and retrosternal mobilization and stabilization with metal struts; they reported 98 percent success, 1.8 percent major recurrences, and 2.7 percent minor recurrences.[102] Shamberger and Welch reported a 12-year experience of 152 pectus carinatum repairs utilizing bilateral resection of costal cartilages and osteotomy, with satisfactory results in all patients and only a 3.9 percent complication rate, including pneumothorax, wound infection, atelectasis, and local tissue necrosis. Experience at our own institution has been similar, with virtually no recurrence in patients corrected after maximal growth.[101]

Table 6-8	Key components of pectus carinatum repair
1. Transverse or midline incision	
2. Skin subcutaneous and muscle flaps	
3. Excision of all elevated cartilages	
4. Contralateral cartilage resection (if unilateral)	
5. Anterior sternal osteotomy to depress sternum to neutral position	
6. Bone wedge to hold sternum in neutral position	
7. Wound closure with closed drainage	

OTHER CHEST WALL ANOMALIES

POLAND'S SYNDROME

Alfred Poland, as a medical student affiliated with Guy's hospital, is credited with having described, in 1841, the congenital absence of pectoralis major and minor muscles, although this had previously been reported in the French and German literature in 1826 and 1839, respectively. Poland's finding was attributed to his name in 1962 by Clarkson of the same hospital.[104] This disease is a spectrum of deficiency or absence of components of the chest wall, including the pectoralis major, pectoralis minor, serratus anterior, ribs 2 to 5, and the breast and areolar complex.[105] Associated hand deformities include brachydactyly, syndactyly, and ectromelia.

The incidence of this disease is approximately 1 in 30,000 live births.[106,107] Shamberger and associates recently reported a 33-year 75-patient experience with Poland's syndrome.[108] Of these patients, 40 were male and 35 female; 44 were right-sided, 30 left-sided, and 1 bilateral. Absence of the pectoralis major and minor muscles or their significant hypoplasia was described in all patients. The spectrum of chest wall involvement included 41 patients with normal chest walls, 10 with hypoplasia of the ribs, 11 with major depression deformities and 5 with minor depression deformities of the ribs, and 8 with complete aplasia of the ribs.

In its most severe form, the classic presentation of Poland's syndrome involves herniation of the lung through the chest wall defect during coughing or crying

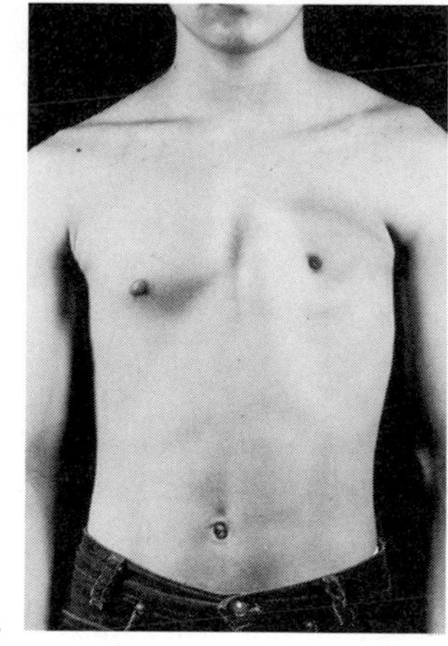
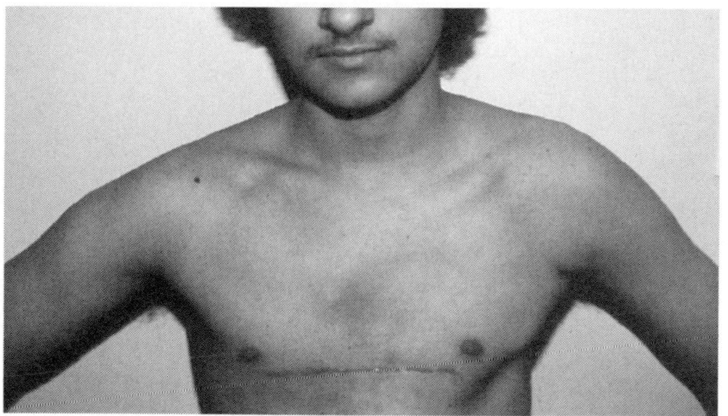

Figure 6-10 A and B. Teenager with right-sided Poland's syndrome; pre- and postoperative views.

in a newborn. For this flail segment, prompt repair is necessary. Without lung herniation, toddlers with this syndrome can be observed until adolescence, when the remaining muscles of the chest wall have reached a size sufficient to facilitate repair. Repair should be timed based on clinical symptoms, cosmetic abnormalities, and the age and physical build of child.

Successful surgical repair using autologous rib grafts,[108] latissimus muscle flaps,[109] synthetic mesh,[110] or a combination of these modalities has been described. CT is an acceptable means of evaluating these patients after surgical repair. Figure 6-10 shows a typical patient before and after repair. Postoperative recurrence is unlikely and can be repaired with rewiring of the original bone or cartilage grafts to the sternum and native rib cage or with autologous grafts and mesh similar to the procedure in primary repair.

PENTALOGY OF CANTRELL

A syndrome of lower sternal cleft, epigastric or high omphalocele, anterior diaphragmatic defect, absent pericardium, and an intracardiac anomaly was originally described in 1958 by Cantrell.[10] The developmental etiology is unknown, but it has been suggested to relate to anomalies in defined subunits of a ventral midline developmental field.[111] As with all developmental syndromes, a spectrum of clinical manifestations can be found. The heart is usually found within the omphalocele defect and, if the omphalocele ruptures, an ectopia cordis can be created (Fig. 6-11). Regardless, immediate surgical attention is warranted in any case of pentalogy of Cantrell. Staged repair is usually required to first close the epigastric omphalocele, repair the diaphragmatic defect, and effect skin coverage of the heart. Secondary procedures to obtain bony coverage of the heart may be delayed for 2 to 3 years to allow for adequate growth. Repair of the intracardiac defect is usually deferred until after somatic closure, although in rare instances simultaneous repair can be accomplished.

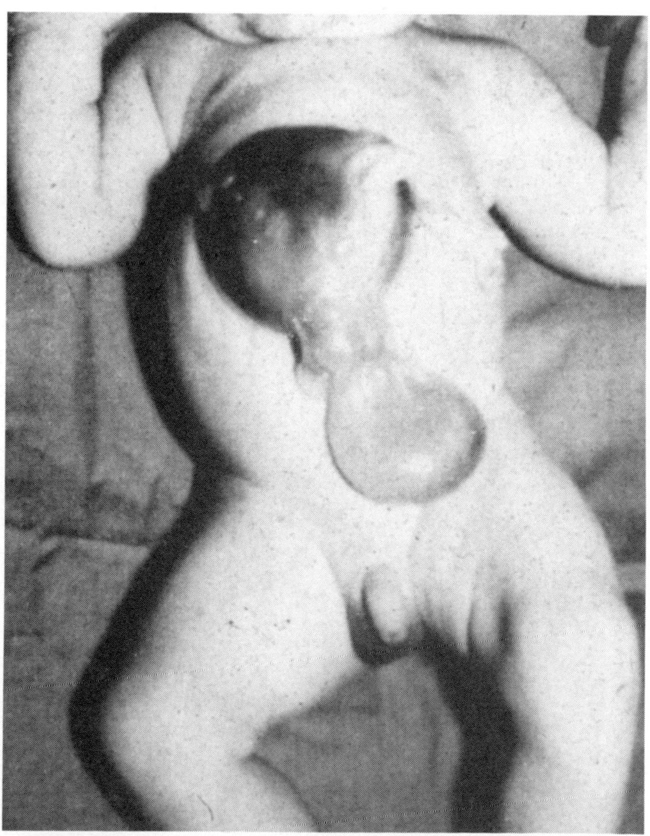

Figure 6-11 Photograph of newborn infant with pentalogy of Cantrell. Note the upper omphalocele, foreshortened sternum with defect, and pericardial defect.

JEUNE'S SYNDROME

Originally described by Jeune in 1954,[9] the syndrome of asphyxiating thoracic chondrodystrophy ranges from a lethal condition at birth to a survivable and surgically treatable disorder.[112] The original patient described had a narrow, rigid chest wall and multiple cartilagenous anomalies and died early in the perinatal period from respiratory insufficiency. An autosomal recessive pattern of inheritance has been described, but not in association with known chromosomal abnormalities.[113]

Clinical features include a narrow thorax along both the transverse and sagittal axes, protuberant abdomen, little respiratory movement of the chest wall, short and wide ribs, costochondral junctions that are splayed and barely reach the anterior axillary line, and irregular costal cartilage. Associated findings include short extremities with relatively wide bones, fixed and elevated clavicles, and a small hypoplastic pelvis (Fig. 6-12A and B). Pulmonary development can also be abnormal; findings vary from patient to patient.[114]

Operative repair offers limited success and is usually performed when children are on oxygen and may be ventilator-dependent. Available modalities for surgical chest wall expansion include sternal splitting, anterior chest wall release, autologous grafts, artificial ribs, stainless steel support struts, and mesh and other prostheses. After axial growth, further procedures may be required to facilitate chest wall expansion. The limiting factor for survival following surgical correction is not the chest wall itself but the underlying pulmonary hypoplasia.

STERNAL CLEFT

Failure of ventral fusion of the thoracic wall causing cleft sternum is extremely rare, and the largest series in the literature comprise fewer than 10 patients each.[115–117] Associated malformations include congenital cardiac abnormalities, maxillofacial hemangiomata, and omphalocele.[115,118] The goals of surgical correction of the split sternum are bony protection of the heart, great vessels, and other mediastinal structures as well as anterior thoracic stability to maintain normal physiologic pressures for the support of respiratory function and circulation.[118,119]

Repair of sternal clefts is best performed in the neonatal period, where primary repair is possible.[115,117,118,120,121] Isolated reports have demonstrated some success of surgical correction in adults as well, using bone grafts, muscle flaps, sliding chondrotomies, posterior sternal wall repairs, posterior periosteal flaps, sternal bars, chondral grafts.[117,118,121–124]

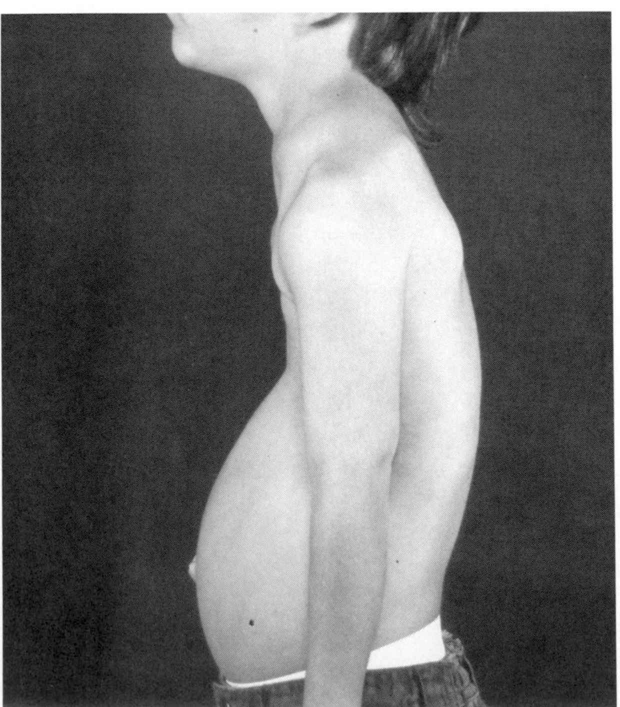

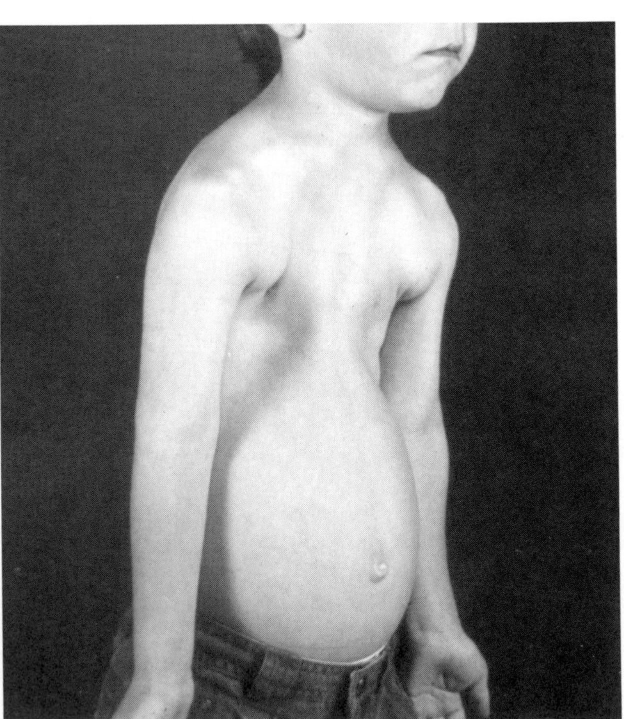

Figure 6-12 A and B. Patient with congenital Jeune's syndrome. Lateral view (A) shows marked decrease in AP diameter of chest, while anterolateral view (B) shows marked undergrowth of ribs.

Acastello and coworkers recently reviewed their experience with 8 patients over a 14-year period, 6 (75 percent) of whom were female, who underwent surgical correction of sternal cleft with 1- to 8-year follow-up.[115] Three methods were used: (1) primary closure; (2) partial resection of the upper three costal cartilages and disruption of the sternoclavicular junction, followed by closure of the sternal bars with wire; and (3) mobilization and approximation of sternocleidomastoid muscles with costal homograft and mesh. All three groups fared relatively well, although one patient in group 3 had an unsatisfactory result and required reoperation with the technique of group 2. The patients corrected with primary repair had the best outcomes, although mild pectus excavatum developed in some in the long term.

MINOR ANOMALIES

A number of chest wall anomalies may occur that usually require specific diagnosis but may not require operative intervention. Rib anomalies include fusion, partial absence, and growth deformities. Similar findings may occur with the costal cartilages, particularly in the costal margin area of the lower chest. Most of these anomalies do not require surgical intervention unless there is instability of the chest wall or significant body image issues exist. Most anomalies for which operative repair is contemplated should be observed until children reach school age or complete teenage growth.

References

1. Shamberger RC. Congenital chest wall deformities. *Curr Probl Surg* 1996;33(6):469–542.
2. Golladay ES, Golladay GJ. Chest wall deformities. *Indian J Pediatr* 1997;64(3):339–350.
3. Ayres JG, Pope FM, Reidy JF, Clark TJ. Abnormalities of the lungs and thoracic cage in the Ehlers-Danlos syndrome. *Thorax* 1985;40(4):300–305.
4. Golladay ES, Char F, Mollitt DL. Children with Marfan's syndrome and pectus excavatum. *South Med J* 1985;78(11): 1319–1323.
5. Meyer L. Zur chirurgischen Behandlung der angeborenen Trichterbrust. *Verh Berl Med Ges* 1911;42:364.
6. Ravitch MM. The operative treatment of pectus excavatum. *Ann Surg* 1949;129:929.
7. Nuss D, Kelly RE Jr, Croitoru DP, Katz ME. A 10-year review of a minimally invasive technique for the correction of pectus excavatum. *J Pediatr Surg* 1998;33(4):545–552.
8. Ravitch MM. Unusual sternal deformity with cardiac symptoms: Operative correction. *J Thorac Surg* 1952; 23:138.
9. Jeune M, Carron R, Beraud CL. Polychondrodystrophie avec blocage thoracique d'evolution fatale. *Pediatrie* 1954;9:390.
10. Cantrell JR, Haller JA, Ravitch MM. A syndrome of congenital defects involving the abdominal wall, sternum, diaphragm, pericardium, and heart. *Surg Gynecol Obstet* 1958;107(5):602–614.
11. Poland A. Deficiency of the pectoralis muscles. *Guys Hosp Rep* 1841;6:191.
12. Froriep R. Beobachtung eines Falles von Mangel der Brustdruse. *Notizen Geb Nat Heilk* 1839;10:9.
13. Lallemand LM. Absence de trots cotes simulant un enforcement accidental. *Epherm Med Montpellier* 1826;1:144.
14. Shamberger R, Hendren WH III. Congenital deformities of the chest wall and sternum. In: Pearson FG, Cooper J, Deslauriers J, et al (eds). *Thoracic Surgery.* Philadelphia: Elsevier, 2002.
15. Moore KL. *The Developing Human: Clinically Oriented Embryology.* Philadelphia: Saunders, 1988.
16. Skandalakis JE, Gray SW, Ricketts R, Skandalakis LJ. The anterior body wall. In: Skandalakis JE, Skandalakis GSW (eds). *Embryology for Surgeons: The Embryological Basis for the Treatment of Congenital Defects,* 4th ed. Baltimore: Williams & Wilkins, 1994.
17. Feng J, Hu T, Liu W, et al. The biomechanical, morphologic, and histochemical properties of the costal cartilages in children with pectus excavatum. *J Pediatr Surg* 2001;36(12):1770–1776.
18. Fonkalsrud EW. Current management of pectus excavatum. *World J Surg* 2003;27(5):502–508.
19. Leung AK, Hoo JJ. Familial congenital funnel chest. *Am J Med Genet* 1987;26(4):887–890.
20. Wachtel FW, Ravitch MM, Grishman A. The relation of pectus excavatum to heart disease. *Am Heart J* 1956; 52(1):121–137.
21. Waters P, Welch K, Micheli LJ, et al. Scoliosis in children with pectus excavatum and pectus carinatum. *J Pediatr Orthop* 1989;9(5):551–556.
22. Shamberger RC, Welch KJ. Cardiopulmonary function in pectus excavatum. *Surg Gynecol Obstet.* 1988;166(4): 383–391.
23. Shamberger RC. Cardiopulmonary effects of anterior chest wall deformities. *Chest Surg Clin North Am* 2000; 10(2):245–252, v–vi.
24. Morshuis WJ, Folgering HT, Barentsz JO, et al. Exercise cardiorespiratory function before and one year after operation for pectus excavatum. *J Thorac Cardiovasc Surg* 1994;107(6):1403–1409.
25. Kaguraoka H, Ohnuki T, Itaoka T, et al. Degree of severity of pectus excavatum and pulmonary function in preoperative and postoperative periods. *J Thorac Cardiovasc Surg* 1992;104(5):1483–1488.
26. Borowitz D, Cerny F, Zallen G, et al. Pulmonary function and exercise response in patients with pectus excavatum after Nuss repair. *J Pediatr Surg* 2003;38(4):544–547.
27. Lacquet LK, Morshuis WJ, Folgering HT. Long-term results after correction of anterior chest wall deformities. *J Cardiovasc Surg (Torino)* 1998;39(5):683–688.
28. Derveaux L, Clarysse I, Ivanoff I, Demedts M. Preoperative and postoperative abnormalities in chest x-ray indices and in lung function in pectus deformities. *Chest* 1989;95(4):850–856.
29. Derveaux L, Ivanoff I, Rochette F, Demedts M. Mechanism of pulmonary function changes after surgical correction for funnel chest. *Eur Respir J* 1988;1(9):823–825.
30. Sigalet DL, Montgomery M, Harder J. Cardiopulmonary effects of closed repair of pectus excavatum. *J Pediatr Surg* 2003;38(3):380–385; discussion 380–385.

31. Wynn SR, Driscoll DJ, Ostrom NK, et al. Exercise cardiorespiratory function in adolescents with pectus excavatum. Observations before and after operation. *J Thorac Cardiovasc Surg* 1990;99(1):41–47.
32. Quigley PM, Haller JA Jr, Jelus KL, Loughlin GM, Marcus CL. Cardiorespiratory function before and after corrective surgery in pectus excavatum. *J Pediatr* 1996;128(5 Pt 1):638–643.
33. Haller JA Jr, Loughlin GM. Cardiorespiratory function is significantly improved following corrective surgery for severe pectus excavatum. Proposed treatment guidelines. *J Cardiovasc Surg (Torino)* 2000;41(1):125–130.
34. Blickman JG, Rosen PR, Welch KJ, et al. Pectus excavatum in children: Pulmonary scintigraphy before and after corrective surgery. *Radiology* 1985;156(3):781–782.
35. Castile RG, Staats BA, Westbrook PR. Symptomatic pectus deformities of the chest. *Am Rev Respir Dis* 1982;126(3):564–568.
36. Cahill JL, Lees GM, Robertson HT. A summary of preoperative and postoperative cardiorespiratory performance in patients undergoing pectus excavatum and carinatum repair. *J Pediatr Surg* 1984;19(4):430–433.
37. Kowalewski J, Barcikowski S, Brocki M. Cardiorespiratory function before and after operation for pectus excavatum: Medium-term results. *Eur J Cardiothorac Surg* 1998; 13(3):275–279.
38. Beiser GD, Epstein SE, Stampfer M, et al. Impairment of cardiac function in patients with pectus excavatum, with improvement after operative correction. *N Engl J Med* 1972;287(6):267–272.
39. Malek MH, Fonkalsrud EW, Cooper CB. Ventilatory and cardiovascular responses to exercise in patients with pectus excavatum. *Chest* 2003;124(3):870–882.
40. Peterson RJ, Young WG Jr, Godwin JD, et al. Noninvasive assessment of exercise cardiac function before and after pectus excavatum repair. *J Thorac Cardiovasc Surg* 1985;90(2):251–260.
41. Kowalewski J, Brocki M, Dryjanski T, et al. Pectus excavatum: Increase of right ventricular systolic, diastolic, and stroke volumes after surgical repair. *J Thorac Cardiovasc Surg* 1999;118(1):87–92; discussion 92–93.
42. Einsiedel E, Clausner A. Funnel chest. Psychological and psychosomatic aspects in children, youngsters, and young adults. *J Cardiovasc Surg (Torino)* 1999;40(5):733–736.
43. Ravitch MM. Asymmetric congenital deformity of the ribs. Collapse of the right side of the chest. *Ann Surg* 1980;191(5):534–538.
44. Fonkalsrud EW, Dunn JC, Atkinson JB. Repair of pectus excavatum deformities: 30 years of experience with 375 patients. *Ann Surg* 2000; 231(3):443–448.
45. Mansour KA, Thourani VH, Odessey EA, et al. Thirty-year experience with repair of pectus deformities in adults. *Ann Thorac Surg* 2003;76(2):391–395; discussion 395.
46. Haller JA Jr, Peters GN, Mazur D, White JJ. Pectus excavatum. A 20-year surgical experience. *J Thorac Cardiovasc Surg* 1970;60(3):375–383.
47. Sidden CR, Katz ME, Swoveland BC, Nuss D. Radiologic considerations in patients undergoing the Nuss procedure for correction of pectus excavatum. *Pediatr Radiol* 2001;31(6):429–434.
48. Shamberger RC, Welch KJ. Surgical repair of pectus excavatum. *J Pediatr Surg* 1988;23(7):615–622.
49. Haller JA Jr, Kramer SS, Lietman SA, Use of CT scans in selection of patients for pectus excavatum surgery: A preliminary report. *J Pediatr Surg* 1987;22(10):904–906.
50. Daunt SW, Cohen JH, Miller SF. Age-related normal ranges for the Haller index in children. *Pediatr Radiol* 2004.
51. Fonkalsrud EW, DeUgarte D, Choi E. Repair of pectus excavatum and carinatum deformities in 116 adults. *Ann Surg* 2002;236(3):304–312; discussion 312–314.
52. Shamberger RC, Welch KJ, Castaneda AR, et al. Anterior chest wall deformities and congenital heart disease. *J Thorac Cardiovasc Surg* 1988;96(3):427–432.
53. Haller JA Jr. History of the operative management of pectus deformities. *Chest Surg Clin N Am* 2000;10(2): 227–235, v.
54. Haller JA Jr. Severe chest wall construction from growth retardation after too extensive and too early (< 4 years) pectus excavatum repair: An alert. *Ann Thorac Surg* 1995;60(6):1857–1858.
55. Haller JA Jr, Colombani PM, Humphries CT, et al. Chest wall constriction after too extensive and too early operations for pectus excavatum. *Ann Thorac Surg* 1996;61(6):1618–1624; discussion 1625.
56. Haller JA Jr. Complications of surgery for pectus excavatum. *Chest Surg Clin North Am* 2000;10(2): 415–426, ix.
57. Colombani PM. Recurrent chest wall anomalies. *Semin Pediatr Surg* 2003;12(2):94–99.
58. Arn PH, Scherer LR, Haller JA Jr, Pyeritz RE. Outcome of pectus excavatum in patients with Marfan syndrome and in the general population. *J Pediatr* 1989;115(6): 954–958.
59. Hasegawa T, Yamaguchi M, Ohshima Y, et al. Simultaneous repair of pectus excavatum and congenital heart disease over the past 30 years. *Eur J Cardiothorac Surg* 2002;22(6):874–878.
60. Ravitch MM. The operative treatment of pectus excavatum. *J S C Med Assoc* 1955;51(7):244–249.
61. Ravitch MM, The operative treatment of pectus excavatum. *J Pediatr* 1956;48(4):465–472.
62. Ravitch MM. Operation for correction of pectus excavatum. *Surg Gynecol Obstet* 1958;106(5):619–622.
63. Ravitch MM. The operative correction of pectus carinatum. *Bull Soc Int Chir* 1975;34(2):117–120.
64. Moghissi K. Long-term results of surgical correction of pectus excavatum and sternal prominence. *Thorax* 1964;19:350–354.
65. Haller AJ Jr, Katlic M, Shermeta DW, et al. Operative correction of pectus excavatum: An evolving perspective. *Ann Surg* 1976;184(5):554–557.
66. Haller JA Jr, Scherer LR, Turner CS, Colombani PM. Evolving management of pectus excavatum based on a single institutional experience of 664 patients. *Ann Surg* 1989;209(5):578–582; discussion 582–583.
67. Golladay ES, Wagner CW. Pectus excavatum: A 15-year perspective. *South Med J* 1991;84(9):1099–1102.
68. Morshuis WJ, Mulder H, Wapperom G, et al. Pectus excavatum. A clinical study with long-term postoperative follow-up. *Eur J Cardiothorac Surg* 1992;6(6):318–328; discussion 328–329.
69. Ellis DG, Snyder CL, Mann CM. The "re-do" chest wall deformity correction. *J Pediatr Surg* 1997;32(9): 1267–1271.

70. Kamei Y, Torii S, Hasegawa T, et al. Endoscopic correction of pectus excavatum. *Plast Reconstr Surg* 2001; 107(2):333–337.
71. Fonkalsrud EW, Follette D, Sarwat AK. Pectus excavatum repair using autologous perichondrium for sternal support. *Arch Surg* 1978;113(12):1433–1437.
72. Gilbert JC, Zwiren GT. Repair of pectus excavatum using a substernal metal strut within a Marlex envelope. *South Med J* 1989;82(10):1240–1244.
73. Fonkalsrud EW. Management of pectus chest deformities in female patients. *Am J Surg* 2004;187(2): 192–197.
74. Fonkalsrud EW, Bustorff-Silva J. Repair of pectus excavatum and carinatum in adults. *Am J Surg* 1999;177(2): 121–124.
75. Fonkalsrud EW, Salman T, Guo W, Gregg JP. Repair of pectus deformities with sternal support. *J Thorac Cardiovasc Surg* 1994;107(1):37–42.
76. Saxena AK, Schaarschmidt K, Schleef J, et al. Surgical correction of pectus excavatum: The Munster experience. *Langenbecks Arch Surg* 1999;384(2):187–193.
77. Scherer LR, Arn PH, Dressel DA, et al. Surgical management of children and young adults with Marfan syndrome and pectus excavatum. *J Pediatr Surg* 1988; 23(12):1169–1172.
78. Haller JA Jr, Peters GN, White JJ. Surgical management of funnel chest (pectus excavatum). *Surg Clin North Am* 1970;50(4):929–934.
79. Kowalewski J, Brocki M, Zolynski K. Long-term observation in 68 patients operated on for pectus excavatum: Surgical repair of funnel chest. *Ann Thorac Surg* 1999;67(3):821–824.
80. Prevot J. Treatment of sternocostal wall malformations of the child. A series of 210 surgical corrections since 1975. *Eur J Pediatr Surg* 1994;4(3):131–136.
81. Croitoru DP, Kelly RE Jr, Goretsky MJ, et al. Experience and modification update for the minimally invasive Nuss technique for pectus excavatum repair in 303 patients. *J Pediatr Surg* 2002;37(3):437–445.
82. Hebra A, Swoveland B, Egbert M, et al. Outcome analysis of minimally invasive repair of pectus excavatum: Review of 251 cases. *J Pediatr Surg* 2000;35(2):252–257; discussion 257–258.
83. Hosie S, Sitkiewicz T, Petersen C, et al. Minimally invasive repair of pectus excavatum—the Nuss procedure. A European multicentre experience. *Eur J Pediatr Surg* 2002;12(4):235–238.
84. Miller KA, Woods RK, Sharp RJ, et al. Minimally invasive repair of pectus excavatum: A single institution's experience. *Surgery* 2001;130(4):652–657; discussion 657–659.
85. Nuss D, Croitoru DP, Kelly RE Jr, et al. Review and discussion of the complications of minimally invasive pectus excavatum repair. *Eur J Pediatr Surg* 2002;12(4):230–234.
86. Miller KA, Ostlie DJ, Wade K, et al. Minimally invasive bar repair for "redo" correction of pectus excavatum. *J Pediatr Surg* 2002;37(7):1090–1092.
87. Engum S, Rescorla F, West K, et al. Is the grass greener? Early results of the Nuss procedure. *J Pediatr Surg* 2000;35(2):246–251; discussion 257–258.
88. Roberts J, Hayashi A, Anderson JO, et al. Quality of life of patients who have undergone the Nuss procedure for pectus excavatum: Preliminary findings. *J Pediatr Surg* 2003;38(5):779–783.
89. Moss RL, Albanese CT, Reynolds M. Major complications after minimally invasive repair of pectus excavatum: Case reports. *J Pediatr Surg* 2001; 36(1):155–158.
90. Fonkalsrud EW, Beanes S, Hebra A, et al. Comparison of minimally invasive and modified Ravitch pectus excavatum repair. *J Pediatr Surg* 2002;37(3):413–417.
91. Molik KA, Engum SA, Rescorla FJ, et al. Pectus excavatum repair: Experience with standard and minimal invasive techniques. *J Pediatr Surg* 2001;36(2):324–328.
92. De Ugarte DA, Choi E, Fonkalsrud EW. Repair of recurrent pectus deformities. *Am Surg* 2002;68(12)1075–1079.
93. Singh SV. Surgical correction of pectus excavatum and carinatum. *Thorax* 1980;35(9):700–702.
94. Prabhakaran K, Paidas CN, Haller JA, et al. Management of a floating sternum after repair of pectus excavatum. *J Pediatr Surg* 2001;36(1):159–164.
95. Pretorius ES, Haller JA, Fishman EK. Spiral CT with 3D reconstruction in children requiring reoperation for failure of chest wall growth after pectus excavatum surgery. Preliminary observations. *Clin Imaging* 1998;22(2): 108–116.
96. Shamberger RC, Welch KJ. Surgical correction of pectus carinatum. *J Pediatr Surg* 1987;22(1):48–53.
97. Shamberger RC, Welch KJ. Surgical correction of chondromanubrial deformity (Currarino Silverman syndrome). *J Pediatr Surg* 1988;23(4):319–322.
98. Fonkalsrud EW. Pectus carinatum: The undertreated chest malformation. *Asian J Surg* 2003;26(4):189–192.
99. Fonkalsrud EW, Beanes S. Surgical management of pectus carinatum: 30 years' experience. *World J Surg* 2001;25(7):898–903.
100. Pena A, Perez L, Nurko S, Dorenbaum D. Pectus carinatum and pectus excavatum: Are they the same disease? *Am Surg* 1981;47(5):215–218.
101. Pickard LR, Tepas JJ, Shermeta DW, Haller JA Jr. Pectus carinatum: Results of surgical therapy. *J Pediatr Surg* 1979;14(3):228–230.
102. Saxena AK, Willital GH. Surgical repair of pectus carinatum. *Int Surg* 1999;84(4):326–330.
103. Tiller GE, Polumbo PA, Weis MA, et al. Dominant mutations in the type II collagen gene, *COL2A1*, produce spondyloepimetaphyseal dysplasia, Strudwick type. *Nat Genet* 1995;11(1):87–89.
104. Clarkson P. Poland's syndactyly. *Guys Hosp Rep* 1962;111:335–346.
105. Urschel HC Jr. Poland's syndrome. *Chest Surg Clin North Am* 2000;10(2):393–403, viii.
106. McGillivray BC, Lowry RB. Poland syndrome in British Columbia: Incidence and reproductive experience of affected persons. *Am J Med Genet* 1977;1(1):65–74.
107. Freire–Maia N, Chautard EA, Opitz JM, et al. The Poland syndrome: Clinical and genealogical data, dermatoglyphic analysis, incidence. *Hum Hered* 1973;23(2):97–104.
108. Shamberger RC, Welch KJ, Upton J III. Surgical treatment of thoracic deformity in Poland's syndrome. *J Pediatr Surg* 1989;24(8):760–765; discussion 766.
109. Haller JA Jr, Colombani PM, Miller D, Manson P. Early reconstruction of Poland's syndrome using autologous rib grafts combined with a latissimus muscle flap. *J Pediatr Surg* 1984;19(4):423–429.

110. Urschel HC Jr, Byrd HS, Sethi SM, Razzuk MA. Poland's syndrome: Improved surgical management. *Ann Thorac Surg* 1984;37(3):204–211.
111. Carmi R, Boughman JA. Pentalogy of Cantrell and associated midline anomalies: A possible ventral midline developmental field. *Am J Med Genet* 1992;42(1):90–95.
112. Kozlowski K, Masel J. Asphyxiating thoracic dystrophy without respiratory disease: Report of two cases of the latent form. *Pediatr Radiol* 1976;5(1):30–33.
113. Tahernia AC, Stamps P. "Jeune syndrome" (asphyxiating thoracic dystrophy). Report of a case, a review of the literature, and an editor's commentary. *Clin Pediatr (Phila)* 1977;16(10):903–908.
114. Williams AJ, Vawter G, Reid LM. Lung structure in asphyxiating thoracic dystrophy. *Arch Pathol Lab Med* 1984;108(8):658–661.
115. Acastello E, Majluf R, Garrido P, et al. Sternal cleft: A surgical opportunity. *J Pediatr Surg* 2003;38(2):178–183.
116. Daum R, Zachariou Z. Total and superior sternal clefts in newborns: A simple technique for surgical correction. *J Pediatr Surg* 1999;34(3):408–411.
117. de Campos JR, Filomeno LT, Fernandez A. Repair of congenital sternal cleft in infants and adolescents. *Ann Thorac Surg* 1998;66(4):1151–1154.
118. Fokin AA. Cleft sternum and sternal foramen. *Chest Surg Clin North Am* 2000;10(2):261–276.
119. Verska JJ. Surgical repair of total cleft sternum. *J Thorac Cardiovasc Surg* 1975;69(2):301–305.
120. Firmin RK, Fragomeni LS, Lennox SC. Complete cleft sternum. *Thorax* 1980;35(4):303–306.
121. Knox L, Tuggle D, Knott-Craig CJ. Repair of congenital sternal clefts in adolescence and infancy. *J Pediatr Surg* 1994;29(12):1513–1516.
122. Biswas G, Khandelwal NK, Venkatramu NK, Chari PS. Congenital sternal cleft. *Br J Plast Surg* 2001;54(3):259–261.
123. Sarper A, Oz N, Arslan G, Demircan A. Complete congenital sternal cleft associated with pectus excavatum. *Texas Heart Inst J* 2002;29(3):206–209.
124. Suri RK, Sharma RK, Jha NK, Sharma BK. Complete congenital sternal cleft in an adult: Repair by autogenous tissues. *Ann Thorac Surg* 1996;62(2):573–575.

CHAPTER

7 CONGENITAL PULMONARY ANOMALIES

Karen Michiko Kling

BACKGROUND

Overview

The most described congenital pulmonary anomalies include congenital cystic adenomatoid malformations (CCAMs), bronchogenic cysts (BCs), congenital lobar emphysema (CLE), and pulmonary sequestration (PS). Although much less common and less surgically amenable, pulmonary lymphatic malformations, hemangiomas, agenesis, alveolar capillary dysplasia, pleuropulmonary blastoma, bronchial lesions, and arteriovenous malformations should also be included. Congenital lung anomalies are rare and usually limited to one hemithorax. There is no evidence of familial or ethnic preponderance, although there is a slight predilection (1.3:1) for

KEY CONCEPTS

- Epidemiology
  - Congenital pulmonary anomalies include a multitude of clinical entities linked by a common developmental lineage. The prevalence and sex distributions are dependent upon the particular malformation. These anomalies represent different variations of shared embryologic pathways and therefore possess clinical similarities and occasionally present simultaneously.
- Pathophysiology
  - Physiologically, the impact of these lesions, which can be mild or detrimental, depends largely on two factors—pulmonary hypoplasia and fetal hydrops. The mass effect of fetal intrathoracic lesions can impair lung development and decrease cardiac output secondary to mediastinal shift, causing fetal demise or severe compromise. Lesions that replace functional lung parenchyma can also cause pulmonary insufficiency.
- Clinical features
  - Many congenital pulmonary anomalies present postnatally with frequent pulmonary infections, respiratory distress, and hemoptysis, although others are discovered incidentally on plain chest radiography. Prenatal diagnoses of congenital pulmonary malformations are sometimes acquired with prenatal surveillance imaging.
- Diagnostics
  - Prenatal ultrasound is the primary diagnostic modality whereby congenital pulmonary anomalies are identified in utero and the degree of hydrops is assessed. Postnatally, computed tomography, magnetic resonance imaging, or ultrasound can be used to differentiate lesions based on anatomic characteristics; but since surgical resection is the treatment for most mass lesions, additional imaging may be superfluous.
- Treatment
  - Resection often is curative for focal lesions, but outcome is ultimately dependent on residual pulmonary function and associated medical conditions. Fetal intervention is being offered as an alternative for some congenital pulmonary anomalies, although outcomes have been mixed.
- Outcomes
  - Outcomes depend on the particular disease process. Generally excellent survival rates are noted with timely treatment of bronchogenic cysts, pulmonary sequestration, and congenital lobar emphysema. The prognoses of other entities are adversely affected by the presence of fetal hydrops as well as associated congenital developmental anomalies.

boys. Most conditions are recognized within the first 6 months of life because of respiratory symptoms. These pulmonary anomalies create problems by replacing functional lung parenchyma or displacing structures with their mass. This limits the space into which the developing lung can grow and causes hypoplasia with concomitant pulmonary hypertension or decreases venous return, leading to fetal hydrops. Congenital lung lesions can also be seen in association with other congenital malformations and prematurity, thus adding to the management challenge. Resection is recommended as soon as thoracotomy and general anesthesia are well tolerated, and the rapidity of action is governed by the severity of respiratory symptoms. For lesions with mass effect or those that focally replace lung parenchyma, resection is usually curative and may involve a segmental or lobar lung resection. Without comorbidities, resection is well tolerated; occasionally an incidental diagnoses in an asymptomatic adult with preclusive medical comorbidities will warrant observation instead of surgery.[1] For those with diffuse processes throughout the lung, resection is much less successful. Outcomes are most dependent on the degree of pulmonary hypoplasia and the morbidity of associated anomalies such as fetal hydrops, cardiac compromise, renal anomalies, and syndromic defects. Survival varies from greater than 95 percent for isolated lesions to less that 10 percent in those with associated congenital malformations or hydrops; the dismal outcome of hydropic babies has spurned some to attempt to intervene through fetal surgery.

Anatomy and physiology

Pulmonary development has four stages. During the embryonic stage (weeks 0 to 7), the laryngotracheal groove deepens and separates the lung bud from the primitive foregut, forming the tracheobronchial tree; in the pseudoglandular phase (weeks 8 to 16), the more distal airways develop. Errors in lung bud migration during these first two phases are from aberrant mesodermal and endodermal embryogenesis and lead to bronchogenic cysts, sequestrations, CCAMs, and foregut duplications. The timing of developmental mishaps can affect outcome not only by more significantly limiting parenchymal development but also by altering location. For example, a BC that develops early is more central, occurring during formation of the proximal tree; those developing later occur more peripherally. The last two stages of lung development involve growth and development of the alveoli and their supporting vessels. During the canalicular phase (17 to 24 weeks), there is rapid growth of terminal airways and development of alveoli; the terminal air sac stage (25 weeks to term) is for alveolar expansion and maturation. At this point, space-occupying lesions in the chest limit the space into which the ipsilateral lung can expand and cause mediastinal shift, similarly affecting contralateral lung development to varying degrees. Respiratory distress of the newborn is the most urgent clinical scenario and occurs because of airway obstruction from extrinsic mass effect, mediastinal shift, pulmonary hypoplasia, or compression of functional lung. Antenatal sonographic evidence of a thoracic lesion is probably the most common "presentation" in those with prenatal care. Such care affords the opportunity to screen for associated conditions, especially cardiac and chromosomal anomalies that may significantly alter the prognosis for the fetus and expectations of the parents. In older patients, recurrent pulmonary infections, hemoptysis, or dysphagia from adjacent masses are the usual symptoms. With the current prevalence of axial imaging performed readily for many clinical complaints, anomalies are also found incidentally.

The most important imaging study is a chest roentgenogram or an ultrasound (US) that demonstrates the space-occupying lesion, the degree of mediastinal shift, and residual lung. US, computed tomography (CT), and magnetic resonance imaging (MRI) very precisely define the pulmonary and vascular anatomy of the lesion; however, often surgical resection is required regardless of the diagnosis. The timing of resection is determined by the patient's respiratory course; therefore plain radiography may be sufficient. Many anatomic considerations are most accurately and effectively addressed during surgery. Additional invasive and costly imaging should be reserved for those patients in whom the results may obviate operation, alter the timing of operation, or without which safety would be compromised. In addition, many infants require general anesthesia to undergo examination in confining scanners and the complications of assisted ventilation with pulmonary anomalies can be detrimental. The choice of imaging modalities is largely dependent on personal preferences, availability, and the experience of radiologists and surgeons evaluating the studies.

BRONCHOGENIC CYST

Pathophysiology

BCs occur with equal frequency between the sexes and account for 25 percent of congenital pulmonary anomalies.[2] Associated syndromes and chromosomal abnormalities are not reported with BCs, and other defects are unusual. BCs are comprised of nonfunctional pulmonary tissue that stems from abnormal airway buds. They have different characteristics depending on the timing of their appearance with respect to fetal development and can be found in many locations. BCs are usually single, unilateral, and found in the lower lobes; occasionally, bilateral and multiple cysts have been reported. Mediastinal cysts near the trachea, carina, and esophagus are considered most common by some, but others state up to 70 percent of cysts are parenchymal.[3,4] Other locations include the airway wall, chest wall, pericardium, pancreas, adrenal gland,

and tongue. Those that occur before the division of the foregut and bronchopulmonary systems may be densely adherent or, rarely, may communicate with the esophagus. If a cyst develops during the pseudoglandular stage, when proximal airways are being formed, it is usually located near central airways or parenchyma; if a cyst forms during the canalicular (developing alveoli) phase, it is situated peripherally. The cyst wall is composed of both smooth muscle and cartilage and is lined with mucous glands in addition to ciliated columnar or cuboidal cells. Mucoid material can accumulate within the cyst and is often responsible for considerable growth, which usually occurs gradually. Most cysts are between 1 and 10 cm in size and have fibrous connections with surrounding tissues. Extrathoracic cysts do not communicate with adjacent tracheobronchial structures; rarely, however, peripheral lung lesions will communicate with the airway.[5]

Clinical presentation

Infection is the most common presentation for BCs and is noted in up to half of symptomatic patients. Cough, wheezing, fever, or hemoptysis often prompt chest roentgenography, which may demonstrate a mass or cyst. Symptoms related to mass effect such as dysphagia, airway obstruction, or a palpable neck mass account for most of the remaining symptoms. Hemoptysis is unusual but reported. In addition, some BCs are detected with antenatal US or as an incidental mediastinal mass seen on chest roentengraphy for upper respiratory infections. The majority of patients (two-thirds) manifest subacute symptoms and present early in childhood, while those with incidentally noted lesions are typically older children or even adults when the cyst is discovered. The most urgent presentation involves airway obstruction due to extrinsic compression of a major airway; this can lead to hypoventilation, or it can cause hyperinflation, mediastinal shift, decreased venous return, and cardiopulmonary collapse. The airway lumen can also be obstructed by an enlarging cyst within the airway wall, which is an unusual presentation but may mimic a foreign body. Rapid enlargement due to mucus production, hemorrhage, or inflammation can acutely obstruct the airway, so that bronchoscopy may be the only useful diagnostic and therapeutic modality, since a predominant mass visible on radiologic imaging is lacking. Patients with multiple peripheral cysts usually present in the perinatal period due to impaired respiration from displacement of normal lung. If there is an element of peripheral airway obstruction, postobstructive infections or lobar hyperinflation may develop.

Diagnostic modalities

BCs are seen primarily on plain chest roentgenography, CT scans, or US. They can be seen on the chest roentgenogram as an opacified or lucent mass or a cyst with an air-fluid level; or they may simply be suggested by postobstructive emphysematous changes (Fig. 7-1). CT is used to eliminate any nonsurgical diagnoses (abscesses, pneumonias, or lymphatic malformations), localize the mass, and determine the best exposure for resection. On CT, BCs appear cystic with a nonenhancing wall, and air-fluid levels may be present (Fig. 7-2). Differentiating between a BC and a pulmonary abscess can be difficult radiologically, but BCs are more commonly associated with an indolent clinical course, persistent radiographic findings, and limited response to antibiotic treatment. In addition, BCs can occur in association with pulmonary abscess, but prolonged symptoms

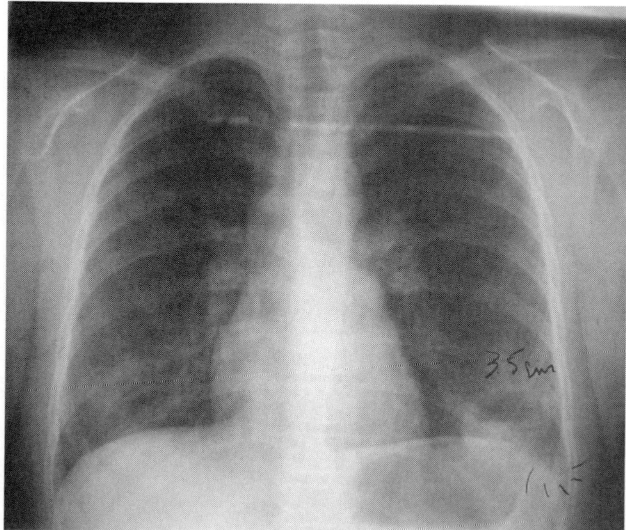

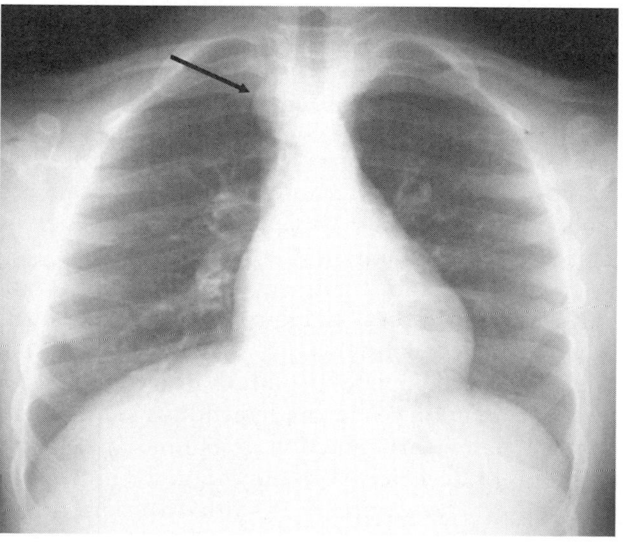

Figure 7-1 Plain chest films of bronchogenic cysts. **A.** The cyst as a left-lower-lobe air-fluid level. **B.** A mass adjacent to the mediastinum on the right.

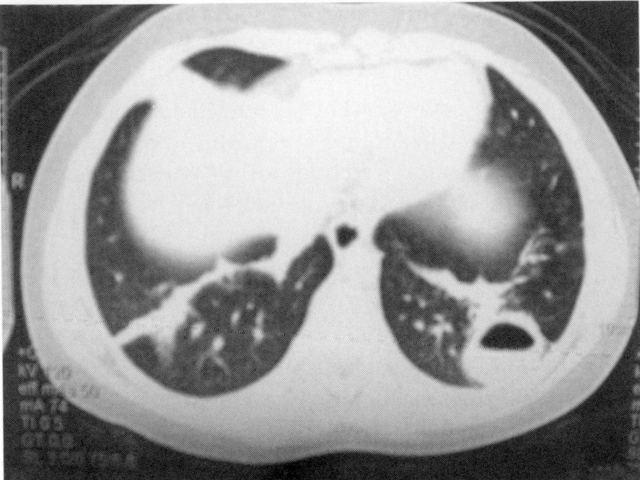

Figure 7-2 Corresponding CT to Fig. 7-1A showing the left-lower-lobe cyst with an air-fluid level.

of systemic infection probably warrant resectional therapy regardless of etiology. Patients with postobstructive or segmental emphysematous changes on chest radiography may require bronchoscopy to rule out an airway foreign body (especially in the age group in which aspiration is common) or extrinsic airway compression. Compression of the esophagus can be seen in patients who present with dysphagia and undergo esophagography. Once compression is identified on one of the above studies, CT scan, other axial imaging, or US should be performed to identify the mass responsible and define its anatomy (Figs. 7-3 and 7-4). Since BCs rarely communicate with the gastrointestinal tract and this can be easily addressed at operation, esophageal contrast studies to rule out gastrointestinal communication are unnecessary.

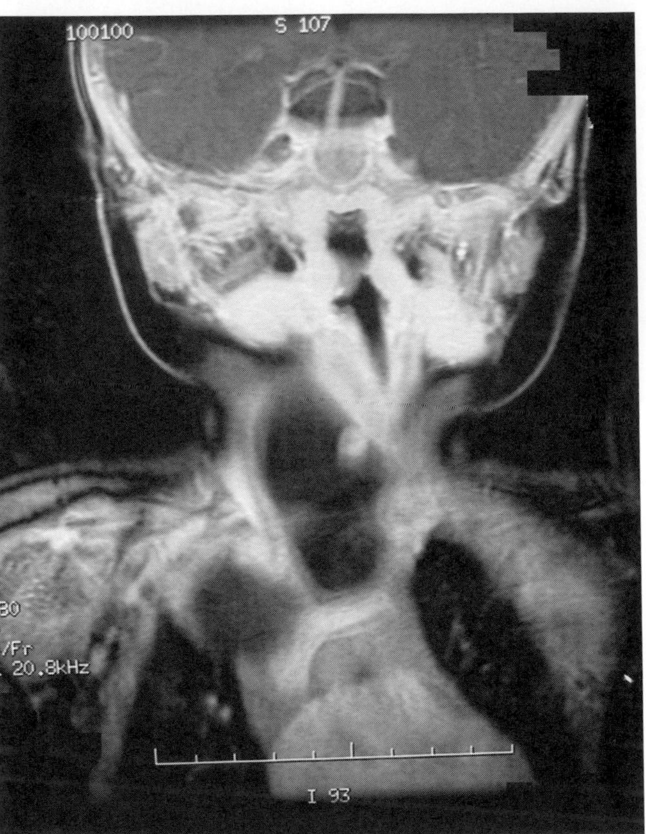

Figure 7-3 MRI coronal section of a large bronchogenic cyst involving the right neck and apical chest cavity. This mass presented as a palpable neck mass and displaced the trachea. The small, solid 1-cm lesion within the neck portion of the cyst represents a cartilaginous remnant densely adherent to the trachea. Note the displacement of neck structures.

Treatment

Complete surgical excision is the treatment of choice for BCs. Usually, this is accomplished via simple enucleation performed with thoracotomy, thoracoscopy, neck exploration, or median sternotomy; however, segmental pulmonary resection may be necessary if the lesion is intraparenchymal. Children who present with infection should first undergo treatment with antibiotics to decrease inflammation and improve pulmonary toilet preoperatively. Obviously, postobstructive phenomena may not permit complete resolution of infections and require intervention when the infection is still present and when pulmonary function is optimized. Airway obstruction or deviation is an indication for urgent or, rarely, emergent resection. Those with dysphagia, mass-related symptoms, or incidental findings should have resection performed electively. Comorbidities that increase anesthetic risk should be resolved preoperatively unless airway obstruction is severe, but resection

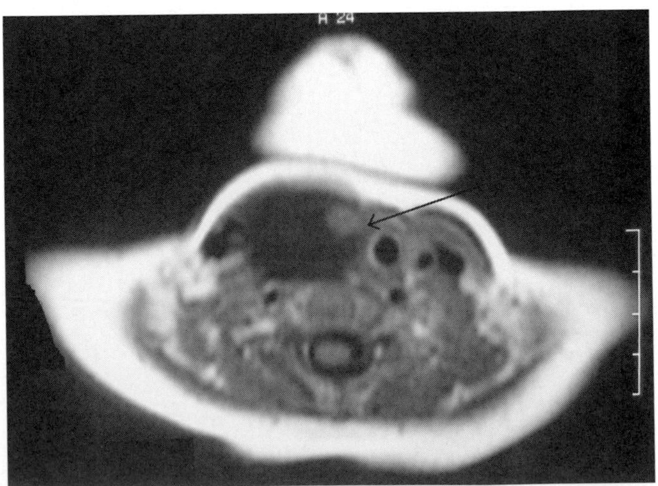

Figure 7-4 Axial section of the MRI in Fig. 7-3, demonstrating the size of the cyst in the upper thoracic cavity. Again, the cartilaginous remnant can be seen (arrow).

should not be delayed more than a few months, as malignancy in preexisting BCs has been reported as early as age 8.[6] Prenatally diagnosed BCs should be followed by sequential US, but as the cysts do not routinely enlarge rapidly in utero, monitoring is not as frequent as with CCAMs. If a large cyst does cause in utero compromise from mediastinal shift or hydrops, decompression can be performed in utero with cyst aspiration or thoracoamniotic shunt placement.[7] Cysts are generally treated after delivery and confirmation of the diagnosis, since other cystic malformations of the newborn appear similar on prenatal US but may require different treatment.

Congenital lung and chest anomalies can occur in association with one another; therefore a surgeon should anticipate rare but possible vascular abnormalities in pulmonary blood supply that may be encountered during resection of BCs. Cysts commonly have fibrous adhesions to important mediastinal structures such as the esophagus or trachea, and the cyst's mass may displace structures, especially nerves, to nonanatomic positions. So as to avoid injury, careful identification to preserve these structures and dissection close to the cyst wall are required (Fig. 7-5). Usually, the maintenance of fluid in the cyst helps to define its borders; however, sometimes, after considerable dissection, depending on the position of the cyst, decompression may be required for exposure or extraction. Areas where the cyst is invested in vital surrounding structures may require fulguration of the small amount of cystic epithelium left behind. Infected cysts are even more adherent and often surrounded by reactive vascular tissue, making anatomic planes difficult to identify and dissect. To decrease this inflammatory reaction and improve pulmonary function, patients with signs of infection should be treated with antibiotics for a few weeks before surgery. A large pulmonary abscess that persists on antibiotic treatment should be percutaneously drained prior to surgery; a small abscess can be debrided or removed with resection of the BC. If infection cannot be cleared, one must proceed with surgery; but this may result in the resection of additional surrounding tissue. Cysts rarely communicate with the gastrointestinal tract or airway; however, during dissection of a cyst near luminal structures, one should make sure that there is no connection and that, if there is luminal communication, it has been divided and the lumen securely closed without narrowing. As mentioned before, a proximal endobronchial lesion that rapidly expands can cause acute airway obstruction and a surgical airway emergency. In this case, emergent rigid bronchoscopy is required to secure the airway and assess whether the lesion is amenable to endoscopic or open sleeve resection of the airway. Small lesions in the proximal airway of a relatively large patient can be resected endoscopically if one can maintain the airway wall's integrity after resection. Residual cyst wall that does not obstruct the airway can be fulgurated with a laser. More distal lesions in smaller airways may require segmental resection of the airway and associated parenchyma. Smaller endobronchial lesions that do not totally occlude the airway do not need emergent intervention, but action should be taken promptly. These lesions may cause intermittent obstruction through a ball-valve effect and allow inspiration but diminish exhalation, resulting in hyperinflation. This, in turn, can lead to mediastinal shift, decreased contralateral ventilation, and decreased venous return. In addition, the trachea may become deviated, making intubation challenging; one should be prepared to use flexible or rigid bronchoscopy to establish an airway at the time of anesthetic induction. Positive-pressure ventilation exacerbates mediastinal shift and should be avoided, as this may have hemodynamic consequences. Positive pressure ventilation should be avoided; it may worsen hyperinflation, mediastinal shift, and respiratory mechanics. Temporarily, mainstem intubation of the contralateral bronchus may be used to ventilate one lung until the obstructing lesion can be removed.

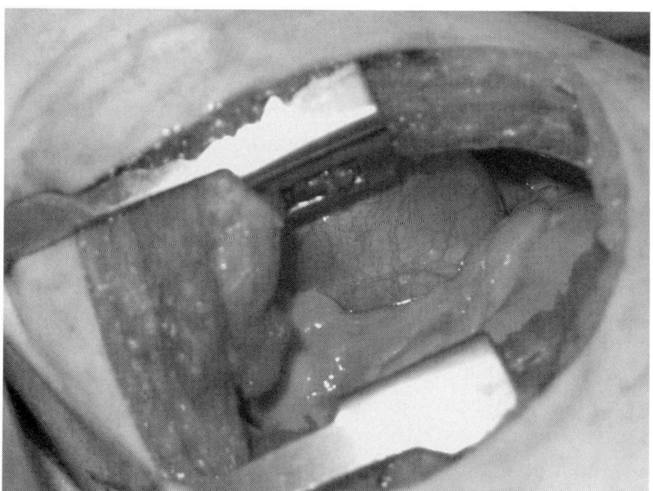

Figure 7-5 Operative photograph through a right-sided thoracotomy showing the bronchogenic cyst depicted in Figs. 7-3 and 7-4. Normal lung can be seen displaced inferiorly, with the large apical cyst seen adjacent to but not involving the lung. After dissection in the chest up to and including the thoracic inlet, the mass was still fixed and a counterincision was necessary in the neck, through which additional dissection was performed. The cyst was then decompressed and pulled out into the neck incision. The point of maximal adhesion was between the cartilaginous remnant and the tracheal wall.

Although not all agree, most pediatric surgeons feel that asymptomatic children should undergo resection of BCs in the absence of prohibitive medical conditions. Malignancy is rare, but since most lesions are resected, the true incidence of malignant degeneration is hard to quantify. Childhood adenocarcinoma and rhabdomyosarcoma have been reported within BCs. A well-differentiated papillary adenocarcinoma was found in a 55-year-old woman explored for abdominal pain who had a retroperitoneal BC.[8–10] Therefore, even in asymptomatic adults, BCs that have been present since birth have had many years of malignant potential and should be resected promptly. The expected longevity, comorbid illnesses, and ability to perform resection through less invasive maneuvers such as bronchoscopy or thoracoscopy factor into the decision whether to undertake resection. Older adults with small, stable, asymptomatic cysts not prone to connection with the tracheobronchial tree or infection may warrant conservative treatment,[11] but malignancy must be excluded via percutaneous or transbronchial cyst fluid and/or cyst wall biopsy. Malignancy, infection, recurrence after aspiration, or an intraparenchymal lesion should prompt complete surgical resection. An additional, practical reason for the removal of asymptomatic BCs is that cysts tend to increase in size due to mucus production and ultimately become symptomatic or inflamed, making subsequent resection more difficult and prone to complications.

Outcomes

The survival after BC resection is essentially 100 percent, as associated conditions are rare. Morbidity includes wound infections, lymphatic leak, and nerve injury and is similar to complications for other procedures in the thoracic or neck region. Inflammation of the cyst can make dissection more difficult and may slightly increase these risks in the hands of an inexperienced operator. Recurrence is also rare unless complete excision of the cyst was not performed; this underscores the importance of total removal and/or fulguration of any remaining mucosa so as to prevent regrowth.

PULMONARY SEQUESTRATION

Pulmonary sequestration (PS) accounts for 30 percent of bronchopulmonary-foregut malformations[4] and was first described by Pryce in 1946. Gender predilection may favor males 1.5:1, but there is no strong preference and evidence of specific genetic etiology is lacking, although male siblings with sequestrations have been reported.[12]

Pathophysiology

Sequestrations represent nonfunctional embryonic lung and lack normal continuity with the tracheobronchial tree. In addition, their blood supply is largely systemic. PS may arise from accessory lung buds that develop dependent on systemic vessels or may be created by systemic blood vessels dragging embryonic lung away from the primary tracheobronchial tree. Arterial supply to the sequestration most often arises from below the diaphragm as a branch of the abdominal aorta, and

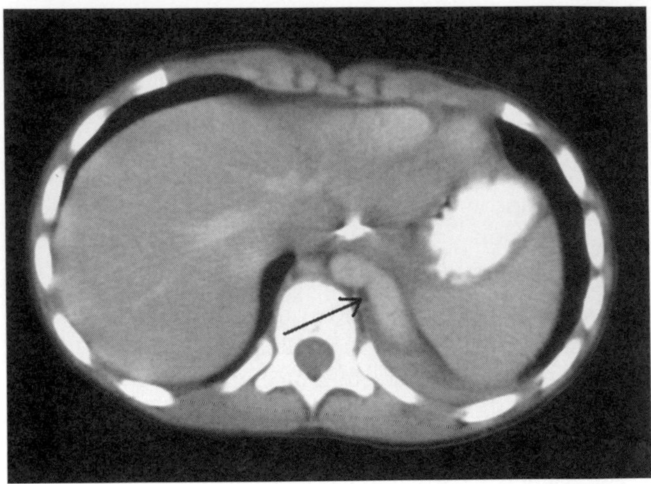

Figure 7-6 Computed tomography of pulmonary sequestration on the left side, demonstrating the infradiaphragmatic aortic blood supply to the mass, which continues into the left thoracic cavity (arrow).

sequestrations can be seen in a subdiaphragmatic location (Fig. 7-6). As foregut and bronchopulmonary development occur closely in time and space, PS are frequently associated with other congenital lung or gastrointestinal malformations, and sequestrations have been seen in conjunction with CCAM, tracheoesophageal fistulas, esophageal cysts, and BCs. It has even been proposed that sequestrations may be variants of CCAMs or BCs that develop an aberrant blood supply.

Sequestrations usually occur in the lower lobes and are unilobar, but they can involve the entire lung[13] or, rarely, both lungs. The distinction between intralobar and extralobar types of sequestration is important not only because the anatomy differs but also because differences in development can be related to their anatomic and clinical differences. If a sequestration develops before the visceral pleura have been completely formed, it will be situated within the normal lung parenchyma and is intralobar; extralobar sequestrations develop after pleural formation of the normal lung is complete. Consequently, extralobar sequestrations are enveloped by their own pleura. Some studies report a 2:1 preponderance of extralobar sequestrations and others a 3:1 ratio in favor of the intralobar kind.

Intralobar sequestrations are most commonly found (80 percent) in the lower lobes, and 70 percent are found on the left side; therefore the left lower posterior and basilar segments are the most common locations.[14,15] Unlike in their counterpart extralobar sequestrations, they rarely include associated anomalies, and communication with the gastrointestinal tract is unusual. Intralobar sequestrations have no pleural covering and are found within the parenchyma of normal lung; they may have abnormal communications with airway structures or surrounding alveoli and therefore some degree of aeration.[16] The majority of intralobar sequestrations (85 percent) derive their blood supply from the abdominal aorta as the vessel courses through the inferior pulmonary ligament into the chest to supply the intraparenchymal sequestration. The thoracic aorta, brachiocephalic artery, and coronary arteries have also been documented as rare sources of systemic arterial supply[14]; in about 15 percent of cases, there are multiple arteries to the mass. The inferior pulmonary veins provide venous drainage for left-sided intralobar sequestrations; right-sided ones drain via the vena cava. This anomalous right-sided vein can create a lucency on plain radiography that looks like the curved sharp-edged blade of a scimitar bordering the right heart; it is known as the "scimitar sign."

Extralobar sequestrations are more often seen in boys (3:1), and associated congenital anomalies occur in up to half the patients. Concomitant congenital anomalies include structural cardiac disease, pectus excavatum, pericardial defects, cervical vertebral anomalies, pulmonary vascular hypoplasia, arteriovenous malformations, intestinal duplications (terminal ileal or colonic), esophageal diverticula, and diaphragmatic hernia. Congenital diaphragmatic hernia or eventration is present in 30 percent of infants with extralobar sequestrations. These, which are reported to represent between 25 and 60 percent of sequestrations, also occur mostly in the lower lobes and predominantly on the left side (75 to 90 percent). They are located largely between the left lower lobe and the diaphragm and can even be found intraabdominally near the adrenal gland. The arterial supply is from the abdominal aorta, venous drainage is via the azygos or hemiazygos vein, and extralobar sequestrations are covered by their own pleural membrane. Extralobar sequestrations are not connected to the tracheobronchial tree; they therefore do not usually become infected, are not aerated, and are often asymptomatic. In addition, diagnosis of intraabdominal sequestrations may be difficult due to lack of contrast in comparison to other solid intraabdominal organs. Often the discovery of extralobar sequestrations in early infancy results from tests and operations for associated conditions.

Clinical presentation

Most commonly, children present with chronic cough or recurrent pneumonia at several years of age. Pulmonary abscess can occur and can cause massive hemoptysis or hemothorax due to the erosion of vessels under systemic arterial pressure; fatality has been reported. Diagnosis and presentation of sequestrations antenatally or in the newborn period is unusual because sequestrations are not cystic, there is no aeration to differentiate them from normal lung patterns, and respiratory distress is uncommon. There are, however, some situations in which sequestrations are discovered in this young age group. Workup of associated anomalies can reveal extralobar sequestrations and is responsible for the incidental discovery of about 15 percent of sequestrations. Infants can present with respiratory distress, but this is unusual unless there is entire lung involvement, significant displacement of functional lung, or lung hypoplasia from in utero mass effect. Rarely, a large sequestration will produce a mediastinal shift with hemodynamic consequences or a sequestration's aberrant vascular supply will cause shunting and congestive failure. Sequestrations communicate with the gastrointestinal tract in about 10 percent of cases, and these present during infancy due to infection. Forty-three percent of these sequestrations were evident in 7 days, 30 percent within the remaining year, 17 percent by age 18, and 10 percent in adulthood.[17]

Diagnostic modalities

The diagnostic workup should begin with a plain chest roentgenogram to look for consolidation (since extralobar sequestrations are not aerated), mass effect, or evidence of lung abscess. Documentation of the aberrant infradiaphragmatic blood supply using US confirms the sequestration (Fig. 7-7); ancillary tests such as CT, MRI, or aortography are not necessary if plain film and US clearly demonstrate a thoracic mass with an infradiaphragmatic aortic blood supply. US is excellent in the hands of a qualified operator, does not require the same degree of stillness as MRI or CT (which may require general anesthesia in a child), and does not require the administration of contrast. Complex tests should be used only if additional information is needed to

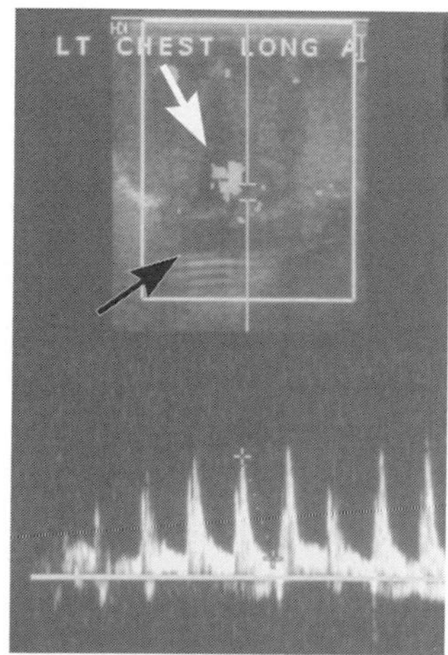

Figure 7-7 Ultrasound showing a sagittal section of the thoracoabdominal region with the aorta (black arrow) as well as the aberrant systemic blood supply originating from the aorta and leading to the sequestration (white arrow). Below is shown the waveform of the vessel proving it to be arterial.

evaluate unusual vasculature, concomitant airway or congenital chest anomalies, or to resolve anatomic questions that cannot be effectively evaluated and treated in the operating room.

Treatment

The treatment for PS is resection. For intralobar sequestration, this requires resection of the segment or lobe involved. Sequestrations that involve the entire lung mandate pneumonectomy. Adhesions from previous infection may make dissection difficult and require resection of additional normal lung to safely remove the sequestration. Any communication between the intralobar sequestration and the tracheobronchial tree is effectively obliterated with staples or sutures to avoid postoperative air leak. Early in the operation, the arterial blood supply should be addressed as it courses through the inferior pulmonary ligament from the abdominal aorta or as it comes directly off of the thoracic aorta. Additional blood supply via hypoplastic or friable pulmonary vessels can also be present and must be ligated, as blood loss from these tributaries can be substantial. Extralobar sequestrations can be intraabdominal, so their absence just above the diaphragm may require exploration of the abdomen.

Communication with the gastrointestinal tract is more common with extralobar sequestrations, although there have been reports involving intralobar sequestrations. When communication occurs, 70 percent is to the lower esophagus and 15 percent is with the stomach, with the middle and upper esophagus representing a few percent of occurrences. In a study of 57 patients with gastrointestinal involvement and extralobar sequestration, 75 percent occurred on the right side and half of these involved the entire right lung; 7 percent were bilateral, some of which included structural esophageal abnormalities; and 25 percent had a dual blood supply with hypoplastic pulmonary arterial supply in addition to systemic aortic supply. In cases where lobar or segmental airways connected to the esophagus, the corresponding airway was absent in conjunction with the tracheobronchial tree.[17] The sequestrations described above, referred to as communicating bronchopulmonary foregut malformations (CBPFMs), were then anatomically classified into four groups.[17] Sequestrations (16 percent) found in conjunction with tracheoesophageal fistula (proximal atresia and distal fistula) were classified as IA. Here, the right main bronchus of a hypoplastic right lung inserts into the esophagus and must be reimplanted into the trachea; although a pulmonary artery and vein are present, there can be accessory systemic blood supply. Type IB cases have the dominant airway of a lobe or segment connected to the esophagus, and this airway is reimplanted into the tracheobronchial tree if technically feasible; resection is performed otherwise. Type II sequestrations represented 33 percent of CBPMFs in the series and have a right main bronchus leading to the esophagus without associated atresia. This bronchus should be reimplanted into the trachea. The pulmonary vasculature is normoanatomic but may be hypoplastic. The most commonly seen CBPFMs (46 percent) are type III sequestrations, in which lobar or segmental airways communicate with a normal esophagus; these are treated with resection. They have the systemic arterial supply typical of sequestrations and may also have an atretic pulmonary blood supply as well as venous drainage via pulmonary, azygos, or portal routes. Type 4 sequestrations (5 percent) are intralobar sequestrations with tracheobronchial connection to the esophagus and should be resected.

Adults who have sequestrations should undergo resection unless there is prohibitive risk from medical comorbidities or their projected survival will not be enhanced. Although conservative management of asymptomatic sequestrations has been discussed in the literature,[18] this was based on the assumption that their clinical behavior would mirror diminution on imaging. There is no evidence for this. All symptomatic lesions should be addressed. Asymptomatic intralobar sequestrations and extralobar sequestrations with gastrointestinal communication carry significant risk of infection and hemorrhage; asymptomatic extralobar sequestrations without connection to the gastrointestinal or tracheobronchial tree pose the potential risk of malignancy.

Outcomes

The outcomes for children with isolated PS are generally excellent. The major morbidity comes from associated pulmonary hypoplasia, as in those patients with concomitant diaphragmatic hernia or congenital cardiac anomalies. In the 15 percent of sequestrations with associated conditions, mortality is 75 percent.[19] However, survival after surgical resection of isolated defects has reached almost 100 percent, even if pneumonectomy is required. Complications occur infrequently and are treatable. Improvements in imaging and understanding of the vascular abnormalities associated with sequestrations make exsanguination from an aberrant artery preventable. The main complications are postoperative pulmonary infection or leak from a gastrointestinal communication. Reflux is also frequently reported in patients who had sequestrations connected at the gastroesophageal junction.

CONGENITAL LOBAR EMPHYSEMA

Congenital lobar emphysema (CLE) is a rare problem that is more prevalent in male infants, with a 3:1 preponderance. It involves hyperinflated histologically normal lung and most frequently occurs in the left upper lobe. Lobes are involved in the following distribution: left upper lobe, 40 percent; right middle lobe, 35 percent; right upper lobe, 20 percent; and bilateral disease, 1 percent.[20] Although a single upper lobe is the most usual site, multiple lobes can be involved. Associated cardiac, renal, and rib abnormalities are present in 20 percent of cases.

Pathophysiology

CLE is caused when the airway collapses on expiration and air is trapped, leading to hyperinflation after stacking of breaths. If the airway also collapses on inspiration, air can still enter the emphysematous segment through pores of Kohn with the adjacent lung and continue to inflate. Over time, large emphysematous air sacs are created by destruction of the septa from the continuous hyperinflation. The reason for airway collapse is most often hypoplasia of airway cartilage; although only documented in 35 percent of cases, it may be present in up to 70 percent. The precise cause of hyperinflation may remain unidentified in up to 50 percent of cases. Any intrinsic or extrinsic cause for airway narrowing can lead to CLE. Intrinsic causes are more often present in infancy and include not only hypoplastic cartilage but also airway torsion, congenital narrowing, excess bronchial mucosa, endobronchial lesions, mucous plugging, and foreign bodies. Extrinsic causes include compression from masses, enlarged cardiac chambers (15 percent), lymphadenopathy, and vascular rings. Extrinsic causes and foreign bodies are an important part of the differential for children after the newborn period. Physiologically, symptoms occur when CLE causes displacement of normal lung, creating mediastinal shift and decreasing venous return. Additionally, normal lung is compressed and impaired by the overexpanded segment. Alveolar fibrosis, alveolar septal destruction, and polyalveolar lobes can also cause congenital lobar hyperinflation. Polyalveolar lobes have an increased number of alveoli, which accumulate air. This anomaly may account for up to 30 percent of congenital hyperinflation syndromes.[21]

Clinical presentation

The characteristics of presentation are governed not only by the degree of hyperinflation but also by the time over which it occurs. With gradual displacement of normal lung and mediastinal shift, compensation can occur, but the physiologic effect is profound with severe and rapid changes. The presentation of CLE can be striking if a sudden increase in hyperinflation acutely causes mediastinal shift and cardiopulmonary collapse. This sort of presentation is characteristic of CLE caused by intrinsic airway obstruction or collapse secondary to cartilage hypoplasia. With extrinsic causes of airway collapse and parenchymal anomalies (i.e., polyalveolar lobes, septal destruction), increases in hyperinflation tend to be gradual and compensated until severe. Crying spells can considerably and rapidly exacerbate hyperinflation and precipitate distress. Infants commonly present at 1 to 2 months of age after respiratory distress has prompted examination and radiographic study. The degree of distress ranges from tachypnea with feeding, to baseline tachypnea, to cyanosis. Perinatal presentation is less common but can occur if the CLE is large or if the infant is undergoing radiographic examination for concomitant anomalies and the segmental hyperinflation is noted. Babies with symptoms noted in the newborn period are more likely to have significant and progressive problems and require resection early on. Half of the infants who have resection of their CLE have been diagnosed at several days of age, with the remaining half not being diagnosed for months. The latter group usually has an insidious presentation, since there is a period during which the airway has not yet reached a critically small size; it may therefore take several months for air trapping to occur. Similarly, for the parenchymal causes of CLE to result in a significant accumulation of air and hyperinflation, some time may be required. This sort of disease may manifest itself as mild tachypnea, failure to thrive, isolated expiratory wheezing, hyperresonance, tracheal deviation, or shifted maximal cardiac impulse point on physical exam.

Diagnostic modalities

Plain chest radiography is the most useful and perhaps only necessary study to diagnose CLE. In utero diagnosis is unusual, as the lungs are not aerated and the discovery is made on radiographic imaging when the infant has symptoms of tachypnea and respiratory distress. Sometimes the diagnosis is made incidentally because of fever or during imaging associated with other medical issues. The characteristic appearance of the chest radiograph includes a hyperlucent area with surrounding atelectasis, ipsilateral diaphragmatic flattening, and possibly mediastinal and tracheal deviation away from the hyperinflated side (Fig. 7-8). Although secondary studies are rarely necessary to diagnose CLE, CT scanning may be helpful in elucidating the exact type of lesion (Fig. 7-9). In addition, CT imaging can sometimes identify the cause of the airway obstruction causing the CLE (i.e., an endobronchial lesion or extrinsic compression). In older children in whom foreign bodies are common or in whom extrinsic causes are more prevalent, MRI or CT should be employed to investigate the causes of airway obstruction, such as a thoracic mass or vascular ring. If there is suspicion of an endobronchial lesion or foreign body, bronchoscopy should be performed. Pulmonary function tests would show slightly decreased flow but are unnecessary. Since hyperinflation can occur only postnatally, all but the segment involved with CLE has developed normally without any in utero compression and there is no lung hypoplasia. Ventilation/perfusion

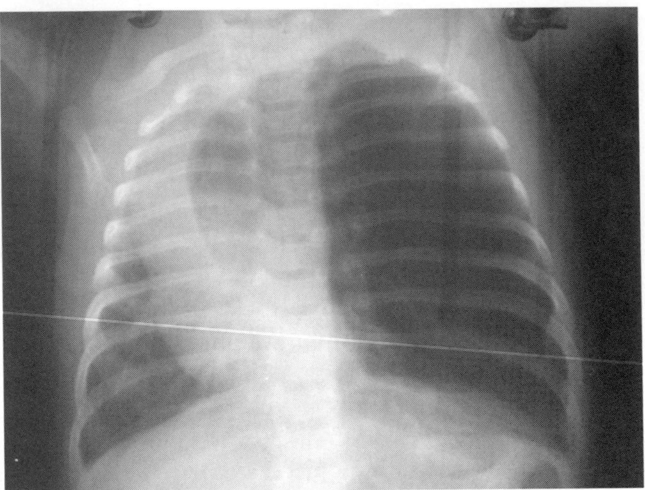

Figure 7-8 Plain chest film of a large left-sided CLE with significant mediastinal shift.

(V/Q) scanning is also unnecessary; it would demonstrate delayed uptake and washout of xenon with decreased flow in the emphysematous area and can occasionally identify some additional small areas of hyperinflation; however, these will otherwise be evident and can be resected at thoracotomy. Echocardiography and renal US should be performed to identify any associated cardiac conditions and renal anomalies, respectively, which will be noted in 20 percent of patients.

Treatment

The treatment for CLE is total resection of the hyperinflated lung. It is curative and should be performed promptly. One must also be sure to investigate and eliminate extrinsic and intrinsic causes of airway obstruction leading to hyperinflation that can masquerade as CLE. If treating these issues leads to resolution of hyperinflation, the diagnosis is not primary CLE and lobectomy can be avoided. Up to half of the cases of CLE have no definite determined etiology; of the remainder, most have hypoplastic cartilage. Therefore, salvage of the lobe is very rarely possible. Occasionally, endobronchial lesions causing a ball-valve effect are amenable to endoscopic removal. However, the narrow caliber of the airway can make this difficult and can require resection of the associated parenchyma if the resulting lumen is not of sufficient caliber or if the airway wall is compromised and collapses. Masses or vascular rings are very rare, but such causes of extrinsic compression can be surgically treated, leading to a normal airway.

Infants with increasing hyperinflation or significant symptoms should remain under medical supervision until expedient surgical resection is performed. Evaluation of potential associated cardiac disease should be performed if respiratory distress is not severe. Supplemental oxygen should be used to treat mild tachypnea and distress and babies should be kept calm, since crying can substantially exacerbate the hyperinflation. Some feel that the presence of mediastinal shift mandates medical observation until resection is done, regardless of the symptomatology. CLE that is diagnosed after a long period of stability without significant symptoms or change in shift is unlikely to decompensate suddenly, and these patients can remain at home for the few weeks it may take to arrange elective surgery. Symptoms, inadequate access to medical care, or unpredictable compliance are indications for admission and prompt excision. The most dramatic presentation of CLE is that of cardiorespiratory collapse from acute mediastinal shift and decreased venous return. In this situation, oxygen should be administered and the baby kept calm. Efforts should be made to avoid intubation and positive-pressure ventilation, since this may worsen hyperinflation and precipitate the need for emergency thoracotomy. If the patient cannot be maintained without intubation, there are several caveats. Intubation may be made more

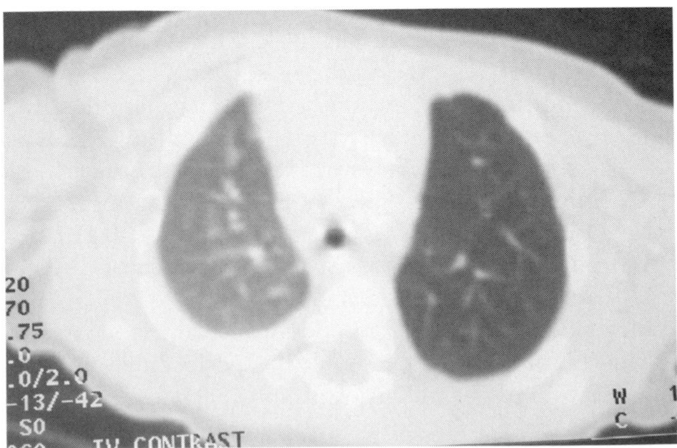

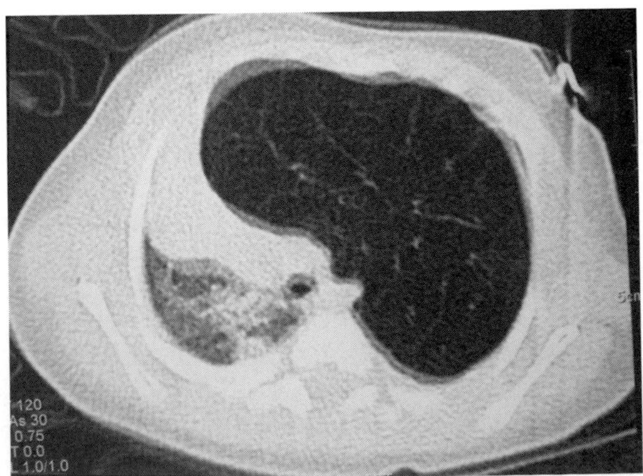

Figure 7-9 Computed tomography of CLE showing hyperexpansion but no mediastinal shift **(A)** or severe mediastinal shift **(B)**.

difficult by tracheal deviation away from the side of the hyperinflation. Efforts should be made to minimize the positive pressure applied. High-frequency or jet ventilation can be useful to ventilate with decreased pressure if spontaneous ventilation is not sufficient. Right mainstem intubation, if the lobar emphysema occurs on the left, may allow selective ventilation of the normal lung and decrease hyperinflation and mediastinal shift. Selective intubation of the left mainstem is difficult due to mediastinal shift and the orientation of the airway. If cardiac output is severely impaired, decompression of the emphysematous lobe via needle can reduce mediastinal shift and hopefully improve cardiovascular function. A large air leak will ensue, however, and jet or high-frequency ventilation may be required to optimize ventilation. By varying the column of water in the thoracostomy collection chamber, one can control the amount of leak. The greater the column of water against which the air leak passively drains, the higher the inspiratory pressure can get before the leak develops and the capacity to distend normal lung is lost. These same emergency considerations apply to elective resections for CLE. With intubation and positive pressure, immediate thoracotomy may become necessary. Therefore the surgical team should be ready to perform emergent thoracotomy before induction of anesthesia. Fiberoptic equipment should be available, since tracheal deviation may be significant. The patient should be anesthetized but left spontaneously breathing, and when positive pressure becomes necessary, low ventilatory pressures should be used, even if one has to tolerate slightly suboptimal parameters, until the lobe is delivered from the chest. Mainstem intubation, if tolerated, may help to reduce hyperinflation of the affected side, but the key is rapid mobilization of the lobe out of the chest so that normal lung can be ventilated and the mediastinum can return to a normal position (Figs. 7-10 and 7-11). Vessels are in normal anatomic orientation but may be friable. To prevent recurrence, resection of the entire involved lobe and any adjacent hyperinflated tissue is essential. Although small residual amounts of hyperinflation may appear insignificant in comparison to the dominant lobe, these areas can become hyperinflated and physiologically significant. Remaining lobes should be positioned to prevent torsion; the right middle lobe is most prone to this, so it should be sutured to adjacent tissues. In addition, release of the inferior pulmonary ligament may allow the lower lobe to more easily occupy the hemithorax. Adults with asymptomatic CLE should not need resection as long as there is no significant mediastinal shift. There is no known risk of malignancy and infectious complications are rare.

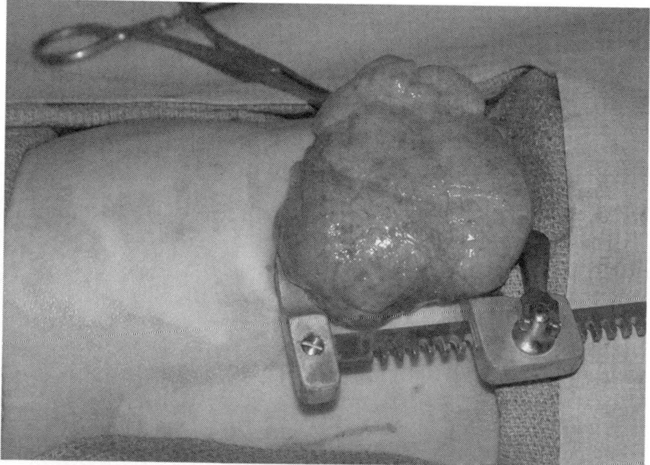

Figure 7-10 Delivery of the emphysematous lobe from the chest to improve respiratory mechanics is the first step in the operation for CLE.

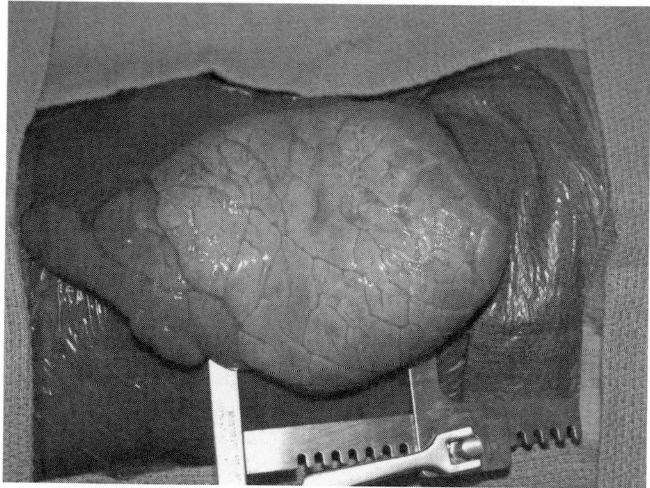

Figure 7-11 Operative photo showing the emphysematous lobe and surrounding normal lung.

Outcomes

Survival for babies with CLE approaches 100 percent even in those who undergo emergent thoracotomy. Associated anomalies of the heart or kidneys are responsible for major morbidity and mortality. In 5 to 10 percent of patients, minor complications such as pneumonia, reintubation, or wound complications occur. The surrounding atelectatic lung expands to fill the hemithorax after resection of CLE, and children continue to increase the size and number of their alveoli substantially until age 4; lung growth does not cease until age 8. Pulmonary function tests obtained years after resection demonstrate equal lung volumes on both sides. At least 90 percent of these patients are without any functional impairment.[2]

CONGENITAL CYSTIC ADENOMATOID MALFORMATION

Congenital cystic adenomatoid malformation (CCAM) is a result of abnormal mesenchymal growth between weeks 1 and 6 of gestation, resulting in a benign lung tumor of dysplastic overgrown bronchioles. CCAM probably occurs in 1:30,000 pregnancies. CCAMs occur equally in male and female infants; there is no known association with chromosomal defects or teratogens, but additional congenital defects occur in about 25 percent of fetuses. These include diaphragmatic hernia, cardiac anomalies, intestinal atresias, renal agenesis, and pectus deformities. Most CCAMs occupy a part of one lobe, the lower lobes being most commonly affected. Type I CCAMs are the most common and occur mostly on the right side; types II and III do not demonstrate side predisposition.

Pathophysiology

During development, a defect occurs in switching from the canalicular phase of lung development to the terminal sac phase, and this leads to the histologic appearance of CCAMs in the fetal lung at 20 weeks' gestation.[22] Examination of lung sections reveals a mass of abnormal and overgrown bronchioles that do not form channels or proper airways, although there is continuity of the CCAM with the tracheobronchial tree. The abnormal bronchioles are lined by cuboidal or columnar epithelial cells, and the occasional presence of skeletal muscle suggests a hamartomatous type of lesion. CCAMs are typically classified by the cyst size as type I (macrocystic disease), type II (mixed), and type III (microcystic).[23] Type I CCAM represent 60 to 70 percent of CCAMs and usually consist of one to four cysts, each of which is larger than 2 cm. Half of the type I lesions occur on the left, 35 percent on the right, and 2 to 14 percent bilaterally.[24,25] Cyst walls are lined with ciliated pseudostratified columnar epithelium but may also have smooth muscle cells. The type II mixed CCAM (20 percent) has the poorest prognosis, owing to its high association with prematurity (75 percent) and other congenital anomalies, which occur in up to 70 percent of type II CCAMs.[22] This defect involves a combination of adenomatoid areas and small and medium-sized cysts about 1 cm in size. Alveolar-type tissue is found among cysts lined with ciliated cuboidal or columnar epithelium in type II CCAM. Type III microcystic CCAM accounts for 10 percent of lesions and is a firm mass, which usually occupies an entire lobe. This subtype presents more often in boys. It has a significant solid component, which makes its appearance on US echogenic; it is composed of adenomatoid bronchioalveolar tissue with a few small cysts and no normal lung. There is also a classification system that divides CCAMs into only two types: macrocystic (>5 mm) cysts and microcystic (<5 mm) cysts combined with solid components.[26]

Clinical presentation

The most common symptom of CCAM is respiratory distress secondary to compression of normal lung and hypoplasia of the surrounding lung. Again, mediastinal shift and decreased cardiac output can exacerbate the cardiorespiratory situation. In utero, mass effect can lead not only to lung hypoplasia but also to hydrops. Esophageal compression by the mass can also result in polyhydramnios. Infants with hydrops have severe lung hypoplasia; in the past, essentially all fetuses with hydrops died. Some 70 percent of the fetuses died in utero and 90 percent of those that were delivered did not survive. In addition, hydrops precipitates preeclampsia and premature delivery, thus further exacerbating the situation by adding prematurity and all its inherent pulmonary complications to already hypoplastic lungs. The degree of hypoplasia determines the presentation as well as the projected outcome. Newborns with large CCAMs that developed early in utero have significant shift and in utero compression, leading to severe associated hypoplasia. These newborns usually present with significant respiratory distress. Most infants, however, have varying degrees of respiratory symptoms at birth, and half of CCAMs will be discovered in the newborn period because of symptoms or prenatal screening. The diagnosis is almost always made by 6 months of age, and the majority of diagnoses (60 percent) are made within the first month of life. Many infants have prenatal diagnoses now, and even those born without symptoms are followed. Occasionally, there will be radiologic regression of the mass; however, disappearance of the mass histologically is difficult to prove and, with long-standing disease, bronchoalveolar cancer and rhabdosarcoma have been reported.[27] If the CCAM is small and demonstrates little mass effect during development, lung function may be normal and children will present with recurrent infections when they are older. The infants that present after the newborn period (50 percent) fare much better and have milder CCAMs. Their lesions may not cause respiratory distress at rest, but they may become symptomatic during upper respiratory infections, increased activity or feeding; thus such infants may develop tachypnea, wheezing, decreased breath sounds over the CCAM, or failure to thrive. A pattern of recurrent infection can also prompt workup with plain chest radiography, leading to the diagnosis, but it may take recurrent infiltrates in the same lobe to finally raise enough suspicion to diagnose an underlying CCAM. Sometimes an incidental diagnosis is made as patients undergo unrelated imaging.

Diagnostic modalities

The cystic nature of CCAMs makes them easily identifiable on prenatal US by 12 weeks' gestation; this is therefore the most commonly diagnosed congenital pulmonary anomaly. In conjunction with the features of the mass itself (i.e., macrocystic, microcystic, or solid), displacement of the heart and/or diaphragm may be apparent. In 65 percent of cases, there is polyhydramnios, and hydrops and ascites are present in up to

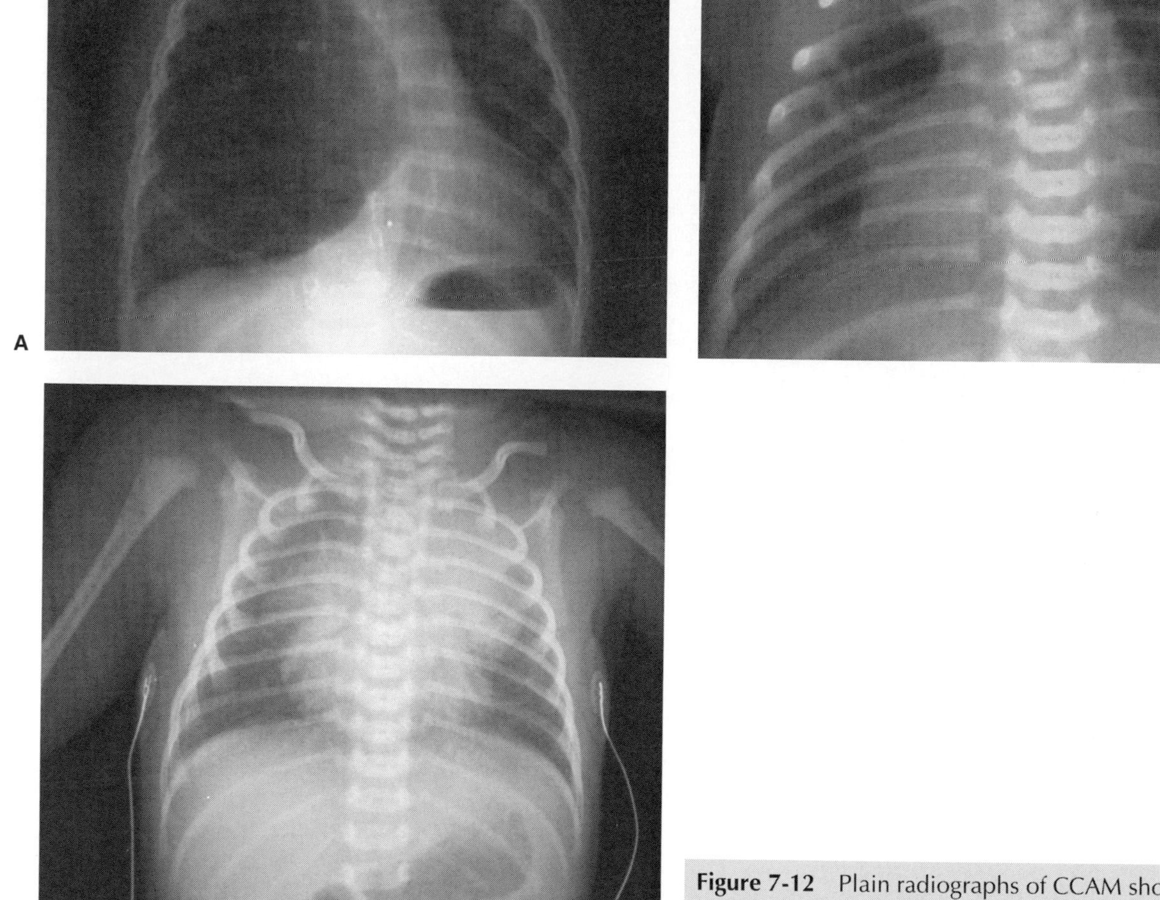

Figure 7-12 Plain radiographs of CCAM showing macrocystic, mixed, and microcystic variations **(A,B,** and **C).**

45 percent; these are ominous signs. Most infants are diagnosed prenatally or as newborns; however, 15 percent are not recognized until after 6 months of age. Prenatally diagnosed CCAMs should be confirmed postnatally, as some CCAMs seen on prenatal sonography are no longer apparent on postnatal imaging. In babies diagnosed after delivery, respiratory distress, unequal breath sounds, prematurity, or associated anomalies have prompted plain film or other imaging that reveals the CCAM pathology. The mass on chest film typically appears cystic, solid, or mixed, and there is usually some degree of mediastinal shift (Fig. 7-12). Sometimes plain film findings can mimic other conditions. One frequent example is congenital diaphragmatic hernia, which obviously has a very different treatment algorithm. A nasogastric tube seen in the chest proves it to be diaphragmatic hernia. In the newborn period, US may be the only study necessary to confirm the diagnosis of CCAM, and it can differentiate macrocystic from microcystic types, which may have prognostic value. In addition, the rare vascular abnormalities that can occur with CCAM can be demonstrated nicely on US. US or CT imaging helps assess the degree of lung involvement and differentiates CCAM from other mediastinal and lung lesions, such as sequestration, BCs, diaphragmatic hernia, and lymphangiectasis. Chest CT plays a more prominent role in the diagnosis of CCAMs as the age at presentation increases, probably being more effective at deciphering the growing differential of infectious etiologies, malignancies, and foreign bodies that can affect older children. Many surgeons also prefer CT imaging because of their own ease at interpreting axial images (Fig. 7-13).

Treatment

CCAMs are resected even in asymptomatic patients; the goal is to perform resection before the development of infectious or malignant complications. Although mass effect does exist and the clinical condition may be somewhat improved with resection, pulmonary hypoplasia is the predominant lung issue and therefore governs the patient's respiratory prognosis. Prenatal US should be performed at least every 2 weeks to detect hydrops,

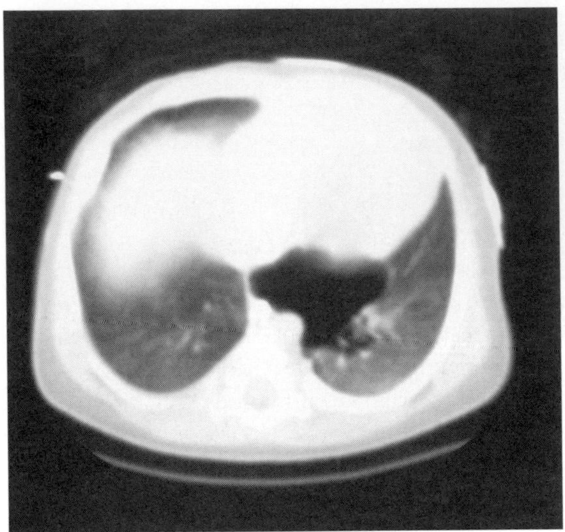
A

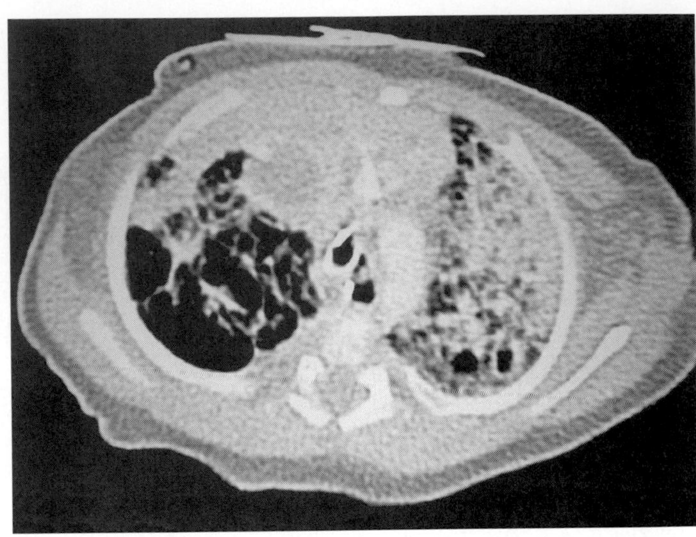
B

Figure 7-13 Computed tomography of CCAM showing macrocystic and mixed variations (**A** and **B**).

which is the most ominous sign of poor outcome. Babies with hydrops should immediately be referred to a tertiary center. Fetal echocardiography should be employed to identify associated cardiac defects and thereby provide more prognostic information.

Currently, there are several options for the management of CCAMs with severely hypoplastic lungs: traditional postnatal care and cardiorespiratory support, fetal intervention, or termination. Even in cases with hydrops, regression (presumably due to maturation) of the CCAM can occur in up to 15 percent of cases, and this should be taken in consideration in weighing the risks and benefits of fetal intervention and termination. Prenatal steroid administration has been postulated to accelerate the involution process in utero. In a study of three patients all with second-trimester diagnoses of fetal hydrops, hydrops resolved after betamethasone administration, and all babies were delivered without significant respiratory compromise, making further investigation of steroid manipulation of CCAMs intriguing.[28] Obviously the degree of lung development, hypoplasia, and resultant pulmonary hypertension will contribute heavily to the decision on how to proceed, as will the presence or absence of hydrops. For fetuses without hydrops, modern resuscitation, prepartum steroids, ventilatory techniques, and extracorporeal membrane oxygenation (ECMO) yield almost 100 percent survival. Therefore fetal intervention cannot be routinely recommended for this group of patients but should be reserved for those with early development of hydrops. Fetal intervention via cyst aspiration or thoracoamniotic shunting to decrease mass effect was described as early as 1988.[29] Cyst aspiration is not a long-term solution, as repeated drainage is required because of the rapid reaccumulation of fluid.[26] If a dominant large cyst is present, thoracoamniotic shunting has been reported to be successful in a small number of hydropic patients; shunt dislodgement or occlusion, however, can be problematic. In 6 fetuses with hydrops and a predominant large cyst, 5 of 6 patients treated with thoracoamniotic shunting survived, the one death having been due to premature delivery from rupture of membranes. This emphasizes the point that even less invasive fetal procedures disturb the intrauterine environment enough to pose the risk of premature delivery.[30]

The use of fetal thoracotomy for CCAM resection continues to evolve. In a review of 134 fetuses with CCAM over a 15-year period, the outcomes of 120 were analyzed: 14 fetuses were terminated, 19 had fetal procedures of some kind, and 6 (mentioned above) had thoracoamniotic shunting. Between gestational ages 21 and 29 weeks, 13 hydropic fetuses underwent hysterotomy, fetal thoracotomy, and lobectomy. Survival for these 13 patients was 62 percent, hydrops resolved in 2 weeks, mediastinal shift resolved in 3 weeks, and there was lung growth. The five deaths in this group were all due to inability to maintain the pregnancy during the procedure or perioperatively.[26] Preterm labor combined with pulmonary hypoplasia is responsible for most of the morbidity and mortality associated with this technique. Of the 101 fetuses for which traditional management with delivery followed by postnatal resection was chosen, every hydropic fetus died in utero or the infant expired shortly after birth, but all of the 76 nonhydropic fetuses survived (4 required ECMO). These data verify that nonhydropic fetuses have good prognoses without fetal procedures but that CCAM with hydrops is almost always lethal without prenatal intervention. Without hydrops, the risk of fetal intervention outweighs the benefit; these infants should be treated after delivery with an attempt to carry the fetus to term; fetal procedures should be limited to those with hydrops. Other studies support these data.[30–33] If "mirror" syndrome (maternal hyperdynamic state) or placentomegaly developed, fetal interventions did not yield any survivors due to the inability to maintain pregnancy. Therefore fetal interventions are not indicated in these situations or in the face of other lethal anomalies. Some families in this situation have opted for termination. After 32 weeks, if hydrops develops or if the biophysical profile of a viable fetus deteriorates (at least 24 weeks' gestation without lethal conditions), early delivery is indicated.

Preterm delivery occurs in up to half of patients with CCAM, and prenatal steroids should be given to those of less than 32 weeks' gestation to enhance lung maturity. Most of these infants will require immediate intubation and resuscitation. Infants of less than 29 weeks' gestation have not only CCAM related lung hypoplasia but also lung disease of prematurity; many may not tolerate early thoracotomy, as they will be dependent on high ventilator settings to sustain marginal respiratory parameters. If mass effect seems to be the predominant cause of respiratory failure, resection should be done promptly, whereupon the condition may improve. However, if pulmonary insufficiency is secondary to lung hypoplasia or prematurity, the positioning or retraction necessary for surgery may be more than the baby can tolerate. For very premature and low-birth-weight babies whose primary lung disease is the main cause of respiratory failure, resection should wait until the infant can tolerate a thoracotomy. Remember also that, as with in utero CCAM, these lesions may decrease in size postnatally. To improve respiratory mechanics, one can place the child with the symptomatic side down to limit its aeration and possibly decrease distention on the affected side. Jet or high-frequency ventilation minimizes hyperinflation and decreases traumatic airway pressures. Cardiac conditions must be addressed aggressively and congestive failure must be treated with inotropes and diuresis. For babies in whom hypoplasia is severe, ECMO can be used for support if the infant weighs more than 2 kg and can tolerate systemic heparinization. Surgical resection of the CCAM can be performed while the child is on ECMO or after improvement allows reasonable conventional ventilator settings. Postoperative inability to wean from bypass after 2 to 3 weeks indicates hypoplasia so severe that the infant is unsalvageable and bypass support is withdrawn.

For more stable newborns with a prenatal diagnosis of CCAM, confirmatory chest films should be obtained, as there may be regression of the mass. A mass not evident on plain film should be investigated by US or CT; patients with no evidence of mass on these studies are followed with serial US. Almost half the patients who have "regression/involution" of their CCAM based on imaging studies will ultimately manifest symptoms or plain film findings warranting excision.[34] Excision should be performed when a mass becomes evident on subsequent exams. Infants who clearly have CCAM but in whom symptoms are mild or absent can undergo elective resection as long as no mediastinal shift develops over the first 48 hours. Tachypnea, mediastinal shift, oxygen requirement, or ventilator dependence mandates resection as soon as preoperative preparation can be completed. Associated cardiac lesions are common, especially in type II lesions, and should be anticipated and studied with echocardiogram prior to surgery. Asymptomatic or incidental CCAMs should be resected electively, since there is a documented risk of malignancy,[27] and to avoid the infectious complications that would likely develop. In addition, resection in infancy affords better compensatory lung growth than surgery done later on.

Significant anesthetic difficulties regarding airway deviation or hyperinflation are rare as compared with CLE; however, they must be anticipated. Resection of CCAMs usually entails lobectomy, but pneumonectomy may be required in up to 15 percent of cases (Figs. 7-14 and 7-15). This occurs more commonly with type III CCAM, which may involve the entire lung, and is also more difficult to distinguish from normal lung tissue due to its diffuse and microscopic nature. Rarely, segmental resection of the CCAM is possible. There may be additional systemic arterial supply similar to that in sequestration, although the main vessels and airways have a normal anatomic configuration.

Outcomes

Prematurity and pulmonary hypoplasia are the most important factors in determining outcome, and the variations in presentation account for the tremendous range in survival (11 to 95 percent),[24] with fetal hydrops portending the poorest prognosis. Fetal lung/transverse thoracic area (L/T ratio) has also been

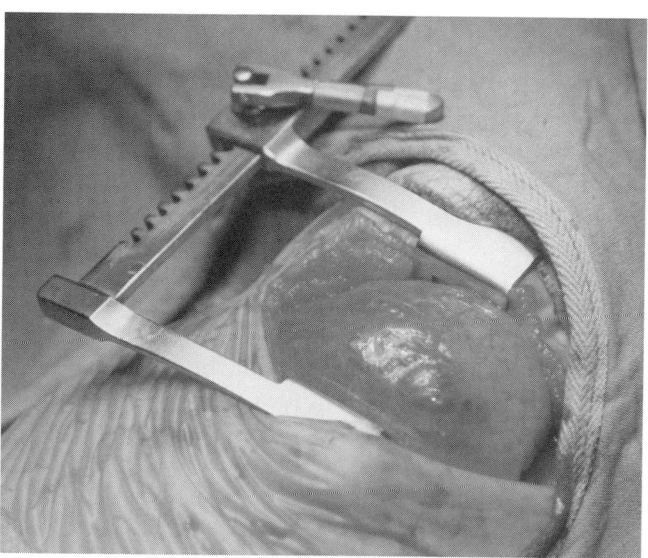

Figure 7-14 Operative photo of CCAM with large predominant cyst.

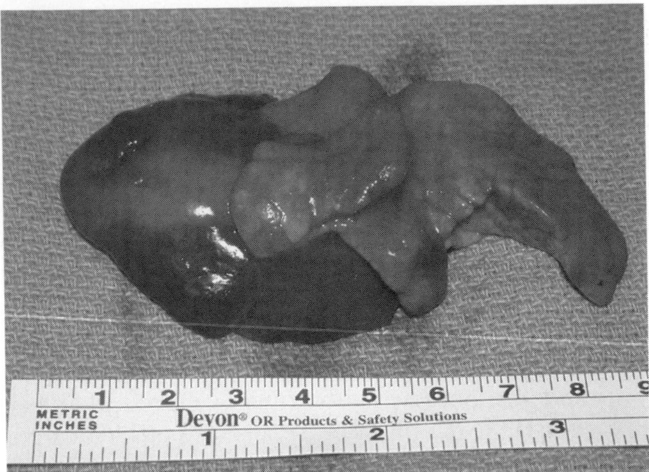

Figure 7-15 Postoperative specimen demonstrating the CCAM (cyst decompressed) and surrounding normal lung.

used to estimate the severity of disease; a value below 0.25 suggests a poorer prognosis.[35] Type I macrocystic CCAM is associated with survival rates of 70 to 95 percent. Type II and III CCAMs have poorer prognosis (<50 percent survival)[22] due to associated cardiac defects, lung hypoplasia, a higher incidence of prematurity in type II lesions, and more frequent diffuse lung involvement in type III. Additionally, hydrops and polyhydramnios, which both independently worsen prognosis, occur more frequently with type II CCAM. Fetal hydrops is a grave prognosticator and is seen in up to 45 percent of fetuses with CCAM; 68 percent of these will suffer fetal demise; of the remaining 32 percent that are delivered, 89 percent succumb, making the outcome with hydrops almost universally fatal. Fetal surgery shows promise for CCAM causing fetal hydrops, in which demise used to be almost certain; some reports quote survival rates for hydropic fetuses as high as 74 percent with fetal intervention.[26] Unfortunately, preterm delivery still leads to fetal demise 25 percent of the time.[26] Cases without hydrops have a more favorable prognosis. All nonhydropic fetuses analyzed in the literature survived without fetal intervention; fetal techniques can therefore not be recommended for nonhydrops cases at this point. The ability to prevent surgically induced preterm delivery may expand the indications for fetal surgery in the future. Of all CCAMs diagnosed in the prenatal period, up to 60 percent will die in utero or shortly after birth, since a significant number of cases have hydrops or polyhydramnios. Polyhydramnios alone carries a 50 percent mortality.[24] However, among the infants who come to delivery, 80 to 100 percent survival has been documented, since this group (1) has a low incidence of hydrops and (2) comprises mainly favorable CCAM subtypes.[4,36] Infants without hydrops, without prematurity, infants, and those without concomitant anomalies have up to 90 percent survival. Children with delayed presentation due to infection fare best, with essentially 100 percent survival.

CONGENITAL PULMONARY LYMPHATIC MALFORMATIONS

Congenital pulmonary lymphangiectasis

Congenital pulmonary lymphangiectasis or lymphangectasia (CPL) is a very rare and often fatal condition that is twice as common in male as in female infants. The bronchovascular space, pleura, and septa are filled with dilated lymphatics because, during the fifth month of gestation, the interstitial connective tissue does not regress and lymphatic channels become occluded. This obstruction leads to diffusely dilated cystic lymphatics[37] and there is concomitant pulmonary hypoplasia. Lymphedema has been seen in association, as have congenital cardiac malformations and Noonan, Ullrich-Turner, and Down's syndromes.[38] The neonatal presentation and dismal clinical course distinguish primary congenital lymphangiectasis from a secondary form of the disease. Many fetuses do not survive, and newborns present with respiratory failure and pleural effusion. Plain chest roentgenography demonstrates effusions with prominent interstitium, diffusely granular parenchyma (Fig. 7-16), and variable hyperinflation.[38] The diagnosis is supported by aspiration of lymph from effusions and confirmed by biopsy (Fig. 7-17). Treatment is supportive and aimed at draining effusions and minimizing lymphatic volume. A low-fat, high-protein diet with medium-chain triglycerides is employed in hopes of diminishing lymphatic fluid and emptying the

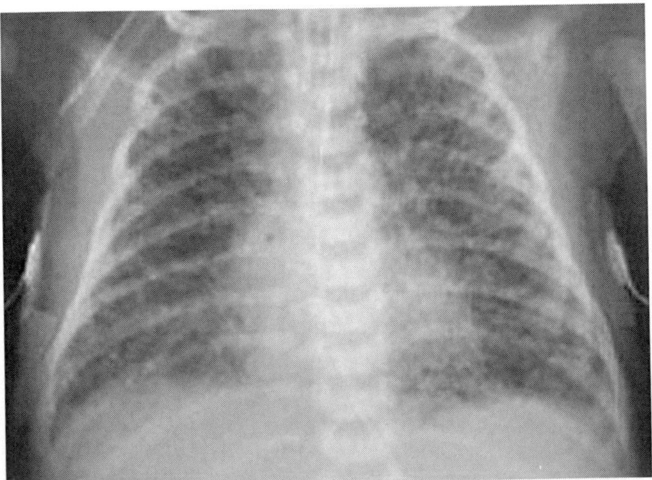

Figure 7-16 Plain film of congenital pulmonary lymphangiectasis demonstrating the ground-glass, diffuse pattern on radiography.

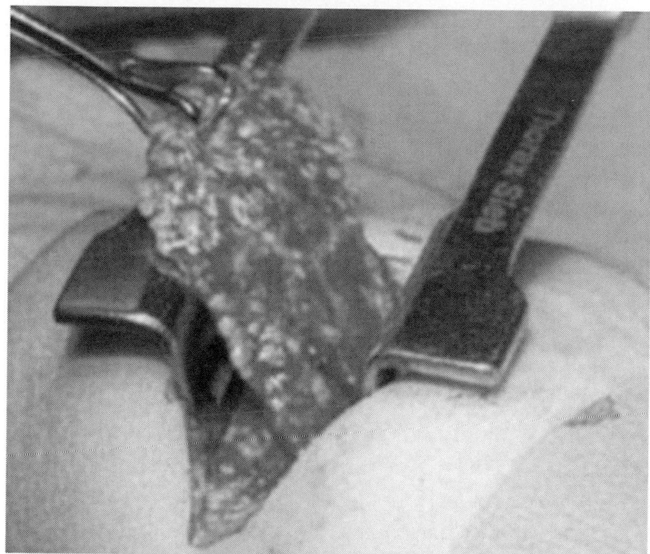

Figure 7-17 Clinical appearance of congenital pulmonary lymphangiectasis.

congested parenchymal lymphatics. Higher mean airway pressures for ventilation may help decrease the accumulation of pleural fluid, although reports of success in this endeavor are only anecdotal. Octreotide may decrease chylous effusions, minimize lymphatic volume, and alleviate some symptoms of lymphangiectasis. There are also two patients (one adolescent and one adult) with elevated plasma fibrinolytic activity in whom antiplasmin therapy significantly decreased symptoms.[39] Although heart and lung transplantation has been reported, results have been discouraging.[37] Theoretically, there may be a possibility that the regression of lymphatics that was supposed to occur in utero could continue postnatally and lead to diminution of symptoms. There is at least one case report of spontaneous recovery from this condition in the neonatal period. This report does not include biopsy confirmation of the diagnosis, however, and could therefore represent a simple chylous pleural effusion instead.[40] Unfortunately, CPL is often rapidly fatal due to significant pulmonary hypoplasia, especially in infants who present with antenatal or immediate postnatal diagnosis. There are scant reports of older children or even adults diagnosed later in life with pulmonary lymphangiectasis who have a milder clinical course.

Pulmonary lymphangiomatosis

Pulmonary lymphangiomatosis is rare and occurs equally in both male and female children. It can be distinguished from lymphangiectasis, as there are multiple well-defined lymphangiomas within the lung parenchyma; in addition, there are other lymphatic disorders in up to 75 percent of cases.[37] Increased proliferation of lymphatics in the mediastinum and lung tissue occurs, but there is normal surrounding lung parenchyma. The developmental pathway for these lymphangiomata is unknown. Histologically the cells are all benign, although clinically the disease can appear quite diffuse and invasive or may demonstrate isolated lymphangiomas. The lymphangiomas are located bilaterally in the mediastinum, pleura, chest wall, parenchyma, or bone. The presentation is usually later in childhood, with respiratory distress, wheezing, chylous effusions (pleural, pericardial, or peritoneal), protein loss, failure to thrive, lymphopenia, associated infections, chyloptysis, or even disseminated intravascular coagulation (DIC). On chest film, there are bilateral interstitial infiltrates, pleural effusions, and pericardial effusions; CT scanning demonstrates thickened pulmonary septa and possibly encasement of the mediastinal and perihilar regions. Pulmonary function tests can demonstrate both an obstructive and/or restrictive pattern. Lymphangiomata can be seen on lymphangiography near the thoracic duct, in the lung, and in bone. The presence of chylothorax with lytic bone lesions is highly suggestive of pulmonary lymphangiomatosis.[37] Biopsy can be performed and is diagnostic, with special endothelial stains such as factor VIII–related antigen and CD31 used to identify this lesion.[37] This is prognostic only, as progression is unavoidable. Lesions continue to progress and ultimately grow and cause compression phenomena. Palliative treatment is focused at decreasing lymphatic volume and obstruction. Drainage of chylous effusions should be performed to treat symptoms and careful monitoring for nutrition and infection is important due to loss of lymphocytes in the effusions. Sclerotherapy with doxycycline is often useful in palliating effusions and minimizing protein losses. Resection is generally met with high recurrence because complete excision without destroying essential structures is unlikely. This process remains mostly fatal.

PULMONARY HEMANGIOMATOSIS

Pulmonary hemangiomatosis is a very rare benign vascular tumor of the lung that is locally invasive but has no metastatic potential. There are few reported cases. On microscopic study, there is proliferation of capillaries of the thin-walled vessels in the pulmonary interstitium. Pulmonary hypertension can be severe and patients present with respiratory distress and/or desaturation. There can also be an associated consumptive coagulopathy (Kasabach-Merritt syndrome) or hemolytic anemia from sequestration or destruction related to the hemangiomas. Treatment once again is supportive and includes aggressive pulmonary toilet, control of associated infections, and nutritional support. Steroids, cytotoxic agents, radiation, laser ablation, embolization or resection of localized disease, and cryotherapy have all been tried to ablate hemangiomatosis; none, unfortunately, has shown much promise. Doxycycline has been used in a young adult patient with some abatement of symptoms and improvement of pulmonary function tests.[41] There have recently been some encouraging results with interferon alpha as an antiangiogenesis factor to prevent proliferation of smooth muscle, endothelium, and fibroblasts; although there can be hemodynamic effects in the first 48 h, side effects are otherwise minimal.[42] Lung transplantation has also been reported in a few cases in which the disease progressed to unrecoverable pulmonary failure, but long-term results are not available.[43] Owing to the advent of interferon and potentially lung transplantation, there may be some success in treating this previously universally fatal condition.

PRIMARY PULMONARY HYPOPLASIA AND AGENESIS

Pulmonary hypoplasia can be primary or secondary, occurs rarely, and is without gender preference. Secondary hypoplasia occurs after conditions mechanically restrict lung development by (1) occupying the thoracic cavity, by (2) limiting development of the thorax (thoracic dystrophies), or by (3) impeding amniotic fluid return (renal impairment or neuromuscular dysfunction of diaphragmatic excursion). Primary hypoplasia or its most extreme form, agenesis, in which there is complete absence of parenchymal and bronchial structures on one side, is very rare and probably develops when there is failure of bronchial budding from the trachea. Agenesis is extremely rare, with a worldwide experience of only several hundred cases. Many congenital anomalies have been seen with primary pulmonary hypoplasia/agenesis; these are mostly intracardiac defects, esophageal atresia, and genitourinary anomalies. Lung hypoplasia can affect one or both sides to varying degrees. With unilateral hypoplasia there seems to be no side predilection. Agenesis is clearly unilateral or incompatible with life; it, however, can be associated with contralateral hypoplasia. Left-sided agenesis is slightly more common and right-sided agenesis is more frequently associated with other congenital defects, which exist in up to 50 percent of these patients.

Presentation is variable and some infants are asymptomatic, being diagnosed only due to investigation of another condition or on the basis of a physical exam that demonstrates decreased breath sounds or mediastinal/tracheal displacement. After a time, older children may develop chest wall asymmetry or scoliosis, which prompts radiographic evaluation and diagnosis. Antenatal diagnosis is more frequently being made with routine antenatal US. The most predominant presentation is pulmonary infection, although no anatomic cause is identified for postobstructive phenomena. It is suspected that decreased clearance mechanisms play a role.[2] The diagnosis is obvious on plain film and reveals an empty hemithorax with contralateral lung hypertrophy displacing the mediastinum to the affected side. Vertebral abnormalities are also commonly seen on plain film.[44] In agenesis, the mediastinal structures are deviated toward the hyperlucent side and not contralaterally, as with a tension pneumothorax. Severe atelectasis from a variety of causes, such as mainstem occlusion, can appear similar. Therefore confirmation that the bronchus is absent must be obtained bronchoscopically. A normal trachea and contralateral bronchus will be seen without evidence of airway structures on the affected side. If the anesthetic or surgical risk is unacceptable (i.e., respiratory compromise from infection, coagulopathy, associated cardiac disease), imaging studies such as CT, US, or MRI may be used as confirmatory studies. However, since bronchoscopy is otherwise mandatory and conclusive, these tests are usually unnecessary. Bronchography with contrast has been utilized in the past, but it poses significant risk to the contralateral lung, and the other studies mentioned have largely replaced it. Diagnostic studies in pulmonary aplasia are more important in identifying other causes of lung collapse than merely diagnosing absent lung. In patients with pulmonary aplasia who undergo echocardiography or cardiac catheterization, there is pathognomonic absence of the ipsilateral pulmonary artery.

The treatment of primary hypoplasia and agenesis is focused on the prevention of infection in the solitary lung and meticulous pulmonary toilet, since infections of the lone lung are life-threatening. Infections must be aggressively treated with antibiotics, any necessary bronchodilators, chest physiotherapy, and nutritional support. Surgical involvement is usually limited to bronchoscopic confirmation of agenesis, maintenance of the contralateral bronchus, or correction of associated anomalies. It is important to consolidate procedures to minimize general anesthesia and optimize lung performance. This can be challenging in the face of other associated anomalies that may require procedures. An example is tracheoesophageal fistula (TEF) repair, which requires displacement of the solitary lung. Obviously it would be advantageous to perform thoracotomy on the side with absent lung if feasible, and expeditious surgery is a necessity. Although usually not necessary, cardiopulmonary bypass can be used to support a patient temporarily. Alternatives to intrathoracic procedures should be employed whenever possible; an example would be transabdominal occlusion of the gastroesophageal junction via ligature with concomitant gastrostomy for TEF (J.C.Y. Dunn, personal communication). Lung transplantation has not been reported for pulmonary agenesis.[2]

Half of the children born with pulmonary agenesis used to die before age 5 from pulmonary infections or associated anomalies[4,45]; infants with right-sided agenesis fared worse owing to the increased incidence of additional defects. With more powerful antibiotics and sophisticated ventilation, survival seems to be improving. With respect to secondary pulmonary hypoplasia, the intervention is usually respiratory support. In a few cases of hypoplasia caused by thoracic dystrophy, thoracoplasty to distract and enlarge the thorax may be helpful, but most of these patients die because of insurmountable associated congenital conditions.

ALVEOLAR CAPILLARY DYSPLASIA

Alveolar capillary dysplasia (ACD) is very rare and uniformly fatal. This entity involves abnormal pulmonary capillaries coupled with abnormal pulmonary lobules. There is an increased distance separating the pneumocytes and vessels and there may be absence of pulmonary veins or misalignment of the veins within the pulmonary intralobular septa. Most cases are sporadic, although there has been a report of one familial case with potential autosomal dominant inheritance.[46] The condition is rare, with less than 70 cases reported in the literature. In over half of reported ACD cases, associated cardiac, intestinal, or urologic abnormalities are present. Infants have persistent and severe pulmonary hypertension and perish, although not necessarily immediately. A diagnosis of ACD can be made on histopathologic review of the lung biopsy; this can be of prognostic significance in that the family can be counseled regarding the grim prognosis. Infants are treated for pulmonary hypertension, and it is the persistence of this finding in the absence of other causative factors that prompts a search for ACD. Treatment for the pulmonary hypertension usually utilizes the standard measures of alkalinization, sophisticated ventilation, nitric oxide, and ECMO. Prostacyclin administration and inhaled nitric oxide both decrease pulmonary vascular hypertension and increase oxygen saturation in ACD, but there is no known treatment that has been shown to affect survival.[47] Often, treatment is continued until the infant succumbs to refractory pulmonary hypertension or infection, and postmortem examination makes the diagnosis. If a child with pulmonary hypertension is showing no improvement despite maximal therapy, some advocate early biopsy to establish a diagnosis of ACD, so that the family can be counseled and offered termination for this fatal condition. There is not significant experience with lung transplantation for ACD.

PULMONARY ARTERIOVENOUS FISTULA

Congenital pulmonary arteriovenous fistulas are extremely rare; less than 20 reports of newborn cases exist in the literature.[48] They exist in two varieties. There is a capillary form with multiple capillary telangiectasias, which is inherited in an autosomal dominant pattern and expressed with variable penetrance. It is associated with Osler-Weber-Rendu syndrome in 60 percent of cases. There is also a cavernous type, in which one or more branches of the pulmonary artery feed a cavernous angioma.[49] Patients present with a spectrum of symptoms of respiratory distress ranging from mild tachypnea to clubbing, polycythemia, cyanosis, and cardiac failure from intrapulmonary shunting; only 15 percent are diagnosed in infancy. The degree of distress depends on the number of vessels involved in the fistula process and the size of the fistulas. When small peripheral arterioles are involved, there is minimal if any respiratory and hemodynamic effect, whereas when more proximal larger vessels or more numerous small vessels are involved, symptoms may be profound and life-threatening. Significant pulmonary hemorrhage can occur, however; this is fairly common in the capillary form. In addition, cerebral infections are thought to develop secondary to emboli that bypass the natural alveolar filter of the lung by flowing through the fistulas.

Diagnostic imaging with chest x-ray demonstrates increased vascular markings or interstitial infiltrates; however, these are very nonspecific findings. V/Q scans are abnormal, and arterial blood gases show right-to-left shunting. On CT scan, there may be a high-attenuation signal in the lung parenchyma, and one may see a confluence of vessels suggestive of arteriovenous fistulas. These findings can be confirmed by echocardiography, nuclear medicine study, or pulmonary angiography. Echocardiography can also be employed in the following manner. Using agitated microbubbles, an injection is administered; the bubbles that would usually be caught in the natural capillary alveolar barrier travel instead through fistulas and therefore enter the left heart and can be seen on echocardiographic imaging of the left atrium. Albumin labeled with radioactive tracer can also be injected and would normally be caught by the capillary alveolar filter and appear in the lung parenchyma. The appearance of albumin-labeled tracer in the systemic circulation indicates shunting. The parenchyma where the tracer is absent defines the location where the tracer has bypassed the usual system, and this localizes the arteriovenous fistula. Pulmonary angiography is the "gold standard" and not only demonstrates the capillary network of abnormally shaped vessels but also serves as an avenue for treatment via embolization. Embolization is extremely successful for focal lesions and immediately results in improvement of arterial blood oxygen saturation.[49] For diffuse disease, recurrent fistulas, or fistulas where embolization has failed, resection should be performed and can be curative if the degree of lung resection can be tolerated. Interferon may have application in cases where the disease is too diffuse for surgical resection; it has been used in attempts to control the growth and proliferation of arteriovenous fistulas, but there is no documented evidence of its success.

PLEUROPULMONARY BLASTOMA

Pleuropulmonary blastoma (PPB) is a thoracic neoplasm involving a mixture of primitive sarcomatous and blastematous elements involving the pulmonary and/or pleural tissues. As such, it is in the category of dysembryonic malignancies, which occur only in children. In up to 25 percent of cases, PPB occurs in association with other neoplastic or dysplastic conditions, and there can be familial presence of other dysplastic lesions.[50] PPB can be classified into three types. Type I is purely cystic, type II is mixed solid and cystic, and type III is purely solid. Histologically, there are multiloculated cysts with thin septa lined with ciliated columnar epithelium; beneath this is a network of dense, primitive sarcomatous tumor cells.

The presentation is usually due to respiratory difficulty, fever, or malaise. A recent study of 50 patients[50] suggests that type I lesions are least frequent and present within the first year of life, sometimes being diagnosed in the newborn period (mean age, 10 months at presentation). Type II lesions (most common) present at about 3 years of age and type III lesions at about 4 years of age. Diagnosis is made largely with plain films or CT scanning, which demonstrates cystic or solid masses and possibly pleural effusion. The lesion may resemble a pneumonic process or postpneumonic empyema and infectious etiologies have prompted surgery, only to discover that malignancy was truly the cause.

The treatment for PPB is surgical resection of the affected lobe(s) and pleura. There are no reports of bilateral disease. Lower lobes tend to be involved more frequently and an extensive inflammatory process with adhesions is frequently present, making the dissection painstaking and hemorrhagic. In a minority of cases, the tumor is exclusively extrapulmonary. Extension into the mediastinum may make total resection infeasible in a minority of cases. Recurrence is seen 14 to 46 percent of the time and is more problematic with type II and III lesions. Postresection chemotherapy is employed in most patients, and although no standard regimen has been agreed on, most regimens include vincristine. Radiotherapy is also often added for extensive or residual disease. Outcome is dependent on the type of PPB and its metastatic potential. For type I disease, there has been no evidence of metastasis, recurrence rates are the lowest, and survival is about 80 percent over 5 years. Pleural and mediastinal disease confers a poor prognosis. Distant metastases in the above-mentioned study occurred only in type II and III patients and in a total of 26 percent of all PPB cases. The most common sites of metastasis were bone, spinal cord, and brain. Types II and III disease are associated with more frequent recurrence and metastasis, which portends a lower 5-year survival of about 40 percent.[49]

BRONCHIAL LESIONS

Bronchial lesions are rare in children but have been reported in pediatric patients and include adenomas, chondromas, lipomas, endobronchial sarcomas, and hamartomas. The presentation is often due to respiratory distress, hyperinflation syndromes, or recurrent pneumonia due to postobstructive complications; the diagnosis can be obscured by pneumonia initially. At least one report details a neonate presenting with respiratory distress in whom chondroma lesions involved the pleura, mainstem airways, and parenchyma, requiring sleeve resection to remove the airway obstruction and involved parenchyma.[50] Plain films may demonstrate a nonspecific infiltrate or hyperinflation secondary to airway obstruction. CT scanning (Fig. 7-18) may demonstrate the endobronchial lesion. Bronchoscopy is essential in diagnosis and treatment. Some lesions can be resected endoscopically using shaving techniques or neodymium-YAG laser ablation. In patients with small airways or wide-based tumors involving substantial amounts of the airway wall, endoscopic techniques may be inadequate. In this situation, thoracotomy with sleeve resection or lobar resection may be necessary. Some advocate open thoracotomy in all cases, since the recurrence for incompletely resected lesions is high and one rarely knows the malignant potential of the tumor at the time of resection.[51] This also provides access for lymph node sampling. Proponents state that the wide base of these lesions makes complete endoscopic resection difficult; therefore endoscopic resection is not appropriate for malignant tumors. In addition, benign lesions that are incompletely resected can have local recurrence and redevelopment of airway symptoms.

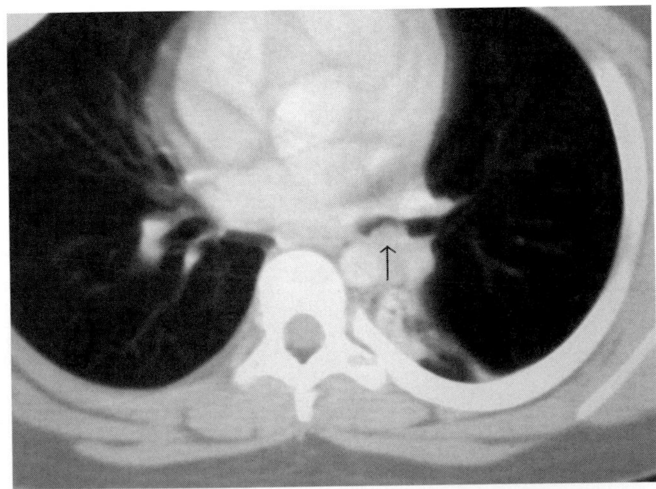

Figure 7-18 CT scan of bronchial chondroma with mass (arrow) protruding into the left mainstem bronchus.

References

1. Bromley B, Parad R, Estroff JA, et al. Fetal lung masses: Prenatal course and outcome. *J Ultrasound Med* 1995;14(12):927–936.
2. Oldham KT. Lung. In: Oldham KT, Colombani PM, Foglia PR (eds). *Surgery of Infants and Children: Scientific Principles and Practice.* Philadelphia: Lippincott-Raven, 1997:935–970.
3. Haller JA, Golladay ES, Pickard LR, et al. Surgical management of lung bud anomalies: Lobar emphysema, bronchogenic cyst, cystic adenomatoid malformation, and intralobar pulmonary sequestrations. *Ann Thorac Surg* 1979;28(1):33–43.
4. DeLorimer AA. Congenital malformations and neonatal problems of the respiratory tract. In: Welch KJ, Randolph JG, Ravitch MM, et al (eds). *Pediatric Surgery.* Chicago: Year Book, 1986:631–651.
5. Crawley-Coha T. Congenital lung malformations, In: Wise BV, McKenna C, Garvin G, et al (eds). *Nursing Care of the General Pediatric Surgery Patient.* Gaithersburg, MD: Harmon Aspen, 2000:176–187.
6. Suen HC, Mathisen DJ, Grillo HD, et al. Surgical management and radiological characteristics of bronchogenic cysts. *Ann Thorac Surg* 1993;55(2):467–481.
7. Kitano Y, Flake AW, Crombleholme TM, et al. Open fetal surgery for life-threatening fetal malformations. *Semin Perinatol* 1999;23(6):448–461.
8. Sullivan SM, Okada S, Kudo M, et al. A retroperitoneal bronchogenic cyst with malignant change. *Pathol Int* 1999;49(4):338–341.
9. Krous HF, Sexauer CL. Embryonal rhabdomyosarcoma arising within a congenital bronchogenic cyst in a child. *J Pediatr Surg* 1981;16:506–508.
10. Murphy JJ, Blair GK, Fraser GC, et al. Rhabdomyosarcoma arising within congenital pulmonary cysts: Report of three cases. *J Pediatr Surg* 1992;27:1364–1367.
11. Bolton JW, Shahian DM. Asymptomatic bronchogenic cysts: What is the best management? *Ann Thorac Surg* 1992;53:1134–1137.
12. Abuhamad A, Bass T, Katz M, et al. Familial recurrence of pulmonary sequestration. *Obstset Gynecol* 1996;87(5):843–845.
13. Jona JZ, Raffensperger JG. Total sequestration of the right lung. *J Thorac Cardiovasc Surg* 1975;69(3):361–364.
14. Savic B, Birttel F, Tholen W, et al. Lung sequestration: Report of seven cases and review of 540 published cases. *Thorax* 1979;334:96–101.
15. Buntain WL, Woolley MM, Mahour GH, et al. Pulmonary sequestration in children: A 23-year experience. *Surgery* 1977;81(4):413–420.
16. Carter R. Pulmonary sequestration. *Ann Thorac Surg* 1969;7(1):68–68.
17. Srikanth MS, Ford EG, Stanley P, et al. Communicating bronchopulmonary foregut malformations: Classification and embryogenesis. *J Pediatr Surg* 1992;27(6):732–736.
18. MacGillivray TE, Harrison MR, Goldstein RB, et al. Disappearing fetal lung lesions. *J Pediatr Surg* 1993;28(10):1321–1324.
19. Chan V, Greenough A, Nicolaides K. Antenatal and postnatal treatment of pleural effusion and extra lobar pulmonary sequestration. *J Perinat Med* 1996;24:335–338.
20. Cremin BJ, Movsowitz H. Lobar emphysema in infants. *Br J Radiol* 1971;44(525):692–696.
21. de Lorimier AA. Respiratory problems related to the airway and lung. In: O'Neill AJ, Rowe MI, Grosfeld JL, et al (eds). *Pediatric Surgery.* St. Louis: Mosby, 1998:873–897.
22. Borowitz D, Huday B. Congenital lung malformations. In: Glick PL, Pearl HR, Irish MS, Caty MS (eds). *Pediatric Surgery Secrets.* Philadelphia: Hanley & Belfus, 2001:47–52.
23. Stocker JT, Madewell JE, Drake RM. Congenital cystic adenomatoid malformation of the lung. Classification and morphologic spectrum. *Hum Pathol* 1977;8:155–171.
24. Thorpe-Beeston JG, Nicolaides KH. Cystic adenomatoid malformation of the lung: Prenatal diagnosis and outcome. *Prenat Diagn* 1994;14(8):677–688.
25. Miller RK, Sieber WK, Yunis EJ. Congenital cystic adenomatoid malformation of the lung: A report of 17 cases and review of the literature. *Pathol Annu* 1980;15:387–402.
26. Adzick NS, Harrison MR, Crombleholme TM. Fetal lung lesions: Management and outcome. *Am J Obstet Gynecol* 1998;179:884–889.
27. Benjamin DR, Cahill JL. Bronchioalveolar carcinoma of the lung and congenital cystic adenomatoid malformation. *Am J Clin Pathol* 1991;95(6):889–892.
28. Tsao K, Hawgood S, Vu L, et al. Resolution of hydrops fetalis in congenital cystic adenomatoid malformation after prenatal steroid therapy. *J Pediatr Surg* 2003;38(3):508–510.
29. Rodeck CH, Firsk NM, Fraser, DI, et al. Long-term in utero drainage of fetal hydrothorax. *N Engl J Med* 1998;319:1135–1138.
30. Adzick NS, Harrison MR, Flake AW, et al. Fetal surgery for cystic adenomatoid malformation of the lung. *J Pediatr Surg* 1993;28:806–812.
31. Brown MF, Lewis D, Brouillette RM, et al. Successful prenatal management of hydrops, caused by congenital cystic adenomatoid malformation, using serial aspirations. *J Pediatar Surg* 1995;30(7):1098–1099.
32. Evans MG. Hydrops fetalis and pulmonary sequestration. *J Pediatr Surg* 1996;31(6):761–764.
33. Miller JA, Corteville JE, Langer JC. Congenital cystic adenomatoid malformation in the fetus: Natural history and predictors of outcome. *J Pediatr Surg* 1996;31(6):805–808.
34. Davenport M, Warne SA, Cacciaguerra S, et al. Current outcome of antenatally diagnosed cystic lung disease. *J Pediatr Surg* 2004;39(4):549–556.
35. Kamata U, Sawai T, Kamiyama M, et al. Outcome predictors for infants with cystic lung disease. *J Pediatr Surg* 2004;39(4):603–606.
36. Ryckman FC, Rosenkrantz JG. Thoracic surgical problems in infancy and childhood. *Surg Clin North Am* 1985;65:1423–1454.
37. Faul JL, Berry GJ, Colby TV, et al. Thoracic lymphangiomas, lymphangiectasis, lymphangiomatosis, and lymphatic dysplasia syndrome. *Am J Respir Crit Care Med* 2000;161(3):1037–1046.
38. Moerman P, Vandenberghe K, Devlieger H, et al. Congenital pulmonary lymphangiectasis with chylothorax: A heterogeneous lymphatic vessel abnormality. *Am J Med Genet* 1993;47(1):54–58.

39. MacLean JE, Cohen E, Weinstein M. Primary intestinal and thoracic lymphangectasia: A response to antiplasmin therapy. *Pediatrics* 2002;109(6):1177–1180.
40. Scott C, Wallis C, Dinwiddie R, et al. Primary pulmonary lymphangiectasis in a premature infant: Resolution following intensive care. *Pediatr Pulmonol* 2003;35(5):405–406.
41. Ginns LC, Roberts DH, Mark EJ, et al. Pulmonary capillary hemangiomatosis with atypical endotheliomatosis: Successful antiangiogenic therapy with doxycycline. *Chest* 2003;124(5):2017–2022.
42. White CW. Treatment of hemangiomatosis with recombinant interferon alfa. Semin Hematol 1990;27:15–22.
43. Eltorky MA, Headley AS, Winer-Muram H, et al. Pulmonary capillary hemangiomatosis: A clinicopathologic review. *Ann Thorac Surg* 1994;57(3):772–776.
44. Swischuk LE, Richardson CH, Nichols MM, et al. Primary pulmonary hypoplasia in the neonate. *J Pediatr* 1979;95(4):573–577.
45. Booth JB, Berry CL. Unilateral pulmonary agenesis. *Arch Dis Child* 1967;42(224):361–374.
46. Boggs S, Harris MC, Hoffman DJ, et al. Misalignment of pulmonary veins with alveolar capillary dysplasia: Affected siblings and variable phenotypic expression. *J Pediatr* 1994;124(1):125–128.
47. Steinhorn RH, Cox PN, Fineman JR, et al. Inhaled nitric oxide enhances oxygenation but not survival in infants with alveolar capillary dysplasia. *J Pediatr* 1997;130(3):417–422.
48. Olgunturk R, Oguz D, Tunaoglu S, et al. Pulmonary arteriovenous fistula in the newborn: A case report of Rendu-Osler-Weber syndrome and a review of the literature. *Turk J Pediatr* 2001;43(4):332–337.
49. Priest JR, Mc Dermott MB, Bhatia S, et al. Pleuropulmonary blastoma: A clinicopathologic study of 50 cases. *Cancer* 1997;80(1):147–161.
50. Hoekstra MO, Bertus PM, Nikkels PG, et al. Multiple pulmonary chondromata. A rare cause of neonatal respiratory distress. *Chest* 1994;105(1):301–302.
51. Morini F, Quattruci S, Cozzi DA, et al. Bronchial adenoma: An unusual cause of recurrent pneumonia in childhood. *Ann Thorac Surg* 2003;76(6):2085–2087.

CHAPTER

8 TRACHEAL DISEASES

Todd S. Weiser, Douglas J. Mathisen

BACKGROUND

HISTORICAL PERSPECTIVE

Early in the evolution of tracheal surgery, it was believed that the amount of trachea that could be excised safely was four rings or approximately 2 cm. Because of this belief, much of the early work in this area focused on the use of prosthetics for tracheal replacement. To this date, while some results achieved in the laboratory appear promising,[1,2] consistent success has not yet been attained for replacement of the airway.

In parallel with the efforts to find a suitable prosthetic device, efforts were under way to determine the possibilities of resection and primary reconstruction. Grillo and colleagues[3–5] systematically investigated the limits of resection of the trachea that might permit primary reconstruction without excessive tension and without destruction of its vital blood supply. These experiments in human cadavers demonstrated that the blood supply of the trachea entered in its lateral pedicles and that mobilization of the trachea is best accomplished by anterior and posterior dissection only. These experiments concluded that a median length of 4.5 cm or approximately seven rings could be resected and primarily reconstructed with an acceptable amount of tension. Dedo and Fishman utilized laryngeal release to allow greater resections with less tension.[6]

These anatomic experiments and others[7,8] in tracheal mobilization have served as the rationale behind the surgical approaches utilized today in tracheal surgery. Lesions of the cervical trachea are resected and reconstructed predominantly with only pretracheal dissection and neck flexion. Resections for pathology of the

KEY CONCEPTS

- Epidemiology
  - Primary tracheal tumors are rare, with an estimated 2.7 new cases diagnosed per million persons per year. The many remaining tracheal pathologies comprise heterogeneous epidemiologies.
- Pathophysiology
  - Congenital tracheal stenosis may present as a web-like diaphragm, most often at the subcricoid level. Primary tracheal tumors are largely (about two-thirds) made up of adenoid cystic and squamous cell carcinomas with roughly equal histologic frequency. Other tumors include pleomorphic adenomas, leiomyomas, chondromas, carcinoid tumors, mucoepidermoid tumors, and sarcomas. The laryngotracheal junction is the most frequent location of injury in airway trauma. Most tracheoesophageal fistulas are complications from mechanical ventilation.
- Clinical features
  - Patients with tracheal pathology usually present with signs and symptoms of upper airway obstruction: dyspnea on exertion, wheezing, stridor, and obstructive pneumonia. Tracheal tumors most commonly present with cough, hemoptysis and signs of progressive airway obstruction, although signs and symptoms vary with tumor histology. Tracheoesophageal fistulas typically manifest as a sudden increase in tracheal secretions and ingested material in the trachea.
- Diagnostics
  - Anteroposterior and lateral tomography is useful to define upper tracheal pathology. Fluoroscopy demonstrates functional vocal cord asymmetry and

other details (e.g., airway collapse with malacia). Computed tomography is helpful in malignant disease to assess extramural extent and lymphadenopathy. Inspiratory/expiratory computed tomography is the easiest, most accurate noninvasive method to diagnose tracheomalacia. Flexible and rigid bronchoscopy is critical in the definitive assessment of the trachea.

- Treatment
  - Tracheal resection can be performed using a cervical or transthoracic approach, depending on the location and extent of the lesion. Tracheal release maneuvers are primarily intended to prevent excessive tension on the anastomosis and avoid the need for excessive tracheal dissection.
  - Laryngotracheal injuries should be treated with airway establishment (e.g., tracheostomy). Traumatic lacerations of the lower trachea can be approached via partial or full sternotomy or right posterolateral thoracotomy.
  - Congenital tracheal stenoses may be treated with anterior tracheoplasty and patch repair or slide tracheoplasty.
  - Most tracheoesophageal fistulas require tracheal resection. Anastomotic complications are reduced if definitive single-stage correction of the fistula is delayed until after the patient has been successfully weaned from mechanical ventilation. Fistula control can be achieved by placing a tracheostomy with the balloon placed below the fistula, draining gastrostomy, and feeding jejunostomy.
  - Idiopathic laryngotracheal stenoses have been treated with complex, multistaged procedures or single-stage procedures involving partial resection of the subglottic larynx and immediate plastic reconstruction.
- Outcomes/prognosis
  - At the Massachusetts General Hospital, operative mortality for primary tracheal tumor resection has improved from 21 percent in the 1960s to 3 percent in the last decade. The overall 1-, 5-, and 10-year survival rates for primary tracheal carcinoma have been reported to be 84, 45, and 25 percent respectively. All tracheal surgery is subject to anastomotic complications, including suture line granulomas, stenosis, and tracheal separation. Predictors of anastomotic complications include reoperation, diabetes, lengthy resections, laryngotracheal resections, age 17 years or less, and preoperative tracheostomy. Anastomotic complications are associated with a 7.4 percent mortality, compared to 0.06 percent in patients who did not experience anastomotic complications.

intrathoracic trachea can be performed with hilar release with or without bronchial reimplantation along with pretracheal dissection and cervical flexion.

As the issues of extent of resection, methods of mobilization, limits of acceptable tension, and preservation of blood supply were established, primary resection and reconstruction became the accepted mode of managing most diseases that involved the trachea. Reports followed of resection and primary reconstruction of lengths of the trachea that had been thought previously to be impossible.[9–11]

ANATOMY

The adult trachea measures 11 cm in average length from the anterior border of the cricoid cartilage to the carinal spur. There are 18 to 22 cartilaginous rings in the human trachea, with approximately two rings per centimeter. The only complete cartilaginous ring in the normal airway is the cricoid cartilage of the larynx. The remainder of the rings are C-shaped, connected posteriorly by the membranous portion of the trachea. The blood supply of the trachea is shared with the esophagus laterally and with the main bronchi below. Above, the blood supply originates from the inferior thyroid artery, and vessels to the lower trachea are derived from the bronchial vessels (Fig. 8-1). Importantly, branches of these vessels enter the trachea laterally.

PATHOLOGY

CONGENITAL LESIONS

Congenital tracheal stenosis may present as a web-like diaphragm, most often at subcricoid level. More lengthy stenoses may involve the entire trachea, sometimes with a normal larynx and main bronchi, or they may involve variable lengths of the trachea (Fig. 8-2). Funnel-like narrowing is sometimes seen, with gradual narrowing to the stenotic segment. Segmental stenosis of the lower trachea may be accompanied by bronchial anomalies such as origin of all or part of the right upper lobe bronchus from the trachea just above the stenotic segment. Most often the cartilaginous rings are circular in the area of stenosis. Other developmental anomalies may occur in a patient with congenital tracheal stenosis.

TRAUMA

External trauma

The trachea, carina, and main bronchi may be damaged by either blunt or penetrating trauma. Blunt cervical injury may result in injury to the airway at any level from the hyoid bone to the carina.[12] The presentation of these injuries may be subtle. Subcutaneous emphysema may be detected in the neck or, if the injury involves the more

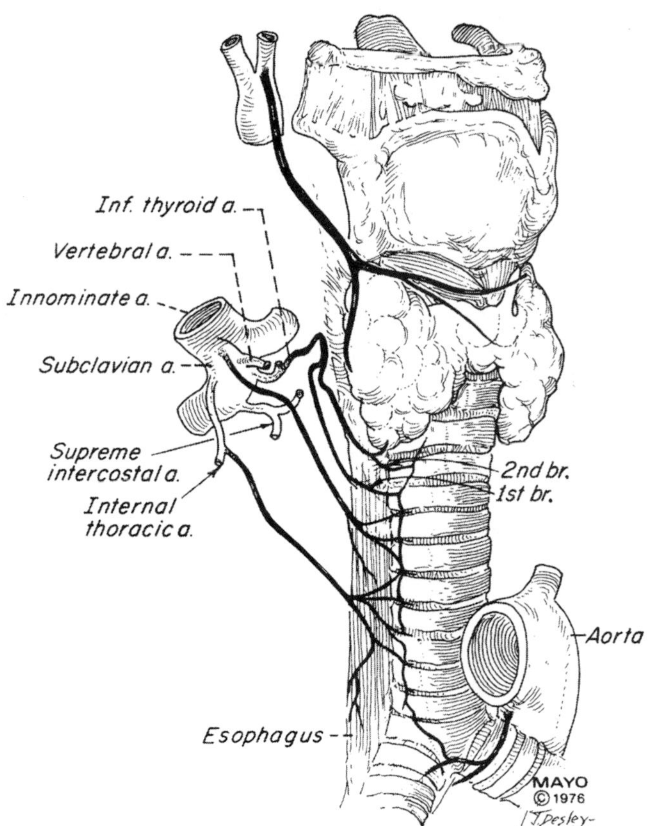

Figure 8-1 Arterial supply to the thoracic trachea. Inf = inferior; a = artery; br = branch. [From Salassa JR, Pearson BW, Payne WS. Gross and microscopical blood supply to the trachea. Reprinted with permission from the Society of Thoracic Surgeons (*Ann Thorac Surg* 1977;24:100–107). By permission of Mayo Clinic.]

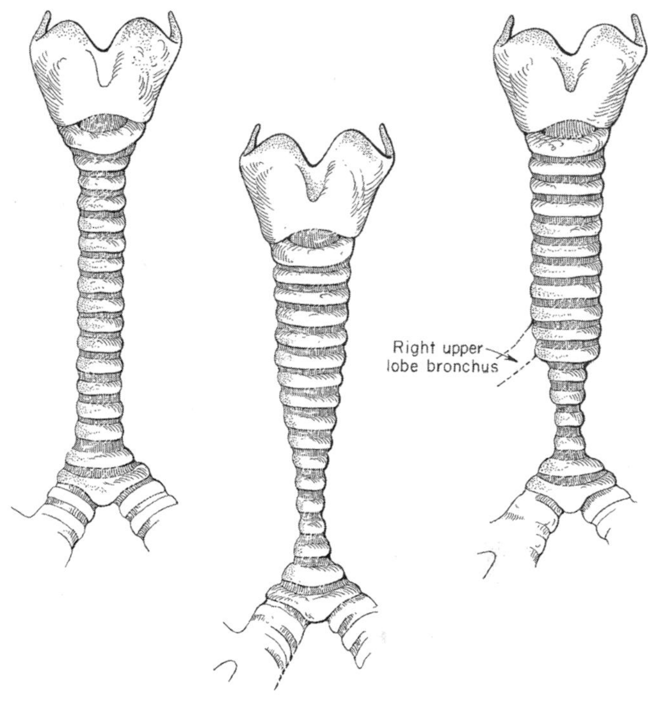

Figure 8-2 Congenital tracheal stenosis. Type I (left): Generalized hypoplasia of the trachea. The airway has a normal caliber at the level of the cricoid cartilage and also in the main bronchi. Type II (center): Funnel-like narrowing. The trachea has a normal caliber immediately below the cricoid cartilage but funnels to its narrowest point, most frequently above the carina. Type III (right): Segmental stenosis may be accompanied by bronchial anomalies. The segmental stenosis may vary in length and may be at various levels. (From Cantrell JR, Guild HC. Congenital stenosis of the trachea. *Am J Surg* 1964;108:297. With permission.)

distal trachea, air may be seen on x-ray to dissect mediastinal tissues. Pneumothorax may result from tracheal injury within the chest cavity. Patients may present with varying severities of dyspnea from airway obstruction caused by these injuries or from tracheal transection. A patient with an initially satisfactory airway may rapidly decompensate while under observation or as intubation or examination of the airway is attempted.

If the airway is partially separated, a flexible bronchoscope with an endotracheal tube threaded over it is the best way to assess it. If difficulty is encountered, emergency tracheostomy should be quickly performed before the airway is lost. A completely transected trachea may retract into the mediastinum but is easily located by finger palpation and grasped by clamps and delivered into the field.

When the lower trachea is damaged, prominent injuries to the chest, typical of high-impact trauma, are often seen. Injuries to the carina and the main and lobar bronchi may occur from crushing injuries to the chest.[13] These tend to occur more frequently than tracheal injuries.

Inhalational injuries

Tracheal injury may also occur in the form of thermal or chemical damage by inhalation. Inhalation burns of the larynx, trachea, and bronchi may be particularly difficult injuries. The degree of inflammatory change, granulation tissue response, and scarring will depend on the depth of mucosal injury. In most cases the tracheal rings are not destroyed. Resection is generally precluded, as lengthy injuries often occur. A number of cases of airway obstruction caused by burns have been managed initially by a tracheostomy placed at the second or third ring, typically within the area of burn injury, followed later by placement of a silicone T tube to span the injured area.[14]

IATROGENIC INJURIES

Acute intubation injuries

Lacerations of the trachea during intubation occur most often in the membranous wall. These may be long and may also damage the esophagus, resulting in a

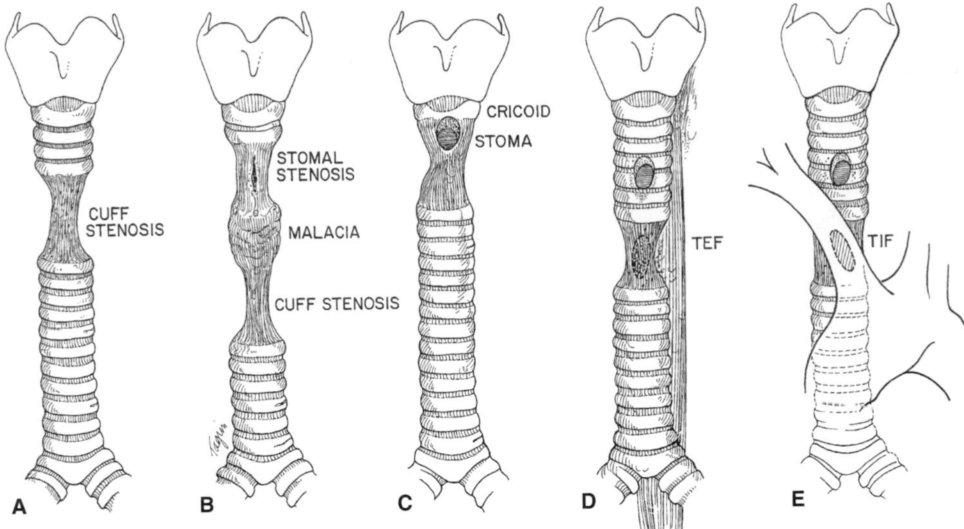

Figure 8-3 Diagrams of principal postintubation tracheal lesions. A. Cuff stenosis from the cuff of an endotracheal tube. B. Cuff stenosis from the cuff of a tracheostomy tube, usually lower in the trachea than that from an endotracheal tube. Stomal stenosis also occurs at the site of the tracheostomy itself. Malacia may occur either at the level of the cuff or in the segment between the stoma and the cuff stenosis. C. Cuff stenosis at the site of a high tracheostomy stoma, which has eroded into the lower margin of the cricoid cartilage. In older patients, this may erode back further into the subglottic larynx, producing a laryngotracheal stenosis. D. Tracheoesophageal fistula (TEF) produced by pressure of the cuff against the membranous wall, often abetted by an indwelling firm nasogastric tube. E. One type of tracheoinnominate fistula (TIF), the result of a high-pressure cuff erosion. The more common type, but also rare, is that seen with a low-placed tracheostomy stoma, which rests against the innominate artery itself. Not shown here are the lesions that occur in the larynx as a result of endotracheal tubes. (From Grillo HC. Surgical management of postintubation tracheal injuries. *J Thorac Cardiovasc Surg* 1979;78:860. With permission.)

tracheoesophageal fistula. Associate respiratory symptoms and concomitant esophageal injuries are indications for immediate repair.

Postintubation injuries

Postintubation injuries to the trachea include granulomas, strictures, malacia, and tracheoesophageal and tracheoinnominate artery fistulas (Fig. 8-3).

Tracheal strictures represent the most common postintubation injuries. These occur principally either at the level of the tracheal stoma or that of the tracheal cuff. Both result from proliferative and cicatricial responses to tracheal injury. Granulomas result from erosion by the tip of a tracheostomy or endotracheal tube and can also occur at the site of a healed tracheostomy. Stomal stenosis results from the gradual enlargement of a tracheal stoma and its eventual healing by contraction. This pulls the sides of the defect together, distorting the tracheal lumen to a triangular configuration with the base of the triangle located posteriorly, consisting of the uninjured membranous wall. The instigating large stoma may result from overzealous excision of tracheal wall at the time of the initial tracheostomy, from erosive infection around the margins of the stoma, or most commonly from erosion secondary to leverage by equipment attached to the tracheostomy tube during ventilation. The stenotic process may extend into the subglottic larynx if the previous tracheostomy was placed inappropriately high in the trachea.

Cuff stenosis, on the other hand, is caused by circumferential erosion of the trachea by excessive pressure exerted by the sealing cuff. In the healing process, cicatricial connective tissue is formed, which contracts in a circumferential fashion. The route of entry of the ventilatory tube does not affect the occurrence of cuff injury, only its level. These lesions are seen in patients who have had only endotracheal intubation as well as those with previous tracheostomy. Cuff injuries have been observed in patients with only 48 h of exposure to a high-pressure cuff.[15] However, since the length of exposure increases the risk of injury, these lesions are seen more frequently in patients after prolonged ventilation.

The development of the large-volume, low-pressure cuff for tracheostomy and endotracheal tubes for ventilation has greatly lowered the incidence of cuff stenoses.

However, since the compliance curve of the plastic from which these cuffs are made is unsatisfactory when the cuff is inflated beyond its normal filled volume, pressure rises rapidly with additional filling. Therefore overinflation of these cuffs converts them to high-pressure cuffs. This fact leads to a continued incidence of cuff stenosis.

Malacia of the trachea rather than stenosis may also occur at the level of cuff injury. The mucosa generally reveals squamous metaplasia in contrast to the scar tissue seen in the stenotic lesion. It is not clear why some patients develop malacic lesions rather than stenosis. Areas of malacia can also be seen between the level of a tracheal stoma and a cuff stenosis.

Tracheoesophageal fistulas occur most often in patients who have a ventilating cuff in the trachea for a long period of time concomitant with a feeding tube in the esophagus. These may represent large fistulas that can extend from one cartilaginous margin to the other. In most cuff fistulas, there is a circumferential injury to the trachea at the level of the fistula. Smaller fistulas are occasionally seen, which may be related to the tip of the tube pointing against the membranous wall. These variations must be considered in surgical repair.

Anterior injuries of the trachea may lead to the development of tracheoinnominate artery fistulas. These are most often due to direct erosion of the inner elbow of the tracheostomy tube in an inferiorly placed stoma. Placement of the tracheal stoma at the conventional level of the second or third tracheal ring prevents these fistulas.

Radiation therapy can produce late stenosis of the larynx and trachea. Because of the intrinsic damage to these tissues, surgical repair is hazardous. Laryngeal injuries are best managed by dilatation provided that the interval between dilatations is long enough to be tolerated. Tracheal stenosis due to irradiation may be treated with T-tube placement or carefully considered reconstruction with omental transfer to augment healing.[16] Unfortunately, radiation injury to the airway may be impossible to correct.

IDIOPATHIC LARYNGOTRACHEAL STENOSIS

A rare patient will present with stenosis of the airway at various levels without history of trauma, infection, inhalation injury, or airway intubation. This diagnosis is one of exclusion and is characterized by an inflammatory cicatricial stenosis at the level of the subglottic larynx, cricoid, and upper trachea. An overwhelming majority of these patients are female and typically present with signs and symptoms of upper airway obstruction.[17,18] This process is confined intrinsically to the wall of the airway and the immediately surrounding connective tissue.

It is impossible to predict the future course of the disease. When airway obstruction becomes severe and does not respond for sufficiently long intervals to dilatation, surgery may be entertained, with, however, the clear caveat that the disease may progress. Most patients, in our experience, are best treated with definitive laryngotracheal resection and primary reconstruction.[17,18] Since the stenosis often involves the subglottic larynx, complete removal of all inflammatory tissue is often impossible.

TRACHEOBRONCHOMALACIA

Acquired tracheomalacia may result from postintubation injury. However, in patients with chronic obstructive pulmonary disease, malacia may develop in the lower trachea, main bronchi, and sometimes the more distal bronchi in the absence of prior intubation. When the patient attempts to expire or to cough, the membranous wall approximates to the anterior, softened cartilaginous wall, causing nearly total obstruction. Consequently, the posterior membranous wall elongates and becomes redundant. It is possible to ameliorate the deformity by pulling the ends of the cartilages toward one another posteriorly, restoring a more circular shape to the airway. The redundant membranous wall must be tacked to the posterior splinting material to prevent it from falling forward into the lumen.[19] Various materials have been used for splinting, none with complete success. These have included fascia lata, pericardium, lyophilized bone, polytetrafluoroethylene, and rigid plastic splints. We currently utilize sheets of polypropylene mesh to plicate the membranous wall as described by Rainer.[20]

TRACHEAL TUMORS

Primary tracheal tumors are rare. It is estimated that tracheal tumors occur in about 2.7 new cases per million per year.[21] The rarity of these tumors and their often insidious presentation frequently leads to a delay in diagnosis and inappropriate treatment until the definitive diagnosis is made.

Tumor classification

About two-thirds of primary tracheal tumors are of two histologic types: squamous cell carcinoma (SCC) and adenoid cystic carcinoma (ACC), formally known as "cylindroma." These two types occur with equal frequency. The remaining third of the tumors are widely distributed in a heterogeneous group, both malignant and benign. A variety of secondary tumors involve the trachea. These include carcinomas of the larynx, thyroid, lung, and esophagus. Rarely, tumors may metastasize to the submucosa of the trachea or to the mediastinum, with secondary invasion of the trachea. Thus, carcinoma of the breast and mediastinal lymphoma may invade the trachea.

SCC may be either exophytic or ulcerative. It may also be multiple and extend over a considerable length of trachea. The tumor metastasizes to the regional lymph nodes and, in its more aggressive and late forms, invades mediastinal structures. In general, its progress appears to be relatively rapid in comparison with that of ACC. A number of these patients have returned with a second SCC of the lung or oropharynx. SCC occurs predominantly in men, usually cigarette smokers.[22]

ACC often has a very prolonged course of clinical symptoms, sometimes extending for years. Following treatment, many years may pass before a recurrence is noted. ACC may extend over long distances submucosally in the airways and also perineurally. It spreads to regional lymph nodes, although less characteristically than does squamous cell carcinoma. Although it may invade the thyroid or muscular coats of the esophagus by contiguity, ACC that has not been surgically interfered with frequently displaces mediastinal structures before actually invading them. Metastases to the lungs are not uncommon. These may grow very slowly over a period of many years and remain asymptomatic until they become quite large. Metastases to bone and other organs occur. In contrast to tracheal squamous cell carcinoma, the male to female ratio of ACC is essentially equal and the smoking history of these patients appears to be incidental.[21]

The group of tumors other than SCC and ACC, although representing only about one-quarter of the population, is composed of a multitude of tumor types and varying degrees of malignancy, including both epithelial and mesenchymal neoplasms. This list includes pleomorphic adenomas, leiomyomas, chondromas, carcinoid tumors, mucoepidermoid tumors, and sarcomas.

Secondary tumors involving the trachea should be briefly noted. Both papillary and follicular carcinoma of the thyroid and mixed varieties of the two may invade the trachea primarily, usually at the level of the isthmus.[23] Invasion of the trachea by thyroid carcinoma is best managed by resection with airway reconstruction. Localized extension of tumor may also require partial esophageal resection or radical resection, including laryngectomy with mediastinal tracheostomy. More commonly invasion is seen after thyroidectomy for carcinoma, in cases where the surgeon was aware that he or she was "shaving off" the tumor from the trachea. In such cases, concurrent or early resection of the involved trachea should be considered.

CLINICAL FEATURES

Patients with pathologic lesions of the trachea usually present with signs and symptoms of upper airway obstruction: dyspnea on exertion, wheezing, stridor, and obstructive pneumonia. The most common presentation, wheezing and dyspnea on exertion, is frequently misinterpreted as adult-onset asthma. It is not uncommon for the symptoms in these patients to become progressively worse and correspondingly be treated with corticosteroids before the correct diagnosis is finally made. It should be a diagnostic rule that any patient who presents with such symptoms who has been intubated and ventilated must be considered to have organic stenosis unless proven otherwise.

Tumors of the trachea may also present insidiously. Their most common signs and symptoms are cough (37 percent), hemoptysis (41 percent), and the signs of progressive airway obstruction, including shortness of breath on exertion (54 percent), wheezing and stridor (35 percent), and, less commonly, dysphagia or hoarseness (7 percent).[21] Signs and symptoms may vary with the histology of the tumor. Hemoptysis is prominent in patients with squamous cell carcinoma and usually leads to earlier diagnosis. ACC more commonly presents with wheezing or stridor as a predominant symptom, often leading to delay in diagnosis. In one study, the mean duration of symptoms prior to diagnosis in patients with SCC of the trachea was only 4 months, whereas in those with ACC, it was 18 months.[24]

Tracheoesophageal fistula will be manifest by a sudden increase in tracheal secretions and, of course, the appearance of any ingested material in the trachea. If the patient is on a respirator, gastric distention may appear. Tracheoinnominate arterial fistulas are rare but may be announced by a premonitory hemorrhage. In treating bleeding from a tracheostomy, it is important to differentiate between erosion of tracheal granulations or mucosa and arterial fistula. Any suspicious hemorrhage from a tracheal stoma should be immediately investigated.

DIAGNOSTIC MODALITIES

RADIOGRAPHIC ASSESSMENT

Definitive diagnosis of airway problems is often delayed because of an apparently normal chest radiograph. Closer inspection will often reveal abnormality of the tracheal air column. Lesions can frequently be seen on overpenetrated views or tomograms of the larynx and trachea.[25,26] The location of the lesion, its linear extent, extratracheal involvement, and the amount of airway uninvolved can be determined. Lateral neck views, using soft tissue technique with the patient swallowing and the neck hyperextended to bring the trachea up above the clavicles, are useful to define pathology in the upper trachea. Fluoroscopy not only demonstrates functional asymmetry of the vocal cords if present but may give additional information about the extent of the lesion and collapse of the airway if malacia is present. In some cases, polytomography (AP and lateral views) give additional detail, particularly of mediastinal involvement. Computed tomography (CT) offers little over standard radiologic techniques for benign disease but is especially helpful in malignant disease to assess extramural extent and enlarged lymph nodes. A combination of inspiratory and expiratory images from a CT is currently the easiest and most accurate noninvasive method of diagnosing tracheomalacia.[27] The exact role of magnetic resonance imaging (MRI) has yet to be defined. Sagittal and coronal views, however, have been helpful in certain cases and may provide more accurate detail than standard radiographic techniques.

BRONCHOSCOPY

Certainly the role of both flexible and rigid bronchoscopy in the diagnosis of tracheal pathology cannot be overstated. Biopsy specimens of both benign and malignant lesions of the trachea are made with these techniques. In planning surgical resections, bronchoscopy is invaluable. Definitive assessment of the airway is performed by meticulous endoscopic measurements with a rigid bronchoscope. Measurement of the carina, bottom of the lesion, top of the lesion, and level of the vocal cords will determine the extent of the disease process and likelihood of reconstruction. At the time of bronchoscopy, it is important to assess the adequacy of the larynx and degree of inflammation of the mucosa.

Airway management and endoscopy

Crucial to the management of all problems of the trachea is the ability to control the airway. Tracheal trauma, tumors, and postintubation stenosis may present with acute airway obstruction.[28] Endotracheal intubation may be impossible and even dangerous, especially in patients with high tracheal lesions. Simple maneuvers to elevate the head of the patient, administration of cool mist, oxygen, and careful sedation may allow control of the airway to be accomplished in a semielective manner. Control is best accomplished in the operating room, where an assortment of rigid bronchoscopes, dilators, biopsy forceps, and instruments to perform emergency tracheostomy are available. Anesthesia, as in elective tracheal operations, is best accomplished by inhalation technique to allow spontaneous ventilation.[29] Muscle-relaxing agents should not be used to avoid the lethal combination of airway obstruction and an apneic patient.

Initial evaluation should be performed with a rigid bronchoscope carefully inserted through the vocal cords, stopping just proximal to the level of obstruction. This can be passed beyond most tumors, even those causing nearly total obstruction. Once the status of the distal airway has been assessed, the tumor can be partially removed with biopsy forceps to determine its consistency and vascularity. For most tumors, the tip of the rigid bronchoscope can be used to core out most of the tumor.[29] The tumor can then be grasped with biopsy forceps and removed. If bleeding ensues, the bronchoscope may be passed into the distal airway for ventilation, and this will also serve to tamponade bleeding.

Postintubation stenoses pose a slightly different problem in airway control. Bronchoscopy is invaluable in determining the extent of airway involvement and, just as importantly, the amount of uninvolved airway. As accurate measurements as possible should be recorded. The quality of the mucosa should be carefully assessed. Marked inflammation and erythema may dictate delay of definitive surgical correction to a time when this has subsided. Flexible and rigid bronchoscopes are both utilized in these situations.

Caution must be taken with flexible bronchoscopy in the assessment of critical airway stenosis. The flexible bronchoscope may precipitate airway obstruction in patients with critical stenoses by increasing secretions or causing bleeding or edema. If the physician performing the endoscopy is unprepared to dilate the patient emergently, acute airway obstruction may develop and death ensue. Whenever severe airway stenosis is encountered, it is best not to manipulate the stenosis with the flexible bronchoscope. Proper evaluation should be performed in the operating room with facilities available to dilate the stenosis if necessary. In nonemergent cases, endoscopy is best performed as part of the planned surgical procedure.

As a general rule, the rigid bronchoscope is much more valuable in assessing airway pathology. Attempting to pass a large rigid bronchoscope beyond a tough, inflammatory stricture may be impossible, may result in tracheal rupture, or may cause total airway obstruction secondary to bleeding or edema. Jackson dilators passed through the rigid bronchoscope under direct vision and an assortment of graduated rigid bronchoscopes can be used to serially dilate postintubation and idiopathic strictures. By gradually dilating these tight, rigid strictures, the risk of perforation and bleeding is minimized. Racemic epinephrine and steroids are often used for 24 to 48 h to minimize subsequent reactive edema.

It is important to understand that dilation or endoscopic removal of malignant or inflammatory strictures is often only a temporizing measure. In the case of inflammatory stricture, restenosis usually develops within days to weeks. The use of these techniques in emergent situations allows more thorough evaluation of the patient and enables surgery to be performed electively. Many patients are on corticosteroids at the time of presentation and, by improving the airway, these may be tapered and discontinued. This will enable the operation to be performed at a later time without the threat of impaired healing.

The above maneuvers are also used in an elective operation when the patient has presented with a narrowed but not critical airway. Dilation with rigid bronchoscopy permits assessment of the distal airway, placement of an endotracheal tube, and provision of an adequate lumen to prevent carbon dioxide accumulation early in the procedure.

Tracheostomy may be necessary in some patients as the only method to secure an airway. If feasible, this should be placed through the most damaged portion of the trachea in order to preserve the maximal amount of normal trachea for subsequent reconstruction. If tracheostomy is contemplated at the completion of tracheal resection, which is rarely necessary, it should be placed at least two rings away from the anastomosis. The anastomosis should then be protected with the thyroid gland or strap muscles to avoid contamination of the suture line. This will lessen the likelihood of subsequent dehiscence or stenosis. A tracheostomy tube should never be placed through an anastomosis.

SURGICAL THERAPY

Anesthesia

Anesthesia for tracheal reconstruction, especially where there is a high degree of airway obstruction distally, is best administered by inhalational agents.[29] A slow, patient induction may be necessary if there is a high degree of airway obstruction. This is preferable and safer than paralysis of respiration with a consequent urgent need to establish an airway.

The surgeon should be available with an array of rigid bronchoscopes from pediatric to adult sizes as the induction commences. The residual airway through which the patient is breathing may measure as little as 2 or 3 mm in diameter. In most cases, tumors are not circumferential. After bronchoscopy, a small endotracheal tube can often be insinuated past a highly obstructive tumor. In other cases the tube is left above the tumor. This contrasts with the circumferential stenoses seen in some inflammatory lesions. In rare cases, it may be necessary to resect portions of tumor with biopsy forceps in order to enlarge the channel for passage of a tube.

At the time of tracheal division, this tube is pulled back or removed and a sterile cuffed, flexible, armored endotracheal tube is inserted into the distal airway across the operative field. Sterile connecting tubing is passed to the anesthesiologist to allow ventilation of the patient. This armored tube is removed whenever necessary for suctioning or placement of sutures. Toward the completion of the operation, the original endotracheal tube is advanced into the distal airway and the anastomotic sutures are tied. The patient should be breathing spontaneously at the end of the procedure so that extubation can be performed in the operating room. High-frequency ventilation has been used with equal success intraoperatively, but we have been quite satisfied with the technique described. High-frequency ventilation is especially useful in certain complex carinal reconstructions.

Ideally, the patient should be extubated and breathe spontaneously at the conclusion of the procedure. Particularly where the trachea has been greatly shortened, it is desirable not to have even a low-pressure cuff lying in contact with the anastomosis for any period of time. The use of cardiopulmonary bypass is not usually necessary in adult tracheal surgery, even in complex carinal reconstructions. However, it may be requisite in repairing congenital airway lesions in the pediatric population, especially in the presence and correction of cardiac anomalies.[30]

MANEUVERS TO MINIMIZE TENSION

Most tracheal operations can be performed without complex tracheal release maneuvers. The location of the lesion is an important factor in determining which procedures will be of benefit. Certain maneuvers are more effective for achieving additional length in performing surgery for disease in the cervical trachea, whereas others are more effective for the intrathoracic trachea. A release maneuver is primarily performed to prevent unnecessary tension on the anastomosis and avoid the need for excessive dissection of the trachea, which might jeopardize the lateral blood supply.

The simplest maneuver to minimize tension after tracheal resection for cervical pathology is flexion of the neck and mobilization of the pretracheal plane, avoiding the lateral blood supply to the trachea. Flexion of the neck between 15 and 35 degrees may result in downward movement of the trachea by as much as 4.5 cm, or the equivalent of seven tracheal rings. Flexion beyond this may achieve up to 1.5 cm of added length. The amount of trachea that may be removed with simple flexion varies greatly with the patient's age and physical habitus as well as other conditions. When these simple maneuvers fail to provide sufficient length, a Montgomery suprahyoid laryngeal release can be performed, generally before the anastomosis is completed.[31] This is accomplished by dividing the muscles that insert on the superior aspect of the hyoid bone. The hyoid bone is then divided just medial to the lesser cornua. When this maneuver is performed, an additional 1.5 cm of length can be obtained.

Flexion of the head and mobilization of the anterior surface of the trachea is also important for lower tracheal lesions. Laryngeal release has not been helpful in gaining additional length for intrathoracic tracheal lesions. Mobilization of the right hilum and inferior pulmonary ligament should be completed first. A U-shaped incision in the pericardium below the inferior pulmonary vein will allow the hilar structures and bronchus to advance in a cephalad fashion.[32] Additional length may be obtained by completely incising the pericardium around the hilar vessels.

TRACHEAL RESECTION

Cervical approach

The cervical or upper cervicomediastinal approach is used for limited tumors of the upper trachea and for almost all benign strictures of the trachea at any level.[33] The patient is usually anesthetized by inhalation and a

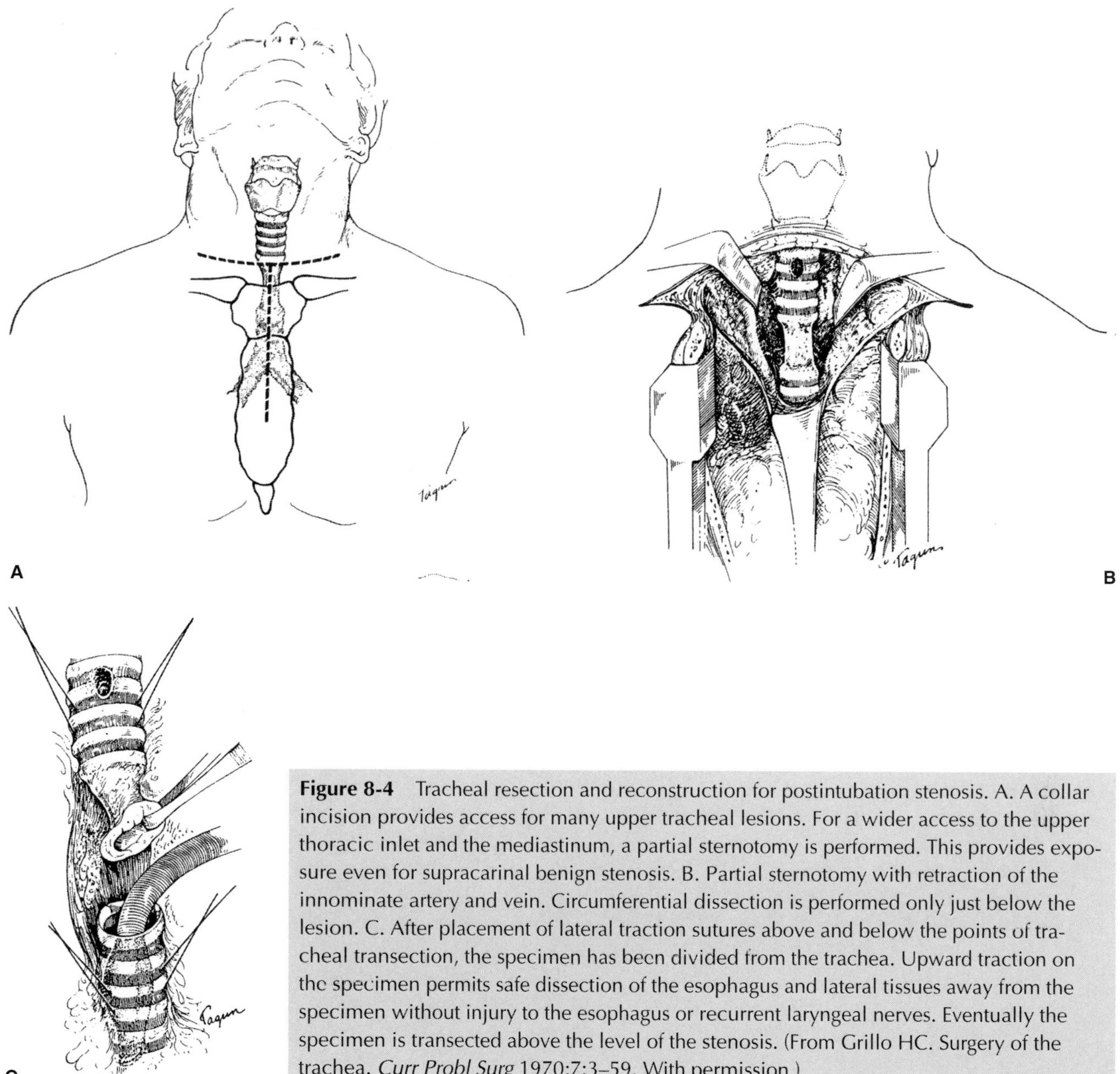

Figure 8-4 Tracheal resection and reconstruction for postintubation stenosis. A. A collar incision provides access for many upper tracheal lesions. For a wider access to the upper thoracic inlet and the mediastinum, a partial sternotomy is performed. This provides exposure even for supracarinal benign stenosis. B. Partial sternotomy with retraction of the innominate artery and vein. Circumferential dissection is performed only just below the lesion. C. After placement of lateral traction sutures above and below the points of tracheal transection, the specimen has been divided from the trachea. Upward traction on the specimen permits safe dissection of the esophagus and lateral tissues away from the specimen without injury to the esophagus or recurrent laryngeal nerves. Eventually the specimen is transected above the level of the stenosis. (From Grillo HC. Surgery of the trachea. *Curr Probl Surg* 1970;7:3–59. With permission.)

rigid bronchoscope is passed. A stricture less than 6 mm in diameter is dilated under direct vision with rigid pediatric bronchoscopes. If the stricture is greater than 6 mm in diameter, an endotracheal tube may be placed just above the lesion. If the lesion is subglottic, the stricture must be dilated and a small endotracheal tube passed through it. An endotracheal tube may be slipped past most tumors or through the cored center of the rare circumferential tumor. If jet ventilation is employed, a tube as small as 14F suffices.

The trachea is explored through a collar incision, which may circumcise an existing tracheal stoma (Fig. 8-4A). The anterior surface of the trachea is exposed from the cricoid cartilage to the carina. The thyroid isthmus is then divided, dissected from the trachea, and retracted laterally with sutures. In inflammatory lesions, it is essential to keep the dissection close against the trachea to avoid the risk of injury to the back wall of the innominate artery. If the lesion extends below the sternal notch, making it easily accessible through the collar incision, the exposure is increased by making a "T" incision, the vertical arm extending downward to a point 1 cm below the sternal angle (Fig. 8-4B). The sternum is divided to that point only and separated with a small chest spreader. Exposure is not improved with a full median sternotomy, since the carina lies at the level of the angle of Louis, and the great vessels, lying anteriorly, inhibit better visualization.

In cases of inflammatory stenosis, meticulous dissection is performed along the lateral aspects of only the involved trachea. If there is difficulty in identifying the level of the lesion, intraoperative bronchoscopy will facilitate its recognition. The position of the bronchoscope light is identified at the upper and then the lower extent of the lesion while an assistant pushes a #25 needle through the tracheal wall for precise localization. Dissection close to the tracheal wall or the scar replacing it avoids injury to the recurrent laryngeal nerves, which lie in the tracheoesophageal groove on either side. The nerves are intentionally not exposed. This is a particularly important point if the stenosis is located just below the cricoid cartilage, since the recurrent nerves enter the larynx just medial to the inferior cornua of the thyroid cartilages.

The trachea is then circumferentially dissected at the level immediately below the distal margin of the lesion (Fig. 8-4C). Sterile anesthesia equipment is assembled on the field prior to division of the trachea. Lateral traction sutures of 2-0 Vicryl are placed on either side of the trachea in the midlateral portion approximately 1 cm below the anticipated level of transection. These pass vertically through the full thickness of the tracheal wall and around one or more rings (Fig. 8-5A). The trachea is opened anteriorly just distal to the lesion, staying close to the lesion if it is benign. If the wall is still diseased at this point, a second incision is made one ring lower until good tissue is identified; then the trachea is transected. After the transection, an assistant maintains tension on the two lateral traction sutures and holds the flexible armored ventilating tube in the distal trachea. Circumferential dissection of the residual distal trachea is limited to its first 1 to 2 cm to protect the segmental blood supply. Devascularization invites necrosis and a possibly irreparable restenosis.

In the case of tumors of the upper trachea, since there is no peritracheal inflammation, the recurrent laryngeal nerves are usually identified and followed to above the level chosen for tracheal transection. This permits excision of paratracheal lymph nodes immediately adjacent to the tumor-bearing segment. To determine the appropriate level of tracheal transection, the trachea is initially opened through a tumor-free area at the level of the tumor.

Lateral traction sutures are placed proximally 1 cm above the proposed proximal level of transection. Again, no more than 1 cm of trachea is freed circumferentially. If the upper level of transection is at the inferior border of the cricoid cartilage, no attempt is made to dissect more cephalad posteriorly, since this would involve the zone of fusion between the upper esophagus and the cricoid, risking esophageal injury. To test the ease with which the tracheal ends can be brought together, the anesthetist flexes the patient's neck and the proximal and distal traction sutures are crossed, bringing the tracheal ends together. Importantly, the length of trachea that may be safely removed must be determined prior to division. Whether resection is feasible is usually based on radiologic and bronchoscopic measurements made prior to skin incision and rarely on surgical exploration.

Once it has been demonstrated that the anastomosis can be performed without excessive tension, the neck is again hyperextended. The first anastomotic suture—we prefer 4-0 coated Vicryl—is placed in the posterior midline with the lie outside, and the suture is clipped to the drapes above. The next suture is placed lateral to this and clipped to the drapes just caudad to the previous one. The sutures are thus serially inserted until a point is reached just posterior to the midlateral tracheal traction suture (Fig. 8-5A). The same placement of sutures is now carried out on the opposite side, from the posterior midline to the midlateral suture. Serial sutures are placed anteriorly, proceeding from the lateral traction sutures to the midline (Fig. 8-5B). The cross-field ventilatory tube may have to be removed intermittently for the placement of difficult sutures or drawn to one side as the sutures are inserted.

When all sutures have been placed, the oral endotracheal tube is advanced from above until the end is visible in the wound. The distal trachea is suctioned, the tube in it is withdrawn, and anesthesia is now resumed via the original endotracheal tube, which is advanced into the distal trachea beyond the anastomosis. The patient's head is firmly supported on blankets in full flexion and then the lateral traction sutures are crossed, pulled together on either side, and tied. The tracheal ends are apposed end-to-end, not deliberately intussuscepted.

The anterior anastomotic sutures are tied first, without tension, and the ends are cut after tying each. The assistant now rotates the trachea by gently drawing medially on the traction sutures on the surgeon's side of the table. The suture just posterior to the lateral traction suture is tied, as then are the rest of the posterior sutures. This is then repeated on the opposite side (Fig. 8-5C). The ends of traction sutures are removed, leaving their knotted loops in place to guard against tension on the anastomotic sutures. The integrity of the anastomosis is checked under saline. Flat, closed suction drains are placed in the pretracheal and substernal spaces, and the strap muscles are approximated in the midline.

After the incision has been closed, a heavy suture is placed through the skin crease beneath the chin and through the presternal skin. Two sutures, one on each side, may be used if a midline incision was necessary. These sutures are tied with the patient's neck in flexion to guard against sudden hyperextension of the neck in the first week following operation.

The patient is usually extubated as he or she awakens. An unsatisfactory airway at this point is not likely to improve unless the problem is secondary to laryngeal edema. If this is the case, a small endotracheal tube can be left in position until the problem subsides. It is preferable to leave the cuff deflated if possible.

Transthoracic approach

The transthoracic approach utilizing a posterolateral thoracotomy through the fourth intercostal space is used for tumors of the lower trachea and carina and for a few

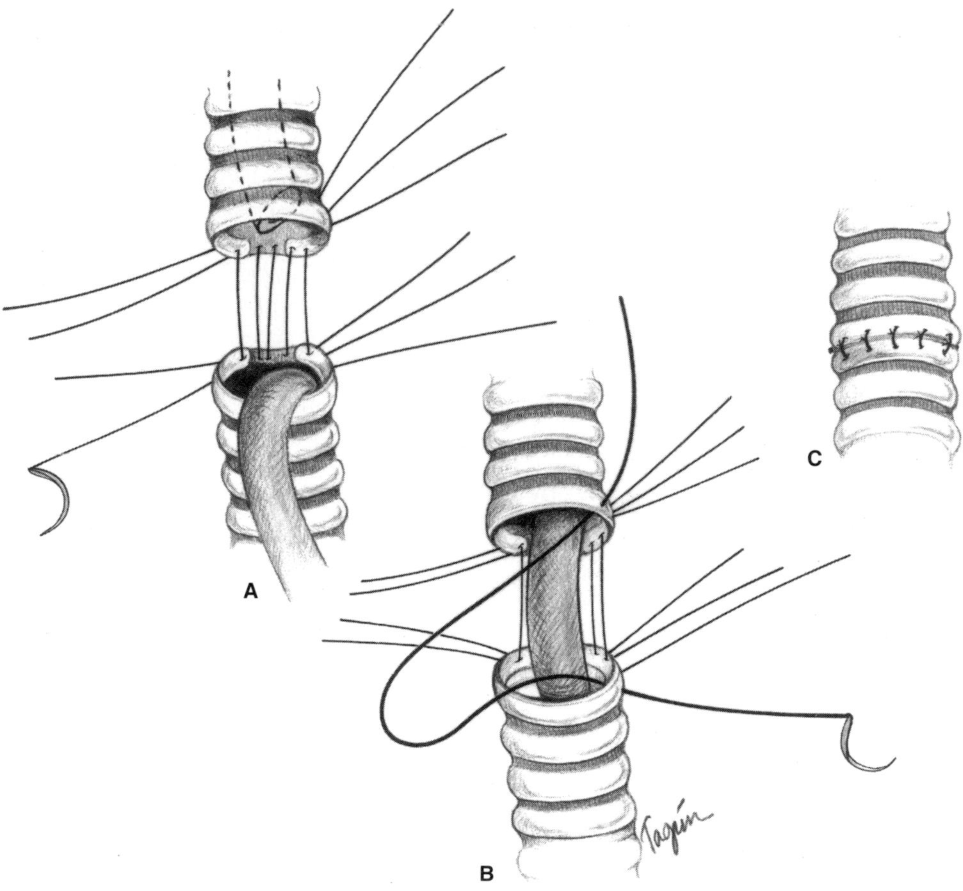

Figure 8-5 A. Tracheal anastomosis. Sutures are placed individually, beginning in the midline posteriorly and ranging anteriorly on either side. B. After the sutures have been placed on either side up to the level of the midlateral traction sutures, the anterior sutures are placed. Frequently, the endotracheal tube is not advanced from above until after all sutures have been placed. C. The neck is placed in the flexed position and the lateral traction sutures are tied on either side (not shown) to remove tension from the anastomotic sutures. After this, anastomotic sutures are tied from anterior to posterior on either side. The completed anastomosis is airtight. (From Grillo HC. Surgery of the trachea. *Curr Probl Surg* 1970;7:3–59. With permission.)

inflammatory lesions. The right arm is draped free, and the neck and anterior chest are included in the field. This allows for alteration of the incision or the addition of a cervical component should laryngeal release or other maneuvers be necessary. An extra long, single lumen endotracheal tube with sufficient diameter is used to intubate a main bronchus.

Dissection of the thoracic trachea is carried out in a similar fashion to that for more proximal pathology. In cases of malignancy, an effort is made to resect surrounding tissues with the tumor. Eventually, the trachea is dissected circumferentially below the tumor and sometimes above it, although the upper portion of the dissection can be completed after division of the trachea below. Traction sutures are placed in the midlateral tracheal wall distal to the tumor. If the transection is close to the carina, the sutures are placed in the lateral walls of the right and left main bronchi. Again, anesthesia tubing brought across the field is joined to a flexible armored tube placed in the distal trachea or, preferably, the left main bronchus to allow collapse of the right lung for better exposure during the anastomosis. If this results in significant intrapulmonary shunting, the right pulmonary artery may be gently clamped.

Flexion of the neck, even with the patient in the lateral thoracotomy position, delivers the proximal trachea into the thorax. Dissection anterior to the trachea and both main bronchi will provide additional mobility. These are important maneuvers in obtaining a tension-free anastomosis. In the resection of a malignant tumor, paratracheal and subcarinal lymph nodes that are not in proximity to the mass should not be radically resected for fear of devascularizing the airway. The technique of anastomosis is similar to that used in the upper trachea.

LARYNGOTRACHEAL TRAUMA

The laryngotracheal junction is the most frequent location of injury in airway trauma. The most important initial aspect of treating a laryngotracheal injury is the establishment and maintenance of an airway. The wound is debrided and those familiar with the techniques of tracheal repair may directly anastomose the trachea. If the surgeon lacks experience or if other life-threatening injuries demand, it is preferable to anchor the distal trachea to the base of the neck and place a tracheostomy tube in the distal separated end. In this case, distal tracheostomy should not be done, as it will only further injure tracheal tissue and provide no advantage over a tube placed in the already divided end. Secondary repair can be performed at a later date. If tracheal repair is performed, it will be necessary in most cases to place a small protective tracheostomy approximately 2 cm below the anastomosis. This serves to compensate for severely impaired glottic function due to concurrent injuries to the recurrent laryngeal nerve.

Traumatic lacerations of the lower trachea can often be repaired through an anterior approach. This can be achieved either through a partial sternotomy or, if addressing cardiac injuries, through a full sternotomy with additional exposure obtained using anterior and posterior pericardiotomies between the superior vena cava and aorta. For those less familiar with this approach, the lowermost trachea as well as carinal and bronchial ruptures are best approached through a right posterolateral thoracotomy.

SLIDE TRACHEOPLASTY

Three surgical techniques have been described for correction of congenital tracheal stenoses. First, tracheal resection and reconstruction in children has been described.[34,35] This has limited utility in the pediatric population, as only a finite length of trachea, approximately 25 to 30 percent, can be resected and followed by end-to-end suture before excessive anastomotic tension may result in separation.[36] To address this issue, patients with long congenital stenoses have been treated with an anterior tracheoplasty and patch repair with costal cartilage or pericardium.[37,38] The latter must be suspended to the mediastinum, and all patch techniques require prolonged stenting with intubation during early healing. This approach has also been complicated by the formation of excessive granulation tissue arising from the mesenchymal surface of the patches, often requiring multiple bronchoscopic debridements. These patches can also suffer from necrosis and or collapse, necessitating reoperation. Goldstraw introduced slide tracheoplasty as an alternative to the management of patients with long-segment congenital tracheal stenosis.[39]

The surgical approach for these lesions is similar to that utilized for tracheal pathology in adults. The upper and lower ends of the stenotic segment are precisely identified, so that the lesion might be divided horizontally at its midpoint (Fig. 8-6A). Dissection is carried circumferentially around the midpoint of the stenotic segment only. It is helpful to place traction sutures of 3-0 Vicryl in the midlateral point of the tracheobronchial junction on either side or in the proximal right and left main bronchi (Fig. 8-6B). Following transection of the trachea, intubation and ventilation are carried out across the operative field.

Vertical divisions of the proximal and distal segments are next carried out (Fig. 8-6B and C). It is essential that the full length of stenosis be incised. The right-angled corners of tracheal wall represented by the meeting points of the vertical and horizontal incisions are trimmed to make a gently sloping corner (Fig. 8-6D). The lateral blood supply is hardly disturbed for the lower segment, as the vertical incision is based anteriorly. For the upper segment, however, somewhat more circumferential dissection is necessary. A single 3-0 Vicryl suture is placed through and through the tracheal wall close to the distal tip of the upper flap for traction (Fig. 8-6C). The anastomosis is created using techniques similar to those described earlier (Fig. 8-6D and E).

TRACHEOESOPHAGEAL FISTULAS

We have proposed a conservative approach to the management of acquired, nonmalignant tracheoesophageal fistulas.[40] As stated previously, the majority of these result from complications of mechanical ventilation and most are actually diagnosed while patients are being mechanically ventilated. This important fact dictates our approach to this problem.

It is known from our experience with tracheal reconstruction for postintubation tracheal stenosis that postoperative mechanical ventilation is associated with a higher incidence of anastomotic complications.[41] Most tracheoesophageal fistulas require tracheal resection because of circumferential injury to the trachea or size of the fistula. We have therefore adopted an approach that delays definitive correction of the fistula until patients have been successfully weaned from mechanical ventilation.

The devastating pulmonary complications from tracheoesophageal fistulas can be minimized by a few simple maneuvers. A new tracheostomy tube should be placed so that the balloon is below the fistula, so as to minimize soiling of the tracheobronchial tree. A draining gastrostomy tube should be placed to minimize gastroesophageal reflux, and a feeding jejunostomy tube should be placed for nutritional supplementation. These measures should obviate the need for esophageal diversion and ligation of the gastroesophageal junction. Esophageal diversion should be reserved for continued soilage of the tracheobronchial tree despite the previously mentioned measures or for supracarinal fistulas that

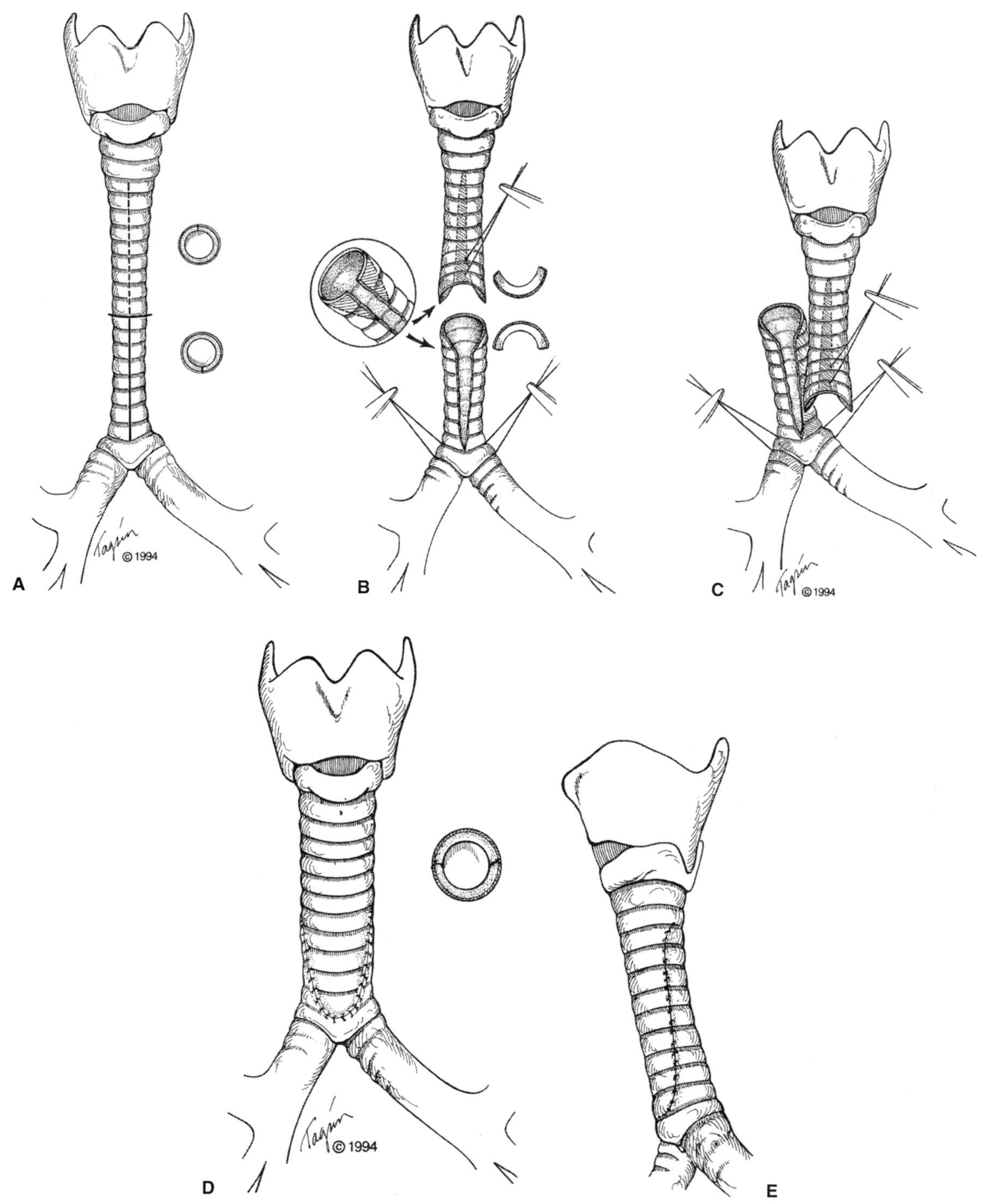

Figure 8-6 Technique of slide tracheoplasty. A. The extent of stenosis is precisely identified. The stenotic segment is divided transversely in its midpoint after circumferential dissection at that locus only. The upper stenotic segment is incised vertically posteriorly, and the lower segment is incised anteriorly for the full length of stenosis. B. The right-angled corners produced by these divisions are trimmed above and below. A stay suture near the tip of the superior flap and traction sutures at the tracheobronchial angles or main bronchi are both helpful. Minimal dissection of lateral blood supply is performed. C. The two ends are pulled together after placement of individual anastomotic sutures around the entire oblique circumference of the tracheoplasty. D and E. The circumference is doubled, resulting in a fourfold increase in cross-sectional area. (From Grillo HC. Slide tracheoplasty for long segment tracheal congenital stenosis. *Ann Thorac Surg* 1994;59:613–621. Reprinted by permission from the Society of Thoracic Surgeons.)

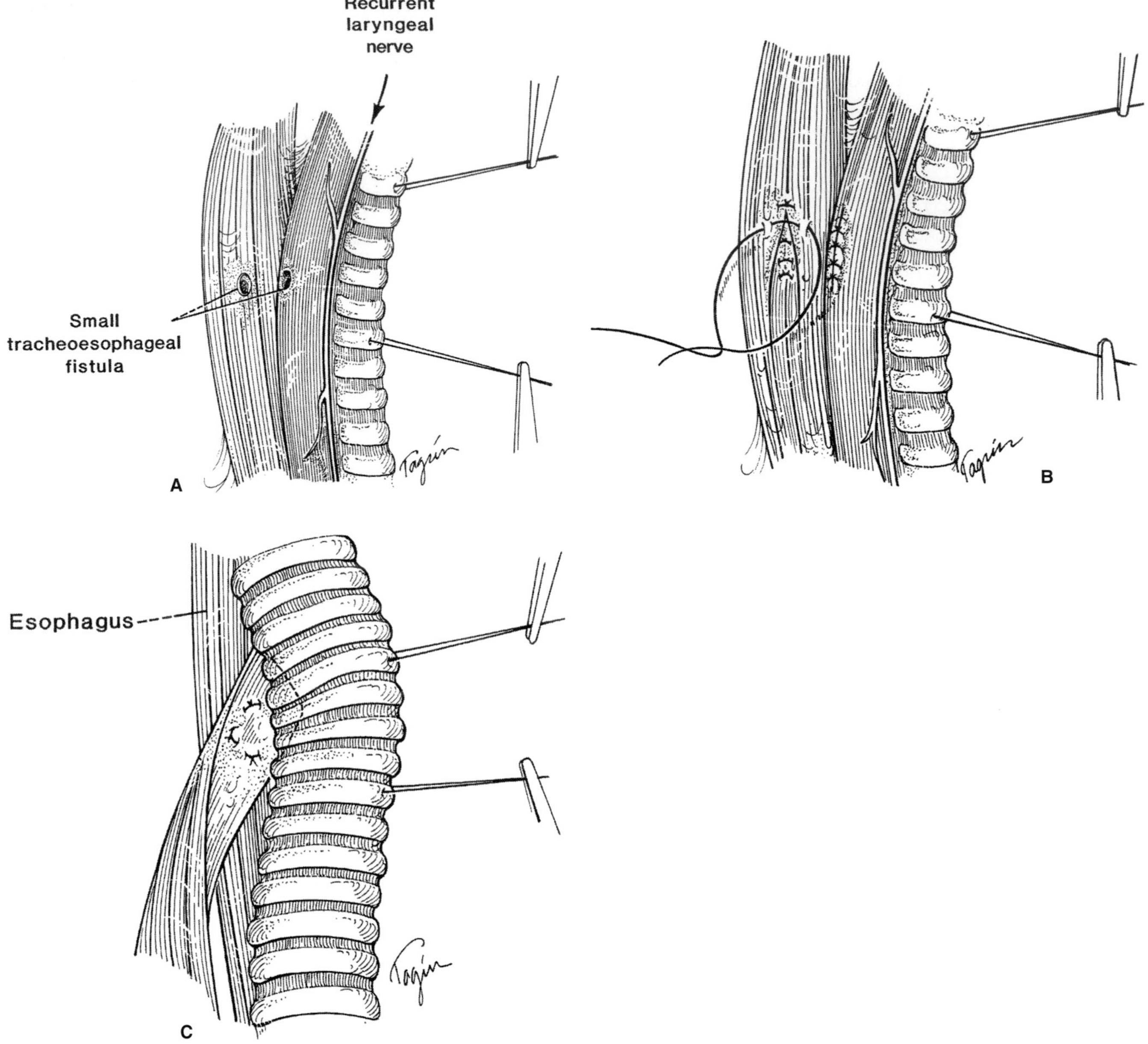

Figure 8-7 A and B. Small tracheoesophageal fistula treated by division and local repair. The recurrent laryngeal nerve is elevated with the trachea. The esophagus is closed in two layers. C. A strap muscle is used to cover the esophageal suture line and separate it from the tracheal suture line. (From Mathisen DJ, Grillo HC, Wain JC, Hilgenberg AD. Management of acquired nonmalignant tracheoesophageal fistula. *Ann Thorac Surg* 1991;52:759–765. Reprinted with permission from the Society of Thoracic Surgeons.)

cannot be controlled otherwise. Once the patient is weaned from mechanical ventilation, single-stage repair can be undertaken without the risks of postoperative ventilation.

The principles of tracheal surgery must be closely followed, since many of these cases are reoperations or associated with more than the usual amount of inflammation. The most important initial decision is to determine whether the fistula can be simply resected and closed or whether tracheal resection and reconstruction will be required.

Most tracheoesophageal fistulas are approached through a low collar incision often including the tracheostomy stoma if present. A right lateral thoracotomy through the fourth interspace is preferable for fistulas at or just above the carina or in the case of a reoperation if the previous procedure was performed through the chest.

The small tracheoesophageal fistula that does not require tracheal resection poses unique technical problems (Fig. 8-7A). Care must be taken to avoid injury to the recurrent laryngeal nerves, as local inflammation may make their identification difficult. In these circumstances, it is best to identify the nerves at a location remote from the fistula. The nerves should be elevated with the trachea during exposure of the fistula.

Once the fistula is identified, it should be divided. We prefer to close the tracheal defect with absorbable suture material (4-0 Vicryl). The esophageal defect is then closed in two layers (Fig. 8-7B). A local strap muscle is mobilized to buttress and separate the tracheal and esophageal suture lines (Fig. 8-7C). This should minimize the risk of recurrent fistula.

The fistula that requires tracheal resection, although technically more complicated, provides significantly improved exposure. Circumferential dissection above and below the fistula should be very close to the trachea to avoid injury to the recurrent nerves. Resection of the damaged portion of the trachea gives excellent exposure of the esophageal defect (Fig. 8-8A). The esophageal defect is closed longitudinally in two layers (Fig. 8-8B). It is essential to separate the esophageal suture line with a local strap muscle to help prevent recurrent tracheoesophageal fistula (Fig. 8-8C). Tracheal reconstruction is performed as detailed earlier (Fig. 8-8D).

IDIOPATHIC LARYNGOTRACHEAL STENOSIS

Inflammatory stenosis of the upper trachea, which also involves the subglottic larynx, cannot be treated by simple circumferential resection, since this would destroy the function of the recurrent laryngeal nerves. Many complex and multistaged procedures have been devised to solve this problem. In an effort to improve the results obtained by such operations, single-stage procedures involving partial resection of the subglottic larynx and immediate plastic reconstruction by varying techniques have evolved. Systematic approaches to this problem have been made by Ogura and Roper,[42] Gerwat and Bryce,[43] Pearson and coworkers,[44] Couraud and associates,[45] and Grillo.[17] All reported surprisingly good results using single-stage laryngotracheoplastic procedures.

In those patients in whom the stenotic process involves only the anterior portion of the subglottic larynx, resection of this portion of the cricoid arch is sufficient (Fig. 8-9). The posterior margin of resection is along the lower border of the cricoid cartilage.

In patients with circumferential subglottic lesions extending in front of the posterior plate of the cricoid, the line of posterior mucosal resection is incised above the level of stenosis, approaching the arytenoid cartilages (Fig. 8-10A). All involved mucosa and scar tissue is excised from the front of the posterior cricoid plate, leaving the cartilage intact posteriorly to be surfaced by a broad-based flap of membranous trachea advanced from below (Fig. 8-10B). The posterior cricoid plate itself is usually not significantly involved. The plane between mucosa and cartilage can be dissected with a scalpel or bluntly with a fine dental spatula. One must stop short of the superior border of the cricoid plate, which lies immediately below the arytenoid cartilages. No attempt is made to groove or otherwise alter the posterior cricoid cartilage itself. Division of the trachea is also carried out differently. Posteriorly, a flap of membranous wall is fashioned (Fig. 8-10C). When the anastomosis is made, the posterior mucosal sutures pass only through the full thickness of mucosa and submucosa of the posterior wall of the larynx and then through the full thickness of the membranous wall of the trachea (Figure 8-10D).

The margin of the anterior defect in the subglottic larynx is sutured in both types of resection to a prow-shaped segment of one distal tracheal ring (Fig. 8-9D). The midline of the thyroid cartilage is approximated to the midline of the peak of the most proximal cartilage of the trachea. The traction sutures are tied and followed by the individual anastomotic sutures.

RESULTS

CONGENITAL STENOSIS

We have generally followed a conservative therapeutic approach to airway lesions in infants and small children. As indicated earlier, the juvenile trachea tolerates anastomotic tension less well than the adult. Furthermore, following anastomosis, a small amount of edema in a small airway may cause more significant obstruction than a similar thickness of edema in the adult. While growth of a stenosis is in general proportional to that of the normal tissues and does not actually correct congenital stenosis, sufficient improvement may obviate the need for correction or permit the patient to grow, so that surgical reconstruction can be performed with less risk. As described earlier, most cases of congenital tracheal stenosis are best addressed with slide tracheoplasty.

On completion of this procedure, the circumference of the trachea is doubled, the cross-sectional area is quadrupled, and the stenotic segment is shortened by half. It is clearly advantageous to have the trachea repaired with the tracheal wall containing native cartilages and normal tracheal epithelium. It has been demonstrated that this repair provides a permanent enlargement of the airway diameter and does not inhibit subsequent tracheal growth.[46]

Since the introduction of slide tracheoplasty at the Massachusetts General Hospital in 1991, we have treated eight patients ranging in age from 10 days to 19 years with stenoses varying in length and location as well as other associated congenital lesions.[47] All patients survived and obtained a widely patent and stable airway. In all juvenile patients, the repaired tracheal segment continued to grow. Given the intolerance of tension in juvenile tracheal anastomosis, slide tracheoplasty should, in our opinion, be considered for all but the shortest stenotic segments.

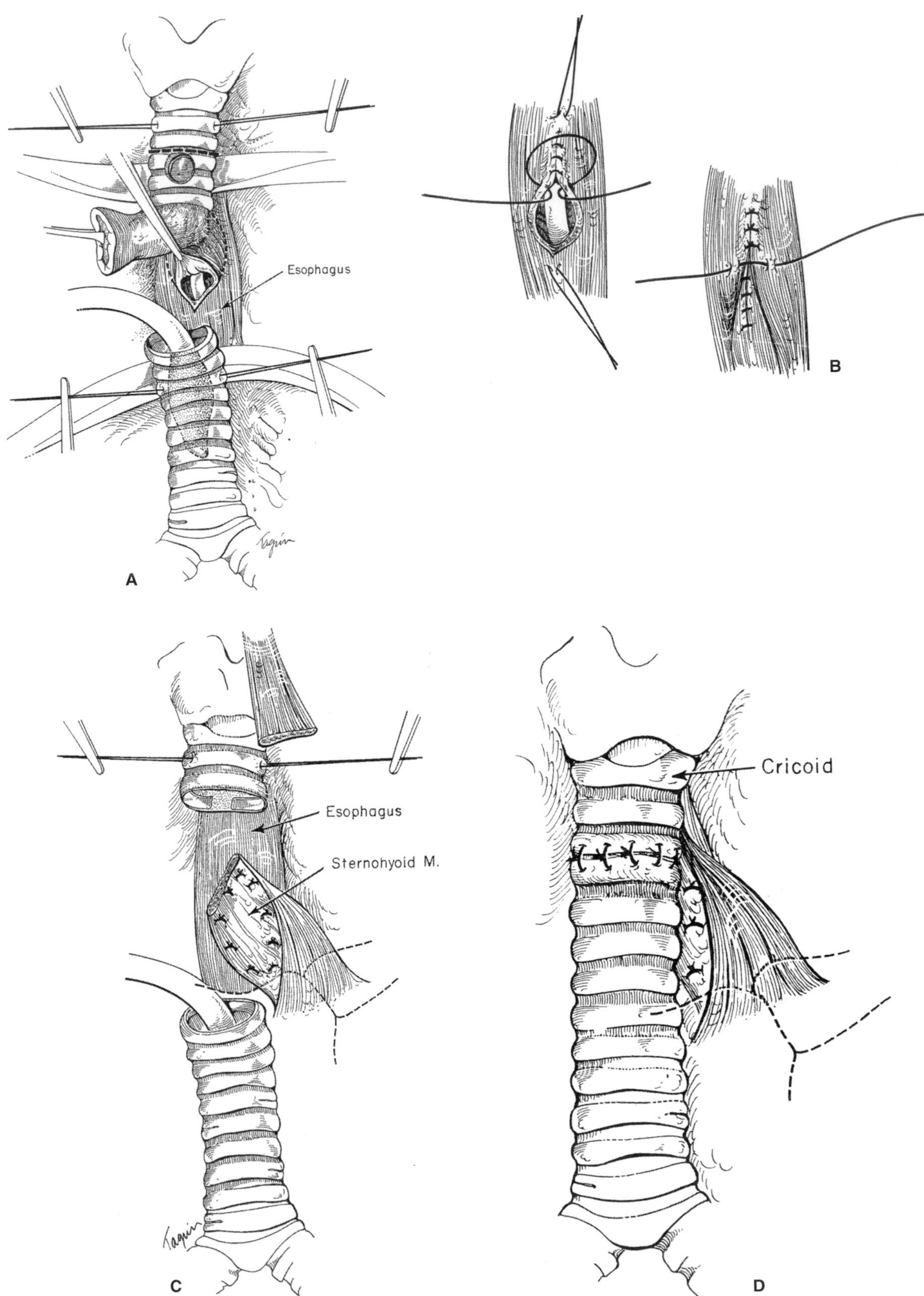

Figure 8-8 A. Circumferential dissection above and below the fistula is near the trachea to avoid injury to the recurrent nerves. Division of damaged trachea gives excellent exposure to the esophageal defect. B. The esophageal defect is closed in two layers. C. A local strap muscle is used to buttress the esophageal closure and separate it from the tracheal suture line. M = muscle. D. Completed tracheal anastomosis, with strap muscle posterior to it separating it from the esophageal suture line. (From Mathisen DJ, Grillo HC, Wain JC, Hilgenberg AD. Management of acquired nonmalignant tracheoesophageal fistula. *Ann Thorac Surg* 1991;52:759–765. Reprinted with permission from the Society of Thoracic Surgeons.)

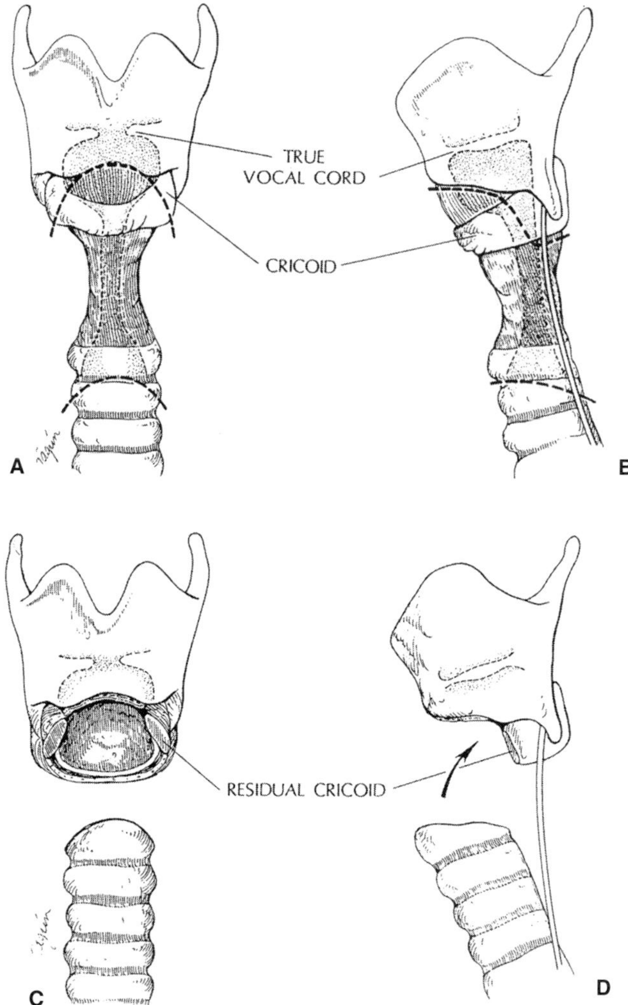

Figure 8-9 Operative repair of anterolateral stenosis of the subglottic larynx and upper trachea. A. Anteroposterior view. B. Lateral view. The figures demonstrate the extent of stenosis and ultimate lines of transection. The stenosis extends into the subglottic larynx well above the border of the cricoid anteriorly. There is, however, no involvement of the posterior mucosal wall of the subglottic larynx or of the upper trachea. The proximal line of transection is centered in the midline to divide the larynx from the trachea posteriorly at the lower border of the posterior cricoid lamina or cricoid plate. Inferiorly, the most proximal tracheal ring of residual trachea is cut backward to posterior ends. C and D. Larynx and trachea after removal of the specimen. The recurrent laryngeal nerves have been left intact but are not dissected out, as might be suggested by the diagrammatic representation. The mucous membrane of the larynx has been transected sharply at the same level of division as the cartilage.

POSTTRAUMATIC STENOSIS

Earlier we published our experience in treating traumatic injuries to the airway.[12] In this series, 10 patients with acute injuries and 17 with delayed traumatic laryngotracheal stenosis were evaluated and treated. All 10 of the acute injuries had excellent airway preservation; voice was preserved and successful repair of the esophagus made in one. Repair of delayed stenosis was successful in 16 of 17 patients. All but one patient had preservation of voice, despite the presence of vocal cord paralysis in 14 patients preoperatively. The cases of concomitant esophageal injury, present in four patients, were successfully repaired without development of tracheoesophageal fistula.

POSTINTUBATION STENOSIS

Postintubation tracheal injuries remain the most common indication for tracheal resection and reconstruction, despite definition of the etiology of these lesions and development of techniques for their avoidance. We reported 503 patients who underwent tracheal resection and reconstruction for postintubation lesions.[41] The balloon cuff of an endotracheal or tracheostomy tube accounted for 251 lesions; 178 lesions were at the site of a tracheostomy, and 38 patients had evidence of both lesions. In 36 patients, the exact site was uncertain, often due to prior attempts at treatment including multiple tracheostomies. Of the 503 patients, 441 had lesions that were isolated to the trachea, while 62 had concomitant involvement of the subglottic larynx.

Many patients had undergone prior attempts at surgical treatment before referral. These included resection (n = 53); tracheal operations such as wedge resection, splinting, or fissure (n = 31); and laryngeal procedures such as stenting, grafting, or fissure (n = 20). Sixty patients had had T tubes placed and at least 45 had had laser treatment. Eight patients had prior repairs of tracheoesophageal fistula, three of which had failed.

The initial procedure was carried out through a cervical incision in 350 patients. In 145 patients a partial upper sternal division through the sternal angle was used, with 2 more patients requiring the addition of right anterior thoracotomy to this approach. Six patients underwent repair via a high posterolateral thoracotomy. The amount of trachea resected ranged from 1.0 to 7.5 cm and was most commonly between 2 and 4 cm.

Of the 503 initial operations, 324 involved a trachea-to-trachea anastomosis and 117 patients had reconstructions involving partial resection of the cricoid cartilage with laryngotracheal anastomosis. In the total series of 503 patients 9.7 percent underwent laryngeal releases. However, only 8 percent of the 450 patients who had not undergone tracheal resection and reconstruction previously were deemed to need laryngeal release to reduce anastomotic tension, in comparison with 24.5 percent of the 53 who had prior resection and reconstruction. Many in the former group represent our earlier experience in tracheal surgery. Only one patient required intrapericardial hilar release.

The results have been classified as good, satisfactory, failure, and death. The result is described as good if the patient is functionally able to perform usual activities and

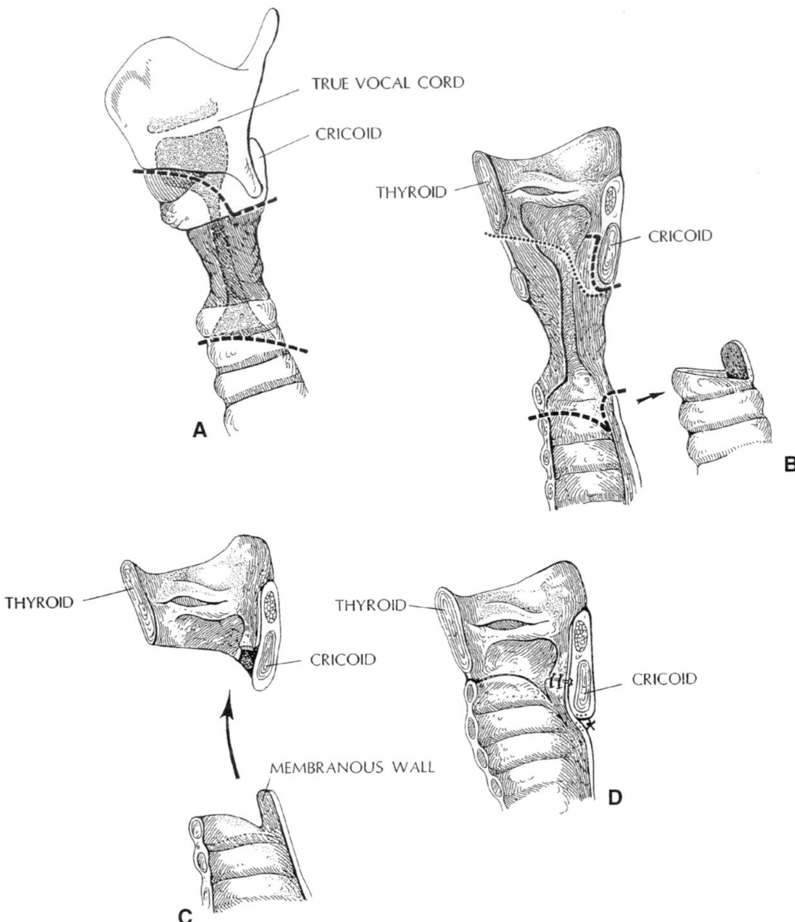

Figure 8-10 Resection and reconstruction of circumferential stenosis of the subglottic larynx and upper trachea. A. External line of cartilaginous division of both larynx and trachea is the same as for anterolateral stenosis. B. Interior views of the larynx and trachea demonstrate modifications necessary when the stenosis involves the mucosa and submucosa just in front of the posterior cricoid plate. The superior dotted line indicates that the mucosa with its scarring will be cut back to within a short distance, if necessary, of the arytenoid cartilages. Inferiorly, the posterior membranous wall has been retained as a broad-based flap. C. Resected specimen, leaving a bare area of the intraluminal portion of the lower part of the cricoid posterior lamina. The flap of membranous wall of the trachea will be fitted into this defect to provide prompt and complete mucosal coverage. D. The mucosa of the larynx has been anastomosed to the mucosa of the membranous wall of the trachea. External to the lumen, connective tissue of the membranous wall has been fixed with four sutures to the inferior margin of the cricoid cartilage, ensuring that the flap will stay firmly applied to the surface. (From Grillo HC. Reconstruction after subglottic laryngeal and upper tracheal stenosis resection. *Ann Thorac Surg* 1982;33:3–18. Reprinted with permission from the Society of Thoracic Surgeons.)

postoperative roentgenograms or bronchoscopic examinations show an anatomically good airway. Patients are placed in the satisfactory category if they can perform normal activities but are stressed on exercise. In the absence of symptoms, this is also applied to those with abnormalities involving the vocal cords or those with significant airway narrowing evident on either endoscopic or roentgenologic examination. Failure indicates the need for a permanent tracheostomy or T tube.

The average length of follow-up was 3 years. The results were categorized as good in 440 patients and satisfactory in 31 patients; there were 20 failures and

12 deaths. Failure was treated with tracheostomy (n = 11), T tube (n = 7), or dilations (n = 2).

IDIOPATHIC LARYNGOTRACHEAL STENOSIS

In experienced hands, laryngotracheal resection and reconstruction is associated with excellent results and minor complications. The experience in treating this rare entity at the Massachusetts General Hospital in 35 patients was published by Grillo,[17] with a subsequent update including 73 patients by Ashiku et al.[18]

All but two patients were female. The duration of symptoms before evaluation varied between 4 months to 32 years, with the greatest number reporting 1 to 3 years of symptoms. At the time of referral, a total of at least 75 procedures had been performed on 28 of the 73 patients. The extent of surgical resection ranged from 1 to 5 cm with an average of 2.6 cm. Resection of the entire anterior cricoid was performed in 59 patients, while only partial or no cricoid resection was necessary in 10 and 4 patients, respectively. Thirty-six patients required mucosal resection from the posterior cricoid plate, with tracheal membranous wall advancement flap reconstruction.

Extubation in the operating room was possible in 67 of the 73 patients. These patients did not require further airway intervention during their initial hospital stay. Immediate protective tracheostomies were placed in five patients; however, only one was used in the last 30 patients of this series. One patient had a negative reexploration for postoperative cervical subcutaneous emphysema. Six patients underwent early dilation for obstructing granulation tissue.

In long-term follow-up, 66 (92 percent) of 72 patients had either excellent (n = 19) or good (n = 47) results. Of the remainder, 5 required only occasional dilations. A poor result was seen in one patient in whom at least yearly dilations became necessary. No patients in this series have required permanent tracheostomies or T tubes. Additionally, there was no perioperative mortality.

TRACHEOESOPHAGEAL FISTULA

We have reported our results on the treatment of benign acquired tracheoesophageal fistulas in 38 patients.[40] The vast majority resulted from the combined effects of a nasogastric tube and either an endotracheal tube or a tracheostomy tube. The remainder were secondary to laryngotracheal trauma (n = 5) and complications of radiation therapy (n = 2) and anterior spinal fusion (n = 2).

Eight patients had undergone attempted repair at other institutions. Many had more than one attempted repair. The reasons for failure included the need for postoperative mechanical ventilation and failure to interpose tissue between tracheal and esophageal suture lines. Seven patients from other institutions underwent esophageal diversion with cervical esophagostomy or pharyngostomy and three had ligation or interruption of the gastroesophageal junction.

Tracheal resection and reconstruction was performed in 31 patients. This was done to address the presence of full-thickness circumferential damage at the level of the tracheal pathology or when the defect in the membranous tracheal wall was too large for direct closure. Six of these patients additionally had longitudinal closure of the membranous wall of the trachea where the fistula had been located. The amount of injured trachea would have been too excessive to allow reconstruction otherwise. Five patients had laryngotracheal resection because of pathology involving the subglottic larynx. Tracheal damage was too extensive in one patient to allow tracheal resection; therefore a T tube was placed following repair of the fistula. There has been no recurrence of the fistula in this patient and a good airway is maintained in this fashion.

Thirty-three patients had direct closure of the esophageal fistula utilizing a two-layer closure as described. Some narrowing of the esophageal lumen is inevitable in this situation but is well tolerated by most patients. Because of prior cervical esophagostomy, five patients underwent end-to-end esophageal anastomosis. Thirty-four patients had interposition of a local strap muscle between the esophageal and tracheal suture lines. Cervicomediastinal exenteration with creation of a mediastinal tracheostomy and a substernal colon bypass was required for a tracheoesophageal fistula following laryngectomy and irradiation.

Four patients died following repair of tracheoesophageal fistulas (10.5 percent). Three of these died following attempted transthoracic repair of very distal tracheoesophageal fistulas. All had extensive mediastinal sepsis at the time of repair and required mechanical ventilation after surgery. The fourth death occurred in a young man who underwent extensive tracheal resection with laryngeal release. Tracheal separation occurred on the sixth postoperative day and the patient could not be resuscitated.

Two patients developed small recurrent tracheoesophageal fistulas requiring reoperation. Both had previous cervical esophagostomies and required end-to-end anastomoses. Theses recurrent fistulas were small and were successfully managed by short tracheal resection and closure of the esophageal defect. Tracheal stenosis developed at the level of the retained stoma in one patient and was corrected by a second tracheal resection.

Of the 34 surviving patients, 33 were able to take aliment orally. Five patients required esophageal dilatation for narrowing at the level of the repair of the esophageal fistula. None still require dilation. The one patient who does not take aliment orally is also one of two patients requiring a tracheal appliance to provide an airway.

Another patient requires a T tube because of the extent of injury to her airway.

Single-stage repair of a tracheoesophageal fistula gives excellent results, with a low incidence of recurrent fistulas. These results continue to support the approach outlined for management of acquired nonmalignant tracheoesophageal fistulas.

PRIMARY TRACHEAL TUMORS

Gaissert[22] has recently presented our 40-year cumulative experience at Massachusetts General Hospital of treating primary adenoid cystic carcinomas (ACCs) and squamous cell carcinomas (SCCs) of the trachea. During this time, 270 patients were evaluated, with histologic distribution equally distributed between ACC and SCC. Resection was performed in 191 (71 percent) patients, with an operative mortality of 7.3 percent (14 of 191). Importantly, both rates of resection and hospital mortality have improved with each decade (Table 8-1). As our experience has grown, operative mortality has decreased from 21 percent in the 1960s to 3 percent in this last decade.

Resection was not performed in 79 patients, 34 in those with ACC (25 percent) and 45 patients with SCC (33 percent). Contraindications to resection have included tumor length (67 percent) and locoregional extent (24 percent) in the vast majority of cases, with distant metastases only rarely present (7 percent). The determination of unresectability was made during operative exploration in 17 of 208 patients (8 percent). ACCs tended to be longer lesions and were also associated with more significant locoregional extension. This explains the more frequent observation of ACC resection with positive microscopic tracheal and radial margins (59 percent) as compared with SCCs (18 percent).

The overall survival for all patients with primary tracheal carcinoma was 84 percent at 1 year, 45 percent at 5 years, and 25 percent at 10 years. Mean survival was 38 months in resected SCCs, 8.8 months in resectable SCCs, 69 months in resected ACCs, and 41 months in unresectable ACCs. Notably, survival after incomplete resection of ACCs was still 14.5 percent at 15 years. Multivariate analysis identified ACCs and complete resection to be associated with 5-year survival and ACCs, complete resection, and age to be associated with 10-year survival. Tumor length, lymph node status, or type of resection did not influence long-term survival.

The presence of tumor at the resection margins of ACCs, even by frozen section during operation, has particular importance in airway reconstruction. The surgeon must often compromise complete resection for the sake of safety, and the above data indicate that a small though not statistically significant survival benefit exists in these patients. All these patients now receive postoperative irradiation. Suture line recurrence thus far has been rare, and late recurrence has been that of distant disease. In contrast, irradiation of unresected tumor is all but uniformly characterized by local recurrence in 3 to 5 years despite a good response early.

The analysis of this 40-year experience with surgical management of primary tumors of the trachea appears to confirm and extend conclusions based on previously reported experiences.[48] Primary ACCs and SCCs of the trachea are best treated by resection when primary reconstruction may be safely accomplished. Resection should be followed by full-dose mediastinal irradiation in most cases.

COMPLICATIONS

Complications following tracheal surgery are similar regardless of the problem for which resection and reconstruction is performed. Wright and colleagues[49] recently presented the most complete analysis of anastomotic complications after tracheal resection. This review of 901 patients identifies relevant risk factors for the development of these problems and further describes their management. Anastomotic complications include granulations at the suture line, stenosis, and tracheal separation.

A significant reduction in suture granuloma formation has been seen since the conversion to absorbable suture material used for the anastomosis. In fact, the use of absorbable Vicryl sutures since 1978 has all but eliminated suture-related granulations. These can be successfully managed with bronchoscopic suture removal and local steroid injection. More extensive processes may require reoperation for resection, T-tube placement, or tracheostomy.

Table 8-1 Experience with primary tracheal carcinoma over four decades at Massachusetts General Hospital[a]

Decade	Total patients (N)	ACC patients (N)	SCC patients (N)	Resections performed (N)	Resection rate (%)	Hospital mortality (%)
1962–1971	19	7	12	13	68	21
1972–1981	54	29	25	33	61	11
1982–1991	107	54	53	71	66	5
1992–2001	88	43	45	72	82	3
Total	268	133	135	189	71	7

ACC = adenoid cystic carcinoma; SCC = squamous cystic carcinoma.

[a]Two patients operated on in 2002 were excluded from the table.

Stenosis and separation of a tracheal, carinal, or bronchial anastomosis are feared complications of airway reconstructive surgery. Excessive tension on an anastomosis is probably the most frequent cause of technical failures. Dangerous tensions may appear after resection of more than 50 percent of the trachea in the adult and of more than 30 to 40 percent in the child. These are very general percentages and do not apply to specific individuals, who may vary widely with respect to age, body habitus, pathology, prior surgery, and other comorbidities. Carinal resections are particularly at risk because of the complex nature of the reconstructions required and the fact that primary tumors may involve a considerable length of trachea as well as of main bronchi.

Several predictors of anastomotic complications were demonstrated: reoperation, diabetes, lengthy (≥ 4 cm) resections, laryngotracheal resections, age ≤ 17 years, and need for a tracheostomy before operation. The frequency of anastomotic complications was higher in patients undergoing operations for tracheoesophageal fistula than in those being treated for tracheal tumors, postintubation stenoses, and idiopathic laryngotracheal stenoses. Of note, corticosteroid use was not associated with an increase in complication rate. This is most likely secondary to the management strategy of our group, which is to defer tracheal operations in the presence of high-dose steroids until such drugs can be effectively tapered.

Overall, 81 patients experienced anastomotic complications in this series. Thirty-seven patients had separation of the suture line, another 37 patients developed anastomotic stenosis, and 7 had airway obstruction from granulation tissue formation.

Complications were treated with multiple dilations (n = 2), temporary tracheostomy (n = 7) or T-tube (n = 16) placement, permanent tracheostomy (n = 14) or T-tube (n = 20) placement, and reoperation (n = 16). The mortality of patients who had anastomotic complications was 7.4 percent (6 of 81), compared with 0.06 percent (5 of 820) in those without anastomotic complications. In this series, no patient has died due to their anastomotic complications since 1988. This success is attributed to the routine use of postoperative bronchoscopy and the early recognition and subsequent definitive management of anastomotic complications.

With attention to detail, even complications can be successfully managed. Successful management can not only save a life but also preserve the airway and voice.

References

1. Shaha A, DiMaio T, Money S, et al. Prosthetic reconstruction of the trachea. *Am J Surg* 1988;156:306–309.
2. Kim J, Suh SW, Shin JY, et al. Replacement of a tracheal defect with a tissue-engineered prosthesis: Early results from animal experiments. *J Thorac Cardiovasc Surg* 2004;128:124–129.
3. Grillo HC, Dignan EF, Miura T. Extensive resection and reconstruction of mediastinal trachea without prosthesis or graft: An anatomical study in man. *J Thorac Cardiovasc Surg* 1964;48:741.
4. Mulliken J, Grillo HC. The limits of tracheal resection with primary anastomosis: Further anatomical studies in man. *J Thorac Cardiovasc Surg* 1968;55:418.
5. Miura T, Grillo HC. The contribution of the inferior thyroid artery to the blood supply of the human trachea. *Surg Gynecol Obstet* 1966;123:99–102.
6. Dedo HH, Fishman NH. Laryngeal release and sleeve resection for tracheal stenosis. *Ann Otol Rhinol Laryngol* 1969;78:285.
7. Ferguson DJ, Wild JJ, Wangensteen OH. Experimental resection of the trachea. *Surgery* 1950;28:597.
8. Michelson E, Solomon R, Maun L, Ramierz J. Experiments in tracheal reconstruction. *J Thorac Cardiovasc Surg* 1961;41:748.
9. Miscall L, McKittrick JB, Giordano RP, Nolan RG. Stenosis of the trachea; resection and end-to-end anastomosis. Report of two cases. *Arch Surg* 1963;87:726.
10. Barclay RS, McSwan N, Welsh TM. Tracheal reconstruction without the use of grafts. *Thorax* 1957;12:177.
11. Grillo HC, Bendixen HH, Gephart T. Resection of the carina and lower trachea. *Ann Surg* 1963;158:889.
12. Mathisen DJ, Grillo HC. Laryngotracheal trauma. *Ann Thorac Surg* 1987;43:254–262.
13. Kelly JP, Webb WR, Moulder PV, et al. Management of airway trauma I: Tracheobronchial injuries. *Ann Thorac Surg* 1985;40:551–555.
14. Gaissert HA, Lofgren RH, Grillo HC. Upper airway compromise after inhalation injury: Complex strictures of larynx and trachea and their management. *Ann Surg* 1993;218;672–678.
15. Grillo HC. Surgical treatment of postintubation tracheal injuries. *J Thorac Cardiovasc Surg* 1979;78:860–875.
16. Muehrcke DD, Grillo HC, Mathisen DJ. Reconstructive airway surgery after irradiation. *Ann Thorac Surg* 1995;59:14–18.
17. Grillo HC, Mark EJ, Mathisen DJ, Wain JC. Idiopathic laryngotracheal stenosis: The entity and its management. *Ann Thorac Surg* 1993;56:80–87.
18. Ashiku SK, Kuzucu A, Grillo HC, et al. Idiopathic laryngotracheal stenosis: Effective definitive treatment with laryngotracheal resection. *J Thorac Cardiovasc Surg* 2004;127:99–107.
19. Herzog H, Heitz M, Keller R, Graedel E. Surgical therapy for expiratory collapse of the trachea and large bronchi. In: Grillo HC, Eschapasse H (eds). *International Trends in General Thoracic Surgery: Major Challenges.* Philadelphia: Saunders, 1987:74–90.
20. Rainer WG, Newby JP, Kelbe DC. Long-term results of tracheal support surgery for emphysema. *Dis Chest* 1968;53:765–774.
21. Grillo HC, Mathisen DJ. Primary tracheal tumors: Treatment and results. *Ann Thorac Surg* 1990;49:69–77.
22. Gaissert HG, Grillo HC, Shadmehr HB, et al. Long-term survival after resection of adenoid cystic and squamous cell carcinoma of the trachea and carina. *Ann Thorac Surg* 2004;78:1889–1896.

23. Grillo HC, Suen HC, Mathisen DJ, Wain JC. Resectional management of thyroid carcinoma invading the airway. *Ann Thorac Surg* 1992;54:3–10.
24. Weber AL, Grillo HC. Tracheal tumors: Radiological, clinical and pathological evaluation. *Adv Otorhinolaryngol* 1978;24:170.
25. Weber AL, Grillo HC (ed). Symposium on the larynx and trachea. *Radiol Clin North Am* 1978;16:291–308.
26. Felson B, Neoplasms of the trachea and mainstem bronchi. *Semin Roentgenol* 1983;18:23–37.
27. Acquino SL, Shepard JAO, Ginns LC, et al. Acquired tracheomalacia: Ddetection by expiratory CT scan. *J Comp Assis Tomog* 2001;25:394–399.
28. Mathisen DJ, Grillo HC. Endoscopic relief of malignant airway obstruction. *Ann Thorac Surg* 1989;48:469–475.
29. Wilson RS. Tracheal resection. In: Marshall BE, Longnecker DE, Fairley HB (eds). Anesthesia for thoracic procedures. Boston: Blackwell Scientific, 1988;415–432.
30. Rutter MJ, Cotton RT, Azizkhan RG, Manning PB. Slide tracheoplasty for the management of complete tracheal rings. *J Pediatr Surg* 2003;38:928–934.
31. Montgomery WW. Suprahyoid release for tracheal anastomosis. *Arch Otolaryngol* 1974;99:255–260.
32. Newton JR, Grillo HC, Mathisen DJ. Main bronchial sleeve resection with pulmonary conservation. *Ann Thorac Surg* 1991;52:1272–1280.
33. Grillo HC. Surgery of the trachea. In: Keen G (ed). *Operative Surgery and Management*, 2d ed. Bristol, UK: Wright, 1987:776–784.
34. Delorimer AA, Harrison MR, Hardy K, et al. Tracheobronchial obstruction in infants and children: Experience with 45 cases. *Ann Surg* 1990;212:277–289.
35. Grillo HC, Zannini P. Management of obstructive tracheal disease in children. *J Pediatr Surg* 1984;19:414–416.
36. Maeda M, Grillo HC. Effect of tension on tracheal growth after resection and anastomosis in puppies. *J Thorac Cardiovasc Surg* 1973;65;658–668.
37. Tsugawa C, Kimura K, Muraji T, et al. Congenital stenosis involving a long segment of the trachea: Further experience in reconstructive surgery. *J Pediatr Surg* 1988; 23:471–475.
38. Idriss FS, DeLeon SY, Ilbawi MN, et al. Tracheoplasty with pericardial patch for extensive tracheal stenosis in infants and children. *J Thorac Cardiovasc Surg* 1984;88:527–536.
39. Tsang V, Murday A, Gilbe C, Goldstraw P. Slide tracheoplasty for congenital funnel-shaped stenosis. *Ann Thorac Surg* 1989;48:632–635.
40. Mathisen DJ, Grillo HC, Wain JC, Hilgenberg AD. Management of acquired nonmalignant tracheoesophageal fistula. *Ann Thorac Surg* 1991;52:759–765.
41. Grillo HC, Donahue DM, Mathisen DJ, et al. Postintubation tracheal stenosis: Treatment and results. *J Thorac Cardiovasc Surg* 1995;109:486–493.
42. Ogura JH, Roper CL. Surgical correction of traumatic stenosis of the larynx and pharynx. *Laryngoscope* 1962;72:468–480.
43. Gerwat J, Bryce DP. The management of subglottic stenosis by resection and direct anastomosis. *Laryngoscope* 1974;84:940–947.
44. Pearson FG, Cooper JD, Nelems JM, van Nostrand AWP. Primary tracheal anastomosis after resection of the cricoid cartilage with preservation of recurrent laryngeal nerves. *J Thorac Cardiovasc Surg* 1975;70:806–816.
45. Couraud L, Brichon PY, Velly JF. The surgical treatment of inflammatory and fibrous laryngotracheal stenosis. *Eur J Cardiothor Surg* 1988;2:410–415.
46. Macchiarini DE, deMontpreville V, Mazmanian GM, Dartevelle P. Tracheal growth after slide tracheoplasty. *J Thorac Cardiovasc Surg* 1997;113:558–566.
47. Grillo HC, Wright CD, Vlahakes GJ, MacGillivray TE. Management of congenital tracheal stenosis by means of slide tracheoplasty or resection and reconstruction, with long-term follow-up of growth after slide tracheoplasty. *J Thorac Cardiovasc Surg* 2002;123:145–152.
48. Pearson FG, Todd TRJ, Cooper JD. Experience with primary neoplasms of the trachea and carina. *J Thorac Cardiovasc Surg* 1984;88:511–518.
49. Wright CD, Grillo HC, Wain JC, et al. Anastomotic complications after tracheal resections: Prognostic factors and management. *J Thorac Cardiovasc Surg* 2004;128: 731–739.

CHAPTER

9 BENIGN DIFFUSE PULMONARY DISORDERS

Micah Fisher, Jonathan B. Orens

INTRODUCTION

Diffuse benign pulmonary disorders cover a broad range of primary lung diseases and may also be associated with systemic disorders. These range from idiopathic pulmonary fibrosis with a chronic presentation and poor survival to hypersensitivity pneumonitis with an acute presentation and a good response to treatment. Some of these diseases have unique clinical findings while others share similar radiographic changes, symptoms, or pulmonary function abnormalities. Therapy differs for many of the diffuse benign pulmonary diseases; therefore accurate diagnosis is paramount.

Each of these disorders may be categorized on the basis of several findings. First, diseases may be due to intrinsic or extrinsic injury. For instance, the pneumoconioses are due to the inhalation of damaging foreign material into the lung, while hypersensitivity pneumonitis is due to an allergic response to foreign material or medications. On the other hand, interstitial lung diseases such as idiopathic pulmonary fibrosis (IPF), sarcoidosis, lymphangioleiomyomatosis (LAM), eosinophilic granulomatosis (EG), and the pulmonary disorders associated with collagen vascular disease are believed to be due to intrinsic lung injury/inflammation. The benign diffuse lung diseases may also be categorized based on their

KEY CONCEPTS

- Epidemiology
  - Diffuse benign pulmonary disorders cover a broad range of primary lung diseases and can be associated with systemic disorders.
- Pathophysiology
  - Most benign pulmonary disorders are derived from intrinsic or extrinsic injury. Such injury can take the form of cellular and/or humoral immunologic injury triggered by inhaled antigens, infectious agents, or autoimmune processes. Chemical injury from smoking or certain drugs has also been implicated.
- Clinical features
  - Most presenting symptoms include progressive dyspnea and cough. Other symptoms include chest pain, wheezing, and hemoptysis. Physical signs include heavy use of accessory muscles of breathing, cyanosis, and clubbing. Systemic signs of illness seen with some illnesses include fatigue, weight loss, and malaise.
- Diagnostics
  - Most diffuse benign disorders are characterized by plain chest radiography, computed tomography, and open or video-assisted thoracoscopic lung biopsy. Most of these disorders have characteristic radiologic pulmonary parenchymal patterns, adenopathy (e.g., sarcoidosis), and histologic characteristics. Bronchoscopy with transbronchial biopsies/bronchoalveolar lavage, fine-needle aspiration biopsies, and sputum cultures and/or cytologies are also helpful in many cases. Finally, a complete blood count with differential (e.g., eosinophilic processes), and serum chemistries are helpful in some cases.
- Treatment
  - Although treatment recommendations vary with the particular pulmonary process, many are corticosteroid-based while others are predicated on removal of an inciting agent (e.g., drug, tobacco smoke).
- Outcomes
  - Clinical outcomes vary widely according to the particular process.

physiologic presentation, particularly the type of change seen by pulmonary function studies. Some of the disorders are associated with an obstructive ventilatory defect (LAM, EG) or restrictive ventilatory defect [IPF, nonspecific interstitial pneumonitis (NSIP), asbestosis], while others may present with combined obstruction and restriction [sarcoid, bronchiolitis obliterans with organizing pneumonia (BOOP)]. Finally, the diseases may be categorized based on their individual radiographic findings (i.e., diffuse interstitial infiltrates, patchy alveolar infiltrates, cystic lesions, or honeycombing). This chapter reviews the common benign pulmonary disease including clinical presentation, diagnosis, and treatment.

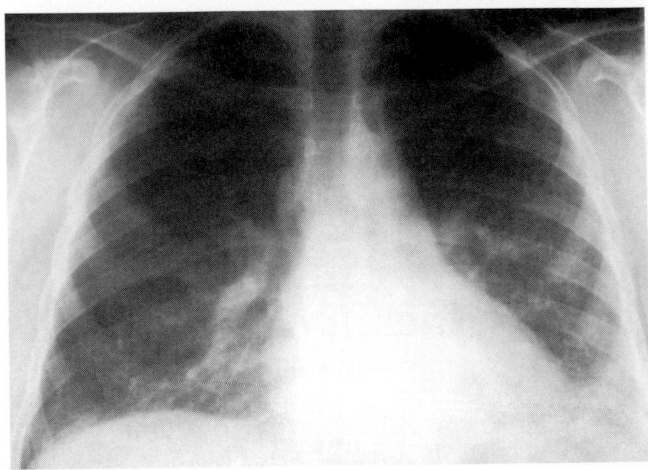

Figure 9-1 PA chest x-ray of a patient with IPF. Note small lung volumes and lower lobe interstitial infiltrates.

IDIOPATHIC PULMONARY FIBROSIS (IPF)/ USUAL INTERSTITIAL PNEUMONITIS (UIP)

Idiopathic pulmonary fibrosis (IPF) is a progressive, fatal disease without a known cause. It is manifest by diffuse interstitial lung scarring with a predominance of fibrosis in the subpleural and lower lung zones.[1] This disease has carried several different names, including cryptogenic fibrosing alveolitis, usual interstitial pneumonitis, and others. In a euphemistic way, IPF is considered the "mother" of all interstitial lung disorders. The reason for this distinction is because of its progressive nature, refractoriness to any form of therapy, and miserable clinical course, culminating in death. Indeed, a diagnosis of true IPF portends a relentless course that usually leads to death within 5 years of diagnosis.[2–5] Most patients present with the insidious onset of worsening dyspnea and nonproductive cough. The typical patient is in his or her sixties or above, but young patients have been affected, particularly in familial forms of the disease. IPF is frequently misdiagnosed initially as "pneumonia" because symptoms include cough and dyspnea associated with pulmonary infiltrates. The disease is distinguished from pneumonia because there is usually a long-term course of symptoms, and fever and purulent sputum production are lacking. Physical examination typically shows bilateral "Velcro-like" rales, predominantly in the lung bases. Resting or exercised-induced hypoxemia is invariably present, depending on the stage of the disease. Digital clubbing is a frequent finding. Chest x-rays show small lung volumes with interstitial infiltrates predominantly in the lower and peripheral lung zones (Fig. 9-1). High-resolution computed tomography (HRCT) of the chest is an invaluable tool to help distinguish the diagnosis of IPF from other interstitial lung disorders. Typical findings include peripheral and lower lung zone interstitial thickening with honeycombing and traction bronchiectasis[6,7] (Fig. 9-2A and B). The fibrosis and honeycomb-

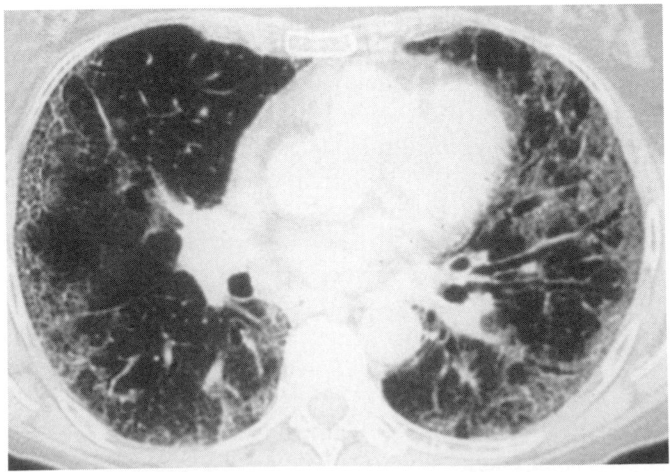

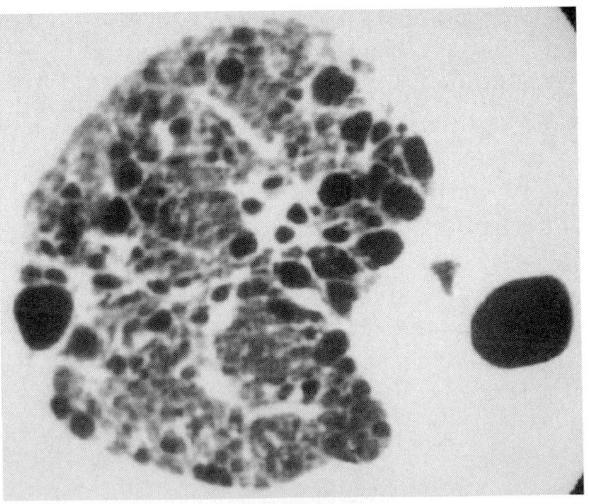

Figure 9-2 A. High-resolution chest CT of IPF showing peripheral interstitial fibrotic infiltrates with areas of traction bronchiectasis interspersed with areas of normal lung parenchyma. (Courtesy of Stanley Siegelman, MD.) B. Close-up view of HRCT showing marked honeycombing and interstitial fibrotic changes in a patient with IPF.

ing may be interspersed with relatively normal-appearing lung parenchyma. Pulmonary function studies show a restrictive ventilatory defect with a low diffusing capacity for carbon monoxide (DLCO).[7] As the disease progresses, the total lung capacity, vital capacity, and DLCO fall, indicative of worsening fibrosis. In the early stages of the disease, oxygen desaturation may occur only with exercise; but as the disease progresses, severe resting hypoxemia is a common finding.[7]

The diagnosis of IPF is established by open lung biopsy together with appropriate clinical and radiographic findings.[1,7] Transbronchial bronchoscopic biopsies are frequently performed by many practitioners for interstitial lung disease and may be useful to exclude other diagnoses such as sarcoidosis, BOOP, eosinophilic pneumonia, or extrinsic allergic alveolitis. However, transbronchial biopsies are inadequate to establish the diagnosis of IPF because a larger tissue sample is necessary in order to visualize the geographic changes seen in this condition. These include areas of fibrosis and honeycombing interposed between areas of normal-appearing lung[1,7] (Fig. 9-3). Thus, video-assisted thoracoscopic surgical (VATS) biopsy has become the routine approach if a tissue diagnosis is warranted. It is important to note that there is controversy regarding the need to establish a tissue diagnosis when all clinical and radiographic findings suggest the diagnosis of IPF.[8] This is particularly true for older patients and those with far advanced disease. For those with atypical findings and in particular for younger patients, open biopsy should be seriously considered. The one diagnosis that has frequently been confused with IPF on clinical grounds is NSIP, which is discussed in greater detail in its own section. Importantly, NSIP tends to carry a much better prognosis than IPF, with many patients responding well to therapy with corticosteroids.

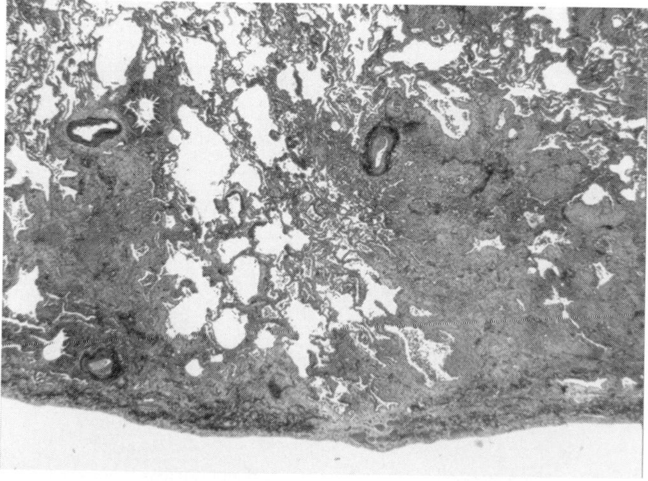

Figure 9-3 Histologic appearance of IPF from an open lung biopsy. Note areas of honeycombing with interstitial thickening and fibrosis.

Treatment for IPF with medical therapy is of limited value. High-dose corticosteroids (1 mg/kg methylprednisolone) given for several weeks and followed by a very protracted taper has been the mainstay of therapy for many years, with few patients improving.[7] One study showed minimal improvement with a combination of prednisone and azathioprine,[9] but widespread success with this approach has not been reported. Other potent agents such as cyclophosphamide have been used, also with limited success.[7] Gamma interferon has been the drug most recently studied for the treatment of IPF; data with regard to efficacy are still limited. In a small pilot study, some patients responded to daily subcutaneous injections with improvement in vital capacity.[10] A larger multicenter randomized study sponsored by the drug's manufacturer failed to show improvement in vital capacity, which was the primary endpoint of the trial. However, in a post hoc subgroup analysis, a survival benefit was noted.[11] At present, it is unclear whether this drug will prove to be beneficial for IPF; further study is necessary to settle the question of its utility for this disease. For patients below age 65 who are otherwise healthy, lung transplantation remains the only viable treatment option for IPF.

NONSPECIFIC INTERSTITIAL PNEUMONITIS

After Liebow and Carrington proposed the first major classification scheme for the idiopathic interstitial *pneumonias*,[12] several investigators found that a significant number of biopsies did not fit into the described subtypes.[13,14] The term *nonspecific interstitial pneumonitis* (NSIP), first used by Katzenstein, represents a distinct histologic type of interstitial *pneumonitis* with clinical characteristics that differ from UIP/IPF.

Although NSIP and IPF can be clinically indistinguishable, there are some differences that may help to differentiate these two diagnoses. In a study comparing patients with NSIP and those with IPF, the former typically had a subacute onset rather than the insidious onset typical of IPF.[15] There was no gender predominance. Fever was a common complaint of patients with NSIP and is rare in IPF.

Radiographically, NSIP is typically described as showing diffuse bilateral ground-glass opacities on HRCT.[16] Honeycombing is a hallmark feature of IPF but should not be present in NSIP in any greater amount than microscopic honeycombing. Alveolar infiltrates and occasionally nodules have also been described in NSIP, but these are not the predominant abnormalities.

The diagnosis of NSIP is made by open or thoracoscopic lung biopsy (Fig. 9-4). Katzenstein originally divided biopsies among three groups based on the amount of fibrosis present.[14] Group I consisted of interstitial infiltrates with predominant lymphocytes, occasional plasma cells, and minimal fibrosis. The infiltrates

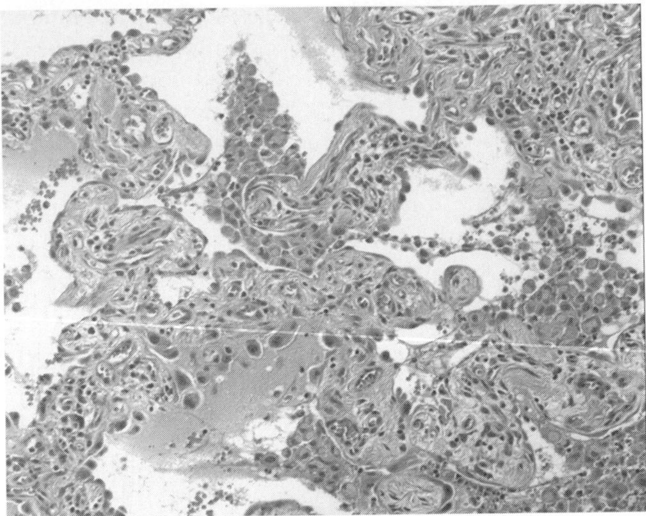

Figure 9-4 Open lung biopsy specimen from a patient with nonspecific interstitial pneumonitis showing diffuse interstitial thickening with inflammatory cells and collagen. (Courtesy of Rubin Tuder, MD.)

were noted to be temporally uniform, in contrast to the lesion of UIP, which is temporally heterogeneous. Group II contained the interstitial infiltrates but had marked amounts of associated fibrosis. Group III included marked distortion of the lung architecture from collagen deposition, scarring, and occasional honeycombing.

The prognosis for NSIP is much better than that for IPF. The majority of patients will improve or recover (74 percent in one series).[15] However, the likelihood of improvement is dependent on the severity of fibrosis. Patients with Katzenstein group III NSIP (severe fibrosis) have the least favorable prognosis. Corticosteroids with or without other immunosuppressive agents are the mainstay of therapy. However, it is important to note that there are no randomized controlled trials proving benefit for any form of therapy, and a number of patients have improved without specific treatment.

CRYPTOGENIC ORGANIZING PNEUMONIA/ BRONCHIOLITIS OBLITERANS ORGANIZING PNEUMONIA

First described in 1983[17] and then again in 1985[18] under the name bronchiolitis obliterans organizing pneumonia (BOOP), cryptogenic organizing pneumonia (COP) is an increasingly recognized cause of pulmonary disease. Disagreement continues to exist regarding the name for this process, thus both names are used interchangeably.[19] Although the term *BOOP* is more commonly used in the United States, *COP* is preferred, as designated by the American Thoracic Society and European Respiratory Society. COP specifically refers to the idiopathic form of the disease. However, organizing pneumonia, the histologic correlate, has been identified in association with a variety of diseases as well as drug and inhalational exposures.

COP can present in a variety of forms.[20–23] The most common is as a nonresolving pneumonia.[18,20–23] Patients typically complain of fevers, cough, and malaise. Myalgias have also been described in a number of patients. The symptoms will usually have been going on for several months at the time of presentation, and such patients may have been treated with one or multiple courses of antibiotics with no significant improvement.

Clinical testing is nonspecific.[18,20–23] A mild leukocytosis is common, as well as an elevated erythrocyte sedimentation rate, sometimes over 100. Pulmonary function tests almost invariably show some degree of restriction and a reduced diffusion capacity. Frank hypoxemia is rare.[18]

Chest radiography typically shows multiple areas of patchy alveolar infiltrates bilaterally.[18] CT scans will most commonly show areas of consolidation with air bronchograms; however, a variety of other patterns have also been described[18,21] (Fig. 9-5). These range from a diffuse nodular pattern to band-like areas of consolidation. Pleural effusions are uncommon.

The diagnosis of COP requires lung biopsies showing the histologic features of organizing pneumonia[18,20–24] (Fig. 9-6). Although transbronchial biopsies are sometimes sufficient, clinicians must understand that the small biopsies obtained by this procedure may be insufficient to completely distinguish the process from other underlying pathology.[19,23,24] It is important to exclude other processes, since organizing pneumonia can sometimes be found in association with other entities, such as fibrotic disease. Thoracoscopic or open lung biopsy may in some circumstances be necessary to establish a firm diagnosis.

Treatment consists of glucocorticoids for 6 to 12 months.[18,20–24] Patients typically have a good response,

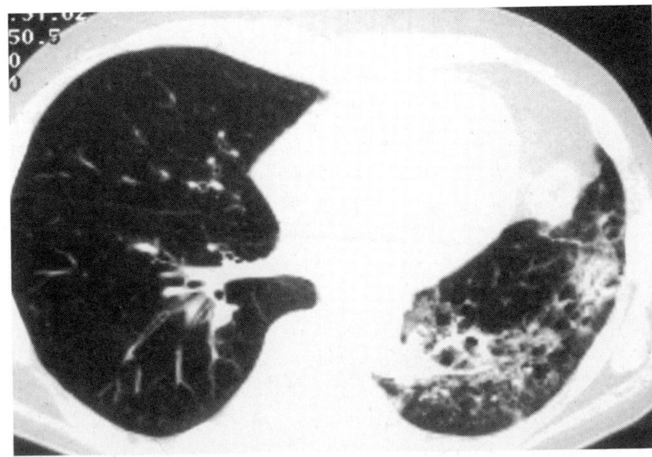

Figure 9-5 Chest CT scan showing the patchy infiltrates characteristic of BOOP.

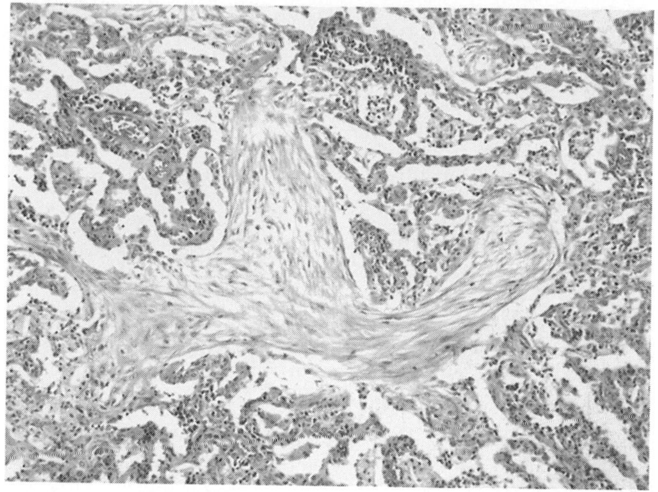

Figure 9-6 Histopathologic specimen from a patient with BOOP. Note tufts of loose collagen plugging the airway.

with close to two-thirds having clinical remission within a short time. However, relapses while tapering steroids are common. Relapses typically respond to reinstitution of higher doses of glucocorticoids and do not appear to affect the long-term course of the disease.

COP has had other notable presentations.[18,20–24] Focal lesions resembling solitary lung nodules have been described by a number of authors. The diagnosis was typically found after surgical resection, which stemmed from the concern that the nodules were a malignant process. The patients tended to do well without any further treatment. A rapidly progressive form of COP has also been described.[25] This form advances much more rapidly, with a fulminant course and high mortality.

OTHER IDIOPATHIC INTERSTITIAL PNEUMONIAS

Idiopathic pulmonary fibrosis, NSIP, and COP make up the majority of the idiopathic interstitial pneumonias (IIP) encountered in clinical practice. There are other forms of IIP that are less common and are dealt with briefly below.

Acute interstitial pneumonia (AIP)

AIP is a rapidly progressive interstitial disease with typically a fulminant course.[19] It typically presents with a viral-like prodrome of myalgias, fever, chills, and malaise. Patients usually present within 3 weeks of onset of the illness and most require mechanical ventilation. CT reveals diffuse ground-glass opacification and, to a lesser extent, basilar airspace consolidation. The histologic lesion is that of diffuse alveolar damage. Mortality is high, well over 50 percent, and there is no proven effective therapy.

Respiratory bronchiolitis-associated interstitial lung disease (RB-ILD) and desquamative interstitial pneumonia (DIP)

Respiratory bronchiolitis is a pathologic lesion found in cigarette smokers; it is characterized by pigmented macrophages in the lumens of the first- and second-order respiratory bronchioles.[19] These lesions are most often seen incidentally on biopsies done for unrelated reasons and rarely cause symptoms. However, a small percentage of patients do present with clinically significant interstitial disease with this lesion on biopsy; the clinical condition is then termed RB-ILD.

The clinical spectrum runs from minimal complaints to severe dyspnea.[19] The most common complaints are gradually progressive dyspnea and new or worsening cough. There is a male predominance with a ratio of 2:1. CT typically reveals centrilobular nodules, thickened airways, and sometimes ground-glass opacification. Patients almost universally improve with cessation of smoking.

The pathologic lesion of DIP is an accumulation of macrophages in the alveolar spaces.[19] Because of its similar male predominance, association with cigarette smoking, and the presence of macrophages, DIP is thought to represent one end of a spectrum of disease, where the other end would be RB-ILD. However, there are some differences, such as the uniform presence of ground-glass opacification seen in DIP. Honeycombing can be seen in DIP, but only in a minority of patients, and it tends to be very limited in extent. As with RB-ILD, the prognosis is good, with smoking cessation thought to be important. Patients with DIP are commonly treated with corticosteroids, but there have been no treatment trials proving benefit.

Lymphoid interstitial pneumonia (LIP)

LIP is the last of the idiopathic interstitial pneumonias included in the recent consensus classification.[19] This disease is most often seen in combination with other diseases such as Sjögren's syndrome, acquired immunodeficiency syndrome, various autoimmune diseases, and Castleman's disease.[19,26,27] The disease tends to affect women more than men. Initial presentations include slowly progressive shortness of breath, cough, and weight loss. CT typically reveals a pattern of bilateral diffuse or patchy ground-glass opacification, with poorly defined centrilobular nodules.[27] Thickening of the peribronchiovascular bundles and irregular septal thickening are also common.[27] Cystic changes are noted in a majority of patients, but honeycombing is less common.

The histology of LIP is marked by a dense infiltration with lymphocytes and plasma cells.[19,26] The infiltration is especially marked in the alveolar septum. Lymphoid follicles and germinal centers are commonly seen.

The prognosis is highly variable, with the majority of patients remaining stable or improving; however, over one-third of patients may have progressive disease.[19,26,27]

Treatment usually consists of corticosteroids with or without other immunosuppressive agents.

INTERSTITIAL LUNG DISEASE ASSOCIATED WITH COLLAGEN VASCULAR DISEASE

The collagen vascular diseases present with a wide range of symptoms and findings, and they have variable courses. Given the systemic nature of the diseases, it is not unexpected to find that patients commonly develop pulmonary pathology. The full range of known complications is beyond the scope of this chapter and have been described in detail elsewhere.[28] The complications are not limited to the lung parenchyma but rather include all aspects of the respiratory system as well as the respiratory muscles, pleural space, upper airway, and pulmonary vasculature. The complications also do not always represent a direct injury caused by the underlying collagen vascular disease. Some of the therapies for these diseases have pulmonary side effects, such as methotrexate-induced lung injury in patients being treated for rheumatoid arthritis or pulmonary infections from immunosuppression. Bibasilar fibrosis from repeated aspirations due to esophageal dysmotility from scleroderma has been well described.

Histologically, the types of interstitial disease found include those that have been previously mentioned. These comprise nonspecific interstitial pneumonia, UIP, and BOOP.[28,29] Other forms of interstitial disease have also been described, including lymphocytic interstitial pneumonia and diffuse alveolar damage.[28,29] Prognosis depends on the histologic type of interstitial disease and is largely similar to that seen in patients without underlying collagen vascular disease.

SARCOIDOSIS

Sarcoidosis is a multiorgan disease with almost all cases having pulmonary manifestations at some point during its course.[30] Pulmonary manifestations range from asymptomatic hilar adenopathy, to endobronchial involvement with airflow limitation to diffuse nodules to end-stage lung fibrosis.

Sarcoidosis has a worldwide distribution and affects different racial and ethnic groups variably. In the United States, annual incidence estimates are 10.9 cases per 100,000 whites and 35.5 cases per 100,000 blacks.[31] The etiology remains unknown, but some epidemiologic research supports an infectious etiology whereas other evidence suggests an environmental exposure.[30]

The clinical presentation of pulmonary sarcoidosis is highly variable. Probably the most common is asymptomatic hilar adenopathy found on chest radiography done for an unrelated reason.[30,32] Common pulmonary symptoms include cough, dyspnea, and retrosternal chest pain.

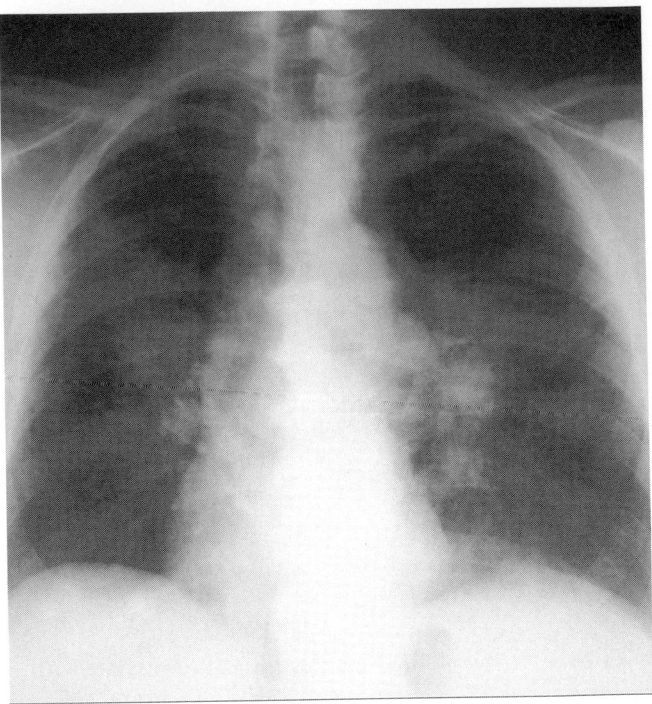

Figure 9-7 Chest x-ray showing bilateral hilar adenopathy without pulmonary infiltrates, depicting stage I pulmonary sarcoidosis.

Systemic symptoms include fatigue, weight loss, and malaise.[30,32] Löfgren's syndrome is a notable acute presentation of sarcoidosis characterized by the triad of hilar lymphadenopathy, polyarthralgias, and erythema nodosum.

Sarcoidosis is staged by chest radiographs.[33] Stage I disease is defined as the presence of hilar lymphadenopathy without other parenchymal infiltrates (Fig. 9-7), whereas stage II includes hilar lymphadenopathy with infiltrates. In stage III disease there are infiltrates without hilar lymphadenopathy, and stage IV disease is defined by the presence of end-stage fibrosis (Fig. 9-8).

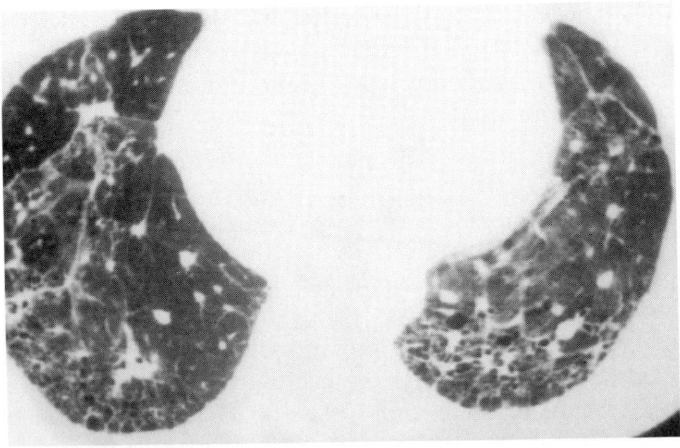

Figure 9-8 Bilateral fibrotic changes as seen in stage IV pulmonary sarcoidosis.

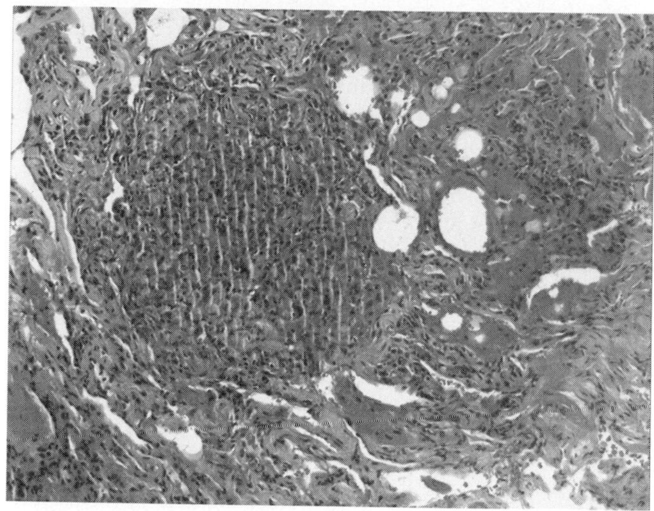

Figure 9-9 Transbronchial lung biopsy showing typical noncaseating granuloma from a patient with pulmonary sarcoidosis. (Courtesy of Rubin Tuder, MD.)

Classically, sarcoidosis has an upper and midlung zone predominance. Small nodules ranging in size from 2 mm to 1 cm in diameter are the most common finding.[33] The nodules are typically found around the bronchovascular bundles. Patchy areas of airspace consolidation can also be seen, leading to the term *alveolar sarcoidosis*.[33] Mediastinal adenopathy is very common on CT, with calcification present in approximately 50 percent of patients, typically in a focal or "eggshell" pattern.[33]

Histologically the lesion of sarcoidosis is the noncaseating granuloma. Granulomas are tightly packed and composed of epithelioid cells, including multinucleated giant cells and lymphocytes[30–32,34] (Fig. 9-9). These lesions can be found in lymph nodes, the lung parenchyma, and airway mucosa. However, noncaseating granulomas are not unique to sarcoidosis and other etiologies must be excluded clinically and pathologically, including fungal and mycobacterial disease, hypersensitivity pneumonitis, pneumoconiosis such as beryllium disease, and drug reactions.[34]

No treatment is needed for asymptomatic patients with hilar adenopathy. The majority of these patients and patients with Löfgren's syndrome will have complete spontaneous remissions.[32] Corticosteroids are the mainstay of treatment for symptomatic sarcoidosis. Other immunosuppressive agents such as cyclophosphamide, methotrexate, and azathioprine are reserved for patients with chronic non-steroid-responsive disease, although there is little literature to fully support their use.[32]

PULMONARY ALVEOLAR PROTEINOSIS

Pulmonary alveolar proteinosis (PAP) is a rare disease first described by Rosen and colleagues in 1958.[35] The hallmark of this disorder is the thick, proteinaceous material that fills the alveolar spaces and impairs gas exchange. The disease is now recognized to exist in three forms: acquired, congenital, and secondary.[36] The acquired form represents over 90 percent of all reported cases[36] and is the type mainly discussed here.

Acquired PAP typically affects men more than women, and these patients are about 40 years of age on average.[35,36] Symptoms tend to be gradual in onset, with a median of 7 months before diagnosis.[36] Common complaints include progressive dyspnea, cough, and fatigue.[37] Low-grade fevers have been reported, but higher temperatures suggest a superimposed infection.[37] Physical exam findings are nonspecific and frequently normal despite significant hypoxemia.[36] The radiographic appearance is nonspecific, with typically a bilateral alveolar filling process, but interstitial patterns can coexist or predominate.[36] High-resolution CT scans show ground-glass opacification in a geographic pattern.[36] CT may also show interlobular thickening of the septa, producing a "crazy paving" pattern[36] (Fig. 9-10).

Historically, open lung biopsy was required for diagnosis.[36] However, more recent experience has shown that bronchoscopic techniques can reliably diagnose the majority of patients.[36,37] Bronchoalveolar lavage (BAL) produces a characteristic "milky" return, which represents the proteinaceous material that accumulates in the alveolar spaces.[36,37] Transbronchial biopsies have a high diagnostic yield as well.[37]

Treatment of PAP has been with whole-lung lavage under general anesthesia with a double-lumen endotracheal tube.[36,37] This procedure produces significant and durable improvements in clinical, physiologic, and radiographic parameters. However, the majority of patients will need repeated lavages over time.

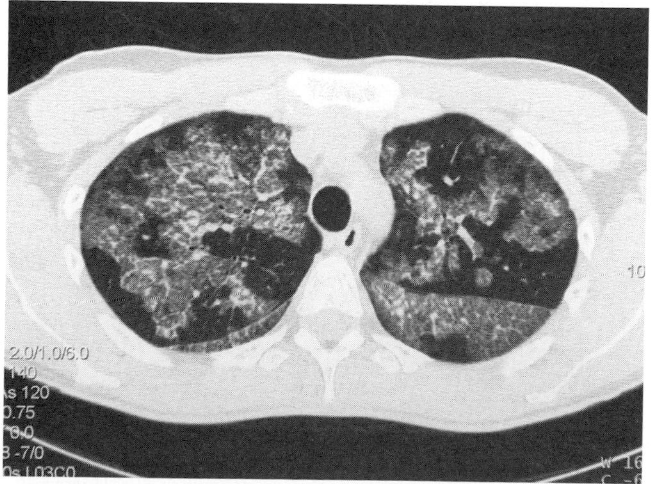

Figure 9-10 Pulmonary alveolar proteinosis. Note bilateral infiltrates with a distinct appearance that has been described as "crazy paving."

Recent studies have found a link between granulocyte-macrophage colony-stimulating factor (GM-CSF) and PAP.[36] Initial studies found that GM-CSF "knockout" mice develop a lung disease similar to PAP. Further studies have found that most patients with acquired PAP have blocking antibodies to GM-CSF in lavage fluid and serum. These findings have led to the novel approach of using exogenous GM-CSF as treatment, with some success in small case series.

EOSINOPHILIC LUNG DISEASES

The eosinophilic lung diseases constitute a wide range of processes with a common finding of eosinophils in serum, lavage fluid, and/or on histology.[38] Early classifications included the syndrome of pulmonary infiltrates with eosinophilia (PIE); however, peripheral eosinophilia is variable in some processes and thus is not inclusive of the full range of diseases. Since their first description, authors have used a variety of names, which has added confusion to the terminology. The most current terminology is used here for a review of the important processes likely to be encountered. These include eosinophilic pneumonia, acute and chronic eosinophilic pneumonia, Churg-Strauss syndrome, and allergic bronchopulmonary aspergillosis. A discussion of all the other diseases included in this category is beyond the scope of this chapter.

Simple eosinophilic pneumonia (Löffler's syndrome)

Löffler's syndrome was first described in 1932.[39] It consists of migratory pulmonary infiltrates and blood eosinophilia. Patients are typically asymptomatic or have only minimal symptoms.[39] Chest x-ray findings are usually described as a combination of interstitial and alveolar patterns that are migratory and peripherally located and often based in the pleura.[40] Infiltrates can be unilateral or bilateral.[40]

The underlying etiology, when found, has usually been linked to a parasitic infection.[38] *Ascaris* infection has classically been described. Drug reactions have also been found.

Patients typically have full resolution of radiographic and blood abnormalities within 1 month.[38] This resolution is usually spontaneous and rarely requires treatment with corticosteroids. Pathologic specimens are seldom required to confirm the diagnosis.

Idiopathic acute eosinophilic pneumonia

Idiopathic acute eosinophilic pneumonia (IAEP) is a rare disease that has typically been reported to occur in otherwise young, healthy individuals. Since the first reports in 1989, around 100 cases have been described.[41–43] This is a diagnosis of exclusion with a characteristic presentation that includes an acute febrile illness (usually of less than 5 days' duration), bilateral infiltrates, hypoxemic respiratory failure, and significant BAL eosinophilia (> 25 percent).[38,41–43] IAEP can easily mimic atypical pneumonia and acute respiratory distress syndrome (ARDS).

The typical presentation is that of a febrile illness with dyspnea, cough, myalgias, pleuritic chest pain, and respiratory distress.[38,41–43] Mechanical ventilation is frequently required. Chest x-rays invariably show bilateral infiltrates, which are usually diffuse and can be alveolar, interstitial, or a mixture of both. Only a minority of patients present with peripheral eosinophilia. However, the subsequent development of eosinophilia has been reported in as many as 68 percent of patients in one series.[43]

BAL is recommended in suspected cases to demonstrate the characteristic eosinophilia in the lavage fluid.[38,41–43] Eosinophil counts representing 40 to 50 percent of the differential is typical. When done, transbronchial biopsies and open lung biopsies have found varying stages of diffuse alveolar damage, including with marked interstitial and alveolar infiltration with eosinophils.[44] Because IAEP is a diagnosis of exclusion, the second role for lavage and/or biopsy is to rule out the presence of an underlying infectious etiology.

Treatment generally consists of corticosteroids with a relatively short duration. Patients will generally have a rapid response, with improvement within 1 to 2 days.[38] Relapse after discontinuation of steroids is not characteristic, and the absence of relapse has been suggested as a diagnostic criterion.[38] In one series, almost 25 percent of patients improved spontaneously without the use of corticosteroids.[43]

Chronic eosinophilic pneumonia

Although this process was originally described by Christoforidis and Molnar in 1960,[45] most authors give the credit to Carrington and coworkers, who published the first large series in 1969.[46] As compared with acute eosinophilic pneumonia, chronic eosinophilic pneumonia (CEP) has a more subacute presentation and causes milder symptoms.

In one series of 107 patients, the average duration of symptoms before diagnosis was 7.7 months.[47] Patients tend to be in their fourth or fifth decade at presentation. A 2:1 female-to-male ratio has been noted.[47,48] A history of atopy occurs in one-half of patients, with asthma being the most common form.[47,48] Presenting complaints have included cough (90 percent), fever (87 percent), dyspnea (57 percent), and weight loss (57 percent).[47] Other notable symptoms seen in approximately one-third of patients include sputum production, wheezing, and night sweats.[47]

Diagnostic tests can be very helpful in the diagnosis of CEP. Peripheral eosinophilia is very common, occurring in 88 to 95 percent of patients, with a mean value of 26

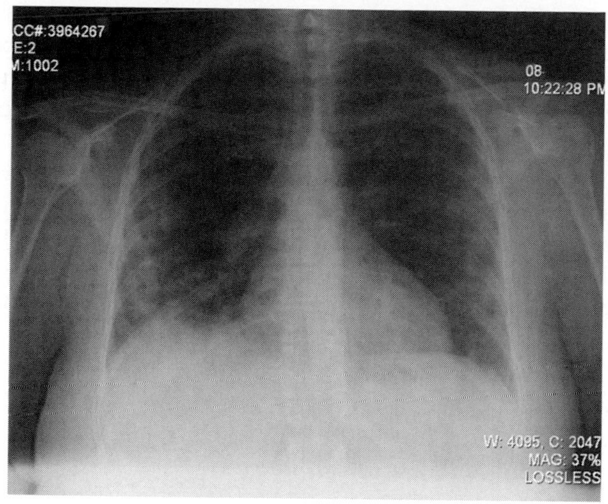

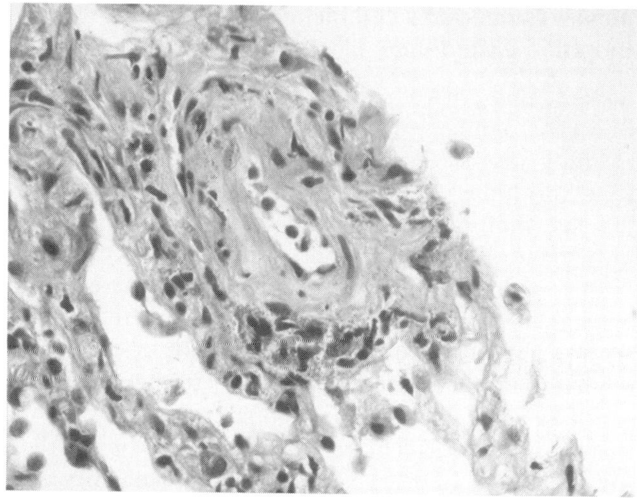

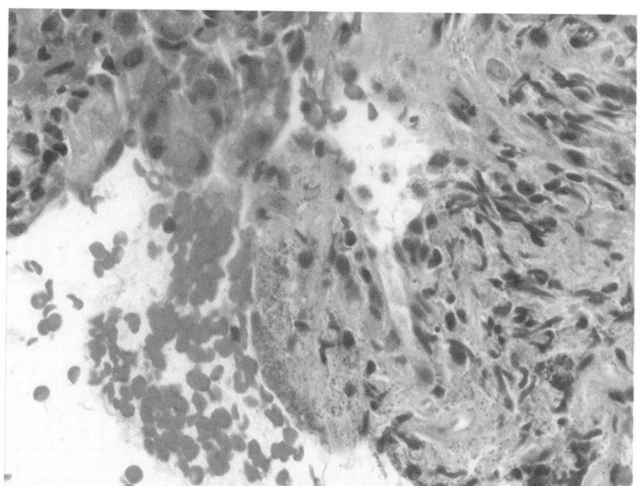

Figure 9-11 A. PA chest x-ray of a 43-year-old patient with eosinophilic pneumonia. Note the peripheral infiltrates, which are characteristic of this process. B and C. Transbronchial biopsy of eosinophilic pneumonia stained with hematoxylin and eosin. Note the scattered eosinophils (B) within the interstitium. C. Dense eosinophilic granules in the interstitium.

to 32 percent.[47,48] Other laboratory values are also elevated, including erythrocyte sedimentation rates and serum IgE levels.[47,48] *Bronchoalveolar lavage* contains very high levels of eosinophils, representing 25 percent to over 40 percent of the total cells.[38,48]

Chest radiography has classically been reported as showing the "photographic negative of pulmonary edema"[46] (Fig. 9-11A). However, a more recent series of patients have shown that only 25 percent have this finding.[47] The most common findings are peripheral bilateral infiltrates that were described as consolidated, ground-glass, or a mixture of both.[38,47–48] Upper lobe predominance is more common than lower lobe.[48] Migratory opacities, pleural effusions, and cavitation are uncommon.[38,47–48] CT sometimes helps to show the peripheral nature of the infiltrates.[38] Mediastinal adenopathy has been shown in 3 of 6 patients in one series[49] and 7 of 40 patients in another.[48]

Biopsy typically reveals intraalveolar exudates rich with eosinophils and histiocytes.[38,46–48] The surrounding interstitium is frequently also infiltrated with eosinophils and histiocytes[38,46–48] (Fig. 9-11B). Approximately 50 percent of patients may also have interstitial fibrosis.[38,46–48] At times, mild vasculitis is seen.[38,46–48] Coexisting BOOP is also a frequent finding.[46–48]

Some authors suggest that patients with a typical clinical presentation and typical radiographic findings can be treated empirically.[47] Others would favor the addition of bronchoscopy with lavage to confirm the presence of increased eosinophils.[38] However, most favor empiric trials of corticosteroids. Patients typically show rapid improvement in symptoms, usually within 24 to 48 h, followed in time by radiographic resolution.[46–48] This rapid response is felt to be characteristic and confirms the diagnosis. The lack of a prompt response should suggest an alternative diagnosis and consideration of a biopsy.

Unlike acute eosinophilic pneumonia, CEP is characterized by a high rate of relapse when patients are weaned off of steroids.[46–48] Most authors have recommended prolonged courses of steroids, on the order of 6 months to 1 year. Although relapses are common, they respond well to increased doses of steroids.

Pulmonary Langerhans cell histiocytosis (eosinophilic *granuloma*)

Pulmonary Langerhans cell histiocytosis (PLCH), also know as eosinophilic *granuloma* (EG), is a rare form of diffuse lung disease. Although most commonly found affecting the lungs solely, Langerhans cell histiocytosis can involve multiple organs including the bone, skin, pituitary gland, and other organs.[50] Langerhans cells are normally found in small numbers in the lung, where they function as antigen-presenting cells. In PLCH, the population of Langerhans cells is expanded, with destructive consequences for the parenchyma. The etiology for the expansion of this cell population is unknown.

Affected individuals tend to be in their third or fourth decade at the time of diagnosis.[51–52] The vast majority of patients diagnosed with PLCH are current smokers.[50–52] At presentation, approximately one-fourth of patients will be asymptomatic.[50,51] Common symptoms include nonproductive cough, dyspnea with exertion, and pleuritic chest pain.[51] In one series, 11 percent of patients had experienced spontaneous pneumothorax.[51] Chest radiography typically reveals bilateral reticulonodular and interstitial infiltration with upper- and middle-lobe predominance.[50] Cystic changes are common and may be the predominant lesion in later stages of the disease.[50] Similar findings on CT, in the proper clinical context, are felt to be diagnostic, thus obviating the need for open lung biopsy.[50,53]

The course of the illness is highly variable. Most patients will have resolution of symptoms and radiographic abnormalities with smoking cessation, but a small percentage will go on to end-stage lung disease.[50,51] Corticosteroids have been variably used, but there is no consensus as to their utility. Lung transplantation has been advocated for patients with end-stage disease; however, there are reports of recurrence in the transplanted lung.[54]

ALLERGIC BRONCHOPULMONARY ASPERGILLOSIS

Allergic bronchopulmonary aspergillosis (ABPA) occurs in up to 28 percent of patients with steroid dependent asthma and 15 percent of patients with cystic fibrosis.[55–57] The disease occurs when patients have a complex immune response to antigens expressed by *Aspergillus* that is colonizing the bronchial mucosa. Although most commonly associated with the ubiquitous fungus *Aspergillus fumigatus*, this allergic process has been described with other fungi including *Candida*, *Penicillium*, and other species of *Aspergillus*, including *A. flavus*.[55] The diagnosis of ABPA is based on a variety of clinical, radiographic, and laboratory findings. Suggested criteria include a history of asthma or cystic fibrosis, immediate cutaneous reactivity to *Aspergillus* species, an elevated total IgE (> 1000 ng/mL), elevated serum IgE and IgG antibodies to *Aspergillus fumigatus*, precipitating antibodies to *Aspergillus fumigatus*, central bronchiectasis, and chest x-ray infiltrates. Striking peripheral blood eosinophilia is common as well as sputum cultures that grow *Aspergillus* species.

Symptoms commonly include wheeze, cough, fever, and anorexia.[55,57] Sputum production is also common with "dirty green" plugs. During an exacerbation chest radiography may reveal fleeting pulmonary infiltrates as well as dense infiltrates in central bronchioles giving rise to a "gloved finger" appearance.

Corticosteroids are the cornerstone of therapy as they not only treat exacerbations but also decrease their frequency.[55–57] Most authors recommend initial treatment for several months followed by a slow taper. Some patients will go into clinical remission but the majority will require continued long-term therapy for intermittent exacerbations. Recently several studies have suggested a role for the oral antifungal itraconazole as a steroid sparing adjunct.[58,59]

HYPERSENSITIVITY PNEUMONITIS

Hypersensitivity pneumonitis (HP) is a clinically diverse disease process that results from the inhalation of a variety of antigens.[60–62] Farmer's lung is the classic example first described in 1932 by Campbell,[63] but since then numerous other examples of HP, also known as extrinsic allergic alveolitis, have been described.[60–62] The hallmark of this disease is an individual's immunologic response to an inhaled antigen. Therefore, for HP to develop, several steps are required. First, the patient must be exposed to a potential antigen; second, the antigen must be of sufficiently small size (usually < 3 μm) to travel through the respiratory tract and be deposited in an alveolus and distal bronchial tree; and last, there must be an immune response resulting in an inflammatory reaction.[60–62]

A multitude of exposures to a variety of antigens have been documented and described. Most forms of HP have been associated with antigens from fungi and bacteria such as *Mucor stolonifer*, which causes paprika slicer's lung in people who work with moldy paprika pods, and *Thermoactinomyces vulgaris*, which causes bagassosis in people who work with moldy sugar cane.[60] Pigeon breeder's lung is caused by exposure to animal proteins found in bird droppings, feathers, and serum.[60] A variety of chemicals have been implicated in HP, including hydrophthalic anhydride, which causes epoxy resin lung in people who work with heated epoxy resin.[60]

Although many people may be exposed to an antigen because of their occupations or hobbies, typically only a small percentage will go on to develop HP.[60–62] For example, in one study, only 8 percent of pigeon breeders in the Canary Islands were found to meet the criteria for pigeon breeders' lung.[64] In most studies, only 5 to 15 percent of exposed people go on to develop features of HP.[61] The host factors that determine whether an individual will develop an inflammatory reaction have yet to be determined.

Hypersensitivity pneumonitis has classically been subdivided into three forms: acute, subacute, and chronic.

Acute hypersensitivity pneumonitis

The acute form of HP is thought to occur after a large inhalational exposure to an antigen. Characteristic symptoms include fever, chills, dyspnea, chest tightness, cough, and malaise.[60–62] Symptoms usually begin within 4 to 8 h of exposure and resolve 24 to 48 h later.[60–62] Patients typically describe similar symptoms after repeated exposures. Chest radiography can show diffuse ground-glass opacification or reticulonodular infiltrates[62] (Fig. 9-12). A lower-lobe predominance is common.[62] Lung function tests can reveal a restrictive defect as well as impaired diffusion.[61]

Subacute and chronic hypersensitivity pneumonitis

Unlike acute HP, subacute and chronic forms have an insidious onset of cough and dyspnea.[60–62] Other common symptoms include fatigue, malaise, and weight loss. Few authors make a distinction between subacute and chronic forms other than to suggest that patients with subacute HP can experience episodes of symptoms similar to acute HP.[61] A major difference between acute and other forms is the tendency to develop parenchymal fibrosis in some cases leading to end-stage lung disease. These patients can also develop right heart failure and digital clubbing.[60] Chest x-rays and CT in chronic forms

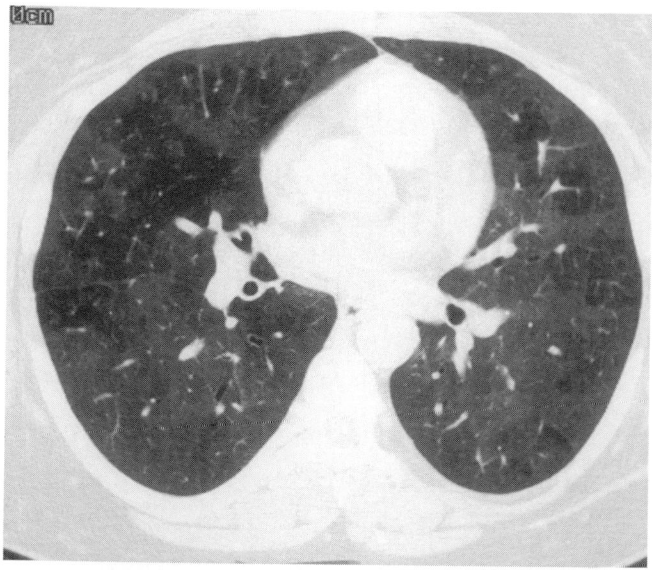

Figure 9-12 Chest CT of a 45-year-old woman with acute hypersensitivity pneumonitis from exposure to a pet bird. Note bilateral "ground-glass" opacifications.

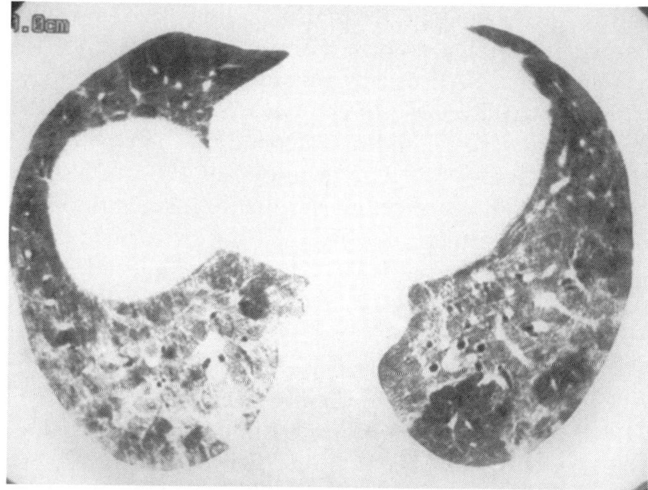

Figure 9-13 Chest CT scan showing bilateral diffuse interstitial fibrosis with interspersed ground-glass opacifications from a patient with chronic hypersensitivity pneumonitis.

have marked fibrosis and ground glass attenuation[60–62] (Fig. 9-13). Centrilobular poorly defined micronodules are very suggestive of HP in both the acute and chronic forms.[60] Pulmonary function testing usually reveals restriction and decreased diffusion but a small percentage of patients have also been shown to develop an obstructive defect regardless of a smoking history.[60–62,65]

As there are no definitive tests, the diagnosis of hypersensitivity pneumonitis is largely based on clinical presentation and history.[60–62,66] Suggested diagnostic criteria typically include (1) a history of exposure to a known antigen, (2) serum precipitating antibodies to the suspected antigen, (3) a history of common symptoms temporally related to antigen exposure, (4) an appropriate response to an inhalation challenge, (5) compatible results from radiographic and pulmonary function tests, and (6) granulomatous interstitial pneumonitis.[60–62,66] With this framework, several key points need further discussion.

A thorough history of possible exposures, occupational and domestic, is vitally important to discern possible antigens. However, in regard to subacute and chronic forms, the insidious nature of the disease may prevent the identification of likely antigen.

Although supportive, the finding of precipitating antibodies is not diagnostic as a high number of exposed people will develop antibody responses but will not have detectable disease.[60–62] Alternatively, the absence of antibodies does not rule out HP owing to the lack of standardized antigen testing in laboratories.

Inhalational challenges, exposing the patient to the suspected antigen in either the natural environment or in a hospital setting and monitoring for a clinical response, has been used in the research setting.[60] Whether it will be readily usable in the clinical setting remains to be seen.

Invasive diagnostic testing, including BAL and lung biopsy, is typically used in cases where the diagnosis is less apparent. BAL usually reveals a marked lymphocytosis with an inversion of the CD4 to CD8 ratio; however, this is variable and may depend on the type of HP and host factors.[60,62] The histology of HP can also be variable. Findings of cellular bronchiolitis, lymphoplasmacytic interstitial infiltrates, and poorly formed granulomas are considered typical.[62] However, multiple other patterns including UIP and NSIP have also been described.[60,62]

Most experts agree that the first goal of treatment is eliminating exposure to the inciting antigen.[60–62] However, repeated exposure to inhaled antigens does not necessarily lead to a chronic form with fibrosis but currently there is no way to predict which patients will have a progressive form of the disease.[60–62] There is no consensus for the use of corticosteroids.[60–62] A randomized controlled trial using corticosteroids in farmer's lung showed that corticosteroids lead to a more rapid improvement in pulmonary function, but there was no difference in outcomes at 5 years.[67] Interestingly, patients who were treated with corticosteroids tended to have more frequent episodes.[67]

DRUG-INDUCED LUNG DISEASE

A review from 1986 indicates that at that time 37 commonly used drugs had established pulmonary parenchymal toxicities.[68,69] Since then, more toxicities have been described. The true incidence of drug-induced injury is unknown, owing to the absence of definitive diagnostic studies and the high rate of underlying pulmonary diseases as well as other drugs and treatments with known pulmonary toxicities. Thus it is difficult to establish definitive causal relationships. Histologically, the majority of the injury patterns resemble those of disorders already discussed.[68–70] These include nonspecific interstitial pneumonia, organizing pneumonia, eosinophilic pneumonia, and hypersensitivity pneumonitis. Other patterns of injury include diffuse alveolar damage, pulmonary hemorrhage, and edema. Two of the more common clinically encountered drug toxicities are discussed below.

Methotrexate-induced lung injury

The spectrum of methotrexate pulmonary toxicity is wide, including interstitial disease, pleural effusions, fibrosis, and noncardiogenic pulmonary edema.[68,71] The most commonly reported toxicity is an interstitial pneumonitis, which has been variably termed methotrexate pneumonitis, acute interstitial pneumonitis, and hypersensitivity pneumonitis. The true frequency is unknown, with reports ranging from 2.1 to 7.6 percent of patients. It usually presents in a subacute fashion, with cough, dyspnea, and low-grade fevers. Peripheral eosinophilia has been reported in up to 40 percent of patients. Pulmonary function tests typically reveal a restrictive pattern with a reduced diffusion capacity. Chest radiographs have usually shown a bilateral, predominantly basilar interstitial pattern. Alveolar and nodular patterns as well as pleural effusions and adenopathy have also been reported (Fig. 9-14). Lung biopsy reveals lymphocytic infiltration of the interstitium; granulomas and eosinophilia are seen in some cases (Fig. 9-15).

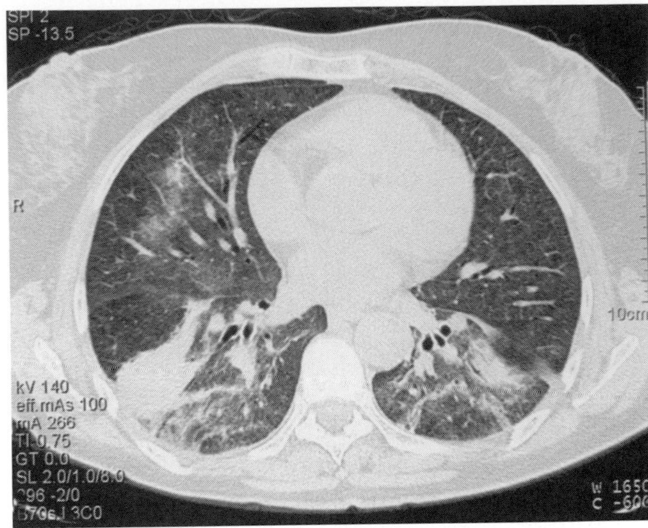

Figure 9-14 Methotrexate-induced lung injury showing bilateral pulmonary infiltrates with areas of consolidation on a background of increased interstitial markings.

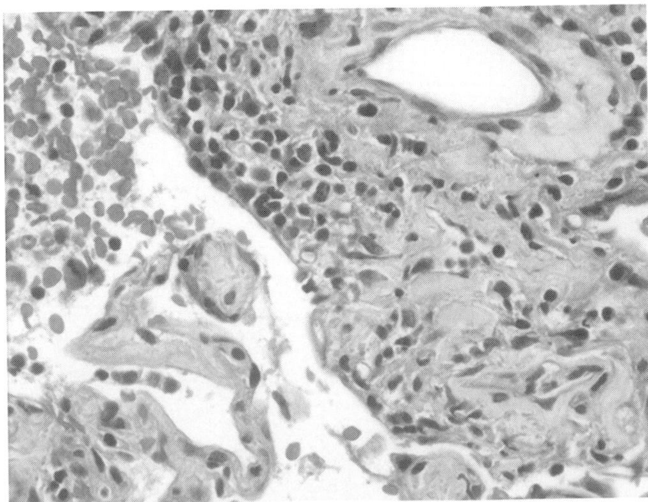

Figure 9-15 Biopsy specimen of methotrexate-induced lung injury showing lymphocytic interstitial infiltrates with occasional eosinophils.

Methotrexate pneumonitis can occur at any time during therapy, and dose and route of therapy do not appear to predict its occurrence.[68,71] Most people will recover completely after cessation of the methotrexate. Corticosteroids are generally recommended for patients with significant impairment.

Amiodarone pulmonary toxicity

Four clinical presentations of amiodarone pulmonary toxicity have been described: interstitial pneumonitis, acute respiratory distress syndrome ARDS, BOOP, and pulmonary nodules.[69,72] The most common is interstitial pneumonitis. The presentation is typically subacute, and it tends to occur after several months of therapy. Although it can occur at any dose, it does so usually in the context of a higher daily dosage (> 400 mg/day). Patients' complaints frequently include cough, dyspnea, fever, and pleuritic chest pain.

There are no diagnostic studies for amiodarone pulmonary toxicity.[69,72] Laboratory studies are nonspecific but can show leukocytosis and elevated erythrocyte sedimentation rates. Pulmonary function studies reveal decreased diffusion capacity. Chest radiographs reveal patchy bilateral interstitial infiltrates. Lung biopsy is of limited value, as the findings are nonspecific. Alveolar accumulation of foamy macrophages occurs in people on amiodarone with or without clinical disease. Other findings include type II pneumocyte hyperplasia and alveolar septal thickening.

Treatment consists of discontinuing amiodarone.[69,72] The majority of cases slowly resolve due in part to the prolonged half-life of the agent. Corticosteroids have had anecdotal success in some cases. For some patients in whom the use of alternative antiarrhythmic agents was not possible, a strategy of low-dose corticosteroids while continuing amiodarone has had some success.

References

1. Katzenstein AL, Myers JL. Idiopathic pulmonary fibrosis: Clinical relevance of pathologic classification. *Am J Respir Crit Care Med* 1998;157(4 Pt 1):1301–1315.
2. Schwartz DA, Helmers RA, Galvin JR, et al. Determinants of survival in idiopathic pulmonary fibrosis. *Am J Respir Crit Care Med* 1994;149(2 Pt 1):450–454.
3. Gay SE, Kazerooni EA, Toews GB, et al. Idiopathic pulmonary fibrosis: Predicting response to therapy and survival. *Am J Respir Crit Care Med* 1998;157(4 Pt 1): 1063–1072.
4. Bjoraker JA, Ryu JH, Edwin MK, et al. Prognostic significance of histopathologic subsets in idiopathic pulmonary fibrosis. *Am J Respir Crit Care Med* 1998;157(1):199–203.
5. King TE Jr, Tooze JA, Schwarz MI, et al. Predicting survival in idiopathic pulmonary fibrosis: Scoring system and survival model. *Am J Respir Crit Care Med* 2001;164(7): 1171–1181.
6. Gross TJ, Hunninghake GW. Idiopathic pulmonary fibrosis. *N Engl J Med* 2001;345(7):517–525.
7. American Thoracic Society. Idiopathic pulmonary fibrosis: Diagnosis and treatment. International consensus statement. American Thoracic Society (ATS), and the European Respiratory Society (ERS). *Am J Respir Crit Care Med* 2000;161(2 Pt 1):646–664.
8. Hunninghake GW, Zimmerman MB, Schwartz DA, et al. Utility of a lung biopsy for the diagnosis of idiopathic pulmonary fibrosis. *Am J Respir Crit Care Med* 2001;164(2): 193–196.
9. Raghu G, Depaso WJ, Cain K, et al. Azathioprine combined with prednisone in the treatment of idiopathic pulmonary fibrosis: A prospective double-blind, randomized, placebo-controlled clinical trial. *Am Rev Respir Dis* 1991; 144(2):291–296.
10. Ziesche R, Hofbauer E, Wittmann K, et al. A preliminary study of long-term treatment with interferon gamma-1b and low-dose prednisolone in patients with idiopathic pulmonary fibrosis. *N Engl J Med* 1999;341(17):1264–1269.
11. Raghu G. Gamma interferon for the treatment of idiopathic pulmonary fibrosis: Results of a multicenter trial. Presented at the ATS meeting, Seattle, WA,. 2003.
12. Liebow AA, Carrington CB. The interstitial pneumonias. In: Simon M, Potchen EJ, LeMay M (eds). *Frontiers of Pulmonary Radiology*. New York: Grune & Stratton, 1969:102–141.
13. Kitaichi M. Pathologic features and the classification of interstitial pneumonia of unknown etiology. *Bull Chest Dis Res Inst Kyoto Univ* 1990;23(1–2):1–18.
14. Katzenstein AL, Fiorelli RF. Nonspecific interstitial pneumonia/fibrosis. Histologic features and clinical significance. *Am J Surg Pathol* 1994;18(2):136–147.
15. Nagai S, Kitaichi M, Itoh H, et al. Idiopathic nonspecific interstitial pneumonia/fibrosis: Comparison with idiopathic pulmonary fibrosis and BOOP. *Eur Respir J* 1998; 12(5):1010–1019.
16. Cottin V, Donsbeck AV, Revel D, et al. Nonspecific interstitial pneumonia. Individualization of a clinicopathologic entity in a series of 12 patients. *Am J Respir Crit Care Med* 1998;158(4):1286–1293.
17. Davison AG, Heard BE, McAllister WA, Turner-Warwick ME. Cryptogenic organizing pneumonitis. *Q J Med* 1983;52(207):382–394.
18. Epler GR, Colby TV, McLoud TC, et al. Bronchiolitis obliterans organizing pneumonia. *N Engl J Med* 1985;312(3):152–158.
19. American Thoracic Society/European Respiratory Society International Multidisciplinary Consensus Classification of the Idiopathic Interstitial Pneumonias. *Am J Respir Crit Care Med* 2002;165(2):277–304.
20. Epler GR. Bronchiolitis obliterans organizing pneumonia. *Arch Intern Med* 2001;161(2):158–164.

21. Oikonomou A, Hansell DM. Organizing pneumonia: The many morphological faces. *Eur Radiol* 2002;12(6): 1486–1496.
22. Cordier JF, Loire R, Brune J. Idiopathic bronchiolitis obliterans organizing pneumonia. Definition of characteristic clinical profiles in a series of 16 patients. *Chest* 1989; 96(5):999–1004.
23. Lohr RH, Boland BJ, Douglas WW, et al. Organizing pneumonia. Features and prognosis of cryptogenic, secondary, and focal variants. *Arch Intern Med* 1997;157(12): 1323–1329.
24. Cordier JF. Update on cryptogenic organizing pneumonia (idiopathic bronchiolitis obliterans organizing pneumonia). *Swiss Med Wkly* 2002;132(41–42):588–591.
25. Cohen AJ, King TE Jr, Downey GP. Rapidly progressive bronchiolitis obliterans with organizing pneumonia. *Am J Respir Crit Care Med* 1994; 149(6):1670–1675.
26. Strimlan CV, Rosenow EC III, Wieland LH, Brown LR. Lymphocytic interstitial pneumonitis. Review of 13 cases. *Ann Intern Med* 1978;88(5):616–621.
27. Johkoh T, Muller NL, Pickford HA, et al. Lymphocytic interstitial pneumonia: Thin-section CT findings in 22 patients. *Radiology* 1999;212(2):567–572.
28. Freemer MM, King TE. Connective tissue diseases. In: Scharz MI, King TE (eds). *Interstitial Lung Disease.* Hamilton, Ontario: BC Decker, 2003.
29. Kim EA, Lee KS, Johkoh T, et al. Interstitial lung diseases associated with collagen vascular diseases: Radiologic and histopathologic findings. *Radiographics* 2002;22(Spec No):S151–S165.
30. Newman LS, Rose CS, Maier LA. Sarcoidosis. *N Engl J Med* 1997;336(17):1224–1234.
31. Rybicki BA, Major M, Popovich J Jr, et al. Racial differences in sarcoidosis incidence: A 5-year study in a health maintenance organization. *Am J Epidemiol* 1997;145(3): 234–241.
32. Thomas KW, Hunninghake GW. Sarcoidosis. *JAMA* 2003;289(24):3300–3303.
33. Chiles C. Imaging features of thoracic sarcoidosis. *Semin Roentgenol* 2002;37(1):82–93.
34. Statement on sarcoidosis. Joint Statement of the American Thoracic Society (ATS), the European Respiratory Society (ERS) and the World Association of Sarcoidosis and Other Granulomatous Disorders (WASOG). *Am J Respir Crit Care Med* 1999;160(2):736–755.
35. Rosen SH, Castleman B, Liebow AA. Pulmonary alveolar proteinosis. *N Engl J Med* 1958;258(23):1123–1142.
36. Seymour JF, Presneill JJ. Pulmonary alveolar proteinosis: Progress in the first 44 years. *Am J Respir Crit Care Med* 2002;166(2):215–235.
37. Wang BM, Stern EJ, Schmidt RA, Pierson DJ. Diagnosing pulmonary alveolar proteinosis. A review and an update. *Chest* 1997;111(2):460–466.
38. Allen JN, Davis WB. Eosinophilic lung diseases. *Am J Respir Crit Care Med* 1994;150(5 Pt 1):1423–1438.
39. Loffler W. Zur differential—Diagnose der Lungeninfiltrierungen: II. Uber fluchtige succedan—Infiltrate (mit eosinophilie). *Beitr Klin Tuberk* 1932;79: 368–392.
40. Citro LA, Gordon ME, Miller WT. Eosinophilic lung disease (or how to slice P.I.E.). *Am J Roentgenol Radium Ther Nucl Med* 1973;117(4):787–797.
41. Allen JN, Pacht ER, Gadek JE, Davis WB. Acute eosinophilic pneumonia as a reversible cause of noninfectious respiratory failure. *N Engl J Med* 1989; 321(9): 569–574.
42. Badesch DB, King TE Jr, Schwarz MI. Acute eosinophilic pneumonia: A hypersensitivity phenomenon? *Am Rev Respir Dis* 1989;139(1):249–252.
43. Philit F, Etienne-Mastroianni B, Parrot A, et al. Idiopathic acute eosinophilic pneumonia: A study of 22 patients. *Am J Respir Crit Care Med* 2002;166(9):1235–1239.
44. Tazelaar HD, Linz LJ, Colby TV, et al. Acute eosinophilic pneumonia: Histopathologic findings in nine patients. *Am J Respir Crit Care Med* 1997;155(1):296–302.
45. Christoforidis AJ, Molnar W. Eosinophilic pneumonia. Report of two cases with pulmonary biopsy. *JAMA* 1960; 173:157–161.
46. Carrington CB, Addington WW, Goff AM, et al. Chronic eosinophilic pneumonia. *N Engl J Med* 1969;280(15): 787–798.
47. Jederlinic PJ, Sicilian L, Gaensler EA. Chronic eosinophilic pneumonia. A report of 19 cases and a review of the literature. *Medicine (Baltimore)* 1988;67(3):154–162.
48. Marchand E, Reynaud-Gaubert M, Lauque D, et al. Idiopathic chronic eosinophilic pneumonia. A clinical and follow-up study of 62 cases. The Groupe d'Etudes et de Recherche sur les Maladies "Orphelines" Pulmonaires (GERM"O"P). *Medicine (Baltimore)* 1998;77(5): 299–312.
49. Mayo JR, Muller NL, Road J, et al. Chronic eosinophilic pneumonia: CT findings in six cases. *AJR* 1989;153(4): 727–730.
50. Vassallo R, Ryu JH, Colby TV, et al. Pulmonary Langerhans'-cell histiocytosis. *N Engl J Med* 2000;342(26): 1969–1978.
51. Friedman PJ, Liebow AA, Sokoloff J. Eosinophilic granuloma of lung. Clinical aspects of primary histiocytosis in the adult. *Medicine (Baltimore)* 1981;60(6):385–396.
52. Travis WD, Borok Z, Roum JH, et al. Pulmonary Langerhans cell granulomatosis (histiocytosis X). A clinicopathologic study of 48 cases. *Am J Surg Pathol* 1993;17(10):971–986.
53. Brauner MW, Grenier P, Tijani K, et al. Pulmonary Langerhans cell histiocytosis: Evolution of lesions on CT scans. *Radiology* 1997;204(2):497–502.
54. Gabbay E, Dark JH, Ashcroft T, et al. Recurrence of Langerhans' cell granulomatosis following lung transplantation. *Thorax* 1998;53(4):326–327.
55. Vlahakis NE, Aksamit TR. Diagnosis and treatment of allergic bronchopulmonary aspergillosis. *Mayo Clin Proc* 2001;76(9):930–938.
56. Hanley-Lopez J, Clement LT. Allergic bronchopulmonary aspergillosis in cystic fibrosis. *Curr Opin Pulm Med* 2000;6(6):540–544.
57. Greenberger PA. Allergic bronchopulmonary aspergillosis. *J Allergy Clin Immunol* 2002;110(5):685–692.
58. Stevens DA, Schwartz HJ, Lee JY, et al. A randomized trial of itraconazole in allergic bronchopulmonary aspergillosis. *N Engl J Med* 2000;342(11):756–762.
59. Wark PA, Hensley MJ, Saltos N, et al. Anti-inflammatory effect of itraconazole in stable allergic bronchopulmonary aspergillosis: A randomized controlled trial. *J Allergy Clin Immunol* 2003;111(5):952–957.

60. Selman M. Hypersensitivity pneumonitis. In: Scharz MI, King TE (eds). Interstitial Lung Disease. Hamilton, Toronto: BC Decker, 2003.
61. Bourke SJ, Dalphin JC, Boyd G, et al. Hypersensitivity pneumonitis: Current concepts. *Eur Respir J* 2001;2(Suppl):81s–92s.
62. Glazer CS, Rose CS, Lynch DA. Clinical and radiologic manifestations of hypersensitivity pneumonitis. *J Thorac Imaging* 2002;17(4):261–272.
63. Campbell J. Acute symptoms following work with hay. *BMJ* 1932;2:1143–1166.
64. Rodriguez DC, Carrillo T, Castillo R, et al. Relationships between characteristics of exposure to pigeon antigens. Clinical manifestations and humoral immune response. *Chest* 1993;103(4):1059–1063.
65. Erkinjuntti-Pekkanen R, Kokkarinen JI, Tukiainen HO, et al. Long-term outcome of pulmonary function in farmer's lung: A 14 year follow-up with matched controls. *Eur Respir J* 1997;10(9):2046–2050.
66. Rose C, King TE Jr. Controversies in hypersensitivity pneumonitis. *Am Rev Respir Dis* 1992;145(1):1–2.
67. Kokkarinen JI, Tukiainen HO, Terho EO. Effect of corticosteroid treatment on the recovery of pulmonary function in farmer's lung. *Am Rev Respir Dis* 1992;145(1):3–5.
68. Cooper JA Jr, White DA, Matthay RA. Drug-induced pulmonary disease. Part 1: Cytotoxic drugs. *Am Rev Respir Dis* 1986;133(2):321–340.
69. Cooper JA Jr, White DA, Matthay RA. Drug-induced pulmonary disease: Part 2. Noncytotoxic drugs. *Am Rev Respir Dis* 1986;133(3):488–505.
70. Rossi SE, Erasmus JJ, McAdams HP, et al. Pulmonary drug toxicity: Radiologic and pathologic manifestations. *Radiographics* 2000;20(5):1245–1259.
71. Cannon GW. Methotrexate pulmonary toxicity. *Rheum Dis Clin North Am* 1997;23(4):917–937.
72. Pollak PT. Clinical organ toxicity of antiarrhythmic compounds: Ocular and pulmonary manifestations. *Am J Cardiol* 1999;84(9A):37R–45R.

CHAPTER

10 SURGICAL MANAGEMENT OF BULLOUS EMPHYSEMA AND SPONTANEOUS PNEUMOTHORAX

Geoffrey Cousins, Terri L. Jordan, Jon Kiev

SURGICAL MANAGEMENT OF BULLOUS EMPHYSEMA

The surgical treatment of bullous emphysema has evolved over the last century as the understanding of the pathophysiology of this disease has been redefined. Initial surgical efforts to either augment or restrict the thoracic cavity were unsuccessful. These early procedures were followed by tracheoplasty and other procedures in an effort to decrease dead-space volume. It was not until 1959 that Brantigan first recognized and described parenchymal plication, allowing compressed but otherwise normal lung tissue to reexpand.[1] Since Brantigan's seminal investigations, efforts have grown to refine surgical approaches to these critically ill patients.[2]

KEY CONCEPTS

- Epidemiology
  - Spontaneous pneumothoraces affect more than 20,000 people in the United States per year. Primary spontaneous pneumothoraces occur most commonly in male smokers in early adulthood. Bullous disease is most prevalent in patients with severe emphysematous disease.
- Pathophysiology
  - Pneumothoraces can be broadly classified into spontaneous or acquired types. Spontaneous pneumothoraces arise most commonly from rupture of an apical bleb, with secondary causes including chronic obstructive pulmonary disease, cystic fibrosis, *Pneumocystis carinii* pneumonia, and lung carcinoma. Acquired pneumothoraces are generally related to iatrogenic or traumatic causes, including thoracic tumor biopsies, central line placement, thoracocentesis, and barotrauma from positive-pressure ventilation.
  - Bullous disease arises from emphysematous disease, histologically classified as proximal acinar, panacinar, and distal acinar emphysema. Chronic expiratory airflow obstruction leads to structural changes in lung parenchyma and the formation of bullae; bullae are histologically composed of trabeculations of destroyed fibrous septa devoid of blood vessels.
- Clinical features
  - Spontaneous pneumothoraces are often heralded by the sudden onset of chest pain and shortness of breath. Signs of tension pneumothorax include unilateral decreased breath sounds, hypotension and/or shock, jugular venous distention, and tracheal deviation contralateral to the affected side.
  - Patients with bullous disease present with signs and symptoms of chronic obstructive pulmonary disease predicated on dyspnea, resting hypoxemia, and significant functional impairment. The chest is hyperresonant with percussion.
- Diagnostics
  - Pneumothorax is most readily diagnosed with plain chest radiography. Although not necessary for diagnosis, spiral high-resolution computed tomography is useful to define pathologic lung states and surgical planning.

- Plain radiographic changes associated with bullous disease include diaphragm flattening, increasing radiolucency, increased anteroposterior diameter, and increased retrosternal air. Computed tomography reliably delineates the size, location, and extent of bullous formations. Spirometry usually reflects a declining FEV_1/FVC ratio (FEV_1 typically < 0.8), marginal DLCO, and increased functional residual capacity, consistent with chronic airflow obstruction and pulmonary hyperinflation. Arterial blood gases indicate hypoxemia and hypercapnia.
- Treatment
  - Tube thoracostomy effectively reexpands the collapsed lung and is definitive therapy for most pneumothoraces. Surgery is necessary for persistent air leaks, failure of lung reexpansion, recurrent pneumothoraces, and bilateral pneumothoraces. Surgical procedures include pleural abrasion and pleural stripping.
  - Ideal surgical candidates for the resection of bullae are those with localized (apical) disease, reduced forced vital capacity, low P_{CO_2}, and minimal inflammation and sputum production. Other surgical indications include recurrent pneumothoraces, bronchopleural fistulas, and bullae associated with infection, chest pain, or hemoptysis. Surgical treatment consists of video-assisted thoracic surgical bullectomy, Monaldi intracavitary drainage, and open bullectomy.
- Outcomes/prognosis
  - Tube thoracostomy and pleural abrasion/stripping are associated with extremely low rates of morbidity and mortality.
  - Persistent air leak is the most common complication following bullectomy. Surgical mortality should be 5 percent or less. Patients who are younger and otherwise healthy with rapidly progressing dyspnea, normal forced vital capacity, FEV_1 greater than 40 percent, and normal diffusion capacity fare best.

Although bullous emphysema has generally been managed medically, especially in regard to complications such as pneumothorax, hemoptysis, and infection, the thoracic community is beginning to recognize the benefits of surgical intervention in selected patients. At present, although objective results are difficult to quantify, specific patients who are properly selected benefit from surgery.

DEFINITION

Emphysema is defined by an abnormal enlargement of the air spaces distal to the terminal nonrespiratory bronchiole. Airway obstruction and its flow characteristics are defined by both dilatation and parenchymal destruction.[3] A bulla is formed as overdistention and destruction of the secondary lobule occurs. Bullae have thin, fibrous walls; lack pulmonary vessels; and contain air-filled spaces that act to compress other, normal areas of lung. They are recognized radiographically by the absence of vasculature and relative radiolucency, easily seen on plain films. Bullae should be distinguished from blebs, or smaller subpleural air collections, which are separated from the underlying parenchyma by a thin pleural covering. Blebs usually occur at the apices and result from subpleural alveolar rupture. They occasionally coalesce to form larger blebs.

HISTORY

The current tenets of emphysema surgery are based on a myriad of fascinating early surgical procedures that were developed but eventually abandoned.[4] Although the first human anatomic description of emphysema occurred in the 1780s, it was not until 100 years later that surgical solutions were sought.[5] It is important to explain these failed procedures briefly so as to understand and recognize the pathophysiology of this complex, poorly understood disease.

1. Costochondrectomy: an effort to increase the flexibility of the noncompliant thorax by resecting costal cartilage. This early chest wall operation was thought to reduce rib-cage restriction and allow room for pulmonary expansion.
2. Thoracoplasty: an attempt to restore the shape of the thoracic cavity surgically and decrease thoracic volumes, although it ultimately worsened respiratory function in most patients.
3. Tracheoplasty: an attempt to minimize the airway collapse seen in emphysema, and tracheostomy was done to minimize dead space and improve pulmonary toilet.
4. Phrenicectomy: by inducing a paralyzed and elevated diaphragm, this procedure was intended to minimize lung volumes and prevent lung overdistention, again reducing the volume of the thorax.
5. Pneumoperitoneum: produced objective pulmonary improvement but caused severe abdominal pain and cramping.
6. Pleurectomy and pleurodesis procedures were thought to improve parenchymal blood flow via collateral circulation.
7. Sympathectomies were performed to minimize bronchospasm and vasodilate underperfused areas.

CLASSIFICATION OF EMPHYSEMA

In evaluating emphysema patients for surgery, a basic pathophysiologic understanding is needed so that the disease can be classified on physiologic, morphologic, and therapeutic grounds. The surgeon is responsible for recognizing these categories in order to assess the morbidity and benefit to a potential patient in whom surgery for bullous emphysema is being offered. By summarizing these classifications, the surgeon is enabled to select the subgroups of patients who should be surgical candidates.

The physiologic classification uses spirometric data to grade, in a reproducible fashion, the severity of the disease. Based on FEV_1 and FVC, patients are deemed stage I through stage III, based on the severity of their lung dysfunction.

Morphologic classifications of chronic obstructive pulmonary disease (COPD) consider the pulmonary lobule as a unit composed of a terminal bronchiole and alveoli.[6] The three subgroups are centrilobular, panlobular, and distal acinar disease. The three pathologic varieties of emphysema are distinguished in the early phases of the disease but later become difficult to differentiate.[7] All varieties are associated with the formation of bullae.

Proximal acinar emphysema is associated with smoking and is caused by inflammation of the distal airways, most commonly in the upper lung fields. The respiratory bronchioles are enlarged and destroyed.

Panacinar or diffuse emphysema involves the entire acinus, causing uniform destruction. Commonly in association with $alpha_1$ antitrypsin deficiency, there is progressive enlargement of the airspaces, with the lower lobes predominant. A low diffusion capacity and pruning of the pulmonary vasculature are typical features in these dyspneic patients.

Distal acinar emphysema involves the distal part of the ducts, sacs, and acinus and leads to pulmonary fibrosis. Its subpleural location leads to its characteristic formation of bullae and spontaneous pneumothorax, and it is the form of emphysema that surgeons will most commonly deal with successfully.[8]

Finally, the therapeutic classification of COPD allows candidate selection for therapies other than surgery. These include but are not limited to smoking cessation, pulmonary rehabilitation, lung transplantation, and lung volume reduction surgery.

PATHOPHYSIOLOGY

The expiratory airflow obstruction typical of COPD is caused by the chronic pathologic changes that occur from the central airway to the lung parenchyma. Cigarette smoke accounts for 90 percent of emphysema in the United States. The airway remodeling and fibrotic process, along with parenchymal destruction, lead to dyspnea.[9] The adverse changes in pulmonary function, exercise capacity, and pulmonary vascularity become limiting over the course of the patient's life.

Through spirometry, declining FEV_1/FVC acts as a sentinel indicator of airflow obstruction. As functional residual capacity increases owing to loss of lung parenchyma and elasticity, pulmonary hyperinflation occurs. Specific radiologic changes like diaphragmatic flattening, increasing radiolucency, and increased retrosternal air become obvious. These changes are clinically evident with an increase in the anteroposterior (AP) diameter of the chest and hyperresonance during percussion.

Similarly, as COPD progresses, resting hypoxemia leads to severe functional impairment. Exercise capacity becomes limited, with respiratory muscles requiring maximal oxygen consumption. As the alveolar-arterial oxygen gradient widens, hypercapnia ensues, further contributing to the associated degrees of pulmonary hypertension, which are inevitable with advancement of the disease.

Bullous emphysema is characterized by the formation of either bullae or blebs. The walls of the bullae are composed of the trabeculations of destroyed fibrous septa devoid of blood vessels. Successful surgery for bullous emphysema depends on the character and quality of the underlying lung. Although a large bulla with a narrow neck is easily resected, the structural changes in the nonbullous parenchyma ultimately determine the effectiveness of the resection. At the same time, the degree to which bullae contribute to dyspnea depends on the amount of lung they displace and the character of the underlying lung. In broad terms, patients with diffuse emphysema with complete loss of parenchyma and with well-demarcated bullae do not fare as well as those with normal underlying parenchyma. Although patients with a giant bullae and normal underlying parenchyma perform most favorably, this type of patient is in the minority.

CLINICAL PRESENTATION AND INDICATIONS FOR SURGERY

The degree of dyspnea in patients with bullous emphysema is difficult to quantitate, and the degree to which the bulla itself is causing impairment versus the underlying parenchymal issues is equally difficult to determine. Prophylactic bullectomy in asymptomatic patients has been performed, but its efficacy is unknown because the natural history of the asymptomatic bulla patient is unknown.[10] The resection of bullae occupying greater than 50 percent of a hemithorax results in clinical improvement in disabled dyspneic patients.[11] Additionally, patients with pulmonary artery hypertension also benefit from pneumonectomy, as vascular crowding is eliminated by the removal of the compressive bulla.

Patients with minimal inflammation and minimal sputum production benefit most from the resection of localized bullous disease. Other surgical indications include recurrent pneumothoraces as well as the presence of bronchopleural fistulas.[12] In nondyspneic patients, those with infection or hemoptysis attributed to a bulla and patients with severe chest pain or an underlying suspicion of lung cancer may benefit from resection.

In the broadest terms, patients with severe dyspnea, increased residual volume, decreased diffusing capacity of the lung (DLCO), and scant sputum production fare better surgically than those with diffuse parenchymal abnormalities defined by severe bronchitis and copious sputum production. Younger patients with rapid progression of dyspnea and who have given up smoking are better surgical candidates.[13] Additionally, those patients with reduced FVC and low P_{CO_2} with apical bullous disease fare best surgically.

Exercise testing has been used to define the patients who will have postoperative improvement. However, no single test will determine which patient will benefit from bullectomy. The surgeon who treats patients with emphysema will learn to rely on clinical judgment in the selection of patients for bullectomy, again emphasizing the surgical dictum to remove as little functional lung as possible.

PREOPERATIVE MANAGEMENT

Although chest x-ray is a useful screening modality to define bullous disease and offers comparison to previous studies, the computed tomography (CT) scan is a more sensitive as well as a mandatory study to delineate the size, location, and extent of the space-occupying lesion. The CT reliably details the bulla in regard to other thoracic pathology. CT offers three-dimensional assessment of the dominant bulla and shows the degree of vascular crowding, mediastinal shift, and lung herniation. Although these factors may not correlate with patients' symptoms, CT allows the surgeon to target specific lung areas for resection.[14]

Ventilation/perfusion (V/Q) scanning provides a functional assessment of the vascular and parenchymal integrity of the lung, but it is more useful in evaluating patients with emphysema who are being considered for lung volume reduction surgery. V/Q scanning offers little useful information to the surgeon planning to resect a known, nonfunctioning bulla.

Pulmonary function tests and arterial blood gases are important parameters in selecting patients for preoperative evaluation; unfortunately, however, they have little predictive value. Ideal surgical candidates will have normal FEV_1, preserved DLCO, and no hypercapnia. Patients like these are rare. More typically, surgeons will operate on patients with $FEV_1 < 0.8$ and marginal diffusion capacities.

Additional clinical evaluation includes therapy for smoking cessation and pulmonary rehabilitation. Abstinence from smoking combined with progressive preoperative conditioning are prerequisites for elective bullectomy. Additionally, all patients should undergo bronchoscopy to evaluate and clear the airways and rule out any possibility of an underlying lung cancer. Formal bronchoscopy can be done at the time of surgery to confirm endotracheal tube placement.

OPERATIVE STRATEGIES

The surgical approach to bullous lung disease is designed to remove all space-occupying, nonfunctioning airspaces and thereby decrease both dead space and residual volume. The surgeon must preserve as much normal lung as possible; major anatomic resections are discouraged.[15] Similarly, segmental resections are rarely indicated because bullous disease is seldom confined to an anatomic segment. With these parameters in mind, three general approaches to bullectomy have emerged, including VATS, intracavitary drainage, and open bullectomy.

Video-assisted thoracic surgery (VATS)

Bullectomy with VATS is currently the most widely performed procedure for bullous emphysema.[16] High-risk patients with marginal pulmonary function are ideal candidates for VATS. Performed under general anesthesia, VATS bullectomy requires placement of a double-lumen endotracheal tube and lateral decubitus positioning. The first 1-cm incision is placed in the midaxillary line in the fifth intercostal space for camera access. Using a 30-degree thoracoscope, the entire hemithorax can be examined, and two additional port sites can be planned to allow maximum maneuverability. Adhesions are lysed in an avascular plane and the bullae are identified. Endoscopic staplers with commercially available bovine pericardial strips for staple-line reinforcement are used to ligate and resect the bullae at their bases. Care is taken to preserve functioning lung parenchyma. Hemostasis and pneumostasis are critical in these patients. Although air leaks are expected, minimizing them at the time of surgery is the best preventive measure available.

Intracavitary Drainage

Intracavitary drainage (Monaldi procedure) for bullous disease was derived from a technique to drain refractory tuberculous cavitary disease. This technique has been modified and currently involves resecting a small portion of the rib overlying the bulla. A purse-string suture is placed to incorporate the parietal and visceral pleura and the wall of the bulla. Next, the bulla is opened within the purse string and a Foley catheter is inserted and inflated with air. The purse-string suture is then tightened and the catheter placed under water to suction. Talc pleurodesis of the pleural cavity and bulla may also be performed and has been shown to be effective. This technique has proven useful in high-risk patients who may not tolerate bullectomy. Results are gratifying, with a marked improvement in FEV_1 and *VC*.

Open Bullectomy

Unilateral bullectomy is performed through a posterolateral thoracotomy in patients with large, compressive bullae. The walls of the bulla are opened and the trabeculae excised. The bulla's wall is then folded over the remaining raw lung surface and the stapler fired across the base of the bulla (Fig. 10-1). Some surgeons advocate the use of bovine pericardial strips to provide additional pneumostasis. Pleurodesis may be performed and chest tubes are placed. If bilateral bullectomies are necessary, a median sternotomy or a clamshell incision may be considered. Median sternotomy has been shown to be superior in maintaining pulmonary function in the postoperative period.

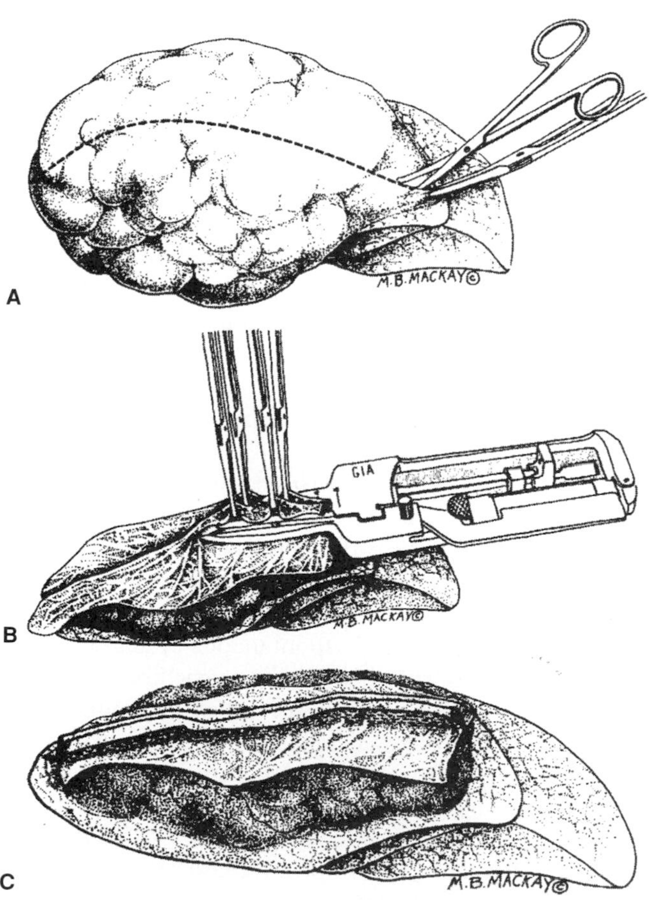

Figure 10-1 Operative technique for open bullectomy. A. Longitudinal opening of the bulla. B. Folding of the visceral pleura over the raw lung surface and stapling of the entire base of the cyst. C. Completed bullectomy. (From Deslauriers J, Leblanc P, McClish A. *General Thoracic Surgery,* 3d ed. Philadelphia: Lea & Febiger, 1989. With permission.)

Lung Volume Reduction Surgery (LVRS)

Lung volume reduction surgery (LVRS) was begun in 1957 by Brantigan, but it was not until the mid 1990s that it became accepted in the thoracic community. By resecting only the most diseased portions of lung, the elastic recoil of the remaining lung is improved, thereby improving respiratory mechanics. Multiple parenchymal plications were thought to restore the circumferential pull on the collapsed smaller airways and vessels. Cooper and associates at Washington University demonstrated significant objective and clinical improvements in pulmonary function and respiratory mechanics.[17] Surgical approaches to lung volume reduction are performed through median sternotomy or thoracoscopy.[18] Patient outcomes are being examined by the National Emphysema Treatment Trial (NETT).

Patients selected for LVRS generally have FEV_1 of less than 35 percent, with marked hyperinflation and evidence of moderate to severe emphysema.[19] Heterogeneous disease is the hallmark radiologic finding to allow targeted resection of diseased tissue. Both high-resolution CT scanning and V/Q scans are useful in the radiologic evaluation of the potential surgical patient. Patients must be motivated to participate in pulmonary rehabilitation and preoperative smoking cessation.

Postoperatively, patients are extubated as soon as possible and mobilized aggressively; pulmonary rehabilitation is also restarted. Marked improvement in FEV_1 and clinical function is seen within the first 6 months after surgery.[20] Many patients are weaned from oxygen and resume activities of daily living with minimal restriction.

POSTOPERATIVE MANAGEMENT

Postoperative pulmonary rehabilitation is critical in this patient population. Every effort must be made to extubate these patients at the end of the surgical procedure. Clear communication with the anesthesia team is important, combining an epidural catheter with the judicious use of fluids allows for a rapid transition through the critical postoperative period.

Proper staple-line closure and reinforcement minimizes the expected air leak, which may not be evident until the completion of the surgical procedure. Chest tube management is often debated. We typically employ tubes with 10 cm of water, no suction. If the patient collapses his or her lung or adequate reexpansion was not obtainable at the time of surgery, low continuous suction may be indicated. Additionally, if subcutaneous emphysema becomes disabling, chest tubes on suction may be of benefit.

Patients are sitting upright in the immediate postoperative period. Incentive spirometry, early ambulation, and chest physiotherapy are encouraged in both the pre- and postoperative periods. Daily chest x-rays should be obtained over the first few days to look for any sign of infiltrate, signaling an early pneumonia. Patients receive prophylactic antibiotic coverage along with protection against deep venous thrombosis in the form of subcutaneous heparin and pneumatic compression devices. Preoperative smoking cessation therapy is continued. As their exercise tolerance improves, many patients are weaned to lower oxygen requirements. Nutrition is begun once bowel function returns. All efforts are made to provide enteral nutrition early so as to maintain a positive nitrogen balance. Steroids that were weaned preoperatively are used sparingly and only when necessary. Bedside bronchoscopy is used liberally for those patients who are unable to clear their secretions or if an infectious etiology is suspected.

Postoperative complications are expected in this group of patients; however, careful patient selection and an efficient operation seem to minimize these. Persistent air leak is the most common complication and may last for many days. Massive air leaks require immediate reexploration. Every effort should be made to extubate at the end of the surgical procedure. Minimizing positive-pressure ventilation will minimize air leaks and promote pulmonary toilet in the early postoperative period.

Surgical mortality should be 5 percent or less. Careful patient selection is the cornerstone of minimizing patient morbidity and mortality. Results are fairly predictable on the patient's clinical presentation, pulmonary function testing, and CT scan. Patients who are younger and otherwise healthy with rapidly progressing dyspnea, normal forced vital capacity, FEV_1 greater than 40 percent, and normal diffusion capacity perform better in the postoperative period and have a lower overall morbidity.

SURGICAL TREATMENT OF SPONTANEOUS PNEUMOTHORAX

DEFINITION

Spontaneous pneumothoraces affect more than 20,000 people in the United States per year. Because "free air" in the chest may be life-threatening, a search for the underlying cause of the pneumothorax should proceed urgently. Pneumothoraces can be classified as spontaneous or acquired. This chapter focuses on spontaneous pneumothorax from both primary and secondary causes. Acquired pneumothoraces are generally related to iatrogenic causes or trauma and are more easily linked to their antecedent causes.

HISTORY

The term *pneumothorax* was first introduced in 1803 by Etard on postmortem examination. At that time, tuberculosis was considered the primary cause of pneumothorax. Later, Kjaergaard described apical bleb rupture as the predominant cause of pneumothorax development.[21] Additionally, he clearly defined the bimodal age distribution, male predominance, and specific physical characteristics of those patients most likely to sustain a spontaneous pneumothorax.

Initial historical treatment involved prolonged bed rest. Thoracotomy and bleb resection became popular in the early 1950s followed by thoracostomy tube placement for the initial presentation of patients with spontaneous pneumothorax. Surgeons added parietal pleurectomy and mechanical abrasion techniques to minimize pneumothorax recurrence rates.

Since the early 1990s, VATS has been used to perform apical bullectomy and parietal pleurectomy, with improved patient outcomes and lower recurrence rates. As thoracic surgeons gravitate toward more minimally invasive procedures in order to facilitate shorter hospital stays and less operative morbidity, VATS has allowed older and sicker patients, who were formerly not considered surgical candidates, to be managed more aggressively.

PATHOPHYSIOLOGY

Although there are numerous classifications, the most common cause of spontaneous pneumothorax is rupture of an apical bleb (Fig. 10-2). There are numerous physiologic theories regarding bleb formation; they are, however, of little significance to the surgeon. Spontaneous primary pneumothoraces occur more commonly in male smokers in early adulthood. Other common etiologies of pneumothorax include iatrogenic causes such as subclavian line insertion for intravenous or parenteral access and pacemaker insertion. Various thoracic interventions such as percutaneous lung or mediastinal tumor biopsies, transthoracic needle aspiration, and thoracentesis are other common iatrogenic causes of pneumothorax.

Secondary causes of spontaneous pneumothorax include chronic obstructive disease, cystic fibrosis, tuberculosis (Fig. 10-3), *Pneumocystis carinii* pneumonia in immunocompromised patients, and lung cancers. Spontaneous pneumothoraces occur in patients receiving positive-pressure ventilation (Fig. 10-4). Barotrauma resulting in pneumothorax occurs during bronchoscopy as well, as elevated levels of positive end-expiratory pressure (PEEP) are generated.

CLINICAL PRESENTATION

The sudden onset of chest pain and shortness of breath is the typical hallmark of spontaneous pneumothorax in the specific patient population of tall, thin males. Physical examination may be normal and chest x-ray

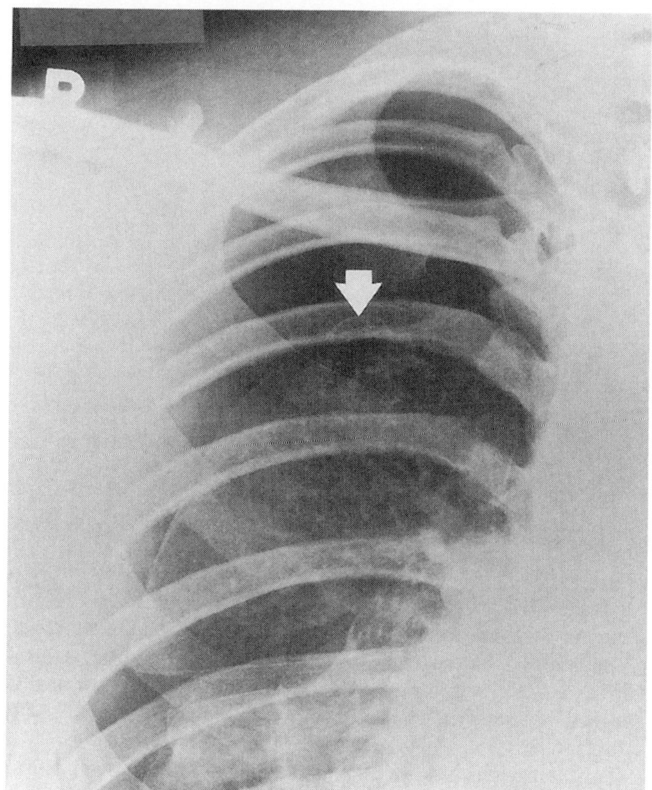

Figure 10-2 Primary spontaneous pneumothorax. The visceral pleural line is clearly demonstrated, together with a lateral avascular space. There is a pleural bleb at the apex of the lung (arrow), a common finding. Such blebs are usually not detectable when the lung reexpands. (From Hansell. *Imaging Diseases of the Chest,* 4th ed. Philadelphia: Mosby, 2005. With permission.)

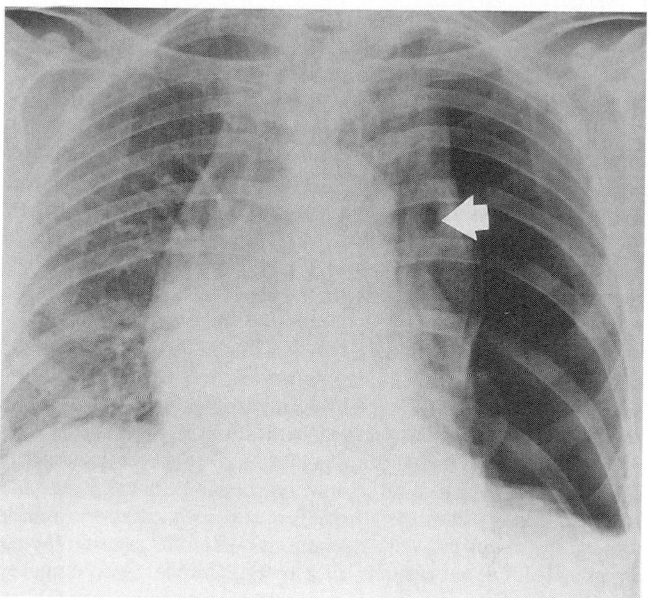

Figure 10-3 Left pneumothorax caused by a tuberculous bronchopleural fistula. Anteroposterior chest radiograph of a 58-year-old man with acute dyspnea and pain in the left side of the chest. The lung, prevented from complete collapse by intrapleural adhesions, contains a cavity (arrow). (From Hansell. *Imaging Diseases of the Chest,* 4th ed. Philadelphia: Mosby, 2005. With permission.)

usually confirms the diagnosis. If a significant collapse is present, signs such as diminished tactile fremitus, hyperresonance to percussion, and decreased breath sounds on the affected side may be present. CT scan is generally not necessary for diagnosis; however, spiral and high-resolution CT scans (Fig. 10-5) are useful to delineate various pathologic lung states. Specifically, *lymphangioleiomyomatosis* (LAM), histiocytosis X, interstitial lung diseases, and blebs and bullae are most easily seen by CT. Additionally, CT may assist with potential surgical planning. Although radiologists estimate the percentage of pneumothorax seen radiographically, these numbers are not reproducible and should not be relied on for surgical purposes.

Tension pneumothorax is a clinical diagnosis; it should never be diagnosed radiographically (Fig. 10-6). Signs of tension pneumothorax include unilateral decreased breath sounds with tympany to percussion, hypotension and other signs of shock, jugular venous distention, and tracheal deviation away from the involved side. The presentation of tension pneumothorax is usually dramatic. Such patients are dusky, cyanotic,

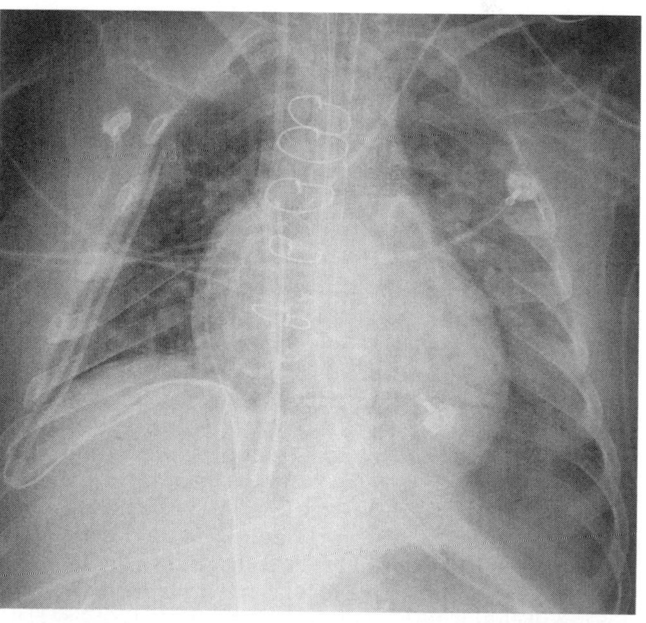

Figure 10-4 Spontaneous pneumothorax in a mechanically ventilated patient with acute respiratory distress syndrome. Supine plain chest radiography reveals increased lucency over the left upper abdomen due to air in the anterior costophrenic sulcus. There is increased sharpness of the left heart border. (From Hansell. *Imaging Diseases of the Chest,* 4th ed. Philadelphia: Mosby, 2005. With permission.)

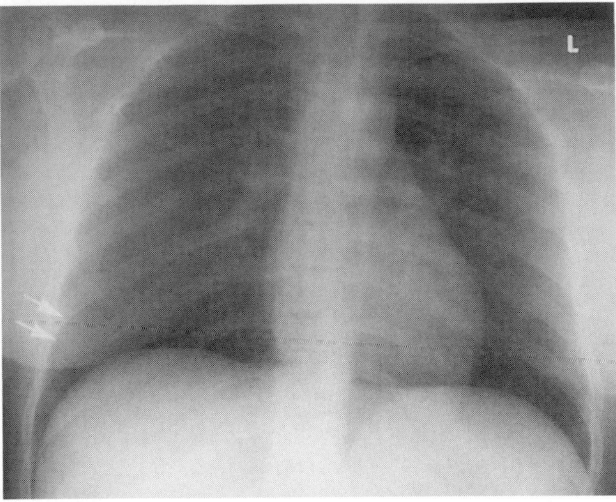

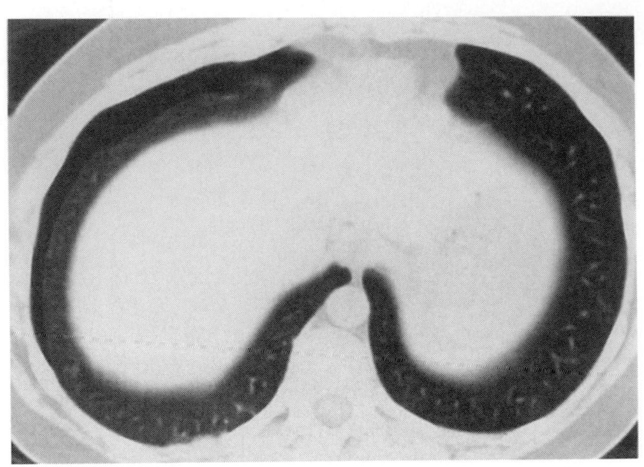

Figure 10-5 Pneumothorax in a supine patient as seen with plain film and computed tomography. A. Supine chest radiograph shows a deep lateral costophrenic sulcus on the right side with a subtle lateral line indicating a pneumothorax (*arrow*). B. Supine computed tomography of the chest shows air in the anterior and lateral costophrenic sulci and air in contact with the anterior mediastinal fat. (From Hansell. *Imaging Diseases of the Chest,* 4th ed. Philadelphia: Mosby, 2005. With permission.)

and generally tachycardic. The reduced preload caused by tension pneumothorax causes sweating and stimulates the sympathetic nervous system. Immediate decompression with an Angiocath is justified without x-ray, followed by chest-tube insertion.

TREATMENT OF SPONTANEOUS PNEUMOTHORAX

Tube thoracostomy

Lung reexpansion is the goal of treatment for pneumothorax. Small asymptomatic pneumothoraces may be observed and followed in the outpatient setting provided that the patient is reliable and medical care is available nearby. However, patients with underlying lung disease (e.g., COPD) may not tolerate observation of even small pneumothoraces; these patients may need thoracostomy-tube placement even in the face of tiny pneumothoraces.

Chest-tube diameter and selection depends on operator experience. Generally, any tube placed in the proper location with proper technique will suffice. Larger-caliber tubes are needed when fluid collections are present. Local anesthetic infiltration with 1% lidocaine is necessary for local pain control. Inexperienced residents will tend to place tubes before anesthetics have taken effect, causing patient anxiety and making insertion of the thoracostomy tube difficult. There is rarely a need for conscious sedation in a cooperative, well-informed patient.

Drainage systems are also varied. Outpatient treatment of spontaneous pneumothorax can be managed with the Heimlich valve, while inpatients are typically

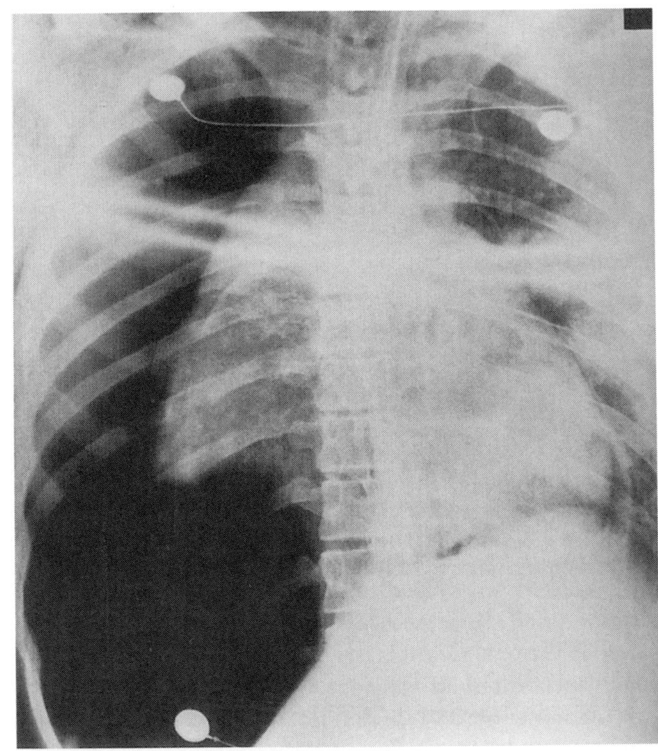

Figure 10-6 Right tension pneumothorax. There is marked deepening of the right hemidiaphragm and contralateral mediastinal shift, indicated by the position of the heart and endotracheal tube. Complete right lung collapse is prevented by consolidation. A small left pneumothorax is also noted. (From Hansell. *Imaging Diseases of the Chest,* 4th ed. Philadelphia: Mosby, 2005. With permission.)

managed with disposable underwater-seal bottles. Most simple pneumothoraces respond to these management modalities. Chest tubes are removed once the lung is fully reexpanded. Some surgeons use provocative maneuvers (e.g., chest-tube clamping) to make sure that the pneumothorax will not recur before the thoracostomy tube has been removed. If there is repeated lung collapse, pleurodesis should be considered. Occasionally a persistent air leak will require further, more aggressive intervention.

Estimates regarding the recurrence of pneumothorax are variable and depend on the nature of the underlying lung tissue, cause, resolution, and management of the initial episode as well as the factors that have prompted the recurrence. Patients must be made aware that ipsilateral or contralateral pneumothorax recurrence is possible at any time.

OPERATIVE STRATEGIES

Surgery should be considered and offered to patients with recurrent pneumothoraces and to those individuals remote from medical care. Other surgical indications include persistent air leaks (i.e., bronchopleural fistulas), failure of lung reexpansion, and bilateral pneumothoraces. Patients with previous contralateral pneumonectomy or those engaged in specialized occupations (pilots, scuba divers) should also be considered for surgery.

The preferred surgical approach (open thoracotomy vs. VATS) is hotly debated, although the ultimate goals of pneumothorax resolution and the minimization of recurrence are accomplished through either technique. Specific surgical procedures for pneumothorax include pleural abrasion and pleural stripping. By mechanically irritating the parietal pleura, a pleural symphysis can be created. A surgical sponge, cautery scratch pad, or Kitner are all useful for this technique. A layer of blood created following the mechanical abrasion is enough to promote the formation of adhesions. At the same time, fibrin glue, talc slurry, and doxycycline may be used to reinforce the mechanical abrasion, although many surgeons consider these additive therapies unnecessary.

Apical parietal pleurectomy (stripping) is another very effective procedure to eliminate pneumothorax. Care must be taken during pleurectomy around major vasculature at the lung apex, and the correct nonvascular plane must be achieved proximal to the endothoracic fascia. Pleurectomy is very effective and can be extended beyond the apex to include the entire hemithorax, creating a superior pleural symphysis. If lung pathology is present (e.g., blebs or bullae) this should be addressed simultaneously. Suture lines should be buttressed if underlying parenchyma is friable.

The surgeon is responsible for complete lung reexpansion at the end of the procedure. In the operating room, the lung parenchyma and mechanics of respiration must be closely observed. Barotrauma should be minimized by the anesthesiologist. Chest tubes are placed appropriately and strategically. Bronchoscopy should be completed to clear airway secretions, and pain control must be adequate to allow aggressive pulmonary toilet in the postoperative period.

Postoperative chest x-rays must be checked and followed. Chest tube outputs and air leaks must resolve prior to chest tube removal. Patients are ambulated on the first postoperative evening, and their diets are advanced as tolerated. A baseline AP and lateral chest x-ray is taken prior to discharge. Patients are encouraged to resume full activities as their tolerance permits.

References

1. Brantigan O, Mueller E. Surgical treatment of pulmonary emphysema. *Am Surg* 1957;789–804.
2. Brantigan O, Mueller E, Kress MB. A surgical approach to pulmonary emphysema. *Am Rev Respir Dis* 1959;80: 194–202.
3. Fletcher C, Peto R. The natural history of chronic airflow obstruction. *BMJ* 1977;1(6077):1645–1648.
4. Naef AP. History of emphysema surgery. *Ann Thorac Surg* 1997;64(5):1506–1508.
5. Cooper JD, Trulock EP, Triantafillou AN, et al. Bilateral pneumectomy (volume reduction) for chronic obstructive lung disease. *J Thorac Cardiovasc Surg* 1995;109:106–116
6. Heppleston AG, Leopold JG. Chronic pulmonary emphysema anatomy and pathogenesis. *Am J Med* 1961;31: 279–291.
7. Heard BE. A pathological study of emphysema of the lungs with chronic bronchitis. *Thorax* 1958;13:136–149.
8. Kim WD, Eidelman DH, Izquierdo JL, et al. Centrilobular and panlobular emphysema in smokers. Two distinct morphologic and functional entities. *Am Rev Respir Dis* 1991;144:1385–1390.
9. Saetta MP, Kim WD, Izquierdo JL, et al. Extent of centrilobular and panacinar emphysema in smokers' lungs: Pathological and mechanical implications. *Eur Respir J* 1994;7:664–671.
10. Morgan MD, Edwards CW, Morris J, Mathews HR. Origin and behavior of emphysematous bullae. *Thorax* 1989;44(7):533–538.
11. Mehran RJ, Deslauriers J. Indications for surgery and patient work-up for bullectomy. *Chest Surg Clin North Am* 1995;5(4):717–734.
12. DeVries WC, Wolfe WG. The management of spontaneous pneumothorax and bullous emphysema. *Surg Clin North Am* 1980;60:851.

13. Gaensler EA, Jederlinic PJ, FitzGerald MX. Patient work-up for bullectomy. *J Thorac Imaging* 1986;1(2): 75–93.
14. Dartevelle P, Macchiarini P, Chapelier A. Operative technique of bullectomy. *Chest Surg Clin North Am* 1995;5(4): 735–749.
15. Goldstraw P, Petrou M. The surgical treatment of emphysema. The Brompton approach. *Chest Surg Clin North Am* 1995;5(4):777–796.
16. Wakabayashi A. Thoracoscopic technique for management of giant bullous lung disease. *Ann Thorac Surg* 1993;56: 708–712.
17. Cooper JD, Patterson JA, Sundaresen RS, et al. Results of 150 consecutive bilateral lung volume reduction procedures in patients with severe emphysema. *J Thorac Cardiovasc Surg* 1996;112:1319–1330.
18. Kotloff RM, Tino G, Bavaria JE, et al. Bilateral lung volume reduction surgery for advanced emphysema: A comparison of median sternotomy and thoracoscopic approaches. *Chest* 1996;110:1399–1406.
19. Szekely LA, Oelberg DA, Wright CD, et al. Preoperative predictors of operative morbidity and mortality in COPD patients undergoing bilateral lung volume reduction surgery. *Chest* 1997; 111:550–558.
20. O'Brien GM, Furukawa S, Kuzma AM, et al. Improvements in lung function, exercise, and quality of life in hypercapnic COPD patients after lung volume reduction surgery. *Chest* 1999;115:75–84.
21. Beauchamp G. Spontaneous pneumothorax and pneumomediastinum. In: Pearson FG, Deslauriers J, Ginsberg RJ (eds). *Thoracic Surgery*. New York: Churchill Livingstone, 1995:1037–1054.

CHAPTER

11 THERAPIES FOR BENIGN AND MALIGNANT PLEURAL DISEASES

Denis Aleksandrovich Tereb, Joseph LoCicero III

INTRODUCTION

Historical background

For centuries the pleura remained a closed page for physicians. Observation of quick and lethal outcomes in patients with pleural injury defined its limits. Death from spontaneous pneumothorax, hemothorax, or empyema in the preanesthesia and preantibiotic eras was the norm. Before the Common Era, physicians achieved few successes with pleural conditions. However, Hippocrates himself dared approach this lethal problem, achieving a mortality rate of only 50 percent for loculated empyema.[1] He used careful observation, physical examination, and accurately timed incision and drainage. Since that time, the slow development of understanding of the basic physiology of lung expansion and pleural anatomy coupled with the rapid advances in anesthesia, the development of successful surgical approaches to the treatment of pulmonary diseases, and the development of antibiotics opened a new page in the mitigation of pleural morbidity. Gradually over time,

KEY CONCEPTS

- Epidemiology
  - Pleural diseases encompass a broad range of both benign and malignant pathologic processes. The peak age for the development of diffuse malignant mesothelioma is in the sixth decade of life.
- Pathophysiology
  - Pleural effusions are generally categorized into transudates and exudates; transudates are thought to be caused by increased hydrostatic pressures or decreased oncotic pressures, whereas exudates result from increased permeability. Effusions can also be caused by a breach in the integrity of the pleural membrane with contamination of the space by foreign or infective substances (i.e., parapneumonic effusions). Pleura-based masses or thickening can arise from many processes, including benign fibrous tumors, primary malignant mesothelioma, or metastatic disease.
- Clinical features
  - Chest pain, dyspnea, fever, weight loss, and hypoglycemia are frequent symptoms associated with primary malignant pleural tumors. Hypertrophic pulmonary osteoarthropathy can affect more than 20 percent of benign localized fibrous pleural tumors.
- Diagnostics
  - Plain chest radiography often gives an accurate assessment of effusions and air in pleural cavities as well as pleural thickening. Computed tomography aids in evaluating pleural effusions and differentiating pleural, lung, and bone pathology. Magnetic resonance imaging has 100 percent sensitivity and 93 percent specificity in the detection of pleural malignancy. Needle aspiration, needle biopsy, limited thoracotomy, and video-assisted thoracoscopic surgery are the main invasive diagnostic tools available to diagnose pleural disorders. Quantification of pleural fluid glucose, amylase, lactate dehydrogenase, cell count, microbiologic studies, and cytology are often useful in characterizing an unknown exudative pleural effusion.
- Treatment
  - Most benign pleural effusions and pneumothoraces are treated by evacuation of the excess fluid or air, often with tube thoracostomy, and treatment of the

underlying process. Pleurodesis is used for recurrent or persistent effusions; thoracic duct ligation may be required for severe chylous leaks. Localized mesotheliomas require complete en bloc resection (e.g., extrapleural pneumonectomy), with adjuvant or neoadjuvant therapies. Diffuse malignant mesothelioma has no widely accepted therapy; multimodality treatment is the most commonly applied approach.

- Outcomes
  - For localized mesothelioma, local recurrence often develops at surgical sites within the first 24 months after resection. For diffuse malignant mesothelioma, multimodal therapies lead to survival times of 16 and 24 months after diagnosis, depending on the extent of disease and the histologic subtype.

physicians improved the management of pleural injuries and infections. In the last century, a whole new set of pleural diseases—such as human immunodeficiency virus and complications after cardiac, lung, and esophageal surgery—arose, and protocols for management developed. A better understanding of the development of primary and secondary malignancies of the pleura gave rise to the evolution of surgical and nonsurgical therapies for those conditions (Fig. 11-1).

Embryology and anatomy of the pleural space

The pleural space is the area between the parietal and visceral pleural layers, which normally contains about 5 to

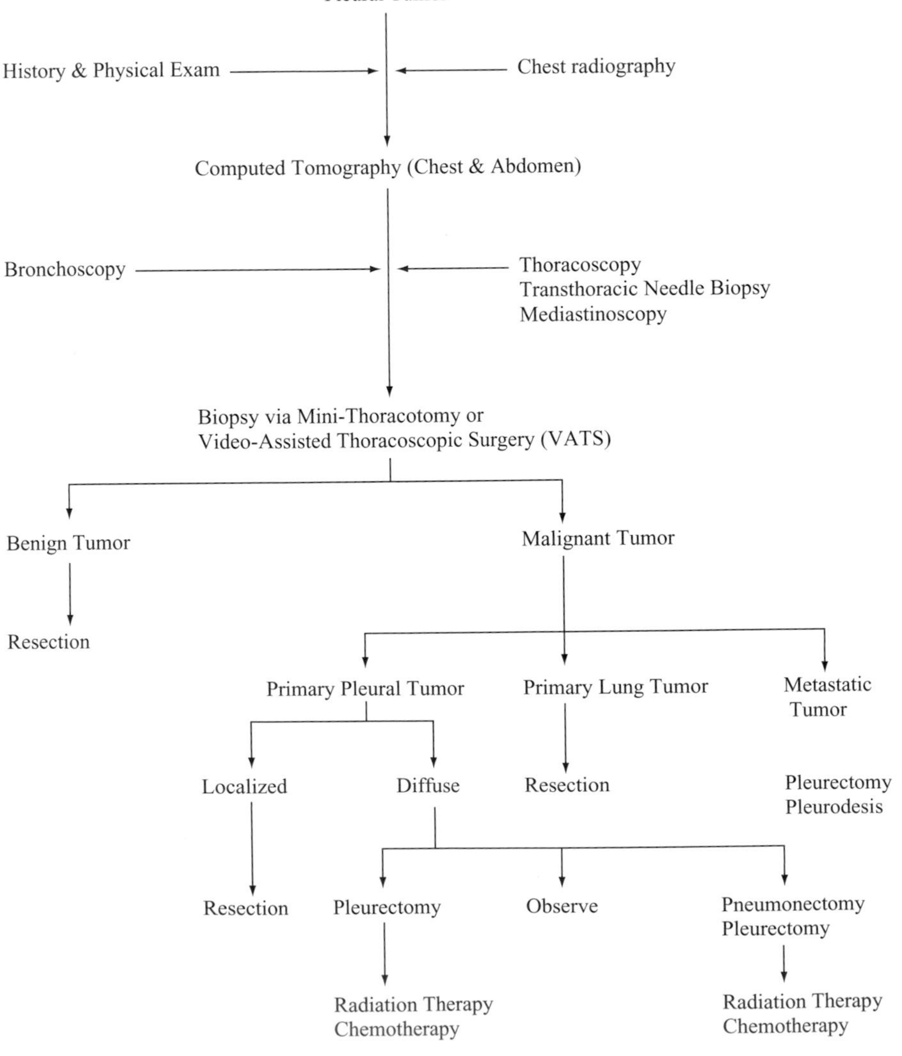

Figure 11-1 Decision-making flowchart.

20 mL of pleural fluid.[2] The parietal pleura covers the chest wall, diaphragm, and mediastinum. Each lung is invested and enclosed within the pleura. During embryonic development, the growth of lung buds into the coelom leads to investment of the lungs by a mesothelial lining. The parietal pleura is divided into four areas: (1) the costal pleura lining the ribs and intercostal muscles, (2) the diaphragmatic pleura covering the thoracic surfaces of the diaphragm and containing tiny channels connecting pleural and peritoneal cavities, (3) the mediastinal pleura adjacent to the mediastinum, and (4) the cervical pleura covering the superior aspect of the pleural space in the plane of the first rib. Two important surgical structures of the parietal pleura are the costodiaphragmatic sinus and the costomediastinal sinus, which represent the junction of the corresponding pleural surfaces and are considered safe sites of entry into the pleural space during surgical procedures. The transition point between the parietal and visceral pleura is around the root of the lung, which consists of the main bronchus, the pulmonary artery and veins, the bronchial artery and veins, and associated lymph nodes and autonomic nerves. Extension of the anterior and posterior reflections of the pleura from the inferior border of the lung root to the diaphragmatic surface forms the pulmonary ligament. The blood supply of the parietal pleura arises from the posterior intercostal, internal mammary, superior phrenic, and anterior mediastinal arteries. The venous course corresponds to the arterial course. Intercostal and phrenic nerves provide innervation to the parietal pleura. Lymphatics of the parietal pleura drain to regional lymph nodes: costals drain into intercostals and substernal nodes, diaphragmatics drain into phrenic nodes, mediastinals drain into anterior and posterior mediastinal nodes, and some of the cervicals drain into axillary lymph nodes.

The visceral pleura is tightly adherent to the lung parenchyma. It receives its blood supply from the branches of the bronchial and pulmonary arteries. Veins of the visceral pleura are part of the pulmonary veins. Bronchial veins do not drain the visceral pleura. There is no somatic innervation of the visceral pleura; visceral innervation consists of vagal and sympathetic branches of the pulmonary plexus. Lymphatic capillaries located under the mesothelial cells in the connective tissue combine with the superficial efferent lymphatics of the lung to form an extensive subpleural lymphatic plexus, which drains into the mediastinal lymph nodes. The majority of the pleural cavity lining is formed by mesenchymal tissue, mesothelial precursors, and cells. A small percentage of cells arise from epithelial tissue, lipoid tissue, neural cells, and endothelial and smooth muscle cells of the lymphatic and blood vessels.[3–5]

The pleura is in direct or indirect contact with multiple organs including heart, lungs, esophagus, and the abdominal organs. Injury to these organs or pathologic conditions affecting them will directly or indirectly influence the pleura.

NORMAL PHYSIOLOGY OF THE PLEURA

Fluid dynamics enable the pleura to perform its functions. The rate of entry of fluid into the pleural space is approximately 0.01 mL/kg/h.[6] Starling's law best describes the movement of fluid across the pleural membrane:

$$Qf = Lp \times A\,(Pcap - Ppl) - Gd\,(Ncap - Npl)$$

Where Qf = fluid movement
Lp = filtration coefficient
A = surface area of the pleural membrane

P and N = hydrostatic and oncotic pressures, respectively, of the capillary (cap) and pleural (pl) space

Gd = the solute reflection coefficient for protein, which is approximately 0.80 in humans[7]

The hydrostatic pressure gradient of the parietal pleura is approximately 30 cmH_2O, and the pleural pressure is approximately −5 cmH_2O. The net hydrostatic pressure gradient therefore is about 35 cmH_2O. Oncotic pressures oppose hydrostatic forces and are about 29 cmH_2O, whereas plasma oncotic pressure is approximately 34 cmH_2O and the pleural fluid pressure is approximately 5 cmH_2O (34 − 5 = 29 cmH_2O). The total net result is 35 cmH_2O − 29 cmH_2O or 6 cmH_2O (Fig. 11-2). Because of the low-pressure blood supply to the visceral pleura via the bronchial artery, the net gradient fluid movement across visceral pleura is close to zero.[8]

Wang has described pleural fluid dynamics.[9] Pleural fluid originates from lymphatic drainage and is reabsorbed through the parietal pleural stomal openings of lymphatic capillaries. Since no such capillaries exist in the visceral pleura, it does not participate in reabsorption.[10] Lymphatic clearance of pleural fluid has a linear pattern with a maximal rate of 0.28 mL/kg/h. This is approximately 28 times higher than the rate of pleural fluid accumulation.[11] The presence of direct stomal openings on the diaphragmatic surface of the parietal pleura explains the abdominal origin of pleural fluid formation. Accumulation of pleural fluid develops when the formation of pleural fluid exceeds its clearance. This can be due to an increase in pleural fluid formation, a decrease in lymphatic clearance, or a combination of the two.

DIAGNOSIS OF PLEURAL DISORDERS

Imaging, invasive diagnostic procedures, and direct inspection are important in the diagnosis of the abnormalities of the pleura. Invasive procedures are almost always necessary. These can be done by needle aspiration of the pleural effusion, needle biopsy of pleural tumors, open-technique surgical biopsy of the pleura, or video-assisted minimally invasive surgical pleural visualization and directed sampling.

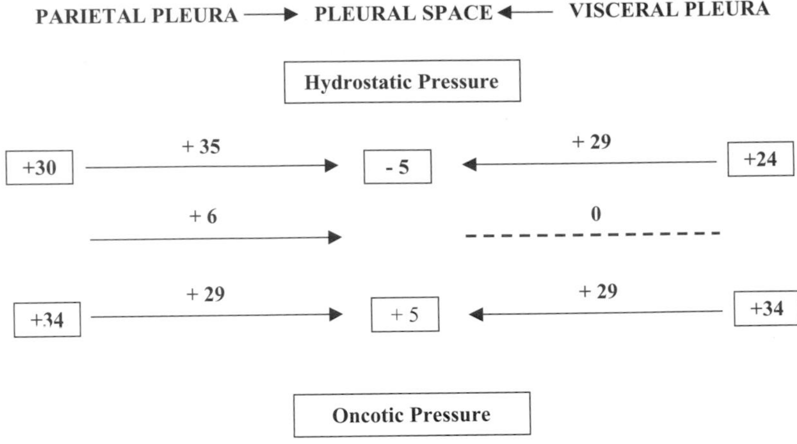

Figure 11-2 Diagram of the pressures influencing the intrapleural pressure. (From Light RW. *Pleural Diseases,* 3d ed. Baltimore: Williams & Wilkins, 1995:9. With permission.)

Radiologic evaluation

Radiographic methods of diagnosis are extremely important and are the initial steps in the clinical evaluation of pleural diseases. After physical examination, plain chest radiography is the most useful initial screening test. Chest radiography is sensitive for the assessment of pleural effusions and air in pleural cavities. Radiography does not provide information about the origin of pleural fluid. With the patient in the upright position, pleural fluid initially accumulates in the costodiaphragmatic space, resulting in blunting of the costodiaphragmatic angle. There must an accumulation of about 175 mL of pleural fluid if it is to be detected radiographically. In cases of subpulmonic or intrapulmonic effusion, the costodiaphragmatic angle may be clear. On upright radiograph, changes of more than 2 cm in the position of the diaphragm and separation of the lower border of the lung on the left side from the stomach bubble indicate a subpulmonic effusion. A diagonal fissure shadow indicates loculated pleural fluid. Posteroanterior and lateral radiographs are the usual screening tests. For ill or immobile patients, a supine film is an alternative. On a supine radiograph, the pleural effusion presents as a diffuse shadow in the corresponding pleural space. It is sometimes difficult to estimate the presence and amount of pleural fluid on a supine film. In these cases lateral decubitus or semisupine oblique radiographs are informative in evaluating free pleural fluid. Radiographs may demonstrate thickening of the pleura. Chest radiographs are an important follow-up in evaluating the treatment of pleural pathology and its results.

Computed tomography (CT) of the chest is the most widely used test for the evaluation and follow-up of treatment of pleural effusions. The CT scan helps to differentiate pleural pathology from lung pathology, as in distinguishing a lung abscess from pleural empyema with pneumothorax. It also can show bone pathology, such as metastases or tuberculosis. However, the CT scan does not differentiate types of pleural fluids or the presence of pleural symphysis.

Ultrasound is a useful test in the study of pleural diseases. It can be used in several situations: to identify loculated effusions; for assistance in attempted thoracentesis, pleural biopsy, or tube thoracostomy placement; and to differentiate effusion from pleural thickening. It is relatively inexpensive, can be done faster than a CT scan, and can be done at the bedside of seriously ill patients. The technology employs 5– to 7.5-MHz transducers, and real-time scanning is utilized. However, ultrasound is operator-dependent. Color Doppler ultrasound provides even better resolution than gray-scale examination by demonstrating the color signal of pleural fluid and showing the neovascularization of a pulmonary lesion. Transthoracic needle biopsy under ultrasound guidance is an effective and safe way to evaluate thoracic disorders.[12]

Magnetic resonance imaging (MRI) does not provide additional benefits over standard radiologic techniques for the examination of pleural masses and pleural effusions. However, recent data indicate that MRI has a sensitivity of 100 percent and a specificity of 93 percent in the detection of pleural malignancy, making it more useful and superior to CT in differentiating malignant from benign pleural disease.[13]

Positron emission tomography (PET) is a new modality in the diagnosis of pleural tumors. Early reports show that PET has a high sensitivity in the diagnosis of malignant mesothelioma.[14] It can be helpful in differentiating malignant effusions and identifying nodal or other metastases that are not otherwise apparent.

Invasive diagnostic tools

There are several ways to obtain samples of pleural fluid or pleural tissue: needle aspiration, needle biopsy, limited thoracotomy, video-assisted minimally invasive thoracic surgery, and thoracotomy. Pleural fluid can usually be obtained by thoracocentesis with or without radiologic guidance. Pleural fluid may also be obtained during surgical intervention performed for other reasons.

Characteristics of pleural effusions (transudates/exudates)

It is important to differentiate the type of pleural effusion. The two types, transudates and exudates, are based on theories regarding the formation and reabsorption of pleural fluid as modified by Broaddus and others.[15] From this viewpoint, transudates are the result of increased hydrostatic pressures or decreased oncotic pressures, whereas exudative effusions result from increased permeability. Three classic criteria, described by Light in 1972,[16] help to distinguish between the two. Meeting at least one of the following criteria defines an exudative effusion, whereas a transudative effusion meets none: (1) ratio of pleural fluid protein to serum protein greater than 0.5; (2) ratio of pleural fluid lactate dehydrogenase (LDH) to serum LDH greater than 0.6; and (3) pleural fluid LDH greater than two-thirds of the upper normal limit for serum. New methods of categorization based on a Bayesian approach have led to an improvement of Light's criteria. Heffner and Light evaluated 1448 patients for the following data: pleural fluid LDH, ratio of pleural fluid LDH to serum LDH, and ratio of pleural fluid to serum protein, pleural fluid protein, ratios of pleural fluid to serum cholesterol, pleural fluid cholesterol, and gradient of pleural fluid to serum albumin.[17] They compared this with the clinician's suspicion for the type of exudate and found that this approach markedly improved the diagnostic accuracy of discriminating between exudative and transudative pleural effusions. It eliminated confusing terms such as "pseudoexudates."

In the case of an unknown exudative pleural effusion, the pleural fluid should be tested for glucose, amylase, LDH, differential cell count, microbiologic studies, and cytology. Other studies such as pH, adenosine deaminase (ADA) level, interferon-gamma level, polymerase chain reaction (PCR) for tuberculous DNA, or lipid analysis may be performed but should be based on the index of suspicion for specific conditions. Data suggest that serum levels of interleukin-1a (IL-1a) and tumor necrosis factor alpha (TNF-α) can distinguish exudates from transudates, while pleural fluid IL-6 levels could be useful as an additional marker in the differential diagnosis of tuberculosis as well as malignant and parapneumonic exudates.[18] In the case of a suspected malignant origin of pleural effusion, cytologic examination including cell morphology, number of mitotic figures, and number of cells in S phase is important.

In the case of a suspected pleural mass or thickening, the most informative data are obtained by sampling the diseased pleura or the pleural mass. Pleural fluid aspiration cytology and transcutaneous pleural biopsy provide very low yields of sensitivity. However, thoracocentesis is usually performed as the initial test. In the case of malignancy, pleural fluid cytology is positive in only 30 to 50 percent of cases. As little as 10 mL of pleural fluid was equivalent to larger volumes for diagnosing pleural malignancy.[19] Pleural fluid samples may be informative in the case of pleural thickening with pleural effusion of infectious origin. Pleural biopsy is indicated if there is a need to characterize an unexplained pleural effusion or to evaluate focal or diffuse pleural thickening or pleural masses. A bleeding abnormality is a relative contraindication for pleural biopsy and should be corrected prior to the procedure. Percutaneous pleural biopsy is diagnostic in only one-third of the cases involving pleural tumors and does not provide sufficient tissue for immunohistochemical or electron microscopic studies. CT-directed pleural biopsy has been shown to be superior to closed Abrams' needle biopsy in the setting of cytology-negative unilateral pleural effusions suspicious for malignancy. Maskel and colleagues showed that there is a 40 percent difference in sensitivity in favor of CT-guided biopsy. Patients with parietal pleural thickening of < 5 mm and > 5 mm underwent biopsy by CT guidance with 75 and 100 percent diagnostic sensitivities respectively.[20] Previously, the traditional way of sampling the pleura was limited thoracotomy with pleural biopsy. Usually a small incision was made in line with a possible subsequent extended thoracotomy with resection of a short segment of overlying rib, along with sampling of the abnormal pleura. Extended thoracotomy should not be performed for diagnostic purposes because it exposes the patient with metastatic adenocarcinoma to the unnecessary morbidity of a large operation and complicates subsequent surgical resection in patients with malignant mesothelial tumors. The negative side of "open" pleural biopsy is significant morbidity of a major procedure in a patient debilitated by disease. Now, minimally invasive video-assisted thoracoscopy (VATS) has become the "gold standard" for the diagnosis of pleural lesions. This method provides good observation of the pleura, allows for multiple pleural biopsies from different sites under direct visual control, delivers a sufficient amount of tissue for laboratory diagnosis, and carries a smaller percentage of morbidity and mortality. Thoracoscopy is indicated in two situations. In the first, when thoracocentesis and closed pleural biopsy (CPB) have failed to yield a diagnosis, VATS often establishes one. In the second, when these procedures have established a diagnosis of pleural malignancy, VATS helps to stage the disease more precisely or, in some cases, to perform definitive therapy. Thoracoscopy is the only procedure that can provide a diagnosis of early stage (IA) mesothelioma. The diagnostic value of thoracoscopy is as high as 93.3 percent, and it appears to be a relatively safe technique. VATS is diagnostic in at least 80 percent of pleural malignancies. Application of a semirigid thoracoscope may improve the method's sensitivity.[21] However, pleural adhesions can lower its diagnostic value.[22]

PRIMARY PLEURAL DISORDERS

Defined by Scharifker and Kaneko as disorders originating from histologic elements of visceral and parietal pleural linings, primary pleural disorders may be benign or malignant.[23]

Benign primary pleural disorders

Benign fibrous tumors of the pleura may arise from any portion of the pleura; however, the majority originate from the visceral pleura. These tumors are usually ovoid or round, grow on a pedicle, and are almost always solitary. Calcifications or cystic components may be found within the tumor. In half of these cases, the tumors have a membranous capsule. The usual histologic pattern is disorderly fibroblast-like cells with collagen and elastin bundles. Other patterns enumerated by Moran include storiform, herringbone, and mixed forms or patterns resembling a leiomyoma or neurofibroma.[24] Benign fibrous tumors affect both sexes equally, may occur at any age, and are more common in the fifth to eighth decades of life. The majority of affected patients are asymptomatic. For those who are symptomatic, chronic cough, dyspnea, clubbing, and chest pain are the usual presentations. Chest pain is usually related to parietal pleural involvement. Hypertrophic pulmonary osteoarthropathy can affect more than 20 percent of benign localized fibrous tumors of the pleura. This is significantly higher than in bronchial carcinoma, where such osteoarthropathy is present in 5 percent of the cases. The clinical presentation of hypertrophic pulmonary osteoarthropathy includes arthralgia with stiffness and edema of the joints, usually the ankles. Bone pain is most commonly bilateral, affecting the ulna and radius. Periosteal thickening is seen radiologically. Another significant finding in symptomatic patients with benign fibrous tumors of the pleura is severe hypoglycemia, which may affect 3 to 4 percent of patients with large tumors. Although several explanations were postulated by Nelson,[25] the theory focusing on insulin-like growth hormone as described by Bunn, Cole, and Strom and their associates is currently the most popular.[26–28]

Malignant primary pleural disorders

Primary pleural malignancies can be divided into two major groups: malignant localized fibrous tumors and diffuse malignant mesotheliomas. This division is important because of the difference in treatment approach and clinical prognosis.

Malignant localized fibrous tumors

The incidence of localized malignant pleural tumors compared to that of benign tumors is unclear. Different estimates range from 12 to 36 percent, as reported by Briselli, Okike, and England and their associates.[29–31] These tumors have a tendency to be large, to originate from the parietal pleura, to show areas of calcification and necrosis, and to grow into the pulmonary parenchyma. They are part of a continuum moving from benign to malignant. Compared to benign fibrous tumors, they show cellular pleomorphism and a larger number of mitotic figures. The immunohistochemical characteristics of both benign and malignant fibrous tumors are similar.

Patients with malignant localized pleural tumors are usually symptomatic at clinical presentation. Chest pain, dyspnea, fever, and hypoglycemia are common presentations. However, osteoarthropathy is rarely seen with malignant tumors. A malignant localized tumor of the pleura can be suspected if there is adjacent organ invasion. However, final diagnosis is established on the basis of histologic examination. As reported by Okike and England and their colleagues, long-term survival is poor, ranging between 12 and 45 percent.[30,31] Prognosis depends on the complete surgical removal of tumor. Pleural effusion is a poor prognostic sign, but chest wall and pericardial invasion does not influence long-term outcome if complete excision is achieved. Recurrences are primarily at the site of prior excision. Blood- and lymph-borne metastases are seen in patients with persistent or recurrent disease. Metastases to the liver and the central nervous systems are the most common.

Malignant diffuse mesothelioma

Reports of pleural tumors were published as early as the eighteenth century. However, the first definitive pathologic description was documented in 1937 by Klemperer and Rabin.[32] Cellular origins were described by Stout and Murray in 1942.[33] The wide use of asbestos between the 1930s and 1960s led to the exposure of a large number of people. The most studied lethal pleural malignancy is diffuse malignant mesothelioma. Its relation to asbestos exposure was clearly shown by Wagner and associates in 1960.[3] They reported on 33 cases of asbestosis in mine workers from Northern Cape Province, South Africa. Further reports by Selikoff[34] and Whitwell[35] in the United States elicited wide interest among scientists, physicians, and the general public. Exposure to asbestos leads to a number of benign and malignant diseases. Asbestos diseases are dose-dependent. In the United States, exposure is now limited to 0.1 fibers per cubic centimeter. Exposure to other toxic substances, radiation, viruses, and hereditary predisposition may play a role. Patients who smoke are not at higher risk to develop mesothelioma but are at higher risk for the development of lung cancer. The molecular basis of asbestos-mediated disease is under active investigation.[36]

The peak age for the development of diffuse malignant mesothelioma is the sixth decade of life. Mesothelioma can occur in young adulthood or even childhood, but it usually has a latency period of at least 20 years following a significant exposure to asbestos. The clinical presentation of diffuse malignant mesothelioma is nonspecific. In the early stages, dyspnea is the usual sign and is due to the related pleural effusion. In the later stages, the presence of chest discomfort and severe chest pain is due to the ingrowth of tumor into the chest wall and intercostal nerves. Notably, in the later stages of development, symptoms of dyspnea may improve due to fusion of the pleural surfaces with the elimination of the effusion. Dyspnea returns in the final stages of the disease in conjunction with intolerable chest pain.

Mesothelioma can grow into surrounding tissue, leading to secondary symptoms based on the site of invasion.[37,38] Weight loss is present in only 30 percent of the patients. Fever, anorexia, hemoptysis, hoarseness, and Horner's syndromes are uncommon, as are paraneoplastic syndromes. Thrombocytosis with platelet counts over 400,000/mL was described by Olesen and Torshauge in 30 to 40 percent of patients.[39] Ruffle described hypercalcemia, hypoglycemia, inappropriate secretion of antidiuretic hormone, autoimmune hemolytic anemia, and hypercoagulability in relation to mesothelioma.[26] Diffuse dullness on percussion and decreased breath sounds on the affected side are usually the only findings on physical examination and are attributed primarily to the development of a pleural effusion. Chest and abdominal CT scans are usually the only tests indicated unless specific symptoms are present. Bronchoscopy is of value only to exclude primary endobronchial tumor in highly suspicious circumstances. Heelan and associates in 1999 showed that MRI improves the diagnosis of chest wall and diaphragmatic invasion.[40] However, it is not better than CT in defining the local extent of the tumor. PET is a promising technique in the diagnosis and staging of diffuse malignant mesothelioma, as shown by Benard and associates.[14] The combination of CT and the PET images can be beneficial in determining the pretherapy staging of malignant mesothelioma (Figs. 11-3 and 11-4).

Although needle aspiration of the pleural effusion with cytology is informative in 30 to 50 percent of cases, minimally invasive video-assisted thoracoscopy, as described by Boutin, provides a diagnosis in 80 percent of studies.[41] These two approaches are useful in the early stages of disease, which are characterized by the presence of pleural effusions and unobliterated pleural space. Later stages usually present with fusion of pleural surfaces or filling of the pleural space with tumor mass. At this point limited incisional thoracotomy with excision of a tumor sample is required. As a general rule, the biopsy incision is made in line with a possible future thoracotomy incision. Exploratory thoracotomy should be avoided. Biopsy material must be freshly submitted to allow for appropriate histochemical and electron microscopic diagnosis.

Mesothelioma has different histologic patterns, but it is difficult to make a definitive histologic diagnosis based on light microscopy alone. Immunohistochemical and electron microscopic evaluation is required for a definitive conclusion. Malignant mesothelioma is characterized by staining for calretinin (88 percent) and vimentin (58 percent), while adenocarcinomas typically lack these markers and are positive for carcinoembryonic antigen (84 percent), CD 15 (77 percent), and Ber-EP4 (82 percent).[42] Tumor markers are not used routinely in the diagnosis

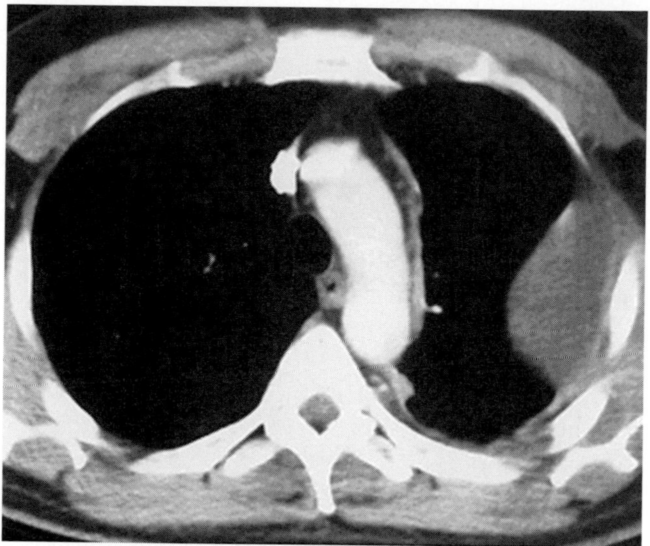

Figure 11-3 Computed tomographic image from a patient with mesothelioma showing a loculated pleural effusion and calcified pleura against the mediastinum.

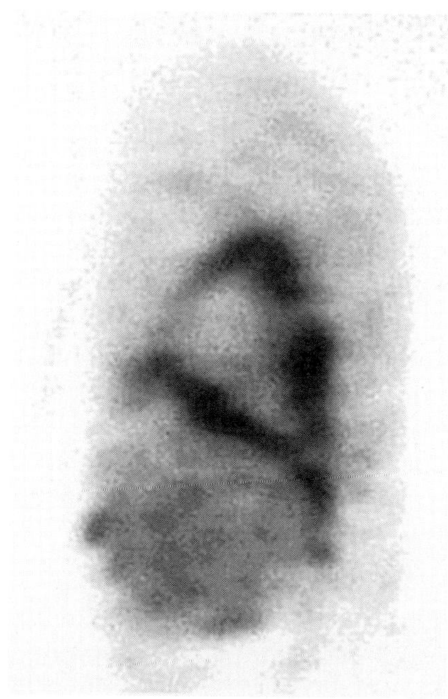

Figure 11-4 Positron emission tomography image from the same patient shown in Fig. 11-3, demonstrating localized disease.

Table 11-1 Staging of mesothelioma: tumor description

Primary tumor (T)	
TX	Primary tumor cannot be assessed
T0	No evidence of primary tumor
T1	Tumor involves ipsilateral parietal pleura, with or without focal involvement of visceral pleura
T1a	Tumor involves ipsilateral parietal (mediastinal, diaphragmatic) pleura. No involvement of visceral pleura
T1b	Tumor involves ipsilateral parietal (mediastinal, diaphragmatic) pleura, with focal involvement of visceral pleura
T2	Tumor involves any of the ipsilateral pleural surfaces with at least one of the following: • Confluent visceral pleural tumor (including fissure) • Invasion of diaphragmatic muscle • Invasion of lung parenchyma
T3[a]	Tumor involves any of the ipsilateral pleural surfaces with at least one of the following: • Invasion of the endothoracic fascia • Invasion into mediastinal fat • Solitary focus of tumor invading the soft tissues of the chest wall • Nontransmural involvement of the pericardium
T4[b]	Tumor involves any of the ipsilateral pleural surfaces with at least one of the following: • Diffuse or multifocal invasion of soft tissues of the chest wall • Any involvement of rib • Invasion through the diaphragm to the peritoneum • Invasion of any mediastinal organ(s) • Direct extension to the contralateral pleura • Invasion into the spine • Extension to the internal surface of the pericardium • Pericardial effusion with positive cytology • Invasion of the myocardium • Invasion of the brachial plexus

[a]T3 describes locally advanced but potentially resectable tumor.
[b]T4 describes locally advanced, technically unresectable tumor.

of diffuse malignant mesothelioma. Mesothelioma staging allows for a more accurate prognosis. The present staging system was proposed at the International Mesothelioma Interest Group by Rusch and associates.[43] Tables 11-1, 11-2, and 11-3 list the staging system as currently utilized. The epithelioid subtype has the best prognosis.[44]

SECONDARY PLEURAL DISORDERS

These disorders affect pleural linings or the pleural space because of the influence of pathologic conditions related to other organs or as a result of external factors. As with primary pleural disorders, they can be benign or malignant.

Table 11-2 Staging of mesothelioma: nodal disease and metastasis

Regional lymph nodes (N)	
NX	Regional lymph nodes cannot be assessed
N0	No regional lymph node metastases
N1	Metastases in the ipsilateral bronchopulmonary and/or hilar lymph node(s)
N2	Metastases in the subcarinal lymph node(s) and/or the ipsilateral internal mammary or mediastinal lymph node(s)
N3	Metastases in the contralateral mediastinal, internal mammary, or hilar lymph node(s), and/or the ipsilateral or contralateral supraclavicular or scalene lymph node(s)
Distant metastasis (M)	
MX	Distant metastases cannot be assessed
M0	No distant metastasis
M1	Distant metastasis

Benign secondary pleural disorders

Secondary benign disease can be subdivided based on macroscopic or microscopic disruption of anatomic barriers and be complicated by bacterial, fungal, parasitic, or viral infection.

Pneumothorax

Spontaneous pneumothorax, which occurs in the absence of thoracic trauma, is classified as primary or secondary. Primary spontaneous pneumothorax affects patients who do not have significant underlying lung disease. Secondary pneumothorax affects people with significant lung disease. The most common condition is chronic obstructive pulmonary disease (COPD). Diagnosis of a pneumothorax should be made based on a history and physical examination. However, a chest roentgenogram is obtained to confirm suspicions. Assessment of the size of a pneumothorax remains problematic. However, in general, a distance of less than 3 cm from apex to cupola is considered small, and more than 3 cm large. The condition of the patient plays an important role in choosing a plan of management. Patients whose respiratory rate is more than 24 breaths per minute, heart rate less than 60 beats

Table 11-3 Staging of mesothelioma

	Stage grouping		
I	T1	N0	M0
IA	T1a	N0	M0
IB	T1b	N0	M0
II	T2	N0	M0
III	T1, T2	N1	M0
	T1, T2	N2	M0
	T3	N0, N1, N2	M0
IV	T4	Any N	M0
	Any T	N3	M0
	Any T	Any N	M1

per minute or more than 120 beats per minute, whose blood pressure is abnormal (high or low), whose room-air saturation is less than 90 percent, or who are unable to speak whole sentences between breaths are considered unstable.[45]

Patients with acquired immunodeficiency syndrome (AIDS) can develop spontaneous pneumothorax in the setting of *Pneumocystis carinii* pneumonia (PCP); this occurs in approximately 6 percent of the cases.[46] PCP is characterized by the development of necrotizing pneumonia and diffuse subpleural blebs, causing pneumothoraces that are frequently refractory, recurrent. and bilateral.[47] Mechanical ventilation leads to additional barotrauma, especially when positive-pressure ventilation is used. This leads to 90 percent mortality in hospitalized HIV-positive patients with PCP.[48,49] Treatment with oral trimethoprim/sulfamethoxazole in dosages that produce adequate systemic blood levels has virtually eliminated pneumothorax secondary to PCP. The most common causes of AIDS-related problems are parapneumonic effusions or empyemas and Kaposi's sarcoma.[50]

Mechanical injury to the pleura and lungs occurs mostly as a result of trauma. External chest wounds lead to the entry of air and blood into the pleural cavity and the consequent development of pneumo- and hemothorax. Injury to lung parenchyma can lead to simple or tension pneumothorax, hemothorax, or pneumohemothorax. Trauma to the heart, great vessels, major lymphatics, trachea, or esophagus leads to collections of blood, lymph, or air in the pleural space. Escaping air leads to an increase in pressure in the pleural cavity, lung collapse, and mediastinal shift. These changes can acutely affect cardiac hemodynamics and quickly lead to death if left untreated. In most cases knowledge of the mechanism of injury, patient complaints, and physical examination are sufficient to suspect pleural injury, which is then confirmed radiologically. The pleura is capable of reabsorbing significant amounts of fluid from the pleural space. Also, the pleura can reabsorb intrapleural air at the rate of approximately 1.25 percent a day. Therefore, as suggested by Clark and colleagues, small pleural effusions and small nonexpanding pneumothoraces may be treated expectantly by controlled observation and repeated x-ray examinations.[51]

Pleural effusions

Effusions constitute the most common secondary benign disorder of the pleura. Benign pleural effusion can originate from parietal and visceral pleural capillaries, interstitial space of the lung, or the peritoneum. There are four types of benign pleural reactions: effusions, plaques, local fibrosis of the parietal pleura, and diffuse pleural fibrosis. Transudative pleural effusions are complications of a large number of disorders. Pleural effusions occur in conjunction with congestive heart failure in 38 percent of the cases. They occur in post-cardiac injury syndrome in 1 to 68 percent of patients, depending on the cause of injury. Pleural effusions also occur in 5 percent of patients with rheumatoid arthritis, 50 percent of patients with systemic lupus erythematosus, and 4 to 20 percent of patients with acute pancreatitis.[52] Damage to the mechanism of lymphatic clearance of pleural fluid is another mechanism of pleural fluid accumulation and plays a role in the development mostly of malignant effusions.

Additional noninfectious and nonneoplastic causes of pleural effusions include sympathetic effusions and pleural ascites. Sympathetic effusions occur in association with acute lung deflation, such as atelectasis secondary to a bronchial mucus plug or obstructing tumor. The lung collapses and the increased negative pressure in the pleural cavity leads to an increase in the production of pleural fluid to rapidly equalize the pressure in the pleural cavity. In these cases, evacuation of the pleural fluid does not result in lung reexpansion unless the underlying bronchial obstruction is corrected. This often requires bronchoscopy to relieve the obstruction. In patients with significantly large collections of ascites, fluid can be drawn into the pleural space. The patient develops defects in the diaphragm, probably due to abdominal distention. The negative intrapleural pressure draws fluid into the chest. In these cases, tube thoracostomy is contraindicated because it does not correct the underlying problem and will result in significant fluid losses. If the underlying condition can be treated, that should be accomplished. For example, in patients who have this condition secondary to cirrhosis, a transcutaneous intrahepatic portocaval shunt or liver transplant will correct the problem.[53]

Hemothorax is usually the result of trauma. Sources of hemorrhage vary depending on the organ or vessel injured, and blood, which may accumulate slowly or rapidly, will compress normal lung. Bleeding may continue and even cause mediastinal shift (Fig. 11-5). If blood remains in the chest for a longed time, it may clot and cause scarring, which will entrap the lung. Even a

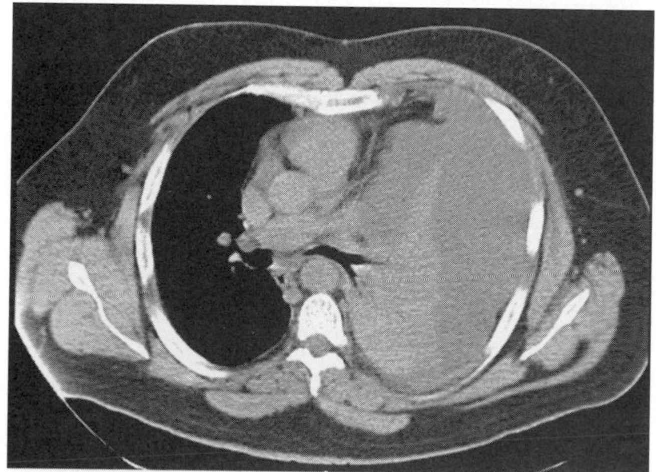

Figure 11-5 Computed tomography image from a patient with a large hemothorax, demonstrating compression of the lung and mediastinal shift.

small amount of blood in the chest will cause the accumulation of additional pleural fluid over time, thus causing the effusion to increase.

Parapneumonic effusions develop as a result of lung parenchymal inflammation or inflammatory disease at or near the diaphragm and are characterized as exudates. They develop in 36 to 66 percent of hospitalized patients with bacterial pneumonia.[54] Three variables—pleural space anatomy, pleural fluid bacteriology, and pleural fluid chemistry—were used by Light and coworkers in 1995 to classify parapneumonic effusions into seven classes: small parapneumonic effusions, typical parapneumonic effusions, borderline complicated parapneumonic effusions, simple complicated parapneumonic effusions with positive Gram's stain and culture and no overt purulence, complex complicated parapneumonic effusions with loculation, simple empyema, and complex empyema.[54] The simplified classification of parapneumonic effusions commonly used in clinical practice is exudative, fibrinopurulent and organizing stages. The exudative stage is the earliest phase and is the product of increased fluid release from the inflamed lung. It is characterized by free-flowing fluid that may be clear or turbid. The fibrinopurulent phase is characterized by thickening of the fluid to a creamy state that becomes more organized and gelatinous with time and begins within hours to days after the appearance of the parapneumonic effusion. An example is given in Fig. 11-6. The organizing state is characterized by firm granulation tissue that becomes hard and densely adherent to the lung over time. This phase begins as early as 7 to 10 days after the development of the effusion. Figure 11-7 shows one of the hallmark signs of an early organizing phase, with the dense tissue adherent to the lung presenting as a dense area on the edge of the lung. The American College of Chest Physicians Parapneumonic Effusions Panel divided patients with parapneumonic effusions by the categories based on the risk for poor outcomes.[55] Parapneumonic effusions can develop as a result of bacterial, fungal, viral, or parasitic contamination. Patients with pleural effusions uniformly present with dyspnea and pleuritic pain. Patients with complicated effusions and empyema usually present with fever and general malaise in addition to the above symptoms. The presence of copious amounts of sputum may indicate the development of a bronchopleural fistula, which complicates few pneumonias but occurs in approximately 1.5 percent of lobectomy cases and 4.6 percent of pneumonectomy cases. Clinical signs include pyrexia, hemoptysis, cough, and expectoration of brown fluid. Preoperative radiation, devascularization of the bronchial stump, prolonged high-pressure ventilation, immunosupression, and infection (particularly tuberculosis) are associated with a high incidence of postoperative bronchopleural fistula formation.[56]

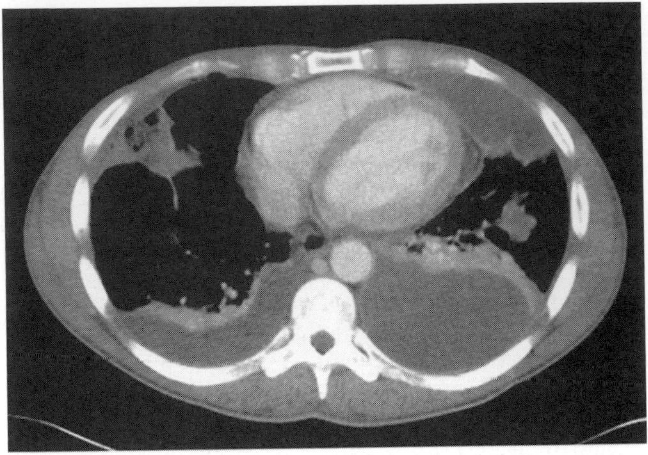

Figure 11-7 Computed tomographic image from a patient with multiple pulmonary abscesses who developed bilateral empyema. Note the proteinaceous deposits, appearing as hyperdense areas at the edge of the effusions.

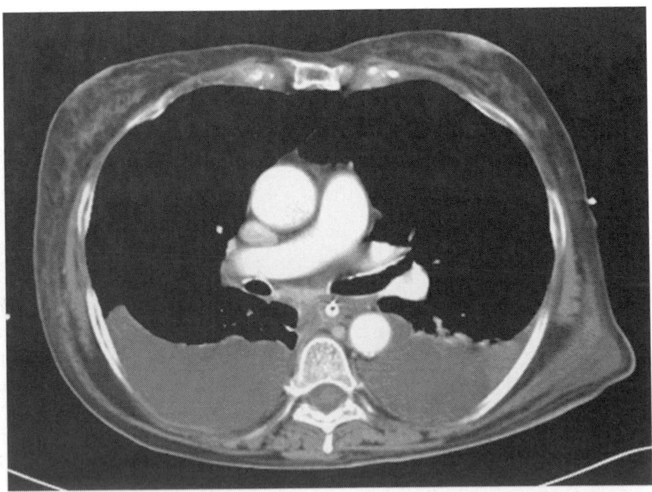

Figure 11-6 Computed tomographic image from a patient with bilateral early empyema secondary to an esophageal perforation and mediastinal abscess.

Mycobacterial and fungal infections of the pleura are uncommon in the United States. Primary tuberculosis of the lung caused by *Mycobacterium tuberculosis* produces pleural effusions and pleuritis in only 4 to 8 percent of cases and rarely requires surgical intervention. Diagnosis is based on sputum or gastric content positive for *M. tuberculosis*, pleural fluid positive for *M. tuberculosis*, and pleural tuberculous granuloma diagnosed by resection or tissue biopsy of the pleura. Mixed infection with *M. tuberculosis* and other bacteria is difficult to manage. Medical management is the mainstay of treatment in the early stages of tuberculous pleural involvement. Treatment usually requires quadruple drug therapy and removal of pleural fluid. Treatment of tuberculous empyema depends upon the stage of the disease and includes drug therapy, tube thoracostomy, decortication, possible parenchymal lung resection, and obliteration of the pleural space. The usual presentation after partial lung resection is persistent air leak, fluid drainage, fever, and weight loss.

Rarely, fungal diseases cause pleural effusions. Diagnosis relies on the identification of fungus in pleural fluid. Treatment requires pleural sterilization and complete obliteration of the pleural space. In cases of chronic *Aspergillus* empyema, all efforts should be made to save the underlying lung, because morbidity and mortality after pneumonectomy are high in patients with preexisting empyema. The presence of a pleural effusion contaminated by *Candida albicans* strongly suggests an esophagopleural fistula, especially in immunocompromised patients, as detailed by Emery and associates.[57] The diagnosis and initial treatment are established by placement of a chest tube and analysis of the pleural fluid. Definitive treatment for patients without recurrent or advanced esophageal cancer involves repair of the defect reinforced by myoplasty or omentoplasty and obliteration of the pleural space.

Malignant secondary pleural disorders

Malignant secondary pleural disorders predominantly become manifest as malignant pleural effusions.

Pleural effusions

Twenty-five percent of all pleural effusions in a general hospital setting are secondary to cancer. The most common primary histology for patients with metastatic pleural effusion secondary to a solid tumor includes non-small lung cancer, breast cancer, and ovarian cancer. Neoplastic diseases of the lungs and airways can involve the pleura directly by tumor extension or hematogenous spread. Neoplastic involvement of the pleura often results in malignant pleural effusion. Breast cancer is the second most common malignancy causing approximately 25 percent of all malignant pleural effusions. Nearly all cancers can metastasize to the pleura.

The median life expectancy associated with malignant pleural effusions is markedly different depending on primary pathology.[58] For lung cancer, the median life expectancy after development of a pleural effusion is 6 weeks, while for breast cancer the life expectancy is 2 years. Nearly all hematologic malignancies can present with or develop pleural effusions during the clinical course of the disease. Among the most common disorders are Hodgkin's and non-Hodgkin lymphomas, with a frequency of 20 to 30 percent, especially if mediastinal involvement is present. Acute and chronic leukemias and myelodysplastic syndromes are rarely accompanied by pleural involvement. An increasingly important cause of effusion is immunocompromised lymphoproliferative disorder, as may be seen in HIV-positive patients and transplant patients. In most cases, pleural fluid responds to treatment of the primary disease, whereas resistant or relapsing cases may necessitate pleurodesis.[59]

TREATMENT OF PLEURAL DISORDERS

Spontaneous pneumothorax

For spontaneous pneumothorax, management decisions vary between patients with primary or secondary spontaneous pneumothoraces.[45] A clinically stable patient with a small primary pneumothorax may be observed for 3 to 6 h and can be discharged home if repeat chest radiographs exclude progression of the pneumothorax. These patients should have follow-up as outpatients within 12 to 48 h for repeat chest radiography. Needle aspiration or insertion of a chest tube is not recommended unless progression of the pneumothorax is noted. Presence of symptoms for more than 24 h does not affect the treatment recommendations. A clinically stable patient with a large pneumothorax requires a lung reexpansion procedure and hospitalization in the majority of the cases. The lung reexpansion can be accomplished by placement of a small-bore (< 14F) catheter or tube thoracostomy. Catheters or tubes may be attached to a water seal or one-way valve until the lung is completely reexpanded and the air leak has resolved. If the lung does not reexpand, connection to suction is required. Primary spontaneous pneumothorax can be managed by manual pleurocentesis as an alternative to chest-tube thoracostomy drainage. A recent prospective multicenter pilot study by Noppen and colleagues noted no difference in immediate success, 1-week success, length of stay, 1-year pneumothorax recurrence, or urgent readmissions between the two groups.[60] Most of these patients require hospitalization. Reliable, stable patients may be discharged with a catheter or tube connected to a one-way valve. Recommended follow-up is every 2 days until the problem is resolved. Clinically unstable patients with a large pneumothorax require hospitalization after placement of a chest tube. Patients with a bronchopleural fistula, a large air leak, or those on positive-pressure ventilation should have a large-bore (28F) chest tube inserted. Application of water seal or suction follows the same criteria as for stable patients. Removal of chest tubes requires confirmation of lung reexpansion by chest x-ray, absence of air leak, and discontinuation of suction. Chest radiographs should be completed within 12 h after resolution of the air leak. For patients with persistent air leaks, observation for a maximum of 4 days is recommended. Patients with air leaks persisting beyond 4 days should be evaluated for operative intervention. Currently, thoracoscopy is the preferred method of management. Placement of additional chest tubes and bronchoscopy with an attempt to seal endobronchial sites are not indicated. A minithoracotomy is an alternative to the thoracoscopic approach. Surgical intervention should address two principles: (1) removal of the bullae or defects that led to the air leak and (2) prevention of future lung collapse by mechanical pleurodesis. Intraoperative pleurodesis should be performed by parietal pleural abrasion limited to the upper half of the hemithorax. Parietal pleurectomy is an acceptable alternative.

Chemical pleurodesis with talc is acceptable for patients refusing surgery or who are not surgical candidates. The success rate with chemical pleurodesis is 78 to 91 percent, compared to success rates of 95 to 100 percent with surgical interventions.[61] Talc slurry is a preferred agent if chemical pleurodesis is to be performed. Recurrent pneumothorax prevention is indicated in patients with a second episode of spontaneous pneumothorax or in a patient with a first episode and a persistent air leak.

In patients with a first-time pneumothorax, surgical intervention is indicated for those with a contralateral pneumonectomy or tension pneumothorax, those who live or will be far from medical care, and those whose jobs entail being exposed to rapid changes in high or low atmospheric pressure (e.g., professional pilots, flight attendants, or commercial divers). In addition, there is growing support for performing a CT scan after lung reexpansion in order to look for bullous disease (Fig. 11-8). If significant bullae are found, it is justifiable to operate during that admission because of the increased likelihood of a second pneumothorax. Patients should be hospitalized for a second spontaneous pneumothorax. These individuals require surgical intervention owing to their underlying lung disease. Traumatic pneumothoraces should be treated according to trauma management protocol and usually require placement of 28 to 36F chest tubes.

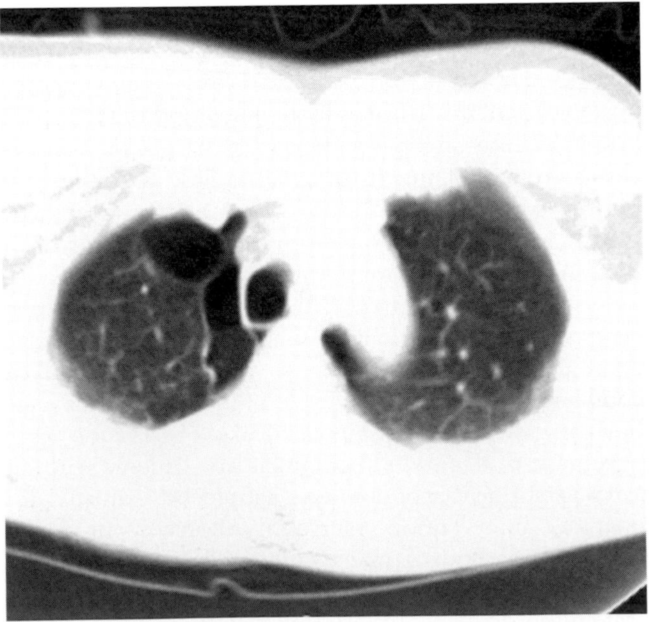

Figure 11-8 Computed tomographic image from a patient with a primary first-time pneumothorax, demonstrating several large bullae in the right apex.

Pleural effusions

The management of pleural effusions is predicated on the cause. In patients with transudates, the underlying process should be identified and treated. Large, clinically significant transudative pleural effusions may require thoracocentesis or tube thoracostomy. Practically all transudative pleural effusions should be treated conservatively. Treatment should be directed toward the cause of the effusion. Nonsteroidal anti-inflammatory medications are the usual treatment for effusions associated with postcardiotomy syndromes. Diuretic treatment is directed toward hydrostatic resolution of effusions. Occasionally, thoracentesis or more invasive thoracic procedures are required to control large symptomatic effusions.

Removal of the chest tube placed to drain a pleural effusion is indicated when the daily drainage decreases to a rate comparable with the pleural cavity's resorptive capacity, the cause of the effusion is treated and controlled, and the patient's physical condition has improved. One randomized study showed that there was no difference in drainage time, hospital stay, fluid reaccumulation rates, or thoracentesis rates among patients with their chest tubes removed with a daily threshold output rate of 200 mL/day or less.[62] Another study evaluating the manner of chest-tube removal demonstrated no difference in the rate of complications whether chest tubes were removed during end-inhalation or end-exhalation.[63]

Hemothorax

The management of a hemothorax includes initial fluid resuscitation and tube thoracostomy with blood evacuation. If hemorrhage continues, VATS or thoracotomy may be required to control bleeding and remove all the blood from the pleural cavity. In general, initial drainage of more than 1200 mL or continued hemorrhage of more than 250 mL/h requires exploration. Nonexpansion of the lung after evacuation of the hemothorax may require decortication and lung reexpansion via thoracotomy or VATS.

Parapneumonic effusions

Treatment of parapneumonic effusions is based on clinical judgment and depends on the stage of the process and amount of free fluid. Neoplastic pleural effusions should be treated symptomatically or, if complicated by infection, aggressively. Asymptomatic pleural effusions may be observed. If the patient is symptomatic, simple and complete drainage for diagnosis and relief of dyspnea may be performed as an initial approach. Without adequate drainage, the patient will be subject to one or more of the following: prolonged hospitalization, prolonged evidence of systemic toxicity, increased morbidity, increased risk of residual ventilatory impairment, risk of local spread of the inflammatory reaction, and increased mortality.[64] The American College of Chest Physicians Parapneumonic Effusions Panel grouped management approaches into six categories: no drainage performed, therapeutic thoracocentesis, tube thoracostomy, fibrinolytics, VATS, and open surgery (including thoracotomy with or without decortication and rib resection).[55] Fibrinolytic therapy requires a chest tube for drug delivery. VATS requires a postprocedural tube thoracostomy. Surgery requires a postprocedural tube thoracostomy. Every approach requires treatment of the underlying cause, including appropriate systemic medications. The lowest mortality rates for the treatment of parapneumonic effusion were achieved with thoracotomy (1.9 percent), fibrinolytic therapy (4.3 percent), and VATS (4.8 percent). The requirement for a second intervention in the management of parapneumonic effusion was highest for no drainage (49.2 percent) and therapeutic thoracentesis (46.3 percent) and lowest for VATS (0 percent) and surgery (10.7 percent). Low-risk patients with parapneumonic effusions may not require drainage, while those in the advanced categories require drainage by thoracentesis or tube thoracostomy. Fibrinolytics, VATS, and thoracotomy are recommended approaches in the management of advanced parapneumonic effusions or empyema. The VATS technique for thoracic empyema in the fibrinopurulent stage is the recommended approach and is more effective when applied primarily rather than after attempted fibrinolytic therapy.[65] Patients treated in the organizing stage of empyema with antibiotics and fibrinolytics have demonstrated considerable improvement.[66]

During the preantibiotic era, techniques of open drainage of loculated empyemas were developed; these are still used today. The first, described by Shede, was resection of two or more ribs with marsupialization accomplished by sewing the skin to the pleura. This allows local cleaning and healing of the cavity from inside out. Once the infection is under control, the hole rapidly closes over in a few weeks. In 1935, Eloesser described a procedure to treat tuberculous empyema. A skin flap is created, sections of two ribs underlying the flap are resected, and the flap is folded into the thorax to create an opening into the chest.[67] This procedure is rarely used now for the treatment of tuberculosis, although it has found use in the treatment of postpneumonectomy empyema and bronchopleural fistula.[68] The Eloesser procedure is used in conjunction with various tissue flaps that can obliterate the thoracic cavity and close the fistula.[69]

Recurrent pleural effusions require one or more of the following: drainage of the pleural space, apposition of the visceral and parietal pleural surfaces with complete expansion of the lung, dispersion of extrapleural sclerosing agent throughout the pleural space, and maintenance of pleural apposition until chemical or inflammatory pleuritis occurs in order to allow the pleural surfaces to fuse. Treatment options include thoracentesis or repeat thoracocentesis; tube thoracostomy; drainage and sclerosis with talc, bleomycin, or other material; a chronic indwelling pleural catheter (Pleurx, Denver Biomedical, Golden CO)[70]; pleuroperitoneal shunt[71]; or thoracoscopy with drainage and talc instillation.[72]

Occasionally after drainage of a pleural effusion, the underlying lung may remain collapsed, creating a "trapped lung." Radiographically this can be misinterpreted as a pneumothorax. Catheter drainage does not reexpand the lung. The standard approach for management of this problem is to perform a thoracotomy and decortication with removal of the pleural inflammation trapping the lung. This procedure is not indicated in cases of malignant pleural disease due to the shortened life expectancy and significant morbidity associated with the procedure. It is indicated for patients with benign disease who have objective evidence of restriction of ventilation with progressive and refractory dyspnea.

Tuberculous effusions

Primary tuberculous effusions resolve spontaneously within 2 to 4 months in most individuals. However, if untreated with antituberculous chemotherapy, 65 percent of these patients will develop pulmonary or extrapulmonary tuberculosis within 5 years.[73] The current recommendation for tuberculous effusions consists of isoniazid, rifampin, and pyrazinamide for 2 months, followed by isoniazid and rifampin for the next 4 months.[74] Corticosteroids have been advocated as an adjunct to medical therapy of tuberculous pleural effusions. The presumed role of steroids is to speed up resolution of symptoms, increase reabsorption of pleural fluid, and prevent residual pleural thickening. A large, randomized placebo-controlled study did not confirm the benefit of steroids in the management of tuberculous pleural effusions.[75] Therefore steroids should be used only if acute symptoms—such as fever, chest pain, or dyspnea—affect the patient's quality of life. Early pleural fluid drainage has been suggested to improve outcomes in patients with tuberculous pleural effusions. A recent randomized study noted that the only difference between patients treated with multiple medications versus those treated with pleural fluid aspiration plus medical treatment was more rapid resolution of dyspnea in the drainage group of 4 days versus 8 days.[76] Decortication in tuberculous pleural effusions is an indicated surgical procedure in cases of failure of pleural drainage or extension of pleural involvement to more than one-third of the hemithorax. Decortication should be accomplished as early as 2 to 4 weeks after the initiation of drug therapy. An algorithm for management is provided in Fig. 11-9.

Chylothorax

The initial management of patients with chylothorax depends on the etiology. Selle and colleagues in 1997

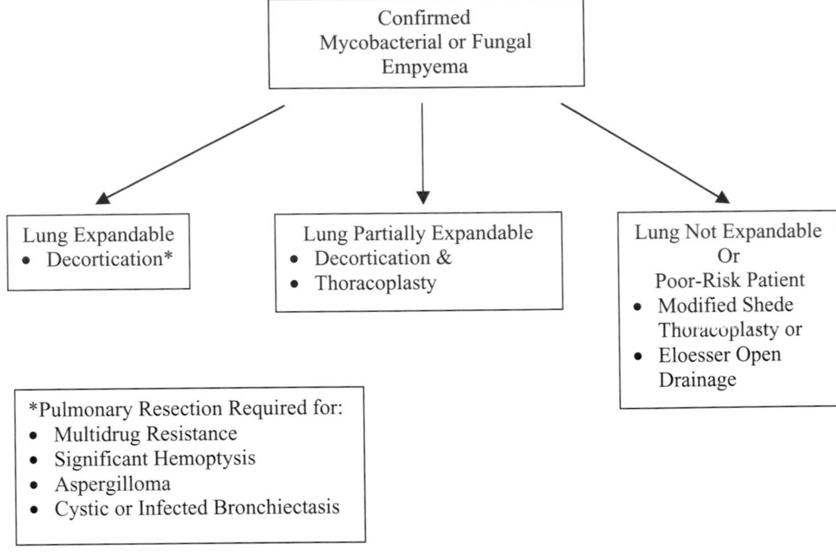

Figure 11-9 Simplified algorithm for the management of patients with mycobacterial or fungal empyemas.

established guidelines for the approach to the patient with chylothorax.[77] Conservative therapy consists of maintaining effective thoracostomy tube drainage with good lung expansion and adequate nutrition. This is coupled with restricted fat intake, or nothing by mouth and hyperalimentation (Fig. 11-10). No optimal time for duration of therapy is established. In approximately 50 percent of the patients the leak will close spontaneously within 2 weeks of therapy. When chest-tube output is more than 500 mL/day, surgical therapy is recommended. Surgical therapy for the control of a chylous fistula includes direct ligation of thoracic duct injury, mass ligation of the thoracic duct low in the chest, pleuroperitoneal shunting, pleurectomy, and occasional decortication. With unilateral chylothorax, the affected side is explored. When the chylothorax is bilateral, the right side is explored. Some advocate preoperative feeding of the patient with 100 to 200 mL of olive oil or heavy

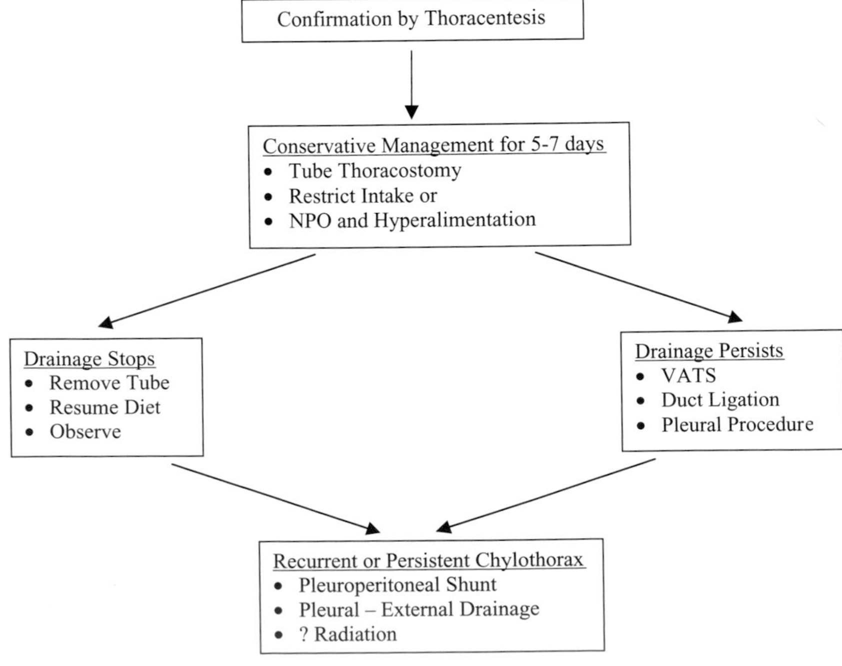

Figure 11-10 Simplified algorithm for the management of patients with chylothorax.

cream 2 to 3 h prior to the operation. An alternative method of visualization is the injection of a 1% aqueous solution of Evans blue dye into the leg, which leads to staining of the thoracic duct in 5 min and may last up to 12 min. These maneuvers are rarely necessary. Ligation of the thoracic duct just above diaphragm is the most commonly accepted approach. Supradiaphragmatic ligation of the duct is performed low in the right chest above the right crus of the diaphragm, where the duct lies on the vertebral column between the aorta and the azygos vein. This approach obviates the need for visualization of the duct leak. The pleuroperitoneal one-way Denver shunt and fibrin glue are alternatives in the treatment of persistent leak after surgical duct ligation.

Nontraumatic chylothorax, exclusive of the neonatal group, usually suggests widespread fatal illness. In nontraumatic chylothorax, the cause must be determined. If it is neoplastic in origin, radiation and chemotherapy are the prime treatment modalities; occasionally surgical treatment may be required. Radiation therapy is especially effective in cases of chylothorax caused by mediastinal lymphoma or carcinoma. Irradiation of the thoracic duct and lymphatics with 20 Gy promotes closure of the thoracic duct leak in most cases. Idiopathic causes in the neonate usually respond well to thoracentesis and diet restriction. In cases resulting from trauma, an initial trial of nonoperative therapy is indicated. Transthoracic ligation of the duct is indicated when the average daily chyle loss exceeds 1500 mL/day in adults for more than 5 days. If the chyle flow has not diminished within 14 days or if nutritional complications appear imminent, surgery is indicated.

Malignant pleural effusions

The treatment of malignant pleural effusions is complex. Chest-tube drainage, pleurodesis, pleural sclerosis, and drainage with a chronic indwelling pleural catheter are the most common modes of therapy. Talc is the most effective sclerosing agent used and is often administered as a slurry.[78] Almost all sclerosing agents can produce fever, tachycardia, chest pain, and nausea. Narcotic premedication to control pain symptoms prior to instillation of the sclerosing agent is the current best medical practice. After drainage of pleural fluids, the slurry (4 to 6 g of talc in a solution of 100 mL saline with or without lidocaine) is usually instilled. Rotation of patients treated with intrapleural talc suspension is unnecessary.[79] Tetracycline, popular in the past, is no longer available for pleurodesis. Doxycycline has replaced tetracycline as an alternative sclerosant; however, it is not as effective as talc. Bleomycin is as effective as talc for pleurodesis, but it is expensive and produces systemic toxicity. The pleuroperitoneal shunt is an effective alternative. It requires placement of a fenestrated catheter intracorporeally via a subcutaneous tunnel connecting the pleural space with the peritoneal cavity. A one-way valve within a subcutaneous pumping chamber allows the patient to self-drain the pleural cavity on a daily basis. Another type, the Pleurx catheter is a soft Silastic chronic indwelling catheter. The patient or caregiver drains the pleural fluid periodically by connecting the tubing to a disposable vacuum container to provide relief of dyspnea and potentially achieve spontaneous pleurodesis. The primary benefits of the Pleurx catheter drainage compared to chest tube and doxycycline sclerosis in patients with malignant effusions are the improved quality of life, reduced medical costs, improved function, treatment in an outpatient setting, and occasionally spontaneous pleurodesis.[70] The recommended limits of drainage are 1000 to 1500 mL of fluid removed from one hemithorax during a single procedure to prevent the reexpansion of pulmonary edema.

Mesothelioma

Localized mesothelioma

Solitary fibrous tumors of the pleura require complete en bloc surgical resection. Resection margins should comprise 1 to 2 cm of healthy tissue. For pedunculated tumors, resection of the involved pleura, chest wall, or lung parenchyma is called for. This sometimes requires lobectomy or pneumonectomy. VATS techniques have been successfully used to remove smaller pedunculated tumors located on the visceral or parietal pleura. Extreme caution should be used to avoid contaminating thoracoscopic sites, because contact metastasis and recurrence of tumor at surgical sites have been recorded.[80] Staging by de Perrot and colleagues combines both benign and malignant tumors into one system[81] (Table 11-4). Adjuvant therapy may be beneficial in the management of localized fibrous tumors, especially for the control of tumor recurrence at incision sites. Neoadjuvant therapy can be helpful in the case of large solitary malignant tumors; however, its application is complicated by the absence of hard evidence for effectiveness. New therapies—such as photodynamic therapy, immunotherapy, and gene therapy—resemble those used

Table 11-4 Classification of solitary fibrous tumors of the pleura

Stage	0	Pedunculated tumor without signs of malignancy
Stage	I	Sessile or "inverted" tumor without signs of malignancy
Stage	II	Pedunculated tumor with histologic signs of malignancy
Stage	III	Sessile or "inverted" tumor with histologic signs of malignancy
Stage	IV	Multiple synchronous metastatic tumors

Malignancy is recognized by the presence of the following features: high cellularity with crowding and overlapping of nuclei, cellular pleomorphism, high mitotic count (more than four per 10 high-power fields), necrosis, or stromal/vascular invasion.
Source: de Perrot et al.[81] With permission.

for diffuse malignant mesothelioma. Most recurrences are seen at surgical sites within the first 24 months after the initial resection; therefore quarterly follow-up is necessary.

Diffuse mesothelioma

There is no widely accepted curative approach for diffuse malignant mesothelioma.[82] Despite intensive investigation, the prognosis associated with this malignancy remains bleak. Surgical treatment of mesothelioma remains the most effective modality. Newer approaches allow sicker groups of patients to be diagnosed and treated earlier in the course of the disease, with less morbidity and mortality. Despite these advances, the treatment of diffuse malignant mesothelioma is controversial and difficult to evaluate owing to the absence of randomized prospective studies. The goal of treatment is local control.

Mesothelioma is unresponsive to most chemo- and radiotherapy regimens and typically has a high rate of recurrence even after the most aggressive surgical approaches. The average survival of patients with or without treatment is 6 to 8 months.[83,84] Multimodality therapy is the most commonly applied approach and has some benefit in prolonging the survival of a very select group of patients. New modalities—such as photodynamic therapy, immunotherapy, and gene therapy—are currently under intensive investigation and may lead to improvement of survival in patients with this deadly disease. Single-agent and combination trials of chemotherapy have not shown significant benefit in the treatment of mesothelioma. The best responses were observed with antimetabolites and anthracyclines. Although mortality was unaffected, response rates were shown to be in the range of 15 to 35 percent.[85] Some newer agents have been used in the management of mesothelioma. Paclitaxel or docetaxel, when used as single agents, showed some benefit, mostly acting as radiosensitizers. P-30 protein showed a similar response rate, with limited side effects. Multidrug treatment with doxorubicin, cisplatin, bleomycin, and mitomycin has been shown to be of some benefit and is the most commonly used regimen in conjunction with surgery. Despite this, however, there is as yet no hard evidence of significant benefit associated with chemotherapy.

Intracavitary application of chemotherapeutic agents provides some benefit in the treatment of intraperitoneal mesothelioma but did not display the same effect in pleural disease. The average survival associated with this modality was 21 months.[86] External-beam radiation therapy, like chemotherapy, has been ineffective in prolonging survival in mesothelioma patients, although occasional studies have shown some degree of regression. More than 50 Gy has been administered to provide palliation. Because of the wide target field and the proximity of multiple radiosensitive vital organs, radiation therapy of the pleura is problematic. Complications of radiotherapy for mesothelioma include nausea, vomiting, radiation hepatitis, esophagitis, myelitis, myocarditis, pneumonitis, and bilateral deterioration of pulmonary function.[87] Radiation therapy, delivered by external beam or brachytherapy, may be effective as an adjunct to surgical resection to control local disease. Radioactive colloid, such as chromic phosphate (P32), which has low tissue permeability, is effective in delivering high doses of radiation to a large volume of pleural space. Its best use is in controlling recurrent pleural effusions in patients with diffuse pleural involvement. Radiation therapy is successful in controlling chest wall implants following invasive procedures.[88]

By default, surgery is the main treatment approach for the management of malignant mesothelioma. There are three primary roles for surgical intervention: (1) diagnosis, usually approached by VATS or limited thoracotomy; (2) extirpation in patients with early-stage, potentially resectable disease, usually approached by pleurectomy or pleuropneumonectomy; and (3) palliation for patients with late-stage unresectable disease, usually effected by pleurodesis. An assessment of each patient's stage and condition is necessary to define suitable surgical candidates. Tables 11-2, 11-3, and 11-4 define the staging of diffuse malignant mesothelioma. The patient's overall patient health, functional status, nutritional status, and cardiopulmonary function must be evaluated. The postoperative predicted FEV_1 should be calculated; this may require a ventilation/perfusion scan. CT, MRI, and PET scans are diagnostic imaging studies utilized in the evaluation of resectability. Relative contraindications for extrapleural pneumonectomy include a history of myocardial infarction within 3 months, life-threatening arrhythmias, $PaO_2 < 55$ mmHg, $PCO_2 > 45$ mmHg, postoperative predicted $FEV_1 < 1$ L, or evidence of pulmonary hypertension. The presence of distant metastasis; absence of extrapleural fat planes; substantial involvement of the chest wall, major vascular structures, or the esophagus; or diffuse lesions of the pericardium or diaphragm all connote unresectability.

The first report of an attempted complete resection of diffuse mesothelioma was made in 1922 by Eiselsberg, from Germany. An extrapleural pneumonectomy was first performed by Mason in 1949.[89] Parietal pleurectomy is performed through a posterolateral thoracotomy with stripping of the pleura and pericardium from the apex of the lung to the diaphragm. Most of the parietal pleura can be removed, but the diaphragmatic pleura and much of the mediastinal pleura usually cannot be resected completely. The operative mortality is 2 percent in a highly select group of patients. The median survival time using this approach ranges from 9.0 to 18.3 months. As a purely palliative measure, parietal pleurectomy is the most effective means of reducing the recurrence of pleural effusions in mesothelioma. Complications include bronchopleural fistulas with prolonged air leak, hemorrhage, pneumonia, subcutaneous emphysema, incomplete tumor removal, and, rarely, empyema.

Extrapleural pneumonectomy is a radical procedure that includes en bloc removal of the parietal pleura, ipsilateral lung, pericardium, and ipsilateral diaphragm.

Currently, extrapleural pneumonectomy is indicated for patients with technically resectable tumors contained within the pleural envelope, with no involvement of mediastinal lymph nodes.[91] This procedure carries significant morbidity and an operative mortality of 5 to 35 percent. The average survival after extrapleural pneumonectomy ranges between 4 and 21 months, based on the results of several studies. Local recurrence generally develops after pleurectomy/decortication and distant metastasis develops after extrapleural pneumonectomy. Supraventricular arrhythmia is the most common complication after extrapleural pneumonectomy, at a rate of 20 to 40 percent.[92] Other complications include bronchopleural fistula, empyema, chylothorax, myocardial infarction, and congestive heart failure.

Multimodality therapy combining surgical resection, chemotherapy, and adjuvant radiation therapy is the most aggressive approach in the management of diffuse malignant mesothelioma. Survival after such trimodal therapies ranges between 16 and 24 months and depends on the extent of disease and the histologic subtype.[93] The sites of tumor recurrence are the ipsilateral hemithorax (35 percent), the peritoneal cavity (26 percent), and the contralateral hemithorax (17 percent). Only 4 percent of patients develop distant metastasis.[94] Pleurectomy/decortication combined with chemotherapy did not show significant survival benefit in several studies.[95] An evaluation of factors relating to the survival of patients with malignant mesothelioma by the Cancer and Leukemia Group between 1984 and 1994 showed that the best survival (13.9 months) was in groups of patients who were younger than 49 years and had an Eastern Cooperative Oncology Group (ECOG) performance status of 0 as well as in patients who were older than 49 years with a performance status of 0 and a hemoglobin > 14.6 g/dL. The worst survival (1.4 months) occurred in patients with a white blood cell count $> 15.6/\text{mm}^3$ and an ECOG performance status of 1 or 2.[96] The most common sites of metastasis are the liver and the contralateral lung.

Newer modalities in the management of malignant mesothelioma include intracavitary photodynamic adjuvant therapy after extrapleural pneumonectomy, immunotherapy, and gene therapy. Despite initial reports, no improvement in survival or local tumor control was demonstrated for photodynamic therapy in larger studies.[97] Newer sensitizers are under investigation. Like most malignancies, pleural mesothelioma appears to be resistant to mechanisms of immune-mediated destruction. However, in vitro studies and experiments in animal models have shown that high concentrations of immunotherapeutic agents can overcome this resistance. High levels of transforming growth factor beta, interleukin-2, interferon alpha, and interferon gamma were evaluated as treatment modalities. No conclusive clinical trials are complete at this time. Gene therapy may offer another adjunctive treatment. One promising approach in current experimental cancer gene therapy is the introduction of a toxic or "suicide" gene into mesothelioma cells, facilitating their destruction. This method of mesothelioma management is currently being developed in multiple centers in the United States; however, clinical application of this treatment is not yet developed. Palliative therapy includes different approaches for pain control and control of malignant pleural effusions.

References

1. Hippocrates. Aphorism 44. In: Adams LB Jr (ed). *The Genuine Works of Hippocrates: The Classics of Surgery.* Birmingham, AL: Gryphon Editions, 1985:768–771.
2. Miserocchi G. Physiology and pathophysiology of pleural fluid turnover. *Eur Respir J* 1997;10:219–225.
3. Wagner JC, Slegg CA, Marchand P. Diffuse pleural mesotheliomas and asbestosis exposure in Northwestern Cape Province. *Br J Ind Med* 1960;17:260.
4. Wagner JC. The discovery of the association between blue asbestos and mesotheliomas and the aftermath. *Br J Ind Med* 1991;48:399.
5. Musk AW, Dolin PJ, Armstrong BK, et al. The incidence of malignant mesothelioma in Australia. 1947–1980. *Med J Aust* 1989;150:242.
6. Matthay MA, Callen PW, Filly RA, et al. relationship of pleural effusions to pulmonary hemodynamics in patients with congestive heart failure. *Am Rev Respir Dis* 1985;132:1253.
7. Kinasewitz GT, Groome LJ, Marshall RP, et al. Role of pulmonary lymphatics and interstitium in visceral pleural fluid exchange. *J Appl Physiol* 1984;56:355.
8. Albernine KH, Wiener-Kronish JP, Staub NC. The structure of the parietal pleura and its relationship to pleural liquid dynamics in sheep. *Anat Rec* 1984;208:401.
9. Wang NS. The preformed stomas connecting the pleural cavity and the lymphatics in the parietal pleura. *Am Rev Respir Dis* 1975;111:12.
10. Gaudio E, Rendina EA, Pannarale L, et al. Surface morphology of the human pleura. A scanning electron microscopic study. *Chest* 1988;92:149.
11. Wiener-Kronish JP, Broaddus VC, Albertine KH, et al. Removal of pleural fluid and protein by lymphatics in awake sheep. *J Appl Physiol* 1988;64:384.
12. Yang PC. Ultrasound-guided transthoracic biopsy of the chest. *Radiol Clin North Am* 2000;38:323–343.
13. Hierholzer J, Luo L, Bittner RC, et al. MRI and CT in the differential diagnosis of pleural disease. *Chest* 2000;118: 604–609.
14. Benard F, Sterman D, Smith RJ, et al. Metabolic imaging of malignant pleural mesothelioma with fluorodeoxyglucose positron emission tomography. *Chest* 1998;114:713.
15. Broaddus VC, Light RW. What is the origin of pleural transudates and exudates? (Editorial.) *Chest* 1992;102: 658.
16. Light RW, Macgregor MI, Luchsinger PC, Ball WC Jr. Pleural effusions: The diagnostic separation of transudates and exudates. *Ann Intern Med* 1972;77:507.

17. Heffner JE, Sahn SA, Brown LK. Multilevel likelihood ratios for identifying exudative pleural effusion. *Chest* 2002;121:1916–1920.
18. Xirouchaki N, Tzanakis N, Bouros D, et al. Diagnostic value of interleukin-$_1$alpha, interleukin-6, and tumor necrosis factor in pleural effusions. *Chest* 2002;121:815–820.
19. Sallach SM, Sallach JA, Vasquez E, et al. Volume of pleural fluid required for diagnosis of pleural malignancy. *Chest* 2002;122:1913–1917.
20. Maskell NA, Gleeson FV, Davies RJO. Standard pleural biopsy vs. CT-guided needle biopsy for diagnosis of malignant pleural effusions: Randomized controlled trial. *Lancet* 2003;361:1326–1331.
21. Ernst A, Hersh CP, Herth F, et al. A novel instrument for the evaluation of the pleural space: An experience in 34 patients. *Chest* 2002;122:1530–1534.
22. Blanc FX, Atassi K, Bignon J, Housset B. Diagnostic value of medical thoracoscopy in pleural disease: A 6-year retrospective study. *Chest* 2002;121:1677–1683.
23. Scharifker D, Kaneko M. Localized fibrous "mesothelioma" of pleura (submesothelial) fibroma: A clinicopathologic study of 18 cases. *Cancer* 1979;43:627.
24. Moran CA, Suster S, Koss MN. the spectrum of histologic growth patterns in benign and malignant fibrous tumors of pleura. *Semin Diagn Pathol* 1992;9:169.
25. Nelson R, Burman SO, Kiani R, et al. Hypoglycemic coma associated with benign pleural mesothelioma. *J Thorac Cardiovasc Surg* 1975;69:306.
26. Bunn PA Jr, Ridgway EC. Paraneoplastic syndromes. In: DeVita VT Jr, Hellman S, Rosenberg SA (eds). *Cancer: Principles and Practice of Oncology*, 3d ed. Philadelphia: Lippincott, 1989:1896.
27. Cole FH, Ellis RA, Goodman RC, et al. Benign fibrous pleural tumor with elevation of insulin-like growth factor and hypoglycemia. *South Med J* 1990;83:690.
28. Strom EH, Skjorten F, Aarseth LB, Haug E. Solitary fibrous tumors of pleura. An immunohistochemical, electron-microscopic and tissue culture of a tumor producing insulin-like growth factor I in a patient with hypoglycemia. *Pathol Res Pract* 1991;187:109.
29. Briselli M, Mark EJ, Dickerson R. Solitary fibrous tumors of pleura: Eight new cases and review of 360 cases in the literature. *Cancer* 1981;47:2678.
30. Okike N, Bernatz PE, Woolner LB. Localized mesothelioma of the pleura. Benign and malignant variants. *J Thorac Cardiovasc Surg* 1978;75:363.
31. England DM, Hochholzer L, McCarthy MJ. Localized benign and malignant fibrous tumors of the pleura: A clinicopathologic review of 223 cases. *Am J Surg Pathol* 1989;13:640.
32. Klemperer P, Rabin CB. Primary neoplasms of the pleura. A report of five cases. *Arch Pathol* 1937;11:385.
33. Stout AP, Murray MR. localized pleural mesothelioma. *Arch Pathol* 1942;34:951.
34. Selikoff IJ, Churg J, Hammond EC. Relation between exposure to asbestos and mesothelioma *N Engl J Med* 1965;272:560.
35. Whitwell F, Rawcliffe RM. Diffuse malignant pleural mesothelioma and asbestosis exposure. *Thorax* 1971;26:6.
36. Carbone M, Fisher S, Powers A, et al. New molecular and epidemiological issues in mesothelioma: Role OF SV-40. *J Cell Physiol* 1999;180:167–172.
37. Elmes PC, Simpson MJC. The clinical aspect of mesothelioma. *QJM New Series* 1976;45:427.
38. Ruffie R, Feld R, Minkin S, et al: Diffuse malignant mesothelioma of the pleura in Ontario and Quebec: A retrospective study of 332 patients. *J Clin Oncol* 1989;7:1157.
39. Olesen LL, Thorshauge H. Thrombocytosis in patients with malignant pleural mesothelioma. *Cancer* 1988;62: 1194.
40. Heelan RT, Rusch VW, Begg CB, et al. Staging of malignant pleural mesothelioma: Comparison of CT and MR imaging. *AJR* 1999;172:1039–1047.
41. Boutin C, Viallat JR, Aelony Y. *Practical Thoracoscopy.* Berlin: Springer-Verlag, 1991.
42. Kamp DW, Mossman BT. Asbestosis associated cancers: Clinical spectrum and pathogenic mechanisms. *Clin Occup Environ Med* 2002;2:753–757.
43. Rusch VW and The International Mesothelioma Interest Group. A proposed new International TNM staging system for malignant pleural mesothelioma. *Chest* 1995;108:1122.
44. Boutin C, Schlesser M, Frenay C, Astoul P. Malignant pleural mesothelioma. *Eur Respir J* 1998;12:972–981.
45. Baumann MH, Strange C, Heffner JE, et al and the AACP Pneumothorax Consensus Group. Management of spontaneous pneumothorax: An American College of Chest Physicians Delphi consensus statement. *Chest* 2001;119: 590–602.
46. Sepkowitz KA. Pneumothorax in AIDS. *Ann Intern Med* 1991;24:12, 455–459.
47. Crawford BK. Treatment of AIDS-related bronchopleural fistula by pleurectomy. *Ann Thorac Surg* 1992;54(2): 214–215.
48. Byrnes TA. Pneumothorax in patients with acquired immunodeficiency syndrome. *J Thorac Cardiovasc Surg* 1989;98(4):546–550.
49. Walker WA. AIDS-related bronchopleural fistula. *Ann Thorac Surg* 1993;55:1048.
50. Trejo O, Giron JA, Perez-Guzman E, et al. Pleural effusion in patients infected with the human immunodeficiency virus. *Eur J Clin Microbiol Infect Dis* 1997;16:807–815.
51. Clark TA. Spontaneous pneumothorax. *Am J Surg* 1972;124 (6):728–731.
52. Bedford DE, Lovibond JL. Hydrothorax in heart failure. *Br Heart J* 1941;3:93–111.
53. Strauss RM, Martin LG, Kaufman SL, Boyer TD. Transjugular intrahepatic portal systemic shunt for the management of symptomatic cirrhotic hydrothorax. *Am J Gastroenterol* 1994;89(9):1520–1522.
54. Light RW, Girad WM, Jenkinson SG, et al. Parapneumonic effusions. *Am J Med* 1980;69:507–512.
55. Colice GL, Curtis A, Deslauriers J, et al for the American College of Chest Physicians Parapneumonic Effusions Panel. Medical and surgical treatment of parapneumonic effusions, an evidence-based guideline. *Chest* 2000;118: 1158–1171.
56. Cerfolio RJ. The incidence, etiology and prevention of postresectional bronchopleural fistula. *Semin Thorac Cardiol Surg* 2001;13:3–7.
57. Emery RW, Graif JL, Hale K, et al. Treatment of end-stage chronic obstructive pulmonary disease with double lung transplantation. *Chest* 1991;99:533.
58. Burrows CM, Mathews WC, Colt HG. Predicting survival in patients with recurrent symptomatic malignant pleural

effusions: An assessment of the prognostic values of physiologic, morphologic, and quality of life measures of extent of disease. *Chest* 2000;117:73–78.
59. Alexsandrakis MG, Passam FH, Kyriakou DS, Bouros D. Pleural effusion in hematologic malignancies. *Chest* 2004; 125:1546–1555.
60. Noppen M, Alexander P, Driesen P, et al. Manual aspiration vs. chest tube drainage in first episode of primary spontaneous pneumothorax: A multicenter, prospective, randomized pilot study. *Am J Respir Crit Care Med* 2002;165:1240–1244.
61. Baumann MH, Strange C. Treatment of spontaneous pneumothorax: A more aggressive approach? *Chest* 1997;112:789–804.
62. Younes RN, Gross JL, Aguiar S, et al. When to remove a chest tube? A randomized study with subsequent consecutive validation *J Am Coll Surg* 2002;195:658–662.
63. Bell RL, Ovadia P, Abdullah F, et al. Chest tube removal: End-inspiration or end-expiration? *J Trauma* 2001;50: 674–677.
64. Colice GL, Curtis A, Deslauriers J, et al. Medical and surgical treatment of parapneumonic effusions: An evidence-based guideline. *Chest* 2000;118:1158–1171.
65. Petrakis IE, Kogerakis NE, Drositis IE, et al. Video-assisted surgery for thoracic empyema: Primary, or after fibrinolytic therapy failure? *Am J Surg* 2004;187: 471–474.
66. Simpson G, Roomes D, Reeves B. Successful treatment of empyema thoracis with human recombinant deoxyribonuclease. *Thorax* 2003;58:365–366.
67. Eloesser L. An operation for tuberculous empyema. *Surg Gynecol Obstet* 1935;60:1096–1097.
68. Halling JD, Johnson FE. Eloesser procedure for postpneumonectomy bronchopleural fistula. *Am J Surg* 2004;187: 100–101.
69. Molnar JA, Pennington DG. Management of postpneumonectomy broncho-cutaneous fistula with a single free flap. *Ann Plast Surg* 2002;48:88–91.
70. Putnam JB Jr, Light RW, Rodriguez RM, et al. A randomized comparison of indwelling pleural catheter and doxycycline pleurodesis in the management of malignant pleural effusions. *Cancer* 1999;86:1992–1999.
71. Lee KA, Harvey JC, Reich H, Beattie EJ. Management of malignant pleural effusions with pleuroperitoneal shunting. *J Am Coll Surg* 1994;178:586–588.
72. Mager HJ. Distribution of talc suspension during treatment of malignant pleural effusion with pleurodesis. *Lung Cancer* 2002;36:77–81.
73. Chan CH, Arnold M, Chan CY, et al. Clinical and pathological features of tuberculous pleural effusion and its long-term consequences. *Respiration* 1991; 58:171–175.
74. Bass JB, Farer LS, Hopewell PC, et al. Treatment of tuberculosis and tuberculosis infection in adults and children. *Am J Respir Crit Care Med* 1994;149:1359–1374.
75. Wyser C, Walzl G, Smedema JP, et al. Corticosteroids in the treatment of tuberculous pleurisy: A double-blind, placebo-controlled, randomized study. *Chest* 1996;110:333–338.
76. Lai YF, Chao TY, Wang YH, Lin AS. Pigtail drainage in the treatment of tuberculous pleural effusions: Randomized study. *Thorax* 2003;58:149–152.
77. Selle JG, Synder WA, Schreiber JT. Chylothorax. *Ann Surg* 1971;177:245.
78. Jacobi CA, Wenger FA, Schmitz-Rixen T, Muller JM. Talc pleurodesis in recurrent pleural effusions. *Langenbecks Arch Surg* 1998;383:156–159.
79. Anthony VB. Pathogenesis of malignant pleural effusions and talc pleurodesis. *Pneumologie* 1999;53:493–498.
80. Cardillo G, Facciolo F, Cavazzana AO, et al. Localized (solitary) fibrous tumors of pleura: An analysis of 55 patients. *Ann Thorac Surg* 2000;70:1808–1812.
81. de Perrot M, Fischer S, Bundler MA, et al. Solitary fibrous tumors of pleura. *Ann Thorac Surg* 2002;74:285–293.
82. Sterman D, Kaiser LR, Albelda SM. Advances in the treatment of malignant pleural mesothelioma. *Chest* 1999;116: 504–520.
83. Brenner J, Sordillo PP, Magill GB, Golbey RB. Malignant mesothelioma of pleura: Review of 123 patients. *Cancer* 1982;49:2431–2435.
84. Huncharek M, Kelsey K, Mark EJ, et al. Treatment and survival in diffuse malignant pleural mesothelioma: A study of 83 cases from Massachusetts General Hospital. *Anticancer Res* 1996;16:1265–1268.
85. Ong ST, Vogelzang NJ. Chemotherapy in malignant pleural mesothelioma: A review. *J Clin Oncol* 1996;14:1007–1017.
86. Aisner J. Current approach to malignant mesothelioma of pleura. *Chest* 1995;107:332S–344S.
87. Maasilta P, Kivisaari L, Holsti LR, et al. Radiographic chest assessment of lung injury following hemithorax irradiation for pleural mesothelioma. *Eur Respir J* 1991;4: 76–83.
88. Boutin C, Rey F, Viallat JR. Prevention of malignant seeding after invasive diagnostic procedures in patients with pleural mesothelioma: A randomized trial of local radiotherapy. *Chest* 1995;108:754–758.
89. Kittle CF. Treatment: I. The surgical treatment of mesothelioma. In: Kittle, CF (ed). *Mesothelioma: Diagnosis and Management.* Chicago: Year Book, 1987:61–72.
90. Pass HI, Pogrebniak HW. Malignant pleural mesothelioma. *Curr Probl Surg* 1993;30:921–1012.
91. Jaklitsch MT, Grondin SC, Sugarbaker DJ. Treatment of malignant mesothelioma. *World J Surg* 2001;25:210–217.
92. Harpole DH, Liptay MJ, DeCamp MM, et al. Prospective analysis of pneumonectomy: Risk factors for major morbidity and cardiac dysrhythmias. *Ann Thorac Surg* 1996;61:977–982.
93. Sugarbaker DJ, Norberto JJ. Multimodality management of malignant pleural mesothelioma. *Chest* 1998;113: 61S–65S.
94. Baldini EH, Recht A, Strauss GM, et al. Patterns of failure after trimodality therapy for malignant pleural mesothelioma. *Ann Thorac Surg* 1997;63:334–338.
95. Lee JD, Perez S, Wang HJ, et al. Intrapleural chemotherapy for patients with incompletely resected malignant mesothelioma: The UCLA experience. *J Surg Oncol* 1995; 60:262–267.
96. Herndon JE, Green MR, Chahinian AP, et al. Factors predictive of survival among 337 patients with mesothelioma treated between 1984 and 1994 by the Cancer and Leukemia Group B. *Chest* 1998;113:723–731.
97. Pass HI, Temeck BK, Kranda K, et al. Phase III randomized trial of surgery with or without intraoperative photodynamic therapy and postoperative immunochemotherapy for malignant pleural mesothelioma. *Ann Surg Oncol* 1997;4:628–633.

CHAPTER

12 LUNG CARCINOMA

Nishant Patel, Torin P. Fitton, Richard F. Heitmiller

INTRODUCTION AND EPIDEMIOLOGY

Lung cancer is the leading cause of cancer-related mortality in both males and females, accounting for 173,770 new cases and 160,440 deaths in 2003. Despite numerous investigations and aggressive multimodality therapy, the death rate from lung cancer has declined by only a modest 1.8 percent since 1991. The high cost, considerable morbidity, and poor outcomes associated with lung cancer mandate prompt investigation when it is suspected.

RISK FACTORS FOR THE DEVELOPMENT OF LUNG CANCER

Smoking

Smoking is the single most reversible cause of lung cancer. The precise mechanism by which smoking promotes carcinogenesis is unknown, although numerous studies have suggested that it promotes base-pair mutations and paralyzes cellular repair mechanisms.[1] Although all forms

KEY CONCEPTS

- Epidemiology
  - Lung cancer is the leading cause of cancer-related mortality in both males and females, accounting for 173,770 new cases and 160,440 deaths in 2003. Despite numerous investigations and aggressive multimodality therapy, the death rate from lung cancer has declined by only 1.8 percent since 1992.
- Pathophysiology
  - Smoking remains the single most reversible cause of lung cancer. Although the exact mechanism by which smoking promotes carcinogenesis is unknown, many studies suggest that it promotes base-pair mutations and paralyzes cellular repair mechanisms. The incidence of lung cancer is significantly higher among African Americans versus Caucasians, perhaps related to increased genetic susceptibility or smoking exposure. Although there have been studies relating exposure to a variety of compounds, including polycyclic aromatic hydrocarbons, the carcinogenic effect of these substances has not been identified. Early work with genetic mapping suggests that certain families are at risk to develop lung cancer.
- Clinical features
  - Approximately 90 to 95 percent of all lung cancer patients are symptomatic at the time of presentation. Presenting symptoms are determined by the stage, location, histology, and intrinsic biology of the tumor. Pulmonary symptoms include cough, dyspnea, wheezing and stridor, hemoptysis, pleuritic chest pain, and obstructive pneumonia. Nonpulmonary symptoms result from a primary tumor or a large metastatic lymph node that invades or compresses adjacent structures. Such symptoms may stem from chest wall invasion, diaphragm invasion, phrenic nerve invasion, recurrent laryngeal nerve dysfunction, superior vena cava syndrome and pericardial effusion, esophageal invasion, and vertebral body invasion.
- Diagnostics
  - Diagnosis of lung cancer includes a thorough history and physical examination and radiology examinations, including chest x-ray, computed tomography, magnetic resonance imaging, and positron emission tomography. It also includes cytologic evaluation and invasive examinations, including fine-needle

aspiration, bronchoscopy, mediastinoscopy, thoracoscopy, and thoracotomy.

- Treatment
  - Although patients with stage I and II disease are best treated with curative surgery, some patients either refuse surgery or are inoperable due to comorbidities. Curative radical primary radiotherapy may be an option for these patients. Radiotherapy can therefore be applied as the primary treatment in inoperable patients, as an adjunct to surgery, or as palliative treatment. It can be combined with chemoradiotherapy and is used postoperatively in the majority of patients who have mediastinal lymph node metastases. The use of chemotherapy is controversial in the treatment of lung cancer. Neoadjuvant chemotherapy has been shown in some studies to improve survival time and reduce recurrence as compared with surgery alone. Surgical therapy is contingent on preoperative patient assessment, which includes pulmonary function tests, evaluation of comorbidities, and a functional assessment test that measures the maximum oxygen consumption of a patient with compromised lung function. Operative procedures include pneumonectomy, lobectomy, segmentectomy, and wedge resection.
- Outcomes
  - Patients with T1N0M0 disease have a better prognostic outlook than any other subset. Sixty-one percent of patients with stage IA disease and 38 percent of those with stage IB disease are expected to survive at least 5 years after diagnosis and treatment. Survival diminishes with each TNM subset and staging, with stage IIIA showing a 5-year survival rate of 9 percent.

of smoking are associated with an increased lifetime risk of developing lung cancer, cigarette smokers have twice the risk.[2–4] Government-mandated reductions in tar and nicotine concentrations over the last 30 years have reduced the incidence of lung cancer, but several studies have demonstrated that smokers of low-tar cigarette increase consumption, largely negating the benefit.[3] Studies comparing smoking intensity versus duration have demonstrated that length of exposure is a more significant risk factor.[4] Although smoking cessation should be strongly encouraged in all patients, the risk of developing lung cancer among ex-smokers is not reduced over time but remains equivalent to the time point at which smoking cessation occurred.

Diet

Dietary factors play a significant role in the pathogenesis of breast and gastrointestinal cancer, but little is known about their role with respect to lung cancer. Several studies have found that diets rich in fruits, vegetables, and vitamin A seem to confer a protective effect, but the patient populations studied had a much lower incidence of smoking. The absolute effect of diet on lung cancer remains unknown.

Race

The incidence of lung cancer was significantly higher among African Americans versus Caucasians (81.2 vs. 63.2 per 100,000) between 1996 and 2002. Five-year survival rates for African Americans were significantly decreased versus Caucasians (12 versus 15 percent) during the same period. Racial disparities in the incidence of lung cancer may represent an increased genetic susceptibility or smoking exposure and differences in socioeconomics affecting access to health care.

Occupational factors

Longitudinal prospective studies of patient populations exposed to radon gas, asbestos, polycyclic aromatic hydrocarbons, arsenic, chromate, and bis (chloromethyl) ether demonstrate an increased risk for the development of lung cancer. The carcinogenic effect of each of these substances has not been identified.

Air pollution

Exposure to air pollution may increase the risk of lung cancer. Metanalysis has demonstrated a significant increase in percentage of damaged DNA adducts in heavily exposed industrial workers versus urban workers, but the absolute effect of this damage on the eventual development of lung cancer is unknown.[5]

Family history

Multiple incidences of lung cancer among family members even with minimal to moderate exposure to risk factors supports the hypothesis that genetic susceptibility plays a role in the development of lung cancer.[6] Studies of patients occupationally exposed to asbestos and polycyclic aromatic hydrocarbons found that metabolizers of the drug debrisoquin showed a fourfold increase in lung cancer risk compared with poor metabolizers.[7] Segregation analysis of 337 families with a high incidence of lung cancer demonstrated that a codominant inheritance of a rare autosomal gene seemed to correlate with an earlier onset of lung cancer in smokers.[8] However, each of these studies on genetic polymorphisms linked with lung cancer found significant heterogeneity.[9] Recent studies have focused on CYP2D6 and the cytochrome P450 (CYP) 1A1 gene as markers of lung cancer susceptibility. CYP2D6 metabolizes tobacco nitrosamine products into mutagenic products inducing carcinogenesis.[10] The cytochrome P450 (CYP) 1A1 gene encodes an aryl-hydrocarbon hydroxylase that activates polycyclic hydrocarbons in the presence of electrophilic metabolites. Polymorphisms in CYP1A1 seem to correlate with increased risk of lung cancer, but the exact mechanism is unknown.

BIOLOGY OF LUNG CARCINOMA

Identification of a reproducible and reliable biological marker pointing to patients at risk for the development of lung cancer would represent a major advancement in understanding of the molecular biology of this disease. Numerous molecular aberrations have been found with increased incidence in lung cancer, but none are sensitive or specific enough for clinical application.

THE *p53* GENE

Mutations in *p53* constitute the most common genetic alterations associated with cancer. This gene is activated in response to numerous environmental and cellular insults and plays an important role in regulating transcription, cell division, and apoptosis. Loss of *p53* expression is catastrophic, allowing genetically damaged cells to proliferate without inhibition, possibly leading them to develop into aberrant precancerous tumor cells. Recent studies show a dose-response relationship between tobacco consumption and the frequency of *p53* mutations.[11]

THE P16^{INK4A}CYCLIN D1-CDK4-RB PATHWAY

The *p16*^{INK4A}cyclin D1-CDK4-RB pathway is another growth-regulatory pathway that has been found to be inactivated in lung cancer. The *p16*^{INK4A}cyclin D1-CDK4-RB regulates the phase transition of the cell cycle and prevents cell division in the presence of damaged nuclear components. RB has been found to be inactivated in both small cell lung carcinomas (90 percent) and less commonly in non-small cell lung carcinomas (15 to 30 percent).[12,13]

THE *RAS* ONCOGENE

The *RAS* oncogene family, consisting of *KRAS*, *HRAS*, and *NRAS*, encodes genes for proteins regulating GTPase activity, which is necessary for signal transduction. *RAS* genes locked in the "on" position by point mutations at codons 12, 13, and 61 can lead to uncontrolled cell division. *RAS* mutations characterize 20 to 30 percent of adenocarcinomas and 15 to 20 percent of non-small cell lung carcinomas but are very uncommonly seen in small cell lung carcinomas.[14]

THE *MYC* GENE FAMILY

MYC, a basic helix-loop-helix leucine-zipper (bHLHZ) class of transcription factor, is activated following signal transduction down the *RAS* cascade. *MYC* and *MAX* form the heterodimer *MYC-MAX*, which increases transcription of specific downstream genes. Amplification of the *MYC* gene family is more common in small cell lung cancer than non-small cell lung cancer (SCLC).[14] Figure 12-1 schematically represents the major pathways involved in lung cancer cells.

PATHOLOGY

Table 12-1 lists the 1999 World Health Organization's histopathologic classification for lung cancer. Lung cancer can be divided into three categories: non-SCLC, comprising approximately 75 percent of all cases; SCLC, comprising 20 percent of cases; and 5 percent comprised of rare mixed epithelial types and tumors that arise in bronchial glands or other tissues.[15]

NON-SMALL CELL LUNG CANCER (NSCLC)

SCLCNSCLC is subdivided into squamous cell carcinoma, adenocarcinoma, and undifferentiated large cell carcinoma.

Squamous cell carcinoma

Squamous cell carcinoma has recently been supplanted by adenocarcinoma as the most common lung cancer type.[16,17] Squamous cell carcinoma arises from bronchial epithelium[18] and develops into a polypoid or sessile mass primarily in the major bronchi, thus obstructing the airway lumen. As a result, obstructive pneumonia often accompanies squamous cell carcinoma. Furthermore, squamous cell carcinoma accounts for approximately half of all superior sulcus tumors (Pancoast tumors)[19] and commonly shows liver and small intestinal metastases.

Morphologically, squamous cell carcinoma appears to have an irregular, gray-white cut surface with a spiculated shape due to the mass's tethering to the surrounding pulmonary parenchyma. Central necrosis is common and may include cavitation. Under the microscope, squamous cell carcinoma appears similar to stratified squamous epithelium except that it is architecturally disordered. Additionally, well-differentiated squamous cell carcinomas show anucleate keratinization and squamous pearls. Variants of poorly differentiated squamous cell carcinoma that have been identified include

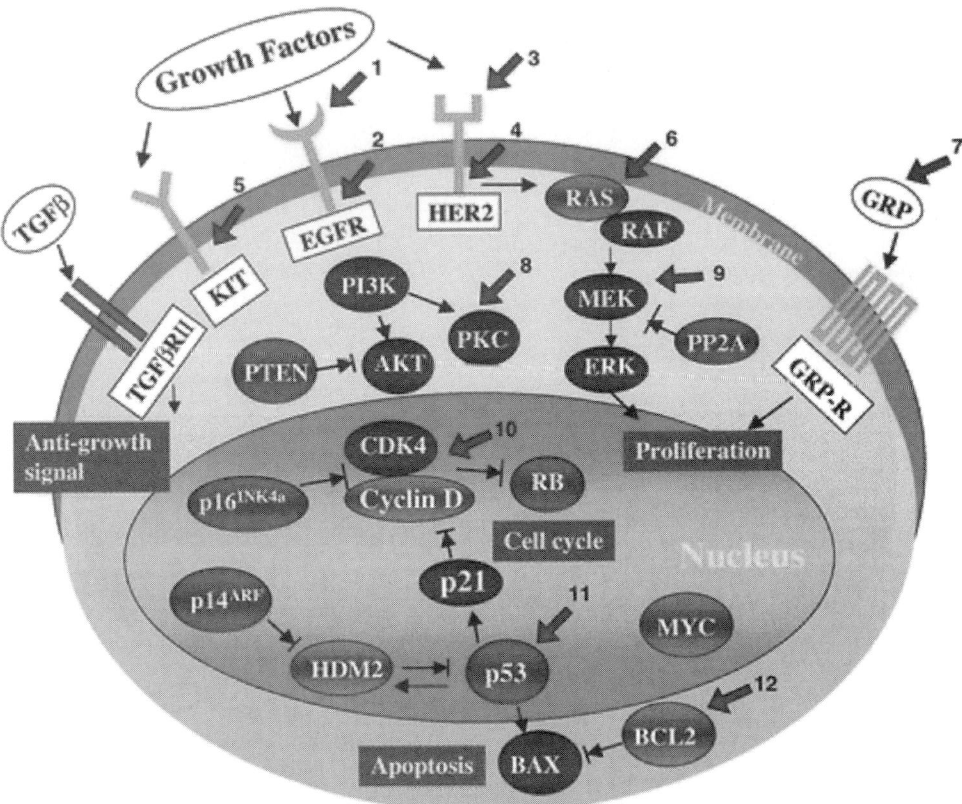

Figure 12-1 Schematic representation of the common growth-stimulatory and inhibitory cascades involved in lung cancer cells. (From Sekido Y, et al. Molecular Genetics of Lung Cancer. *Annu Rev Med* 2003;54:73-87. With permission.) Molecules in green denote activation, whereas molecules in red denote inactivation. Purple arrows indicate the potential sites for targeted therapy. Examples include #1, monoclonal antibodies against EGFR (IMC-C225 and ABX-EGF); #2, inhibitors of EGFR (ZD1839, OSI-774, and PKI166); #3, monoclonal antibody against HER2 (trastuzumab); #4, inhibitor of HER2 (CI-1033); #5, inhibitor of KIT (imatinib); #6, inhibitor of RAS (SCH66336 and R115777); #7, monoclonal antibody against GRP (2A11); #8, inhibitor of PKC (ISIS3521); #9, inhibitor of MEK (CI1040); #10, inhibitor of CDKs (flavopiridol); #11, replacing wild-type p53 (adenovirus p53); #12, inhibitor of BCL2 (G3139). CDK4 =\, cyclin-dependent kinase-4; EGFR = epidermal growth factor receptor; ERK = extracellular signal-regulated kinase; MEK = MAP kinase/ERK-activating kinase; GRP = gastrin-releasing peptide; GRP-R = GRP-receptor; PI3K = phosphatidylinositol 3 kinase; PKC = protein kinase C; PP2A = protein phosphatase 2A; RB = retinoblastoma protein; TGFβ = transforming growth factor beta; TGFRII = transforming growth factor beta type II receptor.

papillary, clear cell, small cell, and basaloid subtypes. These variants present microscopic differences but do not indicate clinical significance.

Adenocarcinoma

Adenocarcinoma, the most common lung cancer type and the one occurring most frequently in nonsmokers, originates in the bronchioloalveolar epithelium or the mucous glands, commonly as a peripheral mass. Adenocarcinoma tumors usually involve pleura, remain asymptomatic, and metastasize before the primary lesion becomes symptomatic or a diagnosis is made. The scalene lymph nodes seem to be the most frequent site of metastasis. Adenocarcinoma nodules that arise in other sites may appear similar to primary nodules in the lung. Cytokeratins assist in distinguishing between lung adenocarcinomas and adenocarcinomas arising in other sites. In lung adenocarcinoma, cytokeratin 7 shows up positive, while cytokeratin 20 shows up negative. Another marker, thyroid transcription factor-1 (TTF-1), is solely found in lung adenocarcinoma and thyroid cancer and also distinguishes metastatic adenocarcinoma from an unknown primary site.[20]

Table 12-1 World health organization classification of lung and pleural tumors

1. Epithelial tumors
1.1. Benign
1.1.1. Papillomas
1.1.1.1. Squamous cell papilloma
Exophytic
Inverted
1.1.1.2. Glandular papilloma
1.1.1.3. Mixed squamous cell and glandular apilloma
1.1.2. Adenomas
1.1.2.1. Alveolar adenoma
1.1.2.2. Papillary adenoma
1.1.2.3. Adenomas of salivary-gland type
Mucous gland adenoma
Pleomorphic adenoma
Others
1.1.2.4. Mucinous cystadenoma
1.1.2.5. Others
1.2. Preinvasive lesions
1.2.1. Squamous dysplasia/Carcinoma in situ
1.2.2. Atypical adenomatous hyperplasia
1.2.3. Diffuse idiopathic pulmonary neuroendocrine cell hyperplasia
1.3. Malignant
1.3.1. Squamous cell carcinoma
Variants
1.3.1.1. Papillary
1.3.1.2. Clear cell
1.3.1.3. Small cell
1.3.1.4. Basaloid
1.3.2. Small cell carcinoma
Variant
1.3.2.1. Combined small cell carcinoma
1.3.3. Adenocarcinoma
1.3.3.1. Acinar
1.3.3.2. Papillary
1.3.3.3. Bronchioloalveolar carcinoma
1.3.3.3.1. Nonmucinous (Clara/pneumocyte type II)
1.3.3.3.2. Mucinous
1.3.3.3.3. Mixed mucinous and nonmucinous or intermediate cell type
1.3.3.4. Solid adenocarcinoma with mucin
1.3.3.5. Adenocarcinoma with mixed subtypes
1.3.3.6. Variants
1.3.3.6.1. Well-differentiate fetal adenocarcinoma
1.3.3.6.2. Mucinous (colloid) adenocarcinoma
1.3.3.6.3. Mucinous cystadenocarcinoma
1.3.3.6.4. Signet-ring adenocarcinoma
1.3.3.6.5. Clear cell adenocarcinoma
1.3.4. Large cell carcinoma
Variants
1.3.4.1. Large cell neuroendocrine carcinoma
1.3.4.1.1. Combined large cell neuroendocrine carcinoma
1.3.4.2. Basaloid carcinoma
1.3.4.3. Lymphoepithelioma-like carcinoma
1.3.4.4. Clear cell carcinoma
1.3.4.5. Large cell carcinoma with rhabdoid phenotype
1.3.5. Adenosquamous carcinoma
1.3.6. Carcinomas with pleomorphic, sarcomatoid or sarcomatious elements
1.3.6.1. Carcinomas with spindle and/or giant cells
1.3.6.1.1. Pleomorphic carcinoma
1.3.6.1.2. Spindle cell carcinoma
1.3.6.1.3. Giant cell carcinoma
1.3.6.2. Carcinosarcoma
1.3.6.3. Pulmonary blastoma
1.3.6.4. Others
1.3.7. Carcinoid tumor
1.3.7.1. Typical carcinoid
1.3.7.2. Atypical carcinoid
1.3.8. Carcinomas of salivary-gland type
1.3.8.1. Mucoepidermoid carcinoma
1.3.8.2. Adenoid cystic carcinoma
1.3.8.3. Others
1.3.9. Unclassified carcinoma

2. Soft tissue tumors
2.1. Localized fibrous tumor
2.2. Epitheloid hemangioendothelioma
2.3. Pleuropulmonary blastoma
2.4. Chondroma
2.5. Calcifying fibrous pseudotumor of the pleura
2.6. Congenital peribronchial myofibroblastic tumor
2.7. Diffuse pulmonary lymphangiomatosis
2.8. Desmoplastic small round cell tumor
2.9. Other

3. Mesothelial tumors
3.1. Benign
3.1.1. Adenomatoid tumor
3.2. Malignant
3.2.1. Epitheloid mesothelioma
3.2.2. Sarcomatoid mesothelioma
3.2.2.1. Desmoplastic mesothelioma
3.2.3. Biphasic mesothelioma
3.2.4. Other

4. Miscellaneous tumors
4.1. Hamartoma
4.2. Sclerosing hemangioma
4.3. Clear cell tumor
4.4. Germ cell neoplasms
4.4.1. Teratoma, mature or immature
4.4.2. Malignant germ cell tumor
4.5. Thymoma
4.6. Melanoma
4.7. Others

5. Lymphoproliferative Disease
5.1. Lymphoid interstitial pneumonia
5.2. Nodular lymphoid hyperplasia
5.3. Low-grade marginal zone B-cell lymphoma of the mucosa-associated lymphoid tissue
5.4. Lymphomatoid granulomatosis

6. Secondary Tumors

7. Unclassified Tumors

8. Tumor-like Lesions
8.1. Tumorlet
8.2. Multiple meningothelioid nodules
8.3. Langerhans cell histiocytosis
8.4. Inflammatory pseudotumor (inflammatory myofibroblastic)

(*Continued*)

Table 12-1 World health organization classification of lung and pleural tumors (*continued*)

8.5. Organizing pneumonia	8.9. Multifocal micronodular pneumocyte hyperplasia
8.6. Amyloid tumor	8.10. Endometriosis
8.7. Hyalinizing granuloma	8.11. Bronchial inflammatory polyp
8.8. Lymphangioleiomyomatosis	8.12. Others

Source: From Brambilla E, et al. The new World Health Organization classification of lung tumors. *Eur Respir J* 2001;18:1059–1068. With permission.

Morphologically, peripheral adenocarcinomas have a gray-white cut surface with an irregularly lobulated shape. Anthracotic pigment in the tumor mass is common. Necrosis and hemorrhage are present only in lesions greater than 5 cm. Lung adenocarcinoma also displays a pseudomesotheliomatous form, where a rind of tumor tissue forms around the lung due to growth of extremely peripheral tumors into the pleura. As a result, radiographic imaging and intraoperative observation of lung adenocarcinoma give the appearance of mesothelioma.[21–22]

Microscopic study of adenocarcinoma reveals four major subtypes: acinar, papillary, bronchioloalveolar, and solid. Minor variants also classified include sarcomatoid,[23] well-differentiated mucinous or colloid,[24] signet-ring cell,[25] clear cell,[26] and enteric.[27]

Bronchioloalveolar carcinoma (BAC) originates from nonciliated bronchiolar epithelial cells (Clara cells) and usually presents as a peripheral lesion that was once thought to be associated with preexisting scars.[28,29] Recent studies now claim that central fibrosis follows tumor initiation and is the product of the tumor itself.[30] BAC tends to occur in the elderly and is evenly distributed among males and females.[31,32] Patients with BAC who are radiologically and clinically relevant include patients with radiographs and complaints that suggest pneumonia, patients with a solitary lesion located in the periphery, or patients with multiple dense nodules throughout one or both lungs, representing metastases from a distant neoplasm.[33]

Morphologic findings of BAC distinguish between mucinous and nonmucinous subtypes that differ in clinical appearance and outcome. Mucinous BAC appears multifocal or multinodular with an unfavorable prognosis due to inoperability, while nonmucinous BAC usually exists as a solitary lesion and shows a more favorable clinical outcome.[34] Furthermore, in comparing nodules of the same size and stage, mucinous tumors are more prone to metastasize from the lung than nonmucinous BACs, thus further worsening the prognosis of mucinous BAC.[32]

Large cell undifferentiated carcinoma

Some 15 percent of all lung cancers are large cell undifferentiated carcinomas (LCUCs).[35] LCUCs arise centrally or peripherally and are at least 5 cm in diameter. They appear lobulated, with a white-gray cut surface, and are commonly associated with necrosis. Microscopic study reveals large polygonal cells that show vesiculated chromatin, nucleoli, and clearly outlined cytoplasmic borders. Furthermore, no keratinization or glandular differentiation occurs. Giant cell and clear cell carcinomas are two variants of LCUCs.

Under the microscope, giant cell carcinomas appear as large pleomorphic tumor cells that are frequently multinucleate. Microscopic investigation of giant cell neoplasms often reveals cannibalistic behavior, where the tumors appear to engulf one another. Primary clear cell carcinomas of the lung are diagnosed only in the event that other clear cell neoplasms of the lung are omitted. Clinically, clear cell carcinoids,[36] metastatic renal cell carcinoma,[37] metastatic glycogen-rich balloon cell melanoma,[38] and benign clear cell "sugar" tumors[39] should all be considered using radiography, electron microscopy, and immunohistology before primary clear cell carcinoma of the lung is diagnosed.

SMALL CELL LUNG CANCER (SCLC)

SCLC comprises 20 percent of all lung cancers.[40] Most small cell lung cancers arise centrally; approximately 10 percent are found in the periphery.[41] Small cell lung cancer lesions are typically small hyperchromatic cells with a molded white-tan appearance. Histology reveals the absence of cytoplasm and inconspicuous nucleoli. Necrosis is common due to the rapid growth and scarce cytoplasm of these tumors. A majority of SCLC cells contain dense-core granules and are positive for neuron-specific enolase, chromogranin A, Leu-7, and synaptophysin; less frequently, they are positive for carcinoembryonic antigen (CEA) and ACTH. SCLCs tend to manifest paraneoplastic syndromes due to the release of polypeptide hormones. These tumors frequently invade lymphatic and vascular tissue, often resulting in mediastinal adenopathy. Metastasis is early and frequent; metastasis can invade almost every organ, and is present in approximately 70 percent of patients at diagnosis. Historically, SCLC was subdivided into oat cell, intermediate, and combined variants. The World Health Organization has dropped these classifications and currently recognizes only the combined SCLC variant. Less than 10 percent of SCLCs are combined small cell with non-small cell components. Of these, 4 to 6 percent are admixed with large cell undifferentiated lung cancer and 1 to 3 percent with adenocarcinoma or squamous cell carcinoma.[42]

NEUROENDOCRINE TUMORS

Neuroendocrine tumors of the lung are classified into SCLCs, typical carcinoid tumors, atypical carcinoid tumors, and large cell neuroendocrine tumors.

Typical carcinoid tumors

Typical carcinoid tumors, or bronchial carcinoid tumors, are found equally among males and females and are most often seen in young to middle-aged adults. Typical carcinoid tumors are similar to GI tract tumors and frequently arise centrally, where they are associated with cartilaginous airways, leading to obstruction and potential wheezing, coughing, or pneumatic symptoms. Some have been reported to arise in the peripheral lung.[43]

Morphologically, typical carcinoid tumors grow to 2 to 4 cm as polyploid masses that are tan to dark red in color with no apparent mitotic activity, necrosis, or hemorrhaging. These tumors display organoid growth that has a trabecular, nested, solid sheet or ribbon-like pattern. Electron microscopy reveals dense-core granules in the cytoplasm. Immunohistologic studies indicate that typical carcinoid tumors are often positive for neurone-specific enolase (NSE), chromogranin A, Leu-7, synaptophysin, bombesin, CEA, ACTH, calcitonin, and keratin.[44] The release of ectopic hormones, in particular ACTH, vasopressin, insulin, and 5-hydroxytryptophan, may be attributable to these tumors. The rate of metastasis is low for typical carcinoid tumors, allowing for complete excision and a more favorable clinical outcome.

Atypical carcinoid tumors

Atypical carcinoids, first described in 1972,[46] are pleomorphic tumors with hyperchromatic nuclei that are larger than typical carcinoids and usually grow to more than 3 cm in diameter. Unlike typical carcinoids, atypical carcinoids display increased mitotic activity and evidence of necrosis and hemorrhaging. Electron microscopy shows a disruption of the organoid growth pattern. Atypical carcinoids metastasize more frequently than typical carcinoids. In the original study describing atypical carcinoids, 70 percent of lesions metastasized, with a mortality rate of 30 percent.[45]

Large cell neuroendocrine carcinomas

Large cell neuroendocrine carcinomas are most often found among heavy smokers and arise commonly as peripheral masses. Histologic studies reveal that these tumors are at least three times the size of small cell cancers. Furthermore, large cell neuroendocrine carcinomas show an organoid growth pattern, cellular palisading, necrosis, a mitotic activity similar to that of small cell cancers, and a varying granular pattern of chromatin.[46] Clinically, large cell neuroendocrine carcinomas are extremely aggressive. Many studies have demonstrated poor prognosis despite the fact that, pathologically, most of these tumors are T1 or T2. Recent studies have shown a poor 2-year follow-up with all patients either deceased or with distant metastases.[47,47] The 5-year survival rate for patients with large cell neuroendocrine lesions is 18 percent in those with stage I disease and a 13 percent for those with disease of any stage disease.[48]

RARE CARCINOMAS

Adenosquamous carcinoma

Adenosquamous carcinoma accounts for 1.8 percent of all lung cancers and is subdivided into a glandular type that may derive from squamous metaplasia in preexisting adenocarcinoma, mixed types that may originate from undifferentiated carcinomas transitioning into other elements, and a squamous type that resembles mucoepidermoid carcinoma.[49] Clinical, radiographic, and pathologic evidence of adenosquamous carcinoma reveals a striking similarity to that of pure adenocarcinoma. Although the malignancy of these tumors is a topic of controversy, the prognosis remains poor, with a 5-year survival rate of 35 percent.[50]

Sarcomatoid carcinomas, carcinosarcomas, and pulmonary blastomas

Sarcomatoid carcinomas, carcinosarcomas, and pulmonary blastomas account for approximately 1 percent of all pulmonary cancers.[50] These tumors show a male-to-female ratio of 2:1 and are usually found in smokers complaining of dyspnea, hemoptysis, or cough. Most lesions of these types are large, between 1.5 and 12 cm in diameter, and appear irregularly shaped or spiculated on radiographs. Necrosis and hemorrhaging are common. Microscopic study of these lesions reveals a variety of histologic appearances. These include sarcoma-like monodifferentiated spindle-cell and pleomorphic lesions, biphasic lesions consisting of carcinomas and nondescript spindle-cell components, biphasic tumors with heterologous differentiation of components resembling sarcomas, biphasic neoplasms admixing fetal-like glands with nondescript blastema-like small cells, and tumors that appear similar to inflammatory pseudotumors of the lung.[52–55]

CLINICAL PRESENTATION AND DIAGNOSTIC MODALITIES

Approximately 90 to 95 percent of all lung cancer patients are symptomatic; of these, 27 percent display symptoms secondary to the primary tumor, 32 percent

Table 12-2 Pulmonary and nonpulmonary symptoms associated with lung cancer

Pulmonary symptoms
Cough
Dyspnea
Wheezing and stridor
Hemoptysis
Lung abscess
Nonpulmonary symptoms
Chest wall invasion
Diaphragm invasion
Mediastinal invasion
Phrenic nerve invasion
Recurrent laryngeal nerve dysfunction
Superior vena cava syndrome
Pericardial effusion
Esophageal invasion
Vertebral body invasion
Paraneoplastic syndromes
Metastatic symptoms

present symptoms secondary to metastatic spread, and 34 percent show nonspecific symptoms.[51] The signs and symptoms of lung carcinoma depend on the stage at diagnosis and the location, histology, and intrinsic biology of the tumor. These factors are critical to understanding the pulmonary, nonpulmonary, and metastatic symptoms associated with lung cancer. Nonspecific symptoms, such as weight loss and fatigue, are also common in lung cancer patients. Pulmonary and nonpulmonary symptoms associated with lung cancer are listed in Table 12-2.

PULMONARY SYMPTOMS

Pulmonary symptoms associated with lung cancer result from tumor involvement in the lung, bronchi, or metastatic lymph nodes. These symptoms include cough, dyspnea, wheezing and stridor, hemoptysis, pneumonic symptoms, and lung abscess.

Cough

Cough, occurring in 75 percent of patients, is the most common symptom associated with lung cancer and is due to bronchial irritation or compression.[52] However, cough is a common pulmonary manifestation of other diseases and is characteristic of cigarette smokers. Nevertheless, the cough's severity worsens and persists when a patient develops lung cancer.

Dyspnea

Dyspnea is the second most common symptom associated with lung cancer and occurs in 50 to 60 percent of patients.[57] It may result from a central tumor or may spread from a hilar lymph node owing to bronchial obstruction. The obstruction may be complete or partial and may or may not include atelectasis. Dyspnea may also result from peripheral tumors causing lymph node spread, lymphatic occlusion, lymphangitic spread, or diffuse alveolar spread of the tumor.

Wheezing and stridor

Wheezing occurs when a partial blockage of a proximal bronchus narrows the airway to less that half the normal diameter. An inspiriting stridor may occur instead of a wheeze when the proximal mainstem bronchus is partially occluded.

Hemoptysis

Hemoptysis, the coughing up of blood, occurs in 25 to 40 percent of lung cancer patients. Hemoptysis is also a common manifestation of bronchitis, tuberculosis, and other pathologic conditions. As a symptom of lung cancer, hemoptysis frequently occurs from degenerating central tumors or central tumors that invade adjoining bronchial tissue. Hemoptysis warrants immediate follow-up with bronchoscopy and a chest x-ray (CXR).

Pneumonic symptoms may follow bronchitis, atelectasis, or postobstructive pneumonia. Cough, excessive sputum production, fever, and pleuritic chest pain due to contact of an inflamed lung with the parietal pleura are common symptoms of patients with postobstructive atelectasis or pneumonia. Bronchoscopy should be performed on patients with a history of pneumonia that exceeds 2 months.

Lung abscess

Lung abscess is due to postobstructive pneumonia and is often seen in squamous or large cell carcinomas as a result of secondary infection of a tumor's necrotic site or cavity.

NONPULMONARY SYMPTOMS

Nonpulmonary symptoms of lung cancer result from a primary tumor or an enlarged metastatic lymph node that invades or compresses adjacent structures.

Chest wall invasion

Tumors that invade the chest wall often present as chest pain. Peripheral adenocarcinomas are most frequently associated with invasion or contact with the parietal pleura or deeper structures such as the intercostal muscles, ribs, and neurovascular bundle. Tumor invasion into the intercostal muscles and ribs creates a gnawing chest pain. Invasion into the neurovascular bundle produces a radial chest wall pain. Superior sulcus tumors may cause chest and shoulder pain from invasion into the intercostal muscles and ribs, radiating arm pain from invasion into the C8 and T1 roots of the brachial plexus, and pain associated with Horner's syndrome that is due to invasion of the stellate sympathetic ganglion. Horner's syndrome manifests itself as unilateral enophthalmos, ptosis, myosis, and anhidrosis of the face. The combination of these three symptoms of superior sulcus tumors is called Pancoast's syndrome.

Invasion of the diaphragm

Invasion of the diaphragm may lead to diaphragmatic dysfunction and augment dyspnea on exertion or pleural effusion. The diaphragm's lymph is extensive; therefore early lymphatic spread can occur if it is invaded by a tumor.

Mediastinal invasion

Mediastinal invasion of a tumor leads to varying symptoms that may precipitate from invasion into the phrenic nerve, laryngeal nerve, superior vena cava, pericardium, esophagus, or vertebral body.

Phrenic nerve invasion

Phrenic nerve invasion is usually diagnosed by a CXR that illustrates the elevation of the right or left hemidiaphragm. Patients with phrenic nerve invasion often present with diaphragmatic paralysis or hiccups and dyspnea on exertion. Patients may also experience referred pain in the shoulders from phrenic nerve invasion or diaphragmatic involvement.

Recurrent laryngeal nerve dysfunction

Dysfunction of the left recurrent laryngeal nerve results from invasion by tumors located in the left upper lobe at the point where the nerve loops around the aortic arch. Laryngeal nerve paralysis occurs when a left-upper-lobe tumor intrudes into the vagus nerve. Mediastinal adenopathy may also lead to invasion or compression of the vagus nerve, causing paralysis. A third mechanical stress that leads to laryngeal paralysis is invasion or compression of the recurrent laryngeal nerve itself by a hilar mass.

Recurrent laryngeal nerve dysfunction and paralysis abducts the vocal cords, leading to effects ranging from minor changes in tone to hoarseness. Pulmonary consequences resulting from insufficient coughing and a diminished positive end-expiratory pressure have also been noted.

Superior vena cava syndrome

Superior vena cava syndrome may occur from invasion or compression of the superior vena cava by a tumor medially located in the right upper lobe, from venous thrombosis, or from mediastinal adenopathy. Superior vena cava syndrome presents in 4 percent of all lung cancer patients and occurs predominantly in patients with SCLC pathology.

The increase in pressure in the upper thorax and head is the basis for the associated signs and symptoms. These may include flushing of the face, headache, dyspnea, cough, disruption of vision, and less commonly edema in the upper extremities, pain, dysphagia, and syncope. Patients may also present with facial cyanosis due to the slowing of venous drainage.

Pericardial effusion

Pericardial effusion results from pericardial involvement by a primary tumor. Pericardial tamponade occasionally accompanies pericardial effusion and presents as dyspnea or as sinus tachycardia or atrial fibrillation. Diagnosis of pericardial effusion depends on the location and size of the primary tumor as seen on radiographic images and echocardiography. A diagnosis of pleural effusion is usually made prior to recognition of pericardial effusion, but when a patient presents with persisting dyspnea or worsening cough after treatment for pleural effusion, management of pericardial effusion is necessary.

Esophageal invasion

Dysphagia due to primary tumor invasion into the esophagus is rare. A more common sighting is compression of the esophagus by subcarinal or posterior mediastinal lymphadenopathy associated with advanced lower lobe tumors. Cancerous subcarinal lymph nodes may erode the esophagus and produce a tracheoesophageal fistula that results in aspirations, pneumonitis, and/or hemoptysis.

Vertebral body invasion

Invasion into a vertebral body by a posterior tumor causes a persisting localized back pain. If the tumor invades the epidural space, patients present with symptoms associated with spinal cord compression. Signs and symptoms depend on the area of the spinal cord compressed, but they tend to include numbness, tingling, or weakness.

Paraneoplastic syndromes

Paraneoplastic syndromes occur in approximately 2 percent of all lung cancer patients and are predominantly characteristic of SCLCs and squamous cell carcinoma. Moreover, paraneoplastic syndromes tend to precede the diagnosis of the primary lung tumor. Table 12-3 lists the most common paraneoplastic syndromes associated with lung cancer.

Hypertrophic pulmonary osteoarthropathy

Although many paraneoplastic syndromes are seen in SCLC, hypertrophic pulmonary osteoarthropathy (HPO) is a rarity. Periostisis of distal ends of long bones is the keynote characteristic of HPO, with the tibia, fibula, and radius being the bones most commonly afflicted. Periostisis causes bone tenderness and leads to swelling;

Table 12-3 Paraneoplastic syndromes associated with lung cancer

Hypertrophic pulmonary osteoarthropathy
Clubbing of digits
SIADH
Hypercalcemia
Ectopic ACTH syndrome
Neuropathies
Lambert-Eaton myasthenic syndrome
Thrombophlebitis

SIADH = syndrome of inappropriate antidiuretic hormone secretion; ACTH = adrenocorticotropic hormone.

patients with HPO are symptomatically debilitated. If the disease progresses, it is common to see metacarpal/metatarsal involvement and acute polyarthritis. Clubbing of digits is always associated with HPO. Periostisis is easily seen on radiographs and leads to elevated levels of alkaline phosphatase. Symptomatic relief is usually achieved on resection of the primary lung tumor.

Clubbing of digits

Patients with NSCLCs often exhibit clubbing of digits independent of hypertrophic pulmonary osteoarthropathy. A recent study found that 31 of 88, or 35 percent, of patients with NSCLC presented with clubbing.[53] The same study showed that men and women with NSCLC show clubbing of digits more frequently than men and women with SCLC.[58]

Syndrome of inappropriate antidiuretic hormone secretion

Although hypersecretion of antidiuretic hormone (ADH) is frequent in patients with lung cancer, the syndrome of inappropriate antidiuretic hormone (SIADH) secretion is diagnosed only when patients present with hyponatremia. Hyponatremia is associated with a serum osmolarity less than 275 mOsm/kg, excretion of sodium into the urine that exceeds 25 meq/L, and a urine osmolarity that surpasses the serum osmolarity. Furthermore, patients with SIADH may present with symptoms of anorexia, nausea, vomiting, confusion, lethargy, and seizures.

Symptoms associated with SIADH usually resolve when the small cell tumor is chemotherapeutically or radiotherapeutically treated. Patients who present with recurrent small cell disease and continue to present with SIADH require alternative treatments. Demeclocycline, an ADH blocker that prevents the action of ADH on the distal renal tubule, is commonly used in the medical treatment of patients with recurrent disease.

Similar signs and symptoms are characteristic of hyponatremia from inappropriate secretion of atrial natriuretic peptide.[54] Like patients with SIADH, patients with inappropriate secretion of atrial natriuretic factor present with high urine sodium concentrations and excessive antidiuresis that can be treated by chemoradiotherapy of the small cell tumor. However, patients with atrial natriuretic peptide secretion do not indicate abnormal levels of ADH.

Hypercalcemia

Hypercalcemia occurs in approximately 10 percent of all patients with lung cancer. The most common cause of hypercalcemia in lung cancer patients is the ectopic production of parathyroid hormone (PTH), most often associated with squamous cell carcinoma. Approximately 15 percent of all hypercalcemia in lung cancer patients is etiologically due to factors secondary to PTH and humoral secretion.[55] Diagnosis of ectopic parathyroid hormone production is made by hypophosphatemia and excessive levels of serum PTH along with the exclusion of metastatic bone disease. In a clinical setting, hypercalcemia due to elevated levels of PTH causes dehydration and neurologic symptoms such as lethargy and a diminished level of consciousness. Treatment for hypercalcemia is achieved on resection of the tumor. However, recurrence of the tumor and associated hypercalcemia is frequent.

Ectopic adrenocorticotropic syndrome

A significant portion of patients with small cell cancers exhibit elevated levels of adrenocorticotropic hormone (ACTH). Nevertheless, a diagnosis of Cushing's syndrome is rare, less than 5 percent, because of the promptness of the ACTH elevation that occurs.[56] Instead, symptoms of elevated ACTH levels are attributed to hypokalemia, with potassium levels dropping below 3 mmol/L, hyperglycemia, and metabolic alkalosis. Diagnosis of ectopic ACTH syndrome can also be made by the presence of elevated ACTH levels in the blood or elevated 17-hydroxycorticosteroids in the urine.

Peripheral and central neuropathies

SCLC and squamous cell carcinoma are the most common causes of peripheral and central neuropathies in lung cancer patients. Peripheral neuropathies include sensory, sensorimotor, and autonomic dysfunctions and are the most common paraneoplastic syndrome associated with lung cancer. Central neuropathies consist of cerebellar degeneration, dementia, brainstem encephalitis, and encephalomyelitis and are less common. Although the paraneoplastic syndromes mentioned earlier involve hormones and hormone-like secretions, neurologic paraneoplastic syndromes are mediated by the immune system because of the irregular expression of antigens by cancer cells that are supposed to be expressed only by the nervous system. The aberrant expression of antigens activates an immune response whereby antibodies proliferate and interfere with neurologic function. In some cases antibodies to these antigens may also lead to neurologic destruction.[57]

Furthermore, neuropathies tend to have a later onset and to occur in patients with significant weight loss. The late onset makes it difficult to distinguish neuromuscular weakness secondary to neuropathy from disability due to metastatic disease. Central nervous system metastasis should be ruled out by MRI or computed tomography (CT) prior to diagnosing neuropathy as the cause of neurologic and muscular dysfunction.

Lambert-eaton myasthenic syndrome

Lambert-Eaton myasthenic syndrome most often occurs in SCLC and is associated with deficient neuromuscular conduction produced by immunoglobulin IgG antibodies that target omega conotoxin-sensitive voltage-gated calcium channels found in tumor cells and at the end-plates of neurons.[58] As a result, calcium influx is disrupted and acetylcholine release severely reduced.

Patients who present with Lambert-Eaton myasthenic syndrome are symptomatic for muscle weakness and fatigue, hyporeflexia, autonomic dysfunction, and dry mouth. The thighs are particularly affected, causing patients to walk in a wobbly manner. These symptoms usually precede the onset of symptoms of the primary tumor itself. A recent study has shown that symptoms of this disease have an onset that may occur up to 4 years prior to attaining radiographic evidence of the lesion.[59] Successful treatment of patients with Lambert-Eaton myasthenic syndrome has been achieved with resection of the tumor, chemotherapy, and radiotherapy.

Thrombophlebitis

Migratory thrombophlebitis, also known as Trousseau's syndrome, is associated with excess thromboplastin-like substances, due to lung cancer, in the circulation. Treatment with warfarin is often unsuccessful; subcutaneous unfractionated or low-molecular-weight heparin treatment is necessary to prevent recurring thromboses.[60]

METASTATIC SYMPTOMS

The brain and spinal cord, bones, liver and adrenal glands, and skin and soft tissue are the most common sites of metastases seen in patients with lung cancer.

Central nervous system metastases occur in 10 percent of lung cancer patients and reveal symptoms that result from increased intracranial pressure-namely headache, vomiting, nausea, and a diminished level of consciousness. Seizures are uncommon.

Bone metastases tend to produce localized pain and require radiologic study. Some 25 percent of lung cancer patients develop bone metastases, of which 55 percent occur in the axial skeleton and 12 percent in the appendicular skeleton.[61]

Liver and adrenal metastases are discovered routinely on CT scans and are usually asymptomatic. Liver metastases occur in 3 to 6 percent of lung cancer patients; metastases to the adrenal gland occur in 3 to 7 percent of lung cancer patients.[62]

Skin and soft tissue metastases are found in only 8 percent of lung cancer patients and have a late onset. Patients present with painless masses in the subcutaneous or intramuscular layers, occasionally followed by necrosis and the formation of a wound due to tumor erosion through the skin. In the latter circumstance, excision is necessary.

DIAGNOSIS

Diagnosis of lung cancer includes a thorough history and physical examination; radiographic examinations including CXR, CT, MRI, and PET; cytologic evaluation; and invasive examinations including fine-needle aspiration, bronchoscopy, mediastinoscopy, thoracoscopy, and thoracotomy.

History and physical examination

The history and physical examination is the first and most important step in evaluating a patient with lung cancer. Key elements that may help in diagnosing lung cancer are the etiologic factors mentioned earlier. These include smoking history, secondhand smoke exposure, and industrial exposure to carcinogens such as asbestos and polycyclic aromatic hydrocarbons. Physical manifestations of lung cancer should also be noted. These include cough, dyspnea, hemoptysis, wheezing on auscultation and pleural effusion revealed by percussion, lung abscess, or tenderness on palpitation of the thorax due to chest wall invasion. Evidence of paraneoplastic syndromes such as clubbing of digits; the ptosis, myosis, and anhydrosis associated with Horner's syndrome; or tenderness of bones due to hypertrophic pulmonary osteoarthropathy should also be documented. Other relevant assessments include weight loss and muscle wasting, leading to debilitation; and examination of the oral cavity, neck, and supraclavicular areas for other tumors and lymph node metastases.

Preoperative assessment should include pulmonary function tests to assess operative risk. Patients with vital capacities below 50 percent, FEV_1 (forced expiratory volume in 1 s) less than 50 percent or less than 2 L (most significantly less than 0.8 L), and reductions in maximum voluntary ventilation (MMV) are at significant risk and should not be operated on. Preoperative risk has also been associated with hypercapnea and hypoxemia.[63]

Radiography

Chest X-ray

A CXR is the most important diagnostic test for lung cancer. A review of old chest radiographs is essential in determining operability. Therefore records of old CXRs should be kept for diagnostic workup. A posteroanterior and lateral CXR may reveal a malignant, benign, or indeterminate lesion. Malignant masses appear large and spiculated with evidence of rib invasion or destruction and widening of the mediastinum. Benign masses, however, appear small and smooth. These masses are concentrically calcified and do not require further workup. A considerable percentage of lesions are classified as indeterminate and requires further workup. A CXR that is completely normal provides evidence against lung cancer; as a result, lung cancer can be ruled out as a diagnosis. Rarely, tiny lesions may be hidden behind other structures.

A CXR may also detect hilar and mediastinal adenopathy, but one cannot confirm metastases without biopsy or mediastinoscopy to prove lymph node metastases. A radiographic image that shows hemidiaphragmatic elevation is evidence of volume loss due to atelectasis or phrenic nerve involvement by a primary tumor. Vertebral body invasion is also identifiable. Furthermore, pleural effusion is readily seen on a CXR. Malignancy, however, should be diagnosed only on the basis of cytologic examination.

Computed tomography

CT of the chest and upper abdomen is a standard assessment tool for patients diagnosed or documented with lung cancer. CT illustrates the size, shape, and location of the mass. CT may also indicate invasion into contiguous structures, such as ribs or vertebral bodies. Lesions that are unidentifiable on CXR may be observed in CT, along with any unsuspected pleural effusion. A CT of the upper abdomen is essential to monitor for potential metastases to the liver and adrenal glands.

The most beneficial information from CT assessment of lung cancer patients regards possible metastasis to mediastinal lymph nodes. A recent study highlighted the fact that CT is the most effective way to assess for mediastinal adenopathy.[64] However, histologic confirmation is necessary to diagnose metastatic involvement for nodes that look positive on the CT scan.

Magnetic resonance imaging

MRI has not proved to offer an improvement over CT, but it provides high-quality images that can be useful in assessing lung cancers adjacent to the vertebral body or spinal canal and in evaluating tumors associated with vascular structures. MRI is superior to CT in detailing the changes in bone marrow that may suggest cancer involvement and in the imaging of blood flow without contrast enhancement. Nevertheless, the high rate of false-positives clearly indicates that MRI overdiagnoses mediastinal involvement.[65]

Positron emission tomography

PET detects specific positron-emitting isotopes of low-molecular-weight atoms. Isotopes of carbon, fluorine, oxygen, and nitrogen are more commonly detected. PET scanning uses a D-glucose analogue, fluorodeoxyglucose (FDG), with radiolabeled fluorine 18 (^{18}F). Malignant cells have a higher rate of glucose metabolism than normal cells. FDG is taken up by cells and phosphorylated into FDG-6-PO_4, which cannot be metabolized any further. As a result, the radiolabeled FDG-6-PO_4 accumulates in malignant cells and is an excellent visual marker that can help identify metastases, nodal stage, recurrence, and response to medical therapy. Furthermore, PET offers the advantage of imaging the entire body after injection of FDG, allowing the clinician to simultaneously monitor the primary tumor, nodal metastases, and distant metastases. Limitations of PET include its inability to assess invasion of a lesion into contiguous structures and or to determine tumor size. Furthermore, false-positive results because of inflammatory lesions and false-negative results in small- or low-metabolism neoplasms render PET inappropriate for these scenarios.[66] PET should be used as a complementary imaging study to CXR, CT, and/or MRI. Nevertheless, some studies have shown that PET is superior to CT in evaluating mediastinal staging in NSCLCs.[67,68]

Cytology

Sputum cytology is less often used for diagnostic evaluation, given the advancements in bronchoscopy and biopsy. Nevertheless, sputum cytology is a relatively simple test that depends on tumor size, location, and sputum production. Sputum samples should be fixed and stained immediately or collected over at least 3 days and preserved in 50 percent ethanol and 2 percent polyethylene glycol (Saccamanno's solution).

Central tumors have the highest diagnostic yield, since these tumors are more likely to shed cancer cells into sputa. Central tumors show a diagnostic yield of approximately 77 percent, compared with 47 percent for peripheral tumors and only 20 percent for peripheral tumors less than 3.0 cm in maximum diameter.[69] A more recent study found an average sensitivity of 66 percent and a specificity of 99 percent for sputum cytology.[70] Squamous cell carcinomas tend to have the highest diagnostic yield among non-small cell carcinomas because of their predominant central location.

Invasive diagnostic procedures

Invasive diagnosis may involve fine-needle aspiration, bronchoscopy, mediastinoscopy, biopsy, video-assisted thoracoscopy, and/or thoracotomy.

Fine-needle aspiration

CT-guided transthoracic needle aspiration (TNA) is an effective method of diagnosing peripheral lesions that are not anatomically adjacent to large vascular structures or are not situated under ribs. TNA obtains useful histologic and cytologic information that successfully determines malignancy. However, because of the high rate of false-negatives, a positive diagnosis of a benign tumor must be made before malignancy is ruled out. If no such diagnosis is made, the tumor should be classified as indeterminate and must undergo further evaluation. TNA is the method of choice for patients who present with poor lung function and/or those who reject thoracotomy. Complications that arise due to TNA include pneumothorax, hemoptysis, and air embolism.

A second strategy for fine-needle aspiration is endoscopic ultrasound fine-needle aspiration (EUS-FNA). EUS-FNA is commonly used to assess enlarged subcarinal and posterior mediastinal lymph nodes, with results comparable to those from CT-guided FNA but without the risk pneumothorax.[71] However, EUS-FNA is limited in its ability to determine resectability and should therefore be used with care.

A transbronchial approach can also be implemented and is discussed below.

Bronchoscopy

Bronchoscopy of the trachea and bronchi is a standard invasive procedure that should follow CXR and CT in the workup of patients suspected of having lung cancer. Bronchoscopy utilizes a flexible fiberoptic bronchoscope that can be used to examine awake or mildly sedated patients. Bronchoscopy may reveal lung cancer and the staging of a tumor as well as providing an assessment of the bronchial tree.

Bronchoscopic diagnosis of lung carcinoma can be achieved using any one of many different methods: biopsy, transbronchial FNA, saline lavage, or fluoroscopic brushing.

Bronchoscopy may diagnose a tumor, distortion of the bronchial tree, or indicate the absence of pathology. A tumor is diagnosed in 25 to 50 percent of patients, most of who are afflicted with small cell and squamous cell tumors because of their central location. Distortion of the bronchial tree due to compression or thickening and blunting of the trachea or minor carina can be analyzed using transbronchial needle aspiration (TBNA), where a 20- or 22-gauge needle is passed through the fiberoptic bronchoscope. The needle then punctures the airway wall at the location of interest, revealing lymph node or tumor aspirates. TBNA has limited application in staging because of frequent false-positive results. Furthermore, mediastinoscopy is a better method than TBNA for staging mediastinal lymph nodes for disease.

Bronchoscopic evaluation often reveals normal findings with peripheral lesions. Fluoroscopic brushings and transbronchial biopsies are implemented in assessing peripheral lesions; their success rate is approximately 66 percent.[72]

As a staging tool, bronchoscopy provides information relating to the tumor's location. Furthermore, bronchoscopy also denotes the length of normal bronchus located proximal to the tumor, the tumor's relationship to the tracheal carina, and any evidence of airway compression due to extrinsic tumors or adenopathy. Studies have also found that transbronchial needle aspiration reveals submucosal or peribronchial metastases.[73]

Mediastinoscopy

Cervical mediastinoscopy is considered the "gold standard" for staging superior mediastinal lymph nodes; it does so with a sensitivity greater than 90 percent, a specificity of 100 percent, and an accuracy in diagnosing mediastinal disease greater than 90 percent.[74] Scenarios that unquestionably necessitate mediastinoscopy include lymph nodes larger than 1 cm prior to thoracotomy and patients likely to enter neoadjuvant therapy. A debate over the use of mediastinoscopy still exists. Proponents of selective mediastinoscopy for patients with negative CT scans argue that mediastinoscopy has a high rate of negative findings. Proponents of routine mediastinoscopy following negative CT argue that mediastinoscopy has few complications and that CT has a high false-negative rate. We argue for a more selective application of mediastinoscopy.

In the event that CT does not show mediastinal adenopathy at lymph node station 5 or 6 for patients with left hilar tumors or left-upper-lobe nodules, extended cervical mediastinoscopy is suggested. Extended cervical mediastinoscopy is particularly effective in staging lymph nodes and masses located in the paraaortic zones or the aortopulmonary window.[75]

Video-assisted thoracoscopy

Video-assisted thoracoscopy (VATS) uses three or four 1- to 2-cm incisions in the chest wall. Two to three of the holes are used for instruments while a thorascope with a camera is inserted into the last one. Unlike other staging techniques, VATS allows complete visualization and biopsy of lesions located in the lung parenchyma, chest wall, diaphragm, and mediastinal structures. VATS is particularly effective in sampling lymph nodes in stations 5 and 6 and was found useful in staging T3 and T4 disease (TNM staging is discussed below).[76] Drawbacks of VATS include the general anesthesia required and the inability to evaluate nodules located deep in the parenchyma of the lung. These deep masses are impalpable, making them difficult to locate and sample.

Thoracotomy

Because of the advent of less invasive diagnostic techniques, thoracotomy is less frequently used for diagnosing and staging lung cancer. Nevertheless, some patients require thoracotomies to ensure diagnosis of lung cancer. FNA or biopsy followed by analysis of a frozen section at the time of thoracotomy reveals the diagnosis. Mediastinal lymph node sampling or dissection is required if a diagnosis of lung cancer is made at the time of thoracotomy.

STAGING AND PROGNOSIS

Staging

Accurate and reproducible staging of lung cancer is imperative for appropriate patient management and

Table 12-4 TNM Descriptors

Primary tumor (T)	
TX	Primary tumor cannot be assessed, or tumor proved by the presence of malignant cells in sputum or bronchial washes but not visualized by imaging or bronchoscopy
T0	No evidence of primary tumor
Tis	Carcinoma in situ
T1	Tumor 3 cm or less in greatest dimension, surrounded by lung or visceral pleura, without bronchoscopic evidence of invasion more proximal than the lobar bronchus
T2	Tumor with any of the following features of size or extent: More than 3 cm in greatest dimension; involves main bronchus, 2 cm or more distal to the carina; invades the visceral pleura; associated with atelectasis or obstructive pneumonitis that extends to the hilar region but does not involve the entire lung
T3	Tumor of any size that directly invades any of the following: chest wall, diaphragm, mediastinal pleura, parietal pericardium; or tumor in the main bronchus less than 2 cm distal to the carina, but without involvement of the carina; or associated atelectasis or obstructive pneumonitis of the entire lung
T4	Tumor of any size that invades any of the following: mediastinum, heart, great vessels, trachea, esophagus, vertebral body, carina; or tumor with a malignant pleural or pericardial effusion, or satellite tumor nodule(s) within the ipsilateral primary tumor lobe of the lung
Regional lymph nodes (N)	
NX	Regional lymph nodes cannot be assessed
N0	No regional lymph node metastasis
N1	Metastasis to ipsilateral peribronchial and/or ipsilateral hilar lymph nodes, and the intrapulmonary nodes involved by direct extension of the primary tumor
N2	Metastasis to ipsilateral mediastinal and/or subcarinal lymph nodes
N3	Metastasis to contralateral mediastinal, contralateral hilar, ipsilateral or contralateral scalene, or supraclavicular lymph nodes
Distant metastasis (M)	
MX	Presence of distant metastasis cannot be assessed
M0	No distant metastasis
M1	Distant metastasis present

Source: From Mountain CF. A new international staging system for lung cancer. *Chest* 1997;111:1710–1717. With permission.

progress in research. Staging involves classifying a patient based on TNM descriptors into different stages that have therapeutic and prognostic relevance. T stands for the size of the primary tumor, N for regional lymph node involvement, and M for metastases (Table 12-4). Once the T, N, and M have been assessed, a patient is assigned a stage: IA, IB, IIA, IIB, IIIA, IIIB, or IV (Table 12-5; Figs. 12-2 to 12-7).

The process of staging occurs at three different points during patient care. First, a cTNM, or clinical TNM, is hypothesized based on diagnostic techniques including history and physical examination, noninvasive imaging, and invasive procedures. A second TNM that confirms or revises cTNM is determined on the basis of surgical findings. Finally, a pTNM, or pathologic TNM, is determined postoperatively on the basis of pathologic results.

Knowledge of the lymph node mapping scheme is essential for understanding regional node involvement. The lymph node mapping scheme has been revised and is shown in Fig. 12-8.

An understanding of TNM classification and the lymph node scheme reveals the different stages assigned to lung cancer patients. The stages directly influence prognosis and treatment.

PROGNOSTIC IMPLICATIONS

Patients with T1N0M0 disease have a better prognostic outlook than any other subset.[77] Some 61 percent of patients with stage IA disease and 38 percent with stage IB

Table 12-5 TNM stages

Stage	TNM subset		
Stage 0			
	Carcinoma in situ		
Stage IA	T1 N0 M0		
Stage IB	T2 N0 M0		
Stage IIA	T1 N1 M0		
Stage IIB	T2 N1 M0		
	T3 N0 M0		
Stage IIIA	T3 N1 M0		
	T1 N2 M0	T2 N2 M0	T3 N2 M0
Stage IIIB	T4 N0 M0	T4 N1 M0	T4 N2 M0
	T1 N1 M0	T2 N3 M0	T3 N2 M0
	T4 N3 M0		
Stage IV	Any T Any N M1		

Source: From Mountain CF. A new international staging system for lung cancer. *Chest* 1997;111:1710–1717. With permission.

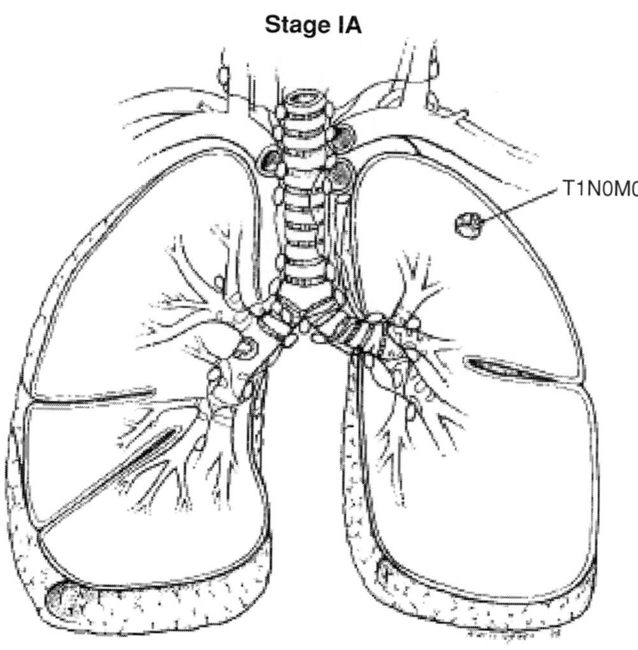

Figure 12-2 Stage IA. (From Mountain CF. The international system for staging lung cancer. *Semin Surg Oncol* 2000;18:106–115. With permission.)

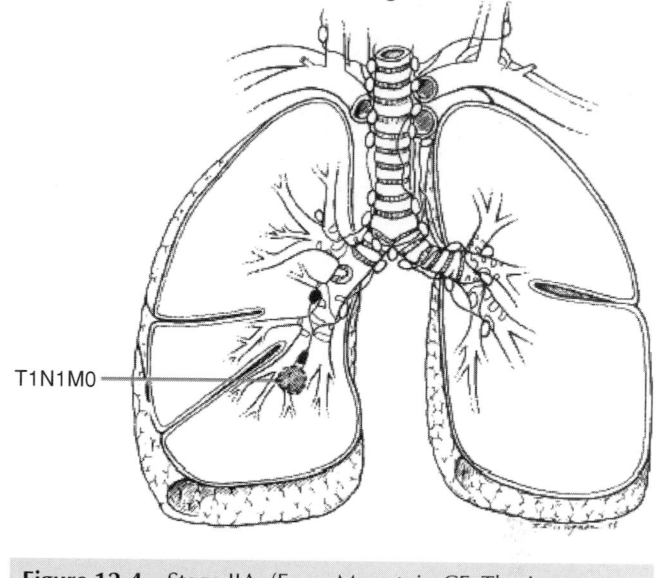

Figure 12-4 Stage IIA. (From Mountain CF. The international system for staging lung cancer. *Semin Surg Oncol* 2000;18:106–115. With permission.)

disease are expected to survive at least 5 years after diagnosis and treatment.[78] Of all patients with pathologic stage IA disease, 67 percent survive at least 5 years after resection, versus 57 percent of those with pathologic stage IB.[83] These results are expected, given that stages IA and IB diseases show no indication of lymph node or distant metastases. Stage IA and IB disease is almost always surgically resectable, with procedures varying depending on the location of the primary nodule. In medically inoperable patients, radiotherapy is currently the treatment of choice.

T1N1M0 stage IIA disease is a rarity. Nevertheless, the need to revise the staging system to include IIA and IIB is warranted owing to different survival data for each. The 5-year survival rate for patients with cT1N1M0 stage IIA disease is 34 percent; it is only 24 and 22 percent for patients with cT2N1M0 and cT3N0M0 stage IIB disease, respectively.[83] After resection, the 5-year survival rate for patients with pT1N1M0 stage IIA disease was 55 percent, versus 38 and 39 percent for patients with pT2N1M0 and pT3N0M0 stage

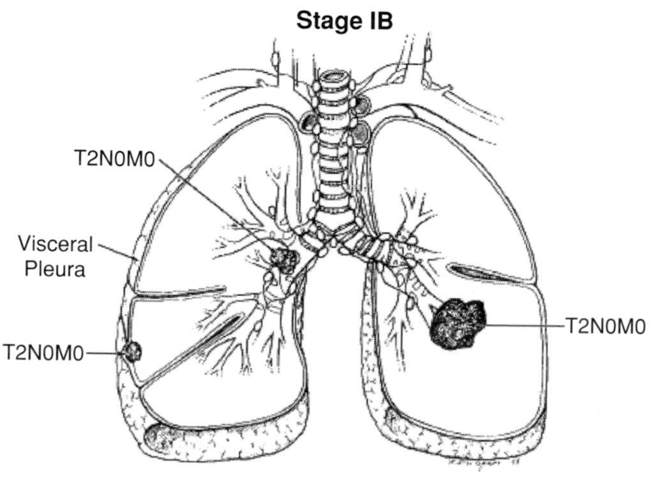

Figure 12-3 Stage IB. (From Mountain CF. The international system for staging lung cancer. *Semin Surg Oncol* 2000;18:106–115. With permission.)

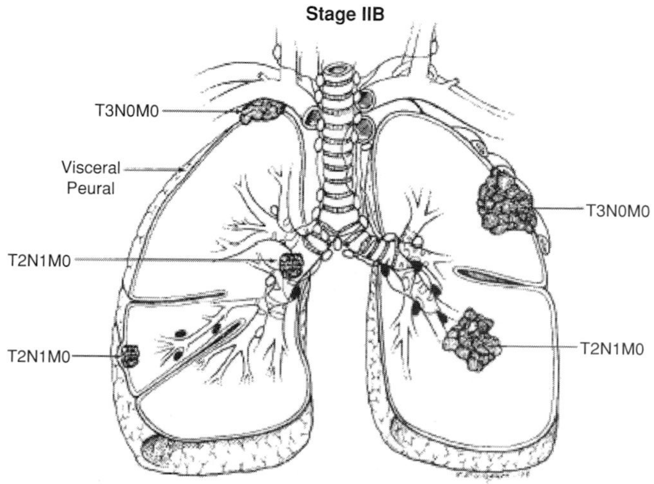

Figure 12-5 Stage IIB. (From Mountain CF. The international system for staging lung cancer. *Semin Surg Oncol* 2000;18:106–115. With permission.)

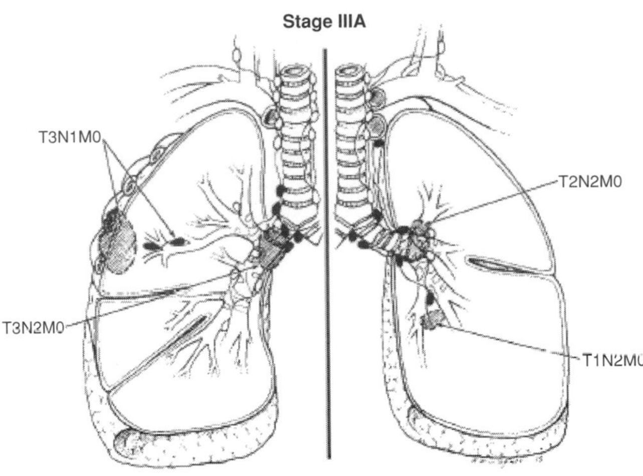

Figure 12-6 Stage IIIA. (From Mountain CF. The international system for staging lung cancer. *Semin Surg Oncol* 2000;18:106–115. With permission.)

IIB disease, respectively.[83] Stage IIA and IIB disease involves resectable tumors, and the surgical procedure depends on the location of the tumor. Radiotherapy is the treatment of choice in medically inoperable patients.

Stage IIIA disease includes T3N1M0, T1N2M0, T2N2M0, and T3N2M0 subsets. Patients diagnosed with cT3N1M0 stage IIIA disease have the worst prognosis, with a 5e-year survival rate of 9 percent, compared with the combined 5-year survival rate of 13 percent for patients with cT1N2M0, cT2N2M0, and cT3N2M0 stage IIIA disease.[83] After resection, the 5-year survival rate for pT3N1M0 stage IIIA disease was 25 percent,

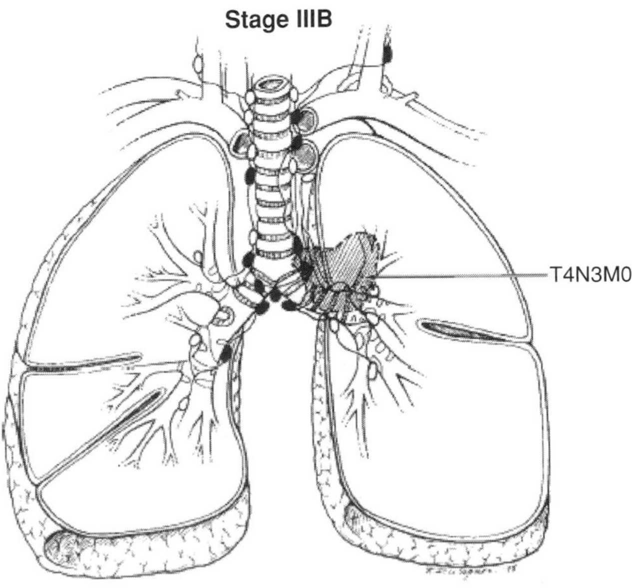

Figure 12-7 Stage IIIB. (From Mountain CF. The international system for staging lung cancer. *Semin Surg Oncol* 2000;18:106–115. With permission.)

contrasted with 23 percent for patients with pT1-2-3N2M0 stage IIIA disease.[83] Stage IIIA tumors are surgically resectable, but studies have shown that preoperative chemotherapy followed by postoperative chemotherapy or radiotherapy provides the best chance for long-term survival.

Stage IIIB includes T4N0-1-2-3M0, T1N3M0, T2N3M0, and T3N3M0 subsets. Patients with cT4N0-1-2M0 had a 5-year survival rate of 6 to 8 percent, versus 3 percent for patients with cT1-2-3-4N3M0.[83] Stage IIIB disease is inoperable, because it is not possible to eradicate all of the disease, and no survival advantage has been shown from surgical resection. The treatment of choice is chemoradiotherapy.

Patients with the poorest prognosis are those with stage IV disease that includes any T, any N, M1 subsets. Because of distant metastases and inoperability, these patients have a 5-year survival rate of only 1 percent.[83] Treatment of stage IV disease focuses on palliative care and quality-of-life issues. Surgery is rarely a treatment option owing to metastatic disease. Chemotherapy is the common treatment modality for stage IV disease, although radiotherapy and adjuvant therapy have also been implemented.

MEDICAL AND SURGICAL THERAPY

MEDICAL TREATMENT

Radiotherapy

The goal of radiotherapy or any medical treatment is to increase the chance of survival by reducing the survival rate of cancerous cells. The response to radiotherapy depends on factors that influence a cancer cell's radiosensitivity, including the ability to repair itself from radiation damage, the ability of the cancer cell to reoxygenate, the redistribution of cells during the cell cycle, and the repopulation of cells between radiotherapy fractions. Larger tumors do not respond as well to radiotherapy because they have more cells, requiring a higher dose. However, dosage is dependent on tissue tolerance and often limits the amount that is clinically applicable. Radiotherapy can be applied as the primary treatment in inoperable patients, as an adjunct to surgery, or as a palliative treatment.

Primary radiotherapy

Although patients with stage I and stage II disease are best treated with curative surgery, some patients either refuse surgery or are inoperable because of comorbidities. Curative radical primary radiotherapy may be an option for these patients. A recent retrospective review of patients with stage I or II NSCLC that received a median dose of 60 Gy with 2 Gy five times a week showed recurrence in 53 percent.[79] Metanalyses found survival benefits from radiotherapy in patients with unresectable stage I

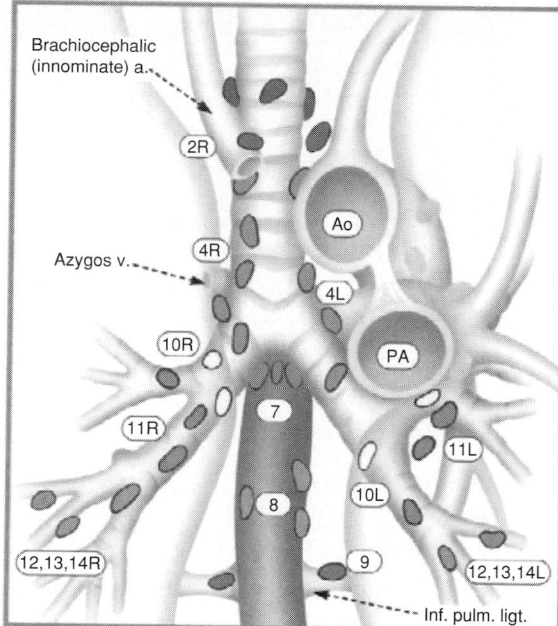

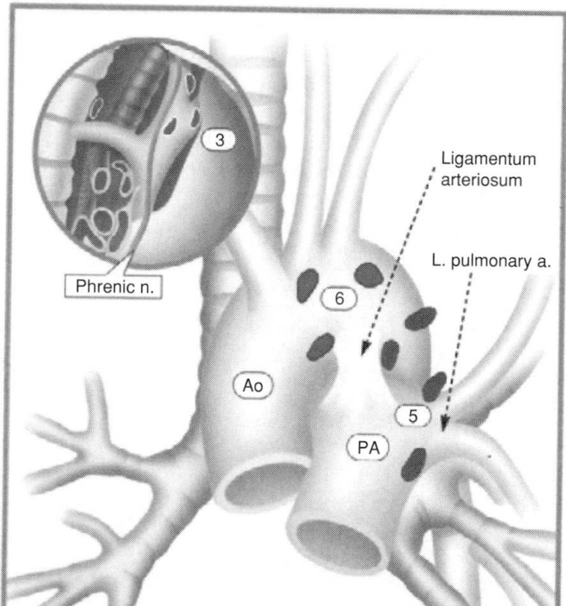

Superior Mediastinal Nodes

- **1** Highest Mediastinal
- **2** Upper Paratracheal
- **3** Pre-vascular and Retrotracheal
- **4** Lower Paratracheal (including Azygos Nodes)

N_2 = single digit, ipsilateral
N_3 = single digit, contralateral or supraclavicular

Aortic Nodes

- **5** Subaortic (A-P window)
- **6** Para-aortic (ascending aorta or phrenic)

Inferior Mediastinal Nodes

- **7** Subcarinal
- **8** Paraesophageal (below carina)
- **9** Pulmonary Ligament

N_1 Nodes

- **10** Hilar
- **11** Interlobar
- **12** Lobar
- **13** Segmental
- **14** Subsegmental

Figure 12-8 Lymph node mapping scheme. (From Mountain CF, Dresler CM. Regional lymph node classification for lung cancer staging. *Chest* 1997;111:1718–1723. With permission.)

and II disease, with a 5-year survival rate of 15 to 20 percent.[80] A recent report illustrates poor local control of stage III disease in 17 percent of patients treated with primary radiotherapy.[81]

Chemoradiotherapy

For treating stage III disease, improvements in the medical treatment of lung cancer are seen with concomitant or sequential chemoradiotherapy. A recent study compared primary radiotherapy with chemoradiotherapy (cisplatin on days 1 and 29 and five weekly cycles of vinblastine) and found that the combined modality improved survival time. Radiotherapy alone showed a survival time of 9.6 months, while the combined therapy showed a survival time of 13.7 months. The same study also indicated that the 5-year survival rate for chemoradiotherapy was 17 percent, compared with 7 percent for radiotherapy alone.[82] Other studies have found more modest results in patients diagnosed with stage IIIA and IIIB disease.[83,84] A recent randomized trial has contrasted concurrent chemoradiotherapy with sequential chemoradiotherapy and found that concurrent treatment resulted in an improved response rate (84 vs. 66 percent), median survival time (16.5 vs. 13.3 months), and 3-year survival rate (27 vs. 12.5 percent).[85]

Hyperfractionated radiotherapy

Improvements in radiotherapy have also involved altering the fractionation schemes, where smaller radiation doses are used to limit late tissue damage. Studies have shown that hyperfractionation treatment produces an improved survival time and rate.[86-87] Another study compared standard primary radiotherapy with hyperfractionated radiotherapy (69.6 Gy at 1.2 Gy twice a day) and combined chemoradiotherapy (100mg/m^2 cisplatin on days 1 and 29, 5mg/m^2 vinblastine once a week for 5 weeks, and 60 Gy at 2.0 Gy per day) and found that the chemoradiotherapy approach showed the most favorable 1-year survival rate, 60 percent, followed by hyperfractionated radiotherapy at 51 percent and standard radiotherapy at 46 percent.[88]

Surgical adjuvant radiotherapy

Radiotherapy can be implemented preoperatively or postoperatively in an attempt to improve survival rate and time. Surgical adjuvant radiotherapy may also utilize chemotherapy.

Preoperative radiotherapy

Preoperative radiotherapy was first suggested in the 1960s as a method to prevent the postoperative persistence of tumors. Nevertheless, studies have highlighted that preoperative radiotherapy does not provide any survival benefit.[89,90]

Preoperative chemoradiotherapy

The lack of improvement observed in preoperative radiotherapy has led to studies involving preoperative chemoradiotherapy. The toxicity associated with this treatment is managed by splitting the radiation course over a longer period of time. A recent study implemented 5-fluorouracil, etoposide, and cisplatin with radiotherapy and found improved resectability and survival, although the 30 percent survival rate was still too low.[91] Overall, adjuvant chemoradiotherapy is a promising treatment for improving resectability and diminishing recurrence in patients with stage III disease.

Postoperative radiotherapy

Studies have shown that no survival benefit is gained from postoperative radiotherapy in lung cancer patients who do not have mediastinal lymph node metastases. However, in lung cancer patients with mediastinal lymph node involvement, a survival benefit has been documented,[92] along with a diminished rate of recurrence. Histologically, squamous cell carcinomas respond better to postoperative radiotherapy than adenocarcinoma, although both cell types indicate better survival.

Palliative radiotherapy

Radiotherapy appears to palliate symptoms associated with lung cancer. Irradiation of a primary tumor has been documented to relieve hemoptysis, chest pain, dyspnea, superior vena cava syndrome, and vocal cord paralysis.[93] Improved prognosis for patients with brain metastases has also been found following whole-brain irradiation. Symptoms due to metastases, such as certain paraneoplastic syndromes, respond less frequently to radiotherapy.

Table 12-6 Risks associated with radiotherapy
Spinal cord damage
Radiation pneumonitis
Fibrosis
Radiation esophagitis
Skin irritation
Fatigue

Radiotherapy risks

Radiotherapy involves many risks, including spinal cord damage, which are listed in Table 12-6.

Spinal cord damage Irradiation of the hilar and mediastinal lymph nodes is usually approached using an anteroposterior/posteroanterior parallel-pair technique. The risk of spinal cord damage increases with this technique; the use of multiple beams also elevates risk.

Radiation pneumonitis and lung fibrosis Patients with radiation pneumonitis present with fever, dyspnea, cough, and pleuritic chest pain approximately 6 weeks after radiotherapy. Radiographic imaging indicates changes in the radiation field, but these rarely extend outside of this area. Grade 3 (significant) pneumonitis arises in approximately 5 percent of radiotherapy patients and is more prominent in patients with larger radiation fields and higher daily and total dosages.[94]

Lung fibrosis is a long-term effect that commonly damages areas of the lung that receive fractionated treatment of 20 to 25 Gy. Patients with poor lung function should not receive higher doses. Patients should also not receive higher doses for large sections of lung.[95]

Radiation esophagitis Radiation fields that target the hilar or mediastinal lymph nodes will include the esophagus, often leading to radiation esophagitis 3 weeks into radical radiotherapy. Patients present with a chief complaint of difficulty in swallowing food; they report that food sticks to the esophagus and may therefore refuse food and drink. Aggressively treated patients, such as those receiving chemoradiotherapy, experience radiation esophagitis more frequently than patients treated solely with radiotherapy.[91] Symptoms associated with radiation esophagitis normally resolve 2 to 4 weeks after radiotherapy.[101]

Fatigue and skin damage Patients undergoing radiation treatment will appear fatigued toward the end of the regimen and after therapy. The skin at the entry and exit sites of the radiation beams often reddens because of irritation, which can be assuaged with hydrocortisone cream.

Brain metastases Postoperative irradiation of the brain, typically consisting of 30 Gy in 10 fractions, has improved the survival time to 11 months in patients with brain metastases, although 30 percent relapse at the site of resection and 30 percent relapse at a new site in the brain.[96] Patients with unresectable brain tumors or with multiple brain metastases survive 3 to 6 months.[97,98]

Chemotherapy

The use of chemotherapy is a controversial topic in the treatment of lung cancer, varying from one of strong belief in chemotherapy for all patients to another equally strong belief in the inappropriateness of chemotherapy outside of clinical test trials.[99,100] A variety of chemotherapeutic drugs have been studied for potential benefits in single-agent treatment, combined drug treatment, and either neoadjuvant therapy, adjuvant chemotherapy, or chemotherapy for advanced nonresectable disease.

Single versus combination chemotherapy

Studies have shown that combination chemotherapy elicits a higher response than single-agent chemotherapy.[101] A complete clinical response is generally observed in only 10 to 15 percent of patients with local disease. Therefore most patients respond only partially to chemotherapy.

Neoadjuvant chemotherapy

Although neoadjuvant chemotherapy may allow previously unresectable tumors to be resected, the primary goal is to prolong survival by reducing micrometastases. Studies have shown that neoadjuvant chemotherapy improves survival time and reduces recurrence versus surgery alone.[102,103]

Adjuvant chemotherapy

The poor survival rates following resection of stage II and IIIA disease warrant improved treatment. Many studies have shown modest improvement in survival time and survival rates in patients treated with adjuvant chemotherapy.[104,105] The results are unspectacular; more studies are required to determine whether adjuvant chemotherapy provides any long-term benefits.

Chemotherapy for advanced disease

Chemotherapy may limit micrometastases and improve local control in patients with advanced disease stage IIIA and IIIB. Chemotherapy for stage IV advanced disease, however, focuses on prolonging survival and palliating symptoms. Recent studies have illustrated that chemotherapy for advanced stage IV disease improves survival time and survival rates.[106–107] More trials are required and a focus on palliation of symptoms must be emphasized to reduce toxicity.

Treatment of small cell lung cancer

Radiotherapy of SCLC

Historically, radiotherapy was the primary method for the treatment of SCLC. Owing to the realization that SCLC is a systemic disease and because of the advent of chemotherapy, the role of radiotherapy has changed. Radiotherapy is now commonly used to serve two purposes: locoregional irradiation and prophylactic cranial irradiation.

The goal of locoregional irradiation is to minimize relapse and enhance local control. Many studies have shown that radiotherapy decreases relapse, but they have not found a significant survival benefit. Modest improvements have been found using combined chemoradiotherapy for SCLC. Metanalysis consisting of 2100 SCLC patients found that the combined chemoradiotherapy arm showed a 14 percent decrease in death rate and a 5.4 percent improvement in the three-year survival rate versus chemotherapy alone.[108]

Prophylactic cranial irradiation (PCI), typically 20 to 40 Gy in 2- to 2.5-Gy fractions,[109] is commonly used to limit brain metastases associated with SCLC. Studies have effectively shown a decrease in brain metastases with PCI treatment but no improvements in survival.[110,111]

Chemotherapy for SCLC

Chemotherapy is the cornerstone for the medical treatment of SCLC. The most common agents employed include etoposide, cisplatin, cyclophosphamide, doxorubicin, and vincristine. Potentially active agents include gemcitabine, paclitaxel, and docetaxel.

Combination chemotherapy results in improved survival versus single-agent chemotherapy. The two most common combination chemotherapy regimens used are etoposide-cisplatin and cyclophosphamide-doxorubicin-vincristine. Patients receiving etoposide-cisplatin treatment showed improved response but not significant improvement in survival over the cyclophosphamide-doxorubicin-vincristine combination.[112] Furthermore, the alternating regimen of etoposide-cisplatin and cyclophosphamide-doxorubicin-vincristine did not provide a therapeutic advantage for extensive SCLC.[121] Table 12-7 lists common single agents and combinations for SCLC.

Increasing dose intensity of most drugs does not appear to improve survival. A study that compared a standard dose to a high dose of etoposide-cisplatin treatment found no benefits with the higher-dose treatment but did find heightened toxicity.[113] Aggressive treatments implementing higher-dose chemotherapy also results in a high risk of myelosuppression.

Alternating non-cross resistant chemotherapy and anticoagulant implementation are two new efforts to improve chemotherapy of SCLC. Alternating non-cross resistant chemotherapy is based on the idea that alternating two combinations of non-cross resistant drugs reduces the likelihood of tumor resistance. A recent review, however, did not show major advantages over standard chemotherapy. The study concluded that non-cross resistant chemotherapy resulted in similar responses and toxicity without notable improvement in survival.[114] Some studies have shown improvements

Table 12-7 Single-agent and combination chemotherapy for small cell lung cancer

Established single agents
Carboplatin
Cisplatin
Cyclophosphamide
Doxorubicin
Etoposide (intravenous)
Etoposide (oral)
Vincristine
Promising single agents
Docetaxel
Gemcitabine
Paclitaxel
Combination therapy
Cylophosphamide–doxorubicin
Doxorubicin–etoposide
Cyclophosphamide–doxorubicin–vincristine–etoposide
Etoposide–carboplatin
Ifosfamide–cisplatin–etoposide
Cisplatin–vincristine–doxorubicin-etoposide

Source: Adapted from Feld R, et al. Small cell lung cancer. In: Pearson FG et al (eds). *Thoracic Surgery.* Philadelphia: Churchill Livingston, 2002:925–946. With permission.

associated with non-cross resistant regimens, but the literature is rife with conflicting results.

Recent studies have evaluated the effects of anticoagulants, most notably warfarin, on patient survival. A recent study found that patients treated with chemoradiotherapy and warfarin had a median survival of 50 weeks, compared with 24 weeks for patients receiving chemoradiotherapy alone. Furthermore, the warfarin-treated arm experienced a later onset of disease progression, suggesting that the anticoagulant influenced metastasis of the tumor.[115] Despite these results, warfarin treatment increases the risk of hemorrhage. Further experimental trials are necessary to elucidate the use of anticoagulants.

SURGICAL THERAPY

Surgical treatments of lung cancer include pneumonectomy, lobectomy, segmentectomy, and wedge resection. The decision to operate must be contingent on preoperative patient assessment, which should include a pulmonary function test, an evaluation of comorbidities, and a functional assessment test that measures the maximal oxygen consumption (Vo2) in a patient with compromised lung function. Figure 12-9 represents an algorithm for preoperative assessment to determine operability.

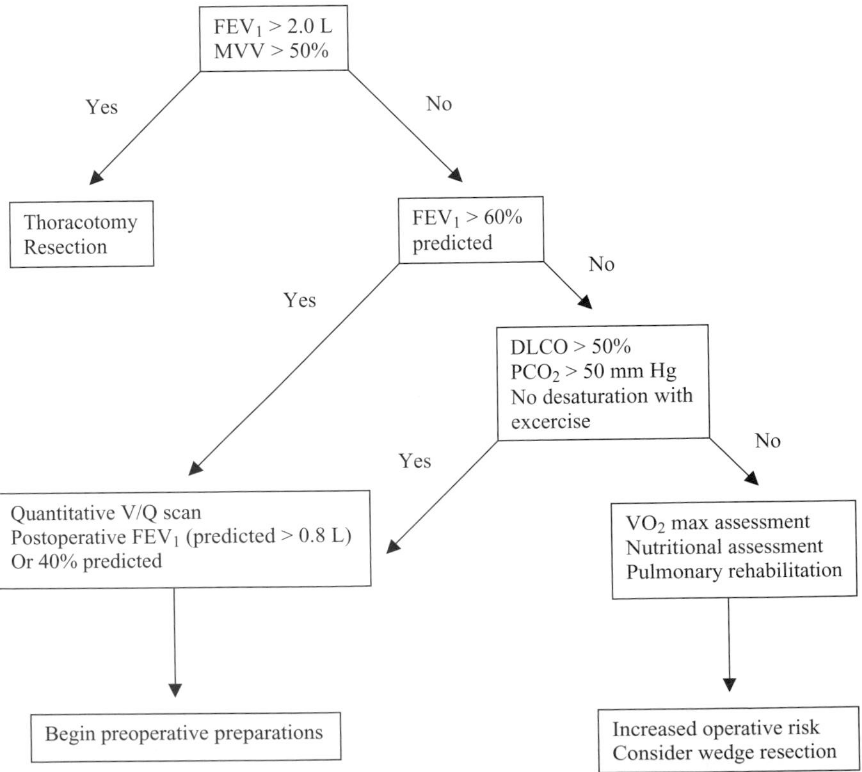

Figure 12-9 Assessing preoperative risk in patients with lung cancer. (Adapted from Kaiser LR. Right-sided pulmonary resections. In: Kaiser LR, et al. (eds). *Mastery of Cardiothoracic Surgery.* Philadelphia: Lippincott-Raven, 1998:38–52. With permission.)

Pneumonectomy

Because of the high mortality and morbidity associated with the removal of a lung, pneumonectomy should be considered the final surgical procedure of choice. Moreover, patients with poor pulmonary function or with unresectable disease and elderly patients should undergo extensive pulmonary function tests to predict pulmonary reserve following pneumonectomy.

Pneumonectomy is the procedure of choice in patients who cannot be treated with curative intent by lobectomy. The indications for performing pneumonectomy depend on the size, pathology, and location of the tumor, which can be assessed preoperatively or intraoperatively. Because of the risk associated with pneumonectomy, the surgeon should always consider a lesser resection with the same curative outcome a viable option.

Clear communication between the surgeon and anesthesiologist is essential for pneumonectomy. Upon deciding on pneumonectomy, it is the surgeon's duty to inform the anesthesiologist so that he or she can place a double-lumen endobronchial tube into the patient's bronchus opposite the side of pneumonectomy.

Right pneumonectomy

incision Right pneumonectomy proceeds with a right posterolateral thoracotomy via the fifth intercostal space. This approach provides the best access to both the anterior and posterior areas of the lung. Rib excision is unnecessary and may actually compromise the closure of the incision in the event of dehiscence due to empyema and infection. A muscle-sparing incision can also be made at the fourth intercostal space.

Operative technique

Posterior retraction of the lung and dissection of the pleura at the anterior hilum is the initial operative step. The pleura is incised superiorly over the bronchus and inferiorly to the inferior pulmonary vein, which is subsequently encircled after the inferior pulmonary ligament is dissected up to the level of the vein. The superior pulmonary vein and the right pulmonary artery are identified. The artery is encircled at the point where it lies posterior to the vena cava, although the location of the tumor or lymph node involvement may necessitate pericardial dissection to isolate the proximal artery. In the event of pericardial dissection, the surgeon should incise anterior to the phrenic nerve and proceed along the hilum. At this point the surgeon also assesses the superior and inferior pulmonary veins for encirclement. Pericardial dissection may function as a useful tool for determining central tumor resectability.

If pericardial dissection is unnecessary for resection, the superior pulmonary vein is isolated and encircled. At this point the lung is retracted anteriorly and the bronchus is dissected. Depending on the tumor location, bronchus dissection may be aided by division of the azygos vein as it passes the bronchus on its way to the right upper lobe, providing a clear anatomic landmark.

The order in which the vasculature is divided depends on the tumor location. If artery involvement is present, the veins and bronchus should be divided first to maximize artery exposure. It may also benefit the surgeon to divide the bronchus first, allowing for improved exposure of arteries and veins. The arteries and veins are closed with a vascular stapler or with nonabsorbable monofilament suture. The bronchus can be closed with a stapler or with absorbable suture. If the bronchus is sewn closed, sutures should be interrupted and placed approximately 1 mm apart. After closure, the surgeon should test for air leaks, which require additional suture. Furthermore, the surgeon may utilize pericardium, pleura, or other vascularized tissue to patch the suture line.

The contents of the subcarinal and superior mediastinal spaces are appropriately removed following mediastinal lymph node dissection. If the pericardial sac has been incised or excised, the surgeon must reapproximate the pericardial edges or close the pericardium with a prosthetic material that will keep the heart in place. The material must also be porous for drainage, and the surgeon must take care not to overconstrict the heart and cause any tamponade.

Following pneumonectomy, the mediastinum is repositioned. Introducing a needle into the chest and evacuating air from the postpneumonectomy space until met with resistance effectively repositions the mediastinum. A chest tube can also be placed in the postpneumonectomy space for 12 to 24 h to drain any bleeding and to equilibrate the mediastinum.

Left pneumonectomy

Incision The standard approach for left pneumonectomy is a posterolateral thoracotomy via the fifth intercostal space. A muscle-sparing incision can also be made at the fourth intercostal space. Tumor involvement and resectability is then assessed.

Operative technique Hilar involvement warrants pericardial dissection along the hilum in order to evaluate the extent of atrial involvement, convergence of the pulmonary veins, and proximal involvement of the pulmonary artery. The pericardial incision should be made anterior to the phrenic nerve with care to prevent nerve damage. Major proximal invasion of the atrium is problematic because the amount of atrium resectable is limited. The posterior hilum should be assessed for involvement by running a finger around it.

The left main pulmonary artery is short in length, justifying pericardial dissection to evaluate a centrally located tumor as well as division of the ligamentum arteriosum in order to assess the entire length of the artery.

If the tumor is resectable and pneumonectomy is the operative choice, the pulmonary artery and superior and inferior pulmonary veins are encircled within the pericardium (if pericardial dissection was necessary). If possible, the lung is retracted posteriorly while the hilar pleura is incised anteriorly and superiorly. A blunt clamp or a finger is used to encircle the left main pulmonary artery. The inferior pulmonary ligament is cut, allowing for encirclement of the inferior pulmonary vein; the superior pulmonary vein is encircled. As in right pneumonectomy, the order in which the hilar structures are divided depends on the location of the tumor. Furthermore, the same closure methods used in right pneumonectomy are used in left pneumonectomy: the main pulmonary artery, the superior pulmonary vein, and the inferior pulmonary vein can be divided using two rows of staples or with monofilament suture. Division of the left main bronchus is difficult because of the anatomic location of the aortic arch. Moreover, the carina is not visible, as in right pneumonectomy, and cannot be mobilized. The bronchus is retracted toward the direction of the incision placement. This adequately facilitates stapler placement and division. If a stapler is unavailable, division of the bronchus can be achieved with incision and closure using interrupted absorbable suture.

If pericardial dissection was implemented, closure of the postpneumonectomy space using a fenestrated patch is required to prevent the heart from shifting out of place. As in right pneumonectomy, if the pericardium only has been incised, suture can be used to close the space. The surgeon must avoid constricting the heart in reapproximating the pericardium with a patch so as to prevent tamponade.

A chest tube is introduced into the postpneumonectomy space to equilibrate the position of the mediastinum and to allow drainage of any bleeding. The chest tube must be removed within 24 h. An alternative method to equilibrate the mediastinum is to evacuate the air present in the postpneumonectomy space with a needle in order to restore negative pressure in the pleural cavity.

Lobectomy

Lobectomy is the procedure of choice for resecting early-stage disease. In contrast to limited resection, lobectomy evaluates lobar lymph nodes and provides adequate parenchymal margins. A recent study compared lobectomy to limited pulmonary resection and found that lessser resections do not improve morbidity, mortality, or pulmonary function. Because of the higher rate of mortality and the rate of relapse associated with lesser resection, lobectomy is the surgical procedure of choice in resecting peripheral T1N0 NSCLCs.[116] Lobectomy is also the choice for peripheral tumor resection, while pneumonectomy is generally reserved for centrally located tumors. Despite better outcomes and less frequent recurrences of disease, some patients are unable to undergo lobectomy and must settle for a lesser resection. Patients with borderline pulmonary function or those who have a history of pulmonary resection should be considered for segmentectomy, which removes the artery and vein, bronchus segment, and accompanying lymph nodes. Wedge resection is more of a compromise because it does not isolate the vasculature associated with the wedge.

The different lobes of the lung have defining characteristics that distinguish the operative technique required for resection. Prior to resection, an endobronchial double-lumen tube is placed into the bronchus opposite to the side of lobectomy to initiate one-lung ventilation.

Right upper lobectomy

Incision A posterolateral incision is made at the fifth intercostal space with the patient lying in the left lateral decubitus position. This approach allows for the best access to all areas of the lung. A muscle-sparing incision can also be made at the fourth intercostal space.

Operative technique Anterior and superior incision of the hilar pleura occurs with the lung retracted posteriorly. The surgeon dissects the superior pulmonary vein distally toward the lung parenchyma and proximally to the pericardial reflection. Upon dissection, the vein is encircled with a finger. The middle lobe venous branch, which drains to the superior pulmonary vein, is recognized and preserved. The right main pulmonary artery lies superior and posterior to the vein and is dissected and followed proximally as it passes posteriorly to the superior vena cava. The surgeon encircles the artery when the appropriate dissection plane is deciphered, followed by placement of a Rumel tourniquet. The surgeon then dissects the artery distally until the apical anterior arterial branch is identified.

The pulmonary artery's strength comes from the intimal layer, given that a muscular layer does not exist. This makes the pulmonary artery very weak and fragile, requiring extremely careful handling by the surgeon. After identifying the plane of dissection, the surgeon dissects the artery superiorly along the hilum. The azygos vein crosses the right mainstem bronchus just superior to the right-upper-lobe bronchus, providing a clear anatomic landmark. If the vein is invaded by a tumor, the azygos vein must be divided. The surgeon dissects the pulmonary artery from the bronchus. The pleura overlying the bronchial bifurcation is incised. At this point, the surgeon encircles the bronchus.

Division usually proceeds with the artery, followed by the veins and the bronchus; it can be performed with a vascular stapler or suture. Generally the order in which the surgeon divides structures is based on removing the structure whose absence will enhance the exposure of other structures. In closing the bronchus, the surgeon should allow for a small stump to staple in order to avoid impingement on the main or other lobar bronchi. Margins should always be clear of tumor and inflammation. It may be necessary to oversew the suture line with absorbable suture or to patch the suture line with vascular tissue such as pleura or pericardium so as to avoid fistula formation.

Right middle lobectomy

Incision The standard approach to right middle lobectomy is a posterolateral thoracotomy via the fifth intercostal space. A muscle-sparing incision can also be made via the fourth intercostal space.

Operative technique Two general methods of right middle lobectomy are practiced. The first relies on visualization of the pulmonary artery within the fissure. If the artery is not seen, the fissure is divided to expose the artery, creating air leaks. A more versatile method does not rely on the visibility of the pulmonary artery within the fissure. The surgeon retracts the lung posteriorly. The hilar pleura over the superior pulmonary vein is dissected and the middle lobe vein observed. The middle lobe vein is then ligated and divided, revealing the connective tissue of the middle lobe bronchus just posterior to the vein. Careful dissection of the bronchial connective tissue reveals the bronchus. The middle lobe artery lies slightly posterior and superior to the middle lobe bronchus. The surgeon then clamps the middle lobe bronchus, taking care not to damage the arterial branch, and the bronchus is divided using a scalpel. The surgeon can close the bronchus with interrupted sutures or a stapler.

Division of the bronchus clearly reveals the middle lobe arterial branch, which is then ligated and divided. Upon division of the artery, vein, and bronchus, the surgeon divides the minor and oblique fissures using a linear stapler, effectively removing the lobe. Following middle lobe resection, mediastinal lymph node dissection is performed to determine pathologic TNM staging.

Right lower lobectomy

Incision As in right middle lobectomy, right lower lobectomy is approached either by a posterolateral thoracotomy via the fifth intercostal space or using a muscle-sparing incision via the fourth intercostal space.

Operative technique As in right middle lobectomy, right lower lobectomy depends on the ability to identify the pulmonary artery within the fissure. If disease is discovered within the fissure or if hilar involvement is observed, the hilar pleura should be incised anteriorly and posteriorly to identify and encircle the pulmonary artery lateral to the superior vena cava.

The surgeon then identifies the arterial branch supplying the lower lobe's superior segment and the arterial branch supplying the middle lobe. Posterior dissection along the branch to the superior segment bifurcates the upper lobe bronchus and bronchial intermediate. The surgeon retracts the lung anteriorly, incises the pleura overlying the bifurcation, and uses a stapler from the superior segmental arterial branch to the bifurcation. Next, the surgeon identifies the posterior segmental located on the superior aspect of the artery and divides the posterior aspect of the fissure.

The surgeon divides the pulmonary artery to reveal the bronchus lying medial to the artery. Retraction of the pulmonary artery superiorly identifies the origin of the middle lobe bronchus and the location for division of the lower lobe bronchus. The lower lobe bronchus is divided and closed with a stapler or is dissected with a scalpel and closed with interrupted absorbable sutures.

Following division of the bronchus, the surgeon retracts the lung toward the apex of the chest and divides the inferior pulmonary ligament to the level of the inferior pulmonary vein. The surgeon should also dissect the inferior pulmonary lymph node to assess pathologic staging. The surgeon dissects the superior pulmonary vein and passes a finger around it where division is to take place. Division can proceed with a stapler or with clamping or division with a scalpel, followed by running monofilament sutures. The vein is closed with suture. Last, a stapler is used to remove the lobe.

Bilobectomy

A lesion located in the bronchus intermedius or in the bronchus's external aspect warrants a bilobectomy to remove the right middle and lower lobes. In the event that a bilobectomy is warranted, the vasculature should be divided for each lobe as described above. Upon division of the pulmonary arterial branches, the surgeon divides the bronchus just distal to the upper lobe takeoff above the origin of the middle lobe bronchus.

Left upper lobectomy

Left upper lobectomy is technically challenging because of the anatomic relationship between the aortic arch and the pulmonary artery. Furthermore, the superior mediastinum is not easily accessible owing to the position of the aortic arch relative to the left main bronchus, thus limiting the extent of lymph node sampling in the paratracheal area. Mediastinoscopy is useful in assessing the paratracheal area, since access through the thoracotomy is limited.

Incision Left upper lobectomy proceeds through posterolateral thoracotomy via the fifth intercostal space or by a muscle-sparing incision via the fourth intercostal space.

Operative technique With the left upper lobe retracted posteriorly, the hilar pleura is incised anteriorly and superiorly. The pulmonary artery, located superior and posterolateral to the superior pulmonary vein, is identified as it passes beneath the aortic arch. Division of the venous branch first may be warranted in the event that the apical segmental branch of the vein crosses the artery and obscures the pulmonary artery's apical posterior segmental trunk. The left pulmonary artery is dissected and encircled with a finger while a C clamp is used to pass umbilical tape around the artery. The surgeon should place a Rumel tourniquet in the event that proximal occlusion of the artery should be required. The superior pulmonary vein, including the lingular branch, is dissected and divided using a stapler. The pulmonary artery is dissected in the distal direction toward the fissure. The surgeon identifies the superior segmental branch to the lower lobe and staples the posterior portion of the fissure. The anterior segmental arterial branch to the upper lobe, which lies proximal and opposite to the origin of the superior segmental branch, is divided. The surgeon then identifies the lingular branches by following the pulmonary artery further distally; they are then ligated and divided. Finally, the stapler is used to complete the anterior portion of the fissure.

The bifurcation of the left main bronchus of the upper lobe is visualized by reflecting the artery inferiorly. Division of bronchus supplying the left upper lobe should be performed carefully to avoid damage to the branch supplying the left lower lobe. Division of the left-upper-lobe bronchus is completed with a stapler and should occur as close to the bifurcation as possible. The surgeon may also divide the bronchus using a scalpel and then close with 3-0 or 4-0 monofilament or braided nonabsorbable sutures. The closure should be assessed to repair any air leaks.

Paraaortic and aortopulmonary window lymph node dissection is essential. Furthermore, the surgeon removes the contents of the subcarinal space.

Patients with borderline pulmonary function may undergo a lingula-sparing upper lobectomy instead.

Left lower lobectomy

Left lower lobectomy is a much simpler procedure than the other resections described. As in left upper lobectomy, mediastinoscopy is vital for assessing lesions and lymph nodes on the left side that are obscured owing to the relative positions of the aortic arch and left main bronchus.

Incision Left lower lobectomy proceeds through posterolateral thoracotomy via the fifth intercostal space or using a muscle-sparing incision via the fourth intercostal space. Thoracotomy via the sixth intercostal space provides no advantage.

Operative technique Dissection begins with the upper lobe retracted posteriorly. The pleura is dissected anteriorly and superiorly to the pulmonary artery. The artery is identified and encircled with a finger. As in upper lobectomy, umbilical tape is passed around the artery and a Rumel tourniquet is placed to provide proximal control. Once the pulmonary artery is visible within the fissure, the surgeon incises and dissects the pleura over the pulmonary artery and then anteriorly and posteriorly along the artery. The artery supplying the lower lobe is identified and stapled or doubly ligated. Upon identification of the superior segmental arterial branch, the surgeon incises the pleura overlying the pulmonary artery in the posterior direction to the point where the artery enters the parenchyma of the lung. The surgeon then completes the fissure using a stapler.

The lower lobe is tethered medially by the inferior pulmonary ligament, which is electrocauterized, and then divided to the inferior pulmonary vein. The vein is encircled with a finger or right-angled clamp and then ligated and divided with a stapler or clamped and sutured. The surgeon retracts the proximal pulmonary artery stump superiorly, revealing the lower lobe bronchus bifurcating off the left main bronchus. Division of the lower lobe bronchus must include the superior segmental bronchus and is optimally performed as close to the bifurcation as possible.

The surgeon should assess and remove the contents of the paraaortic, aortopulmonary window, and subcarinal lymph nodes and also the inferior pulmonary ligament node to complete staging. Anteriorly retracting the lung and posteriorly incising the pleura inferior to the left main bronchus provides access to the subcarinal space.

With all lobectomy procedures, the surgeon must place chest tubes to evacuate air and drain fluid. For upper lobectomy, a chest tube is placed in the apex; lower lobectomy necessitates a chest tube just superior to the diaphragm.

Segmentectomy and limited resections

Pulmonary resections that involve the removal of less than a lobe are classified into anatomic segmental resections or nonanatomic wedge resections. For patients with limited pulmonary function, segmentectomy and wedge resection provide alternatives to lobectomy.

Segmentectomy

Bronchoscopic evaluation is necessary prior to segmentectomy to ensure that the segmental bronchi are disease-free. The presence of extrinsic compression, inflammatory changes, and tumors requires more extensive procedures. Furthermore, intraoperative assessment of mediastinal and lobar lymph nodes is essential, making segmentectomy the procedure of choice to rule out lobectomy. If nodes are positive, segmentectomy is unlikely to be curative. Tumor size and location are also important considerations. Ideally, tumors should be peripherally located and less than 3 cm in maximum diameter.

Commonly, the segments of the right upper lobe (anterior, apical, and posterior) and right lower lobe (four superior and medial basal segments) lend themselves to segmentectomy of the right lung. The right middle lobe has minimal preserved lung and therefore does not undergo segmentectomy. The left-upper-lobe segments (anterior, apicoposterior, and lingular) are resectable along with the superior, anteromedial, and basal segments of the left lower lobe.

Incision As in lobectomy, the approach of choice is a posterolateral thoracotomy via the fifth intercostal space. Once again, a muscle incision via the fourth intercostal space is an alternative.

Operative technique The order in which the hilar structures are divided varies. Typically, the segmental arterial branches are divided first to expose the segmental bronchus. The lobar and segmental bronchi are dissected and lobar node dissection is completed to test for metastases. The segmental bronchus is then divided and closed with absorbable suture. The bronchus may also be stapled.

The veins are typically the last vascular structures divided. The intersegmental veins delineate the intersegmental plane. The surgeon should identify, dissect, and divide the appropriate veins, taking care to spare the intersegmental vein to allow for venous drainage of other segments and thus reduce postoperative complications.

With the lung inflated, the parenchyma of the lung is divided. The visceral pleura is then divided and the segment removed by stapling along the intersegmental plane, ensuring appropriate margins of about 2 cm. Potential air leaks should be assessed and repaired and chest tubes placed (one in the apex to evacuate air and a basal tube placed posteriorly for drainage).

Wedge resections

Wedge resection, a nonanatomic resection, is commonly used for biopsy of a lung with interstitial pneumonitis, sarcoidosis, or radiation injury. In patients with lung cancer, wedge resections are performed in the presence of small peripheral nodules. Anatomic segmentectomy is preferred over wedge resection because intrasegmental lymph node resection provides better margins and the removal of lymph nodes with segmental bronchi provides better staging.

Incision The approach of choice is a posterolateral thoracotomy via the fifth intercostal space, although a muscle-incision via the fourth intercostal space is an alternative.

Operative technique Once the nodule to be resected has been identified, a wedge resection can be performed by clamping and cutting out the nodule with margins and then sewing with running suture. Alternative methods include stapling, electrocautery, and laser photoablation followed by excision, using a 40- to 50-W free beam or a 10- to 15-W contact tip to excise the tumor. To minimize invasiveness, video-assisted thoracoscopy is yet another method that can be used.

Video-assisted thoracic surgery

Video-assisted thoracic surgery (VATS) is a minimally invasive approach that avoids retraction of the ribs in order to minimize postoperative pain and debilitation; it uses the same surgical principles as those employed in thoracoscopic procedures. VATS is an option for patients with peripherally located nodules less than 3 cm in maximum diameter.

Patients undergoing a VATS procedure are anesthetized with a double-lumen endotracheal tube. Because of single-lung ventilation, hemodynamics are monitored with an arterial pressure line.

The patient is placed in the lateral position, in the same way as when a posterolateral thoracotomy is being performed,, and the three working ports are positioned in an inverted triangle configuration.

Wedge resection is the most common surgical procedure utilizing VATS. Some hospitals have begun to use VATS for lobectomy, but the practice has not been extensively studied. For VATS lobectomy, two incisions are made: one at the seventh and one at the eighth intercostal spaces. These incisions are used for chest tube placement once the procedure is completed. A third 6-cm utility incision is made along the anterior axillary line in the fifth intercostal space. For upper lobectomies, a fourth 10-mm port at the third intercostal space helps to gain access to the superior aspect of the hilum when the pulmonary artery's apical posterior branch is being dissected.

In lower lobectomy, the inferior pulmonary ligament is divided first, followed by division of the inferior pulmonary vein. The rest of the hilar structures are approached posteriorly. The lower lobe bronchus is isolated and divided with a stapler, exposing the pulmonary arteries, which are subsequently isolated and divided with an endoscopic vascular stapler. The fissure is then divided and removed through the 6-cm utility incision, followed by removal of the lobe.

Upper lobectomies using VATS tend to be more difficult than lower lobectomies. The pulmonary vein is isolated and divided first. However, unlike the case in lower lobectomy, the anterior and apical posterior segmental pulmonary arteries are divided instead of the bronchus. The bronchus is then divided, followed by the fissure. The lobe is removed via the utility incision.

After completion of upper or lower lobectomies using VATS, the lungs are reinflated, potential air leaks are assessed and repaired, and chest tubes are placed in the two lower incisions.

Surgical management of small cell lung cancer

Chemotherapy is the standard therapy for SCLC. However, patients who present with a single pulmonary nodule undergo resection, often combined with combination chemotherapy with or without radiotherapy and prophylactic cranial irradiation.

CONCLUSION

Lung cancer is the leading cause of cancer-related death among men and women in the United States. Therefore, any indication of carcinoma warrants immediate and thorough investigation and appropriate TNM staging. With the advent of minimally invasive surgery, new radiographic imaging modalities, and advances in chemotherapy regimens, the treatment of lung cancer has progressed considerably. Nevertheless, the most pivotal component in reducing lung cancer incidence is minimizing risk factors, the most significant of which is smoking.

References

1. Denissenko MF, Pao A, Tang M, et al. Preferential formation of benso[a]pyrene adducts at lung cancer mutational hotspots in p54. *Science* 1996;274:430.
2. IARC Monographs on the evaluation of the carcinogenic risk of chemicals to humans, vol 38. Lyons, France: International Agency for Research on Cancer, 1986.
3. Gritz ER. Cigarette smoking: The need for action by health professionals. *CA Cancer J Clin* 1988;38:194.
4. Flanders WD, Lally CA, Zhu BP, et al. Lung cancer mortality in relation to age, duration of smoking, and daily cigarette consumption: Results from Cancer Prevention Study II. *Cancer Res* 2003;63:6556.
5. Peluso M, Ceppi M, Munnia A, et al. Analysis of 13 ^{32}P-DNA postlabelling studies onoccupational cohorts exposed to air pollution. *Am J Epidemiol* 2001;153:546.
6. Law MR. Genetic predisposition to lung cancer. *Br J Cancer 1990;*61:195.
7. Caporaso N, Hayes RB, Dosemeci M, et al. Lung cancer risk, occupational exposure, and the debrisoquin metabolic phenotype. *Cancer Res* 1989;49:3675.
8. Sellers TA, Bailey-Wilson JE, Elston RC, et al. Evidence for mendelian inheritance in the pathogenesis of lung cancer. *J Natl Cancer Inst* 1990;82:1272.
9. d'Errico A, Taioli E, Chen X, Vineis P. Genetic metabolic polymorphisms and the risk of cancer: A review of the literature. *Biomarkers* 1996;1:149.
10. Crespi CL, Penman BW, Gelboin HV, et al. A tobacco smoke-derived nitrosamine, 4-(methylnitrosamino)-1-(3 pyridyl)-1-butanonone, is activated by multiple human cytochrome p450s including the polymorphic human cytochrome p4502D6. *Carcinogenesis* 1991;12:1197.
11. Kondo K, Tsuzuki H, Sasa M, et al. A dose-response relationship between the frequency of p53 mutations and tobacco consumption in lung cancer patients. *J Surg Oncol* 1996;61:20.
12. Reissmann PT, Koga H, Takahashi R, et al. Inactivation of the rentinoblastoma susceptibility gene in non-small cell lung cancer. *Oncogene* 1993;8:1913.
13. Cagle PT, El-Naggar AK, Xu H-J, et al. Differential retinoblastoma protein expression in neuroendocrine tumors of the lung. *Am J Pathol* 1997;150:393.
14. Richardson GE, Johnson BE. The biology of lung cancer. *Semin Oncol* 1993;20:105.
15. Salgia R, Blank R, Skarin A. Heart and mediastinum. In: Skarin A (ed). *Atlas of Diagnostic Oncology,* 3[d] ed. London: Mosby, 2002:62.
16. Vincent RG, Pickren JW, Lane NVW, et al. The changing histopathology of lung cancer: A review of 1682 cases. *Cancer* 1977;39:1617.
17. Fraire AE, Cooper SP, Greenberg SD, Buffler PA. Carcinoma of the lung: Changing cell distribution and histopathologic cell types. *Prog Surg Pathol* 1992;12:129.
18. McDowell EM. The respiratory epithelium. V. Histogenesis of lung carcinoma in the human. *J Natl Cancer Inst* 1978;61:587.
19. Paulson DL. Superior sulcus tumor: Results of combined therapy. *NY State J Med* 1971;71:2050.
20. Ordonez NG. Value of thyroid transcription factor-1 immunostaining in distinguishing small cell lung carcinomas from other small cell carcinomas. *Am J Surg Pathol* 2000;24:1217.
21. Dessy E, Pietra GG. Pseudomesotheliomatous adenocarcinoma of the lung: An immunohistochemical and ultrastructural study of three cases. *Cancer* 1991;68:247.
22. Lin JI, Tseng CH, Tsung SH. Pseudomesotheliomatous carcinoma of the lung. *South Med J* 1980;73:655.
23. Nakatani Y, Kitamura H, Inayama Y, et al. Pulmonary adenocarcinomas of the fetal lung type: A clinicopathologic study indicating differences in histology, epidemiology, and natural history of low-grade and high-grade forms. *Am J Surg Pathol* 1998;22:399.
24. Moran CA, Hochholzer L, Fishback N, et al. Mucinous (so-called colloid) carcinomas of the lung. *Mod Pathol* 5:634, 1992.
25. Hayashi H, Kitamura H, Nakatani Y, et al. Primary signet-ring-cell carcinoma of the lung: Histochemical and immunohistochemical characterization. *Hum Pathol* 1999;30:378.
26. Gaffey MJ, Mills SE, Ritter JH. Clear cell tumors of the lower respiratory tract. *Semin Diagn Pathol* 1997;14:222.
27. Weidner N. Pulmonary adenocarcinoma with intestinal-type differentiation. *Ultrastruct Pathol* 1992;16:7.
28. Meyer EC, Liebow AA. Relationship of interstitial pneumonia, honeycombing and atypical proliferation to cancer of the lung. *Cancer* 1965;18:322.
29. Fraire AE, Greenberg SD. Carcinoma and diffuse interstitial fibrosis of the lung. *Cancer* 1973;31:1078.
30. Barsky SH, Huang SJ, Bhuta S. The extracellular matrix of pulmonary scar carcinomas is suggestive of a desmoplastic origin. *Am J Pathol* 1996;124:412.
31. Clayton F. The spectrum of significance of bronchioloalveolar carcinomas. *Pathol Annu* 1988;23:361.
32. Schulze ES, Mattia AR, Chew FS. Bronchioloalveolar carcinoma. *Am J Roentgenol* 1994;162:1294.
33. Sutton LN, Morrison JF, Rees MR. Radiographic features and prognosis in bronchioloalveolar carcinoma: A local experience. *Respir Med* 1989;83:471.
34. Manning JT Jr, Spjut HJ, Tschen JA. Bronchioloalveolar carcinoma: The significance of two histopathologic types. *Cancer* 1984;54:525.
35. Carter D, Patchefsky AS. *Tumors and Tumor-like Conditions of the Lung.* Philadelphia: Saunders, 1998:266.
36. Gaffey MJ, Mills SE, Frierson HF Jr, et al. Pulmonary clear cell carcinoid tumor: Another entity in the differential diagnosis of pulmonary clear cell neoplasia. *Am J Surg Pathol* 1998;22:1020.

37. Yoshida J, Nagai K, Hasebe T, et al. Pulmonary metastasis of renal cell carcinoma resected sixteen years after nephrectomy. *Jpn J Clin Oncol* 1995;25:20.
38. Nowak MA, Fatteh SM, Campbell TE. Glycogen-rich malignant melanomas and glycogen-rich balloon cell malignant melanomas: Frequency and pattern of PAS positivity in primary and metastatic melanomas. *Arch Pathol Lab Med* 1998;122:353.
39. Bonetti F, Pea M, Martignoni G, et al. Clear cell ("sugar") tumor of the lung is a lesion strictly related to angiomyolipoma—The concept of a family of lesions characterized by the presence of the perivascular epithelioid cell (PEC). *Pathology* 1994;26:230.
40. Cook RM, Miller YE, Bunn PA Jr. Small cell lung cancer: Etiology, biology, clinical features, staging, and treatment. *Curr Probl Cancer* 1993;30:42.
41. Gephardt GN, Grady KJ, Ahmad M, et al. Peripheral small cell undifferentiated carcinoma of the lung: Clinicopathologic features of 17 cases. *Cancer* 1988;61:1002.
42. Salgia R, Blank R, Skarin A. Heart and mediastinum. In: Skarin A (ed). *Atlas of Diagnostic Oncology*, 3[d] ed. London: Mosby, 2002:62.
43. Abdi EA, Goel R, Bishop S, Bain GO. Peripheral carcinoid tumors of the lung: A clinicopathologic study. *J Surg Oncol* 1988;39:190.
44. Salgia R, Blank R, Skarin A. Heart and mediastinum. In: in Skarin A (ed). *Atlas of Diagnostic Oncology*, 3[d] ed. London, Mosby, 2002:62.
45. Arrigoni MG, Woolner LB, Bernatz PE. Atypical carcinoid tumors of the lung. *J Thorac Cardiovasc Surg* 1972;64:413.
46. Travis WD, Rush W, Flieder DB, et al. Survival analysis of 200 pulmonary neuroendocrine tumors with clarification of criteria for atypical carcinoid and its separation from typical carcinoid. *Am J Surg Pathol* 1998;22: 934.
47. Travis WD, Linnoila RI, Tsokos MG, et al. Neuroendocrine tumors of the lung with proposed criteria for large-cell neuroendocrine carcinoma: An ultrastructural, immunohistochemical, and flow cytometric study of 35 cases. *Am J Surg Pathol* 1991;15:529.
48. Dresler CM, Ritter JH, Patterson GA, et al. Clinical-pathologic analysis of 40 patients with large cell neuroendocrine carcinoma of the lung. *Ann Thorac Surg* 1997;63:180.
49. Ishida T, Kaneko S, Yokohama H, et al. Adenosquamous carcinoma of the lung: Clinicopathologic and immunohistochemical features. *Am J Clin Pathol* 1992;97:678.
50. Nappi O, Glasner SD, Swanson PE, Wick MR. Biphasic and monophasic sarcomatoid carcinomas of the lung: A reappraisal of "carcinosarcomas" and "spindle cell carcinomas." *Am J Clin Pathol* 1994;102:331.
51. Carbone PP, Frost JK, Feinstein AR, et al. Lung cancer: Perspective and prospects. *Ann Intern Med* 1970;73:1024.
52. Cromartie RS, Parker EF, May JE, et al. Carcinoma of the lung: A clinical review. *Ann Thorac Surg* 1980;30:30.
53. Sridhar KS, Lobo CF, Altman RD. Digital clubbing and lung cancer. *Chest* 1998;114:1535.
54. Campling BG, Sarda IR, Baer KA, et al. Secretion of atrial natriuretic peptide and vasopressin by small cell lung cancer. *Cancer* 1995;75:2442.
55. Cryer PE, Kissaine JM. Clinicopathologic conference: Malignant hypercalcemia. *Am J Med* 1979;65:486.
56. Shepard FA, Laskey J, Evans WK, et al. Cushing's syndrome associated with ectopic corticotrophin production and small cell lung cancer. *J Clin Oncol* 1992;10:21.
57. Posner JB. Paraneoplastic syndromes. *Curr Opin Neurol* 1997;10:471.
58. Lennon VA, Lambert EH. Autoantibodies bind solubilized calcium channel-omega-conotoxin complexes from small cell lung carcinoma: A diagnostic aid for Lambert-Eaton myasthenic syndrome. *Mayo Clin Proc* 1989;64:1498.
59. McEvoy KM. Diagnosis and treatment of Lambert-Eaton myasthenic syndrome. *Neurol Clin* 1994; 12:387.
60. Zuger M, Demarmels-Biasitutti F, Wuillemin WA, et al. Subcutaneous low-molecular weight heparin for treatment of Trousseau's syndrome. *Ann Hematol* 1997;75:165.
61. Krishnamurthy GT, Tubi M, Miss J, et al. Distribution pattern of metastatic bone disease: A need for total body skeletal imaging. *JAMA* 1977;237:2504.
62. Pagani JJ. Non-small cell lung carcinoma adrenal metastases: Computed tomography and percutaneous needle biopsy in their diagnosis. *Cancer* 1984;53:1058.
63. Evans SE, Scanlon PD. Current practice in pulmonary function testing. *Mayo Clin Proc* 2003;78:758.
64. McCloud TC, Bourgouin PM, Greenberg RW, et al. Bronchogenic carcinoma: Analysis of staging in the mediastinum with CT by correlative lymph node mapping and sampling. *Radiology* 1992;182:319.
65. Stiglbauer R, Schurawitzki H, Klepetko W, et al. Contrast-enhanced MRI for the staging of bronchogenic carcinoma: Comparison with CT and histopathologic staging: Preliminary results. *Clin Radiol* 1991;44:293.
66. Line BR, White CS. Positron emission tomography scanning for the diagnosis and management of lung cancer. *Curr Treat Options Oncol* 2004;5:63.
67. von Haag DW, Follette DM, Roberts PF, et al. Advantages of positron emission tomography over computed tomography in mediastinal staging of non-small cell cancer. *J Surg Res* 2002;103:160.
68. Toloza EM, Harpole L, McCrory DC. Noninvasive staging of non-small cell lung cancer: A review of the current evidence. *Chest* 2003;123:137S.
69. Kato H, Konako C, Ono J, et al. *Cytology of the Lung: Techniques and Interpretation*. Tokyo: Igaku-Shoin, 1983.
70. Rivera MP, Detterbeck F, Mehta AC. Diagnosis of lung cancer: The guidelines. *Chest* 2003;123:129S.
71. Savage C, Zwischenberger JB. Image-guided fine needle aspirate strategies for staging of lung cancer. *Clin Lung Cancer* 2000;2:101.
72. Radke JR, Conway WA, Eyler WR, Kvale PA. Diagnostic accuracy in peripheral lung lesions: Factors predicting success with flexible fiberoptic bronchoscopy. *Chest* 1979;76:176
73. Shure D, Fedullo F. Transbronchial needle aspiration in the diagnosis of submucosal and peribronchial bronchogenic carcinoma. *Chest* 1985;88:49.
74. Hsu HS, Wang LS, Hsieh CC, et al. The role of mediastinoscopy in the evaluation of thoracic disease and lung cancer. *J Chin Med Assoc* 2003;66:231.

75. Rodriguez P, Santana N, Gamez P, et al. Mediastinoscopy in the diagnosis of mediastinal disease. An analysis of 181 explorations. *Arch Bronconeumol* 2003;39:29.
76. Sebastian-Quetglas F, Molins L, Baldo X, et al and the Spanish Video-assisted Thoracic Surgery Study Group: Clinical value of video-assisted thoracoscopy for preoperative staging of non-small cell lung cancer. *Lung Cancer* 2003;42:297.
77. Harpole DH Jr, Herndon JE II, Wolfe WG, et al, A prognostic model of recurrence and death in stage I non–small cell lung cancer utlizing presentation, histopathology and oncoprotein expression. *Cancer Res* 1995;55:51.
78. Mountain CF. Revisions in the international system for staging lung cancer. *Chest* 1997;111:1710.
79. Zierhut D, Bettscheider C, Schubert K, et al. Radiation therapy of stage I and II non-small cell lung cancer. *Lung Cancer* 2001;34:S39.
80. Sirzen F, Kjellen E, Sorenson S, Cavallin-Stahl E. A systematic overview of radiation therapy effects in non–small cell lung cancer. *Acta Oncol* 2003;42:493.
81. Arriagada R, le Chevalier T, Quoix E, et al. ASTRO Plenary: Effective chemotherapy on locally advanced non-small cell lung cancer: A randomized study of 353 patients. *Int J Radiat Oncol Biol Phys* 1991;20:1183.
82. Dillman RO, Herndon J, Seagren SL, et al. Improved survival in stage III non–small cell lung cancer: Seven-year follow-up of cancer and leukemia group B (CALB) 8433 trial. *Natl Cancer Inst* 1996;88:1210.
83. Sause W, Kolesar P, Taylor S, et al. Five-year results: phase III trial of regionally advanced, unresectable non-small cell lung cancer, ROG 8808, ECOG 4588, SWOG 8992 [abstr 1743]. *Proc ASCO* 1998;17:435a.
84. Planting A, Helle P, Drings P, et al. A randomized study of high-dose split course radiotherapy preceded by high-dose chemotherapy versus high-dose radiotherapy only in locally advanced non–small cell lung cancer. An EORTC Lung Cancer Cooperative Group trial. *Ann Oncol* 1996;7:139.
85. Furuse K, Fukuoka Y, Takada Y, et al for the West Japan Lung Cancer Group: A randomized phase III study of concurrent versus sequential thoracic radiotherapy (TRT) in combination with mitomycin (M), vindesine (V), cisplatin (P) in unresectable stage III non-small cell lung cancer (NSCLC) (Abstract No. 1649). *Proc Am Soc Clin Oncol* 1997;16:459a.
86. Byhardt RW. The evolution of radiation therapy oncology group (RTOG) protocols for non–small cell lung cancer. *Int J Radiat Oncol Biol Phys* 1995;32:1513.
87. Komaki R, Scott C, Lee JS, et al. Impact of adding concurrent chemotherapy to hyperfractionated radiotherapy for locally advanced non-small cell lung cancer (NSCLC): Comparison of RTOG 83-11 and RTOGH 91-06. *Am J Clin Oncol* 1997;20:435.
88. Sause WT, Scott C, Taylor S, et al. Preliminary results of a phase III trial in regionally advanced, unresectable non-small-cell lung cancer. *J Natl Cancer Inst* 1995;87:198.
89. Shields TW. Preoperative radiation therapy in the treatment of bronchial carcinoma. *Cancer* 1972;30:1388.
90. Warram J. Preoperative irradiation of cancer of the lung: Final report of a therapeutic trial. A collaborative study. *Cancer* 1975;36:914.
91. Pincus M, Reddy S, Lee MS, et al. Preoperative combined modality therapy for Stage III M_0 non-small cell lung carcinoma. *Int J Radiat Oncol Biol Phys* 1988; 15:189.
92. Kirsh MM, Sloan H. Mediastinal metastases in bronchogenic carcinoma: Influence of postoperative irradiation, cell type and location. *Ann Thorac Surg* 1982; 33:459.
93. Slawson RG, Scott RM. Radiation therapy in bronchogenic carcinoma. *Radiology* 1979;132:175.
94. Komaki R, Scott C, Lee JS, et al. Impact of adding concurrent chemotherapy to hyperfractionated radiotherapy for locally advanced non–small cell lung cancer: Comparison ofRTOG 83-11 and RTOG 91-06. *Am J Clin Oncol* 1997;20:435.
95. Prager D, Cameron R, Ford J, Figlin R. Bronchogenic carcinoma. In: Murray JF, Nadel JA (eds). *Textbook of Respiratory Medicine*. Philadelphia: Saunders, 2000:1415.
96. Wronski M, Arbit E, Burt M, et al. Survival after surgical treatment of brain metastases from lung cancer: A follow-up study of 231 patients treated between 1976 and 1991. *J Neurosurg* 1995;83:605.
97. Coia L. The role of radiation therapy in the treatment of brain metastases. *Int J Radiat Oncol Biol Phys* 1992;23:229.
98. Kurtz JM, Gelber R, Brady LW. The palliation of brain metastases in a favorable patient population: A randomized clinical trial by the radiation oncology group. *Int J Radiat Oncol Biol Phys* 1981;7:891.
99. Vokes EE, Bitran JD, Vogelzang NJ. Chemotherapy for non–small cell lung cancer. The continuing challenge. *Chest* 1991;99:1326.
100. Haskell CM. Chemotherapy and survival of patients with non–small cell lung cancer. A contrary view. *Chest* 1991;99:1325.
101. Donnadieu N, Paesmans M, Sculier JP. Chemotherapy of non-small cell bronchial cancers. Meta-analysis of the literature as a function of the extent of the disease. *Rev Mal Respir* 1991;8:197.
102. Rosell R, Gomez-Codina J, Camps C, et al. A randomized trial comparing preoperative chemotherapy plus surgery with surgery alone in patients with non-small–cell lung cancer. *N Engl J Med* 1994;330:153.
103. Roth JA, Atkinson EN, Fossella F, et al. Long-term follow-up of patients enrolled in a randomized trial comparing perioperative chemotherapy and surgery with surgery alone in resectable stage IIA non–small cell lung cancer. *Lung Cancer* 1998;21:1.
104. Niiranen A, Niitamo-Korhonen S, Kouri A, et al. Adjuvant chemotherapy after radical surgery for non-small-cell lung cancer: A randomized study. *J Clin Oncol* 1992;10:1927.
105. Wada H, Hitomi S, Teramatsu T. Adjuvant chemotherapy after complete resection in non–small cell lung cancer. *J Clin Oncol* 1996;14:1048.
106. Perrone F, Rossi A, Ianniello GP, et al. Vinorelbine plus best supportive care (BSC) versus BSC in the treatment of advanced non-small cell lung cancer patients: Results of phase III randomized trial [abstr 1752]. *Proc ASCO* 1998;17.
107. Non-Small Cell Lung Cancer Collaborative Group: Chemotherapy in non-small cell lung cancer: A meta-

analysis using updated data on individual patients from 52 randomized clinical trials. *Br Med J* 1995;311:899.
108. Pignon JP, Arriagada R, Ihde DC, et al. A meta-analysis of thoracic radiotherapy for small-cell lung cancer. *N Engl J Med* 1992;327:1618.
109. Turrisi AT. Brain irradiation and systemic chemotherapy for small cell lung cancer: Dangerous liaisons? *J Clin Oncol* 1990;8:196.
110. Arriagada R, Le Chevalier T, Riviere A, et al. Patterns of failure after prophylactic cranial irradiation in small-cell lung cancer: Analysis of 505 randomized patients. *Ann Oncol* 2002;13:748.
111. Cao K, Huang H, Tu M. Clinical study of prophylactic cranial irradiation for small-cell lung cancer. *Zhonghua Zhong Liu Za Zhi* 2000;22:336.
112. Roth BJ, Johnson DH, Einhorn LH, et al. Randomized study of cyclophosphamide, doxorubicin, and vincristine versus cisplatin and etoposide versus alternation of these two regimens in extensive small-cell lung cancer: A phase III trial of the Southeastern Cancer Study Group. *J Clin Oncol* 1992;10:282.
113. Ihde DC, Mulshine J, Kramer B, et al. Randomized trial of high vs. standard dose etoposide (VP16) and cisplatin in extensive small cell lung cancer (SCLC) (Abstr). Presented at the 6th World Conference on Lung Cancer, Melbourne, November 10–14, 1991. *Proc Am Soc Clin Oncol* 1991;10:240.
114. Elliot JA, Osterlind K, Hansen HH. Cyclic alternating "non-cross resistant" chemotherapy in the management of small cell anaplastic carcinoma of the lung. *Cancer Treat Rev* 1984;11:103.
115. Zacharski LR, Henderson WG, Rickles FR, et al. Effect of warfarin in small cell carcinoma of the lung. *JAMA* 1981;205:831.
116. Ginsberg RJ, Rubinstein LV. Randomized trial of lobectomy versus limited resection for T1 N0 non-small cell lung cancer. Lung Cancer Study Group. *Ann Thorac Surg* 1995;60:615.

CHAPTER

13 GASTROESOPHAGEAL REFLUX AND PRIMARY ESOPHAGEAL MOTILITY DISORDERS

Malcolm V. Brock

GASTROESOPHAGEAL REFLUX

INTRODUCTION

Gastroesophageal (GE) reflux is the movement of gastric contents including acid, pepsin, and bile salts from the stomach into the esophagus. The term *GE reflux*, as the abbreviated description of an ailment, is a misnomer since everyone refluxes. In fact, most people experience asymptomatic reflux of gastric contents from the stomach into the esophagus several times daily as a normal physiologic process. When reflux does occur, gravity, peristalsis, normal swallowing of saliva, and secretions from esophageal glands help return the gastric contents back into the stomach. A distinction must be made, therefore, between physiologic GE reflux and GE reflux disease (GERD). It is common practice among physicians to diagnose GERD when reflux becomes sympto-

KEY CONCEPTS

- Epidemiology
  - Gastroesophageal reflux disease (GERD) affects nearly 10 percent of the population daily, 14 percent weekly, and 15 percent monthly. Achalasia has an incidence of 1 to 2 per 200,000 persons, with both sexes equally affected.
- Pathophysiology
  - GERD results from excessive movement of gastric contents—including acid, pepsin, and bile salts—from the stomach into the esophagus. It arises from several factors, including compromise of the antireflux barrier, defective esophageal peristalsis, abnormal production of bile salts and gastric acid, and inadequate gastric emptying.
  - Achalasia is a motility disorder of the esophagus characterized by the loss of neurons from the myenteric plexus, which results in aperistalsis of the esophageal body, failure of the lower esophageal sphincter (LES) to relax with swallowing, and elevated LES pressures. This condition arises from inflammation of the myenteric plexus and associated fibrosis, depletion, and loss of ganglion cells.
- Clinical features
  - GERD symptoms include gastrointestinal and/or respiratory symptoms. Typical gastrointestinal symptoms consist of heartburn, chest pain, acid regurgitation, and dysphagia. Less common respiratory features include chronic asthma, refractory cough, laryngitis, and wheezing. Complications include esophagitis, ulceration, strictures, bleeding, and carcinoma.
  - Achalasia is characterized by dysphagia progressing from solid to liquid foods. Regurgitation and chest pain can also occur, sometimes leading to weight loss, a sign of advanced disease.
- Diagnostics
  - Diagnostics for GERD include 24-h intraesophageal and intragastric pH monitoring, 24-h intraesophageal and intragastric bilimetry, esophageal manometry, vectometry of the LES, gastric scintigraphy, endoscopy, and barium swallow studies.

- Barium swallow has a 75 percent sensitivity in diagnosing achalasia, mainly because it misses early disease; a "bird's beak" narrowing of the distal esophagus and proximal dilatation are suggestive of achalasia. Manometry is the "gold standard" test for achalasia, revealing incomplete relaxation of the LES upon swallowing; the esophageal body exhibits isobaric pressure waves.
- Treatment
  - Initial conservative management of GERD consists of antacid therapies, including proton-pump inhibitors; elevating the head of the bed during sleeping; avoiding tight clothing, bending or stooping; smoking cessation; and avoidance of certain foods. Antireflux operations are indicated in cases refractory to medical therapy, complications, and reflux due to mechanical problems. Operations include the Nissen fundoplication, Toupet partial fundoplication, and Collis gastroplasty.
  - For achalasia, the four palliative measures commonly employed include medication, botulinum toxin injection, mechanical dilation, and surgical (Heller) myotomy. All of these approaches attempt to reduce the tone of the LES.
- Results/outcomes
  - The outcomes of antireflux surgery are generally favorable, but long-term follow-up studies have pointed to the persistence or return of GERD symptoms in about one-third of patients. The most common early postoperative symptom after laparoscopic antireflux surgery is dysphagia, occurring in about 20 percent of patients; 6 percent complain of long-term dysphagia. Long-term postoperative complications include early satiety (49 percent), abdominal bloating (36 percent), inability to vomit (31 percent), diarrhea (20 percent), nausea (8 percent), and recurrent reflux (8 percent).
  - Approximately two-thirds of patients undergoing Heller myotomy experience good to excellent late outcomes. Late complications of the procedure include GERD, the development of Barrett's esophagus, peptic strictures, high-grade dysphagia, and frank carcinoma.

matic or if there are histopathologic alterations in the esophagus or respiratory tract due to refluxed gastroduodenal contents. DeMeester, who over the last three decades has contributed enormously to our understanding of GERD, argues that the best workable definition for clinicians in diagnosing GERD involves the presence of symptoms (either typical or atypical, see below) as well as one or two objective measures that document the abnormal reflux, such as endoscopically visible changes, abnormal pH readings, or evidence on esophageal biopsies.[1] Although there is no "gold standard" of criteria whereby GERD may be recognized, simply stated, two factors must be present: (1) acid-peptic or pancreaticobiliary secretions must reach the esophagus with increased frequency and (2) the esophagus must be unable to clear those refluxed materials back into the stomach.

GERD, and its most common symptom, heartburn, affects nearly 10 percent of the population daily, 14 percent weekly, and 15 percent monthly.[2] The chronicity of GERD symptoms also produces complications that are disease entities themselves. Reflux esophagitis, a condition in GERD patients manifest by endoscopically evident lesions in the esophageal mucosa, may be prevalent in close to 80 percent of GERD patients.[3,4] Barrett's metaplasia was found at autopsy to be six times more prevalent than would have been recognized clinically prior to death.[5] Although GERD is distributed equally among men and women, both reflux esophagitis and Barrett's metaplasia are predominantly diseases of men, with a male:female ratio in the former of 2:1 to 3:1 and a ratio as high as 10:1 in the latter.[6]

PATHOPHYSIOLOGY

GERD results when the homeostatic balance between the erosive nature of refluxed gastric contents and the reparative efforts of the esophageal epithelia is shifted in favor of the GE reflux. This can produce histopathologic injury, acute and chronic symptoms, or both. There are myriad considerations including excessive GE reflux events, prolonged exposure of the esophageal epithelia to gastric contents, decreased epithelial resistance, decreased gastric clearance from the esophagus, and other dietary, behavioral, and emotional factors.[7] Since the abdominal cavity in general has a higher pressure than the thoracic cavity, GE reflux would occur continuously without an effective barrier between the two compartments. But GERD is multifactorial in its pathogenesis and many factors—not only abnormalities of the antireflux barrier but also the presence of hiatal hernias, defects in peristaltic function of the esophageal body, and gastric factors such as bile salts, acid, volume of refluxed contents, and adequacy of emptying—all play a role in producing GERD. Each of these contributing factors must be considered in turn.

Antireflux barrier

The antireflux barrier is not one distinct anatomic structure but rather a functional unit that derives its integrity from many different parts. The principal components constituting this barrier include (1) the intrinsic pressure of the lower esophageal sphincter (LES), (2) the intraabdominal location of the LES, (3) the crural diaphragm, (4) the phrenoesophageal membrane, and (5) maintenance of the acute angle of His between the distal esophagus and the proximal stomach. Further complicating the matter is the fact that different components of the barrier predominate during different physiologic circumstances.[8] When an individual is lying down, for instance, the intrinsic pressure of the LES plays a major role in preventing reflux, while the intraabdominal location of the LES becomes critical during swallowing. Similarly, the diaphragmatic crus predominates during episodes of increased intraabdominal pressure, as during a vasovagal maneuver. Additionally, each component of the antireflux barrier influences another. Indeed, manometric readings of the LES are taken by convention at mid- or end-expiration because the diaphragmatic contribution of the LES increases the lower esophageal pressure during inspiration. This interdependence of its parts inures the antireflux barrier to catastrophic loss of all functional integrity, since failure of one or more parts can be compensated to a degree by other barrier components.

The lower esophageal sphincter

The LES corresponds to a 3- to 4-cm segment of circular smooth muscle in the wall of the distal esophagus, which—although morphologically indistinct from the surrounding esophageal body—has a specialized function. Importantly, this muscle's unique properties include:

1. Maintenance of a resting pressure about 10 to 30 mmHg higher than that of the stomach.[9]
2. An ability to develop spontaneous tension on stretching.[8]
3. An ability to respond to transmural electrical stimulation with relaxation.[8]
4. A swallowing reflex that lasts for 5 to 8 s to accommodate a passing food bolus. The intrinsic esophageal muscles, usually in a tonic state of contraction, relax as a response to normal physiologic swallowing.

The physiologic consequence is that the LES creates an area or a zone of high pressure, identified by manometry, just cephalad to the anatomic GE junction. To perform the actual measurement, a pressure transducer is pulled back from the stomach into the esophagus and a rise in pressure is observed over the gastric baseline at the LES. If continuous monitoring of the LES is performed, there is a normal, large physiologic temporal and individual variance of its pressure. Larger increases up to 80 mmHg can occur with lesser fluctuations during sleep. In an individual without GERD, there are two situations in which the high-pressure zone is not usually present[1]: (1) during the swallowing reflux and (2) during a belch, when air is vented from an overly distended stomach. Either physiologically or pathophysiologically, it is the loss of this high-pressure zone that is critical for GERD to occur so that gastroduodenal juice can reach the esophagus.

In normal individuals, the vast majority of reflux events result from the transient incompetence of the LES rather than a reduced basal tone of the sphincter.[10] These transient relaxations occur without any temporal relationship to swallowing, are not accompanied by esophageal peristalsis for subsequent clearance of any refluxed contents, and persist longer than the physiologic swallow-induced LES relaxations.[11] There is some evidence that early GERD involves more frequent transient LES relaxations.[12]

Certain common foods and medicines have profound effects on the LES and its ability to maintain the pressure zone (Table 13-1). This fact is not lost on most GERD sufferers, who quickly learn how to exacerbate and alleviate their symptoms solely through diet.

Table 13-1 Foods, medications, and hormones that influence resting LES pressure

	Resting LES pressure	
	Increased	**Decreased**
Food	Protein	Chocolate Fatty meals Yellow onions Smoking Coffee Alcohol Peppermint Gastric acidification
Medications	Cisapride Prostaglandin $F_{2\alpha}$ AlphaAdrenergics (metoclopramide) Domperidone Cholinergics (Bethanecol)	Nitrates Calcium channel blockers Theophylline Meperidine Anticholinergics (Atropine) Diazepam Barbiturates Morphine Nicotine Progesterone Antispasmotics Antidepressants
Hormones	Gastrin Motilin Substance P	Cholecystokinin Secretin Vasoactive Intestinal Polypeptide Somatostatin Gastric inhibitory polypeptide Glucagon

Length and intraabdominal location of the lower esophageal sphincter

In addition to incompetence of the gastroesophageal junction due to transient dysfunction of the LES, more permanent disability of the LES can occur. In fact, the most common reason for permanent LES dysfunction remains a decreased intrinsic LES pressure.[13] In addition to intrinsic LES pressure, however, the total LES length as well as intraabdominal length and position of the sphincter contribute to LES competency.[14] These principles are not to be glossed over by the surgeon, since they form a firm basis from which surgical repair of this complex, multifactorial disease is undertaken. The shorter the total LES length, the higher the pressure that must be maintained in the high-pressure zone to effectuate resistance to refluxed contents (Fig. 13-1). A short LES with an overall length less than 2 cm would then not be competent with an intrinsic sphincter pressure of 10 mmHg, an LES pressure commonly observed in patients with reflux esophagitis who are sitting upright.[15] If the stomach is distended, the length of the LES is further compromised. This is analogous to the way in which the neck of a balloon shortens as the balloon is inflated.[1] Factors that promote gastric dilation, such as overeating and increased aerophagia, can both contribute to increased esophageal reflux. The former is a common consequence of living in affluent western societies, and the latter results from attempts to neutralize caustic gastroduodenal refluxed contents with repetitive swallowing of alkaline saliva.

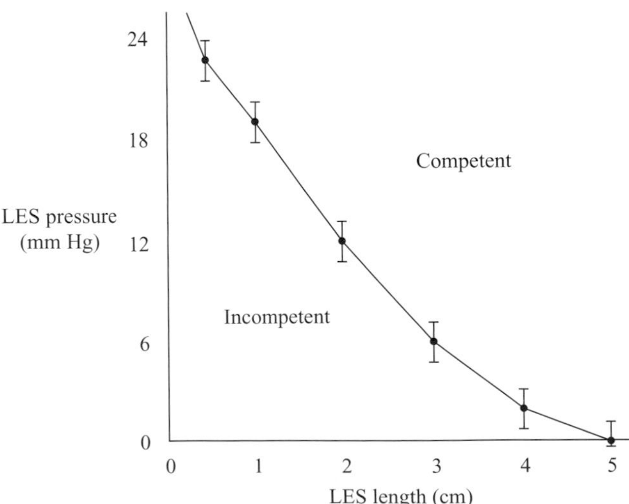

Figure 13-1 The relationship of the magnitude of pressure in the high-pressure zone and the overall length of the zone to resistance to the flow of fluid through the zone. LES = lower esophageal sphincter, competent = no flow, incompetent = flow of varied volumes. (From DeMeester TR, Peters JH, Bremner CG, Chandrasoma P. Biology of gastroesophageal reflux disease: Pathophysiology relating to medical and surgical treatment. *Annu Rev Med* 1999;50:469–506. With permission.)

An LES securely located in the abdomen has a higher transmural pressure than a LES that has slipped higher into the thorax. At least a portion of the LES needs exposure to intraabdominal pressure, especially during periods of high intraabdominal pressure, or else an effective barrier against reflux is lost. Again, DeMeester draws an apt analogy by likening this concept to the futility of attempting to sip soda from a large bottle with a fragile straw that keeps collapsing due to both the hydrostatic pressure of the surrounding liquid and the negative pressure induced by sucking on the straw.[1]

It is worthwhile to note that normal LES pressure can be substantially curtailed by both a short overall LES length and an abnormal LES position. Adding to this complexity are the wide ranges of LES and gastric pressures that can occur with changes of body position,[15] suggesting that early symptoms may occur episodically due to a patient's position. The symptoms then are difficult to reproduce in the formal clinical setting.

Angle of his and hiatal hernias

The anatomic relationship between the cardia of the stomach and the left side of the esophagus (known as the angle of His) contributes to the prevention of reflux. This acute angle can be thought of as functioning much like a one-way valve prohibiting duodenogastric juice from reaching the chest. The clinical significance of the angle of His pertains to its anatomic disruption due to a type 1 or sliding hiatal hernia. Hiatal hernias, or the prolapsing of the stomach through the diaphragmatic/esophageal hiatus into the chest, are very common. Although there are wide variations in the reported prevalence of these axial hernias, it is estimated that over half of the U.S. population over 50 years of age have hiatal hernias,[16,17] implying a relationship of the latter with age and obesity.

In the early postwar era, Allison in the United Kingdom was among the first to suspect an association between GERD and hiatal hernias.[18,19] In the mid-1980s, this concept gained credence when a series of papers highlighting endoscopic and radiographic data showed that a vast majority of patients with GERD have an associated hiatal hernia.[16,20–23] Sloan and colleagues, in a series of provocative maneuvers, established a relationship between the increasing size of a hiatal hernia, the resultant decrease in LES pressure, and an increased susceptibility to GERD.[24] Of note, the authors found a high correlation between the size of the hiatal hernia and the degree of susceptibility to reflux.[25] The mechanism that underlies the interrelationship between the presence of a hiatal hernia and reduced LES pressure has also recently been reviewed.[26] One hypothesis is that gastric distention is a potent stimulus of transient LES relaxations, and that hiatal hernias, with their resultant altered stomach anatomy, lower the threshold at which transient

LES relaxations can occur and incite GERD.[26] A second hypothesis involves a more mechanical explanation that implicates the large gaping hiatus resulting after a hiatal hernia as an important contributor to reflux, especially during periods of abrupt increases in intraabdominal pressure.[26] The significance of both hypotheses is that the anatomic disruption due to hiatal hernias is progressive and that the reflux can become increasingly abnormal as the size of the hernia enlarges. Moreover, large hiatal hernias also reduce esophageal clearance, leading to increased exposure of the esophagus to gastroduodenal juice. It is useful to stress that, in this anatomically and functionally complex area of the gastroesophageal junction, the presence of a hiatal hernia is just one variable of multiple possible factors that can render an individual vulnerable to GERD.

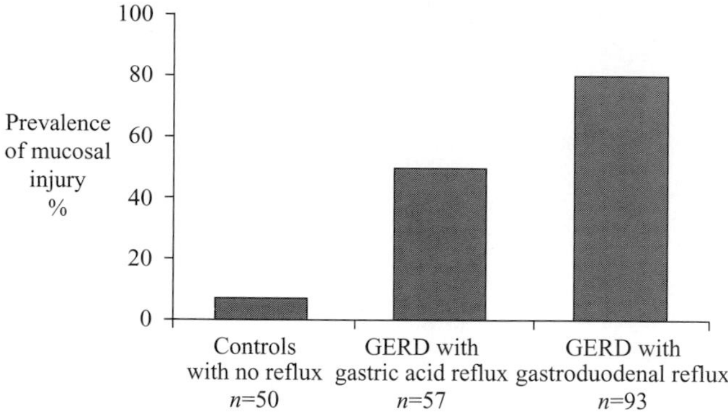

Figure 13-3 The relationship between the composition of the gastric juice refluxed and the prevalence of mucosal injury. (From DeMeester TR, Peters JH, Bremner CG, Chandrasoma P. Biology of gastroesophageal reflux disease: Pathophysiology relating to medical and surgical treatment. *Annu Rev Med* 1999;50:469–506. With permission.)

Defects in esophageal clearance, mucosal resistance, gastric contents, exposure to acid and bile salts

Figures 13-2 and 13-3 illustrate the concept that subjective complaints and objective complications of GERD are due to esophageal mucosal injuries resulting from both the failure of the esophageal antireflux barrier and the irritating nature of the refluxed contents themselves. It has long been known that although peptic secretions from the stomach are often implicated in such mucosal injury, bile and pancreatic secretions, irrespective of pH, are equally corrosive.[27] Moreover, up to 42 percent of patients who have an ineffective high-pressure zone of the lower esophagus do not sustain mucosal injury, suggesting a vigorous clearance of these corrosive gastroduodenal secretions by a well-functioning esophageal contractile body.[28] How long the esophageal mucosa remains in contact with refluxed gastroduodenal contents depends not only on esophageal peristalsis but also on gravity, salivation, and bicarbonate secretion from the submucosal glands of the esophagus.[8] Most of the acid is cleared by gravity and peristalsis.[29] Neutralization with saliva and bicarbonate secretion plays a smaller role.[30,31] Prolonged exposure to gastroduodenal contents, however, results in injury of the esophageal mucosa. This is especially significant at night, when sleeping diminishes both salivation and esophageal motility, resulting in increased nocturnal exposure to esophageal acid.

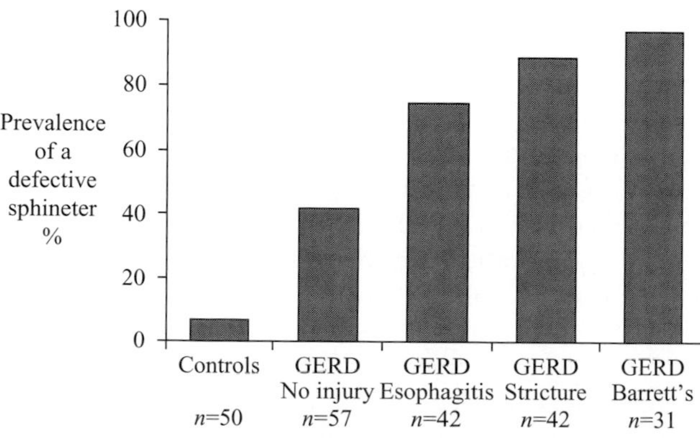

Figure 13-2 The relationship between various degrees of mucosal injury and the prevalence of a defective LES. (From DeMeester TR, Peters JH, Bremner CG, Chandrasoma P. Biology of gastroesophageal reflux disease: Pathophysiology relating to medical and surgical treatment. *Annu Rev Med* 1999;50:469–506. With permission.)

Repetitive exposure of the esophagus to these secretions leads not only to damage of the overlying mucosa but also to inflammatory changes of the underlining esophageal muscle;[32] since these inflammatory changes lead to fibrosis, the esophageal body's contractility is lost, producing a vicious cycle of more contact with gastroduodenal contents in the distal esophagus and inciting more injury.[33] In addition, there is some evidence to suggest that the loss of esophageal contractility can even potentiate gastroesophageal regurgitation and aspiration.[34]

Finally, esophageal clearance can also be retarded by other factors, such as cigarette smoking and large hiatal hernias. Smoking increases the frequency of acid reflux events and decreases the amount of saliva available for acid neutralization.[35,36] Patients with large hiatal hernias suffer "retrograde flow" when the normal antegrade flow of esophageal contents is disrupted by the hernial sac and the pooled contents are forced back into the esophagus.[37]

It is clear that the specific chemical composition of the refluxate plays a major role in GERD. The classic paradigm holds that GERD is primarily a disease of gastroesophageal acid reflux; however, this has been taken over by the realization that although the stomach has

Table 13-2 Evidence implicating both gastric and duodenal secretions in gastroesophageal reflux disease

Study Findings	Authors	Date
Improvement of both esophagitis and patient symptoms after removal of only the biliary component of gastroesophageal reflux	Salminen et al.[155]	1997
Larger probability of mucosal injury if patient had gastroduodenal reflux rather than either gastric acid or duodenal reflux alone	Fein et al.[39]	1997
Esophageal bile acid concentration is significantly higher in patients with mucosal injury than normal subjects	Nehra et al.[156]	1998
Time of acid exposure is significantly higher in patients with mucosal injury than in normal subjects	Nehra et al.[156]	1998

acid and pepsin as its main caustic agents, the duodenum—with its bile salts, lysolecithin, and pancreatic enzymes—also plays a primary role in the etiology of esophageal mucosal injury. In physiologic concentrations, both gastric acid and duodenal juice are not as noxious alone as they are together.[38,39] Multiple experiments in various animal models have established the importance of both acid and bile salts in eliciting severe esophageal mucosal injury.[34,40] In humans, the accumulated evidence that acid and bile synergism is critical to the mucosal injury inherent in GERD is equally as compelling (Table 13-2).

There is some controversy about the association of refluxed biliary contents and the development of columnar lined esophagus with intestinal metaplasia, the so-called Barrett's esophagus. The prevalence of Barrett's esophagus is closely related to GERD, and Barrett's esophagus is the starting point for a sequence of esophageal mucosal changes that can lead to esophageal adenocarcinoma in particular.[41] The incidence of diagnosed Barrett's esophagus and esophageal adenocarcinoma has increased dramatically over the last three decades. Although the cause of this increase is unknown, DeMeester emphasizes the striking parallels between the rise of Barrett's and adenocarcinoma and the more frequent use, starting in the 1970s, of potent acid-suppression therapy.[1] He suggests that before 1970, complications of Barrett's esophagus were primarily acid-related ulcers and strictures; but because of the lowering of gastric pH, bile salts now function as mutagens, contributing to the development of malignancy.[42]

Relative to the stomach and duodenum, the esophageal mucosa is quite vulnerable to injury from gastroduodenal juices.[43] The main reason is that the esophageal mucosa lacks a thick mucosal coat as rich in bicarbonate as that seen in the stomach; instead, it has only a thin mucosal covering that offers little protection. Moreover, the squamous epithelium of the esophagus is devoid of reparative processes such as "rapid restitution," the mechanism by which the stomach and duodenum can quickly repair minor peptic lesions.[8] As mentioned previously, normal individuals must weather intermittent periods of gastroesophageal reflux. The barriers that the esophagus uses to accomplish this involve cell membranes resistant to low concentrations of hydrogen ions and tight junctions between adjacent cell membranes to limit movement of these ions through intercellular spaces. Squamous cell membranes also have the capacity, via ionic exchange mechanisms, to rid a cell of hydrogen ions.[8]

CLINICAL FEATURES

Classically, symptoms can usually be divided into symptoms that are either gastrointestinal (GI) (typical) or respiratory (atypical) in nature. GI symptoms are by far, the more common presenting complaints. Typical GI symptoms consist of heartburn (pyrosis) or chest pain, acid regurgitation, and dysphagia. Heartburn often occurs within an hour of eating, during exercise, or while an individual is lying recumbent, especially postpriandially. A patient's quality of life is adversely affected if such heartburn occurs three or more times a week.[44] The heartburn associated with GERD has also been variously described as a dull discomfort, localized pressure, or even a severe squeezing pain across the middle of the chest. This type of pain has been postulated to be the result of acid-induced esophageal spasm. Patients with GERD and angina-like chest pain pose difficult diagnostic challenges; often in these patients, the possibility of cardiac ischemia cannot be safely ruled out during an abbreviated stay in the emergency department.

Acid regurgitation, on the other hand, is often a silent process marked only by the spontaneous taste of acid or bitterness in the mouth or pharynx. It can be precipitated by any movement that increases intraabdominal pressure, such as bending or belching. A less frequent manifestation of regurgitation is water brash, a vagally mediated hypersalivation response to esophageal acidification that may produce up to 10 mL of saliva in 1 min. Dysphagia and odynophagia are insidious markers of more complicated pathology, such as peptic strictures, peristaltic dysfunction, or esophageal ulcers. About 30 percent of all patients with GERD complain of some degree of dysphagia.[45]

GE reflux has long been associated with respiratory diseases and so-called atypical symptoms such as chronic asthma, refractory cough, laryngitis, or wheezing.[46,47] In fact, the prevalence of GE reflux in asthmatics and patients with chronic cough can be as high as 80 and 40 percent, respectively.[48–50] Furthermore, asthmatics tend not to exhibit the classic GI symptoms of GE reflux; GE reflux is, in fact, clinically silent in 24 percent of patients with difficult-to-control asthma.[49] Although both asthma and GERD coexist in many individuals, it is difficult to identify GERD as the etiology of the asthma. Chronic coughing either alone or in combination with other symptoms is estimated to occur in some 10 to 40 percent of GERD patients.[47,51] The pathophysiologic principle in effect here is that the dysfunction of one compartment of the GI tract (in this case the stomach and GE junction) disrupts the function of the more proximal compartment with symptoms that are referable to the pharynx and larynx.[1,52] Further, the cause of this cough can be macro- or microaspiration, an increased bronchial hyperresponsiveness, or a vagally mediated esophageal-tracheobronchial reflex.[10] The latter predominates in patients whose chronic cough remains unexplained even after a thorough systematic evaluation and is postulated to be due to acid stimulation of esophageal nerve endings, with the consequent activation of the cough center.[10]

Other less common atypical symptoms are otolaryngologic in nature due to the refluxed food entering the proximal esophagus and the adjacent hypopharynx.[53,54] These symptoms include laryngeal and tracheal stenosis, globus sensation (a feeling of fullness or a lump in the throat that does not seem to clear despite swallowing), dysphonia, and even chronic coughing. Remarkably, an estimated 4 to 10 percent of patients evaluated by otolaryngologists have GERD.[55] Erosions of dental enamel with concomitant loss of tooth substance and the development of caries are the most frequent oral manifestations of GERD.

Clinical presentation

Typically a patient seeks medical attention for GERD after suffering for 1 to 3 years with the disease.[56] Although some authors suggest that there is no consistent disease progression in GERD or that there is no way to predict a relationship between duration of symptoms and incidence of complications such as esophagitis, ulceration, strictures and bleeding,[57,58] progressive loss of esophageal clearance of gastric contents is commonly associated clinically with severe mucosal injury, repetitive regurgitation, aspiration, and eventually pulmonary failure.[34,59] Stein and colleagues argue that once the antireflux barrier is lost, a relationship does exist between the degree of esophageal mucosal injury sustained and the prevalence of the ineffective barrier[1] (Fig. 13-2). Once the reflux then exceeds the tolerance of the organ's vulnerable epithelium, complications occur. This epithelium, however, does not have to be limited to that of the esophagus, but may be vulnerable epithelium of the larynx, pharynx, or airways.[26] Some frequent complications of GERD are shown in Table 13-3.

Table 13-3 Complications of gastroesophageal reflux disease
Esophagitis
Esophageal ulcers
Peptic strictures
Hemorrhage
Esophageal peristaltic dysfunction
Barrett's metaplasia and dysplasia
Esophageal adenocarcinoma
Noncardiac chest pain
Pulmonary, ear, nose, or throat complaints

When esophagitis does occur, most cases are healed temporarily by medical therapy; however, 80 percent recur chronically when conservative therapy is discontinued.[60] With the exception of esophageal adenocarcinoma, mortality from GERD is uncommon, being estimated at close to 0.1 per 100,000 cases.[56]

Other clinical features

In theory, delayed gastric emptying may have profound deleterious effects and can also exacerbate GERD. It can increase the gastroesophageal pressure gradient; increase gastric volume, which would allow a greater volume of gastric contents to be refluxed; it could increase the frequency of transient LES relaxations; and it can increase the secretion of gastric acid.[11] In reality however, the vast majority of patients do not seem to have delayed gastric emptying. A metanalysis of 30 published studies makes this clear, also indicating that, in some patients, accelerated gastric emptying can occur.[61] Kahrilas and Paldofino also remind us that most patients with gastroparesis do not have esophagitis, which, the authors conclude, suggests that gastric emptying probably has only limited effects on the pathophysiology of GERD.[25]

Selected conditions involving gastroparesis (e.g., gastroparesis diabeticorum, scleroderma, collagen-vascular disease) may be factors contributing to GERD. GERD is observed in 90 percent of patients with scleroderma with a concomitant incompetence of the LES.[25] In addition, scleroderma patients have poor esophageal wall muscle tone and a loss of propulsive and emptying mechanisms to clear esophageal contents. As the disease progresses, there is a resultant atrophy of esophageal wall smooth muscle, with fibrous infiltration making esophageal body contractility even more difficult. GERD in this situation tends to be more recalcitrant and surgical treatments, such as antireflux procedures, are not as effective as they tend to be in patients without scleroderma.[62]

About 50 to 80 percent of pregnant women report heartburn.[63] In addition to the anatomic change caused by a growing uterus, factors associated with increased reflux are also precipitated, such as decreasing LES pressure and slower gastric emptying. Zollinger-Ellison syndrome is another disease entity that may lead to increased GERD, although typically these patients have a primary change in the nature of the refluxate rather than abnormalities of their antireflux barrier.[25] About 42 percent of patients with Zollinger-Ellison syndrome have been found to have endoscopic evidence of reflux esophagitis.[64]

Helicobacter pylori is not associated with GERD; in fact, most epidemiologic studies actually suggest that infection with *H. pylori* has a protective effect for both the development of severe GERD as well as its complications of Barrett's esophagus, dysphagia, and esophageal adenocarcinoma.[65] Moreover, after antibiotic eradication of *H. pylori* infection, there is an increased incidence of both esophagitis[66] and GERD.[67] The theory suggesting a protective effect due to *H. pylori* is further substantiated by data showing improvement in the efficacy of antisecretory therapy for esophagitis and in the maintenance of the remission in the presence of *H. pylori* infection.[68,69]

DIAGNOSTIC MODALITIES

A general approach to the patient presenting with GERD is outlined in Fig. 13-4, a decision-making flowchart. Empiric therapy with proton-pump inhibitors (PPIs) has emerged as an appealing approach to the evaluation of GERD among gastroenterologists, especially since no single test is truly diagnostic of GERD. PPIs were introduced to the United States in 1989 with the promotion of omeprazole.[70] These drugs reduce acid production by as much as 80 to 90 percent in both the basal and postprandial states.[71] This occurs via inhibition of the final common pathway of acid secretion at the H^+, K^+-adenosine triphosphatase (ATPase pump).[72] This was a dramatic improvement over the popular histamine (H_2) antagonists, which had decreased acid secretion by only 30 to 50 percent.[71] The net effect was that medical therapy went from controlling symptoms only in the milder forms of GERD[73] to alleviating symptoms and healing esophagitis in the vast majority of GERD sufferers.[74] Several well-controlled prospective studies have recently examined empiric therapy with PPIs.[75–77] These studies used either endoscopy or pH monitoring as measures of PPI efficacy and reported a 68 to 80 percent sensitivity of diagnosing GERD due to improvement in endoscopy or esophageal pH monitoring. Fass and coworkers even purported the use of omeprazole to be as effective as pH monitoring in diagnosing GERD and stressed the significant cost reductions of this "omeprazole test" versus either endoscopic or pH monitoring modes of diagnosis.[75]

Empiric therapy is recommended to young patients (below 50 to 60 years of age) with clinically suspicious GERD who have no associated "alarm signs or symptoms" (such as bleeding, nausea, vomiting, dysphagia, weight loss, or iron deficiency).[25] It is usually given once a day for 2 to 4 weeks to allow adequate dosing and to provide a reliable response.[25] The response time of empiric PPIs to atypical GERD symptoms is longer than that to typical symptoms, sometimes taking up to 3 months.[25] The PPIs currently on the market include omeprazole (Prilosec), esomeprazole (Nexium), lansoprazole (Prevacid), pantoprazole (Protonix), and rabeprazole (Acidphex). The most frequently reported adverse events with PPIs include headache, diarrhea, and abdominal pain. Symptomatic response to therapy usually occurs in 4 to 8 weeks, but this does not preclude the presence of an esophageal malignancy. In fact, this masking of the symptoms of malignancy and/or Barrett's metaplasia by PPIs does not allow the clinician to diagnose these disorders if they are present. In summary, Kahrilas is correct when he states that knowing the therapeutic response of a GERD patient is useful information, but it does not establish, in and of itself, the correct diagnosis or the best therapeutic option.[26]

For the surgeon who is referred a patient with GERD, preoperative diagnostic studies are imperative not only to verify the diagnosis, but also to detect any confounding functional disorders of the esophagus or stomach that may be contributing factors to GERD as well as to provide information that will be helpful in choosing the most appropriate operative approach. The diagnostic choices have expanded dramatically over the last decade to include 24-h intraesophageal and intragastric pH monitoring, 24-h intraesophageal and intragastric bilimetry, conventional esophageal manometry, vectometry of the lower esophageal sphincter, gastric scintigraphy, upper digestive tract endoscopy, and barium swallow studies.[78] Most surgeons require some combination of the above preoperatively; in our hospital, this usually involves a barium swallow, 24-h pH monitoring, endoscopy, manometry, and gastric scintigraphy.

Barium esophagogram

Although nonspecific, a double-contrast barium esophagogram or "barium swallow" has emerged as a useful initial screening test for GERD. This study is proficient in detecting mucosal alterations, anatomic abnormalities, gross motility disorders, and esophageal wall complications often observed with GERD. It is most useful in demonstrating the presence and length of structural abnormalities such as strictures and hiatal hernia and can give data about the length of the entire esophagus. It is often invaluable in patients who present with dysphagia. It should not be used as the sole diagnostic test preoperatively, since it fails to detect many cases of esophagitis and Barrett's metaplasia, especially in view of the fact that reflux can occur in more than 25 percent of asymptomatic patients.

Figure 13-5 shows a barium swallow of a normal esophagus for reference. Figure 13-6 depicts a patient

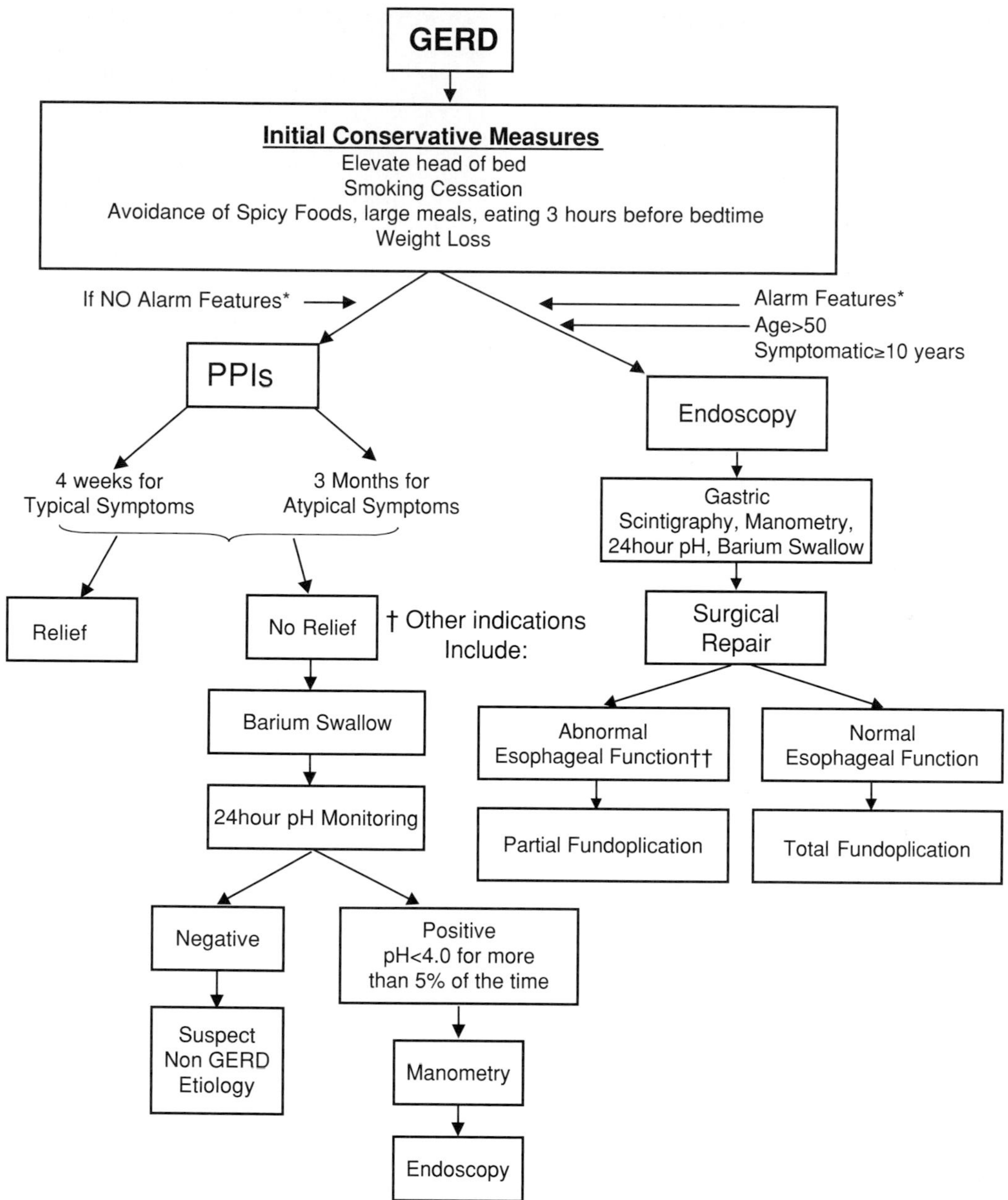

Figure 13-4 Decision-making flowchart.

with GERD who has both a hiatal hernia and a Schatzki B ring.

pH monitoring

Twenty-four-hour pH monitoring is among the most sensitive and specific tests for diagnosing GERD. Ambulatory monitoring for 24 h with an esophageal pH probe involves positioning a thin pH electrode (diameter ~1.2 mm) via the nares to about 5 cm above the manometrically determined GE junction and measuring the changes in pH during normal daily activities. A log is maintained to document symptomatic GERD exacerbations and to correlate these episodes with the patient's activities.

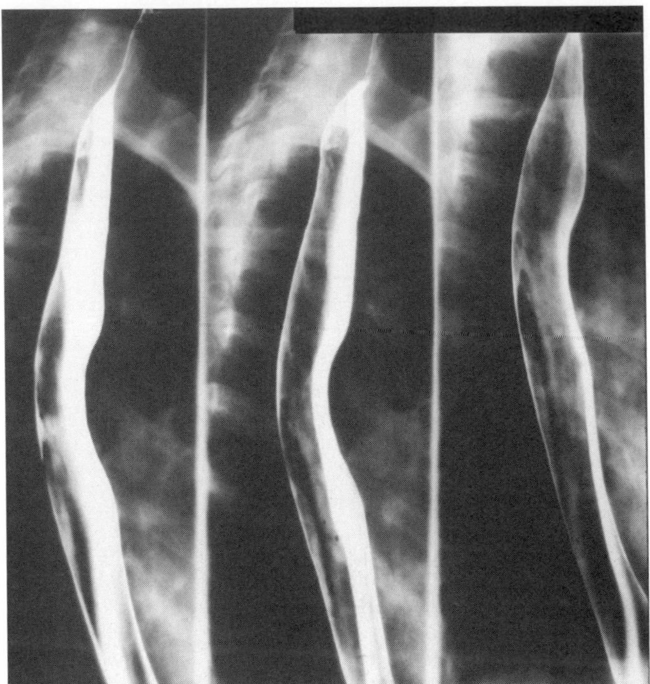

Figure 13-5 Barium esophagogram of a normal esophagus. (Courtesy of Bronwyn Jones, MD, Johns Hopkins Medical Institutions.)

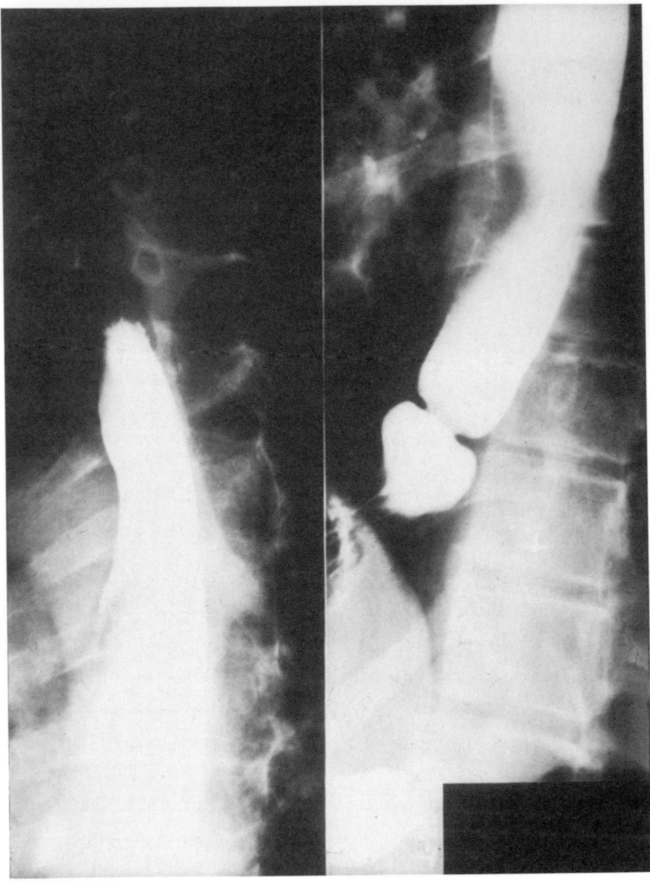

Figure 13-6 Barium esophagogram of a patient with GERD complications of a hiatal hernia and a Schatzki B ring. (Courtesy of Bronwyn Jones, MD, Johns Hopkins Medical Institutions.)

Bielefeldt and associates remind us that it is important for the clinician to realize that pH recordings are directly affected by body position, activity level, certain foods and fluid (especially alcohol), smoking, coughing, vomiting, and so on.[79] Although patients are encouraged to continue with normal diet and activities during monitoring, foods that interfere with the pH probe, such as frozen or exceedingly hot foods, should be avoided.[79] Adverse effects of the probe are minimal except belching and coughing, which are both self-limiting.

A pH test is deemed positive when the pH value is less than 4 for greater than 3.5 to 5 percent of the recording time.[79,80] It is important to realize that since there are no absolute cutoff thresholds, pH testing has limitations on sensitivity, so that up to 25 to 30 percent of patients with GERD are missed because their pH test results are within the normal range.[81–83] In addition, nondiagnostic tests occur in as many as 5 percent of recordings due to failure of the equipment, probe dislocation, or inadvertently wrong probe placement.[79] The pH probe can detect and quantify both acid and alkaline GERD and can, in theory, predict patients most at risk for future complications. Long-term monitoring of esophageal pH can be used not only for diagnostic purposes but also as a means of measuring response to therapy.[84]

Normal individuals typically have less than 50 episodes of reflux in 24 h; each event is short and ends abruptly, with the total reflux time being less than 5 percent of the total recording time. In a typical abnormal 24-h pH study, the classic features of increased number of reflux events are evident, so that the esophageal mucosa is bathed in a pH of less than 4 for over 5 percent of the recording time. Recordings such as these are typically seen in the postprandial period.

Endoscopy

If erosive esophagitis is present, endoscopy is diagnostic of GERD with a specificity almost 90 percent.[25] However, since only 30 to 40 percent of patients even have erosive esophagitis,[25,85,86] the corollary is that endoscopy is a technique with poor sensitivity in GERD.[87,88] Only about 50 percent of patients who complain of heartburn are found to have esophagitis by endoscopic evaluation.[89] Spechler cautions that clinicians should be wary that an endoscopic evaluation does not invariably answer the question, "Does the patient have GERD?"[8] A normal endoscopic exam, for example, does not exclude GERD as the etiology of the symptom complex. He suggests that endoscopy is useful, however, in answering four other questions, "Is there reflux esophagitis? Is the esophagitis severe? Is there an esophageal stricture? Is there Barrett's esophagus?"[8]

Table 13-4	Indications for early endoscopy in patients with suspected gastroesophageal reflux disease
Fever	
Anorexia	
Weight loss	
Dysphagia	
Odynophagia	
Bleeding	

Practice guidelines for the use of endoscopy in GERD were last updated in June 1999; at that time, it was recommended that if empiric therapy is unsuccessful or if patients have symptoms suggesting complicated disease, they should undergo further diagnostic testing such as endoscopy.[90] Furthermore, the guidelines emphasize ruling out Barrett's esophagus in these patients. Spechler suggests that symptoms typical of complicated disease may indicate early endoscopy[8]; these symptoms are listed in Table 13-4. If, on endoscopy, there are findings consistent with severe esophagitis, peptic stricture, Barrett's epithelium, or ulceration, multiple biopsies should be obtained to rule out Barrett's high-grade dysplasia or malignancy. Figures 13-7 and 13-8 depict endoscopic images of typical and severe esophagitis, respectively. The typical histologic appearance of esophagitis is shown in Fig. 13-9.

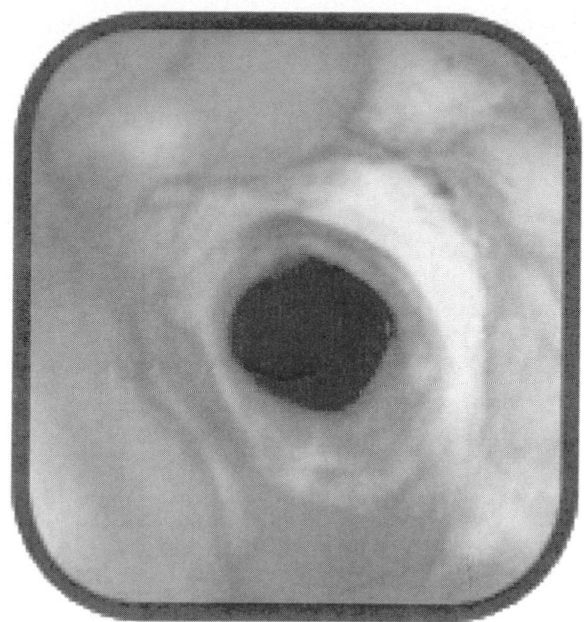

Figure 13-8 Endoscopic appearance of a patient with complications of GERD. (From www.gicare.com. With permission.)

Gastric scintigraphy and manometry

Gastroparesis, especially in combination with other esophageal motility disorders, can lead to an increased risk of GERD and erosive esophagitis. Gastric scintigraphy is the modern diagnostic standard for monitoring both the solid and liquid phases of gastric emptying. A test meal is labeled with a gamma marker and the transit time for this marker to exit the stomach is measured using a gamma camera. As mentioned previously, since the normal peristaltic motility of the tubular esophagus aids in clearance of refluxed gastroduodenal contents, manometric recordings to document motility disturbances are often performed. Most surgeons require

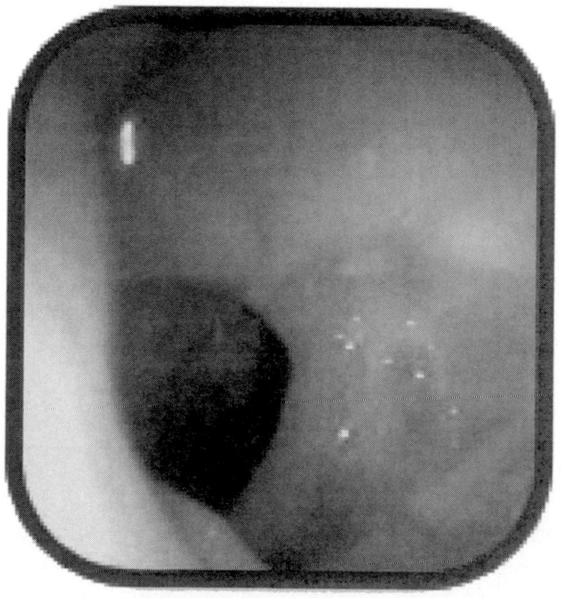

Figure 13-7 Typical endoscopic appearance of a patient with GERD. (From www.gicare.com. With permission.)

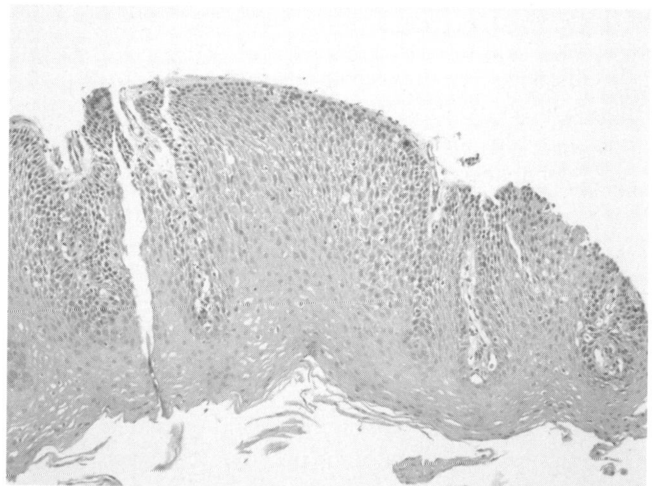

Figure 13-9 Typical histologic section from a patient with GERD. (Courtesy of Elizabeth Montgomery, MD, Johns Hopkins Medical Institutions.)

manometry preoperatively, since a 360-degree fundoplication in the presence of abnormal contractile function may lead to significant postoperative complications such as dysphagia. A 270-degree fundoplication creates a looser fit that should not only adequately prevent gastroduodenal contents from refluxing, but also allow the patient to belch and vomit.

Finally, there are new diagnostic techniques that may, in the near future, translate into the clinic and have a significant impact on medical practice. The Bilitec 2001 (Synectics, Stockholm, Sweden) is a portable spectrophotometer that measures nonacid reflux by monitoring bilirubin as a surrogate marker for bile reflux. Multichannel intraluminal impedance (MII) (Sandhill Scientific Inc., Highlands Ranch, CO) is a new technique allowing the measurement of esophageal volume refluxate. Both techniques assess the role of nonacidic esophageal reflux. Precise evaluation of the competence of the lower esophageal sphincter by esophageal vectometry may permit the identification of patients who are liable to experience recurrence of their reflux symptoms on discontinuing medical therapy.

MEDICAL THERAPY

General conservative measures for GERD include elevating the head of bed when going to sleep, avoiding sleeping within 3 h after eating, not wearing tight clothing, and avoiding bending or stooping. Patients should be encouraged to lose weight (a practical recommendation is 20 lb per 6-month period); to stop smoking and drinking alcohol; to eat small, frequent meals; to avoid spicy foods and citrus fruits, which irritate the esophageal mucosa; as well as to avoid fast foods and drugs that can lower LES pressure (Table 13-1). Most of these maneuvers promote esophageal clearance or limit the actual occurrence of the gastroesophageal reflux event. Smoking cessation, for example, enhances the clearance of acid by increasing salivation and reducing the frequency of reflux.[7]

In addition, many patients now self-medicate, a trend recently enhanced by large, aggressive marketing campaigns to promote H_2 receptor antagonists as medications to relieve "heartburn." Over-the-counter Pepcid AC, Tagamet HB, and Zantac are all big sellers. Although they can offer symptomatic relief, patients may achieve the same result by eating fewer processed, fatty foods and adhering to other conservative measures. For mild heartburn, the use of chewing gum or oral lozenges may augment salivation and help minimize acid reflux.[7]

Medical therapy has often precipitated heated discussions in the past between surgeons and gastroenterologists, with the former arguing that only surgery prevents both gastric acid and pancreaticobiliary reflux, while medical therapy only inhibits acid reflux. In the modern therapeutic era of PPIs, however, the clinical observation has been that previously difficult-to-heal esophagitis, esophageal ulcers, or reflux symptoms are now successfully managed medically, albeit with high-frequency dosing.[91] Two important studies have improved our understanding of this paradox. Using omeprazole, both Champion and associates and Marshall and coworkers found that omeprazole was equally effective in preventing both gastric and biliary reflux.[92,93]

Table 13-5	Common reasons for treatment failures in gastrointestinal reflux disease ("golden rule")
Incorrect diagnosis	
Inadequate acid suppression (much less common with use of proton pump inhibitors)	
Noncompliance with drug regimen (cost versus psychosocial issues)	
Pill-induced injury	
Hypersecretor of acid (Zollinger-Ellison syndrome)	
Delayed gastric emptying	

This has led Richter to state that, as a clinical gastroenterologist, he has become so enamored with PPIs that he has evolved a "golden rule" contending that any lack of improvement in a patient on PPIs strongly suggests that a disease other than GERD is present (Table 13-5).[72] Although many patients do obtain symptomatic relief of GERD and healing of their esophagitis with present medical therapy, the long-term risks of these expensive medications are unknown. Richter reminds surgeons that although an operation offers a potential "cure" for GERD, paradoxically patients who respond best to PPIs have the most favorable surgical outcomes.[77] Clearly, both gastroenterologists and surgeons must work together in treating this disease and openly discuss with each patient the unique, individual circumstances specific to his or her case that may indicate either long-term medical therapy or a surgical correction.

SURGICAL THERAPY

Indications for antireflux procedure

Most indications for an antireflux procedure are relative indications since, in the absence of surgery, the condition rarely results in serious morbidity or mortality.[94] These relative indications are usually due to mechanical problems, intractable medical therapy issues, or due to complications of GERD. They are outlined in Table 13-6.

The surgeon's most challenging decision about operative therapy for this disorder concerns the patient without mechanical considerations or GERD complications. In the era of PPIs, those patients with uncomplicated reflux must make a decision about whether or not to have surgery based usually on their lack of current symptomatic relief, reduced quality of life, or the inconvenience of medical therapy. The surgeon must be clear to

Table 13-6 Relative indications for antireflux surgery

Large mechanical defect, such as a hiatal hernia
Paraesophageal hiatal hernia
Poorly controlled symptoms, especially after 3 months of medical therapy
Persistent mucosal injury: esophagitis, stricture, aspiration, bleeding, Barrett's, ulcer
As an alternative to long-term medical therapy

these patients when giving informed consent for the procedure that there are no valid data adequately comparing modern medical and surgical therapy and that, even with laparoscopic or robotic techniques and in experienced hands, surgical intervention is accompanied by a small mortality rate of 0.2 percent.[7,95] Ironically, patients who respond well to PPIs are also the same patients who fare well with antireflux surgery.[72] At any rate, the newer laparoscopic or robotic approaches are allowing for earlier operations on younger patients who choose not to endure lifelong medical therapy. Decreased median hospital stays and reduced postoperative pain[97] as compared with the open surgical equivalent, further beguile both patients and referring physicians.

Antireflux operations: principles

Two decades ago, it was relatively rare for a patient with early GE reflux to be referred for surgical intervention. The introduction of laparoscopic fundoplication by Dallemagne[98] has changed this significantly. Although long-term durability of results remains to be proven, laparoscopic Nissen fundoplication has become the gold standard for most surgeons contemplating surgical treatment of GERD. Although controversies still exist,[99] Catarci and colleagues, in their metanalysis of 25 randomized controlled trials and 41 papers published from 1974 to 2002, found that the benefits of the laparoscopic approach involved significantly lower operative morbidity, shorter postoperative stays, and less time away from work.[100] Important outcome measures such as the incidence of recurrence, reoperation due to failure of the fundoplication, operative mortality, incidence of dysphagia, and bloating did not differ between open and laparoscopic techniques. The popularity of this procedure continues to increase, and the reduced operative morbidity has attracted even more patients. Most of the pioneering "open" operations for GERD are now of historical interest only (Table 13-7). Especially innovative work was performed by Ronald Belsey and Lucius Hill, of Bristol, England, and Seattle, Washington, respectively. Both men developed effective procedures for hiatus hernias and GERD through the open thoracic and abdominal approaches, respectively.

The surgical principles of the open procedures, however, have remained unchanged in the laparoscopic setting.

Table 13-7 Old and new antireflux procedures for gastroesophageal reflux disease

Old terminology	New terminology
Nissen	Complete fundoplication
Nissen-Rosetti	Complete fundoplication
Hill	Complete fundoplication
Belsey	Partial fundoplication
Dor	Partial fundoplication
Toupet	Partial fundoplication

1. Restore the anatomic and physiologic relationships of the LES at the gastroesophageal junction. If there is a hiatal hernia, this involves reducing the hernia.
2. Increase the intraabdominal esophageal length.
3. Tighten the hiatus to prevent recurrent herniation of the gastroesophageal junction.
4. Protect the vagus nerve.
5. Create an antireflux valve that will prevent reflux but allow physiologic functions such as swallowing, vomiting, and belching. This is done with a complete 360-degrees wrap (normal esophageal motility) or a partial 270-degrees wrap (dysfunctional esophagus).
6. Esophageal resection should be performed rarely.

Esophageal resection is reserved for (1) end-stage GERD with a totally unyielding (fibrotic) esophagus, (2) Barrett's esophagus with high-grade dysplasia or frank malignancy, and (3) patients with a history of multiple unsuccessful antireflux procedures.

In addition, Ginsberg and Pearson advocate that performance of the correct surgical procedure is also predicated on consideration of whether or not significant esophageal shortening has occurred.[94] Esophageal shortening is typically the esophageal response to chronic panmural inflammation. It is also commonly seen with Barrett's esophagus.[101] If there is esophageal shortening, an intraoperative decision must be made as to whether or not fundoplication can be done tension-free with or without an esophageal lengthening procedure.[94]

Operative approach for laparoscopic nissen fundoplication

Before beginning, the stomach is fully decompressed with a nasal or orogastric tube. After positioning the patient in a modified lithotomy position and establishing a pneumoperitoneum of 15 mmHg intraabdominal pressure, five trocar sites are placed (three 10-mm and two 5-mm). The operation is begun by effectuating adequate exposure of the right and left crus. On the right, a fan retractor is deployed to retract the left hepatic lobe, the gastrohepatic ligament is incised, and the right crus and esophagus are revealed with sharp and blunt dissection (Fig. 13-10). Pitfalls here include failure to identify the crus and damage to adjoining structures in the lesser omentum, such as an aberrant left hepatic artery.[102] Identification of the left crus is done by incising the

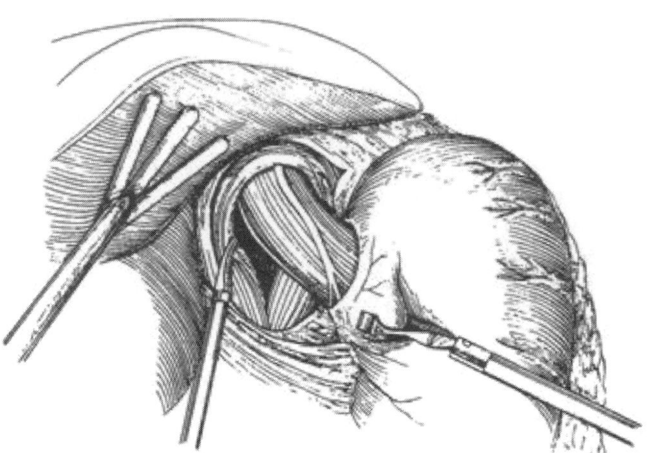

Figure 13-10 Exposure of the right and left crus. (Reprinted from Freeman et al. Ed. Mark Ferguson. Laparoscopic Nissen Fundoplication. www.ctsnet.org. Accessed August 30, 2004.)

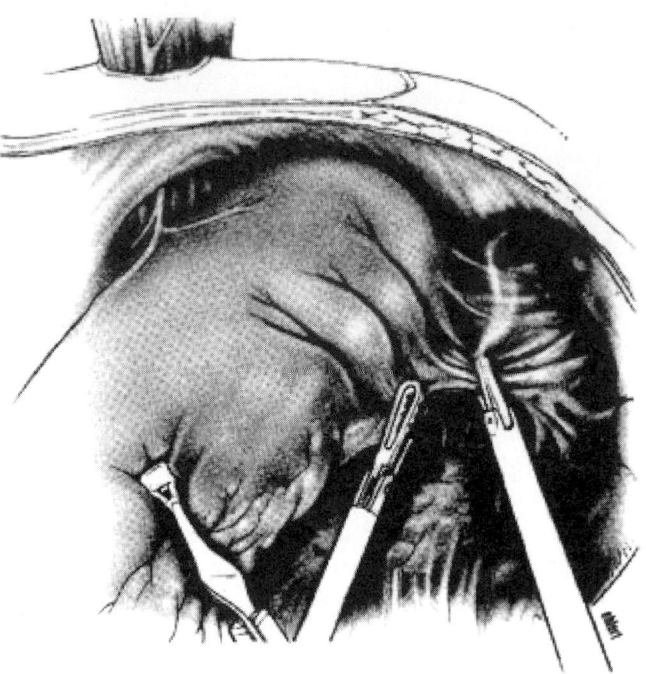

Figure 13-11 Using the harmonic scalpel, the gastric fundus is mobilized by dividing the short gastrics. (From Townsend et al. Hiatal hernia and gastroesophageal reflux disease. In: *Sabiston Textbook of Surgery: The Biological Basis of Modern Surgical Practice,* 16th ed. Philadelphia: Saunders; 2000:761. With permission.)

phrenoesophaeal ligament and peritoneum overlying the esophagus followed by blunt dissection. Blunt dissection is carried out circumferentially and the esophagus is mobilized and circled with a Penrose drain, with care given to the posterior vagus. Once the crura have been adequately exposed, any hiatal hernias are reduced and the esophageal hiatus is closed. The closure of the crura is a critical step and can be done with 2-0 Prolene sutures after the orogastric tube has been removed and replaced with a 56F Maloney bougie.[102] Bites of the crura must be sufficient but not so deep as to injure the aorta on the left or the inferior vena cava on the right. The closure should be snug but not too tight. The fundus of the stomach is then mobilized by dividing the short gastric vessels, usually using a harmonic scalpel (Fig. 13-11). The fundus must be able to be brought tension-free behind the esophagus with a Babcock clamp and graspers (Fig. 13-12). A tension-free fundoplication is created by suturing the anterior and posterior fundus for a length of about 2 cm using 3-0 or 4-0 silk sutures (Fig. 13-13). In order to minimize the chance of esophageal perforation, one must avoid using sutures from the wrap to the lower esophagus (even pledgeted sutures) or rough manipulation of the lower esophagus using the grasping laparoscopic instruments.

Discharge of the patient usually occurs after 2 days if the patient remains on the normal postoperative pathway. Any complaints of dysphagia are normally temporary and resolve within weeks postoperatively.

Complete versus partial fundoplication

If there is preoperative evidence of abnormal esophageal motility on manometric studies or of end-stage GERD such as strictures or Barrett's esophagus, many surgeons have preferred to perform a partial fundoplication because

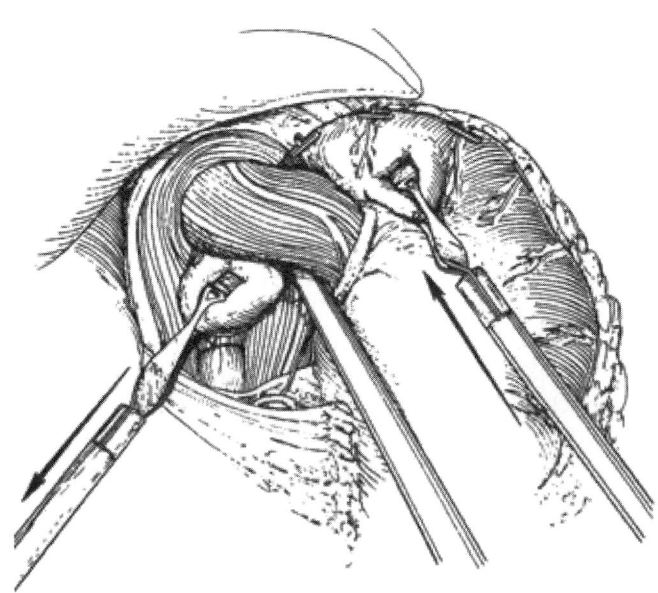

Figure 13-12 Creating the fundoplication (From Freeman et al. Ed. Mark Ferguson. Laparoscopic Nissen Fundoplication. www.ctsnet.org, August 30, 2004.)

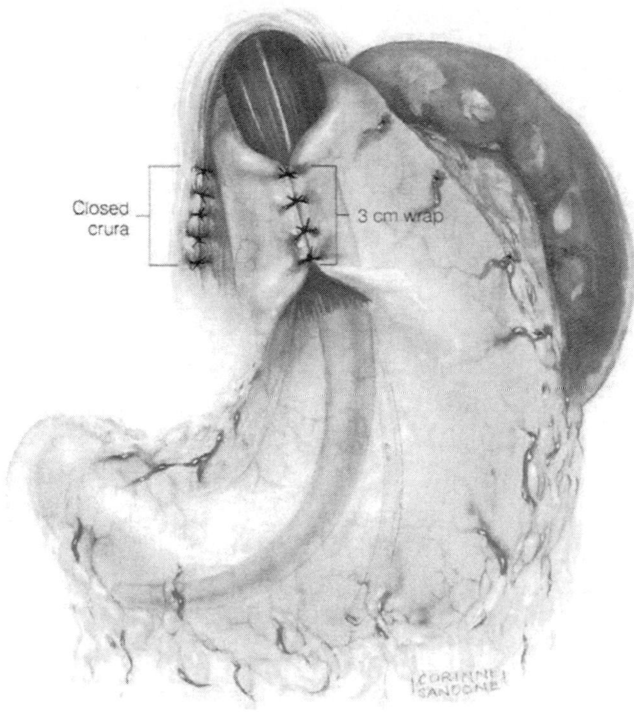

Figure 13-13 The completed Nissen complete fundoplication. (From Cameron JL, Sandone C. Atlas of Surgery: The Esophagus, the Stomach, the Duodenum, the Spleen, Laparoscopic Cholecystectomy December 1994. With permission.)

of the worry that a complete fundoplication would be obstructive and result in clinically evident symptoms of delayed esophageal emptying. A laparoscopic partial fundoplication (Toupet), which involves a partial posterior fundoplication (Fig. 13-14) has been the surgery of choice in this scenario. But since preoperative manometric abnormalities are not predictive of postoperative dysphagia,[103] there has been a search for evidence-based reasoning behind the operative approach to these patients. Data are accumulating from randomized controlled clinical trials (RCT) comparing partial and total fundoplications.[100] In a recent large RCT of laparoscopic complete (Nissen) versus laparocopic partial (Toupet) fundoplication procedures, there were no differences in recurrent GERD symptoms or postoperative 24-h pH tests in these patients.[104,105] There were more postoperative manometric abnormalities as well as more new-onset dysphagia, however, in the Nissen group. Since the follow-up of only 4 months in the trial is too short to yield definitive findings, evidence-based decisions must wait for a longer period to draw conclusions on the real efficacy of laparoscopic Nissen versus Toupet in these patients.

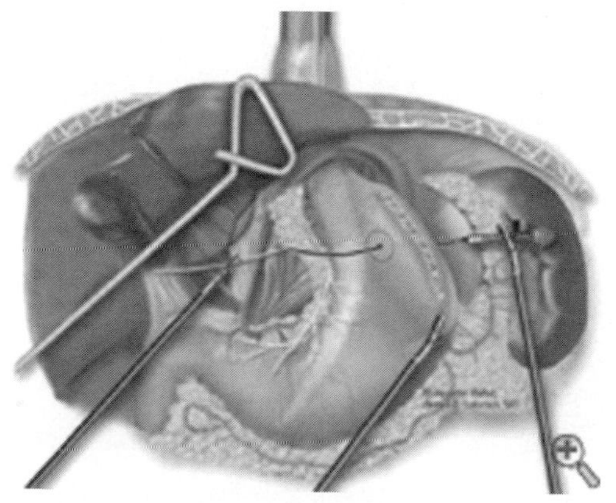

Figure 13-14 The completed Toupet partial fundoplication (From www.laparoscopyhospital.com.)

Operative approach for laparoscopic toupet partial fundoplication

The surgical approach involves the same steps as a laparoscopic Nissen procedure except that the posterior wrap of the stomach is only 270 degrees and not the full 360 degrees (Fig. 13-14). The fixation of the fundus to the left and right crura provides both the stability and strength for the wrap. This is performed with 1-cm bites of seromuscular layers of the gastric fundus to the anterior aspect of the crura. Usually three sutures are placed into each crus at approximately 1-cm intervals. Although this wrap also involves fixing the esophagus to the wrap with one or two sutures, these esophageal sutures should not be full-thickness or used to provide "strength" to the repair.

Collis gastroplasty

Since many fundoplications fail due to acquired esophageal shortening, the Collis gastroplasty technique should be in the thoracic surgeon's armamentarium. Yau and associates, in examining 100 patients, compared esophageal length and found that those with the shortest esophagi had a recurrence rate of 8 percent, versus 2 percent in those with longer esophagi.[106] A Collis gastroplasty "lengthens" the esophagus and allows the fundoplication to be performed tension-free around the new "neoesophagus." During laparoscopy, however, it may be difficult to appreciate a shortened esophagus due to diaphragmatic elevation from carbon dioxide insufflation. Shortening of the esophagus is usually a result of fibrosis from long-standing severe reflux and is not present in patients with symptoms of only short duration. Important factors identified to be associated with the presence of esophageal shortening and thus predictive of the need for a Collis gastroplasty include redo antireflux procedure, a paraesophageal hernia, Barrett's esophagus, an irreducible hernia, and a stricture.[107,108]

Operative approach for laparoscopic collis gastroplasty

The procedure begins as with the Nissen fundoplication except that with the laparoscopic Collis, it is absolutely

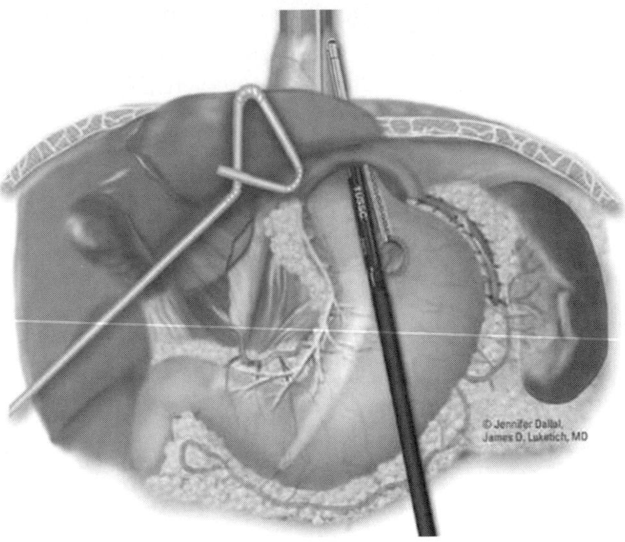

Figure 13-15 Laparoscopic Collis gastroplasty stapled window step. (www.laparoscopy.net)

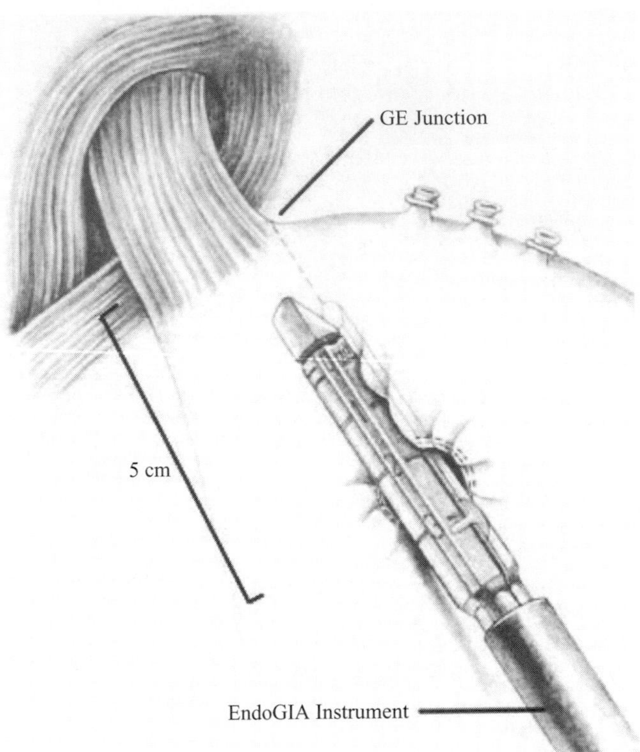

Figure 13-16 Laparoscopic Collis gastroplasty linear stapler step. (www.laparoscopy.net)

critical that the exact location of the esophageal junction be determined. Since the stomach must be very mobile, the short gastric vessels are taken, and extensive dissection of both the lesser curvature as well as the posterior aspect of the stomach is encouraged. A bougie (no. 54 or 60) is inserted into the esophagus and through to the stomach in order to guide the placement of a surgical stapling device capable of performing a circular anastomosis. As shown in Fig. 13-15, the stapling instrument is pushed right against the bougie, the anterior and posterior gastric walls are secured in the instrument, and the stapler is fired, leaving a 2.5-cm round stapled window. An endoscopic linear stapling device is then inserted into the newly formed circular window, positioned along the bougie parallel to the lesser curve, and fired (Fig. 13-16). In this way a 5-cm gastric tube of neoesophagus from the esophageal junction can be created to allow a tension-free fundoplication to be performed. A standard Nissen fundoplication technique is then used to complete the procedure.

Endoscopic approaches

The endoscopic full-thickness plication device is designed to inhibit reflux with a single plication near the gastroesophageal junction. These first-generation endoscopic instruments, introduced by Swain in 1986, are essentially sewing devices attached to the ends of video endoscopes.[109] They allow the endoscopist to perform a full-thickness plication of the proximal stomach by placing stitches below the LES (Fig. 13-17). This may improve the competency of the gastroesophageal barrier by restoring the valvular mechanism of the gastroesophageal junction and helping to reduce the pressure against the LES. General anesthesia is not used, there are no surgical incisions, and—in pilot studies—these procedures have proved to reduce symptoms and medication use in patients with GERD.[110,111]

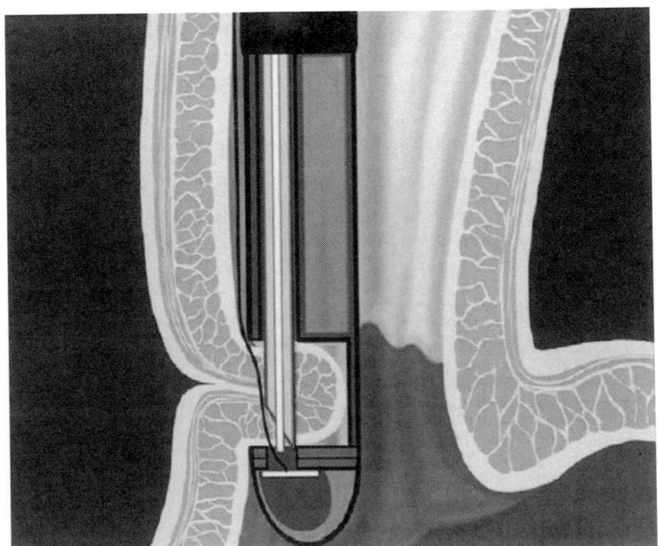

Figure 13-17 The endoscopic cinch placing a suture below the gastroesophageal junction. (From Oleynikov et al.[112] With permission.)

Other alternatives to laparoscopic surgery include the use of endoscopic radiofrequency energy and the injection of silicon-type polymer into the gastroesophageal junction.[112] The former, known, as the Stretta procedure, has been pioneered by Utley and is based on augmenting the LES due to scar formation from multiple radiofrequency-induced thermal lesions.[113] The latter, first reported by O'Conner and Lehman,[114] creates a sclerosed, stronger LES after endoscopic polymer injection.

OUTCOMES/PROGNOSIS

Antireflux surgery outcomes are generally favorable, but long-term follow-up studies have pointed to the persistence or return of GERD symptoms (to prompt daily PPIs) in about one-third of patients.[115,116] The most common early postoperative symptom after laparoscopic antireflux surgery appears to be dysphagia, occurring in about 20 percent of patients.[117] In fact, the existence of symptomatic dysphagia preoperatively was the best predictor of postoperative dysphagia.[79] As time elapsed from the date of surgery, however, only 6 percent of patients complained of long-term dysphagia.[117] Over 90 percent of patients with postoperative dysphagia can be treated expectantly, with recalcitrant patients being reserved for either endoscopic dilation or surgical revision (<1 percent).[117] Other long-term complications after antireflux surgery include early satiety in 49 percent of patients, abdominal bloating in 36 percent, an inability to vomit in 31 percent, diarrhea in 20 percent, nausea in 8 percent, and recurrent reflux in 8 percent.[118,119] In the majority of cases, these symptoms occur within the first 2 years postoperatively.[118,120] The management of persistent symptoms postoperatively begins with a careful evaluation of the postoperative neoanatomy along with its resultant physiology to determine whether acid reflux is indeed controlled. Often recurrent or persistent GERD in the presence of an anatomically pristine fundoplication indicates the reintroduction of medical therapy. The most frequent causes of reoperation for failure of a fundoplication is the disruption of the wrap, followed by breakdown of the crural repair, slipped wrap, and finally a too loosely or too tightly wrapped fundoplication.[118]

In general, redo surgery is approached via open technique, although there are many reports of successful redo laparoscopic approaches.[121–123] In almost all cases, the wrap is densely adherent to the liver; often, identifying and preserving the vagus is extremely challenging, since it can be anatomically displaced. Avoiding iatrogenic perforations of the stomach and esophagus are challenging yet critical, since this can affect operative mortality directly.[118] Outcomes of redo surgery are in the main poorer than for the initial surgery.

Table 13-8 Motility disorders that can cause esophageal dysphagia
Achalasia
Diffuse esophageal spasm
Nutcracker esophagus

PRIMARY ESOPHAGEAL DYSMOTILITY DISORDERS

INTRODUCTION

Most commonly with esophageal dysmotility disorders, the patient presents with dysphagia. These dysmotility disorders can either be primary or secondary in etiology. The former denote no relation to any systemic disease, whereas the latter are always associated with another condition. Primary motility disorders usually associated with esophageal dysphagia are listed in Table 13-8.

The main diagnostic tools used to evaluate esophageal motility disorders continue to be fluoroscopy, barium swallow, and manometry as well as endoscopy, especially to rule out the presence of malignancy. Manometry in particular is critical to our ability to diagnose and understand esophageal motility. It involves the recording of pressure within the esophagus and can evaluate the action of pressure waves produced by smooth muscle in the main body of the esophagus as well as at the LES.

The apparatus consists of thin tubing, inserted via nose or mouth, with openings at various locations in the esophagus. A pH probe is also part of the equipment.

The openings in the tubing sense the esophageal pressure in various locations and transmit information to a computer that records pressures on moving graph paper. Wave patterns are compared to normalized samples and evaluated for abnormalities. Patients have nothing by mouth for 8 h before the test; the procedure itself is usually safe, with minimal discomfort such as gagging. During normal esophageal peristalsis, there is an ordered, progressive esophageal pressure wave that propulses food down the length of the esophagus.

ACHALASIA

Achalasia is a motility disorder of the esophagus characterized by the loss of neurons from the myenteric plexus, which results in aperistalsis of the esophageal body, failure of the LES to relax with swallowing, and elevated LES pressures. The cardinal finding of this disease entity is the absence of peristalsis in the esophageal body; this alone is sufficient to make the diagnosis of achalasia. The incidence of this disorder is approximately 1 to 2 persons per 200,000 population,[124] with both sexes equally affected. Familial cases comprise less than 1 percent of the total disease prevalence.[125]

This disorder has a colorful past, with one of the first recorded descriptions attributed to Thomas Willis, who wrote the following of achalasia in 1679[126]: "the mouth of the stomach [cardia] being always closed either by a tumor or palsie, nothing could be admitted into the ventricle [stomach] unless it were violently opened."

Willis's prescribed treatment consisted of dilating the dysfunctional LES with a whalebone fitted with a piece of sponge at the end. His patient fared well, using the device daily for 15 years.[126]

Dilatation, with occasional modifications such as the transgastric approach of Mikulicz, remained the mainstay of therapy until the early twentieth century, when cardioplasty became the procedure of choice.[126] Despite Heller's development of the esophageal myotomy procedure in 1913, cardioplasty did not fall into disfavor until 1949, when Barrett and Franklin pointed out the late reflux-related complications in patients who had undergone these procedures. The modern surgical approach is a modification of the Heller myotomy as developed in 1923 by Zaaijer, who simplified the technique from a double to a single extramucosal myotomy.[126]

Pathophysiology

Under the microscope, patients with achalasia have inflammation of the myenteric plexus with associated fibrosis, depletion, and eventual loss of ganglion cells. On careful inspection, the infiltrate consists of activated T-cell lymphocytes surrounding degenerating nerve fibers[131,132] and inhibitory ganglion cells.[133,134] Electron microscopy reveals Wallerian degeneration of myelin sheaths and disruption of axonal membranes.[135] The exact etiology of achalasia is unknown. It is uncertain, for example, whether the inflammatory process results in secondary destruction of ganglion cells/neurons or if it is due to an infectious or autoimmune process. Suffice it to say that a loss of inhibitory ganglion cells in the region of the LES results in the latter's dysfunction and that prolonged LES dysfunction is accompanied by esophageal aperistalsis and dilation presumably due to degeneration of ganglion cells in the esophageal body itself.[127] This aperistalsis is not reversible with known medical therapy.

Clinical features

The clinical history is often misleading, since patients usually adapt well to this slow, progressive disease and may not seek medical treatment for 5 to 6 years after onset of symptoms. Patients typically present between 20 and 40 years of age. Almost all have dysphagia, especially to solid foods, and this is progressive, with liquid dysphagia developing in as many as two-thirds of patients.[127] In fact, the presence of the two symptoms together has been shown to have some utility diagnostically, especially in differentiating achalasia from obstructive strictures or tumors.[128] Another diagnostic pearl involves the ability of some patients to tolerate a meal and alleviate retrosternal fullness with slow, deliberate swallowing of their food.[127] In addition to dysphagia, regurgitation and chest pain can occur; the three symptoms in combination can eventually lead to weight loss, usually a sign of advanced disease. Other symptoms can include nocturnal coughing as well as bronchopulmonary complications.[129] There is about a 5 percent chance of developing esophageal squamous carcinoma of the midesophagus (presumably due to chronic inflammation and esophagitis), but this usually occurs late, with the best study to date showing a mean interval between the onset of dysphagia and esophageal cancer of nearly 20 years.[130]

Diagnostic modalities

Physical findings are mostly unremarkable. A chest radiograph is usually normal, but it can be useful if the disease is more advanced. In these cases, a megaesophagus with vertical shadow along the length of the mediastinum, an air-fluid level in the posterior mediastinum, or aspiration pneumonitis, may be present, and there may be no gastric bubble.

A barium swallow has a sensitivity of approximately 75 percent, mainly because it misses early disease.[136] When positive, it will demonstrate narrowing of the distal esophagus (the so-called bird's beak, because it resembles the beak of the common North American songbirds) and dilation of the proximal esophagus (Fig. 13-18). Concomitant administration of amyl nitrate may

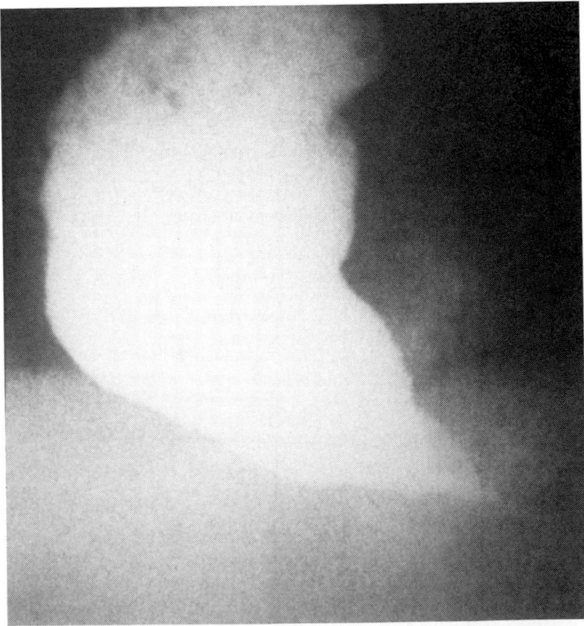

Figure 13-18 Barium esophagogram of a patient with achalasia. (Courtesy of Bronwyn Jones, MD, the Johns Hopkins Medical Institutions.)

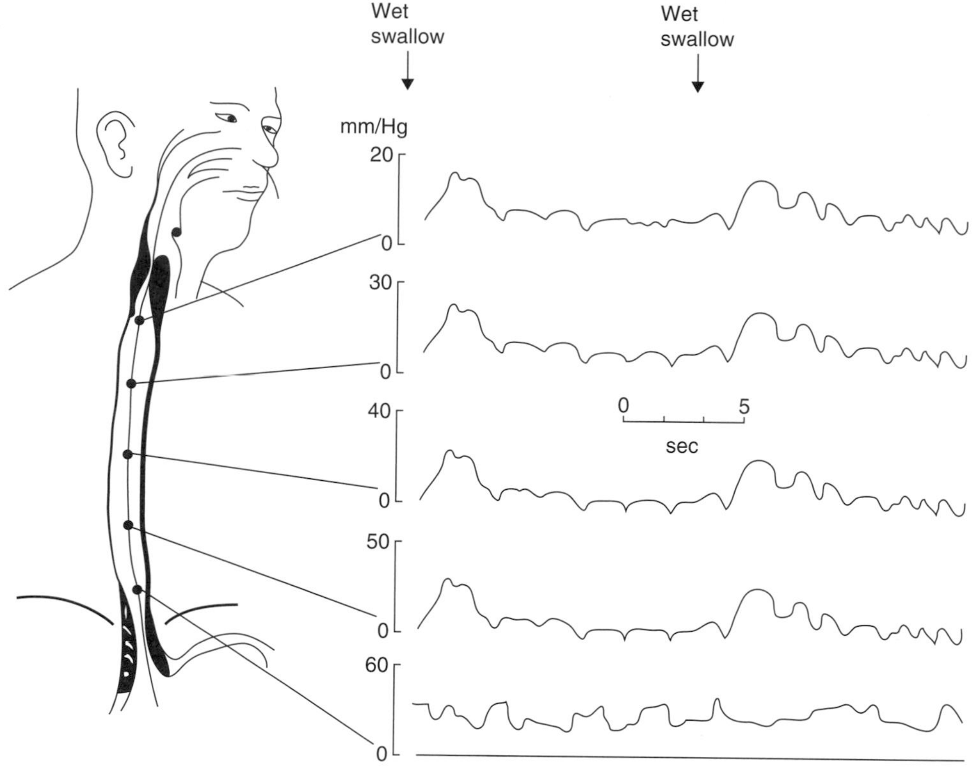

Figure 13-19 Manometry tracing of a patient with achalasia. (From www.ctsnet.org)

help in differentiating achalasia from pseudoachalasia during an upper GI series. Endoscopy for achalasia is often normal but should be pursued to exclude the presence of distal esophageal cancer. There should be some resistance at the LES, but not enough to prevent passage of the endoscope. If the latter is encountered, another diagnosis should be considered, such as pseudoachalasia or malignancy. All abnormal mucosal findings should be biopsied. Manometry, however, is the gold standard for diagnostic tests of achalasia. The LES, due to its incomplete relaxation with swallowing, has a high pressure, usually in excess of 26 mmHg. The esophageal body proper exhibits simultaneous isobaric pressure waves (Fig. 13-19). In addition, there is a more vigorous form of the disease featuring high-amplitude (>50 mmHg) simultaneous pressure waves in the esophageal body.

The differential diagnosis of achalasia is broad. Table 13-9 lists these disorders along with their distinguishing diagnostic features.

Medical therapy

At present, the degenerative defect of achalasia that pertains to the neuronal destruction of ganglia and neurons in the myenteric plexus cannot be restored. Medical and surgical treatment is therefore directed mainly toward palliation of symptoms and the prevention of complications.[127] Overall, treatment centers on the relief of LES obstruction. The four palliative measures commonly employed include medication, botulinum toxin injection, mechanical dilatation, and surgical myotomy.

In general, these measures work by their direct effect of relaxing the smooth muscle of the LES and they do alleviate symptoms in approximately 70 percent of patients.[137] Long-term administration of pharmacologic agents has limited utility; this treatment modality is reserved for those unable to benefit from more invasive therapies, such as the elderly or patients with debilitating

Table 13-9 Differential diagnosis of achalasia
Benign disorders
Strictures, rings, hiatal hernia, diverticula, benign tumors
–Identified with cine esophagram or esophagoduodenoscopy (EGD)
Pseudoachalasia
–Functional obstruction of LES by direct tumor invasion of muscle
Paraneoplastic syndromes
–Bronchogenic, gastric, pancreatic
Chagas' disease
–*T. cruzi* parasite can be found in blood and serology
–Cardiac, GI, GU, respiratory abnormalities
Other motility abnormalities
–Manometry
Malignancy
–Identified with esophagoduodenoscopy (EGD)

comorbidities. Perhaps the most effective agents are either the nitrates, such as isosorbide dinitrate 5 to 10 mg given sublingually before meals, or calcium channel blockers, such as nifedipine 10 to 30 mg taken orally a half hour before meals. An alternative is nitroglycerin 0.4 mg, again given sublingually and shortly before meals as well as at night. Relief of symptoms tends to occur in those with minimal esophageal dilation (< 5 cm).[138] The main side effect of the nitrates, in particular, is headache, which can prevent continued use of these agents in as many as one-third of patients.[127]

Botulinum toxin injection

The endoscopic injection of 80 to 100 U of botulinum toxin type A (Botox, from *Clostridium botulinum*) in the LES is effective in as many as 75 percent of patients.[139] Its mechanism of action depends on its ability to bind to presynaptic cholinergic receptors and irreversibly block the release of acetylcholine. This is usually a temporary effect (new axonal sprouts gradually form), with most patients requiring a second injection within a year.[140,141] Complications of the procedure are generally minimal and may include chest discomfort and occasional rash.[127] A disadvantage of the technique is an increased perforation rate when a subsequent myotomy is performed for more permanent symptom relief. This is presumably due to an obscure submucosal plane that makes dissection in this area difficult at best.

Endoscopic balloon dilatation

Pneumatic dilatation involves the inflation of a balloon at the gastroesophageal junction with a forcible rupture of the LES. There is no consensus concerning the ideal inflation pressure or duration of inflation, although, in general, dilation to at least 3 cm is necessary to tear the circular muscle to effectuate any long-term reduction in LES pressure.[127] A Gastrografin swallow is performed immediately after the procedure to look for mucosal tears or perforation. Since delayed perforations do occur, an observation period of approximately 6 h is mandatory in most centers. Response rates generally exceed 85 percent, with older patients who have a longer duration of symptoms faring better than younger ones.[142] Response rates do not seem to be determined by the degree of esophageal dilation achieved during the procedure.[143] About 17 percent of patients need repeat dilatations, and the efficacy of these retreatments is only half that of the original procedure.[144]

Since the risk of perforations is low (1 to 3 percent) and mortality is a rare event, occurring in 0.3 percent, endoscopic pneumatic dilatation has become the most common initial treatment of achalasia.[145–147] Furthermore, unlike the injection of botulinum toxin, it does not adversely affect later myotomy.

Surgical therapy

The most commonly performed surgical procedure for achalasia is a modified Heller myotomy, or an esophagomyotomy with an antireflux procedure. Usually this is performed through a transthoracic approach with a partial fundoplication. In recent years, however, thoracoscopic and laparoscopic techniques have gained more popularity and have achieved comparable outcome results. The modified Heller myotomy involves a limited division of the LES muscle in a controlled fashion. The main controversies surrounding the procedure include the exact approach, extent of myotomy, and whether or not an antireflux procedure is required.

A brief description of the procedure follows. After the insertion of a double-lumen endotracheal tube to deflate the left lung, a left posterolateral thoracotomy is employed. The inferior pulmonary ligament is divided and the lung is retracted anterosuperiorly. Opening of the mediastinal pleura then exposes the esophagus, which is encircled with a 0.25-in. Penrose drain. The phrenoesophageal membrane is incised circumferentially and the esophageal smooth muscle layer separated from its mucosa laterally for a distance of about 10 cm. The distal end of the myotomy extends about 1 cm onto the stomach. The cardia is reconstructed with a modified Belsey or Dor partial fundoplication. If an epiphrenic diverticulum is present, it should be excised and a myotomy performed on the opposite side of the esophagus.

Outcomes/prognosis

A recent metanalysis of the modified Heller myotomy in three series with a 10-year follow-up reported that 66 percent of patients had good to excellent late outcomes.[148–150] Late complications of the procedure include GERD, the development of Barrett's esophagus, peptic strictures, high-grade dysphagia, and frank carcinoma. Only 10 to 15 percent of patients required additional surgery. Rarely is a complete esophageal resection indicated for achalasia. Patients contemplated for surgery usually present with large, dilated, tortuous esophagi that respond poorly to either dilatation or surgical myotomy. Other indications for surgical resection include multiple prior failed myotomies, reflux injury caused either by an incomplete wrap or too much wrap, and the persistence of significant reflux symptoms in patients after surgical myotomy or dilatation.

OTHER MOTILITY DISORDERS OF THE ESOPHAGUS

Diffuse esophageal spasm (DES)

Pathophysiology and clinical features

This is a motor disorder with an excess number of large-amplitude, long-duration, repetitive contractions of esophageal smooth muscle in the distal esophagus. It usually occurs in the absence of coordinated peristalsis. Although clinically a patient may have chest pain and

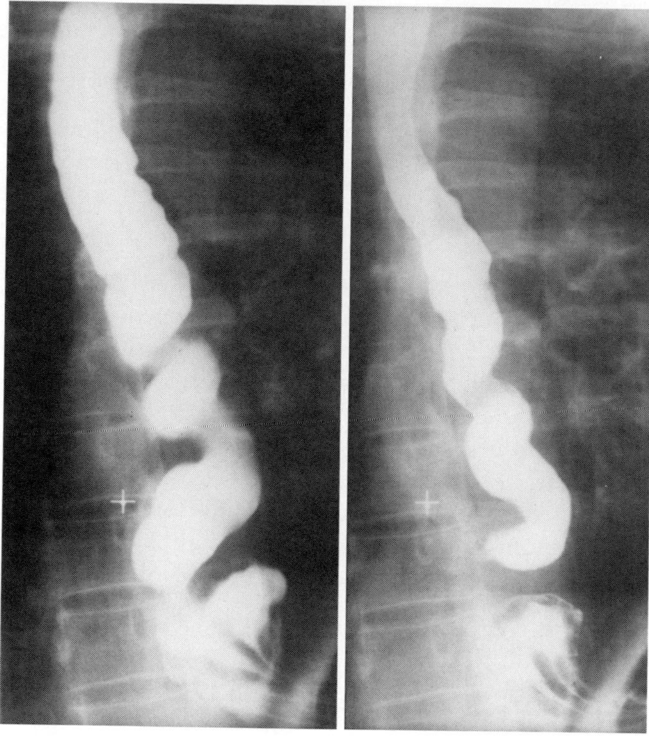

Figure 13-20 Barium esophagogram of a patient with diffuse esophageal spasm and hiatal hernia (Courtesy of Bronwyn Jones, MD, the Johns Hopkins Medical Institutions.)

dysphagia, DES represents only 3 percent of all cases of dysphagia. One-third of patients also have a poorly relaxing LES. Chest pain is a common complaint, and in these cases it is imperative to rule out angina and coronary artery disease. Symptoms of DES may be precipitated by stress, esophageal reflux, hot/cold food, and carbonated beverages, to name only a few. No specific pathology or pathophysiology has yet been described. There is some suggestion that the disorder may be the result of either a hypersensitivity of the esophagus to cholinergic stimulation, a defect in nitric oxide neuromuscular communication, or a combination of both.[126]

Diagnostic modalities

Classically, a barium swallow shows a corkscrew appearance, which is due to the contrast being held up within the segments of the esophagus (Fig. 13-20). The most important diagnostic evaluation is based primarily on manometric and clinical findings. In general, the manometric readings show that 20 percent or more of all contractions occur simultaneously, with amplitudes exceeding 30 mmHg (Fig. 13-21). The LES pressures are normal, and although there are some uncoordinated contractions, there is also some normal peristaltic activity.

Medical and surgical therapy

The most effective treatment is yet to be defined. Medical reassurance alone often results in improved symptoms.[151] Other medical therapy is similar to that

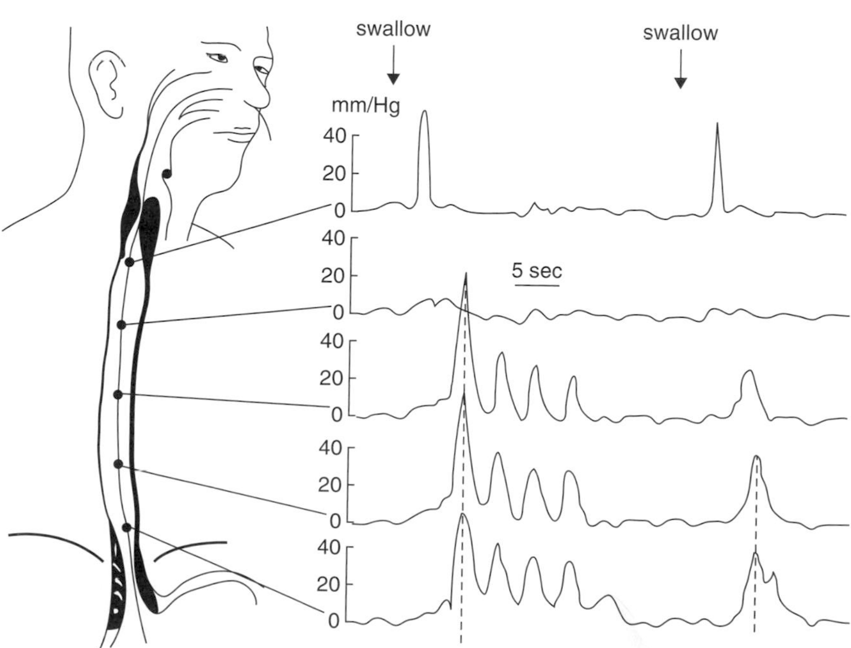

Figure 13-21 Manometry tracing of a patient with diffuse esophageal spasm. (From www.ctsnet.org)

outlined for achalasia—that is, nitrates, pneumatic dilatation, and the injection of botulinum toxin. Surgery is mainly indicated if medically refractory symptoms such as pain or dysphagia persist.

Nutcracker esophagus

Pathophysiology and clinical features

In this condition, episodic, sharp chest pain is the main symptom that brings the patient to presentation. It is characterized manometrically by esophageal contraction waves of high amplitude, normally in the distal esophagus. The terminology used to describe this motility disorder has led to much confusion. In addition to "nutcracker esophagus," proposed by Benjamin and associates in 1979, it has also been known as "super-squeeze esophagus"[152] (as coined by Gelfand and Botoman[153]) or hypertensive peristalsis. Although the etiology is unknown, nutcracker esophagus probably belongs to a spectrum of motility disorders and sits somewhere in between DES and achalasia.[126]

Diagnostic modalities

Diagnostically, both barium swallows and endoscopic examination are usually normal. Manometry again is the diagnostic study of choice and reveals intermittent contraction amplitudes that exceed 180 mmHg.

Medical and surgical therapy

In controlled trials, only diltiazem has been shown to be efficacious in symptom relief.[154] No similar data exist for dilation or surgical therapy with long myotomy or partial fundoplication.[152] In fact, surgery may not only fail to alleviate the symptoms but also add the complication of dysphagia, thus exacerbating the patient's symptoms.[126] Since this condition is rare, concise recommendations about surgery in patients with nutcracker of the esophagus will probably not be forthcoming.

References

1. DeMeester TR, Peters JH, Bremner CG, Chandrasoma P. Biology of gastroesophageal reflux disease: Pathophysiology relating to medical and surgical treatment. *Annu Rev Med* 1999;50:469–506.
2. Nebel OT, Fornes MF, Castell DO. Symptomatic gastroesophageal reflux: Incidence and precipitating factors. *Am J Dig Dis* 1976;21(11):953–956.
3. DeMeester TR, Wang CI, Wernly JA, et al. Technique, indications, and clinical use of 24 hour esophageal pH monitoring. *J Thorac Cardiovasc Surg* 1980;79(5):656–670.
4. Johnsson F, Joelsson B, Gudmundsson K, Greiff L. Symptoms and endoscopic findings in the diagnosis of gastroesophageal reflux disease. *Scand J Gastroenterol* 1987;22(6):714–718.
5. Cameron AJ, Zinsmeister AR, Ballard DJ, Carney JA. Prevalence of columnar-lined (Barrett's) esophagus: Comparison of population-based clinical and autopsy findings. *Gastroenterology* 1990;99(4):918–922.
6. Wienbeck M, Barnert J. Epidemiology of reflux disease and reflux esophagitis. *Scand J Gastroenterol Suppl* 1989; 156:7–13.
7. Kahrilas PJ. Gastroesophageal reflux disease and its complications, including Barrett's metaplasia. In: Feldman MFL, Sleisenger MH (eds). *Sleisenger and Fordtran's Gastrointestinal and Liver Disease*, 7th ed. St. Louis: Saunders; 2002:599–618.
8. Spechler SJ. Medical treatment of gastroesophageal reflux disease. In: Griffith Pearson JDC, Deslauriers J, Ginsberg R, et al (eds). *Esophageal Surgery*. Philadelphia: Churchill-Livingstone; 2002:234–244.
9. Holloway RH, Dent J. Pathophysiology of gastroesophageal reflux: Lower esophageal sphincter dysfunction in gastroesophageal reflux disease. *Gastroenterol Clin North Am* 1990;19(3):517–535.
10. Ing AJ, Ngu MC. Cough and gastro-oesophageal reflux. *Lancet* 1999;353(9157):944–946.
11. Holloway RH, Hongo M, Berger K, McCallum RW. Gastric distention: A mechanism for postprandial gastroesophageal reflux. *Gastroenterology* 1985;89(4): 779–784.
12. Dent J, Dodds WJ, Friedman RH, et al. Mechanism of gastroesophageal reflux in recumbent asymptomatic human subjects. *J Clin Invest* 1980;65(2):256–267.
13. Zaninotto G, DeMeester TR, Schwizer W, et al. The lower esophageal sphincter in health and disease. *Am J Surg* 1988;155(1):104–111.
14. DeMeester TR, Wernly JA, Bryant GH, et al. Clinical and in vitro analysis of determinants of gastroesophageal competence: A study of the principles of antireflux surgery. *Am J Surg* 1979;137(1):39–46.
15. Iwakiri K, Sugiura T, Kotoyori M, et al. Effect of body position on lower esophageal sphincter pressure. *J Gastroenterol* 1999;34(3):305–309.
16. Ott DJ, Gelfand DW, Chen YM, et al. Predictive relationship of hiatal hernia to reflux esophagitis. *Gastrointest Radiol* 1985;10(4):317–320.
17. Wright RA, Hurwitz AL. Relationship of hiatal hernia to endoscopically proved reflux esophagitis. *Dig Dis Sci* 1979;24(4):311–313.
18. Allison PR. Reflux esophagitis, sliding hiatal hernia, and the anatomy of repair. *Surg Gynecol Obstet* 1951;92(4): 419–431.
19. Allison P. Peptic ulcer of the esophagus. *J Thorac Surg* 1946;15:308.
20. Sontag SJ, Schnell TG, Miller TQ, et al. The importance of hiatal hernia in reflux esophagitis compared with lower esophageal sphincter pressure or smoking. *J Clin Gastroenterol* 1991;13(6):628–643.
21. Kaul B, Petersen H, Myrvold HE, et al. Hiatus hernia in gastroesophageal reflux disease. *Scand J Gastroenterol* 1986;21(1):31–34.
22. Berstad A, Weberg R, Froyshov Larsen I, et al. Relationship of hiatus hernia to reflux oesophagitis: A

prospective study of coincidence, using endoscopy. *Scand J Gastroenterol* 1986;21(1):55–58.

23. Pearson FG. Hiatal hernia, gastroesophageal reflux, and other conditions. In: Griffith Pearson JDC, Deslauriers J, Ginsberg R, et al (eds). *Esophageal Surgery*. Philadelphia: Churchill-Livingstone; 2002:223–233.
24. Sloan S, Rademaker AW, Kahrilas PJ. Determinants of gastroesophageal junction incompetence: Hiatal hernia, lower esophageal sphincter, or both? *Ann Intern Med* 1992;117(12):977–982.
25. Kahrilas PJ. Gastroesophageal reflux disease and its complications, including Barrett's metaplasia. In: Feldman MFL, Sleisenger MH (eds). *Sleisenger and Fordtran's Gastrointestinal and Liver Disease*, 7th ed. St. Louis: Saunders; 2002:599–618.
26. Kahrilas PJ. Supraesophageal complications of reflux disease and hiatal hernia. *Am J Med* 2001;111(Suppl) 8A:51S–55S.
27. Pairolero PTV, Payne S. Esophagus and diaphragmatic hernias. In: Schwartz SST, Spencer F (eds). *Principles of Surgery*. New York: McGraw-Hill; 1989:1103–1156.
28. Joelsson BE, DeMeester TR, Skinner DB, et al. The role of the esophageal body in the antireflux mechanism. *Surgery* 1982;92(2):417–424.
29. DeMeester SR, DeMeester TR. Columnar mucosa and intestinal metaplasia of the esophagus: Fifty years of controversy. *Ann Surg* 2000;231(3):303–321.
30. Helm JF, Dodds WJ, Pelc LR, et al. Effect of esophageal emptying and saliva on clearance of acid from the esophagus. *N Engl J Med* 1984;310(5):284–288.
31. Meyers RL, Orlando RC. In vivo bicarbonate secretion by human esophagus. *Gastroenterology* 1992;103(4): 1174–1178.
32. Zaninotto G, DeMeester TR, Bremner CG, et al. Esophageal function in patients with reflux-induced strictures and its relevance to surgical treatment. *Ann Thorac Surg* 1989;47(3):362–370.
33. Rakic S, Stein HJ, DeMeester TR, Hinder RN. Role of esophageal body function in gastroesophageal reflux disease: Implications for surgical management. *J Am Coll Surg* 1997;185(4):380–387.
34. Johnson WE, Hagen JA, DeMeester TR, et al. Outcome of respiratory symptoms after antireflux surgery on patients with gastroesophageal reflux disease. *Arch Surg* 1996;131(5):489–492.
35. Kahrilas PJ, Gupta RR. The effect of cigarette smoking on salivation and esophageal acid clearance. *J Lab Clin Med* 1989;114(4):431–438.
36. Kahrilas PJ, Gupta RR. Mechanisms of acid reflux associated with cigarette smoking. *Gut* 1990;31(1):4–10.
37. Sloan S, Kahrilas PJ. Impairment of esophageal emptying with hiatal hernia. *Gastroenterology* 1991;100(3): 596–605.
38. Kauer WK, Peters JH, DeMeester TR, et al. Mixed reflux of gastric and duodenal juices is more harmful to the esophagus than gastric juice alone: The need for surgical therapy re-emphasized. *Ann Surg* 1995;222(4):525-531; discussion 531–533.
39. Fein M, Ireland AP, Ritter MP, et al. Duodenogastric reflux potentiates the injurious effects of gastroesophageal reflux. *J Gastrointest Surg* 1997;1(1): 27–33.
40. Marshall RE, Anggiansah A, Owen WA, Owen WJ. The relationship between acid and bile reflux and symptoms in gastro-oesophageal reflux disease. *Gut* 1997;40(2): 182–187.
41. Prach AT, MacDonald TA, Hopwood DA, Johnston DA. Increasing incidence of Barrett's oesophagus: Education, enthusiasm, or epidemiology? *Lancet* 1997;350(9082):933.
42. Theisen J, Oberg S. Surgical and medical therapies for GERD—Can we see into the future? *Am J Gastroenterol* 1998;93(6):1008–1009.
43. Orlando RC. Why is the high grade inhibition of gastric acid secretion afforded by proton pump inhibitors often required for healing of reflux esophagitis? An epithelial perspective. *Am J Gastroenterol* 1996;91(9):1692–1696.
44. Carlsson R, Dent J, Bolling-Sternevald E, et al. The usefulness of a structured questionnaire in the assessment of symptomatic gastroesophageal reflux disease. *Scand J Gastroenterol* 1998;33(10):1023–1029.
45. Jacob P, Kahrilas PJ, Vanagunas A. Peristaltic dysfunction associated with nonobstructive dysphagia in reflux disease. *Dig Dis Sci* 1990;35(8):939–942.
46. Sontag SJ. Gastroesophageal reflux and asthma. *Am J Med* 1997;103(5A):84S–90S.
47. Harding SM, Richter JE. The role of gastroesophageal reflux in chronic cough and asthma. *Chest* 1997;111(5): 1389–1402.
48. Sontag SJ, Schnell TG, Miller TQ, et al. Prevalence of oesophagitis in asthmatics. *Gut* 1992;33(7):872–876.
49. Irwin RS, Curley FJ, French CL. Difficult-to-control asthma: Contributing factors and outcome of a systematic management protocol. *Chest* 1993;103(6): 1662–1669.
50. Mello CJ, Irwin RS, Curley FJ. Predictive values of the character, timing, and complications of chronic cough in diagnosing its cause. *Arch Intern Med* 1996;156(9): 997–1003.
51. Irwin RS, French CL, Curley FJ, et al. Chronic cough due to gastroesophageal reflux: Clinical, diagnostic, and pathogenetic aspects. *Chest* 1993;104(5):1511–1517.
52. DeMeester TR, Ireland AP. Gastric pathology as an initiator and potentiator of gastroesophageal reflux disease. *Dis Esophagus* 1997;10(1):1–8.
53. Jacob P, Kahrilas PJ, Herzon G. Proximal esophageal pH-metry in patients with "reflux laryngitis." *Gastroenterology* 1991;100(2):305–310.
54. Shaker R, Milbrath M, Ren J, et al. Esophagopharyngeal distribution of refluxed gastric acid in patients with reflux laryngitis. *Gastroenterology* 1995;109(5): 1575–1582.
55. Ormseth EJ, Wong RK. Reflux laryngitis: Pathophysiology, diagnosis, and management. *Am J Gastroenterol* 1999;94(10):2812–2817.
56. Brunnen PL, Karmody AM, Needham CD. Severe peptic oesophagitis. *Gut* 1969;10(10):831–837.
57. Isolauri J, Luostarinen M, Isolauri E, et al. Natural course of gastroesophageal reflux disease: 17–22 year follow-up of 60 patients. *Am J Gastroenterol* 1997;92(1): 37–41.
58. Sonnenberg A, El-Serag HB. Clinical epidemiology and natural history of gastroesophageal reflux disease. *Yale J Biol Med* 1999;72(2–3):81–92.

59. Stein HJ, Eypasch EP, DeMeester TR, et al. Circadian esophageal motor function in patients with gastroesophageal reflux disease. *Surgery* 1990;108(4):769–777; discussion 777–778.
60. Hetzel DJ, Dent J, Reed WD, et al. Healing and relapse of severe peptic esophagitis after treatment with omeprazole. *Gastroenterology* 1988;95(4):903–912.
61. Scarpignato C. Gastric emptying in gastroesophageal reflux disease and other functional esophageal disorders. In: Scarpignato C, Galmuche JP (eds). *Functional Investigation in Esophageal Disease*. Basel: Karger; 1994:223–259.
62. Martin JFP, Duranceau A. Secondary esophageal motor disorders. In: Griffith Pearson JDC, Deslauriers J, Ginsberg R, et al (eds). *Esophageal Surgery*. Philadelphia: Churchill-Livingstone; 2002:551–568.
63. Bainbridge ET, Temple JG, Nicholas SP, et al. Symptomatic gastro-oesophageal reflux in pregnancy: A comparative study of white Europeans and Asians in Birmingham. *Br J Clin Pract* 1983;37(2):53–57.
64. Miller LS, Vinayek R, Frucht H, et al. Reflux esophagitis in patients with Zollinger-Ellison syndrome. *Gastroenterology* 1990;98(2):341–346.
65. Napierkowski J, Wong R. Gastroesophageal reflux disease. In: Rakel RBE, (ed). *Conn's Current Therapy 2004*. Philadelphia: Saunders; 2003:573–578.
66. Labenz J, Blum AL, Bayerdorffer E, et al. Curing *Helicobacter pylori* infection in patients with duodenal ulcer may provoke reflux esophagitis. *Gastroenterology* 1997;112(5):1442–1447.
67. Feldman M, Cryer B, Sammer D, et al. Influence of *H. pylori* infection on meal-stimulated gastric acid secretion and gastroesophageal acid reflux. *Am J Physiol* 1999;277(6 Pt 1):G1159–G1164.
68. Verdu EF, Armstrong D, Idstrom JP, et al. Effect of curing *Helicobacter pylori* infection on intragastric pH during treatment with omeprazole. *Gut* 1995;37(6):743–748.
69. Labenz J, Tillenburg B, Peitz U, et al. *Helicobacter pylori* augments the pH-increasing effect of omeprazole in patients with duodenal ulcer. *Gastroenterology* 1996;110(3):725–732.
70. Sontag SJ, Hirschowitz BI, Holt S, et al. Two doses of omeprazole versus placebo in symptomatic erosive esophagitis: The U.S. Multicenter Study. *Gastroenterology* 1992;102(1):109–118.
71. Maton PN. Omeprazole. *N Engl J Med* 1991;324(14): 965–975.
72. Richter JE. Indications for surgical referral for hiatal hernia and gastroesophageal reflux: A Gastroenterologist's Viewpoint. In: F. Griffith Pearson JDC, Deslauriers J, Ginsberg R, et al; (eds). *Esophageal Surgery*. Philadelphia: Churchill-Livingstone; 2002:245–249.
73. Sontag SJ. The medical management of reflux esophagitis: Role of antacids and acid inhibition. *Gastroenterol Clin North Am* 1990;19(3):683–712.
74. Porro GB, Pace F, Peracchia A, et al. Short-term treatment of refractory reflux esophagitis with different doses of omeprazole or ranitidine. *J Clin Gastroenterol* 1992;15(3): 192–198.
75. Fass R, Ofman JJ, Gralnek IM, et al. Clinical and economic assessment of the omeprazole test in patients with symptoms suggestive of gastroesophageal reflux disease. *Arch Intern Med* 1999;159(18):2161–2168.
76. Schenk BE, Kuipers EJ, Klinkenberg-Knol EC, et al. Hypergastrinaemia during long-term omeprazole therapy: Influences of vagal nerve function, gastric emptying and *Helicobacter pylori* infection. *Aliment Pharmacol Ther* 1998;12(7):605–612.
77. Neville PMMP, Edwards A. Response to pantoprazole is an effective diagnostic test for gastroesophageal reflux disease: Results of a randomized double-blind placebo-controlled pilot study (abstr). *Gastroenterology* 1998;114(Suppl):A242.
78. Collard JM. New insights into the assessment of gastro-oesophageal reflux disease. *Acta Chir Belg* 1996;96(4): 144–149.
79. Bielefeldt K, Gupta P, Aggarwal A. Gastroesophageal reflux disease and esophageal motility. *Virtual Hospital-*Esophageal function: A primer for clinicians (see www.vh.org) 2001.
80. Kahrilas PJ, Quigley EM. Clinical esophageal pH recording: A technical review for practice guideline development. *Gastroenterology* 1996;110(6):1982–1996.
81. Johnsson F, Joelsson B. Reproducibility of ambulatory oesophageal pH monitoring. *Gut* 1988;29(7):886–889.
82. Wiener GJ, Morgan TM, Copper JB, et al. Ambulatory 24-hour esophageal pH monitoring: Reproducibility and variability of pH parameters. *Dig Dis Sci* 1988;33(9): 1127–1133.
83. Younes Z, Johnson DA. Diagnostic evaluation in gastroesophageal reflux disease. *Gastroenterol Clin North Am* 1999;28(4):809–830, v.
84. Campbell DPMD. Gastroesophageal reflux in infants and children. In: F. Griffith Pearson JDC, Deslauriers J, Ginsberg R, et al (eds). *Esophageal Surgery*. Philadelphia: Churchill-Livingstone; 2002:255–265.
85. Venables TL, Newland RD, Patel AC, et al. Omeprazole 10 milligrams once daily, omeprazole 20 milligrams once daily, or ranitidine 150 milligrams twice daily, evaluated as initial therapy for the relief of symptoms of gastro-oesophageal reflux disease in general practice. *Scand J Gastroenterol* 1997;32(10):965–973.
86. Armstrong D. Endoscopic evaluation of gastro-esophageal reflux disease. *Yale J Biol Med* 1999;72(2–3):93–100.
87. Richter JE. Severe reflux esophagitis. *Gastrointest Endosc Clin N Am* 1994;4(4):677–698.
88. Richter JE, Castell DO. Gastroesophageal reflux: Pathogenesis, diagnosis, and therapy. *Ann Intern Med* 1982;97(1):93–103.
89. Johansson KE, Ask P, Boeryd B, et al. Oesophagitis, signs of reflux, and gastric acid secretion in patients with symptoms of gastro-oesophageal reflux disease. *Scand J Gastroenterol* 1986;21(7):837–847.
90. DeVault KR, Castell DO. Updated guidelines for the diagnosis and treatment of gastroesophageal reflux disease. The practice parameters Committee of the American College of Gastroenterology 1999. *Am J Gastroenterol* 1999;94(6):1434–1642.
91. Sampliner RE. New treatments for Barrett's esophagus. *Semin Gastrointest Dis* 1997;8(2):68–74.
92. Champion G, Richter JE, Vaezi MF, et al. Duodenogastroesophageal reflux: Relationship to pH and importance in Barrett's esophagus. *Gastroenterology* 1994;107(3):747–754.
93. Marshall JK, Thompson AB, Armstrong D. Omeprazole for refractory gastroesophageal reflux disease during

pregnancy and lactation. *Can J Gastroenterol* 1998;12(3): 225–227.

94. Ginsberg R, Pearson FG. Indications for surgery for hiatal hernia and gastroesophageal reflux: The surgeon's perspective. F. Griffith Pearson JDC, Deslauriers J, Ginsberg R, et al (eds). *Esophageal Surgery.* Philadelphia: Churchill-Livingstone; 2002:250–254.
95. Perdikis G, Hinder RA, Lund RJ, et al. Laparoscopic Nissen fundoplication: Where do we stand? *Surg Laparosc Endosc* 1997;7(1):17–21.
96. Deleted in press.
97. Peters JH, DeMeester TR, Crookes P, et al. The treatment of gastroesophageal reflux disease with laparoscopic Nissen fundoplication: Prospective evaluation of 100 patients with "typical" symptoms. *Ann Surg* 1998;228(1): 40–50.
98. Dallemagne B, Weerts JM, Jehaes C, et al. Laparoscopic Nissen fundoplication: Preliminary report. *Surg Laparosc Endosc* 1991;1(3):138–143.
99. Darling G, Deschamps C. Technical controversies in fundoplication surgery. *Thorac Surg Clin* 2005;15(3): 437–444.
100. Catarci M, Gentileschi P, Papi C, et al. Evidence-based appraisal of antireflux fundoplication. *Ann Surg* 2004; 239(3):325–337.
101. Gastal OL, Hagen JA, Peters JH, et al. Short esophagus: Analysis of predictors and clinical implications. *Arch Surg* 1999;134(6):633–636; discussion 637–638.
102. Freeman ME, Huguet KL, Hinder RA. Mark Ferguson (ed). *Laparoscopic Nissen Fundoplication.* Available at: www.ctsnet.org/ Accessed August 30, 2004.
103. Wills VL, Hunt DR. Dysphagia after antireflux surgery. *Br J Surg* 2001;88(4):486–499.
104. Zornig C, Strate U, Fibbe C, et al. Nissen vs Toupet laparoscopic fundoplication. *Surg Endosc* 2002;16(5): 758–766.
105. Fibbe C, Layer P, Keller J, et al. Esophageal motility in reflux disease before and after fundoplication: A prospective, randomized, clinical, and manometric study. *Gastroenterology* 2001;121(1):5–14.
106. Yau P, Watson DI, Jamieson GG, et al. The influence of esophageal length on outcomes after laparoscopic fundoplication. *J Am Coll Surg* 2000;191(4):360–365.
107. Urbach DR, Khajanchee YS, Glasgow RE, et al. Preoperative determinants of an esophageal lengthening procedure in laparoscopic antireflux surgery. *Surg Endosc* 2001;15(12):1408–1412.
108. Mittal SK, Awad ZT, Tasset M, et al. The preoperative predictability of the short esophagus in patients with stricture or paraesophageal hernia. *Surg Endosc* 2000;14(5): 464–468.
109. Swain CP, Mills TN. An endoscopic sewing machine. *Gastrointest Endosc* 1986;32(1):36–38.
110. Chuttani R, Sud R, Sachdev G, et al. A novel endoscopic full-thickness plicator for the treatment of GERD: A pilot study. *Gastrointest Endosc* 2003;58(5):770–776.
111. Filipi CJ, Lehman GA, Rothstein RI, et al. Transoral, flexible endoscopic suturing for treatment of GERD: A multicenter trial. *Gastrointest Endosc* 2001;53(4):416–422.
112. Oleynikov D, Oelschlager B. New alternatives in the management of gastroesophageal reflux disease. *Am J Surg* 2003;186(2):106–111.
113. Triadafilopoulos G, Utley DS. Temperature-controlled radiofrequency energy delivery for gastroesophageal reflux disease: The Stretta procedure. *J Laparoendosc Adv Surg Tech A* 2001;11(6):333–339.
114. O'Connor KW, Madison SA, Smith DJ, et al. An experimental endoscopic technique for reversing gastroesophageal reflux in dogs by injecting inert material in the distal esophagus. *Gastrointest Endosc* 1984;30(5): 275–280.
115. Spechler SJ, Lee E, Ahnen D, et al. Long-term outcome of medical and surgical therapies for gastroesophageal reflux disease: Follow-up of a randomized controlled trial. *JAMA* 2001;285(18):2331–2338.
116. Vakil N, Shaw M, Kirby R. Clinical effectiveness of laparoscopic fundoplication in a U.S. community. *Am J Med* 2003;114(1):1–5.
117. Perdikis GH, Wetscher GJ. Nissen fundoplication for gastroesophageal reflux disease: Laparoscopic Nissen fundoplication-technique and results. *Dis Esophagus* 1996;9:272–277.
118. Hinder RA, Klingler PJ, Perdikis G, Smith SL. Management of the failed antireflux operation. *Surg Clin North Am* 1997;77(5):1083–1098.
119. Hinder RA, Filipi CJ, Wetscher G, et al. Laparoscopic Nissen fundoplication is an effective treatment for gastroesophageal reflux disease. *Ann Surg* 1994;220(4): 472–481; discussion 481–483.
120. Jamieson GG. The results of anti-reflux surgery and reoperative anti-reflux surgery. *Gullet* 1993;3:41–45.
121. Curet MJ, Josloff RK, Schoeb O, Zucker KA. Laparoscopic reoperation for failed antireflux procedures. *Arch Surg* 1999;134(5):559–563.
122. O'Reilly MJ, Mullins S, Reddick EJ. Laparoscopic management of failed antireflux surgery. *Surg Laparosc Endosc* 1997;7(2):90–93.
123. Granderath FA, Kamolz T, Schweiger UM, et al. Is laparoscopic refundoplication feasible in patients with failed primary open antireflux surgery? *Surg Endosc* 2002;16(3):381–385.
124. Mayberry JF, Atkinson M. Studies of incidence and prevalence of achalasia in the Nottingham area. *Q J Med* 1985;56(220):451–456.
125. Allgrove J, Clayden GS, Grant DB, Macaulay JC. Familial glucocorticoid deficiency with achalasia of the cardia and deficient tear production. *Lancet* 1978;1(8077): 1284–1286.
126. Wood MG, Hagen JA. Primary esophageal motor disorders. In: Griffith Pearson JDC, Deslauriers J, Ginsberg R, et al (eds). *Esophageal Surgery.* Philadelphia: Churchill-Livingstone; 2002: 515–535.
127. Clouse RE; Diamant NE. Esophageal motor and sensory function and motor disorders of the esophagus. In: Feldman M, Friedman L, Sleisenger MH (eds). *Sleisenger and Fordtran's Gastrointestinal and Liver Disease.* St. Louis: Saunders; 2002:577–584.
128. Cattau EL Jr. Symptoms of esophageal dysfunction. In: Castell DO, Johnson LF (eds). *Esophageal Function in Health and Disease.* New York: Elsevier Biomedical; 1983:31–46.
129. Vantrappen G, Hellemans J, Deloof W, et al. Treatment of achalasia with pneumatic dilatations. *Gut* 1971;12(4): 268–275.

130. Meijssen MA, Tilanus HW, van Blankenstein M, et al. Achalasia complicated by oesophageal squamous cell carcinoma: A prospective study in 195 patients. *Gut* 1992; 33(2):155–158.
131. Raymond L, Lach B, Shamji FM. Inflammatory aetiology of primary oesophageal achalasia: An immunohistochemical and ultrastructural study of Auerbach's plexus. *Histopathology* 1999;35(5):445–453.
132. Clark SB, Rice TW, Tubbs RR, et al. The nature of the myenteric infiltrate in achalasia: An immunohistochemical analysis. *Am J Surg Pathol* 2000;24(8):1153–1158.
133. Cassella RR, Brown AL Jr, Sayre GP, Ellis FH Jr. Achalasia of the esophagus: Pathologic and etiologic considerations. *Ann Surg* 1964;160:474–487.
134. Csendes A, Smok G, Braghetto I, et al. Gastroesophageal sphincter pressure and histological changes in distal esophagus in patients with achalasia of the esophagus. *Dig Dis Sci* 1985;30(10):941–945.
135. Cassella RR, Ellis FH Jr, Brown AL Jr. Fine-structure changes in achalasia of esophagus. II. Esophageal smooth muscle. *Am J Pathol* 1965;46:467–475.
136. Fuller L, Huprich JE, Theisen J, et al. Abnormal esophageal body function: Radiographic-manometric correlation. *Am Surg* 1999;65(10):911–914.
137. Bassotti G, Annese V. Review article: Pharmacological options in achalasia. *Aliment Pharmacol Ther* 1999;13(11):1391–1396.
138. Bortolotti M. Medical therapy of achalasia: A benefit reserved for few. *Digestion* 1999;60(1):11–16.
139. Pasricha PJ, Rai R, Ravich WJ, et al. Botulinum toxin for achalasia: Long-term outcome and predictors of response. *Gastroenterology* 1996;110(5):1410–1415.
140. Prakash C, Freedland KE, Chan MF, Clouse RE. Botulinum toxin injections for achalasia symptoms can approximate the short term efficacy of a single pneumatic dilation: A survival analysis approach. *Am J Gastroenterol* 1999;94(2):328–333.
141. Vaezi MF, Richter JE, Wilcox CM, et al. Botulinum toxin versus pneumatic dilatation in the treatment of achalasia: A randomised trial. *Gut* 1999;44(2): 231–239.
142. Clouse RE, Abramson BK, Todorczuk JR. Achalasia in the elderly: Effects of aging on clinical presentation and outcome. *Dig Dis Sci* 1991;36(2):225–228.
143. Khan AA, Shah SW, Alam A, et al. Massively dilated esophagus in achalasia: Response to pneumatic balloon dilation. *Am J Gastroenterol* 1999;94(9):2363–2366.
144. Parkman HP, Reynolds JC, Ouyang A, et al. Pneumatic dilatation or esophagomyotomy treatment for idiopathic achalasia: Clinical outcomes and cost analysis. *Dig Dis Sci* 1993;38(1):75–85.
145. Vaezi MF, Richter JE. Current therapies for achalasia: Comparison and efficacy. *J Clin Gastroenterol* 1998;27(1): 21–35.
146. Spiess AE, Kahrilas PJ. Treating achalasia: From whalebone to laparoscope. *JAMA* 1998;280(7):638–642.
147. Reynolds JC, Parkman HP. Achalasia. *Gastroenterol Clin North Am* 1989;18(2):223–255.
148. Di Simone MP, Felice V, D'Errico A, et al. Onset timing of delayed complications and criteria of follow-up after operation for esophageal achalasia. *Ann Thorac Surg* 1996;61(4):1106–1110; discussion 1110–1111.
149. Ellis FH Jr, Watkins E Jr, Gibb SP, Heatley GJ. Ten to 20-year clinical results after short esophagomyotomy without an antireflux procedure (modified Heller operation) for esophageal achalasia. *Eur J Cardiothorac Surg* 1992;6(2):86–89; discussion 90.
150. Malthaner RA, Tood TR, Miller L, Pearson FG. Long-term results in surgically managed esophageal achalasia. *Ann Thorac Surg* 1994;58(5):1343–1346; discussion 1346–1347.
151. Richter JE, Wu WC, Johns DN, et al. Esophageal manometry in 95 healthy adult volunteers: Variability of pressures with age and frequency of "abnormal" contractions. *Dig Dis Sci* 1987;32(6):583–592.
152. Heitmiller R. Surgery of achalasia and other motility disorders. In: Kaiser L KI, Spray T (eds). *Mastery of Cardiothoracic Surgery*. Philadelphia: Lippincott-Raven; 1998:151–159.
153. Gelfand MD, Botoman VA. Esophageal motility disorders: A clinical overview. *Am J Gastroenterol* 1987;82(3): 181–187.
154. Cattau EL Jr, Castell DO, Johnson DA, et al. Diltiazem therapy for symptoms associated with nutcracker esophagus. *Am J Gastroenterol* 1991;86(3):272–276.
155. Salminen JT, Salo JA, Tuominen JA, et al. pH-Metric analysis after successful antireflux surgery: Comparison of 24-hour pH profiles in patients undergoing floppy fundoplication or Roux-en-Y duodenal diversion. *J Gastrointest Surg* 1997;1(6):494–498.
156. Nehra D, Howell P, Pye JK, Beynon J. Assessment of combined bile acid and pH profiles using an automated sampling device in gastro-oesophageal reflux disease. *Br J Surg* 1998;85(1):134–137.

CHAPTER

14 ESOPHAGEAL PERFORATION

Firas F. Mussa, Steven R. DeMeester

INTRODUCTION

In 1724, Hermann Boerhaave published the presentation, clinical course, and autopsy findings of spontaneous rupture of the esophagus in his patient Lord van Wassenaer, High Admiral of the Dutch Navy. He described the clinicopathologic correlation between esophageal perforation and a fatal outcome. This outcome

KEY CONCEPTS

- Epidemiology
  - Iatrogenic instrumentation (e.g., endoscopy, dilatation, tube passage) has replaced spontaneous rupture as the leading cause of esophageal perforation and accounts for 60 to 75 percent of esophageal injuries.
- Pathophysiology
  - Esophageal perforation results in leakage of esophageal and gastric contents into the mediastinum, producing a chemical burn and superinfection. Left untreated, this leads to a severe inflammatory response and sepsis.
  - Esophageal perforations are broadly divided into intraluminal and extraluminal types. Intraluminal injuries are caused by instrumentation, foreign bodies, caustic ingestion, esophagitis, carcinoma, infection, or barotrauma. Extraluminal causes include stab or gunshot sounds, blunt trauma, and operative injuries.
- Clinical features
  - Patients sustaining a cervical esophageal perforation typically present with cervical pain, odynophagia, subcutaneous emphysema, and neck tenderness and crepitus. Dysphagia, pain, tachycardia, and fever usually occurs shortly after iatrogenic perforation. Intraabdominal esophageal perforation usually presents with peritonitis. Late manifestations of untreated perforations often include hypoxia, sepsis, and shock.
- Diagnostics
  - An antecedent history of instrumentation or vomiting often points to the etiology and possibility of esophageal perforation. Plain chest radiography may show pneumomediastinum, subcutaneous emphysema, or subdiaphragmatic air. Diagnosis is usually confirmed with esophagography, which demonstrates a leak in 50 to 60 percent of cervical and 80 to 90 percent of thoracic esophageal perforations. Esophagoscopy and computed tomography are other diagnostic modalities used in selected circumstances.
- Treatment
  - The initial management of patients presenting with esophageal perforations includes cessation of oral intake, fluid resuscitation, and broad-spectrum antibiotics. Definitive treatment of perforations is divided into nonoperative and operative management. Nonoperative management may be undertaken in selected patients with limited perforations that drain back into the esophagus and are not associated with distal obstruction, communication with the abdominal cavity, or systemic sepsis. Operative treatment is predicated on adequate debridement, reinforced primary repair, wide drainage, and distal feeding tube placement. In the absence of underlying esophageal disease, there is a trend toward primary reinforced repair regardless of the perforation's duration. Underlying esophageal disease is best addressed before or at the time of perforation repair.
- Outcomes
  - Esophageal perforation has an associated mortality rate of 20 percent.

remained inevitable for nearly 200 years, and perforation of the esophagus still represents a true surgical emergency. In 1946, Barrett[1,2] and Olsen and Claggett[3] in 1947 described the first successful repair of esophageal perforation. Although spontaneous esophageal rupture is uncommon, the dramatic increase in the use of invasive diagnostic procedures for the diagnosis and treatment of gastrointestinal diseases has resulted in a significant increase in the incidence of esophageal perforation.

PATHOPHYSIOLOGY

Depending on its location, esophageal perforation may take a catastrophic course rapidly unless the diagnosis is prompt and treatment is instituted immediately. Subsequent to perforation, esophageal and gastric contents are sucked into the mediastinum by negative intrathoracic pressure, producing a chemical burn. The presence of oral bacteria in saliva and digestive enzymes in gastric fluid initiate a mixed necrotizing superinfection adjacent to vital organs in the mediastinum and upper abdomen. This combination of insults leads to a severe inflammatory response and sepsis. Perforation of the esophagus can be divided into intraluminal or extraluminal causes.

Intraluminal causes

Instrumental injuries

These account for 60 to 75 percent of esophageal perforations[4–14] and can occur during endoscopy, dilatation, or tube passage. The actual risk of perforation during routine endoscopy alone is estimated at 0.03 percent with flexible esophagoscopes (compared with 0.11 percent with the now almost obsolete rigid esophagoscopes). However, the risk increases considerably with therapeutic intervention. It ranges from 0.3 percent after balloon dilatation to 25 percent after palliative stent placement for cancer.[15,16] In the absence of a diseased esophagus, iatrogenic injuries occur most commonly in Killian's triangle, which is formed by the inferior constrictor and the cricopharyngeus muscles. Perforation of the esophagus also occurs at areas of normal anatomic narrowing, such as the distal esophagus just proximal to the gastroesophageal junction and the impingement of the aortic arch and left mainstem bronchus.

Foreign bodies

Fish bones, impacted food, or solid objects (e.g., coins), in rare circumstances, cause acute perforation in areas of anatomic esophageal narrowing. This circumstance is more common in children and is often associated with a delay in diagnosis; it can lead to the development of mediastinal abscess or empyema.

Caustic ingestion, retained pills, severe peptic esophagitis, and Barrett's ulceration

Prior to the widespread availability of proton pump inhibitors, reflux esophagitis with esophageal ulcer was a relatively common cause of esophageal perforation. Currently, reflux disease alone rarely leads to perforation of the esophagus.

Esophageal carcinoma

Perforation associated with esophageal cancer usually results from instrumentation of a bulky or locally advanced tumor; it is associated with a poor prognosis.

Infection

Severe esophageal infections with human immunodeficiency virus (HIV), herpes simplex virus (HSV), *Candida* species, and tuberculosis all have been reported to cause esophageal perforation.

Spontaneous perforation or barotrauma

Perforation of the esophagus may be related to a rapid increase in intraluminal pressure (e.g., emesis, coughing, weight lifting, seizures). If the upper esophageal sphincter fails to relax, the increase in intraabdominal pressure may lead to a tremendous pressure rise within the esophagus, resulting in perforation.

Extraluminal causes

Penetrating injuries

Esophageal perforation from stab or gunshot wounds typically involves the cervical esophagus and is rarely fatal by itself.[17]

Blunt trauma

Esophageal perforation secondary to blunt trauma is rare. It can occur secondary to compression of the esophagus between the sternum and spine in motor vehicle accidents.[18]

Operative injuries

Perforation of the esophagus has been reported with thyroid surgery, operations on the anterior cervical spine, pulmonary resections, and laparoscopic fundoplication or myotomy procedures.

CLINICAL FEATURES

The clinical presentation of esophageal perforation depends on three factors: location, degree of containment, and elapsed time since injury. The differential diagnosis includes myocardial infarction, peptic ulcer disease, pancreatitis, aortic dissection, spontaneous pneumothorax, and pneumonia. Cervical perforation typically presents with cervical pain, odynophagia, and subcutaneous emphysema with neck tenderness and crepitus on palpation. The diagnosis may be suspected from the patient's history. Iatrogenic perforation usually presents shortly after the procedure, with dysphagia, pain, tachycardia, and fever. If left untreated, this progresses to hypoxia, sepsis, and shock. Pleural effusion may develop after 24 h.

Spontaneous esophageal rupture or Boerhaave's occurs more commonly outside the hospital setting. The typical patient is an elderly male with a history of recent emesis. These patients tend to present late and have a worse prognosis. Intraabdominal perforations usually present with peritonitis and rapidly deteriorate into shock and sepsis.

DIAGNOSTIC MODALITIES

An antecedent history of instrumentation or vomiting can be elicited from most patients with esophageal perforation. Plain chest radiography may show pneumomediastinum, subcutaneous emphysema, or air under the diaphragm within the first hour of perforation, but pleural effusion often takes 24 h to develop. The chest film is normal in 10 percent of patients.[19] The diagnosis is usually confirmed with an esophagogram—a swallow study with water-soluble (e.g., Gastrografin) contrast. Esophagograms will demonstrate the leak in 50 to 60 percent of cervical and 80 to 90 percent of thoracic perforations[20,21] (Figs. 14-1 to 14-3). Such studies should be performed with the patient in the right lateral decubitus position so as to avoid rapid transit of contrast into the stomach, in which case a small leak may be missed. Esophagoscopy is the diagnostic option in unstable or mechanically ventilated patients. Any discoloration or submucosal hematoma on upper endoscopy should be considered highly suspicious for perforation.

Computed tomography (CT) of the chest and abdomen is useful in selected patients when esophagography is unavailable or the findings from such studies are nondiagnostic. Abnormalities on chest CT may include mediastinal free air, esophageal thickening, or an air-fluid level adjacent to the esophagus, representing a mediastinal abscess cavity.[22,23]

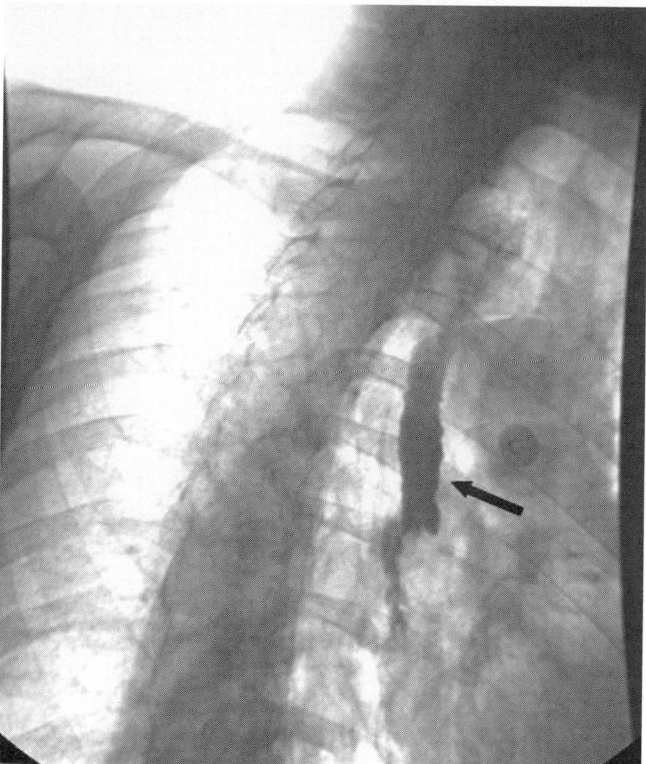

Figure 14-2 Lateral view of Gastrografin contrast study. The arrow points to contrast extravasation in the midesophagus.

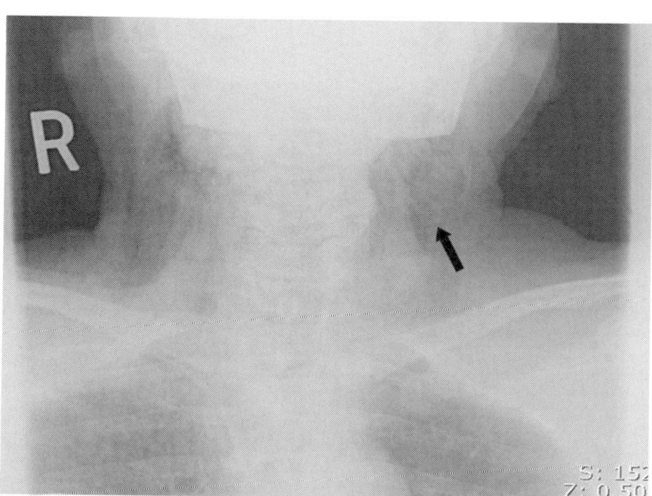

Figure 14-1 Anteroposterior view of neck radiograph. The arrow points to subcutaneous air.

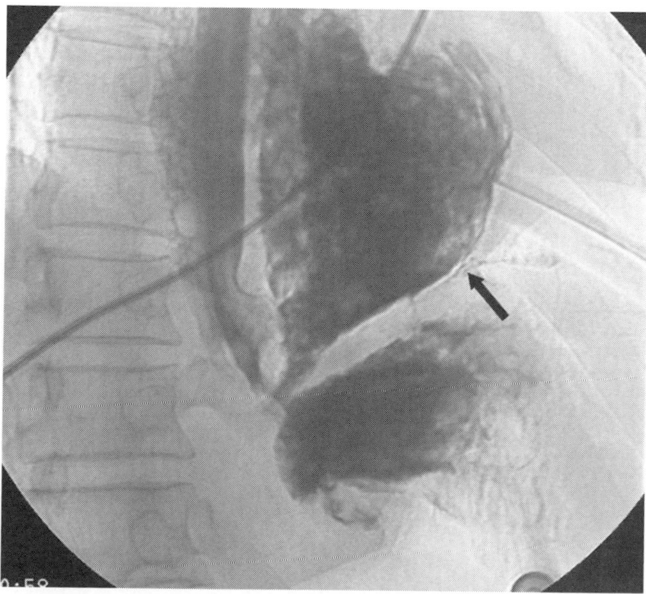

Figure 14-3 Lateral view of Gastrografin contrast study. The arrow points to contrast extravasation in the distal esophagus at the gastroesophageal junction.

THERAPY

The overriding consideration in the treatment of esophageal perforation is the status of the native (preperforation) esophagus and, in particular, the presence of cancer, achalasia, or stricture.[24] Other considerations include contained versus free leak, the patient's clinical status, time since perforation, and location of the perforation. The treatment principles are based on (1) debridement of necrotic tissues to control infection and to prevent continued soilage, (2) elimination of any distal esophageal obstruction, (3) secure closure of the perforation with appropriate drainage, and (4) establish enteral access. Treatment options are operative and nonoperative.

Nonoperative management

In 1979, Cameron published the criteria for nonoperative management of esophageal perforation,[25] updated by Altorjay in 1997.[5] These criteria include (1) intraluminal dissection, (2) transmural perforation that drains back into the esophagus, (3) no associated obstruction in the distal esophagus, (4) no perforation within the abdominal cavity, and (5) no evidence of systemic sepsis. Once esophageal perforation is suspected, oral intake is stopped, fluid resuscitation is instituted, and broad-spectrum antibiotics are initiated. Acid secretion is reduced with proton pump inhibitors, and patients are sustained on total parenteral nutrition. Mediastinal and pleural collections should be drained via tube thoracostomy or percutaneously by catheters placed under CT guidance. The importance of continued monitoring for any clinical deterioration cannot be overemphasized. Operative intervention should be performed immediately upon any such deterioration.

Perforation of the cervical esophagus is usually treated nonoperatively, stopping any oral intake (e.g., NPO), instituting broad-spectrum antibiotics, and providing frequent oral suctioning.[26] An algorithm outlining the current management of esophageal perforation is shown in the decision-making flowchart (Fig. 14-4).

Operative management

Perforation of the cervical esophagus

Perforation of the cervical esophagus and the development of an abscess above the aortic arch can be managed with drainage alone through a cervical approach. An incision is made along the anterior border of the left sternocleidomastoid muscle (SCM). The omohyoid and strap muscles are divided. The carotid sheath is identified and mobilized laterally, and the inferior thyroid artery is ligated. The recurrent laryngeal nerve can be found as it courses in the tracheoesophageal groove, just anterior to the inferior thyroid artery. The esophagus is identified and a search is made for the site of perforation. Closure of the perforation is not mandatory, especially when severe inflammation is present and there is no distal obstruction.

However, closure of an accessible early perforation may be carried out provided that minimal dissection is performed. In such repairs, the esophageal mucosa is approximated with interrupted fine absorbable sutures and the muscle layer closed separately. An associated mediastinal abscess can often be drained by blunt dissection

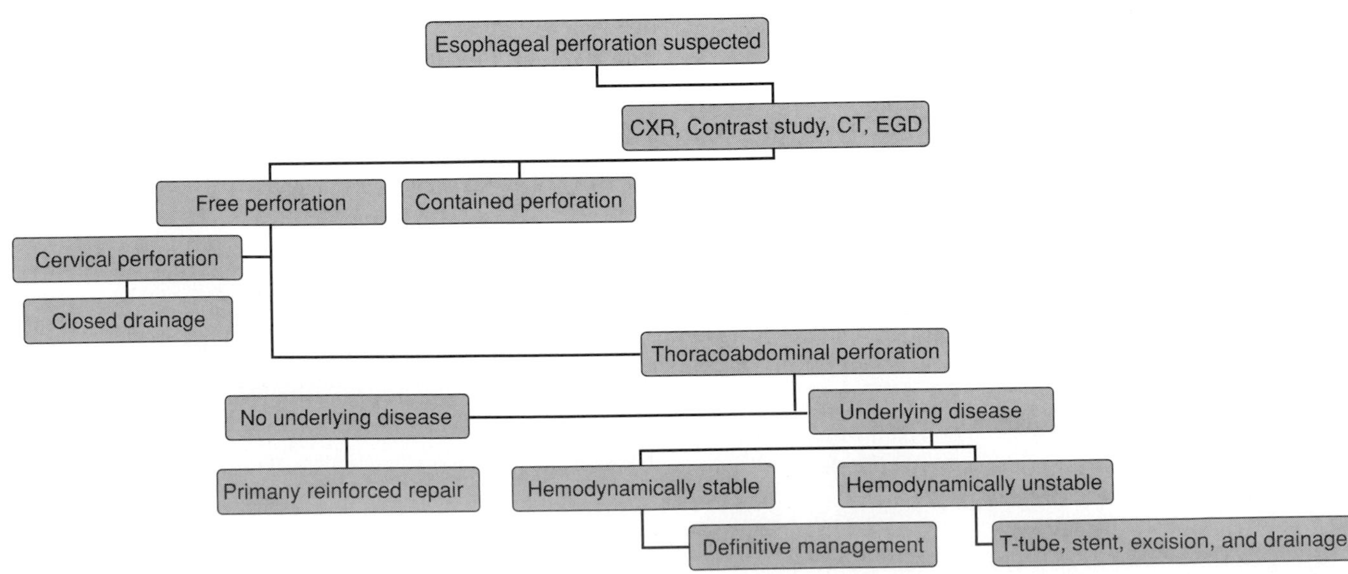

Figure 14-4 Decision-making flowchart. An algorithm outlining the current management of esophageal perforation.

through the thoracic inlet down into the abscess. Placement of a closed suction drain in the abscess cavity and closing the wound complete the procedure. Regardless of whether simple drainage or surgical closure is used for cervical perforations, most patients recover promptly and have a low mortality rate. A repeat swallow study is necessary prior to resuming oral intake.

Intrathoracic and abdominal esophageal perforation

The mortality rates of intrathoracic esophageal perforation are almost three times those of cervical esophageal injuries.[27] The most favorable outcomes are obtained after primary repair of such perforations within 24 h. However, accumulating experience suggests that, regardless of the duration of the injury, primary repair should be attempted in patients without an underlying abnormality of the esophagus and with stable hemodynamics.[28] Perforations of the middle third of the esophagus are best approached through a right thoracotomy, while a left thoracotomy is best for perforations of the lower esophagus. Perforations should be approached on the side of pleural contamination. Abdominal esophageal perforation without significant intrapleural contamination may be approached through an upper midline incision.

After surgical exposure has been gained, contaminated fluid is drained and mediastinal and esophageal devitalized tissues are debrided. Next, the location of the perforation is sought. When this has been identified, exposure is facilitated by incising the muscle layers proximally and distally. Once well exposed, the mucosal defect is trimmed and closed using interrupted fine monofilament absorbable suture. Subsequently, the muscle layer is approximated over the mucosal closure. It is important to buttress the repair with adjacent tissues in order to reduce the rate of leak. The choice of buttressing tissue depends on the approach used for the repair. During a thoracic approach, a pleural[29,30] intercostal muscle or an elevated diaphragmatic pedicle flap[30] can be used to bolster the primary repair. Wide mediastinal drainage is mandatory in addition to the repair. Drainage is achieved by opening the mediastinal pleura above and below the level of the tear from the thoracic inlet to the diaphragm and then irrigating and draining the mediastinum with well-positioned chest tubes and drains. If a laparotomy is performed for perforation of the lower esophagus, the repair can be reinforced with omentum[31] or a fundoplication.

Late esophageal perforation

Esophageal perforation with a delayed presentation or diagnosis results in increased mediastinal contamination, inflammation, tissue destruction, and hemodynamic instability. In the absence of underlying esophageal disease, many believe that a primary reinforced repair is the procedure of choice regardless of the perforation's duration. Drainage alone is acceptable in selected cases of cervical perforations. Unstable patients represent a unique challenge and are best served with either resection, control of the esophageal fistula with a T tube and wide pleural drainage, or endoscopic placement of a removable self-expandable Silastic stent and drainage. Esophageal exclusion and diversion is rarely necessary or appropriate with the number of options currently available.

Esophageal perforation associated with esophageal diseases

Primary repair is ill advised in the presence of preexisting esophageal disease such as cancer or stricture, since the underlying process remains[32] and is associated with a high likelihood of repair breakdown and subsequent mortality.[33] In most circumstances, the best option for distal malignant obstruction is resection with delayed reconstruction.[34] In selected patients with an early diagnosis of esophageal perforation and minimal pleural and mediastinal contamination, gastrointestinal continuity may be reestablished at the time of the primary resection.[6,34,35]

Patients with achalasia who develop a perforation during balloon dilatation should undergo mucosal closure of the perforation with closure of the overlying muscle, followed by a complete myotomy on the opposite side of the esophagus.[36] The repair is buttressed with a partial fundoplication.

When perforation occurs in the presence of severe gastroesophageal reflux, an antireflux procedure is indicated both to buttress the repair and to treat the reflux. In the setting of severe caustic injuries, primary repair is rarely undertaken. The injured esophagus and/or stomach are resected through a transhiatal approach. The esophageal hiatus is closed to avoid herniation of intraabdominal organs into the chest. The contaminated chest is drained, and a gastrostomy or feeding jejunostomy tube is placed. Patients are returned to the operating room at a later date for definitive reconstruction.

SUMMARY

Esophageal perforation continues to pose a diagnostic and therapeutic challenge and has an associated mortality rate of 20 percent. Instrumentation has replaced spontaneous rupture as the leading cause of esophageal perforation. Nonoperative management is appropriate in selected patients, but patients with evidence of systemic illness require prompt intervention. In the absence of cancer or an undilatable stricture, reinforced primary repair is the preferred treatment for patients who require an operation. Selection of treatment must be individualized and take into account many variables, including cause, duration, underlying esophageal disease, and the patient's condition.

References

1. Barrett N. Spontaneous perforation of the esophagus: Review of the literature and a report of three new cases. *Thorax* 1946;1(48).
2. Barrett N. Report of a case of spontaneous rupture of the esophagus successfully treated by operation. *Br J Surg* 1947;35:216–217.
3. Olsen ACO. Spontaneous rupture of the esophagus: Report of a case with immediate diagnosis and successful surgical repair. *Postgrad Med* 1947;2:417–419.
4. Iannettoni MD, Vlessis AA, Whyte RI, et al. Functional outcome after surgical treatment of esophageal perforation. *Ann Thorac Surg* 1997;64(6):1606–1609; discussion 1609–1610.
5. Altorjay A, Kiss J, Voros A, et al. Nonoperative management of esophageal perforations: Is it justified? *Ann Surg* 1997;225(4):415–421.
6. Altorjay A, Kiss J, Voros A, et al. The role of esophagectomy in the management of esophageal perforations. *Ann Thorac Surg* 1998;65(5):1433–1436.
7. Attar S, Hankins JR, Suter CM, et al. Esophageal perforation: A therapeutic challenge. *Ann Thorac Surg* 1990;50(1):45–49; discussion 50–51.
8. Bufkin BL, Miller JI Jr, Mansour KA. Esophageal perforation: Emphasis on management. *Ann Thorac Surg* 1996;61(5):1447–1451; discussion 1451–1452.
9. Kotsis L, Kostic S, Zubovits K. Multimodality treatment of esophageal disruptions. *Chest* 1997;112(5):1304–1309.
10. Okten I, Cangic AK, Ozdemir N, et al. Management of esophageal perforation. *Surg Today* 2001;31(1):36–39.
11. Salo JA, Isolauri JO, Heikkila LJ, et al. Management of delayed esophageal perforation with mediastinal sepsis: Esophagectomy or primary repair? *J Thorac Cardiovasc Surg* 1993;106(6):1088–1091.
12. Shaffer HA Jr, Valenzuela G, Mittal RK. Esophageal perforation: A reassessment of the criteria for choosing medical or surgical therapy. *Arch Intern Med* 1992;152(4): 757–761.
13. Tilanus HW, Bossuyt P, Schattenkerk ME, et al. Treatment of oesophageal perforation: A multivariate analysis. *Br J Surg* 1991;78(5):582–585.
14. Wang N, Razzouk AT, Safari A, et al. Delayed primary repair of intrathoracic esophageal perforation: Is it safe? *J Thorac Cardiovasc Surg* 1996;111(1):114–121; discussion 121–122.
15. Acunas B, Rozanes I, Akpinar S, et al. Palliation of malignant esophageal strictures with self-expanding nitinol stents: Drawbacks and complications. *Radiology* 1996;199(3):648–652.
16. Kinsman KJ, DeGregorio BT, Katon RM, et al. Prior radiation and chemotherapy increase the risk of life-threatening complications after insertion of metallic stents for esophagogastric malignancy. *Gastrointest Endosc* 1996;43(3): 196–203.
17. Weiman DS, Walker WA, Brosnan KM, et al. Noniatrogenic esophageal trauma. *Ann Thorac Surg* 1995;59(4):845–859; discussion 849–850.
18. Beal SL, Pottmeyer EW, Spisso JM. Esophageal perforation following external blunt trauma. *J Trauma* 1988; 28(10):1425–1432.
19. Han SY, McElvein RB, Aldrete JS, et al. Perforation of the esophagus: Correlation of site and cause with plain film findings. *AJR Am J Roentgenol* 1985;145(3):537–540.
20. Foley MJ. Ghahremani GG, Rogers LF. Reappraisal of contrast media used to detect upper gastrointestinal perforations: Comparison of ionic water-soluble media with barium sulfate. *Radiology* 1982;144(2):231–237.
21. Sarr MG, Pemberton JH, Payne WS. Management of instrumental perforations of the esophagus. *J Thorac Cardiovasc Surg* 1982;84(2):211–218.
22. Maher MM, Lucey BC, Boland C, et al. The role of interventional radiology in the treatment of mediastinal collections caused by esophageal anastomotic leaks. *AJR Am J Roentgonol* 2002;178(3):649–653.
23. Backer CL, Lo Cicero J III, Hartz RS, et al. Computed tomography in patients with esophageal perforation. *Chest* 1990;98(5):1078–1080.
24. White RK. Diagnosis and management of esophageal perforation. *Am Surg* 1992;58:112–119.
25. Cameron JL, Kieffer RF, Hendrix TR, et al. Selective nonoperative management of contained intrathoracic esophageal disruptions. *Ann Thorac Surg* 1979;27(5):404–408.
26. Nesbitt JC, Sawyers JL. Surgical management of esophageal perforation. *Am Surg* 1987;53(4):183–191.
27. Sandrasagra FA, English TA, Milstein BB. Esophageal intubation in the management of perforated esophagus with stricture. *Ann Thorac Surg* 1978;25(5):399–401.
28. Whyte RI, Iannettoni MD, Orringer MB. Intrathoracic esophageal perforation: The merit of primary repair. *J Thorac Cardiovasc Surg* 1995;109(1):140–144; discussion 144–146.
29. Grillo HC, Wilkins EW Jr. Esophageal repair following late diagnosis of intrathoracic perforation. *Ann Thorac Surg* 1975;20(4):387–399.
30. Kotsis L, Agocs L. The effectiveness of diaphragmatic pedicled grafts in esophageal injuries and wall reconstruction. *Eur J Cardiothorac Surg* 1998;14(2):218–220.
31. Sabanathan S, Eng J, Richardson J. Surgical management of intrathoracic oesophageal rupture. *Br J Surg* 1994; 81(6):863–865.
32. Skinner DB, Little AG, DeMeester TR. Management of esophageal perforation. *Am J Surg* 1980;139(6):760–764.
33. Moghissi K, Pender D. Instrumental perforations of the oesophagus and their management. *Thorax* 1988;43(8): 642–646.
34. Orringer MB, Stirling MC. Esophagectomy for esophageal disruption. *Ann Thorac Surg* 1990;49(1):35–42; discussion 42–43.
35. Matthews HR, Mitchell IM, McGuigan JA. Emergency subtotal oesophagectomy. *Br J Surg* 1989;76(9):918–920.
36. Urbani M, Mathisen DJ. Repair of esophageal perforation after treatment for achalasia. *Ann Thorac Surg* 2000;69(5): 1609–1611.

CHAPTER

15 SURGICAL MANAGEMENT OF ESOPHAGEAL CANCER

Avedis Meneshian, Richard F. Heitmiller

INTRODUCTION

Considerable progress has been made in the management of esophageal cancer in the past two decades. The epidemiologic shift in incidence from squamous cell cancer to adenocarcinoma of the esophagogastric junction, coupled with a growing understanding of Barrett's esophagus as a precursor to adenocarcinoma, has allowed earlier detection of this disease and improved options for successful therapeutic intervention. Moreover, the advent of evidence-based medicine and its emphasis on outcomes of surgical (e.g., anastomotic) techniques and postsurgical care has paved the way for patient care pathways that have significantly decreased surgical morbidity and mortality, as well as length of hospital stay and cost, thereby allowing the focus of therapy to shift from merely surviving an operation to a more complete emphasis on cancer treatment and patient quality of life. Finally, the adoption of multimodality (chemo-, radio-, immuno- and surgical) therapy and the growing utility of molecular biomarkers has and will provide the next great front upon which to expand our growing therapeutic armamentarium. This chapter emphasizes the current strategies employed for the surgical management of esophageal cancer.

KEY CONCEPTS

- Epidemiology
  - Historically and internationally, squamous cell carcinoma of the esophagus has been the most common epithelial esophageal malignancy. However, over the past two or three decades, the United States, United Kingdom, and western Europe have witnessed a major epidemiologic shift wherein the incidence of adenocarcinoma has risen sixfold, making it now the most common malignant histologic cell type. The incidence of esophageal cancer within the United States is 3.2 in 100,000 persons, and 14,500 new cases are diagnosed on a yearly basis.
- Pathophysiology
  - The precise etiology of esophageal cancer remains unknown. Data suggest that epithelial cancers arise as a result of chronic irritation of the esophagus from a wide range of sources, including tobacco, alcohol, or refluxed gastric contents, and patients who are immunosuppressed may be at increased risk. The strongest correlation remains that between esophageal adenocarcinoma and Barrett's esophagus (BE). Data support the notion of a tumor progression model, wherein the normal stratified squamous epithelium of the esophagus is transformed into a columnar-lined epithelium extending from the esophagogastric junction upward (BE), then on to dysplasia and ultimately invasive adenocarcinoma. However, many important questions remain, such as why and how Barrett's mucosa progresses into adenocarcinoma, why it tends to occur predominantly in white men, precisely how long it takes for this transformation to occur, and what might be done to retard this process. The genetic changes involved in this transformation remain an area of intensive investigation.
- Clinical features
  - Progressive dysphagia remains the hallmark presenting complaint of patients with esophageal cancer. Associated odynophagia or substernal or epigastric discomfort are less common symptoms. Patients

with squamous cell cancers report a history of extensive tobacco and/or alcohol use, and most will present with some degree of weight loss. On the other hand, those with adenocarcinomas (predominantly white men of middle to upper socioeconomic status) will report a long-standing history of reflux disease with attendant chronic antacid use; weight loss is less commonly noted. Findings of hoarseness, supraclavicular adenopathy, or a tracheoesophageal fistula suggest advanced disease.

- Diagnosis
  - Any complaint of dysphagia should prompt a barium esophagogram, which may reveal a characteristic narrowing of the esophagus. However, endoscopy and biopsy are critical for a tissue diagnosis. Once confirmed, a computed tomography (CT) scan of the chest and abdomen should be obtained to evaluate the lung parenchyma, mediastinal structures, and liver for metastatic disease or local invasion, and an endoscopic ultrasound (EUS) should be obtained to accurately stage the depth of invasion of the primary tumor and the status of locoregional lymph nodes. Positron emission tomography (PET) and combined PET/CT are gaining popularity as adjuncts with which to detect small distant metastases and are particularly useful as a means to follow patients undergoing neoadjuvant therapy. Diagnostic laparoscopy or thoracoscopy may be used to exclude advanced disease or lymph node involvement when sufficient information is not obtained with CT, EUS, or PET.
- Treatment
  - Selection of appropriate treatment depends upon tumor stage and the patient's overall condition. Surgery remains the best single-modality therapy for those with localized disease, such as superficial tumors with no regional lymph node involvement. Multimodality therapy with preoperative (neoadjuvant) chemoradiation followed by surgery may provide the best outcomes for patients with large primary tumors, those with greater depth of invasion of the esophageal wall, or those with regional lymph node involvement. Palliation for symptoms of malignant dysphagia in those with unresectable disease can be achieved with chemoradiation or with lasers, stents, or photodynamic therapy.
- Outcomes
  - Long-term outcomes are stage-specific, but cumulative 5-year survival after esophagectomy rarely exceeds 25 percent. Randomized, controlled trials assessing the impact of multimodality (particularly neoadjuvant) therapy on survival have had mixed results. Improvements in therapy will undoubtedly require earlier detection with improved, cost-effective (possibly genetic) surveillance programs and a combination of surgical, chemo-, radio-, and immunotherapies.

CLASSIFICATION

Esophageal cancers can be classified as epithelial tumors, metastatic tumors, lymphomas, or sarcomas, with epithelial cancers (squamous cell and adenocarcinoma in particular) accounting for more than 90 percent of these malignancies. Each of these tumor types tends to cluster along certain segments of the esophagus, a fact that has important implications for their surgical management. For example, more than half of squamous cell cancers develop in the middle third of the esophagus,[1] whereas more than two-thirds of adenocarcinomas are located in the lower third.[2] The more rare epithelial tumors, such as small cell cancers, occur with equal frequency in the middle and lower thirds,[3] and both primary esophageal malignant melanomas and choriocarcinomas, although rare, are most commonly encountered in the lower third. Esophageal sarcomas can occur anywhere along the esophagus,[4] as can lymphomas or metastases. This discussion focuses entirely on the common epithelial tumors, squamous cell carcinoma and adenocarcinoma, and addresses the surgical options available for their management.

INCIDENCE

The incidence of esophageal cancer varies considerably from country to country and even from region to region within the same country.[5] This disparity highlights the multifactorial etiology of esophageal cancer and the consequent difficulty in assessing true and meaningful trends in incidence worldwide. Within the United States, the reported incidence of esophageal cancer is 3.2 in 100,000 persons,[6] and 14,500 new cases are diagnosed on a yearly basis.[7] With regard to their ethnic and geographic distribution, squamous cell cancers have been found to occur with equal frequency in Caucasian and African-American patients, whereas esophageal adenocarcinomas are almost exclusively a disease of Caucasian men. Although squamous cell cancer remains the most common malignant histologic cell type worldwide, the overall incidence of esophageal adenocarcinoma in western countries has been steadily increasing, particularly within the United States, the United Kingdom, and western Europe.[6,8–10]

For example, between 1973 and 1982, a 74 percent increase in esophageal adenocarcinoma was noted in Caucasian men in the United States,[6] while there was no increase in squamous cell tumors in Caucasian men during that same period and only a 30 percent overall increase in squamous cell cancers in women and African Americans.[6] More recently, from 1975 to 2001, the incidence of esophageal adenocarcinoma has increased sixfold, while that of squamous cell cancer has trended slightly downward.[7] As compared with the incidence of other common malignancies in the same relative time period, the incidence of esophageal and esophagogastric adenocarcinomas rose at a rate exceeding that of cutaneous melanoma, non-Hodgkin's lymphoma, and lung cancer.[10] A similar rise in the incidence of esophageal adenocarcinomas has been reported in the United Kingdom[11,12] and western Europe.[13] A review of the prevalence of esophageal carcinomas from 1959 to 1994 at one high-volume tertiary care center in the United States revealed that, although squamous cell cancers were the most common cell type overall, adenocarcinomas, which were rare prior to 1978, had surpassed squamous cell tumors as the most prevalent esophageal neoplasm by 1992.[14] The cause of this remarkable shift in esophageal cancer cell type has yet to be fully determined, but the answer must rest, at least in part, in understanding the multifactorial pathogenesis of esophageal epithelial tumors.

PATHOGENESIS

The precise etiology of esophageal cancer remains unknown. The more common epithelial tumors are believed to arise as a result of chronic irritation of the esophagus from a wide range of sources, such as tobacco, alcohol, carcinogens, dietary factors, lye, radiation, stasis, and refluxed gastric contents. Moreover, the likelihood of developing cancer may be increased in patients with impaired host immune defenses.[15] The geographic, ethnic, and demographic distribution of esophageal cancer varies widely, and whether this variance can be explained solely by environmental factors or whether a genetic component exists as well remains unclear.

Squamous cell cancer

Tobacco and alcohol use

Tobacco use has been clearly associated, in a dose-dependent manner, with the development of squamous cell esophageal cancer,[16–22] and this risk appears to decrease with smoking cessation. Even smokeless tobacco products have been found to increase the risk of cancers of the mouth, larynx, pharynx, and esophagus.[23] However, unlike the case with squamous cell cancers, it is less clear to what extent smoking contributes to the development of esophageal adenocarcinomas. Although epidemiologic studies suggest that cigarette consumption is far less common in patients with esophageal adenocarcinomas than in those with squamous tumors,[21,24] a link does appear to exist.[24] Numerous studies have documented the relationship between alcohol consumption and squamous cell esophageal cancer.[18–22,25,26] This cancer risk is also dose-dependent, and the combined risks of alcohol and smoking appear to be additive.

Dietary factors

A number of nutritional and dietary factors have been evaluated in an attempt to explain the worldwide variability in the incidence of esophageal cancer, but no clear association has been made. Some studies suggest that the populations with the highest incidence of squamous cell esophageal cancer share certain dietary characteristics, such as the consumption of high-starch/low fruit and vegetable-containing diets.[27] Certain reports have actually found that diets rich in fruit might protect against esophageal cancer.[28] Still others have reported that dietary fungal contaminants may produce mycotoxins, which are carcinogenic and may promote the development of squamous cell cancers of the esophagus.[29] Despite these interesting associations, no definitive causal relationships have been demonstrated.

Achalasia

It remains a matter of debate whether an association exists between achalasia and squamous cell cancer of the esophagus, and definitive studies have proven difficult to coordinate. The considerable delay between the onset of achalasia and the development of esophageal cancer predisposes studies evaluating the risk of cancer in patients with achalasia to underestimate the actual risk,[30] as a prolonged follow-up period is required to demonstrate an association. Nevertheless, it is clear that 70 percent of patients with achalasia who go on to develop cancer are males and that the vast majority of those who progress to malignancy develop squamous cell cancers.[31]

Other etiologic factors

Other factors associated with an increased risk of squamous cell esophageal cancer include lye ingestion, radiation therapy, the Plummer-Vinson syndrome, and previous head and neck squamous cell cancer. The interval between the injury and the development of cancer may be considerable in patients who sustain lye ingestion or who are irradiated. Some evidence supports the hypothesis that impaired host defenses might increase the risk of developing esophageal cancer.[15] Both vitamin and mineral deficiencies have been cited as explanations for the high cancer rates seen in endemic regions, and the risk of esophageal cancer appears to be elevated in patients with pernicious anemia.[32]

Adenocarcinoma

Barrett's esophagus

Barrett's esophagus (BE) is a condition in which the normal stratified squamous mucosa of the esophagus is replaced by a columnar-lined epithelium that extends to varying degrees upward from the esophagogastric junction. This is an acquired, metaplastic process that occurs in response to esophageal mucosal injuries which heal in the setting of continued gastroesophageal reflux. The precise incidence of BE is not known, although reports suggest that it might afflict up to 2 percent of the general population.[33] Moreover, although the incidence of BE appears to have increased over the past two decades,[33,34] this may reflect an overall increase in the number of endoscopies performed rather than a true increase in the incidence or prevalence of the disease.[33–35]

There is a well-documented association between BE and esophageal adenocarcinoma, with an estimated annual risk of transformation of 0.4 percent[36] and a lifetime risk of adenocarcinoma in 8 to 15 percent of patients, irrespective of medical or surgical antireflux therapy. Barrett's mucosa is detected in more than 60 percent of pathologic specimens from patients who undergo esophagectomy for adenocarcinoma[9]; many investigators believe that all esophageal adenocarcinomas arise from underlying BE and that when BE is not identified in the pathologic specimens, it is because it has been replaced entirely by carcinoma. There are a number of studies suggesting that dysplasia in the setting of BE is the immediate precursor to esophageal adenocarcinoma.[35,37–40] In one study, 81 patients with documented BE were followed prospectively for a mean of 3.6 (0.5 to 8) years. Three of these patients developed adenocarcinoma, two with antecedent high-grade and one with low-grade dysplasia. No patient without intervening dysplasia developed adenocarcinoma.[39] Others have confirmed that dysplasia is a prerequisite for adenocarcinoma and that, whereas low-grade dysplasia is potentially reversible, progression to invasive adenocarcinoma is inevitable once the threshold of high-grade dysplasia is reached.[40]

Although there is a well-documented association between BE, dysplasia, and esophageal adenocarcinoma, many important issues remain unresolved, such as why and how Barrett's mucosa progresses to adenocarcinoma, why it tends to occur predominantly in white males, precisely how long it takes for this progression to occur, and whether there is any therapy that may retard or halt this progression. The genetic changes involved in the transformation from BE to invasive adenocarcinoma have been studied extensively over the past two decades. Early genetic events involved in the neoplastic progression of this disease include a number of well-studied tumor suppressors and protooncogenes, such as *p16, p53, APC, Rb,* and *DCC.*[41] To date, no single genetic marker has proven sufficient to predict which patients will progress to invasive adenocarcinoma and when. Additionally, a number of biomarkers and potential therapeutic targets are currently under review; these include epidermal growth factor receptor, HER-2/Neu, cyclooxygenase-2, cyclin D1, bcl-2, and E-cadherin, among others.[42,43]

SCREENING

Esophageal cancer remains a devastating disease, due in large part to its aggressive nature and the fact that most patients present with stage III disease, where surgery is less apt to provide a long-term cure. Earlier detection would undoubtedly translate into improved survival in this patient population, but difficulty remains in adequately identifying the subgroup at risk and providing a cost-effective screening strategy for this relatively rare disease.[44–46]

For example, although esophageal adenocarcinoma is frequently accompanied by Barrett's metaplasia, only 5 percent of patients who present with esophageal adenocarcinoma carry an antecedent diagnosis of BE[35,45,46] for which they have been followed endoscopically. Therefore it follows that the vast majority of patients with adenocarcinoma would not have benefited from endoscopic surveillance strategies unless these had been applied to the general population (which for such a rare disease would never prove cost-effective) or unless a subgroup at particularly high risk could be identified (which, to date, has not been achieved). It is quite possible that our best hope for early detection (and therefore improved therapeutic outcomes) might lie with the identification of molecular biomarkers for esophageal adenocarcinoma that can be assayed from readily available biological samples (such as serum or urine) from patients who are considered to be at high risk from an epidemiologic perspective. This subset may then be entered into an endoscopic surveillance program with the goal of capturing early-stage patients in a more cost-effective manner. Such biomarkers are currently under intensive investigation, but none has proven clinically useful to date.[42,43]

DIAGNOSIS AND WORKUP

Clinical presentation

The typical patient with a squamous cell carcinoma of the esophagus is a man in the sixth or seventh decade of life who complains of difficulty swallowing and weight loss extending over several months. Cigarette smoking and alcohol consumption are usually a part of the patient's social history. Pain on swallowing (odynophagia) or substernal or epigastric pain are less common complaints. The findings of hoarseness from recurrent laryngeal nerve involvement, supraclavicular adenopathy, or a tracheoesophageal fistula indicate advanced, generally unresectable disease.

On the other hand, the typical patient with an adenocarcinoma of the distal esophagus, esophagogastric junction, or cardia presents at a younger age (in the fifth or sixth decade) and is usually a white man of middle or upper socioeconomic status. Although progressive dysphagia is again the primary complaint, significant weight loss at presentation is far less common than for patients with squamous cell cancers, and a history of cigarette smoking or alcohol abuse is less frequently reported. More often, a history of a hiatal hernia and reflux with attendant chronic antacid use is elicited.

Diagnostic evaluation

Any complaint of dysphagia merits a barium esophagogram, which may reveal a characteristic narrowing of the esophagus suggestive of an esophageal carcinoma. However, endoscopic assessment and biopsy of the lesion are essential for a histopathologic confirmation of the diagnosis. Endoscopic biopsies and brushings of the lesion will yield the diagnosis in over 90 percent of patients.[47,48] Multiple biopsies may be necessary to confirm the diagnosis of an invasive malignancy in a lesion that is submucosal or necrotic.[47] Nondiagnostic studies or in situ carcinoma in the face of a large lesion seen on radiographic or endoscopic studies and in the appropriate clinical setting should not be accepted, and biopsies should be repeated.

Table 15-1 American joint committee on cancer (AJCC) TNM classification for esophageal carcinoma

T0	No evidence of primary tumor
T1	Invades lamina propria or submucosa
T2	Invades muscularis propria
T3	Invades adventitia
T4	Invades adjacent structures
N0	No regional lymph node metastasis
N1	Regional lymph node metastasis
M0	No distant metastasis
M1	Distant metastasis
M1a	Invasion of celiac or cervical lymph nodes
M1b	Other distant metastasis
Stage 0	Tis N0 M0
Stage I	T1 N0 M0
Stage IIA	T2 N0 M0; T3 N0 M0
Stage IIB	T1 N1 M0; T2 N1 M0
Stage III	T3 N1 M0; T4 Any N M0
Stage IV	Any T Any N M1

Staging

TNM Classification

Assessment of the extent of disease at the time of initial diagnosis has traditionally been considered (and still is) critical for guiding optimal management and delivering a prognosis. Accurate determination of the extent of disease has a major impact on such therapeutic variables as single- versus multimodality treatment or curative versus palliative intent. Moreover, because many patients now receive preoperative (neoadjuvant) therapies that effectively downstage a tumor, it has been suggested that postoperative pathologic findings may not reflect the initial stage at diagnosis, thereby underscoring the need for accurate pretherapy staging. However, this school of thought has recently been challenged, as some authors suggest that it is the postoperative pathologic stage that serves as the best predictor of survival in patients who are treated with neoadjuvant chemoradiotherapy followed by esophagectomy.[49]

In 1987, the tumor-node-metastasis (TNM) staging system for esophageal cancer, developed by the American Joint Committee on Cancer (AJCC), was revised to consist of pathologic staging only, so that stage would more accurately reflect prognosis and therefore predict survival.[50,51] The most recent revision of this system is presented in Table 15-1.[52] In the current AJCC staging system, the T designator is divided into T1 to T4, according to the depth of tumor penetration into the wall of the esophagus. A T1 tumor is one that penetrates up to but not through the submucosa; a T2 tumor penetrates into but not through the muscularis propria; and a T3 tumor is transmural, with growth into the periesophageal tissues. If the tumor invades an adjacent structure, such as the aorta or spine, it is classified as T4. However, this remains an imperfect system; as data from several centers now suggest that the muscularis mucosa, which separates the mucosa from the submucosa, is an important anatomic boundary in that the likelihood of lymph node metastases increases significantly once tumors invade beyond this point.[53,54] Moreover, the likelihood of regional lymph node metastases increases with the depth of tumor penetration into the wall of the esophagus.[53,55–58] These factors are not accurately reflected in the current TNM staging system. Another shortcoming of the current AJCC staging system is that lymph node involvement is staged as either N0 (no involved nodes) or N1 (one or more involved nodes). However, recent evidence suggests that with esophageal adenocarcinoma, the likelihood of long-term survival correlates closely with the number of regional lymph node metastases. Patients with four or fewer lymph nodes involved with tumor after esophagectomy and lymphadenectomy have a better overall survival than those with five or more lymph node metastases.[55,56,58,59] In addition, the ratio of involved to total resected lymph nodes provides information on the extent of disease and the likelihood of recurrence, with those patients having greater than 25 percent nodal involvement being at particularly high risk for systemic recurrence.[55,60]

Finally, the M designator is used to classify patients as being without (M0) or with (M1) evidence of systemic metastases. Patients with systemic metastases (M1) are further subdivided into those with nonregional lymph node metastases (M1a) and those with true systemic or visceral metastases (M1b). Controversy remains regarding whether celiac nodal involvement represents extended locoregional disease or true systemic metastases.[61] Experience at several centers suggests that survival in patients who have only nonregional lymph node metastases (M1a) exceeds that of patients with visceral metastases (M1b),[56] whereas others have found that patients with celiac node involvement behave as if they had systemic or visceral metastases.[62,63] Still others have reported that it is the number of regional lymph nodes involved which serves as the best predictor, and not the differentiation between M1a and M1b disease.[55] A clear resolution to this debate has yet to be achieved.

Molecular staging

Several studies have found that the presence of a methylated adenomatous polyposis coli gene in the serum of patients with esophageal adenocarcinoma correlates with a more advanced disease stage and worse survival.[64] Similarly, patients with a mutation in the *p53* gene appear to have a worse prognosis as compared with stage-matched controls.[65,66] Additionally, panels of tumor markers are currently under investigation in an attempt to provide prognostic information after resection, and molecular markers have been used to predict the response to chemotherapy in patients with esophageal cancer.[67–69] As the molecular biology of this disease becomes better understood, the utility of these molecular strategies, both for staging purposes and potentially for therapy, holds great promise.

Clinical staging

Once a tissue diagnosis has been established, evaluation to determine the extent of disease (Fig. 15-1) should include a CT scan of the chest and abdomen. The chest CT is useful for evaluating the lung parenchyma and mediastinal structures.[70] Lymph nodes greater than 1 cm in diameter with necrotic centers are suggestive of metastatic involvement. The chest CT is also helpful for assessing aortic or pericardial involvement with tumor, which would preclude esophagectomy. The accuracy of identifying metastases to the liver and celiac axis by abdominal CT depends on the bulk of the disease. Small liver metastases, peritoneal studding, and abdominal nodes are often undetectable.[70,71]

Although a CT scan of the chest and abdomen is useful for identifying patients with distant metastases and unresectable disease due to tumor invasion or adherence to critical structures such as the aorta, pericardium, and tracheobronchial tree, it is less useful in determining the depth of the primary lesion and/or regional lymph node involvement, two critical factors with implications for prognosis and management.[72] There are now a number of studies documenting the utility of transesophageal endoscopic ultrasonography (EUS), laparoscopy, and thoracoscopy as preoperative staging tools. The greatest experience is with EUS,[72–78] with which the depth of the primary tumor can be determined with an overall accuracy of 89 percent.[72,78] Regional lymph node involvement can also be determined with an overall accuracy of 81 percent.[72,73] Additionally, EUS-guided fine-needle aspiration can distinguish benign from malignant lymph nodes with 92 percent accuracy as compared with surgery.[76] This is

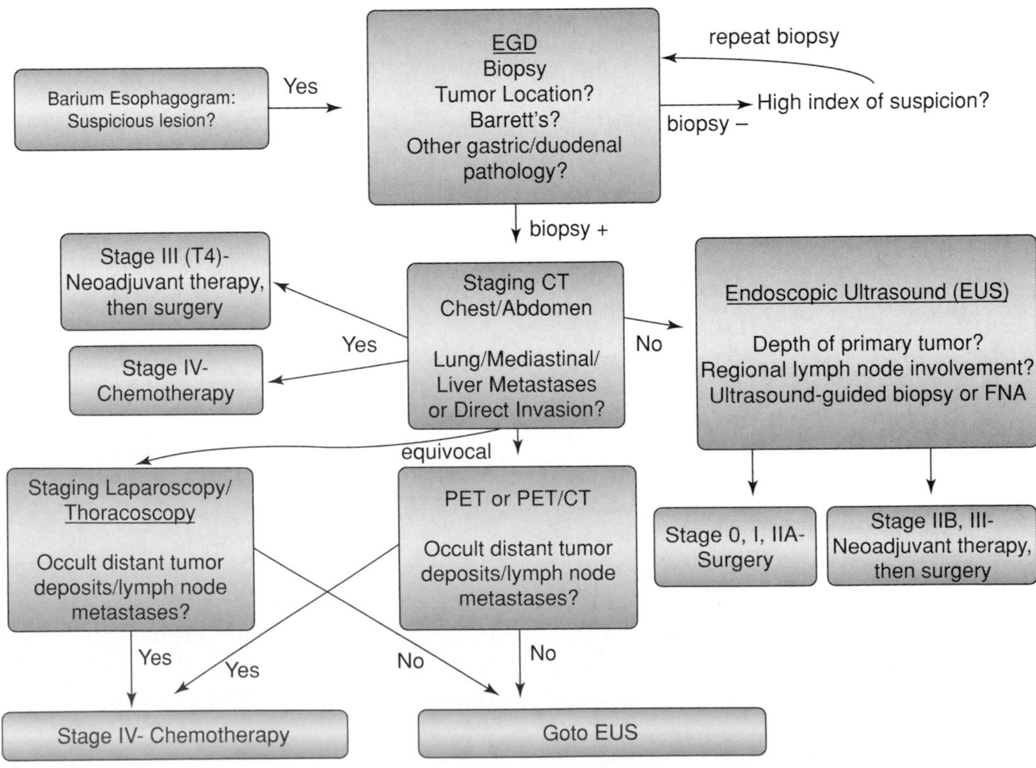

Figure 15-1 Basic diagnostic and staging algorithm for the workup of esophageal carcinoma.

particularly important for assessing celiac lymph node involvement, where EUS with or without FNA can predict the subset of patients who may best be treated as having advanced disease.[62,63] However, because of the low depth of penetration of ultrasound, EUS is not a reliable technique for diagnosing liver and peritoneal metastases.[73] Therefore laparoscopic evaluation of the peritoneal cavity to assess abdominal lymph node involvement or to exclude liver metastases or peritoneal implants should be utilized when a high yield of staging information is not obtainable with CT and EUS alone. The staging accuracy of laparoscopy for nodal involvement exceeds 95 percent.[79–84] Unsuspected findings such as liver metastases or peritoneal studding, which alter treatment and save the patient a laparotomy, also occur in 12 to 17 percent of patients.[80–82,84] Thoracoscopy has a high level of accuracy (95 percent) for detecting regional node involvement[80,85] within the chest. PET and combined PET/CT are additional staging techniques that are gaining popularity. The main niche for PET will likely be for the detection of distant metastases (sensitivity 81 percent, specificity 91 percent)[86] likely to be missed with routine CT scanning rather than for the detection of small locoregional nodal metastases, where EUS is so sensitive.[86,87] Bronchoscopy is an important adjunct for upper- and middle-third tumors to exclude the possibility of direct extension of an esophageal cancer into the tracheobronchial tree.

In summary, although accurate pretherapy TNM staging remains critical for the initial management of esophageal malignancies, posttherapy pathologic staging appears to correlate best with prognosis after neoadjuvant therapy and surgery. EUS is vital for accurate TN staging of all lesions of either histologic type following a CT evaluation that has excluded distant metastases or tracheal or aortic involvement. PET may provide additional information, particularly for distant disease missed by CT, and laparoscopy appears to be most useful for evaluating the abdominal spread of disease in patients with distal-third or gastroesophageal junction tumors in whom sufficient information is not obtained with CT or PET (Figs. 15-1 and 15-2). One algorithm for the stage-based management of esophageal cancer is presented in Fig. 15-3.

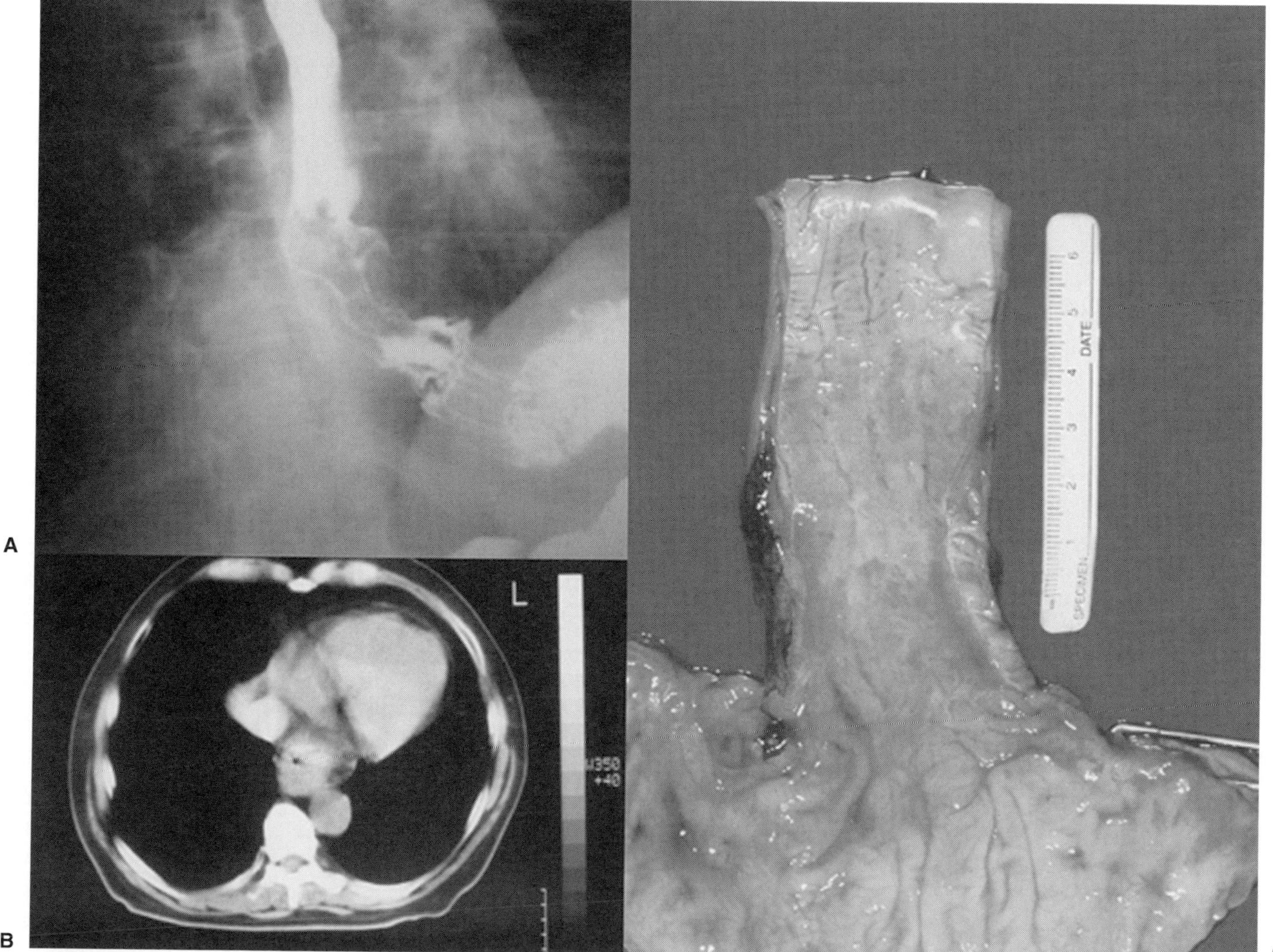

Figure 15-2 (A) Barium esophagogram, (B) computed tomography, and (C) gross pathology of esophageal adenocarcinoma.

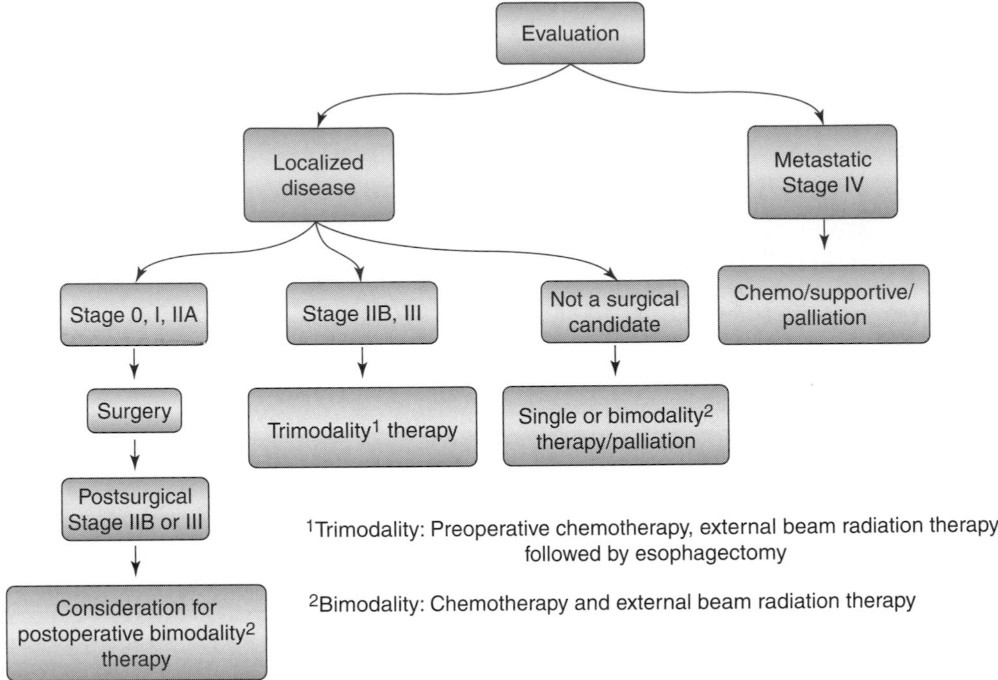

Figure 15-3 Mayo Clinic strategy for the treatment of esophageal carcinoma. (Adapted from Deb SJ, Deschamps C. Esophageal tumors. In: Cameron JL (ed). *Current Surgical Therapy*, 8th ed. Philadelphia:. Elsevier-Mosby; 2004:44–49. With permission.)

SURGICAL THERAPY

The goal of any therapy designed to manage patients with esophageal cancer should be to relieve symptoms (predominantly dysphagia) and treat the underlying cancer. An ideal therapy would accomplish both, safely and effectively. Currently, four main treatment strategies exist: surgery as a single modality with curative intent, chemo/radiotherapy as an independent modality with curative intent, multimodality therapy with surgery combined with pre- or postoperative chemo- and/or radiotherapy with curative intent, and finally surgical and nonsurgical means of palliative therapy. Of these, surgery remains the most effective means of achieving a long-term cure. This discussion focuses primarily on the surgical management of esophageal carcinoma, with salient discussion of the relevant features of adjuvant, neoadjuvant, and nonsurgical palliative therapy.

Preoperative preparation

Once the decision has been made to proceed with surgery in the management of esophageal cancer, a number of steps must be taken to optimize patients for the enormous physiologic stress involved and to minimize the risks of perioperative complications. As perioperative pulmonary complications are by far the most common (and perhaps most preventable), vigorous preoperative pulmonary physiotherapy—consisting of regular use of incentive spirometry and a flutter valve, a regimen of daily ambulation, and absolute discontinuation of smoking—are strongly encouraged. Moreover, it has been suggested that the use of epidural catheters for pain control in this patient population might decrease the risk of postoperative pulmonary complications.[88–90]

Preoperative nutritional support should be instituted, with liquid diet supplements or a nasoenteric feeding tube if needed, particularly in patients with high-grade esophageal obstruction. A preoperative jejunostomy feeding tube can be considered in severely malnourished patients in whom other means of enteral nutrition have been exhausted or in those who will undergo neoadjuvant therapy. Although most authors report that the routine use of preoperative gastrostomy tubes for enteral alimentation does not have an adverse impact on the subsequent creation of a gastric conduit,[91] the theoretical possibility of localized gastric fibrosis and/or compromise of the gastroepiploic arcade, which might preclude the future use of a gastric conduit, must be acknowledged.

Finally, since many patients now undergo neoadjuvant therapy, careful attention should be given to the normalization of their hematocrit and immunologic status before embarking on a major procedure. Additionally, all patients with esophageal cancer must undergo a careful assessment of their cardiac status before resection, and recommendations such as the need for cardiac stress testing and intervention or perioperative heart rate control with beta blockade should be considered.

Preoperative endoscopy

Before the incision is made, a careful endoscopic assessment of the upper gastrointestinal tract should be performed by the operating surgeon in order to confirm the location of the tumor, its length (from the incisors and the cardia), the cephalad extent of Barrett's mucosa or radiation changes above the tumor, whether there is any extension of the tumor into the stomach (or other gastric pathology), the ease of passage of the endoscope through the pylorus, and whether there is evidence of preexisting duodenal ulcer disease. This information is gathered best by the operating surgeon immediately before the operation and occasionally leads to a change in the planned operative approach.

Surgical principles

The basic principles of surgery—which include the gentle handling of tissues, meticulous hemostasis, avoidance of dead space, and the creation of a tension-free anastomosis—are critical to successful surgical outcomes. These basic principles must be applied to the management of esophageal disease. The integrity of an esophagogastric anastomosis after resection of an esophageal carcinoma is predicated on the observation of a set of specific principles. Careful adherence to these details ensures a successful anastomosis.

Regardless of the reconstructive conduit selected, maintenance of an adequate arterial supply to and venous drainage from the conduit is mandatory. For example, the right gastroepiploic artery must be preserved in order to ensure the viability of a gastric conduit.[92] Venous return is perhaps just as essential, as its interruption can result in venous infarction. This applies not only to the conduit but also to the proximal esophagus, which should not be dissected out of its bed more than is necessary to perform the anastomosis; excessive dissection can increase the risk of local tissue ischemia. Adequate conduit length should always be planned to allow for a tension-free anastomosis. Finally, when a gastric conduit is utilized, adequate gastric decompression should be provided, especially in the event that gastric dysmotility results in retention. Vomiting exerts undue force against the suture line and should be avoided. For this reason, a nasogastric tube is left in place after the operation, and appropriate gastric emptying procedures, such as a pyloromyotomy or a pyloroplasty, should be included when gastric tube reconstruction is chosen. Although a number of studies suggest that there is no significant difference in long-term outcome with or without a pyloric drainage procedure, others have found that a pyloromyotomy does decrease the risk of delayed gastric emptying in the immediate postoperative period.[93] Moreover, as a pyloric drainage procedure takes relatively little operating time and is generally considered of extremely low risk, one should consider its routine use in conjunction with a gastric pull-up procedure.

The operation: partial esophagogastrectomy with regional lymphadenectomy

The standard operation to resect an esophageal cancer with curative intent includes resecting the involved portion of the esophagus, the proximal stomach, and the regional lymph nodes. Therefore the surgical resection is most aptly termed a partial esophagogastrectomy (Fig. 15-4) with regional lymphadenectomy. The resected esophagus is replaced with a conduit created from the stomach or a segment of small or large intestine, which is

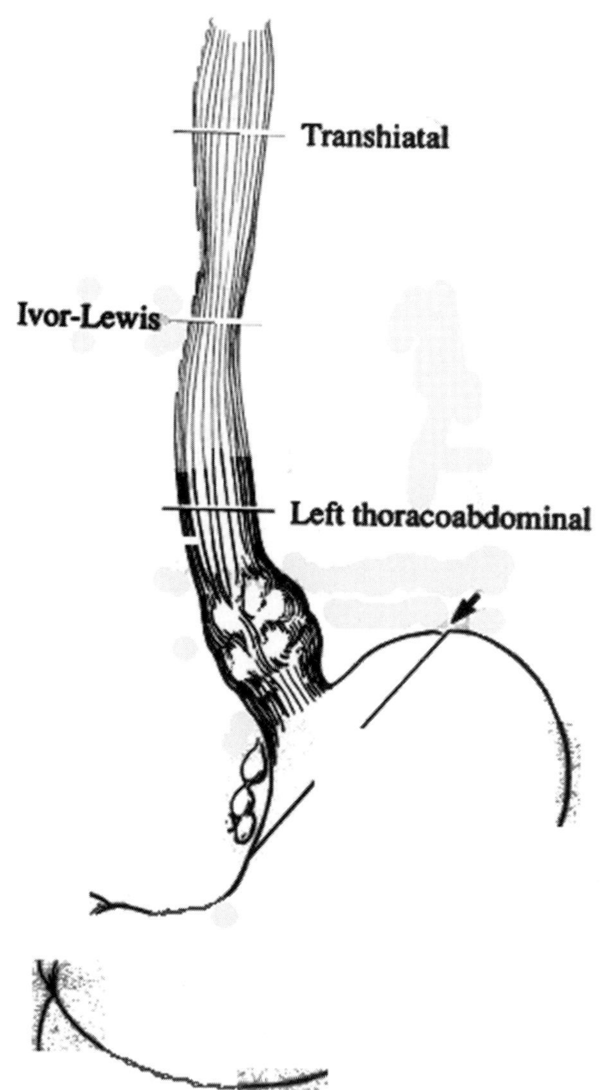

Figure 15-4 Regardless of the surgical approach utilized, a partial esophagogastrectomy is performed to resect esophageal tumors. Depending upon the approach used, different lengths of esophagus are removed. (Adapted from Heitmiller RF. Carcinoma of the esophagus. In: Bayless TM (ed). *Current Therapy in Gastroenterology and Liver Disease,* 4th ed. St. Louis: Mosby–Year Book; 1994:81. With permission.)

mobilized as a vascularized pedicle and anastomosed to the remaining proximal esophagus.

Although a number of incisional approaches have been used to perform this partial esophagogastrectomy—including transhiatal, Ivor-Lewis (combined right thoracotomy and laparotomy), left thoracoabdominal, three-incision, and minimally invasive techniques—the underlying operation and oncologic principles remain the same. The specific incisional approach used largely determines how much esophagus is removed and where the esophageal anastomosis will be located. In the past, proponents have argued in support of their preferred technique, giving the impression that these were uniquely different procedures. However, all of the incisional techniques basically utilize the same conceptual partial esophagogastrectomy and regional lymphadenectomy, and the results reported are similar in terms of surgical morbidity, mortality, and oncologic outcome[94–97] regardless of the incisional approach. Perhaps most importantly, survival is clearly related to pathologic tumor stage and appears to be entirely independent of the surgical esophagectomy technique utilized.[94,98]

In general, the principal variables faced by the surgeon performing a partial esophagogastrectomy—such as which incision(s) to use, the length of esophagus to resect, the extent of lymphadenectomy, the choice of conduit, where to perform the anastomosis, and which route through the chest the conduit will take—have very little impact on the overall surgical and oncologic outcomes; many of these decisions are ultimately a function of surgeon and/or patient preference. The choice of which type of incisional approach is most suitable takes several factors into consideration, including tumor location, the patient's condition and body habitus, previous operations, prior irradiation, the replacement conduit organ of choice, the extent of nodal dissection, and, perhaps most prominently, the particular surgeon's preference. Typically, an experienced esophageal surgeon has a strong bias toward utilizing one particular approach, usually based on the approach used during training. However, there are benefits and limitations to each approach, and the technique chosen should be tailored to meet the particular needs of the individual patient.

Transhiatal approach

Transhiatal esophagectomy (THE) is an increasingly popular surgical approach wherein the distal portion of the intrathoracic esophagus is mobilized through the esophageal hiatus and the proximal portion through a cervical incision. The increasing prevalence of adenocarcinomas in the distal esophagus and esophagogastric junction has been responsible in large part for the widespread use of the transhiatal approach, since these tumors are readily accessible for dissection under direct vision through the esophageal hiatus. Moreover, the regional lymph nodes for these distal tumors are in the parahiatal and proximal lesser curvature regions,[99] both of which are accessible via laparotomy. The resected esophagus is reconstructed using stomach or long-segment colon, which is passed up into the neck as a vascularized graft to be anastomosed to the proximal cervical esophagus.[100–102]

The esophageal replacement conduit is passed through the chest and into the neck by either the subcutaneous, substernal, or posterior mediastinal routes, with the posterior mediastinal being the preferred route when possible. The theoretical advantages of the THE include avoiding postthoracotomy discomfort, providing a wide proximal esophageal margin to ensure complete resection of the tumor, a cervical anastomosis (where the consequences of an anastomotic leak are theoretically minimized), and an esophageal reconstruction that results in an excellent quality of swallowing. However, no significant differences in outcomes (surgical or oncologic) have been born out when compared to transthoracic approaches in randomized controlled trials.[94–97]

It has been well documented that the THE approach is acceptable for both benign and malignant esophageal diseases.[103,104] Indications for THE in patients with benign disease include esophageal neuromotor dysfunction, esophageal stricture, and BE with high-grade dysplasia. In addition, previous esophageal surgery does not necessarily preclude the transhiatal approach, as more than 50 percent of patients referred with benign diseases who undergo THE have previously undergone one or more esophageal or periesophageal procedures, including previous antireflux repair, esophagomyotomy, or vagotomy. Although contiguity of the esophageal tumor with the aorta or prevertebral fascia on CT is not synonymous with invasion and is not an absolute contraindication to using this approach, tracheobronchial invasion by upper- or middle-third esophageal tumors, confirmed by preoperative bronchoscopy, is an absolute contraindication to THE.[105]

The disadvantages of THE include an inability to visualize middle- or proximal-third tumors or to perform high intrathoracic regional lymphadenectomy under direct vision, the potential for injury to intrathoracic structures, and the need for long-segment esophageal replacement. Although the technique is generally safe and well tolerated, it is associated with an incidence of recurrent laryngeal nerve injury in 6 percent and major respiratory complications in 10 percent of patients, as well as anastomotic leak rates of 0.8 to 20 percent. Mortality rates of 0 to 3 percent have been reported in large series.[102,106–110]

Ivor-Lewis approach

A partial esophagogastrectomy using a combined transabdominal and right thoracotomy approach (Ivor-Lewis technique) was designed to optimize the exposure of the intrathoracic esophagus, which passes through the upper two-thirds of the chest along the right posterior mediastinum.[106] Once the involved intrathoracic esophagus is mobilized, a partial esophagogastrectomy is performed and the esophagus is replaced by stomach, colon, or (less frequently) jejunum, which is passed into the chest along the esophageal bed and anastomosed to the proximal esophagus usually at the level of the azygos arch. The theoretical advantages of this technique include the excellent exposure of the mid- to upper thoracic esophagus the ability to perform a regional lymphadenectomy under direct vision, while the disadvantages are related to the use of thoracotomy and an intrathoracic anastomosis, with the potential consequences of an intrathoracic anastomotic leak. Reported complications (just as with the THE approach) include respiratory problems in 11 percent, anastomotic leak in 3 to 12 percent, and wound infections in 5 percent. Operative mortality ranges from 0 to 4 percent.[98,108,111–116]

Three-incision approach

The three-incision esophagectomy combines all of the advantages of the Ivor-Lewis approach with regard to access to upper- and middle-third tumors and the intrathoracic lymph nodes, with the additional advantage of the cervical anastomosis. Of all of the incisional approaches, this one affords the best direct access to all areas of dissection, as no portion of the operation is performed without direct visualization. Accordingly, it is conceptually the safest approach for a young and/or less experienced esophageal surgeon to utilize but is by nature a slightly more cumbersome operative approach, with the need for patient repositioning intraoperatively and three separate fields of dissection.

Left Thoracoabdominal approach

The left thoracoabdominal approach utilizes a single incision extending from the left chest to the abdomen. This technique is ideal for patients with tumors near the gastroesophageal junction, especially when the extent of gastric invasion is unclear, because it yields superb exposure and maximizes reconstructive options of the lower third of the esophagus.[117] Its disadvantages include the need for costal arch division, a perception of more postoperative pulmonary complications, the limitation of length of proximal esophagus that is resected, and poor visualization of the middle third of the esophagus due to the presence of the aortic arch. Again, randomized controlled trials have not revealed a significant difference in oncologic or surgical outcomes as compared with other incisional approaches.[94–97] Respiratory complications are the most common postoperative problem. Pulmonary complications are reported in up to 24 percent of cases. Anastomotic leaks occur in 0 to 12 percent of cases. The reported operative mortality is 0 to 6.2 percent.[118,119]

Minimally invasive esophagectomy (MIE)

As minimally invasive surgery continues to advance, the application of techniques learned from laparoscopy and VATS to the management of esophageal cancer naturally follows. A number of studies have now documented the safety and feasibility of these minimally invasive approaches, which include hybrid operations, such as laparotomy combined with VATS, or laparoscopy combined with open thoracotomy, the entirely transhiatal laparoscopic esophagectomy, or the equivalent of a three-incision approach, which combines separate laparoscopic and thoracoscopic mobilization with a cervical incision and anastomosis.[120]

This last technique was recently reported in a series of 222 patients managed with minimally invasive esophagectomy (MIE) for malignancy or high-grade dysplasia in the setting of BE. In this series, MIE was successfully completed in 206 patients (92.8 percent), with an operative mortality of 1.4 percent. Anastomotic leaks were reported in 11.7 percent, and hospital stay was 7 days.[120] Quality-of-life scores were similar to preoperative levels and age-matched population norms. Overall, these early studies reveal that MIE provides results for partial esophagogastrectomy and regional lymphadenectomy similar to those of the open operative approaches.

Extent of lymphadenectomy

Much debate remains regarding the appropriate extent of lymphadenectomy for esophageal cancer. The rationale for the development of radical or en bloc esophagectomy techniques rests on the facts that the majority of patients present with locally advanced cancers, that postesophagectomy survival in this setting is poor, and that recent advances in surgical results have not been associated with improved postoperative survival by stage. Moreover, even among patients with suspected early-stage disease, nearly 20 percent are found to have regional lymph node involvement at the time of surgery.[121] Two general treatment approaches have developed in an attempt to improve posttreatment survival. One is to combine surgery with chemotherapy and radiation therapy; the neoadjuvant chemoradiation therapy protocols discussed further on are the most notable of these combination therapies. The other approach attempts to improve postsurgical survival by adding radical or en bloc esophageal lymphadenectomy.[122]

The esophagus has an extensive regional lymphatic drainage. Arbitrarily, the lymphatic drainage has been divided into three zones or fields: cervical, intrathoracic, and abdominal. Standard esophagectomy techniques involve regional, or one-field, lymphadenectomy. Radical approaches advocate two- or three-field lymphadenectomy in conjunction with esophageal resection and replacement. Proponents of radical lymph node resection for esophageal cancer have paved the way to understanding the lymphatic drainage patterns of metastases to local and regional lymph nodes. Most notably, these investigators have found that for squamous cell cancers, there is a significant incidence of local and regional lymph node involvement and skip metastases, even in lesions that previously were considered early-stage disease,[123–128] thereby leading to the impetus for extensive lymph node dissections. However, such skip lesions have not been found with early-stage adenocarcinomas, which present with only locoregional lymph node involvement.[121]

The oncologic benefit of the more extensive and potentially morbid radical lymph node dissections (particularly for early-stage adenocarcinomas) has yet to be determined. Although many nonrandomized single-institution series have been published claiming improved long-term survival and decreased local recurrence with radical lymph node dissections,[129] no definitive randomized studies have been performed to date. Radical esophagectomy is a significantly more complex procedure than most standard techniques. This is reflected in reported morbidity rates as high as 58 percent.[130] Nevertheless, 30-day mortality rates as low as 1.6 to 4.3 percent have been reported.[129–132] Survival data using radical esophagectomy techniques are conflicting. One study found that there was improved survival in early-stage tumors using en bloc esophagectomy compared to a standard transhiatal technique.[129] Although prospective, this trial was not randomized; because earlier-stage patients were selected for the en bloc approach, the results and conclusions might have been biased. In another nonrandomized, single-institution series, improved survival was noted in patients with stage III disease using radical esophagectomy compared with standard surgical techniques.[132] Some have reported an overall 5-year survival rate as high as 40 percent using extended radical esophagectomy for esophageal cancer,[130] whereas others have found no difference in overall survival between standard transhiatal and radical transhiatal esophagectomy in which two-field lymphadenectomy is added.[131] Moreover, despite the wide surgical dissection performed during radical techniques, reports have still documented a 21 percent locoregional cancer recurrence rate.[133] The determination of which cell type and tumor stage, if any, will benefit from radical surgical techniques, has yet to be resolved. At present, no definitive randomized trials exist to address this question on an evidence-based platform. Therefore the type of lymph node dissection performed for esophageal cancer remains controversial and depends on the practicing surgeon's (and patient's) preferences.

Reconstruction conduit

Esophageal reconstruction can be achieved by the creation of a gastric tube or by performing a colonic or jejunal interposition. A tube constructed from the greater curvature of the stomach and vascularized by the right gastroepiploic arcade, for anatomic and physiologic reasons, conceptually remains the ideal and most commonly employed method for esophageal replacement after curative resection for esophageal cancer.[134] In adults, preexisting colonic disease or prior colon resection may prohibit the use of a colon conduit, and anomalous arterial patterns or a poor marginal artery can make colon interposition less appealing. In contrast, the stomach has an excellent and predictable arterial supply. Moreover, the gastroepiploic arcade, which runs outside the greater curvature of the stomach, lengthens when a gastric tube is created and therefore does not limit the length of the conduit. The colon and jejunum, with their fan-shaped mesenteries, are longer than their respective vascular supplies and tend to be redundant when interposed between the esophagus and stomach. Finally, the creation of a gastric tube conduit after esophageal resection requires only a single (esophagogastric) anastomosis, whereas the use of a colonic conduit requires three such anastomoses, making for a longer and often more technically arduous operation.

In constructing a gastric conduit for a cervical anastomosis after esophagectomy, the gastric tube must be fashioned wide enough to allow the passage of solid foods yet narrow enough to facilitate emptying without stasis and to fit in the limited space of the upper neck. A tube based on the greater curvature of the stomach that is 4 to 5 cm in diameter appears to accomplish these goals.[135]

In most situations the stomach remains the conduit of choice for esophageal replacement in adults. However, indications for the use of colonic interposition remain; these include prior gastric resection and/or gastric outlet obstruction, as well as the need for long-segment esophageal replacement in patients who have previously undergone distal gastrectomy or who presently require complete removal of the esophagus and the stomach. In such patients, the insufficient length of the gastric conduit precludes its use. Additionally, when a short segmental resection of the distal esophagus is performed, usually in benign disease, reconstruction with colon or jejunum serves the dual purpose of preserving gastric function and acting as an effective barrier to reflux. In all cases, the ultimate goal is to restore the function of swallowing as close to normal as possible with minimal morbidity and mortality.

When a colon interposition is planned, a colonoscopy or barium enema should be performed to detect any significant colonic lesion that would preclude using the colon, such as carcinoma, extensive diverticulosis, or inflammation. Arteriography or CT angiography of the abdominal aorta and its visceral branches is reserved for patients with a history of previous abdominal vascular or colonic surgery, or patients at risk for vascular lesions from systemic diseases such as diabetes or hyperlipidemia. All patients require a mechanical bowel preparation prior to surgery. Overall, results from a number of studies using colon or stomach for esophageal replacement have found no significant differences in functional outcomes, morbidity, or mortality,[107,110,136–142] and the incidence of anastomotic leak (0 to 14 percent) or graft ischemia (0 to 10 percent) was comparable across studies.

The jejunum is commonly ranked third after stomach and colon and is often reserved for reconstruction after partial, rather than total, esophageal resection. The reason for this preference is the finite length of the mesenteric pedicle, which hinders mobilization of the jejunum on its own blood supply from the abdomen to the neck. In the appropriate situation, however, the jejunum may provide a durable and entirely satisfactory conduit with good long-term swallowing function. There are three indications for small bowel interposition: reconstruction of the distal esophagus and esophagogastric junction with a pedicled graft for undilatable strictures or unremitting reflux disease; replacement with a free graft after circumferential resection of pharynx, larynx, and cervical esophagus; and total esophageal replacement with or without vascular augmentation when other options, such as stomach or colon, are unavailable. Contraindications to its use are short-gut syndrome and inflammatory bowel disease.

Anastomotic techniques

Irrespective of the conduit chosen for esophageal reconstruction, the anastomosis can be fashioned using hand-sewn (running or interrupted, one- or two-layer, absorbable or permanent suture, knots within or outside the esophageal lumen), stapled, or "semimechanical" techniques. One prospective randomized study comparing 21 single-layered interrupted to 21 single-layered continuous cervical anastomoses found no significant difference in leak rate.[143] Another compared a single-layer continuous hand-sewn anastomosis to one fashioned with a circular stapling device in a prospective, nonrandomized study of 580 patients. Comparable leak rates of 5 percent in the hand-sewn group and 3.8 percent in the stapled group ($p = 0.69$) were documented.[144] Some reports using the semimechanical anastomosis have also documented leak rates as low as 2.7 percent.[109,145–147] Moreover, although a number of recent, nonrandomized studies have touted the superiority of stapled anastomoses, with reported leak rates as low as 2.7 percent,[109,148] these results are in fact not significantly different from those in earlier reports of hand-sewn cervical esophagogastric anastomoses with leak rates of 0.8 percent.[110] Finally, a recent metanalysis of randomized controlled trials revealed no significant difference in leak rates regardless of the anastomotic technique employed.[149]

As for anastomotic strictures and the need for dilatation, some reports have suggested that rates of anastomotic stricture are lower in totally mechanically stapled anastomoses (18 percent) versus hand-sewn or semimechanical anastomoses (45 percent).[146] However, in a metanalytic review of randomized, controlled trials, no statistically significant differences were borne out.[149] The most significant finding was that, compared with historical controls, the rates of leak and stricture have declined dramatically in the past two decades (irrespective of anastomotic method employed)—a testament to improved techniques and instrumentation as well as improved peri- and postoperative care, which has undoubtedly played a major role in the reduction in morbidity and mortality in surgery for esophageal cancer.

EXPECTED POSTOPERATIVE COURSE

Strict adherence to predefined patient care pathways combined with centralization of esophageal surgery at high-volume centers of excellence have clearly contributed to recent improvements in postoperative morbidity and mortality.[150–153] With the advent of improved pulmonary physiotherapy and epidural pain control as well as the implementation of uniform patient care pathways,[106,150] postoperative complications (pulmonary complications in particular) have been minimized. Although many variations on such care plans exist, general guidelines for postesophagectomy care might be as follows: most patients are extubated on the night of surgery or the following morning and are encouraged to be out of bed and to ambulate with assistance on postoperative day 1. The nasogastric tube is generally removed between days 3 to 5, and jejunostomy feeding is begun the same day. A postoperative barium or Gastrografin swallow is obtained between days 4 to 6; if the anastomosis is intact, the patient's diet is advanced and chest tubes, if present, are removed thereafter. Patients are discharged when they can tolerate a soft diet but often still require supplemental jejunostomy feeds at night. This is typically on postoperative day 7 or 8. The jejunostomy tube is removed 4 weeks after surgery. Recent studies comparing the quality of life (QOL) of postesophagectomy patients with that of age-matched normal controls using well-validated QOL assessment tools suggest no significant differences in outcomes between such patients and the normal population.[154]

PREVENTION/MANAGEMENT OF COMPLICATIONS

Anastomotic leak

Despite significant advances over the past two decades, an anastomotic leak remains among the most dreaded complications of esophageal surgery and accounts for nearly 40 percent of the operative mortality in many series. Overall reported anastomotic leak rates, whether the anastomosis was stapled or hand-sewn, range from 0 to 25 percent.[98,107–112,155] Although many earlier reports suggested a higher incidence of cervical than of intrathoracic leaks, more recent data suggest that, in experienced hands, equally low leak rates can be achieved with cervical anastomoses.[94,109,110] Prevention remains the hallmark of the management of this complication. Attention to meticulous technique, the gentle handling of tissues, the preservation of arterial supply and venous drainage, and a tension-free anastomosis are integral to minimizing the risks of postoperative anastomotic leak.

An asymptomatic cervical anastomotic leak that is detected on a routine postoperative barium swallow and appears to drain back into the esophageal lumen usually heals without intervention. Larger or uncontained leaks require adequate drainage. Cervical esophageal leaks generally occur between the fifth and eight postoperative days and present with fever, subcutaneous emphysema, or signs of a local cervical wound infection. Clinical manifestations of sepsis mandate prompt opening of the cervical incision and wound packing, with the cessation of oral intake and maintenance of enteral nutrition through a jejunostomy tube until the leak heals. Attempts to repair or revise the anastomosis should not be made, particularly because the vast majority of cervical leaks will heal with local wound management.

Traditionally, intrathoracic anastomotic leaks posed a more formidable problem, with associated mortality rates as high as 50 to 71 percent.[98,108,156] However, more recent data suggest that the modern era of surgical therapy has brought about a significant reduction in mortality after an intrathoracic leak, from 43 to 3.3 percent.[157] These leaks are generally clinically evident after postoperative day 7, when fever, leukocytosis, or signs of systemic sepsis become apparent. The diagnosis and extent of the leak can be determined with a Gastrografin swallow or contrast-enhanced CT scan, and prompt drainage is generally advocated. Depending on the degree of contamination and size of the leak, this may involve image-guided pigtail catheter drainage, chest tube placement, or formal reexploration and open drainage.

Small, well-drained leaks can be managed conservatively if the lung is well expanded and there is no local sepsis, as first described for the management of traumatic esophageal perforation.[158] Larger leaks without evidence of conduit or esophageal remnant necrosis can be managed with surgical repair and tissue flap (pleural, pericardial, omental, or myocutaneous) coverage.[155,159,160] However, if there is extensive necrosis, the safest plan is resection of the conduit, replacement of the gastric remnant within the abdomen, and a diverting cervical esophagostomy with delayed reconstruction.[157,161] Enteral nutrition via the jejunostomy feeding tube that is placed routinely after esophagectomy has proven critical to the improved survival of patients facing the devastating consequences of a large anastomotic disruption.[157]

Anastomotic stricture

Anastomotic strictures occur regardless of the conduit utilized (gastric, colonic, or jejunal), the anastomotic technique utilized (hand-sewn or stapled), or the incisional approach used. In many reports, 10 to 30 percent of patients develop a stricture at the anastomosis. Risk factors include a previous anastomotic leak (nearly 50 percent of these patients develop anastomotic stricture as fibrosis with anastomotic healing occurs), varying degrees of conduit ischemia, or neoadjuvant therapy.[136]

Initial management should be dilation of the stricture. This can be accomplished with balloon endoscopic dilatation, soft-tapered Maloney dilators, or wire-guided Savory dilators. Most strictures can be managed with repeated dilatations without the need for surgical revision. Maintenance of a tension-free anastomosis with an unencumbered arterial supply and venous drainage is critical to minimizing the risk of anastomotic stricture.

Conduit necrosis

Conduit necrosis is an uncommon event (0.5 to 5 percent) but carries a mortality of up to 50 to 70 percent.[107,110,136–142] Patients present with signs of sepsis, acidosis, and respiratory failure, often within the first few hours after surgery. The diagnosis can be confirmed by the appearance of mucosal cobblestoning on a Gastrografin swallow, a CT scan of the chest, or a careful endoscopic evaluation. Management requires prompt resection of the necrosed segment, return of the remaining viable conduit to the abdominal cavity, and creation of a cervical esophagostomy for diversion.[161] Enteral nutrition is maintained through the jejunostomy tube and reconstruction is delayed. Again, this complication can be prevented by ensuring there is no torsion of the conduit as it traverses the chest, ensuring adequate arterial supply and venous drainage, and minimizing perioperative periods of relative hypotension or hypoxemia.

Reflux

Reflux after an esophagectomy is probably far more common than is generally recognized but is less frequently studied or addressed in the literature, since it is often readily managed with conservative therapy. Recommendations include the avoidance of liquid with meals, eating smaller-volume meals more frequently during the day, remaining upright after meals, and avoiding meals close to bedtime. Some patients require the use of a sleeping wedge when recumbent. Surgically, reflux can be minimized by creating the esophageal anastomosis at or above the level of the azygos vein.

Delayed gastric emptying

Clinically significant delayed gastric emptying is uncommon and generally occurs early in the postoperative setting. These early cases can be minimized with a pyloroplasty or pyloromyotomy performed at the time of the original operation,[93] although most studies have found no significant differences in long-term outcomes with or without such pyloric drainage procedures. Other causes of ineffective gastric emptying might include obstruction at a narrowed esophageal hiatus or a redundant intrathoracic conduit. Endoscopy and balloon dilation of the pylorus can be attempted, in addition to the use of promotility agents such as metoclopramide and erythromycin. If conservative management fails, the patient may require reoperation.

Pulmonary complications

Respiratory complications, which include aspiration, pneumonia or a failure to wean from the ventilator for more than 48 h, account for the most common causes of postoperative morbidity after esophageal resection and reconstruction. Risk factors for pulmonary complications include advanced age, malnutrition (serum albumin < 3.5 g/dL), chronic obstructive pulmonary disease, and an operative blood loss of more than 1 L.[94] Although not borne out definitively in randomized controlled trials, active cigarette smoking also portends a poor postoperative pulmonary recovery.

The best way to manage pulmonary complications is prevention, which is contingent upon early extubation and rapid mobilization with concomitant use of incentive spirometry and flutter valves. Optimization of preoperative nutrition and smoking cessation are critical albeit theoretical factors. The use of epidural catheters for pain control has been found to significantly decrease the risk of postoperative pulmonary complications and is recommended for all patients undergoing esophageal resection and reconstruction.[88–90] Additionally, vigilance for patients at risk for aspiration is a must. Studies have found that up to two-thirds of patients undergoing an esophagectomy develop new and transient swallowing dysfunction within the first week after surgery.[162] This generally resolves within 1 month. These patients are most prone to aspirate at the time of extubation and again at the onset of oral alimentation. Ensuring that such patients are ready for extubation and careful observation (with head-of-bed elevation) at the initiation of feeds are critical to minimizing this complication. Finally, appropriate antimicrobial prophylaxis initiated immediately prior to and continued during the operation has been found to decrease the risk of perioperative pneumonia.[163]

ONCOLOGIC OUTCOMES (SURVIVAL)

Survival after surgical resection is discussed separately from the description of individual operative techniques in order to emphasize the fact that postesophagectomy survival is a function of stage (Fig. 15-5) and not the incisional approach utilized or the extent of lymphadenectomy performed. Several points concerning postesophagectomy survival have now become clear. The first is that the cumulative postoperative 5-year survival after resection remains approximately 15 to 25 percent (Fig. 15-6) irrespective of the surgical technique employed.[95–98] The second fact is that the majority of patients who present for surgery are found to have stage III disease, and survival for these patients, even with surgery, is poor (approximately 10 to 15 percent) (Fig. 15-5). The third point is that postsurgical survival is little

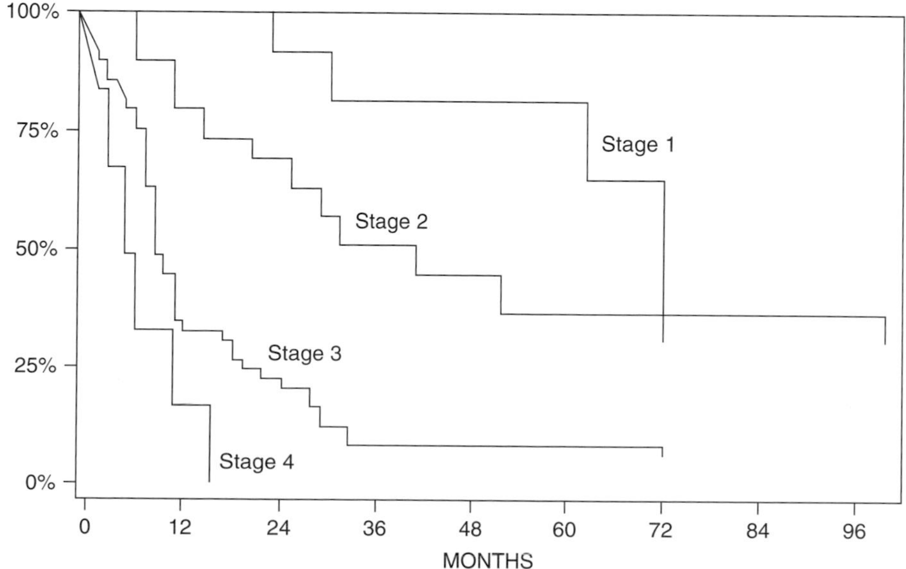

Figure 15–5 Kaplan-Meier survival by stage for patients treated with esophagectomy alone. Both squamous cell carcinoma and adenocarcinoma are included. (Adapted from Salazar et al.[164] With permission.)

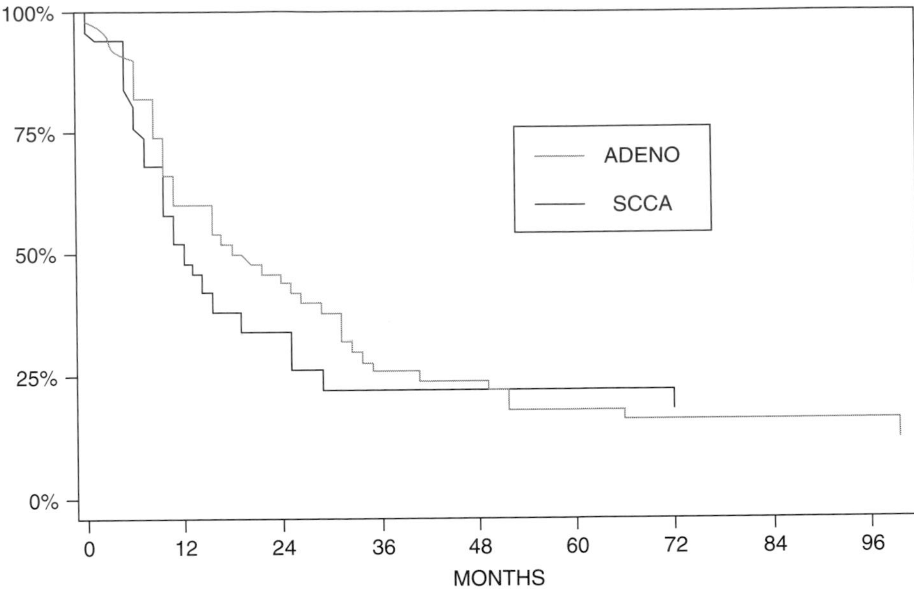

Figure 15–6 Cumulative (all stages included) Kaplan-Meier postesophagectomy survival. Survival at 5 years is 18 percent. (Adapted from Salazar et al.[164] With permission.)

influenced by whether the lesion is a squamous cell cancer or an adenocarcinoma[164,165] (Fig. 15-6). Finally, despite advances in surgical techniques, morbidity, mortality, and perioperative care, postesophagectomy survival has remained remarkably stable over time. Wilkins made this same point almost a decade ago after reviewing postoperative survival figures for the years 1952 to 1986. On the basis of his review, he queried whether surgery had "gone as far as it could go" and speculated that further improvement in survival figures would require combination therapy regimens that included systemic chemotherapy.[166]

ADJUVANT AND NEOADJUVANT THERAPY

Overall outcomes in the management of esophageal cancer remain suboptimal; poor long-term survival and local recurrences are the rule. However, improved perioperative morbidity and mortality have allowed a shift in the emphasis for these patients from surviving the operation to a more holistic approach to cancer therapy. The late stage of presentation of most patients with carcinoma of the esophagus, combined with a rich lymphatic network, make esophageal cancer a systemic disease, which is rarely cured with surgery alone despite a seemingly curative resection. In fact, the best available data for single-modality surgical therapy report 5-year survival rates that rarely exceed 25 percent, despite resection with curative intent. Therefore adjuvant therapy with radiation for local control and/or chemotherapy for local and/or distant eradication of micrometastases has been studied extensively, and is discussed in great detail in Chap. 16.

Despite early enthusiasm, neither radiation nor chemotherapy alone, nor the combination of the two (in conjunction with surgery) in the adjuvant setting has been found to improve survival in patients with cancer of the esophagus. However, the use of combined chemoradiotherapy in the neoadjuvant or preoperative setting appears to hold some promise. The rationale for the use of neoadjuvant chemoradiotherapy is based on a number of important albeit theoretical factors.[167] First, combined multimodality chemoradiotherapy maximizes the potential therapeutic benefits of each modality without compounding toxicity and may in fact have a synergistic therapeutic effect. Second, such therapy is often better tolerated preoperatively than in the postoperative setting. Third, there is some evidence to suggest that neoadjuvant therapy allows a greater percentage of patients to be deemed resectable. Finally and perhaps most importantly, there are some promising data suggesting that preoperative chemoradiotherapy may be the only adjunct to surgical resection that actually improves survival, particularly in the subset of patients who have a complete response to neoadjuvant treatment (i.e., no residual tumor found at the time of resection).

Although several well-conducted randomized controlled trials have been performed to compare surgery alone against surgery with neoadjuvant chemoradiotherapy, much debate remains regarding the interpretation of these trials and the neoadjuvant algorithm that might be most effective. The only trial to date that found a statistically significant difference in survival was the 1996 Irish study, in which 3-year survival was 32 percent in patients who received surgery with neoadjuvant chemoradiotherapy as compared with 6 percent in those receiving surgery alone.[168] However, critics have argued that the poor survival (compared with published historical controls) in the surgery-alone group suggests that preoperative staging accuracy may have been an issue, thereby bringing the validity of their results into question. A second study from the University of Michigan found that surgery in combination with neoadjuvant chemoradiotherapy improved survival (30 percent) versus surgery alone (16 percent), but this study was not powered so as to yield statistical significance.[169] A third trial from France failed to find a survival difference with neoadjuvant therapy versus surgery alone[170] but has been criticized as having employed a neoadjuvant regimen with minimal efficacy. Although these studies are promising, definitive answers await rigorous randomized controlled trials.

NONSURGICAL PALLIATION FOR ESOPHAGEAL CANCER

The management of the symptoms of esophageal cancer (dysphagia in particular) remains a challenge. Even after successful surgical resection with curative intent, a large proportion of patients treated surgically eventually develop recurrence. As the morbidity and mortality associated with palliative surgery are high, surgical palliative approaches have largely been replaced by nonsurgical techniques. Malignant dysphagia results from partial or complete occlusion of the esophageal lumen. The goals of treatment are to maintain esophageal luminal patency, minimize hospitalization, and provide adequate pain relief. Current therapeutic options for palliation include chemo/radiotherapy or the use of lasers, stents, or photodynamic therapy (PDT).

Laser therapy

Laser therapy is a well-accepted form of palliation for esophageal tumors. Laser treatment has been found to be superior to dilation or other methods of thermal destruction, especially in the setting of proximal esophageal lesions, where stent placement may not be feasible. The overall success rate of laser therapy varies from 62 to 93 percent. Advantages of laser therapy include the prolonged duration of dysphagia relief (2 to 4 months) and the low complication rate. A distinct disadvantage is that multiple laser sessions are often required to achieve adequate and durable palliation. Complications include tracheoesophageal fistula formation (0.7 to 6.3 percent), bleeding, and perforation (1 to 5.8 percent).[171]

Esophageal stents

Self-expanding metal stents (SEMS) are composed of tightly wound wire coils or mesh that is wrapped around a small delivery device, making endoscopic placement simple and often obviating the need for aggressive predeployment dilation and its attendant risk of perforation. On deployment, SEMS radially expand to a predetermined diameter and generally bring immediate relief of dysphagia. Successful stent deployment and improvement in swallowing has been reported in 90 to 100 percent of patients with malignant esophageal obstruction.[172]

Relative contraindications to the use of SEMS include soft or noncircumferential stenoses or markedly angulated strictures, which may prevent adequate anchoring of the SEMS. Early minor complications include chest pain, stent misplacement (minimized by choosing a stent 4 cm longer than the length of the stricture), and migration (which can result from using stents with suboptimal radial expansion). Early major complications include perforation or bleeding, which occurs in 6 percent of patients. Life-threatening long-term complications of gastrointestinal bleeding, perforation, or tracheoesophageal fistulas occur in 4 to 7 percent of patients. Tumor ingrowth is a late complication that has been reduced with the advent of silicone-covered or polyurethane-covered SEMS. Treatment options for the management of tumor ingrowth include laser therapy, electrocoagulation, PDT, argon plasma coagulation, and the placement of an overlapping second SEMS.[171]

Photodynamic therapy (PDT)

PDT is a nonthermal ablative technique that results in local and specific necrosis of malignant esophageal tissue. A photosensitive chemical (Photofrin) with a relative specificity for malignant tissue is administered to the patient intravenously 2 to 3 days before drug activation. An endoscopically placed laser is then utilized to generate a monochromatic beam, thereby activating porfimer sodium and generating cytotoxic singlet oxygen radicals. These reactive oxygen species cause rapid vascular stasis and hemorrhage, thus triggering direct and anoxia-induced tumor necrosis.[171]

The tissue-specific effects of PDT are based on the relative specificity of the photosensitizer for malignant tissue, the directed application of the light source, the transmission depth of the wavelength of the light, and the oxygen content of the tissue. Because there is no cumulative toxicity to surrounding tissue, PDT can be repeated without interfering with or precluding other forms of therapy. Contraindications to the use of PDT include known porphyria (or hypersensitivity to porphyrins), tumor infiltration into the respiratory tract, the presence of a tracheoesophageal fistula, symptomatic pleural or pericardial effusions, or unstable arrhythmias.

CONCLUSIONS

The increasing incidence of esophageal adenocarcinoma, coupled with a growing understanding of BE and dysplasia as its immediate precursors, have opened new doors for earlier detection and more effective therapeutic intervention for esophageal cancer. Moreover, improved surgical outcomes and perioperative care have allowed a more holistic approach to the care of the cancer patient. As molecular biomarkers and gene and immunotherapies continue to evolve, the multimodality therapy of esophageal carcinoma should bring increasing promise to patients afflicted with this disease.

References

1. Postlethwaite R. Squamous cell carcinoma of the esophagus, In: *Surgery of the Esophagus*, 2d ed. Stamford, CT: Appleton-Century; 1986:369.
2. Ming S. Adenocarcinoma and other epithelial tumors of the esophagus. In: Ming S, Goldman H (eds). *Pathology of the Gastrointestinal Tract.* Philadelphia: Saunders; 1992:459.
3. Ibrahim N, Briggs J, Corbishley C. Extrapulmonary oat cell carcinoma. *Cancer* 1984;54:1645–1661.
4. Choh J, Khazei A, Ihm H. Leiomyosarcoma of the esophagus: Report of a case and review of the literature. *J Surg Oncol* 1986;32:223–226.
5. Paymaster JC, Sanghvi LD, Gangadharan P. Cancer in the gastrointestinal tract in Western India. *Cancer* 1968;21:279–288.
6. Yang PC, Davis S. Incidence of cancer of the esophagus in the U.S. by histologic type. *Cancer* 1988;61:612–617.
7. Jemal A, Murray T, Ward E, et al. Cancer statistics, 2005. *CA Cancer J Clin* 2005;55:10–30.
8. Hesketh PJ, Clapp RW, Doos WG, Spechler SJ. The increasing frequency of adenocarcinoma of the esophagus. *Cancer* 1989;64:526–530.
9. Pera M, Cameron AJ, Trastek VF, et al. Increasing incidence of adenocarcinoma of the esophagus and esophagogastric junction. *Gastroenterology* 1993;104:510–513.
10. Blot WJ, Devesa SS, Kneller RW, Fraumeni JF Jr. Rising incidence of adenocarcinoma of the esophagus and gastric cardia. *JAMA* 1991;265:1287–1289.
11. Powell J, McConkey CC. Increasing incidence of adenocarcinoma of the gastric cardia and adjacent sites. *Br J Cancer* 1990;62:440–443.
12. Johnston BJ, Reed PI. Changing pattern of oesophageal cancer in a general hospital in the UK. *Eur J Cancer Prev* 1991;1:23–25.
13. Reed PI, Johnston BJ. The changing incidence of oesophageal cancer. *Endoscopy* 1993;25:606–608.
14. Heitmiller RF, Sharma RR. Comparison of prevalence and resection rates in patients with esophageal squamous cell carcinoma and adenocarcinoma. *J Thorac Cardiovasc Surg* 1996;112:130–136.
15. Oka M, Attwood SE, Kaul B, et al. Immunosuppression in patients with Barrett's esophagus. *Surgery* 1992;112:11–17.
16. Newcomb PA, Carbone PP. The health consequences of smoking: Cancer. *Med Clin North Am* 1992;76:305–331.
17. Hiyama T, Sato T, Yoshino K, et al. Second primary cancer following laryngeal cancer with special reference to smoking habits. *Jpn J Cancer Res* 1992;83:334–339.
18. Choi SY, Kahyo H. Effect of cigarette smoking and alcohol consumption in the etiology of cancers of the digestive tract. *Int J Cancer* 1991;49:381–386.
19. Franceschi S, Talamini R, Barra S, et al. Smoking and drinking in relation to cancers of the oral cavity, pharynx, larynx, and esophagus in northern Italy. *Cancer Res* 1990;50:6502–6507.
20. De Stefani E, Munoz N, Esteve J, et al. Mate drinking, alcohol, tobacco, diet, and esophageal cancer in Uruguay. *Cancer Res* 1990;50:426–431.
21. Gray JR, Coldman AJ, MacDonald WC. Cigarette and alcohol use in patients with adenocarcinoma of the gastric cardia or lower esophagus. *Cancer* 1992;69:2227–2231.
22. Vaughan TL, Davis S, Kristal A, Thomas DB. Obesity, alcohol, and tobacco as risk factors for cancers of the esophagus and gastric cardia: Adenocarcinoma versus squamous cell carcinoma. *Cancer Epidemiol Biomarkers Prev* 1995;4:85–92.
23. Christen AG, McDonald JL Jr, Olson BL, Christen JA. Smokeless tobacco addiction: A threat to the oral and systemic health of the child and adolescent. *Pediatrician* 1989;16:170–177.
24. Gammon MD, Schoenberg JB, Ahsan H, et al. Tobacco, alcohol, and socioeconomic status and adenocarcinomas of the esophagus and gastric cardia. *J Natl Cancer Inst* 1997;89:1277–1284.
25. Adami HO, McLaughlin JK, Hsing AW, et al. Alcoholism and cancer risk: A population-based cohort study. *Cancer Causes Control* 1992;3:419–425.
26. Kato I, Nomura AM, Stemmermann GN, Chyou PH. Prospective study of the association of alcohol with cancer of the upper aerodigestive tract and other sites. *Cancer Causes Control* 1992;3:145–151.
27. Ghadirian P, Ekoe JM, Thouez JP. Food habits and esophageal cancer: An overview. *Cancer Detect Prev* 1992;16:163–168.
28. Block G, Patterson B, Subar A. Fruits, vegetables, and cancer prevention: A review of the epidemiological evidence. *Nutr Cancer* 1992;18:1–29.
29. Liu GT, Qian YZ, Zhang P, et al. Etiological role of *Alternaria alternata* in human esophageal cancer. *Chin Med J(Engl)* 1992;105:394–400.
30. Aggestrup S, Holm JC, Sorensen HR. Does achalasia predispose to cancer of the esophagus? *Chest* 1992;102:1013–1016.
31. Chuong JJ, DuBovik S, McCallum RW. Achalasia as a risk factor for esophageal carcinoma: A reappraisal. *Dig Dis Sci* 1984;29:1105–1108.
32. Hsing AW, Hansson LE, McLaughlin JK, et al. Pernicious anemia and subsequent cancer: A population-based cohort study. *Cancer* 1993;71:745–750.
33. van Blankenstein M, Looman CW, Johnston BJ, Caygill CP. Age and sex distribution of the prevalence of Barrett's esophagus found in a primary referral endoscopy center. *Am J Gastroenterol* 2005;100:568–576.

34. Pohl H, Welch HG. The role of overdiagnosis and reclassification in the marked increase of esophageal adenocarcinoma incidence. *J Natl Cancer Inst* 2005;97: 142–146.
35. Conio M, Cameron AJ, Romero Y, et al. Secular trends in the epidemiology and outcome of Barrett's oesophagus in Olmsted County, Minnesota. *Gut* 2001;48: 304–309.
36. Shaheen NJ, Crosby MA, Bozymski EM, Sandler RS. Is there publication bias in the reporting of cancer risk in Barrett's esophagus? *Gastroenterology* 2000;119:333–338.
37. DeMeester SR, DeMeester TR. Columnar mucosa and intestinal metaplasia of the esophagus: Fifty years of controversy. *Ann Surg* 2000;231:303–321.
38. Rudolph RE, Vaughan TL, Storer BE, et al. Effect of segment length on risk for neoplastic progression in patients with Barrett esophagus. *Ann Intern Med* 2000;132: 612–620.
39. Miros M, Kerlin P, Walker N. Only patients with dysplasia progress to adenocarcinoma in Barrett's oesophagus. *Gut* 1991;32:1441–1446.
40. Tytgat GN, Hameeteman W. The neoplastic potential of columnar-lined (Barrett's) esophagus. *World J Surg* 1992;16:308–312.
41. Koppert LB, Wijnhoven BP, van Dekken H, et al. The molecular biology of esophageal adenocarcinoma. *J Surg Oncol* 2005;92:169–190.
42. Tew WP, Kelsen DP, Ilson DH. Targeted therapies for esophageal cancer. *Oncologist* 2005;10:590–601.
43. McManus DT, Olaru A, Meltzer SJ. Biomarkers of esophageal adenocarcinoma and Barrett's esophagus. *Cancer Res* 2004;64:1561–1569.
44. Sharma P, Sidorenko EI. Are screening and surveillance for Barrett's oesophagus really worthwhile? *Gut* 2005; 54(Suppl 1):i27–i32.
45. Dulai GS, Guha S, Kahn KL, et al. Preoperative prevalence of Barrett's esophagus in esophageal adenocarcinoma: A systematic review. *Gastroenterology* 2002;122: 26–33.
46. Corley DA, Levin TR, Habel LA, et al. Surveillance and survival in Barrett's adenocarcinomas: A population-based study. *Gastroenterology* 2002;122:633–640.
47. Kobayashi S, Kasugai T. Brushing cytology for the diagnosis of gastric cancer involving the cardia or the lower esophagus. *Acta Cytol* 1978;22:155–157.
48. Winawer SJ, Sherlock P, Belladonna JA, et al. Endoscopic brush cytology in esophageal cancer. *JAMA* 1975;232: 1358.
49. Chirieac LR, Swisher SG, Ajani JA, et al. Posttherapy pathologic stage predicts survival in patients with esophageal carcinoma receiving preoperative chemoradiation. *Cancer* 2005;103:1347–1355.
50. Iizuka T, Isono K, Kakegawa T, Watanabe H. Parameters linked to ten-year survival in Japan of resected esophageal carcinoma. Japanese Committee for Registration of Esophageal Carcinoma Cases. *Chest* 1989;96:1005–1011.
51. Ellis FH Jr. Treatment of carcinoma of the esophagus or cardia. *Mayo Clin Proc* 1989;64:945–955.
52. American Joint Committee on Cancer. *AJCC Cancer Staging Manual*, 5th ed. Philadelphia: Lippincott Williams & Wilkins; 1997:65–68.
53. Nigro JJ, Hagen JA, DeMeester TR, et al. Occult esophageal adenocarcinoma: Extent of disease and implications for effective therapy. *Ann Surg* 1999;230:433–438.
54. Rice TW, Blackstone EH, Goldblum JR, et al. Superficial adenocarcinoma of the esophagus. *J Thorac Cardiovasc Surg* 2001;122:1077–1090.
55. Nigro JJ, DeMeester SR, Hagen JA, et al. Node status in transmural esophageal adenocarcinoma and outcome after en bloc esophagectomy. *J Thorac Cardiovasc Surg* 1999;117:960–968.
56. Korst RJ, Rusch VW, Venkatraman E, et al. Proposed revision of the staging classification for esophageal cancer. *J Thorac Cardiovasc Surg* 1998;115:660–669.
57. Rice TW, Zuccaro G Jr, Adelstein DJ, et al. Esophageal carcinoma: Depth of tumor invasion is predictive of regional lymph node status. *Ann Thorac Surg* 1998;65:787–792.
58. Hagen JA, DeMeester SR, Peters JH, et al. Curative resection for esophageal adenocarcinoma: Analysis of 100 en bloc esophagectomies. *Ann Surg* 2001;234:520–530.
59. Ellis FH Jr, Heatley GJ, Balogh K. Proposal for improved staging criteria for carcinoma of the esophagus and cardia. *Eur J Cardiothorac Surg* 1997;12:361–364.
60. Holscher AH, Bollschweiler E, Bumm R, et al. Prognostic factors of resected adenocarcinoma of the esophagus. *Surgery* 1995;118:845–855.
61. Eloubeidi MA, Wallace MB, Hoffman BJ, et al. Predictors of survival for esophageal cancer patients with and without celiac axis lymphadenopathy: Impact of staging endosonography. *Ann Thorac Surg* 2001;72:212–219.
62. Christie NA, Rice TW, DeCamp MM, et al. M1a/M1b esophageal carcinoma: Clinical relevance. *J Thorac Cardiovasc Surg* 1999;118:900–907.
63. Hiele M, De Leyn P, Schurmans P, et al. Relation between endoscopic ultrasound findings and outcome of patients with tumors of the esophagus or esophagogastric junction. *Gastrointest Endosc* 1997;45:381–386.
64. Kawakami K, Brabender J, Lord RV, et al. Hypermethylated APC DNA in plasma and prognosis of patients with esophageal adenocarcinoma. *J Natl Cancer Inst* 2000;92: 1805–1811.
65. Ireland AP, Shibata DK, Chandrasoma P, et al. Clinical significance of p53 mutations in adenocarcinoma of the esophagus and cardia. *Ann Surg* 2000;231:179–187.
66. Schneider PM, Stoeltzing O, Roth JA, et al. P53 mutational status improves estimation of prognosis in patients with curatively resected adenocarcinoma in Barrett's esophagus. *Clin Cancer Res* 2000;6:3153–3158.
67. Aloia TA, Harpole DH Jr, Reed CE, et al. Tumor marker expression is predictive of survival in patients with esophageal cancer. *Ann Thorac Surg* 2001;72:859–866.
68. Samejima R, Kitajima Y, Yunotani S, Miyazaki K. Cyclin D1 is a possible predictor of sensitivity to chemoradiotherapy for esophageal squamous cell carcinoma. *Anticancer Res* 1999;19:5515–5521.
69. Heeren PA, Kloppenberg FW, Hollema H, et al. Predictive effect of p53 and p21 alteration on chemotherapy response and survival in locally advanced adenocarcinoma of the esophagus. *Anticancer Res* 2004; 24:2579–2583.
70. Quint LE, Glazer GM, Orringer MB, Gross BH. Esophageal carcinoma: CT findings. *Radiology* 1985; 155:171–175.

71. Becker CD, Barbier P, Porcellini B. CT evaluation of patients undergoing transhiatal esophagectomy for cancer. *J Comput Assist Tomogr* 1986;10:607–611.
72. Tio TL, Coene PP, Hartog Jager FC, Tytgat GN. Preoperative TNM classification of esophageal carcinoma by endosonography. *Hepatogastroenterology* 1990;37:376–381.
73. Heintz A, Mildenberger P, Georg M, et al. Endoscopic ultrasonography in the diagnosis of regional lymph nodes in esophageal and gastric cancer: Results of studies in vitro. *Endoscopy* 1993;25:231–235.
74. Botet JF, Lightdale CJ, Zauber AG, et al. Preoperative staging of esophageal cancer: Comparison of endoscopic US and dynamic CT. *Radiology* 1991;181:419–425.
75. Dittler HJ, Siewert JR. Role of endoscopic ultrasonography in esophageal carcinoma. *Endoscopy* 1993;25:156–161.
76. Wiersema MJ, Vilmann P, Giovannini M, et al. Endosonography-guided fine-needle aspiration biopsy: Diagnostic accuracy and complication assessment. *Gastroenterology* 1997;112:1087–1095.
77. Tio TL, Cohen P, Coene PP, et al. Endosonography and computed tomography of esophageal carcinoma: Preoperative classification compared to the new (1987) TNM system. *Gastroenterology* 1989;96:1478–1486.
78. Rice TW, Boyce GA, Sivak MV. Esophageal ultrasound and the preoperative staging of carcinoma of the esophagus. *J Thorac Cardiovasc Surg* 1991;101:536–543.
79. Krasna MJ. Advances in staging of esophageal carcinoma. *Chest* 1998;113:107S–111S.
80. Luketich JD, Schauer P, Landreneau R, et al. Minimally invasive surgical staging is superior to endoscopic ultrasound in detecting lymph node metastases in esophageal cancer. *J Thorac Cardiovasc Surg* 1997;114:817–821.
81. Bemelman WA, van Delden OM, van Lanschot JJ, et al. Laparoscopy and laparoscopic ultrasonography in staging of carcinoma of the esophagus and gastric cardia. *J Am Coll Surg* 1995;181:421–425.
82. Rau B, Hunerbein M, Reingruber B, et al. Laparoscopic lymph node assessment in pretherapeutic staging of gastric and esophageal cancer. *Recent Results Cancer Res* 1996;142:209–215.
83. van Delden OM, de Wit LT, Bemelman WA, et al. Laparoscopic ultrasonography for abdominal tumor staging: Technical aspects and imaging findings. *Abdom Imaging* 1997;22:125–131.
84. Gouma DJ, de Wit LT, Nieveen VD, et al. Laparoscopic ultrasonography for staging of gastrointestinal malignancy. *Scand J Gastroenterol Suppl* 1996;218:43–49.
85. Krasna MJ, Flowers JL, Attar S, McLaughlin J. Combined thoracoscopic/laparoscopic staging of esophageal cancer. *J Thorac Cardiovasc Surg* 1996;111:800–806.
86. Lowe VJ, Booya F, Fletcher JG, et al. Comparison of positron emission tomography, computed tomography, and endoscopic ultrasound in the initial staging of patients with esophageal cancer. *Mol Imaging Biol* 2005;1–9.
87. Luketich JD, Schauer PR, Meltzer CC, et al. Role of positron emission tomography in staging esophageal cancer. *Ann Thorac Surg* 1997;64:765–769.
88. Nan DN, Fernandez-Ayala M, Farinas-Alvarez C, et al. Nosocomial infection after lung surgery: Incidence and risk factors. *Chest* 2005;128:2647–2652.
89. Hansdottir V, Philip J, Olsen MF, et al. Thoracic epidural versus intravenous patient-controlled analgesia after cardiac surgery: A randomized controlled trial on length of hospital stay and patient-perceived quality of recovery. *Anesthesiology* 2006;104:142–151.
90. Norris EJ, Beattie C, Perler BA, et al. Double-masked randomized trial comparing alternate combinations of intraoperative anesthesia and postoperative analgesia in abdominal aortic surgery. *Anesthesiology* 2001;95:1054–1067.
91. Margolis M, Alexander P, Trachiotis GD, et al. Percutaneous endoscopic gastrostomy before multimodality therapy in patients with esophageal cancer. *Ann Thorac Surg* 2003;76:1694–1697.
92. Thomas DM, Langford RM, Russell RC, Le Quesne LP. The anatomical basis for gastric mobilization in total oesophagectomy. *Br J Surg* 1979;66:230–233.
93. Urschel JD, Blewett CJ, Young JE, et al. Pyloric drainage (pyloroplasty) or no drainage in gastric reconstruction after esophagectomy: A meta-analysis of randomized controlled trials. *Dig Surg* 2002;19:160–164.
94. Rentz J, Bull D, Harpole D, et al. Transthoracic versus transhiatal esophagectomy: A prospective study of 945 patients. *J Thorac Cardiovasc Surg* 2003;125:1114–1120.
95. Goldminc M, Maddern G, Le Prise E, et al. Oesophagectomy by a transhiatal approach or thoracotomy: A prospective randomized trial. *Br J Surg* 1993;80:367–370.
96. Hulscher JB, van Sandick JW, de Boer AG, et al. Extended transthoracic resection compared with limited transhiatal resection for adenocarcinoma of the esophagus. *N Engl J Med* 2002;347:1662–1669.
97. Walther B, Johansson J, Johnsson F, et al. Cervical or thoracic anastomosis after esophageal resection and gastric tube reconstruction: A prospective randomized trial comparing sutured neck anastomosis with stapled intrathoracic anastomosis. *Ann Surg* 2003;238:803–812.
98. Muller JM, Erasmi H, Stelzner M, et al. Surgical therapy of oesophageal carcinoma. *Br J Surg* 1990;77:845–857.
99. Feith M, Stein HJ, Siewert JR. Pattern of lymphatic spread of Barrett's cancer. *World J Surg* 2003;27:1052–1057.
100. Shriver CD, Burt M. Transhiatal esophagectomy. *Semin Thorac Cardiovasc Surg* 1992;4:307–313.
101. Orringer MB. Technical aids in performing transhiatal esophagectomy without thoracotomy. *Ann Thorac Surg* 1984;38:128–132.
102. Orringer MB. Surgical options for esophageal resection and reconstruction with stomach. In: Baue AE, Geha AS, Hammond GL, et al (eds). *Glenn's Thoracic and Cardiovascular Surgery*, 6th ed. Stamford, CT: Appleton & Lange; 1996:899–922.
103. Orringer MB, Marshall B, Stirling MC. Transhiatal esophagectomy for benign and malignant disease. *J Thorac Cardiovasc Surg* 1993;105:265–276.
104. Davis EA, Heitmiller RF. Esophagectomy for benign disease: Trends in surgical results and management. *Ann Thorac Surg* 1996;62:369–372.
105. Iannettoni M, Chang A. Transhiatal esophagectomy. In: Yang SC, Cameron DE (eds). *Current Therapy in Thoracic and Cardiovascular Surgery*. Philadelphia: Mosby; 2004:373–377.

106. Gillinov AM, Heitmiller RF. Strategies to reduce pulmonary complications after transhiatal esophagectomy. *Dis Esoph* 1998;11:43–47.
107. Orringer MB, Marshall B, Iannettoni MD. Transhiatal esophagectomy: Clinical experience and refinements. *Ann Surg* 1999;230:392–400.
108. Giuli R, Gignoux M. Treatment of carcinoma of the esophagus: Retrospective study of 2,400 patients. *Ann Surg* 1980;192:44–52.
109. Orringer MB, Marshall B, Iannettoni MD. Eliminating the cervical esophagogastric anastomotic leak with a side-to-side stapled anastomosis. *J Thorac Cardiovasc Surg* 2000;119:277–288.
110. Heitmiller RF, Fischer A, Liddicoat JR. Cervical esophagogastric anastomosis: Results following esophagectomy for carcinoma. *Dis Esoph* 1999;12:264–269.
111. Sauvanet A, Baltar J, Le Mee J, Belghiti J. Diagnosis and conservative management of intrathoracic leakage after oesophagectomy. *Br J Surg* 1998;85:1446–1449.
112. Whooley BP, Law S, Alexandrou A, et al. Critical appraisal of the significance of intrathoracic anastomotic leakage after esophagectomy for cancer. *Am J Surg* 2001; 181:198–203.
113. King RM, Pairolero PC, Trastek VF, et al. Ivor Lewis esophagogastrectomy for carcinoma of the esophagus: Early and late functional results. *Ann Thorac Surg* 1987; 44:119–122.
114. Mathisen DJ, Grillo HC, Wilkins EW Jr, et al. Transthoracic esophagectomy: A safe approach to carcinoma of the esophagus. *Ann Thorac Surg* 1988;45: 137–143.
115. Mitchell RL. Abdominal and right thoracotomy approach as standard procedure for esophagogastrectomy with low morbidity. *J Thorac Cardiovasc Surg* 1987;93:205–211.
116. Allen MS. Ivor Lewis esophagectomy. In: Loop FD, Mathisen DJ (eds). *Seminars in Thoracic and Cardiovascular Surgery*, 4th ed. Philadelphia: Saunders; 1992:320.
117. Heitmiller RF. The left thoracoabdominal incision. *Ann Thorac Surg* 1988;46:250–253.
118. Heitmiller RF. Results of standard left thoracoabdominal esophagogastrectomy. *Semin Thorac Cardiovasc Surg* 1992;4:314–319.
119. Shahian DM, Neptune WB, Ellis FH Jr, Watkins E Jr. Transthoracic versus extrathoracic esophagectomy: Mortality, morbidity, and long-term survival. *Ann Thorac Surg* 1986;41:237–246.
120. Luketich JD, Alvelo-Rivera M, Buenaventura PO, et al. Minimally invasive esophagectomy: Outcomes in 222 patients. *Ann Surg* 2003;238:486–494.
121. Stein HJ, Feith M, Bruecher BL, et al. Early esophageal cancer: Pattern of lymphatic spread and prognostic factors for long-term survival after surgical resection. *Ann Surg* 2005;242:566–573.
122. Lerut T, Coosemans W, Decker G, et al. Extended surgery for cancer of the esophagus and gastroesophageal junction. *J Surg Res* 2004;117:58–63.
123. Tajima Y, Nakanishi Y, Ochiai A, et al. Histopathologic findings predicting lymph node metastasis and prognosis of patients with superficial esophageal carcinoma: Analysis of 240 surgically resected tumors. *Cancer* 2000;88:1285–1293.
124. Kato H, Tachimori Y, Mizobuchi S, et al. Cervical, mediastinal, and abdominal lymph node dissection (three-field dissection) for superficial carcinoma of the thoracic esophagus. *Cancer* 1993;72:2879–2882.
125. Matsubara T, Ueda M, Abe T, et al. Unique distribution patterns of metastatic lymph nodes in patients with superficial carcinoma of the thoracic oesophagus. *Br J Surg* 1999;86:669–673.
126. Igaki H, Kato H, Tachimori Y, Nakanishi Y. Cervical lymph node metastasis in patients with submucosal carcinoma of the thoracic esophagus. *J Surg Oncol* 2000;75:37–41.
127. Fujita H, Sueyoshi S, Yamana H, et al. Optimum treatment strategy for superficial esophageal cancer: Endoscopic mucosal resection versus radical esophagectomy. *World J Surg* 2001;25:424–431.
128. Kodama M, Kakegawa T. Treatment of superficial cancer of the esophagus: A summary of responses to a questionnaire on superficial cancer of the esophagus in Japan. *Surgery* 1998;123:432–439.
129. Hagen JA, Peters JH, DeMeester TR. Superiority of extended en bloc esophagogastrectomy for carcinoma of the lower esophagus and cardia. *J Thorac Cardiovasc Surg* 1993;106:850–858.
130. Nishimaki T, Suzuki T, Suzuki S, et al. Outcomes of extended radical esophagectomy for thoracic esophageal cancer. *J Am Coll Surg* 1998;186:306–312.
131. Bumm R, Feussner H, Bartels H, et al. Radical transhiatal esophagectomy with two-field lymphadenectomy and endodissection for distal esophageal adenocarcinoma. *World J Surg* 1997;21:822–831.
132. Altorki NK, Girardi L, Skinner DB. En bloc esophagectomy improves survival for stage III esophageal cancer. *J Thorac Cardiovasc Surg* 1997;114:948–955.
133. Bhansali MS, Fujita H, Kakegawa T, et al. Pattern of recurrence after extended radical esophagectomy with three-field lymph node dissection for squamous cell carcinoma in the thoracic esophagus. *World J Surg* 1997;21: 275–281.
134. Gawad KA, Hosch SB, Bumann D, et al. How important is the route of reconstruction after esophagectomy: A prospective randomized study. *Am J Gastroenterol* 1999; 94:1490–1496.
135. Heitmiller RF. Impact of gastric tube diameter on upper mediastinal anatomy after transhiatal esophagectomy. *Dis Esoph* 2000;13:288–292.
136. Briel JW, Tamhankar AP, Hagen JA, et al. Prevalence and risk factors for ischemia, leak, and stricture of esophageal anastomosis: Gastric pull-up versus colon interposition. *J Am Coll Surg* 2004;198:536–541.
137. Davis PA, Law S, Wong J. Colonic interposition after esophagectomy for cancer. *Arch Surg* 2003;138:303–308.
138. Peracchia A, Bardini R, Ruol A, et al. Esophagovisceral anastomotic leak: A prospective statistical study of predisposing factors. *J Thorac Cardiovasc Surg* 1988;95: 685–691.
139. DeMeester TR, Johansson KE, Franze I, et al. Indications, surgical technique, and long-term functional results of colon interposition or bypass. *Ann Surg* 1988; 208:460–474.
140. Gaissert HA, Mathisen DJ, Grillo HC, et al. Short–segment intestinal interposition of the distal esophagus. *J Thorac Cardiovasc Surg* 1993;106:860–866.

141. Cerfolio RJ, Allen MS, Deschamps C, et al. Esophageal replacement by colon interposition. *Ann Thorac Surg* 1995;59:1382–1384.
142. Mansour KA, Bryan FC, Carlson GW. Bowel interposition for esophageal replacement: Twenty-five-year experience. *Ann Thorac Surg* 1997;64:752–756.
143. Bardini R, Bonavina L, Asolati M, et al. Single-layered cervical esophageal anastomoses: A prospective study of two suturing techniques. *Ann Thorac Surg* 1994;58: 1087–1089.
144. Fok M, Ah-Chong AK, Cheng SW, Wong J. Comparison of a single layer continuous hand-sewn method and circular stapling in 580 oesophageal anastomoses. *Br J Surg* 1991;78:342–345.
145. Collard JM, Romagnoli R, Goncette L, et al. Terminalized semimechanical side-to-side suture technique for cervical esophagogastrostomy. *Ann Thorac Surg* 1998;65:814–817.
146. Ercan S, Rice TW, Murthy SC, et al. Does esophagogastric anastomotic technique influence the outcome of patients with esophageal cancer? *J Thorac Cardiovasc Surg* 2005;129:623–631.
147. Santos RS, Raftopoulos Y, Singh D, et al. Utility of total mechanical stapled cervical esophagogastric anastomosis after esophagectomy: A comparison to conventional anastomotic techniques. *Surgery* 2004;136:917–925.
148. Behzadi A, Nichols FC, Cassivi SD, et al. Esophagogastrectomy: The influence of stapled versus hand-sewn anastomosis on outcome. *J Gastrointest Surg* 2005;9:1031–1040.
149. Urschel JD, Blewett CJ, Bennett WF, et al. Handsewn or stapled esophagogastric anastomoses after esophagectomy for cancer: Meta-analysis of randomized controlled trials. *Dis Esoph* 2001;14:212–217.
150. Cerfolio RJ, Bryant AS, Bass CS, et al. Fast tracking after Ivor Lewis esophagogastrectomy. *Chest* 2004;126: 1187–1194.
151. Zehr KJ, Dawson PB, Yang SC, Heitmiller RF. Standardized clinical care pathways for major thoracic cases reduce hospital costs. *Ann Thorac Surg* 1998;66: 914–919.
152. Dimick JB, Pronovost PJ, Cowan JA, Lipsett PA. Surgical volume and quality of care for esophageal resection: Do high-volume hospitals have fewer complications? *Ann Thorac Surg* 2003;75:337–341.
153. Dimick JB, Cattaneo SM, Lipsett PA, et al. Hospital volume is related to clinical and economic outcomes of esophageal resection in Maryland. *Ann Thorac Surg* 2001;72:334–339.
154. Deschamps C, Nichols FC III, Cassivi SD, et al. Long-term function and quality of life after esophageal resection for cancer and Barrett's. *Surg Clin North Am* 2005;85:649–656, xi.
155. Urschel JD. Esophagogastrostomy anastomotic leaks complicating esophagectomy: A review. *Am J Surg* 1995;169:634–640.
156. Patil PK, Patel SG, Mistry RC, et al. Cancer of the esophagus: Esophagogastric anastomotic leak: A retrospective study of predisposing factors. *J Surg Oncol* 1992;49:163–167.
157. Martin LW, Swisher SG, Hofstetter W, et al. Intrathoracic leaks following esophagectomy are no longer associated with increased mortality. *Ann Surg* 2005;242:392–399.
158. Cameron JL, Kieffer RF, Hendrix TR, et al. Selective nonoperative management of contained intrathoracic esophageal disruptions. *Ann Thorac Surg* 1979;27: 404–408.
159. Crestanello JA, Deschamps C, Cassivi SD, et al. Selective management of intrathoracic anastomotic leak after esophagectomy. *J Thorac Cardiovasc Surg* 2005;129: 254–260.
160. Paul S, Bueno R. Section VI: Complications following esophagectomy: Early detection, treatment, and prevention. *Semin Thorac Cardiovasc Surg* 2003;15:210–215.
161. Iannettoni MD, Whyte RI, Orringer MB. Catastrophic complications of the cervical esophagogastric anastomosis. *J Thorac Cardiovasc Surg* 1995;110:1493–1500.
162. Heitmiller RF, Jones B. Transient diminished airway protection after transhiatal esophagectomy. *Am J Surg* 1991;162:442–446.
163. Bratzler DW, Houck PM. Antimicrobial prophylaxis for surgery: An advisory statement from the National Surgical Infection Prevention Project. *Clin Infect Dis* 2004;38:1706–1715.
164. Salazar JD, Doty JR, Lin JW, et al. Does cell type influence post-esophagectomy survival in patients with esophageal cancer? *Dis Esoph* 1998;11:168–171.
165. Holscher AH, Bollschweiler E, Schneider PM, Siewert JR. Prognosis of early esophageal cancer: Comparison between adeno- and squamous cell carcinoma. *Cancer* 1995;76:178–186.
166. Wilkins EW Jr. Perspective. In: Delarue NC, Wilkins EW Jr, Wong J (eds). *International Trends in General Thoracic Surgery*, 4th ed. St. Louis: Mosby; 1988:440.
167. Brock MV. Neoadjuvant and adjuvant therapy of esophageal cancer. In: Cameron JL (ed). *Current Surgical Therapy*, 8th ed. Philadelphia: Elsevier–Mosby; 2004:55–57.
168. Walsh TN, Noonan N, Hollywood D, et al. A comparison of multimodal therapy and surgery for esophageal adenocarcinoma. *N Engl J Med* 1996;335:462–467.
169. Urba SG, Orringer MB, Turrisi A, et al. Randomized trial of preoperative chemoradiation versus surgery alone in patients with locoregional esophageal carcinoma. *J Clin Oncol* 2001;19:305–313.
170. Bosset JF, Gignoux M, Triboulet JP, et al. Chemoradiotherapy followed by surgery compared with surgery alone in squamous-cell cancer of the esophagus. *N Engl J Med* 1997;337:161–167.
171. Jagannath S, Canto MI. Lasers, stents, and photodynamic therapy in esophageal cancer. In: Yang SC, Cameron DE (eds). *Current Therapy in Thoracic and Cardiovascular Surgery*. Philadelphia: Mosby; 2004:366–369.
172. Portwood GL, Reed CE. Use of lasers and stents in malignant esophageal disease. In: Franco KL, Putnam JB Jr (eds). *Advanced Therapy in Thoracic Surgery*. Hamilton, Ontario: Decker; 1998:441.

CHAPTER

16 NEOADJUVANT AND PRIMARY CHEMORADIATION STRATEGIES IN THE TREATMENT OF ESOPHAGEAL CANCER

Michael K. Gibson

INTRODUCTION

Esophageal cancer comprises a small percentage (1.5 percent) and low incidence (~14,000) of total cancer cases in the United States; however, the mortality rate remains high.[1] Overall 5-year survival despite aggressive treatment in large, multidisciplinary oncology centers ranges between 15 and 25 percent.[2] This rate likely reflects both the late stage of disease at diagnosis as well as inadequacy of therapy. Fully 50 percent of cases are metastatic

KEY CONCEPTS

- Epidemiology
  - Esophageal cancer comprises 1.5 percent of total cancer cases in the United States. The mortality rate is high, with overall survival rates between 15 and 25 percent despite aggressive therapies. Approximately 50 percent are metastatic at diagnosis; cure rates with multimodality therapy for locally advanced disease do not exceed 40 percent. It is one of the fastest-rising cancer types in the United States.
- Pathophysiology
  - Most esophageal cancers comprise squamous cell cancer or adenocarcinoma. Squamous cell carcinoma derives from the esophageal epithelial lining, occurring mostly in the upper and middle esophagus. It is the most common subtype worldwide and thought to be caused by environmental carcinogens. Adenocarcinoma makes up most cases in the United States. The major risk factor is the presence of Barrett's esophagus (intestinal form), a premalignant condition characterized by metaplastic transformation of normal esophageal mucosa to columnar epithelium from chronic exposure of the gastroesophageal junction and distal esophagus to gastric contents.
- Clinical features
  - Most patients present with dysphagia, loss of appetite, and weight loss; other symptoms include odynophagia, asthenia, fatigue, cough, and retrosternal and abdominal discomfort. Physical signs are uncommon and nonspecific; some include cachexia, cervical and supraclavicular adenopathy, and abdominal masses. Laboratory findings are also nonspecific; no specific tumor markers are available.
- Diagnostics
  - Imaging modalities include upper gastrointestinal series, esophagograms, and computed tomography (CT). Diagnosis is confirmed by endoscopic biopsy. Metastatic disease is detected with CT or positron emission tomography (PET) imaging.
- Treatment
  - Curative treatment of locally advanced esophageal cancer includes various combinations of surgical resection and chemoradiotherapy.
- Outcomes
  - Accumulated experience with multiple chemotherapeutic regimens combined with radiotherapy and surgery results in overall survival of no more than 40 percent, pathologic cure rates between 25 and 35 percent, and frequent distant recurrences.

at diagnosis, and cure rates with multimodality therapy for locally advanced disease do not exceed 40 percent. Compounding this high mortality rate is the rising incidence of esophageal cancer. While the overall number of cases is small relative to other cancers of the gastrointestinal (GI) tract, esophageal cancer is distinguished in being among the fastest-rising types of cancer in the United States, mostly due to the shift in histology from squamous cell carcinoma to adenocarcinoma.

These sobering numbers regarding both incidence and mortality provide ample justification for continued efforts to improve early diagnosis, staging, and treatment of esophageal cancer. This chapter aims to provide a review and synopsis of current multimodality approaches to locally advanced esophageal cancer. The goal is to confirm the standards of care while also reviewing areas currently under investigation and in need of improvement. A separate chapter in this text focuses on diagnosis, staging, and primary surgical management of this disease.

Definitions

Performance status

Performance status is determined by a categorical scale used to indicate a patient's overall health and functional status. It is one clinical measure used to determine the potential for chemotherapy to cause side effects in a given patient.

Neoadjuvant treatment

This is treatment given *before* surgery. An example is neoadjuvant chemoradiotherapy, which is concomitant chemotherapy and radiotherapy given *prior to* surgical resection. Other terms for this include "induction treatment" and "preoperative therapy."

Chemoradiotherapy

Chemoradiotherapy comprises the combination of chemotherapy and radiation therapy given simultaneously.

Adjuvant

Treatment given *after* surgery is designated adjuvant therapy. An example is adjuvant chemotherapy, which is chemotherapy given *after* the patient has been rendered free of disease by surgical resection.

Response

This describes the effect of treatment on the tumor and the patient. Primarily measured on bidimensional imaging (CT, MRI), it can be categorized as complete response (no tumor seen), partial response (tumor shrinkage), stable disease (no change in tumor), or progression (tumor growth). The RECIST criteria are a commonly used set of rules for evaluating response.[3]

Tumor stage

Tumor stage defines the extent of tumor, both primary and metastatic. It is typically described with both the tumor-node-metastasis (TNM) and American Joint Committee on Cancer (AJCC) criteria.[4]

Clinical stage

This is the tumor stage as determined by multiple imaging [computed tomography (CT), positron emission tomography (PET)] and invasive modalities [endoscopy, endoscopic ultrasound (EUS) and laparoscopic inspection of the peritoneal cavity] but without pathologic inspection of the resected tumor specimen. For esophageal cancer, clinical staging is defined by the depth of tumor invasion into the esophageal wall as determined by EUS.

Pathologic stage

This is the tumor stage as determined by pathologic inspection of the resected specimen. This is the "gold standard" for staging of the primary tumor in esophageal cancer.

Historical background

Surgery was the first treatment and continues to be one of the standard treatment options for locally advanced, resectable esophageal cancer, although local control and survival are disappointing. In perhaps the largest published series to date of primary transhiatal esophagectomy for esophageal cancer, survival was clearly related to stage at diagnosis, with the highest survival in patients with stage 1 disease (Fig. 16-1).[5,6]

In a U.S. intergroup trial that enrolled 234 patients (52 percent adenocarcinoma) to a control arm treated with surgery alone, median survival was 16.1 months.[7] Although preoperative studies suggested that all patients had resectable disease, only 59 percent underwent a total resection with negative margins. Further, an additional 17 percent had local failure as a first site of recurrence, resulting in an overall 58 percent rate of failure to control local disease. Distant recurrence was seen in 50 percent of the curatively resected patients.

Similar results were observed in the 50-patient surgery-alone control arm of a single institution trial of esophageal cancer (68 percent adenocarcinoma) carried out at the University of Michigan.[8] Median survival was 17.6 months; 10 percent did not undergo resection and 38 percent of the remainder developed local failure. Distant failure as a component of first failure occurred in 60 percent.

Because this historical standard of care using surgical resection remains largely ineffective for higher stages of locally advanced disease, various combinations of chemotherapy and radiotherapy given with and without surgery continue to be investigated. These multimodality approaches are categorically reviewed later in the chapter.

Anatomic considerations

Although esophageal anatomy is most important in the setting of surgical management, it does have implications for staging and the use of multimodality therapy. The

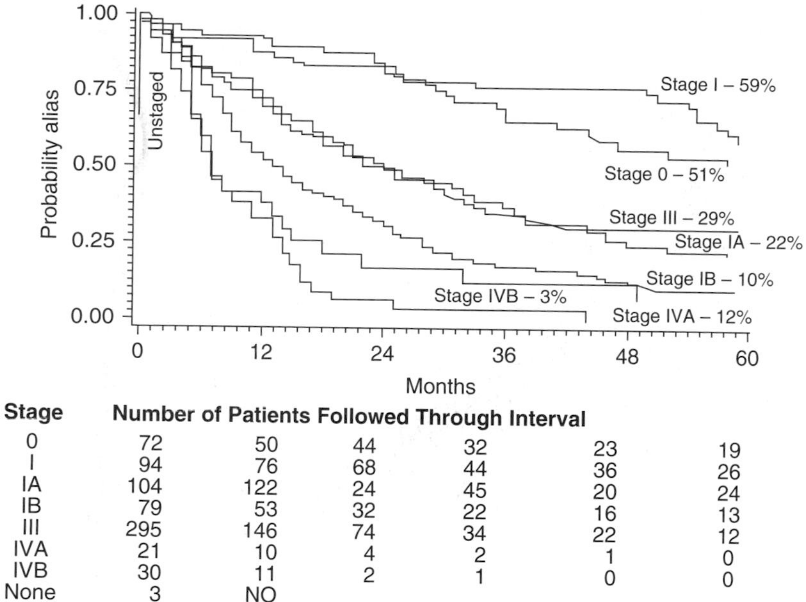

Stage	Number of Patients Followed Through Interval					
0	72	50	44	32	23	19
I	94	76	68	44	36	26
IA	104	122	24	45	20	24
IB	79	53	32	22	16	13
III	295	146	74	34	22	12
IVA	21	10	4	2	1	0
IVB	30	11	2	1	0	0
None	3	NO				

Figure 16-1 Stage-dependent Kaplan-Meier survival in patients undergoing transhiatal esophagectomy for carcinoma of the intrathoracic esophagus and cardia. (From Orringer et al. *Ann Surg* 2003;230(3). With permission.)

esophagus is unique in possessing no adventitial layer, and it does have a rich network of mucosal and submucosal lymphatics that drain longitudinally (Fig. 16-2). Tumors of the cervical and middle esophagus tend to drain to upper mediastinal lymph nodes, while those of the lower esophagus and gastroesophageal junction (GEJ) tend to drain to lower mediastinal nodes and, in particular, nodal groups of the celiac basin. Anatomic knowledge of draining lymph node regions relative to primary tumor location is important for staging, surgical approach, and the construction of radiation ports with adequate inclusiveness and margins.

The rich lymphatic drainage is also of note in considering the addition of systemic chemotherapy to multimodality management. Tumors as early as pathologic stage T2 have access to draining lymphatics, providing a route for early systemic spread. The addition of chemotherapy to surgery and/or radiation may improve outcome by targeting early micrometastatic disease that occurs via these anatomic routes.

An additional anatomic consideration is the distinction between distal esophagus, GEJ, and gastric cardia. Although lesions in this area are closely linked by location and histology, controversy exists regarding similarities and differences related to both clinical behavior and treatment. Stein and Siewart describe a helpful classification system that defines three distinct tumor entities in this transition region—defined as adenocarcinoma of the esophagogastric junction types I, II, and III. Type I tumors involve the distal esophagus and may approach the GEJ from above. Type II lesions involve the true cardia, and type III lesions are subcardial gastric cancers that may infiltrate the GEJ from below. Type I lesions seem to differ from types II and III in that they more often arise in the setting of gastroesophageal reflux disease (GERD) and Barrett's esophagus, are not related to *Helicobacter pylori*, and drain to mediastinal and celiac nodal regions as opposed to celiac, splenic, and paraaortic nodes.

These authors also suggest alternative surgical approaches to these three groups. Lesions are treated with complete removal of primary tumor and lymphatics (R0) via radical transmediastinal esophagectomy for type I lesions and via extended total gastrectomy for types II and III lesions, usually following preoperative chemotherapy or chemoradiotherapy.[9,10]

PATHOPHYSIOLOGY

Histology

By far the majority of esophageal cancers represent one of two histologic types. Squamous cell carcinoma

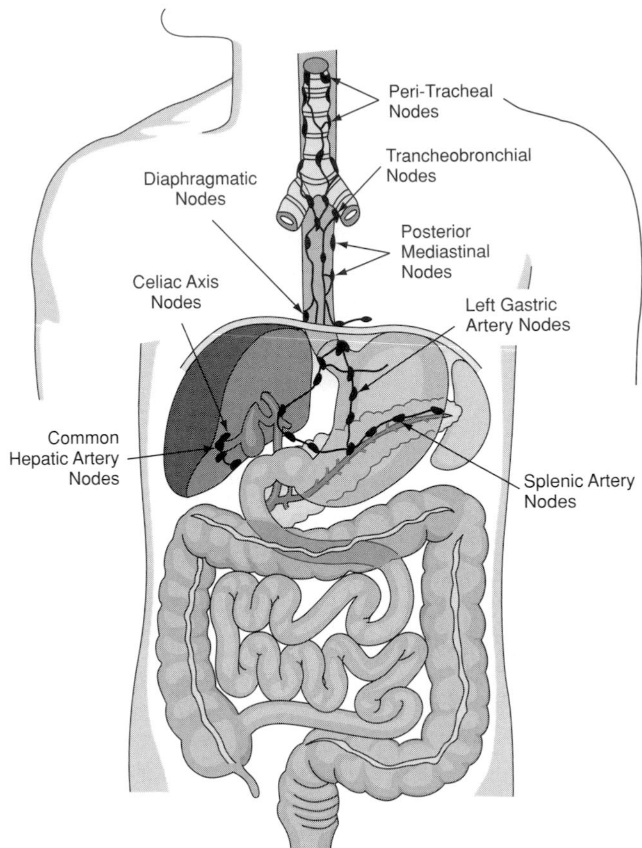

Figure 16-2 Major lymphatic drainage areas of the esophagus. (From Esophageal cancer. In: Devita et al. *Principles and Practice of* Oncology, Lippincott Williams & Wilkins, 2005. with permission)

(Fig. 16-3A) is characterized by varying degrees of differentiation of the squamous cells that form the normal epithelial lining of the esophagus. This type most commonly occurs in the upper (cervical) and middle esophagus. Worldwide, this remains the most common subtype of esophageal cancer and is thought to be caused by environmental carcinogens present in tobacco and alcohol.[11]

Adenocarcinoma (Fig. 16-3B) now makes up the majority of cases in the United States.[12,13] In contrast to squamous cell carcinoma, the major risk factor for adenocarcinoma is the presence of Barrett's esophagus (BE). This premalignant condition is thought to arise via metaplastic transformation of normal esophageal mucosa to columnar epithelium as a result of chronic exposure of the GEJ and distal esophagus to gastric contents. Only the intestinal form of BE is thought to be associated with the development of adenocarcinoma; however, the molecular mechanisms of malignant transformation are still under active investigation.

Barrett's esophagus

Underlying the tremendous increase in esophageal adenocarcinoma in the United States and parts of Europe is a possible increase as well in the incidence of BE. It remains unclear, however, whether this might represent detection bias. Further complicating the role of BE is the finding that it is associated with but not required for the formation of adenocarcinoma. Nevertheless, it remains the most important risk factor for this disease. It is associated with a relative risk of adenocarcinoma 40 to 125 times greater than that in persons without BE, resulting in an incidence of approximately 0.5 percent per year in patients with BE.[14,15]

Risk factors for the development of BE include chronic GERD and obesity. The pathogenic pathway is thought to start with chronic esophageal epithelial inflammation, then leading in an ordered progression from metaplasia through dysplasia to in situ cancer and eventually invasive cancer. The molecular and cytogenetic changes associated with each step in this malignant progression are under active study.[16] A representative diagram of this process is provided in Fig. 16-4.

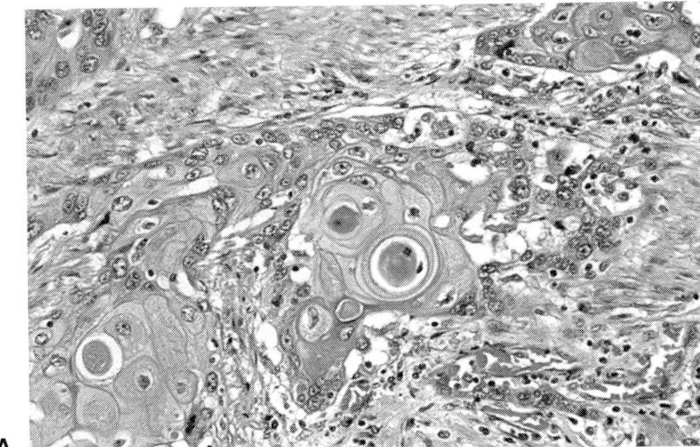

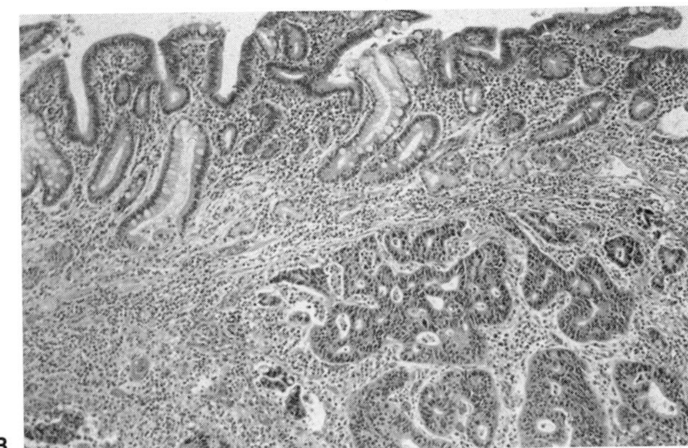

Figure 16-3 Representative histologic samples of esophageal cancer. A. Adenocarcinoma. B. Squamous cell carcinoma. (Courtesy of Elizabeth Montgomery, MD.)

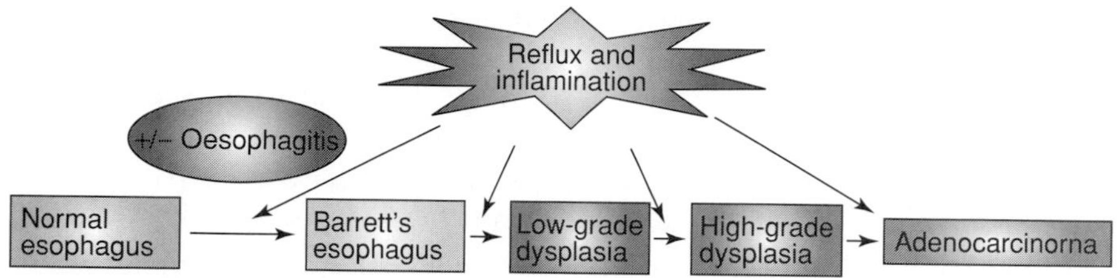

Figure 16-4 Proposed carcinogenic pathway of esophageal adenocarcinoma indicating progression from esophagitis through several stages of Barrett's esophagus to invasive adenocarcinoma. (From Wild and Hardie.[16] With permission.)

CLINICAL FEATURES

Epidemiology

The epidemiology of esophageal cancer is notable for geographic, ethnic, and histologic variation. It is the eighth most common cancer worldwide, with the majority consisting of squamous cell carcinoma (SCC), and the sixth leading cause of cancer death.[17] The areas of highest incidence include Turkey, northern Iran, southern republics of the former Soviet Union, and northern China.[17] Although rare in the United States, it is highly fatal, occupying a position as the seventh leading cause of cancer death in men in the United States. It is much more common in men, particularly African Americans, than in women.[1]

In contrast to the worldwide preponderance of SCC, notable in the United States as well as countries such as Australia and the United Kingdom is the shift in epidemiology from SCC to adenocarcinoma histology. Although the incidence of gastric adenocarcinoma continues to decline, adenocarcinomas of the distal esophagus and GEJ are steadily rising, particularly among white males.[12,13,18] Although there has been a slight decrease in mortality for this disease, fully half of these patients present with advanced disease, and the majority of cases prove fatal.

Clinical presentation

Each of the common histologic types of esophageal cancer presents with similar symptoms. Most often, patients develop dysphagia and weight loss. Nutritional deficits are likely related to both inability to swallow and loss of appetite. Undigested food may be regurgitated, and patients also experience worsening of acid reflux as well as odynophagia. Additional common symptoms include systemic complaints such as asthenia and fatigue as well as cough and retrosternal and abdominal discomfort.

Physical signs are uncommon and nonspecific. Cachexia may be found, and occasionally cervical and supraclavicular lymph enlargement, abdominal masses, and hepatomegaly are detected. Laboratory findings are nonspecific, and no tumor markers are available. Detection of the primary tumor is made with imaging modalities including upper GI series, esophagograms, and CT scans. Diagnosis is confirmed by endoscopic biopsy. Metastatic disease is detected with CT or PET imaging, and occasionally tumor tissue is obtained from distant sites of disease.

THERAPY

There are two currently accepted standards of care for curative treatment of locally advanced esophageal cancer: surgery and chemoradiotherapy. Similar cure rates are seen with each approach for both histologies (SCC and adenocarcinoma); however, the outcome remains poor. As a result, other combinations and sequences of the three major therapeutic categories—surgery, chemotherapy, and radiation therapy—continue to be actively investigated. The most current studies incorporate targeted biological agents. The overall goal is to improve survival by increasing the pathologic response rate and decreasing distant recurrence.

Primary surgery

Esophagectomy was the first curative therapy for esophageal cancer and remains one standard of care for treatment of locally advanced, resectable disease. Several approaches to resection are available, including the transthoracic (Ivor-Lewis), trans-hiatal, and en bloc methods. Selection of method is determined by the surgeon based on technical experience, patient factors, and location of tumor. Major differences in these approaches include location and number of lymph nodes removed as well as surgical morbidity and mortality.

A number of studies have investigated the relative merits of each type of procedure. A persistent concern for both esophagectomies and gastrectomies is the relationship between the number of lymph nodes and extent of margin removed and survival.[19,20] While the removal of lymph nodes and nearby tissues is more extensive with the transthoracic and en bloc approaches, it remains unclear whether overall survival is improved with the more extensive surgeries. The issue of transhiatal versus transthoracic esophagectomy has also been studied in several randomized trials and metanalyses. Although complications are more frequent with the latter, overall survival is equivalent between the two.[21,22]

Primary chemoradiotherapy

Primary chemoradiotherapy (CRT) is the other standard of care for locally advanced disease. In addition to offering a nonsurgical curative option for resectable lesions, it is also the only curative treatment for T4 (invading local structures such as pericardium and aorta) disease and the preferred management for cervical esophageal tumors. Although cervical tumors may be resected, a complete tracheoesophagectomy is required. Because this approach is disfiguring and function-altering for swallowing and speaking, CRT is preferred.

The benchmark is the Intergroup (RTOG 85-01) study first published in 1992, then with further follow-up in 1999.[23,24] Patients with locally advanced SCC (90 percent of the patients) or adenocarcinoma were randomized to either radiotherapy (RT) alone or RT with cisplatin and infusional 5-fluorouracil (5-FU). Radiotherapy was given in once-daily fractions of 200 cGy to a total dose of 5000 cGy in the combined group and 6400 cGy in the RT-alone group. Patients also received four monthly cycles of cisplatin (day 1) and infusional 5-FU (days 1 to 4), with the first two cycles given concomitantly with RT. Five-year survival was 27 percent in the CRT group and 0 percent in the radiation-alone group.

The RTOG 85-01 study established CRT as a curative option, provided an approach for patients who could not or did not want to have surgery, and confirmed that radiation alone was not curative. Given the clear albeit low cure rate as well as a 46 percent occurrence of local failure, several follow-up studies were carried out with the goal of improving survival and decreasing local failure.

The first follow-up study, Intergroup 0122, was a phase II study that intensified both the RT and the chemotherapy used in RTOG 85-01. Thirty-eight patients with SCC received three cycles of induction chemotherapy with cisplatin and a 5-day infusion of 5-FU followed by two more cycles of chemotherapy concomitant with RT to 6480 cGy. Six patients died from treatment-related complications, a sizable number of patients did not complete the chemoradiotherapy portion, and efficacy was not better than demonstrated in RTOG 85-01.[25] As such, this approach was not pursued subsequently through the Intergroup/RTOG mechanism.

To improve on locoregional control while avoiding the additional toxicity associated with induction chemotherapy, a modified phase III randomized study, RTOG 94-05 (Intergroup 0123), was instead initiated.[26] This study compared the RTOG 85-01 regimen of 5040 cGy of RT with a regimen containing the same dose and schedule of chemotherapy but a total RT dose of 6480 cGy in patients with SCC and adenocarcinoma. Toxicity was higher in the intensified arm, and the study was terminated early by the data safety and monitoring committee owing to a low likelihood (< 5 percent) that the investigational regimen would be found to be superior. As such, based on this series of studies of primary CRT, the current standard remains the RTOG 85-01 regimen. Of note, as in the prior two studies of primary chemoradiotherapy, ROTG 94-05 contained few patients with adenocarcinoma and confirmed the high rate of locoregional recurrence in patients who do not undergo subsequent surgery.

Neoadjuvant chemotherapy

An additional multimodality approach under active study, particularly in the United Kingdom, is the combination of pre- and postoperative chemotherapy with surgery. Two large, published, randomized trials of patients with both adenocarcinoma and SCC of the esophagus provide conflicting results. In the U.S. study, led by Kelsen, patients were randomized to either three cycles of preoperative 5-FU and cisplatin followed by surgery and two more cycles of postoperative chemotherapy or surgery alone.[7] There was no difference in 3-year survival (23 vs. 26 percent). The U.K. Medical Research Council (MRC) study, led by Cunningham, evaluated two cycles of 5-FU and cisplatin followed by surgery versus surgery alone. In contrast to the U.S. study, the MRC trial found a better 3-year survival with the addition of preoperative chemotherapy to surgery (32 vs. 25 percent).[27] There was a similar rate of R0 resection (59 Kelsen, 54 percent MRC) in each study, but patients in the U.S. study received more chemotherapy. Nevertheless, given the difficulty in resolving these opposing results, preoperative chemotherapy alone should still be considered investigational.

More recently, investigators with the U.K. MRC conducted a second study of preoperative chemotherapy. In contrast to the previously mentioned MRC study, which involved only esophageal cancer, the majority of patients in the second study had resectable gastric (74 percent) and GEJ (15 percent) cancers. Distal esophageal (11 percent) adenocarcinomas accounted for only 11 percent of the tumors. Treatment consisted of three pre- and three postoperative cycles of ECF (epirubicin, cisplatin, and infusional 5-FU) chemotherapy. Although 88 percent of patients completed preoperative chemotherapy, only 40 percent completed their postoperative cycles of ECF. Curative resection was higher in the chemotherapy group (79 versus 69 percent), pathologic stage was lower in the chemotherapy group, and there was a trend toward better survival in the patients treated with chemotherapy. Generalization of these results to esophageal adenocarcinoma must be done with care, as only 26 percent of patients had this disease.[28]

Adjuvant chemotherapy

Another approach to combining surgery with chemotherapy is to give the chemotherapy postoperatively (adjuvant chemotherapy) only. Several trials by the Japan Clinical

Oncology Group randomized patients with intrathoracic SCC to esophageal resection with extended lymphadenectomy alone or followed by chemotherapy. In the earlier study, in which adjuvant chemotherapy consisted of two cycles of cisplatin and vindesine, there was no difference in 5-year survival.[29] The latter study updated the adjuvant chemotherapy to two cycles of cisplatin and infusional 5-FU for patients with an R0 transthoracic resection of intrathoracic SCC.[30] At a median follow-up of 62.8 months, the 5-year disease-free survival favored the combined-therapy group, mostly for patients with node-positive disease. There was a statistically nonsignificant trend toward better overall survival as well.

A more recent study was carried out by the Eastern Cooperative Oncology Group in patients with adenocarcinoma.[31] This phase II trial (E8296) evaluated adjuvant cisplatin and paclitaxel every 3 weeks for four courses in patients with completely resected, node-positive adenocarcinoma of the esophagus, gastroesophageal junction, and cardia. Eligible patients had surgically staged $T_2N_1M_0$ or $T_{3-4}N_{0-1}M_0$ margin-negative disease and had not undergone preoperative therapy. A total of 55 eligible patients were analyzed, of whom 49 (89 percent) had lymph node involvement. The regimen was tolerable, and 46 (84 percent) of patients completed all four cycles of chemotherapy. After a median follow-up for surviving patients of 2.9 years (minimum follow-up of 2 years), the actual 2-year survival rate was 60 percent.[31] These results are encouraging and favorable when compared with historical controls treated with surgery alone.

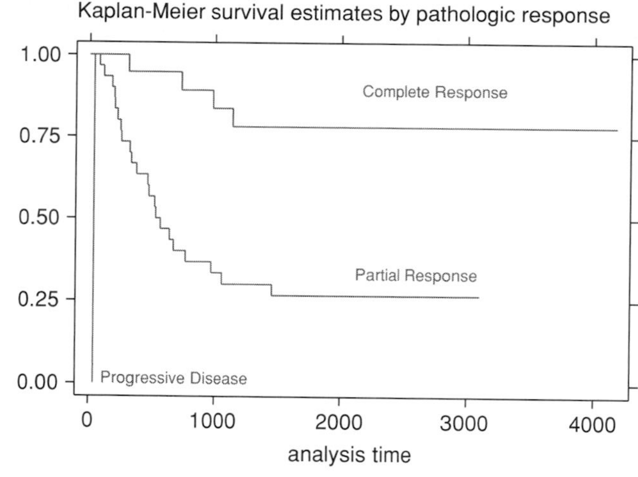

Figure 16-5 Kaplan-Meier survival stratified by pathologic response to induction and concomitant chemoradiotherapy in patients with esophageal squamous cell cancer and adenocarcinoma.

Chemoradiotherapy followed by surgery

Given the encouraging but not overwhelming survival results obtained with primary chemoradiotherapy or chemotherapy plus surgery, the logical subsequent combination involved adding surgery after chemoradiotherapy. As reviewed above, primary CRT in (mostly) SCC achieved cure rates approaching 27 percent, with failures involving a mixture of locally persistent disease and subsequent distant metastases. Escalating the RT dose in RTOG 94-05 did not improve local control, so subsequent studies added esophagectomy after CRT to remove residual tumor. An additional benefit of surgery is the availability of a pathologic specimen, which provides the "gold standard" for response to neoadjuvant therapy. Chemotherapy, in addition to providing radiosensitization, may also reduce systemic micrometastatic disease.

Phase II studies that used cisplatin/5-FU-based regimens demonstrated an encouraging pathologic complete response rate (pCR) of approximately 25 percent and survival approaching 40 percent.[32,33] There was often an apparent improvement in survival and local control compared with historical controls treated with surgery alone. In addition, pathologic response became a surrogate for postoperative survival. Pathologic complete response was associated with a 70 percent cure rate, while residual disease portended a much poorer survival of 30 percent (Fig. 16-5). Subsequent randomized trials assessing the value of preoperative cisplatin/5-FU/RT versus surgery alone, however, showed disparate results.

Preoperative chemoradiotherapy versus surgery alone

There are at least four randomized trials of preoperative chemoradiotherapy versus surgery alone. They are summarized in Table 16-1. The two trials by Urba and Walsh and their coworkers showed benefit, while the two by LePrise and Bosset and their associates did not.[34–37] Although the results are conflicting, no trial is considered definitive or without fault.

In the trial by Walsh and colleagues, 113 patients with adenocarcinoma were randomized to surgery alone or surgery combined with preoperative chemoradiotherapy. Radiation involved 40 Gy in 15 fractions.[37] Chemotherapy, which began on the first day of radiotherapy, consisted of 5-FU 15 mg/kg by continuous infusion on days 1 to 5 and cisplatin 75 mg/m^2 on day 1. Each drug was repeated during week 6 after the completion of RT. The pathologic complete response rate to neoadjuvant therapy was 25 percent, and the incidence of positive nodes in the surgical specimen was reduced from 82 to 42 percent ($p < 0.001$). The median survival was improved from 11 to 16 months ($p = 01$). Survival at 1, 2, and 3 years improved from 44 to 52 percent; 26 to 37 percent; and 6 to 32 percent, respectively. Despite the striking results, the trial was criticized because of the unexpectedly

Table 16-1 Summary of major trials evaluating multimodality treatment of locally advanced esophageal cancer

	RO, resection surgery only arm	3-year survey, surgery	3-year survey, CMT[a]	Median follow-up for survivors	Histology	Schedule
Preoperative chemoradiotherapy						
Le Prise	Not available (total n = 86)	47%[b]	47%[b]	Not available	Squamous	Sequential to 20 Gy
Bosset	69% (94/137)	34%	36%	55.2 months	Squamous	Sequential, Interrupted (no 5-FU) to 37 Gy
Urba	88% (44/50)	16%	30%	8.2 years	Both	Concurrent to 45 Gy
Walsh	Not available (total n = 113)	6%	32%	> 5 years	Adeno	Concurrent to 40 Gy
Preoperative chemotherapy						
Kelsen	59% (135/227)	26%	23%	46.5 months	Both	N/A
MRC	54% (215/402)	25%	32%	37.9 months	Both	N/A
Primary chemoradiotherapy (CRT), 5-year survival						
Herskovic	N/A	CRT, 27%	R only, 0 %	12.5 months	Both	CRT, 64 Gy R, 50 Gy

[a]Combined-modality therapy.
[b]Survival at 1 year (3-year results not available).

poor results achieved with surgery alone and the relatively small sample size.

In the University of Michigan study by Urba and colleagues, 100 patients (68 percent adenocarcinoma) were randomized to surgery alone or neoadjuvant cisplatin, 5-FU, and vinblastine concomitant with 45 Gy of radiotherapy.[8] The pathologic complete response rate was 28 percent (24 percent for adenocarcinoma). Median survival was 17.6 months with neoadjuvant therapy and 16.9 months with surgery alone. Three-year survival reached 30 versus 16 percent ($p = 0.18$). Unfortunately this study did not have the statistical power to detect a modest but clinically significant improvement in survival. It is noteworthy, however, that the improvement in 3-year survival was similar to the outcome observed in the trial reported by Walsh and associates.

A French multicenter randomized trial led by Bosset examined the role of preoperative chemoradiotherapy in 282 patients with stage I and II SCC.[34] Although no survival benefit was seen, disease-free survival and local recurrence-free survival were prolonged. Several issues may explain the negative result. The radiotherapy regimen was unconventional, given as 18.5 Gy in five fractions over 1 week, and repeated after a 2-week break for a total dose of only 37 Gy. Further, single-agent cisplatin (80 mg/m^2 given 0 to 2 days prior to each week of RT) was given nonconcurrently with RT.

The study by LePrise and colleagues randomized 86 patients with SCC to two cycles of sequential 5-FU and cisplatin interrupted by radiotherapy given as 20 Gy over 10 fractions. Median survival was no different between the two groups in these patients, who were treated with a substandard dose of radiotherapy.

There are several possible explanations for these conflicting results. Comparing the four studies is difficult because of differences in such factors as sequencing of chemotherapy and radiation; doses, types, and schedules of chemotherapy; and radiation and surgical outcome. While the results of these trials and other phase II studies have led to the adoption of preoperative chemoradiotherapy as accepted treatment within community practice, the results are mixed. This approach cannot be considered standard of care and is best used in the confines of a clinical trial.

A U.S. intergroup trial was designed to test definitively whether preoperative cisplatin, 5-FU, and radiotherapy improve outcome compared with surgery alone. Unfortunately, this trial was terminated as a result of poor accrual. Although the cause of the disappointing accrual is undoubtedly multifactorial, a contributing factor may have been the lack of consensus about an optimal regimen of preoperative chemoradiotherapy, especially with the shift to an increasing incidence of adenocarcinoma.

Metanalyses

There are two recently published metanalyses of randomized controlled trials comparing neoadjuvant chemoradiation followed by surgery with surgery alone. The first study evaluated 1116 patients enrolled in nine trials.[38] Compared to surgery alone, the odds ratios showed a nonsignificant trend toward improved survival with neoadjuvant chemoradiotherapy (0.79, 0.77, and 0.66 for 1-, 2-, and 3-year survival, respectively); however, the improvement in 3-year survival reached the level of statistical significance only when the analysis was restricted to those trials using concurrent chemotherapy and radiation (OR 0.45, 95 percent CI, 0.26 to 0.79).

The second study evaluated six randomized controlled trials of 764 patients (all were included in the above analysis as well) that compared preoperative chemoradiotherapy plus surgery versus surgery alone.[39] Most patients had SCC, and in at least four of the six trials, radiation and chemotherapy were given concurrently. Compared with surgery alone, preoperative chemoradiotherapy again significantly improved 3-year survival (OR 0.53, 95 percent CI 0.31 to 0.93).

SUMMARY OF PRIOR STUDIES

Results from selected randomized trials and two metanalyses suggest the promise of neoadjuvant concomitant chemoradiotherapy followed by surgery for improving survival in patients with locally advanced resectable esophageal cancer. However, despite these encouraging results, the sobering fact remains that far less than half of this group of highly selected patients treated with this aggressive approach are cured. To determine the reasons for continued failure to achieve cure in most patients, our group recently reviewed the experience at Johns Hopkins in two phase II trials that provided intensive regimens of double-agent cisplatin-based chemotherapy combined with radiotherapy prior to surgical resection.[40]

Combined trial results demonstrated that 93 percent (86 of 92) of those underwent surgery (one refused, two died preoperatively, and three developed metastatic disease) and 87 percent (80 of 92) were completely resected with negative margins (three had positive margins and three had distant metastasis at surgery). The pathologic complete response rate was 33 percent (30 of 92). At a median follow-up of 42 months, median survival of all enrolled patients was 35 months, and 4-year survival was 43 percent. As expected, patients with a pathologic complete response did better—73 percent survival at 4 years (median not reached)—whereas the remainder of the patients had 4-year survival of 28 percent (median 20 months) ($p < 0.001$). The pattern of initial failure was locoregional alone in 6 percent (5 of 90), locoregional plus distant in 3 percent (3 of 90), and distant alone in 38 percent (34 of 90). Although survival and local control were improved by preoperative therapy, suboptimal pathologic complete responses and failure as manifest by distant metastases remain troublesome.

RECENT APPROACHES

Given the problems of both inadequate pathologic complete response and postsurgery systemic recurrence, investigators are more recently focusing on ways to intensify treatment. Newer approaches are combining more efficacious preoperative regimens with more tolerable adjuvant therapy. Variations on this theme include using newer chemotherapy agents that are active in adenocarcinoma, adding several cycles of induction chemotherapy prior to preoperative chemoradiation, increasing the number of cytotoxic agents administered concurrent with radiation therapy, and adding adjuvant chemotherapy.

Newer chemotherapy

Recently developed treatment strategies that involved doublets of either cisplatin and paclitaxel or cisplatin and irinotecan have shown promise in an era in which esophageal adenocarcinoma is increasing.[41,42] These drugs in combination with radiotherapy may be better tolerated, and this approach has a response rate at least equal to that attained by cisplatin/5-FU-based regimens. In these two studies, done at Memorial Sloan-Kettering Cancer Center (MSKCC), the pCR rate with weekly bolus of cisplatin/irinotecan was 27 percent; with weekly infusional paclitaxel plus bolus cisplatin, it was 24 percent.

Induction chemotherapy

Several other studies evaluated the addition of induction chemotherapy prior to concomitant chemoradiotherapy and subsequent surgery. In one trial at the M.D. Anderson Cancer Center (MDACC), 38 patients with resectable (82 percent adenocarcinoma) cancer of the esophagus received induction chemotherapy consisting of two courses of 5-FU, cisplatin, and paclitaxel followed by radiotherapy to 45 Gy with concurrent 5-FU and cisplatin and then surgery. Potentially curative resection was possible in 35 patients, and a complete pathologic response rate was noted in 8 (23 percent). With a median follow-up of 58 months, 3- and 5-year survival estimates were 63 and 39 percent, respectively.[43,44]

In two other trials, one from MDACC and the other from MSKCC, induction chemotherapy with weekly cisplatin and irinotecan was followed by either 5-FU, paclitaxel, and concurrent radiation (MDACC) or cisplatin, irinotecan, and concurrent radiation (MSKCC) in patients with mostly adenocarcinoma.[41,45] In the preliminary report from the dose-escalation portion of the MSKCC study, a pCR rate of 27 percent was found in the 15 patients who underwent surgery. The final analysis of the MDACC study reported a pCR rate of 26 percent and a median survival of 22.1 months after a minimum follow-up of 28 months.

Intensified chemotherapy

Increasing the number of cytotoxic agents combined with radiotherapy, with the goal of intensifying neoadjuvant therapy in order to achieve higher pCR and survival, was also studied in at least three recent trials. In the largest study, investigators from the Minnie Pearl Cancer Research Network treated 129 patients with localized esophageal cancer (both histologies) with concurrent radiation to 45 Gy and every-3-week paclitaxel, carboplatin, and infusional 5-FU followed by resection.[46] The pCR rate was 36 percent (47 of 129) for all patients entered into the study, and 57 percent of patients required hospitalization. At a median follow-up of 45 months, the 3-year estimated survival rate was 41 percent. These results indicate added toxicity without substantial incremental survival improvement.

A phase II single-institution study just published in abstract form also evaluated the regimen of paclitaxel, carboplatin, and 5-FU with RT to 45Gy followed by surgery in patients with esophageal or gastric cancer. Of 36 patients treated, 33 underwent surgery, resulting in a pCR rate of 30 percent. This intensified three-drug regimen was better tolerated than in the prior study, perhaps because paclitaxel was given weekly instead of every 3 weeks. While the pCR rate was not much higher than seen with prior regimens, survival data are not yet available.[47]

A third study, from the University of Michigan and also in abstract form, evaluated preoperative infusional 5-FU, weekly cisplatin, paclitaxel, and RT to 45 Gy followed by two cycles of monthly adjuvant chemotherapy with infusional 5-FU, cisplatin, and paclitaxel. Of 65 enrolled patients, 60 had surgery but only 40 percent tolerated the planned dose of adjuvant chemotherapy. The pCR rate was 17 percent and, at a median follow-up of 2.2 years, 3-year survival was 50 percent, with a median survival of 2.8 years.[48]

Adjuvant chemotherapy

At least two studies added postoperative chemotherapy following neoadjuvant, concomitant chemoradiotherapy with the goal of reducing recurrence from systemic, micrometastatic disease. In the study (cited above) by Urba and colleagues, only 40 percent of patients received the adjuvant chemotherapy. In a second study, patients were to receive three cycles of postoperative every-3-week paclitaxel and cisplatin.[49] Few (15 of 35 eligible) patients completed a full course of adjuvant therapy because of physical and psychological fatigue. Specific toxicities included neutropenia in 69 percent of patients as well as significant orthostatic hypotension and nutritional deficits. The idea that adjuvant chemotherapy improves survival may be valid, but testing the theory remains technically difficult because of the toxicity of the therapy.

Although each of these four approaches to improve pCR and survival are reasonable in principle and feasible in application, none provided a marked improvement in either outcome when compared with historical experience with 5-FU and cisplatin-based regimens used in the randomized trials. Further, these approaches have not yet been compared with surgery alone or neoadjuvant 5-FU, cisplatin, and RT. Although such comparisons are planned and perhaps under way, until they are completed we favor treatment with 5-FU and cisplatin combined with radiation to 45 Gy prior to surgery.

Primary chemoradiotherapy versus neoadjuvant chemoradiotherapy followed by surgery

Whether the addition of surgery after concurrent chemoradiotherapy adds additional survival benefit compared with chemoradiotherapy or surgery alone remains controversial. Data from several patterns-of-care (PCS) surveys and randomized trials are conflicting. A survival benefit from the trimodal approach was suggested in a survey involving 400 patients treated between 1992 and 1994.[50] For these patients with thoracic adenocarcinoma or SCC, preoperative chemoradiotherapy was associated with a higher 2-year survival rate compared with definitive chemoradiotherapy without surgery (63 vs. 39 percent). Although the difference was not statistically significant, trimodal therapy also resulted in a significant reduction in locoregional failure at 2 years (22 vs. 30 percent).

A follow-up PCS study reviewed findings in 414 patients treated between 1996 and 1999.[51] Compared with the initial study, more patients overall were treated with preoperative concurrent chemoradiotherapy (27 vs. 10 percent) and more patients with adenocarcinoma received the trimodal approach compared to those with SCC (46 vs. 19 percent). Fifty-five percent were treated with definitive concurrent chemoradiotherapy alone. Survival data, however, were not presented in this second study.

While the PCS studies suggest a benefit to surgery following chemoradiotherapy, two randomized trials did not conclusively support this approach. In one trial, 177 patients with SCC were randomly assigned to two treatment groups. The first group received three cycles of 5-FU, leucovorin, etoposide, and cisplatin followed by concomitant chemoradiotherapy (to 40 Gy) followed by surgery. The second group received the same chemotherapy followed by definitive chemoradiotherapy (to 60 Gy) without surgery. The surgically treated patients approached better local control (site of first relapse was local in 64 vs. 81 percent, $p = 0.08$), but the 3-year overall (28 vs. 20 percent) and median (16 vs. 15 months) survival durations were not different.[52]

In the second study, 455 patients with esophageal SCC or adenocarcinoma received induction chemoradiotherapy with either protracted or split-course radiation plus two courses of 5-FU and cisplatin chemotherapy. Patients with at least a partial response and without a contraindication to surgery or continued chemoradiotherapy (n = 259) were then randomly assigned to continue chemoradiotherapy or to undergo surgery. In a preliminary report,

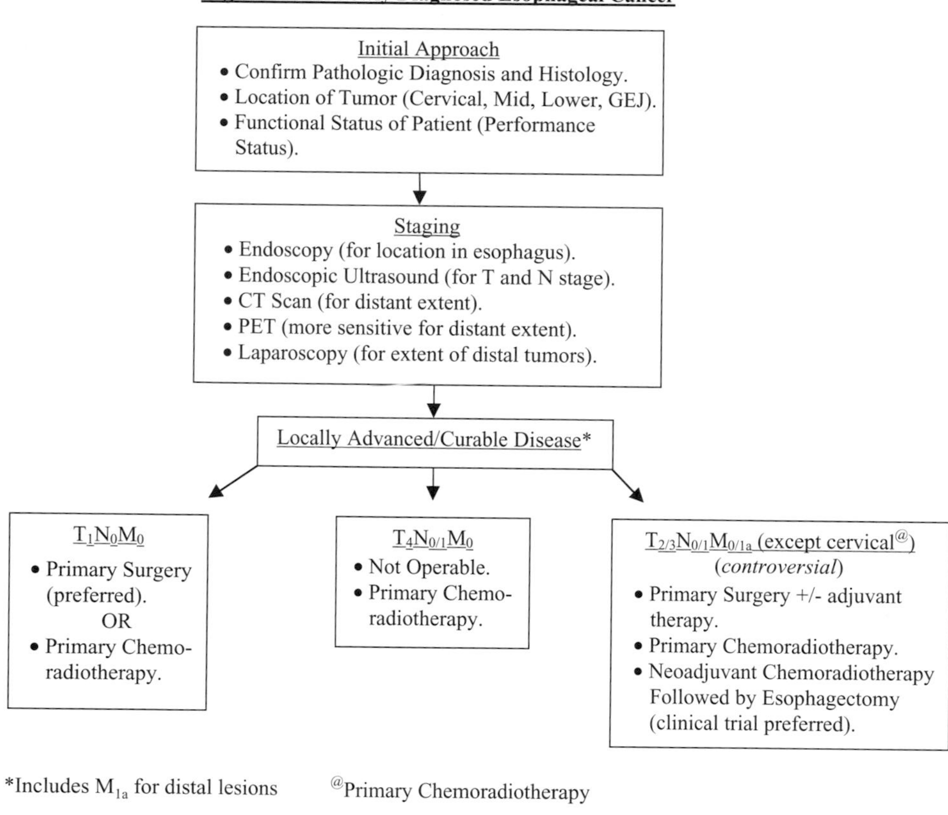

Figure 16-6 Algorithm for newly diagnosed esophageal cancer.

continued chemoradiotherapy was associated with similar 2-year survival (40 vs. 34 percent) and median survival (19.3 vs. 17.7 months) compared with surgery. Surgically treated patients were significantly less likely to require esophageal stents (13 vs. 27 percent, $p = 0.005$) or repeated dilation (22 vs. 32 percent, $p = 0.07$).[53]

Although the sum of these results is conflicting, several trends emerge. First, locally persistent/recurrent disease after chemoradiotherapy alone is frequent. Second, there is a lack of data for nonsurgical management of patients with adenocarcinoma. Third, the use of trimodal therapy is increasing for patients with adenocarcinoma, in an era in which this histologic type of esophageal cancer is increasing. This information, in concert with the results of two randomized studies and two metanalyses, suggests that neoadjuvant chemoradiotherapy prior to surgery is emerging as a better option than surgery alone for patients with locally advanced, resectable esophageal cancer.[36–39,54] Controversy remains, however, as to whether trimodal therapy or primary chemoradiotherapy is the better option for resectable (not T4 or cervical) disease. An algorithm that summarizes management options is provided in the decision-making flowchart (Fig. 16-6).

FUTURE AND ONGOING STUDIES

With the multiple approaches outlined above, the accumulated experience with multiple cytotoxic drugs combined in several schedules with radiotherapy and surgery continues to demonstrate overall survival of no more than 40 percent, pathologic CR of 25 and 35 percent, and mostly distant recurrences. In order to surmount this survival barrier, future approaches must incorporate modern staging, radiotherapy, and surgical techniques with directed regimens and drug therapy based on individual tumor characteristics. Recent advances in individual tumor profiling based on such markers as methylation and protein expression make this a promising possibility.[55,56] Perhaps the planned and ongoing studies—including such targeted agents as tyrosine kinase and angiogenesis inhibitors in the treatment of high-risk patients—will achieve the control of distant disease that is crucial to improving survival for patients with esophageal cancer.

ACKNOWLEGMENTS

To Arlene Forastiere for suggestions, continued mentoring, and friendship.

References

1. Jemal A, Tiwari RC, Murray T, et al. Cancer statistics, 2004. *CA Cancer J Clin* 2004;54:8–29.
2. Salazar JD, Doty JR, Lin JW, et al. Does cell type influence post-esophagectomy survival in patients with esophageal cancer? *Dis Esoph* 1998;11:168–171.
3. Therasse P, Arbuck SG, Eisenhauer EA, et al. New guidelines to evaluate the response to treatment in solid tumors. European Organization for Research and Treatment of Cancer, National Cancer Institute of the United States, National Cancer Institute of Canada. *J Natl Cancer Inst* 2000;92:205–216.
4. Esophagus. In: Greene F, Page D, Fleming I, et al (eds). *AJCC Cancer Staging Manual*, 6th ed. New York: Springer; 2002:91–98.
5. Orringer MB, Marshall B, Iannettoni MD. Transhiatal esophagectomy: Clinical experience and refinements. *Ann Surg* 1999;230:392–400; discussion 400–403.
6. Rice TW, Blackstone EH, Rybicki LA, et al. Refining esophageal cancer staging. *J Thorac Cardiovasc Surg* 2003;125:1103–1113.
7. Kelsen DP, Ginsberg R, Pajak TF, et al. Chemotherapy followed by surgery compared with surgery alone for localized esophageal cancer. *N Engl J Med* 1998;339:1979–1984.
8. Urba SG, Orringer MB, Turrisi A, et al. Randomized trial of preoperative chemoradiation versus surgery alone in patients with locoregional esophageal carcinoma. *J Clin Oncol* 2001;19:305–313.
9. Siewert JR, Stein HJ, Sendler A, et al. Surgical resection for cancer of the cardia. *Semin Surg Oncol* 1999;17:125–131.
10. Stein HJ, Siewert JR. Improved prognosis of resected esophageal cancer. *World J Surg* 2004;28:520–525.
11. Schottenfeld D. Epidemiology of cancer of the esophagus. *Semin Oncol* 1984;11:92–100.
12. Devesa SS, Blot WJ, Fraumeni JF Jr. Changing patterns in the incidence of esophageal and gastric carcinoma in the United States. *Cancer* 1998;83:2049–2053.
13. el-Serag HB. The epidemic of esophageal adenocarcinoma. *Gastroenterol Clin North Am* 2002;31:421–440, viii.
14. Shaheen N, Ransohoff DF. Gastroesophageal reflux, Barrett esophagus, and esophageal cancer: Scientific review. *JAMA* 2002;287:1972–1981.
15. Staba MJ, Mauceri HJ, Kufe DW, et al. Adenoviral TNF-alpha gene therapy and radiation damage tumor vasculature in a human malignant glioma xenograft. *Gene Ther* 1998;5:293–300.
16. Wild CP, Hardie LJ. Reflux, Barrett's oesophagus and adenocarcinoma: Burning questions. *Nat Rev Cancer* 2003;3:676–684.
17. Pisani P, Parkin DM, Bray F, et al. Estimates of the worldwide mortality from 25 cancers in 1990. *Int J Cancer* 1999;83:18–29.
18. Brown LM, Devesa SS. Epidemiologic trends in esophageal and gastric cancer in the United States. *Surg Oncol Clin N Am* 2002;11:235–256.
19. Bonenkamp JJ, Hermans J, Sasako M, et al. Extended lymph-node dissection for gastric cancer. Dutch Gastric Cancer Group. *N Engl J Med* 1999;340:908–914.
20. Hartgrink HH, van de Velde CJ, Putter H, et al. Extended lymph node dissection for gastric cancer: Who may benefit? Final results of the randomized Dutch gastric cancer group trial. *J Clin Oncol* 2004;22:2069–2077.
21. Hulscher JB, van Sandick JW, de Boer AG, et al. Extended transthoracic resection compared with limited transhiatal resection for adenocarcinoma of the esophagus. *N Engl J Med* 2002;347:1662–1669.
22. Hulscher JB, Tijssen JG, Obertop H, et al. Transthoracic versus transhiatal resection for carcinoma of the esophagus: A meta-analysis. *Ann Thorac Surg* 2001;72: 306–313.
23. Herskovic A, Martz K, al-Sarraf M, et al. Combined chemotherapy and radiotherapy compared with radiotherapy alone in patients with cancer of the esophagus. *N Engl J Med* 1992;326:1593–1598.
24. Cooper JS, Guo MD, Herskovic A, et al. Chemoradiotherapy of locally advanced esophageal cancer: Long-term follow-up of a prospective randomized trial (RTOG 85–01). Radiation Therapy Oncology Group. *JAMA* 1999;281: 1623–1627.
25. Minsky BD, Neuberg D, Kelsen DP, et al. Final report of Intergroup Trial 0122 (ECOG PE-289, RTOG 90–12): Phase II trial of neoadjuvant chemotherapy plus concurrent chemotherapy and high-dose radiation for squamous cell carcinoma of the esophagus. *Int J Radiat Oncol Biol Phys* 1999;43:517–523.
26. Minsky BD, Pajak TF, Ginsberg RJ, et al. INT 0123 (Radiation Therapy Oncology Group 94–05) phase III trial of combined-modality therapy for esophageal cancer: High-dose versus standard-dose radiation therapy. *J Clin Oncol* 2002;20:1167–1174.
27. Surgical resection with or without preoperative chemotherapy in oesophageal cancer: A randomised controlled trial. *Lancet* 2002;359:1727–1733.
28. Allum W, Cunningham D, Weeden S. Perioperative chemotherapy in operable gastric and lower oesophageal cancer: A randomized, controlled trial (the MAGIC trial, ISRCTN 93793971). *Proc ASCO* 2003.
29. Ando N, Iizuka T, Kakegawa T, et al. A randomized trial of surgery with and without chemotherapy for localized squamous carcinoma of the thoracic esophagus: The Japan Clinical Oncology Group Study. *J Thorac Cardiovasc Surg* 1997;114:205–209.
30. Ando N, Iizuka T, Ide H, et al. Surgery plus chemotherapy compared with surgery alone for localized squamous cell carcinoma of the thoracic esophagus: A Japan Clinical Oncology Group Study—JCOG9204. *J Clin Oncol* 2003; 21:4592–4596.
31. Armanios M, Xu R, Forastiere A, et al. Phase II adjuvant chemotherapy for resected adenocarcinoma of the esophagus, gastro-esophageal (GE) junction and cardia (E8296): A trial of the Eastern Cooperative Oncology Group. *Proc ASCO* 2003.
32. Forastiere AA, Orringer MB, Perez-Tamayo C, et al. Preoperative chemoradiation followed by transhiatal esophagectomy for carcinoma of the esophagus: Final report. *J Clin Oncol* 1993;11:1118–1123.
33. Forastiere AA, Heitmiller RF, Lee DJ, et al. Intensive chemoradiation followed by esophagectomy for squamous cell and adenocarcinoma of the esophagus. *Cancer J Sci Am* 1997;3:144–152.

34. Bosset JF, Gignoux M, Triboulet JP, et al. Chemoradiotherapy followed by surgery compared with surgery alone in squamous-cell cancer of the esophagus. *N Engl J Med* 1997;337:161–167.
35. Le Prise E, Etienne PL, Meunier B, et al. A randomized study of chemotherapy, radiation therapy, and surgery versus surgery for localized squamous cell carcinoma of the esophagus. *Cancer* 1994;73:1779–1784.
36. Urba SG, Orringer MB, Turrisi A, et al. Randomized trial of preoperative chemoradiation versus surgery alone in patients with locoregional esophageal carcinoma. *J Clin Oncol* 2001;19:305–313.
37. Walsh TN, Noonan N, Hollywood D, et al. A comparison of multimodal therapy and surgery for esophageal adenocarcinoma. *N Engl J Med* 1996;335:462–467.
38. Urschel JD, Vasan H. A meta-analysis of randomized controlled trials that compared neoadjuvant chemoradiation and surgery to surgery alone for resectable esophageal cancer. *Am J Surg* 2003;185:538–543.
39. Fiorica F, Di Bona D, Schepis F, et al. Preoperative chemoradiotherapy for oesophageal cancer: A systematic review and meta-analysis. *Gut* 2004;53:925–930.
40. Kleinberg L, Knisely JP, Heitmiller R, et al. Mature survival results with preoperative cisplatin, protracted infusion 5-fluorouracil, and 44-Gy radiotherapy for esophageal cancer. *Int J Radiat Oncol Biol Phys* 2003;56:328–334.
41. Ilson DH, Bains M, Kelsen DP, et al. Phase I trial of escalating-dose irinotecan given weekly with cisplatin and concurrent radiotherapy in locally advanced esophageal cancer. *J Clin Oncol* 2003;21:2926–2932.
42. Brenner B, Ilson DH, Minsky BD, et al. Phase I trial of combined-modality therapy for localized esophageal cancer: Escalating doses of continuous-infusion paclitaxel with cisplatin and concurrent radiation therapy. *J Clin Oncol* 2004;22:45–52.
43. Swisher SG, Ajani JA, Komaki R, et al. Long-term outcome of phase II trial evaluating chemotherapy, chemoradiotherapy, and surgery for locoregionally advanced esophageal cancer. *Int J Radiat Oncol Biol Phys* 2003;57:120–127.
44. Ajani JA, Komaki R, Putnam JB, et al. A three-step strategy of induction chemotherapy then chemoradiation followed by surgery in patients with potentially resectable carcinoma of the esophagus or gastroesophageal junction. *Cancer* 2001;92:279–286.
45. Ajani JA, Walsh G, Komaki R, et al. Preoperative induction of CPT-11 and cisplatin chemotherapy followed by chemoradiotherapy in patients with locoregional carcinoma of the esophagus or gastroesophageal junction. *Cancer* 2004;100:2347–2354.
46. Meluch AA, Greco FA, Gray JR, et al. Preoperative therapy with concurrent paclitaxel/carboplatin/infusional 5-FU and radiation therapy in locoregional esophageal cancer: Final results of a Minnie Pearl Cancer Research Network phase II trial. *Cancer J* 2003;9:251–260.
47. Anne P, Axelrod E, Rosato E, et al. A phase II trial of preoperative paclitaxel, carboplatin, 5-FU and radiation in patients with resectable esophageal or gastric cancer (Ca). *Proc ASCO* 2004.
48. Urba SG, Hayman J, Ianettonni M, et al. Pre-operative chemoradiation with cisplatin (CDDP), 5-fluorouracil (5FU), and paclitaxel (Tax), followed by surgery and adjuvant chemotherapy, for loco-regional esophageal carcinoma. *Proc ASCO* 2004.
49. Heath EI, Burtness BA, Heitmiller RF, et al. Phase II evaluation of preoperative chemoradiation and postoperative adjuvant chemotherapy for squamous cell and adenocarcinoma of the esophagus. *J Clin Oncol* 2000;18:868–876.
50. Coia LR, Minsky BD, Berkey BA, et al. Outcome of patients receiving radiation for cancer of the esophagus: Results of the 1992–1994 Patterns of Care Study. *J Clin Oncol* 2000;18:455–462.
51. Suntharalingam M, Moughan J, Coia LR, et al. The national practice for patients receiving radiation therapy for carcinoma of the esophagus: Results of the 1996–1999 Patterns of Care Study. *Int J Radiat Oncol Biol Phys* 2003;56:981–987.
52. Stahl M, Wilke H, Walz M, et al. Randomized phase III trial in locally advanced squamous cell carcinoma (SCC) of the esophagus: Chemoradiation with and without surgery. *Proc ASCO* 2003.
53. Bedenne L, Michel P, Bouche O, et al. Randomized phase III trial in locally advanced esophageal cancer: Radiochemotherapy followed by surgery versus radiochemotherapy alone (FFCD 9102). *Proc ASCO* 2002.
54. Walsh TN, Grennell M, Mansoor S, et al. Neoadjuvant treatment of advanced stage esophageal adenocarcinoma increases survival. *Dis Esoph* 2002;15:121–124.
55. Gibson M, Abraham S, Wu TT, et al. Epidermal growth factor receptor, p53 mutation and pathologic response predict survival in patients with locally advanced esophageal cancer treated with pre-operative chemoradiotherapy. *ASCO Proc* 2003.
56. Brock M, Gou M, Akiyama Y, et al. Prognostic importance of promoter hypermethylation of multiple genes in esophageal adenocarcinoma. *Clin Cancer Res* 2003;9:2912–2919.

CHAPTER

17 THORACIC TRAUMA

Edward E. Cornwell III, David Efron, David C. Chang

INTRODUCTION

Over 15,000 Americans die of major chest wounds each year. On presentation, evidence of thoracic trauma may be obvious, as is the case with bullet holes, subcutaneous emphysema, or sucking chest wounds; or evidence may be more subtle, as with a mild increase in respiratory rate. All patients who present with thoracic trauma, regardless of the mechanism or injury, are best approached utilizing guidelines promoted by the Advanced Trauma Life Support (ATLS) course offered by the American College of Surgeons. Control of airway, breathing, and circulation is of paramount importance to the successful management of thoracic trauma and is often integral to the diagnostic workup of these injuries.

With an airway ensured, the chest is inspected (front and back) and auscultated to assess for breath sounds. Tracheal position is noted, heart sounds are identified, and jugular venous status is assessed. Electrocardiographic leads are placed and rhythm is determined. For all patients

KEY CONCEPTS

- Epidemiology
  - Over 15,000 Americans die of major chest injuries each year.
- Pathophysiology
  - Thoracic trauma can be broadly classified into blunt and penetrating injuries. Structures that can be injured include the bony thorax (e.g., spinal column, ribs, sternum, scapula), lung, trachea, heart, great vessels, esophagus, and diaphragm.
- Clinical features
  - Clinical presentations of thoracic trauma vary according to the structure-specific injury or injuries. Potential signs and symptoms include dyspnea/tachypnea, hypotension, entry and exit wounds, contusions, subcutaneous emphysema, diminished breath and/or heart sounds, tracheal shift, and jugular venous distention.
- Diagnostics
  - All patients with thoracic trauma should undergo upright plain chest and cervical spine radiography to rapidly identify injuries to the bony thorax, hemopneumothorax, and possible structural injuries to the mediastinum. Other diagnostic tests are dictated by the patient's clinical status, the trauma mechanism, and the examiner's suspicion of a particular injury. Ultrasonography can be useful in identifying pericardial fluid and cardiac motion. Computed tomography, esophagography/esophagoscopy, aortography, bronchoscopy, and thoracoscopy are often very useful in diagnosing thoracic injury. In some cases, thoracotomy in the emergency department may ultimately reveal a particular injury.
- Treatment
  - All trauma patients are best treated initially by utilizing Advanced Trauma Life Support guidelines. These are predicated on assuring airway control, breathing, and circulation in the setting of potential multisystem trauma. Further management is predicated on the structure-specific injury.
- Outcomes/prognosis
  - Clinical outcomes of thoracic trauma vary according to the patient's presentation and site-specific injury or injuries.

with suspected chest trauma, a chest x-ray is obtained (upright where possible).

A number of other diagnostic tests are employed in the workup of thoracic trauma, the use of which is dictated by the patient's clinical status, the mechanism of trauma, and the examiner's suspicion of a particular injury. Ultrasonographic imaging in the trauma room is a simple and rapid method of identifying acute pericardial fluid and cardiac motion. Thoracic computed tomography (CT), aortography, esophagography/esophagoscopy, and transesophageal ultrasonography may also play a role in the diagnosis of thoracic injury. Ultimately, thoracotomy may be necessary for both diagnosis and therapy. Patients with thoracic trauma frequently demonstrate multisystem trauma, and the workup must be tailored to this reality: the most life-threatening injuries are addressed first.

This chapter discusses common problems encountered in patients with thoracic trauma. The management of structure-specific problems (e.g., heart injury, lung injury, etc.) is presented, as well as specific diagnostic and therapeutic considerations that may arise owing to the presence of so many physiologically important structures in the chest cavity.

STRUCTURE-SPECIFIC DIAGNOSES

Injuries to the bony thorax

The bony thorax comprises the sternum and manubrium anteriorly, a solid rib cage anterolaterally, and the vertebral column posteriorly. The upper thorax is also superficially covered by the scapulae posteriorly, and the clavicles are in position along the anterior apices bilaterally. These structures combine to confer substantial protection to the underlying soft tissues. The vast majority of information regarding injuries to the bony thorax can be gleaned from physical examination and initial chest x-ray, to be followed as needed by further radiographic investigation.

Rib fractures

Injury to the rib cage runs a spectrum from simple rib fractures to actual volume loss of the thoracic cavity. Simple rib fractures are common and generally well tolerated. In the absence of underlying pathology, the treatment consists of pain control, incentive spirometry, and aggressive pulmonary toilet. Patients with rib fractures at multiple levels (usually greater than three) pose a greater challenge in pain control. In these patients and especially in the elderly, high thoracic epidural analgesia has been shown to be an important adjunct to therapy.[1] Appropriate analgesia allows the patient to better expand the lung, it also prevents significant atelectasis and helps the patient clear secretions, thereby reducing the risk of pneumonia. In addition to epidural and intercostal blocks, nonsteroidal anti-inflammatory drugs (including COX-2 inhibitors) and opioid analgesics play an important role.

The location of the rib fractures is very important in the workup of the multiply injured patient. Fracture of the upper ribs (1, 2, and 3) suggests a significant force transmitted to the thorax and a risk of concomitant great vessel injury. Fracture of the lower ribs (8, 9, and 10) should raise suspicion of injury to solid abdominal organs, especially if there is simultaneous abdominal discomfort.

A flail chest describes a segment of chest wall that is fractured in multiple places, resulting in an area of the bony thorax that is "free" from rigid fixation. Small flail segments may be tolerated with good analgesia. Flail segments of larger area may compromise pulmonary function by blunting the negative inspiratory force of spontaneous respiration. That is, the negative pressure of the descending diaphragm preferentially collapses the chest wall, preventing aeration of the lung. In these cases, the treatment is positive-pressure ventilation until chest wall mechanics can improve. Oxygenation is often additionally impaired by the underlying pulmonary contusion that nearly always accompanies such an injury. Occasionally the flail segment (especially a large one) must be surgically fixed in place to maintain the integrity of the chest wall and allow ventilation and healing.

Injuries to the thoracic spine

Whereas fractures of the vertebral body or transverse process are common, unstable fractures of the thoracic spine are not. Indeed, vertebral column instability from gunshot wounds is exceedingly rare.[2] The entire spinal column is inspected and palpated on secondary survey. Radiographic assessment is tailored to physical findings, neurologic examination, and, in some cases, suspicion as a result of the mechanism of injury. Initial films include anteroposterior (AP) and cross-table lateral x-rays of the thoracic spine. CT scans of the vertebral columns in patients with fractures are helpful to identify the integrity of the three-column (anterior, posterior, and middle) architecture of the spine (Fig. 17-1). Unstable fractures require spinal precautions and eventual fixation. Assessment of the spinal canal and injury of the cord often requires magnetic resonance imaging (MRI).

Patients with neurologic deficits following blunt spinal injuries (neurologic loss or an "incomplete" exam in the awake patient) receive a bolus of methylprednisolone at a dose of 30 mg/kg over 1 h.[3] If the diagnosis is made within 3 h of injury, an infusion of methylprednisolone is continued for 23 h at a dose of 5.4 mg/kg/h. If the steroid is started between 3 and 8 h, the infusion is maintained for 48 h. There is no role for steroids if the diagnosis is made greater than 8 h postinjury or in patients with penetrating trauma.

Other thoracic bony injuries

Sternal fractures are most often treated conservatively. Such fractures, however, can be strong indicators of severe force injury and should raise awareness for associated

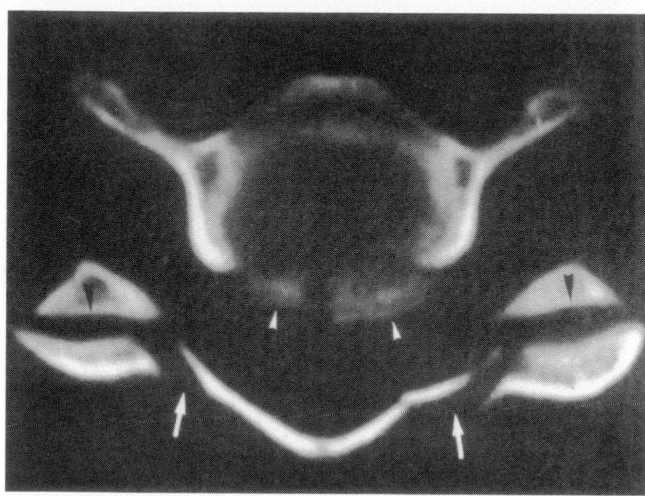

Figure 17-1 CT of unstable fracture demonstrating disruption of middle and posterior column elements.

injuries, such as blunt aortic, cardiac, and pulmonary injuries.

Scapular fractures are generally a source of significant patient discomfort. Although they contribute very little to the life-threatening nature of chest trauma, the presence of a scapular fracture is a strong indicator of severe force injury that must raise suspicion of simultaneous injury to the great vessels.

Lung injuries

Pulmonary contusion

Contusion of the lung parenchyma may occur from both blunt and penetrating injury. With blunt trauma, it occurs secondary to the transmission of force across the bony thorax. As such, children may present with large pulmonary contusions in the face of little evidence of bony thoracic injury, given the fairly elastic nature of immature bone. Penetrating injury results in contusion from the dissipation of the kinetic energy of the missile or from injury to peripheral pulmonary vasculature.

Pulmonary contusions cause embarrassment of oxygenation, with hypoxemia worsening over 24 to 48 h following injury. Older patients are particularly susceptible to complication following pulmonary contusion.[4] Treatment consists of aggressive pulmonary toilet and support of oxygenation to the degree necessary. To this end, aggressive analgesia is often vital because of concomitant painful injury to the chest wall. Small contusions often require only minimal oxygen supplementation. Larger contusions may necessitate mechanical ventilation with positive end-expiratory pressure as well as pressure-controlled ventilation.

Penetrating lung injury

Although the majority of patients with penetrating lung injury may be managed with tube thoracostomy alone (including over 80 percent of patients with injury to the right chest), the greatest evolution of thought has occurred regarding patients with more severe lung injuries requiring emergency lifesaving surgery. The life-threatening complications of massive hemorrhage, air embolism, and large intrapulmonary shunt require careful attention of physicians in emergency medicine, trauma surgery, anesthesiology, and surgical critical care.

One of the underappreciated and potentially devastating consequences of thoracotomy for ongoing thoracic bleeding is systemic air embolism. When one considers the clinical circumstances, perhaps it is surprising that this complication is not seen more frequently: (1) the patient typically has major ongoing hemorrhage that leads to depressed intravascular volumes and pressures; (2) the most common scenario is that of a bullet injury that has destroyed much of the pulmonary parenchymal architecture; and (3) shortly after intubation, the patient has a high positive airway pressure combined with low intravascular pressure in the face of abnormal communication between these two components of the pulmonary anatomy. The resulting scenario of air escaping the small airways and entering the bronchial veins and ultimately the pulmonary vein becomes understandable, producing systemic air embolism. Because the above-mentioned contributing factors are all unavoidable, the one modification that might be offered is a heightened sense of urgency and, where possible, rapid transport of these patients to the operating room before intubation. At this point, positioning, rapid preparation, and draping of the patient should occur first, reserving intubation for a point as close in time as possible to the actual incision. This practice decreases the length of time when increased airway pressures are present in combination with ongoing pulmonary bleeding. If the injury is to the left chest, advancing the tube down into the right mainstem bronchus and keeping the left lung collapsed may also be of benefit if the collapse can be tolerated by the patient. When the thorax is entered, occlusion of the pulmonary hilum with a vascular clamp or with the surgeon's fingers can impede the continuous passage of air into the coronary, cerebral, and other systemic arteries. In this regard, one of the major advances in trauma surgery in the 1990s was the use of the stapling device to facilitate pulmonary tractotomy for hemorrhage control and to minimize the introduction of systemic air.

Stapled pulmonary tractotomy has been shown in several series to provide rapid and effective exposure to bleeding pulmonary parenchymal vessels and transected bronchi.[5] The technique can be performed with either single- or double-lumen endotracheal intubation, with a Duval lung clamp placed parallel to the tract of the bullet. The stapling device is positioned so that one of the arms is placed through the entrance and exit wounds of the lungs (Fig. 17-2). When the stapler fires, the bullet tract is exposed fully, allowing the surgeon to directly suture bleeding vessels and transected bronchi (Fig. 17-3).

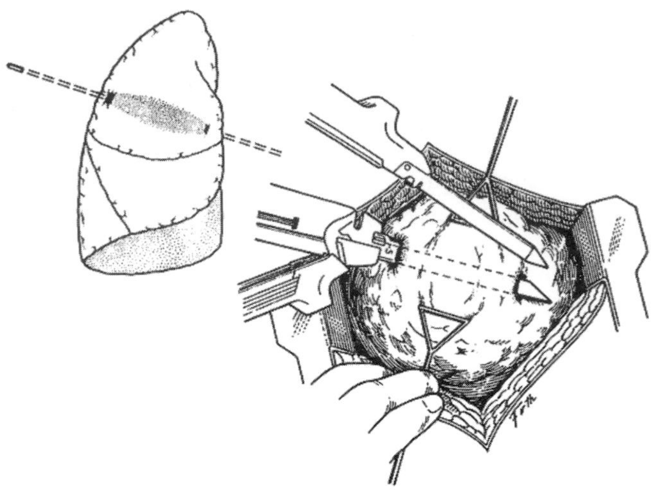

Figure 17-2 Placement of stapler through bullet tract.

Pulmonary tractotomy for hemorrhage has dramatically decreased the number of patients requiring anatomic resection for trauma.

There is a common local inflammatory response in the lung following gunshot injuries consisting of vasodilatation. When this is combined with the hypoventilation associated with local contusion, atelectasis, and intraparenchymal hemorrhage, a ventilation/perfusion (V/Q) mismatch and hypoxemia may occur. Accordingly, the aforementioned advances introduced by stapled tractotomy in providing lung-sparing surgery has occasionally produced the unintended consequence of delivering patients to the intensive care unit with severe hypoxemia following lifesaving thoracotomy for hemorrhage control. The irony is that patients undergoing the substantially more morbid procedure of pneumonectomy for hemorrhage control would less likely present with severe hypoxemia (although the acute right heart dysfunction exacerbating the hemorrhagic shock produces prohibitive mortality).

CASE A 20-year old male presented in hemorrhagic shock following gunshot injuries to the left upper lobe, lingula, left lower lobe, proximal intercostals branching off of the distal thoracic aorta, as well as injuries to the diaphragm, stomach, small bowel, and lumbar veins. Emergency surgery for hemorrhage control included left thoracotomy, left-upper-lobe and left-lower-lobe tractotomy, ligation of bleeding intercostals, as well as exploratory laparotomy for "damage control." The sequelae of hemorrhagic shock included coagulopathy, requiring reevacuation of blood in the chest and abdomen in the early postoperative period. Massive transfusion of blood and blood products finally achieved hemostasis in this patient, but his severe hypoxemia was refractory to numerous manipulations in the surgical intensive care unit. The patient's repeated desaturations, cardiopulmonary arrests, and instability precluded transport or even manipulation of his endotracheal tube. A desperation maneuver of advancing his endotracheal tube into the right mainstem bronchus to exclude the V/Q-mismatched left lung yielded only transient improvement (Fig. 17-4). This patient ultimately died of severe hypoxemia despite the fact that hemostasis was finally achieved, prompting the authors to wonder whether he would have had a better chance of survival with a pneumonectomy.

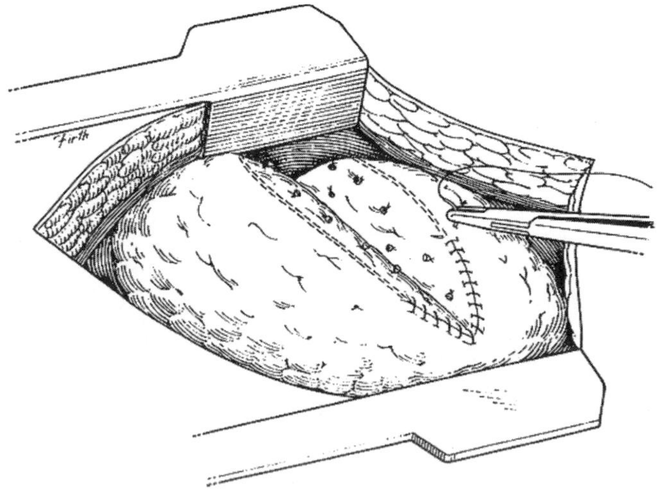

Figure 17-3 Opening the tract, individually ligating vessels, and, if necessary, oversewing the staple line.

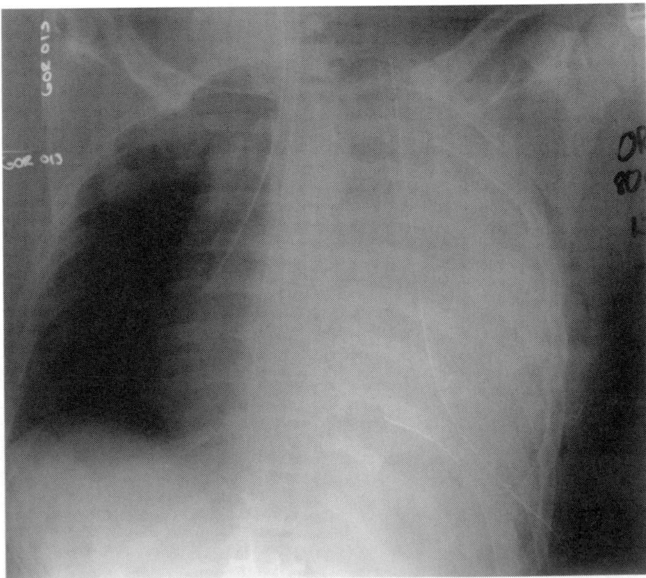

Figure 17-4 Massive hemothorax, parenchymal hemorrhage, atelectasis on the left, with endotracheal tube advanced toward the right mainstem bronchus.

In general, pneumonectomy is far more morbid than pulmonary tractotomy, but the case presented here represents the most extreme example of how V/Q mismatch after lung-sparing surgery can produce an unexpected dilemma.

Tracheobronchial injuries

Disruption of the tracheobronchial tree may be fatal due to loss of airway prior to transport from the scene. Subcutaneous emphysema, pneumothorax, or massive air leak after tube thoracostomy or hemoptysis may be suggestive of tracheobronchial disruption. Injury to the cervical esophagus may also result in dysphagia, pain, and cough and often occurs just distal to the cricoid cartilage.

Treatment is initiated with 100% oxygen and bronchoscopy. For bronchial laceration, placement of the endotracheal tube into the uninjured side facilitates repair and improves oxygenation. The operative approach depends on the location of injury. Posterior tracheal injury is repaired via a right posterolateral thoracotomy. The anterior and superior aspects of the trachea are best approached via median sternotomy, while the left and right bronchi are best addressed by their respective thoracotomies. Repair is performed with nonabsorbable sutures, with care taken to reapproximate the mucosa (Fig. 17-5).

Cardiac injuries

Historically, the absence of a diagnostic "gold standard" has made it difficult to assess the incidence of blunt cardiac injuries (BCI, formally called myocardial contusions) among patients sustaining chest trauma. Electrocardiography (ECG), cardiac enzyme analysis, and echocardiography have all been employed inconsistently in pursuing the diagnosis, thus making the literature difficult to interpret.

Practice management guidelines created by the Eastern Association for the Surgery of Trauma (EAST) have provided a great service in identifying patients at risk for complications from blunt cardiac injuries. Key recommendations and their levels of support include the following[6]:

Level I

- An admission ECG should be performed on all patients with a suspicious mechanism.

Level II

- A normal admission ECG in a hemodynamically stable patient should end pursuit of the diagnosis.
- Patients with abnormal ECGs (arrhythmia, ST-segment changes, ischemia, heart block) should be admitted for monitoring for 24 to 48 h.
- If the patient is hemodynamically unstable, an echocardiogram should be performed.
- Nuclear medicine studies are of little benefit.

Level III

- Sternal fracture is not predictive of BCI.
- CPK or cardiac troponin T are not useful in identifying patients who will develop complications related to BCI.
- Patients with cardiac disease, an abnormal ECG, and hemodynamic instability may be operated on if they are appropriately monitored.

The presentation of patients with penetrating injuries of the heart may range from "dead on arrival" or "in extremis" for patients with exsanguination to dyspnea or orthopnea in patients who are fortunate enough to have cardiac tamponade.[7] The classic triad of tamponade

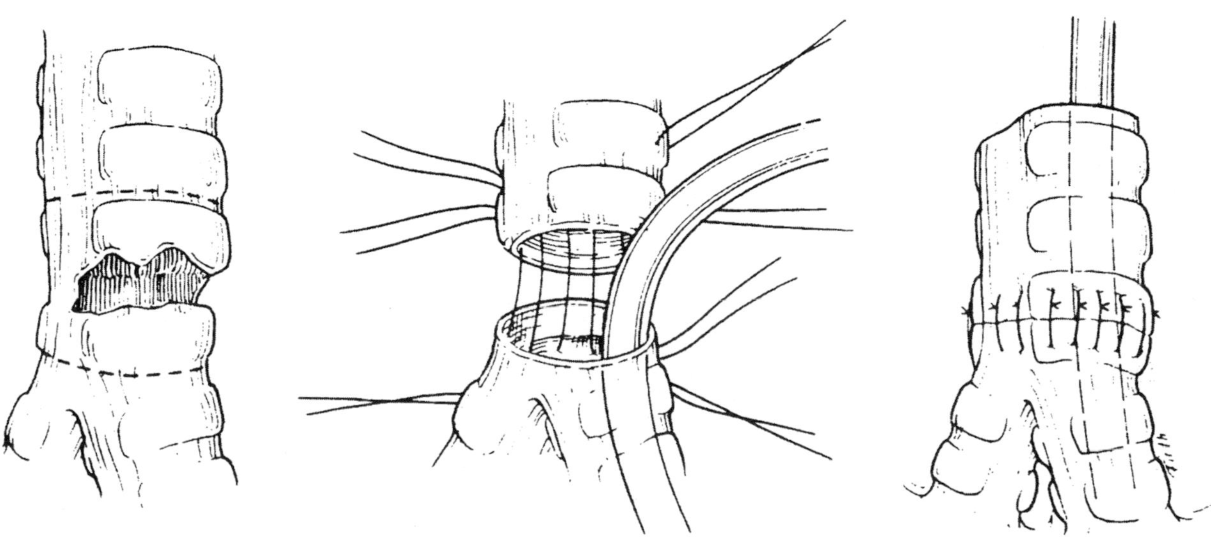

Figure 17-5 Repair of tracheobronchial injuries.

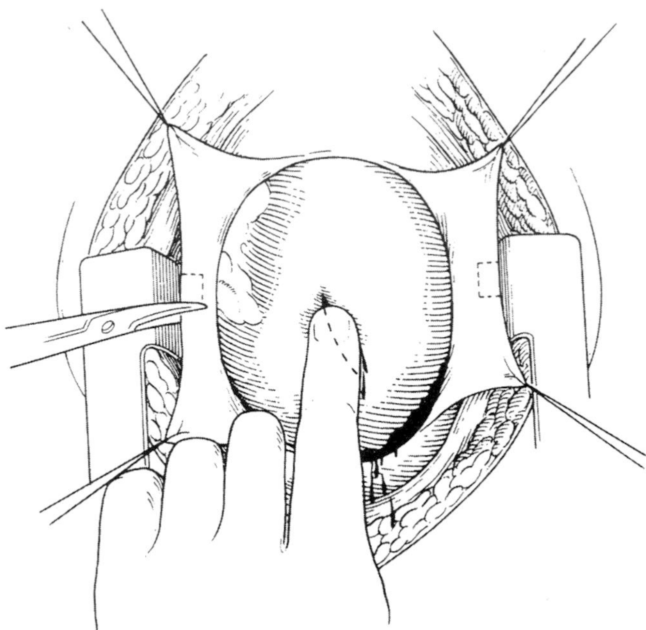

Figure 17-6 Finger occlusion of cardiac laceration.

(hypotension, muffled heart tones, jugular venous distention) is identified in only about one-third of patients with the diagnosis.

The diagnosis of cardiac injury should be entertained in any patients with a precordial penetrating wound. The pericardial view of the rapid emergency department (ED) sonogram (focused abdominal sonography for trauma, or FAST) is the most expeditious way to secure the diagnosis in the nonmoribund patient. Patients with thoracoabdominal injuries requiring laparotomy should be prepped and draped as though sternotomy were to be undertaken. The patients with heart injuries in addition to abdominal injuries may be identified by intraoperative transdiaphragmatic pericardial window. Patients arriving at the trauma center with vital signs who receive a prompt diagnosis and surgical intervention have substantially better survival rates. Other factors predicting improved survival include stab wounds versus gunshot wounds, single-chamber versus multiple-chamber injury, and the location of thoracotomy (operating room vs. ED).[8,9]

Pericardial tamponade due to a penetrating heart injury is the desired lesion every surgeon looks for when executing the heroic maneuver of ED thoracotomy. Once access is gained to the left chest, a craniocaudad incision is made along the pericardium in order to deliver the heart and evacuate hemopericardium while avoiding transection of the phrenic nerve. In this scenario, potential survivors are the patients who regain cardiac activity and blood pressure. Finger occlusion of the cardiac laceration (Fig. 17-6) allows for transport to the operating room for definitive repair.

We prefer to utilize a 3-0 polypropylene suture on a large (SH or MH) needle to achieve definitive repair (Fig. 17-7). The use of Teflon pledgets (Fig. 17-8) facilitates reapproximation of the laceration and is crucial in the repair of lacerations adjacent to coronary vessels. Survivors of cardiac injuries have a small but significant percentage of valvular and septal defects and warrant postoperative echocardiography.[10]

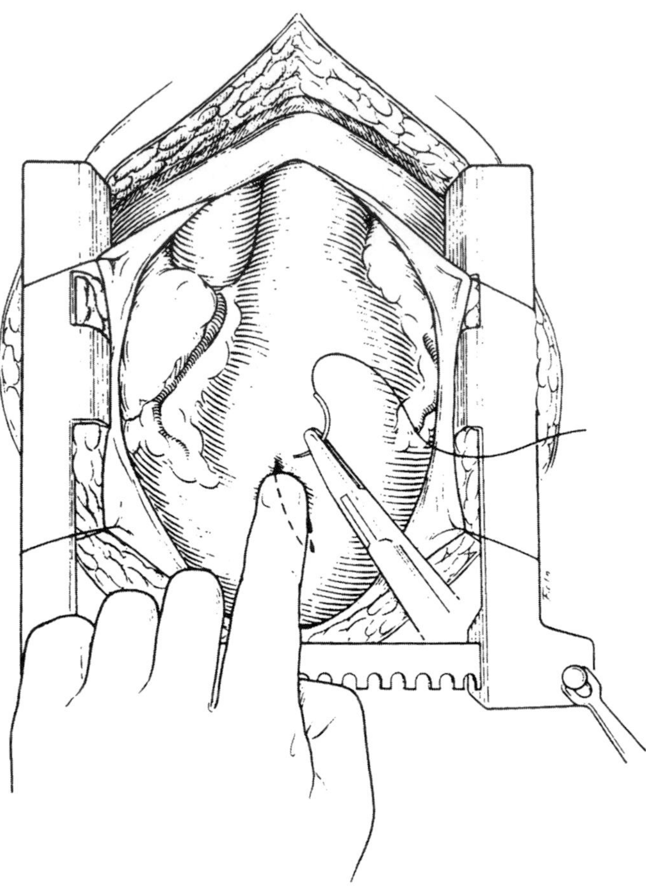

Figure 17-7 Suture repair of a cardiac laceration.

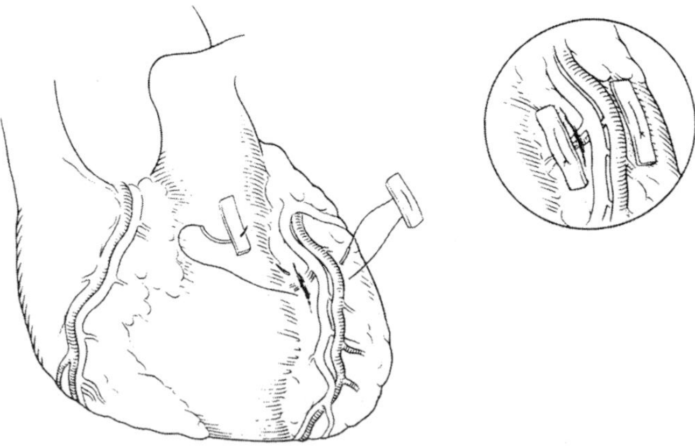

Figure 17-8 The use of Teflon pledgets to reapproximate a cardiac laceration adjacent to coronary vessels.

Aortic injuries

Unfortunately the overwhelming majority of patients with gunshot injury to the thoracic aorta present with exsanguination, thus offering little hope for salvage in even the most efficient trauma system or trauma center.[11] There has been a considerable evolution of thought, however, regarding patients who sustain blunt aortic injuries (BAIs).

Blunt injury to the thoracic aorta is responsible for approximately 8000 deaths a year in the United States. The vast majority of these injuries are produced from the deceleration mechanism encountered in a motor vehicle collisions, but they may also occur in falls from heights, pedestrian accidents, and crushing chest wounds. Aortic rupture is a common cause of death in commercial airline disasters.

The majority of patients sustaining BAIs are dead at the scene. Early diagnosis and treatment are paramount to realizing high survival rates in patients reaching the hospital alive. These patients have typically sustained deceleration forces concentrated at the junction of the fixed and nonfixed segments of the thoracic aorta (just distal to the left subclavian artery). This results in disruption of the intima and the media of the vessel; vascular flow is maintained because the thin adventitial layer is preventing complete vessel disruption, extravasation, and exsanguination. This emphasizes the importance of medical control of blood pressure in these patients once the diagnosis has been secured and while the surgical team is being mobilized. Many clinicians have been fooled into performing a "blind thoracotomy" in the unstable, multiply injured trauma patient with a mechanism of injury and chest x-ray suspicious for a BAI, only to realize that extrathoracic injuries are far more likely than a BAI to produce a dropping hematocrit or hemodynamic instability. Simply put, BAI with complete rupture produces rapid death, not hemodynamic instability.

The nature of this diagnosis and its associated injuries makes it unlikely for randomized controlled trials or large single-center experiences to be generated. However, significant class II multi-institutional data have been produced and compiled by EAST and the American Association for the Surgery of Trauma (AAST) in order to create practice management guidelines.[12,13]

BAI should be considered in all patients sustaining injuries due to motor vehicle accidents, and a chest x-ray should be the initial screening tool. The most common finding prompting further diagnostic workup includes widened mediastinum, obscure aortic knob (Fig. 17-9), deviation of the left mainstem bronchus, or opacification of the aortopulmonary window. Aortography is a highly sensitive, specific, and accurate gold standard for the diagnosis of BAI (Fig. 17-10). Spiral or helical CT scans are extremely sensitive and may be used alone to rule out BAI. A growing number of patients are undergoing aortic repair on the basis of classic findings on helical CT (pseudoaneurysm, intimal disruption, periaortic hemorrhage) (Fig. 17-11). Transesophageal echocardiography is also a sensitive and specific test. It does, however, require training and expertise, which may not be as readily available as angiography.

Prompt repair of the blunt aortic injury is preferred. If the patient has more immediately life-threatening injuries

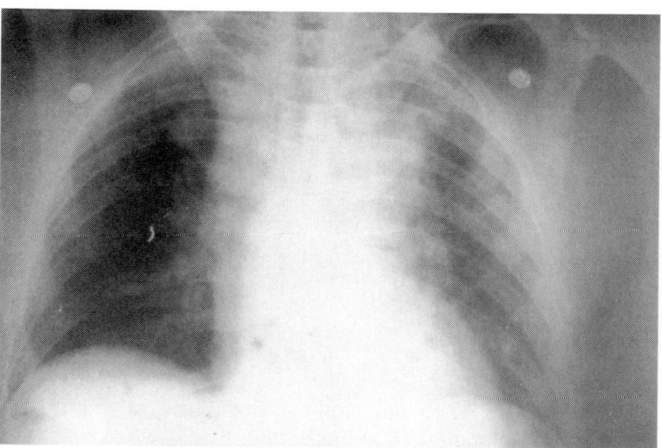

Figure 17-9 Chest x-ray demonstrating widened mediastinum and obscure aortic knob.

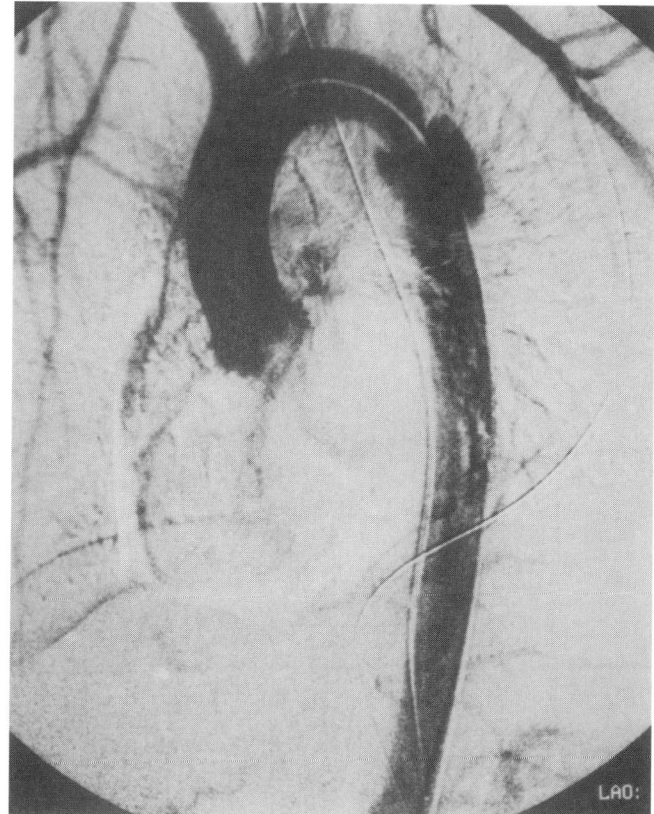

Figure 17-10 Aortogram with injury distal to the left subclavian artery.

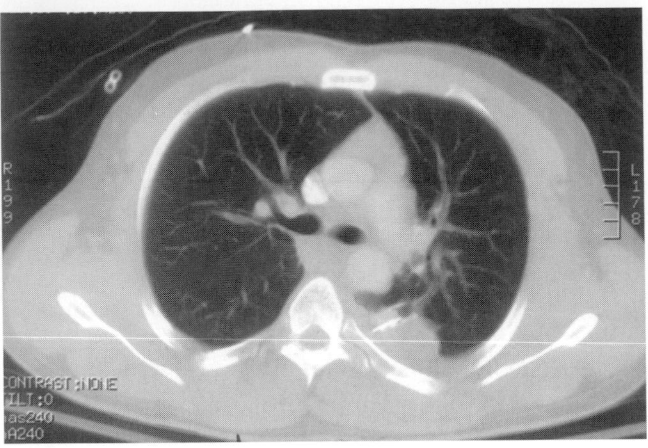

Figure 17-11 CT scan of blunt aortic injuries, showing pseudoaneurysm and periaortic hemorrhage.

that require intervention, such as emergent laparotomy or craniotomy, or if the patient is a poor operative candidate due to age or comorbidities, the aortic repair may be delayed. Medical control of blood pressure with beta blockers and nitroprusside is advised until surgical repair can be accomplished. Repair of the aortic injury is best accomplished with some method of distal perfusion, either bypass or shunt. Neurologic complications appear to correlate with ischemia time; therefore this time should be kept to a minimum.

Injuries to other great vessels

Most injuries of the great vessels are the result of penetrating trauma and require immediate intervention. Diagnostic investigation aimed at precise anatomic localization of the injury is appropriate only for hemodynamically stable patients. Proximal vessel injuries (pulmonary hilar, innominate, and superior vena caval injuries) are often diagnosed at exploration for massive bleeding. More distal vessels (neck, subclavian, and axillary) may be visualized with duplex ultrasonography, CT angiography, and traditional arteriography. Unequal pulses, asymmetrical ankle-brachial indices, and expanding hematomas should all raise suspicion for arterial injury. Massive bleeding may be seen with both arterial and venous injury. Minimizing time between injury and definitive operative management is key for reducing mortality.

Because of the fixed nature of many vital structures in the mediastinum, suspicion as to which structures are injured is very important to the choice of surgical incision. Timely exposure is crucial for a successful outcome. Injury to the great vessels of the left chest (including the left subclavian artery and vein and proximal aorta) will likely result in massive hemothorax. Depending on the track of injury, it is often difficult to accurately predict the bleeding source. Left lateral thoracotomy is the incision of choice for lung parenchymal injuries as well as access to the descending aorta. A right thoracotomy is the exposure for similar injuries on that side. The subclavian vessels are best approached via an incision directly over the medial third of the clavicle extending from the clavicular head and curving down toward the deltopectoral groove.[14] The medial clavicle is stripped of its muscular attachments (a periosteal elevator of some sort is helpful) and resected. If the injury is more proximal, this is combined with a median sternotomy (Fig. 17-12). The median sternotomy provides excellent exposure to the most proximal branches of the aortic arch.

An ED thoracotomy may have been performed, given the massive blood loss; however, this incision alone all but prohibits operative access to the upper thorax, especially the subclavian vessels. One proposed solution is a trapdoor type of incision, made by extending the medial edge of the incision along the sternum to the sternal notch and laterally just superior to the left clavicle, which is also divided within the middle third (Fig. 17-12). With the segment retracted laterally, access to the distal aortic arch and subclavian vessels is facilitated. However, this highly morbid incision carries a significant blood loss due to extensive muscle division and the need for iatrogenic rib fracture; moreover, it does not provide a significantly better exposure than the median sternotomy with clavicular extension. Care must be taken to avoid injury to the brachial plexus and phrenic nerves with these approaches.

All subclavian and axillary arterial injuries should undergo repair except in the most severely unstable patients. Temporary shunting may be necessary in these patients. Repair may be achieved by primary anastomosis, autologous vein graft or patch, or interposition of a

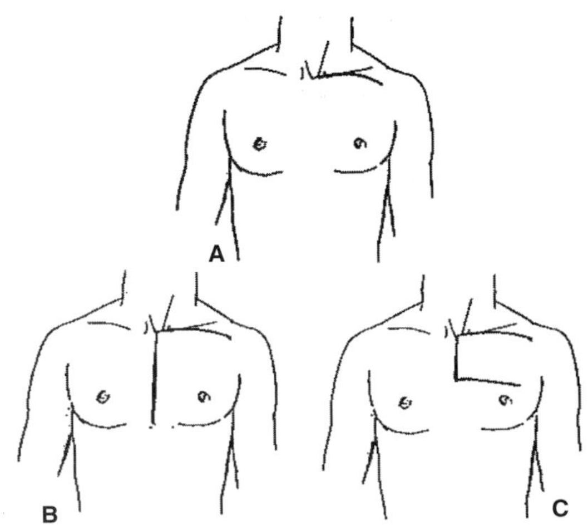

Clavicular incision (A), combined clavicular incision and median sternotomy (B), and trap door incision (C).

Figure 17-12 Incisions for approaches to injuries of the great vessels.

prosthetic graft. Subclavian vein injuries are repaired only if simple (no significant narrowing of the vessel or need for interposition or patch): otherwise ligation of the vein is generally well tolerated. Close monitoring of the ensuing limb edema and vigilance for compartment syndrome avoid the need for prophylactic forelimb fasciotomy.

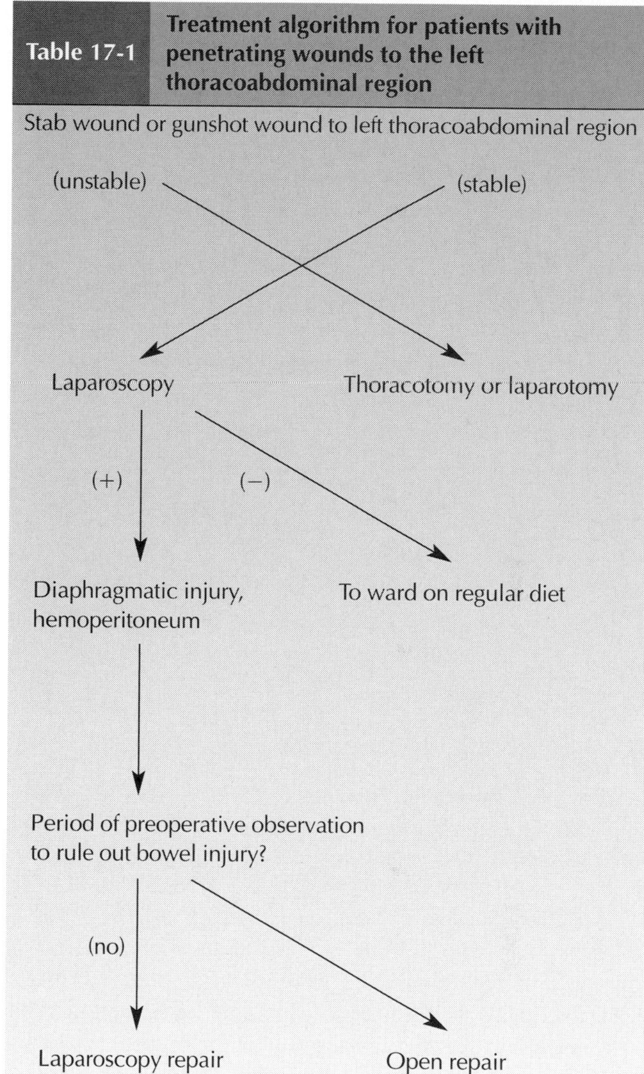

Table 17-1 Treatment algorithm for patients with penetrating wounds to the left thoracoabdominal region

Esophageal injuries

The esophagus, which runs along the length of the posterior mediastinum, is most frequently injured by penetrating trauma. In the unstable patient, esophageal injury is identified at thoracotomy. For stable patients, esophagoscopy and esophagography detect 90 percent of injuries to the esophagus. Other findings may include subcutaneous emphysema, mediastinal air, pleural effusion, or unexplained persistent fever for more than 24 h following injury. It should be noted that a stable patient with a transmediastinal gunshot wound is far more likely to have an esophageal injury than an aortic injury.

As with other structures in the mediastinum, the level of injury dictates the operative approach. For proximal thoracic esophageal injury, a right posterolateral thoracotomy is used. Injury to the distal thoracic esophagus is best addressed via a left posterolateral thoracotomy.

Esophageal injuries identified early are repaired primarily (in layers if possible) and often reinforced with tissue-flap coverage (pleural tissue, intercostals muscle, or fundoplication). Those repaired in a delayed manner (> 12 h) require wide drainage with multiple tube thoracostomies. Esophageal diversion is considered especially if there is evidence of mediastinitis.

Diaphragmatic injuries

It is clear that some stable patients with gunshot or stab wounds to the left thoracoabdominal region (between the nipple and costal margin) have diaphragmatic injuries that go unappreciated. These patients typically are admitted for a period of observation or chest tube placement for a hemopneumothorax. The small diaphragmatic laceration may remain clinically occult and cause no problem. Alternatively, it may enlarge with Valsalva maneuvers over the ensuing weeks, months, years, or decades to a size large enough to admit abdominal viscera (colon or stomach). Given the poor follow-up with trauma patients, it is impossible to know how many will experience a diaphragmatic hernia (DH). However, it is known that DH with incarcerated bowel represents a potentially lethal sequela of diaphragmatic injury.[15]

Two prospective series performed where *all* patients with penetrating left thoracoabdominal trauma underwent surgical evaluation (laparotomy or thoracotomy for unstable patients, laparoscopy for stable patients) established the incidence of occult diaphragmatic injuries in stable patients at approximately 25 percent.[16,17] One might expect a similar incidence with a right-sided injury, but the liver protects against the subsequent development of DH. Thus we recommend an algorithm utilizing laparoscopy as a tool to visualize the left hemidiaphragm and inspect for hemoperitoneum and any concomitant abdominal injuries (Table 17-1). We employ a running nonabsorbable suture (i.e., 2-0 Prolene) for our open diaphragmatic repairs.

SPECIAL CONSIDERATIONS

Pneumothorax

Pneumothorax is a frequent complication of both blunt and penetrating chest trauma. Air allowed into the pleural space results in partial or total collapse of the lungs. On auscultation, breath sounds are distant or absent. Subcutaneous emphysema identified by crepitus over the injured side may be detected. Chest x-ray demonstrates opacity and absence of lung markings. If there is an

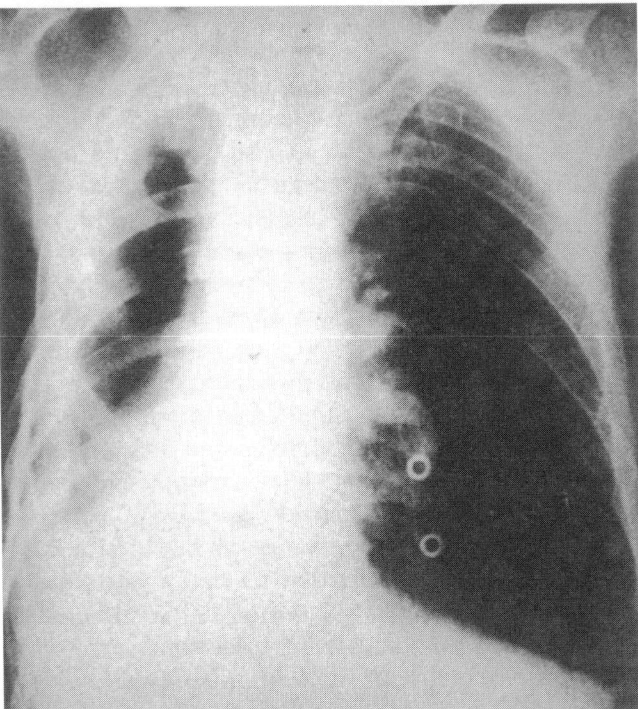

Figure 17-13 The chest x-ray that should not exist. Most tension pneumothoraces should be clinically obvious. Note the absence of air markings, the flattened diaphragm, and the shift of the mediastinal structures to the right.

ongoing air leak from the lung parenchyma, a tension pneumothorax may develop. This may be accelerated by intubation and positive-pressure ventilation provided to a patient with an initially small air leak. Massive overinflation of the affected side causes shift of the relatively pliable mediastinal structures toward the opposite side of the chest as well as flattening of the diaphragm. This may be clinically evident with a trachea that deviates toward the opposite side. The increase in intrathoracic pressure causes an embarrassment of venous return to the heart and a subsequent drop in blood pressure. The striking clinical picture associated with tension pneumothorax should prompt immediate decompression without a chest x-ray in most cases (Fig. 17-13). If a chest tube is not immediately available, a large-bore IV catheter is used to access the chest cavity in the second intercostal space in the midclavicular line. This is followed by expeditious placement of a thoracostomy tube, most often in the fifth intercostal space in the anterior axillary line.

Simple pneumothorax is treated by tube thoracostomy alone. For uncomplicated pneumothorax, moderate-sized (28F) tubes are appropriate. The patient with an open pneumothorax ("sucking" chest wound) should have the wound sterilely dressed with occlusive gauze taped on three sides prior to chest tube placement. Unfortunately, traumatic pneumothorax is often accompanied by intrapleural hemorrhage.

Table 17-2 Indications for thoracotomy
Injury with hemodynamic instability (< 80 mmHg systolic) unresponsive to adequate resuscitation
>1500 mL of blood evacuated initially on chest tube insertion
Ongoing blood loss (>200–300 mL/h for 4 h)
Persistent hemothorax despite adequate drainage two chest tubes

Hemothorax

Any structure in the chest can bleed and cause hemothorax. In addition, intraabdominal bleeding in patients with diaphragmatic injury can also manifest as hemothorax. As with pneumothoraces, hemothorax is treated initially by tube thoracostomy. Whereas a smaller-bore tube may be appropriate for the treatment of pneumothorax, 36 to 40F chest tubes are more effective at successfully evacuating intrapleural blood. If the bleeding is self-limited (low in volume, with declining chest tube output) and the blood is well evacuated, this is the only intervention required. If the hemothorax is massive or the bleeding is ongoing, then the patient is taken to the operating room for prompt thoracotomy and hemostasis. The indications for thoracotomy for hemothorax are outlined in Table 17-2. It should be remembered that a chest x-ray following insertion of a chest tube is vital. A potential pitfall exists in patients who do not meet operative criteria based on chest tube output alone. Rapid accumulation of clotted blood in the pleural space may clog the tube and give the false impression that ongoing bleeding is minimal. This may be the source of confusion in the multiply injured patient with persistent hypotension (Fig. 17-14). In addition, the simple maneuver of

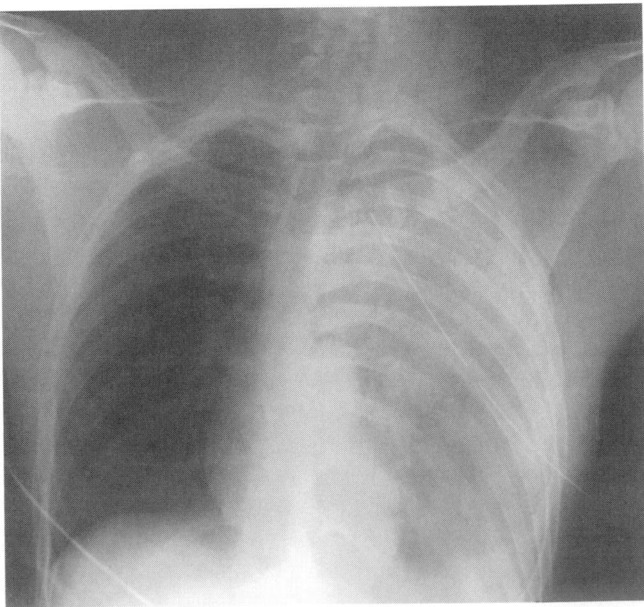

Figure 17-14 Large left hemothorax despite well-placed chest tube.

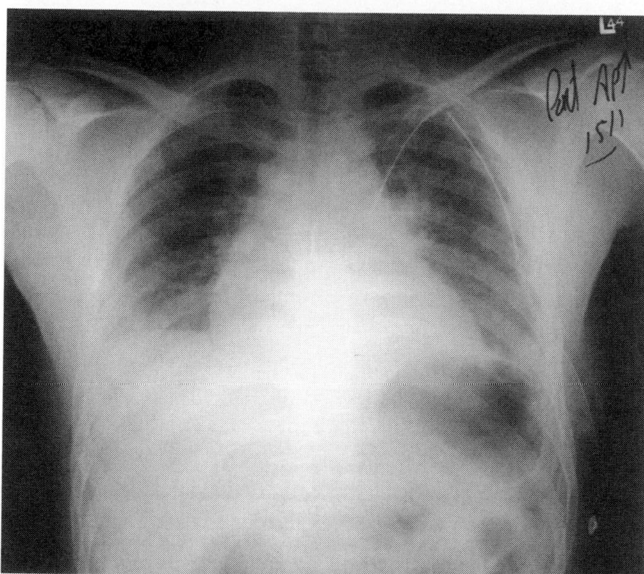

Figure 17-15 One could not possibly spin this kinked chest tube without encountering resistance. If spinning is not possible, the tube should be slowly and sterilely withdrawn and readvanced before it is secured.

spinning the chest tube before securing it in place eliminates the possibility of kinking and makes tubal occlusion less likely (Fig. 17-15).

Chest tube management

A few specific principles are important in the management of chest tubes in trauma patients. When a bullet or knife invades the pleural space, bacterial contamination occurs before antibiotics are administered; thus the use of antibiotics constitutes early presumptive therapy rather than true prophylaxis. Evidence-based guidelines generated by EAST recommend that a first-generation cephalosporins be given at the time of chest tube placement for traumatic hemopneumothorax and continued for no longer than 24 h.[18] Longer courses of therapy do not yield any benefit in terms of reduction of septic complications. Interestingly, the data suggest there may be a reduction in the incidence of pneumonia but not empyema (which is surprisingly uncommon) in trauma patients receiving prophylactic antibiotics when the chest tube is placed.

For patients with hemopneumothoraces, we choose to remove the tube when the output has dropped to less than 200 mL/24 h and there is no recurrence of pneumothorax on water seal. The management of persistent hemothorax is discussed later in this chapter.

Emergency department thoracotomy

Thoracotomy performed in the ED is a heroic lifesaving measure reserved for patients with penetrating injury to the torso who have lost vital signs in transport to or shortly after arriving at the hospital. Greatest survival rates are achieved in the subset of patients with stab wounds to the right ventricle and with pericardial tamponade.[19]

A generous incision is made from the left sternal border in the fourth of or fifth intercostal space and extended to the midaxilla posterolaterally. The intercostal muscles are divided sharply, with care not to injure the underlying lung parenchyma. A right chest tube is placed simultaneously by another member of the trauma team. A Finochetto retractor is placed and the intercostal space is widened for exposure. The pericardium is easily identified medially and inspected. A bulging pericardium is suggestive of pericardial tamponade and requires immediate decompression. The pericardial sac is opened via a craniocaudad incision anteriorly along the pericardial sac. Care is taken to avoid injury to the left phrenic nerve, which runs along the lateral aspect of the pericardium. If there is no evidence of tamponade, the hemothorax is evacuated and the left hemithorax is thoroughly inspected for sites of bleeding and injury, with special attention to the injury tract.

In order to optimize blood flow to the carotid and coronary circulations, the thoracic aorta is occluded either by an atraumatic vascular clamp or by direct compression against the vertebral column. The former method has the advantage of freeing the surgeon's hands for other procedures (such as cardiac massage) as well as keeping the confined space of the hemithorax clear; however, the esophagus may easily be injured in the process. The latter method avoids the risk of esophageal injury but necessitates an additional hand in the field.

Open cardiac massage, defibrillation, or temporary hemostatic measures are taken; if a blood pressure and pulse are reestablished, the patient is brought immediately to the operating room to complete repairs and achieve closure of the thoracotomy.

Transmediastinal gunshot wounds

Hemodynamically unstable patients with transmediastinal gunshot wounds typically receive rapid tube thoracostomy and transport to the operating room. Because victims of gunshot wounds to the esophagus are much more commonly stable from a hemodynamic standpoint than their counterparts with aortic injuries, it is worthwhile to reexamine the role of aortography in the immediate workup of stable patients with transmediastinal gunshot wounds.[20] Although aortography should not be omitted from the workup completely, it should follow other diagnostic studies, particularly esophagography, which can proceed while the interventional angiography team is being mobilized. Bronchoscopy and echocardiography may also be performed, although patients with tracheobronchial and heart injuries have more obvious clinical presentations. Moreover, aortography may be safely postponed until after operative repair of esophageal injuries, where delay can result in increased morbidity and mortality.

Thoracoscopy for residual hemothorax

Although the majority of traumatic hemothoraces are adequately managed by tube thoracostomies, residual posttraumatic hemothorax may occur in about 5 percent of cases. Surgical evacuation via thoracoscopy decreases the risk of contamination of the residual blood, empyema, or fibrothorax requiring open decortication. Thoracoscopic evacuation is best accomplished within 5 days after injury, when the semisolid clot can easily be suctioned.[21] Patients being considered for thoracoscopic evacuation of persistent hemothorax should be evaluated by a CT of the chest, as this has been shown to be superior to chest x-ray in distinguishing free intrapleural blood from contusion, atelectasis, and intra-parenchymal hemorrhage.[22]

An interesting phenomenon may arise when patients look clinically worse in the immediate postoperative period following elective thoracoscopic evacuation of residual hemothorax. This is explained by (1) the fact that double-lumen endotracheal tubes are frequently employed and reinflation of the lung on the surgical side is not immediate, giving a picture of radiographic deterioration, and (2) the previously described inflammatory response involving vasodilatation following a gunshot injury may still be present during operative lung collapse, causing worsened V/Q mismatch and desaturation. Thus, in addition to the x-ray looking worse, the patient cannot be extubated and is transported to the surgical intensive care unit. Patience is advised, as both the radiographic and clinical picture typically improve in the first 24 h.

Bullet emboli

Bullet emboli are unusual complications of gunshot injuries to the chest. Bullets may enter the circulation directly either through the heart or through a blood vessel.[23] In addition, the architecture of the lung parenchyma offers another possible entry point; bullets in the lung may migrate into the pulmonary venous circulation and ultimately into the left heart and arterial circulation. This explains the observation that bullets initially seen on chest x-ray may disappear on subsequent films. These bullets may ultimately become lodged in the brachial, carotid, or iliac arteries or other branching points within the arterial system. Symptoms are due to arterial obstruction caused by the lodged bullet, requiring surgical excision.

A unique diagnostic feature of migrating bullets in the circulatory system occurs when a bullet lodges in the heart.[24] Because of heart motion, intracardiac bullets will appear "fuzzy" on chest x-rays, with indistinct borders (Fig. 17-16).

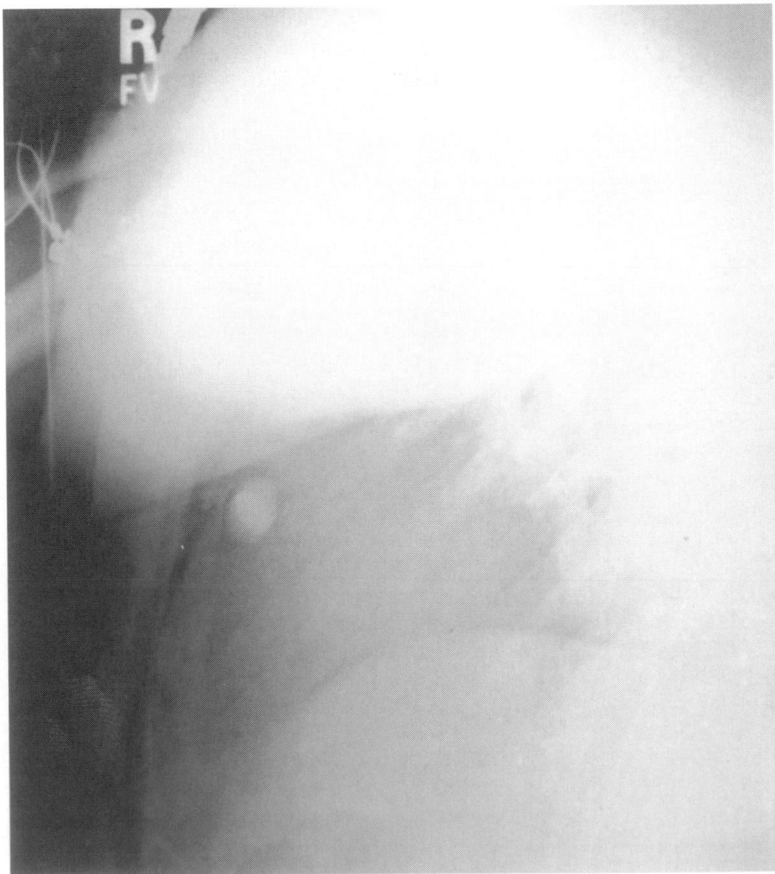

A

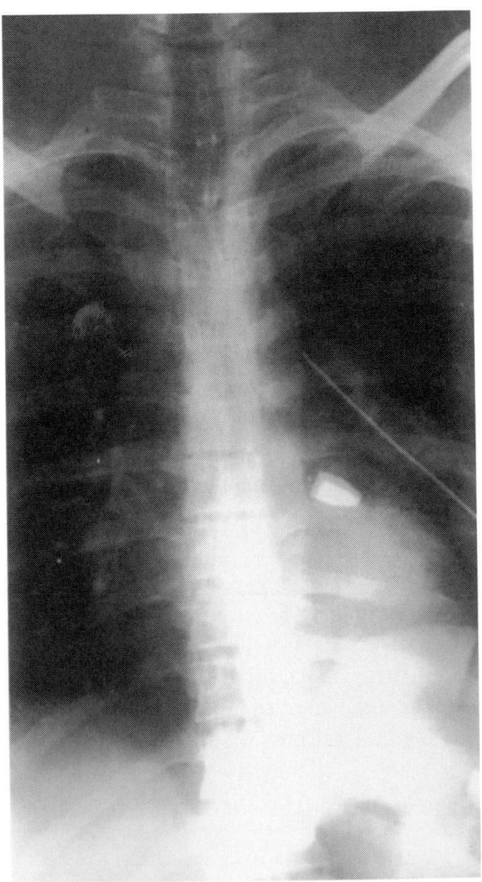
B

Figure 17-16 "Fuzzy" heart sign of an intracardiac bullet.

References

1. Moon MR, Luchette FA, Gibson SW, et al. Prospective, randomized comparison of epidural versus parenteral opioid analgesia in thoracic trauma. *Ann Surg* 1999;229:684–692.
2. Cornwell EE, Chang DC, Bonar JP, et al. Thoracolumbar immobilization for trauma patients with torso gunshot wounds. *Arch Surg* 2001;136:324–327.
3. Bracken MB, Shepard MJ, Holford TR, et al. Administration of methylprednisolone for 24 or 48 hours of tirilazad mesylate for 48 hours in the treatment of acute spinal cord injury. *AMA* 1997;277:1597–1604.
4. Kollmorgen DR, Murray Kam Sullivan JJ, et al. Predictors of mortality in pulmonary contusion. *Am J Surg* 1994;168: 659–664.
5. Velmahos GC, Baker C, Demetriades D, et al. Lung-sparing surgery after penetrating trauma using tractotomy, partial lobectomy, and pneumorrhaphy. *Arch Surg* 1999;134: 186–189.
6. Pasquale MD, Nagy K, Clarke J. *Practice Guideline for Screening of Blunt Cardiac Injury.* Eastern Association for the Surgery of Trauma, 1998. Available at: www.east.org/tpg/chap2.pdf.
7. Porter JM, Ivatury RR. Unwillingness to lie supine? A sign of pericardial tamponade. *Am Surg* 1997;63(4):365–366.
8. Asensio JA, Berne JD, Demetriades D, et al. One hundred five penetrating cardiac injuries: A 2-year prospective evaluation. *J Trauma* 1998;44(6):1073–1082.
9. Tyburski JG, Astra L, Wilson RF, et al. Factors affecting prognosis with penetrating wounds of the heart. *J Trauma* 2002;48(4):587.
10. Demetriades D, Charalambides C, Pantanowitz D. Late sequelae of penetrating cardiac injuries. *Br J Surg* 1990; 77(7):813–814.
11. Cornwell EE, Kennedy F, Berne TV, et al. Gunshot wounds to the thoracic aorta in the '90s: Only prevention will make a difference. *Am Surg* 1995;61(8):721–723.
12. Fabian TC, Richardson JD, Croce MA, et al. Prospective study of blunt aortic injury: Multicenter trial of the American Association for the Surgery of Trauma. *J Trauma* 1997;42:374–383.
13. Nagy K, Fabian T, Rodman G, et al. Guidelines for the diagnosis and management of blunt aortic injury: An EAST practice management guidelines work group. *J Trauma* 2000;48(6):1128–1143.
14. Demetriades D, Asensio JA. Subclavian and axillary vascular injuries. *Surg Clin North Am* 2001;81(6):1357–1373.
15. Murray J, Demetriades D, Ashton K. Acute tension diaphragmatic herniation: Case Report. *J Trauma* 1997;43: 698–700.
16. Murray J, Demetriades D, Cornwell EE, et al. Penetrating left thoracoabdominal trauma: The incidence and clinical presentation of diaphragm injuries. *J Trauma* 1997;43: 624–626.
17. Murray J, Demetriades D, Asensio JA, et al. Occult injuries to the diaphragm: Prospective evaluation of laparoscopy in penetrating injuries to the left lower colon. *J Am Coll Surg* 1998;187:626–630.
18. Luchette FA, Barrie PS, Oswanski MF, et al. Practice management guidelines for prophylactic antibiotic use in tube thoracostomy for traumatic hemopneumothorax: The EAST practice management guidelines work group. Eastern Association for Trauma. *J Trauma* 2000;48(4): 753–757.
19. Branney SW, Moore EE, Feldhaus KM, et al. Critical analysis of two decades of experience with post-injury emergency department thoracotomy in a regional trauma center. *J Trauma* 1998;45:87–95.
20. Cornwell EE, Kennedy F, Ayad IA, et al. Transmediastinal gunshot wounds. A reconsideration of the role of aortography. *Arch Surg* 1996;131:949–953.
21. Vassiliu P, Velmahos G, Toutouzas KG. Timing, safety, and efficacy of thoracoscopic evacuation of undrained post-traumatic hemothorax. *Am Surg* 2001;67:1165–1169.
22. Velmahos G, Demetriades D, Chan L, et al. Predicting the need for thoracoscopic evacuation of residual traumatic hemothorax: Chest radiograph is insufficient. *J Trauma* 1999;46(1):65–70.
23. Shen P, Mirzayan R, Jain T, et al. Gunshot wound to the thoracic aorta with peripheral arterial bullet embolization: Case report and literature review. *J Trauma* 1998;44(2): 394–397.
24. Kronson JW, Demetriades D. Retained cardiac missile: An unusual case report. *J Trauma* 2000;48(2):312–313.

CHAPTER

18 PACING OF THE DIAPHRAGM

John A. Elefteriades, George J. Koullias

INTRODUCTION

The concept of using electricity to stimulate artificial respiration, recommended by Beard and Rockwell in 1875, dates back to a suggestion by Cavallo, in his 1777 treatise on the application of electricity for human ailments, for using electrical stimulation of the phrenic nerve as a technique for cardiopulmonary resuscitation. A few years later, Hufeland recommended electrical stimulation of the phrenic nerve to induce contraction of the

KEY CONCEPTS

- Epidemiology
  - Central alveolar hypoventilation and high cervical spinal cord injury (quadriplegia) account for the vast majority of clinical cases of diaphragmatic pacing.
- Pathophysiology
  - Central alveolar hypoventilation stems from a malfunction of the respiratory control center in the medulla, with a resultant deficiency in respiratory drive. Etiologies include ischemia, trauma, infection, neoplasm, iatrogenic causes, and idiopathic etiologies. High cervical spinal cord injuries resulting in quadriplegia are caused by motor vehicle accidents, sports injuries and accidental falls, infections, neoplasms, vascular abnormalities, and infarctions. Spinal cord injury at or above the C3-C5 levels, where the lower motor neurons of the phrenic nerve are located, causes partial or complete phrenic nerve paralysis.
- Clinical features
  - Criteria for diaphragmatic pacing include complete respiratory paralysis for at least 3 months with structurally intact phrenic nerves and a functionally intact diaphragm as well as absence of severe chest wall deformities and intrinsic pulmonary pathology.
  - Prolonged hypoxia and hypoventilation can lead to cor pulmonale from chronic hypoxic pulmonary vasoconstriction and cerebral dysfunction.
- Diagnostics
  - Phrenic nerve and diaphragmatic stimulation serve to assess phrenic nerve conduction velocity and diaphragmatic action potential. Fluoroscopic imaging of diaphragmatic excursion is done to assess diaphragmatic function.
- Treatment
  - Pacemaker electrode can be implanted via a minithoracotomy or a cervical or thoracoscopic approach. Device implantation varies according to the device selected. Pulse-train stimulation is employed for diaphragmatic skeletal muscle.
- Outcomes
  - Review of worldwide experience reveals that diaphragmatic pacing has been completely successful in meeting the ventilatory needs of 47 percent of patients, partially successful in 35 percent, and unsuccessful in 17 percent; 27 percent were paced full-time and 61 percent part-time. Complications include electrode dysfunction, infection, diaphragm fatigue, bloody pleural effusions, and phrenic nerve damage. Although no comparative trials have demonstrated the superiority of diaphragmatic pacing over prolonged mechanical ventilation, several advantages are inferred from experience, including physical independence and fewer complications associated with prolonged tracheal cannulation.

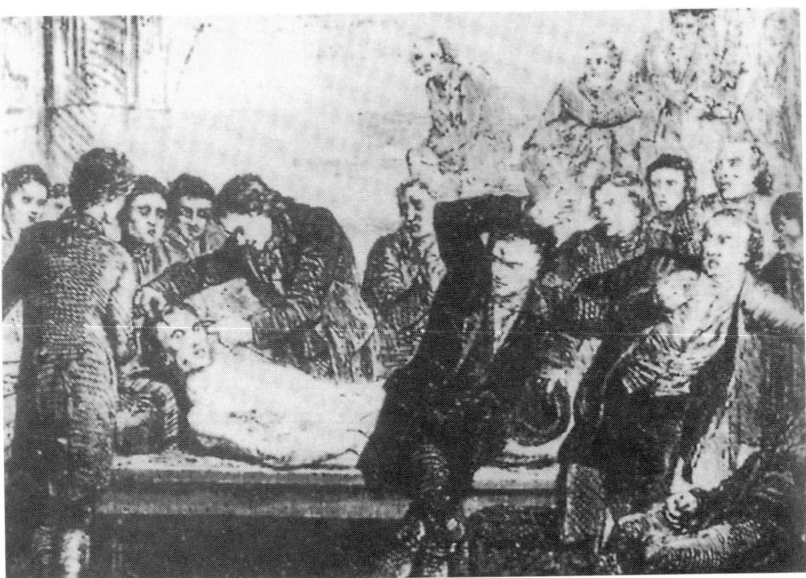

Figure 18-1 Induction of artificial respiration by galvanic phrenic nerve stimulation by Ure (1818) in a "freshly hung criminal." (From Ure.[2])

diaphragm.[1] In 1818, Ure demonstrated the feasibility of electrical stimulation of the phrenic nerve in "a freshly hung criminal": "The success of it was truly wonderful. Full . . . breathing instantly commenced. The chest heaved and fell; the belly was protruded and again collapsed, with the relaxing and retiring diaphragm"[2] (Fig. 18-1). Electrical stimulation of the phrenic nerve was popularized by Duchenne de Boulogne during a cholera epidemic in 1849 as a technique for cardiopulmonary resuscitation in treating asphyxia.[3] In 1927, Israel reported on the use of transcutaneous stimulation of the phrenic nerves for ventilation of six apneic newborns, all of whom survived.

Long-term continuous diaphragmatic pacing as it exists today became possible through the work of Glenn and associates at Yale (1964–1986).[4] Complete ventilatory support of a quadriplegic patient was first achieved in 1972.[5] In 1980, continuous bilateral low-frequency stimulation of the conditioned diaphragm for complete respiratory support was advocated by the same group. Owing to the rather small number of patients in need of diaphragmatic pacing, advances in pacer technology have been relatively slow. Nevertheless, new developments in pacing techniques continue to evolve into clinical practice. Recent examples include intercostal muscle recruitment and intramuscular diaphragm pacing.

INDICATIONS

The currently established indications for diaphragmatic pacing as a mode of ventilatory support include (1) central alveolar hypoventilation and (2) high cervical spinal cord injury (quadriplegia). These two indications account for the vast majority of clinical cases of diaphragmatic pacing (Fig. 18-2).

The use of diaphragmatic pacing has been studied in several additional conditions: intractable hiccups, end-

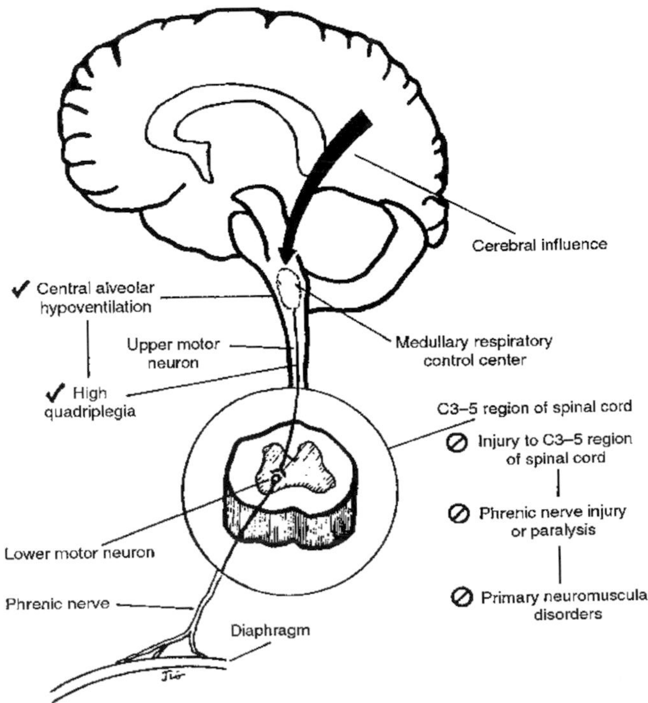

Figure 18-2 Respiratory control system for determining appropriate or inappropriate indications for diaphragmatic pacing. Check marks indicate appropriate indications for diaphragmatic pacing. International "verboten" signs indicate inappropriate indications.

stage chronic obstructive pulmonary disease, brainstem tumors or infarction, and basilar meningitis.[6] The use of diaphragmatic pacing has been found by Glenn and the senior author of this chapter to be effective in treating patients with intractable hiccups; however, the number of patients who have truly intractable hiccups, resistant to modern medical therapy, is very low. Diaphragmatic pacing has also been used in patients with severe end-stage chronic obstructive pulmonary disease in whom ventilatory drive is based on hypoxia rather than hypercarbia.[6] In this very limited group of patients, diaphragmatic pacing can provide an oxygen-protected mode of ventilation, since pacing ensures adequate ventilation despite the loss of hypoxic drive.

CENTRAL ALVEOLAR HYPOVENTILATION

The various sleep apnea syndromes should be differentiated, since different types of sleep apnea require different treatment modalities. The basic differentiation, as elucidated by Shneerson, is between obstructive and central sleep apnea.[7] In obstructive sleep apnea, there is adequate respiratory drive, but the defect is anatomic; that is, collapse of the upper airway prevents adequate ventilation during inspiration. Etiologies of obstructive sleep apnea include pharyngeal tumors and inflammatory lesions, pharyngeal muscle discoordination, and, most frequently, obesity and aging (with consequent tissue laxity).

Distinct from obstructive sleep apnea is central sleep apnea, in which the principal pathogenic mechanism involves malfunction of the respiratory control center in the medulla, with a resultant deficiency in respiratory drive. The upper airway in these patients is normal and patent. The primary causes of central sleep apnea include ischemic, traumatic, infectious, neoplastic, iatrogenic, and idiopathic etiologies. Patients suffering from central sleep apnea often demonstrate a characteristic Pickwickian habitus, are frequently somnolent during the day, and progressively develop chronic hypoxia, pulmonary vasoconstriction, secondary fixed pulmonary hypertension, and right-sided heart failure. It has recently been recognized that many sleep apnea patients also demonstrate clinical or subclinical changes in their response to hypoxia and hypercarbia during the day, not only during sleep. This has led to the more appropriate description of this condition as *central alveolar hypoventilation* instead of *central sleep apnea*. Standard spirometric pulmonary function testing can readily distinguish between central hypoventilation and other disorders affecting respiratory muscle strength. Central alveolar hypoventilation is an appropriate indication for diaphragmatic pacing.

QUADRIPLEGIA

The other more common indication for diaphragmatic pacing is high quadriplegia from cervical spinal cord injury.[5] This patient population has increased in recent years owing to improvements in emergency care delivery systems, widespread availability of positive-pressure ventilation, and improved long-term respiratory care. Causes of quadriplegia include motor vehicle accidents, sports injuries and accidental falls, infections, neoplasms, vascular abnormalities, and infarctions.

The lower motor neurons of the phrenic nerve are located in the spinal cord at the levels of C3–C5. Injury to the spinal cord below these levels causes quadriplegia but does not usually disrupt ventilation. Injury at the C3-C5 levels, where cell bodies of the phrenic nerve are located, may produce a partially injured phrenic nerve with upper motor neuron communication. In this case, the decision to insert a diaphragmatic pacer is more difficult, since the patient may retain a substantial spontaneous ability to ventilate; also, the addition of diaphragmatic pacing may not lead to respiratory improvement because the phrenic nerve is compromised from degeneration. In patients with spinal cord injury at a level higher than C3-C5, the capacity for spontaneous ventilation is eliminated by virtue of neural isolation of the cell bodies of the phrenic nerve from efferent stimuli from the brain, but phrenic nerve integrity is usually preserved.[8] In addition, with the exception of the sternocleidomastoid and trapezius muscles, intercostal (T1-T12), abdominal (T7-L1), and pelvic (L1-S2) accessory muscles are also denervated. These individuals with high quadriplegia and preserved phrenic nerves are ideal candidates for diaphragmatic pacing.

CHARACTERISTICS OF CANDIDATE PATIENTS FOR DIAPHRAGMATIC PACING

Several criteria apply to patient selection and successful application of diaphragmatic pacing (Fig. 18-3).[9] Requirements include:

1. Relatively normal cognitive function and the absence of severe compromising central nervous system pathology.
2. Presence of a supportive network of family members and friends.
3. Complete respiratory paralysis without recovery for at least 3 months after the injury or the onset of apnea.
4. Intact phrenic nerves. Direct nerve injury from trauma, tumor invasion, degenerative disease, or injury after cardiac surgery contraindicates diaphragmatic pacing.
5. An inherently sound diaphragm with no muscular disorder. In the case of central hypoventilation, the patient should demonstrate at least a 5-cm maximum excursion of the diaphragm with spontaneous breathing. Quadriplegic patients are not required to exhibit the same degree of excursion; however, some brisk downward deflection of the diaphragm with

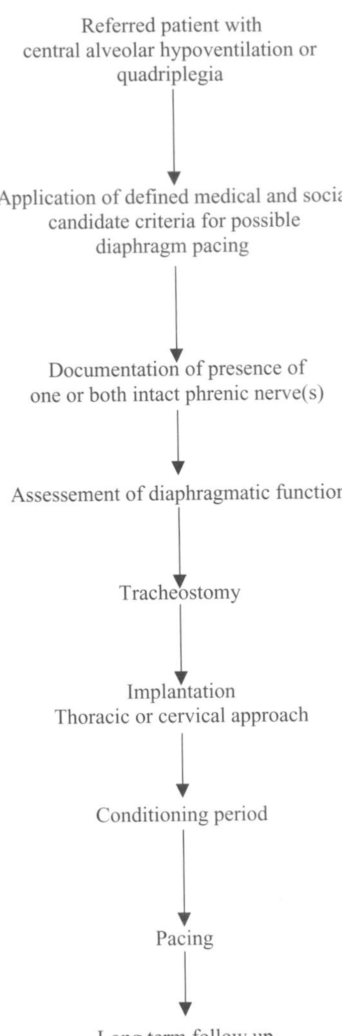

Figure 18-3 Decision-making flowchart.

percutaneous stimulation of the phrenic nerve should be observed in these patients.

6. Absence of severe intrinsic pulmonary pathology.
7. Absence of severe chest wall deformity.
8. Presence of a professional team of health care providers familiar with pacing techniques and the long-term aftercare.

ASSESSMENT OF PHRENIC NERVE AND DIAPHRAGMATIC FUNCTION

The presence of intact phrenic nerves and diaphragms is of paramount importance. The phrenic nerve and its conduction time are assessed with either transcutaneous or rarely open nerve stimulation (Fig. 18-4). The transcutaneous testing method is essentially a phrenic nerve conduction test. A thimble electrode aimed posteriorly is placed at the motor point of the nerve, which is located medial to the lateral edge of the clavicular head of the sternocleidomastoid muscle. The muscle is retracted medially and stimulation is applied. We look for a brisk visible and palpable ipsilateral hemidiaphragmatic contraction.[9] The diaphragmatic action potential and the phrenic nerve conduction time are also measured by placing percutaneous electrodes at the level of the eighth intercostal space, one at the anterior axillary line and one at the posterior axillary line. A ground electrode is applied at the xiphoid. Phrenic nerve conduction times between 7.5 and 10.0 ms are normal; however, slightly prolonged times (11 to 14 ms) do not necessarily preclude pacing.

A cervical magnetic stimulation method for the evaluation of phrenic nerve function has also been described

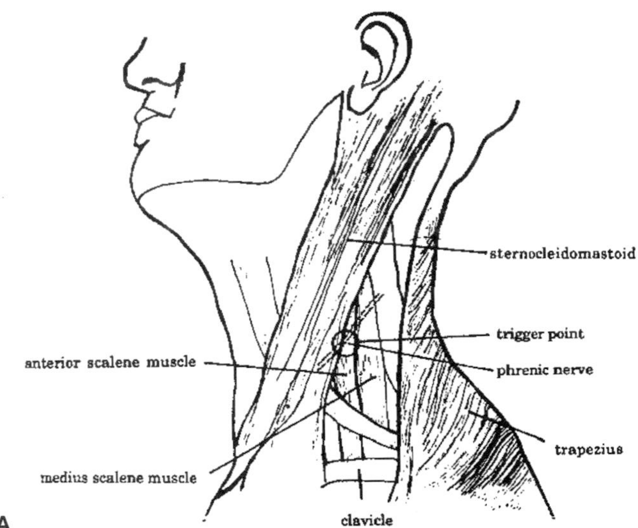

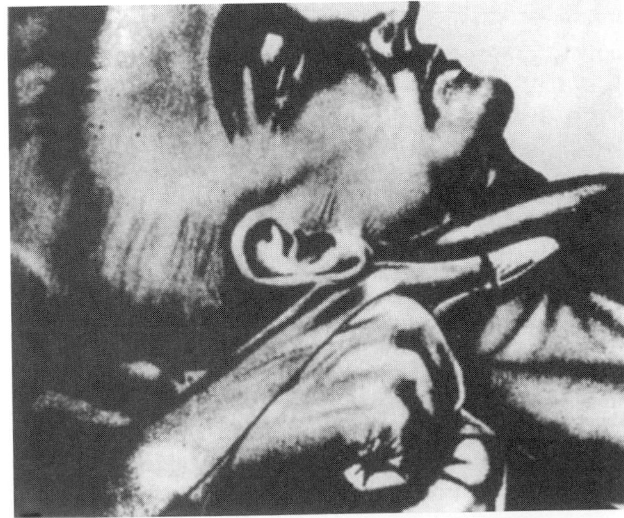

Figure 18-4 Percutaneous assessment of the phrenic nerve by electrical stimulation. **A.** Anatomic location of the phrenic nerve trigger point for percutaneous stimulation. **B.** Application of the thimble electrode.

and involves placement of a magnetic coil on the neck, which causes depolarization of the infraforaminal segments of cervical nerve roots C3-C5.[10] Bilateral phrenic nerve stimulation is usually performed by this means. Careful interpretation of the derived results is needed, because cross stimulation of additional muscles can be observed with this method. Overall, the number of candidate patients evaluated with this method is small, and the application of this technique for phrenic nerve assessment is not standard.

The clinical response of the diaphragm is paramount. Simple clinical inspection and palpation of the brisk contraction often suffice. Fluoroscopy can be used to quantify the degree of hemidiaphragmatic contraction. Failure to elicit a strong contraction almost invariably indicates a nonviable phrenic nerve. In rare instances, nerve viability cannot be ascertained by noninvasive methods. In this case, if pacing is still strongly considered, operative exploration and direct stimulation of the nerve should ensue.[9]

Patients with spinal cord injury occasionally manifest delayed recovery of respiratory function; an initially ventilator–dependent patient may regain spontaneous breathing. Accordingly, we recommend a minimal 3-month waiting period before the final decision for diaphragmatic pacing is made. This waiting period also allows for many other serious issues related to the acute injury to resolve. The patient finds time to adjust psychologically, establish rehabilitation regimens, adjust to altered bowel and bladder function, and prevent or treat decubitus ulcer formation.

PULSE TRAIN STIMULATION

Unlike cardiac muscle, the diaphragm is a skeletal muscle and thus not an electrical syncytium. Consequently, a single electrical impulse, such as that delivered by a cardiac pacemaker, cannot propagate through the entire diaphragm muscle. Rather, a series of multiple stimuli is required to produce a mechanically effective diaphragmatic contraction.[11] This series of electrical impulses is termed a *pulse train*. The pulse train is characterized by several parameters. The *rate* of the pulse train refers to the number of pulse trains delivered by the pacemaker per minute and corresponds to the desired respiratory rate. The *duration* of the pulse train refers to the length of time of the pulse train, which essentially determines the duration of paced inspiration. The *pulse width* refers to the duration of each individual impulse within the pulse train. The *frequency* refers to the number of individual impulses within the pulse train delivered per second. The *amplitude* represents the voltage of each stimulus within the pulse train. The amplitude, frequency, and pulse width determine the strength of the induced diaphragmatic contraction and thus the resultant tidal volume.[11]

Phrenic nerve stimulation can be conducted in a unipolar or bipolar mode, depending on the number of electrodes in contact with the phrenic nerve. Within the last decade, experimental studies have achieved intramuscular stimulation of the phrenic nerve within the diaphragm muscle; such intramuscular stimulation of the diaphragm has been attempted in a limited number of patients (see below).

PACING EQUIPMENT AND COMMERCIALLY AVAILABLE DEVICES

Unlike cardiac pacemakers, which are totally implantable, diaphragmatic pacemakers have an extracorporeal generator, approximately the size of a clock radio, in addition to the implantable components, which include nerve electrodes and receivers. Electrical output is transmitted through an antenna, the coil of which is taped securely on the patient's skin over the receiver site. The radiofrequency signal from the antenna is transmitted by inductive coupling to the receiver and from there through the nerve electrode to the phrenic nerve (Fig. 18-5). This system was designed by Glenn and colleagues at Yale and is the prototype for the three commercially available diaphragmatic pacing systems currently in use.[5] Although a totally implantable pacemaker system has been designed by Hogan and coworkers[11] and Landmuller and associates,[13] the need for a battery adequate to power the energy-demanding pulse-train stimulation and the relatively low numbers of diaphragmatic pacemakers required annually have contributed to the slowness technical engineering progress.

Currently, three diaphragmatic pacing systems are in use. Each varies slightly with respect to design. The Avery system (Avery Laboratories, Glen Cove, NY) uses the half cuff or 180-degree electrode originally developed at Yale. The system is also used for other applications of skeletal muscle stimulation. Currently, the Jukka Astrostim model (Atrotech OY, Tampere, Finland) is used by our group and others, with favorable results. This model differs from the Avery device by virtue of a quadripolar electrode. Two Teflon strips, each carrying two electrodes, are apposed to the nerve, one anteriorly and the other posteriorly. Stimulation of the phrenic nerve occurs through any of the electrode contacts at any given time, permitting incomplete stimulation of the phrenic nerve fascicles and associated diaphragmatic muscle bundles. Such selective stimulation allows some bundles to contract as others rest, a concept that seems to resemble natural respiratory patterns more closely than do other methods. At regular time intervals, the generator provides an increased pulse train, which leads to a higher tidal-volume breath and also contributes to better conditioning of the diaphragm muscle. Like the Astrostim device, the Vienna phrenic pacemaker (Medimplant, Inc., Vienna, Austria) stimulates the

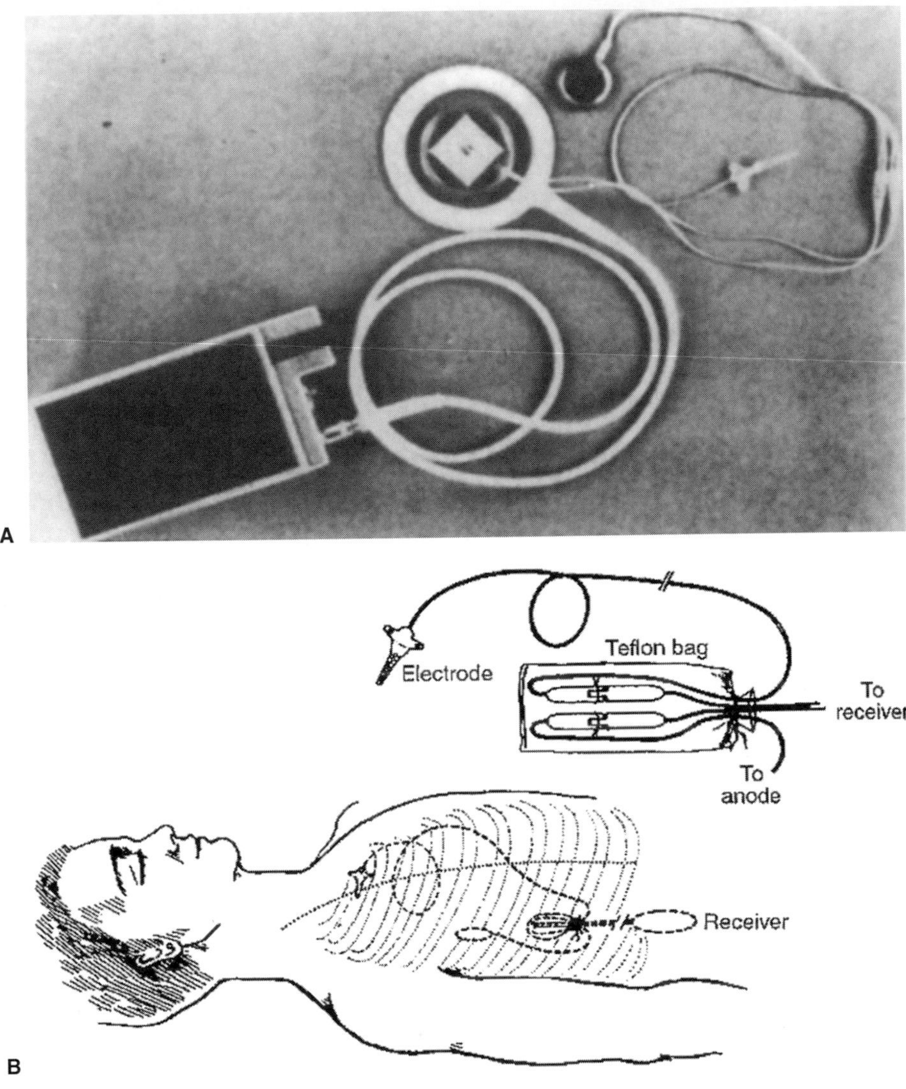

Figure 18-5 Apparatus for diaphragmatic pacing. **A.** The hardware includes the transmitter, external antenna, implantable receiver, and phrenic nerve electrode. **B.** Inserted equipment. The phrenic nerve electrode is placed at the upper thoracic part of the nerve and the receiver is located over a flat part of the lower anterolateral chest wall.

phrenic nerve by using multiple electrode contacts and incomplete stimulation of the nerve.[14]

IMPLANTATION TECHNIQUE

Implantation of the pacing electrode can be performed via a thoracotomy, a cervical incision, or a recently developed thoracoscopic approach. During implantation by any approach, extreme caution should be taken in placing the electrode on the phrenic nerve, because damage to this nerve during implantation would essentially preclude pacing.

The open minithoracotomy is currently our preferred approach (Fig. 18-6). The operation is conducted through a limited anterior incision in the second or third intercostal space. Implantations of the right and left pacemaker systems are usually performed 2 weeks apart. The internal mammary artery and vein are divided deliberately to avoid accidental disruption. The phrenic nerve is identified anterior to the pulmonary hilum. A location superior to the heart is chosen, where the nerve is accessible and the electrode can sit perfectly flat and with no tension beneath the nerve. The mediastinal pleura is incised several millimeters away from and parallel to the nerve, anteriorly and posteriorly. The electrode is slipped atraumatically behind the phrenic neurovascular bundle in such a way that the bundle rests on the half cuff platinum contact of the unipolar electrode. The Silastic support of the electrode is sutured to the adjacent pleura. We usually do not

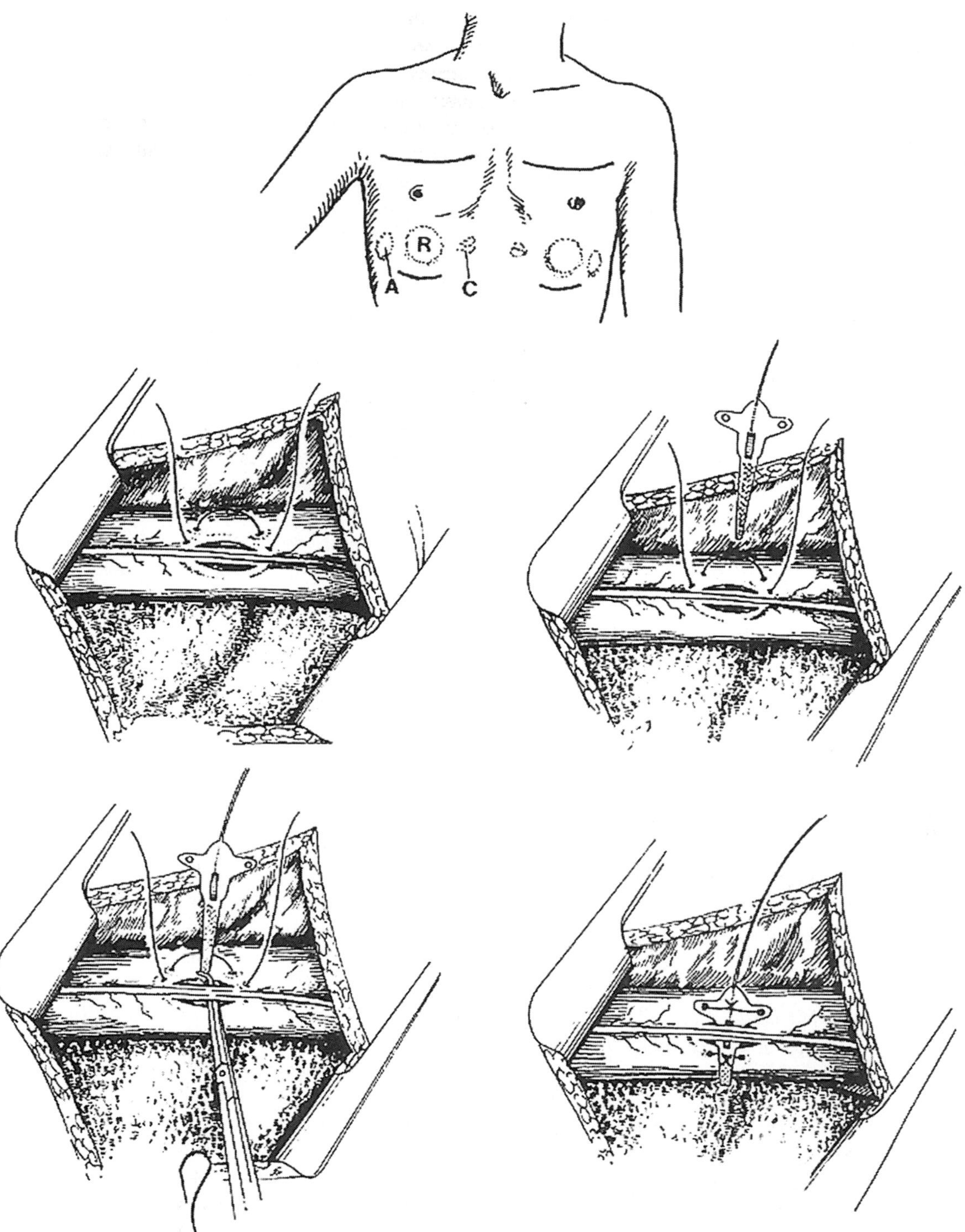

Figure 18-6 Transthoracic approach to the phrenic nerves for diaphragmatic pacing. (Modified from Glenn WWL. The diaphragm. In: Glenn WWL (ed). *Thoracic and Cardiovascular Surgery,* 4th ed. Stamford, CT: Appleton-Century-Crofts, 1983:363. With permission.)

treat minor bleeding in the area of the bundle, since it usually stops quickly, and we discourage any use of electrocautery because of the danger of injury to the phrenic nerve. The electrode is left in a redundant fashion on the lung in order to avoid tension during lung excursion and is passed through the chest wall inside a chest tube. A subcutaneous pocket is created at a point in the lower anterolateral chest wall to house the receiver.

The cervical approach for electrode placement avoids the creation of a thoracotomy. In our institution, however, this approach has been discouraged for several reasons, the most important being the existence of accessory phrenic nerve radicals that originate below the C3-C5 level and consequently do not join the nerve until the mediastinum; a cervically placed electrode would not stimulate these fibers. In the event that a cervical approach is chosen, as in the case of presence of pulmonary parenchymal pathology or a mildly deformed thorax, a 5-cm incision is made above and parallel to the midclavicle. The lateral edge of the sternocleidomastoid muscle is retracted medially and the phrenic nerve is seen overlying the scalenus anticus muscle. An electrical probe is placed in contact with the nerve and a 2- to 10-mA current is applied. A brisk ipsilateral diaphragmatic contraction confirms nerve identification; further dissection and placement of the permanent pacing electrode proceeds thereafter in a fashion similar to that used in the transthoracic approach. The pocket housing the subcutaneous receiver is placed in the infraclavicular region by blunt dissection through the existing cervical incision. For the cervical approach, both sides can be performed during the same operation. If a tracheostomy is not already present, the patient should be temporarily intubated. When a tracheostomy is present, the site is covered with an occlusive dressing to decrease the risk of contamination during electrode placement.

Placement of the Medimplant device and intraoperative testing are usually done through a median sternotomy, as both electrodes use the same receiver. In general, pacing that requires high threshold values or failure to pace at all should be evaluated immediately for improper lead placement, lead dislodgement, lead damage, or injury to the phrenic nerve itself.

DEVICE SETTINGS AND CONDUCT OF PACING

Fluoroscopy, performed at the initial evaluation of the diaphragm and at pacemaker implantation is used to determine proper threshold current settings.[11] A radiopaque ruler is placed with the numeral "1" at the dome of the diaphragm to calculate diaphragmatic descent during adjustments of pacemaker current. The fluoroscopy tube is always kept at 30 cm for all diaphragm evaluations. Maximal voluntary diaphragmatic descent is determined for patients with central hypoventilation. The currents needed to produce a discernible and also a maximal contraction of the diaphragm are recorded. For clinical pacing, the current is set just above that needed for maximal excursion. Reassessment of the diaphragm with respect to current settings is performed at intervals thereafter. The pacing rate is individualized for each patient; in general, however, for bilateral pacing, six to ten breaths per minute usually suffice. Unilaterally paced adults and children usually require higher rates. Pacemaker default settings for inspiratory duration and pulse width are usually preset by the manufacturer. The inspiratory duration is usually 1.3 s for adults and 0.9 s for children. Pulse width is set at 150 ms. Pacing is not begun until 2 weeks after implantation; earlier initiation has led to the development of bloody pleural effusions, most probably as a result of disruption of immature adhesions by the strong diaphragmatic contractions elicited by pacing.[11]

Although unilateral, bilateral, or alternating intermittent pacing is available, the preference of the Yale group in most cases is to condition the diaphragm for low-frequency, continuous bilateral pacing.[14] No skeletal muscle, including the diaphragm, is able to contract maximally and continuously. Although the diaphragm contracts incessantly to provide respiration, activation of the individual nerve fascicles and corresponding muscle fibers is staggered such that during any given breath, a percentage of dormant motor units is allowed metabolic recovery from previous activation. Because pulse-train stimulation of the phrenic nerve activates most or all of the nerve fascicles and nerve bundles, individual motor units are not allowed to rest, and the unconditioned diaphragm tires easily.

Because of these issues, a program of gradual conditioning is used to allow the diaphragm to acclimate to pulse-train electrical stimulation and, in the case of quadriplegia, to restore the diaphragm that has atrophied from disuse. The pacing schedule usually begins with 15 minutes of pacing per hour, in the supine position, for several hours a day. The number of minutes per hour and the number of hours per day are gradually increased in a systematic fashion until full-time pacing is achieved. The adaptive process may require weeks to months, depending on the condition of the diaphragm at the inception of pacing. Quadriplegic patients with atrophied diaphragms require longer conditioning times than patients with central hypoventilation. Along with progressive increases in the duration of the pacing period, the frequency of stimuli in the pulse train and the number of breaths per minute that provide adequate ventilation are gradually decreased, both measures aiming at minimizing diaphragmatic fatigue. Fatigue is usually manifest as a decrease in tidal volume or increase in end-tidal carbon dioxide pressure in the absence of specific pulmonary problems. In this case, the patient is rested temporarily on mechanical ventilation and pacing is resumed with a shorter pacing period. The fully conditioned diaphragm demonstrates a high percentage of slow-twitch oxidative fibers, which provides histologic and biochemical evidence reflecting its capacity to perform sustained work.

Patients with central hypoventilation who require only part-time nocturnal pacing of 8 to 12 h can implement their full pacing plan immediately; the period of time during the day that the patient is not paced is adequate to prevent diaphragm fatigue. These patients usually require

6 to 10 breaths per minute, with a frequency of 20 to 25 MHz, and pulse intervals of 40 to 50 ms.[11]

COMPLICATIONS

Diaphragm pacemakers mandate a thorough understanding of the device and its limitations as well as the principles of pacing to produce a successful pacing outcome. Because of the limited application of these devices, it is very important that the patient have access to a professional team of health care providers with implantation experience, familiarity with diaphragmatic pacing and its complications, as well as long-term aftercare.[14]

Potential complications of diaphragmatic pacing include receiver and electrode failure. Based on a study by Weese-Mayer and colleagues, the most common complication is receiver failure, occurring, on average, at 56.3 months after implantation. Receiver failure may occur as a result of breakdown of the insulating cover or electrical short circuiting of the receiver's internal components. In patients with cardiac pacemakers, there have also been cases of cross-talk between the two devices. Placement of the electrode at the cervical area has also been associated with transmission of impulses to the brachial plexus, with rhythmic muscle contractions of the upper extremity.

Other potential complications include bloody pleural effusions in cases of premature initiation of conditioning, acute and chronic phrenic nerve injury, diaphragm fatigue, and device infection. Systemic or other temporary or chronic physiologic stresses occurring in quadriplegic patients usually increase the pacing requirements. The currently available devices, unfortunately, do not monitor or correct for such circumstances. In these cases, careful assessment of the patient's condition and readjustment of the pacemaker is required to avoid the disastrous situation in which a paced patient under physiologic stress is returned to mechanical ventilation and maintained on it unnecessarily.

LAPAROSCOPIC INTRAMUSCULAR DIAPHRAGMATIC PACING

In order to mitigate inconvenience and length of stay after thoracotomy, a group from University Hospitals of Cleveland has developed a method of phrenic nerve activation with laparoscopic insertion of intramuscular diaphragmatic electrodes.[15] The procedure uses standard laparoscopic techniques to locate the motor points of the diaphragm by means of a mapping technique. By *motor point*, the authors connote an area of the diaphragm muscle contained within the space defined by the entrance points of the phrenic nerve into the diaphragm. To locate this motor point, the patient is temporarily taken off mechanical ventilation, a suction electrode is applied at the area of the diaphragm under investigation, and electrical currents from 0 to 24 mA are applied. Mathematical analysis of the derived data from several stimulation sides allows prediction of the approximate location of the motor points in each hemidiaphragm. The implantation of a total of four electrodes follows and the electrodes are subsequently tunneled to the right supraclavicular region. Two weeks later, a four-channel electrical stimulator is connected directly with the electrodes and pacing is implemented over a conditioning period of approximately 20 to 50 weeks. Relatively encouraging initial early and midterm results of this technique were recently published for a small group of 6 patients with quadriplegia.[16] There was one failure to place electrodes among these patients; 3 patients were weaned completely off the ventilator;, and the other 2 patients were progressively increasing their time off the ventilator with conditioning. No patients with central hypoventilation have yet received this device. The device, up to this point, does not use a receiver, requires an intact phrenic nerve, and is not successful in patients with lower motor neuron disease or muscular disorders. The device depends on an intact phrenic nerve, as it stimulates the radicles of the nerve in the diaphragm.[16] Our group is skeptical toward the laparoscopic approach. We believe that the putative negative impact of the traditional minithoracotomy approach is exaggerated. The thoracic approach is certain to capture all the radicles of the phrenic nerve. Above all, the laparoscopic system *passes the wires permanently through to the outside of the body*. Experience with other externalized devices would suggest that infection must ultimately follow; for infection to ascend to the nerve would be disastrous.

RESULTS

The review by Glenn and colleagues of the worldwide experience with 477 patients who had undergone diaphragmatic pacemaker insertion of any type clearly demonstrates the feasibility and effectiveness of this technique.[9] Of these patients, 165 had detailed follow-up. Pacing in these patients was completely successful in meeting ventilatory needs in 47 percent of patients, partially successful in 35 percent, and unsuccessful in 17 percent. Twenty-seven percent were paced full-time and 61 percent were paced part-time. Several smaller studies have examined long-term outcomes in groups of patients of different age groups and with different device types placed for different indications.

At last follow-up, 6 of the original 14 full-time, bilateral, low-frequency quadriplegic patients of the Yale group continued to pace full time; all have done so for over 10 years. Two patients have died. Six patients who failed pacing or paced intermittently did so for various reasons, including insufficient nursing and supportive care, progressive disability from quadriplegia, insufficient funds to continue pacing, and noncompliance.[17] Of note, the Yale long-term study determined that chronic pacing had no negative effects on the phrenic nerve or diaphragm. Furthermore, tidal volume and pacing thresholds did not deteriorate at all over time. Pacing was shown to be fully capable of meeting full-time ventilatory requirements continuously, for years at a time, including durations of more than a decade in certain patients.

Weese-Mayer and associates reviewed results in 64 patients, including 35 children, who underwent quadripolar electrode pacing. At a mean follow-up of 2 years for children, pacing was successful in 94 percent. Successful pacing without complications, however, was substantially lower in adults (60 percent). At a mean follow-up of 2.2 years for the adults, the success rate and complication-free success rates were 86 and 52 percent respectively. Electrode dysfunction was the most common overall complication (19 percent); infection occurred in 2.9 percent; and phrenic nerve damage developed in 3.8 percent.[18] Favorable results in smaller patient groups were also published for the Medimplant device and the Vienna pacemaker.[14]

Hunt[19] and Brouillette[20] and their associates have clarified certain characteristics specific to pacing of infants and young children. Their experience in 32 patients with predominant congenital central hypoventilation demonstrated that pacing can be effective; 25 of 32 patients survived and the vast majority were rehabilitated adequately to allow return home. because of the immaturity of the pediatric musculoskeletal system, diaphragmatic pacing should always be intermittent in this population.

At present, no prospective trial has been performed to compare diaphragmatic pacing with mechanical ventilation or other modes of ventilatory support, nor is one foreseen. The number of patients who require or qualify for pacing is limited and this population is heterogeneous. It has been the experience of the group at Yale that, at least in patients with central hypoventilation, progressive respiratory deterioration is common and death from hypoventilation is possible in the untreated individual. Moreover, the sequelae of prolonged hypoventilation and hypoxia include cor pulmonale from chronic hypoxic vasoconstriction and permanent cerebral dysfunction. In this regard, diaphragmatic pacing in properly selected patients is thought to retard the decline in overall function that would otherwise result from untreated hypoxia.

In a similar fashion, although no comparative trials have established the superiority of pacing over mechanical ventilation in patients with quadriplegia, some inferences may be drawn from accumulated data in the literature. It is our opinion that, in carefully selected patients, diaphragmatic pacing offers a number of advantages over positive-pressure ventilation. In properly selected quadriplegic patients, diaphragmatic pacing offers a much-needed sense of increased geographic independence. Paced patients attest to the increased ease with which they are able to travel, whether for work, study, or pleasure. In addition to increased freedom, paced patients have more natural phonation and speech. The advent of tracheal buttons has decreased the risk for tracheal complications associated with prolonged tracheal cannulation, such as secretion management, infections, tracheal stenosis, erosion, and fistulization.[5,8]

Patients who undergo successful diaphragmatic pacing have reduced health care costs, since many of them are able to reside at home or outside of an institutionalized setting. The duration of life is often quite limited in quadriplegic patients on long-term mechanical ventilation. The excellent longevity of the Yale patients followed on long-term pacing stands in marked contrast to the expected poor survival with conventional means. Above all, the technical components of diaphragmatic pacing systems need updating to mirror the tremendous advances in cardiac pacing. Fully implantable pacing devices that can respond to varying physiologic requirements are sorely needed.

References

1. Hufeland CW. Usum uis electriciae in asphyxia experimentis illustratum. Göttingen, Germany: Dissertatio Inauguralis Medica, 1783.
2. Ure A. An account of some experiments made on the body of a criminal immediately after execution, with physiological and practical observations. *J Sci Arts (Lond)* 1819;6:283.
3. Duchenne GBA. De l'ectrisation localisee et de son application a la pathologie et a le therapeutique par courant induits et par courants galvaniques interrompus et continues par le Dr. Duchenne. Paris: Bailliere, 1872.
4. Glenn WWL. The treatment of respiratory paralysis by diaphragm pacing. *Ann Thorac Surg* 1980;30:106.
5. Glenn WWL, Holcomb WG, McLaughlin AJ et al. Total ventilatory support in a quadriplegic patient with radiofrequency electrophrenic respiration. *N Engl J Med* 1972; 286:513.
6. Glenn WWL, Gee BL, Schachter EN. Diaphragm pacing: Application to a patient with chronic obstructive pulmonary disease. *J Thorac Cardiovasc Surg* 1978;75:273.
7. Shneerson, JM. *Disorders of Ventilation.* Oxford, UK: Blackwell Scientific, 1988.
8. Glenn WWL, Holcomb WG, Shaw RK, et al. Long-term ventilatory support by diaphragm pacing in quadriplegia. *Ann Surg* 1976;183:566.
9. Glenn WWL, Brouillette RT, Dentz B, et al. Fundamental considerations in pacing of the diaphragm for chronic ventilatory insufficiency: A multicenter study. *PACE* 1988;11:2121.

10. Mills GH, Kyroussis D, Hamnegard CH, et al. Unilateral magnetic stimulation of the phrenic nerve. *Thorax* 1995;50:1162.
11. Hogan JF, Koda H, Glenn WWL. Electrical techniques for stimulation of the phrenic nerve to pace the diaphragm: Inductive coupling and battery powered total implant in asynchronous and demand modes. *PACE* 1989;12:847.
12. Hogan JF, Holcomb WG, Glenn WWL. A programmable, totally implantable, battery powered diaphragm pacemaker: Design characteristics. In: Saha S, (ed). *Proceedings of the Fourth New England Bioengineering Conference.* Elmsford, NY: Pergamon, 1976:221.
13. Lanmuller H, Bijak M, Mayr W, et al. Useful applications and limits of battery powered implants in functional electrical stimulations. *Artif Organs* 21;210, 1997.
14. Glenn WWL, Phelps ML, Elefteriades JA, et al. Twenty years of experience in phrenic nerve stimulation to pace the diaphragm. *PACE* 1986;9:780.
15. DiMarco AF, Onders RP, Kowalski KE, et al. Phrenic nerve pacing in a tetraplegic patient via intramuscular diaphragm electrodes. *Am J Resp Crit Care Med* 2002; 166:1604.
16. Onders RP, DiMarco AF, Ignagni AR, et al. Mapping the phrenic nerve motor unit: The key to a successful laparoscopic diaphragm pacing system in the first human series. *Surgery* 2004;136(4):819.
17. Elefteriades JA, Hogan JF, Handler A, et al. Long-term follow-up of bilateral pacing of the diaphragm in quadriplegia. *N Engl J Med* 1992;326:1433.
18. Weese-Mayer DE, Silvestri JM, Kenny AS, et al. Diaphragm pacing with quadripolar phrenic nerve electrode: An international study. *PACE* 1996;19: 1311.
19. Hunt CE, Matalon SV, Thompson TR, et al. Central hypoventilation syndrome: Experience with bilateral phrenic nerve pacing in 3 neonates. *Am Rev Respir Dis* 1978;118:23.
20. Brouillette RT, Ilbawi MN, Klemka-Walden L, et al. Stimulus parameters for phrenic nerve pacing in infants and children. *Pediatr Pulmonol* 1988;4:33.

PART II

ADULT CARDIAC SURGERY

CHAPTER

19 CARDIOVASCULAR FUNCTION AND PHYSIOLOGY

Jeffrey M. Dodd-O

BASIC MYOCYTE PHYSIOLOGY

Myocyte depolarization

Cardiac myocytes possess the capacity to contract because they contain a series of protein filaments (myofibrils) oriented along the longitudinal axis of the cell (see below). For myocytes to shorten, these myofibrils must be stimulated to slide. The impetus for the stimulation originates on the myocyte's surface membrane (sarcolemma) and is transmitted to the intracellular myofibrils. Aspects of the composition of the sarcolemma allow it to assume this function. The intra- and extracellular fluid is predominantly water. The ionic components within the intra- and extracellular fluids differ because the cell's surface membrane serves to maintain some compounds intracellularly and exclude other compounds extracellularly. This segregating function is possible because water-insoluble components of the membrane prevent free passage of water-soluble components through the membrane. The initial creation of a concentration gradient between extra- and intracellular ions is achieved by energy-dependent ion pumps located within the membrane. These pumps can move ions across the membrane against a concentration gradient. Because of the uneven concentrations of charged ions in the intra- and extracellular fluids separated by the cell membrane, there is an electrical gradient across the membrane (i.e., a transmembrane potential).

KEY CONCEPTS

- Membrane potentials are created by energy-dependent ion pumps which segregate charged ions on either side of hydrophobic cell membrane.
- Cell depolarization possible because channels open within the hydrophobic membrane to allow charged ions, driven by concentration gradients, to cross the membrane.
- Trigger for the opening of transmembrane ion channel is typically a change in the membrane potential. Different channels are triggered to open at different membrane potentials.
- The sarcomere is the contractile element of the myocyte. Each sarcomere is composed of a series of parallel myofilaments. Coaxial movement of these myofilaments, some of which are tethered to the ends of the sarcomere, result in sarcomere shortening.
- The strength of contraction is influenced by resting length of the myocyte, sudden stretch of the myocyte, or rapidly repeated contraction of the myocyte. Speed of shortening is influenced by afterload.
- A ventricle exposed chronically to high afterload will adapt by concentric hypertrophy because this reduces wall stress according to the law of Laplace.
- Myocardium receiving insufficient energy supply will either die (infarction), become dysfunctional (ischemia), or reduce its energy needs (hibernate). Reperfused tissue is termed "stunned" if it does not contract up to its potential in spite of adequate energy supply.
- Diastole is more energy-demanding than systole, and diastolic dysfunction can be more difficult to treat than systolic dysfunction
- Dysfunctional endothelium leads to vascular occlusion by: (1) exposing underlying tissue factor to circulating factor VII, initiating thrombosis; (2) does not allow for the interaction of thrombin with thrombomodulin and the subsequent activation of protein C to its anticoagulant form; (3) does not produce nitric oxide, important to help decrease platelet activation, decrease vasospasm, and decrease vascular inflammation

Physiology of the myocyte cell membrane

The human body is composed predominantly of salts and water. This pool of salts and water is segregated into functional units (cells and their intracellular components) that locally alter the concentration of the salts they contain. Hydrophobic phospholipid membranes surrounding the cells (and intracellular compartments) prevent the exit/entrance of water-soluble salts and allow the cells to maintain this individualized environment.[1] Units within these phospholipid membranes allow continued adjustment of the ion content within the cell (or intracellular compartment). For example, an energy-dependent Na^+,K^+ pump extrudes Na^+ ions from the cell and takes K^+ ions into the cell at an exchange of three Na^+ ions extruded per two K^+ ions taken in. This allows cells to raise intracellular potassium concentrations and lower intracellular sodium. Another pump extrudes calcium in exchange for sodium, increasing intracellular calcium concentrations in relation to the extracellular fluid, although it allows Na^+ (extruded by the Na^+,K^+ pump) to reenter the cell. This pump is driven by the Na gradient created by the energy-dependent Na^+,K^+ pump. Similarly, intracellular compartments called the sarcoplasmic reticulum (SR) contain energy-dependent ion pumps in their surrounding membranes that allow them to collect the majority of the intracellular calcium. Other channels within the membrane act as passages that intermittently open to allow transit of a specific ion through the cell membrane. Regulation of pump activation and channel opening is vital for the proper functioning of the cell.

Moving ions against their concentration gradient to create a relative intracellular deficit or abundance requires energy. In the cell, this energy is supplied in the form of ATP. This segregation of ions, along with the imbalance of ionic charge that is associated, creates a potential (energy) gradient across the membrane, which drives the rapid flux of ions that occurs if and when a transmembrane ion channel is opened. In the cell, the trigger to opening the ion channels is often the potential or ionic concentration gradient of the surrounding milieu. Thus, transmembrane channels are frequently described as being either voltage-gated (opening probability is increased if the transmembrane potential of the surrounding membrane is within certain parameters) or ion-gated (opening probability is increased if there is a sudden change in the concentration of an ion in the surrounding fluid).

T Tubules and sarcoplasmic reticulum

The cell-surface change initiating myofibril movement is a flux of charged ions across some point of the sarcolemma.[1] This ion flux disrupts the balance of charged particles present in the baseline (resting) state, and a new transmembrane electrical gradient develops at that point on the sarcolemma. Ion channels traversing the adjacent sarcolemma, closed to the passage of ions under resting transmembrane potentials, become exposed to the new transmembrane potential of the adjacent sarcolemma. Exposure to this new transmembrane potential increases the open probability of these nearby channels. The passage of ions through these newly open channels changes the membrane potential surrounding the channel, exposing an additional section of the cell membrane to a different transmembrane potential. In this way, the new transmembrane potential propagates along the surface of the myocytes. Invaginations in the cell membrane, called T tubules, penetrate into the cell into close proximity to the myocyte contractile proteins. These T tubules act as extensions off of the surface membrane and allow changes in the cell surface to effect changes deep within the myocyte.

Physiology of the conduction system

Relative to the extracellular fluid, the intracellular fluid in the resting state has higher concentrations of sodium, lower concentrations of K^+ and of Ca^{2+}, and a relatively negative charge. When ion channels in the cell membrane are opened under these conditions, Na^+ and Ca^{2+} tend to enter the cell rapidly.[2] They are driven both by ion concentrations and electrical potential. By contrast, K^+ tends to leave the cell owing to its concentration gradient, although the electrical potential gradient reduces its speed of exit. When the cell is depolarized so that the transmembrane gradient is less negative intracellularly, the rate of K^+ exit is higher.

When the transmembrane electrical potential, usually −90 mV at rest, becomes less negative, sodium channels on the cell membrane are triggered to open (Fig. 19-1). Also triggered in these channels by cell membrane depolarization is the closing of the channel, although this process is (of course) delayed until after the channel has been opened. Other channels, like L-type calcium chan-

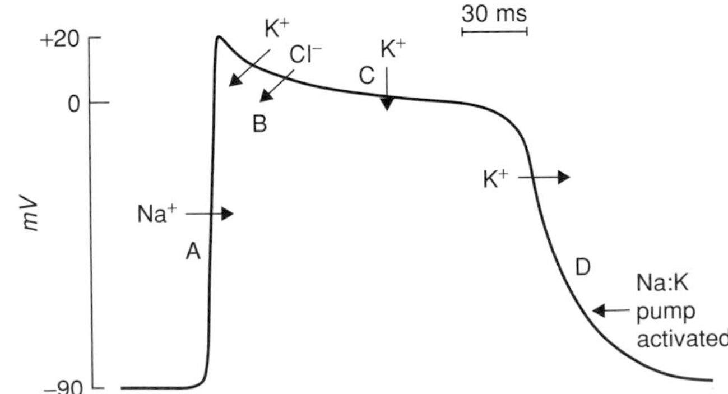

Figure 19-1 Correlation between the changes in ion conductance and the resultant changes in transmembrane potential during the various phases of the cardiac myocyte action potential. A. depolarization; B. rapid repolarization; C. plateau phase; D. late repolarization. (Modified from Rubart M, Zipes DP. Mechanisms of sudden cardiac death. *J Clin Invest* 2005;115(9):2305–2315. With permission.)

nels, also open when the cell membrane has begun to depolarize. The initiation of ion passage through calcium channels is delayed until after the Na^+ channels have begun to close. The opening of these Na^+ and Ca^{2+} channels results in the entrance of cations into the cell, decreasing the magnitude of the membrane potential. As the membrane potential reaches a nadir, K^+ channels are triggered to open. Their opening increases the rate of exit of K^+ from the intracellular space into which it had been concentrated. The loss of cations from the intracellular space helps return the transmembrane potential back to the resting state. This K^+ channel is inwardly rectified (i.e., turned off when cell is depolarized) and is the channel responsible for maintaining the resting membrane potential. This basic sequence is somewhat modified by channels for Cl^- and transiently open channels for K^+ (activated after depolarization to allow Cl^- entrance into cell and K^+ efflux from cell, beginning to reverse to return the transmembrane potential toward −90 mV).

Compared with the membrane on the surface of the cell, the membrane of T tubules has a relatively high concentration of L-type calcium channels. As stated earlier, these T tubules extend to close approximation with the myofibrils—the contractile apparatus of the myocyte. Also located intracellularly near the junction of the myofibrils and the T tubules are compartments known as SR. The membrane of the SR contains ion pumps that concentrate calcium within the SR. The membrane of the SR also contains channels that, when open, allow the sequestered calcium to exit the SR. The stimulus for opening of the calcium channels on the SR is a rise in calcium in the cytoplasm surrounding the SR. Thus, as membrane depolarization propagates from the cell surface down the invaginations known as the T tubules, it stimulates L-type calcium channels in the T tubules to open. This allows calcium to enter the cell at a site near the SR, raising cytosolic calcium concentrations near the SR. These high calcium concentrations near the SR stimulate calcium release from the SR, a phenomenon known as calcium-induced calcium release. The rise in calcium concentrations near the myofibrils results in reorientation of the troponin in the thin filaments, moving the tropomyosin (attached to the troponin) and making it sterically possible for the actin of the thin filament to bind to myosin. Contraction is terminated (and relaxation initiated) by the closing of calcium channels in the SR and the reuptake of calcium by the SR as a result of pumps activated on the SR. The drop in calcium concentrations surrounding the thin/ thick filaments results in the return of tropomyosin filaments to a position preventing the interaction of actin and myosin filaments.

Ion channel activity is somewhat complex. The impetus to open a channel may also initiate the process to close the channel after a set period of time. Furthermore, a channel which has opened and closed may need an additional stimulus to transform it back to a state where it can again be stimulated to be opened. Thus, channels can be described as being in the resting state (closed and capable of being opened), the open state, or the inactive state (closed and incapable of being opened until modified by an intermediary stimulus (Fig. 19-2).

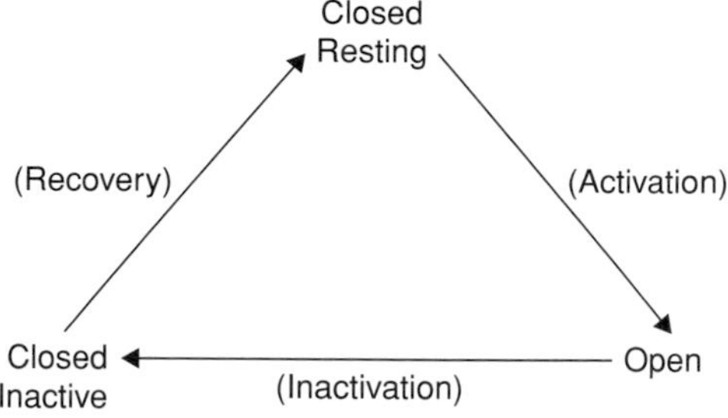

Figure 19-2 The three states of a voltage-gated ion channel. Two closed and one open state are shown, along with the transitions between these states that open the channel (activation), close the channel (inactivation), and end its refractoriness (recovery). [From Katz AM. Cardiac ion channels. *N Engl J Med* 328(17):1244-1251,1993. With permission.]

Furthermore, as ions pass rapidly through a channel, the electrical and ion gradient in the fluid surrounding the channel is rapidly changing. Some channels, described as rectified channels, alter the resistance imposed by the channel to ion flow through the channel as the surrounding electrical or ion potential is changing. In speaking of K^+ channels, an ion whose exit from the depolarized cell tends to restore the resting membrane potential (by increasing the relative concentration of negatively charged ions intracellularly), outward rectified channels increase the resistance to K^+ passage as the membrane potential returns to resting state. This type of channel tends to promote restoration of the repolarized state. By contrast, inward rectifiying K^+ channels are relatively more resistant to ion passage as the membrane is depolarized. This type of channel tends to promote the maintenance of the depolarized state.

The ion channel predominating in different cell sites of the heart (atria/ventricles vs. sinus node/AV node) differ.[3] This difference in predominating ion channel helps explain the special features of different sites of the heart. Fast-conducting sodium channels predominate in the atria and ventricles, allowing for rapid depolarization and expediting conduction. These channels are less prominent in the SA node and AV node, reducing rate of conduction through these sites.

Additional features of the SA and AV node are responsible for the automaticity (i.e., spontaneous depolarization) that is characteristic of these cells. The resting membrane potential of contracting atria and ventricular myocytes is maintained by an inward rectifying (i.e., shuts off when cell is depolarized) potassium channel that maintains resting membrane potential of around –90 mV. In the nodal tissues, additional channels (voltage-dependent slow Na channel that allows Na to slowly enter cell as depolarization reaches –70 to –90 mV and, possibly an outward rectifying K channel that reduces K flow as repolarization progresses) result in an unstable "resting" membrane potential. Thus, the resting membrane potential of nodal cells will spontaneously diminish from about −70 mV to about −50 mV, at which time voltage-dependent Ca^{2+} channels will open and allow complete depolarization.

Finally, nodal tissue (predominantly AV node) contains a K^+ channel that is central to pharmacologic interventions commonly used to treat dysrhythmias. This channel, activated by adenosine and by acetylcholine ($I_{Kach,Ado}$), allows K^+ to exit the cell upon stimulation by either adenosine or acetylcholine. The exit of K^+ makes the membrane potential more negative, hyperpolarizing the cell and making depolarization more difficult. Thus, acetylcholine reduces sinus node spontaneous depolarization and adenosine blocks transmission through the AV node (Fig. 19-3).

As suggested earlier, intracellular calcium concentrations regulate myocyte contraction by controlling the steric relationship between myosin and actin myofilaments through the interaction of calcium with troponin. Cell membrane depolarization stimulates the cascade responsible for changing intracellular calcium concentrations around the contractile myofibrils. Excitation-contraction coupling refers to the interdependence of cell-membrane depolarization (cellular excitation), and the cascade of events leading to cellular concentration changes locally within the cell.

Phase 1 depolarization, mediated by opening of voltage-gated fast Na channels, depolarizes the membrane to a point at which L-type Ca^{2+} channels can open (Fig. 19-4). The influx of calcium through these (dihydropyridine-sensitive) voltage-gated channels, especially through those located along the T tubules, increases intracellular calcium concentration in the vicinity of the SR. (The calcium channels on the SR are termed ryanodine-sensitive calcium channels because the compound ryanodine induces their opening). This triggers the opening of calcium channels in the SR membrane, releasing calcium stored in the SR. The result of calcium entrance into the cell via L-type calcium channel opening combined with release of calcium from SR stores is a dramatic increase in calcium concentration of the cytoplasm surrounding the contractile myofilaments. High concentrations of calcium allows binding of calcium to troponin C of the thin filament, modulating the troponin such that tropomyosin (attached to troponin) gets moved from its position of preventing interaction between actin (of the thin filament) and myosin. The strength of bond between actin and myosin is decreased by acidosis, high

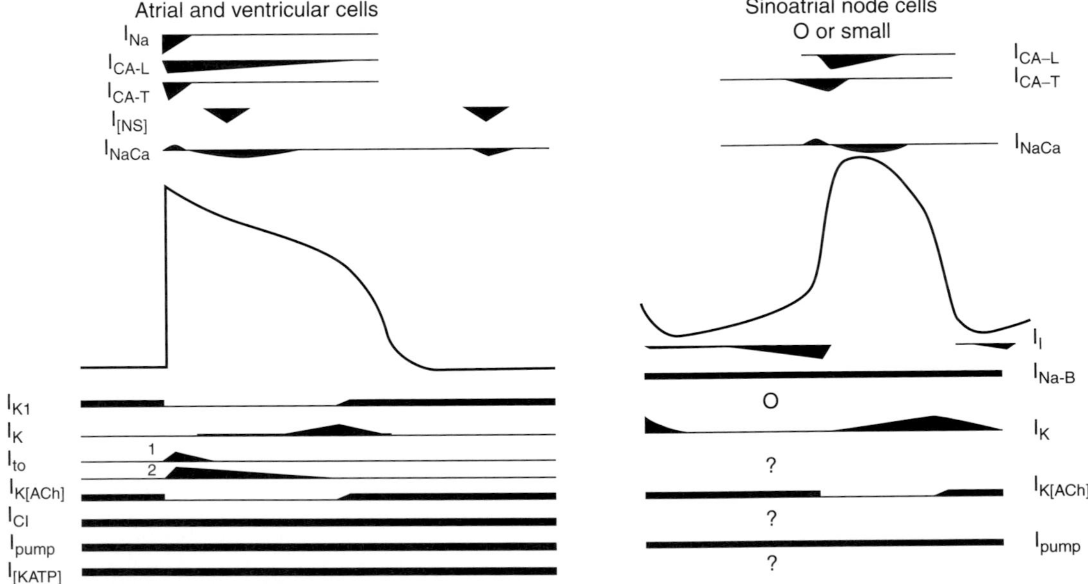

Figure 19-3 A comparison of the stylized action potential of atrial and ventricular cells (left) vs sinoatrial node cells (right) as well as the ionic currents whose contribution to each action potential is confirmed. Other ion channels may exist. Ion current bar deflections depict only the approximate time course (not the magnitude) of the current. Brackets around channel names indicate the current is active only under pathologic conditions. Question mark indicates the uncertain presence of this channel in the sinoatrial node. I_{NS} = Calcium gated channel, sodium inward current; I_{NaCa} = electrogenic Na^+-Ca2$^+$ exchange current; $I_{k(ACh)}$ = acetylcholine dependent potassium current I_{NS} = I_{Cl} = Chloride current; I_{pump} = electrogenic pump; I_f = sodium dependent inward current; $I_{Na\text{-}B}$ = inward background sodium current. (From Sicilian Gambit: a report of the Task Force of The Working Group on Arrythmia of the European Society of Cardiology. *Circulation.* 84:1831–1851, 1991 P1835, Figure 2)

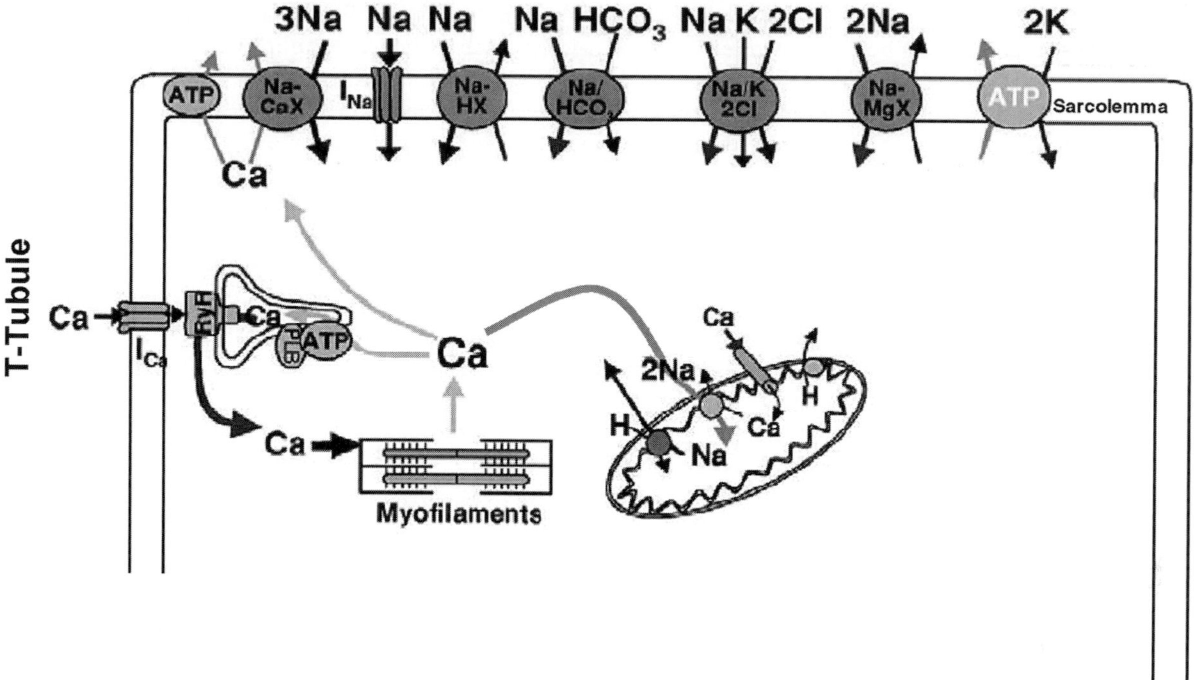

Figure 19-4 Calcium transport in ventricular myocyte. PLB = phospholambam, RyR = Ryanodine Receptor, X = Exchanger.

concentrations of Mg^{2+}, or high concentrations of phosphate. This bond is enhanced by caffeine and by beta-adrenergic stimulation. Beta-adrenergic stimulation increases actin-myosin bonding through a cascade that results in the activation of myosin binding protein C.

Regulation of myocyte function by the myocyte cell-surface receptor

Beta receptors

How can beta stimulation result in so many divergent effects (e.g., increased inotropy, increased lusitropy)? The beta receptor is a protein which is incorporated within the cell membrane, spans the entire depth of the membrane, and has components which extend into the cytoplasm as well as components exposed on the surface of the cell.[4,5] When an extracellular agonist stimulates the portion of the receptor exposed on the cell surface, a conformational change in the beta receptor allows the portion of the receptor protruding into the cytoplasm to bind to a G protein (i.e., it is a G protein–coupled receptor). G proteins have multiple components and stimulation of the G protein causes dissociation of the subunits so that each subunit is free to regulate its particular effector. One such effector is adenylate cyclase, which is activated to increase intracellular concentrations of cAMP and thereby activate protein kinase A (PKA). Activated PKA is then capable of phosphorylating multiple intermediaries of excitation-contraction. For example, it increases intracellular calcium concentrations by facilitating calcium entrance into the cell (via L-type calcium channels) as well as calcium release from compartments within the cell (i.e., the SR).

Beta-agonist stimulation also expedites relaxation. Relaxation results from a drop in cytosolic calcium concentrations, decreasing calcium binding to troponin C and allowing tropomyosin to return to a position that inhibits interaction between actin and myosin. Although some cytosolic calcium leaves the myocyte through the sodium-calcium exchanger on the cell surface, the predominant method of lowering cytosolic calcium levels is reuptake by the SR. The pump mediating calcium reuptake by the SR is dependent upon ATP and regulated by the phosphorlylation of phospholamban. Beta stimulation facilitates relaxation by two mechanisms. First, it results in phophorylation of troponin I by PKA, expediting dissociation of calcium from troponin C. Beta stimulation also results in phosphorylation of phospholamban, which speeds up calcium reuptake into the SR.

Muscarinic receptors

Muscarinic receptors sensitive to acetylcholine are also present on the myocardium. In particular, the heart contains the m2 subtype of muscarinic receptor.[6,7] Like beta receptors, muscarinic receptors appear to be incorporated within the cell membrane, span the entire depth of the membrane, contain components exposed to the extracellular fluid and components exposed to the intracellular fluid, and coupled to a G protein. The G protein to which the m2 receptor is coupled has inhibitory effects upon adenylate cyclase and is sensitive to pertussis toxin. In fact, the negative inotropic effects of m2 receptor stimulation appear to be indirect; i.e., they can be demonstrated only in the setting of baseline stimulation adenylate cyclase. It therefore appears that their negative inotropy results entirely from this inhibitory effect on adenylate cyclase.

In the atria and nodal myocytes, m2 receptors appear to have a direct effect (i.e., not dependent on baseline stimulation) on the inward rectifying potassium channel that maintains phase 4 (resting) membrane potential. By opening this channel though a direct action of the G protein upon the channel, m2 receptor stimulation hyperpolarizes the resting membrane to slow the automaticity rate of the cells.

Adenosine receptors

Another G-protein receptor found to by physiologically important in the heart is the adenosine receptor. There are three basic subtypes of adenosine receptors (A_1, A_2, A_3), with A_1 and A_1 subtypes inhibiting adenylate cyclase–inhibitory G proteins while A_2 receptors increase adenylate cyclase via stimulatory G proteins.[8] These receptors also regulate other pathways via G proteins. Thus, A_1 and A_1 subtypes mediate the catabolism of phospholipids while A_2 receptors regulate phosphoinositide metabolism.

Two clinical effects of exogenous adenosine can be traced back to distribution and effects of various adenosine receptors. A_1 receptors are located with high concentration in the nodal tissues. Stimulation of these receptors opens the inward rectifying potassium channel that maintains phase 4 (resting) membrane potential. Like the effects of m2 receptor stimulation, opening this channel through a direct action of the G protein on the channel, stimulation of the m2 receptor hyperpolarizes the resting membrane to slow the automaticity rate of the cells. In the coronary vasculature, A_2 receptors predominate. Their stimulation results in vasodilation, likely through G protein–mediated activation of intracellular adenylate cyclase.

Alpha-adrenergic receptors

There is growing evidence that alpha, adrenergic stimulation of myocytes results in a positive inotropic effect.[9] The mechanism and clinical importance of this is unclear. It may also be coupled to myocardial hypertrophy.

MYOCARDIAL CONTRACTILE FUNCTION

The sarcomere as a contractile element

Contractile apparatus

Like all muscle cells, cardiac myocytes have the capacity to contract and relax. This capacity is conveyed by a series of protein filaments (myofibrils) oriented along the longitudinal axis of the cell. The alignment of myofibrils is consistent and repetitive, resulting in a characteristic pattern visible by electron microscopy.[1,10] Using electron microscopy, early investigators identified within myocytes parallel bands that appeared to move toward each other as the myocyte shortened. These bands were defined as the ends of the contractile unit of the myocyte and given the name "sarcomeres." The integrated shortening of a series of sarcomeres results in myocyte contraction.

The sarcomere contains two types of coaxially aligned filaments that differ in their component protein (myosin vs. actin/tropomyosin/troponin) as well as in thickness (myosin myofibrils are thicker, actin/tropomyosin/troponin myofilaments are thinner). The myosin filaments composing the thick myofilament is a mixture of "heavy" and "light" chains. Specifically, each thick filament contains two heavy myosin chains and each heavy myosin chain is associated with two light myosin chains. Each thick filament is itself composed of an actin polymer as well as tropomyosin and troponin proteins bound to each other.

Thin and thick filaments are aligned as follows. Each thin filament is aligned end-to-end with another thin filament. Each pair of thin myofibrils is straddled by a single thick filament lying parallel to it. Within the myocyte, the contractile unit containing a pair of thin myofilaments and their associated thick myofilament is bound on the ends by a Z band. The Z band (for *Zuckung,* the German word for "contraction") is a dark band visible by electron microscopy and corresponding to the site to which the ends of a series of parallel units of myosin with their paired actin thin filaments are anchored. This is considered to define the ends of a sarcomere, the contractile unit of the myocyte. Under appropriate stimulation, the myofibrils of a thin-filament pair will move closer to each other through an interaction with the adjacent thick filament. Because each member of a thin-filament pair is anchored to Z bands, this coaxial movement draws the Z bands within the cell closer to one another and the cell shortens.

The thick myosin filament is attached to the Z band by a protein called titin or connectin. This protein contains a nonmalleable portion that anchors the filament to the Z band as well as a distensible portion that enfolds on itself if the sarcomere is not stretched. On stretching, the Z bands are pulled farther apart from one another and the enfolded portion of the titin protein is extended. When stretching is relieved, the elastic recoil of the titin molecule helps to actively restore the sarcomere to its resting length (Fig. 19-5).

The movement of thin filaments is an energy-requiring process regulated by local calcium concentrations within the cell. Two thin filaments move toward each other in the longitudinal plane by each "pulling" itself along a shared myosin filament. Under "resting" conditions, physical contact between actin and myosin filaments is prohibited by the tropomyosin component of the thin filament. Tropomyosin is a protein strand that can interdigitate between actin and myosin, preventing their physical contact. Tropomysin can be moved out of place by

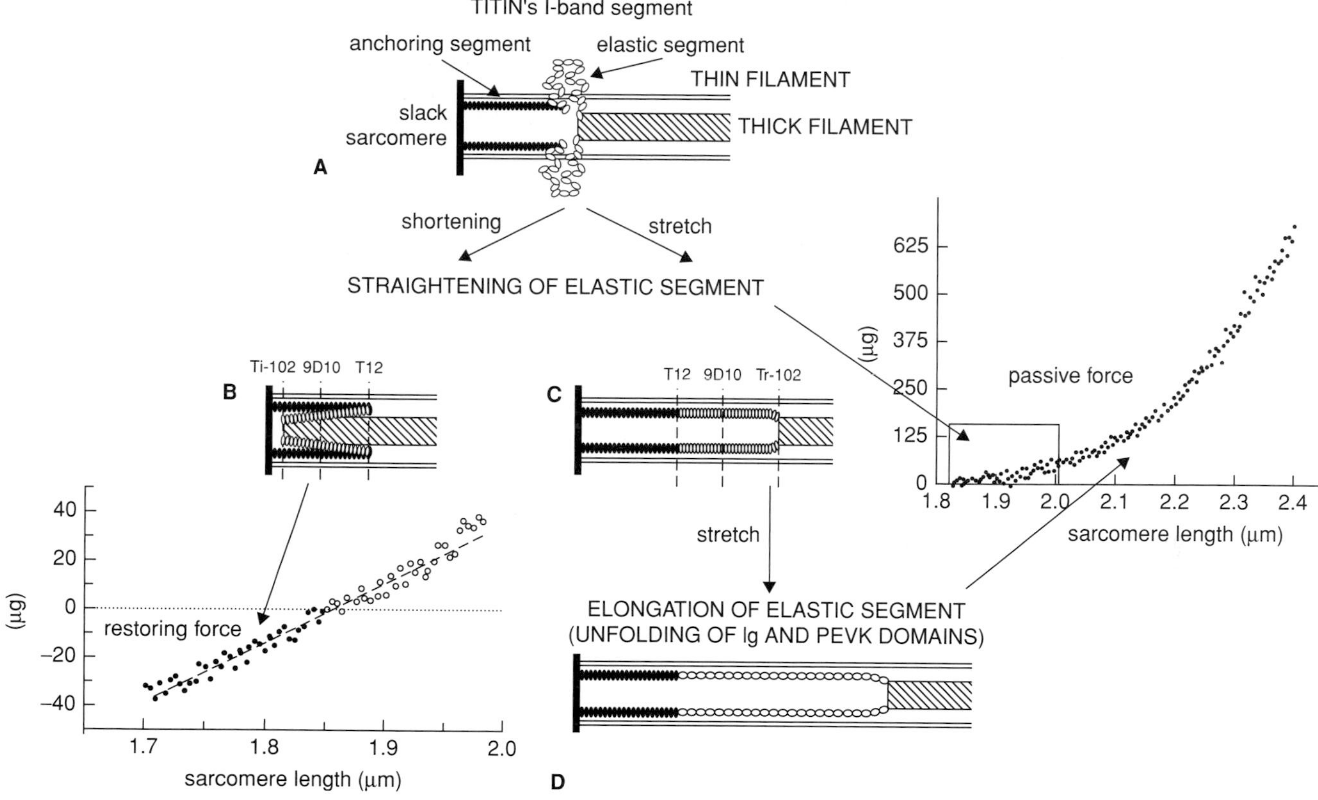

Figure 19-5 Working hypothesis force generation (passive and active) by titin. The black beads = nonelastic component of titin's I band; white beads = elastic (force-generating) component of titin. A, Slack sarcomere: the elastic component is highly folded. B, Shortened sarcomere: elastic component straightened to develop restoring forces. C, Stretched sarcomere: elastic component straightened to develop passive force. D, Further sarcomere stretch unfolds the molecular subdomains of titin's elastic component, generating high levels of passive force.

the actions of the third protein of the thin filament, the troponin protein. The presence of calcium sterically alters the troponin, causing it to reorient itself within the thin filament and thereby moving the tropomyosin strand to which it is attached. The movement of the tropomyosin strand removes the physical barrier preventing actin-myosin interaction and allows the thin filaments to move closer to each other along a shared myosin chain.

Myocardial contractile physiology

Contractility is the ability of a myocyte to shorten, measured at a given preload and a given afterload. Changing the preload will alter contractility due to the length-tension relationship. Changing the afterload will alter contractility because it mandates generation of a different wall stress to achieve shortening.

Length-tension (Frank-Starling) relationships

The force of contraction of a cardiac myocyte increases when the sarcomere is stretched (within the lengths of 1.7 to 2.4 μm).[11,12] Mechanistically, this increased contractility can be divided into two parts: (1) an immediate increase in force that is unaccompanied by a change in intracellular calcium concentration and (2) an additional increase in force of delayed (minutes) onset which is associated with an increase in intracellular calcium. The increase in intracellular calcium causing the second phase is probably mediated by changes in the cell membrane. The first phase, which apparently involves a change in myofilament sensitivity to calcium, is the Frank-Starling phenomenon (named for Otto Frank and Ernest Starling, who initiated the concept based upon experimental findings they made at the beginning of the twentieth century). Although it was initially hypothesized that sarcomere stretching improved myosin-actin, the increase in force of contraction is observed even when the sarcomere is stretched to distances that would begin to reduce the potential for actin and myosin cross-bridge formation. An alternative explanation is that stretching the myocyte narrows the sarcomere, reducing the spacing between myosin and actin filaments. This facilitates myosin-actin interaction. Studies in which the interfilament distance is reduced by cellular dehydration result in an increased calcium sensitivity of contractile strength, as is seen by myocyte stretch.[12] A stretch-induced change in myofilament sensitivity to calcium by a yet unexplained mechanism remains a third possible explanation.

Force-velocity relationships

To measure contractile force free of compounding influences from preload, afterload, or heart rate, the concept of measuring the velocity of shortening in a myocyte with no afterload has been developed.[13,14] In such a scenario, the maximal velocity of shortening (V_{max}) would be a measure of the inotropy of a myocyte. Practically speaking, it is difficult to completely remove external resistance from a contracting myocyte. The value of V_{max} must therefore be extrapolated from the maximal velocities observed when a myocyte is made to contract against a series of different afterloads. At one extreme of this series would be the minimal afterload at which the myocyte is no longer able to shorten at all ($V_{max} = 0$). This relationship is hyperbolic rather than linear. Although the reason for this hyperbolic relationship remains unclear, it is felt to be due in part to shortening inactivation and in part to elastic forces that passively resist stretch (at long sarcomere length) or shortening (at short sarcomere length). Such passive elastic forces could be contributed by titin (Fig. 19-6).

"Anrep effect"

As stated above, there is a two-phase response of myocytes to an abrupt stretch.[15] The first phase is an increase in contractility, which occurs without a change in cytosolic calcium. This is known as the Frank-Starling effect. There is a delayed second phase, which is associated with an increase in cytosolic calcium. The change in intracellular calcium seems to be independent of the SR, although the exact mechanism behind the rise remains obscure.

"Treppe effect"

Increasing heart rate increases the strength of contraction. This phenomenon, termed the Treppe effect (*Treppe*, German for "step") is associated with an increase in intracellular calcium concentrations.[16] This is suggested to be due to an inability of the SR and myocyte calcium extruding pumps to completely return cytosolic calcium to baseline levels between sequential cell depolarizations. The result is a buildup of calcium within the cell.

CARDIAC PUMP FUNCTION

Myocyte cytoskeleton

Synchronized contraction of cardiac myocytes is necessary for most efficient pumping function of the heart.[10] This requires tight adhesion of cells along the axis of their shortening as well as organized propagation of the

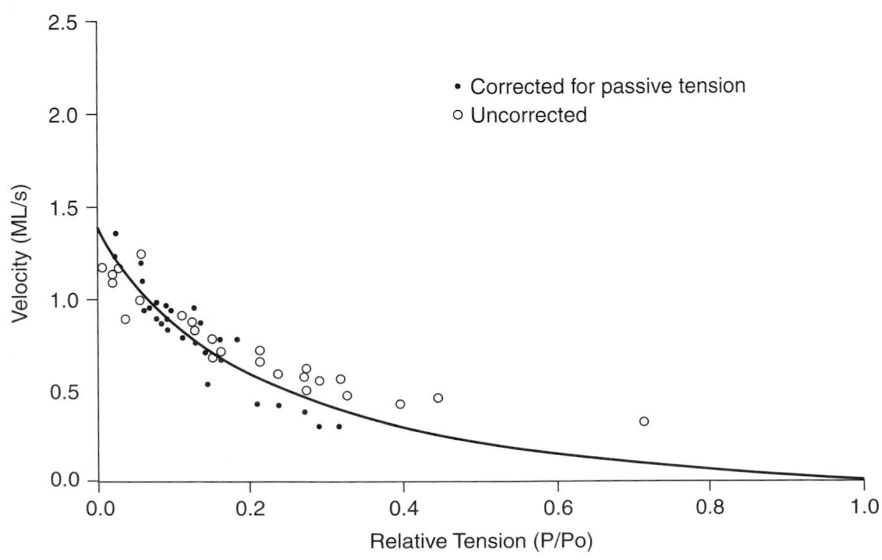

Figure 19-6 The influence of resting tension on the shortening velocity of isolated myocytes. The general relationship of faster shortening velocity observed when resting external tension is decreased can be seen whether passive (intra-myocyte) tension is present (open circles) or mathematically excluded from the calculations (closed circles). Figure 7 from Sweitzer NK and Moss RL. Determinants of loaded shortening velocity in single cardiac myocytes permeabilized with alpha-hemolysin. *Circ Res.* 73:1150-1162, 1993

contractile stimulus. To accomplish this, the basic structure of the myocyte is one of contractile myofibrils attached, via fascia adherens, to cadherin anchors at the ends of the myocyte. The myofibrils are held in alignment by an intracellular scaffold-like network consisting of the protein desmin. These desmin "scaffolds," traversing the myocyte at intervals along its longitudinal axis, are anchored to the lateral sarcolemmal wall by plaques called costameres. These plaques, rich in the protein vinculin, act both to maintain the spatial interval between the desmin scaffolds as well as to mechanically link the cells laterally to the sarcolemmal membrane and extracellular matrix. The desmins are anchored to the cadherins at the longitudinal end of the myocyte by desmosomes.

The site of end-to-end adherence between two myocytes is called the intercalated disk. This site functions to physically anchor two myocytes as well as allow for intercellular continuity of action potential propagation and chemical signaling between these myocytes. The physical anchor is maintained by junctions between cadherins of adjacent cells. The communication between myocytes connected in the longitudinal axis is made possible by channels composed of two connexons. Each channel is comprised of two connexons aligned coaxially, and each connexon is comprised of six connexin molecules arranged in a circle. There are different types of connexin and different densities of connexon channels among different myocytes.

The characteristics of these intercalated disks are quite important in determining the ease of communication between myocytes in the longitudinal plane. Consistent with this, the composition and number of connexons varies with the electrophysiologic requirements of the myocytes involved. Myocytes of the atria and ventricles, serving principally a contractile function, contain a fair abundance of connexon channels, with connexin 43 being the most abundant connexin present. In the sinus node and atrioventricular node, there are few connexon channels joining cells longitudinally. In the sinus node, this allows the natural depolarization of the cells to occur without inhibition by the hyperpolarizing effects of the surrounding contractile myocytes. In the atrioventricular node, the girth of connexon channels slows communication between cells, slowing transmission of the electrical impulse. By contrast, the cells of the Purkinje system contain high numbers of large connexon channels composed of the high-conductance connexin 40. This allows rapid transmission of electrical impulses throughout the Purkinje system.

Cardiac mechanics

Frank-Starling model

The ability of the heart to contract is influenced by the resting volume within the heart in much the same way as the contractility of its component sarcomeres (and myocytes) is influenced by the resting length to which they are stretched. This has led physiologists to view the heart as a series of sarcomeres demonstrating length-tension relationships—the model conceptualized by Frank and Starling. In this regard, the capacity of the heart to eject blood against a given resistance increases as the volume within the heart immediately prior to initiating systole (i.e., the end-diastolic volume) increases. This relationship, and its analogy to the length-tension relationship of individual sarcomeres, is demonstrated in Fig. 19-7A and B. Because the volume within equally compliant hearts is directly proportional to the pressure within the heart, this Frank-Starling model can also be displayed as an effect of pulmonary capillary wedge pressure on the stroke volume or ejection fraction of the ventricle.

Preload and diastolic compliance

Filling of the ventricular chamber with blood distends the ventricle, stretching the individual sarcomeres of the component myocytes. The magnitude of force that must be overcome to stretch a sarcomere to a given length varies with the recoiling forces of the sarcomere. Analogously, the magnitude of the three-dimensional force (i.e., pressure) needed to distend the ventricular chamber to a given volume varies with the compliance of the chamber. Distending two ventricles with the same volume of blood will result in a higher intraventricular pressure within the less compliant ventricle. Furthermore, the compliance of a chamber tends to decrease as the chamber is filled. Thus, adding 20 mL to a nearly empty ventricle increases the intraventricular pressure much less than does adding 20 mL to the same ventricle already containing 200 mL of blood.

Afterload

Under normal circumstances, the pressure preventing a ventricular chamber from contracting (i.e., afterload) is the pressure required to sufficiently distend an arterial bed to accept the blood ejected by the contracting ventricle. Thus, the afterload to the left ventricle (LV) is the pressure within the systemic arterial system. As with all elastic chambers, the compliance of the arterial bed decreases as it fills with blood. Thus, the afterload of the LV increases as the ventricle empties and ejects blood into the aorta. At some point, the ventricle stops ejecting because the pressures required to further distend the systemic arterial system exceed those that the ventricle is capable of generating. This point marks the end of physiologic ventricular systole.

The cardiac cycle

Pressure-volume loops The above discussion emphasizes three points: (1) the extent to which ventricular contractility is facilitated by optimizing sarcomere length at any point in its pressure-generating cycle is reflected by the intraventricular volume at any point during contraction; (2) the compliance of the LV is reflected by the pressure generated within the LV for any increase in LV volume

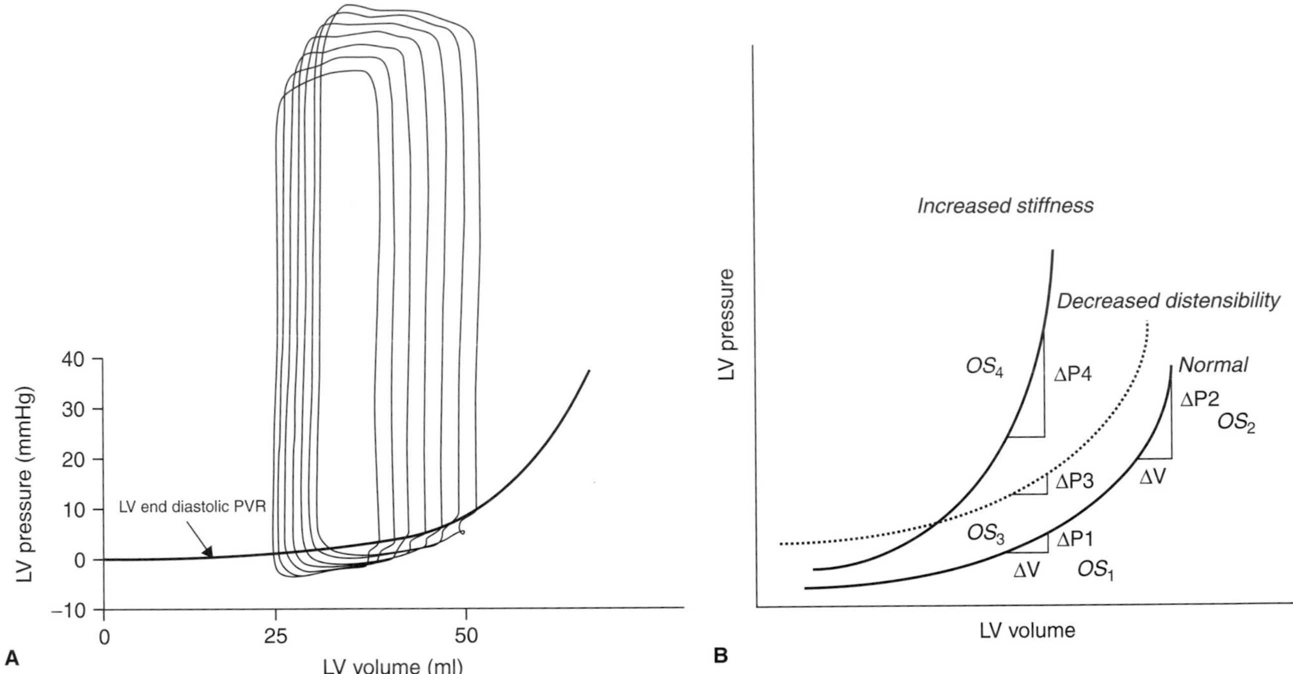

Figure 19-7 A: Determining left ventricular compliance by changing left ventricular volume to define end-diastolic pressure-volume relationship. The curvilinear nature of ED-PVR suggests that normal LV becomes more resistant to filling as end diastolic volume increases B: Illustration of the effect of different left ventricular operant stiffness (OS) conditions on end-diastolic pressure-volume relationship increasing slope of ED-PVR suggests decreasing compliance of myocardium/intercellular components decreasing slope of ED-PVR = lusitropy parallel shift up of ED-PVR (with same slope) suggests extramyocardial forces (RV loading/interventricular forces; pericardial constraint)

during relaxation; and (3) the capacity of the LV to eject blood depends on its ability to generate enough pressure to overcome afterload. This illustrates the utility of evaluating ventricular performance in terms of the relationship between the pressure and volume within the ventricle at any point in time.

Active contraction of the ventricle is indicated by the bottom right-hand corner of the pressure-volume square. At this point, intraventricular volume stops increasing (marking the end of diastole) and intraventricular pressure begins to rise rapidly. At the top right-hand corner of this relationship, the aortic valve opens. Thus, by generating a constant pressure, the ventricle is able to continually eject blood into the aorta. The volume within the ventricle thereby decreases, myocytes subsequently contract, and the sarcomere shortens from its ideal length for force generation. The myocyte shortens until sarcomere length has been reduced so much that it is no longer able to generate the force needed to further shorten. This point, indicated by the top left-hand corner of the pressure-volume loop, is termed the end-systolic pressure-volume point and represents the dependence of ventricular shortening on the volume of the LV and its capacity to generate pressure. From this point, the ventricle ceases generating force and the intraventricular pressure decreases as is represented by the vertical line marking the left side of the pressure-volume loop. Finally, the mitral valve opens and blood starts filling the ventricle. Although the ventricle has not yet begun to contract, the pressure within it slowly increases as blood enters across the mitral valve prior to initiation of myocyte shortening (Fig. 19-8).

Contractility As indicated above, the end-systolic pressure-volume point on the pressure-volume loop indicates the limit to the pressure-generating capacity of the ventricle at a given preload. By changing the afterload experimentally, a series of pressure-volume loops can be generated such that the minimal preload required to generate any given pressure can be determined. The straight line connecting the end-systolic pressure-volume points of this series of loops is termed the end-systolic pressure-volume relationship (ESPVR). This relationship is an indication of the strength of contraction of the ventricle. A more vertical line or one shifted more to the left indicates greater contractility. A more horizontal line or one shifted more to the right indicates less contractility (Fig. 19-9).

Compliance Similar to its usefulness in evaluating LV contractility, the pressure-volume loop can be used to monitor the diastolic function of the heart. The bottom-right corner of the pressure-volume loop marks the point at which diastole ends and systole begins for the ventricle.

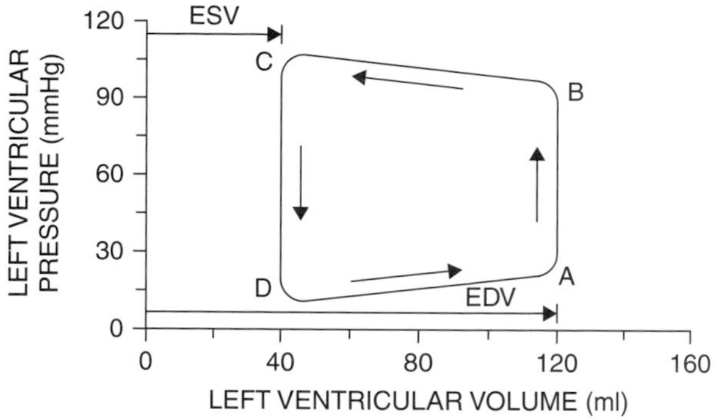

Figure 19-8 Schematic depiction of left ventricular pressure-volume relationship. A = end diastole; *upward arrow* = isovolumetric contraction; B = Aortic valve open; *leftward arrow* = ventricular ejection; C = aortic valve closure; *downward arrow* = isovolumetric relaxation; D = mitral valve opening; *rightward arrow* = diastolic ventricular filling

This point, the end-diastolic pressure-volume point, indicates the pressure required to fill the noncontracting ventricle with a given volume of blood. A series of pressure-volume loops can experimentally be created to evaluate the pressure generated within the noncontracting heart as it is filled with greater or lesser volumes of blood. The line connecting the end-diastolic pressure-volume points of this series of loops is termed the end diastolic pressure-volume relationship (EDPVR). Unlike the ESPVR, the EDPVR tends to be curvilinear because the compliance of elastic containers tends to decrease as the container is filled. Nevertheless, an EDPVR line that is more vertical or raised higher along the vertical axis suggests decreased compliance of the ventricle. An EDPVR line that is more horizontal or lowered along the vertical axis suggests an increased compliance of the ventricle (Fig. 19-7A).

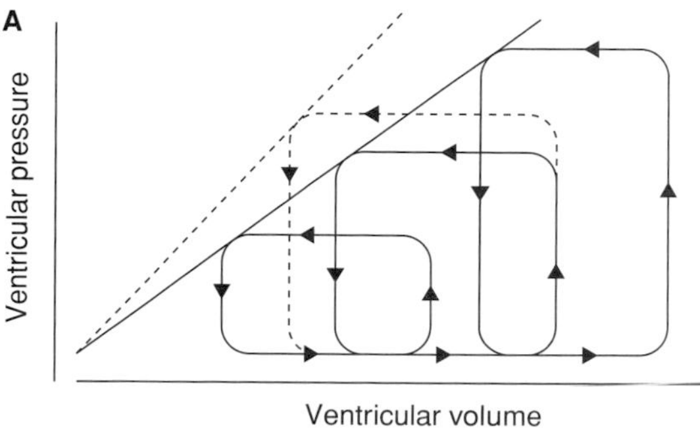

Figure 19-9 The Frank-Starling law of the heart–End-systolic pressure is determined by end-systolic volume and is independent of end-diastolic volume. The end-systolic pressure-volume relationship is altered by the ventricular contractile state. As indicated by dashed line, increased inotropy increases the ejection volume and end systolic pressure at any given end-diastolic ventricular volume.

Myocardial wall stress

A circular object is envisioned as a series of 360 straight lines each offset from one another by 1 degree and each tangential to the radius of the circle. The stress on the wall of a distended, elastic circle can then be viewed as the force distending each of these tangential lines. In the case of the heart, the stress on the wall of the ventricle can be thought of as the force stretching each of the mocytes of the wall. The interrelationship of the factors composing this force is a physical principle explained by the law of Laplace. This law states that the tension in the wall is related to the pressure gradient across the wall (P), the radius of the ventricle (R), and the wall thickness (th) as follows:

$$T = [(P)(R)] / [(2)(th)]$$

Thus distending the ventricle (increasing the radius R) increases the stress on the ventricular myocytes. By contrast, hypertrophy of the ventricle (increasing wall thickness th) decreases tension on the wall. This explains why ventricular hypertrophy is a natural adaptation of the LV to hypertension.

Cardiac energetics

Molecules consist of positively charged protons and negatively charged electrons in close proximity. The close proximity of the positively and negatively charged particles is maintained by electromagnetic force or "bonds." According to the first law of thermodynamics, the energy of these bonds must be converted to another form if the bond is broken. By breaking these bonds under controlled conditions, living organisms can harness the energy of the bonds and use if for doing work (moving objects over distance).

The energy form most efficiently utilized by cells of living organisms is that contained in the bonds joining phosphate residues to certain organic compounds in the form of adenosine triphosphate (ATP), adenosine diphosphate (ADP), or creatine phosphate (CP). The energy ingested by organisms is often in the form of fatty acids, proteins, and carbohydrates (having few ATP molecules). To convert the energy from the nonphosphate bonds ingested by organisms to a form that can be utilized by cells of living organisms (the phosphate bonds of ATP), a cascade of enzyme-mediated reactions is utilized. This cascade is driven by the energy released from the transfer of electrons when reduced (containing electrons that can be donated) forms of the intermediaries nicotinamide adenine dinucleotide (NADH) and flavin adenine dinucleotide (FADH) are oxidized (give up the electrons they can donate). The NADH and FADH donate these electrons to oxygen, forming water and releasing energy.[17,18]

The ingested form of energy (glucose, amino acids, fatty acid) is converted to a form that can be utilized by the cell (ATP) through a series of reactions involving conversion of glucose, amino acids, and fatty acids to acetyl CoA (glycolysis converts glucose to acetyl CoA via pyruvate as an intermediary; diverse processes convert amino acids to acetyl CoA; beta oxidation converts fatty acid to acetyl CoA). The Kreb cycle allows acetyl CoA to donate the electron-containing hydrogen ions needed to reduce FAD to $FADH_2$ and reduce NAD to NADH + H^+. The subsequent enzyme-mediated transfer of electrons from $FADH_2$ and NADH + H^+ to oxygen initially creates initially creates a high concentration of electrons within the intermembrane space of the mitochondria. This gradient then drives the formation of ATP from ADP and inorganic phosphate.

Under normal circumstances, 60 to 80 percent of the ATP utilized by the heart is generated from fatty acids; the remainder is generated predominantly from glucose. Paradoxically, the ATP production from fatty acids is less sensitive to ischemia than is the production from glucose. Ischemia therefore results in a reduction of the conversion of pyruvate to acetyl CoA, thereby increasing the conversion of pyruvate to lactate by an alternative pathway. The increased lactate production results in cellular acidosis. The lack of oxygen available to accept hydrogen ions liberated by the Kreb cycle increases intracellular $[H^+]$, further exacerbating intracellular acidosis. Finally, the lack of oxygen reduces the cellular capacity to bind phosphate to ADP. Phosphate residues are sequentially removed from ADP, degrading it first to adenosine monophosphate (AMP) and then to adenosine. The adenosine exits the myocyte to stimulate adenosine receptors, causing pain (angina).

As an alternative to oxidative phosphorylation, the body can also restore ATP levels by transferring a phosphate moiety from phosphocreatine (PC) to ADP. This phosphate transfer is utilized by the heart, skeletal muscle, and brain [the three organs containing the enzyme creatinine phosphokinase (CPK) under conditions of inadequate perfusion]. The phosphocreatine is formed by the transfer of phosphate from ATP to creatine, a transfer occurring most readily under conditions of adequate tissue perfusion.

CORONARY BLOOD FLOW

Normal coronary blood flow

Coronary blood flow supplies 60 to 90 mL/min of blood per 100 g of resting myocardium. The energy driving this perfusion is the pressure gradient between the proximal aorta (the origin of the coronary arteries) and the intraventricular pressure.[19] The influence of the intraventricular pressure derives from the fact that the same wall stresses responsible for generating intraventricular pressure also act to compress the coronary vessels traveling through the myocardial wall. Because the gradient between intraaortic pressure and intraventricular pressure is greatest when the ventricle is not contracting, the majority of coronary blood flow occurs during ventricular diastole. Coronary blood flow is both autoregulated and influenced by changing energy demands of the myocardial tissue. The factors affecting flow during periods of increased metabolic demand likely include neurohumoral factors as well as the factors responsible for autoregulation.

Autoregulatory mechanisms of coronary blood flow

Coronary blood flow is autoregulated.[19] That is, factors intrinsic to the heart and its vasculature assure that flow to the heart is kept constant in spite of changes in perfusion pressure of the heart. It is felt that the majority of the vascular resistance to coronary blood flow is supplied by vessels smaller than 100 to 150 μm in diameter and that these vessels represent the site of vascular autoregulation. Although the exact mechanisms responsible for this autoregulation remain a mystery, it is felt that a mixture of metabolic products, myogenic factors, and extrinsic compression from surrounding tissue play a role.

Metabolic products felt to be candidates for regulating coronary control include adenosine, prostaglandin, oxygen carbon monoxide, carbon dioxide, and potassium concentrations in the tissue. Adenosine is an obvious candidate because insufficient oxygen delivery raises tissue adenosine levels as inorganic phosphate moieties are sequentially removed from ATP in an attempt to harvest the energy of their bonds during hypoxia. However, removal of adenosine from interstitial spaces does not prevent coronary autoregulation, leaving other candidates as contributors. Prostaglandins can also cause dilation through stimulation of G protein–coupled receptors. This influence may be more pronounced in scenarios when nitric oxide is less abundant, as in severe atherosclerotic disease. Partial pressure of oxygen in the circulating blood or surrounding tissue may play a direct role by stimulating the opening of vascular smooth muscle cell K channels, which are coupled to the hypoxia-sensitive cytochrome b_{558}. Similarly, dropping levels of ATP can stimulate the opening of ATP-sensitive K channels in smooth muscle cells, causing vascular dilation. Nitric oxide is known to dilate coronary vasculature through a mechanism involving the activation of soluble guanylate cyclase. The release of nitric oxide is stimulated by hypoxia. Carbon monoxide can also activate soluble guanylate cyclase, making carbon monoxide (produced from the breakdown of heme to biliverdin) a possible mediator. Similarly, carbon dioxide has been shown to cause coronary dilation, possibly through a mechanism involving nitric oxide and/or cyclic guanosine monophosphate (GMP).

Myogenic contributions to autoregulation involve the ability of smooth muscle cells to "sense" flow and alter tone to maintain flow constant. Mechanisms by which smooth muscle cells accomplish this are both unclear and difficult to evaluate in vitro. Still, it is apparent that the majority of this response is contributed by vessels between 30 and 70 μm in diameter. The cascade probably involves the sensing of altered intraluminal pressure or shear stress, the activation of nonspecific ion channels in the smooth muscle cell, and the phosphorylation of myosin light chains in the smooth muscle cell by myosin light chain kinase.

External compression of the coronary microvasculature by contraction of the surrounding tissue can also act as a feedback control of coronary blood flow. As coronary blood flow becomes inadequate, the force of myocyte contraction decreases due to limited energy supplies. This decreases the magnitude of the external forces acting to compress small coronary microvasculature, facilitating coronary blood flow.

Physiologic consequences of coronary insufficiency

Myocardial ischemia

Myocardial ischemia is the condition whereby the myocardial blood flow and/or oxygen supply is insufficient to satisfy the demands of the myocardial tissue. This can reflect either an inappropriate limitation to blood flow (i.e., low-flow ischemia), an inappropriate excess in myocardial demand (i.e., high-flow ischemia), or low blood oxygen content such that oxygen delivery is insufficient in spite of appropriate blood supply and tissue demand (i.e., hypoxia). Myocytes respond by shifting their energy metabolism from aerobic (mitochondrial) to anaerobic (glycolytic) pathways. Alternative sources of stored energy (other than ATP) are utilized, such as creatine phosphate. These stores, however, are quite limited. As a result, metabolites of the complete breakdown of ATP (such as adenosine), metabolites of glycolysis (such as lactate), and a host of other substances (such as bradykinin and angiotensin) are released into the interstitial fluid.

When myocardial energy demands exceed the supply, energy reserves begin to decrease. This can result in dysfunction of any of the energy-dependent activities commonly attributed to the myocyte. Thus diastolic function, systolic function, automaticity, and/or intercellular communication can each be impaired. Diastolic dysfunction impairs relaxation, making it more difficult to fill the ventricle with blood. Diastole, driven by ATP-dependent calcium uptake by the SR, is more sensitive to limited energy supplies than is systole. Still, insufficient energy impairs force generation by the sarcomeres, limiting ventricular contraction. The lack of ventricular filling resulting from diastolic dysfunction hinders compensation by the Frank-Starling mechanism. With more dramatic imbalances between myocardial oxygen supply and demand, all contractile capacity of the ventricle is lost. Whether this loss of contractile function is temporary or permanent depends in part upon the severity of the energy supply-demand mismatch as well as the duration of its existence. Finally, insufficient energy impairs maintenance of membrane potentials by the nodal cells. This compromises the normal development of automaticity by SA node cells as well as conduction through AV node and Purkinje cells.

Myocardial infarction

An insufficient myocardial oxygen supply, if maintained too long, results in the utilization of all energy reserves by the myocardium. This leads to irreversible myocyte damage and begins to be seen after 20 min to 2 h of ischemia. With no energy, even the basic requirements for cell survival (i.e., exclusive of contractile function) cannot be maintained. Transmembrane ion concentrations are lost, and osmotic forces cause cell expansion to the point of membrane disruption as well as lysis of intracellular organelles. The tight junctions of intercalated disks between cells are disrupted, and cell-to-cell communication is lost. Recovery cannot occur following such catastrophic changes.

"Stunned" myocardium

Reperfusion of ischemic myocardium does not always result in the return of normal myocyte function.[20,21] There is often a persistent dysfunction of reperfused tissue in spite of blood and energy delivery capable of supporting much greater energy expenditure by the myocytes. The dysfunction that persists under these conditions is termed "stunning," an important characteristic of which is that it persists in the setting of a relative abundance of energy delivery. Other characteristics include the retained capacity of stunned myocardium to increase the force of contraction on exposure to inotropes as well as the lack of influence of beta agonists or beta blockers on the rate of recovery of stunned myocardium. The duration of stunning depends on factors such as the severity and duration of ischemia as well as the adequacy and immediacy of return of normal blood flow.

The cascade responsible for stunning is incompletely understood. Still, it is felt to involve oxygen-derived free radicals released during the early moments of reperfusion. Furthermore, it can be attenuated by utilizing iron chelators such as deferoxamine. This suggests that hydroxyl radicals, generated from superoxide by an iron-catalyzed reaction, mediate at least part of the reaction. There is speculation that nitric oxide released during reperfusion may contribute through the formation of peroxynitrite after binding with the superoxide radicals. Unfortunately, free-radical scavengers have thus far been only inconsistently beneficial in preventing myocardial stunning. In any case, altered availability of calcium or sensitivity of myocyte myofibrils to calcium are chief suspects as to the mechanism by which contractile function is impaired.

"Hibernating" myocardium

Myocardial hibernation is another state of reversible myocyte dysfunction related to an insufficient blood supply.[22] In contrast to myocardial stunning, which occurs following reperfusion, myocardial hibernation occurs while impaired blood delivery is ongoing. Thus, it is felt to be a way by which the myocyte preserves itself through decreasing energy expenditures to meet the energy supply available. The mechanism of myocardial hibernation is also unclear. Light-microscopically, there is a decrease in contractile elements, an increase in glycogen accumulation, and an alteration in the morphology of both the mitochondria and the T tubules. These changes are reversible, and contractile function is restored with the return of a normal blood supply.

Coronary endothelial function

Rather than serving as a passive lining between the blood and vascular smooth muscle, coronary endothelial cells play an active role in preventing the development of myocardial ischemia.[23–25] Thus the endothelium promotes anticoagulation, fibrinolysis, and vasodilation. It inhibits inflammation, platelet aggregation, leukocyte adhesion, and smooth muscle cell proliferation. It also provides antioxidant effects. The healthy endothelium accomplishes these roles through the release of a series of mediators. These include the antithrombotics (i.e., fibrin deposition inhibitors); antithrombin; protein C, protein S, thrombomodulin, and tissue factor pathway inhibitor; and the fibrinolytic tissue plaminogen activator. In addition, nitric oxide produced by healthy endothelium provides a wide range of anti-ischemic actions from vasodilation, to antithrombosis, to antiproliferation.

Antithrombin is a serine protease inhibitor which neutralizes thrombin and inhibits activated factor Xa and factor IXa. This three-pronged approach to the inactivation of thrombin helps ensure the inability of thrombin to convert fibrinogen to a fibrin clot. The activity of antithrombin is increased several thousandfold by the presence of heparin, another endothelial product. This suggests that most of the effects of antithrombin likely occur on vascular surfaces. The protein C–protein S-thrombomodulin system works to destroy activated coagulation factors Va and VIIIa. Thus thrombin binds to thrombomodulin, which both removes the thrombin and allows the thrombomodulin to activate protein C. The protein C destroys coagulation factors Va and VIIIa in a reaction that is accelerated by the vitamin K–dependent glycoprotein protein S. Tissue plasminogen activator, a serine protease released by the endothelium, is responsible for the conversion of inactive plasminogen to plasmin, which mediates fibrinolysis (Fig. 19-10).

The vasodilatory effects of nitric oxide result from its stimulation of soluble guanylate cyclase, leading to a decrease in intracellular calcium. Nitric oxide's anti-inflammatory effect results principally from its ability to inhibit nuclear factor K-B, a transcription factor important in the regulation of many inflammatory proteins. It inhibits platelet aggregation by decreasing intraplatelet concentrations of calcium through a cascade similar to that by which nitric oxide causes vasodilation. It reduces leukocyte adhesion by decreasing the expression of vascular cell adhesion molecule via inhibition of nuclear factor K-B. Nitric oxide's capacity to inhibit smooth muscle cell proliferation is poorly understood but may involve its activation of PKA. The effects of nitric oxide on free radical balance is complex, although it is a potent inhibitor of

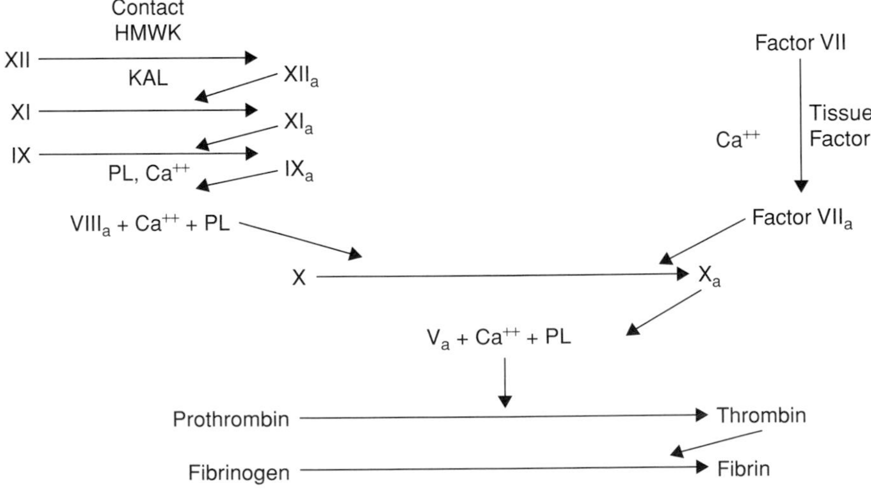

Figure 19-10 Intrinsic (Contact HMWK)/Extrinsic (Factor VII) pathways are laboratory classifications within the body, clotting initiated by exposure of Tissue Factor to factor VII (Extrinsic Pathway). The subsequent cascade results in production of Thrombin and Fibrin. HMWK = high molecular weight kininogen; kal = kallidrein; PL = phospholipid; Ca^{++} = ionic calcium.

free fatty acid, phosphatidylcholine, and low-density lipoprotein (LDL) oxidation.

The production of nitric oxide can be stimulated by neurohumoral mediators (e.g., acetylcholine), by products released by circulating cells (e.g., bradykinin, serotonin), or by mechanical forces (e.g., shear stress). Nitric oxide production is impaired in the presence of atherosclerosis through a series of mechanisms. First, atherosclerotic plaques physically exclude endothelial cells from the stimulants for its release (e.g., shear stress). Second, there is a direct effect of cholesterol components (e.g., lysophosphatidylcholine, a component of oxidized LDL) on the nitric oxide signaling pathway [i.e., protein kinase C, G proteins, and caveolin–endothelial nitric oxide synthase (eNOS) interaction]. Finally, cholesterol enhances the activity of the superoxide-producing NADPH (reduced nicotinamide adenine dinucleotide phosphate) oxidase and xanthine oxidase enzyme systems within the vascular wall. Since oxygen radicals scavenge nitric oxide, this effectively decreases the bioavailability of the decreased amounts of nitric oxide produced.

PHYSIOLOGY OF HEART FAILURE

Systolic dysfunction

Systolic dysfunction is the impaired ability of the ventricle to generate force and shorten.[26,27] This leads to failure when the compromise results in dyspnea, fatigue, and/or fluid retention. The precipitating events can be ischemic or idiopathic. Although infiltrative (e.g., amyloidosis) processes may cause systolic dysfunction, these usually lead primarily to diastolic dysfunction. Symptoms of systolic dysfunction lead to progressive deterioration in health-related quality of life and increased mortality. Prognosis is worse when the etiology is ischemic rather than nonischemic in origin.

The cascade leading to systolic dysfunction and its progression is likely multifactorial. Endothelial dysfunction leads to the loss of beneficial products (nitric oxide, prostacyclin) and an increase in deleterious products (endothelin, angiotensin) from the endothelial cells. Decreasing blood pressure, a consequence of decreasing cardiac output, stimulates the adrenergic, the renin-angiotensin-aldosterone, and hypothalamic-neurohypophyseal systems as well as the natriuretic peptide pathways. Increased beta stimulation increases heart rate and may impair the ability of the SR to efficiently gather released calcium. Chronic beta stimulation also increases the production of tumor necrosis factor alpha, interleukin-6, and other inflammatory cytokines that exacerbate inflammation, apoptosis, and fibrosis. Norepinephrine can exacerbate myocardial ischemia, promote myocyte hypertrophy, and affect apoptosis. Stimulation of the renin-angiotensin-aldosterone system increases cellular hypertrophy, interstitial fibrosis, and vascular myocyte mitogenesis. The neurohypophysis releases vaopressin, stimulating vasoconstriction and thus exacerbating the demands on the dysfunctional myocytes. There is decreased sensitivity to atrial and brain natriuretic peptides, probably as a result of receptor downregulation as well as increased activity of cyclic guanosine monophosphodiesterase. The loss of vasodilatory effects, a result of decreased sensitivity to these peptides, compounds the vasoconstrictive influence of angiotensin II and vasopressin.

A series of randomized placebo-controlled studies have documented the beneficial effects of various medication classes in the progression and mortality of systolic dysfunction. Beta blockers, likely due (at least in part) to their inhibition of the adrenergic pathway, improve both clinical status and overall mortality. Angiotensin-converting enzyme (ACE) inhibitors, likely due to their effect upon the renin-angiotensin-aldosterone system, show benefits similar to those of beta blockade. The effects of ACE inhibitors may be additive to those of beta blockers. There is growing evidence that angiotensin-receptor antagonists demonstrate benefits similar to those of ACE inhibitors, also likely through inhibition of the renin-angiotensin-aldosterone system. The effects of this class of medications may be additive to those of both beta blockers and ACE inhibitors. Although growing evidence as well as our current understanding of the pathophysiology of systolic dysfunction suggests that the role of angiotensin II receptor blockers will be similar to that of ACE inhibitors in the therapy of systolic dysfunction, they are currently not recommended as an alternative to ACE inhibitors except in those patients who cannot tolerate the latter. Similarly, although hydralazine with a nitrate may help to reduce the progression of abnormal myocardial/vascular growth, there is currently not enough evidence to recommend this combination as an alternative to ACE inhibitors except in those patients who cannot tolerate the latter. Digoxin has been shown to improve symptoms, but it does not alter mortality. Calcium channel blockers may actually worsen mortality in patient with compromised LV systolic function.

Diastolic dysfunction

Diastolic dysfunction is an inability of the myocardium to stop generating force and shortening as well as to completely return to its unstressed force and length in the normal time period.[28,29] This can occur in combination with or in the absence of systolic dysfunction. Unfortunately there is no consensus definition of normal systolic function. It is also difficult to determine what the normal time interval is for the myocardium to revert from a force-generating, contracting state to a state of unstressed force and length. Thus, although it is increasingly appreciated that isolated diastolic dysfunction can cause symptomatic heart failure, this diagnosis requires verification of the presence of heart failure, the absence of systolic dysfunction, and the exclusion of other processes (e.g., anemia, pulmonary dysfunction, hypothyroidism) that can masquerade as heart failure.

Isolated diastolic heart failure may account for up to one-third of the cases of congestive heart failure. It appears more prominent in older patient than younger ones, hypertensive (particularly isolated systolic hypertension) patients, and females rather than males. It dramatically reduces health-related quality of life. Acute exacerbations can lead to hospital admission, and mortality in the recently hospitalized or elderly is similar to that of systolic heart dysfunction. The mechanism leading to its development is unclear, although increasing interest is being directed at the role of aldosterone. Aldosterone also acts via mineralocorticoid receptors to stimulate deposition of collagen and extracellular matrix. The RALES (Randomized ALdactone Evaluation Study) trial showed that the aldosterone inhibitor spironolactone, at doses devoid of blood pressure effects and having little or no effect on LV mass, prevents cardiac collagen accumulation in renovascular hypertension with high aldosterone levels. This cascade may be responsible for the benefits of ACE inhibitors and angiotensin II receptor antagonists, which also reduce extracellular matrix and collagen deposition. Angiotensin I stimulation, reduced by ACE inhibition and by angiotensin receptor inhibition, promotes aldosterone release. Furthermore, aldosterone can have a positive feedback effect to stimulate angiotensin II receptors.

There are no randomized double-blind prospective studies to guide our therapy of this disease process. The potential role of the renin-angiotensin-aldosterone pathway suggests that ACE inhibitors, angiotensin II receptor blockers, and a reduction in aldosterone may each be helpful. The role of beta blockade has been debated. Although myocardial relaxation is more energy-dependent than is contraction, canine studies suggest that early diastolic relaxation is impaired by beta-adrenergic inhibition. Furthermore, a lack of reduction of episodes of pulmonary edema following coronary revascularization in patients with isolated diastolic dysfunction suggests that ischemia does not play a predominant role. Still, the general long-term benefits of beta blockade combined with its ability to reverse LV hypertrophy make it difficult to exclude. Few data exist as to the effects of calcium channel blockade, particularly utilizing dihydropyridine calcium channel antagonists, in this process.

Adaptive changes in chronic congestive heart failure

Chronic heart failure results in myocardial adaptations teleologically consistent with optimizing distribution of wall stress as explained by Laplace's law. Thus when pressure overload increases wall stress, the myocyte wall thickens through parallel hypertrophy to reduce the tension sensed by each myocyte back down to normal levels. Although volume overload also increases the stresses on individual myocytes, the changes in wall thickness mandated to compensate for this appear to be less dramatic. Whether this represents influence from the Frank-Starling effect is unclear. Nevertheless, the myocyte's replication is predominantly serial, with some parallel replication when volume overload is the predominant stimulus.

The pathways leading to these changes seem to involve a number of mediators. There is reexpression of fetal proteins which, although they increase myocyte mass, contract less effectively than their adult counterparts. There is an increase in collagen and fibrous tissue deposition, both interstitial and perivascular. This may decrease diastolic compliance (to limit the use of Frank-Starling means to compensate for myocardial dysfunction) as well as to limit dilatory reserve of the coronaries. There is a paucity of mitochondrial and vascular growth relative to myocyte replication, decreasing the vascularity and energy available relative to the number of myocytes. Calcium handling deteriorates, due both to a relative decrease in the amount of SR and in the function of the calcium pumps on the SR. Finally, the composition of the myosin light chains in the ventricular sarcomeres changes, decreasing the effectiveness of the actin-myosin unit and possibly its sensitivity to calcium. As stated earlier, the cascades leading to this remodeling appear to involve the adrenergic system, the renin-angiotensin-aldosterone system, neurohumeral pathways, and dysfunction of the endothelial system. This understanding has led to our current therapy profile to prevent the progression of remodeling from beneficial to maladaptive. In addition, there is anecdotal evidence suggesting that mechanical unloading of decompensated hearts may lead to a regression of the maladaptive changes by a yet unclear mechanism.

Cardiac chamber remodeling after surgical correction

Coronary artery bypass grafting

Revascularization is felt to improve regional and global ventricular function in addition to reducing infarct size.[30–33] Thus, complete revascularization of patients with recent heart failure, left ventricle ejection fraction (LVEF) below 40 percent, and large areas of myocardium at risk (as evidenced by thallium imaging or nitrate-enhanced 99m-technetium sestamibi) increases LVEF and decreases LV end-systolic volume. This correlates with a significant trend toward improved 40-month survival. Although the mechanism of this salutary effect on remodeling is unclear, it is felt that revascularization, by recapturing maximal function in previously hibernating and stunned myocardium through reestablishment of the proper relationship between myocardial oxygen supply and demand, will reduce wall stress on individual myocytes and thereby help reduce/reverse the cascade leading to remodeling. Furthermore, vascular stenosis leads to thickening and perivascular fibrosis of arteries and small vessels distal to the stenosis. This process is felt to limit the vasodilatory reserve of these vessels, compounding the limitations to blood flow that are associated with vascular remodeling.

Aortic valve replacement

Aortic stenosis Aortic valve replacement (AVR) surgery is currently recommended for patients with symptomatic aortic stenosis and hemodynamic evidence that their aortic stenosis is severe (i.e., with an aortic valve area < 0.9 cm^2). It is recommended for otherwise asymptomatic patients who have a hypotensive response to exercise or evidence of progressive LV dysfunction or who are undergoing another cardiovascular surgery. LV dysfunction can be systolic or diastolic in nature.

The hemodynamic response to AVR is quite dramatic when it is performed to relieve aortic stenosis.[34–39] Complete recovery of both systolic and diastolic function is possible, although recovery of systolic function usually precedes recovery of diastolic function and recovery is more likely if preoperative impairment is less severe. Still, the elevated LV mass characteristic of severe aortic stenosis is reduced 18 months following AVR and almost completely resolved by 5 years following AVR. Regression may be more rapid when stentless aortic valves are used. Because the renin-angiotensin system appears to play a prominent role in the LV hypertrophy associated with aortic stenosis, some patients may be more (e.g., deletion/deletion polymorphism for the angiotensin-converting enzyme gene) or less (e.g., insertion/insertion polymorphisms for the angiotensin-converting enzyme gene) predisposed to left ventricular hypertrophy (LVH) with aortic stenosis. These patients may also be more or less likely, respectively, to experience regression of LVH following surgical alleviation of aortic stenosis. Furthermore, although operative mortality is higher and complete functional recovery less likely if preoperative contractile function is severely depressed [New York Heart Association (NYHA) class III or IV], the poor prognosis of these patients with medical treatment alone often makes AVR the most advisable option.

Aortic insufficiency Surgical repair of aortic valvular insufficiency is indicated in symptomatic patients as well as asymptomatic patients with evidence of progressive deterioration of LV function. This can be defined as LVEF less than 50 percent or an increase in the LV end-diastolic diameter greater than 5.5 cm. Surgery in asymptomatic patients is encouraged, because awaiting the development of severe LV dysfunction worsens the prognosis following AVR.

Like AVR for stenotic disease, AVR for insufficiency results in a regression of the adaptive changes precipitated by the insufficiency.[36,38,40–42] Thus, myocardial hypertrophy is regressing toward normal at 1.6 years following surgery and is often normal by 8.1 years. Regression is delayed and less complete in patients with severe preoperative dysfunction, as evidenced by NYHA classification III or IV or LV ejection fraction below 25 percent.

Mitral valve replacement and repair

Mitral stenosis Mitral valve surgery for mitral stenosis involves either dilation (i.e., commissurotomy), repair (i.e., reconstruction), or replacement. The relative benefits of mitral commissurotomy versus mitral valve replacement (MVR) vary among investigators.[25,43,44] Universally, however, commissurotomy is associated more frequently with a higher likelihood of traumatic insufficiency as well as higher reoperation rates (for insufficiency as well as for restenosis). On the other hand, commissurotomy can often be performed with equal success transvenously rather than surgically, dramatically reducing early postprocedure morbidity and recovery time. This makes transvenous commissurotomy an attractive alternative for the older patient with limited life expectancy.

The inconsistent benefit of MVR for mitral stenosis may reflect the fact that rheumatic mitral valvular stenosis varies both in its pathology and its progression. Additionally, however, it is becoming appreciated that maintenance of an intact subvalvular apparatus (i.e., mitral ring, chordae, and papillary muscles) is both possible and important in MVR surgery for mitral stenosis. This apparatus can be responsible for 25 percent of LV contractile function. Although long-term follow-up is lacking, early hemodynamic results suggest that modification of prosthetic valves to more closely duplicate the native valve in form and function (e.g., quadricusp mitral valve) as well as facilitate maintenance of the subvalvular apparatus is possible.

Mitral insufficiency Mitral valve surgery for insufficiency can involve either repair (e.g., reconstructive) or replacement. Options for repair include annuloplasty (often including the rigid Carpentier or pliable Duran prosthetic rings), resection of the prolapsing segment, and repair (i.e., shortening, elongating, reimplanting, replacing) of dysfunctional chordae tendineae or papillary muscle. Such procedures are more likely to be successful when patients are younger (more pliable valves), the procedure requires chordal/papillary muscle shortening (rather than lengthening), and the etiology is endocarditis or ischemia. They are less likely to be successful when the patient is older, the valves are deformed, or the disease process is rheumatic heart disease.

The increasing interest in mitral valve repair rather than replacement surgery stems from incomplete satisfaction with the effects of replacement surgery upon LV function.[45,46] It has long been recognized that LV contractile function, as depicted by LVEF, is depressed following MVR for mitral insufficiency. This was initially felt to represent an unmasking, by the removal of the low pressure "pop-off" of regurgitant flow into the low-pressure left atrium, of preexisting LV dysfunction. It is more recently appreciated, however, that disruption of the subvalvular apparatus (i.e., annulus, chordae, and papillary muscle structure) contributed to this deterioration in LV function. Thus, the subvalvular apparatus is felt to prepare the LV for normal contraction and to account for up to 25 percent of the LV systolic function. As such, conservation of an intact subvalvular apparatus is becoming more of a priority when mitral valve surgery is undertaken.

Long-term results of surgical intervention for mitral insufficiency vary significantly with the age of the patient, the severity of the preoperative ventricular dysfunction, and the capacity to preserve subvalvular structures intact. Thus, unlike remodeling following AVR for aortic stenosis, the left ventricle typically does not improve its contractile function following MVR for mitral insufficiency. Although the majority of patients improve symptomatically, their left ventricular ejection fraction often deteriorates. Preoperative predictors of poor outcomes include NYHA classification III or IV, age above 60 years, end-systolic left ventricular diameter greater than 5.2 cm, and LVEF less than 50 percent. For patients below age 60 in NYHA classification I or II, with end-systolic left ventricular diameter less than 4.5 cm and LVEF greater than 60 percent, functional survival is excellent. The likelihood of improving left ventricular contractile function is greater both in patients without severe preoperative dysfunction and in those capable of having their subvalvular apparatus maintained intact.

References

1. Walker CA, Spinale FG. The structure and function of the cardiac myocyte: A review of fundamental concepts. *J Thorac Cardiovasc Surg* 1999;118:375–382.
2. Katz AM. Selectivity and toxicity of antiarrhythmic drugs: Molecular interactions with ion channels. *Am J Med* 1998;104: 179–195.
3. Albrecht CA. Proarrhythmia with non-antiarrhythmics. A review. *Cardiology* 2004;102:122–139.
4. Bers DM. Cardiac excitation-contraction coupling. *Nature* 2002;415:198–205.
5. Scoote M, Poole-Wilson PA, Williams AJ. The therapeutic potential of new insights into myocardial excitation-contraction coupling. *Heart* 2003;89:371–376.
6. Dhein S, van Koppen CJ, Brodde OE. Muscarinic receptors in the mammalian heart. *Pharmacol Res* 2001;44:161–182.
7. Felder CC. Muscarinic acetylcholine receptors: Signal transduction through multiple effectors. *FASEB J* 1995; 9:619–625.
8. Mubagwa K, Flameng W. Adenosine, adenosine receptors and myocardial protection: An updated overview. *Cardiovasc Res* 2001;52:25–39.
9. Brodde OE, Bruck H, Leineweber K, Seyfarth T. Presence, distribution and physiological function of adrenergic and muscarinic receptor subtypes in the human heart. *Basic Res Cardiol* 2001;96:528–538.
10. Severs NJ. The cardiac muscle cell. *Bioessays* 2000; 22:188–199.
11. Fuchs F, Smith SH. Calcium, cross-bridges, and the Frank-Starling relationship. *News Physiol Sci* 2001; 16:5–10.
12. McDonald KS, Moss RL. Osmotic compression of single cardiac myocytes eliminates the reduction in Ca^{2+} sensitivity of tension at short sarcomere length. *Circ Res* 1995;77:199–205.
13. Landesberg A. Molecular control of myocardial mechanics and energetics: The chemo-mechanical conversion. *Adv Exp Med Biol* 1997;430:75–87.
14. Sweitzer NK, Moss RL. Determinants of loaded shortening velocity in single cardiac myocytes permeabilized with alpha-hemolysin. *Circ Res* 1993;73:1150–1162.
15. Alvarez BV, Perez NG, Ennis IL, et al. Mechanisms underlying the increase in force and Ca(2+) transient that follow stretch of cardiac muscle: A possible explanation of the Anrep effect. *Circ Res* 1999;85:716–722.
16. Alpert NR, Leavitt BJ, Ittleman FP, et al. A mechanistic analysis of the force-frequency relation in non-failing and progressively failing human myocardium. *Basic Res Cardiol* 93(Suppl 1):23–32.
17. Stanley WC. Cardiac energetics during ischaemia and the rationale for metabolic interventions. *Coron Artery Dis* 2001;12(Suppl 1):S3–S7.
18. Zhang J. Myocardial energetics in cardiac hypertrophy. *Clin Exp Pharmacol Physiol* 2002;29:351–359.
19. Jones CJ, Kuo L, Davis MJ, Chilian WM. Regulation of coronary blood flow: Coordination of heterogeneous control mechanisms in vascular microdomains. *Cardiovasc Res* 1995;29:585–596.
20. Kloner RA, Jennings RB. Consequences of brief ischemia: Stunning, preconditioning, and their clinical implications: Part 1. *Circulation* 2001;104:2981–2989.
21. Kloner RA, Jennings RB. Consequences of brief ischemia: Stunning, preconditioning, and their clinical implications: Part 2. *Circulation* 2001;104:3158–3167.
22. Heusch G, Schulz R. The biology of myocardial hibernation. *Trends Cardiovasc Med* 2000;10:108–114.
23. Behrendt D, Ganz P. Endothelial function. From vascular biology to clinical applications. *Am J Cardiol* 2002;90: 40L–48L.
24. Bonetti PO, Lerman LO, Lerman A. Endothelial dysfunction: A marker of atherosclerotic risk. *Arterioscler Thromb Vasc Biol* 2003;23:168–175.
25. Onnasch JF, Schneider F, Mierzwa M, Mohr FW. Mitral valve repair versus mitral valve replacement. *Z Kardiol* 2001;90(Suppl 6):75–80.
26. Klein L, O'Connor CM, Gattis WA, et al. Pharmacologic therapy for patients with chronic heart failure and reduced systolic function: Review of trials and practical considerations. *Am J Cardiol* 2003;91:18F–40F.
27. Zannad F, Dousset B, Alla F. Treatment of congestive heart failure: Interfering the aldosterone-cardiac extracellular matrix relationship. *Hypertension* 2001;38: 1227–1232.
28. Zile MR, Brutsaert DL. New concepts in diastolic dysfunction and diastolic heart failure: Part I: Diagnosis, prognosis, and measurements of diastolic function. *Circulation* 2002;105:1387–1393.
29. Zile MR, Brutsaert DL. New concepts in diastolic dysfunction and diastolic heart failure: Part II: Causal mechanisms and treatment. *Circulation* 2002;105:1503–1508.
30. Mule JD, Bax JJ, Zingone B, et al. The beneficial effect of revascularization on jeopardized myocardium: Reverse remodeling and improved long-term prognosis. *Eur J Cardiothorac Surg* 2002;22:426–430.

31. Sutton MG, Sharpe N. Left ventricular remodeling after myocardial infarction: Pathophysiology and therapy. *Circulation* 2000;101:2981–2988.
32. Yousef ZR and Marber MS. The open artery hypothesis: Potential mechanisms of action. *Prog Cardiovasc Dis* 2000;42:419–438.
33. Yousef ZR, Redwood SR, Bucknall CA, et al. Late intervention after anterior myocardial infarction: Effects on left ventricular size, function, quality of life, and exercise tolerance: Results of the Open Artery Trial (TOAT Study). *J Am Coll Cardiol* 2002;40:869–876.
34. Beyerbacht HP, Lamb HJ, van der LA, et al. Aortic valve replacement in patients with aortic valve stenosis improves myocardial metabolism and diastolic function. *Radiology* 2001;219:637–643.
35. Dellgren G, Eriksson MJ, Blange I, et al. Angiotensin-converting enzyme gene polymorphism influences degree of left ventricular hypertrophy and its regression in patients undergoing operation for aortic stenosis. *Am J Cardiol* 1999;84:909–913.
36. Krayenbuehl HP, Hess OM, Monrad ES, et al. Left ventricular myocardial structure in aortic valve disease before, intermediate, and late after aortic valve replacement. *Circulation* 1989;79:744–755.
37. Lee JW, Choi KJ, Lee SG, et al. Left ventricular muscle mass regression after aortic valve replacement. *J Korean Med Sci* 1999;14:511–519.
38. Monrad ES, Hess OM, Murakami T, et al. Time course of regression of left ventricular hypertrophy after aortic valve replacement. *Circulation* 1988;77:1345–1355.
39. Walther T, Schubert A, Falk V, et al. Left ventricular reverse remodeling after surgical therapy for aortic stenosis: Correlation to renin-angiotensin system gene expression. *Circulation* 2002;106:I23–I26.
40. Chaliki HP, Mohty D, Avierinos JF, et al. Outcomes after aortic valve replacement in patients with severe aortic regurgitation and markedly reduced left ventricular function. *Circulation* 2002;106:2687–2693.
41. Moidl R, Simon P, Chevtchik O, et al. Reversal of ventricular dilatation after correction of aortic incompetence: Mechanical prosthesis compared with biological procedures. *Thorac Cardiovasc Surg* 1998; 46:188–191.
42. Tarasoutchi F, Grinberg M, Filho JP, et al. Symptoms, left ventricular function, and timing of valve replacement surgery in patients with aortic regurgitation. *Am Heart J* 1999;138:477–485.
43. Arora R, Kalra GS, Singh S, et al. Percutaneous transvenous mitral commissurotomy: Immediate and long-term follow-up results. *Catheter Cardiovasc Intervent* 2002;55: 450–456.
44. Hamasaki N, Nosaka H, Kimura T, et al. Ten-years clinical follow-up following successful percutaneous transvenous mitral commissurotomy: Single-center experience. *Catheter Cardiovasc Intervent* 2000;49:284–288.
45. Kumar AS, Choudhary SK, Mathur A, et al. Homograft mitral valve replacement: Five years' results. *J Thorac Cardiovasc Surg* 2000;120:450–458.
46. Rothenburger M, Rukosujew A, Hammel D, et al. Mitral valve surgery in patients with poor left ventricular function. *Thorac Cardiovasc Surg* 2002;50:351–354.

CHAPTER

20 COAGULATION AND HEMOSTASIS

Ala' Sami Haddadin, Nauder Faraday

INTRODUCTION

Bleeding is a common problem in cardiac surgery; as many as 80 percent of patients will require blood transfusion. Management is complicated by the wide differential diagnosis of post–cardiopulmonary bypass (CPB) bleeding, the limited utility of standard laboratory tests for diagnosis in this setting, and the narrow time window available for diagnosis and treatment of the bleeding patient. In approximately 5 percent of patients, hemorrhage will persist and require surgical exploration for definitive correction.[1] In one large series, reoperation for bleeding was associated with a longer ICU stay, greater need for an intraaortic balloon pump, and higher risk of death.[2] Pericardial tamponade also occurs more commonly in bleeding patients, being seen in approximately 2 percent of cardiac surgical patients.[3] Pericardial tamponade in cardiac surgical patients often presents in atypical fashion and is associated with hemodynamic instability and the need for surgical exploration.[3] A thorough understanding of normal and abnormal hemostasis, anticoagulant and procoagulant drugs, and coagulation testing is required to effectively manage the cardiac surgical patient.

NORMAL AND ABNORMAL HEMOSTASIS: THE ROLE OF CARDIOPULMONARY BYPASS (CPB)

Hemostasis is the process of blood clot formation at the site of vessel injury. It is an exquisitely well-regulated process that involves cellular elements (primarily platelets and endothelial cells) and plasma components (procoagulant, anticoagulant, and fibrinolytic proteins). Under normal physiologic conditions, blood flowing throughout the vasculature remains in a fluid state. Fluidity is maintained by (1) inhibition of platelets by endothelial

KEY CONCEPTS

- Artificial surfaces of the cardiopulmonary bypass (CPB) circuit disrupt normal homeostatic mechanisms that keep blood fluid by activating platelets, coagulation factors, and fibrinolytic proteins.
- High dose heparin (300–400 U/kg) is used to prevent blood clotting during CPB and the anticoagulant effect of heparin is reversed by protamine sulfate after CPB is complete.
- Bleeding during and after cardiac surgery is common and has may be caused by many different abnormalities. The most common causes of bleeding are: platelet dysfunction, excessive fibrinolysis, insufficient concentrations of coagulation factors, residual heparin, and hypothermia. Surgical causes of bleeding should be considered when bleeding is brisk despite visible clot formation and/or normal or mildly abnormal coagulation tests.
- Prophylactic administration of antifibrinolytic agents (aprotinin, epsilon amino caproic acid, and tranexamic acid) reduces blood loss, transfusion volume, and the proportion of cardiac surgical patients who require transfusion by 30%.
- Pericardial tamponade occurs in 2% of cardiac surgical patients and should be suspected in all patients who exhibit hemodynamic compromise in the presence of high central filling pressures.

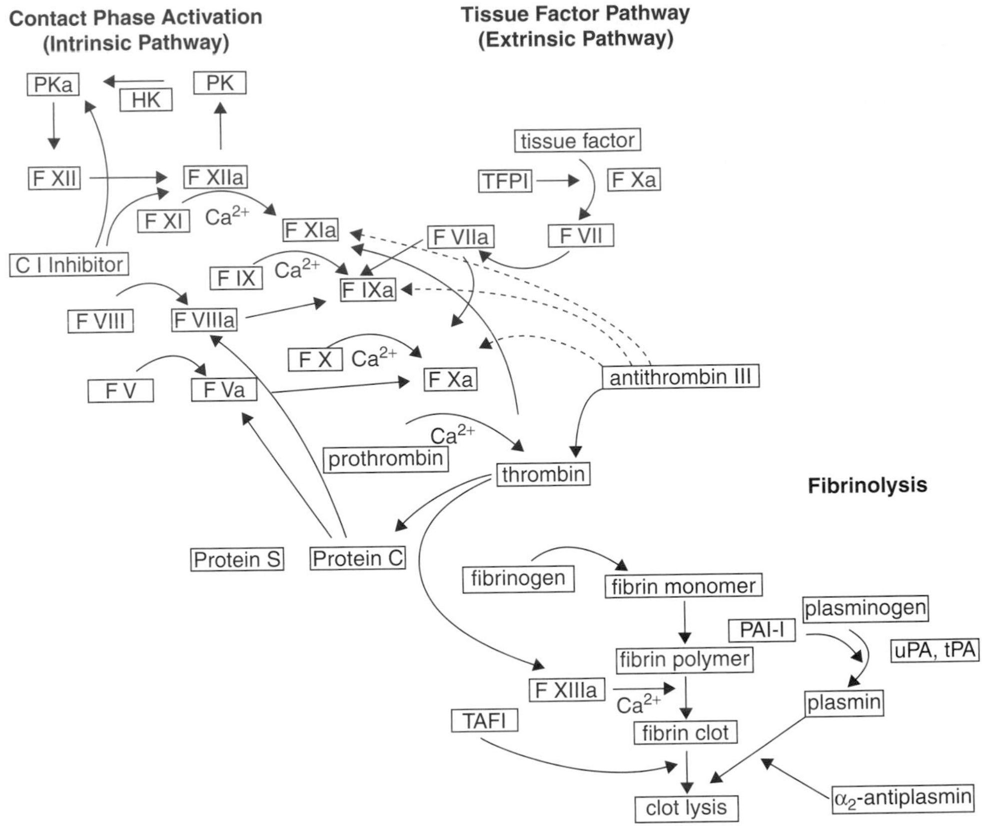

Figure 20-1 The coagulation cascade. F = factor, HK = high-molecular-weight kininogen, PAI-1 = plasminogen activator inhibitor-1, PK = plasma kallikrein, TAFI = thrombin activatable fibrinolysis inhibitor, TFPI = tissue factor pathway inhibitor, tPA = tissue-type plasminogen activator, uPA = urokinase-type plasminogen activator. (Adapted from Tapper H, Herwald H. Modulation of hemostatic mechanisms in bacterial infectious diseases. *Blood* 2000;96(7):2329–2337. With permission.)

release products (e.g., prostacyclin and nitric oxide), (2) endothelial heparinoids, and (3) circulating soluble anticoagulants (e.g., tissue factor pathway inhibitor and antithrombin). It is also important to recognize that platelets and procoagulant proteins circulate, for the most part, in an inactive state, and that an activating stimulus is required to initiate clot formation. In the absence of such a stimulus, blood remains fluid because there is no signal to induce clot formation.

Under normal circumstances, clot formation is initiated when the integrity of the endothelium is breached. This causes the exposure of subendothelial collagen, to which von Willebrand factor and platelets rapidly adhere. Subendothelial tissue factor is also exposed, and the binding of tissue factor to trace amounts of circulating activated factor VII (FVIIa) activate the coagulation cascade through the tissue factor ("extrinsic") pathway (Fig. 20-1). Under ordinary in vivo conditions, the coagulation proteins of the contact activation ("intrinsic") pathway play a very minor role in thrombus formation.

From the initial steps of hemostasis, both platelet and coagulation activation are amplified. Adherent platelets become activated through engagement of a variety of agonist receptors (e.g., collagen, thrombin, ADP), and then bind fibrinogen and to each other. This recruitment process of platelets is called aggregation. Simultaneously, the binding of tissue factor to factor VII generates more FVIIa, and in the presence of other coagulation enzymes (V, VIII, and X) and cofactors (Ca^{2+}) as well as platelet phospholipid, thrombin is generated (see Fig. 20-1). Thrombin plays a central role in hemostasis because it is a key activator of multiple pathways: (1) It is a potent platelet activator, (2) it catalyzes the conversion of fibrinogen to fibrin en route to formation of an insoluble fibrin clot, (3) it activates anticoagulant proteins through its action on thrombomodulin and protein C, and (4) it activates fibrinolysis by inducing endothelial cells to release tissue plasminogen activator (t-PA). The end result of the normal hemostatic process is formation of a thrombus localized to the site of vascular injury, limitation of clot propagation, and initiation of the time-delayed process of fibrinolysis/vessel recanalization.

The extracorporeal surfaces of the CPB circuit disrupt the normal homeostatic mechanisms that maintain blood

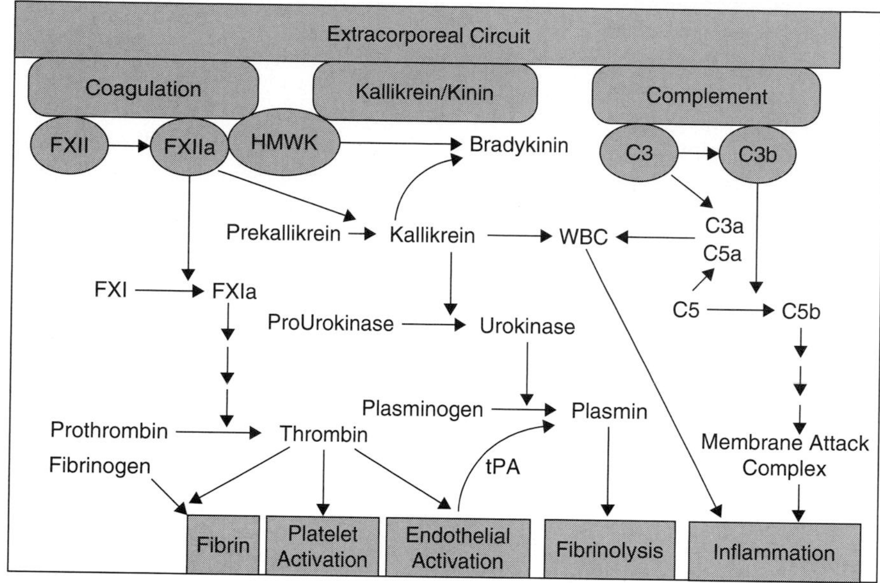

Figure 20-2 Extracorporeal circuitry activates coagulation and inflammation. HMWK = high-molecular-weight kinongen, tPA = tissue-type plasminogen activator.

fluidity (Fig. 20-2). CPB surfaces lack endothelial cells and as such lack tonic platelet inhibition. Furthermore, the positively charged surfaces of the circuit allow the binding and autoactivation of several plasma coagulation proteins, including fibrinogen, prekallikrein, and high-molecular-weight kininogen. To prevent activation of hemostatic elements during CPB, systemic anticoagulation with heparin is employed (see discussion on heparin below). Although heparin is extremely effective at preventing clinical clot formation, inhibition of coagulation is not complete and trace amounts of thrombin are generated.[4,5] As a result, platelets become activated by exposure to thrombin, circuit-bound fibrinogen, and shear forces, and the coagulation cascade becomes activated[4,5] through the contact activation pathway (see Fig. 20-2). Platelets activated during CPB become refractory to subsequent stimuli and are dysfunctional after CPB.[6–8]. Endothelial t-PA and activated kallikrein promote fibrinolysis by accelerating the conversion of plasminogen to plasmin.[9,10] In addition to activating coagulation, proinflammatory proteins such as kallikrein and complement become activated by the extracorporeal circuit, which in turn leads to activation of leukocytes, endothelial cells, and the systemic release of cytokines. The induction of systemic inflammation may enhance abnormal hemostasis[11] and is believed to play a role in the development of multisystem organ dysfunction as well (see Laffey[12] for full review). The use of more biocompatible extracorporeal circuits is associated with decreased platelet activation, fibrinolysis, and thrombin generation.[13] However, these circuits are not sufficiently biocompatible that they lead to improved clinical hemostasis in cardiac surgery.[14]

HEPARIN

Heparin is a heterogeneous glycosaminoglycan that ranges from 5,000 to 30,000 Da in molecular weight. It is closely related to heparan sulfate, an endogenous glycosaminoglycan, which is found on the surface of endothelial cells and in extracellular matrix. Heparin is a highly sulfated, negatively charged molecule that is bound by plasma and endothelial proteins. It can be obtained from porcine intestinal mucosa or bovine lung. Both preparations have similar biological activity. Heparin's anticoagulant effect begins immediately after intravenous injection. Its half-life is directly proportional to the dose administered—i.e. larger doses are cleared more slowly than smaller doses—with a dose of 400 U/kg having a half-life of approximately 2.5 h. Heparin is actively taken up by reticuloendothlial cells. These cells can store and later release heparin and are the major pathway through which heparin is eliminated. A small amount of unfractionated heparin is cleared by the kidneys, but smaller heparin molecules (e.g., low-molecular-weight heparin) are cleared primarily through renal mechanisms. Heparin exerts its anticoagulant effect by accelerating (approximately 1000 times) the ability of antithrombin (formerly "antithrombin III") to neutralize thrombin (factor IIa) and factor Xa. Each heparin molecule has a pentasaccharide segment that binds to a specific sequence on antithrombin and is required for anticoagulant activity. Heparin molecules less than 18 saccharide units in length (less than 5000 Da) do not inactivate thrombin but retain their anti-Xa activity.

High-dose heparin (300 to 400 U/kg) is routinely used to establish anticoagulation prior to the initiation of CPB. The intensity of thrombogenic stimuli posed by the

CPB circuit mandates a level of anticoagulation 10 times greater than that used in other settings (plasma heparin concentrations of 3 to 5 U/mL vs. 0.3 to 0.7 U/mL for CPB vs. treatment of deep venous thrombosis or pulmonary embolism). It is important to recognize that heparin dosing for CPB was derived empirically based on the activated clotting time (ACT) at which clot formation was not observed on CPB circuitry. Bull and colleagues[15] found clot formation at an ACT less than 180 s but none at an ACT greater than 300 s. These authors advocate an ACT of 480 s as a way of providing a margin of anticoagulation safety. The minimal dose of heparin and ACT level required to safely conduct CPB has not been the subject of prospective randomized trials; based on observational work in the 1970s, most centers aim for an ACT greater than 400 s. However, a number of authors have reported good results at lower ACTs.[16]

PROTAMINE

Protamine is a polypeptide composed primarily of arginine. It has a molecular weight of approximately 4300 Da and is highly positively charged. DNA contains large quantities of protamine, and the primary commercial source of protamine is salmon sperm. Protamine is used to neutralize heparin's anticoagulant effect. Positively charged arginine moieties on protamine form ionic bonds with negatively charged sulfate groups on heparin and neutralize heparin's effect. After intravenous injection, all free heparin is immediately and irreversibly bound to protamine. Protamine neutralizes the anti–factor IIa effect of heparin far more than its anti–factor Xa effect. Thus protamine is less effective at neutralizing low-molecular-weight heparin than standard unfractionated heparin. Protamine can produce an antihemostatic effect by inhibiting platelet function and inducing the release of t-PA from endothelial cells. In addition, rapid injection of protamine causes histamine release and hypotension, and protamine administration can produce life-threatening pulmonary hypertension.

The dose of protamine required to neutralize heparin after CPB is controversial. Because protamine has many untoward side effects, administration of the lowest possible effective dose is desirable. In practice, heparin reversal after CPB can be effectively accomplished using fixed protamine dosing or protamine-heparin titration. Bull advocates the use of a fixed protamine dose of 1.3 mg for every 100 U of heparin used for CPB.[15] However, in vitro, as little as 0.3 mg of protamine is capable of reversing 100 U of unfractionated heparin.[17] Because the ACT is universally used to monitor anticoagulation during CPB, most centers assess the ACT after protamine administration to determine the adequacy of protamine's reversal effect. An ACT less than 130 s or within 10 percent of pre-CPB levels is considered adequate reversal. Unfortunately, the ACT is a very poor test for residual heparinization after protamine administration because it is insensitive to low levels of heparin and does not correlate with plasma heparin levels. Automated heparin-protamine titration systems are available that determine the amount of circulating heparin activity and the appropriate neutralizing dose of protamine. Although the dose of protamine given after CPB is lowered with the use of these devices, clinical bleeding after CPB is not reduced.[18]

DEFINITION AND DIFFERENTIAL DIAGNOSIS OF EXCESSIVE BLEEDING AFTER CARDIAC SURGERY

Identification of the bleeding patient begins in the operating room and continues in the postoperative care unit. Assessment of the adequacy of hemostasis begins a few minutes after protamine is administered. The definition of bleeding is empiric and varies to some extent from institution to institution. In the OR, excessive bleeding is often defined as diffuse bleeding from multiple tissue surfaces without an identifiable surgical source and in the absence of visible clot formation. In the ICU, excessive bleeding is defined in terms of chest tube drainage. Common definitions of excessive bleeding are as follows: greater than 200 mL/h in any hour, greater than 150 mL/h for two consecutive hours, greater than 100 mL/h for three consecutive hours, or any sudden increase in chest tube drainage to a level greater than 100 mL/h.

The differential diagnosis of excessive bleeding after CPB is wide and based on the pathologic disturbances attendant on CPB. In addition to the issues associated with the artificial surfaces of the bypass circuitry and those of heparin/protamine, CPB is associated with other physiologic disturbances that can affect coagulation. These disturbances include hemodilution with CPB priming solutions, hemodilution associated with massive transfusion, and the use of systemic hypothermia for organ protection. As in all surgical procedures, the potential for a surgical cause for excessive bleeding must always be considered, especially in the presence of persistent brisk bleeding and visible clot (in the surgical field or chest tubes). Similarly, preoperative hematologic abnormalities should be considered; however, in most cases these should have been identified during the preoperative history and physical exam. A list of the potential causes of excessive bleeding after CPB is given in Table 20-1.

Diagnosis of the specific cause of bleeding is particularly challenging after cardiac surgery because traditional laboratory tests have poor predictive value in this setting. In vitro abnormalities in coagulation testing are ubiquitous in these patients and are poorly correlated with the presence or absence of clinical bleeding.[19–21]. Nonetheless, algorithms that incorporate laboratory testing in the management of bleeding patients do reduce blood loss and transfusion of blood products.[22–24]

Table 20-1	Causes of excessive bleeding after cardiopulmonary bypass
Surgical factors	Arterial or large venous bleeding
Bypass-related factors	Platelet dysfunction Thrombocytopenia Excessive fibrinolysis Depletion of coagulation factors Residual heparin/heparin rebound Hypothermia Disseminated intravascular coagulation
Patient factors	Congenital bleeding diathesis Concurrent systemic diseases (e.g.. renal or hepatic failure) Medications (e.g., thrombolytics, antiplatelet agents)
Transfusion-related factors	Hemodilution

LABORATORY TESTS OF HEMOSTASIS

Tests of the coagulation cascade

Activated coagulation time (ACT)

The ACT is a bedside test of coagulation that measures the time to clot formation in whole blood that is activated by either celite or kaolin. The celite or kaolin activates the contact activation pathway (see Fig. 20-1), and thus the ACT measures the function of the enzymes/inhibitors in that pathway. The normal range for ACT is 107 ± 13 s[25] (Table 20-2). Predictably, the ACT is prolonged in the presence of heparin. Prolongation of the ACT in response to heparin is fairly linear at heparin concentrations greater than 1 U/mL, and observational studies demonstrate that it is an effective monitor for adequacy of heparin anticoagulation during CPB. However, it is insensitive to heparin at lower concentrations, including concentrations in the therapeutic range (i.e., 0.3–0.7 U/mL). Therefore return of the ACT to baseline after protamine administration does not ensure that heparin is entirely neutralized.[26] Conversely, thrombocytopenia, hemodilution, hypothermia, and circulating nonheparin anticoagulants can also prolong the ACT. Therefore prolongation of the ACT does not necessarily diagnose residual heparinization.

Prothrombin time (PT)

The prothrombin time is used to assess the tissue factor pathway (see Fig. 20-1), which consists of tissue factor and factor VII, and coagulation factors in the common pathway (factors II, V, X, and fibrinogen). In this test, clotting is initiated by recalcifying citrated patient plasma in the presence of thromboplastin (tissue factor). The endpoint for the PT is the formation of a fibrin clot, which is detected by visual, optical, or electromechanical means. Congenital or acquired deficiencies in proteins involved in the tissue factor pathway will prolong the PT. These conditions include warfarin therapy, vitamin K deficiency, and severe liver disease. Differences among commercially available reagents (e.g., thromboplastin) result in variable sensitivity to alterations in these coagulant proteins. In order to promote standardization for

Table 20-2 Tests of hemostatic function (average normal values given)

Test (normal range)	Significance of abnormal test
Coagulation system	
ACT (< 130 s)	Heparin present, insufficient coagulation proteins or platelet number
Prothrombin time (PT) (10–13 s)	Deficiencies or inhibitors of tissue factor pathway and common pathways: VII, X, V (< 50%), II(< 30%), fibrinogen (< 100 mg/dL)
International normalized ratio (1.0)	
Activated partial thromboplastin time (25–40 s)	Deficiencies or inhibitors of contact activation and common pathways: XII, HMW kininogen, prekallikrein, XI(< 20%), X, V, II (< 30–50%), fibrinogen (< 100 mg/dL)
Platelets	
Platelet count (150,000–400,000/μL)	Quantitative abnormalities of platelets
Bleeding time (< 7 min)	Impaired platelet function, thrombocytopenia, deficiency of von Willebrand factor (vWF), severe anemia, improper technique
Aggregation (qualitative)	Impaired platelet function
Platelet function analyzer 100	Impaired platelet function, thrombocytopenia, (> 180 s) vWF deficiency
Fibrinolysis	
Fibrinogen (150–400 mg/dL)	Deficiency of fibrinogen
D-dimer test	Positive test indicates ongoing fibrinolysis
Whole-blood hemostasis	
Thromboelastograph	
MA (50–60 mm)	Hypofibrinogenemia, thrombocytopenia, platelet dysfunction
Clot lysis time	Accelerated fibrinolysis
SonoClot	Hypofibrinogenemia, thrombocytopenia, hypercoagulable states

monitoring oral anticoagulant therapy, an international reference thromboplastin was developed. The international normalized ratio (INR) is an expression of the PT that adjusts for differences in the sensitivities of the reagents used in each local lab with the international reference standard (see Table 20-2).

Activated partial thromboplastin time (aPTT)

The aPTT is used to assess the integrity of the contact pathway (see Fig. 20-1). The test is performed by recalcifying citrated plasma in the presence of a negatively charged substance such as kaolin and a thromboplastic material that does not have tissue factor activity (hence the name "partial thromboplastin"). Like that for the PT, the endpoint for the aPTT is the formation of a fibrin clot, which is detected by visual, optical, or electromechanical means. Deficiencies in contact activation proteins, common pathway proteins, and anticoagulants such as heparin will prolong test results (see Table 20-2).

Tests of platelet function

Platelet count

Platelet count can be determined by automated cell counting or manual examination of a peripheral blood smear. The normal concentration of platelets in circulating blood is 150,000 to 400,000/μL (see Table 20-2). However, fewer cells are required for adequate surgical hemostasis (50,000 to 100,000/μL) provided that platelet function is normal. In nonsurgical patients, spontaneous bleeding does not usually occur until the platelet count is below 10,000/μL. In cardiac surgical procedures, in which platelet function is commonly abnormal, a platelet count greater than 100,000/ μL is considered adequate for hemostasis.

Platelet aggregometry

The "gold standard" test for assessing platelet function is platelet aggregometry (see Table 20-2). Abnormalities in platelet function are common after cardiac surgery. However, platelet aggregometry is too cumbersome and time-consuming for clinical use in cardiac surgery.

Bleeding time

Although classically described as a test of platelet function, the bleeding time is an in vivo test of global hemostatic function in which platelets (and endothelial cells) play a significant role. The test is performed by creating a standardized skin incision and measuring the time it takes for bleeding to cease. Normal bleeding times range between 4 and 10 min (see Table 20-2). Numerous prospective blinded investigations have demonstrated that this test has very limited ability to predict risk of perioperative bleeding, whether it is used before or after surgery.[27,28] Even in patients given therapeutic doses of aspirin, an increase in bleeding time was not associated with clinically significant bleeding after cardiac surgery.[29,30] The American College of Pathologists does not recommend the bleeding time as a screening tool to assess risk of bleeding in surgical patients.[31]

Platelet function analyzer-100 (PFA-100)

The PFA-100 uses citrated whole blood to test platelet adhesion and aggregation in a high-shear environment. The test measures the time required for platelets to plug a hole in a collagen-coated cartridge through which blood is forced to flow. Closure time is prolonged with thrombocytopenia and platelet function abnormalities (see Table 20-2), particularly those due to vWF and aspirin. The test is now clinically employed as an in vitro "bleeding time." Like investigations using the bleeding time, studies in cardiac surgery demonstrate that the PFA-100 has limited ability to predict which patients will have significant bleeding complications.[32]

Tests of fibrinolysis

Fibrinogen

Fibrinogen is factor I in the coagulation cascade and is converted to fibrin by thrombin (factor IIa) en route to becoming an insoluble clot. Fibrinogen is also a required cofactor for platelet aggregation. The concentration of soluble fibrinogen in the plasma can be directly measured. The normal concentration of fibrinogen in circulating plasma is 150 to 400 mg/dL. A fibrinogen concentration greater than 100 mg/dL is considered adequate for hemostasis (see Table 20-2). Hemodilution, excessive consumption, or inadequate hepatic production can all lead to abnormal fibrinogen levels.

D-Dimer

Insoluble fibrin is formed when adjacent fibrin molecules are cross-linked. Fibrinolysis is a process in which plasmin cleaves cross-linked fibrin in a way that produces dimeric units (D-dimer) from each of two adjacent fibrin units. An increase in D-dimer is universally observed during CPB (see Table 20-2), indicating the presence of fibrinolysis, and excessive fibrinolysis is related to bleeding after cardiac surgery.[10]

Tests of whole-blood hemostasis

Thromboelastograph (TEG)

The TEG measures the overall hemostatic response from initial activation of coagulation to clot formation, retraction, and lysis. It uses unanticoagulated whole blood to produce a tracing that reflects various components of the hemostatic process. The reaction time (R; normal range, 7.5 to 15 min) is a measure of the time to initial clot formation (see Table 20-2). The R value is comparable to the whole-blood clotting time and may be accelerated by adding a contact activator to the sample cuvette. Prolongation of the R value is consistent with a deficiency in one or more plasma coagulation factors. The maximum amplitude (MA; normal range, 50 to 60 mm) provides a measure of clot strength and may be decreased by qualitative or quantitative platelet dysfunction or by hypofibrinogenemia. Both the alpha angle and the clot formation time (K) provide measures of the rate of clot growth. Any factors that slow the kinetic rate of clot formation would prolong these variables. Available data suggest that the TEG has limited ability to predict blood loss in cardiac surgery[33] but may be useful when it is integrated with other tests into an algorithm for hemostatic management.[23,24]

SonoClot

The SonoClot (Sienco, Inc., Morrison, CO) is a device that measures the viscoelastic strength of clot as it forms in unanticoagulated whole blood. The device generates a curve that can be divided into several parts, termed "waves," based on the rate of increase of impedance with time[34] (see Table 20-2). The time to peak impedance is often used as a measure of hemostatic competence. Abnormalities in platelet number and function and fibrinogen concentration can alter SonoClot parameters. Limited data are available that evaluate the utility of this device for identifying clinically meaningful abnormalities in coagulation after cardiac surgery.

PROPHYLACTIC STRATEGIES FOR POST-CPB HEMORRHAGE

Aprotinin

Aprotinin is a 58–amino acid polypeptide that has inhibitory activity against a wide variety of serine proteases, most notably plasmin and kallikrein. The antiplasmin action of aprotinin is approximately four times as great as its antikallikrein action. Aprotinin was first introduced for clinical use in surgery as an anti-inflammatory agent, where an in vivo hemostatic effect was serendipitously observed. Because aprotinin inhibits the activity of both kallikrein and plasmin, it inhibits both the production of plasmin and its enzymatic fibrinolytic activity (see Fig. 20-1). This antifibrinolytic action is the most likely mechanism through which aprotinin exerts its hemostatic benefit; however, other mechanisms (e.g., platelet preservation, anti-inflammation[35]) may also play a role. Aprotinin is eliminated primarily by the kidney and has an elimination half-life of approximately 7 h in patients with normal renal function.

Aprotinin is indicated for prophylaxis of bleeding in patients undergoing coronary artery bypass grafting (CABG). Dosing regimens in cardiac surgical procedures have varied. The most effective regimen appears to be 2 million kallikrein inhibitor units (KIU) administered intravenously prior to CPB, another 2 million units in the pump prime, plus a continuous infusion of 500,000 KIU/h.[36,37] Efficacy at half this dosage has been reported in some studies[38]; however, higher dosages appear to provide no additional hemostatic benefit.[39] Aprotinin was shown to reduce postoperative bleeding in patients undergoing repeat CABG surgery,[40,41] in patients with bacterial endocarditis,[42] and those taking aspirin.[43] Two metanalyses have verified the efficacy of aprotinin[44,45] for reducing blood loss and transfusion (30 to 50 percent reduction) in cardiac surgical procedures. Effective treatment of bleeding patients with aprotinin after cardiac surgery has been reported as salvage therapy in some case reports, but the efficacy of this use has not been verified in prospective trials.

Several potential adverse consequences of aprotinin therapy are noteworthy. First, aprotinin use is associated with prolongation of the celite ACT in vitro. Prolongation of this test is due to the inhibitory action of aprotinin on the serine proteases of the coagulation cascade.[41] To account for this in vitro phenomenon, some authors have suggested increasing the minimally acceptable celite ACT to 750 s during management of CPB. Alternatively, the kaolin ACT can be monitored and maintained at the usual level (ACT greater than 400 s) during CPB because this test is not significantly affected by aprotinin.[46] Second, because aprotinin is a bovine-derived protein, it is associated with a significant incidence of anaphylactoid reactions, particularly upon reexposure. The incidence of anaphylactoid reactions with aprotinin therapy within 6 months of initial exposure is reported as 4.5 percent, but this incidence decreases to 1.5 percent after 6 months.[47] Thus reexposure to aprotinin within 6 months is not recommended. Third, aprotinin has the potential for inducing a prothrombotic state. A high incidence of premature coronary graft thrombosis was reported in one series when aprotinin was first introduced in cardiac surgery, but this prothrombotic tendency was not observed in prospective randomized trials or metanalyses.[44,45]

Epsilon aminocaproic acid (eaca) and tranexamic acid (TA)

Epsilon aminocaproic acid and tranexamic acid are small straight-chain or cyclic structures that resemble lysine. Fibrinolysis requires the binding of plasmin to fibrinogen and of t-PA to plasmin through lysine recognition sites. EACA and TA exert an antifibrinolytic action by competitively inhibiting the binding of plasmin to fibrinogen/fibrin and of t-PA to plasmin. TA is approximately 10 times more potent than EACA.[48] Elimination of EACA is primarily through renal mechanisms, and the plasma half-life for EACA is 1 to 5 h. Dosage should be reduced 15 to 25 percent in patients with significant renal dysfunction or oliguria.

Lysine analogues are indicated for the treatment of bleeding in a number of conditions but are not approved by the FDA for use in CPB. Nonetheless, these agents are widely used and have proven efficacy in cardiac surgery.[44,45] When administered prior to CPB, both EACA and TA reduce bleeding and transfusion by approximately 30 percent.[49–52] EACA is administered as a loading dose of 75 to 150 mg/kg at the beginning of surgery followed by a continuous infusion at 10 to 15 mg/kg/h. Dosage of TA is one-tenth that of EACA.[48] EACA and TA are associated with the development of a prothrombotic state, and venous thrombosis has been reported with their use in some cases.

Desamino-8-arginine vasopressin (DDAVP)

DDAVP is a vasopressin analogue that replaces R-arginine with the L-isomer. It is devoid of the vasoconstrictive properties of vasopressin while maintaining (or increasing) its antidiuretic and hemostatic actions. Administration of DDAVP improves hemostasis by increasing the plasma concentration of vWF and factor VIII, in part by inducing their release from endothelial cells. The drug can be administered intravenously, subcutaneously, or intranasally. Its elimination half-life is 1 to 2 h, although increased circulating concentrations of vWF and factor VIII may persist for several hours.

DDAVP is indicated for prophylaxis and treatment of bleeding in patients with hemophilia A, von Willebrand's disease, and uremia. The dose of DDAVP is 0.3 μg/kg. Although initial reports indicated that DDAVP might reduce bleeding in cardiac surgery,[53] subsequent investigations did not confirm this benefit.[54] The inability of DDAVP to improve hemostasis when used routinely in cardiac surgery is consistent with the observation that vWF activity increases in these patients with or without DDAVP administration. Thus, use of this drug in cardiac surgery should be reserved for those patients with hemophilia, von Willebrand's disease, or other conditions in which factor VIII- or vWF-mediated hemostasis are known to be impaired.

Prophylactic platelet transfusion

Abnormalities in platelet function after CPB are very common. This functional deficit has been characterized as a CPB-related activation of platelets that leads to platelet degranulation,[6] loss of cell-surface adhesive receptors,[7] and refractoriness to agonist stimulation.[8] Prophylactic administration of antifibrinolytic agents is reported to preserve platelet function and reduce the need for perioperative transfusion.[35] Prophylactic platelet transfusion is not effective.[55]

Acute normovolemic hemodilution

Acute normovolemic hemodilution (ANH) is a procedure in which blood is removed intraoperatively and replaced with a noncellular fluid to maintain intravascular volume. The blood is collected in standard blood bags containing anticoagulant, stored at room temperature, and reinfused after major blood loss has ceased, or sooner if indicated. ANH was reported to reduce allogeneic blood transfusion in cardiac surgery.[56] However, the potential advantage of this technique is mitigated by the high prevalence of preoperative anemia in cardiac surgical patients, the potential to induce myocardial ischemia in patients with coronary artery disease, and conflicting reports about the benefit of ANH. A few studies have demonstrated that ANH, when combined with preoperative erythropoietin, can reduce the need for allogeneic blood transfusion in cardiac surgery.[57] However, data are too limited to advocate routine use of this technique.

Intraoperative blood salvage

This term describes the technique of salvaging and reinfusing the patient's own blood lost during surgery. The technique has appeal for its potential to limit exposure to allogeneic blood products. Unfortunately, a number of clinical trials have failed to demonstrate a reduction in allogeneic transfusion requirements when this technique is used in cardiac surgery.[58,59]

On-pump versus off-pump coronary artery bypass surgery

Hemostatic abnormalities in cardiac surgery are closely related to the use of CPB. Avoidance of CPB in cardiac surgery is a potential method to reduce perioperative bleeding and the need for transfusion. A prospective randomized trial of conventional coronary revascularization versus off-pump coronary grafting demonstrated lower blood loss and transfusion requirements in patients randomized to the off-pump procedure.[60]

MANAGEMENT OF POSTOPERATIVE HEMORRHAGE

Even in the presence of effective preventive therapies, bleeding can still occur both in the OR and postoperative care area. As described in the preceding section, there are numerous causes of bleeding after CPB, and narrowing the diagnosis to a single cause poses a significant challenge. The initial steps are supportive: assuring adequate intravascular volume and circulating red cell mass to maintain perfusion and tissue oxygen delivery. Communication among surgical, anesthesia, and ICU providers should occur early for all patients who experience significant bleeding. Efforts to restore normothermia should be aggressively pursued.

In cases where bleeding is brisk, the clinician is forced to treat empirically while waiting for results of diagnostic studies. Treatment should focus on the most likely causes of bleeding and those easiest to correct. Additional protamine sulfate to reverse residual heparin is the usual first step. Increments of 50 to 100 mg can be given, but the total dose of protamine should not exceed 1.3 mg/100 U heparin administered for CPB.

Table 20-3 General treatment guidelines for diagnostic laboratory abnormalities

Hemostatic test/result	Suggested therapy
Platelet count < 100,000	Transfuse 4–6 U of platelets
PT > 1.5 times normal	Transfuse 2–4 U of FFP
aPTT > 1.5 times normal	Additional protamine (if PT is not elevated), transfuse 2–4 U of FFP (if PT is elevated)
Fibrinogen < 100 mg/dL	Transfuse cryoprecipitate
TEG MA < 45 mm	Transfuse 4–6 U platelets or DDAVP 0.3 U/kg

PT = prothrombin time; aPTT = activated partial thromboplastin time; TEG MA = thromboelastogram maximum angle; FFP = fresh frozen plasma; DDAVP = desamino-8-arginine vasopressin.

Transfusion of platelets should follow and then fresh frozen plasma (FFP) if bleeding has not subsided. Under ideal circumstances and in cases where bleeding is not life-threatening, treatment should proceed based on results of diagnostic testing. A number of treatment algorithms have used a variety of laboratory tests to help guide management of the bleeding patients. Algorithm-driven strategies have reduced blood loss and transfusion in a number of studies, despite the fact that the strategies have all used different diagnostic tests and threshold values to guide therapy.[22–24] Anecdotal reports suggest that antifibrinolytic agents may have some role for salvage therapy in bleeding patients, but prospective trials do not support this use. Emerging evidence suggests that administration of recombinant activated factor VIIa may be effective for treatment of postoperative hemorrhage[61,62]; however, data are too limited to recommend its use in cardiac surgery at this time. General guidelines that link specific diagnostic test results with therapies are shown on Table 20-3.

It is important to recognize that most patients will have abnormal laboratory test results after CPB and many will not bleed. An abnormal laboratory test does not mandate therapy. Treatment should be reserved for those patients whose abnormal test result is obtained in the presence of clinically significant bleeding.

PERICARDIAL TAMPONADE

Pericardial tamponade is a condition in which increased pressure in the pericardial space compresses one or more cardiac chambers and causes hemodynamic abnormalities (see Spodick[63] for a recent review). Cardiac tamponade is usually caused by fluid that fills the entire pericardial space and surrounds the heart. However, in some instances the fluid may be localized and may compress only a portion of the heart. Tamponade caused by localized cardiac compression from an expanding pericardial hematoma is the type of tamponade frequently encountered in the first 24 h after cardiac surgery.[3] It is an important cause of low-cardiac-output syndrome, occurring in 2 percent of all cardiac surgical patients and more commonly in those requiring multiple transfusion for hemorrhage.[3] Delayed tamponade may occur 1 to 2 weeks after cardiac surgery, and is associated with systemic anticoagulation.[64] Tamponade should be considered in any cardiac surgical patient who has evidence of hemodynamic compromise with high filling pressures.

The fundamental pathophysiologic abnormality in pericardial tamponade is inadequate cardiac preload. As intrapericardial pressure rises, the transcardiac pressure gradient (i.e., the difference in pressure between inside and outside the heart) decreases and cardiac filling is impaired. When pericardial pressure is high enough, cardiac chamber collapse can occur. The highly compliant right heart chambers are more susceptible to collapse, classically with right atrial collapse occurring in late diastole and right ventricular collapse in early diastole. Reduction in cardiac preload leads to a reduction in stroke volume. Compensatory sympathetic activation ensues, which leads to tachycardia and vasoconstriction in an attempt to maintain cardiac output and blood pressure. When compensatory mechanisms are exhausted, hemodynamic collapse can follow.

Diagnosis of pericardial tamponade in cardiac surgical patients requires a high index of suspicion. In late tamponade, classical signs and symptoms may be present, including tachycardia, tachypnea, dyspnea, hypotension, and signs of systemic hypoperfusion: cool, mottled extremities, low urine output, and narrow pulse pressure. However, the presentation of early postoperative tamponade in the sedated, mechanically ventilated patient can be much more subtle, sometimes appearing only as a steady increase in pressor requirements in patients with ongoing blood loss. In either case, hemodynamic instability, usually in the presence of high central filling pressures, should alert the clinician to the possibility of cardiac tamponade. Pulsus paradoxus, a reduction in arterial blood pressure of >10 mmHg with inspiration, is a key finding in pericardial tamponade that can often be discerned by palpation or observation of the arterial blood pressure tracing. The electrocardiogram shows low voltage and may show electrical alternans from the heart swinging in pericardial fluid. Chest x-ray may show widening of the cardiac silhouette and mediastinum. The central venous pressure is almost always high (except in patients with concurrent hypovolemia), and equalization of diastolic pressures in the right atrium, right ventricle, pulmonary artery, and pulmonary capillary bed is classically observed. Echocardiography can be quite helpful in establishing the diagnosis of tamponade. Visualization of pericardial effusion or clot with cardiac chamber compression, usually diastolic collapse of the right atrium or ventricle, is a sensitive and specific test for tamponade.[65,66]

Definitive treatment of cardiac tamponade almost always requires evacuation of pericardial fluid. In cardiac surgical patients, pericardial fluid can be drained in one of three ways: (1) via percutaneous needle drainage, (2) by opening the inferior aspect of the sternotomy incision (performed emergently in the ICU), or (3) by intraoperative exploratory median sternotomy. Prior to definitive correction, supportive management includes intravascular volume expansion to augment preload and inotropic/pressor support, which is best accomplished with epinephrine infusion. The appropriate definitive therapy depends on the severity of hemodynamic compromise and the urgency with which therapy is required. Intraoperative exploratory median sternotomy is the most desirable option in patients who develop early postoperative tamponade, but this option may not be feasible in the patient with imminent hemodynamic collapse. In such a case, hemodynamic stabilization may be achieved through percutaneous or direct drainage prior to definitive mediastinal exploration. Indeed, such measures can be performed at the bedside, may be lifesaving, and should even be considered prior to the induction of anesthesia for intraoperative mediastinal exploration in those patients who exhibit severe hemodynamic instability. Patients who develop late tamponade (1 to 2 weeks or more after cardiac surgery) may be best managed by percutaneous catheter drainage. Patients who develop recurrent late effusions (i.e., those with postpericardiotomy syndrome) may need a pericardial window for definitive management of their effusion and tamponade.

References

1. Shroyer AL, Coombs LP, Peterson ED, et al. The Society of Thoracic Surgeons: 30-day operative mortality and morbidity risk models. *Ann Thorac Surg* 2003;75:1856–1864.
2. Unsworth-White MJ, Herriot A, Valencia O, et al. Resternotomy for bleeding after cardiac operation: A marker for increased morbidity and mortality. *Ann Thorac Surg* 1995;59:664–647.
3. Russo AM, O'Connor WH, Waxman HL. Atypical presentations and echocardiographic findings in patients with cardiac tamponade occurring early and late after cardiac surgery. *Chest* 1993;104:71–78.
4. Slaughter TF, Lebleu TH, Douglas JM, et al. Characterization of prothrombin activation during cardiac surgery by hemostatic molecular markers. *Anesthesiology* 1994;80:520–526.
5. Tanaka K, Takao M, Yada I, et al. Alterations in coagulation and fibrinolysis associated with cardiopulmonary bypass during open heart surgery. *J Cardiothorac Anesth* 1989;3:181–188.
6. Harker LA, Malpass TW, Branson HE. Mechanism of abnormal bleeding in patients undergoing cardiopulmonary bypass: Acquired transient platelet dysfunction associated with selective a-granule release. *Blood* 1980;56:824.
7. Rinder CS, Mathew JP, Rinder HM. Modulation of platelet surface adhesion receptors during cardiopulmonary bypass. *Anesthesiology* 1991;75:563.
8. Ferraris VA, Ferraris SP, Singh A, et al. The platelet thrombin receptor and postoperative bleeding. *Ann Thorac Surg* 1998;65:352–358.
9. Stibbe J, Kluft C, Brommer EJP, et al. Enhanced fibrinolytic activity during cardiopulmonary bypass in open-heart surgery in man is caused by extrinsic (tissue-type) plasminogen activator. *Eur J Clin Invest* 1984;14:375–382.
10. Gram J, Janetzko T, Jespersen J, et al. Enhanced effective fibrinolysis following the neutralization of heparin in open heart surgery increases the risk of post-surgical bleeding. *Thromb Haemostas* 1990;63:241–245.
11. Khuri SF, Wolfe JA, Josa M, et al. Hematologic changes during and after cardiopulmonary bypass and their relationship to the bleeding time and nonsurgical blood loss. *J Thorac Cardiovasc Surg* 1992;104:94–107.
12. Laffey JG, Boylan JF, Cheng DCH. The systemic inflammatory response to cardiac surgery. *Anesthesiology* 2002;97:215–252.
13. Reubens FD, Labow RS, Lavallee GR, et al. Hematologic evaluation of cardiopulmonary bypass circuits prepared with a novel block copolymer. *Ann Thorac Surg* 1999;67:989–996.
14. Kuitunen AH, Heikkila LJ, Salmenpera MT. Cardiopulmonary bypass with heparin-coated circuits and reduced systemic anticoagulation. *Ann Thorac Surg* 1997;63:438–444.
15. Bull BS, Korpman RA, Huse BD. Heparin therapy during extracorporeal circulation: I. Problems inherent in existing heparin protocols. *J Thorac Cardiovasc Surg* 1975;69:674–684.
16. Metz S, Keats AS. Low activated coagulation time during cardiopulmonary bypass does not increase postoperative bleeding. *Ann Thorac Surg* 1990;49:440.
17. Dutton DA, Hotersall AP, McLaren AD. Protamine activation after cardiopulmonary bypass. *Anaesthesia* 1983;38:264–269.
18. Shore-Lesserson L, Reich DL, DePerio M. Heparin and protamine titration do not improve haemostasis in cardiac surgical patients. *Can J Anaesth* 1998;45:10–18.
19. Gravlee GP, Arora S, Lavender SW, et al. Predictive value of blood clotting tests in cardiac surgical patients. *Ann Thorac Surg.* 1994;58:216–221.
20. Ray MJ, Hawson GAT, Just SJE, et al. Relationship of platelet aggregation to bleeding after cardiopulmonary bypass. *Ann Thorac Surg* 1994;57:981–986.
21. Faraday N, Guallar E, Sera VA, et al. Utility of whole blood hemostatometry using the clot signature analyzer for assessment of hemostasis in cardiac surgery. *Anesthesiology* 2002;96:1115–1122.
22. Despotis GJ, Grishaber JE, Goodnough LT. The effect of an intraoperative treatment algorithm on physicians' transfusion practice in cardiac surgery. *Transfusion* 1994;34:290–296.
23. Shore-Lesserson L, Manspeizer HE, DePerio M, et al. Thromboelastography-guided algorithm reduces transfusions in complex cardiac surgery. *Anesth Analg* 1999;88:312–319.

24. Nuttall GA, Oliver WC, Santrach PJ, et al. Efficacy of a simple intraoperative transfusion algorithm for nonerythrocyte component utilization after cardiopulmonary bypass. *Anesthesiology* 2001;94:773–781.
25. Hattersley PG. Activated coagulation time of whole blood. *JAMA* 1966;196:436.
26. Culliford AT, Gitel SN, Starr N. Lack of correlation between activated clotting time and plasma heparin during cardiopulmonary bypass. *Ann Surg* 1981;193:105.
27. Pilgram-Larsen J, Wisloff F, Jorgensen JJ. Effect of high dose ampicillin and cloxacillin on bleeding time in open-heart surgery. *Scand J Thorac Cardiovasc Surg* 1985;19:45–48.
28. Burns ER, Billet HH, Frater RW, et al. The preoperative bleeding time as a predictor of postoperative hemorrhage after cardiopulmonary bypass. *J Thorac Cardiovasc Surg* 1986;92:319–312.
29. Weksler BB, Pett SB, Alonso D, et al. Differential inhibition by aspirin of vascular and platelet prostaglandin synthesis in atherosclerotic patients. *N Engl J Med* 1983;308:800–805.
30. Reich DL, Patel GC, Vela-Cantos F, et al. Aspirin does not increase homologous blood requirements in elective coronary bypass surgery. *Anesth Analg* 1994;79:4–8.
31. Peterson P, Hayes TE, Arkin CF, et al. The preoperative bleeding time test lacks clinical benefit: College of American Pathologists' and American Society of Clinical Pathologists' position article. *Arch Surg* 1998;133:134–139.
32. Lasne D, Fiemeyer A, Chatellier G, et al. A study of platelet functions with a new analyzer using high shear stress (PFA 100) in patients undergoing coronary artery bypass graft. *Thromb Haemost* 2000;84:794–799.
33. Nuttall GA, Oliver WC, Ereth MH, et al. Coagulation tests predict bleeding after cardiopulmonary bypass. *J Cardiothorac Vasc Anesth* 1997;11:815–823.
34. Hett DA, Walker D, Pilkington SN, et al. Sonoclot analysis. *Br J Anaesth* 1995;75:771–776.
35. Van Oeveren W, Harder MP, Roozendaal KJ. Aprotinin protects platelets against the initial effect of cardiopulmonary bypass. *J Thorac Cardiovasc Surg* 1990;99:788.
36. Bidstrup BP, Royston D, Sapsford RN. Reduction in blood loss after cardiopulmonary bypass with high dose aprotinin (Trasylol). *J Thorac Cardiovasc Surg* 1989; 97:364.
37. Royston D. High-dose aprotinin therapy: A review of the first five years' experience. *J Cardiothorac Anesth* 1992;6:76.
38. Levy JH, Pifarr R, Schaff H, et al. A multicenter, placebo-controlled double-blind trial of aprotinin in patients undergoing repeat coronary artery bypass grafting. *Circulation* 1995;92:2236–2244.
39. Hardy JF, Desroches J. Natural and synthetic antifibrinolytics in cardiac surgery. *Can J Anaesth* 1992;3: 353–365.
40. Royston D, Bidstrup BP, Taylor KM. Effect of aprotinin on the need for blood transfusion after repeat open heart surgery. *Lancet* 1987;2:1289.
41. Royston D, Bidstrup BP, Sapsford RN. Reduced blood loss after open heart surgery with aprotinin is associated with an increase in the activated clotting time (ACT). *J Cardiothorac Anesth* 1989;3:80.
42. Royston D. The serine antiprotease aprotinin (Trasylol): A novel approach to reducing postoperative bleeding. *Blood Coag Fibrinol* 1990;1:55.
43. Bidstrup BP, Royston D, McGuiness C. Aprotinin in aspirin treated patients. *Perfusion* 1990;5:77.
44. Munoz JJ, Birkmeyer NJO, Birkmeyer JD, et al. Is e-amiocaproic acid as effective as aprotinin in reducing bleeding with cardiac surgery? A meta-analysis. *Circulation* 1999;99:81–89.
45. Levi M, Cromheecke ME, de Jonge E, et al. Pharmacological strategies to decrease excessive blood loss in cardiac surgery: A meta-analysis of clinically relevant endpoints. *Lancet* 1999;354:1940–1947.
46. Dietrich W, Dilthey G, Spannagl M. Influence of high-dose aprotinin on anticoagulation, heparin requirement, and celite- and kaolin-activated clotting time in heparin pretreated patients undergoing open-heart surgery: A double-blind, placebo-controlled study. *Anesthesiology* 1995;83:679.
47. Dietrich W, Spath P, Ebell A. Prevalence of anaphylactic reactions to aprotinin: analysis of two hundred forty-eight reexposures to aprotinin in heart operations. *J Thorac Cardiovasc Surg* 1997;113:194.
48. Horrow JC, Van Riper DF, Strong MD. The dose-relationship of tranexamic acid. *Anesthesiology* 1995;82: 383–392.
49. Horrow JC, Van Riper DF, Strong MD. The hemostatic effects of tranexamic acid and desmopressin during cardiac surgery. *Circulation* 1991;84:2063–2070.
50. DelRossi AJ, Cernaianu AC, Botros S. Prophylactic treatment of post-perfusion bleeding using EACA. *Chest* 1989; 96:27–30.
51. Shore-Lesserson L, Reich DL, Vela-Cantos F. Tranexamic acid reduces transfusions and mediastinal drainage in repeat cardiac surgery. *Anesth Analg* 1996;83:18–26.
52. Reid RW, Zimmerman AA, Laussen PC. The efficay of tranexamic acid versus placebo in decreasing blood loss in pediatric patients undergoing repeat cardiac surgery. *Anesth Analg* 1997;84:990–996.
53. Salzman EW, Weinstein MJ, Weintraub RM. Treatment with desmopressin acetate to reduce blood loss after cardiac surgery. *N Engl J Med* 1986;314:1402–1406.
54. Hackmann T, Gascoyne RD, Naiman SC. A trial of desmopressin (1-desamino-8-D-arginine vasopressin) to reduce blood loss in uncomplicated cardiac surgery. *N Engl J Med* 1989;321:1437.
55. Simon TL, Akl BF, Murphy W. Controlled trial of routine administration of platelet concentrates in cardiopulmonary bypass surgery. *Ann Thorac Surg* 1984;37: 359–364.
56. Petry AF, Jost T, Sievers H. Reduction of homologous blood requirements by blood pooling at the onset of cardiopulmonary bypass. *J Thorac Cardiovasc Surg* 1994;107:1210–1214.
57. Sowade O, Warneke H, Scigalla P. Avoidance of allogeneic blood transfusions by treatment with recombinant human erythropoietin in patients undergoing open heart surgery. *Blood* 1997;89:411–418.
58. Bell K, Stott K, Sinclair CJ. A controlled trial of intraoperative autologous transfusion in cardiothoracic surgery measuring effect on transfusion requirements and clinical outcomes. *Transf Med* 1992;2:295–300.

59. Body SC, Birmingham J, Parks R. Safety and efficacy of autotransfusion of shed mediastinal blood after cardiac surgery: A multicenter analysis. *J Cardiothorac Vasc Anesth* 1999;13:410–416.
60. Ascione R, Williams S, Lloyd CT, et al. Reduced postoperative blood loss and transfusion requirement after beating-heart coronary operations: A prospective randomized study. *J Thorac Cardiovasc Surg.* 2001;121:689–696.
61. Al Douri M, Shafi T, Al Khudairi D, et al. Effect of the administration of recombinant activated factor VII (rFVIIa; NovoSeven) in the management of severe uncontrolled bleeding in patients undergoing heart valve replacement. *Blood Coagul Fibrinolysis.* 2000;11(Suppl 1):S121–S127.
62. Tanaka KA, Waly AA, Cooper WA, et al. Treatment of excessive bleeding in Jehovah's Witness patients after cardiac surgery with recombinant factor VIIa (NovoSeven). *Anesthesiology* 2003;98:1513–1515.
63. Spodick DH. Acute cardiac tamponade. *N Engl J Med* 2003;349:684–690.
64. Borkon AM, Schaff HV, Gardner TJ. Diagnosis and management of postoperative pericardial effusions and late cardiac tamponade following open heart surgery. *Ann Thorac Surg* 1981;31:512.
65. Gillam LD, Guyer DE, Gibson TC. Hydrodynamic compression of the right atrium: A new echocardiographic sign of cardiac tamponade. *Circulation*1983;68:294.
66. Leimgruber P, Klopfenstein HS, Wann LS. The hemodynamic derangement associated with right ventricular diastolic collapse in cardiac tamponade: An experimental echocardiographic study. *Circulation* 1983;68:612.

CHAPTER

21 CARDIOPULMONARY BYPASS

Edward H. Kincaid, John W. Hammon

Cardiopulmonary bypass (CPB) has developed into an invaluable tool for operations on the thoracic viscera. By interfacing with the cardiovascular system, total CPB completely replaces the function of the heart and lungs for a short time. Modifications of CPB have been designed to partially replace or control more specific aspects of the cardiopulmonary systems. To fully utilize the tremendous flexibility available with "the pump," one must understand its components, operation, and potential for complications.

HISTORY

The development of CPB is a testament to personal perseverance and collaboration and demonstrates how cardiac surgery has truly evolved as a science. Initial progress in the field of extracorporeal circulation required mastery of the principles of total-body oxygen delivery and consumption. Later, further refinements in the understanding of metabolic demands at the cellular level served to enhance the safety and flexibility of circulatory support. Undoubtedly the most important milestone in the development of CPB is John Gibbon's use of the first clinical application of CPB. In 1953, after devoting most of his career to this work, he successfully repaired an atrial septal defect in a young woman with a pump-oxygenator. Additional milestones include the work of Bigelow, who, in the early 1950s, reported on systemic hypothermia with topical cooling as a means to reduce oxygen demand during the periods of reduced oxygen delivery inevitably encountered during operations on the heart. Shortly thereafter, Lillehei began performing congenital repairs using "cross circulation," employing a parent's cardiopulmonary system to support a child's during cardiac surgery. Finally, in the mid-1950s, Kirklin and colleagues at the Mayo Clinic ushered in the era of routine congenital repairs using the Mayo-Gibbon pump-oxygenator. Modern refinements in equipment and techniques have subsequently evolved as a consequence of the proliferation of coronary revascularization surgery and increased industrial interest.

COMPONENTS OF THE CPB CIRCUIT

Current-generation CPB circuits maintain much of the simplicity of older perfusion equipment but have much more flexibility and ability to more precisely control various perfusion parameters. Core components of any circuit include cannulas, tubing, a pump, and an oxygentator (Fig. 21-1). In reality, however, even basic circuits used in routine clinical practice include many other features such as additional pump heads for suction, venting of the heart, and delivery of cardioplegia. Venous reservoirs are also needed to maintain adequate circuit volume and remove air. Filters are required at various levels to prevent embolic complications. Finally, a heat exchanger facilitates systemic and myocardial cooling and rewarming.

CANNULAS

Arterial cannulation

Cannulation for CBP is typically performed centrally with an inflow cannula in the ascending aorta and outflow cannula(s) in the right atrium. Basic requirements for an arterial cannula include a size large enough to permit adequate flows without creating excessive back pressure at the pump head. At the same time, the size and design of the cannula must allow for easy placement with minimal vessel trauma. Beyond these basic requirements, a multitude of other aspects of cannula design may arguably affect performance. Such features include tip angle, size and number of end or side holes, wire reinforcement, and filters. Most arterial

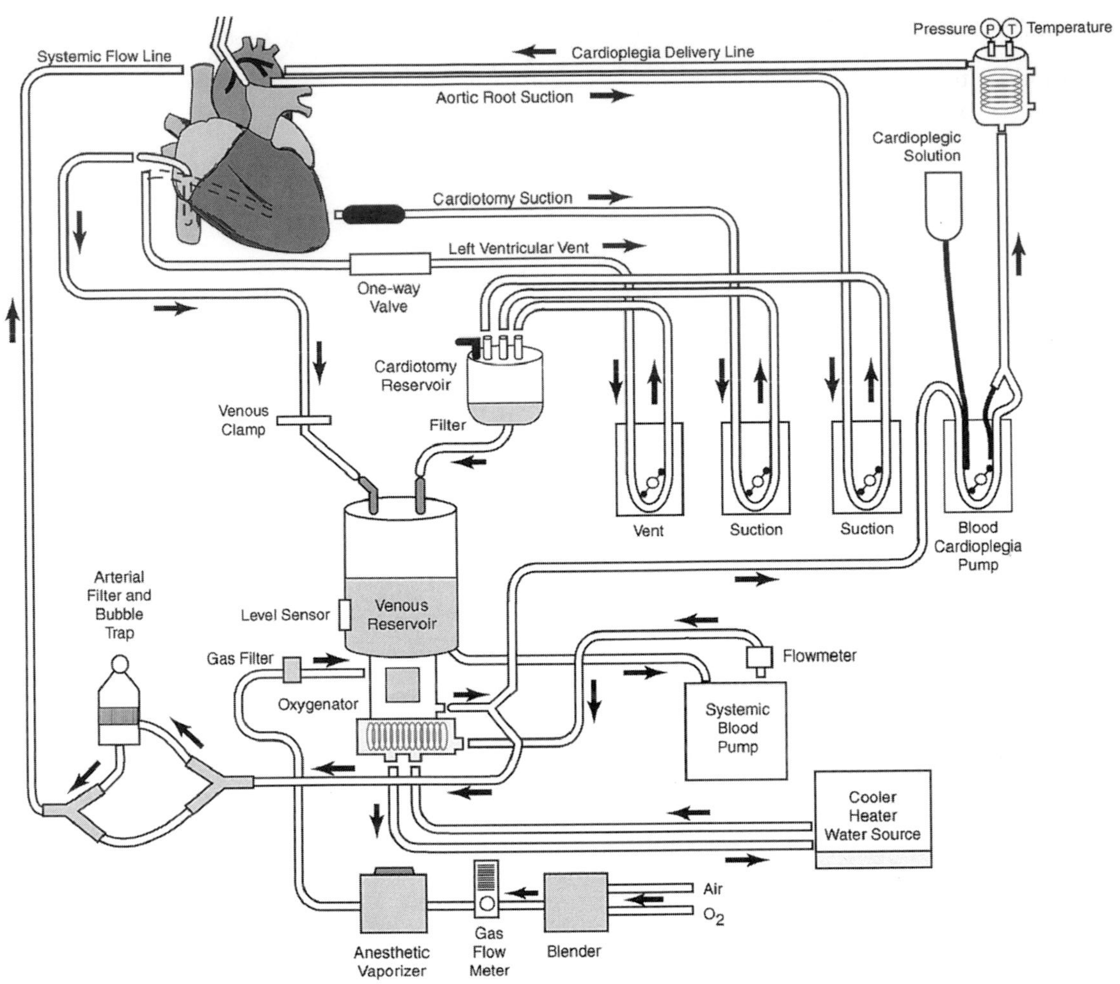

Figure 21-1 Schematic of typical CPB circuit. (Reprinted with permission from Cohn LH, Edmunds LD Jr (eds). *Cardiac Surgery in the Adult*, 2d ed. New York: McGraw-Hill, 2003. With permission.)

catheters are rated by a performance index, which relates external diameter, flow, and pressure differential. High-velocity jets may damage the aortic wall, dislodge atheroemboli, produce dissections, disturb flow to nearby vessels and cause cavitation and hemolysis. Aortic catheters with only side ports are designed to minimize jet effects and better distribute arch vessel perfusion and pressure; they may be associated with fewer strokes.[1]

Aortic cannulation

Various locations on the ascending aorta and aortic arch are most often used as sites for insertion of the arterial cannula because of simplicity and maintenance of antegrade blood flow. In patients with no significant ascending aortic atherosclerosis, this location is also associated with the least risk of inflow-related complications in routine cardiac cases. However, multiple other locations can be good alternatives, including the common femoral, axillary, and innominate arteries; descending thoracic aorta; and rarely the left ventricular (LV) apex. The choice is influenced by the planned operation and the distribution of atherosclerotic disease.

To cannulate the ascending aorta, most surgeons place two purse-string sutures with or without pledgets partially through the aortic wall to encompass a diameter of approximately 1 to 1.5 cm. Next, with a systolic blood pressure preferably less than 100 mmHg, a 4- to 5-mm full-thickness stab wound is made, occasionally dilated, and then controlled under finger or forceps pressure. The cannula is then inserted under the finger or forceps approximately 1 to 2 cm into the lumen of the aorta. Backbleeding is detected to ensure that the tip is completely within the lumen and positioned to direct flow to the midtransverse aorta. A long catheter with the tip placed beyond the left subclavian artery may also be used. Proper cannula placement is critical and is confirmed by noting pulsatile pressure in the aortic line monitor and equivalent pressure in the radial artery.

Complications of ascending aortic cannulation include bleeding from tears in the aortic wall, malposition of the cannula tip, atheromatous or air emboli, and aortic dissection. It is essential to monitor aortic line and radial artery pressures and to carefully observe the aorta for possible cannula-related complications during the onset of CPB and placement of aortic clamps. Asymmetrical cooling of the face or neck may suggest a problem with cerebral perfusion. Late bleeding and infected or uninfected false aneurysms are delayed complications of aortic cannulation.

Femoral artery cannulation

The common femoral artery is probably the second most common location for CPB inflow. Reasons for cannulating the femoral artery include inadequacy or inavailability of the ascending aorta in cases such as aortic dissection, reoperation, descending aortic surgery, and minimally invasive cardiac procedures. Severe atherosclerosis of the ascending aorta is generally not a good indication for femoral cannulation because of the likely coexistence of severe disease in distal segments of the aorta and iliac arteries. Alternative strategies for CPB in this scenario are discussed later in this chapter.

Exposure of the femoral artery is through a small oblique incision just below the inguinal ligament. Only the anterior surface of the vessel need be exposed. After placement of a 5-0 monofilament purse-string suture, the common femoral artery is punctured and a guidewire is passed to the aorta. Transesophageal echocardiography (TEE) guidance can be used to confirm the location of the wire. A long, thin-walled cannula is then passed over the wire into the distal aorta. Most adult men can be perfused adequately with a 21F cannula; in women, a 19F cannula usually suffices.

Disadvantages of femoral cannulation include local complications such as vessel injury or groin wound complications and perfusion-related problems. These include abdominal aortic dissection or perforation, embolic phenomena from retrograde flow through a diseased abdominal aorta, and malperfusion of aortic branches in acute aortic dissection. Additionally, ischemic complications of the distal leg may occur during prolonged retrograde perfusions; these may result in the release of myoglobin and subsequent renal injury. Finally, some speculate that retrograde flow to the cerebral and coronary arteries may result in lower perfusion pressures or oxygen saturation of blood at the end of the perfusion stream.

Other sites of arterial cannulation

The axillary subclavian artery is increasingly used for cannulation.[2,3] Advantages include freedom from atherosclerosis, antegrade flow into the arch vessels, and protection of the arm and hand by collateral flow. Because of these advantages and the dangers of retrograde perfusion in patients with aortic dissection, some surgeons prefer this cannulation site for this and other conditions involving the aortic arch. The right axillary artery is usually used and is approached through a subclavicular incision, taking care not to damage the adjacent brachial plexus. In order to prevent injury to the fragile axillary or subclavian artery, some prefer to anastamose a small-caliber graft end to side to the axillary artery followed by insertion of the cannula into the graft.

Venous cannulation

In most applications, venous blood enters the circuit through negative pressure generated by siphonage. Thus, venous return flow rates are determined largely by the height differential between the right atrium and venous reservoir. Venous return can be impeded by resistance in cannulas, tubing, and connectors and may cease completely with entrainment of significant amounts of air into the venous line, creating an "air lock." This situation can be managed by correcting the source of air entrainment (e.g., with a loose purse-string suture) and then elevating the venous tubing such that the air rises in the direction of the venous reservoir. Continued arterial inflow from the pump creates positive central venous pressure, which will eventually drive the air into the reservoir, where it evacuates. Venous cannulas are usually made of flexible plastic, which may be stiffened against kinking by wire reinforcement. The size required is determined by the patient's size, the anticipated flow rate, and cannula flow characteristics, such as resistance. Catheters are typically inserted through purse string–guarded incisions in the right atrial appendage, lateral atrial wall, or directly in the superior vena cava (SVC) and inferior vena cava (IVC).

Two basic approaches for central venous cannulation are used. For coronary artery or aortic valve operations, single venous cannulation of the right atrium alone suffices. In adults, this is usually performed with a 40F to 46F "two-stage" device that has a set of drainage holes in the distal portion and a second set located more proximally (Fig. 21-2). The distal end is positioned in the IVC while the proximal side holes drain the right atrium. This cannula may provide for better drainage than a single-stage cannula, especially when positioning of the heart may kink the venae cavae. Bicaval cannulation is used primarily for isolating the right atrium when surgery dictates opening this chamber. Caval tourniquets are also necessary in this situation to prevent bleeding and air entry into the system.

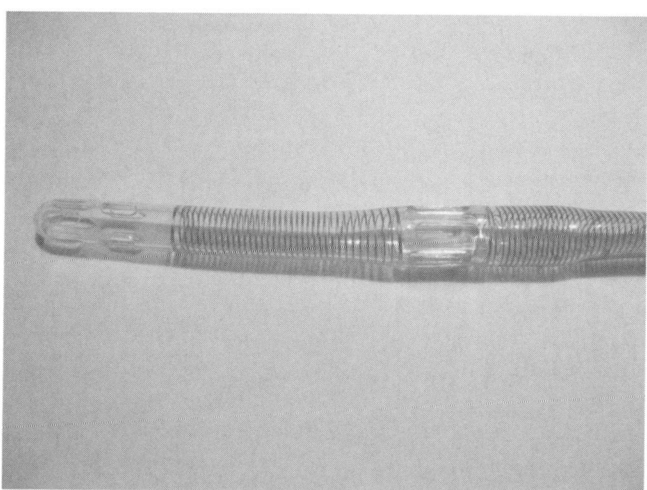

Figure 21-2 Two-stage venous cannula with separate drainage holes for the inferior vena cava and right atrium.

Because of coronary sinus return, caval tourniquets should not be tightened without decompressing the right atrium. Bicaval cannulation is often preferred to facilitate venous return during exposure of the left atrium and mitral valve, mainly because of the potential for obstruction of the SVC or IVC during exposure. Using both techniques, the operative team should carefully monitor central venous pressure to prevent obstruction of the SVC.

Placement of a single venous cannula is most easily accomplished through the right atrial appendage. After application of a vascular clamp, the right atrial appendage is excised, or it may be opened longitudinally when the appendage is small. A purse-string suture is then placed just below the free edges, which are controlled with forceps. After release of the clamp, the cannula is inserted towards the IVC. The height of blood within the unclamped cannula is a good measure of central venous pressure. During bicaval cannulation, the IVC cannula is generally placed on the lateral wall of the right atrium near the junction with the IVC. During placement of the purse-string suture, the right atrium is gently retracted with the assistant's hand or forceps while monitoring hemodynamics. A stab incision is made in the middle of the purse-string, the defect is dilated with a curved clamp, and the cannula, either straight or right-angled, is then directed into the IVC. The cannula should not be inserted with the proximal side holes located too distally within the IVC, as this may impede hepatic venous drainage. SVC cannulation is typically accomplished with either a straight cannula placed through the lateral wall of the atrium, as in IVC cannulation, or with a right-angled cannula placed directly into the SVC. In this procedure, the anterior surface of the SVC is exposed by dividing the pericardial reflection overlying its superior border. An oval-monofilament purse-string suture oriented longitudinally is placed, and an incision is made along the length of the purse-string suture while controlling the free edges with forceps. The tip of the cannula is then directed superiorly, taking care to avoid tip placement in the azygos vein.

Access to the central venous system for blood return can also be obtained through the common femoral or internal jugular veins. Remote cannulation for CPB is particularly beneficial for reoperative cardiac procedures, minimally invasive "on-pump" cardiac procedures such as mitral valve repair via right thoracotomy/thoracoscopy, and aortic surgery through a left thoracotomy. Depending on the size of the cannula, either open or percutaneous methods can be used. Most surgeons would recommend a maximum size of 21F to 22F for percutaneous venous access without the need for direct vessel repair after decannulation. Typically, a long, wire-reinforced cannula with an ultrathin wall is advanced over a guidewire through the femoral vein to the right atrium under transesophageal TEE guidance. For bicaval drainage, some femoral venous cannulas are designed to be advanced into the SVC; multiple levels of side holes subsequently drain both venae cavae individually. An alternative strategy for bicaval drainage employs two individual venous cannulas, one in the femoral vein to drain the IVC and one in the right internal jugular vein to drain the SVC.

As an adjunct to remote cannulation for venous drainage, most surgeons employ some means of active assist over the standard gravity or siphonage power for blood return. "Assisted venous return" can be achieved by applying a regulated vacuum to a closed hard-shell venous reservoir or by kinetically assisting return via a centrifugal pump placed in the venous return line. Assisted venous return is also useful in cases using standard central cannulation sites but where the use of smaller cannulas may be beneficial, such as a MAZE procedure or operation through a ministernotomy. The most significant disadvantage of assisted venous drainage is an increased risk of air entrainment and subsequent microembolization to the arterial circulation.[4,5]

TUBING AND CONNECTORS

The various components of the heart-lung machine are connected by polyvinyl tubing and fluted polycarbonate connectors. Medical-grade polyvinyl chloride (PVC) tubing is universally used because it is flexible, compatible with blood, inert, smooth, transparent, resistant to kinking and collapse, and can be heat-sterilized. In adults, 1/2-in. tubing is generally used for inflow and 5/8-in. tubing for outflow. Wider tubing improves flow dynamics but also increases priming volume. Tubing lengths between patient and pump should also be minimized so as to reduce priming volume.

One controversy that continues over tubing is the use of herparin bonding to the interior surfaces, a technique that has many theoretical advantages associated with a reduced blood-plastic interface. The use of heparin-coated circuits during CPB has some proven advantages,[6–8] such as reduced activation of complement pathways. However, there is only weak evidence that heparin-coated perfusion circuits reduce the need for systemic heparin or reduce bleeding or thrombotic problems associated with CPB, and the overall inflammatory response to CPB is not reduced.

PUMPS

Two types of pumps can by used, and each has its own set of advantages and disadvantages. Centrifugal pumps consist of a vaned impeller or of nested, smooth plastic cones, which, when rotated rapidly, propel blood by centrifugal force. An arterial flowmeter is required to determine forward blood flow, which varies with the speed of rotation and the afterload of the arterial line. Centrifugal pumps produce pulseless flow and generate less negative pressure; therefore they may produce less cavitation and fewer gaseous microemboli. They can pump small amounts of air but become "deprimed" if more than 30 to 50 mL of air enters the blood chamber.

Centrifugal pumps are probably superior for temporary extracorporeal assist devices, left-heart bypass, for assisting venous return. They are often used as the arterial inflow pump on the CPB circuit.

Roller pumps consist of two rollers situated 180 degrees apart inside a curved raceway. Forward flow is generated by roller compression of tubing, which can be sized from 1/4 to 5/8 in., ID depending on flow requirements. Flow rate depends on the diameter of the tubing, rate of rotation, length of the compression raceway, and completeness of compression, which is adjusted to be barely nonocclusive against a standing column of fluid that produces 45 to 75 mmHg of back pressure. At this degree of compression, hemolysis and tubing wear are minimal. Flow rate is determined from calibration curves for each pump for different tubing sizes and rates of rotation. Roller pumps are inexpensive, reliable, safe; they are insensitive to afterload, have small priming volumes, but can produce high negative pressures and may shed microparticles from compressed tubing. Roller pumps are used almost exclusively for vents, sucker systems, and the delivery of cardioplegia.

One advantage roller pumps have is the ability to produce pulsatile blood flow. Normally, standard roller pumps produce a sine-wave pulse of around 5 mmHg, but they can be set to generate pulse pressures above 20 mmHg as detected on peripheral arterial pressure monitors. Theoretically, pulsatile perfusion delivers more energy to cells and may result in improvements in peripheral resistance, renin release, and cellular hypoxia. However, studies on the clinical benefits of pulsatile perfusion are inconclusive. Complications that may occur during operation of either type of pump include loss of electricity; loss of the ability to control pump speed, producing "runaway pump" or "pump creep" when turned off; loss of the flowmeter or revolutions per minute (RPM) indicator; rupture of tubing in the roller pump raceway; and reversal of flow by improper tubing in the raceway. A means to provide pumping manually in case of electrical failure should always be available.

VENOUS RESERVOIR

The venous reservoir serves as a receiving chamber for venous return; facilitates gravity drainage; is a venous bubble trap; provides a convenient place to add drugs, fluids, or blood; and adds storage capacity for the perfusion system. During full CPB, as much as 1 to 3 L of blood may be stored in the reservoir, depending somewhat on the patient's preoperative volume status. Reservoirs may be rigid (hard) plastic canisters ("open" types) or soft, collapsible plastic bags ("closed" types). The rigid canisters facilitate volume measurements and the management of venous air, often have larger capacity, are easier to prime, permit suction for vacuum-assisted venous drainage, and may be less expensive. Soft bag reservoirs minimize the blood-gas interface and reduce the risk of pumping massive air emboli. A closed system is preferred to avoid the large amount of air-blood contact in open systems.

OXYGENATORS

Membrane oxygenators are most commonly used and imitate the natural lung by interspersing a thin membrane of either microporous polypropylene (0.3- to 0.8-μm pores) or silicone rubber between the gas and blood phases. Compared with bubble oxygenators, membrane oxygenators are safer, produce less particulate and gaseous microemboli, are less reactive to blood elements, and allow superior control of blood gases. The plasma-filled pores prevent gas from entering blood but facilitate transfer of both oxygen and CO_2. The most popular design uses sheaves of hollow fibers (120 to 200 μm) connected to inlet and outlet manifolds within a hard-shell jacket. Arterial PCO_2 is controlled by gas flow, and PO_2 is controlled by the fraction of inspired oxygen (FIO_2) produced by an air-oxygen blender, which also adds in variable amounts of volatile anesthetics. Modern membrane oxygenators add up to 470 mL of O_2 and remove up to 350 mL of CO_2 at 1 to 7 L of flow with priming volumes of 220 to 560 mL. Most units combine a venous reservoir, heat exchanger, and hollow-fiber membrane oxygenator into one compact unit.

Bubble oxygenators are obsolete in most western countries but are used elsewhere for short-term CPB because of their low cost and good efficiency. Because each bubble presents a new foreign surface to which blood elements react, bubble oxygenators cause progressive injury to blood elements and entrain more gaseous microemboli. In bubble oxygenators, venous blood drains directly into a chamber into which oxygen is infused through a diffusion plate that produces thousands of small oxygen bubbles within the blood. Gas exchange occurs across a thin film at the blood-gas interface around each bubble. Bubbles and blood are separated by settling, filtration, and defoaming surfactants in a reservoir. Commercial bubble oxygenators incorporate a reservoir and heat exchanger within the same unit and are placed upstream to the arterial pump.

HEAT EXCHANGERS

Heat exchangers control body temperature by heating or cooling blood passing through the perfusion circuit. Frequently hypothermia is used during cardiac surgery to reduce oxygen demand or facilitate operative exposure by temporary circulatory arrest. Gases are more soluble in cold than in warm blood; therefore rapid rewarming of cold blood in the circuit or body may cause the formation of bubble emboli. Most membrane oxygenator units incorporate a heat exchanger upstream of the oxygenator so as to minimize bubble emboli. Blood is not heated above 40°C to prevent denaturation of plasma proteins, and temperature differences within the body and perfusion circuit are limited to 5 to 10°C to prevent bubble emboli. The heat exchanger may be supplied by hot and cold tap water, but separate heater/cooler units with convenient temperature-regulating controls are preferred.

FILTERS

Filters are universally used within CPB circuits to prevent both macro- and microemboli, which, in both gaseous and particulate form, likely produce much of the morbidity associated with cardiac operations using CPB. As compared with no filter, studies indicate that all commercially available filters effectively remove gaseous and particulate emboli. Most investigations find that the Dacron wool depth filter is most effective, particularly in removing micro- and macroscopic air. Pressure differences across filters vary between 24 and 36 mmHg at a flow of 5 L/min. Filters cause slight hemolysis and tend to trap some platelets.

Because of significant debris present within cardiotomy suction blood, the need for microfilters in the cardiotomy suction reservoir is universally accepted, and most commercial units contain an intergrated micropore filter. Most circuits also contain an arterial line filter of some type, although efficacy in this location remains unsettled. These filters are usually also of the Dacron wool type and must be used with a bypass line during priming to purge trapped air. Leukocyte-depleting arterial filters have not been proven effective at limiting the inflammatory response or other complications.

CARDIOTOMY RESERVOIR AND FIELD SUCTION

Blood aspirated from the surgical wound may be directed to the cardiotomy reservoir for defoaming, filtration, and storage before it is added directly to the perfusate. A sponge impregnated with a surfactant removes bubbles by reducing surface tension at the blood interface, and macro-, micro-, or combined filters remove particulate emboli. Negative pressure is generated by either a roller pump or by vacuum applied to the rigid outer shell of the reservoir. The degree of negative pressure and blood level must be monitored to avoid excessive suction or introducing air into the perfusate.

The cardiotomy suction and reservoir is a major source of hemolysis, particulate and gaseous microemboli, fat globules, cellular aggregates, platelet injury and loss, cytokine-generated thrombin formation, and fibrinolysis. Air aspirated with wound blood contributes to blood activation and destruction and is difficult to remove because of the high proportion of nitrogen, which is poorly soluble in blood. High suction volumes and the admixture of air are particularly destructive of platelets and red cells. Commercial reservoirs are designed to minimize air entrainment and excessive injury to blood elements. The removal of air and microemboli is also facilitated by allowing aspirated blood to settle within the reservoir before it is added to the perfusate.

An alternative method for recovering field-aspirated blood is to dilute the blood with saline and then remove the saline to return only packed red cells to the perfusate. Centrifugal cell washers automate this process and remove air, thrombin, and nearly all biological and nonbiological microemboli from the aspirate at the cost of discarding plasma. A third alternative is to discard all field-aspirated blood. Increasingly, field-aspirated blood is recognized as a major contributor to the thrombotic, bleeding, and inflammatory complications of CPB.

VENTS AND DECOMPRESSION OF THE HEART

During CPB, blood escaping atrial or venous cannulas and from the coronary sinus and thebesian veins may pass through the unopened right heart into the pulmonary circulation. This blood plus bronchial venous blood, blood regurgitating through the aortic valve, and blood from undiagnosed abnormal sources (patent foramen ovale, patent ductus, etc.) may distend the left ventricle. Venting of the heart during CPB aids in myocardial protection by preventing ventricular distention and keeping warm blood out of the heart during hypothermic cardioplegic arrest. Ventricular overdistention can be a particularly serious problem in the presence of severe aortic valvular insufficiency.

There are several methods for venting the left heart during cardiac arrest. The most common techniques include placement of a multihole catheter from the right superior pulmonary vein across the mitral valve; use of an aortic root vent, often in combination with an antegrade cardioplegia catheter; placement of a suction catheter in the main pulmonary artery, which decompresses the left atrium across the pulmonary capillary bed; and, less commonly, placement of a suction catheter directly into left ventricular apex. Vent catheters are drained to the cardiotomy reservoir, usually by a dedicated roller pump. The most common complication of left heart venting is residual air when

Table 21-1 Strategies for management of intracardiac air

Preventive measures
Limited use of vents
Vents off or on low suction while aorta or heart chamber is open
Instillation of CO_2 into the operative field
De-airing maneuvers
Aortic venting during and after cross-clamp release
Needle aspiration of left ventricular apex
Valsalva breaths
Rotation of operating table
Manual dislodgment, e.g., inversion of left atrial appendage
Maintenance of partial cardiopulmonary bypass with left ventricular ejection

the heart is filled and begins to contract. De-airing maneuvers (Table 21-1)—such as manual displacement, Valsalva breaths, and TEE detection of residual pockets—are important methods for ensuring its removal.

CARDIOPLEGIA DELIVERY SYSTEMS

Cardioplegic solutions are delivered through a separate perfusion system that includes a reservoir, heat exchanger, roller pump, bubble trap, and perhaps microfilter. The system may be completely independent of the main perfusion circuit, or it may branch from the arterial line. The system may also be configured to vent the aortic root between infusions.

HEMOCONCENTRATORS

Hemoconcentrators, like oxygenators, contain one of several available semipermeable membranes (typically hollow fibers) that transfer water, electrolytes (e.g., potassium), and molecules up to 20 kDa out of the blood compartment. Hemoconcentrators may be connected to either venous or arterial lines or a reservoir in the main perfusion circuit, but they require high pressure in the blood compartment to effect fluid removal. Thus a roller pump is needed unless the unit is connected to the arterial line. Suction may or may not be applied to the air side of the membrane to facilitate filtration. At flows from 500 mL/min, up to 180 mL/min of fluid can be removed. Hemoconcentrators conserve platelets and most plasma proteins as compared to centrifugal cell washers and may allow greater control of potassium concentrations than is possible with the use of diuretics. Aside from cost, disadvantages are few and adverse effects rare.

CONDUCT OF CARDIOPULMONARY BYPASS

The performance of CPB requires constant interaction between the surgeon, perfusionist, and anesthesiologist, especially during periods of transition to and from artificial perfusion. Although frequent dialogue is important, often a member of the team, usually the surgeon, may be focused on other aspects of the operation and unavailable to discuss nonemergent aspects of perfusion in a particular case. For this reason, written protocols and procedures developed in a multidisciplinary fashion are important for ensuring the safe conduct of CPB.

ASSEMBLY OF THE CPB CIRCUIT

The perfusionist is responsible for setting up and preparing the heart-lung machine and all components necessary for the proposed operation. Most perfusionists use commercial, sterile, preprepared, customized tubing packs, which are connected to the various components that constitute the heart-lung machine. This dry assembly takes about 10 to 15 min; the unit can then be kept in standby for up to 7 days. Once the system is primed with fluid, which takes about 15 min, it should be used within 8 h. After assembly, the perfusionist conducts a safety inspection and completes a written prebypass checklist.

PRIMING

Adult extracorporeal perfusion circuits require 1.5 to 2.0 L of balanced electrolyte solution (lactated Ringer's solution, Normosol-A, or Plasma-Lyte). Before connections are made to the patient, the prime is recirculated through a micropore filter to remove particulates and air emboli. The priming volume represents approximately 30 to 35 percent of the patient's blood volume and reduces the hematocrit to about two-thirds of the preoperative value. Hemodilution is an important cause of intraoperative and postoperative anemia. Priming requirements can be reduced by using smaller-diameter and shorter tubing lengths and operating the machine with minimal perfusate in the venous and cardiotomy reservoirs. Autologous blood prime, usually with retrograde venous blood into the pump, is another method to reduce crystalloid priming volume, but this risks hypovolemic sequelae prior to the initiation of CPB. Improvements in clinical outcomes have not been definitively proven with these techniques.

The use of colloids (albumin, gelatins, dextrans, and hetastarches) in the priming volume is controversial. Colloids reduce the fall in colloid osmotic pressure and may reduce the amount of fluid entering the extracellular space. However, prospective clinical studies have failed to document significant clinical benefits with albumin, which is expensive and may have adverse effects.[9,10] Hetastarch may contribute to postoperative bleeding.

ANTICOAGULATION AND REVERSAL

Porcine heparin (300 to 400 U/kg IV) is given before arterial or venous cannulas are inserted, and CPB is not started until anticoagulation is confirmed by activated clotting time (ACT). Most would agree that the minimum ACT to begin CPB is 400 s, but many groups prefer a goal of 480 s because heparin only partially inhibits thrombin formation during CPB. Inadequate anticoagulation risks thrombosis of the circuit at the extreme end of the spectrum, but it may also result in less dramatic consumption of clotting factors and postoperative coagulopathy. Excessively high concentrations of heparin (ACT > 1000 s) may cause remote bleeding away from operative sites.

Failure to achieve a satisfactory ACT may be due to inadequate heparin or to low concentrations of circulating antithrombin. If a total of 500 U/kg of heparin fails to prolong ACT adequately, fresh frozen plasma or recombinant antithrombin is needed to increase antithrombin concentrations and overcome "heparin resistance," a phenomenon more commonly seen in patients on preoperative intravenous heparin therapy.

Antifibrinolytic agents such as aminocaproic acid or tranexamic acid are routinely used during cardiopulmonary bypass and have been shown to improve postoperative chest tube drainage but not clinical outcome. Another pharmacologic strategy to reduce bleeding complications is the use of aprotinin, a serine-protease inhibitor with general anti-inflammatory properties. Extensive literature exists on the beneficial effects of aprotinin on a variety of clinical outcome measures, especially with reoperative cardiac surgery.[11] The most important of these benefits may be a reduction in the risk of stroke, noted in a large retrospective analysis.[12] Drawbacks to aprotinin include significant cost and possibly an adverse effect on renal function in the presence of angiotensin converting enzyme inhibitors.[13] With aprotinin use, ACT should be measured using kaolin as opposed to celite, as celite artifactually and erroneously increases ACT.

During CPB, the ACT is measured every 30 min. If the ACT goes below the target level, more heparin is given. Usually one-third of the initial heparin bolus is given every hour even when the ACT is within the normal range. Hepcon tests, which measure heparin concentration, may also be used; although their results are more reproducible than ACT, ACT is less time-consuming and provides satisfactory monitoring of anticoagulation.

One milligram of protamine (not to exceed 3 mg/kg) is given for each 100 U of heparin injected in the initial bolus dose. The heparin-protamine complex activates complement and often causes acute hypotension, which may be attenuated by adding calcium (2 mg/1 mg protamine). After one-third of the planned protamine dose has been administered, blood must not be returned to the cardiotomy reservoir from the surgical field. Rarely, protamine may cause an anaphylactic reaction in patients with antibodies to protamine insulin. Neutralization of heparin is usually confirmed by an ACT or Hepcon test, and more protamine (50 mg) is given if either test remains prolonged and bleeding is a problem. "Heparin rebound" is the term used to describe a delayed heparin effect due to the release of tissue heparin after protamine is cleared from the circulation. Although protamine is a mild anticoagulant, one or two supplemental 25- to 50-mg doses can be given empirically if heparin rebound is suspected. In most instances the heart-lung machine should be available for immediate use until the patient leaves the operating room.

STARTING CPB

CPB is started at the surgeon's request with concurrence of the anesthesiologist and perfusionist. As venous return enters the machine, the perfusionist progressively increases arterial flow while monitoring the patient's blood pressure and volume levels in all reservoirs. Important observations include adequacy of venous drainage, acceptable flow rates, acceptable arterial line pressure, oxygenation of arterial blood, appropriate systemic arterial pressure, and adequate decompression of the heart. Once full stable cardiopulmonary bypass is established, lung ventilation is discontinued, systemic cooling may begin, and the aorta may be clamped for arresting the heart.

CARDIOPLEGIA

After aortic cross-clamping, cardiac arrest is usually achieved with antegrade blood or crystalloid cardioplegia administered directly into the aortic root by a dedicated cardioplegia roller pump. The heart usually arrests within 30 to 60 s. A delay may indicate problems with delivery of the solution, incomplete aortic occlusion, or unrecognized aortic regurgitation. Retrograde cardioplegia is often given after an antegrade dose to facilitate cardioplegia delivery distal to atherosclerotic stenoses of the coronary arteries. In contrast to antegrade cardioplegia, epicardial and intracardiac procedures are not much hindered by delivery of retrograde cardioplegia. The usual flow of retrograde cardioplegia is 200 to 400 mL/min at coronary sinus pressures between 30 and 50 mmHg. Induction of electrical arrest is slower (2 to 4 min) than with antegrade, and retrograde cardioplegia may provide incomplete protection of the right ventricle.

DETERMINANTS OF SAFE PERFUSION

Blood flow rate

The generally accepted flow rate at 35 to 37°C and hematocrit of 25 percent is approximately 2.4 L/min/m^2 in deeply anesthetized and muscle-relaxed patients. Hemodilution reduces blood oxygen content and dictates that flow rate must increase over resting normal cardiac output or oxygen demand must decrease. As long as mean arterial pressure remains above 50 to 60 mmHg (i.e., above the autoregulatory range), cerebral blood flow is preserved even if systemic flow is less than normal. However, as total systemic flow is progressively reduced, there is a hierarchal reduction of flow to other organs. First skeletal muscle flow falls, then flow to the abdominal viscera and bowel, and finally flow to the kidneys.

Arterial pressure

Systemic arterial blood pressure is a function of flow rate, blood viscosity (hematocrit), and vascular tone. Perfusion of the brain is normally protected by autoregulation, which appears to be lost somewhere between 55 and 60 mmHg during CPB at moderate hypothermia and hematocrit 24 percent. This pressure is thus generally regarded to be the lowest safe pressure for routine CBP. In older patients, who may have vascular disease and/or hypertension, mean arterial blood pressure is generally maintained between 70 and 80 mmHg at 37°C. Higher pressures are undesirable because collateral blood flow to the heart and lungs increases blood in the operative field. Hypotension during CPB may be due to low pump flow, aortic dissection, measurement error, or vasodilatation. Phenylephrine is most often used to elevate blood pressure, but arginine vasopressin (0.05 to 0.1 U/min) may also be used. If anesthesia is adequate, hypertension is generally treated by nitroprusside or nitroglycerin.

Mean blood pressure is an important perfusion parameter in nonpulsatile CPB, the most common mode of perfusion. Pulsatile CPB theoretically reduces vasocontrictive reflexes and neuroendocrine responses and may increase oxygen consumption, reduce acidosis, and improve organ perfusion. Effective generation of pulse pressure, however, requires a larger-diameter aortic cannula and higher nozzle velocities, which may increase trauma to blood elements.

Hematocrit

The ideal hematocrit during CPB remains controversial because of competing advantages and disadvantages.[14,15] Low hematocrits reduce blood viscosity and hemolysis, reduce oxygen-carrying capacity, and reduce the need for blood transfusion. Hypothermia reduces oxygen consumption and permits perfusion at 26 to 28°C with hematocrits between 18 and 22 percent; at higher temperatures, however, limits on pump flow may not satisfy oxygen demand. Neurologic and renal function appear to be most susceptible to damage with low hematocrits, a problem that may be overcome with increasing pump flows to maintain adequate oxygen delivery.[16] A good generalization is that hematocrit should not be maintained below 22 to 24 percent.

Temperature

The ideal temperature for uncomplicated adult cardiac surgery is controversial, although most routine adult cardiac operations are performed with mild systemic hypothermia (28 to 32°C). This allows for some organ protection by means of reduced cellular metabolism but avoids complications associated with lower temperatures, such as interference with enzyme and organ function, increased systemic vascular resistance, delays in cardiac recovery, lengthened duration of CPB, and increased risk of cerebral hyperthermia with rewarming. Increasingly, efforts are made to avoid cerebral hyperthermia during and after operation.

Acid/Base management

There are two strategies for managing blood pH during hypothermia: pH stat and alpha stat. In adults, alpha stat may be better for neurologic protection, as the microembolic burden may be lessened. pH stat maintains temperature-corrected pH 7.40 at all temperatures and requires the addition of CO_2 as the patient is cooled. Alpha stat allows the pH to increase during cooling, so that blood becomes alkalotic. Cerebral blood flow is higher, while pressure is passive and uncoupled from cerebral oxygen demand with pH stat. With alpha stat, cerebral blood flow is lower, autoregulated, and coupled to cerebral oxygen demand.

PATIENT MONITORING

Systemic arterial pressure is typically monitored by radial, brachial, or femoral arterial catheter; central venous pressure is routinely monitored by a jugular venous catheter. Routine use of a Swan-Ganz pulmonary arterial catheter is controversial and not necessary for uncomplicated operations in low-risk patients. Bladder or rectal temperature is usually used to estimate the temperature of the main body mass but does not reflect brain temperature, which is estimated by nasopharyngeal or tympanic membrane sensors. The jugular venous bulb temperature is considered the best surrogate for brain temperature but is more difficult to obtain.

TEE examination is an important monitor during most applications of CPB[17,18] to assess catheter and vent insertion and location, severity of aortic atherosclerosis, myocardial injury, infarction, dilatation, contractility, thrombi and residual air, valve function after repair or replacement, diagnosis of dissection, and adequacy of deairing at the end of CPB.

Mixed venous oxygenation (SvO_2), which assesses the relationship between DO_2 and $\dot{V}O_2$, is monitored on the CPB circuit. SvO_2 below 60 percent indicates inadequate oxygen delivery; but because of differences in regional vascular tone, higher SvO_2 does not assure adequate oxygen delivery to all vascular beds. When adequacy of perfusion is questionable, more frequent blood gas monitoring should be performed to assess for metabolic acidosis.

TERMINATION OF CPB

Discontinuation of CPB involves a complex interplay of physiologic manipulation and operating room personnel. Requirements for termination of CPB include physiologic systemic temperature, adequate heart and lung function, acceptable acid-base and electrolyte status, and no trapped intracardiac air. De-airing maneuvers are important to prevent coronary embolization and cardiac failure (Table 21-1). Once preparations are completed, surgeon, anesthesiologist, and perfusionist begin to wean the patient off CPB. The perfusionist gradually occludes the venous line and simultaneously reduces pump input as cardiac rate and rhythm, arterial pressure and pulse, and central venous pressure are monitored and adjusted. Initially blood volume within the pump is kept constant, but as pump flow approaches zero, volume is added or removed from the patient to produce arterial and venous pressures within the physiologic ranges. During weaning, cardiac filling and contractility is often monitored by TEE, and intracardiac repairs and regional myocardial contractility are assessed. Pulse oximetry saturation near 100 percent, end-tidal CO_2 greater than 25 mmHg, and mixed venous oxygen saturation greater than 65 percent confirm satisfactory ventilation and circulation. When cardiac performance is satisfactory and stable, all catheters and cannulas are removed, protamine is given to reverse heparin, and blood return from the surgical field is discontinued. Once the patient is hemodynamically stable as determined by surgeon and anesthesiologist and after starting wound closure, the perfusate may be returned to the patient in several ways. The entire perfusate may be washed and returned as packed cells, or excess fluid may be removed by a hemoconcentrator. At least some of the perfusate, which still contains heparin and coagulation factors, is gradually pumped into the patient to maintain intravascular volume, which can fluctuate significantly after separation from CPB. Occasionally some of the perfusate must be bagged and given later. The circuit should not be completely disassembled until the chest is closed and the patient is ready for transfer.

CIRCUIT COMPLICATIONS

Life-threatening incidents occur in 0.4 to 2.7 percent of operations with CPB. Massive air embolism, aortic dissection, dislodgement of cannulas, and clotting within the circuit during perfusion are the principal causes of serious injury or death. Malfunction of the heater-cooler, oxygenator, pumps, and electrical supply are the most common threatening incidents related to equipment. Other threatening incidents include premature takedown or clotting within the perfusion circuit. Complications related to connections to and from the heart-lung machine and perfusion during operation are described above, with descriptions of the various components of the perfusion circuit.

METABOLIC COMPLICATIONS AND ORGAN INJURY

Depending on the degree of investigation, untoward systemic and organ-specific effects of CPB can be found in essentially all patients placed on the pump. Minor complications predominate, but in 0.1 to 0.5 percent, serious and life-threatening events can be attributed to the effects of CPB (Table 21-2).

Table 21-2 Adverse manifestations of CPB

	Common and mild	Uncommon and severe
Systemic	SIRS	Multiorgan failure
Cardiac	Tachycardia, atrial arrythmias	Low-cardiac-output state, ventricular arrhythmias
Pulmonary	Mild hypoxia, tachypnea	ARDS
Neurologic	Anxiety, drowsiness, neuropsychological deficit	Delirium, encephalopathy, stroke
Renal	Oliguria, <50% increase in serum creatinine	Acute renal failure
Gastrointestinal	Nausea, vomiting, anorexia	Ileus, perforation, stress gastritis, pancreatitis
Hepatic	Mild serum transaminase and bilirubin elevation	Jaundice, fulminant liver failure
Hematologic	Anemia, mild thrombocytopenia, leukocytosis	HIT with thrombosis, disseminated intravascular consumption

SIRS = systemic inflammatory response syndrome; ARDS = acute respiratory distress syndrome; HIT = heparin-induced thrombocytopenia

GENERAL MECHANISMS AND THE SYSTEMIC INFLAMMATORY RESPONSE SYNDROME

Cardiopulmonary bypass preempts normal reflex and chemoreceptor control of the circulation, initiates coagulation, generates vasoactive and cytotoxic substances, and produces a variety of microemboli. Ischemia/reperfusion is also an important cause of reversible and irreversible cell injury and may not be detected because regional hypoperfusion may not be evident. Regional perfusion is also influenced by acid-base relationships during cooling and may affect postoperative organ function. Temperature differences within the body and within organs produce regional temperature-perfusion mismatch, which can precipitate regional hypoperfusion and acidosis due to inadequate oxygen delivery. There is no method to monitor regional perfusion during cardiopulmonary bypass, and even direct temperature surveillance of vital organs may fail to detect temperature differences within the organ.

The subsequent inflammatory response produces the terminal complement attack complex, anaphylactoxins, cytotoxic proteases, collagenases, metalloproteinases, reactive oxidants, endotoxin, and activated neutrophils and monocytes, which can destroy nonhost organisms but also tissue cells. These agents directly access the specialized cells of every organ by passing between endothelial cell junctions to reach the interstitial compartment. Reduced plasma colloid osmotic pressure, elevated venous pressure, and widened endothelial cell junctions increase the volume of the interstitial space during CPB in proportion to the duration of bypass, magnitude of the dissection, transfusions, and other factors. In prolonged bypass runs, the interstitial compartment may increase 18 to 33 percent, but intracellular water does not increase during CPB.

The systemic inflammatory response syndrome (SIRS) can be detected to some degree in nearly all patients subjected to a pump-oxygenator. Clinically, this is manifest as fevers, leukocytosis, tachypnea, tachycardia in the non beta-blocked heart, as well as fatigue, malaise, anorexia, and nausea. Elevated levels of circulating catecholamines are also present and contribute to the development of atrial and ventricular arrhythmias. Besides exposure to the circuit, other factors contributing to the development of SIRS include anemia and blood transfusions, hypotension, surgical trauma, pain, and preexisting patient factors such as infection or advanced heart failure. Strategies to limit the severity of SIRS are thus aimed at minimizing time on pump, avoiding other precipitating factors, and medical optimization of the patient prior to surgery. No pharmacologic strategies are effective in prevention.

MICROEMBOLIZATION

Microemboli, which are defined as particles less than 500 μm in diameter, that enter the circulation during CPB are important causes of regional ischemia. Air entry into the perfusion circuit produces the most dangerous gas emboli because nitrogen is poorly soluble in blood and is not a metabolite. Carbon dioxide is rapidly soluble in blood and is sometimes used to flood the surgical field to displace air. Foreign emboli, largely generated in the surgical wound, reach the circulation from the surgical field via the cardiotomy reservoir. The cardiotomy reservoir is the primary source of foreign emboli and the major source of blood-generated emboli, particularly fat emboli.[19] Extensive activation and physical damage to blood elements produce a wide variety of emboli, which tend to increase with the duration of perfusion.

The principal methods for reducing circulating microemboli include the following: adequate anticoagulation, membrane oxygenator, washing blood aspirated from the surgical wound,[20] filter in the cardiotomy reservoir, secure purse-string sutures around cannulas, strict control of all air entry sites within the perfusion circuit, removal of residual air from the heart and great vessels, and avoidance of atherosclerotic emboli.

Many intraoperative strategies are available to reduce cerebral atherosclerotic embolization. These include routine epicardial echocardiography of the ascending aorta to detect both anterior and posterior atherosclerotic plaques and sites free of atherosclerosis for placing the aortic cannula. Recently, special catheters with or without baffles or screens have been developed to reduce the number of atherosclerotic emboli that reach the cerebral circulation.[21,22] In patients with moderate or severe ascending aortic atherosclerosis, a single application of the aortic clamp as opposed to partial or multiple applications is strongly recommended and has been shown to reduce postoperative neuronal and neurocognitive deficits in a large clinical series.[23] In these patients, retrograde cardioplegia is preferred over antegrade cardioplegia to avoid a sandblasting effect of the cardioplegic solution. No aortic clamp may be safe or even possible in some patients with severe atherosclerosis or "porcelain aorta," and other techniques may be required (see "Special Topics," below). Filter placement within the CPB circuit is likely an important step to prevent emboli. However, air and fat can pass through filters and air and atherosclerotic emboli may enter the circulation downstream of the filter.

SPECIFIC ORGAN INJURY

Cardiac injury

It is difficult to separate postoperative cardiac dysfunction from injury due to CPB, ischemia/reperfusion, direct surgical trauma, the disease being treated, and inadequate myocardial protection. The heart, like all organs and tissues, is subject to microemboli, protease and chemical cytotoxins, activated neutrophils and monocytes, and regional hypoperfusion during CPB. Some degree of myocardial "stunning" during the period when coronary blood flow is interrupted is inevitable, as is some degree of reperfusion injury after ischemia. Both myocardial edema and distention of the flaccid cardioplegic heart during aortic cross-clamping reduce myocardial contractility. Last, if myocardial contractility is weak, excessive preload or high afterload during weaning from CPB will increase ventricular end-diastolic volume, myocardial wall stress, and oxygen consumption. Thus the postoperative performance of the heart depends on many variables and not just the injuries produced by CPB.

Neurologic injury

The brain is the most sensitive organ exposed to damage by CPB and also the most important organ to protect. Even small injuries may produce detectable, functional losses that are not detectable or important in other organs. Regional hypoperfusion, edema, microemboli, and circulating cytotoxins may cause subtle losses in cognitive function, behavioral patterns, and physiologic and physical function that can pass unnoticed, be accepted and dismissed, or profoundly compromise the patient's quality of life. The most obvious neuropsychologic abnormalities are coma, delirium, and confusion, but often transitory episodes of delirium and confusion are dismissed as due to anesthesia or medications. More subtle losses are determined by comparison of preoperative and postoperative performance using a standard battery of neuropsychological tests.

Advancing age increases the risk of stroke or cognitive impairment, especially after the age of 60, at least in part because other risk factors for neurologic injury also increase with age. Hypertension and diabetes occur in approximately 55 and 25 percent of cardiac surgical patients, respectively. Fifteen percent have carotid stenosis of 50 percent or greater, and up to 13 percent have had a transient ischemic attack or prior stroke. The severity of atherosclerosis in the ascending aorta as detected by epiaortic ultrasound scanning adds to the risk of stroke or cognitive dysfunction. Palpable ascending aortic atherosclerotic plaques markedly increase the risk of right carotid arterial emboli as detected by Doppler ultrasound.[24] The incidence of severe aortic atherosclerosis is 1 percent in cardiac surgical patients less than 50 years old and is 10 percent in those of age 75 to 80.

Mechanisms of cerebral injury during CPB are microemboli and hypoperfusion, which are to some extent mutually exclusive. Microemboli are distributed in proportion to blood flow; thus reduced cerebral blood flow reduces microembolic injury but increases the risk of hypoperfusion.[25] In clinical practice, air, atherosclerotic debris, and fat are the major types of microemboli causing brain injury and all cause neuronal necrosis by blocking small cerebral vessels. Massive air embolism causes a large ischemic injury, but gaseous cerebral microemboli may directly damage endothelium in addition to blocking blood flow.

Besides protecting against embolic events, recommended conditions for protecting the brain during CPB include mild hypothermia (32° to 34°C) and a hematocrit above 25 percent. Temporary increases in cerebral venous pressure caused by SVC obstruction and excessive rewarming above blood temperatures of 37°C should be avoided. Barbiturates reduce cerebral metabolism by decreasing spontaneous synaptic activity and provide a definite neuroprotective effect during clinical cardiac surgery using CPB. Unfortunately, these agents delay emergence from anesthesia and prolong ICU stays. Although the use of aprotinin has been associated with fewer strokes in retrospective analysis, currently no agent is strongly recommended for protection of the central nervous system during CPB.

Off-pump myocardial revascularization theoretically avoids many of the causes of cerebral injury due to CPB, but, as noted above, many causes of neuronal injury are independent of CPB and related to atherosclerosis and the entry of air into the circulation. Measurements of carotid emboli by Doppler ultrasound indicate fewer emboli and improved neurocognitive outcomes in patients who have off-pump surgery as compared to those with on-pump revascularization.[26,27] Unfortunately, metanalyses of randomized trials comparing on- and off-pump CABG have not demonstrated a definitive reduction in stroke risk.[28,29]

Lung injury

Hypoxia of some degree is a nearly universal finding after CPB. Patient factors and the separate effects of operation and CPB combine to compromise lung function early after operation. Chronic smoking and emphysema are the most common patient factors, but muscular weakness, chronic bronchitis, occult pneumonia, preoperative pulmonary edema, and unrelated respiratory disease are other contributors to postoperative pulmonary dysfunction. Incisional pain, lack of movement, shallow respiratory sighs, reduced pulmonary compliance, weak cough, increased pulmonary arteriovenous shunting, and interstitial edema, to some degree, are consequences of anesthesia and any operation. CPB significantly adds to this injury.

During CPB, the lungs are supplied by the bronchial arteries and pulmonary arterial blood flow may be absent or minimal. Whether or not alveolar cells suffer an ischemia/reperfusion injury is unclear, but the lungs are subject to many insults that combine to increase pulmonary capillary permeability and interstitial lung water. Hemodilution, reduced plasma oncotic pressure, and temporary elevation of left atrial or pulmonary venous pressure during CPB or during weaning from CPB increase extravascular lung water. Microemboli and circulating cellular, vasoactive, and cytotoxic mediators of the inflammatory response reach the lung via bronchial arteries during CPB and with resumption of the pulmonary circulation during weaning. These agents increase pulmonary capillary permeability, perivascular edema, and bronchial secretions and perhaps cause observed changes in alveolar surfactant. All of these changes combine to enhance regional atelectasis, increase susceptibility to infection, and increase the physiologic arteriovenous shunt, which reduces systemic arterial PaO_2.

Postoperative respiratory care is based on restoring normal pulmonary capillary permeability and interstitial lung volume, preventing atelectasis, reinflating atelectatic segments, maintaining normal arterial blood gases, preventing infection, and facilitating removal of bronchial mucus. Improved postoperative respiratory care, an understanding of the mechanisms of lung injury during CPB, and efforts to prevent or control the causes of injury can markedly reduce the incidence of pulmonary complications.

Renal injury

Some degree of renal injury is inevitable during CPB, and postperfusion proteinuria occurs in all patients. The incidence of acute renal failure requiring dialysis after CPB is 1 to 5 percent, depending on the complexity of surgery and preoperative factors. As with other organs, the preoperative health of the kidneys is a major factor in the ability of that organ to withstand the microembolic, cellular, and regional malperfusion injuries caused by CPB. Risk factors for postoperative renal dysfunction include age over 70, diabetes mellitus, previous cardiac surgery, congestive heart failure, and a complex, prolonged operation. Hemoglobin is toxic to renal tubules and its precipitation can block both blood and urine flow to the tubules. Hemodilution dilutes plasma hemoglobin; improves flow to the outer renal cortex; improves total renal blood flow; increases creatinine, electrolyte, and water clearance; and increases glomerular filtration and urine volume.

Perioperative periods of low cardiac output and/or hypotension added to the microembolic, cellular and cytotoxic injuries of CPB and to any preoperative renal disease are the major cause of postoperative renal failure. Low cardiac output reduces renal perfusion pressure and causes angiotensin II production and renin release, which further decreases renal blood flow. Kidneys, already compromised by preoperative disease and the CPB injury, are particularly sensitive to ischemic injury secondary to low cardiac output and hypotension. Thus perioperative management includes efforts to maximize cardiac output using dopamine or dobutamine if necessary, avoiding renal arterial vasoconstrictive drugs, providing adequate crystalloid infusions to maintain urine volume, and alkalinizing urine to minimize the precipitation of tubular hemoglobin if excessive hemolysis has occurred. Unfortunately, no pharmacologic strategies have proven beneficial in protecting renal function after CPB.

Pancreatic injury

Less than 1 percent of patients develop clinical pancreatitis after CPB, but approximately 30 percent develop a transitory, asymptomatic increase in plasma amylase and/or lipase. A history of recurrent pancreatitis, perioperative circulatory shock or hypotension, excessively prolonged CPB, and continuous, high doses of inotropic agents are risk factors for the development of postoperative clinically relevant pancreatitis. Experimentally and clinically, high doses of calcium increase intracellular trypsinogen activation and histologic evidence of pancreatitis. Fulminant pancreatits is very rare but often fatal.

SPECIAL TOPICS

THE "BAD AORTA"

Some degree of atherosclerosis of the ascending aorta is a common finding during cardiac surgery. Simple palpation can often detect local areas of plaque that must be avoided ien cannulating, clamping, or manipulating the aorta. Epiaortic scanning is more sensitive for the detection of ascending aortic atherosclerosis and is preferred for all patients who have a history of transient ischemic attack, stroke, severe peripheral vascular disease, palpable calcification in the ascending aorta, calcified aortic knob on chest radiograph, age above 50 to 60 years, or TEE findings of moderate aortic atherosclerosis.[30]

Some findings on examination of the aorta can dramatically alter the conduct of an operation. Calcified aorta (porcelain aorta), which occurs in 1 to 4 percent of patients, is one such finding. This condition increases the risks of dislodgement of atheromatous debris from the aortic wall due to manipulation, cross-clamping, or the sandblasting effect of the cannula jet and greatly increases the risks of perioperative stroke, aortic dissection, and postoperative renal dysfunction.[31] Many strategies exist for patient management in this setting; these depend on the surgeon's preference and the cardiac condition being treated (Fig. 21-3). For coronary artery bypass, a first question one must ask is "Is the pump necessary?" Conversion from on-pump to off-pump CABG is a good alternative, especially when manipulation of the ascending aorta can be completely avoided. In this scenario, pedicled single or sequential arterial grafts, T or Y grafts from a pedicled mammary artery, or vein grafts anastomosed to arch vessels can be used.

If CPB is deemed necessary, minimal manipulation of the aorta should remain a primary focus. Initially, the best site for cannulation must be determined. Femoral cannulation in this setting is usually not a good alternative because of the likely coexistence of severe atherosclerosis in the aortoiliac and femoral circulations. In contrast, the axillary artery is usually free of significant disease and is often a good alternative. Another option is cannulation of a "soft spot," if one exists, atraumatically on the ascending aorta or aortic arch.

Next, one must decide whether aortic cross-clamping is necessary. Many coronary operations can be performed without a cross clamp on the empty, beating heart. Alternatively, ventricular fibrillation can be induced electrically or with hypothermia for coronary or mitral valve operations with cross-clamping. Finally, deep hypothermic circulatory arrest (DHCA) can be used to replace the aortic valve without ever placing a clamp.[32] If aortic cross-clamping is deemed necessary, DHCA can be used initially to replace the ascending aorta with a graft using an open technique. The graft can then be clamped for reinstitution of CPB and maintenance of cardiac arrest.

Severe aortic atherosclerosis is a risk factor for the still rare but dramatic complication of intra- or postoperative aortic dissection. The first clues may be discoloration beneath the adventitia near the cannula site, proximal vein anastomosis or clamp location, an increase in arterial line pressure, or a sharp reduction in return to the venous reservoir. TEE may be helpful in confirming the diagnosis,

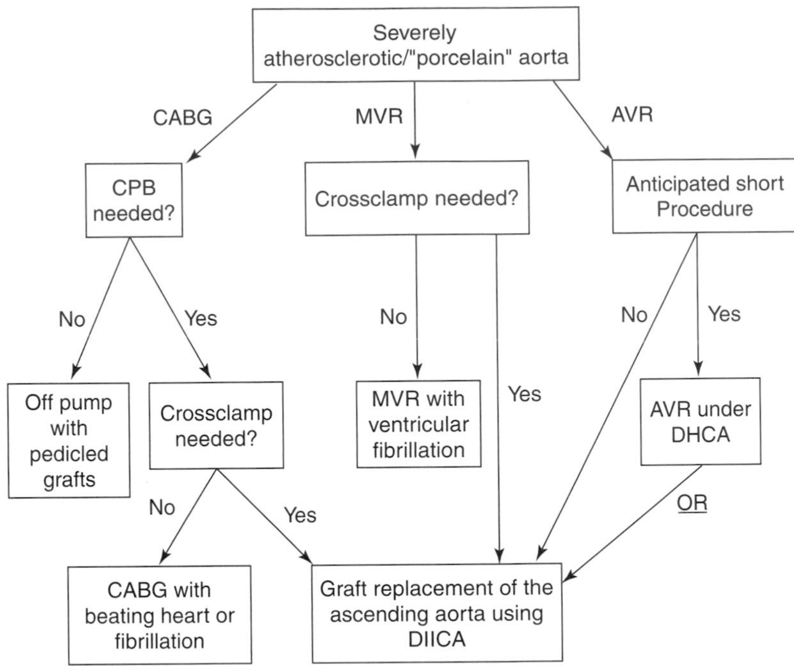

Figure 21-3 Algorithm for management of the severely atherosclerotic ascending aorta.

but prompt action is necessary to limit the dissection and maintain perfusion. If a localized dissection occurs immediately upon removing the cross clamp, the clamp should be reapplied to limit proximal and distal extension of the dissection flap. Local suture or partial graft repair is then performed. For more extensive dissections, the cannula must be promptly transferred to a peripheral artery or uninvolved distal aorta. Blood pressure should be controlled pharmacologically and perfusion cooling to temperatures less than 20°C initiated. During hypothermic circulatory arrest, the aorta is opened at the original site of cannulation and repaired by direct suture, patch, or circumferential graft. When dissection is recognized early, survival rates range from 66 to 85 percent, but when this problem occurs late or is discovered after operation, survival is approximately 50 percent.

PERSISTENT LEFT SUPERIOR VENA CAVA

The presence of a persistent left superior vena cava (PLSVC) is rare but should be suspected when the left innominate vein is small or absent and a large coronary sinus or the PLSVC itself is seen on baseline TEE, as the PLSVC usually drains into the coronary sinus. A PLSVC may thus complicate retrograde cardioplegia or entry into the right heart. For epicardial operations, standard single- or two-stage venous cannulation remains effective, although retrograde cardioplegia cannot be used. For other cases, if an adequate-sized innominate vein is present (30 percent of patients), the PLSVC can simply be occluded during CPB and cerebral venous return will not be impeded. If the innominate vein is absent or small (about 75 percent of patients) or if the right SVC is not present, occlusion of the PLSVC may cause venous hypertension and possible cerebral injury. In these patients, the SVC may be cannulated directly or through the coronary sinus ostium. Alternatively, for simple cases such as repair of a secundum atrial septal defect, standard cannulation can be performed and a sump suction cathether placed into the coronary sinus while the right atrium is open.

MASSIVE AIR EMBOLISM

Massive air embolism during perfusion is a rare but catastrophic event. When this is detected, perfusion should stop immediately and clamps should be placed on both venous and arterial lines. Air in the circuit should be removed rapidly by recirculation and entrapment of all air in a reservoir or bubble trap. The patient should immediately be placed in steep Trendelenburg and blood and air at the site of entry should be aspirated until no air is retrieved. TEE should rapidly be employed to search for air, but perfusion must resume promptly, depending on body temperature, to prevent ischemic brain damage. Cooling to deep hypothermia should be considered to protect the brain and other organs while the air is located and removed. As soon as possible, retrograde perfusion of the brain should be undertaken while the aortic arch is simultaneously aspirated with the patient in steep Trendelenburg. Corticosteroids and/or barbiturates may be considered. Depending on circumstances and availability, hyperbaric oxygen therapy may be helpful if patients can be treated within 5 h of operation.[33]

DEEP HYPOTHERMIC CIRCULATORY ARREST (DHCA)

DHCA is used for operations involving the aortic arch, porcelain aorta, thoracoabdominal aneurysms, pulmonary thrombendarterectomy, selected uncommon cardiovascular and neurologic procedures, and certain complex congenital heart procedures. The technology involves reducing body temperature to less than 20°C, arresting the circulation for a short period and then rewarming to 37°C. Most surgical teams cool to either electroencephalographic (EEG) silence, jugular venous saturation above 95 percent, or for at least 30 min before stopping circulation at nasopharyngeal or tympanic membrane temperatures below 20°C. Perfusion cooling is usually supplemented by surface cooling using hypothermia blankets and/or packing the head in ice. During rewarming, hyperthermia is avoided by keeping the arterial inflow temperature below 37°C.

Changes in temperature affect acid-base balance, which must be monitored and managed during deep hypothermia. In adults, the pH-stat protocol (CO_2 is added to maintain temperature corrected blood pH at 7.4) is often used during cooling instead of the alpha-stat protocol, which allows cold blood to become alkalotic. Compared with alpha-stat, pH-stat increases the rate and uniformity of brain cooling and slows the rate of brain oxygen consumption by 30 to 40 percent. pH-stat is even more commonly used in pediatric DHCA applications. Alpha-stat management is often substituted during rewarming when more potential microemboli may be present. Hyperglycemia appears to increase brain injury and is avoided during deep hypothermia. The value of high-dose corticosteroids or barbiturates remains unproven.

The "safe" duration of circulatory arrest during deep hypothermia is unknown. In adults, arrest times as short as 25 min are associated with reduced performance on neuropsychological tests of fine motor function and memory.[34] At 18°C, cerebral metabolism and oxygen consumption are 17 to 40 percent of normothermia, and abnormal EEG patterns and cerebrovascular responses can be detected after 30 min of circulatory arrest. Most investigators report increased mortality and adverse neurologic outcomes after 40 to 65 min of circulatory arrest. Thus, the maximal "safe" duration of DHCA is considered by most surgeons to be approximately 45 min. Advanced age or a preoperative history of stroke may leave less safety margin for brain injury.

Cerebral perfusion can often be maintained during DHCA in either antegrade or retrograde fashion. Interval resumption of normal circuit flow is ideal but is usually not technically possible except in cases not involving open work on the aortic arch, i.e., pulmonary thromboendarterectomy. Antegrade cerebral perfusion, which appears to have more clinical benefit than retrograde perfusion, is most easily applied after cannulation of the right axillary artery. The innominate artery can then be occluded to achieve corporeal circulatory arrest while maintaining flow to the brain via the right carotid artery. Flows usually range between 8 and 12 mL/kg to keep mean pressure in the range of 40 to 70 mmHg in the right radial artery or pressure sensor on the end of the cannula. Less commonly, the cerebral vessels can be cannulated separately. Selective antegrade cerebral perfusion risks dislodging atheromatous emboli, air embolism, cerebral edema, or injury from excessive perfusion pressure.

Retrograde cerebral perfusion is achieved by placing a perfusion cannula (often a retrograde coronary sinus catheter) into the SVC, which is then perfused at flows between 250 to 400 mL/min and blood pressures usually between 25 to 40 mmHg. A snare is usually placed around the SVC catheter cephalad to the azygos vein to reduce runoff. Because minimal cortical perfusion has been detected with this technique, its main theoretical benefit is the retrograde flush of air and debris from the cerebral vessels. After increased use in the 1980s, retrograde cerebral perfusion was not widely employed because many studies had failed to demonstrate clinical benefit.

CANNULATION FOR MINIMALLY INVASIVE SURGERY

Peripheral cannulation sites as described above may be used for minimal-access cardiac surgery, but often central cannulation of the aorta, atrium, or central veins is accomplished using specially designed or smaller cannulas placed through the small operative incision or through a separate small incision in the chest wall. Venous return is often augmented by applying negative pressure (see "Venous Cannulation," above). Specially designed cross clamps, some with flexible handles, can also be used through small incisions. Other options include complete cannulation by remote access, using equipment such as the Port Access System, which provides a means for full CPB, cardioplegia administration, and aortic cross clamping without exposing the heart and can be used for both valvular and coronary artery operations.[35] Separate transcutaneous catheters are inserted through the right internal jugular vein into the coronary sinus for retrograde cardioplegia and the pulmonary artery for left heart venting. A multilumen catheter is inserted through the femoral artery and, using TEE and/or fluoroscopy, is positioned in the ascending aorta for arterial pump inflow, for balloon occlusion of the ascending aorta, and for administration of antegrade cardioplegia into the aortic root. Venous return is captured by a femoral venous catheter advanced into the right atrium.

Minimally invasive surgery using CPB is associated with potential complications that include perforation of vessels or cardiac chambers, aortic dissection, incomplete de-airing, systemic air embolism, and failure of the balloon aortic clamp. Because CO_2 is heavier than air and more soluble in blood, the surgical field is sometimes flooded with CO_2 at a flow of 5 to 10 L/min to displace air when the heart is open. The balloon clamp can leak, prolapse through the aortic valve, or move distally to occlude arch vessels. Early use of the balloon clamp appeared to be associated with higher risks of aortic dissection; with more experience, however, this complication appears less common. For safety, the position of the occluding balloon is closely monitored by TEE, bilateral radial arterial pressures, and occasionally transcranial Doppler ultrasound.

References

1. Weinstein GS. Left hemispheric strokes in coronary surgery: Implication for end-hole aortic cannulas. *Ann Thorac Surg* 2001;71:128–132.
2. Gerdes A, Joubert-Hubner E, Esders K, Sievers H-H. Hydrodynamics of aortic arch vessel during perfusion through the right subclavian artery. *Ann Thorac Surg* 2000;69:1425–1430.
3. Neri E, Massetti M, Capannini G, et al. Axillary artery cannulation in type A aortic dissection operations. *J Thorac Cardiovasc Surg* 1999;118:324–329.
4. Willcox TW, Mitchell SJ, Gorman DF. Venous air in the bypass circuit: A source of arterial line emboli exacerbated by vacuum–assisted venous drainage. *Ann Thorac Surg* 1999; 1285–1289.
5. La Pietra A, Groggi EA, Pua BB, et al. Assisted venous drainage presents the risk of undetected air microembolism. *J Thorac Cardiovasc Surg* 2000;120:856–863.
6. Hsu L-C. Heparin-coated CPB circuits: Current status. *Perfusion* 2001;16:417–428.
7. Ovrum E, Mollnes TE, Fosse E, et al. High and low heparin dose with heparin-coated cardiopulmonary bypass: Activation of compliment and granulocytes. *Ann Thorac Surg* 1995; 60:1755–1761.
8. Aldea GS, Soltow LO, Chandler WL, et al. Limitation of thrombin generation, platelet activation, and inflammation by elimination of cardiotomy suction in patients undergoing coronary artery bypass grafting heated with heparin-bonded circuits. *J Thorac Cardiovasc Surg* 2002;123: 742–755.
9. Cochrane Injuries Group Albumin Reviews. Human albumin administration in critically ill patients: Systemic review of randomized controlled trials. *BMJ* 1998;317: 235–240.
10. Wilkes MM, Navicks RJ. Patient survival after human albumin administration. A meta-analysis of randomized, controlled trials. *Ann Intern Med* 2001;135:149–164.
11. Levi M, Cromheecke ME, de Jonge E, et al. Pharmacological strategies to decrease excessive blood loss in cardiac surgery: A meta-analysis of clinically relevant endpoints. *Lancet* 1999;354:1940–1947.
12. Sedrakyan A, Treasure T, Elefteriades JA. Effect of aprotinin on clinical outcomes in coronary artery bypass graft surgery: A systematic review and meta-analysis of randomized clinical trials. *J Thorac Cardiovasc Surg* 2004;128: 442–448.
13. Kincaid EH, Ashburn DA, Hoyle JR, et al. Does the combination of aprotinin and ACE inhibitor cause renal failure after cardiac surgery? *Ann Thorac Surg* 2005;80: 1388–1393.
14. DeFoe GR, Ross CS, Olmstead EM, et al. Lowest hematocrit on bypass and adverse outcomes associated with coronary artery bypass grafting. *Ann Thorac Surg* 2001;71:769–776.
15. Groom RC. High or low hematocrits during cardiopulmonary bypass for patients undergoing coronary artery bypass graft surgery? An evidence-based approach to the question. *Perfusion* 2002;17:99–102.
16. Ranucci M, Romitti F, Isgro G, et al. Oxygen delivery during cardiopulmonary bypass and acute renal failure after coronary operations. *Ann Thorac Surg* 2005;80: 2213–2220.
17. Shanewise JS, Cheung AT, Aronson S, et al. ASE/SCA guidelines for performing a comprehensive intraoperative multiplane transesophageal echocardiography examination. Recommendation of the American Society of Echocardiography Council for Intraoperative Echocardiography and the Society of Cardiovascular Anesthesiologists Task Force for Certification in Perioperative Echocardiography. *Anesth Analg* 1999:99: 870–884.
18. Lucina MG, Savage RM, Hearm C, Kraenzler EJ. The role of transesophageal echocardiography on perfusion management. *Semin Cardiothorac Vasc Anesth* 2001;5: 321–334.
19. Brooker RF, Brown WR, Moody DM, et al. Cardiotomy suction: A major source of brain lipid emboli during cardiopulmonary bypass. *Ann Thorac Surg* 1998;65: 1651–1655.
20. Kincaid EH, Jones TJ, Stump DA, et al. Processing scavenged blood with a cell saver reduces cerebral lipid microembolization. *Ann Thorac Surg* 2000;70: 1296–1300.
21. Reichenspurner H, Navia JA, Benny G, et al. Particulate embolic capture by an intra-aortic filter device during cardiac surgery. *J Thorac Cardiovasc Surg* 2000119:233–244.
22. Cook DJ, Zehr KJ, Orszulak TA, et al. Profound reduction in brain embolization using an endoaortic baffle during bypass in swine. *Ann Thorac Surg* 2002;73:198–202.
23. Hammon JW, Stump DA, Kon ND, et al. Risk factors and solutions for the development of neurobehavioral changes after coronary artery bypass grafting. *Ann Thorac Surg* 1998:63:1613–1618.
24. Stump DA, Brown WR, Moody DM, et al. Microemboli and neurologic dysfunction after cardiovascular surgery. *Semin Cardiothorac Vasc Anesth* 1999;3:47–54.
25. Jones TJ, Stump DA, Deal D, et al. Hypothermia protects the brain from embolization by reducing and redirecting the embolic load. *Ann Thorac Surg* 1999;68:1465.

26. Dijk DV, Jansen EWL, Hijman R, et al. Cognitive outcome after off-pump and on-pump coronary artery bypass graft surgery. *JAMA* 2002;287:1405–1412.
27. Diegeler A, Hirsch R. Schneider F, et al. Neuromonitoring and neurocognitive outcome in off-pump versus conventional coronary bypass operation. *Ann Thorac Surg* 2000;1162–1166.
28. van der Heijden GJ, Nathoe HM, Jansen EW, et al. Meta-analysis on the effect of off-pump coronary bypass surgery. *Eur J Cardiothorac Surg* 2004;26:81–24.
29. Wijeysundera DN, Beattie WS, Djaiani G, et al. Off-pump coronary artery surgery for reducing mortality and morbidity: Meta-analysis of randomized and observational studies. *J Am Coll Cardiol* 2005;46:872–882.
30. Beique FA, Joffe D, Tousignant G, et al. Echocardiographic-based assessment and management of atherosclerotic disease of the thoracic aorta. *J Cardiothorac Vasc Anesth* 1998;12:206–220.
31. Davila-Roman VG, Kouchoukos NT, Schechtman KB, et al. Atherosclerosis of the ascending aorta is a predictor of renal dysfunction after cardiac operations. *J Thorac Cardiovasc Surg* 1999; 117:111–116.
32. Aranki SF, Nathan M, Shekar P, et al. Hypothermic circulatory arrest enables aortic valve replacement in patients with unclampable aorta. *Ann Thorac Surg* 2005;80:1679–1686.
33. Ziser A, Adir Y, Lavon H, et al. Hyperbaric oxygen therapy for massive arterial air embolism during cardiac operations. *J Thorac Cardiovasc Surg* 1999;117: 818–821.
34. Reich DL, Uysal S, Sliwinski M, et al. Neuropsychological outcome following deep hypothermia circulatory arrest in adults. *J Thorac Cardiovasc Surg* 1999;117:156–163.
35. Galloway AC, Shemin RJ, Glower DD. et al. First report of the Port Access International Registry. *Ann Thorac Surg* 1999;67:51–58.

CHAPTER

22 MYOCARDIAL PROTECTION

Constantine L. Athanasuleas, Gerald D. Buckberg

INTRODUCTION

A successful outcome after cardiac surgery depends on many factors. Accurate recognition of the pathology and the judicial choice of methods to achieve cardiac repair are essential. Equally important are the physiologic consequences of the operation. Ventricular function must be preserved or improved during cardiac procedures. Myocardial protection is therefore the crucial component of success in cardiac surgery.

This chapter is a brief "state of the art" review of myocardial protection as currently applied in the vast majority of cardiac operations worldwide. The mainstay of myocardial protection is cardioplegia. We offer a brief review of the components of cardioplegia and their effects on cardiac metabolism and function, followed by a detailed description of "how to do it."

Much has been written about cardioplegia regarding (1) route of delivery (antegrade vs. retrograde or both), (2) method of delivery (continuous vs. intermittent), and (3) temperature (warm vs. cold). This has often led to confusion and adversarial positions. Surgeons appropriately want to keep things simple, but as Einstein once said, "Everything should be made as simple as possible, but not simpler." In this chapter we present a method of cardioplegia that has been extensively applied clinically. It is called the "integrated method" of protection because it combines the salient features of the above elements in a manner that suits the ongoing physiologic needs of the heart during the course of an operation and expedites the time phase of the procedure.

BASIS OF CARDIOPLEGIA

Cardioplegia markedly reduces oxygen demand in the arrested heart and must be delivered uniformly in sufficient quantity to match this low demand (Fig. 22-1). These requirements are met by antegrade and retrograde delivery, cold-blood cardioplegia to reduce oxygen demands, and warm cardioplegia perfusion for induction and resuscitation. "Integrated myocardial protection" is a strategy that addresses each of these requirements in a manner that allows the operation to be performed without interruption.[1] This method (1) provides a bloodless operative field, (2) avoids unnecessary ischemia and cardioplegia overdose, and (3) permits aortic unclamping and discontinuation of bypass shortly after cardiac repair.

Electromechanical activity of the heart raises oxygen demand during arrest. Hypothermia reduces this demand and ischemic damage when coronary flow is interrupted in the course of the revascularization procedure provided that the cardioplegic perfusate is distributed adequately with reinfusions. Hypothermia alone, however, does not completely avoid injury in chronically "energy depleted" (ischemic) hearts (Fig. 22-2).

TYPES OF CARDIOPLEGIA

Blood cardioplegia consists of four parts of blood to one part crystalloid solution. It is a natural buffering agent, maintains oncotic pressure, has advantageous rheologic properties, and is a free-radical scavenger. Blood cardioplegia replenishes substrate in vulnerable hearts, limits reperfusion injury, and reverses ischemia/reperfusion changes in the acutely ischemic myocardium. Complete myocardial recovery occurs after 4 h of ischemia in normal hearts when protected with cold-blood cardioplegia. However, it is uncommon to address normal hearts. The sequences described below were developed experimentally and are now clinically used routinely in the jeopardized hearts that are currently commonplace in cardiac surgical practice.

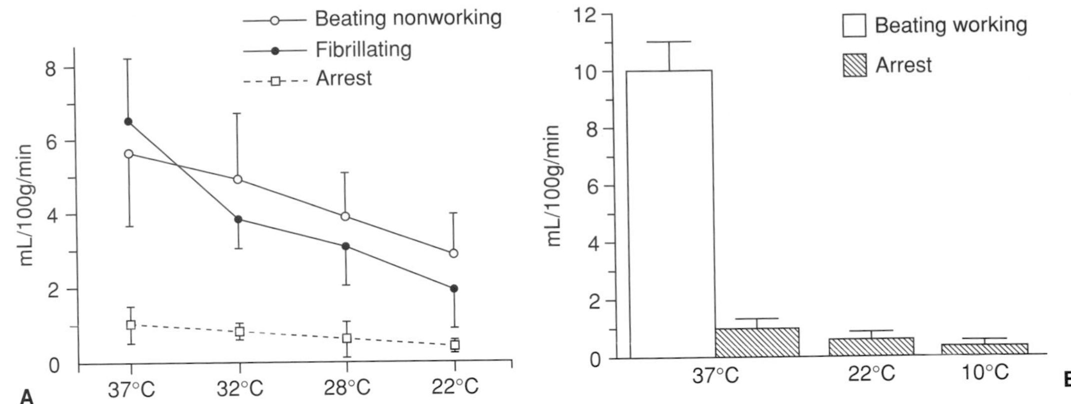

Figure 22-1 Left ventricular (LV) oxygen requirements of the beating, empty, fibrillating, arrested heart from 37°C to 22°C. Note in (A) the low oxygen demands of arrest and the negligible change between 22°C and 10°C as the heart rewarms from collateral flow. (B) Higher demands exist if electromechanical activity returns when systemic perfusate washes out the cardioplegic solution.

Cold-crystalloid cardioplegia does not have the rheologic advantages of blood cardioplegia. When administered in multiple doses, it often results in systemic hemodilution. Crystalloid cardioplegia also shifts the oxyhemoglobin dissociation curve leftward, retarding Na^+/K^+ adenosine triphosphatase and thereby producing edema and activation of platelets, leukocytes, and complement.[2]

COMPONENTS OF BLOOD CARDIOPLEGIA

Blood cardioplegia consists of four parts of blood to one part crystalloid solution. The components (Table 22-1) of blood cardioplegia have been well described in detail previously and are reviewed briefly here.[3] Other more concentrated constituent dilutions (1:8 to 1:50) may be

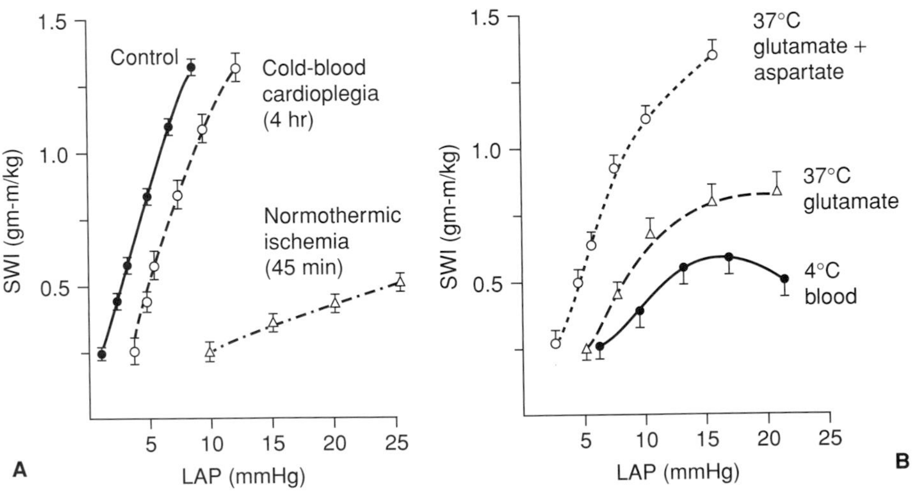

Figure 22-2 (A) LV function every 20 min in normal hearts subjected to 4 h of aortic clamping with blood cardioplegia compared with depressed function after 45 min of normothermic arrest without cardioplegia. (B) LV function when jeopardized hearts undergoing 45 min of normothermic ischemia are subjected to 2 h more of aortic clamping. Note (1) no further improvement when only cold cardioplegic perfusate is given over the 45-min arrest period and (2) progressively increased recovery when the cardioplegic solution is supplemented with warm glutamate and aspartate during induction of cardioplegia and reperfusion with intermittent cold doses of blood every 20 min of supplemental aortic clamping. These data suggest the value of amino acid enrichment in jeopardized hearts. LAP = left atrial pressure; SWI = stroke-work index.

Table 22-1 Induction and terminal "hot shot" cardioplegia (bag 1)

Cardioplegia additive	Volume added (mL)	Component modified	Concentration delivered[a]
Potassium chloride (2 meq/mL)	15	Potassium ion	16–20 meq/L
Tromethamine (THAM) (0.3 mol/L)	225	pH	pH 7.5–7.7
Citrate-phosphate-dextrose	225	Calcium ion	0.2–0.4 mmol/L
Aspartate, glutamate	250	Substrate	13 mmol/L each
50% Dextrose in water	40	Glucose	< 400 mg/dL
5% Dextrose in water	200	Osmolarity	380–400 mOsm

[a]When mixed in a 4:1 ratio with blood.

used if the crystalloid component is appropriately varied to create the desired blood:crystalloid composition described in this chapter (Tables 22-2, 22-3, and 22-4).

A high level of potassium maintains cardiac arrest and prevents sudden intracellular calcium accumulation and disruption of the sarcolemma, as observed when reoxygenation occurs. A low level of calcium is used to limit calcium loading during the conditions of impaired ionic balance in the early period of reperfusion. The amino acid substrates aspartate and glutamate increase the energy-depleted heart's ability to utilize oxygen and hasten ionic recovery. Hyperosmolarity reduces edema. Alkalosis with tromethamine (THAM) is used in preference to bicarbonate, which yields more CO_2 and acidosis, to (1) limit the evolution of acidosis during ischemia and (2) hasten enzymatic recovery.

We routinely use two formulations of cardioplegia (bags 1 and 2) during elective cardiac operations and switch between them based on the metabolic requirements of the heart during specific phases of the operation. Bag 1 is called "induction/terminal" cardioplegia and is a high-potassium (20 meq/L), aspartate- and glutamate-enriched solution (Table 22-1). It is infused as a cold solution after aortic cross-clamping to arrest the heart and then infused as a warm solution just prior to the release of aortic cross-clamping after all cardiac repairs are completed in order to resuscitate the energy-depleted ischemic myocardium ("hot shot"). Bag 2 is called "maintenance" cardioplegia and consists of a low-potassium (7 to 10 meq/L) mixture without the amino acid additives (Table 22-2). It is administered as a cold solution intermittently during the operation. A third cardioplegia (bag 3) is called "rescue" cardioplegia and is used following myocardial infarction as a controlled reperfusate (Table 22-3). Its rationale and use are described further on.

DELIVERY OF CARDIOPLEGIA

Cardioplegia is effective only if it is well distributed. Adding retrograde perfusion via transatrial cannulation of the coronary sinus improves subendocardial perfusion, avoids ostial cannulation during aortic valve procedures, limits the removal of retractors during mitral procedures, and permits flushing of air and atheromas during coronary reoperations. Experimentally, right ventricular nutritive flow is limited by retrograde perfusion. Clinical studies show that switching from antegrade to retrograde perfusion raises oxygen uptake and lactate washout, indicating that each modality perfuses different areas.[4] Therefore both antegrade and retrograde perfusion is required for complete protection (Fig. 22-3). Recent studies have shown that combined benefits occur by *simultaneous* delivery of retrograde and antegrade cardioplegia in coronary bypass procedures.[5,6] After vein grafting to a coronary artery, cardioplegia may be given through the graft in an antegrade manner and simultaneously through the coronary sinus. Myocardial venous hypertension is prevented by drainage through the thebesian veins.

Noncoronary collateral flow from mediastinal collaterals displaces cardioplegia with warmer systemic blood. Topical hypothermia slows rewarming but may cause pulmonary complications (phrenic palsy) without supplementing the cardioprotective effects. Hence continuous or intermittent cardioplegia is required. Continuous cardioplegic perfusion has been advocated to avoid

Table 22-2 Cold maintenance cardioplegia (bag 2)

Cardioplegia additive	Volume added (mL)	Component modified	Concentration delivered[a]
Potassium chloride (2 meq/mL)	10	Potassium ion	8–10 meq/L
Tromethamine (THAM) (0.3 mol/L)	200	pH	pH 7.6–7.8
Citrate-phosphate-dextrose	50	Calcium ion	0.5–0.6 mmol/L
5% Dextrose in water 1/4 isotonic saline solution	550	Osmolarity	340–360 mOsm

[a]When mixed in a 4:1 ratio with blood.

Table 22-3 "Rescue" warm-blood cardioplegia reperfusate[a] (bag 3)

Cardioplegia additive	Volume added (mL)	Component modified	Final concentration
Potassium chloride (2 meq/mL)	40	K^+	20–25 meq/L
Tromethamine (THAM) (0.3 mol/L)	225	pH	7.5–7.6
Citrate-phosphate-dextrose	225	Ca^+	0.1–0.25 mmol/L
Glucose	$40D_{50}W$	Glucose	> 400 mg/dL
Osmolarity	—	Osmolarity	380–400 mOsm
Glutamate	125	Substrate	13 mmol/L
Aspartate	125	Substrate	13 mmol/L
5% Dextrose and H_2O	250	—	—
Diltiazem	300 μg/kg body weight		

[a]When mixed in a 4:1 ratio with blood.

ischemia, but adequate protection may not be achieved at usual flow rates, and the surgeon's vision becomes obscured during infusion. Intermittent cardioplegia, delivered at 10- to 20-min intervals maintains arrest, slows rewarming, and restores substrates depleted during ischemia. In addition, it flushes accumulated metabolites and counteracts acidosis and edema.

TEMPERATURE OF CARDIOPLEGIA

Integrated myocardial management also addresses the special needs of the myocardium based on nutritive needs and underlying pathology. Hence both cold and warm cardioplegia is used in this method at various times.

During routine elective operations in patients with good ventricular function, cardioplegic arrest is done with cold-blood cardioplegia (bag 1). If ventricular function is impaired or there is active ischemia, induction is carried out with warm bag 1 cardioplegia. In both cases, cardioplegia is first given antegrade and then retrograde. If the heart is arrested with a warm induction, low potassium nonenriched cardioplegia (bag 2) is then given antegrade and retrograde to cool the heart. Temperature is always monitored in the septum to assure optimal cooling and distribution.

Warm-blood cardioplegia (37°C) given initially (induction) limits reperfusion damage in ischemic hearts.[7] It enhances metabolic repair by channeling aerobic adenosine triphosphate production to reparative processes. Other cardioplegic components, citrate-phosphate-dextrose (CPD), and buffers (THAM) limit calcium influx and acidosis. Clinical studies confirm our experimental findings and show that warm-blood cardioplegia ("hot shot") after ischemia improves recovery. Warm cardioplegic induction and reperfusion solutions are augmented with the amino acids glutamate and aspartate to replenish key Krebs cycle intermediates depleted by ischemia. These additions enhance the reparative processes after a period of myocardial ischemia.

A modified warm cardioplegia known as "rescue" cardioplegia may be used to resuscitate the arrested heart after acute myocardial infarction or cardiac arrest occurring soon after bypass surgery.[8] The solution (bag 3, Table 22-3) contains the amino acid–enriched solutions with the addition of diltiazem, which limits calcium influx into the injured myocardium. This solution may be infused for 20 min selectively into the infarcted artery via a saphenous vein bypass prior to its attachment to the aorta. During this phase, the ventricle is vented via the right superior pulmonary vein. Rescue cardioplegia may also be used globally (antegrade and retrograde, alternating 5 min each for 20 min). We have observed marked rhythm and hemodynamic improvement after witnessed cardiac arrest of up to 120 min with this approach.

Table 22-4 Modified noncardioplegic cold blood (bag 4)

Solution additive	Volume added (mL)	Component modified	Concentration delivered[a]
Tromethamine (THAM) (0.3 mol/L)	50	pH	pH 7.5–7.6
Citrate-phosphate-dextrose	50	Calcium ion	0.5–0.6 mmol/L
Magnesium chloride (2 meq/mL)	10	Magnesium ion	4–6 mg/L
5% Dextrose in water 1/4 isotonic saline solution	1000	Osmolarity, glucose	340–360 mOsm
Mannitol (25%)	50	Osmolarity, oxygen-radical scavenger	340–360 mOsm

[a]When mixed in a 4:1 ratio with blood.

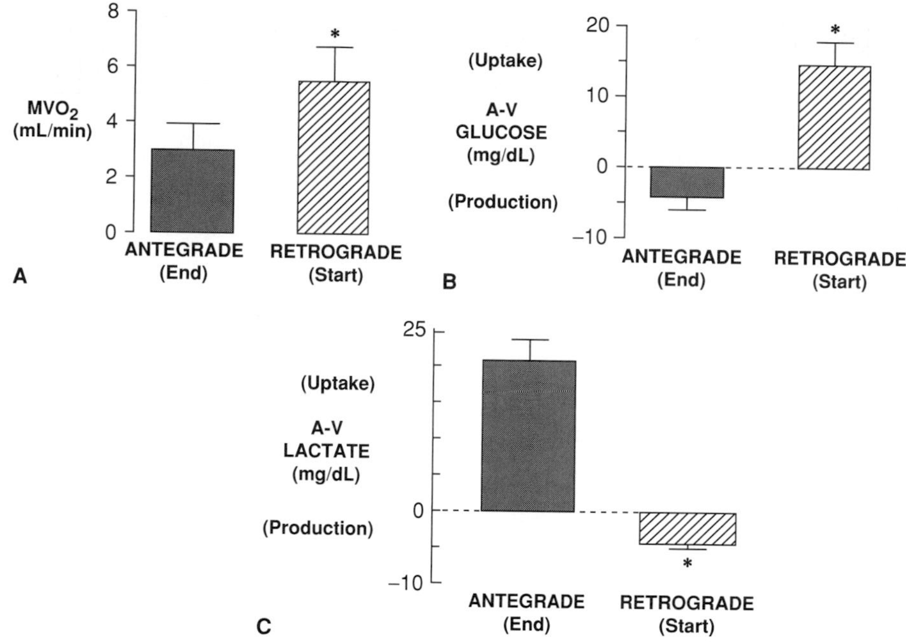

Figure 22-3 Myocardial metabolic changes in coronary patients when cardioplegic induction solution is converted from antegrade to retrograde. Note the increase in myocardial oxygen uptake (MVO_2), glucose uptake, and lactate production, suggesting different areas of perfusion by the antegrade and retrograde methods of delivery. This implies an advantage to both methods.

AORTIC CLAMPING

Coronary artery bypass grafting (CABG) is the most common cardiac operation, and the risk of intraoperative cerebral atheroemboli is increased among elderly patients undergoing revascularization. Atherosclerotic emboli are more likely after repeated aortic tangential clamping for proximal anastomoses. The integrated approach of myocardial protection permits bypass grafting and all cardiac procedures to be performed with single clamping of the aorta. The use of single aortic cross-clamping has been avoided by some owing to concern that this method will extend the ischemic time. There is evidence that morbidity and cost are reduced despite a longer aortic clamp time when integrated protection is applied.[9] These findings contradict the notion that surgeons must battle the clock when the aorta is clamped. The extent of cardiac damage is related to *how* the heart is protected rather than *how long* the aorta is clamped. Blood cardioplegia provides sufficient cardiac nourishment during aortic clamping to permit excellent myocardial protection.

CARDIOPLEGIC TECHNIQUE

This is a general overview of how cardioplegia is used in typical operations. Special situations and details pertaining to specific operations are reviewed further on.

Cardiopulmonary bypass is initiated with core cooling to about 34°C. The aorta is clamped and cold bag 1 is infused antegrade at a flow of 300 mL/min over a 2-min period. Then cold bag 1 is infused via a retrograde cannula into the coronary sinus at a flow of 200 mL/min for 2 min. Septal temperature is monitored throughout. A temperature below 14°C indicates good distribution of cardioplegia and adequate cooling. All cardiac repairs are done while the aorta is clamped, including proximal anastomosis. Intermittent maintenance cardioplegia, bag 2, is given at 15-min intervals, both antegrade and retrograde. After cardiac repairs are completed, a warm reperfusate ("hot shot") is infused antegrade for 2 min (150 mL/min) and then retrograde (150 mL/min). This is followed by a continuous infusion of warm noncardioplegic blood antegrade into the aortic root while the cross clamp is still in place at a flow of 300 to 350 mL/min at a pressure equal to or less than 80 mmHg. The aortic clamp is released usually within 3 to 5 min after adequate contractility is observed. The aortic vent is activated and the patient tilted with the head down slightly to evacuate any air while the heart is ejecting.

Alternatively, bag 1 ("warm induction") is used initially to arrest the heart where acute ischemia is present or in cases of severely depressed systolic function. The administration of substrates in this situation has been proven to improve postoperative function. After the warm induction, bag 2 maintenance cold-blood cardioplegia is infused antegrade and retrograde as above.

CARDIOPLEGIA DELIVERY SYSTEMS

All operations include the use of a heat exchanger to cool or warm the cardioplegia (Fig. 22-4), cannulas for antegrade and retrograde delivery, and a monitoring-infusion system. The system we use is shown in Fig. 22-5. The three controls are color-coded and easily within reach.

1. A stopcock, which switches between antegrade and retrograde infusion. Attached to these infusion lines are thinner ones for infusion pressure monitoring.
2. A flow clamp to activate the aortic vent.
3. Flow clamps on the retrograde line and on a line attached to this line. The latter can be used to deliver cardioplegia through a vein graft or directly into the coronary ostia via a handheld cannula during aortic valve operations (Fig. 22-5).

An *antegrade* cannula is placed high in the right ascending aorta and slightly to the right side. This cannula contains a pressure line and vent port to suction air and blood between infusions. Since we use a single aortic clamping for all operations, when proximal grafting of vein is performed, blood can be vented from the aorta while giving continuous retrograde cold noncardioplegia blood. Placing this cannula slightly to the side of the aorta away from the anterior surface allows pooled blood to be effectively suctioned, thereby permitting good visualization of the anterior surface of the aorta for grafting. This site is not used for proximal grafting and is secured with a purse-string suture at the end of the operation.

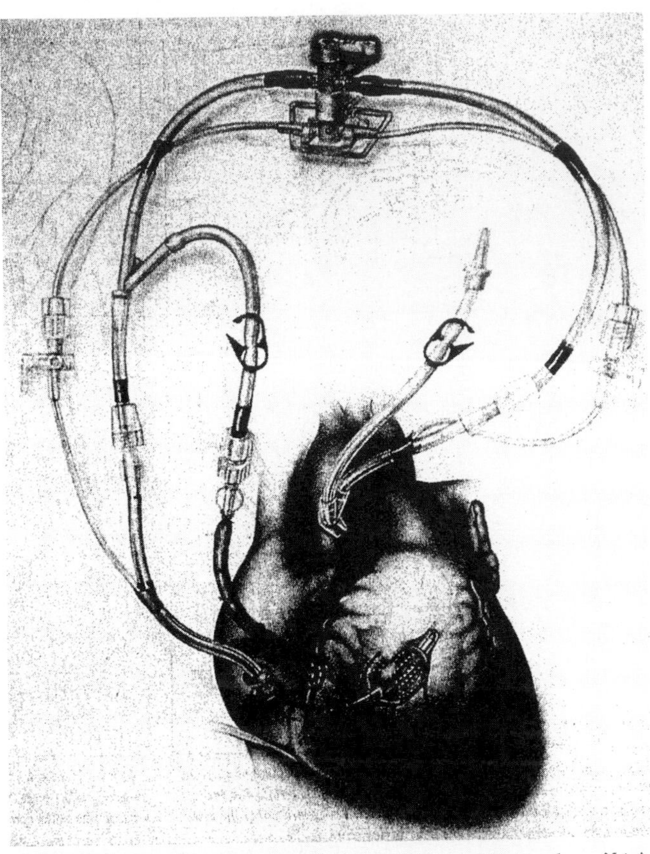

Figure 22-5 Tubing use for antegrade, retrograde, and vein perfusion connected to the retrograde arm. Note the stopcock that allows simultaneous delivery of cardioplegic perfusate and monitoring of arterial or coronary sinus pressure. The tubing connected to the retrograde limb allows simultaneous retrograde/antegrade perfusion down the vein graft or right coronary ostium during aortic valve replacement.

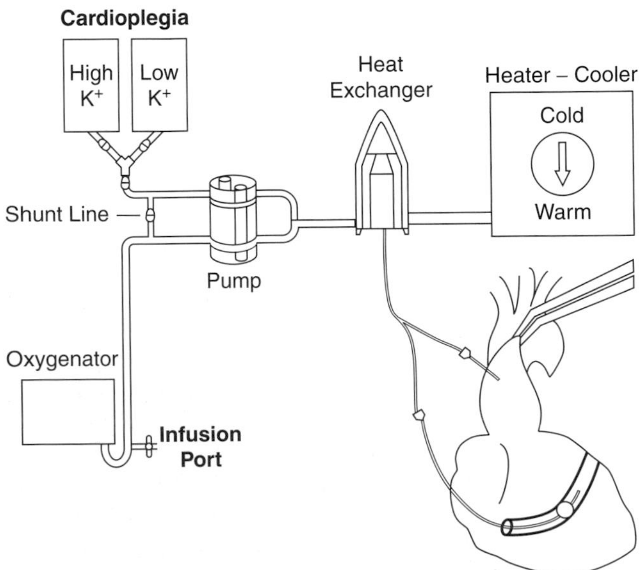

Figure 22-4 Blood cardioplegic delivery system for high-dose (bag 1) and low-dose (bag 2) cardioplegia solutions. These are mixed 4:1 with blood from the oxygenator. The shunt line allows delivery of blood through the roller head of the pump after the warm reperfusate is given.

The *retrograde* cannula has a self-inflating or manually inflated balloon at its tip; it also contains a line for monitoring infusion pressure. It is placed low in the right atrium anterior to the venous cannula and just above the caval junction. It is directed into the coronary sinus by aiming at the left shoulder. The cannula is advanced until it meets resistance within the coronary sinus, usually adjacent to the left atrial appendage (Figs. 22-6 and 22-7).

The coronary sinus can be injured by forceful cannulation or continued administration of cardioplegia when coronary sinus pressure exceeds 50 mmHg. This can occur while the heart is elevated during circumflex artery grafting. The perfusionist notes high pressure, then low pressure as a consequence of acute perforation, or the surgeon sees red blood accumulate in the pericardial well. Perforation can be repaired directly with 5-0

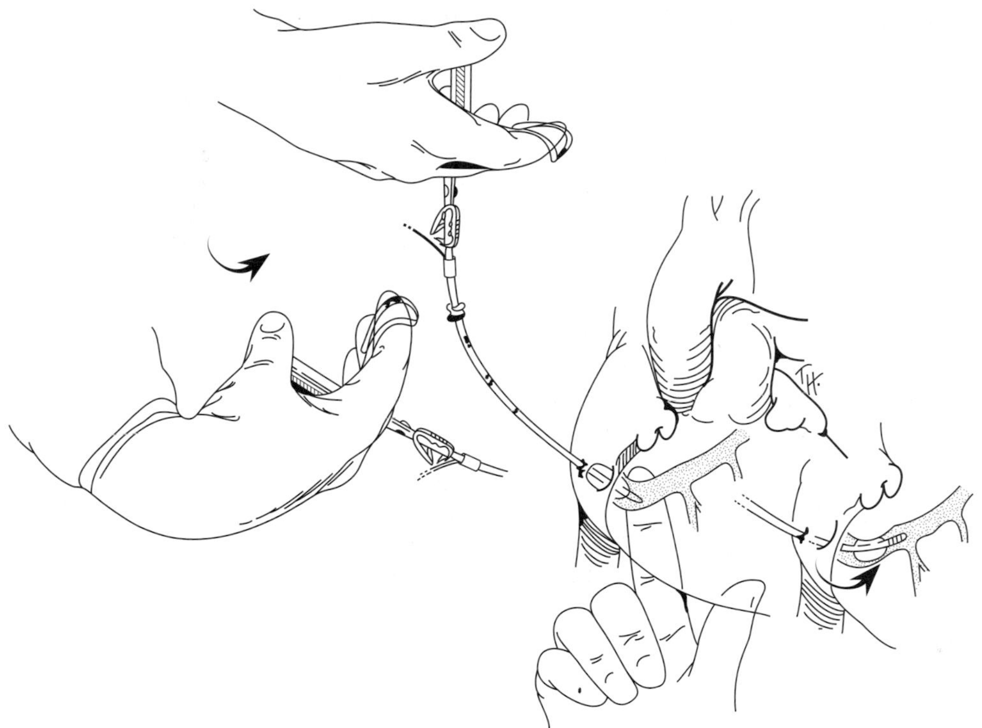

Figure 22-6 Method for introducing the retrograde cannula. Note that the cannula is rotated anteriorly and toward the left shoulder to follow the course of the coronary sinus.

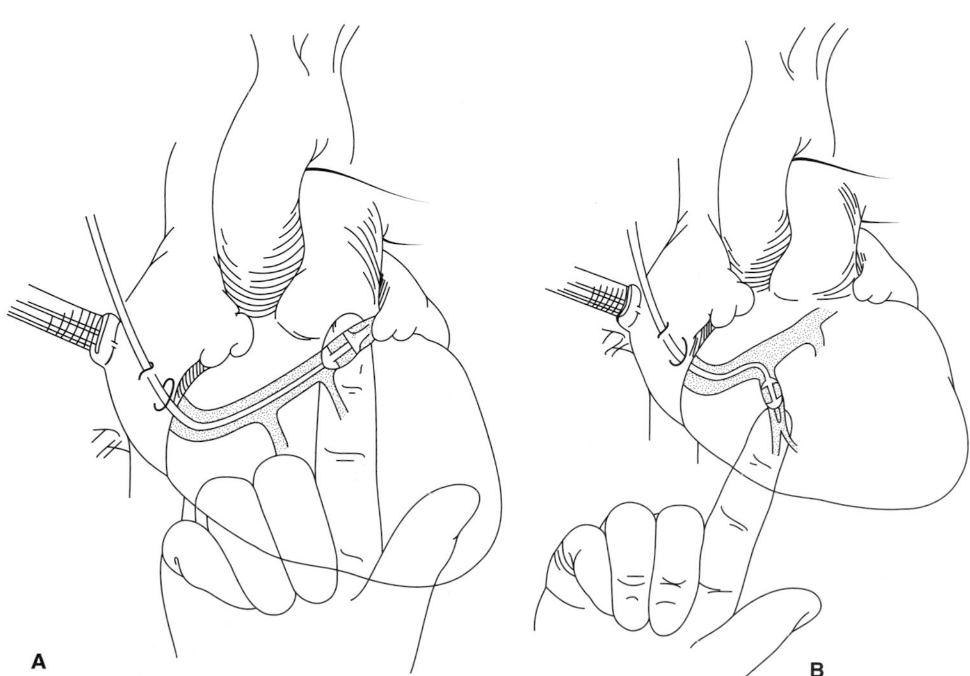

Figure 22-7 (A) Correct placement of retrograde catheter. (B) Incorrect placement of catheter into coronary vein, confirmed by palpation.

polypropylene sutures or pericardial pledgets if the tear site is not distinct. Hematomas are often self-contained after heparin reversal.

MONITORING CARDIOPLEGIA LINE PRESSURE

The regulation of cardioplegia infusion pressure avoids edema and endothelial damage. It also detects aortic insufficiency produced by distortion of the noncoronary aortic cusp by the venous cannula or clinically insignificant regurgitation. Slight manual compression of the right ventricular outflow tract will push the septum against the posterior left ventricle and close the aortic valve, allowing adequate root pressure. During retrograde infusion, measurement of pressure verifies correct placement of the coronary sinus cannula.

During antegrade infusion, aortic root pressure is maintained between 60 and 80 mmHg at a flow rate of 200 mL/min or, in hypertrophied hearts, 250 mL/min. Blood cardioplegia is given over time to ensure maximal oxygen delivery. Failure to arrest means inadequate systemic venous drainage (full heart), incomplete aortic clamping, or aortic insufficiency. Aortic pressure of below 30 mmHg means that antegrade flow is insufficient and only retrograde infusion should be used. High aortic pressure (greater than 100 mmHg) may occur with extensive obstructive coronary disease. If this happens, the infusion rate should be slowed to give the correct dose over time. During the final warm cardioplegia infusion ("hot shot"), the aortic root pressure should not exceed 50 mmHg to avoid endothelial dysfunction.

During retrograde infusion, coronary sinus pressure is maintained between 20 and 40 mmHg at a flow of 200 mL/min. A coronary sinus pressure greater than 50 mmHg means improper positioning or cardiac retraction. This is treated by reducing the flow rate immediately, repositioning the catheter, and then resuming flow. Textured balloons should not be moved during infusion because of coronary sinus wall traction and possible injury. A coronary sinus pressure below 20 mmHg indicates that the balloon is not inflated or not occluding the coronary sinus. The cannula tip and balloon should then be repositioned by palpation. Added maneuvers to improve retroperfusion include compressing the junction of the coronary sinus and right atrium or placing a snared suture around the coronary sinus, thus fixing it in place and preventing regurgitation of cardioplegia into the atrium. Other rarer causes of low pressure include persistent left superior vena cava (SVC) and left atrial unroofing of the coronary sinus. The presence of a left SVC is usually determined before cardiopulmonary bypass and the vessel occluded with a tourniquet only if an intact innominate vein is present. If the innominate vein is absent, only antegrade cardioplegia is used to avoid myocardial underperfusion.

APPLICATIONS OF CARDIOPLEGIA

Coronary artery bypass grafting

During CABG operations the body is cooled to 34°C. The heart is arrested with high-potassium *cold* blood cardioplegia (bag 1) in elective low-risk operations with good ventricular function. For simplicity, this solution is enriched with aspartate and glutamate, rather than preparing another solution without these. Cardioplegia is delivered antegrade (300 mL/min for 2 min), then retrograde (200 mL/min for 2 min). Alternatively, this same potassium-enriched *warm*-blood cardioplegia ("warm induction") is used initially to arrest the heart in cases of acute ischemia or severely depressed systolic function. After the warm induction, maintenance low-potassium cold-blood cardioplegia (bag 2) is infused into the aortic root and retrograde into the coronary sinus. This same solution is used intermittently during the course of the grafting.

Following cardioplegic arrest, all anastomoses are constructed in a dry operative field using distal/proximal grafting in sequence. The right coronary is first grafted because retrograde nutritive perfusion is limited. Maintenance cardioplegia (bag 2) is then given simultaneously retrograde via the coronary sinus cannula and its side-arm antegrade into the newly grafted vessel at a flow rate of 200 mL/min for 1 min. Air is purged from the graft as the distal coronary suture is tied. This maneuver protects the right ventricle by antegrade direct coronary perfusion. The left ventricle is simultaneously protected by retrograde perfusion. The aortic vent is temporarily closed to distend the aortic root. While cardioplegia is infusing retrograde and simultaneously through the unattached vein graft, determination of graft length in the distended vein becomes quite easy.

During proximal grafting of vein to the aorta, retrograde cold noncardioplegic blood is infused at 200 mL/min. Cold blood maintains arrest and limits potassium overdose. This solution can be enhanced with CPD, THAM, magnesium, and mannitol, which prevent resumption of low-level electromechanical activity (bag 4, Table 22-4). The aorta is vented by active suction during proximal grafting, allowing good visualization. When proximal grafting is completed, cardioplegia infusion is then switched to the antegrade mode. Air is evacuated from the aortic root as the proximal suture line is secured. Air is also evacuated from the grafts during antegrade infusion with a 27-gauge needle.

Newly constructed grafts perfuse the heart after each proximal connection. The next distal graft is then constructed in a dry operative field while the heart is vented. The sequence is repeated for each distal and proximal anastomosis, leaving one proximal graft to be connected to the aorta after the final distal left internal mammary artery (LIMA) anastomosis is constructed. While the LIMA anastomosis is begun, systemic rewarming is started and the cardioplegic solution is rewarmed.

After the LIMA is grafted, antegrade warm enriched cardioplegia (bag 1) is delivered for two minutes at a flow of 150 mL/min, followed by retrograde warm cardioplegia, also at a flow of 150 mL/min. During the retrograde infusion, the last proximal vein graft is sewn to the aorta, followed immediately by infusion of warm noncardioplegia blood at a flow of 250 to 300 mL/min until the proximal grafting is complete. The heart usually begins contracting and systolic compression of the capillary bed raises coronary sinus pressures, but this is of no concern. Antegrade flow is started to de-air the aortic root, as before, and the grafts are de-aired with the 27-gauge needle to prevent air embolus.

Combined operations

In combined valve/coronary procedures, distal coronary grafting is performed first. The valve is then replaced or repaired. Every 15 to 20 min, maintenance cold cardioplegia (bag 2) is delivered through the unattached vein grafts and simultaneously into the coronary sinus. All proximal anastomoses are then constructed while the aorta is clamped. The proximal right graft is sewn last to maximize right ventricular perfusion. Warm cardioplegic reperfusion (bag 1, "hot shot") is started at the end of the next to the last proximal anastomosis. The perfusionist then delivers retrograde warm blood and the aorta is vented gently while the final right graft is sewn to the aorta. By this point the high-potassium cardioplegia is washed out and the heart begins contracting slowly. The stopcock is switched to antegrade infusion of warm blood as described above. When good contractility is observed, the aortic clamp is removed and the patient weaned from cardiopulmonary bypass, usually with minimal inotropic support. Phenylephrine infusion at 0 to 2 μg/kg/min is often needed, since the enriched solutions tend to cause a transient vasodilatation.

Evolving myocardial infarction

The procedure is slightly modified for patients with acute evolving myocardial infarction and total occlusion of a coronary artery. Cardiopulmonary bypass is instituted in the usual manner with systemic cooling to 34°C. The left ventricle is vented via the right superior pulmonary vein to minimize myocardial oxygen demands. The aorta is clamped and the heart arrested with a warm induction (bag 1), as previously described, followed by maintenance cold cardioplegia (bag 2). The noninfarct vessels are grafted first, as described previously for treating high-risk coronary patients. All proximal anastomoses are made except for one graft, which will be connected to the aorta during the 20-min interval for infarct vessel reperfusion described below. The whole heart receives a final "hot shot" cardioplegia, followed by retrograde warm blood infusion as in the standard CABG operation.

Following completion of distal and proximal grafting of the compensating remote muscle (except one graft to remote noninfracted muscle), the infarct-related artery is grafted last, following perfusion with warm "rescue cardioplegia" (bag 3) at 50 mL/min (≤50 mmHg pressure) for 20 min (Table 22-3). This is a substrate-enriched, hyperosmotic, hypocalcemic, alkalotic, diltiazem-containing solution. Connection of the last proximal graft going to remote muscle is made during prolonged infarct graft perfusion. This interval allows ongoing surgical activity during this 20-min warm infusion via the infarct vessel.

The last proximal anastomosis (from the infarct region) is made after the prolonged reperfusion via the infarct graft. Warm retrograde normal blood perfusion is distributed to the infarct region during this interval of making the aortic connection so as to avoid additional ischemia. Cardiopulmonary bypass with the vented heart is continued for 30 more min to allow recovery of the newly revascularized infarcted myocardium. We have observed significant return of regional contractility despite more than 6 h of ischemia. The details and outcome of this technique have been previously described.[8]

Cardiac reoperations

The integrated cardioplegia method described above has been found to be particularly useful in repeat operations. In coronary bypass operations, a generally accepted rule is that old grafts should be left undisturbed. This "no touch" technique prevents embolization of friable atherosclerotic debris into the distal vasculature.

Following sternotomy, only the aorta and right atrium are dissected free of surrounding adhesions. Following cannulation and institution of cardiopulmonary bypass, cardioplegia is delivered as in nonrepeat operations. The aorta is vented to decompress the heart, and only then is the heart freed of surrounding pericardial adhesions. This avoids compression of old vein grafts and embolization. Distal and proximal grafts are constructed in sequence, as with all coronary operations. The single aortic cross-clamping technique avoids compression of old grafts and ischemia, which can be induced by the side-biting aortic clamping method, where graft flow is temporarily interrupted.

Clinical outcomes with this method in repeat CABG have demonstrated no increased mortality, even in patients with markedly reduced systolic function preoperatively.[10]

Myocardial protection during aortic root replacement

The myocardium must be carefully protected during repair of ascending aortic aneurysm or dissection. The coronary ostia are often isolated for reimplantation into a graft. Intermittent cardioplegia can be administered directly into the unattached ostia, but care must be taken to avoid injury, particularly in cases of aortic dissection. An approach we have found useful is to first graft the right coronary artery with saphenous vein. The proximal right coronary artery is temporarily occluded with a Silastic vascular loop. Cardioplegia can then be administered intermittently antegrade via the right coronary artery and simultaneously retrograde into the coronary sinus. This permits maximum distribution throughout the myocardium and does not interfere with the operation. The aortic root and ascending aorta can be repaired with ease in a dry field. After the root has been reconstructed, the ostia are reimplanted into the graft and the saphenous vein graft ligated at the anastomosis to the right coronary artery, either with a running suture or a large clip. This method assures global myocardial protection and avoids injury to the friable coronary ostia.

CONCLUSIONS

"Integrated myocardial management" as described above allows cardiac procedures to proceed smoothly and rapidly, since there is no interruption or delay for infusion of cardioplegia. The duration of cardiopulmonary bypass is actually shortened while simultaneously taking advantage of the benefits of different methods. Ongoing studies will likely lead to the incorporation of additional cardioprotective methods, such as preconditioning agents, white blood cell filters, oxygen-radical scavengers, endothelium-enhancing agents, and molecular factors that will further improve the safety of ischemic intervals and limit reperfusion damage.

References

1. Buckberg GD, Beyersdorf F, Allen BS, Robertson JM. Integrated myocardial management: Background and initial application. *J Card Surg* 1995;10:68–89.
2. Guyton RA. Oxygenated crystalloid cardioplegia. *Semin Thorac Cardiovasc Surg* 1993;5:114–121.
3. Robertson JM, Vinten-Johansen J, Buckberg GD, et al. Safety of prolonged aortic clamping with blood cardioplegia. I. Glutamate enrichment in normal hearts. *J Thorac Cardiovasc Surg* 1984;88:395–401.
4. Buckberg GD. Antegrade/retrograde blood cardioplegia to ensure cardioplegic distribution: Operative techniques and objectives. *J Card Surg* 1989;4:216–238.
5. Ihnken K, Morita K, Buckberg GD, et al. The safety of simultaneous arterial and coronary sinus perfusion: Experimental background and initial clinical results. *J Card Surg* 1994;9:15–25.
6. Noyez L, van Son JA, van der WT, et al. Retrograde versus antegrade delivery of cardioplegic solution in myocardial revascularization. A clinical trial in patients with three-vessel coronary artery disease who underwent myocardial revascularization with extensive use of the internal mammary artery. *J Thorac Cardiovasc Surg* 1993;105:854–863.
7. Beyersdorf F, Allen BS, Buckberg GD, et al. Studies on prolonged acute regional ischemia: I. Evidence for preserved cellular viability after 6 hours of coronary occlusion. *J Thorac Cardiovasc Surg* 1989;98:112–126.
8. Beyersdorf F, Sarai K, Maul FD, et al. Controlled reperfusion during emergency coronary artery bypass surgery after angioplasty failure restores immediate segmental contractility. *J Interven Cardiol* 1991;4:53–62.
9. Loop FD, Higgins TL, Panda R, et al. Myocardial protection during cardiac operations: Decreased morbidity and lower cost with blood cardioplegia and coronary sinus perfusion. *J Thorac Cardiovasc Surg* 1992;104:608–618.
10. Athanasuleas CL, Riemer DW, Buckberg GD. The role of integrated myocardial management in reoperative coronary surgery. *Semin Thorac Cardiovasc Surg* 2001;13:33–37.

CHAPTER

23 POSTOPERATIVE MANAGEMENT OF THE CARDIAC SURGICAL PATIENT

Ala' Sami Haddadin, Nauder Faraday

INTRODUCTION

Patients undergoing cardiac surgery today are older and have more comorbid illnesses than patients in previous years. The average cardiac surgical patient has less reserve in each organ system to compensate for the obligate organ injury that occurs as part of surgery and cardiopulmonary bypass (CPB). As a result, patients are at greater risk to suffer clinical complications of cardiac surgical procedures than ever before. Yet despite this increase in risk, overall morbidity and mortality have not increased substantially over the past 25 years, in large part owing to improvements in intra- and postoperative management strategies. Prevention of complications requires a thorough understanding of the pathophysiologic basis for the development of organ dysfunction after cardiac surgery, the ability to identify high-risk patients, and the ability to execute therapeutic strategies that prevent complications from developing. In those patients in whom complications develop, early diagnosis and treatment can prevent further deterioration and limit subsequent morbidity and mortality.

Effective management of today's cardiac surgical patient requires a team of dedicated clinicians who provide a continuum of care that begins preoperatively, continues intraoperatively, and proceeds into the postoperative period. Early postoperative care (first 12 to 24 h) can be regarded as an extension of the intraoperative period and focuses on resolving any issues that develop intraoperatively. The emphasis during this early postoperative phase is primarily on restoring cardiopulmonary stability and normal hemostasis. For the majority of patients, sufficient stability can be achieved within the first 12 to 24 h that the patient can be safely discharged

KEY CONCEPTS

- Cardiac surgery involves unique anatomic and physiologic stresses that tax the reserve of every organ system. Continuous postoperative surveillance is required for early recognition of pathology and for rapid institution of organ and life preserving therapies.
- Cardiac surgery causes transient (lasting 12–24 hours) myocardial injury, sympathetic hyper-reactivity, and the systemic inflammatory response syndrome (SIRS) in nearly all patients. As a result, hemodynamic instability requiring transient pressor and/or vasodilator infusions and intravascular volume expansion should be expected in all patents during the first 6-24 postoperative hours.
- Atrial fibrillation/flutter occurs in 20-60% of patients after cardiac surgery, and its incidence can be reducted by half through prophylactic administration of beta blockers, amiodarone, or sotalol.
- Significant pulmonary compromise should be expected in all cardiac surgical patients postoperatively, with 5% of patients experiencing overt respiratory failure. Diuresis should be instituted as soon as SIRS abates to limit fluid accumulation in the injured post-CPB lung.
- Liberation from mechanical ventilation should be sought at the earliest possible time in all patients. Extubation in most patients can be achieved as soon as they are awake enough to maintain airway patency and achieve adequate spontaneous gas exchange. In patients with significant respiratory compromise, daily assessment of a spontaneous breathing trial is the best method to assess readiness for extubation.
- Aggressive glucose control with a goal of 80-110 mg/dL within 24 hours of ICU arrival reduces the incidence of death, sepsis, and renal failure after cardiac surgery.

from the ICU. However, in a sizable minority of patients, significant dysfunction in one or more organ systems persists past 24 h. In the second phase of care, which has similarities with noncardiac surgical intensive care, management focuses on establishing specific diagnoses and treatment strategies for postsurgical complications. Regardless of phase, the hallmark of effective postoperative management is early recognition of pathology and rapid institution of therapy to prevent further clinical deterioration or the development of overt morbidity.

PATHOPHYSIOLOGY OF ORGAN DYSFUNCTION AFTER CARDIAC SURGERY

Cardiac surgery involves a number of unique anatomic and physiologic stresses that tax the reserve of every organ system and increase the likelihood that clinical morbidity will develop. A list of these stressors and their pathophysiologic and clinical sequelae is shown in Table 23-1.

GENERAL MANAGEMENT ISSUES IN THE EARLY POSTOPERATIVE PERIOD

The early postoperative period is characterized by instability in a number of organ systems, including cardiac, pulmonary, hematologic, and renal/electrolyte. This instability is a direct result of the anatomic and physiologic disturbances that take place intraoperatively (see Table 23-1). If significant organ injury was not sustained during intraoperative events, instability tends to be brief, resolving in the first 12 to 24 h after surgery. Resolution is rapid because the primary stressors causing instability (i.e., insults related to CPB) are confined to the intraoperative period. Once removed from these intraoperative influences, the patient can recover rapidly if organ reserve was not exhausted. Intensive monitoring of vital organ system function and rapid intervention for patients that deviate from predefined physiologic parameters are required during this early phase.

Transfer of care and monitoring

The transport and transfer of care from the OR to the ICU is an inherently dangerous process. To reduce risk, hemodynamic stability should be assured prior to leaving the OR. The ventilatory strategy required to achieve adequate gas exchange intraoperatively should be noted, and manual bag ventilation should be initiated with 100 percent O_2 with a respiratory frequency appropriate for CO_2 exchange. Monitoring during transfer should be at a level comparable to that used intraoperatively and should include at a minimum the following: electrocardiogram, arterial blood pressure (BP), and pulse oximetry.

On arrival in the ICU, all care providers should initially focus on assuring the adequacy of cardiopulmonary function. Manual ventilation should be replaced with mechanical ventilation at the earliest possible time. Ventilator settings [FIO_2, positive end-expiratory pressure (PEEP), mode, tidal volume, and rate] should be guided by the OR team on the basis of intraoperative gas exchange, acid/base balance, and anatomic concerns. Pulse oximetry and end-tidal CO_2 should be monitored continuously. Hemodynamic monitoring should be reestablished at the intraoperative level. All patients should have arterial BP monitoring unless technically unfeasible. In addition, continual electrocardiographic (ECG) monitoring with ST-segment analysis is standard. Continual ECG monitoring allows for early detection of arrhythmias and ischemia. The combination of leads allowing the most sensitive detection of ischemia is somewhat controversial. Some authors advocate monitoring leads II/V_5[1,2] while more recent data supports the use of II/V_3 or V_4.[3] Full 12-lead ECG analysis should occur on arrival to the ICU and every 4 to 8 h for the first 12 to 24 h postoperatively.

Routine surveillance labs should include hemoglobin or hematocrit, sodium and potassium, glucose, and arterial blood gas; these should be obtained every 4 to 8 h or more frequently when clinically indicated. Additional hematologic and chemistry tests need not be routine but should be obtained based on clinical signs/symptoms. Chest x-ray is mandatory in all patients to verify the positioning of invasive tubes and catheters and to evaluate for chest pathology (e.g., hemothorax, pneumothorax, infiltrate/edema).

A central venous catheter is mandatory for the administration of vasoactive drugs. However, the need for a central venous catheter versus a pulmonary artery (PA) catheter remains controversial. Although the PA catheter can provide hemodynamic information about a patient's status that might otherwise be unknown, it has yet to be clearly demonstrated that this information, or changes in patient management resulting from it, improve patient outcome. Two prospective cohort studies have reported greater morbidity and mortality in patients who received PA catheters as part of their treatment.[4,5] Two prospective randomized trials in vascular surgical patients and one in critically ill patients failed to demonstrate a benefit of PA catheter–directed management compared to a central venous catheter alone[6–8]; however, there was no increase in morbidity or mortality in the PA catheter groups. Prospective randomized trials that evaluate the use of the PA catheter in cardiac surgery have not been performed. Although it is possible that PA catheters may benefit certain high-risk patients, such as those undergoing cardiac surgery, it is not possible to make a strong recommendation for their routine use. If a PA catheter is indicated in a patient whose hemodynamic status is uncertain, it should ideally be left in place for as short a time as is necessary to obtain the diagnostic information needed to guide therapy.

Table 23-1 Anatomic, physiologic, and clinical consequences of cardiac surgery and cardiopulmonary bypass

Stressor	Pathophysiologic sequelae	Clinical sequelae
Anatomic		
Aortic cannulation/decanulation	Aortic athero-embolism	Stroke (large vessel)
Aortic cross-clamping/unclamping	Myocardial ischemia/reperfusion injury	LV and RV dysfunction/low CO
		Atrial and ventricular arrhythmias
	Aortic athero-embolism	Stroke (large vessel)
Cardiac manipulation/positioning	Aortic athero-embolism	Stroke (large vessel)
	Decreased cardiac output (OPCAB)	Pre-renal azotemia, hepatic, mesenteric insufficiency
Atrial cannulation	Atrial trauma	Atrial arrhythmias
Pericardiotomy	Pericardial inflammation	Atrial arrhythmias
Valve replacement	Septal trauma	AV conduction block
	Cordal attachment to valve severed (mitral only)	LV dysfunction/low CO
Physiologic		
Extracorporeal circulation	Activation of contact activation pathway of coagulation	Need for heparin/protamine coagulopathy
	Activation of fibrinolytic systems	Coagulopathy
	Activation of systemic inflammation (complement, leukocytes, cytokines)	SIRS
		Capillary leak syndrome
		Inflammatory end organ damage to brain, heart, lung, and kidney
	Microembolization	Stroke (small vessel)
Controlled hypotension (MAP = 40–60 mm-Hg)	Systemic hypoperfusion	Stroke (watershed)
	Sympathetic activation	Arrhythmias
	Renin-angiotensin release	BP lability
		Pre-renal azotemia, hepatic, mesenteric insufficiency
Non-pulsatile blood flow	Systemic hypoperfusion	Stroke (watershed)
	Sympathetic activation	Arrhythmias
	Renin-angiotensin release	BP lability
		Pre-renal azotemia, hepatic, mesenteric insufficiency
Hypothermia	Decreased efficiency of coagulation cascade	Coagulopathy
	Shivering/increased O_2 consumption and CO_2 production	Hypercarbia/ventilatory insufficiency
	Sympathetic activation	Arrhythmias
		BP lability

LV = left ventricular; RV = right ventricular; CO = cardiac output; OPCAB = off-pump coronary artery bypass; AV = atrioventricular; SIRS = systemic inflammatory response syndrome; MAP = mean arterial pressure; BP = blood pressure.

Hypothermia

Hypothermia is commonly deliberately induced intraoperatively to protect organs from ischemic injury during periods of diminished blood flow. The ability of hypothermia to reduce ischemic organ damage, particularly in the brain, has been shown in a number of animal models and clinical settings. In a prospective randomized trial of hypothermic (28° to 32°C) versus normothermic (37°C) CPB for coronary revascularization, normothermia was associated with a worse neurologic outcome.[9] In patients who have sustained global injury to the central nervous system (CNS) injury during cardiac arrest, induction of hypothermia after the arrest improves neurologic recovery.[10,11] The decrement in temperature required to confer this protective effect is controversial and may be as little as a few degrees Celsius. It is appropriate that some degree of deliberate hypothermia remain a part of cardiac surgical procedures in which ischemic organ damage is a risk.

Unfortunately, hypothermia has adverse physiologic consequences as well (see Table 23-1). It may contribute to postoperative hemorrhage by decreasing the efficiency of the coagulation cascade.[12] Hypothermia stimulates sympathetic nervous discharge, contributes to postoperative hemodynamic lability and hypertension, and may promote myocardial ischemia.[13,14] Shivering in response to hypothermia increases O_2 consumption and CO_2 production, thus increasing the workload of the pulmonary system. A sedated postoperative patient may not produce adequate respiratory compensation for this increase in work, and respiratory acidosis may ensue unless mechanical ventilation is maintained at appropriate levels. Finally, perioperative hypothermia is associated with an increased risk of wound infection in noncardiac surgical procedures.[15] To mitigate the adverse effects of hypothermia in the postoperative period, active warming should be initiated postoperatively with a goal of restoring temperature to between 36° and 37°C. Although a number of warming methods are available, forced-air warming devices appear to be the most effective.[16]

Cardiovascular system

Hemodynamic instability commonly occurs in the early postoperative phase of cardiac surgery. Intraoperative insults (see Table 23-1) can have an adverse impact on each of the major physiologic determinants of cardiovascular function (Fig. 23-1). For example, ischemia, ischemia-reperfusion injury, and CPB-related inflammation can all contribute to depressed myocardial contractility after cardiac surgery. Indeed, biventricular dysfunction has been documented in as many as 90 percent of patients following cardiac surgery.[17,18] In most patients this dysfunction resolves within 24 h; however, inotropic support may be required until this transient dysfunction resolves. Those patients with ventricular dysfunction prior to surgery are more likely to require inotropic support and for a longer duration than patients with normal ventricular function. Similarly, hypovolemia leads to inadequate preload in a large number of patients after surgery. Hypovolemia can be caused by bleeding and/or third-space losses, which in turn are sequelae of CPB-induced abnormalities in hemostasis and systemic inflammation. Intravascular volume resuscitation is required to maintain adequate perfusion and BP for at least the first 6 to 12 h after surgery. Finally, vascular tone can be excessively high from adrenergic hyperactivation or low from CPB-induced systemic inflammatory response syndrome (SIRS). Thus, transient infusions of vasodilators or vasoconstrictors may be needed until vascular stability returns, usually within 24 h of surgery.

The goal of hemodynamic management in the early postoperative phase is to maintain adequate BP and perfusion (i.e., cardiac output) and ensure oxygen delivery to the tissues. It is important to recognize that there is no strong evidence to support one management regimen over another; therefore diagnosis and therapy must be guided by physiologic and pharmacologic principles.

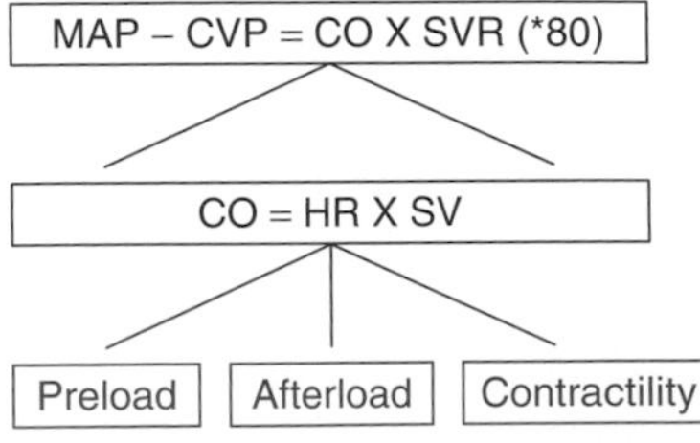

Figure 23-1 Determinants of cardiac output and blood pressure.

Cardiac index in normal healthy volunteers ranges from 2.4 to 4.2 L/min/m^2. However, "normal" cardiac performance in patients after cardiac surgery is not clearly defined; indeed, ventricular dysfunction is nearly ubiquitous even though most patients do not suffer long-term consequences. Adequacy of BP and perfusion is a clinical diagnosis determined by frequent monitoring of vital signs and physical findings. Targets for therapy are a mean arterial pressure (MAP) of 65 to 85; strong, palpable peripheral pulses (particularly in the lower extremities); and urine output of 0.5 mL/kg/h. Invasive monitors can be useful to confirm clinical findings and when these are inadequate or unreliable [e.g., patients with significant preoperative left ventricular (LV) dysfunction, renal failure, or peripheral vascular disease]. A cardiac index of 2.0 to 2.2 L/min/m^2 is generally adequate immediately following cardiac surgery and should be a minimal target in most patients. Monitoring of mixed venous oxygen saturation, from either intermittent blood sampling or continuous invasive cooximetry, can provide data to complement other information, but insufficient data are available to advocate routine use of these technologies. As a general guideline, a mixed venous saturation of 60 to 70 percent is adequate, 50 to 60 percent is borderline adequate, and below 50 percent suggests inadequate oxygen delivery.

Patients who do not meet the criteria for adequacy of BP and perfusion ("low-cardiac-output syndrome") should be identified, the cause of hemodynamic insufficiency diagnosed, and treatment initiated prior to the development of end-organ compromise. In this subset of patients, direct cardiac output and pressure monitoring can be particularly useful to diagnose the patient's condition and guide therapy. Information from a pulmonary artery catheter can readily provide a physiologic diagnosis for inadequate hemodynamics [e.g., poor cardiac contractility, inadequate preload, or low/high systemic vascular resistance (SVR)]. However, a pathologic diagnosis often requires correlation with additional historical and laboratory findings to make a definitive diagnosis and plan treatment (e.g., operative report and ECG findings for diagnosis of myocardial ischemia). Echocardiographic analysis can also be useful in these patients when anatomic abnormalities—such as pericardial effusion/tamponade, ventricular wall motion abnormalities, or valvular dysfunction—are in the differential diagnosis.

Once a diagnosis is made, a large number of inotropic and vasoactive agents are available to support the circulation until definitive correction of the underlying abnormality occurs. Each of these agents has particular pharmacokinetic and pharmacodynamic properties that may be advantageous or disadvantageous in any single patient (Table 23-2). Without evidence indicating a difference in patient outcome based on selection of vasoactive drug, the astute clinician should be familiar with each agent to enable selection of the appropriate drug(s) in each clinical circumstance. In addition to pharmacologic agents, a number of mechanical devices (e.g., intraaortic balloon pump, ventricular assist device, etc.) to support the circulation also need to be considered and employed in the appropriate clinical setting.

Myocardial ischemia

ECG and echocardiographic evidence of myocardial ischemia appears in up to 50 percent of patients in the first several hours after coronary revascularization and is associated with adverse outcome.[19,20] However, in the majority of patients who undergo cardiac surgery, early ECG changes are nonspecific and do not represent clinically meaningful ischemia. Significant ischemia can often be distinguished from incidental ECG findings by the concurrent presence of ventricular dysrhythmias and/or hemodynamic insufficiency. Hypotension or low CO in the presence of high central filling pressures is a particularly ominous finding. The presence of regional wall motion abnormalities on ECG also supports the diagnosis of significant myocardial ischemia.

Patients with ongoing myocardial ischemia in the early postoperative period must be treated promptly. Beta blockade and antiplatelet/anticoagulant therapy, the therapeutic mainstays for myocardial ischemia in other settings, are generally not useful immediately after cardiac surgery because of ongoing bleeding and hemodynamic instability. Intravenous infusion of nitroglycerin or a calcium channel antagonist (nicardipine) may be useful, particularly in cases of internal mammary artery spasm[21,22]; however, hemodynamic instability often precludes their use. Furthermore, randomized trials that support the use of these agents after cardiac surgery are lacking.

Medical management of myocardial ischemia after cardiac surgery is limited to physiologic manipulations

Table 23-2 Vasoactive agents, dosing, hemodynamic and adverse effects

	Vaso-constrict	Vaso-dilate	Contractility	HR	BP	CO	$t_{1/2}$	Adverse effects
VAP 0.01–0.04 (U/min)	+++ VAP-R	—	—	0/↓	↑	↓	10–20 min	Organ ischemia
PNE 0.1–2.0 (μg/kg/min)	++/+++ α_1-R	—	—	0/↓	↑	↓	150 min	Organ ischemia
NE 0.01–0.5 (μg/kg/min)	++++ α_1-R	0/+ β_2-R	+++/++++ β_1-R	0/↓	↑↑	0/↓	1.45–2.90 min	Organ ischemia Arrhythmias
EPI 0.01–0.5 (μg/kg/min)	++++ α_1-R	++++ β_2-R	++++ β_1-R	↑	↑↑	↓/0/↑	Approx 2 min	Organ ischemia Arrhythmias
DA 1.0–20 (μg/kg/min)	+++ α_1-R	+ β_2-R +++ DA_1-R	+++ β_1-R	↑	↑	↓/0/↑	2 min	Organ ischemia Arrhythmias
DOB 1.0–20 (μg/kg/min)	—	+++ β_2-R	+++ β_1-R	0/↑	0/↓	↑	2 min	Hypotension Arrhythmias
ISOP 0.01–0.5 (μg/kg/min)	—	++++ β_2-R	++++ β_1-R	↑↑	↓↓	↑↑	2.5–5 min	Hypotension Arrhythmias Myocardial ischemia
MIL 0.3–0.8* (μg/kg/min)	—	+++ PDEI	+++ PDEI	0/↑	↓	↑	2–3 h	Hypotension
NES 0.01–0.03* (μg/kg/min)	—	++ ANP	-	0	↓	↑	18–23 min	Hypotension
FEN 0.03–0.16 (μg/kg/min)	—	+++ DA_1-R	-	0	↓	↑	9.8 min	Hypotension

ANP = atrial natriuretic peptide; BP = blood pressure; CO = cardiac output; DA = dopamine; DOB = dobutamine; EPI = epinephrine; FEN = fenoldopam; HR = heart rate; ISOP = isoproterenol; MIL = milrinone; NE = norepinephrine; NES = nesiritide; PDEI = phosphodiesterase inhibition; PNE = phenylephrine; R = receptor; $t_{1/2}$ = plasma half-life; VAP = vasopressin; ↑ = increase; 0 = no effect; ↓ = decrease; *loading dose required.

aimed at optimizing myocardial O_2 supply and demand. Hemodynamic improvement should be sought with optimization of preload. Inotropic/vasoconstrictive agents should be reduced as much as possible while maintaining minimally acceptable BP and CO. Recent epidemiologic evidence supports transfusion of red blood cells to a hemoglobin of 10 to 11 in patients above 65 years of age with ongoing myocardial ischemia.[23] If conservative measures fail to reverse ischemia, invasive therapy is warranted. Insertion of an intraaortic balloon pump may be useful to stabilize the patient while more definitive steps are taken. Percutaneous coronary intervention or surgical reexploration and coronary bypass grafting are often required in patients who have persistent myocardial ischemia and hemodynamic instability.

Arrhythmias

Supraventricular and ventricular arrhythmias are common after cardiac surgery. A number of factors associated with an increased risk of postoperative arrhythmias have been identified: advanced age, preoperative history of arrhythmia, history of congestive heart failure, use of bicaval venous cannulation, and longer duration of CPB.[24] In addition to arrhythmogenic intraoperative events (see Table 23-1), a number of postoperative conditions can incite arrhythmias as well (e.g., sympathetic hyperactivity, myocardial ischemia, electrolyte disturbances, atrial distention, and drug therapies). Effective therapies for the prevention of atrial tachyarrhythmias have been described, but pharmacologic prophylaxis against ventricular arrhythmias is unproved. As in all clinical settings, hemodynamically unstable arrhythmias (supraventricular or ventricular) require immediate attention and treatment, often including cardioversion/defibrillation.

Bradycardia Sinus bradycardia, junctional rhythm, and atrioventricular (AV) conduction disturbances comprise the majority of bradycardic rhythms after cardiac surgery. Perioperative drug therapies (beta blockers, digoxin, or amiodarone), hypothermia, electrolyte disturbances, and direct trauma to conductive tissue may all contribute to the development of bradycardia. Among bradycardic rhythm disturbances, high-grade conduction blockade (i.e., new bifascicular or trifascicular block and complete heart block) is the most serious because it usually leads to significant hemodynamic compromise and injury to the conduction system that may be permanent. Infusion of β_1 agonists (see Table 23-2) can effectively increase heart rate and perfusion with mild bradycardia and conduction disturbances. However, pacing is required for more serious bradycardia. Whenever possible, atrial contraction should be preserved because it improves cardiac output and reduces the potential for atrial clot formation. Furthermore, ventricular contractile force is greater when the electrical impulse is generated at or above the AV node instead of at the ventricular level. Thus, in patients with sinus or junctional bradycardia who require pacing, atrial pacing is favored over AV sequential pacing, which is favored over ventricular pacing. In patients with AV conduction block, AV sequential (or DDD) pacing is favored over ventricular pacing. Most patients who have significant AV conduction block that persists 5 to 7 days after surgery require permanent pacemaker placement.

Supraventricular arrhythmias Supraventricular tachycardia occurs in 20 to 60 percent of patients undergoing cardiac surgery and is more frequent after valve surgery than coronary artery bypass grafting (CABG).[24–26] The vast majority of supraventricular tachycardia after cardiac surgery is atrial fibrillation or flutter.[26] Atrial fibrillation most commonly develops between postoperative days 1 and 4, with peak incidence on days 2 and 3.[26] It is associated with an increased length of hospital stay, higher cost, and increased risk of stroke; it can lead to hemodynamic compromise in some high-risk patients.[24,26] The incidence of atrial fibrillation can be reduced by 50 to 60 percent by prophylactic treatment with beta blockers, amiodarone, or sotalol.[27] Preoperative loading with amiodarone is more effective than postoperative loading; however, both methods reduce the incidence of atrial fibrillation.[28] Daily magnesium started preoperatively and continued for 4 days postoperatively was also shown to reduce the incidence of atrial fibrillation after CABG.[29] When atrial fibrillation does develop, therapy should first be directed at assuring hemodynamic stability and rate control. Cardioversion should be used in patients who are hemodynamically unstable. In others, rate can be controlled with intravenous beta or calcium blockers, although beta blockers may be superior in the perioperative period.[30] Intravenous amiodarone may be preferable for rate control in patients with reduced LV function (ejection fraction below 40 percent) because it offers hemodynamic stability superior to that provided by beta or calcium blockers. Once heart rate has been controlled, amiodarone loading is useful for conversion to and maintenance of sinus rhythm.[31]

Ventricular arrhythmias Ventricular ectopy is common after cardiac surgery, but sustained ventricular tachycardia (VT) and fibrillation (VF) are not. The presence of frequent ventricular ectopy is associated with increased risk for sudden cardiac death in patients with structural heart disease (e.g., history of myocardial infarction, ejection fraction below 40 percent), but not in those without heart disease.[32] However, prophylactic suppression of ectopy with antiarrhythmic agents except beta blockers has not been shown to improve clinical outcome in acute or chronic settings.[32,33] Indeed, available data indicate no benefit of lidocaine suppression in the short term[34] and increased mortality with class I antiarrhythmic suppression (as with encainide or flecainide) in the long-term.[35] Thus, management of ventricular ectopy after cardiac surgery should follow the guidelines set forth in other clinical settings: prophylactic suppression of ventricular ectopy is not indicated in asymptomatic individuals. Patients who develop sustained ventricular tachycardia (i.e., more than 30 s of VT or symptomatic VT) or ventricular fibrillation should be cardioverted and/or defibrillated and treated with an antiarrhythmic agent. Amiodarone is the agent of first choice according to present American Heart Association guidelines. An underlying cause for the arrhythmia (e.g., electrolyte disturbance, myocardial ischemia) should be identified and corrected. In those patients who do not have a reversible cause for VT/VF, implantation of an automatic internal cardiodefibrillator has been shown to improve survival (with or without electrophysiologic studies).[32,36,37]

Pulmonary system

Cardiac surgery is associated with a marked reduction in pulmonary function that peaks 24 h after surgery and gradually improves over the next several weeks.[38–40] The pulmonary defect is characterized by a 30 to 50 percent reduction in forced vital capacity and forced expiratory volume (FEV_1), creating a restrictive lung defect in all patients.[38–40] There is an increase in lung edema,[41,42] an increase in atelectasis[43] (primarily affecting the left lower lobe), a decrease in pulmonary compliance,[44] widening of the alveolar-arterial O_2 gradient,[45] and increase in the work of breathing.[46] The clinical significance of these gas exchange and restrictive lung defects is dependent on the degree of pulmonary compromise present prior to surgery. For patients with normal pulmonary function, the reduction in pulmonary mechanics and gas exchange usually has limited clinical consequences; but for those with significant preexisting pulmonary deficits, the new abnormalities can lead to respiratory failure. Although a reduction in pulmonary mechanics is ubiquitous, only about 5 to 6 percent of patients will suffer postoperative respiratory failure (defined as the need for mechanical ventilation for more than 72 h).[47] Less than 2 percent will develop acute respiratory distress syndrome (ARDS).[48]

The causes of postoperative pulmonary dysfunction are both anatomic and physiologic and are influenced by both intraoperative and postoperative events. Pain and splinting from median sternotomy are contributory, particularly in young patients. Diaphragmatic dysfunction from phrenic nerve injury may occur in some patients; it is caused intraoperatively during topical cardiac cooling with ice-slush solution.[49,50] However, significant respiratory insufficiency does not usually occur unless there has been bilateral diaphragmatic injury or significant preoperative respiratory compromise.[51] Parenchymal lung injury from CPB-related SIRS and ischemia/reperfusion injury contributes substantially to postoperative lung dysfunction, and the development of respiratory failure is related to the duration of CPB[47] (see Table 23-1). Pulmonary capillary leak from inflammatory injury resembles oleic acid injury and promotes the formation of pulmonary edema,[42] even at normal filling pressures. Patients with poor LV function are at particular risk for the development of postoperative pulmonary complications[52] because the combination of high LV filling pressures and pulmonary capillary leak enhances the formation of pulmonary edema. In addition, patients who develop extrapulmonary complications (e.g., sepsis, renal failure, stroke, gastrointestinal bleeding, and infection) are at increased risk for respiratory failure.[47]

Therapies for the prevention and treatment of pulmonary complications after cardiac surgery are limited. Prophylaxis with steroids prior to CPB, in an attempt to reduce systemic inflammation, has not been shown to reduce pulmonary complications.[53,54] The importance of postoperative analgesia in thoracic surgery is well recognized. Pain after median sternotomy is usually moderate and can be effectively controlled with a combination of narcotic analgesics and anti-inflammatory agents. Intravenous patient-controlled analgesia can be useful to achieve adequate analgesia in patients with more severe pain. Endotracheal extubation should be sought at the earliest possible time it can be safely achieved after surgery (see "Ventilatory Management," below).

The efficacy of lung expansion maneuvers, such as incentive spirometry, deep breathing exercises, and intermittent-positive pressure ventilation is controversial, with some but not all studies showing a reduction in pulmonary complications.[55,56] However, in those studies that do show a benefit, there appears to be no advantage of one therapy over the others.[55,56] Because the CBP-injured lung is susceptible to edema formation, even at relatively low filling pressures, fluid management is a key component of strategies designed to reduce pulmonary complications. The astute clinician must balance the hemodynamic benefits of preload augmentation against the risks of pulmonary edema formation. As a general rule, postoperative fluids should be administered in a way that assures adequate hemodynamics at the lowest possible filling pressures; when postoperative SIRS abates, diuresis should begin, usually on postoperative day 1. However, caution must be exercised to avoid overt hypovolemia and systemic hypoperfusion in an overzealous attempt to limit intravascular volume.

Ventilator management

The vast majority of patients who undergo cardiac surgery are transferred from the operating room to the ICU with an endotracheal tube in place. In the early postoperative period (first 24 h), the need for endotracheal intubation and mechanical ventilatory support is based on the following principles: (1) assure airway protection in an anesthetized patient who may not be capable of maintaining airway patency; (2) assure adequacy of

Table 23-3 Ventilator weaning and extubation criteria

General criteria	Clinical status improving Hemodynamically stable[a] (MAP > 65, CI >2 L/min/m^2) Chest tube drainage < 50 mL/h 36°C > temp < 38°C No shivering
Airway protection criteria	Awake, follows commands Cough and gag intact Muscle strength adequate (patient capable of 5 s head lift) Pulmonary secretions manageable
Gas exchange criteria	pH >7.32 P_{CO_2} < 52 mm-Hg Pa_{O_2} > 70 mm-Hg on 40% O_2, PEEP 5 cm-H_2O
Ventilatory reserve criteria	f/TV < 80 during spontaneous breathing trial on pressure support of 5 cm-H_2O or T-piece Respiratory rate < 30 Negative inspiratory force > −25 cm-H_2O Forced vital capacity > 10 mL/kg

MAP = mean arterial pressure; CI = cardiac index; f/TV = frequency of breathing (i.e., respiratory rate)/tidal volume (expressed as liters).
[a]Pressors/inotropes and circulatory assist devices (e.g., intraaortic balloon pump) are permitted if doses are not escalating and active titration is not required.

oxygenation and ventilation in an anesthetized patient who may have inadequate respiratory drive and/or respiratory muscle function and significant ventilation/perfusion mismatching; and (3) provide a margin of safety for patients who may encounter significant challenges from hemodynamic instability, acute hemorrhage, and acid/base abnormalities. Each of these problems is a direct result of intraoperative events (see Table 23-1); in most patients, these problems will resolve in the first 4 to 12 h after surgery. Weaning from mechanical ventilation in this early period is a matter of providing appropriate support for the pulmonary system until these acute issues resolve and then rapidly decreasing mechanical support to minimal levels (e.g., 40 percent oxygen, PEEP of 5 cmH_2O, and pressure support of 5 cmH_2O or T piece). Those patients who are capable of maintaining airway patency and adequate gas exchange and who demonstrate adequate ventilatory reserve on minimal support can then be safely extubated (Table 23-3).

The use of endotracheal intubation and mechanical ventilation, although often life-sustaining, is associated with significant complications (see Tobin[57,58] and Kollef[59] for reviews). These complications include baro- and volutrauma, oxygen toxicity, glottic and tracheal injury, decreased cardiac output, and pneumonia.[59] Liberation from mechanical ventilatory support should be sought at the earliest possible time in all patients. This principle applies to patients who follow a routine postoperative course as well as those who develop significant complications, although the actual time course of successful extubation will vary from a few hours in routine cases to several days or weeks in the sickest of patients. Conversely, those patients who are extubated prematurely and require reintubation have an increased risk of nosocomial pneumonia[60] and a sixfold increased risk of mortality over those who are successfully extubated.[61] The challenge for the clinician is to recognize those patients ready for weaning and to time their extubation appropriately.

In contrast to patients who follow a routine postoperative course, weaning must be delayed in patients who suffer perioperative complications, particularly when injury to the brain, heart, kidneys, or lungs has occurred or when severe SIRS or sepsis has developed. These patients will need additional time before weaning criteria are met. In those patients who have sustained significant lung injury, as occurs with ARDS, ventilatory strategies that reduce tidal volumes (≤6 mL/kg) and inspiratory pressures (plateau pressure below 35 cmH_2O) have been shown to shorten recovery time and improve survival.[62] The fraction of inspired oxygen (F_{IO_2}) should be reduced to 0.5 as quickly as tolerated to reduce potential for oxygen toxicity. Increasing PEEP improves V/Q matching in most patients and facilitates reduction in F_{IO_2}. To reduce the incidence of ventilator-associated pneumonia due to the aspiration of gastric contents, patients should be placed in a semirecumbent position (i.e., head of bed elevated to 30 degrees).[63]

Once the patient's underlying injury or disease process improves, weaning can be contemplated. Traditional strategies for ventilator weaning include a gradual reduction in the rate of intermittent mandatory ventilation (IMV) or in the level of pressure-support ventilation. Some studies suggest a benefit of pressure-support weaning over

IMV weaning.[64] Esteban and coworkers[65] reported more rapid liberation from mechanical ventilation with a single daily trial of spontaneous breathing than with either a gradual decrease in IMV or pressure support. In the Esteban study, those patients who could successfully complete a spontaneous breathing trial for 2 h (defined as respiratory rate below 35, O_2 saturation above 90 percent, heart rate below 140 or without a 20 percent increase or decrease from baseline, SBP $\geq 90 \leq 180$, and no agitation, diaphoresis, or anxiety) were extubated, and those who failed were rested for 24 h before another spontaneous breathing trial was attempted. All weaning methods are associated with failure rates (i.e., reintubation) of 15 to 20 percent. It is likely that overall success may improve by combining daily spontaneous weaning trials with useful elements from other weaning modalities and highly predictive extubation criteria (i.e., respiratory rate/tidal volume [liters] < 80),[66] but verification of such a management strategy requires additional clinical trials.

Renal system

Half of all patients who undergo cardiac surgery will experience a significant reduction in renal function (defined as an increase in serum creatinine greater than 25 percent).[67] Although deterioration in renal function is common, acute renal failure that requires dialysis occurs in only 4 to 5 percent of patients.[68] Analogous to postoperative pulmonary dysfunction, the development of clinically significant renal dysfunction is directly linked to the severity of preoperative renal impairment.[69] Additional preoperative risk factors for the development of renal insufficiency include valve surgery (vs. CABG), reduced LV function, peripheral vascular disease, chronic obstructive pulmonary disease (COPD), and the use of an intraaortic balloon pump. Despite improvements in renal replacement therapy over the past 25 years, mortality for patients who develop acute renal failure remains approximately 50 percent,[70] with mortality now largely attributable to respiratory, infectious, and bleeding complications instead of renal failure per se.

The overwhelming majority of cases of acute renal insufficiency that develop after cardiac surgery are due to acute tubular necrosis (ATN), (see Thadhani[71] for a review of acute renal failure). The pathophysiologic basis for ATN in cardiac surgery is from a combination of prerenal causes that progress to frank renal ischemia. Systemic inflammation, renal atheroembolization, and nephrotoxins also contribute to the development of renal dysfunction in this setting. As can be seen in Table 23-1, a variety of intraoperative events (e.g., CPB, controlled hypotension, nonpulsatile blood flow, aortic cross clamping, etc.), can promote the development of renal insufficiency. Postoperatively, renal dysfunction can be exacerbated by persistent hemodynamic instability (i.e., low cardiac output and/or hypotension).

Management of perioperative renal insufficiency can be divided into two overlapping processes: strategies to prevent the development of renal insufficiency and strategies to treat established renal dysfunction. The mainstay of therapy in both processes is to maintain adequate hemodynamics, and in so doing, prevent or treat prerenal azotemia. In particular, cardiac index (CI) and BP must be maintained in a range consistent with adequate renal perfusion. Generally, a CI greater than 2.2 L/min/m^2 and MAP greater than 65 to 70 mmHg is adequate. Intravascular volume expansion is mandated in hypovolemic patients. Inotropic support should be provided for patients with low CI due to ventricular dysfunction, and pressors should be titrated to maintain adequate BP in vasodilated states (e.g., SIRS/sepsis). Management can be assisted by central venous pressure monitoring and/or cardiac output monitoring when a patient's hemodynamic status is unclear. In addition to hemodynamic management, nephrotoxins should be discontinued whenever possible. Nonsteroidal anti-inflammatory agents and angiotensin converting enzyme inhibitors are two commonly used drugs that should be avoided in the setting of acute renal dysfunction. Aminoglycosides and amphotericin are classically included as agents to avoid in patients with renal insufficiency. Although it is reasonable to avoid exposure to these agents when possible, they should not be withheld from patients who have an underlying infectious process that these agents can effectively treat, because effective treatment of the underlying infection will usually lead to improved renal function.

A number of agents are purported to be renal protectants and are in clinical use to prevent the development of acute perioperative renal insufficiency. These include diuretics (furosemide, mannitol), dopamine, and, more recently, fenoldopam (a selective dopamine$_1$ receptor agonist). Despite the widespread use of these agents, current data do not support their routine use for prophylaxis of renal failure in cardiac surgery. Indeed, in prospective, randomized, placebo-controlled trials in cardiac surgery, prophylactic administration of furosemide was associated with a worse renal outcome, and prophylactic low-dose dopamine showed no benefit.[72] Similarly, in critically ill patients with SIRS, prophylactic administration of low-dose dopamine did not improve renal outcome or shorten ICU and hospital length of stay.[73] Although fenoldopam was reported to preserve renal function in a case series of cardiac surgical patients[74] and in one prospective randomized placebo-controlled trial in abdominal aortic surgery,[75] data are too limited to support its routine use for renal protection in cardiac surgery. To date the only agent of proven utility in the prophylaxis of renal insufficiency is acetylcysteine[76]; its efficacy was shown in patients with significant renal impairment who underwent procedures involving the use of radiographic contrast agents, not cardiac surgery.

Unfortunately there are no specific therapies for the amelioration of renal dysfunction in those patients who develop postoperative renal insufficiency; treatment is supportive only. The atrial natriuretic peptide anaratide initially showed promise for the treatment of ATN,[77] but subsequent investigations showed no benefit.[78] Another natriuretic peptide, nesiritide, has proven to be of benefit in the treatment of decompensated heart failure[79] and may have benefit in the treatment of postoperative patients with congestive heart failure and concurrent renal dysfunction,[80] but use for this indication has not yet been proved in clinical trials. Supportive therapy begins by ensuring adequate hemodynamics and avoiding nephrotoxins, as described above. Once prerenal azotemia and postrenal obstruction have been ruled out, management of established renal insufficiency is focused on attempting to maintain appropriate fluid and electrolyte balance. Fluid intake should be kept to a minimum. In oliguric patients, diuretics should be administered to facilitate fluid management and treat hyperkalemia. Although nonoliguric renal failure has a better prognosis than oliguric renal failure, data are limited that the use of diuretics to induce a nonoliguric state changes the overall outcome. Nonetheless, fluid and electrolyte management is simplified in patients in whom diuretics improve urine output.

Dialysis

The indications for dialysis in renal failure following cardiac surgery are the same as in other settings: fluid overload, hyperkalemia, acidosis, and uremia. Renal replacement therapy can be provided as conventional intermittent hemodialysis (IHD) or as continuous hemodialysis (usually as veno-veno hemodialysis, or CVVHD). A comparison of the two modes is shown in Table 23-4. The major advantage of IHD—rapidity of clearance and fluid removal—is also its major disadvantage, because it can lead to hemodynamic instability. In patients who have significant hemodynamic instability, CVVHD is the preferred therapy. When IHD is chosen for stable patients, recent data demonstrate that daily hemodialysis improves renal recovery and survival better than every-other-day dialysis.[81]

Gastrointestinal system and glucose management

GI complications occur in 0.5 to 1.5 percent of patients undergoing cardiac surgery.[82,83] The most common complication is upper GI bleeding, usually from duodenal or gastric ulceration. Ileus, pancreatitis, and mesenteric ischemia may also occur. Splanchnic hypoperfusion during CPB is purported to be the pathophysiologic mechanism underlying these complications,[84] and the duration of CPB is associated with the development of GI complications. Embolization to the splanchnic bed during intraoperative aortic manipulation may also play a role. In those patients who develop acute mesenteric ischemia, mortality is high.[85] Patients undergoing cardiac surgery should receive stress ulcer prophylaxis. Therapy should continue for at least as long as the patient remains mechanically ventilated; however, the appropriate duration of prophylaxis in this patient population has not been well studied.

Nutritional support

Cardiac surgery patients who develop significant postoperative complications are at risk for the development of malnutrition in the same way as other critically ill patients. The acute stress response to critical injury/illness includes the development of a catabolic state characterized by (1) increased glycogenolysis and gluconeogenesis (often with hyperglycemia and insulin resistance), (2) increased proteolysis and nitrogen wasting, and (3) alterations in micronutrients. The extent of muscle wasting and weight loss in the ICU is inversely correlated with long-term survival. Malnutrition is associated with a number of deleterious consequences, including infection, poor wound healing, the formation of decubitus ulcers, overgrowth of bacterial flora, and immune system dysfunction.[86,87]

Although the presence of malnutrition is clearly associated with adverse outcome, the impact of nutritional support on outcome in the critically ill patient is more controversial. Data that specifically address the utility of nutritional support in cardiac surgery patients are extremely sparse. In one metanalysis of randomized trials in patients who have undergone general surgery, total

Table 23-4 Comparison of renal replacement therapy modes

	Urea clearance	CV stability	Osmolar stability	Fluid balance	Cytokine clearance
IHD	200 mL/min 22 L/day (4 H x 3/week)	–	–	–	–
CVVHD	25 mL/min 36 L/day	+	+	+	+

CV = cardiovascular; CVVHD = continuous veno-veno hemodialysis; IHD = intermittent hemodialysis; – = disadvantage; + = advantage.

parenteral nutrition did not change overall mortality but was associated with fewer major complications than standard care (i.e., oral diet and dextrose infusion).[88] In surgical patients with protein-calorie malnutrition, parenteral nutrition reduced both mortality and infectious complications compared to standard care.[89] A number of studies have compared parenteral to enteral nutritional support. Enteral support is associated with an even lower risk of infectious complications than parenteral support[89] and is therefore preferred if at all possible.

Glucose management

Hyperglycemia is common in cardiac surgery patients. High levels of serum epinephrine and cortisol contribute to hyperglycemia by producing a state of insulin resistance.[90,91] Hyperglycemia in critically ill patients, including patients undergoing cardiac surgery, is associated with adverse outcome,[92,93] although the mechanistic link between hyperglycemia and the development of complications is unclear. Intensive, rapid glucose control with insulin infusion to maintain serum glucose between 80 and 110 mg/dL (within 24 h of ICU arrival) markedly reduces the incidence of death, sepsis, and acute renal failure in mechanically ventilated surgery patients compared with standard glucose management.[94] Thus, aggressive glucose control with intravenous insulin should be standard therapy in virtually all cardiac surgery patients.

Infection

Patients undergoing cardiac surgery are at risk for infection of the sternal wound and mediastinum. Like other critically ill patients, they are also at risk for infection of the lung, urinary tract, and central venous catheters; these infections may progress to sepsis. In addition, patients with indwelling intravascular hardware (e.g., valve replacement and ventricular assist devices) are at risk for infection of their hardware, which commonly becomes seeded during bacteremia originating from a central venous catheter.

Infection after cardiac surgery often presents in atypical fashion. Rarely do patients present with a complete constellation of classic findings for an infectious process: fever, leukocytosis, and definitive evidence for a source (e.g., purulent drainage from a sternal wound and unstable sternum or purulent sputum and chest x-ray diagnostic for pneumonia). More typically, patients present with signs and symptoms of sepsis without a definitive infectious source. Tachypnea with or without overt respiratory distress and oliguria (or increasing serum creatinine) are common nonspecific indicators of postoperative infection. Similarly, an acute change in hemodynamic status, particularly the development of hypotension or a deterioration in mental status, often manifesting as delirium, should raise concern for infection to a high level. A high index of suspicion, rapid diagnosis, and institution of definitive antibiotic and/or surgical management are required to improve outcome from infectious complications. New therapies for the treatment of sepsis have emerged; these also appear to improve outcome.

Sternal wound infection/mediastinitis

Deep sternal wound infection occurs in 1.5 to 7 percent of patients after median sternotomy for cardiac surgery.[95–97] This is often a late complication diagnosed in 1.5 percent of patients at discharge, 4.6 percent of patients at 30 days, and 7.3 percent at 90 days.[97] Risk factors for the development of sternal wound infection include diabetes, obesity, peripheral vascular disease, surgical reexploration (for bleeding), use of the internal mammary artery, and prolonged postoperative ventilation and ICU stay.[95,98] The development of sternal wound infection is associated with an increase in perioperative mortality, length of hospitalization, and hospital costs.[99] *Staphylococcus* species (*S. aureus* and coagulase-negative *Staph.*) are causative in the majority of cases, but cultures may be negative in a large proportion of patients.[96,100] Classic signs and symptoms of wound infection are chest pain, purulent wound drainage, sternal instability, fever, and leukocytosis, but findings may be absent in some patients. Effective therapy requires aggressive wound debridement and a prolonged antibiotic course.[101]

Venous catheter infections

The presence of central venous catheters in cardiac surgery patients is nearly universal. These catheters are useful for administering medications that cannot be safely given peripherally and for monitoring hemodynamic status. However, they are associated with the development of mechanical (pneumothorax, bleeding, venous thrombosis) and infectious complications that occur with an overall frequency of between 5 and 20 percent (see Merrer and coworkers[102] and McGee and Gould[103] for full reviews). Subclavian catheterization is associated with a lower complication rate (except pneumothorax) than either femoral[102] or internal jugular[104,105] catheterization; therefore the subclavian site is preferred. Because the incidence of complications from central venous catheters is so alarmingly high and it increases over time, the need for ongoing central venous access should be evaluated on a daily basis. All central venous catheters should be removed at the earliest possible time.

A variety of strategies to prevent infectious complications from central venous catheters have been tested. Table 23-5 distinguishes between those strategies that have proven benefit from those shown to be ineffective. In brief, full barrier protection (i.e., sterile gown and gloves, cap and mask, full-body sterile drape) during catheter insertion[106] and skin preparation with chlorhexidine[107] have proven efficacy in reducing catheter-related infectious complications and should be the standard of care. Antiseptic-coated catheters are effective at reducing

Table 23-5 Strategies for the prevention of catheter-related infection

Effective	Ineffective
Use of subclavian site	Antibiotic ointment used at exit site
Full barrier protection	Silver-impregnated subcutaneous cuffs
Chlorhexidine skin prep	Needleless access devices
Antiseptic-coated catheters and hub connectors	Routine scheduled catheter changes

infectious complications and are cost-effective when the rate of catheter-related bloodstream infection is greater than 2 percent.[108–110] Routine scheduled replacement of catheters over a guidewire or placement at a new site does not decrease infectious complications and is associated with an increased risk of mechanical complications.[111]

Catheters should be replaced only when there is clinical suspicion of infection. An algorithm for the management of suspected catheter-related infection has been developed by McGee and Gould.[103] Briefly, catheter-related infection should be suspected in any patient who has had a central venous catheter in place for 3 days or more and who displays evidence of infection without a confirmed source. The catheter site should be inspected. If an exit-site infection is present, the catheter should be removed and a new one placed at a new site. If the exit site is not clearly infected, the catheter should be exchanged over a guidewire and the intracutaneous portion sent for culture. If the catheter culture is positive, the indwelling catheter should be removed and a new one placed at a new site. If the catheter culture is negative, a catheter-related infection is unlikely.

Sepsis

Sepsis is a systemic response to infection that is defined by (1) a white blood cell count above 12,000 or below 4000 or more than 10 percent bands and (2) two or more of the following: temperature above 38.5°C or below 36.0°C, heart rate above 90 beats per minute, respiratory rate above 20 breaths per minute, or $PaCO_2$ below 32 mmHg.[112] Septic shock is defined as sepsis-induced hypotension (systolic BP less than 90 mmHg or greater than 40 mmHg reduction from baseline) or the requirement for vasopressors/inotropes despite adequate fluid resuscitation and evidence of organ hypoperfusion (e.g., altered mental status, oliguria, lactemia).[112] Severe sepsis is common in ICU patients and is associated with a mortality of 30 percent.[113]

The key components of successful management are rapid, effective hemodynamic resuscitation and early administration of appropriate antibiotics. A recent study showed that rapid institution of goal-directed therapy (fluids to maintain central venous pressure at 8 to 12 mmHg, vasopressors to maintain MAP above 65, vasodilators to maintain MAP below 90, and red cell transfusion and or dobutamine to achieve mixed venous O_2 saturation above 70 percent) in septic emergency department patients improved in-hospital survival from 30 to 45 percent.[114] These recent findings contrast with older studies that failed to show a benefit of hemodynamic optimization strategies,[115,116] but these older studies began goal-directed therapy much later in the septic process. Early, rapid resuscitation appears to be vital to improved outcome.

Recently two additional therapies have proved effective in the treatment of patients with severe sepsis: activated protein C and steroids. In a prospective randomized placebo-controlled trial including 1690 patients, a 96-h infusion of activated protein C reduced mortality from 30.8 to 24.7 percent.[117] However, there was an increased incidence of serious bleeding in the group receiving activated protein C. The safety and efficacy of activated protein C has not been tested in patients receiving concurrent anticoagulant therapy, which is commonly needed in septic cardiac surgery patients because of AF or mechanical cardiac valves. In another prospective randomized placebo-controlled trial in patients with septic shock, a 7-day course of hydrocortisone (50 mg IV every 6 h) plus fludrocortisone (50 μg daily PO) improved survival and reduced the need for vasopressor therapy in patients with relative adrenal insufficiency (defined as failure to increase serum cortisol by at least 10 μg/dL during the ACTH stimulation test). No benefit of steroid therapy was observed in patients without adrenal insufficiency.[118]

References

1. London MJ, Hollenberg M, Wong MG, et al. Intraoperative myocardial ischemia: Localization by continuous 12-lead electrocardiography. *Anesthesiology* 1988;69:232–241.
2. Kaplan JA, King SB. The precordial electrocardiographic lead (V5) in patients who have coronary-artery disease. *Anesthesiology* 1976;45:570–574.
3. Landesberg G, Mosseri M, Wolf Y, et al. Perioperative myocardial ischemia and infarction: Identification by continuous 12-lead electrocardiogram with online ST-segment monitoring. *Anesthesiology* 2002;96: 264–270.
4. Connors AF, Speroff T, Dawson NV, et al. The effectiveness of right heart catheterization in the initial care of critically ill patients. SUPPORT Investigators. *JAMA* 1996;276:889–897.
5. Polanczyk CA, Rohde LE, Goldman L, et al. Right heart catheterization and cardiac complications in patients

undergoing noncardiac surgery: An observational study. *JAMA* 2001;286:309–314.
6. Bender JS, Smith-Meek MA, Jones CE. Routine pulmonary artery catheterization does not reduce morbidity and mortality of elective vascular surgery: Results of a prospective, randomized trial. *Ann Surg* 1997;226: 229–236.
7. Valentine RJ, Duke ML, Inman MH. Effectiveness of pulmonary artery catheters in aortic surgery: A randomized trial. *J Vasc Surg* 1998;27:203–211.
8. Rhodes A, Cusack RJ, Newman PJ, et al. A randomised, controlled trial of the pulmonary artery catheter in critically ill patients. *Intens Care Med* 2002;28:256–264.
9. Martin TD, Craver JM, Gott JP. Prospective, randomized trial of retrograde warm blood cardioplegia: Myocardial benefit and neurologic threat. *Ann Thorac Surg* 1994;57:298–302.
10. Hypothermia after Cardiac Arrest Study Group T. Mild therapeutic hypothermia to improve the neurologic outcome after cardiac arrest. *N Engl J Med* 2002;346: 549–556.
11. Bernard SA, Gray TW, Buist MD. Treatment of comatose survivors of out-of-hospital cardiac arrest with induced hypothermia. *N Engl J Med* 2002;346:557–563.
12. Rohrer MJ, Natale AM. Effect of hypothermia on the coagulation cascade. *Crit Care Med* 1992;20:1402–1405.
13. Frank SM, Cattaneo CG, Wieneke-Brady MB, et al. Threshold for adrenomedullary activation and increased cardiac work during mild core hypothermia. *Clin Sci (Lond)* 2002;102:119–125.
14. Frank SM, Fleisher LA, Breslow MJ, et al. Perioperative maintenance of normothermia reduces the incidence of morbid cardiac events: A randomized clinical trial. *JAMA* 1997;277:1127–1134.
15. Kurz A, Sessler DI, Lenhardt R. Perioperative normothermia to reduce the incidence of surgical-wound infection and shorten hospitalization. Study of Wound Infection and Temperature Group. *N Engl J Med* 1996;334:1209–1215.
16. Kurz A, Kurz M, Poeschl G, et al. Forced-air warming maintains intraoperative normothermia better than circulating-water mattresses. *Anesth Analg* 1993;77:89–95.
17. Mangano DT. Biventricular function after myocardial revascularization in humans: Deterioration and recovery patterns during the first 24 hours. *Anesthesiology* 1985;62:571.
18. Breisblatt WM, Stein KL, Wolfe CJ. Acute myocardial dysfunction and recovery: A common occurrence after cardiopulmonary bypass surgery. *J Am Coll Cardiol* 1990;15:1261.
19. Leung JM, O'Kelly B, Browner WS. Prognostic importance of postbypass regional wall-motion abnormalities in patients undergoing coronary artery bypass graft surgery. *Anesthesiology* 1989;71:16.
20. Jain U, Laflamme CJA, Aggarwal A. Electrocardiographic and hemodynamic changes and their association with myocardial infarction during coronary artery bypass surgery. *Anesthesiology* 1997;86:576.
21. Engelman RM, Harji-Rovsov I, Breyer RH. Rebound vasospasm after coronary revascularization. *Ann Thorac Surg* 1984;37:469.
22. Apostolidou I, Skubas NJ, Bakola A, et al. Effects of nicardipine and nitroglycerine on perioperative myocardial ischemia in patients undergoing coronary artery bypass surgery. *Semin Thorac Cardiovasc Surg* 1999; 11:77–83.
23. Wu WC, Rathore SS, Wang Y, et al. Blood transfusion in elderly patients with acute myocardial infarction. *N Engl J Med* 2001;345:1230–1236.
24. Matthew JP, Parks R, Savino JS, et al. Atrial fibrillation following coronary artery bypass graft surgery. Predictors, outcomes, and resource utilization. *JAMA* 1996;276:300–306.
25. Creswell LL, Schuessler RB, Rosenbloom M, et al. Hazards of postoperative atrial arrhythmias. *Ann Thorac Surg* 1993;56:539–349.
26. Ommen SR, Odell JA, Stanton MS. Atrial arrhythmias after cardiothoracic surgery. *N Engl J Med* 1997;336: 1429–1434.
27. Crystal E, Connolly SJ, Sleik K, et al. Interventions on prevention of postoperative atrial fibrillation in patients undergoing heart surgery: A meta-analysis. *Circulation* 2002;106:75–80.
28. White CM, Giri S, Tsikouris JP, et al. A comparison of two individual amiodarone regimens to placebo in open heart surgery. *Ann Thorac Surg* 2002;74:69–74.
29. Toraman F, Karabulut EH, Alhan HC, et al. Magnesium infusion dramatically decreases the incidence of atrial fibrillation after coronary artery bypass grafting. *Ann Thorac Surg* 2001;72:1256–1261.
30. Balser JR, Martinez EA, Winters BD, et al. β-adrenergic blockade accelerates conversion of postoperative supraventricular tachyarrhythmias. *Anesthesiology* 1998;89:1052–1059.
31. Hilleman DE, Spinler SA. Conversion of recent-onset atrial fibrillation with intravenous amiodarone: A meta-analysis of randomized controlled trials. *Pharmacotherapy* 2002;22:66–74.
32. Cannom DS, Prystowsky EN. Management of ventricular arrhythmias: Detection, drugs, and devices. *JAMA* 1999;281:172–179.
33. Kendall MJ, Lynch KP, Hjalmarson A, et al. β-blockers and sudden cardiac death. *Ann Intern Med* 1995;123: 358–367.
34. Hine LK, Laird N, Hewitt P, et al. Meta-analytic evidence against prophylactic use of lidocaine in acute myocardial infarction. *Arch Intern Med* 1989;149:2694–2698.
35. The Cardiac Arrhythmia Suppression Trial (CAST) Investigators. Preliminary report: Effect of encainide and flecainide on mortality in a randomized trial of arrhythmia suppression after myocardial infarction. *N Engl J Med* 1989;321:406–412.
36. Buxton AE, Lee KL, Fisher JD, et al. A randomized study of the prevention of sudden death in patients with coronary artery disease. *N Engl J Med* 1999;341:1882–1890.
37. Moss AJ, Zareba W, Hall WJ, et al. Prophylactic implantation of a defibrillator in patients with myocardial infarction and reduced ejection fraction. *N Engl J Med* 2002;346:877–883.
38. Stock MC, Downs JB, Weaver D, et al. Effect of pleurotomy on pleural function after median sternotomy. *Ann Thorac Surg* 1986;42:441–444.
39. Johnson D, Hurst T, Thomson D, et al. Respiratory function after cardiac surgery. *J Cardiothorac Vasc Anesth* 1996;10:571–577.

40. van Belle AF, Wesseling GJ, Penn OC, et al. Postoperative pulmonary function abnormalities after coronary artery bypass surgery. *Respir Med* 1992;86:195–199.
41. Boldt J, Zickmann B, Dapper F, et al. Does the technique of cardiopulmonary bypass affect lung water content? *Eur J Cardiothorac Surg* 1991;5:22–26.
42. Barnas GM, Watson RJ, Green MD, et al. Lung and chest wall mechanical properties before and after cardiac surgery with cardiopulmonary bypass. *J Appl Physiol* 1992;73:1040–1046.
43. Magnusson L, Zemgulis V, Wicky S. Atelectasis is a major cause of hypoxemia and shunt after cardiopulmonary bypass. *Anesthesiology* 1997;87:1153–1163.
44. Chaney MA, Nikolov MP, Blakeman B. Pulmonary effects of methylprednisolone in patients undergoing coronary artery bypass grafting and early tracheal extubation. *Anesth Analg* 1998;87:27–33.
45. MacNaughton PD, Braude S, Hunter DN. Changes in lung function and pulmonary capillary permeability after cardiopulmonary bypass. *Crit Care Med* 1992;20: 1289–1294.
46. Wilson RS, Sullivan SF, Malm JR. The oxygen cost of breathing following anesthesia and cardiac surgery. *Anesthesiology* 1973;39:387–393.
47. Canver CC, Chanda J. Intraoperative and postoperative risk factors for respiratory failure after coronary artery bypass. *Ann Thorac Surg* 2003;75:853–857.
48. Asimakopoulos G, Smith PL, Ratnatunga CP. Lung injury and acute respiratory distress syndrome after cardiopulmonary bypass. *Ann Thorac Surg* 1999;68: 1107–1115.
49. Rousou JA, Parker T, Engelman RM, et al. Phrenic nerve paresis associated with the use of iced slush and the cooling jacket for topical hypothermia. *J Thorac Cardiovasc Surg* 1985;89:921.
50. Curtis JJ, Nawarawong W, Walls JT. Elevated hemidiaphragm after cardiac operations: Incidence, prognosis, and relationship to the use of topical ice slush. *Ann Thorac Surg* 1989;48:764.
51. Chandler KW, Rozas CJ, Kory RC, et al. Bilateral diaphragmatic paralysis complicating local cardiac hypothermia during open heart surgery. *Am J Med* 1984;77:243.
52. Bando K, Sun K, Binford RS. Determinations of long duration of endotracheal intubation after cardiac operations. *Ann Thorac Surg* 1997;63:1026–1033.
53. Coffin LH, Shinozaki T, DeMeules JE, et al. Ineffectiveness of methylprednisolone in the treatment of pulmonary dysfunction after cardiopulmonary bypass. *Am J Surg* 1975;130:555–559.
54. Chaney MA, Durazo-Arvizu RA, Nikolov MP, et al. Methylprednisolone does not benefit patients undergoing coronary artery bypass grafting and early tracheal extubation. *J Thorac Cardiovasc Surg* 2001;121:561–569.
55. Celli BR, Rodriguez KS, Snider GL. A controlled trial of intermittent positive pressure breathing, incentive spirometry, and deep breathing exercises in preventing pulmonary complications after abdominal surgery. *Am Rev Respir Dis* 1984;130:12–15.
56. Overend TJ, Anderson CM, Lucy SD, et al. The effect of incentive spirometry on postoperative pulmonary complications: A systematic review. *Chest* 2001;120:971–978.
57. Tobin MJ. Mechanical ventilation. *N Engl J Med* 1994;330:1056–1061.
58. Tobin MJ. Advances in mechanical ventilation. *N Engl J Med* 2001;344:1986–1996.
59. Kollef MH. The prevention of ventilator-associated pneumonia. *N Engl J Med* 1999;340:627–634.
60. Torres A, Gatell JM, Aznar E. Re-intubation increases the risk of nosocomial pneumonia in patients needing mechanical ventilation. *Am J Respir Crit Care Med* 1995;152:137–141.
61. Epstein SK, Ciubotaru RL, B. WJ. Effect of failed extubation on the outcome of mechanical ventilation. *Chest* 1997;112:186–192.
62. The Acute Respiratory Distress Syndrome Network. Ventilation with lower tidal volumes as compared with traditional tidal volumes for acute lung injury and the acute respiratory distress syndrome. *N Engl J Med* 2000;342:1301–1308.
63. Torres A, Serra-Batles J, Ros E. Pulmonary aspiration of gastric contents in patients receiving mechanical ventilation: The effect of body position. *Ann Intern Med* 1992;116:540–543.
64. Brochard L, Rauss A, Benito S, et al. Comparison of three methods of gradual withdrawal from ventilatory support during weaning from mechanical ventilation. *Am J Respir Crit Care Med* 1994;150:896–903.
65. Esteban A, Frutos F, Tobin MJ, et al. A comparison of four methods of weaning patients from mechanical ventilation. *N Engl J Med* 1995;332:345–350.
66. Yang KL, Tobin MJ. A prospective study of indexes predicting the outcome of trials of weaning from mechanical ventilation. *N Engl J Med* 1991;324:1445–1450.
67. Tuttle KR, Worrall NK, Dahlstrom LR, et al. Predictors of ARF after cardiac surgical procedures. *Am J Kidney Dis* 2003;41:76–83.
68. Shroyer AL, Coombs LP, Peterson ED, et al. The Society of Thoracic Surgeons: 30-day operative mortality and morbidity risk models. *Ann Thorac Surg* 2003;75:1856–1864.
69. Chertow GM, Lazarus JM, Christiansen CL. Preoperative renal risk stratification. *Circulation* 1997;95:878–884.
70. Lange HW, Aeppli DM, Brown DC. Survival of patients with acute renal failure requiring dialysis after open heart surgery: Early prognostic indicators. *Am Heart J* 1987;113:1138.
71. Thadhani R, Pascual M, Bonventre JV. Acute renal failure. *N Engl J Med* 1996;334:1448–1460.
72. Lassnigg A, Donner E, Grubhofer G, et al. Lack of renoprotective effects of dopamine and furosemide during cardiac surgery. *J Am Soc Nephrol* 2000;11:97–104.
73. The ANZICS Clinical Trials Group. Low-dose dopamine in patients with early renal dysfunction: a placebo-controlled randomised trial. *Lancet* 2000;356:2139–2143.
74. Garwood S, Swamidoss CP, Davis EA, et al. A case series of low-dose fenoldopam in seventy cardiac surgical patients at increased risk of renal dysfunction. *J Cardiothorac Vasc Anesth* 2003;17:17–21.
75. Halpenny M, Rushe C, Breen P, et al. The effects of fenoldopam on renal function in patients undergoing elective aortic surgery. *Eur J Anaesthesiol* 2002;19:32–39.
76. Tepel M, van der Giet M, Schwarzfeld C, et al. Prevention of radiographic-contrast-agent-induced

reductions in renal function by acetylcysteine. *N Engl J Med* 2000;343:180–184.
77. Allgren RL, Marbury TC, Rahman SN, et al. Anaritide in acute tubular necrosis. *N Engl J Med* 1997;336:828–834.
78. Lewis J, Salem MM, Chertow GM, et al. Atrial natriuretic factor in oliguric acute renal failure. *Am J Kidney Dis* 2000;36:767–774.
79. The VMAC (Vasodilation in the Management of Acute CHF) Investigators. Intravenous nesiritide vs. nitroglycerine for the treatment of decompensated congestive heart failure: A randomized controlled trial. *JAMA* 2002;287:1531–1540.
80. Moazami N, Damiano RJ, Bailey MS, et al. Nesiritide (BNP) in the management of postoperative cardiac patients. *Ann Thorac Surg* 2003;75:1974–1976.
81. Schiffl H, Lang SM, Fischer R. Daily hemodialysis and the outcome of acute renal failure. *N Engl J Med* 2002;346:305–310.
82. Ohri SK, Desai JB, Gaer JAR, et al. Intraabdominal complications after cardiopulmonary bypass. *Ann Thorac Surg.* 1991;52:82–84.
83. Johnston G, Vitikainen K, Knight R, et al. Changing perspective on gastrointestinal complications in pateints undergoing cardiac surgery. *Am J Surg* 1992;163.
84. Christenson JT, Schmuziger M, Maurice J, et al. Postoperative visceral hypotension the common cause for gastrointestinal complications after cardiac surgery. *Thorac Cardiovasc Surg* 1994;42.
85. Venkateswaran RV, Charman SC, Goddard M, et al. Lethal mesenteric ischaemia after cardiopulmonary bypass: A common complication? *Eur J Cardiothorac Surg* 2002;22:534–538.
86. Kinney JM, Weissman C. Forms of malnutrition in stressed and unstressed patients. *Clin Chest Med* 1986;7:19.
87. Mainous MR, Deitch EA. Nutrition and Infection. *Surg Clin North Am* 1994;74:659.
88. Heyland DK, Montalvo M, MacDonald S, et al. Total parenteral nutrition in the surgical patient: a meta-analysis. *Can J Surg* 2001;44:102–111.
89. Braunschweig CL, Levy P, Sheean PM, et al. Enteral compared with parenteral nutrition: A meta-analysis. *Am J Clin Nutr* 2001;74:534–542.
90. Mizock BA. Alterations in carbohydrate metabolism during stress: A review of the literature. *Am J Med* 1995; 98:75–84.
91. McCowen KC, Malhotra A, Bistrian BR. Stress-induced hyperglycemia. *Crit Care Clin* 2001;17:107–124.
92. Fietsam RJ, Bassett J, Glover JL. Complications of coronary artery surgery in diabetic patients. *Am Surg* 1991; 57:551–557.
93. O'Neill PA, Davies I, Fullerton KJ, et al. Stress hormone and blood glucose response following acute stroke in the elderly. *Stroke* 1991;22:842–847.
94. Van den Berghe G, Wouters P, Weekers F, et al. Intensive insulin therapy in critically ill patients. *N Engl J Med* 2001;345:1359–1367.
95. Gummert JF, Barten MJ, Hans C, et al. Mediastinitis and cardiac surgery–An updated risk factor analysis in 10,373 consecutive adult patients. *Thorac Cardiovasc Surg* 2002;50:87–91.
96. Fowler VG, Kaye KS, Simel DL, et al. *Staphylococcus aureus* bacteremia after median sternotomy. Clinical utility of blood culture results in the identification of postoperative mediastinitis. *Circulation* 2003;108:73–78.
97. Jonkers D, Elenbaas T, Terporten P, et al. Prevalence of 90-days postoperative wound infections after cardiac surgery. *Eur J Cardiothorac Surg* 2003;23:97–102.
98. Ridderstolpe L, Gill H, Granfeldt H, et al. Superficial and deep sternal wound complications: Incidence, risk factors, and mortality. *Eur J Cardiothorac Surg* 2001;20: 1168–1175.
99. Kirkland KB, Briggs JP, Trivette SL, et al. The impact of surgical-site infections in the 1990s: attributable mortality, excess length of hospitalization, and extra costs. *Infect Control Hosp Epidemiol* 1999;20:725–730.
100. Kutsal A, Ibrisim E, Catav Z, et al. Mediastinitis after open heart surgery. Analysis of risk factors and management. *J Cardiovasc Surg* 1991;32:38–41.
101. Pairolero PC, Arnold PG, Harris JB. Long-term results of pectoralis major muscle transposition for infected sternotomy wounds. *Ann Surg* 1991;213:583–590.
102. Merrer J, De Jonghe B, Golliot F, et al. Complications of femoral and subclavian venous catheterization in critically ill patients. A randomized controlled trial. *JAMA* 2001;286:700–707.
103. McGee DC, Gould MK. Preventing complications of central venous catheterization. *N Engl J Med* 2003;348: 1123–1133.
104. McKinley S, Mackenzie A, Finfer S, et al. Incidence and predictors of central venous catheter related infection in intensive care patients. *Anaesth Intens Care* 1999;27:164–169.
105. Timsit JF, Farkas JC, Boyer JM. Central vein catheter-related thrombosis in intensive care patients: Incidence, risk factors, and relationship with catheter-related sepsis. *Chest* 1998;114:207–213.
106. Raad I, Hohn DC, Gilbreath BJ, et al. Prevention of central venous catheter–related infections by using maximal sterile barrier precautions during insertion. *Infect Control Hosp Epidemiol* 1994;15:231–238.
107. Maki DG, Ringer M, Alvarado CJ. Prospective randomised trial of povidone-iodine, alcohol, and chlorhexidine for prevention of infection associated with central venous and arterial catheters. *Lancet* 1991;338:339–343.
108. Maki DG, Stolz SM, Wheeler S, et al. Prevention of central venous catheter-related bloodstream infection by use of an antiseptic-impregnated catheter: A randomized, controlled trial. *Ann Intern Med* 1997;127:257–266.
109. Veenstra DL, Saint S, Saha S, et al. Efficacy of antiseptic-impregnated central venous catheters in preventing catheter-related bloodstream infection. A meta-analysis. *JAMA* 1999;281:261–267.
110. Veenstra DL, Saint S, Sullivan SD. Cost-effectiveness of antiseptic-impregnated central venous catheters for the prevention of catheter-related bloodstream infection. *JAMA* 1999;282:554–560.
111. Cook D, Randolph A, Kernerman P, et al. Central venous catheter replacement strategies: A systematic review of the literature. *Crit Care Med* 1997;25:1417–1424.
112. The American College of Chest Physicians/Society of Critical Care Medicine Consensus Conference. Definitions for sepsis and organ failure and guidelines for the use of innovative therapies in sepsis. *Crit Care Med* 1992;20:864–874.

113. Angus DC, Linde-Zwirble WT, Lidicker J, et al. Epidemiology of severe sepsis in the United States: Analysis of incidence, outcome, and associated costs of care. *Crit Care Med* 2001;29:1303–1310.
114. Rivers E, Nguyen B, Havstad S, et al. Early goal-directed therapy in the treatment of severe sepsis and septic shock. *N Engl J Med* 2001;345:1368–1377.
115. Hayes MA, Timmins AC, Yau EHS, et al. Elevation of systemic oxygen delivery in the treatment of critically ill patients. *N Engl J Med* 1994;330:1717–1722.
116. Gattinoni L, Brazzi L, Pelosi P, et al. A trial of goal-oriented hemodynamic therapy in critically ill patients. SvO_2 Collaborative Group. *N Engl J Med* 1995;333:1025–1032.
117. Bernard GR, Vincent JL, Laterre PF, et al. Efficacy and safety of recombinant human activated protein C for severe sepsis. *N Engl J Med* 2001;344:699–709.
118. Annane D, Sebille V, Charpentier C, et al. Effect of treatment with low doses of hydrocortisone and fludrocortisone on mortality in patients with septic shock. *JAMA* 2002;288:862–871.

CHAPTER

24 POSTOPERATIVE THERAPIES TO REDUCE LONG-TERM CARDIOVASCULAR RISK

Ty J. Gluckman, Richard A. Lange, Roger S. Blumenthal

INTRODUCTION

Cardiac surgery plays an important role in the management of patients with a wide range of cardiovascular disorders. Over the last decade, the number of cardiac surgical procedures performed annually in the United States has steadily increased.[1] For patients who have undergone successful cardiac surgery, close attention should be directed to reducing the risk of subsequent cardiovascular events. Accordingly, this chapter focuses on therapies that should be offered to patients following coronary artery bypass grafting (CABG), valve replacement, or surgical correction of adult congenital heart disease (Table 24-1). Levels of recommendation, both in terms of the weight and source of evidence, are provided when available (Table 24-2). An "ABC" format, similar to that introduced by the American College of Cardiology (ACC) and the American Heart Association (AHA),[2] is used to present recommendations in a manner that makes them easy to recall and apply.

ASPIRIN

Aspirin irreversibly inhibits the cyclooxygenase enzyme involved in the production of thromboxane, a potent promoter of platelet aggregation. After CABG, maintenance of graft patency is important in preventing future adverse cardiovascular events.[3] Saphenous vein grafts are used more frequently than arterial grafts and are more likely to experience early thrombotic occlusion.[4] Exposure of saphenous vein grafts to arterial pressure leads to decreased levels of thrombomodulin (a potent anticoagulant that inhibits local thrombin generation[5,6]) and an intense inflammatory response, with endothelial injury, platelet activation, and fibrin deposition.[7,8]

KEY CONCEPTS

- Epidemiology
  - Over the last decade the number of cardiac surgery procedures performed in the United States has steadily increased.
- Problem
  - In spite of benefits conferred by cardiac surgery, most patients remain at increased risk for subsequent cardiovascular events. This is due in part to an underutilization of risk-reducing therapies following cardiac surgery.
- Approach
  - Current guidelines recommend a number of therapies following coronary artery bypass grafting, valve replacement, or surgical correction of adult congenital heart disease in order to reduce cardiovascular risk. Because many physicians perceive guidelines as lengthy and complex, recommendations should be presented in a manner that makes them easy to recall and apply.
- Conclusion
  - In order to reduce cardiovascular morbidity and mortality following cardiac surgery, efforts should be made to increase adherence to guideline recommendations through simplified approaches to risk reduction.

Table 24-1 Recommended therapies following CABG, valve replacement, or surgical correction of adult congenital heart disease

Therapy	CABG	Valve replacement	Congenital heart disease
Aspirin	Lifelong	Low dose after 3 months (bioprosthetic valves) Low dose with anticoagulation (mechanical valves)	Systemic to pulmonary shunt Controversial in plexogenic arteriopathy and pulmonary vascular obstructive disease
ADP receptor antagonists	Clopidogrel, if aspirin intolerant	No data	No data
Anticoagulation	Not recommended unless there is another indication	Up to 3 months (bioprosthetic valves) Long-term (mechanical valves)	Right-to-left shunt with a thromboembolic event Controversial, but may be used after Fontan operation
ACE inhibitors or ARBs	Lifelong	Not recommended unless there is another indication	Not recommended unless there is another indication
Aldosterone inhibitors	Recommended for the patient with heart failure or left ventricular systolic dysfunction on maximal medical therapy	Recommended for the patient with heart failure or left ventricular systolic dysfunction on maximal medical therapy	Recommended for the patient with heart failure or left ventricular systolic dysfunction on maximal medical therapy
Antibiotic prophylaxis	Not recommended unless there is another indication	Recommended	Recommended for many repaired congenital defects
Beta-adrenergic blockers	Perioperative use for all patients Long-term use for all patients following an MI	Perioperative use for all patients	Perioperative use for all patients
Blood pressure control	< 130/85 mmHg	<130/85 mmHg	< 130/85 mmHg
Cholesterol reduction	A statin to lower LDL-C to < 100 mg/dL	A statin to lower LDL-C based on ATP III guidelines[154]	A statin to lower LDL-C based on ATP III guidelines[154]
Cigarette smoking/ tobacco cessation	All patients	All patients	All patients
Diabetes mellitus control	Strict glycemic control (HbA1c < 7.0%)	Strict glycemic control (HbA1c < 7.0%)	Strict glycemic control (HbA1c < 7.0%)
Diet and weight management	Caloric reduction with a balanced diet restricted in sodium, saturated fat, and cholesterol	Caloric reduction with a balanced diet restricted in sodium, saturated fat, and cholesterol	Caloric reduction with a balanced diet restricted in sodium, saturated fat, and cholesterol
Digoxin	Recommended for the patient with heart failure or left ventricular systolic dysfunction on maximal medical therapy	Recommended for the patient with heart failure or left ventricular systolic dysfunction on maximal medical therapy	Recommended for the patient with heart failure or left ventricular systolic dysfunction on maximal medical therapy
Exercise	Cardiac rehabilitation or structured exercise program	Cardiac rehabilitation or structured exercise program	Cardiac rehabilitation or structured exercise program

ACE = angiotensin converting enzyme; ADP = adenosine diphosphate; ARBs = angiotensin receptor blockers; ATP = adult treatment panel; CABG = coronary artery bypass grafting; HbA1c = Serum glycosylated hemoglobin concentration; LDL-C = low-density lipoprotein cholesterol; MI = myocardial infarction.

Administration of aspirin early after CABG (< 48 h) is associated with a reduction in the incidence of graft occlusion,[3,9–13] in-hospital myocardial infarction (MI),[14] stroke,[14] and death.[14] Therefore current guidelines recommend that it be given within 6 to 24 h of CABG and continued lifelong unless contraindicated [American College of Chest Physicians (ACCP), grade 1A; European Society of Cardiology (ESC), grade 1A].)[15–17]

In the patient who has undergone prosthetic valve implantation, the presence of a foreign surface and increased shear forces may lead to activation of circulating platelets[18] and thromboembolism. Thus, warfarin is usually prescribed postoperatively. In the case of bioprosthetic valves, endothelialization of the valve occurs within 3 months of implantation, at which time the risk of thrombosis is attenuated. Warfarin may then be discontinued and low-dose (75 to 100 mg/day) aspirin alone prescribed (ACC/AHA, class I; ACCP, grade 2C)[19,20] unless additional risk factors for thromboembolism are present (i.e., atrial fibrillation, left ventricular

Table 24-2 ACC/AHA/ESC/ACCP[a] Levels of recommendation and evidence

Class I	Class II	Class IIa	Class IIb	Class III
Clear evidence and/or general agreement that a treatment or diagnostic approach is useful and effective	Conflicting evidence and/or a differing opinion about the use and efficacy of a given treatment or diagnostic procedure	Weight of evidence and/or opinion suggests useful and efficacious	Usefulness and efficacy is less well established by evidence/opinion	Evidence or general agreement that the treatment or diagnostic approach is either useless or harmful

A (highest)	B (intermediate)	C (lowest)
Data derived from multiple randomized clinical trials involving large numbers of patients	Data derived from a limited number of randomized clinical trials involving small numbers of patients or with important limitations or from analyses of nonrandomized trials or observational registries[b]	Data derived from expert consensus opinion or observational studies (C+ for overwhelming observational studies)[c]

[a]ACC = American College of Cardiology; AHA = American Heart Association; ESC = European Society of Cardiology; ACCP = American College of Chest Physicians.
[b]Derived from ACC/AHA/ESC.
[c]Derived from ACCP.

systolic dysfunction, left atrial enlargement, previous thromboembolism, or a known hypercoagulable state). For the patient with a bioprosthetic valve in the aortic position, low-dose aspirin may be used in lieu of warfarin immediately after surgery,[21] as the thromboembolic risk remains low throughout the postoperative period.[21–23]

Unlike bioprosthetic valves, mechanical valves are at greater risk for thromboembolic complications even 3 months after implantation. Aspirin therapy alone is inadequate for preventing thromboembolic events in the patient with a mechanical valve (ACC/AHA, class III).[19] However, coadministration of low-dose (75 to 100 mg/day) aspirin with warfarin should be considered (ACC/AHA, class IIa; ACCP, grade 2A to 2C),[19,20] as studies have demonstrated a reduction in the incidence of systemic thromboembolic events and death with only a small, incremental risk of major bleeding with such therapy.[24] Combination therapy can also facilitate a dose reduction in anticoagulation, as the use of aspirin in the patient with an international normalized ratio (INR) of 2.5 to 3.5 is as efficacious in preventing systemic emboli as anticoagulation alone with an INR of 3.5 to 4.5.[25] For patients who experience an embolic event despite "adequate" antithrombotic therapy, the addition of low-dose aspirin (75 to 100 mg) or an increase in the dose should be considered (ACCP, grade 1C+).[20]

There are currently no consensus guidelines on the use of aspirin following surgery for congenital heart disease. Although there are limited data suggesting that low-dose aspirin is beneficial in the patient with pulmonary vascular obstructive disease (i.e., plexogenic arteriopathy),[26] its use is controversial, as such patients are at increased risk of pulmonary hemorrhage and massive hemoptysis. In those who have undergone placement of a systemic-to-pulmonary shunt,[27–29] aspirin likely reduces the risk of shunt thrombosis early after implantation; however, the benefit from long-term treatment once the shunt has endothelialized is not known. Because thrombocytopenia and abnormal platelet function may occur in the perioperative period, use of aspirin should largely be restricted to the patient with a clear indication for its use.[30]

Many patients referred for cardiac surgery have concomitant peripheral or cerebral vascular disease. In a metanalysis of 195 trials involving 135,640 patients with vascular disease, the Antiplatelet Trialists' Collaboration demonstrated a significant reduction in the incidence of serious vascular events (MI, stroke, or vascular death) with aspirin as compared to placebo (10.7 vs. 13.2 percent, respectively; $p < 0.0001$).[31] Thus, aspirin should be administered to all patients with vascular disease unless contraindicated (ACC/AHA, class A).[2]

ADP RECEPTOR ANTAGONISTS (THIENOPYRIDINES)

The thienopyridine drugs—ticlopidine and clopidogrel—irreversibly inhibit platelet aggregation by blocking the adenosine diphosphate (ADP) receptor on the platelet surface. When used as an alternative to aspirin, these agents reduce adverse outcomes in patients with known cardiovascular disease.[32,33] When combined with aspirin, they are beneficial in patients with an acute coronary syndrome[34] and in those undergoing percutaneous coronary intervention.[35–37] In the patient undergoing cardiac surgery, however, concurrent use of a thienopyridine increases the risk of postoperative bleeding and the need for transfusion.[38,39] Thus, in the patient who has recently taken a thienopyridine, elective cardiac surgery is usually delayed for several days until the antiplatelet effects have waned.

There are few studies of thienopyridine use in patients undergoing CABG. Two randomized trials have demonstrated a higher rate of saphenous vein graft patency in patients receiving ticlopidine versus those receiving placebo[40,41]; however, ticlopidine is rarely used because it has been associated with severe hematologic complications.[42,43] Clopidogrel has an excellent track record of safety and tolerability, but its use in the cardiac surgery patient has not been prospectively studied. In a post hoc analysis of the Clopidogrel versus Aspirin in Patients at Risk of Ischemic Events (CAPRIE) trial,[44] patients receiving clopidogrel after CABG had a 31 percent relative reduction in adverse cardiovascular events compared to those taking aspirin. Its efficacy, however, was predominantly limited to those who had already had an ischemic event on aspirin (e.g., aspirin failures).[45] More recently, in a post hoc analysis of the Clopidogrel in Unstable angina to prevent Recurrent ischemic Events (CURE) trial, patients receiving clopidogrel and aspirin after CABG had no greater improvement in clinical outcomes than those taking aspirin alone (odds ratio of 0.97; 95 percent confidence interval, 0.74 to 1.26) and a strong trend toward a higher rate of life-threatening or major bleeding (odds ratio of 1.3; 95 percent confidence interval, 0.93 to 1.71).[46] Thus, thienopyridines should not be used as first-line agents in the management of patients following cardiac surgery. Instead, they should be used as an alternative to aspirin for those who are intolerant of it or unable to take it (ACCP, grade 2C for clopidogrel; ACCP, grade 2B for ticlopidine).[15,47]

ANTICOAGULATION

Warfarin is the most commonly used anticoagulant and achieves its effect predominantly by antagonizing the vitamin K–dependent carboxylation of several procoagulant proteins (factors II, VII, IX, X and proteins C and S). Warfarin therapy is associated with a modest improvement in clinical outcome late (> 7 years) after CABG,[48] but it is no more effective at maintaining saphenous vein graft patency than aspirin[10,49,50] or placebo.[9,49] Accordingly, current guidelines suggest that warfarin be used after CABG only if there is another indication for anticoagulation (ACCP, grade 2C).[15]

In the patient who has undergone valve replacement, warfarin therapy is typically initiated a few days after surgery (ACCP, grade 1C to 2C)[20] with continuation for at least 3 months (ACC/AHA, class I).[19] The level and duration of anticoagulation beyond this period varies and is largely determined by (1) the type of valve, (2) the location of the valve, and (3) the presence or absence of risk factors for thromboembolism (table 24-3).

No consensus guidelines currently exist regarding the use of anticoagulants in patients with surgically corrected congenital heart disease. Although patients who have undergone the Fontan operation are often placed on warfarin because of an increased risk of pulmonary and central nervous system emboli,[51–53] its use in these patients remains controversial.[51] In contrast, warfarin should be used indefinitely for the patient with a right-to-left shunt who has experienced a thromboembolic event. An exception to this is the patient with Eisenmenger's syndrome, where the risk of hemoptysis and pulmonary hemorrhage outweighs the potential benefit of anticoagulation.

Some patients who undergo successful cardiac surgery develop conditions that warrant anticoagulation. Atrial fibrillation is the most common of these, as it occurs in 20 to 50 percent of patients postoperatively.[54–58] Anticoagulation (e.g., intravenous heparin) should be used for atrial fibrillation persisting more than 48 h after

Table 24-3 Anticoagulation (warfarin sodium) recommendations 3 months after prosthetic valve replacement

Valve and modifiers	INR goal	ACC/AHA class	ACCP grade
Mechanical valve			
Aortic and no thrombotic risk factor(s)[a]			
Bileaflet (St. Jude Medical)	2.0–3.0	I	1A
Bileaflet (Carbomedics)	2.0–3.0	I	1C+
Medtronic Hall type	2.0–3.0	I	1C+
Starr-Edwards type	2.5–3.5	I	
Other disk valve	2.5–3.5	I	
Tilting disk unable to take aspirin	3.5–4.5	IIa	
Aortic and thrombotic risk factor(s)[a]	2.5–3.5	I	1C+
Mitral and no thrombotic risk factor(s)[a]	2.5–3.5	I	1C+
Bioprosthetic valve			
Aortic and thrombotic risk factor(s)[a]	2.0–3.0	I	1C+
Mitral and thrombotic risk factor(s)[a]	2.5–3.5	I	1C+ (2.0–3.0 INR)

[a]Atrial fibrillation, left ventricular dysfunction, left atrial enlargement, previous thromboembolism, and hypercoagulable condition.
INR = international normalized ratio [prothrombin time].

surgery to reduce the risk of stroke[59,60] (ACC/AHA/ESC class IIa, level B).[61] Other postoperative conditions that warrant anticoagulation include (1) a left atrial or ventricular thrombus and (2) a significant left ventricular wall motion abnormality in the setting of a recent anterior MI.[16] Whether anticoagulation after surgery should also be offered to patients with chronic left ventricular systolic dysfunction is unclear at this time.[62] Current guidelines[63] and the recently released Warfarin and Antiplatelet Therapy in Chronic Heart failure (WATCH) study[64] do not support this strategy (ACC/AHA class IIb, level B or C).

ANGIOTENSIN CONVERTING ENZYME INHIBITORS AND ANGIOTENSIN RECEPTOR BLOCKERS

Angiotensin converting enzyme (ACE) inhibitors and angiotensin receptor blockers (ARBs) are potent inhibitors of the renin-angiotensin system. In select patients with cardiovascular disease, use of these agents significantly reduces the incidence of adverse cardiovascular events, including death, MI, and hospitalization for heart failure. Although current surgical guidelines do not comment on the long-term use of these agents postoperatively,[16] there is strong evidence to support their use in the patient undergoing cardiac surgery. That is, the benefits associated with their use outweigh the potential risks, which include renal insufficiency,[65,66] cough (predominantly with ACE inhibitors),[67,68] hyperkalemia,[66,69] and angioedema.[67,70] Because these agents may cause renal agenesis in the fetus, they should not be administered to the female patient who is or may become pregnant.[71,72]

In addition to their blood pressure–lowering effects, ACE inhibitors reduce vascular inflammation,[73,74] improve endothelial function,[75] and limit adverse ventricular remodeling.[76] In clinical trials, ACE inhibitor therapy has reduced adverse cardiovascular events in patients (1) with vascular disease,[77,78] (2) with heart failure or left ventricular systolic dysfunction,[79–84] or (3) undergoing CABG.[85,86] Accordingly, an ACE inhibitor should be considered for long-term postoperative use based on current guideline recommendations (ACC/AHA, class IIa, level B for patients with vascular disease and ACC/AHA, class I, level A; ESC, level A for patients with heart failure or left ventricular systolic dysfunction).[2,63,87]

Although ARBs benefit the patient with heart failure or left ventricular systolic dysfunction,[66,88–91] current guidelines recommend limiting their use to the patient who is intolerant of an ACE inhibitor (ACC/AHA, class IIa, level A; ESC, level C).[63,87] This recommendation is based on studies showing a greater reduction in mortality among patients treated with an ACE inhibitor as compared to those treated with an ARB.[87,89,92,93] More recently, findings from the Valsartan In Acute Myocardial Infarction Trial (VALIANT)[94] have challenged this notion. In this study, valsartan was as efficacious as captopril in reducing mortality in patients with ischemic left ventricular systolic dysfunction; however, there was no additional benefit to taking both agents. This latter finding is in keeping with current guideline recommendations (ACC/AHA, class IIb, level B)[63] but differs from other studies suggesting that the addition of ARBs to ACE inhibitors may be of particular benefit to patients with chronic heart failure or left ventricular systolic dysfunction[95] (ESC, level B).[87]

ALDOSTERONE INHIBITORS

Aldosterone production increases in proportion to heart failure severity[96] and leads to (1) activation of the renin-angiotensin system,[97] (2) cardiac fibrosis,[98,99] and (3) potassium excretion, which increases the risk of arrhythmias.[100] The aldosterone antagonists spirinolactone and eplerenone have been shown to improve survival in the patient with heart failure due to left ventricular systolic dysfunction.[101,102] Current guidelines recommend their use in the patient with left ventricular systolic dysfunction and symptomatic heart failure despite maximal medical therapy (ACC/AHA, class IIa, level B; ESC, level B).[63,87] Gynecomastia or breast pain (10 percent incidence with spironolactone)[101] and hyperkalemia (5.5 percent incidence with eplerenone)[102] are among the more common adverse effects of these drugs.

ANTIBIOTIC PROPHYLAXIS

Infective endocarditis occurs in 20,000 Americans each year.[103] Most cases of infective endocarditis occur because bacteria adhere to the surface of previously damaged endocardium following transient bacteremia.[104] Although any intracardiac structure exposed to the bloodstream may be affected, valvular involvement predominates.[105] The presence of foreign intracardiac material increases an individual's risk of infective endocarditis,[104] largely by providing a nidus for initial bacterial adherence. This is of particular importance among patients who have undergone cardiac surgery for valvular or congenital heart disease.

The mainstay of infective endocarditis prevention is to (1) avoid conditions that predispose to "unnecessary" bacteremia (i.e., skin piercings, tattoos, etc.) and (2) administer prophylactic antibiotics to the patient considered to be at "high risk" for endocarditis. The cardiac conditions and medical procedures for which antibiotic prophylaxis is indicated are presented in Table 24-4. Several factors affect the recommended antibiotic prophylaxis regimen, including the anticipated risk of bacteremia with the medical procedure, the microorganisms

Table 24-4 Postoperative cardiac conditions and medical procedures warranting antibiotic prophylaxis for infective endocarditis[30,106,107]

Surgically corrected cardiac conditions
- Prosthetic cardiac valves[a]
- Surgically constructed systemic to pulmonary shunts or conduits[a]
- Corrected congenital heart defects or procedures
  - Atrioventricular septal defect, complete
  - Atrioventricular septal defect, partial if left residual AV-valve regurgitation
  - Aortic coarctation
  - Fontan
  - Marfan's syndrome (aortic surgery)
  - Tetralogy of Fallot[a]
  - Transposition of the great vessels (postoperative and congenitally corrected)[a]
  - Ventricular septal defect, residual[b]
- Noncoronary vascular grafts (initial 6 months after surgery)

Medical procedures
- Dental
  - Extractions and implants
  - Periodontic, endodontic, subgingival, or intraligamentary instrumentation
  - Prophylactic cleaning where bleeding is anticipated
- Respiratory
  - Tonsillectomy and/or adenoidectomy
  - Surgical operations of the respiratory mucosa
  - Rigid bronchoscopy
- Gastrointestinal
  - Variceal sclerotherapy
  - Esophageal stricture dilation
  - Open or endoscopic procedures for biliary obstruction
  - Surgical operations of the intestinal mucosa
- Genitourinary
  - Prostatic or urinary tract surgery
  - Cystocopy
  - Urethral instrumentation or dilation
  - Lithotripsy
  - Gynecologic procedures in the presence of an infection

[a]At higher risk for infective endocarditis.
[b]Questionable need for prophylaxis if no residual shunt after closure.[30]

Table 24-5 Prophylactic antibiotic regimens[106, 107]

Dental, respiratory, and gastrointestinal (esophageal) procedures
- Not allergic to penicillin
  - Amoxicillin 2.0 g PO 1 h before the procedure or ampicillin 2.0 g IM or IV 30 min before the procedure
- Allergic to penicillin
  - Clindamycin 600 mg PO 1 h before the procedure or
  - Cephalexin 2.0 g PO 1 h before the procedure or
  - Cefadroxil 2.0 g PO 1 h before the procedure or
  - Azithromycin 500 mg PO 1 h before the procedure or
  - Clarithromycin 500 mg PO 1 h before the procedure or
  - Clindamycin 600 mg IV 30 min before the procedure or
  - Cefazolin 1.0 g IV 30 min before the procedure

Gastrointestinal (nonesophageal) and genitourinary procedures—higher risk
- Not allergic to penicillin
  - Ampicillin 2.0 g IM or IV plus gentamicin 1.5 mg/kg IV 30 min before the procedure followed by amoxicillin 1.0 g PO or ampicillin 1.0 g IM 6 h after the procedure
- Allergic to penicillin
  - Vancomycin 1.0 g IV (over 1–2 h) plus gentamicin 1.5 mg/kg IM or IV 30 min before the procedure

Gastrointestinal (nonesophageal) and genitourinary procedures—not higher risk
- Not allergic to penicillin
  - Amoxicillin 2.0 g PO 1 h before the procedure or
  - Ampicillin 2.0 g IM or IV 30 min before the procedure
- Allergic to penicillin
  - Vancomycin 1.0 g IV (over 1–2 h) 30 min before the procedure

g = grams; IM = intramuscular; IV = intravenous; kg = kilogram; mg = milligrams; PO = oral.

involved, the level of risk attributed to the patient's underlying condition, and the route of antibiotic delivery (Table 24-5).[106,107]

BETA-ADRENERGIC BLOCKERS

By inhibiting the effects of catecholamines on beta-adrenergic receptors, beta-adrenergic blockers have antiarrhythmic, antianginal, and sympatholytic effects on the cardiovascular system. They have been shown to significantly improve cardiovascular outcomes in patients with a history of MI[108–110] or congestive heart failure,[111–114] prompting current guidelines to recommend their long-term use in these conditions (ACC/AHA, class I, level B, and ESC, level B for MI; ACC/AHA, class I, level A or B, and ESC, level A for congestive heart failure).[63,87,115] As antihypertensive agents, beta-adrenergic blockers have similar efficacy to other commonly used agents (i.e., ACE inhibitors, diuretics, etc.),[116–118] but they appear to offer greater cardiovascular protection.[119,120] Although generally well tolerated, beta-adrenergic blockers may cause fatigue,[121] sexual dysfunction,[121] and short-term exacerbation of heart failure symptoms.[122]

The postoperative use of beta-adrenergic blockers is strongly indicated for most patients who have undergone cardiac surgery. When administered in the early postoperative period, beta-adrenergic blockers inhibit sympathetic outflow,[57,58,123–126] thereby blunting the hyperadrenergic stress response commonly seen after surgery.[123] This reduces the incidence of postoperative atrial fibrillation,[57,58,124–128] stroke,[129,130] and heart failure.[131] By comparison, long-term postoperative use of beta-adrenergic blockers is of greatest benefit in the patient who has undergone CABG, particularly if he or she has had a previous MI.[132] This likely reflects the ability of beta-adrenergic blockers to reduce ischemia, particularly in regions of the myocardium that have been incompletely revascularized.[133] Based on this, current guidelines strongly recommend the perioperative use of a beta-adrenergic blocker in all patients undergoing cardiac surgery (ACC/AHA/ESC, class I, level A)[61] and their long-term use in the patient who has undergone CABG following an MI (ACC/AHA, class I, level C).[115]

BLOOD PRESSURE CONTROL

Because systemic arterial hypertension is associated with an increased risk of numerous adverse cardiovascular events,[134–139] close attention to blood pressure control should be a primary focus for the patient following cardiac surgery. Current guidelines recommend a blood pressure below 130/85 mmHg for the patient with known congestive heart failure (ACC/AHA, class I, level A)[2] and below 130/80 mmHg for the patient with diabetes mellitus and/or chronic kidney disease.[140] Although lifestyle changes—including restriction of dietary sodium, weight reduction, avoidance of excess alcohol, and regular aerobic exercise—should be recommended as the initial treatment, most patients will require at least two medications to achieve their target blood pressure.[141] For the patient requiring medical therapy, strong consideration should be given to the use of an ACE inhibitor, beta-adrenergic blocker, and/or thiazide diuretic as a first-line agent.

CHOLESTEROL REDUCTION

Low-density-lipoprotein cholesterol (LDL-C) is an atherogenic particle that is strongly linked to the development of vascular disease. In both its native and oxidized forms, it causes endothelial cell injury and dysfunction,[142,143] promotes the formation of an atherosclerotic plaque,[144] and increases the risk of cardiovascular events.[145] By blocking cholesterol synthesis, the 3-hydroxy-3-methylglutaryl-coenzyme A (HMGCoA) reductase inhibitors—so-called statins—improve cardiovascular outcomes, as demonstrated in studies of primary[146–148] and secondary[149–153] prevention. Current guidelines recommend a statin as first-line therapy for most patients with cardiovascular disease, with the goal of achieving a LDL-C at least less than 100 mg/dL.[154]

The use of statins after cardiac surgery is indicated to reduce the risk of subsequent cardiovascular events, especially for the patient who has undergone CABG.[16] Aggressive LDL-C reduction is associated with a higher rate of saphenous vein graft patency,[155] a lower need for revascularization,[48] and a reduction in all-cause mortality.[156] These effects occur independent of atherosclerotic regression,[157–159] suggesting that statins may provide benefit largely through their favorable effects on endothelial function, inflammation, plaque stability, and/or thrombosis.[160] In the patient undergoing surgical repair of valvular or congenital heart disease, statin administration is largely dictated by his or her cardiovascular risk and serum LDL-C level.[154] For the patient who is prescribed a statin, close attention must be paid to potential side effects, including myopathy,[161] myositis,[162] rhabdomyolysis,[163] and hepatitis.[164]

CIGARETTE SMOKING/TOBACCO CESSATION

Smoking promotes the development and progression of cardiovascular disease[165] and is an important predictor of future cardiovascular events.[166] Individuals who continue to smoke after cardiac surgery have higher rates of saphenous vein graft occlusion,[167,168] MI,[169] bioprosthetic valve degeneration,[170] congestive heart failure,[171] cardiac reoperation,[169,172] stroke,[173] and death.[172,174,175] Early cessation of smoking can significantly reduce these risks[176]; however, therapies to assist with this are infrequently offered to patients prior to hospital discharge.[177] Since fewer than 10 percent of cigarette smokers achieve long-term success with smoking cessation without assistance,[178] current guidelines recommend that therapies to promote smoking cessation be provided to all smokers immediately after surgery (ACC/AHA, grade 1).[16] Buproprion (with or without nicotine replacement)[179,180] and behavioral support[181,182] have the greatest efficacy; however, rimonabant, a medication currently under investigation, may be of particular benefit among patients who are obese.[183] Because combination therapy has the greatest success,[184,185] two or more treatment options should be provided to smokers after surgery to maximize the likelihood of long-term smoking cessation.

DIABETES MELLITUS CONTROL

Diabetes mellitus is an independent risk factor for the development[186,187] and progression of cardiovascular disease[188] and an important predictor of perioperative stroke,[137] rehospitalization,[189] need for revascularization,[190] and death.[174,190–193] In the United Kingdom Prospective Diabetes Study,[194] each 1 percent reduction in mean glycosylated hemoglobin (HbA1c) serum concentration was associated with a 14 percent reduction in the incidence of nonfatal MI ($p < 0.0001$). Similar findings have been demonstrated in patients who have undergone CABG,[195] with a strong inverse correlation between saphenous vein graft endothelial function and mean HbA1c serum concentration.[196] Because of this, current efforts should focus on strict postoperative glycemic control[197] with a long-term target serum concentration of HbA1c < 7.0 percent.[198]

DIET AND WEIGHT MANAGEMENT

In the early postoperative period, obesity is associated with an increased risk of sternal dehiscence and hospital readmission, but it does not appear to increase the risk of MI, stroke, or death.[199] Long term failure to maintain an ideal body weight, however, increases the risk of coronary artery disease,[200] stroke,[201] congestive heart failure,[202] death,[203] and other comorbid conditions (i.e., diabetes mellitus, hypertension, and hypercholesterolemia).[200] To reduce these risks, obese patients should institute caloric reductions of at least 500 kcal/day until they are at their ideal body weight.[204] This is best achieved with a diet enriched with protein (15 percent of calories), complex carbohydrates (50 to 60 percent of calories), omega-3 fatty acids, fruits, vegetables, nuts, and whole grains and restricted in saturated fat (< 7 percent total calories), cholesterol (< 200 mg/day), and sodium (< 2.4 g/day).[154,204–207]

DIGOXIN

Historically, digoxin was routinely used to prevent postoperative arrhythmias following cardiac surgery.[208,209] Recent data, however, have shown that prophylactic administration of digoxin postoperatively does not prevent arrhythmias[58,125,210,211] and, in fact, may actually increase the risk of their development.[57,210,212] Based on this, current guidelines do not recommend the routine use of digoxin following cardiac surgery.[61]

In contrast, digoxin should be considered for use in the patient with symptomatic left ventricular dysfunction receiving maximal medical therapy (ACC/AHA, class I, level A).[63] Support for this comes from the Digitalis Investigation Group, which demonstrated a 28 percent reduction in the rate of hospitalization for congestive heart failure in patients with left ventricular systolic dysfunction who received digoxin ($p < 0.001$).[213] Although no mortality benefit was demonstrated in this study, subsequent post hoc analyses have reported an association between improved mortality with lower serum levels of digoxin (0.5 to 0.8 ng/mL)[214] and higher mortality in women treated with digoxin.[215] Although the mechanisms underlying these findings are not completely known, they underscore the idea that there is a narrow therapeutic window for digoxin and raise concern that there may be gender-specific effects. In addition, intermittent monitoring of digoxin levels should be considered, given the possibility of drug-drug interactions that may alter the serum digoxin concentration.

EXERCISE

Because regular physical activity has been shown to have long-term cardiovascular benefit,[216–219] current guidelines recommend participation in moderate levels of aerobic and weight-training exercise for at least 30 min/day most days of the week.[220,221] For patients who have had recent cardiac surgery, close supervision in a structured home exercise program[222–225] or cardiac rehabilitation program[226,227] is desirable. If available, cardiac rehabilitation is preferable to home exercise because it provides more intensive risk-factor management, physical activity counseling, and intensive nutritional modification.[228] This translates into reduced rates of hospitalization,[229] greater functional capacity,[222, 230-233] improved quality of life,[234–236] and better autonomic function.[233,237,238] Therefore early referral[239,240] to a cardiac rehabilitation program should be recommended to all patients after CABG[16] and to most patients following surgical correction of valvular[227] or congenital heart disease.[222]

CONCLUSION

Given the importance of postoperative cardiovascular risk reduction, physicians and healthcare providers must possess a comprehensive knowledge of available therapies that should be offered to the patient who has undergone cardiac surgery. The therapies discussed in this review have strong data supporting their use in a wide range of patients with cardiovascular disease and offer particular benefit in those who have undergone CABG, valve replacement, or surgical repair of congenital heart disease. By offering these recommendations in an "ABC" format, a simple framework is provided to more effectively develop disease management protocols and individual therapeutic courses of action that should increase adherence to current guidelines and reduce cardiovascular morbidity and mortality following cardiac surgery.

References

1. Society of Thoracic Surgeons. Adult CV surgery national database—Fall 2003 executive summary contents. Available at: www.sts.org. Accessed January 26, 2004.
2. Gibbons RJ, Abrams J, Chatterjee K, et al. ACC/AHA 2002 guideline update for the management of patients with chronic stable angina—Summary article: A report of the American College of Cardiology/American Heart Association Task Force on Practice Guidelines (Committee on the Management of Patients with Chronic Stable Angina). *Circulation* 2003;107(1):149–158.

3. Chesebro JH, Fuster V. Pathogenesis and prevention of aortocoronary bypass graft occlusion. *Int J Clin Pharmacol Res* 1986;6(4):261–267.
4. Israel DH, Adams PC, Stein B, et al. Antithrombotic therapy in the coronary vein graft patient. *Clin Cardiol* 1991;14(4):283–295.
5. Kim AY, Walinsky PL, Kolodgie FD, et al. Early loss of thrombomodulin expression impairs vein graft thromboresistance: Implications for vein graft failure. *Circ Res* 2002;90(2):205–212.
6. Sperry JL, Deming CB, Bian C, et al. Wall tension is a potent negative regulator of in vivo thrombomodulin expression. *Circ Res* 2003;92(1):41–47.
7. Unni KK, Kottke BA, Titus JL, et al. Pathologic changes in aortocoronary saphenous vein grafts. *Am J Cardiol* 1974;34(5):526–532.
8. Nwasokwa ON. Coronary artery bypass graft disease. *Ann Intern Med* 1995;123(7):528–545.
9. Pantely GA, Goodnight SH Jr, Rahimtoola SH, et al. Failure of antiplatelet and anticoagulant therapy to improve patency of grafts after coronary-artery bypass: A controlled, randomized study. *N Engl J Med* 1979; 301(18):962–966.
10. van der Meer J, Hillege HL, Kootstra GJ, et al. Prevention of one-year vein-graft occlusion after aortocoronary-bypass surgery: A comparison of low-dose aspirin, low-dose aspirin plus dipyridamole, and oral anticoagulants. The CABADAS Research Group of the Interuniversity Cardiology Institute of The Netherlands. *Lancet* 1993;342(8866):257–264.
11. Lorenz RL, Schacky CV, Weber M, et al. Improved aortocoronary bypass patency by low-dose aspirin (100 mg daily). Effects on platelet aggregation and thromboxane formation. *Lancet* 1984;1(8389):1261–1264.
12. Meister W, von Schacky C, Weber M, et al. Low-dose acetylsalicylic acid (100 mg/day) after aortocoronary bypass surgery: A placebo-controlled trial. *Br J Clin Pharmacol* 1984;17(6):703–711.
13. Collaborative overview of randomised trials of antiplatelet therapy—II: Maintenance of vascular graft or arterial patency by antiplatelet therapy. Antiplatelet Trialists' Collaboration. *BMJ* 1994;308(6922):159–168.
14. Mangano DT. Aspirin and mortality from coronary bypass surgery. *N Engl J Med* 2002;347(17):1309–1317.
15. Stein PD, Dalen JE, Goldman S, Theroux P. Antithrombotic therapy in patients with saphenous vein and internal mammary artery bypass grafts. *Chest* 2001;119(1 Suppl):278S–282S.
16. Eagle KA, Guyton RA, Davidoff R, et al. ACC/AHA Guidelines for Coronary Artery Bypass Graft Surgery: A Report of the American College of Cardiology/American Heart Association Task Force on Practice Guidelines (Committee to Revise the 1991 Guidelines for Coronary Artery Bypass Graft Surgery). American College of Cardiology/American Heart Association. *J Am Coll Cardiol* 1999;34(4):1262–1347.
17. Patrono C, Bachmann F, Baigent C, et al. Expert consensus document on the use of antiplatelet agents. The task force on the use of antiplatelet agents in patients with atherosclerotic cardiovascular disease of the European society of cardiology. *Eur Heart J* 2004;25(2): 166–181.
18. Bluestein D, Rambod E, Gharib M. Vortex shedding as a mechanism for free emboli formation in mechanical heart valves. *J Biomech Eng* 2000;122(2):125–134.
19. Bonow RO, Carabello B, de Leon AC Jr, et al. Guidelines for the management of patients with valvular heart disease: Executive summary. A report of the American College of Cardiology/American Heart Association Task Force on Practice Guidelines (Committee on Management of Patients with Valvular Heart Disease). *Circulation* 1998;98(18):1949–1984.
20. Stein PD, Alpert JS, Bussey HI, et al. Antithrombotic therapy in patients with mechanical and biological prosthetic heart valves. *Chest* 2001;119(1 Suppl): 220S–227S.
21. Gherli T, Colli A, Fragnito C, et al. Comparing warfarin with aspirin after biological aortic valve replacement: A prospective study. *Circulation* 2004;110(5):496–500.
22. Babin-Ebell J, Schmidt W, Eigel P, Elert O. Aortic bioprosthesis without early anticoagulation—Risk of thromboembolism. *Thorac Cardiovasc Surg* 1995;43(4): 212–214.
23. Joyce LD, Nelson RM. Comparison of porcine valve xenografts with mechanical prostheses. A 7 1/2 year experience. *J Thorac Cardiovasc Surg* 1984;88(1): 102–113.
24. Little S, Massel D. Antiplatelet and anticoagulation for patients with prosthetic heart valves. *Cochrane Database Syst Rev* 2003;4:CD003464.
25. Meschengieser SS, Fondevila CG, Frontroth J, et al. Low-intensity oral anticoagulation plus low-dose aspirin versus high-intensity oral anticoagulation alone: A randomized trial in patients with mechanical prosthetic heart valves. *J Thorac Cardiovasc Surg* 1997;113(5): 910–916.
26. Fuster V, Steele PM, Edwards WD, et al. Primary pulmonary hypertension: Natural history and the importance of thrombosis. *Circulation* 1984;70(4):580–587.
27. Reller MD. Congenital heart disease: Current indications for antithrombotic therapy in pediatric patients. *Curr Cardiol Rep* 2001;3(1):90–95.
28. Motz R, Wessel A, Ruschewski W, Bursch J. Reduced frequency of occlusion of aorto-pulmonary shunts in infants receiving aspirin. *Cardiol Young* 1999;9(5): 474–477.
29. Al Jubair KA, Al Fagih MR, Al Jarallah AS, et al. Results of 546 Blalock-Taussig shunts performed in 478 patients. *Cardiol Young* 1998;8(4):486–490.
30. Deanfield J, Thaulow E, Warnes C, et al. Management of grown up congenital heart disease. *Eur Heart J* 2003;24(11):1035–1084.
31. Collaborative meta-analysis of randomised trials of antiplatelet therapy for prevention of death, myocardial infarction, and stroke in high risk patients. *BMJ* 2002; 324(7329):71–86.
32. Bellavance A. Efficacy of ticlopidine and aspirin for prevention of reversible cerebrovascular ischemic events. The Ticlopidine Aspirin Stroke Study. *Stroke* 1993; 24(10):1452–1457.
33. A randomised, blinded, trial of clopidogrel versus aspirin in patients at risk of ischaemic events (CAPRIE). CAPRIE Steering Committee. *Lancet* 1996;348(9038): 1329–1339.

34. Yusuf S, Zhao F, Mehta SR, et al. Effects of clopidogrel in addition to aspirin in patients with acute coronary syndromes without ST-segment elevation. *N Engl J Med* 2001;345(7):494–502.
35. Goods CM, al-Shaibi KF, Liu MW, et al. Comparison of aspirin alone versus aspirin plus ticlopidine after coronary artery stenting. *Am J Cardiol* 1996;78(9):1042–1044.
36. Mehta SR, Yusuf S, Peters RJ, et al. Effects of pretreatment with clopidogrel and aspirin followed by long-term therapy in patients undergoing percutaneous coronary intervention: The PCI-CURE study. *Lancet* 2001; 358(9281):527–533.
37. Steinhubl SR, Berger PB, Mann JT III, et al. Early and sustained dual oral antiplatelet therapy following percutaneous coronary intervention: A randomized controlled trial. *JAMA* 2002;288(19):2411–2420.
38. Hongo RH, Ley J, Dick SE, Yee RR. The effect of clopidogrel in combination with aspirin when given before coronary artery bypass grafting. *J Am Coll Cardiol* 2002;40(2):231–237.
39. Yende S, Wunderink RG. Effect of clopidogrel on bleeding after coronary artery bypass surgery. *Crit Care Med* 2001;29(12):2271–2275.
40. Chevigne M, David JL, Rigo P, Limet R. Effect of ticlopidine on saphenous vein bypass patency rates: A double-blind study. *Ann Thorac Surg* 1984;37(5):371–378.
41. Limet R, David JL, Magotteaux P, et al. Prevention of aorta-coronary bypass graft occlusion. Beneficial effect of ticlopidine on early and late patency rates of venous coronary bypass grafts: A double-blind study. *J Thorac Cardiovasc Surg* 1987;94(5):773–783.
42. Love BB, Biller J, Gent M. Adverse haematological effects of ticlopidine. Prevention, recognition and management. *Drug Saf* 1998;19(2):89–98.
43. Bennett CL, Kiss JE, Weinberg PD, et al. Thrombotic thrombocytopenic purpura after stenting and ticlopidine. *Lancet* 1998;352(9133):1036–1037.
44. Bhatt DL, Chew DP, Hirsch AT, et al. Superiority of clopidogrel versus aspirin in patients with prior cardiac surgery. *Circulation*. Jan 23 2001;103(3):363–368.
45. Verheugt FW. Clopidogrel versus aspirin after cardiac surgery. *Circulation* 2001;104(13):E76.
46. Fox KA, Mehta SR, Peters R, et al. Benefits and risks of the combination of clopidogrel and aspirin in patients undergoing surgical revascularization for non-ST-elevation acute coronary syndrome: The Clopidogrel in Unstable angina to prevent Recurrent ischemic Events (CURE) Trial. *Circulation* 2004;110(10):1202–1208.
47. Stein PD, Dalen JE, Goldman S, Theroux P. Antithrombotic therapy in patients with saphenous vein and internal mammary artery bypass grafts. *Chest* 1998;114(5 Suppl):658S–665S.
48. Knatterud GL, Rosenberg Y, Campeau L, et al. Long-term effects on clinical outcomes of aggressive lowering of low-density lipoprotein cholesterol levels and low-dose anticoagulation in the post coronary artery bypass graft trial. Post CABG Investigators. *Circulation* 2000;102(2):157–165.
49. McEnany MT, Salzman EW, Mundth ED, et al. The effect of antithrombotic therapy on patency rates of saphenous vein coronary artery bypass grafts. *J Thorac Cardiovasc Surg* 1982;83(1):81–89.
50. Yli-Mayry S, Huikuri HV, Korhonen UR, et al. Efficacy and safety of anticoagulant therapy started pre-operatively in preventing coronary vein graft occlusion. *Eur Heart J* 1992;13(9):1259–1264.
51. Monagle P, Cochrane A, McCrindle B, et al. Thromboembolic complications after Fontan procedures—The role of prophylactic anticoagulation. *J Thorac Cardiovasc Surg* 1998;115(3):493–498.
52. Shirai LK, Rosenthal DN, Reitz BA, et al. Arrhythmias and thromboembolic complications after the extracardiac Fontan operation. *J Thorac Cardiovasc Surg* 1998;115(3): 499–505.
53. Rosenthal DN, Friedman AH, Kleinman CS, et al. Thromboembolic complications after Fontan operations. *Circulation* 1995;92(9 Suppl):II287–II293.
54. Creswell LL, Schuessler RB, Rosenbloom M, Cox JL. Hazards of postoperative atrial arrhythmias. *Ann Thorac Surg* 1993;56(3):539–549.
55. Zaman AG, Archbold RA, Helft G, et al. Atrial fibrillation after coronary artery bypass surgery: A model for preoperative risk stratification. *Circulation* 2000;101(12):1403–1408.
56. Aranki SF, Shaw DP, Adams DH, et al. Predictors of atrial fibrillation after coronary artery surgery. Current trends and impact on hospital resources. *Circulation* 1996;94(3):390–397.
57. Mathew JP, Fontes ML, Tudor IC, et al. A multicenter risk index for atrial fibrillation after cardiac surgery. *JAMA* 2004;291(14):1720–1729.
58. Andrews TC, Reimold SC, Berlin JA, Antman EM. Prevention of supraventricular arrhythmias after coronary artery bypass surgery. A meta-analysis of randomized control trials. *Circulation*.1991;84(5 Suppl): III236–III244.
59. Reed GL III, Singer DE, Picard EH, DeSanctis RW. Stroke following coronary-artery bypass surgery. A case-control estimate of the risk from carotid bruits. *N Engl J Med* 1988;319(19):1246–1250.
60. Taylor GJ, Malik SA, Colliver JA, et al. Usefulness of atrial fibrillation as a predictor of stroke after isolated coronary artery bypass grafting. *Am J Cardiol* 1987;60(10): 905–907.
61. Fuster V, Ryden LE, Asinger RW, et al. ACC/AHA/ ESC guidelines for the management of patients with atrial fibrillation: Executive summary. A Report of the American College of Cardiology/ American Heart Association Task Force on Practice Guidelines and the European Society of Cardiology Committee for Practice Guidelines and Policy Conferences (Committee to Develop Guidelines for the Management of Patients with Atrial Fibrillation): Developed in Collaboration with the North American Society of Pacing and Electrophysiology. *J Am Coll Cardiol* 2001;38(4): 1231–1266.
62. Diet F, Erdmann E. Thromboembolism in heart failure: Who should be treated? *Eur J Heart Fail* 2000;2(4): 355–363.
63. Hunt SA, Baker DW, Chin MH, et al. ACC/AHA guidelines for the evaluation and management of chronic heart failure in the adult: Executive summary. A Report of the American College of Cardiology/American Heart Association Task Force

on Practice Guidelines (Committee to Revise the 1995 Guidelines for the Evaluation and Management of Heart Failure): Developed in Collaboration with the International Society for Heart and Lung Transplantation; Endorsed by the Heart Failure Society of America. *Circulation* 2001;104(24): 2996–3007.

64. Massie B. Final Results of the Warfarin and Antiplatelet Trial in Chronic Heart Failure (WATCH): A Randomized Comparison of Warfarin, Aspirin, and Clopidogrel. Paper presented at the American College of Cardiology 2004 Scientific Sessions, 2004; New Orleans.
65. Mimran A, Ribstein J, DuCailar G. Converting enzyme inhibitors and renal function in essential and renovascular hypertension. *Am J Hypertens* 1991;4(1 Pt 2):7S–14S.
66. Pfeffer MA, Swedberg K, Granger CB, et al. Effects of candesartan on mortality and morbidity in patients with chronic heart failure: The CHARM-Overall programme. *Lancet* 2003;362(9386):759–766.
67. Israili ZH, Hall WD. Cough and angioneurotic edema associated with angiotensin-converting enzyme inhibitor therapy. A review of the literature and pathophysiology. *Ann Intern Med* 1992;117(3):234–242.
68. Weber MA. Comparison of type 1 angiotensin II receptor blockers and angiotensin converting enzyme inhibitors in the treatment of hypertension. *J Hypertens Suppl* 1997;15(6):S31–S36.
69. Reardon LC, Macpherson DS. Hyperkalemia in outpatients using angiotensin-converting enzyme inhibitors. How much should we worry? *Arch Intern Med* 1998; 158(1):26–32.
70. Warner KK, Visconti JA, Tschampel MM. Angiotensin II receptor blockers in patients with ACE inhibitor-induced angioedema. *Ann Pharmacother* 2000;34(4): 526–528.
71. Hanssens M, Keirse MJ, Vankelecom F, Van Assche FA. Fetal and neonatal effects of treatment with angiotensin-converting enzyme inhibitors in pregnancy. *Obstet Gynecol* 1991;78(1):128–135.
72. Blum N, Kamens C, Mayo H, Holt J. What treatments are safe and effective for mild to moderate hypertension in pregnancy? *J Fam Pract* 2004;53(6):492–494.
73. Brull DJ, Sanders J, Rumley A, et al. Impact of angiotensin converting enzyme inhibition on post-coronary artery bypass interleukin 6 release. *Heart* 2002; 87(3):252–255.
74. van Haelst PL, Tervaert JW, van Geel PP, et al. Long-term angiotensin converting enzyme-inhibition in patients after coronary artery bypass grafting reduces levels of soluble intercellular cell adhesion molecule-1. *Eur J Vasc Endovasc Surg* 2003;26(4):387–391.
75. Ko L, Maitland A, Fedak PW, et al. Endothelin blockade potentiates endothelial protective effects of ACE inhibitors in saphenous veins. *Ann Thorac Surg* 2002;73(4):1185–1188.
76. Kjoller-Hansen L, Steffensen R, Grande P. Beneficial effects of ramipril on left ventricular end-diastolic and end-systolic volume indexes after uncomplicated invasive revascularization are associated with a reduction in cardiac events in patients with moderately impaired left ventricular function and no clinical heart failure. *J Am Coll Cardiol* 2001;37(5):1214–1220.
77. Yusuf S, Sleight P, Pogue J, et al. Effects of an angiotensin-converting-enzyme inhibitor, ramipril, on cardiovascular events in high-risk patients. The Heart Outcomes Prevention Evaluation Study Investigators. *N Engl J Med* 2000;342(3):145–153.
78. Fox KM. Efficacy of perindopril in reduction of cardiovascular events among patients with stable coronary artery disease: Randomised, double-blind, placebo-controlled, multicentre trial (the EUROPA study). *Lancet* 2003;362(9386):782–788.
79. Effects of enalapril on mortality in severe congestive heart failure. Results of the Cooperative North Scandinavian Enalapril Survival Study (CONSENSUS). The CONSENSUS Trial Study Group. *N Engl J Med* 1987;316(23):1429–1435.
80. Effect of enalapril on survival in patients with reduced left ventricular ejection fractions and congestive heart failure. The SOLVD Investigators. *N Engl J Med* 1991;325(5):293–302.
81. Effect of ramipril on mortality and morbidity of survivors of acute myocardial infarction with clinical evidence of heart failure. The Acute Infarction Ramipril Efficacy (AIRE) Study Investigators. *Lancet* 1993;342(8875):821–828.
82. Cohn JN, Johnson G, Ziesche S, et al. A comparison of enalapril with hydralazine-isosorbide dinitrate in the treatment of chronic congestive heart failure. *N Engl J Med* 1991;325(5):303–310.
83. Kober L, Torp-Pedersen C, Carlsen JE, et al. A clinical trial of the angiotensin-converting-enzyme inhibitor trandolapril in patients with left ventricular dysfunction after myocardial infarction. Trandolapril Cardiac Evaluation (TRACE) Study Group. *N Engl J Med* 1995;333(25):1670–1676.
84. Pfeffer MA, Braunwald E, Moye LA, et al. Effect of captopril on mortality and morbidity in patients with left ventricular dysfunction after myocardial infarction. Results of the survival and ventricular enlargement trial. The SAVE Investigators. *N Engl J Med* 1992;327(10):669–677.
85. Oosterga M, Voors AA, Pinto YM, et al. Effects of quinapril on clinical outcome after coronary artery bypass grafting (The QUO VADIS Study). QUinapril on Vascular Ace and Determinants of Ischemia. *Am J Cardiol* 2001;87(5):542–546.
86. Kjoller-Hansen L, Steffensen R, Grande P. The Angiotensin-converting Enzyme Inhibition Post Revascularization Study (APRES). *J Am Coll Cardiol* 2000;35(4):881–888.
87. Remme WJ, Swedberg K. Guidelines for the diagnosis and treatment of chronic heart failure. *Eur Heart J* 2001;22(17):1527–1560.
88. Sharma D, Buyse M, Pitt B, Rucinska EJ. Meta-analysis of observed mortality data from all-controlled, double-blind, multiple-dose studies of losartan in heart failure. Losartan Heart Failure Mortality Meta-analysis Study Group. *Am J Cardiol* 2000;85(2):187–192.
89. McKelvie RS, Yusuf S, Pericak D, et al. Comparison of candesartan, enalapril, and their combination in congestive heart failure: Randomized evaluation of strategies for left ventricular dysfunction (RESOLVD) pilot study. The RESOLVD Pilot Study Investigators. *Circulation* 1999;100(10):1056–1064.

90. Mazayev VP, Fomina IG, Kazakov EN, et al. Valsartan in heart failure patients previously untreated with an ACE inhibitor. *Int J Cardiol* 1998;65(3):239–246.
91. Pitt B, Segal R, Martinez FA, et al. Randomised trial of losartan versus captopril in patients over 65 with heart failure (Evaluation of Losartan in the Elderly Study, ELITE). *Lancet* 1997;349(9054):747–752.
92. Pitt B, Poole-Wilson P, Segal R, et al. Effects of losartan versus captopril on mortality in patients with symptomatic heart failure: Rationale, design, and baseline characteristics of patients in the Losartan Heart Failure Survival Study—ELITE II. *J Card Fail* 1999;5(2): 146–154.
93. Jong P, Demers C, McKelvie RS, Liu PP. Angiotensin receptor blockers in heart failure: Meta-analysis of randomized controlled trials. *J Am Coll Cardiol* 2002;39(3):463–470.
94. Pfeffer MA, McMurray JJ, Velazquez EJ, et al. Valsartan, captopril, or both in myocardial infarction complicated by heart failure, left ventricular dysfunction, or both. *N Engl J Med* 2003;349(20):1893–1906.
95. McMurray JJ, Ostergren J, Swedberg K, et al. Effects of candesartan in patients with chronic heart failure and reduced left-ventricular systolic function taking angiotensin-converting-enzyme inhibitors: The CHARM-Added trial. *Lancet* 2003;362(9386): 767–771.
96. Zannad F. Aldosterone and heart failure. *Eur Heart J* 1995;16(Suppl N):98–102.
97. Harada E, Yoshimura M, Yasue H, et al. Aldosterone induces angiotensin-converting-enzyme gene expression in cultured neonatal rat cardiocytes. *Circulation* 2001;104(2):137–139.
98. Lijnen P, Petrov V. Induction of cardiac fibrosis by aldosterone. *J Mol Cell Cardiol* 2000;32(6):865–879.
99. Fullerton MJ, Funder JW. Aldosterone and cardiac fibrosis: In vitro studies. *Cardiovasc Res* 1994;28(12): 1863–1867.
100. Cooper HA, Dries DL, Davis CE, et al. Diuretics and risk of arrhythmic death in patients with left ventricular dysfunction. *Circulation* 1999;100(12):1311–1315.
101. Pitt B, Zannad F, Remme WJ, et al. The effect of spironolactone on morbidity and mortality in patients with severe heart failure. Randomized Aldactone Evaluation Study Investigators. *N Engl J Med* 1999; 341(10):709–717.
102. Pitt B, Remme W, Zannad F, et al. Eplerenone, a selective aldosterone blocker, in patients with left ventricular dysfunction after myocardial infarction. *N Engl J Med* 2003;348(14):1309–1321.
103. (*AHA*) *AHA*. Heart disease and stroke statistics: 2004 update. Available at: www.americanheart.org. Accessed January 26, 2004.
104. Moreillon P, Que YA. Infective endocarditis. *Lancet* 2004;363(9403):139–149.
105. Mylonakis E, Calderwood SB. Infective endocarditis in adults. *N Engl J Med* 2001;345(18):1318–1330.
106. Dajani AS, Taubert KA, Wilson W, et al. Prevention of bacterial endocarditis. Recommendations by the American Heart Association. *Circulation* 1997;96(1):358–366.
107. Horstkotte DFF, Gutschik E, Lengyel M, et al. Guidelines on prevention, diagnosis and treatment of infective endocarditis executive summary. *Eur Heart J* 2004;00:1–10.
108. Timolol-induced reduction in mortality and reinfarction in patients surviving acute myocardial infarction. *N Engl J Med* 1981;304(14):801–807.
109. A randomized trial of propranolol in patients with acute myocardial infarction. II. Morbidity results. *JAMA* 1983;250(20):2814–2819.
110. Gottlieb SS, McCarter RJ, Vogel RA. Effect of beta-blockade on mortality among high-risk and low-risk patients after myocardial infarction. *N Engl J Med* 1998;339(8):489–497.
111. Dargie HJ. Effect of carvedilol on outcome after myocardial infarction in patients with left-ventricular dysfunction: The CAPRICORN randomised trial. *Lancet* 2001;357(9266):1385–1390.
112. Effect of metoprolol CR/XL in chronic heart failure: Metoprolol CR/XL Randomised Intervention Trial in Congestive Heart Failure (MERIT-HF). *Lancet* 1999;353(9169):2001–2007.
113. The Cardiac Insufficiency Bisoprolol Study II (CIBIS-II): A randomised trial. *Lancet* 1999;353(9146):9–13.
114. Packer M, Coats AJ, Fowler MB, et al. Effect of carvedilol on survival in severe chronic heart failure. *N Engl J Med* 2001;344(22):1651–1658.
115. Braunwald E, Antman EM, Beasley JW, et al. ACC/AHA 2002 guideline update for the management of patients with unstable angina and non-ST-segment elevation myocardial infarction—Summary article: A report of the American College of Cardiology/American Heart Association task force on practice guidelines (Committee on the Management of Patients with Unstable Angina). *J Am Coll Cardiol* 2002;40(7):1366–1374.
116. Wilhelmsen L, Berglund G, Elmfeldt D, et al. Beta-blockers versus diuretics in hypertensive men: Main results from the HAPPHY trial. *J Hypertens* 1987;5(5):561–572.
117. Furberg CD, Cutler JA. Diuretic agents versus beta-blockers. Comparison of effects on mortality, stroke, and coronary events. *Hypertension* 1989;13(5 Suppl):I57–I61.
118. Hansson L, Lindholm LH, Niskanen L, et al. Effect of angiotensin-converting-enzyme inhibition compared with conventional therapy on cardiovascular morbidity and mortality in hypertension: The Captopril Prevention Project (CAPPP) randomised trial. *Lancet* 1999; 353(9153):611–616.
119. Wikstrand J, Warnold I, Tuomilehto J, et al. Metoprolol versus thiazide diuretics in hypertension. Morbidity results from the MAPHY Study. *Hypertension* 1991;17(4): 579–588.
120. Psaty BM, Koepsell TD, LoGerfo JP, et al. Beta-blockers and primary prevention of coronary heart disease in patients with high blood pressure. *JAMA* 1989;261(14): 2087–2094.
121. Ko DT, Hebert PR, Coffey CS, et al. Beta-blocker therapy and symptoms of depression, fatigue, and sexual dysfunction. *JAMA* 2002;288(3):351–357.
122. Jessup M, Brozena S. Heart failure. *N Engl J Med* 2003;348(20):2007–2018.
123. Oka Y, Frishman W, Becker RM, et al. Clinical pharmacology of the new beta-adrenergic blocking drugs. Part 10. Beta-adrenoceptor blockade and coronary artery surgery. *Am Heart J* 1980;99(2):255–269.

124. Kowey PR, Taylor JE, Rials SJ, Marinchak RA. Meta-analysis of the effectiveness of prophylactic drug therapy in preventing supraventricular arrhythmia early after coronary artery bypass grafting. *Am J Cardiol* 1992;69(9):963–965.
125. Rubin DA, Nieminski KE, Reed GE, Herman MV. Predictors, prevention, and long-term prognosis of atrial fibrillation after coronary artery bypass graft operations. *J Thorac Cardiovasc Surg* 1987;94(3):331–335.
126. Fuller JA, Adams GG, Buxton B. Atrial fibrillation after coronary artery bypass grafting. Is it a disorder of the elderly? *J Thorac Cardiovasc Surg* 1989;97(6):821–825.
127. Janssen J, Loomans L, Harink J, et al. Prevention and treatment of supraventricular tachycardia shortly after coronary artery bypass grafting: A randomized open trial. *Angiology* 1986;37(8):601–609.
128. Maisel WH, Rawn JD, Stevenson WG. Atrial fibrillation after cardiac surgery. *Ann Intern Med* 2001;135(12):1061–1073.
129. Likosky DS, Leavitt BJ, Marrin CA, et al. Intra- and postoperative predictors of stroke after coronary artery bypass grafting. *Ann Thorac Surg* 2003;76(2):428–434; discussion 435.
130. Murdock DK, Rengel LR, Schlund A, et al. Stroke and atrial fibrillation following cardiac surgery. *WMJ* 2003;102(4):26–30.
131. Ghai A, Harris L, Harrison DA, et al. Outcomes of late atrial tachyarrhythmias in adults after the Fontan operation. *J Am Coll Cardiol* 2001;37(2):585–592.
132. Chen J, Radford MJ, Wang Y, et al. Are beta-blockers effective in elderly patients who undergo coronary revascularization after acute myocardial infarction? *Arch Intern Med* 2000;160(7):947–952.
133. Geraci SA, Haan CK. Effect of beta blockers after coronary artery bypass in postinfarct patients: What can we learn from available literature? *Ann Thorac Surg* 2002;74(5):1727–1732.
134. Wilson PW. Established risk factors and coronary artery disease: The Framingham Study. *Am J Hypertens* 1994;7(7 Pt 2):7S–12S.
135. Staessen JA, Fagard R, Thijs L, et al. Randomised double-blind comparison of placebo and active treatment for older patients with isolated systolic hypertension. The Systolic Hypertension in Europe (Syst-Eur) Trial Investigators. *Lancet* 1997;350(9080):757–764.
136. Levy D, Larson MG, Vasan RS, et al. The progression from hypertension to congestive heart failure. *JAMA* 1996;275(20):1557–1562.
137. Bucerius J, Gummert JF, Borger MA, et al. Stroke after cardiac surgery: A risk factor analysis of 16,184 consecutive adult patients. *Ann Thorac Surg* 2003;75(2):472–478.
138. Boucher JM, Dupras A, Jutras N, et al. Long-term survival and functional status in the elderly after cardiac surgery. *Can J Cardiol* 1997;13(7):646–652.
139. Domanski MJ, Borkowf CB, Campeau L, et al. Prognostic factors for atherosclerosis progression in saphenous vein grafts: The postcoronary artery bypass graft (Post-CABG) trial. Post-CABG Trial Investigators. *J Am Coll Cardiol* 2000;36(6):1877–1883.
140. Chobanian AV, Bakris GL, Black HR, et al. The Seventh Report of the Joint National Committee on Prevention, Detection, Evaluation, and Treatment of High Blood Pressure: The JNC 7 report. *JAMA* 2003;289(19):2560–2572.
141. Cushman WC, Ford CE, Cutler JA, et al. Success and predictors of blood pressure control in diverse North American settings: The antihypertensive and lipid-lowering treatment to prevent heart attack trial (ALLHAT). *J Clin Hypertens (Greenwich)* 2002;4(6):393–404.
142. Ross R. Atherosclerosis—An inflammatory disease. *N Engl J Med* 1999;340(2):115–126.
143. Libby P. Current concepts of the pathogenesis of the acute coronary syndromes. *Circulation* 2001;104(3):365–372.
144. Stary HC, Chandler AB, Dinsmore RE, et al. A definition of advanced types of atherosclerotic lesions and a histological classification of atherosclerosis. A report from the Committee on Vascular Lesions of the Council on Arteriosclerosis, American Heart Association. *Circulation* 1995;92(5):1355–1374.
145. Kannel WB, Castelli WP, Gordon T, McNamara PM. Serum cholesterol, lipoproteins, and the risk of coronary heart disease. The Framingham study. *Ann Intern Med* 1971;74(1):1–12.
146. Shepherd J, Cobbe SM, Ford I, et al. Prevention of coronary heart disease with pravastatin in men with hypercholesterolemia. West of Scotland Coronary Prevention Study Group. *N Engl J Med* 1995;333(20):1301–1307.
147. Downs JR, Clearfield M, Weis S, et al. Primary prevention of acute coronary events with lovastatin in men and women with average cholesterol levels: Results of AFCAPS/TexCAPS. Air Force/Texas Coronary Atherosclerosis Prevention Study. *JAMA* 1998;279(20):1615–1622.
148. Sever PS, Dahlof B, Poulter NR, et al. Prevention of coronary and stroke events with atorvastatin in hypertensive patients who have average or lower-than-average cholesterol concentrations, in the Anglo-Scandinavian Cardiac Outcomes Trial—Lipid Lowering Arm (ASCOT-LLA): A multicentre randomised controlled trial. *Lancet* 2003;361(9364):1149–1158.
149. MRC/BHF Heart Protection Study of cholesterol lowering with simvastatin in 20,536 high-risk individuals: A randomised placebo-controlled trial. *Lancet* 2002;360(9326):7–22.
150. Randomised trial of cholesterol lowering in 4444 patients with coronary heart disease: The Scandinavian Simvastatin Survival Study (4S). *Lancet* 1994;344(8934):1383–1389.
151. Sacks FM, Pfeffer MA, Moye LA, et al. The effect of pravastatin on coronary events after myocardial infarction in patients with average cholesterol levels. Cholesterol and Recurrent Events Trial investigators. *N Engl J Med* 1996;335(14):1001–1009.
152. Prevention of cardiovascular events and death with pravastatin in patients with coronary heart disease and a broad range of initial cholesterol levels. The Long-Term Intervention with Pravastatin in Ischaemic Disease (LIPID) Study Group. *N Engl J Med* 1998;339(19):1349–1357.
153. Shepherd J, Blauw GJ, Murphy MB, et al. Pravastatin in elderly individuals at risk of vascular disease (PROSPER): A randomised controlled trial. *Lancet* 2002;360(9346):1623–1630.

154. Executive Summary of The Third Report of The National Cholesterol Education Program (NCEP) Expert Panel on Detection, Evaluation, and Treatment of High Blood Cholesterol in Adults (Adult Treatment Panel III). *JAMA* 2001;285(19):2486–2497.
155. The effect of aggressive lowering of low-density lipoprotein cholesterol levels and low-dose anticoagulation on obstructive changes in saphenous-vein coronary-artery bypass grafts. The Post Coronary Artery Bypass Graft Trial Investigators. *N Engl J Med* 1997;336(3):153–162.
156. Flaker GC, Warnica JW, Sacks FM, et al. Pravastatin prevents clinical events in revascularized patients with average cholesterol concentrations. Cholesterol and Recurrent Events CARE Investigators. *J Am Coll Cardiol* 1999;34(1):106–112.
157. Brown G, Albers JJ, Fisher LD, et al. Regression of coronary artery disease as a result of intensive lipid-lowering therapy in men with high levels of apolipoprotein B. *N Engl J Med* 1990;323(19):1289–1298.
158. Blankenhorn DH, Azen SP, Kramsch DM, et al. Coronary angiographic changes with lovastatin therapy. The Monitored Atherosclerosis Regression Study (MARS). The MARS Research Group. *Ann Intern Med* 1993; 119(10):969–976.
159. Fuster V, Badimon JJ. Regression or stabilization of atherosclerosis means regression or stabilization of what we don't see in the arteriogram. *Eur Heart J* 1995;16(Suppl E):6–12.
160. Rosenson RS, Tangney CC. Antiatherothrombotic properties of statins: Implications for cardiovascular event reduction. *JAMA* 1998;279(20):1643–1650.
161. Phillips PS, Haas RH, Bannykh S, et al. Statin-associated myopathy with normal creatine kinase levels. *Ann Intern Med* 2002;137(7):581–585.
162. Pasternak RC, Smith SC, Jr, Bairey-Merz CN, et al. ACC/AHA/NHLBI clinical advisory on the use and safety of statins. *J Am Coll Cardiol* 2002;40(3): 567–572.
163. Staffa JA, Chang J, Green L. Cerivastatin and reports of fatal rhabdomyolysis. *N Engl J Med* 2002;346(7): 539–540.
164. Gotto AM Jr. Safety and statin therapy: Reconsidering the risks and benefits. *Arch Intern Med* 2003;163(6): 657–659.
165. Waters D, Lesperance J, Gladstone P, et al. Effects of cigarette smoking on the angiographic evolution of coronary atherosclerosis. A Canadian Coronary Atherosclerosis Intervention Trial (CCAIT) Substudy. CCAIT Study Group. *Circulation* 1996;94(4):614–621.
166. Tofler GH, Muller JE, Stone PH, et al. Comparison of long-term outcome after acute myocardial infarction in patients never graduated from high school with that in more educated patients. Multicenter Investigation of the Limitation of Infarct Size (MILIS). *Am J Cardiol* 1993; 71(12):1031–1035.
167. FitzGibbon GM, Leach AJ, Kafka HP. Atherosclerosis of coronary artery bypass grafts and smoking. *Can Med Assoc J* 1987;136(1):45–47.
168. Solymoss BC, Nadeau P, Millette D, Campeau L. Late thrombosis of saphenous vein coronary bypass grafts related to risk factors. *Circulation* 1988;78(3 Pt 2): I140–I143.
169. Voors AA, van Brussel BL, Plokker HW, et al. Smoking and cardiac events after venous coronary bypass surgery. A 15-year follow-up study. *Circulation* 1996;93(1):42–47.
170. Nollert G, Miksch J, Kreuzer E, Reichart B. Risk factors for atherosclerosis and the degeneration of pericardial valves after aortic valve replacement. *J Thorac Cardiovasc Surg* 2003;126(4):965–968.
171. Ruel M, Rubens FD, Masters RG, et al. Late incidence and predictors of persistent or recurrent heart failure in patients with aortic prosthetic valves. *J Thorac Cardiovasc Surg* 2004;127(1):149–159.
172. van Domburg RT, Meeter K, van Berkel DF, et al. Smoking cessation reduces mortality after coronary artery bypass surgery: A 20-year follow-up study. *J Am Coll Cardiol* 2000;36(3):878–883.
173. Butchart EG, Moreno de la Santa P, Rooney SJ, Lewis PA. The role of risk factors and trigger factors in cerebrovascular events after mitral valve replacement: Implications for antithrombotic management. *J Card Surg* 1994;9(2 Suppl):228–236.
174. Herlitz J, Brandrup-Wognsen G, Haglid M, et al. Predictors of death during 5 years after coronary artery bypass grafting. *Int J Cardiol* 1998;64(1):15–23.
175. Cen YY, Glower DD, Landolfo K, et al. Comparison of survival after mitral valve replacement with biologic and mechanical valves in 1139 patients. *J Thorac Cardiovasc Surg* 2001;122(3):569–577.
176. Ockene JK, Kuller LH, Svendsen KH, Meilahn E. The relationship of smoking cessation to coronary heart disease and lung cancer in the Multiple Risk Factor Intervention Trial (MRFIT). *Am J Public Health* 1990;80(8):954–958.
177. Steffenino G, Galliasso M, Gastaldi C, et al. Nurses' observational study on the practice of secondary prevention in a cardiovascular department. *Ital Heart J* 2003;4(7): 473–478.
178. Data and Statistics, Trends in Tobacco Use 2003. *American Lung Association*. Available at: http://www.lungusa.org/data/.
179. Jorenby DE, Leischow SJ, Nides MA, et al. A controlled trial of sustained-release bupropion, a nicotine patch, or both for smoking cessation. *N Engl J Med* 1999;340(9): 685–691.
180. Woolacott NF, Jones L, Forbes CA, et al. The clinical effectiveness and cost-effectiveness of bupropion and nicotine replacement therapy for smoking cessation: A systematic review and economic evaluation. *Health Technol Assess* 2002;6(16):1–245.
181. Lancaster T, Stead LF. Individual behavioural counselling for smoking cessation. *Cochrane Database Syst Rev* 2002(3):CD001292.
182. Fiore MC. US public health service clinical practice guideline: Treating tobacco use and dependence. *Respir Care* 2000;45(10):1200–1262.
183. Anthenelli R. Late breaking clinical trials II. Effects of rimonabant in the reduction of major cardiovascular risk factors. Results from the STRATUS-US trial (smoking cessation is smokers motivated to quit) and the RIO-LIPIDS trial (weight reducing and metabolic effects in overweight/obese patients with dyslipidemia). Paper presented at the Annual Scientific Session, American College of Cardiology, 2003; New Orleans.

184. Stitzer ML. Combined behavioral and pharmacological treatments for smoking cessation. *Nicotine Tob Res* 1999;1(Suppl 2):S181–S187; discussion S207–S110.
185. Molyneux A, Lewis S, Leivers U, et al. Clinical trial comparing nicotine replacement therapy (NRT) plus brief counselling, brief counselling alone, and minimal intervention on smoking cessation in hospital inpatients. *Thorax* 2003;58(6):484–488.
186. Coutinho M, Gerstein HC, Wang Y, Yusuf S. The relationship between glucose and incident cardiovascular events. A metaregression analysis of published data from 20 studies of 95,783 individuals followed for 12.4 years. *Diabetes Care* 1999;22(2):233–240.
187. Kannel WB, McGee DL. Diabetes and glucose tolerance as risk factors for cardiovascular disease: The Framingham study. *Diabetes Care* 1979;2(2):120–126.
188. Geiss LSSP. *Diabetes in America*. Bethesda, MD: National Diabetes Data Group. National Institutes of Health, National Institute of Diabetes and Digestive and Kidney Disease, 1995.
189. Whang W, Bigger JT Jr. Diabetes and outcomes of coronary artery bypass graft surgery in patients with severe left ventricular dysfunction: Results from The CABG Patch Trial database. The CABG Patch Trial Investigators and Coordinators. *J Am Coll Cardiol* 2000;36(4):1166–1172.
190. Thourani VH, Weintraub WS, Stein B, et al. Influence of diabetes mellitus on early and late outcome after coronary artery bypass grafting. *Ann Thorac Surg* 1999;67(4):1045–1052.
191. Mathew V, Holmes DR. Outcomes in diabetics undergoing revascularization: The long and the short of it. *J Am Coll Cardiol* 2002;40(3):424–427.
192. Carson JL, Scholz PM, Chen AY, et al. Diabetes mellitus increases short-term mortality and morbidity in patients undergoing coronary artery bypass graft surgery. *J Am Coll Cardiol* 2002;40(3):418–423.
193. Clough RA, Leavitt BJ, Morton JR, et al. The effect of comorbid illness on mortality outcomes in cardiac surgery. *Arch Surg* 2002;137(4):428–432; discussion 432–433.
194. Stratton IM, Adler AI, Neil HA, et al. Association of glycaemia with macrovascular and microvascular complications of type 2 diabetes (UKPDS 35): Prospective observational study. *BMJ* 2000;321(7258):405–412.
195. Lazar HL, Chipkin SR, Fitzgerald CA, et al. Tight glycemic control in diabetic coronary artery bypass graft patients improves perioperative outcomes and decreases recurrent ischemic events. *Circulation* 2004;109(12):1497–1502.
196. Lorusso R, Pentiricci S, Raddino R, et al. Influence of type 2 diabetes on functional and structural properties of coronary artery bypass conduits. *Diabetes* 2003;52(11):2814–2820.
197. Hoogwerf BJ. Postoperative management of the diabetic patient. *Med Clin North Am* 2001;85(5):1213–1228.
198. Standards of medical care for patients with diabetes mellitus. *Diabetes Care* 2003;26(Suppl 1):S33–S35.
199. Rock MA, Fox SA, Stitt LW, et al. Is obesity a predictor of mortality, morbidity and readmission after cardiac surgery? *Can J Surg* 2004;47(1):34–38.
200. Wilson PW, D'Agostino RB, Sullivan L, et al. Overweight and obesity as determinants of cardiovascular risk: The Framingham experience. *Arch Intern Med* 2002;162(16):1867–1872.
201. Rexrode KM, Hennekens CH, Willett WC, et al. A prospective study of body mass index, weight change, and risk of stroke in women. *JAMA* 1997;277(19):1539–1545.
202. Kenchaiah S, Evans JC, Levy D, et al. Obesity and the risk of heart failure. *N Engl J Med* 2002;347(5):305–313.
203. Stevens J, Cai J, Pamuk ER, et al. The effect of age on the association between body-mass index and mortality. *N Engl J Med* 1998;338(1):1–7.
204. Nawaz H, Katz DL. American College of Preventive Medicine Practice Policy statement. Weight management counseling of overweight adults. *Am J Prev Med* 2001;21(1):73–78.
205. Appel LJ, Moore TJ, Obarzanek E, et al. A clinical trial of the effects of dietary patterns on blood pressure. DASH Collaborative Research Group. *N Engl J Med* 1997;336(16):1117–1124.
206. Hu FB, Willett WC. Optimal diets for prevention of coronary heart disease. *JAMA* 2002;288(20):2569–2578.
207. Kotchen TA, McCarron DA. Dietary electrolytes and blood pressure: A statement for healthcare professionals from the American Heart Association Nutrition Committee. *Circulation* 1998;98(6):613–617.
208. Johnson LW, Dickstein RA, Fruehan CT, et al. Prophylactic digitalization for coronary artery bypass surgery. *Circulation* 1976;53(5):819–822.
209. Csicsko JF, Schatzlein MH, King RD. Immediate postoperative digitalization in the prophylaxis of supraventricular arrhythmias following coronary artery bypass. *J Thorac Cardiovasc Surg* 1981;81(3):419–422.
210. Tyras DH, Stothert JC Jr, Kaiser GC, et al. Supraventricular tachyarrhythmias after myocardial revascularization: A randomized trial of prophylactic digitalization. *J Thorac Cardiovasc Surg* 1979;77(2):310–314.
211. Weiner B, Rheinlander HF, Decker EL, Cleveland RJ. Digoxin prophylaxis following coronary artery bypass surgery. *Clin Pharm* 1986;5(1):55–58.
212. Rose MR, Glassman E, Spencer FC. Arrhythmias following cardiac surgery: Relation to serum digoxin levels. *Am Heart J* 1975;89(3):288–294.
213. The effect of digoxin on mortality and morbidity in patients with heart failure. The Digitalis Investigation Group. *N Engl J Med* 1997;336(8):525–533.
214. Rathore SS, Curtis JP, Wang Y, et al. Association of serum digoxin concentration and outcomes in patients with heart failure. *JAMA* 2003;289(7):871–878.
215. Rathore SS, Wang Y, Krumholz HM. Sex-based differences in the effect of digoxin for the treatment of heart failure. *N Engl J Med* 2002;347(18):1403–1411.
216. Leon AS, Connett J. Physical activity and 10.5 year mortality in the Multiple Risk Factor Intervention Trial (MRFIT). *Int J Epidemiol* 1991;20(3):690–697.
217. Lee CD, Folsom AR, Blair SN. Physical activity and stroke risk: A meta-analysis. *Stroke* 2003;34(10):2475–2481.
218. Wannamethee SG, Shaper AG, Walker M. Physical activity and mortality in older men with diagnosed coronary heart disease. *Circulation* 2000;102(12):1358–1363.

219. Hambrecht R, Niebauer J, Marburger C, et al. Various intensities of leisure time physical activity in patients with coronary artery disease: Effects on cardiorespiratory fitness and progression of coronary atherosclerotic lesions. *J Am Coll Cardiol* 1993;22(2):468–477.
220. Smith SC Jr, Blair SN, Bonow RO, et al. AHA/ACC Scientific Statement: AHA/ACC guidelines for preventing heart attack and death in patients with atherosclerotic cardiovascular disease: 2001 update: A statement for healthcare professionals from the American Heart Association and the American College of Cardiology. *Circulation* 2001;104(13):1577–1579.
221. Fletcher GF. How to implement physical activity in primary and secondary prevention. A statement for healthcare professionals from the Task Force on Risk-reduction, American Heart Association. *Circulation* 1997;96(1): 355–357.
222. Longmuir PE, Tremblay MS, Goode RC. Postoperative exercise training develops normal levels of physical activity in a group of children following cardiac surgery. *Pediatr Cardiol* 1990;11(3):126–130.
223. Arthur HM, Smith KM, Kodis J, McKelvie R. A controlled trial of hospital versus home-based exercise in cardiac patients. *Med Sci Sports Exerc* 2002;34(10):1544–1550.
224. Kodis J, Smith KM, Arthur HM, et al. Changes in exercise capacity and lipids after clinic versus home-based aerobic training in coronary artery bypass graft surgery patients. *J Cardiopulm Rehabil* 2001;21(1):31–36.
225. Stevens R, Hanson P. Comparison of supervised and unsupervised exercise training after coronary bypass surgery. *Am J Cardiol* 1984;53(11):1524–1528.
226. Ades PA. Cardiac rehabilitation and secondary prevention of coronary heart disease. *N Engl J Med* 2001;345(12):892–902.
227. Stewart KJ, Badenhop D, Brubaker PH, et al. Cardiac rehabilitation following percutaneous revascularization, heart transplant, heart valve surgery, and for chronic heart failure. *Chest* 2003;123(6):2104–2111.
228. Balady GJ, Ades PA, Comoss P, et al. Core components of cardiac rehabilitation/secondary prevention programs: A statement for healthcare professionals from the American Heart Association and the American Association of Cardiovascular and Pulmonary Rehabilitation Writing Group. *Circulation* 2000;102(9):1069–1073.
229. Hedback B, Perk J, Hornblad M, Ohlsson U. Cardiac rehabilitation after coronary artery bypass surgery: 10-year results on mortality, morbidity and readmissions to hospital. *J Cardiovasc Risk* 2001;8(3):153–158.
230. Sire S. Physical training and occupational rehabilitation after aortic valve replacement. *Eur Heart J* 1987;8(11): 1215–1220.
231. Newell JP, Kappagoda CT, Stoker JB, et al. Physical training after heart valve replacement. *Br Heart J* 1980; 44(6):638–649.
232. Pasquali SK, Alexander KP, Coombs LP, et al. Effect of cardiac rehabilitation on functional outcomes after coronary revascularization. *Am Heart J* 2003;145(3): 445–451.
233. Tygesen H, Wettervik C, Wennerblom B. Intensive home-based exercise training in cardiac rehabilitation increases exercise capacity and heart rate variability. *Int J Cardiol* 2001;79(2–3):175–182.
234. Milani RV, Lavie CJ. Prevalence and effects of cardiac rehabilitation on depression in the elderly with coronary heart disease. *Am J Cardiol* 1998;81(10):1233–1236.
235. Muller-Nordhorn J, Kulig M, Binting S, et al. Change in quality of life in the year following cardiac rehabilitation. *Qual Life Res* 2004;13(2):399–410.
236. Simchen E, Naveh I, Zitser-Gurevich Y, et al. Is participation in cardiac rehabilitation programs associated with better quality of life and return to work after coronary artery bypass operations? The Israeli CABG Study. *Isr Med Assoc J* 2001;3(6):399–403.
237. Takeyama J, Itoh H, Kato M, et al. Effects of physical training on the recovery of the autonomic nervous activity during exercise after coronary artery bypass grafting: Effects of physical training after CABG. *Jpn Circ J* 2000;64(11):809–813.
238. Lucini D, Milani RV, Costantino G, et al. Effects of cardiac rehabilitation and exercise training on autonomic regulation in patients with coronary artery disease. *Am Heart J* 2002;143(6):977–983.
239. Carrel T, Mohacsi P. Optimal timing of rehabilitation after cardiac surgery: The surgeon's view. *Eur Heart J* 1998;19(Suppl O):O38–O41.
240. Dubach P, Myers J, Wagner D. Optimal timing of phase II rehabilitation after cardiac surgery. The cardiologist's view. *Eur Heart J* 1998;19(Suppl O):O35–O37.

CHAPTER

25 PRIMARY CORONARY ARTERY BYPASS SURGERY

Tain-Yen Hsia, David D. Yuh

INTRODUCTION

Coronary artery disease represents a spectrum of clinical syndromes caused by insufficient coronary blood flow to the myocardium. It is almost always due to subintimal atheroma deposition, leading to arterial luminal stenosis or occlusion and wall thickening. Affecting more than 1.5 million Americans annually, it is the most common form of heart disease, and its complications are the leading cause of death in both men and women. According to the American Heart Association,[1] someone in the United States suffers from a coronary artery disease-related event about every 29 s, with a subsequent death every minute. This prevalence has fueled rapid advances in the medical, interventional, and surgical management of this disease since the first coronary cineangiography was performed in 1962.

KEY CONCEPTS

- Epidemiology
  - Affecting more than 1.5 million Americans annually, coronary artery disease is the most common form of heart disease, and its complications are the leading cause of death in both men and women.
- Pathophysiology
  - Coronary artery disease is generally caused by atherosclerotic luminal narrowing, resulting in insufficient coronary blood flow to the myocardium. The process consists of subintimal atheroma deposition, leading to arterial luminal stenosis or occlusion and wall thickening.
- Clinical features
  - Typically, significant coronary atherosclerosis becomes manifest as angina, but it can also present with angina-equivalent symptoms, including dyspnea, dizziness, syncope, and pulmonary edema. Malignant coronary disease leading to ischemic cardiomyopathy is associated with congestive symptoms. Identified factors that contribute to severe atherosclerotic coronary artery disease include obesity, hypercholesterolemia, obesity, diabetes, tobacco use, and sedentary lifestyle.
- Diagnostics
  - Twelve-lead electrocardiography is initially used to diagnose myocardial ischemia. Further investigation consists of exercise stress testing, evaluation of myocardial enzymes (i.e., CPK-MB, troponin), echocardiography, and coronary angiography.
- Treatment
  - Initial medical management of acute myocardial ischemia consist of beta blockade, nitrates, and supplemental oxygen. After precise delineation of coronary arteriopathy, definitive treatment consists of coronary artery bypass grafting or percutaneous angioplasty and stenting.
- Outcomes/prognosis
  - Coronary artery bypass grafting carries an overall mortality of about 3 percent; elective primary coronary bypass carries a mortality rate of approximately 1.7 percent. Complications associated with coronary artery bypass grafting consists of renal failure, neurologic injury, heart failure, hemorrhage, renal failure, respiratory failure, and renal dysfunction. Overall, coronary artery bypass grafting achieves excellent outcomes with respect to angina relief and resumption of normal activities. In general, completeness and durability of revascularization is superior with surgical revascularization versus percutaneous interventions.

Introduced in 1962 by Sabiston at Johns Hopkins and later by Garrett and DeBakey, coronary artery bypass grafting (CABG) has evolved into the "gold standard" therapy for patients with multivessel coronary artery disease. Despite advances in percutaneous interventional techniques, CABG remains among the most frequently performed operations in the United States, resulting in approximately $50 billion in annual health care expenditures.

NORMAL CORONARY ANATOMY[2,3] AND PHYSIOLOGY

The right and left coronary arteries originate from the ascending aorta behind their respective aortic valve leaflets, usually in the upper third of the sinuses of Valsalva. The left coronary orifice is superior and lateral to the right. The left coronary arterial system is divided into the left anterior descending (LAD) and circumflex arteries after a short combined course as the left main coronary artery. The *dominance* of the coronary arteries depends on whether the posterior descending coronary artery is derived from the *right* versus the *left* coronary artery. The coronary is *right dominant* in 85 to 90 percent of normal individuals. The right coronary departs the aorta anterolaterally and courses within the right atrioventricular groove, curving around the acute margin of the heart. In this course, the main right coronary artery supplies the right atrium, sinus and atrioventricular nodes, and right ventricular free wall. It almost always bifurcates distally into the posterior descending and right posterolateral coronary arteries. The posterior descending coronary artery traverses the posterior interventricular groove toward the apex of the heart to perfuse the posterior ventricular septum, while the posterolateral branch(es) supply the posterior surface of the left ventricle.

The left main coronary artery courses anterosuperiorly for 10 to 20 mm from the left sinus of Valsalva and bifurcates into the nearly equal sized LAD and circumflex coronary arteries. The LAD traverses the anterior interventricular groove toward the apex of the heart, giving off diagonal, septal perforating, and right ventricular branches before terminating at the apex. Occasionally, the LAD may collateralize with the posterior descending artery or replace it to supply the posterior interventricular groove. The diagonal branches supply the anterolateral wall of the left ventricle. The first diagonal branch may occasionally be referred to as the ramus intermedius artery when it originates directly from the left main artery, resulting in a trifurcation between the LAD, circumflex, and ramus intermedius coronary arteries. The septal perforators supply the anterior two-thirds of the ventricular septum, extending perpendicularly from the LAD. The right ventricular branches supply the anterior surface of the right ventricle.

The circumflex coronary artery courses along the left atrioventricular groove, giving off marginal branches to supply the lateral wall of the left ventricle, the left atrium, and the posteromedial papillary muscle. In 85 to 95 percent of patients, the circumflex coronary artery terminates near the obtuse margin of the left ventricle; in the remaining patients, (i.e., *left dominance*), it may continue and give rise to the posterior descending coronary artery.

Because the contracting ventricular wall compresses intramyocardial vessels, coronary blood flow occurs primarily during diastole, when the aortic valve is closed, the myocardium relaxes, and the aortic diastolic pressure is transmitted through the sinuses of Valsalva to the coronary ostia. The ascending aorta and sinuses maintain uniform coronary flow throughout diastole. The main coronary arteries and branches that course through the epicardium of the heart act as conductance vessels, offering minimal resistance to blood flow. There is no detectable pressure drop along the epicardial coronary arteries, even at the highest levels of flow. The major resistance vessels are the arterioles and the rich network of capillaries that form interregional collaterals and may provide compensatory perfusion in chronic coronary insufficiency. Therefore metabolic, endothelial, humoral/neural, and autoregulatory mechanisms intended to match blood flow to oxygen consumption and perfusion pressure regulate coronary vascular resistance.

As an aerobic organ, the normal heart requires the oxidation of substrates for energy generation and can tolerate only a small oxygen debt even at basal resting states. Therefore myocardial metabolism dictates oxygen consumption. Because oxygen stores in the heart are small and low oxygen saturations in coronary venous blood (25 to 30 percent at rest) do not allow further extraction, changes in myocardial oxygen requirements lead to rapid changes in coronary vascular resistance. Myocardial ischemia and hypoxia stimulate potent vasoactive substances, such as adenosine and nitric oxide, to recruit resistance vessels and increase coronary blood flow. Because the epicardial arteries and arterioles are extensively innervated by autonomic nervous fibers, the intricate balance between sympathetic (vasoconstrictive) and parasympathetic (vasodilatory) mechanisms exerts additional control.[4]

Autoregulatory vasodilatation of the coronary arterial circulation maintains myocardial perfusion even during abrupt changes in perfusion pressures. Studies in humans have shown that myocardial perfusion can be maintained with reduced perfusion pressures as low as 45 mmHg distal to a stenotic segment.[5] However, this compensatory response to the obstruction of a proximal epicardial vessel may be compromised in the setting of chronic hypertension and left ventricular hypertrophy. Given the heart's dependence on an uninterrupted oxygen supply, conditions that cause increased metabolic activity and oxygen requirements are quickly compensated by obligatory autoregulatory coronary vasodilatation and increased perfusion to ensure adequate oxygen delivery. This is why the heart is particularly vulnerable to occlusive arterial disease.

PATHOPHYSIOLOGY OF MYOCARDIAL ISCHEMIA/INFARCTION

Coronary atherosclerosis is a slow, complex disease process that typically starts in childhood and often progresses with age. Its precise cause remains incompletely understood. It is generally agreed that local damage to the endothelium that produces migration and aggregation of platelets and monocytes is a prerequisite event. Proposed mechanisms of this initial endothelial injury include shear stress from turbulent flow, infectious and immunologic factors, and noxious chemicals. With the release of various chemotactic growth factors and vasoconstrictors such as thromboxane A_2, migration and proliferation of smooth muscle cells results in the accumulation of collagen, elastic fibers, proteoglycan, calcium, complex carbohydrates, and other connective tissues in the intimal and subintimal areas. Infiltration of lipoproteins due to altered endothelial permeability further increases the fibrolipoid accumulation, which, with repeated injuries, can progress to an atheromatous plaque.[6] Hypercholesterolemia and other risk factors may precipitate or accelerate the process of coronary atherosclerosis. The identified controllable risk factors are:

Hypercholesterolemia (especially low-density lipoprotein > 100 mg/dL)
Smoking or exposure to tobacco smoke
High blood pressure
Diabetes mellitus
Obesity
Physical inactivity

Coronary atherosclerosis is a dynamic process. Focal intimal fibrolipoid accumulations can initially narrow the coronary arteries. As these lipoid foci or atheromas convert into plaques of fibrous connective tissues, producing stenotic lesions, further deposition of new layers of plaques can result in complete coronary occlusion. Within an atherosclerotic plaque, newly formed small vessels can suddenly bleed, causing plaque hemorrhage and rupture, which can worsen the degree of stenosis and precipitate a myocardial infarction. Aggregation of platelets within the narrowed vessel lumen with decreased flow can induce thrombosis and sudden complete occlusion.[7] It is believed that most acute myocardial infarctions result from acute thrombotic occlusion. Furthermore, fissuring or rupture of atherosclerotic plaques can complicate or initiate occlusive thrombosis, adding to the unstable state.[8]

Coronary atherosclerosis usually involves the proximal portions of larger coronary arteries, especially at or just beyond branching sites. Therefore stenoses of the LAD, circumflex, and right coronary arteries often involve the first of the secondary branchings (i.e., first diagonal, obtuse marginal, and posterior descending branches). When the disease is more severe, origins and main trunks may be involved. The left main coronary artery is significantly diseased in 10 to 20 percent of patients. Diffuse distal disease severe enough to render a coronary artery unsuitable for bypass grafting is relatively uncommon.

With coronary artery disease, myocardial ischemia and necrosis occur when coronary blood flow, impaired by atherosclerotic stenosis, is insufficient to meet oxygen demand. Because the heart has virtually no reserve stores of oxygen and relies entirely on aerobic metabolism, its high rate of energy expenditure results in a sudden, striking decline of oxygen tension and left ventricular functional impairment within seconds of coronary occlusion. Coronary occlusion can cause myocardial ischemia in as little as 60 s, and depressed function, or myocardial stunning, in less than 20 min.[9] The subendocardium is most vulnerable to myocardial ischemia because its collateral blood flow is lowest and oxygen consumption highest.[10] Thus, myocardial necrosis progresses toward the epicardium with continued ischemia and is accelerated when there is little collateral flow, marked arterial hypotension (e.g., cardiogenic shock), and elevated oxygen demand caused by inotropic stimulation or tachycardias. Thus blood pressure control and the prevention of tachyarrhythmias are vital during the early postinfarction interval to limit the spread of myocardial damage. With continued waves of necrosis, transmural infarction involving the entire thickness of the ventricular wall can occur.[11] The recognition of this time-dependent progression of infarct and the conditions necessary for functional recovery of salvaged myocardium constituted the basis for rapid reperfusion interventions, including thrombolysis and angioplasty. Studies have shown that reperfusion within 6 h from the onset of symptoms decreases infarct size, better preserves ventricular function, and improves survival.[12]

CLINICAL CORONARY SYNDROMES

Stable angina

Angina pectoris is the development of chest discomfort or pain with exertion that ceases with rest. It is typically described as a substernal heavy, dull, or crushing pain with frequent radiation to the left shoulder, arm, and/or neck. It is not an inevitable symptom nor does its absence indicate freedom from coronary artery disease; however, it does signify the presence of reversible myocardial ischemia without cellular necrosis. Since angina is due to a reduction in coronary flow reserve, the greater the reduction, the more severe the angina. The severity of angina is categorized into the four Canadian Cardiovascular Society Functional classifications:

Class 1: Angina occurring with strenuous activity. There is no limitation to ordinary activity.
Class 2: Angina occurring with fast-paced walking or walking up an incline or stairs. There is only slight limitation to ordinary activity.

Class 3: Angina occurring when walking less than two blocks on level ground or climbing one flight of stairs. There is significant limitation to ordinary activity.

Class 4: Angina occurring with mild activity. May occur at rest but lasts less than 15 min (beyond which the angina is unstable). There is inability to carry out mild activity.

The clinical presentation of patients with angina varies considerably. Furthermore, as chest pain in general tends to be nonspecific, the differential diagnosis is broad and includes gastrointestinal reflux, biliary colic, peptic ulcer disease, aortic dissection, esophageal disorders, lower respiratory tract infection, pneumonitis, and a variety of musculoskeletal discomforts. Once other differential diagnoses are ruled out, evaluation with electrocardiography (ECG), exercise or stress testing, and myocardial enzyme levels is necessary to confirm the diagnosis of myocardial ischemia. In general, patients with class 1 and 2 stable angina can be managed medically with coronary angiography as an option following provocative testing for ischemia. Coronary angiography is recommended for patients with class 3 and 4 angina.

Atypical anginal equivalents

In some patients, even with severe coronary artery disease, myocardial ischemia does not lead to typical anginal chest pain. Instead, such patients present with the so-called *anginal equivalent* complaints, whereby myocardial ischemia is suggested by symptoms including dyspnea, dizziness, syncope, and pulmonary edema and is later confirmed by ECG criteria. Usually these symptoms are due to left ventricular systolic or diastolic dysfunction whenever the myocardium becomes ischemic under stress. Furthermore, a small number of patients exhibit "silent" or asymptomatic ischemia that can be discovered only by continuous ECG monitoring.

Acute coronary syndromes

Acute coronary syndromes (ACS) include unstable angina, postinfarction angina, and Prinzmetal's angina. They represent a spectrum of symptomatic and prognostic worsening of coronary artery disease over a short period. Prinzmetal's angina is caused by coronary arterial spasm and is diagnosed by ECG during an episode of pain. Postinfarct angina is angina or myocardial ischemia occurring less than 2 weeks following an acute myocardial infarction. Unstable angina represents spontaneous pain, even at rest, and signifies an acute change in the severity, character, or triggering threshold of stable angina. The term *unstable angina* actually describes several subgroups of syndromes that carry the same clinical outcomes. Patients may present with persistent anginal pain, ECG criteria indicating myocardial ischemia, and mild enzyme elevations. The cause of unstable angina is now recognized to be a sudden change in the coronary arterial circulation, such as plaque rupture or acute thrombosis. This clinical situation remains reversible but tends to recur either as further episodes of unstable angina or a fulminant acute myocardial infarction. Under these circumstances, the 1-year mortality rates range between 8 to 10 percent, while the 1-year nonfatal myocardial infarction rate ranges from 12 to 14 percent.[14]

All patients presenting with ACS are initially managed medically to alleviate ongoing ischemia and to prevent an acute myocardial infarction. More than 80 percent of treated patients become asymptomatic within 48 h. Myocardial infarction is ruled out by ECG and enzymatic evaluations. In general, patients who present with unstable or postinfarct angina nearly always require coronary angiography and revascularization.

Acute myocardial infarction[15]

Prolonged myocardial ischemia without reperfusion ultimately leads to irreversible cellular necrosis and myocardial infarction. Most acute myocardial infarctions result from subtotal or total coronary artery occlusion by a thrombus associated with acute rupture of an atherosclerotic plaque. Although the acutely occluded coronary artery often was not previously severely stenotic, the mere presence of significant coronary artery disease clearly increases the risk for acute myocardial infarction. For example, patients with severe proximal LAD coronary lesions are particularly prone to suffer acute and often fatal myocardial infarctions. Increased numbers of coronary arteries with stenotic disease also lead to higher probabilities of acute myocardial infarction.

Following an infarction, the location of the coronary arterial occlusion, presence of other diseased vessels, and extent of collateral perfusion will determine the extent of myocardial injury in the early period. Additional detrimental effects of postinfarct arrhythmias, hypotension, left ventricular distention, and increased wall stress can further reduce the viability of borderline regions and increase the ultimate infarct size.

According to the World Health Organization (WHO) definition, the diagnosis of myocardial infarction is based on the presence of at least two of the following three criteria: (1) a clinical history of ischemic-type chest discomfort, (2) changes on serially obtained ECG tracings, and (3) a rise and fall in serum cardiac markers.[16] Typically, patients present with a sudden onset of severe chest pain or their anginal equivalent that is not relieved by rest or sublingual nitroglycerin. Often, there is associated shortness of breath, nausea, diaphoresis, and general malaise. Subendocardial or nontransmural infarctions usually demonstrate new ST-segmental depressions and T-wave inversions on the 12-lead ECG. As the infarction progresses, ST segments may become elevated and later evolve into Q waves that indicate a transmural infarct.

Since less than 25 percent of patients admitted to the hospital with ischemic-type chest discomfort are subsequently diagnosed as having had an acute myocardial infarction and about half of all patients with acute myocardial infarction do not exhibit diagnostic ST-segment changes, myocardial enzyme markers play an essential role in establishing the diagnosis. The classic myocardial creatine kinase isoenzyme CK-MB, which appears within hours after injury and peaks at 8 to 24 h after infarction, lacks sufficient sensitivity and specificity but remains an efficient means of early detection. Levels of troponin, with its cardiac specific subunits I and C, are more sensitive and specific for myocardial infarction. Furthermore, because troponin release is stoichiometrically correlated with the amount of myocardial necrosis, these enzymes can also be used to estimate infarct size and prognosis. Since serum troponin levels may present up to 14 days after infarction, detection of recurrent acute infarction requires concomitant CK-MB measurements.

EARLY COMPLICATIONS

Death

About 70 to 80 percent of patients with coronary artery disease who seek medical advice will ultimately die of cardiac-related causes. Most of these patients present with acute or subacute heart failure, often within a short time after an acute myocardial infarction or precipitated by a ventricular dysrhythmia. Others will deteriorate slowly, with chronic heart failure secondary to myocardial scarring resulting from past myocardial infarctions. The overall survival of patients with clinically evident coronary artery disease is 75 percent at 5 years after the initiation of medical treatment, 60 percent at 10 years, and 45 percent at 15 years.[17]

Approximately 20 percent of patients sustaining an acute myocardial infarction will die suddenly within hours of the event. Presumably, the cause of death is ventricular fibrillation, asystole, or acute severe ventricular failure. Many survivors will have persistent postinfarct arrhythmias or conduction abnormalities; arrhythmogenic foci are known to arise from myocardial scars. Early hospital death (i.e., less than 3 months) after surviving the initial event is thought to vary between 10 to 50 percent. However, the size of the infarct is an important prognosticator: the larger the infarct, the higher the mortality. Also, additional infarctions and the development of cardiogenic shock, ventricular perforation/aneurysm, or valvular regurgitation will increase the likelihood of early death.

Cardiogenic shock

Within minutes of coronary occlusion, a striking impairment of left ventricular function occurs. Heart failure follows when uninvolved myocardium can no longer sustain the normal hemodynamic requirements. With loss of 40 percent or more of the left ventricular myocardial mass, severe systolic failure ensues and cardiogenic shock develops.[4] Clinically, there is hemodynamic instability in the absence of hypovolemia with associated tachycardia, mental status changes, and reduced urinary output. The cardiac index generally falls to less than 2 L/min/m^2 of body surface area and the pulmonary capillary wedge pressure is typically higher than 18 mmHg.

Cardiogenic shock remains the most common cause (80 percent) of in-hospital mortality following an acute myocardial infarction. Occurring in approximately 8 percent of all patients with myocardial infarction, its management requires prompt treatment to reduce myocardial oxygen demand, maintain circulatory support, and minimize myocardial damage. At present, the treatment of choice is aggressive medical resuscitation and mechanical support with early revascularization. Mechanical support, including intraaortic balloon pump counterpulsation and ventricular assist devices, not only rests the stunned myocardium and facilitates recovery but also minimizes irreversible end-organ injury resulting from prolonged shock. Early surgical revascularization has been shown to reduce mortality, especially when performed within 4 to 6 h of the onset of symptoms.

Postinfarct ventricular rupture and ventricular septal defect

During the period immediately following an acute myocardial infarction, the newly infarcted myocardium can become thin and necrotic; it may then rupture under the stress of the ventricular pressure load. Because the left ventricle generates greater wall stress than the right ventricle, perforation of the left ventricular free wall and interventricular septum can complicate an acute myocardial infarction.

Approximately 20 percent of early deaths after acute myocardial infarction are due to acute rupture of the left ventricular free wall.[18] Perforation of the ventricular wall usually occurs within the first week following an acute myocardial infarction but may occur at any time within 2 weeks. It is usually heralded by abrupt deterioration of a patient after a recent myocardial infarction, leading to massive hemopericardium, tamponade, and sudden death. In some patients, the perforation is more gradual, with formation of a hematoma at the site of the necrosed myocardium. When this condition is diagnosed promptly, urgent operation is the only modality that confers long-term survival and is indicated if the patient is not moribund. The classic infarctectomy and patch closure technique has not been completely satisfactory because it often leaves such a large defect that ventricular function is irreparably diminished. Recently, the introduction of a sutureless technique using a polytetrafluoroethylene (PTFE) patch without the use of cardiopulmonary bypass has demonstrated early promising results.[19]

When a patient suffering from a recent myocardial infarction develops a new pansystolic murmur and acute symptoms of heart failure or cardiogenic shock, a postinfarct ventricular septal defect (VSD) is almost always the culprit. Complicating 1 to 2 percent of cases of acute myocardial infarction, postinfarct VSD is a frequent cause of early cardiac death, with a 4-week survival rate less than 20 percent.[20] These defects most often occur in the anterior or apical portion of the interventricular septum and are due to a transmural anterior infarction involving occlusion of the LAD coronary artery. The defect allows for left-to-right shunting with increased pulmonary blood flow, pulmonary venous hypertension, and right-sided heart failure. An oxygen saturation measurement taken from the pulmonary artery is higher than that from the right atrium due to mixing of saturated and desaturated blood at the ventricular level. The diagnosis can be readily confirmed by echocardiography, with Doppler flow showing right-to-left shunting across the interventricular septum. Further evaluations with right heart catheterization, left ventriculography, or coronary angiography may be performed if the patients is stable, but this is often unnecessary if the echocardiogram is adequate. Surgical repair is mandatory but is technically difficult owing to the extensive myocardial necrosis that is inevitably present. Recent techniques that do not require extensive necrotectomy have demonstrated improved results.

Postinfarct mitral insufficiency

Mitral incompetence in the setting of coronary artery disease can follow a myocardial infarction due to rupture or disruption of an ischemic papillary muscle. Chronic mitral regurgitation due to ischemic papillary muscle dysfunction is relatively uncommon; however, acute incompetence complicates the outcome of 40 percent of patients sustaining a myocardial infarction and is a major predictor of mortality.[21] With acute postinfarct mitral insufficiency, the posteromedial papillary muscle is ruptured in 75 percent of cases, correlating with an inferoposterior left ventricular infarction. Typically, the mitral leaflet becomes flail and prolapses into the left atrium during systole. Sometimes papillary muscle necrosis alone without rupture can result in enough dysfunction to produce severe mitral regurgitation.

Acute postinfarct mitral incompetence is a life-threatening complication; almost two-thirds of patients will die within the first 24 h after its onset if surgical intervention is delayed.[22] Survival is better when the papillary muscle is intact; a complete rupture carries the worst outcome. Clinically, patients present with an insidious onset of pulmonary edema, acute hemodynamic deterioration, and cardiogenic shock, typically 2 to 7 days after a myocardial infarction. A new apical systolic murmur is not uniformly present because with severe mitral regurgitation and the profound shock that ensues, the cardiac output may be too low to generate adequate flow across the mitral valve. Right heart catheterization demonstrates elevated right ventricular and pulmonary arterial pressures without the right atrial-to-pulmonary artery oxygen saturation step-up otherwise associated with a postinfarct VSD. In addition, the pulmonary capillary wedge pressure is elevated and often shows prominent "*v*" waves on the pressure tracing. Definitive diagnosis with Doppler transesophageal echocardiography allows assessment of the severity of mitral valvular incompetence and can also define areas of impaired left ventricular contraction. Although aggressive medical resuscitation and the use of intraaortic balloon pump counterpulsation are invaluable in the initial management of these patients, surgical repair or replacement of the mitral valve remains the definitive treatment of this condition.

LATE COMPLICATIONS

Left ventricular scarring and aneurysm

After an acute myocardial infarction, the zone of myocardial necrosis eventually demarcates into an area of thin fibrous scar that is devoid of myocytes and is either akinetic or dyskinetic. Although the actual prevalence is likely lower because of the widespread use of thrombolytic therapy and early angioplasty, in about 10 to 30 percent of these patients, the infarction and the subsequent scar is large and weak enough to make the fibrous wall bulge outward, forming a true left ventricular aneurysm. About 85 percent of left ventricular aneurysms are located near the apex of the heart as the result of a transmural anterolateral infarction.[23] Small or moderate-sized aneurysms (i.e., < 5 cm diameter) are often asymptomatic. Congestive heart failure and recurrent angina are the most frequent clinical manifestations of significant left ventricular aneurysms, whereby the large dyskinetic wall reduces ventricular function and increases the wall stress of the uninvolved myocardium. Other complications stemming from left ventricular aneurysms include mural thromboembolism and intractable ventricular tachyarrhythmias. The 5-year survival of patients with untreated symptomatic left ventricular aneurysms is around 60 percent. Many modalities can diagnose a left ventricular aneurysm, but left ventriculography is quite sensitive and can often clearly demarcate the aneurysm from the rest of the ventricular wall segments. Surgical resection of the aneurysm followed by ventricular reconstruction offers improved survival compared with medical therapy and is often accompanied by concomitant CABG.

Extensive left ventricular scarring and aneurysm formation predispose to intractable ventricular tachyarrhythmias. These patients generally also suffer from global left ventricular dysfunction and the tachyarrhythmias are typically unresponsive to antiarrhythmic therapy. Management of these patients is a continuing area of intense investigation, where advances are being made in new ablative electrophysiologic techniques to eradicate the arrhythmogenic foci. Many of these patients, however, will require implantation of automatic implantable cardiac defibrillators to prevent sudden death.

Chronic ischemic heart disease

Some patients with progressive coronary artery disease suffer from chronic, recurrent myocardial ischemic episodes as opposed to a single devastating infarction. Consequently these patients develop symptoms of chronic ischemic cardiomyopathy and congestive heart failure. As noted previously, myocardial ischemia impairs left ventricular function and increases the workload on the normal myocardium. The larger the area of dyskinesis or akinesis from repeated insults, the greater the gradual reduction in both global systolic and diastolic function. Often, these patients exhibit symptoms of heart failure associated with recurrent myocardial ischemia. Furthermore, right ventricular function can also be expected to be impaired in patients with chronic ischemic heart disease. This can be due to occlusive disease of the right coronary artery, pulmonary arterial hypertension, dyskinesis of the ventricular septum, and left ventricular dilatation.

There is a great deal of physiologic and functional variability among patients with depressed ventricular function from chronic ischemic heart disease. Therefore preoperative prediction of the efficacy of surgical intervention can be difficult. Some patients have moderately increased left ventricular end-diastolic pressures and reduced exercise capacity but minimal cardiomegaly. Although these patients often have marked ischemic dysfunction, revascularization is indicated to rescue or protect viable myocardium and improve functional capacities. In some cases, poor left ventricular function is due to myocardial "hibernation" or "stunning" and therefore may benefit from revascularization. In general, patients with recurrent heart failure and reversible ischemic episodes are likely to improve after CABG.

In some patients, chronic myocardial ischemia leads to ischemic cardiomyopathy. This is signified clinically by moderate to severe cardiomegaly, reduced cardiac output, significantly elevated right-sided venous pressures, hepatomegaly, ascites, and peripheral edema. The advanced left ventricular dysfunction is the result of extensive myocardial scarring due to a sustained reduction in coronary perfusion. These patients tend to have diffuse small vessel coronary disease and are therefore not expected to benefit from revascularization.

INDICATIONS FOR CORONARY ARTERY BYPASS GRAFTING

Indications for coronary artery bypass surgery are predicated on improving the patient's quality of life, (i.e., relief of symptoms, increased exercise tolerance, prolonged survival). There is general agreement from several randomized trials that CABG provides a survival advantage as compared with medical therapy in patients with (1) left main stenosis, (2) triple-vessel disease, (3) double-vessel disease with proximal left anterior descending (LAD) stenosis, (4) impaired left ventricular function, and (5) severe ischemia and multivessel disease.[24]

There is a large body of literature comparing percutaneous coronary interventional techniques with surgical revascularization. Although useful, the data must be interpreted critically in the context of the selection and exclusion criteria of patients within the trials. Recent technological advances have enlarged the pool of patients with single- or multi-vessel disease where percutaneous intervention is a reasonable alternative or even a preferred initial approach. However, patients and cardiologists must take into consideration the incidence of recurrent angina and need for repeat revascularization procedures. For patients who are not suitable for percutaneous intervention or when percutaneous intervention has failed, surgery should be strongly considered.

Based on an extensive review of the literature in 1999, a joint task force from the American College of Cardiology and American Heart Association revised the original 1991 guidelines for coronary artery bypass surgery (Table 25-1).[25] Nominally, based on several studies showing improved myocardial function following operative reperfusion, emergency surgical revascularization is generally preferred over medical/percutaneous intervention after acute myocardial infarction. Patients presenting within 6 h of chest pain and an evolving myocardial infarction should be considered for early operation. However, owing to its rapidity in restoring vessel patency, percutaneous intervention has replaced surgery in most centers except in cases of associated mechanical complications (i.e., postinfarct ventricular septal defect, acute mitral insufficiency). An additional subgroup that may benefit from emergency CABG includes patients with acute proximal LAD occlusion and refractory/recurrent angina, since persistent pain reflects continued ischemia of viable myocardium. Emergency CABG is necessary when occlusive complications develop during percutaneous intervention. The majority of these complications result from coronary artery dissections that begin as intimal defects caused by a guidewire or balloon dilatation. In general, in performing emergency coronary artery bypass for these patients or those in cardiogenic shock, the initial goal is to quickly initiate cardiopulmonary bypass support, cardioplegic arrest, and cooling to reduce further myocardial damage. Not surprisingly, operative mortality and morbidity rates associated with emergency coronary bypass are greater than those occurring after elective or even urgent operations. This increased operative

Table 25-1 American College of Cardiology/American Heart Association guidelines for coronary artery bypass graft surgery: indications

Asymptomatic or mild angina

Class I

1. CABG should be performed in patients with asymptomatic or mild angina who have significant left main coronary artery stenosis. (*Level of Evidence: A*)
2. CABG should be performed in patients with asymptomatic or mild angina who have left main equivalent: significant (greater than or equal to 70%) stenosis of the proximal LAD and proximal left circumflex artery. (*Level of Evidence: A*)
3. CABG is useful in patients with asymptomatic ischemia or mild angina who have 3-vessel disease. (Survival benefit is greater in patients with abnormal LV function; e.g., EF less than 0.50 and/or large areas of demonstrable myocardial ischemia.) (*Level of Evidence: C*)

Class IIa

CABG can be beneficial for patients with asymptomatic or mild angina who have proximal LAD stenosis with 1- or 2-vessel disease. (This recommendation becomes a Class I if extensive ischemia is documented by noninvasive study and/or LVEF is less than 0.50.) (*Level of Evidence: A*)

Class IIb

CABG may be considered for patients with asymptomatic or mild angina who have 1- or 2-vessel disease not involving the proximal LAD (If a large area of viable myocardium and high-risk criteria are met on noninvasive testing, this recommendation becomes Class I). (*Level of Evidence: B*)

Stable angina

Class I

1. CABG is recommended for patients with stable angina who have significant left main coronary artery stenosis. (*Level of Evidence: A*)
2. CABG is recommended for patients with stable angina who have left main equivalent: Significant (greater than or equal to 70%) stenosis of the proximal LAD and proximal left circumflex artery. (*Level of Evidence: A*)
3. CABG is recommended for patients with stable angina who have 3-vessel disease. (Survival benefit is greater when LVEF is less than 0.50.) (*Level of Evidence: A*)
4. CABG is recommended in patients with stable angina who have 2-vessel disease with significant proximal LAD stenosis and either EF less than 0.50 or demonstrable ischemia on noninvasive testing. (*Level of Evidence: A*)
5. CABG is beneficial for patients with stable angina who have 1- or 2-vessel CAD without significant proximal LAD stenosis but with a large area of viable myocardium and high-risk criteria on noninvasive testing. (*Level of Evidence: B*)
6. CABG is beneficial for patients with stable angina who have developed disabling angina despite maximal noninvasive therapy, when surgery can be performed with acceptable risk. If angina is not typical, objective evidence of ischemia should be obtained. (*Level of Evidence: B*)

Class IIa

1. CABG is reasonable in patients with stable angina who have proximal LAD stenosis with 1-vessel disease. (This recommendation becomes Class I if extensive ischemia is documented by noninvasive study and/or LVEF is less than 0.50). (*Level of Evidence: A*)
2. CABG may be useful for patients with stable angina who have 1- or 2-vessel CAD without significant proximal LAD stenosis but who have a moderate area of viable myocardium and demonstrable ischemia on noninvasive testing. (*Level of Evidence: B*)

Class III

1. CABG is not recommended for patients with stable angina who have 1- or 2-vessel disease not involving significant proximal LAD stenosis, patients who have mild symptoms that are unlikely due to myocardial ischemia, or patients who have not received an adequate trial of medical therapy and
   a. have only a small area of viable myocardium or (*Level of Evidence: B*)
   b. have no demonstrable ischemia on noninvasive testing. (*Level of Evidence: B*)
2. CABG is not recommended for patients with stable angina who have borderline coronary stenoses (50% to 60% diameter in locations other than the left main coronary artery) and no demonstrable ischemia on noninvasive testing. (*Level of Evidence: B*)
3. CABG is not recommended for patients with stable angina who have insignificant coronary stenosis (less than 50% diameter reduction). (*Level of Evidence: B*)

Table 25-1 American College of Cardiology/American Heart Association guidelines for coronary artery bypass graft surgery: indications (*continued*)

Unstable angina/non–ST-segment elevation MI (NSTEMI)

Class I

1. CABG should be performed for patients with unstable angina/NSTEMI with significant left main coronary artery stenosis. (*Level of Evidence: A*)
2. CABG should be performed for patients with unstable angina/NSTEMI who have left main equivalent: significant (greater than or equal to 70%) stenosis of the proximal LAD and proximal left circumflex artery. (*Level of Evidence: A*)
3. CABG is recommended for unstable angina/NSTEMI in patients in whom revascularization is not optimal or possible, and who have ongoing ischemia not responsive to maximal nonsurgical therapy. (*Level of Evidence: B*)

Class IIa

CABG is probably indicated for patients with unstable angina/NSTEMI who have proximal LAD stenosis with 1- or 2-vessel disease. (*Level of Evidence: A*)

Class IIb

CABG may be considered in patients with unstable angina/NSTEMI who have 1- or 2-vessel disease not involving the proximal LAD when percutaneous revascularization is not optimal or possible. (If there is a large area of viable myocardium and high-risk criteria are met on noninvasive testing, this recommendation becomes Class I.) (*Level of Evidence: B*)

ST-segment elevation MI (STEMI)

Class I

Emergency or urgent CABG in patients with STEMI should be undertaken in the following circumstances:

a. Failed angioplasty with persistent pain or hemodynamic instability in patients with coronary anatomy suitable for surgery. (*Level of Evidence: B*)

b. Persistent or recurrent ischemia refractory to medical therapy in patients who have coronary anatomy suitable for surgery, who have a significant area of myocardium at risk, and who are not candidates for PCI. (*Level of Evidence: B*)

c. At the time of surgical repair of postinfarction ventricular septal rupture or mitral valve insufficiency. (*Level of Evidence: B*)

d. Cardiogenic shock in patients less than 75 years old with ST-segment elevation or left bundle-branch block or posterior MI who develop shock within 36 hours of MI and are suitable for revascularization that can be performed within 18 hours of shock, unless further support is futile because of patient's wishes or contraindications/unsuitability for further invasive care (*Level of Evidence: A*)

e. Life-threatening ventricular arrhythmias in the presence of greater than or equal to 50% left main stenosis and/or triple-vessel disease (*Level of Evidence: B*)

Class IIa

1. CABG may be performed as primary reperfusion in patients who have suitable anatomy and who are not candidates for or who have had failed fibrinolysis/PCI and who are in the early hours (6 to 12 hours) of evolving STEMI. (Level of Evidence: B)
2. In patients who have had an STEMI or NSTEMI, CABG mortality is elevated for the first 3 to 7 days after infarction, and the benefit of revascularization must be balanced against this increased risk. Beyond 7 days after infarction, the criteria for revascularization described in previous sections are applicable. (*Level of Evidence: B*)

Class III

1. Emergency CABG should not be performed in patients with persistent angina and a small area of myocardium at risk who are hemodynamically stable. (*Level of Evidence: C*)
2. Emergency CABG should not be performed in patients with successful epicardial reperfusion but unsuccessful microvascular reperfusion. (*Level of Evidence: C*)

Poor LV function

Class I

1. CABG should be performed in patients with poor LV function who have significant left main coronary artery stenosis. (*Level of Evidence: B*)
2. CABG should be performed in patients with poor LV function who have left main equivalent: significant (greater than or equal to 70%) stenosis of the proximal LAD and proximal left circumflex artery. (*Level of Evidence: B*)
3. CABG should be performed in patients with poor LV function who have proximal LAD stenosis with 2- or 3-vessel disease. (*Level of Evidence: B*)

Table 25-1 American College of Cardiology/American Heart Association guidelines for coronary artery bypass graft surgery: indications (*continued*)

Class IIa

CABG may be performed in patients with poor LV function with significant viable noncontracting, revascularizable myocardium and without any of the above anatomic patterns. (*Level of Evidence: B*)

Class III

CABG should not be performed in patients with poor LV function without evidence of intermittent ischemia and without evidence of significant revascularizable viable myocardium. (Level of Evidence: B)

Life-threatening ventricular arrhythmias

Class I

1. CABG should be performed in patients with life-threatening ventricular arrhythmias caused by left main coronary artery stenosis. (*Level of Evidence: B*)
2. CABG should be performed in patients with life-threatening ventricular arrhythmias caused by 3-vessel coronary disease. (*Level of Evidence: B*)

Class IIa

1. CABG is reasonable in bypassable 1- or 2-vessel disease causing life-threatening ventricular arrhythmias. (This becomes a Class I recommendation if the arrhythmia is resuscitated sudden cardiac death or sustained ventricular tachycardia.) (*Level of Evidence: B*)
2. CABG is reasonable in life-threatening ventricular arrhythmias caused by proximal LAD disease with 1- or 2-vessel disease. (This becomes a Class I recommendation if the arrhythmia is resuscitated sudden cardiac death or sustained ventricular tachycardia). (*Level of Evidence: B*)

Class III

CABG is not recommended in ventricular tachycardia with scar and no evidence of ischemia. (*Level of Evidence: B*)

CABG after failed PTCA

Class I

1. CABG should be performed after failed PTCA in the presence of ongoing ischemia or threatened occlusion with significant myocardium at risk. (*Level of Evidence: B*)
2. CABG should be performed after failed PTCA for hemodynamic compromise. (*Level of Evidence: B*)

Class IIa

1. It is reasonable to perform CABG after failed PTCA for a foreign body in crucial anatomic position. (*Level of Evidence: C*)
2. CABG can be beneficial after failed PTCA for hemodynamic compromise in patients with impairment of the coagulation system and without previous sternotomy. (*Level of Evidence: C*)

Class IIb

CABG can be considered after failed PTCA for hemodynamic compromise in patients with impairment of the coagulation system and with previous sternotomy. (*Level of Evidence: C*)

Class III

1. CABG is not recommended after failed PTCA in the absence of ischemia. (*Level of Evidence: C*)
2. CABG is not recommended after failed PTCA with inability to revascularize due to target anatomy or no-reflow state. (*Level of Evidence: C*)

Patients with previous CABG

Class I

1. Coronary bypass should be performed in patients with prior CABG for disabling angina despite optimal nonsurgical therapy. (If angina is not typical, then objective evidence of ischemia should be obtained.) (*Level of Evidence: B*)
2. Coronary bypass should be performed in patients with prior CABG without patent bypass grafts but with Class I indications for surgery for native-vessel CAD (significant left main coronary stenosis, left main equivalent, 3-vessel disease). (*Level of Evidence: B*)

Table 25-1 American College of Cardiology/American Heart Association guidelines for coronary artery bypass graft surgery: indications (*continued*)

Class IIa
1. Coronary bypass is reasonable in patients with prior CABG and bypassable distal vessel(s) with a large area of threatened myocardium by noninvasive studies. (*Level of Evidence: B*)
2. Coronary bypass is reasonable in patients who have prior CABG if atherosclerotic vein grafts with stenoses greater than 50% supplying the LAD coronary artery or large areas of myocardium are present. (*Level of Evidence: B*)

Class I: Conditions for which there is evidence and/or general agreement that a given procedure or treatment is useful and effective.
Class II: Conditions for which there is conflicting evidence and/or a divergence of opinion about the usefulness/or efficacy of a procedure.
Class IIa: Weight of evidence/opinion is in favor of usefulness/efficacy.
Class IIb: Usefulness/efficacy is less well established by evidence/opinion.
Class III: Conditions for which there is evidence and/or general agreement that the procedure/treatment is not useful/effective and in some cases may be harmful.

risk is often outweighed by the poorer outcome of nonsurgical treatment.

PREOPERATIVE DATA

Comprehensive evaluation of the patient referred for CABG is obligatory. The cardiac surgeon's attention to detail leads to optimal risk assessment, preoperative preparation, operative planning, and postoperative care; these are all equally critical to the ultimate success of the operation. A complete history and physical is performed by the operative surgeon, with special attention to signs of congestive heart failure, extracardiac organ dysfunction, concomitant valvular or peripheral vascular disease, previous conditions that may limit vascular conduit availability, and other comorbidities. Standard laboratory investigations include a complete blood count, electrolyte panel, renal and liver function tests, urinalysis, coagulation profile, and blood type and cross. Recent (e.g., within 1 month) anteroposterior and lateral plain chest radiography is reviewed, with particular attention to the cardiac silhouette, vascular calcifications, and pulmonic processes. At Johns Hopkins, when a plain chest film demonstrates aortic calcification, chest computed tomography is performed to further evaluate the ascending aorta for atherosclerotic plaques. A 12-lead ECG is obtained to establish conduction and ST-segmental baselines. Preoperative myocardial perfusion and viability studies—such as nuclear scintigraphy, stress tests, and magnetic resonance imaging—are reviewed to assist operative strategy and to assess the likelihood of surgical success. When a radial artery conduit is considered, Doppler evaluation of the nondominant hand is performed to assess ulnar artery collateralization. We routinely obtain bilateral carotid artery ultrasonography prior to coronary artery bypass to screen for hemodynamically significant carotid stenosis.

Coronary angiograms are reviewed by all surgeons involved in the case. The coronary "road map" permits detailed examination of the coronary vessels for size, suitability, and priority for bypass. In addition, the relationships between the diseased vessels and regional wall motion abnormalities must be ascertained. Suggestions of aortic valvular insufficiency and mitral valvular regurgitation on left ventriculography should be further investigated with an echocardiogram.

Preoperative protection of the heart to minimize further myocardial damage is of utmost importance. Administration of beta blockers, nitrates, angiotensin converting enzyme (ACE) inhibitors, and calcium antagonists is continued to the operative date. For patients with unstable angina or intramural thrombus, intravenous heparin is continued up to 4 h prior to the operation. Placement of an intraaortic balloon pump is indicated when medical management fails to relieve angina or in cases of ischemic cardiogenic shock. Patients who come to surgery having received thrombolytics, such as alteplase, streptokinase, reteplase, face a heightened risk of perioperative hemorrhage. More recently, the use of antiplatelet-aggregation drugs—such as abciximab (ReoPro), eptifibatide (Integrilin), tirofiban (Aggrastat), and clopidogrel (Plavix)—has become popular. If the patient's coronary syndrome is stable, it is advisable to discontinue these medications at an appropriate time (each has a different half-life) before the operation. At Johns Hopkins, we continue aspirin up to the date of surgery owing to recent data showing improved operative outcomes.

Although potential comorbid conditions affecting CABG outcomes are many, the patient's overall state of health and the potential for complete revascularization remain critically important. Incomplete revascularization due to severe distal disease or inadequate conduit leads to higher mortality and a poor long-term prognosis. A multivariate analysis of over 13,000 patients identified seven adverse factors that influence survival: advanced age, ejection fraction, clinical status (e.g., shock, emergency surgery), female sex, diabetes, previous coronary artery bypass surgery, and congestive heart failure. Other cormorbid conditions that should be addressed include previous stroke, history of significant bleeding, hypertension, angina class, concurrent infection (e.g., urinary tract, dental), chronic obstructive pulmonary disease (COPD), and hepatic and renal insufficiencies. Since 1989, the Society of Thoracic Surgeons has established a database of coronary and valvular cardiac operations performed in the United States. Surgeons can now obtain immediate risk stratification data for a given patient simply by entering clinical data online at http://www.sts.org.

SURGICAL TECHNIQUES

The primary goal of coronary artery bypass surgery is to completely revascularize all significantly stenosed (i.e., 50 percent luminal narrowing or more) coronary arterial trunks and branches with a diameter of at least 1 mm. In patients with multivessel disease with a number of stenosed branches, sequential distal anastomoses may be required to conserve conduit length. The sequence of distal anastomoses usually entails grafting the most ischemic region first to allow early intraoperative administration of cardioplegia. However, pedicled grafts, such as the internal mammary artery, are usually anastomosed last to prevent inadvertent injury to these comparatively fragile tissues. Retrograde delivery of cardioplegia, in addition to antegrade delivery, is often prudent in the setting of significant left main coronary disease, severe triple-vessel disease, and aortic insufficiency. When retrograde cardioplegia is used, it may be prudent to perform the right coronary artery distal anastomosis initially for early delivery of antegrade cardioplegia, since there is some evidence that retrograde delivery does not provide optimal right ventricular protection. We use a standard anastomotic sequence consisting of the right/inferior wall (i.e., right or posterior descending coronary) first, the lateral wall (i.e., circumflex marginal) second, and the anterior wall (e.g., LAD) last.

At Johns Hopkins, approximately 80 percent of primary coronary bypass operations are performed with cardiopulmonary bypass support under cardioplegic arrest. Over the last decade, much attention has been given to the application of minimally invasive approaches to coronary artery bypass surgery. Although robot-assisted cardiac surgery remains largely investigational and limited-access techniques on the arrested (e.g., Port-Access, Heartport) or beating heart [minimally invasive direct coronary artery bypass (MIDCAB)] have not been fully embraced, coronary revascularization on the beating heart without the use of cardiopulmonary bypass has

Table 25-2 Coronary artery bypass conduit indications, contraindications, and graft failure rate

	Indication	Contraindication	Failure rate
Left internal mammary artery	Whenever feasible	Emergency surgery Poor flow or injury Subclavian artery stenosis/occlusion	3–8% at 1 year 4–12% at 5 years 7–12% at 10 years
Right internal mammary artery	Young patient	Diabetes (relative)	
Free internal mammary artery graft	When internal mammary artery cannot be used as pedicled graft	Atherosclerotic or dissection	8–25% intermediate term
Radial artery	Arterial conduit	Positive Allen test Incomplete palmer arch Prior carpal tunnel operation Prior radial arterial cannulation (relative)	15% at 3 months further 7% during next 6 months
Gastroepiploic artery	Additional arterial conduit	Prior gastric resection Atherosclerosis of celiac axis Emergency surgery Large heart Severe LV dysfunction	4% at 2 months 8% between 2 and 5 years
Inferior epigastric artery	Lack of other conduits Prior use of internal Mammary artery	Paramedian abdominal incision Atherosclerosis Previous groin incision (relative)	21% at 5 years
Greater saphenous vein	Best venous conduit	Too small (< 2 mm)	10–15% in first month 2–3% per year between 1 and 5 years 5% per year after 5 years 50% in 10 years + 25% with stenosis

gained popularity. In some centers, off-pump coronary artery bypass (OPCAB) has become the primary method of surgical revascularization. Despite the theoretical benefit of avoiding the sequelae of cardiopulmonary bypass, convincing data demonstrating superior or equivalent graft patency rates as compared with conventional techniques, reduced morbidity and mortality, faster recovery, and lower health care costs are still lacking. OPCAB techniques are discussed elsewhere in this textbook.

Choice of graft conduits

Table 25-2 lists graft conduit options, their indications and contraindications, and patency rates. Multiple studies clearly demonstrate early and late survival benefits with the use of a pedicled internal mammary artery as a graft to the LAD; this pedicled graft should be used whenever possible. The right pedicled internal mammary artery graft can be used to bypass the right coronary artery or, when sufficiently long, can be tunneled through the transverse sinus to reach targets in the proximal left lateral wall. In patients less than 50 years of age, we routinely use bilateral mammary artery grafts unless the patient has diabetes, is obese, or suffers from severe COPD. There is some evidence to suggest that these conditions predispose to sternal wound complications if both mammary arteries are used. If the internal mammary artery is injured or has suboptimal flow, it can still be used as a free arterial graft.

The greater saphenous vein remains the primary source of free grafts. If it is absent or inadequate, the lesser saphenous vein is an option. When the saphenous vein is preoperatively anticipated to be inadequate, bilateral radial artery grafts should be evaluated and prepared for harvesting as free grafts. Cephalic veins should be used only as a last resort. The inferior epigastric and gastroepiploic arteries can also be used as free grafts; however, limitations on length, inconsistent availability due to early branching and small caliber, and tedious dissection have made these infrequently used conduits. In our practice, we rarely use such unusual pedicled arterial conduits. Certainly such grafts should be avoided in emergency operations or with excessive cardiac enlargement. Alternative sources of graft conduits include cryopreserved human saphenous vein allografts, bovine internal mammary and sacral arteries, and various small-diameter synthetic (i.e., polyurethane, PTFE) conduits. All these alternative conduits exhibit unacceptably low patency rates or are not in active clinical use.

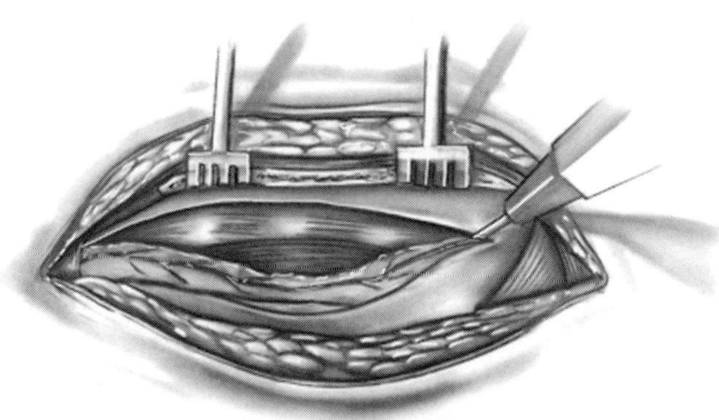

Figure 25-1 Harvesting of left internal thoracic artery. An asymmetrical retractor is used to elevate the left hemisternum. The parietal pleura and endothoracic fascia medial and lateral to the internal thoracic artery and accompanying veins are incised with the electrocautery and then, using a combination of blunt and electrocautery dissection, the pedicle of the internal thoracic artery is separated from the chest wall. Metal clips are used to secure the larger branches. The pedicle can be harvested from the level of the subclavian vein down to the bifurcation of the superior epigastric and musculophrenic arteries. After systemic heparinization, the pedicle is divided distally and flow is assessed. [From Woo YJ, Gardner TJ. Myocardial revascularization with cardiopulmonary bypass. In: Cohn LH, Edmunds LH Jr (eds). *Cardiac Surgery in the Adult.* New York: McGraw-Hill; 2003:581–607. With permission.]

Operative technique

The median sternotomy is followed by internal mammary artery dissection (Fig. 25-1). We routinely inject the internal mammary artery with intraluminal papaverine and wrap the pedicled graft in a papaverine-soaked sponge. A full therapeutic dose of heparin (300 U/kg) is given at this time to achieve an activated clotting time (ACT) of 480 s (550 s if aprotinin is used). After confirming that the internal mammary artery and saphenous vein grafts are satisfactory, a standard pericardial well is created. At this time, the ascending aorta is palpated to detect potential plaques and select a cannulation site. Obvious calcified plaques are avoided. The aorta and pulmonary artery reflection is divided, obtaining adequate space in the aortopulmonary window to permit aortic cross clamping. We use two 2-0 braided purse-string sutures placed in the adventitial layer for aortic cannulation; the preferred position is just inferior to the innominate artery takeoff along the lesser curvature of the aorta. For most adults, a 20F Soft-Flo aortic cannula (Sarns, Inc., Ann Arbor, MI) provides maximal flow rates of up to 5800 mL/min. Once the position of the aortic cannula tip is confirmed, the arterial limb of the cardiopulmonary bypass circuit is connected. For uncomplicated, isolated coronary artery bypass, we prefer using a single dual-stage cannula for venous drainage. Usually a 32/34F cannula is adequate, especially if vacuum assistance is used. Larger patients may require larger cannulas. The venous cannula is placed through a purse-string stitch consisting of 2-0 braided suture placed in the right atrial appendage. For primary elective coronary artery

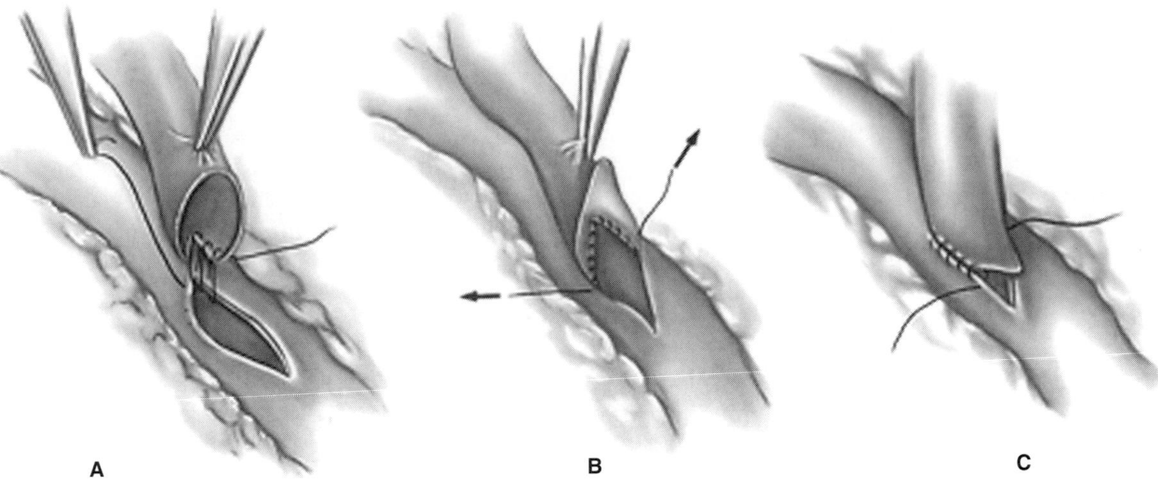

Figure 25-2 Distal anastomosis. A. A fine polypropylene suture is passed through the conduit and coronary artery in a running fashion toward and around the anastomotic heel. B. After several throws, the conduit is gently parachuted down to the coronary artery. C. A suture is continued toward and around the anastomotic toe until the other end of the suture is reached. [From Woo YJ, Gardner TJ. Myocardial revascularization with cardiopulmonary bypass. In: Cohn LH, Edmunds LH Jr (eds). *Cardiac Surgery in the Adult.* New York: McGraw-Hill; 2003:581–607. With permission.]

bypass, cardiotomy suction is no longer used to reduce the risk of particulate emboli returning to the bypass circuit. Shed mediastinal blood is returned to the patient via cell-saver recovery. A 4-0 polypropylene horizontal mattress stitch is placed in the mid-ascending aorta to secure the antegrade cardioplegia cannula.

Once a satisfactory ACT is confirmed and the cardiopulmonary bypass lines have been checked for kinks or clamps, cardiopulmonary bypass is initiated and conducted with nonpulsatile flow of 1.8 to 2.2 L/min/m^2 with a target mean arterial peripheral pressure of 50 mmHg, or higher if the patient has significant peripheral vascular disease. The pulmonary artery is routinely vented. The systemic temperature is allowed to drift initially, then is lowered to 34°C or lower when prolonged bypass time is expected. The cardioplegia line is flushed free of air. We primarily employ antegrade blood cardioplegia with or without retrograde supplementation. At Johns Hopkins, a 2:1 mixture of blood to high-potassium crystalloid solution (50 meq sodium bicarbonate and 60 meq potassium) is administered approximately every 20 min. If retrograde cardioplegia is used, the coronary sinus pressure is monitored and maintained at 35 mmHg during infusion.

To initiate arrest, the distal ascending aorta is cross-clamped proximal to the arterial cannula and 800 to 1000 mL of cardioplegia is administered in an antegrade manner. The surgeon confirms an adequate aortic root pressure and the absence of left ventricular distention. Additional myocardial cooling is provided by continuous topical irrigation with cold saline instilled into the peri-

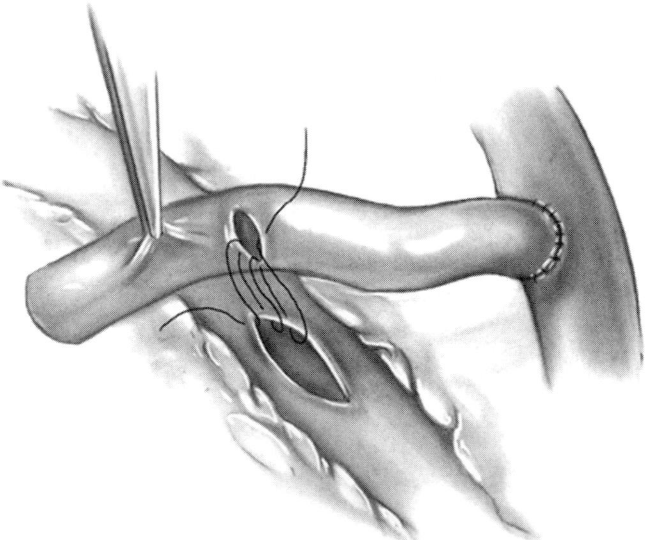

Figure 25-3 Sequential distal anastomosis. After determination of the appropriate geometric alignment of the conduit and coronary artery, a coronary arteriotomy and conduit venotomy or arteriotomy are created and, in a manner similar to that described for distal anastomosis, a polypropylene suture is used in continuous fashion beginning near the heel. [From Woo YJ, Gardner TJ. Myocardial revascularization with cardiopulmonary bypass. In: Cohn LH, Edmunds LH Jr (eds). *Cardiac Surgery in the Adult.* New York: McGraw-Hill; 2003:581–607. With permission.]

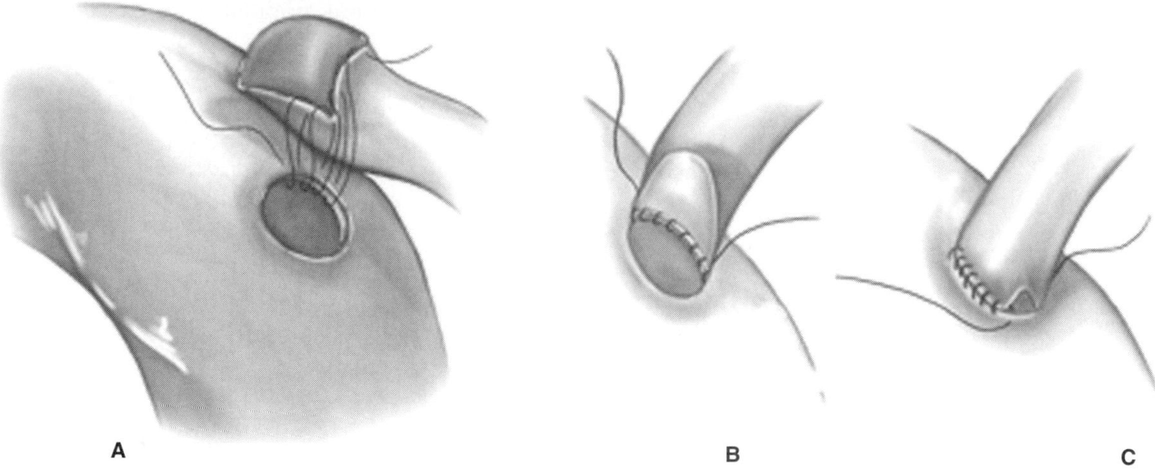

Figure 25-4 Proximal anastomosis. A. The technique of single cross-clamping is demonstrated. An aortotomy is created with a knife and punch. Appropriate conduit length and orientation are established and a fine polypropylene suture is used in a running fashion towards and around the anastomotic heel. B. The conduit is then carefully parachuted down onto the aorta. C. The suture is continued toward and around the anastomotic toe. [From Woo YJ, Gardner TJ. Myocardial revascularization with cardiopulmonary bypass. In: Cohn LH, Edmunds LH Jr (eds). *Cardiac Surgery in the Adult.* New York: McGraw-Hill; 2003:581–607. With permission.]

cardial well; the irrigant is cleared by a discard suction device. Once cardiac arrest is achieved, the heart is elevated to inspect the coronary artery's anatomy and distal graft sites.

Silastic loops are placed proximal and distal to the intended site of the coronary arteriotomy to facilitate anastomosis. The arteriotomy, made at an axial plane to the course of the target artery, is constructed in a standard end-to-side manner with a running 7-0 Prolene suture (Fig. 25-2). Many surgeons elect to perform sequential anastomoses to perfuse two or more coronary arteries with a graft. This entails the construction of one or more side-to-side anastomoses (Fig. 25-3). Besides conserving graft conduit length, this technique augments graft outflow (i.e., lower resistance to flow), which many believe tends to provide greater graft patency. After each free graft distal anastomosis is constructed, the graft is flushed with approximately 100 mL of blood cardioplegia. Bleeding sites on the vein graft and at the anastomosis can then be easily identified and repaired. After all of the distal free graft anastomoses are completed, the mammary artery is dissected free from its pedicle and the tip prepared for anastomosis. Adequate flow in the internal mammary artery is confirmed and the distal anastomosis, usually to the LAD, is constructed in an end-to-side fashion.

Free graft proximal anastomoses are generally performed with the cross clamp in place. Some surgeons prefer to use a partial occluding clamp to permit coronary perfusion during performance of the proximal anastomoses; others prefer to minimize manipulation of the aorta. Small 4.0-mm aortotomies are created with an aortic punch. Proximal anastomoses are generally constructed with 6-0 Prolene in an end-to-side fashion (Fig. 25-4). Prior to securing the final proximal anastomosis, the pulmonary vent is turned off and the heart is filled with blood. Air is then evacuated from the ascending aorta through the last unsecured proximal suture line, which is subsequently tied. The aortic cross clamp is then removed. The pulmonary vent is removed and its site oversewn. Once the surgeon elects to wean from cardiopulmonary bypass, the anesthesiologist is asked to restart ventilation. Cardiopulmonary bypass is then gradually weaned to off, the heart is decannulated, and heparin reversal with protamine is initiated. Appropriate mediastinal and pleural drains are placed and the chest is closed.

SPECIAL CONSIDERATIONS

The atherosclerotic aorta

Embolization of atherosclerotic debris from a severely atherosclerotic aorta is generally considered the primary cause of perioperative stroke in CABG patients. Aortic plaque can be assessed initially with manual palpation; however, this method can easily miss noncalcified atheromas. The most sensitive modality whereby aortic atherosclerosis can be assessed is epiaortic ultrasonographic scanning.

In some cases of patchy ascending aortic disease, "safe" sites for application of the cross clamp and construction of proximal anastomoses can be identified. In these cases, side-biting partial aortic clamps should be avoided. When extensive aortic calcification is identified (e.g., "porcelain" aorta), OPCAB is a reasonable alternative to avoid cross clamping the aorta. Proximal anastomoses can be constructed in this setting with one of several commercial anastomotic device systems. Other alternatives include conducting the surgery under fibrillatory arrest, replacement of the ascending aorta with a Dacron graft, or basing free grafts on the internal mammary artery pedicle.

Failure to wean from cardiopulmonary bypass

When the patient cannot be successfully weaned from cardiopulmonary bypass, an assessment of the reasons for failure must be efficiently conducted. A review of existing biventricular contractility, adequacy of inotropic/pharmacologic support, optimal cardiac function (e.g., adequate volume and heart rate), metabolic conditions (e.g., acidosis, hyperkalemia), and bypass graft patency must be carefully performed.

Manual palpation of bypass grafts can be misleading, as an occluded graft can display accentuated pulsatility. Doppler ultrasonography with a flow probe can provide an accurate assessment of the patency of either venous or arterial graft conduits. Poor flow in a newly constructed bypass graft is almost always due to technical error; such grafts should be revised prior to further attempts at weaning from cardiopulmonary bypass. It is often prudent to re-review the preoperative coronary angiogram to determine whether nongrafted territories should be addressed. Transesophageal echocardiography is an important modality to (1) identify new or old regional wall abnormalities that may be relieved by additional revascularization and (2) recognize any intracardiac factor, such as valvular dysfunction or previously undetected shunting, that may be contributing to the failure to wean.

If, despite optimization of all correctable parameters, separation from cardiopulmonary bypass remains impossible, mechanical assistance is indicated. Intraaortic balloon pump counterpulsation is usually the initial option to improve coronary perfusion and reduce ventricular afterload. Its use and contraindications are discussed elsewhere in this book. Further inability to wean will require the use of formal ventricular assist devices if the patient meets the criteria for their implantation.

POSTOPERATIVE RECOVERY

Early postoperative management of CABG patients does not differ significantly from that of other cardiac surgical patients and is not covered in detail here. In general, patients who undergo primary coronary artery bypass are quickly weaned off mechanical ventilatory support and extubated. Parenteral inotropes and intraaortic balloon pumps are weaned as appropriate. We do not routinely use pulmonary artery catheterization in this patient population; however, when indicated, it can assist in the management of hemodynamic performance in the early postoperative period. A 12-lead ECG is obtained early after the patient arrives in the intensive care unit and compared with a preoperative ECG. Serial ECGs are obtained to detect new ischemia. We do not routinely obtain postoperative cardiac enzyme markers. On the first postoperative day, mediastinal and pleural chest tubes are removed if drainage is less than 30 mL/h for 4 consecutive hours. Beta blockers and aspirin are administered early if there are no hemodynamic or coagulation issues. We now routinely load our patients orally with amiodarone (400 mg/day for 5 days, followed by 200 mg/day) as prophylaxis for atrial dysrhythmias. Some surgeons elect to administer clopidogrel along with aspirin in the early postoperative period to address growing evidence for aspirin resistance in some patients. Since several trials have demonstrated that an aggressive lipid-lowering strategy confers beneficial effects on graft patency, we now routinely administer lovastatin or an equivalent drug postoperatively.

Once deemed stable, patients are transferred from the intensive care unit to a monitored step-down unit and are actively ambulated with the assistance of physical therapists. If pacing wires have been placed and there are no concerning arrhythmias, they are removed by the second postoperative day. A coordinated program of physical therapy and dietary management should be initiated as soon as the patient leaves the hospital. Inpatient or outpatient rehabilitation and physical therapy are arranged as needed. Patients who smoke must give up tobacco; this may require pharmacologic nicotine replacement. Preoperative emphasis on smoking cessation can be invaluable. Other modifiable risk factors for coronary atherosclerosis, such as hypertension and hyperlipidemia, should be monitored and controlled in a comprehensive program to promote graft patency.

Acute postoperative myocardial ischemia/infarction

Early postoperative myocardial ischemia and/or infarction, especially when associated with hemodynamic disturbances, can have a major adverse effect on operative outcomes. A postoperative myocardial infarction, defined by new Q waves on the postoperative ECG, occurs in 4 to 5 percent of patients. A new Q-wave myocardial infarction is usually attributed to poor distal perfusion, but it can be also be due to incomplete revascularization, technical graft failure, inadequate myocardial preservation, or inadequate resuscitation in the early postoperative period. Cardiomegaly, prolonged cardiopulmonary bypass, reoperative coronary artery bypass surgery, and bypass grafting combined with other cardiac operations are known risk factors for postoperative myocardial infarction. Other factors identified from the Coronary Artery Surgery Study

(CASS) trial predictive of postoperative myocardial infarction include female gender, severe preoperative angina pectoris, severe left main coronary stenosis, and three-vessel disease.[26]

Accurate diagnosis of a myocardial infarction after cardiac surgery requires an integrated approach that combines laboratory and clinical findings. While new, persistent Q-waves on ECG are suggestive of postoperative myocardial infarction, nonspecific ST-T-segment abnormalities on ECG and typical postoperative elevations of biochemical markers (e.g., creatinine kinase, troponin) often make this diagnosis difficult. Nevertheless, when suspicious ECG changes are associated with hemodynamic and/or rhythm disturbances, postoperative myocardial ischemia should be ruled out. Patients with ST-T-segment elevations and a low cardiac index should prompt consideration of intraaortic balloon pump support. Bedside transthoracic or, when necessary, transesophageal echocardiography can provide valuable supportive data if regional wall motion abnormalities are seen, especially if they correlate with ECG findings. When an integrated review of these diagnostic modalities and clinical indications are highly suggestive of an acute postoperative myocardial ischemia/infarction, immediate coronary angiography is indicated. Subsequent percutaneous intervention or operative rescue is determined based on the clinical situation.

OUTCOMES

Historically, coronary artery bypass surgery has been one of the most scrutinized operations. There is a tremendous amount of literature analyzing, comparing, and modifying CABG outcomes. Below, we focus upon the nature of early post-CABG mortality, important postoperative complications, and positive outcome variables.

Perioperative mortality

Early in-hospital mortality from primary coronary artery bypass surgery has seen a steady decline from the 1970s into the 1990s. Recently, however, the patient population referred for coronary artery bypass has become increasingly complex, hence the decline has plateaud in recent years. Older patients, more advanced and diffuse coronary artery disease, worsening left ventricular function, failure of multiple previous percutaneous manipulations, more serious comorbidities, and a greater frequency of reoperation have contributed to an increase in perioperative risk. Therefore only risk-adjusted outcome data can be truly informative. Currently, the overall operative mortality rate for CABG is about 3 percent; elective primary coronary artery bypass carries a mortality rate of 1.7 percent, according to the database of the Society of Thoracic Surgeons.

Perioperative morbidity

As a consequence of CABG performed on higher-risk patients, most cardiac surgeons have witnessed an increase in the rate of postoperative complications. Perioperative myocardial infarction has been covered previously; this section reports other common operative morbidities.

Hemorrhage

Coagulopathy, platelet dysfunction/depletion, and the release of proinflammatory factors are recognized consequences of cardiopulmonary bypass. Even with OPCAB and the use of antifibrinolytics, such as aminocaproic acid (Amicar) and aprotinin (Trasylol), significant bleeding still occurs. The rate of reexploration for bleeding following conventional coronary artery bypass ranges from 2 to 5 percent. Risks for bleeding include older age, preoperative aspirin and other antiplatelet agents, reoperation, prolonged cardiopulmonary bypass time, and bilateral internal mammary artery grafts.

Mediastinitis

Deep sternal wound infections occur in 1 to 4 percent of primary coronary artery bypass patients. This complication clearly increases mortality and may bring long-lasting morbidity to the patient. Obesity, the use of bilateral internal mammary grafts, diabetes, prolonged operation, and prior coronary artery bypass are all risk factors for mediastinitis. Appropriate and timely administration of perioperative antibiotics, meticulous skin preparation, and attention to sterile technique can help minimize this troublesome complication.

Respiratory insufficiency

Prolonged ventilator dependence (e.g., more than 1 day) occurs in approximately 6 percent of CABG patients. Many factors contribute to postoperative respiratory failure, but preexisting pulmonary disease is the most important predictor. When patients undergo coronary artery bypass with a preoperative forced expiratory volume in 1 s (FEV_1) less than 1.5 L or an FEV_1/forced vital capacity (FVC) ratio of less than 0.65, the rate of postoperative pulmonary complications can be as high as 29 percent.[27] Coronary artery bypass patients with severe COPD have significantly higher mortality rates (19 percent) than those with mild to moderate or no COPD.

Neurologic complications

Adverse neurologic outcome following coronary artery bypass surgery is the subject of ongoing investigation. It is a dreaded complication that can manifest in numerous ways. Nearly three-quarters of coronary artery bypass patients experience some degree of neuropsychological derangement, which tends to be transient. However, persistent or permanent significant neurologic deficits are important causes of postoperative mortality and morbidity. In general, a *type I deficit* is associated with a major focal deficit and/or stupor or coma; a *type II deficit* is characterized by a measurable deterioration of intellectual function and memory. In a review of nearly 2200 patients, both type I and type II deficits occurred in about 3 percent of coronary artery bypass patients.[28] Known factors contributing to type I deficits include older age, ascending aortic atherosclerosis, history of stroke, use of intraaortic balloon pump, diabetes, hypertension, and unstable angina.

Atrial fibrillation

Up to 40 percent of CABG patients will experience at least one episode of atrial fibrillation. It is the most frequent postoperative rhythm disturbance and usually occurs on the second or third postoperative day. Although mostly benign and self-terminating, atrial fibrillation is associated with prolonged hospitalization, hemodynamic instability, and thromboembolism. The stroke risk in patients experiencing postoperative atrial fibrillation is increased threefold.[29] The exact mechanism behind this dysrhythmia is likely multifactorial, including increased endogenous catecholamine levels, atrial ischemia, and atrial reentrant pathways. The recent routine use of beta blockade has significantly reduced its incidence. At Johns Hopkins, we routinely use amiodarone to prevent postoperative atrial fibrillation.

Renal dysfunction

Up to 8 percent of CABG patients develop postoperative renal dysfunction. In a multi-institutional review, 7.7 percent of patients had postoperative serum creatinine levels equal to or greater than 2.0 mg/dL or an increase of 0.7 mg/dL or more from preoperative levels. Nearly 18 percent of these patients required hemodialysis, associated with a 30-day mortality rate of 63 percent.[30] Predictors of renal dysfunction include advanced age, baseline renal disease, diabetes, poor cardiac function, previous coronary artery bypass surgery, peripheral vascular disease, and use of the intraaortic balloon pump.

Angina relief

Coronary artery bypass surgery is highly effective in relieving anginal symptoms and improving quality of life. Randomized trials consistently show that surgical revascularization confers more durable symptomatic relief than medical therapies. Approximately 80 percent of coronary artery bypass patients are angina-free at 5 years and 63 percent at 10 years.[31] Detailed statistical analysis reveals that the hazard function for the return of angina has an early phase that peaks at about 3 months postoperatively and a late phase that peaks at 3 years. The early phase is likely due to incomplete revascularization and graft failure, while late phase results from progression of native coronary artery disease and late stenosis/occlusion of bypass grafts. Recurrent angina, whether early or late, indicates repeat coronary angiography to dictate whether percutaneous intervention or reoperation is necessary. Predictors of angina recurrence include female sex, obesity, hypertension, incomplete revascularization, and absence of the internal mammary artery graft.

Return to work

The ability to return to employment is another important endpoint in CABG outcome analyses. There is no universal agreement on whether coronary artery bypass surgery confers an advantage in obtaining gainful employment. Clearly, those patients employed prior to surgery are most likely to return to work after surgery. Also, CABG patients in the middle of their professional productive years are more inclined to continue working. In general, among patients employed shortly before CABG, 80 percent are back to work a year later. Among patients with unfavorable factors—such as older age, return of angina, and preoperative unemployment or disability—less than 20 percent returned to work.[32]

Long-term survival

After an early nadir within the first 6 postoperative months, mortality rates after CABG increase steadily after 1 year. The increase in the hazard ratio at 15 years is twice that at 5 years. Late death is mostly due to noncardiac causes; however, progression of native coronary disease and graft atherosclerosis continues to plague these patients. Recent data obtained from the CASS registry shows that 97 percent of CABG patients are alive at 1 year, 90 to 92 percent at 5 years, 74 to 81 percent at 10 years, and 56 to 66 percent at 15 years.[33]

SUMMARY

Primary coronary artery bypass surgery remains the cornerstone of treatment for ischemic heart disease. For patients with advanced multivessel coronary artery disease or those with left ventricular functional impairment, surgical revascularization still provides greater symptomatic relief and superior survival rates than medical or percutaneous interventional therapies. Although minimally invasive techniques and OPCAB have generated much investigation and controversy, over three-quarters of all CABGs performed in the United States are performed with conventional cardiopulmonary bypass support. Employment of an all-arterial versus saphenous vein-supplemented conduit strategy is still an active arena of debate.

Despite a steady increase in the proportion of older or "high-risk" patients being referred for surgery, major perioperative mortality and morbidity continues to be low, and long-term outcomes are excellent. Years of surgical innovation and experience have set the standard against which future advances in percutaneous coronary interventions, molecular therapeutics, and novel surgical approaches will be compared.

References

1. American Heart Association website. www.aha.org.
2. Anderson RH, Becker AE. *Cardiac Anatomy.* London: Churchill Livingstone; 1980.
3. Cho PW, Finney S, Gardner TJ. Ischemic heart disease and its complications. In: Baumgartner WA, Owen S, Cameron D, Reitz BA (eds). *The Johns Hopkins Manual of Cardiac Surgical Care.* St Louis: Mosby; 1994.
4. Ganz P, Ganz W. Coronary blood flow and myocardial ischemia. In: Braunwald E (ed). *Heart Disease: A Textbook of Cardiovascular Medicine*, 6th ed. Philadelphia: Saunders; 2001.
5. Pijls NHJ, De Bruyne B. *Coronary Pressure.* Dodrecht, The Netherlands: Kluwer; 1997:12–13.
6. Roberts WC. Does thrombosis play a major role in the development of symptom-producing atherosclerotic plaques? *Circulation* 1973;48:1161.
7. Stary HC, Chandler AB, Dinsmore RE, et al. A definition of advanced types of atherosclerotic lesions and a histological classification of atherosclerosis: A report from the Committee on Vascular Lesions of the Council on Arteriosclerosis, American Heart Association. *Circulation* 1995;92:1355–1374.
8. Falk E. Coronary thrombosis: Pathogenesis and clinical manifestations. *Am J Cardiol* 1991;68:28B.
9. Tennant R, Wiggers CJ. The effect of coronary occlusion on myocardial contractions. *Am J Physiol* 1935;112:351.
10. Hoffman JI. Transmural myocardial perfusion. *Prog Cardiovasc Dis* 1987;29:429–464.
11. Fibrinolytic Therapy Trialists (FTT) Collaborative Group. Indications for fibrinolytic therapy in suspected acute myocardial infarction: Collaborative overview of early mortality and major morbidity results from all randomised trials of more than 1000 patients. *Lancet* 1994;343:311–322.
12. Hand M, Brown C, Horan M, Simons-Morton D. The National Heart Attack Alert Program: Progress at 5 years in educating providers, patients and the public, and future directions. *J Thromb Thrombol* 1998;6:9–17.
13. Campeau L. Grading of angina pectoris (letter). *Circulation* 1976;54:522.
14. American Heart Association. *Heart and Stroke Facts: 1995 Statistical Supplement.* Dallas: American Heart Association; 1996.
15. Antman E, Braunwald E. Acute myocardial infarction. In: Braunwald E (ed). *Heart Disease: A Textbook of Cardiovascular Medicine*, 6th ed. Philadelphia: Saunders; 2001.
16. Pedoe-Tunstall H, Kuulasmaa K, Amouyel P, et al. Myocardial infarction and coronary deaths in the World Health Organization MONICA Project. *Circulation* 1994;90:583–612.
17. Stenotic atherosclerotic coronary artery disease. In: Kouchoukos N, Blackstone E, Doty D, et al (eds). *Cardiac Surgery*, 3d ed. London: Churchill Livingstone; 2003:360.
18. Reardon MJ, Carr CL, Diamond A, et al. Ischemic left ventricular free wall rupture: Prediction, diagnosis, and treatment. *Ann Thorac Surg* 1997;64:1509.
19. Padro JM, Mesa JM, Silvestre, et al. Subacute cardiac rupture: Repair with a sutureless techniques. *Ann Thorac Surg* 1993;55:20.
20. Crenshaw BS, Granger CB, Birnbaum Y, et al. Risk factors, angiographic patterns, and outcomes in patients with ventricular septal defect complicating acute myocardial infarction. *Circulation* 2000;101:27.
21. Lamas GA, Mitchell GF, Flaker GC, et al. Clinical significance of mitral regurgitation after acute myocardial infarction. *Circulation* 1997;96:827.
22. Hickey MS, Smith LR, Muhlbaier LH, et al. Current prognosis of ischemic mitral regurgitation: Implications for future management. *Circulation* 1988;78:151.
23. Left ventricular aneurysm. In: Kouchoukos N, Blackstone E, Doty D, (eds). *Cardiac Surgery*, 3d ed. London, Churchill Livingstone; 2003:438.
24. Yusuf S, Zucker D, Peduzzi P, et al. Effect of coronary artery bypass graft surgery on survival: Overview of ten-year results from randomized trials by the Coronary Artery Bypass Graft Surgery Trialist Collaboration. *Lancet* 1994;344:563.
25. Eagle KA, Guyton RA, Davidoff R, et al. ACC/AHA guidelines for coronary artery bypass graft surgery: Executive summary and recommendations: A report of the American College of Cardiology/American Heart Association Task Force on Practice Guidelines (Committee to Revise the 1991 Guidelines for Coronary Artery Bypass Graft Surgery). *Circulation* 1999;100:1464.
26. Schaff HV, Gersh BJ, Fisher LD, et al. Detrimental effect of perioperative myocardial infarction on late survival after coronary artery bypass. Report from the Coronary Artery Surgery Study-CASS. *J Thorac Cardiovasc Surg* 1984;88:972.
27. Kroenke K, Lawrence VA, Theroux JF, et al. Operative risk in patients with severe obstructive pulmonary disease. *Arch Intern Med* 1992;152:967.
28. Roach GW, Kanchuger M, Mangano CM, et al. Adverse cerebral outcomes after coronary bypass surgery. *N Engl J Med* 1996;335:1857.
29. Aranki SF, Shaw DP, Adams DH, et al. Predictors of atrial fibrillation after coronary artery surgery: Current trends and impact on hospital resources. *Circulation* 1996;94:390.
30. Mangano CM, Diamondstone LS, Ramsay JG, et al. Renal dysfunction after myocardial revascularization: Risk factors, adverse outcomes, and hospital resource utilization. *Ann Intern Med* 1998;128:194.
31. Cameron AA, Davis KB, Rogers WJ. Recurrence of angina after coronary artery bypass surgery: Predictors and prognosis (CASS Registry). Coronary Artery Surgery Study. *J Am Coll Cardiol* 1995;26:895.
32. Rogers WG, Coggin CJ, Gersh BJ, et al. Ten-year follow-up of quality of life in patients randomized to receive medical therapy or coronary artery bypass graft surgery: The Coronary Artery Surgery Study (CASS). *Circulation* 1990;82:1647.
33. Gersh BJ, Braunwald E, Bonow RO. Chronic coronary artery disease. In: Braunwald E (ed). *Heart Disease: A Textbook of Cardiovascular Medicine*, 6th ed. Philadelphia: Saunders; 2001:1306.

CHAPTER

26 OFF-PUMP CORONARY ARTERY BYPASS

Eric A. Peck, Paul Sergeant

INTRODUCTION

The pathophysiology, diagnosis, and treatment of coronary artery disease are presented in Chapter 25. This chapter will focus on a somewhat controversial treatment option for patients with coronary atherosclerosis: off-pump coronary artery bypass (OPCAB). This technique has been practiced to some degree for many years, but it has regained popularity only recently with the development of devices that allow for superb exposure and stabilization of the anastomotic area. With the spectrum of patients presenting with coronary disease becoming more complex and higher-risk, surgeons have been looking for surgical options that may reduce complications. OPCAB has this potential because it avoids cardiopulmonary bypass (CPB) and the associated morbidity.

OPCAB is not simply the standard coronary bypass operation performed without the assistance of a cardiopulmonary bypass. Rather, it is a concept whose primary goal should be the reduction of morbidity and mortality. The technical result should be identical to that for a standard coronary artery bypass graft (CABG) operation: the same number, location, and quality of anastomoses. Further, OPCAB must be a reproducible technique, allowing it to be taught to other surgeons and incorporated into the training of cardiothoracic surgical residents. This aspect is something that is being studied in a scientific fashion at Gasthuisberg Hospital in Belgium (study in progress). For OPCAB to be a successful strategy, it should be applicable to the entire spectrum of patients.

In Leuven a practical algorithm is used to determine whether a particular patient has a bypass performed with or without CPB (Fig. 26-1). Obviously, for any patient in extremis, receiving cardiac compressions, or with malignant arrhythmias, emergent institution of CPB is lifesaving and necessary. In this patient subset, the authors perform CABG on CPB, but with a beating heart to minimize further ischemia. In more stable patients, the next branch in the decision tree involves whether the

KEY CONCEPTS

- Team approach
  - Although all cardiac surgery requires a multidisciplinary approach to the surgical procedure, this is especially true for off-pump coronary artery bypass grafting (CABG). Close and clear communication with the anesthesiologist is critical for the safe performance of the procedure. Similarly, the nursing staff should be included in the dialogue so that it can anticipate each step in the operation and prepare instruments, shunts, and sutures as necessary and in a timely fashion.
- Minimization of risk
  - Off-pump CABG has the potential to reduce morbidity and mortality significantly. However, if done improperly, it can lead to higher complication rates. This is best avoided by minimizing potential intraoperative risk at every possible step.
- Reengineering
  - To achieve optimal results with this technique, it must be realized that this procedure is not just a CABG performed without the assistance of cardiopulmonary bypass. Instead, it requires a complete reengineering of the operative technique and physiologic concepts, including optimizing oxygen supply and demand and maintaining hemodynamic stability before, during, and after cardiac manipulation.

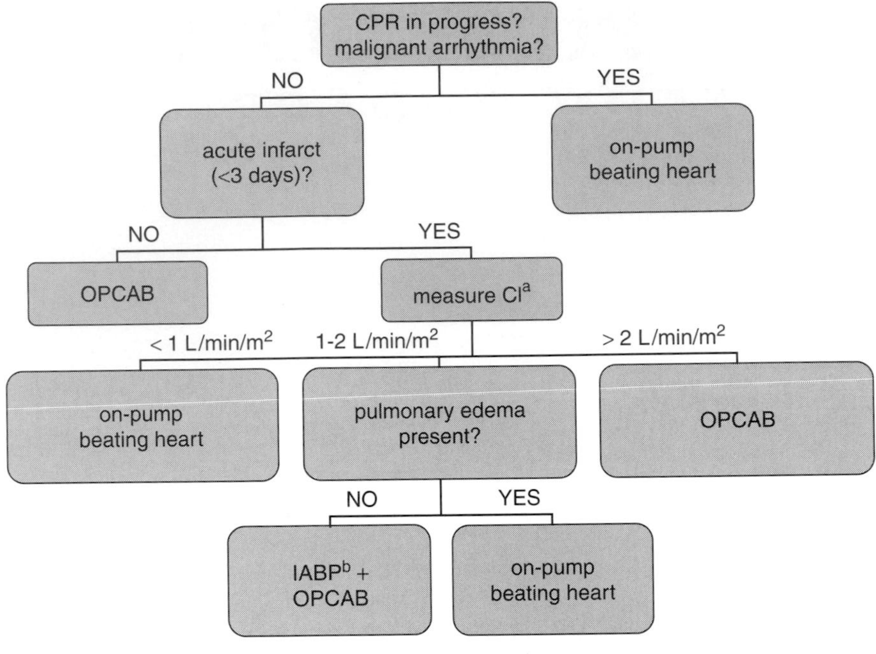

Figure 26-1 (From Peck EA, Sergeant PL. Leuven, Belgium.)

patient has had an acute infarct (within 3 days of surgery). Regardless of other risk factors or comorbidities (e.g., complexity of coronary lesions, cardiomegaly, redo surgery, ejection fraction), if the infarct is more than 3 days old, the procedure is performed off-pump. For an acute infarct, a pulmonary artery catheter is placed and the cardiac index (CI) is measured. If the CI is less than 1 $L/min/m^2$, the patient is placed on CPB and the revascularization is completed with the heart beating. For patients with a CI greater than 2 $L/min/m^2$, procedures are performed off-pump. In patients with a CI between 1 and 2 $L/min/m^2$, a determination is made as to the presence or absence of pulmonary edema. The authors believe that pulmonary vascular congestion is an indication of severe left ventricular dysfunction and indicates a patient who probably will not tolerate cardiac manipulation and may need assistance with oxygenation. These patients undergo CABG with CPB, but with the heart beating.

A less evident component of a successful OPCAB program is the ability to perform these procedures without undue stress on the operating team: surgeons, anesthesiologists, and nurses. Many teams feel averse to performing OPCAB because of the level of anxiety that results from conducting this technique under suboptimal conditions. Hemodynamic instability, ischemia, unpredictability, and perhaps an open confrontation between the anesthetic and surgical teams all contribute to this. The structured environment and organized, stepwise technique developed by one of the authors (Dr. Sergeant) has created an atmosphere of collegiality and open communication, eliminating these stressful triggers and leading to a pleasant operating environment.

This approach involves a number of factors geared toward minimizing risk and enhancing the safety of the procedure. The key to this is the optimization of intraoperative patient hemodynamics (i.e., heart rate/rhythm, blood pressure, cardiac filling pressures, electrolytes, and body temperature) before cardiac manipulation. This provides a stable platform that allows the surgeon to enucleate the heart from the pericardium safely during the anastomotic period. Further, it optimizes the myocardium to tolerate any transient ischemia that is produced. Without proper anesthetic conditioning, the entire concept of OPCAB is unsafe and the operation should not be performed. Each step in the authors' technique is designed to eliminate or reduce the risk associated with off-pump revascularization. Not all steps are essential for every coronary anastomosis in every patient. However, the authors are unable to predict which circumstances will produce instability for any specific patient and/or anastomosis, and it is for this reason that the authors use the safeguards in every patient and for every anastomosis. Without such stringent controls, a certain percentage of patients will require urgent/emergent conversion to on-pump CABG, which clearly has been shown to result in significant morbidity and mortality.[1–3]

Surgeons also must be able to perform anastomoses in smaller spaces and on vessels that may be at unfamiliar angles. To maintain hemodynamic stability, the heart must be manipulated so that mitral insufficiency is not created or worsened and the right heart may fill properly.

In many cases this leads to the anastomoses being more technically challenging than what is encountered on-pump. It is important that the OPCAB surgeon retrain to become competent in creating high-quality anastomoses that are durable and achieve patency rates equivalent to those of anastomoses completed with CPB and an arrested heart. Methods to accomplish this are discussed later in this chapter.

REENGINEERING

"Changing minds"

In evaluating whether to use a new technique in one's practice, it is important to identify the "drivers" that influence the decision. Inappropriate drivers probably will lead to failure of the reengineering process. This topic will be addressed briefly here. Examples of inappropriate drivers include greed, ambition, and excitement about a novel technique. In the authors' early experience with OPCAB, we did not have the proper motivation and for that reason did not perform more than about 10 percent of CABGs off-pump. Further, these cases were very stressful and unpredictable in light of the authors' desire to try out a new technique.

Coronary bypass surgery has achieved unparalleled long-term results that have been studied more extensively perhaps than the results of any other surgical procedure. Although surgeons have relied on this record to maintain patient referrals, the advent of drug-eluting intracoronary stents has produced excellent results as well. Percutaneous stenting, however, is associated with vastly reduced early morbidity and mortality. It was this realization that led the authors to the proper "driver" toward OCPAB surgery: the goal of eliminating early complications while maintaining the outstanding long-term results expected for CABG surgery. With this goal in mind, a technique was developed that minimizes risk for the patient at every possible step.

Although this reengineering process has been described briefly and simply in this text, it was a lengthy and difficult process. In changing one's practice to embrace a new concept, well-defined behavioral processes take place in the mind that may inhibit or facilitate such change. Howard Gardner closely examines these entities in *Changing Minds.*[4] He describes seven important elements that influence whether an individual is likely to change his or her mind on a particular subject: reason, research, resonance, representational redescriptions, resources and rewards, real-world events, and resistances. The first six elements facilitate mind change, whereas the final one serves as a barrier. These will be detailed below according to Gardner's explanations.

Reason implies that an individual is able to see a logical, rational approach to the pertinent issue and weigh each consideration appropriately. A surgeon should be able, for example, to evaluate each risk and benefit of the OPCAB procedure as it compares to conventional CABG surgery and make an honest assessment of whether he or she should change his or her belief.

Research refers to factual, objective data that can be presented to support the argument for change, including statistical evidence. This chapter stands as an example of this, and the authors hope it will change erroneous preconceptions of OPCAB.

Resonance describes a more esoteric phenomenon by which the idea of change somehow appeals to an individual cognitively, an affective response to that individual's set of standards and moral beliefs. If a surgeon has a preconceived sense that avoiding CPB will benefit his or her patients, he or she probably will be more accepting of a change to OPCAB surgery.

Representational redescriptions are related to the number of different forms in which a potential change can be described; the greater the number, the more influential the argument. One is much more likely to change others' minds about OPCAB by presenting information in multiple contexts: verbal, textual, graphical, illustrative, and live visual presentations.

Resources and rewards is perhaps the most simple of these concepts to understand. When presented with the materials needed to implement change or when receiving actual compensation for effecting change, an individual is more likely to do so. For example, if unique OPCAB surgical supplies will be provided at cost or free of charge or if the surgeon receives a larger professional fee for performing OPCAB, it seems likely that many surgeons will accept change more readily.

Real-world events can influence minds in a larger sense, affecting large groups of people or entire societies. For instance, if a high judicial court created a legal precedent that put surgeons performing conventional CABG surgery more at risk for litigation, the motivation for change to OPCAB would be great.

Resistances are many and will be described here in some detail, but they all have in common a psychological or behavioral mechanism that acts as a barrier to change. Roxburgh describes a number of mechanisms that impede the process of change, specifically as related to business managers.[5] However, these ideas are relevant to medical decision making and thus are important in reengineering toward OPCAB. The *status quo bias* refers to the idea that individuals are more concerned about the risk of loss than they are excited by the prospect of gain associated with a change. The term *endowment effect* reflects a strong desire to keep what we own, such as our knowledge and skill with a particular surgical technique. It is human nature to become reluctant to discard failing projects in which we have invested a large amount of time and resources: the *sunk-cost effect.* The *herding instinct* describes the desire of a person to conform to the behavior and opinions of others even if a more successful strategy requires breaking away from the trend.

Roxburgh[5] also states that people are prone to *misestimating future hedonic states.* In other words, when confronted with potential changing circumstances, people are not able to predict accurately the "pleasure or pain" they will feel afterward. However, as it turns out, people adjust surprisingly quickly to the new environment. There are other resistances that fall under the category of *false consensus*: confirmation bias, selective recall, biased evaluation, and groupthink. Biased evaluation refers to the quick acceptance of evidence that supports hypotheses, and contradictory evidence is subjected to rigorous evaluation and almost certain rejection.

Economic impact

It is important to discuss the impact of the OPCAB approach on the real costs of surgical coronary revascularization. There are two methods by which OPCAB may influence cost. The first is a "production line" effect that involves eliminating over 50 CPB-related instruments in the CPB circuit and reducing operating room personnel (e.g., no perfusionist, fewer surgeons/nurses). A second effect is realized in terms of reduced morbidity as a consequence of the new technique. This effect (e.g., reducing stroke or renal failure rates) may apply only to a very small number of patients but constitutes a huge cost benefit. Combined, these effects lead to dramatic overall cost reductions once a complete reengineering toward OPCAB has been realized. This cost benefit has been reported consistently in the OPCAB literature.[6–9]

Team approach

A successful OPCAB program requires that all operating room staff (surgeons, anesthesiologists, and nurses) work together as a team with open lines of communication. This ensures that all members are able to anticipate each step and its potential complications so that they are prepared to correct any abnormalities. The authors also believe that it is essential for the surgeon and the anesthesiologist to have frequent collegial communication during the procedure so that both parties agree as each step in the operation is performed. This has the added benefit of producing a stress-free environment for all members of the operating team and leads to improved multidisciplinary care for the patient. If at any point and for any reason the anesthetist does not feel that the patient is stable enough to proceed, the manipulation is delayed until the hemodynamics have been optimized.

SURGICAL TECHNIQUES

The authors' OPCAB technique has evolved over time. Since 1999, new devices have become available and the authors' experience with optimal anesthetic management and surgical manipulation has improved greatly. This goal of safe OPCAB and zero tolerance for conversion to CPB requires that every effort be made to ensure safety.

Patient conditioning

The first step in a successful OPCAB procedure begins before the incision is made. It is critical that the patient's hemodynamics be optimized to tolerate the stresses that surgical intervention will apply. To this end, patient hemodynamics must be "conditioned" adequately before any surgical manipulation of the heart. Thus, patients must have a normal heart rate (50 to 70 beats per minute), normal systemic and pulmonary arterial pressures, normothermia, and normal electrolytes. For these reasons, monitoring in the authors' institution includes radial arterial catheterization, central venous and Swan-Ganz catheterization, and transesophageal echocardiography (TEE) for all OPCAB cases. TEE permits the detection of new wall motion abnormalities that may indicate early myocardial ischemia. Pulmonary artery monitoring is used to follow diastolic pressures as an early indicator of cardiac ischemia; alternatives include direct left atrial or pulmonary arterial pressure monitoring. It is the role of the anesthesiologist to adjust the patient's filling pressures to achieve pulmonary arterial diastolic (PAD) pressures between 10 and 15 mmHg (Fig. 26-2). In patients with certain preoperative conditions (e.g., atrial fibrillation, left ventricular hypertrophy), higher PADs are tolerated, reflecting the need for higher filling pressures. This is the exception, however, and the vast majority of patients will have the safest operation with PADs in the lower range. As will be described below, during most of the anastomotic period the heart lies outside the pericardium and the triangle of Einthoven, making detection of ischemia by electrocardiography (ECG) and TEE more difficult. Hence, the authors use the Swan-Ganz catheter as the primary mechanism to detect, treat, and follow this occurrence.

Another important role of the anesthesiologist is to optimize myocardial oxygen metabolism; this is achieved primarily by maintaining a normal heart rate. Patients are beta-blocked adequately before surgery, with heart rates

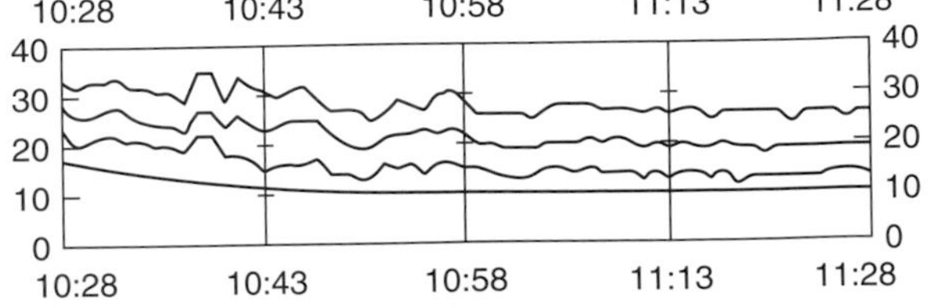

Figure 26-2 Anesthesia conditioning for OPCAB. Note that the pulmonary artery (PA) diastolic pressure is lowered from 18 to 10 before cardiac manipulation takes place. This tracing is from a PA catheter during mammary artery harvesting. (From Sergeant PL. Leuven, Belgium.)

usually maintained around 60 beats per minute (bpm). However, if a patient has a heart rate greater than 80 bpm, intravenous metoprolol is given to ensure that the heart is well protected from catecholamine surges. Any patient whose heart rate is below 60 bpm has atrial pacing wires placed and is paced atrially throughout the procedure. Atrioventricular sequential pacing is used for patients with additional conduction abnormalities. Oxygen demand is optimized through the strict avoidance of any inotropic medications, maintenance of filling pressures by leg elevation without Trendelenburg and volume infusion, and nitrates and alpha$_1$ agonists as needed to optimize coronary perfusion pressure.

Serum electrolytes and acid-base balance also must be normalized to minimize triggers of arrhythmias. Serum potassium levels are checked hourly and repleted if they are less than 4.0 meq/L as a protective measure against extrasystoles, atrial fibrillation, ventricular tachycardia, and ventricular fibrillation. In the authors' concept, extrasystoles [premature ventricular contractions(PVCs)] are considered abnormal and should never occur. When a PVC does occur, its etiology must be determined. The surgeon may have caused the PVC by touching the heart, and if this is the case, the anesthesiologist is notified and the operation proceeds. However, if the PVC was spontaneous, the patient's potassium level is checked. Levels below 4.0 meq/L are repleted, but if they already are in the normal range, the abnormal beat is considered ischemic in origin until proved otherwise. The ECG ST segments should be evaluated, as should the pulmonary artery (PA) diastolic pressure and TEE for wall motion abnormalities. Only when all the members of the team are convinced that there is no ongoing ischemia does the operation continue. The authors have noticed, for instance, that a slightly misplaced stabilizer device may occlude coronary vessels, causing ischemia, which manifests as multiple PVCs. Only by adhering to these stringent principles can problems be identified and corrected in a timely fashion, avoiding hemodynamic compromise in the patient.

The patient's body temperature is regulated by two means. First, the room is kept warm until the patient is prepped and draped. Subsequently, it may be lowered to a comfortable temperature for the surgical staff. Second, a heated water blanket is placed underneath the patient and maintained at 40°C throughout the procedure. With these techniques, it is rare for a patient to leave the operating theater with a core temperature below 36.3°C.

Incision

A median sternotomy is the incision of choice to perform OPCAB. This approach provides the most complete exposure for completion of all potential anastomoses while optimizing technical precision. Any coronary artery may be grafted with this exposure, and complex arterial reconstructions may be performed. Minimally invasive coronary artery bypass (MIDCAB) permits the use of a smaller minithoracotomy but is limited mainly to isolated revascularization of the anterior wall. More complex reconstructions are not possible. There also is concern that the quality of these anastomoses is reduced; this may translate into poorer long-term graft patency. For all these reasons, the authors strongly advocate a full median sternotomy for the optimal performance of OCPAB in all situations.

After the internal mammary artery (IMA) is mobilized from the chest wall, the pericardium is opened longitudinally, extending to the apex of the heart and completely along the diaphragm. The left pericardial edge is suspended from the retractor/drapes, but the right pericardial edge is left alone. This serves to rotate the heart slightly to the right, bringing the left anterior descending artery (LAD) closer to the midline of the operating field.

Conduit harvest

It is the standard of care to use at least one IMA for coronary revascularization. Usually the left IMA is harvested, but there are certain circumstances in which either right or bilateral IMA grafting is indicated. Patients with a patent dialysis shunt in the left upper extremity are at risk for a steal syndrome if a left IMA conduit is used. Also, an IMA should not be harvested ipsilateral to a subclavian artery stenosis. Patients with extensive atherosclerosis may benefit from angiography of the IMAs and the subclavian arteries during cardiac catheterizations. For younger patients who are not diabetic, many surgeons choose to use both IMAs to provide two pedicled arterial grafts; this technique has demonstrated long-term patency. The specific technique for taking the IMA off the chest wall is beyond the scope of this chapter. The authors routinely open the pleura during IMA harvest, but this is a matter of surgeon preference. The authors routinely leave the right pleura intact and do not place the heart into the right chest.

A reversed saphenous vein is the most common conduit for the remaining grafts. This conduit is easy to harvest, is usually in good supply, is easy to work with, and has well-documented long-term patency in most situations. Newer techniques of endoscopic harvesting have further popularized the use of the saphenous vein because this technique reduces lower extremity wound complications and discomfort dramatically.

Alternative choices for a conduit are generally more difficult to harvest, are often more difficult to work with, and have lower long-term patency rates. These choices include the lesser saphenous vein, the cephalic/basilic vein, a radial artery, the gastroepiploic artery, and cryopreserved vein. Only in situations in which conduit availability is severely limited should these other choices be considered.

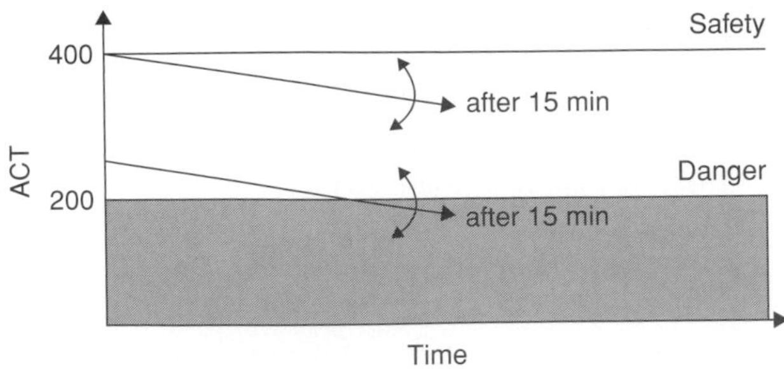

Figure 26-3 Anticoagulation safety. If an adequate level of heparinization is not maintained, the risk of thrombosis increases substantially. This can be exacerbated by infrequent monitoring of the activated clotting time during the anastomotic period. (From Sergeant PL. Leuven, Belgium.)

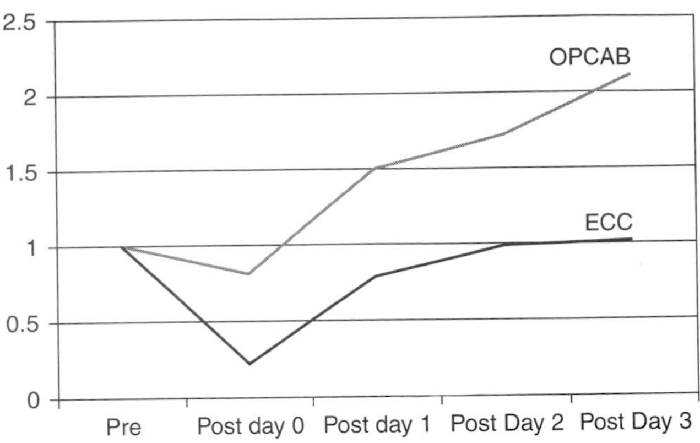

Figure 26-4 Hypercoagulable profile of OPCAB patients. These data represent coagulation indices (CI) compared to baseline for patients undergoing standard CABG surgery (ECC group) compared with OPCAB. As expected, the group on-pump has a reduction of the coagulation index perioperatively (more likely to bleed) secondary to the effects of cardiopulmonary bypass. This returns to normal by POD#3. In contrast, the OPCAB group does not have a perioperative reduction in the CI but ends up being significantly hypercoagulable. These results were obtained by thromboelastography. (Adapted from Quigley and associates.[14])

Anticoagulation

Anticoagulation consists of an intravenous heparin bolus administered at the completion of IMA harvesting to achieve a target activated clotting time (ACT) of 400 s or more; the heparin dose is usually 300 U/kg. ACT measurements are repeated every 20 min, and additional heparin is administered as necessary. Many authors in the OPCAB literature routinely use a target ACT of 250 s[10,11] despite a lack of evidence that this level is safe or prevents graft thrombosis. If the ACT level is too low to begin with or is not measured with adequate frequency, there is the potential for graft thrombosis (Fig. 26-3). Furthermore, some data suggest that patients undergoing OPCAB have intrinsic hypercoagulable states[12,13] (Fig. 26-4). The authors feel that full-dose heparin should be used in all circumstances during the anastomotic period to maximize graft patency. Because OPCAB patients do not develop coagulopathies related to cardiopulmonary bypass, the authors feel strongly that performing vascular anastomoses with only partial anticoagulation confers a significant risk of thrombotic complications. Full protamine reversal is instituted at the completion of all anastomoses.

Enucleation

In contrast to conventional CABG surgery, the left IMA to left anterior descending coronary artery is usually the first graft anastomosis performed in OPCAB procedures. This is the case because it is often the easiest to complete, requires minimal cardiac manipulation, and provides revascularization of the most critical myocardial region, conferring added protection from hemodynamic stability and arrhythmias during the remainder of the operation. The details of exposure for this anastomosis are described later in this chapter. After this step, the heart is enucleated from the pericardium so that the other coronaries may be visualized, stabilized, and grafted. This process is simple and consists of two parts.

First, a deep pericardial anchor stitch is placed with a long, heavy monofilament suture. The location of this stitch is of the utmost importance (Fig. 26-5). It should lie adjacent to the right inferior pulmonary vein, as far to the right as possible. This serves to lift the heart very effectively up out of the pericardium, bringing the

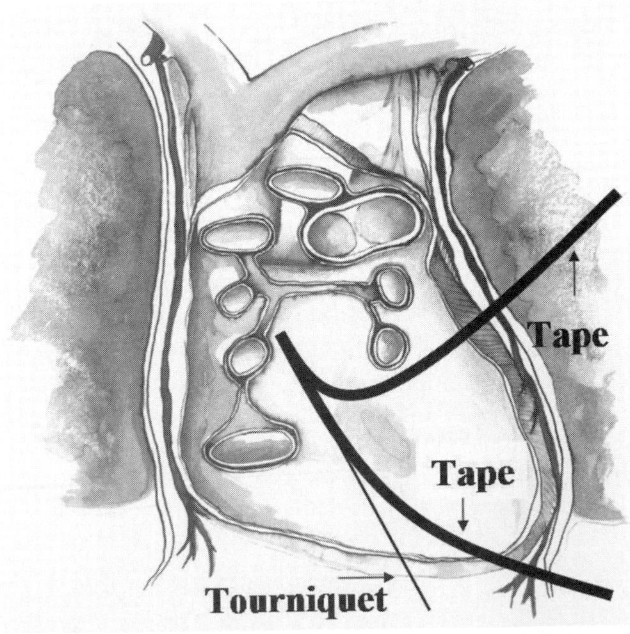

Figure 26-5 Position of anchor stitch. The anchor stitch should be placed as far to the right side as possible, adjacent to the right inferior pulmonary vein. (From Sergeant PL. Leuven, Belgium.)

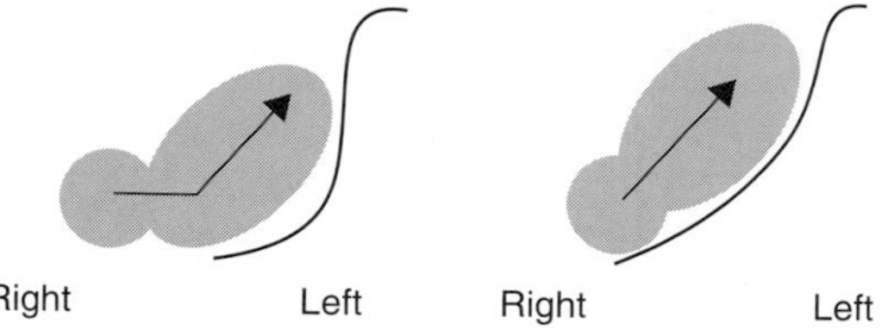

Figure 26-6 Axis between left atrium and left ventricle. Accurate placement of the anchor stitch ensures that the mitral valve remains competent during the enucleation process. (From Sergeant PL. Leuven, Belgium.)

atrioventricular groove closer to the surgeon. Even more important, however, is the fact that this position prevents any distortion of the atrioventricular axis so that mitral insufficiency is not created or worsened if it is already present (Fig. 26-6). A long sponge (opened up lengthwise) then is passed through the suture (Fig. 26-7), and a tourniquet is advanced until the sponge is at the anchor stitch.

Second, the two "arms" of the sponge are used to lift the heart up and out of the pericardium. The assistant slowly pulls up and toward the patient's left with both arms of the sling, making sure to keep the mass of the heart supported (Fig. 26-8). It is critical that this step be performed slowly (about 2 mm with each cardiac contraction) to ensure stable hemodynamics. If at any time the filling pressures rise or the sponge appears to be constricting the left ventricle, the arms are lowered and the process is repeated. It is very unusual for any problems to occur during this procedure, and in fact, the authors have noticed that the heart functions in a superb manner when elevated in this fashion. It is important after enucleation to readjust the right atrial filling pressures by means of leg elevation and volume infusion. The right ventricle should be inspected to make sure it does not distend as a result of malposition of the sling or the anchor stitch. Finally, the position of the sling on the left ventricular mass is checked and adjusted as needed; this may require subtle repositioning of the sling arms.

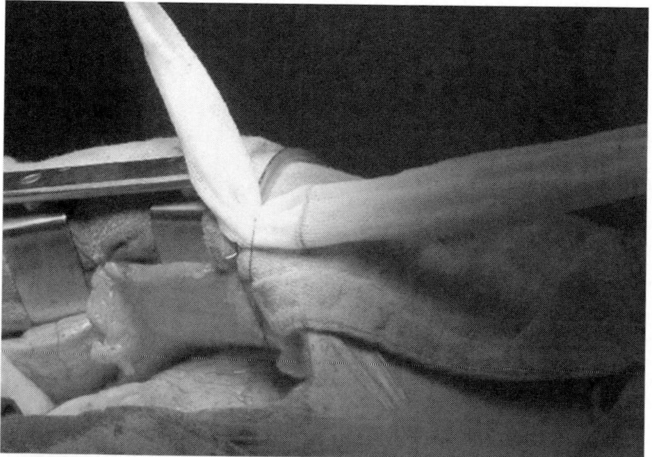

Figure 26-7 Sponge and tourniquet for enucleation. The tourniquet is advanced until the sponge rests at the anchor stitch against the posterior pericardium. (From Sergeant PL. Leuven, Belgium.)

Visualization

After successful enucleation, visualization is optimized in two steps: table rotation and apical suction. The operating table is rotated 30 degrees toward the surgeon (the patient's right), ensuring that the patient's right leg is protected from falling by a secured padded block (Fig. 26-9). A standard safety strap or belt would serve the same function. This table rotation causes the heart to move slightly toward the patient's right side, opening the space between the retractor and the lateral wall of the heart. Usually the circumflex marginal branches become visible after this step. It is important to remind the anesthesiologist to rezero the pulmonary arterial catheter transducer after this maneuver.

Next, the apical suction device is placed near the ventricular apex in an area devoid of coronary vessels to prevent occlusive ischemia (Fig. 26-10). Care must be taken to avoid the diaphragmatic surface of the heart, where the device may entrain air and become dislodged. With the apical suction device used in conjunction with the sling support, the authors have found that only 200 mmHg of suction is required to maintain contact with the heart. This low degree of suction has the added benefit of reducing epicardial trauma. The function of the apical device is threefold: axial stabilization, reformatting of the ventricle, and axial displacement. Axial stabilization occurs once the device is secured in the desired position while preserving the ability of the heart for rotational contractility. After suction is applied to the apical suction device, the ventricular shape is reformatted from a globular to a more normal configuration (Fig. 26-11) by gently pulling the heart anteriorly. Unpublished data from sheep hearts have demonstrated that the combination of the apical suction device and sling support increases both contractility and relaxation by 20 percent (Fig. 26-12). While the ventricle is maintained in its optimal configuration, the axis is displaced both superiorly and to the patient's right (in the direction of the patient's right shoulder). This allows adequate exposure of lateral wall vessels while avoiding right-sided filling impairment from kinking or compression.

Stabilization

The final preparation before the first coronary arteriotomy is made involves stabilization of the specific target coronary vessel. This has become much easier with the development of newer stabilizing devices over the last 4 to 5 years. These devices usually require 450 mmHg of

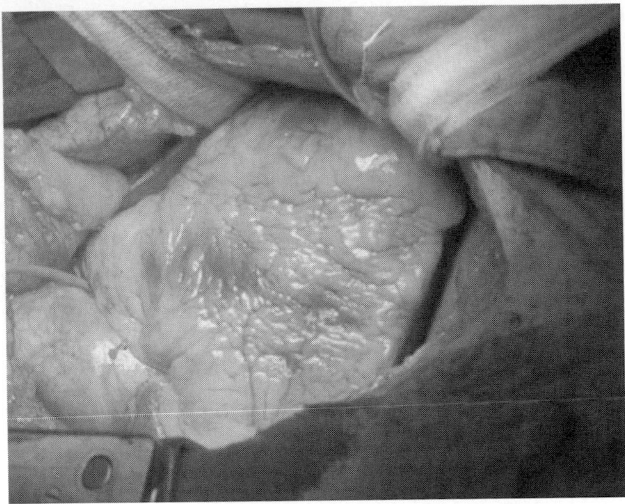

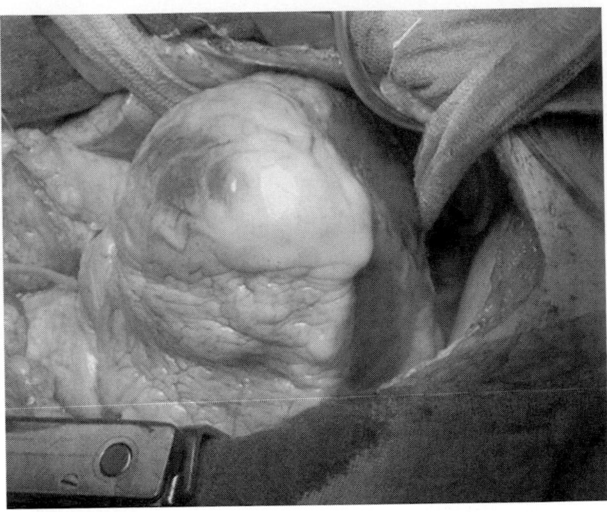

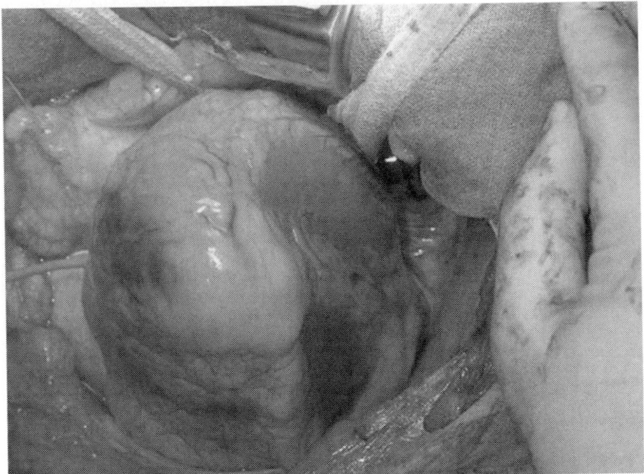

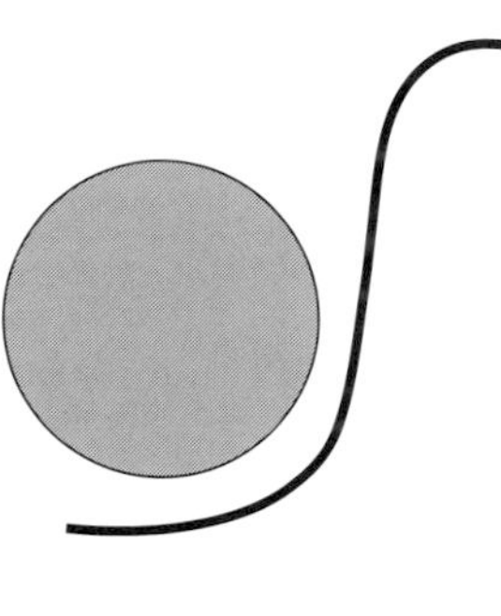

Figure 26-8 Enucleation of the heart from the pericardium. As the arms of the sponge are pulled to the left, the heart rises out of the pericardium. This should be done slowly and should proceed without difficulty even with enlarged hearts or in patients with reduced ejection fractions. Note that the heart is globular and not in its normal configuration. (From Sergeant PL. Leuven, Belgium.)

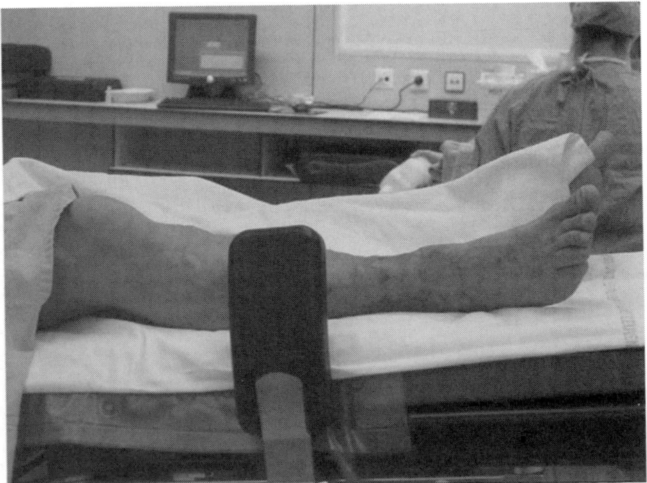

Figure 26-9 Protective leg block. This padded block is fastened securely to the operating table and prevents the patient's right leg from falling during table rotation toward the surgeon. A safety strap could serve in a similar fashion. (From Peck EA, Sergeant PL. Leuven, Belgium.)

suction to stabilize the heart for a technically perfect anastomosis. In addition to the stabilizer, 4-0 braided sutures can be placed superficially in the epicardium adjacent to the coronary artery target and placed under gentle traction with hemostats to enhance the stabilization. A number of strategies may be employed in light of the particular anatomy confronted during this step (Fig. 26-13). It is important not to apply suction directly over a coronary artery, however, as this may result in ischemia. A technique that often helps prevent this problem involves placing bone wax in one or two of the suction holes that must lie atop a coronary artery (Fig. 26-14).

Exposure of all target coronaries is identical with the exception of the LAD and the right coronary proximal to the take-off of the posterior descending artery. Because the LAD anastomosis is performed first, the sling support and apical suction are not placed initially. After the pericardium is suspended, additional horizontal sutures are placed along the lateral aspect of the left pericardium from cephalad to caudad, pulled anteriorly, and fastened to the surgical drapes (Fig. 26-15). This rotates the heart about 15 degrees toward the midline and

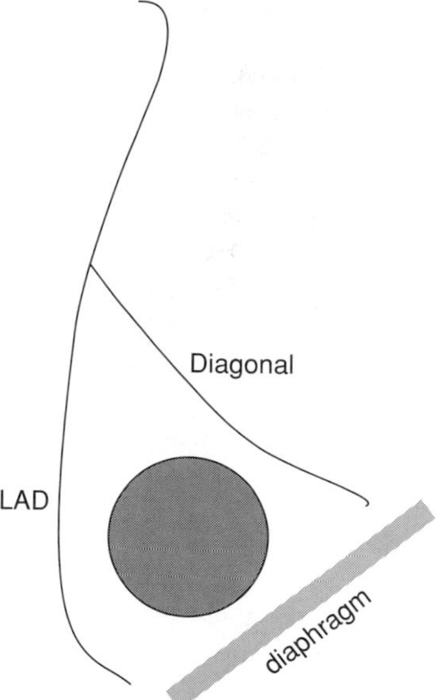

Figure 26-10 Placement of an apical suction device. The device should be placed near the apex, ensuring that no coronary vessel is occluded and avoiding the diaphragmatic surface of the heart, where it is prone to sucking air and becoming dislodged. (From Sergeant PL. Leuven, Belgium.)

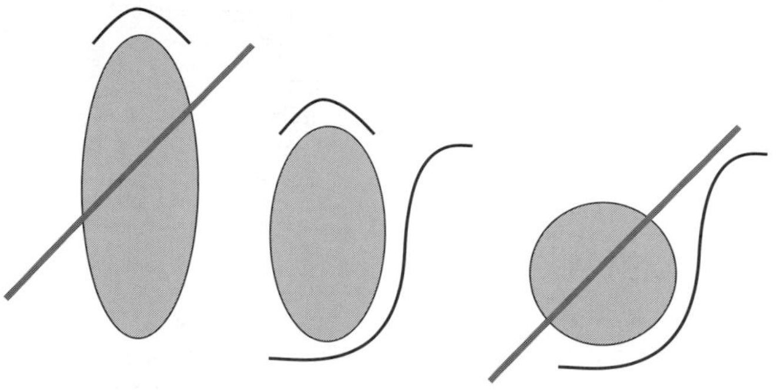

Figure 26-11 Ventricular reformatting with the apical suction device. The combination of sling support and apical suction provides the optimal ventricular format, translating into normal contractility and relaxation. (From Sergeant PL. Leuven, Belgium.)

brings the LAD into the middle of the operative field. At this point, target stabilization may proceed, followed by coronary shunting and completion of the graft anastomosis. In certain circumstances, diagonal vessels also may be revascularized using this exposure. However, if they lie more toward the lateral wall, the standard enucleation exposure is preferred.

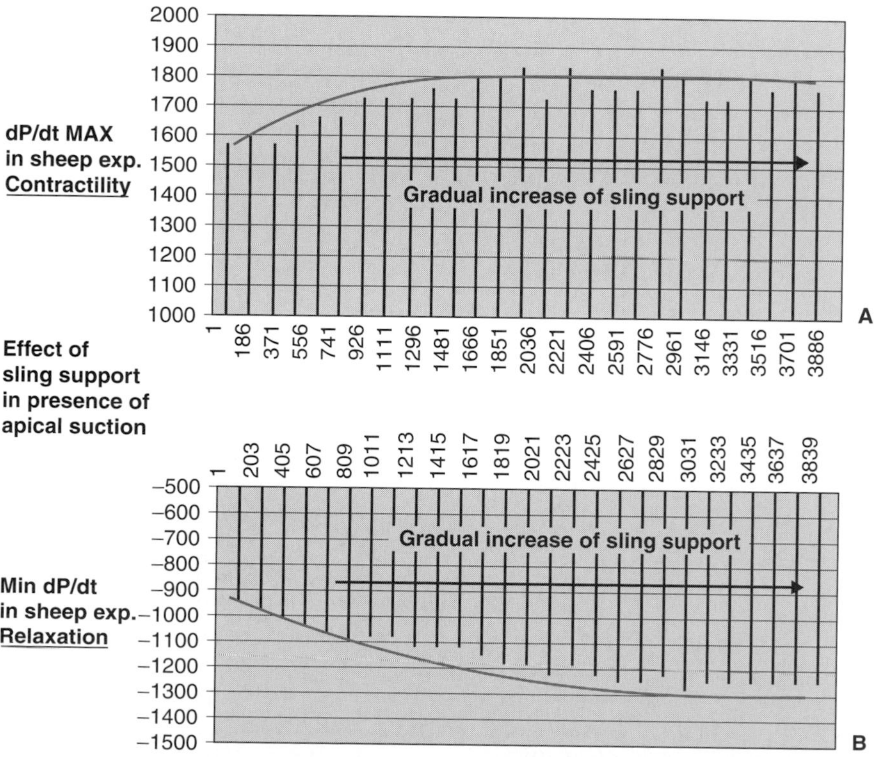

Figure 26-12 Improved ventricular function with the combination of apical suction and sling support. Apical suction alone does not provide for optimal ventricular performance. As demonstrated in an in vivo sheep model, there is a 20 percent improvement in both contractility and relaxation when sling support is added to apical suction. (From unpublished data from Sergeant PL. Leuven, Belgium.)

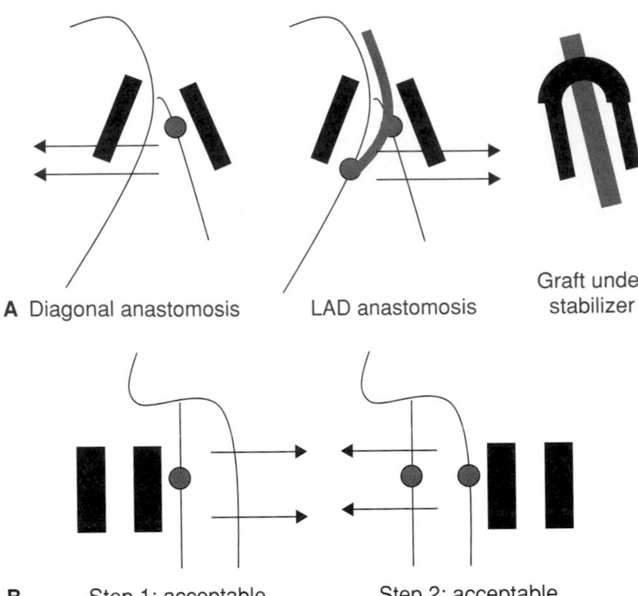

Figure 26-13 Stabilization strategies with a combination of a suction device and epicardial traction sutures. Both parts demonstrate various combinations of stabilizer placement/configuration and epicardial retraction sutures to stabilize the target coronary while avoiding compressive ischemia. (From Sergeant PL. Leuven, Belgium.)

The exposure of the right coronary proximal to the posterior descending coronary artery is also unique. Similar to exposure of the LAD, this is performed without the sling support or the apical suction device. Epicardial traction sutures are placed on the inferior wall near the acute margin and pulled in a cephalad direction, bringing the right coronary more anteriorly and into view (Fig. 26-16). This allows for target coronary stabilization with a combination of the suction stabilizer and additional epicardial traction sutures (Fig. 26-17).

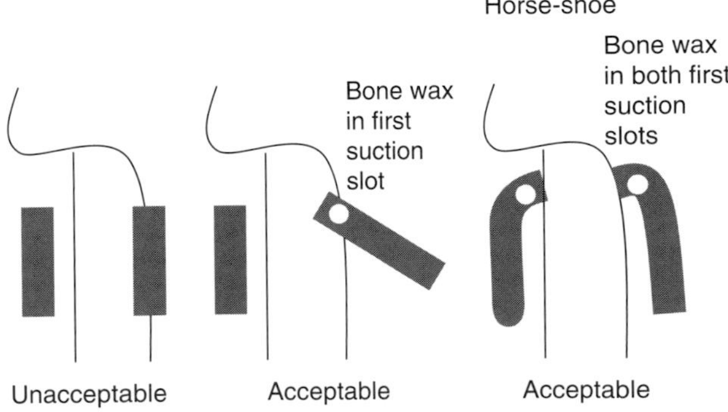

Figure 26-14 Use of bone wax to prevent suction over coronary artery during stabilization. Selective use of bone wax to occlude suction holes on the stabilizer allows optimal stabilization for complex anatomical situations. (From Sergeant PL. Leuven, Belgium.)

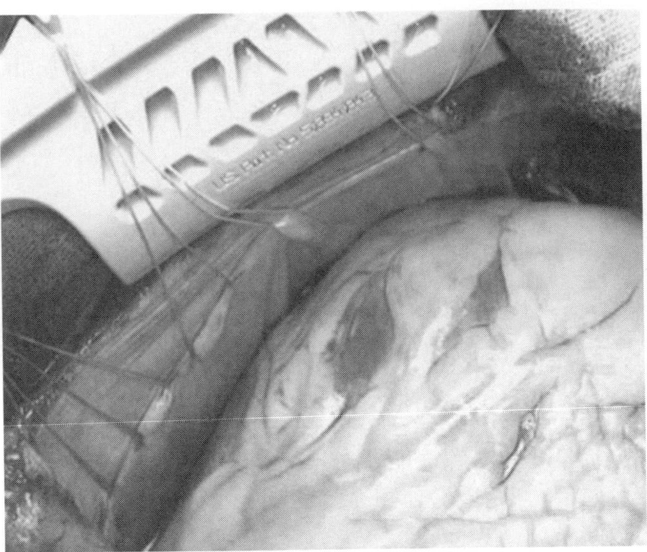

Figure 26-15 Placement of pericardial sutures for left anterior descending artery (LAD) exposure. Placement of lateral sutures in the left pericardium will rotate the heart so that the LAD is in the middle of the operative field and ready for stabilization. (From Sergeant PL. Leuven, Belgium.)

Shunt insertion

The primary objective of placing an intracoronary shunt during anastomotic construction is the avoidance or minimization of ischemia. Some surgeons never shunt,

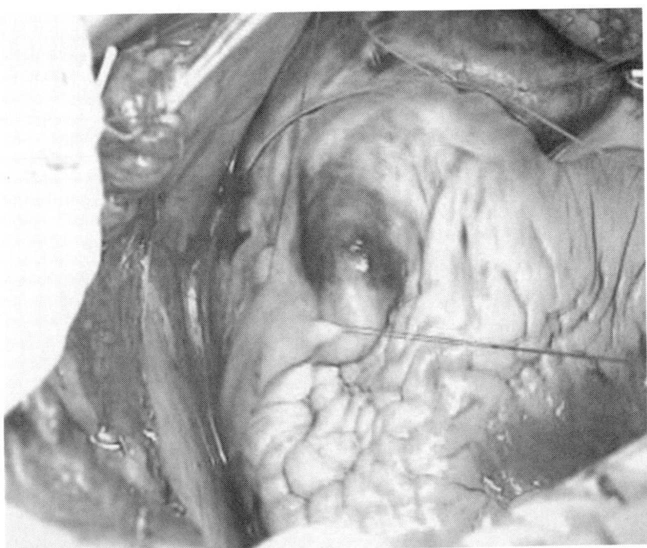

Figure 26-16 Placement of epicardial sutures to expose the right coronary artery. Epicardial sutures placed near the acute margin and placed under traction elevate the proximal right coronary into view for stabilization. (From Sergeant PL. Leuven, Belgium.)

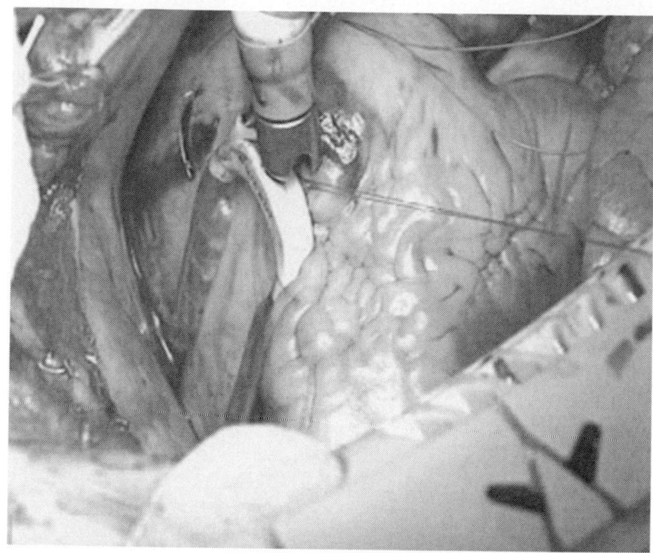

Figure 26-17 Stabilization of the right coronary artery. This image demonstrates stabilization of the right coronary artery proximal to the posterior descending. Note the combination of epicardial traction sutures and target vessel stabilizer. There is no sling support for this exposure. (From Sergeant PL. Leuven, Belgium.)

some do selectively, and some shunt with every anastomosis.[14,15] The authors firmly believe in the third approach. The techniques described in this chapter are focused on reducing risk at every step to avoid hemodynamic instability and conversion to CPB. Thus, a shunt should be used for every anastomosis. The majority of coronary anastomoses probably can be completed safely without shunting. However, it is not possible to predict when shunting will be needed to avoid ischemic complications; thus, the only way to minimize risk fully is to shunt every time.

Flow through a shunt varies according to its internal diameter. All shunt sizes greater than 1.00 mm provide adequate blood flow to the distal coronary territory[16] (Fig. 26-18). The maintenance of distal coronary flow has been further demonstrated to preserve myocardial function compared with temporary coronary occlusion.[17–20] This translates into a more stable operative environment and lower stress for the surgical team and also facilitates the construction of a technically perfect coronary anastomosis.

A frequently unmentioned advantage of placing intracoronary shunts is the improved visibility and exposure of the coronary artery walls. The shunt not only serves to keep blood out of the anastomotic area, it also keeps the vessel open to prevent suturing the back wall and improves visualization of the toe and heel areas. Furthermore, careful manipulation of the shunt can facilitate technically challenging anastomoses by opening space between the coronary wall and the shunt itself.

The main criticism of routine shunt placement during OPCAB is concern about endothelial damage; this concern is supported in the literature.[15,21] For surgeons who choose not to shunt, the alternative is to occlude the

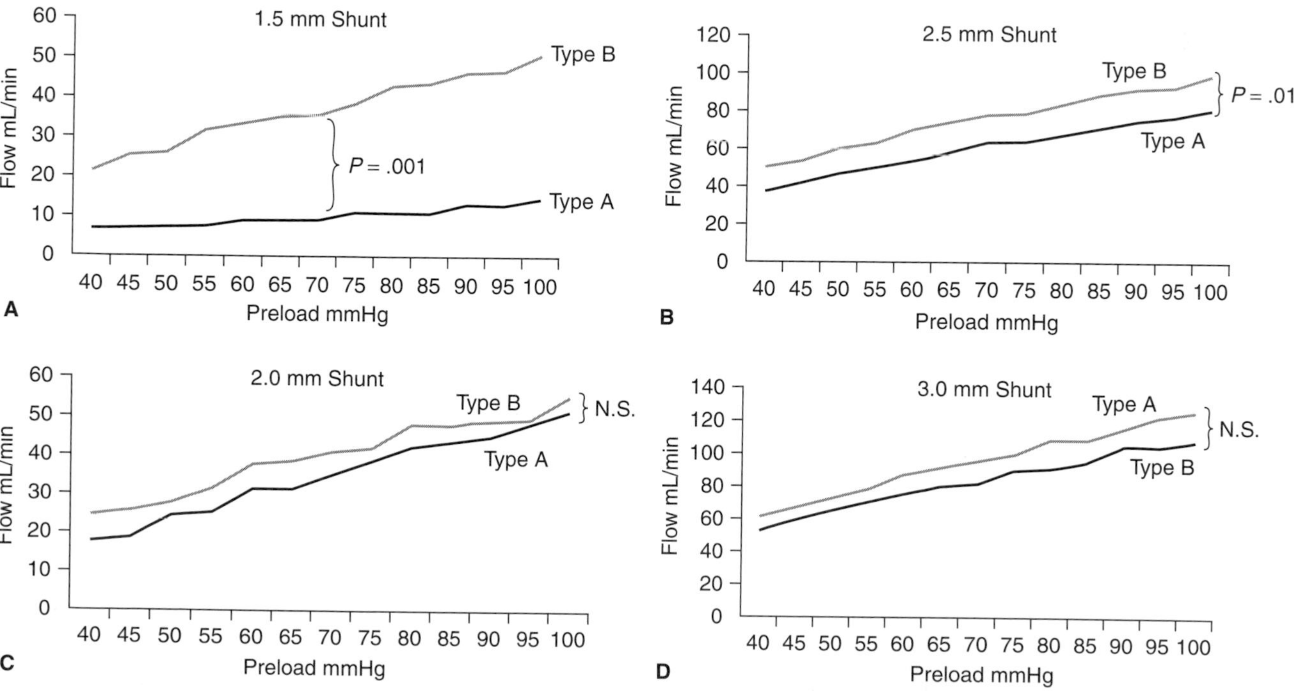

Figure 26-18 Effect of internal shunt diameter on flow. These graphs depict flow through a shunt with a given diameter at various levels of preload (pressure). Shunts A and B are from different manufacturers. Data for shunts of 1.00 mm are not shown as only minimal flow was measured across all levels of preload. (From Grunenfelder and associates.[16])

coronary with Silastic slings and use a CO_2 blower/mister. However, when studies have compared endothelial damage resulting from shunts with damage from vessel occlusion, shunts appear to be less traumatic.[22] In addition, the blower/mister device has been associated with severe complications, including endothelial damage and air embolism.[23] In considering all the risks and benefits of shunting for OPCAB, the authors believe the data firmly support the routine use of shunts to facilitate a safer procedure and the creation of technically perfect anastomoses.

Certainly, it also is reasonable to expect that the shunt insertion technique influences the degree of intimal disruption. The tip of the shunt should be placed in a "gooseneck" orientation rather than being pushed directly in, minimizing intimal trauma. The longer of the two shunt ends always is inserted first. The direction, whether proximal or distal, in which to insert the long end depends on the coronary anatomy. It should be placed away from coronary branches so that it will not lead to selective perfusion. These techniques are not part of routine surgical training, often need to be performed with the surgeon's nondominant hand, and can be challenging. For this reason, it is recommended that this technique be practiced in a model, re-creating the various angles and narrow spaces that will be encountered during OPCAB surgery (Fig. 26-19). This enhances the surgeon's skill and ease at placing shunts so that the risks will be minimized during an actual operation.

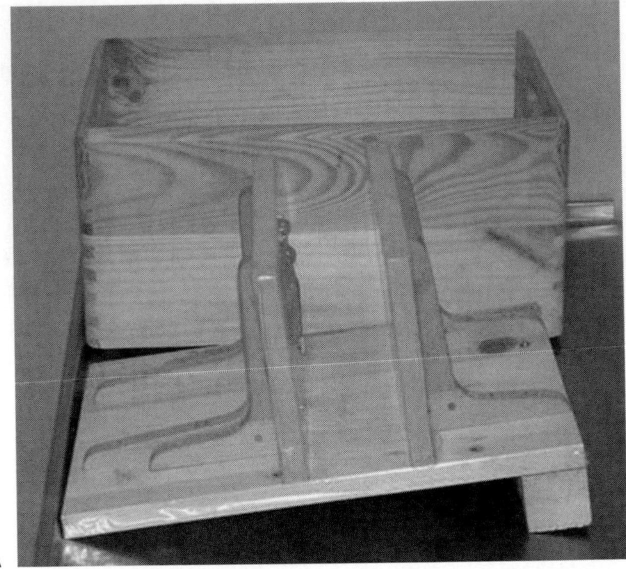

A

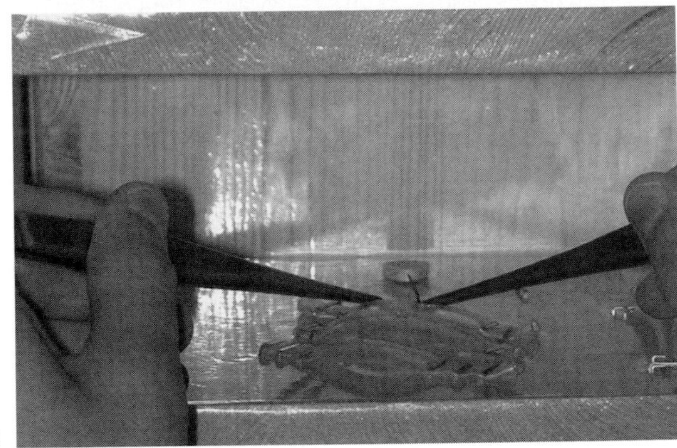

B

Figure 26-19 Use of training box to learn shunt insertion technique. This box allows the learning of shunt insertion technique. It re-creates the angles and narrow spaces encountered during OPCAB surgery. The authors' practice is to perform at least 1000 shunt insertions in this box before placement in a human. (From Sergeant PL. Leuven, Belgium.)

Distal anastomoses

This is the final common step for each target vessel. For IMA conduits the authors recommend 8-0 polypropylene sutures and use 7-0 polypropylene for saphenous vein conduits. In the following paragraphs, a brief summary of the exposure and graft technique is given.

The LAD most often is revascularized first as it is the easiest to perform and, once completed, permits OPCAB to proceed more safely. Good exposure of lateral wall coronary targets requires that the heart be enucleated after placement of the deep pericardial anchoring stitch and sling support. Visualization is enhanced with table rotation and axial stabilization/displacement with the apical suction device, facilitating stabilization of the circumflex marginal vessels, although in a somewhat narrow space (Fig. 26-20). This space can be optimized by refinements in positioning the axial stabilizer, further widening of the sternal retractor, and adjustment of the vessel stabilizer itself. Opening of the right pleura with placement of the heart in the right chest is not only unnecessary but potentially harmful if venous return is impeded.

The inferior wall vessels (posterolateral and posterior descending arteries) are performed similarly, usually after completion of lateral wall grafts. The heart is enucleated, and apical suction is applied with displacement of the heart superiorly and to the right. This brings the inferior wall into a vertical alignment away from the diaphragm and allows for target vessel stabilization. The exposure of the right coronary proximal to the posterior descending (mid-right coronary artery) has been described and does not require enucleation or apical suction (Fig. 26-16).

Proximal anastomoses

Standard techniques of partial aortic occlusion for construction of the proximal graft anastomoses suffice for OPCAB as well. These connections are completed with 6-0 polypropylene suture in the standard fashion and will not be discussed further here.

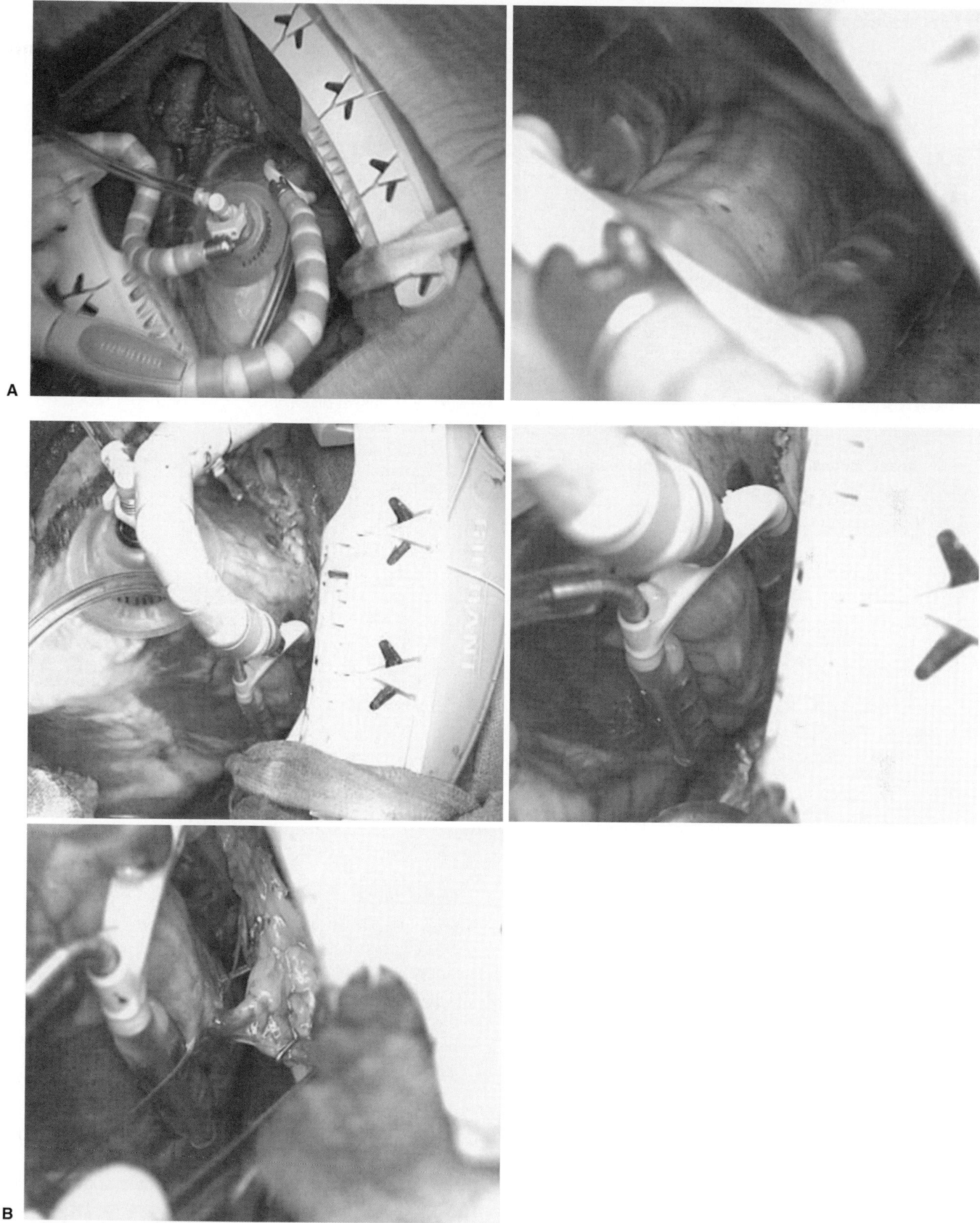

Figure 26-20 Exposure, stabilization, and anastomosis of lateral wall vessels. A. These represent operative field and close-up views of the first obtuse marginal branch being stabilized for subsequent grafting. Note the nearly vertical orientation of the coronary and the narrow space between the vessel and the sternal retractor. These anastomoses are technically more challenging but can be facilitated by practice in a training box that re-creates this environment. B. These represent exposure and stabilization of the second obtuse marginal branch. The last picture in this series shows the end of a free right internal mammary artery graft anastomosed to the coronary. (From Sergeant PL. Leuven, Belgium.)

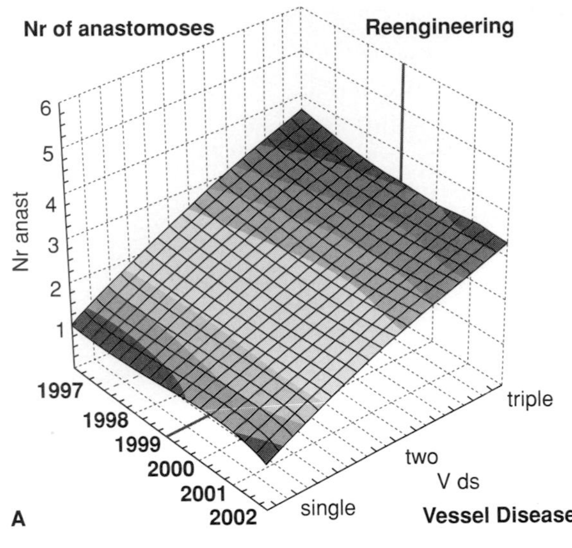

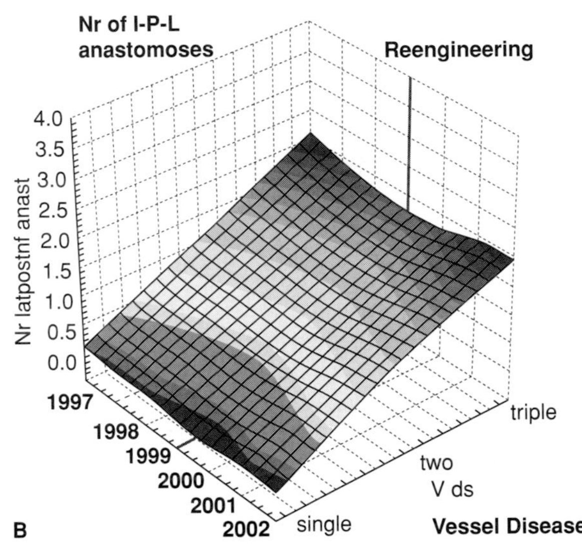

Figure 26-21 A. Number of anastomoses, including lateral wall, with OPCAB. The number of anastomoses per patient has not changed since the conversion to OPCAB in mid-1999. B. Although there was an early decrease in lateral wall anastomoses after the transition to OPCAB, that number has returned to the previous level. I-P-L: inferior, posterior, and lateral wall. (From Sergeant PL. Leuven, Belgium.)

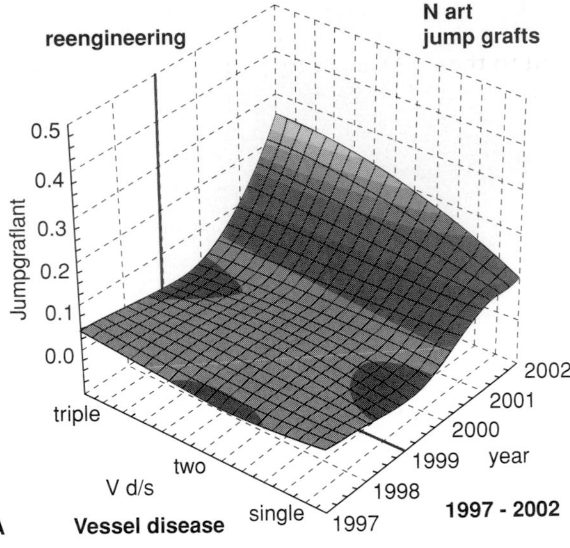

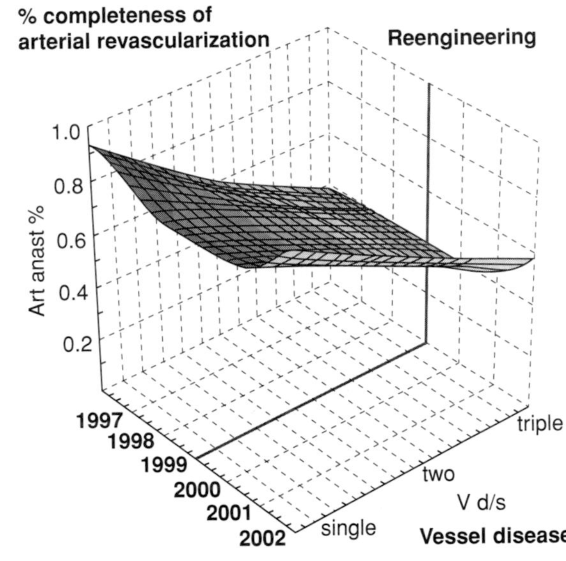

Figure 26-22 Use of arterial grafts and all-arterial revascularization. A. This graph shows that the use of sequential arterial grafts has increased dramatically at KU Leuven since the reengineering of the unit toward OPCAB. B. These data demonstrate that all-arterial grafting did not suffer from the switch to OPCAB. In fact, in the most recent year this percentage increased significantly. (From Sergeant PL. Leuven, Belgium.)

Revascularization strategies

A frequent criticism of OPCAB is that fewer anastomoses are performed, especially on the lateral wall. In inexperienced hands this may be true, but with a technique that is safe and effective, all potential coronary targets should be accessible. Figure 26-21 shows data from KU Leuven pertaining to this issue before and after the transition to OPCAB.

The performance of OPCAB also does not preclude the surgeon from completing an all-arterial revascularization. In contrast, the concept of reducing complications while maximizing benefit in OPCAB is concordant with this strategy, and it is technically feasible to do so. Unless a patient is extremely morbidly obese or older than age 80 years, the authors prefer to use bilateral IMAs with the right mammary artery being a free graft, sequentially grafted around the lateral and inferior walls. Since the authors' transition to OPCAB surgery, the percentage of arterial anastomoses and all-arterial revascularization has increased dramatically (Fig. 26-22).

At KU Leuven, the authors avoid all manipulation of the aorta whenever possible to reduce the risk of embolic stroke. For this reason, the standard coronary revascularization scheme consists of the left IMA grafted to the LAD and a free right IMA graft taken off the proximal left IMA and sequentially anastomosed around the lateral and inferior walls. If there is a contraindication for the use of bilateral IMA grafts, the saphenous vein is used. In an elderly patient with significant comorbid conditions and a good-quality small-caliber vein, this also may be taken off the proximal left IMA before being sequenced around the lateral and inferior walls. When the left IMA is used as an inflow source for a free graft, the anastomosis is placed as proximal on the left IMA as possible, where the vessel caliber is maximal; a shunt also is placed to ensure a technically perfect anastomosis. There has been no increased incidence of LIMA-to-LAD graft failure as a consequence of this strategy. In some cases, though, there is no alternative to placing a graft on the ascending aorta. In this situation, the surgeon can avoid placing a partial occlusion clamp by using novel technologies such as HeartString or other connector devices that are less likely to shower emboli.

OUTCOMES

Literature

It is important to remember that in reviewing the literature regarding a specific surgical technique, the data represent the specific technique described and must be powered adequately for the reader to draw conclusions. It is easy to make any technique appear unsuccessful if it is performed by inexperienced surgeons or if the components of the operation are not the most effective. Furthermore, outcomes cannot be evaluated if the specific technique has not involved all measures to eliminate risk. Conclusions pertain only to the exact circumstances that existed in the study.

A large proportion of the data that follow are from KU Leuven and represent a comparison between two groups: before and after reengineering to OPCAB. The data are representative of the entire surgical unit, not a particular surgeon, but the OPCAB technique is identical for each one by protocol. These data indicate how good outcomes are possible when a good, safe technique is employed in a large number of patients by an experienced team. Simple modifications such as using lower heparin dosing and selective rather than routine shunting probably would lead to less favorable outcomes. Most of the figures shown below depict data that trend toward benefit but do not achieve statistical significance unless noted. This does not imply that the data are not significant. Instead, with the small differences between outcomes that occur only in a small percentage of patients, the power calculations would require each group to have as many as 10,000 or 100,000 patients.

Mortality

A number of studies have documented a significant improvement in mortality in OPCAB patients compared with on-pump CABG,[24–28] as do data from KU Leuven (Figs. 26-23 and 26-24). Risk cannot be reduced when none is present. Therefore, low-risk patients tend not to have a mortality benefit from OPCAB. However, for patients with increasing risk, here defined by Euroscore,

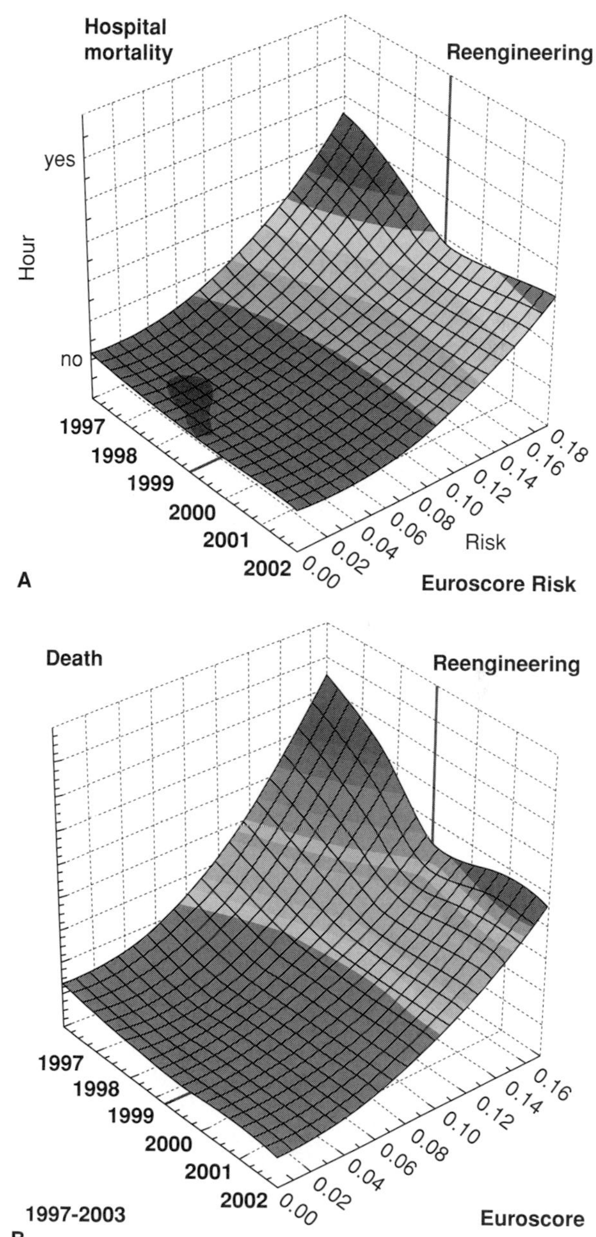

Figure 26-23 Improved mortality with OPCAB compared with CABG on-pump. A. In-hospital mortality has improved since the conversion to OPCAB for patients at higher risk. B. Three-month mortality also has improved (20 percent relative risk reduction) for these patients. (From Sergeant PL. Leuven, Belgium.)

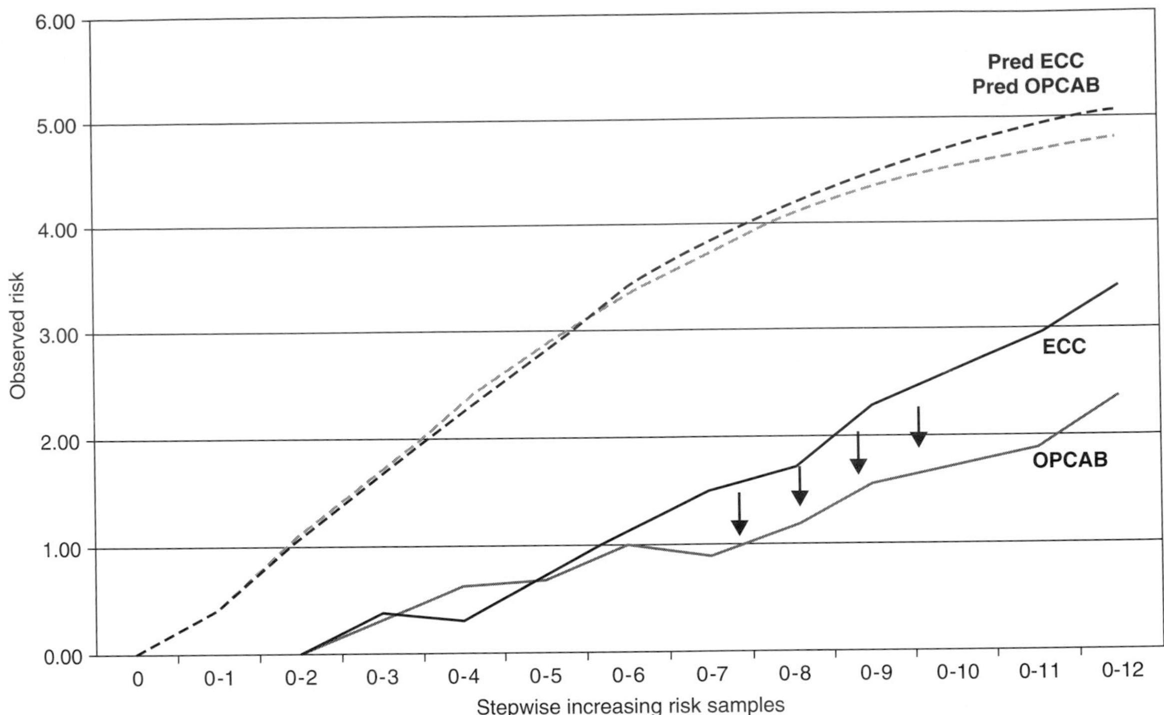

Figure 26-24 Comparison of expected to observed mortality. This graph shows that patients with CABG on-pump (ECC) have much better mortality than predicted on the basis of risk. Observed mortality in OPCAB patients is even better than that for the ECC group in patients with increasing risk. Note: Expected mortality was the same for both groups. (From Sergeant PL. Leuven, Belgium.)

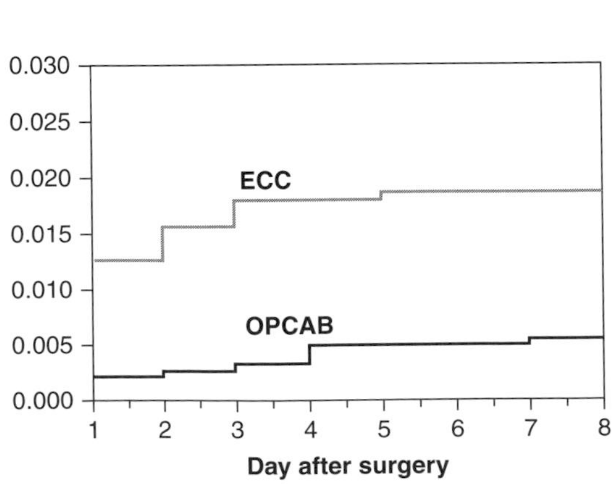

Figure 26-25 Incidence of stroke by postoperative day. Stroke still occurs in patients undergoing OPCAB, but the number of events occurring within surgery is reduced dramatically. Postoperative strokes probably occur secondary to hypotension and atrial fibrillation with cerebral embolization. (From Sergeant PL. Leuven, Belgium.)

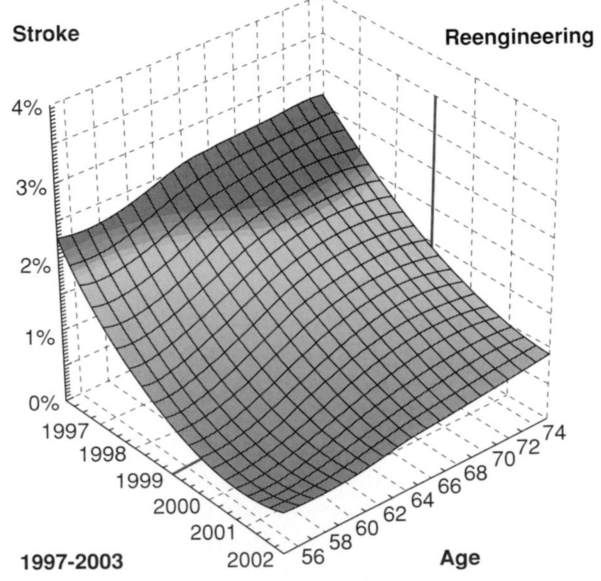

Figure 26-26 Incidence of stroke by age. The incidence of stroke has declined across all age groups (60 percent relative risk reduction) since reengineering to OPCAB. (From Sergeant PL. Leuven, Belgium.)

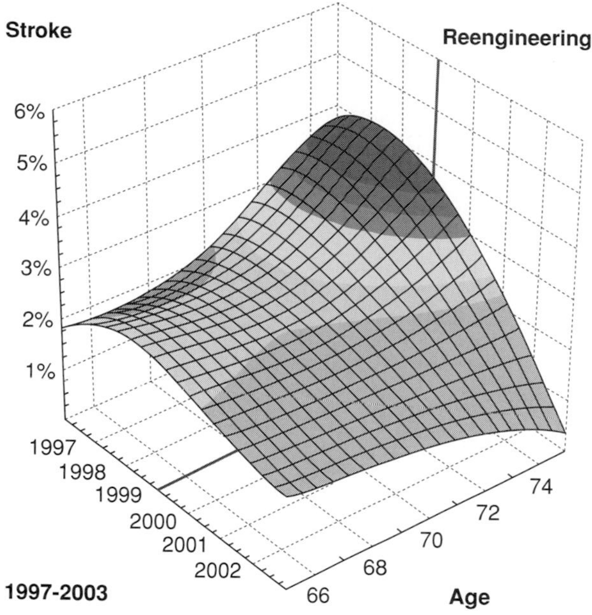

Figure 26-27 Stroke rate in high-risk patients. These data represent patients with preoperative carotid stenosis greater than 80 percent. This cohort consists of 200 patients in each group and achieves statistical significance ($p = 0.02$) with a relative risk reduction of 68 percent. (From Sergeant PL. Leuven, Belgium.)

the improvement in mortality, both in hospital and at 3 months, is substantial.

Morbidity

Avoidance of cardiopulmonary bypass and its associated complications tends to result in improvements in outcomes for all organ systems. Below is a summary of the literature pertaining to this along with data from KU Leuven.

Neurologic

This category includes two distinct areas of injury: stroke and neurocognitive dysfunction. Stroke is a more clearly defined outcome, and because of its low incidence, it is difficult to demonstrate an improvement without very large patient cohorts. Nonetheless, various studies in the literature have demonstrated either equivalent[29–31] or reduced[32–36] stroke rates for patients undergoing OPCAB compared with those receiving on-pump CABG. Similarly, data from KU Leuven show that intraoperative stroke essentially has been eliminated by the routine performance of OPCAB. Postoperative strokes still occur as a result of hypotension and atrial fibrillation with cerebral embolization (Fig. 26-25). Lower stroke risk is also evident when stroke is stratified according to patient age (Fig. 26-26). These data become statistically significant when patients at high risk for stroke are compared (Fig. 26-27).

Pulmonary

This category often is represented by the "time to extubation" metric. Many OPCAB centers have demonstrated significantly reduced extubation times that translate into shorter lengths of stay in the intensive care unit (ICU).[37–39] Furthermore, a number of reports have advocated the safe extubation of OPCAB patients in the operating room at the conclusion of the procedure.[40,41]

Cardiac

These complications can be separated into myocardial infarction (MI) and enzyme release not associated with acute infarction. Graft failure also can be included in this

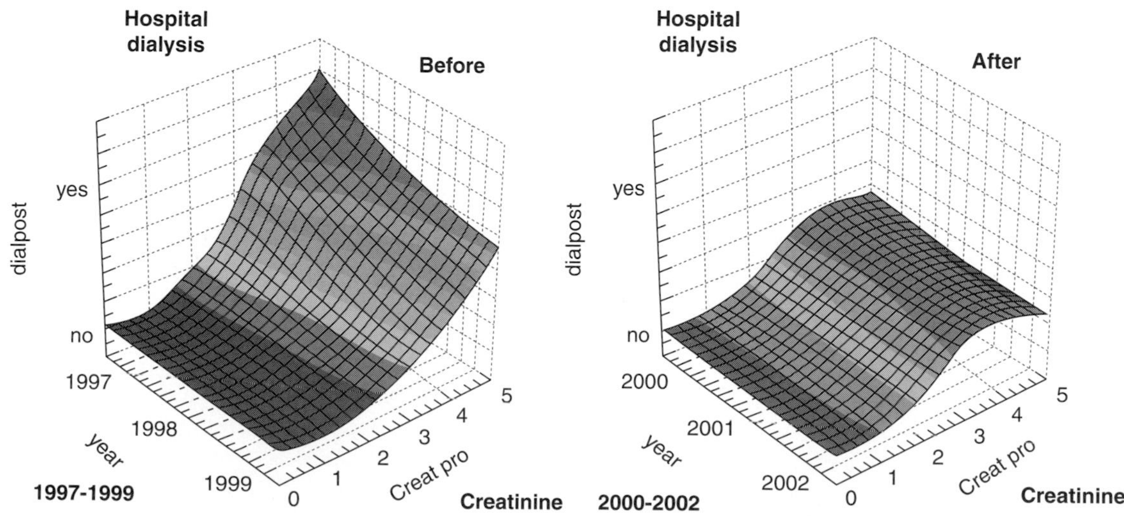

Figure 26-28 Reduction in renal complications with OPCAB. Since the reengineering to OPCAB, patients have experienced a 26 percent relative risk reduction in the need for hemodialysis or ultrafiltration. For this level of benefit to achieve statistical significance, 11,000 patients would be needed in each group. Notice, however, that for patients most at risk (creatinine 4 to 5 mg/dL), the incidence of postop dialysis is reduced up to 50 percent. (From Sergeant PL. Leuven, Belgium.)

subsection because acute graft occlusion often leads to infarction. Although many studies have demonstrated no difference in the incidence of perioperative MI[42–44] with OPCAB, some authors have found a reduction in this event in patients undergoing OPCAB.[26,45] Logic dictates that avoiding ischemic cardioplegic arrest will reduce myocardial injury during CABG procedures. Data from KU Leuven do not reveal any reduction in the incidence of MI in OPCAB patients.

The significance of elevated troponin values after OPCAB remains uncertain. Certainly, no data about the "normal" levels of troponin after this procedure are conclusive. A few studies have investigated enzyme release after OPCAB,[42,46–52] and the results seem to indicate a trend toward reduced troponin levels but no specific correlation with reduced infarct rates.

Graft failure rates with OPCAB generally seem to be equivalent to those for conventional on-pump CABG.[53,54] One article that placed international focus on poor graft patency in OPCAB[10] demonstrated only that the specific technique used by those authors and performed by those surgeons was less than satisfactory. This finding should not be generalized to a belief that all OPCAB procedures are doomed to similarly poor outcomes with respect to graft failure. Only by minimizing risk and maximizing safety (e.g., full anticoagulation, use of intracoronary shunts) can the full benefits of OPCAB be realized.

Renal

Perhaps the area of greatest benefit in OPCAB patients is the renal system. Patients with preexisting renal dysfunction who undergo conventional CABG have a significant propensity for postoperative renal complications, including temporary or permanent hemodialysis. For patients with normal kidney function, the risks are quite low, and thus, OPCAB results suggest no benefit. However, in high-risk cohorts it has been proved clearly that avoiding CPB leads to dramatically reduced renal complications.[55–59] This is in agreement with data from KU Leuven, which have shown a 26 percent reduction in the relative risk for postoperative hemodialysis or ultrafiltration (Fig. 26-28).

Hematologic

The literature supports the notion that OPCAB patients experience less blood loss from surgery in addition to having lower transfusion requirements.[24,60–62] Presumably, this is a result of less severe coagulation disturbances in these patients, most notably with respect to platelet dysfunction.

Length of stay

The performance of OPCAB has been shown to reduce the length of stay of cardiac surgical patients.[63–65] This probably is a result of reduced systemic inflammation, decreased fluid requirements, and quicker time to extubation. Furthermore, lower morbidity rates also lead to earlier patient discharge from the hospital. Evidence from KU Leuven supports these findings as well, especially when patients are stratified by age or Euroscore (Fig. 26-29).

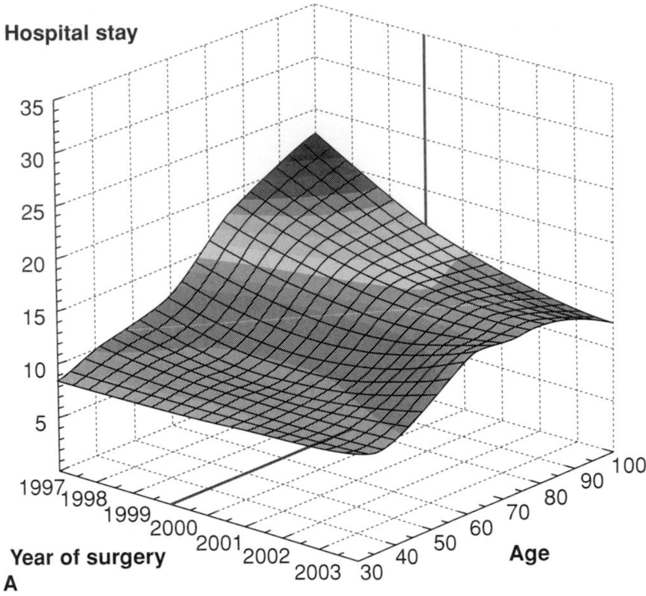

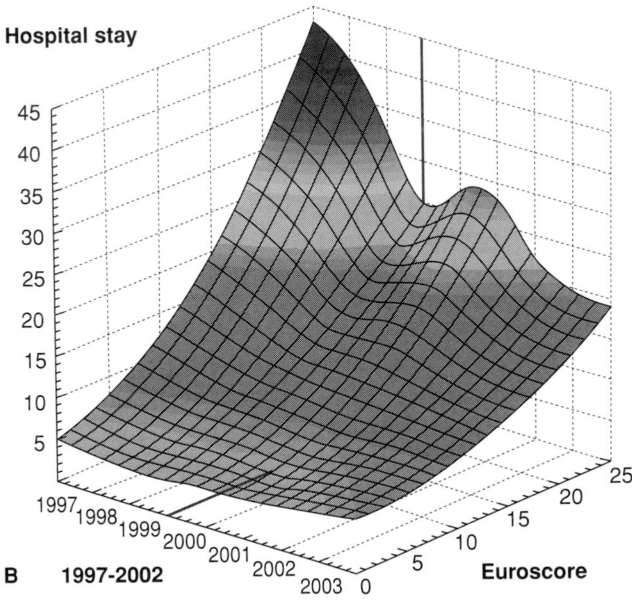

Figure 26-29 Length of stay as a function of patient age and Euroscore. A. There is a statistically significant improvement in length of stay ($p = 0.02$) in patients undergoing OPCAB. This is only a 5 percent improvement for the entire cohort, but with hospital discharge being an outcome present for all patients, small differences can be significant. B. Similarly, when stratified by Euroscore, the transition to OPCAB has reduced hospital stay as well. (From Sergeant PL. Leuven, Belgium.)

Cost

Economic savings in OPCAB patients are realized by two means: (1) small, production-line advantages that result from every patient undergoing surgery (e.g., reduced operating room charges, reduced personnel charges) and (2) large savings in a small number of patients who avoid severe complications (e.g., reduced incidence of stroke and renal failure). Therefore, OPCAB can lead to dramatic cost savings. The literature supports this.[6,7,66–68]

SUMMARY

OPCAB is much more than a simple alternative to conventional CABG surgery without the assistance of CPB. It is a concept that emphasizes patient safety and long-term benefit. To achieve this, a multidisciplinary approach must be employed, involving nursing, anesthesia, and surgery. When all efforts are made to minimize risk and provide a stress-free operating room environment, great benefit for the patient may be achieved. Although there is some disagreement in the literature about short- and long-term outcomes with OPCAB, one must be cognizant of the specific techniques used and the experience of the surgeons involved in a study. There is surely more than one successful OPCAB technique. With perseverance and diligent training and retraining, OPCAB should become applicable to the entire spectrum of patients presenting for surgical coronary revascularization.

References

1. Edgerton JR, Dewey TM, Magee MJ, et al. Conversion in off-pump coronary artery bypass grafting: An analysis of predictors and outcomes. *Ann Thorac Surg* 2003;76: 1138–1142.
2. Mujanovic E, Kabil E, Hadziselimovic M, et al. Conversions in off-pump coronary surgery. *Heart Surg Forum* 2003;6: 135–137.
3. Soltoski P, Salerno T, Levinsky L, et al. Conversion to cardiopulmonary bypass in off-pump coronary artery bypass grafting: Its effect on outcome. *J Cardiovasc Surg (Torino)* 1998;13:328–334.
4. Gardner H. *Changing Minds*. Boston: Harvard Business School Press; 2004.
5. Roxburgh C. Hidden flaws in strategy. *McKinsey Quart* 2003;2:27.
6. Ascione R, Lloyd CT, Underwood MJ, et al. Economic outcome of off-pump coronary artery bypass surgery: A prospective randomized study. *Ann Thorac Surg* 1999;68: 2237–2242.
7. Boyd WD, Desai ND, Del Rizzo DF, et al. Off-pump surgery decreases postoperative complications and resource utilization in the elderly. *Ann Thorac Surg* 1999;68:1490–1493.
8. Cartier R. Current trends and technique in OPCAB surgery. *J Cardiovasc Surg (Torino)* 2003;18:32–46.
9. Lancey RA, Soller BR, Vander Salm TJ. Off-pump versus on-pump coronary artery bypass surgery: A case-matched comparison of clinical outcomes and costs. *Heart Surg Forum* 2000;3:277–281.
10. Khan NE, De Souza A, Mister R, et al. A randomized comparison of off-pump and on-pump multivessel coronary-artery bypass surgery. *N Engl J Med* 2004;350: 21–28.
11. Ascione R, Narayan P, Rogers CA, et al. Early and midterm clinical outcome in patients with severe left ventricular dysfunction undergoing coronary artery surgery. *Ann Thorac Surg* 2003;76:793–799.
12. Donias HW, D'Ancona G, Pande RU, et al. Heparin dose, transfusion rates, and intraoperative graft patency in minimally invasive direct coronary artery bypass. *Heart Surg Forum* 2003;6:176–180.
13. Quigley RL, Fried DW, Pym J, Highbloom RY. Off-pump coronary artery bypass surgery may produce a hypercoagulable patient. *Heart Surg Forum* 2003;6:94–98.
14. Balkhy HH, Quinn CC, Lois KH, Munsch CM. Routine intracoronary shunting in multivessel off-pump coronary artery bypass: A retrospective review of in-hospital outcomes in 550 consecutive cases. *Heart Surg Forum* 2003;6: E32–E35.
15. Demaria RG, Fortier S, Malo O, et al. Influence of intracoronary shunt size on coronary endothelial function during off-pump coronary artery bypass. *Heart Surg Forum* 2003;6:160–168.
16. Grunenfelder J, Comber M, Lachat M, et al. Validation of intracoronary shunt flow measurements for off-pump coronary artery bypass operations. *Heart Surg Forum* 2004;7:26–30.
17. Dapunt OE, Raji MR, Jeschkeit S, et al. Intracoronary shunt insertion prevents myocardial stunning in a juvenile porcine MIDCAB model absent of coronary artery disease. *Eur J Cardiothorac Surg* 1999;15:173–178.
18. Lucchetti V, Capasso F, Caputo M, et al. Intracoronary shunt prevents left ventricular function impairment during beating heart coronary revascularization. *Eur J Cardiothorac Surg* 1999;15:255–259.
19. Sepic J, Wee JO, Soltesz EG, et al. Intraluminal coronary shunting preserves regional myocardial perfusion and function. *Heart Surg Forum* 2003;6:E120–E125.
20. Yeatman M, Caputo M, Narayan P, et al. Intracoronary shunts reduce transient intraoperative myocardial dysfunction during off-pump coronary operations. *Ann Thorac Surg* 2002;73:1411–1417.
21. Gerosa G, Bottio T, Valente M, et al. Intracoronary artery shunt: An assessment of possible coronary artery wall damage. *J Thorac Cardiovasc Surg* 2003;125:1160–1162.
22. Wippermann J, Albes JM, Brandes H, et al. Acute effects of tourniquet occlusion and intraluminal shunts in beating heart surgery. *Eur J Cardiothorac Surg* 2003;24:757–761.
23. Mair H, Sergeant P. Air embolism caused by blower mister. *J Thorac Cardiovasc Surg* 2004;127:897.
24. Akpinar B, Guden M, Sanisoglu I, et al. Does off-pump coronary artery bypass surgery reduce mortality in high risk patients? *Heart Surg Forum* 2001;4:231–236.
25. Al Ruzzeh S, Ambler G, Asimakopoulos G, et al. Off-pump coronary artery bypass (OPCAB) surgery reduces risk-stratified morbidity and mortality: A United Kingdom Multi-Center Comparative Analysis of Early Clinical Outcome. *Circulation* 2003;108(Suppl 1):II1–II8.

26. Al Ruzzeh S, Nakamura K, Athanasiou T, et al. Does off-pump coronary artery bypass (OPCAB) surgery improve the outcome in high-risk patients? A comparative study of 1398 high-risk patients. *Eur J Cardiothorac Surg* 2003;23: 50–55.
27. Al Ruzzeh S, George S, Yacoub M, Amrani M. The clinical outcome of off-pump coronary artery bypass surgery in the elderly patient. *Eur J Cardiothorac Surg* 2001;20: 1152–1156.
28. Ascione R, Reeves BC, Rees K, Angelini GD. Effectiveness of coronary artery bypass grafting with or without cardiopulmonary bypass in overweight patients. *Circulation* 2002;106:1764–1770.
29. Arom KV, Emery RW, Flavin TF, et al. OPCAB surgery: A critical review of two different categories of pre-operative ejection fraction. *Eur J Cardiothorac Surg* 2001;20: 533–537.
30. Cheng W, Denton TA, Fontana GP, et al. Off-pump coronary surgery: Effect on early mortality and stroke. *J Thorac Cardiovasc Surg* 2002;124:313–320.
31. D'Ancona G, Saez I, Baillot R, et al. Determinants of stroke after coronary artery bypass grafting. *Eur J Cardiothorac Surg* 2003;24:552–556.
32. Abraham R, Karamanoukian HL, Jajkowski MR, et al. Does avoidance of cardiopulmonary bypass decrease the incidence of stroke in diabetics undergoing coronary surgery? *Heart Surg Forum* 2001;4:135–140.
33. Ascione R, Reeves BC, Chamberlain MH, et al. Predictors of stroke in the modern era of coronary artery bypass grafting: A case control study. *Ann Thorac Surg* 2002;74:474–480.
34. Athanasiou T, Al Ruzzeh S, Kumar P, et al. Off-pump myocardial revascularization is associated with less incidence of stroke in elderly patients. *Ann Thorac Surg* 2004;77:745–753.
35. Bucerius J, Gummert JF, Borger MA, et al. Stroke after cardiac surgery: A risk factor analysis of 16,184 consecutive adult patients. *Ann Thorac Surg* 2003;75:472–478.
36. Demaria RG, Carrier M, Fortier S, et al. Reduced mortality and strokes with off-pump coronary artery bypass grafting surgery in octogenarians. *Circulation* 2002;106:I5–I10.
37. Aldea GS, Goss JR, Boyle EM Jr, et al. Use of off-pump and on-pump CABG strategies in current clinical practice: The Clinical Outcomes Assessment Program of the state of Washington. *J Cardiovasc Surg (Torino)* 2003;18:206–215.
38. Jarvinen O, Laurikka J, Tarkka MR. Off-pump versus on-pump coronary bypass: Comparison of patient characteristics and early outcomes. *J Cardiovasc Surg (Torino)* 2003;44: 167–172.
39. Zamvar VY, Khan NU, Madhavan A, et al. Clinical outcomes in coronary artery bypass graft surgery: Comparison of off-pump and on-pump techniques. *Heart Surg Forum* 2002;5:109–113.
40. Cumpeeravut P, Visudharom K, Jotisakulratana V, et al. Off-pump coronary artery bypass surgery: Evaluation of extubation time and predictors of failed early extubation. *J Med Assoc Thai* 2003;86(Suppl 1):S28–S35.
41. Straka Z, Brucek P, Vanek T, et al. Routine immediate extubation for off-pump coronary artery bypass grafting without thoracic epidural analgesia. *Ann Thorac Surg* 2002;74:1544–1547.
42. Ascione R, Lloyd CT, Gomes WJ, et al. Beating versus arrested heart revascularization: Evaluation of myocardial function in a prospective randomized study. *Eur J Cardiothorac Surg* 1999;15:685–690.
43. Calafiore AM, Di Mauro M, Canosa C, et al. Early and late outcome of myocardial revascularization with and without cardiopulmonary bypass in high risk patients (EuroSCORE>=6). *Eur J Cardiothorac Surg* 2003;23: 360–367.
44. Calafiore AM, Di Mauro M, Canosa C, et al. Myocardial revascularization with and without cardiopulmonary bypass in multivessel disease: Impact of strategy on midterm outcome. *Ann Thorac Surg* 2003;76:32–36.
45. Bouchard D, Cartier R. Off-pump revascularization of multivessel coronary artery disease has a decreased myocardial infarction rate. *Eur J Cardiothorac Surg* 1998;14(Suppl 1):S20–S24.
46. Baker RA, Andrew MJ, Ross IK, Knight JL. The Octopus II stabilizing system: Biochemical and neuropsychological outcomes in coronary artery bypass surgery. *Heart Surg Forum* 2001;4(Suppl 1):S19–S23.
47. Bennetts JS, Baker RA, Ross IK, Knight JL. Assessment of myocardial injury by troponin T in off-pump coronary artery grafting and conventional coronary artery graft surgery. *Aust N Z J Surg* 2002;72:105–109.
48. Birdi I, Caputo M, Hutter JA, et al. Troponin I release during minimally invasive coronary artery surgery. *J Thorac Cardiovasc Surg* 1997;114:509–510.
49. Bonatti J, Hangler H, Hormann C, et al. Myocardial damage after minimally invasive coronary artery bypass grafting on the beating heart. *Ann Thorac Surg* 1998;66: 1093–1096.
50. Chang PP, Sussman MS, Conte JV, et al. Postoperative ventricular function and cardiac enzymes after on-pump versus off-pump CABG surgery. *Am J Cardiol* 2002;89: 1107–1110.
51. Crescenzi G, Cedrati V, Landoni G, et al. Cardiac biomarker release after CABG with different surgical techniques. *J Cardiothorac Vasc Anesth* 2004;18:34–37.
52. Czerny M, Baumer H, Kilo J, et al. Inflammatory response and myocardial injury following coronary artery bypass grafting with or without cardiopulmonary bypass. *Eur J Cardiothorac Surg* 2000;17:737–742.
53. Al Ruzzeh S, George S, Bustami M, et al. The early clinical and angiographic outcome of sequential coronary artery bypass grafting with the off-pump technique. *J Thorac Cardiovasc Surg* 2002;123:525–530.
54. Contini M, Iaco A, Iovino T, et al. Current results in off pump surgery. *Eur J Cardiothorac Surg* 1999;16(Suppl 1): S69–S72.
55. Ascione R, Nason G, Al Ruzzeh S, et al. Coronary revascularization with or without cardiopulmonary bypass in patients with preoperative nondialysis-dependent renal insufficiency. *Ann Thorac Surg* 2001;72:2020–2025.
56. Riess FC, Moshar S, Bader R, et al. Clinical outcome of patients with and without renal impairment undergoing a minimally invasive LIMA-to-LAD bypass operation. *Heart Surg Forum* 2000;3:313–318.
57. Ascione R, Lloyd CT, Underwood MJ, et al. On-pump versus off-pump coronary revascularization: Evaluation of renal function. *Ann Thorac Surg* 1999;68:493–498.
58. Hayashida N, Teshima H, Chihara S, et al. Does off-pump coronary artery bypass grafting really preserve renal function? *Circ J* 2002;66:921–925.

59. Loef BG, Epema AH, Navis G, et al. Off-pump coronary revascularization attenuates transient renal damage compared with on-pump coronary revascularization. *Chest* 2002;121:1190–1194.
60. Ascione R, Williams S, Lloyd CT, et al. Reduced postoperative blood loss and transfusion requirement after beating-heart coronary operations: A prospective randomized study. *J Thorac Cardiovasc Surg* 2001;121:689–696.
61. Baumgartner FJ, Yokoyama T, Gheissari A, et al. Effect of off-pump coronary artery bypass grafting on morbidity. *Am J Cardiol* 2000;86:1021–1022, A10.
62. Haase M, Sharma A, Fielitz A, et al. On-pump coronary artery surgery versus off-pump exclusive arterial coronary grafting: A matched cohort comparison. *Ann Thorac Surg* 2003;75:62–67.
63. Deuse T, Detter C, Samuel V, et al. Early and midterm results after coronary artery bypass grafting with and without cardiopulmonary bypass: Which patient population benefits the most? *Heart Surg Forum* 2003;6:77–83.
64. Hernandez F, Cohn WE, Baribeau YR, et al. In-hospital outcomes of off-pump versus on-pump coronary artery bypass procedures: A multicenter experience. *Ann Thorac Surg* 2001;72:1528–1533.
65. Novick RJ, Fox SA, Stitt LW, et al. Effect of off-pump coronary artery bypass grafting on risk-adjusted and cumulative sum failure outcomes after coronary artery surgery. *J Cardiovasc Surg (Torino)* 2002;17: 520–528.
66. Arom KV, Emery RW, Flavin TF, Petersen RJ. Cost-effectiveness of minimally invasive coronary artery bypass surgery. *Ann Thorac Surg* 1999;68:1562–1566.
67. Nomura F, Mukai S, Tamura K, et al. Cost performance and efficacy of off-pump coronary artery bypass grafting. *Hiroshima J Med Sci* 2002;51:85–87.
68. Puskas JD, Thourani VH, Marshall JJ, et al. Clinical outcomes, angiographic patency, and resource utilization in 200 consecutive off-pump coronary bypass patients. *Ann Thorac Surg* 2001;71:1477–1483.

CHAPTER

27 REOPERATIVE CORONARY ARTERY BYPASS SURGERY

Christopher J. Barreiro, Anshuman Bansal

INTRODUCTION

Coronary artery bypass (CAB) surgery is the most common cardiac surgical procedure, with nearly 350,000 operations performed annually in the United States. Reoperative coronary artery bypass surgery accounts for approximately 5 percent of all isolated CAB procedures and is often the result of graft failure, progression of native coronary disease, or incomplete revascularization. Recent data from the Society of Thoracic Surgeons database show that there has been a decrease in the number and percentage of redo-CAB (2000, N = 8929, or 6.1

KEY CONCEPTS

- Epidemiology
  - Among the 350,000 coronary bypass operations performed annually in the United States, reoperative coronary artery bypass surgery (redo-CAB) accounts for approximately 5 percent of all isolated coronary artery bypass grafting (CABG) procedures. Recent data from the Society of Thoracic Surgeons database show that there has been a decrease in the number and percentage of redo-CAB procedures (2000, N = 8929, or 6.1 percent; 2004, N = 6654, or 4.7 percent).
- Pathophysiology
  - Reoperative coronary artery surgery is performed for patients in whom there is definite demonstrated myocardial viability with associated symptomatology. A multivariate analysis demonstrated that preoperative angina, use of vein grafts only, previous myocardial infarction, incomplete revascularization, female gender, and smoking at a younger age were independent risk factors for recurrent angina and a potential need for reoperation.
- Clinical features
  - In more recent years, the reoperative candidate population has evolved to include older patients, with diminished left ventricular function, triple-vessel coronary artery disease, and graft failure becoming the predominant etiologic factors. Recently, however, there appears to have been an increasing number of reoperative candidates with progression of their native disease distal to their patent conduit graft sites.
- Diagnostics
  - Diagnostic tests include those used to assess viable myocardium and those used for planning the operation. The tests frequently used for detecting viable myocardium include thallium scintigraphy, dobutamine echocardiography, magnetic resonance imaging, and positron emission tomography. Coronary angiography is the gold standard for determining the need for revascularization and the appropriate targets. Standard computed tomography (CT) can be used to assess the substernal structures. However, with the development of multislice CT and three-dimensional (3-D) reconstruction, accurate pictures of the cardiac anatomy and the relationships of bypass grafts to mediastinal structures as well as the sternum can be demonstrated vividly.
- Treatment
  - Reoperative surgery for coronary artery disease requires knowledge of mediastinal structures and a staged entry into the chest with the use of an oscillating saw and scissors for division of the outer and inner tables, respectively. Femoral

artery and vein cannulation may be necessary if it is anticipated that cardiac structures are in jeopardy of being injured upon reentry. Careful dissection in the area of previous vein grafts that may be atherosclerotic is important, as downstream debris from these vein grafts is the most common cause of mortality in this high-risk group of patients.

- Outcomes
  - Overall operative mortality rates for patients undergoing reoperative coronary artery surgery range from approximately 4 to 11 percent. They are higher for patients undergoing emergency reoperation. Five- and 10-year survival rates for reoperation have been reported at approximately 75 percent and 55 percent, respectively.

percent; 2004, $N = 6654$, or 4.7 percent). There are probably many reasons for this trend, including better medical management and interventional cardiology. Most redo-CAB procedures today are performed more than 10 years after the primary CAB and are technically more challenging because of the difficulty of sternal reentry, the presence of patent bypass grafts, and limitations of potential bypass conduits. In addition to the technical complexities, the risk profile of reoperative candidates continues to increase. These patients are older, have a greater extent of coronary artery disease, and have worse left ventricular function. However, these obstacles have been offset by improvements in operative techniques and perioperative care, resulting in improved survival and postoperative outcomes in redo-CAB patients.

PREDICTORS OF REOPERATION

Surgical reintervention rates and recurrent symptoms are two of the primary outcomes that are used to measure the success of the initial CAB procedure. In a large cohort of patients, freedom from redo-CAB at 1, 5, 10, and 15 years was 99 percent, 97 percent, 89 percent, and 72 percent, respectively.[1] In addition, freedom from recurrent angina after initial CAB surgery has been demonstrated to be approximately 80 percent at 10 years.[2] In a multivariate analysis, preoperative angina, use of vein grafts only, previous myocardial infarction, incomplete revascularization, female gender, smoking, and younger age were found to be independent risk factors for recurrent angina.[3]

Reoperative candidates include patients with recurrent ischemic symptoms who have evidence of viable myocardium at risk as a result of progression of their coronary disease or graft failure. Studies have demonstrated that predictors of redo-CAB include young age at initial operation, absence of internal mammary artery (IMA) grafts, incomplete revascularization, impaired functional status, and multivessel disease.[4] Initially, a majority of redo-CAB surgeries were performed because of incomplete revascularization or worsening atherosclerosis of the native coronary arteries. As the reoperative candidate population evolved to include older patients with increased left ventricular dysfunction and triple-vessel disease, graft failure became the predominant etiologic factor. More recently, however, there has been an increasing number of reoperative candidates with progression of their native disease distal to their patent arterial graft sites.[5,6]

The choice of a graft conduit at the primary operation has been shown to be a significant factor in determining the need for reoperation. The increased use of arterial conduits, including IMA and radial artery grafts, in place of venous conduits has reduced the rate of reoperation significantly in recent years. IMA patency rates after primary CAB surgery are higher than 90 percent at 10 years, in contrast to saphenous vein grafts (SVGs), which begin to deteriorate rapidly after 5 years and have a 50 percent patency rate at 10 years.[7,8] In fact, up to 15 to 20 percent of SVGs become occluded by 1 year.[9] IMA grafts also have been shown to reduce the incidence of late myocardial infarction (MI), rehospitalization, and redo-CAB compared with patients receiving only vein grafts.[10] Similar benefits have been realized with radial and gastroepiploic arterial free grafts.[11,12] Because of the improved patient survival and patency rates of arterial grafts, the IMA graft has become the conduit of choice for primary CAB as well as for redo-CAB surgery for SVG stenosis.

Early SVG stenosis within the first year of primary CAB often is due to intimal hyperplasia. The increased intimal thickness presumably is due to exposure of the vein to arterial pressures. This proliferative lesion ultimately results in vein graft atherosclerosis, which is the leading cause of late occlusion and accelerates dramatically after 5 years. SVG atherosclerosis has a worse prognosis than does native vessel atherosclerosis. The lesion in a vein graft is often more diffuse and prone to plaque rupture, leading to increased rates of thromboembolic events. As a result, even minimal manipulation of SVGs or antegrade cardioplegia during redo-CAB surgery can dislodge atheromatous emboli and result in MI. This represents the most common cause of operative mortality in patients undergoing redo-CAB surgery. Arterial grafts are much less prone to occlusion, although they can develop a neointimal proliferation, most commonly at the distal anastomotic site.

PREOPERATIVE CONSIDERATIONS

Preoperative planning is of even greater importance in redo-CAB surgery than it is in primary procedures. For

Table 27-1 Preoperative assessment

Chest x-ray	Thallium scintigraphy
Computed tomography	Dobutamine echocardiography
Coronary angiography	Magnetic resonance imaging
Positron emission tomography	Vascular Doppler imaging

the reoperation to proceed safely, adequate preoperative assessment and analysis are critical (Table 27-1). The patient's history must be reviewed thoroughly, with close attention paid not only to any previous cardiac surgery but also to any relevant procedures or comorbidities that may affect the surgeon's approach to the reoperation. For example, a patient with a previous history of mediastinitis should be considered for a thoracotomy incision as an alternative to redo-sternotomy if the coronary anatomy is favorable for this approach. Medications should be reviewed carefully so that any drugs affecting platelet function or coagulation can be discontinued at least 1 week before the operation. Most important, it is essential to have a clear and complete understanding of the patient's native coronary and bypass graft anatomy before any reoperation. This information can be gathered from previous operative records and coronary angiograms. It also must be determined whether bypassing the potentially graftable vessels will improve perfusion to viable myocardium. Obviously, revascularization of nonviable myocardium will provide no benefit to the patient. In addition to determining the feasibility of beneficial revascularization, adequate bypass conduits must be available.

Chest X-ray and computed tomography

The surgeon can evaluate the risk of sternal reentry by means of radiography. A posteroanterior and lateral chest x-ray can give the surgeon an idea of the proximity of important cardiac structures to the sternum. Steel clips that are visible on a chest radiograph also can be used to trace the path of patent IMA grafts. CT can be used to give a more detailed view of substernal structures if necessary. CT scans can determine the size and position of cardiac chambers as well as the path of bypass conduits. This information can be used to guide the sternal reentry. In patients at high risk for hemorrhage or injury to substernal structures, femoral dissection should be performed to allow for peripheral cardiopulmonary bypass (CPB). Alternative incisions should be considered if they are deemed necessary on the basis of this evaluation. In addition to standard CT scanning, intravenous angiography multislice CT and 3-D reconstruction is a recent technological advancement that has been found to be extremely accurate in detecting coronary artery bypass graft patency and occlusion.[13] It also provides clear and accurate pictures of the cardiac anatomy and the relationships of bypass grafts to mediastinal structures (Fig. 27-1).

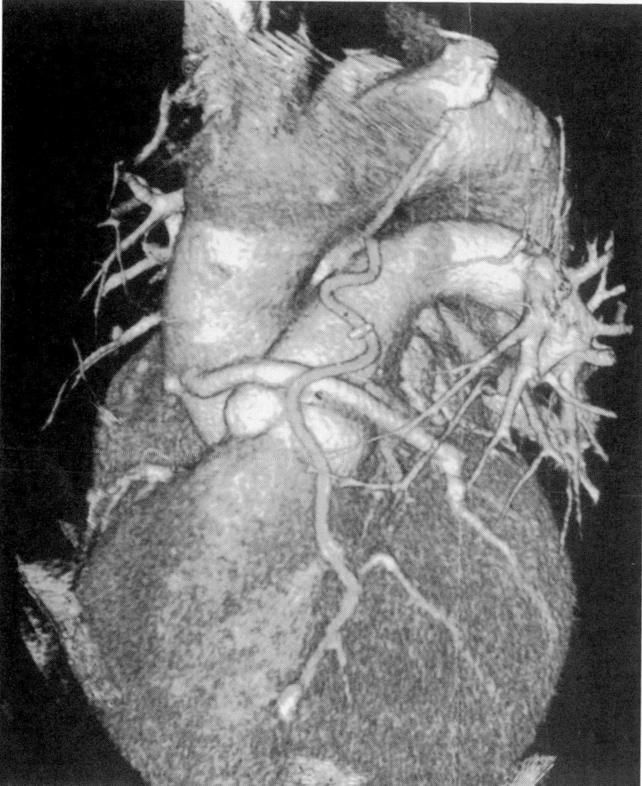

Figure 27-1 Multislice computer tomography illustrating the relationship of the internal thoracic artery and saphenous vein graft to other cardiac structures.

Coronary angiography

Coronary angiography is a necessary step in the complete preoperative assessment of potential redo-CAB patients. To gain a better understanding of the patient's coronary anatomy, previous angiograms and operative notes should be reviewed and are invaluable tools for the reoperative surgeon as well as the interventional cardiologist performing the angiogram. The coronary angiogram can be used to estimate the severity of atherosclerotic and thrombotic lesions. The severity of native coronary and SVG stenosis often is underestimated on the basis of a single angiographic view. Therefore, multiple projections are required to visualize the entire coronary arterial tree as well as the previously placed bypass grafts. The angiogram also can help determine whether graftable vessels are present. To ensure that this is done accurately, the angiographer must inject all relevant branches and allow enough time for the filling of the coronaries by collaterals. Of course, angiography must be used in conjunction with the surgeon's intraoperative assessment of the patient's coronary anatomy.

Assessing viable myocardium

Impaired left ventricular function secondary to ischemic heart disease is not always irreversible and may improve considerably after revascularization. Restoration of blood flow to chronically underperfused and recurrently ischemic myocardium often can lead to the recovery of contractile function. However, revascularization of scar tissue will not result in functional improvement. In light of the considerable operative morbidity and mortality among patients with left ventricular (LV) dysfunction undergoing surgical revascularization, especially redo-CAB, it is essential to differentiate between viable and nonviable myocardium. Several noninvasive imaging modalities are used to identify physiologic markers of myocardial viability in regions with contractile dysfunction. The most commonly used techniques to ascertain viability include positron emission tomography (PET), thallium scintigraphy, dobutamine echocardiography, and magnetic resonance imaging (MRI). PET is an established method for demonstrating preserved metabolic activity through the use of ^{18}F-fluorodeoxyglucose as a marker of myocardial glucose utilization. Thallium scanning is used to assess myocardial perfusion and membrane integrity, whereas the myocardial contractile reserve is best evaluated by using dobutamine echocardiography or MRI.[14] Dobutamine echocardiography increasingly is being employed in the evaluation of viable myocardium.

Bypass conduits

The surgeon should have a preoperative plan for the selection of bypass conduits. Venous Doppler studies often are used to determine the adequacy of saphenous vein segments. Vein mapping is a simple, accurate, and noninvasive way to predict the course of the vein and demonstrate venous anomalies. On occasion, venous mapping can influence the surgeon's choice of the venectomy site.[15] Arterial Doppler studies can assess the radial arteries. In addition, Allen's test can help ensure that the fingers will receive proper flow if the radial artery is to be used as a potential graft. Abnormalities in the IMA also can be seen on Doppler studies. IMA ultrasound assessment may reduce the need for invasive preoperative testing for patency and length and allow for postoperative assessment of coronary artery flow reserve.[16] However, IMA angiography provides a more complete evaluation of these arteries and should be used whenever possible.

TECHNICAL STRATEGIES

The increased complexity of redo-CAB surgery is due to a variety of unique anatomic considerations that result in an increased risk for perioperative MI. For this reason, perioperative MI remains the leading cause of in-hospital mortality in this patient population.[17] The major anatomic considerations include the risks of sternal reentry, potential injury to stenotic or patent bypass grafts, difficulty with cannulation of the reoperative aorta, an increased risk of embolic phenomena, and a limitation of remaining bypass conduits (Table 27-2).

Table 27-2 Technical challenges of redo-CAB surgery
Sternal reentry
Potential injury to patent grafts
Cannulation of atherosclerotic aorta
Embolization from atheromatous saphenous vein grafts
Bypass conduit availability

The significant amount of sternal adhesions often encountered during sternal reentry increases the risk of hemorrhage as well as injury to underlying structures.[18] Native structures that are often adherent to the posterior sternum can include the right ventricle, right atrium, aorta, innominate vein, and lung. In addition, functioning venous and arterial bypass conduits from the initial operation can be placed at risk. If difficulty with the sternotomy is anticipated, preparations for peripheral CPB should be instituted. Harvesting and preparation of the new venous and arterial conduits should be undertaken before resternotomy. Arterial cannulation for peripheral CPB can be performed through the femoral artery, or it can be performed through the axillary artery if the patient has significant aorto-iliac disease. The femoral vein is used most commonly for venous cannulation.

The use of a sagittal oscillating saw is often considered the safest approach during resternotomy (Fig. 27-2). Sternal wires should be cut anteriorly but left in place.[19] The oscillating saw then is used to divide the outer table of the sternum, using the wires as a guide for the depth of the cut. In this way, the intact wires posterior to the sternum provide added protection to underlying structures during sternal reentry but are removed as the inner table is divided. The inner table is divided with Mayo scissors (Fig. 27-2). After the sternum has been opened, meticulous dissection must be employed to separate adherent mediastinal structures from the chest wall (Fig. 27-3). Care must be taken to avoid excessive manipulation of venous bypass grafts because this can lead to the dissemination of atheromatous emboli. Intrapericardial dissection then continues in preparation for cannulation. Once the aorta is dissected out, it must be examined for the presence of significant atherosclerotic disease, which could lead to embolic phenomena upon cannulation.[20] This is accomplished through palpation and epiaortic scanning to identify the most disease-free portions of the aorta. If the degree of atherosclerotic disease of the aorta is thought to be too great, the femoral or axillary arteries are other possible cannulation sites, as was mentioned above.

Myocardial protection can be provided through a combination of both antegrade and retrograde cardioplegia during redo-CAB surgery. Although antegrade cardioplegia alone may be adequate during a primary CAB, this is not the case during reoperations. Antegrade cardioplegia may be ineffective in providing protection

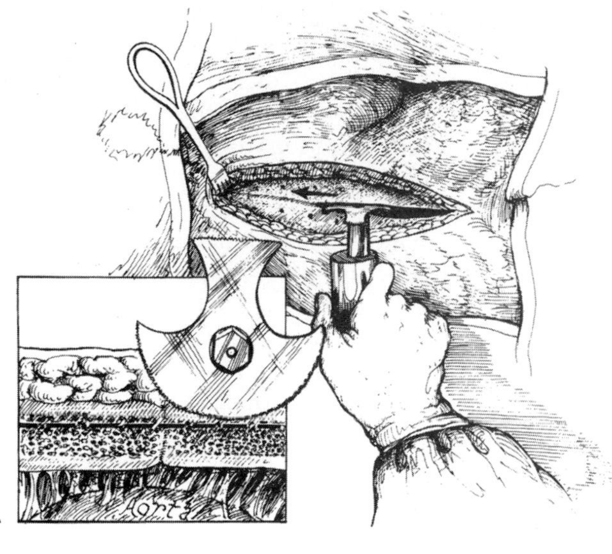

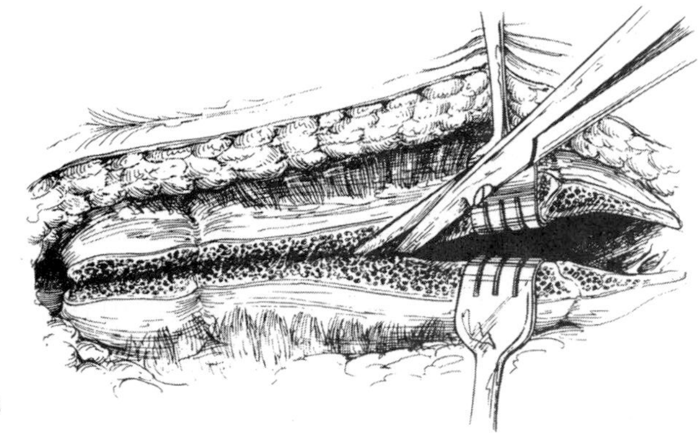

Figure 27-2 **A.** Use of the oscillating saw to divide the outer table and **(B)** the straight Mayo scissors to divide the inner table.

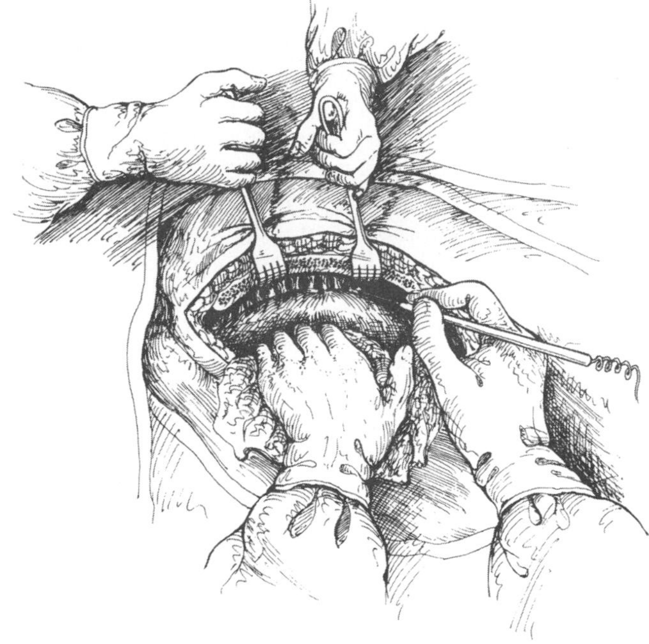

Figure 27-3 Use of the electrocautery unit to separate adhesions from the sternum and chest wall.

to areas of the myocardium supplied by in situ arterial grafts and also can increase the risk of dislodging atheromatous debris from previously placed SVGs. In contrast, retrograde cardioplegia is delivered via the coronary sinus and the coronary venous system and can avoid the problems associated with antegrade cardioplegia. However, the adequacy of retrograde cardioplegia must be assessed in terms of the coronary sinus pressure, uniformity of myocardial cooling, and distention of the coronary venous system.[21] To ensure uniform cardioplegic protection, patent in situ arterial grafts also must be occluded.

Once intrapericardial dissection of the heart is complete, the native coronary vasculature and initial bypass conduits are assessed. In conjunction with preoperative angiographic data, an operative strategy is formulated. The vessels to be bypassed and the SVGs to be replaced are determined. As was mentioned above, SVG atherosclerosis is present in a large majority of vein grafts. For this reason, replacement of all older SVGs must be considered. However, this often is not feasible because of the limitation of available bypass conduits. Unnecessary manipulation of SVGs must be avoided to prevent atheroemboli from forming. Therefore, the operative plan must be individualized, and relatively disease-free SVGs will be left in place even if they are more than 5 years old.

Many technical decisions must be made to revascularize ischemic myocardium that is being perfused by a stenotic SVG: The present SVG can be left alone or divided, and it can be replaced with a new SVG or an arterial graft. Every effort must be made to bypass left anterior descending artery (LAD) disease with the left IMA if this was not done at the initial operation because of the superior long-term patency rates. However, studies have shown that when new arterial grafts are used and the old vein grafts are interrupted, a hypoperfusion syndrome may develop, resulting in worsened myocardial ischemia or infarction. In addition to being a risk factor for hypoperfusion, an IMA-to-LAD graft with interruption of an old SVG was found to be an independent predictor of operative mortality.[22,23] This is due to an initial period of decreased flow through the arterial graft compared with the previous vein graft. The risk of hypoperfusion outweighs the risk of atheroemboli from an old SVG; therefore, old SVGs should be left in place when a new arterial graft is used to bypass the same coronary vessel. However, hypoperfusion is often not an issue when an old SVG is replaced with another SVG. Therefore, the old SVG should be interrupted in those situations.

The site of both the distal and proximal anastomoses is another challenge faced by the surgeon during redo-CAB surgery. The distal anastomosis site from the primary operation often can be reused when one is replacing an old SVG with a new one. However, progression of native vessel disease distal to this site may require the placement of a second bypass conduit on this more distal vessel. A challenge to the proximal anastomosis is posed by the often limited sites available on the reoperative aorta. This can be avoided by using sequential vein grafts that have multiple distal anastomoses but only one proximal anastomosis. In situ arterial grafts are optimal not only because they have excellent long-term patency but also because they have no proximal anastomoses. The proximal anastomosis of arterial free grafts can be sewn to the hood of an old SVG graft, which is often free from atherosclerosis. Arterial free grafts also can be anastomosed proximally to another arterial graft to form a composite T- or Y-type anastomosis.[24,25]

ALTERNATIVE MANAGEMENT

Nonsurgical interventions

Various nonsurgical approaches to revascularization, such as percutaneous transluminal coronary angioplasty (PTCA) and intracoronary stenting, are becoming more widespread. In fact, after the late 1990s, the number of PTCA surgeries began to exceed the number of CAB surgeries performed each year. As the line begins to blur between candidates for surgical versus nonsurgical revascularization, many studies have been performed to compare these two techniques for primary revascularization. However, the data are more limited in patients in need of reintervention who already have undergone CAB surgery. One retrospective review analyzed 632 patients with previous CAB who underwent elective redo-CAB or PTCA. The results demonstrated equivalent overall survival, event-free survival, and relief of angina between the two groups. PTCA also was found to have a lower risk of procedural morbidity and mortality. However, redo-CAB is associated with greater success in providing complete revascularization as well as a reduced need for subsequent revascularization procedures.[26] Similar survival results were found in a more recent randomized trial of PTCA versus redo-CAB in which overall 3-year survival was 76 percent and 73 percent, respectively.[27] In a review of patients referred for reoperation versus PTCA at the Cleveland Clinic, those undergoing redo-CAB were more likely to be male and have diabetes, hypertension, valvular disease, and severe LV systolic dysfunction. These patients generally had fewer functioning venous and arterial grafts and a larger region of myocardium in jeopardy. Although reoperation is associated with a higher risk of in-hospital complications than is angioplasty, it has potential long-term benefit when there is a lack of functioning bypass grafts or a lack of a patent arterial graft to the LAD.[28]

Current percutaneous techniques rely heavily on the implantation of intracoronary stents as opposed to the previously used dilating balloon devices. SVG stenosis also can be treated with stenting; however, stenting usually is limited to grafts with focal or discrete disease. Outcomes are much poorer for diffusely degenerated SVGs. The risk of embolization from SVG atherosclerosis to the distal coronary bed is also greater compared with intracoronary or arterial graft stenting. Recent advances in percutaneous techniques include catheter-based systems designed to capture atheromatous debris as well as drug-coated stents.[29] These advances are believed to decrease procedural morbidity and long-term graft restenosis rates. However, further studies are necessary to compare the long-term outcomes of these newer techniques with the outcomes from operative revascularization.

Surgical interventions

In an effort to minimize the potential complications associated with cardiopulmonary bypass and median sternotomy, alternative surgical treatments have become more prevalent in recent years. Off-pump redo-CAB has been shown in some studies to decrease mortality without altering the risk of perioperative MI, stroke, renal failure, or reoperation for bleeding.[30,31] In a study performed on patients with single-vessel disease who required reoperation, traditional on-pump patients were shown to have a higher rate of postoperative transfusions, longer periods of ventilatory support, and a higher rate of postoperative arterial fibrillation than those undergoing off-pump CAB (OPCAB). Patients who had on-pump surgery also had longer hospital stays and higher in-hospital mortality.[32] The potential disadvantages of re-OPCAB must be noted. The operation becomes technically more challenging with the need to graft intramyocardial vessels on a beating heart. There is a greater risk for emboli to occur from atherosclerotic but patent vein grafts during dissection of a beating heart. The risk of aortic dissection during OPCAB has been shown to be greater than it is in traditional CAB surgery, and the need for the use of a partial occluding clamp on the aorta is also a disadvantage of the off-pump method.[33] In addition, re-OPCAB has been observed to be less effective at relieving symptoms. In one study, patients undergoing re-OPCAB surgery had a higher rate of recurrence of angina and an increased use of nitrates at follow-up.[34] Until more studies are available to substantiate the benefits of re-OPCAB, it should be used selectively after an individualized risk assessment is performed.

In patients with a previous history of mediastinitis, resternotomy can be a risky method to gain access for reoperation. In some patients there is also a significant risk of damaging a patent graft running across the midline during resternotomy. If it is not necessary to revascularize several vessels, a left thoracotomy incision can be a viable alternative to gain access to specific vessels.

Other indications for considering a thoracotomy include cardiac structures adherent to the sternum, previous mediastinal radiation therapy, calcification in the ascending aorta, diffuse atherosclerosis, and the need for blood conservation.[35] Patients are placed in the lateral decubitus position, and a posterolateral thoracotomy is performed through the fourth or fifth intercostal space. Redo-CAB through a left-sided thoracotomy often was performed in conjunction with peripheral CPB in the past. More recently, however, there has been a trend toward performing this type of reoperation without CPB. Studies have shown that off-pump surgery through a thoracotomy does not increase the risk and reduces mortality and postoperative complications.[35,36] To gain access to vessels of the lateral wall and the circumflex and distal right coronary branches, a left posterolateral thoracotomy is the incision of choice, and the operation often can be performed off-pump. The proximal anastomosis to the aorta is done with a partial occluding aortic clamp. The graft then is anastomosed to the coronary, using a stabilizer. This technique has been shown to be a safe method to revascularize the lateral wall.[37] A left anterior thoracotomy will provide access to the distal LAD. If a vein graft or radial artery graft is used, the proximal anastomosis to the axillary/subclavian artery is performed through a separate incision and routed to the LAD. Since complete revascularization is usually not possible via the thoracotomy incision, this approach should be used only in patients at considerable risk with a resternotomy who require only one or two grafts.

Minimally invasive direct coronary artery bypass (MIDCAB) is performed under direct vision without sternotomy or cardiopulmonary bypass. The technique is used in reoperative patients through various incisions to revascularize one or two areas of the heart. The procedure is best suited to access anterior coronary vessels through a small anterior thoracotomy. MIDCAB can be combined with PTCA to provide revascularization to less severely diseased vessels. It also can be done with CPB if a multivessel bypass is to be performed. Anterior coronary vessels are grafted with the left IMA if it has not been used previously. However, harvesting of the IMA is technically more difficult with the limited exposure offered by the minithoracotomy incision. Additional small incisions allow access to individual regions of the heart. A midline epigastric incision is made to graft posterior vessels, using the gastroepiploic artery as the bypass conduit. Lateral coronaries can be bypassed with radial artery or SVGs via a posterior minithoracotomy. The proximal aortic anastomosis can be very difficult without the access provided by a median sternotomy. Despite its limitations, a 3-year study showed that reoperative MIDCAB grafting had lower rates of supraventricular arrhythmia and transfusion than did traditional redo-CAB. MIDCAB also avoids the risks of resternotomy, aortic manipulation, and cardiopulmonary bypass but does not offer an advantage for mortality, stroke, or MI. In cases in which single-territory revascularization is indicated, MIDCAB can offer a safer alternative to traditional redo-CAB surgery.[38,39]

REOPERATIVE CORONARY OUTCOMES

Survival

Redo-CAB is much more hazardous than primary revascularization because of the increased surgical complexity as well as the vulnerable patient population undergoing reoperation. Redo-CAB patients are a substantially higher-risk subgroup than patients undergoing a primary operation in terms of perioperative morbidity and mortality, relief of cardiac symptoms, and long-term survival. Overall operative mortality rates have been reported to be from 2.0 to 3.2 percent for primary coronary bypass compared with a rate of 6.9 to 11.4 percent for redo-CAB surgery.[40–42] Operative mortality rates are even higher for patients undergoing an emergency reoperation at 16.4 to 25 percent.[43,44] The main reason for a higher operative mortality with reoperations is an increased risk of perioperative infarction. Causes of MI include incomplete revascularization as a result of distal coronary disease, vein graft thrombosis, IMA graft failure, emboli from vein grafts, injury to patent grafts, and hypoperfusion from inadequate arterial grafting (Table 27-3). Similarly, the late results for redo-CAB are less favorable than those for a primary operation. In a retrospective study of 2030 patients at Emory University, 5- and 10-year survival rates for reoperation were 76 percent and 55 percent, respectively.[44] In contrast, 56 percent of patients were alive at 15 years after primary CAB surgery in the Coronary Artery Surgery Study (CASS) of 8221 patients.[45] In another study of 6591 primary CAB patients, 5- and 10-year actuarial survival was 90 percent and 75 percent, respectively. This is in contrast to the 5- and 10-year actuarial survival of 80 percent and 65 percent, respectively, in 508 redo-CAB patients.[40]

Predictors of mortality

Preoperative characteristics of redo-CAB patients associated with an increased operative mortality include a history of peripheral vascular disease, diabetes, anginal

Table 27-3 Etiology of perioperative myocardial infarction
Incomplete revascularization
Vein graft thrombosis
Internal mammary artery graft failure
Embolic phenomena from saphenous vein grafts
Injury to patent grafts
Hypoperfusion syndrome

status, and preoperative MI.[46] Abnormal left ventricular function, a large number of patent but atherosclerotic grafts, the absence of IMA grafts, and preoperative New York Heart Assoication (NYHA) class III or IV status are also factors that increase the operative risk. Risk factors that correlate with reduced *long-term* survival after redo-CAB surgery are older age, impaired left ventricular function, hypertension, diabetes, congestive heart failure, emergency surgery, and female sex.[44]

The time interval between the primary operation and redo-CAB surgery has also been shown to be a significant factor in operative risk and mortality. Very early reoperation (1 year or less) can be correlated with a much higher mortality rate than later reoperation. Studies demonstrate mortality rates between 21 and 28 percent in patients after very early reoperation versus 8.4 to 8.9 percent in those reoperated on more than 1 year after the initial operation.[40,47,48] However, as the time interval becomes greater than 10 years, increased mortality rates have been observed. In one study, patients with a reoperative interval of 1 to 10 years had a 6.0 percent (18 of 312) mortality rate, compared with 17.6 percent (13 of 74) for those in whom the interval between operations was more than 10 years.[40]

In a study of over 800 patients undergoing redo-CAB, those receiving retrograde coronary sinus cardioplegia had an in-hospital mortality rate of 2.5 percent versus 5.4 percent in patients receiving antegrade cardioplegia.[49]

Multiple reoperations

A number of patients have required a third or fourth coronary revascularization procedure. However, the complexity of disease and the difficulty of the surgery also increase. In addition, the availability of potential bypass conduits becomes a major concern. The indications for additional operative revascularization remain the same, and patients often come to attention because of disabling angina that is unresponsive to medical therapy. As expected, perioperative mortality and MI rates in these patients are higher than they are in first-time redo patients. In a study of 102 patients undergoing a third or fourth CAB, the in-hospital mortality rate was 9.8 percent, with a perioperative MI rate of 8.8 percent. Actuarial survival of these patients at 5 years was found to be between 76 and 79 percent. At 10 years, survival dropped to 59 percent.[50] Consistent predictors of increased mortality in the patients after a third operation include age greater than 65 years and left ventricular dysfunction with an ejection fraction less than 40 percent.[51,52] Despite the increased perioperative risks involved, these patients have reasonable long-term survival and symptomatic improvement after multiple redo-CAB procedures. In more recent years, many of these patients have been treated by interventional cardiology with the use of angioplasty and stents.

SUMMARY

Redo-CAB surgery will continue to be an alternative for a number of patients, especially as the time from their initial procedures lengthens. The treatment modalities available to patients experiencing the recurring symptoms of ischemic heart disease also continue to increase. In addition to the improvements in surgical technique, the cardiac surgeon must remain acquainted with advances in percutaneous catheter interventions to devise the most appropriate treatment strategy for each patient. The surgeon performing the reoperation must recognize the unique challenges involved. The differences between primary and reoperative procedures cannot be underestimated, and preoperative assessment and analysis of each patient's anatomy are critical. With an awareness of the technical complexities and risk profile of the patients, redo-CAB surgery can be performed with relatively low morbidity and mortality and good long-term relief of symptoms. With the advancements in operative technique and improved surgical technology, the outlook for patients with repeat coronary revascularizations continues to be promising.

References

1. Sergeant P, Blackstone E, Meyns B, et al. First cardiological or cardiosurgical reintervention for ischemic heart disease after primary coronary artery bypass grafting. *Eur J Cardiothorac Surg* 1998;14:480–487.
2. Risum O, Abdelnoor M, Svennevig JL, et al. Risk factors of recurrent angina pectoris and of non-fatal myocardial infarction after coronary artery bypass surgery. *Eur J Cardiothorac Surg* 1996;10:173–178.
3. Cameron AA, Davis KB, Rogers WJ. Recurrence of angina after coronary artery bypass surgery: Predictors and prognosis (CASS Registry). *J Am Coll Cardiol* 1995;26:895–899.
4. Cosgrove DM, Loop FD, Lytle BW, et al. Predictors of reoperation after myocardial revascularization. *J Thorac Cardiovasc Surg* 1986;92:811–821.
5. Akins CW, Buckley MJ, Daggett WM, et al. Reoperative coronary grafting: Changing patient profiles, operative indications, techniques, and results. *Ann Thorac Surg* 1994;58:359–364.
6. Yau TM, Borger MA, Weisel RD, et al. The changing pattern of reoperative coronary surgery: Trends in 1230 consecutive reoperations. *J Thorac Cardiovasc Surg* 2000;120:156–163.
7. Loop FD, Lytle BW, Cosgrove DM, et al. Influence of the internal-mammary-artery graft on 10-year survival and other cardiac events. *N Engl J Med* 1986;314:1–6.
8. Fitzgibbon GM, Kafka HP, Leach AJ, et al. Coronary bypass graft fate and patient outcome: Angiographic follow-up of 5,065 grafts related to survival and reoperation

in 1,388 patients during 25 years. *J Am Coll Cardiol* 1996;28:616–626.
9. Canos DA, Mintz GS, Berzingi CO, et al. Clinical, angiographic, and intravascular ultrasound characteristics of early saphenous vein graft failure. *J Am Coll Cardiol* 2004;44:53–56.
10. Christenson JT, Vala D, Faidutti B, et al. Choice of graft material at primary CABG influences cardiac death and reintervention rates. *Med Princ Pract* 2002;11:141–146.
11. Zacharias A, Habib RH, Schwann TA, et al. Improved survival with radial artery versus vein conduits in coronary bypass surgery with left internal thoracic artery to left anterior descending artery grafting. *Circulation* 2004;109:1489–1496.
12. Albertini A, Lochegnies A, El Khoury G, et al. Use of the right gastroepiploic artery as a coronary artery bypass graft in 307 patients. *Cardiovasc Surg* 1998;6:419–423.
13. Yamakami S, Toyama J, Okamoto M, et al. Noninvasive detection of coronary artery bypass graft patency by intravenous electron beam computed tomographic angiography. *Jpn Heart J* 2003;44:811–822.
14. Bax JJ, van der Wall EE, Harbinson M. Radionuclide techniques for the assessment of myocardial viability and hibernation. *Heart* 2004;90:26–33.
15. Head HD, Brown MF. Preoperative vein mapping for coronary artery bypass operations. *Ann Thorac Surg* 1995;59:144–148.
16. Ehrsam JE, Spittell PC, Seward JB. Internal mammary artery: 100% visualization with new ultrasound technology. *J Am Soc Echocardiogr* 1998;11:10–12.
17. Grinda JM, Zegdi R, Couetil JP, et al. Coronary reoperations: Indications, techniques and operative results: Retrospective study of 240 coronary reoperations. *J Cardiovasc Surg* 2000;41:703–708.
18. Follis FM, Pett SB, Miller KB, et al. Catastrophic hemorrhage on sternal re-entry: Still a dreaded complication? *Ann Thorac Surg* 1999;68:2215–2219.
19. Baumgartner WA: Reoperation. In: Jamieson SW, Shumway NE (eds). *Cardiac Surgery*, 4th ed. St. Louis: Butterworths; 1986:606–611.
20. Blauth CI, Cosgrove DM, Webb BW, et al. Atheroembolism from the ascending aorta: An emerging problem in cardiac surgery. *J Thorac Cardiovasc Surg* 1992;103:1104–1111.
21. Lytle BW. Coronary artery reoperations. In: Cohn L, Edmund LH (eds). *Cardiac Surgery in the Adult,* 2d ed. McGraw-Hill; 2003:659.
22. Navia D, Cosgrove DM, Lytle BW, et al. Is the internal thoracic artery the conduit of choice to replace a stenotic vein graft? *Ann Thorac Surg* 1994:57:40–43.
23. Otaki M, Lust RM, Sun YS, et al. Experimental supplemental vein grafting and hypoperfusion syndrome. *Ann Thorac Surg* 1995;59:1423–1428.
24. Lytle BW. Reoperation for coronary artery disease. In: Yang SC, Cameron DE (eds). *Current Therapy in Thoracic and Cardiovascular Surgery.* Philadelphia: Mosby; 2004:665.
25. Tector AJ, Kress DC, Amundsen SM, et al. Reoperation in patients with closed SVG and patent LITA-LAD graft: T-graft approach. *Ann Thorac Surg* 1995;59:1509–1512.
26. Stephan WJ, O'Keefe JH, Piehler JM, et al. Coronary angioplasty versus repeat coronary artery bypass grafting for patients with previous bypass surgery. *J Am Coll Cardiol* 1996;28:1140–1146.
27. Morrison DA, Sethi G, Sacks J, et al. Percutaneous coronary intervention versus repeat bypass surgery for patients with medically refractory myocardial ischemia: AWESOME randomized trial and registry experience with post CABG patients. *J Am Coll Cardiol* 2002;40:1951–1954.
28. Brener SJ, Loop FD, Lytle BW, et al. Profile of candidates for repeat myocardial revascularization: Implications for selection of treatment. *J Thorac Cardiovasc Surg* 1997;114:153–161.
29. Mulvihill NT, Marco J. Percutaneous intervention for atherosclerotic disease in saphenous vein grafts. *Int J Cardiol* 2002;83:103–110.
30. Dewey TM, Magee MJ, Acuff T, et al. Beating heart surgery reduces mortality in the reoperative bypass patient. *Heart Surg Forum* 2002;5:S301–S316.
31. Alamanni F, Pompilio G, Polvani G, et al. Off-pump redo coronary artery bypass grafting: Technical aspects and early results. *Heart Surg Forum* 2002;5:S432–S444.
32. Stamou SC, Pfister AJ, Dangas G, et al. Beating heart versus conventional single-vessel reoperative coronary artery bypass. *Ann Thorac Surg* 2000;69:1383–1387.
33. Chavanon O, Carrier M, Cartier R, et al. Increased incidence of acute ascending aortic dissection with off-pump aortocoronary bypass surgery? *Ann Thorac Surg* 2001;71:117–121.
34. Czerny M, Zimpfer D, Kilo J, et al. Coronary reoperations: Recurrence of angina and clinical outcome with and without cardiopulmonary bypass. *Ann Thorac Surg* 2003;75:847–852.
35. Azoury FM, Gillinov AM, Lytle BW, et al. Off-pump reoperative coronary artery bypass grafting by thoracotomy: Patient selection and operative technique. *Ann Thorac Surg* 2001;71:1959–1963.
36. Lajos TZ, Akhter M, Bergsland J, et al. Limited access left thoracotomy for reoperative coronary artery disease: On or off pump. *J Card* Surg 2000;15:291–295.
37. D'Ancona G, Karamanoukian H, Lajos T, et al. Posterior thoracotomy for reoperative coronary artery bypass grafting without cardiopulmonary bypass: Perioperative results. *Heart Surg Forum* 2000;3:18–22.
38. Doty JR, Salazar JD, Fonger JD, et al. Preoperative MIDCAB grafting: 3-year clinical experience. *Eur J Cardiothorac Surg* 1998;13:641–649.
39. Pascucci S, Gunkel L, Zietak T, et al. Use of MIDCAB procedure for redo coronary artery bypass. *J Cardiovasc Surg* 2002;43:143–146.
40. Salomon NW, Page US, Bigelow JC, et al. Reoperative coronary surgery: Comparative analysis of 6591 patients undergoing primary bypass and 508 patients undergoing reoperative coronary artery bypass. *J Thorac Cardiovasc Surg* 1990;100:250–259.
41. Christenson JT, Schmuziger M, Simonet F. Preoperative coronary artery bypass procedures: Risk factors for early mortality and late survival. *Eur J Cardiothorac Surg* 1997;11:129–133.
42. Merlo C, Aidala E, La Scala E, et al. Mortality and morbidity in reoperation comparing to first intervention in coronary revascularization. *J Cardiovasc Surg (Torino)* 2001;42:713–717.
43. Machiraju VR. How to avoid problems in redo coronary artery bypass surgery. *J Cardiovasc Surg (Torino)* 2004;19:284–290.

44. Weintraub WS, Jones EL, Craver JM, et al. In-hospital and long-term outcome after reoperative coronary artery bypass graft surgery. *Circulation* 1995;92(Suppl):II-50–57.
45. Myers WO, Blackstone EH, Davis K, et al. CASS registry: Long term surgical survival. *J Am Coll Cardiol* 1999;33:488–498.
46. Noyez L, Skotnicki SH, Lacquet LK.Morbidity and mortality in 200 consecutive coronary reoperations. *Eur J Cardiothorac Surg* 1997;11:528–532.
47. Christenson JT, Simonet F, Schmuziger M. The impact of a short interval (< or = 1 year) between primary and reoperative coronary artery bypass grafting procedures. *Cardiovasc Surg* 1996;4:801–807.
48. Schmuziger M, Christenson JT, Maurice J, et al: Reoperative myocardial revascularization: An analysis of 458 reoperations and 2645 single operations. *Cardiovasc Surg* 1994;2:623–629.
49. Kaul TK, Fields BL, Wyatt DA, et al. Reoperative coronary artery bypass surgery: Early and late results and management in 1300 patients. *J Cardiovasc Surg (Torino)* 1995;36:303–312.
50. Craver JM, Hodakowski GT, Shen Y, et al. Third-time coronary artery bypass operations: Surgical strategy and results. *Ann Thorac Surg* 1996;62:1801–1807.
51. Brenowitz JB, Johnson WD, Kayser KL, et al. Coronary artery bypass grafting for the third time or more: Results of 150 consecutive cases. *Circulation* 1988;78:1166–1170.
52. Lytle BW, Navia JL, Taylor PC, et al: Third coronary artery bypass operations: Risks and costs. *Ann Thorac Surg* 1997;64:1287–1295.

CHAPTER

28 MANAGEMENT OF CONCOMITANT CAROTID AND CORONARY ARTERY DISEASE

Daniel J. Durand, David D. Yuh

INTRODUCTION

The relation between atherosclerotic coronary artery disease and carotid disease is an intuitive association that is well supported by clinical data. These two regions of the vasculature are close to each other and have important similarities in structure and embryologic origin. In a specific individual, these vascular beds have a common genetic background

KEY CONCEPTS

- Epidemiology
  - Stroke is a major complication of cardiac surgery, with an incidence ranging from 2.1 to 5.2 percent. As many as 22 percent of coronary artery bypass graft (CABG) candidates have hemodynamically significant carotid disease, which is a risk factor for perioperative stroke. This percentage is likely to increase as the population continues to age and coronary artery bypass grafting is used in increasingly older patients. Although carotid disease is associated with an increase in perioperative stroke risk, it is responsible for only a minority of strokes associated with CABG.
- Pathophysiology
  - Several mechanisms have been proposed for perioperative strokes after CABG; the most important are arterial emboli and cerebral hypoperfusion. It is theoretically possible for carotid lesions to act through either mechanism, showering emboli though plaque rupture or causing hypoperfusion via thrombosis and/or obstruction of arterial flow.
- Diagnostics
  - On physical examination, the most important finding is the presence of a carotid bruit. Although a carotid bruit is not pathognomonic for carotid stenosis, studies at the authors' center suggest a 40 percent positive predictive value for carotid stenosis (in excess of 70 percent) in CABG populations. From a demographic perspective, increased age, cerebrovascular disease, and peripheral vascular disease also greatly increase the likelihood of carotid disease. For patients at risk for carotid disease, duplex ultrasound represents a noninvasive means of assessing carotid disease quantitatively. Magnetic resonance angiography, cerebral angiography, and computed tomography (CT)-angiography represent more costly and/or invasive methods of assessing the degree of stenosis that may be useful in confirming duplex findings and in instances in which duplex results are vague.
- Treatment
  - Treatment of patients with combined coronary and carotid disease centers on medical management with antiplatelet therapy and/or cholesterol-lowering agents and carotid endarterectomy (CEA). Patients who are candidates for CABG in whom CEA also is indicated can be approached with one of three strategies: "staged" but separate procedures with CEA performed before CABG, the "combined" procedure with CEA and CABG performed under the same anesthesia, and "reverse-staged" procedures with CABG performed before CEA. In their

practice, the authors advocate treating the symptomatic territory (i.e., carotid or coronary) first and reserving combined procedures for patients with severe symptoms in both territories. Percutaneous carotid angioplasty with or without stenting is an emerging technique that is being applied in concert with CABG in a similar fashion at select centers.

- Outcomes
  - In the absence of large prospective randomized trials, there is no high-grade evidence to support the contention that CEA lowers perioperative stroke risk. However, the most recent meta-analyses indicate that MI is more common in patients undergoing the staged procedure and stroke rates are higher in those undergoing the reverse-staged procedure. The risk of stroke and myocardial infarction (MI) is similar for the combined procedure, although overall mortality is higher than for either the staged or reverse-staged procedures. However, the North American Symptomatic Carotid Endarterectomy Trial (NASCET) and the Asymptomatic Carotid Atherosclerosis Study (ACAS) trials have provided strong evidence that CEA reduces long-term stroke risk in symptomatic patients with stenosis greater than 50 percent and asymptomatic patients with stenosis greater than 60 percent. Generally, the tighter the carotid stenosis, the greater the benefit from CEA on long-term stroke risk.
- Screening
  - Many centers now screen all or a majority of CABG patients for carotid disease despite strong evidence suggesting that most perioperative strokes are caused by unrelated mechanisms. Such that mandatory screening is difficult to justify in light of the current lack of evidence on concomitant CEA/CABG and the costs associated with performing duplex ultrasound. Based on research at the Johns Hopkins Hospital, the authors advocate screening only patients who are over age 65, have a carotid bruit, or have physical symptoms of cerebrovascular disease [i.e., transient ischemic attack (TIA) or stroke].

and are subject to virtually the same environment throughout the individual's lifetime. It is therefore no surprise that the finding of coronary artery disease virtually assures that there is some degree of carotid pathology and vice versa. From the standpoint of the cardiothoracic surgeon, this means that up to 22 percent of candidates for coronary artery bypass surgery have significant carotid disease.[1] This number is likely to increase as the population continues to age and CABG is used in more elderly patients.

Although the importance of combined coronary and carotid disease is intuitive, its treatment is complex and controversial. Historically, the procedures to address each condition were developed separately and were evaluated with different metrics. The clinical benefits of CABG have been measured as reductions in myocardial infarction, reintervention, and mortality rates, whereas those of CEA have been measured as reductions in stroke and mortality rates. Complicating the picture, each operation is associated with complications that the other is intended to prevent; myocardial infarction and stroke are well-recognized complications of CEA and CABG, respectively. Furthermore, one must consider that although carotid disease is often present in coronary bypass patients, the majority of those patients experience no symptoms from their cerebrovascular disease (CVD). In deciding which operations are appropriate for each subpopulation, one must bear in mind their impact on all endpoints (e.g., myocardial infarction, stroke, death) weighed against the likelihood of all complications. Finally, less invasive procedures such as percutaneous angioplasty and carotid stenting have become more widespread in recent years, adding a further layer of complexity to treatment options. This chapter will guide cardiothoracic surgeons through the challenges of identifying and managing carotid disease in coronary bypass patients and review the evidence for and against current treatment options.

CAROTID DISEASE AND PERIOPERATIVE STROKE ASSOCIATED WITH CORONARY ARTERY BYPASS SURGERY

Stroke is one of the most prevalent and debilitating complications of coronary artery bypass surgery and frequently negates the benefits of coronary revascularization. Clinically, perioperative stroke is defined as an acute neurologic event that is secondary to circulatory impairment lasting more than 24 h and occurring within a specified period after surgery. Nearly all centers define stroke in this manner, and most obtain radiologic imaging [i.e., CT or magnetic resonance imaging (MRI)] to delineate the distribution and extent of cerebral injury after a perioperative stroke. Although there is variability in the definition of a perioperative stroke (e.g., 14 versus 28 days), most strokes present within the first 3 days after coronary bypass surgery. Over the last two decades, the incidence of perioperative stroke has remained fairly constant, ranging from 2.1 to 5.2 percent.[2,3] A variety of risk factors have been identified for perioperative stroke in CABG patients (Table 28-1), and several closely related mechanisms have been proposed (Table 28-2), the most important of which are arterial emboli and cerebral hypoperfusion. It is theoretically possible for carotid lesions to affect strokes by either of these mechanisms in the postoperative period, creating emboli through plaque rupture, thrombosis, or diminished arterial flow.

Table 28-1 Risk factors for perioperative stroke in coronary bypass patients

Demographic	Preoperative	Intraoperative
Age >65 Retired	Hypertension Mean systolic blood pressure Diabetes mellitus Carotid bruit Prior CVA Prior CVD (CVA or TIA) Left main disease >50 Tobacco use >10 pack-years	Cardiopulmonary bypass time Use of intraaortic balloon pump Mean cross-clamp time Use of membrane oxygenator

CVA = cerebrovascular accident; CVD = cerebrovascular disease; TIA = transient ischemic attack.

However, since the carotid arteries are not manipulated surgically during CABG and since carotid thrombi rarely are found on radiographic imaging, it has been postulated that carotid stenosis and/or occlusion cause strokes primarily through cerebral hypoperfusion during low-cardiac-output states (e.g., while the patient is on cardiopulmonary bypass or in the early postoperative period).

A recent meta-analysis concluded that less than half of CABG patients who suffered perioperative strokes had significant carotid disease, defined as either significant stenosis or occlusion.[4] An extensive retrospective study from the authors' practice at the Johns Hopkins Hospital yielded similar results.[5] In addition, carotid disease is a fairly specific risk factor for aortic arch atherosclerosis,[6] which is widely believed to be the most important source of arterial emboli in CABG-related strokes. As a result, it remains uncertain whether the link between carotid disease and perioperative stroke is truly causal, because carotid disease alone never has been proved to be an independent risk factor for perioperative stroke, controlling for aortic atherosclerosis. At the same time, there are reports of individuals in whom the finding of preoperative stenosis preceded a "watershed" stroke in the distribution of a stenotic carotid artery.[7] In summary, carotid disease is associated with an increased stroke risk in CABG patients, but less than half of CABG-related strokes occur in patients with carotid disease and it is likely that only a subset of those strokes are due to carotid stenosis per se rather than to related conditions.

Table 28-2 Mechanisms of perioperative stroke in coronary bypass patients

Mechanism of stroke	% of perioperative strokes in coronary artery bypass
Embolic	62.1
Unclassified	13.9
Multiple etiologies	10.1
Hypoperfusion	8.1
Lacunar	1
Thrombotic	1

Source: Data from Likosky DS, et al. Determination of etiologic mechanisms of strokes secondary to coronary artery bypass graft surgery. *Stroke* 2003;34:2830.

Although the effect of carotid disease on perioperative stroke risk remains uncertain, the effect on long-term stroke risk is well documented. Carotid disease is thought to cause 20 to 30 percent of strokes.[8] With regard to long-term stroke risk, the natural history of carotid disease in CABG patients is presumably similar to that of nonsurgical patients in large prospective studies of carotid stenosis such as the North American Symptomatic Carotid Endarterectomy Trial and the Asymptomatic Carotid Atherosclerosis Study.[9,10] No large prospective studies have addressed the long-term impact of carotid stenosis or occlusion in CABG patients specifically. A final point to consider is that there is probably a small degree of mechanistic overlap between "long-term" and "perioperative" strokes; there are bound to be CABG patients with carotid stenosis who by chance have strokes caused by carotid plaque rupture that is not related to the operation itself within the perioperative period. It is not known what percentage of perioperative strokes occur by this mechanism.

CORONARY ARTERY DISEASE AND MYOCARDIAL INFARCTION ASSOCIATED WITH CAROTID ENDARTERECTOMY

It has long been known that vascular lesions outside the coronary vascular bed can be "index lesions" of myocardial infarction. Indeed, MI is a well-documented complication of several commonly performed peripheral vascular interventions, such as aortic and infrainguinal procedures. The mechanism is thought to be embolic, as fragments of plaque from the diseased vascular bed are mobilized during surgical manipulation and become lodged in already stenosed coronary arteries. Nonfatal and fatal myocardial infarctions remain devastating postoperative complications of carotid endarterectomy, although the incidence of MI in ACAS was less than 1 percent.[11] These numbers seem surprisingly low when one considers that up to 50 percent of patients with carotid disease have some degree of coronary artery disease. Of course, MI rates are likely to be somewhat higher in CABG patients, all of whom have significant coronary artery disease.

CAROTID DISEASE IN CORONARY ARTERY BYPASS PATIENTS

Previous studies have reported an incidence of carotid disease in CABG patients ranging from 2 to 22 percent.[5]

This range is rather wide because the definition of "significant" carotid disease varies between centers. For example, even ACAS and NASCET stratified their cohorts using different numerica thresholds. Specifically, ACAS defined 60 percent luminal stenosis as significant, whereas NASCET initially employed a 70 percent threshold that later was changed to 50 percent.[9,10] After ACAS showed a significant but underwhelming clinical benefit for carotid endarterectomy using the 60 percent threshold, numerous follow-up studies used greater degrees of carotid stenosis as thresholds to trigger surgical intervention. The heterogeneous nature of "significant" stenosis is equally apparent in studies of carotid disease in CABG populations, in which thresholds routinely have ranged from 50 percent to 80 percent luminal narrowing.

Regardless of the threshold one uses to define significant carotid disease, there are several ways to identify and quantify carotid lesions. Ideally, the process begins by including questions in the history that are designed to identify patients at high risk for carotid disease. Because the etiologies of carotid artery disease and coronary artery disease are so similar, it is best to focus on risk factors that have been validated in previous studies of carotid disease in CABG populations (Table 28-3). On physical examination, the most important finding is the presence of a carotid bruit. Although a carotid bruit is not pathognomonic for carotid stenosis, at the authors' center nearly 40 percent of CABG patients with a bruit had carotid stenosis in excess of 70 percent as measured by carotid duplex ultrasound.[5] In addition, any examination findings indicative of CVD (e.g., focal neurologic deficits) or peripheral vascular disease (e.g., weak distal extremity pulses, popliteal bruits) greatly increase the likelihood of carotid disease.

For patients identified as being at high risk for carotid disease, screening by duplex ultrasound represents a noninvasive means of quantitatively assessing carotid disease. Duplex ultrasonographic measurements are obtained from peak blood flow velocities measured across the proximal internal carotid artery that are correlated to the gold standard of percentage luminal occlusion derived from digital subtraction angiography. For example, the authors' institution uses the criteria listed in Table 28-4 to translate measurements from duplex studies to percentage luminal stenosis. Equivocal cases can be evaluated further by means of MRI and/or conventional carotid angiography. With angiography, the authors define percentage stenosis according to the NASCET criteria:

$$100 \times \left(1 - \frac{\text{carotid luminal diameter at point of stenosis}}{\text{Normal carotid luminal diameter distal to stenosis}}\right)$$

It is important to note that different measurement criteria were used in the past. The MRC European Carotid Surgery Trial used an estimate of the unseen carotid bulb wall instead of the distal carotid luminal diameter.[12] Still another "common carotid method" uses the diameter of the common carotid instead of the luminal diameter of the distal carotid. Although there are advantages and disadvantages to each method, what matters most is consistency.

Table 28-3 Risk factors for carotid disease in coronary bypass patients

Highly significant ($p < 0.01$)	Significant ($p < 0.05$)
Prior CVA	Tobacco *use*[a]
Prior CVD (CVA or TIA)[a]	Left main disease > 50
Carotid bruit[a]	Hypertension[a]
Peripheral vascular disease	Prior CEA
Age > 65[a]	

CVA = cerebrovascular accident; CVD = cerebrovascular disease; TIA = transient ischemic attack.

[a]Shared risk factors for stroke and cerebrovascular disease in coronary artery bypass patients.

Table 28-4 Duplex correlation criteria in use at the Johns Hopkins Hospital

Carotid luminal stenosis, %	Criteria
0–49	No spectral broadening Peak systolic velocity < 140 cm/s End diastolic velocity < 100 cm/s ICA/CCA ratio < 2.0
50–69	Spectral broadening throughout systole Peak systolic velocity > 140 cm/s End diastolic velocity <= 100 cm/s; ICA/CCA ratio >= 2.0
70–99	Spectral broadening throughout systole Peak systolic velocity > 250 cm/s End diastolic velocity > 100 cm/s ICA/CCA ratio > = 4.0
100	No detectable flow Look for low or reversed flow component in CCA Proximal ICA may have characteristic "thump flow" or "flow reversal"

ICA = internal carotid artery; CCA = common carotid artery.

TREATMENT OF SEVERE CAROTID STENOSIS

When a patient is diagnosed with carotid stenosis (i.e., nonocclusive carotid disease), two treatment strategies are available: (1) medical management with antiplatelet therapy and/or cholesterol-lowering agents and (2) carotid endarterectomy or percutaneous angioplasty with or without carotid stenting. The choice of therapy is typically guided by the presence or absence of cerebrovascular symptoms (i.e., prior stroke or transient ischemic attack) and the extent of stenosis based on the results of several large multicenter prospective randomized clinical trials conducted in the 1980s and 1990s.

Carotid endarterectomy

NASCET compared CEA with medical management (aspirin) and identified a 15 percent absolute reduction in stroke risk (i.e., 25 percent versus 10 percent) at 2 years in symptomatic patients with carotid stenosis in excess of 70 percent.[9] Further analysis showed a more modest benefit in patients with carotid stenosis in excess of 50 percent.[13] Among the three largest studies on asymptomatic cohorts, the Carotid Artery Surgery Asymptomatic Narrowing versus Aspirin (CASANOVA) and Veterans Affairs (VA) trials found no significant benefit for CEA.[14,15] ACAS identified an absolute stroke risk reduction of just 5 percent (i.e., 10 percent to 5 percent).[10] Since the degree of benefit patients receive from CEA is directly proportional to their preoperative stroke risk, there has been a great deal of research into models that incorporate a variety of risk factors in addition to the degree of carotid stenosis to expand indications for CEA to all patients who are likely to benefit from surgery. Critics of ACAS and NASCET maintain that CEA is now less effective because medical therapies have evolved whereas the majority of CEAs are performed by surgeons with higher complication rates than those at the centers of excellence used in the landmark studies. The net result is that CEA is indicated strongly in symptomatic patients with carotid stenosis in excess of 70 percent. The role of CEA is more controversial in asymptomatic patients with carotid stenosis, but it generally is recommended in cases of severe or critical (e.g., 80 to 90 percent) carotid disease. It is not known how these results extrapolate to CABG patients, in whom operative complications such as MI and/or death are likely to be much higher to the extent that they may negate the stroke-risk benefits of CEA.

Carotid angioplasty and stenting

This is an era of expanding applications for endovascular interventions. Although carotid angioplasty and stenting certainly have become more widespread over the last decade, they remain investigational procedures. At most centers, carotid angioplasty has been supplanted by stenting because carotid artery dissections during balloon inflation are less likely to occur with stenting. A recent meta-analysis conducted for the Cochrane collaboration looked across all studies comparing angioplasty and stenting to conventional CEA and found few significant differences between the two approaches.[16] Although the endovascular approach clearly avoids minor surgical complications such as cranial neuropathy, the rates of major complications such as stroke, death, and MI are similar to those observed in NASCET. Furthermore, data on long-term stroke rates with percutaneous techniques remain unclear. In general, these recent studies have used the same indications for carotid stenting that were previously applied to CEA. However, there has been substantial heterogeneity between studies, making it difficult to compare carotid stenting to CEA. Toward this end, several trials of stenting versus CEA and medical therapy are under way and will provide further guidance.

SURGICAL TREATMENT OF COMBINED CORONARY AND CAROTID DISEASE

Surgical treatment for concomitant coronary and carotid disease varies between centers, primarily because there are no large multicenter prospective randomized trials to guide therapy. Consequently, surgeons have been forced to rely on small studies and meta-analyses, many of which are contradictory. In their practice, the authors advocate treating the symptomatic territory (i.e., carotid or coronary) first and reserving combined procedures for patients with symptoms in both territories. The reasoning for that recommendation is summarized below.

Staged carotid endarterectomy–coronary artery bypass grafting

In the staged approach, the carotid lesion is addressed first by CEA, followed by CABG at a later point. The time interval between the procedures has varied in the literature from days to months. The rationale behind this sequence is predicated on a reduction in perioperative stroke risk resulting from prophylactic treatment of the carotid lesion. This strategy is most appropriate in patients whose carotid disease is equally or more advanced than their coronary disease, as those patients must forego CABG for some period. Conversely, this strategy is inappropriate for patients with critical coronary stenosis or severe multiple-vessel disease, since the heightened risk of perioperative myocardial infarction remains unaddressed.

The two large meta-analyses[17,18] of combined procedures to date have shared the intuitive conclusion that MI is more common relative to stroke in patients undergoing staged procedures (Table 28-5). These studies had differing results regarding the absolute incidence of either complication, but in general, the risk of MI with the staged approach is over 5 percent, whereas the incidence of stroke is about 5 percent or less. Mortality rates do not appear to be higher with staged procedures compared with combined approaches.

Reversed staged coronary artery bypass grafting–carotid endarterectomy

In patients whose coronary disease is more critical than their carotid disease, a reversed staged approach may be

Table 28-5 Summary of meta-analyses of combined coronary bypass–carotid endarterectomy operations

			Combined[a]			Staged[a]		
Meta-analysis	Year	N (Publications)	Stroke	MI	Death	Stroke	MI	Death
Moore et al.[17]	1995	56	6.2	4.7	5.6	5.3	11.5	9.4
Borger et al.[19]	1999	16	6.0	—	4.7	3.2	—	2.9
Das et al.[20]	2000	58	3.9	—	4.5	1.5	—	5.9
Naylor et al.[18]	2003	97	4.6	3.6	4.6	2.7	6.5	3.9

[a]Outcome in percent.
MI = myocardial infarction.
Source: Huh J, Wall MJ, Soltero ER. Treatment of combined coronary and carotid artery disease. *Curr Opin Cardiol* 2003;18(6):447–453.

appropriate. Myocardial infarction was the most common complication associated with CEA in the ACAS study and has been shown to occur with greater frequency in patients with unstable angina and coronary artery disease. Patients who have undergone CABG recently have reduced their risk of perioperative MI and thus are thought to be better candidates for subsequent CEA. As one would expect, the results of the reversed staged approach are the converse of those with conventional staged approach (Table 28-5); stroke rates are higher than perioperative myocardial infarction rates with this approach. In general, mortality rates are diminished with this approach, although there is not enough evidence to draw firm conclusions.

Combined carotid endarterectomy–coronary artery bypass grafting

For patients experiencing symptoms from both coronary disease and carotid disease, it may be advantageous to operate on both territories simultaneously. Because the prospect of addressing both lesions and their associated complications is so appealing, there has been a disproportionate number of papers studying this combined approach. Various techniques have been demonstrated: (1) CEA before opening the thorax, (2) CEA after opening the thorax but before cannulation, and (3) CEA while the patient is on cardiopulmonary bypass. The first is by far the most popular.

The results of the combined approach have varied widely. In the meta-analyses conducted to date (Table 28-5), the incidences of stroke, MI, and death have been around 5 percent.[17–20] These numbers probably are skewed by the fact that combined procedures are more likely to be offered to sicker patients. At the same time, there are indications that the technical complexity of operating on both territories has poor reproducibility and may even be dangerous when attempted outside centers of excellence. For example, a study of 226 patients treated with concomitant procedures at community-based hospitals demonstrated a combined stroke/mortality rate of 17.7 percent.[21]

RISK STRATIFICATION MODELS FOR PREOPERATIVE CAROTID SCREENING IN CABG PATIENTS

Based on the issues discussed above, CEA is indicated in only about 5 percent of the total CABG population. Screening all CABG patients for carotid disease with duplex ultrasonography requires significant economic resources, causes inconvenience to patients, and creates a potential delay in performing CABG. An alternative approach is to use a selective screening approach based on identified risk factors for carotid disease. The authors' institution selectively screens patients at "high risk" for both carotid disease and stroke: patients with cerebrovascular symptoms, a carotid bruit, or age in excess of 65 years. The authors' algorithm (Fig. 28-1) has a sensitivity in excess of 80 percent and a specificity of 40 percent in identifying significant operable carotid disease (greater

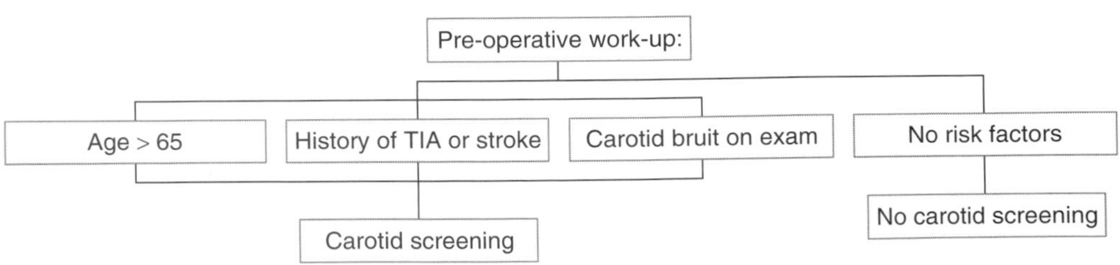

Figure 28-1 Preoperative carotid duplex screening algorithm in use at Johns Hopkins Hospital. (Durand DJ, Perler BA, Roseborough GS, et al: Mandatory versus selective preoperative carotid screening: A retrospective analysis. *Ann Thorac Surg 2004*;78:159–166)

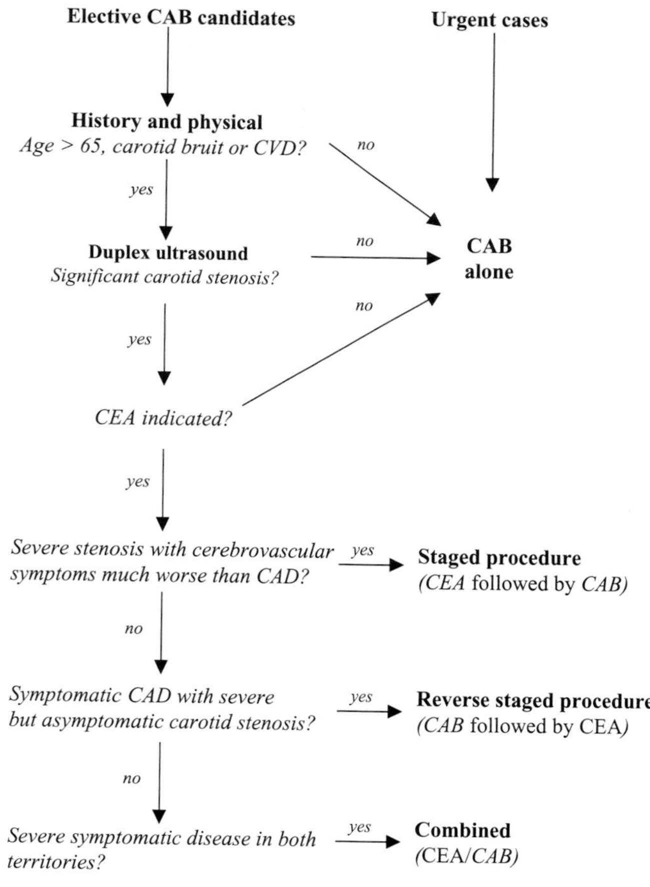

Figure 28-2 Treatment algorithm for coronary bypass patients with concomitant carotid and coronary disease.

than 70 percent stenosis) and has reduced screening loads by 40 percent.[5] Furthermore, a post hoc retrospective analysis indicates that all CABG patients evaluated at the authors' center over a 2-year period who were found to have significant carotid disease and had perioperative strokes would have been identified as "high risk" for carotid stenosis according to the authors' selective screening criteria (Fig. 28-2). The incidence of asymptomatic carotid disease in "low-risk" patients who would have gone unscreened was only 5 percent, and CEA would have been indicated in only 1 percent of those patients. The authors advocate this screening algorithm or one that incorporates additional stroke risk factors (e.g., peripheral vascular disease) to optimize preoperative carotid screening. However, all CABG patients should be informed that they are at increased risk for carotid disease, which may warrant future evaluation after surgery.

SUMMARY

Carotid disease is strongly associated with coronary disease and occurs in a significant number of CABG patients. Patients with carotid disease who undergo CABG are at increased risk for perioperative stroke, although it is unclear whether carotid disease causes these strokes or whether they are due to related vascular pathology such as aortic arch disease. At the same time, myocardial infarction is a rarer but frequently fatal complication of carotid endarterectomy. Treating patients with dual disease therefore requires that one weigh the risks and benefits of treatment options with regard to stroke, myocardial infarction, and death. Although the ACAS and NACSET trials showed convincingly that CEA can benefit well-defined groups of patients in terms of long-term stroke rates, indications for CEA in patients with coronary artery disease are more complex because there have been no large-scale randomized clinical trials comparing the various treatment options available. Surgical treatment options include staged CEA/CABG, reverse-staged CABG/CEA, and simultaneous CEA/CABG. Generally, the best approach is to treat the more symptomatic territory first by performing CEA/CABG in patients with more severe cerebrovascular symptoms and CABG/CEA in those with predominantly coronary symptoms. Although some authors have advocated using the combined approach because it limits the use of anesthesia, some evidence suggests that these patients fare poorly outside the few centers that have a wealth of experience combining these techniques.

References

1. Schwartz LB, Bridgman AH, Kieffer RW, et al. Asymptomatic carotid artery stenosis and stroke in patients undergoing cardiopulmonary bypass. *J Vasc Surg* 1995;21:146–153.
2. McKhann GM, Goldsborough MA, Borowicz LM Jr, et al. Predictors of stroke risk in coronary artery bypass patients. *Ann Thorac Surg* 1997;63:516–521.
3. D'Ancona G, Saez de Ibarra JI, Baillot R, et al. Determinants of stroke after coronary artery bypass grafting. *Eur J Cardiothorac Surg* 2003;24:552–556.
4. Naylor AR, Mehta Z, Rothwell PM, Bell PR. Carotid artery disease and stroke during coronary artery bypass: A critical review of the literature. *Eur J Vasc Endovasc Surg* 2002;23:283–294.
5. Durand DJ, Perler BA, Roseborough GS, et al. Mandatory versus selective preoperative carotid screening: A retrospective analysis. *Ann Thorac Surg* 2004;78:159–166.
6. Fukuda I, Gomi S, Watanabe K, Seita J. Carotid and aortic screening for coronary artery bypass grafting. *Ann Thorac Surg* 2000;70:2034–2039.
7. Hise JH, Nipper ML, Schnitker JC. Stroke associated with coronary artery bypass surgery. *Am J Neuroradiol* 1991;12:811–814.
8. Timsit SG, Sacco RL, Mohr JP, et al. Early clinical differentiation of cerebral infarction from severe atherosclerotic stenosis and cardioembolism. *Stroke* 1992;23:486–491.
9. North American Symptomatic Carotid Endarterctomy Trial Collaborators. Beneficial effect of carotid endarterec-

tomy in symptomatic patients with high-grade stenosis. *N Engl J Med* 1991;325:445–453.

10. Asymptomatic Carotid Atherosclerosis Study Group. Carotid endarterectomy for patients with asymptomatic internal carotid artery stenosis. *JAMA* 1995;273:1421–1428.
11. Young B, Moore WS, Robertson JT, et al. for the ACAS Investigators. An analysis of perioperative surgical mortality and morbidity in the asymptomatic carotid atherosclerosis study. *Stroke* 1996;27:2216–2224.
12. European Carotid Surgery Trialists' Collaborative Group. MRC European Carotid Surgery Trial: Interim results for symptomatic patients with severe (70-99 percent) or with mild (0-29 percent) carotid stenosis. *Lancet* 1991;337:1235–1243.
13. Barnett HJ, Taylor DW, Eliasziw M, et al. Benefit of carotid endarterectomy in patients with symptomatic moderate or severe stenosis: North American Symptomatic Carotid Endarterectomy Trial Collaborators. *N Engl J Med* 1998;339:1415–1425.
14. CASANOVA Study Group. Carotid surgery versus medical therapy in asymptomatic carotid stenosis. *Stroke* 1991;22:1229–1235.
15. Hobson RW 2nd, Weiss DG, Fields WS, et al. Efficacy of carotid endarterectomy for asymptomatic carotid stenosis. The Veterans Affairs Cooperative Study Group. *N Engl J Med* 1993;328(4):221–227.
16. Coward LJ, Featherstone RL, Brown MM. Percutaneous transluminal angioplasty and stenting for carotid artery stenosis. *Cochrane Database Syst Rev* 2004(2):CD000515.
17. Moore WS, Barnett HJ, Beebe HG, et al. Guidelines for carotid endarterectomy: A multidisciplinary consensus statement from the Ad Hoc Committee, American Heart Association. *Circulation* 1995;91(2):566–579.
18. Naylor AR, Cuffe RL, Rothwell PM, Bell PR. A systematic review of outcomes following staged and synchronous carotid endarterectomy and coronary artery bypass. *Eur J Vasc Endovasc Surg* 2003;25:380–389.
19. Borger MA, Fremes SE, Weisel RD, et al. Coronary bypass and carotid endarterectomy: Does a combined approach increase risk? A metaanalysis. *Ann Thorac Surg* 1999;68:14–21.
20. Das SK, Brow TD, Pepper J. Continuing controversy in the management of concomitant coronary and carotid disease: An overview. *Int J Cardiol* 2000;74:47–65.
21. Brown KR, Kresowik TF, Chin MH, et al. Multistate population-based outcomes of combined carotid endarterectomy and coronary artery bypass. *J Vasc Surg* 2003;37:32–39.

CHAPTER

29 MECHANICAL COMPLICATIONS OF MYOCARDIAL INFARCTION

Ryan R. Davies, Michael A. Coady

OVERVIEW

The first clinical description of myocardial infarction (MI) was reported by Herrick in 1912.[1] He concluded from the clinical history that "while sudden death often does occur, yet at times it is postponed for several hours or even days, and in some instances, a complete, that is functionally complete, recovery ensues." In the current era, a complete recovery after an acute MI has become the norm rather than the exception. Unfortunately, however, the mortality for some patients remains devastatingly high. In particular, patients with cardiogenic shock after an acute MI have less than a 50 percent chance of surviving their hospital stay.[2,3]

KEY CONCEPTS

- Epidemiology
  - Six to 10 percent of patients develop cardiogenic shock after myocardial infarction.
  - Mortality rates remain high (40 percent hospital survival).
- Pathophysiology
  - Spiral of worsening ventricular function leads to decreased coronary perfusion, worsening ischemia, and an enlarging infarct zone.
- Clinical features
  - Symptoms of systemic and coronary hypoperfusion, including cold clammy extremities, cyanosis, oliguria, and altred sensorium.
  - Often occurs in patients without previous infarction or revascularization.
- Diagnostics
  - Invasive hemodynamic monitoring important in optimizing both coronary and systemic perfusion.
  - ECG confirms cardiac ischemia; chest X-ray rules out pneumothorax.
  - Emergent echocardiography to rule out other mechanical causes of shock, including papillary muscle or ventricular rupture.
- Treatment
  - Medical
    - No pharmacologic agent has been shown to have survival benefit inotopes/vasodilators/vasopressors should be used to stabilize the patient in preparation for definitive therapy.
    - Thrombolysis of unproven benefit for patients in cardiogenic shock.
  - Surgical
    - Intraaortic balloon pump improves effectiveness of systemic thrombolysis; may improve outcomes in patients with cardiogenic shock; excellent option for hemodynamic stabilization.
    - Percutaneous coronary intervention (PCI). Clear long-term benefit to revascularization in patients with cardiogenic shock (SHOCK trial). Successful angioplasty associated with significant improvements in 30 day mortality.
    - Emergent CABG improves survival in most studies of cardiogenic shock; optimal indications unclear but important treatment where PCI is unsuccessful or inappropriate.
    - Left ventricular assist device and orthotopic heart transplantation are options when revascularization is not possible or ineffective.
- Outcomes and prognosis
  - Hospital mortality rates 60 percent vs 8 percent for those without cardiogenic shock.
  - Emergent revasularization improves survival in nearly all patient groups.

Cardiogenic shock in acute MI may result from a variety of mechanical complications. Most commonly it results from ventricular infarction and dysfunction alone, but other mechanical processes may contribute to the syndrome: ventricular septal rupture, ventricular free wall rupture, and ischemic mitral regurgitation.[4] Although surgical therapies for these three conditions have long been recognized, the importance of timely revascularization in patients with cardiogenic shock in the absence of ventricular rupture or mitral regurgitation has received increased attention recently (see the Decision-Making Flowchart).

The topics covered in this chapter include (1) post–MI cardiogenic shock and ventricular dysfunction, (2) ischemic mitral valve disease, (3) postinfarction ventricular septal rupture, (4) postinfarction ventricular free wall rupture, and (5) ventricular aneurysms.

POSTMYOCARDIAL INFARCTION, CARDIOGENIC SHOCK, AND VENTRICULAR DYSFUNCTION

INTRODUCTION

Cardiogenic shock is a clinical syndrome that is characterized by hypotension and systemic hypoperfusion in the setting of ineffective cardiac function. Although the first report of circulatory collapse secondary to MI may have occurred as early as 1794 with Sir Everald Home's description of the life of the British surgeon Sir John Hunter, Herrick first recognized the clinical signs of cardiogenic shock: cold clammy extremities, oliguria, and an altered mental status.[5,6] These clinical signs are accompanied by alterations in hemodynamic parameters: systolic blood pressure less than 90 mmHg, cardiac index less than 2.2 L/min/m^2, and pulmonary capillary wedge pressure greater than 15 mmHg indicating inadequate cardiac function despite adequate preload.

PATHOPHYSIOLOGY

Myocardial ischemia and infarction

With progressive atherosclerosis of the coronary arteries, normal intraluminal diameter is preserved initially through compensatory outward remodeling; however, eventually these stenoses become functionally important and coronary artery disease becomes symptomatic.[7] Plaque rupture may occur at any time, leading to intraluminal thrombosis.[8] Usually this occurs in angiographically insignificant arteries, but it may cause total occlusion of epicardial arteries, resulting in myocardial hypoperfusion and ischemia. Occlusion of coronary arteries for less than 15 min results in reversible myocardial injury; longer periods result in irreversible damage.[9,10] Brief periods of ischemia correspond clinically to periods of angina (stable or unstable) and may occur on a daily basis[11]; longer periods result in MI.

Stunned myocardium

Within the first few minutes of ischemia, hypoxic myocytes stop contracting, resulting in regions of akinesia and dyskinesia.[11] After reperfusion (whether by relaxation of coronary artery spasm, cessation of exercise in stable angina, or pharmacologic or mechanical reperfusion), regions of viable postischemic myocardium may take hours to days to return to normal function; this delay has been termed myocardial stunning.[12–14] It originally was described in canine models of coronary occlusion and reperfusion and represents contractile dysfunction after *acute* ischemic injury. It includes left ventricular dysfunction after thrombolysis or angioplasty and may be involved in unusual cases of coronary spasm and severe exercise-induced ischemia. The pathogenesis of myocardial stunning is not completely understood. The primary mechanism is thought to be liberation of oxygen free radicals and myocyte adenosine triphosphate (ATP) depletion during reperfusion, but alterations in calcium homeostasis (including excitation-contraction decoupling resulting from sarcoplasmic reticulum dysfunction, calcium overload, and decreased responsiveness of myofilaments to calcium) may play a significant role.[11,15] Although investigators have suggested that calcium channel blockers or free radical scavengers may be useful in the treatment of myocardial stunning, inotropic support of the stunned myocardium until spontaneous recovery occurs remains the mainstay of treatment. Whatever the cause, stunned myocardium results in regions of reperfused, viable, but temporarily dysfunctional myocardium after an acute ischemic event. With sustained reperfusion, there is the potential for recovery of function.

Hibernating myocardium

Historically, it was thought that ventricular wall dysfunction in patients with coronary artery disease results from regions of infarcted myocardium. However, with the advent of reperfusion therapies, it came to be recognized that some dysfunctional myocardium can recover after the return of blood flow to ischemic regions.[16,17] It is thought that these regions of *chronically* ischemic myocardium go into a state of "hibernation" in which metabolic activity is downregulated. This represents an adaptive process that reduces oxygen consumption and prevents irreversible ischemic damage.[16–18] Identification of patients with hibernating myocardium is important, because regions of hibernating myocardium consist of viable cells and revascularization may reverse the dysfunction and ameliorate left ventricular failure.

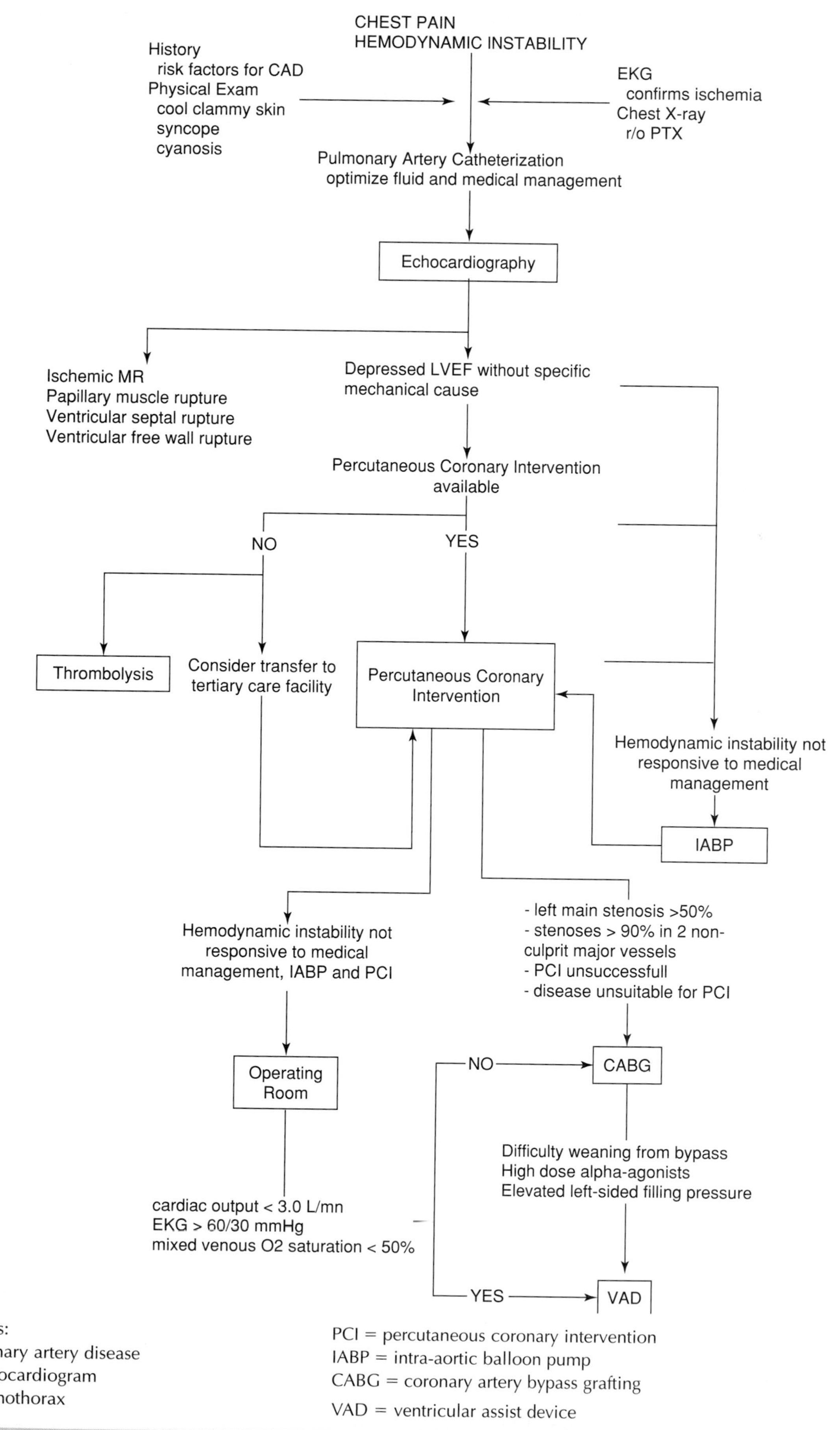

Abbreviations:
CAD = coronary artery disease
EKG = electrocardiogram
PTX = pneumothorax
PCI = percutaneous coronary intervention
IABP = intra-aortic balloon pump
CABG = coronary artery bypass grafting
VAD = ventricular assist device

Decision-making flowchart: Management of patients in cardiogenic shock.

Cardiogenic shock

Acute MI leads to cardiogenic shock through ischemic dysfunction of myocytes and loss of effective contractility. The poor outcomes associated with this syndrome are due, at least in part, to the progressive nature of the dysfunction, in which worsening hypoperfusion leads to increasing ischemic and infarcted regions of myocardium. Cessation of this "vicious cycle" must occur early to increase survival rates in patients who present in cardiogenic shock after MI (Fig. 29-1).

Cardiac function depends on a complex interplay of a variety of factors: myocyte contractility, preload, afterload, and electrical coordination. After myocardial damage, ischemic myocytes lose contractile function. This results in a decrease in stroke volume and cardiac output. To compensate for this loss, sympathetic tone is increased, and this results in tachycardia, systemic vasoconstriction, and increased contractile function in the remaining, nonischemic myocardium. Although these mechanisms help maintain both systemic and coronary perfusion, they also lead to increasing cardiac workload and oxygen consumption in the remaining myocytes.

If the remaining portions of the heart are able to maintain cardiac output and blood pressure, a compensated state may develop that allows for systemic and coronary perfusion without extension of the infarct. However, if the compensatory mechanisms cannot meet the increased demand, the area of ischemic and infarcted myocardium increases, leading to a downward spiral in cardiac function and ultimately to shock. Once mean arterial blood pressure falls below 70 mmHg, coronary blood flow becomes severely restricted.[19] This spiral toward shock and ultimately death is supported by autopsy studies that have shown that infarcted regions of myocardium contain varying degrees of progression, suggesting an initial insult followed by multiple subsequent infarction events.[20] Traditionally, cardiogenic shock was thought to occur after the loss of approximately 40 percent of left ventricular muscle mass.[21] Although studies have varied in the precise definition of hemodynamic variables, most would include systolic blood pressure (SBP) less than 90 mmHg, cardiac index (CI) less than 2.2 L/min/m^2, and pulmonary capillary wedge pressure (PCWP) less than 15 mmHg.[22,23]

Right ventricular dysfunction

Most patients with cardiogenic shock related to ventricular dysfunction have primarily left ventricular failure; in the SHOCK (SHould we emergently revascularize Occluded Coronaries in cardiogenic shoCK) trial, nearly 80 percent of patients presented with shock resulting from predominant left ventricular (LV) failure.[24] In contrast, less than 3 percent of patients presented with isolated right ventricular (RV) failure. However, despite younger age and a lower incidence of multivessel disease, a similar mortality rate was observed in the group with RV infarcts.[4] A variety of factors may contribute to this phenomenon, including RV dependence on atrial filling

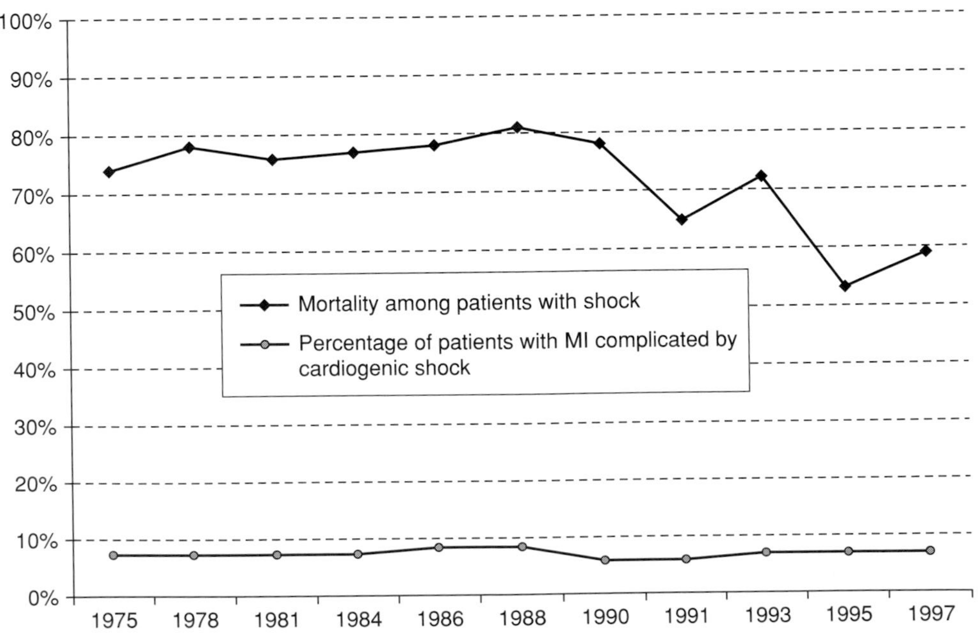

Figure 29-1 Temporal trends in the incidence of cardiogenic shock after myocardial infarction and in mortality among those patients. [Data from Goldberg RJ, Samad NA, Yarzebski J, et al. Temporal trends in cardiogenic shock complicating acute myocardial infarction. *N Engl J Med* 1999;340(15):1162–1168. Permission pending.]

that may be compromised by atrioventricular (AV) dissynchrony, poor RV compensation for ischemia secondary to the large surface area and thin free wall, and concomitant LV dysfunction with loss of septal assistance to RV systole.

Peripheral effects

Traditionally, the vicious cycle of ventricular dysfunction was thought to be the primary pathophysiologic process involved in the development of ventricular dysfunction and cardiogenic shock. More recently, data have begun to suggest that the pathophysiology of cardiogenic shock may be more complicated.[25] Patients in the SHOCK trial and registry have been found to have a wide range of ejection fractions with a mean of approximately 30 percent, and systemic vascular resistance was not universally elevated despite the use of vasopressors.[23,25–27] Based on studies of nitric oxide species, Hochman[25] concluded that some patients may have a significant component of systemic hypoperfusion related to a systemic inflammatory response caused by the release of inflammatory cytokines, and the SHOCK-2 (SHould we inhibit nitric Oxide synthase in patients with Cardiogenic Shock) trial was designed to evaluate additional medical therapies directed toward the inhibition of inflammatory and vasodilatory mediators of shock.[25]

CLINICAL FEATURES

Precise estimates of the incidence of cardiogenic shock after acute MI are difficult to obtain because many patients die before reaching medical care. Furthermore, varying definitions of cardiogenic shock may contribute to variation among studies. The early report by Griffith and associates[28] had an incidence of nearly 20 percent; however, more recent studies have shown a consistent incidence of 6 to 10 percent.[2,29–31] The high incidence reported by Griffith may have been due in part to the inclusion of patients with underresuscitated hypovolemic shock in an era before invasive hemodynamic monitoring.[5] Despite advances in the diagnosis and treatment of patients with MI, the incidence of cardiogenic shock in this population over the last three decades has remained relatively constant.[2] Although mortality rates have improved (Figure 29-1), patients diagnosed with cardiogenic shock during an admission for MI still have a substantially higher in-hospital mortality rate than do those without shock (59 percent versus 8 percent).[2,23] Overall cardiogenic shock accounts for more than 55 percent of the in-hospital mortality of MI.[30] In addition, long-term survival of patients with cardiogenic shock remains significantly lower than that in patients without it even after hospital discharge.[32]

Interestingly, although patients may present to the hospital in cardiogenic shock, a significant proportion (anywhere from 44 to 90 percent) develop shock after admission.[30,33] In-hospital mortality is similar in both groups, although there may be a long-term survival advantage among patients who develop shock after hospital admission.[30,34,35] Median time to the development of shock has varied in reported series from 5 h to nearly 24 h.[24,30,33] This raises the question of whether initial therapies may contribute to the development of cardiogenic shock in some patients and, in light of the high mortality associated with the development of shock (independent of time to onset), suggests the importance of initiating early preventive measures.

The clinical presentation begins with the classic symptoms of MI. With the onset of cardiogenic shock, physical signs of hypoperfusion begin to predominate as oxygen delivery to vital organs becomes impaired: cold and clammy extremities, ashen or cyanotic skin, oliguria, and an altered sensorium.[1] Risk factors for the development of cardiogenic shock include age, diabetes, and a previous MI.[30,36] In addition, studies have demonstrated a correlation between large infarct size (as measured by peak cardiac enzyme levels), anterior MI, a depressed LV ejection fraction, and the development of shock.[36,37] Those who had undergone coronary artery bypass grafting in the past, however, were less likely to develop shock during their admission.[30]

DIAGNOSTIC MODALITIES

Assessment of a patient with systemic hypoperfusion should begin with the exclusion of noncardiac causes. Other causes of shock include hypovolemia, sepsis, pericardial tamponade, aortic rupture, tension pneumothorax, and anaphylaxis (Table 29-1). In light of the poor outcomes associated with the onset of cardiogenic shock after MI, initiation of therapies to improve systemic perfusion should not be delayed.

An electrocardiogram should be performed immediately. Absence of electrocardiographic changes associated with ischemia essentially excludes the diagnosis of post-MI cardiogenic shock. A chest x-ray will rule out pneumothorax as a cause of circulatory collapse. History and physical examination also should assist in differentiating cardiogenic shock from other causes, such as sepsis, anaphylaxis, and neurogenic. In fact, despite the vast armamentarium of advanced diagnostic tests, physical findings remain significant predictors of in-hospital mortality. In the global utilization of streptokinase and t-PA for occluded arteries (GUSTO) trials, subjective signs of hypoperfusion were among the most significant predictors of 30-day mortality: altered sensorium [odds ratio 1.68, 95 percent confidence interval (CI) 1.19 to 2.39], cold clammy skin (1.68, 95 percent CI 1.15 to 2.46), and decreased urine output (2.25, 95 percent CI 1.61 to 3.15).[35]

Initial laboratory investigations should focus on evaluating perfusion and oxygenation by measuring arterial

Table 29-1 Clinical presentation of different etiologies of shock

Cardiogenic shock	Septic shock	Anaphylactic shock	Hypovolemic shock	Hemorrhagic shock	Pericardial tamponade	Tension pneumothorax	Massive pulmonary embolism
Signs and Symptoms							
Pallor, fainting Cold, clammy skin Arrythmias Oliguria	Fever, chills Warm skin Tachycardia Oliguria	Urticaria, hives Warm skin Tachycardia Oliguria Respiratory distress	Pallor, fainting Cold, clammy skin Tachycardia Oliguria	Pallor, fainting Cold, clammy skin Tachycardia Oliguria	Pallor, fainting Cold, clammy skin Tachycardia Oliguria	Pallor, fainting Cold, clammy skin Respiratory distress Tachycardia Oliguria	Pallor, fainting Tachycardia Respiratory distress
Laboratory							
Elevated cardiac enzymes	Elevated white blood cells (+) blood cultures	Eosinophilia		Decreased hemoglobin, hematocrit			
Electrocardiogram							
Ischemic changes	Sinus tachycardia	Sinus tachycardia	Sinus tachycardia	Sinus tachycardia	Low-voltage electrical alterans		Right axis deviation right axis strain
Chest x-ray							
Pulmonary vascular congestion					Pulmonary vascular congestion	Pneumothorax	

blood gas as well as assessing levels of cardiac enzymes and electrolytes and doing a complete blood count. Levels of cardiac enzymes and hematocrit in particular have prognostic significance in patients with acute MI.[38–42] Invasive monitoring of blood pressure should be initiated rapidly, as noninvasive cuff pressures may underestimate actual pressure significantly in the setting of peripheral vasoconstriction. In the absence of evidence of pulmonary edema (on physical examination or chest x-ray), volume status may be assessed by the patient's response to intravenous fluid resuscitation. Perhaps most important in the final determination of cardiac function and etiology are pulmonary artery catheterization and echocardiography.

Echocardiography

Rapid echocardiography is an important tool in the diagnosis and management of patients with cardiogenic shock. It allows for rapid assessment of cardiac function. Multiple studies have shown that the ejection fraction is an important predictor of outcome even when it is measured within 24 h of presentation.[26,43] In addition, it can exclude other causes of circulatory collapse unrelated to ventricular dysfunction such as pericardial tamponade, ischemic mitral regurgitation, and ventricular free wall or septal rupture, which may require different therapies.

Pulmonary artery catheterization

Placement of a pulmonary artery catheter allows direct measurement of right-sided cardiac pressures and extrapolation to left-sided filling pressures. Patients in cardiogenic shock are expected to have poor cardiac function, with adequate ventricular preload leading to depressed cardiac output and hypotension (Table 29-2). In the setting of ventricular infarction, diastolic dysfunction may contribute to impaired ventricular filling, requiring an even higher PCWP to maintain cardiac output. Even in the absence of hypotension, some patients may have evidence of systemic hypoperfusion (and its accompanying clinical signs); their in-hospital mortality, although lower than that of patients with hypotension (43 percent versus 66 percent), is high. Although clinical characteristics are important, hemodynamic monitoring should be initiated rapidly to obtain measurements of ventricular preload and cardiac output.

MEDICAL THERAPIES

As was noted above, therapies should not be delayed while one awaits diagnostic test results. Initial management should be directed immediately toward improving systemic and coronary perfusion and oxygenation. Supplemental oxygen should be delivered, and mechanical

Table 29-2 Hemodynamic measurements with different etiologies of shock

	Cardiogenic shock								
	Biventricular failure	LV failure	RV failure	Septic	Anaphylactic	Hypovolemic or hemorrhagic	Pericardial tamponade	Tension pneumothorax	Massive pulmonary embolism
BP	⇓	⇓	⇓	⇓	⇓	⇓	⇓	⇓	⇓
CO/CI	⇓⇓	⇓⇓	⇓⇓	⇑⇑ or normal	⇑ or normal	⇓	⇓	⇓	⇓⇓
HR	⇑	⇑	⇑	⇑	⇑	⇑	⇑	⇑	⇑
SV	⇓	⇓	⇓	⇑ or normal	⇑ or normal	⇑ or normal	⇓⇓	⇓	⇓
SVR	⇑ or normal	⇑ or normal	⇑ or normal	⇓⇓	⇓⇓	⇑ or normal	⇑	⇑	⇑
CVP	⇑	⇑ or normal	⇑⇑	⇓ or normal	⇓ or normal	⇓⇓	⇑⇑	⇑	⇑⇑
PAP	⇑	⇓	⇓	⇓	⇓	⇓	⇑⇑	⇓	⇑⇑
PCWP	⇑	⇑⇑	normal or ⇓	⇓ or normal	⇓ or normal	⇓⇓	⇑⇑	⇓	normal or ⇓

LV = left ventricular; RV = right ventricular; BP = blood pressure; CO = cardiac output; CI = cardiac index; HR = heart rate; SV = stroke volume; SVR = systemic vascular resistance; CVP = central venous pressure; PAP = pulmonary artery pressure; PCWP = pulmonary capillary wedge pressure.

ventilation should be initiated when appropriate. Electrical complications of acute MI are common and before the development of coronary care units constituted the most common cause of death.[44] Depending on the location of the infarct, a variety of rhythm disturbances may occur, including tachy- and bradyarrythmias in both the atria and the ventricles. Therefore, telemetry monitoring should be initiated to screen for electrical dysfunction and allow for early treatment. Rapid correction of rhythm disturbances with antiarrythmic agents or cardioversion may be required, as atrioventricular dissynchrony may contribute to poor cardiac function. The use of analgesics (morphine sulfate or fentanyl) to control pain is also an important tool in reducing sympathetic tone and thus decreasing preload, afterload, and myocardial work.

Volume resuscitation and electrolyte replacement

Although cardiac dysfunction accounts for most of the decreased cardiac output and systemic hypoperfusion, relative hypovolemia may coexist in as many as 20 percent of patients with cardiogenic shock.[45] Hemodynamic parameters measured with a pulmonary artery catheter should guide resuscitation efforts. Optimal ventricular filling pressures may vary among patients. Initial infusion with either normal saline or Ringer's lactate is appropriate, although blood products should be used early. In patients over 65 years of age with a hematocrit below 33 percent, blood transfusion during admission with MI is associated with a decrease in 30-day mortality (conversely, patients with an admission hematocrit above 36 percent who received a transfusion had a higher mortality rate).[42] Among patients with a hematocrit below 27 percent who do not receive a transfusion, the mortality rate has been shown to be approximately 50 percent, three times higher than that of patients with a normal hematocrit (above 37 percent).[42] Cardiac myocyte dysfunction is worsened by alterations in the electrolyte and acid-base environment.

Vasodilators

Pharmacologic therapies such as nitrates, angiotensin-converting enzyme inhibitors, and beta blockers have proven effectiveness in reducing mortality in patients with MI. However, all these agents have the potential to cause systemic hypotension; their use should be limited in patients in cardiogenic shock. Nitroglycerin has been shown to improve myocardial oxygen delivery and reduce oxygen demand as well as augment the antiaggregatory effects of aspirin on platelets.[46–48] Nitroglycerin also has been shown to reduce ischemia and infarct size. Although it has been difficult to demonstrate a survival benefit among patients treated with nitrates in large trials such as the Grupo Italiano per lo Studio della Sopravivenza nell'infarto Miocardico (GISSI) 3 study,[49] as many as half the patients in the placebo group received off-label nitrates, probably diluting the detection of a real benefit. Also, seven smaller studies demonstrated an impressive reduction (41 percent) in post-MI mortality with the use of nitroglycerin.[50]

Although intravenous nitroprusside has many of the same pharmacologic effects as nitroglycerin, some differences make it less useful in patients with acute MI; most important, it may exacerbate coronary steal by failing to promote collateral blood flow to ischemic myocardium.[51] In light of the salutary effects of nitrates on cardiac work and the potential decrease in mortality, intravenous nitrate therapy (preferably with nitroglycerin) should be started when systemic arterial blood pressure allows. The initial doses should be low (5 to 10 mg/min) with rapid titration upward to optimize arterial blood pressure and left ventricular filling pressures (PCWP between 15 and 22 for patients in severe cardiac failure).

Inotropic support

If optimization of ventricular filling pressures fails to ameliorate systemic hypoperfusion and hypotension, the use of inotropic support and intraaortic balloon counterpulsation should be considered. A variety of inotropic agents are available, and the choice of a specific drug should be tailored to the specific clinical and hemodynamic status of the patient, particularly the degree of systemic hypotension.

Dopamine

In patients with an SBP below 80, dopamine should be the first-line cathecholamine because it has both inotropic and vasoconstrictive effects. Dopamine interacts with a variety of receptors in a dose-dependent manner. These receptors include the dopamine (DA)-1 receptors in the renal vasculature that mediate renal vasodilatation,[52] $beta_1$-adrenergic receptors in the heart leading to increased inotropy and chronotropy, and alpha-adrenergic receptors in the peripheral vasculature leading to increased vascular resistance. As the dose increases, the predominant effect changes; however, there are no precise cutoffs, and the response to dopamine may vary between patients.[52]

At low doses (0.5 to 3.0 μg/kg/min) it acts primarily as a dopaminergic agonist, increasing renal blood flow. At higher doses (3 to 5 μg/kg/min) beta-adrenergic effects become noticeable, though dopaminergic effects still dominate. At these doses, improvement in renal perfusion depends primarily on the increase in cardiac output rather than on dilatation of the renal arterial bed.[53,54] Between 5 and 10 μg/kg/min, beta-adrenergic effects become dominant and alpha-adrenergic effects become noticeable. Finally, in the range of 10 to 20 μg/kg/min, dopamine functions primarily as an alpha-adrenergic agent, leading to significant peripheral vasoconstriction. At doses above 20 μg/kg/min, coronary vasoconstriction may predominate.[50]

Many of the presumed renal protective effects of low-dose dopamine have come under attack recently.[52,55] The renal vasodilatation thought to be related to dopaminergic stimulation actually may be due to augmentation of cardiac output through both increased stroke volume and increased heart rate.[56] Thus, dopamine should be used with care in patients in cardiogenic shock, in whom the increased inotropy may increase myocardial oxygen demand beyond the increase in oxygen delivery, leading to further ischemia; this is particularly of concern at high doses, in which case coronary vasoconstriction may lead to infarction of at-risk myocardium. The dose should be titrated carefully to the desired effect. Dopamine remains an important agent in the initial management of hypotension unresponsive to fluid resuscitation, but the necessity for high-dose dopamine should lead to the insertion of an intraaortic balloon pump to protect myocardium at risk for further ischemia and infarction.

Dobutamine

In contrast to dopamine, dobutamine causes peripheral vasodilatation in association with its inotropic effects. Therefore, it is best used in patients with SBP greater than 80. Dobutamine originally was thought to be a selective $beta_1$-adrenergic agonist, but it now is recognized that it also has alpha- and $beta_2$-adrenergic effects. As with dopamine, the relative importance of these effects changes with the dose.[5] At rates between 2.5 and 15 mg/kg/min, dobutamine increases cardiac output without significantly affecting peripheral vascular resistance (probably as a result of stimulation of both $alpha_1$-mediated vasoconstriction and $beta_2$-mediated vasodilatation).[57] At higher doses, $alpha_1$-adrenergic effects may begin to predominate with an increase in heart rate, left ventricular afterload, and myocardial oxygen demand. In contrast, at lower doses, myocardial oxygen demand may remain constant despite increased contractility because of the reduction in peripheral vascular resistance, ventricular volumes, and wall stress.[58]

Isoproterenol

Isoproterenol is a beta-adrenergic agonist used primarily in the treatment of postcardiotomy cardiogenic shock. It has both an inotropic and a chronotropic effect on the heart and results in systemic vasodilatation. The increase in cardiac output seen with isoproterenol infusion is due largely to a resultant increase in heart rate.[59] Because heart rate is a major determinant of myocardial oxygen demand, isoproterenol infusion may increase myocardial oxygen consumption.[60] In addition, it has been shown to shunt blood from ischemic myocardium to nonischemic areas.[61] This also results in an increase in ventricular instability that may result in ventricular arrhythmias even at relatively low doses.[60] In light of these problems, the use of isoproterenol in the setting of post-MI cardiogenic shock largely has been abandoned. It may have some application in a hypotensive patient with bradycardia, but transvenous pacing is preferred.

Phosphodiesterase inhibitors

Milrinone and amrinone are nonadrenergic inotropic agents. In addition, they have peripheral and pulmonary vasodilatory effects. Although they have minimal chronotropic and arrhythmogenic actions compared with the cathecholamines,[61] they also have long half-lives. This mitigates their usefulness in the acute post-MI setting. Therefore, they are used only when other agents have proved ineffective.[62,63] Most commonly, this occurs in the setting of right-sided heart failure, in which the increased pulmonary vasodilation of these agents has added benefit.

Vasopressors

In patients without adequate arterial blood pressure, vasopressor agents may be required to maintain systemic perfusion.

Norepinephrine

Norepinephrine is a combined alpha- and beta-adrenergic agonist. At low doses, its effects include primarily increased cardiac output and arterial blood pressure (mainly beta-adrenergic-mediated).[64] At higher doses, vascular resistance is markedly increased and cardiac output actually may fall. Treatment with norepinephrine in patients with cardiogenic shock results in rapid increases in blood pressure, vascular resistance, and the left ventricular stroke work index.[60] The last effect presents the main downside to norepinephrine in the setting of post-MI shock. Although the increased blood pressure improves myocardial oxygen supply through increased coronary blood flow,[65] the increase in the stroke work index increases oxygen demand in a potentially ischemic heart. While a shift from anaerobic to aerobic metabolism was observed with norepinephrine infusion in patients with cardiogenic shock, myocardial oxygen extraction remained abnormally high.[65] Other side effects of norepinephrine infusion include aggravation of oliguria through constriction of the renal arterial supply, increased risk of ventricular arrhythmias, and peripheral ischemia and limb loss. Despite these drawbacks, norepinephrine is a potent vasopressor with a rapid onset; its use may be appropriate in severely hypotensive patients to maintain mean arterial pressure in the range of 70 to 80 mmHg while other therapies are instituted.

Vasopressin

Arginine vasopressin has been used frequently in patients with vasodilatory shock. In a variety of circumstances that include septic shock and postcardiotomy vasodilatory shock, an endogenous vasopressin deficiency exists.[66,67] Although that deficiency has not been seen in small series of patients in cardiogenic shock,[66] the recent recognition of a possible vasodilatory component in some patients in the SHOCK trial[25] may indicate a role for vasopressin in this setting. Traditionally, vasopressin was thought to have a negative impact on coronary perfusion; however, this was based on experimental data in normotensive dogs. Data in hypotensive models suggest that vasopressin increases coronary perfusion.[68,69] In addition, clinical trials in critically ill patients with vasodilatory shock suggest that the use of a vasopressin infusion results in decreased norepinephrine requirements, an improved cardiac index, a decreased stroke work index, and better preservation of gastric perfusion.[70] Although further study is necessary, vasopressin may provide a useful adjunct to norephinephrine in the maintenance of systemic blood pressure during the initial phase of cardiogenic shock before the institution of more definitive therapies.

None of the pharmacologic agents listed above has been shown to have a survival benefit in the treatment of cardiogenic shock. They all have significant side effects, and any attempt to increase cardiac output or systemic blood pressure in an attempt to increase coronary perfusion carries a risk of increasing myocardial ischemia. The use of vasopressors should be limited to keep mean arterial pressure at 70 to 80 mmHg, not to return patients to a normotensive state, and inotropes should be used sparingly and under careful monitoring of hemodynamic parameters. In all cases, the most appropriate uses of these agents are as temporizing measures until the initiation of intraaortic balloon pumping, mechanical circulatory support, and revascularization.

Thrombolysis

The improvement in outcome with thrombolysis in patients with acute MI has been well established,[71–73] but in patients with cardiogenic shock, the benefits of this therapy are less clear. Many studies explicitly excluded patients with cardiogenic shock, and even more failed to describe the inclusion or exclusion of those patients.[71,74,75] Thrombolytics may decrease the incidence of the subsequent development of cardiogenic shock,[72,73,76] but no trial has demonstrated a convincing reduction in mortality in patients with already established cardiogenic shock.

Mathey and associates reported the survival of three patients with cardiogenic shock treated with streptokinase in 1980.[77,78] In a larger series of 44 patients, however, mortality remained at 66 percent.[79] The GISSI-1 trial randomized a total of 280 patients with cardiogenic shock. Overall mortality in that group was 70.0 percent and did not differ between those treated with streptokinase (69.9 percent)and controls receiving placebo (70.1 percent).[72] Mortality rates were similar in trials comparing various thrombolytic regimens: The International Study Group reported mortality rates of 78.1 percent and 64.9 percent among 246 patients with cardiogenic shock treated with tissue plasminogen activator (tPA) or streptokinase[80]; the GUSTO trial also had a high 30-day mortality among 2972 patients treated with streptokinase (51 percent) or tPA (57 percent).[30]

Interestingly, among the 44 patients in the Society for Cardiac Angiography registry, arterial patency was achieved in only 19 patients (44 percent versus 71 percent

Table 29-3 Indications and contraindications for thrombolysis

Indications
Clinical history and presentation strongly suggestive of myocardial infarction within 6 h plus one or more of the following:
1 mm ST elevation in two or more contiguous limb leads
2 mm ST elevation in two or more contiguous chest leads
New left bundle branch block
2 mm ST depression in V_{1-4} suggestive of true posterior myocardial infarction
Patients presenting with above within 7–12 h of onset with persistent chest pain and ST-segment elevation
Patients age < 75 years presenting within 6 h of anterior wall myocardial infarction should be considered for recombinant tissue plasminogen activator
Contraindications
Absolute
Aortic dissection
Previous cerebral hemorrhage
Known history of cerebral aneurysm or arteriovenous malformation
Known intracranial neoplasm
Recent (within 6 monhs) thromboembolic stroke
Active internal bleeding (excluding menstruation)
Patients previously treated with streptokinase or anisolated plasminogen streptokinase activator complex (APSAC or anistreplasse) shoud receive tissue plasminogen activator, reteplase, or tenecteplase
Relative
Severe uncontrolled hypertension (blood pressure > 180/110 mmHg) on presentation or chronic severe hypertension
Current use of anticoagulants or known bleeding diathesis
Recent (within past 2–4 weeks) trauma, including head injury or traumatic or prolonged (>10 min) cardiopulmonary resuscitation
Recent (within 3 weeks) major surgery, organ biopsy, or puncture of noncompressible vessel
Recent (within past 6 months) gastrointestinal or genitourinary or other internal bleeding
Pregnancy
Active peptic ulcer disease

Adapted from Lip GY, Chin BS, Prasad N. ABC of antithrombotic therapy: Antithrombotic therapy in myocardial infarction and stable angina. *BMJ* 2002;325(7375):1287–1289.

in the registry as a whole), among whom mortality dropped to 42 percent (versus 84 percent in patients without reperfusion, $p = 0.0005$). In the GUSTO trial, lytic therapy was less likely to be successful in patients with cardiogenic shock [Thrombolysis in Myocardial Infarction (TIMI) 0 or 1 flow 42.9 percent versus 27.7 percent, $p < 0.001$].[34] However, with successful reperfusion, mortality can be decreased significantly.[34,79,81] Thus, the poor performance of thrombolysis in the setting of cardiogenic shock may be secondary to an inability to achieve patency.

The decreased ability of thrombolysis to achieve successful reperfusion in the setting of cardiogenic shock is not completely understood and probably involves a combination of hemodynamic, metabolic, and mechanical factors.[82] Hypotension and coronary hypoperfusion probably play a significant role: In the setting of cardiogenic shock, research in canine models has suggested that the rate and degree of thrombolysis after intracoronary injection of tPA are depressed compared with those in normotensive controls,[83,84] and in clinical trials, hypotension was associated with lower TIMI flow grades after thrombolysis.[85] The augmentation of blood pressure through vasopressors or an intraaortic balloon pump may improve the success rate of thrombolysis in patients with cardiogenic shock.[84,86,87]

Despite these limitations, thrombolysis remains an important treatment for acute ST-elevation MI when percutaneous catheter-based interventions are not available. Indications and contraindications for thrombolytic therapy are well established (Table 29-3).[88] However, recent data suggest that even when percutaneous catheter-based interventions are unavailable, transport to a facility with those services improves survival and decreases complications.[89] Furthermore, the use of intraaortic balloon pumps (see below) to stabilize patients for transport to a tertiary care facility has been shown to be a safe alternative to treatment with thrombolytics.[63] Although thrombolysis is an option in limited circumstances, mechanical revascularization delivers the best outcomes in acute MI patients.

Intraaortic balloon counterpulsation

In 1958, Harken described a mechanism for diastolic augmentation of blood flow.[90,91] However, initial attempts to use femoral–femoral bypass to augment diastolic flow met with technical difficulties, including the need for bilateral femoral arteriotomies and problems with the extracorporeal pump. Efforts at demonstrating increased cardiac perfusion failed. However, after work by Moulopoulos and associates[92,93] in 1968, Kantrowitz

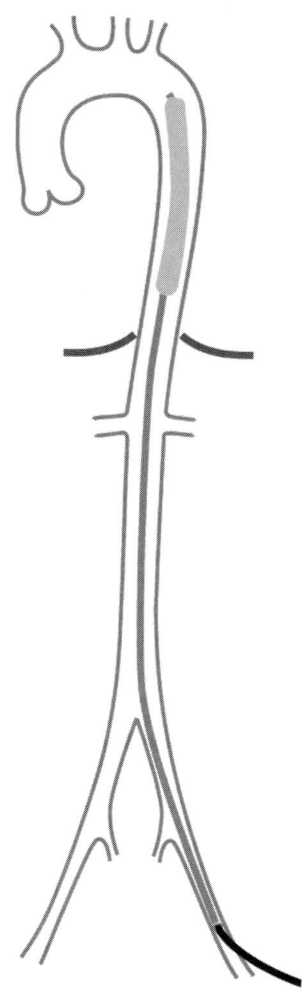

Figure 29-2 Schematic diagram of intraaortic balloon pump placement. The balloon tip should be placed distal to the take-off of the left subclavian artery.

and coworkers described the first use of an intraaortic balloon pump (IABP) to provide diastolic flow augmentation in patients with cardiogenic shock.[94] Initial models required operative placement via a femoral arteriotomy, but in 1979 Bregman and Casarella introduced a percutaneously placed model inserted through a 12F sheath.[95] Further refinements have included a dual-lumen design, wire-guided placement, reduced sheath sizes (8F or 9F for 30-mL to 50-mL balloons), and the use of helium to inflate and deflate the balloon rapidly.[96,97]

Most commonly, the IABP is inserted percutaneously into the femoral artery, using a modified Seldinger technique. After puncture of the artery, a J-wire is advanced into the aorta. The needle is removed, and the IABP catheter is inserted over the wire into the descending aorta. When properly placed, the balloon should lie immediately distal to the origin of the left subclavian artery (Fig. 29-2). In specialized cases such as pediatric patients and those with significant peripheral vascular disease that precludes the use of the femoral artery, other insertion sites may be used, including the ascending aorta, aortic arch, and subclavian, axillary, and iliac arteries.[98–104]

After insertion, the balloon is connected to a pump console that controls its inflation and deflation. The timing of these events is synchronized to the patient's cardiac cycle through the use of either electrocardiographic or aortic pressure-sensitive timing. The balloon inflates with the onset of diastole, displacing blood both proximally and distally and increasing intraaortic pressure (diastolic augmentation). Immediately before systole, the balloon deflates, reducing obstruction to left ventricular ejection (decreased afterload). With electrocardiographic timing, balloon inflation occurs (Fig. 29-3).

The decreased afterload results in a reduction in end-diastolic left ventricular diameter and volume and a reduction in ventricular wall stress; a slight decrease in heart rate also is seen.[105] Multiple studies have shown that, as expected, the reductions in wall stress and heart rate, lead to a decrease in myocardial oxygen demand and consumption.[106] Through diastolic augmentation, the IABP increases coronary perfusion and myocardial oxygen delivery.[107] This increase in coronary blood flow has been observed in both hypotensive animals and patients with cardiogenic shock.[106,108] (Fig. 29-3). Overall, these effects lead to improved hemodynamics (increased cardiac output, decreased PCWP, improved arterial blood pressure, and improved urine output)[109–111] along with improvement in myocardial metabolism (as reflected in decreasing oxygen extraction and a shift toward aerobic metabolism).[65]

Despite these improvements in hemodynamic performance and myocardial metabolism, initial results with the IABP alone in the treatment of cardiogenic shock failed to demonstrate improvement in survival.[112,113] In a small randomized trial (30 patients) that compared optimal medical therapy for cardiogenic shock with intraaortic balloon pumping, in-hospital mortality was similar in both groups (50 percent with IABP versus 44 percent with medical management).[112] However, when IABP is combined with revascularization (via thrombolysis, angioplasty, or surgery), it appears that IABP improves both short- and long-term survival, though patient selection remains a confounding factor in these trials. As was noted above, in the setting of cardiogenic shock or hypotension, the rate and degree of thrombolysis are depressed.[84] Additional work with canine models demonstrated improvement in the rate and degree of thrombolysis as well as the time to reperfusion when IABP was added to thrombolytic therapy.[86,87] Observational studies in humans confirmed an advantage for IABP when it was used with thrombolytics.[114,115]

The GUSTO-1 trial was a large randomized trial that investigated the benefits of thrombolysis. In this trial, analysis of patients with cardiogenic shock who had an IABP placed on hospital day 0 or 1 showed a trend toward improved short-term survival (30-day mortality

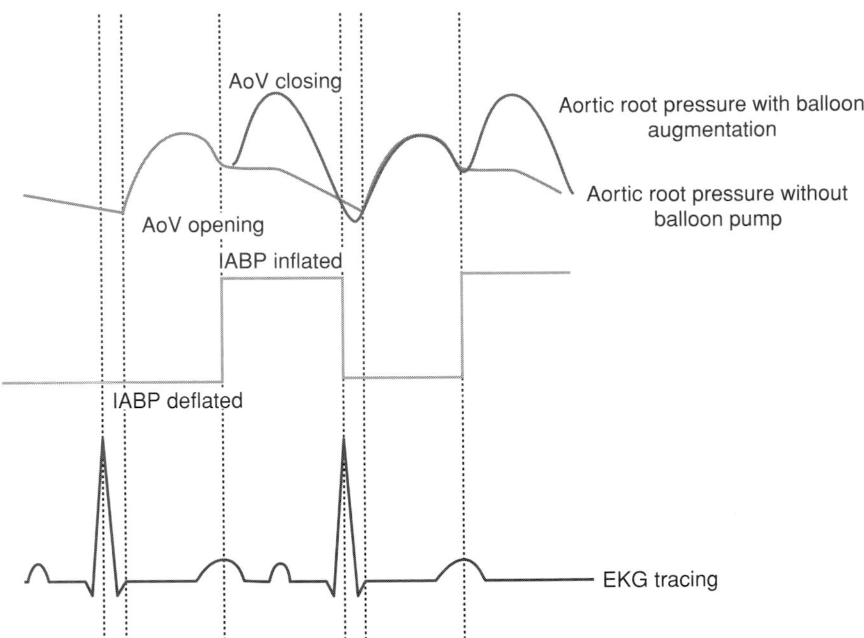

Figure 29-3 Timing of balloon pump inflation and deflation. Deflation is timed to occur just before the QRS complex to reduce afterload maximally as the aortic valve opens. Inflation occurs at the dicrotic notch (corresponding to the peak of the T wave on the ECG). Augmentation of diastolic aortic pressure with balloon inflation is shown by the dark red tracing.

48 percent versus 59 percent) when IABP was used and a significant reduction in 1-year mortality (57 percent versus 67 percent, $p = 0.04$).[116] The trend toward improved 30-day mortality with IABP remained when only patients undergoing revascularization were analyzed (47 percent versus 64 percent).[116] However, the 310 patients included were not randomized to IABP therapy, and the IABP group had significantly higher use of inotropes, pacemakers, pulmonary artery catheters, diagnostic angiography, and revascularization (both percutaneous and surgical). Most of the difference in survival occurred in the first days; this might have been due to earlier use of IABP but also might have resulted from selection of patients with a better prognosis for more aggressive interventions (including IABP and revascularization).

The larger SHOCK registry included nearly 900 patients who were collected prospectively but not randomized. Analysis of this group showed that patients with IABP use had lower in-hospital mortality than did those without it whether thrombolysis was used (47 percent versus 63 percent) or not (52 percent versus 77 percent).[117] Unfortunately, these data also were subject to significant selection bias, and the groups that had the best outcomes were those which underwent revascularization regardless of the adjunctive treatment (thrombolysis with or without IABP support) they received. These results were supported by an analysis of the 23,180 patients with cardiogenic shock enrolled in the National Registry of Myocardial Infarction-2. In this group, use of IABP improved 30-day survival in patients receiving thrombolytics (adjusted odds ratio 0.82; 95 percent confidence interval 0.72 to 0.93), but a slight increase in mortality was noted in patients undergoing percutaneous coronary angioplasty (PTCA) who had placement of an IABP.

These data suggest that the improvement in thrombolysis noted in the canine models when IABP was used for patients in cardiogenic shock may result in a real improvement in outcomes in those patients.[86,87] For patients not receiving thrombolysis, significant patient selection bias exists in all these studies; however, it is clear that IABP alone does not improve survival over medical therapy. Its use, as with inotropic support, should be as an adjunct to maintain systemic and coronary perfusion and minimize infarct expansion before revascularization. Thus, in hospitals without cardiac catheterization capability, stabilization with IABP and transfer to a tertiary care facility may be the best option.[63] Although selection bias is again a confounding factor, retrospective analysis has suggested improvement in community hospital survival (93 percent versus 37 percent, $p = 0.0002$), transfer to a tertiary care center (85 percent versus 37 percent), and 1-year survival (67 percent versus 32 percent, $p = 0.019$) with the use of IABP in this setting.[118] After revascularization, prophylactic use of IABP for 48 h has been shown to maintain patency of revascularized arteries.[119]

Weaning of the IABP should be performed before weaning from inotropic and pressor support except when limb ischemia intervenes.

SURGICAL THERAPIES

Multiple studies have shown that the patency of an infarct-related artery is an important predictor of left ventricular function and mortality after acute MI.[120–126] In addition, most studies have demonstrated worse outcomes with increasing time between symptom onset and reperfusion.[71,72,120,127] These findings were extrapolated to patients with cardiogenic shock, supporting an aggressive approach to early *mechanical* reperfusion for patients in shock after MI. Recently, prospective, randomized data in patients with post-MI cardiogenic shock have become available to define further the indications for and outcomes with emergent revascularization.

Angioplasty

The SHOCK trial enrolled 302 patients with post-MI cardiogenic shock resulting from left ventricular dysfunction and randomized them to receive either optimal medical management (including IABP and thrombolysis) or emergent mechanical revascularization (either percutaneous coronary intervention [PTCA with or without stenting] or coronary artery bypass surgery). Revascularization in this group occurred on average within 1 h of randomization for patients undergoing PTCA and within 3 h for those undergoing coronary artery bypass grafting (CABG). There was a trend toward improved 30-day mortality in the revascularization group (46.7 percent versus 56.0 percent, $p = 0.11$) and a significant reduction in 6-month mortality (50.3 percent versus 63.1 percent, $p = 0.027$) and 1-year mortality (53 percent versus 66 percent, $p = 0.025$) (Fig. 29-4).[23,43,128] Patients who had successful angioplasty (TIMI grade 2 or 3[129]) had very low mortality rates at 30 days (38 percent versus 79 percent, $p = 0.003$), and no patient who had a postpercutaneous coronary intervention (PCI) occluded infarct artery survived (Fig. 29-5).[23,130] The only group that did not appear to benefit from a strategy of emergent revascularization were those over age 75 (30-day mortality 75.0 percent versus 53.1 percent, $p = 0.01$), although these results may have been affected by patient selection and a 25 percent revascularization rate before discharge among medically treated patients[23] and have been called into question by results from other studies.[131] The importance of reducing time to reperfusion in patients with cardiogenic shock after MI has been reinforced by other nonrandomized studies.[132,133] Significant predictors of poor outcomes in all patients include severity of mitral regurgitation,[26] initial TIMI flow, and culprit vessels other than the right coronary artery.[43]

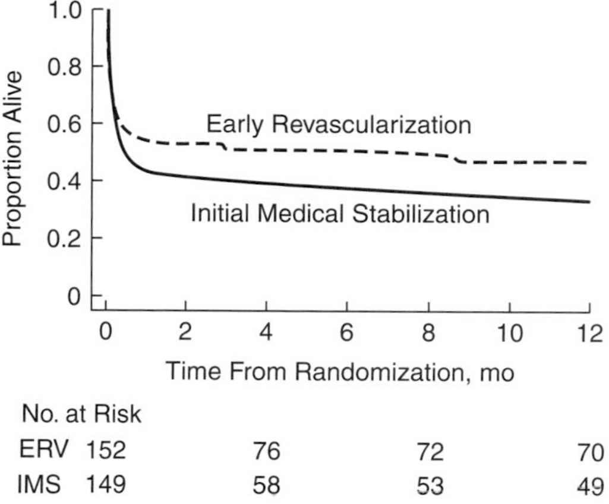

Figure 29-4 Kaplan-Meier survival curve 1 year after randomization to medical therapy or emergent revascularization for cardiogenic shock in the SHOCK trial. [From Hochman JS, Sleeper LA, White HD, et al. One-year survival following early revascularization for cardiogenic shock. *JAMA* 2001;285(2):190–192. Permission pending.]

Stenting

Percutaneous coronary stenting has been shown to improve outcomes and reduce angiographic restenosis during elective PTCA.[134–137] Although there was initial reluctance to use stents in the setting of a potentially unstable coronary thrombus, randomized studies have demonstrated that stenting in the setting of acute MI can be performed safely.[138] Unfortunately, the largest studies have failed to demonstrate a survival benefit from the use of stenting in the setting of MI and instead have shown a trend toward increased mortality with the use of primary stenting (although some have shown reductions in combined endpoints such as recurrent ischemia, infarction, and angina).[137,139,140] However, none of these studies included patients with post-MI cardiogenic shock.

Among patients with cardiogenic shock, Antoniucci and associates described a short- and long-term survival advantage to stent placement over angioplasty alone; however, again, selection bias may have played a role in those patients.[141] Similar results to those for MI alone have been obtained in other nonrandomized trials.[142] The Global Registry of Acute Coronary events has provided observational data that suggest an improvement in outcomes (PCI with stenting predicted hospital survival: odds ratio 3.99, 95 percent confidence interval 2.41 to 6.62).[143] Thus, some evidence exists to support the use of stents in patients with cardiogenic shock; even without strong prospective evidence, it has become common practice (as many as 85 percent of the patients enrolled in the SHOCK trial between 1997 and 1998[130]). Further prospective, randomized investigations are needed to define the indications for stent placement in patients with MI and cardiogenic shock.

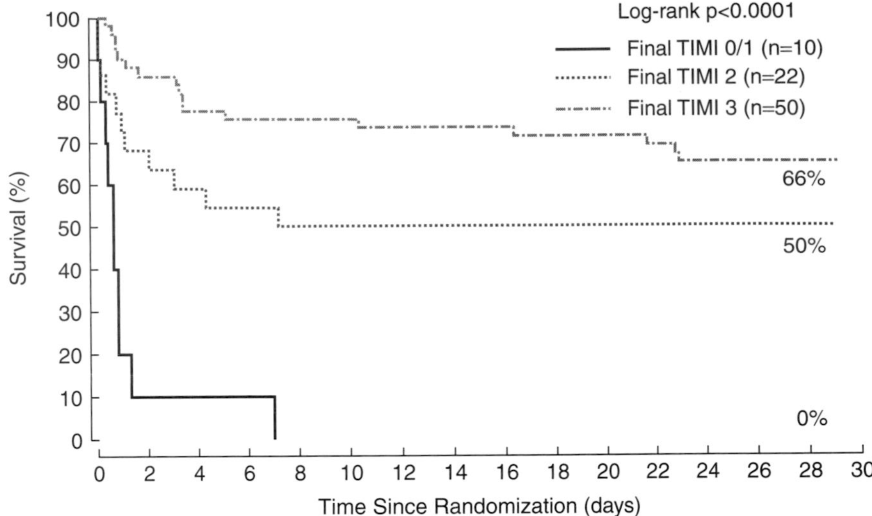

Figure 29-5 Mortality after emergent percutaneous coronary intervention for postinfarction cardiogenic shock stratified by Thrombolysis in Myocardial Infarction (TIMI) flow grade. [From Webb JG, Lowe AM, Sanborn TA, et al. Percutaneous coronary intervention for cardiogenic shock in the SHOCK trial. *J Am Coll Cardiol* 2003;42(8):1380–1386. Permission pending.]

Antiplatelet agents

Among patients who have stents placed after MI, antiplatelet agents have become standard practice, as they appear to reduce short-term restenosis and the need for repeat revascularization.[144–147] In nonrandomized trials, combination treatment with abciximab (a glycoprotein IIb/IIIa inhibitor) decreased 1-month overall mortality (18 percent versus 42 percent, $p = 0.020$) and improved TIMI flow in the infarcted artery compared with stenting alone.[148,149] However, these mortality rates are low, suggesting that the population studied may have been selected for more aggressive treatment. Additional large randomized trials are needed to assess the impact of adding antiplatelet agents to percutaneous stenting of stenosed arteries in patients with acute MI with cardiogenic shock.

Coronary artery bypass

Early outcomes with CABG in the setting of acute MI were poor,[150,151] but surgical revascularization within 6 h improved survival compared with medically treated patients.[152–157] These reports, however, were published as medical management was changing: Randomized trials were evaluating the efficacy of thrombolysis and percutaneous coronary interventions in post-MI patients.[72,73,158] Unfortunately, CABG was not included in these studies. Furthermore, subsequent improvements in both interventional and surgical techniques may make comparisons to contemporary populations and treatments meaningless. Thus, the appropriate use of CABG in the setting of MI in general and cardiogenic shock in particular remains a matter of debate.

The results of the SHOCK trial demonstrated that early revascularization improved survival, and despite more severe disease, mortality in the group receiving CABG (guidelines for the use of emergent CABG included left main stenosis equal to or greater than 50 percent, stenoses greater than 90 percent in two nonculprit major vessels, and patients in whom PCI was unsuccessful or who had disease unsuitable for PCI) was similar to that in patients undergoing percutaneous interventions.[23] Large observational studies support the selective use of CABG in patients with cardiogenic shock; although patients in Killip class IV have seven times the CABG-associated mortality of those in Killip class I, mortality in this group is 27 percent, substantially lower than that in patients who do not receive revascularization and comparable to survival in patients undergoing PCI.[159] Although surgery within 3 days of transmural and 6 h of nontransmural MI has been associated with a higher mortality rate (Table 29-4),[160,161] Lee and associates documented decreased early mortality rates when operation occurs before 18 h in patients with cardiogenic shock (7 percent versus 31 percent).[162] Thus, in patients with ongoing ischemia or cardiogenic shock that is not amenable to medical stabilization, early revacularization with CABG is indicated; however, when possible, surgery should be delayed, especially in patients with transmural infarction.

Unfortunately, randomized data are not available, and the optimal indications for CABG in the setting of MI and cardiogenic shock remain ill defined. In light of the

Table 29-4 Comparison of hospital mortality with respect to time of operation

Time between CABG and MI	Mortality: Transmural MI, %	Mortality: Nontransmural MI, %
< 6 h	12.1	11.5
6–23 h	13.6	6.2[a]
1–7 days	4.3	3.5
8–14 days	2.4	2.7
≥ 15 days	2.6	2.7

Adapted from Lee DC, Oz MC, Weinberg AD, et al. Optimal timing of revascularization: Transmural versus nontransmural acute myocardial infarction. *Ann Thorac Surg* 2001;71(4):1197–1202; discussion 202–204.

CABG = coronary artery bypass grafting; MI = myocardial infarction.

[a] $p = 0.006$ nontransmural versus transmural.

excellent results obtained with thrombolysis and percutaneous revascularization, CABG probably will not become a primary therapy after MI whether or not cardiogenic shock intervenes; instead, it is best reserved for specific indications for which percutaneous revascularization is unsuccessful or inappropriate.

Perioperative considerations

When emergent revascularization by CABG is indicated, timing is important and rapid transport to the operating room is critical; however, some techniques are available to assist in maintaining coronary and systemic perfusion during transport. As was noted above, the use of IABP is preferable to the use of inotropes and vasopressors because of the improvement in myocardial oxygenation and workload. In patients with circulatory collapse, percutaneous cardiopulmonary bypass may be initiated via the femoral artery and vein. Flow rates of 3.5 to 5.0 L have been obtained with this method.[163]

Once the patient is in the operating room, anesthetic induction may lead to catastrophic hypotensive circulatory collapse. It is important that both surgery and perfusion teams be prepared for decompensation before the onset of anesthesia. Although the specific type of anesthetic agent used does not appear to alter myocardial oxygen utilization efficiency significantly,[164] a rapid narcotics-based regimen has been recommended.[165] Rapid institution of cardiopulmonary bypass to provide perfusion to threatened myocardium is essential.

Patients undergoing emergent CABG have high mortality rates; bleeding may contribute to that rate by decreasing myocardial oxygen delivery. In addition, release of cytokines in response to large-volume transfusions as well as thromboxane A_2 release during cardiopulmonary bypass may worsen coagulopathy and pulmonary hypertension, worsening right ventricular ischemia. Aprotinin has been shown to reduce the need for transfusion and can be used safely in patients undergoing emergent CABG,[166,167] even those who have undergone thrombolysis.[168]

The choice of a conduit should not be altered from that for elective cases. Although most surgeons use saphenous vein grafts (SVGs) to minimize bypass time, internal mammary artery (IMA) grafting has not been associated with increased complications compared with saphenous vein grafting even in the setting of cardiogenic shock, and late results with IMA grafts are significantly better than those with SVG.[169–171] To reduce MI, harvesting of the IMA can be performed after the initiation of cardiopulmonary bypass, cross-clamping, and cardioplegia.

In all cases, both antegrade and retrograde cardioplegia should be used for myocardial protection to ensure the delivery of cardioplegia to ischemic areas. Both antegrade and retrograde catheters can be placed before placement of the aortic cross-clamp to ensure rapid delivery of cardioplegia to the entire myocardium. The placement of a "bail-out" catheter across stenotic regions during percutaneous coronary intervention may assist in the delivery of cardioplegia to ischemic regions.[163] Various authors have advocated a variety of techniques for myocardial protection, including hypothermic fibrillatory arrest,[172,173] oxygenated crystalloid cardioplegia,[172,174] blood cardioplegia,[175,176] and substrate-enriched blood cardioplegia.[172,175] However, in a series of experimental studies, Buckberg and coauthors developed specific modifications of the reperfusion process that reduce myocardial oxygen demand and reperfusion injury in ischemic myocardium. These experimental studies subsequently were validated clinically.[176] Conditions favoring recovery of ischemic myocardium include the following: Decompression of the heart, which reduces myocardial oxygen demand by approximately 50 percent[177]; cardioplegic arrest reduces oxygen demand by approximately 90 percent compared with a beating heart[178]; myocardial metabolism is enhanced by warm blood cardioplegia, which maintains normal energy production while decreasing energy demands[179]; low perfusion pressure reduces postischemic edema[180]; and prolonged reperfusion with cardioplegic arrest permits resuscitation of energy-depleted myocardium.[181] Therefore, the standard Buckberg protocol should be used to maximize myocardial protection in patients undergoing CABG who are in cardiogenic shock. This includes induction of cardioplegia with substrate-enriched warm blood cardioplegia for 3 to 5 min, followed by cold blood cardioplegia for 2 to 3 min and then by periodic small-volume infusions. In addition, an infusion of warm blood cardioplegia before removal of the cross-clamp ("hot shot") may improve myocardial recovery.[182]

The occluded artery supplying the largest region of ischemic but viable myocardium should be reperfused first. When vein grafts are used, after completion of the distal anastomosis, regional blood cardioplegia can be delivered to the ischemic area through a side branch of the graft while the proximal anastomosis is completed.

Ventricular assist devices and heart transplantation

In patients with cardiogenic shock refractory to maximal medical management and unimproved by percutaneous intervention or an intraaortic balloon pump, implantation of a ventricular assist device (VAD) is a potentially livesaving maneuver. Two classes of patients may benefit from the use of a VAD: (1) patients with stunned myocardium as a bridge to recovery and (2) patients with extensive infarction requiring a bridge to heart transplantation. Outside clinical trials, VADs are approved for use in patients pending transplantation; therefore, all patients should fulfill the general criteria for transplant recipient selection (Table 29-5).[183] Although complete evaluation is usually impossible in the acute setting, patients with obvious contraindications to transplantation (irreversible neurologic defects, coexisting active neoplasm, etc.) should not be considered for VAD implantation.

Table 29-5 Indications and contraindications for heart transplantation in the acute setting
Indications
Indications for cardiac transplantation determined by severity of heart failure despite optimal therapy
Definite indications
VO_2max < 10 mL/kg/min
NYHA class IV
History of recurrent hospitalization for congestive heart failure
Refractory ischemia with inoperable coronary artery disease and left ventricular ejection fraction < 20%
Recurrent symptomatic ventricular arrythmias
Probable indications
VO_2max < 14 mL/kg/min (or higher with multiple other risk factors)
NYHA class III–IV
Recent hospitalizations for congestive heart failure
Unstable angina not amenable to coronary artery bypass grafting or percutaneous transluminal coronary angioplasty with left ventricular ejection fraction < 0.25%
Contraindications
General contraindications
Presence of any noncardiac condition that would shorten life expectancy or increase the risk of death from rejection or complications of immunosuppression
Specific contraindications[a]
Age > 65 years (varies with the program)
Active infection
Active ulcer disease
Severe diabetes mellitus with end-organ damage
Severe peripheral vascular or cerebrovascular disease
Coexisting neoplasm
Morbid obesity
Creatine clearance < 40–50 mL/min, effective renal plasma flow (ERPF) < 200 mL/min[b]
Bilirubin > 2.5 mg/dL transaminases > 2_ normal[c]
Severe pulmonary dysfunction with FVC and FEV_1 < ~40% of predicted, especially with intrinsic lung disease
Pulmonary artery systolic pressure > 60 mmHg, mean transpulmonary gradient > 15 mmHg, or pulmonary vascular resistance > 5 Wood units[d]
Acute pulmonary thromboembolism
Acute diverticulitis
High risk of life-threatening noncompliance

Source: Adapted from Kirklin JK, McGiffin DC, Pinderski LJ, Tallaj J. Selection of patients and techniques of heart transplantation. *Surg Clin North Am* 2004;84(1):257–287. Permission pending.

[a] Contraindications may be either relative or absolute, depending on severity and program preference.

[b] May be suitable for cardiac transplantation if inotropic support and hemodynamic management produce creatinine below 2 mg/100 mL and creatinine clearance above 50 mL/min. Transplantation may be advisable as a combined heart-kidney transplant.

[c] Requires liver biopsy to exclude cirrhosis or other intrinsic liver disease.

[d] Apply only if the increased resistance is largely nonreactive (fixed).

Table 29-6 Current ventricular assist devices

External centrifugal pump	External pulsatile pump	Internal pusher plate pump	Internal axial flow pump	Total artificial hearts
Biomedicus ECMO	Abiomed BVS 500 Thoratec VAD	Heartmate LVAD Novacor LVAD	Nimbus Intra-Corporeal Assist Device (Heartmate II) Jarvik 2000 DeBakey Micromed	Abiomed TAH Penn State TAH CardioWest TAH

ECMO = extracorporeal membrane oxygenation; VAD = ventricular assist device; LVAD = left ventricular assist device; TAH = total artificial heart.

When used as a bridge to recovery for myocardial stunning, VAD implantation should be accompanied or preceded by mechanical revascularization, whether percutaneous or surgical. In this setting, the use of short-term VAD devices is appropriate. VADs suitable for short-term implantation include the Bio-medicus centrifugal pump and the Abiomed and Thoratec pumps. Although the centrifugal pump is easy to insert, it has a significant incidence of thromboembolic complications despite systemic heparinization, and its use largely has been supplanted by use of the pump devices.[184] The Abiomed VAD (BVS 5000) is a pulsatile asynchronous device that is suitable for use in right, left, or biventricular support for up to 4 weeks; however, because of its size, it largely precludes patient ambulation. Therefore, removal and replacement with a chronic device is indicated if recovery does not occur within 7 to 10 days. The Thoratec pneumatically driven extracorporeal pump is also suitable for left, right, or biventricular short-term support and has the advantage of allowing significant patient mobility. Both devices require systemic anticoagulation.

In patients with large infarcts without the potential for myocardial recovery, the insertion of a longer-term VAD is required as a bridge to transplantation. The two most commonly used devices are the Heartmate VE and Novacor pumps. Both are wearable, pulsatile intracorporeal VADs with only a driveline traversing the skin. The Heartmate has the advantage of requiring only aspirin for antiplatelet activity, not systemic anticoagulation; this is achieved through the use of textured blood contact surface that forms a stable biological lining that is resistant to thrombus formation.[185] Direct comparison of these two devices in randomized trials is ongoing. Other devices with different pump mechanisms are also available (Table 29-6). After clinical stabilization of the patient, a complete evaluation for heart transplantation can proceed. In light of the potential for discovery of contraindications to transplantation after emergent placement of a VAD, consideration—including discussions with patients and families—must be given to the potential need to withdraw support in patients who are found to be unsuitable recipients for heart transplantation.

OUTCOMES AND PROGNOSIS

Survival after CABG for patients in cardiogenic shock or those receiving cardiopulmonary resuscitation (CPR) remains poor; 1-year and 10-year survival rates are 59.4 percent and 47.5 percent.[186] However, these rates compare favorably to medical therapy alone, in which mortality rates in excess of 65 percent at 1 year have been reported.[128] Predictors of poor outcomes after CABG in this population include extent of coronary disease, presence of drug-treated diabetes, and lower arterial pH at entry into the operating room.[186]

SUMMARY

Cardiogenic shock after MI continues to occur in approximately 10 percent of patients who reach the hospital. Though improving slightly, mortality rates remain approximately 60 percent. Patients with hypoperfusion after acute MI should be evaluated rapidly with electrocardiography (ECG), chest x-ray, and echocardiography to determine the cause of shock. In those with cardiogenic shock, therapies should be directed toward stabilization of patients with intravenous fluid resuscitation, pharmacologic therapy as indicated, and rapid placement of an IABP to support coronary and systemic perfusion. Emergent revascularization with PCI or CABG is associated with improved long-term outcomes. Ventricular assist devices provide an important adjunct to revascularization by supporting circulation through the period of myocardial stunning and providing a bridge to transplantation when appropriate.

ISCHEMIC MITRAL VALVE DISEASE

INTRODUCTION

Ischemic mitral regurgitation is a disease of the ventricle and papillary muscles that leads to valvular dysfunction;

KEY CONCEPTS

- Epidemiology
  - Depending on modality, Mitral regurgitation (MR) occursin 8 to 50 percent of patients after Myocardial Infarction
- Pathophysilolgy
  - Three primary pathophysiologic mechanisms
    - Papillary muscle rupture
    - Acute ischemic MR
    - Chronic ischemic MR
  - Papillary muscle rupture results from infarction of the muscle itself and leads to acute cardiovascular decompensation.
  - Acute and chronic MR both result from ischemia to the ventricular wall with distortion of the mitral valve apparatus and failure of leaflet coaptation.
- Clinical Features
  - Pulmonary edema, chest pain, shortness of breath.
  - New holosystolic murmur best heard at the apex.
  - Acuity ranges from sudden collapsee with papillary muscle rupture to gradual onset of congestive heart failure.
- Diagnostics
  - Echocardiography allows evaluation of left ventricular (LV) function and mitral apparatus; can accurately diagnose pulmonary muscle (PM) rupture as well as exclude other mechanical causes of cardiovascular collapse.
- Treatment
  - Medical
    - Medical therapy for acute MR and papillary muscle rupture is supportive only.
    - Chronically, angiotensin-converting enzyme inhibitors and AT_1-recepior blockers improve LV volume and decrease regurgitant fraction.
  - Surgical
    - Indications
      - PM rupture
      - Acute, severe MR not improved by percutaneous coronary intervention or thrombolysis.
      - Chronic 3+ to 4+ MR and symptomatic coronary disease.
      - Other indications: LVESVI ≥ 80 ml/m^2, regurgitant fraction50% greater than forward ejection fraction, estimated regurgitant orifice > 20 mm^2
    - Techniques
      - Repair of PM (rarely).
      - Mitral valve replacement.
      - Mitral valve repair probably best option in most patients with chronic MR.
- Outcomes and Prognosis
  - Operative mortality in acute severe MR (with or without PM rupture) ~20 percent.
  - Chronic MR operative mortality ~13 percent.
  - Repair failure occurs rarely (<10 percent at 5 years).
  - Long-term survival poor (55 to 60 percent at 5 years).

by definition, the leaflets and valvular apparatus are normal. The frequent coexistence of nonischemic mitral valve disease and coronary artery disease has led to a poor understanding of the natural history and optimal treatment of ischemic mitral regurgitation (MR). In addition, chronic MR may develop after postinfarct LV dilatation, resulting in annular dilatation[187–190]; this may be difficult to differentiate from "functional" MR resulting from dilated cardiomyopathy. Mitral regurgitation occurs frequently after acute MI; precise rates have varied from 8 percent to 50 percent, depending on the modality used to detect the disease.[191–205] This reflects the heterogeneity of ischemic MR. It ranges from clinically silent disease that is identifiable only on Doppler echocardiography or angiography to severe disease that leads to cardiogenic shock and hemodynamic collapse; it may present acutely within hours of the infarct or develop insidiously over years with worsening congestive heart failure.

Anatomic considerations

Normal mitral valve function

Normal mitral valve function requires the coordinated and proper functioning of all components of the valve structure: the valvular leaflets, the annulus, the chordae tendineae, the papillary muscles, the left ventricular wall, and the left atrium. The complex interaction of these components can be analyzed through division of the cardiac cycle into four periods: systole, diastole, isovolemic relaxation, and isovolemic contraction (Fig. 29-6).

Ischemia and mitral valve components

As was noted above, in ischemic MR, the leaflets and annulus usually function normally. The chordae tendineae are also not affected by ischemia. However, the papillary muscles (PMs) contain functioning myocardium that is dependent on end-artery perfusion and are thus sensitive to ischemic insult. There are two PMs: the anterolateral and posteromedial papillary muscles. The anterolateral PM often is supplied by two arteries, most often the first circumflex marginal artery and the first diagonal branch of the left anterior descending artery.[206] Ischemia is uncommon in this location and in the surrounding high lateral wall of the LV because of the extensive collateral system. In contrast, the posteromedial PM lies in the watershed of the right coronary and circumflex arteries and more often is supplied by only a single artery; it is therefore highly sensitive to ischemic insult.[206–208] Variations in PM anatomy may lead to increased sensitivity

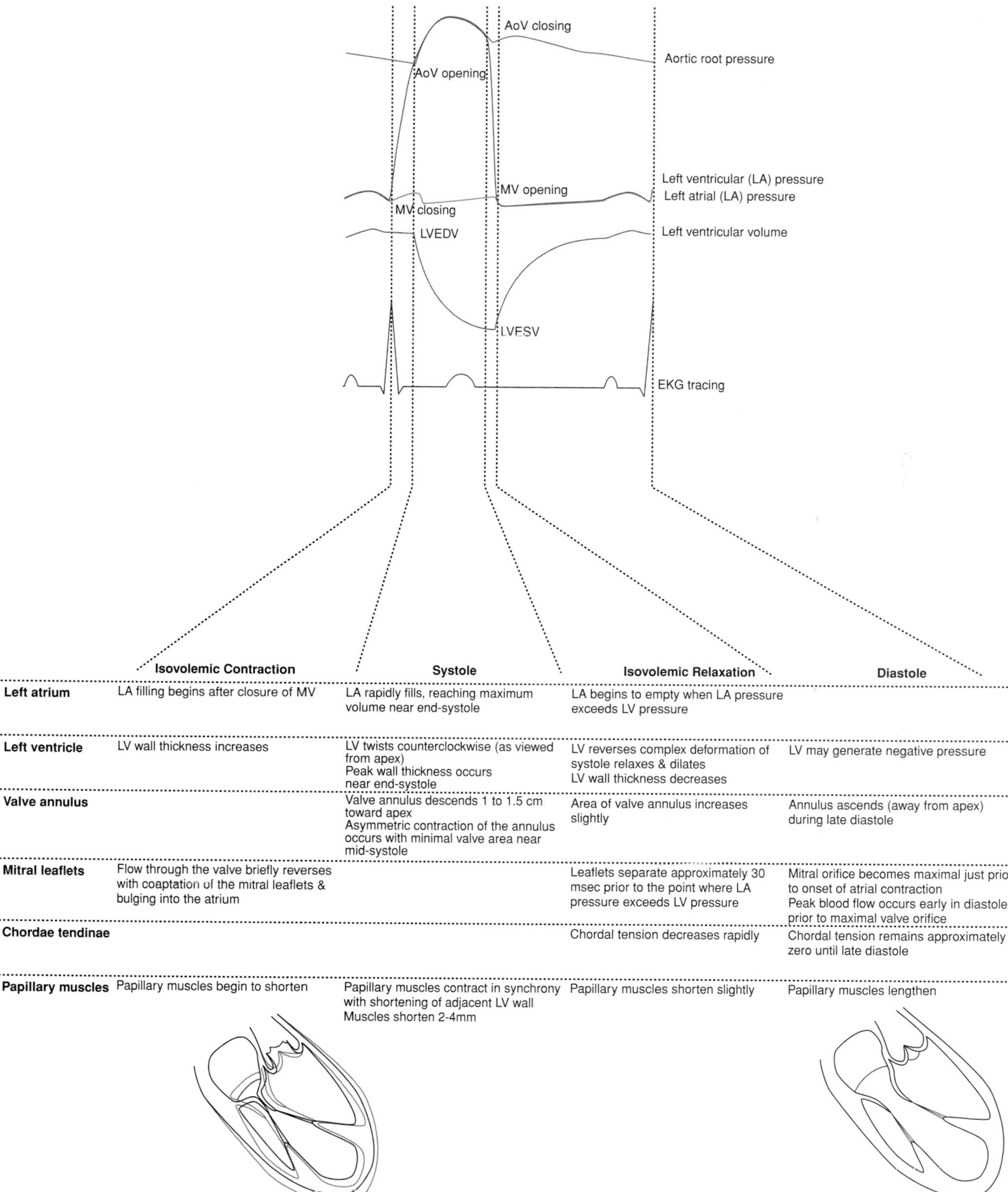

	Isovolemic Contraction	Systole	Isovolemic Relaxation	Diastole
Left atrium	LA filling begins after closure of MV	LA rapidly fills, reaching maximum volume near end-systole	LA begins to empty when LA pressure exceeds LV pressure	
Left ventricle	LV wall thickness increases	LV twists counterclockwise (as viewed from apex) Peak wall thickness occurs near end-systole	LV reverses complex deformation of systole relaxes & dilates LV wall thickness decreases	LV may generate negative pressure
Valve annulus		Valve annulus descends 1 to 1.5 cm toward apex Asymmetric contraction of the annulus occurs with minimal valve area near mid-systole	Area of valve annulus increases slightly	Annulus ascends (away from apex) during late diastole
Mitral leaflets	Flow through the valve briefly reverses with coaptation of the mitral leaflets & bulging into the atrium		Leaflets separate approximately 30 msec prior to the point where LA pressure exceeds LV pressure	Mitral orifice becomes maximal just prior to onset of atrial contraction Peak blood flow occurs early in diastole prior to maximal valve orifice
Chordae tendinae			Chordal tension decreases rapidly	Chordal tension remains approximately zero until late diastole
Papillary muscles	Papillary muscles begin to shorten	Papillary muscles contract in synchrony with shortening of adjacent LV wall Muscles shorten 2-4mm	Papillary muscles shorten slightly	Papillary muscles lengthen

Figure 29-6 Normal mitral valve function requires the coordinated motion of all components of the mitral valve apparatus, including the atrial and ventricular walls.

to ischemia; in particular, narrow PMs supplied by a single central artery are vulnerable to ischemia.[209]

Ischemic MR occurs most commonly in association with transmural posteroinferior infarctions.[189,210,211] The location and size of the infarct influence the occurrence and acuity of MR after MI. In a sheep model, ligation of the two most distal circumflex arteries resulted in 21 percent LV mass infarct and gradual development of MR over 8 weeks; ligating the posterior descending artery as well increased infarct size to 32 percent and led to immediate MR.[211,212] Similar-sized infarcts in other portions of the heart did not lead to MR.[213]

PATHOPHYSIOLOGY

Ischemic MR can be classified broadly into three categories: (1) papillary muscle rupture, (2) acute MR, and (3) chronic MR. These conditions result in a variety of disorders of mitral valve function. Carpentier's functional categorization of mitral valve dysfunction has been applied to the ischemic mitral valve to guide operative management (Fig. 29-7). In this system, MR is categorized by the derangement in leaflet function: normal leaflet motion (type I), prolapsing leaflets (type II), and restricted leaflet motion during either diastole (type IIIa, not seen in ischemic MR) or systole (type IIIb). In the setting of ischemic MR, type I dysfunction occurs when ischemia leads to dilatation of the posterior muscular portion of the valve annulus; this type of deformation may occur with either acute or chronic MR. Type II dysfunction results from papillary muscle rupture in the acute setting or may result from chronic ischemia that leads to papillary muscle elongation. Type IIIb occurs when ischemia results in dilatation of the left ventricle with systolic tethering of the papillary muscles and failure of mitral valve coaptation.

Papillary muscle rupture

Rupture of papillary muscles results in a loss of leaflet tethering, leading to flail mitral leaflets and mitral regurgitation (Carpentier type II). The more commonly affected posteromedial PM consists of one or two large common trunks and multple heads, all of which give off chordae tendineae to both the anterior and the posterior leaflets of the mitral valve. Acute complete rupture of the common trunk leads to massive mitral regurgitation and hemodynamic collapse. In contrast, partial rupture of the

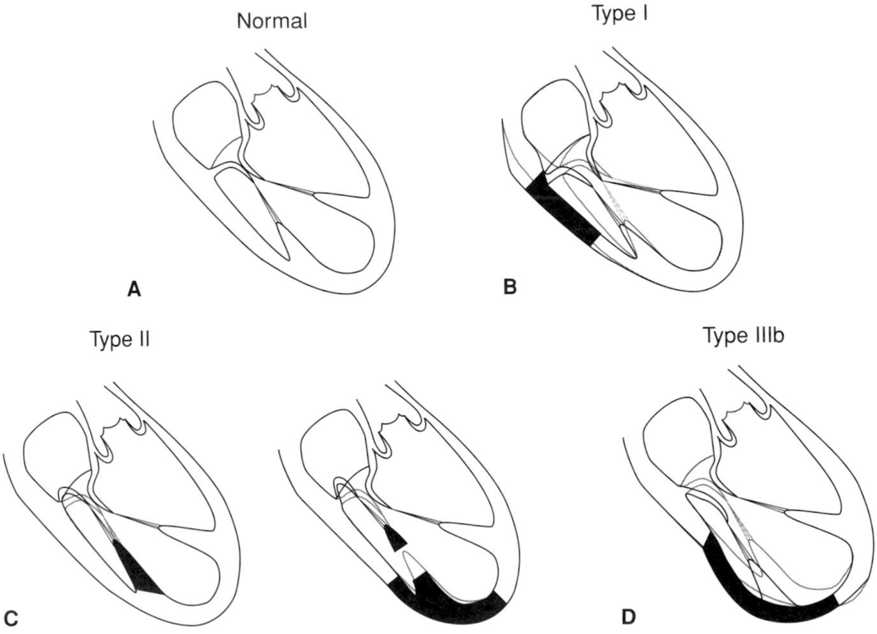

Figure 29-7 Classification of ischemic mitral regurgitation with diagrams of systolic function. **A.** Normal valve function with coaptation of mitral leaflets during systole. **B.** Type I: normal leaflet motion, regurgitation resulting from annular dilatation from ischemia of the adjacent ventricular wall. This results in a central leak. **B.** Type II: prolapsing leaflets. Regurgitation results from either papillary muscle rupture *(left)* in the acute setting or papillary muscle elongation *(right)* secondary to chronic ischemia. This usually results in an asymmetric leak. **C.** Type IIIb: restricted leaflet motion resulting from dysfunction of the ventricular wall and papillary muscle tethering. This may result in either a central or an asymmetric leak, depending on the nature of the ventricular dysfunction.

common trunk or rupture of one of the heads may lead to more moderate (and better tolerated) regurgitation.[214] However, partial rupture may progress to complete rupture, leading to subsequent acute decompensation.[215,216]

Acute mitral regurgitation

When not associated with PM rupture, acute mitral regurgitation results from discoordination of the mitral valve complex. Traditionally, it was thought that PM dysfunction, which is caused by poor systolic shortening of the ischemic PM, leads to mitral valve (MV) prolapse and regurgitation in the acute setting. However, studies have not demonstrated MV prolapse in acute ischemic MR.[217,218] Loss of PM systolic shortening alone does not account for the MR seen after MI. Rather, dysfunction of the left ventricular wall resulting from myocardial ischemia with hibernation or stunning or from infarction may lead to failure of valve coaptation. Depending on the location of the infarct, this may result primarily from annular dilatation (Carpentier type I), as was demonstrated by Miller's group, among others,[189,219,220] or by changes in the interaction between the ischemic and nonischemic papillary muscles during systolic contraction, leading to papillary muscle tethering and restricted leaflet motion (Carpentier type IIIb).[212,221,222] When not repaired in the acute phase, MR unrelated to PM rupture may disappear, remain unchanged, or become more severe.[223]

Chronic mitral regurgitation

Chronic ischemic MR also results from a complex of abnormalities in the valvular apparatus. However, in constrast to acute MR, in which changes may be small and difficult to visualize with current imaging techniques, chronic MR usually results in larger changes that are easily apparent on echocardiography. Although some authors have described lengthening of the PM resulting in MV prolapse (Carpentier type II),[188,224] pathologic studies suggest that PM atrophy and scarring are more common.[211,217,225] This results in leaflet tethering during systole, preventing proper coaptation. This phenomenon has been observed in animal models.[226] LV remodeling in general and dilatation in particular (resulting in both dislocation of the PM apically and laterally and dilatation of the valve annulus) further contribute to leaflet tethering through apical displacement of the PM during systole.[227–231] Three-dimensional modeling of changes in mitral valve and ventricular function demonstrates that all these changes—posterior papillary muscle displacement, annular dilatation, and apical restriction of the posterior leaflet—are associated with the development of IMR (Fig. 29-8).

Ideally, operative therapy should be directed toward the causes of MR in each patient. When tethering and apical displacement are responsible for poor leaflet coaptation (Carpentier type IIIb), lengthening of the PM

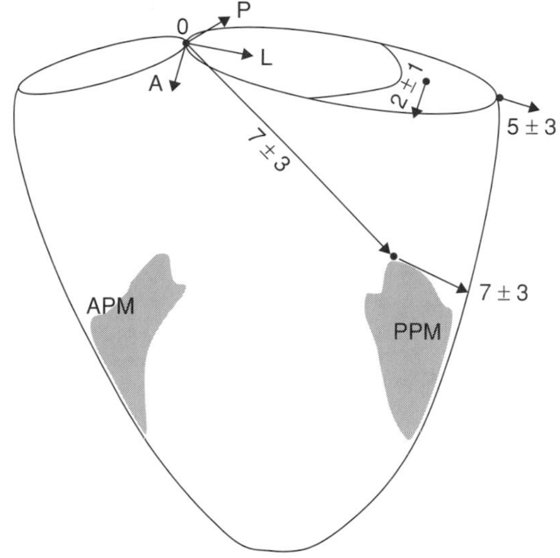

Figure 29-8 Comparison of ischemic changes in mitral valve geometry with and without mitral regurgitation in an ovine model. Arrows represent changes from baseline in the group of animals developing mitral regurgitation that were significantly different from changes occurring in animals that did not develop regurgitation despite similarly located and sized infarcts. Animals developing ischemic mitral regurgitation had more severe displacement of the posterior papillary muscle, septal-lateral dilatation of the annulus, and apical tethering of the posterior leaflet. APM = anterior papillary muscle; PPM = posterior papillary muscle. [From Tibayan FA, Rodriguez F, et al. Geometric distortions of the mitral valvular-ventricular complex in chronic ischemic mitral regurgitation. *Circulation* 2003;108(Suppl 1):116–121. Permission pending.]

theoretically should ameliorate MR by displacing the attachment points of the chordae toward the valve. In contrast, when annular dilatation is the primary abnormality (Carpentier type I), mitral valve repair would be the most appropriate surgical option.

Episodic ischemic mitral regurgitation

A small but important subset of patients may present with chronic *episodic* mitral regurgitation. Patients with this entity develop episodes of dyspnea or flash pulmonary edema with or without associated angina.[232] The murmur of MR will appear during these episodes and subsequently resolve during asymptomatic periods.[233] In these patients, MR is an anginal equivalent caused by transient ischemic dyskinesia of the left ventricular wall that results in apical displacement of the mitral leaflets (Carpentier type IIIb).[234] Because the regurgitation is caused by ischemia of the ventricular wall, treatment should be directed toward ischemia rather than mitral valve function; revascularization without mitral valve surgery should be performed.

CLINICAL FEATURES

Papillary muscle rupture

Papillary muscle rupture usually leads to acute and rapid hemodynamic collapse with massive MR. Severe pulmonary edema is almost invariably present. It occurs a median of 1 day (and nearly invariably within 14 days) after the onset of infarction.[235] The murmur of MR (a holosytolic murmur best heard over the apex) may be mild or absent. This probably is due to three factors: (1) The wide regurgitant orifice causes a minimum of turbulence, (2) the pressure gradient between the left atrium (LA) and the LV normalizes rapidly, reducing turbulence, and (3) the auscultatory findings of severe pulmonary edema may mask the murmur entirely.[236–238] PM rupture is a rare (occurring in 0.3 to 5 percent of patients with acute MI)[215,239,240] but devastating complication of MI. Mortality rises rapidly in patients with PM rupture: 50 percent at 24 h and 75 percent at 48 h.[215] Median survival in medically managed patients ranges from 1 to 4 days in various series.[215,216]

Acute and chronic mitral regurgitation

Depending on the severity of MR that occurs in association with MI, the presentation may range from a new murmur to severe pulmonary edema. Patients who present with mild asymptomatic MR acutely after an MI may be managed as if the MR were not present. When it is not related to papillary muscle rupture, acute MR becomes apparent a median of 7 days after infarction.[216,235] However, a subset of patients (approximately 0.1 percent of those with symptomatic coronary disease) will develop acute severe MR.[241] These patients invariably require surgery for survival. Patients present with symptoms of acute coronary syndromes, including acute onset of chest pain and/or shortness of breath. Pulmonary edema, systemic hypotension, and ultimately cardiogenic shock may ensue rapidly.

As was noted above, infarct size may affect the acuity of the presentation, with chronic MR resulting from smaller LV infarcts. Unlike organic MR,[242] the murmur of ischemic MR correlates poorly with the severity of the regurgitant volume, partly as a result of the low flow present in an ischemic heart.[243] In addition, as many of 50 percent of patients with moderate or severe MR may be missed on physical examination alone.[196] Therefore, even low-intensity murmurs in patients who present with acute MI should be investigated to rule out mitral valve pathology, especially in patients in whom cardiogenic shock or pulmonary edema is associated with well-preserved LV function.[236,243]

The literature on chronic ischemic MR is confounded by the inclusion of patients with nonischemic organic mitral disease in most large series. However, patients with MR appear to have more severe congestive heart failure (CHF) and are more likely to have renal failure than are those without MR.[244] Data from the Cleveland Clinic excluded patients with nonischemic MR. Of the 482 patients undergoing isolated mitral valve surgery for ischemic MR, 80 percent had chronic mitral valve disease. Although separate analyses were not performed for that population, heart failure was common, with 32 percent, 30 percent, and 36 percent of patients in New York Heart Association (NYHA) class II, III, and IV functional status, respectively.[210]

Overall, MR is found in 15 to 20 percent of patients after MI.[196,198] Multiple investigators have demonstrated the association between MR in the setting of acute MI and poor outcomes.[195,245] Barzilai and associates showed a twofold increase in mortality (36 percent versus 15 percent), but that difference disappeared when it was controlled for comorbid conditions.[245] More recent studies, however, though confirming the association between MR and multiple predictors of poor outcomes (including older age, multivessel disease, and severe LV dysfunction),[196,198] have shown an independent effect of MR on cardiovascular mortality. In the 727 patients involved in the Survival and Ventricular Enlargement (SAVE) study, the presence of mild or moderate MR was associated with a twofold increase in cardiovascular mortality in multivariate analysis (median follow-up 3.5 years).[198] Tcheng and colleagues found a similar effect at 1 year (odds ratio 1.5) in patients with moderate or severe MR.[196] Grigioni and associates found that the degree of MR [as measured by estimated regurgitant orifice (ERO)] correlated with mortality in a population of 303 patients operated on more than 16 days after MI with either mitral repair or replacement (risk ratio for ERO less than 20mm^2 1.65, for ERO equal to or greater than 20 mm^2 2.23).[246] Similar results were seen in a series of 4221 patients undergoing percutaneous coronary interventions remote from an MI; the 53 patients with moderate or severe MR had 3-year survival of 68.6 percent versus 92.3 percent for those without any MR.[244] This difference was even more pronounced among those with a left ventricular ejection fraction (LVEF) less than 40 percent. Similarly, in the SHOCK trial, both severe MR and depressed LVEF were predictors of increased 1-year mortality regardless of treatment assignment.[26]

In summary, ischemic mitral valve disease consists of a spectrum of clinical presentations that ranges from acute to chronic and from mild to severe. However, it is associated with poor outcomes regardless of severity.

DIAGNOSTIC MODALITIES

Echocardiography

Echocardiography provides useful diagnostic and prognostic information in both acute and chronic MR. Acutely, transthoracic echocardiography (TTE) is the diagnostic study of choice in evaluating patients with hemodynamic instability after MI. TTE enables the detection of wall motion abnormalities, quantitation of the degree of MR, and assessment for other mechanical causes of circulatory collapse, including septal or free wall rupture; it also may demonstrate flail mitral leaflets or other evidence of PM rupture.

When TTE does not provide adequate information, transesophageal echocardiography (TEE) may be required; some authors recommend routine TEE because of the failure of TTE to detect MR and PM rupture in up to 80 percent of patients.[239] Because of the high mortality rate associated with PM rupture without operation, detection of this uncommon complication as part of the evaluation of patients with MI is imperative. Traditionally, PM rupture was identified by locating a mobile mass attached to the mitral leaflet prolapsing into the right atrium; however, even with TEE this may fail to detect PM rupture in as many as 35 percent of patients; a complete evaluation of the LV is also necessary to evaluate for large-amplitude erratic motion of the PM head in the LV that is indicative of rupture (Fig. 29-9).[208]

In chronic MR, echocardiography can be used to follow progression of disease as well as distinguish ischemic from organic pathology. Doppler echocardiography allows identification and quantification of mitral regurgitant flow (Fig. 29-10), and two-dimensional echocardiography can be used to examine LV structure and identify abnormalities in leaflet and chordal morphology and function. TEE is superior to TTE in the evaluation of valvular pathology, particularly in identifying sequelae of endocarditis such as vegetations, leaflet perforations, and inflammatory changes.

Angiography

The increased diagnostic accuracy of echocardiography has allowed it to replace angiography in the assessment of MR. Thus, angiography remains clinically useful primarily in delineating coronary anatomy and treating stenotic lesions when appropriate. Despite hemodynamic instability, most patients who present with MR in association with acute MI will receive an angiogram.

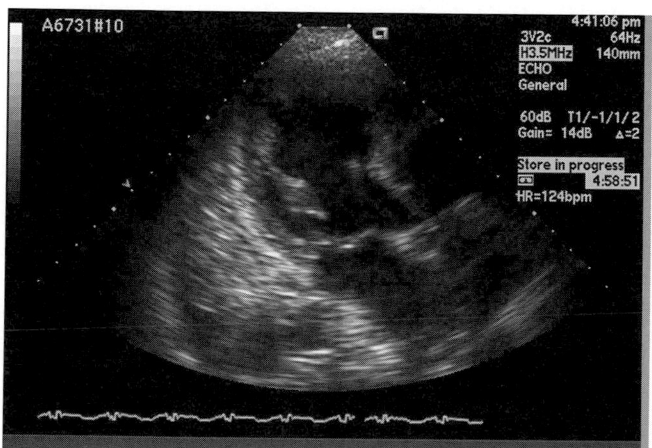

Figure 29-9 Echocardiography of mitral regurgitation caused by papillary muscle rupture with mobile mass attached to the mitral leaflet.

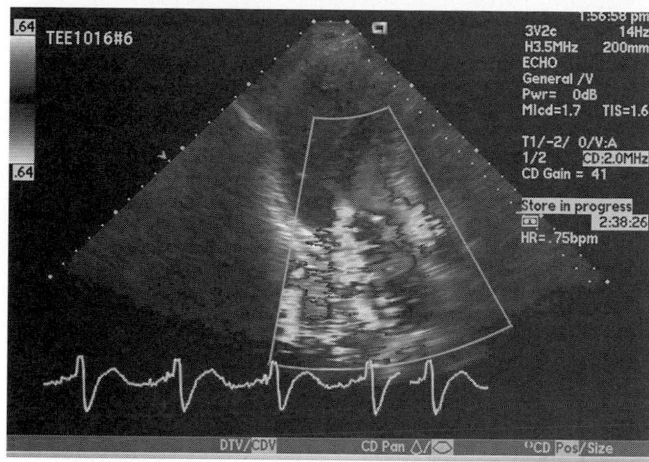

Figure 29-10 Echocardiography of mitral regurgitation demonstrating regurgitant jet using Doppler imaging.

In chronic MR patients, a preoperative angiogram also is used to delineate coronary anatomy and plan the operative procedure and approach. Measurement of intracardiac and intravascular pressures as well as cardiac output assists in the assessment of LV function. However, in light of the high incidence of renal failure in this population,[210] a ventriculogram should be avoided because it provides little information beyond that obtainable by echocardiography.

MEDICAL THERAPY

Acute mitral regurgitation

Therapies directed at patients with acute MR after MI depend largely on the degree of regurgitation and the patient's hemodynamic status. In most patients, the presence of MR will not affect the management of acute infarction; however, a minority of patients will develop 3+ or 4+ MR with heart failure and cardiogenic shock. These patients with acute severe MR should be admitted to the intensive care unit (ICU) until definitive therapy (surgery or, rarely, catheter-based interventions) can be instituted.

Diagnostic studies should be initiated to determine the cause of the decompensation; patients with PM rupture in particular must receive rapid operative therapy. In the ICU, patients should be monitored with arterial pressure and pulmonary artery catheters. Fluid resuscitation should be directed by measurements of central venous and pulmonary wedge pressure as both hypovolemia and volume overload may impair cardiac function significantly. Patients in cardiogenic shock may require inotropic therapy and, when inotropic therapy is inadequate, placement of an intraaortic balloon pump. In the setting of MR, intraaortic balloon pumping has been shown to decrease the regurgitant fraction and increase systemic cardiac output and carotid blood flow, all without changing left ventricular function.[247]

Telemetry monitoring should be used to assess for arrhythmias, which are common in postinfarction MR. The antiarrhythmic agents used should be those least likely to cause hypotension or impair myocardial contractility. Electrical cardioversion may be the best choice for patients with tachyarrhythmias, and transcutaneous or transjugular pacing may be required to control bradyarrhythmias in this setting.

Chronic mitral regurgitation

A variety of pharmacologic agents are available for treating patients with chronic mitral regurgitation. Vasodilators and angiotensin-converting enzyme (ACE) inhibitors or angiotensin-1 (AT1) receptor blockers improve left ventricular volume and decrease the regurgitant fraction through a reduction in afterload. However, no trial has demonstrated an improvement in survival with these treatments. In patients with left ventricular systolic dysfunction, beta blockers have a positive effect on ventricular remodeling and the ejection fraction and have been shown to reduce the volume of MR. Combined use of vasodilators and beta blockade may be particularly useful in patients with MR and left ventricular dysfunction.

SURGICAL THERAPY

Operative indications

Papillary muscle rupture

Operation is the only effective therapy for PM rupture. Although mortality rates are high,[248,249] the rates for nonoperative management are higher. Depending on the location of the rupture, different operative techniques may be indicated. In the setting of PM trunk rupture, mitral valve replacement is recommended. When rupture of the PM head occurs but the adjacent head and body remain viable, repair of the PM may be an option. However, these repairs should be attempted only when the patient's clinical condition allows. Commonly, PM rupture combined with ongoing cardiac motion leads to entanglement of the muscle within the other chordal structures; complete disentangling must be performed before repair to preserve ventricular and valvular function.[250] When the clinical situation does not allow for repair of the PM, mitral valve replacement should be performed.

Acute mitral regurgitation

Most patients with acute MR after MI are managed with medical therapy and percutaneous coronary intervention (PCI). However, in addition to those with PM rupture, at least four subsets of patients may require operative therapy in the acute setting: (1) patients with coronary artery disease requiring surgical revascularization, (2) patients with acute postinfarct angina, (3) patients with acute postinfarction angina and 1+ to 2+ MR, and (4) those with acute severe MR in association with progressive heart failure and cardiogenic shock.

In the first group are patients in whom percutaneous intervention does not achieve adequate revascularization and patients with important left main or severe three-vessel coronary artery disease. Revascularization should be performed first in this population; if postbypass echocardiography continues to demonstrate significant (2+ or greater) MR, valve repair or replacement should be performed. ‘

Patients with postinfarct angina should be managed initially with emergent medical or percutaneous revascularization to relieve angina and prevent extension of the infarct, which might result in heart failure, worsening MR, and cardiogenic shock. Although CABG rarely is completed in time to prevent reinfarction in patients with postinfarct angina, it may decrease eventual infarct size.[251–253] In these patients, exposure of the mitral valve should not be performed unless intraoperative TEE demonstrates 3+ or 4+ MR.

Patients with acute severe MR with hemodynamic instability require emergent revascularization, usually surgical. Although there have been reports of resolution of MR with thrombolysis alone, the results have been inconsistent.[196,199,254,255] Rapid (within 4 h of symptom onset) percutaneous revascularization also has demonstrated occasional dramatic resolution of severe MR in settings where viable myocardium remains in the distribution of the culprit artery.[196,255,256] However, even with successful medical or percutaneous revascularization, mortality rates remain high, and most of these patients continue to have 3+ to 4+ MR.[257]

Indications for operative management of acute severe MR vary between institutions but include pulmonary edema, LV failure, and failure of nonsurgical revascularization to abolish MR; the urgency of mitral valve management depends on the presence or absence of cardiogenic shock.[257] In these patients, medical therapy alone has nearly universal mortality.[216,258,259] Operation for acute severe MR should consist of valve repair or replacement with or without myocardial revascularization.

Both mitral valve repair (MVr) and mitral valve replacement (MVR) are options in these patients. Although long-term results appear to be similar within matched cohorts,[210,260] patients undergoing repair for acute severe MR have higher reoperation rates as a result of valve failure.[260] The difficulty of assessing the viability and long-term strength of the valvular apparatus may play a role in these failure rates. MVr may best be reserved for patients in whom Carpentier type I valve dysfunction predominates; in patients with a significant component of leaflet tethering or prolapse, replacement provides a more secure repair. During replacement, whether mechanical or biological prosthetic valves are chosen, it is important to preserve chordal attachments to preserve LV geometry.[261]

Bypass grafts shold be placed to revascularize all significantly obstructed coronary vessels that are remote from the infarct. Although the survival benefit of revascularization of the infarct-related artery after more than 4 to 6 h of symptoms is not clear, even in completed infarctions revascularization appears to improve left ventricular remodeling.[252,253,262] In contrast, blind revascularization of coronary arteries in patients without preoperative angiograms is not likely to be of benefit: Fewer than 50 percent of patients with acute severe MR have multivessel disease,[258,263] and a prolonged operation may increase mortality further in this critically ill population.

Chronic mitral regurgitation

Patients with chronic MR after MI form the largest group of patients who require MV surgery for ischemia. Patients who require surgical revascularization may have MR that ranges from mild to severe with a corresponding range of symptoms (Fig. 29-11).[264] At the ends of this spectrum, management of patients is relatively clear.

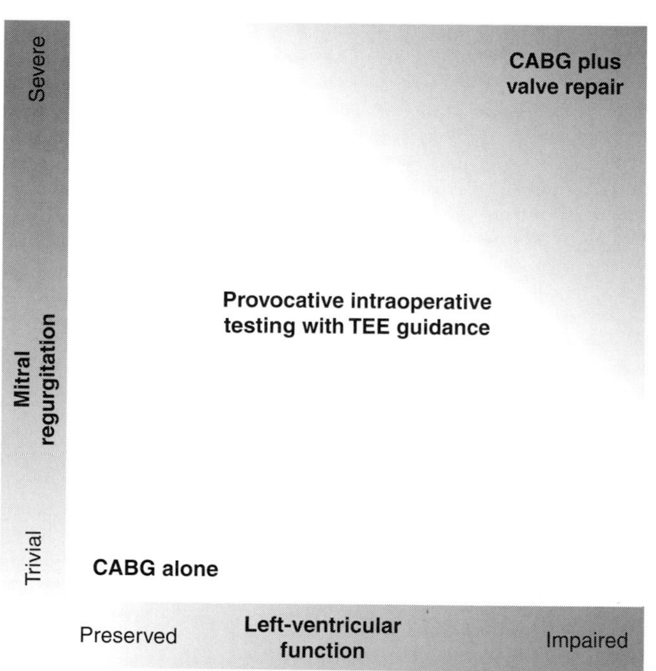

Figure 29-11 Diagram of operative management of chronic mitral regurgitation. Patients with minimal mitral regurgitation and good ventricular function should be managed with CABG alone; those with severe ventricular dysfuction and severe MR warrant mitral valve surgery. Management of patients falling in the intermediate area remains controversial. CABG = coronary artery bypass grafting; MR = mitral regurgitation. [From Byrne JG, Aklog L, Adams DH. Assessment and management of functional or ischaemic mitral regurgitation. *Lancet* 2000;355(9217): 1743–1744.]

In those with only trace or mild MR and few symptoms of heart failure, CABG alone should be performed; in those with severe (3+ to 4+) MR and significant sequelae, concomitant mitral valve surgery is indicated.

Management of patients in the middle of this spectrum remains controversial, with few data to guide therapy. Some series suggest that long-term outcomes in these patients are equivalent whether CABG or CABG with mitral valve surgery is performed.[265] However, CABG alone does not treat MR,[266] and MR even of only mild or moderate severity has been associated with increased long-term mortality.[198,246] Intraoperative assessment of mitral valve function in these patients should include preload and aferload challenges to mitigate the unloading effects of general anesthesia.[187,210,267,268] If provocative testing fails to unmask significant (3+ or 4+) MR or if the resultant MR is associated with focal wall motion abnormalities from the development of ischemia, CABG can be performed without inspection of the mitral valve. However, if these tests demonstrate regurgitation, mitral valve repair or replacement should be considered.

Some patients with ischemic MR may not have viable myocardium that is amenable to surgical revascularization. In these patients, indications for surgical intervention are the same as those for patients with functional nonischemic regurgitation (Fig. 29-12). In contrast to patients undergoing concomitant CABG and valve surgery, in this population the increased afterload after MV surgery is not balanced by improved ventricular function after revascularization; therefore, operative intervention may be poorly tolerated, and many patients may go on to require heart transplantation.

Perioperative considerations

Acute severe mitral regurgitation

Overall surgical management of these patients is similar to the management of those with cardiogenic shock in the absence of MR (see above). Cardiopulmonary bypass should be initiated via direct cannulation of the ascending aorta and bicaval cannulation via the right atrium. Bicaval cannulation maintains decompression during the mitral repair, particularly when exposure of the mitral valve causes superior vena caval obstruction. After aortic cross-clamping and myocardial protection via retrograde and antegrade cardioplegia, the left atrium is opened via a 2-cm-deep dissection of the interatrial groove. Coronary arteries should be grafted before valve surgery. It is important to ensure that all grafts are secure before beginning the valve surgery, as it may be difficult or dangerous to retract the heart after implantation of the prosthetic ring or valve because of the risk of dehiscence or LV rupture.

Chronic mitral regurgitation

Preoperative preparation in these patients is similar to that for other cardiac operations. The surgical approach and the institution of cardiopulmonary bypass are the same as those described for acute MR and include bicaval

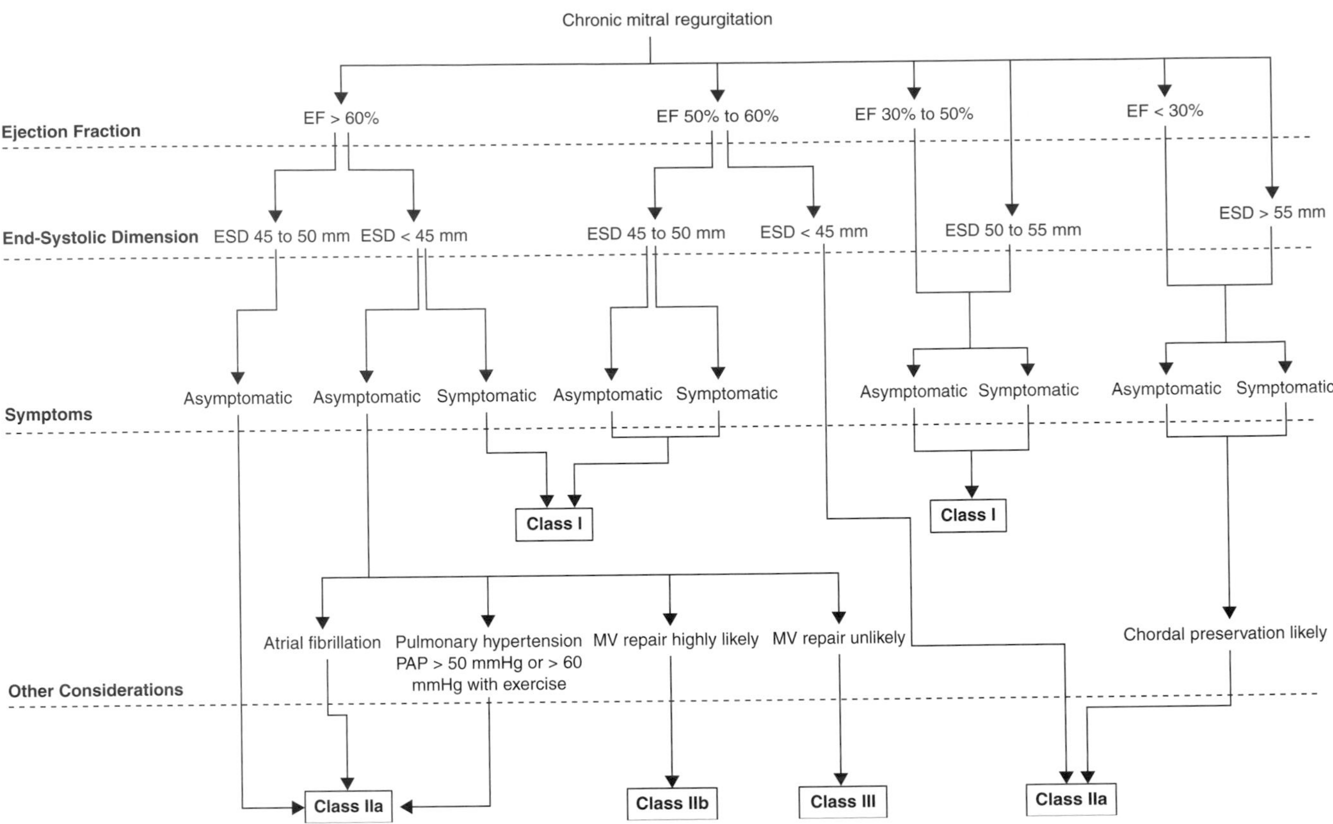

Figure 29-12 Flowchart indicating recommended management of chronic nonischemic mitral regurgitation or chronic ischemic mitral regurgitation without viable myocardium for reperfusion therapy. Class I = evidence and/or agreement that surgery is useful and effective; class IIa = divergence of opinion: weight of evidence/opinion favors usefulness; class IIb = divergence of opinion: usefulness less well established; class III = not indicated or harmful. [Based on the recommendations of the American College of Cardiology/American Heart Association as published in Bonow RO, Carabello B, de Leon AC, et al. ACC/AHA Guidelines for the Management of Patients with Valvular Heart Disease: Executive Summary: A report of the American College of Cardiology/American Heart Association Task Force on Practice Guidelines (Committee on Management of Patients with Valvular Heart Disease). *J Heart Valve Dis* 1998;7(6):672–707.]

cannulation, the use of retrograde and antegrade cardioplegia, and the construction of arterial grafts before the valve procedure. After the induction of anesthesia, the mitral valve should be assessed carefully with TEE to evaluate whether valve surgery is required; if doubt exists, provocative testing should be performed after placement of the arterial cannula.

Operative technique

Repair of rupture of the papillary muscle head

Double-armed, pledgeted 4-0 polypropylene sutures are passed through the viable PM trunk and then into the PM head, where another pledget is used to buttress the knot (Fig. 29-13). The addition of gelatin-resorcinol-formalin glue may help strengthen the repair.[257] In the case of avulsion of the primary chordae, chordal transfer may be performed with a segment of posterior chord. Alternatively, new artificial chordae constructed from extended polytetrafluoroethylene (ePTFE) sutures may be used.[269]

Mitral valve repair versus replacement

The use of repair versus replacement in ischemic MR remains controversial. Because randomized studies are not available to answer this question, large retrospective cohorts provide the only guidance. Gillinov and associates recommend valve repair in most patients. Among the low-risk matched cohorts, MVr had a trend toward improved short- and long-term survival (30-day, 1-year, and 5-year survival 94 percent, 82 percent, and 58 percent versus 81 percent, 56 percent, and 36 percent).[210] However, in the high-risk group, outcomes were similar.[210] When MVr was performed, outcomes were improved with the use of internal thoracic artery graft and the use of a formal annuloplasty band or ring (rather than a pericardial strip).[210] Grossi and associates reported similar results with repair.[260] Patients who may benefit from replacement rather than repair include elderly patients with severe LV dysfunction who may not tolerate a prolonged operation[257] and patients with severe ventricular and PM dysfunction that causes significant type III regurgitation. In

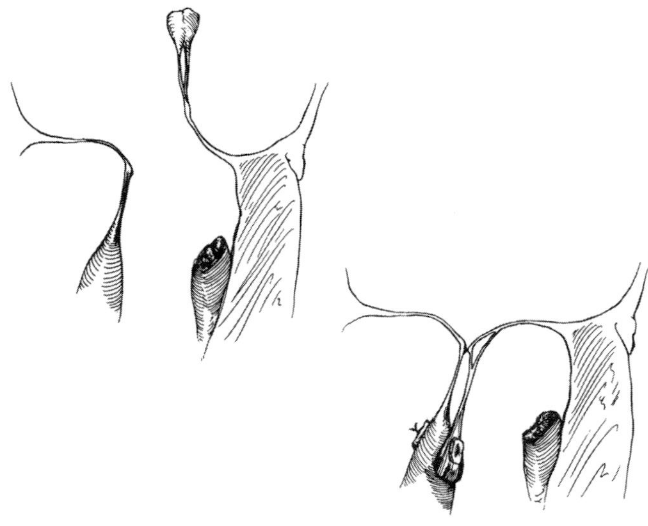

Figure 29-13 Illustration of reimplantation of the ruptured papillary muscle head onto the trunk of the viable adjacent papillary muscle. [Adapted from Figure 32-8 in Kaiser LR, Kron IL, Spray TL (eds). *Mastery of Cardiothoracic Surgery*. Philadelphia: Lippincott-Raven; 1998.]

these patients, repair may not lead to functional coaptation of the mitral leaflets.[210,243,260] Whichever surgical treatment is preferred, careful inspection of the valve should be performed after cardiotomy to identify abnormalities in the papillary muscles and chordae as well as defective leaflet tissue to direct appropriate therapy.

Chordal-sparing mitral valve replacment

Chordal sparing techniques should be used for valve replacement in all patients with ischemic MR. This can be performed by securing the chordae to the valve annulus as described by Khonsari and colleagues (Fig. 29-14).[257] This technique permits resuspension of the chordae with preservation of subvalvular anatomy while allowing for sufficient resection of the anterior leaflet to avoid obstruction of the left ventricular outflow tract. The anterior leaflet is excised, and the rim of leaflet containing the chordal attachment is reattached to the anterior annulus with pledgeted sutures (Khonsari I) (Fig. 29-14A). When the leaflet is calcified, it may be necessary to subdivide the leaflet into two to four segments and reattach each segment to the annulus in an anatomic fashion. If the anterior leaflet is soft and pliable, a central ellipse may be excised and the leaflet free edge may be reattached to the annulus (Khonsari II) (Fig. 29-14B). The posterior leaflet can simply be plicated using horizontal mattress sutures to secure the chordal-leaflet junction to the posterior annulus. The stitches should be placed through the chordal-leaflet junction to elevate the chordae to the level of the valve and preserve the chordal contribution to normal LV geometry as much as possible (Fig. 29-14C).

The decision to use bioprosthetic or mechanical valves should be individualized to the patient on the basis of life expectancy and the risks of anticoagulation. Patients at high risk for anticoagulation or with a life expectancy less than 5 or 6 years are candidates for bioprosthetic valves at most centers.

Mitral valve repair

A wide variety of techniques for MVr have been reported; however, 98 percent of patients in the study by Gillinov and associates[270] underwent annuloplasty, and this is the most common and most consistently effective method. Sizing of the valve should be performed as with standard mitral valve surgery, using the the intertrigonal distance and the area of the anterior leaflet; an undersized annuloplasty is generally preferred. In the Gillinov series, 79 percent of patients had annuloplasties of less than 30 mm, and other series have reported excellent results using undersized annuloplasty for MVr.[210,267,268] Both complete annuloplasty rings and posterior annuloplasty bands have been used, and the results appear similar.[210] However, the additional time required for insertion of a complete ring argues against their continued use.

The annuloplasty ring is sutured into place with 2-0 Dacron horizontal mattress sutures from the left fibrous trigone to the right fibrous trigone along the LV free wall (Fig. 29-15).[257] The sutures should be spaced so that the medial 50 percent of sutures are placed into only 40 percent of the circumference of the annuloplasty ring; this plicates the medial aspect of the annulus and enhances leaflet coaptation.[257] Suture annuloplasty has been reported to enhance coaptation of the leaflets, as has commissuroplasty. Although suture annuloplasty is simple and rapid, the long-term results are poor. Commissuroplasty has significant disadvantages, including instability, partial dehiscence, and the potential to narrow the mitral valve.[257]

Postrepair intraoperative TEE is essential to the operative management of patients undergoing MVr, and its use is associated with improved long-term outcomes after repair.[270] The degree of MR on intraoperative TEE correlates well with early and late postoperative results.[271,272] Although trace to mild residual MR is frequently present and is not associated with decreased survival, it portends a higher reoperation rate.[273] Moderate to severe residual regurgitation at discharge is associated with poor long-term survival[274] and, when identified intraoperatively, necessitates a return to cardiopulmonary bypass and reevaluation of the valve. Redo of the repair has been successful in some populations,[275] but in patients undergoing prolonged procedures with concomitant CABG valve replacement it should not be delayed. In large series, reinstitution of bypass and redo of the valve surgery are required in approximately 2 to 7 percent of cases.[276,277]

In addition to identifying residual MR after repair, TEE is important in detecting dynamic left ventricular outflow tract (LVOT) obstruction caused by systolic anterior motion (SAM) of the anterior mitral leaflet into the LVOT (Fig. 29-16). A variety of factors are associated with the development of SAM after MVr: excessive anterior leaflet

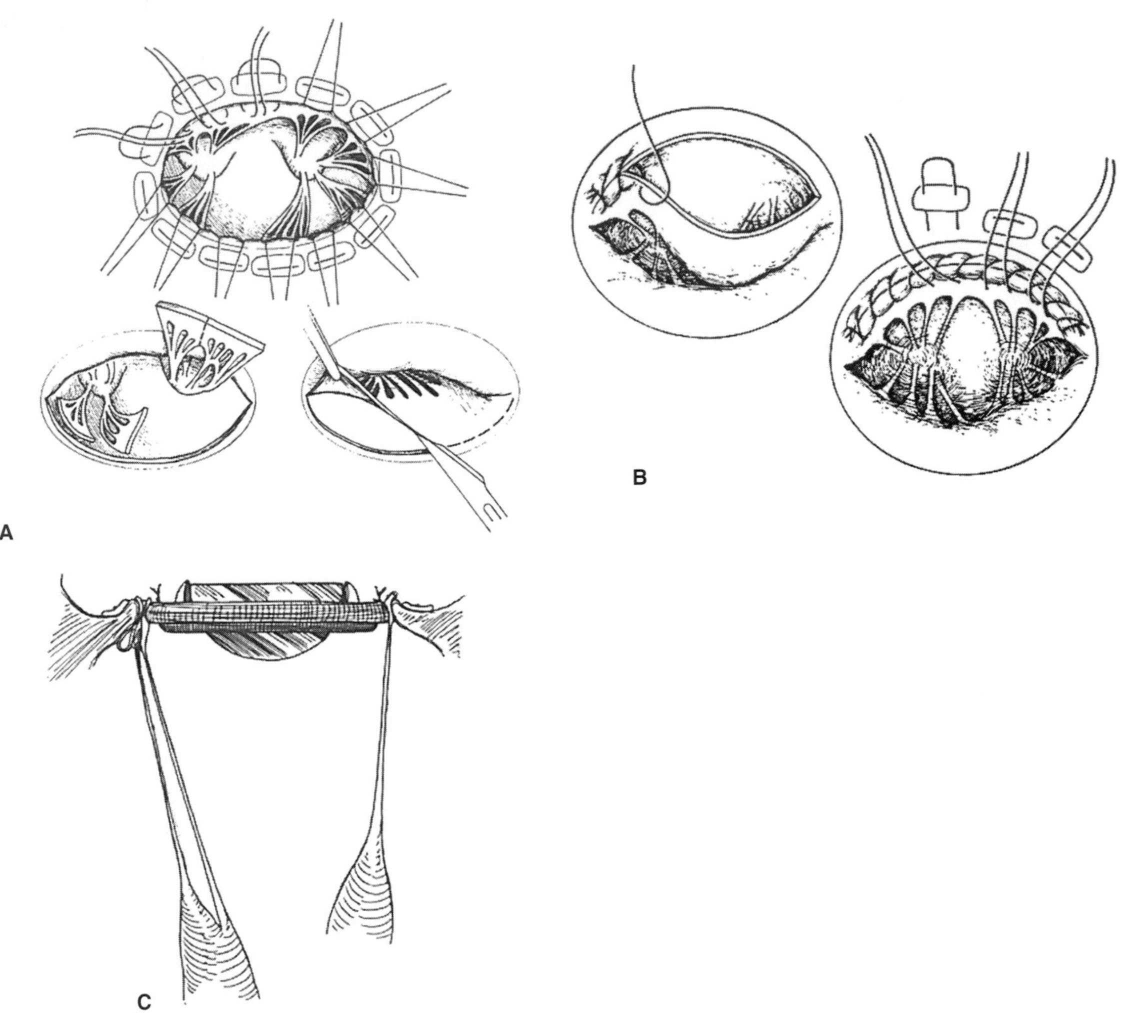

Figure 29-14 Illustration of techniques for chordal preservation during mitral valve replacement. A. Khonsari I technique. The anterior leaflet is excised from the annulus while preserving the leaflet-chordal junction. The leaflet then is divided if necessary, and the chordae are resuspended in their normal anatomic positions surrounding the annulus. B. Khonsari II technique. When the valve leaflet is soft and pliable (as is common in ischemic mitral regurgitation), a central ellipse of the anterior leaflet is excised, and the free edge is reattached to the annulus, using the valve sutures. C. Cross-sectional image. The relationship of the excised anterior leaflet and plicated posterior leaflet to the valve structure is clearly indicated. [Adapted from Figures 34-10 through 34-12 in Kaiser LR, Kron IL, Spray TL (eds). *Mastery of Cardiothoracic Surgery*. Philadelphia: Lippincott-Raven; 1998.]

tissue, increased posterior leaflet height, a hyperkinetic heart, a prominent interventricular septum, a narrow aortic-mitral angle, too small an annuloplasty ring or inaccurate ring orientation, and extensive quadrangular resection of the posterior leaflet.[278] In general, these factors bring leaflet coaptation and the anterior leaflet closer to the septum, resulting in LVOT obstruction. In early series, SAM occurred in approximately 5 to 10 percent of cases of MVr.[279,280] Improvements in operative technique (including the sliding leaflet technique of Carpentier[281,282]) have reduced this incidence in more recent series.

On TEE, SAM can be seen as protrusion of the free edge of the anterior leaflet into the LVOT. It often is associated with deviation of the coaptation point toward the septum as well as a small left ventricle and a bulging septum.[283] Changes in LV geometry with changes in volume status may play a significant role in the development and presentation of SAM; therefore, not all patients will have abnormal postrepair TEEs. In these patients, the postoperative onset of SAM and LVOT obstruction may be heralded by a rapid onset of hypotension, near syncope, and arrhythmias.[283]

The initial treatment of SAM should be directed at optimization of LV volume to displace the anterior leaflet away from the septum. The use of inotropes should be minimized to reduce hyperdynamic left ventricular contractility. Phenylephrine may be used to increase systemic vascular resistance; the reflex bradycardia increases LV size through an increase in diastolic

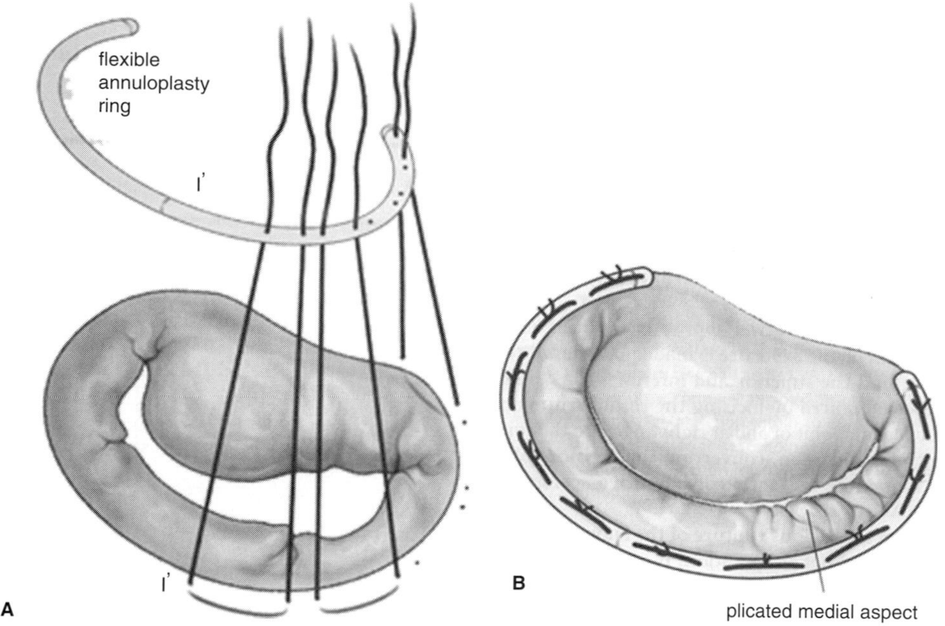

Figure 29-15 Placement of a flexible annuloplasty ring for mitral regurgitation. **A.** The sutures are placed into the annulus in an asymmetric manner so that 50 percent of the sutures along the medial aspect are placed into only 40 percent of the annuloplasty ring. **B.** This results in preferential plication of the region of the posteromedial commissure and enhances coaptation between the anterior and posterior leaflets. [Adapted from Figure 23.8A and B in Buxton BF, Frazier OH, Westaby S (eds). *Ischemic Heart Disease Surgical Management.* Philadelphia: Mosby; 1999.]

filling.[278] Beta blockade may be useful in increasing diastolic filling as well as treating superimposed tachyarrhythmias.[283] Finally, initiation of atrioventricular pacing and adjustment of the pacing intervals have eliminated SAM in some cases.[278] Most patients will respond to medical therapy alone,[280] but patients who require large alterations in hemodynamics with phenylephrine and beta blockade should be considered for reoperative mitral valve surgery.

Other techniques

Because annuloplasty and other techniques of MVr do not address the pathology of ischemic MR (which involves dysfunction of the LV wall that leads to failure of leaflet coaptation), attempts have been made to address ischemic MR at the ventricular level. Two techniques have been validated in animal models but have not been evaluated in humans. LV remodeling through plication of the infarct region reduces the distance between the papillary muscles and the mitral annulus; this reduces systolic tenting and decreases the regurgitant volume.[284] A reduction in tenting and an improvement in MR were noted with selective cutting of a limited number of basal chordae tendineae involved in incomplete valve closure.[285] The applicability of these techniques in humans remains to be seen.

OUTCOMES AND PROGNOSIS

Early results

Few studies have separately addressed the risks and results of mitral valve surgery for acute MR. Historical series report 30-day mortality rates from 10 percent to 70 percent,[258,263,286,287] but they do not have significant applicability to contemporary series, and the wide range probably reflects differences in patient selection rather than operative technique. Outcomes have improved, and operative mortality for acute severe MR in most contemporary series (whether limited to PM rupture or inclusive of all types of acute MR) is approximately 20 percent.[288,289] Patients in cardiogenic shock have higher early mortality in all series.[210,259,260,289] Although patient selection may play a role, the 40 percent mortality reported after surgery for acute MR still improves on the 71 percent mortality seen with medical therapy in the SHOCK registry by a wide margin.[288] Early operation in the absence of hemodynamic compromise does not appear to have an effect on operative mortality.[210,260] There is not a clear consensus about the benefits of repair versus replacement in the acute MR population, and large series suggest that the outcomes are probably similar, although many authors continue to recommend replacement in the acute setting.[260,290]

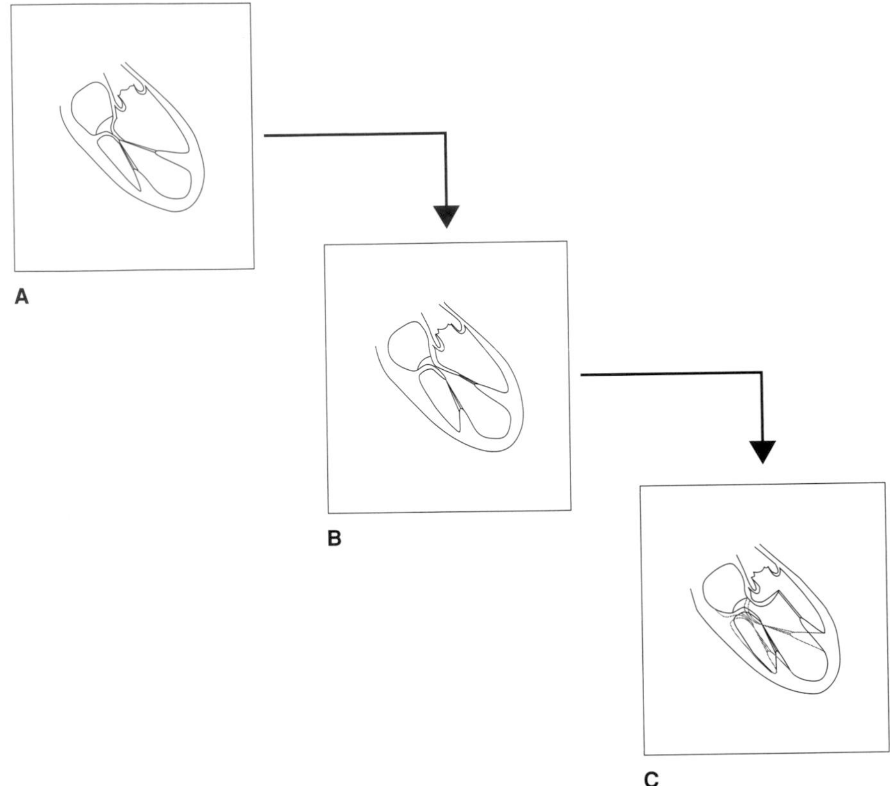

Figure 29-16 Systolic anterior motion of the anterior mitral leaflet and left ventricular outflow tract (LVOT) obstruction. A. Normal heart in systole. B. Displacement of the anterior mitral leaflet toward the ventricular septum and into the LVOT may be precipitated by the posterior portion of the annuloplasty ring pushing the anterior leaflet too far forward, excessive shortening of chordae or papillary muscles during the operative procedure, left ventricular hypertrophy, or a variety of other factors. C. Intermittently, the mitral leaflet may get drawn into the LVOT, causing dynamic obstruction and sudden onset of hypotension.

In three large recent reports limited to mitral valve surgery in ischemic MR, operative mortality was 13 percent.[210,260,289] Previous series had a wide spectrum of operative results that ranged from 3.0 percent to 29.4 percent; this may have been affected by the variable inclusion of patients with chronic non-ischemic MR as well as the heterogeneous population undergoing MR in the setting of coronary artery disease.[187] Similar mortality was observed in the series by Cohn and associates that dealt with patients undergoing concomitant CABG and MVR for ischemic MR.[248] Although multiple studies have demonstrated the negative impact of concomitant CABG on operative mortality during MV surgery,[289,291–293] this probably reflects the underlying pathology rather than the choice of operative procedure. The large series reported by Grossi and associates[260] and Gillinov and coworkers[210] attempted to control for patient selection in order to compare valve replacement with valve repair. Those authors have initiated an emerging consensus that suggests that valve repair is superior to replacement in this population. Risk factors for early mortality after mitral valve surgery include older age, cardiac dysfunction, complex jet direction (for patients undergoing repair), and severe wall motion abnormalities.[210,260]

Late results

Patients undergoing valve replacement rarely require reoperation for valve failure.[294,295] Although there have been concerns about durability of valve repair for ischemic MR, long-term freedom from repair failure requiring reoperation is excellent: 98 percent at 30 days, 96 percent at 1 year, and 91 percent at 5 years.[210] However, many patients with recurrent MR may not reach reoperation or may not be operative candidates at the time of repair failure. Severe MR may recur in up to 5 percent of patients, and mild to moderate MR in 50 percent.[296]

Despite improvements in technique and operative care, only 55 to 60 percent of patients survive 5 years after surgery. In Gillinov's series, among the lowest-risk patients, survival with repair was 58 percent (replacement only, 36 percent), but the highest-risk patients had 5-year survival below 50 percent regardless of the procedure performed.[210] Similar results were obtained by Grossi and coworkers.[260] Risk factors for poor outcomes in these groups included poor preoperative cardiac function, previous cardiac surgery, use of suture rather than ring annuloplasty, inferior or lateral wall motion abnormalities, and preoperative atrial fibrillation.[210,260] The poor outcomes probably reflect the impact of large MIs and progressive LV failure on survival and will not be ameliorated by improvements in mitral surgical techniques.

SUMMARY

There are three forms of ischemic mitral regurgitation: papillary muscle rupture, acute MR, and chronic MR. Papillary muscle rupture requires emergent operative repair, usually with mitral valve replacement, after resection of the ruptured portion. In patients with acute severe MR secondary to ischemia, indications for operation vary between institutions, but emergent revascularization is indicated. When revascularization via thrombolysis or PCI is ineffective, surgical revascularization and mitral valve surgery (usually replacement) are indicated. In patients with chronic MR, mitral valve repair appears to have outcomes equivalent to or better than those of replacement in most populations. Indications for repair include 3+ to 4+ MR in patients needing revascularization. In patients not requiring revascularization, operative decision making is more complex, but in general, symptomatic patients or those with depressed LV function [ejection fraction less than 50 percent or electrostatic discharge (ESD) greater than 50 mm] should be considered for isolated mitral valve procedures. Operative mortality in patients with ischemic MR is approximately 13 percent. Although long-term freedom from reoperation (even with valve repair) exceeds 90 percent at 5 years, survival at 5 years is only 55 to 60 percent. Poor outcomes reflect the impact of large infarctions and extensive coronary disease rather than problems with the mitral surgery.

VENTRICULAR SEPTAL RUPTURE

INTRODUCTION

First described at autopsy in 1845 by Latham,[297] ventricular septal rupture is a rare but highly lethal complication of MI. The first antemortem diagnosis was not made until 1923,[298] and it would be another 30 years before Cooley and associates[299] performed the first successful repair. Since that time, rapid diagnosis and prompt surgical repair represent the best chance for survival.

Although earlier reports described septal rupture in 1 to 3 percent of cases of MI,[300,301] the advent of reperfusion and aggressive strategies of revascularization have reduced

KEY CONCEPTS

- Epidemiology
  - Occurs in <0.5 percent of MI patients.
  - Only 24 percent of medically treated patients with ventricular septal defect (VSR) survive 30-days.
- Pathophysiology
  - Rupture follows large transmural infarction with weakening of the septal wall.
  - Results in left-to-right shunt of variable magnitude with diversion of blood flow from systemic to pulmonary circulation and low-cardiac-output state, ultimately into cardiogenic shock.
- Clinical Features
  - Usually patients first present with MI or angina.
  - Occurs 5 to 6 days after MI.
  - Recurrence of chest pain, shortness of breath, harsh pansystolic murmur.
- Diagnostics
  - Location of infarct of ECG correlates with location of VSR.
  - Echocardiography important to differentiate VSR from acute, servere mitral regurgitation (sensitivity and specificity ~100 percent).
  - Angiography allows delineation of coronary anatomy and guided placement of Intraaortic baloon pump (IABP).
- Treatment
  - Medical
    - Pharmacologic and mechnical support of end-organ perfusion.
    - IABP only method that can improve both systemic and coronary perfusion while reducing systemic vascular resistance to minimize left-to-right shunt.
  - Surgical
    - Rarely patients may remain stable without hemodynamic consequences of a small shunt; these patients may have surgery delayed.
    - Others required urgent or emergent operative repair; repair should not be delayed to await improvement with medical therapy.
    - Multiple techniques described, including apical amputation, path closure, and infarct exclusion.
    - Concomitant coronary artery bypass graft should be performed as indicated.
- Outcomes and Prognosis.
  - Operative mortality remains high (though better than medical therapy): 20 to 50 percent.
  - Impact of different repairs on outcomes not clear.
  - Hospital survivors have excellent long-term survival (61 percent at 8 years).

that rate to less than 0.5 percent.[302] However, mortality remains high, and with only 24 percent of medically treated patients (none of them with cardiogenic shock) surviving to 30 days,[303] surgical repair affords an improvement in outcomes, although long-term survivors remain rare.

PATHOPHYSIOLOGY

Pathology

Ventricular septal rupture (VSR) occurs after a large transmural infarction when enough necrosis occurs to weaken the septal wall. Infarctions complicated by VSR are larger than those which are not,[304,305] and patients with rupture appear less likely to have diffuse coronary artery disease[303,306,307] (though this has not been found in all reports[308]), to have had previous episodes of angina or MI,[300,307,309–312] and to demonstrate evidence of collateral circulation.[306,309,312] This suggests that large infarctions in myocardial regions that are poorly supplied with collateral perfusion may be at particular risk, but otherwise the reason some hearts rupture and others do not is not clear.

There are two types of VSR: simple and complex (Fig. 29-17). Simple ruptures are discrete lesions with defects at a similar level in both ventricles. The path between the ventricles follows a straight path through the infarcted

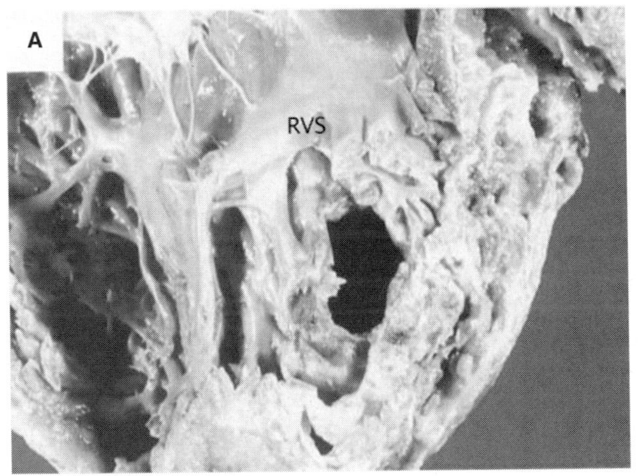

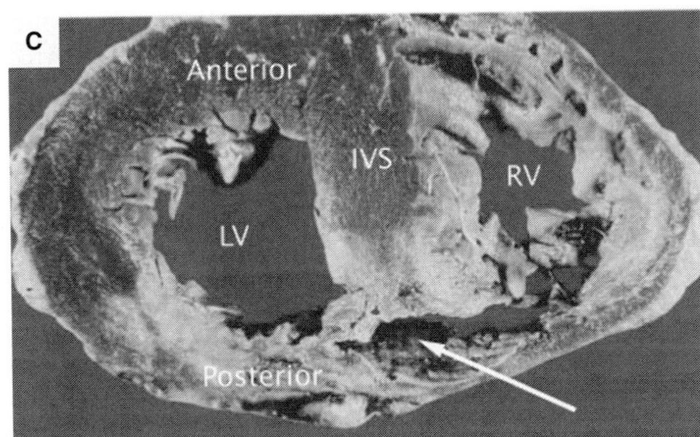

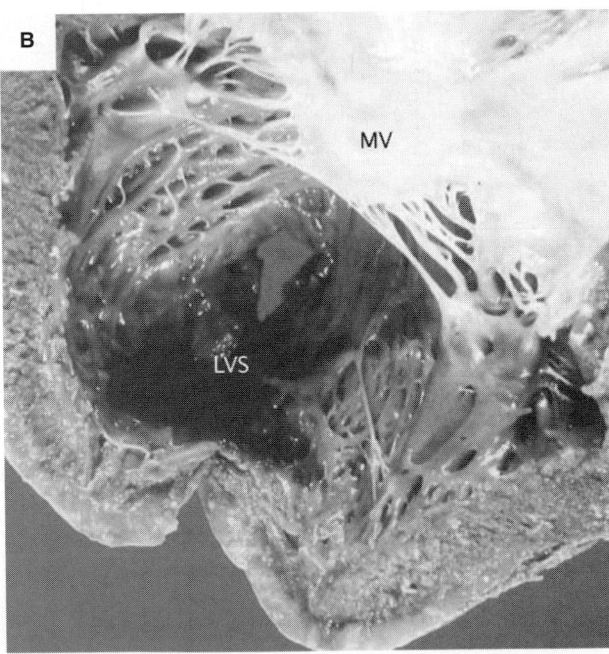

Figure 29-17 Pathologic specimens of ventricular septal rupture. A and B. Simple ventricular septal rupture with a direct through-and-through connection across the septum. The perforation is at the same level on both sides of the septum. C. Complex septal rupture (*arrow*) after infarction of the basal inferior septum and adjacent ventricular wall. LVS = left ventricular aspect of the ventricular septum; RVS = right ventricular aspect of the interventricular septum; MV = mitral valve; IVS = interventricular septum; LV = left ventricle. [From Birnbaum Y, Fishbein MC, Blanche C, Siegel RJ. Ventricular septal rupture after acute myocardial infarction. *N Engl J Med* 2002;347(18):1426–1432. Permission pending.]

myocardium. In contrast, complex ruptures have a convoluted dissection path between the ventricles with regions of extensive hemorrhage and may include areas remote from the primary infarction site. Complex morphology occurs more commonly with inferior infarcts, whereas anterior infarcts are associated with simple VSR.[308]

Anterior VSR usually occurs after acute occlusion of the left anterior descending coronary artery (LAD) and most often is located where the septum joins the free wall. Infarcted myocardium occupies a large section of the anterior portion of the septum. Inferior VSRs occur after occlusion of the right coronary artery. They may be located near the base of the heart, abutting the mitral valve annulus, midway between the base and apex, or, less commonly, near the apex. Midseptal defects, usually resulting from occlusion of a large septal perforating artery, are rarer.

The size of the rupture varies considerably, from millimeters to centimeters, and in 5 to 11 percent of cases, multiple defects are present.[313] VSR may occur in combination with other mechanical defects, including PM or ventricular free wall rupture.[314] Mitral regurgitation occurs in approximately 33 percent of cases but more often results from LV dysfunction than from PM rupture.[315]

Pathophysiology

Interventricular rupture results in a left-to-right shunt of variable magnitude and a significant biventricular hemodynamic load on an already ischemic heart. In most patients, this leads to progressive clinical deterioration, although small ruptures with small shunts may be better tolerated. Initially, the shunt manifests primarily as RV volume overload and increased pulmonary blood flow. Secondary LV volume overload then results. The diversion of blood flow from the systemic to the pulmonary circulation ultimately leads to a low-output cardiac state; this may be more severe in patients with normally compliant right ventricles.[301] Systemic vasoconstriction in response to peripheral hypotension and hypoperfusion results in a worsening of the left-to-right shunt. A progressive spiral in cardiac function results, leading to worsening myocardial perfusion, increased myocardial workload, infarct extension, and ultimately end-organ hypoperfusion and cardiogenic shock. As the LV fails and systemic pressure declines, the volume of the shunt ultimately decreases as cardiovascular collapse ensues.

CLINICAL FEATURES

Changes in the incidence of VSR after MI with the advent of reperfusion therapies have been associated with a change in the timing of presentation. Historically, most patients presented approximately 5 to 6 days after MI.[316] In the current era, the median time to rupture after MI is less than 24 h.[307] Risk factors for VSR after MI include advanced age, hypertension, and the absence of a history of MI or angina.[300,305,307,309–312,317,318] The influence of gender on the incidence of VSR is not clear. Many surgical series contain a preponderance of men,[319,320] and larger series have documented a higher incidence of rupture among women.[302,307]

The symptoms associated with VSR are those of myocardial ischemia, low cardiac output, and shock, particularly when these symptoms occur after resolution of the initial symptoms. Recurrence of chest pain and shortness of breath are common.[311] A harsh pansystolic murmur heard loudest at the left lower sternal border or a palpable parasternal thrill may be present in up to 50 percent of patients with acute VSR; however, the onset of cardiogenic shock may lead to a decrease in turbulent flow and a loss of the murmur.[303] Electrocardiography often demonstrates new ST-segment elevation.[311] The location of the infarct on ECG correlates well with the location of the septal rupture.[321]

DIAGNOSTIC MODALITIES

In a patient with acute cardiovascular collapse after MI, the differential includes VSR, free wall rupture, and mitral regurgitation (with or without PM rupture) as well as acute ventricular dysfunction (Table 29-7).[314] Because free wall rupture has a very different presentation dominated by the signs of pericardial tamponade, the primary diagnostic dilemna with VSR is differentiating patients with MR from those with VSR; this can be made more difficult by the coexistence of these entities in up to 20 percent of patients.[322–324] Differentiation based on clinical examination is difficult, although clues to the existence of VSR include a palpable thrill that generally is not evident in MR and the lack of the severe pulmonary edema common to MR. However, in low-output states, these clues may not allow differentiation between the two complications.

Historically, right heart catheterization was the diagnostic tool of choice for distinguishing these entities.[325] In VSR, right ventricular oxygen saturation is increased, whereas the increase in MR is confined to the pulmonary artery vasculature. However, advances in both transthoracic and transesophageal echocardiography have led to their supplanting right heart catherization in the diagnosis of VSR. Doppler echocardiography can identify the site and size of left-to-right shunts through the septal defect accurately, and sensitivity and specificity as high as 100 percent have been reported in the differentiation of VSR from MR (Fig. 29-18).[326,327] In addition, echocardiography can be used to assess the degree of both right and left ventricular impairment in these patients.

Left ventricular catheterization with angiography has both advantages and disadvantages. Angiography is time-consuming, and the load of contrast dye may be detrimental to both renal and ventricular function; in patients with significant end-organ hypoperfusion, this is an important concern. However, when concomitant coronary revascu-

Table 29-7 Clinical characteristics of ventricular septal rupture, rupture of the ventricular free wall and papillary muscle rupture

Characteristic	Ventricular septal rupture	Rupture of ventricular free wall	Papillary muscle rupture
Incidence	1–3% without reperfusion therapy, 0.2–0.34% with thrombolytic therapy, 3.9% among patients with cardiogenic shock	0.8–6.2%; thrombolytic therapy does not reduce risk; primary PTCA seems to reduce risk	About 1%
Time course	3–7 days without reperfusion therapy; median, 24 h with thrombolysis	1–7 days without reperfusion therapy; mean, 2.7 days with thrombolysis	Median, 1 day (range 1–14 days)
Clinical manifestations	Chest pain, shortness of breath	Anginal, pleuritic, or pericardial chest pain, syncope, hypotension, arrhythmias, nausea, restlessness, hypotension, sudden death	Abrupt onset of shortness of breath and pulmonary edema; hypotension
Physical findings	Harsh holosystolic murmur, thrill (+), S_3, accentuated second heart sound, pulmonary edema, RV and LV failure, cardiogenic shock	Jugulovenous distention (29% of patients), pulsus paradoxus (47%), electromechanical dissociation, cardiogenic schock	A soft murmur in some cases, no thrill, variable signs of RV overload, severe pulmonary edema, cardiogenic shock
Echocardiographic findings	Ventricular septal rupture, left-to-right shunt on color flow Doppler echocardiography through the ventricular septum, pattern of RV overload	> 5 mm pericardial effusion not visualized in all cases, layered, high-acoustic echoes within the pericardium (blood clot), direct visualization of tear, signs of tamponade	Hypercontractile LV, torn papillary muscle or chordae tendineae, flail leaflet, severe mitral regurgitation on color flow Doppler echocardiography
Right heart catherization	Increase in oxygen saturation from RA to RV, large V waves	Ventriculography insensitive, classic signs of tamponade not always present (equalization of diastolic pressures among the chambers)	No increase in oxygen saturation from RA to RV, large V waves, very high pulmonary capillary wedge pressures

From Birnbaum, Birnbaum Y, Fishbein MC, et al. Ventricular septal rupture after acute myocardial infarction. *N Engl J Med* 2002;347(18): 1426–1432. Permission pending.

PTCA = percutaneous transluminal coronary angioplasty; RA = right atrium; RV = right ventricle; LV = left ventricle.

larization is being considered, angiography helps delineate coronary anatomy. As many as 60 percent of patients with VSR may have significant disease in coronary arteries other than the one perfusing the affected portion of the septum, and revascularization may improve long-term survival.[328] Therefore, if the patient's condition permits, preoperative coronary angiography should be performed.

MEDICAL THERAPY

Medical therapy consists of both mechanical and pharmacologic support of cardiac function and end-organ perfusion. In most cases, after the diagnosis of VSR, these therapies are merely temporizing measures. They may allow for the performance of further diagnostic procedures (including cardiac catheterization when appropriate) and maintenance of perfusion en route to the operating room, but operation remains the only definitive treatment.

The goals of medical therapy in this setting are (1) maintenance of end-organ perfusion, (2) optimization of coronary perfusion, (3) reduction in myocardial oxygen demand, and (4) reduction in systemic vascular resistance (SVR) to minimize the left-to-right shunt. In patients without hypotension, vasodilators such as nitroprusside may be useful in reducing SVR; however, they may cause a significant decrease in coronary perfusion as well as end-organ compromise if hypotension occurs.[51] Diuretics may help reduce SVR and preload without similar effects on coronary perfusion. Although inotropic agents may be required to maintain systemic blood flow (and nearly all patients with cardiogenic shock and VSR require them),[307] the increase in systemic pressure may worsen shunting and exacerbate the shift in blood flow from the systemic to the pulmonary circulation. IABP remains the only method that can accomplish all these goals. Counterpulsation decreases left ventricular afterload, which reduces the right-to-left shunt while augmenting cardiac output and

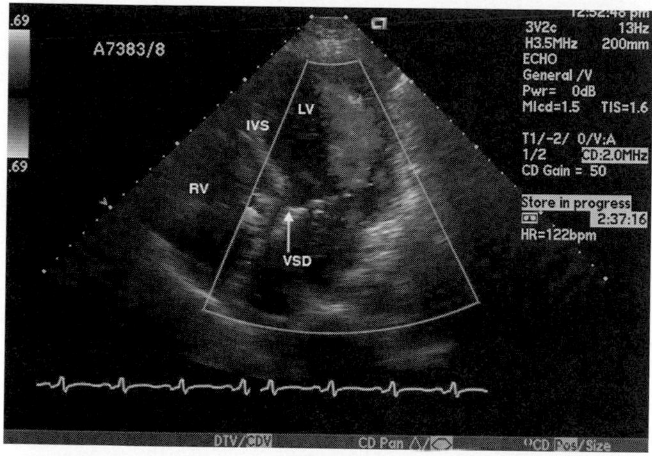

Figure 29-18 Doppler echocardiography demonstrating an ischemic ventricular septal rupture with flow through the ventricular septum during systole. LV = left ventricle; RV = right ventricle; IVS = interventricular septum; VSD = ventricular septal defect.

end-organ perfusion. Through diastolic augmentation, coronary perfusion is maximized. The advantages of IABP suggest that an IABP should be inserted into all patients with VSR and hemodynamic compromise. Although it cannot treat VSR in the long term, it may provide enough time to perform cardiac catheterization, and it optimizes the patient's hemodynamic status before the induction of anesthesia. IABP improves hemodynamics in all patients with VSR, and those patients tolerate counterpulsation well without loss of the beneficial effect with insertion times longer than 24 h.[329]

SURGICAL THERAPY

Timing of surgery

The first successful repairs of VSR were performed in patients more than 1 month after the rupture event.[299–331] It was felt at that time that patients would not tolerate earlier repair both because of their poor hemodynamic status and because it was felt that recently necrosed myocardium would not hold sutures. Those successes, as well as the abrupt acute decompensation and clinical deterioration in other patients, led to the belief that patients with VSR should not be operated on for 1 month after rupture. However, delayed surgery after rupture probably simply selected out patients with smaller defects and relatively preserved hemodynamics whereas patients with more severe disease died during the delay.[332,333] Patients who were not operated on were unlikely to survive the hospital stay, and many patients underwent operative repair only after cardiovascular collapse; 4-week mortality without operation is 80 to 90 percent, and 1-year mortality approaches 100 percent.[302,333,334] More recent data from the SHOCK registry confirm the poor outcomes in critically ill patients with VSR who do not reach operative repair. The registry followed 55 patients with cardiogenic shock secondary to VSR; 24 were managed medically, and 31 underwent high-risk surgery. Overall survival was 28.6 percent among those treated surgically but only 4.2 percent among those treated medically.[307] Because of these dismal outcomes, attempts were made to operate earlier, and in 1977, Daggett and associates reported increased survival in 43 patients operated on early for VSR.[332] Early operation also may decrease the risk of subsequent free wall rupture, which often is preceded by VSR.[311] Since that time, other authors have confirmed the relative survival advantage of early operation in these patients, and operation within 24 to 48 h has become the standard.[335]

Patients presenting after VSR can be grouped broadly into four groups on the basis of hemodynamic status at the time of diagnosis. The first group consists of the few patients who remain hemodynamically stable and in whom a small left-to-right shunt is well tolerated without hemodynamic support or end-organ compromise. These patients may be managed medically until it is convenient to perform the repair, but operative repair should be performed before hospital discharge. The second group consists of patients in cardiogenic shock. This is the largest group of patients with VSR.[302,336] Another large group of patients occupies an intermediate position between those in the first two groups; these patients require operation within 12 to 24 h. Their clinical stability on initial presentation should not lead to medical management or an attempt to delay operation; further deterioration will result, and the patient will require emergent and risky surgical repair. The final group consists of patients who present after the onset of end-organ damage or sepsis. These patients are not likely to survive surgery, and there are case reports of survival using long-term IABP support until they can tolerate operative repair.[337]

Operative technique

General considerations

After median sternotomy, cardiopulmonary bypass is initiated swiftly with bicaval cannulation. Left ventricular venting is not required, as the LV should vent spontaneously via the septal defect and insertion of a vent may dislodge any mural thrombus present in the LV. For the same reason, manipulation of the heart before clamping should be minimized. As with other patients undergoing cardiac operations in proximity to myocardial ischemia, both retrograde and antegrade cardioplegia should be used. Distal coronary anastomoses should be performed before ventriculotomy; this both maximizes myocardial protection and minimizes manipulation of the fragile ventriculotomy repair.

The surgeon often is challenged by the weak and friable myocardium in both the septum and the infarcted regions of the ventricular free wall. These regions have a tendency to weaken, fail, and lead to a residual defect. The use of a generous pericardial patch is important in reducing tension and decreasing the risk of a residual or recurrent septal defect. The closure of the left ventriculotomy, particularly when large free wall infarcts are present, must be performed with large 1-cm bites of tissue and extensive use of felt buttressing to decrease the risk of postoperative free wall rupture.

Surgical approach to interventricular septal rupture

The first repair by Cooley and associates[299] involved a right ventriculotomy for access to the interventricular septum, as was used in the approach to congenital VSR. Unfortunately, this approach has multiple disadvantages: (1) Exposure of the defect is not optimal, (2) damage occurs to the normal myocardium of the right ventricle, (3) collateral blood flow from the right coronary circulation is cut off, and (4) it fails to address the portion of infarcted LV wall that results in paradoxic bulging during ventricular systole. With these weaknesses in mind, Heimbecker and coworkers[338] developed the technique of left ventriculotomy; this allows simultaneous repair of the septal defect along with infarctectomy and aneurysmectomy. This has become the standard surgical approach to most VSR repairs.

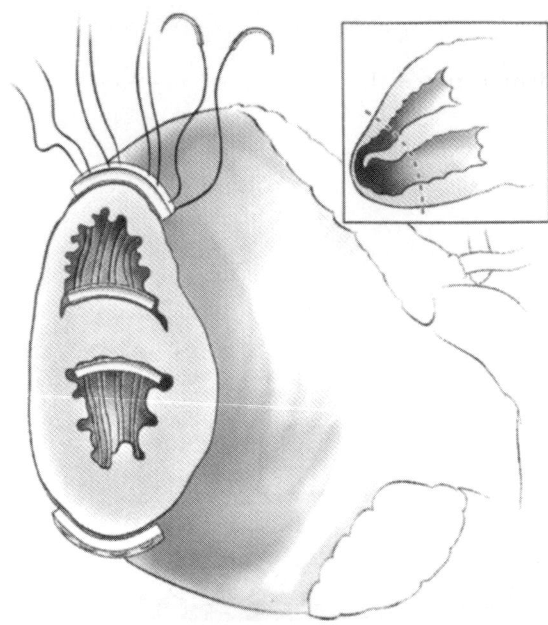

Figure 29-19 Amputation of an apical septal rupture with biventricular closure using pledgeted sutures. [Adapted from Figure 22.11 in Buxton BF, Frazier OH, Westaby S (eds). *Ischemic Heart Disease Surgical Management.* Philadelphia: Mosby; 1999.]

Apical septal rupture

The technique of apical rupture repair is perhaps the most simple, but apical VSRs are rare. Daggett and coworkers first described the technique of apical amputation in 1970.[339] An incision is made through the necrotic left ventricular apex and through the septum and the right ventricular free wall. This results in amputation of the apex of the heart. The repair is completed by approximating the ventricular free walls to the septum, using Teflon felt strips and horizontal mattress sutures (Fig. 29-19).

Anterior septal rupture

The initial approach to anterior septal rupture is via a transinfarct left ventriculotomy with infarct excision. Some small anterior defects may be closed without a prosthetic patch by approximating the free anterior edge of the septum to the right ventricular free wall with mattress sutures of Tevdek over strips of felt. However, most defects require the insertion of a patch to obtain a tension-free repair.

The classical technique involves debridement of the VSR and if necessary slight enlargement of the defect. This permits the placement of horizontal mattress sutures from the right ventricular side of the defect through a thick felt patch and then through the septum. The sutures then are passed through the patch approximately 8 mm from the edge and tied into place. The patch is brought out through the venticulotomy incision, and the incision is closed. Wide bites of viable left ventricular wall are taken, and the closure is buttressed with large felt patches. In this technique, if there is not sufficient anterior septum to anchor the anterior portion of the patch, horizontal mattress sutures may be passed from the epicardial to the endocardial surface of the right ventricle to complete the repair.

As surgical repair has occurred earlier, the strength of the myocardium holding the patch sutures has become a significant issue. Although sutures should be placed into viable myocardium, in the first 24 h after infarct it may be difficult to differentiate viable from nonviable regions. The addition of tissue adhesives to repair techniques adds strength and theoretically reduces the risk of postoperative dehiscence of the septal patch. Seguin and associates described the first use of fibrin sealant in reinforcing patch closure of VSR in three patients.[340] Refinements in technique and biological adhesive have led some authors to advocate the repair of VSR with a pericardial patch and gelatin-resorcinol-formaldehyde (GRF) biological glue.[341] In this technique, placement of the patch is similar to that in the classic approach. However, the sutures anchoring the patch to the septum are placed at a wider radius to ensure attachment to viable myocardium. This suture is a running suture without pledgets. GRF glue is applied over the septal side of the pericardial patch through to the ventriculotomy closure. Excellent results have been obtained with this technique, and successful repair of cardiac rupture without the use of sutures has been reported.[342–345] There has been theoretical concern that the formaldehyde might inhibit ventricular remodeling and growth of fibrous tissue into the patch area. Although autopsy studies have not demonstrated that problem,[343] the next generation of glues promises to alleviate this theoretical concern.

Posterior septal rupture

The repair of inferoposterior septal defects is made more difficult by exposure of the posterior of the heart as well as the proximity of both the posterior descending artery (PDA) and, on the endocardial surface, the posteromedial PM. After cross-clamping, the heart is retracted out of the cardiac well and the posterior surface is exposed. A left ventriculotomy is made through the infarct approximately 1 cm lateral to the PDA, with care taken to leave the papillary muscles undamaged. The patch then is cut and secured with running 4-0 monofilament sutures. As with anterior defects, the patch then may be brought out through the ventriculotomy and secured.

Inferior infarctions with significant LV free wall enlargement require additional techniques. In these cases the infarcted ventricular wall often is thinned out. Use of this weakened myocardium for closure increases the risk of rupture. To strengthen the repair, the ventriculotomy is closed with a Dacron free wall patch backed with pericardium. The patch is secured to the ventricular wall with interposed felt strips on both the epicardial and the endocardial surfaces to strengthen the attachment points.

Repair by infarct exclusion

Athough emergent operative treatment for VSR provided an improvement over the nonoperative management of these patients, mortality rates remained high, exceeding 30 percent in nearly all large series.[301,333,346] The recognition of the importance of LV geometry to appropriate LV function led to a desire to avoid resection of infarcted myocardium as much as possible. This is especially important because patients with higher shunt flow, and therefore better ventricular function, have improved survival rates after VSR repair.[346] David and colleagues[347] and others[348–351] developed the technique of infarct exclusion to exclude the defect and infarcted myocardium from the high-pressure LV system without resection of regions of myocardium, thus preserving normal left ventricular function as much as possible.

As with the techniques discussed above, bicaval cannulation is performed and antegrade and retrograde cardioplegia is given. Occluded coronaries are bypassed before the venticulotomy is begun. For anterior septal defects, an incision is made in the apex of the LV and extended toward the base of the heart approximately 1 cm lateral to the left anterior descending coronary artery through the ventriculotomy. Stay sutures are placed into the ventricular wall to provide exposure, and the endocardial surface is examined. A glutaraldehyde-fixed pericardial patch is cut to fit over the entire extent of infarcted myocardium (in most patients this is approximately 4 by 6 cm[347]). Starting at the lowest and most proximal part of the septum, the patch is secured to healthy myocardium with 3-0 polypropylene sutures in a running fashion (Fig. 29-20). Another suture starting at the same point secures the opposite side of the patch to the noninfarcted portions of the anterolateral LV wall. When the two suture lines meet, the sutures are tied to each other, and the infarcted myocardium becomes excluded from the left ventricle. Closure of the ventriculotomy then proceeds with a buttressed repair of horizontal mattress stitches.

If the infarction extends into the base of the anterior PM, it may not be able to exclude the infarct completely from the LV cavity. In this case, the suture line is brought through the myocardium and buttressed on the epicardial surface with Teflon or pericardial strips. Other authors recommend passing all sutures through to the epicardial surface; in the region of the defect, the suture is passed through the septum and then through the right ventricular free wall to allow buttressing at the epicardial surface.[348]

Repair of a posterior VSR is performed with a similar goal—exclusion of the infarct region from the left ventricular cavity—although as with patch repairs, the proximity of the papillary muscles increases the difficulty of these repairs. The initial incision is made through the posterior wall of the left ventricle, 1 to 2 cm lateral to the PDA, and extended to within 1 cm of the mitral annulus. The incision also is extended toward the apex and the base of the posterior PM. Stay sutures are secured to the ventricular wall; in particular, a suture securing the apex of the heart in the direction of the upper part of the sternotomy facilitates adequate exposure.[352]

The posterior patch is cut in the shape of a triangle to encompass all of the infarct (usually approximately 4 by 7 cm). The base of this triangular patch is secured to the fibrous annulus of the mitral valve, beginning at the middle of the posterior leaflet and extending toward the medial commissure until healthy septal myocardium is reached. The patch is trimmed as needed and sutured to healthy endocardium, using a continuous 3-0 polypropylene suture extending toward the apex of the heart. Finally, the medial side of the patch is sutured to the posterior wall of the left ventricle, using interrupted full-thickness bites buttressed on the epicardial side with a Teflon strip. This excludes the infarct zone from the left ventricular cavity, and the ventriculotomy is closed with buttressed interrupted sutures.

A recent modification of infarct-exclusion included the use of a double-patch technique in which the VSR is closed with a small pericardial patch before insertion of the infarct-excluding patch.[342,353] The inter-"patch" space then is filled with glue. The theoretical advantages of this technique include a more physiologic reconstruction of the interventricular septum, avoidance of contact between tissue adhesive and the systemic circulation, and decreased tension on the infarct-excluding suture lines.[342]

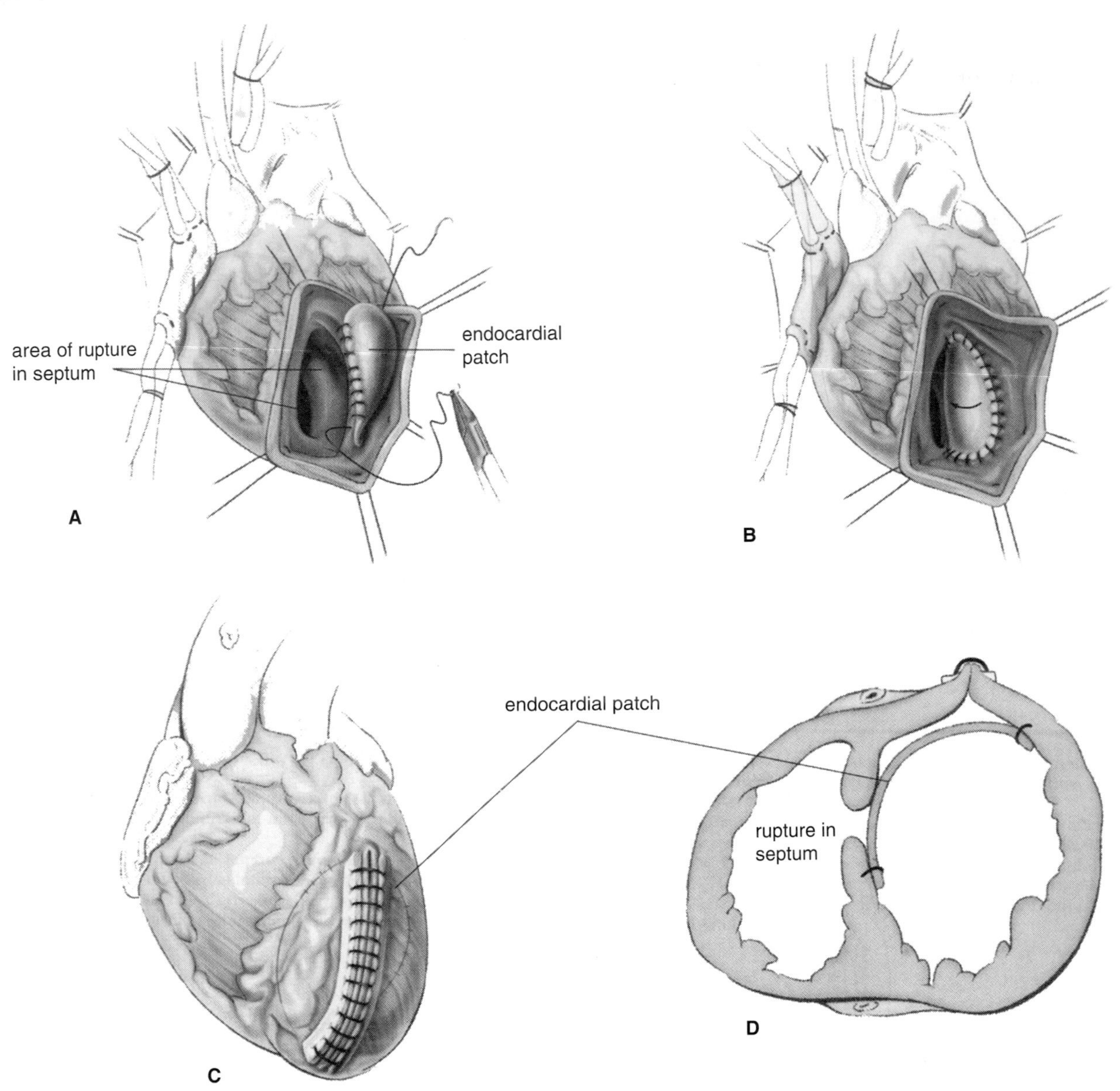

Figure 29-20 Repair of an anterior septal rupture with an endocardial patch and infarct exclusion. An oval pericardial patch is sutured to the septum and lateral wall to exclude the infarcted muscle from the left ventricular cavity. [Adapted from Figure 22.15 in Buxton BF, Frazier OH, Westaby S (eds). *Ischemic Heart Disease Surgical Management.* Philadelphia: Mosby; 1999.]

Whether these benefits are worth the extra time required for placement remains to be established.

Concomitant coronary artery bypass

Reports of coronary artery bypass during repair of VSR describe conflicting results. The disadvantages of concomitant CABG include risk of preoperative left heart catheterization in hemodynamically compromised patients and the prolonged operative and cardiopulmonary bypass times. Although some authors have reported decompensation among approximately 5 percent of patients undergoing angiography,[354] more recent reports suggest that preoperative angiography is not associated with adverse changes in hemodynamics or clinical status.[336,355] Other authors question the value of angiography in the setting of VSR. Although in many series most patients have single-vessel disease,[354,356,357] this is not universally true,[336] and even when it is, as many as 45 percent of patients have multivessel disease. Even patients with anterior infarction and without a previous history of ischemic heart disease do not *invariably* have single-vessel disease.[336] Thus, routine angiography in this population appears to carry little additional risk and may provide useful information; in addition, it allows guided placement of an IABP for hemodynamic stabilization.

Independent of the risk of angiography, some authors question the utility of coronary revascularization in this population. The data in this respect are not clear; however, although many studies have not shown a survival advantage among patients undergoing concomitant CABG, they also have not shown a detrimental effect of CABG despite longer operative and bypass times.[356,358] Other studies have shown improvements in middle- and long-term survival with concomitant CABG.[336, 359] Data do not demonstrate a definitive survival advantage, but no disadvantage to preoperative angiography and concomitant CABG has been demonstrated. The authors recommend routine angiography and bypass of severe proximal stenoses in these patients.

Percutaneous closure of septal rupture

Because of the poor clinical status of patients with VSR, percutaneous closure of the defect offers notable advantages in that it does not require operation and cardiopulmonary bypass and does not have the potential for dehiscence of the ventriculotomy closure that results in rupture. Several case reports have described the successful use of the Amplatzer atrial septal closure device in residual defects after surgical repair.[360–365] The use of percutaneous devices in the acute postinfarct period has been less successful, and all survivors who had not had previous surgeries had transcatheter closure remote from their infarcts.[365,366] It is likely that the soft, friable edges of the defect do not provide an adequate anchor for the device, leading to residual shunting and hemodynamic deterioration. Further refinements in techniques are necessary before percutaneous closure of VSR becomes routine, although its use in closure of residual postsurgical defects appears warranted.

Ventricular assist devices

The use of VADs for hemodynamic support in these patients as a bridge to transplantation is challenging. It may be difficult to secure the cannulas to the postischemic necrotic heart. There are case reports of VAD placement as early as 7 days after MI for postrepair residual defects.[367] However, the use of VADs in the provision of hemodynamic support for patients with an unrepaired VSR has been less successful. One concern particular to patients with VSR is an increase in right-to-left shunting that results in hypoxia and cerebral hypoperfusion.[368] VADs also may be helpful as a bridge to recovery in patients who cannot be weaned from cardiopulmonary bypass. Biventricular support may be required both in patients with right ventricular infarction and in those with residual defect (to prevent an increase in right-to-left shunting).

OUTCOMES AND PROGNOSIS

Postoperative mortality

Several large series have examined outcomes in surgery for VSR. In-hospital and 30-day mortality rates are between 20 percent and 50 percent even in recent series.[301,320,333,336,346,347,355,356,358,369–373] Preoperative characteristics significantly affect the risk of negative outcomes after surgery. The most important predictor of postoperative survival remains preoperative hemodynamic status.[336,347,355,356,372,373] Although measured in a variety of ways (including the presence of cardiogenic shock,[347,356,372,373] the need for inotropic support,[336,355] and the presence of renal failure[347]), increased mortality invariably is seen in patients with poor preoperative cardiac function. Other variables that affect early postoperative survival include posterior infarct location,[370,372] total occlusion of the infarct-related artery,[336] and right ventricular infarction[355] or failure.[347] The poor prognosis of patients with posterior infarcts and VSRs has been attributed to the coexistence of MR in those patients, the increased technical difficulty of repair, and the associated RV infarction.[332,358,374,375] Older age, particularly in patients with poor preoperative clinical status, predicts poor outcomes in some studies,[313,332] but this has been a variable finding.

Impact of operative technique

Mortality rates vary widely among reported series. Other groups have had difficulty replicating the outcomes of the Toronto group with infarct-exclusion. In their experience, no deaths occurred in patients without cardiogenic shock, and overall mortality was only 14 percent.[347] Unfortunately, others have had mortality rates ranging from 30 to 60 percent with similar repairs.[313,376] Similarly, the publication by Skillington before the development of infarct-exclusion reported an overall early mortality rate of only 20.8 percent (mortality in the 2 years immediately before the report had declined to 11.1 percent)[377]; other groups using similar techniques have been unable to duplicate those excellent results.

In light of the small samples in even the largest retrospective studies, changes in practice over time that make any single series unlikely to contain a single operative repair, a wide variety in referral patterns, differences in criteria for operative candidates, and the timing of operation, comparison between series is of little value. These rather than other factors probably explain differences in outcomes even when similar repairs are used.

Causes of early mortality

In most series approximately 5 to 10 percent of patients cannot be weaned from cardiopulmonary support in the operating room.[347,356,370,373] Progressive cardiac failure with a low-output state is the most common cause of postoperative death (50 percent of early mortality), and some degree of failure is present in nearly all patients during the postoperative period.[320,355,356,370] Other causes of death include postoperative free wall rupture, recurrent VSR, severe mitral regurgitation, bleeding, sepsis, cardiac arrest, respiratory failure, and multiple organ system failure (each accounts for 5 to 10 percent of mortality, depending on the series).[355,356,370,373,378] The type of repair performed does not appear to affect the relative frequencies of these causes of postoperative mortality.

Other complications

In most series, recurrence of the VSR occurs in approximately 20 to 30 percent of patients,[320,336,356,373] although the Toronto series of infarct-exclusion contains only a single recurrence with a small residual shunt in 44 cases.[347] The range of recurrence depends on the modality used to detect it. Close echocardiographic follow-up may detect recurrence in nearly 50 percent of patients, but most of these events are not clinically significant and may not influence survival.[356] Patients with small residual defects who are hemodynamically stable may be managed conservatively. In the large series reported by Deja and associates, 14 patients out of the 44 with echocardiographically detected shunts required reoperation.[356] Mortality in patients with clinically significant recurrence approaches 10 percent.[356,377] The double-patch technique has been reported to decrease the recurrence rate in some series,[355] but as with mortality, comparisons between series have little value and further experience with this technique is required. As was noted above, some patients may benefit from percutaneous closure of recurrent or residual defects.[360–365] Mitral regurgitation occurs in approximately 2 percent of patients.[356] Other complications are those common to all emergent cardiac surgery, including sternal dehiscence (2 percent), reoperation for bleeding (6 percent), renal failure requiring hemodialysis (25 percent), arrhythmias requiring temporary (27 percent) or permanent pacemakers (1 percent), and stroke (5 percent).[356]

Late results

Although operative mortality and 30-day mortality are high, hospital survivors have excellent long-term outcomes, especially when their baseline medical status is accounted for (Fig. 29-21[356]). Overall 5-year survival has been approximately 50 to 60 percent in recent series.[336,355,356] However, among hospital survivors, 2-, 5-, and 8-year survival of 85 percent, 63 percent, and 61 percent has been reported.[355] Functional status is also impressive: The majority of long-term survivors (70 to 95 percent) are in NYHA class I or II.[347,355] Late results of earlier repairs are equally impressive: Davies and coworkers reported 37 percent survival at 14 years. with 82 percent of the survivors in NYHA class I or II.[379]

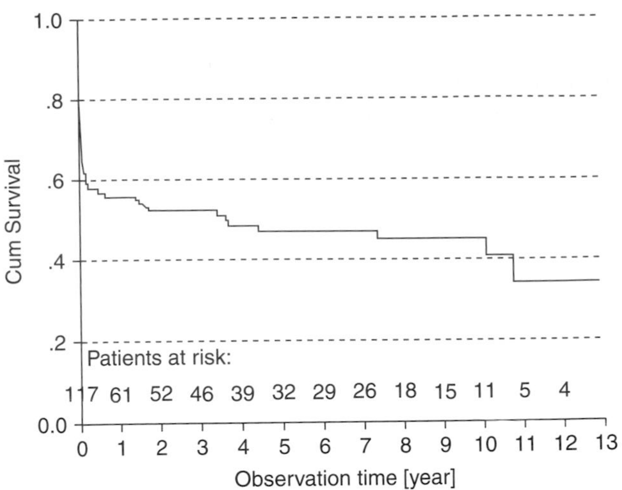

Figure 29-21 Kaplan-Meier survival curve illustrating long-term survival after surgical treatment of ventricular septal rupture. [From Deja MA, Szostek J, Widenka K, et al. Post infarction ventricular septal defect—can we do better? *Eur J Cardiothorac Surg* 2000;18(2):194–201. Permission pending.]

SUMMARY

Ventricular septal rupture occurs in the week after a large MI that results in a necrotic and weakened portion of the ventricular septum. The patients at highest risk are those who angiographically have single-vessel coronary disease without significant collateralization. Clinically, patients present with recurrence of chest pain, and a new harsh pansystolic murmur may be audible. Medical therapy should be used to stabilize the patient and allow for the performance of a diagnostic workup that includes an echocardiogram. Placement of an IABP improves outcomes through reduction in afterload and improvement in shunt dynamics. Although some patients with small, well-tolerated shunts may be managed conservatively, most patients should undergo urgent operative repair. Multiple repairs have been advocated; postoperative mortality ranges from 20 to 50 percent, and comparisons between repairs have not been useful.

VENTRICULAR FREE WALL RUPTURE

INTRODUCTION

William Harvey first described ventricular free wall rupture (VFWR) in 1647. Subsequent authors, including Morgagni,[380] Malmsten and Duben,[381] Winsor,[382] Steven,[383] and Krumbhaar and Crowell,[384] further refined the understanding of cardiac rupture, including its relation to coronary occlusive disease, weakening of the myocardium, and recent MI. Despite this early

KEY CONCEPTS

- Epidemiology
  - In autopsy series, 30 percent of MI accompanied by ventricular free wall rupture (VFWR).
  - One to 4 percent incidence among patients surviving to hospital admission.
  - Accounts for 6 to 17 percent of in-hospital mortality (second leading cause of death).
- Pathophysiology
  - Occurs after large, transmural MI in myocardium without collaterals.
  - Process of infarct expansion results in period of myocardial weakness at approximately 1 to 4 days.
  - If increased wall tension overcomes the tensile strength of the weakened wall, rupture results.
- Clinical Features
  - Eighty percent of ruptures occur within 7 days after infarct.
  - Acute rupture leads to immediate cardiovascular collapse and death due to pencardial tamponade and pulseless electrical activity (PEA)
  - Subacute rupture results in pericardial effusion and hypotension without pulseless electrical activity and cardiac arrest.
    - Signs and symptoms include marked juguler venous distention, pulsus paradoxus, transient electromechanical dissociation (EMD), arrythmias, chest pain, hypotension, and shock.
  - Pseudoaneurysm formaton occurs approximately 3 months after MI with variable symptomatology.
- Diagnostics
  - Rapid pericardiocentesis is both diagnostic and therapeutic.
  - Echocardiography identifies effusion with pericardial clots; Doppler evaluation may identify rupture site.
  - MRI may be useful in evaluating pseudoaneurysms.
- Treatment
  - Medical
    - Optimization of hemodynamic status.
    - Pericardiocentesis.
  - Surgical
    - Subacute rupture
      - Path closure with biological glue or sutures most commonly performed.
      - Glue allows closure without the use of cardiopulmonary bypass.
      - Importance of concomitant CABG not clear.
    - Pseudoaneurysm
      - Repair primarily by closure of neck or patch repair similar to true aneurysms.
- Outcomes and Prognosis
  - Operative survival ~75 percent with onlay patch technique.
  - Similar operative survival for those with pseudoaneurysms.

description, the first successful operation was not performed until 1970. In that year, Hatcher and colleagues[385] reported successful repair of a right VFWR; this was followed shortly by successful left ventricular repairs reported by FitzGibbon and associates[386] and Montegut.[387] However, despite improvements in cardiac care, survival after VFWR remains dismal. Although an uncommon complication of MI, it is the second leading cause of in-hospital death after cardiogenic shock.[388,389]

PATHOPHYSIOLOGY

Left VFWR commonly occurs on the anterior or lateral wall of the ventricle at the midpapillary level.[390,391] The endocardial tear is within 1 cm of the base of one of the papillary muscles in 80 percent of cases.[390] Increased mechanical stress in this location probably results from the countering forces of systolic contraction and PM stretch. Rupture usually occurs at the boundary between viable and necrotic myocardium.[391] Most of these patients have multivessel coronary artery disease with complete occlusion or inadequate revascularization of a major coronary vessel.[392] Collateral circulation is usually absent.

Pathologically, Perdigao and associates[393] described four types of rupture:

Type I: almost direct trajectory without extensive dissection or bloody infiltration of the myocardium
Type II: multicanalicular trajectory and widespread myocardial dissection and bloody infiltration
Type III: orifice of rupture protected by intraventricular thrombus or pericardial adhesions
Type IV: incomplete epicardial, endocardial, or intramyocardial rupture in which the trajectory does not penetrate all layers

However, the division by Becker and van Mantgem[394] of rupture into three types may be more useful clinically:

Type I: an abrupt slitlike tear
Type II: erosion of the infarcted myocardium at the border with viable muscle tissue
Type III: early aneurysm formation

These types correspond with the clinical division of ventricular rupture into acute, subacute, or chronic with pseudoaneurysm formation. Acute rupture occurs with sudden massive hemorrhage into the pericardial space and leads to circulatory collapse and death, often within minutes. Subacute rupture, a term first used by O'Rourke,[395] occurs after a smaller tear in the myocardium that may be sealed temporarily with thrombus or adhesions (Perdigao type III). Finally, chronic rupture occurs when blood leaks slowly from the ventricle. In this case, pericardial adhesions form and contain the rupture, resulting in a false aneurysm. The different time courses of these entities may be affected by infarction location, as fatal cardiac ruptures tend to occur in the anterior and lateral walls, whereas pseudoaneurysm formation is more likely in the inferoposterior walls.[396] The pathogenesis of VFWR is not completely understood. However, increasing knowledge about myocardial repair after infarction provides some insights. After infarction, remodeling begins initially with leukocyte infiltration and clearance of necrotic debris; this leads to a process termed infarct expansion. Clearance of necrotic debris leads to regional thinning and dilatation of the infarcted region of myocardium.[397] Thinning leads to a reduction in the number of myocytes crossing the infarct zone and a corresponding decrease in the tensile strength of the ventricular wall. Dilatation causes increased wall tension (Laplace effect). Thus, infarct expansion results in a period of myocardial weakness (usually 1 to 4 days post-MI) when the myocardium becomes particularly susceptible to rupture. The importance of remodeling to the pathogenesis of rupture is demonstrated by reduced rupture rates in animal models with inhibition of the plasminogen/matric metalloproteinase system that is responsible for ventricular remodeling.[398,399] This period of weakness may be required for eventual scar tissue formation, as these mice also have poor long-term angiogenesis and scar formation in the infarct region.[398,399]

CLINICAL FEATURES

Acute and subacute rupture

The incidence of VFWR peaks during the first week after MI. Autopsy studies suggest that 80 percent of ruptures occur within 7 days of MI,[391] and most acute rupture events occur within 48 h of admission.[400] In large retrospective studies, acute VFWR resulted in death a median of approximately 3 days after the onset of symptoms of MI.[388] Risk factors for VFWR include older age (usually more than 60 years),[391,401] female sex,[317,391,401–404] a history of systemic hypertension[391] without left ventricular hypertrophy[391] or sustained hypertension during admission,[317] the presence of a pericardial rub or pericardial effusion,[401,405] sustained chest pain,[317,403] and the absence of previous MI or angina.[391,403]

The overall incidence after MI varies in reported series, as many patients are unlikely to be identified in clinical series because of prehospital death. In autopsy series, as many as 30 percent of MIs may be accompanied by VFWR.[402] In contrast, much lower rates (1 to 4 percent) are reported among patients surviving to hospital admission for MI.[317,388,389,403,406–409] However, even in these series, it accounts for 6 to 17 percent of in-hospital mortality.[388,403]

Acute rupture is characterized by the sudden onset of chest pain with rapid cardiovascular collapse and pulseless electrical activity caused by pericardial tamponade. These are accompanied by severe jugular venous distention with cyanosis. Death nearly invariably occurs within minutes.[410]

The distinction between these patients and those with subacute rupture has not been defined clearly, but in general, patients with subacute rupture are those in whom pericardial effusion and hypotension of variable severity are not accompanied by pulseless electrical activity and cardiac arrest.[395,411] This subacute form of VFWR occurs in approximately 30 percent of in-patient ruptures,[403,412,413] and early recognition may allow operative repair and increase survival. In this group, the gradual onset of symptoms of pericardial tamponade may be appreciated before the onset of cardiovascular collapse; however, marked jugular venous distention and pulsus paradoxus have been found in only approximately 30 percent[414] and 50 percent[411,415] of patients, respectively. A variety of other signs and symptoms may be present in these patients: arrhythmias (including transient pulseless electrical activity, bradycardias, tachycardias and ventricular fibrillation, syncope, hypotension, shock, and chest pain, which may be transient, prolonged, or recurrent.[395,411,414–418] The sensitivity and specificity of these signs vary (Table 29-8[415]). Particularly in diabetic patients, VFWR may present with sudden collapse from pericardial tamponade even in the absence of antecedent chest pain.[419] Sudden onset of cardiogenic shock in the post-MI period should prompt rapid echocardiographic evaluation to differentiate infarct extension from the various mechanical causes: mitral regurgitation, VSR, and VFWR. Especially in cases of right heart failure or when there are signs and symptoms of pericardial tamponade, rapid diagnostic pericardiocentesis may be indicated.

Chronic rupture with pseudoaneurysm

Chronic VFWR with false aneurysm formation is a rare entity that usually develops within 3 months of MI.[420] Traditionally, this was thought to carry a high rupture risk, and immediate operative therapy was recommended.[421–423] However, in a review of 52 patients, Yeo and associates found no deaths caused by cardiac rupture in the 6 patients with post-MI pseudoaneurysm who were managed medically.[396] In another series, 1-year mortality among nine patients who were managed medically was only 22 percent and no patients had rupture of the pseudoaneurysm.[424] Similar results were obtained in a review by Natarajan and colleagues of the 66 cases reported in the literature.[425] Unfortunately, because of its rarity, the natural history of chronic VFWR with pseudoaneurysm formation has not been defined clearly; the increasing use of echocardiography after MI may allow for the earlier diagnosis of more patients with this disease and allow for better evaluation of the need for operative therapy.

Impact of reperfusion therapy

Reperfusion, whether spontaneous or induced, reduces infarct expansion and decreases infarct size.[253,262,426,427]

Table 29-8 **Sensitivity, specificity, and positive predictive value of different variables used alone or in combination for diagnosing a postinfarction ventricular free wall rupture**

	Sensitivity, %	Specificity, %	Positive predictive value, %
Infarct site			
Anterior	25	70	3.9
Inferior	68	54	6.7
Lateral	7.1	90	3.3
Prior myocardial infarction	3.5	75	0.6
Bundle branch block	32	74	5.7
Pulsus paradoxus	46	99	72
ST-T-wave deviations	32	85	10
Syncope	64	91	26
Hemodynamic signs of cardiac tamponade (CT_H)[a]	85	99	0.9
Pericardial effusion (PE)	100	77	17
Intrapericardial echoes (IE)[b]	93	99	81
Echocardiographic signs of cardiac tamponade (CT_E)[c]	93	99	93
Combinations of signs			
Hemopericardium (Hp)[d]	21	99	85
PE + type I IE	7.1	99	28
Syncope or shock + PE + type II IE + CT_{E+H}	53	100	100
Syncope or shock + PE + type I IE + CT_{E+H}	32	100	100
Syncope or shock + PE + Hp + CT_{E+H}	7.1	100	100

[a] Hemodynamic signs of cardiac tamponade were the presence of an increase in right atrial pressure and characteristic profile of right atrial pressure waveform (depressed *x* descent and blunted *y* descent).

[b] Intrapericardial echoes could be of two types: type I, a wide, thick undulating band overlying the heart suspended in a moderate to large pericardial effusion, and type II, a massive, homogeneous, and immobile structure impinging on adjacent cardiac chambers.

[c] Echocardiographic evidence of cardiac tamponade was present when right atrial diastolic and/or right ventricular early diastolic collapse was associated with either or both of the following findings: Doppler ultrasound findings of exaggerated tricuspid and pulmonic flow velocities and reduction of peak mitral flow velocity with the onset of inspiration and the opposite changes after the onset of expiration or inferior vena caval plethora with blunted respiratory variation.

[d] Pericardial fluid with hematocrit < 25.

CT_H = hemodynamic evidence of cardiac tamponade; CT_E = echocardiographic evidence of cardiac tamponade; IE = intrapericardial echoes; Hp = hemopericardium; CT_{E+H} = echocardiographic and hemodynamic evidence of cardiac tamponade; PE = pericardial effusion.

This would be expected to reduce the incidence of VFWR; however, in the case of thrombolysis, there has been concern that the transformation of bland infarcts into hemorrhagic infarcts may increase the risk of rupture.[428–430] In a metanalysis of four studies, Honan and associates demonstrated a reduction in the risk of rupture when thrombolysis occurred within 7 h but an increased risk after late thrombolysis (after 17 h).[431] Becker and colleagues studied 5711 patients, and although patients who did have a rupture incurred it earlier (between 6 and 12 h), overall there was no difference in the incidence of rupture when thrombolysis occurred between 6 and 24 h.[389] Thus, early thrombolysis appears to have a beneficial effect by limiting infarct size and related necrosis and minimizing regions of transmurality.

In contrast, outcomes after percutaneous revascularization have been uniformly positive.[389,432,433] Comparing 762 patients undergoing angioplasty with 613 receiving thrombolysis, Moreno and associates showed a significant reduction in the incidence of cardiac rupture (odds ratio 0.46, 95 percent CI 0.22 to 0.96).[434] Importantly, increasing time to reperfusion is an independent risk factor for cardiac rupture, reinforcing the importance of timely delivery to the catheterization laboratory.[410] The superiority of percutaneous interventions probably results from improved perfusion without the hemorrhagic or fibrinolytic side effects of thrombolysis.[435]

DIAGNOSTIC MODALITIES

A high index of suspicion in cases of arrhythmias before cardiogenic shock or the sudden onset of shock or severe chest pain is essential to initiating the diagnostic workup of and initial therapy for VFWR.

Electrocardiography, clinical evaluation, and right heart catheterization

Oliva and associates evaluated 70 patients with cardiac rupture and found that patients with rupture were more likely to have persistent, progressive, or recurrent ST elevation (61 percent) than were those with MI without rupture (22 percent, $p \leq 0.002$).[436] Failure of the T wave to invert or reversal of an inverted T wave was also more common among the group with rupture (94 percent versus 34 percent, $p \leq 0.02$).[436] Unfortunately, because rupture is a rare event, the positive predictive value of these ECG signs was only 58 percent and 66 percent, respectively.[436] The best predictors of rupture were clinical symptoms such as pericarditis, repetitive emesis, and restlessness or agitation; when two or more symptoms were present, the positive predictive value for rupture was 95 percent.[436] Other criteria for predicting rupture have been proposed: tachycardia greater than 100 beats per minute with ST-segment elevation equal to or greater than 0.1 mV in lead V_5 (for inferior MI) or lead II (for anterior MI),[437] generalized ST-segment elevation (odds ratio for rupture 9.2),[300] and ST elevation in aVL (odds ratio for rupture 5.4).[438] Unfortunately, because of the relative rarity of cardiac rupture, the positive predictive value of all these criteria tends to be minimal.

Classically, the pericardial tamponade of VFWR should lead to equalization of pressures across the cardiac chambers. Pulmonary artery catheter pressures usually demonstrate evidence of right heart failure: elevated right atrial pressures, the possibility of equalization of right atrial and pulmonary capillary wedge pressures (although pericardial clot may prevent the expected equalization of pressures[439]), and alterations in the right atrial pressure waveform (deep *x* descent and blunted *y* descent).[435] Any of these changes should prompt rapid echocardiography to rule out pericardial tamponade and rupture.

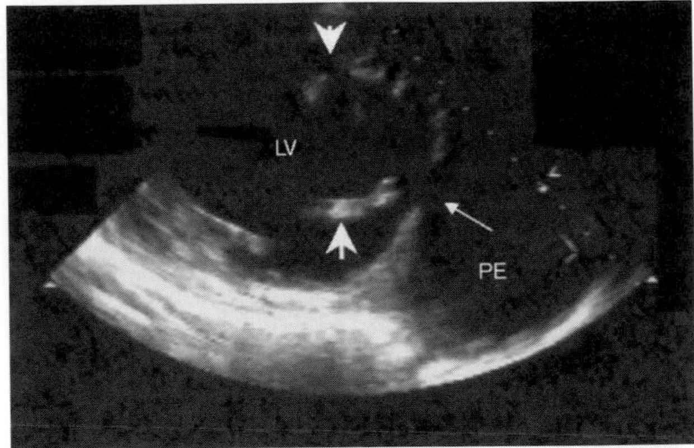

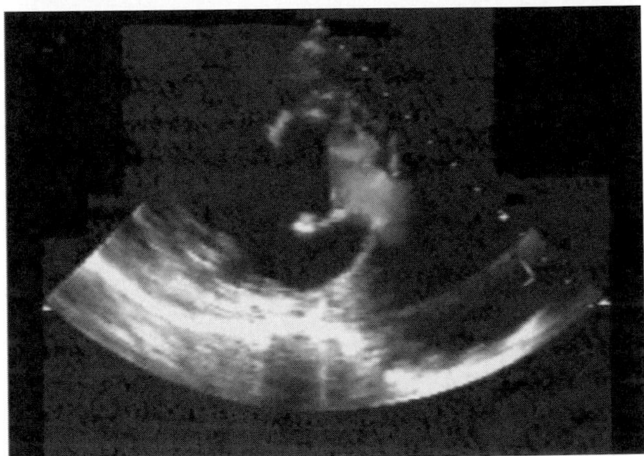

Figure 29-22 Transesophageal two-dimensional (**A**) and Doppler (**B**) echocardiography illustrating ventricular free wall rupture (*white arrow*) into the pericardium from the left ventricle. White arrowheads mark the papillary muscles. Doppler imaging shows flow into the pericardium. PE = pericardial effusion; LV = left ventricle. [From Birnbaum Y, Chamoun AJ, Anzuini A, et al. Ventricular free wall rupture following acute myocardial infarction. *Coron Artery Dis* 2003;14(6):463–470. Permission pending.]

Echocardiography

Echocardiography is the diagnostic study of choice in patients with suspected VFWR. It is noninvasive, safe, easy to perform even at the bedside, and widely available. However, it does have limitations. As many as one-third of patients without rupture will develop pericardial effusions after MI,[440] and so the positive predictive value of pericardial effusion alone is relatively low (27.5 percent).[411] However, the absence of pericardial effusion virtually excludes VFWR as a possibility (Fig. 29-22A).[411] The presence of intrapericardial echoes consistent with blod clots increases the sensitivity and specificity for VFWR, but the positive predictive value is still only 70 percent, as those findings also may occur after infarction fibrinous endocarditis.[411,441] Echocardiography is also useful in ruling out other mechanical causes of acute hemodynamic collapse after MI, including papillary muscle or ventricular septal rupture.

The addition of Doppler measurements and contrast agents has increased opportunities to identify the site of ventricular wall rupture (Fig. 29-22B). Doppler may demonstrate flow from the ventricle into the pericardial sac (although as tamponade progresses, this becomes less evident). Contrast agents (such as air bubbles) may be seen in the pericardial space.[442]

Angiography

In the case of subacute rupture, few data support the use of preoperative angiography. Few long-term survivors undergo concomitant coronary procedures,[443,444] and many angiograms demonstrate normal coronaries other than the infarct-related artery.[445] Transfer to the operating room should not be delayed by cardiac catheterization, as outcomes depend on operative repair of the rupture rather than on concomitant coronary procedures.

Magnetic resonance imaging

Currently, magnetic resonance imaging (MRI) has little use in the setting of acute MI or subacute rupture because it is time-consuming and patients become relatively inaccessible inside the scanner. However, MRI is used with increasing frequency in the evaluation of pseudoaneurysms (Fig. 29-20). Its advantages include high resolution and image quality as well as excellent anatomic definition made possible by three-dimensional (3-D) reconstruction techniques.[446–448]

MEDICAL THERAPY

Acute or subacute rupture

Once the diagnosis of VFWR has been made, medical management is directed toward hemodynamic stabilization. Initial therapies include aggressive intravenous (IV) fluid resuscitation and blood products as needed.[449] After initial stabilization, bed rest and beta blockade with maintenance of systolic blood pressure (SBP) between 100 and 120 may be helpful.[449] There are reports of long-term survivors without surgical repair, but those reports are rare.[449–451]

Percutaneous treament

Pericardiocentesis is both diagnostic and therapeutic. It usually is performed with echocardiographic guidance. When pericardiocentesis demonstrates a serous pericardial effusion, rupture is excluded.[411] Therapeutically, pericardiocentesis decompresses the pericardium and decreases the threat of tamponade.[449] Despite this benefit, tamponade often recurs and proper drainage may be prevented by blood clots in the drainage catheter.[415,449] IABP placement may stabilize patients through improvements in both systemic and myocardial perfusion.[452] Murata and associates[453] described a novel technique for nonoperative management of VFWR. In two cases, injection of fibrin-glue into the pericardial space successfully stabilized patients, with resolution of pericardial effusion. Long-term follow-up of one patient treated with this technique revealed no restriction of LV motion.[454] Further experience with glue-based techniques will define the appropriate indications for such interventions, but it may be particularly applicable in patients with acute rupture, who previously would not have survived operative repair.

Chronic rupture with pseudoaneurysm

Traditionally, the risk of rupture led most patients with pseudoaneurysm to the operating room soon after diagnosis. However, increasing numbers of reports have described conservative management of some patients.[396,424,425] Unfortunately, no specific medical therapy has been recommended for those patients, although in light of a high incidence of stroke in the reported cases, some authors have recommended anticoagulation.[455]

SURGICAL THERAPY

Acute or subacute rupture

In patients with acute or subacute rupture, immediate operative repair is indicated. Anesthetic induction in patients with cardiac tamponade may lead to sudden cardiovascular collapse as a result of peripheral vasodilatation. The patient should be prepared and draped before anesthetic induction. When necessary, mechanical cardiopulmonary support may be initiated via femoral cannulation before induction.[456,457] After induction, the chest and pericardium are opened rapidly, relieving the tamponade. The site of rupture is identified rapidly, although in most cases the tear is sealed with clot and active bleeding will not be seen.

Several surgical approaches to the repair of left ventricular free wall rupture (LVFWR) have been advocated, including infarctectomy and patch closure, simple mattress suturing backed with felt, and an overlay patch sutured or glued into place with or without primary closure of the defect. Although many case reports describe acceptable outcomes with simple closure with pledgeted sutures,[418,458–460] in this repair the sutures are placed into necrotic myocardium; postoperative rupture would be a significant concern. Infarctectomy and patch closure do not have this shortcoming because the friable, infarcted myocardium is resected and sutures are placed into healthy tissue.[461–463] Early reports included simple closure of the defect after infarctectomy[386,445,452,464]; however, this may lead to a significant reduction in LV size and changes in LV geometry, in which case closure with a prosthetic patch is preferred. The disadvantages of this technique include the need for cardiopulmonary bypass and, at least theoretically, changes in LV geometry that may have negative long-term consequences in ventricular function, as has been seen in repair of VSR with infarctectomy.[347]

Nunez and associates were able to avoid the infarctectomy through primary closure of the defect with pledgeted sutures followed by placement of an onlay patch sutured to healthy myocardium (Fig. 29-23).[465] This technique provided good control of ventricular hemorrhage, and those authors reported survival out to 10 months.[465] Others have used similar onlay patches but have chosen not to close the myocardial tear; the patch can be secured with biological glue or sutures.[345,411,444,463,466–473]

With the advent of biological glue, many surgeons have begun to avoid the use of cardiopulmonary bypass in these patients. In posterior ruptures, cardiopulmonary bypass (CPB) often is required, but with anterior

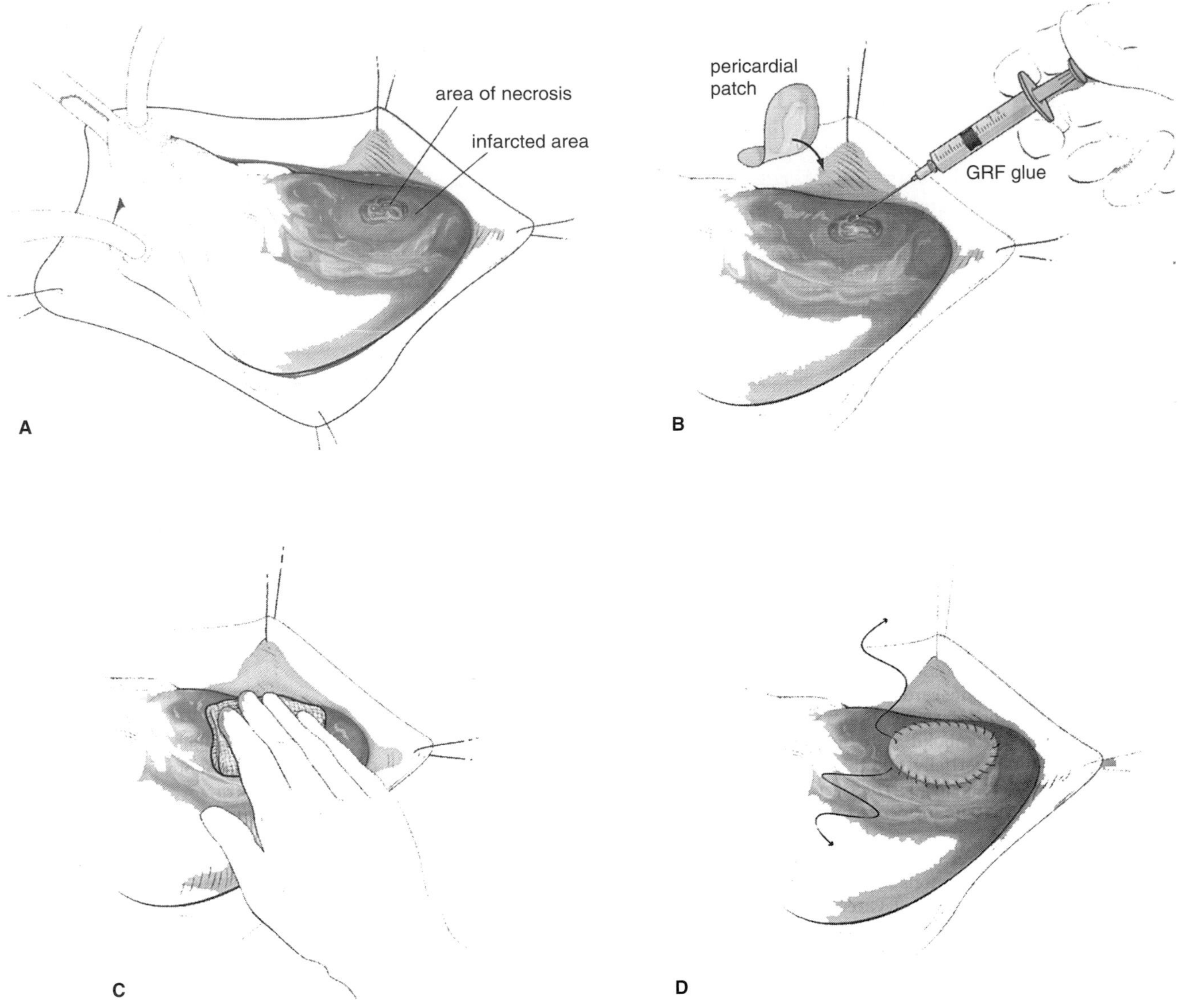

Figure 29-23 Operative technique for onlay patch repair of ventricular free wall rupture. Adapted from Figures 21.1–21.4 in Buxton BF, Frazier OH, Westaby S (eds). *Ischemic Heart Disease Surgical Management.* Philadelphia: Mosby; 1999.]

ruptures, adequate closure can be obtained on the beating heart by using onlay patches secured with glue.[470] In contrast, CPB is required when concomitant cardiac procedures are planned. Opinions about the need to perform CABG during repair of VFWR vary. Because 80 percent of ruptures occur in patients with multivessel coronary disease,[391] some authors advocate initiation of CPB and bypass of all major vessels before repair of the rupture.[458] However, as was noted above, preoperative angiography is not likely to be possible, and most reported long-term survivors have not undergone concomitant bypass procedures.[443–445] The experience with this disease is too limited to make definitive recommendations, and surgeons will have to be guided by the clinical condition of the patient; some authors recommend a "middle ground" of bypassing palpable or clinically evident disease.[435]

Chronic rupture with pseudoaneurysm

As was noted above, the natural history and risk of rupture with pseudoaneurysm are not clearly defined, and the timing of surgery depends on the perceived risk of rupture. In particular, chronic smaller pseudoaneurysms that are stable in terms of size may have a lower propensity for rupture, and patients may do well with conservative management.[396] However, surgical therapy remains the treatment of choice in patients likely to tolerate the operation. Since many patients with chronic pseudoaneurysms will be identified during a workup for coronary artery or mitral valve disease, the decision to operate may be based on the coexistent disease.

Pseudoaneurysms may be repaired with either primary closure of the (usually thin) neck[447,474] or endocardial patch repair[447,475–477] similar to that used in a true LV aneurysm (see below). In the acute setting, the neck may not have sufficient fibrosis to provide an anchor for sutures, and so patch repair is probably a better option. When the myocardial defect is large, patch repair is preferred to minimize changes in LV geometry and relieve tension on the repair.

OUTCOMES

Acute and subacute rupture

The short- and middle-term results of onlay patch operations appear to be excellent. Lopez-Sendon and associates reported the results of 33 operations for ventricular rupture repaired with an onlay patch secured with either glue or sutures; 76 percent of the patients survived the operation, and long-term survival (mean follow-up 30 months) was 48.5 percent.[411] Canovas and associates recently reported middle-term outcomes for 17 patients with glued onlay patches: operative (30-day) mortality was 23.5 percent (4 of 17 patients), with one death resulting from patch failure.[470] Middle-term follow-up revealed only two additional deaths, and echocardiography revealed good ventricular function in the survivors.[470] Others have reported operative survival as high as 100 percent, although patient selection probably played a large role.[444]

Chronic rupture with pseudoaneurysm

Because of its rarity, outcomes after surgical repair of ventricular pseudoaneurysm have been variable. The largest series, examining the 266 cases reported in the literature, found operative mortality of 23 percent; however, medical therapy had a 48 percent mortality rate.[455] Unfortunately, since this was a review of all *reported* cases, publication bias makes these numbers difficult to interpret. Outcomes from ventricular aneurysms may have to be relied on in estimating operative risk in this population.

SUMMARY

Ventricular free wall rupture is a devastating complication of MI; although it occurs uncommonly, it is the second leading cause of in-hospital death after MI. Clinical prediction of patients likely to have rupture is poor; echocardiograms should be obtained when there is any degree of suspicion. When rupture does occur, pericardiocentesis may be both diagnostic and therapeutic and may allow time for operative repair. Survival without operative repair in the setting of acute rupture is uncommon. Operative techniques include closure of the defect with or without an onlay patch. Many authors advocate sutureless repair with biological glue to adhere the patch to the epicardium. The results of onlay patch operations are excellent, with operative mortality of approximately 25 percent and little longer-term mortality. Rarely, patients also may present with chronic rupture and pseudoaneurysm formation. The natural history of this entity is poorly defined, but most authors recommend repair. Techniques include primary closure of the ventricular defect and extensive repairs, as advocated for true ventricular aneurysm (see below)

LEFT VENTRICULAR ANEURYSM

INTRODUCTION

Although earlier reports had described enlargements of other cardiac chambers, the earliest reports of ventricular aneurysms found during autopsy were made by Galeati[478] and Hunter[479] in 1757.[480] Theories about their etiology abounded, but it was not until 1880 to 1900 that many authors independently recognized the correct relationship between coronary thrombosis, MI, ventricular scarring, and aneurysm formation.[480] The surgical correction of postinfarction ventricular aneurysm began with the use of a fascia lata graft by Beck in 1942.[481] Likoff and Bailey[482] reported the first successful aneurysm excision using a Satinsky clamp on a beating heart in 1955; that was followed by the work of Cooley and associates, who in 1958 performed the first modern aneurysm excision using cardiopulmonary bypass.[483] Since that time, repairs have been improved by a series of surgeons who have recognized the importance of normal ventricular geometry to ventricular function.[332,484–488]

Traditionally, LV aneurysm was defined as a region of myocardium exhibiting an abnormal diastolic contour with systolic dyskinesia and paradoxic bulging. However, growing experience with ventricular aneurysm as well as ischemic cardiomyopathy has led to the recognition that even large regions of akinesis without the traditional paradoxic systolic bulging can have deleterious effects on ventricular function (so-called functional aneurysm).[489] Several authors have proposed that any region of myocardial asynergy (akinesia or dyskinesia) large enough to reduce LV function be treated as an LV aneurysm.[490–492]

PATHOPHYSIOLOGY

The formation of LV aneuryms (whether traditional or functional) results from the remodeling process that occurs after transmural MI. This process has been

KEY CONCEPTS

- Epidemiology
  - Incidence depends on exact definition; 10 to 35 percent of patients will develop region of systolic akinesia or dyskinesia after transmural MI.
- Pathophysiology
  - Traditionally ventricular aneurysm is defined as region of myocardium exhibiting abnormal diastolic contour with systolic dyskinesia and paradoxic bulging.
  - Recently clear that even large regions of akinesis may have similar impact on left ventricular function.
  - Ventricular remodeling after large transmural infarct leads to infract expansion and aneurysm formation.
  - Late remodeling involves global LV response to changes in wall stress and strength: chamber dilatation, mural hypertrophy, and changes in LV geometry resulting in poor LV contractile function.
- Clinical Features
  - Commonly presents with congestive heart failure.
  - Other symptoms include angina, dyspnea.
  - Mural thrombus present in 50 percent of patients at surgery.
- Diagnostics
  - Echocardiography identifies valvular disease, differentiates true aneurysms from false.
  - Angiography
    - Gold standard.
    - Estimation of LV aneurysm size and evaluation of coronary anatomy and cardiac function.
- Treatment
  - Medical
    - Aimed at minimizing deleterious effects of LV remodeling ACE inhibitors and beta blockade.
  - Surgical
    - Asymptomatic patients with small aneurysms can be managed medically.
    - Others require operative repair.
    - Multiple techiniques described: plication, linear repair, variety of geometric repairs.
    - Geometric repairs (Dor, Jalene, Cooley) have advantage of restoring LV geometry and preserving long-term LV function.
- Outcomes and Prognosis
  - Operative mortality 2 to 13 percent.
  - Five-year survival from 20 to 42 percent.
  - Survival (short and long trom) probably lower with geometric repairs than with linear repairs.
  - Measurements of LV function improved after repair and improvement are maintained over the long term.

divided arbitrarily into an early phase and a late phase. The early phase (less than 72 h after an infarct) is characterized by infarct expansion that may result in ventricular rupture or ventricular aneurysm.[493] The late phase (more than 72 h) involves global ventricular responses to changes in wall stress and strength, including chamber dilatation, mural hypertrophy, and changes in LV geometry that lead to poor contractile function.[494]

Early remodeling

Early remodeling results primarily from the effects of migration of inflammatory cells into the infarct zone. Necrotic myocytes initiate complement activation and free radical generation, which leads to a cytokine cascade and the migration of neutrophils into the infarct zone.[495] Neutrophil-mediated proteolysis leads to degradation of the intermyocyte collagen struts, resulting in infarct expansion within hours of infarction.[397,496]

The wall thinning and dilatation of infarct expansion lead to elevations in both diastolic and systolic wall stress (LaPlace effect). This causes a further increase in muscle fiber tension. Combined with the greater tendency for infarcted and ischemic myocytes to stretch under a constant load, progressive dilatation results until fibrosis and scarring supervene.[497] Deformation of the border zone and noninfarcted remote myocardium lead to alterations in Starling forces with adaptive changes in ventricular function, including augmented systolic shortening, activation of the sympathetic adrenergic system, and stimulation of natriuretic peptides.[494] When the region of viable myocardium is large enough, these mechanisms result in maintenance of cardiac output and systemic perfusion. However, in the longer term these mechanisms also result in the development of ventricular hypertrophy and higher myocardial oxygen demand in the remainder of the ventricle.

Infarct expansion occurs rapidly after MI. In more than 55 percent of cases, aneurysms are evident within 48 h of MI; the remainder develop within the first 2 weeks.[489] This period forms the vulnerable period in which defects resulting from ventricular wall weakness (including rupture and aneurysm) are most likely to occur because the necrotic myocytes have not been replaced with scar. In cases in which viable, hibernating myocardium is present in the infarct zone, aneurysms seen on initial angiography may resolve over the course of several weeks.[498] Furthermore, reperfusion of the infarct zone may halt the remodeling process and prevent aneurysm formation, as reperfusion has been associated with a lower incidence of ventricular aneurysm.[498,499]

Late remodeling

The late phase of remodeling in the setting of ventricular aneurysm is dominated by the response of the functioning myocardium to the presence of the aneurysm.

During that time, the aneurysm becomes composed primarily of scar tissue. This leads to both systolic and diastolic dysfunction. During systole, the aneurysm fails to contract, leading to reduced ejection fraction and cardiac output. In diastole, the aneurysm wall does not undergo normal distention, resulting in elevated left ventricular diastolic pressure.

The normal myocardium attempts to compensate for these changes primarily with two mechanisms: myocyte hypertrophy and changes in ventricular geometry that attempt to redistribute the wall stress more evenly across the ventricle.[494] Reduction of ventricular wall stress with nitrates between 2 and 8 weeks after an infarct reduces hypertrophy,[500,501] and similar effects as well as decreased ventricular dilatation can be seen with ACE inhibitors.[502–504] Because these compensatory mechanisms may maintain cardiac output and coronary perfusion, ventricular aneurysms may remain asymptomatic for long periods. However, unless the aneurysm is small, progressive dilatation and hypertrophy ultimately result in increasing myocardial oxygen demand with progressive heart failure. The development of heart failure may occur (as it does in aortic regurgitation) with a sudden and profound presentation as the ventricle finally decompensates.[505,506]

CLINICAL FEATURES

The incidence of LV aneurysm depends on the definition and diagnostic techniques used, but approximately 10 to 35 percent of patients develop a region of systolic akinesia or dyskinesia after transmural MI.[480,489,507] Ninety percent of aneurysms occur on the anterior portion of the LV, approximately 25 percent of which occur near the apex.[508–510] Patients with ventricular aneurysm are more likely to have had a previous MI, to have a decreased ejection fraction (less than 50 percent), and to have increased left ventricular end-diastolic pressure (LVEDP) (>21 mmHg) compared with post-MI controls.[507]

Patients with ventricular aneurysm commonly present with CHF. Angina is also a common symptom, occurring in 44 to 98 percent of patients, usually related to obstruction of non-infarct-related arteries as oxygen demand in the dilated LV exceeds oxygen supply.[505,511,512] Other presenting symptoms include dyspnea and other symptoms of CHF as the LV decompensates and can no longer maintain the additional workload required to compensate for the aneurysm. Arrhythmias may occur in the scar tissue, leading to symptoms such as syncope, palpitations, and aggravation of angina or dypnea. Significant ventricular arrhythmias occur in 20 percent of large aneurysms but only 3 percent of smaller ones.[513] Finally, mural thrombus is found in 50 percent of patients undergoing surgery and is especially common in larger aneurysms.[480,505,514] Although this is rare, patients may present with symptoms of embolic disease, including stroke and peripheral arterial occlusion.

DIAGNOSTIC MODALITIES

Historically, electrocardiographic changes (Q waves and persistent ST changes in the anterior leads) and chest roentgenogram findings (LV enlargement and cardiomegaly) have been described in LV aneurysm, as have a variety of physical signs. However, these findings are not specific and play little role in the modern diagnosis of this disease.[480]

Echocardiography

Echocardiography is useful as a noninvasive test for mechanical complications in patients with coronary symptomatology and coronary artery disease. It can identify valvular disease, including mitral regurgitation, that may mimic the vague symptoms of ventricular aneurysm. In addition, it can differentiate true aneurysms from false aneurysms and evaluate for mural thrombus (Fig. 29-24).

Angiography and ventriculography

Although echocardiography has advantages as a test that is noninvasive and easy to perform, ventriculography remains the gold standard for the diagnosis and preoperative evaluation of ventricular aneurysms (Fig. 29-25). In addition to defining cardiac function, it permits determination of coronary anatomy, allowing for optimal operative planning. Di Donato and associates[491] described a method for estimating LV aneurysm size accurately by using the centerline method. Previously, estimates of LV function and aneurysm size were made qualitatively by the cineangiographer. In their study, the extent of asynergy (A percent) was calculated as the percent length of the LV perimeter showing fractional shortening less than 2 standard deviations from the normal mean value. Surgical outcome correlated with A percent rather than with the presence or absence of dyskinetic motion.

Other modalities

Cardiac-gated MRI provides highly accurate delineation of LV geometry and size and can identify mural thrombi. However, it cannot assess coronary anatomy or cardiac function adequately and therefore is not likely to supplant angiography in the near future.

MEDICAL THERAPY

Medical therapy for LV aneurysm consists predominantly of agents directed at minimizing the deleterious aspects of LV remodeling. Nitrates have been shown to reduce myocyte hypertrophy but have not been shown to have a beneficial effect on mortality in clinical trials.[49,515] ACE inhibitors also may inhibit infarct expansion and reduce

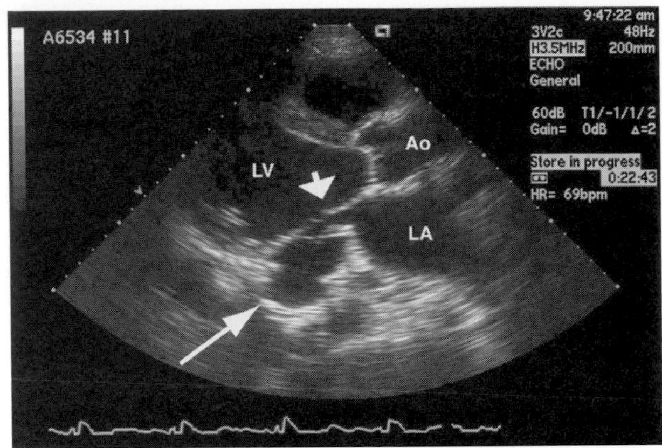

A

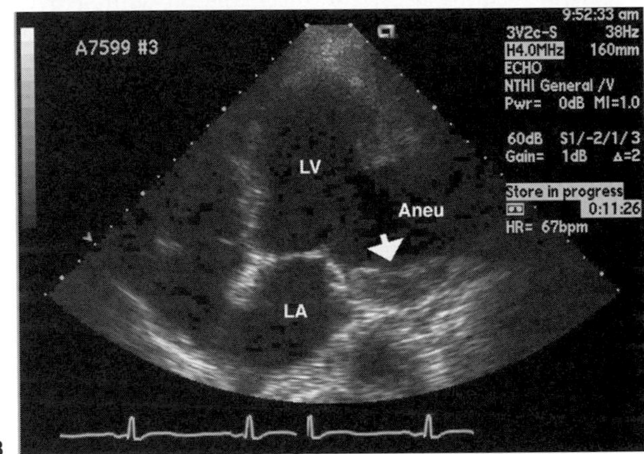

B

Figure 29-24 Two-dimensional echocardiograms. A. Left ventricular pseudoaneurysm (*white arrow*) just inferior to the mitral valve annulus. The ventricular wall continues across the mouth of the pseudoaneurysm (*large white arrowheads*). Small white arrowhead indicates the mitral valve leaflets. B. In contrast, in a true left ventricular aneurysm, the ventricular wall forms the lateral margin of the aneurysm. Mural thrombus (*white arrowhead*) is visible along the aneurysm wall. Ao = aorta; MV = mitral valve; LV = left ventricle; LA = left atrium; PsA = pseudoaneurysm; Aneu = aneurysm.

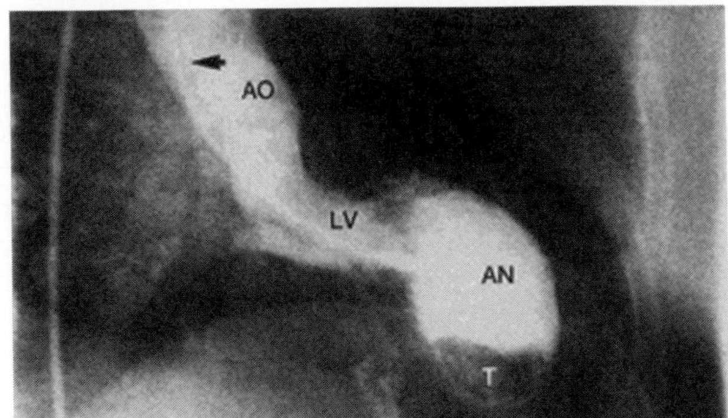

A

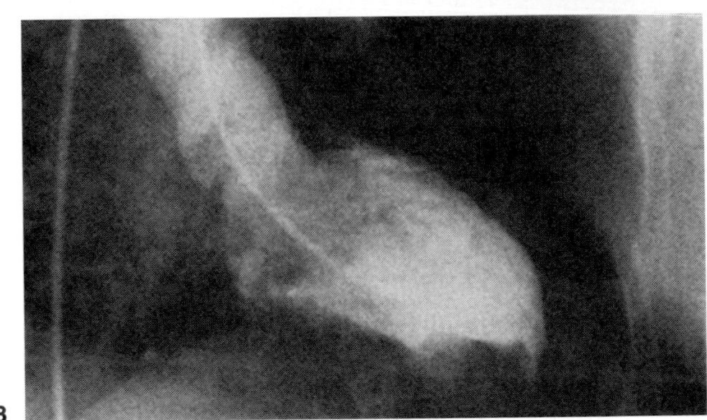

B

Figure 29-25 Angiography of left ventricular aneurysm. The systolic image (A) clearly shows the large region of apical dyskinesia with mural thrombus, whereas the diastolic image (B) appears relatively normal. AN = aneurysm; LV = left ventricle; AO = aorta. [From Patel R, Shenoy MM. Images in clinical medicine: Left ventricular aneurysm. *N Engl J Med* 1993; 329(4):246 Permission pending.]

the incidence of aneurysm. Multiple studies have shown survival benefits in all patients with MI and in those with LV dysfunction.[49,515–517] Although studies have not addressed medical therapy for ventricular aneurysms specifically, standard treatments for LV dysfunction, including beta blockade and ACE inhibitors, should be used as indicated.

SURGICAL THERAPY

Indications for operative repair

Many asymptomatic patients can be managed medically with excellent results. In 18 patients with asymptomatic ventricular aneurysms, Grodin and coworkers noted 90 percent survival at 10 years with a stable clinical course over that time; this contrasts with the 22 symptomatic patients who had 10-year survival below 50 percent.[518] However, the presence of an aneurysm involving more than 25 percent of the LV surface puts a significant strain on the remaining healthy myocardium.[505] In these circumstances it is likely that as with aortic regurgitation, a stable clinical course may be followed by abrupt decompensation with an abrupt increase in operative risk; these patients should receive operative therapy before decompensation.[505,519] However, small asymptomatic aneurysms in patients without elevated LVEDP and without the need for coronary revascularization may be managed medically. Frequent follow-up is important, as any deterioration in LV function or increase in aneurysm size should lead to surgical repair.[520] In addition, asymptomatic patients with comorbid conditions, including operative coronary artery disease and mitral valve dysfunction, should be considered for concomitant aneurysm repair.[520]

Symptomatic patients should be evaluated for operative repair of a ventricular aneurysm; whether the aneurysm is primarily akinetic or dyskinetic, outcomes are similar.[491] Few aneurysms are too large for surgical repair. In the absence of involvement of the papillary muscles, there is almost invariably enough ventricular muscle to sustain cardiac output.[505] Even when the contractile ejection fraction is between 0.25 and 0.30, aneurysms may be treated successfully with surgery provided that the mean pulmonary artery pressure is less than 40 mmHg and the cardiac index is greater than 2.1 L/min; if these conditions are not met, the patient should be considered for transplantation, especially when right ventricular dysfunction, permanent mitral regurgitation, and poor targets for coronary revascularization coexist.[505,513,519] Before surgery these patients should undergo right and left heart catheterization with delineation of the coronary anatomy. Mitral regurgitation should be evaluated, and appropriate treatment planned.

Operative technique

A median sternotomy is performed, saphenous vein or arterial conduits are harvested as needed, and the heart is cannulated for coronary bypass. Except in cases in which the right ventricle must be entered, a single two-stage right atrial cannula is usually sufficient. If indicated, epicardial mapping should be performed. To produce asystole and myocardial relaxation, most authors recommend cold anterograde cardioplegia with a solution containing potassium chloride.[520] A linear left ventriculotomy is then made approximately 3 to 4 cm lateral to the LAD. Mural thrombus then is removed, and blood is aspirated from the ventricle to identify positively the transition zone between viable myocardium and fibrotic scar. A variety of techniques have been described for repair of the LV after aneurysm excision.

Plication

Plication consists of direct closure of the defect without aneurysm excision. Buttressed two-layer monofilament is used to plicate the scar and should be oriented to maintain normal LV geometry. It should be reserved for very small aneurysms without mural thrombus in cases in which LVEDP and LV function are largely preserved.[505]

Linear repair

In 1958, Cooley described the first successful aneurysmectomy using a linear repair with cardiopulmonary bypass. It remains a popular repair, although surgeons (including Cooley)[520] increasingly are turning to geometric repair (see below). A linear repair consists of excision of the aneurysm, leaving a 3-cm rim of scar tissue for fixation of the suture line. The defect then is closed with buttressed mattress sutures placed through the fibrous base. Although it is simple in concept and technique, this procedure leads to alterations in LV geometry that may have a significant impact on long-term function. In particular, the suture line approximates the lateral wall and medial (septal) wall of the LV at a point where they usually would be separated by at least a few centimeters, decreasing LV size and distorting LV geometry. Furthermore, there is no exclusion of septal paradox when the septum is involved in the scarred region.[505]

Geometric reconstructions

A number of surgeons noted high mortality after the linear repair and were troubled by the deformity in the ventricular cavity that resulted. Hutchins and Brawley[521] first brought significant attention to the problem of LV geometry after linear repair and recommended a repair described by Stoney and associates[484] in which the lateral myocardial wall was advanced down the septum to create greater curvature and volume in the LV. Early attempts to ameliorate the problem of LV geometry after aneurysm resection included those of Daggett and associates,[332] who performed an external patch technique, and those of Komeda and associates,[522] who used an inverted T closure of the ventriculotomy to preserve the normal conical shape of the LV.

Circular patch technique

The circular patch technique is most suitable for aneurysms of the posterior portion of the heart.[523] After debridement of the ventriculotomy rim and removal of thrombus, a Dacron patch is cut to a size 2 cm larger in diameter than the defect. Pledgeted 0 horizontal mattress sutures then are used to secure the patch, with the pledgets remaining outside the ventricular cavity. Hemostasis is obtained with a second layer of sutures as required.

Endoventricular patch technique

Subsequently, Jatene,[524] Dor and colleagues,[492,525,526] and Cooley and coworkers[488] described techniques for ventricular reconstruction, all of which involve placement of an endocardial patch in an attempt to maintain normal LV and septal geometry. The technique advocated by Jatene involves the placement of a pursestring suture around the orifice of the aneurysm on a beating heart. Those sutures are used to bring the orifice down to a size estimated to be close to that of the original infarcted area.[505] If the aneurysm is small, it is possible simply to close the defect at this point (although this differs from a linear repair in that the pursestring brings the ventricular wall together with minimal alteration in geometry). More commonly, the aneurysm is resected and a patch is secured to the endoventricular side of the orifice. Although operating on a beating heart makes appropriate placement of the sutures easier, the large amount of prosthetic material left in contact with the pericardium increases the risk of postoperative infection and makes reoperation more difficult secondary to adhesions.[505]

Dor's technique involves slight modifications, including the invariable use of a patch for closure and extension of the patch to exclude scarred septum rather than septal plication as described by Jatene.[527] Finally, in the technique advocated by Cooley and coworkers, the sac is not excised but instead is sutured closed over the patch to augment hemostasis[488] (Fig. 29-26). The advantages of

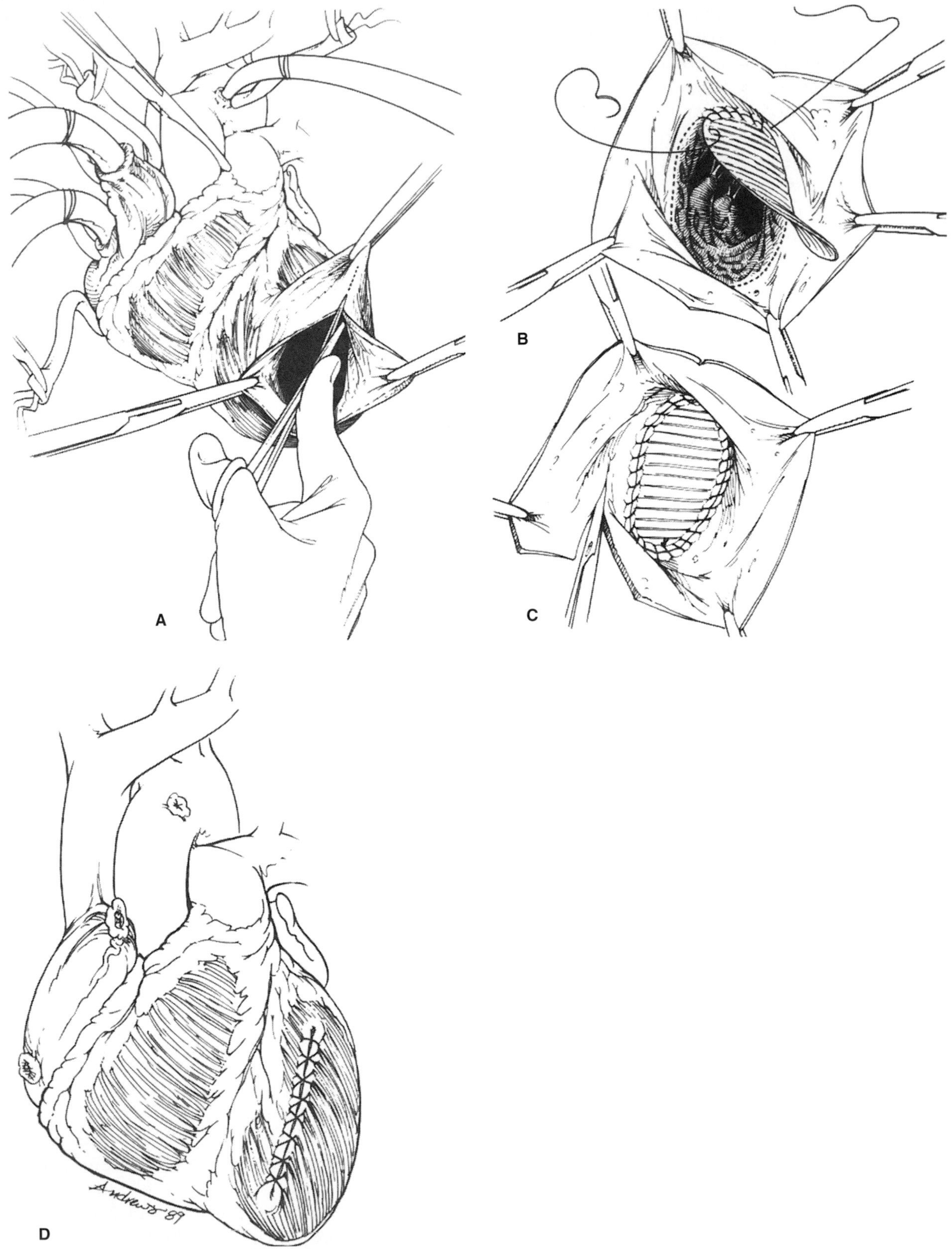

Figure 29-26 Endoaneurysmorrhaphy as advocated by Cooley and associates.[488]

these techniques include applicability to early aneurysms when infarct tissue is friable, preservation of the LAD, and separation of prosthetic material from the sternum when the aneurysmal sac is closed over the defect. In addition, these techniques facilitate patching of infarcted interventricular septum. Recently, Alonni and associates published excellent results with endoaneurysm repair via port access surgery in seven patients.[528]

Concomitant procedures

Valve surgery should be performed in patients with mitral valve disease. Repair or replacement can be performed via the ventriculotomy or by using a standard left atriotomy. Preoperative catheterization should identify patients who require concomitant CABG. Complete myocardial revascularization should be performed if possible. In patients undergoing linear repairs, the distal LAD generally is occluded by the repair. If patients have adequate distal targets, bypass may be performed, although most of these patients have significant distal disease, making bypass impossible.

Other techniques

The injection of a variety of stem cells (including fetal smooth muscle cells and bone marrow cells), as well as autotransplantation of healthy cardiomyocytes, has been reported to improve cardiac function and prevent LV dilatation in animal models.[529–532] This work has been extended to the use of bioengineered vascular smooth muscle grafts during endoventricular aneurysm repair.[533] Although experimental, this work holds promise for providing short-term recovery of normal LV geometry and preventing long-term deleterious LV remodeling.

Postoperative considerations

Postoperatively, patients frequently require inotropic support to facilitate weaning from CPB. Dopamine may be particularly useful for its inotropic and chronotropic effects. Abnormal ventricular compliance and an increased risk for postoperative ventricular arrhythmias in this population may decrease the effectiveness and increase the risk of higher doses of inotropes. Low-level resting tachycardia (heart rate between 100 and 120) may be required to maintain the cardiac index. If pharmacologic agents are ineffective, an intraaortic balloon pump may be required in the short term.

OUTCOMES AND PROGNOSIS

Early Results

Operative mortality in recent series of both linear repair and ventricular reconstruction procedures are approximately 2 to 13 percent, with most series at the lower end.[505,508,522,534–537] Multiple authors have sought to compare linear repair and ventricular reconstruction techniques; although no one has used a randomized trial, most results suggest that ventricular reconstruction provides improved results.[491,535,538,539] In a recent study of 149 patients operated on for LV aneurysm, Lundblad and associates found linear repair to be an independent predictor of both early and overall mortality (odds ratio 4.4, 95 percent CI 1.0 to 16.0).[535]

Other risk factors for early mortality include advanced age,[522,535] three-vessel coronary disease,[535] previous coronary artery bypass,[522] emergency operation,[536] poor preoperative ejection fraction (< 0.20),[491, 522] preoperative severe heart failure (NYHA class IV),[491,522,536,540] nonuse of the IMA,[491,540] mitral regurgitation,[491] and a history of malignant ventricular arrhythmias.[535] Cardiac failure constitutes the most common cause of postoperative death,[536] but ventricular arrhythmias and multiorgan system failure are also important.[536]

Late results

Long-term mortality also appears to be improved with the use of ventricular reconstruction versus linear repair.[535] Five-year mortality varies from 20 to 42 percent.[508,535,541,542] Ten-year survival is only approximately 30 percent[536,541]; however, survival in medical patients is probably worse, and although medical treatment of heart failure has improved, the mechanical dysfunction at the heart of ventricular aneurysm still must be addressed.[543] Most of these patients die of progressive heart failure or recurrent MI or experience sudden death.[536] Risk factors for long-term mortality are advanced age,[535] three-vessel disease,[535] low LVEF or preoperative heart failure,[508,535,536] high PCWP,[536] use of an IABP,[536] more than one previous MI,[535] 2+ or 3+ mitral regurgitation,[508] and a history of malignant ventricular arrhythmia.[508,535]

Left ventricular function

Most measures of left ventricular function are improved after linear repair or ventricular reconstruction. The large study by Di Donato and colleagues demonstrated a significant increase in LVEF after surgery (from 36 percent to 50 percent) with decreased pulmonary pressures and end-diastolic volume index (EDVI).[491] Even patients with large akinetic scars (who had the worst preoperative function) benefited significantly (ejection fraction increased from 25 percent to 41 percent).[491] Similar improvements in left ventricular ejection fraction (LVEF),[508,542,544,545] left ventricular end-diastolic volume (LVEDV),[544] myocardial oxygen consumption,[545] and exercise tolerance[488,544] have been reported by others regardless of the technique used.

There is continuing controversy about the relative advantages of linear repair and ventricular reconstruction. No randomized data exist, and the retrospective data are plagued by problems of comparisons across different time periods, surgeons, and patient populations. Several experienced groups have published large series reporting improvement in postoperative function with the switch to ventricular reconstruction techniques.[509,510,546–548] However, other groups have reported no difference, and some have reported an increase in operative mortality.[539,549] It appears that acceptable results can be obtained with either technique, and the most important determinant of improvement in LV function may be the appropriate size of the LV cavity rather than the specific technique used.[509,521,550] The persistence of improvements in LV function over the long term has not been studied extensively, but in humans only mild worsening of hemodynamic variables and cardiac function has been noted 7 years after surgery.[551] This suggests that although mortality remains high, it may result more from baseline coronary disease than from worsening pump function.

SUMMARY

Ventricular aneurysms result from regions of infarcted myocardium that are either akinetic or dyskinetic. This has profound effects on ventricular remodeling and in most patients results in progressive heart failure in the long term. Most aneurysms develop within 2 weeks of the inciting MI, and approximately 10 to 35 percent of patients develop an aneurysm after transmural MI. Most patients present with congestive heart failure, and the gold standard for evaluation remains angiography and ventriculography; this allows for evaluation of coronary disease and optimal operative planning. Patients with asymptomatic aneurysms may be managed medically, but those with symptoms or with extremely large aneurysms (more than 25 percent of LV surface) merit operative repair. Multiple techniques for repair have been described. The most commonly used in the modern era is a geometric repair with a patch closure of the site of aneurysm resection, optimizing LV geometry and minimizing long-term alterations in LV function. Operative mortality is approximately 10 percent, and 5-year mortality ranges from 20 to 42 percent. However, most patients have significant improvements in LV function and clinical status after aneurysm resection, and the high long-term mortality probably is related to the baseline medical condition rather to than failure of the surgical repair.

References

1. Herrick JB. Clinical features of sudden obstruction of the coronary arteries. *JAMA* 1912;59:2015–2020.
2. Goldberg RJ, Samad NA, Yarzebski J, et al. Temporal trends in cardiogenic shock complicating acute myocardial infarction. *N Engl J Med* 1999;340(15):1162–1168.
3. Bengtson JR, Kaplan AJ, Pieper KS, et al. Prognosis in cardiogenic shock after acute myocardial infarction in the interventional era. *J Am Coll Cardiol* 1992;20(7): 1482–1489.
4. Jacobs AK, Leopold JA, Bates E, et al. Cardiogenic shock caused by right ventricular infarction: A report from the SHOCK registry. *J Am Coll Cardiol* 2003;41(8): 1273–1279.
5. Moscucci M, Bates ER. Cardiogenic shock. *Cardiol Clin* 1995;13(3):391–406.
6. Hunter J. A treatise on the blood, inflammation, and gunshot wounds by the late John Hunter. To which is prefixed a short account of the author's life, by his brother-in-law, Everald Home. In: Willius FA, Keis TE (eds). *Classics of Cardiology*. New York: Dover; 1961:269.
7. Boersma E, Mercado N, Poldermans D, et al. Acute myocardial infarction. *Lancet* 2003;361(9360):847–858.
8. Rauch U, Osende JI, Fuster V, et al. Thrombus formation on atherosclerotic plaques: Pathogenesis and clinical consequences. *Ann Intern Med* 2001;134(3):224–238.
9. Kloner RA, Ganote CE, Whalen DA Jr, Jennings RB. Effect of a transient period of ischemia on myocardial cells: II. Fine structure during the first few minutes of reflow. *Am J Pathol* 1974;74(3):399–422.
10. Jennings RB, Murry CE, Steenbergen C Jr, Reimer KA. Development of cell injury in sustained acute ischemia. *Circulation* 1990;82(Suppl 3):II2–12.
11. Kloner RA, Jennings RB. Consequences of brief ischemia: Stunning, preconditioning, and their clinical implications: Part 1. *Circulation* 2001;104(24): 2981–2989.
12. Braunwald E, Kloner RA. The stunned myocardium: Prolonged, postischemic ventricular dysfunction. *Circulation* 1982;66(6):1146–1149.
13. Heyndrickx GR, Millard RW, McRitchie RJ, et al. Regional myocardial functional and electrophysiological alterations after brief coronary artery occlusion in conscious dogs. *J Clin Invest* 1975;56(4):978–985.
14. Bolli R, Zhu WX, Thornby JI, et al. Time course and determinants of recovery of function after reversible ischemia in conscious dogs. *Am J Physiol* 1988;254 (1 Pt 2):H102–114.
15. Bolli R. Basic and clinical aspects of myocardial stunning. *Prog Cardiovasc Dis* 1998;40(6):477–516.
16. Rahimtoola SH. A perspective on the three large multicenter randomized clinical trials of coronary bypass surgery for chronic stable angina. *Circulation* 1985;72 (6 Pt 2):V123–135.
17. Rahimtoola SH. The hibernating myocardium. *Am Heart J* 1989;117(1):211–221.
18. Braunwald E, Rutherford JD. Reversible ischemic left ventricular dysfunction: Evidence for the "hibernating myocardium." *J Am Coll Cardiol* 1986;8(6): 1467–1470.
19. Mosher P, Ross J Jr, McFate PA, Shaw RF. Control of coronary blood flow by an autoregulatory mechanism. *Circ Res* 1964;14:250–259.
20. Alonso DR, Scheidt S, Post M, Killip T. Pathophysiology of cardiogenic shock: Quantification of myocardial

necrosis, clinical, pathologic and electrocardiographic correlations. *Circulation* 1973;48(3):588–596.
21. Page DL, Caulfield JB, Kastor JA, et al. Myocardial changes associated with cardiogenic shock. *N Engl J Med* 1971;285(3):133–137.
22. Hasdai D, Topol EJ, Califf RM, et al. Cardiogenic shock complicating acute coronary syndromes. *Lancet* 2000;356(9231):749–756.
23. Hochman JS, Sleeper LA, Webb JG, et al. Early revascularization in acute myocardial infarction complicated by cardiogenic shock: SHOCK Investigators: SHould we emergently revascularize Occluded Coronaries for cardiogenic shocK? *N Engl J Med* 1999;341(9):625–634.
24. Hochman JS, Buller CE, Sleeper LA, et al. Cardiogenic shock complicating acute myocardial infarction—etiologies, management and outcome: A report from the SHOCK Trial Registry: SHould we emergently revascularize Occluded Coronaries for cardiogenic shocK? *J Am Coll Cardiol* 2000;36(3 Suppl A):1063–1070.
25. Hochman JS. Cardiogenic shock complicating acute myocardial infarction: Expanding the paradigm. *Circulation* 2003;107(24):2998–3002.
26. Picard MH, Davidoff R, Sleeper LA, et al. Echocardiographic predictors of survival and response to early revascularization in cardiogenic shock. *Circulation* 2003;107(2):279–284.
27. Menon V, Slater JN, White HD, et al. Acute myocardial infarction complicated by systemic hypoperfusion without hypotension: Report of the SHOCK trial registry. *Am J Med* 2000;108(5):374–380.
28. Griffith GC, Wallace WB, Cochran B Jr, et al. The treatment of shock associated with myocardial infarction. *Circulation* 1954;9(4):527–532.
29. Goldberg RJ, Gore JM, Thompson CA, Gurwitz JH. Recent magnitude of and temporal trends (1994-1997) in the incidence and hospital death rates of cardiogenic shock complicating acute myocardial infarction: The second national registry of myocardial infarction. *Am Heart J* 2001;141(1):65–72.
30. Holmes DR Jr, Bates ER, Kleiman NS, et al. Contemporary reperfusion therapy for cardiogenic shock: The GUSTO-I trial experience. *J Am Coll Cardiol* 1995; 26(3):668–674.
31. Killip T 3rd, Kimball JT. Treatment of myocardial infarction in a coronary care unit: A two year experience with 250 patients. *Am J Cardiol* 1967;20(4):457–464.
32. Goldberg RJ, Gore JM, Alpert JS, et al. Cardiogenic shock after acute myocardial infarction: Incidence and mortality from a community-wide perspective, 1975 to 1988. *N Engl J Med* 1991;325(16):1117–1122.
33. Barbash IM, Hasdai D, Behar S, et al. Usefulness of pre- versus postadmission cardiogenic shock during acute myocardial infarction in predicting survival. *Am J Cardiol* 2001;87(10):1200–1203.
34. Berger PB, Tuttle RH, Holmes DR Jr, et al. One-year survival among patients with acute myocardial infarction complicated by cardiogenic shock, and its relation to early revascularization: Results from the GUSTO-I trial. *Circulation* 1999;99(7):873–878.
35. Hasdai D, Holmes DR Jr, Califf RM, et al. Cardiogenic shock complicating acute myocardial infarction: Predictors of death: GUSTO Investigators: Global utilization of streptokinase and tissue-plasminogen activator for occluded coronary arteries. *Am Heart J* 1999;138 (1 Pt 1):21–31.
36. Leor J, Goldbourt U, Reicher-Reiss H, Kaplinsky E, et al. Cardiogenic shock complicating acute myocardial infarction in patients without heart failure on admission: Incidence, risk factors, and outcome: SPRINT Study Group. *Am J Med* 1993;94(3):265–273.
37. Hands ME, Rutherford JD, Muller JE, et al. The in-hospital development of cardiogenic shock after myocardial infarction: Incidence, predictors of occurrence, outcome and prognostic factors: The MILIS Study Group. *J Am Coll Cardiol* 1989;14(1):40–46; discussion 7–8.
38. Antman EM, Tanasijevic MJ, Thompson B, et al. Cardiac-specific troponin I levels to predict the risk of mortality in patients with acute coronary syndromes. *N Engl J Med* 1996;335(18):1342–1349.
39. Heidenreich PA, Alloggiamento T, Melsop K, et al. The prognostic value of troponin in patients with non-ST elevation acute coronary syndromes: A meta-analysis. *J Am Coll Cardiol* 2001;38(2):478–485.
40. Matetzky S, Sharir T, Domingo M, et al. Elevated troponin I level on admission is associated with adverse outcome of primary angioplasty in acute myocardial infarction. *Circulation* 2000;102(14):1611–1616.
41. Ohman EM, Armstrong PW, Christenson RH, et al. Cardiac troponin T levels for risk stratification in acute myocardial ischemia: GUSTO IIA Investigators. *N Engl J Med* 1996;335(18):1333–1341.
42. Wu WC, Rathore SS, Wang Y, et al. Blood transfusion in elderly patients with acute myocardial infarction. *N Engl J Med* 2001;345(17):1230–1236.
43. Sanborn TA, Sleeper LA, Webb JG, et al. Correlates of one-year survival in patients with cardiogenic shock complicating acute myocardial infarction: Angiographic findings from the SHOCK trial. *J Am Coll Cardiol* 2003;42(8):1373–1379.
44. Lee TH, Goldman L. The coronary care unit turns 25: Historical trends and future directions. *Ann Intern Med* 1988;108(6):887–894.
45. Griepp RB, Ergin MA, Galla JD, et al. Looking for the artery of Adamkiewicz: A quest to minimize paraplegia after operations for aneurysms of the descending thoracic and thoracoabdominal aorta. *J Thorac Cardiovasc Surg* 1996;112(5):1202–1213; discussion 13–15.
46. Bassenge E, Zanzinger J. Nitrates in different vascular beds, nitrate tolerance, and interactions with endothelial function. *Am J Cardiol* 1992;70(8):23B–29B.
47. Goldstein RE, Bennett ED, Leech GL. Effect of glyceryl trinitrate on echocardiographic left ventricular dimensions during exercise in the upright position. *Br Heart J* 1979;42(3):245–254.
48. Thadani U. Oral nitrates: More than symptomatic therapy in coronary artery disease? *Cardiovasc Drugs Ther* 1997;11(Suppl 1):213–218.
49. Gruppo Italiano per lo Studio della Sopravvivenza nell'infarto Miocardico (GISSI). GISSI-3: Effects of lisinopril and transdermal glyceryl trinitrate singly and together on 6-week mortality and ventricular function after acute myocardial infarction. *Lancet* 1994;343(8906): 1115–1122.

50. Yusuf S, Collins R, MacMahon S, Peto R. Effect of intravenous nitrates on mortality in acute myocardial infarction: An overview of the randomised trials. *Lancet* 1988;1(8594): 1088–1092.
51. Lavie CJ, Gersh BJ. Acute myocardial infarction: Initial manifestations, management, and prognosis. *Mayo Clin Proc* 1990;65(4):531–548.
52. Debaveye YA, Van den Berghe GH. Is there still a place for dopamine in the modern intensive care unit? *Anesth Analg* 2004;98(2):461–468.
53. Schaer GL, Fink MP, Parrillo JE. Norepinephrine alone versus norepinephrine plus low-dose dopamine: Enhanced renal blood flow with combination pressor therapy. *Crit Care Med* 1985;13(6):492–496.
54. Stevens PE, Bolsin S, Gwyther SJ, et al. Practical use of duplex Doppler analysis of the renal vasculature in critically ill patients. *Lancet* 1989;1(8632):240–242.
55. Perdue PW, Balser JR, Lipsett PA, Breslow MJ. "Renal dose" dopamine in surgical patients: Dogma or science? *Ann Surg* 1998;227(4):470–473.
56. Duke GJ, Briedis JH, Weaver RA. Renal support in critically ill patients: Low-dose dopamine or low-dose dobutamine? *Crit Care Med* 1994;22(12):1919–1925.
57. Ruffolo RR Jr. The pharmacology of dobutamine. *Am J Med Sci* 1987;294(4):244–248.
58. Gillespie TA, Ambos HD, Sobel BE, Roberts R. Effects of dobutamine in patients with acute myocardial infarction. *Am J Cardiol* 1977;39(4):588–594.
59. Litwak RS, Kuhn LA, Gadboys HL, et al. Support of myocardial performance after open cardiac operations by rate augmentation. *J Thorac Cardiovasc Surg* 1968;56(4): 484–496.
60. Bourdarias JP, Dubourg O, Gueret P, et al. Inotropic agents in the treatment of cardiogenic shock. *Pharmacol Ther* 1983;22(1):53–79.
61. Cohen MV, Sonnenblick EH, Kirk ES. Coronary steal: Its role in detrimental effect of isoproterenol after acute coronary occlusion in dogs. *Am J Cardiol* 1976;38(7): 880–888.
62. Califf RM, Bengtson JR. Cardiogenic shock. *N Engl J Med* 1994;330(24):1724–1730.
63. Hollenberg SM. Cardiogenic shock. *Crit Care Clin* 2001;17(2):391–410.
64. Laks M, Callis G, Swan HJ. Hemodynamic effects of low doses of norepinephrine in the conscious dog. *Am J Physiol* 1971;220(1):171–173.
65. Mueller H, Ayres SM, Giannelli S Jr, et al. Effect of isoproterenol, l-norepinephrine, and intraaortic counterpulsation on hemodynamics and myocardial metabolism in shock following acute myocardial infarction. *Circulation* 1972;45(2):335–351.
66. Landry DW, Levin HR, Gallant EM, et al. Vasopressin deficiency contributes to the vasodilation of septic shock. *Circulation* 1997;95(5):1122–1125.
67. Morales DL, Gregg D, Helman DN, et al. Arginine vasopressin in the treatment of 50 patients with postcardiotomy vasodilatory shock. *Ann Thorac Surg* 2000;69(1): 102–106.
68. Ericsson BF. The effect of vasopressin on the distribution of cardiac output in the early phase of haemorrhagic shock in the anesthetized dog. *Acta Chir Scand* 1972;138(2):119–123.
69. Ericsson BF. Hemodynamic effects of vasopressin during haemorrhagic hypotension in the anesthetized dog. *Acta Chir Scand* 1972;138(3):227–233.
70. Dunser MW, Mayr AJ, Ulmer H, et al. Arginine vasopressin in advanced vasodilatory shock: A prospective, randomized, controlled study. *Circulation* 2003;107(18): 2313–2319.
71. AIMS Trial Study Group. Effect of intravenous APSAC on mortality after acute myocardial infarction: Preliminary report of a placebo-controlled clinical trial. *Lancet* 1988;1(8585):545–549.
72. Gruppo Italiano per lo Studio della Streptochinasi nell'Infarto Miocardico (GISSI). Effectiveness of intravenous thrombolytic treatment in acute myocardial infarction. *Lancet* 1986;1(8478):397–402.
73. The GUSTO Investigators. An international randomized trial comparing four thrombolytic strategies for acute myocardial infarction. *N Engl J Med* 1993;329(10): 673–682.
74. Col NF, Gurwitz JH, Alpert JS, Goldberg RJ. Frequency of inclusion of patients with cardiogenic shock in trials of thrombolytic therapy. *Am J Cardiol* 1994;73(2): 149–157.
75. ISIS-2 (Second International Study of Infarct Survival) Collaborative Group. Randomised trial of intravenous streptokinase, oral aspirin, both, or neither among 17,187 cases of suspected acute myocardial infarction: ISIS-2. *Lancet* 1988;2(8607):349–360.
76. Wilcox RG, von der Lippe G, Olsson CG, et al. Trial of tissue plasminogen activator for mortality reduction in acute myocardial infarction. Anglo-Scandinavian Study of Early Thrombolysis (ASSET). *Lancet* 1988;2(8610): 525–530.
77. Mathey D, Kuck KH, Remmecke J, et al. Transluminal recanalization of coronary artery thrombosis: A preliminary report of its application in cardiogenic shock. *Eur Heart J* 1980;1(3):207–212.
78. Mathey DG, Kuck KH, Tilsner V, et al. Non surgical coronary artery recanalization in acute transmural myocardial infarction. *Circulation* 1981;63(3):489–497.
79. Kennedy JW, Gensini GG, Timmis GC, Maynard C. Acute myocardial infarction treated with intracoronary streptokinase: A report of the Society for Cardiac Angiography. *Am J Cardiol* 1985;55(8):871–877.
80. The International Study Group. In-hospital mortality and clinical course of 20,891 patients with suspected acute myocardial infarction randomised between alteplase and streptokinase with or without heparin. *Lancet* 1990;336(8707):71–75.
81. Berger PB, Holmes DR Jr, Stebbins AL, et al. Impact of an aggressive invasive catheterization and revascularization strategy on mortality in patients with cardiogenic shock in the Global Utilization of Streptokinase and Tissue Plasminogen Activator for Occluded Coronary Arteries (GUSTO-I) trial: An observational study. *Circulation* 1997;96(1):122–127.
82. Becker RC. Hemodynamic, mechanical, and metabolic determinants of thrombolytic efficacy: A theoretic framework for assessing the limitations of thrombolysis in patients with cardiogenic shock. *Am Heart J* 1993;125(3): 919–929.

83. Werier J, Ducas J, Gu S, et al. Effect of low-molecular-weight heparin on recombinant tissue plasminogen activator-induced thrombolysis in canine pulmonary embolism. *Chest* 1991;100(2):464–469.
84. Prewitt RM, Gu S, Garber PJ, Ducas J. Marked systemic hypotension depresses coronary thrombolysis induced by intracoronary administration of recombinant tissue-type plasminogen activator. *J Am Coll Cardiol* 1992;20(7):1626–1633.
85. Gibson CM, Murphy S, Menown IB, et al. Determinants of coronary blood flow after thrombolytic administration: TIMI Study Group: Thrombolysis in Myocardial Infarction. *J Am Coll Cardiol* 1999;34(5):1403–1412.
86. Prewitt RM, Gu S, Schick U, Ducas J. Intraaortic balloon counterpulsation enhances coronary thrombolysis induced by intravenous administration of a thrombolytic agent. *J Am Coll Cardiol* 1994;23(3):794–798.
87. Gurbel PA, Anderson RD, MacCord CS, et al. Arterial diastolic pressure augmentation by intra-aortic balloon counterpulsation enhances the onset of coronary artery reperfusion by thrombolytic therapy. *Circulation* 1994;89(1):361–365.
88. Lip GY, Chin BS, Prasad N. ABC of antithrombotic therapy: Antithrombotic therapy in myocardial infarction and stable angina. *BMJ* 2002;325(7375):1287–1289.
89. Topol EJ. Current status and future prospects for acute myocardial infarction therapy. *Circulation* 2003;108(16 Suppl 1):III6–13.
90. Harken DE. Presentation at International College of Cardiology, Brussels, Belgium; 1958.
91. Oberwalder PJ. Intra-aortic balloon pump (IABP) counterpulsation: Theory and clinical applications. *J Thorac Cardiovasc Surg* 1999;2(2). (Available online at http://www.ispub.com/journals/IJTCVS/Vol2N2/iabp.htm.)
92. Moulopoulos SD, Topaz SR, Kolff WJ. Extracorporeal assistance to the circulation and intraaortic balloon pumping. *Trans ASAIO* 1962;8:85–89.
93. Moulopoulos SD, Topaz S, Kolff WJ. Diastolic balloon pumping (with carbon dioxide) in the aorta—a mechanical assistance to the failing circulation. *Am Heart J* 1962;63:669–675.
94. Kantrowitz A, Tjonneland S, Freed PS, et al. Initial clinical experience with intraaortic balloon pumping in cardiogenic shock. *JAMA* 1968;203(2):113–118.
95. Bregman D, Casarella WJ. Percutaneous intraaortic balloon pumping: Initial clinical experience. *Ann Thorac Surg* 1980;29(2):153–155.
96. Leinbach RC, Goldstein J, Gold HK, et al. Percutaneous wire-guided balloon pumping. *Am J Cardiol* 1982;49(7):1707–1710.
97. Low R. Intra-aortic balloon counterpulsation in acute myocardial infarction: Too few or too many?[comment]. *J Am Coll Cardiol* 2003;41(11):1946–1947.
98. Veasy LG, Blalock RC, Orth JL, Boucek MM. Intra-aortic balloon pumping in infants and children. *Circulation* 1983;68(5):1095–1100.
99. Rubenstein RB, Karhade NV. Supraclavicular subclavian technique of intra-aortic balloon insertion. *J Vasc Surg* 1984;1(4):577–578.
100. Mayer JH. Subclavian artery approach for insertion of intra-aortic balloon. *J Thorac Cardiovasc Surg* 1978;76(1):61–63.
101. Lamberti JJ, Cohn LH, Collins JJ Jr. Iliac artery cannulation for intra-aortic balloon counterpulsation. *J Thorac Cardiovasc Surg* 1974;67(6):976–977.
102. Shirkey AL, Loughridge BP, Lain KC. Insertion of the intraaortic balloon through the aortic arch. *Ann Thorac Surg* 1976;21(6):560–561.
103. Salerno TA. Insertion of the intra-aortic balloon through the ascending aorta and its removal under local anesthesia. *Can J Surg* 1983;26(1):69.
104. Bonchek LI, Olinger GN. Direct ascending aortic insertion of the "percutaneous" intraaortic balloon catheter in the open chest: Advantages and precautions. *Ann Thorac Surg* 1981;32(5):512–514.
105. Weber KT, Janicki JS. Intraaortic balloon counterpulsation: A review of physiological principles, clinical results, and device safety. *Ann Thorac Surg* 1974;17(6):602–636.
106. Powell WJ Jr, Daggett WM, Magro AE, et al. Effects of intra-aortic balloon counterpulsation on cardiac performance, oxygen consumption, and coronary blood flow in dogs. *Circ Res* 1970;26(6):753–764.
107. Kusiak VM, Goldberg S. Percutaneous intra-aortic balloon counterpulsation. *Cardiovasc Clin* 1985;15(1):281–302.
108. Kern MJ, Aguirre FV, Tatineni S, et al. Enhanced coronary blood flow velocity during intraaortic balloon counterpulsation in critically ill patients. *J Am Coll Cardiol* 1993;21(2):359–368.
109. Leinbach RC, Buckley MJ, Austen WG, et al. Effects of intra-aortic balloon pumping on coronary flow and metabolism in man. *Circulation* 1971;43(Suppl 5):I77–81.
110. Leinbach RC, Nyilas E, Caulfield JB, et al. Evaluation of hematologic effects of intra-aortic balloon assistance in man. *Trans ASAIO* 1972;18(0):493–500.
111. Willerson JT, Watson JT, Curry GC, et al. Mechanical circulatory assistance with intra-aortic balloon. *Tex Med* 1973;69(12):54–58.
112. O'Rourke MF, Norris RM, Campbell TJ, et al. Randomized controlled trial of intraaortic balloon counterpulsation in early myocardial infarction with acute heart failure. *Am J Cardiol* 1981;47(4):815–820.
113. Scheidt S, Wilner G, Mueller H, et al. Intra-aortic balloon counterpulsation in cardiogenic shock: Report of a co-operative clinical trial. *N Engl J Med* 1973;288(19):979–984.
114. Waksman R, Weiss AT, Gotsman MS, Hasin Y. Intra-aortic balloon counterpulsation improves survival in cardiogenic shock complicating acute myocardial infarction. *Eur Heart J* 1993;14(1):71–74.
115. Stomel RJ, Rasak M, Bates ER. Treatment strategies for acute myocardial infarction complicated by cardiogenic shock in a community hospital. *Chest* 1994;105(4):997–1002.
116. Anderson RD, Ohman EM, Holmes DR Jr, et al. Use of intraaortic balloon counterpulsation in patients presenting with cardiogenic shock: Observations from the GUSTO-I Study:. Global Utilization of Streptokinase and TPA for Occluded Coronary Arteries. *J Am Coll Cardiol* 1997;30(3):708–715.
117. Sanborn TA, Sleeper LA, Bates ER, et al. Impact of thrombolysis, intra-aortic balloon pump counterpulsation, and their combination in cardiogenic shock complicating

acute myocardial infarction: A report from the SHOCK Trial Registry: SHould we emergently revascularize Occluded Coronaries for cardiogenic shocK? *J Am Coll Cardiol* 2000;36(3 Suppl A):1123–1129.
118. Kovack PJ, Rasak MA, Bates ER, et al. Thrombolysis plus aortic counterpulsation: Improved survival in patients who present to community hospitals with cardiogenic shock. *J Am Coll Cardiol* 1997;29(7):1454–1458.
119. Ohman EM, George BS, White CJ, et al. Use of aortic counterpulsation to improve sustained coronary artery patency during acute myocardial infarction: Results of a randomized trial: The Randomized IABP Study Group. *Circulation* 1994;90(2):792–799.
120. The GUSTO Angiographic Investigators. The effects of tissue plasminogen activator, streptokinase, or both on coronary-artery patency, ventricular function, and survival after acute myocardial infarction. *N Engl J Med* 1993;329(22):1615–1622.
121. Vogt A, von Essen R, Tebbe U, et al. Impact of early perfusion status of the infarct-related artery on short-term mortality after thrombolysis for acute myocardial infarction: Retrospective analysis of four German multicenter studies. *J Am Coll Cardiol* 1993;21(6):1391–1395.
122. Lincoff AM, Topol EJ, Califf RM, et al. Significance of a coronary artery with thrombolysis in myocardial infarction grade 2 flow "patency" (outcome in the thrombolysis and angioplasty in myocardial infarction trials): Thrombolysis and Angioplasty in Myocardial Infarction Study Group. *Am J Cardiol* 1995;75(14):871–876.
123. Gibson CM, Murphy S, Menown IB, et al. Determinants of coronary blood flow after thrombolytic administration: TIMI Study Group: Thrombolysis in Myocardial Infarction. *J Am Coll Cardiol* 1999;34(5):1403–1412.
124. Stone GW, Cox D, Garcia E, et al. Normal flow (TIMI-3) before mechanical reperfusion therapy is an independent determinant of survival in acute myocardial infarction: Analysis from the primary angioplasty in myocardial infarction trials. *Circulation* 2001;104(6):636–641.
125. Cura FA, L'Allier PL, Kapadia SR, et al. Predictors and prognosis of suboptimal coronary blood flow after primary coronary angioplasty in patients with acute myocardial infarction. *Am J Cardiol* 2001;88(2):124–128.
126. Dibra A, Mehilli J, Dirschinger J, et al. Thrombolysis in myocardial infarction: Myocardial perfusion grade in angiography correlates with myocardial salvage in patients with acute myocardial infarction treated with stenting or thrombolysis. *J Am Coll Cardiol* 2003;41(6):925–929.
127. Milavetz JJ, Giebel DW, Christian TF, et al. Time to therapy and salvage in myocardial infarction. *J Am Coll Cardiol* 1998;31(6):1246–1251.
128. Hochman JS, Sleeper LA, White HD, et al. One-year survival following early revascularization for cardiogenic shock. *JAMA* 2001;285(2):190–192.
129. Chesebro JH, Knatterud G, Roberts R, et al. Thrombolysis in Myocardial Infarction (TIMI) Trial, Phase I: A comparison between intravenous tissue plasminogen activator and intravenous streptokinase: Clinical findings through hospital discharge. *Circulation* 1987;76(1):142–154.
130. Webb JG, Lowe AM, Sanborn TA, et al. Percutaneous coronary intervention for cardiogenic shock in the SHOCK trial. *J Am Coll Cardiol* 2003;42(8):1380–1386.
131. Antoniucci D, Valenti R, Migliorini A, et al. Comparison of impact of emergency percutaneous revascularization on outcome of patients > or = 75 to those < 75 years of age with acute myocardial infarction complicated by cardiogenic shock. *Am J Cardiol* 2003;91(12):1458–1461.
132. Brodie BR, Stuckey TD, Muncy DB, et al. Importance of time-to-reperfusion in patients with acute myocardial infarction with and without cardiogenic shock treated with primary percutaneous coronary intervention. *Am Heart J* 2003;145(4):708–715.
133. Ellis SG, O'Neill WW, Bates ER, et al. Implications for patient triage from survival and left ventricular functional recovery analyses in 500 patients treated with coronary angioplasty for acute myocardial infarction. *J Am Coll Cardiol* 1989;13(6):1251–1259.
134. Rodriguez A, Bernardi V, Fernandez M, et al. In-hospital and late results of coronary stents versus conventional balloon angioplasty in acute myocardial infarction (GRAMI trial): Gianturco-Roubin in Acute Myocardial Infarction. *Am J Cardiol* 1998;81(11):1286–1291.
135. Stone GW, Brodie BR, Griffin JJ, et al. Prospective, multicenter study of the safety and feasibility of primary stenting in acute myocardial infarction: In-hospital and 30-day results of the PAMI stent pilot trial: Primary Angioplasty in Myocardial Infarction Stent Pilot Trial Investigators. *J Am Coll Cardiol* 1998;31(1):23–30.
136. Suryapranata H, van't Hof AW, Hoorntje JC, et al. Randomized comparison of coronary stenting with balloon angioplasty in selected patients with acute myocardial infarction. *Circulation* 1998;97(25):2502–2505.
137. Antoniucci D, Santoro GM, Bolognese L, et al. A clinical trial comparing primary stenting of the infarct-related artery with optimal primary angioplasty for acute myocardial infarction: Results from the Florence Randomized Elective Stenting in Acute Coronary Occlusions (FRESCO) trial. *J Am Coll Cardiol* 1998;31(6):1234–1239.
138. Stone GW, Marsalese D, Brodie BR, et al. A prospective, randomized evaluation of prophylactic intraaortic balloon counterpulsation in high risk patients with acute myocardial infarction treated with primary angioplasty: Second Primary Angioplasty in Myocardial Infarction (PAMI-II) Trial Investigators. *J Am Coll Cardiol* 1997;29(7):1459–1467.
139. Grines CL, Cox DA, Stone GW, et al. Coronary angioplasty with or without stent implantation for acute myocardial infarction: Stent Primary Angioplasty in Myocardial Infarction Study Group. *N Engl J Med* 1999;341(26):1949–1956.
140. Maillard L, Hamon M, Khalife K, et al. A comparison of systematic stenting and conventional balloon angioplasty during primary percutaneous transluminal coronary angioplasty for acute myocardial infarction: STENTIM-2 Investigators. *J Am Coll Cardiol* 2000;35(7):1729–1736.
141. Antoniucci D, Valenti R, Santoro GM, et al. Systematic direct angioplasty and stent-supported direct angioplasty therapy for cardiogenic shock complicating acute myocardial infarction: In-hospital and long-term survival. *J Am Coll Cardiol* 1998;31(2):294–300.

142. Yip HK, Wu CJ, Chang HW, et al. Comparison of impact of primary percutaneous transluminal coronary angioplasty and primary stenting on short-term mortality in patients with cardiogenic shock and evaluation of prognostic determinants. *Am J Cardiol* 2001;87(10): 1184–1188.
143. Dauerman HL, Goldberg RJ, White K, et al. Revascularization, stenting, and outcomes of patients with acute myocardial infarction complicated by cardiogenic shock. *Am J Cardiol* 2002;90(8):838–842.
144. The EPIC Investigators. Use of a monoclonal antibody directed against the platelet glycoprotein IIb/IIIa receptor in high-risk coronary angioplasty: The EPIC Investigation. *N Engl J Med* 1994;330(14):956–961.
145. Schomig A, Kastrati A, Dirschinger J, et al. Coronary stenting plus platelet glycoprotein IIb/IIIa blockade compared with tissue plasminogen activator in acute myocardial infarction: Stent versus Thrombolysis for Occluded Coronary Arteries in Patients with Acute Myocardial Infarction Study Investigators. *N Engl J Med* 2000;343(6):385–391.
146. Neumann FJ, Kastrati A, Schmitt C, et al. Effect of glycoprotein IIb/IIIa receptor blockade with abciximab on clinical and angiographic restenosis rate after the placement of coronary stents following acute myocardial infarction. *J Am Coll Cardiol* 2000;35(4):915–921.
147. Tcheng JE, Kandzari DE, Grines CL, et al. Benefits and risks of abciximab use in primary angioplasty for acute myocardial infarction: The Controlled Abciximab and Device Investigation to Lower Late Angioplasty Complications (CADILLAC) trial. *Circulation* 2003;108(11):1316–1323.
148. Antoniucci D, Valenti R, Migliorini A, et al. Abciximab therapy improves survival in patients with acute myocardial infarction complicated by early cardiogenic shock undergoing coronary artery stent implantation. *Am J Cardiol* 2002;90(4):353–357.
149. Chan AW, Chew DP, Bhatt DL, et al. Long-term mortality benefit with the combination of stents and abciximab for cardiogenic shock complicating acute myocardial infarction. *Am J Cardiol* 2002;89(2):132–136.
150. Dawson JT, Hall RJ, Hallman GL, Cooley DA. Mortality in patients undergoing coronary artery bypass surgery after myocardial infarction. *Am J Cardiol* 1974;33(4):483–486.
151. Levine FH, Gold HK, Leinbach RC, et al. Safe early revascularization for continuing ischemia after acute myocardial infarction. *Circulation* 1979;60(2 Pt 2):5–9.
152. Phillips SJ, Kongtahworn C, Zeff RH, et al. Emergency coronary artery revascularization: A possible therapy for acute myocardial infarction. *Circulation* 1979;60(2): 241–246.
153. DeWood MA, Spores J, Notske R, et al. Prevalence of total coronary occlusion during the early hours of transmural myocardial infarction. *N Engl J Med* 1980;303(16): 897–902.
154. Berg R Jr, Selinger SL, Leonard JJ, et al. Immediate coronary artery bypass for acute evolving myocardial infarction. *J Thorac Cardiovasc Surg* 1981;81(4): 493–497.
155. DeWood MA, Spores J, Berg R Jr, et al. Acute myocardial infarction: A decade of experience with surgical reperfusion in 701 patients. *Circulation* 1983;68(3 Pt 2): II8–16.
156. Phillips SJ, Kongtahworn C, Skinner JR, Zeff RH. Emergency coronary artery reperfusion: A choice therapy for evolving myocardial infarction: Results in 339 patients. *J Thorac Cardiovasc Surg* 1983;86(5):679–688.
157. DeWood MA, Notske RN, Berg R Jr, et al. Medical and surgical management of early Q wave myocardial infarction: I. Effects of surgical reperfusion on survival, recurrent myocardial infarction, sudden death and functional class at 10 or more years of follow-up. *J Am Coll Cardiol* 1989;14(1):65–77.
158. Lee L, Bates ER, Pitt B, et al. Percutaneous transluminal coronary angioplasty improves survival in acute myocardial infarction complicated by cardiogenic shock. *Circulation* 1988;78(6):1345–1351.
159. Zaroff JG, diTommaso DG, Barron HV. A risk model derived from the National Registry of Myocardial Infarction 2 database for predicting mortality after coronary artery bypass grafting during acute myocardial infarction. *Am J Cardiol* 2002;90(1):1–4.
160. Lee DC, Oz MC, Weinberg AD, et al. Optimal timing of revascularization: Transmural versus nontransmural acute myocardial infarction. *Ann Thorac Surg* 2001;71(4): 1197–1202; discussion 202–204.
161. Lee DC, Oz MC, Weinberg AD, Ting W. Appropriate timing of surgical intervention after transmural acute myocardial infarction. *J Thorac Cardiovasc Surg* 2003;125(1):115–119; discussion 9–20.
162. Lee L, Erbel R, Brown TM, et al. Multicenter registry of angioplasty therapy of cardiogenic shock: Initial and long-term survival. *J Am Coll Cardiol* 1991;17(3): 599–603.
163. Lazar H. Methods of reducing myocardial necrosis after failed percutaneous transluminal coronary angioplasty in patients undergoing emergent coronary artery bypass surgery. In: Lazar H (ed). *Current Therapy for Acute Coronary Ischemia*. Mount Kisko, NY: Futura; 1993:167–186.
164. Hoeft A, Sonntag H, Stephan H, Kettler D. The influence of anesthesia on myocardial oxygen utilization efficiency in patients undergoing coronary bypass surgery. *Anesth Analg* 1994;78(5):857–866.
165. Lee DC, Ting W, Oz M. Myocardial revascularization after acute myocardial infarction. In: Cohn LH, Edmunds LH Jr (eds). *Cardiac Surgery in the Adult*, 2d ed. New York: McGraw-Hill; 2003:639–658.
166. Lemmer JH Jr, Stanford W, Bonney SL, et al. Aprotinin for coronary bypass operations: Efficacy, safety, and influence on early saphenous vein graft patency: A multicenter, randomized, double-blind, placebo-controlled study. *J Thorac Cardiovasc Surg* 1994;107(2):543–551; discussion 51–53.
167. Murkin JM, Lux J, Shannon NA, et al. Aprotinin significantly decreases bleeding and transfusion requirements in patients receiving aspirin and undergoing cardiac operations. *J Thorac Cardiovasc Surg* 1994;107(2): 554–561.
168. Efstratiadis T, Munsch C, Crossman D, Taylor K. Aprotinin used in emergency coronary operation after streptokinase treatment. *Ann Thorac Surg* 1991;52(6): 1320–1321.

169. Sergeant P, Blackstone E, Meyns B. Early and late outcome after CABG in patients with evolving myocardial infarction. *Eur J Cardiothorac Surg* 1997;11(5):848–856.
170. Caes FL, Van Nooten GJ. Use of internal mammary artery for emergency grafting after failed coronary angioplasty. *Ann Thorac Surg* 1994;57(5):1295–1299.
171. Zapolanski A, Rosenblum J, Myler RK, et al. Emergency coronary artery bypass surgery following failed balloon angioplasty: Role of the internal mammary artery graft. *J Card Surg* 1991;6(4):439–448.
172. Beyersdorf F, Mitrev Z, Sarai K, et al. Changing patterns of patients undergoing emergency surgical revascularization for acute coronary occlusion: Importance of myocardial protection techniques. *J Thorac Cardiovasc Surg* 1993;106(1):137–148.
173. Akins CW. Early and late results following emergency isolated myocardial revascularization during hypothermic fibrillatory arrest. *Ann Thorac Surg* 1987;43(2):131–137.
174. Guyton RA, Arcidi JM Jr, Langford DA, et al. Emergency coronary bypass for cardiogenic shock. *Circulation* 1987;76(5 Pt 2):V22–27.
175. Beyersdorf F, Sarai K, Maul FD, et al. Immediate functional benefits after controlled reperfusion during surgical revascularization for acute coronary occlusion. *J Thorac Cardiovasc Surg* 1991;102(6):856–866.
176. Rosenkranz ER, Buckberg GD, Laks H, Mulder DG. Warm induction of cardioplegia with glutamate-enriched blood in coronary patients with cardiogenic shock who are dependent on inotropic drugs and intra-aortic balloon support. *J Thorac Cardiovasc Surg* 1983;86(4):507–518.
177. Allen BS, Okamoto F, Buckberg GD, et al. Reperfusion conditions: Critical importance of total ventricular decompression during regional reperfusion. *J Thorac Cardiovasc Surg* 1986;92(3 Pt 2):605–612.
178. Allen BS, Rosenkranz ER, Buckberg GD, et al. High oxygen requirements of dyskinetic cardiac muscle. *J Thorac Cardiovasc Surg* 1986;92(3 Pt 2):543–552.
179. Rosenkranz ER, Vinten-Johansen J, Buckberg GD, et al. Benefits of normothermic induction of blood cardioplegia in energy-depleted hearts, with maintenance of arrest by multidose cold blood cardioplegic infusions. *J Thorac Cardiovasc Surg* 1982;84(5):667–677.
180. Okamoto F, Allen BS, Buckberg GD, et al. Reperfusion conditions: Importance of ensuring gentle versus sudden reperfusion during relief of coronary occlusion. *J Thorac Cardiovasc Surg* 1986;92(3 Pt 2):613–620.
181. Allen BS, Okamoto F, Buckberg GD, et al. Effects of "duration" of reperfusate administration versus reperfusate "dose" on regional functional, biochemical, and histochemical recovery. *J Thorac Cardiovasc Surg* 1986;92(3 Pt 2):594–604.
182. Teoh KH, Christakis GT, Weisel RD, et al. Accelerated myocardial metabolic recovery with terminal warm blood cardioplegia. *J Thorac Cardiovasc Surg* 1986;91(6):888–895.
183. Kirklin JK, McGiffin DC, Pinderski LJ, Tallaj J. Selection of patients and techniques of heart transplantation. *Surg Clin North Am* 2004;84(1):257–287.
184. Kirklin JK, Young JB, McGiffin DC, et al. Mechanical support of the failing heart. In: Kirklin JK, Young JB, McGiffin DC (eds). *Heart Transplantation.* Philadelphia: Churchill Livingstone; 2002:252–289.
185. Dasse KA, Chipman SD, Sherman CN, et al. Clinical experience with textured blood contacting surfaces in ventricular assist devices. *ASAIO Trans* 1987;33(3):418–425.
186. Sergeant P, Meyns B, Wouters P, et al. Long-term outcome after coronary artery bypass grafting in cardiogenic shock or cardiopulmonary resuscitation. *J Thorac Cardiovasc Surg* 2003;126(5):1279–1286.
187. Dion R, Benetis R, Elias B, et al. Mitral valve procedures in ischemic regurgitation. *J Heart Valve Dis* 1995;4(Suppl 2):S124–129; discussion S9–31.
188. Rankin JS, Hickey MS, Smith LR, et al. Ischemic mitral regurgitation. *Circulation* 1989;79(6 Pt 2):I116–121.
189. Izumi S, Miyatake K, Beppu S, et al. Mechanism of mitral regurgitation in patients with myocardial infarction: A study using real-time two-dimensional Doppler flow imaging and echocardiography. *Circulation* 1987;76(4):777–785.
190. Kaul S, Pearlman JD, Touchstone DA, Esquival L. Prevalence and mechanisms of mitral regurgitation in the absence of intrinsic abnormalities of the mitral leaflets. *Am Heart J* 1989;118(5 Pt 1):963–972.
191. Maisel AS, Gilpin EA, Klein L, et al. The murmur of papillary muscle dysfunction in acute myocardial infarction: Clinical features and prognostic implications. *Am Heart J* 1986;112(4):705–711.
192. Barzilai B, Davis VG, Stone PH, Jaffe AS. Prognostic significance of mitral regurgitation in acute myocardial infarction: The MILIS Study Group. *Am J Cardiol* 1990;65(18):1169–1175.
193. Barzilai B, Gessler C Jr, Perez JE, et al. Significance of Doppler-detected mitral regurgitation in acute myocardial infarction. *Am J Cardiol* 1988;61(4):220–223.
194. Bhatnagar SK, al Yusuf AR. Significance of a mitral regurgitation systolic murmur complicating a first acute myocardial infarction in the coronary care unit—assessment by colour Doppler flow imaging. *Eur Heart J* 1991;12(12):1311–1315.
195. Lehmann KG, Francis CK, Dodge HT. Mitral regurgitation in early myocardial infarction: Incidence, clinical detection, and prognostic implications: TIMI Study Group. *Ann Intern Med* 1992;117(1):10–17.
196. Tcheng JE, Jackman JD Jr, Nelson CL, et al. Outcome of patients sustaining acute ischemic mitral regurgitation during myocardial infarction. *Ann Intern Med* 1992;117(1):18–24.
197. O'Connor CM, Hathaway WR, Bates ER, et al. Clinical characteristics and long-term outcome of patients in whom congestive heart failure develops after thrombolytic therapy for acute myocardial infarction: Development of a predictive model. *Am Heart J* 1997;133(6):663–673.
198. Lamas GA, Mitchell GF, Flaker GC, et al. Clinical significance of mitral regurgitation after acute myocardial infarction: Survival and Ventricular Enlargement Investigators. *Circulation* 1997;96(3):827–833.
199. Lehmann KG, Francis CK, Sheehan FH, Dodge HT. Effect of thrombolysis on acute mitral regurgitation during evolving myocardial infarction: Experience from the Thrombolysis in Myocardial Infarction (TIMI) Trial. *J Am Coll Cardiol* 1993;22(3):714–719.

200. Vicente Vera T, Valdes Chavarri M, Garcia Alberola A, et al. Mitral valve insufficiency in acute myocardial infarction: Assessment with pulsed and coded Doppler color. *Arch Inst Cardiol Mex* 1991;61(2):117–121.
201. Ma HH, Honma H, Munakata K, Hayakawa H. Mitral insufficiency as a complication of acute myocardial infarction and left ventricular remodeling. *Jpn Circ J* 1997;61(11):912–920.
202. Alam M, Thorstrand C, Rosenhamer G. Mitral regurgitation following first-time acute myocardial infarction—early and late findings by Doppler echocardiography. *Clin Cardiol* 1993;16(1):30–34.
203. Neskovic AN, Marinkovic J, Bojic M, Popovic AD. Early predictors of mitral regurgitation after acute myocardial infarction. *Am J Cardiol* 1999;84(3):329–332.
204. Van Dantzig JM, Delemarre BJ, Koster RW, et al. Pathogenesis of mitral regurgitation in acute myocardial infarction: Importance of changes in left ventricular shape and regional function. *Am Heart J* 1996;131(5): 865–871.
205. Feinberg MS, Schwammenthal E, Shlizerman L, et al. Prognostic significance of mild mitral regurgitation by color Doppler echocardiography in acute myocardial infarction. *Am J Cardiol* 2000;86(9):903–907.
206. Voci P, Bilotta F, Caretta Q, et al. Papillary muscle perfusion pattern: A hypothesis for ischemic papillary muscle dysfunction. *Circulation* 1995;91(6):1714–1718.
207. Dion R. Ischemic mitral regurgitation: When and how should it be corrected? *J Heart Valve Dis* 1993;2(5): 536–543.
208. Moursi MH, Bhatnagar SK, Vilacosta I, et al. Transesophageal echocardiographic assessment of papillary muscle rupture. *Circulation* 1996;94(5): 1003–1009.
209. Ranganathan N, Burch GE. Gross morphology and arterial supply of the papillary muscles of the left ventricle of man. *Am Heart J* 1969;77(4):506–516.
210. Gillinov AM, Wierup PN, Blackstone EH, et al. Is repair preferable to replacement for ischemic mitral regurgitation? *J Thorac Cardiovasc Surg* 2001;122(6): 1125–1141.
211. Llaneras MR, Nance ML, Streicher JT, et al. Large animal model of ischemic mitral regurgitation. *Ann Thorac Surg* 1994;57(2):432–439.
212. Gorman RC, McCaughan JS, Ratcliffe MB, et al. Pathogenesis of acute ischemic mitral regurgitation in three dimensions. *J Thorac Cardiovasc Surg* 1995;109(4): 684–693.
213. Gorman JH 3rd, Gorman RC, Plappert T, et al. Infarct size and location determine development of mitral regurgitation in the sheep model. *J Thorac Cardiovasc Surg* 1998;115(3):615–622.
214. Nishimura RA, Gersh BJ, Schaff HV. The case for an aggressive surgical approach to papillary muscle rupture following myocardial infarction: "From paradise lost to paradise regained." *Heart* 2000;83(6):611–613.
215. Wei JY, Hutchins GM, Bulkley BH. Papillary muscle rupture in fatal acute myocardial infarction: A potentially treatable form of cardiogenic shock. *Ann Intern Med* 1979;90(2):149–152.
216. Nishimura RA, Schaff HV, Shub C, et al. Papillary muscle rupture complicating acute myocardial infarction: Analysis of 17 patients. *Am J Cardiol* 1983;51(3): 373–377.
217. Sharma SK, Seckler J, Israel DH, et al. Clinical, angiographic and anatomic findings in acute severe ischemic mitral regurgitation. *Am J Cardiol* 1992;70(3): 277–280.
218. Kono T, Sabbah HN, Rosman H, et al. Mechanism of functional mitral regurgitation during acute myocardial ischemia. *J Am Coll Cardiol* 1992;19(5):1101–1105.
219. Lai DT, Tibayan FA, Myrmel T, et al. Mechanistic insights into posterior mitral leaflet inter-scallop malcoaptation during acute ischemic mitral regurgitation. *Circulation* 2002;106(12 Suppl 1):I40–I45.
220. Lai DT, Timek TA, Tibayan FA, et al. The effects of mitral annuloplasty rings on mitral valve complex 3-D geometry during acute left ventricular ischemia. *Eur J Cardiothorac Surg* 2002;22(5):808–816.
221. Gorman JH 3rd, Jackson BM, Gorman RC, et al. Papillary muscle discoordination rather than increased annular area facilitates mitral regurgitation after acute posterior myocardial infarction. *Circulation* 1997; 96(Suppl 9):II-124–127.
222. Glasson JR, Komeda M, Daughters GT, et al. Early systolic mitral leaflet "loitering" during acute ischemic mitral regurgitation. *J Thorac Cardiovasc Surg* 1998; 116(2):193–205.
223. Otsuji Y, Handschumacher MD, Liel-Cohen N, et al. Mechanism of ischemic mitral regurgitation with segmental left ventricular dysfunction: Three-dimensional echocardiographic studies in models of acute and chronic progressive regurgitation. *J Am Coll Cardiol* 2001;37(2):641–648.
224. Hendren WG, Nemec JJ, Lytle BW, et al. Mitral valve repair for ischemic mitral insufficiency. *Ann Thorac Surg* 1991;52(6):1246–1251; discussion 51–52.
225. Roberts WC, Cohen LS. Left ventricular papillary muscles: Description of the normal and a survey of conditions causing them to be abnormal. *Circulation* 1972;46(1):138–154.
226. Messas E, Guerrero JL, Handschumacher MD, et al. Paradoxic decrease in ischemic mitral regurgitation with papillary muscle dysfunction: Insights from three-dimensional and contrast echocardiography with strain rate measurement. *Circulation* 2001;104(16):1952–1957.
227. Kono T, Sabbah HN, Stein PD, et al. Left ventricular shape as a determinant of functional mitral regurgitation in patients with severe heart failure secondary to either coronary artery disease or idiopathic dilated cardiomyopathy. *Am J Cardiol* 1991;68(4):355–359.
228. Godley RW, Wann LS, Rogers EW, et al. Incomplete mitral leaflet closure in patients with papillary muscle dysfunction. *Circulation* 1981;63(3):565–571.
229. Kinney EL, Frangi MJ. Value of two-dimensional echocardiographic detection of incomplete mitral leaflet closure. *Am Heart J* 1985;109(1):87–90.
230. Yiu SF, Enriquez-Sarano M, Tribouilloy C, et al. Determinants of the degree of functional mitral regurgitation in patients with systolic left ventricular dysfunction: A quantitative clinical study. *Circulation* 2000; 102(12):1400–1406.
231. Tibayan FA, Rodriguez F, Zasio MK, et al. Geometric distortions of the mitral valvular-ventricular complex in

chronic ischemic mitral regurgitation. *Circulation* 2003;108(Suppl 1):116–121.
232. Fehrenbacher G, Schmidt DH, Bommer WJ. Evaluation of transient mitral regurgitation in coronary artery disease. *Am J Cardiol* 1991;68(9):868–873.
233. Cosnay P, Fauchier JP, Raynaud P, et al. Paroxysmal mitral insufficiency caused by ischemic dysfunction of the papillary muscles: Apropos of 39 cases [French]. *Arch Mal Coeur Vaiss* 1985;78(1):81–90.
234. Brody W, Criley JM. Intermittent severe mitral regurgitation. *N Engl J Med* 1970;283(13):673–676.
235. Calvo FE, Figueras J, Cortadellas J, Soler-Soler J. Severe mitral regurgitation complicating acute myocardial infarction: Clinical and angiographic differences between patients with and without papillary muscle rupture. *Eur Heart J* 1997;18(10):1606–1610.
236. Birnbaum Y, Chamoun AJ, Conti VR, Uretsky BF. Mitral regurgitation following acute myocardial infarction. *Coron Artery Dis* 2002;13(6):337–344.
237. Schreiber TL, Fisher J, Mangla A, Miller D. Severe "silent" mitral regurgitation: A potentially reversible cause of refractory heart failure. *Chest* 1989;96(2):242–246.
238. Goldman AP, Glover MU, Mick W, et al. Role of echocardiography/Doppler in cardiogenic shock: Silent mitral regurgitation. *Ann Thorac Surg* 1991;52(2): 296–299.
239. Iwasaki K, Matsuo N, Hina K, et al. Transesophageal echocardiography for detection of mitral regurgitation due to papillary muscle rupture or dysfunction associated with acute myocardial infarction: A report of five cases. *Can J Cardiol* 2000;16(10):1273–1277.
240. Figueras J, Calvo F, Cortadellas J, Soler-Soler J. Comparison of patients with and without papillary muscle rupture during acute myocardial infarction. *Am J Cardiol* 1997;80(5):625–627.
241. Hickey MS, Smith LR, Muhlbaier LH, et al. Current prognosis of ischemic mitral regurgitation: Implications for future management. *Circulation* 1988;78(3 Pt 2): I51–59.
242. Desjardins VA, Enriquez-Sarano M, Tajik AJ, et al. Intensity of murmurs correlates with severity of valvular regurgitation. *Am J Med* 1996;100(2):149–156.
243. Iung B. Management of ischaemic mitral regurgitation. *Heart* 2003;89(4):459–464.
244. Ellis SG, Whitlow PL, Raymond RE, Schneider JP. Impact of mitral regurgitation on long-term survival after percutaneous coronary intervention. *Am J Cardiol* 2002;89(3):315–318.
245. Barzilai B, Davis VG, Stone PH, Jaffe AS. Prognostic significance of mitral regurgitation in acute myocardial infarction: The MILIS Study Group. *Am J Cardiol* 1990;65(18):1169–1175.
246. Grigioni F, Enriquez-Sarano M, Zehr KJ, et al. Ischemic mitral regurgitation: Long-term outcome and prognostic implications with quantitative Doppler assessment. *Circulation* 2001;103(13):1759–1764.
247. Dekker AL, Reesink KD, van der Veen FH, et al. Intraaortic balloon pumping in acute mitral regurgitation reduces aortic impedance and regurgitant fraction. *Shock* 2003;19(4):334–338.
248. Cohn LH, Rizzo RJ, Adams DH, et al. The effect of pathophysiology on the surgical treatment of ischemic mitral regurgitation: Operative and late risks of repair versus replacement. *Eur J Cardiothorac Surg* 1995;9(10): 568–574.
249. David TE. Techniques and results of mitral valve repair for ischemic mitral regurgitation. *J Card Surg* 1994; 9(Suppl 2):274–277.
250. Chitwood WRJ. Mitral valve repair: Ischemic. In: Kaiser LR, Kron IL, Spray TL (eds). *Mastery of Cardiothoracic Surgery*. Philadelphia: Lippincott-Raven; 1998:309–321.
251. Bates ER, Califf RM, Stack RS, et al. Thrombolysis and Angioplasty in Myocardial Infarction (TAMI-1) trial: Influence of infarct location on arterial patency, left ventricular function and mortality. *J Am Coll Cardiol* 1989;13(1):12–18.
252. Marino P, Zanolla L, Zardini P. Effect of streptokinase on left ventricular modeling and function after myocardial infarction: The GISSI (Gruppo Italiano per lo Studio della Streptochinasi nell'Infarto Miocardico) Trial. *J Am Coll Cardiol* 1989;14(5):1149–1158.
253. Pfeffer MA, Braunwald E. Ventricular remodeling after myocardial infarction: Experimental observations and clinical implications. *Circulation* 1990;81(4):1161–1172.
254. Le Feuvre C, Metzger JP, Lachurie ML, et al. Treatment of severe mitral regurgitation caused by ischemic papillary muscle dysfunction: Indications for coronary angioplasty. *Am Heart J* 1992;123(4 Pt 1):860–865.
255. Shawl FA, Forman MB, Punja S, Goldbaum TS. Emergent coronary angioplasty in the treatment of acute ischemic mitral regurgitation: Long-term results in five cases. *J Am Coll Cardiol* 1989;14(4):986–991.
256. Heuser RR, Maddoux GL, Goss JE, et al. Coronary angioplasty for acute mitral regurgitation due to myocardial infarction: A nonsurgical treatment preserving mitral valve integrity. *Ann Intern Med* 1987;107(6):852–855.
257. Tatoulis J. Ischemic mitral valve disease: Surgical repair. In: Buxton BF, Frazier OH, Westaby S (eds). *Ischemic Heart Disease Surgical Management*. Philadelphia: Mosby; 1999:306–313.
258. Loisance DY, Deleuze P, Hillion ML, Cachera JP. Are there indications for reconstructive surgery in severe mitral regurgitation after acute myocardial infarction? *Eur J Cardiothorac Surg* 1990;4(7):394–397.
259. Thompson CR, Buller CE, Sleeper LA, et al. Cardiogenic shock due to acute severe mitral regurgitation complicating acute myocardial infarction: A report from the SHOCK Trial Registry: SHould we use emergently revascularize Occluded Coronaries in cardiogenic shocK? *J Am Coll Cardiol* 2000;36(3 Suppl A):1104–1109.
260. Grossi EA, Goldberg JD, LaPietra A, et al. Ischemic mitral valve reconstruction and replacement: Comparison of long-term survival and complications. *J Thorac Cardiovasc Surg* 2001;122(6):1107–1124.
261. Okita Y, Ando M, Minatoya K, et al. Early and long-term results of surgery for aneurysms of the thoracic aorta in septuagenarians and octogenarians. *Eur J Cardiothorac Surg* 1999;16(3):317–323.
262. Hochman JS, Choo H. Limitation of myocardial infarct expansion by reperfusion independent of myocardial salvage. *Circulation* 1987;75(1):299–306.
263. Tepe NA, Edmunds LH Jr. Operation for acute postinfarction mitral insufficiency and cardiogenic shock. *J Thorac Cardiovasc Surg* 1985;89(4):525–530.

264. Byrne JG, Aklog L, Adams DH. Assessment and management of functional or ischaemic mitral regurgitation. *Lancet* 2000;355(9217):1743–1744.
265. Duarte IG, Shen Y, MacDonald MJ, et al. Treatment of moderate mitral regurgitation and coronary disease by coronary bypass alone: Late results. *Ann Thorac Surg* 1999;68(2):426–430.
266. Aklog L, Filsoufi F, Flores KQ, et al. Does coronary artery bypass grafting alone correct moderate ischemic mitral regurgitation? *Circulation* 2001;104(12 Suppl 1): I68–75.
267. Czer LS, Maurer G, Trento A, et al. Comparative efficacy of ring and suture annuloplasty for ischemic mitral regurgitation. *Circulation* 1992;86(Suppl 5):II46–52.
268. Bolling SF, Pagani FD, Deeb GM, Bach DS. Intermediate-term outcome of mitral reconstruction in cardiomyopathy. *J Thorac Cardiovasc Surg* 1998;115(2): 381–386; discussion 7–8.
269. Komeda M, Glasson JR, Miller DC. Pathophysiologic geometry of the mitral apparatus during ischemic mitral regurgitation—rationale toward a more anatomic repair. In: Buxton BF, Frazier OH, Westaby S (eds). *Ischemic Heart Disease Surgical Management*. Philadelphia: Mosby; 1999:303–306.
270. Gillinov AM, Cosgrove DM, Blackstone EH, et al. Durability of mitral valve repair for degenerative disease. *J Thorac Cardiovasc Surg* 1998;116(5):734–743.
271. Reichert SL, Visser CA, Moulijn AC, et al. Intraoperative transesophageal color-coded Doppler echocardiography for evaluation of residual regurgitation after mitral valve repair. *J Thorac Cardiovasc Surg* 1990;100(5):756–761.
272. Saiki Y, Kasegawa H, Kawase M, et al. Intraoperative TEE during mitral valve repair: Does it predict early and late postoperative mitral valve dysfunction? *Ann Thorac Surg* 1998;66(4):1277–1281.
273. Fix J, Isada L, Cosgrove D, et al. Do patients with less than "echo-perfect" results from mitral valve repair by intraoperative echocardiography have a different outcome? *Circulation* 1993;88(5 Pt 2):II39–48.
274. Dahlberg PS, Orszulak TA, Mullany CJ, et al. Late outcome of mitral valve surgery for patients with coronary artery disease. *Ann Thorac Surg* 2003;76(5):1539–1587; discussion 47–48.
275. Agricola E, Oppizzi M, Maisano F, et al. Detection of mechanisms of immediate failure by transesophageal echocardiography in quadrangular resection mitral valve repair technique for severe mitral regurgitation. *Am J Cardiol* 2003;91(2):175–179.
276. Koch CG, Milas BL, Savino JS. What does transesophageal echocardiography add to valvular heart surgery? *Anesthesiol Clin North America* 2003;21(3): 587–611.
277. Sheikh KH, de Bruijn NP, Rankin JS, et al. The utility of transesophageal echocardiography and Doppler color flow imaging in patients undergoing cardiac valve surgery. *J Am Coll Cardiol* 1990;15(2):363–372.
278. Milas BL, Bavaria JE, Koch CG, Troianos CA. Case 8-2001: Resolution of systolic anterior motion after mitral valve repair with atrial pacing. *J Cardiothorac Vasc Anesth* 2001;15(5):641–648.
279. Schiavone WA, Cosgrove DM, Lever HM, et al. Long-term follow-up of patients with left ventricular outflow tract obstruction after Carpentier ring mitral valvuloplasty. *Circulation* 1988;78(3 Pt 2):I60–65.
280. Grossi EA, Galloway AC, Parish MA, et al. Experience with twenty-eight cases of systolic anterior motion after mitral valve reconstruction by the Carpentier technique. *J Thorac Cardiovasc Surg* 1992;103(3):466–470.
281. Jebara VA, Mihaileanu S, Acar C, et al. Left ventricular outflow tract obstruction after mitral valve repair: Results of the sliding leaflet technique. *Circulation* 1993;88(5 Pt 2):II30–34.
282. Perier P, Clausnizer B, Mistarz K. Carpentier "sliding leaflet" technique for repair of the mitral valve: Early results. *Ann Thorac Surg* 1994;57(2):383–386.
283. Charls LM. SAM—systolic anterior motion of the anterior mitral valve leaflet post-surgical mitral valve repair. *Heart Lung* 2003;32(6):402–406.
284. Liel-Cohen N, Guerrero JL, Otsuji Y, et al. Design of a new surgical approach for ventricular remodeling to relieve ischemic mitral regurgitation: Insights from 3-dimensional echocardiography. *Circulation* 2000;101(23):2756–2763.
285. Messas E, Pouzet B, Touchot B, et al. Efficacy of chordal cutting to relieve chronic persistent ischemic mitral regurgitation. *Circulation* 2003;108(Suppl 1):II111–115.
286. Clements SD Jr, Story WE, Hurst JW, et al. Ruptured papillary muscle, a complication of myocardial infarction: Clinical presentation, diagnosis, and treatment. *Clin Cardiol* 1985;8(2):93–103.
287. Panos A, Christakis GT, Lichtenstein SV, et al. Operation for acute postinfarction mitral insufficiency using continuous oxygenated blood cardioplegia. *Ann Thorac Surg* 1989;48(6):816–819.
288. Tavakoli R, Weber A, Vogt P, et al. Surgical management of acute mitral valve regurgitation due to postinfarction papillary muscle rupture. *J Heart Valve Dis* 2002;11(1): 20–25; discussion 6.
289. Thourani VH, Weintraub WS, Craver JM, et al. Influence of concomitant CABG and urgent/emergent status on mitral valve replacement surgery. *Ann Thorac Surg* 2000;70(3):778–783; discussion 83–84.
290. Gillinov AM, Faber C, Houghtaling PL, et al. Repair versus replacement for degenerative mitral valve disease with coexisting ischemic heart disease. *J Thorac Cardiovasc Surg* 2003;125(6):1350–1362.
291. Lytle BW. Impact of coronary artery disease on valvular heart surgery. *Cardiol Clin* 1991;9(2):301–314.
292. Angell WW, Pupello DF, Bessone LN, et al. Influence of coronary artery disease on structural deterioration of porcine bioprostheses. *Ann Thorac Surg* 1995;60(Suppl 2):S276–281.
293. Christakis GT, Weisel RD, David TE, et al. Predictors of operative survival after valve replacement. *Circulation* 1988;78(3 Pt 2):I25–34.
294. Angell WW, Oury JH, Shah P. A comparison of replacement and reconstruction in patients with mitral regurgitation. *J Thorac Cardiovasc Surg* 1987;93(5):665–674.
295. Oury JH, Cleveland JC, Duran CG, Angell WW. Ischemic mitral valve disease: Classification and systemic approach to management. *J Card Surg* 1994;9(Suppl 2):262–273.
296. Tahta SA, Oury JH, Maxwell JM, et al. Outcome after mitral valve repair for functional ischemic mitral regurgitation. *J Heart Valve Dis* 2002;11(1):11–18; discussion 8–9.

297. Latham PM. Lectures on Subjects Connected with Clinical Medicine Comprising Diseases of the Heart. London: Longman Rees; 1845.
298. Brunn F. Diagnostik der erworbenen ruptur der kammerscheidewand des herzens. *Wien Arch Inn Med* 1923;6:533.
299. Cooley DA, Belmonte BA, Zeis LB, Schnur S. Surgical repair of ruptured interventricular septum following acute myocardial infarction. *Surgery* 1957;41:930.
300. Pohjola-Sintonen S, Muller JE, Stone PH, et al. Ventricular septal and free wall rupture complicating acute myocardial infarction: Experience in the Multicenter Investigation of Limitation of Infarct Size. *Am Heart J* 1989;117(4):809–818.
301. Moore CA, Nygaard TW, Kaiser DL, et al. Postinfarction ventricular septal rupture: The importance of location of infarction and right ventricular function in determining survival. *Circulation* 1986;74(1):45–55.
302. Crenshaw BS, Granger CB, Birnbaum Y, et al. Risk factors, angiographic patterns, and outcomes in patients with ventricular septal defect complicating acute myocardial infarction: GUSTO-I (Global Utilization of Streptokinase and TPA for Occluded Coronary Arteries) Trial Investigators. *Circulation* 2000;101(1):27–32.
303. Lemery R, Smith HC, Giuliani ER, Gersh BJ. Prognosis in rupture of the ventricular septum after acute myocardial infarction and role of early surgical intervention. *Am J Cardiol* 1992;70(2):147–151.
304. Hutchins GM. Rupture of the interventricular septum complicating myocardial infarction: Pathological analysis of 10 patients with clinically diagnosed perforations. *Am Heart J* 1979;97(2):165–173.
305. Cummings RG, Reimer KA, Califf R, et al. Quantitative analysis of right and left ventricular infarction in the presence of postinfarction ventricular septal defect. *Circulation* 1988;77(1):33–42.
306. Skehan JD, Carey C, Norrell MS, et al. Patterns of coronary artery disease in postinfarction ventricular septal rupture. *Br Heart J* 1989;62(4):268–272.
307. Menon V, Webb JG, Hillis LD, et al. Outcome and profile of ventricular septal rupture with cardiogenic shock after myocardial infarction: A report from the SHOCK Trial Registry: SHould we emergently revascularize Occluded Coronaries in cardiogenic shocK? *J Am Coll Cardiol* 2000;36(3 Suppl A):1110–1116.
308. Edwards BS, Edwards WD, Edwards JE. Ventricular septal rupture complicating acute myocardial infarction: Identification of simple and complex types in 53 autopsied hearts. *Am J Cardiol* 1984;54(10):1201–1205.
309. Radford MJ, Johnson RA, Daggett WM Jr, et al. Ventricular septal rupture: A review of clinical and physiologic features and an analysis of survival. *Circulation* 1981;64(3):545–553.
310. Mann JM, Roberts WC. Acquired ventricular septal defect during acute myocardial infarction: Analysis of 38 unoperated necropsy patients and comparison with 50 unoperated necropsy patients without rupture. *Am J Cardiol* 1988;62(1):8–19.
311. Figueras J, Cortadellas J, Soler-Soler J. Comparison of ventricular septal and left ventricular free wall rupture in acute myocardial infarction. *Am J Cardiol* 1998;81(4):495–497.
312. Pretre R, Rickli H, Ye Q, et al. Frequency of collateral blood flow in the infarct-related coronary artery in rupture of the ventricular septum after acute myocardial infarction. *Am J Cardiol* 2000;85(4):497–499.
313. Agnihotri AK, Madsen JC, Daggett WM. Surgical treatment for complications of acute myocardial infarction: Postinfarction ventricular septal defect and free wall rupture. In: Cohn LH, Edmunds LH Jr (eds). *Cardiac Surgery in the Adult.* New York: McGraw-Hill; 2003:681–714.
314. Birnbaum Y, Fishbein MC, Blanche C, Siegel RJ. Ventricular septal rupture after acute myocardial infarction. *N Engl J Med* 2002;347(18):1426–1432.
315. Miller SW, Dinsmore RE, Greene RE, Daggett WM. Coronary, ventricular, and pulmonary abnormalities associated with rupture of the interventricular septum complicating myocardial infarction. *AJR Am J Roentgenol* 1978;131(4):571–577.
316. Topaz O, Taylor AL. Interventricular septal rupture complicating acute myocardial infarction: From pathophysiologic features to the role of invasive and noninvasive diagnostic modalities in current management. *Am J Med* 1992;93(6):683–688.
317. Shapira I, Isakov A, Burke M, Almog C. Cardiac rupture in patients with acute myocardial infarction. *Chest* 1987;92(2):219–223.
318. Oskoui R, Van Voorhees LB, DiBianco R, et al. Timing of ventricular septal rupture after acute myocardial infarction and its relation to thrombolytic therapy. *Am J Cardiol* 1996;78(8):953–955.
319. Massetti M, Babatasi G, Le Page O, et al. Postinfarction ventricular septal rupture: Early repair through the right atrial approach. *J Thorac Cardiovasc Surg* 2000;119 (4 Pt 1):784–789.
320. Pretre R, Ye Q, Grunenfelder J, et al. Operative results of "repair" of ventricular septal rupture after acute myocardial infarction. *Am J Cardiol* 1999;84(7): 785–788.
321. Daggett WM, Buckley MJ, Akins CW, et al. Improved results of surgical management of postinfarction ventricular septal rupture. *Ann Surg* 1982;196(3):269–277.
322. Smyllie JH, Sutherland GR, Geuskens R, et al. Doppler color flow mapping in the diagnosis of ventricular septal rupture and acute mitral regurgitation after myocardial infarction. *J Am Coll Cardiol* 1990;15(6):1449–1455.
323. Amico A, Iliceto S, Rizzo A, et al. Color Doppler findings in ventricular septal dissection following myocardial infarction. *Am Heart J* 1989;117(1):195–198.
324. Gowda KS, Loh CW, Roberts R. The simultaneous occurrence of a ventricular septal defect and mitral insufficiency after myocardial infarction. *Am Heart J* 1976;92(2): 234–236.
325. Meister SG, Helfant RH. Rapid bedside differentiation of ruptured interventricular septum from acute mitral insufficiency. *N Engl J Med* 1972;287(20):1024–1025.
326. Smyllie JH, Sutherland GR, Geuskens R, et al. Doppler color flow mapping in the diagnosis of ventricular septal rupture and acute mitral regurgitation after myocardial infarction. *J Am Coll Cardiol* 1990;15(6):1449–1455.
327. Fortin DF, Sheikh KH, Kisslo J. The utility of echocardiography in the diagnostic strategy of postinfarction ventricular septal rupture: A comparison of two-dimensional

echocardiography versus Doppler color flow imaging. *Am Heart J* 1991;121(1 Pt 1):25–32.
328. Blanche C, Khan SS, Matloff JM, et al. Results of early repair of ventricular septal defect after an acute myocardial infarction. *J Thorac Cardiovasc Surg* 1992;104(4): 961–965.
329. Thiele H, Lauer B, Hambrecht R, et al. Short- and long-term hemodynamic effects of intra-aortic balloon support in ventricular septal defect complicating acute myocardial infarction. *Am J Cardiol* 2003;92(4): 450–454.
330. Payne WS, Hunt JC, Kirklin JW. Surgical repair of ventricular septal defect due to myocardial infarction: Report of a case. *JAMA* 1963;183:603.
331. Effler DB, Tapia FA, McCormack LJ. Rupture of the ventricular myocardium and perforation of the interventricular septum complicating acute myocardial infarction. *Circulation* 1959;20:128.
332. Daggett WM, Guyton RA, Mundth ED, et al. Surgery for post-myocardial infarct ventricular septal defect. *Ann Surg* 1977;186(3):260–271.
333. Deville C, Fontan F, Chevalier JM, et al. Surgery of postinfarction ventricular septal defect: Risk factors for hospital death and long-term results. *Eur J Cardiothorac Surg* 1991;5(4):167–174; discussion 75.
334. Sanders RJ, Kern WH, Blount SG Jr. Perforation of the interventricular septum complicating myocardial infarction: A report of eight cases, one with cardiac catheterization. *Am Heart J* 1956;51(5):736–748.
335. Ryan TJ, Antman EM, Brooks NH, et al. 1999 update: ACC/AHA guidelines for the management of patients with acute myocardial infarction: A report of the American College of Cardiology/American Heart Association Task Force on Practice Guidelines (Committee on Management of Acute Myocardial Infarction). *J Am Coll Cardiol* 1999;34(3):890–911.
336. Barker TA, Ramnarine IR, Woo EB, et al. Repair of post-infarct ventricular septal defect with or without coronary artery bypass grafting in the northwest of England: A 5-year multi-institutional experience. *Eur J Cardiothorac Surg* 2003;24(6):940–946.
337. Baillot R, Pelletier C, Trivino-Marin J, Castonguay Y. Postinfarction ventricular septal defect: Delayed closure with prolonged mechanical circulatory support. *Ann Thorac Surg* 1983;35(2):138–142.
338. Heimbecker RO, Lemire G, Chen C. Surgery for massive myocardial infarction: An experimental study of emergency infarctectomy with a preliminary report on the clinical application. *Circulation* 1968;37(Suppl 4):II3–11.
339. Daggett WM, Burwell LR, Lawson DW, Austen WG. Resection of acute ventricular aneurysm and ruptured interventricular septum after myocardial infarction. *N Engl J Med* 1970;283(27):1507–1508.
340. Seguin JR, Frapier JM, Colson P, Chaptal PA. Fibrin sealant for early repair of acquired ventricular septal defect. *J Thorac Cardiovasc Surg* 1992;104(3):748–751.
341. Musumeci F, Shukla V, Mignosa C, et al. Early repair of postinfarction ventricular septal defect with gelatin-resorcin-formol biological glue. *Ann Thorac Surg* 1996;62(2):486–488.
342. Tanaka H, Hasegawa S, Sakamoto T, Sunamori M. Postinfarction ventricular septal perforation repair with endoventricular circular patch plasty using double patches and gelatin-resorcinol-formaldehyde biological glue. *Eur J Cardiothorac Surg* 2001;19(6):945–948.
343. Hata M, Shiono M, Orime Y, et al. Pathological findings of tissue reactivity of gelatin resorcin formalin glue: An autopsy case report of the repair of ventricular septal perforation. *Ann Thorac Cardiovasc Surg* 2000;6(2): 127–129.
344. Da Silva JP, Cascudo MM, Baumgratz JF, et al. Postinfarction ventricular septal defect: An efficacious technique for early surgical repair. *J Thorac Cardiovasc Surg* 1989;97(1):86–89.
345. Lachapelle K, deVarennes B, Ergina PL, et al. Sutureless patch technique for postinfarction left ventricular rupture. *Ann Thorac Surg* 2002;74(1):96–101.
346. Cummings RG, Califf R, Jones RN, et al. Correlates of survival in patients with postinfarction ventricular septal defect. *Ann Thorac Surg* 1989;47(6):824–830.
347. David TE, Dale L, Sun Z. Postinfarction ventricular septal rupture: Repair by endocardial patch with infarct exclusion. *J Thorac Cardiovasc Surg* 1995;110(5):1315–1322.
348. De Boer HD, de Boer WJ. Early repair of postinfarction ventricular septal rupture: Infarct exclusion, septal stabilization, and left ventricular remodeling. *Ann Thorac Surg* 1998;65(3):853–854.
349. Cooley DA. Repair of the difficult ventriculotomy. *Ann Thorac Surg* 1990;49(1):150–151.
350. Cooley DA. Repair of postinfarction ventricular septal defect. *J Card Surg* 1994;9(4):427–429.
351. Alvarez JM, Brady PW, Ross DE. Technical improvements in the repair of acute postinfarction ventricular septal rupture. *J Card Surg* 1992;7(3):198–202.
352. David TE. Ventricular septal rupture: Repair by infarct exclusion. In: Buxton BF, Frazier OH, Westaby S (eds). *Ischemic Heart Disease Surgical Management.* London: Mosby; 1999:298–302.
353. Tabuchi N, Tanaka H, Arai H, et al. Double-patch technique for postinfarction ventricular septal perforation. *Ann Thorac Surg* 2004;77(1):342–343.
354. Cox FF, Plokker HW, Morshuis WJ, et al. Importance of coronary revascularization for late survival after postinfarction ventricular septal rupture: A reason to perform coronary angiography prior to surgery. *Eur Heart J* 1996;17(12):1841–1845.
355. Labrousse L, Choukroun E, Chevalier JM, et al. Surgery for post infarction ventricular septal defect (VSD): Risk factors for hospital death and long term results. *Eur J Cardiothorac Surg* 2002;21(4):725–732.
356. Deja MA, Szostek J, Widenka K, et al. Post infarction ventricular septal defect—can we do better? *Eur J Cardiothorac Surg* 2000;18(2):194–201.
357. Leavey S, Galvin J, McCann H, Sugrue D. Post-myocardial infarction ventricular septal defect: An angiographic study. *Ir J Med Sci* 1994;163(4):182–183.
358. Dalrymple-Hay MJ, Langley SM, Sami SA, et al. Should coronary artery bypass grafting be performed at the same time as repair of a post-infarct ventricular septal defect? *Eur J Cardiothorac Surg* 1998;13(3):286–292.
359. Muehrcke DD, Daggett WM Jr, Buckley MJ, et al. Postinfarct ventricular septal defect repair: Effect of coronary artery bypass grafting. *Ann Thorac Surg* 1992;54(5):876–882; discussion 82–83.

360. Lee EM, Roberts DH, Walsh KP. Transcatheter closure of a residual postmyocardial infarction ventricular septal defect with the Amplatzer septal occluder. *Heart* 1998;80(5):522–524.
361. Lowe HC, Jang IK, Yoerger DM, et al. Compassionate use of the amplatzer ASD closure device for residual postinfarction ventricular septal rupture following surgical repair. *Catheter Cardiovasc Interv* 2003;59(2): 230–233; discussion 4.
362. Goldstein JA, Casserly IP, Balzer DT, et al. Transcatheter closure of recurrent postmyocardial infarction ventricular septal defects utilizing the Amplatzer postinfarction VSD device: A case series. *Catheter Cardiovasc Interv* 2003; 59(2):238–243.
363. Mullasari AS, Umesan CV, Krishnan U, et al. Transcatheter closure of post-myocardial infarction ventricular septal defect with Amplatzer septal occluder. *Catheter Cardiovasc Interv* 2001;54(4):484–487.
364. Pesonen E, Thilen U, Sandstrom S, et al. Transcatheter closure of postinfarction ventricular septal defect with the Amplatzer septal occluder device. *Scand Cardiovasc J* 2000;34(4):446–448.
365. Landzberg MJ, Lock JE. Transcatheter management of ventricular septal rupture after myocardial infarction. *Semin Thorac Cardiovasc Surg* 1998;10(2):128–132.
366. Pienvichit P, Piemonte TC. Percutaneous closure of postmyocardial infarction ventricular septal defect with the CardioSEAL septal occluder implant. *Catheter Cardiovasc Interv* 2001;54(4):490–494.
367. Faber C, McCarthy PM, Smedira NG, et al. Implantable left ventricular assist device for patients with postinfarction ventricular septal defect. *J Thorac Cardiovasc Surg* 2002;124(2):400–401.
368. Kuhn LA. Management of shock following acute myocardial infarction: I. Drug therapy. *Am Heart J* 1978;95(4):529–534.
369. Lowe JE, Gall SA Jr. (As originally published in 1989.) Correlates of survival in patients with postinfarction ventricular septal defect. *Ann Thorac Surg* 1997;63(5): 1508–1509.
370. Killen DA, Piehler JM, Borkon AM, et al. Early repair of postinfarction ventricular septal rupture. *Ann Thorac Surg* 1997;63(1):138–142.
371. Pretre R, Ye Q, Grunenfelder J, et al. Role of myocardial revascularization in postinfarction ventricular septal rupture. *Ann Thorac Surg* 2000;69(1):51–55.
372. Skillington PD, Davies RH, Luff AJ, et al. Surgical treatment for infarct-related ventricular septal defects: Improved early results combined with analysis of late functional status. *J Thorac Cardiovasc Surg* 1990;99(5):798–808.
373. Cox FF, Morshuis WJ, Plokker HW, et al. Early mortality after surgical repair of postinfarction ventricular septal rupture: Importance of rupture location. *Ann Thorac Surg* 1996;61(6):1752–1757; discussion 7–8.
374. Jones MT, Schofield PM, Dark JF, et al. Surgical repair of acquired ventricular septal defect: Determinants of early and late outcome. *J Thorac Cardiovasc Surg* 1987;93(5):680–686.
375. Zehender M, Kasper W, Kauder E, et al. Right ventricular infarction as an independent predictor of prognosis after acute inferior myocardial infarction. *N Engl J Med* 1993;328(14):981–988.
376. Cooley DA. Postinfarction ventricular septal rupture. *Semin Thorac Cardiovasc Surg* 1998;10(2):100–104.
377. Skillington PD, Davies RH, Luff AJ, et al. Surgical treatment for infarct-related ventricular septal defects: Improved early results combined with analysis of late functional status. *J Thorac Cardiovasc Surg* 1990;99(5): 798–808.
378. Pretre R, Benedikt P, Turina MI. Experience with postinfarction left ventricular free wall rupture. *Ann Thorac Surg* 2000;69(5):1342–1345.
379. Davies MJ. Aortic aneurysm formation: Lessons from human studies and experimental models. *Circulation* 1998;98(3):193–195.
380. Morgagni JB. *The Seat and Causes of Disease Investigated by Anatomy.* London: A. Millau & T. Cadell; 1769.
381. Malmsten HB, Duben GWJ. *Case of Rupture of the Heart.* Dublin, Ireland: Medical Press; 1861.
382. Winsor F. Angina pectoris with rupture of the heart: Extracts from the records of the Middlesex East District Medical Society. *Boston Med Search J* 1880;103: 398–400.
383. Steven JL. Cases of spontaneous rupture of the heart and remarks on the pathology of the condition. *Glasgow Med J* 1884;22:412–427.
384. Krumbhaar EB, Crowell C. Spontaneous rupture of the heart: A clinical pathologic study based on 22 unpublished cases and 632 from the literature. *Am J Med Sci* 1925;170:828–856.
385. Hatcher CR Jr, Mansour K, Logan WD Jr, et al. Surgical complications of myocardial infarction. *Am Surg* 1970;36(3):163–170.
386. FitzGibbon GM, Hooper GD, Heggtveit HA. Successful surgical treatment of postinfarction external cardiac rupture. *J Thorac Cardiovasc Surg* 1972;63(4):622–630.
387. Montegut FJ Jr. Left ventricular rupture secondary to myocardial infarction: Report of survival with surgical repair. *Ann Thorac Surg* 1972;14(1):75–78.
388. Becker RC, Gore JM, Lambrew C, et al. A composite view of cardiac rupture in the United States National Registry of Myocardial Infarction. *J Am Coll Cardiol* 1996;27(6):1321–1326.
389. Becker RC, Charlesworth A, Wilcox RG, et al. Cardiac rupture associated with thrombolytic therapy: Impact of time to treatment in the Late Assessment of Thrombolytic Efficacy (LATE) study. *J Am Coll Cardiol* 1995;25(5):1063–1068.
390. Veinot JP, Walley VM, Wolfsohn AL, et al. Postinfarct cardiac free wall rupture: The relationship of rupture site to papillary muscle insertion. *Mod Pathol* 1995;8(6): 609–613.
391. Batts KP, Ackermann DM, Edwards WD. Postinfarction rupture of the left ventricular free wall: Clinicopathologic correlates in 100 consecutive autopsy cases. *Hum Pathol* 1990;21(5):530–535.
392. Cheriex EC, de Swart H, Dijkman LW, et al. Myocardial rupture after myocardial infarction is related to the perfusion status of the infarct-related coronary artery. *Am Heart J* 1995;129(4):644–650.
393. Perdigao C, Andrade A, Ribeiro C. [Cardiac rupture in acute myocardial infarction: Various clinico-anatomical types in 42 recent cases observed over a period of 30 months]. *Arch Mal Coeur Vaiss* 1987;80(3):336–344.

394. Becker AE, van Mantgem JP. Cardiac tamponade: A study of 50 hearts. *Eur J Cardiol* 1975;3(4):349–358.
395. O'Rourke MF. Subacute heart rupture following myocardial infarction: Clinical features of a correctable condition. *Lancet* 1973;2(7821):124–126.
396. Yeo TC, Malouf JF, Oh JK, Seward JB. Clinical profile and outcome in 52 patients with cardiac pseudoaneurysm. *Ann Intern Med* 1998;128(4):299–305.
397. Eaton LW, Weiss JL, Bulkley BH, et al. Regional cardiac dilatation after acute myocardial infarction: Recognition by two-dimensional echocardiography. *N Engl J Med* 1979;300(2):57–62.
398. Heymans S, Luttun A, Nuyens D, et al. Inhibition of plasminogen activators or matrix metalloproteinases prevents cardiac rupture but impairs therapeutic angiogenesis and causes cardiac failure. *Nat Med* 1999;5(10): 1135–1142.
399. Hayashidani S, Tsutsui H, Ikeuchi M, et al. Targeted deletion of MMP-2 attenuates early LV rupture and late remodeling after experimental myocardial infarction. *Am J Physiol Heart Circ Physiol* 2003;285(3):H1229–1235.
400. Becker RC, Hochman JS, Cannon CP, et al. Fatal cardiac rupture among patients treated with thrombolytic agents and adjunctive thrombin antagonists: Observations from the Thrombolysis and Thrombin Inhibition in Myocardial Infarction 9 Study. *J Am Coll Cardiol* 1999;33(2):479–487.
401. Sugiura T, Nagahama Y, Nakamura S, et al. Left ventricular free wall rupture after reperfusion therapy for acute myocardial infarction. *Am J Cardiol* 2003;92(3): 282–284.
402. Hutchins KD, Skurnick J, Lavenhar M, Natarajan GA. Cardiac rupture in acute myocardial infarction: A reassessment. *Am J Forensic Med Pathol* 2002;23(1): 78–82.
403. Dellborg M, Held P, Swedberg K, Vedin A. Rupture of the myocardium: Occurrence and risk factors. *Br Heart J* 1985;54(1):11–16.
404. Oblath RW, Levinson DC, Griffith GC. Factors influencing rupture of the heart after myocardial infarction. *JAMA* 1952;119(14):1276–1281.
405. Figueras J, Juncal A, Carballo J, et al. Nature and progression of pericardial effusion in patients with a first myocardial infarction: Relationship to age and free wall rupture. *Am Heart J* 2002;144(2):251–258.
406. London RE, London SB. Rupture of the heart: A critical analysis of 47 consecutive autopsy cases. *Circulation* 1965;31:202–208.
407. Friedman HS, Kuhn LA, Katz AM. Clinical and electrocardiographic features of cardiac rupture following acute myocardial infarction. *Am J Med* 1971;50(6):709–720.
408. Bates RJ, Beutler S, Resnekov L, Anagnostopoulos CE. Cardiac rupture—challenge in diagnosis and management. *Am J Cardiol* 1977;40(3):429–437.
409. Rasmussen S, Leth A, Kjoller E, Pedersen A. Cardiac rupture in acute myocardial infarction: A review of 72 consecutive cases. *Acta Med Scand* 1979;205(1–2): 11–16.
410. Yip HK, Wu CJ, Chang HW, et al. Cardiac rupture complicating acute myocardial infarction in the direct percutaneous coronary intervention reperfusion era. *Chest* 2003;124(2):565–571.
411. Lopez-Sendon J, Gonzalez A, Lopez de Sa E, et al. Diagnosis of subacute ventricular wall rupture after acute myocardial infarction: Sensitivity and specificity of clinical, hemodynamic and echocardiographic criteria. *J Am Coll Cardiol* 1992;19(6):1145–1153.
412. Figueras J, Cortadellas J, Soler-Soler J. Left ventricular free wall rupture: Clinical presentation and management. *Heart* 2000;83(5):499–504.
413. Feneley MP, Chang VP, O'Rourke MF. Myocardial rupture after acute myocardial infarction: Ten year review. *Br Heart J* 1983;49(6):550–556.
414. Pollak H, Diez W, Spiel R, et al. Early diagnosis of subacute free wall rupture complicating acute myocardial infarction. *Eur Heart J* 1993;14(5):640–648.
415. Purcaro A, Costantini C, Ciampani N, et al. Diagnostic criteria and management of subacute ventricular free wall rupture complicating acute myocardial infarction. *Am J Cardiol* 1997;80(4):397–405.
416. Ennix CL Jr, Ecker RR, Iverson LI, et al. Early detection and management of left ventricular free wall rupture during acute myocardial infarction. *Am J Cardiol* 1989;63(1): 151–152.
417. Carey JS, Cukingnan RA, Eugene J. Myocardial rupture in expanded infarcts: Repair using pericardial patch. *Clin Cardiol* 1989;12(3):157–160.
418. Kendall RW, DeWood MA. Postinfarction cardiac rupture: Surgical success and review of the literature. *Ann Thorac Surg* 1978;25(4):311–315.
419. Zahger D, Milgalter E, Pollak A, et al. Left ventricular free wall rupture as the presenting manifestation of acute myocardial infarction in diabetic patients. *Am J Cardiol* 1996;78(6):681–682.
420. Figueras J, Cortadellas J, Domingo E, Soler-Soler J. Survival following self-limited left ventricular free wall rupture during myocardial infarction: Management differences between patients with or without pseudoaneurysm formation. *Int J Cardiol* 2001;79(2–3): 103 111; discussion 11–12.
421. Van Tassel RA, Edwards JE. Rupture of heart complicating myocardial infarction: Analysis of 40 cases including nine examples of left ventricular false aneurysm. *Chest* 1972;61(2):104–116.
422. Davidson KH, Parisi AF, Harrington JJ, et al. Pseudoaneurysm of the left ventricle: An unusual echocardiographic presentation: Review of the literature. *Ann Intern Med* 1977;86(4):430–433.
423. Vlodaver Z, Coe JI, Edwards JE. True and false left ventricular aneurysms: Propensity for the latter to rupture. *Circulation* 1975;51(3):567–572.
424. Moreno R, Gordillo E, Zamorano J, et al. Long term outcome of patients with postinfarction left ventricular pseudoaneurysm. *Heart* 2003;89(10):1144–1146.
425. Natarajan MK, Salerno TA, Burke B, et al. Chronic false aneurysms of the left ventricle: Management revisited. *Can J Cardiol* 1994;10(9):927–931.
426. Touchstone DA, Beller GA, Nygaard TW, et al. Effects of successful intravenous reperfusion therapy on regional myocardial function and geometry in humans: A tomographic assessment using two-dimensional echocardiography. *J Am Coll Cardiol* 1989;13(7):1506–1513.
427. Brodie BR, Stuckey TD, Hansen C, Muncy D. Benefit of coronary reperfusion before intervention on outcomes

after primary angioplasty for acute myocardial infarction. *Am J Cardiol* 2000;85(1):13–18.

428. Peuhkurinen KJ, Risteli L, Melkko JT, et al. Thrombolytic therapy with streptokinase stimulates collagen breakdown. *Circulation* 1991;83(6):1969–1975.
429. Yasuno M, Endo S, Takahashi M, et al. Angiographic and pathologic evidence of hemorrhage into the myocardium after coronary reperfusion. *Angiology* 1984;35(12):797–801.
430. Richardson SG, Allen DC, Morton P, et al. Pathological changes after intravenous streptokinase treatment in eight patients with acute myocardial infarction. *Br Heart J* 1989;61(5):390–395.
431. Honan MB, Harrell FE Jr, Reimer KA, et al. Cardiac rupture, mortality and the timing of thrombolytic therapy: A meta-analysis. *J Am Coll Cardiol* 1990;16(2): 359–367.
432. Kinn JW, O'Neill WW, Benzuly KH, et al. Primary angioplasty reduces risk of myocardial rupture compared to thrombolysis for acute myocardial infarction. *Catheter Cardiovasc Diagn* 1997;42(2):151–157.
433. Solodky A, Behar S, Herz I, et al. Comparison of incidence of cardiac rupture among patients with acute myocardial infarction treated by thrombolysis versus percutaneous transluminal coronary angioplasty. *Am J Cardiol* 2001;87(9):1105–1108.
434. Moreno R, Lopez-Sendon J, Garcia E, et al. Primary angioplasty reduces the risk of left ventricular free wall rupture compared with thrombolysis in patients with acute myocardial infarction. *J Am Coll Cardiol* 2002;39(4):598–603.
435. Birnbaum Y, Chamoun AJ, Anzuini A, et al. Ventricular free wall rupture following acute myocardial infarction. *Coron Artery Dis* 2003;14(6):463–470.
436. Oliva PB, Hammill SC, Edwards WD. Cardiac rupture, a clinically predictable complication of acute myocardial infarction: Report of 70 cases with clinicopathologic correlations. *J Am Coll Cardiol* 1993;22(3):720–726.
437. Wehrens XH, Doevendans PA, Widdershoven JW, et al. Usefulness of sinus tachycardia and ST-segment elevation in V(5) to identify impending left ventricular free wall rupture in inferior wall myocardial infarction. *Am J Cardiol* 2001;88(4):414–417.
438. Yoshino H, Yotsukura M, Yano K, et al. Cardiac rupture and admission electrocardiography in acute anterior myocardial infarction: Implication of ST elevation in aVL. *J Electrocardiol* 2000;33(1):49–54.
439. Abel RM, Buckley MJ, Friedlich AL, Austen WG. Survival following free rupture of left ventricular aneurysm: Report of a case. *Ann Thorac Surg* 1976;21(2):175–179.
440. Wunderink RG. Incidence of pericardial effusions in acute myocardial infarctions. *Chest* 1984;85(4): 494–496.
441. Martin RP, Bowden R, Filly K, Popp RL. Intrapericardial abnormalities in patients with pericardial effusion: Findings by two-dimensional echocardiography. *Circulation* 1980;61(3):568–572.
442. Waggoner AD, Williams GA, Gaffron D, Schwarze M. Potential utility of left heart contrast agents in diagnosis of myocardial rupture by 2-dimensional echocardiography. *J Am Soc Echocardiogr* 1999;12(4): 272–274.
443. Raitt MH, Kraft CD, Gardner CJ, et al. Subacute ventricular free wall rupture complicating myocardial infarction. *Am Heart J* 1993;126(4):946–955.
444. Padro JM, Mesa JM, Silvestre J, et al. Subacute cardiac rupture: Repair with a sutureless technique. *Ann Thorac Surg* 1993;55(1):20–23; discussion 3–4.
445. Coletti G, Torracca L, Zogno M, et al. Surgical management of left ventricular free wall rupture after acute myocardial infarction. *Cardiovasc Surg* 1995;3(2): 181–186.
446. Harrity P, Patel A, Bianco J, Subramanian R. Improved diagnosis and characterization of postinfarction left ventricular pseudoaneurysm by cardiac magnetic resonance imaging. *Clin Cardiol* 1991;14(7):603–606.
447. March KL, Sawada SG, Tarver RD, et al. Current concepts of left ventricular pseudoaneurysm: Pathophysiology, therapy, and diagnostic imaging methods. *Clin Cardiol* 1989; 12(9):531–540.
448. Duvernoy O, Wikstrom G, Mannting F, et al. Pre- and postoperative CT and MR in pseudoaneurysms of the heart. *J Comput Assist Tomogr* 1992;16(3):401–409.
449. Figueras J, Cortadellas J, Evangelista A, Soler-Soler J. Medical management of selected patients with left ventricular free wall rupture during acute myocardial infarction. *J Am Coll Cardiol* 1997;29(3):512–518.
450. Blinc A, Noc M, Pohar B, et al. Subacute rupture of the left ventricular free wall after acute myocardial infarction: Three cases of long-term survival without emergency surgical repair. *Chest* 1996;109(2):565–567.
451. Sherer Y, Levy Y, Shahar A, et al. Survival without surgical repair of acute rupture of the right ventricular free wall. *Clin Cardiol* 1999;22(4):319–320.
452. Pifarre R, Sullivan HJ, Grieco J, et al. Management of left ventricular rupture complicating myocardial infarction. *J Thorac Cardiovasc Surg* 1983;86(3):441–443.
453. Murata H, Masuo M, Yoshimoto H, et al. Oozing type cardiac rupture repaired with percutaneous injection of fibrin-glue into the pericardial space: Case report. *Jpn Circ J* 2000;64(4):312–315.
454. Joho S, Asanoi H, Sakabe M, et al. Long-term usefulness of percutaneous intrapericardial fibrin-glue fixation therapy for oozing type of left ventricular free wall rupture: A case report. *Circ J* 2002;66(7):705–706.
455. Frances C, Romero A, Grady D. Left ventricular pseudoaneurysm. *J Am Coll Cardiol* 1998;32(3): 557–561.
456. Scholz KH, Werner GS, Schorn B, et al. Postinfarction left ventricular rupture: Successful surgical intervention after percutaneous cardiopulmonary support during mechanical resuscitation. *Am Heart J* 1994;127(1):210–211.
457. Sakakibara T, Matsuwaka R, Shintani H, et al. Successful repair of postinfarction left ventricular free wall rupture: New strategy with hypothermic percutaneous cardiopulmonary bypass. *J Thorac Cardiovasc Surg* 1996;111(1):276.
458. Sutherland FW, Guell FJ, Pathi VL, Naik SK. Postinfarction ventricular free wall rupture: Strategies for diagnosis and treatment. *Ann Thorac Surg* 1996;61(4): 1281–1285.
459. Stryjer D, Friedensohn A, Hendler A. Myocardial rupture in acute myocardial infarction: Urgent management. *Br Heart J* 1988;59(1):73–74.

460. Chemnitius JM, Schmidt T, Wojcik J, et al. Successful surgical management of left ventricular free wall rupture in the course of myocardial infarction. *Eur J Cardiothorac Surg* 1991;5(1):51–55.
461. Reardon MJ, Carr CL, Diamond A, et al. Ischemic left ventricular free wall rupture: Prediction, diagnosis, and treatment. *Ann Thorac Surg* 1997;64(5):1509–1513.
462. Yamazaki Y, Eguchi S, Miyamura H, et al. Replacement of myocardium with a Dacron prosthesis for complications of acute myocardial infarction. *J Cardiovasc Surg (Torino)* 1989;30(2):277–280.
463. McMullan MH, Maples MD, Kilgore TL Jr, Hindman SH. Surgical experience with left ventricular free wall rupture [see comment]. *Ann Thorac Surg* 2001;71(6): 1894–1898; discussion 8–9.
464. Eisenmann B, Bareiss P, Pacifico AD, et al. Anatomic, clinical, and therapeutic features of acute cardiac rupture: Successful surgical management fourteen hours after myocardial infarction. *J Thorac Cardiovasc Surg* 1978; 76(1):78–82.
465. Nunez L, de la Llana R, Lopez Sendon J, et al. Diagnosis and treatment of subacute free wall ventricular rupture after infarction. *Ann Thorac Surg* 1983;35(5):525–529.
466. Coma-Canella I, Lopez-Sendon J, Nunez Gonzalez L, Ferrufino O. Subacute left ventricular free wall rupture following acute myocardial infarction: Bedside hemodynamics, differential diagnosis, and treatment. *Am Heart J* 1983;106(2):278–284.
467. Pappas PJ, Cernaianu AC, Baldino WA, et al. Ventricular free-wall rupture after myocardial infarction: Treatment and outcome. *Chest* 1991;99(4):892–895.
468. Almdahl SM, Hotvedt R, Larsen U, Sorlie DG. Postinfarction rupture of left ventricular free wall repaired with a glued-on pericardial patch: Case report. *Scand J Thorac Cardiovasc Surg* 1993;27(2):105–107.
469. Padro JM, Caralps JM, Montoya JD, et al. Sutureless repair of postinfarction cardiac rupture. *J Card Surg* 1988;3(4):491–493.
470. Canovas SJ, Lim E, Dalmau MJ, et al. Midterm clinical and echocardiographic results with patch glue repair of left ventricular free wall rupture. *Circulation* 2003; 108(Suppl 1):II237–240.
471. Mantovani V, Vanoli D, Chelazzi P, et al. Postinfarction cardiac rupture: Surgical treatment. *Eur J Cardiothorac Surg* 2002;22(5):777–780.
472. Alamanni F, Fumero A, Parolari A, et al. Sutureless double-patch-and-glue technique for repair of subacute left ventricular wall rupture after myocardial infarction [see comment]. *J Thorac Cardiovasc Surg* 2001;122(4): 836–837.
473. Imagawa H, Nakano S, Akagi H, et al. Pericardial hood repair of cardiac rupture secondary to extended myocardial infarction. *Ann Thorac Surg* 2000;69(6):1959–1960.
474. Muller I, Andrassy P, Firschke C. Left ventricular pseudoaneurysm: A mechanical complication of acute myocardial infarction. *Heart* 2002;87(6):569.
475. Ropers D, Achenbach S, Pfeiffer S. Left ventricular pseudoaneurysm following myocardial infarction. *Heart* 2004;90(5):555.
476. Kocak H, Becit N, Ceviz M, Unlu Y. Left ventricular pseudoaneurysm after myocardial infarction. *Heart Vessels* 2003;18(3):160–162.
477. Park WM, Connery CP, Hochman JS, et al. Successful repair of myocardial free wall rupture after thrombolytic therapy for acute infarction. *Ann Thorac Surg* 2000;70(4): 1345–1349.
478. Galeati DG. De bononiensi scientiarum et artium instituto atque academia commentarii. *De morbus duobus* 1757;IV:26.
479. Hunter J. An account of the dissection of morbid bodys (manuscript). In: *Library of the Royal College of Surgeons* 1757:30–32.
480. Schlicter J, Hellerstein HK, Katz LN. Aneurysm of the heart: A correlative study of one hundred and two proved cases. *Medicine (Baltimore)* 1954;33:43–86.
481. Beck CS. Operation for aneurysm of the heart. *Ann Surg* 1944;120:34–40.
482. Likoff W, Bailey CP. Ventriculoplasty: Excision of myocardial aneurysm: Report of a successful case. *JAMA* 1955;158(11):915–920.
483. Cooley DA, Collins HA, Morris GC Jr, Chapman DW. Ventricular aneurysm after myocardial infarction: Surgical excision with use of temporary cardiopulmonary bypass. *JAMA* 1958;167(5):557–560.
484. Stoney WS, Alford WC Jr, Burrus GR, Thomas CS Jr. Repair of anteroseptal ventricular aneurysm. *Ann Thorac Surg* 1973;15(4):394–404.
485. Dor V, Saab M, Coste P, et al. Left ventricular aneurysm: A new surgical approach. *Thorac Cardiovasc Surg* 1989;37(1):11–19.
486. Jatene AD. Left ventricular aneurysmectomy: Resection or reconstruction. *J Thorac Cardiovasc Surg* 1985;89(3): 321–331.
487. Cooley DA. Ventricular endoaneurysmorrhaphy: A simplified repair for extensive postinfarction aneurysm. *J Card Surg* 1989;4(3):200–205.
488. Cooley DA, Frazier OH, Duncan JM, et al. Intracavitary repair of ventricular aneurysm and regional dyskinesia. *Ann Surg* 1992;215(5):417–423; discussion 23–24.
489. Meizlish JL, Berger HJ, Plankey M, et al. Functional left ventricular aneurysm formation after acute anterior transmural myocardial infarction: Incidence, natural history, and prognostic implications. *N Engl J Med* 1984;311(16): 1001–1006.
490. Buckberg GD. Defining the relationship between akinesia and dyskinesia and the cause of left ventricular failure after anterior infarction and reversal of remodeling to restoration. *J Thorac Cardiovasc Surg* 1998;116(1): 47–49.
491. Di Donato M, Sabatier M, Dor V, et al. Akinetic versus dyskinetic postinfarction scar: Relation to surgical outcome in patients undergoing endoventricular circular patch plasty repair. *J Am Coll Cardiol* 1997;29(7): 1569–1575.
492. Dor V, Sabatier M, Di Donato M, et al. Efficacy of endoventricular patch plasty in large postinfarction akinetic scar and severe left ventricular dysfunction: Comparison with a series of large dyskinetic scars. *J Thorac Cardiovasc Surg* 1998;116(1):50–59.
493. Erlebacher JA, Weiss JL, Weisfeldt ML, Bulkley BH. Early dilation of the infarcted segment in acute transmural myocardial infarction: Role of infarct expansion in acute left ventricular enlargement. *J Am Coll Cardiol* 1984;4(2):201–208.

494. Sutton MG, Sharpe N. Left ventricular remodeling after myocardial infarction: Pathophysiology and therapy. *Circulation* 2000;101(25):2981–2988.
495. Frangogiannis NG, Smith CW, Entman ML. The inflammatory response in myocardial infarction. *Cardiovasc Res* 2002;53(1):31–47.
496. Cleutjens JP, Kandala JC, Guarda E, et al. Regulation of collagen degradation in the rat myocardium after infarction. *J Mol Cell Cardiol* 1995;27(6):1281–1292.
497. Glower DD, Schaper J, Kabas JS, et al. Relation between reversal of diastolic creep and recovery of systolic function after ischemic myocardial injury in conscious dogs. *Circ Res* 1987;60(6):850–860.
498. Iwasaki K, Kita T, Taniguchi G, Kusachi S. Improvement of left ventricular aneurysm after myocardial infarction: Report of three cases. *Clin Cardiol* 1991;14(4): 355–360.
499. Chen JS, Hwang CL, Lee DY, Chen YT. Regression of left ventricular aneurysm after delayed percutaneous transluminal coronary angioplasty (PTCA) in patients with acute myocardial infarction. *Int J Cardiol* 1995; 48(1):39–47.
500. Jugdutt BI. Effect of nitrates on myocardial remodeling after acute myocardial infarction. *Am J Cardiol* 1996; 77(13):17C–23C.
501. Mahmarian JJ, Moye LA, Chinoy DA, et al. Transdermal nitroglycerin patch therapy improves left ventricular function and prevents remodeling after acute myocardial infarction: Results of a multicenter prospective randomized, double-blind, placebo-controlled trial. *Circulation* 1998;97(20):2017–2024.
502. Sharpe N, Murphy J, Smith H, Hannan S. Treatment of patients with symptomless left ventricular dysfunction after myocardial infarction. *Lancet* 1988;1(8580): 255–259.
503. Pfeffer MA, Lamas GA, Vaughan DE, et al. Effect of captopril on progressive ventricular dilatation after anterior myocardial infarction. *N Engl J Med* 1988;319(2):80–86.
504. Sharpe N, Smith H, Murphy J, et al. Early prevention of left ventricular dysfunction after myocardial infarction with angiotensin-converting-enzyme inhibition. *Lancet* 1991;337(8746):872–876.
505. Mills NL, Everson CT, Hockmuth DR. Technical advances in the treatment of left ventricular aneurysm. *Ann Thorac Surg* 1993;55(3):792–800.
506. Cox JL. Left ventricular aneurysms: Pathophysiologic observations and standard resection. *Semin Thorac Cardiovasc Surg* 1997;9(2):113–122.
507. Faxon DP, Ryan TJ, Davis KB, et al. Prognostic significance of angiographically documented left ventricular aneurysm from the Coronary Artery Surgery Study (CASS). *Am J Cardiol* 1982;50(1):157–164.
508. Mickleborough LL, Carson S, Ivanov J. Repair of dyskinetic or akinetic left ventricular aneurysm: Results obtained with a modified linear closure. *J Thorac Cardiovasc Surg* 2001;121(4):675–682.
509. Sinatra R, Macrina F, Braccio M, et al. Left ventricular aneurysmectomy: Comparison between two techniques: Early and late results. *Eur J Cardiothorac Surg* 1997;12(2):291–297.
510. Shapira OM, Davidoff R, Hilkert RJ, et al. Repair of left ventricular aneurysm: Long-term results of linear repair versus endoaneurysmorrhaphy. *Ann Thorac Surg* 1997;63(3):701–705.
511. Jones EL, Craver JM, Hurst JW, et al. Influence of left ventricular aneurysm on survival following the coronary bypass operation. *Ann Surg* 1981;193(6):733–742.
512. Burton NA, Stinson EB, Oyer PE, Shumway NE. Left ventricular aneurysm: Preoperative risk factors and long-term postoperative results. *J Thorac Cardiovasc Surg* 1979;77(1):65–75.
513. Fiore AC, Jatene AD. Surgical treatment of left ventricular aneurysm. In: Baue AE, Geha AS, Laks H, et al (eds.) *Glenn's Thoracic and Cardiovascular Surgery*, 6th ed. Stamford, CT: Appleton & Lange; 1996:2131–2140.
514. Rao G, Zikria EA, Miller WH, et al. Experience with sixty consecutive ventricular aneurysm resections. *Circulation* 1974;50(Suppl 2):II149–153.
515. ISIS-4 (Fourth International Study of Infarct Survival) Collaborative Group. ISIS-4: A randomised factorial trial assessing early oral captopril, oral mononitrate, and intravenous magnesium sulphate in 58,050 patients with suspected acute myocardial infarction. *Lancet* 1995; 345(8951):669–885.
516. Pfeffer MA, Braunwald E, Moye LA, et al. Effect of captopril on mortality and morbidity in patients with left ventricular dysfunction after myocardial infarction: Results of the survival and ventricular enlargement trial: The SAVE Investigators. *N Engl J Med* 1992;327(10): 669–677.
517. The Acute Infarction Ramipril Efficacy (AIRE) Study Investigators. Effect of ramipril on mortality and morbidity of survivors of acute myocardial infarction with clinical evidence of heart failure. *Lancet* 1993;342(8875): 821–828.
518. Grondin P, Kretz JG, Bical O, et al. Natural history of saccular aneurysms of the left ventricle. *J Thorac Cardiovasc Surg* 1979;77(1):57–64.
519. Dor V. Surgery for left ventricular aneurysm. *Curr Opin Cardiol* 1990;5(6):773–780.
520. Cooley DA. Ventricular aneurysms. In: Buxton BF, Frazier OH, Westaby S (eds.) *Ischemic Heart Disease Surgical Management*. London: Mosby; 1999:321–326.
521. Hutchins GM, Brawley RK. The influence of cardiac geometry on the results of ventricular aneurysm repair. *Am J Pathol* 1980;99(1):221–230.
522. Komeda M, David TE, Malik A, et al. Operative risks and long-term results of operation for left ventricular aneurysm. *Ann Thorac Surg* 1992;53(1):22–28; discussion 8–9.
523. Glower DD, Lowe JE. Left ventricular aneurysm. In: Cohn LH, Edmunds LH Jr (eds.) *Cardiac Surgery in the Adult*. New York: McGraw-Hill; 2003:771–788.
524. Jatene AD. Left ventricular aneurysmectomy: Resection or reconstruction. *J Thorac Cardiovasc Surg* 1985;89(3): 321–331.
525. Dor V. Reconstructive left ventricular surgery for post-ischemic akinetic dilatation. *Semin Thorac Cardiovasc Surg* 1997;9(2):139–145.
526. Dor V, Saab M, Coste P, et al. Endoventricular patch plasties with septal exclusion for repair of ischemic left ventricle: Technique, results and indications from a series of 781 cases. *Jpn J Thorac Cardiovasc Surg* 1998;46(5): 389–398.

527. Dor V. Left ventricular aneurysms: The endoventricular circular patch plasty. *Semin Thorac Cardiovasc Surg* 1997;9(2):123–130.
528. Alloni A, Rinaldi M, Gazzoli F, et al. Left ventricular aneurysm resection with port-access surgery: A new mini-invasive surgical approach. *Ann Thorac Surg* 2003;75(3):786–789.
529. Li RK, Weisel RD, Mickle DA, et al. Autologous porcine heart cell transplantation: Improved heart function after a myocardial infarction. *J Thorac Cardiovasc Surg* 2000;119(1):62–68.
530. Li RK, Jia ZQ, Weisel RD, et al. Cardiomyocyte transplantation improves heart function. *Ann Thorac Surg* 1996;62(3):654–660; discussion 60–61.
531. Li RK, Jia ZQ, Weisel RD, et al. Smooth muscle cell transplantation into myocardial scar tissue improves heart function. *J Mol Cell Cardiol* 1999;31(3):513–522.
532. Tomita S, Li RK, Weisel RD, et al. Autologous transplantation of bone marrow cells improves damaged heart function. *Circulation* 1999;100(Suppl 19):II247–256.
533. Matsubayashi K, Fedak PW, Mickle DA, et al. Improved left ventricular aneurysm repair with bioengineered vascular smooth muscle grafts. *Circulation* 2003;108(Suppl 1):II219–225.
534. Trehan N, Kohli V, Meharwal ZS, et al. Surgical treatment of post infarction left ventricular aneurysms: Our experience with double breasting and Dor's repair. *J Card Surg* 2003;18(2):114–120.
535. Lundblad R, Abdelnoor M, Svennevig JL. Repair of left ventricular aneurysm: Surgical risk and long-term survival. *Ann Thorac Surg* 2003;76(3):719–725.
536. Bolooki H, DeMarchena E, Mallon SM, et al. Factors affecting late survival after surgical remodeling of left ventricular aneurysms. *J Thorac Cardiovasc Surg* 2003;126(2):374–383; discussion 83–85.
537. Raman JS, Sakaguchi G, Buxton BF. Outcome of geometric endoventricular repair in impaired left ventricular function. *Ann Thorac Surg* 2000;70(3):1127–1129.
538. Soloman NA, Sathyamurthy I, Jayanthi K, et al. Surgical repair of left ventricular aneurysms: A comparative evaluation of linear versus Dor's repair. *Indian Heart J* 2001;53(6):736–739.
539. Vicol C, Rupp G, Fischer S, et al. Linear repair versus ventricular reconstruction for treatment of left ventricular aneurysm: A 10-year experience. *J Cardiovasc Surg* 1998;39(4):461–467.
540. Stahle E, Bergstrom R, Nystrom SO, et al. Surgical treatment of left ventricular aneurysm—assessment of risk factors for early and late mortality. *Eur J Cardiothorac Surg* 1994;8(2):67–73.
541. Couper GS, Bunton RW, Birjiniuk V, et al. Relative risks of left ventricular aneurysmectomy in patients with akinetic scars versus true dyskinetic aneurysms. *Circulation* 1990;82(Suppl 5):IV248–256.
542. Elefteriades JA, Solomon LW, Salazar AM, et al. Linear left ventricular aneurysmectomy: Modern imaging studies reveal improved morphology and function. *Ann Thorac Surg* 1993;56(2):242–250; discussion 51–52.
543. McCarthy PM. Ventricular aneurysms, shock, and late follow-up in patients with heart failure. *J Thorac Cardiovasc Surg* 2003;126(2):323–325.
544. Kawachi K, Kitamura S, Kawata T, et al. Hemodynamic assessment during exercise after left ventricular aneurysmectomy. *J Thorac Cardiovasc Surg* 1994;107(1):178–183.
545. Kawachi K, Kitamura S, Kawashima Y, et al. Changes in myocardial oxygen consumption and coronary sinus blood flow before and after resection of left ventricular aneurysm after myocardial infarction. *J Thorac Cardiovasc Surg* 1987;94(4):566–570.
546. Vural KM, Sener E, Ozatik MA, et al. Left ventricular aneurysm repair: An assessment of surgical treatment modalities. *Eur J Cardiothorac Surg* 1998;13(1):49–56.
547. Turkay C, Mete A, Yilmaz M, et al. Comparative methods of repairing left ventricular aneurysms. *Tex Heart Inst J* 1997;24(4):343–348.
548. Doss M, Martens S, Sayour S, Hemmer W. Long term follow up of left ventricular function after repair of left ventricular aneurysm: A comparison of linear closure versus patch plasty. *Eur J Cardiothorac Surg* 2001;20(4):783–785.
549. Pasini S, Gagliardotto P, Punta G, et al. Early and late results after surgical therapy of postinfarction left ventricular aneurysm. *J Cardiovasc Surg* 1998;39(2):209–215.
550. Salati M, Paje A, Di Biasi P, et al. Severe diastolic dysfunction after endoventriculoplasty. *J Thorac Cardiovasc Surg* 1995;109(4):694–701.
551. Di Mattia DG, Di Biasi P, Salati M, et al. Surgical treatment of left ventricular postinfarction aneurysm with endoventriculoplasty: Late clinical and functional results. *Eur J Cardiothorac Surg* 1999;15(4):413–418.
552. Bonow RO, Carabello B, de Leon AC, et al. ACC/AHA Guidelines for the Management of Patients With Valvular Heart Disease: Executive Summary: A report of the American College of Cardiology/American Heart Association Task Force on Practice Guidelines (Committee on Management of Patients With Valvular Heart Disease). *J Heart Valve Dis* 1998;7(6):672–707.

CHAPTER

30 AORTIC VALVE REPLACEMENT

John R. Barbour, John S. Ikonomidis

HISTORICAL BACKGROUND

Aortic valvotomy

The first attempt to open a stenotic aortic valve in a patient was performed by Theodore Tuffier on July 13, 1912.[1] This procedure was accomplished by invaginating the ascending aortic wall with a finger and pushing the aorta through the valve. The 26-year-old male patient recovered and returned to his home in Belgium. Russell Brock dilated calcified aortic valves in humans in the late 1940s with instruments passed from the innominate artery or another arterial source.[2] His results were initially poor, and he[3] as well as Bailey and associates[4] later used different dilators in various approaches with somewhat better results. The mortality among those patients remained high, however. Horace Smithy, a South Carolina surgeon, had severe rheumatic aortic stenosis. Having achieved national acclaim for the development and successful use of a valvulotome for closed commissurotomy in patients with rheumatic mitral disease, he developed an aortic valvulotome[5] and enlisted Dr. Alfred Blalock to perform the operation on him. Dr. Blalock agreed as long as he and Dr. Smithy performed the procedure together on another patient first. A patient was scheduled but died of ventricular fibrillation during the induction of anesthesia. Shortly

KEY CONCEPTS

- Epidemiology
  - Approximately 100,000 aortic valve replacement procedures have been performed in the United States in the last 10 years. Most patients present with aortic valve pathology that requires replacement between ages 60 and 80. Replacement for aortic stenosis is performed much more commonly (85 percent) than is replacement for aortic insufficiency.
- Pathophysiology
  - With aortic stenosis, there is a decrease in the effective valve orifice area, resulting in progressive obstruction of the left ventricle. The ventricle adapts through concentric hypertrophy, which increases diastolic stiffness and impairs the efficacy of diastolic coronary blood flow. Diastolic dysfunction precedes systolic dysfunction. With aortic insufficiency, gradual ventricular dilatation occurs, causing an increase in wall stress. This, in conjunction with the decrease in diastolic pressure, reduces diastolic coronary blood flow. With continued dilatation, fibrosis occurs, increasing ventricular stiffness and impairing diastolic relaxation. Eventually, the preload reserve of the ventricle is reached and further dilatation and fibrosis results in a decline in systolic function that may not be recoverable after aortic valve replacement.
- Clinical features
  - Aortic stenosis patients complain of combinations of symptoms of chest pain, syncope, and congestive heart failure. The life expectancy of patients with untreated aortic stenosis who present with angina is 50 percent at 5 years, 50 percent at 3 years with syncope, and 50 percent at 2 years with congestive heart failure symptoms. A small proportion of patients with aortic stenosis present with sudden death. Aortic insufficiency has a more insidious onset and usually is characterized by the development of slow congestive heart failure and fatigue symptoms. Angina pectoris and syncope are rare in these patients. These

patients may be managed on medical therapy for protracted periods with an acceptable quality of life.

- Diagnostics
  - The work-up for candidates for aortic valve replacement includes echocardiography to estimate ventricular function and the degree of stenosis or insufficiency and cardiac catheterization to measure cardiac output, calculate aortic valve area, and image the coronary arteries for significant lesions. A careful oral examination or dental consultation is very important to prevent postoperative prosthetic valve infection.
- Treatment
  - Aortic valve replacement options include homograft, stented and stentless xenograft tissue, and mechanical valves. The decision to use each of these is dependent on patient age and valve preference, comorbid conditions, and contraindications to the use of anti-coagulants. A variety of options are available to manage potential patient-prosthesis mismatch at the time of surgery.
- Outcomes
  - The outcomes of tissue valve replacement show 80 to 93 percent freedom from structural valve failure at 10 to 14 years. Bleeding and thromboembolic events complicate mechanical valve replacement at a rate of approximately 4 percent per patient year. Homograft valve replacements have the highest freedom from structural valve deterioration, with rates of 81 to 93 percent at 15 years. Survival after aortic valve replacement is dependent more on patient comorbidities than on the requirement for valve replacement. Postoperative complications specific for aortic valve replacement include complete heart block (1 percent) and perivalvular leaks (1 to 2 percent).

afterward, Dr. Smithy died of complications related to his severely stenotic aortic valve before the operation could be carried out.

Mechanical prostheses

In the early 1950s, Charles Hufnagel[6] and J. M. Campbell[7] independently developed and implanted artificial valves in the descending thoracic aorta of dogs. In a paper published in 1954, Hufnagel reported a series of 23 patients starting in September 1952 who had this operation for aortic insufficiency.[8] Those efforts preceded the evolution of the most successful of the caged ball valves: the Starr-Edwards prosthesis. That valve, created by M. Lowell Edwards, a retired engineer, and Albert Starr, a cardiac surgeon in Portland, Oregon, originally was implanted in the mitral position in August 1960. The first clinical Starr-Edwards aortic valve implantation was performed in September 1961.[9] Shortly after the introduction of the cage ball concept, a number of similar designs appeared in clinical use that are beyond the scope of this chapter. However, excellent reviews are available.[9,10]

The concept of the tilting disk valve arose from concerns that cage ball valves were bulky and that the hemodynamics were less than ideal. In an attempt to reduce the profile of those valves, a flat disk instead of a ball was used as an occluder. The earliest examples of the tilting disk concept were flat valves. Those valves had a ring with a straight segment on which a disk was hinged much like the lid of a toilet seat. Other modifications included free-floating polypropylene disks such as the one introduced by Melrose and colleagues[11] and other interesting designs such as those produced by Water and McLeod in Edinburgh.[12] In 1969, Bjork and Shiley produced a valve in which a free-floating disk was restrained by two low-profile M-shaped struts.[13,14] The first implantation of the Bjork-Shiley prosthesis was done in 1975. In 1978, the disk profile was changed from plano convex to convexo concave (C-C model) and struts were modified so that the disk moved 2.5 mm downstream as it tilted.[14] In 1981, the valve ring was altered and a single heavier hook replaced the outlet strut, all of which was machined from one piece of metal with no welds (the monostrut valve).[15] Other examples of tilting disk valves included the Lillehei-Caster, Omniscience, and Omni Carbon valves. Some were removed from use because of the high incidence of thrombotic obstruction[16] and others, such as the Medtronic-Hall D16 Valve and the Bjork-Shiley C-C valves, because of an unacceptable incidence of strut fractures.[17]

The earliest bileaflet mechanical valve designs were introduced by Gott and coworkers,[18] Kalke and colleagues,[19] and Wada and coworkers[20] in the early to middle 1960s. Those prostheses failed because of mechanical malfunctions and high thrombogenicity. However, from those failures there arose the realization that bileaflet prostheses had hemodynamic characteristics superior to those of all the prostheses available at that time. In 1976, the bileaflet design was modified, and those valves were manufactured entirely from pyrolytic carbon.[21] Subsequent studies showed that the bileaflet design was very durable and that, in addition, pyrolytic carbon was quite biocompatible and thromboresistant. The prototype pyrolytic carbon bileaflet valve, the St. Jude Medical Prosthesis, was implanted clinically in 1977.[22] That valve has undergone a number of modifications since the original standard St. Jude valve was introduced, including the lower-profile Hemodynamic Plus (HP) Valve,[22] the Masters Valve (which allows internal rotation of the leaflets to get a better seating once the valve is implanted),[23] and the Regent Valve (with a modified external profile to create an even larger internal orifice area for each valve size).[24] Other bileaflet valves are currently in use, such as the Carbomedics[25] (released for clinical use in December 1986) and Sorin Bicarbon[26] (released in 1990) models.

Bioprostheses

With the introduction of glutaraldehyde for the fixation of biological tissue by Carpentier and colleagues in 1969,[27] the use of bioprosthetic material, both porcine valves and bovine pericardium, became feasible alternatives to mechanical designs for valve replacement. The University of Padua has the most extensive experience with the Hancock standard porcine bioprosthesis, which was implanted clinically in the aortic position in March 1970.[28] The Hancock modified orifice (MO) valve was introduced in the wake of concerns about high postimplantation gradients with small valve sizes in the aortic position. That problem, which was due to the bulky muscle bar under the right coronary cusp of the valve, was reconciled with the design of the MO valve, a composite valve that replaces the right coronary cusp with a cusp from another valve that does not contain the muscle bar. The Carpentier-Edwards standard porcine bioprosthesis was introduced in 1975.[29] Second-generation bioprostheses include the Carpentier-Edwards supraannular (SAV) porcine bioprosthesis, which has been available since 1981;[30] the Hancock II porcine bioprosthesis, which was introduced in 1982;[31] and the Medtronic intact porcine bioprosthesis, which has been available since 1985.[32] In general, these valves offer improved zero-pressure fixation that preserves subtle but important histologic features of the valve leaflets along with antimineralization treatments to reduce calcific degeneration of the valve tissue. Additionally, more flexible, lower-profile stent materials and reduced sewing rings are employed to create a larger effective orifice area. Numerous other porcine bioprosthesis are under evaluation.

The first bovine pericardial bioprosthesis was the Ionescu-Shiley valve developed by Marian I. Ionescu and G. Wooler in 1971.[33] In 1981, a low-profile model was released, but it had a much higher rate of failure than the standard Ionescu valve. A final model III was implanted and used clinically before Shiley decided to end the production of pericardial valves in October 1977.[34] The Mitroflow pericardial valve was designed by Siegel and Totten and first was implanted clinically in 1982.[35] The most commonly used pericardial valve currently, the Carpentier-Edwards pericardial valve, was clinically implanted in Paris, France, in July 1980.[36] This valve has undergone a number of modifications, including the Perimount RSR[37] and Magna series.

The first clinically applicable bioprosthetic stentless aortic valve was the Toronto stentless porcine valve (SPV valve) introduced by Dr. Tirone David at the University of Toronto in 1991.[38] This valve offered an increased effective orifice area of the valve by minimizing the sewing ring and eliminating the supporting struts. The stentless valve design consisted of a native porcine valve reinforced by a small amount of fabric sewn to the patient's annulus in a planar fashion, followed by the implantation of a small amount of porcine aorta around the valve commissures directly into the patient's native aorta. Other stentless valves currently in use include the Medtronic Freestyle porcine prosthesis[39] and the Edwards Prima Plus porcine prosthesis.[40] Other stentless valves, such as the 3F Therapeutics stentless equine bioprosthesis,[41] are being evaluated in clinical trials.

The first experimental animal studies involving homograft aortic tissue were performed by Lamb and associates in 1952; they implanted an allograft aortic valve into the descending aorta of a dog.[42] That was followed within 3 years by the clinical reimplantation of the allograft aortic valve into the human descending aorta by Murray[43] and subsequently by Heimbecker and associates in Toronto.[44] The technique for subcoronary implantation of allograft tissue using the single-suture method was reported by Duran and Gunning in 1962[45] and implemented in the same year by Donald Ross[46] in patients with a freeze-dried aortic valve, a feat performed shortly afterward by Barrett-Boyes.[47] Sterilization of homograft valves has undergone a number of changes from formaldehyde, chlorhexidine, propiolactone, methylene oxide, gamma radiation, and storage using a carbon dioxide freezer at −70°C. Currently, most homograft valves are cryopreserved with low-dose antibiotics.

EMBRYOLOGY AND ANATOMY

The aortic valve develops from three swellings or ridges of endomyocardial tissue at the proximal orifice of the septating truncus arteriosus. Those ridges become hollowed out and reshaped to form three thin-walled cusps or pockets at approximately the sixth to seventh week of development.[48] The three aortic valve cusps are semilunar in shape and are named in accordance with whether the sinuses they subtend give rise to coronary artery ostia. Therefore, a right and a left coronary aortic cusp and one noncoronary cusp exist. The base (semilunar point of attachment to the aorta) of the leaflet is approximately one and a half times as long as its free margin. Portions of the noncoronary cusp and a portion of the left coronary cusps are in continuity with the anterior leaflet of the mitral valve (the aortomitral continuity); this is an anatomic consideration that can become very important in valve replacement for endocarditis. The aortic valve annulus is variable in its definition but is toughest in approximately the noncoronary section, constituting tissue between the left and right fibrous trigones of the heart. The ascent of the aortic attachment of the noncoronary cusp toward the right coronary-noncoronary commissure lies directly over the atrioventricular conduction system, which sits in the right fibrous trigone, or the central fibrous body of the heart. Sutures placed too deeply in this area during valve replacement result in atrioventricular conduction block. It is important to understand that the aortic valve leaflets are attached to the aortic root in a scalloped fashion. Most techniques of valve replacement involve conversion of this scalloped aortic annulus to a relatively planar orientation, and this can have important anatomic implications. Certain stented bioprostheses are designed to maintain some of the scalloped architecture when implanted. Each aortic valve leaflet has a small nodular excrescence at its midportion called the node of Arantius or the nodulus Arantii.[49]

An aortic valve leaflet has three layers: the fibrosa or arteriosa (arterial side), the spongiosa (middle), and the ventricularis (ventricular side). These layers are composed of varying proportions of elastin, collagen, and glycosaminoglycans. The outer layers of the valve cusps are covered in endothelial cells that are oriented perpendicularly to the direction of blood flow.[50]

ETIOLOGY AND PATHOPHYSIOLOGY

Aortic valve replacement is performed in patients in whom there is an underlying morphologic or anatomic abnormality of the aortic valve independent of its supporting structures that causes it to become stenotic or regurgitant.

Aortic stenosis

Aortic stenosis arises typically as a result of degenerative calcification in the elderly or as a result of rheumatic degeneration in individuals who have a history of rheumatic fever. Certain congenital conditions also predispose to aortic stenosis. The most common is congenital bicuspid aortic valves, which occur in approximately 5 percent of the population.[49] It is thought that a bicuspid aortic valve creates abnormally turbulent flow in systole, which in turn causes recession of the leaflet's intimal lining and predisposes the patient to calcification and the development of stenosis.

Whatever the cause, the pathophysiology of aortic stenosis relates to a decrease in the effective valve orifice. Changes in flow patterns across the valve result in further valve deterioration. The decreased valve orifice area results in progressive obstruction of the left ventricle. The ventricle adapts through concentric hypertrophic changes in response to increased wall stress. The greater wall thickness increases diastolic stiffness and impairs the efficacy of diastolic coronary blood flow, thus reducing or eliminating coronary flow reserve despite an increase in oxygen requirements by the larger cardiomyocyte mass. As a result of these responses, patients may have congestive heart failure in the absence of systolic ventricular dysfunction. Diastolic dysfunction is followed by systolic dysfunction. Here the worsening valvular stenosis creates a condition of increasing afterload that over time cannot be compensated for by hypertrophy alone. In addition, severe hypertrophy may create intracavitary gradients proximal to the valve that compound the issue and may not be correctable with aortic valve replacement.

Aortic insufficiency

Isolated aortic insufficiency usually develops as a consequence of structural abnormalities of the aortic valve, causing leaflet elongation and prolapse, as seen with myxomatous degeneration or in various connective tissue disorders, such as Marfan's syndrome. Other causes include infective endocarditis, traumatic disruption of a valve leaflet from severe acceleration-deceleration injuries, rheumatoid arthritis, Reiter's syndrome, ankylosing spondylitis, psoriasis, and Takayasu's disease. Patients with calcified degenerative aortic valves may undergo leaflet perforation or tearing, especially in the belly of the leaflet, that results in combined stenosis and regurgitation.

Acute severe incompetence of the aortic valve causes a large volume of diastolic flow reversal into the left ventricle. The ventricle does not have time to adapt to that sudden event, and a rapid rise in diastolic pressure occurs, causing the pulse pressure to decrease and forcing early mitral valve closure to prevent backflow into the left atrium. There is a concomitant increase in heart rate and a decrease in cardiac output. The result is a rapid onset of congestive heart failure.

Chronic, progressive valve incompetence allows time for the accommodation of a smaller gradation in flow reversal. Thus, gradual ventricular dilatation occurs, with preservation of diastolic compliance so that end-diastolic pressure is not elevated in well-compensated aortic insufficiency. The enlarging ventricular chamber causes an increase in wall stress (as an extension of LaPlace's law) that results in some ventricular hypertrophy, but overall the ratio of chamber diameter to wall thickness continues to increase. These events, in conjunction with the decrease in diastolic pressure, reduce diastolic coronary blood flow. With continued dilatation, fibrosis occurs, which increases ventricular stiffness further and impairs diastolic relaxation. Eventually, the preload reserve of the ventricle is reached and further dilatation and fibrosis result in a decline in systolic function that may not be recoverable with aortic valve replacement.

CLINICAL FEATURES

Aortic stenosis

Patients with aortic stenosis typically present to physicians in their sixties and seventies. These patients

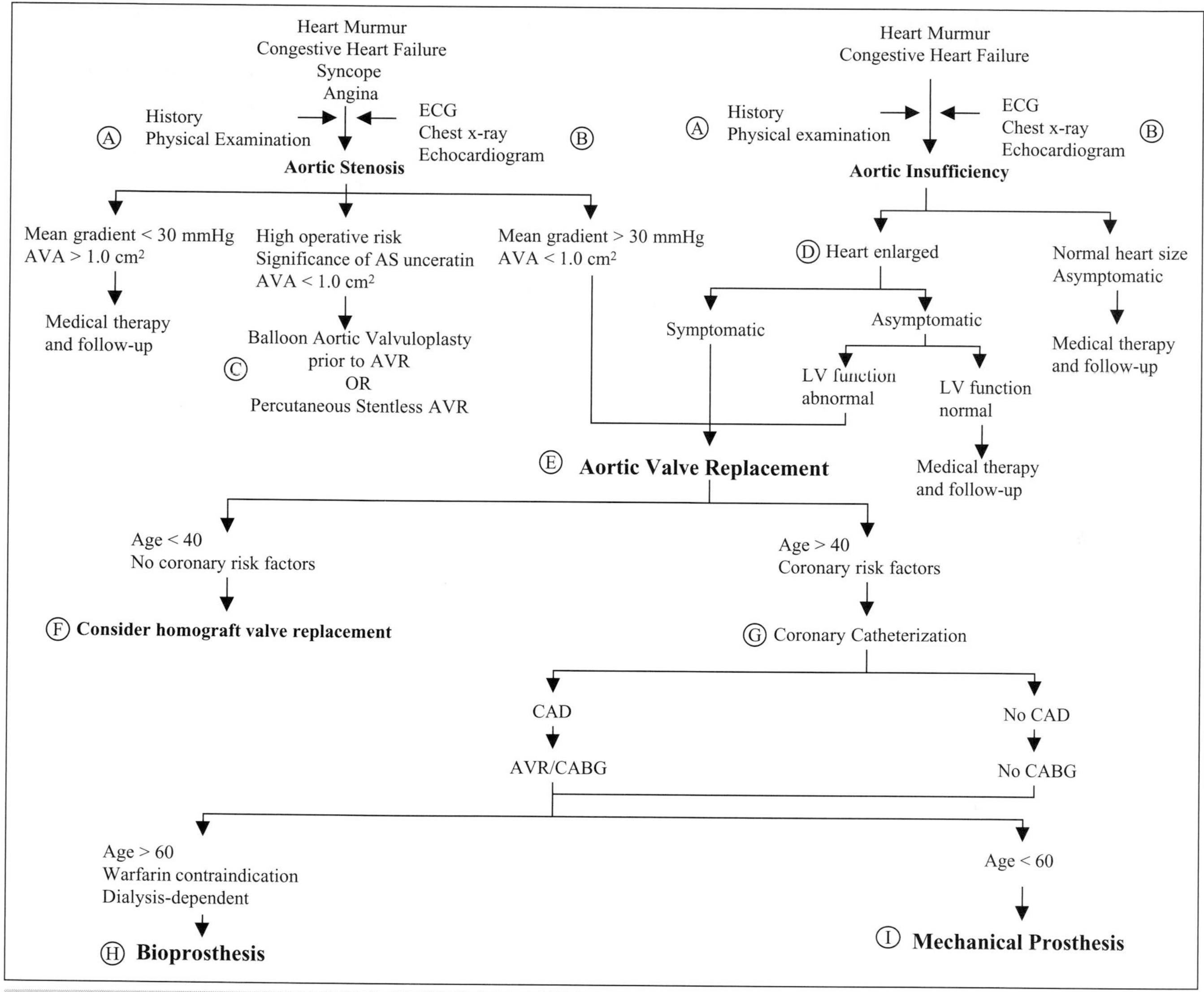

Figure 30-1 Decision-making flowchart.

A. Patients with aortic stenosis complain of combinations of symptoms that constitute the classic triad of chest pain, syncope, and congestive heart failure. A small proportion of patients with aortic stenosis present with sudden death. The murmur of aortic stenosis is of a blowing crescendo-decrescendo type that is best heard in the left sternal border with radiation to both carotid arteries. The heart is hypertrophied but not enlarged, and palpation of the pulse reveals low volume and a delayed upstroke (pulsus parvus et tardus).

Aortic insufficiency is characterized by the development of slow congestive heart failure and fatigue symptoms. Left ventricular dilatation is observed on physical examination. On cardiac auscultation, an early diastolic murmur radiates to the point of maximal intensity (apex) and may be associated with a middiastolic murmur caused by fluttering of the anterior mitral valve leaflet (Austin-Flint murmur). Other physical examination signs include "water-hammer" (Corrigan's) pulses, de Musset's sign (bobbing of the head), Muller's sign (wobbling of the uvula), pistol shots, Duroziez's sign (a murmur heard over the femoral arteries), and Quincke's sign (cyclical blanching of the nail beds).

A dental examination is a very important part of the evaluation of patients with aortic valve disease.

B. With aortic stenosis, the chest radiograph shows calcification of the aortic valve. The electrocardiogram shows left ventricular hypertrophy and left or right bundle branch block if the calcific process involves the conduction system. Echocardiography shows the calcified valve with poorly mobile leaflets and indicates whether it is bi- or tricuspid. Continuous-wave Doppler is used to calculate valve gradients and valve area.

With aortic insufficiency, the chest radiograph may show cardiomegaly and signs of pulmonary congestion. The degree of AI can be estimated by echocardiography, where a diastolic pressure half-time less than 300 ms, a short mitral deceleration time (less than 150 ms), and premature closure of the mitral valve all indicate severe insufficiency. Left ventricular cavity dilatation also is assessed.

Decision-making flowchart (*continued*).

C. In patients with aortic stenosis who have a high operative risk or in whom the clinical significance of the valve lesion is uncertain, balloon valvuloplasty may be useful as a diagnostic and short-term therapeutic tool. Stentless aortic valve replacement performed percutaneously or via left ventricular apical access may be beneficial.

D. Significant left ventricular enlargement is defined as an end-systolic dimension greater than 55 mm or an end-diastolic dimension less than 75 mm.

E. Aortic valve replacement is the treatment of choice for clinically significant aortic valve pathology. Consideration should be given to avoidance of patient-prosthesis mismatch. Techniques for this include the use of a small stented prosthesis, mechanical dilatation of the aortic root, implantation of stentless tissue valves, supraannular positioning of the valve replacement device, implementation of an annulus-enlarging procedure (Nicks, Manouguian, Konno-Rastan), and in certain cases application of the apicoaortic conduit technique.

F. Adults age less than 40 years may be candidates for a subcoronary homograft aortic valve replacement. Although this procedure is technically demanding, it offers extended durability without the need for oral anticoagulant therapy.

G. Coronary catheterization is indicated for age over 40 years or in the presence of coronary artery disease risk factors. Significant coronary artery disease should be bypassed at the time of aortic valve replacement. In addition, the degree of stenosis or insufficiency can be calculated at the time of catheterization.

H. Bioprosthetic valves are clearly indicated for patients over age 70, but in light of the improved longevity of the latest-generation tissue valves, this age limit may be reduced to 60 years. Concomitant significant coronary disease effectively decreases the acceptable age for bioprosthetic valve replacement by a further 5 to 10 years. Dialysis-dependent patients and those in whom warfarin is contraindicated also should receive bioprosthetic valves.

I. Patients less than 60 years of age who do not wish to risk reoperative valve replacement because of structural valve deterioration and are prepared to accept the risks and commitment associated with long-term warfarin administration should be considered for mechanical valve replacement.

complain of combinations of symptoms composing the classic triad of chest pain, syncope, and congestive heart failure. Chest pains in the form of classic angina pectoris are the initial symptom in 50 to 70 percent of patients. Syncope is the presenting symptom in 15 to 30 percent of patients. The life expectancy of patients with untreated aortic stenosis who present with angina is 50 percent at 5 years, 50 percent at 3 years with syncope, and 50 percent at 2 years with congestive heart failure symptoms such as exertional dyspnea, peripheral edema, orthopnea, and paroxysmal nocturnal dyspnea.[51] A small proportion of patients with aortic stenosis present with sudden death, most likely caused by life-threatening arrhythmias resulting from severe left ventricular hypertrophy. In patients who have congenital conditions that predispose them to aortic stenosis, such as congenital bicuspid aortic valves, presentation may occur 10 to 15 years earlier (see Fig. 31-1 on page 563.

Aortic insufficiency

Aortic insufficiency has a more insidious onset and usually is characterized by the development of slow congestive heart failure and fatigue symptoms.[52] Angina pectoris and syncope are rare in these patients. The patients may be managed on medical therapy for protracted periods with an acceptable quality of life. It is possible (but becoming less common) for patients with aortic insufficiency to be managed nonoperatively to the point where the myocardium becomes so decompensated that surgical treatment is untenable.

DIAGNOSTIC MODALITIES

Physical examination

Aortic stenosis

Patients with aortic stenosis present with a typical murmur, which consists of a blowing crescendo-decrescendo–type pattern best heard in the left sternal border with radiation to both carotid arteries. The heart is hypertrophied but not enlarged, and so typically patients with this condition do not have palpable enlarged hearts. Palpation of the pulse reveals low volume and a delayed upstroke (pulsus parvus et tardus) owing to the severity of the stenosis.

Aortic insufficiency

In patients with aortic insufficiency, gradual left ventricular dilatation is observed. On cardiac auscultation, an early diastolic murmur radiates to the point of maximal intensity (apex) and may be associated with a middiastolic murmur caused by fluttering of the anterior mitral valve leaflet (Austin-Flint murmur). In addition, a number of interesting physical examination signs have been noted in these patients, including "water-hammer" (Corrigan's) pulses with wide pulse pressures and low diastolic pressure, de Musset's sign (bobbing of the head), Muller's sign (wobbling of the uvula), pistol shots, Duroziez's sign (a murmur heard over the femoral arteries), and Quincke's sign (cyclical blanching of the nail beds).

An extremely important aspect of the physical examination in patients who are being considered for aortic valve surgery is the examination of the mouth and teeth. Dental disease is a major cause of prosthetic valve endocarditis, and no aortic valve replacement, except in extremely urgent circumstances, should be performed without appropriate dental clearance when that is deemed necessary. Aortic stenosis and insufficiency are not associated with any specific serum laboratory abnormalities.

Diagnostic studies

Aortic stenosis

The chest radiograph shows calcification of the aortic valve and a subtle convexity of the left ventricular silhouette caused by left ventricular hypertrophy. The electrocardiogram shows left ventricular hypertrophy and left or right bundle branch block if the calcific process causing stenosis involves the conduction system significantly. Transthoracic echocardiography shows the calcified valve with poorly mobile leaflets in the parasternal long-axis view. A short-axis view of the valve may show whether the valve is bi- or tricuspid. Continuous-wave Doppler is used to calculate valve gradients and valve area. The peak valve gradient is calculated as a function of the highest measured flow velocity (defined as peak gradient $= 4V^2$, where $V =$ velocity), which often is demonstrated in the four-chamber view. The mean gradient is calculated as a function of the area of the continuous-wave flow velocity curve. Valve area is calculated by the continuity equation and uses both continuous-wave and pulse-wave Doppler. It is calculated by multiplying the left ventricular outflow tract (LVOT) area by the LVOT flow velocity as measured by pulse-wave Doppler and dividing that value by the continuous-wave velocity. The accuracy of echocardiographic measurements is confounded by the presence of extensive calcification, basal septal hypertrophy, and probe orientation. In addition to these factors, severe left ventricular hypertrophy may manifest with subvalvular intracavitary gradients. If present, this may present a significant challenge to the surgeon at operation.

Aortic valve area is estimated at cardiac catheterization by using the Gorlin formula, which in the simplified version is defined as valve area = cardiac output/gradient.[52–54] The Gorlin equation is very sensitive to flow. Therefore, patients who have a reduced ejection fraction may have a falsely reduced valve area as calculated by the Gorlin equation. In these cases, correlation to the echocardiographic calculation is helpful.

Aortic insufficiency

The degree of aortic insufficiency (AI) can be estimated by echocardiography, where the rapidity of equilibration of aortic and left ventricular (LV) diastolic pressure determines the degree of insufficiency. Accordingly, a diastolic pressure half-time less than 300 ms, a short mitral deceleration time (less than 150 ms), and premature closure of the mitral valve all indicate severe AI. Left ventricular cavity dilatation also is assessed.

At catheterization, the degree of AI can be estimated by the degree of leakage of contrast into the left ventricle in diastole. However, this is relied on less frequently because of the increased use of the echocardiographic methods described above.

Patients with aortic stenosis and insufficiency should be evaluated initially with transthoracic echo. If the transthoracic echo is positive for the suspected diagnosis and the patient's symptoms warrant operation, it is logical to proceed with coronary catheterization to rule out the presence of coronary artery disease. In females less than 40 years of age and males less than 35 years of age with no cardiac risk factors, coronary catheterization can be omitted relatively safely.

MEDICAL (NONSURGICAL) THERAPY

Aortic stenosis

There is no acceptable medical therapy for symptomatic aortic stenosis. Antihypertensives and angiotensin-converting enzyme inhibitors must be used with caution because of the risk of profound hypoperfusion. The use of beta blockade may slow the heart rate and provide for a longer systolic interval, potentially resulting in higher stroke volume in patients with stenotic valves. Digitalis glycosides may provide a mild positive inotropic effect that may be beneficial. Percutaneous valvotomy[55] will reduce tight stenosis to moderate stenosis with a final valve area between 0.7 and 1.1 cm^2; this is still inferior to the valve area obtained with a prosthetic valve replacement, which usually provides a valve area over 1.5 cm^2. Hospital mortality varies from 3.5 to 13.5 percent, and within 24 h, 20 to 25 percent of these patients have at least one serious complication, in particular vascular complications at the puncture site. Despite a relatively modest improvement in valve function, the benefit to quality of life rarely lasts beyond a year. This technique is useful for improving the clinical status of patients with severe aortic stenosis as a preamble to open valve replacement.[56] Without valve replacement, however, the prognosis is poor. Currently, it generally is felt that valvotomy alone does not change the natural course of the disease. The poor middle-term results are due mainly to the clinical status of the patients and the moderate and transient improvement in valve function obtained from valvotomy.[57] More recently, percutaneous valve deployment has been employed successfully in patients deemed too high-risk for surgery.[58] These valves consist of pericardial valve substitutes that are mounted on expandable stents. The results of these procedures have been encouraging, but significant long-term results are not available for this technology.

Aortic insufficiency

Therapy for aortic valve regurgitation consists primarily of afterload reduction with vasodilating agents to discourage regurgitation and prevent pathologic remodeling of the myocardium.[59]

INDICATIONS FOR SURGERY

Aortic stenosis

Operation should be considered for aortic stenosis that is considered moderate to severe (aortic valve area less than 1 cm^2) associated with a mean gradient of 30 to 40 mmHg or higher.[59] Asymptomatic patients who meet these criteria also should also be considered because of the small but real incidence of sudden death associated with the natural history of this lesion.

Aortic insufficiency

Severe AI associated with gradual ventricular dilatation and at least New York Heart Association class II symptoms of fatigue and congestive heart failure are considered appropriate indications for surgery. In addition, patients with symptomatic moderate AI with mild to moderate (ejection fraction less than 25 percent) left ventricular dysfunction should be referred for aortic valve replacement (AVR). A symptomatic patient should be considered for surgery if there is LV systolic dysfunction or severe LV dilatation (end-diastolic dimension greater than 75 mm or end-systolic dimension greater than 55 mm).[59–63]

SURGICAL THERAPY

Positioning, incisions, and cardiopulmonary bypass

The patient is placed in the supine position. Monitoring lines such as a radial arterial catheter and a pulmonary arterial catheter can be placed in the holding area under sedation or after the patient is brought into the operating room. Despite excellent advances in cardiothoracic anesthesia, the occasional patient with severe aortic stenosis will experience cardiac arrest during anesthetic induction. In cases of severe aortic stenosis, it therefore is advisable for the surgeon to be immediately available from the time the patient is brought into the operating room. The patient's chest, abdomen, perineum, and lower extremities are prepped and draped in sterile fashion. Median sternotomy is the classic mode of access to the heart, but minimally invasive approaches such as upper hemisternotomy[64] and right parasternotomy[65] have been described. Tacking only the right side of the incised pericardium to the retractor or skin allows the ventricular mass to rotate posteriorly and improves access to the aortic root. The patient is heparinized systemically to reach a blood activated clotting time (ACT) of 400 s. Cardiopulmonary bypass is established by using dual-stage or bicaval cannulation with a left ventricular vent placed across the mitral valve via the right superior pulmonary vein or through a stab incision in the left ventricular apex. Mild to moderate systemic cooling (30°C) is used. If the valve is not regurgitant, cold blood cardioplegia should be delivered antegrade via the aortic root for more uniform myocardial distribution and then intermittently via a retrograde coronary sinus catheter for the duration of the cross-clamp period. If the retrograde catheter cannot be inserted blindly, options include bicaval cannulation and insertion of the retrograde coronary sinus catheter across the visualized coronary sinus orifice and the delivery of antegrade cardioplegia via perfusion catheters positioned or sewn into the coronary ostia.

Numerous approaches to aortotomy have been described, with the most common being oblique aortotomy and near transection aortotomy (Fig. 30-2). Oblique aortotomy begins in the anterior midline of the ascending aorta or just along the left anterior side and extends to the right and inferoposterior into the midportion of the noncoronary sinus. The near-transecting aortotomy should be made 1.0 to 1.5 cm above the origin of the right coronary artery for the best visualization. Therefore, added dissection is required on the anterior surface of the aorta to identify the right coronary artery take-off; this occasionally can result in damage to the right coronary artery and necessitate either repair or vein graft bypass of the right coronary artery. The near-transecting aortotomy is relatively easy to close, but troublesome bleeding may occur posteriorly and can be difficult to manage. In addition, if a small aortic root is encountered so that annulus enlargement is necessary, a right-angle incision must be made in the aorta and extended across the annulus; this can be very challenging to close later. Finally, since the sinotubular junction is 10 to 15 percent smaller in diameter than the annulus, occasionally it is very difficult to pass an appropriately sized aortic valve across the aortotomy to the annulus, especially if the aorta has lost some of its elastic properties as a result of calcification. The oblique aortotomy eliminates many of these concerns and is recommended by the authors. The aortic valve is inspected, and the locations of the coronary ostia are identified.

The valve is carefully excised, taking care not to buttonhole the aorta or damage the aortomitral continuity by incising too deeply. Careful debridement of all calcific matter is undertaken when necessary, followed by irrigation with cold saline to remove particulate matter (Fig. 30-3). The choice of valve and techniques of implantation are discussed below. Systemic rewarming is begun at an appropriate point in the implantation procedure to avoid imposing extra time waiting for the patient to reach normothermia before separation from cardiopulmonary bypass. After valve implantation, a careful inspection is done to confirm correct seating of the valve and ensure that both coronary ostia are unobstructed. A final check for the absence of residual particulate matter

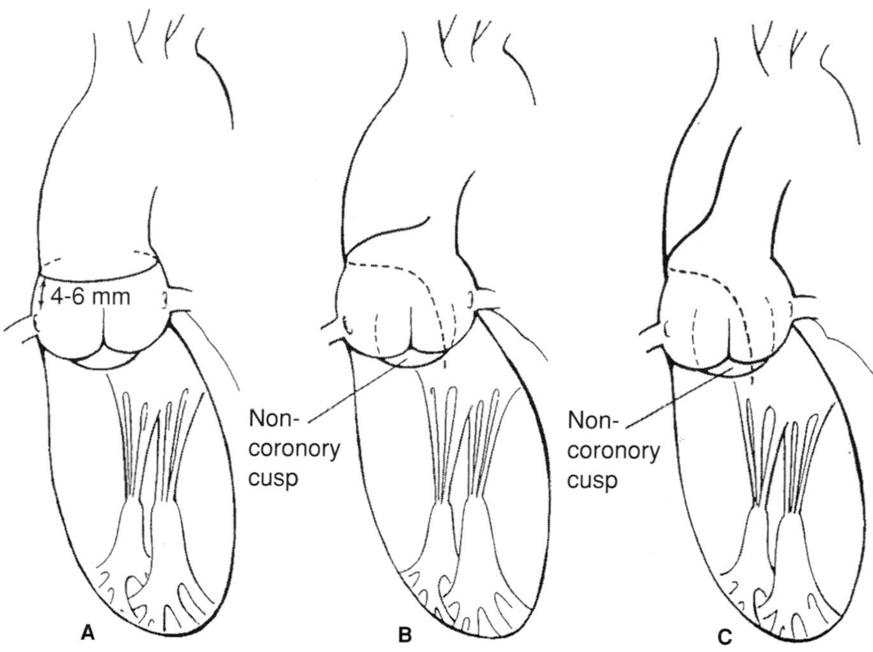

Figure 30-2 Aortotomy incisions. [Reproduced with permission from David TE. Mechanical and bioprosthetic aortic valve replacement. In: Edmunds LH (ed). *Cardiac Surgery in the Adult.* New York: McGraw-Hill; 1997:859–910.]

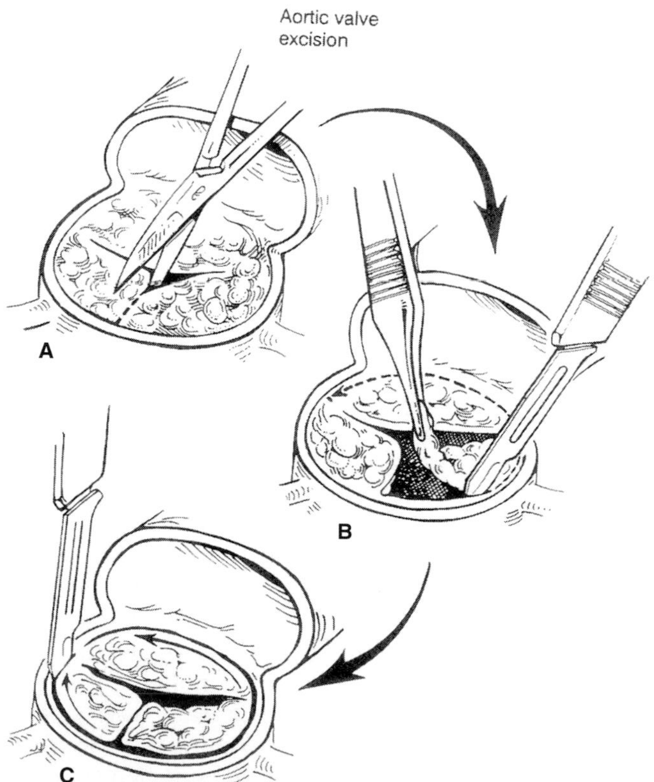

Figure 30-3 Technique of excision of the aortic valve. [Reproduced with permission from David TE. Mechanical and bioprosthetic aortic valve replacement. In: Edmunds LH (ed). *Cardiac Surgery in the Adult.* New York: McGraw-Hill; 1997:859–910.]

should be undertaken. The aortotomy is closed with running polypropylene sutures, and a de-airing vent is placed in the most anterior portion of the ascending aorta. The ventricular vent is removed. A warm cardioplegic infusion is given, and the cross-clamp is removed with the patient placed in the Trendelenburg position. Ventricular and atrial pacing wires are placed, and mechanical ventilation is resumed. De-airing maneuvers such as lung hyperinflation, side-to-side shaking of the chest, and manual agitation of the heart are performed with the heart partially ejecting. Transesophageal echocardiography is very helpful in the assessment of de-airing and in the interrogation of the valve for correct leaflet function and absence of perivalvular leaks. The patient is weaned from bypass at a systemic temperature of 36.5°C with good ventilation parameters. Protamine is given slowly by the surgeon directly into the ascending aorta, and the patient is decannulated. Meticulous hemostasis is obtained, a midline mediastinal drain (36F thoracostomy tube) is placed, and the patient is closed in the standard fashion.

Which type of valve to use

Subcoronary homograft aortic valves are technically more difficult to implant than are stented and stentless bioprostheses and should be considered for younger patients in centers that have extensive experience with homograft valve replacement.

Prosthetic valves have the advantage of relative ease of implantation. Bioprosthetic valves have no requirement for anticoagulation postoperatively, but two drawbacks are associated with these valves. The first is the introduction of a residual transvalvular gradient (especially with smaller valve sizes), which may impede the rapidity and extent of left ventricular mass regression after valve replacement The second drawback, the true Achilles' heel of tissue bioprostheses, is structural valve deterioration that requires reoperation for valve re-replacement. The latest-generation tissue bioprosthesis, such as the Carpentier-Edwards bovine pericardial[66–68]and the Hancock II[31,69] porcine valves, are comparable in results and have 80 to 93 percent freedom from structural valve failure at 10 to 14 years. These failure rates are accelerated in younger patients and patients with renal failure. This type of valve is clearly most appropriate for older patients (i.e., over 70 years of age). However, concomitant cardiac disease (e.g., coronary artery disease) lowers the age at which one tissue valve will suffice for the patient's lifetime by 5 to 10 years.[70] Also, concomitant use of oral lipid-lowering agents appears to have an important protective effect, with reduction of valve deterioration.[71,72] However, the risk of operative mortality with isolated aortic valve reoperation is only 5 to 10 percent,[73–75] making tissue valve replacement a reasonable option even in younger patients who are not interested in taking oral anticoagulants and in centers that do not perform a high volume of more complex aortic valve and root procedures.

Mechanical valves leave significant residual transvalvular gradients in smaller sizes as with stented bioprostheses, and all these patients require oral anticoagulation. The use of oral warfarin is associated with a significant incidence of bleeding and thromboembolic complications.[76,77] Thus, a younger individual who requires aortic valve replacement has to make a choice between the risk of an aortic valve reoperation with bioprosthetic valves and the risk of bleeding and thromboembolic complications related to long-term oral use of warfarin.

Valve implantation techniques and results

Stented aortic valve replacement

After excision of the native aortic valve, the annulus is sized by using the sizers provided by the company that makes the valve type that is selected. Valve sutures are placed in horizontal mattress fashion across the remaining aortic annulus and sequentially placed across the sewing ring of the prosthesis. The prosthetic valve is carefully seated to avoid obstructing the coronary artery ostia; this is followed by the tying and cutting of all the sutures and closure of the aorta. Certain valves are designed to be implanted in an intraannular position (such as certain St. Jude models), necessitating placement of everting (aorta to ventricle) sutures, and others are designed for supraannular seating (such as the Carpentier-Edwards pericardial prostheses), requiring placement of noneverting (ventricle to aorta) sutures. Pledgeted or nonpledgeted sutures are used; there are no conclusive data supporting the superiority of one over the other. In addition, some surgeons implant the prosthesis with a continuous running suture (Fig. 30-4). Although it is intuitively obvious that the largest valve size possible should be implanted, patients with severe LV hypertrophy resulting in intracavitary (i.e., subannular) gradients actually may be reliant on the stenotic native valve to impose sufficient afterload to prevent systolic ventricular collapse before ejection of an adequate stroke volume. In this uncommon situation, it may be appropriate to implant a *smaller* valve to impose a higher residual transvalvular gradient to encourage proper emptying of the ventricle. Alternatively, an interventricular septal myectomy/myotomy may help eliminate the intracavitary gradients in these unusual situations.[78]

The results with stented tissue prostheses continue to improve with each iteration. The latest-generation tissue bioprosthesis, such as the Carpentier-Edwards bovine pericardial[66–68] and the Hancock II[31,69] porcine valves, are comparable in results and have 80 to 93 percent freedom from structural valve failure at 10 to 14 years.

The results with mechanical valves relate more to the risk of bleeding and thromboembolic events. The longest data are available for the St. Jude mechanical prosthesis, with which actuarial freedom (at 10 and 20 years) from reoperation was 93 percent ± 1 percent and 90 percent ± 2 percent; from thromboembolism, 82 percent ± 3 percent and 68 percent ± 8 percent (linearized rate of 2.0 percent per patient-year); and from bleeding events, 77 percent ± 3 percent and 66 percent ± 6 percent (linearized rate of 2.5 percent per patient-year).[76]

The St. Jude stentless valve

This valve usually is implanted via a transecting aortotomy approximately 1.0 to 1.5 cm distal to the origin of the right coronary ostium. After the native valve is excised, the sewing ring is attached in planar fashion at the aortic annular level with simple interrupted sutures. After this procedure (since this valve has no supporting stent), the valve is fixed to the patient's aorta by sewing the rim of porcine aorta to the patient's aorta. The valve therefore must be seated carefully with the first set of interrupted sutures so that the second suture line orients the valve leaflets so that the coronary ostia are not obstructed. This valve is therefore more challenging to implant than are stented prostheses but offers the advantage of lower valve gradients, especially with smaller valve sizes.[79] The most recent data show freedom from hemodynamically significant valve insufficiency to be 82.5 percent at 9 years with 90.1 percent freedom from reoperation.[80] Anticoagulation is not required with this valve.

Medtronic freestyle prosthesis

The Medtronic Freestyle prosthesis preserves most of the porcine aortic root and is not reinforced by stented

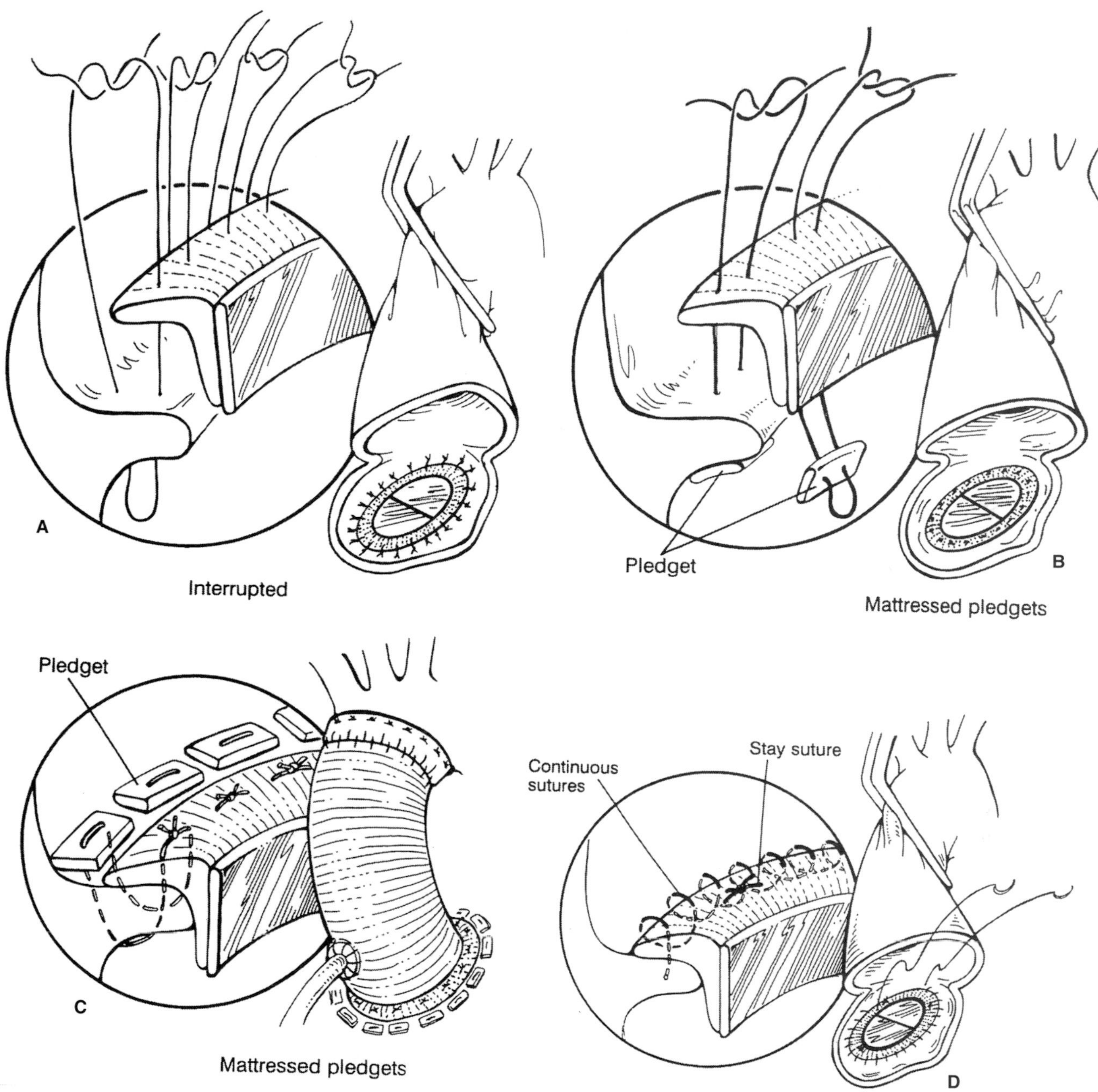

Figure 30-4 Annular suturing techniques. **A.** Interrupted sutures **B.** Noneverting mattressed pledgets **C.** Everted mattress pledgets with replacement of ascending aorta and aortic valve. **D.** Continuous running suture. [Reproduced with permission from David TE. Mechanical and bioprosthetic aortic valve replacement. In: Edmunds LH (ed). *Cardiac Surgery in the Adult.* New York: McGraw-Hill; 1997:859–910.]

or prosthetic fabric. This prosthesis offers the advantage of tailoring to multiple operations, including full aortic root replacement and trimming of the prosthesis for subcoronary valve replacement. The subcoronary operative technique is similar to that for the St. Jude stentless aortic valve except that the Freestyle aorta is scalloped to allow for coronary ostia on the left and right sinuses but typically is not scalloped over the noncoronary sinus. The results from the Medtronic Freestyle prosthesis used as a full aortic root replacement are available to 8 years.[81] At that time, freedom from aortic insufficiency was 100 percent and no cases of structural valve deterioration were observed, with 100 percent freedom from reoperation.[81] Comparison with the St. Jude stentless valve suggests less insufficiency and lower transvalvular gradients with the Freestyle prosthesis.[82] Anticoagulation is not required with this valve.

Subcoronary homograft aortic valve replacement

For the insertion of a homograft, it generally is recommended that a transecting or near-transecting aortotomy be used, though some authors have described the use of a lazy incision starting anteriorly and going to the patient's right but ending at a level well above the expected top of the allograft commissure. After resection of the aortic valve, the aortic annulus can be sized with a Hagar dilator or any convenient prosthetic valve sizer. Correcting for the thickness of the LV outflow tract muscle, generally, the allograft should be 2 to 3 mm smaller than the measured size of the annulus. At this point, the allograft ventricular outflow tract muscle should be trimmed to debulk it, but leaving enough support for suturing and attachment of the valve cusps. Approximately 5 to 7 mm of outflow tract should be left below the valve cusps to allow adequate suturing to the annulus. In addition, if there is residual anterior leaflet of the mitral valve, it can be excised in a planar fashion. Some authors recommend that the homograft not be implanted in anatomic fashion but instead that it be rotated 120 degrees counterclockwise so that the outflow tract muscle does not abut onto the interventricular septum of the recipient. After this, stay sutures usually are placed at 120-degree intervals in the graft, corresponding to the nadirs of the commissures for orientation.

Suturing of the homograft to the annulus can be performed in continuous fashion with running 4-0 polypropylene sutures or in interrupted fashion with running 4-0 polyester sutures placed in simple interrupted fashion. This can be facilitated by inverting the entire homograft into the left ventricular outflow tract of the recipient, making visualization of the suture technique much easier. After this the homograft sinuses are trimmed away to avoid obstructing the left and right coronary ostia, and the residual homograft aorta around the commissures is sutured to the native aortic wall with a running 4-0 polypropylene sutures. The aortic wall in the area of the noncoronary sinus can be left untrimmed to facilitate implantation. Although homograft aortic valve placement can be technically challenging, the results with this technique are excellent, with freedom from reoperation rates in adults of 81 to 93 percent at 15 years[83] and with no anticoagulation required.

Postoperative care and surgical results

Immediate postoperative care should focus on control of hypertension (for which intravenous sodium nitroprusside is used most commonly) and maintenance of adequate filling pressures (central venous pressure 10 to 15 mmHg, pulmonary capillary wedge pressures in the range of 15 to 18 mmHg). Dual-chamber pacing is required in a small proportion of patients who leave the operating room with conduction block. Often this resolves within 24 to 48 h. If conduction block persists longer than 4 to 5 days, permanent pacemaker insertion should be considered. In patients with no conduction disturbances, pacemaker wires can be removed on the third or forth postoperative day. The patient should be placed on telemetry for the duration of the hospital stay, however. The mediastinal tube is removed for outputs less than 150 mL per 24-h.

Patients with mechanical valves are started on oral warfarin on the second postoperative day. The use of daily aspirin coupled with a target International Normalized Ratio (INR) of 2.0 to 2.5 provides satisfactory anticoagulation and minimizes long-term bleeding and thrombotic events. Patients with bioprosthetic valves can be managed with aspirin alone, with no warfarin required.

The 30-day (early) mortality for aortic valve replacement varies from 2 to 5 percent. This number is approximately doubled with redo operations. Preoperative variables that are independently predictive of early mortality include advanced age, renal insufficiency, New York Heart Association class III or IV status, poor ventricular function, concomitant coronary artery disease, and aortic cross-clamp time.

Reoperation for mediastinal hemorrhage should be required in less than 5 percent of cases. Perivalvular leaks occur in 1 to 2 percent. Complete heart block requiring pacemaker insertion occurs in about 1 percent in most series. Stroke occurs in approximately 1 to 2 percent of these patients. There is no practical pharmacologic strategy for the prevention of postoperative atrial fibrillation, which occurs up to one-third of the time (in patients with no previous history). Careful correction of electrolytes and chemical cardioversion with intravenous and oral amiodarone are preferred and are successful 90 to 95 percent of the time. Patients then should be maintained on oral amiodarone for approximately 1 month, by which time the threat of recurrent atrial fibrillation should be resolved. In patients who require warfarin, the use of amiodarone will make it very difficult to manage the INR, and consideration should be given to alternative antiarrhythmics such as procainamide and sotalol. Patients with persistent atrial fibrillation despite attempts at chemical and electrical cardioversion should be maintained on oral warfarin until the arrhythmia resolves.

Patient-prosthesis mismatch

The important objectives of aortic valve replacement are to minimize postoperative gradients and optimize and accelerate the normalization of LV mass regression. Occasionally, a situation arises in which the implanted prosthetic valve has a gradient that is sufficiently severe to prevent a resolution of the physiology associated with valvular disease, resulting in "patient-prosthesis mismatch." This mismatch is expressed in terms of the effective orifice area (EOA) obtained from charts published by each valve company. The EOA is standardized to body surface area [effective orifice area index (EOAI)] and is suggested to be present for EOAI less than 0.85 to 0.90 cm^2/m^2.[84] A number of studies have attempted to investigate whether insertion of a small prosthesis influences short- and long-term survival. In light of the fact that early and late survival after aortic valve replacement usually is related more to concomitant disease processes in the valve itself, it is not surprising that many studies have not found a relationship between early and late survival and aortic valve prosthesis size. A very large study from the Cleveland Clinic by Medallion and colleagues was unable to detect an adverse impact on survival of moderate patient-prosthesis mismatch.[85] In contrast, a study by Kratz and colleagues suggested that patients with a body surface area greater than 1.9 mm who received the St. Jude valve in a size 19 mm or 21 mm had a greater probability of late sudden death.[86] A study by Adams and colleagues found that the insertion of a 19-mm stented bioprosthesis or mechanical valve in elderly males with aortic stenosis was associated with higher operative mortality and therefore recommended that an annulus-enlarging procedure be performed in those patients.[87] However, it is important to remember that the performance of an annulus-enlarging procedure increases the mortality and morbidity associated with aortic valve replacement, and this should be kept in mind when one is considering that procedure. More recently, three large studies have helped clarify the survival effect of patient-prosthesis mismatch on survival. Rao and associates[88] examined a cohort of 2981 patients undergoing aortic valve replacement; they observed that smaller prosthesis-patient size was associated with greater operative mortality but did not affect overall 12-year survival. In a study of 1129 patients, Hanayama and colleagues found that prosthesis-patient size did not influence survival, New York Heart functional class, or LV mass index.[89] Finally, Blackstone and associates examined data on 13,258 aortic valve replacements from nine data sources to address the question of prosthesis-patient size and mortality after aortic valve replacement. In that study, 30-day mortality increased 1 to 2 percent when the indexed orifice area decreased to less than 1.2 cm^2/m^2 or the standardized orifice size decreased to less than −2.5 Z. However, no expression of prosthesis-patient size was associated with reduced intermediate-term (0.5 to 5 years) or late-term (5 to 15 years) survival. In contrast, patient risk factors such as age had a profound effect on survival.[90]

Compared with the impact of valve prosthesis on survival, efficacy of regression of LV hypertrophy may be a more sensitive indicator of the adequacy of a prosthesis. Regression of LV mass after AVR is demonstrated within the first few weeks after surgery and extends out to about 6 months postoperatively.[91,92] The effective prosthesis size on regression of the LV mass has, however, proved somewhat controversial, as some authors have found that insertion of 19-mm and 21-mm stented and mechanical valves was associated with regression at a rate similar to that seen with larger prostheses.[93,94] However, other studies have shown slower regression of LV mass.[95] These controversies are confounded by the fact that the labeling of prosthetic valves and valve sizes do not bear a consistent relationship to the internal diameter of the valve orifice, which is probably the most important hemodynamically significant dimension in terms of postoperative gradients.[96] For example, the internal diameter of a St. Jude standard mechanical valve, which is labeled as 21 mm, is actually 16.7 mm, and the internal diameter of the modified orifice Hancock II porcine valve, which is labeled as 21 mm, is 18 mm. These discrepancies are particularly important in the management of a small aortic root in which insertion of an unnecessarily small prosthesis may result in very high postoperative gradients. In addition, comparison of the hemodynamic characteristics of various valve types becomes very difficult to judge on the basis of these parameters.

In the light of the information presented above, the impact of patient-prosthesis mismatch on postoperative outcomes after AVR is somewhat controversial. The EOAI may be used to identify patients with a "small aortic root" in the operating room, thus helping the surgeon plan the appropriate valve replacement strategy. After calculation of the patient's body surface area, excision of the diseased aortic valve, and annular debridement, the aortic annulus is sized by using the appropriate sizer for the valve intended for use. The EOA for this valve size is taken from a chart published by the valve company. If the EOAI is less than 0.85 to 0.90, the aortic root may be considered small.

Management of a small aortic root

The fundamental goal of the management of a small aortic root is to avoid insertion of an unnecessarily small prosthesis. In general, the surgical options include the use of a small stented prosthesis, mechanical dilatation of the aortic root, implantation of stentless tissue valves, supraannular positioning of the valve replacement device, implementation of an annulus-enlarging procedure, and in certain cases application of the apicoaortic conduit technique. A useful rule of thumb is that increasing the valve size by two increments in general results in a reduction of cardiac stroke work of approximately 40 percent, roughly equivalent to the insertion of an intraaortic balloon counterpulsation device.

Use of a small stented prosthesis

In light of the discussion above, in certain situations it may be appropriate to accept implantation of a small prosthesis that by calculation would result in a patient-prosthesis mismatch. Examples of such situations include elderly inactive patients, patients with multiple comorbidities in whom a fast and relatively simple operation is mandatory for the best outcome, and an aortic root that is so calcified that other valve replacement options may be technically impossible.

Mechanical dilatation of the aortic root

Anecdotal reports have documented successful insertion of larger prosthesis after mechanical dilatation of the aortic root.[97] However, there are very few data regarding the overall safety of this procedure and the amount of annulus enlargement achievable. Caution must be exercised in considering this option.

Implantation of stentless tissue valves

Compared with stented bioprostheses, stentless bioprostheses in general have been confirmed to be hemodynamically superior in various valve sizes. Because of the obliteration of the thick stent with stentless tissue valves, it is often possible to implant a larger valve with a larger internal orifice area than would be the case if a stentless valve were used, resulting in lower postoperative gradients.[98,99] For example, in patients in whom a 19-mm Carpentier-Edwards supraannular pericardial valve fits tightly into the annulus, it is usually possible to fit a 21- or 23-mm St. Jude stentless valve. Successful implantation of this valve is also dependent on the aortic root tissue being pliable and not extensively calcified so that suturing to it is possible.

Supraannular positioning of the valve prosthesis

Because the noncoronary sinus at its nadir may be lower than the nadir of the left and right aortic sinuses, the prosthesis sometimes can be implanted in the supraannular position within the noncoronary sinus.[100] The prosthesis then is sutured along the aortic annulus and the left and right coronary sinuses but attached by pledgeted mattress sutures, with the pledgets outside the aorta in the noncoronary sinus. This technique may allow implantation of a prosthesis that is one size larger than the size of the aortic annulus. Because the prosthesis crosses the aortic annulus, improper debridement of the annulus in this area may result in paravalvular leaks.

Annulus-enlarging procedure

The Nicks[101] procedure allows for the implantation of a prosthesis that is approximately two sizes larger than the measured size of the aortic annulus. This involves the extension of the aortotomy into the nadir of the noncoronary sinus and into the basal third of the anterior leaflet of the mitral valve. An autologous pericardial patch or Dacron patch is fashioned in a teardrop shape, and the wide portion of the teardrop, 3 to 4 cm in transverse diameter, is positioned downward into the mitral valve. Valve sutures or polypropylene sutures then are used to suture the patch along the anterior leaflet of the mitral valve, across the annulus, and up the ascending aorta. Valve implantation sutures are placed across the patch itself in addition to the remainder of the annulus, and the remainder of the aortotomy is closed, incorporating the Dacron patch (Fig. 30-5).

A second type of annulus-enlarging procedure known as the Manouguian[102] procedure involves extension of the aortotomy more posteriorly to the commissure of the noncoronary and left coronary cusps. The incision then is carried through the aortic mitral septum and onto the anterior leaflet of the mitral valve for up to 2 cm; this also opens the roof of the left atrium. A pericardial patch is sutured along the mitral valve incision and the aortotomy as with the Nicks procedure. The prosthesis then is secured to the patch with horizontal mattress sutures that may first be placed through the opened roof of the left atrium, thus closing the atriotomy in the process. Alternatively, the atriotomy can be sutured to the patch with a second suture line. The remainder of the aortotomy then may be closed.

A third, more radical approach to a small aortic root is known as the Konno-Rastan procedure or aortoventriculoplasty.[103] Its use in a small aortic root associated with aortic valve disease is becoming rare, and in general this technique is reserved for enlargements in patients with congenital aortic stenosis who present later in life for aortic valve replacement and patients with other forms of complex congenital heart disease. Here the enlarging incision is made to the left side of the right coronary artery and into the ventricular septum and the free wall of the right ventricle. Next, a patch is used to repair the intraventricular septum and a second patch is used to close the right ventricular free wall defect as well as completing the annular enlargement.

As was stated previously, it is important to remember that the operative risk with aortic valve replacement may be increased with an annulus-enlarging procedure, with one series quoting a 3.5 percent operative risk without annulus enlargement compared with 7.1 percent with annulus enlargement.[104]

Ventricular apicoaortic conduit

In patients in whom it is not possible to deal with an excessively small aortic root, such as those with fibrous tunnel formation, tubular hypoplasia of the ascending aorta, and recurrent aortic valve stenosis that is not relieved by aortic root repair or a valvotomy, ventricular apical aorta conduits have been used as a procedure of last resort.[105,106] The patient is approached by a left lateral thoracotomy based on the fifth intercostal space. A valved conduit then is sutured in end-to-side fashion to the descending thoracic aorta. After this, cardiopulmonary bypass is established and a second graft is sutured to the apex of the left ventricle with the aid of induced fibrillation. The two conduits then are trimmed to length and sutured together, completing the operation (Fig. 30-6). The transthoracic approach provides direct access to the descending aorta and avoids the need for redo sternotomy. The technique, which is relatively simple to perform, does not compromise major coronary arteries, the conduction system, or other valves and may be useful in patients who are not good candidates for other, more conventional procedures.

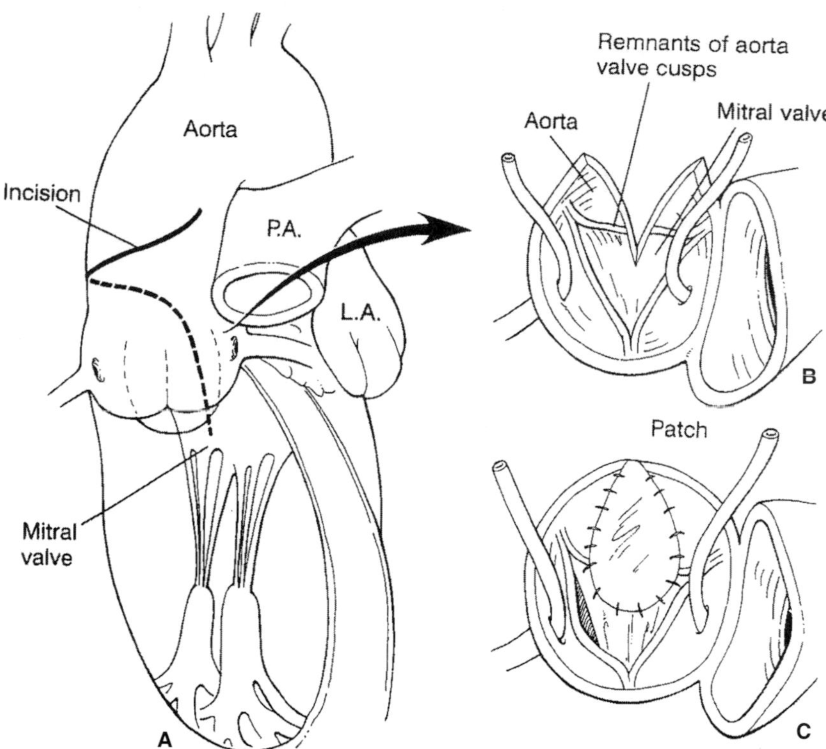

Figure 30-5 Patch enlargement of the aortic annulus at the noncoronary sinus (Nicks procedure). **A.** The aortotomy incision continues downward toward the middle noncoronary sinus. **B.** The incision crosses the aortic annulus into the midmitral portion of the anterior mitral leaflet to the roof of the right atrium. **C.** The incision has extended into the upper third of the mitral leaflet. The width of the patch should not exceed twice the length of the incision into the anterior mitral leaflet. [Reproduced with permission from David TE. Complex operations of the aortic root. In: Edmunds LH (ed). *Cardiac Surgery in the Adult.* New York: McGraw-Hill; 1997:939–957.]

Aortic valve replacement with concomitant coronary artery disease

Many patients with aortic valvular disease have concomitant coronary artery disease (CAD), but the data are limited regarding optimal strategies for the diagnosis and treatment of CAD in those patients. Ischemic symptoms in patients with aortic valvular disease may have multiple causes, such as LV chamber enlargement, increased wall stress or wall thickening with subendocardial ischemia, and right ventricular hypertrophy. Because angina is a poor marker of CAD in these patients, coronary arteriography is recommended in symptomatic patients before aortic valve replacement, especially in males older than age 35 years, premenopausal females older than age 35 years with coronary risk factors, and postmenopausal females.[59]

More than one-third of patients with aortic stenosis who undergo aortic valve replacement surgery have concomitant CAD. Population studies have shown that more than 50 percent of patients over 70 years old have CAD. Combined coronary artery bypass surgery at the time of aortic surgery or aortic valve replacement has had little or no adverse effect on operative mortality. Additionally, coronary bypass grafting at the time of AVR reduces the rates of perioperative myocardial infarction, operative mortality, and late mortality and morbidity compared with patients with significant CAD who do not undergo revascularization at the time of AVR. Incomplete revascularization is associated with greater postoperative systolic dysfunction and reduced survival rates after surgery compared with patients who receive complete revascularization.[107,108] Over the last decade, improved anesthesia and myocardial preservation techniques have been associated with reduced overall operative mortality,[109] and it has become standard practice to bypass all significant coronary artery stenoses surgically when possible in patients undergoing aortic valve surgery.

It is well agreed on that all patients undergoing coronary artery bypass surgery who have severe aortic stenosis,

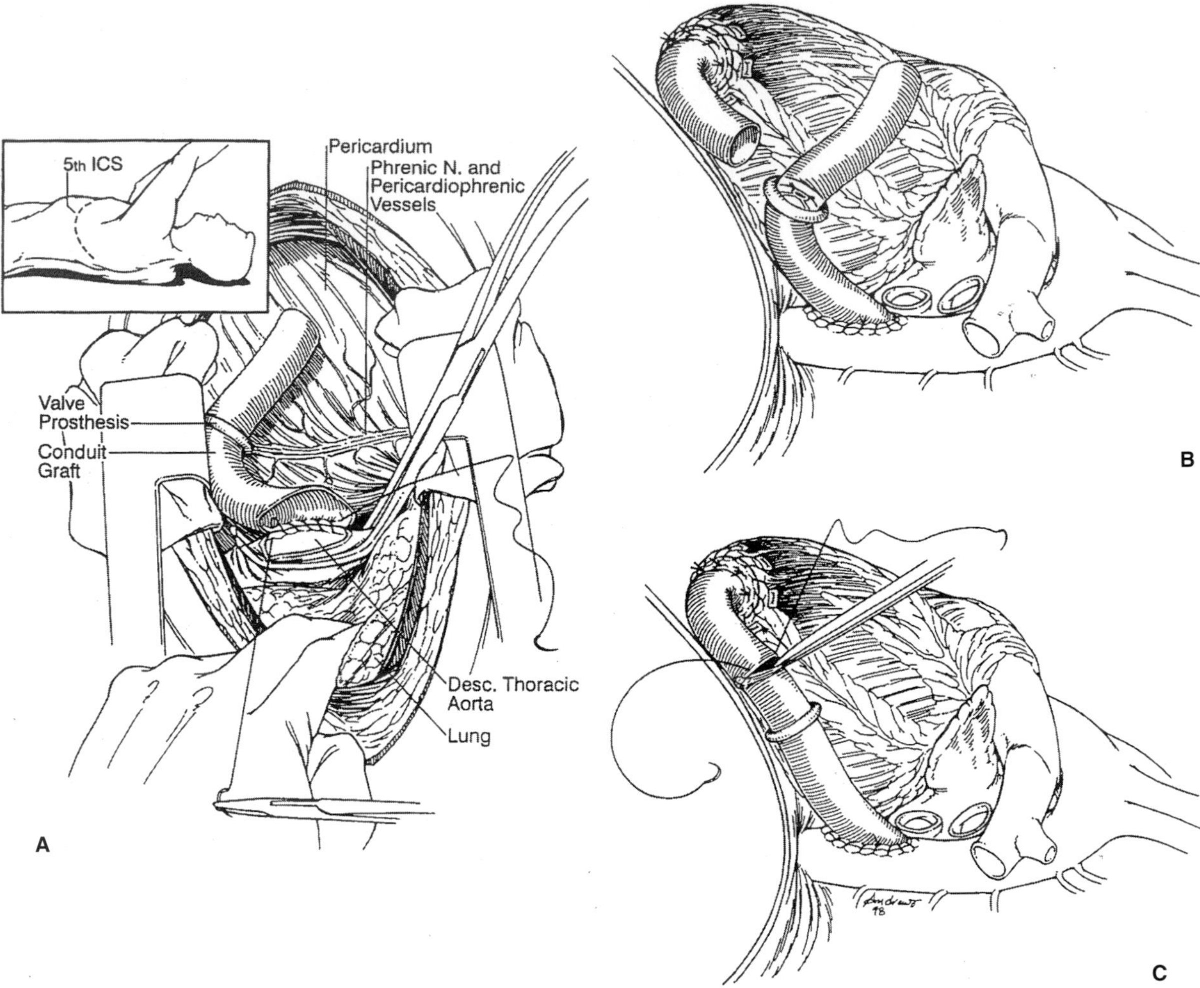

Figure 30-6 Placement of an apicoaortic conduit. **A.** After the patient has been put in the right lateral decubitus position, the left hemithorax is entered through the fifth intercostal space. The descending thoracic aorta is partially occluded, and the valved conduit is anastomosed with continuous 3-0 or 4-0 polypropylene sutures. **B.** Under cardiopulmonary bypass, the rigid prosthesis is attached to the apex of the left ventricular via interrupted pledgeted mattress and continuous sutures. Ventricular fibrillation is induced to facilitate the ventricular attachment. Temporary occluding clamps are used on the grafts during completion of the anastomoses. **C.** The prostheses are connected with a continuous suture. (Reproduced with permission from Cooley DA, Lopez RM, Absi TS. Apicoaortic conduit for left ventricular outflow tract obstruction: Revisited. *Ann Thorac Surg* 2000;69:1511–1514.)

symptomatic or not, should undergo aortic valve replacement at the time of revascularization.[59] Decision making is more difficult in patients with mild to moderate aortic stenosis who have coronary artery disease that requires coronary bypass surgery. Controversy persists regarding the indications for so-called prophylactic valve replacements at the time of coronary bypass surgery in such patients.

It is difficult to predict whether a specific patient with CAD and mild aortic stenosis (AS) is likely to develop clinically significant AS after revascularization. The natural history of mild AS is variable, with some patients manifesting a rapid progression of their disease, with a decrease in valve area of up to 0.3 cm^2 per year and an increase in pressure gradient of 15 to 19 mmHg per year.[110] The average rate of reduction of valve area is 0.12 cm^2 per year,[111] but the rate of change in an individual patient is difficult to foresee. Phillips and associates[112] reviewed 100 patients who underwent AVR after previous coronary artery bypass grafting (CABG) in whom the mean valve gradient was less than 25 mmHg at the time of initial operation. The mean time interval to reoperation was 9.0 years (range 1.4 to 21 years), and overall operative mortality was 7.0 percent. The authors concluded that in light of the relatively long interval between the two operations and the significant decline in the reoperative mortality rate in recent years, an expectant approach to concomitant AVR-CABG is warranted.[112] Karagounis and associates reviewed 200 patients requiring CABG who all had AS with peak gradients less than or equal to 40 mmHg. Among those patients, 46 underwent combined AVR-CABG at first operation. Over a median follow-up period of 4.2 years, none of the patients who had CABG only at first operation required reoperation for AVR. From these data, those authors recommended CABG only for patients with mild aortic stenosis.[113] In contrast, Ahmed and colleagues followed 40 patients with mild to moderate AS who underwent CABG without AVR. Eleven patients (27 percent) in that study group required reoperation for AVR.[114] Similarly, Hochrein and associates noted a 24.3 percent AVR reoperation rate over a 6-year period in patients receiving CABG alone versus 3 percent in patients who underwent AVR-CABG at initial operation.[115] The results of these two studies suggest that AVR is a reasonable option at the time of initial CABG in this patient population. Smith and associates[116] performed a decision analysis that was based on the Society of Thoracic Surgeons national database and submitted the following recommendations. For patients under 70 years old, AVR for mild aortic stenosis is recommended if the peak valve gradient is 25 to 30 mmHg. For older patients, the threshold gradient increases by 1 to 2 mmHg per year of age. Also, CABG is favored only in patients with slow (less than 3 mmHg/year) progression of aortic stenosis, in contrast to those with rapid progression (more than 10 mmHg/year), who should have combined AVR/CABG, with the possible exception of patients over 80 years old who have valve gradients less than 25 mmHg at the time of surgery.[116] The choice of prosthesis does not influence overall survival, but a bioprosthetic valve is probably more appropriate in this setting because of increased complications related to the requirement for anticoagulation with mechanical valves[116] and because the decreased longevity in patients with significant coronary artery disease undergoing AVR with CABG makes structural valve deterioration much less likely.[70]

Aortic valve replacement in end-stage renal disease

Aortic stenosis is common in patients who are undergoing maintenance dialysis. Abnormalities include annular and valvular thickening and calcification of one or more of the heart valves, leading to stenosis with or without concomitant regurgitation.

Many predisposing factors are associated with valvular disease in dialysis patients, with the most noteworthy being secondary hyperparathyroidism.[117,118] Valvular calcification is associated with an elevated calcium-phosphorus product, hypercalcemia, vascular calcification, and elevated phosphate levels; these all are findings that can occur in patients with marked secondary hyperparathyroidism. Valvular calcification also may be found in the absence of secondary hyperparathyroidism, particularly among those with bone disease, older patients, and those who have undergone dialysis for a longer period. The association with adynamic bone disease may be related to the increasing utilization of calcium-containing phosphate binders and the subsequent development of hypercalcemia.[119] Additional factors that may enhance the development of valvular heart disease in this patient population include the presence of one or more of the following conditions: hypertension, hyperlipidemia, LV hypertrophy, hypertrophic cardiomyopathy, mitral valve prolapse, high-cardiac-output states, anemia, and infective endocarditis.

The use of bioprosthetic valves in hemodialysis patients was classified as a class III indication by the 1998 American College of Cardiology/American Heart Association Task Force on Practice Guidelines, with valve replacement with a mechanical prosthesis classified as a class II or IIa indication.[59] This recommendation is based on the widely held opinion that the risk of accelerated bioprosthetic valve failure mandates the use of mechanical prosthetic valves in hemodialysis patients. In a study of over 95,000 patients, Byrne and colleagues reported the survival of all Medicare patients with end-stage renal failure in the United States from 1982 to 1987.[120] The average survival of a patient between 55 and 65 years old from the time dialysis was started was 52 percent at 3 years and 33 percent at 5 years. This suggests that life expectancy among these patients is so poor that there is little need for a prosthetic valve that will endure more than a few years in this population.

Lucke and coworkers[121] reviewed their experience with 19 patients on long-term dialysis undergoing valve replacement from 1979 to 1994. Nine patients received bioprosthetic valves, and 10 received mechanical valves. At a mean follow-up of 32 months, no patient required reoperation for bioprosthesis degeneration; however, patients who received mechanical valves had a higher incidence of thromboembolism and bleeding, leading the authors to conclude that bioprosthetic valve replacement was preferable. Kaplon and associates[122] reviewed 42 patients on chronic preoperative dialysis who underwent valve replacement, of whom 17 received mechanical valves and 25 received bioprostheses. Survival at 3 and 5 years was 50 percent and 33 percent after mechanical valve replacement and 36 percent and 27 percent after bioprosthetic valve replacement ($p = 0.3$). Four patients with bioprostheses required reoperation: three for allograft endocarditis and one at 10 months for bioprosthesis degeneration. One patient who received a mechanical valve required reoperation. Those authors concluded that since the life expectancy of patients on dialysis is limited, bioprosthesis degeneration will be uncommon and therefore surgeons should not hesitate to implant bioprosthetic valves in those patients.[122] More recently, Brinkman and associates[123] reviewed 72 patients on chronic dialysis undergoing valve replacement. In the 46 patients with reliable long-term (greater than 30 days) follow-up data, significant bleeding or stroke was documented in 17 of 34 patients with a mechanical valve and 1 of 12 patients with a bioprosthetic valve. The type of valve implanted did not influence early and late survival. Those authors concluded that the sixfold higher incidence of late bleeding or stroke in patients on dialysis with a mechanical valve requiring warfarin suggested that bioprosthetic valves are the valve substitute of choice in patients on chronic dialysis. Herzog and colleagues[124] studied dialysis patients from the U.S. Renal Data System database who were hospitalized for heart valve replacement surgery from 1978 to 1998. The in-hospital mortality of 5858 dialysis patients (of whom 3415 underwent AVR) undergoing valve surgery was 20.7 percent. There was no significant difference in survival related to the type of prosthetic valve. Those authors concluded that there was no significant difference in survival of dialysis patients after cardiac valve replacement with tissue versus nontissue prosthetic valves.

These data indicate that valvular replacement in patients undergoing hemodialysis has a poor prognosis, and although either type of prosthesis is a viable option, the weight of evidence tends to support the use of bioprosthetic valves in these patients.

Aortic valve replacement in infective endocarditis

Infective endocarditis is a highly lethal disease in which a microorganism colonizes a site in the heart and produces a variety of manifestations, including fever, sepsis, splenomegaly, and embolic events. With aortic valve endocarditis, cardiac abnormalities such as congenitally bicuspid, degenerative, and rheumatic valve disease create endocardial "jet lesions" that promote seeding by microorganisms. Common microorganism sources include dental extractions, endoscopy, urinary tract infections, chronic intravenous drug use, and requirements for long-term, frequently intravenous access such as with chronic chemotherapy, parenteral nutrition, and hemodialysis.

More than 80 percent of native endocarditis cases are due to streptococci (50 percent) and staphylococci (20 percent). The first-line treatment for subacute endocarditis (usually caused by less virulent strains such as *Streptococcus viridans*) is antimicrobial therapy, which in endocarditis patients is guided by identification of the infective organism. The much more fulminant cases of acute endocarditis (often caused by *Staphylococcus aureus*) do not respond well to antibiotics, and early surgery almost always is recommended if feasible. Prosthetic valve endocarditis also has subacute and acute forms, and a wide spectrum of organisms can be responsible. In "early" prosthetic valve endocarditis, or endocarditis within the first 2 months after surgery, *Staphylococcus epidermidis* is the most common organism. Late-onset prosthetic valve endocarditis more closely follows the profile of native valve endocarditis. *Enterococcus faecalis* and *Enterococcus faecium* account for 90 percent of cases of enterococcal endocarditis, usually associated with malignancy or manipulation of the genitourinary or gastrointestinal tract. Recently, microorganisms in the HACEK group (*Haemophilus, Actinobacillus, Cardiobacterium, Eikenella,* and *Kingella* species) have become important causes of endocarditis. In addition to bacteria, fungi, especially *Candida,* are important causes of endocarditis in patients with prosthetic valves, compromised immune systems, or intravenous drug abuse.

Indications for surgical intervention in patients with endocarditis include new-onset unmanageable congestive heart failure and cardiogenic shock secondary to treatable valvular heart disease with or without an established diagnosis of endocarditis. Prompt intervention should not be delayed in acute infective endocarditis patients with congestive heart failure. Surgery is indicated in patients with life-threatening hemodynamic instability caused by surgically treatable valvular heart disease only if a patient's prospects for recovery are reasonable, with satisfactory quality of life after the operation. Surgery is not indicated if complications (such as severe embolic cerebral damage) or comorbid conditions make the prospect of recovery dismal. Additional indications for surgical intervention in a hemodynamically stable patient with documented infective endocarditis include prolonged failure of antimicrobial therapy demonstrated by cultures persistently positive for bacteria, patients with annular or aortic abscesses, pericarditis, fungal and gram-negative endocarditis (antimicrobial therapy is not efficacious), new-onset heart block, evidence of systemic embolism, and vegetation size. Patients with a vegetation diameter greater than 10 mm have a significantly higher incidence of embolization than do those with a vegetation diameter equal to or less than 10 mm.[125]

Aortic valve endocarditis is associated with the highest rate of complications, and surgical intervention most often is indicated. Treatment consists of excision of the infected valve, adequate debridement of perivalvular abscesses, and valve replacement. If the endocarditis appears to be confined to the valve leaflets, prosthetic valve replacement may suffice. In this setting, there are no data supporting the superiority of either bioprosthetic or mechanical valves. If the disease extends into the annulus with or without abscess formation, full debridement followed by tissue allograft is required to reduce postoperative reinfection.[126] Involvement of the aortomitral continuity may mandate excision of this area and reconstruction with bovine pericardium in addition to valve replacement (Fig. 30-7).[127] If possible, it is recommended that the patient have at least 2 days of broad-spectrum intravenous antibiotics to clear microorganisms from the bloodstream.

Operative mortality for infection limited to the aortic valve leaflets is comparable to the operative mortality of

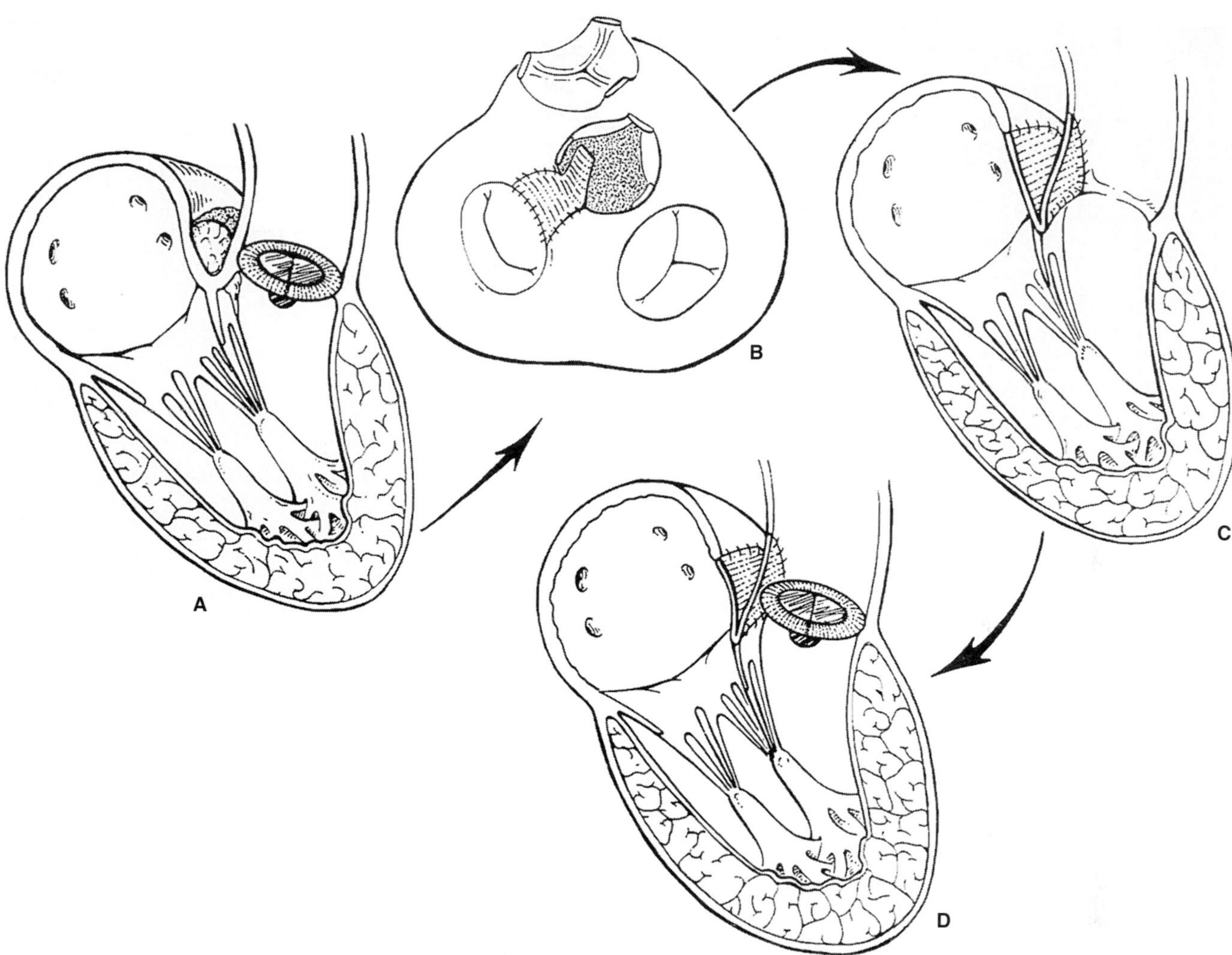

Figure 30-7 Excision of endocardial abscess within fibrous trigone with pericardial patch reconstruction. **A.** Diagram of periprosthetic valvular abscess extending into the fibrous trigone and roof of the left atrium. **B.** Cross-sectional view of the base of the heart with a pericardial patch sutured to the fibrous trigone along the mitral annulus, the roof of the left atrium, and the aortic root. **C.** Sagittal view of patch reconstructing the aortomitral continuity, the roof of the left atrium, and the aortic root. **D.** New prosthetic implant inserted. [Reproduced with permission from David TE. Complex operations of the aortic root. In Edmunds LH (ed). *Cardiac Surgery in the Adult.* New York: McGraw-Hill; 1997:939–957.]

isolated uninfected aortic valve replacement; however, mortality is higher in those with aortic root abscesses or prosthetic valve endocarditis.[127] Published results show an operative mortality for native valve endocarditis of less than 10 percent, and for prosthetic valve endocarditis mortality is between 20 and 25 percent[128,129] David and associates studied 62 patients undergoing valvular intervention for active endocarditis and reported an operative mortality rate of zero for native valve endocarditis and 12.5 percent for prosthetic valve endocarditis.[130] Valve replacement in hemodynamically stable patients results in a favorable outcome in over 80 percent of cases; however, a reinfection rate of 1 to 13 percent can be expected.

Prosthetic valve endocarditis (PVE), as previously discussed, usually involves a clinical course that begins with antibiotic therapy and ends with valvular replacement. Patients with documented PVE who are treated with antibiotic therapy alone generally experience very poor outcomes. Survival rates without surgery are in the range of 20 to 30 percent.[128] Long-term survival of PVE patients after valve replacement is approximately 60 percent at 10 years,[131] with a significant risk of recurrent endocarditis. Recent use of aortic root homografts as the first option for replacement have produced improved early and late survival, and this has become the preferred choice of valve for PVE patients.[132]

SUMMARY

Aortic valve replacement can be performed in patients in whom there is an underlying anatomic or functional abnormality of the aortic valve that causes it to become stenotic or regurgitant. Surgical treatment for aortic valve disease has evolved since its initiation nearly 100 years ago. From the initial attempt to correct aortic stenosis via valvotomy to the mechanical and biological prostheses used today, much progress has been made, and aortic valve replacement has become an excellent method of treating aortic valve disease.

Aortic insufficiency initially may be treated medically with afterload reduction, and failure of this treatment is an indication for surgical valve replacement. Aortic stenosis, however, cannot be treated medically and improves only with intervention. Surgical indications for aortic valve replacement involve the severity of symptoms, the nature of the valve disorder (regurgitant or stenotic), the cause of the disorder, and cardiac function.

For patients in whom surgical replacement of the aortic valve is indicated, clinical decisions involve the correct positioning of the patient, appropriate incision placement, and the use of cardiopulmonary bypass. In addition, the surgeon must choose the appropriate type of valve replacement device, including deciding whether to use a stented aortic valve replacement, a St. Jude stentless valve, or other options, such as the Medtronic Freestyle Prosthesis, or to use a subcoronary homograft aortic valve replacement.

In addition, selected patients have circumstances that involve special surgical considerations regarding surgical aortic valve replacement such as prosthesis-patient mismatch and management of the small aortic root. Certain patients have concomitant conditions such as coronary artery disease, end-stage renal disease, and infective endocarditis, all of which pose specific difficulties for the surgeon.

References

1. Tuffier T: Etat actuel de le chirurgie intrathoracique. *Trans Int Congr Med* 1913 (London 1914);7:249.
2. Brock R. The arterial route to the aortic and pulmonary valves: The mitral route to the aortic valves. *Guys Hosp Rep* 1950;99:236.
3. Brock R. Aortic subvalvular stenosis: Surgical treatment. *Guys Hosp Rep* 1957;106:221.
4. Bailey CP, Bolton HE, Nichols HT et al. Commissurotomy for rheumatic aortic stenosis. *Circulation* 1954;9:22.
5. Smithy HG, Parker EF. Experimental aortic valvulotomy: A preliminary report. *Surg Gynecol Obstet* 1947;84:625–628.
6. Hufnagel CA: Aortic plastic valvular prostheses. *Bull Georgetown Med Center* 1953;4:128.
7. Campbell JM: Artificial aortic valve. *J Thorac Cardiovasc Surg* 1938;19:312.
8. Hufnagel CA, Harvey WP, Rabil PJ, et al. Surgical correction of aortic insufficiency. *Surgery* 1954;33:673.
9. Lefrak EA, Starr A. Caged ball valves. In: Lefrak EA, Starr A (eds). *Cardiac Valve Prostheses.* New York: Appleton-Century-Crofts; 1979:67–166.
10. Fann JI, Moreno-Cabral, Miller DC. Caged-ball valves: The Starr-Edwards and Smeloff-Cutter prosthesis. In: Bodnar E, Frater RWM (eds). *Replacement Cardiac Valves.* New York: Pergammon; 1991:149–186.
11. Melrose DG, Bentall HH, McMillam IKR, et al. The evolution of a mitral valve prosthesis. *Lancet* 1964;2:623.
12. Knight CJ, McLeod N. Taylor DEM. Physical principles of the Edinburgh prosthetic heart valve. *Med Biol Eng Comput* 1977;14:264–272.
13. Bjork VO. The central-flow tilting disc valve prosthesis (Bjork-Shiley) for mitral valve replacement. *Scand J Thorac Cardiovasc Surg* 1970;4:15–23.
14. Bjork VO. The improved Bjork-Shiley tilting disc valve prosthesis. *Scand J Thorac Cardiovasc S*urg 1978;12:81–89.
15. Vogel JHK. The monostrut Bjork-Shiley heart valve. *J Am Coll Cardiol* 1985;6:1142.
16. Chun PKC, Nelson WP. Common cardiac prosthetic valves. *JAMA* 1977;238:401.
17. Cortina J, Martinell J, Artiz V, et al. Comparative clinic results with Omniscience (STM1), Medtronic-Hall and Bjork-Shiley convexo-concave (70 degrees) prostheses in mitral valve replacement. *J Thorac Cardiovasc Surg* 1986;91:174–183.
18. Gott VL, Daggett, RL, Mantini EL, et al. A hinged leaflet valve for total replacement of the human aortic valve. *J Thorac Cardiovasc S*urg 1964;48:713.
19. Kalke BR, Mantini EL, Kaster RL, et al. Hemodynamic features of a double-leaflet prosthetic heart valve of new design. *Trans Am Soc Artif Intern Organs* 1967;13:105.
20. Wada J, Komatau S, Ikeda K, et al. A new hingeless valve. In: Brewer LA (ed). *Prosthetic Heart Valves.* Springfield IL: Charles C. Thomas; 1969:304–314.
21. Emery RW, Palmquist WE, Mettler E, et al. A new cardiac valve prosthesis: In vitro results. *Trans Am Artif Intern Organs* 1978;24:550.
22. Carrel T, Zingg U, Jenni R, et al. Early in vivo experience with the Hemodynamic Plus St. Jude Medical heart valves in patients with narrowed aortic annulus. *Ann Thorac Surg* 1996;61:1418–1422.
23. Zingg U, Aeschbacher B, Seiler C, et al. Early experience with the new Masters series of St. Jude Medical heart valve: In vivo hemodynamic and clinical results in patients with narrowed aortic annulus. *J Heart Valve Dis* 1997;6:535–541.
24. Bach DS, Goldbach M, Sakwa MP, et al. Hemodynamics and early performance of the St. Jude Medical Regent aortic valve prosthesis. *J Heart Valve Dis* 2001;10:436–442.
25. Santini F, Casali G, Viscardi F, et al. The CarboMedics prosthetic heart valve: Experience with 1,084 implants. *J Heart Valve Dis* 2002;11:121–126.
26. Whitaker DC, James SE, Walesby RK. A single-center experience of the Sorin Bicarbon heart valve prosthesis: Long-term clinical, hematological and hemodynamic results. *J Heart Valve Dis* 2004;13:97–102.
27. Carpentier A, Lemaigre G, Ladislas R, Dubost C: Biological factors affecting long-term results of valvular heterografts. *J Thorac Cardiovasc S*urg 1969;58:467.

28. Cevese PO, Gallucci V, Morea M, et al. Heart valve replacement with the Hancock bioprosthesis: Analysis of long-term results. *Circulation* 1977;56(Suppl II):II-111–II-116.
29. Cohn LH, DiSesa VJ, Collins JJ Jr. The Hancock modified-orifice porcine bioprosthetic valve: 1976–1988. *Ann Thorac Surg* 1989;48(Suppl 3):S81–82.
30. Jamieson WRE, Janusz MT, Miyakishima RT, et al. The Carpentier-Edwards standard porcine bioprosthesis—Long-term evaluation of the high pressure glutaraldehyde fixed prostheses: Proceedings of the Fourth International Symposium–Cardiac Bioprosthesis. *J Card Surg* 1988;3(Suppl I):321–336.
31. David TE, Ivanov J, Armstrong S, et al. Late results of heart valve replacement with the Hancock II bioprosthesis. *J Thorac Cardiovasc* Surg 2001;121(2):268–277.
32. Jaffe WM, Barratt-Boyes BG, Sadri A, et al. Early follow-up of patients with the Medtronic Intact porcine valve: A new cardiac bioprosthesis. *J Thorac Cardiovasc Surg* 1989;98:181–192.
33. Ionescue MI, Silverton NP, Tandon AP. The pericardial xenograft valve in the mitral position. In: Ionescu M, Cohn LH (eds). *Mitral Valve Disease*, London, Butterworths; 1985:253–269.
34. Duran CG. The pericardial heart valve: An open question. In: Bodnar E, Frater RWM (eds). *Replacement Cardiac Valves*. New York: Pergammon; 1991:149–186.
35. Anderson DR, Deverall PB, Revuelta JM, et al. Early results of the Mitroflow valve. In: Bodnar E, Yacoub M (eds): *Biologic and Bioprosthetic Valves*. New York: Yorke Medical Books; 1986:725–730.
36. Relland J, Perier P, Lecointe B. The third generation Carpentier-Edwards "bioprosthesis": Early results. *J Am Coll Cardiol* 1985;6:1149–1154.
37. Banbury MK, Cosgrove DM 3rd, Thomas JD, et al. Hemodynamic stability during 17 years of the Carpentier-Edwards aortic pericardial bioprosthesis. *Ann Thorac Surg* 2002;73:1460–1465.
38. Del Rizzo DF, Goldman BS, Christakis GT, David TE. Hemodynamic benefits of the Toronto Stentless Valve. *J Thorac Cardiovasc Surg* 1996;112:1431–1445.
39. Kon ND, Riley RD, Adair SM, et al. Eight-year results of aortic root replacement with the freestyle stentless porcine aortic root bioprosthesis. *Ann Thorac Surg* 2002;73(6):1817–1821.
40. Jin XY, Ratnatunga C, Pillai R. Performance of Edwards prima stentless aortic valve over eight years. *Semin Thorac Cardiovasc Surg* 2001;13(4 Suppl 1):163–167.
41. Sadowski J, Kapelak B, Bartus K, et al. Stentless 3F Therapeutics Aortic Bioprosthesis—a new alternative to aortic valve replacement. *Acta Cardiol* 2004;59:231–232.
42. Lamb CR, Aram HH, Mennell ER. An experimental study of aortic valve homografts. *Surg Gynecol Obstet* 1952;94:129–131.
43. Murray G. Homologous aortic valve segment transplants as surgical treatment for aortic and mitral insufficiency. *Angiology* 1956;7:446–451.
44. Heimbecker RO, Baird RJ, Lajos RJ, et al. Homograft replacement of the human valve: A preliminary report. *Can Med Assoc J* 1962:86:805.
45. Duran CG, Gunning AJ. A method for placing a total homologous aortic valve into the subcoronary position, *Lancet* 1962;2:488.
46. Ross DN. Homograft replacement of the aortic valve. *Lancet* 1962;2:447.
47. Barrat-Boyes BG. Homograft aortic valve replacement in aortic incompetence and stenosis. *Thorax* 1964;19: 131–135.
48. Moore KL. The circulatory system In: Moore KL, ed. *The Developing Human*. Toronto: Saunders; 1982:298–343.
49. Mill MR, Wilcox BR, Anderson RH. Surgical anatomy of the heart. In: Edmunds, KL Jr (ed). *Cardiac Surgery in the Adult*. New York: McGraw-Hill; 1997:35–57.
50. Deck JD. Endothelial cell orientation on aortic valve leaflets. *Cardiovasc Res* 1986:20:760.
51. Frank S, Ross J Jr: The natural history of severe, acquired valvular aortic stenosis. *Am J Cardiol* 1967;19:128.
52. Bonow RO, Lakatos E, Maron BJ, et al. Serial long-term assessment of the natural history of asymptomatic patients with chronic aortic regurgitation and normal left ventricular systolic function. *Circulation* 1991;84:1625.
53. Gorlin R, Gorlin SG. Hydraulic formula for calculation of the area of the stenotic mitral valve, other cardiac valves, and central circulatory shunts. *Am Heart J* 1951;41:1–29.
54. Hakki AH, Iskandrian AS, Bemis CE, et al. A simplified valve formula for the calculation of stenotic cardiac valve areas. *Circulation* 1981;63:1050–1055.
55. Cribier A, Savin T, Berland J, et al. Percutaneous transluminal balloon valvuloplasty of adult aortic stenosis: Report of 92 cases. *J Am Coll Cardiol* 1987;9:381.
56. Johnson RG, Dhillon JS, Thurer RL, et al. Aortic valve operation after percutaneous aortic balloon valvuloplasty. *Ann Thorac Surg* 1990;49:740.
57. DiMario C, Beatt KJ, de Feyter P, et al. Percutaneous aortic balloon dilatation for calcific aortic stenosis in elderly patients: Immediate hemodynamic results and short term follow-up. *Br Heart J* 1987;58:644.
58. Cribier A, Eltchaninoff H, Bash A, et al. Percutaneous transcatheter implantation of an aortic valve prosthesis for calcific aortic stenosis: First human case description. *Circulation* 2002;106:3006–3008.
59. Bonow RO, Carabello B, DeLeon AC, et al. ACC/AHA guidelines for the management of patients with valvular heart disease. *J Am Coll Cardiol* 1998;32: 1486–1582.
60. Bonow RO, Rosing DR, McIntosh CL, et al. The natural history of asymptomatic patients with aortic regurgitation and normal left ventricular function. *Circulation* 1983;68:509.
61. Bonow RO. Asymptomatic aortic regurgitation: Indications for operation. *J Card Surg* 1994;24:1046.
62. Bonow RO. Timing of operation for chronic aortic regurgitation: Influence of left ventricular function on clinical management. *Herz* 1984;9:319.
63. Bonow RO, Picone AL, McIntosh CL, et al. Survival and functional results after valve replacement for aortic regurgitation from 1976 to 1983: Impact of preoperative left ventricular function. *Circulation* 1985;72:1244.
64. Gillinov AM, Banbury MK, Cosgrove DM. Hemisternotomy approach for aortic and mitral valve surgery. *J Card* Surg 2000;15:15–20.
65. Byrne JG, Adams DH, Couper GS, et al. Minimally-invasive aortic root replacement. *Heart Surg Forum* 1999;2:326–329.
66. Banbury MK, Cosgrove DM 3rd, Lytle BW, et al. Long-term results of the Carpentier-Edwards pericardial aortic

valve: A 12-year follow-up. *Ann Thorac Surg* 1998;66 (Suppl 6):S73–76.

67. Poirer NC, Pelletier LC, Pellerin M, Carrier M. 15-year experience with the Carpentier-Edwards pericardial bioprosthesis. *Ann Thorac* Surg 1998;66(Suppl 6):S57–61.
68. Dellgren G, David TE, Raanani E, et al. Late hemodynamic and clinical outcomes of aortic valve replacement with the Carpentier-Edwards Perimount pericardial bioprosthesis. *J Thorac Cardiovasc Surg* 2002;124(1):146–154.
69. Rizzoli G, Bottio T, Thiene G, et al. Long-term durability of the Hancock II porcine bioprosthesis. *J Thorac Cardiovasc Surg* 2003;126(1):66–74.
70. Cohen G, David TE, Ivanov J, et al. The impact of age, coronary artery disease, and cardiac comorbidity on late survival after bioprosthetic aortic valve replacement. *J Thorac Cardiovasc Surg* 1999;117(2):273–284.
71. Farivar RS, Cohn LH. Hypercholesterolemia is a risk factor for bioprosthetic valve calcification and explantation. *J Thorac Cardiovasc Surg* 2003;126(4):969–975.
72. Antonini-Canterin F, Zuppiroli A, Popescu BA, et al. Effect of statins on the progression of bioprosthetic aortic valve degeneration. *Am J Car*diol 2003;92(12): 1479–1482.
73. Vogt PR, Brunner-LaRocca H, Sidler P, et al. Reoperative surgery for degenerated aortic bioprostheses: Predictors for emergency surgery and reoperative mortality. *Eur J Cardiothorac Surg* 2000;17(2):134–139.
74. Gill IS, Masters RG, Pipe AL, et al. Determinants of hospital survival after reoperative single valve replacement. *Can J Cardiol* 1999;15(11):1207–1210.
75. Akins CW, Buckley MJ, Daggett WM, et al. Risk of reoperative valve replacement for failed mitral and aortic bioprostheses. *Ann Thorac Surg* 1998;65(6):1545–1551.
76. Ikonomidis JS, Kratz JM, Crumbley AJ 3rd, et al. Twenty-year experience with the St Jude Medical mechanical valve prosthesis. *J Thorac Cardiovasc Surg* 2003;126(6):2022–2031.
77. Emery RW, Arom KV, Kshettry VR, et al. Decision-making in the choice of heart valve for replacement in patients aged 60–70 years: Twenty-year follow up of the St. Jude medical aortic valve prosthesis. *J Heart Valve Dis* 2002;11(Suppl 1):S37–44.
78. Tasca G, Amaducci A, Parrella PV, et al. Myectomy-myotomy associated with aortic valve replacement for aortic stenosis: Effects on left ventricular mass regression. *Ital Heart J* 2003;12:865–871.
79. Del Rizzo DF, Goldman BS, Christakis GT, David TE. Hemodynamic benefits of the Toronto Stentless Valve. *J Thorac Cardiovasc Surg* 1996;112(6):1431–1445.
80. Bach DS, Goldman B, Verrier E, et al. Toronto SPV Valve Study Group: Durability and prevalence of aortic regurgitation nine years after aortic valve replacement with the Toronto SPV stentless bioprosthesis. *J Heart Valve Dis* 2004;13:64–72.
81. Kon ND, Riley RD, Adair SM, et al. Eight-year results of aortic root replacement with the freestyle stentless porcine aortic root bioprosthesis. *Ann Thorac Surg* 2002;73(6):1817–1821.
82. Riley RD, Hammon JW Jr, Adair SM, et al. Stentless aortic valve replacement with Freestyle or Toronto SPV: An early comparison. *Ann Thorac Surg* 2000;70(1):48–51.
83. O'Brien MF, Harrocks S, Stafford EG, et al. The homograft aortic valve: A 29-year, 99.3% follow up of 1,022 valve replacements. *J Heart Valve Dis* 2001;10(3):334–344.
84. Pibarot P, Dumesnil JG. Hemodynamic and clinical impact of prosthesis-patient mismatch in the aortic valve position and its prevention. *J Am Coll Cardiol* 2000;36: 1131–1141.
85. Medalion B, Blackstone EH, Lytle BW, et al. Aortic valve replacement: Is valve size important? *J Thorac Cardiovasc Surg* 2000;119(5):963–974.
86. Kratz JM, Sade RM, Crawford FA Jr, et al. The risk of small St. Jude aortic valve prostheses. *Ann Thorac Surg* 1994;57:1114–1119.
87. Adams DH, Chen RH, Kadner A, et al. Impact of small prothetic valve size on operative mortality in elderly patients after aortic valve replacement for aortic stenosis: Does gender matter? *J Thorac Cardiovasc Surg* 1999;118: 815–822.
88. Rao V, Jamieson WRE, Ivanov J, et al. Prosthesis-patient mismatch affects survival after aortic valve replacement. *Circulation* 2000;102:III-5–III-9.
89. Hanayama H, Christakis GT, Mallidi HR, et al. Patient prosthesis mismatch is rare after aortic valve replacement: Valve size may be irrelevant. *Ann Thorac Surg* 2002;73: 1822–1829.
90. Blackstone EH, Cosgrove DM, Jamieson WR, et al. Prosthesis size and long-term survival after aortic valve replacement. *J Thorac Cardiovasc Surg* 2003;126:783–796.
91. Christakis GT, Joyner CD, Morgan CD, et al. Left ventricular mass regression early after aortic valve replacement. *Ann Thorac Surg* 1996;62:1084–1089.
92. De Paulis R, Sommariva L, De Matteis GM, et al. Extent and pattern of regression of left ventricular hypertrophy in patients with small size Carbomedics aortic valves. *J Thorac Cardiovasc Surg* 1997;113:901–909.
93. Khan SS, Siegel RJ, DeRobertis MA, et al. Regression of hypertrophy after Carpentier-Edwards pericardial aortic valve replacement. *Ann Thorac Surg* 2000;69: 531–535.
94. Anderson WA, Ilkowski DA, Eldredge J, et al. The small aortic root and the Medtronic-Hall valve: Ultrafast computed tomography assessment of left ventricular mass following aortic valve replacement. *J Heart Valve Dis* 1996;5(Suppl III):S329–35.
95. Sim FKW, Orsulak TA, Schaff HV, Shub C. Influence of prosthesis size on change in left ventricular mass following aortic valve replacement. *Eur J Cardiothorac Surg* 1994;8:193–197.
96. Christakis GT, Buth KJ, Goldman BS, et al. Inaccurate and misleading valve sizing: A proposed standard for valve size nomenclature. *Ann Thorac Surg* 1998;66: 1198–1203.
97. Bartels C, Sievers HH. Successful dilatation of the small aortic root for implantation of a larger valve prosthesis. *J Heart Valve Dis* 1999;8:507–508.
98. David TE, Puschmann R, Ivanov J, et al. Aortic valve replacement with stentless and stented porcine valves: A case-match study. *J Thorac Cardiovasc Surg* 1998;116: 236–241.
99. Rao V, Christakis G, Sever J, et al. A novel comparison of stentless versus stented valves in the small aortic root. *J Thorac Cardiovasc Surg* 1999;117:431–438.

100. Matar AF. Combined annular and supraannular prosthetic implantation for the small aortic annulus. *Ann Thorac Surg* 1984;37:258–260.
101. Nicks R, Cartmill T, Bernstein L. Hypoplasia of the aortic root—the problem of aortic valve replacement. *Thorax* 1970;25:339–346.
102. Manouguian S, Seybold-Epting W. Patch enlargement of the aortic valve ring by extending the aortic incision into the anterior mitral leaflet—new operative technique. *J Thorac Cardiovasc Surg* 1979;78:402–412.
103. Konno S, Imai Y, lida T, et al. A new method for prosthetic valve replacement in congenital aortic stenosis associated with hypoplasia of the aortic valve ring. *J Thorac Cardiovasc Surg* 1975;70:909–917.
104. Sommers KE, David TE. Aortic valve replacement with patch enlargement of the aortic annulus. *Ann Thorac Surg* 1997;63:1608–1612.
105. Norman JC, Nihill MR, Cooley DA. Valved apico-aortic composite conduits for left ventricular outflow tract obstructions. *Am J Cardiol* 1980;45:1265–1271.
106. Cooley DA, Lopez RM, Absi TS. Apicoaortic conduit for left ventricular outflow tract obstruction: Revisited. *Ann Thorac Surg* 2000;69:1511–1514.
107. Del Rizzo DF, Freed D, Abdoh A, et al. Midterm survival of stented versus stentless valves: Does concomitant coronary artery bypass grafting impact survival? *Semin Thorac Cardiovasc Surg* 2001;13(4 Suppl 1):148–155.
108. Iwahashi K, Shida T, Asada T, et al. Management of coronary artery disease combined with aortic stenosis: How to do with mild aortic stenosis. *Kyobu Geka* 2000;53 (Suppl 8):617–621.
109. Brunvand H, Offstad J, Nitter-Hauge S, Svennevig JL. Coronary artery bypass grafting combined with aortic valve replacement in healthy octogenarians does not increase postoperative risk. *Scand Cardiovasc J* 2002;36: 297–301.
110. Otto CM, Pearlman AS, Gardner CL. Hemodynamic progression of aortic stenosis in adults assessed by Doppler echocardiography. *J Am Coll Cardiol* 1989;13: 545–550.
111. Otto CM, Barwash IG, Legget, et al. Prospective study of asymptomatic valvular aortic stenosis: Clinical, echocardiographic, and exercise predictors of outcome. *Circulation* 1997;95:2262–2270.
112. Phillips BJ, Karavas AN, Aranki SF, et al. Management of mild aortic stenosis during coronary artery bypass surgery: An update, 1992–2001. *J Card Surg* 2003;18:507–511.
113. Karagounis A, Valencia O, Chandrasekaran V, et al. Management of patients undergoing coronary artery bypass graft surgery with mild to moderate aortic stenosis. *J Heart Valve Dis* 2004;13:369–373.
114. Ahmed AA, Graham AN, Lovell D, O'Kane HO. Management of mild to moderate aortic valve disease during coronary artery bypass grafting. *Eur J Cardiothorac Surg* 2003;24:535–539.
115. Hochrein J, Lucke JC, Harrison JK, et al. Mortality and need for reoperation in patients with mild-to-moderate asymptomatic aortic valve disease undergoing coronary artery bypass graft alone. *Am Heart J* 1999;138:791–797.
116. Smith WT 4th, Ferguson TB Jr, Ryan T, et al. Should coronary artery bypass graft surgery patients with mild or moderate aortic stenosis undergo concomitant aortic valve replacement? A decision analysis approach to the surgical dilemma. *J Am Coll Cardiol* 2004;44(6):1241–1247.
117. Forman MB, Virmani R, Robertson RM, et al. Mitral annular calcification in chronic renal failure. *Chest* 1984;85:367–371.
118. Abrahams C, D'Cruz I, Kathpalia S. Abnormalities in the mitral valve apparatus in patients undergoing long-term hemodialysis: Autopsy and echocardiographic correlation. *Arch Intern Med* 1982;142:1796–1800.
119. Goldsmith D, Ritz E, Covic A. Vascular calcification: A stiff challenge for the nephrologist: Does preventing bone disease cause arterial disease? *Kidney Int* 2004;66: 1315–1333.
120. Byrne C, Vernon P, Cohen JJ, Effect of age and diagnosis on survival of older patients beginning chronic dialysis. *JAMA* 1994;271:34–36.
121. Lucke JC, Samy RN, Atkins BZ et al. Results of valve replacement with mechanical and biological prostheses in chronic renal dialysis patients. *Ann Thorac Surg* 1997;64:129–133.
122. Kaplon RJ, Cosgrove DM III, Gillinov AM, et al. Cardiac valve replacement in patients on dialysis: Influence of prosthesis on survival. *Ann Thorac Surg* 2000;70:438–441.
123. Brinkman WT, Williams WH, Guyton RA, et al. Valve replacement in patients on chronic renal dialysis: Implications for valve prosthesis selection. *Ann Thorac Surg* 2002;74:37–42.
124. Herzog CA, Ma JZ, Collins AJ. Long-term survival of dialysis patients in the United States with prosthetic heart valves: Should ACC/AHA practice guidelines on valve selection be modified? *Circulation* 2002;105:1336–1341.
125. Mugge A, Daniel WG, Frank G, et al. Echocardiography in infective endocarditis: Reassessment of prognostic implications of vegetation size determined by the transthoracic and the transesophageal approach. *J Am Coll Cardiol* 1989;14:631–638.
126. Sabik JF, Lytle BW, Blackstone EH, et al. Aortic root replacement with cryopreserved allograft for prosthetic valve endocarditis. *Ann Thorac Surg* 2002;74:650–659.
127. David T. Complex operations of the aortic root. In: Edmunds L (ed). *Cardiac Surgery in the Adult*. New York: McGraw Hill; 1997:945–947.
128. Calderwood SB, Swinski LA, Karchmer AW, et al. Prosthetic valve endocarditis: Analysis of factors affecting outcome of therapy. *J Thorac Cardiovasc Surg* 1986;92: 776–783.
129. Baumgartner WA, Miller DC, Reitz BA, et al. Surgical treatment of prosthetic valve endocarditis. *Ann Thorac Surg* 1983;35:87–104.
130. David TE, Bos J, Christakis GT, et al. Heart valve operations in patients with active infective endocarditis. *Ann Thorac Surg* 1990;49:701–705.
131. D'Udekem Y, David TE, Feindel CM, et al. Long term results of surgery for active infective endocarditis. *Eur J Cardiothorac Surg* 1997;11:46–52.
132. Lytle BW, Sabik JF, Blackstone EH, et al. Reoperative cryopreserved root and ascending aorta replacement for acute aortic prosthetic valve endocarditis. *Ann Thorac Surg* 2002;74:S1754–1757.

CHAPTER

31 AORTIC ROOT REPLACEMENT

John R. Barbour, John S. Ikonomidis

HISTORICAL BACKGROUND

The first thoracic aortic replacements were performed with homograft tissue primarily in the descending thoracic aorta. Notable surgeons included Henry Bahnson,[1] DeBakey and Cooley,[2] and Lam and Aranm.[3] Attempts were made to develop artificial fabric grafts for use for aortic replacement, culminating with Michael DeBakey's discovery of Dacron.[4] During the late 1950s, the Houston group led by Michael DeBakey systematically developed operations for resection and graft replacement of the ascending aorta,[5] followed by the descending and thoracoabdominal aorta.[6] In 1963, Starr and associates reported replacing the supracoronary ascending aorta

KEY CONCEPTS

- Epidemiology
  - Aortic aneurysms were the fifteenth most common cause of death in the United States in the year 2000. Among patients who die of thoracic aortic aneurysms (TAAs), rupture is the cause of death in about 80 percent of cases. Approximately 50 percent of thoracic aneurysms involve the root and the ascending aorta. The estimated growth rate for TAAs has been calculated to be 1.2 to 4.2 mm per year. Aneurysms that are larger than 6 cm can be associated with a yearly rate of rupture or dissection of at least 6.9 percent and a death rate of 11.8 percent.
- Pathophysiology
  - Annuloaortic ectasia is a term used to describe an increase in diameter of the aortic annulus coupled with an increase in the diameter of the aortic root. This type of situation is seen in patients with Marfan's syndrome, Ehlers-Danlos syndrome, osteogenesis imperfecta, and pseudoxanthoma elasticum. Annuloaortic ectasia may have familial origins or may be idiopathic. Recently, a significant body of research has focused on the involvement of endogenous extracellular matrix–degrading enzymes in aneurysms and aortic remodeling. Of greatest interest are the matrix metalloproteinases (MMPs), particularly those of the gelatinase class (MMP-2, MMP-9). Another important cause of aortic root destruction is acute infective endocarditis with aggressive organisms such as *Staphylococcus aureus*. A central common theme in the development of aortic root aneurysms is cystic medial degeneration, in which gradual disruption of the media of the aorta occurs, with the creation of small acellular spaces within it. This process weakens the aortic wall, and a slow remodeling of the aortic root and ascending aorta results in aneurysm formation.
- Clinical features
  - Most patients with aortic root pathology are asymptomatic, with the exception of patients who present with endocarditis (sepsis, congestive heart failure) or aortic root destruction secondary to acute type A aortic dissection (severe chest pains, asymmetric pulses, congestive heart failure). The age range of presentation is very broad (twenties to eighties) and is dependent on the underlying pathology. Certain patients will have characteristic stigmata of connective tissue diseases such as Marfan's syndrome.
- Diagnostics
  - The workup for candidates for aortic root replacement includes echocardiography to estimate ventricular function and assess for the possibility of aortic valve preservation. Coronary catheterization is usually necessary to rule out coronary artery

disease. Thin-slice computed tomography (CT) or magnetic resonance imaging (MRI) scanning will provide the necessary information about the anatomy of the aneurysm. A careful oral examination or dental consultation is very important to prevent postoperative prosthetic valve infection.

- Treatment
  - Aortic root replacement options include composite valve-graft, separate valve-graft, xenograft tissue, homograft, pulmonary autograft (Ross procedure), and valve-sparing aortic root replacement. The decision to use each one of these options is dependent on patient age and valve preference, comorbid conditions, the condition of the native aortic valve, and contraindications to the use of anticoagulants.
- Outcomes
  - Operative (30-day) mortality runs in the range of 4 to 10 percent. Reoperation for mediastinal hemorrhage should be required in less than 10 percent of cases. Complete heart block requiring pacemaker insertion occurs in about 1 to 2 percent in most series. Stroke occurs in approximately 1 to 4 percent of these patients. Approximately 30 percent of patients who present for aortic root replacement are candidates for a valve-sparing procedure, which offers improved freedom from bleeding and thromboembolic complications and obviates the need for oral anticoagulation.

and the aortic valve at the same time.[7] In 1968, Bentall and DeBono published a landmark article on replacement of the entire aortic root with anastomoses of the coronary ostia to the replacement graft.[8] The description of this technique included side-to-side anastomoses of the coronary arteries to the graft. The aneurysm sac then was closed completely around the graft. A common complication of this operation was pseudoaneurysmal development at the level of the coronary ostia, presumably caused by the tension placed on the coronary anastomoses. A subsequent modification of this technique by Kouchoukos and coworkers[9] included complete excision of the aneurysm and aortic root, leaving both coronary arteries suspended by only a small "button-shaped" circular portion of aorta that then would be anastomosed directly into a hole created in the side of the Dacron graft, thus eliminating pseudoaneurysm formation. An extended ascending aortic replacement was described by Wheat and associates, effectively excluding most of the ascending aorta but leaving the coronary arteries attached to the remaining aortic root tissue in continuity.[10]

In 1979, acting on the observation that many patients presenting for aortic root replacement have normal aortic valve morphology, Sir Magdi Yacoub and colleagues at Harefield Hospital in the United Kingdom developed a strategy for aortic root replacement in which the aortic valve was preserved.[11] In 1988, Tirone David introduced a different technique for valve-sparing aortic root replacement.[12] Since that time, a number of authors have introduced different variations on these themes.[13–15]

Interest in homograft aortic root replacement began in the 1950s. At that time, Norman Shumway and colleagues at Stanford University were experimenting with excision of the right ventricular outflow tract, the pulmonary valve, and the proximal portions of the pulmonary artery in continuity in dogs and translocating this to the aortic root, with subsequent reconstruction of the pulmonary artery with homograft or tube graft material.[16] The operation in this iteration ultimately would be doomed to failure because of right ventricular failure resulting from the lack of a pulmonary valve, but Donald Ross, building on that experience, later performed the first pulmonary autograft aortic root replacements in humans.[17]

EMBRYOLOGY AND ANATOMY

The aortic root and the ascending aorta develop as part of a common truncus arteriosus that partitions itself into the ascending aorta and the aortic root and the pulmonary artery at approximately the fifth and sixth weeks of development.[18] The aortic root is a tripartite structure owing to the presence of coronary sinuses. The aortic valve proper has no true fibrous annulus, although surgeons use the term *aortic annulus* to describe the junction of the aorta and the ventricle. The noncoronary sinus of the aortic valve tends to be the largest of the three sinuses, and therefore the size of the aortic valve leaflets reflects this, with the noncoronary leaflet generally being the largest. The length of the distance from the basal attachment of each aortic valve leaflet to the aorta is approximately 1.5 times the length of the free margin of the leaflet (Fig. 31-1). The commissures of each of the aortic valves extend right to or just below the sinotubular junction, which marks the anatomic ridge between the end of the aortic root and the beginning of the ascending aorta. In general, the sinotubular ridge is approximately 10 to 15 percent smaller in diameter than the aortic annulus (Fig. 31-1). Anatomic disease states that cause dilatation of the sinotubular junction or dilatation of the aortic annulus will cause insufficiency of the aortic valve. There is an aortic mitral continuity, which is a fibrous tissue attachment between the aorta and the mitral valves that constitutes approximately 55 percent of the circumference of the aortic root. The left side of the aortic root toward the pulmonary artery is

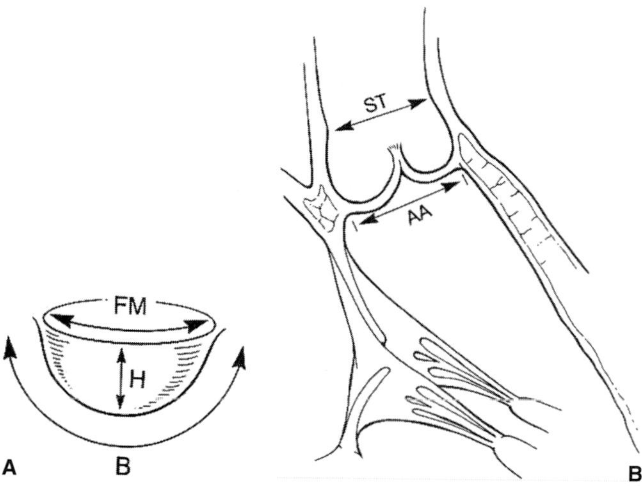

Figure 31-1 Anatomic features of the aortic root. **A.** Normal aortic valve leaflet. **B.** Aortic root demonstrating the smaller diameter of the sinotubular junction compared with the aortic annulus. [Reproduced with permission from David TE. Complex operations of the aortic root. In: Edmunds LH (ed). *Cardiac Surgery in the Adult.* New York: McGraw-Hill; 1997:939–957.]

attached to the ventricular muscle, corresponding to approximately 45 percent of the circumference.

EPIDEMIOLOGY

The exact extent of occurrence of thoracic aortic aneurysms is unknown. Bickerstaff and associates[19] found the prevalence of TAAs to be 5.9 per 100,000 per year in the Rochester, Minnesota, area. Among a total of 72 patients with TAAs studied by Bickerstaff and colleagues, 51 percent, or 37 of the aneurysms in those patients, involved the ascending aorta, 8 (11 percent) the aortic arch, and 27 (38 percent) the descending thoracic aorta.

According to the National Center for Health Statistics, aortic aneurysms (AAs) were the fifteenth most common cause of death in the United States in the year 2000; approximately 0.6 percent of all females and 1.1 percent of all males die of aortic aneurysmal disease. Thoracic aortic aneurysm deaths occur in about 0.7 per 100,000 population per year.[20] Among patients who die of thoracic aortic aneurysms, rupture is the cause of death in about 80 percent of cases.[20]

The estimated growth rate for TAAs has been calculated to be 1.2 to 4.2 mm per year,[21–24] and enlargement accelerates as an aneurysm gets larger.[24] Risk factors for accelerated growth include the presence of dissection in the enlarged segment,[21] synchronous arch[22] or abdominal[25] aortic aneurysm, smoking,[24] no beta-blocker therapy,[26] renal failure,[23] and diastolic hypertension.[23] Rupture is much more likely to occur when the aneurysm exceeds 5 cm in diameter, and the risk of rupture increases as the aneurysm increases in size. Aneurysms larger than 6 cm can be associated with a yearly rate of rupture or dissection of at least 6.9 percent and a death rate of 11.8 percent.[27]

PATHOPHYSIOLOGY

Annuloaortic ectasia[28] is a term used to describe an increase in the diameter of the aortic annulus coupled with an increase in the diameter of the aortic root. This ectasia tends to occur along the fibrous tissue of the ventricle, with the ventricular muscular portion of the aortic root generally preserved. This type of situation is seen in patients with Marfan's syndrome, Ehlers-Danlos syndrome, osteogenesis imperfecta, and pseudoxanthoma elasticum. It may have other familial origins or may be idiopathic. In these syndromes, the aortic sinuses become thinner and dilated and the sinotubular junction increases in diameter. When this happens, the aortic valve leaflets are not allowed to coapt properly because of separation of the commissures. These patients develop central jets of aortic insufficiency on echocardiographic assessment. Degenerative diseases of the aorta may cause dilatation of the ascending aorta and aortic sinuses with minimal or no dilatation of the aortic annulus. The aortic root also may be destroyed in the setting of acute or chronic aortic dissection and other congenital syndromes, such as those associated with bicuspid aortic valves. Recently, a significant body of research has focused on the involvement of endogenous extracellular matrix–degrading enzymes in the involvement of aneurysms and aortic remodeling. Of greatest interest are the matrix metalloproteinases, particularly those of the gelatinase class (MMP-2, MMP-9).[29–31] Another important cause of aortic root destruction is acute infective endocarditis with aggressive organisms such as *Staphylococcus aureus.*

Histologic features

A central common theme in the development of aortic root aneurysms is a condition referred to as cystic medial degeneration or simply medial degeneration. Histologically, the aorta is made up of three layers. The adventitia is composed primarily of a collagen-rich network. The tunica media, or media, is composed of alternating layers of vascular smooth muscle and elastin. Each successive pairing of smooth muscle cells and elastin is referred to as a lamellar unit. In humans, the media of the aortic root is composed of approximately 50 lamellar units. The third layer of the aorta is referred to as the intima and is composed of a single layer of epithelial cells. In many cases of aortic aneurysm, one sees gradual disruption of the media of the aorta, with the creation of small acellular spaces within it. This process of medial degeneration results ultimately in weakening of the aortic wall and inability to sustain the normal shear stresses associated with systole. As a result, a slow remodeling of the aortic root and ascending aorta occurs, leading to aneurysm formation.

CLINICAL PRESENTATION AND DIAGNOSTIC MODALITIES

Patients present for aortic root replacement in a number of circumstances (See the decision-making flowchart). The most acute circumstance is a patient with a Stanford type A aortic dissection in whom the aortic root is virtually destroyed by the proximal extent of the dissection. The condition of these patients constitutes a surgical emergency, and as a result, aortic root replacement in these circumstances is associated with more morbidity and a higher mortality than is standard aortic root replacement. A second acute situation occurs with infective endocarditis. The most common situation in which patients present for aortic root replacement is an aortic root aneurysm. The age range of presentation is wide and starts in the twenties and thirties in patients with hereditary connective tissue disorders and extends into the seventies and even eighties in those with degenerative aneurysms. Other than a family history of aortic aneurysms and connective tissue disorders, risk factors for aortic aneurysms include hypertension and atherosclerosis. Patients with isolated aortic root aneurysms are usually asymptomatic. Those conditions are identified as a result of a workup for another disease process, such as a respiratory tract infection, that results in a chest x-ray. The chest x-ray may identify an abnormality in the mediastinum, resulting in a CT scan or an MRI scan that illustrates the aortic root aneurysm. Alternatively, other patients with aortic aneurysms have significant aortic valve pathology, such as stenosis or insufficiency. Symptoms from these conditions result in referral to a physician. An echocardiogram is performed and shows evidence of aortic stenosis or insufficiency, and often a dilated aortic root is identified. This often leads to a further imaging study, such as a CT scan or an MRI scan, that shows the aortic root aneurysm.

The workup in patients with an aortic root aneurysm involves a careful history and physical examination, assessing for a history of bleeding problems and a history of significant dental work. In addition, a family history of aortic aneurysm should be elicited. The physical examination is generally unremarkable apart from the features of aortic insufficiency and aortic stenosis. Patients with Marfan's syndrome have a very characteristic appearance. They tend to be tall and thin, with joint laxity, pectus excavatum, and very characteristic facial features. After physical examination, patients should have standard blood work and be crossed and typed for 4 to 6 units of red blood cells. Clotting studies should be performed. The electrocardiogram shows no abnormalities specific to the aortic root aneurysm. Chest x-ray often reveals a prominent right mediastinal border, which represents an outpouching of the aortic root and the ascending aorta into the right chest. Transthoracic echocardiography is valuable in showing features of aortic stenosis and aortic insufficiency in addition to allowing assessment of the potential for valve preservation. The most useful test for the evaluation of aortic root aneurysms is a contrast CT scan or MRI, especially scans with three-dimensional reconstructions; this allows precise assessment of the aortic root and its dimensions (Fig. 31-2). Females older than 40 years and males older than 35 years with coronary risk factors should undergo coronary angiography to rule out the presence of coronary artery disease before surgery. In addition, patients with significant neck bruits should have carotid vascular studies and those with a substantial history of smoking should have pulmonary function tests. Finally, a dental examination is critical whenever a prosthetic valve replacement is considered in a patient since bacterial seeding from dental disease is a very important cause of prosthetic valve endocarditis and graft infections.

MEDICAL (NONSURGICAL) THERAPY

At the present time, there is no medical therapy for aortic root dilatation that directly addresses the underlying etiology. Some treatment strategies have focused on the use of broad-spectrum MMP inhibitors to reduce or prevent aneurysm expansion. Franklin and associates administered 500 mg of tetracycline, a global MMP inhibitor, as an intravenous bolus to patients during anesthetic induction for abdominal AA repair.[32] At aortic cross-clamping, aneurysm biopsies were taken and cultured. MMP-9 assay showed a reduction in culture supernatant proteinase values in an increasing serum tetracycline-dependent manner. Thompson and Baxter gave doxycycline 100 mg twice a day for 7 days to five patients before abdominal AA repair, and aneurysm biopsy showed a threefold reduction in MMP-2 and a fourfold reduction in MMP-9 expression compared with nontreated controls in whom those two enzymes were expressed abundantly.[33] After this, a multi-institutional phase II prospective randomized trial was undertaken to assess the safety and potential efficacy of long-term doxycycline administration in 36 patients. Thirty-three patients completed the study, and significant treatment-related side effects occurred in 5, or 13.9 percent, of those patients. There was no significant increase in aneurysm size at 6 months, and plasma MMP-9 levels dropped so that only 21 percent of the patients in the drug arm had MMP-9 that was considered to be elevated compared with 47 percent in the control arm.[34] No similar studies

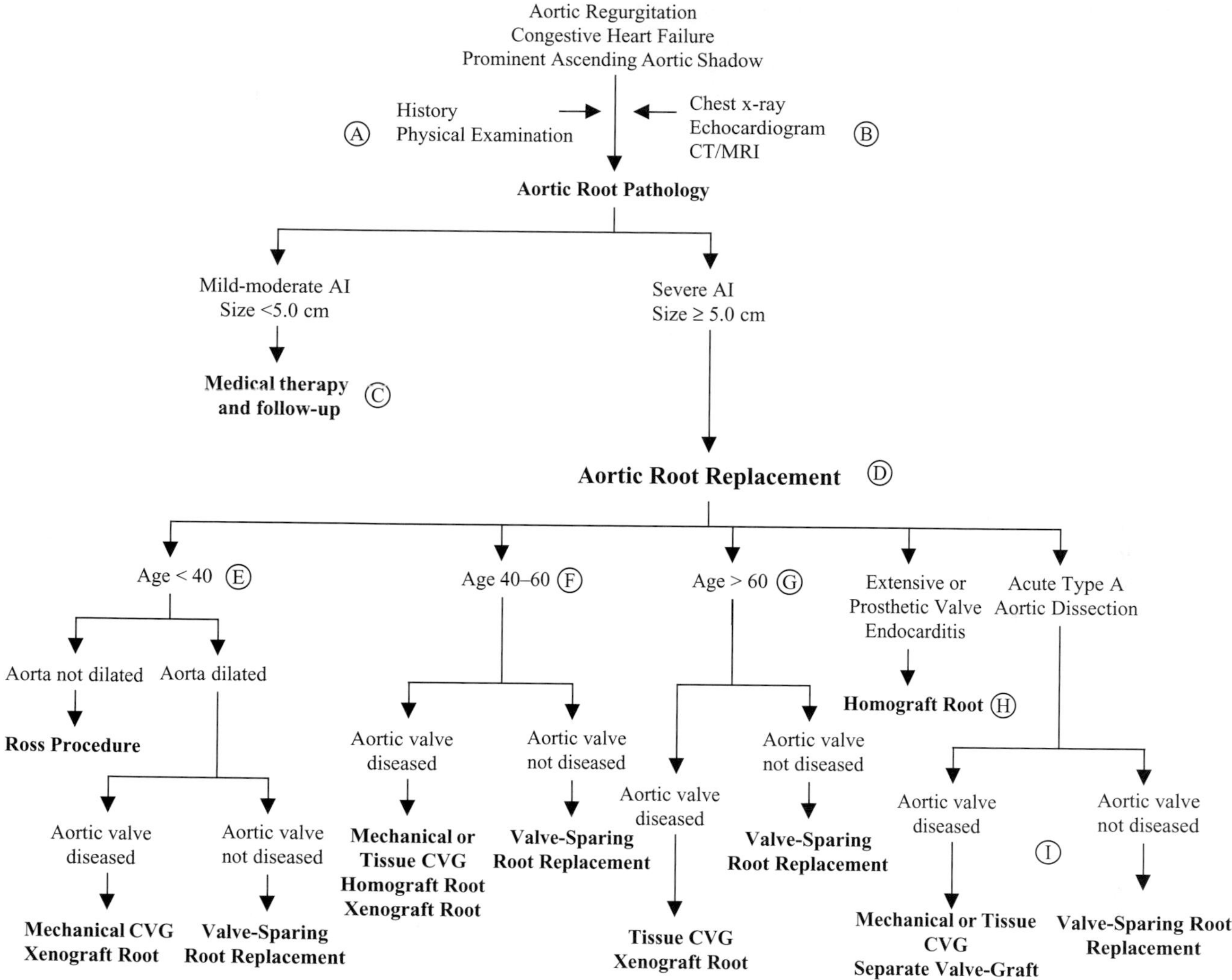

A. Most patients with aortic root aneurysms are asymptomatic. When the aneurysm is associated with significant aortic insufficiency, congestive heart failure symptoms will be a feature. Aortic dissection presents with severe chest pain, asymmetric pulses, and congestive heart failure symptoms. Patients with acute endocarditis will have signs of sepsis and congestive heart failure symptoms. Physical examination may be unremarkable with the exception of a murmur of aortic insufficiency or stenosis. A dental examination is a very important part of the evaluation of patients with aortic valve disease.

B. The chest radiograph often shows a prominent right mediastinal contour. The electrocardiogram is usually unremarkable. Echocardiography allows assessment of aortic valvular stenosis or insufficiency and assessment of whether the valve is bi- or tricuspid. Thin-slice CT or MRI scanning provides important anatomic information about the aortic root that aids in planning surgical therapy.

C. In patients who have only mild to moderate aortic insufficiency or aortic stenosis and in whom the aortic root does not exceed 5 cm in diameter, it is appropriate to follow up with serial imaging studies every 6 to 12 months.

D. Aortic root replacement is indicated in patients with severe aortic valvular pathology in association with significant aortic root pathology.

E. In patients less than 40 years of age, if the aortic valve is not bicuspid and the root is not dilated, the Ross procedure is appropriate. If the aorta is dilated and the valve is diseased, surgical options include xenograft root and mechanical composite valve-graft replacement, depending on the patient's preference for oral anticoagulation. If the valve is morphologically normal, a valve-sparing root replacement technique should be considered.

F. Adults between 40 and 60 years old have as an additional option homograft root replacement.

G. Adults age over 60 years are less likely to require a mechanical valve; therefore, tissue replacement options should be considered first. Older, frailer patients may benefit from the faster, less technically demanding separate valve-graft procedure.

H. Severe native aortic endocarditis with abscess or prosthetic valve endocarditis is best treated with extensive debridement of infected tissue and replacement with homograft tissue to reduce the risk of recurrent infection.

I. Acute type A aortic dissection constitutes a surgical emergency. If the aortic root is relatively intact, a separate valve-graft procedure is appropriate. Extensive destruction of the aortic root requires composite valve-graft reconstruction. Younger patients with morphologically intact aortic valves may benefit from valve-sparing aortic root replacement.

Decision-making flowchart

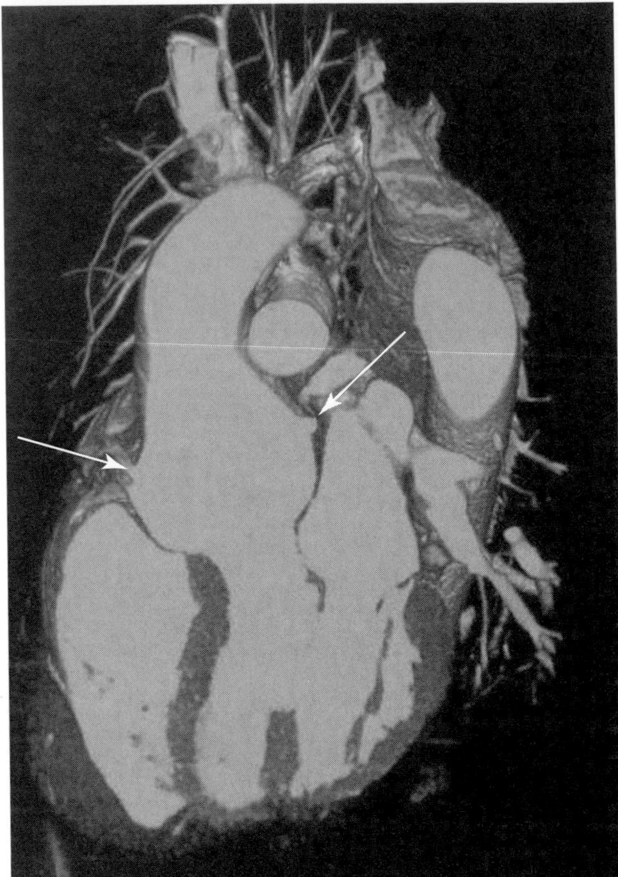

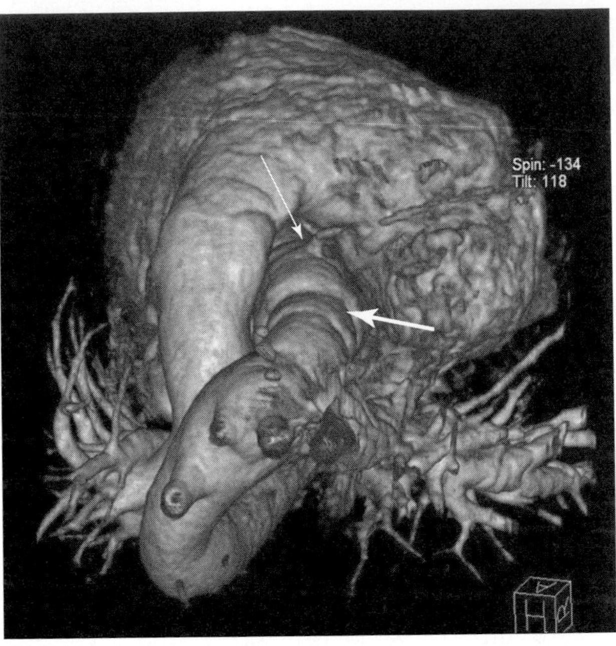

Figure 31-2 Thin-slice three-dimensional computed tomographic reconstructions of aortic root aneurysm before surgery (*left;* arrows denote left and right coronary ostia) and after David-V valve-sparing aortic root replacement (*right;* thin arrow: reimplanted right coronary artery; thick arrow: neosinotubular junction.)

have been performed in patients with thoracic aortic aneurysms. At present, the mainstays of management of aortic root aneurysms are judicious hypertension control in conjunction with regular follow-up with CT scans and transthoracic echocardiography to assess for interval changes in aortic diameter and follow the characteristics of the aortic valve.

INDICATIONS FOR SURGERY

Generally, resection of an aortic root aneurysm is indicated in patients in whom the aortic root diameter exceeds 5 to 5.5 cm[21,35,36] or becomes twice the size of a comparable normal aortic segment. In addition, a patient with an aortic root aneurysm that is seen to grow more than 0.5 cm in a 6-month period also should be considered for operation. Some latitude is given for patients with connective tissue disorders in whom it is known that the aorta is inherently weak and more susceptible to rapid dilatation. The clinical situation often also arises when patients have significant aortic valve pathology in association with an aortic aneurysm that does not quite meet the size criteria for resection. In these circumstances, aortic root replacement is indicated, since isolated replacement of the aortic valve in patients with a large aortic root and ascending aorta can pose technical difficulties in terms of closing the aorta after the aortic valve procedure and may predispose those patients to aortic dissections. In addition, a complicated redo operation for aortic root replacement may be necessary, since the ascending aorta continues to dilate. As was stated earlier, aortic root replacement occasionally is indicated in patients with type A aortic dissections with destruction of the aortic root and also in younger patients with significant aortic valve pathology who have a normal aortic root and ascending aorta and who are undergoing homograft root replacement or a Ross procedure to benefit from the increased durability of the aortic valve associated with this operation. Finally, severe aortic valve endocarditis with abscess or prosthetic valve endocarditis may be best treated with homograft aortic root replacement.

SURGICAL THERAPY

Conduct of the operation

The patient is placed in the supine position under general anesthesia. The chest, abdomen, perineum, and lower extremities are prepped and draped in sterile fashion. Standard median sternotomy and exposure of the heart are performed. The orientation of the aortic root is visualized more easily if only the right side of the pericardium is tacked upward. This rotates the heart counterclockwise and allows the apex of the heart to sink into the left chest, thus improving the exposure of the aortic root. Arterial and venous cannulation is undertaken, and appropriate connections are made to the pump oxygenator. If the patient has no significant aortic insufficiency, an antegrade cardioplegia tack is placed, and in all cases a retrograde cardioplegia cannula also is placed. When everything is in readiness for the initiation of cardiopulmonary bypass, careful dissection is undertaken to separate as much of the aortic root from the pulmonary artery and right ventricular outflow tract as possible. Care must be taken in dissecting anteriorly to avoid injury to the right coronary artery. A careful dissection at this point can result in significant exposure of the aortic root and therefore decrease the amount of time needed to perform the aortic root replacement when the aorta is cross-clamped. After confirmation of an activated clotting time (ACT) longer than 400 s, cardiopulmonary bypass is performed and the aorta is cross-clamped. Whenever possible, the heart should be arrested with antegrade cardioplegia to promote better and faster distribution of the cardioplegia, with a switch to retrograde cold blood cardioplegia throughout the remainder of the surgical procedure. The authors give intermittent shots of 250 mL every 20 min during the cross-clamp period. This is supplemented with a cold saline-infused cooling jacket placed around the left ventricle. A left ventricular apical vent is placed, and a temperature probe is inserted in the interventricular septum to monitor its temperature during the operation, keeping the temperature between 10 and 15°C as long as possible.

The ascending aorta is transected approximately 3 to 4 cm above the right coronary ostium. The aortic valve is inspected at this point, and if the situation is appropriate for valve preservation, the valve is not excised. If the valve is diseased so that its successful preservation is not possible, it is excised and debridement of the annulus is carried out if necessary. At this point, both the left and the right coronary button are dissected free, taking care not to mobilize them significantly. Significant mobilization may result in disorientation and kinking of the button after anastomosis to the Dacron graft. Specific techniques and choices for aortic root replacement are discussed below.

Systemic rewarming is begun at an appropriate point in the implantation procedure to avoid imposing extra time waiting for the patient to reach normothermia before separation from cardiopulmonary bypass. After root replacement, the ventricular vent is removed, and it is useful to give the final shot of cardioplegia antegrade to inspect for significant bleeding points that can be repaired before removal of the cross-clamp and also as an initial test of valve competence. The cross-clamp is removed with the patient placed in the Trendelenburg position and with an ascending aortic vent on. Ventricular and atrial pacing wires are placed, and mechanical ventilation is resumed. De-airing maneuvers such as lung hyperinflation, side-to-side shaking of the chest, and manual agitation of the heart are performed with the heart partially ejecting. Transesophageal echocardiography is very helpful in the assessment of de-airing and also in the interrogation of the valve for correct leaflet function. The patient is weaned from bypass at a systemic temperature of 36.5 to 37°C with good ventilation parameters. Protamine is given slowly by the surgeon directly into the ascending aorta, and the patient is decannulated. Meticulous hemostasis is obtained, a midline mediastinal drain (36F thoracostomy tube) is placed, and the patient is closed in the standard fashion.

Aortic root replacement: choices and results

Composite valve-graft

The current gold standard for aortic root replacement is the composite valve-graft replacement. Typically this consists of a mechanical valve that is annealed to a double-velour woven Dacron graft at the factory. The most commonly used version is the St. Jude composite valve-graft, although other brands are available. The operation consists of removal of the aortic root in its entirety except for the coronary ostia, which are left surrounded by a small circular rim of native aorta. The aortic valve also is excised. After appropriate sizing, pledgeted horizontal mattress nonabsorbable sutures are placed across the annulus in everting fashion (i.e., from aorta to ventricle) and are placed across the sewing ring of the composite valve-graft. The composite valve-graft is seated, and the sutures are tied and cut. For an extra measure of hemostasis, it is useful to suture the remaining rim of the aortic root directly to the sewing ring of the composite valve-graft in running fashion with 3-0 polypropylene sutures. Small holes are made just above the valve in the graft with ophthalmic cautery to allow suture implantation of the right and left coronary buttons. The authors use a small amount of albumin-glutaraldehyde biological glue to seal the interstices of these suture lines to aid in achieving hemostasis, but with the understanding that this step is not a substitute for meticulous surgical technique. A distal anastomosis of the Dacron graft to the ascending aorta then is performed (Fig. 31-3). In the operation originally described by Bentall and Debono in 1968,[8] the aortic root was not excised and the coronary

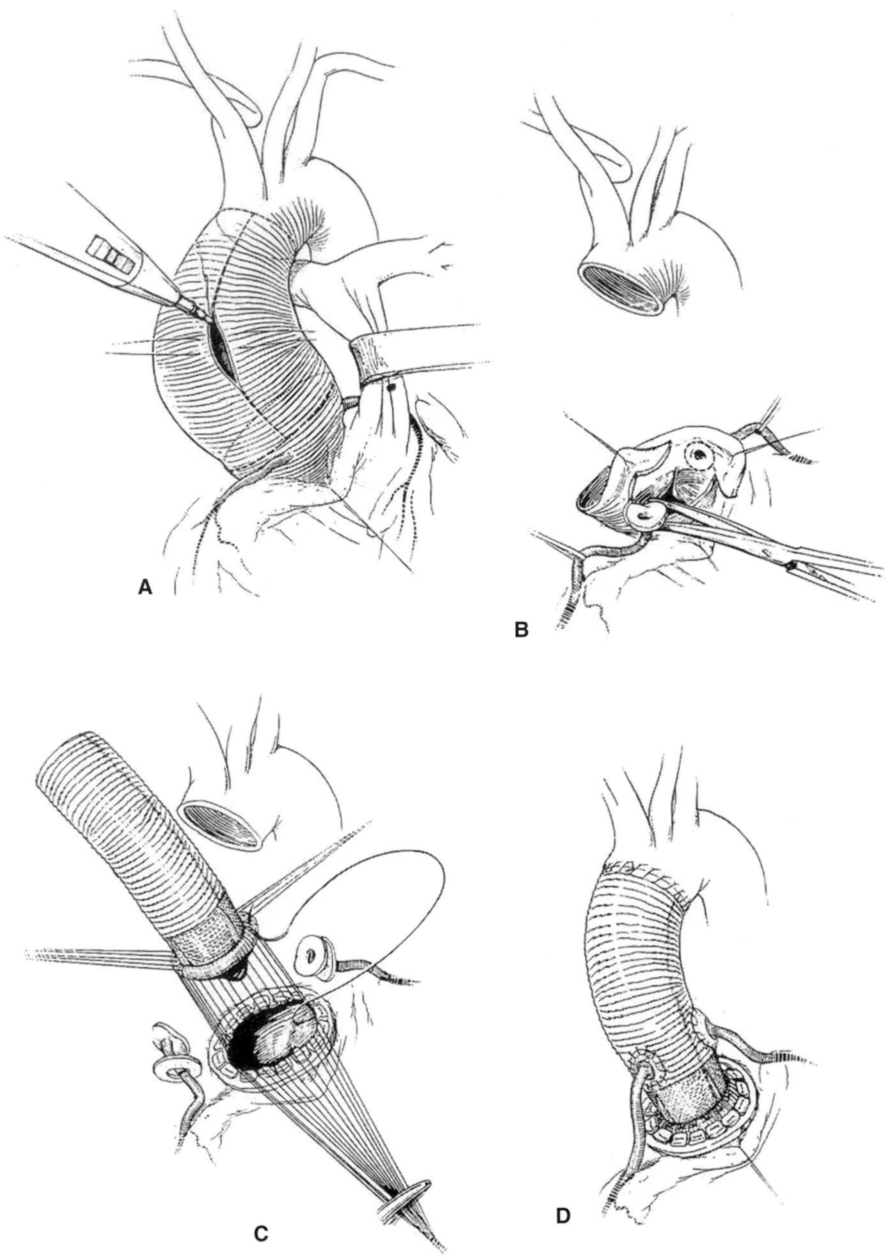

Figure 31-3 Insertion of a composite graft with the button technique. The aorta is opened vertically (**A**), and the coronary ostia are mobilized sufficiently (**B**) before the valve is seated (**C**). The coronary buttons are sewn to the graft (**D**) to complete the repair. (Reproduced with permission from Svensson LG, Crawford ES. Aortic dissection and aortic aneurysm surgery: Clinical observations, experimental investigations, and statistical analyses: Part III. *Curr Probl Surg* 1993;30:1–72.)

ostia were sewn side to side to the Dacron graft. Subsequently, Kouchoukos and coworkers excised the native aorta, leaving the coronary ostia surrounded by a small circular rim of native aorta ("Carrel buttons") for direct end-to-side reimplantation.[9] This constitutes the standard operation performed today. It is therefore not academically appropriate to refer to the latter procedure simply as a Bentall operation; instead, it is a modification of that operation.

Younger individuals may opt for a replacement of a composite graft containing a mechanical valve, accepting the potential complications associated with warfarin administration. In older patients (i.e., those above 65 to 70 years of age) a composite graft consisting of a stented bioprosthetic valve sewn to the Dacron graft by the surgeon at the time of operation may be used.[37] Although these valves are not commercially available, the surgeon can select the appropriate bioprosthetic valve by sizing the annulus after the native valve is excised and then suture it to an appropriately selected Dacron graft. The operation then proceeds as for a composite mechanical valve graft.

During redo aortic root replacements, the tissues around the aortic root, especially posteriorly, can be very difficult to dissect; therefore, mobilization of the coronary artery may be difficult or dangerous. The Cabrol technique[38] of coronary reimplantation involves the placement of 8- or 10-mm tube grafts to each coronary ostium with a side-to-side connection to the main aortic graft (Fig. 31-4). This procedure can be complicated by kinking of the right or left limb of the side graft if it is not oriented correctly in addition to the long-term risk of right coronary artery occlusion.[28,39] An alternative approach involves direct reimplantation of the right coronary button (which almost always can be mobilized sufficiently) and reimplantation of the left coronary artery with an interposition graft between the aortic graft and the left coronary ostium (Fig. 31-5).[39]

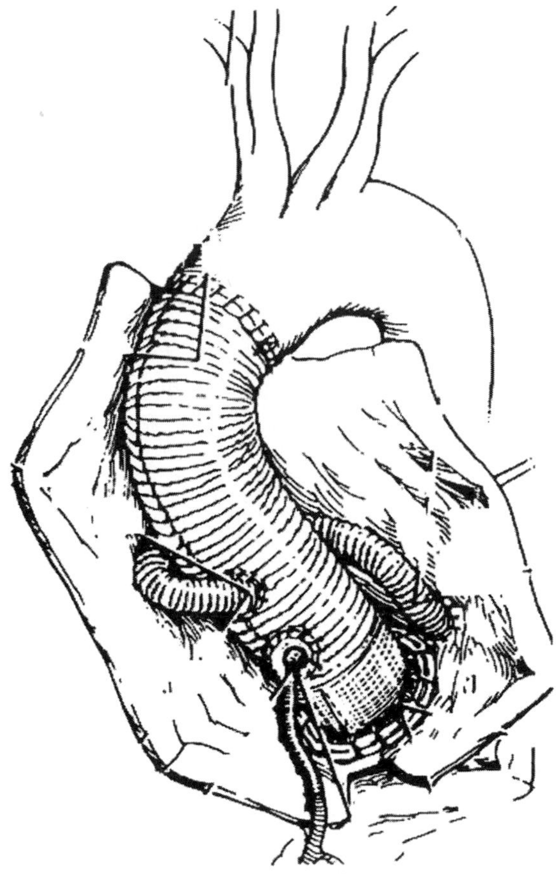

Figure 31-5 Insertion of a composite graft with the use of an interposition graft to the left main coronary artery (coursing behind the ascending aorta) and an aortic button to the right coronary artery. (Reproduced with permission from Svensson LG, Crawford ES. *Cardiovascular and Vascular Disease of the Aorta*. Philadelphia: Saunders; 1997:272.)

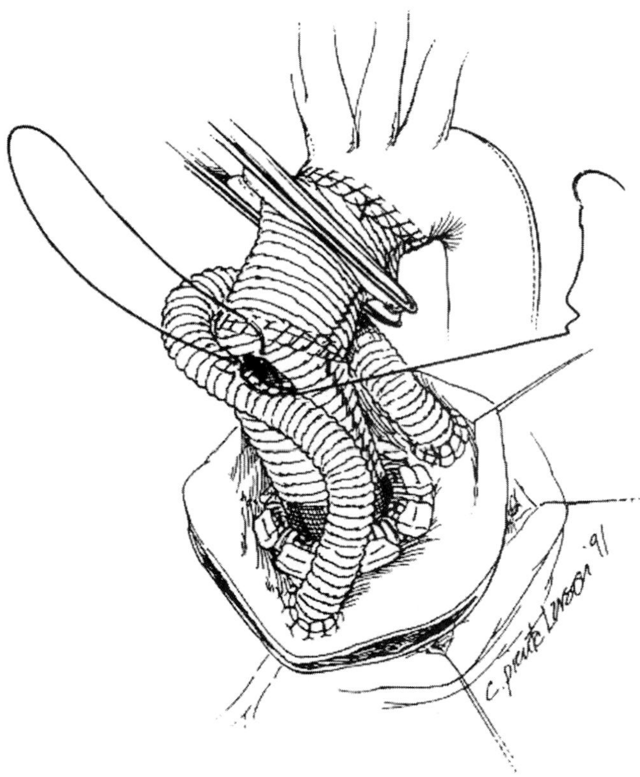

Figure 31-4 Composite valve-graft insertion with the Cabrol technique. The tube graft to the left main ostium is brought behind the composite graft, and the composite graft is sutured to the aortic arch or to the graft that has been used for arch replacement. Finally, the coronary interposition graft is sutured to the right coronary artery ostium and the anastomosis (side-to-side) is completed. (Reproduced with permission from Svensson LG, Crawford ES. Aortic dissection and aortic aneurysm surgery: Clinical observations, experimental investigations, and statistical analyses: Part III. *Curr Probl Surg* 1993;30:1–72.)

The results of composite valve-graft aortic root replacement operations are generally very good but are dependent on the indication for operation. For example, Dossche and colleagues[40] reviewed a cohort of 244 patients (of whom 85 percent had degenerative aneurysm etiology) who underwent aortic root replacement with a composite valve-graft. The hospital mortality rate was 7.8 percent, and the cumulative survival at 5, 10, and 20 years was 76 percent, 62 percent, and 33 percent. Gott and associates reviewed the extensive experience at Johns Hopkins with aortic root replacement in Marfan's syndrome patients over a 24-year

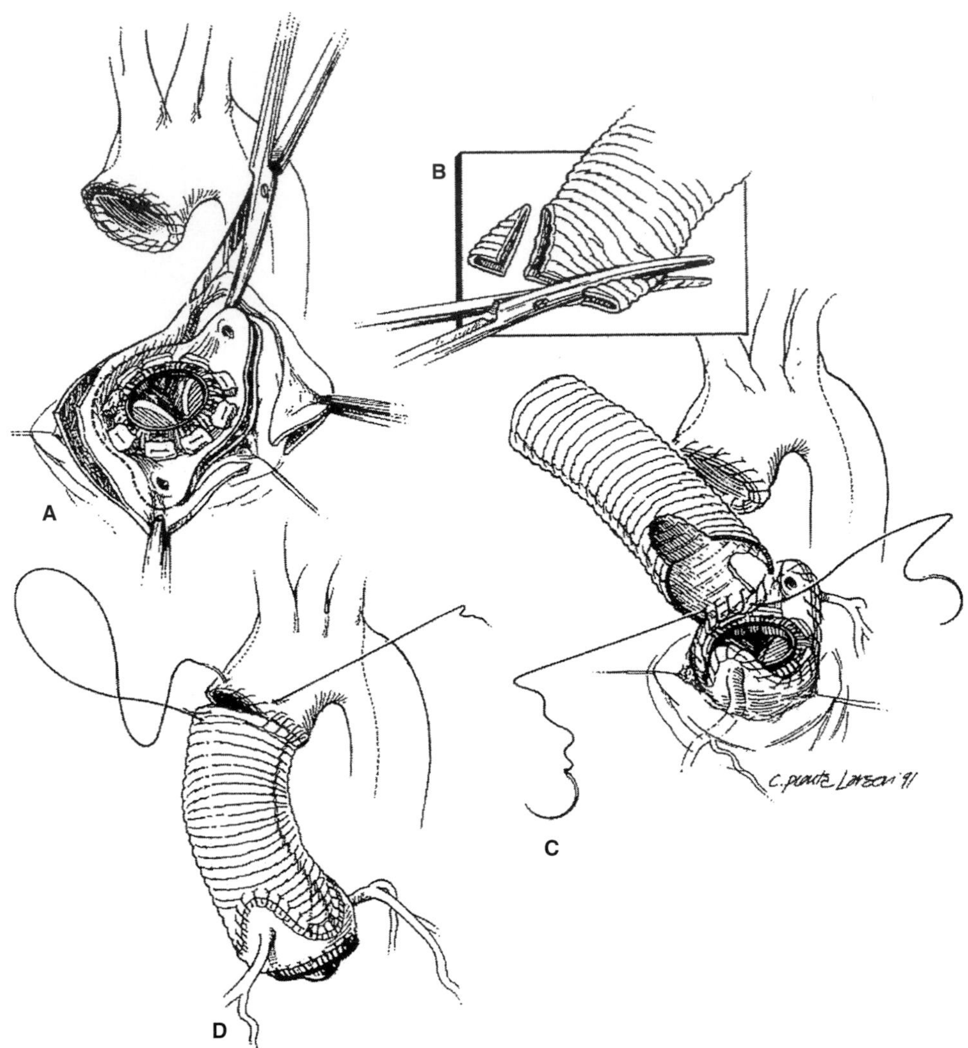

Figure 31-6 Proximal aortic repair using the Wheat method. **A.** The aortic valve is seated, and the aorta is transected circumferentially, with the aortic ostia being preserved carefully and the aortic layers being reapproximated with running sutures. **B.** Scallops are removed from the graft to match the coronary ostia. **C.** The graft is sewn into position, with sutures placed across the valve sewing ring whenever possible. **D.** The distal anastomosis is completed. [Reproduced with permission from Svensson LG, Crawford ES. Aortic dissection and aortic aneurysm surgery: Clinical observations, experimental investigations, and statistical analyses: Part II. *Curr Probl Surg* 1993;29(12):923–1011.]

period.[41] Two hundred thirty-five Marfan's patients underwent elective aortic root replacement with no 30-day mortality. The actuarial freedom from thromboembolism, endocarditis, and reoperation on the residual aorta 20 years postoperatively was 93 percent, 90 percent, and 74 percent, respectively. Lai and associates reviewed the Stanford experience with composite valve-graft (CVG) replacement for acute type A aortic dissection.[42] Thirty-day, 1-year, and 6-year survival estimates of 86 ± 8 percent, 81 ± 9 percent, and 65 ± 16 percent were seen with composite valve-graft replacement, with a 6-year freedom from reoperation of 100 percent. Niederhauser and colleagues reviewed their experience with 181 consecutive CVG patients operated on between 1983 and 1993 with a mean follow-up of 28 months.[43] Overall survival was 75 percent after 7 years; that rate was decreased significantly in patients who had acute aortic dissection (p = 0.0019). Reoperation-free survival was 69 percent at 7 years and significantly decreased after acute dissection (p = 0.0421).

Ehrlich and coworkers[44] reported on 84 patients older than 65 years of age (median age was 74 years with a range of 66 to 89 years) who underwent CVG aortic root replacement over an 11-year period. Hospital mortality was 8.3 percent (7 of 84), with 16 late deaths (19 percent) noted during a median follow-up of 3.2 years (range 0 to 10 years). The authors concluded that composite valve-graft replacement in elderly patients results in low operative mortality, has excellent long-term survival, and averts fatal aneurysm rupture even in that higher-risk population.

The composite valve-graft versus separate valve-graft controversy

In many cases an acceptable alternative to full CVG aortic root replacement is ascending aortic replacement starting at the sinotubular junction in association with separate aortic valve replacement [separate valve-graft (SVG)], leaving an intervening segment of the patient's own aortic root from which the coronary ostia originate. The SVG procedure is less technically demanding and is useful when the sinotubular junction is not effaced and the aortic root is not dilated. It is useful in elderly patients in whom a shorter cross-clamp time may limit morbidity, especially those with acute type A without significant annuloaortic ectasia. A relatively common problem is significant ascending aortic dilatation associated with aortic valve replacement for a bicuspid aortic valve. It is well known that patients with bicuspid aortic valves are predisposed to the development of ascending and root aneurysm. The cause is multifactorial and includes hemodynamic factors and heredity.[45] The decision to pursue CVG replacement to exclude all potentially diseased aortic root tissue is tempered by an increased operative (30-day) mortality rate (4 to 10 percent)[46,47] compared with a 2 to 5 percent operative mortality rate for isolated aortic valve replacement. The SVG technique may provide a reasonable compromise between these two procedural extremes, especially if concomitant procedures must be performed in the same setting; however, there is a risk of aneurysmal dilatation of the intervening aorta over time. McCready and associates[48] observed an approximately 15 percent incidence of significant root dilatation an average of 6.5 years after the SVG procedure. Karck and associates[49] reoperated on 3 of 17 patients (18 percent) an average of 7.8 years after the initial SVG procedure because of recurrent degenerative root aneurysms. Yun and colleagues documented no differences in operative mortality between the CVG and SVG techniques but found a 6 percent reoperation rate after CVG in contrast to a 19 percent reoperation rate after SVG.[47] Similarly, Houel and coworkers[50] found mortality rates of 7.7 percent with CVG versus 11 percent with SVG (p = not significant). Actuarial survival at 10 years postoperatively in these groups was 77.7 ± 5.6 percent versus 75.8 ± 6.9 percent (p = not significant). However, freedom from late complications of the ascending aorta was significantly different (97.3 ± 1.9 percent CVG versus 68.3 ± 9.0 percent SVG at 10 years postoperatively). The SVG technique was identified as a risk factor for late complications of the ascending aorta by multivariate analysis ($p = 0.01$; odds ratio 9). In light of these data, an aggressive approach to CVG replacement in this population is recommended in patients with acceptable risk. When the sinotubular junction and aortic root are intact so that SVG is considered appropriate, the procedure first described by Wheat and associates[10] may be useful to maximize exclusion of as much native aortic root tissue as possible without incurring the extra technical challenge of a full CVG implantation (Fig. 31-6).

Medtronic freestyle prosthesis

The Freestyle aortic root bioprosthesis (Medtronic, Inc., Minneapolis, MN) is a stentless porcine aortic root prepared with low-pressure and zero-pressure fixation processes and alpha-aminooleic acid leaflet anticalcification treatment, with the aim of optimizing both hemodynamics and bioprosthesis durability (Fig. 31-7). The device can be implanted as a subcoronary or modified subcoronary valve replacement, as a complete aortic root replacement (total root), or as a root inclusion. Initial implantations in human subjects began in 1992, and the device has been approved for clinical use in the United States since 1997. The implantation technique of this prosthesis is similar to that for CVG replacement described above. Bach and colleagues[51] reported the 8-year results of a multicenter cohort of 700 patients

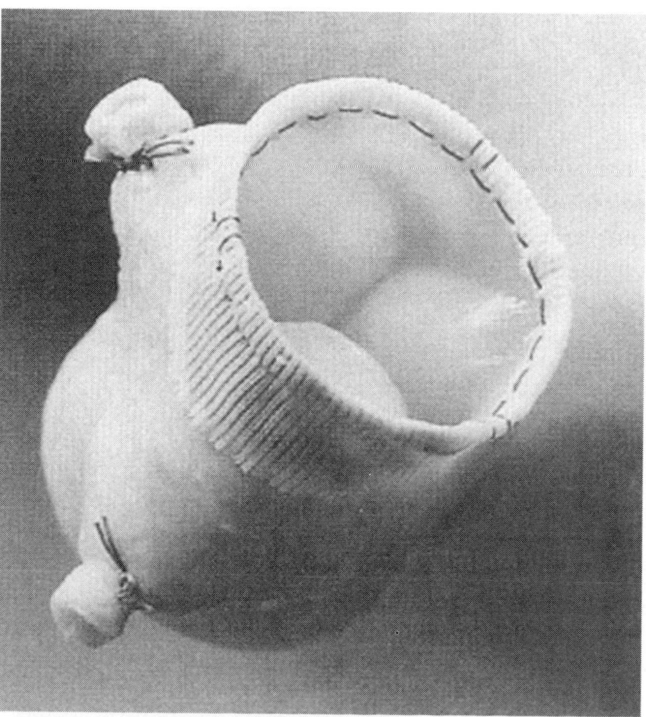

Figure 31-7 Medtronic Freestyle prosthesis. [Reproduced with permission from David TE. Mechanical and bioprosthetic aortic valve replacement In: Edmunds LH (ed). *Cardiac Surgery in the Adult.* New York: McGraw-Hill: 1997:859–910.]

(of whom 93 percent were over 60 years of age) followed prospectively who received various configurations of this prosthesis. A total root replacement was performed in 162 of those patients, with actuarial freedom from valve-related death of 92.3 percent, freedom from structural deterioration of 100 percent, and freedom from moderate or more aortic regurgitation of 98.7 percent. Oral anticoagulation is not required postoperatively.

Homograft aortic root replacement

Aortic root replacement can be performed with a cryopreserved homograft aortic root. This operation is more technically demanding because of the less rigid nature of the tissue used. The operative technique is similar to the techniques described above except that many authors advocate a continuous running suture for the implantation of the left ventricular outflow tract side to the annulus. In addition, this proximal suture line must be planar; that is, it should not follow the scallops of the aortic annulus but should run somewhat under the commissures. This operation is particularly well suited for patients in the age range of 40 to 60 years (e.g., those with congenital bicuspid aortic valve pathology) who require aortic root replacement but do not wish to take oral anticoagulants. The analysis by McGiffin and associates[52] showed that the use of homografts in patients under 40 years of age was associated with an unacceptably high incidence of valve failure over a 15-year period (Fig. 31-8). In addition, homograft root replacement is the operation of choice for extensive native and prosthetic valve endocarditis (PVE). Previous work by McGiffin and associates[53] demonstrated improved freedom from recurrent endocarditis when allograft tissue was used for aortic valve replacement compared with the use of prosthetic valve material. Grinda and colleagues[54] evaluated the short- and long-term results of cryopreserved aortic viable homograft (CAVH) in the treatment of active aortic endocarditis. One hundred four patients underwent CAVH replacement for active aortic valve endocarditis; 73 percent of those operations involved the native aortic valve, and 27 percent involved a prosthetic aortic valve. CAVHs were inserted using the aortic root replacement technique in 89 percent of those patients. Actuarial survival at 10 years was 83 percent, with 93 percent of the patients free from cardiac death. At 10 years, the actuarial rate for freedom from reoperation was 76 percent and that for freedom from recurrent endocarditis was 93 percent. No thromboembolic complications were observed. The results are not as encouraging if one looks only at PVE, however. Lytle and coworkers[55] reviewed 27 patients with aortic valve PVE after previous ascending aortic replacement who underwent reoperation for aortic root replacement with a cryopreserved aortic allograft and prolonged intravenous antibiotic therapy. Survival at 1, 2, 5, and 7.5 years was 92 percent, 88 percent, 70 percent, and 56 percent, respectively, with one patient requiring reoperation for recurrent PVE 8 months after the operation.

Ross procedure

The Ross procedure consists of removal of the native aortic valve and root with preservation of the coronary buttons, followed by excision of the patient's own pulmonary valve encased in the pulmonary artery distally and a small rim of right ventricular outflow tract muscle proximal to the annulus. The pulmonary valve then is translocated to the aortic position as a root replacement, with sewing of the right ventricular muscle to the aortic annulus in a planar fashion, reimplantation of the coronary ostia, and a distal anastomosis between the pulmonary arterial end of the autograft and the ascending aorta. The right ventricle–pulmonary artery side then is reconstructed with a valved pulmonary homograft (Fig. 31-9). This procedure should be performed by surgeons who are extremely competent at aortic root operations. Although the procedure is very demanding technically, the results are outstanding, with 80 percent freedom from reoperation at 20 years,[56] with the failures roughly evenly distributed between the autograft and allograft sides. The operation holds promise for the treatment of infective endocarditis.[57] A very common indication for the performance of this procedure has been for bicuspid aortic valve disease. However, recent reports have shown early dilatation of the autograft with neoaortic valve insufficiency (Fig. 31-10).[58] Histologic analysis shows evidence of medial degeneration in both the aorta (Fig. 31-11) and the pulmonary artery (Fig. 31-12) of patients with bicuspid compared with tricuspid aortic valves.[59] This is not surprising since embryologically the aorta and the pulmonary artery develop from a common truncus. Over time, gradual dilatation of the neosinuses of Valsalva is observed (Fig. 31-13).[60] In light of these more recent data, many surgeons have tempered their enthusiasm for the Ross procedure in this patient population and reserve it for young patients who are not predisposed to aortic or pulmonary artery dilatation.

Valve-sparing aortic root replacement

Approximately 30 percent of patients who require aortic root replacement have a normal aortic valve that leaks because of sinotubular junction effacement and/or aortic annular dilatation secondary to degenerative causes or connective tissue diseases such as Marfan's syndrome. Rather than excising the aortic valve and replacing the root with prosthetic valve material, an operation that encloses the native valve within normal aortic root geometry should restore competency. In 1979, Sir Magdi Yacoub introduced an aortic valve-sparing root replacement ("remodeling," David-II) procedure consisting of excision of all the native aortic tissue except for a small rim around the valve leaflets.[11] An appropriately sized Dacron graft then is fashioned into three scallops at one end and sutured to the residual aortic tissue, followed by coronary reimplantation (Fig. 31-14).

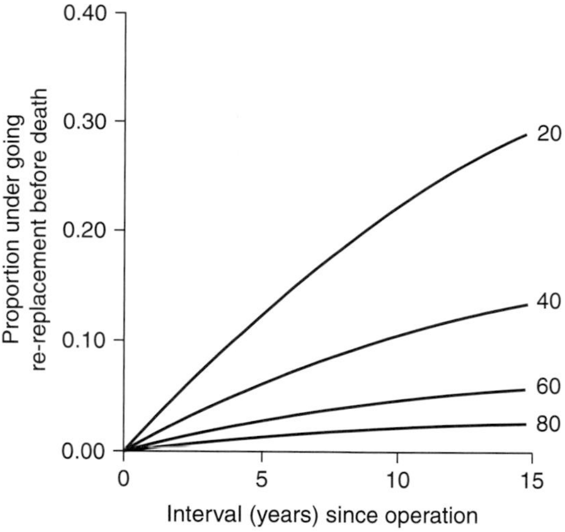

Figure 31-8 Nomogram of the time-related proportion of patients with cryopreserved allograft valves (299 patients, 14 reoperations) who actually will require valve re-replacement for any reason before death according to the age of the patient. (Reproduced with permission from McGiffin DC, Galbraith AJ, O'Brien, et al. An analysis of valve re-replacement after aortic valve replacement with biologic devices. *J Thorac Cardiovasc Surg* 1997;311–318.)

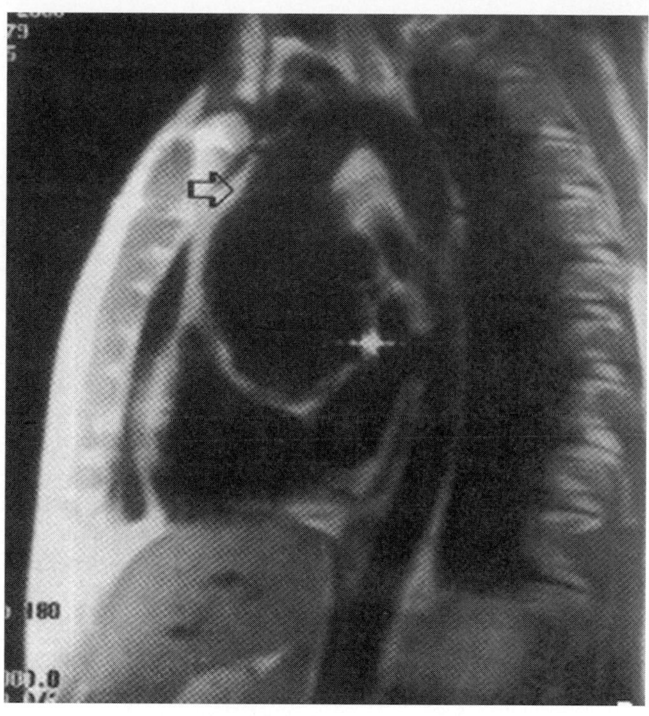

Figure 31-10 Magnetic resonance image of the neoaortic root demonstrating dilatation of the pulmonary autograft and an abrupt transition to normal diameter at the distal suture line, as shown by the arrow. [Reproduced with permission from Sundt TM, Moon MR, Xu H. Reoperation for dilatation of the pulmonary autograft after the Ross Procedure. *J Thorac Cardio Surg* 2001;122(6):1249–1252.]

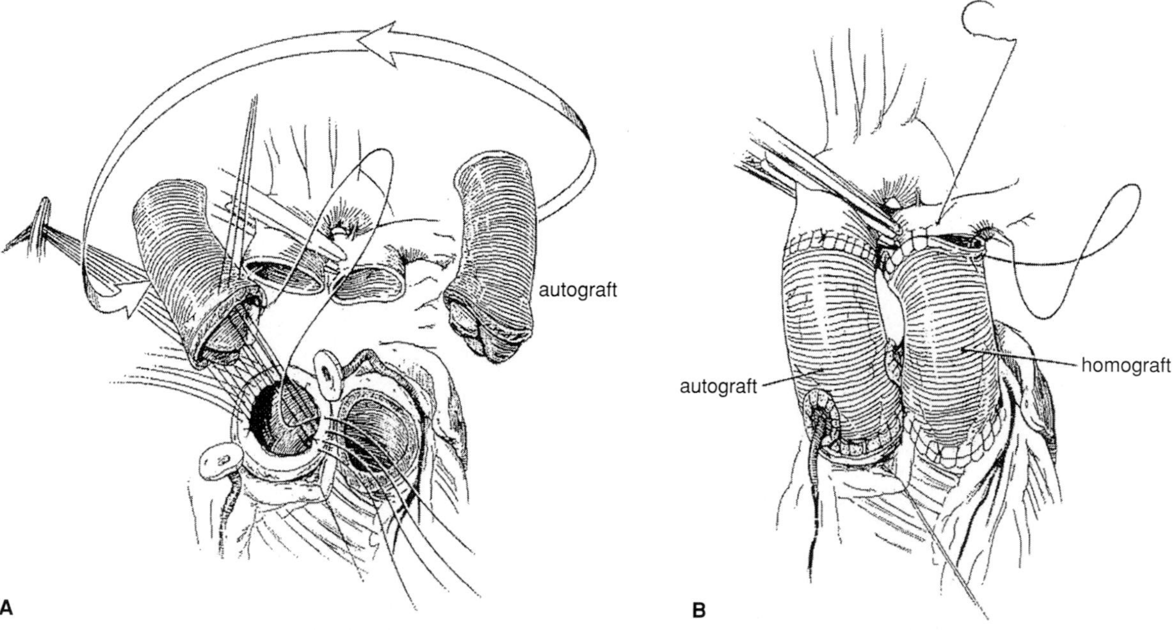

Figure 31-9 Insertion of a pulmonary autograft into the aortic position (Ross procedure). The pulmonary autograft is seated in the aortic annulus with interrupted simple sutures (*left*). Attention is paid to ensure that the valve is properly seated, as the pulmonary valve does not have the differences in valve cusp edge lengths that the aortic valve has. The homograft is sutured into position in the native pulmonary outflow tract to complete the procedure (*right*). (Reproduced with permission from Svensson LG, Crawford ES. Aortic dissection and aortic aneurysm surgery: Clinical observations, experimental investigations, and statistical analyses: Part III. *Curr Probl Surg* 1993;30:1–72.)

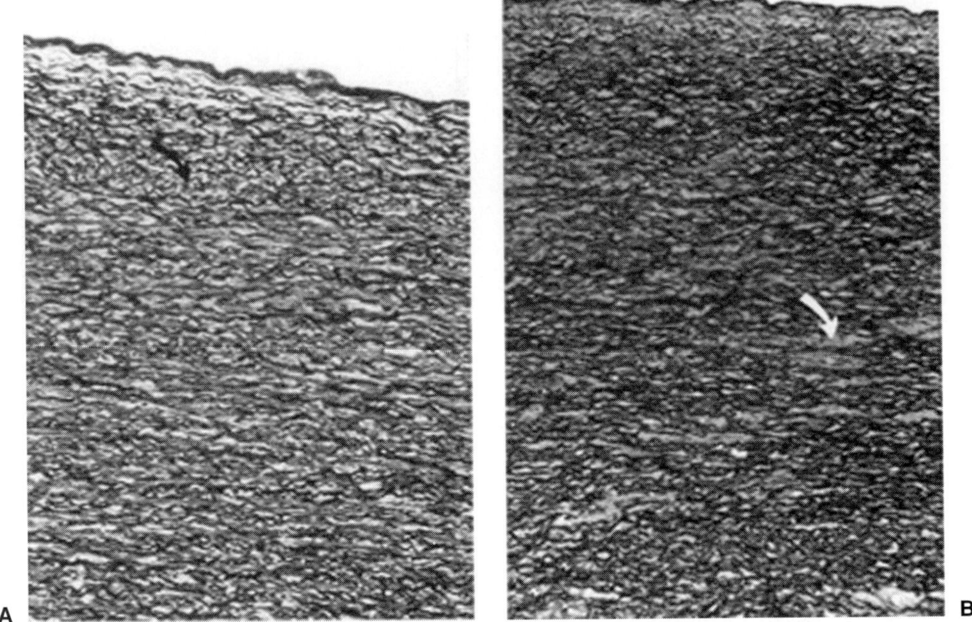

Figure 31-11 **A.** Histologic features of aortic section from a patient with normal trileaflet aortic valve. There are no intimal changes. **B.** Histologic features of the ascending aorta from a 33-year-old patient with bicuspid aortic valve disease. Note the significant medial destruction and the accumulation of mucoid material (*arrow*). There is a marked fragmentation of elastic tissue. [Reproduced with permission from de Sa, M, Moshkovitz Y, Butany T, David TE. Histological abnormalities of the ascending aorta and pulmonary trunk in patients with bicuspid aortic valve disease. *J Thorac Cardiovasc Surg* 1999; 118(4):588–594.]

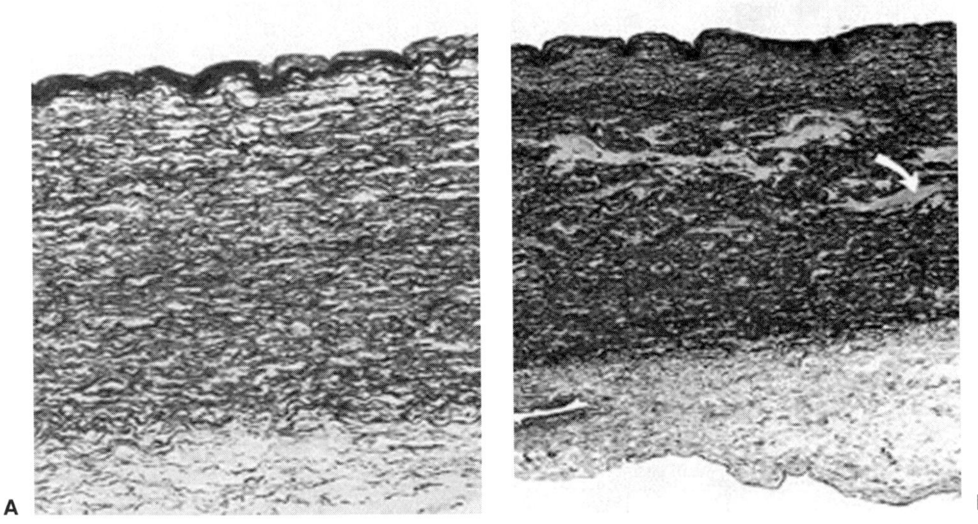

Figure 31-12 **A.** Normal histologic structure of a pulmonary trunk from a 42-year-old patient with tricuspid aortic valve disease. Elastic tissue and smooth muscle cells run circumferentially. Small areas of collagen can be identified (*pale yellow*). **B.** Histologic structure from a 40-year-old patient with bicuspid aortic valve disease. Note the disorganized media with large pools of polysaccharide (*pale blue*) and collagen deposition (*pale yellow*). There is also smooth muscle disorientation and elastic tissue fragmentation. [Reproduced with permission from de Sa M, Moshkovitz Y, Butany J, David TE. Histological abnormalities of the ascending aorta and pulmonary trunk in patients with bicuspid aortic valve disease. *J Thorac Cardiovasc Surg* 1999; 118(4):588–594.]

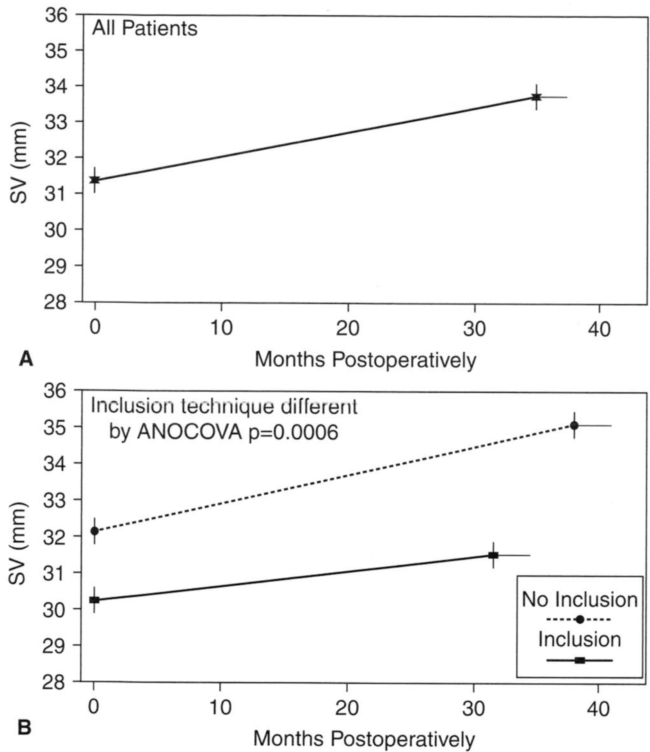

Figure 31-13 Time-related changes in the sinus of Valsalva in the neoaortic root after the Ross procedure. *Upper panel*: The diameter of the sinuses of Valsalva (SV) increased with time ($p = 0.01$). *Lower panel*: Analysis of covariance (ANOCOVA) showed that the increase in the diameter of the sinuses of Valsalva was significantly greater in patients who had aortic root replacement (*dotted line*) than in those who had aortic root inclusion (*solid line*). [Reproduced with permission from David TE, Omran A, Ivanov J. Dilation of the pulmonary autograft after the Ross procedure. *J Thorac Cardiovasc Surg* 1995; 119(2):210–220.]

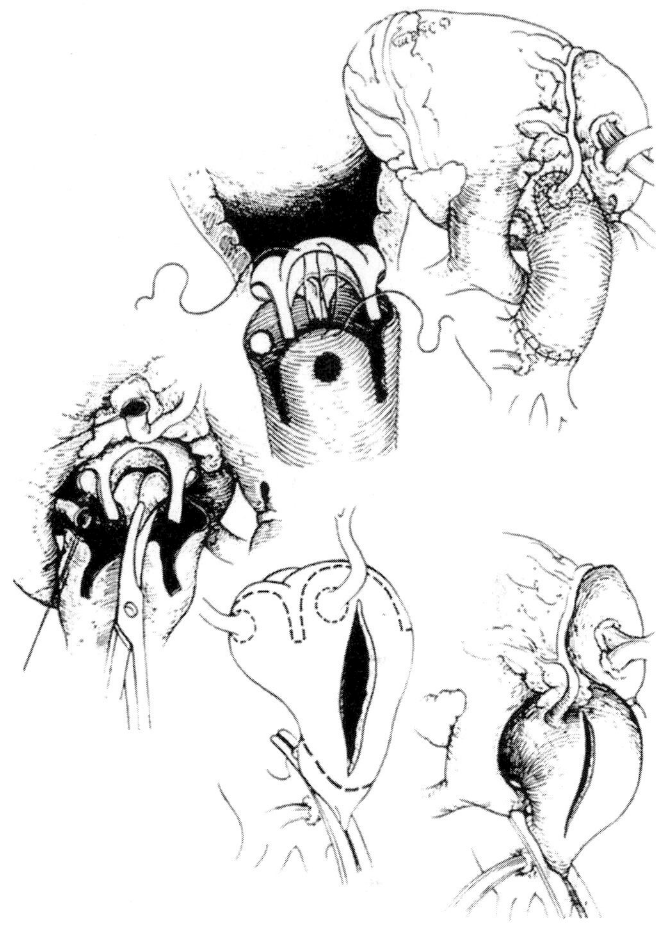

Figure 31-14 Operative technique of the remodeling (Yacoub) valve-sparing aortic root replacement. [Reproduced with permission from Yacoub MH, Gehle P, Chandrasekaran V. Late results of a valve-preserving operation in patients with aneurysms of the ascending aorta and root. *J Thorac Cardiovasc Surg* 1998:115(5);1080–1089.]

In approximately 1988, Dr. Tirone David introduced the valve-sparing "reimplantation" (David-I) procedure,[12] in which sutures placed *proximal to* the aortic valve annulus are sewn to the Dacron graft. In this way, when the graft is seated, the valve sits entirely inside the graft and is attached to it from the inside with a second suture line after coronary reimplantation (Figs. 31-15 to 31-18). The appropriate graft size is selected by measuring the average aortic valve leaflet height in millimeters, multiplying this value by 4/3, and adding 4 to 6 mm to this number to account for the thickness of the left ventricular outflow tract under the aortic annulus.[12]

The Yacoub remodeling procedure does not protect the aortic annulus and leaves it susceptible to dilatation and hence valvar insufficiency over time (Fig. 31-19).[11] David addressed this problem by placing a Teflon felt buttress under the fibrous portion of the annulus (David-III) but abandoned that modification in favor of the reimplantation procedure. If reoperation is required because of valvar incompetence after the remodeling procedure, a full aortic root replacement is necessary because of the persistence of unprotected native aortic root tissue. In contrast, with the David reimplantation procedure, the entire aortic root and annulus are enclosed in graft material, preventing dilatation over time. If reoperation is required, the graft can be opened, the native valve can be excised, and a stented or stentless valve of choice may be sutured directly into the graft,[61] obviating the need for a much more difficult root re-replacement.

With the original David operation, isolated case reports described native valve failure with fibrotic, retracted aortic leaflets seen at reoperation, perhaps consistent with repeated trauma to the leaflets secondary to the lack of "neosinuses" produced with the Yacoub procedure.[61,62] The David procedure has undergone two iterations to address this issue. The first (David-IV) involved the selection of a graft 4 to 6 mm larger in diameter than the calculation dictates and plication of

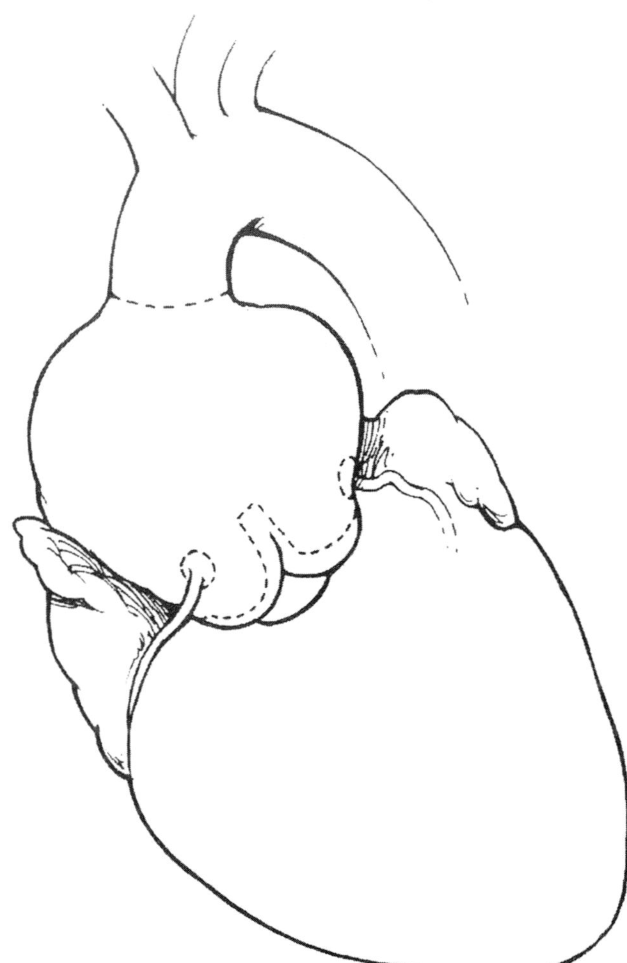

Figure 31-15 Reimplantation (David-I) valve-sparing aortic root replacement. The dotted lines indicate the resection lines along the arterial wall. [Reproduced with permission from Cochran RP, Kunzelman KS. Valve-sparing operations for dilated aortic root. In: Franco KL, Verrier ED (eds). *Advanced Therapy in Cardiac Surgery*, 2d ed. Hamilton, Ontario, Canada: BC Elsevier; 2003:311–322.]

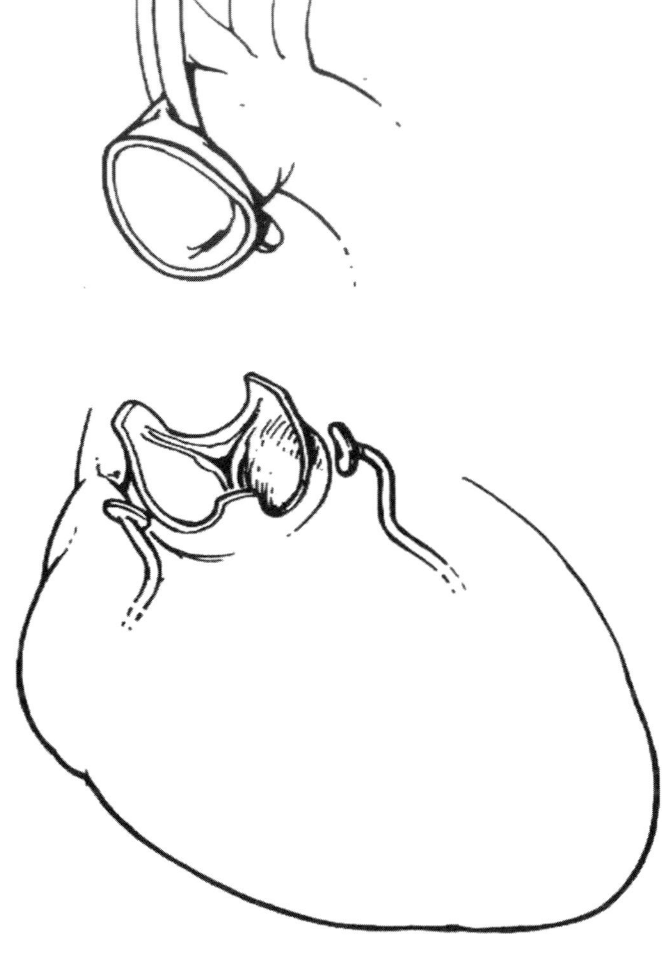

Figure 31-16 Reimplantation (David-I) valve-sparing aortic root replacement. The aortic valve and a small portion of arterial wall are left attached to the left ventricular outflow tract. [Reproduced with permission from Cochran RP, Kunzelman KS. Valve-sparing operations for dilated aortic root. In Franco KL, Verrier ED (eds). *Advanced Therapy in Cardiac Surgery*, 2d ed. Hamilton, Ontario, Canada: BC Elsevier; 2003:311–322.]

the neosinotubular junction down to the correct size. With the current (David-V) modification, the Dacron graft used for the aortic root replacement is oversized by 6 to 8 mm in diameter and then pleated at the annular and new sinotubular junction.[63,64] The graft will billow outward when it is subjected to arterial pressure, thus creating neosinuses (Figs. 31-20 to 31-23). Other authors have described modifications such as the use of a large and a small graft to facilitate the creation of neoaortic sinuses,[65] graft scalloping (Fig. 31-24),[13] and the use of a graft (Fig. 31-25) designed with sinuses of Valsalva already incorporated.[14] Still other modifications have been described.[66]

The results of the David operation have been excellent, with 100 percent freedom from reoperation in Dr. David's hands.[67] Similar excellent results have been reported by other investigators.[68–72] In addition, the indications for this procedure are expanding to include bicuspid aortic valves[73] and type A aortic dissection.[74,75] Patients benefit from the long-term durability associated with preservation of their own valves, and anticoagulation is not required postoperatively.[67,76]

Postoperative care and surgical results

Immediate postoperative care should focus on control of hypertension (for which intravenous sodium nitroprusside is used most commonly) and maintenance of adequate filling pressures (central venous pressure 10 to 15 mmHg, pulmonary capillary wedge pressures in the range of 15 to 18 mmHg). Dual-chamber pacing is required in a small proportion of patients who leave the

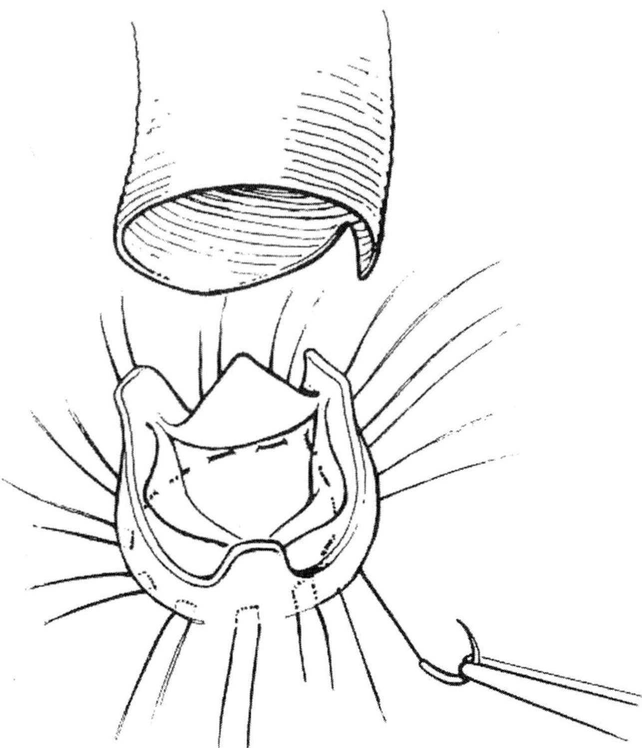

Figure 31-17 Reimplantation (David-I) valve-sparing aortic root replacement. Multiple horizontal mattress sutures are run from inside to outside the left ventricular outflow tract just below the aortic valve on the left side and through a single horizontal plane on the right side. [Reproduced with permission from Cochran RP, Kunzelman KS. Valve-sparing operations for dilated aortic root. In Franco KL, Verrier ED (eds). *Advanced Therapy in Cardiac Surgery*, 2d ed. Hamilton, Ontario, Canada: BC Elsevier; 2003:311–322.]

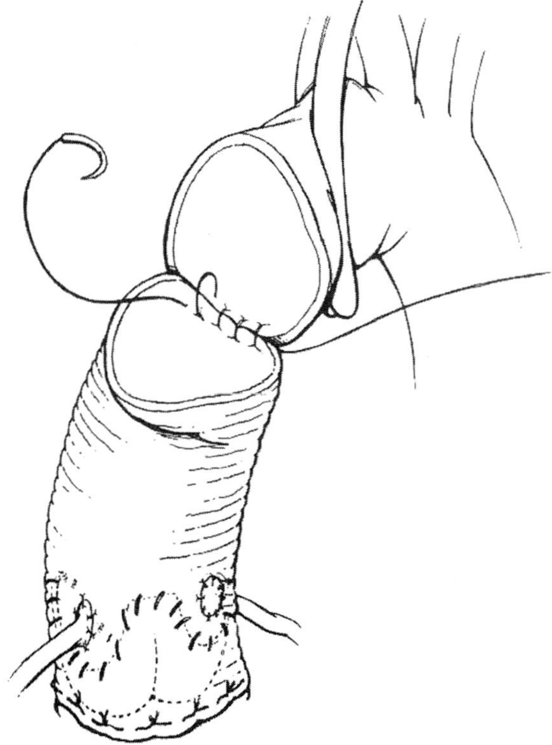

Figure 31-18 Reimplantation (David-I) valve-sparing aortic root replacement. The aortic valve is reimplanted into the Dacron graft. It is secured at two separate levels below the leaflets by the horizontal mattress sutures and above the leaflets by suturing the remnants of arterial wall to the Dacron graft. The coronary arteries also are reimplanted. [Reproduced with permission from Cochran RP, Kunzelman KS. Valve-sparing operations for dilated aortic root. In Franco KL, Verrier ED (eds). *Advanced Therapy in Cardiac Surgery*, 2d ed. Hamilton, Ontario, Canada: BC Elsevier; 2003:311–322.]

operating room in conduction block. Often this resolves within 24 to 48 hours. If conduction block persists longer than 4 to 5 days, permanent pacemaker insertion should be considered. In patients with no conduction disturbances, pacemaker wires can be removed on the third or fourth postoperative day. The patient should be placed on telemetry for the duration of the hospital stay, however. The mediastinal tube is removed for outputs less than 150 mL per 24 h.

Patients with mechanical valves are started on oral warfarin on the second postoperative day. The use of daily aspirin coupled with a target International Normalized Ratio (INR) of 2.0 to 2.5 provides satisfactory anticoagulation and minimizes long-term bleeding and thrombotic events. Patients with bioprosthetic valves can be managed with aspirin alone, with no warfarin required.

The 30-day (early) mortality for aortic root replacement varies from 4 to 10 percent.[46,47] This number is approximately doubled with redo operations. Reoperation for mediastinal hemorrhage should be required in less than 10 percent of cases. Complete heart block requiring pacemaker insertion occurs in about 1 to 2 percent in most series. Stroke occurs in approximately 1 to 4 percent of these patients. There is no practical pharmacologic strategy for the prevention of postoperative atrial fibrillation, which occurs up to one-third of the time (in patients with no previous history). Careful correction of electrolytes and chemical cardioversion with intravenous and oral amiodarone are preferred and are successful 90 to 95 percent of the time. Patients should be maintained on oral amiodarone for approximately 1 month, by which time the threat of recurrent atrial fibrillation should be resolved. In patients who require warfarin, the use of amiodarone makes it very difficult to manage the INR, and consideration should be given to alternative antiarrhythmics such as sotalol and procainamide. Patients with persistent atrial fibrillation despite attempts at chemical and electrical cardioversion should be maintained on oral warfarin until the arrhythmia resolves.

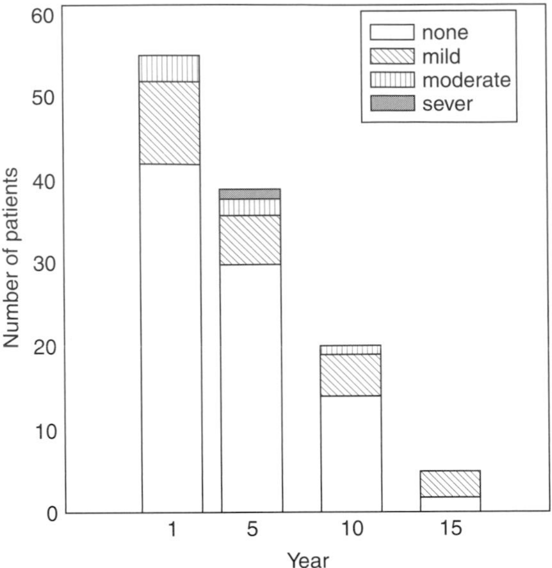

Figure 31-19 Presence or absence of aortic regurgitation and its degree postoperatively after remodeling (Yacoub) valve-sparing aortic root replacement. [Reproduced with permission from Yacoub MH, Gehle P, Chandrasekaran V. Late results of a valve-preserving operation in patients with aneurysms of the ascending aorta and root. *J Thorac Cardiovasc Surg* 1998:115(5);1080–1089.]

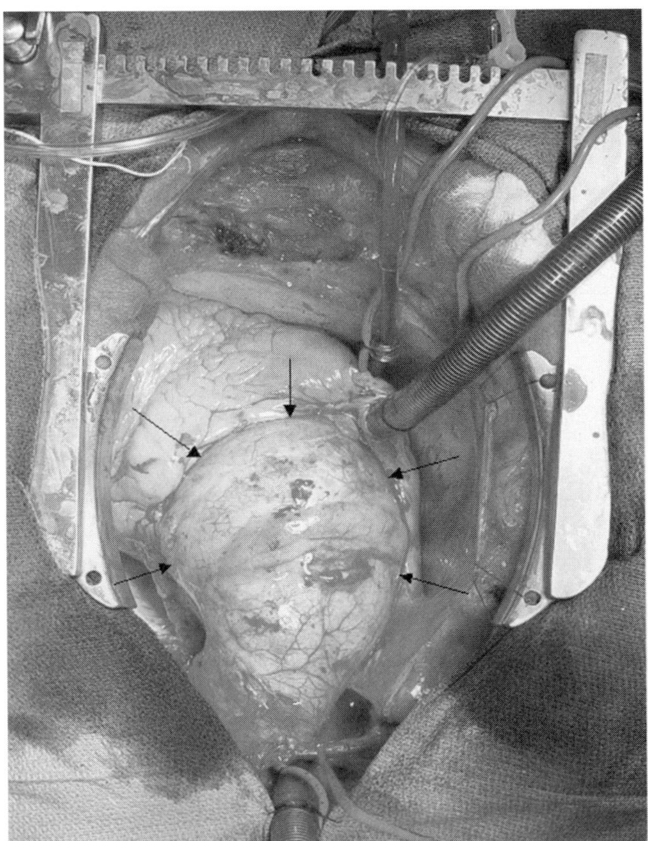

Figure 31-20 Reimplantation (David-V) valve-sparing aortic root replacement. Intraoperative photograph of ascending and root aortic aneurysm (*arrows*).

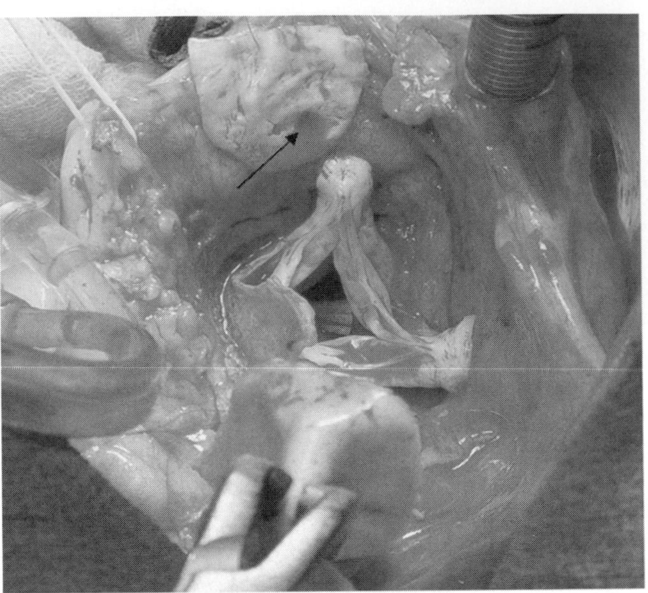

Figure 31-21 Reimplantation (David-V) valve-sparing aortic root replacement. The diseased aortic tissue is excised, leaving the aortic valve (*center of picture*) surrounded by a small rim of native aorta. The right main coronary artery ostium is shown (*arrow*). The left coronary ostium is obscured by the aortic cross-clamp (*bottom center of picture*).

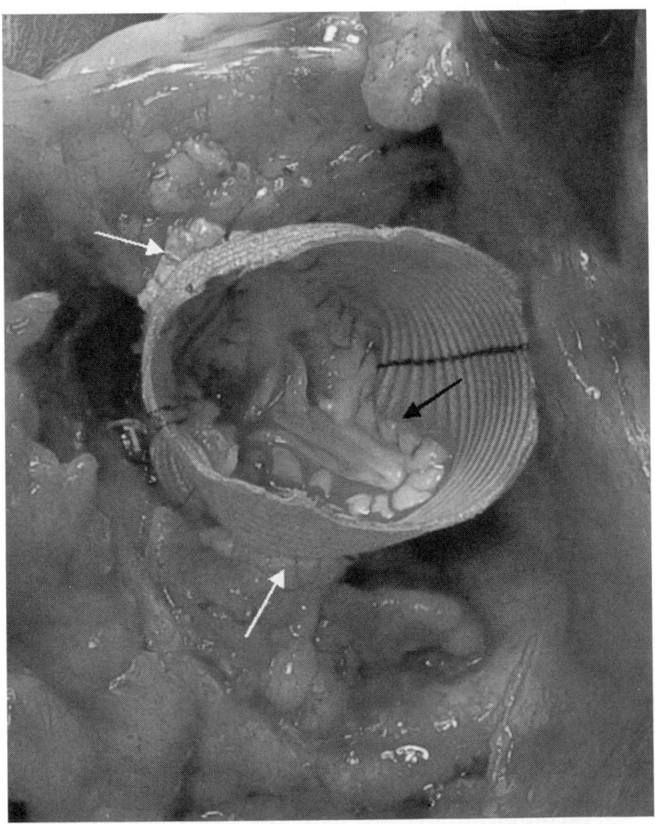

Figure 31-22 Reimplantation (David-V) valve-sparing aortic root replacement. The aortic valve is now reimplanted inside the Dacron graft (*dark arrow*). The right (*top white arrow*) and left (*bottom white arrow*) main coronary arteries are reimplanted separately into the graft.

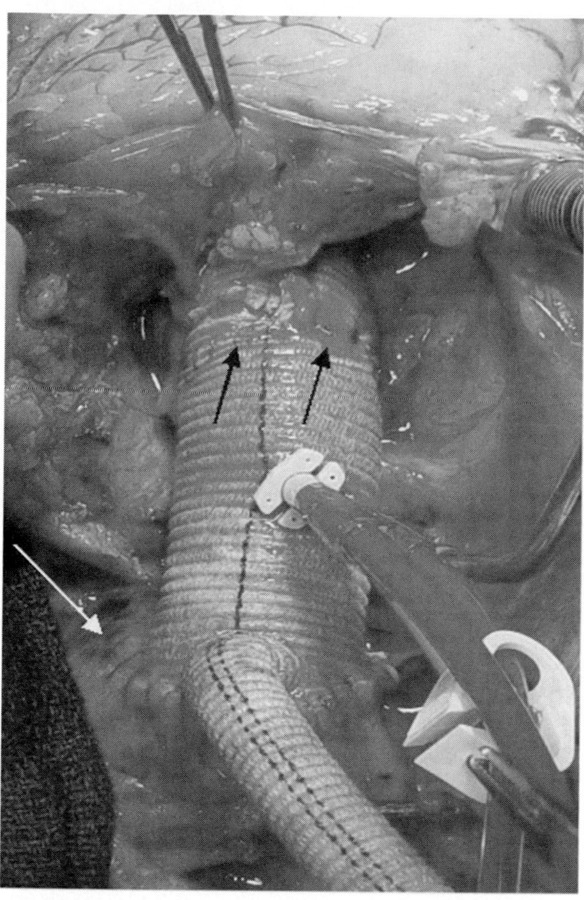

Figure 31-23 Reimplantation (David-V) valve-sparing aortic root replacement. The completed procedure is shown. Note the new sinotubular junction (*dark arrows*) and the hemiarch replacement suture line (*white arrow*).

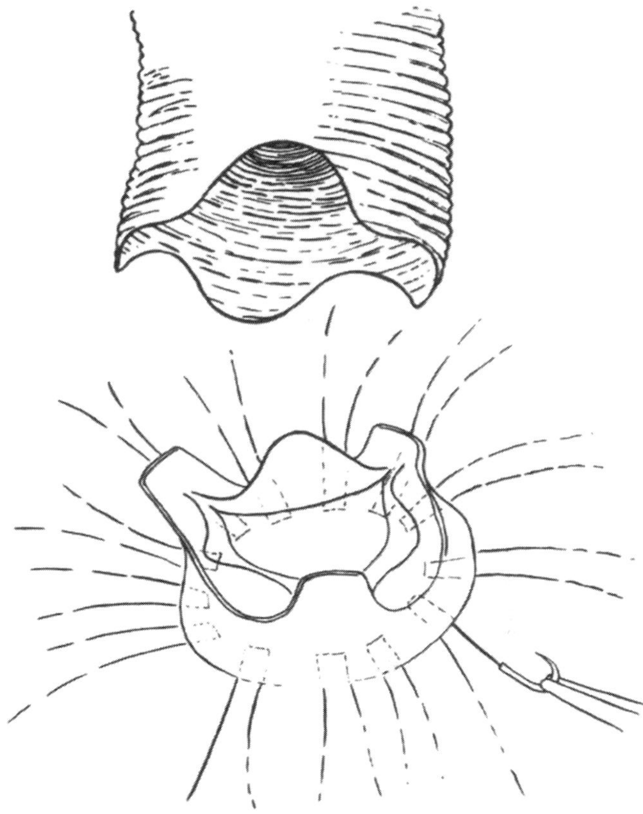

Figure 31-24 Valve-sparing aortic root replacement (Cochran modification). Creation of three completely symmetric scallops in the proximal conduit and circumferential subvalvular suture placement. [Reproduced with permission from Cochran RP, Kunzelman KS, Eddy AC, et al. Modified conduit preparation creates a pseudosinus in an aortic valve-sparing procedure for aneurysm of the ascending aorta. *J Thorac Cardiovasc Surg* 1995;109(6):1049–1057.]

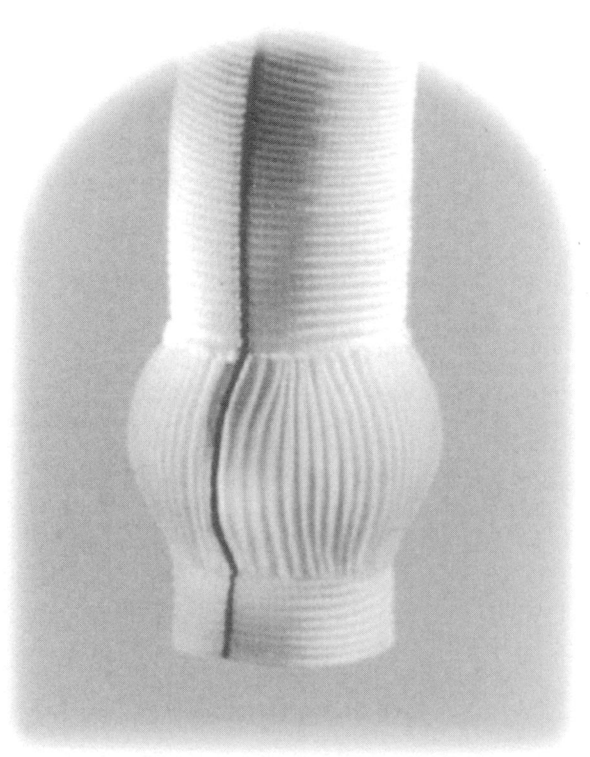

Figure 31-25 The DePaulis aortic Dacron conduit. [Reproduced with permission from De Paulis, De Matheis, et al. One-year appraisal of a new aortic root conduit with sinuses of Valsalva. *J Thorac Cardiovasc Surg* 2002;123(4):33–39.]

SUMMARY

Improvements in surgical technique, modifications of the procedure, and the development of specialized graft materials have improved the outcomes of aortic root replacement significantly.

Risk factors for the development or accelerated growth of ascending aortic aneurysms include aortic dissection, aneurysmal disease elsewhere in the aortic wall, smoking, renal failure, and diastolic hypertension. Ascending aortic dilatation can result from genetic conditions such as Marfan's syndrome, congenital bicuspid aortic valve, and osteogenesis imperfecta as well as from excessive extracellular matrix degradation caused by unregulated activity of enzymes such as matrix metalloproteinases, as seen in inflammatory conditions. Aneurysmal enlargement of the aortic root can occur with an increase in the diameter of the aortic annulus (annuloaortic ectasia) or without dilatation of the aortic annulus (degenerative disease).

Although certain patients may present with associated symptoms such as onset of pain from acute aortic dissection, the majority of these patients do not present with any specific physical abnormality, and many ascending aortic aneurysms are detected as an incidental finding. Contrasted computed tomography scans or magnetic resonance images, particularly those with three-dimensional reconstructions, have become the most useful diagnostic tests for evaluating the aortic root. There is no medical therapy for ascending aortic root aneurysms, and beyond therapy for blood pressure reduction and careful follow-up, including frequent radiologic imaging, surgical replacement of the aortic root is the only treatment.

For patients in whom surgical replacement of the aortic root is indicated, the surgeon must choose the appropriate ascending aortic root replacement device. Current options for aortic root replacement include composite synthetic xenograft valve-conduit prostheses and homograft replacement. Additional options include using the patient's own pulmonary valve after transposition to the aortic position (Ross procedure) and valve-sparing aortic root replacement.

References

1. Bahnson HT. Definitive treatment of saccular aneurysms of the aorta with excision of sac and aortic suture. *Surg Gynecol Obstet* 1953;96:383.
2. DeBakey ME, Cooley DA. Successful resection of aneurysm of thoracic aorta and replacement by graft. *JAMA* 1953;152:673.
3. Lam C, Aram HA. Resection of the descending thoracic aorta for aneurysm: A report of the use of a homograft in a case and an experimental study. *Am Surg* 1951;134:743.
4. DeBakey ME, Cooley DA, Carwford ES, et al. The clinical application of new flexible knitted dacron arterial substitute. *Arch Surg* 1958;77:713–714.
5. Cooley DA, DeBakey ME. Resection of entire ascending aorta in fusiform aneurysm using cardiac bypass. *JAMA* 1956;162: 1158.
6. DeBakey ME, Creech O Jr, Morris GC Jr. Aneurysm of the thoracoabdominal aorta involving the celiac superior mesenteric, and renal arteries: Report of four cases treated by resection and homograft replacement. *Ann Surg* 1956;144:549.
7. Starr A, Edwards WL, McCord MD, et al. Aortic replacement. *Circulation* 1963;27:779.
8. Bentall H, De Bono A. A technique for complete replacement of the ascending aorta. *Thorax* 1968;23:338.
9. Kouchoukos NT, Marshall WG Jr, Wedige-Stecher TA. Eleven-year experience with composite graft replacement of the ascending aorta and aortic valve. *J Thorac Cardiovasc Surg* 1986;92:691–705.
10. Wheat MW Jr, Wilson JR, Bartley TD. Successful replacement of the entire ascending aorta and aortic valve. *JAMA* 1964;188:717.
11. Yacoub MH, Gehle P, Chandrasekaran V, et al. Late results of a valve-preserving operation in patients with aneurysms of the ascending aorta and root. *J Thorac Cardiovasc Surg* 1998;5:1080–1090.
12. David TE, Feindel CM. An aortic valve-sparing operation for patients with aortic incompetence and aneurysm of the ascending aorta. *J Thorac Cardiovasc Surg* 1992;103: 617–621.
13. Cochran RP, Kunzelman KS, Eddy AC, et al. Modified conduit preparation creates a pseudosinus in an aortic valve-sparing procedure for aneurysm of the ascending aorta. *Thorac Cardiovasc Surg* 1995;109(6):1049–1057.
14. De Paulis R, De Matteis GM, Nardi P, et al. Analysis of valve motion after the reimplantation type of valve-sparing procedure (David I) with a new aortic root conduit. *Ann Thorac Surg* 2002;74(1):53–57.
15. Zehr KJ, Thubrikar MJ, Gong GG, et al. Clinical introduction of a novel prosthesis for valve-preserving aortic root reconstruction for annuloaortic ectasia. *J Thorac Cardiovasc Surg* 2000;120(4):692–698.
16. Pillsbury RC, Shumway NE. Replacement of the aortic valve with the autologous pulmonic valve. *Surg Forum* 1966;17:176–177.
17. Ross DN. Replacement of aortic and mitral valves with a pulmonary autograft. *Lancet* 1967;2(7523):956–958.
18. Moore, KL. The circulatory system In: Moore KL (ed). *The Developing Human*. Toronto: Saunders; 1982: 298–343.
19. Bickerstaff LK, Pairolero PC, Hollier LH, et al. Thoracic aortic aneurysms: A population based study. Surgery 1982:92:1103–1109.
20. Lilienfield DE, Gunderson PD, Sprafka JM, Vargas C. Epidemiology of aortic aneurysms: Mortality trends in the United States, 1952 to 1981. *Arteriosclerosis* 1987:7: 637–643.
21. Coady MA, Rizzo JA, Hammond GL, et al. What is the appropriate size criterion for resection of thoracic aortic aneurysms? *J Thorac Cardiovasc Surg* 1997;113: 476–491.
22. Hirose Y, Hamada S, Takayima M, et al. Aortic aneurysms: Growth rates measured with CT. *Radiology* 1992;185: 249–252.

23. Masuda Y, Takanasji K, Takasu J, et al. Expansion rate of thoracic aortic aneurysms and influencing factors. *Chest* 1992;102:461–466.
24. Dapunt OE, Galla JD, Sadeghi AM, et al. The natural history of thoracic aortic aneurysms. *J Thorac Cardiovasc Surg* 1994;107:1006–1009.
25. Hirose Y, Hamada S, Takamiya M. Predicting the growth of aortic aneurysms: A comparison of linear versus exponential models. *Angiology* 1995;46:413–419.
26. Shores J, Berger KR, Murphy EA, Pyeritz RE. Progression of aortic dilataion and the benefit of long-term beta-adrenergic blockade in Marfan's syndrome. *N Engl J Med* 1994; 330:1335–1341.
27. Davies RR, Goldstein LJ, Coady MA, et al. Yearly rupture or dissection rates for thoracic aortic aneurysms: Simple prediction based on size. *Ann Thorac Surg* 2002;73:17–27.
28. Svensson LG, Crawford ES, Hess KR, et al. Composite valve graft replacement of the proximal aorta: Comparison of techniques in 348 patients. *Ann Thorac Surg* 1992;54:427–437.
29. Absi TS, Sundt TM 3rd, Tung WS, et al. Altered patterns of gene expression distinguishing ascending aortic aneurysms from abdominal aortic aneurysms: Complementary DNA expression profiling in the molecular characterization of aortic disease. *J Thorac Cardiovasc Surg* 2003;126:344–357.
30. Fedak PW, de Sa MP, Verma S, et al. Vascular matrix remodeling in patients with bicuspid aortic valve malformations: Implications for aortic dilatation. *J Thorac Cardiovasc Surg* 2003;126:797–806.
31. Boyum J, Fellinger EK, Schmoker JD, et al. Matrix metalloproteinase activity in thoracic aortic aneurysms associated with bicuspid and tricuspid aortic valves. *J Thorac Cardiovasc Surg* 2004;127:686–691.
32. Franklin IJ, Harley SL, Greenhalgh RM, Powell JT. Uptake of tetracycline by aortic aneurysm wall and its effect on inflammation and proteolysis. *Br J Surg* 1999;86: 711–775.
33. Thompson RW, Baxter BT. MMP inhibition in abdominal aortic aneurysms: Rationale for a prospective randomized clinical trial. *Ann NY Acad Sci* 1999;878:159–178.
34. Baxter BT, Pearce WH, Waltke EA, et al. Prolonged administration of doxycycline in patients with small asymptomatic abdominal aortic aneurysms: Report of a prospective (phase II) multicenter study. *J Vasc Surg* 2002;36:1–12.
35. Coady MA, Rizzo JA, Hammond GL, et al. Surgical intervention criteria for thoracic aortic aneurysms: A study of growth rates and complications. *Ann Thorac Surg* 1999;67:1922–1926.
36. Elefteriades JA. Natural history of thoracic aortic aneurysms: Indications for surgery and surgical versus nonsurgical risks. *Ann Thorac Surg* 2002;74:S1877–1880.
37. Hilgenberg AD, Mora BN. Composite aortic root replacement with a bovine pericardial valve conduit. *Ann Thorac Surg* 2003;75(4):1338–1339.
38. Cabrol C, Pavie A, Gandjbakhch I, et al. Complete replacement of the ascending aorta with reimplantation of the coronary arteries: New surgical approach. *J Thorac Cardiovasc Surg* 1981;81:309–315.
39. Svensson LG. Approach to the insertion of composite valve graft. *Ann Thorac Surg* 1992;54:376–378.
40. Dossche KM, Schepens MA, et al. A 23-year experience with composite valve graft replacement of the aortic root. *Ann Thorac Surg* 1999;67:1070–1077.
41. Gott VL, Cameron DE, Alejo DE, et al. Aortic root replacement in 271 Marfan patients: A 24-year experience. *Ann Thorac Surg* 2002;73:438–443.
42. Lai DT, Miller DC, Mitchell RS, et al. Acute type A aortic dissection complicated by aortic regurgitation: Composite valve graft versus separate valve graft versus conservative valve repair. *J Thorac Cardiovasc Surg* 2003;126:1978–1986.
43. Niederhauser U, Kunzli A, Genoni M, et al. Composite graft replacement of the aortic root: Long-term results, incidence of reoperations. *Thorac Cardiovasc Surg* 1999; 47(5):317–321.
44. Ehrlich MP, Ergin MA, McCullough JN, et al. Favorable outcome after composite valve-graft replacement in patients older than 65 years. *Ann Thorac Surg* 2001;71: 1454–1459.
45. Fedak PW, Verma S, David TE, et al. Clinical and pathophysiological implications of a bicuspid aortic valve. *Circulation* 2002;106:900–904.
46. Borger MA, Preston M, Ivanov J, et al. Should the ascending aorta be replaced more frequently in patients with bicuspid aortic valve disease? *J Thorac Cardiovasc Surg* 2004;128:677–683.
47. Yun KL, Miller DC, Fann JI, et al. Composite valve graft versus separate aortic valve and ascending aortic replacement: Is there still a role for the separate procedure? *Circulation* 1997;96:II-368–375.
48. McCready RA, Pluth JR. Surgical treatment of ascending aortic aneurysms associated with aortic valve insufficiency. *Ann Thorac Surg* 1979;28:307–316.
49. Karck M, Laas J, Heinemann M, Borst HG. Long-term follow-up after separate replacement of the aortic valve and ascending aorta. *Herz* 1992;17:394–397.
50. Houel R, Soustelle C, Kirsch M, et al. Long-term results of the Bentall operation versus separate replacement of the ascending aorta and aortic valve. *J Heart Valve Dis* 2002;11: 485–491.
51. Bach DS, Kon ND, Dumesnil JG, et al. Eight-year results after aortic valve replacement with the Freestyle stentless bioprosthesis. *J Thorac Cardiovasc Surg* 2004;127:1657–1663.
52. McGiffin DC, Galbraith AJ, O'Brien MF, et al. An analysis of valve re-replacement after aortic valve replacement with biologic devices. *J Thorac Cardiovasc Surg* 1997;113:311–318.
53. McGiffin DC, Galbraith AJ, McLachlan GJ, et al. Aortic valve infection: Risk factors for death and recurrent endocarditis after aortic valve replacement. *J Thorac Cardiovasc Surg* 1992;104:511–520.
54. Grinda JM, Mainardi JL, D'Attellis N, et al. Cryopreserved aortic viable homograft for active aortic endocarditis. *Ann Thorac Surg* 2005;79:767–771.
55. Lytle BW, Sabik JF, Blackstone EH, et al. Reoperative cryopreserved root and ascending aorta replacement for acute aortic prosthetic valve endocarditis. *Ann Thorac Surg* 2002;74:S1754–1757.
56. Oury JH, Hiro SP, Maxwell JM, et al. The Ross Procedure: Current registry results. *Ann Thorac Surg* 1998;66(Suppl 6):S162–165.
57. Birk E, Sharoni E, Dagan O, et al. The Ross procedure as the surgical treatment of active aortic valve endocarditis. *J Heart Valve Dis* 2004;13:73–77.
58. Sundt TM, Moon MR, Xu H. Reoperation for dilatation of the pulmonary autograft after the Ross procedure. *J Thorac Cardiovasc Surg* 2001;122:1249–1252.

59. De Sa M, Moshkovitz Y, Butany J, David TE. Histologic abnormalities of the ascending aorta and pulmonary trunk in patients with bicuspid aortic valve disease: Clinical relevance to the Ross procedure. *J Thorac Cardiovasc* Surg 1999;118:588–594.
60. David TE, Omran A, Ivanov J, et al. Dilation of the pulmonary autograft after the Ross procedure. *J Thorac Cardiovasc* Surg 2000;119:210–220.
61. Ikonomidis JS, Miller DC. Stentless bioprosthetic aortic valve replacement after valve-sparing aortic root replacement. *J Thorac Cardiovasc Surg* 2002;124:848–851.
62. Leyh RG, Fischer S, Kallenbach K, et al. High failure rate after valve-sparing aortic root replacement using the "remodeling technique" in acute type A aortic dissection. *Circulation* 2002;106:I229–233.
63. Demers P, Liang D, Miller DC. Images in cardiovascular medicine:Simultaneous "Tirone David-V" valve-sparing aortic root replacement and radical mitral valve repair for the Marfan syndrome with Barlow syndrome. *Circulation* 2003;108(16):116–117.
64. Miller DC. Valve-sparing aortic root replacement in patients with the Marfan syndrome. *J Thorac Cardiovasc Surg* 2003;125:773–778.
65. Demers P, Miller DC. Simple modification of "T. David-V" valve-sparing aortic root replacement to create graft pseudosinuses. *Ann Thorac Surg* 2004;78:1479–1481.
66. Zehr KJ, Thubrikar MJ, Gong GG, et al. Clinical introduction of a novel prosthesis for valve-preserving aortic root reconstruction for annuloaortic ectasia. *J Thorac Cardiovasc Surg* 2000;120(4):692–698.
67. De Oliveira NC, David TE, Ivanov J, et al. Results of surgery for aortic root aneurysm in patients with Marfan syndrome. *J Thorac Cardiovasc Surg* 2003;125(4): 789–796.
68. Ikonomidis JS, Bradley SM, Crawford FA Jr. Valve-sparing aortic root replacement: Experience at MUSC. *J SC Med Assoc* 2004;100:274–277.
69. Bethea BT, Fitton TP, Alejo DE, et al. Results of aortic valve-sparing operations: Experience with remodeling and reimplantation procedures in 65 patients. *Ann Thorac Surg* 2004;78:767–772.
70. Gelsomino S, Frassani R, Morocutti G, et al. A short-term experience with the Tirone David I valve sparing operation for the treatment of aneurysms of the ascending aorta and aortic root. *J Cardiovasc Surg* 2003;11(3): 189–194.
71. Kallenbach K, Hagl C, Walles T, et al. Results of valve-sparing aortic root reconstruction in 158 consecutive patients. *Ann Thorac Surg* 2002;74(6):2026–2032.
72. Aybek T, Wohleke T, Simon A, et al. Five-year experience with valve sparing surgery for aortic root aneurysms. *Thorac Cardiovasc Surg* 2002;50(1):35–39.
73. Aicher D, Langer F, Kissinger A, et al. Valve-sparing aortic root replacement in bicuspid aortic valves: A reasonable option? *J Thorac Cardiovasc Surg* 2004;128:662–668.
74. Kallenbach K, Leyh RG, Salcher R, et al. Acute aortic dissection versus aortic root aneurysm: Comparison of indications for valve sparing aortic root reconstruction. *Eur J Cardiothorac Surg* 2004;25:663–670.
75. Erasmi AW, Stierle U, Bechtel JF, et al. Up to 7 years' experience with valve-sparing aortic root remodeling/reimplantation for acute type A dissection. *Ann Thorac Surg* 2003;76:99–104.
76. Karck M, Kallenbach K, Hagl C, et al. Aortic root surgery in Marfan syndrome: Comparison of aortic valve-sparing reimplantation versus composite grafting. *J Thorac Cardiovasc Surg* 2004;127: 391–398.

CHAPTER

32 MITRAL VALVE DISEASE

John R. Doty, Tomasz Timek

INTRODUCTION

Historical overview

Surgical treatment of mitral valve disease has been investigated for over a century, beginning with Brunton's initial observations about the potential for operative relief of mitral stenosis in 1902.[1] In 1922, Cutler and Levine[2] were the first to resect a portion of a stenotic mitral valve successfully, and mitral commissurotomy was introduced by Souttar in 1925.[3] However, it was not until the work of Harken and Bailey with closed mitral commissurotomy in the late 1940s that a more predictable operation became available.[4,5]

KEY CONCEPTS

- Epidemiology
  - Mitral valve stenosis usually results from rheumatic heart disease; females are affected more often than males, with a 2:1 to 3:1 ratio. Mitral insufficiency has many causes but most commonly results from myxomatous degeneration.
- Pathophysiology
  - Rheumatic mitral disease is characterized by thickened attenuated valve leaflets, often with shortened chordae and annular calcification, resulting in a narrowed valvular orifice or incomplete leaflet coaptation as a result of restriction. Myxomatous disease is characterized by redundant leaflet tissue and elongated chordae, leading to valvular prolapse and insufficiency. Idiopathic or ischemic dilated cardiomyopathy often leads to mitral annular dilatation, insufficient leaflet coaptation, papillary muscle dysfunction, and central mitral insufficiency.
- Clinical features
  - Patients with mitral insufficiency or stenosis usually have an initial extended asymptomatic period. Signs and symptoms common to both entities include congestive heart failure (e.g., dyspnea, orthopnea, easy fatigability), atrial fibrillation, hemoptysis, and thromboembolism (more common with stenosis). Cardiac auscultation reveals a presystolic murmur and an apical diastolic rumble with mitral stenosis. With mitral insufficiency, multiple systolic preejection "clicks" from mitral prolapse and a holosystolic murmur radiating to the left axilla can be heard.
- Diagnostics
  - Chest radiography reveals left atrial enlargement and pulmonary vascular congestion (Kerley B lines) in mitral stenosis and insufficiency. Electrocardiography may reveal atrial fibrillation and criteria for right ventricular hypertrophy (e.g., right axis deviation, large R waves in V_1). Transesophageal echocardiography (TEE) provides excellent visualization of the mitral valve. Thickened, restricted leaflets typically are noted with rheumatic mitral stenosis, the severity and direction of regurgitant jet, and pulmonary vein flow reversal in mitral insufficiency seen on Doppler echocardiography. Mean and maximal transvalvular gradients and mean mitral valve area are assessed on TEE, as well as ruptured chordae, left atrial size, left atrial thrombus, and left ventricular segmental wall motion.
- Treatment
  - Rheumatic mitral disease usually is best treated with mitral valve replacement; bioprosthetic valves are used in the elderly and patients who cannot or do not desire long-term anticoagulation, and mechanical prostheses are used in younger patients and/or

patients with chronic atrial fibrillation who already require anticoagulation. The treatment for significant mitral insufficiency is guided by the etiology; however, mitral repair generally is favored over replacement because it preserves the subvalvular apparatus and eliminates the need for long-term anticoagulation.

- Outcomes
  - Hospital mortality for isolated mitral valve replacement and repair in the United States is 6 percent and 1 to 2 percent, respectively. Concomitant coronary artery bypass grafting increases mortality rates to 10 percent and 7 percent, respectively. Risk factors for operative and early postoperative mortality include stroke, infection, hemorrhage, organ failure, advanced age and New York Heart Association functional class, concomitant coronary artery disease, and respiratory insufficiency. Long-term survival after mitral valve repair generally is more favorable than is the case with mitral valve replacement.

The advent of cardiopulmonary bypass in 1953 permitted direct visualization of the mitral valve, and a number of operations were developed to repair mitral insufficiency. Starr and Edwards[6] performed the first mitral valve replacement in 1961, and that quickly became the treatment of choice for all types of mitral valve disease that were not amenable to open commissurotomy.

Since the early days of mitral valve surgery, some surgeons have attempted to repair and preserve the mitral valve.[7] Those investigators continued the pioneering efforts of Lillehei[8] in an ever stronger effort to repair rather than replace the mitral valve. Kay, Reed, Wooler, and others continued to explore techniques for repairing insufficient valves during that period.[9–11] In the early 1970s, Carpentier introduced a new classification system for mitral insufficiency and described operations for correcting leaflet abnormalities as well as annuloplasty techniques.[12] Duran, Cosgrove, and others have built on those repair techniques with the use of reduction ring annuloplasty.[13,14]

Anatomic considerations

The mitral valve has two leaflets and is located at the junction of the left atrium and the left ventricle. The anterior leaflet is larger, is sail-like, and traverses approximately one-third of the annular circumference. The height of the anterior leaflet often is used clinically to size mitral valve prostheses. The posterior leaflet is smaller, is more rectangular, and typically has three scallops, denoted P1, P2, and P3. The posterior leaflet traverses about two-thirds of the annular circumference. The free edge of the leaflets is called the bare or membranous zone, with the remainder of the leaflets being termed the rough zone. The leaflets are separated by the anterolateral and posteromedial commissures (Fig. 32-1). Nutrients for leaflet tissue are supplied by annular and ascending chordal vessels. The leaflets have long been thought to be passive, inert structures that are at the hemodynamic mercy of the ebb and flow of ventricular contraction, but recent data refute that view. Leaflet tissue is richly innervated, has intrinsic contractile properties, has a complex heterogeneous ultrastructure, and may be important in modulating timely and efficient valve closure.[15,16]

The mitral annulus is a poorly defined structure without a clear "ring" configuration that anchors the base of the leaflets. It has two major fibrous components that are termed the trigones. The right fibrous trigone is part of

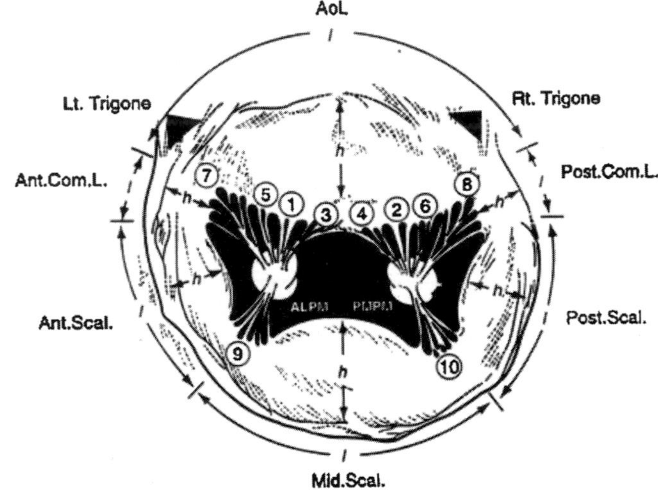

Figure 32-1 Mitral valve and subvalvular apparatus, showing anterolateral papillary muscle (ALPM), posteromedial papillary muscle (PMPM), aortic leaflet (AoL), anterior commissural leaflet (Ant.Com.L.), posterior commissural leaflet (Post.Com.L.), anterior scallop (Ant.Scal.), middle scallop (Mid.Scal.), height of leaflet (h), length of attachment of leaflet (l), left posterior scallop (Post.Scal.), right fibrous trigone (Rt.Trigone), left fibrous trigone (Lt.Trigone), anterior main chorda (1), posterior main chorda (2), anterior paramedial chorda (3), posterior paramedial chorda (4), anterior paracommissural chorda (5), posterior paracommissural chorda (6), anterior commissural chorda (7), posterior commissural chorda (8), anterior cleft chorda (9), and posterior cleft chorda (10). (Reproduced with permission from Sakai T, Okita Y, Ueda Y, et al. Distance between mitral annulus and papillary muscles: Anatomic study in normal human hearts. *J Thorac Cardiovasc Surg* 1999;118:636.)

the central fibrous body of the heart, being in continuity with the aortic valve, the tricuspid valve, and the membranous septum. The portion of the annulus that anchors the anterior mitral leaflet is in direct continuity with portions of the left and noncoronary aortic valve leaflets. The intertrigonal distance defines the fibrous, or anterior, portion of the mitral annulus and is an important clinical marker for valve and annuloplasty sizing because the fibrous annulus is thought to remain unchanged across the spectrum of mitral disease. However, this surgical dogma is being challenged in ischemic and functional mitral regurgitation, where the aortomitral continuity indeed may remodel.[17–19] The posterior, or lateral, annulus is mostly muscular and confirms most of the dynamic shape and area change of the mitral opening during the cardiac cycle. The normal mitral valve area ranges between 4 and 6 cm^2, and the normal annular diameter ranges between 5 and 11 cm and maintains a 3:4 ratio of the anterior-posterior distance to the commissure-commissure distance. The annulus increases in size during early diastole and decreases rapidly during late diastole and early systole, with most of size reduction occurring before ventricular contraction.[20] The annulus is saddle-shaped, with the highest points located anteriorly and posteriorly and the lowest points located at the commissures. The three-dimensional (3-D) structure of the annulus may be important for proper leaflet stress distribution and effective valve closure.[21]

Two major papillary muscles support the mitral valve. Both papillary muscles provide chordae tendineae to both mitral leaflets. The anterolateral papillary muscle usually has one major head and is larger; the posteromedial papillary muscle is flatter and can have two or more heads. Vascular supply to the anterolateral papillary muscle usually comes from both the left anterior descending and circumflex arteries, whereas the posterolateral papillary muscle often is supplied only by the posterior descending artery. The chordae tendineae are classified into three groups. First-order chordae arise near the tips of the papillary muscles and insert on the leading edge of the leaflets. The first-order chordae prevent prolapse of the leaflet tips. Second-order chordae also arise from the tips of the papillary muscles but insert farther back on the leaflet, either on the rough zone or at the junction between the rough zone and the clear zone. The second-order chordae are larger and thicker and serve to stabilize the valve, maintain valvular-ventricular continuity, and aid ventricular systolic performance. Third-order chordae arise from ventricular wall trabeculations and insert near the annulus. The chordae also serve as scaffolding for nutrient vessels to supply leaflet tissue, and their ultrastructural composition has been found to be related to their function.[22]

The mitral valve is surrounded by numerous important structures that must be considered during surgery. The circumflex artery and the coronary sinus lie near the mitral annulus in the posterior atrioventricular groove. As was mentioned previously, the aortic valve is located near the right fibrous trigone and the anterior leaflet. The bundle of His is also near the right fibrous trigone.

PATHOPHYSIOLOGY

Mitral stenosis

Mitral valve stenosis is typically a result of rheumatic fever. Although the incidence has declined in the United States, this etiology remains a significant problem around the world. Rheumatic heart disease is the result of antigen cross-reactivity from group A beta-hemolytic *Streptococcus* and is a pancarditis, affecting valve leaflets, endocardium, and myocardium to varying degrees. Mitral valve involvement is most common, followed by combined mitral and aortic involvement. The classic findings of rheumatic mitral valve disease are commissural fusion, chordal fusion and shortening, and leaflet fibrosis and retraction (Fig. 32-2). Calcification can be quite severe, particularly in older patients. Other, less common causes of mitral stenosis include severe annular and leaflet calcification (see below), congenital deformities, carcinoid syndrome, neoplasm, and atrial thrombus.

Mitral stenosis results in an elevated transvalvular gradient during diastole between the left atrium and the left ventricle. A mean valve area less than 1.0 cm^2 and a mean transvalvular gradient more than 10 mmHg are considered

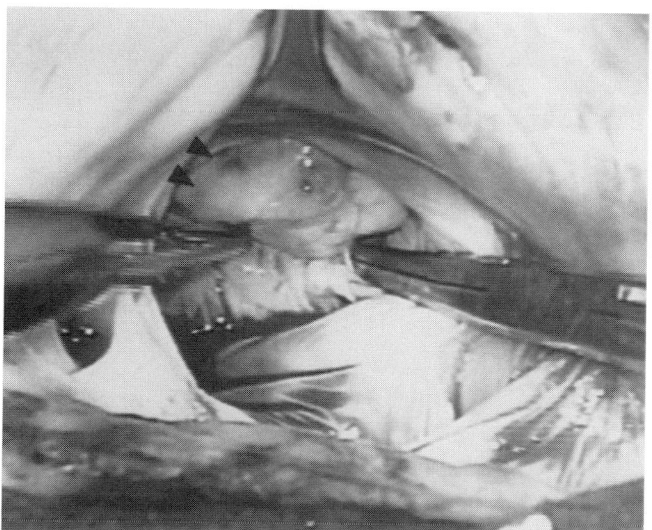

Figure 32-2 Intraoperative photograph of mitral stenosis as a result of rheumatic heart disease. The mitral leaflets are markedly restricted. The arrowheads point to the anterior leaflet near the anterolateral commissure. (Reproduced with permission from Fann JI, Ingels NB, Miller DC. Pathophysiology of mitral valve disease. In: L. Henry Edmunds, L. H. Cohn (eds). *Cardiac Surgery in the Adult*, 2d ed. New York: McGraw-Hill; 2003:901–931.)

severe mitral stenosis. The gradient value may rise considerably with exertion concurrent with the onset of symptoms that patients may not experience at rest. With chronic mitral stenosis, the patient will develop increasing left atrial pressure and left atrial dilatation. The dilated atrium becomes prone to fibrillation and the development of intraarterial thrombus from stagnant flow within the enlarged chamber. Elevated left atrial pressures eventually are reflected to the right heart, resulting in increased pulmonary vascular resistance and pulmonary hypertension.

Mitral insufficiency

A wide range of diseases can result in mitral valve insufficiency; they generally are categorized into the four broad groups of rheumatic, degenerative, infectious, and ischemic causes. Degenerative causes are the most common, followed by rheumatic and ischemic and finally infectious. Other, less common disorders include congenital deformities, endocardial lesions, cardiomyopathies, and collagen vascular diseases.

Carpentier classified mitral insufficiency into three pathoanatomic types according to motion of the leaflets and chordae (Fig. 32-3). Type I mitral insufficiency describes normal leaflet and chordal function; this group includes insufficiency from isolated annular dilatation and insufficiency from leaflet perforation from endocarditis, dilated cardiomyopathy, and ischemic heart disease complicated by ischemic mitral insufficiency. Type II insufficiency consists of leaflet prolapse or excessive leaflet motion; this group includes ischemic papillary muscle rupture as well as a "floppy" mitral valve that is associated with chordal elongation or rupture. Type III mitral insufficiency encompasses leaflet restriction; this group includes rheumatic valvular disease and endocardial fibrosis. Type III mitral insufficiency is further subdivided into a and b, based on leaflet restriction during diastole (type IIIa) or systole (type IIIb). Type IIIb insufficiency is observed with ischemic mitral insufficiency (with or without annular dilatation) and dilated cardiomyopathy (with annular dilatation).

Degenerative mitral insufficiency

Degenerative mitral valve disease is the leading cause of mitral insufficiency in the United States. Also known as myxomatous degeneration, this process results in a wide range of pathoanatomic conditions, including floppy mitral valve, mitral valve prolapse, and severe mitral regurgitation. Mitral valve prolapse is most common in young females and can have a familial component; the more severe forms of insufficiency are more common in males.

In myxomatous disease, the mitral leaflets become thickened and opaque, and the degenerative process may extend down the chordae and out onto the annulus. A minority of patients with mitral valve prolapse actually progress to symptomatic mitral insufficiency; those patients can be placed in three categories: isolated chordal rupture, isolated annular dilatation, and combined chordal rupture and annular dilatation (the most common). Chordal rupture can result in acute mitral insufficiency and should be suspected in patients with no previous clinical history of coronary artery disease or acute myocardial infarction.

Rheumatic mitral insufficiency

Most commonly, rheumatic heart disease results in isolated mitral stenosis or combined stenosis and insufficiency

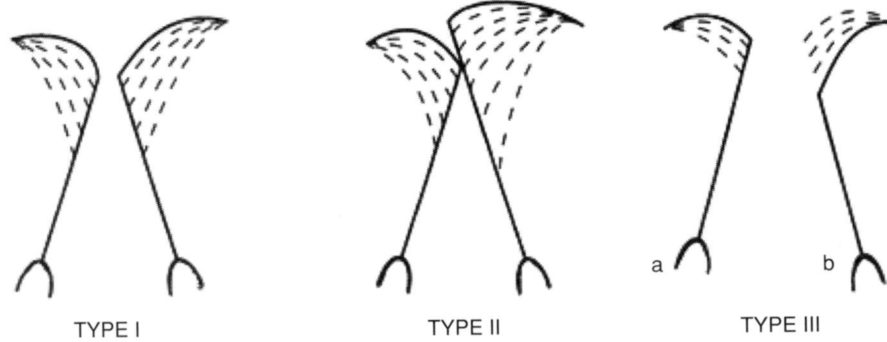

Figure 32-3 Carpentier's functional classification of the types of leaflet and chordal motion associated with mitral regurgitation. In type I, the leaflet motion is normal. Type II mitral regurgitation is due to leaflet prolapse or excessive motion. Type III (restricted leaflet motion) is subdivided into restriction during diastole (a) and systole (b). Type IIIb typically is seen in patients with ischemic mitral regurgitation. The course of the leaflets during the cardiac cycle is represented by the dashed lines. (Modified with permission from Carpentier A. Cardiac valve surgery: The "French correction." *J Thorac Cardiovasc Surg* 1983;86:323.)

resulting from fusion and fixation of the leaflets. Occasionally, a patient will develop isolated rheumatic mitral insufficiency, which differs in that there is no commissural fusion or involvement of the chordae tendineae. The leaflets, however, show the typical thickening and fibrosis of rheumatic heart disease.

Endocarditis

The mitral valve can be involved by bacterial or fungal infective processes and can present in either an acute or a chronic form. *Streptococcus* and *Staphylococcus* are the most common organisms and can cause leaflet perforation, vegetations, chordal rupture, and annular abscesses. These patients are at risk for systemic embolization of vegetations with the subsequent development of mycotic aneurysms and stroke.

Ischemic mitral insufficiency

Ischemic mitral insufficiency is a complex process in which several factors combine to result in mitral regurgitation. It is most easily regarded as two separate entities according to the time of presentation: acute and chronic.

Acute ischemic mitral insufficiency is caused by papillary muscle dysfunction. Ischemia to the posteromedial papillary muscle and the underlying ventricular wall is more likely to result in insufficiency than in left anterior descending artery (LAD)-based anterior myocardial infarctions.[23] Patients with ischemic papillary muscle dysfunction demonstrate varying amounts of mitral insufficiency that generally is related to the overall area of left ventricular (LV) akinesia or dyskinesia around the affected papillary muscle. Experimental studies have shown that isolated ischemia of papillary muscles does not lead to significant mitral insufficiency,[24] and papillary muscle dysfunction actually may decrease the degree of insufficiency during acute posterolateral ischemia.[25] Acute infarction and rupture of a papillary muscle is rare but results in severe mitral insufficiency and heart failure. This event typically occurs between 48 h and 7 days after the initial myocardial infarction, and patient survival is very low without surgical intervention.

Chronic ischemic mitral insufficiency is caused by papillary muscle fibrosis, annular dilatation, and ventricular remodeling. Infarction and chronic ischemia result in scarring and elongation of the papillary muscle and, most important, misalignment of the papillary muscle as a result of changes in ventricular geometry. Ventricular remodeling thus leads to changes in leaflet coaptation and mitral insufficiency. In particular, leaflet tethering most often is associated with ischemic mitral insufficiency caused by posterolateral myocardial infarction, whereas normal leaflet motion may be seen with the significant annular dilatation observed in end-stage heart failure. Combined, these two processes typically lead to chronic ischemic mitral insufficiency, which in the current research and clinical paradigm is considered a "ventricular" disease.

CLINICAL FEATURES

Epidemiology

Mitral stenosis usually is derived from rheumatic heart disease, although a definite history of rheumatic fever can be elicited in only 50 to 60 percent of patients. Females are affected more often than males by a 2:1 to 3:1 ratio. Although the onset of rheumatic heart disease usually occurs before the second decade, valvular manifestations become clinically evident 10 to 30 years later in life. Nonrheumatic causes of mitral stenosis include severe mitral annular and/or leaflet calcifications (e.g., chronic hemodialysis patients), congenital mitral malformations, malignant carcinoid syndrome, neoplasm, endocarditis, and prior mitral valve procedures.

Unlike mitral stenosis, mitral insufficiency has many causes. The most common etiology of systolic mitral insufficiency is myxomatous degeneration, more commonly referred to as "flail" leaflet, "floppy" mitral valve, or mitral valve prolapse, which accounts for 30 to 70 percent of cases. Other causes include ischemic heart disease, dilated cardiomyopathy, rheumatic disease, endocarditis, chordal rupture, congenital malformations, and collagen vascular disorders.

Mitral stenosis

A patient with mitral stenosis typically remains asymptomatic for many years. With increasing severity, however, symptoms of pulmonary venous congestion become more apparent, including orthopnea and paroxysmal nocturnal dyspnea. Reduced LV output results in dyspnea on exertion and easy fatigability. Further chronic elevation of left atrial pressure will result in pulmonary hypertension and right ventricular failure characterized by tricuspid regurgitation, ascites, peripheral edema, and hepatic congestion.

Patients with significant mitral stenosis may have acute worsening of their symptoms during episodes of atrial fibrillation, and this further reduces LV filling. Frank hemoptysis is uncommon in these patients and results from either submucosal varices in the pulmonary bed or pulmonary infarction. Acute pulmonary edema presents with frothy pink-colored sputum from alveolar capillary rupture.

Up to 20 percent of patients with mitral stenosis present with systemic thromboembolism, and nearly half of these conditions affect the cerebral circulation. Usually this is due to the development of intraatrial thrombus, most commonly in patients with an enlarged left atrium, atrial fibrillation, or chronic heart failure. Less commonly, embolism results from infective endocarditis.

Physical examination typically reveals a presystolic murmur and an apical diastolic rumble on cardiac auscultation. The patient is often thin and weak ("cardiac cachexia"), and manifestations of pulmonary hypertension can be noted easily by the presence of a right ventricular heave along the left side of the sternum.

Mitral valve replacement for mitral stenosis generally is indicated in patients with symptoms and a mean valve area of 1.0 cm^2 or less. It should be appreciated that symptoms can occur in patients with combined mitral stenosis and insufficiency with a valve area as large as 1.5 cm^2. Other indications for replacement include new-onset atrial fibrillation, pulmonary hypertension, early signs of right ventricular failure, hemoptysis, and non-streptococcal endocarditis. Balloon mitral valvotomy provides a less invasive option for selected patients, with good long-term outcomes, although the creation of mitral insufficiency continues to be a concern.[26] Significant pulmonary hypertension often is associated with mitral stenosis; however, judicious diuretic and pulmonary vasodilator therapies usually can be titrated to avoid acute right ventricular failure. Historically, pulmonary artery hypertension arising from mitral stenosis usually was ameliorated both early and late after mitral valve replacement. The surgical risk for valvular procedures, however, increases significantly in the presence of pulmonary hypertension, and intervention is recommended before the onset of this pathophysiology.[27]

Mitral insufficiency

Patients with chronic mitral insufficiency also have an initial extended asymptomatic period. As with mitral stenosis, the development of dyspnea on exertion, orthopnea, paroxysmal nocturnal dyspnea, and breathlessness denote elevated left atrial pressures. Progressive regurgitant volumes in the left atrium predispose the patient to atrial fibrillation and the eventual development of right-sided heart failure. A patient with acute mitral insufficiency from infective endocarditis or acute papillary muscle rupture can present in septic or cardiogenic shock. Hemoptysis and thromboembolism are less common in mitral insufficiency than they are in mitral stenosis.

Typical findings on physical examination of patients with chronic mitral insufficiency include a normal or enlarged body habitus resulting from a lack of physical activity. Multiple systolic preejection "clicks" from mitral valve prolapse can be heard on cardiac auscultation. Patients who have progressed to actual mitral insufficiency demonstrate a holosystolic murmur that radiates to the left axilla.

Mitral valve repair or replacement for mitral insufficiency is indicated for moderate to severe symptoms (3+ to 4+ mitral insufficiency on echocardiography or cardiac catheterization), the onset of congestive heart failure symptoms, new-onset atrial fibrillation, reduced LV ejection fraction with exercise, LV dilatation (LV end-systolic diameter greater than 40 to 50 mm), endocarditis refractory to antibiotic therapy, and papillary muscle rupture associated with cardiogenic shock. The optimal timing for surgical intervention in asymptomatic patients with significant mitral regurgitations has not been defined. Surgical indications for functional ischemic mitral insufficiency are somewhat controversial. Patients undergoing coronary artery bypass grafting with 3+ to 4+ mitral insufficiency despite optimal medical therapy generally should undergo valve repair. Moderate mitral regurgitation associated with ventricular ischemia is the major source of debate, with current clinical practice favoring valvular intervention at the time of myocardial revascularization.[28] Functional improvement also has been noted in selected patients with ischemic cardiomyopathy undergoing mitral valve reduction annuloplasty, in which an undersized annuloplasty band is used to correct type I insufficiency and compensate for abnormally dilated LV geometry.

DIAGNOSTICS

Chest radiography

Patients with mitral stenosis demonstrate enlargement of the left atrium characterized by straightening of the left mainstem bronchus and a double shadow along the right heart border. Both mitral stenosis and mitral insufficiency can produce pulmonary vascular congestion that is seen on chest radiography as enlarged pulmonary lymphatics known as Kerley B lines.

Electrocardiography

Atrial fibrillation is the most common electrocardiographic finding in patients with either mitral stenosis or mitral insufficiency. Right ventricular hypertrophy and pulmonary hypertension are suggested by right axis deviation and large R waves in lead V_1. Most patients, however, present with a normal electrocardiogram (ECG).

Echocardiography

Transesophageal echocardiography is superior to transthoracic echocardiography for evaluation of the mitral valve. Characteristics of rheumatic mitral stenosis, such as thickening and reduced movement of the leaflets with a "hockey stick" appearance of the valve, are seen easily on two-dimensional echocardiography. Doppler echocardiography should be employed to determine mean and maximal transvalvular gradients as well as mean mitral valve area. In patients with mitral insufficiency, careful attention is paid to the duration, amount, and direction of the regurgitant jet on Doppler echocardiography. Severe mitral insufficiency is characterized by a pansystolic jet, a larger area of regurgitation, and flow that reaches into the pulmonary veins, resulting in transient flow reversal.

For patients with both mitral insufficiency and mitral stenosis, the heart should be evaluated for the presence of ruptured chordae, left atrial size, and the presence of left atrial thrombus. In addition, regional wall motion function of the left ventricle should be noted carefully before surgical intervention.

Cardiac catheterization

Echocardiography is more precise and accurate in delineating the nature of mitral valvular disease, making routine left heart catheterization and ventriculography unnecessary in the majority of patients. Cardiac catheterization may be needed to determine the degree of mitral stenosis, based on the Gorlin formula, if clinical data and echocardiography are discordant. Older patients and patients with a history of coronary artery disease should undergo coronary angiography for evaluation of possible significant coronary artery disease, which can be addressed percutaneously or concomitantly in the operating room.

SURGICAL THERAPY

Selection of bioprosthetic versus mechanical mitral valve prosthesis

Mechanical mitral valve prostheses usually are selected for younger patients, patients with chronic atrial fibrillation requiring long-term anticoagulation, and any patient who wishes to minimize the chances of reoperation. Patients of any age in sinus rhythm who wish to avoid or whose lifestyle or medical condition (e.g., gastrointestinal bleeding) prohibits long-term anticoagulation are considered for a bioprosthetic valve. It must be recognized, however, that bioprosthetic valves are subject to structural valvular deterioration and generally should be avoided in patients younger than 35 to 40 years of age, in whom such valve failure is accelerated. An exception to this is young females who wish to become pregnant and hence must avoid Coumadin during early pregnancy. Bioprosthetic valves generally are selected for patients older than 70 years of age in normal sinus rhythm, since these valves deteriorate more slowly in the elderly and are therefore less likely to require re-replacement. Conversely, bioprosthetic valves usually should be avoided in patients with chronic renal failure and hypercalcemia secondary to hyperparathyroidism because of the possibility of accelerated valve deterioration. In general, patient survival is not affected by the choice of a mechanical prosthesis or a bioprosthesis,[29,30] but the risk of valvular complications changes with time. Valve complications are initially higher with a mechanical prosthesis, with a subsequent cross-over at approximately 7 years to more valvular-related morbidity with bioprostheses (Fig. 32-4)

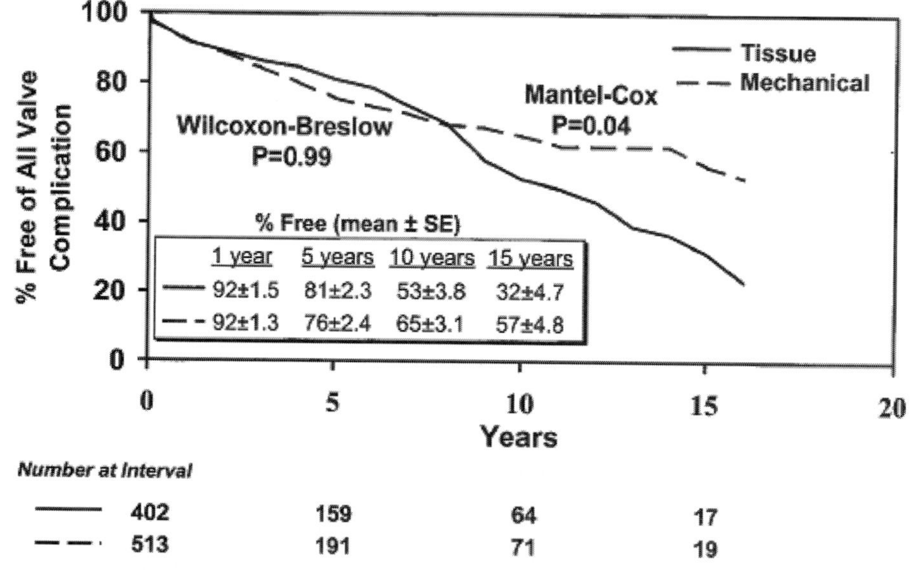

Figure 32-4 Freedom from all valve complications, including valve thrombosis, embolism, hemorrhage, perivalvular leak, structural failure, endocarditis, pannus formation, annular erosion, reoperation, valve-related death, death within 30 days of reoperation, valve failure, and hemolysis, in mitral valve recipients. Two statistical tests are shown; the Wilcoxon-Breslow test gives greater weight to early events, and the Mantel-Cox test weights early and late events equally. (Reproduced with permission from Khan SS, Trento A, DeRobertis M, et al. Twenty-year comparison of tissue and mechanical valve replacement. *J Thorac Cardiovasc Surg* 2001;122(2):257–269.)

dictated by structural degeneration and the need for late reoperation.[30]

Cardiopulmonary bypass and operative exposure

Routine intraoperative monitoring for mitral valve surgery should include arterial and venous pressure lines and a pulmonary artery catheter. Inhaled nitric oxide occasionally is useful in selectively reducing pulmonary vascular resistance in patients with pulmonary hypertension. Median sternotomy with central aortic and bicaval cannulation is the preferred operative approach for most patients. A right thoracotomy incision and femoro-femoral cannulation also can be used and may be advantageous in patients with previous surgery, patent bypass grafts, or previous mediastinitis. Femoro-femoral cardiopulmonary bypass also is employed when one is using minimally invasive, thoracoscopic, or robotic approaches to the mitral valve.

The inferior approach through the left atrium is the most common method of exposure (Fig. 32-5). The left atrium is incised behind the interatrial groove and carried cephalad toward the left atrial appendage and posteriorly behind the inferior vena cava. This approach provides good exposure for almost all operations on the mitral valve.

The superior approach requires mobilization of the superior vena cava and incision through the dome of the left atrium. The incision is extended behind the aorta and the superior vena cava to provide satisfactory visualization.

The transseptal approach requires occlusion of the superior and inferior venae cavae with caval snares to work through the right atrium. First, an oblique incision is made into the right atrium, extending from a point medial to the right atrial appendage toward the interatrial groove. Next, the interatrial septum is incised at the foramen ovale and extended superiorly to meet the right atrial incision. This approach provides excellent exposure of the mitral valve and is particularly useful in the reoperative setting and in patients in whom tricuspid valve surgery also is required. It is important to remember that the right atrial incision often will transect the sinus node artery, interrupting sinus rhythm.

Regardless of the type of atrial incision, a vent should be placed into the left atrium through the right superior pulmonary vein. Bicaval cannulation is advantageous in that it keeps the venous cannulae from obstructing the surgeon's view of the operative field. Handheld retractors

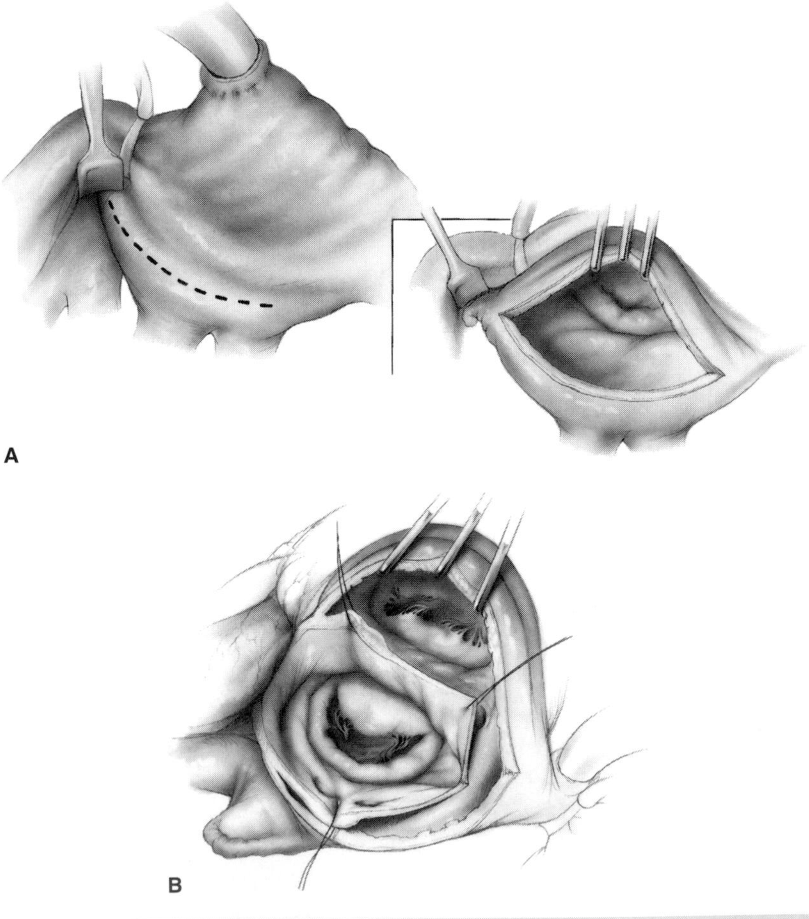

Figure 32-5 Inferior approach to left atrium. (From Doty DB. *Cardiac Surgery: Operative Technique*. St. Louis: Mosby; 1997:261.)

or self-retaining retractors are employed to pull the right ventricle anteriorly and further expose the valve.

Mitral valve replacement

In excising mitral valve tissue in anticipation of valve replacement, the chordae tendineae and papillary muscles should be preserved, if possible, as it has been demonstrated clearly that maintaining the inherent structure of the subvalvular apparatus improves LV performance both early and late after mitral valve replacement. The anterior leaflet is grasped with forceps and incised sharply with a scalpel approximately 2 to 3 mm from the mitral annulus. The anterior leaflet is excised from the mitral annulus, leaving a small rim of leaflet tissue attached to the annulus and preserving all normal chordal attachments. Thickened or elongated chordae should be excised at the level of the papillary muscles.

The posterior leaflet generally should be left in place unless it is grossly thickened, as in severe rheumatic disease, or very redundant, as in severe myxomatous disease. If it is thought that the posterior leaflet will impinge on the prosthetic valve, it should be resected carefully in a manner similar to that used for the anterior leaflet. Caution should be used in dividing chordal attachments to the posterior leaflet, as it is easy to injure the underlying myocardium and disrupt the atrioventricular groove. Several chordal-sparing techniques have been described that preserve normal chordal attachments while debulking diseased leaflet tissue (Fig. 32-6).

Extensive resection or debridement of annular calcium deposits generally should be avoided unless the deposits preclude passing the suture needles through the mitral annulus. Debridement should be carried out cautiously, for extensive removal of calcium can separate the annulus, creating atrioventricular discontinuity. If a large area of ventricular myocardium or atrioventricular groove is left exposed, it should be covered by suturing a patch of pericardium at the edge of the debridement area. Copious irrigation should be employed to flush out any remaining debris to avoid embolization.

The most common method for prosthetic valve insertion is to place interrupted pledgeted mattress sutures around the entire circumference of the mitral annulus (Fig. 32-7). The sutures should be placed accurately through the mitral annulus, taking care to avoid penetrating the atrioventricular groove or the ventricular myocardium. For bileaflet or tilting disk mechanical prostheses, the valve sutures should be placed in an everting fashion (atrium to ventricle) to minimize tissue interference with the valve mechanism. For bioprosthetic valves, a noneverting (ventricle to atrium) suture pattern may be used. It generally is easier to place all the sutures through the annulus first and then place them through the sewing ring of the prosthesis. Once all the sutures are placed, gentle traction is used to slide the prosthetic valve down to the annulus.

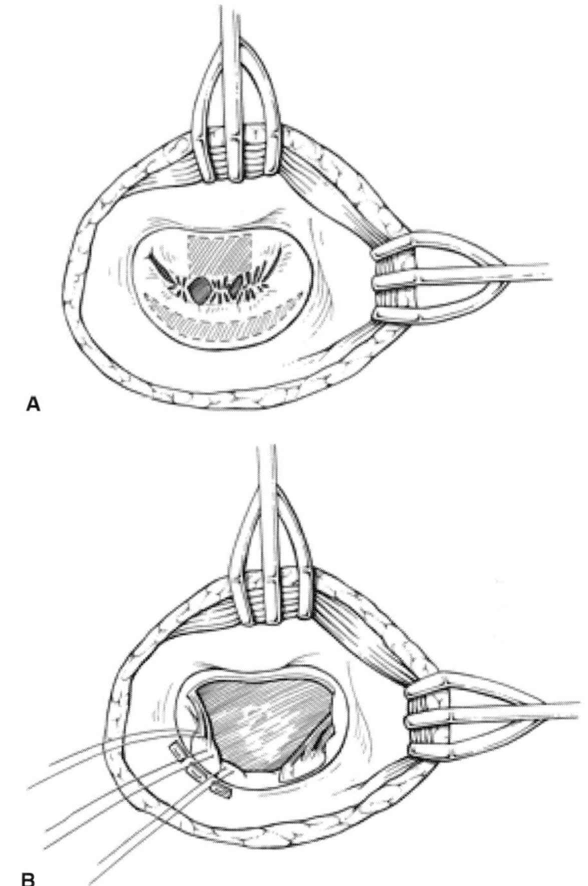

Figure 32-6 Techniques to maintain annular–papillary muscle continuity. A. An ellipse is removed from the posterior leaflet, and a flap is cut from the central portion of the anterior leaflet. The anterior flap is flipped to the posterior annulus and tacked to the caudad edge of the posterior leaflet and the posterior annulus. Sutures anchoring the prosthesis include the annulus and the anterior and posterior leaflet remnants, to which chordae are attached.
B. The anterior leaflet is partially excised, and remnants are "furled" to the annulus by sutures used to insert the prosthesis. (Reproduced with permission from Gudbjartsson T, Aranki S, Cohn LH. Mechanical/bioprosthetic mitral valve replacement. In: L. Henry Edmunds, L. H. Cohn (eds). *Cardiac Surgery in the Adult,* 2d ed. New York: McGraw-Hill; 2003:951–986.)

Care should be taken to avoid pulling up on the annulus and to keep the sutures under gentle tension to prevent loops of suture from being trapped below the prosthetic valve. The sutures then are tied securely to complete the valve insertion.

Mitral valve homografts are used infrequently but are useful for replacing portions of or entire valves that have been destroyed by endocarditis in young patients or females of childbearing age who wish to become pregnant. The papillary muscles of the homograft are

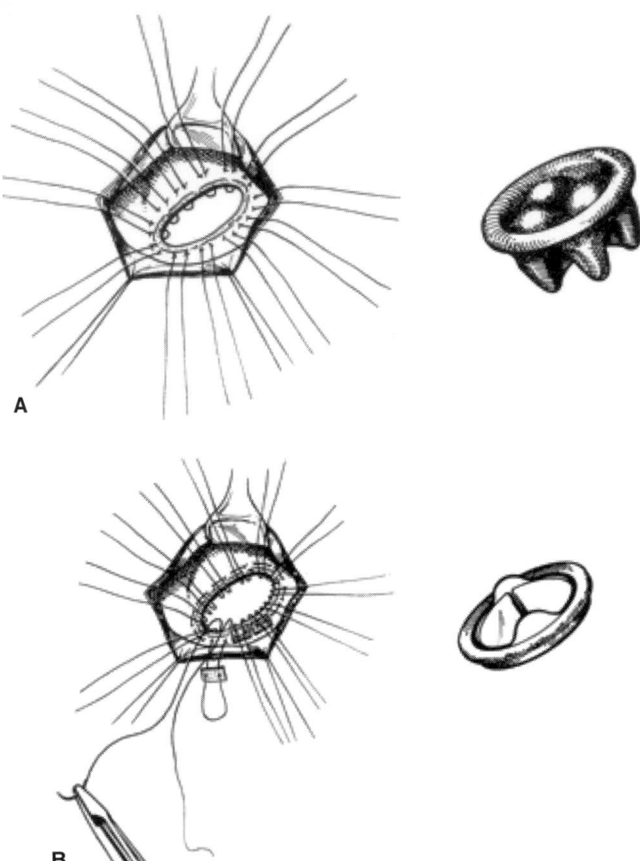

Figure 32-7 Suturing techniques for prosthetic mitral valve implantation. Noneverting (subannular) sutures placed from ventricle to atrium for bioprosthetic valves. Everting (supraannular) sutures placed from atrium to ventricle for bileaflet or tilting-disk valves. (Reproduced with permission from Gudbjartsson T, Aranki S, Cohn LH. Mechanical/bioprosthetic mitral valve replacement. In: L. Henry Edmunds, L. H. Cohn (eds). *Cardiac Surgery in the Adult*, 2d ed. New York: McGraw-Hill; 2003:951–986.)

attached to the native papillary muscles, using multiple fine polypropylene sutures. The homograft annulus then is attached to the native annulus, using a continuous polypropylene suture, and the entire repair is supported with a complete ring annuloplasty. The outcomes of homograft replacement in specialized centers approach those of bioprosthetic valves,[31] but other investigators have reported less satisfactory results. The Achilles' heel of homograft replacement is proper sizing and homograft papillary muscle positioning within the patient's ventricle. A recently introduced bovine pericardium stentless mitral valve[32] holds promise for overcoming those obstacles, but long-term performance data are lacking.

After the prosthetic valve has been seated and checked for adequate leaflet mobility, the left atrial appendage is ligated by suture or stapler to prevent thrombus formation in patients with chronic atrial fibrillation. If desired, intraoperative ablation for atrial fibrillation may be attempted while the atrium is open. The inferior left atrial, superior left atrial, and right atrial incisions are closed with continuous 3-0 polypropylene sutures. If those sutures are used, the transseptal incision is closed with continuous 4-0 polypropylene sutures. Multiple deairing maneuvers are employed before removal of the aortic cross-clamp.

Concomitant cardiac procedures are necessary in many cases of mitral valve replacement. Coronary artery bypass is the most common of these procedures and should be performed before valve replacement, as this minimizes manipulating and possibly injuring the heart (i.e., myocardial or atrioventricular groove rupture) after the rigid mitral prosthetic is in place. Furthermore, it permits cardioplegia to be delivered through the bypass grafts. Tricuspid valve repair or replacement usually is conducted after the performance of mitral valve replacement (often through the transseptal approach), since this portion of the operation can be performed after removal of the aortic cross clamp. In cases of concomitant aortic and mitral valve replacement, most surgeons excise the aortic valve before addressing the mitral valve; the aortic valve then is seated after the mitral valve is in place. Of note, care should be taken to avoid injuring the aortic annulus and aortic-mitral continuity while one is excising the anterior mitral valve leaflet.

Mitral valve repair

After the initiation of cardiopulmonary bypass, cardioplegic arrest, and exposure of the left atrium, the mitral valve is evaluated systematically for suitability for repair. The annulus should be inspected for dilatation, mobility, calcification, and contraction. Both leaflets then are examined for thickening, pliability, coaptation, prolapse, and restriction of motion. Both commissures should be inspected for evidence of fusion. The chordae are evaluated for shortening or elongation as well as thickening and fusion. Finally, the papillary muscles are examined for evidence of rupture or elongation. In considering valve repair, it is useful to recall the Carpentier classification to determine whether there is normal leaflet motion (annular dilatation or leaflet perforation), prolapsed leaflet motion (chordal or papillary muscle rupture or elongation), or restricted leaflet motion (rheumatic disease or ventricular dilatation).

Reduction annuloplasty

When the mitral valve leaflets have normal motion but do not coapt properly as a result of annular dilatation, the mitral annulus can be reduced in size to push the leaflets closer together and provide a greater area of leaflet coaptation. Ring annuloplasty provides a symmetric method to reduce annular size and can be performed as either a complete annuloplasty or a posterior (partial) annuloplasty.

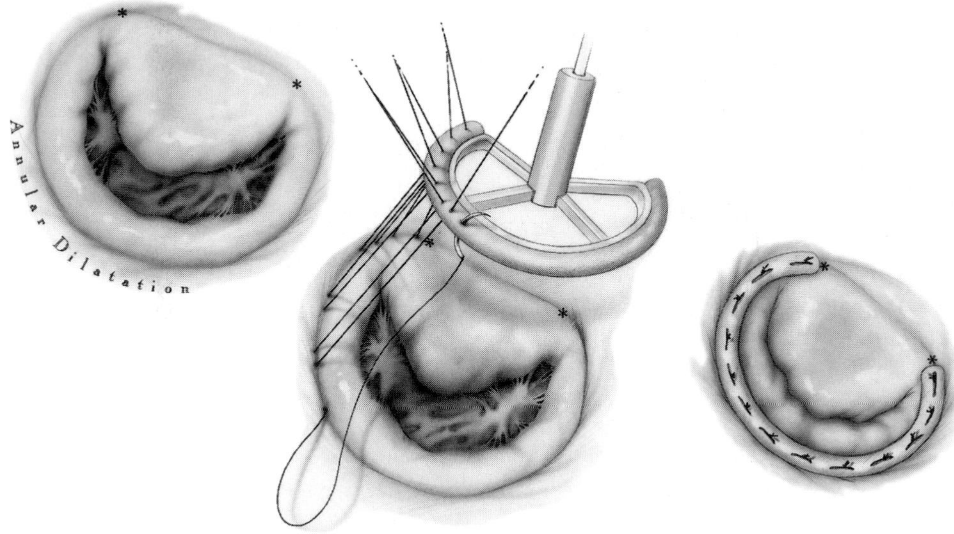

Figure 32-8 Posterior ring annuloplasty. (From Doty DB. *Cardiac Surgery: Operative Technique*. St. Louis: Mosby; 1997:255.)

The mitral annulus is measured according to the size of the anterior leaflet, using the commissures or fibrous trigones as reference points. Interrupted mattress sutures then are placed through the mitral annulus and into the ring prosthesis (Fig. 32-8). As with prosthetic valve replacement, the ring is lowered to the annulus and the sutures are tied to plicate the annulus gently. Mitral annuloplasty is a key component of the reparative armamentarium and is included almost routinely with most repair techniques to reduce annular size and stabilize the repair. At this time, no clear superiority of one ring type, whether rigid, semirigid, flexible, partial, or complete, has been demonstrated clinically in terms of repair durability or LV function. However, custom-made pericardial "annuloplasty strips" have been associated with higher mitral regurgitation (MR) recurrence rates. Regardless of type, annuloplasty prostheses alter normal annular dynamics, restrict motion of the posterior leaflet, and flatten the 3-D shape of the native annulus.[33,34] Ischemic and functional mitral regurgitation represents a particular clinical challenge as the valve is structurally normal yet significant regurgitation is present. Currently, implantation of an undersized annuloplasty ring alone has been the procedure of choice for this vexing clinical entity, yet it is not a panacea, as short-term MR recurrence rates may be as high as 30 percent.[35] Annular septal-lateral reduction, papillary muscle repositioning, device-based alteration of ventricular shape, ventricular plication, and chordal severing are all experimental procedures aimed at addressing the "ventricular" etiology of functional MR.[36–40]

Repair of mitral leaflet perforation

Perforations of the mitral valve leaflets caused by endocarditis should be repaired with autologous tissue if possible. The perforation is debrided carefully to remove all infected and fibrinous material. Very small perforations may be closed primarily with single 5-0 polypropylene sutures. If pledgets are required, they should be constructed of autologous pericardium to avoid placing foreign material in the repair. Larger defects should be reconstructed with a patch of pericardium, using a continuous 4-0 polypropylene suture.

Posterior leaflet excision and repair

When a segment of the posterior leaflet has become elongated and prolapsed, segmental excision and repair can be performed. The prolapsed segment and any chordae that insert only into that segment of the posterior leaflet are resected back to the level of the annulus. Interrupted braided sutures with pledgets are placed horizontally through the annulus at both edges of the defect in the posterior leaflet and tied to reapproximate the annulus. The leaflet edges then are approximated, using a continuous 4-0 polypropylene suture, beginning at the free edge of the leaflet and running back to the annulus. The repair is supported with a posterior annuloplasty ring.

Ruptured chordae tendineae repair

Rupture of chordae that support the anterior leaflet represents a more complex problem than do ruptures of chordae that support the posterior leaflet, as attempts to resect portions of the anterior leaflet may render the valve incompetent as a result of the loss of surface area. In general, surgical correction of anterior leaflet pathology requires mature surgical judgment and is technically complex. Consequently, anterior leaflet prolapse is frequently the "deal breaker" that leads many surgeons to replace rather than repair an incompetent valve.

Chordal transfer from the posterior leaflet can be employed to reconstruct these valves. The ruptured chordae

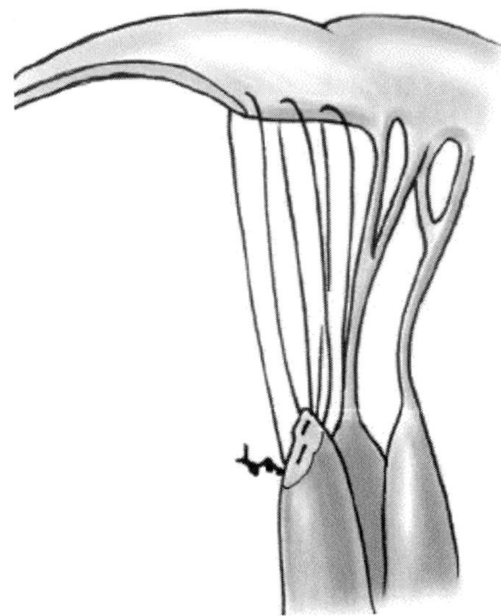

Figure 32-9 Operative technique to replace ruptured chordae tendineae with Gore-Tex sutures. A single suture is passed successively through the papillary muscle and the free margin of the leaflet to create several pairs of artificial chordae. (Reproduced with permission from David TE. Artificial chordae. *Semin Thorac Cardiovasc Surg* 2004;16:163.)

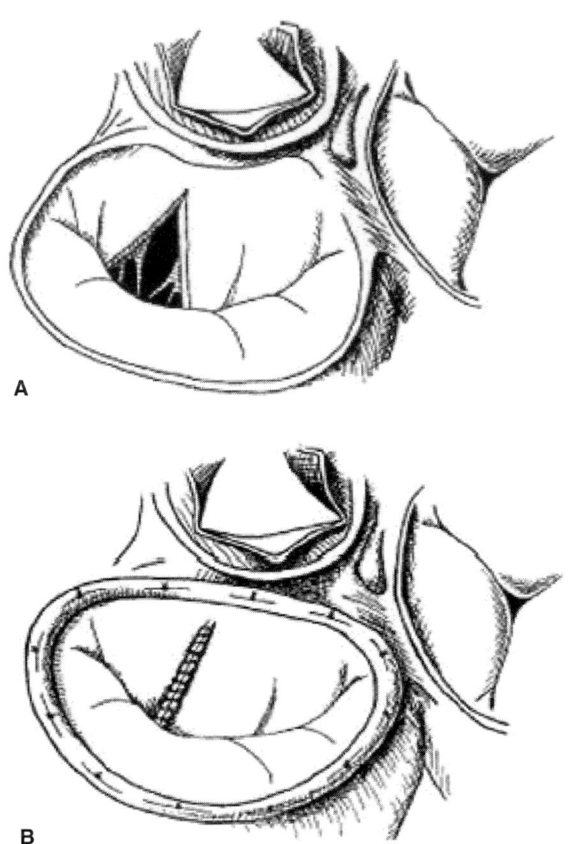

Figure 32-10 Surgical technique for anterior leaflet resection. A. Boundaries of resection of anterior leaflet. B. Completed anterior leaflet resection with ring annuloplasty. (Reprinted with permission from Galloway AC, Grossi EA, Bizekisc LS, et al. Evolving techniques for mitral valve reconstruction. *Ann Surg* 2002;236:291.)

tendineae and a small portion of the unsupported free edge of the anterior leaflet are resected. A segment of the posterior leaflet directly opposite the unsupported area of the anterior leaflet is selected and incised back to the level of the posterior annulus, retaining the chordal attachments. This segment of posterior leaflet then is transposed anteriorly and used to repair the defect in the anterior leaflet, using a continuous 5-0 polypropylene suture. The defect in the posterior leaflet then is reconstructed as previously described for posterior excision. The entire repair is supported with a ring annuloplasty. Alternatively, ruptured chordae can be replaced, using Gore-Tex sutures (Fig. 32-9), with good long-term durability, although considerable experience is needed to judge chordal length properly.[41] Other surgeons report durable and reproducible results with triangular resection of the affected segment of the anterior leaflet (Fig. 32-10), usually as a result of myxomatous disease, and subsequent ring annuloplasty.[42] Leaflet resection also may have the advantage of reducing systolic anterior motion (SAM) and the resulting LV outflow obstruction. Shortening or retraction of the anterior leaflet, a challenging problem seen in rheumatic or radiation valvulitis, can be treated successfully with autologous pericardial patch augmentation of the anterior leaflet.[43]

Sliding valvuloplasty

Certain patients, such as those with Barlow's syndrome or long-standing myxomatous disease, may have excessive posterior leaflet tissue, resulting in a leaflet that is both too long and too wide. These valves may require excision and reduction of the amount of leaflet tissue to achieve a competent repair.

With "sliding" valvuloplasty, the central (P2) segment is resected as with a standard posterior excision (Fig. 32-11). The incision is extended laterally to each side to create wedge-shaped resections along the posterior annulus. The base of the leaflet then is reapproximated to the mitral annulus from either side, and the central area of resection is reapproximated as with a standard posterior excision. The entire repair is supported with a posterior ring annuloplasty.

OUTCOMES AND PROGNOSIS

Mitral valve replacement

According to the Society of Thoracic Surgeons (STS) database in 2002, hospital mortality after isolated mitral valve replacement in the United States is approximately 6 percent. If concomitant coronary artery bypass grafting

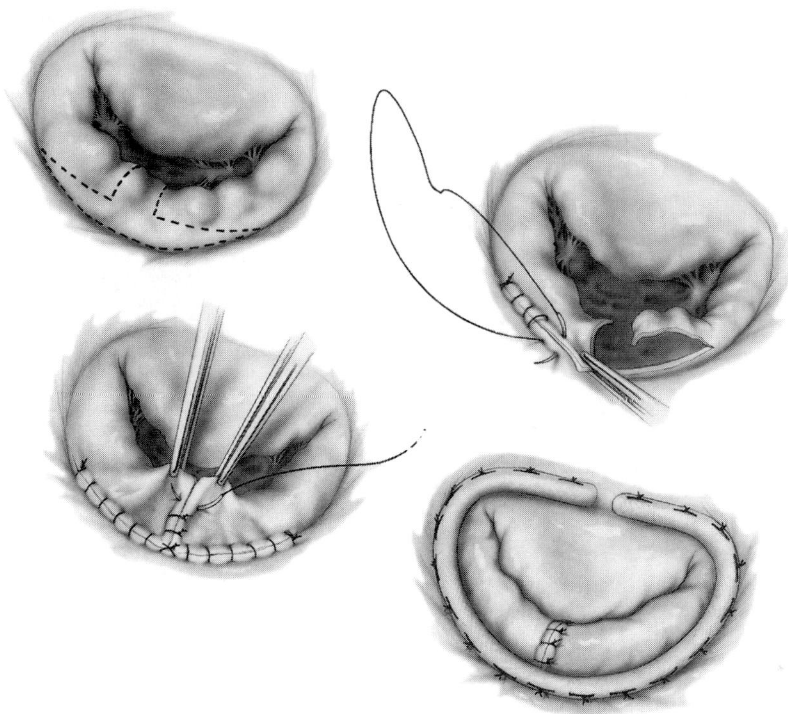

Figure 32-11 Sliding valvuloplasty. (From Doty DB. *Cardiac Surgery: Operative Technique*. St. Louis: Mosby; 1997:259.)

is required, the early mortality rises to 10 percent. Risk factors for early mortality after mitral valve replacement include stroke, infection, hemorrhage, organ failure, and respiratory insufficiency. Older age, advanced New York Heart Association functional class, and concomitant coronary artery disease all are associated with an increased risk for operative mortality.[29,30,44–49]

Long-term survival after mitral valve replacement with either a mechanical or a bioprosthetic valve is approximately 50 percent at 10 years. Determinants of late death include thromboembolism, hemorrhage from anticoagulation, heart failure, and coronary artery disease. Patients with atrial fibrillation are at higher risk for both thromboembolism and anticoagulant-associated hemorrhage.

Other complications after mitral valve replacement include structural deterioration of the bioprosthesis, which occurs in over 50 percent of these valves after 15 years. Endocarditis is uncommon with either mechanical or bioprosthetic valves but can be aggressive and life-threatening. Perivalvular leak is also uncommon.

Mitral valve repair

According to the STS database, hospital mortality after isolated mitral valve repair in the United States in 2002 was between 1 and 2 percent. The addition of coronary artery bypass grafting increases the early mortality to approximately 7 percent. Risk factors for operative mortality include advanced age and repair for ischemic mitral insufficiency.

Long-term outcomes after mitral valve repair have been excellent, with survival rates at 13 to 15 years ranging from 72 to 90 percent. Freedom from reoperation approaches 90 percent in several series at 10 years. Rates of thromboembolism, anticoagulant-related hemorrhage, and endocarditis are very low.[50–53] Mitral valve repair may provide a better outcome in selected patients with ischemic mitral regurgitation, although both valve repair and valve replacement generally are associated with a poor long-term prognosis in this difficult patient population.[54,55]

EVOLVING TECHNOLOGIES

The last decade has witnessed the rapid evolution of new technologies in cardiothoracic surgery, with an emphasis on minimally invasive procedures. Valvular surgery has been at the forefront of this change. The introduction of Heartport technology (Johnson & Johnson Corp, New Brunswick, NJ) in 1994 began the era of minimally invasive cardiac surgery. The technology has been used successfully by selected centers for totally endoscopic mitral valve repair with excellent results and high patient satisfaction.[56,57] However, as a

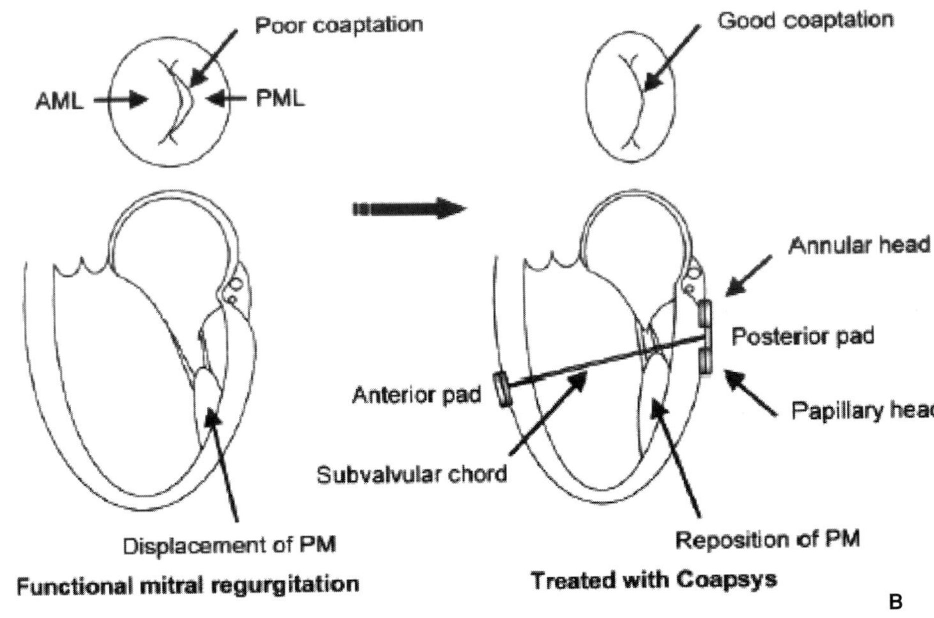

Figure 32-12 Functional mitral regurgitation results from dilatation of the mitral valve annulus or lateral papillary muscle displacement in dysfunctional left ventricles. With the Coapsys device, the mitral leaflets are drawn together by the annular head of the posterior pad to increase valve coaptation, and papillary muscles are repositioned by the papillary head of the posterior pad. AML = anterior mitral leaflet; PM = papillary muscle; PML = posterior mitral leaflet. (Reproduced with permission from Fukamachi K, Inoue M, Popovic ZB, et al. Off-pump mitral valve repair using the Coapsys device: A pilot study in a pacing induced mitral regurgitation model. *Ann Thorac Surg* 2004;77:689.)

result of complications stemming mainly from endovascular aortic occlusion, the initial enthusiasm for this technology has waned. Clinical experience with robotic mitral valve repair in the United States has been encouraging,[58] but a steep learning curve, prolonged operative time, and high costs are still significant hurdles to the widespread use of such advanced techniques. The Coapsys device (Fig. 32-12) designed to address functional MR[37] is a further advancement, permitting off-pump valve repair. The device consists of a transventricular suture with two epicardial pads and is designed to reduce annular size, alter ventricular geometry, and reposition the papillary muscles. Percutaneous valvular interventions represent yet another technological leap. The feasibility of catheter-based Alfieri edge-to-edge, or double-orifice, valve repair with a catheter-delivered clip (Fig. 32-13) used to approximate the central edges of the mitral leaflets has been demonstrated.[59] Successful percutaneous repair of chronic ovine ischemic mitral regurgitation with an endovascularly placed coronary sinus annuloplasty ring also has been reported.[60] Needless to say, these interventions, alone or in combination, may serve to replace traditional reparative techniques of mitral insufficiency in selected patients, but clinical data are lacking at this time.

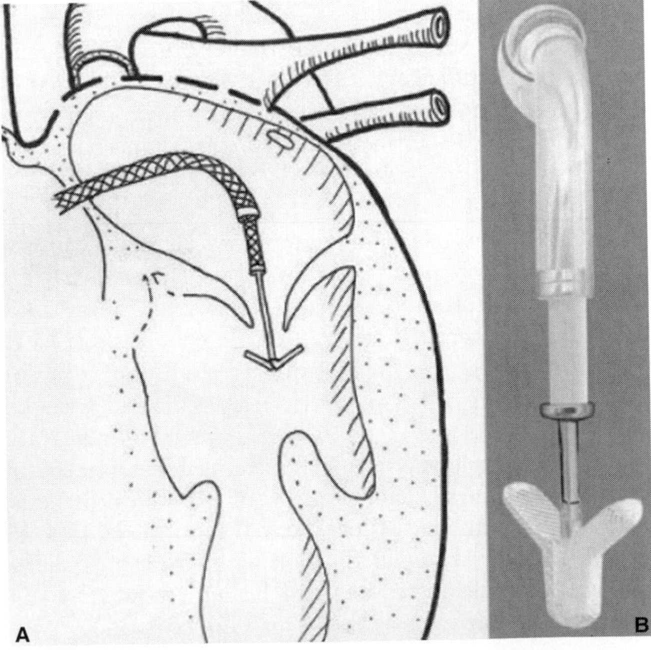

Figure 32-13 A. Schematic of the CVRS guide catheter across the atrial septum. The clip delivery system is positioned through the guide. The clip is in the open position in the left ventricle, ready to be retracted to grasp the mitral leaflets. B. The distal end of the delivery system and the polyester-covered clip shown in the open position. (Reproduced with permission from St. Goar FG, Fann JI, Komtebedde J, et al. *Circulation* 2003;108:1991.)

References

1. Brunton L. Preliminary note on the possibility of treating mitral stenosis by surgical methods. *Lancet* 1902 1:352.
2. Cutler EC, Levine SA. Cardiotomy and valvulotomy for mitral stenosis: Experimental observations and clinical notes concerning an operated case with recovery. *Boston Med Surg J* 1923;188:1023.
3. Souttar H. The surgical treatment of mitral stenosis. *Br Med J* 1925;2:603–606.
4. Harken DE, Ellis LB, Ware PF, Norman LR. The surgical treatment of mitral stenosis: Valvuloplasty. *N Engl J Med* 1948;239:801.
5. Bailey CP. The surgical treatment of mitral stenosis (mitral commissurotomy). *Dis Chest* 1949;15:377.
6. Starr A, Edwards ML. Mitral replacement: Clinical experience with a ball valve prosthesis. *Ann Surg* 1961;154:726.
7. McGoon DC. Repair of mitral insufficiency due to ruptured chordae tendinae. *J Thorac Cardiovasc Surg* 1960;39:357–363.
8. Lillehei CW, DeWall RA. Surgical correction of pure mitral insufficiency by annuloplasty under direct vision. *Lancet* 1957;77:446.
9. Kay JH, Zubiate P, Mendez MA, et al. Mitral valve repair for significant mitral insufficiency. *Am Heart J* 1978;96:253.
10. Reed GE, Tice DA, Clauss RH. Asymmetric exaggerated mitral annuloplasty: Repair of mitral insufficiency with hemodynamic predictability. *J Thorac Cardiovasc Surg* 1965;49:752.
11. Wooler GH, Nixon PG, Grimshaw VA, et al. Experiences with the repair of the mitral valve in mitral incompetence. *Thorax* 1962;17:49.
12. Carpentier A, Deloche A, Dauptain J, et al. A new reconstructive operation for correction of mitral and tricuspid insufficiency. *J Thorac Cardiovasc Surg* 1971;61:1.
13. Duran DG, Pomar JL, Revuelta JM, et al. Conservative operation for mitral insufficiency: Critical analysis supported by postoperative hemodynamic studies in 72 patients. *J Thorac Cardiovasc Surg* 1980;79:326.
14. Cosgrove DM, Stewart WJ. Mitral valvuloplasty. *Curr Probl Cardiol* 1989;14:359.
15. Grand-Allen KJ, Calabro A, Gupta V, et al. Glycosaminoglycans and proteoglycans in normal mitral valve leaflets and chordae: Association with regions of tensile and compressive loading. *Glycobiology* 2004;14:621–633.
16. Marron K, Yacoub MH, Polak JM, et al. Innervation of human atrioventricular and arterial valves. *Circulation* 1996;94:368–375.
17. Tibayan FA, Rodriguez F, Langer F, et al. Annular remodeling in chronic ischemic mitral regurgitation: Ring selection implications. *Ann Thorac Surg* 2003;76:1549–1555.
18. Timek TA, Dagum P, Lai DT, et al. Tachycardia-induced cardiomyopathy in the ovine heart: Mitral annular dynamic three-dimensional geometry. *J Thorac Cardovasc Surg* 2003;125:315–324.
19. Hueb AC, Jatene FB, Moreira LF, et al. Ventricular remodeling and mitral valve modifications in dilated cardiomyopathy: New insights from anatomic study. *J Thorac Cardiovasc Surg* 2002;124:1216–1224.
20. Glasson JR, Komeda M, Daughters GT, et al. Most ovine mitral annular three-dimensional size reduction occurs before ventricular systole and is abolished with ventricular pacing. *Circulation* 1997;96:II-115–122.
21. Salgo IS, Gorman JH, Gorman RC, et al. Effect of annular shape on leaflet curvature in reducing mitral leaflet stress. *Circulation* 2002;106:711–717.
22. Ritchie J, Warnock JN, Yoganathan AP. Structural characterization of the chordae tendineae in native porcine mitral valves. *Ann Thorac Surg* 2005;80:189–197.
23. Timek TA, Lai DT, Tibayan F, et al. Ischemia in three left ventricular regions: Insights into the pathogenesis of acute ischemic mitral regurgitation. *J Thorac and Cardiovasc Surg* 2003;125:559–569.
24. Kaul S, Spotnitz WD, Glasheen WP, Touchstone DA. Mechanism of ischemic mitral regurgitation: An experimental study. *Circulation* 1992;84:2167–2180.
25. Messas E, Guerrero JL, Handschumacher MD, et al. Paradoxical decrease in ischemic mitral regurgitation with papillary muscle dysfunction: Insights from three-dimensional and contrast echocardiography with strain rate measurement. *Circulation* 2001;104:1952–1957.
26. Kang DH, Park SW, Song SJ, et al. Long-term clinical and echocardiographic outcome of percutaneous mitral valvuloplasty: Randomized comparison of Inoue and double balloon techniques. *J Am Coll Cardiol* 2000;35:169–175.
27. Vincens JJ, Temizer D, Post JR, et al. Long-term outcome of cardiac surgery in patients with mitral stenosis and severe pulmonary hypertension. *Circulation* 1995;92(Suppl):II-137–II-142.
28. Lam BK, Gillinow AM, Blackstone EH, et al. Importance of moderate ischemic mitral regurgitation. *Ann Thorac Surg* 2005;79:462–470.
29. Khan SS, Trento A, DeRobertis M, et al. Twenty-year comparison of tissue and mechanical valve replacement. *J Thorac Cardiovasc Surg* 2001;122(2):257–269.
30. Cen YY, Glower DD, Landolfo K, et al. Comparison of survival after mitral valve replacement with biologic and mechanical valves in 1139 patients. *J Thorac Cardiovasc* Surg 2001;122:569–577.
31. Ali M, Iung B, Lansac E, et al. Homograft replacement of the mitral valve: Eight year results. *J Thorac Cardiovasc Surg* 2004;128:529–534.
32. Mohr FW, Lehman S, Falk V, et al. Clinical experience with stentless mitral valve replacement. *Ann Thorac Surg* 2005;79:772–775.
33. Green GR, Dagum P, Glasson JR, et al. Restricted posterior leaflet motion after mitral ring annuloplasty. *Ann Thorac Surg* 1999;68(6):2100–2106.
34. Glasson JR, Green GR, Nistal JF, et al. Mitral annular size and shape in sheep with annuloplasty rings. *J Thorac Cardiovasc Surg* 1999;117(2):302–309.
35. McGee EC, Gillinow AM, Blackstone EH, et al. Recurrent mitral regurgitation after annuloplasty for functional ischemic mitral regurgitation. *J Thorac Cardiovasc Surg* 2004;128:916–924.
36. Timek TA, Lai DT, Tibayan F, et al. Septal-lateral annular cinching ("SLAC") abolishes acute ischemic mitral regurgitation. *J Thorac Cardiovasc Surg* 2002;123:881–888.
37. Fukamachi K, Inoue M, Popovic ZB, et al. Off-pump mitral valve repair using the Coapsys device: A pilot study in a pacing induced mitral regurgitation model. *Ann Thorac Surg* 2004;77:688–693.
38. Kron IL, Green GR, Cope JT. Surgical relocation of the posterior papillary muscle in chronic ischemic mitral regurgitation. *Ann Thorac Surg* 2002;74:600–601.

39. Messas E, Pouzet B, Touchot B, et al. Efficacy of chordal cutting to relieve chronic persistent ischemic mitral regurgitation. *Circulation* 2003;108:II-111–II-115
40. Liel-Cohen N, Guerrero JL, Otsuji Y, et al. Design of a new surgical approach for ventricular remodeling to relieve ischemic mitral regurgitation: Insights from 3-dimensional echocardiography. *Circulation* 2000;101:2756–2763.
41. David TE. Artificial chordae. *Semin Thorac Cardiovasc Surg* 2004;16:161–168.
42. Saunders PC, Grossi EA, Schwrats CF, et al. Anterior leaflet resection of the mitral valve. *Semin Thorac Cardiovasc Surg* 2004;16:188–193.
43. Romano MA, Patel HJ, Pagani FD, et al. Anterior leaflet repair with patch augmentation for mitral regurgitation. *Ann Thorac Surg* 2005;79:1500–1504.
44. Corbineau H, Du Haut Cilly FB, Langanay T, et al. Structural durability in Carpentier Edwards standard bioprosthesis in the mitral position: A 20-year experience. *J Heart Valve Dis* 2001;10(4):443–448.
45. Fiore AC, Barner HB, Swartz MT, et al. Mitral valve replacement: Randomized trial of St. Jude and Medtronic Hall prostheses. *Ann Thorac Surg* 1998;66(3):707–712; discussion 712–713.
46. Kuntze CE, Blackstone EH, Ebels T. Thromboembolism and mechanical heart valves: A randomized study revisited. *Ann Thorac Surg* 1998;66(1):101–107.
47. Mangoni AA, Koelling TM, Meyer GS, et al. Outcome following mitral valve replacement in patients with mitral stenosis and moderately reduced left ventricular ejection fraction. *Eur J Cardiothorac Surg* 2002;22(1):90–94.
48. Mehta RH, Eagle KA, Coombs LP, et al. Society of Thoracic Surgeons National Cardiac Registry: Influence of age on outcomes in patients undergoing mitral valve replacement. *Ann Thorac Surg* 2002;74(5):1459–1467.
49. Thourani VH, Weintraub WS, Craver JM, et al. Influence of concomitant CABG and urgent/emergent status on mitral valve replacement surgery. *Ann Thorac Surg* 2000;70(3):778–783; discussion 783–784.
50. Yau TM, El-Ghoneimi YA, Armstrong S, et al. Mitral valve repair and replacement for rheumatic disease. *J Thorac Cardiovasc Surg* 2000;119(1):53–60.
51. Braunberger E, Deloche A, Berrebi A, et al. Very long-term results (more than 20 years) of valve repair with Carpentier's techniques in nonrheumatic mitral valve insufficiency. *Circulation* 2001;104(12 Suppl 1): I8–I11.
52. Mohty D, Orszulak TA, Schaff HV, et al. Very long-term survival and durability of mitral valve repair for mitral valve prolapse. *Circulation* 2001;104(12 Suppl 1):I-1–II7
53. Savage EB, Ferguson TB Jr, DiSesa VJ. Use of mitral valve repair: Analysis of contemporary United States experience reported to the Society of Thoracic Surgeons National Cardiac Database. *Ann Thorac Surg* 2003;75(3):820–825.
54. Grossi EA, Goldberg JD, LaPietra A, et al. Ischemic mitral valve reconstruction and replacement: Comparison of long-term survival and complications. *J Thorac Cardiovasc Surg* 2001;122:1107–1124.
55. Gillinov AM, Wierup PN, Blackstone EH, et al. Is repair preferable to replacement for ischemic mitral regurgitation? *J Thorac Cardiovasc Surg* 2001;122(6):1125–1141.
56. Casselman FP, Van Slycke S, Dom H, et al. Endoscopic mitral valve repair: Feasible, reproducible, and durable. *J Thorac Cardiovasc Surg* 2003;125:273–282.
57. Grossi EA, Galloway AC, LaPietra A, et al. Minimally invasive mitral valve surgery: A 6-year experience with 714 patients. *Ann Thorac Surg* 2002;74(3):660–663.
58. Nifong LW, Chitwood WR, Pappas PS, et al. Robotic mitral valve surgery: A United States multicenter trial. *J Thorac Cardiovasc Surg* 2005;129:1395–1404.
59. Fann JI, St Goar FG, Komtebedde J, et al. Beating heart catheter-based edge-to-edge mitral valve procedure in a porcine model. *Circulation* 2004;110:988–993.
60. Daimon M, Shiota T, Gillinow AM, et al. Percutaneous mitral valve repair for chronic ischemic mitral regurgitation: A real-time three-dimensional echocardiographic study in an ovine model. *Cirulation* 2005; III(17):2183–2189.

CHAPTER

33 TRICUSPID VALVE DISEASE

David L. Joyce

INTRODUCTION

Definitions

Diseases of the tricuspid valve can be subdivided in several ways. The broadest distinction separates congenital lesions (e.g., Ebstein's anomaly, tricuspid atresia) from those which are acquired. This chapter focuses primarily on acquired lesions, which can be divided into functional disease and organic disease. Functional disease typically occurs in the setting of an anatomically normal valve and results from pulmonary artery hypertension and right ventricular dilatation. This condition most often is secondary to left-sided valvular disease but also may result

KEY CONCEPTS

- Epidemiology
  - Tricuspid stenosis is rare in North America and Europe, is more common in Latin America and India, and is associated with rheumatic heart disease (4 of 100,000 people). Tricuspid regurgitation is common among patients with right heart failure, with an incidence of 0.9 percent in the United States and less than 1 percent internationally. Tricuspid disease does not appear to have a race or age predilection.
- Pathophysiology
  - The etiologies of tricuspid valve disease include rheumatic disease, endocarditis, carcinoid, papillary muscle dysfunction, trauma, and congenital anomalies. It also is associated with right heart failure and pulmonary hypertension.
- Clinical features
  - Tricuspid valve disease often is detected incidentally during evaluation of left heart conditions. Signs and symptoms are often consistent with congestive heart failure and can include dyspnea on exertion, orthopnea, jugular venous distention, ascites, and peripheral edema. Advanced disease also can present with hemoptysis and paroxysmal nocturnal dyspnea. Physical examination reveals a pansystolic (tricuspid regurgitation) or presystolic (tricuspid stenosis) murmur in the fourth and fifth intercostal spaces at the left sternal border or epigastrium. Hepatojugular reflux, pulsatile liver, and signs of hepatic dysfunction also may be present. Tricuspid endocarditis often presents with pneumonia or manifestations of septic emboli.
- Diagnostics
  - Electrocardiographic features include peaked P waves or a Q wave in V_1 as a result of right atrial volume overload and enlargement. Plain chest radiography may demonstrate cardiomegaly with right-sided chamber enlargement. Doppler and two-dimensional echocardiography confirms the diagnosis, revealing structural abnormalities and measures of pulmonary arterial pressures, the degree of stenosis/regurgitation, and right ventricular dysfunction. Cardiac catheterization usually reveals elevated right atrial and ventricular end-diastolic pressures in tricuspid regurgitation. A diastolic pressure–atrioventricular pressure gradient that increases with respiration is found in patients with significant tricuspid stenosis. For tricuspid endocarditis, major diagnostic criteria include valvular vegetations and pyrexia, with positive blood cultures, septic pulmonary emboli, and a murmur constituting minor criteria.
- Treatment
  - Tricuspid valve repair or replacement is indicated for tricuspid stenosis and moderate to severe tricus-

pid regurgitation, usually associated with New York Heart Association class III or IV symptoms. Tricuspid stenosis usually is treated with commissurotomy. Surgical techniques for tricuspid regurgitation include bicuspidization, DeVega suture annuloplasty (moderate tricuspid insufficiency), Carpentier ring annuloplasty (moderate to severe tricuspid insufficiency), and prosthetic valve replacement. Tricuspid endocarditis is treated primarily with intravenous antibiotics, with surgical correction reserved for treatment failures. For tricuspid endocarditis, nominal surgical therapy consists of debridement and valvular repair.

- Outcomes
  - The DeVega suture annuloplasty for tricuspid regurgitation is associated with a 4 percent operative mortality, a 5 percent recurrence rate, and an actuarial survival rate of 71.5 percent at 14 years. Carpentier ring annuloplasty is associated with an actuarial survival of 68.3 percent at 10 years.

from Eisenmenger's syndrome, right ventricular (RV) infarction, or primary pulmonary hypertension. These types of disease typically manifest in the clinical presentation of tricuspid regurgitation (TR). Organic disease (in which there is an anatomic abnormality of the valve) is associated most frequently with rheumatic fever but also may occur in the setting of infective endocarditis, trauma, carcinoid syndrome, Libman-Sacks endocarditis, eosinophilic leukemia, and diffuse collagen disorders. Tricuspid stenosis (TS) is the most common manifestation of organic disease, although insufficiency can occur alone or in combination with stenosis. A summary of the disorders implicated in tricuspid valve disease is given in Fig. 33-1.

Historic highlights

Starr and colleagues[1] reported the first surgical experience with tricuspid valve replacement (TVR) in a series of 13 patients who had undergone multiple valve replacement; one of those patients underwent replacement of the aortic, mitral, and tricuspid valves on February 21, 1963. Although the paucity of indications for TVR limited its implementation, the recognition of tricuspid valve endocarditis as an epidemic among heroin addicts in Detroit between 1966 and 1968 rejuvenated interest in tricuspid valve surgery. Valve replacement combined with intravenous antibiotics failed to control the severe gram-negative sepsis, yielding a mortality rate of 100 percent. In search of a more efficacious treatment strategy, Agustin Arbulu began performing experimental removal of the tricuspid valve in dogs. Six of the seven experimental animals survived the manipulation (performed in 1969), prompting Arbulu to translate his findings to the clinical realm.[2] In a series of 55 patients with tricuspid endocarditis secondary to *Pseudomonas aeruginosa*, Arbulu removed the tricuspid valve, with a 61 percent survival rate at 25 years.[3,4]

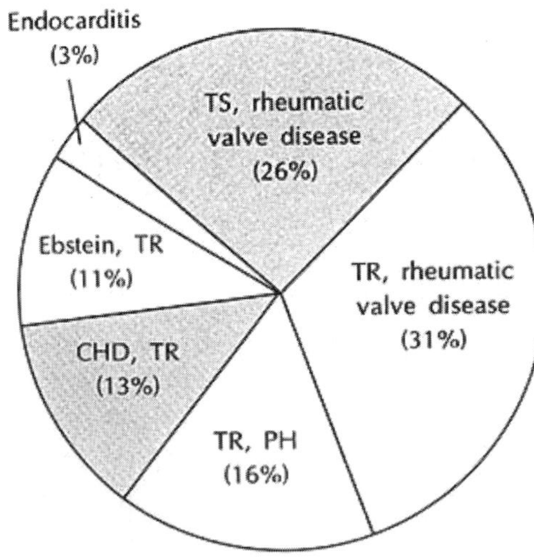

Figure 33-1 Summary of disorders implicated in tricuspid valve disease. [From Virmani R et al. Burke AP. Pathology of valvular heart diseases. In: Rahimtoola SH, (ed). *Atlas of heart disease.* Philadelphia: Mosby; 1997:116, with permission.]

Anatomic considerations

As its name implies, the tricuspid valve contains three leaflets. The anterior leaflet is the largest and is attached to the dominant papillary muscle by chordae tendineae. The posterior leaflet is the smallest and, along with the septal leaflet, attaches directly to the parietal and septal walls of the right ventricle via chordae. The adult valve is typically 36 +/− 4.5 mm in diameter and covers a surface area of 10.5 cm^2. In the setting of dilated cardiomyopathy, the valve diameter can increase to 45 mm in some cases. Important anatomic considerations for the surgeon include the presence of the conducting system near the base of the septal leaflet and the relationships of the annulus to the base of the aortic valve, the membranous septum, the central fibrous body, the right coronary artery, the lateral atrioventricular junction, the coronary sinus, and the bundle of His (Fig. 33-2).[5]

PATHOPHYSIOLOGY

Disorders of the tricuspid valve can result from structural abnormalities or changes in ventricular geometry in the setting of a normal valve. The etiology of TS is due to rheumatic heart disease in over 90 percent of cases.[6]

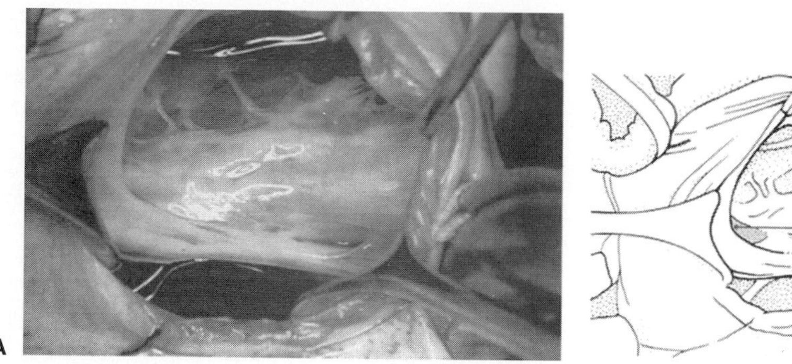

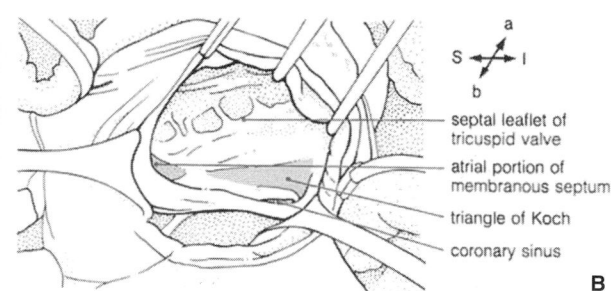

Figure 33-2 Anatomic features of the normal tricuspid valve. [From Cohn LH, Edmunds LH Jr, eds. *Cardiac Surgery in the Adult.* New York: McGraw-Hill; 2003:1001–1015, with permission.]

Conversely, pure TR is usually a consequence of RV dilatation and failure.

Tricuspid stenosis

The surgical pathology of TS can be divided into four categories: rheumatic disease, congenital anomalies, metabolic disorders, and infective endocarditis.[6] On gross pathology, stenotic tricuspid valves are found to have fibrous thickening of the leaflets with shortening and thickening of the chordae tendineae (Fig. 33-3). Fusion of the commissures leads to obstruction of blood flow and the resultant symptoms of TS. Histologic examination of the valvular tissue reveals deposition of collagen and elastic fibers.[6]

Tricuspid regurgitation

Regurgitation of the tricuspid valve results from a wide array of entities. Organic causes include rheumatic heart disease, endocarditis, prolapse, carcinoid, papillary muscle dysfunction, trauma, connective tissue disorders, rheumatoid arthritis, and radiation therapy.[7] Functional disease results from any condition that predisposes to elevated right heart pressures. Gross pathologic features of the regurgitant tricuspid valve include fibrous thickening of the leaflets, minimal calcification, and dilatation of the annulus.[7] In contrast to TS, there is no fusion of the commissures or shortening of the chordae.

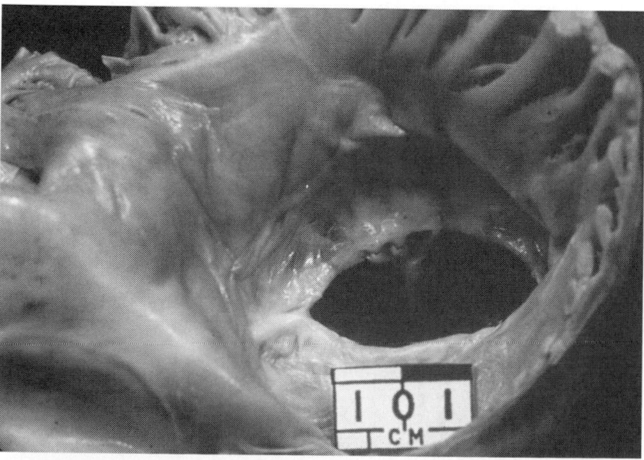

Figure 33-3 Gross pathology of a stenotic tricuspid valve secondary to rheumatic heart disease. [From Waller BF, Howard J, Fess S. Pathology of tricuspid valve stenosis and pure tricuspid regurgitation: Part I. *Clin Cardiol* 1995;18(2):97–102, with permission.]

CLINICAL FEATURES

Epidemiology

Tricuspid stenosis is rare in North America and Europe. It is more common in Latin America and India, where it typically is associated with rheumatic heart disease, which affects 4 of 100,000 people. In patients with coexisting mitral stenosis, the rate of TS is approximately 5 to 10 percent, and it typically is associated with some degree of TR.[8] The various etiologies of tricuspid valve disease are shown in Fig. 33-1. Tricuspid regurgitation is common among patients with right heart failure and has an incidence of 0.9 percent in the United States (less than 1 percent internationally). Tricuspid valve disease does not have a predilection for race or age.

Typical clinical presentation

Tricuspid valve disease usually is brought to the attention of the medical practitioner during evaluation of left-sided conditions. A history of rheumatic heart disease or an abnormality detected on cardiac auscultation may alert the clinician, but frequently these patients present with dyspnea on exertion, orthopnea, and other symptoms of left-sided failure. In advanced cases, hemoptysis and paroxysmal nocturnal dyspnea may occur.[9]

Physical examination symptoms and signs

Signs of tricuspid valve disease are related to the onset of right heart failure and include jugular venous distention, ascites, and peripheral edema. Patients also may complain of vague abdominal discomfort associated with hepatomegaly. In light of the high rate of concordant left-sided disease, most patients are detected on the basis of congestive heart failure. Physical examination is notable for the presence of a murmur, which can be auscultated at the left sternal edge at the fourth and fifth intercostal spaces or in the epigastrium. The murmur of TR is pansystolic and may be high-pitched, often increasing on inspiration (Carvallo's sign). TS produces a presystolic murmur that also increases with inspiration. This feature permits its differentiation from murmurs associated with mitral valve disease. Atrial fibrillation is a common finding. Hepatojugular reflux or a pulsatile liver may be demonstrated in cases of TR, and clinical signs of hepatic dysfunction also may be present.

Hallmark primary laboratory abnormalities

Routine laboratory tests may aid in the diagnosis of the underlying condition, with leukocytosis commonly seen in the setting of infective endocarditis. Renal and hepatic impairment also may be present in cases of chronic ventricular dysfunction.

DIAGNOSTIC MODALITIES

Electrocardiographic findings include peaked P waves (caused by right atrial overload) or a Q wave in V_1 (resulting from an enlarged right atrium). Posteroanterior and lateral plain chest radiography may demonstrate cardiomegaly with enlargement of the right-sided cardiac structures. A pleural effusion also may be present along with upward displacement of the diaphragm resulting from ascites. Doppler and two-dimensional echocardiography is required to confirm the diagnosis, showing structural abnormalities of the valve and allowing measurement of pulmonary artery pressures, the degree of regurgitation, and right ventricular function (Fig. 33-4).

Cardiac catheterization provides useful information for evaluating the anatomy and functionality of the tricuspid valve. In the setting of TR, right atrial and ventricular end-diastolic pressures usually are elevated. Tricuspid stenosis is characterized by a diastolic pressure gradient between the right atrium and the right ventricle that increases during inspiration and decreases with expiration. By providing a visual image of flow through the tricuspid valve, angiography can demonstrate the degree of retrograde filling of the right atrium, the superior and inferior caval veins, and the hepatic veins as well as the functional activity of the right ventricle.[10]

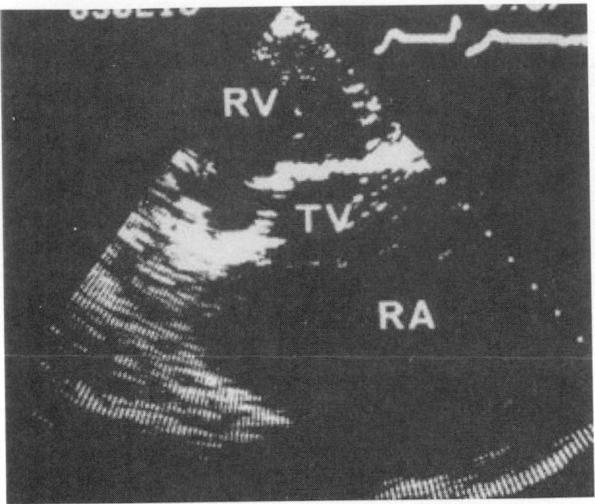

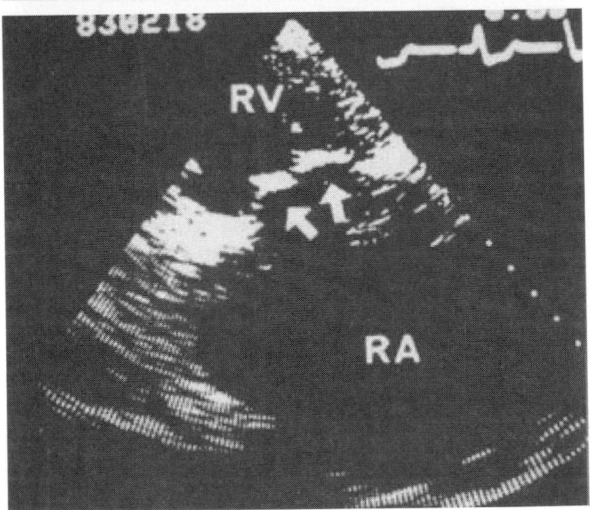

Figure 33-4 Echocardiographic features of tricuspid regurgitation (From Shimada R et al: Diagnosis of tricuspid stenosis by M-mode and two-dimensional echocardiography. *Am J Cardiol* 1984;53:164, with permission.)

MEDICAL THERAPY

Acquired disease of the tricuspid valve represents a structural abnormality for which there is no effective pharmacotherapy. In general, tricuspid insufficiency is well tolerated in the absence of elevated pulmonary pressures. For example, echocardiograms performed in 95 healthy women revealed some degree of TR in 52 of the subjects.[11] Nevertheless, elevation of the pulmonary vascular resistance may dictate surgical repair in selected patients.

SURGICAL DECISION MAKING

Indications for repair include the diagnosis of either TS or moderate to severe TR (Table 33-1). Some have advocated performing annuloplasty when the valve diameter exceeds twice the normal distance (typically

Table 33-1 Indications for surgery involving the tricuspid valve

Diagnosis of tricuspid stenosis
New York Heart Association classes III and IV
Moderate and severe tricuspid regurgitation
Annulus dilatation > 100% (70 mm)
Lesser degrees of tricuspid regurgitation (controversial)

70 mm), whereas others have recommended prophylactic annuloplasty in patients with minimal or mild TR to prevent progression of the disease in those undergoing left-sided valve surgery. Among patients undergoing mitral valve surgery, 5 to 20 percent also require tricuspid annuloplasty.[12] Most patients who require surgery of the tricuspid valve fall into New York Heart Association (NYHA) classes III and IV.

OPERATIVE TECHNIQUES

Surgical management of acquired diseases of the tricuspid valve has evolved from reparative techniques to prosthetic replacement and back again after greater experience with and modifications of each of those techniques. Since operative repair of tricuspid valve lesions is performed almost universally in the setting of concomitant cardiac surgical procedures, median sternotomy is typically the approach of choice.

Tricuspid stenosis: commissurotomy

For tricuspid stenosis, surgical management is straightforward and involves commissurotomy of the diseased valve. Successful commissurotomy requires adequate visualization of the valve and careful attention to the surrounding anatomic structures.[13] It is usually unnecessary to open all three commissures, since such maneuvers are likely to result in significant tricuspid insufficiency that is difficult to correct. Instead, separation of the fused commissures on either side of the septal leaflet results in a straight (septal) and a curved (mural) leaflet with excellent hemodynamic properties.[14]

Tricuspid regurgitation

Surgical techniques for addressing TR include bicuspidization, purse-string reduction of the annulus, placement of rigid or flexible annuloplasty rings, and prosthetic replacement. Selection of the appropriate treatment depends on the extent of dysfunction and the condition of the native valve. The goals of therapy include restoration of normal valve function through the use of an easily reproducible technique that yields consistent results.[15]

Bicuspidization

The posterior annulus of the tricuspid valve is the only structurally unsupported area of the tricuspid valve annulus, making this area particularly susceptible to dilatation and subsequent TR.[16] Various annuloplasty techniques have been described that are based on the principle of correcting this abnormality.[17] Bicuspidization for tricuspid insufficiency is performed using one or two pledgeted 0 Prolene sutures to obliterate the annular segment corresponding to the posterior leaflet (Fig. 33-5).[2] This technique is generally satisfactory in patients with moderate TR.

DeVega Suture Annuloplasty

Owing to its simplicity, the DeVega repair has gained popularity for the management of moderate to severe TR. This technique involves running a single pledgeted 0 Prolene suture between the anterior and septal leaflets at the level of the commissure.[18] Two sequential sutures are placed in this fashion, running clockwise through the annulus. These sutures are tightened to obliterate the portion of the annulus that has been plicated (Fig. 33-6). On the basis of some estimates, up to 26 percent of patients undergoing surgery of the mitral or aortic valve may require tricuspid annuloplasty.[19] Operative mortality after DeVega annuloplasty is 4 percent.[20] Recurrence of tricuspid insufficiency has been demonstrated in 5 percent of

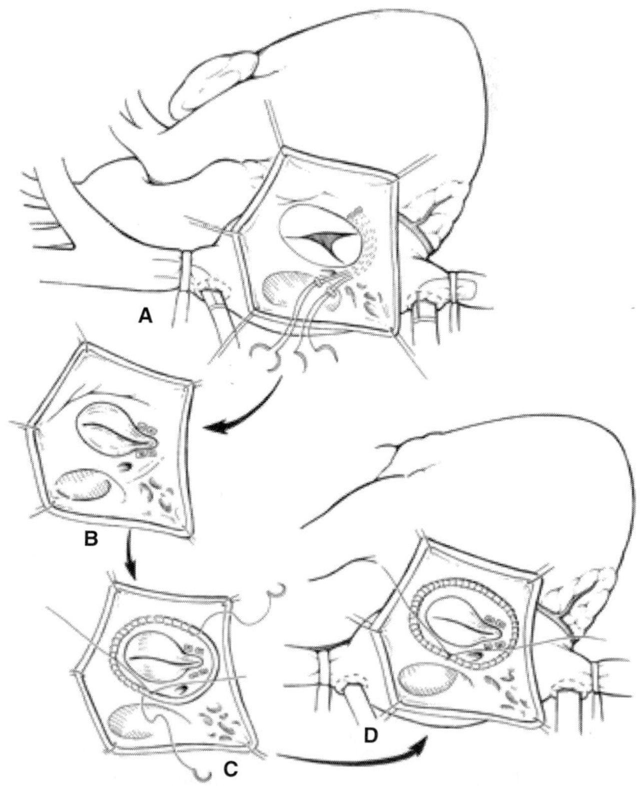

Figure 33-5 Tricuspid valve bicuspidization. (From Cohn LH, Edmunds LH Jr, eds. *Cardiac Surgery in the Adult.* New York: McGraw-Hill; 2003:1001–1015, with permission.)

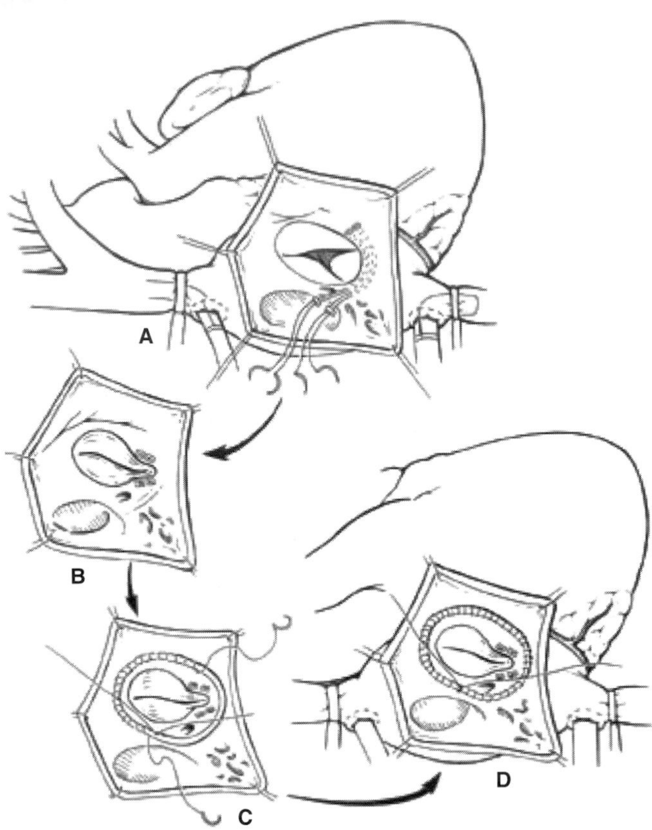

Figure 33-6 A modified DeVega annuloplasty technique is shown. (From Cohn LH, Edmunds LH Jr, eds. *Cardiac Surgery in the Adult.* New York: McGraw-Hill; 2003:1001–1015, with permission.)

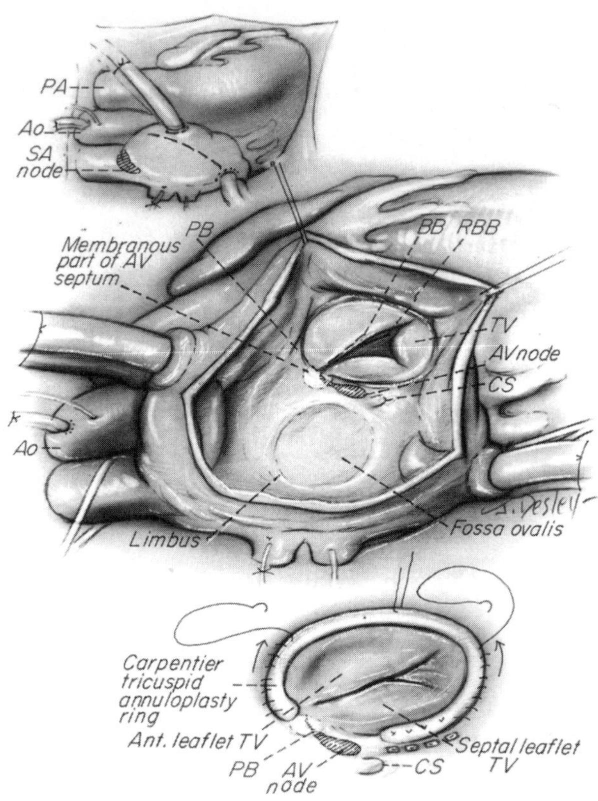

Figure 33-7 Technique for tricuspid annuloplasty using a Carpentier-Edwards ring. (From Kirklin JW, Barratt-Boyer BG. *Cardiac surgery,* second edition. New York: Churchill Livingstone, 1993:592, with permission.)

patients undergoing this procedure and has been attributed to an inadequate mitral valve procedure or left ventricular failure.[21] Long-term follow-up of this procedure shows an actuarial survival rate of 71.5 ± 8.2 percent at 14 years.[22]

Carpentier ring annuloplasty

In cases of severe TR, rigid or flexible ring annuloplasty is well accepted as optimal therapy. The principles of repair are similar to those for suture annuloplasty with respect to reducing the size of the valve orifice. However, the increase in dilatation seen in cases of severe TR mandates greater stability with the repair. A sizer is used to measure the area of the septal leaflet to allow selection of the appropriate ring. Tricuspid rings are designed with an opening that corresponds to the region of the atrioventricular (AV) node to minimize damage to the conducting system during surgery. Interrupted pledgeted 2-0 Ticron sutures are placed through the annulus and then passed through the ring, securing it in place (Fig. 33-7). First described by Carpentier and colleagues,[23] this procedure has had several subsequent modifications. Nevertheless, the principles of repair remain the same regardless of the type of ring used. This technique has been estimated to be suitable in up to 96 percent of cases of acquired tricuspid valve disease and is associated with a hospital mortality rate of 9 to 10 percent in patients undergoing concomitant left-sided valve surgery (nonvalve-related deaths).[24,25] Actuarial survival from this procedure at 10 years is 68.3 percent.[26] A recent study comparing several different suture and ring annuloplasty techniques demonstrated an increase in recurrent TR over time with the DeVega annuloplasty.[27] These findings have led to the recommendation that suture annuloplasties be abandoned in favor of various types of ring annuloplasties to reduce the rate of reoperation, which has an associated hospital mortality rate of 37 percent.[27]

TRICUSPID VALVE REPLACEMENT

After tricuspid valve repair, assessment of persistent insufficiency can be determined by one or more of the following techniques: (1) injection of saline into the right ventricle with a clamp occluding the pulmonary artery, (2) manual palpation for regurgitant flow performed by inserting a finger through the right atrial appendage, and (3) external palpation of the right atrium.[2] Valve replacement should be performed in cases of persistent tricuspid insufficiency. Predictors for the need for valve replacement include jugular venous distention, increased severity of tricuspid valve incompetence, previous cardiac surgery, and the presence of TS.[12] Because of the increased rate of thromboembolism and valve thrombosis associated with mechanical valve replacement, tissue valves are preferred in most cases. In a metanalysis of 1160 prosthetic valves, the pooled survival hazard ratio of mechanical prosthesis versus bioprosthesis was found to be 1.07.[28] The freedom from reoperation hazard ratio was 1.24 in that study.[28] Survival rates are similar between the two types of valve replacement.[29–31] The surgical technique involves placement of interrupted pledgeted 0 Ticron imbricating sutures that are passed initially through the leading edge of the valve leaflets and subsequently through the prosthetic valve sewing ring (Fig. 33-8).[2] Paying careful attention to the regional anatomy and leaving the native valve leaflets in place reduce the likelihood of injury to the conduction system.

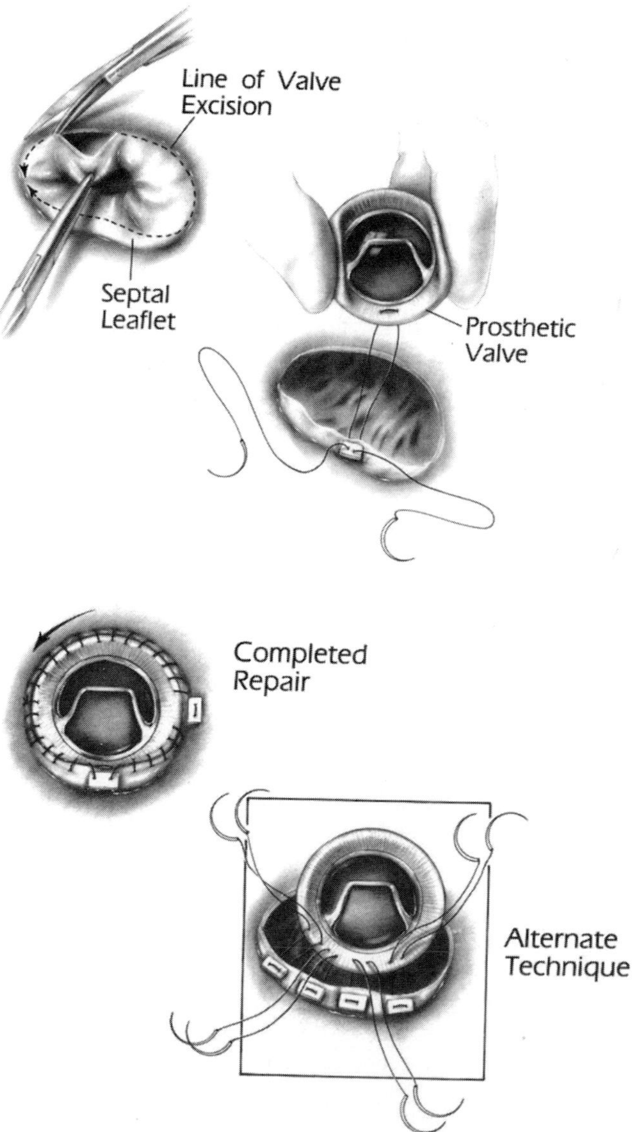

Figure 33-8 Technique for tricuspid valve replacement. (From Doty DB. *Cardiac Surgery: Operative Technique.* St. Louis: Mosby; 1997, with permission.)

TRICUSPID ENDOCARDITIS

Pathophysiology and epidemiology

Infective endocarditis (IE) of the tricuspid valve has become more widespread because of the increase in intravenous drug abuse. Tricuspid valve endocarditis (TVE) results from the showering of infectious particulate matter after intravenous puncture. Risk factors include parenteral drug abuse (e.g., heroin, amphetamines, cocaine), alcoholism, burns, and immunodeficiency.[31] A variety of pathogenic microorganisms are involved (Table 33-2). The incidence of polymicrobial disease is increasing, adding to the challenge of treating this condition.[32] TVE accounts for 5 to 10 percent of all patients with infective endocarditis. However, this is the most commonly affected valve in intravenous drug users. Several factors account for the greater prevalence of IE in the left heart: a higher frequency of left-sided congenital lesions, lower right-sided pressures that lead to a decrease in valve stress, and reduced right heart blood oxygen content.[31]

Clinical presentation

Patients with TVE typically present with symptoms of pneumonia or septic pulmonary emboli rather than the congestive signs and symptoms often seen with left-sided lesions. A murmur of tricuspid regurgitation is often present, with cardiomegaly occurring rarely in progressive disease. Plain chest radiography demonstrates segmental infiltrates that tend to be more common in the lower lobes. Echocardiography is useful in diagnosing TVE, with a sensitivity between 80 and 100 percent.[31] The presence of a vegetation and pyrexia constitute the major criteria for diagnosis, with multiple positive blood cultures, septic pulmonary emboli, absence of systemic emboli, and TVR murmur qualifying as minor criteria.[31] A definitive diagnosis of endocarditis requires that two major criteria or one major criterion and three minor criteria be present.

Table 33-2 Microorganisms involved in tricuspid valve endocarditis

Pathogen	Percentage
Staphylococcus aureus	50–80
Pseudomonas aeruginosa	10–40
Streptococcus alpha	10–20
Candida	3–5
Other	10–20
Polymicrobial	10–20

Source: Chan P, Ogilby JD, Segal B. Tricuspid valve endocarditis. *Am Heart J* 1989;117(5):1140–1146, with permission.

Treatment Options

Most cases of TVE can be managed medically with intravenous antibiotics. However, treatment failures secondary to drug resistance, progressive hemodynamic compromise, septic emboli, or renal failure resulting from drug toxicity often necessitate surgical correction.[33] Surgical correction is indicated in cases of severe congestive heart failure or persistent sepsis.[31] In some cases of large vegetations, left-sided valve involvement, or gram-negative or *Candida* infections, surgery may be warranted as primary therapy.[31] However, fever, recurrent pulmonary embolizations, and polymicrobial infections are not in and of themselves indications for surgery.[31] Surgical therapy is aimed at removal of the infected tissue while maintaining valve function. This can be accomplished by means of debridement followed by either concomitant repair or valve replacement in a staged procedure. Tricuspid valvulectomy without replacement also has been shown to represent a viable alternative to valve replacement in many cases.[34] Valve replacement in the setting of drug abuse–related TVE is of questionable value in light of those patients' tendency to relapse in their addiction. However, valvectomy without replacement is limited by the regurgitation and right heart failure that often follow this procedure. This strategy can result in hepatic congestion that complicates subsequent valve replacement, when necessary. Therefore, a reconstructive valvuloplasty with autogenous pericardial tissue has been proposed as a method that can provide adequate hemodynamic outcomes without the need for a prosthetic material.[35] The long-term results of this approach are not available. Aggressive counseling is mandatory to prevent recurrence of drug abuse.

References

1. Starr A, McCord CW, Wood J, et al. Surgery for multiple valve disease. *Ann Surg* 1964;160:596–613.
2. Edmunds LH. *Cardiac Surgery in the Adult.* New York: McGraw-Hill, 2004.
3. Arbulu A, Thoms NW, Wilson RF. Valvulectomy without prosthetic replacement: A lifesaving operation for tricuspid pseudomonas endocarditis. *J Thorac Cardiovasc Surg* 1972;64(1):103–107.
4. Arbulu A, Holmes RJ, Asfaw I. Surgical treatment of intractable right-sided infective endocarditis in drug addicts: 25 years experience. *J Heart Valve Dis* 1993;2(2):129–137.
5. Sabiston DC, Spencer FC. Surgery of the chest. In: Karp, RB (ed) *Acquired Disease of the Tricuspid Valve.* Philadelphia: Saunders; 2004:1667–1672.
6. Waller BF, Howard J, Fess S. Pathology of tricuspid valve stenosis and pure tricuspid regurgitation: Part I. *Clin Cardiol* 1995;18(2):97–102.
7. Waller BF, Howard J, Fess S. Pathology of tricuspid valve stenosis and pure tricuspid regurgitation: Part II. *Clin Cardiol* 1995;18(3):167–174.
8. Kasper D , Braunwald E, Fauci F, et al. *Harrison's Principles of Internal Medicine.* New York: McGraw-Hill; 2004:490–491.
9. Kratz J. Evaluation and management of tricuspid valve disease. *Cardiol Clin* 1991;9(2):397–407.
10. Cha SD, Desai RS, Gooch AS, et al. Diagnosis of severe tricuspid regurgitation. *Chest* 1982;82(6):726–731.
11. Michelsen S, Hurlen M, Otterstad JE. Prevalence of tricuspid and pulmonary regurgitation diagnosed by Doppler in apparently healthy women: Possible influence on their physical performance? *Eur Heart J* 1988;9 (1):61–67.
12. McGrath LB, Gonzalez-Lavin L, Bailey BM, et al. Tricuspid valve operations in 530 patients: Twenty-five-year assessment of early and late phase events. *J Thorac Cardiovasc Surg* 1990;99(1):124–133.
13. Revuelta JM, Garcia-Rinaldi R, Duran CM. Tricuspid commissurotomy. *Ann Thorac Surg* 1985;39(5):489–491.
14. Victor S, Nayak VM. Bicuspidization for tricuspid stenosis. *Ann Thorac Surg* 1998;65(5):1468–1470.
15. Carpentier A, Deloche A, Hanania G, et al. Surgical management o*f acquired tricuspid valve disease.* J Thorac Cardiovasc Surg 1974;67(1):53–65.
16. Deloche A, Guerinon J, Fabiani JN, et al. [Anatomical study of rheumatic tricuspid valve diseases: Application to the study of various valvuloplasties]. *Ann Chir Thorac Cardiovasc* 1973;12(4):343–349.
17. Cohn LH. Tricuspid regurgitation secondary to mitral valve disease: When and how to repair. *J Card Surg* 1994;9(Suppl 2):237–241.
18. DeVega NG. La anuloplastia selectiva reguable y permanente. *Rev Esp Cardiol* 1972;25:6.
19. Wei J, Chang CY, Lee FY, Lai WY. De Vega's semicircular annuloplasty for tricuspid valve regurgitation. *Ann Thorac Surg* 1993;55(2):482–485.
20. Duran CM, Kumar N, Prabhakar G, et al. Vanishing De Vega annuloplasty for functional tricuspid regurgitation. *J Thorac Cardiovasc Surg* 1993;106(4):609–613.
21. Boyd AD, Engelman RM, Isom OW, et al. Tricuspid annuloplasty: Five and one-half years' experience with 78 patients. *J Thorac Cardiovasc Surg* 1974;68(3):344–351.
22. Chidambaram M, Abdulali SA, Baliga BG, Ionescu MI. Long-term results of DeVega tricuspid annuloplasty. *Ann Thorac Surg* 1987;43(2):185–188.
23. Carpentier A, Deloche A, Dauptain J, et al. A new reconstructive operation for correction of mitral and tricuspid insufficiency. *J Thorac Cardiovasc Surg* 1971;61(1):1–13.
24. Carpentier A, Deloche A, Hanania G, et al. Surgical management of acquired tricuspid valve disease. *J Thorac Cardiovasc Surg* 1974;67(1):53–65.
25. Gatti G, Maffei G, Lusa AM, Pugliese P. Tricuspid valve repair with the Cosgrove-Edwards annuloplasty system: Early clinical and echocardiographic results. *Ann Thorac Surg* 2001;72(3):764–767.
26. Onoda K, Yasuda F, Takao M, et al. Long-term follow-up after Carpentier-Edwards ring annuloplasty for tricuspid regurgitation. *Ann Thorac Surg* 2000;70(3):796–799.
27. McCarthy PM, Bhudia SK, Rajeswaran J, et al. Tricuspid valve repair: Durability and risk factors for failure. *J Thorac Cardiovasc Surg* 2004;127(3):674–685.

28. Rizzoli G, Vendramin I, Nesseris G, et al. Biological or mechanical prostheses in tricuspid position? A meta-analysis of intra-institutional results. *Ann Thorac Surg* 2004;77(5):1607–1614.
29. Carrier M, Hebert Y, Pellerin M, et al. Tricuspid valve replacement: An analysis of 25 years of experience at a single center. *Ann Thorac Surg* 2003;75(1):47–50.
30. Mangoni AA, DiSalvo TG, Vlahakes GJ, et al. Outcome following isolated tricuspid valve replacement. *Eur J Cardiothorac Surg* 2001;19(1):68–73.
31. Chan P, Ogilby JD, Segal B. Tricuspid valve endocarditis. *Am Heart J* 1989;117(5):1140–1146.
32. Atkinson JB, Virmani R. Infective endocarditis: Changing trends and general approach for examination. *Hum Pathol* 1987;18(6):603–608.
33. Yee ES, Khonsari S. Right-sided infective endocarditis: Valvuloplasty, valvectomy or replacement. *J Cardiovasc Surg (Torino)* 1989;30(5):744–748.
34. Arbulu A, Holmes RJ, Asfaw I. Tricuspid valvulectomy without replacement: Twenty years' experience. *J Thorac Cardiovasc Surg* 1991;102(6):917–922.
35. Yee ES, Ullyot DJ. Reparative approach for right-sided endocarditis: Operative considerations and results of valvuloplasty. *J Thorac Cardiovasc Surg* 1988;96(1):133–140.

CHAPTER

34 SURGICAL MANAGEMENT OF ENDOCARDITIS

Christina M. Vassileva, David D. Yuh

INTRODUCTION

Early theories of the pathogenesis of IE centered on the misconception that cardiac valves are valscularized with an extensive network of capillaries that allow microorganisms to gain access to the microcirculation of the valves after an episode of bacteremia and establish infection.[1,2] Gross[3] was the first to refute this misconception by demonstrating that the presence of blood vessels in the cardiac valves is a result of an inflammatory process and that normally cardiac valves are not vascularized.

KEY CONCEPTS

- Epidemiology
  - The incidence of infective endocarditis (IE) in the general population is estimated to be 3.2 to 11.6 cases per 1,000,000 person-years. It is more common in males and in the elderly. In over 75 percent of these patients, there is an identifiable cardiac lesion, with valvular heart disease being the most common (42.1 percent), followed by prosthetic valves (21.7 percent) and congenital heart disease (11.7 percent).
- Pathophysiology
  - The sequence of events leading to the development of native valve IE can be broken down into five steps: (1) damage to the endocardial surface of the valve, (2) accumulation of platelets and thrombi, leading to the formation of nonbacterial thrombotic endocarditis (NBTE), (3) transient bacteremia of any source, (4) adherence of bacteria to the NBTE, and (5) survival and multiplication of the bacteria with subsequent growth of the vegetation.
- Clinical features
  - The symptoms associated with subacute bacterial endocarditis are insidious. They can include persistent low-grade fever, malaise, anorexia, weight loss, fatigue, and general myalgias, especially low back pain. The initial manifestation of this subcaute disease may be reflective of embolic complications associated with IE. Active bacterial endocarditis generally involves the left side of the heart and often is associated with high-grade fevers, chills, lethargy, and profound malaise and rapidly progresses to severe sepsis and circulatory collapse.
- Diagnostics
  - A thorough history and a physical examination are very important for diagnosing IE. A comprehensive history can provide clues. There are classic physical findings associated with IE. Leukocytosis is more common with acute endocarditis. Anemia is frequently present, and proteinuria and/or hematuria are seen commonly in the urine. Although a chest x-ray is important as a first imaging procedure, echocardiography is the modality of choice for the diagnosis of IE. A transesophageal echocardiogram is often most diagnostic of IE, especially in patients with prosthetic valves.
- Treatment
  - Medical
    - The cornerstone of medical treatment for IE is proper antimicrobial therapy. Successful antibiotic treatment of IE is influenced by a number of factors, including the type of organism, the duration of infection, the specific valve involved, and patient characteristics.

- Surgical:
  - There are well-defined indications for surgical intervention that are emergent or urgent. The surgical principles include excision or removal of all infected tissue, secure repair with nonprosthetic material, and continued postoperative antibiotic therapy. Mitral and tricuspid valves should be repaired if possible. Aortic valve endocarditis generally is treated with prosthetic aortic valve replacement, but in situations in which there is extensive annular damage, a homograft or autograft procedure is recommended. This is seen most commonly in patients with prosthetic valve endocarditis with an annular abscess.
- Outcomes:
  - Operative mortality rates vary between 3 and 14.5 percent in most series, with higher mortality rates observed in patients who are preoperatively moribund and patients with prosthetic valve endocarditis. Significant risk factors for early mortality include age, staphylococcal endocarditis, preoperative New York Heart Association (NYHA) class, and preoperative renal failure. Overall 5-year survival is between 75 and 88 percent, and 10-year survival is 63 to 81 percent. Overall recurrence rates range from 4.5 to 12.3 percent, with recurrence being defined as IE occurring more than 6 months after the original presentation. Relapse, which is defined as IE occurring within 6 months of the first manifestation, ranges from 2.7 to 3.3 percent. Patients who survive 1 year after the initial episode of IE are more than three times as likely to die than is the general population.

PATHOGENESIS

Early models of experimental IE were cumbersome and not always reproducible. Significant advances in the pathogenesis of IE followed the development of a simple and reproducible model of IE. Garrison and Freedman[4,5] were the first to describe an elegant model of rabbit endocarditis by introducing a polyethylene catheter containing a bactrial innoculum via the femoral vein into the right side of the heart or via the right carotid artery into the left side of the heart. Their model was modified by Durack and Beeson[6] to approximate the clinical scenario more closely by introducing the bacteria intravenously via an ear vein after catheter placement. This model proved highly reliable and 100 percent reproducible,[6] allowing important insight into the pathogenesis of this clinical entity to be gained.

The sequence of events leading to the development of native valve IE can be broken down into five distinct steps: (1) damage to the endocardial surface of the valve, (2) accumulation of platelets and thrombi, leading to the formation of NBTE, (3) transient bacteremia of any source, (4) adherance of bacteria to the NBTE, and (5) survival and multiplication of the bacteria with subsequent growth of the vegetation.

Damage to the endocardial surface of the valve

This is the first step toward the pathogenesis of IE. The valve surface may become damaged in a variety of ways, including normal wear and tear with age, congenital malformations that produce turbulent flow, and iatrogenic catheters or wires placed in the heart chambers.

Deposition of fibrin and platelets (NBTE)

Normal endothelial cells are nonthrombogenic.[7] However, after endothelial damage, the subendothelium becomes exposed to the circulation, initiating a sequence of events that may result in thrombus formation. Valvular endothelium seems to be particularly susceptible to this process.[8] When a plastic catheter is used to produce experimental damage to healthy aortic valves and the adjacent aortic endothelium, both show denudation of endothelium, whereas only the cardiac valve shows a lesion consisting of platelets and fibrin, showing the particular tendency of valvular endothelium to promote the development of NBTE compared with other vascular endothelium.[8] Chino and associates[9] performed an autopsy study of 3404 atomic bomb survivors and found NBTE in 2.4 percent. Interestingly, the lesions were almost exclusively on the left side of the heart, suggesting that hemodynamic stress plays a major role in the development of endothelial trauma.[9] Similarly, Lepeschkin[10] performed 1024 autopsies of patients with IE and found that the mitral valve was most commonly involved (86 percent), followed by aortic (55 percent), tricuspid (19.6 percent), and pulmonary valve (1.1 percent) involvement. He postulated that this incidence was reflective of the pressures to which the different valves were exposed.[10] Rodbard[11] performed an elegant study demonstrating that the localization of endocariditis could be explained by the hemodynamic effect of a high-pressure gradient across a narrow orifice, that is, the heart valve. When nebulized suspensions of bacteria were blown in a uniform-caliber agar tube, few colonies were noted to appear randomly. When the same experiment was performed through an agar tube, abundant bacterial deposition occurred just distal to the narrowed orifice.[11] Since the left side of the heart is subjected to higher pressures, the anatomic predisposition of endocarditis to occur on the left side of the heart could be explained on the basis of this experimental model.[11] In addition, congenital valvular abnormalities as well as rheumatic heart disease (which was very common at that time) predominate on the left side, creating altered hemodynamics, that is, turbulent flow that damages the endothelial surface over time, allowing for the formation of NTBE.

Transient bacteremia

Transient bacteremia has been documented by multiple investigators after manipulations of the oral cavity (dental extractions, tooth brushing), upper airway (rigid bronchoscopy), gastrointestinal tract (colonoscopy), and genitourinary tract (cystoscopy, childbirth) as well as various percutaneous biopsies. The degree of bacteremia clearly is related to the extent of the trauma produced by a procedure, and so more invasive procedures lead to a higher degree of bacteremia.[12] In turn, the amount of bacteria that adhere to heart valves is directly proportional to the duration and magnitude of the bacteremia, as suggested by in vitro experiments.[13,14]

Bacterial adherence to NBTE

The vegetation of IE forms once bacteria adhere to the NBTE. On gross pathologic examination, the vegetation consists of bacteria embedded in a matrix of fibrin and platelets. Angrist and Oka[15] were the first to suggest that bacterial attachment is most likely to occur to a damaged valve with NBTE. This subsequently was proved in the rabbit experimental model of IE[4–6] and shown to be true with human valves as well.[14] Bacterial strains differ in their ability to adhere to heart valves. For example, gram-negative bacilli frequently cause transient bacteremia yet are an unusual cause of endocarditis.[8] When various strains of *Streptococcus viridans*, enterococci, coagulase-negative and coagulase-positive staphylococci, pseudomonas, *Escherichia coli*, and *Klebsiella pneumoniae* are studied in vitro, the bacteria that most commonly cause endocarditis are found to adhere more readily to human heart valves in vitro.[13] Ample evidence has been produced showing that dextran plays a major role in the adherence process. When in vitro adherence of oral streptococci to platelet-fibrin matrix is studied, higher production of dextran correlates with better adherence.[16] Further in vivo experiments showed that rabbits with NBTE were more likely to develop IE when injected with a strain of *Streptococcus sanguis* that produced high levels of dextran than they were when injected with a mutant strain that produced less dextran.[16] In addition, pretreating the dextran-producing strain with dextrinase decreased its ability to cause IE in this animal model.[16] Interestingly, various bacterial strains differ with respect to their dependence on dextran for adherence. For example, both glucan-positive and glucan-negative streptococci show increased adherence to damaged compared with normal canine and human valves in vitro, yet the increased adherence to damaged valve leaflets was found to be dependent on dextran production only for the glucan-positive strains.[14] When glucan-positive strains were grown in sucrose-deficient medium or pretreated with dextrinase, impairing their ability to produce dextran, they were equally adherent to normal and to damaged valves.[14] Adding exogenous dextran restored their increased adherence to the damaged valves.[14] In contrast, the increased adherence of glucan-negative strains was not dependent on dextran production.[14] Thus, other factors probably play a role.

Platelets also appear to be important in this process. Endocarditis-causing strains of bacteria were found to bind to and activate platelets in the presence of plasma proteins, whereas gram-negative bacilli, a rare cause of endocarditis, did not.[17] Compared with control animals, thrombocytopenic rabbits exhibit smaller vegetations but higher density of streptococci within the vegetations [colony-forming units (CFU) per gram of vegetation], suggesting that platelets inhibit bacterial proliferation and thus may limit disease progression in patients with endocarditis.[18] One mechanism by which platelets may accomplish that is the release of thrombin-induced platelet-microbicidal proteins (tPMPs) by activated platelets.[18,19] tPMPs act by causing permeabilization of the bacterial membrane and interfering with macromolecular synthesis.[20] tPMPs, which first were described in the rabbit model of IE, possess potent antistaphylococcal activity.[19] When strains of *Staphylococcus aureus* susceptible versus resistant to tPMPs are compared in their endocarditis characteristics, it appears that the susceptible strain produces more limited disease, as shown by lower bacteremia rates, smaller vegetations, and lesser degree of valvular damage and perivalvular inflammation as well as clinically relevant parameters such as later onset of valvular incompetence and increased preservation of ventricular function.[21] Bacteria could trigger the secretion of tPMPs via direct activation of platelets[17] or by induction of tissue factor, leading to thrombin formation, which in turn is a potent platelet agonist.[18] Human equivalents of tPMPs have been identified as well, termed thrombocidins.[22]

Growth of vegetation

Gross pathologic examination of the formed vegetation shows bacteria embedded in a matrix of fibrin and platelets, with a paucity of polymorphonuclear leukocytes (PMNs). Once the vegetation has formed on the valve surface, local proliferation of bacteria occurs, leading to an increase in size (Fig. 34-1). In addition, sustained bacteremia allows for reseeding of the vegetation.[23]

HISTORICAL BACKGROUND

Pelletier and Petersdorf[24] are credited with the first attempt to devise a schema of diagnostic criteria for IE. Their original classification included cases of definite, probable, and possible IE. To satisfy the definite criteria for diagnosis, histologic confirmation during surgery or

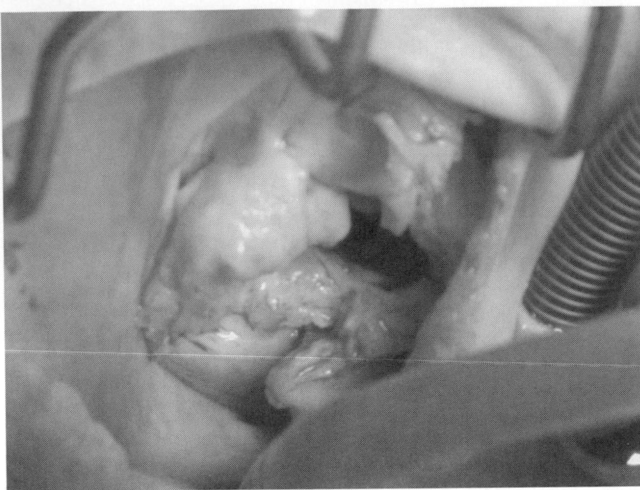

Figure 34-1 Intraoperative photograph of tricuspid endocarditis.

autopsy was required, excluding the majority of patients treated medically. The other two categories required persistently positive blood cultures so that patients with one negative culture among many positive ones were excluded, reducing the sensitivity of the diagnosis based on these criteria[24] (Table 34-1).

Von Reyn and associates retrospectively analyzed 123 cases with a discharge diagnosis of IE.[25] They classified those cases into definite, probable, possible, and rejected IE by modifying the criteria of Pelletier and Petersdorf, thus improving the sensitivity and specificity of the diagnosis. As with Pelletier and Petersdorf, the definite diagnosis of IE still required histologic confirmation. The two major modifications they introduced were (1) the idea of persistently positive instead of uniformly positive blood cultures (allowing for an occasional negative blood culture) and (2) the strict definition of heart conditions predisposing to endocarditis (definite valvular or congenital heart disease or a cardiac prosthesis).[25] All the cases that did not fit one of those diagnostic categories were rejected. Based on their definition system in this retrospective review, 15.4 percent (19 of 123) of cases were classified as definite, 35.8 percent (44 of 123) as probable, and 33.3 percent (41 of 123) as possible; 15.4 percent (19 of 123) were rejected. Within the rejected category, in 15 of the 19 patients, an alternative diagnosis was found, and in only 4 patients the diagnosis of IE could not be excluded definitively[25] (Table 34-2).

Table 34-1 The Pelletier and Petersdorf criteria for the diagnosis of infective endocarditis

1. *Definite infective endocarditis:* histologic evidence of infected endocardial vegetation(s) from examination of tissue obtained from cardiac surgery, embolectomy, or autopsy
2. *Probable infective endocarditis:* either uniformly positive blood cultures with known underlying heart disease *and* evidence of emboli to the skin or viscera or negative blood cultures in individuals with fever (>38°C), new regurgitant valvular heart murmurs, and embolic phenomena
3. *Possible infective endocarditis:* either uniformly positive blood cultures with known underlying heart disease *or* embolic phenomena or negative blood cultures with fever, known underlying heart disease, and embolic episodes

Source: From Pelletier and Petersdorf,[24] with permission.

Table 34-2 The Von Reyn criteria for the diagnosis of infective endocarditis

Definite
- Direct evidence of infective endocarditis based on histology from surgery or autopsy or on bacteriology (Gram stain or culture) of valvular vegetation or peripheral embolus

Probable
- A. Persistently positive blood cultures[a] plus one of the following:
  1. New regurgitant murmur or
  2. Predisposing heart disease[b] and vascular phenomena[c]
- B. Negative or intermittently positive blood cultures[d] plus all three of the following:
  1. Fever
  2. New regurgitant murmur
  3. Vascular phenomena

Possible
- A. Persistently positive blood cultures plus one of the following:
  1. Predisposing heart disease
  2. Vascular phenomena
- B. Negative or intermittently positive blood cultures with all three of the following:
  1. Fever
  2. Predisposing heart disease
  3. Vascular phenomena
- C. For streptococcus viridans cases only: at least two positive blood cultures without an extracardiac source, and fever

Rejected
- A. Endocarditis unlikely; alternative diagnosis generally apparent
- B. Endocarditis likely; empiric antibiotic therapy warranted
- C. Culture-negative endocarditis diagnosed clinically but excluded by postmortem

Source: From von Reyn et al,[25] with permission.

[a] At least two blood cultures obtained with two of two positive, three of three positive, or at least 70% of culture positive if four or more cultures obtained.

[b] Definite valvular or congenital heart disease or a cardiac prosthesis (excluding permanent pacemakers).

[c] Petechiae, splinter hemorrhages, conjunctival hemorrhages, Roth's spots, Osler's nodes, Janeway lesions, aseptic meningitis, glomerulonephritis, and pulmonary, central nervous system, coronary, or peripheral emboli.

[d] Any rate of blood culture positivity that does not meet the definition of persistently positive.

In 1994, the Duke Endocarditis Service published new criteria for the diagnosis of IE, utilizing specific echocardiographic findings.[26] Their diagnostic categories included definite, possible, and rejected IE. On the basis of those criteria, a definite diagnosis could be established by pathologic evidence of IE or clinically, using strictly defined major and minor criteria. Either two major, one major and three minor, or five minor criteria are required to establish the diagnosis. Major criteria include positive blood cultures for IE (either isolation of a typical organism for IE from two separate blood cultures or evidence of persistent bacteremia with an organism consistent with IE) and evidence of endocardial involvement (by echocardiography or detection of a new regurgitant murmur on clinical examination). Various minor criteria were proposed that, although nonspecific, when present in combination provide some supporting evidence for the diagnosis of suspected IE. Most of them are based on the various clinical manifestations of IE (fever, vascular phenomena, etc.) and the risk factors associated with it, such as predisposing heart conditions and intravenous drug use[26] (Table 34-3A and B).

Table 34-3 The Duke criteria for the diagnosis of infective endocarditis

A. Proposed New Criteria for Diagnosis of Infective Endocarditis

Definite infective endocarditis
- Pathologic criteria
  - Microorganisms: demonstrated by culture or histology in a vegetation, *or* in a vegetation that has embolized, *or* in an intracardiac abscess *or*
  - Pathologic lesions: vegetation or intracardiac abscess present, confirmed by histology, showing active endocarditis
- Clinical criteria, using specific definitions listed part B of this table
  - 2 major criteria *or*
  - 1 major criterion and 3 minor criteria *or*
  - 5 minor criteria

Possible infective endocarditis
- Findings consistent with infective endocarditis that fall short of "definite " but not "rejected"

Rejected
- Firm alternate diagnosis for manifestations or endocarditis, *or*
- Resolution of manifestations of endocarditis, with antibiotic therapy for 4 days or less, *or*
- No pathologic evidence of infective endocarditis at surgery or autopsy after antibiotic therapy for 4 days or less

B. Definitions of Terminology Used in the Proposed New Criteria

Major criteria
- Positive blood culture for infective endocarditis
  - Typical microorganism for infective endocarditis from two separate blood cultures
  - *Streptococcus viridans,*[a] *streptococcus bovis,* HACEK group, *or* community-acquired *Staphylococcus aureus* or enterococci in the absence of a primary focus, *or*
  - Persistently positive blood cultures, defined as recovery of a microorganism consistent with infective endocarditis from
    - (1) Blood cultures drawn more than 12 h apart *or*
    - (2) All three or a majority of four or more separate blood cultures, with first and last drawn at least 1 h apart
- Evidence of endocardial involvement
  - Positive echocardiogram for infective endocarditis
    - (1) Oscillating intracardiac mass on valve or supporting structures, *or* in the path of regurgitant jets, *or* on implanted material in the absence of an alternate anatomic explanation, *or*
    - (2) Abscess *or*
    - (3) New partial dehiscence of prosthetic valve *or*
  - New valvular regurgitation (increase or change in preexisting murmur not sufficient)

Minor criteria
- Predisposition: predisposing heart condition *or* intravenous drug use
- Fever: ≥38.0°C (100.4°F)
- Vascular phenomena: major arterial emboli, septic pulmonary infarcts, mycotic aneurysm, intracarnial hemorrhage, conjunctival hemorrhages, Janeway lesions
  - Immunologic phenomena: glomerulonephritis, Osler's nodes, Roth's spots, rheumatoid factor
- Microbiological evidence: positive blood culture but not meeting major criterion as noted previously[b] *or* serologic evidence of active infection with an organism consistent with infective endocarditis
- Echocardiogram: consistent with infective endocarditis but not meeting major criterion as noted previously

Source: Durack et al,[26] with permission.

HACEK=*Haemophilus* spp., *Actinobacillus actinomycetemcomitans, Cardiobacterium hominis, Eikenella* spp., and *Kingella kingae.*
[a]Including nutritional variant strains.
[b]Excluding single positive cultures for coagulase-negative staphylococci and organisms that do not cause endocarditis.

Dajani and associates ranked the risk of the various cardiac conditions for the development of IE as high, intermediate, and low.[27] The Duke criteria include only conditions that pose a high or intermediate risk and exclude those which confer only a low risk.[26] Using a subset of their patient population (n = 69) that had pathologically confirmed evidence of endocarditis, the investigators from the Duke Endocarditis Service applied their criteria as well as the older Von Reyn criteria and concluded that the Duke criteria had 80 percent (55 of 69) sensitivity compared with the 51 percent (35 of 69) sensitivity of the Von Reyn criteria.[26] The Duke criteria are also highly specific.[28–30] In a study of 100 patients with fever of unknown origin, the specificity of the Duke criteria was 99 percent.[30] In addition, the negative predictive value of the Duke criteria also approaches 100 percent, as was suggested by a study that followed a number of patients in whom the diagnosis of IE was rejected by the Duke criteria and found that none of them developed endocarditis during follow-up.[31] After their introduction, the Duke criteria were validated by multiple investigators.[28,29,31–37]

EPIDEMIOLOGY

Incidence

The incidence of IE in the general population is estimated to be between 3.2 and 11.6 cases per 100,000 person-years.[38–40] Endocarditis is more common in males and in the elderly (more than 65 years old).[41] Although predisposing factors usually are found in patients with IE, about a quarter of those patients do not have any identifiable cardiac lesion.[42,43] Valvular heart disease is the most common underlying condition (42.1 percent), followed by prosthetic valves (21.7 percent) and congenital heart disease (11.7 percent), cardiac pacemakers (1.3 percent), and hypertrophic cardiomyopathy (0.7 percent).[42] No previous heart disease is evident in 22.1 percent of cases.[42]

Risk factors

Congenital heart disease

Congenital cardiac malformations significantly increase the risk of IE. In one study, the incidence of IE among patients with a variety of heart defects was 120 per 100,000 person-years compared with the much lower incidence in the general population cited above.[44] The more common lesions predisposing to endocarditis include ventricular septal defects, transposition of the great vessels, tetralogy of Fallot, patent ductus arteriosus, and coarctation of the aorta. Among those lesions, cyanotic lesions are associated with a greater risk.[45]

In older patients, two important congenital lesions are bicuspid aortic valves and mitral valve prolapse. The presence of mitral valve prolapse is estimated to increase the risk of endocarditis 5.3- to 8.2-fold.[46,47] This increase is attributed to mitral valve prolapse associated with a regurgitant murmur, as the presence of mitral valve prolapse without a systolic murmur was not a risk factor.[46,47] In one study, the incidence of IE in patients with mitral valve prolapse associated with a systolic murmur was estimated to be 52 per 100,000 person-years, compared with 4.6 per 100,000 person-years in patients with mitral valve prolapse without a murmur; the latter incidence was similar to the incidence in the general population.[48] Congenital lesions not associated with turbulent flow usually do not contribute to an increased risk of IE. For example, the risk of an isolated atrial septal defect (ASD) without mitral regurgitation is low.[45]

Acquired heart disease

Rheumatic heart disease, which once was an important risk factor for endocarditis, has given way to other acquired cardiac diseases, many iatrogenic, such as intravenous drug use (IVDU) and nosocomial endocarditis associated with increasing use of intravascular catheters and intracardiac devices such as pacemakers and automatic implanted cardiac defibrillators (AICDs). Degenerative heart disease continues to be an important risk factor, especially with aging of the population. Commonly encountered abnormalities are sclerosis or calcification of the aortic valve and mitral annular or chordal calcification.[43] Other risk factors include a previous episode of endocarditis[49,50] and valvular surgery, especially replacement with prosthetic valves.

CLINICAL PRESENTATION

Subacute bacterial endocarditis

Symptoms usually occur within 2 weeks of the initial infection, and an incubation period longer than 1 month is rare. The initial presentation is that of nonspecific symptoms that are mild and subtle in nature, leading to a delay in diagnosis as a result of both patient reluctance to seek medical attention and physician failure to include IE in the differential diagnosis. A high index of suspicion is therefore necessary for the prompt diagnosis of this condition. The most common presenting symptoms are persistent low-grade fever, malaise, anorexia, weight loss, fatigue, and generalized myalgias, especially low back pain. Arthralgias and arthritis are produced by immune complex deposition in the various joints. Arthritis tends to be asymmetric and oligoarticular. Most of these manifestations disappear promptly on initiation of appropriate antimicrobial therapy. On occasion, subacute bacterial endocarditis may present as a chronic wasting illness that may mimic cancer or HIV.[51]

Many of the initial manifestations of subacute disease are caused by the various complications of IE, with a prolonged course secondary to a delay in diagnosis. Embolic phenomena may result in (1) sudden onset of neurologic symptoms, depending on the territory of the occluded cerebral vessel, (2) acute arterial insufficiency, especially in the lower extremities, (3) sudden onset of left or right upper quadrant pain after embolic infarction of the kidney or spleen, (4) acute unilateral blindness after occlusion of a retinal artery, (5) myocardial infarction after embolization into a coronary artery, (6) embolic pulmonary infarcts with right-sided endocarditis leading to symptoms resembling pneumonia, (7) painless hematuria induced by multiple small renal infarcts, and (8) dyspnea or chest pain secondary to septic pulmonary emboli. Progressive scarring or destruction of the infected valve may lead to new-onset congestive heart failure (CHF). Renal disease could be a part of the initial presentation in the form of interstitial nephritis, proliferative glomerulonephritis, or, rarely, renal failure secondary to renal emboli. Mycotic aneurysms are usually asymptomatic but may present with symptoms of an expanding mass or, if rupture occurs, with headache and other symptoms of intracranial hemorrhage.

Acute bacterial endocarditis

The initial manifestations in acute disease are different from those in subacute disease. Acute bacterial endocarditis usually involves the left side of the heart. Patients present early in the course of infection with high-grade fevers, chills, lethargy, and profound malaise and rapidly progress to severe sepsis and circulatory collapse. Thus, it is crucial to establish the diagnosis quickly to institute an appropriate antimicrobial therapy. Complications are common and usually occur within a week of disease onset. Destruction of the valves occurs rapidly, leading to symptoms of CHF. Symptoms related to embolic events are common, especially with involvement of the aortic valve (see "Subacute Bacterial Endocarditis," above).

Prosthetic valve endocarditis

Prosthetic valve endocarditis is divided into early and late depending on whether it occurs within 60 days or more than 60 days after valve replacement.[51] Early prosthetic valve endocarditis is related to either intraoperative contamination or postoperative complications that increase the risk of developing prosthetic valve endocarditis, such as reoperation for bleeding and prolonged intubation secondary to pulmonary complications,[51] as discussed previously in the material on risk factors. The clinical presentation is similar to that of acute bacterial endocarditis. Late prosthetic valve endocarditis, in contrast, presents more like subacute bacterial endocarditis and commonly is caused by the same pathogenic organisms.[51]

Complications of IE

Complication rates are high at above 80 percent.[52] Although discussed separately in this section for the sake of completeness, they frequently are part of the initial presentation of the disease. The most common complications of IE are CHF, embolic events (especially stroke), and perivalvular abscess formation.

Congestive heart failure

CHF is the most common cause of death in patients with IE. It most commonly results from destruction of intracardiac valves, leading to acute volume overload. Other rare causes of CHF include (1) embolization of vegetation components into the coronary arteries, leading to a myocardial infarction (MI) that subsequently may be complicated by CHF if it is large, (2) functional valve stenosis caused by very large vegetations, typically fungal, but also possibly by staphylococci and even vancomycin-resistant enterococci (VRE), and (3) rupture of the papillary muscles of the mitral valve from infection, resulting in acute mitral valve regurgitation (MVR). Patients with aortic valve involvement are at especially high risk of developing acute-onset CHF.[53,54]

Intracardiac abscess

Abscess formation occurs when the necrotic process extends from the base of the vegetation into the surrounding myocardium. The incidence of perivalvular abscess ranges from 13 percent in one clinical series to 30 percent at autopsy to as high as 41 percent when the aortic valve is involved.[55–57] In patients with prosthetic valve endocarditis at the aortic position, the incidence of abscess formation is exceedingly high, reaching 78 percent in one large series, with many of the abscesses being multiple.[58] The abscesses most commonly involve the aortic valve and may extend to the anterior mitral valve leaflet or the interventricular or intraatrial septum. Previously undetected atrioventricular or right bundle branch block strongly suggests the presence of an abscess.[59] Aortic valve involvement combined with IVDU increases the relative risk of abscess formation by a factor of 2.5.[60] Other clinical parameters that increase the suspicion that an abscess has formed include the presence of pericarditis, CHF, a prosthetic valve, valvular regurgitation, and *Staph. aureus* endocarditis.[61] Abscess formation is associated with high mortality: 57 percent cumulative mortality at 4.5 years of follow-up in one small study.[62] Transesophageal echocardiography (TEE) is the study of choice for the diagnosis of perivalvular abscess, with a sensitivity of 80 percent compared with 36 percent for transthoracic echocardiography (TTE).[63] Echocardiographic signs of perivalvular abscess formation include (1) anterior or posterior aortic root thickness greater than 9 mm, (2) perivalvular density greater than 14 mm in the interventricular septum, (3) sinus of Valsalva defects or aneurysms, and (4) abnormal rocking motility of prosthetic valves.[54]

Pseudoaneurysm (mycotic aneurysm)

Liquefaction of abscess contents within cardiac structures may lead to a contained rupture. The resulting cavity is exposed to high pulsatile pressures, and over time, pseudoanurysm formation occurs. This may occur in the aortic root, in the ventricular wall, or in rare cases in the anterior leaflet of the mitral valve. The incidence of pseudoaneurysm is between 2 and 10 percent.[64] Extension of the necrosis also can result in leaflet perforation, chordal or papillary muscle rupture, rupture of the interventricular septum or the ventricular free wall, and dehiscence of prosthetic valves.

Purulent pericarditis

Suppurative pericarditis results from the extension of a myocardial or annular abscess into the pericardial space. It is characterized by high fever and a high white blood cell (WBC) count, severe chest pain, and rapid deterioration in the patient's condition.

Extracardiac mycotic aneurysms

Extracardiac mycotic aneurysms may develop in distant blood vessels when the vessel wall becomes the focus of infection from the persistent bacteremia or as a result of embolization of a valvular vegetation. Intracranial mycotic aneurysms usually involve the distal branches of the middle cerebral artery. Leakage or rupture of these aneurysms can present with stroke or subarachnoid hemorrhage.

Fistulas

Both abscesses and pseudoaneurysms may rupture into the surrounding structures, forming fistulas. This type of rupture can occur in one of the cardiac chambers, leading to intracardiac shunt, or in the pericardium, leading to tamponade, worsening the already poor hemodynamics. Fistula formation is a rare complication of IE, with an incidence ranging from less than 1 to 9 percent in the different studies, with the higher incidence occurring in studies limited to prosthetic valve endocarditis.[58,63,65–67] Mortality exceeds 50 percent.[65]

Conduction abnormalities

Extension of the infectious process to conduction tissues results in various conduction abnormalities, with a reported incidence between 14 and 26 percent in various studies.[68–71] The most commonly observed abnormality is first-degree atrioventricular (AV) block.[68] The development of electrocardiographic (ECG) changes is not associated with any particular microorganism.[68] New-onset ECG changes should raise suspicion for invasive infection, especially abscess formation. In one prospective study, patients with new conduction defects had twofold higher mortality compared with patients without them.[68]

Cerebrovascular accident

Embolic complications are common in patients with IE. They are more common in younger patients than in the elderly.[72,73] The main embolic complications are stroke, splenic or renal infarcts, and septic pulmonary emboli.

Stroke is a common complication of IE. It occurs when a vegetation or a part of one embolizes to a distant blood vessel in the brain. Among patients with left-sided endocarditis, mitral valve vegetations are more common, are larger, and are three times more likely to result in stroke compared with vegetations on the aortic valve.[74] For prosthetic valve endocarditis, there does not appear to be a difference in the rate of stroke between mitral valve and aortic valve vegetations.[74] However, when native valve infections are compared, the risk of stroke is approximately five times higher in patients with mitral valve versus aortic valve involvement.[74] Important predictors of stroke in patients with left-sided endocarditis are mitral valve (MV) vegetation and size greater than 7 mm.[74] Similarly, vegetation size is an important predictor of death, although the difference in the risk of death in patients with MV versus AV involvement is not statistically significant.[74] Therefore, stroke remains a major morbidity issue. Hemorrhagic stroke is considered a relative contraindication for valve replacement.[75] With ischemic strokes, there is a risk of conversion to hemorrhagic stroke after the initiation of cardiopulmonary bypass (CPB). However, in patients with stroke and CHF, the risk of further neurologic compromise must be weighed against the risk of death from CHF.[75]

Metastatic abscess

Abscesses can migrate and develop virtually anywhere in the body and most frequently present with persistent fever despite adequate antimicrobial therapy.[75] The spleen is a common site of abscess formation. Although some abscesses can be managed by percutaneous drainage, when they occur in the spleen, they are best managed with splenectomy. A small study investigated mortality in patients with endocarditis complicated by splenic abscess and found that those who underwent splenectomy had 18 percent mortality compared with 100 percent mortality among those who were treated conservatively.[76]

Septic arthritis

Patients with prosthetic joints are particularly likely to experience this complication. In a small prospective study (n = 53), 34 percent of patients with prosthetic joints and *Staph. aureus* bacteremia developed infection of their prostheses.[77] Management is usually conservative unless frank purulent fluid collections, fistulas, or prosthetic instability develops.[75]

Renal failure

Renal insufficiency may result from emboli, severe sepsis, or immune complex–mediated processes such as glomerulonephritis.

Septic pulmonary emboli

Septic pulmomary emboli are common in intravenous drug users who present with tricuspid valve endocarditis. These emboli may undergo necrosis with cavitation. During the initial presentation, septic pulmonary emboli may be mistaken for pneumonia, especially if IVDU is not immediately obvious.

DIAGNOSIS

History and physical examination

Obtaining a thorough history is a very important part of the diagnostic process. The examining physician should elicit the presence of absence of the major presenting symptoms of IE. On physical examination, cardiac murmur is the cornerstone finding of IE. It almost always is present in patients with subacute disease but may be absent in those with right-sided endocarditis or acute disease. In contrast, the appearance of a new regurgitant murmur is most common with aortic involvement by acute endocarditis with rapid destruction of the valve. The wide pulse pressure characteristic of chronic aortic regurgitation is typically absent with acute aortic regurgitation. Fever, tachycardia, and anemia may lead to a systolic ejection murmur caused by an increase in cardiac output that may be difficult to distinguish from a pathologic murmur. With tricuspid valve endocarditis, the pulmonary artery pressure is often normal and the murmur of tricuspid regurgitation is a soft crescendo-decrescendo murmur that may be difficult to detect unless right ventricular failure has occurred with elevated right ventricular systolic pressures resulting in the typical pansystolic murmur. Fever frequently is detected and is more commonly present in patients with positive cultures than in patients with culture-negative endocarditis (80.7 percent versus 50.0 percent).[78]

Physical examination may reveal signs of CHF or evidence of emboli such as deficits on neurologic examination, decreased peripheral pulses from arterial occlusion, and pericardial rub with pericardial involvement by the disease process. Pallor of the skin and mucous membranes is almost always present and results from anemia. Splenomegaly, petechiae, and clubbing of the fingers may be present with long-standing untreated disease. Splenomegaly is seen more commonly in patients with acute disease. Petechiae occur commonly in groups on the palate, conjunctivae, buccal mucosa, and upper extremities and usually are seen in the setting of long-standing disease. Various cutaneous manifectations of IE have been described. They may be present in various combinations. Their etiology (vascular versus immunologic) often is debated. None are pathopneumonic, but all are fascinating and usually are discussed out of proportion to their clinical utility. Osler's nodes are exquisitely tender, painful raised erythematous lesions with a central area of pallor. They usually measure 0.5 to 1.5 cm and typically occur on the tips of the fingers but also may be present on the tips of the toes, the thenar and hypothenar area of the hands, and the lower arms. They last for hours to days (typically a day) and then spontaneously disappear. Janeway lesions are irregular, painless, slightly nodular erythematous lesions, 2 to 5 mm in size, that typically present on the palms of the hands and the soles of the feet and slowly disappear. Splinter hemorrhages are longitudinal dark red streaks under the nail beds. Although they may be seen in IE patients, they also may occur as a result of trauma. Petechiae may be found, typically on the soft palate, the buccal mucosa, and the extremities. They usually appear in crops and then fade away in 2 to 3 days. Roth's spots are oval retinal hemorrhages with a central area of pallor.

Laboratory data

Multiple laboratory abnormalities may be present in patients with IE; none are specific for the disease, but together they provide support for the suspected diagnosis. Leukocytosis is often absent but may be marked with acute endocarditis. It may be seen more commonly in the elderly (over 65 years of age) (61.2 percent versus 40.2 percent).[79] Anemia is almost always present and is of the normochromic normocytic variety. Creatinine may be elevated if renal damage has occurred. On urinalysis, proteinuria and/or hematuria are common. Other laboratory abnormalities include an elevated erythrocyte sedimentation rate (ESR), the presence of rheumatoid factor, and decreased levels of serum complement.

The cornerstone laboratory abnormality in IE is the presence of persistent bacteremia. To maximize the information obtained from the blood cultures, it is essential that the skin be prepped adequately to avoid contamination by skin microflora. This is especially important in patients with suspected prosthetic valve endocarditis, in whom the leading causative pathogen is coagulase-negative *Staphylococcus*, which is also the major skin pathogen and thus the major cause of false-positive cultures.[80] Blood should not be obtained from indwelling catheters, which may be contaminated, thus making it impossible to distinguish between bacteremia caused by IE and that caused by a line infection. An adequate amount of blood must be obtained, especially to make an accurate diagnosis of subacute endocarditis, which typically causes low-grade bacteremia with only 1 to 10 CFU per milliliter of venous blood.[81] According to the Duke criteria, blood cultures aid in the diagnosis of IE if there are two positive blood cultures for the same organism drawn 12 or more hours apart or all of three or the majority of four blood cultures are positive for the same organism, with the first and last drawn at least 1 h apart.[26]

With rare organisms such as *Brucella* spp., *Bartonella* spp., *Legionella* spp., *Mycobacterium* spp., *Nocardia* spp., and rickettsial species, one positive blood culture is acceptable.[82] The amount of blood drawn is also important. Current recommendations suggest that 20 mL of blood be obtained per two-bottle blood culture set (one aerobic and one anaerobic medium). Each set is defined as blood obtained from a single venipuncture.[80] For pediatric patients, the amount of blood needed per blood culture set is 10 to 20 mL for adolescents, 3 to 5 mL for older children, 2 to 3 mL for infants age 1 month to 2 years, and 1 to 2 mL for neonates.[80] The diagnosis of fungal endocarditis can be challenging. Although the same methods for obtaining blood cultures are used, the sensitivity of preoperative blood cultures for establishing the diagnosis was only 45 percent in one study.[83] If routine blood cultures remain negative but the clinical suspicion is high, blood cultures should be obtained by using a specialized medium that optimally supports fungal growth. In addition, serologic testing for fungi may be used to establish the diagnosis of histoplasmosis or cryptococcosis endocarditis.[84] Routine cultures usually are incubated for 5 to 7 days, after which a final result is reported by the microbiology laboratory. If the presence of fastidious organisms is suspected, the incubation period may be extended to a total of 2 to 3 weeks.

Newer methods are available to aid in the diagnosis of IE when traditional blood culture systems do not provide the causative pathogen. Molecular biological techniques such as DNA amplification methods are useful in cases of culture-negative endocarditis or when traditional blood culture methods yield a pathogen with unusual characteristics that evades correct taxonomic positioning. Polymerase chain reaction (PCR) is a widely available method. The amplification of highly conserved genetic sequences that are present in all bacteria can be used to identify nonculturable pathogens.[82] The bacterial 16S ribosomal gene contains highly conserved regions and has emerged as one such target.[82] In addition, specific primers are available for many bacterial genera, including most of the causative pathogens of culture-negative endocarditis.[85] Another novel method is the detection of bacterial antigens in urine samples. Currently available for pneumoccocal antigen, this technique has promise as a rapid method of diagnosing IE.[84]

Imaging studies

Plain chest radiography

Findings on plain chest x-ray (CXR) are nonspecific but nevertheless may provide supportive evidence for the diagnosis of IE. Cardiomegaly may indicate CHF or pericardial involvement. Pulmonary congestion also may be seen with CHF. Prosthetic valves may be visualized and their position may be determined if patients cannot recall their history. Multiple nodular infiltrates may be seen, suggestive of septic pulmonary emboli, especially in patients with IVDU. On serial radiographs, some of these infiltrates may disappear as new ones appear. Cavitation with air-fluid levels also may be present. In endocarditis complicated by a splenic infarct, a left pleural effusion may be seen.

Other imaging modalities, such as computed tomography (CT), magnetic resonance imaging (MRI), and nuclear medicine imaging, have a limited role in the diagnosis of IE and rarely offer any information beyond that provided by CXR and echocardiography.

Echocardiography

Echocardiography is the imaging modality of choice for the diagnosis of IE. The hallmark finding is the detection of a vegetation, which is defined as an irregularly shaped echogenic mass on the surface of the involved cardiac structure (valve, myocardium, or intracardiac device) that moves in an oscillating fashion throughout the cardiac cycle (Fig. 34-2). Vegetations typically occur on the

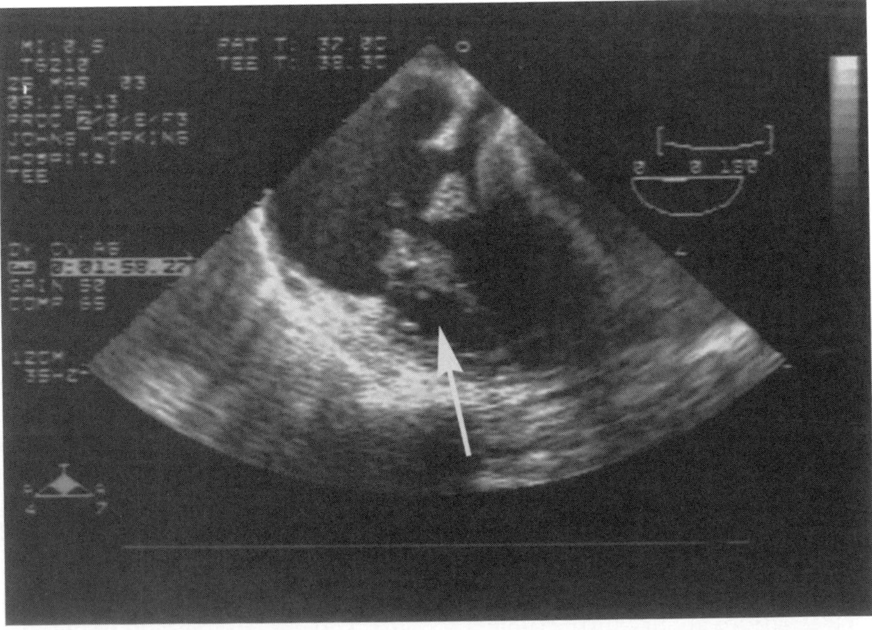

Figure 34-2 Transthoracic echocardiographic image of tricuspid valve vegetations resulting from infective bacterial endocarditis.

atrial side of mitral and tricuspid valves and on the ventricular side of aortic and pulmonary valves, as originally described by Rodbard.[11] Although cardiac valves are the most commonly involved, vegetations also may occur on the atrial and venricular endothelium, typically at the site of impact of a high-velocity jet or shunt, as well as on intracardiac devices such as atrial or ventricular pacing leads. Echocardiography is also the primary modality for the detection and characterization of cardiac complications that result from endocardial infection.[86–89] Prosthetic valve dehiscence is characterized by a rocking motion with excursion greater than 15 degrees in at least one direction.[61] Rarely, gross separation of the prosthetic annulus may be detected.

Abscesses have a variable appearance on echocardiography. They may appear as echogenic, echolucent, or heterogeneous masses or areas of thickening within the myocardium or valve annulus. An echo-free space suggests that complete liquefaction of the abscess contents has occurred. A pseudoaneurysm is detected as flow within the abscess cavity after its rupture. Fistulas appear as shunting of a high-velocity jet of blood during systole. Leaflet perforation is seen as a defect in the leaflet accompanied by the flow of blood through it. Ruptured chords are seen as independently moving strands attached to leaflets or papillary muscles. Rheumatic valvular lesions, a rare cause of endocarditis in the modern era, are seen as a restricted valve opening secondary to diffuse thickening of the valve leaflets with or without concomitant commissural thickening.

Transthoracic versus transesophageal echocardiography

The original Von Reyn criteria for the diagnosis of IE, although very specific, were not very sensitive. The introduction of the Duke criteria into clinical practice made the diagnosis of IE easier, partly because of the inclusion of echocardiographic findings as part of the major criteria. More recently, a new diagnostic dilemma has emerged with the advent of TTE. Transthoracic echocardiography is an excellent diagnostic modality with a specificity approaching 98 percent.[90] The sensitivity of TTE varies with the size of the vegetation (almost zero for vegetations less than 5 mm, 50 percent for vegetations 5 to 10 mm, and 84 percent for vegetations larger than 10 mm).[91] Overall, the sensitivity of TEE has been shown to be superior to that of TTE by many investigators.[90–97] The specificity of TEE is high (88 to 100 percent), and the sensitivity of TEE approaches 100 percent on native valves and 86 to 94 percent on prosthetic valves.[57,95,96,98,99] This compares well with the overall sensitivity of TTE for the detection of IE of less than 60 percent.[90,91,97,98,100] The improved sensitivity of TEE compared with TTE is the result of several factors. First, the utilization of the transesophageal approach allows decreased distance between the probe and the heart, with the subsequent opportunity to use higher-frequency probes, which offer better spatial resolution. Second, in the setting of prosthetic valves, the anterior approach offered by TTE does not allow visualization of the posterior aspects of the mitral valve because of the acoustic shadows created by the prosthetic material. Mitral regurgitation is visualized better from the atrial aspect offered by TEE. In addition, the various complications of endocarditis are better visualized via TEE. Several patient-related factors compromise the ability to obtain a technically adequate TTE study as a result of marked attenuation of sound conduction. These factors include obesity, chest wall deformities, and pulmonary processes that result in hyperinflated lungs [emphysema, chronic obstructive pulmonary disease (COPD), mechanical ventilation]. In the elderly, the differentiation of vegetations from the degenerative valvular changes that are encountered commonly in this age group may be facilitated by TEE images.[98] Lambl's excrescences are thin filamentous echodense mobile strands composed of collagen that are detected frequently on prosthetic valves but also may be associated with native valves.[101–104] Their clinical significance is unclear, but they have been accepted as a normal variant.

Several factors should be considered when one is deciding to obtain TTE versus TEE to diagnose IE. The advantages and disadvantages of each modality must be compared. Although more sensitive, TEE is invasive in nature and more expensive. In addition, it may not be immediately available. Although frequently performed when IE is suspected, echocardiography may not always be necessary to confirm the diagnosis. In the Duke criteria, echocardiography is one of two ways to provide evidence of endocardial involvement, and that is only one of the major criteria. The higher sensitivity of TEE certainly offers an advantage over TTE for the detection of vegetations; however, in the face of a lack of other clinical findings to support a diagnosis of IE, the detection of a vegetation may merely indicate a thrombus and cannot be used to establish the diagnosis.

Roe and associates[94] studied 112 patients who had undergone both TTE and TEE to determine the incremental benefit of obtaining TEE compared with TTE. In that study, TTE initially was used as part of the Duke criteria, and a diagnostic category was assigned on the basis of the findings of TTE examination. Reassignment of the diagnostic category then was evaluated when TEE was used instead of TTE in the same cohort of patients.[94] When the pretest likelihood of IE was high, category reassignment rarely occurred and a TTE was usually sufficient to establish the diagnosis.[94] Diagnostic reassignment occurred mainly in patients with an intermediate pretest likelihood of a positive diagnosis and more often in patients with prosthetic valves (11 percent of episodes of suspected IE with native valves and 34 percent of episodes with prosthetic valves).[94] In those patients, the majority of negative TTE studies followed by a positive TEE necessitated a reassignment from possible to definite endocarditis and only rarely from rejected to possible endocarditis.[94] This study did not evaluate the quality of the TTE exams, and it is possible that some of the negative TTE studies were technically inadequate, thus underestimating the utility of TTE.

A conservative approach to the use of TEE uses the pretest likelihood of having IE to determine which test to obtain in pursuit of the diagnosis. Patients with a low clinical suspicion of endocarditis who are at low risk of complications if endocarditis is present are candidates for the use of TTE as an initial study. A technically adequate negative study may direct the investigation in another direction, assuming a noncardiac etiology of the patient's presentation. If the clinical picture changes later, TEE may be obtained.[90,98] In patients with a high pretest likelihood of the disease, TTE usually is sufficient to establish a definite diagnosis of IE.[94] TTE may be particularly useful for the evaluation of the tricuspid valve, as the physical proximity of that valve to the chest wall allows excellent visualization. However, for patients with an intermediate likelihood of having IE, TEE may be used as the initial study of choice, especially in patients who are difficult to image with TTE and those with a high risk of complications.

For patients with prosthetic valves, TEE should be obtained first as it repeatedly has been shown to be superior to TTE in this patient population.[95,105,106] Despite the high sensitivity of TEE, false-negative studies occur with this modality as well.[98] The vegetation size may be below the limit of resolution, the vegetation may have embolized and therefore no longer is present, and inadequate study or acoustic shadowing may interfere with the detection of the vegetation.[98] Therefore, if the clinical suspicion persists in the face of negative TEE study, another study should be obtained in 7 to 10 days.[98] However, a negative TEE virtually excludes the diagnosis of IE in a patient with native valves in whom the diagnosis is suspected.[94]

MEDICAL MANAGEMENT

The cornerstone of medical management for IE is proper antimicrobial therapy. It is therefore crucial to identify the causative organism to guide therapy. When patients present with the subacute syndrome, there is no urgency to initiate empiric therapy and risk further inability to isolate the causative pathogen. Instead, the proper blood cultures should be obtained to establish the diagnosis, and then therapy should be initiated on the basis of the microbiological susceptibility data. This ideal clinical scenario may not be feasible if the patient presents late with advanced disease and a grave clinical condition or with acute endocarditis caused by highly virulent pathogens. In this situation, two to three culture sets should be obtained from separate venipuncures within 5 min[80] and empiric therapy should initiated, based on an assessment of the risk factors present as well as the clinical findings, to postulate the most likely organism.

In patients with native valves who are not intravenous drug users, streptococci cause more than half of cases of IE, with the majority of these cases caused by *S. viridans*, followed by staphylococci (with *Staph. aureus* 5 to 10 times more common than *Staphylococcus epidermidis*) and enterococci.[107] *Haemophilus aphrophilus, Actinobacillus actinomycetemcomitans, Cardiobacterium hominis, Eikenella corrodens,* and *Kingella kingae* (HACEK) organisms are members of the oropahryngeal flora that have emerged as an important cause or endocarditis.[107] They typically cause subacute disease and are difficult to isolate, necessitating continued empiric therapy.[107] For patients with native valve endocarditis who present with subacute disease, antibiotic therapy should be delayed until blood cultures are drawn and microbiological data become available as long as a patient is stable and monitored. If empiric therapy must be initiated, a combination of penicillin and gentamicin is reasonable as it is aimed toward the majority of the causative pathogens. If staphylococcal involvement is suspected, penicillinase-resistant penicillins such as nafcillin (or oxacillin) plus gentamicin may be used unless there is high suspicion for the presence of methicillin-resistant *Staphylococcus aureus* (MRSA) or the patient is allergic to beta-lactam. If the cultures remain negative and the patient's clinical status is not improving, ampicillin may be added to cover the HACEK group of organisms, as they are difficult to isolate from blood. Endocarditis caused by *S. viridans* and *Streptococcus bovis* can be cured by a 2-week course of a beta-lactam plus aminoglycoside combination provided that certain condition are fulfilled (Table 34-4).[108]

In injection drug users, the most commonly isolated pathogen is *Staph. aureus*, which accounts for more than half of cases of infective endocarditis, followed by streptococci and enterococci.[109] The choice of empiric antimicrobial agents in this patient population should take into account the usual pathogens encountered in a particular community, the prevalence of MRSA in isolated pathogens, the patient's allergy profile, and resistance data from the hospital's microbiology department. If the prevalence of MRSA is low and the patient is not allergic

Table 34-4 Criteria favoring the use of short-course, 2-week beta-lactam plus aminoglycoside combination therapy for penicillin-sensitive streptococcal endocarditis

1. Penicillin-sensitive oral (viridans group) streptococcus or *streptococcus bovis* (minimum inhibitory concentration $\leq$ 0.125 mg/L)
2. Native valve endocarditis
3. No heart failure, no aortic insufficiency, no conduction abnormalities
4. No evidence of extracardiac metastatic septic foci
5. Vegetation size $\leq$ 10 mm in diameter
6. Favorable clinical response within 7 days, including resolution of fever

Source: Adapted from Hoen,[108] with permission.

Table 34-5 Native valve endocarditis involving penicillin-susceptible *Streptococcus viridans* and *Streptococcus bovis* (minimum inhibitory concentration ≤ 0.1 μg/mL)[a]

Antibiotic	Dosage and route	Duration, weeks	Comments
Aqueous crystalline penicillin G sodium	12–18 million U/24 h IV either continuously or in 6 equally divided doses	4	Preferred in most patients > 65years and in those with impairment of the eighth nerve or renal function
or			
Cefriaxone sodium	2 g once daily IV or IM[b]	4	
Aqueous crystalline penicillin G sodium with gentamicin sulfate[c]	12–18 million U/24 h IV either continuously or in 6 equally divided doses	2	When obtained 1 h after a 20- to 30-min IV infusion or IM injection, serum concentration of gentamicin of approximately
	1 mg/kg IM or IV every 8 h	2	3 μg/mL is desirable; through concentration should be < 1 μg/mL
Vancomycin hydrochloride[d]	30 mg/kg per 24 h IV in 2 equally divided doses, not to exceed 2 g/24 h unless serum levels are monitored	4	Vancomycin therapy is recommended for patients allergic to beta-lactams; peak serum concentrations of vancomycin should be obtained 1 h after completion of infusion and should be in the range of 30–45 μg/mL for twice-daily dosing

Source: From Wilson et al,[116] with permission.

IV = intravenous; IM = imtramuscular.

[a] Dosages recommended are for patients with normal renal function. For nutritionally variant streptococci, see Table 34-7.

[b] Patients should be informed that IM injection of ceftriaxone is painful.

[c] Dosing of gentamicin on a mg/kg basis will produce higher serum concentrations in obese patients than in lean patients. Therefore, in obese patients, dosing should be based on ideal body weight. (Ideal body weight for males in 50 kg + 2.3kg/in > 5 ft; ideal body weight for females is 45.5 kg + 2.3 kg/in > 5 ft.) Relative contraindications to use of gentamicin are age > 65 years renal impairment, and impairment of the eighth nerve. Other potentially nephrotoxic agents (eg, nonsteroidal anti-inflammatory drugs) should be used cautiously in patients receiving gentamycin.

[d] Vancomycin dose should be reduced in patients with impaired renal function. Vancomycin given on a mg/kg basis will produce higher serum concentrations in obese patients than in lean patients. Therefore, in obese patients, dosing should be based on ideal body weight. Each dose of vancomycin should be infused over ≥ 1 h to reduce the risk of the histamine-release "red man" syndrome.

to beta-lactams, empiric therapy with nafcillin (or oxacillin) plus gentamicin should suffice until microbiology data become available. If the patient is allergic to beta-lactams, the prevalence of MRSA in the community is high, or the patient is hemodynamically unstable, empiric therapy with vancomycin plus gentamicin is reasonable. The use of tripelenamine and pentazocine ("Ts and blues") has been associated with *Pseudomonas aeruginosa* endocarditis,[110] and antipseudomonal coverage may be added to the empiric regimen. Gram-negative bacteria constitute less than 2 percent of bacteria found in this patient population.[111] Thus, their routine empiric coverage is probably unwarranted. IVDU is a major risk factor for fungal endocarditis.[83] In any critically ill patient who is not improving on empiric vancomycin plus gentamicin, the addition of antifungal drugs should be considered pending microbiological data. Other risk factors for fungal endocarditis include dialysis, long-term intravenous catheters, prolonged use of antibiotics, hyperalimentation, immunosuppression, and implantation of prosthetic devices such as heart valves and pacemakers.[112]

For patients with uncomplicated right-sided endocarditis caused by methicillin-susceptible *Staph. aureus*, 2-week therapy with nafcillin plus gentamicin may be adequate to achieve a cure. Chambers and associates[113] compared a 2-week regimen of nafcillin plus aminoglycoside with a 2-week regimen of vancomycin plus aminoglycoside for tricuspid valve *Staph. aureus* endocarditis and found a success rate of 94 percent for the nafcillin arm. The vancomycin arm was stopped early because of a high rate of failure to cure.[113] In this study, patients with left-sided involvement, renal failure, extrapulmonary metastatic infection, and infection caused by MRSA as well as pregnant patients were excluded.[113] These results have been confirmed by others.[114,115] For specific treatment options for various pathogens, refer to Tables 34-5 through 34-11.

SURGICAL MANAGEMENT

The indications for surgical intervention in the setting of IE are summarized below (Table 34-12).[116–119]

Mitral valve endocarditis

Mitral valve repair

The surgical options for mitral valve endocarditis are limited to valve repair and valve replacement. Valve repair

Table 34-6 Native valve endocarditis involving *Streptococcus viridans* and *Streptococcus bovis* relatively resistant to penicillin G (minimum inhibitory concentration > 0.1 μg/mL and < 0.5 μg/mL)[a]

Antibiotic	Dosage and route	Duration, weeks	Comments
Aqueous crystalline penicillin G sodium with gentamicin sulfate[b]	18 million U/24 h IV either continuously or in 6 equally divided doses.	4	Cefazolin or other first-generation cephalosporins may be substituted for penicillin in patients whose penicillin hypersensitivity is not of the immediate type
	1 mg/kg IM/IV every 8 h	2	
Vancomycin hydrochloride[c]	30 mg/kg per 24 h IV in 2 equally divided doses, not to exceed 2 g/24 h unless serum levels are monitored	4	Vancomycin therapy is recommended for patients allergic to beta-lactams

Source: From Wilson et al,[116] with permission.

IV = intravenous; IM = imtramuscular.

[a]Dosages recommended are for patients with normal renal function.

[b]For specific dosing adjustment and issues concerning gentamicin (obese patients, relative contraindications), see Table 34-5 footnotes.

[c]For specific dosing adjustment and issues concerning vancomycin (obese patients, length of infusion), see Table 34-5 footnotes.

offers superior outcomes to valve replacement and is therefore the procedure of choice in patients with mitral valve endocarditis whenever feasible. The infection usually begins on the leaflet surface and subsequently spreads to involve the annulus and the surrounding myocardium. Thus, early operation is advocated by some, especially in patients with more aggressive pathogens such as *Staph. aureus*, even in the setting of active infection, to increase the chance of achieving valve repair.[120] Various techniques have been developed to allow the cardiac surgeon to preserve the mitral valve while achieving complete resection of all infected tissue. Small leaflet perforations can be managed with primary repair. Larger perforations can be repaired with an autologous pericardial patch (Fig. 34-3) soaked in 0.6% glutaraldehyde solution for 10 min and then washed with saline before insertion so that the smooth surface of the pericardium faces the left atrium.[120] With this technique, the entire anterior leaflet can be replaced by an autologous pericardium patch provided that the marginal chordae are free of infection.[120] After complete debridement, posterior leaflet defects can be repaired with a quadrangular resection (Fig. 34-4). If the marginal chordae are involved with the infectious process or are ruptured, resection of the infected tisssue followed by reconstruction with chordal transposition can be used.[120] In this

Table 34-7 Standard therapy for endocarditis caused by Enterococci[a]

Antibiotic	Dosage and route	Duration, weeks	Comments
Aqueous crystalline penicillin G sodium with gentamicin sulfate[b]	18–30 million U/24 h IV either continuously or in 6 equally divided doses	4–6	4-week therapy recommended for patients with symptoms < 3 months in duration, 6-week therapy recommended for patients with symptoms >3 months in duration
	1 mg/kg IM/IV every 8 h	4–6	
Ampicillin sodium with gentamicin sulfate[b]	12 g/24 h IV either continuously or in 6 equally divided doses	4–6	
	1 mg/kg IM or IV every 8 h	4–6	
Vancomycin hydrochloride[c] with gentamicin sulfate[b]	30 mg/kg per 24 h IV in 2 equally divided doses, not to exceed 2 g/24 h unless serum levels are monitored.	4–6	Vancomycin therapy is recommended for patients allergic to beta-lactam; cephalosporins are not acceptable alternatives for patients allergic to penicillin
	1 mg/kg IM/IV every 8 h	4–6	

Source: From Wilson et al,[116] with permission.

IV = intravenous; IM = intramuscular.

[a] All enterococci causing endocarditis must be tested for antimicrobial susceptibility to selected optimal therapy. This table is for endocarditis caused by gentamicin- or vancomycin-susceptible enterococci, *Streptococci viridans* with a minimum inhibitory concentration of >0.5 μg/mL, nutritionally variant *S viridans*, or prosthetic valve endocarditis caused by *S viridans* or *Streptococcus bovis*. Antibiotic dosages are for patients with normal renal function.

[b] For specific dosing adjustment and issues concerning gentamicin (obese patients, relative contraindications), see Table 34-5 footnotes.

[c] For specific dosing adjustments and issues concerning vancomycin (obese patients, length of infusions), see Table 34-5 footnotes.

Table 34-8 Endocarditis caused by staphylococci in the absence of prosthetic material[a]

Antibiotic	Dosage and route	Duration	Comments
Methicillin-susceptible staphylococci			
Regimens for non-beta-lactam-allergic patients			
Nafcillin sodium or oxacillin sodium with optional addition of	2 g every 4 h	4–6 weeks	Benefit of additional aminoglycosides has not been established
gentamycin sulfate[b]	1 mg/kg IM or IV every 8 h	3–5 days	
Regimens for beta-lactam-allergic patients			
Cephazolin (or other first-generation cephalosporins in equivalent dosages) with optional addition of	2 g IV every 8 h	4–6 weeks	Cephalosporins should be avoided in patients with immediate-type hypersensitivity to penicillin
genatamicin sulfate[b]	1 mg/kg IM or IV every 8 h	3–5 days	
Vancomycin hydrochloride[c]	30 mg/kg per 24 h IV equally divided doses, not to exceed 2 g/24 h unless serum levels are monitored	4–6 weeks	Recommended for patients allergic to penicillin
Methicillin-resistant staphylococci			
Vancomycin hydrochloride[c]	30 mg/kg per 24 h IV in 2 equally divided doses, not to exceed 2 g/24 h unless serum levels are monitored	4–6 weeks	

From Wilson et al,[116] with permission.
IV = intravenous; IM = intramuscular.
[a]For treatment of endocarditis caused by penicillin-susceptible staphylococci (minimum inhibitory concentration ≤ 0.1 μg/mL), aqueous crystalline penicillin G sodium (Table 34-5, first regimen) can be used for 4 to 6 weeks instead of nafcillin or oxacillin. Shorter antibiotic courses have been effective in some drug addicts with right-sided endocarditis caused by *Staphylococcus aureus*.
[b]For specific dosing adjustments and issues concerning gentamicin (obese patients, relative contraindications), see Table 34-5 footnotes.
[c]For specific dosing adjustments and issues concerning vancomycin (obese patients, length of infusion), see Table 34-5 footnotes.

Table 34-9 Endocarditis caused by Staphylococci in the presence of a prosthetic valve or other prosthetic material[a]

Antibiotic	Dosage and route	Duration, weeks	Comments
Regimen for methicillin-resistant Staphylococci			
Vancomycin hydrochloride[b]	30 mg/kg per 24 h IV in 2 or 4 equally divided doses, not to exceed 2 g/24 h unless serum levels are monitored.	≥6	
With rifampin[c]	300 mg orally every 8 h	≥6	Rifampin increases the amount of warfarin sodium required for antithrombotic therapy.
With gentamycin sulfate[d]	1 mg/kg IM or IV every 8 h	2 (initial 2 weeks)	
Regimen for methicillin-susceptible Staphylococci			
Nafcillin sodium or oxacillin sodium	2 g IV every 4 h	≥6	First-generation cephalosporins or vancomycin should be used in patients allergic to beta-lactams
With rifampin[c]	300 mg orally every 8 h	≥6	Cephalosporins should be avoided in patients with immediate-type
With gentamicin sulfate[d]	1 mg/kg IM or IV every 8 h	2 (initial 2 weeks)	hypersensitivity to penicillin or with methicillin-resistant staphylococci

From Wilson et al,[116] with permission.
IV = intravenous; IM = imtramuscular.
[a] Dosages recommended are for patients with normal renal function.
[b] For specific dosing adjustment and issues concerning vancomycin (obese patients, length of infusion),see Table 34-5 footnotes.
[c] Rifampin plays a unique role in the eradication of staphylococcal infection involving prosthetic material; combination therapy is essential to prevent rifampin resistance.
[d] For specific dosing adjustment and issues concerning gentamycin (obese patients, relative contraindications), see Table 34-5 footnotes.

Table 34-10 Therapy for endocarditis caused by HACEK microorganisms (*Haemophilus parainfluenzae, Haemophilus aphrophilus, Actinobacillus actinomycetemcomitans, Cardiobacterium Hominis, Eikenella corrodens,* and *Kingella kingae*)[a]

Antibiotic	Dosage and route	Duration, weeks	Comments
Ceftriaxone sodium[b]	2 g once daily IV/IM	4	Cefotaxime sodium or other third-generation cephalosporins may be substituted
Ampicillin sodium[c]	12 g/24 h IV either continuously or in 6 equally divided doses	4	
with gentamicin sulfate[d]	1 mg/kg IM/IV every 8 h	4	

Source: From Wilson et al,[116] with permission.
IV = intravenous; IM = intramuscular.
[a] Antibiotic dosages are for patients with normal renal function.
[b] Patients should be informed that intramuscular injection of ceftriaxone is painful.
[c] Ampicillin should not be used if laboratory tests show beta-lactamase production.
[d] For specific dosing adjustment and issues concerning gentamicin (obese patients, relative contraindications), see Table 34-5 footnotes.

technique, marginal chordae of the posterior leaflet are detached with a small piece of posterior leaflet and then reattached to the anterior leaflet.[120] Ruptured commissural chordae can be managed by leaflet sliding plasty: After removal of all infected tissue, the commissural area of both leaflets is detached from the annulus and the two remnants are approximated and sutured together.[120]

Endocarditis of the commissure is a technically challenging problem. It usually involves both cusps and may extend into the mitral valve annulus, causing an abscess. Vegetations in the commissure can be managed with excision of the infected tissue (up to a quarter to a third of the valve area), followed by commissuroplasty (Fig. 34-5). In this technique, the leaflet remnants are reapproximated at the level of their normal closure, and the residual D-shaped defect is closed primarily if small or with a pericardial patch if large.[121] Fortunately, there is redundancy of the mitral valve tissue, allowing this to be accomplished without narrowing the valve orifice.[121] Annular abscess with limited leaflet loss can be managed with annular reconstruction. This can be accomplished by unroofing the abscess, followed by closure of the defect with a pericardial patch (Fig. 34-6) or construction of a "pseudoannulus" for more extensive annular involvement (Fig. 34-7).[121,122] The avoidance of prosthetic rings to complete the repair is preferable but not always possible, especially when there is preexisting annular dilatation secondary to chronic mitral insufficiency.[120] Early results of mitral valve repair using these techniques even in the setting of active infection demonstrate that mitral valve repair can be accomplished with low operative mortality and a low rate of reoperation.[120,123] This allows preservation of the subvalvular apparatus, restoration of mitral valve competence, and improvement of left heart hemodynamics without an increase in the risk for recurent endocarditis.[120,123]

Table 34-11 Fungal endocarditis and culture-negative endocarditis[a]

Antibiotic	Dosage and route	Duration, weeks
Fungal endocarditis[a]		
Amphotericin B	1 mg/kg per day IV	6–8
with or without	(total dose 2.0–2.5 g)	
flucytosine	150 mg/kg per day orally in 4 divided doses	6–8
Culture-negative endocarditis[b]		
Vancomycin	15 mg/kg IV every 12 h	
plus gentamicin	1 mg/kg IM or IV every 8 h	6

Data from Bonow et al,[118] with permission.

[a] Recommendation for fungal endocarditis were not part of the American Heart Association recommendations on infective endocarditis.[116]

[b] Proposed regimen for culture-negative, presumed bacterial endocarditis.[117]

Mitral valve replacement

When repair is not possible because of massive destruction of the valve, valve replacement is warranted. When the subvalvular apparatus is not affected by the infectious process, valve replacement with preservation of the subvalvular apparatus is preferable. Multiple studies have validated the importance of preserving the subvalvular apparatus for maintenance of left ventricular function.[124–128] In the setting of IE, there is a potential concern for an increased risk of recurrent endocarditis with preservation of the subvalvular apparatus while the valve is replaced with a prosthesis. To investigate this question, Lee and coworkers[123] conducted a retrospective review of patients with IE of the mitral valve and found that preservation of the subvalvular apparatus did not increase the risk of residual or recurrent endocarditis.

When the subvalvular apparatus is involved, as with papillary muscle abscess, valve replacement is necessary.

Table 34-12 Indications for surgery in patients with infective endocarditis

Indication	Evidence-based
Emergency indication for cardiac surgery (same day)	
1. Acute AR with early closure of mitral valve	A
2. Rupture of sinus of Valsalva aneurysm into right heart chamber	A
3. Rupture into pericardium	A
Urgent indication for cardiac surgery (within 1–2 days)	
4. Valvular obstruction	A
5. Unstable prosthesis	A
6. Acute AR or MR with heart failure, NYHA III–IV	A
7. Septal perforation	A
8. Evidence of annular or aortic abscess, sinus or aortic true or false aneurysm, fistula formation, or new-onset conduction disturbances	A
9. Major embolism + mobile vegetation> 10 mm + appropriate antibiotic therapy < 7–10 days	B
10. Mobile vegetation >15 mm + appropriate antibiotic therapy < 7–10 days	C
11. No effective antimicrobial therapy available	A
Elective indication for cardiac surgery (earlier is usually better)	
12. Staphylococcal prosthetic valve endocarditis	B
13. Early prosthetic valve endocarditis (≤ 2 months after surgery)	B
14. Evidence of progressive paravalvular prosthetic leak	A
15. Evidence of valve dysfunction and persistent infection after 7–10 days of appropriate antibiotic therapy, as indicated by presence of fever or bacteremia, provided that there are no noncardiac causes of infection	A
16. Fungal endocarditis caused by a mold	A
17. Fungal endocarditis caused by a yeast	B
18. Infection with difficult to treat organisms	B
19. Vegetation growing larger during antibiotic therapy > 7days	C

Source: From Olaison and Pettersson,[119] with permission.

A=strong evidence or general agreement that cardiac surgery is useful and effective;
B=inconclusive or conflicting evidence or a divergence or opinion about the usefulness/efficacy of cardiac surgery, but weight of evidence/opinion of the majority is in favor; C=inconclusive or conflicting evidence or a divergence of opinion; lack of clear consensus on the basis of evidence/opinion of the majority; AR=aortic regurgitation; MR=mitral regurgitation; NYHA=New York Heart Association classification.

In the mitral position, a mechanical valve is the prosthesis of choice.

Novel techniques

Mitral valve replacement with a cryopreserved mitral homograft has several advantages. It maintains the subvalvular apparatus, does not require anticoagulation, and has a higher resistance to infection. The operative technique for mitral valve replacement with homografts published by Acar and associates in 1996 is discussed here.[129] Proper valve selection is crucial for optimal results. The subvalvular apparatus (the morphologic characteristics of the papillary muscles and the distribution of the chordae) and the valve characteristics (the height of the anterior leaflet, the distance between the annulus and the anterior papillary muscle, and the anteroposterior diameter of the annulus) of the donor and recepient are matched using preoperative echocardiography. The homograft selected is slightly bigger than the recepient valve (measurement plus 3 mm). The operation is accomplished by gaining access to the mitral valve via the left atrium. The homograft is harvested so that approximately 15 mm of papillary muscle tissue remains beyond the origin of the chordae. The recepient papillary muscle is mobilized from the left ventricular wall, creating a slit into which the homograft papillary muscle is inserted. The papillary muscles of the donor and the recepient are sutured side to side without any pledgets and away from the origin of the chordae to prevent chordal or papillary muscle rupture as a result of erosion of these structures. As the homograft papillary muscles undergo necrosis, the strength of the anastomoses is maintained by the formation of fibrotic tissue in the area. Attention must be paid to maintaining the orientation of the papillary heads so that the tension on the leaflets is evenly distributed. This can be accomplished by using the head of the commissural chordae as a reference point. The valve of the homograft then is sutured to the annulus with a continuous suture, starting at the posteromedial commissure

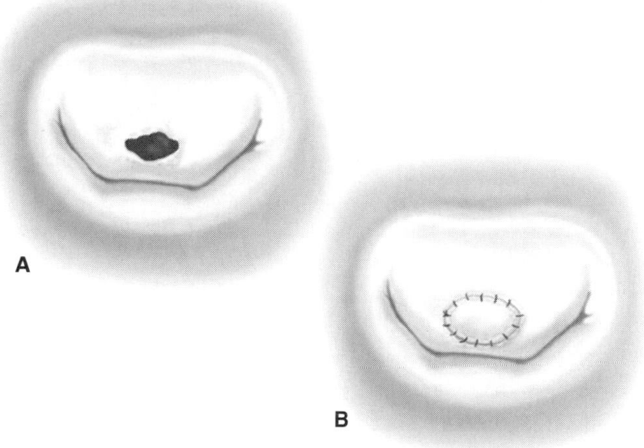

Figure 34-3 Autologous pericardial patch repair of the anterior mitral valve leaflet. [Reprinted with permission from Filsoufi F, Adams DH. Surgical treatment of mitral valve endocarditis. In: Cohn LH, Edmunds LH Jr (eds). *Cardiac Surgery in the Adult.* New York: McGraw-Hill; 2003:987–997.]

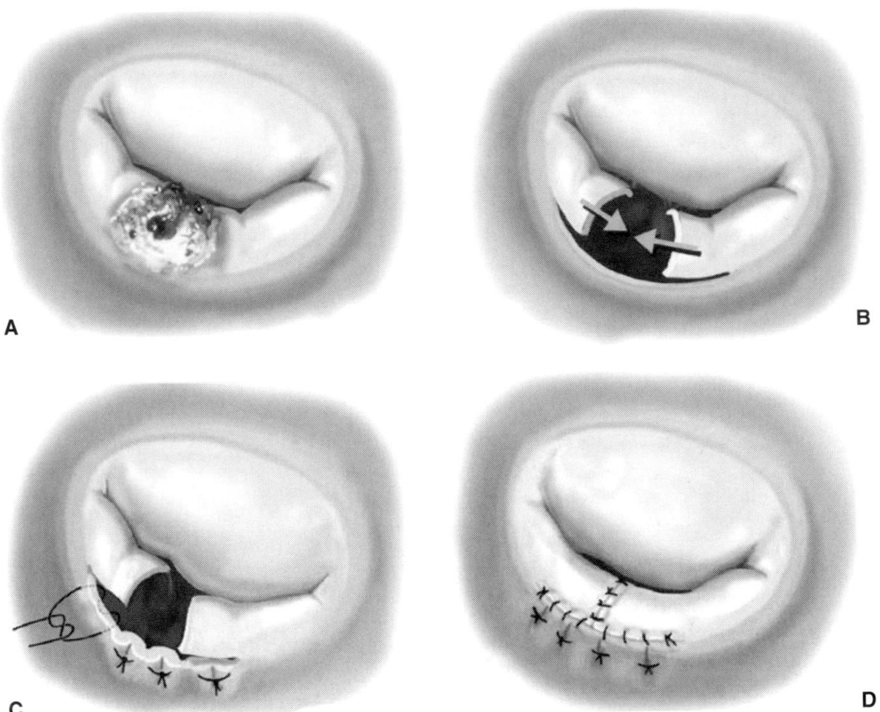

Figure 34-4 Repair of P2 segment of posterior mitral valve leaflet with quadrangular resection and sliding plasty of the P1 and P3 segments. **A.** Posterior leaflet endocarditis with P2 segment prolapse. **B.** Resection of the P2 segment. **C.** Compression mattress sutures placed along the posterior annulus. **D.** Sliding plasty of the P1 and P3 segments. [Reprinted with permission from Filsoufi F, Adams DH. Surgical treatment of mitral valve endocarditis. In: Cohn LH, Edmunds LH Jr (eds). *Cardiac Surgery in the Adult.* New York: McGraw-Hill; 2003:987–997.]

and proceeding to the anterior leaflet, then the anterolateral commissure, and finally the posterior leaflet. The procedure is completed with a prosthetic ring annuloplasty.[129]

The reported results of this operation are conflicting. Some studies report low operative mortality as well as a low need for reoperation,[129,130] whereas in the hands of others this procedure has an unacceptably high early and/or late failure rate.[131,132]

Tricuspid valve endocarditis

Although tricuspid valve endocarditis occurs primarily among intravenous drug users, it can occur in patients with central intravenous catheters and sometimes in patients with congenital heart disease. It also may occur as a community-acquired infection in patients with no known predisposing factors.[133] A high level of suspicion is necessary as the disease can have a rapidly progressive course that is complicated by right heart failure and respiratory insufficiency. In the majority of cases, tricuspid valve endocarditis responds well to medical management. The usual indications for surgical intervention are sepsis unresponsive to antimicrobial therapy, right heart failure from valvular insufficiency, and recurrent pulmonary emboli resulting in severe respiratory failure. Frequently, patients referred for surgery have all three of these indications and subsequently are not the best operative candidates. There are several options available to the cardiac surgeon faced with tricuspid valve endocarditis, including simple vegetectomy, valve excision without replacement, valve repair, and partial or complete valve replacement.

Tricuspid valve excision (without valve replacement)

Tricuspid valvulectomy without subsequent valve replacement removes the infected tissue and achieves cure of the acute endocarditis. The main body of information on this topic comes from the work of Arbulu and associates,[134] who reported the largest series of tricuspid valvulectomies ($n = 53$) with 100 percent follow-up over 22 years and concluded that this procedure was the treatment option of choice for tricuspid endocarditis. The operation is simple, quick, and easy to perform compared with valve replacement and is less expensive. However, several arguments could be made against this

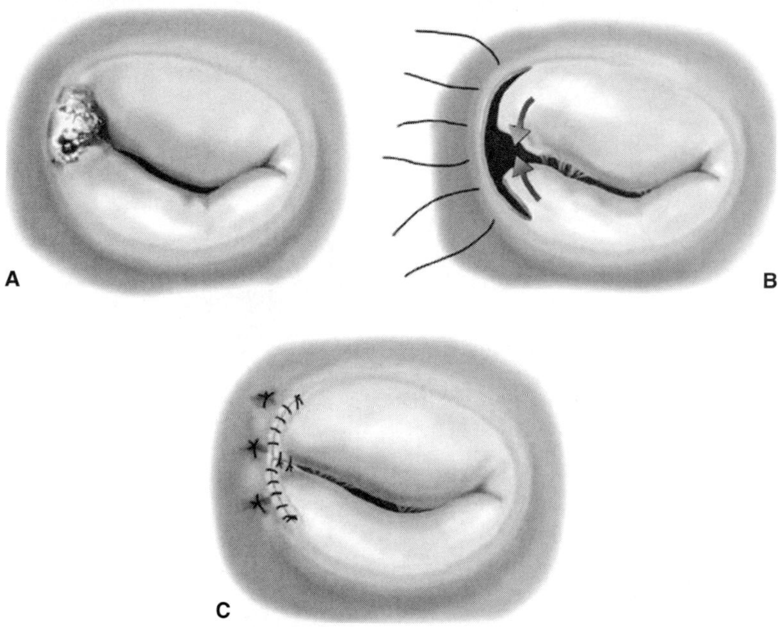

Figure 34-5 Repair strategy for commissural involvement with endocarditis. **A.** Anterior mitral commissure endocarditis with prolapse. **B.** Debridement of infected area followed by annular compression sutures. **C.** Sliding commissuroplasty in the paracommissural area. [Reprinted with permission from Filsoufi F, Adams DH. Surgical treatment of mitral valve endocarditis. In: Cohn LH, Edmunds LH Jr (eds). *Cardiac Surgery in the Adult.* New York: McGraw-Hill; 2003:987–997.]

treatment option. After removal of the tricuspid valve, the right atrial pressure rises in proportion to the right ventricular pressure and rises even higher in the case of elevated pulmonary vascular resistance (PVR). Thus, before committing a patient to valvulectomy, one must ensure that he or she has normal right and left ventricular function as well as normal pulmonary vascular resistance and thus is able to withstand the additional stress imposed on the right heart postoperatively. Although the majority of patients with tricuspid valve endocarditis may fulfill this requirement, patients with congenital heart disease or pacemaker/defibrillator leads as predisposing factors may have compromised right or left ventricular function. Moreover, some patients with tricuspid valve endocarditis may develop pulmonary hypertension immediately as a result of multiple septic pulmonary emboli. In addition, the procedure is contraindicated in patients with left-sided endocarditis. In the drug addict population, one must compare the outcomes of valvulectomy with those when valve replacement or repair is used. In the replacement group of Arbulu and associates,[134] mortality was 100 percent, 80 percent of which was due to inability to control the endocarditis. Superior results have been achieved by multiple investigators.[135,136] In addition, since half or more of these patients return to drug use after discharge from the hospital, valve replacement will put them at a high risk of reinfection.[134] However, those authors do not address valve repair with autologous tissue such as pericardium or fascia lata as a treatment option in this situation. Finally, those authors argue that long-term survival is possible after valvulectomy. In their series, actuarial

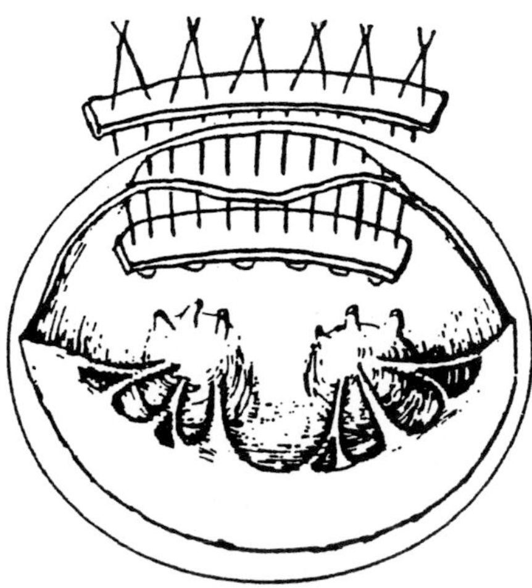

Figure 34-6 Repair of small mitral annular abscesses. After complete debridement, small mitral annular abscess cavities (< 5 mm) can be repaired with a pericardial buttressing strip. (Reprinted with permission from Moon MR, Stinson EB, Miller DC. Surgical treatment of endocarditis. *Prog Cardiovasc Dis* 1997;40:239–264.)

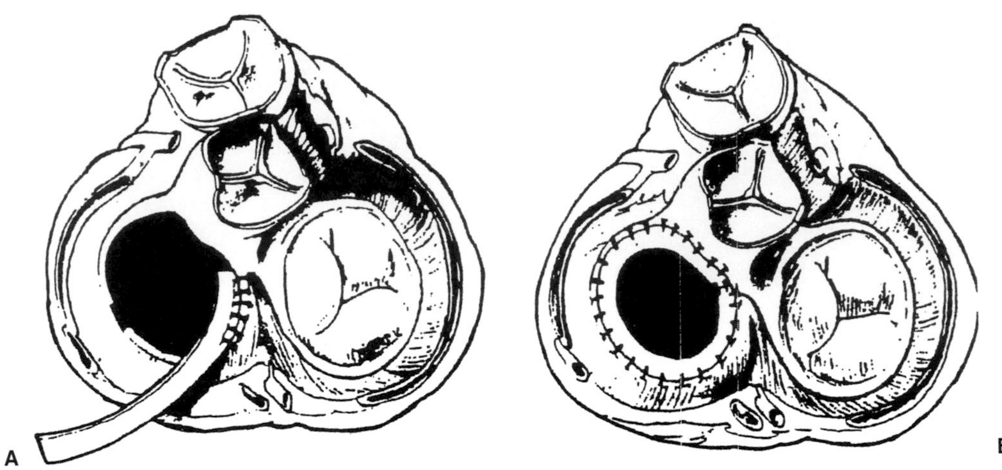

Figure 34-7 Repair of extensive mitral annular involvement with endocarditis. Complete mitral annular replacement may be performed by constructing a "pseudoannulus" with a circumferential pericardial strip. (Reprinted with permission from David TE, Feindel CM, Armstrong S, et al. Reconstruction of the mitral annulus: A ten year experience. *J Thorac Cardiovasc Surg* 1995;110:1323–1332.)

survival at 22 years was 64 percent.[134] Eleven percent of the patients required valve replacement after the valvulectomy operation.[134] However, although extensive follow-up was obtained on this difficult to track patient population, no data were reported on the severity of the right heart failure of the valvulectomy survivors. Other complications can develop as well after tricuspid valve resection, such as centrolobular fibrosis.[137]

Debridement

A more conservative approach to total valvulectomy is simple debridement or "vegetectomy" without subsequent repair of the defect. This procedure removes the infected tissue but preserves the healthy components of the tricuspid valve. Clearly, this approach is not useful when there is significant destruction of the valve. Simple vegectectomy can be performed without CPB. This offers a major advantage in the setting of right-sided endocarditis complicated by pulmonary involvement by avoiding worsening of the respiratory function after CPB. The technique of tricuspid valve vegetectomy without the use of CPB was described first by Raman, Bellomo, and Shah[138] and utilizes a brief period (less than 2 min) of vena caval inflow occlusion to provide a bloodless operative field. The superior and inferior venae cavae are dissected, and slings are placed around them. Stay sutures are placed in the right atrial wall. Ten thousand units of heparin is administered systemically, after which the cavae are clamped, the right atrium is entered, and the vegetation is excised with care not to exceed 2 min of inflow occlusion. The right atrial cavity then is irrigated with an antibiotic solution, a partial occlusion clamp is applied to the atriotomy site, and the caval clamps are released. The atriotomy site is closed by approximating the edges of the atrial incision within the clamp. Because the defect is not repaired, tricuspid regurgitation to various degrees is an inevitable consequence of this procedure. In their series of seven patients, Raman and associates[138] reported that five patients developed trivial and two patients developed moderate tricuspid regurgitation after vegetectomy that was stable on mean follow-up of 19 months. The description of this technique is included for the sake of completeness only, as it generally is not used today.

Tricuspid valve repair

The procedure of choice in the setting of tricuspid endocarditis is valve repair. However, it is of the utmost importance to resect all infected tissue without concern about the feasibility of subsequent repair to free the patient of the infectious process. For repair to be feasible, the annulus and the surrounding myocardium must be free of infection. Tricuspid valve endocarditis most frequently involves the anterior leaflet, followed by the posterior leaflet. The septal leaflet is the least frequently involved. Techniques similar to those applied to mitral valve endocarditis can be used in an attempt to preserve as much of the native tricuspid apparatus as possible. Leaflet perforation can be managed with primary repair if it is small or with an autologous pericardial patch if it is large, as was previously described.[120] Commissural resection followed by commissural reconstruction by leaflet sliding plasty, as previously described, can be used for ruptured commissural chordae[120] (this is an alternative to a bicuspid leaflet). Chordal transposition may not always be an option in tricuspid valve repair, as the chordae are not directly opposite one another and may not always be expendable, such as the chordae to the septal leaflet.[139] The chordae to the posterior leaflet, however, can be used for chordal transposition.[139] Vegetation confined to the central one-half to three-quarters of the anterior leaflet can be managed with standard quadrangular resection of the involved cusp tissue and infected chordae, followed by local annuloplasty or annular plication using pericardial pledgets.[139] Alternatively, the defect can be closed with an autologous pericardial patch.[139] Fixing the pericardial patch in glutaraldehyde solution may reduce the late shrinkage of the patch that results in valve incompetence.[139] When the chordae are not involved in the infectious process, resuspension of the choradae to the patch can be accomplished.[140] When the chordae as well as the accompanying papillary muscle head are infected, basilar chordae inserting near the annulus can be detached and their muscular trabecular attachments can be mobilized by dissecting them off the right ventricular wall to form new papillary muscle.[139] This papillary muscle–chordal apparatus then is attached to the free margin of the pericardial patch.[139] When the posterior half of the anterior leaflet is involved and resection of the vegetation leaves a large defect that cannot be closed primarily, the anterior leaflet can be sutured to the posterior leaflet, producing a bicuspid valve.[139] Alternatively, when the anterior half of the anterior leaflet is involved, a bicuspid valve can be created after resection by suturing the anterior leaflet to the septal leaflet.[140] Monofilament sutures and pledgets constructed from autologous pericardium are simple techniques that can be used to minimize the risk of recurrent infection. Annular plication or De Vega annuloplasty can be used to improve the competence of the valve without the addition of prosthetic material.

The results of tricuspid valve repair are somewhat difficult to interpret from the published literature mainly because of the small numbers in each series, but there is an overall trend toward reduction of right ventricular dimensions, tricuspid regurgitation, and right heart failure.[136,139,140] In addition, recurrent tricuspid regurgitation may be reduced when Carpentier-Edwards (CE) rings are used for annuloplasty after repair, although the risk of recurrent infection must be balanced against the risk of recurrent tricuspid regurgitation.[120,139] The adequacy of the repair can be inspected by injecting saline into the right ventricle as well as by intraoperative TEE, and further adjustments can be made to ensure optimal results.

Tricuspid valve replacement

When the resection of all infected tissue leaves a large valve defect, repair may not be feasible and total replacement of the tricuspid valve may be necessary. There are several options in this situation. The choice of valve for replacement is controversial, reflecting the fact that no solution is ideal. The debate has long centered on mechanical versus bioprosthetic valves. Mechanical valves offer the advantage of durability but are associated with the risk of bleeding complications. In the tricuspid position, a high level of anticoagulation with an International Normalized Ratio (INR) of 3.5 to 4.5 is needed to prevent thrombosis. Bioprosthetic valves are considered by many the valves of choice for tricuspid valve endocarditis. In the setting of infection, they are thought to confer higher resistance to reinfection. Bioprostheses in other positions usually are considered for elderly patients to avoid the risks of anticoagulation while expecting a low rate of reoperation as a result of limited life expectancy. However, the population of patients with tricuspid valve endocarditis usually consists of younger induviduals. The expected life of the bioprostheses at other positions is on the order of 10 to 15 years, but it is postulated that the lower pressures on the right side of the heart may lead to a greater life span at the tricuspid position. Little is known about the long-term durability of bioprostheses in the tricuspid position. In medium-term follow-up of tricuspid valve replacement up to 10 years, it appears that bioprostheses do not offer an advantage over mechanical prostheses in terms of either survival or reoperation rate.[141,142] However, most of these studies did not include patients with endocarditis, in whom bioprosthetic valves may offer a unique advantage over mechanical prostheses. In addition, long-term follow-up beyond 10 to 15 years is limited. One study found that at 18 years of follow-up of tricuspid valve replacement with bioprostheses (n = 98; only 2 patients had tricuspid valve endocarditis), the majority of late deaths were due to CHF and freedom from reoperation was 62.7 +/− 10.7 percent.[143] Fifty percent of the reoperations were due to valve dysfunction, with the main cause of valve dysfunction being pannus formation on the ventricular side of the cusps.[143] Other studies suggest that at 15 years and beyond, the need for reoperation does increase with bioprostheses in the tricuspid position.[144] In addition, calcification of bioprosthetic valves in younger patients may require re-replacement even sooner: within a decade.[139]

Tricuspid valve replacement with a bioprosthesis seems a reasonable option in the setting of a high risk for reinfection, whereas mechanical prosthesis may be considered in younger patients and in those who already have a left-sided mechanical prosthesis.

Novel techniques

Novel techniques have emerged in the management of tricuspid valve destruction by endocarditis. In the recent past, partial or total homograft replacement of the tricuspid valve was added to the surgeon's repertoire. Partial homograft replacement takes advantage of the fact that the infection of the tricuspid valve most frequently involves the anterior leaflet, sometimes the posterior leaflet, but only rarely the septal leaflet.[145] The anterior leaflet is functionally the most important portion of the valve, and if infection is limited to this leaflet, replacement of it alone restores the functional integrity of the valve. A great deal of improvisation is necessary to trim the mitral homograft so that a partial homograft is created to replace the resected portion of the native valve. In one report, 50 percent of the anterior tricuspid leaflet was replaced successfully with a partial mitral homograft consisting of a large portion of the anterior leaflet of the mitral valve along with the commissure, the chordae, and the head of the corresponding papillary muscle. The papillary muscle was sutured side to side to the anterior papillary muscle of the tricuspid valve, and the mitral leaflet was sutured to the annulus and to the remaining portion of the native anterior tricuspid leaflet.[146] A Carpentier prosthetic ring was inserted at the tricuspid annulus for reinforcement.[146] Couetil and associates[145] described another technique for partial mitral homograft replacement of the tricuspid valve. In their series, both the anterior and posterior leaflets of the tricuspid valve were excised. The tricuspid valve was reconstructed using the anterior leaflet of the mitral valve homograft alone; if the tricuspid valve area was enlarged, the anterior leaflet along with the posterior commissure with the adjacent part of the posterior leaflet was used. In the first scenario, the partial homograft was prepared by separating the two leaflets by dividing the commissural areas of cusp tissue and dividing the papillary muscles between the attachments of anterior and posterior leaflet chordae. In the second scenario, the partial homograft was prepared using the anterior leaflet and the posterior commissure with the adjacent part of the posterior leaflet. The partial homograft then was sutured to the tricuspid annulus, starting at the anteroseptal commissure of the tricuspid valve and continuing from left to right. When the middle of the anterior leaflet is reached, the anterior leaflet of the homograft is coapted with the native septal leaflet with a stay suture to determine the correct position of the anterior papillary muscle in the right ventricle. Then a solid base for implantation is created by trimming some of the trabeculations, and the anterior papillary muscle is sutured in place. The remainder of the anterior leaflet of the mitral homograft then is sutured to the tricuspid annulus. When part of the posterior leaflet of the mitral valve homograft is used as well, the coaptation of the valve leaflets is completed by suturing the posterior leaflet remnant side to side to the septal leaflet, expanding its surface. The repair is completed by implantation of the posterior papillary muscle in the right ventricle. If needed, the annulus can be reinforced with a Carpentier rigid tricuspid annuloplasty ring.[145]

The first report of tricuspid valve replacement with mitral homograft was published by Pomar and Mestres in 1993.[147] In their technique, cryopreserved mitral homografts were implanted according to their orientation within the left ventricle, with the anterior leaflet oriented anteriorly and coming into contact with the free right ventricular wall and the posterior one posteriorly coming in contact with the septal part of the AV orifice; no prosthetic ring annuloplasty was used, and the homograft leaflets were sutured directly to the remnant of the tricuspid annulus.[147,148] Six-year follow-up of five HIV-infected patients who underwent this procedure demonstrated good functional status (all in NYHA class I) despite the fact that serial echocardiography demonstrated severe total vascular regeneration (TVR) in three of the five patients and moderate TVR in one of the five.[148] No reoperations were required, and all homografts remained free of both calcification and papillary muscle rupture.[148]

To avoid protrusion of the anterior leaflet of the mitral homograft into the right ventricular outflow tract, Acar and associates[149] modified the technique of Pomar and Mestres by changing the orientation of the mitral homograft so that the anterior leaflet was oriented toward the interventricular septum, and the posterior leaflet toward the right ventricular outflow tract. The anteroposterior papillary muscle was inserted into the right ventricular free wall, and the posteromedial papillary muscle was inserted into a trench created in the interventricular septum.

Miyagishima and associates[150] modified the technique of Acar and associates[149] with regard to the implantation of the papillary muscles while preserving the same leaflet orientation. In this technique, the papillary muscles are exteriorized through the right ventricular wall. The posteromedial papillary muscle exits through the anterior wall of the right ventricle about 4 cm from the tricuspid ring, and the anterolateral papillary muscle is brought out through the inferior wall of the right ventricle between the acute marginal artery and the patent ductus arteriosus (PDA). The procedure was completed with the insertion of a mitral annuloplasty ring (CE) in the antianatomic position, reducing the anterior and posterior portions of the right AV valve but leaving the septal portion corresponding to the anterior leaflet of the mitral homograft intact.[150] Although this is done in the hope of preventing long-term regurgitation, it has the disadvantage of increasing the risk of reinfection through the insertion of prosthetic material and thus may mitigate the benefit of using a mitral homograft. In addition, annular dilatation may not present a problem because of the acute nature of the infectious process. Thus, using this technique routinely may not offer any benefit to the majority of patients who do not have annular dilatation while subjecting them to potential risks. Early results of this technique utilized in five patients demonstrated no early mortality. Three of five patients were available for echocardiography at 1 year, among whom regurgitation was absent in two and trivial in one. Two of the five developed complete heart block that required the insertion of a permanent pacemaker.[150] Hvass and associates[151] compared the two techniques of papillary muscle attachment and found that implantation time was reduced by using the exteriorization technique. The attachment of the papillary muscles inside the right ventricle is technically more challenging. If residual regurgitation is detected by intaoperative echocardiography, this situation must be remedied by repositioning the papillary muscles deeper into the ventricle or moving the homograft leaflets above the level of the tricuspid annulus. This is in contrast to the ease of readjusting the tension of the papillary muscles in the exteriorized approach by simply mobilizing the papillary muscles from outside the right ventricle. In addition, this approach compensates for the discrepancy between the length of the chordae and the anatomy and bulk of the papillary muscles of the homograft and the size of the recipient's right ventricular cavity and the location and size of the tricuspid papillary muscles.[151]

Tricuspid valve replacement using fresh mitral homografts has been described, taking advantage of the potential benefit of fresh human tissue with its higher resistance to infection compared with a cryopreserved mitral homograft.[152] However, the logistics of this option are even more difficult as the mitral valve cannot be preserved indefinitely in an antibiotic solution at 4°C. One of the major limitations of the use of mitral homografts for tricuspid valve replacement in endocarditis patients is the need for accurate preoperative sizing using echocardiography. In addition, the subvalvular apparatus of the tricuspid valve is not very well defined. For example, the chordae to the anteroseptal commissure originate directly from the right venrticular wall without papillary muscle support. The papillary muscles also demonstrate considerable variability in anatomy, and this has major implications for the attachment of the donor papillary muscles. As was pointed out by Cosgrove,[153] this may be a major influencing factor for the development of postoperative valve incompetence. Thus, partial and total homograft replacement of the tricuspid valve at this stage is considered an investigational approach, and further studies are needed to define its utility and compare it with tricuspid valve repair or replacement with a bioprosthesis or a mechanical prosthesis.

Aortic valve endocarditis

Several surgical options are available for aortic valve endocarditis. They include closure of any annular and/or aortic defects with patch, followed by suturing the prosthesis directly to the patch;[154,155] supracoronary placement of the prosthetic valve with closure of the coronary ostia, followed by coronary artery bypass grafting (CABG);[156] the Bentall procedure using composite prosthetic valve conduit;[157] the Ross procedure;[158] and aortic root replacement with an allograft.[142]

Prosthetic aortic valve replacement

Earlier arguments centered on mechanical versus bioprosthetic valves. Recent studies suggest that survival may be similar for both valve types[159] and that recurrence is low with either bioprostheses or mechanical valves as long as adequate debridement of all infected tissue is accomplished.[160] Mechanical valves offer the advantage of durability but require long-term anticoagulation. Recent data indicate that they can be used safely as replacement devices, with an acceptable early mortality rate.[161,162] Secure implantation of the mechanical prosthesis may be compromised if the annulus is destroyed.[161] Medium-term follow-up data, however, suggest that there is a survival benefit from using autografts and homografts for replacement of the aortic valve compared with prosthetic valves (mechanical and bioprostheses).[58,163–165] One study found that long-term survival for patients with standard prostheses is on the order of 50 to 60 percent at 5 years and 30 to 40 percent at 10 years when in-hospital mortality is included, whereas in their series in the long term, when allograft aortic roots were used, survival was 76 percent at 5 years and 53 percent at 10 years.[58] However, it may be too early to see the effects of late allograft structural failure.[58] Current data show that at 10 years, freedom from reoperation for allograft-related complications is greater than 90 percent,[166–168] making the allograft the valve of choice for replacement in aortic valve endocarditis. It has many advantages over prostheses.

Aortic homografts

Aortic valve endocarditis is frequently extensive, destroying the annulus and spreading to involve the anterior mitral valve leaflet and the membranous portion of the interventricular septum, forming fistulas, pseudoaneurysms, and abscesses. Aortic homografts offer the advantage of flexibility, which allows them to be implanted securely in the often distorted aortic annulus; this would be difficult to accomplish with rigid mechanical or stented bioprostheses, possibly resulting in recurrent endocarditis or valve dehiscence.[163]

Moreover, the attached anterior leaflet of the mitral valve can be used as additional tissue to repair defects created by the infectious process.[58] Homografts are more resistant to infection,[58,163,164,169] presumably as a result of the higher ability of postoperative antibiotics to penetrate the entire device, and do not require anticoagulation. Allografts come in the form of aortic valves or roots, and the roots may allow more extensive debridement to be performed. For example, one study noticed higher mortality in patients who received a valve-only replacement compared with the Bentall operation for prosthetic valve endocarditis.[162] This may be explained in part by the opportunity to accomplish wider debridement of all infected tissue, necessitating a root rather than a valve replacement. The risk of recurrent endocarditis is lower when homografts are used to replace infected aortic valves compared with mechanical prostheses and bioprostheses.[169] However, this benefit may extend over the first year or so after valve replacement, as the risk of recurrent endocarditis appears to be low and constant over time when nonstented refrigerated homografts are used, whereas the risk of recurrent endocarditis when prosthetic valves are used peaks initially in the first 2 to 3 months[58,169,170] and then remains at a low constant level comparable to that of homografts.[169] One study found the incidence of prosthetic valve endocarditis after primary valve replacement to be 4.1 percent 4 years postoperatively.[170] The instantaneous risk of infection of the homograft is still fivefold lower than that of prosthetic valves.[58,169]

Aortic homograft/autograft root replacement

The operation is performed through a median sternotomy and on cardiopulmonary bypass.[58] The goals of the operation are to remove all infected tissue and replace the aortic valve, thus restoring the structural integrity of the left ventricular outflow tract. The general principle of the operation is wide aggressive debridement of all infected tissue without regard to factors affecting reconstruction or potential complications such as heart block.[58] Next, the allograft is brought in. To orient the allograft in the proper position, the two fibrous trigones and the anterior mitral leaflet on the homograft are aligned with the patient's fibrous trigones and anterior mitral valve leaflet. The homograft then is sutured to the myocardium proximal to the site of infection, using interrupted or continuous 4-0 polypropylene monofilament sutures. No artificial material is used. Fistulas and ventricular septal defects secondary to the infection are repaired with bovine or autologous pericardium.[58] False aneurysms can be closed directly or with a patch of pericardium.[169] The proximal suture line can be reinforced with either bovine or autologous pericardium or even with a saphenous vein.

Abscess cavities are opened and aggressively debrided of all necrotic material. The most common site of abscess formation is the mitral-aortic intervalvular fibrosa,[58] and this makes inmplantation of the replacement valve difficult because there is limited healthy tissue to sew to. This problem is solved by suturing the attached anterior leaflet of the mitral valve on the aortic homograft to the native anterior leaflet of the mitral valve. When this is done, the abscess cavity is excluded from the circulation while being allowed to drain into the mediastinum, which itself is drained with chest tubes for 48 to 72 h. The coronary ostia are mobilized as buttons and are sewn to the homograft with a 5-0 polypropylene monofilament suture in a running fashion. The distal anastomosis is fashioned end to end with running 4-0 polypropylene monofilament sutures. Various techniques are available to minimize the risk of infection of the homograft. The homografts routinely are soaked in an antibiotic solution. The suture lines may be reinforced with human or bovine pericardium instead of Teflon felt strips.

Multiple studies have shown that homograft root replacements have acceptable operative mortality between 3 and 14.5 percent,[167,168,171–173] with the higher mortality rates related to moribund preoperative status or prosthetic valve endocarditis.[172,173] Heart block is the most common postoperative complication, with complete heart block requiring the placement of a permanent pacemaker occurring in 30 percent of these patients.[58] Other complications include bleeding and renal and respiratory failure. Overall survival rates range from 53 to 92 percent at 5 years[166,167,171] and 85 percent to 91 percent at 10 years.[166,172] Recurrent endocarditis rates are low (0 to 3.5 percent) at 5 to 10 years.[168,169,172] Recurrence or reinfection of the previously replaced aortic valve is associated with a very high mortality rate (approximately 65 percent).[170]

Homografts have disadvantages as well. For example, homografts deteriorate after implantation. Another problem is calcification over time. Although the long-term results have been encouraging, accelerated homograft calcification as early as 3 years after implantation has been described.[174] The mechanism is unclear. Multiple mechanisms have been postulated, from immunologic[175] to cessation of activity of the energy-requiring calcium-extruding pumps in the nonviable homograft cells.[176] Although studies published in the 1980s showed lower freedom from reoperation with the use of homografts,[177,178] more recent studies have shown excellent overall data, with freedom from reoperation at 10 years greater than 90 percent[166–168] unless undersized homografts are used.[172] Another problem is immediate availability in the setting of an urgent or emergent operation. To overcome these problems, the use of autografts has emerged as an option for the treatment of aortic valve endocarditis. Autografts are immediately available for use, have a potentially longer life span than allografts, and may be more resistant to infection since they constitute viable tissue. The need for double-valve replacement is a major drawback of this approach and may preclude its use in certain situations in which the patient may not be stable enough to undergo such an extensive procedure. In addition, the higher friability of the autograft compared with the homograft makes the Ross operation a technically challenging one.

OUTCOMES

Mortality rates from IE continue to be relatively high despite recent advances in diagnosis and treatment. Significant risk factors for early mortality include age, staphyloccocal endocarditis, preoperative NYHA class, and preoperative renal failure.[163] Overall 5-year survival is between 75 and 88 percent,[42,173,179–181] and 10-year survival is between 63 and 81 percent.[52,173,179,181]

Relapse is defined as IE occurring within 6 months of the original attack with the same organism. Overall relapse rates for IE range from 2.7 to 3.3 percent.[42,179] Recurrence is defined as IE occurring more than 6 months after the original attack or with a different organism. Overall recurrence rates range from 4.5 to 12.3 percent.[42,179] For patients with prosthetic valve endocarditis, endocarditis in the first postoperative year is a risk factor for recurrence.[42] Mortality is higher among patients with recurrent endocarditis.[42] Patients who survive 1 year after the initial episode of endocarditis are still more than three times more likely to die than is the general population.[180]

References

1. Luschka H. Das endocardium imd die endocarditis. *Arch Pathol Anat Physiol* 1852;4:171
2. Rosenow EC. Experimental infectious endocarditis. *J Infect Dis* 1912;11:210
3. Gross L. Significance of blood vessels in human heart valves. *Am Heart J* 1937;13:275
4. Garrison PK, Freedman LR. Experimental endocarditis: I. Staphylococcal endocarditis in rabbits resulting from placement of a polyethylene catheter in the right side of the heart. *Yale J Biol Med* 1970;42:394–410.
5. Perlman BB, Freedman LR. Experimental endocarditis: II. Staphylococcal infection of the aortic valve following placement of a polyethylene catheter in the left side of the heart. *Yale J Biol Med* 1971;44:206–213.
6. Durack DT, Beeson PB. Experimental bacterial endocarditis: I. Colonization of a sterile vegetation. *Br J Exp Pathol* 1972;53:44–49.
7. Rodgers GM, Greenberg CS, Shuman MA. Characterization of the effects of cultured vascular cells on the activation of blood coagulation. *Blood* 1983;61: 1155–1162.
8. Johnson CM. Adherence events in the pathogenesis of infective endocarditis. *Infect Dis Clin North Am* 1993; 7(1):21–36.
9. Chino F, Kodama A, Otake M, Dock DS. Nonbacterial thrombotic endocarditis in a Japanese autopsy sample: A series of 80 cases. *Am Heart J* 1975;90:190–198.
10. Lepeschkin E. On the relation between the site of valvular involvement in endocarditis and the blood pressure resting on the valve. *Am J Med Sci* 1952;224:318.
11. Rodbard S. Blood velocity and endocarditis. *Circulation* 1960;27:18–28.
12. Everett ED, Hirschman JV. Transient bacteremia and endocarditis: A review. *Medicine (Baltimore)* 1977; 56:61.
13. Gould K, Ramirez-Ronda CH, Holmes RK, Sanford JP. Adherence of bacteria to heart valves in vitro. *J Clin Invest* 1975;56:1364–1370.
14. Ramirez-Ronda CH. Adherence of glucan-positive and glucan-negative streptococcal strains to normal and damaged heart valves. *J Clin Invest* 1978;62:805–814.
15. Angrist A, Oka M. Pathogenesis of bacterial endocarditis. *JAMA* 1963;183:249–252.
16. Scheld WM, Valone JA, Sande MA. Bacterial adherence in the pathogenesis of endocarditis: Interaction of bacterial dextran, platelets and fibrin. *J Clin Invest* 1978;61: 1394–1404.
17. Clawson CC, White JG. Platelet interactions with bacteria: I. Reaction phases and effects of inhibitors. *Am J Pathol* 1971;82:367–380.
18. Sullam PM, Frank U, Yeaman MR, et al. Effect of thrombocytopenia on the early cause of streptococcal endocarditis. *J Infect Dis* 1993;168:910–914.
19. Yeaman MR, Puentes SM, Norman DC, Bayer AS. Partial characterization and staphylocidal activity of thrombin-induced platelet microbicidal protein. *Infect Immun* 1992;60:1202–1209.
20. Yeaman MR, Bayer AS. Antimicrobial peptides from platelets: Drug resistance updates. *Drug Resist Updat* 1999;2:116–126.
21. Kupferwasser LI, Yeaman MR, Shapiro SM, et al. In vitro susceptibility to thrombin-induced platelet microbicidal protein is associated with reduced disease progression and complication rates in experimental Staphylococcal aureus endocarditis: Microbiological, histopathologic, and echocardiographic analyses. *Circulation* 2002;105:746–752.
22. Krijgsveld J, Zaat SA, Meeldijk J, et al. Thrombocidins, microbicidal proteins from human blood platelets, are C-terminal deletion products of CXC chemokines. *J Biol Chem* 2000;275:20374–20381.
23. Durack DT. Experimental bacterial endocarditis: IV. Structure and evolution of very early lesions. *J Pathol* 1975;45:81–89.
24. Pelletier LL, Petersdorf RG. Infective endocarditis: A review of 125 cases from the University of Washington hospitals, 1963-1972. *Medicine (Baltimore)* 1977;56: 287–313.
25. Von Reyn CF, Levy BS, Arbeit RD, et al. Infective endocarditis: An analysis based on strict case definitions. *Ann Intern Med* 1981;94:505–518.
26. Durack DT, Lukes AS, Bright DK, and the Duke Endocarditis Service. New criteria for diagnosis of infective endocarditis: Utilization of specific echocardiographic findings. *Am J Med* 1994;96: 200–209.
27. Dajani AS, Bisno AL, Chung KJ, et al. Prevention of bacterial endocarditis: Recommendations by the American Heart Association. *JAMA* 1990;264:2919–2922.
28. Nettles RE, McCarty DE, Corey GR, et al. An evaluation of the Duke criteria in 25 pathologically confirmed cases of prosthetic valve infective endocarditis. *Clin Infect Dis* 1997;25:1401–1403.
29. Hoen B, Selton-Suty C, Danchin N, et al. Evaluation of the Duke criteria versus the Beth Israel criteria for the diagnosis of infective endocarditis. *Clin Infect Dis* 1995;21:905–909.
30. Hoen B, Beguinot I, Rabaud C, et al. The Duke criteria for diagnosing infective endocarditis are specific: Analysis of 100 patients with acute fever or fever of unknown origin. *Clin Infect Dis* 1996;23:298–302.
31. Dodds, GA, Sexton DJ, Durack DT, et al. Negative predictive value of the Duke criteria for infective endocarditis. *Am J Cardiol* 1996;77:403–407.
32. Bayer AS, Ward JI, Ginzton LE, et al. Evaluation of new criteria for the diagnosis of infective endocarditis. *Am J Med* 1994;96:211–219.
33. Cecchi E, Parrini I, Chinaglia A, et al. New diagnostic criteria for infective endocarditis: A study of sensitivity and specificity. *Eur Heart J* 1997;18:1149–1156.
34. Gagliardi JP, Nettles RE, McCarty DE. Native valve infective endocarditis in elderly and younger adult patients: Comparison of clinical features and outcomes using the Duke criteria and the Duke Endocarditis Database. *Clin Infect Dis* 1998;26: 1165–1168.
35. Del Pont JM, De Cicco LT, Vartalitis C, et al. Infective endocarditis in children: Clinical analysis and evaluation of two diagnostic criteria. *Pediatr Infect Dis J* 1995;14: 1079–1086.

36. Bayer AS, Bolger AF, Taubert KA, et al. Diagnosis and management of infective endocarditis and its complications. *Circulation* 1998;98(25):2936–2948
37. Habib G, Derumeaux G, Avierinos JF. Value and limitations of the Duke criteria for the diagnosis of infective endocarditis. *J Am Coll Cardiol* 1999;33:2023–2029.
38. Berlin JA, Abrutyn E, Strom BL, et al. Incidence of infective endocarditis in the Delaware Valley 1998-1990. *Am J Cardiol* 1995;76:933–936.
39. Hogevik H, Olaison L, Andersson R, et al. Epidemiologic aspects of infective endocarditis in an urban population. *Medicine (Baltimore)* 1995;74:324–339.
40. Griffin MR, Wilson WR, Edwards, WD, et al. Infective endocarditis: Olmsted County, Minnesota, 1950 through 1981. *JAMA* 1985;254(9):1199–1202.
41. Steckelberg JM, Melton LJ III, Ilstrup D, et al. Influence of referral bias on the apparent clinical spectrum of infective endocarditis. *Am J Med* 1990;88:582–588.
42. Mansur AJ, Dal Bo CMR, Fukushima JT, et al. Relapses, recurrences, valve replacements, and mortality during the long-term follow-up after infective endocarditis. *Am Heart J* 2001;141(1):78–86.
43. McKinsey DS, Ratts TE, Bisno AL. Underlying cardiac lesions in adults with infective endocarditis: The changing spectrum. *Am J Med* 1987;82:681–688.
44. Moller JH, Anderson RC. 1000 consecutive children with a cardiac malformation with 26- to 37-year follow-up. *Am J Cardiol* 1992;70:661–667.
45. Steckelberg JM, Wilson WR. Risk factors for infective endocarditis. *Infect Dis Clin North Am* 1993;7:9–19.
46. Clemens JD, Horwitz RI, Jaffe C, et al. A controlled evaluation of the risk of bacterial endocarditis in persons with mitral valve prolapse. *N Engl J Med* 1982;307: 776–781.
47. Hickey AJ, MacMahon SW, Wilcken DEL. Mitral valve prolapse and bacterial endocarditis: When is antibiotic prophylaxis necessary? *Am Heart J* 1985;109:431–435.
48. MacMahon SW, Roberts JK, Kramer-Fox R, et al. Mitral valve prolapse and infective endocarditis. *Am Heart J* 1987;113:1291–1298.
49. Welton DE, Young JB, Gentry WO, et al. Recurrent infective endocarditis: Analysis of predisposing factors and clinical features. *Am J Med* 1979;66:932–938.
50. Storm BL, Abrutyn E, Berlin JA, et al. Dental and cardiac risk factors for infective endocarditis: A population-based, case-control study. *Ann Intern Med* 1998;129:761–769.
51. Crawford MH, Durack DT. Clinical presentation of infective endocarditis. *Cardiol Clin* 2003;21(2): 159–166.
52. Castillo JC, Anguita MP, Ramirez A, et al. Long term outcome of infective endocarditis in patients who were not drug addicts: A 10 year study. *Heart* 2000;83(5):525–530.
53. Mills J, Utley J, Abbott J. Heart failure in infective endocarditis: Predisposing factors, course and treatment. *Chest* 1974;66:151–159.
54. Moon MR, Stinson EB, Miller DC. Surgical treatment of endocarditis. *Prog Cardiovasc Dis* 1997;40:239–264.
55. Sandre R, Shafran SD. Infective endocarditis: Review of 135 cases over 9 years. *Clin Infect Dis* 1996;22: 276–286.
56. Arnett EN, Roberts WC. Valve ring abscess in infective endocarditis: Frequency, location and clues to clinical diagnosis from the study of 95 necropsy patients. *Circulation* 1976;54:140–145.
57. Daniel WG, Mugge A, Martin RP, et al. Improvement in the diagnosis of abcesses associated with endocarditis by transesophageal echocardiography. *N Engl J Med* 1991; 324:795–800.
58. Sabik JF, Lytle BW, Blackstone EH, et al. Aortic root replacement with cryopreserved allograft for prosthetic valve endocarditis. *Ann Thorac Surg* 2002;74: 650–659.
59. Blumberg E, Karalis D, Chandrasekaran K, et al. Endocarditis-associated paravalvular abscess: Do clinical parameters predict the presence of abscess? *Chest* 1995; 107:898–903.
60. Omari B, Shapiro S, Ginzton L, et al. Predictive risk factors for periannular extension of native valve endocarditis: Clinical and echocardiographic analyses. *Chest* 1989; 96(6):1273–1279.
61. Sachdev M, Peterson GE, Jollis JG. Imaging techniques for diagnosis of infective endocarditis. *Infect Dis Clin North Am* 2002;16(2):319–337.
62. Chan KW. Early clinical course and long-term outcome of patients with infective endocarditis complicated by perivalvular abscess. *CMAJ* 1983;167(1):19–24.
63. Choussat R, Thomas D, Isnard R, et al. Perivalvular abscesses associated with endocarditis: Clinical features and prognostic factors of overall survival in a series of 233 cases. *Eur Heart J* 1999;20:232–241.
64. Modesto KM, Pellikka PA, Malouf JF, et al. Mycotic aneurysm of the left ventricle: Echocardiographic diagnosis. *J Am Soc Echocardiogr* 2003;16(2):191–193.
65. Anguera I, Quaglio G, Miro JM, et al. Aortocardiac fistulas complicating infective endocarditis. *Am J Cardiol* 2001;87(5):652–654.
66. San Roman JA, Vilacosta I, Sarria C, et al. Clinical course, microbiologic profile and diagnosis of periannular complications in prosthetic valve endocarditis. *Am J Cardiol* 1999;83:1075–1079.
67. Sexton DJ, Bashore TM. Infective endocarditis. In Topol EJ (ed). *Comprehensive Cardiovascular Medicine.* Philadelphia: Lippincott-Raven; 1998:637–667.
68. Meine TJ, Nettles RE, Anderson DJ, et al. Cardiac conduction abnormalities in endocarditis defined by the Duke criteria. *Am Heart J* 2001,142(2):280–285.
69. DiNubile MJ, Calderwood SB, Steinhaus DM. Cardiac conduction abnormalities complicating native valve active infective endocarditis. *Am J Cardiol* 1986;58: 1213–1217.
70. Wang K, Gobel F, Gleason DF. Complete heart block complicating bacterial endocarditis. *Circulation* 1972;46: 939–947.
71. Pearce ML, Guze LB. Some factors affecting prognosis in bacterial endocarditis. *Ann Intern Med* 1961;55: 270–282.
72. Selton-Suty C, Hoen B, Grentzinger A, et al. Clinical and bacteriological characteristics of infective endocarditis in the elderly. *Heart* 1997;77(3):260–263.
73. Werner GS, Schulz R, Fuchs JB, et al. Infective endocarditis in the elderly in the era of transesophageal echocardiography: Clinical features and prognosis compared with younger patients. *Am J Med* 1996;100(1): 90–97.

74. Cabell CH, Pond KK, Peterson GE, et al. The risk of stroke and death in patients with aortic and mitral valve endocarditis. *Am Heart J* 2001;142(1): 75–80.
75. Sexton DJ, Spelman D. Current best practices and guidelines: Assessment and management of complications in infective endocarditis. *Infect Dis Clin North Am* 2002;16(2):507–521.
76. Robinson SL, Saxe JM, Lucas CE, et al. Splenic abscess associated with endocarditis. *Surgery* 1992;112:781–786; discussion 786–787.
77. Murdock DR, Roberts SA, Fowler Jr VG,et al. Infection of orthopedic prostheses after *Staph aureus* bacteremia. *Clin Infect Dis* 2001;32:647–649.
78. Zamorano J, Sanz J, Moreno R, et al. Comparison of outcome in patients with culture-negative versus culture-positive active infective endocarditis. *Am J Cardiol* 2001;87(12):1423–1425.
79. Zamorano J, Sanz J, Moreno R, et al. Better prognosis of elderly patients with infective endocarditis in the era of routine echocardiography and non-restrictive indications for valve surgery. *J Am Soc Echocardiogr* 2002;15(7): 702–707.
80. Towns ML, Reller LB. Diagnostic methods: Current best practices and guidelines for isolation of bacteria and fungi in infective endocarditis. *Infect Dis Clin North Am* 2002;16(2)363–376.
81. Werner AS, Cobbs CG, Kaye D, Hook EW. Studies on the bacteremia of bacterial endocarditis. *JAMA* 1967;202: 199–203.
82. Lisby G, Gutschik E, Durack DT. Molecular methods for diagnosis of infective endocarditis. Inf*ect Dis Clin North Am* 2002;16(2):393–412.
83. Ellis ME, Al-Abdely H, Sandridge A, et al. Fungal endocarditis: Evidence in the world literature, 1965-1995. *Clin Infect Dis* 2001;32:50–62.
84. Murray PR, Traynor P, Hopson D. Critical assessment of blood culture techniques: Analysis of recovery of obligate and facultative anaerobes, strict aerobic bacteria, and fungi in aerobic and anaerobic blood culture bottles. *J Clin Microbiol* 1992;30:1462–1468.
85. Lepidi H, Durack DT, Raoult D. Diagnostic methods: Current best practices and guidelines for histologic evaluation in infective endocarditis. *Infect Dis Clin North Am* 2002;16(2):339–361.
86. Bansal RC, Graham BM, Jutzy KR, et al. Left ventricular outflow tract to left atrial communication secondary to rupture of mitral-aortic intervalvular fibrosa in infective endocarditis: Diagnosis by transesophageal echocardiography and color flow imaging. *J Am Coll Cardiol* 1990; 15:499–504.
87. Winslow TM, Friar DA, Larson AW, et al. A rare complication of aortic valve endocarditis: Diagnosis with transesophageal echocardiography. *J Am Soc Echocardiogr* 1995;8:546–550.
88. Nomeir AM, Downes TR, Cordell AR. Perforation of the anterior mitral leaflet caused by aortic valve endocarditis: Diagnosis by two-dimensional, transesophageal echocardiography and color flow Doppler. *J Am Soc Echo*cardiogr 1992;5:195–198.
89. Habib G, Guidon C, Tricoire E, et al. Papillary muscle rupture caused by bacterial endocarditis: Role of transesophageal echocardiography. *J Am Soc Echocardiogr* 1994;7:79–81.
90. Shively BK, Gurule FT, Roldan CA, et al. Diagnostic value of transesophageal compared with transthoracic echocardiography in infective endocarditis. *J Am Coll Cardiol* 1991;18:391–397.
91. Reynolds HR, Jagen MA, Tunick PA, Kronzon I. Sensitivity of transthoracic versus transesophageal echocardiography for the detection of native valve endocarditis in the modern era. *J Am Soc Echocardiogr* 2003;16(1):310–315.
92. Erbel R, Rohmann S, Drexler M, et al. Improved diagnostic value of echocardiography in patients with infective endocarditis by transesophageal approach: A prospective study. *Eur Heart J* 1988;9:43–53
93. Krivokapich J, Child JS. Role of transthoracic and transesophageal echocardiography in diagnosis and management of infective endocarditis. *Cardiol Clin* 1996;14:363–382.
94. Roe MT, Abramson MA, Li J, et al. Clinical information determines the impact of transesophageal echocardiography on the diagnosis of infective endocarditis by the Duke criteria. *Am Heart J* 2000;139(6):945–951.
95. Daniel WG, Muggle A, Grote J, et al. Comparison of transthoracic and transesophageal echocardiography for detection of abnormalities of prosthetic and bioprosthetic valves in the mitral and aortic positions. *Am J Cardiol* 1993;71:210–215.
96. Birmingham GD, Rahko PS, Ballantyne R. Improved detection of endocarditis with transesophageal echocardiography. *Am Heart J* 1992;123:774–781.
97. Shapiro SM, Young E, De Guzman S, et al. Transesophageal echocardiography in diagnosis of infective endocarditis. *Chest* 1994;105:377–382.
98. Ryan EW, Bolger AF. Transesophageal echocardiography in the evaluation of infective endocarditis. *Cardiol Clin* 2000;18(4):773–787.
99. Karalis DG, Bansal RC, Hauck AJ, et al. Transesophageal echocardiographic recognition of subaortic complications in aortic valve endocarditis: Clinical and surgical implications. *Circulation* 1993;86:353–362.
100. Mugge A, Daniel WG, Gunter F, et al. Echocardiography in infective endocarditis: Reassessment of prognostic implications of vegetation size determined by the transthoracic and the transesophageal approach. *J Am Coll Cardiol* 1989;14:631–638.
101. Isada LR, Torelli JN, Stewart WJ, Klein AL. Detection of fibrous strands on prosthetic mitral valves with transesophageal echocardiography: Another potential embolic source. *J Am Soc Echocardiogr* 1994;7: 641–645.
102. Orsinelli, Pearson AC. Detection of prosthetic valve strands by transesophageal echocardiography: Clinical significance in patients with suspected cardiac source of embolism. *J Am Coll Cardiol* 1995;26:1713–1718.
103. Ionescu AA, Newman GR, Butchart EG, Fraser AG. Morphologic analysis of a strand from a prosthetic mitral valve: No evidence of fibrin. *J Am Soc Echocardiogr* 1999;12:766–768.
104. Rozich JD, Edwards WD, Hanna RD, et al. Mechanical prosthetic valve-associated strands: Pathologic correlates to transesophageal echocardiography. *J Am Soc Echocardiogr* 2003;16(1):310–315.

105. Khandheria BK, Seward JB, Oh JK, et al. Value and limitations of transesophageal echocardiography in assessment of mitral valve prostheses. *Circulation* 1991;83:1956–1968.
106. Gueret P, Vignon P, Fournier P, et al. Transesophageal echocardiography for the diagnosis and management of nonobstructive thrombosis of mechanical mitral valve prosthesis. *Circulation* 1995;91:103–110.
107. Kaye D. Infective endocarditis. In: Fauci AS, et al. *Harrison's Principles of Internal Medicine,* 14th ed. New York: McGraw-Hill; 785–786, 1998.
108. Hoen B. Special issues in the management of infective endocarditis caused by Gram-positive cocci. *Infect Dis Clin North Am* 2002;16(2):437–452.
109. Levine DP, Crane LR, Zervos MJ. Bacteremia in narcotic addicts at the Detroit Medical Center: II. Infectious endocarditis: A prospective comparative study. *Rev Infect Dis* 1986;8(3):374–396.
110. Brown PD, Levine DP. Infective endocarditis in the injection drug user. *Infect Dis Clinic North Am* 2002;16(3):645–665.
111. Miro JM, del Rio A, Mestres CA. Infective endocarditis in intravenous drug abusers and HIV-1 infected patients. *Infect Dis Clin North Am* 2002;16(2):273–295.
112. Rubenstein E, Lang R. Fungal endocarditis. *Eur Heart J* 1995;16(Suppl B):84–89.
113. Chambers HF, Miller RT, Newman MD. Right-sided *Staphylococcus aureus* endocarditis in intravenous drug abusers: Two-week combination therapy. *Ann Intern Med* 1988;109(8):619–624.
114. Fortun J, Perez-Molina JA, Anon MT, et al. Right-sided endocarditis caused by *Staphylococcus aureus* in drug abusers. *Antimicrob Agents Chemother* 1995;39(2): 525–528.
115. Ribera E, Gomez-Jimenez J, Cortes E, et al. Effectiveness of cloxacillin with and without gentamycin in short-term therapy for right-sided *Staphylococcus aureus* endocarditis: A randomized, controlled trial. *Ann Intern Med* 1996;125(12);969–974.
116. Wilson WR, Karchmer AW, Dajani, et al. Antibiotic treatment of adults with infective endocarditis due to streptococci, enterococci, staphylococci, and HACEK microorganisms: American Heart Association. *JAMA* 1995;274:1706–1713.
117. Nunley DL, Perlman PE. Endocarditis: Changing trends in epidemiology, clinical and microbiologic spectrum. *Postgrad Med* 1993;93:235–238.
118. Bonow RO, Carabello B, de Leon AC Jr, et al. ACC/AHA guidelines for the management of patients with valvular heart disease: A report of the American College of Cardiology/American Heart Association Task Force on practice guidelines (Committee on management of patients with valvular heart disease). *J Am Coll Cardiol* 1998;32:1486–1582.
119. Olaison L, Pettersson G. Current best practices and guidelines: Indications for surgical intervention in infective endocarditis. *Cardiol Clin* 2003;21:235–251.
120. Dreyfus G, Serraf A, Jebara VA, et al. Valve repair in acute endocarditis. *Ann Thorac Surg* 1990;49:706–713.
121. David TM, Chard RB. Commissuroplasty: A method of valve repair for mitral and tricuspid endocarditis. *Ann Thorac Surg* 1999;68:1727–1730.
122. David TE, Feindel CM, Armstrong S, Sun Z. Reconstruction of the mitral annulus: A ten-year experience. *J Thorac Cardiovasc Surg* 1995;110:1323–1332.
123. Lee EM, Shapiro LM, Wells FC. Conservative operation for infective endocarditis of the mitral valve. *Ann Thorac Surg* 1998;65:1087–1092.
124. David TE, Uden DE, Strauss HD. The importance of the mitral apparatus in left ventricular function after correction of mitral regurgitation. *Circulation* 1983;68:76–82.
125. Horstkotte D, Schulte HD, Bircks W, Strauer BE. The effect of chordal preservation on late outcome after mitral valve replacement: A randomized study. *J Heart Valve Dis* 1993;2:150–158.
126. Hetzer R, Bougiokas G, Franz M, Borst HG. Mitral valve replacement with preservation of papillary muscles and chordae tendineae—revival of a seemingly forgotten concept. *Thorac Cardiovasc Surg* 1983;31:291–296.
127. Komeda M, David TE, Rao V, et al. Late hemodynamic effects of the preserved papillary muscles during mitral valve replacement. *Circulation* 1994;90(Suppl 2):190–194.
128. David TE, Armstrong S, Sun Z. Left ventricular function after mitral valve surgery. *J Heart Valve Dis* 1995;4(Suppl): 175–180.
129. Acar C, Tolan M, Berrebi A, et al. Homograft replacement of the mitral valve: Graft selection, technique of implantation, and results in forty-three patients. *J Thorac Cardiovasc Surg* 1996;111:367–380.
130. Gulbins H. Mitral valve surgery utilizing homografts: Early results. *J Heart Valve Dis* 2000;9:222–229.
131. Doty DB. Cardiac valve replacement with mitral homograft. *Semin Thorac Cardiovasc Surg* 2001;13(Suppl 4): 35–42.
132. Kumar AS. Homograft mitral valve replacement: Five years' results. *J Thorac Cardiovasc Surg* 2000;120:450–458.
133. Shimoni Z. Tricuspid valve endocarditis in adult patients without known predisposing factors. *Eur J Clin Microbiol Infect Dis* 2001;20(1):49–51.
134. Arbulu A, Holmes RJ, Asfaw I. Surgical treatment of intractable right-sided endocarditis in drug addicts: 25 years' experience. *J Heart Valve Dis* 1993;2:129–137.
135. Stern HJ, Sisto DA, Strom JA, et al. Immediate tricuspid valve replacement for endocarditis: Indications and results. *J Thorac Cardiovasc Surg* 1986;91:163–167.
136. Renzulli A, De Feo M, Carozza A, et al. Surgery for tricuspid valve endocarditis: A selective approach. *Heart Vessels* 1999;14(4):163–169.
137. Stern HJ, Sisto DA, Strom JA, et al. Immediate tricuspid valve replacement for endocarditis: Indications and results. *J Thorac Cardiovasc Surg* 1986;91:163–167.
138. Raman J, Bellomo R, Shah P. Avoiding the pump in tricuspid valve endocarditis—egetectomy under inflow occlusion. *Ann Thorac Surg* 2002;8(6):350–353.
139. Allen MD, Slachman F, Eddy C, et al. Tricuspid valve repair for tricuspid valve endocarditis: Tricuspid valve "recycling." *Ann Thorac Surg* 1991;51:593–598.
140. Lange R, De Simone R, Bauernschmitt R, et al. Tricuspid valve reconstruction, a treatment option in acute endocarditis. *Eur J Cardiothorac Surg* 1996;10:320–326.
141. Ratnatunga CP, Edwards MB, Dore CJ, Taylor KM. Tricuspid valve replacement: UK heart valve registry mid-term results comparing mechanical and biological prostheses. *Ann Thorac Surg* 1998;66:1940–1947.

142. Rizzoli G, De Perini L, Bottio T, et al. Prosthetic replacement of the tricuspid valve: Biological or mechanical? *Ann Thorac Surg* 1998;66:S62–67.
143. Nakano K, Ishibashi-Ueda H, Kobayashi J, et al. Tricuspid valve replacement with bioprostheses: Long term results and causes of valve dysfunction. *Ann Thorac Surg* 2001;71:105–109.
144. Scully HE, Armstrong CS. Tricuspid valve replacement: Fifteen years of experience with mechanical prostheses and bioprostheses. *J Thorac Cardiovasc Surg* 1995;109: 1035–1041.
145. Couetil JP, Argyriadis PG, Shafy A, et al. Partial replacement of the tricuspid valve by mitral homografts in acute endocarditis. *Ann Thorac Surg* 2002;73:1808–1812.
146. Ramsheyi A, D'Attellis N, Le Lostec Z, et al. Partial mitral homograft for tricuspid valve repair. *Ann Thorac Surg* 1997;64:1486–1488.
147. Pomar JL, Mestres CA. Tricuspid valve replacemnt using a mitral homograft. Surgical technique and initial results. *J Heart Valve Dis* 1993;2:125–128.
148. Mestres CA, Miro JM, Pare JC, Pomar JL. Six-year experience with cryopreserved mitral homografts in the treatment of tricuspid valve endocarditis in HIV-infected drug addicts. *J Heart Valve Dis* 1999;8(5): 575–577.
149. Acar C, Iung B, Cormier B, et al. Double mitral homograft for recurrent bacterial endocarditis of the tricuspid and mitral valves. *J Heart Valve Dis* 1994;3: 470–472.
150. Miyagishima RT, Brumwell ML, Jamieson WRE, Munt BI. Tricuspid valve replacement using a cryopreserved mitral homograft: Surgical technique and initial results. *J Heart Valve Dis* 2000;9:805–809.
151. Hvass U, Baron F, Fourchy D, Pansard Y. Mitral homografts for total tricuspid valve replacement: Comparison of two techniques. *J Thorac Cardiovasc Surg* 2001;121: 592–594.
152. Katsumata T, Westaby S. Mitral homograft replacement of the tricuspid valve for endocarditis. *Ann Thorac Surg* 1997;63:1480–1482.
153. Cosgrove DM. Mitral homograft for tricuspid valve replacement. *J Heart Valve Dis* 1993;2:124.
154. Symbas PN, Vlasis SE, Zacharopoulos L, Lutz JF. Acute endocarditis: Surgical treatment of aortic regurgitation and aortico-left ventricular discontinuity. *J Thorac Cardiovasc Surg* 1982;84:291–296.
155. David TE, Bos J, Christakis GT, et al. Heart valve operations in patients with active infective endocarditis. *Ann Thorac Surg* 1990;49:701–705.
156. Reitz BA, Stinson EB, Watson DC, et al. Translocation of the aortic valve for prosthetic valve endocarditis. *J Thorac Cardiovasc Surg* 1981;81:212–218.
157. Frantz PT, Murray GF, Wilcox RB. Surgical management of left ventricular-aortic discontinuity complicating bacterial endocarditis. *Ann Thorac Surg* 1980;29:1–7.
158. Joyce F, Tingleff J, Pettersson G. Ross operation in the treatment of prosthetic aortic valve endocarditis. *Semin Thorac Cardiovasc Surg* 1995;7:38–46.
159. Moon MR, Miller DC, Moore KA, et al. Treatment of endocarditis with valve replacement: The question of tissue versus mechanical prosthesis. *Ann Thorac Surg* 2001;71:1164–1171.
160. Aagaard J, Andersen PV. Acute endocarditis treated with radical debridement and implantation of mechanical or stented bioprosthetic devices. *Ann Thorac Surg* 2001; 71:100–104.
161. Bauernschmitt R, Jacob HG, Vahl CF, et al. Operation for infective endocarditis: Results after implantation of mechanical valves. *Ann Thorac Surg* 1998;65:359–364.
162. Hagl C, Galla JD, Lansman SL, et al. Replacing the ascending aorta and aortic valve for acute prosthetic valve endocarditis: Is using prosthetic material contraindicated? *Ann Thorac Surg* 2002;74:S1781–1785.
163. Niwaya K, Knott-Craig CJ, Santangelo K, et al. Advantage of autograft and homograft valve replacement for complex aortic valve endocarditis. *Ann Thorac Surg* 1999;67:1603–1608.
164. McGiffin DC, Galbraith AJ, McLachlan GJ, et al. Aortic valve infection. *J Thorac Cardiovasc Surg* 1992;104: 511–520.
165. Pagano D, Allen SM, Bonser RS. Homograft aortic valve and root replacement for severe destructive native or prosthetic endocarditis. *Eur Cardiothorac Surg* 1994;8: 173–176.
166. Yacoub M, Rasmi NRH, Sundt TM, et al. Fourteen-year experience with homovital homografts for aortic valve replacement. *J Thorac Cardiovasc Surg* 1995;110:186–194.
167. Dearani JA, Orszulak TA, Schaff HV, et al. Results of allograft aortic valve replacement for complex endocarditis. *J Thorac Cardiovasc Surg* 1997;113:285–291.
168. Doty JR, Salazar JD, Liddicoat JR, et al. Aortic valve replacement with cryopreserved aortic allograft: Ten-year experience. *J Thorac Cardiovasc Surg* 1998;115: 371–380.
169. Haydock D, Barratt-Boyes B, Macedo T, et al. Aortic valve replacement for active infectious endocarditis in 108 patients: A comparison of freehand allograft valves with mechanical prostheses and bioprostheses. *J Thorac Cardiovasc Surg* 1992;103:130–139.
170. Ivert TSA, Dismukes WE, Cobbs LG, et al. Prosthetic valve endocarditis. *Circulation* 1984;69:223–232.
171. Dossche KM, Defauw JJ, Ernst SM, et al. Allograft aortic root replacement in prosthetic aortic valve endocarditis: A review of 32 patients. *Ann Thorac Surg* 1997;63:1644–1649.
172. Yankah AC, Klose H, Petzina R, et al. Surgical management of acute aortic root endocarditis with viable homografts: 13-year experience. *Eur J Cardiothorac Surg* 2002;21:260–267.
173. Aranki SF, Santini F, Adams DH, et al. Aortic valve endocarditis: Determinants of early survival and late morbidity. *Circulation* 1994;90:II175–182.
174. Osman A, McCann J, Shemin RJ, Lazar HL. Accelerated allograft degeneration after aortic valve endocarditis. *Ann Thorac Surg* 1999;68:1849–1850.
175. Vogt PR, von Segesser KL, Jenni R, et al. Emergency surgery for acute infective aortic valve endocarditis: Performance of cryopreserved homografts and mode of failure. *Eur J Cardiothorac Surg* 1997;11:53–61.
176. Mitchell RN, Jonas RA, Schoen FJ. Pathology of explanted cryopreserved allograft heart valves: Comparison with aortic valves from orthotopic heart transplants. *J Thorac Cardiovasc Surg* 1998;115: 118–127.

177. O'Brief MF, Stafford EG, Gardner MAH, et al. A comparison of aortic valve replacement with viable cryopreserved and fresh allograft valves with a note on chromosomal studies. *J Thorac Cardiovasc Surg* 1987;94:812–824.
178. Baratt-Boyes GB, Roche MB, Subramanyan R, et al. Long-term follow-up of patients with the antibiotic-sterilized aortic homograft valve inserted freehand in the aortic position. *Circulation* 1987;75:768–777.
179. Netzer RO, Zollinger E, Seiler C, Cerny A. Infective endocarditis: Clinical spectrum, presentation and outcome: An analysis of 212 cases 1980-1995. *Heart* 2000;84(1):25–30.
180. Tornos MP, Permanyer-Miralda G, Olona M, et al. Long-term complications of native valve infective endocarditis in non-addicts: A 15-year follow-up study. *Ann Intern Med* 1992;117(7):567–572.
181. Aranki SF, Adams DH, Rizzo RJ, et al. Determinants of early mortality and late survival in mitral valve endocarditis. *Circulation* 1995;92:II143–149.

CHAPTER

35 ASCENDING AND ARCH ANEURYSMS OF THE AORTA

Anthony D. Caffarelli, Pieter J. A. van der Starre, R. Scott Mitchell

"There is no disease more conducive to clinical humility than aneurysms of the aorta."

—Sir William Osler

INTRODUCTION

Surgical repair of ascending and arch aneurysms of the aorta is one of the most formidable challenges facing the cardiovascular surgeon. The challenges stem from the often catastrophic consequences of rupture of the thoracic aorta, the variegated clinical presentations associated with aortic disruption, and the risk of incurring devastating neurologic injury during aortic arch repair. This chapter describes the epidemiology, pathophysiology, clinical features, diagnosis, treatment, and outcomes of ascending and arch aneurysms of the aorta.

KEY CONCEPTS

- Epidemiology
  - The leading cause of aneurysms of the ascending aorta is medial degeneration, which may be idiopathic or accelerated by heritable disorders of connective tissue; conversely, arch aneurysms are due to chronic dissection or long-standing hypertension and atherosclerosis.
- Pathophysiology
  - Histopathologic investigations of aneurysmal tissue have shown that a majority of ascending aortic and arch aneurysms are associated with medial degeneration in the layers of the aortic wall. This is characterized by a triad of (1) loss of noninflammatory smooth muscle cells, (2) fragmentation of elastic fibers, and (3) accumulation of basophilic ground substance in cell-depleted areas of the medial layer of the vessel wall. This combination of factors weakens the aortic wall, thereby increasing wall tension; this can induce aortic dilatation and aneurysm formation, leading to higher wall stress and eventually resulting in intramural hemorrhage, aortic dissection, or rupture. Medial degeneration can be accelerated by inborn errors of metabolism that affect any component of the aortic connective tissue. Known heritable disorders of connective tissue that commonly manifest as ascending and arch aneurysms of the aorta are Marfan's syndrome, Ehlers-Danlos syndrome, Loeys-Dietz syndrome, familial forms of thoracic aortic aneurysm and dissection, and bicuspid aortic valve disease; Turner's syndrome and Noonan's syndrome occur far less frequently.
- Clinical features
  - Most patients with thoracic aortic aneurysms are asymptomatic at the time of presentation, and aneurysms of the ascending aorta usually are detected as incidental findings during testing for other disorders. In contrast, because of their anatomic location and the space-occupying nature of the aneurysm, aneurysms of the aortic arch may impinge on important mediastinal structures and are therefore symptomatic more often than are aneurysms of the ascending or descending aorta. Symptoms attributable to the aneurysm are cause for concern and consideration for early surgical intervention. Patients with rupture of an ascending or arch aneurysm often present in extremis.
- Diagnostics
  - The most common finding on chest x-ray for a thoracic aortic aneurysm is widening of the superior mediastinum; other findings include displacement

and compression of the mediastinal contents and curvilinear calcification in the aneurysmal wall. Echocardiography is widely available, can be noninvasive (TTE) or minimally invasive (TEE), and is relatively inexpensive. TTE can visualize the aortic root and ascending aorta accurately and is suitable for evaluating the size of moderate aneurysms and assessing cardiac complications such as aortic regurgitation, impaired left ventricular function, and hemopericardium. Intraoperative application of TEE allows continuous monitoring of the surgical procedure without disturbing the sterile field. Because of its speed and wide availability, computed tomography/computed tomography angiography (CT/CTA) is currently the most common diagnostic imaging method for studying the aorta. CTA has the advantage of demonstrating aortic wall thickening, calcification, and luminal thrombus, thus displaying the true axial extent of an aneurysm. Magnetic resonance angiography is emerging as a diagnostic tool but is less readily available and has limited utilization in acute aortic problems because of its limited applicability.

- Treatment
  - Symptomatic patients with ascending or arch aneurysms should be evaluated urgently for surgical repair. Patients presenting with rupture should be operated urgently, since these conditions are almost uniformly fatal without prompt surgical intervention. Operative intervention in a patient with a nonheritable connective tissue disorder should be considered when the ascending aortic aneurysm diameter ranges from 5 to 5.5 cm. For patients with an aneurysm diameter less than 5 cm who are being monitored with serial imaging, an indication for surgical intervention would be a 10 percent increase in size over a 6- to 12-month time course. For patients with a heritable disorder of connective tissue, surgical intervention for the ascending aorta should be considered at a diameter of 4 cm for Loeys-Dietz syndrome, 4 to 4.5 cm for Marfan's syndrome, 4.5 to 5.0 cm for bicuspid aortic valve, and 5.0 cm for Ehlers-Danlos syndrome and thoracic aortic aneurysm and dissection patients. Factors that prompt the recommendation for surgery when the aorta is less than 5.0 cm include rapid growth of the aortic diameter (more than 1 cm per year), a family history of premature aortic dissection (dissection less than 5.0 cm), and the presence of moderate or severe aortic regurgitation. Operative repair varies with the underlying pathology and the quality of the aortic wall, the status of the aortic valve, expected survival, and the general well-being of the patient.
- Outcomes
  - Progress over the last three decades, including improved surgical instrumentation, and advances in perfusion strategies with resultant improvements in myocardial and cerebral protection have augmented the surgical armamentarium significantly, facilitating the management of complex aortic problems. Replacement of the ascending aorta is a safe and effective procedure, with operative mortality rates of 2 to 5 percent. The operative mortality varies with the acuity of the operation, patient age, left ventricular function, and extent of operation. Late survival after operation is approximately 65 percent at 5 years and 55 percent at 7 years. For patients with Marfan's syndrome, a valve-sparing aortic root replacement is a reasonable alternative to a composite vale graft. Survival is excellent with the reimplantation and remodeling techniques and complications are rare, but the long-term durability of this repair has not been established. For aortic arch replacement, the average operative mortality rate is 13 percent, with long-term survival ranging from 61 to 82 percent at 5 years and 31 to 69 percent at 10 years. Despite these advances, providing adequate cerebral protection and preventing cerebral embolization during reconstruction of the calcified and atherosclerotic aorta are a formidable challenge.

Definitions

A *true* aortic aneurysm is defined arbitrarily as a 50 percent enlargement of the normal aorta for a particular body surface area, age, and gender.[1] Clinically, the term usually is reserved for ascending aortic (sinus or tubular) diameters greater than 3.5 to 4.0 cm or aortic arch diameters greater than 4 cm. Some experienced thoracic aortic surgical centers use a ratio of 2× in which the diameter of the enlarged aortic segment is in the numerator and that of the normal contiguous aorta is in the denominator.[2] The combination of dilation of the ascending aorta and dilation of the aortic annulus is termed *annuloaortic ectasia*.[3] A *false* aortic aneurysm is a localized dilation whose wall consists of adventitia, some or all of the media, and compressed periaortic tissue usually associated with trauma, infection, or previous operations on the aorta. The classification of thoracic aortic aneurysms is based on the location, morphologic characteristics, or etiology.[4]

Classification according to location

The location of the aneurysm affects clinical manifestations, natural history, and treatment options as well as providing insight into the etiology of the aneurysm formation. Thoracic aortic aneurysms can involve the ascending aorta, the arch, or the descending aorta. The ascending aorta is the portion of aorta starting at the aortic annulus and ending at the origin of the innominate artery near the pericardial reflection. The ascending aorta

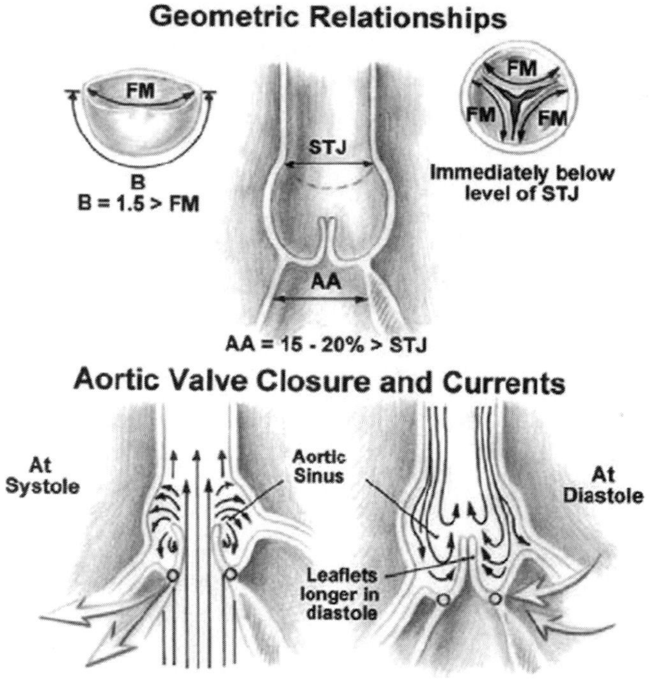

Figure 35-1 The static and basic functional anatomy of the aortic root valve complex. Note that the sinotubular junction diameter is approximately 15 percent less than that of the base of the aorta (putative aortic annulus). The DaVinci sinus currents are depicted; they enhance leaflet closure at the end of systole and protect leaflets from wall impact during systole. In addition, movement of the annulus changes the tension-length relationships of the leaflets to enhance function. It is difficult to demonstrate in a two-dimensional figure the time-dependent expansion of the aortic root that occurs during the first third of systole and the change in its overall configuration from a truncated cone shape with acorn protuberances of the sinuses to a larger, more cylindric form that would offer less impedance to ejection. FM = free margin; B = base of semilunar leaflet insertion; STJ = sinotubular junction; AA = aortic annulus (defined as the base of the aorta, not the semilunar leaflet attachment scalloped edge). (Reproduced, with permission, from Hopkins.[181])

is separated further into a proximal sinus portion, also known as the aortic root, and a distal tubular portion, with the demarcation line occurring at the sinotubular junction, which is at the top of the aortic valve commissures (Fig. 35-1). These distinctions are important in that operations involving the aortic root require repair or replacement of the aortic valve and reimplantation of the coronary arteries. The aortic arch begins at the proximal origin of the innominate artery, traverses in conjunction with the brachiocephalic vessels, and ends at the distal origin of the left subclavian artery, dividing the aortic arch into the proximal, transverse, and distal sections, respectively. Aneurysms of the descending thoracic aorta originate distal to the origin of the left subclavian artery, whereas thoracoabdominal aneurysms originate in the descending thoracic aorta and extend below the diaphragm to involve various extents of the abdominal aorta.

Classification according to morphology

The gross pathoanatomic description of thoracic aortic aneurysms includes fusiform and saccular aneurysms. Fusiform aneurysms involve a long segment of the aorta with uniform dilation involving the whole circumference of the aortic wall, whereas saccular aneurysms usually involve only a localized segment of the aorta with an eccentric dilation that communicates with the main lumen of the aorta by a variable-sized neck.[4]

Classification according to etiology

Classification by etiology provides the most meaningful nomenclature for thoracic aortic aneurysms because of the treatment implications but at the same time is the most difficult to do. This stems from the variety of causes of thoracic aortic aneurysms, which histologically look very similar. The leading cause of aneurysms of the ascending aorta is medial degeneration, which may be idiopathic or accelerated by heritable disorders of connective tissue; conversely, arch aneurysms are due to chronic dissection or long-standing hypertension and atherosclerosis. This is discussed in more detail in the pathophysiology section.

Historical highlights

The first description of arterial aneurysms is attributed to Galen, who observed false aneurysms in gladiators injured during battle in the second century. During that period, Antyllus made the distinction between traumatic and degenerative aneurysms and was the first to attempt surgical treatment of aneurysms with proximal and distal ligation.[5] In 1557, Vesalius[6] is credited with the first correct clinical diagnosis, and Morgagni outlined fascinating and detailed case histories, postmortem findings, and commentaries on three cases of ruptured thoracic aneurysm in young adults in 1769. In his great work *The Seats [Sites] and Causes of Diseases*, he described the graphic case report of a "strumpet [prostitute] of eight-and-twenty years of age" who died suddenly in the act of performing her profession, causing considerable embarrassment to her client.[7]

The early operative treatment of thoracic aneurysms was entirely palliative, consisting of the introduction of wire within the sac to stimulate clot formation or the wrapping of cellophane around the sac to induce periarterial fibrosis. Before the availability of cardiopulmonary bypass, surgical treatment of thoracic aortic aneurysms was limited to resection of discrete saccular aneurysms associated with coarctations.[7] Even though the first isolated thoracic aneurysm of the arch was resected by Monod and Meyer in Paris in 1950,[8] the development of current aortic surgery procedures was contingent on improvements in vascular surgical instruments and the evolution of arterial grafts and bypass procedures in conjunction with cardiopulmonary bypass (CPB) and the various perfusion techniques.

Ascending aneurysms

Cooley and DeBakey[9] are credited with the first resection of an ascending aortic aneurysm and replacement with a graft in 1956; subsequently, a variety of approaches evolved. In 1960, Mueller and colleagues[10] combined supracoronary graft replacement with bicuspidization of an incompetent aortic valve. In 1963, Starr and associates[11] described supracoronary graft replacement and replacement of the aortic valve. In 1964, Wheat and coworkers[12] described a technique of radical resection of the aortic wall that left small buttons of tissue adjacent to the coronary ostia, replacement of the aorta with a graft, and prosthetic replacement of the aortic valve. Bentall and DeBono[13] and, independently, Edwards and Kerr[14] introduced a method of replacing the aortic valve and ascending aorta simultaneously using a composite valve graft (CVG) and reimplanting the coronary ostia into the graft. After 1968, the CVG procedure evolved to include full-thickness end-to-side coronary anastomoses in the

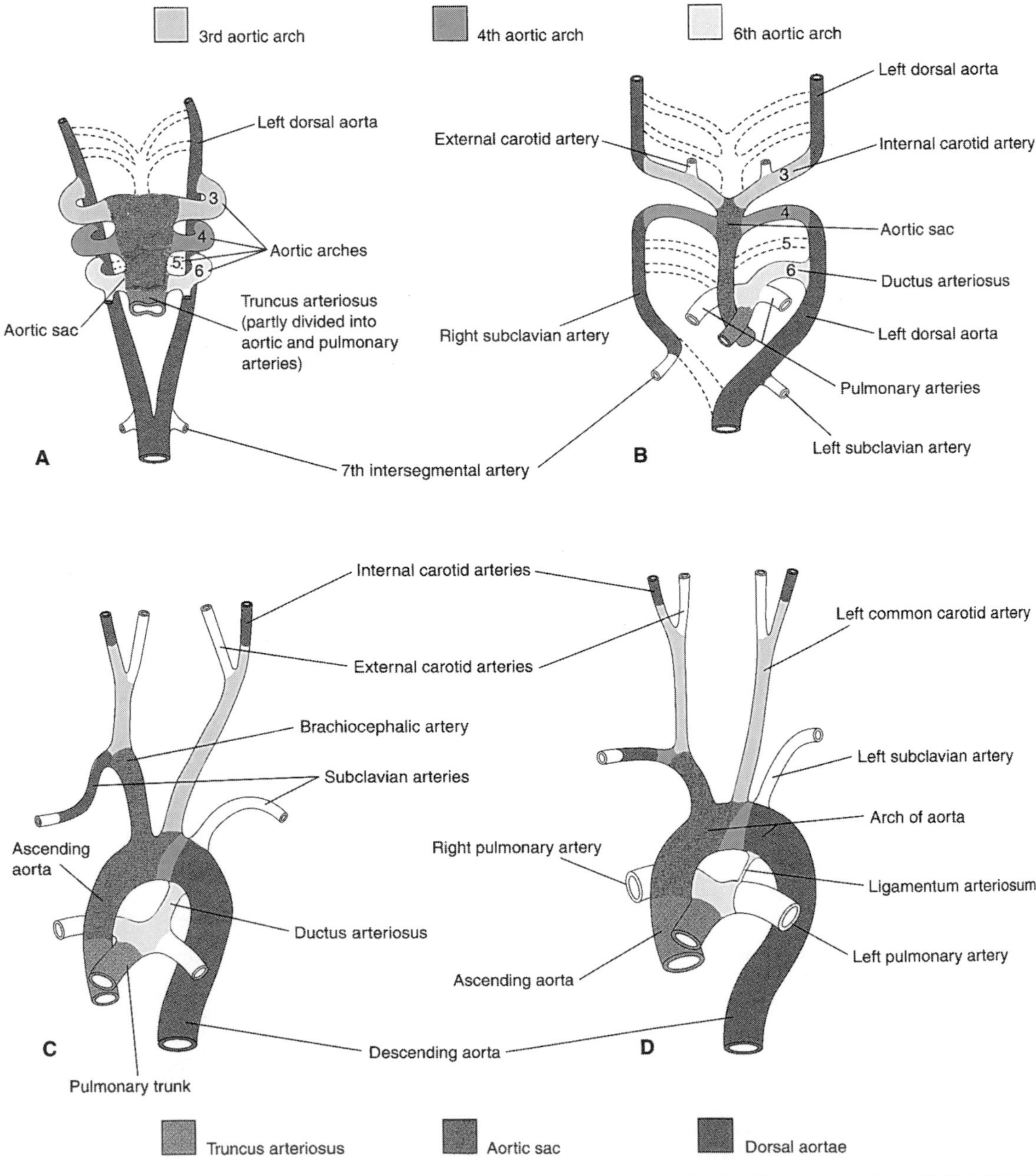

Figure 35-2 Arch development and anomalies. **A.** Diagrams showing transformation of the early aortic arch pattern (6 to 8 weeks) into the adult pattern. (Reproduced, with permission, from Jweied et al.[182])

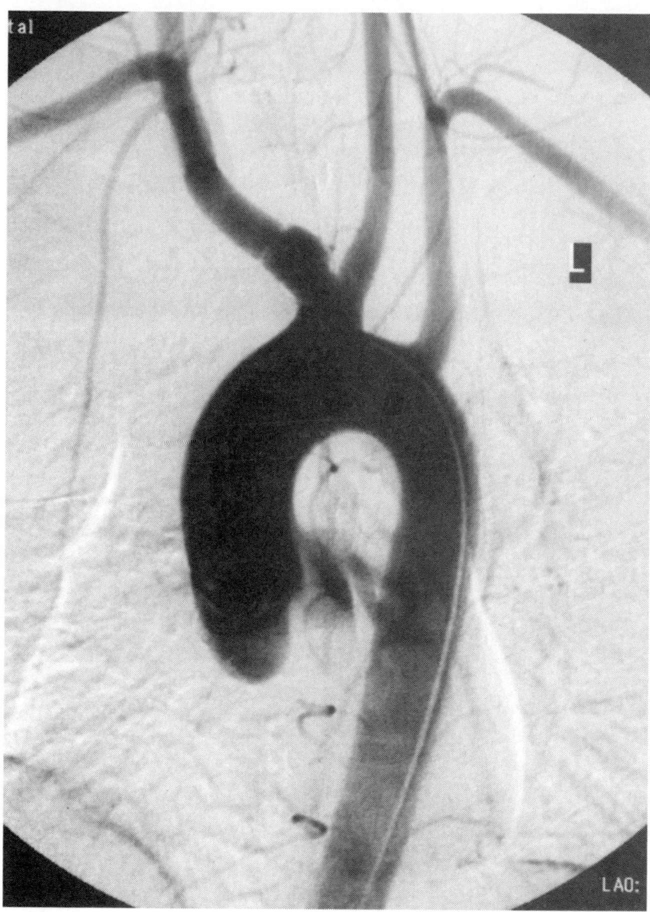

Figure 35-2 (*continued*) Arch development and anomalies. **B.** Aortogram demonstrating a bovine arch with a pseudoaneurysm near the origin of the innominate artery. (Reproduced, with permission, from Junqueira.[183])

form of Carrel "buttons" of aorta and a full-thickness end-to-end distal aortic anastomosis rather than the original "wrap inclusion" or Bentall technique.[2]

Arch aneurysms

Resection of aortic arch aneurysms has remained a more formidable surgical challenge. In 1957, DeBakey and colleagues[15] reported the first successful replacement of an ascending and arch aneurysm with an aortic homograft, using CPB with separate innominate and left common carotid artery perfusion. Bloodwell and associates[16] modified the basic CPB technique in 1968 to perfuse the carotid and vertebral arteries separately and implant the arch vessels together as a single "button." Griepp and associates[17] at Stanford first used the technique of circulatory arrest for complete replacement of the aortic arch in 1975 with implementation of the "open distal." In 1983, the "elephant trunk" technique was introduced by Borst and associates[18] as an alternative for the treatment of patients with extensive aortic aneurysmal disease involving the arch and the descending or thoracoabdominal aorta.

Basic embryology and/or anatomic considerations

At one stage of development, two aortic arches (right and left) are present, with normal development including persistence of the left arch and involution of the right arch. Originating from the aortic arch are branching vessels, with many variations in both the number and the position of those vessels. Permutations may be as few as one or as many as six branches, with these anomalies intimately associated with the development of the fourth arterial arches (Fig. 35-2A). In about 80 percent of people,

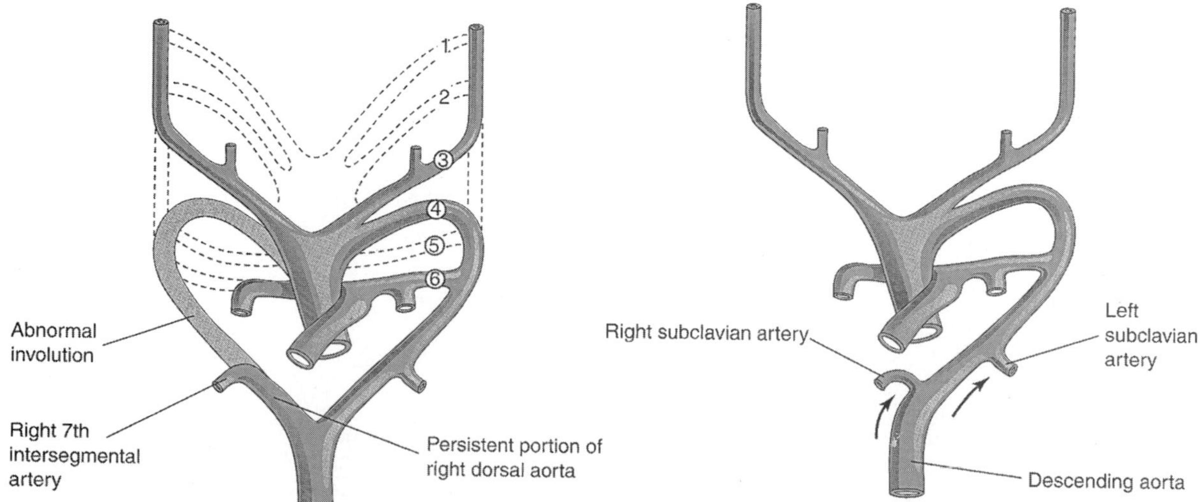

Figure 35-2 (*continued*) Arch development and anomalies. **C.** Diagram showing the embryologic basis of an aberrant right subclavian artery. (Reproduced, with permission, from Jweied et al.[182])

the branching order is innominate, left common carotid, and left subclavian; however, in 11 percent of these patients, a bovine arch exists where the innominate and the left common carotid have a common ostia and the left subclavian arises independently from the arch (Fig. 35-2B).[19,20] Aberrant right subclavian artery (ARSCA) affects approximately 0.1 percent of the population and is often an incidental finding on imaging studies. It occurs when the right fourth aortic arch and the right dorsal aorta involute cranial to the seventh intersegmental artery.[21] The ARSCA arises from the descending aorta or a diverticulum and crosses to the right behind the esophagus (Fig. 35-2C). Surgeons must be aware of the possible variations in the great vessels arising from the aortic arch because misidentification during surgery could be catastrophic.

Table 35-1 Etiology of ascending and arch aortic aneurysms

Medial degeneration
• Idiopathic degeneration
• Heritable disorders of connective tissue
Marfan's syndrome (MFS)
Ehlers-Danlos syndrome (EDS)
Loeys-Dietz syndrome
Familial thoracic aortic aneurysms and dissections (TAAD)
Bicuspid aortic valve (BAV)
Turner's and Noonan's syndromes
Infection
• Mycotic aneurysms
• Syphilitic aneurysms
Inflammatory
• Takayasu's arteritis
• Behçet's disease
• Giant cell arteritis
Chronic aortic dissection

PATHOPHYSIOLOGY

Introduction

The aortic wall is organized into three distinct layers: the intima, media, and adventitia (Fig. 35-3). The media of the aorta is composed of smooth muscle cells within a matrix of elastin, collagen, and other structural proteins, including fibrillin, laminin, glycosaminoglycans, proteoglycans, and fibronectin. The overall strength of the aortic wall is determined by the relative amounts of elastin and collagen; elastin conveys the arterial recoil capabilities, and collagen provides the necessary structural strength. Defects in either protein can cause aortic pathology.[22] Table 35-1 lists the etiology of thoracic aortic aneurysms; these entities and their clinical implications are described in the following section.

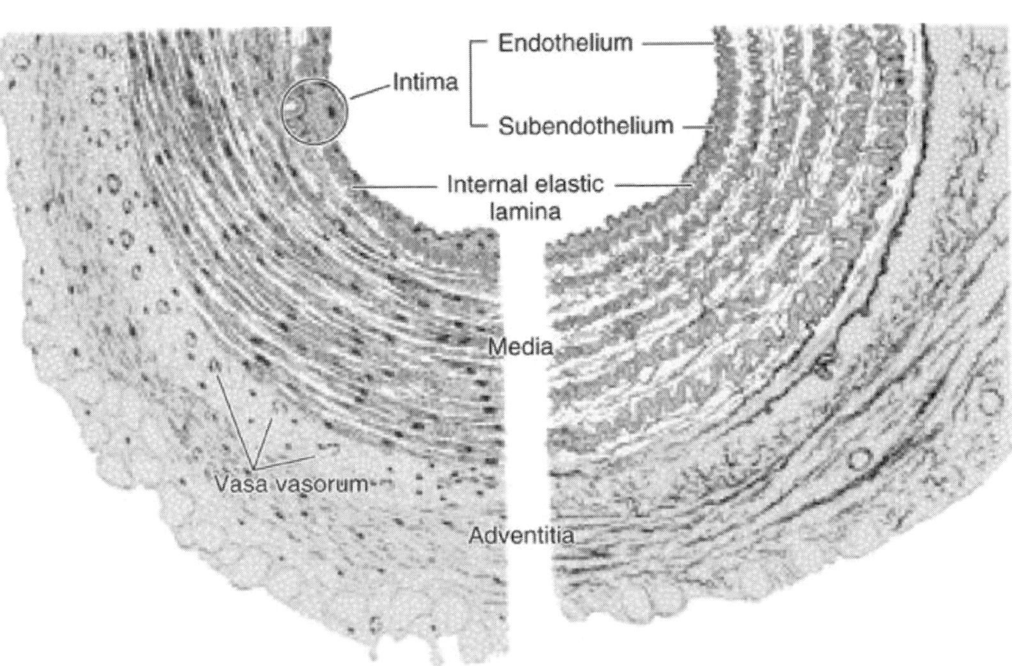

Figure 35-3. Artery wall. Diagrams of a muscular artery prepared by hematoxylin and eosin (H&E) staining (*left*) and an elastic artery stained by Weigert's method (*right*). The tunica media of a muscular artery contains predominantly smooth muscle, whereas the tunica media of an elastic artery is formed by layers of smooth muscle intercalated by elastic laminae. The adventitia and the outer part of the media have small blood vessels (vasa vasorum) and elastic and collagenous fibers. (Reproduced, with permission, from Fedak et al.[183])

Medial degeneration

Idiopathic medial degeneration

Histopathologic investigations of aneurysmal tissue have shown that the majority of ascending aortic and arch aneurysms are associated with medial degeneration in the layers of the aortic wall.[23,24] These degenerative changes within the aortic media, which historically and incorrectly were called medial necrosis or cystic medial necrosis,[25] are characterized by a triad of (1) loss of noninflammatory smooth muscle cells, (2) fragmentation of elastic fibers, and (3) accumulation of basophilic ground substance in cell-depleted areas of the medial layer of the vessel wall. This combination of factors first weakens the aortic wall, thereby increasing the wall tension, which can induce aortic dilatation and aneurysm formation, leading to higher wall stress and eventually resulting in intramural hemorrhage, aortic dissection, or rupture. Medial degeneration occurs normally to some extent with aging, but the process is accelerated by hypertension.[26] In addition, turbulent flow within the aneurysm cavity frequently leads to the formation of laminated thrombus and further atherosclerotic depositions in the aortic wall. The thrombus lining and aortic calcifications, although often substantial, convey no added strength for the prevention of rupture.[22]

Heritable disorders of connective tissue

Medial degeneration is accelerated by inborn errors of metabolism that affect any component of the aortic connective tissue (i.e., ground substance, collagen, elastin, or smooth muscle cells). Known heritable disorders of connective tissue that commonly manifest as ascending and arch aneurysms of the aorta are Marfan's syndrome, Ehlers-Danlos syndrome, Loeys-Dietz Syndrome, familial forms of thoracic aortic aneurysm and dissection, and bicuspid aortic valve disease; Turner's syndrome and Noonan's syndrome occur far less frequently.

Marfan's syndrome Among hereditary diseases, Marfan's syndrome (MFS) is the most prevalent inherited connective tissue disorder, with a prevalence of approximately 1 in 3000 to 5000 individuals. The condition is inherited in an autosomal dominant manner with complete penetrance but demonstrates variable expression with significant intra- and interfamilial variation[2](Fig. 35-4). More than 100 mutations have been identified I the fibrillin-1 gene on chromosome 15, as well as more recently identified missense mutations in TGFBR2 gene which encodes for the TGF-β receptor. As a result, defective coding of fibrillin, the major structural component of elastin, occurs as well as excessive transforming growth factor β (TGF-β) activity. The consequence is both a decrease in the amount of elastin in the aortic wall and a loss of the normally highly organized structure of elastin (Fig. 35-5). In addition, Marfan aortic tissue has enhanced expression of metalloproteinases, which may promote both fragmentation of medial elastic layers and elastolysis.[27] The end result is an aorta that exhibits markedly abnormal elastic properties that lead to progressive increases in stiffness and dilation. Additional cardiovascular complications include mitral valve prolapse and regurgitation and left ventricular dilation, but aortic root dilation is the most common cause of morbidity and mortality.

Ehlers-Danlos syndrome Ehlers-Danlos syndrome (EDS) is a rare autosomal dominant inherited disorder of connective tissue that results from mutations in the *COL3A1* gene, which encodes for type III collagen on chromosome 2. The classification of EDS has been simplified into six major types, including vascular EDS (formerly known as type IV EDS), which carries a substantial risk of rupture of the aorta and its major branches.[28] Arteries in the thorax and abdomen account for 50 percent of the vascular complications,[29] but any anatomic location can be involved, with a predilection for medium-size arteries.

Loeys-Dietz syndrome The Loeys-Dietz syndrome (LDS) is a recently described autosomal dominant aortic aneurysm syndrome that has widespread systemic involvement.[29a] A spectrum of mutations in transforming growth factor β receptors 1 and 2 (*TGFBR1* or *TGFBR2*, respectively) cause the LDS which histologically results in a loss of elastin content and disarrayed elastic fibers in the aortic media.[29b] The phenotype of LDS overlaps with that of Marfan's syndrome (aortic aneurysm, arachnodactyly, dural ectasia), but it also includes distinctive features such as widely spaced eyes (hypertelorism), bifid uvula and/or cleft palate, and generalized arterial tortuosity. The natural history of LDS differs considerably from other connective tissue disorders with the average age at a first cardiovascular event much lower than that for patients with untreated Marfan's syndrome or vascular Ehlers-Danlos syndrome suggesting that mutations in *TGFBR1* or *TGFBR2* predispose to a more aggressive and widespread vascular disease.

Familial thoracic aortic aneurysms and dissections It is coming to be known that patients without genetic syndromes such as Marfan's or Ehlers-Danlos also manifest familial clustering of thoracic aortic aneurysms and dissections (TAAD). In the Yale database of over 1600 patients, detailed family trees of 300 families revealed that 21 percent of aneurysm probands have a first-order relative with a known or likely aortic aneurysm.[30] Most pedigrees suggest an autosomal dominant mode of inheritance, but there is marked variability in the expression and penetrance of the disorder in which some inherit and pass on the gene but show no manifestation of the disease. These nonsyndromic patients have been studied, and to date three genomic loci for nonsyndromic familial TAAD have been elucidated: the TAAD1 locus mapped to the long arm of chromosome 5, with approximately half of the identified families mapping to this locus; the FAA1 locus on the long arm of chromosome

Criterion	Major	Minor
Skeletal system		
Manifestations	Pectus carinatum or pectus excavatum requiring surgery, arm span to height ratio >1.05 or reduced US/LS* <0.86 (adults), positive wrist and thumb sign, scoliosis >20° or spondylolisthesis, limited elbow extension (<170°), pes planus, protrusio acetabuli (by radiography)	Facial appearance, joint hypermobility, pectus excavatum of moderate severity, highly arched palate
Involvement	4 of 7 major present	2 of 7 major present, or 1 of 7 major and 2 of 4 minor present
Ocular system		
Manifestations	Ectopia lentis	Myopia, flat cornea, iris or ciliary muscle hypoplasia
Involvement	Ectopia lentis present	2 of 3 minor present
Cardiovascular system		
Manifestations	Dilation of ascending aorta with or without aortic regurgitation and involving sinuses of Valsalva, dissection of ascending aorta	Mitral valve prolapse, annulus mitralis calcification (age of onset, <40 y), pulmonary artery dilation, dilatation or dissection of descending thoracic or abdominal aorta (age of onset, <50 y)
Involvement	1 of 2 major present	1 of 4 minor present
Pulmonary system		
Manifestations		Pneumothorax, apical blebs (chest radiography)
Involvement		1 of 2 minor present
Skin		
Manifestations		Striae atrophicae (not associated with weight changes or pregnancy), recurrent or incisional hernias
Involvement		1 of 2 minor present
Dura		
Manifestations	Lumbosacral dural ectasia by CT or MRI	
Involvement	Dural ectasia present	
Family		
Involvement	First-degree family member independently fulfilling diagnostic criteria, mutation in *FBN1* known to cause MFS	

*US/LS indicates ratio of upper segment to lower segment.

Figure 35-4 Diagnostic criteria according to the Ghent nosology.[2]

11, which is responsible for aneurysmal disease in one large family; and the MFS2 locus on chromosome 3, which is a rare cause of familial TAAD.[4] Therefore, TAAD is now a recognized heritable disorder of connective tissue.

Turner's and Noonan's syndromes Turner's syndrome is a sex aneuploidy syndrome in which the most common chromosome constitution is 45-X0; it has an incidence of 1 in 5000 live female births. The cardiovascular problems include bicuspid aortic valve (present in one-third of subjects), coarctation of the aorta, hypertension, and TAAD. Aortic root dilation is present in approximately 40 percent of Turner's syndrome patients. Another rare genetic disorder that occasionally predisposes to aortic aneurysms is Noonan's syndrome, an autosomal dominant condition.

Bicuspid aortic valve disease Bicuspid aortic valve (BAV) is the most common congenital heart malformation, with a population prevalence of 1 to 2 percent. It is not clear that BAVs are heritable, but groups have shown that there is a high incidence of familial clustering that is compatible with an autosomal dominant inheritance pattern with reduced penetrance.[31–33] Familial aggregation studies have indicated that 9.1 percent of persons with BAV have a first-degree relative with BAV, with males and females equally affected.[34] The clinical consequences of BAV disease focus on either valvular (stenosis, insufficiency, or infection) or vascular (dilation or dissection) complications. Sabet and coworkers[35] performed a large pathologic review and revealed that BAV disease results in a stenotic lesion in three-quarters of patients, insufficiency in 15 percent, and a mixed lesion in 10 percent. The vascular complications of BAV disease are less well understood, but the presence of BAV is an independent risk factor for progressive aortic dilation, aneurysm formation, and dissection.[36] In fact, BAV disease carries a 9- to 18-fold higher incidence of ascending aortic dilation.[37,38] The cause of this association initially was attributed to "poststenotic dilation,"

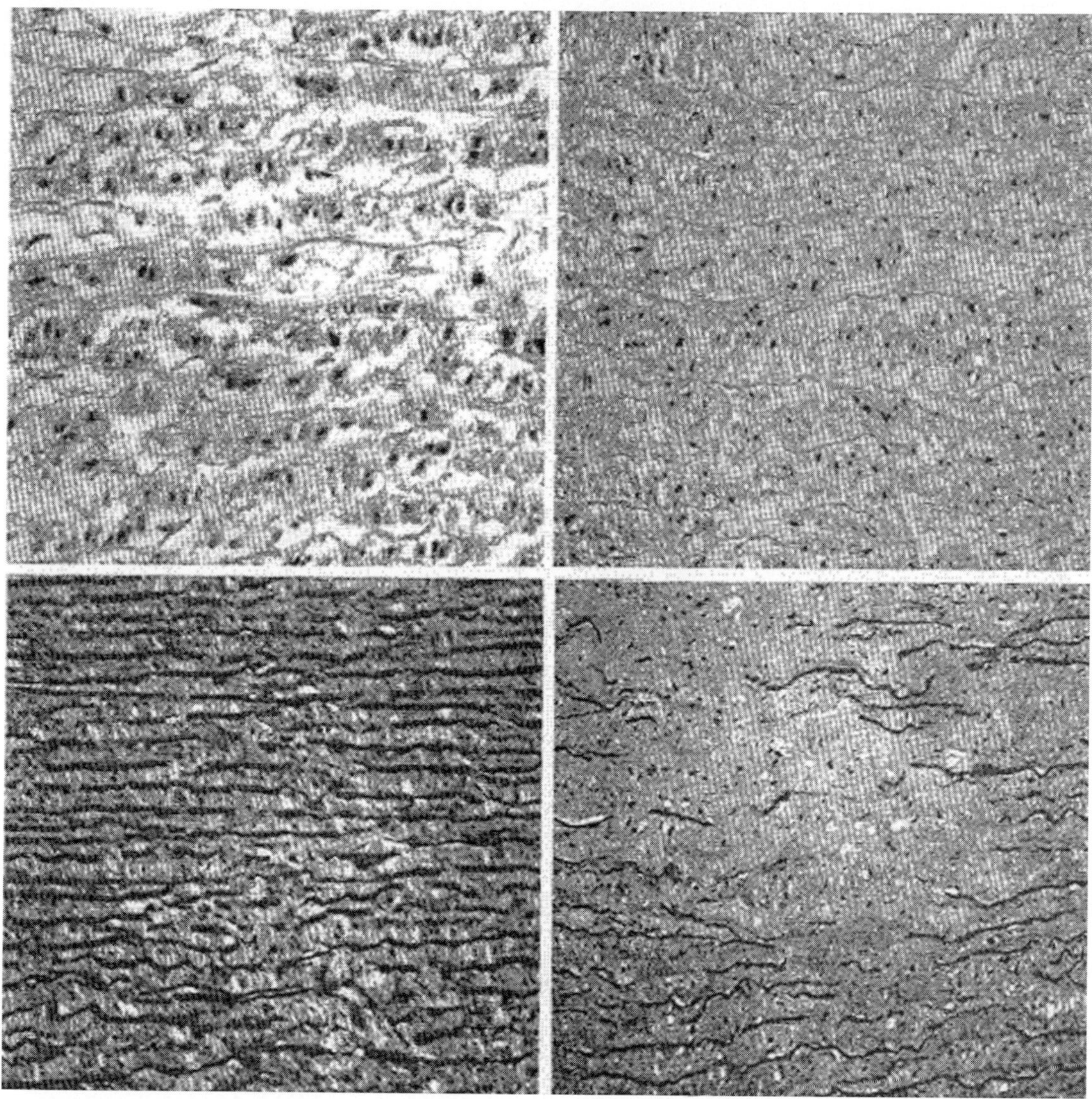

Figure 35-5 Histology. Normal aorta stained with hematoxylin and eosin (H&E) ×120 (*upper left*) showing uniform distribution of elastin layers and fibromyocytes between them and Alcian blue/fuchsin/picric acid stain ×120 (*lower left*) with elastin stained red, fibromyocytes pale khaki-colored, and connective tissue pale gray-blue. Erdheim's disease of the aorta stained with H&E ×120 (*upper right*) shows irregular distribution of fibromyocytes with irregularity and loss of elastic lamellae. In the lower right, Alcian blue/fuchsin/picric acid stain ×120 shows disruption and loss of elastic lamellae (*red*) and a hyperabundance of acidic mucin (*green-blue*).

with high-velocity turbulent flow distal to a stenosis leading to downstream dilation. However, advances in molecular biology have offered new insights that implicate intrinsic abnormalities of the aortic wall as being responsible for the pathologic development of aortic dilation. Embryologically, the aortic valvular cusps and ascending arterial media both arise from common neural crest cells during development. Apoptosis of those neural crest derivatives, specifically premature vascular smooth muscle cell apoptosis within the aortic media, is present in ascending aortic aneurysms of bicuspid aortic valve carriers.[39,40] Additionally, fibrillin-1 deficiency in the aortic media of BAV patients has been implicated in triggering matrix metalloproteinase production, leading to matrix disruption and thus aortic dilation[41] (Fig. 35-6). The cause of bicuspid aortic valves is unknown, but BAV is associated with accelerated degeneration of the aortic media, indicating that BAV disease is an ongoing pathologic process, not a discrete developmental defect.[42]

Chronic aortic dissection

Both Stanford type A and type B chronic aortic dissections tend to dilate over time. The natural history starts with a vulnerable aortic wall at baseline, which is stressed

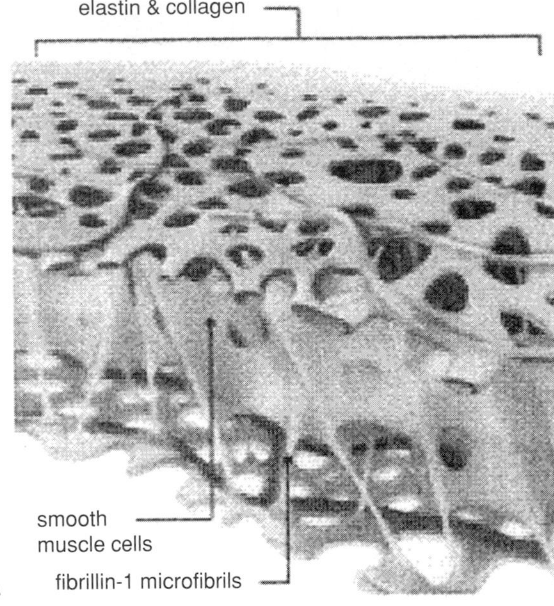

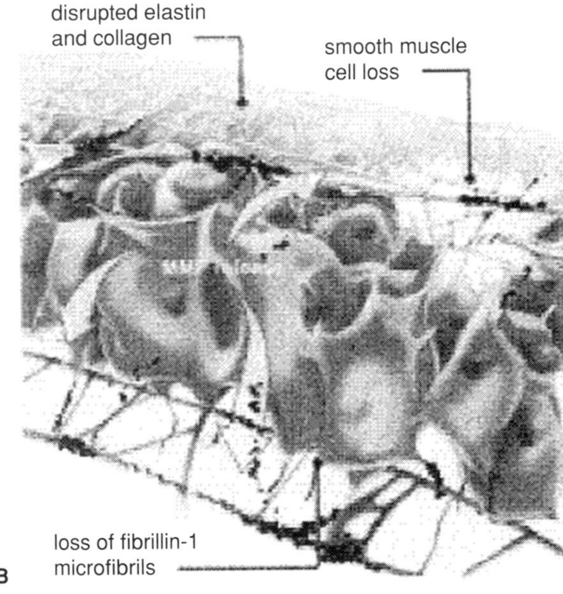

Figure 35-6 The elastic laminae of the aortic media provide structural support and elasticity to the aorta. In normal tricuspid valve patients (**A**), fibrillin-1 microfibrils tether smooth muscle cells to adjacent elastin and collagen matrix components. In patients with BAV (**B**), deficient microfibrillar elements result in smooth muscle cell detachment, matrix metalloproteinase release, matrix disruption, cell death, and a loss of structural support and elasticity. (Reproduced, with permission, from Fedak et al.[42])

with the tearing of the intimal flap, leaving the structural integrity of the aorta destabilized to only the weakened outer wall of the false lumen. Consequently, those with chronic aortic dissection are at high risk for aneurysm formation. Debakey and colleagues found that aneurysms developed in 46 percent of patients with uncontrolled hypertension but in only 17 percent with controlled hypertension.[43] Recently, Griepp and coworkers found that after repair of acute type A dissections, the growth of the distal aorta averaged 0.85 mm a year for the aortic arch and 1.24 mm a year for the descending thoracic aorta.[44]

Infection

Mycotic aneurysms

Osler[45] adopted the term *mycotic* to denote aneurysms originating on the basis of infection.[46] Mycotic aneurysms of the thoracic aorta are rare but can be fatal if they are not diagnosed early. Bacterial seeding of the aortic wall can occur by hematogenous spread to the intima or the vasa vasorum, lymphatic spread, or direct extension from an adjacent infected focus. The thin endothelial intimal lining of the aorta is generally highly resistant to infection, but disruption of this barrier by atherosclerosis reduces resistance to infection.[47] Epidemiologically, this disease, which traditionally has been due to endocarditis, now has an increased tendency to afflict the elderly, possibly as a result of an atherosclerotic load facilitating infection. Aneurysms are usually saccular and well localized, with *Staphylococcus aureus* and *Salmonella* species being the predominant organisms. Surgery with complete excision and debridement of infected tissue with in-line aortic reconstruction is the definitive treatment. Lifelong prophylactic antibiotic therapy may be advisable to prevent recurrences unless there is a clearly identifiable and treatable source of infection.

Syphilitic aneurysms

Syphilis was once perhaps the most common cause of ascending aortic aneurysms, but in an era of aggressive antibiotic treatment, such luetic aneurysms are seen rarely in medical centers.[48] Syphilitic aortitis is a chronic mesarteritis and periarteritis of the aorta, with patchy destruction and scarring of musculoelastic medial tissue and replacement by vascularized connective tissue.[46] The complications of aortitis develop 10 to 20 years after onset of disease in most cases, with the most common manifestation being a localized saccular aneurysm in the ascending aorta.[49]

Inflammatory aneurysms

Walker and colleagues[50] were the first to define the term *inflammatory aneurysm*. Typical histologic examination shows signs of chronic inflammation in the adventitia with a marked lymphoplasmacytic cell infiltrate and granulation or proliferatrion of fibrous tissue. Three inflammatory arteritides affect the ascending and arch of the aorta with aneurysmal disease: Takayasu's arteritis, Behçet's disease, and giant cell arteritis.

Takayasu's arteritis

Takayasu's arteritis is a nonspecific inflammatory disease of unknown etiology that mainly involves media in the elastic arteries such as the pulmonary artery, the subclavian artery, and abdominal branches of the aorta.[51] The inflammatory process results in predominantly chronic arterial occlusive lesion of the main branches of the aortic arch but occasionally results in arterial aneurysmal formation, following a cyclic course.[52] Histologically, thickening of the intima is the normal occurrence, resulting in stenosis and occlusion; however, degeneration of the elastic tissue with proliferation of the connective tissue mainly in the medial layer of the arteries may result in dilatation of the artery and aneurysm formation.[52]

Behçet's disease

Behçet's disease is a multisystemic disorder characterized by recurrent urogenital ulcers, ocular manifestations, and skin lesions, with cardiovascular involvement appearing in only 7 to 29 percent of patients.[53] However, the leading cause of death in patients with Behçet's disease is a rupture of a large aortic or arterial aneurysm.[54] Venous lesions are the norm, with arterial manifestations accounting for only 12 percent of vascular complications in patients with Behçet's disease. The arterial lesion, which develops in the aorta and the pulmonary artery as well as in their major branches, is an aneurysm in 65 percent of patients and an occlusion in 35 percent.[53] At histologic analysis, aortitis is seen in both the active and scar stages. Active aortitis leads to the destruction of the media and fibrosis, predisposing the patient to saccular aneurysms.[55] Perforation of the arterial wall caused by obliterative endarteritis of the vasa vasorum may result in aneurysm formation or rupture.[56]

Giant cell arteritis

Giant cell arteritis (GCA), also known as temporal arteritis, cranial arteritis, granulomatous arteritis, and Horton's disease, is a chronic systemic vasculitis of unknown etiology that affects medium-size and large arteries.[57–59] It has been reported that as many as 15 percent of patients with temporal arteritis may have angiographic evidence of aortic involvement[60] and that patients with GCA are 17.3 times more likely to develop a thoracic aortic aneurysm than is the general population.[61] Typical histopathologic findings are disruption of the internal elastic lamina and an inflammatory cellular infiltrate with giant cells.[59]

Complications of ascending aortic dilation

Dilation of the ascending aorta is currently the most common cause of isolated aortic valvular regurgitation.[62] A normal valve becomes incompetent as a result of the passive stretching of its leaflets and commissures caused by dilation of the sinotubular ridge, the ascending aorta, or the sinuses, although the aortic annulus often remains normal in size in the non-Marfan population.

CLINICAL FEATURES

The decision to recommend surgical therapy is based on the clinical assessment that the potential for complications during observation and the associated consequences are more significant than the morbidity and mortality of surgical repair. This clinical decision must rely on current knowledge of the natural history of ascending and arch aneurysms.

Natural history

Unlike the natural history of untreated abdominal aortic aneurysms, the natural history of thoracic aortic aneurysms is ill defined, mainly because of the asymptomatic course of the disease until dissection, rupture, or the appearance of symptoms. The majority of the published information details the natural history of descending thoracic aneurysms, with substantially less information available for ascending or arch aneurysms. With that caveat, there is comprehensive information available for ascending and arch aneurysms related to MFS, but such data are lacking for other pathologies. It is appreciated that the size and etiology of the aneurysm contribute to the natural history of thoracic aortic aneurysms, which often concludes with patient death because of rupture or dissection.

Size

According to Laplace's law,

$$T = (P * R)/M$$

where T is the tension in the walls, P is the pressure difference across the wall, R is the radius of the cylinder, and M is the thickness of the wall; the combination of an enlarging radius and a thinning wall leads to increased wall tension. This represents the onset of a positive feedback cycle that results in progressive aortic dilation and culminates in rupture or dissection. In all reliable contemporary natural history studies, an ascending aortic diameter of 6 cm emerges as the mean or the median diameter quite consistently.[63] Coady and associates found that a diameter of 6 cm is the "hinge point" beyond which there is a 30 percent increase in the probability of rupture.[64] The 5-year survival rate for patients with ascending aortic aneurysms ranged from 36 to 61 percent in the earlier days[65] and reached 59 to 77 percent in the modern era[66] for aneurysms equal to or greater than 6 cm and less than 6 cm, respectively. Regarding aneurysm growth rates, Hirose and coauthors noted that the growth rate of aneurysms was greater in the arch (0.56 cm per year) than in the descending thoracic (0.42 cm per year) or the abdominal aorta (0.28 cm per year).[67] A more recent review of the Yale database[68] reported an annual growth rate of 0.07 cm for aneurysms in the ascending aorta or aortic arch and found that increasing size is associated more strongly with an increased risk of rupture than with an increased risk of dissection. Additionally, the risk of rupture with time as a function of initial aneurysm size is 11 times worse with an aortic size of 5.0 to 5.9 cm and nearly 27 times worse with a size of 6.0 cm or greater when each is compared with aneurysms less than 4.0 cm.

Etiology

In addition to aneurysm size, the etiology of the aneurysm has a profound impact on rupture, dissection, and death. The most common cardiovascular complication in patients with MFS is progressive aortic root enlargement that initially occurs at the sinuses of Valsalva. Ascending aortic aneurysm can precipitate acute type A dissection, aortic rupture, aortic regurgitation (AR), or all three, and these complications were the primary cause of death before the advent of successful preventive therapies.[2] Currently, aortic dissection is the major cause of premature morbidity and mortality in patients with Marfan's syndrome. In a study by Murdoch and associates[69] that looked at causes of death in MFS patients, cardiovascular manifestations accounted for 93 percent of the deaths (52 of 56), with aortic root complications (dilation, dissection, and regurgitation) accounting for 80 percent of those deaths, with an average age at death of 32 years. This was similar to the findings of Marsalese and coworkers, in which 87 percent of the known causes of death were attributable to the cardiovascular system and 61 percent were the result of aortic dissection, rupture, or sudden cardiac death, with a mean age at death of 35 years.[70]

BAV is also an independent risk factor for progressive aortic dilation, aneurysm formation, and dissection.[71] Dore and associates[72] evaluated 50 adults with BAV with transthoracic echocardiography and found that progressive dilation occurred at all levels [from the basal attachment of the leaflets to 1 cm beyond the sinotubular junction (STJ)], ranging from 0.3 mm per year at the basal attachment within the left ventricular outflow tract to 1.0 mm per year 1 cm beyond the STJ. These rates of dilation are greater than the reported rate of 0.8 mm per decade in the normal population. In fact, BAV disease carries a 9- to 18-fold higher incidence of ascending aortic dilation.[73,74] Furthermore, replacement of BAV for either aortic insufficiency or stenosis does not eliminate the resulting aortic complications. After aortic valve replacement, BAV patients, when compared with tricuspid aortic valve patients, have progressive dilation of the proximal ascending aorta[75] and have a greater incidence of sudden death and aortic events.[76] Thus, the influence of BAV disease on the ascending aorta is a reality; therefore, surgeons should consider valve pathology when making decisions about ascending aortic replacement.

The natural history of Loeys-Dietz syndrome, resulting from a spectrum of mutations in *TGFBR1* or *TGFBR2*, differs considerably from other connective tissue disorders with the average age at a first cardiovascular event much lower than that for patients with untreated Marfan's syndrome or vascular Ehlers-Danlos syndrome. In their cohort of 90 patients[29b], the median survival was 37.0 years, with 27 deaths during the study period with the mean age of death being 26.0 years (range: 0.5 to 47.0), and the mean age at vascular surgery—most often for ascending aortic aneurysm or dissection—was 19.8 years (range: 1.2 to 46.0). Twenty-nine patients (32 percent of the cohort) died before the age of 19 as a result of a vascular dissection or rupture suggesting that Loeys-Dietz syndrome is an aggressive connective tissue disorder with a worse cardiovascular risk profile than classic MFS, including aortic dissection at a young age and at small dimensions.

DIAGNOSTIC MODALITIES

Typical clinical presentations

Symptoms

Most patients with thoracic aortic aneurysms are asymptomatic at the time of presentation, and aneurysms of the ascending aorta usually are detected as incidental findings during testing for other disorders (i.e., widening of the mediastinum or prominence of the aortic knob on routine chest radiography or aortic enlargement on echocardiography, thoracic computed tomography, or magnetic resonance imaging). In contrast, aneurysms of the aortic arch, because of their anatomic location and the space-occupying nature of the aneurysm, may impinge on important mediastinal structures and are therefore symptomatic more often than are aneurysms of the ascending or descending aorta.[24] Hoarseness results from stretching of the left recurrent laryngeal nerve, stridor from compression of the trachea, dysphagia from impingement on the lumen of the esophagus, dyspnea from compression of the lung, and plethora and edema from compression of the superior vena cava.[77] Aneurysms of the ascending aorta associated with dilation of the aortic valve annulus may present with signs and symptoms of aortic regurgitation. Additionally, chest or back pain may indicate acute expansion or leakage of the aneurysm in which the location of discomfort roughly correlates with the involved aortic segment. Precordial pain is associated with involvement of the ascending aorta; radiation to the neck and jaw often accompanies aortic arch involvement, whereas descending thoracic and thoracoabdominal aortic aneurysms tend to produce interscapular and low back pain, respectively. In contrast, the clinical features of aortic dissection are the acute onset of chest and/or back pain of a blunt, severe, and sometimes radiating and migrating nature.[78] Symptoms attributable to the aneurysm are cause for concern and consideration for early surgical intervention. Patients with rupture of an ascending or arch aneurysm often present in extremis (see the decision-making flowcharts).

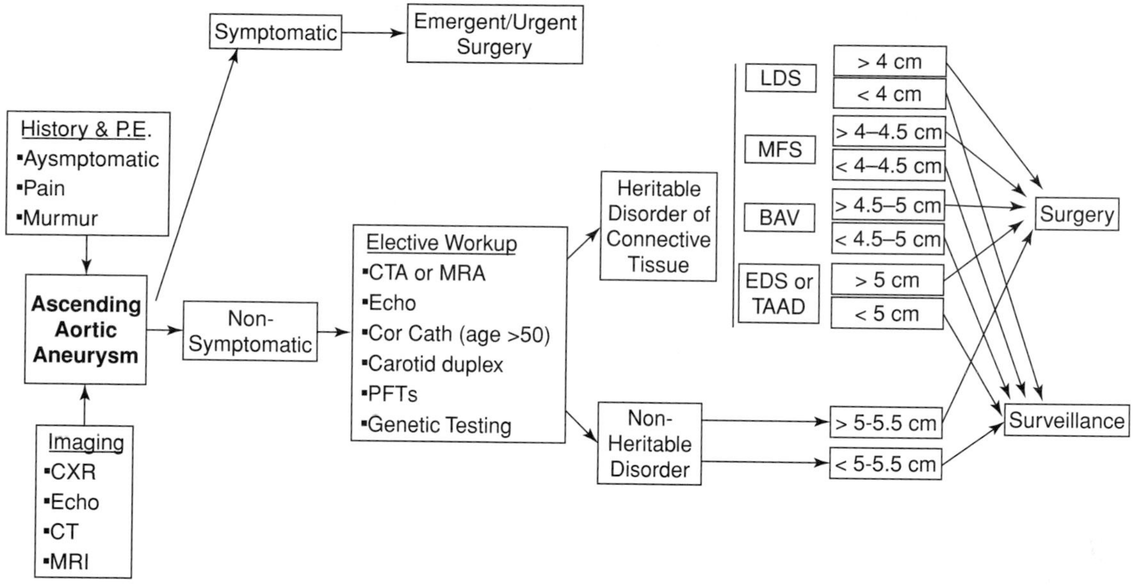

Decision-making flowchart: Ascending aortic aneurysm

Signs

The physical examination is often normal in a patient without rupture of an ascending or arch aneurysm, with the rare exception of a large aneurysm that is palpated in the suprasternal notch. Other physical findings may include venous distention secondary to superior vena caval or innominate vein obstruction. Aneurysms of the ascending aorta associated with dilation of the aortic valve annulus may present with signs of aortic regurgitation (i.e., widened pulse pressure, decrescendo diastolic murmur, bisferiens pulse, "pistol-shot sound," Duroziez's sign, and Quincke's pulse). A thorough vascular examination should be carried out to identify concomitant peripheral vascular disease (abdominal aortic

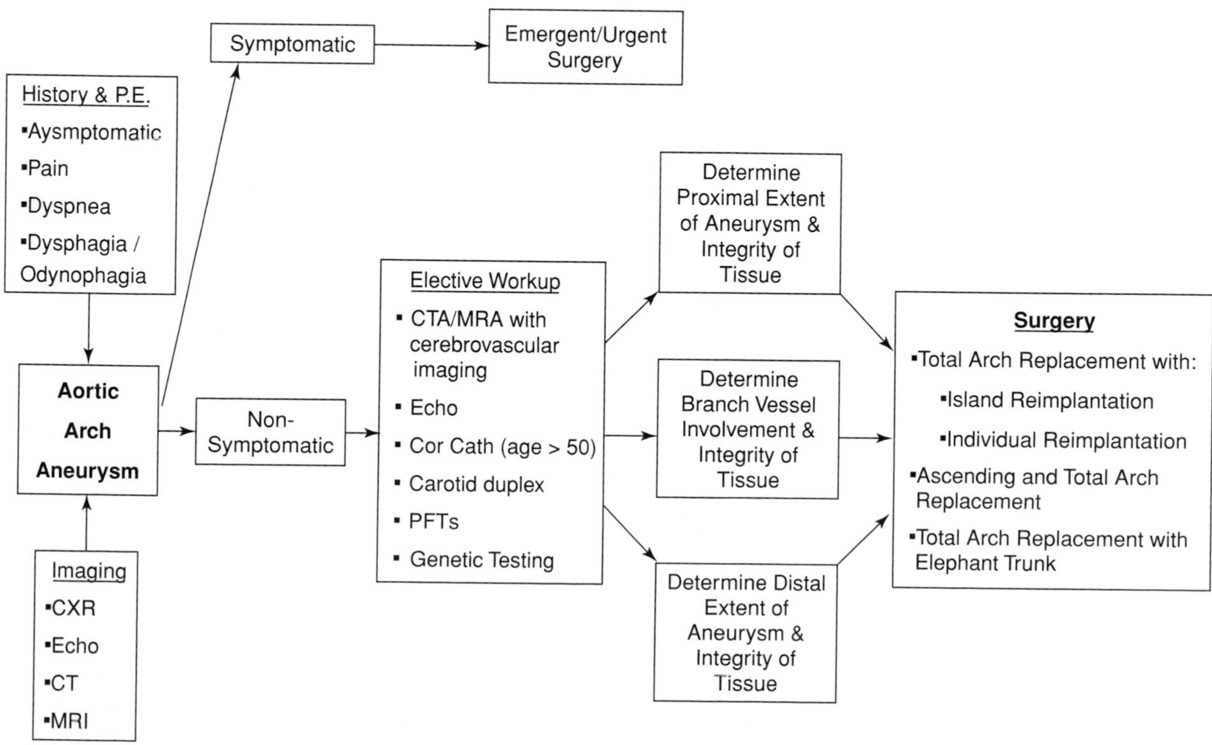

Decision-making flowchart: Aortic arch aneurysm

aneurysms are present in 10 to 20 percent of patients with atherosclerotic involvement of an ascending aortic aneurysm).[79,80] The physical examination also should focus on identifying marfanoid features (Fig. 35-4) as well as phenotypic features of Loeys-Dietz syndrome (blue sclerae, hypotelorism, bifid uvula, malar flattening, retrognathia, camptodactyly, arachnodactyly, and translucency of the skin with visible veins and distended scars[29b]).

Hallmark primary laboratory abnormalities

There are none.

Recommended diagnostic studies

The diagnosis of aortic aneurysms has been revolutionized by developments in cross-sectional imaging. Traditionally, these aneurysms were investigated by contrast angiography, but the last two decades have seen considerable developments in the diagnosis of aortic disease by echocardiography, computed tomography (CT), and magnetic resonance imaging (MRI). These developments have led to a complete change in the way in which aortic disease is evaluated and have contributed to an improvement in treatment outcomes.[81]

When a thoracic aortic aneurysm is detected, it is typically not possible to determine the rate of growth; therefore, if the aneurysm does not meet the criteria for surgical intervention, it is appropriate to obtain a repeat imaging study 6 months after the initial study. If the aneurysm is unchanged in size, it is reasonable to obtain an imaging study on an annual basis in most cases. However, if there is a significant increase in aortic size from one study to the next but surgical intervention is still not indicated, the interval between studies should be decreased to 3 or 6 months. For surveillance to be useful, serial imaging studies should be performed in the same center with the same technique so that direct comparisons can be made between comparable images.[48]

Chest roentgenography

The abnormality of a thoracic aneurysm may be detected on chest radiographs, with the most common finding being widening of the superior mediastinum. Other findings include displacement and compression of the mediastinal contents, such as the trachea and esophagus, and curvilinear calcification in the aneurysmal wall[82] (Fig. 35-7). However, aneurysms that involve the ascending aorta and the aortic arch sometimes cannot be differentiated from tumors or other masses in the mediastinum.[83]

Echocardiography

Both transthoracic echocardiography (TTE) and transesophageal echocardiography (TEE) have an important role in aortic imaging. Echocardiography is widely available, noninvasive (TTE) or minimally invasive (TEE), and relatively inexpensive. TTE can visualize the aortic

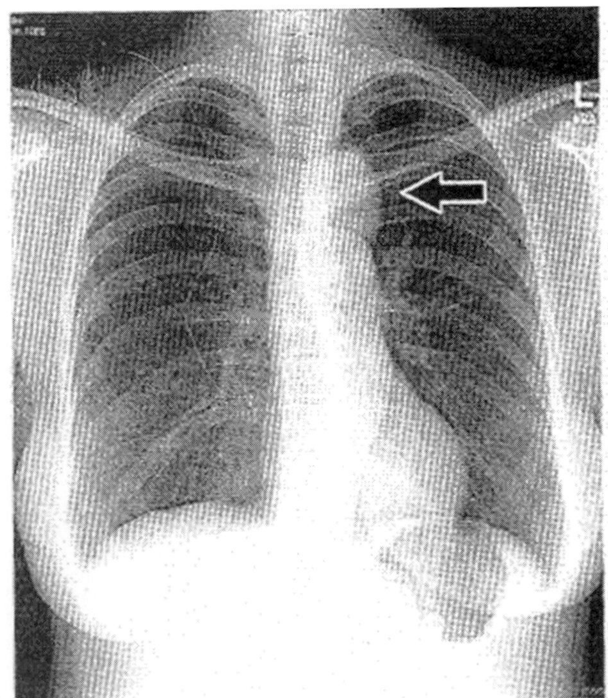

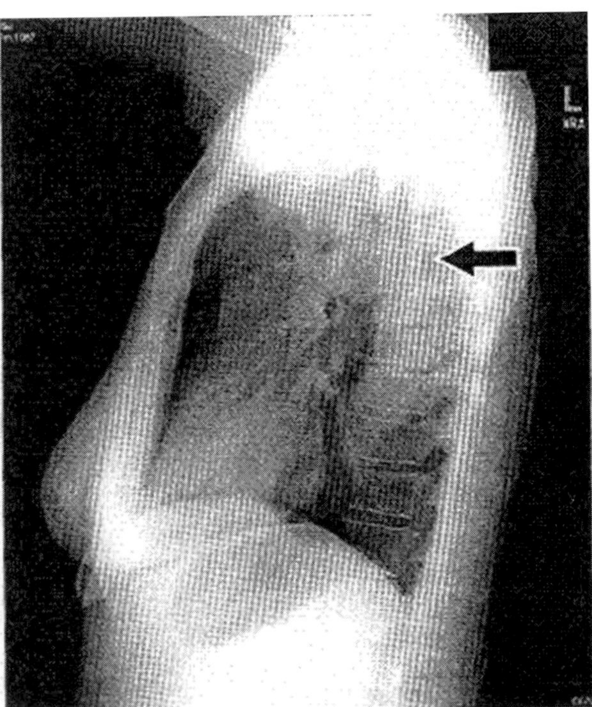

Figure 35-7 Chest roentgenography demonstrating an aortic arch aneurysm (*black arrow*) on both the anterior-posterior film and the lateral film.

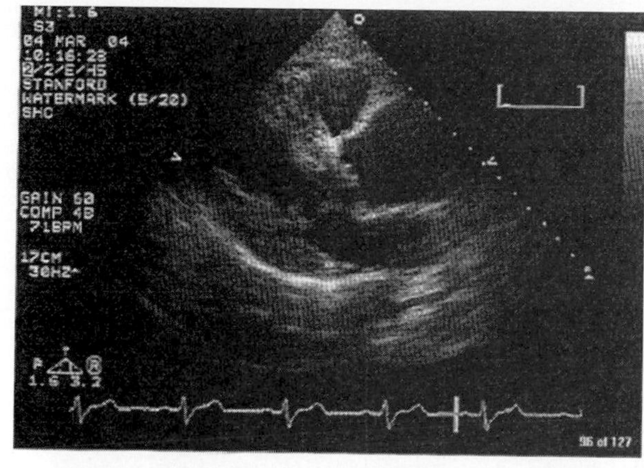

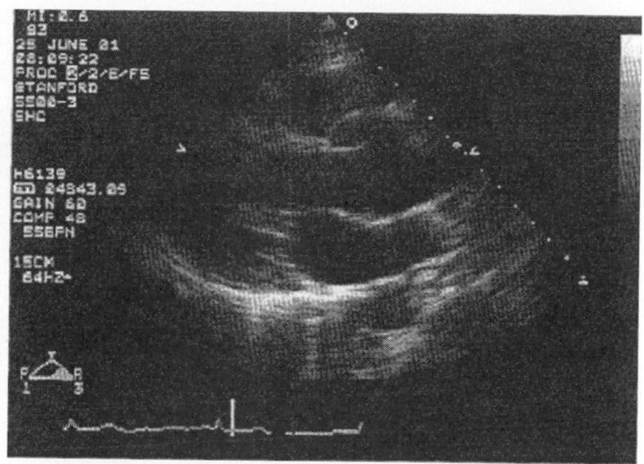

Figure 35-8 Echocardiography. **A.** Long-axis view of a patient with a bicuspid aortic valve and an ascending aortic aneurysm. Note that the ascending aneurysm starts at the level of the sinotubular junction without dilation of the sinuses. **B.** In contrast, note the long-axis view of a Marfan's disease patient with dilation of both the sinuses and the ascending aorta.

root and ascending aorta accurately and is very suitable for evaluating the size of moderate aneurysms and assessing cardiac complications such as aortic regurgitation, impaired left ventricular function, and hemopericardium (Fig. 35-8). It is less than ideal for showing the full extent of the aortic arch and evaluating the origins of head and neck vessels. In contrast, TEE with the current multiplanar transducers has few blind areas (i.e., posterior to the trachea) that limit evaluation. Most important, because of its bedside applicability, TEE is the imaging modality of choice for the diagnosis and exclusion of ascending aortic dissection in an unstable patient, with a European multicenter study reporting a diagnostic sensitivity of 99 percent and a specificity of 98 percent.[84] Combined with color flow imaging, TEE allows not only the identification of the intimal flap with the true and the false lumen and identification of the entry and reentry but also the detection of associated complications such as aortic regurgitation, pericardial and pleural effusions, coronary involvement, and thrombosis in the false lumen. Today in most centers, patients with proximal aortic dissection diagnosed by TEE who are surgical candidates are taken directly to the operating room, saving valuable time. Additionally, intraoperative application of TEE allows continuous monitoring of the surgical procedure without disturbing the sterile field, in contrast to epicardial echocardiography.

Computed tomography and computed tomography angiography

Because of its speed and wide availability, computed tomography/computed tomography angiography (CT/CTA) is currently the most common diagnostic imaging method for studying the aorta. With the advent of multidetector-row scanners, CT can provide the excellent spatial resolution necessary to image the aorta accurately with reasonable doses of iodinated contrast medium in a short acquisition time.[85] Limitations on contrast use because of renal insufficiency or a history of allergy usually can be dealt with, particularly when there is an urgent need to make a definitive diagnosis. CTA combines a rapid bolus intravenous injection using a pressure injector with a timed breath hold and spiral CT acquisition during peak arterial opacification. Curved planar reformations and three-dimensional (3-D) reformations using maximum-intensity projection (MIP) and shaded surface display (SSD) after segmentation and editing of bony and other unwanted structures provide excellent visualization of the aorta and its branch vessels (Figs. 35-9 and 35-10).[86] CTA (axial images) has the advantage of demonstrating aortic wall thickening, calcification, and luminal thrombus, thus displaying the true axial extent of the aneurysm, as the aortography or 3-D MIP and SSD images display only the enhancing lumen of the vessel. In addition, these wall parameters are important in establishing the etiology of the aneurysm and in decision making for further management. However, it should be noted that measurement based purely on the basis of axial images, which may not be orthogonal, can be misleading. Tortuosity of the aorta can lead to a false estimation of aneurysm size; therefore, 3-D SSD reconstruction has facilitated assessment of aneurysm size and extent significantly.

CTA is the imaging study of choice in a suspected leaking aneurysm, in which rapid evaluation is imperative. In elective ascending and arch aneurysm repair, CTA is able to display the origins of aortic branches and their relation to the aneurysm, the proximal and distal extent of the aneurysm, and the adjacent thoracic structures, all of which are critical to operative planning. Currently, 64-bit scanners also are capable of imaging coronary arteries, eliminating the necessity for selective catheter injection for coronary assessment.

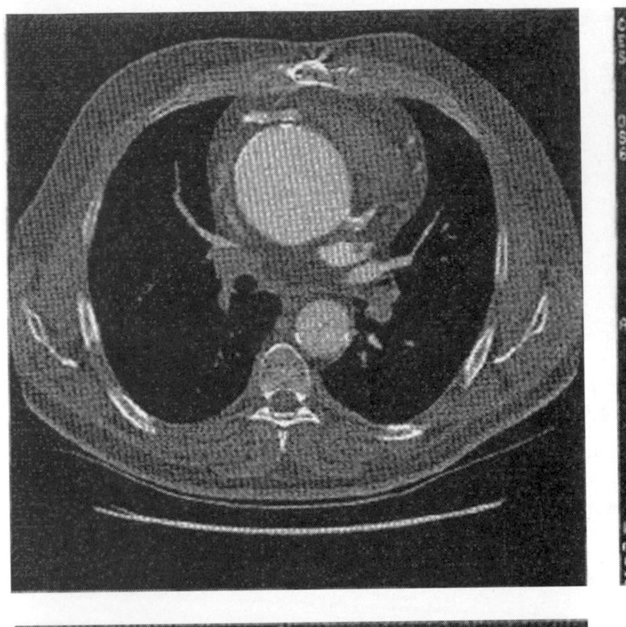
A

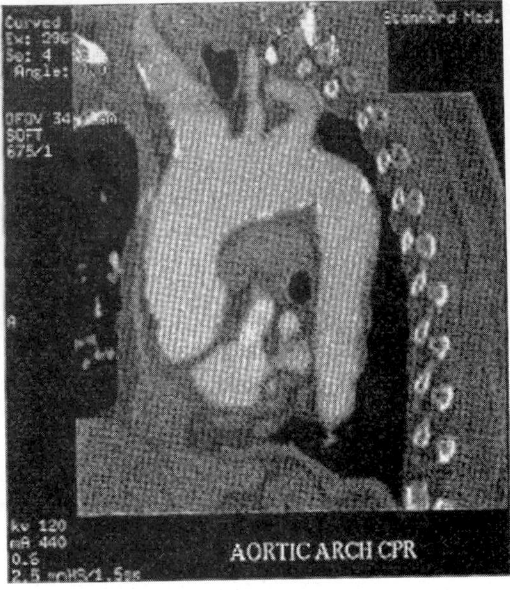

B

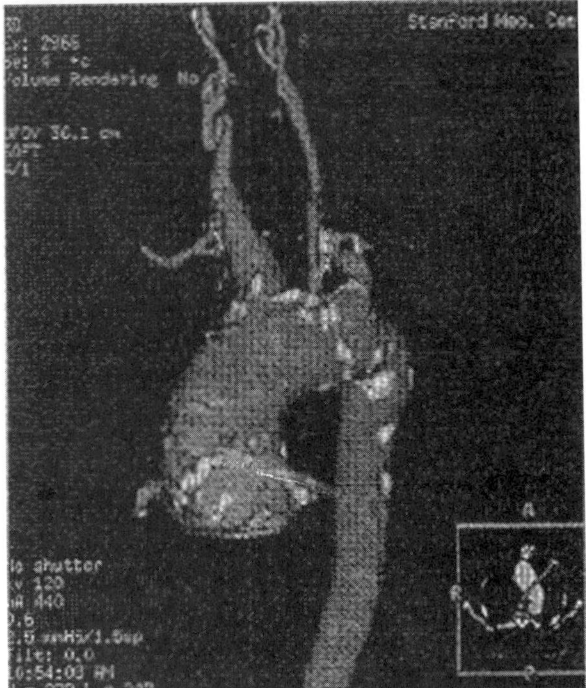

C

Figure 35-9 Computed tomography angiography of the thoracic aorta in a 59-year-old man. A 2.5-cm axial slice (**A**) showing a uniformly dilated ascending aortic aneurysm measuring 7.0 cm in diameter. Curved planar reformation through the aortic arch (**B**) shows extension of the aneurysm into the aortic arch and aneurysmal dilatation of the innominate artery. A volume-rendered image (**C**) displays rotation of the right sinus of Valsalva anteriorly. Both right and left coronary arteries are patent but ectatic.

Magnetic resonance imaging and magnetic resonance angiography

Magnetic resonance imaging is emerging as the premier imaging method for the diagnosis of diseases of the thoracic aorta in stable patients. MRI provides visualization in the sagittal and coronal planes and eliminates the need for noniodinated contrast and radiation exposure. Magnetic resonance angiography (MRA) of the thoracic aorta usually requires a combination of several available MRI methods, each of which has certain advantages and contributes to the diagnostic versatility of the technique. Contrast-enhanced MRA (CE-MRA) is the most widely used MRA method because it is rapid and robust, providing projection images of the aorta similar to those provided by conventional invasive angiography. Black-blood MRI permits assessment of the vessel wall by saturating

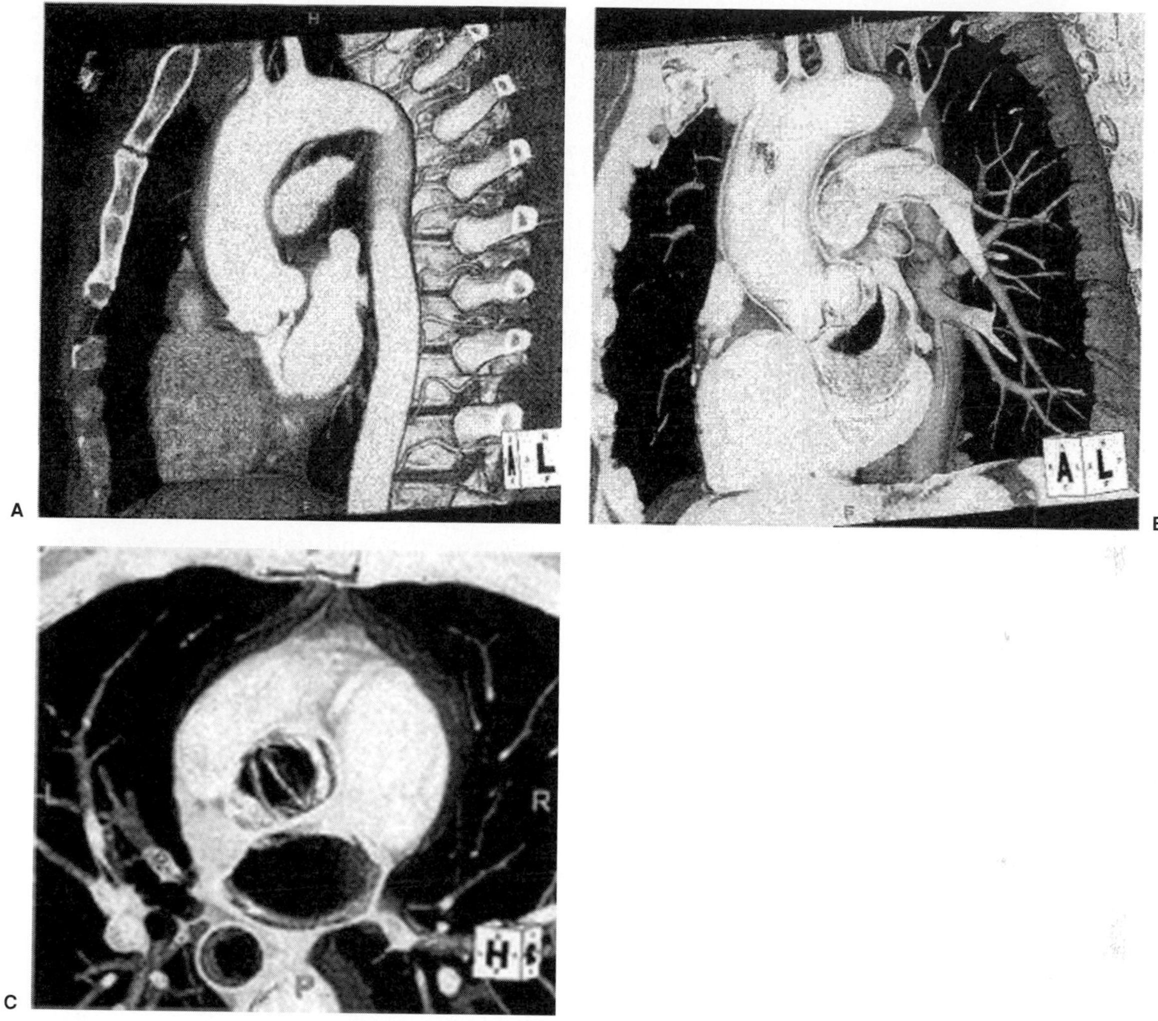

Figure 35-10 Computed tomography angiography of the thorax with retrospective ECG gating in a 53-year-old man with a bicuspid aortic valve. A thick-slab volume-rendered image (**A**) shows aneurysmal dilatation of the ascending aorta with extension into the aortic arch. A volume-rendered image with transparent rendering of the flow lumen (**B, C**) allows visualization of the inner surface of the thoracic aortic aneurysm (**B**) and provides a good three-dimensional view of the bicuspid valve (viewed cranially).

the signal from the lumen. Phase-contrast imaging provides functional information about the flow. Gradient-echo cine images can demonstrate aortic regurgitation in the presence of disease of the ascending aorta. The field continues to develop, and many new MRA methods promise further improvements in acquisition time and resolution.[87] However, MRI/MRA is less readily available and has limited utilization in acute aortic problems because of limited applicability to ventilated and invasively monitored patients. Indwelling pacemaker wires also frequently prevent its use.

MEDICAL TREATMENT

The medical therapies available to slow the growth of thoracic aortic aneurysms and reduce their risk of dissection or rupture are quite limited, and most studies have focused on marfanoid patients. Whether these benefits truly can be extrapolated to the non-Marfan population with thoracic aneurysms is unknown.[48] Some early experimental evidence suggests that oxidative stress may play a role in the pathogenesis of atherosclerotic thoracic aortic aneurysms and that perhaps therapy with statins, matrix metalloproteinase (MMP) inhibitors, and angiotensin II receptor blockers may have a protective effect.[88,89]

Marfan's syndrome

Studies addressing the efficacy of beta-blockade in MFS patients have concluded that such therapy is successful in a subset of individuals.[90,91] Overall, medicated patients showed slower aortic root growth (defined as absolute growth rate or growth rate adjusted for age and body size), fewer cardiovascular endpoints [defined as aortic regurgitation (AR), dissection, or surgery; congestive heart failure; or death], and an improved survival rate.[2] It is important to note that even though abnormal aortic growth was slowed significantly in medicated patients, therapy did not prevent aortic dilation[92–94] or the need for surgical correction. Currently, it is recommended that all patients with MFS be considered for beta-adrenergic blockade to reduce inotropy and chronotropy and thereby reduce both acute and chronic hemodynamic stress on the aortic root. Treatment begins with a low dose, which is titrated to keep the heart rate below 70 in a resting state and below 100 after submaximal exercise. Contraindications to beta-adrenergic blockade include severe diabetes, Raynaud's phenomenon, and bronchospasm. In the setting of beta-blocker intolerance, a trial with a calcium channel blocker is indicated on the basis of a small trial that suggested its efficacy in protecting MFS aorta.[91] Encouraging results in the Marfan rat model with angiotensin-converting enzyme (ACE) inhibitors may warrant a clinical trial.[95,96]

Exercise restriction represents a second approach to reducing hemodynamic stress in MFS patients.[97] Individuals with MFS are encouraged to remain active; aerobic exercise should be performed in moderation, but contact sports should be avoided. Most important, they should avoid isometric exercises, especially weight lifting, because of the marked elevation in blood pressure that occurs during sustained maximal muscle contraction.[2]

Bicuspid aortic valve

The benefit of beta blockers in preventing aortic dilation in BAV disease is not clear; however, hypertension should be monitored and controlled carefully. The role of MMP inhibitors and gene or protein therapy in augmenting deficient extracellular matrix components in the bicuspid aorta is an exciting prospect that warrants further investigation.[98]

Loeys-Dietz syndrome

The mechanism by which mutations in the TGF-β receptor cause the multisystem manifestations of Loeys-Dietz syndrome is complex and poorly understood. TGF-β antagonists have the ability to alleviate or eliminate many manifestations, including aortic aneurysms, in mouse models of Marfan's syndrome.[98a] Although the application of this approach to Loey-Dietz syndrome may prove beneficial, caution is warranted, pending validation in genetically defined animal models.[29b]

SURGICAL TREATMENT

The optimal timing of surgical repair of thoracic aortic aneurysms is somewhat uncertain in light of the limited data on their natural history.[48] The major objectives of surgical treatment are to alleviate symptoms related to the aortic disease, reduce the frequency of complications associated with the specific aortic disease, and, in the case of aortic aneurysm, prevent death from rupture. Extensive aortic disease may require staged operative procedures.[99]

Indications for operation

Symptoms

Symptomatic patients with ascending or arch aneurysms should be evaluated urgently for surgical repair. Patients presenting with rupture should be operated on urgently, since these conditions are almost uniformly fatal without prompt surgical intervention.

Size and growth rate

Current recommendations for elective resection of the ascending aorta are based on the fact that the mean diameter of the aorta at the time of dissection or rupture is around 6 cm, but this actually means that half these patients have experienced a highly lethal complication by the time a diameter of 6 cm is reached.[100] Therefore, with the markedly reduced operative risk today, the authors, as do others,[101,102] recommend ascending aortic operations in nonheritable connective tissue disorder patients when the ascending aortic aneurysm diameter ranges from 5 to 5.5 cm. For patients who have diameters less than 5 cm and are being monitored with serial imaging, an indication for surgical intervention would be a 10 percent increase in size over a 6- to 12-month time course. Additionally, since the majority of ascending aortic aneurysms are discovered in the course of evaluation for aortic insufficiency, progressive aortic valvular regurgitation is another common indication for operation.

Influence of etiology

Patients with a heritable disorder of connective tissue such as MFS, EDS, LDS, BAV, or TAAD who have an ascending or arch aneurysm require earlier surgical intervention than do nonheritable patients. The traditional threshold that prompts the consideration of prophylactic aortic root replacement in patients with MFS has been predicated on aortic size, and replacement is recommended when the diameter reaches 5.0 cm.[103,104] The association between increased aneurysm diameter and the risk for dissection or rupture has been established clearly, and aneurysm size greater than 6 cm portends a fourfold increase in the cumulative risk of aortic rupture or dissection in patients with MFS.[104] Some patients with MFS experience acute dissections when the aortic diameter is less than 5.0 cm.[105] In patients with Loey-Dietz syndrome, aortic dissection often occurred in childhood and in aortas with diameters well under 5 cm.[29b] Therefore, for heritable disorders of connective tissue, surgical intervention for the ascending aorta should be considered at a diameter approaching 4 cm for LDS patients, 4 to 4.5 cm for MFS patients, 4.5 to 5 cm for BAV patients, and 5 cm for EDS or TAAD patients. In addition, young children with LDS should undergo surgical intervention when the maximal dimension of the ascending aorta exceeds the 99th percentile and the diameter of the aortic annulus exceeds 1.8 cm.[29b] For patients with ascending aortic aneurysms below these values, surveillance is warranted. Factors that prompt a recommendation for surgery when the aorta is less than 5.0 cm include rapid growth of the aortic diameter (more than 1 cm per year), a family history of premature aortic dissection (dissection less than 5.0 cm), and the presence of moderate or severe AR.[2]

Choice of operations

Ascending aortic operations

The surgical technique employed for treatment of an ascending aortic aneurysm varies with the underlying pathology and the quality of the aortic wall, the skill of the operating surgeon, the status of the aortic valve, and the age, expected survival, and general well-being of the patient.[23] The primary technical objectives of repair are surgical excision of all aneurysmal segments with graft replacement and restoration of function to the aortic valve.

Choosing the technique most appropriate for the patient and the pathology requires careful consideration of the factors that Ergin and associates[106] have outlined (Table 35-2). Among these factors are the following:

1. *Age and expected survival.* In an older high-risk patient, separate valve and ascending aortic replacement may be the appropriate therapy if life expectancy is limited.[107] Reduction aortoplasty is less technically demanding than is tube graft replacement of the ascending aorta, but the long-term results reveal a significant risk of recurrent dilation.[108,109]
2. *Underlying pathology and quality of the aortic wall.* A weakened aortic wall in a patient with Marfan's syndrome or dissection will require complete excision of the dilated portion of the aorta and the root. The button modification of the Bentall procedure has proved in the authors' hands the most versatile and durable reconstruction.[110] Sparing the aortic valve in MFS patients is controversial[111], although early date with 5 year followup is encouraging.
3. *Anatomic condition of the aortic annulus, the valve leaflets, the sinuses, and the sinotubular ridge.* The anatomic condition of these important elements of aortic valvular integrity usually dictates whether the valve can be spared or whether a separate valve-ascending aortic replacement may be feasible. In the authors' experience, the ideal candidate for a valve-sparing root replacement is a patient with a normal valve and annulus in whom a dilated sinotubular ridge or dilated sinuses leads to aortic insufficiency. A separate valve and ascending aorta replacement that leaves behind thinned, dilated sinuses is a compromise that should be avoided in patients with a relatively long life expectancy.[112]
4. *Condition of the distal aorta.* If the condition of the distal aorta mandates a future operation for associated distal arch or descending aneurysm or dissection, a fail-safe initial repair at the root is of paramount importance. The presence of even modest degrees of aortic regurgitation may complicate an operation on the distal aorta substantially, and this frequently requires the utilization of hypothermic circulatory arrest. In these cases, the authors prefer a composite replacement rather than a valve-sparing procedure, except in the case of an absolutely normal valve with AR secondary to dilation of the STJ.
5. *The risk of anticoagulation.* A young female desirous of childbearing presents a particularly nasty dilemma. A valve-sparing root repair or perhaps a pulmonary autograft may allow long-term durability. Reoperations on a biological composite valve graft undoubtedly will incur more risk than will a simple aortic valve reoperation and should be avoided.
6. *Presence of active annular infection.* First and foremost, total excision of all infected tissue must be achieved. Annular and root reconstruction then can be accomplished with autologous materials, with the considerations for anticoagulation that were outlined above. Although low rates of reinfection may be achieved with conventional prostheses, repairs that avoid prosthetic material such as homografts and pulmonary autografts may be preferable.

Table 35-2 Factors influencing the choice of ascending aortic operations
Age and expected survival
Underlying pathology and quality of the aortic wall
Anatomic condition of aortic annulus, valve leaflets, sinuses, and sinotubular ridge
Condition of the distal aorta
Risk of anticoagulation
Presence of active annular infection

Source: Modified from Ergin et al.[106]

Arch operations

The specific technical aspects of aortic arch replacement depend on the location of the aneurysm within the arch and the extent of involvement of the contiguous ascending and descending aorta.[24] To replace the dilated arch with a prosthetic tube graft, the brachiocephalic vessels must be removed from the arch before its interposition. Traditionally, this involved removing and then reimplanting the brachiocephalic vessels en bloc during hypothermic circulatory arrest. However, many surgeons have adopted a newer surgical technique by using a multilimbed prosthetic arch graft to which each arch vessel is anastomosed individually in turn, thereby reducing the duration of hypothermic circulatory arrest; avoiding the proximal portion of the arch vessels, which is frequently diseased; and allowing inspection of all anastomoses for hemostasis.[48]

Operative technique

Preoperative evaluation

Since myocardial infarction, respiratory failure, renal failure, and stroke are the principal causes of death and morbidity after operations on the thoracic aorta, preoperative assessment of the function of these organ systems is essential.[113]

Anesthetic considerations

Although the anesthetic management of patients undergoing aortic arch surgery includes practices common to most cardiac operations, there are conditions associated with the repair of aortic aneurysmal rupture that warrant special consideration. Anesthetic induction tends to blunt the sympathetically mediated compensatory responses of vasoconstriction and tachycardia that often are associated with acute thoracic aortic disruption. Therefore, acute cardiovascular collapse may result from conventional induction. To avoid this situation, endotracheal intubation and femoral vessel cannulation under local anesthesia with simultaneous institution of general anesthesia and CPB often are instituted in the setting of aneurysmal rupture.

Standard monitoring After induction of anesthesia and intubation with a single-lumen endotracheal tube, venous access is obtained with a large-bore central line and several large-bore peripheral lines. For invasive arterial pressure monitoring and blood sampling, an arterial line is placed, but the location of placement is dependent on the operation that is being performed. If antegrade selective cerebral perfusion will be performed via the right axillary artery, the authors frequently monitor both left and right radial artery pressures. Pulmonary artery pressures, cardiac filling pressures, and output are measured by using a pulmonary artery catheter. Intraoperative TEE is used to estimate both ventricular filling and contractility, assess valvular function, allow selection of cannulation sites free of atherosclerotic disease, and confirm the appropriate advancement of the guidewire and venous cannula from the femoral vein into the superior vena cava. Thermistor probes measure bladder, venous perfusate, and two tympanic temperatures. Five-lead electrocardiography and pulse oximetry are observed. Urine output is measured with a Foley catheter. Both invasive and noninvasive measures of cerebral oximetry also may be beneficial.

Perfusion

In the case of ascending aortic aneurysms, if an aneurysm does not involve the distal ascending aorta or the proximal aortic arch, these sites can be used for cannulation. If this is not possible, the axillary artery or innominate arteries may be used for arterial return from the pump-oxygenator. Femoral cannulation, especially in older patients with diffuse atheromatous disease, risks retrograde embolization to the brain as well as retrograde aortic dissection. Bicaval venous cannulation allows improved myocardial preservation as well as retrograde filling of the superior vena cava as a final flush of particulate or gaseous material from the cerebral circulation before restoration of antegrade perfusion. In the case of arch aneurysms or if clamping of the ascending aorta is not possible, deep hypothermic circulatory arrest with additional cerebral protection is necessary.

Cerebral protection

Because of its location, surgery of the aortic arch requires manipulation and exclusion of the cerebral circulation; therefore, cerebral protection is a primary concern and the utilization of optimal methods for the preservation of cerebral function is necessary to avoid ischemic or embolic brain injury. Over the last three decades, cerebral protection during arch procedures has evolved to avoid both the permanent and the transient neurologic dysfunction (TND) seen after aortic surgery. Initially, simple profound hypothermic circulatory arrest as described by Griepp and associates[17] seemed adequate, but it was associated with both focal and generalized neurologic injury with longer periods of arrest. Retrograde cerebral perfusion was popularized by Ueda and coworkers,[114] but TND was observed commonly with ischemic periods longer than 40 to 60 min. Selective antegrade cerebral perfusion and hypothermia as described by Kazui and colleagues[115] appears to provide cerebral protection for even longer ischemic periods (more than 40 to 60 min).

Deep hypothermia and circulatory arrest The technique of deep hypothermia and circulatory arrest (DHCA) was described by Drew and associates in 1959.[116] Children undergoing surgery for Tetralogy of Fallot were cooled to 12°C (nasopharyngeal), allowing a circulatory arrest time of 1 h. The introduction of DHCA by Griepp and coworkers[17] as an operative tool more than 30 years ago still serves as the basis for the surgical treatment of complex thoracic aortic pathologies. This technique allows the performance of an open distal anastomosis and better visualization of the aortic arch in a relatively bloodless field. The main disadvantages of DHCA include coagulopathy, increased CPB time, and renal and neurologic dysfunction.[117]

The vulnerability of the brain during circulatory arrest has been a great concern. Even at brain temperatures as low as 18°C, the safe arrest time is considered to be no longer than 30 to 40 min. An additional factor in the incidence of cerebral damage is the increasing age of these patients.[118] To protect the brain against ischemia, several different techniques are available, among which hypothermia is a standard, well-accepted application. To be able to establish the precise temperature of the brain, it is important to know which monitoring site is the most accurate for that purpose. The routinely used sites include esophageal, rectal, bladder, nasopharyngeal, pulmonary arterial, and skin temperatures. Several studies have compared the efficacy of the different monitoring sites in indicating the temperature of the brain, particularly in the dynamic phase of cooling and rewarming. Although core temperature sites, in particular bladder and esophageal temperature, may reflect accurately changes in body temperature during moderate hypothermia,[119,120] the accurate estimation of the optimal brain temperature site is still a matter of debate. The only available study in which brain temperature was measured directly during DHCA included patients undergoing surgical clipping of a cerebral aneurysm.[121] Routine monitoring sites, including tympanic temperatures, under- or overestimated brain temperature, with relatively large differences between individual patients. Although the effective time of arrest of cerebral perfusion has been shortened substantially by the application of antegrade low-flow cold blood cerebral perfusion, it is still important to assess cerebral temperature as accurately as possible. In the authors' practice at Stanford, this includes the measurement of bladder temperature, venous perfusate temperature, and two tympanic temperatures.

Since hypothermia is applied for brain protection because it diminishes cerebral oxygen consumption ($CMRO_2$), electroencephalography (EEG) monitoring has been advocated to assess uniform cooling and the degree of depression of the electrical signaling obtained during cooling. However, the EEG records only the postsynaptic potentials of cortical neurons, not the metabolic status of basal structures. During cooling, the EEG becomes isoelectric between 20 and 18°C, but consistency of variation during hypothermia is unproven. The association between intraoperative EEG changes and postoperative neurologic deficits is weak. Still, EEG is used to determine electrical silence before DHCA and assess the effects of additional pharmacologic protective strategies.[122]

The bispectral index (BIS), which is derived from the analysis of phase and frequency interrelationships of EEG waves, was studied in patients undergoing cardiac surgery with CPB. BIS showed a reduced need for anesthetics after the initiation of CPB compared with before CPB.[123] This important observation was confirmed in patients by using the patient state index (PSI), another measure used to detect a patient's level of hypnosis.[124] Monitoring DHCA patients with PSI revealed that after rewarming and termination of CPB, the level of anesthetic sedation might last several hours without any additional administration of anesthetics. This might be due to the combination of deep hypothermia and pharmacologic protection with barbiturates, which is the authors' common practice. Since anesthetics may cause myocardial depression and unwanted hypotension as a result of vasodilatation, monitors such as BIS and PSI have the capacity to improve outcomes by preventing unnecessary anesthetic intervention in the early post-CPB period.

A second monitoring method to assess cerebral cooling and lowering of $CMRO_2$ that has been studied intensively is jugular venous bulb oxygen saturation ($SjVO_2$). $SjVO_2$ is measured by inserting a catheter percutaneously in the internal jugular vein and advancing it in a retrograde fashion into the jugular bulb. The actual measurements of $SjVO_2$ are performed intermittently by sampling from the catheter or continuously by using a fiber-optic catheter.[125] During cerebral cooling, the cerebral metabolic rate and cerebral oxygen extraction both decrease, resulting in an increase in $SjVO_2$. Some authors suggest that cooling during DHCA should continue until $SjVO_2$ has increased to at least 95 percent, indicating sufficient global cerebral hypothermia, although regional differences still will go undetected.[126]

The cerebral protective effect of hypothermia is undisputed,[127] but the specific temperature to guarantee maximal protection during DHCA is unknown. Hypothermia not only lowers the brain energy demands by lowering $CMRO_2$ but also provides protection by reducing excitatory neurotransmitter release, decreasing free radical production, and maintaining cellular integrity.[128] Most authors indicate that DHCA is started at a temperature of 15 to 20°C measured at core, tympanic, or both sites.[118,129,130] The disadvantages of lower temperatures include fewer autoregulatory mechanisms and longer CPB times with resultant coagulopathies and cellular edema. Studies of neurologic deficit after DHCA conclude that an arrest time of 25 to 30 min is probably the maximally tolerated ischemic period, particularly for the brain. The duration of DHCA time and the age of the patients are reported to be the most important risk factors for mortality and postoperative neurologic deficit.[117,118,129]

To diminish cerebral ischemic time, perfusion of the brain during deep hypothermia has been implemented, including retrograde cerebral perfusion (RCP) and antegrade selective cerebral perfusion (ASCP). Recent reports indicate the superiority of ASCP,[131–133] with neurologic deficit rates of 5 to 8 percent[129] and transient brain dysfunction rates of 10 to 30 percent.[117,132] Cerebral autoregulation is significantly better preserved with ASCP than with RCP or with no selective cerebral perfusion.[130] An alternative approach using the axillary artery for antegrade perfusion during DHCA has shown promising results[134] even in emergency conditions.[135] Additionally, this technique of ASCP has allowed the recent trend toward moving away from very low temperatures toward higher systemic temperatures, up to 25°C with selective cold (15°C)[136,137] or even moderate hypothermic (25°C)[138] perfusion of the brain, to prevent temperature-induced coagulopathy and loss of cerebral autoregulation.

In spite of these improvements, the substantial residual neurologic problems after surgery with deep hypothermia have inspired researchers to focus on the rewarming phase after circulatory arrest. Several studies using $SjVO_2$ monitoring have reported significant venous desaturation during rewarming.[139,140] Apparently, there is a discrepancy between oxygen demand and oxygen supply in this crucial phase that was reported to be

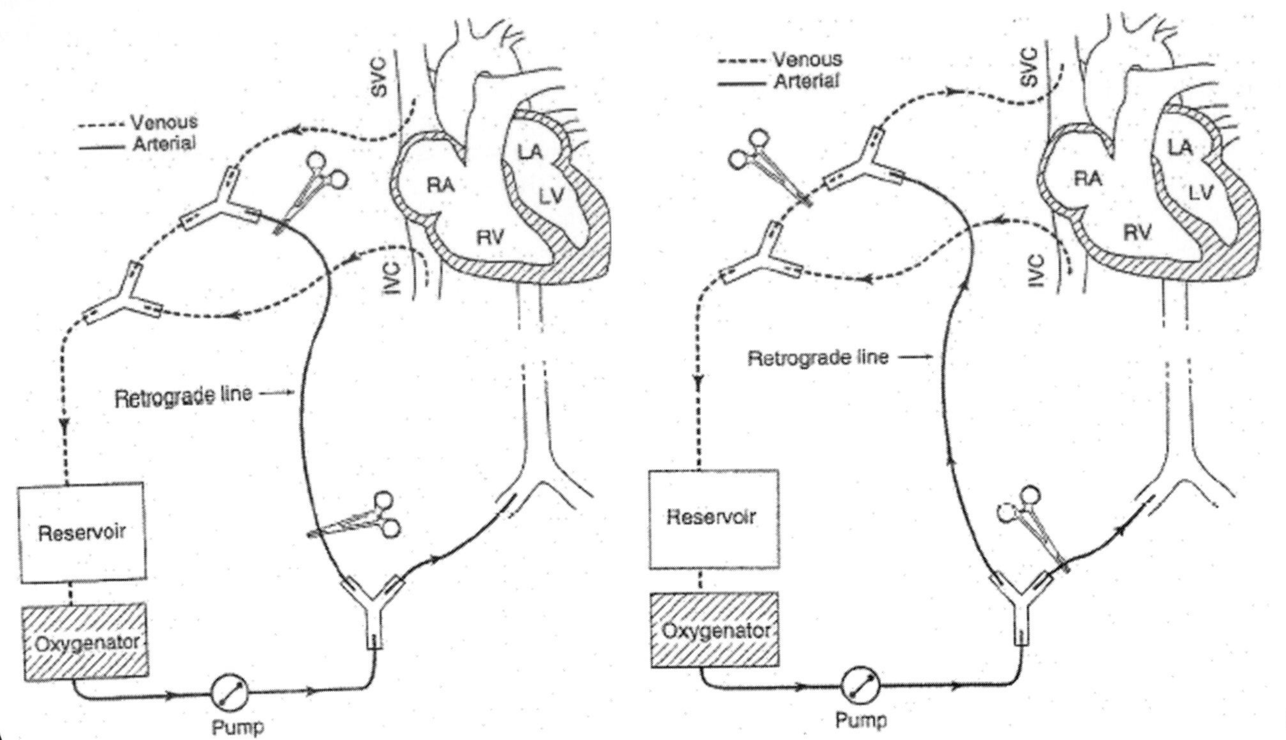

Figure 35-11 Retrograde cerebral perfusion. Schematic for retrograde cerebral perfusion via the superior vena cava. **A.** Cannulation configuration for cardiopulmonary bypass and retrograde cerebral perfusion (RCP). The retrograde line is primed and clamped. **B.** RCP through the superior vena cava (SVC) after arterial return is directed through the retrograde line into the SVC. LA = left atrium; LV = left ventricle; RV = right ventricle; RA = right atrium; IVC = inferior vena cava.

prevented by mild hypercapnia,[141] with a critical limit of desaturation defined as 50 percent.[139] Changing the rate of rewarming had no effect on the reduction of jugular venous saturation, indicating that a relative impairment of cerebral blood flow in the presence of marked hemodilution may be responsible for this phenomenon. Although there are no convincing data showing that jugular venous desaturation is related to postoperative neurologic deficit, a study using preoperative MRI suggested that patients with greater preoperative abnormalities had higher degrees of desaturation during rewarming.[142] Since patients undergoing surgery on the aortic arch may show preoperative impairment of cerebral perfusion, they represent a vulnerable group for venous jugular desaturation during rewarming after DHCA. Large, prospective multicenter studies may show a relationship between these two variables.

Retrograde cerebral perfusion Retrograde cerebral perfusion was described by Mills and Ochsner in 1980 as a treatment for massive air embolism during CPB.[143] Intermittent and later continuous RCP was adopted by Ueda and associates[114] as a method for cerebral protection during procedures involving the aortic arch. Before the emergence of ASCP, RCP was used commonly as an adjunct to DHCA during surgery on the thoracic aorta as a way to improve the neurologic outcome. In RCP, oxygenated blood is delivered to the brain in a retrograde manner via a cannula placed in the superior vena cava (Fig. 35-11). The hypothetical neuroprotective mechanisms of RCP include maintenance of cerebral hypothermia, washout of embolic air or debris, cerebral perfusion, and metabolic support. However, on the basis of human and laboratory investigations, the neuroprotective mechanisms of RCP remain controversial. Compared with ASCP, RCP seems to be less effective but still provides somewhat more brain preservation than does DHCA, probably as a result of the continued cerebral cooling via the venoarterial and venovenous collateral circulations.[144]

Antegrade selective cerebral perfusion The earliest attempts to repair the aortic arch relied on complex methods of extracorporeal cerebral perfusion. In 1957, DeBakey and associates[15] reported a successful resection of an aortic arch aneurysm using normothermic CPB achieved by means of several pumps and bilateral cannulation of both the subclavian and carotid arteries. Eventually, the CPB perfusion technique was simplified by Dubost and associates[145] and Pearce and associates[146] by using a single pump with a Y-connection of the arterial line; however, over the next two decades, extracorporeal cerebral perfusion during aortic arch replacement was overshadowed by the growing interest in and utilization of circulatory arrest and deep hypothermia.[144]

In 1986, Frist and associates[147] from Stanford initiated the new ASCP "era" by incorporating a CPB technique with partial brachiocephalic perfusion, with low CPB flow (30 to 50 mL/kg/min) and moderate systemic cooling (26 to 28°C).[144] The arterial line from a single pump head had a Y-shape to perfuse both the femoral artery and either the innominate or the left carotid artery. In 1991, Bachet and associates[148] introduced a procedure that employed cold blood "cerebroplegia," which was perfused via the innominate and left common carotid arteries through separate pumps and heat exchangers. Kazui and colleagues[115] are credited with advancing the current use of ASCP by introducing the employment of separate arterial pump heads for the cerebral and systemic circulations to provide individual hypothermic perfusion to each system at 25°C (Fig. 35-12). Cerebral perfusion was achieved by means of endoluminal cannulation of the brachiocephalic and left common carotid arteries while the left subclavian artery was clamped or occluded with a Fogarty catheter to avoid the steal phenomenon. In an elegant experimental study, Tanaka and associates[149] provided laboratory evidence supporting the use of ASCP and outlined important perfusion details such as the optimum perfusion flow rate, pressure, and temperature.

Pharmacologic protection Because deep hypothermia, including ASCP, often leads to an unwanted neurologic outcome in patients with circulatory arrest, additional strategies of neuroprotection are applied, including pharmacologic interventions. The cerebral protective effects of barbiturates in global ischemia have been studied in various models, including in humans after cardiac arrest.[150] All the trials failed to demonstrate an improvement in outcome. There are no randomized clinical studies showing advantageous effects of barbiturates in DHCA patients, and it has been suggested that barbiturates may jeopardize the energy state of the brain in patients with these conditions.[151] Still, in a survey on current practice, 35 percent of the respondents believed there was sufficient evidence to support the use of barbiturates in aortic surgery with DHCA.[152] As potential support for the use of barbiturates, it could be stated that barbiturates have been shown to be protective in patients with incomplete, focal ischemia in specific settings such as those which are present during cardiopulmonary bypass because of multiple emboli. In addition, they may be helpful in protecting the brain during rewarming after DHCA, particularly in the early phase, when the observed jugular venous oxygen desaturation mentioned above indicates a lack of oxygen delivery.

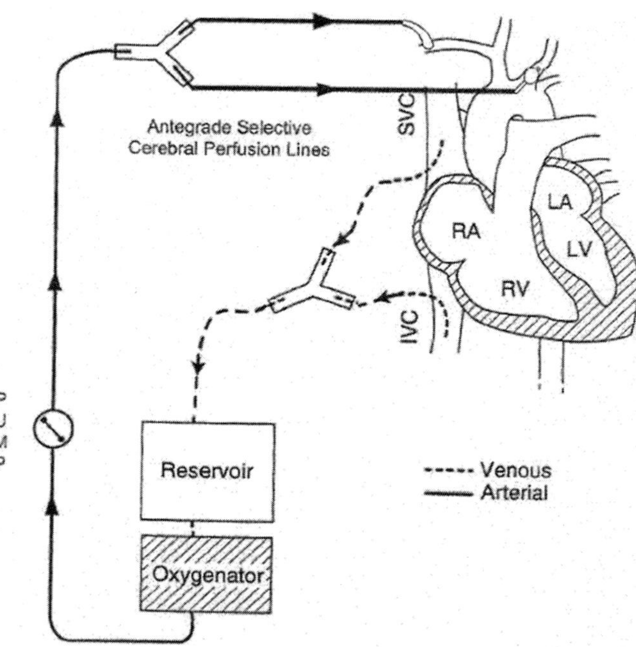

Figure 35-12 Antegrade cerebral perfusion. Schematic for antegrade selective cerebral perfusion via the right axillary artery and the left common carotid artery. LA = left atrium; LV = left ventricle; RV = right ventricle; RA = right atrium; IVC = inferior vena cava.

Steroids, in particular dexamethasone and methylprednisolone, are used routinely during DHCA surgery,[152] mainly because they counteract the systemic inflammatory response (SIRS) during and after cardiopulmonary bypass. Brain ischemia is considered to be a combination of embolization and SIRS, and steroids have been shown to improve the neurologic outcome in DHCA patients.[153]

Specific operative considerations

Replacement of the ascending aorta Once stable CPB has been established, left heart venting is accomplished through either a pulmonary artery vent or a right superior pulmonary venous vent (Fig. 35-13). A balloon-tipped catheter is inserted into the right atrium and positioned in the coronary sinus for the delivery of retrograde cardioplegia. Adjunctive CO_2 perfusion of the operative field may be used. After myocardial protection is assured by instituting intermittent cold coronary sinus perfusion plus topical hypothermia, the ascending aorta is cross-clamped proximal to the origin of the innominate artery. The aorta then is transected completely proximal to the aortic clamp (leaving a cuff of circumferential aortic tissue to suture) and at the STJ. A Dacron tube graft that is selected to match the diameter of the aorta is anastomosed end to end to the distal aortic cuff with running 4-0 Prolene sutures, commencing on the left side, passing along the posterior wall to the right, and being completed along the anterior wall. If the aortic wall integrity is suspect, a 4- to 5-mm strip of polytetrafluoroethylene (PTFE) felt may be incorporated in the distal suture line to minimize blood loss from suture pull-through. If aortic valve replacement or repair is necessary, it is performed. The proximal anastomosis then is performed by trimming the tube graft at the appropriate length, followed by suturing to the proximal aorta with a 4-0 Prolene suture. Once again, if aortic wall integrity is suspect, incorporation of PTFE felt for

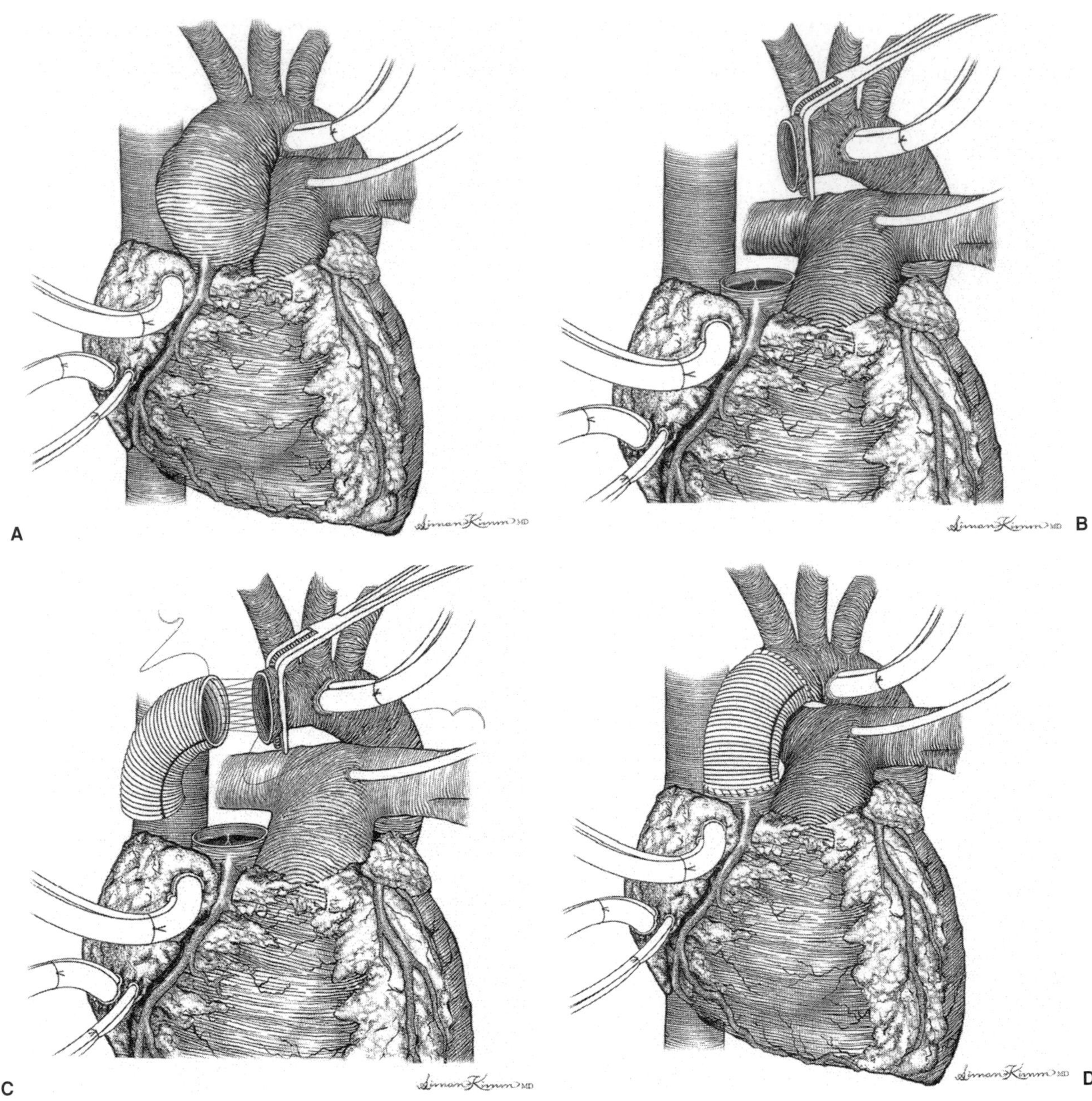

Figure 35-13 Ascending aortic replacement. **A.** Routine cannulation with arterial cannulation in the underside of the midarch. Bicaval cannulation and retrograde cardioplegia are used, as well as a pulmonary artery vent. **B.** After cross-clamping the aorta and instilling cardioplegia, the aortic valve, sinuses of Valsalva, coronary ostia, and sinotubular junction are all ascertained to be normal. **C.** Full-thickness cuffs of proximal and distal aorta are fashioned, and then an end-to-end anastomosis with an appropriately sized woven Dacron graft is constructed, utilizing running 4-0 monofilament sutures. **D.** An aspirating needle in the highest point of the graft allows evacuation of air before discontinuation of the bypass. (Illustration by Simon Kimm, MD.)

reinforcement is recommended. Just before completion of the proximal anastomosis, the pulmonary artery vent is discontinued, the heart is filled with blood, and standard de-airing procedures are carried out. The proximal suture line then is tied; a needle vent is placed in the graft and connected to cardiotomy suction to expel any residual air with the patient in the Trendelenburg position. Finally, the clamp is removed from the graft, allowing reperfusion of the coronary circulation. Strict attention is paid to avoiding left ventricular dilation until cardiac ejection commences. Once rewarming has been completed, CPB is terminated, followed by removal of cannulas and the achievement of hemostasis. Hemorrhage can be a serious problem after repair despite meticulous surgical technique. Consequently, the application of local hemostatic factors (e.g., thrombin-impregnated Gelfoam, Avitene, or Surgicel) in addition to the appropriate administration of procoagulant factors is often necessary.

Replacement of the ascending aorta and aortic root Once stable CPB has been established, a left heart vent is placed and a balloon-tipped catheter is inserted into the right atrium and positioned in the coronary sinus for the delivery of retrograde cardioplegia (Fig. 35-14). After the aorta is cross-clamped proximal to the origin of the innominate artery, the myocardial preservation techniques that were described previously are instituted. The aorta is completely transected proximal to the aortic clamp (leaving a cuff of circumferential aortic tissue to suture) and just above the level of the main coronary artery ostia. The aortic valve then is excised, and a composite valve graft repair commences. For a mechanical valve, a Dacron valved conduit is sutured into the annulus with 2-0 pledgeted horizontal mattress sutures. For a biological valve, a porcine root replacement is instituted with interrupted 3-0 horizontal mattress sutures. The left and right coronary artery orifices are excised from the aorta, leaving a 4- to 5-mm rim of aortic wall. Approximately 1 to 2 cm of the coronary arteries is mobilized carefully to avoid tension, the left coronary button is anastomosed to the valved conduit, us ing a running 5-0 Prolene suture. To avoid traction and subsequent distortion of the right coronary artery, the distal graft anastomosis is completed before the right coronary button anastomosis is performed. Therefore, the valve conduit is measured, transected, and sutured end to end to the distal graft repair with a running 4-0 Prolene suture and allowed to fill retrograde, followed by the right coronary button anastomosis. Just before the completion of this suture line, the heart is filled with blood and standard de-airing maneuvers are performed. A needle vent connected to cardiotomy suction is placed in the graft, and any residual air is expelled with the patient in the Trendelenburg position. Finally, the clamp is removed from the graft, allowing reperfusion of the coronary circulation. Once rewarming has been completed, CPB is terminated, followed by removal of the cannulas and achievement of hemostasis.

Replacement of the ascending aorta and aortic root with a homograft or xenograft In patients with infective endocarditis and aortic root dilation, homograft aortic root replacement is a good option after radical debridement of all infected or devitalized tissue. The proximal end of the graft is sutured to the native aortic annulus with interrupted or continuous 4-0 Prolene sutures. Occasionally, the suture line is reinforced with a strip of pericardium to ensure hemostasis and the aortic homograft is placed in the natural position without rotation. The homograft anterior mitral valve leaflet can be utilized to patch erosions into the septum after meticulous debridement. Anastomosis then is performed from the native left and right coronary artery ostia to the corresponding coronary ostia of the aortic homograft. Extension with a Dacron tube graft sometimes is used to replace the entire diseased aorta. For implantation of a xenograft, refer to Chapter 30.

Reestablishing coronary flow Frequently, with large aneurysms or false aneurysms, the coronary ostia are laterally displaced from the new aortic lumen. This distance can make primary attachment of the coronary ostia-to-ascending graft difficult even after adequate mobilization with full-thickness aortic buttons, especially in redo patients. Therefore, coronary flow can be established with various procedures (Table 35-3 and Fig. 35-15). Cabrol and coworkers[154] originally described connecting the two coronary ostia end to end with a separate Dacron interposition graft that then was anastomosed side to side to the aortic conduit; the entire repair was wrapped in the aneurysm wall to control bleeding. The modified Cabrol technique involves resecting the entire aortic wall and forming coronary ostial buttons, which are mobilized, sutured end to end with a smaller Dacron tube graft, and anastomosed side to side with the aortic conduit.[155] Alternatively, the Kay-Zubiate technique[156] relies solely on autologous tissue; saphenous vein is employed as an interposition graft for the displaced coronary ostia. In the absence of infection and particularly in redo root operations, in which adequate mobilization of the coronary buttons is impossible, a short interposed segment of 6- or 8-mm Dacron™ graft works nicely.

Axillary artery cannulation The axillary artery and innominate arteries are our preferred site of arterial cannulation for CPB when either the ascending aorta or the arch is unsuitable for cannulation and/or to facilitate selective antegrade cerebral perfusion when hypothermic circulatory arrest will be utilized in the performance of an open distal anastomosis (Fig. 35-16). The technique begins with a 6- to 8-cm transverse incision approximately two fingerbreadths below the distal clavicle in the deltopectoral groove. The pectoralis major muscle is divided in the direction of its fibers. The pectoralis minor muscle is retracted laterally or divided. Using sharp dissection, the artery is dissected from the surrounding tissue. Because the axillary artery lies deep to the axillary vein, it is usually necessary to mobilize and retract the vein. Care is taken to preserve elements of the brachial plexus or to avoid disrupting lymphatics, especially in females. Proximal and distal control of the axillary artery is obtained, and 5000 units of heparin is administered intravenously. A longitudinal arteriotomy is performed, and a 6- or 8-mm Dacron side graft is anastomosed with a 5-0 Prolene sutures. The vascular clamps are removed from the artery, restoring flow to the right arm, and the Dacron graft is filled with heparinized saline solution. A 22F Sarns or 21F DLP cannula is inserted into the graft, secured with heavy ligatures, and connected to the CPB circuit. At the termination of CPB, the graft is amputated, leaving a 2- to 3-mm cuff that is oversewn with a double layer of 5-0 Prolene sutures. The clavipectoral fascia, subcutaneous tissue, and skin are closed in three separate layers with a running absorbable suture.

Open distal anastomosis and replacement of the aortic arch The open technique for distal anastomosis is

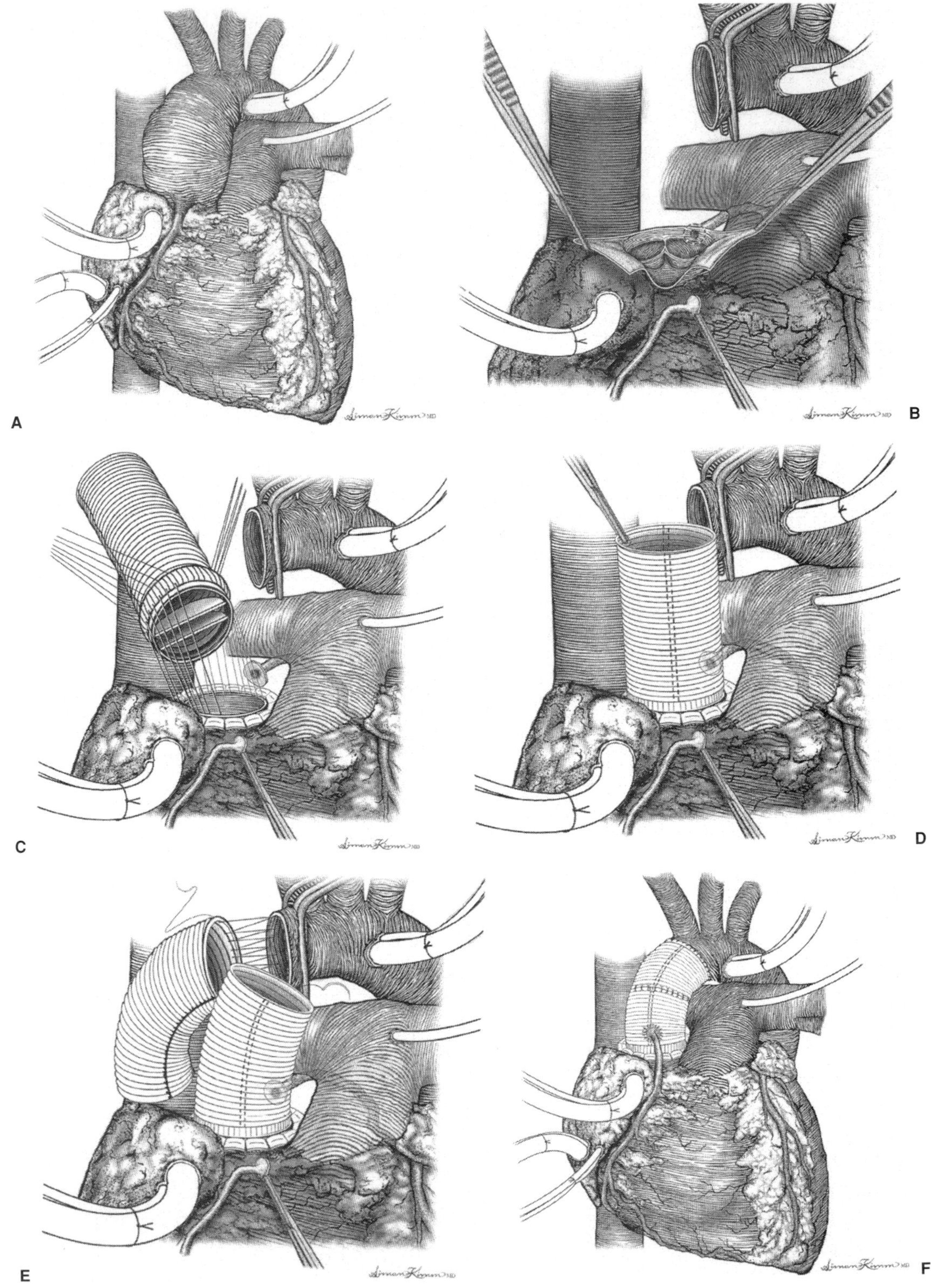

Figure 35-14 Replacement of ascending aorta and aortic root. **A.** An ascending aortic aneurysm that involves the sinuses of Valsalva. Cannulation is as in Figure 35-13, but because of aortic regurgitation, antegrade cardioplegia is delivered via a hand-held cannula. **B.** The dilated coronary sinuses along with the diseased aortic valve are excised. **C.** A composite valve graft is then sewn with interrupted, everting pledgeted 2-0 mattress sutures to the aortic annulus. **D.** Full-thickness coronary buttons are fashioned, with the left button reimplanted first. **E.** The distal anastomosis with a running 4-0 polypropylene suture, utilizing a separate graft, which allows an end-to-end Dacron anastomosis using different size grafting materials for the proximal and distal anastomosis. **F.** The repair is complete after the graft-to-graft anastomosis, and a tension-free reimplantation of the right coronary button is performed. (Illustration by Simon Kimm, MD.)

Table 35-3 Techniques for reestablishing coronary flow in ascending aortic aneurysms

Technique	Description
Classic Cabrol	Two coronary ostia connected in an end-to-end fashion with Dacron interposition graft, then anastomosed side to side with the aortic conduit
Modified Cabrol	Coronary ostial buttons are mobilized, sutured end to end with a smaller Dacron tube graft, and then anastomosed side to side with the aortic conduit
Kay-Zubiate	Individual coronary button anastomosed end to end with an interposition graft of autologous vein, then an end-to-side anastomosis with the aortic conduit
Dacron interposition	Individual coronary button anastomosed end to end with an interposition graft of Dacron, then an end-to-side anastomosis with the aortic conduit

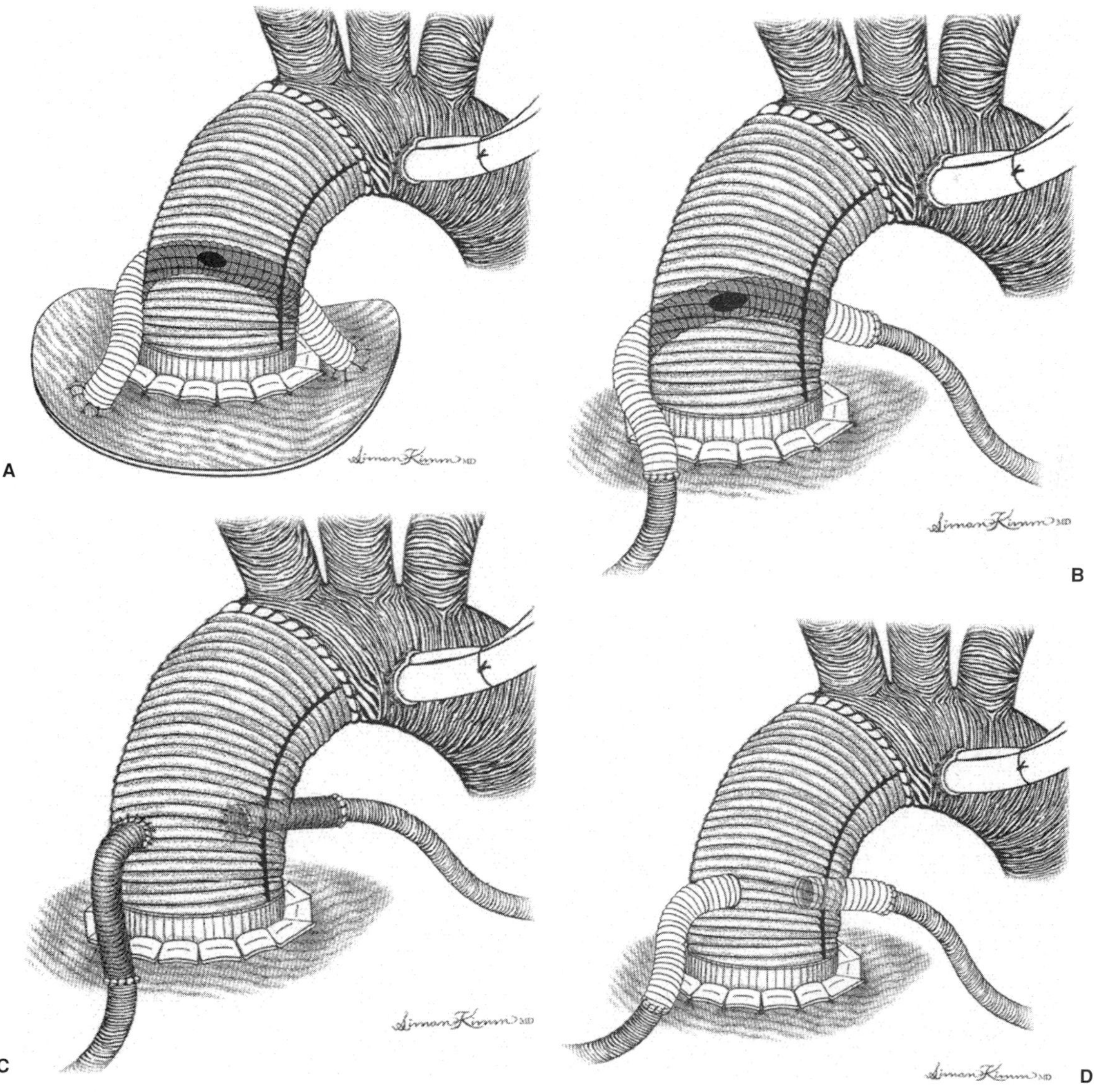

Figure 35-15 Alternative methods for coronary reimplantation. **A.** The classic Cabrol method, with a 6-mm or 8-mm graft sewn end to end to the coronary ostia and side to side to the aortic graft. **B.** Cabrol modification that utilizes the same graft sewn end to end to full-thickness coronary buttons, again with a side-to-side central anastomosis. **C.** Using short segments of saphenous vein graft to sew end to end to full-thickness coronary buttons to allow revascularizing coronaries that are laterally displaced that cannot be mobilized back toward the aortic graft. **D.** An alternative utilizing 6-mm Dacron conduit as an interposition graft. (Illustration by Simon Kimm, MD.)

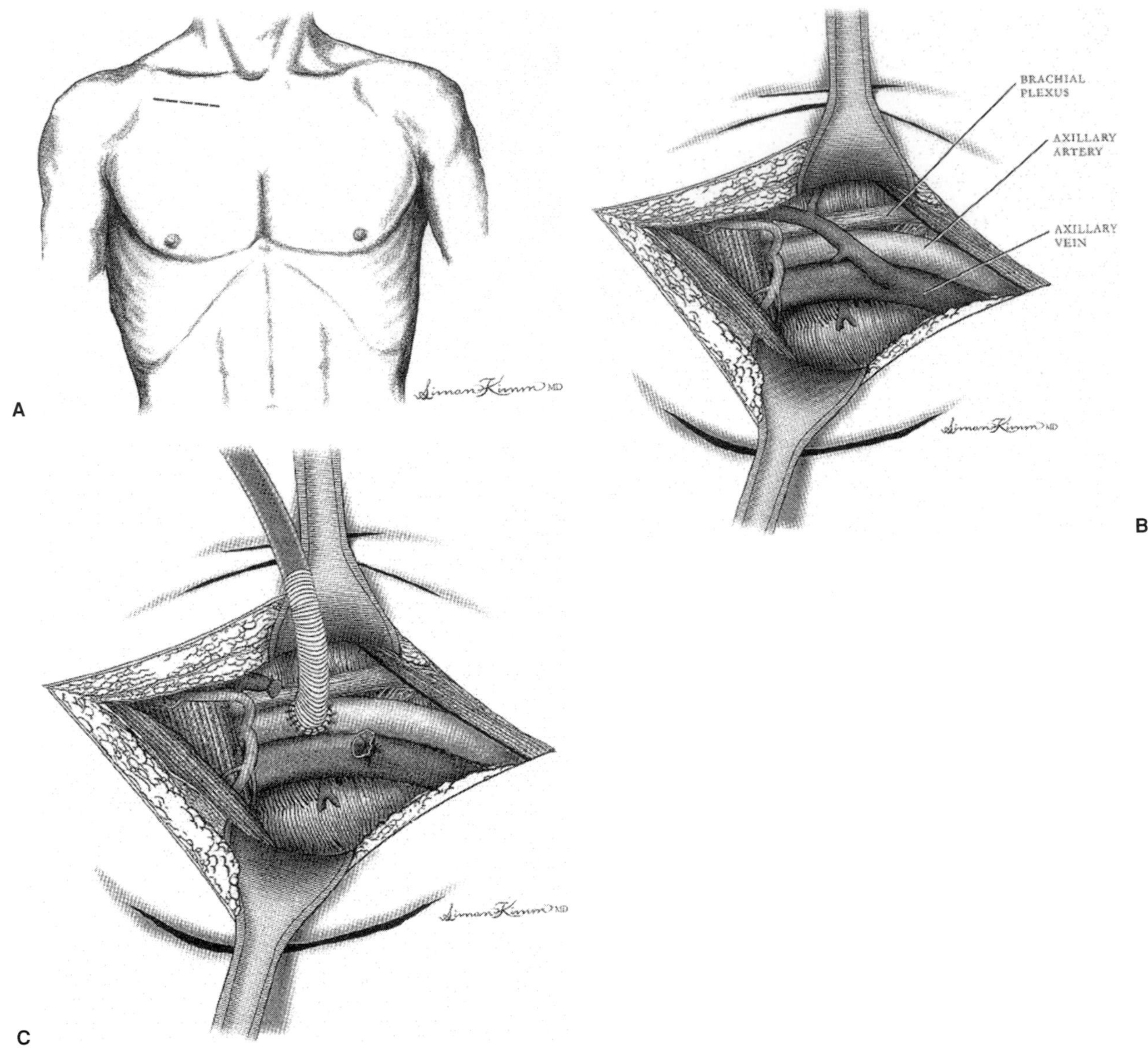

Figure 35-16 Axillary artery cannulation. **A.** Infraclavicular incision on the right in the deltopectoral groove. **B**. Axillary artery is dissected from behind the overlying axillary vein, which then is clamped with a partially occluding side-biting clamp, allowing an end-to-side anastomosis with a 6-mm or 8-mm Dacron graft (**C**). This graft then can be cannulated for an arterial cannulation site. (Illustration by Simon Kimm, MD.)

required when aortic arch or hemiarch reconstruction is indicated. Upon completion of axillary artery cannulation, midline sternotomy, mediastinal dissection (including exposure of the proximal innominate artery and left carotid artery), and venous cannulation (bicaval, two-stage, or femoral), the patient is cooled systemically to a target temperature of approximately 22°C. In the interim, the ascending aorta is fully mobilized and cross-clamped distally. An aortotomy is performed to decompress the aneurysm proximally, and a diastolic arrest of the heart is induced by using cold blood cardioplegia via antegrade, retrograde, and/or handheld delivery in concert with topical hypothermia. The aortic root is dissected further with excision/debridement of aortic valvular elements and dissection/mobilization of the coronary buttons. Replacement of the aortic root and reimplantation of the coronary buttons may proceed at this point or be deferred, based on when the systemic cooling is complete. When the target temperature is achieved, the patient is placed in the Trendelenburg position and the innominate artery is clamped proximally, arresting flow to the body and permitting selective antegrade cerebral perfusion via the right carotid artery and the right vertebral artery to proceed at a flow rate of 5 mL/kg/min. The aortic cross-clamp is removed, and diseased distal ascending and aortic arch tissue is excised. Back bleeding through the left common carotid may be absent, suggesting an incomplete circle of Willis, or may

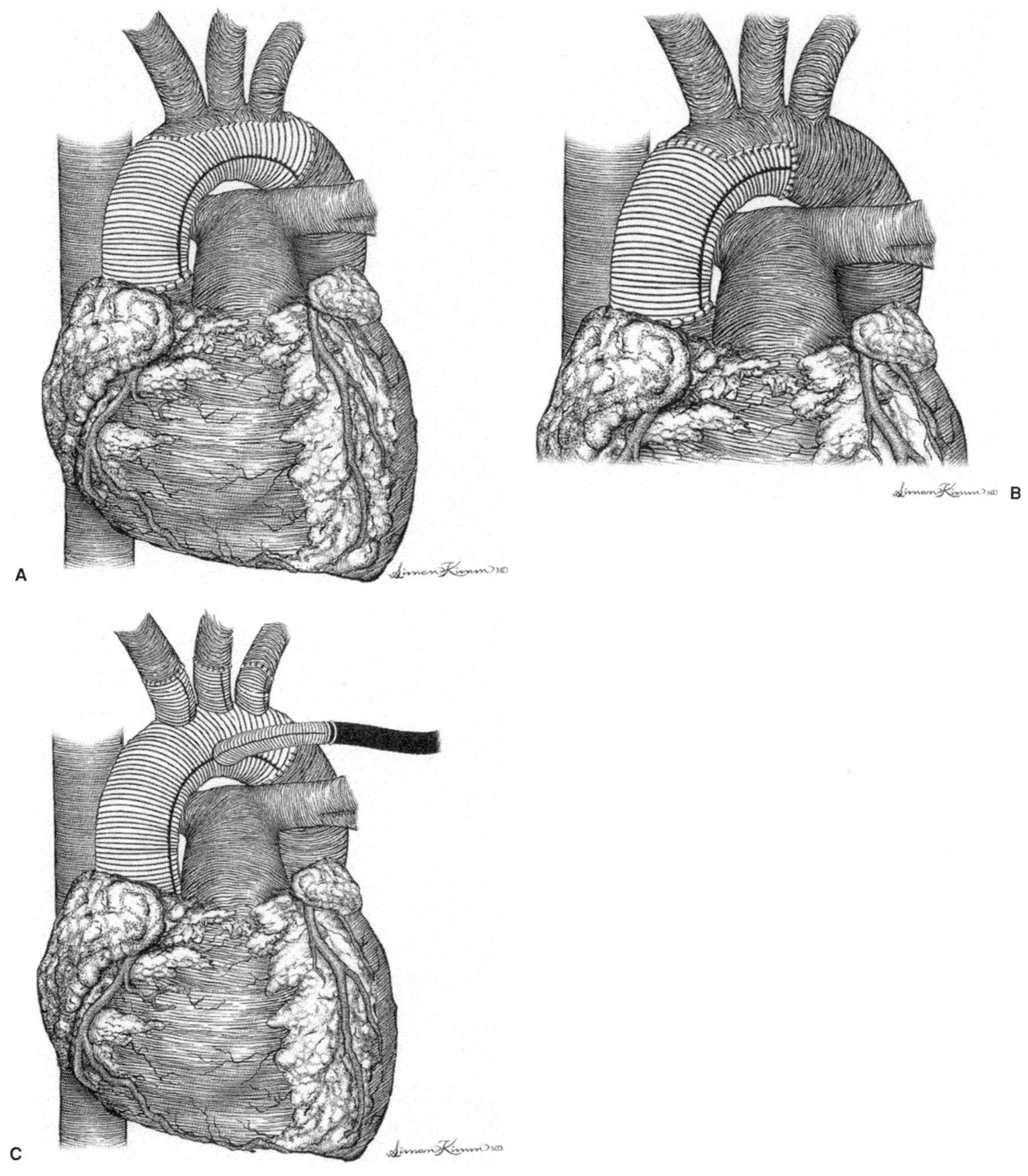

Figure 35-17 Multiple methods for aortic arch reconstructions. **A.** A complete arch replacement with distal end-to-end anastomosis and reimplantation of left subclavian, left common carotid, and innominate arteries as an "island" patch. **B.** The hemiarch or "peninsula" technique. **C.** An alternative method utilizing a multibranch graft with individual anastomoses to the left subclavian, left carotid, and innominate arteries, utilizing the fourth branch as a perfusion port. (Illustration by Simon Kimm, MD.)

be present but falsely reassuring if it is derived from collateral flow via the external carotid system. Therefore, to enhance antegrade cerebral perfusion, an appropriately sized pediatric coronary sinus catheter is placed into the left carotid artery via its takeoff from the aortic arch, secured in place by insufflation of the balloon cuff, and further bolstered by an extrinsic Silastic vessel loop. The loop is connected to the arterial inflow, providing an additional source of antegrade cerebral perfusion at 5 mL/kg/min. Higher cerebral temperatures may require selective antegrade cerebral blood flows of up to 20 mL/kg/min.

Depending on the integrity and caliber of the ostia of the great vessels, they may be reimplanted together as an "island" (Fig. 35-17A) or a "peninsula" (transverse arch or hemiarch replacement; Fig. 35-17B) as well as individually (in the setting of total aortic arch replacement). If chronic dissection is present, the septum between the true and false channels of the descending thoracic aorta is excised, providing a common channel. For total aortic arch replacement, it is often convenient to utilize a prefabricated branch graft, which may provide enhanced flexibility and efficiency in configuring the arch reconstruction (Fig. 35-17C). In any event, the distal aortic anastomosis is constructed by using a felt reinforced 4-0 Prolene suture technique. Great vessel reimplantation is performed with a 6-0 Prolene running suture. After completion of the arch anastomoses, antegrade flow into the graft is commenced and gradual rewarming is initiated while the proximal aortic reconstruction is completed.

In the setting of known descending thoracic aortic disease that is likely to require future operative repair, an "elephant trunk" distal aortic repair should be utilized (Fig. 35-18). In this technique, a 5- to 10-cm cuff of Dacron graft is left in the native descending thoracic aorta to provide a proximal anastomotic site for future intervention (open repair via left thoracotomy or stent graft via an endoluminal approach). An appropriately sized Dacron tube graft is chosen. Stay sutures are placed on the proximal extent, which is intussuscepted into the distal portion of the graft destined to serve as the elephant trunk. The graft in this intussuscepted configuration is inserted into the distal aorta, and a running 4-0 Prolene anastomosis is fashioned between the native aorta and the indwelling double-layer tube graft. The intussuscepted proximal portion of the tube graft is retrieved from the descending thoracic aorta by placing traction on the previously placed stay sutures. The remainder of the aortic arch reconstruction proceeds as was described previously.

Upon completion of the distal aortic reconstruction, the pediatric coronary sinus catheter is removed, a cross-clamp is applied to the graft, and the innominate artery is reopened with full flow to the body restored. The distal graft then may be cannulated (with a right-angle soft flow or a curved metal-tip aortic cannula placed via stab incision or the accessory limb of a prefabricated branch graft) to assist in CPB and rewarming for the remainder of the procedure. At this point, attention is redirected to completion of the aortic root replacement, performance of graft-to-graft anastomosis (running 4-0 Prolene sutures), and completion of coronary reimplantation.

OUTCOMES/PROGNOSIS

Results of operation

Ascending aortic aneurysms

Replacement of the ascending aorta has been demonstrated to be a safe and effective procedure for the treatment of chronic aneurysmal disease of the ascending aorta, with operative mortality rates of 2 to 5 percent in the most successful series.[157–159] The operative mortality varies with the acuity of the operation, patient age, left ventricular function, and the extent of operation.[23] The late survival rate after operation is approximately 65 percent at 5 years and 55 percent at 7 years.[157,160–162]

Marfan's syndrome Before 1968, the outlook for patients with MFS who required surgical repair of aneurysms or dissections involving the aortic root was bleak because of the high operative risk, the nearly prohibitive bleeding rates, and the frequent occurrence of serious postoperative complications.[2] With the advent of composite valve graft repair and valve-sparing aortic root replacement and modern CPB and myocardial protection, survival is excellent when a low-risk and durable procedure is performed in an experienced thoracic aortic surgical center.

Composite valve graft repair In a landmark paper by Gott and associates,[163] the safety and efficacy of aortic root replacement surgery with a composite valve graft technique in MFS patients were outlined. The mortality rate for elective root replacement in 455 patients was a remarkably low 1.5 percent, but the rate was much higher (11.7 percent) in those requiring emergency surgery for acute or chronic type A dissections, emphasizing the importance of early, elective root replacement before ascending dissection. Long-term survival after prophylactic aortic root replacement is also quite favorable, probably because the composite valve graft configuration provides no nidus for clot formation, minimizing the risk of late cerebrovascular accidents. In contrast, MFS patients who have had aortic dissection have a significantly reduced long-term survival, which has been reported at 50 to 70 percent at 10 years.[164,165]

Valve-sparing aortic surgical repair Yacoub and subsequently David pioneered what is termed generically valve-sparing aortic root replacement. The two surgical approaches are distinct: The Yacoub procedure is referred to as the remodeling technique, and the David procedure is called the reimplantation technique. Both procedures are options for almost all patients with aortic root aneurysms if the aortic valve is structurally normal, but the David procedure protects against further annular dilation. If AR is present because of STJ dilation or cusp prolapse, the AR can be corrected by restoring the normal STJ geometry, shortening the cusp free margin, or both. Structurally abnormal cusps are a contraindication for the procedure, as is an aortic annulus greater than 27 to 29 mm, and CVG with a mechanical valve remains the operation of choice for patients who require anticoagulation for other conditions.[2]

Recent outcome reports from both Yacoub's and David's institutions indicate that the operative mortality rate for either procedure is low, but the need to return to the operating room for bleeding was sixfold higher after a Yacoub remodeling than after a David reimplantation (18 percent versus 3 percent).[166,167] Probably this is secondary to the long-exposed suture lines running up the

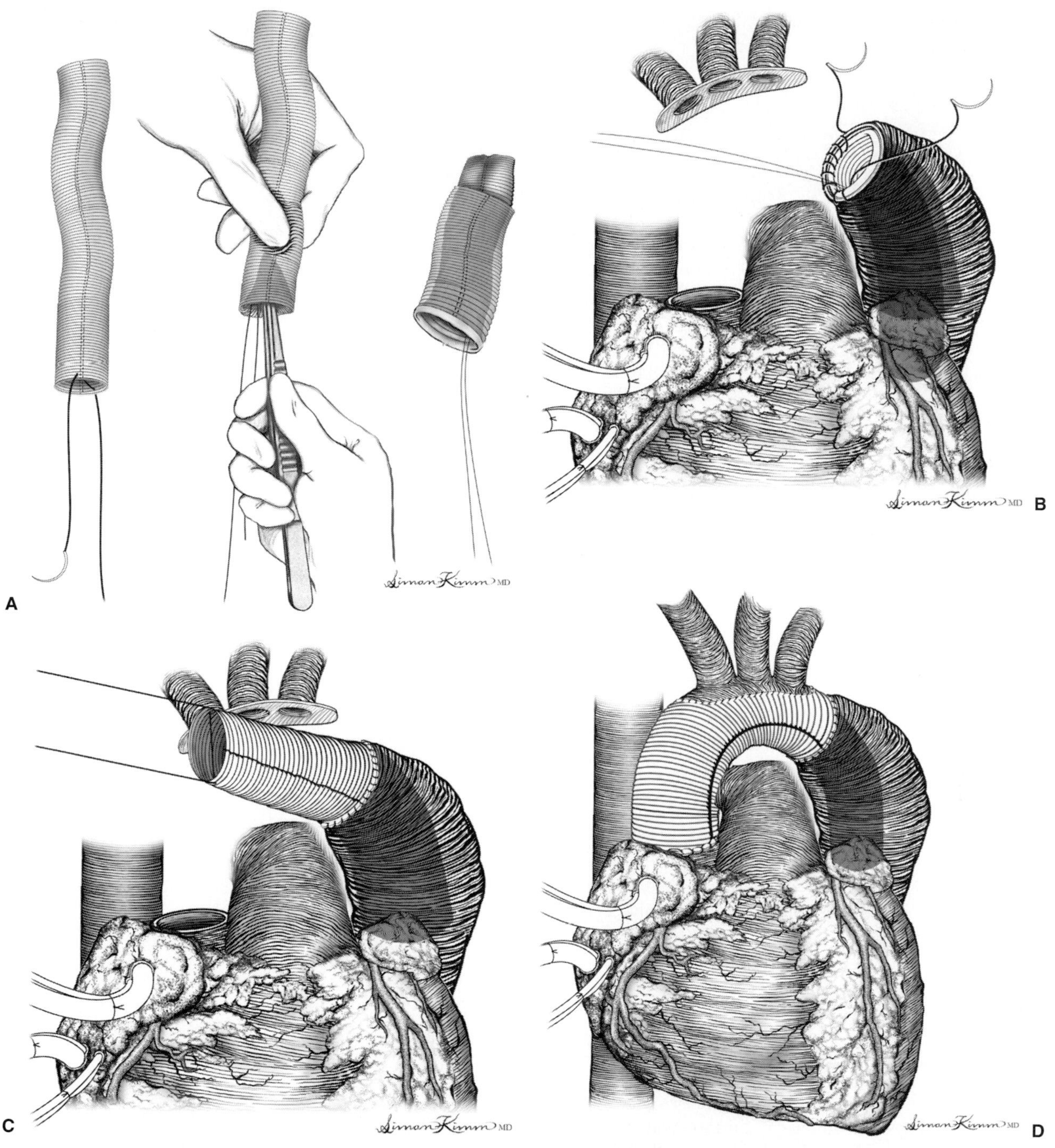

Figure 35-18 Complete arch replacement utilizing the elephant trunk technique. Initially, an appropriate-length graft is intussuscepted into itself (**A**) and then placed into the proximal descending thoracic aortic aneurysm, and the distal anastomosis is constructed to full-thickness aorta (**B**). The arch part of the graft then is withdrawn from the elephant trunk, and the arch vessels are reanastomosed in the preferred manner **(C,D).** This method facilitates subsequent operations, as necessary, on the descending thoracic aorta. (Illustration by Simon Kimm, MD.)

aortic pillars and down into the individual sinuses. For prophylactic aortic repairs, long-term survival is excellent with either technique.

The main issue facing patients and clinicians who are deciding between a mechanical CVG and a valve-sparing technique is the durability of the preserved aortic valve. Data from the Yacoub group indicated that 22 percent of patients had moderate AR at follow-up (median follow-up of 3 years).[167] The presence of mild AR early after surgery portended a progression to more severe AR over time. The prevalence of late AR was lower in David's series, but 25 percent of patients at 10 years had 3+ to 4+ AR.[167] A trend toward less AR favored the David reimplantation technique over the

Table 35-4 A comparison of results with the current technique and a selection of other series of resections of the aortic arch

Authors	*n*	Era	Extent of Resection	Technique of ASCP	Perioperative Mortality, %	Stroke Rate, %	TND Rate, %
Spielvogel et al[185a]	109	1999–2004	All total arch Arch alone 23.9% Arch & Asc 50.5% Arch & Root 15.6% Arch & Desc 2.8%	Initial HCA period, then ASCP via branched graft	4.6	4.6	5.5
Numata et al[186b]	120	1998–2002	All total arch Arch & Desc 5%	Balloon-tipped catheter + right axillary perfusion	5.8	0.8	5.8
Sundt et al[187b]	19	1997–2001	All total arch Arch & Desc 26% Arch & Root 16%	63% ASCP via patch graft to vessels, 53% RCP	11	11	16
Okita et al[132a]	30	1997–1999	All total arch Arch & Desc 6.6% Arch & Root 3.3%	Balloon-tipped catheter ± right axillary perfusion	6.6	6.6	13.3
Di Eusanio et al[188b]	352	1995–2002	All total arch Arch alone 9.1% Arch & Asc 53.1% Arch & Desc 4.5% Total aorta 23.3%	Balloon-tipped catheters	6.8	3.5	5.4
Kazui et al[189b]	220	1990–1999	All total arch Arch alone 1% Arch & Asc 44% Arch & Desc 3% Asc, Desc, Arch 51%	Balloon-tipped catheters	12.7	3.3	6.0
Wozniak et al[190b]	21	1990–1995	Hemiarch 28.6% only (unilateral) Total Arch 71.4% Concomitant Root 100%	Right axillary perfusion	19	9.5	4.8
Kazui et al[191b]	330	1986–2001	Hemiarch 6% Total Arch 94% Asc, Desc, Arch 49%	Balloon-tipped catheters	11.2	2.4	4.2
Bachet et al[173b]	171	1984–1998	All total arch Arch alone 22.2% Arch & Asc 19.2% Asc ± Arch 44.4% Arch & Desc 14%	Direct cannulation, proximal clamps	16.9	12.8	N/A

Source: Modified from Sielvogel et al.[185]
[a]Indicates that the series contains nonemergent cases only.
[b]Indicates that the series contains elective, urgent, and emergent cases.
Asc = ascending; Desc = descending; HCA = hypothermic circulatory arrest; ASCP = antegrade selective cerebral perfusion; TND = transient neurologic dysfunction.

Yacoub technique. Another clinical endpoint reflecting valve durability is reoperation. In David's series, it is remarkable that no valve-sparing patient required reoperation, but only nine patients remained at risk at 8 years. This result was superior to Yacoub's experience, in which 17 percent of patients required reoperation by 10 years (17 patients at risk at 10 years). The low numbers of patients who could be evaluated at the late term make these figures unratable secondary to large standard errors. Larger studies with longer-term follow-up will be necessary to see if it is possible to assess fully the durability of these two procedures. In summary, the valve-sparing aortic root replacement may present patients with MFS with a reasonable alternative to CVG. Survival is excellent with either technique and complications are rare, but the long-term durability of this repair has not been established. Therefore, patients who select a valve-sparing procedure must accept the risk of reoperation in the future.[2]

Aortic arch operations

As various modifications of surgical technique have been introduced, the morbidity and mortality associated with transverse aortic arch replacement have decreased over the last decades.[17,18,168,169] Despite these recent advances, providing adequate cerebral protection and preventing cerebral embolization during reconstruction of a calcified and atherosclerotic aorta remain a formidable challenge.[170] In 10 major series, the average operative mortality rate for aortic arch replacement was 13 percent (6 to 23 percent).[160,171–178] For chronic aneurysms, the operative mortality rate was 11 percent (6 to 22 percent) and was similar for patients with degenerative aneurysms (6 to 22 percent) and those with chronic dissections (6 to 19 percent).[24] Long-term survival has been reported to range from 61 percent to 82 percent at 5 years and from 31 percent to 69 percent at 10 years.[161,179,180] Factors independently associated with a worse long-term outcome included symptomatic presentation, angina, the extent of proximal replacement, a concurrent unoperated aneurysm, cardiac dysfunction, stroke, and renal dysfunction.[161]

Contemporary series of total aortic arch replacements show increasingly impressive results, with low perioperative mortality rates and a low incidence of permanent neurologic injury (Table 35-4). These improvements are a direct result of increasing experience, improved perioperative care, and superior myocardial and cerebral protection strategies; however, there is no consensus about the best line of attack for these complex operations, especially with regard to cerebral protection.

SUMMARY

Ascending aorta and arch pathology represents a continuing challenge for cardiovascular surgeons. Progress over the last three decades, including improved surgical instrumentation, and advances in perfusion strategies with resultant improvements in myocardial and cerebral protection have augmented the surgical armamentarium significantly, facilitating the management of complex aortic problems. Increasingly, it is possible to relieve symptoms and prevent catastrophic dissection and rupture with appropriately timed prophylactic repairs even as surgeons strive to maintain more physiologic conditions with valve preservation techniques and in-line reconstructions. Significant challenges remain as surgeons attempt to increase their understanding of these degenerative processes and refine surgical procedures to allow more complex repairs while minimizing surgical morbidity.

References

1. Johnston KW, Rutherford RB, Tilson MD, et al. Suggested standards for reporting on arterial aneurysms: Subcommittee on Reporting Standards for Arterial Aneurysms, Ad Hoc Committee on Reporting Standards, Society for Vascular Surgery and North American Chapter, International Society for Cardiovascular Surgery. *J Vasc Surg* 1991;13(3):452–458.
2. Milewicz DM, Dietz HC, Miller DC. Treatment of aortic disease in patients with Marfan syndrome. *Circulation* 2005 22;111(11):e150–e157.
3. Ellis PR, Cooley DA, De Bakey ME. Clinical considerations and surgical treatment of annulo-aortic ectasia: Report of successful operation. *J Thorac Cardiovasc Surg* 1961;42:363–370.
4. Hasham SN, Guo DC, Milewicz DM. Genetic basis of thoracic aortic aneurysms and dissections. *Curr Opin Cardiol* 2002;17(6):677–683.
5. Westaby S, Cecil B. Surgery of the thoracic aorta. *Landmarks in Cardiac Surgery.* Oxford: Isis Medical Media; 1997:223.
6. Hirst AE Jr, Johns VJ Jr, KIME SW Jr. Dissecting aneurysm of the aorta: A review of 505 cases. *Medicine (Baltimore)* 1958;37(3):217–279.
7. Hurt R. *The History of Cardiothoracic Surgery from Early Times.* New York: Parthenon; 1996.
8. Monod O, Meyer A. Resection of an aneurysm of the arch of the aorta with preservation of the lumen of the vessel. *Circulation* 1950;1(2):220–224.
9. Cooley DA, DeBakey ME. Resection of entire ascending aorta in fusiform aneurysm using cardiac bypass. *JAMA* 1956;162:1158.
10. Mueller WH, Dammann FJ, Warren WD. Surgical correction of cardiovascular deformities in Marfan's syndrome. *Ann Surg* 1960;152:506.
11. Starr A, Edwards ML, McCord CW, et al Aortic replacement. *Circulation* 1963;27:779.
12. WheatT MW Jr, Wilson JR, Bartley TD. Successful replacement of the entire ascending aorta and aoritc valve. *JAMA* 1964;188:717–719.
13. Bentall H, De Bono A. A technique for complete replacement of the ascending aorta. *Thorax* 1968;23(4):338–339.
14. Edwards WS, Kerr AR. A safer technique for replacement of the entire ascending aorta and aortic valve. *J Thorac Cardiovasc Surg* 1970;59(6):837–839.
15. DeBakey ME, Crawford ES, Cooley DA, Morris GC Jr. Successful resection of fusiform aneurysm of aortic arch with replacement by homograft. *Surg Gynecol Obstet* 1957;(105):657–664.
16. Bloodwell RD, Hallman GL, Cooley DA. Total replacement of the aortic arch and the "subclavian steal" phenomenon. *Ann Thorac Surg* 1968;5(3):236–245.
17. Griepp RB, Stinson EB, Hollingsworth JF, Buehler D. Prosthetic replacement of the aortic arch. *J Thorac Cardiovasc Surg* 1975;70(6):1051–1063.
18. Borst HG, Walterbusch G, Schaps D. Extensive aortic replacement using "elephant trunk" prosthesis. *Thorac Cardiovasc Surg* 1983;31(1):37–40.
19. Bergman RA, Afifi AK, Miyauchi R. Illustrated encyclopedia of human anatomic variation (online). Available at http://www.vh.org/adult/provider/anatomy/AnatomicVariants/Cardiovascular/Text/Arteries/Aorta.html.
20. Liechty JD, Shields TW, Anson BJ. Variations pertaining to the aortic arches and their branches; with comments on surgically important types. *Q Bull Northwest U Med School* 1957;31(2):136–143.
21. Davies M, Guest PJ. Developmental abnormalities of the great vessels of the thorax and their embryological basis. *Br J Radiol* 2003;76(907):491–502.

22. Greenberg R, Risher W. Clinical decision making and operative approaches to thoracic aortic aneurysms. *Surg Clin North Am* 1998;78(5):805–826.
23. Yun KL. Ascending aortic aneurysm and aortic root disease. *Coron Artery Dis* 2002;13(2):79–84.
24. Moon MR, Sundt TM, III. Aortic arch aneurysms. *Coron Artery Dis* 2002;13(2):85–92.
25. Erdheim J. Medionecrosis aortae idiopathica cystica. *Virchows Arch* 1930;276:187.
26. Guo D, Hasham S, Kuang SQ. et al Familial thoracic aortic aneurysms and dissections: Genetic heterogeneity with a major locus mapping to 5q13-14. *Circulation* 2001;103(20):2461–2468.
27. Segura AM, Luna RE, Horiba K, et al. Immunohistochemistry of matrix metalloproteinases and their inhibitors in thoracic aortic aneurysms and aortic valves of patients with Marfan's syndrome. *Circulation* 1998;98(Suppl 19):II331–II337.
28. Pyeritz RE. Marfan syndrome and other disorders of fibrillin. In: Rimoin D, Conner J, Pyeritz RE, Korf B (eds). *Principles and Practice of Medical Genetics,* 4th ed. Edinburgh: Churchill Livingstone; 2002: 3977–4020.
29. Germain DP, Herrera-Guzman Y. Vascular Ehlers-Danlos syndrome. *Ann Genet* 2004;47(1):1–9.
29a. Loeys BL, Chen J, Neptune ER, et al. A syndrome of altered cardiovascular, craniofacial, neurocognitive, and skeletal development caused by mutations in TGFBR1 or TGFBR2. *Nat Genet* 2005;37:275–281.
29b. Loeys BL, Schwarze U, Holm T, et al. Aneurysm syndromes caused by mutations in the TGF-β receptor. *N Engl J Med* 2006;355:788–798.
30. Coady MA, Davies RR, Roberts M, et al. Familial patterns of thoracic aortic aneurysms. *Arch Surg* 1999;134(4): 361–367.
31. Emanuel R, Withers R, O'Brien K, et al. Congenitally bicuspid aortic valves: Clinicogenetic study of 41 families. *Br Heart J* 1978;40(12):1402–1407.
32. Clementi M, Notari L, Borghi A, Tenconi R. Familial congenital bicuspid aortic valve: A disorder of uncertain inheritance. *Am J Med Genet* 1996;62(4): 336–338.
33. Huntington K, Hunter AG, Chan KL. A prospective study to assess the frequency of familial clustering of congenital bicuspid aortic valve. *J Am Coll Cardiol* 1997;30(7):1809–1812.
34. Huntington K, Hunter AG, Chan KL. A prospective study to assess the frequency of familial clustering of congenital bicuspid aortic valve. *J Am Coll Cardiol* 1997;30(7):1809–1812.
35. Sabet HY, Edwards WD, Tazelaar HD, Daly RC. Congenitally bicuspid aortic valves: A surgical pathology study of 542 cases (1991 through 1996) and a literature review of 2,715 additional cases. *Mayo Clin Proc* 1999;74(1):14–26.
36. Hahn RT, Roman MJ, Mogtader AH, Devereux RB. Association of aortic dilation with regurgitant, stenotic and functionally normal bicuspid aortic valves. *J Am Coll Cardiol* 1992;19(2):283–288.
37. Edwards WD, Leaf DS, Edwards JE. Dissecting aortic aneurysm associated with congenital bicuspid aortic valve. *Circulation* 1978;57(5):1022–1025.
38. Liddicoat JE, Bekassy SM, Rubio PA, et al. Ascending aortic aneurysms: Review of 100 consecutive cases. *Circulation* 1975;52(Suppl 2):I202–I209.
39. Bonderman D, Gharehbaghi-Schnell E, Wollenek G, et al. Mechanisms underlying aortic dilatation in congenital aortic valve malformation. *Circulation* 1999;99(16): 2138–2143.
40. Schmid FX, Bielenberg K, Schneider A, et al. Ascending aortic aneurysm associated with bicuspid and tricuspid aortic valve: Involvement and clinical relevance of smooth muscle cell apoptosis and expression of cell death-initiating proteins. *Eur J Cardiothorac Surg* 2003;23(4):537–543.
41. Fedak PW, de Sa MP, Verma S, et al. Vascular matrix remodeling in patients with bicuspid aortic valve malformations: Implications for aortic dilatation. *J Thorac Cardiovasc Surg* 2003;126(3):797–806.
42. Fedak PW, Verma S, David TE, et al. Clinical and pathophysiological implications of a bicuspid aortic valve. *Circulation* 2002;106(8):900–904.
43. DeBakey ME, McCollum CH, Crawford ES, et al. Dissection and dissecting aneurysms of the aorta: Twenty-year follow-up of five hundred twenty-seven patients treated surgically. *Surgery* 1982;92(6):1118–1134.
44. Halstead JC, Meier M, Spielvogel D, et al. The fate of the distal aorta after repair of acute type A dissection: American Association for Thoracic Surgery(abstract). 4-12-2005.
45. Osler W. The Gulstonian lectures on malignant endocarditis. *Br Med J* 1885;1:467.
46. Frist WH, Miller DC. Aneurysms of ascending thoracic aorta and transverse aortic arch. *Cardiovasc Clin* 1987;17(3):263–287.
47. Malouf JF, Chandrasekaran K, Orszulak TA. Mycotic aneurysms of the thoracic aorta: A diagnostic challenge. *Am J Med* 2003;115(6):489–496.
48. Isselbacher EM. Thoracic and abdominal aortic aneurysms. *Circulation* 2005;111(6):816–28.
49. Heggtveit HA. Syphilitic aortitis: A clinicopathologic autopsy study of 100 cases, 1950 to 1960. *Circulation* 1964;29:346–355.
50. Walker DI, Bloor K, Williams G, Gillie I. Inflammatory aneurysms of the abdominal aorta. *Br J Surg* 1972;59(8): 609–614.
51. Weaver FA, Yellin AE, Campen DH, et al. Surgical procedures in the management of Takayasu's arteritis. *J Vasc Surg* 1990;12(4):429–437.
52. Sasaki S, Kubota S, Kunihara T, et al. Surgical experience of the thoracic aortic aneurysm due to Takayasu's arteritis. *Int J Cardiol* 2000;75(Suppl 1):S129–S134.
53. Park JH, Chung JW, Joh JH, et al. Aortic and arterial aneurysms in behcet disease: Management with stent-grafts—initial experience. *Radiology* 2001;220(3): 745–750.
54. Park JH, Han MC, Bettmann MA. Arterial manifestations of Behcet disease. *AJR Am J Roentgenol* 1984;143(4): 821–825.
55. Matsumoto T, Uekusa T, Fukuda Y. Vasculo-Behcet's disease: A pathologic study of eight cases. *Hum Pathol* 1991;22(1):45–51.
56. Vasseur MA, Haulon S, Beregi JP, et al. Endovascular treatment of abdominal aneurysmal aortitis in Behcet's disease. *J Vasc Surg* 1998;27(5):974–976.

57. Evans JM, Hunder GG. Polymyalgia rheumatica and giant cell arteritis. *Rheum Dis Clin North Am* 2000;26(3):493–515.
58. Salvarani C, Cantini F, Boiardi L, Hunder GG. Polymyalgia rheumatica and giant-cell arteritis. *N Engl J Med* 2002;347(4):261–271.
59. Gelsomino S, Romagnoli S, Gori F, et al. Annuloaortic ectasia and giant cell arteritis. *Ann Thorac Surg* 2005;80(1): 101–105.
60. Lie JT. Aortic and extracranial large vessel giant cell arteritis: A review of 72 cases with histopathologic documentation. *Semin Arthritis Rheum* 1995;24(6): 422–431.
61. Evans JM, O'Fallon WM, Hunder GG. Increased incidence of aortic aneurysm and dissection in giant cell (temporal) arteritis: A population-based study. *Ann Intern Med* 1995;122(7):502–507.
62. Olson LJ, Subramanian R, Edwards WD. Surgical pathology of pure aortic insufficiency: A study of 225 cases. *Mayo Clin Proc* 1984;59(12):835–841.
63. Ergin MA, Spielvogel D, Apaydin A, et al. Surgical treatment of the dilated ascending aorta: When and how? *Ann Thorac Surg* 1999;67(6):1834–1839.
64. Coady MA, Rizzo JA, Hammond GL, et al. What is the appropriate size criterion for resection of thoracic aortic aneurysms? *J Thorac Cardiovasc Surg* 1997;113(3): 476–491.
65. Joyce JW, Fairbairn JF, Kincaid OW, Juergen JL. Aneurysms of the thoracic aorta: A clinical study with special reference to prognosis. *Circulation* 1964;29:176–181.
66. Coady MA, Rizzo JA, Hammond GL, et al. What is the appropriate size criterion for resection of thoracic aortic aneurysms? *J Thorac Cardiovasc Surg* 1997;113(3): 476–491.
67. Hirose Y, Hamada S, Takamiya M, et al. [Growth rates of aortic aneurysms as a risk factor in rupture: An evaluation with CT.] *Nippon Igaku Hoshasen Gakkai Zasshi* 1993;53(6):635–640.
68. Davies RR, Goldstein LJ, Coady MA, et al. Yearly rupture or dissection rates for thoracic aortic aneurysms: Simple prediction based on size. *Ann Thorac Surg* 2002; 73(1):17–27.
69. Murdoch JL, Walker BA, Halpern BL, et al. Life expectancy and causes of death in the Marfan syndrome. *N Engl J Med* 1972;286(15):804–808.
70. Marsalese DL, Moodie DS, Vacante M, et al. Marfan's syndrome: Natural history and long-term follow-up of cardiovascular involvement. *J Am Coll Cardiol* 1989;14 (2):422–428.
71. Hahn RT, Roman MJ, Mogtader AH, Devereux RB. Association of aortic dilation with regurgitant, stenotic and functionally normal bicuspid aortic valves. *J Am Coll Cardiol* 1992;19(2):283–288.
72. Dore A, Brochu MC, Baril JF, et al. Progressive dilation of the diameter of the aortic root in adults with a bicuspid aortic valve. *Cardiol Young* 2003;13(6):526–531.
73. Edwards WD, Leaf DS, Edwards JE. Dissecting aortic aneurysm associated with congenital bicuspid aortic valve. *Circulation* 1978;57(5):1022–1025.
74. Liddicoat JE, Bekassy SM, Rubio PA, et al. Ascending aortic aneurysms: Review of 100 consecutive cases. *Circulation* 1975;52(Suppl 2):I202–I209.
75. Yasuda H, Nakatani S, Stugaard M, et al. Failure to prevent progressive dilation of ascending aorta by aortic valve replacement in patients with bicuspid aortic valve: Comparison with tricuspid aortic valve. *Circulation* 2003;108(Suppl 1):II291–II294.
76. Russo CF, Mazzetti S, Garatti A, et al. Aortic complications after bicuspid aortic valve replacement: Long-term results. *Ann Thorac Surg* 2002;74(5):S1773–S1776.
77. Kouchoukos NT, Dougenis D. Surgery of the thoracic aorta. *N Engl J Med* 1997;336(26):1876–1888.
78. Nienaber CA, Eagle KA. Aortic dissection: New frontiers in diagnosis and management: Part I: From etiology to diagnostic strategies. *Circulation* 2003;108(5):628–635.
79. Pressler V, McNamara JJ. Thoracic aortic aneurysm: Natural history and treatment. *J Thorac Cardiovasc Surg* 1980;79(4):489–498.
80. Crawford ES, Svensson LG, Coselli JS, et al. Surgical treatment of aneurysm and/or dissection of the ascending aorta, transverse aortic arch, and ascending aorta and transverse aortic arch: Factors influencing survival in 717 patients. *J Thorac Cardiovasc Surg* 1989;98(5 Pt 1): 659–673.
81. Hartnell GG. Imaging of aortic aneurysms and dissection: CT and MRI. *J Thorac Imaging* 2001;16(1):35–46.
82. Lin JS, Chang SC, Chen FJ, Chern MS. The half-moon sign: A useful roentgen sign of saccular aneurysm of the aortic arch. *Chest* 1996;109(1):127–130.
83. Chen JT. Plain radiographic evaluation of the aorta. *J Thorac Imaging* 1990;5(4):1–17.
84. Erbel R, Engberding R, Daniel W, et al. Echocardiography in diagnosis of aortic dissection. *Lancet* 1989;1(8636): 457–461.
85. Costello P, Ecker CP, Tello R, Hartnell GG. Assessment of the thoracic aorta by spiral CT. *AJR Am J Roentgenol* 1992;158(5):1127–1130.
86. Sharma U, Ghai S, Paul SB, et al. Helical CT evaluation of aortic aneurysms and dissection: A pictorial essay. *Clin Imaging* 2003;27(4):273–280.
87. Tatli S, Yucel EK, Lipton MJ. CT and MR imaging of the thoracic aorta: Current techniques and clinical applications. *Radiol Clin North Am* 2004;42(3):565–585, vi.
88. Thompson MM. Controlling the expansion of abdominal aortic aneurysms. *Br J Surg* 2003;90(8):897–898.
89. Ejiri J, Inoue N, Tsukube T, et al. Oxidative stress in the pathogenesis of thoracic aortic aneurysm: Protective role of statin and angiotensin II type 1 receptor blocker. *Cardiovasc Res* 2003;59(4):988–996.
90. Shores J, Berger KR, Murphy EA, Pyeritz RE. Progression of aortic dilatation and the benefit of long-term beta-adrenergic blockade in Marfan's syndrome. *N Engl J Med* 1994;330(19):1335–1341.
91. Rossi-Foulkes R, Roman MJ, Rosen SE, et al. Phenotypic features and impact of beta blocker or calcium antagonist therapy on aortic lumen size in the Marfan syndrome. *Am J Cardiol* 1999;83(9):1364–1368.
92. Shores J, Berger KR, Murphy EA, Pyeritz RE. Progression of aortic dilatation and the benefit of long-term beta-adrenergic blockade in Marfan's syndrome. *N Engl J Med* 1994;330(19):1335–1341.
93. Yin FC, Brin KP, Ting CT, Pyeritz RE. Arterial hemodynamic indexes in Marfan's syndrome. *Circulation* 1989;79(4):854–862.

94. Reed CM, Alpert BS. Assessment of ventricular performance after chronic beta-adrenergic blockade in the Marfan syndrome. *Am J Cardiol* 1992;70(4):541–542.
95. Nagashima H, Sakomura Y, Aoka Y, et al. Angiotensin II type 2 receptor mediates vascular smooth muscle cell apoptosis in cystic medial degeneration associated with Marfan's syndrome. *Circulation* 2001;104(12 Suppl 1):I282–I287.
96. Nagashima H, Uto K, Sakomura Y, et al. An angiotensin-converting enzyme inhibitor, not an angiotensin II type-1 receptor blocker, prevents beta-aminopropionitrile monofumarate-induced aortic dissection in rats. *J Vasc Surg* 2002;36(4):818–823.
97. Braverman AC. Exercise and the Marfan syndrome. *Med Sci Sports Exerc* 1998;30(Suppl 10):S387–S395.
98. Fedak PW, Verma S, David TE, et al. Clinical and pathophysiological implications of a bicuspid aortic valve. *Circulation* 2002;106(8):900–904.
98a. Habashi J, Judge DP, Holm T, et al. Losartan, an AT1 antagonist, prevents aortic aneurysm in a mouse model of Marfan syndrome. *Science* 2006;312:117–121.
99. Kouchoukos NT, Dougenis D. Surgery of the thoracic aorta. *N Engl J Med* 1997;336(26):1876–1888.
100. Ergin MA, Spielvogel D, Apaydin A, et al. Surgical treatment of the dilated ascending aorta: When and how? *Ann Thorac Surg* 1999;67(6):1834–1839.
101. Coady MA, Rizzo JA, Hammond GL, et al. What is the appropriate size criterion for resection of thoracic aortic aneurysms? *J Thorac Cardiovasc Surg* 1997;113(3): 476–491.
102. Ergin MA, Spielvogel D, Apaydin A, et al. Surgical treatment of the dilated ascending aorta: When and how? *Ann Thorac Surg* 1999;67(6):1834–1839.
103. Gott VL, Greene PS, Alejo DE, et al. Replacement of the aortic root in patients with Marfan's syndrome. *N Engl J Med* 1999;340(17):1307–1313.
104. Davies RR, Goldstein LJ, Coady MA, et al. Yearly rupture or dissection rates for thoracic aortic aneurysms: Simple prediction based on size. *Ann Thorac Surg* 2002;73(1):17–27.
105. Gott VL, Greene PS, Alejo DE, et al. Replacement of the aortic root in patients with Marfan's syndrome. *N Engl J Med* 1999;340(17):1307–1313.
106. Ergin MA, Spielvogel D, Apaydin A, et al. Surgical treatment of the dilated ascending aorta: When and how? *Ann Thorac Surg* 1999;67(6):1834–1839.
107. Yun KL, Miller DC, Fann JI, et al. Composite valve graft versus separate aortic valve and ascending aortic replacement: Is there still a role for the separate procedure? *Circulation* 1997;96(Suppl 9):II-75.
108. Bauer M, Pasic M, Schaffarzyk R, et al. Reduction aortoplasty for dilatation of the ascending aorta in patients with bicuspid aortic valve. *Ann Thorac Surg* 2002;73(3): 720–723.
109. Mueller XM, Tevaearai HT, Genton CY, et al. Drawback of aortoplasty for aneurysm of the ascending aorta associated with aortic valve disease. *Ann Thorac Surg* 1997;63(3):762–766.
110. Kouchoukos NT, Marshall WG Jr, Wedige-Stecher TA. Eleven-year experience with composite graft replacement of the ascending aorta and aortic valve. *J Thorac Cardiovasc Surg* 1986;92(4):691–705.
111. David TE. Current practice in Marfan's aortic root surgery: Reconstruction with aortic valve preservation or replacement? What to do with the mitral valve? *J Card Surg* 1997;12(Suppl 2):147–150.
112. Yun KL, Miller DC, Fann JI, et al. Composite valve graft versus separate aortic valve and ascending aortic replacement: Is there still a role for the separate procedure? *Circulation* 1997;96(Suppl 9):II-75.
113. Kouchoukos NT, Dougenis D. Surgery of the thoracic aorta. *N Engl J Med* 1997;336(26):1876–1888.
114. Ueda Y, Miki S, Kusuhara K, et al. Surgical treatment of aneurysm or dissection involving the ascending aorta and aortic arch, utilizing circulatory arrest and retrograde cerebral perfusion. *J Cardiovasc Surg (Torino)* 1990;31(5): 553–558.
115. Kazui T, Inoue N, Yamada O, Komatsu S. Selective cerebral perfusion during operation for aneurysms of the aortic arch: A reassessment. *Ann Thorac Surg* 1992;53(1): 109–114.
116. Drew CE, Keen G, Benazon DB. Profound hypothermia. *Lancet* 1959;1(7076):745–747.
117. Fleck TM, Czerny M, Hutschala D, et al. The incidence of transient neurologic dysfunction after ascending aortic replacement with circulatory arrest. *Ann Thorac Surg* 2003;76(4):1198–1202.
118. Reich DL, Uysal S, Sliwinski M, et al. Neuropsychologic outcome after deep hypothermic circulatory arrest in adults. *J Thorac Cardiovasc Surg* 1999;117(1):156–163.
119. Ramsay JG, Ralley FE, Whalley DG, et al. Site of temperature monitoring and prediction of afterdrop after open heart surgery. *Can Anaesth Soc J* 1985;32(6):607–612.
120. Robinson J, Charlton J, Seal R, et al. Oesophageal, rectal, axillary, tympanic and pulmonary artery temperatures during cardiac surgery. *Can J Anaesth* 1998;45(4):317–323.
121. Stone JG, Young WL, Smith CR, et al. Do standard monitoring sites reflect true brain temperature when profound hypothermia is rapidly induced and reversed? *Anesthesiology* 1995;82(2):344–351.
122. Stump DA, Jones TJ, Rorie KD. Neurophysiologic monitoring and outcomes in cardiovascular surgery. *J Cardiothorac Vasc Anesth* 1999;13(5):600–613.
123. Lundell JC, Scuderi PE, Butterworth JF. Less isoflurane is required after than before cardiopulmonary bypass to maintain a constant bispectral index value. *J Cardiothorac Vasc Anesth* 2001;15(5):551–554.
124. Edmonds HL Jr. Advances in neuromonitoring for cardiothoracic and vascular surgery. *J Cardiothorac Vasc Anesth* 2001;15(2):241–250.
125. Nakajima T, Kuro M, Hayashi Y, et al. Clinical evaluation of cerebral oxygen balance during cardiopulmonary bypass: On-line continuous monitoring of jugular venous oxyhemoglobin saturation. *Anesth Analg* 1992;74(5):630–635.
126. Griepp RB, Ergin MA, McCullough JN, et al. Use of hypothermic circulatory arrest for cerebral protection during aortic surgery. *J Card Surg* 1997;12(Suppl 2):312–321.
127. Busto R, Dietrich WD, Globus MY, Ginsberg MD. The importance of brain temperature in cerebral ischemic injury. *Stroke* 1989;20(8):1113–1114.
128. Busto R, Globus MY, Dietrich WD, et al. Effect of mild hypothermia on ischemia-induced release of neurotrans-

mitters and free fatty acids in rat brain. *Stroke* 1989;20(7):904–910.

129. Czerny M, Fleck T, Zimpfer D, et al. Risk factors of mortality and permanent neurologic injury in patients undergoing ascending aortic and arch repair. *J Thorac Cardiovasc Surg* 2003;126(5):1296–1301.
130. Neri E, Sassi C, Barabesi L, et al. Cerebral autoregulation after hypothermic circulatory arrest in operations on the aortic arch. *Ann Thorac Surg* 2004;77(1):72–79.
131. Matalanis G, Hata M, Buxton BF. A retrospective comparative study of deep hypothermic circulatory arrest, retrograde, and antegrade cerebral perfusion in aortic arch surgery. *Ann Thorac Cardiovasc Surg* 2003;9(3): 174–179.
132. Okita Y, Minatoya K, Tagusari O, et al. Prospective comparative study of brain protection in total aortic arch replacement: Deep hypothermic circulatory arrest with retrograde cerebral perfusion or selective antegrade cerebral perfusion. *Ann Thorac Surg* 2001;72(1):72–79.
133. Sinatra R, Melina G, Pulitani I, et al. Emergency operation for acute type A aortic dissection: Neurologic complications and early mortality. *Ann Thorac Surg* 2001;71(1):33–38.
134. Kouchoukos NT, Masetti P. Total aortic arch replacement with a branched graft and limited circulatory arrest of the brain. *J Thorac Cardiovasc Surg* 2004;128(2): 233–237.
135. Whitlark JD, Goldman SM, Sutter FP. Axillary artery cannulation in acute ascending aortic dissections. *Ann Thorac Surg* 2000;69(4):1127–1128.
136. Bachet J, Guilmet D, Goudot B, et al. Antegrade cerebral perfusion with cold blood: A 13-year experience. *Ann Thorac Surg* 1999;67(6):1874–1878.
137. Kazui T, Kimura N, Komatsu S. Surgical treatment of aortic arch aneurysms using selective cerebral perfusion: Experience with 100 patients. *Eur J Cardiothorac Surg* 1995;9(9):491–495.
138. Griepp RB. Cerebral protection during aortic arch surgery. *J Thorac Cardiovasc Surg* 2001;121(3):425–427.
139. Croughwell ND, Frasco P, Blumenthal JA, et al. Warming during cardiopulmonary bypass is associated with jugular bulb desaturation. *Ann Thorac Surg* 1992;53(5):827–832.
140. Kiziltan HT, Baltali M, Koca D, et al. Reduced jugular venous oxygen saturation during rewarming from deep hypothermic circulatory arrest: Cerebral overextraction? *Cardiovasc Surg* 2003;11(3):213–217.
141. Hanel F, von Knobelsdorff G, Werner C, Schulte EJ. Hypercapnia prevents jugular bulb desaturation during rewarming from hypothermic cardiopulmonary bypass. *Anesthesiology* 1998;89(1):19–23.
142. Goto T, Yoshitake A, Baba T, et al. Cerebral ischemic disorders and cerebral oxygen balance during cardiopulmonary bypass surgery: Preoperative evaluation using magnetic resonance imaging and angiography. *Anesth Analg* 1997;84(1):5–11.
143. Mills NL, Ochsner JL. Massive air embolism during cardiopulmonary bypass: Causes, prevention, and management. *J Thorac Cardiovasc Surg* 1980;80(5):708–717.
144. Di Eusanio M, Di Eusanio G. Cerebral protection during surgery of the thoracic aorta: A review. *Ital Heart J* 2004;5(12):883–891.
145. Dubost CH, Blondeau PH, Piwinca A, Cachera JP. Surgical treatment of aneurysm of the thoracic aorta: Apropos of 25 cases expored surgically. *J Chronic Dis* 1962;(83):331–359.
146. Pearce CW, Weichert RF III, del Real RE. Aneurysms of aortic arch: Simplified technique for excision and prosthetic replacement. *J Thorac Cardiovasc Surg* 1969;58(6):886–890.
147. Frist WH, Baldwin JC, Starnes VA, et al. A reconsideration of cerebral perfusion in aortic arch replacement. *Ann Thorac Surg* 1986;42(3):273–281.
148. Bachet J, Guilmet D, Goudot B, et al. Cold cerebroplegia: A new technique of cerebral protection during operations on the transverse aortic arch. *J Thorac Cardiovasc Surg* 1991;102(1):85–93.
149. Tanaka H, Kazui T, Sato H, et al. Experimental study on the optimum flow rate and pressure for selective cerebral perfusion. *Ann Thorac Surg* 1995;59(3):651–657.
150. Randomized clinical study of thiopental loading in comatose survivors of cardiac arrest: Brain Resuscitation Clinical Trial I Study Group. *N Engl J Med* 1986;314 (7):397–403.
151. Siegman MG, Anderson RV, Balaban RS, et al. Barbiturates impair cerebral metabolism during hypothermic circulatory arrest. *Ann Thorac Surg* 1992;54(6):1131–1136.
152. Dewhurst AT, Moore SJ, Liban JB. Pharmacological agents as cerebral protectants during deep hypothermic circulatory arrest in adult thoracic aortic surgery: A survey of current practice. *Anaesthesia* 2002;57(10):1016–1021.
153. Langley SM, Chai PJ, Jaggers JJ, Ungerleider RM. Preoperative high dose methylprednisolone attenuates the cerebral response to deep hypothermic circulatory arrest. *Eur J Cardiothorac Surg* 2000;17(3):279–286.
154. Cabrol C, Pavie A, Gandjbakhch I, et al. Complete replacement of the ascending aorta with reimplantation of the coronary arteries: New surgical approach. *J Thorac Cardiovasc Surg* 1981;81(2):309–315.
155. Embrey RP. Modified Cabrol's technique for composite replacement of the aortic valve and ascending aorta. *J Card Surg* 1993;8(5):562–566.
156. Zubiate P, Kay JH. Surgical treatment of aneurysm of the ascending aorta with aortic insufficiency and marked displacement of the coronary ostia. *J Thorac Cardiovasc Surg* 1976;71(3):415–421.
157. Kouchoukos NT, Wareing TH, Murphy SF, Perrillo JB. Sixteen-year experience with aortic root replacement: Results of 172 operations. *Ann Surg* 1991;214(3): 308–318.
158. Cohn LH, Rizzo RJ, Adams DH, et al. Reduced mortality and morbidity for ascending aortic aneurysm resection regardless of cause. *Ann Thorac Surg* 1996;62(2): 463–468.
159. Lewis CT, Cooley DA, Murphy MC, et al. Surgical repair of aortic root aneurysms in 280 patients. *Ann Thorac Surg* 1992;53(1):38–45.
160. Galloway AC, Colvin SB, LaMendola CL, et al. Ten-year operative experience with 165 aneurysms of the ascending aorta and aortic arch. *Circulation* 1989;80(3 Pt 1): I249–I256.
161. Crawford ES, Svensson LG, Coselli JS, et al. Surgical treatment of aneurysm and/or dissection of the ascend-

ing aorta, transverse aortic arch, and ascending aorta and transverse aortic arch: Factors influencing survival in 717 patients. *J Thorac Cardiovasc Surg* 1989;98(5 Pt 1): 659–673.

162. Lawrie GM, Earle N, DeBakey ME. Long-term fate of the aortic root and aortic valve after ascending aneurysm surgery. *Ann Surg* 1993;217(6):711–720.
163. Gott VL, Greene PS, Alejo DE, et al. Replacement of the aortic root in patients with Marfan's syndrome. *N Engl J Med* 1999;340(17):1307–1313.
164. Smith JA, Fann JI, Miller DC, et al. Surgical management of aortic dissection in patients with the Marfan syndrome. *Circulation* 1994;90(5 Pt 2):II235–II242.
165. Yamazaki F, Shimamoto M, Fujita S, et al. Surgical treatment for cardiovascular lesions of patients with Marfan syndrome. *Jpn J Thorac Cardiovasc Surg* 2002;50(9): 366–370.
166. Birks EJ, Webb C, Child A, et al. Early and long-term results of a valve-sparing operation for Marfan syndrome. *Circulation* 1999;100(Suppl 19):II29–II35.
167. De Oliveira NC, David TE, Ivanov J, et al. Results of surgery for aortic root aneurysm in patients with Marfan syndrome. *J Thorac Cardiovasc Surg* 2003;125(4): 789–796.
168. Schepens MA, Dossche KM, Morshuis WJ, et al. The elephant trunk technique: Operative results in 100 consecutive patients. *Eur J Cardiothorac Surg* 2002;21(2): 276–281.
169. Ergin MA, Griepp EB, Lansman SL, et al. Hypothermic circulatory arrest and other methods of cerebral protection during operations on the thoracic aorta. *J Card Surg* 1994;9(5):525–537.
170. Spielvogel D, Strauch JT, Minanov OP, et al. Aortic arch replacement using a trifurcated graft and selective cerebral antegrade perfusion. *Ann Thorac Surg* 2002;74(5): S1810–S1814.
171. Ergin MA, Galla JD, Lansman L, et al. Hypothermic circulatory arrest in operations on the thoracic aorta: Determinants of operative mortality and neurologic outcome. *J Thorac Cardiovasc Surg* 1994;107(3):788–797.
172. Usui A, Abe T, Murase M. Early clinical results of retrograde cerebral perfusion for aortic arch operations in Japan. *Ann Thorac Surg* 1996;62(1):94–103.
173. Bachet J, Guilmet D, Goudot B, et al. Antegrade cerebral perfusion with cold blood: a 13-year experience. *Ann Thorac Surg* 1999;67(6):1874–1878.
174. Livesay JJ, Cooley DA, Reul GJ, et al. Resection of aortic arch aneurysms: A comparison of hypothermic techniques in 60 patients. *Ann Thorac Surg* 1983;36(1):19–28.
175. Borst HG, Buhner B, Jurmann M. Tactics and techniques of aortic arch replacement. *J Card Surg* 1994;9(5):538–547.
176. Coselli JS, Buket S, Djukanovic B. Aortic arch operation: Current treatment and results. *Ann Thorac Surg* 1995;59(1):19–26.
177. Okita Y, Takamoto S, Ando M, et al. Mortality and cerebral outcome in patients who underwent aortic arch operations using deep hypothermic circulatory arrest with retrograde cerebral perfusion: No relation of early death, stroke, and delirium to the duration of circulatory arrest. *J Thorac Cardiovasc Surg* 1998;115(1): 129–138.
178. Ehrlich MP, Ergin MA, McCullough JN, et al. Predictors of adverse outcome and transient neurological dysfunction after ascending aorta/hemiarch replacement. *Ann Thorac Surg* 2000;69(6):1755–1763.
179. Safi HJ, Brien HW, Winter JN, et al. Brain protection via cerebral retrograde perfusion during aortic arch aneurysm repair. *Ann Thorac Surg* 1993;56(2):270–276.
180. Okita Y, Ando M, Minatoya K, et al. Early and long-term results of surgery for aneurysms of the thoracic aorta in septuagenarians and octogenarians. *Eur J Cardiothorac Surg* 1999;16(3):317–323.
181. Hopkins RA. Aortic valve leaflet sparing and salvage surgery: Evolution of techniques for aortic root reconstruction. *Eur J Cardiothorac Surg* 2003;24(6):886–897.
182. Jweied E, Fogelson B, Fishman D, Merlotti G. Blunt injury of the innominate artery associated with a bovine arch. *J Trauma* 2002;52(5):1002–1004.
183. Junqueira. *Histology,* 10th ed. New York: McGraw-Hill; 2004.
184. Fedak PW, Verma S, David TE, et al. Clinical and pathophysiological implications of a bicuspid aortic valve. *Circulation* 2002;106(8):900–904.
185. Spielvogel D, Halstead JC, Meier M, et al. Aortic arch replacement using a trifurcated graft: Simple, versatile, and safe. *Ann Thorac Surg* 2005;80(1):90–95.
186. Numata S, Ogino H, Sasaki H, et al. Total arch replacement using antegrade selective cerebral perfusion with right axillary artery perfusion. *Eur J Cardiothorac Surg* 2003;23(5):771–775.
187. Sundt TM, Moon MR, DeOliviera N, et al. Contemporary results of total aortic arch replacement. *J Card Surg* 2004;19(3):235–239.
188. Di Eusanio M, Schepens MA, Morshuis WJ, et al. Separate grafts or en bloc anastomosis for arch vessels reimplantation to the aortic arch. *Ann Thorac Surg* 2004;77(6):2021–2028.
189. Kazui T, Washiyama N, Muhammad BA, et al. Total arch replacement using aortic arch branched grafts with the aid of antegrade selective cerebral perfusion. *Ann Thorac Surg* 2000;70(1):3–8.
190. Wozniak G, Dapper F, Zickmann B, et al. Selective cerebral perfusion via innominate artery in aortic arch replacement without deep hypothermic circulatory arrest. *Int J Angiol* 1999;8(1):50–56.
191. Kazui T, Yamashita K, Washiyama N, et al. Usefulness of antegrade selective cerebral perfusion during aortic arch operations. *Ann Thorac Surg* 2002;74(5): S1806–S1809.

CHAPTER

36 THORACOABDOMINAL ANEURYSMS

Glenn S. Roseborough

INTRODUCTION

Since its introduction by Michael DeBakey in 1956,[1] thoracoabdominal aneurysm repair generally presents the most technically challenging and controversial issues in vascular surgery. The surgical repair of thoracoabdominal aneurysms is an undertaking that requires substantial preoperative planning and consideration of a wide array of techniques. Each of those techniques has its champions, and several authors have published comparably good results using widely different methods. In this chapter, the common principles that are applicable to all thoracoabdominal

KEY CONCEPTS

- Epidemiology
  - Thoracoabdominal aneurysms (TAAs) develop in patients with atherosclerotic disease, chronic aortic dissection, and connective tissue disorders (e.g., Marfan's syndrome, Ehler-Danlos syndrome).
- Pathophysiology
  - Pathologic processes include chronic inflammation, remodeling of extracellular matrix, and depletion of vascular smooth muscle cells. Elastin depletion in the media layer of the aortic wall is a common finding.
- Clinical features
  - Approximately 80 percent of TAAs are atherosclerotic in nature, associated with smoking, hypertension, hypercholesterolemia, and advanced age. Approximately 20 percent of TAAs develop from chronic aortic dissections and occur in patients with connective tissue disorders. The risk of rupture increases rapidly when aneurysmal diameter reaches or exceeds 6 cm. The most common presentation includes abdominal or back pain, although many TAAs are discovered incidentally.
- Diagnostics
  - TAAs are classified commonly according to the anatomic scheme developed by Crawford (types I through IV). Helical computed tomography and magnetic resonance angiography are the diagnostic modalities of choice, largely having supplanted angiography.
- Treatment
  - Medical therapy includes the reduction of risk factors for aneurysmal expansion (e.g., smoking, hypercholesterolemia) and tight blood pressure control predicated on the use of beta blockers. Interventional therapy includes open surgical and stent graft repair. Surgical repair can take the form of traditional "clamp-and-sew" or newer distal perfusion approaches. Spinal cord protection is of particular concern in open surgical repairs.
- Outcomes
  - In-hospital mortality rates after surgery range between 8 and 15 percent in most series. Common postoperative complications include bleeding, respiratory failure, myocardial infarction or cardiac failure, renal failure, and paraplegia. Operative risk increases with advanced age, aneurysm complexity, emergency operation, coronary and cerebrovascular disease, pulmonary disease, and renal failure. Outcomes may be improved with the distal perfusion approach to repair. Five-year survival rates range between 53 and 73 percent, with significant rates of diminished functional outcomes after open repair in certain populations.

aneurysm surgery are described. In addition, most of the surgical techniques currently in use to repair these aneurysms are discussed, with emphasis on those which are preferred at the Johns Hopkins Hospital.

PATHOPHYSIOLOGY

Insight into the pathophysiology of aortic aneurysm formation at the cellular level has come into focus only recently. The pathologic processes observed in aneurysm development include chronic inflammation, remodeling of the extracellular matrix, and depletion of vascular smooth muscle cells. A basic feature common to all aneurysms is the depletion of elastin, a key structural protein in the media layer of the aortic wall. Normal turnover of matrix proteins is mediated by a family of enzymes called matrix metalloproteinases (MMPs); their activity is regulated by proteins called tissue inhibitors of metalloproteinases (TIMPs). Several MMPs have elastase activity. In separate studies, MMP-2, MMP-3 (stromelysin-1), MMP-9, and MMP-12 [human macrophage elastase (HME)] have been found to have increased activity in aneurysmal tissue.[2,3]

Other components of the inflammatory response appear to play a role in aneurysm formation. The complement fixation pathway seems to be involved in matrix proteolysis, as large amounts of complement-fixing immunoglobulin G (IgG) and complement C3 have been detected in aortic aneurysms.[4] Increased amounts of the inflammatory cytokines tumor necrosis factor-alpha (TNF-alpha), TNF-beta, prostaglandin E_2, and interleukin 6 also have been documented in aneurysm tissue.[5,6] Finally, smooth muscle cells are eliminated at least in part by apoptosis, an active process of cell death associated with increased protein synthesis. This depletes a population of cells that are capable of directing connective tissue repair.[7] All these findings suggest that aortic aneurysm formation is the result of a complex interaction of inflammatory mediators and structural components involved in maintaining the extracellular matrix.

CLINICAL FEATURES

Natural history

A majority of TAAs are atherosclerotic in nature and, as with abdominal aortic aneurysms (AAAs), are related to smoking, hypertension, high cholesterol, and advanced age. TAAs are the most common type of aneurysm to develop in patients previously diagnosed with AAAs, occurring in 6 percent of those patients. Approximately 20 percent of TAAs occur in patients who develop chronic aneurysmal dilatation after an aortic dissection and in patients with connective tissue disorders, most notably Marfan's syndrome and Ehlers-Danlos syndrome. Compared with AAAs, the natural histories of TAAs have not been well documented owing to the lower incidence of TAAs and the fact that the advanced imaging techniques required to diagnose TAAs have been in general use only for the last two decades. In most patients, slow progressive dilatation ultimately leads to death from rupture if it is not treated[8–12] (Fig. 36-1). The other major cause of death in this population of patients is cardiac disease. The rate of aneurysmal dilatation is approximately a 10 percent increase in diameter per year, with higher average rates of growth in patients with TAAs resulting from aortic dissection. The risk of rupture is related to aneurysm size. It is low below 6 cm but increases dramatically with growth in maximum diameter beyond 6 cm; most vascular surgeons recommend conservative therapy for patients with TAAs that are less than 6 cm in diameter and repair if they are more than 6 cm in patients who are acceptable surgical candidates. However, Cambria and coworkers found a higher rate of rupture in patients with TAAs larger than 5 cm.[13] TAAs that result from aortic dissection have been found to be at higher risk for rupture than are atherosclerotic TAAs in separate studies done by Crawford and Denatale and by Pressler and colleagues.[8,14] In addition, Juvonen and colleagues found that patients with TAAs resulting from chronic dissections tended to experience rupture earlier.[15] In that study, the median last known diameter of the aorta in patients who had a rupture was 5.4 cm. Additional risk factors for rupture in that study were chronic obstructive pulmonary disease and poorly controlled hypertension. One therefore may consider repair of a TAA that is less than 6 cm in the setting of chronic dissection, particularly in a patient with poorly controlled hypertension and lung disease.

Classification

TAAs usually are classified according to the anatomic scheme developed by E. Stanley Crawford and coworkers.[16] They are classified as types I through IV. A type I TAA begins in the proximal thoracic aorta and extends to the level of the celiac artery. A type II TAA is the most extensive variety, generally involves the entire thoracic and abdominal aorta, and accounts for a large proportion of TAAs that develop years after an extensive aortic dissection. A type III TAA is defined by its proximal extent in the midthoracic aorta, generally is described in the region of the T6 vertebra or the inferior pulmonary vein, and may involve varying amounts of the abdominal aorta. A type IV TAA begins above the celiac axis and extends into the infrarenal aorta. Huynh and colleagues modified the original Crawford classification to include a type V TAA, which begins in the middescending thoracic aorta and terminates at the level of the renal arteries[17] (Fig. 36-2). This classification not only reflects what is encountered at surgery but is important for reporting results, since more extensive aneurysms generally are associated with more complications. Aneurysms that involve only

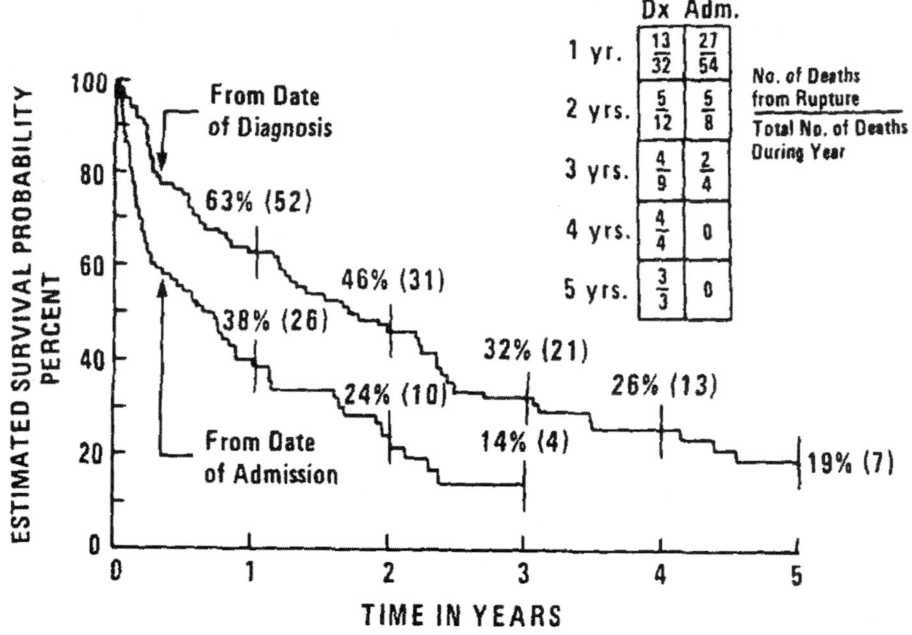

Figure 36-1 Kaplan-Meier probability survival curves from date of diagnosis and date of admission in 94 patients. Numbers of patients at risk at 12, 24, 36, and 48 months are in parentheses. (From Crawford ES, DeNatale RW. Thoracoabdominal aortic aneurysm: Observations regarding the natural course of the disease. *J Vasc Surg* 1986;3:578–582.)

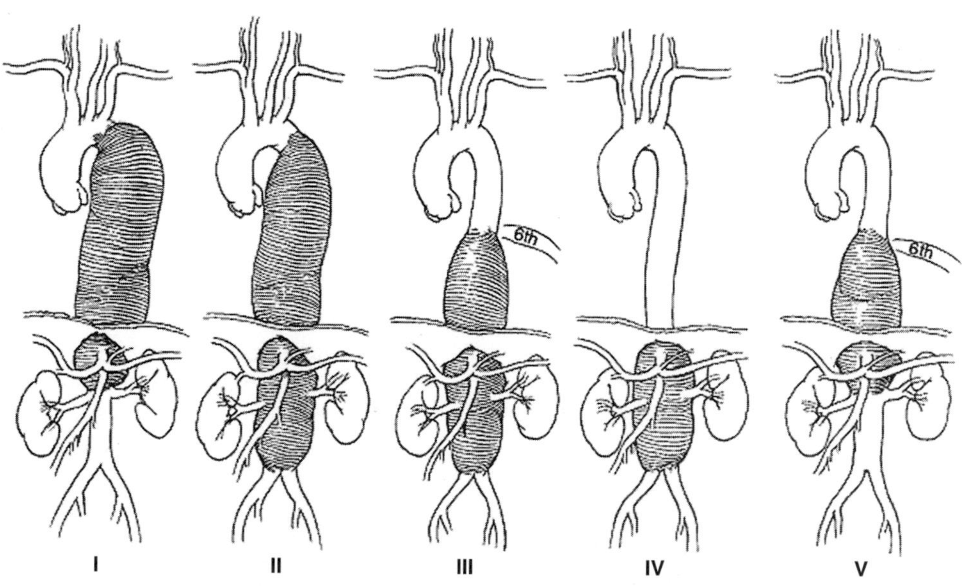

Figure 36-2 Modified Crawford classification of thoracoabdominal aortic aneurysms. *Extent I:* from distal to left subclavian artery to above renal arteries. *Extent II:* from distal to left subclavian artery to aortic bifurcation. *Extent III:* from sixth intercostal space to aortic bifurcation. *Extent IV:* from diaphragm to aortic bifurcation (total abdominal aorta). *Extent V:* from sixth intercostal space to above renal arteries. (From Huynh TTT, Miller CC, Estrera AL, et al. Determinants of hospital length of stay after thoracoabdominal aortic aneurysm repair. *J Vasc Surg* 2002;35:648–653.)

the descending thoracic aorta are not included in this classification and are considered separately, although many of the same principles of TAA repair are used to repair thoracic aneurysms.

Presentation

Most TAAs are discovered as incidental findings on plain x-ray, computed tomography (CT), or magnetic resonance imaging (MRI) studies obtained for other reasons. Up to 40 percent of patients with TAAs become symptomatic.[18] The symptoms commonly include acute abdominal or back pain. The development of severe acute pain is considered indicative of an impending rupture, and urgent repair generally is recommended within 24 h of presentation. However, the author has observed patients with histories of moderate subacute pain that had been present for weeks to months and resolved with surgical repair; it appears that not all patients with pain are at risk for imminent rupture. Less commonly, TAAs also present with gastric outlet obstruction, renal failure, aortic thrombosis, or failure to thrive. Rupture presents as acute pain with manifestations of shock or sudden death.

DIAGNOSTIC MODALITIES

Currently there are no recommended screening tests for TAAs because of to their low incidence (1 per 100,000 population[19]) and substantial diagnostic imaging costs. Aortic aneurysms are found on plain x-ray studies about 25 percent of the time. Ultrasound is not useful since the suprarenal aorta is often difficult to image and the thoracic aorta cannot be imaged with this modality. The main diagnostic modalities used for TAAs are CT scanning, MRI, and angiography. A CT or MRI is mandatory for obtaining reliable data on the outer diameter of the aneurysm. A high-quality axial study may provide adequate information for operative planning in straightforward cases; however, helical CT or MRI angiography with three-dimensional reconstruction is important in defining arch involvement or pathology, especially in visceral branch vessels. Because of the high resolution of these studies, formal angiography rarely is required for preoperative planning (Fig. 36-3). In the author's institution, a helical CT scan with three-dimensional (3-D) reconstructions is the imaging method of choice. It provides virtually all the information required to plan surgical repair with data that are immediately accessible to the surgeon on a digital workstation. The software for 3-D reconstructions is very user-friendly and permits retrieval and manipulation of images with minimal assistance from technicians. In contrast, MRI angiography (MRA) is slow and expensive and requires extensive postprocessing. It is more prone to false positives for occlusive disease of branch vessels, and reviewing the digital images requires extensive technical assistance. In the author's practice, MRA is reserved for patients with contraindications to CT angiography, such as contrast allergy and renal insufficiency. Aortography played an important role in preoperative planning for TAA repairs in the past, but this modality has been replaced to a large extent by the high-quality imaging of CT and MRA. Nevertheless, the author does use aortography to identify and locate the spinal artery of Adamkiewicz (see below). Recently, however, Japanese investigators have been able to identify this elusive but important structure with CT and MRA.[20,21] The author's institution has not been able to reproduce the Japanese experience reliably thus far.

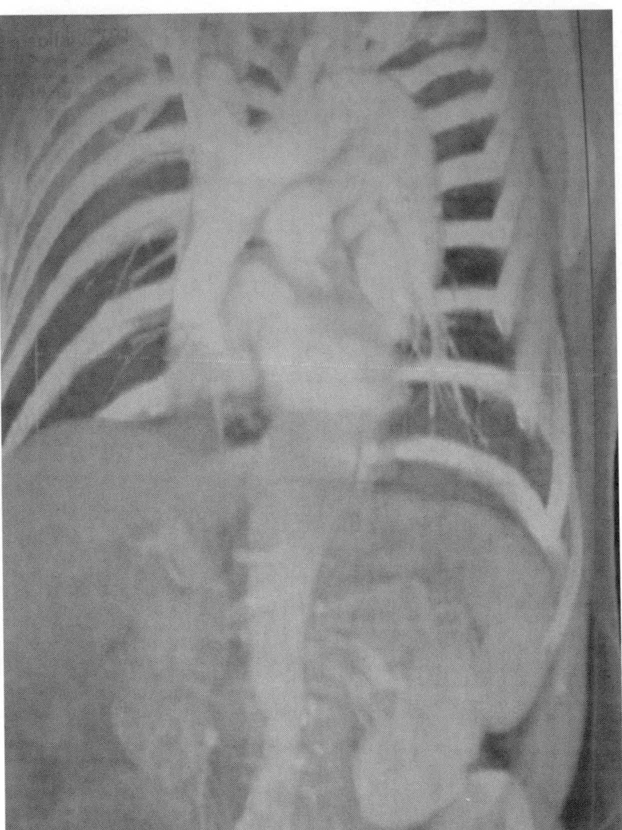

Figure 36-3 Three-dimensional reconstruction of computed tomography angiogram demonstrating the anatomy of the aortic arch and visceral branches in a patient with a Crawford II thoracoabdominal aneurysm.

MEDICAL THERAPY

Medical therapy consists of controlling risk factors for continued aneurysmal expansion. These patients should be advised to quit smoking, and blood pressure and cholesterol should be controlled strictly. Beta blockers have been advocated to decrease the expansion rate of aortic aneurysms, but a randomized controlled trial conducted in Canada did not confirm their effectiveness.[22] Doxycycline, a known metalloproteinase inhibitor, protects against aneurysm expansion in animal models, and one randomized trial demonstrated decreased expansion rates with daily administration of this drug in a phase 2 trial.[23] However, it is premature to recommend chronic doxycycline therapy to all patients with aortic aneurysms.

SURGICAL THERAPY

Preoperative evaluation and planning

Because of the high-risk nature of thoracoabdominal aneurysm repair, appropriate decision making is imperative in the selection of patients for surgery and in the performance of the surgical procedure to obtain good results (see the Decision-Making Flowchart). There are three important components to preoperative evaluation and planning in TAA surgery: determining operative risk, planning the extent and technical sequence of the repair, and selecting surgical adjuncts to minimize morbidity.

The determination that TAA repair is indicated for a patient assumes that the risk of observation is greater than the risk of repair. It is therefore necessary to have a reasonable understanding of a patient's perioperative risk. Postoperative morbidity and mortality is related largely to the cardiac, pulmonary, and renal systems; hence, a thorough evaluation of those systems is imperative. At a minimum, cardiac function should be evaluated with an echocardiogram. An abnormal electrocardiogram (ECG), a history of coronary artery disease or symptoms of chest pain, congestive heart failure, or poor exercise tolerance should prompt evaluation by a cardiologist and some form of stress testing. Dobutamine echocardiography is considered to be contraindicated in patients with aneurysms because of the possibility of precipitating rupture, and so stress thallium scanning and formal exercise testing are the screening diagnostics of choice. Cardiac catheterization should be performed if reconstruction of the ascending aorta or aortic arch is anticipated. Pulmonary function tests, including spirometry and a room air blood gas, should be obtained, since single-lung ventilation usually is required intraoperatively. Renal function and hepatic function are evaluated with blood chemistries. An individualized decision to operate is based on an integration of the estimated risks of rupture and repair for a specific patient after this information has been acquired.

With TAA repair, it is imperative that the surgeon plan the entire operation in advance and anticipate the

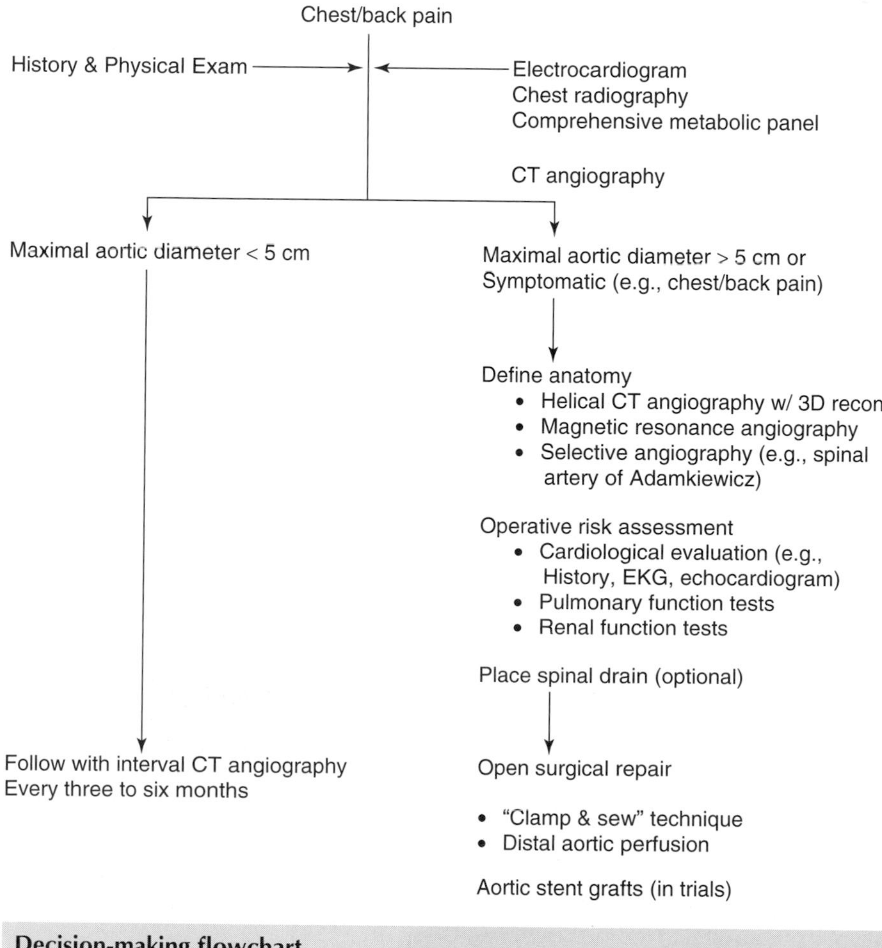

Decision-making flowchart

extent of and steps in the planned repair. This includes the location of the proximal and distal extent of the repair, the location and sequence of aortic clamping, and plans for reimplanting, bypassing, or reconstructing aortic branch vessels. This is important for several reasons. First, the extent of the repair will determine the level of the thoracotomy and the extent of the incision. It also will determine which adjuncts are required intraoperatively, such as cardiopulmonary bypass equipment and neurophysiologic monitoring. The most important consideration in preoperative planning relates to the pathology of the aortic arch. For TAAs involving the proximal descending thoracic aorta, it is crucial that one appreciate the patient's arch anatomy, since arch involvement may warrant the participation of a cardiac surgeon to conduct the cardiopulmonary bypass and hypothermic circulatory arrest. With extensive arch involvement, it may be necessary to perform the repair in stages. For example, in cases in which the aortic arch and the descending thoracic aorta are diseased, the arch can be replaced first, leaving a graft extension (i.e., "elephant trunk") in the descending thoracic aorta. The descending thoracic aorta is repaired several months later, at which time the new graft replacing the descending thoracic aorta is sewn to the elephant trunk proximally. This staged approach obviates the perilous prospect of clamping and anastomosing the graft to a diseased aortic arch.

Spinal cord protection

The next important consideration in preoperative planning is the way one plans to prevent spinal cord and other end-organ damage from intraoperative ischemia. Multiple strategies are available to accomplish this goal. With respect to spinal cord protection, they include (1) spinal artery conservation, (2) selective intercostal artery conservation, (3) intraoperative monitoring with somatosensory evoked potentials (SSEP) or motor evoked potentials (MEP), (4) systemic hypothermia, (5) regional hypothermia, (6) lumbar drainage of cerebrospinal fluid (CSF), (7) distal aortic perfusion, either passive or active, (8) aortic conservation with aortic "tailoring," and (9) pharmacologic manipulation. With respect to visceral protection, the options include regional or systemic hypothermia and distal aortic perfusion.

Selective intercostal artery (spinal artery) ***reimplantation***

The most detrimental form of intraoperative ischemia that can occur during TAA repair is spinal cord ischemia, which can occur in up to 40 percent of TAA repairs. The clinical manifestations include a spectrum of spinal cord deficits that can be observed immediately after surgery or up to 3 days later. The most severe form results in complete paraplegia and usually is associated with a mortality rate over 50 percent. The spinal cord becomes ischemic as critical blood flow through intercostal arteries is interrupted when these intercostal arteries are ligated in the course of the aneurysm repair. Over 100 years ago, it was recognized that in humans, a single intercostal artery often gives rise to a branch that provides a major proportion of blood flow to the anterior spinal cord: the spinal artery or the great radicular artery of Adamkiewicz. This artery usually arises from a left-sided intercostal artery between the eighth thoracic (T8) and the first lumbar (L1) vertebrae and has a characteristic radiographic appearance. Animal studies have suggested that preserving the spinal artery can prevent paraplegia.[24] Clinical experience at the Johns Hopkins Hospital and elsewhere has confirmed that preserving the spinal artery in patients undergoing TAA repair can result in improved neurologic outcomes.[25,26] Therefore, at the author's institution, surgeons make an effort to identify the spinal artery of Adamkiewicz preoperatively by performing selective angiography of patent intercostal arteries in the lower descending thoracic aorta (Fig. 36-4). With careful technique, this blood vessel can be identified in up to 86 percent of cases.[27] All efforts are made to conserve the involved intercostal artery at the time of surgery by reimplanting or bypassing to the aortic segment from which this intercostal arises or by including this area of aorta within the proximal or distal anastomosis. At the author's institution, it has been found that identifying and preserving the spinal artery is particularly beneficial in repairs of atherosclerotic TAAs, in which the spinal artery is more likely to be one of the few intercostals that are not chronically occluded by aortic thrombus.[28] In this subset of patients, spinal artery identification and preservation resulted in no cases of spinal cord injury in a group of 45 patients. Other authors dispute the value of identifying and preserving the spinal artery.[29,30]

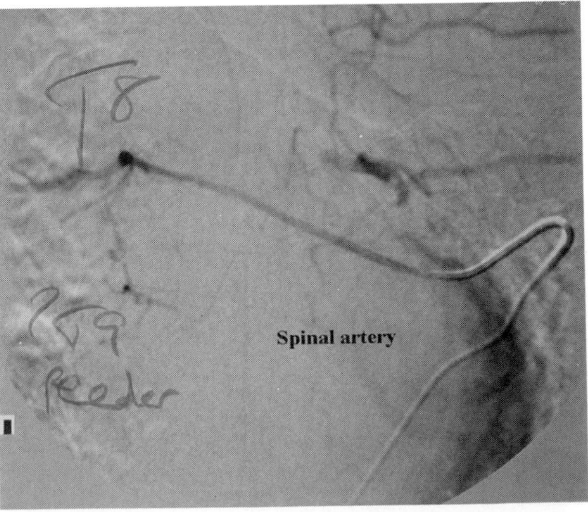

Figure 36-4 Spinal artery angiogram demonstrating characteristic hairpin appearance of spinal artery of Adamkiewicz.

Nonselective intercostal artery reimplantation

If the spinal artery is not identified, consideration still is given to reimplantation of intercostal arteries in the lower thoracic region. Safi and colleagues and Cambria and coworkers have shown in separate studies that intercostal artery reimplantation in the T8 to L1 region improves neurologic outcomes,[31,32] and Jacobs and colleagues have reported outstanding results with intercostal artery reimplantation guided partially by MEP.[33,34] The disadvantage of nonselective intercostal artery reimplantation is that multiple intercostals generally must be reimplanted to assure that adequate spinal cord circulation has been maintained in this scenario. Reimplanting multiple intercostals requires a large intercostal patch, which can become aneurysmal in the future, or multiple small patches. The extra suture lines increase the length and complexity of the operation as well as the risk of bleeding. This approach is particularly unappealing to those who employ the clamp-and-sew method of TAA reconstruction, since without distal aortic perfusion, the time that is devoted to reimplanting intercostals adds to the visceral ischemic time because the visceral branch vessels generally are reimplanted after the intercostals.

Intraoperative neurologic monitoring

To help limit intercostal reimplantation, attempts have been made to use intraoperative neurophysiologic monitoring to identify important intercostals and guide selective reimplantation of those vessels. Initial attempts at neurophysiologic monitoring were performed by measuring SSEPs. Laschinger and associates published early work in dogs[35] showing that SSEP was a sensitive detector of spinal cord ischemia and that distal aortic perfusion could prevent spinal cord ischemia. Subsequent clinical work by that group showed that SSEP loss for more than 30 min predicted spinal cord injury in TAA repair.[36] SSEP is limited in that it detects ischemia primarily in the dorsal spinal cord and can miss ischemic injury in the ventral horns of the spinal cord, where the motor tracts are situated.[37] As a result, intraoperative monitoring of MEPs has been proposed to overcome this limitation,[38] and clinically, MEP monitoring has been shown to be more accurate than SSEP monitoring in detecting spinal cord ischemia.[39,40] Most clinical experience with this technique comes from Holland, where separate groups have had excellent results using MEP to prevent spinal cord ischemia.[33,34,41–43] Using MEP to guide selective intercostal artery reattachment, Jacobs and colleagues achieved paraplegia rates of under 3 percent in a series of almost 200 patients.[34] The author's group has been using MEP since 2000 but has had difficulty reproducing those results. This group has noted a delayed appearance of abnormal MEP signals that can occur with isolated ischemia of the thoracic spinal cord.[44]

Systemic hypothermia

The development of a hypothermic environment around the spinal cord confers at least partial protection from ischemia during TAA repair. In animal experiments, Colon and coworkers demonstrated that systemic hypothermia protected the spinal cord from periods of ischemia up to 45 min.[45] The benefits of hypothermia can be realized at moderate temperatures (32°C) without incurring the risk of cardiac arrhythmias that occurs at lower temperatures, particularly below 30°C. Moderate hypothermia can be achieved passively or actively with a heat exchanger in a cardiopulmonary bypass circuit; the latter technique is preferred since it allows for active rewarming of the patient at the conclusion of the repair. The disadvantages of this approach include a higher propensity for bleeding stemming from the required anticoagulation and coagulopathies associated with cardiopulmonary bypass and variability in the availability of cardiopulmonary bypass support for some vascular surgeons. In the most extreme form of systemic hypothermia, TAA repair can be performed under profound hypothermia (18°C) and circulatory arrest, as advocated by Kouchoukos and coworkers in this country and by others elsewhere.[46–48] Kouchoukos and coworkers reported very low rates of spinal cord injury with this approach.[46] In the author's practice, this strategy is applied selectively to difficult distal aortic arch anatomy, since circulatory arrest is not without significant morbidity, including neurocognitive dysfunction. Safi and colleagues reported that profound hypothermia and circulatory arrest did not offer significant benefit compared with moderate hypothermia and partial bypass.[49]

Regional hypothermia

It is also possible to develop spinal cord hypothermia without systemic cooling by using a regional infusion of a cold solution via an epidural catheter. This technique has been championed by Cambria and colleagues at the Massachusetts General Hospital, who have been able to achieve excellent results with respect to spinal cord injury without systemic hypothermia or distal aortic bypass.[32,50,51] With this technique, it is necessary to protect the viscera during extensive TAA reconstructions with cold regional perfusion of those organs as well. Despite good published results, the technique has not been adapted widely at other centers.

Cerebrospinal fluid drainage

When the proximal thoracic aorta is clamped, the intracranial and CSF pressures rise. Conversely, blood pressure distal to the clamp drops dramatically. Spinal perfusion pressure, which is represented by mean arterial pressure of the spinal cord minus CSF pressure, therefore drops markedly. CSF drainage reduces CSF pressure in the spinal canal and therefore improves spinal perfusion pressure when spinal perfusion is low intraoperatively as well as in the postoperative period, when CSF pressure may rise as a result of the spinal cord edema that accompanies ischemia–reperfusion injury. Blaisdell and Cooley first demonstrated that decreasing spinal fluid pressure (pharmacologically with intravenous urea) can have a beneficial effect on paraplegia rates in dogs.[52] Subsequently, it was found anecdotally to be useful in resolving delayed-onset paraplegia in the early postoperative period.[53] However, a small prospective randomized study performed by Crawford and coworkers found that CSF drainage had no effect on paraplegia rates.[54] Eleven years later at the same institution, Coselli and colleagues found a statistically significant benefit with CSF drainage in a repeat study, lowering neurologic deficits from 13 percent in the control group to 2.6 percent in the treatment group.[55]

Distal aortic perfusion

Two fundamental surgical approaches are employed in TAA repair: (1) the so-called clamp-and-sew approach and (2) distal aortic perfusion techniques. The clamp-and-sew method originally employed by DeBakey and Crawford has been employed for over 40 years and still is used by some accomplished aortic surgeons, particularly in patients with less extensive aneurysms.[56–59] In this approach, the aorta is clamped sequentially during the construction of the proximal anastomosis, the reimplantation of critical branches, and the construction of the distal anastomosis. Repair can be performed quickly by an experienced surgeon with less blood loss, since intraoperative anticoagulation is not necessary with this method. However, this technique can expose the viscera to perilously long ischemic times if technical difficulties are encountered with the proximal anastomosis or intercostal artery reimplantation, resulting in end-organ ischemia.

The distal aortic perfusion strategy maintains perfusion of the aorta and its branches distal to the area where the clamps are placed while an anastomosis is created. Distal perfusion can be passive or active. Examples of passive distal perfusion include the Gott aortic shunt,[60–62] an axillofemoral bypass that is constructed before the thoracotomy is begun,[63] and an "octopus" of catheters whose proximal ends are placed in the Dacron tube graft after the proximal anastomosis is completed and whose distal ends are placed in and perfuse the orifices of the renal and mesenteric arteries while the distal thoracic aorta is repaired.[64] Active distal aortic perfusion involves pumping blood through a centripedal pump into the abdominal aorta while the thoracic aorta is clamped. At the Johns Hopkins Hospital, surgeons believe that this technique is the standard of care in TAA repair as it has several important advantages. A heat exchanger attached to the pump circuit permits active cooling of the patient and, more important, active rewarming at the end of the procedure, when hypothermia contributes to coagulopathy. The advantage of being able to rewarm the patient actively to physiologic temperatures cannot be overstated. The flow in the pump circuit can be adjusted to manipulate the blood pressure proximal and distal to the aortic cross-clamp; typical pump flows range between 1.0 and 2.5 L/min. Proximal hypertension and distal hypotension are corrected by increasing pump flow; proximal hypotension and distal hypertension are corrected by decreasing pump flow. An obstruction to inflow or outflow can be detected by high resistance that is noted in the circuit but would go undetected in a passive shunt. The circuit can be converted quickly to a full cardiopulmonary bypass circuit if the patient experiences cardiac arrest or it becomes apparent intraoperatively that circulatory arrest is required to complete a difficult proximal anastomosis near the aortic arch. Numerous centers have demonstrated improved results in TAA surgery with distal aortic perfusion, and it is the preferred adjunct in most centers.[65–69]

The author's group prefers the use of nonselective distal aortic perfusion, in which the abdominal aorta is perfused via the left femoral artery while the thoracic aortic reconstruction is performed. The patient is cooled to 32°C before spinal cord or visceral ischemia occurs. The mesenteric and renal arteries are clamped and not perfused while the segment of abdominal aorta containing those branches is reconstructed. The author's institution finds that mesenteric and renal revascularization can be accomplished within 30 to 60 min and that renal failure and clinically significant visceral ischemia rarely are encountered with this technique. However, other investigators have shown improved results with selective distal perfusion using direct cannulation of the renal and mesenteric arteries while the visceral abdominal aorta is clamped. Jacobs used selective perfusion (with isothermic blood) in 73 patients and had excellent results, with permanent renal failure occurring in only 1 patient (1.4 percent) and transient dialysis required in 5(6.8 percent). Koksoy and associates[70] and Hassoun and associates[71] independently undertook clinical trials to determine whether intraoperative cold perfusion of the viscera could minimize ischemic injury and improve postoperative outcomes, particularly with respect to renal function. Their techniques and findings differed, but both studies found some benefit to cold visceral perfusion. In the Koksoy trial, the kidneys were perfused with cold crystalloid containing steroids and mannitol, and the mesenteric vessels were perfused with warm blood from the left heart bypass circuit. In that study, renal failure was decreased in the cold perfusion group.[70] In the Hassoun trial, all the visceral vessels were perfused selectively with blood that had been cooled to 4°C by being passed through a heat exchanger. The investigators in that trial found no difference in the rate of renal failure but did find improved survival in the group that received cold perfusion.[71]

Aortic conservation

Occasionally, one encounters a moderately dilated distal thoracic aorta while replacing a large aneurysm of the more proximal thoracic aorta in which formal aortic replacement may not be warranted but it may be desirable to try to prevent aneurysmal degeneration of this distal segment to avoid additional surgery in the future. Similarly, it is sometimes necessary to operate on a nondilated aortic segment to correct malperfusion from an aortic dissection. In these situations, it is often preferable not to replace the involved aorta to avoid spinal cord and visceral ischemia. This can be accomplished by using an aortic "tailoring" procedure developed by G. Melville Williams at the Johns Hopkins Hospital. With this approach, a longitudinal aortotomy is made (in the case of an aortic dissection, the intimal flap subsequently is resected), and the aorta is closed with to a diameter of approximately 2 cm to decrease wall tension and prevent further aneurysmal degeneration. This procedure eliminates the need to sacrifice or reimplant any aortic branches and can be performed with very short cross-clamp times. Williams and colleagues first reported this technique in the treatment of patients with chronic dissecting aneurysms[72] and then applied it to the management of acute aortic dissections complicated by malperfusion.[73] Surgeons at the author's institution routinely tailor a segment of aorta that is up to 4 cm in diameter and occasionally tailor even larger segments. Since Williams began this performing this procedure, reoperation has not been required on any tailored segments for subsequent aneurysmal degeneration, with the exception of patients with connective tissue disorders; such disorders, including Marfan's syndrome and Ehlers-Danlos syndrome, are contraindications to the aortic tailoring approach.

Pharmacologic adjuncts

Most surgeons administer intravenous mannitol before any identified periods of renal ischemia. Mannitol is an osmotic diuretic and free radical scavenger that preserves urine flow after renal ischemia. It does not necessarily prevent ischemic renal failure but promotes a nonoliguric state that is easier to manage clinically.[74–80] Additionally, mannitol can ameliorate pulmonary injury associated with aortic surgery.[81]

Acher and coworkers use the partial opioid agonist naloxone for neuroprotection during TAA reconstruction, which they perform with the clamp-and-sew technique and routine ligation of all intercostal arteries. They reported excellent results, with paraplegia rates of 3 percent,[56] although their experience has not been duplicated elsewhere.

A host of pharmacologic agents that interfere with the ischemia–reperfusion injury process have been tested for their ability to prevent spinal cord injury, and they are reviewed thoroughly by de Haan.[82] There are no uniform recommendations for the use of any of these agents. At the author's institution, it has been found that diazoxide, a mitochondrial potassium–adenosine triphosphate (ATP) channel opener, protects against ischemic spinal cord injury in a rabbit model.[83] Further work has shown that this effect is achieved through decreased production of reactive oxygen species in the mitochondria (unpublished data). Current research in cardiology and neurology has focused on poly-adenosine diphosphate (ADP) ribose polymerase (PARP), an enzyme that participates in multiple cellular pathways involved in DNA repair, apoptosis, and ischemic preconditioning. This area of investigation shows promise for improvement in outcomes with respect to partial or delayed neurologic deficits that result from a modest ischemic (and subsequent reperfusion) injury to the spinal cord.

Operative technique

The author's protocol for surgical TAA repair begins 2 days before surgery with spinal angiography. A spinal drain is placed by the anesthesiologists the day before surgery so that if a bloody tap occurs during drain placement, there is time for the hemorrhage to resolve without postponing or canceling the operation. After anesthetic induction, the patient is intubated with a single-lumen endotracheal tube that then is exchanged for a double-lumen endotracheal tube to permit single-lung ventilation. Proper placement of the tube is confirmed bronchoscopically. A double-lumen endotracheal tube is important not only to collapse the left lung to facilitate exposure of the aorta in the left chest but also to prevent blood and secretions from depositing in the left lung. Bronchial blockers do not provide reliable isolation of the left lung throughout these long operations and are not recommended.

A Swan-Ganz pulmonary artery catheter and additional central venous lines are placed. A radial arterial catheter always should be placed in the right arm, since a catheter in the left radial artery becomes useless if is necessary to clamp the aortic arch between the left carotid artery and the left subclavian artery. A transesophageal echocardiogram probe is placed, and the patient is put in the right lateral decubitus position on a beanbag with the left arm padded on a Kraus retractor. The spinal drain is connected to a drainage apparatus with a pop-off valve set to 5 to 10 cm H_2O. The hips are rotated obliquely to keep the right groin in the surgical field. The left chest is prepped to the axilla superiorly, the spine posteriorly, and the sternum anteriorly. The abdomen is prepped to the right of the midline. Both groins are prepped to provide surgical access to the femoral vessels. A Cell-Saver and a rapid infuser should be readily available in the operating room.

The incision is determined by the proximal extent of the aneurysm. In situations in which the proximal clamp is placed on or just distal to the aortic arch, as in a type I or type II TAA or for chronic dissection arising just beyond the left subclavian artery, a standard posterolateral thoracotomy is done. The chest is entered in the fourth intercostal space to allow satisfactory exposure of the aortic arch. A type III TAA may be approached through a sixth or seventh interspace incision, whereas a type IV TAA may be approached through an eighth or ninth interspace incision. The incision is carried down onto the abdominal wall, across the oblique muscles lateral to the left rectus abdominus muscle. The retroperitoneal plane is entered deep to the transversus abdominus muscle and developed posteriorly to the psoas muscle under the diaphragm. It is easy to enter the peritoneal cavity inadvertently at this point, especially medially by the edge of the rectus abdominus muscle, where the peritoneum is thin and adherent. The costal margin is divided with heavy scissors, connecting the left chest cavity to the retroperitoneum, and the left internal mammary artery is ligated.

A single simple thoracotomy incision rarely provides enough exposure to repair an extensive TAA. The author's preference is to perform a subperiosteal resection of the rib above or below the interspace that is entered, depending on where exposure is needed most. Additional exposure is provided by "notching" an additional rib adjacent to the excised rib; a 2-cm segment is excised subperiosteally near the costispinal junction (Fig. 36-5). This approach usually provides adequate exposure to repair even the most extensive TAA. Other surgeons recommend performing a double thoracotomy through one or two skin incisions or a stepwise thoracotomy, in which two or more ribs are divided vertically to extend the thoracotomy through more than one interspace.[84] A self-retaining retractor is placed in the wound and is critical to maintaining exposure of the large field in these long cases: the Omni, Thompson, and Buchwalter retractors are examples of such retractors.

After the chest is entered, ventilation of the left lung is arrested to collapse the lung. The aneurysm, left lung, and heart are inspected. There can be extensive adhesions between the lung and the aneurysm. Filmy adhesions are taken down to mobilize the lung off the aneurysm. If the adhesions are dense, lysis of them can cause extensive intrathoracic and intrapulmonary hemorrhage, and it may be necessary to work around the lung and even open the aneurysm without mobilizing the lung off it. The diaphragm is divided to expose the entire thoracoabdominal aorta, joining the left pleural cavity and the retroperitoneum into a single operative field. This can be done in two different ways. A radial incision can be made from the anterior edge of the diaphragm where the costal margin is divided directly down to the aortic hiatus. This incision is simple to close but results in paralysis of the diaphragm lateral to the incision. Alternatively, the diaphragm can be taken down peripherally, leaving a 2-cm cuff along the chest wall all the way to the aortic hiatus. This is the preferred incision at the author's institution because it preserves the function of the diaphragm and has a minimal effect on postoperative respiratory function, facilitating repair of TAAs in patients with even marginal respiratory status.

The patient then is placed on partial (left heart) bypass with a Bio-Medicus centripedal pump circuit. The inflow site for the cardiopulmonary bypass pump circuit can be one of three sites: the proximal descending thoracic aorta, the left atrium, or the left inferior pulmonary vein. Aortic cannulation can be hazardous, especially in a diseased aorta, and can lead to extensive bleeding while the cannula is in place or after it is removed. The author never cannulates the ascending aorta or the aortic arch because of difficulty with exposure and the risk of stroke. Atrial cannulation requires a pericardiotomy and manip-

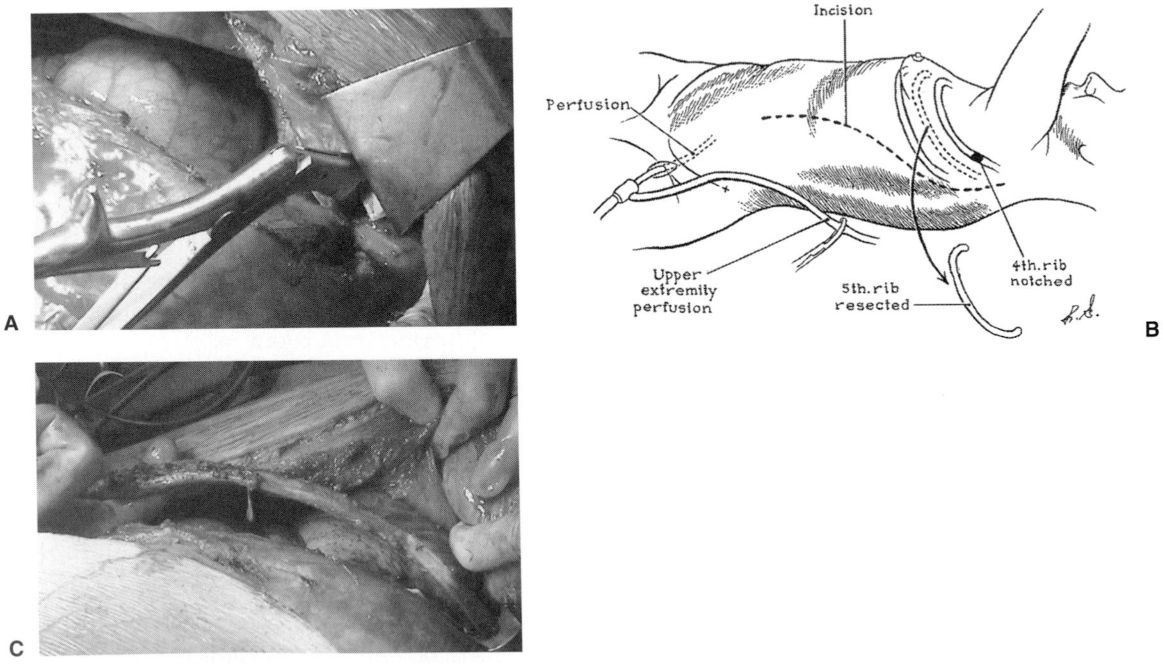

Figure 36-5 Thoracic exposure demonstrating subperiosteal resection of fifth rib and "notching" of fourth rib to gain additional exposure. (Diagram from Williams GM, Schlossberg L. *Atlas of Aortic Surgery*. Baltimore: Williams & Wilkins, 1997, with permission.)

ulation of the heart. The preferred site at the author's institution is the left inferior pulmonary vein, which can be accessed in an extrapericardial location. It is easy to locate after division of the inferior pulmonary ligament and mobilization of the lower lobe of the left lung, although occasionally it cannot be used because of adhesions in this area. The patient is anticoagulated systemically with 100 to 150 U/kg of intravenous heparin, and an activated clotting time (ACT) is checked. A pledgeted purse-string suture of 2-0 Ticron is placed in the left inferior pulmonary vein, and the vein is opened after the anesthesiologist delivers a Valsalva breath to prevent air embolism. An angled Sarns venous cannula (20F to 24F) is placed into the pulmonary vein through the purse-string suture and connected to the inflow limb of the pump circuit.

Outflow of the cardiopulmonary bypass circuit usually is delivered via the left common femoral artery. An oblique groin incision is made, and the left femoral artery is dissected out by an assistant while the thoracotomy is being performed. The artery can be cannulated directly, but the author prefers to isolate the artery and sew an 8-mm Dacron graft end to side onto it. A straight 22F or 24F aortic cannula is inserted into and secured to this graft. This technique decreases the chance of creating a dissection in the iliofemoral system and permits antegrade perfusion of the left leg as well as retrograde perfusion up the left iliac system, eliminating the ischemia of the left leg that results from direct cannulation. It also allows the perfusionist to keep the pump circuit flowing into the left leg at a rate of at least 500 cc/min if it is necessary to clamp the left iliac system during the distal aortic reconstruction.

There are four basic steps in surgical TAA repair: construction of the proximal anastomosis, ligation/reimplantation of thoracic intercostal arteries, reimplantation or bypass of the renal and mesenteric arteries, and construction of the distal anastomosis. One must determine preoperatively if the aortic arch is involved; this will necessitate the involvement of a cardiac surgeon to conduct full cardiopulmonary bypass and circulatory arrest to effect repair. An aneurysm or dissection that begins just beyond the left subclavian artery may be repaired with a proximal cross-clamp on the aortic arch between the left common carotid artery and the left subclavian artery (Fig. 36-6). This is generally safe but does entail a risk of stroke and recurrent laryngeal nerve injury.

The distal cross-clamp is placed just beyond the level of anticipated aortic transection to minimize distal ischemia during the construction of the proximal anastomosis. The anastomosis between an appropriately sized Dacron tube graft and the proximal aorta is constructed in an end-to-end fashion with running 3-0 polypropylene (e.g., Prolene) sutures. The author prefers to reinforce the anastomosis with strips of Teflon felt incorporated circumferentially in the suture line.

Once the proximal anastomosis is completed and tested for hemostasis, the distal thoracic aorta is repaired.

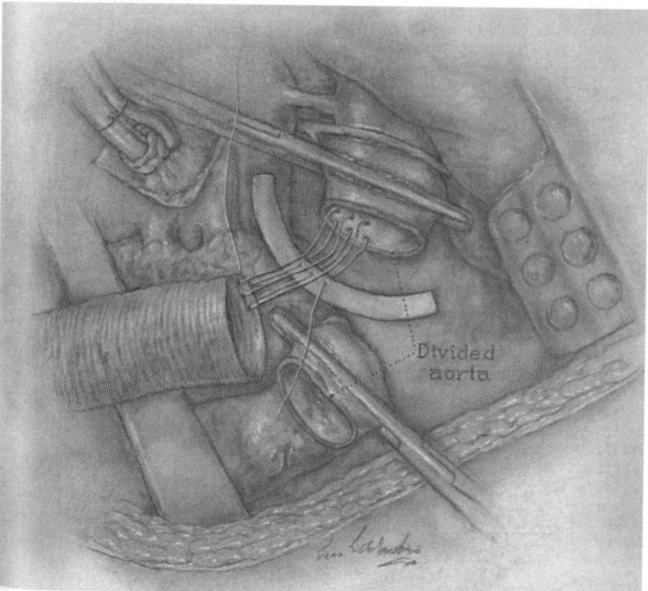

Figure 36-6 Illustration of the construction of the proximal anastomosis during repair of the descending thoracic aorta just beyond the left subclavian artery. The venous cannula for the aortofemoral bypass circuit is shown in the left atrial appendage; the author's standard practice currently is to cannulate the inferior pulmonary vein without violating the pericardium. (Diagram from Williams GM, Schlossberg L. *Atlas of Aortic Surgery*. Baltimore: Williams & Wilkins; 1997, with permission.)

The smooth conduct of this portion of the operation is critical to minimize the risk of paraplegia. Upper left-sided intercostal arteries are ligated before the thoracic aorta is opened if they can be reached behind the aorta, but this can be difficult and can lead to bleeding. The author attempts to dissect out lower left-sided thoracic intercostal arteries and clamp them with atraumatic vascular clamps to prevent back bleeding and steal from the spinal cord circulation, but this is not always possible. The right-sided intercostal arteries are virtually never accessible external to the aorta. The distal clamp is moved to the level of the diaphragm, and the aorta is opened and inspected for patent intercostals branches. The upper intercostal arteries generally can be oversewn safely down to the level of T8 (Fig. 36-7). If the location of the spinal artery is known, the intercostal artery supplying that vessel is reimplanted into the Dacron tube graft with a side-to-side anastomosis or by means of a short interposition graft placed between the Dacron tube graft and a patch of tissue around the relevant intercostal artery; the other intercostal arteries are oversewn. If the spinal artery is not found, serious consideration is given to reimplanting any patent intercostal arteries between the T8 and L1 levels. In this situation, surgeons at the author's institution usually try to reimplant at least one or two pairs of intercostal arteries in the distal thoracic

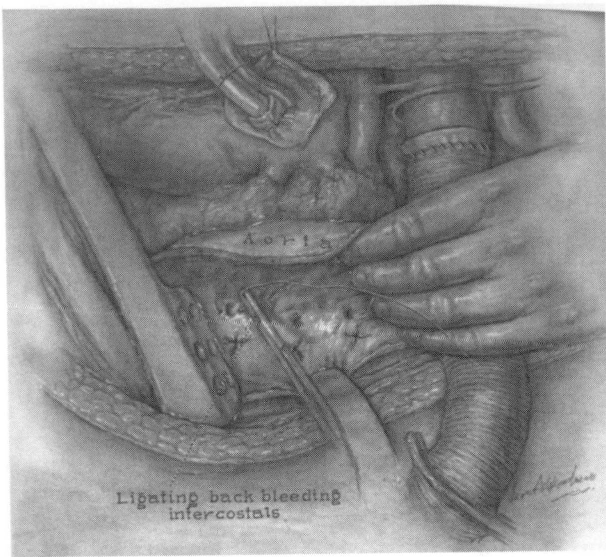

Figure 36-7 Illustration depicting opening of the descending thoracic aorta after a proximal anastomosis has been performed, with ligation of back bleeding intercostal arteries. (Diagram from Williams GM, Schlossberg L. *Atlas of Aortic Surgery.* Baltimore: Williams & Wilkins; 1997, with permission.)

aorta, particularly large ones that back bleed poorly (Fig. 36-8). It may be necessary to thrombectomize or endarterectomize the aorta to identify patent intercostals. Jacobs employs MEP monitoring to guide selective clamping and reimplantation of intercostal arteries that may be critical to spinal cord perfusion and has reported excellent results, with paraplegia rates of 3 percent.[34] Surgeons at the author's institution have employed MEP since 2000 but have found it to be much less accurate in predicting spinal cord injury. Similar efforts using SSEP monitoring have been even less rewarding. This portion of the operation can take an hour or more, resulting in prolonged visceral ischemia if distal aortic perfusion is not employed.

The visceral abdominal aorta is repaired next. The distal clamp is moved to the most proximal location that will permit repair; if the TAA terminates at the celiac artery, the clamp is placed above the renal arteries so that the kidneys are perfused continuously by the left atrial-femoral bypass circuit. Usually, the clamp is placed below the renal arteries, resulting in visceral and renal ischemia. The celiac and superior mesenteric arteries are dissected out and clamped or controlled from within the aorta with Fogarty balloon catheters once the aorta has been opened. The renal arteries do not back bleed significantly and thus do not need to be controlled. If the TAA terminates near those branches, they can be incorporated into the distal anastomosis. If it extends into the infrarenal aorta, they are reimplanted into the side of the graft (Fig. 36-9). The configuration of the reimplantation depends on the amount of dilatation in this region. With less extensive aneurysms, the celiac, superior mesenteric, and renal arteries can be reimplanted into the side of the graft as a single patch. More often, the celiac, superior mesenteric, and right renal arteries are implanted as one patch and the left renal artery is implanted as a second patch. With extensive aneurysms in this region, the mesenteric vessels are implanted as a single patch and the two renal arteries are implanted as separate patches. The left kidney usually is implanted last and therefore is subjected to the longest ischemic times.

Reimplantation of the visceral vessels usually can be accomplished within 30 to 60 min. In these cases, bowel infarction and permanent renal failure are very rare, and so surgeons at the author's institution do not selectively

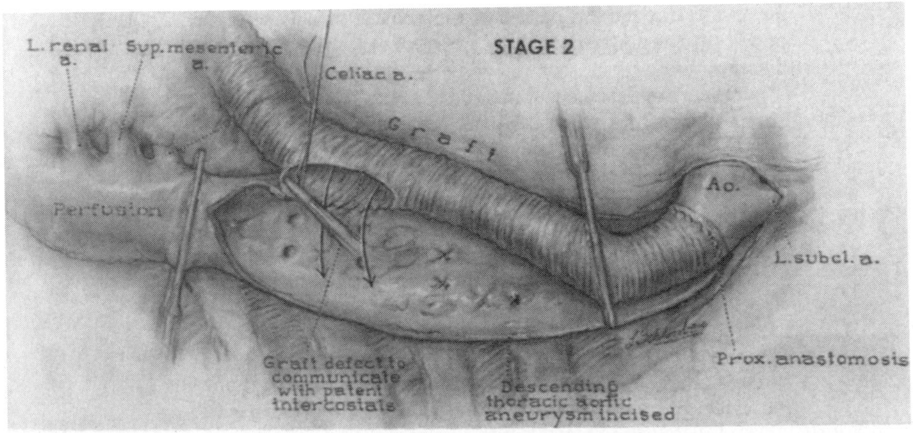

Figure 36-8 Illustration depicting reimplantation of critical intercostal arteries in the side of an aortic graft as a Carrel patch. The abdominal aorta and visceral organs are being perfused during this stage of the procedure by the aortofemoral bypass circuit. (Diagram from Williams GM, Schlossberg L. *Atlas of Aortic Surgery.* Baltimore: Williams & Wilkins; 1997, with permission.)

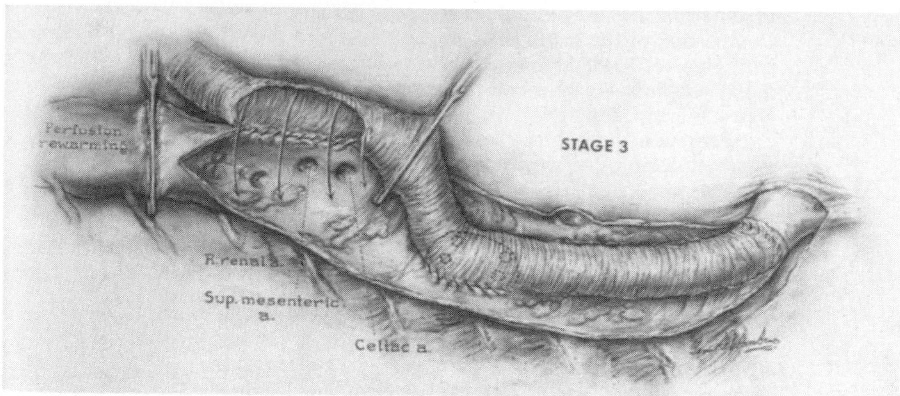

Figure 36-9 Illustration depicting reimplantation of the mesenteric and renal arteries in the side of an aortic graft. Occasionally this can be accomplished as a single patch, but two, three, or even four inclusion patches may be necessary to reimplant the vessels. (Diagram from Williams GM, Schlossberg L. *Atlas of Aortic Surgery*. Baltimore: Williams & Wilkins; 1997, with permission.)

perfuse or shunt the visceral vessels routinely during the visceral vessel reconstruction. Ischemic times increase with the number of patches and can exceed an hour with a difficult reconstruction. If prolonged visceral ischemia is anticipated, consideration should be given to perfusion of the viscera by means of selective catheterization of these vessels and perfusion with either cold blood or crystalloid when the visceral aorta first is opened, as this may reduce the incidence of postoperative renal failure and increase survival rates.[70,71,85] If there is aneurysmal involvement of the branch vessels, interposition grafting from the main Dacron tube graft to those vessels may be required. Surgeons at the author's institution have reported ruptures of aneurysms of the visceral patches, and so they now make every effort to limit patch size, especially in Marfan's disease patients.[86]

Once the visceral patch anastomoses have been completed, the graft is de-aired by back bleeding the mesenteric vessels, and the cross-clamp is placed on the graft at a point distal to the patch anastomoses to permit antegrade visceral perfusion. The distal anastomosis then is performed end to end to the infrarenal aorta if the aneurysm terminates there. If there is iliac artery involvement, a bifurcated graft is sewn to the iliacs first; the proximal end then is anastomosed end to end to the distal aspect of the more proximal Dacron graft. Exposure of the right iliac artery can be difficult from thoracoabdominal incisions and may require a retroperitoneal incision in the right lower quadrant to effect the repair. In cases of iliac artery involvement, every effort is made to revascularize the hypogastric arteries, since spinal cord perfusion may be dependent on the hypogastric circulation after intercostal arteries and lumbar arteries are divided.[34]

After the visceral arteries are reimplanted, the patient is warmed actively with the heat exchanger on the cardiopulmonary bypass circuit while the distal anastomosis is being completed. Once the patient reaches 36.5°C, the bypass circuit is clamped and heparinization is reversed with protamine. The cannula in the pulmonary vein is removed while a Valsalva maneuver is performed. The graft on the femoral artery is clamped and divided, leaving a 1-cm stump of graft on the femoral artery, which then is oversewn. The diaphragm is closed with a heavy running suture after the patient is taken out of the flexed position. The thoracoabdominal and groin incisions are closed in standard fashion. Left apical and basal chest tubes are placed in the left chest, and an Axiom sump drain is placed in the retroperitoneum. The patient's double-lumen endotracheal tube is exchanged for a single-lumen tube before the patient is transported to the intensive care unit. The apical tube is removed on postoperative day 1 if there is no pneumothorax, as is the Axiom drain. The basal chest tube is removed when chest drainage is minimal. The spinal drain is removed on postoperative day 3.

SPECIAL CONSIDERATIONS

Thoracoabdominal aneurysms related to chronic aortic dissection

TAAs related to chronic aortic dissection pose a number of special technical challenges. First, the proximal anastomosis can be very difficult to perform when the dissection originates very close to the left subclavian artery takeoff. Even cross-clamping between the left carotid artery and the left subclavian artery may not permit a satisfactory repair, and circulatory arrest with deep hypothermia may be required. The false lumen must be entered, and it may be necessary to mobilize the back wall of the aorta off the chest wall to ensure that the adventitia of the back wall is included in the anastomosis. Otherwise, one inadvertently

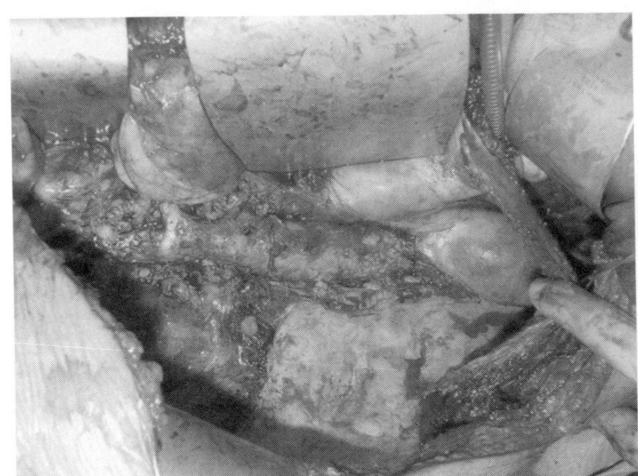

A

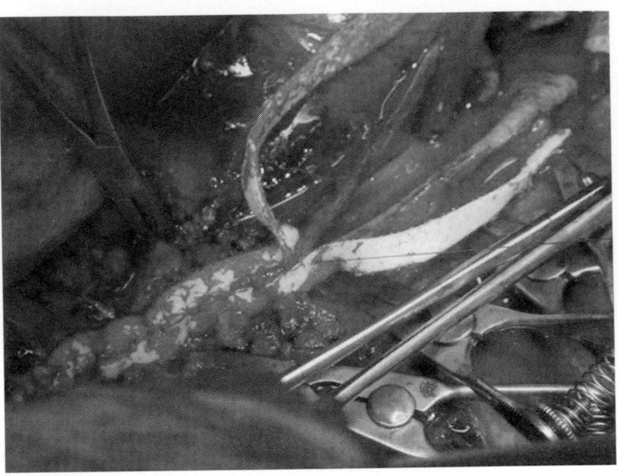

C

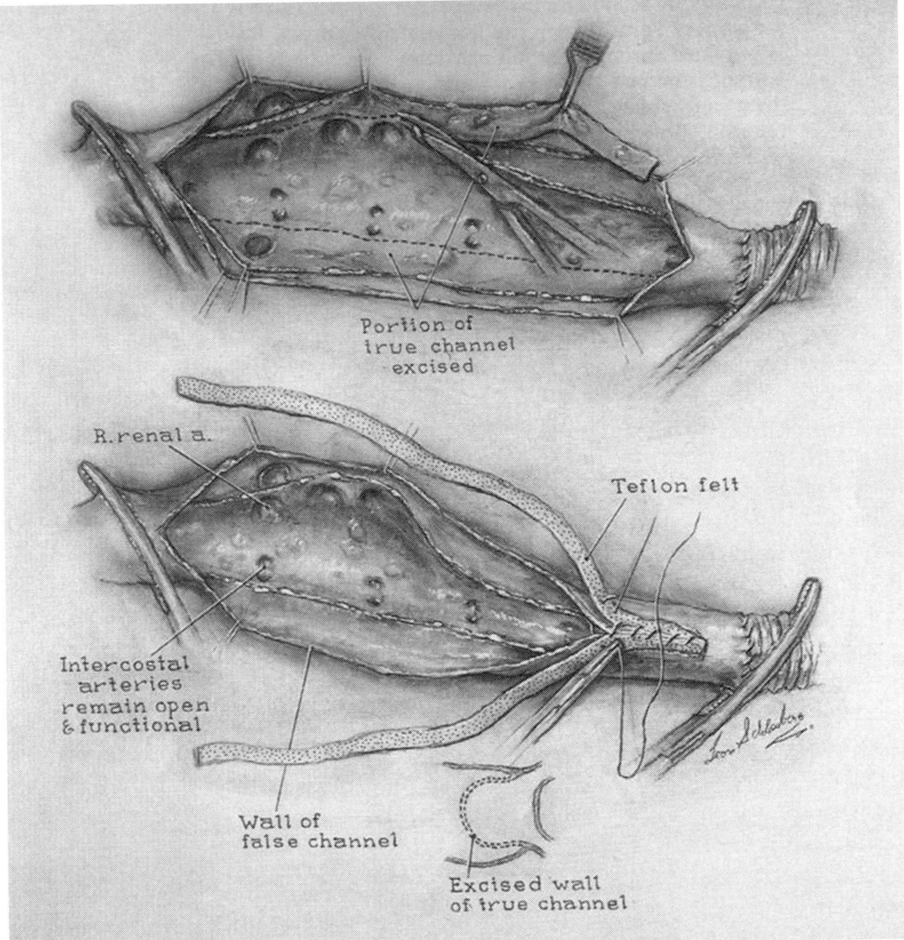

B

Figure 36-10 Repair of an acute aortic dissection arising in an aneurysm of the descending thoracic aorta complicated by malperfusion of the mesenteric circulation. The aneurysm has been replaced proximally, and the malperfusion has been treated by means of a longitudinal aortotomy, resection of the intimal flap, and closure of the aorta to a small diameter. The suture line is buttressed by strips of Teflon felt. (Diagram from Williams GM, Schlossberg L. *Atlas of Aortic Surgery.* Baltimore: Williams & Wilkins; 199, with permission.)

may omit the adventitia from the back wall of the anastomosis, resulting in disastrous bleeding. Once this happens, placement of repair stitches in this area is extremely difficult, and it usually becomes necessary to redo the entire anastomosis.

Second, there are more likely to be more patent intercostal arteries in the descending thoracic aorta than is the case with atherosclerotic aneurysms. Even if the false lumen is thrombosed, it rarely involves the entire posterior wall of the thoracic aorta, leaving many patent intercostal branches. Opening the descending thoracic aorta not only results in massive blood loss from intercostal back-bleeding but also may create a huge steal syndrome from the spinal circulation, increasing the likelihood of paraplegia. In these cases, therefore, attempts are made to get external control of as many intercostal arteries as possible with atraumatic spring-loaded clamps before the descending thoracic aorta is opened. Once bleeding is controlled and the surgeon has decided how much of the aorta must be replaced, it can be determined whether these vessels should be reimplanted or ligated.

A third complicating factor relates to the distal intimal flap found in chronic aortic dissections. Malperfusion may result distal to the area where the intimal flap is excised unless care is taken in managing the flap at that point. If the aneurysm terminates in the infrarenal aorta or the distal thoracic aorta several centimeters above the celiac artery, the bypass is stopped temporarily, the distal clamp is removed briefly, and a V-shaped wedge is cut in the intimal flap through the open end of the aorta to stabilize the flap and turn it into a flow divider. Surgeons at the author's institution have prevented distal malperfusion with this technique.

In some cases of TAAs stemming from chronic dissection, large aneurysms of the proximal descending thoracic or the infrarenal aorta are repaired, leaving a moderately aneurysmal distal thoracic or visceral aorta. In situations in which the maximum diameter of the distal aorta is dilated but less than 4 cm, surgeons at the author's institution perform a longitudinal aortotomy, resect the intimal flap, and close of the aorta to a narrower diameter of 2 cm (Fig. 36-10). This "aortic tailoring" decreases aortic wall tension, reducing the chances of further aneurysmal dilatation. Of note, in the author's experience, this strategy does not appear to be applicable in patients with connective tissue disorders. This simplified technique preserves intercostal arteries in the distal thoracic aortic segment that otherwise would have to be ligated or reimplanted, decreasing the risk of paraplegia. In the visceral segment of the aorta, the longitudinal aortotomy usually can be opened and closed in less than 20 min, a very short ischemic time that the viscera tolerates very well. This technique can be applied to other areas of the aorta but is particularly valuable in the critical areas

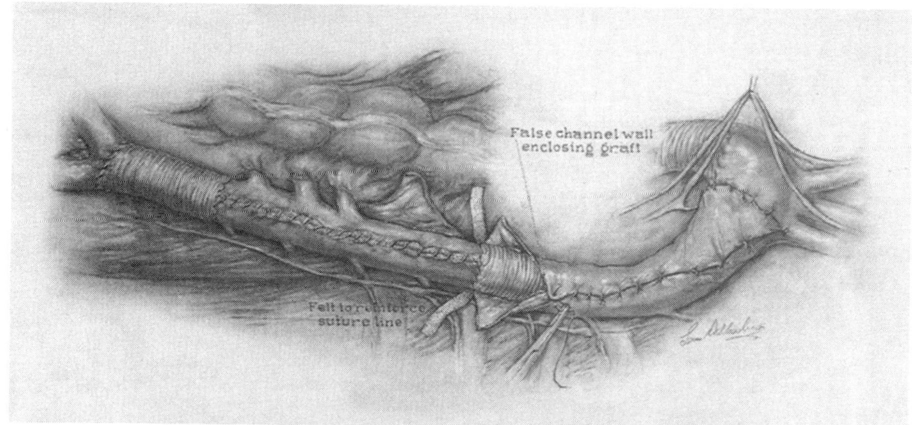

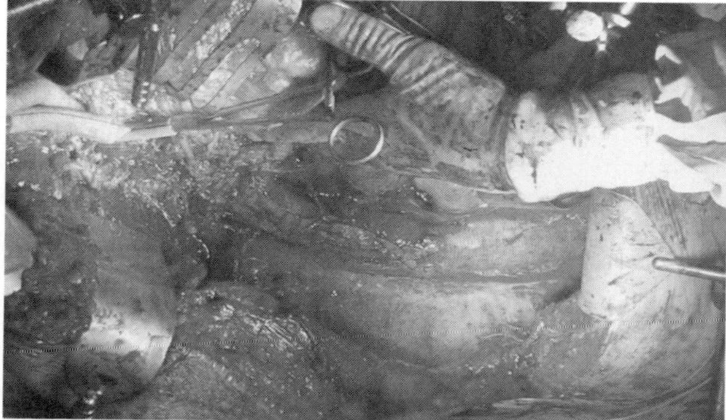

Figure 36-10 (continued)

of the lower thoracic and abdominal aorta. It also may be employed to correct acute branch malperfusion in an acute aortic dissection. In this situation, the aortic intimal flap is resected and any intimal flap that extends into the orifices of branch vessels is tacked down within the orifices.

Ruptured thoracoabdominal aneurysms

Ruptured TAAs usually present formidable technical challenges. The patient's symptoms often suggest whether the rupture occurred in the thoracic or the abdominal aorta. If one discovers intraoperatively that a ruptured abdominal aneurysm is in fact a ruptured TAA, one must first examine the supraceliac aorta at the aortic hiatus. If it is amenable to clamping and the performance of a proximal anastomosis (less than 4 cm in diameter), one should perform a medial visceral rotation to achieve exposure of the suprarenal aorta and control the mesenteric vessels. The infrarenal aorta is controlled distally, and the aorta can be replaced without circulatory bypass. If the supraceliac aorta is too diseased, the laparotomy can be converted to a thoracoabdominal incision across the left costal margin, allowing access to the fifth intercostal space if the costal margin is divided at the level of the xiphoid process. With proximal involvement of the thoracic aorta, consideration should be given to using distal bypass if it is readily available.

More often, the diagnosis of a ruptured TAA is known before exploration. In many such cases, patients have remained stable enough to undergo diagnostic imaging and transfer to a tertiary care center that has the personnel and resources to repair those aneurysms. Selective bias at least partially accounts for the fact that in many published series, the results of repairing ruptured TAAs approach those for repairing ruptured infrarenal AAAs, with survival rates in the range of 40 to 50 percent.[87–93] At the author's center, if surgeons believe the patient is stable enough, they take the additional time to place a spinal drain and neuromonitoring leads if resources are readily available. Needless to say, these judgments are made on an individual basis.

Endovascular thoracoabdominal aneurysm repair

Numerous case reports and small series have documented successful endovascular repair of aneurysms of the descending thoracic aorta.[94–99] Early experience was obtained with "homemade" stent grafts, using investigational protocols. There are now several commercially produced covered stents in clinical trials. They can be delivered through the femoral artery but in some cases may require gaining access through the iliac artery or infrarenal aorta to achieve deployment. Most authors who have experience with homemade devices find the commercially available devices to be superior and preferable. Endovascular repair is not immune to the complication of paraplegia. Investigators at the Mount Sinai Hospital in New York City found that endovascular repair of descending thoracic aneurysms was complicated by spinal cord ischemia in 3 of 53 patients (5.7 percent), with permanent paraplegia resulting in 2 of those individuals.[100]

Branched endovascular stent grafts are being developed in several centers to permit endovascular repair of thoracoabdominal aneurysms as well as aneurysms that involve the aortic arch. Strategies include using devices with prefabricated branches and constructing a branched device in situ by deploying components into branch vessels through holes in the main Dacron graft after it is deployed. The first technique has been employed to reconstruct the aortic arch,[101] and the second technique has been used to repair juxtarenal and suprarenal aneurysms.[102–106] Another option is to perform extraanatomic bypasses to either the arch vessels or the visceral vessels, permitting the coverage of these branch orifices with straight tube endografts, as has been reported by Flye and associates.[107]

Greenberg and coworkers recently reported promising results in repairing juxtarenal aortic aneurysms with a branched endograft in a small series of selected patients,[102] although the follow-up interval was short. This technology presents a formidable technical challenge at the time of repair and is fraught with the potential for malperfusion of critical branch vessels. There is no potential for preserving intercostal blood flow with this technology, and the occlusive disease that is present in up to 30 percent of TAAs can compromise the patency of branch vessel grafts. Over the long term, with extensive TAAs, there are bound to be massive conformational changes after an aneurysm is decompressed, as is seen with infrarenal stent grafts but on a much larger scale. Such changes can lead to "endoleaks" from graft component migration or separation or, worse, branch vessel occlusion and end-organ malperfusion. Intraluminal staplers are being developed to fix the branch stents to the main aortic device. This may help prevent endoleaks at component junctions but would not address branch vessel occlusion. It is the author's opinion that it is unlikely that extensive TAAs will ever be amenable to endovascular repair.

COMPLICATIONS AND RESULTS

Despite advances in surgical technique and perioperative care, the mortality and morbidity associated with TAA repair remain high. In-hospital mortality rates vary from 8 percent to 15 percent in most series and may be considerably higher in subsets of patients with extensive aneurysms or comorbidities. Complications occur in up to 75 percent of these patients. Common major complications include reoperation for bleeding, respiratory failure, myocardial infarction or cardiac failure, renal failure, and paraplegia. These postoperative complications, along with preoperative complicating factors such as emergency operation, extensive aneurysms (particularly Crawford type II TAA), advanced age, renal insufficiency, coronary disease, cerebrovascular disease, and pulmonary disease, generally are associated with adverse outcomes.[16–18,32,59,108–113] Hospital stays in uncomplicated cases are typically 10 to 14 days and may be considerably longer when there are complications.

The pioneering work of Stanley Crawford represents the gold standard for TAA repair with the clamp-and-sew technique. In 1986, Crawford published his experience with TAA repair in 605 patients using this technique.[8] Thirty-day mortality was 8.9 percent; variables predictive of early death were advanced age, prolonged clamp time, chronic obstructive pulmonary disease (COPD), atherosclerotic heart disease, renal failure, and renal artery obstruction. Five-year survival was 60 percent, and a third of late deaths were due to cardiac disease. Renal failure requiring dialysis occurred in 5 percent of patients with normal preoperative renal function and 17 percent of patients with preoperative chronic renal insufficiency. Neurologic deficits in the lower extremities occurred in 11 percent of these patients, with complete paraplegia in 6 percent. The presence of rupture, reattachment of intercostal arteries, the presence of aortic dissection, and the extent of the aneurysm were significant variables associated with neurologic deficits. The last two variables had a particularly strong influence on neurologic outcomes with the clamp-and-sew technique. Neurologic deficits occurred in 30 percent of patients with dissections compared with 7.4 percent of patients without dissections and varied from 2 percent in patients with Crawford IV aneurysms to 28 percent in patients with Crawford II aneurysms (Table 36-1)

Crawford's experience was updated in 1993, by which time his series included 1509 patients.[18] Once again, rupture, dissection, and the extent of aneurysmal disease were particularly predictive of perioperative death, renal failure, and paraplegia. Other groups using the clamp-and-sew approach have published similar results.[58,59] In the series of Schepen and coworkers, the hospital mortality rate was 11.4 percent, neurologic deficit occurred in 13.8 percent of patients, and renal failure occurred in 14.1 percent.[59] In the series of Mauney and colleagues,[58] hospital mortality was 13 percent, neurologic deficit was 10 percent, and renal failure requiring dialysis was 11 percent. Cambria and associates performed a thorough analysis of their series of 337 patients, in whom the clamp-and-sew technique was used in 93 percent and epidural cooling was used in 57 percent. Variables predictive of death in that series were rupture, emergent operation, intraoperative hypotension, a high transfusion requirement, spinal cord injury, major paraplegia, renal failure, and pulmonary complications.[32] Preoperative variables associated with spinal cord injury were rupture, type I and II TAA, and urgent or emergent operation; intraoperative variables included epidural cooling, sacrifice of T9–L1 intercostals, and intraoperative hypotension as well as prolonged operative time, cross-clamp time, and visceral ischemia.

There is evidence that the addition of distal bypass can improve the results obtained with clamp-and-sew techniques, particularly in high-risk patients with extensive aneurysms and aortic dissections. Schepens and colleagues were able to show in their series of 258 patients that left heart bypass reduced mortality, neurologic deficits, and the need for postoperative dialysis.[68] Coselli and coworkers found that left heart bypass was particularly beneficial in patients with type II TAAs, in whom neurologic deficits were reduced from 13 percent to 5 percent.[69].In a separate publication, Coselli and colleagues reported that the selective use of distal bypass eliminated dissection as a risk factor for postoperative neurologic deficits.[114] Safi and coworkers also demonstrated that left heart bypass in conjunction with CSF drainage could be beneficial in preventing neurologic injury in high-risk patients.[115]

Postoperative renal failure consistently has been shown to be a strong predictor of death in all studies of TAA repair. It typically is associated with a mortality rate of approximately 50 percent. Schepens and coworkers found that age, ischemic heart disease, diabetes, and preoperative creatinine were significant predictors of postoperative renal failure by univariate analysis and were able to develop a stepwise logistic regression equation that accurately predicts the risk of postoperative renal failure by using just two variables: age and preoperative creatinine.[116] Safi and colleagues also examined this subject and found that renal failure was associated with preoperative creatinine, the clamp-and-sew technique, left renal artery reimplantation, and visceral perfusion.[117]

Long-term survival after TAA repair varies between 53 and 73 percent at 5 years. The majority of deaths are due to cardiac disease, although Svensson and associates found that aortic dissection, postoperative neurologic deficit, and renal insufficiency also adversely affected long-term survival.[18] Schepens and coworkers found that early or late reoperation for aortic-related pathology was required in 18 percent (31 of 172) of patients.[118] Cambria and associates found on long-term follow up that 11 percent of patients (33 of 333) required reintervention after discharge for additional aortic pathology or graft-related problems.[119] Conversely, many patients develop TAAs after having an aneurysm repaired in either the distal or the proximal aorta. Coselli and colleagues examined their results in patients undergoing TAA repair as a second operation after undergoing surgery on the proximal thoracic or distal infrarenal aorta.[120,121] Surprisingly, they observed a trend toward better results in patients with previous thoracic aortic repair, although that group of patients was younger, had fewer comorbidities, and had fewer emergent repairs than did the group of patients who did not undergo previous thoracic repair. In the patients who underwent TAA repair after distal aortic surgery, the results were quite acceptable, with an in-hospital mortality rate of 12 percent, a paraplegia rate of 4.1 percent, and a renal failure rate of 11.4 percent. Patients also can develop aneurysms of the intercostal or

Table 36-1 Univariate relations between patient clinical variables and postoperative early death, neurologic deficit, and renal failure

Variable	No. cases	30-day death %	30-day death P Value	Neuromuscular deficit %	Neuromuscular deficit P Value	Dialysis %	Dialysis P Value
Age (years)							
17–55	122	2.5	0.0323	16.4	0.0242	6.6	NS
66–65	205	9.3		12.7		8.3	
66–70	148	10.8		10.8		5.4	
71+	130	12.3		4.6		10.0	
Sex							
Male	409	8.3	NS	10.3	NS	9.0	0.0530
Female	196	10.2		13.3		4.6	
Dissection	102	11.8	NS	30.4	0.0000	9.8	NS
Nondissecrtions	503	8.3		7.4		7.2	
Extent of ancurysm replaced							
I	144	9.0	NS	10.4	0.0000	5.6	0.0451
II	159	10.7		28.3		6.3	
III	157	10.8		3.2		12.7	
IV	145	4.8		2.1		5.5	
Ruptrure	26	19.2	NS	26.9	0.0097	15.4	NS
Nonruptrure	579	8.5		10.5		7.3	
Symptomatic	424	10.1	NS	12.5	NS	7.8	NS
Asymptomatic	181	6.1		8.3		7.2	
RAOD	115	15.7	0.0049	7.0	NS	9.6	NS
None	490	7.3		12.2		7.1	
AHD	200	12.5	0.0302	9.0	NS	11.0	0.0268
None	405	7.2		12.3		5.9	
CVA	76	10.5	NS	5.3	NS	15.8	0.0040
None	529	8.7		12.1		6.4	
COPD	170	14.1	0.0051	7.6	NS	10.6	NS
None	435	6.9		12.6		6.4	
HBP	434	9.9	NS	10.4	NS	8.3	NS
None	171	6.4		13.5		5.8	
Previous anecurysm repair	181	7.2	NS	13.3	NS	8.8	NS
None	424	9.7		10.4		7.1	
Renal dysfunction	84	17.9	0.0020	7.1	NS	23.8	0.0000
None	521	7.5		11.9		5.0	
Reattached intercostal	207	10.1	NS	23.2	0.0000	6.8	NS
None	385	7.8		4.9		7.3	
Reattached lumbar	61	6.6	NS	19.7	0.0296	9.8	NS
None	522	8.8		10.3		6.7	
Clamp time (min)							
12–30	75	5.3	0.0154	2.7	0.0000	1.3	NS
31–45	203	8.9		3.9		7.4	
46–60	177	5.1		12.4		7.3	
61+	135	14.8		25.9		11.1	
Concurrent ancurysm repair	51	15.7	NS	3.9	NS	13.7	NS
None	554	8.3		11.9		7.0	

NS = not significant ($p > 0.05$) by chi-square test; RAOD = renal artery occlusive disease; AHD = atherosclerotic heart disease; CVA = cerebrovascular disease; COPD = chronic obstructive pulmonary disease; HBP = hypertension.

[a] Thirteen cases were missing intercostal data.

[b] Twenty-two cases were missing lumbar data.

[c] Fifteen cases were missing clamp time data.

From Crawford ES, Crawford JL, Safi, HJ, et al. Thoracoabdominal aortic aneurysms: Preoperative and intraoperative factors determining immediate and long-term results of operations in 605 patients. *J Vasc Surg* 1986;3:389–404.

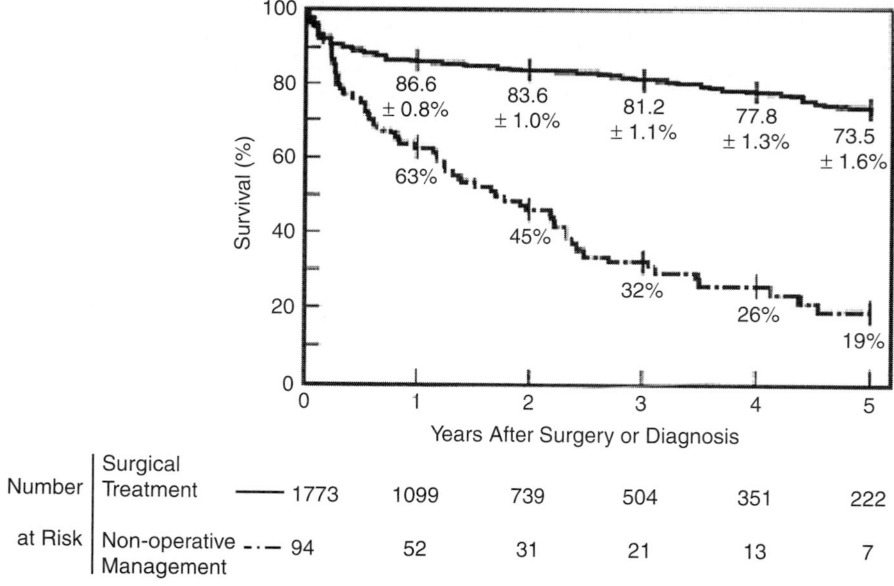

Figure 36-11 Survival curves showing improved survival of a cohort of 1773 patients operated on by Coselli and colleagues compared with the original cohort of 94 nonoperatively treated patients followed by Crawford. (From Coselli JS, Conklin LD, LeMaire SA. Thoracoabdominal aortic aneurysm repair: Review and update of current strategies. *Ann Thorac Surg* 2002;74:S1881–1884.)

visceral inclusion patches of aorta that are reimplanted onto the Dacron tube grafts. In the author's institution, it was noted that aneurysmal expansion of the inclusion patches occurred in 7.5 percent of patients on long-term follow-up, and therefore, surgeons there recommend implanting small patches of aorta onto the side of the graft, particularly in patients with connective tissue disorders.[86]

Because of the considerable intraoperative technical challenges and the complex postoperative management issues these operations present, they are best performed by experienced surgeons in centers that have extensive critical care resources. Cowan and associates studied the effect of experience (as defined by surgeon and hospital volumes) on outcomes and found that both variables had a significant effect on operative outcomes.[122] Mortality was reduced by more than half when the operations were performed by high-volume surgeons compared with low-volume surgeons; similar reductions in mortality were seen when the procedures were performed in high-volume hospitals compared with low-volume hospitals. Further demonstrating this benefit, Girardi and Coselli showed that even octogenarians can undergo TAA repair with reasonable outcomes when it is performed by an experienced surgeon in a high-volume center.[123]

TAA repair does improve long-term survival, as has been demonstrated by Crawford and Denatale[8] and Coselli and coworkers,[124] but this benefit is dependent on satisfactory surgical results (Fig. 36-11). A good functional outcome is even harder to achieve. Rechtenwald and associates retrospectively studied the functional outcomes of 101 patients undergoing TAA repair over a 6-year period.[125] They found that only 63 percent of patients experienced a good functional outcome at the time of discharge, and that number dropped to 52 percent 1 year after discharge. The results were compromised by a hospital mortality rate of 18 percent and a 12 percent incidence of neurologic deficits; the poor 1-year outcomes were due largely to a 1-year mortality rate of 33 percent. Good functional outcomes correlated with good surgical outcomes; predictors of good outcome were elective operation, short visceral ischemic times, normal preoperative and postoperative renal function, use of left atrial-femoral bypass, and absence of postoperative neurologic deficits and pulmonary dysfunction.

SUMMARY

Repair of TAAs is a challenging exercise that requires considerable preoperative planning, intraoperative skill, and meticulous postoperative care. With a combination of surgical adjuncts, good immediate and long-term results can be achieved. Although there are a number of options for surgical management of these patients, the author's preferred approach includes preoperative CT angiography, selective spinal artery angiography, intraoperative neurophysiologic monitoring, selective spinal artery reimplantation when appropriate, empiric intercostal artery reimplantation when no spinal artery is found, aortic conservation with aortic tailoring in select circumstances, and intraoperative distal aortic perfusion to minimize visceral end-organ ischemia. Postoperative mortality and complications such as cardiac, renal, and respiratory failure as well as spinal cord injury continue to be significant problems. Future advances in the pharmacologic manipulation of ischemia–reperfusion injury as well as in endovascular techniques will, one hopes, provide further improvements in the management of these challenging patients.

References

1. DeBakey ME, Creech O, Morris CG. Aneurysms of the thoracoabdominal aorta involving the celiac, superior mesenteric, and renal arteries: Report of four cases treated by resection and homograft replacement. *Ann Surg* 1956;44:549–573.
2. Carrell TW, Burnand KG, Wells GM, et al. Stromelyesin-1 (matrix metalloproteinase-3) and tissue inhibitor of metalloproteinase-3 are overexpressed in the wall of abdominal aortic aneurysms. *Circulation* 2002;105(4):405–407.
3. Elmore JR, Keister BF, Franklin DP, et al. Expression of matrix metalloproteinases and TIMPs in human abdominal aortic aneurysms. *Ann Vasc Surg* 1998;12:221–228.
4. Capella JF, Paik DC, Yin NX, et al. Complement activation and subclassification of tissue immunoglobulin G in the abdominal aortic aneurysm. *J Surg Res* 1996;65: 31–33.
5. Shteinberg D, Halak M, Shapiro S, et al. Abdominal aortic aneurysm and aortic occlusive disease: A comparison of risk factors and inflammatory response. *Eur J Vasc Endovasc Surg* 2000;20:462–465.
6. Armstrong PJ, Johanning JM, Calton WC, et al. Differential gene expression in human abdominal aorta: Aneurysmal versus occlusive disease. *J Vasc Surg* 2002; 35:346–355.
7. Thompson RW, Liao SX, Curci JA. Vascular smooth muscle cell apoptosis in abdominal aortic aneurysms. *Coron Artery Dis* 1997;8:623–631.
8. Crawford ES, Denatale RW. Thoracoabdominal aortic-aneurysm—Observations regarding the natural course of the disease. *J Vasc Surg* 1986;3:578–582.
9. Coselli J, de Figueirido L. Natural history of descending and thoracoabdominal aortic aneurysms. *J Card Surg* 1997; 12(Suppl 2):285–289.
10. Elefteriades JA. Natural history of thoracic aortic aneurysms: Indications for surgery, and surgical versus nonsurgical risks. *Ann Thorac Surg* 2002;74: S1877–S1880.
11. Lobato AC, Puech-Leao P. Predictive factors for rupture of thoracoabdominal aortic aneurysm. *J Vasc Surg* 1998; 27:446–453.
12. Griepp RB, Ergin MA, Galla JD, et al. Natural history of descending thoracic and thoracoabdominal aneurysms. *Ann Thorac Surg* 1999;67:1927–1930.
13. Cambria RA, Gloviczki P, Stanson AW, et al. Outcome and expansion rate of 57 thoracoabdominal aortic-aneurysms managed nonoperatively. *Am J Surg* 1995; 170:213–217.
14. Pressler V, Mcnamara JJ, Chang L. Thoracic aortic-aneurysm—Natural-history and treatment. *Clin Res* 1979;27:A11.
15. Juvonen T, Ergin MA, Galla JD, et al. Risk factors for rupture of chronic type B dissections. *J Thorac Cardiovasc Surg* 1999;117:776–784.
16. ES, Crawford JL, Safi HJ, et al. Thoracoabdominal aortic-aneurysms—Preoperative and intraoperative factors determining immediate and long-term results of operations in 605 patients. *J Vasc Surg* 1986;3:389–404.
17. Huynh TT, Miller CC, Estrera AL, et al. Determinants of hospital length of stay after thoracoabdominal aortic aneurysm repair. *J Vasc Surg* 2002; 35(4):648–653.
18. Svensson LG, Crawford ES, Hess KR, et al. Experience with 1509 patients undergoing thoracoabdominal aortic operations. *J Vasc Surg* 1993; 17(2):357–368.
19. Svensjo S, Bengtsson H, Bergqvist D. Thoracic and thoracoabdominal aortic anerysm and dissection: An investigation based on autopsy. *Br J Surg* 1996; 83:68–71.
20. Yamada N, Okita Y, Minatoya K, et al. Preoperative demonstration of the Adamkiewicz artery by magnetic resonance angiography in patients with descending or thoracoabdominal aortic aneurysms. *Eur J Cardiothorac Surg* 2000; 18(1):104–111
21. Yoshioka K, Niinuma H, Ohira A, et al. MR angiography and CT angiography of the artery of Adamkiewicz: Noninvasive preoperative assessment of thoracoabdominal aortic aneurysm. *Radiographics* 2003; 23: 1215–1225.
22. Laupacis A. Propranolol for small abdominal aortic aneurysms: Results of a randomized trial. *J Vasc Surg* 2002;35:72–79.
23. Baxter BT, Pearce WH, Waltke EA, et al. Prolonged administration of doxycycline in patients with small asymptomatic abdominal aortic aneurysms: Report of a prospective (phase II) multicenter study. *J Vasc Surg* 2002;36:1–12.
24. Wadouh F, Lindemann EM, Arndt CF, et al. The arteria radicularis magna anterior as a decisive factor influencing spinal cord damage during aortic occlusion. *J Thorac Cardiovasc Surg* 1984;88:1–10.
25. Williams GM, Perler BA, Burdick JF, et al. Angiographic localization of spinal-cord blood-supply and its relationship to postoperative paraplegia. *J Vasc Surg* 1991;13: 23–35.
26. Heinemann MK, Brassel F, Herzog T, et al. The role of spinal angiography in operations on the thoracic aorta: Myth or reality? *Ann Thorac Surg* 1998;65:346–351.
27. Kieffer E, Fukui S, Chiras J, et al. Spinal cord arteriography: A safe adjunct before descending thoracic or thoracoabdominal aortic aneurysmectomy. *J Vasc Surg* 2002; 35:262–268.
28. Williams GM, Roseborough GS, Webb TH, et al. Preoperative selective intercostal angiography in patients undergoing thoracoabdominal aneurysm repair. *J Vasc Surg* 2004;39:314–320.
29. Griepp RB, Ergin MA, Galla JD, et al. Looking for the artery of Adamkiewicz: A quest to minimize paraplegia after operations for aneurysms of the descending tho-

racic and thoracoabdominal aorta. *J Thorac Cardiovasc Surg* 1996;112:1202–1213.

30. Minatoya K, Karck M, Hagl C, et al. The impact of spinal angiography on the neurological outcome after surgery on the descending thoracic and thoracoabdominal aorta. *Ann Thorac Surg* 2002;74:S1870–S1872.
31. Safi HJ, Miller CC 3rd, Carr C, et al. Importance of intercostal artery reattachment during thoracoabdominal aortic aneurysm repair. *J Vasc Surg* 1998; 27(2):58–66.
32. Cambria RP, Clouse WD, Davison JK, et al. Thoracoabdominal aneurysm repair: Results with 337 operations performed over a 15-year interval. *Ann Surg* 2002;236:471–479.
33. Jacobs MJ, Meylaerts SA, de Haan P, et al. Strategies to prevent neurologic deficit based on motor-evoked potentials in type I and II thoracoabdominal aortic aneurysm repair. *J Vasc Surg* 1999;29:48–57.
34. Jacobs MJ, de Mol BA, Elenbaas T, et al. Spinal cord blood supply in patients with thoracoabdominal aortic aneurysms. *J Vasc Surg* 2002;35:30–37.
35. Laschinger JC, Cunningham JN, Catinella FP, et al. Detection and prevention of intraoperative spinal cord ischemia after cross-clamping of the thoracic aorta: Use of somatosensory evoked potentials. *Surgery* 1982; 92(6):1109–1116.
36. Cunningham JN Jr, Laschinger JC, Spencer FC. Monitoring of somatosensory evoked potentials during surgical procedures on the thoracoabdominal aorta: IV. Clinical observations and results. *J Thorac Cardiovasc Surg* 1987;94:275–285.
37. De Haan P, Kalkman CJ, Jacobs MJ. Spinal cord monitoring with myogenic motor evoked potentials: Early detection of spinal cord ischemia as an integral part of spinal cord protective strategies during thoracoabdominal aneurysm surgery. *Semin Thorac Cardiovasc Surg* 1998;10:19–24.
38. Laschinger JC, Owen J, Rosenbloom M, et al. Direct noninvasive monitoring of spinal cord motor function during thoracic aortic occlusion: Use of motor evoked potentials. *J Vasc Surg* 1988;7:161–171.
39. Dong CCJ, MacDonald DB, Janusz MT. Intraoperative spinal cord monitoring during descending thoracic and thoracoabdominal aneurysm surgery. *Ann Thorac Surg* 2002;74:S1873–S1876.
40. Meylaerts SA, Jacobs MJ, Van I, et al. Comparison of transcranial motor evoked potentials and somatosensory evoked potentials during thoracoabdominal aortic aneurysm repair. *Ann Surg* 1999;230:742–749.
41. Jacobs MJ, Meylaerts SA, de Haan P, et al. Assessment of spinal cord ischemia by means of evoked potential monitoring during thoracoabdominal aortic surgery. *Semin Vasc Surg* 2000;13:299–307.
42. Jacobs MJ, Mess WH. The role of evoked potential monitoring in operative management of type I and type II thoracoabdominal aortic aneurysms. *Semin Thorac Cardiovasc Surg* 2003;15:353–364.
43. van Dongen EP, Schepens MA, Morshuis WJ, et al. Thoracic and thoracoabdominal aortic aneurysm repair: Use of evoked potential monitoring in 118 patients. *J Vasc Surg* 2001;34:1035–1040.
44. Lips J, de Haan P, Bouma GJ, et al. Delayed detection of motor pathway dysfunction after selective reduction of thoracic spinal cord blood flow in pigs. *J Thorac Cardiovasc Surg* 2002;123:531–538.
45. Colon R, Frazier OH, Cooley DA, McAllister HA. Hypothermic regional perfusion for protection of the spinal cord during periods of ischemia. *Ann Thorac Surg* 1987;43:639–643.
46. Kouchoukos NT, Masetti P, Rokkas CK, Murphy SF. Hypothermic cardiopulmonary bypass and circulatory arrest for operations on the descending thoracic and thoracoabdominal aorta. *Ann Thorac Surg* 2002;74: S1885–S1887.
47. Kieffer E, Koskas F, Walden R, et al. Hypothermic circulatory arrest for thoracic aneurysmectomy through left-sided thoractomy. *J Vasc Surg* 1994;19:457–464.
48. Grabenwoger M, Ehrlich M, Simon P, et al. Thoracoabdominal aneurysm repair: Spinal cord protection using profound hypothermia and circulatory arrest. *J Card Surg* 1994; 9(6):679–684.
49. Safi H, Miller C, Subramaniam M, et al. Thoracic and thoracoabdominal aortic aneurysm repair using cardiopulmonary bypass, profound hypothermia, and circulatory arrest via left side of the chest incision. *J Vasc Surg* 1998; 30(1):591–598.
50. Cambria RP, Davison JK, Zannetti S, et al. Clinical experience with epidural cooling for spinal cord protection during thoracic and thoracoabdominal aneurysm repair. *J Vasc Surg* 1997;25:234–241.
51. Cambria RP, Davison JK, Carter C, et al. Epidural cooling for spinal cord protection during thoracoabdominal aneurysm repair: A five-year experience. *J Vasc Surg* 2000;31:1093–1101.
52. Blaisdell FW, Cooley DA. The mechanism of paraplegia after temporary thoracic aortic occlusion and its relationship to spinal fluid pressure. *Surgery* 1962;51:351–355.
53. Hill AB, Kalman PG, Johnston KW, Vosu HA. Reversal of delayed-onset paraplegia after thoracic aortic surgery with cerebrospinal fluid drainage. *J Vasc Surg* 1994;20:315–317.
54. Crawford ES, Svensson LG, et al. A prospective randomized study of cerebrospinal-fluid drainage to prevent paraplegia after high-risk surgery on the thoracoabdominal aorta. *J Vasc Surg* 1991;13:36–46.
55. Coselli JS, Lemaire SA, Koksoy C, et al. Cerebrospinal fluid drainage reduces paraplegia after thoracoabdominal aortic aneurysm repair: Results of a randomized clinical trial. *J Vasc Surg* 2002;35:631–639.
56. Acher CW, Wynn MM, Hoch JR, et al. Combined use of cerebral spinal-fluid drainage and naloxone reduces the risk of paraplegia in thoracoabdominal aneurysm repair. *J Vasc Surg* 1994;19:236–248.
57. Cambria RP, Davison JK, Zannetii S, et al. Thoracoabdominal aneurysm repair—Perspectives over a decade with the clamp-and-sew technique. *Ann Surg* 1997;226:294–303.
58. Mauney MC, Tribble CG, Cope JT, et al. Is clamp and sew still viable for thoracic aortic resection? *Ann Surg* 1996; 223(5):534–540.
59. Schepens MA, Defauw JJ, Hamerlijinck RP, et al. Surgical treatment of thoracoabdominal aortic aneurysms by simple crossclamping: Risk factors and late results. *J Thorac Cardiovasc Surg* 1994; 107(1): 134–142.

60. Donahoo JS, Brawley RK, Gott VL. The heparin-coated vascular shunt for thoracic aortic and great vessel procedures: A ten-year experience. *Ann Thorac Surg* 1977;23: 507–513.
61. Valiathan MS, Weldon CS, Bender HW Jr, et al. Resection of aneurysms of the descending thoracic aorta using a GBH-coated shunt bypass. *J Surg Res* 1968;8:197–205.
62. Verdant A, Cossette R, Page A, etal. Aneurysms of the descending thoracic aorta: Three hundred sixty-six consecutive cases resected without paraplegia. *J Vasc Surg* 1995;21:385–390.
63. Comerota AJ, White JV. Reducing morbidity of thoracoabdominal aneurysm repair by preliminary axillofemoral bypass. *Am J Surg* 1995;170:218–222.
64. Ballard J, Duensing. RA. Extracorporeal techniques in thoracoabdominal aortic surgery. Semin Vasc Surg 2000; 13(4):331–339.
65. Safi HJ, Campbell MP, Miller CC III, Iliet al. Cerebral spinal fluid drainage and distal aortic perfusion decrease the incidence of neurological deficit: The results of 343 descending and thoracoabdominal aortic aneurysm repairs. *Eur J Vasc Endovasc Surg* 1997;14:118–124.
66. Safi HJ. Role of the BioMedicus pump and distal aortic perfusion in thoracoabdominal aortic aneurysm repair. *Artif Organs* 1996; 20(6):694–699.
67. Bonatti J, Watzka S, Antretter H, et al. Spinal cord protection in descending and thoracoabdominal aortic surgery: The role of distal perfusion. *Thorac Cardiovasc Surg* 1996;44:136–139.
68. Schepens MAAM, Vermeulen FEE, Morshuis WJ, et al. Impact of left heart bypass on the results of thoracoabdominal aortic aneurysm repair. *Ann Thorac Surg* 1999;67:1963–1967.
69. Coselli JS, LeMaire SA. Left heart bypass reduces paraplegia rates after thoracoabdominal aortic aneurysm repair. *Ann Thorac Surg* 1999; 67:1931–1934.
70. Koksoy C, LeMaire SA, Curling PE, et al. Renal perfusion during thoracoabdominal aortic operations: Cold crystalloid is superior to normothermic blood. *Ann Thorac Surg* 2002;73:730–738.
71. Hassoun HT, Miller III, Huynh TTT, et al. Cold visceral perfusion improves early survival in patients with acute renal failure after thoracoabdominal aortic aneurysm repair: 1. *J Vasc Surg* 2004;39:506–512.
72. Williams GM, Robicsek F, Fehrenbacher JW. Treatment of chronic expanding dissecting aneurysms of the descending thoracic and upper abdominal-aorta by extended aortotomy, removal of the dissected intima, and closure. *J Vasc Surg* 1993;18:441–449.
73. Webb TH, Williams GM. Abdominal aortic tailoring for renal, visceral, and lower extremity malperfusion resulting from acute aortic dissection. *J Vasc Surg* 1997;26: 474–480.
74. Baird RJ, Firor WB, Barr HW. Protection of renal function during surgery of the abdominal aorta. *Can Med Assoc J* 1963;89:705–8.:705–708.
75. Barry KG, Cohen A, Knochel JP, et al. Mannitol infusion: II. The prevention of acute functional renal failure during resection of an aneurysm of the abdominal aorta. *N Engl J Med* 1961;264:967–971.
76. Barry KG, Cohen A, Leblanc P. Mannitolization: I. The prevention and therapy of oliguria associated with cross-clamping of the abdominal aorta. *Surgery* 1961; 50:335–340.
77. Beall AC Jr, Hall CW, Morris GC Jr, DeBakey ME. Mannitol-induced osmotic diuresis during renal artery occlusion. *Ann Surg* 1965;161:46–52.
78. Nicholson ML, Baker DM, Hopkinson BR, Wenham PW. Randomized controlled trial of the effect of mannitol on renal reperfusion injury during aortic aneurysm surgery. *Br J Surg* 1996;83:1230–1233.
79. Paul MD, Mazer CD, Byrick RJ, et al. Influence of mannitol and dopamine on renal function during elective infrarenal aortic clamping in man. *Am J Nephrol* 1986; 6:427–434.
80. Payne JH, Wood DL, Goethal JA. Oliguria and renal failure in abdominal aortic surgery: Prophylaxis with mannitol. *Am Surg* 1963;29:713–718.
81. Paterson IS, Klausner JM, Goldman G, et al. Pulmonary edema after aneurysm surgery is modified by mannitol. *Ann Surg* 1989;210:796–801.
82. De Haan P. Pharmacologic adjuncts to protect the spinal cord during transient ischemia. *Semin Vasc Surg* 2000; 13(4):264–271.
83. Caparrelli DJ, Cattaneo SM, Bethea BT, et al. Pharmacological preconditioning ameliorates neurological injury in a model of spinal cord ischemia. *Ann Thorac Surg* 2002;74:838–844.
84. Tsukube T, Yoshimura M, Matsuda H, et al. Rib-cross thoracotomy for replacement of the thoracoabdominal or total descending aorta. *J Vasc Surg* 2003; 37(1): 219–221.
85. Jacobs MJ, Eijsman L, Meylaerts SA, et al. Reduced renal failure following thoracoabdominal aortic aneurysm repair by selective perfusion. *Eur J Cardiothorac Surg* 1998;14:201–205.
86. Dardik A, Perler BA, Roseborough GS, Williams GM. Aneurysmal expansion of the visceral patch after thoracoabdominal aortic replacement: An argument for limiting patch size? *J Vasc Surg* 2001;34:405–409.
87. Bradbury AW, Bulstrode NW, Gilling-Smith G, et al. Repair of ruptured thoracoabdominal aortic aneurysm is worthwhile in selected cases. *Eur J Vasc Endovasc Surg* 1999;17:160–165.
88. Cowan JA, Dimick JB, Wainess RM, et al. Ruptured thoracoabdominal aortic aneurysm treatment in the United States: 1988 to 1998. *J Vasc Surg* 2003;38:319–322.
89. Girardi LN, Krieger KH, Altorki NK, et al. Ruptured descending and thoracoabdominal aortic aneurysms. *Ann Thorac Surg* 2002;74:1066–1070.
90. Lemaire SA, Rice DC, Schmittling ZC, Coselli JS. Emergency surgery for thoracoabdominal aortic aneurysms with acute presentation. *J Vasc Surg* 2002;35: 1171–1178.
91. Lewis ME, Ranasinghe AM, Revell MP, Bonser RS. Surgical repair of ruptured thoracic and thoracoabdominal aortic aneurysms. *Br J Surg* 2002;89:442–445.
92. Mastroroberto P, Chello M. Emergency thoracoabdominal aortic aneurysm repair: Clinical outcome. *J Thorac Cardiovasc Surg* 1999;118:477–481.
93. Velazquez OC, Bavaria JE, Pochettino A, Carpenter JP. Emergency repair of thoracoabdominal aortic aneurysms with immediate presentation. *J Vasc Surg* 1999;30:996–1001.

94. Kato N, Hirano T, Ishida M, et al. Acute and contained rupture of the descending thoracic aorta: Treatment with endovascular stent grafts. *J Vasc Surg* 2003; 37(1): 100–105.
95. Orend KH, Scharrer-Pamler R, Kapfer X, et al. Endovascular treatment in diseases of the descending thoracic aorta: 6-year results of a single center. *J Vasc Surg* 2003; 37(1):91–99.
96. Ellozy SH, Carroccio A, Minor M, et al. Challenges of endovascular tube graft repair of thoracic aortic aneurysm: Midterm follow-up and lessons learned: 1. *J Vasc Surg* 2003;38:676–683.
97. Scharrer-Pamler R, Kotsis T, Kapfer X, et al. Complications after endovascular treatment of thoracic aortic aneurysms. *J Endovasc Ther* 2003;10:711–718.
98. Lambrechts D, Casselman F, Schroeyers P, et al. Endovascular treatment of the descending thoracic aorta. *Eur J Vasc Endovasc Surg* 2003;26:437–444.
99. Najibi S, Terramani TT, Weiss VJ, et al. Endoluminal versus open treatment of descending thoracic aortic aneurysms. *J Vasc Surg* 2002;36:732–737.
100. Gravereaux EC, Faries PL, Burks JA, et al. Risk of spinal cord ischemia after endograft repair of thoracic aortic aneurysms. *J Vasc Surg* 2001;34:997–1003.
101. Schneider DB, Curry TK, Reilly LM, et al. Branched endovascular repair of aortic arch aneurysm with a modular stent-graft system. *J Vasc Surg* 2003;38:855.
102. Greenberg RK, Haulon S, Lyden SP, et al. Endovascular management of juxtarenal aneurysms with fenestrated endovascular grafting: 1. *J Vasc Surg* 2004;39:279–287.
103. Anderson JL, Berce M, Hartley DE. Endoluminal aortic grafting with renal and superior mesenteric artery incorporation by graft fenestration. *J Endovasc Ther* 2001;8: 3–15.
104. Hosokawa H, Iwase T, Sato M, et al. Successful endovascular repair of juxtarenal and suprarenal aortic aneurysms with a branched stent graft. *J Vasc Surg* 2001;33: 1087–1092.
105. Chuter TA, Gordon RL, Reilly LM, et al. Multibranched stent-graft for type III thoracoabdominal aortic aneurysm. *J Vasc Interv Radiol* 2001;12:391–392.
106. Stanley BM, Semmens JB, Lawrence-Brown MMD, et al. Fenestration in endovascular grafts for aortic aneurysm repair: New horizons for preserving blood flow in branch vessels. *J Endovasc Ther* 2001;8:16–24.
107. Flye MW, Choi ET, Sanchez LA, et al. Retrograde visceral vessel revascularization followed by endovascular aneurysm exclusion as an alternative to open surgical repair of thoracoabdominal aortic aneurysm: 1. *J Vasc Surg* 2004;39:454–458.
108. Azizzadeh A, Huynh TTT, Miller CC, et al. Postoperative risk factors for delayed neurologic deficit after thoracic and thoracoabdominal aortic aneurysm repair: A case-control study. *J Vasc Surg* 2003; 37(4):750–754.
109. Cambria RP, Davison JK, Zannetti S, et al. Thoracoabdominal aneurysm repair: Perspectives over a decade with the clamp-and-sew technique. *Ann Surg* 1997; 226(3):294–303.
110. Cina CS, Lagana A, Bruin G, et al. Thoracoabdominal aortic aneurysm repair: A prospective cohort study of 121 cases. *Ann Vasc Surg* 2001; 16(5):631–638.
111. Coselli JS. Thoracoabdominal aortic-aneurysms: Experience with 372 patients. *J Card Surg* 1994;9:638–647.
112. Coselli JS, Lemaire SA, Miller CC, et al. Mortality and paraplegia after thoracoabdominal aortic aneurysm repair: A risk factor analysis. *Ann Thorac Surg* 2000;69:409–414.
113. Hollier LH, Symmonds JB, Pairolero PC, et al. Thoracoabdominal aortic aneurysm repair: Analysis of postoperative morbidity. *Arch Surg* 1988; 123(7): 871–875.
114. Coselli JS, LeMaire SA, de Figueiredo LP, Kirby RP. Paraplegia after thoracoabdominal aortic aneurysm repair: Is dissection a risk factor? *Ann Thorac Surg* 1997; 63(1):28–35.
115. Safi HJ, Bartoli S, Hess KR, et al. Neurologic deficit in patients at high risk with thoracoabdominal aortic aneurysms: The role of cerebral spinal fluid drainage and distal aortic perfusion. *J Vasc Surg* 1994; 20(3):434–444.
116. Schepens MA, Defauw JJ, Hamerlijnck RP, Vermeulen FE. Risk assessment of acute-renal-failure after thoracoabdominal aortic-aneurysm surgery. *Ann Surg* 1994;219:400–407.
117. Safi HJ, Harlin SA, Miller CC, et al. Predictive factors for acute renal failure in thoracic and thoracoabdominal aortic aneurysm surgery. *J Vasc Surg* 1996;24:338–344.
118. Schepens MAAM, Dekker E, Hamerlijnck RPHM, Vermeulen FEE. Survival and aortic events after graft replacement for thoracoabdominal aortic aneurysm. *Cardiovasc Surg* 1996;4:713–719.
119. Clouse WD, Marone LK, Davison JK, et al. Late aortic and graft-related events after thoracoabdominal aneurysm repair: 1. *J Vasc Surg* 2003;37:254–261.
120. Coselli JS, LeMaire SA, Buket S, Berzin E. Subsequent proximal aortic operations in 123 patients with previous infrarenal abdominal aortic aneurysm surgery. *J Vasc Surg* 1995; 22(1):59–67.
121. Coselli JS, Poli de Figueirido LF, LeMaire SA. Impact of previous thoracic aneurysm repair on thoracoabdominal aortic aneurysm management. *Ann Thorac Surg* 1997; 64(3):639–650.
122. Cowan J, Dimick JB, Henke PK, et al. Surgical treatment of intact thoracoabdominal aortic aneurysms in the United States: Hospital and surgeon volume-related outcomes: 1. *J Vasc Surg* 2003;37:1169–1174.
123. Girardi LN, Coselli JS. Repair of thoracoabdominal aortic aneurysms in octogenarians. *Ann Thorac Surg* 1998; 65(2):491–495.
124. Coselli JS, Conklin LD, LeMaire SA. Thoracoabdominal aortic aneurysm repair: Review and update of current strategies. *Ann Thorac Surg* 2002;74:S1881–S1884.
125. Rectenwald JE, Huber TS, Martin TD, et al. Functional outcome after thoracoabdominal aortic aneurysm repair. *J Vasc Surg* 2002;35:640–647.

CHAPTER

37 AORTIC DISSECTION

Jay G. Shake, G. Melville Williams

INTRODUCTION

In the United States, acute aortic dissections are the most common life-threatening disease processes of the aorta, presenting a risk to life roughly double that of ruptured abdominal aortic aneurysms. The diagnosis of aortic dissection is complicated by the fact that other, far more common disease processes occur with similar complaints. Insight into the similarities of these diseases is important since incorrect management of patients with aortic dissection can be fatal. A thorough understanding of the pathophysiology, anatomic classifications, and clinical features, along with knowledge about the constellation of diagnostic techniques, allows one to initiate the appropriate management, either medical or surgical. Advances in each of these areas, along with the ongoing education of medical professionals about this entity, have improved survival in patients with this potentially lethal condition.

KEY CONCEPTS

- Epidemiology
  - The actual incidence of aortic dissection is difficult to determine since many patients probably die without the diagnosis having been made. The incidence is estimated to be 5 to 30 patients per million population per year and continues to increase with the aging of the population. Aortic dissection is the most common life-threatening disease process of the aorta, and its risk to life is roughly double that of a ruptured abdominal aortic aneurysm.
- Pathophysiology
  - The classical theory states that an intimal tear is the primary cause of a dissection, with subsequent hemorrhage within the media portion of the aorta creating two lumens. The etiology of the tear can involve multiple causes, including connective tissue disorders that lead to a diseased aortic media, hypertension, and iatrogenic aortic trauma; recently, a theory has been propounded that states that bleeding from the vasa vasorum into the media causes an intramural hematoma that eventually leads to intimal destruction.
- Clinical features
  - The most crucial factor in identifying a patient with acute aortic dissection is a high degree of suspicion. Patients generally appear with the abrupt onset of chest pain that is usually substernal and often is described as sharp, ripping, stabbing, or tearing; that pain radiates to the back in only a third of these patients. Patients generally appear ill and anxious. Anxiety and pain result in catecholamine release with resultant tachycardia and increased blood pressure above the normal baseline hypertension. This frequently is diagnosed as an acute myocardial infarction and also may be associated with other end-organ complications, such as syncope, cerebrovascular accident, anuria, and acute ischemia of the abdomen or extremities. It also can present with profound hypotension secondary to cardiac tamponade. It is critical to avoid unnecessary delays, as conventional estimates of mortality after ascending aortic dissection have been reported to be 1 to 2 percent per hour during the first 24 to 48 h, 75 percent at 2 weeks, and as high as 90 percent at 3 months.
- Diagnostics
  - The history and physical examination can be very helpful. Connective tissue disorders and/or hypertension can provide a clue to this life-threatening process. Similarly, on physical examination, end-organ disease

can be manifested by the absence of pulses, lack of urine output, and neurologic deficit as well as other end-organ findings. Electrocardiography is obtained to help distinguish a dissection from an acute myocardial infarction. A chest x-ray can show a widened mediastinum as well as a new left-sided pleural effusion, although both of these signs may be absent with dissection. Computed tomography (CT) scanning is currently the most commonly employed image modality for evaluating a patient suspected of having an acute aortic dissection. Transesophageal echocardiography is becoming one of the imaging modalities of choice for making the diagnosis. It does not require dye injection and has a high degree of sensitivity (99 percent) and specificity (89 percent). Aortography has been considered the gold standard but is currently not the diagnostic procedure of choice. Its major value is in assessing individuals with a sudden onset of acute renal failure, mesenteric or limb ischemia, hypertensive crisis, or new-onset neurologic findings.

- Treatment
  - *Medical*: Aggressive medical therapy should be initiated at the first clinical suspicion of an aortic dissection, consisting of management of blood pressure and pain. Patients with type B dissection continue on medical management unless their pain cannot be controlled or there is end-organ involvement.
  - *Surgical*: A standard type A resection requires immediate operation. If there is associated aortic valve regurgitation, it often can be corrected by resuspending the aortic commissures with simple pledgeted sutures. If salvage of the valve seems unlikely, a root replacement using a composite graft is generally the treatment of choice. If the intimal tear originates in the arch or begins in the ascending aorta and extends into the aortic arch, the arch generally has to be replaced.
- Outcomes
  - As published in a longitudinal study by the Stanford group, among patients who survived type A dissection, 1-, 5-, 10-, and 15-year survival was 67 percent, 55 percent, 37 percent, and 24 percent, respectively. In the same series, patients with type B dissections did not fare as well. Their survival with the same follow-up period was 56 percent, 48 percent, 29 percent, and 11 percent, respectively.

Definitions

By convention, an aortic dissection is a potentially life-threatening cardiovascular event that is caused by hemorrhage through an intimal tear (Fig. 37-1) so that with every cardiac ejection, the aortic wall separates, or dissects. This process creates a second lumen that runs parallel to the first. The true lumen is composed of the intima and a thin layer of media, and the false lumen is composed of the remainder of the media and the adventitia. The cleavage plane between the two lumens is the dissection flap. There also have been several case reports of multiple lumens after dissection of previously healed dissection flaps. When the dissection extends proximally from the intimal tear toward the heart, it is referred to as a retrograde dissection, whereas dissections that propagate away from the heart are antegrade dissections. Classically, an acute dissection is one in which the interval between onset and therapeutic intervention is less than 2 weeks, and beyond this period it is called a chronic dissection. A recently added definition—subacute—is used to describe the period between 2 weeks and 2 months, though the classical description is used in this chapter. These definitions arose from data suggesting a higher mortality in the first 14 days and lower attrition rates in those who survive that critical period.[1] It is not surprising, then, that there are major differences between acute and chronic dissections with regard to medical therapy, surgical approach, and prognosis.

Acute dissections must be distinguished clearly from aneurysms of the aorta that are often simple, asymptomatic expansions of the vessel that frequently result from atherosclerosis. Many are discovered incidentally during routine imaging studies. The term *dissecting aortic aneurysm* should be avoided in describing acute dissections, which often may occur in the absence of an aneurysm. However, one frequently sees this phrase used to

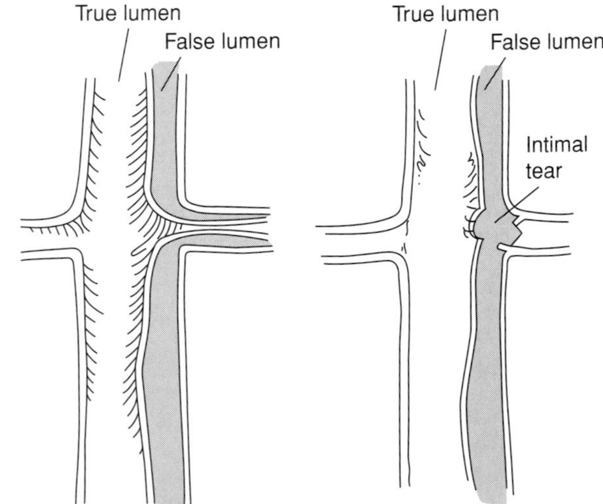

Figure 37-1 Schematic of aortic dissection. An aortic dissection is a hemorrhage within the wall of the aorta and is positively identified when a dissection flap is seen separating the parallel-running true and false lumens. Branch vessel occlusion results from external compression on the true lumen or shearing of the vessel at its origin. [From Green GR, Kron IL. Aortic dissection. In: Edmunds LJ Jr (ed). *Cardiac Surgery in the Adult.* New York: McGraw-Hill; 1997:1095.]

describe chronic dissections with aneurysmal dilatation of the thin-walled false lumen. Because of the confusion this term creates regarding appropriate classifications and management (aneurysm versus dissection), most authors discourage its use.

An intramural hematoma (IMH) is a contained collection of blood within the wall of the aorta (without an intimal tear) that may be a separate pathologic abnormality of the aortic media or, as some have suggested, another step in the cascade that culminates in an aortic dissection or rupture. If an IMH is demonstrated and subsequently an intimal tear is identified, the aortic abnormality is better described as a noncommunicating aortic dissection with a thrombosed false lumen.

Historical highlights

Rupture of the inner layer of the aorta without rupture of the outer layer was described by Nicholls in 1728[2] (Table 37-1). In 1761 he described the first well-documented case of aortic dissection during the autopsy of King George II of England, who reportedly died while straining on a commode. In particular, reference was made to an intimal tear, a hematoma in the wall of the ascending aorta, and blood in the pericardium.[2] A year later Morgagni[3] coined the term *aortic dissection*, yet the underlying pathophysiology was poorly understood and continued to elude investigators for nearly 100 years. The belief held by many surgeons and scientists was that aortic dissections represent an early stage of common saccular aneurysms.[4] One of the first individuals to recognize and draw attention to the lack of understanding of aortic dissections was Peacock in his comprehensive review.[5] Despite that publication, few advances were made for several decades. The understanding of the disease process as it is known today began in 1930 with the work of Erdheim, who accurately described the histologic changes seen in aortic dissection, although he incorrectly introduced the term *cystic medionecrosis*.[6]

Despite advances in the understanding of the disease process and its recognition as an entity separate from aneurysms, aortic dissection continued to be an underrecognized clinical entity. Swaine and Latham[7] are credited with making the first antemortem diagnosis of aortic dissection in 1856, yet it remained predominantly a postmortem diagnosis until the early twentieth century. In fact, in 1934 Shennan[8] reported that the correct antemortem diagnosis was made in only 6 of the 300 cases he reviewed. In 1922, Davy and Gates[9] used an imaging modality to confirm their clinical diagnosis. A probably more important contribution from the field of radiology to the diagnosis of aortic dissections was made in 1948 by Paullin and James when they introduced the concept of contrast angiography.[10]

The first surgical attempt to treat an aortic dissection was made in 1935 by Gurin and associates,[11] who fenestrated a dissection in an iliac artery to treat malperfusion syndrome. Fenestration failed to gain overwhelming support, perhaps because of the disease process and late recognition rather than shortcomings of the technique. Because of the poor outcomes, others offered alternative techniques for treatment. In 1949, Abbott[12] introduced wrapping of the aorta with cellophane to prevent rupture. This and other techniques remained unsatisfying, and it was not until 1955 that DeBakey and coworkers[13] described the first series of patients successfully treated with primary surgical repair. Two years later they refined the surgical technique with the use of extracorporeal circulation during surgical repairs, and this remains a mainstay of contemporary aortic surgery.[14]

A significant advancement in medical therapy for aortic dissections was introduced by Wheat and associates[15] in 1965. Their work demonstrated the relationship of

Table 37-1	Aortic dissection: Important historical events
1760	Nicholls's autopsy of King George II
1761	Morgagni coins the phrase *aortic dissection*
1826	Laennec coins the misnomer *aneurysme dissequant*
1843	Peacock performs first comprehensive review
1856	Swaine and Latham make first antemortem diagnosis
1922	Davy and Gates make first radiographic confirmation of clinical diagnosis
1930	Erdheim describes histologic changes and introduces the term *cystic medionecrosis*
1934	Shennan makes correct antemortem diagnosis in only 6 of 300 cases
1935	Gurin makes first attempt at surgical treatment (fenestration in iliac artery)
1948	Paullin and James introduce contrast angiography for diagnosis
1949	Abbott uses cellophane wrapping to prevent rupture of a dissected aorta
1955	DeBakey and coworkers do first series of surgically treated patients with primary repair
1957	Cooley and colleagues use extracorporeal circulation during descending clamping
	DeBakey makes first use of selective antegrade cerebral perfusion
1961	DeBakey and associates do first anatomic classification of dissection
1965	DeBakey simplifies classification into three basic types
	Wheat and colleagues identify importance of intensive medical treatment to decrease blood pressure and aotic wall stress (dP/dt)
1975	Griepp publishes first successful series using hypothermic circulatory arrest
1979	Miller and coworkers devise Stanford classification
1981	Carpentier introduces thromboexclusion
1984	Larson and Edwards further classify DeBakey III to IIIa and IIIb
1990	Ueda introduces retrograde cerebral perfusion
	Endovascular stents introduced

increased blood pressure to the rate of aortic pressure upstroke during the cardiac cycle, referred to as dP/dt (the derivative of raw blood pressure), to aortic wall stress.[15] Beta-adrenergic blocking agents have a favorable influence on both of these parameters and remain a mainstay in medical management of both acute and chronic dissections.

Anatomic classification

Several classification systems from various medical institutions have been propagated through the medical literature and surgical wards. All are based primarily on anatomic differences with regard to the location of the intimal tear and the length of the false lumen. The distinguishing feature in all the classifications is the distinction between tears of the ascending aorta or aortic arch (DeBakey type 1 or 2, Stanford type A, Massachusetts General proximal, and University of Alabama ascending) and tears distal to the origin of the left subclavian artery (DeBakey 3, Stanford B). The DeBakey and Stanford classifications are used most frequently in clinical practice and are discussed in detail in this chapter.

The original DeBakey classification of aortic dissections was published in 1961[16] and later was simplified into three basic types.[17] A DeBakey type 1 dissection starts at the ascending aorta and continues the entire length of the aorta. A DeBakey type 2 is limited to the ascending aorta, and a type 3 begins below the left subclavian artery, thus sparing the ascending aorta and arch. Larson and Edwards[18] further classified the DeBakey 3 into two subgroups: Type 3a is localized to the thoracic aorta, and 3b continues into the abdominal aorta (Fig. 37-2).

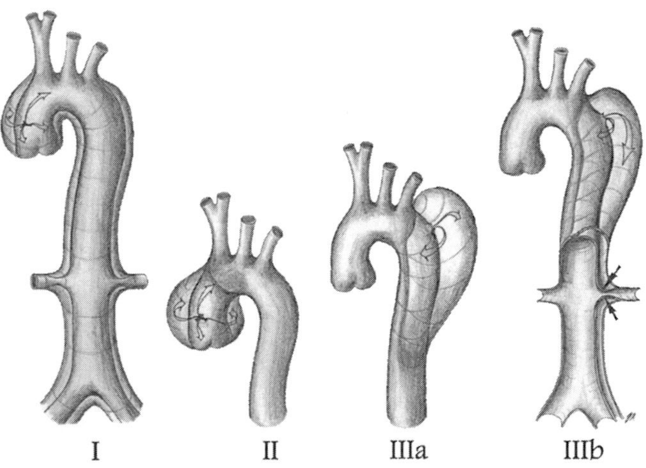

Figure 37–2 DeBakey classification system. I. Type 1 dissections involve the ascending aorta, arch, and descending aorta. II. Type 2 dissections are isolated to the ascending aorta. IIIa. Type 3a dissections involve only the descending aorta. IIIb. Type 3b dissections involve the descending aorta and continue below the diaphragm into the abdominal aorta. The intimal tear site (*light arrows*) and false lumen are noted in each figure. Compression of the true lumen of the left renal artery, as shown in IIIb, demonstrates branch vessel occlusion (*dark arrows*). [From Coady MA, Rizzo JA, Goldstein LJ, Elefteriades JA. Natural history, pathogenesis, and etiology of thoracic aortic aneurysms and dissection. In: Elefteriades JA (ed). *Cardiology Clinics: Diseases of the Aorta*, vol 17. Philadelphia: Saunders; 1999:626.]

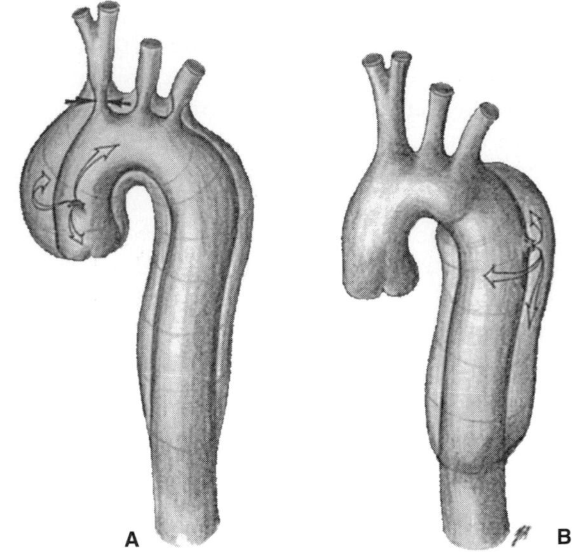

Figure 37-3 Stanford classification system. A. Type A dissections involve the ascending aorta and may or may not continue in the arch and proceed down the descending aorta. This figure demonstrates an intimal tear in the ascending aorta (*light arrows*) and occlusion of the innominate artery by the false lumen (*dark arrows*). B. Type B dissections are isolated in the descending aorta and may or may not involve the visceral or iliac vessels. [From Coady MA, Rizzo JA, Goldstein LJ, Elefteriades JA. Natural history, pathogenesis, and etiology of thoracic aortic aneurysms and dissection. In: Elefteriades JA (ed). *Cardiology Clinics: Diseases of the Aorta*, vol 17. Philadelphia: Saunders; 1999:627.]

The simpler Stanford classification has only two subsets and emphasizes the clinical uniqueness of dissections that involve the ascending aorta.[19] The Stanford type A dissection includes any dissection that involves the ascending aorta (DeBakey 1 and 2) regardless of where the primary intimal tear occurs, and the Stanford type B dissection involves only the descending aorta (DeBakey 3) (Fig. 37-3). Those authors contend that only two subsets are needed since the clinical behavior is determined by whether there is involvement of the ascending aorta. A criticism of the Stanford system is the inability of the simplified classification to define for the reader the extent of the disease process, that is, whether the dissection involves the visceral vessels or extends beyond them. The A and B classification separates patients typically requiring immediate surgery (type A) from those managed medically (type B), reserving surgery for type B patients with complications.

PATHOPHYSIOLOGY

There are numerous theories regarding the process that initiates an aortic dissection. The exact interrelation between two important factors the intimal tear and the medial degeneration has not been established. The classical theory states that the intimal tear is the primary cause of the dissection and that hemorrhage within a normal media occurs as a result of the primary injury. The simplest example of this occurs after iatrogenic aortic trauma from catheterization, cannulation, application of aortic cross clamps, and intraaortic balloon pumps. Another theory suggests that the primary abnormality is related to defective aortic media that subsequently results in an intimal tear, as demonstrated by the higher incidence in patients with connective tissue disorders. A more recent theory is that bleeding from the vasa vasorum into the media creates an intramural hematoma that becomes a localized area of stress, leading to intimal disruption. Finally, atherosclerotic ulcers have been blamed for cases of aortic dissection secondary to intimal disruption and medial necrosis; however, this theory has not gained overwhelming support in a majority of cases.

Intimal tear

An intimal tear is a consistent feature in most aortic dissections since only 2 to 4 percent of dissections present without them, and most of those dissections are confined to the descending aorta. As was mentioned previously, whether the occurrence of the intimal tear is the primary event that leads to the aortic wall separation remains controversial and has not been established scientifically. Intimal tears occur at points of fixation along the aorta, with a majority located within the first few centimeters of the ascending aorta. The next most common site is the initial portion of the descending aorta, then the aortic arch, and finally a few tears below the diaphragm (Fig. 37-4).[19,20] Two-thirds of dissections involve the ascending aorta. The primary tear usually traverses the aortic lumen obliquely and rarely involves more than half the circumference of the aorta. Total disruption of the intima has been reported with intima-intimal intussusception. Once initiated, the dissection progresses either antegrade or retrograde and is usually in the outer third of the media; this is why dissections often rupture into the pleural or pericardial space. The false lumen frequently occupies the right anterior portion of the ascending aorta, and the medial half of the ascending aorta remains intact. In the arch, the false lumen is often along the greater curve and extends into the innominate, left carotid, and left subclavian arteries. In the descending aorta, the false lumen follows the anterolateral wall and therefore frequently involves the left renal artery.[20] Interruption of the blood supply to major branches of the aorta by extrinsic compression by the false lumen or shearing off of the true lumen may lead to malperfusion syndrome with organ and/or limb ischemia. Proximal extension of the dissection can shear the coronary arteries, leading to myocardial ischemia. Rupture into the pleura or pericardium can be seen, depending on the location of the tear, with intrapericardial rupture most commonly from the ascending aorta and rupture into the left pleura most commonly from arch and descending aorta tears. Rupture into the pericardium is the most common cause of death in the first 2 weeks. The endpoint of the dissection is determined by scarring of the aortic wall secondary to atherosclerosis, natural barriers, or reentry into the true lumen. The presence of reentry prevents thrombosis of the false lumen, and its persistence is a negative long-term prognostic indicator because of a higher incidence of aneurysmal dilatation as a result of structural weakness of the thin wall of the false lumen. When a critical point is reached, usually with the aortic diameter greater than 5 cm, ominous consequences are likely.

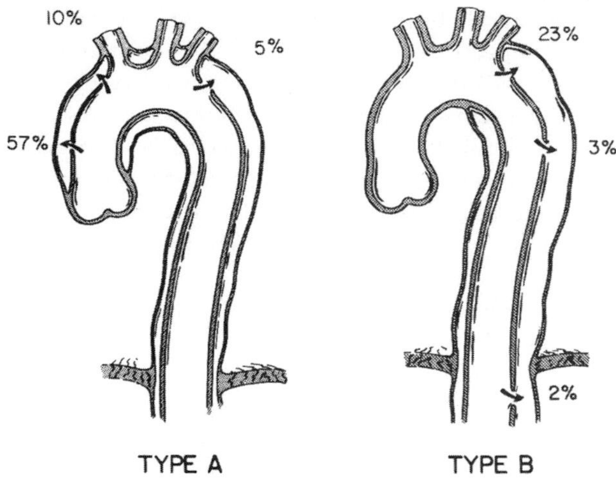

Figure 37-4 Intimal tear site. The intimal tear site of an aortic dissection most frequently is in the ascending aorta. This schematic demonstrates the frequency of intimal disruption when the Stanford classification system is used. [From Erkin MA, Griepp RB. Dissection of the aorta. In: Baue AE, Geha AS, Hammond GL, et al (eds). *Glenn's Thoracic and Cardiovascular Surgery*. Stamford CT: Appleton and Lange; 1991:2273.]

Abnormality of aortic media

The normal aorta contains collagen, elastin, and smooth muscle cells that contribute to its structural integrity, distensibility, and vascular tone, respectively. The adventitia provides a majority of the tensile strength of the aortic wall; however, abnormal constituents of the media, as seen in connective tissue disorders, are associated with an increased incidence of aortic dissection; those disorders include Marfan's syndrome, Ehlers-Danlos syndrome, and other familial forms of connective tissue disorders.

Marfan's syndrome is an autosomal dominant inherited connective tissue disorder that results in a point mutation in the fibrillin-1 gene on chromosome 15. The syndrome involves many organ systems: dura, ocular, pulmonary, cardiovascular, skeletal, integument, and skin. In addition to the molecular analysis for the diagnosis, new stringent criteria require that at least four of eight typical manifestations be present. Particular attention is paid to skeletal involvement. The incidence is approximately 1 per 5000 live births; however, there are many incomplete forms of the disease, and in as many as 25 percent of cases, the disease has a sporadic form. To date, there are more than 100 different mutations of the fibrillin-1 gene. There is no racial or ethnic predisposition.

Type IV Ehlers-Danlos syndrome (EDS) is a disorder of a chain of type III collagen with an incidence of 1 in 5000 births. This disease is characterized by tissue fragility, skin hyperextensibility, and articular hypermobility. Aortic involvement is seen predominantly with EDS type IV, which is transferred in an autosomal dominant fashion.

Other disease processes that are believed to contribute to aortic dissection include all processes that injure the media. Inflammatory states such as autoimmune diseases (rheumatoid arthritis, Takayasu's arteritis, Behçet's disease, Ormond's disease), infectious disease (syphilis, rarely bacterial or fungal), high doses of zinc in animal models, and illicit drugs (cocaine, amphetamines) have been implicated.

Erdheim's first description of the structural change in the dissected aorta wall included the description of "cystic medionecrosis," which was thought to be the histologic sine qua non of aortic dissections, yet no true cysts or necrosis are present.[6] The characteristic microscopic change includes elastic tissue fragmentation and focal separation of the elastic and fibromuscular components of the media. Small spaces form and fill with amorphous material that resembles the extracellular matrix of connective tissue, and this can lead to large-scale loss of elastin, producing overt medial degeneration. Some authors believe there is progressive medial degeneration with aging and long-standing hypertension, laying the groundwork for dissection and medial hemorrhage.

Intramural hematoma

In 1920, Krukenberg first described an IMH of the aorta as a "dissection without an intimal tear." An IMH is thought to result from spontaneous rupture of the vasa vasorum into the media, creating a concentric hematoma (collection of blood) in the wall of the aorta. Further enlargement of the collection results in localized areas of increased stress, leading to further media separation. This actually reaches a steady state or regresses with time. It also can progress to an aortic dissection, an intimal tear, and a false lumen. The belief that this cascade exists is supported by the finding that 10 to 20 percent of patients who are thought to have an acute aortic dissection are found to have an intramural hematoma, suggesting that it may have been a precursor.[21] Later-generation CT and magnetic resonance imaging (MRI) scanners with higher resolution have increased the incidence of this diagnosis and have shown that this entity most frequently is confined to the descending aorta. Whether this pathology is a separate entity from other media abnormalities is not clear.

CLINICAL FEATURES

Epidemiology

In the United States, aortic dissections are the most common acute illness of the aorta, with more than 2000 new cases per year; they are almost twice as common as ruptured abdominal aortic aneurysms. The incidence rate is estimated to be 5 to 30 patients per million population per year and continues to increase with the aging of the population; however, the precise incidence is difficult to determine because many cases are undiagnosed.[22] To put things in perspective, the incidence of acute myocardial infarction is 4400 patients per million population per year. Although the incidence of acute aortic dissection is relatively lower, it is still important to health care providers since the outcome can be fatal after complications of rupture, acute myocardial ischemia, cardiac tamponade, cerebrovascular accident, or severe aortic regurgitation. Aortic dissection can occur in all age groups; however, it is rare in infants and children less than 16 years of age. Most cases affect males between the fourth and seventh decades, with a peak in the age group 50 to 69 years old.[20] The incidence is reported to be low in Asians in the western world, yet it is seen frequently in Japan and China. The incidence is higher in African-Americans, reflecting their increased incidence of hypertension rather than a racial predilection.[20] Males are afflicted two to three times as often as females.

Typical clinical presentation

The most important point in identifying a patient with an acute aortic dissection is suspicion, which is crucial in making an early diagnosis. Patients with acute disease often appear ill and are aware that something is terribly wrong. Anxiety and pain result in catecholamine release, tachycardia, and increased blood pressure above the normal baseline hypertension. The difficulty in making a rapid diagnosis lies in the fact that initial complaints signifying the beginning of the aortic dissection process

Table 37-2 Differential diagnosis of aortic dissection

Acute myocardial infarction
Aortic regurgitation (without dissection)
Aortic aneurysm (without dissection)
Cholecystitis
Embolism (atherosclerosis or cholesterol)
Esophageal pathology
Mediastinal tumors
Musculoskeletal pain
Pleuritis
Pneumonia

often have similarities to the symptoms of more common entities (Table 37-2). It thus is understandable that up to a third of patients found to have an acute aortic dissection initially are suspected of having other conditions, such as acute myocardial infarction, nondissecting aneurysms, pulmonary embolism, and aortic valve disease.[23] A patient's past medical history needs to be investigated since prior episodes of chest pain, coronary artery disease, or chronic aortic dissection will be informative. In addition, a history of prior pulmonary embolism, hypertension, illicit drug use, or aneurysmal disease or a family history of a connective tissue disorder can help direct one to a diagnosis.

A typical patient is a male in his sixties who has a history of hypertension and has an abrupt onset of chest pain that is maximal at onset. The pain is usually substernal and often is described as sharp, ripping, stabbing, or tearing; it may radiate to the back. However, back pain is seen in only a third of these patients, and this suggests that the absence of back pain does not rule out an aortic dissection. The pain may change its location, depending on the extension of the dissection (Table 35-3). The pain is believed to be caused by distention of the aortic wall and may diminish or completely subside in 4 to 5 h, producing a false sense of security. A second attack signifies extension of the dissection and should alert caregivers to the fact that the current management is not working, pointing to a grim clinical outcome if the course is not redirected. A newly diagnosed aortic dissection that is without chest pain or is discovered incidentally by imaging is probably a chronic dissection. Other, less common presentations of an acute aortic dissection include syncope without chest pain, new neurologic changes, and cardiac failure secondary to aortic insufficiency or cardiac tamponade. Oliguria or anuria can be seen with dissection into the renal arteries, with the propensity of involvement of the left kidney greater than that of the right. Persistent abdominal pain secondary to mesenteric ischemia signifies visceral vessel involvement. In contrast, myocardial infarction pain usually starts slowly and intensifies and is often dull in nature. Consequently, acute aortic dissection should be part of the differential diagnosis of patients presenting with syncope, cerebrovascular accident, acute congestive heart failure, or acute ischemia of the abdomen or extremities.

Table 37-3 Common presenting signs and symptoms of aortic dissection

Asymptomatic with abnormal imaging
Cerebrovascular accident
Congestive heart failure
Hematemesis
Hemoptysis
Oliguria (or anuria)
Pain alone
Paraplegia
Pulse loss
Syncope
Vocal cord paralysis

Patients with intramural hematomas are often older than those with classical aortic dissections (74 years versus 56.5 years) and are almost universally hypertensive. The pain mimics that of classical dissections, yet these dissections usually do not produce branch vessel occlusion and therefore do not result in visceral or limb ischemia. This is probably a result of IMH being a localized lesion rather than the lengthy aortic lesion typically seen in a propagated dissection. The disease most frequently involves only the descending aorta and occurs at a more superficial layer in the media. This may explain why there is a higher rupture rate than there is with aortic dissections.

It is critical to avoid unnecessary delays in the diagnosis and treatment of acute aortic dissection. Conventional estimates of mortality after ascending aortic dissection have been 1 to 2 percent per hour during the first 24 to 48 h, 75 percent at 2 weeks, and as high as 90 percent at 3 months. More recent data suggest a more favorable outcome, with only a 58 percent in-hospital mortality rate among high-risk patients managed medically (nonoperative). The results for type B dissections are not as ominous.

Aortic injuries that result from blunt trauma are highly lethal and often are confounded by concomitant injuries. In survivors, the dissection is rarely excessive and often is limited to the aortic isthmus: the most proximal portion of the descending aorta. This portion of the aorta is fixed in the posterior chest, unlike the mobile heart and arch, which are free to move after the chest strikes a stationary object such as the dashboard of an automobile. Although there is debate about how the dissection is initiated, most believe that the difference in mobility plays a large role in this process. It is important to mention that traumatic aortic injuries are not usually classical aortic dissections and that the urgency of repair is related to the fact that they often are contained ruptures rather than simple intimal tears. Patients with traumatic acute dissections also can present with signs of impending rupture or with a "pseudo-coarctation" from circular prolapse of the intima and media that produces aortic obstruction. Other patients are asymptomatic in regard to the aortic trauma because of distracting injuries or have significant neurologic compromise and are diagnosed with standard trauma imaging.

Physical examination

The physical examination frequently reveals an anxious patient aware that something is terribly wrong. Tachycardia is often present from anxiety or pain in conjunction with hypertension or with hypotension if a catastrophic event is evolving. Pulse deficits indicative of malperfusion are found in less than 20 percent of all patients,[24] but among the elderly, half of patients with proximal aortic dissection have missing femoral or brachial pulses.[22] Absence of pulses in the upper extremities is suggestive of ascending involvement, and loss of pulse in the lower extremities is indicative of distal involvement. Transient loss of pulses most likely represents changes in the position of the dissection flap. Neurologic deficits, including delirium, paresis, and loss of consciousness, occur in up to 40 percent of patients with proximal aortic dissection. Fortunately, acute cerebrovascular accidents are the presenting complaint in less than 5 percent of patients. Paraplegia also may be seen after dissection when critical intercostal arteries are separated from the aortic lumen. Rarely, hemoptysis or hematemesis is seen with perforation into the esophagus or the tracheobronchial tree. Superior vena cava syndrome, upper airway compression, and vocal cord paralysis (compression of the left recurrent laryngeal nerve) are more often the result of chronic expansion. A diastolic murmur secondary to aortic insufficiency is seen in half of patients with proximal aortic dissection.[24,25] Signs of pericardial involvement such as jugular venous distention, distant heart sound, and pulsus paradoxus indicate a more ominous extension. Although diagnostic thoracentesis yielding blood indicates the need for emergent surgery, one must remember that a pleural effusion can represent expression of an exudative inflammatory reaction from a dissected aorta that requires no surgical intervention. Furthermore, a pleural effusion and concomitant mediastinal hematoma warrant further investigation and probably emergent surgical intervention.

DIAGNOSTIC MODALITIES

Diagnostic studies

Hallmark primary laboratory abnormalities

Laboratory testing plays a minor role in the evaluation of a patient with a suspected aortic dissection since there is no sensitive or specific diagnostic laboratory test. However, standard chemistry and hematologic tests should be done immediately to establish baseline values and rule out other disease processes. In patients with an aortic dissection, laboratory abnormalities can reflect the distribution of the disease process. For example, an elevation in blood urea nitrogen and serum creatinine may signal renal artery involvement. Metabolic acidosis suggests viscera or lower extremity malperfusion; however, similar to elevations of bilirubin and other liver enzymes, it often is found too late in the clinical course to change the outcome. Extensive acute aortic dissections can involve elevations in C-reactive protein and mild to moderate leukocytosis.[26]

Electrocardiogram

An electrocardiogram must be obtained in all patients to help distinguish an acute myocardial infarction, for which thrombolytic therapy may be lifesaving, from an aortic dissection, in which thrombolytic therapy may be lethal. To complicate the issue, about 20 percent of patients with proximal aortic dissection have electrocardiographic evidence suggestive of an acute myocardial infarction or acute ischemia.[27] Furthermore, a normal electrocardiogram is present in a third of patients with coronary involvement, and a majority of patients with acute coronary occlusion have only nonspecific ST-T wave changes.[27] Therefore, any patient with an acute coronary syndrome who is suspected of having an acute aortic dissection must undergo additional diagnostic testing before receiving thrombolytic drug therapy.

Diagnostic imaging

The demonstration of a dissection flap between two separate lumens is the definitive finding in diagnosing an aortic dissection. Other signs suggestive of a dissection include a thrombosed false lumen, central displacement of an intimal flap, and separation of intimal calcifications. High-quality diagnostic imaging can do more than establish the diagnosis of an aortic dissection (Table 37-4). The information gathered can alter interventional and surgical planning, such as detection and grading of aortic insufficiency and assessment of the involvement of major side branches, particularly the coronary arteries and arch vessels. Furthermore, the urgency of intervention can be altered by detection of contrast extravasation or the identification of periaortic or mediastinal hematomas.

Table 37-4 Diagnostic imaging capabilities
Confirm diagnosis of dissection
Localize intimal tear(s) and extent of disease
Allows classification of the dissection (type A or B)
Distinguish between noncommunicating and communicating dissections
Identify true and false lumens
Determine important branch vessel involvement (arch vessels, visceral vessels, and coronary arteries)
Detect contrast extravasation (rupture) or mediastinal hematoma
Diagnose and grade aortic valve insufficiency

The use of two or even three imaging techniques to diagnose an acute aortic dissection is excessive and lends to unnecessary time loss. The ideal imaging technique should be rapid and easily obtained at any hour of the day and should not expose the patient to undue stress. The two most frequently used techniques in the acute setting are CT and transesophageal echocardiography (TEE). Other techniques are viewed as second-line yet offer distinct benefits and disadvantages that warrant mention in this chapter.

At the authors' institution, a patient with chest pain and a high clinical suspicion of having an acute aortic dissection immediately will have an electrocardiogram (ECG) and a chest x-ray (CXR) to rule out other obvious causes. An unstable patient will be transferred immediately to the operating room for intubation, placement of invasive monitoring lines, and an intraoperative TEE. If no dissection is seen and assuming that the patient becomes hemodynamically stable after resuscitation, the patient is instrumented appropriately for transfer to other areas of the hospital for further workup and monitoring. A stable patient seen in the emergency department usually first undergoes a contrast-enhanced helical CT scan with three-dimensional (3-D) reconstruction and then TEE or MRI if there are diagnostic uncertainties. Aortography is used rarely and is reserved for patients with perfusion abnormalities. In the absence of ominous findings on initial imaging and with no indication for surgery, repeat imaging is carried out within 3 to 5 days of admission to the hospital. If there is an increase in the size of the aorta, a suggestion of rupture, or progression of the dissection, surgery should be considered strongly.

Plain chest radiography

An abnormal chest x-ray is seen in somewhere between 60 percent[24] and 90 percent[25] of patients suspected of having an acute aortic dissection; however, a normal CXR is inadequate to rule out an acute aortic dissection.[28] Signs to look for include a new left-sided pleural effusion, enlarged cardiac silhouette, pleural cap, and separation of the aortic wall calcification. Also, a widened aorta or mediastinum should elevate suspicion enough to prompt investigation with more sensitive and specific imaging techniques.

Computed tomography

Contrast-enhanced helical CT is currently the most commonly employed imaging modality in evaluating patients suspected of having an acute aortic dissection. CT significantly decreased the risk to patients by eliminating the need for direct arterial injection during traditional aortography. The data set can be acquired during a single breath hold and can be used to reconstruct two- and three-dimensional images from virtually any perspective. The diagnosis is based on the identification of a dissection flap separating the true and false lumens (Fig. 37-5A and B). This technique can demonstrate arch and visceral vessel involvement and also allows visualization of the surrounding mediastinal structures rather than just the luminal contours seen with standard aortography. Movement of the aortic wall during the cardiac cycle may create motion artifacts that appear as dissections. It also may limit image resolution, resulting in the misdiagnosis of subtle or discrete dissections. Mural thrombi in fusiform thoracic aneurysms may be mistaken for aortic dissection without reentry. Newer scanners have estimated sensitivities and specificities of more than 95 percent in diagnosing acute dissection. They also have been shown to have 93 percent sensitivity and specificity with regard to diagnosing arch vessel involvement.[29–32] Patients who cannot receive iodinated contrast are not good candidates for CT imaging, though the only absolute contraindication for emergent scanning is significant allergy, particularly anaphylaxis. Pretreatment with steroids is recommended in those patients before the study. Renal insufficiency is a relative contraindication, and a serum creatinine above 2.0 mg/dL is a common laboratory reference point above which iodinated contrast carries a greater risk of serious renal impairment.

Transthoracic/transesophageal echocardiography

The diagnosis of acute aortic dissection by standard M-mode and two-dimensional transthoracic echocardiography (TTE) is reliant on the detection of a dissection flap. The sensitivity and specificity of TTE range from 77 to 80 percent and 93 to 96 percent, respectively, for involvement of the ascending aorta[33–35] and TTE has even more limited success in diagnosing descending dissections (70 percent).[34] This modality is particularly limited in patients who are obese or who have abnormal chest walls, such as those with Marfan's syndrome (pectus carinatum, pectus excavatum) or chronic obstructive pulmonary disease (barrel chest). Therefore, in general, TTE is inadequate to make a diagnosis of aortic dissection reliably.

Transesophageal echocardiography has become one of the imaging modalities of choice for diagnosing acute aortic dissection. Although the technique is very operator-dependent, it has high sensitivity (99 percent) and specificity (89 percent).[36] TEE can demonstrate the origin of intimal tears and evaluate flow in both the true and false lumens (Fig. 37-6). Aortic insufficiency, pericardial effusions, and pleural effusions are easily demonstrated, whereas coronary or arch vessel involvement is not easily visualized. There are two potential shortcomings with this technique. The hypertensive response to probe placement may be dangerous in individuals with acute dissections, yet this danger can be minimized with adequate monitoring and sedation. There is also a "blind spot" in the ascending aorta and arch caused by air in the right mainstem bronchus between the esophagus and the aorta, although it rarely interferes with the appropriate diagnosis. A tortuous aorta also may be difficult to image. Because the dissection is viewed in "real time," a

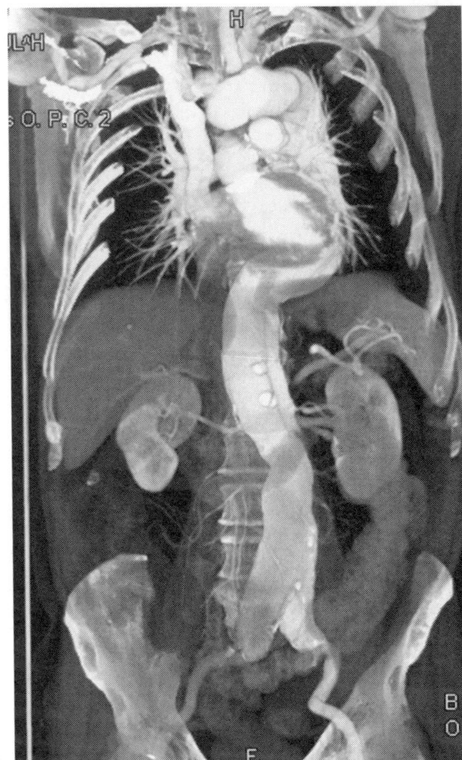

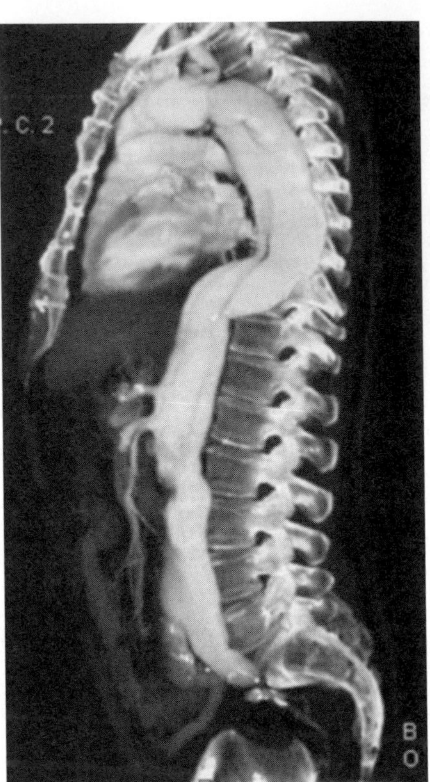

Figure 37-5 Helical computed tomography with three-dimensional reconstruction. Modern high-resolution computed tomography with intravenous contrast and three-dimensional reconstruction allows one to visual the entire aorta from any perspective. Note the dissection flap and the true and false lumens. Furthermore, intimal tear sites, extent of disease, and branch vessel involvement usually can be seen. This information is extremely valuable in planning the surgical approach. A. Coronal view. B. Sagittal view. (Images courtesy of Elliot Fishman, MD, Department of Radiology, Johns Hopkins Hospital.)

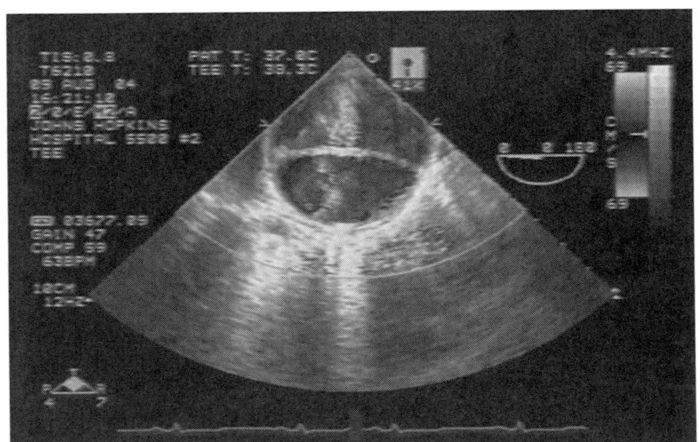

Figure 37-6 Transesophageal echocardiography (TEE). Dissection of descending aorta. This type B dissection is identified in the descending aorta by using standard TEE. Note the linear, echogenic dissection flap separating the true and false lumens. Doppler analysis demonstrates flow in both lumens. (Image courtesy of Mary Corretti, MD, Department of Cardiology, Johns Hopkins Hospital.)

mobile dissection flap sometimes can be visualized (Fig. 37-7A and B).

Magnetic resonance imaging

Magnetic resonance imaging is both highly sensitive and highly specific in diagnosing aortic dissection (nearly 100 percent)[29,31,32] (Fig. 37-8). MRI provides outstanding identification of branch involvement, aortic valve insufficiency, and localization of intimal tears. With newer scanners, images can be obtained with rapid acquisition and have high enough resolution to identify proximal coronary artery involvement. The use of this modality may be limited in potentially unstable patients with acute aortic dissections since MRI scanners often are in remote locations in the hospital, making patient transport a time-consuming and potentially dangerous endeavor. Also, the monitoring devices and mechanical ventilation equipment that accompany this type of patient are often not compatible with the large magnetic fields encountered in the scanner environment. Therefore, in most hospitals, this technique is best used in patients with chronic aortic dissections during follow-up.

A

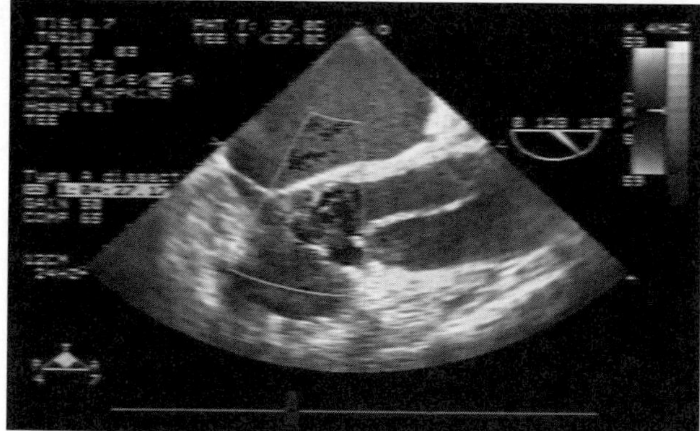

B

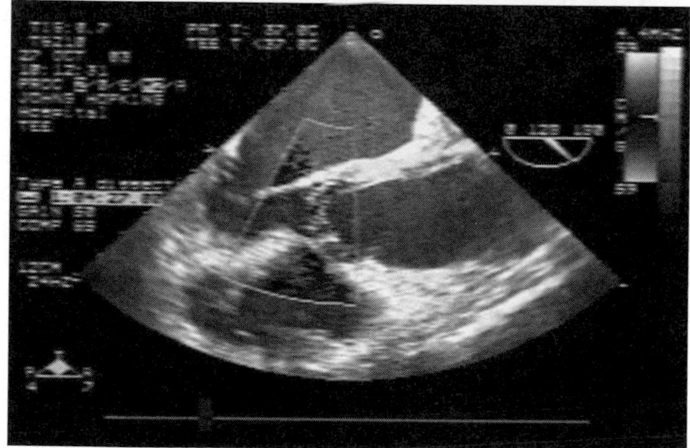

Figure 37-7 Transesophageal echocardiography (TEE). Mobile flap in the ascending aorta. The "real-time" capabilities of TEE allow one to visualize mobile dissection flaps during the cardiac cycle. Note the echogenic flap in the dilated ascending aorta shown here moving during systole (A) to create a false lumen and its approximation with the aortic wall during diastole (B). (Images courtesy of Kelly Grogan, MD, Department of Anesthesia, Johns Hopkins Hospital.)

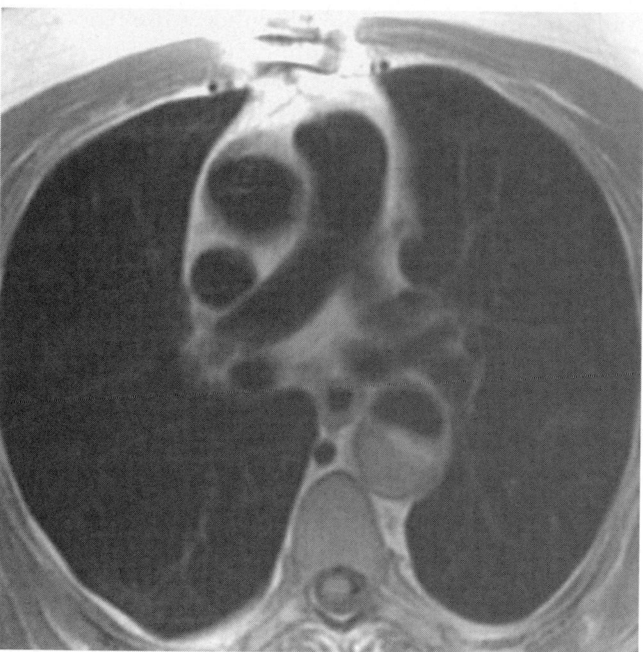

Figure 37-8 Magnetic resonance imaging of aortic dissection. Axial image of the mid-descending thoracic aorta shows the linear signal of a dissection flap. The high sensitivity and specificity of this technique make it a valuable instrument for diagnosing acute dissections and following chronic dissections. (Image courtesy of David Bluemke, MD, Department of Radiology, Johns Hopkins Hospital.)

Aortography

Aortography was the first accurate diagnostic modality for evaluating patients suspected of having an aortic dissection and until recently was considered the gold standard of diagnostic tests. However compared with newer techniques, angiography has low sensitivity and requires a large volume of contrast that can have significant nephrotoxic effects. The low sensitivity of angiography was accepted as other, more accurate methods of investigation were not available. To visualize the entire aorta for signs of dissection, small amounts of contrast were injected at different levels, using different projections. Alternatively, intravenous aortography with digital subtraction may be performed, using less invasive techniques and smaller amounts of contrast media, but it provides lower-resolution images compared with conventional angiography. Injection into the false lumen is characterized by late filling with contrast or absence of branch vessels. The true lumen frequently is compressed and may appear spiral in shape. Aortography clearly identifies branch vessel involvement and is therefore valuable in assessing individuals with a sudden onset of acute renal failure, mesenteric or limb ischemia, hypertensive crisis, or new-onset neurologic findings. A missed diagnosis can occur in patients with a thrombosed false lumen or IMH. Despite these shortcomings, aortography remains a valuable tool to evaluate patients suspected of having aortic dissection. The invasive nature allows interventional procedures such as catheter-based fenestration of the dissection, intravascular ultrasound, and coronary angiography.

Intravascular ultrasound

Intravascular ultrasound (IVUS) was introduced as a technique to complement angiographic investigations of the aorta. The routine use of this technique to diagnose aortic dissections has not been tested; however, the sensitivity and specificity have been reported to be close to 100 percent.[37] This technique directly visualizes the vessel wall by using ultrasound transducers in the aorta lumen. The standard three-layer appearance of the aortic wall can be differentiated from that of the single-layer outer wall of the false lumen. Also, branch involvement can be seen clearly and the precise mechanism of vessel compromise may be visualized: either a dissection narrowing the origin or the ostium covered by a prolapsing intimal flap. Intramural hematomas appear as crescent-shaped or circumferential thickening. However, in regions with aneurysmal dilatation, the whole aorta cannot be seen. This technique may be most valuable in patients who are suspected of having an acute aortic dissection but have a normal aortogram.

Imaging during follow-up

Diagnostic imaging at the time of follow-up is mandatory. Follow-up of most patients is done with noninvasive tests such as helical CT angiography and MRI. Magnetic resonance imaging is probably first-line in following patients with chronic dissections and is particularly useful in those with renal insufficiency who are unable to tolerate the additional nephrotoxic contrast agents needed for CT scanning. An important consideration in ordering serial imaging is the ease with which findings can be compared to those from prior studies. It is therefore logical to use the same imaging modality as in prior studies to allow a one-to-one comparison. The current recommendation for following a dissection in an outpatient is to obtain a baseline study before discharge from the hospital and then at 6-month intervals for the first year and yearly thereafter. Aortic dilatation greater than 0.5 cm in a 6-month period is significant and warrants serial imaging at 3-month intervals if surgery is not yet indicated. Progressive aortic valve insufficiency should be followed with serial TTE.

MEDICAL THERAPY

Acute medical therapy

Aggressive medical therapy should be initiated at the first clinical suspicion of an aortic dissection and continued throughout the workup and treatment phases, including patients who are destined for the surgical arm of therapy. The location of the evaluation and resuscitation is determined by the hemodynamic stability of the patient. An unstable patient belongs in the operating room. A stable patient can undergo a more detailed evaluation, including transport to other areas of the hospital for testing and imaging. Before transport to remote areas of the hospital, the patient should be moved to an intensive care unit for placement of appropriate monitoring: an indwelling arterial catheter, central venous access, and a Foley catheter. Regardless of the progress in the diagnostic process, in any patient suspected of having an aortic dissection, the primary goal of medical therapy is to arrest the dissecting process by means of optimal pain management and blood pressure control. The target systolic blood pressure should be between 100 and 120 mmHg, though this must be modified if oliguria or neurologic symptoms develop. It is preferable to avoid procedures that may precipitate further dissection and possible rupture, such as TEE and insertion of an invasive line in an extremely anxious patient, until pain, anxiolytic therapy, and blood pressure control can be achieved.

The mainstay of medical therapy for aortic dissection began in the 1960s with the landmark paper by Wheat and associates[15] that linked the progression of dissections to both mean arterial pressure and the rate of rise (dP/dt) of the arterial pulse. The class of drugs most successful at controlling both of these factors has been the class of beta-adrenergic blocking agents. The first agent used was the nonselective beta blocker propranolol (0.05 to 0.15 mg/kg every 4 to 6 h). More commonly today, cardiac-specific beta-blocking agents (beta$_1$ selective) are first-line, with other agents added to control blood pressure after the heart rate is suppressed adequately and the inotropic state is decreased. Hemodynamically unstable patients and those potentially intolerant to beta blockers because of bradycardia, heart failure, or asthma may benefit from beta-blocking agents with ultrashort half-lives such as esmolol (loading dose 0.5 mg/kg over 2 to 5 min, followed by an infusion 0.10 to 0.20 mg/kg/min). If compromising effects are seen, the drug infusion can be withheld until the untoward effects are diminished. The loading dose of esmolol can be held to avoid severe hypotension during its introduction. If beta-blocking agents alone do not control blood pressure adequately, vasodilating agents such as sodium nitroprusside (initial dose 0.25 μg/kg/min) should be added. However, since these agents used alone can increase the force of left ventricular ejection (dP/dt), they should be used concomitantly with beta-blocking agents. Another useful drug is labetalol (10 to 20 to 80 mg every 15 min), which has alpha-adrenergic blocking properties in addition to nonselective beta-adrenergic antagonist properties. This reduces the peripheral resistance without significantly decreasing the heart rate or cardiac output. Although there are limited data supporting the use of calcium channel blocking agents (verapamil, diltiazem, nifedipine, nicardipine), it seems reasonable to use these agents in this population to reduce blood pressure if the other agents are not available or are not tolerated.

Changes in peripheral pulses, spinal cord or central nervous system changes, continued pain in spite of adequate blood pressure control, signs of cardiac tamponade, and changes in aortic valve sounds can signify extension of the dissection. Other signs of propagation of the tear include new myocardial ischemia and renal compromise. Patients with significant hemodynamic instability or neurologic impairment may need orotracheal intubation to provide improved safety for travel to diagnostic modalities such as MRI, CT, and angiography. Intubation also allows increased sedation to blunt the hypertension seen with TEE probe insertion.

Long-term medical management

Patients who survive aortic dissection repair and those being medically managed with chronic type A or B dissections begin a lifelong requirement of optimal medical therapy and close follow-up. Meticulous blood pressure control is particularly difficult in hypertensive patients on a multidrug regimen. Recurrence of a dissection, propagation of a current lesion, or aneurysmal dilatation of a chronic dissection is seen in higher percentages of patients with poor blood pressure control [systolic blood pressure(SBP) above 120 mmHg]. Healing of the dissection can be achieved with medical therapy, but this is rare. In these cases, the false lumen disappears and a thickened, scarred wall develops. Physical examination follow-up every 6 months is recommended.

INTERVENTIONAL RADIOLOGY

Surgical therapy has been the mainstay for acute type A dissections and for type B dissections with complications of aortic rupture, impending rupture, or organ malperfusion. However, aortic replacement has not been without significant in-hospital mortality and morbidity. As a result, other, less invasive techniques are under investigation, particularly for the management of type B dissections. Specifically, two percutaneous methods have been investigated to manage those with aortic dissections: balloon fenestration and, more recently, endovascular aortic stent graft placement.

Catheter-based fenestration

Catheter-based balloon fenestration between the true and false lumens essentially creates controlled reentry tears in the dissection flap to reestablish flow to obliterated branches.[38–40] Flow from the aortic lumen with a satisfactory blood pressure (usually the false lumen) to the lumen being compromised (usually a collapsed true lumen) provides blood flow to the branch vessels. It should be noted that the true lumen often stays collapsed several centimeters below the fenestration. Therefore, the fenestration should be at or near the level of the affected branch vessels. Although this minimally invasive approach appears to be desirable, it often requires extended periods in the interventional suite and frequently is followed by severe hypotension related to reperfusion.

Endovascular aortic stent grafting

Upper abdominal balloon fenestration often does not eliminate the transseptal pressure gradient completely, and self-expandable covered stents have to be deployed within the aortic lumen above the compromised branch vessels. This method was reported in 1990, and only a few centers in the United States have significant experience with it. Stenting of the thoracic aorta has been found to be technically complex, particularly for the arch. However, currently the main obstacle to expansion of thoracic aortic stenting is the lack of a clinically available device. Interventionalists have been able to circumvent this problem in patients with small-diameter thoracic aortas by deploying several abdominal aortic covered stents in series. The major theoretical disadvantages of aortic stenting are graft migration, unproven long-term stability, and fear that placement of intraluminal stents will compromise future aortic surgery. There are three situations in which stent placement appears to be preferred to fenestration: when the false lumen cannot be accessed successfully, making fenestration impossible; when significant thrombus is present in the false lumen, risking transseptal embolization; and when there is diffuse, severe true lumen collapse that would require multiple fenestrations.

SURGICAL THERAPY

General points

Indications for surgical repair of an acute dissection include involvement of the ascending aorta (Stanford type A) or failure of medical management of any acute type B dissection as demonstrated by continued pain or hypertension despite appropriate medical therapy, evidence of progression of the dissection, signs of impaired organ or extremity perfusion, and signs of impending rupture. Indications for repair of chronic dissections are similar yet more commonly include recurrent pain or significant aneurysmal dilatation. An aortic diameter of 5 to 5.5 cm warrants surgical intervention. This is particularly true in patients with connective tissue disorders such as Marfan's disease and Ehlers-Danlos syndrome. The decision to operate on a patient with an intramural hematoma or a penetrating atherosclerotic ulcer is very similar to the indications for a classical aortic dissection, including almost universally an emergent procedure if the ascending aorta is involved. The urgency is related to the superficial nature of this disease process and the higher propensity of rupture. A point to keep in mind is that repair is best performed in an elective setting rather than in an emergency setting after rupture or malperfusion.

In general, any patient with a type A dissection requires operative repair unless this is deemed to present an unreasonably high operative risk. This subset of patients probably would not survive an operation or simply would refuse one and require optimized medical management. Differentiating the category a patient is in, high-risk versus inoperable, is not always easy. It has been suggested that interval or permanent nonoperative management of acute type A dissections may be permitted in select patients: those who are referred and those whose conditions are diagnosed several days after presentation and who have survived the early dangerous period. These patients can undergo the surgery semielectively rather than emergently. As a blanket statement, this may be true; however, as a policy, operative management of a type A dissections should not be delayed. There are four patient populations in whom it is probably advisable to delay operative repair: severe head injury, septic, significant burn surface area, and severe pulmonary contusion. For those with severe brain trauma whose prognosis is uncertain, it is best to wait until the patient has made a significant neurologic recovery. Clamping and unclamping of the aorta can cause swings in cerebral perfusion pressure and worsen existing perfusion abnormalities. Infectious complications are too great for septic patients and those at high risk of infection, such as patients with serious burns.

Patients more than 80 years of age have long been known to be at high risk; however, increased age is only a relative contraindication, and experienced aortic surgeons have demonstrated satisfactory results in this population. Patients who are comatose or obtunded are unlikely to improve after surgery, yet there have been numerous reports of miraculous improvements after paralysis or stroke. Some groups recommend early operation in patients with collagen vascular disease, large false aneurysms, medical compliance issues, aortas with large penetrating ulcers, and significant IMHs. Once surgical therapy is indicated, the technique of repair is up to the surgeon: graft replacement of the affected aortic segment, surgical fenestration, or thromboexclusion. Graft replacement is by far the most common choice worldwide.

Operative technique

Anesthesia

Single-lumen endotracheal tubes can be used for procedures performed through a median sternotomy, whereas a double-lumen tube is almost mandatory for procedures performed through a left thoracotomy or thoracoabdominal incision. Arterial monitoring usually includes one or two radial artery catheters, depending on the location of the dissection. Additionally, if femoral artery cannulation is employed for cardiopulmonary bypass, another site of interest is distal to the aortic cross clamp to measure distal (visceral) pressures. This can be accomplished most easily by monitoring femoral artery cannula perfusion pressures. Central venous access is necessary for the delivery of pharmacologic agents, potential rapid administration of crystalloid and blood products, and placement of a pulmonary artery catheter if needed. Upper body temperatures usually are measured with an esophageal probe, and lower body temperatures with a urinary bladder probe at the tip of a Foley catheter or a rectal probe. Tympanic membrane, esophageal, or nasopharyngeal temperatures can be used to estimate brain temperatures in patients who are undergoing hypothermic circulatory arrest.

Cardiopulmonary bypass

There are several arterial and venous cannulation configurations, depending on the location of the dissection. For Stanford type A dissections, the standard cardiopulmonary bypass circuit is from the right atrium, using a two-stage cannula, to the uninvolved distal aortic arch, peformed with TEE guidance. Alternative arterial cannulation sites for antegrade perfusion include the innominate artery and the right axillary artery and, rarely, through the left ventricular apex. Either femoral artery can be used for retrograde perfusion if the descending aorta is not involved. There is some debate about which femoral artery to use in the setting of lower body malperfusion, though intuitively the groin with the weaker pulse would be the artery to cannulate since greater flow, as well as arterial pressure, would be through the contralateral groin artery with the false lumen. Since abdominal dissections often involve the left femoral artery and continue toward the left lower extremity, cannulation often is done through a cut down on the right groin. Perfusion of the false lumen would result in further retrograde dissection and malperfusion of the aortic branch vessels. If this occurs, cardiopulmonary bypass has to be discontinued and the contralateral artery must be used for cannulation. Once bypass is initiated and after approximately 40 min of cooling to reach the target temperature, the heart is unloaded by venous exsanguination to the pump reservoir and the aorta is clamped. Cardiopulmonary bypass is continued with systemic hypothermia (18°C), low flow (1000 to 1500 mL/min/m^2), and low pressure (30 to 50 mmHg). Cardioplegia often is delivered through a retrograde coronary sinus catheter, with additional protection delivered with a handheld cannula down the uninvolved coronary ostia.

Repairs of acute type B dissections are performed routinely with a partial left heart bypass or a full cardiopulmonary bypass. The formally popular clamp-and-sew technique has fallen largely out of favor, though it continues to be used by some surgeons, with acceptable results. Because partial left heart bypass does not require an oxygenator or pump suction, the dose of heparin can be significantly lower (100 units per kilogram) than it is with routine open heart surgery. Furthermore, if proximal extension of the dissection is discovered, conversion to a circuit capable of hypothermic circulatory arrest is relatively simple, involving the addition of an oxygenator and a femoral venous cannula. Venous drainage of oxygenated blood is done through a left inferior pulmonary vein or the left atrium, and arterial cannulation sites include the distal thoracic aorta and the femoral artery. However, rather than directly cannulate the femoral artery, the authors routinely attach a prosthetic graft to allow continued circulation to the leg and preserve vessel integrity. Briefly, an 8-mm Dacron tube graft is sutured end to side to the common femoral artery, using a running 5-0 polypropylene suture. This size graft easily accommodates a 22F arterial cannula. Next, a 16-gauge central venous catheter is inserted through the graft, using the Seldinger technique to allow the perfusionist to measure distal (visceral) pressures continuously.

Cerebral and spinal cord protection

Surgical repair of the aortic arch frequently requires a period of altered blood flow to the brain. Cerebral protection during this critical period can be achieved with continued antegrade or retrograde cerebral perfusion, deep hypothermic circulatory arrest (HCA), or a combination of the two. In 1957, DeBakey was the first to use selective antegrade cerebral perfusion to resect an aortic arch aneurysm; however, worldwide acceptance did not occur because of the initial disappointing results. Repair of these lesions was all but abandoned until 1975, when Griepp and colleagues demonstrated the successful use of HCA alone.[41] The basic concept of this technique is that cerebral cooling reduces neuronal metabolic activity, preventing injury from lethal excitatory neurotransmitters, free radicals, and the triggering of apoptosis (programmed cell death).[42] Currently, the consensus is that 30 to 40 min of hypothermic circulatory arrest at 18°C is relatively safe; however, increased cognitive decline can be expected as the time increases. Although large animal studies offer evidence that profound hypothermia (5 to 7°C) may provide superior cerebral protection,[43] most surgeons use 18 to 20°C because of fear of nonischemic neuron and pneumocyte injury (Table 37-5). An additional advantage of HCA is that it provides a bloodless field and allows the surgeon to excise the aorta at the site of the distal clamp; the technique also is at least conceptually simple to perform. Hypothermia is achieved by slow cooling during cardiopulmonary bypass, with a maximal 10°C temperature gradient between the patient and the perfusate until the ideal temperature is reached. Tympanic membrane or nasopharyngeal temperatures are used to guide theoretical brain temperatures; however, these temperatures are notoriously unpredictable. Electroencephalographic monitoring can be used to identify the absence of brain activity. Additionally, the head routinely is packed in ice during the cooling and hypothermic periods. Steroid and barbiturate administration has some theoretical advantages, though its use has not been shown consistently to provide further neuroprotection. Reinitiation of cardiopulmonary bypass and systemic rewarming proceed without exceeding a 10°C temperature gradient. Mannitol and furosemide are used by many surgeons to promote free radical scavenging and minimize neuronal swelling. Despite numerous successes with HCA, surgical strategies have changed, and at this time most surgeons make every attempt to avoid HCA alone and prefer to provide continuous blood flow to the central nervous system.

Table 37-5 Estimates of safe periods of circulatory arrest at different core temperatures

Temperature, °C	Estimated safe duration of hypothermic circulatory arrest, min
37	5
30	9
25	14
20	21
15	31
10	45

From McCollough JN, Zhang N, Reich, et al. Cerebral metabolic suppression during circulatory arrest in humans. *Ann Thorac Surg* 1999;67:1895.

In 1990, Ueda and associates[44] proposed the use of retrograde cerebral perfusion, a technique previously used to treat large air embolisms during cardiopulmonary bypass, as an adjunct to HCA in an attempt to prolong its safe duration. There is significant debate about how much blood actually reaches the brain, whether cerebral edema occurs, and whether any clinical improvement is seen after its use. As a result, this technique has not been adopted widely. Those who employ retrograde perfusion tend to use it for brief periods during HCA or in cases in which the risk of embolic events is high. The details of the technique depend on the venous cannulation used for cardiopulmonary bypass. If bicaval cannulation is used, reverse flow through the superior vena cava is simple and effective. If a dual-stage venous cannula has been used, a retrograde coronary sinus catheter can be placed similarly in the superior vena cava (SVC) with a purse-string suture. A flow rate in the SVC high enough to maintain a pressure of 15 to 25 mmHg is recommended.

Several large retrospective studies have shown improved neuroprotection with selective antegrade cerebral perfusion, and the largest series to date (413 patients) demonstrated comparable neurologic outcomes after more than 90 min of cerebral perfusion.[45] At the authors' institution, surgeons routinely employ selective antegrade cerebral perfusion, using right axillary cannulation (usually with a 6- or 8-mm Dacron graft and a 22F arterial cannula sewn end to side to the axillary artery) or, less commonly, cannulation of the innominate artery or distal ascending aorta. The axillary arteries are rarely calcified or involved in the dissection process. The concept of antegrade blood flow is appealing and is certainly more physiologic than retrograde flow or circulatory arrest. There is also a trend toward using warmer perfusion temperatures (25°C); this allows shorter cardiopulmonary bypass (CPB) times and a theoretical reduction in coagulation disorders; however, it may risk higher rates of brain and spinal cord injury. Also, one must be aware that manipulation of the aortic arch can cause dislodgement of atheroembolic debris, particularly if the aortic arch is severely calcified.

Spinal cord injury resulting in paraplegia can be a devastating outcome after an aortic dissection or repair.

The incidence of spinal cord ischemia after repair of a type B dissection can be as high as 19 to 36 percent.[46,47] Several techniques have been used for spinal cord protection: pharmacologic agents (steroids, free radical scavengers, adenosine, vasodilators), partial bypass, and cerebrospinal fluid drainage.[48] Preoperative aortography with selective cannulation of the artery of Adamkiewicz can direct surgeons in regard to important intercostal regions to reimplant during the surgical repair.

Hemostasis

Surgical repair of aortic dissections can be associated with large-volume blood loss; thus, immediate access to packed red blood cells, platelets, and fresh frozen plasma is mandatory. Preoperative coagulopathy, prolonged CPB, and hypothermic circulatory arrest all contribute to further difficulties in the maintenance of anastomotic hemostasis. Thin, diseased aortic walls also contribute to the technical difficulties encountered in this patient population. Currently, several types of adhesives have been used to approximate the dissected aortic wall and "condition" the tissue for sutures in an attempt to prevent disruption of the anastomosis. Fibrin glue and gelatin resorcinol formalin biologic glue (GFR) have been used more widely in Europe and Asia, and a glutaraldehyde–bovine serum albumen (BSA) combination is widely accepted in the United States (BioGlue), CryoLife, Kennesaw, GA). Long-term clinical outcome studies and investigations into the materials' carcinogenic potential have not been elucidated fully. Toxicity from components of the glue, formalin in particular, has been reported. Bleeding from graft interstices was a significant problem in older-generation grafts but has been all but eliminated by the use of more recent polyester collagen-impregnated grafts.

Other techniques to prevent bleeding include reinforcement of the suture lines with Teflon felt pledgets, strips, or rings. Many surgeons have described sandwiching the dissected aorta between the graft and the outer Teflon felt strip. The authors occasionally suture the Teflon felt between the wall of the true and false lumens, essentially placing it in the false lumen.

Antifibrinolytic agents such as aprotinin and aminocaproic acid can be useful yet may be most effective when administered before the procedure. The caveat is that many surgeons prefer to administer aprotinin during the rewarming phase after hypothermic circulatory arrest rather than before it is initiated.

Stanford type A dissection

Ascending aortic replacement

Stanford type A dissections are best approached through a median sternotomy. As cardiopulmonary bypass is being initiated, the PA window can be dissected, and the ascending aorta can be freed from the surrounding tissue. A longitudinal aortotomy is done to resect the dissected intima, provide access to the coronary ostia for cold cardioplegia, and allow inspection of the aortic valve for incompetence. Occasionally, one or more of the aortic commissures can be untethered from the aortic wall by the dissection. If this occurs, it is necessary to resuspend the aortic commissures by using simple pledgeted sutures[49] (Fig. 37-9). If salvage of the valve seems unlikely, there is significant involvement or dilatation of the root, or the patient has a known connective tissue disorder, one more likely will need to

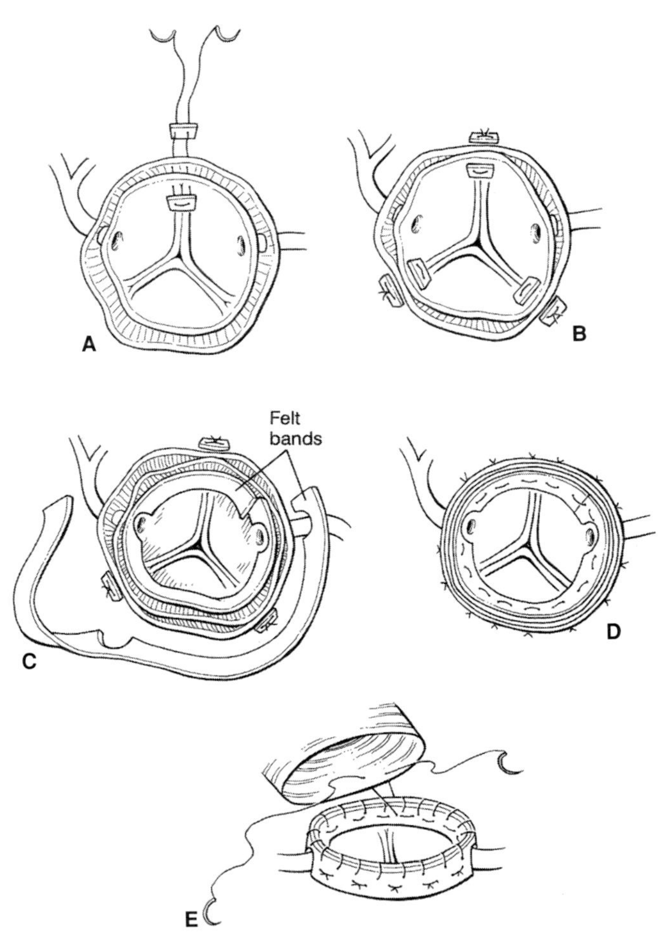

Figure 37-9 Aortic valve resuspension. If the aortic valve commissures become untethered from the aortic wall, it is necessary to reattach them by using simple pledgeted sutures (A and B). If the valve is deemed competent and appears salvageable, further reinforcement is needed to obliterate the false lumen at the aortic root. One technique is to place felt (polytetrafluoroethylene) strips on the inside and outside of the aorta to create a sewing cuff (C and D). The ascending tube graft then can be sewn to the newly created cuff (E). [From Stone C, Borst H. Dissecting aortic aneurysms. In: Edmunds LJ Jr (ed). *Cardiac Surgery in the Adult.* New York: McGraw-Hill; 1997:1125.]

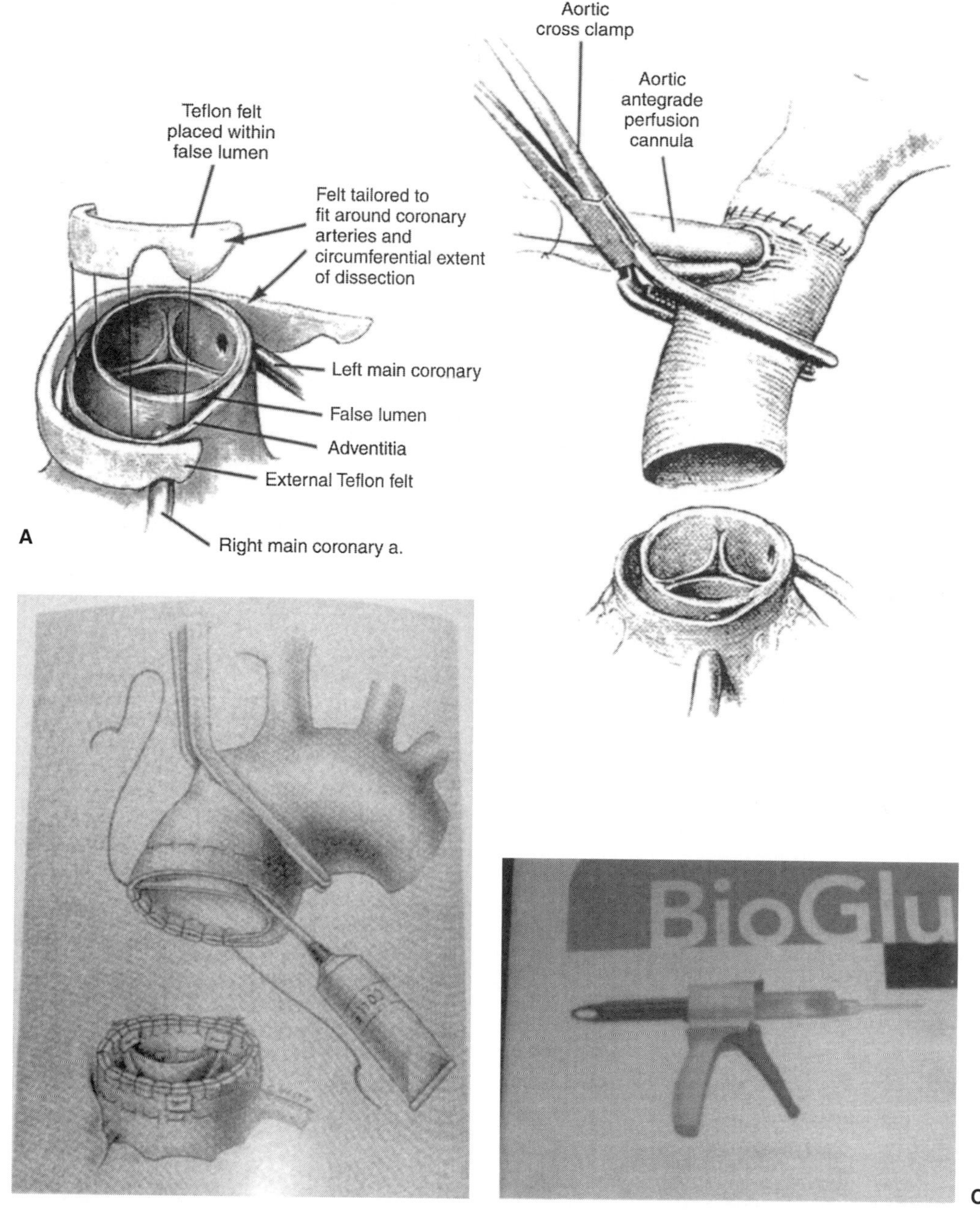

Figure 37-10 Ascending aorta replacement. Preservation of the aortic valve is often possible after Stanford type A dissections. Obliteration of the false lumen with external and internal polytetrafluoroethylene (PTFE) strips often can be achieved with further assistance from new bioadhesives that also "condition" the aorta wall. Patient rewarming after hypothermic circulatory arrest can be aided by graft cannulation and reinstitution of cardiopulmonary bypass while the proximal anastomosis is being completed. (From Yun KL, Miller DC. Technique of aortic valve preservation in acute type A aortic dissection. *Oper Tech Cardiol Thorac Surg* 1996;1:68.)

proceed to root replacement using a composite graft. If the valve is competent, the aorta is transected above the commissures and BioGlue is injected into the false lumen. This area is reinforced with Teflon strips to create a "sewing cuff" at the origin of the aorta, or strips are used during the graft-aorta anastomosis to provide added support. Then attention is directed to the distal segment where it is trimmed at the clamp site and prepared for the anastomosis. A Dacron tube graft then is sutured end to end to the remaining aorta, essentially replacing the diseased aorta (Fig. 37-10). The patient then can be rewarmed and weaned from CPB.

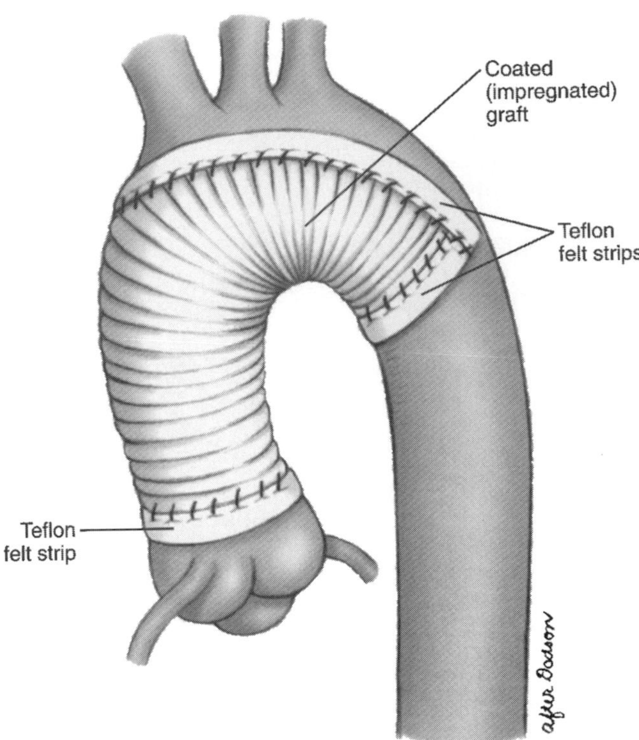

Figure 37-11 Hemiarch replacement. When a Stanford type A dissection extends into the proximal aortic arch, it is possible to replace part of the arch with the ascending aorta. Teflon felt strips frequently are used for further reinforcement. [From Galla JD, McCullough JN, Ergin MA, et al. Surgical techniques, aortic arch and deep hypothermic circulatory arrest: Real-life suspended animation. In: Elefteriades JA (ed). *Cardiology Clinics: Diseases of the Aorta*, vol 17. Philadelphia: Saunders; 1999:767.]

Aortic arch replacement

If the intimal tear originates in the arch or begins in the ascending aorta and extends into the aortic arch, it probably has to be replaced. However, if only part of the arch is involved, the surgical procedure may be limited to a hemiarch, which basically consists of replacement of the inferior wall of the aorta (Fig. 37-11). If the dissection involves the root and the entire arch, it is best replaced using circulatory arrest conditions, with a composite root replacement for the ascending aorta and a Dacron tube graft for the arch. A hole is made in the graft for attachment of the "island" of neck vessels. If those vessels also are dissected, most surgeons advocate individualized attachment rather than the use of a single island. The distal anastomosis is completed first, followed by the arch vessel island (Fig. 37-12). To minimize circulatory arrest time, a clamp can be placed on the transverse arch graft just proximal to the innominate artery to allow the reinitiation of CPB. Then the ascending aorta graft can be anastomosed to the transverse arch graft.

Composite aortic root replacement

Patients with a significantly dilated aortic root, those with severely diseased aortic valves, and those with connective tissue disorders usually need replacement of the aortic root rather than resuspension or repair. Replacement of the separate components of both an aortic valve and a tube graft has not had favorable long-term results. However, composite graft replacement (graft with valve attached), the modified Bentall procedure, has had outstanding short- and long-term results[50,51] (Fig. 37-13). Cannulation, cardioplegia, and cardiopulmonary bypass are as described for conventional

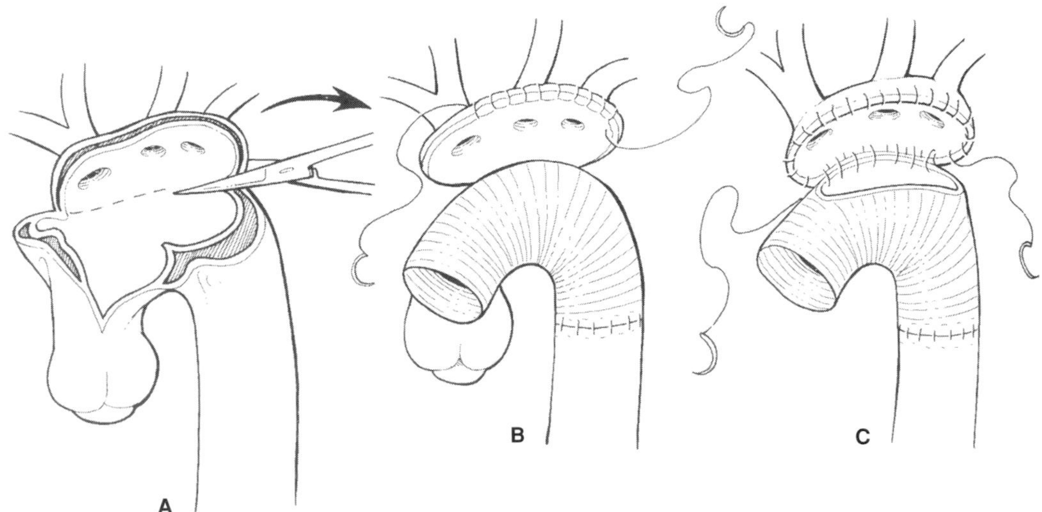

Figure 37-12 Aortic arch replacement. If the entire aortic arch is being replaced, it is often best done as an "island" of neck vessels in a single anastomosis. A. The arch vessels are excised from the dissected aortic arch. B. The aortic walls are reapproximated with a continuous suture or outer and inner layer of polytetrafluoroethylene felt strips, and the distal anastomosis is completed. C. The island is attached to the superior portion of the graft. [From Stone C, Borst H. Dissecting aortic aneurysm. In: Edmunds LJ Jr (ed). *Cardiac Surgery in the Adult.* New York: McGraw-Hill; 1997:1125.]

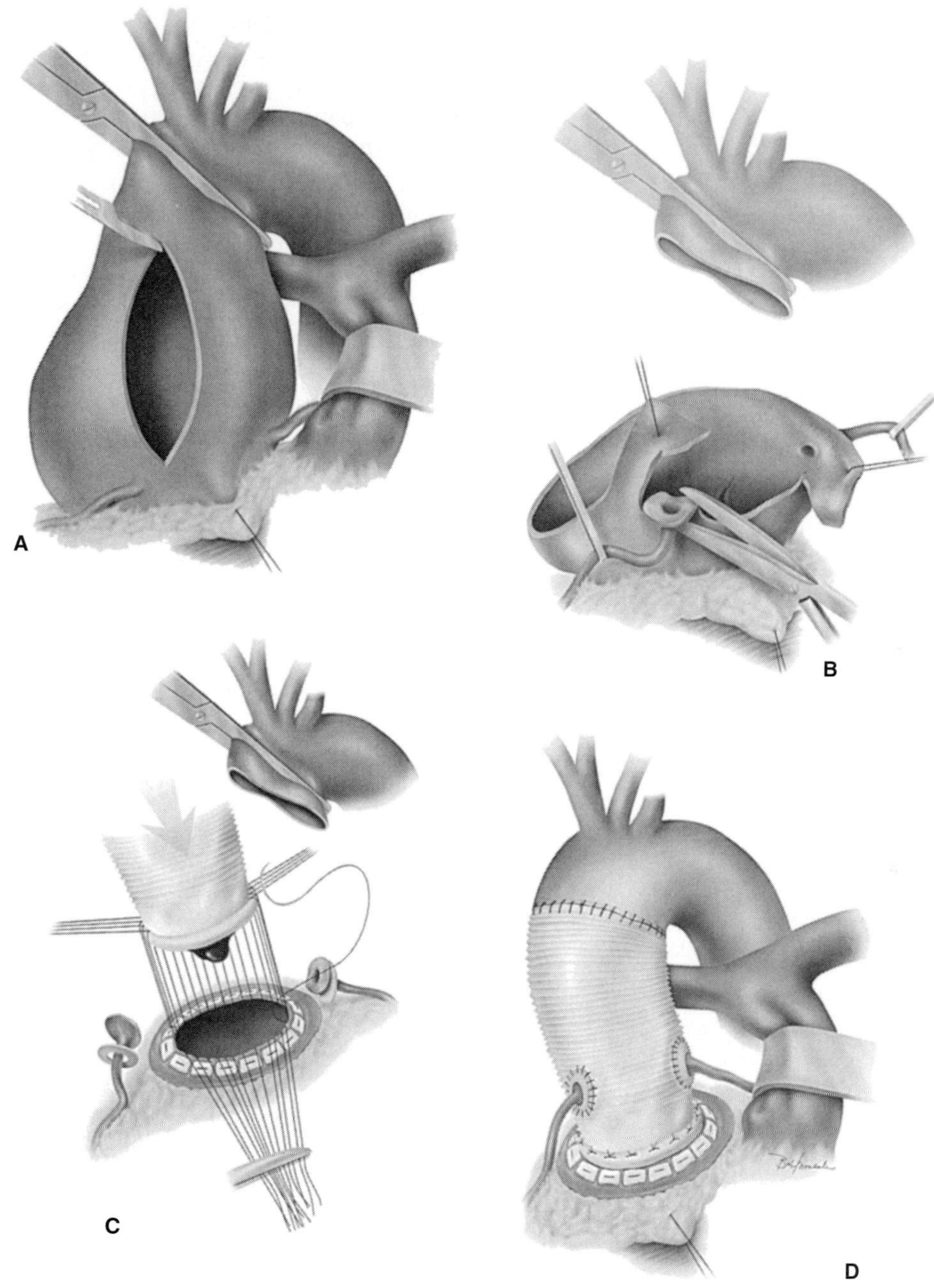

Figure 37-13 Composite aortic root replacement. A. Aorta is cross-clamped, and ascending aorta is opened. B. Aorta is transected, and coronary arteries are excised as buttons. C. The composite graft is sewn to the annulus. D. Distal anastomosis is completed, and the coronary buttons, with polytetrafluoroethylene pledget washers for reinforcement, are attached to the graft. [From Cameron DE. Surgical techniques: Ascending aorta. In: Elefteriades JA (ed). *Cardiology Clinics: Diseases of the Aorta*, vol 17. Philadelphia: Saunders; 1999:739.]

aortic root replacement surgery. The aortic root is excised, along with excision of the aortic leaflets. Interrupted pledgeted 2-0 Tevdek sutures are placed in the annulus and then into the suture ring of the composite prosthesis. If the coronary arteries have migrated more than 12 mm from the annulus, an everting mattress suture is used. If the coronary ostia are low-lying, the mattress sutures are placed below the annulus, allowing the coronary arteries to be anastomosed directly to the graft in an end-to-side fashion. Alternatively, the dissected coronary ostia can be identified and small "coronary buttons" of aortic tissue can be created,

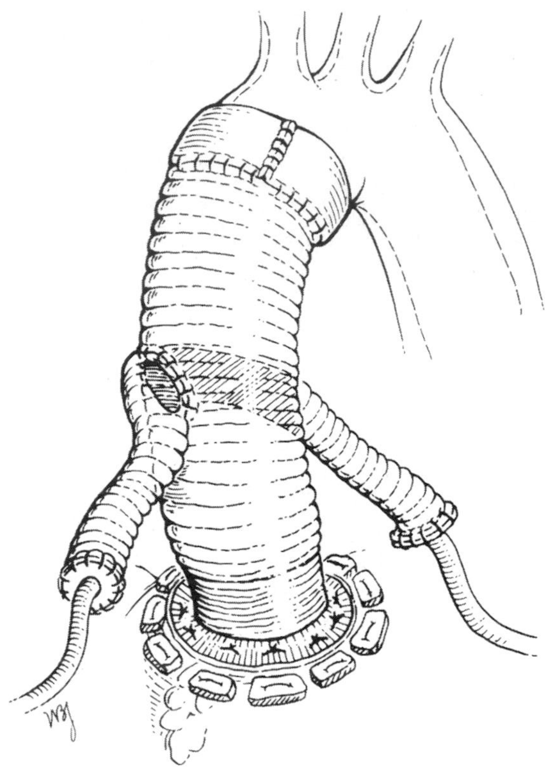

Figure 37-14 Cabrol modification. When mobilization of the coronary ostia is not possible or the length is not sufficient for implantation on the composite graft, other techniques are available to provide flow to the coronary arteries. The Cabrol modification utilizes an interposed graft between the coronary ostia and a side-to-side anastomosis to the composite graft. [Right side from Ergin MA, Griepp RB. Dissections of the aorta. In: Baue AE, Geha AS, Hammond GL, et al (eds). *Glenn's Thoracic and Cardiovascular Surgery*. Stamford CT: Appleton and Lange; 1991:2273.]

allowing an anastomosis with a hole cut in the graft. Usually a circular polytetrafluoroethylene (PTFE) felt washer is used to approximate and reinforce the potentially dissected coronary artery. Alternatively, closure of the coronary ostia with coronary artery bypass grafting has been attempted, although this has had poor long-term results.[52] Another alternative is the Cabrol modification, which utilizes an interposed graft between the coronary ostia and a side-to-side anastomosis to the composite graft[53,54] (Fig. 37-14). Similarly poor results have limited the widespread use of this technique for most composite replacements.

Valve-preserving root replacement

The role of valve-preserving root replacement in routine dilated aortic roots remains to be determined, and some would say it has no role in a patient with an acute aortic dissection. However, Frist and Miller[55] at Stanford University reported preservation of native valves in 84 percent of patients with type A dissections. However, the valves could be salvaged in only 50 percent of patients with chronic dissections because of established pathology.[55] A simple rule to guide the surgeon is that if the root is dilated to more than 36 mm, a composite graft probably is needed. Also, if the dissection continues proximally to include the coronary ostia, the procedure becomes very technically challenging and may present unnecessary risks to the patient unless it is done in the most experienced hands. However, aortic valve preservation in a nondilated root can avoid the complications of valve prosthesis and the anticoagulation required after the placement of a composite graft. Cannulation, cardioplegia, and CPB are as described for conventional aortic root replacement surgery. The aortic root is excised, leaving a 3-mm margin of aortic sinus tissue on the aortic annulus, and the height is approximately two-thirds the diameter of the graft. Then the coronary arteries are freely mobilized. A Dacron graft with a diameter that optimizes leaflet coaptation (28 to 30 mm in adults) then is sewn to the aortic annulus. Three horizontal mattress sutures (4-0 polypropylene) are placed from the inside of the graft to the top of the vertical incisions made for each commissure. One arm of each suture is run in a continuous fashion around the aortic annulus to seat the graft to the annulus. Teflon felt strips can be used to reinforce the suture line and facilitate hemostasis. Holes are cut in the Dacron graft opposite the coronary arteries and then anastomosed with continuous 4-0 polypropylene sutures. A Teflon felt washer can be used to provide further support (Fig. 37-15).

Stanford type B dissections

Acute aortic dissections of the distal arch and those starting distal to the left subclavian artery that extend proximally require emergency surgery, using a median sternotomy and elephant trunk when possible. Dissections clearly beginning distal to the left subclavian artery may require surgery for continued expansion or be at risk for rupture. Chronic type B dissections may have a pronounced dilatation, frequently distorting normal anatomy and thus making cross-clamping below the left subclavian artery difficult, yet that area often is spared. Before surgery, these patients are best evaluated with contrast-enhanced 3-D CT scans to determine the anatomic relationships of the arch branches and determine the possible need for hypothermic circulatory arrest.

The standard incision for a type B dissection is a left thoracotomy or thoracoabdominal incision, depending on the extent of disease, with the hips swiveled to allow femoral access for cannulation. Cannulation and CPB are not different from those described for conventional aortic root replacement surgery and are

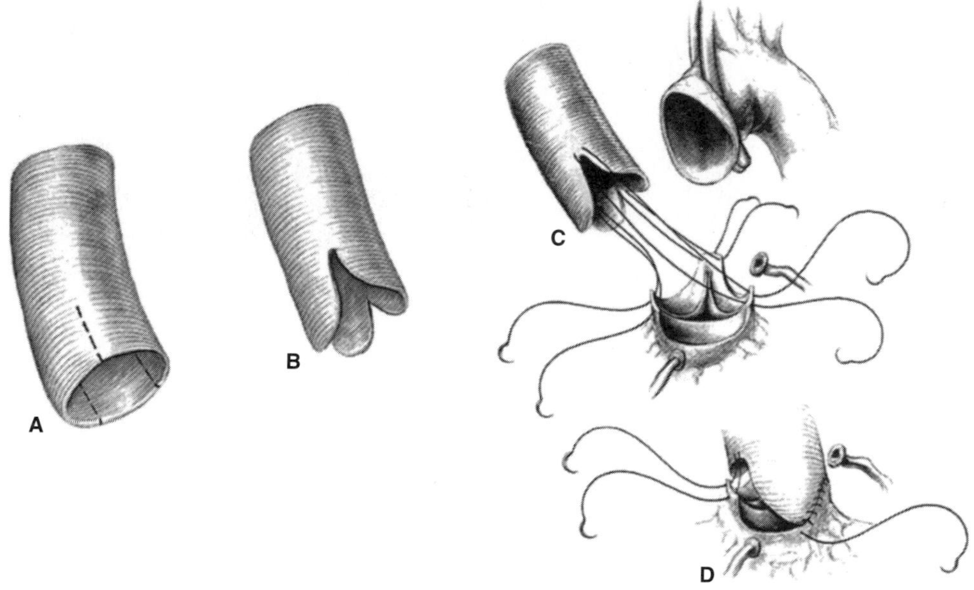

Figure 37-15 Valve-preserving root replacement. A. A Dacron graft size is selected that has a diameter that optimizes leaflet coaptation. B. Vertical incisions are made in the graft for each commissure. C. The coronary arteries are mobilized and the aortic root is excised, leaving a 3-mm margin of aortic sinus tissue on the aortic annulus and a height approximately two-thirds the diameter of the graft. Three horizontal mattress sutures are placed at each commissure and run in a continuous fashion around the annulus, and the coronary buttons are attached to the side of the graft. (From David TE. Remodeling the aortic root and preservation of the native aortic valve. *Oper Tech Card Thorac Surg* 1996;1:44.)

described in the CPB section in this chapter. Briefly, after CPB is initiated, the aorta is clamped to achieve proximal and distal control and then opened proximally to identify clearly the true and false lumens; then it is replaced or repaired segmentally. Every intercostal artery that is not believed to be the source of blood supply to the spinal cord is suture ligated. This can be determined to some extent by preoperative selective injection of the intercostal arteries. To prepare the proximal aorta for suturing, a Teflon felt strip is sutured on each side of the dissected aortic wall, creating a sewing cuff. A Dacron graft of the same diameter is anastomosed end to end to the sewing cuff. The preserved intercostal arteries then are anastomosed with a Carrel patch. The aortic clamp is moved distally, and the visceral vessels are reimplanted (Fig. 37-16). Alternatively, if the dissection extends into the abdomen and the diameter is less than 4 cm, the membrane can be resected and the remaining walls can be approximated (tailored) and reinforced with Teflon felt strips (Fig. 37-17).[56]

Several other techniques have been described to provide distal perfusion with oxygenated blood and unload the left ventricle during cross-clamping, including aortofemoral left heart bypass[57] and heparin-bonded "Gott" shunts.[58]

Surgical fenestration

Surgical fenestration first was performed by Gurin and assoicates[11] in 1935 and was the first surgical treatment for aortic dissection; however, it is seen currently by many surgeons as a procedure worthy of historical mention only. It initially was conceived because it made sense from a physiologic standpoint since it redirects blood back to the true lumen and, perhaps more important, reproduces the decompression of the false lumen seen in spontaneous survivors.

Nevertheless, patients who present with malperfusion symptoms warrant emergent redirection of flow from the false to the true lumen to prevent further ischemia and certain death. In patients with serious malperfusion of the distal aorta such as total obstruction of flow to the iliac vessels or viscera, surgical fenestration in the abdomen is a simple and well-tolerated procedure. It may be particularly valuable in patients with type B dissections who otherwise would not be candidates for proximal repair. The fenestration normally is completed in the infrarenal aorta (Fig. 37-18). Catheter-based fenestration has made this almost a historical procedure. However, knowledge of this technique may be valuable in centers without prompt access to a provider experienced in percutaneous techniques.

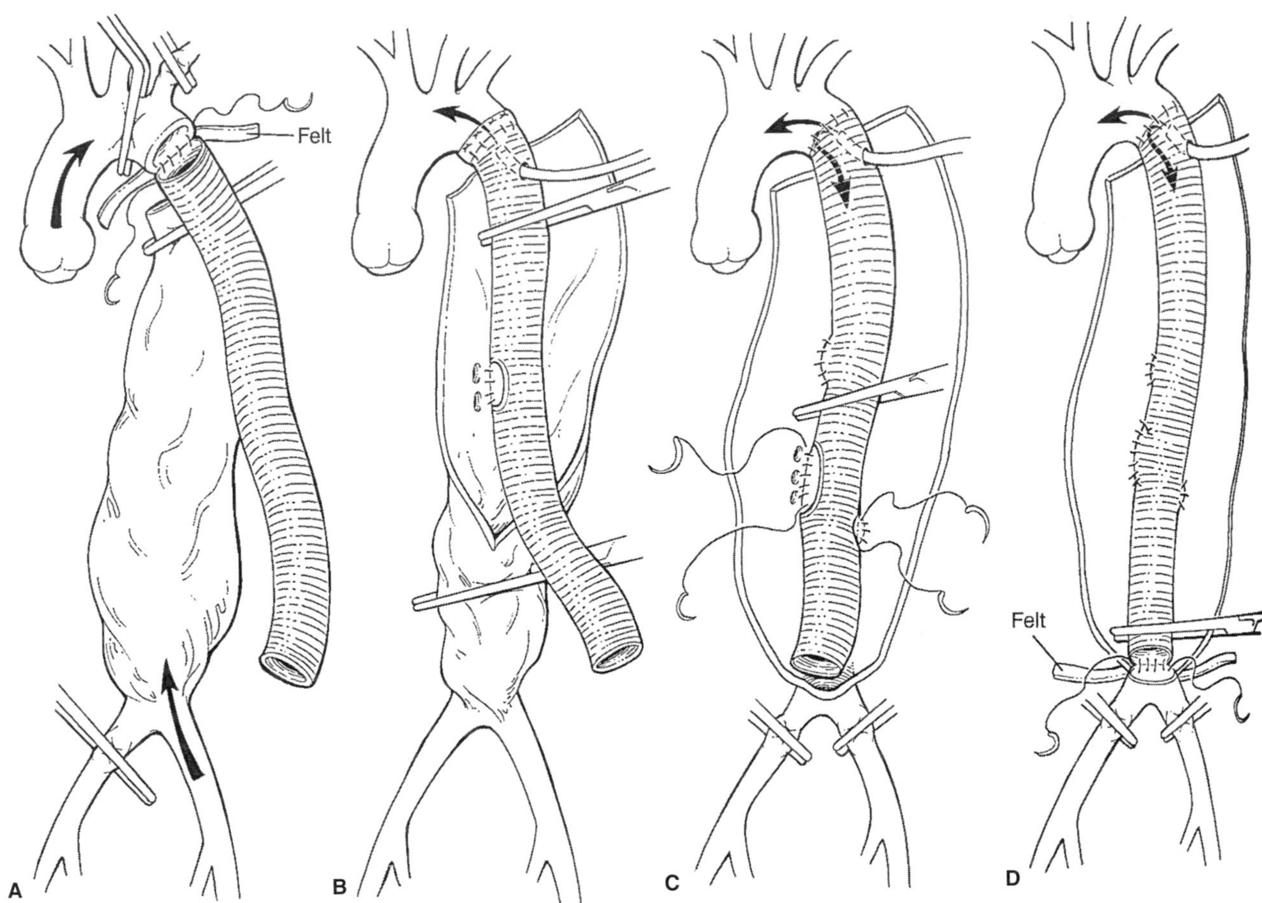

Figure 37-16 Repair of a type B dissection. Replacement of the thoracoabdominal aorta can be accomplished in a stepwise fashion. A. Femoral cannulation perfuses the lower body while the heart continues to eject, providing blood flow to the upper body and head. The aorta is transected just below the subclavian artery, and the aortic arch is inspected for disease. A graft is sewn end to end to the proximal aorta. B. The proximal clamp is moved to the graft, and a second arterial cannula is inserted into the graft to perfuse the head. The aorta is incised longitudinally, and bleeding intercostals of the upper six pairs are oversewn. A group of lower intercostal arteries believed to supply the spinal cord is sutured to the graft. C. The proximal clamp is moved down, and a patch of aorta containing the celiac, superior mesenteric, and right renal arteries is sewn to the graft. The left renal artery is sutured separately to the graft. D. The clamp is moved to below the visceral vessels, and the distal anastomosis is completed. [From Stone C, Borst H. Dissecting aortic aneurysm. In: Edmunds LJ Jr (ed). *Cardiac Surgery in the Adult.* New York: McGraw-Hill; 1997:1125.]

Thromboexclusion

Carpentier and colleagues[59] proposed a new surgical approach to aortic dissection in 1981 in an effort to correct the aortic lesion yet avoid the need to place sutures in the area of the dissection. The basic theoretical principles are as follows: Arterial reconstruction is done with an aortoaortic bypass graft that carries blood from the ascending aorta to a site on the nondissected aorta (usually infrarenal). A permanent clamp then is placed high on the descending aorta, preventing antegrade flow down the aorta and redirecting it down the newly created aortic conduit. Blood stagnates and ultimately thromboses in the false lumen of the segment of descending aorta that is devoid of major branches or is not in continuity with the true lumen receiving flow from the newly created aortic conduit. The progressive nature of the thrombosis allows for a period of circulatory adaptation, minimizing ischemia to the spinal cord (Fig. 37-19).

The thromboexclusion technique has several potential advantages: (1) The procedure can be performed without the use of cardiopulmonary bypass, (2) the entire operation is performed on nondissected aorta, and (3) there is no clamping of the descending aorta (before bypass) requiring cardiac unloading, spinal cord protection, and distal perfusion. One disadvantage is that thromboexclusion cannot be used for an already ruptured dissection. Visceral embolization with intestinal

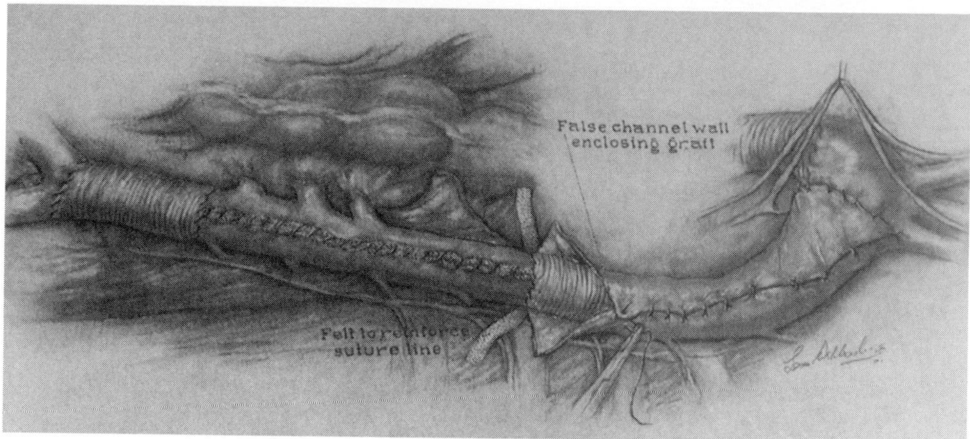

Figure 37-17 Aorta tailoring. If the aortic dissection extends into the abdomen and the diameter is less than 4 cm, the dissection flap can be resected and the remaining walls can be approximated (tailored) and reinforced with Teflon felt strips. [From Stone CD, Greene PS, Gott VL, et al. Single-stage repair of distal aortic arch and thoracoabdominal dissection aneurysms using aortic tailoring and circulatory arrest. *Ann Thorac Surg* 1994;57(3): 580–587.]

infarction and pancreatitis has been seen related to clamping of the aorta. In addition, the risks of paraplegia have not been eliminated.

The procedure is performed through a midline incision from the sternal notch to the pubis. A large-caliber Dacron graft (22 to 26 mm) is sewn end to side to the ascending aorta with the help of a side-biting clamp. The graft is routed through the right chest, usually exiting the diaphragm near the vena cava, and passes either in front of or behind the left lobe of the liver, behind the transverse mesocolon, and finally into the retroperitoneum. The distal anastomosis also is done in an end-to-side fashion to the infrarenal aorta with temporary occlusion of the aorta or a side-biting clamp. After flow is established through the graft, the descending aorta is occluded permanently just beyond the takeoff of the left subclavian artery. Because the Carpentier clamp is not commercially available in the United States, some authors advocate the use of a standard stapling device without reinforcing felt strips to occlude the aorta (TA-55, 4.8 mm, United States Surgical Corp., Norwalk, CT).[60]

RESULTS

The potential for a life-threatening cardiovascular event caused by an aortic dissection cannot be underestimated. In a review from Stanford University, the perioperative mortality rate for acute type A dissections was approximately 7 ± 5 percent and was even higher for chronic type A dissections (11 ± 7 percent). That review also demonstrated the seriousness of emergent repair of acute type B dissections. As others had experienced, they found that this disease process has an extremely high mortality rate (28 to 65 percent) and paraplegia (30 to 35 percent) incidence.[55] Similarly, results from the Yale–New Haven Hospital for type B dissections showed 1-year survival to be 47 percent and 5-year survival to be 28 percent. These relatively poor results are common and can be explained by the fact that many patients presented with or developed life-threatening complications because of the severity of the illness. Much of this is related to visceral or lower extremity ischemia.[61]

Long-term surgical results may be best demonstrated in a series of patients followed by the Stanford group for 30 years. In 174 patients with a type A dissection, 1-, 5-, 10-, and 15-year survival was 67 percent, 55 percent, 37 percent, and 24 percent, respectively. Additionally, that group followed 46 patients with type B dissections, who did not fare as well. Their survival over the same follow-up period was 56 percent, 48 percent, 29 percent, and 11 percent, respectively.[62]

SUMMARY

Acute aortic dissection is the most lethal process of the aorta and involves an intimal tear and layer separation, usually in the outer two-thirds of the media. Dissections are classified according to the origin of the intimal tear and the extent of the false lumen. Untreated dissections of the ascending aorta (Stanford type A) have extremely high mortality rates, with estimated losses of 1 to 2 percent per hour during the first 24 to 48 h, 75 percent at 2 weeks, and as high as 90 percent at 3 months. Some centers

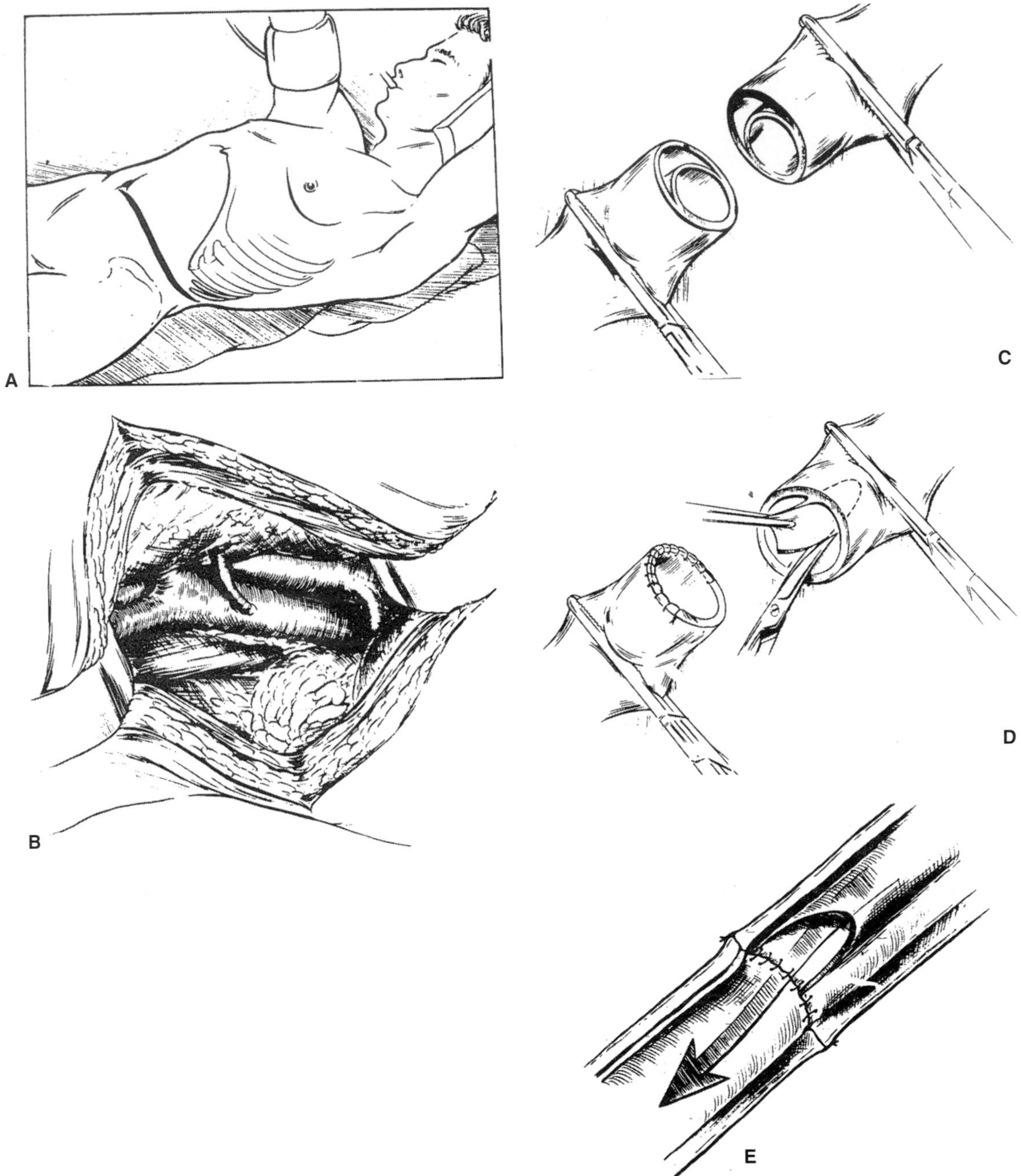

Figure 37-18 Surgical fenestration. A. A flank incision is made with the left side slightly elevated. B. Retroperitoneal dissection exposes the distal abdominal aorta. C. Division of the infrarenal aorta exposes the dissection flap as well as the true and false lumens. D. Excision of the dissection flap from the proximal segment and reapproximation of the layers of the aorta of the distal segment. E. End-to-end anastomosis redirecting flow to the true lumen. (From Elefteriades JA, Hartleroad J, Gusberg RJ, et al. Long-term experience with descending aortic dissection: The complication-specific approach. *Ann Thorac Surg* 1992;53:11–21.)

have demonstrated acceptable early mortality and short-term outcomes compared with historical data with regard to select type A patients cared for with interval surgery (semielective rather than emergent) or permanent nonoperative management. It is doubtful that these results can be achieved in a majority of centers. Type A dissections should be treated with aggressive medical therapy and then emergent surgical repair as soon as a patient is declared a surgical candidate. Operative mortality for acute type A dissection is

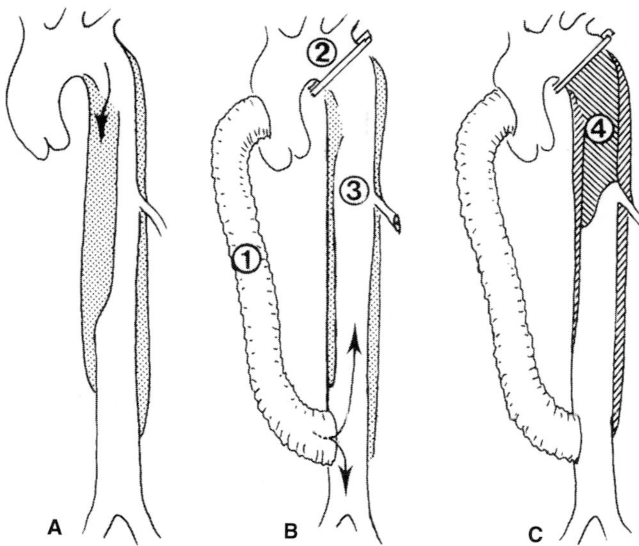

Figure 37-19 Thromboexclusion. The concept of reversal of flow and thromboexclusion is demonstrated in this schematic of an aortic dissection. 1. A Dacron graft is placed to bypass the dissected area of the aorta. 2. A permanent clamp or staple is placed at the upper limit of the dissection. 3. Flow reversal in the aorta returns blood to the true lumen and theoretically obliterates the false lumen. 4. Thrombosis occurs in the remaining false lumen and in areas of the aorta without major branches. (From Carpentier A, Deloche A, Fabiani JN, et al. New surgical approach to aortic dissection: Flow reversal and thromboexclusion. *J Thorac Cardiovasc Surg* 1981;81:659–668.)

approximately 7 percent and is even slightly higher, at about 11 percent, for those with a chronic dissection. Long-term survival after surgery is estimated to be 67 percent, 55 percent, 37 percent, and 24 percent at 1, 5, 10, and 15 years, respectively.

Type B dissections occur less frequently, though they have higher morbidity and mortality rates. Initial management is often medical, in contrast to type A dissections, with surgery reserved for patients with signs or symptoms of malperfusion, rupture, or significant aneurysmal dilatation. The mainstay of medical management is hypertension control, with beta-adrenergic blocking preparations being first-line agents. A particularly beneficial effect seen with this drug class is attenuation of the upstroke of the pulsatile wave within the aorta (dP/dt). Percutaneous methods of fenestration and endoluminal stent placement have been successful in select patients at select centers of excellence. Patients treated with aggressive medical management have estimated survival rates of only 73 percent at 1 year and 58 percent at 5 years. Surgical patients represent a group with more ominous presenting complaints and higher postoperative morbidity. This explains their survival of 56 percent, 48 percent, 29 percent, and 11 percent at 1, 5, 10, and 15 years, respectively.

A thorough understanding of the pathophysiology, anatomic classification, and clinical and radiographic investigations, along with appropriate medical and surgical management of this disease process, is extremely important in patients with this serious condition of the aorta.

References

1. Masuda Y, Yamada Z, Morooka N, et al. Prognosis of patients with medically treated aortic dissections. *Circulation* 1991;84(Suppl5):III-7.
2. Nicholls F. Observations concerning the body of his Late Majesty. *Phil Trans R Soc Lond* 1761;52:265.
3. Morgagni JB. DeSedibus et causis morborum per natomen indagatis (1761). Translated from the Latin by Alexander B, 1769. *iol* 1960;5:94
4. Laennec R. *Traite de l'auscultation mediate et maladies des poumons et du coeur*, vol 2. JS Chaude; 1826:696.
5. Leonard JC. Thomas Bevill Peacock and the early history of dissecting aneurysm. *Br Med J* 2979;2:260.
6. Erdheim J: Medionecrosis aotae idiopathica cystica. *Virchows Arch Pathol Anat Physiol* 1930;276:87.
7. Swaine K, Latham PM. A case of dissecting aneurysm of the aorta. *Trans Pathol Soc Lond* 1855;7:106.
8. Shennan T. *Dissecting Aneurysms Special Report.* Medical Research Council Series. London: His Majesty Stationary Office; 1934.
9. Davey H, Gates M. Case of dissecting aneurysm of the aorta. *Br Med J* 1922;1:471.
10. Paullin JE, James DF. Dissecting aneurysm of aorta. *Postgrad Med* 1948;4:291.
11. Gurin D, Bulmer JW, Derby R. Dissecting aneurysms of the aorta: Diagnosis and operative relief of acute arterial obstruction due to this cause. *NY J Med* 1935;35:1200.
12. Abbott OA. Clinical experiences with application of polythene cellophane upon aneurysms of thoracic vessels. *J Thorac Surg* 1949;18:435.
13. DeBakey ME, Cooley DA, Creech O. Surgical consideration of dissecting aneurysm of the aorta. *Ann Surg* 1955;35:1200.
14. Cooley DA, DeBakey ME, Morris GC Jr. Controlled extracorporeal circulation in surgical treatment of aortic aneurysm. *Ann Surg* 1957;146:473.
15. Wheat MW Jr, Palmer RJ, Bartley TB. Treatment of dissecting aneurysm of the aorta without surgery. *J Thorac Cardiovasc Surg* 1965;50:364.
16. DeBakey ME, Henly WS, Cooley DA, et al. Surgical treatment of dissecting aneurysms of the aorta: Analysis of seventy-two cases. *Circulation* 1961;24:290.
17. DeBakey ME, Henly WS, Cooley DA, et al. Surgical management of dissecting aneurysms of the aorta. *J Thorac Cardiovasc Surg* 1965;49:130.
18. Larson EW, Edwards WD. Risk factors for aortic dissection: A necropsy study of 161 cases. *Am J Cardiol* 1984;53:849.
19. Miller DC, Stinson EB, Oyer PE. Operative treatment of aortic dissections: Experience with 125 patients over sixteen year period. *J Thorac Cardiovasc Surg* 1979;78:365.
20. Hirst AE, Johns VJ Jr, Kine SW. Dissecting aneurysm of the aorta: A review of 505 cases. *Medicine (Baltimore)* 1958;37:217.

21. Coady MA, Rizzo JA, Elefteriades JA. Pathologic variants of thoracic aortic dissection: Penetrating atherosclerotic ulcer and intramural hematomas. *Cardiol Clin* 1999;17:637.
22. Svensson LG, Crawford ES. Aortic dissection and aortic aneurysm surgery: Clinical observations, experimental investigations and statistical analyses: Part II. *Curr Probl Surg* 1992;29:913.
23. Spittell PC, Spittell JAJ, Joyce JW. Clinical features and differential diagnosis of aortic dissection: Experience with 236 cases (1980 through 1990). *Mayo Clin Proc* 1993; 68:642.
24. Hagan PG, Nienaber CA, Isselbacher EM. The international registry of acute aortic dissection (IRAD): New insights into an old disease. *JAMA* 2000;283:897.
25. Slater EE, Desanctis RW. The clinical recognition of dissection aortic aneurysm. *Am J Med* 1976;60:625.
26. Suzuki T, Katoh H, Watanabe M. Novel biochemical diagnostic method for aortic dissection: Results of a prospective study using an immunoassay of smooth muscle myosin heavy chain. *Circulation* 1996;93:1244.
27. Kamp TJ, Goldschmidt-Clemont PJ, Brinker JA, et al. Myocardial infarction, aortic dissection, and thrombolytic therapy. *Am Heart J* 1994;128:1234.
28. Hartnell GG, Wakely CJ, Tottle A, et al. Limitations of chest radiography in discriminating between aortic dissection and myocardial infarction: Implications for thrombolysis. *J Thorac Imaging* 1993;8:152.
29. Nienaber CA, von Kodolitsch Y. Diagnostic imaging of aortic diseases. *Radiologe* 1997;37:402.
30. Nienaber CA, von Kodolitsch Y, Nicolas V. The diagnosis of thoracic aortic dissection by noninvasive imaging procedures. *N Engl J Med* 1993;328:1.
31. Kersting-Sommerhoff BA, Higgins CB, White, et al. Aortic dissection: Sensitivity and specificity of MR imaging. *Radiology* 1988;166:651.
32. Sommer T, Fehske W, Holzknecht N. Aortic dissection: A comparative study of diagnosis with spiral CT, multiplanar transesophageal echocardiography, and MR imaging. *Radiology* 1996;199:347.
33. Mintz GS, Kotter MN, Segal BL, et al. Two-dimensional echocardiographic recognition of the descending thoracic aorta. *Am J Cardiol* 1979;44:232.
34. Iliceto S, Ettorre G, Francioso G, et al. Diagnosis of aneurysm of the thoracic aorta: Comparison between two non invasive techniques: two-dimensional echocardiography and computed tomography. *Eur Heart J* 1984;5:545.
35. Khandheria BK, Tajik AJ, Taylor CL. Aortic dissection: Review of value and limitations of two-dimensional echocardiography in a six-year experience. *J Am Soc Echocardiogr* 1989;2:17.
36. Erbel R, Engberding R, Daniel W, et al. Echocardiography in diagnosis of aortic dissection. *Lancet* 1989;1:457.
37. Yamada E, Matsumura M, Omoto R. Usefulness of a prototype intravascular ultrasound imaging in evaluation of aortic dissection and comparison with angiographic study, transesophageal echocardiography, computed tomography, and magnetic resonance imaging. *Am J Cardiol* 1995; 75:161.
38. Faykus MH, Hiette P, Koopot. Percutaneous fenestration of a type I aortic dissection for relief of lower extremity ischemia. *Cardiovasc Intervent Radiol* 1992;15:183.
39. Saito S, Arai H, Kin K. Percutaneous fenestration of dissecting intima with a transeptal needle: A new therapeutic technique for visceral ischemia complicating acute aortic dissection. *Catheter Cardiovasc Diagn* 1992;26:130.
40. Williams DM, Andrews JC, Marx MV, et al. Creation of reentry tears in aortic dissection by means of percutaneous balloon fenestration: Gross anatomic and histologic considerations. 1993;4:75.
41. Griepp RB, Stinson EB, Hollingsworth JF, et al. Prosthetic replacement of the aortic arch. *J Thorac Cardiovasc Surg* 1975;70(6):1051.
42. Baumgartner WA, Walinsky PL, Salazar JD, et al. Assessing the impact of cerebral injury after cardiac surgery: Will determining the mechanism reduce this injury? *Ann Thorac Surg* 1999;67(6):1871.
43. Gillinov AM, Redmond JM, Zehr KJ, et al. Superior cerebral protection with profound hypothermia during arrest. *Ann Thorac Surg* 1993;55(6):1432.
44. Ueda Y, Miki S, Kusuhara K, et al. Surgical treatment of aneurysms or dissection involving the ascending aorta and aortic arch, utilizing circulatory arrest and retrograde cerebral perfusion. *J Cardiovasc Surg* 1990;31(5):553.
45. Di Eusanio M, Schepens MA, Morshius WJ, et al. Antegrade selective cerebral perfusion during operations on the thoracic aorta: Risk factors influencing survival and neurological outcome in 413 patients. *J Thorac Cardiovasc Surg* 2002;124(6):1080.
46. Coselli JS, LeMarie SA, de Figueiredo LE. Paraplegia after thoracoabdominal aneurysm repair: Is dissection a risk factor? *Ann Thorac Surg* 1997;63:28.
47. Cunningham JN Jr, Laschinger JC, Spencer FC. Monitoring of somatosensory evoked potentials during surgical procedures on the thoracoabdominal aorta: IV. Clinical observations and results. *J Thorac Cardiovasc Surg* 1987;94:275.
48. Safi HJ, Hess KR, Randel M. Cerebrospinal fluid drainage and distal aortic perfusion: Reducing neurologic complications in repair of thoracoabdominal aortic aneurysms types I and II. *J Vasc Surg* 1996;23:223.
49. Najafi H, Dye WS, Javid H. Acute aortic regurgitation secondary to aortic dissection: Surgical management without valve replacement. *Ann Thorac Surg* 1972;14:474.
50. Bentall H, DeBono A. A technique for complete replacement of the ascending aorta. *Thorax* 1968;23:338.
51. Kouchoukos NT, Wareing TH, Murphy SF, et al. Sixteen-year experience with aortic root replacement: Results of 172 operations. *Ann Surg* 1991;214:308.
52. Borst HG, Laas J, Heinemann M. Type A aortic dissection: Diagnosis and management of malperfusion phenomena. *Semin Thorac Cardiovasc Surg* 1991;3:238.
53. Cabrol C, Pavie A, Mesnildrey P. Long-term results with total replacement of the ascending aorta and reimplantation of the coronary arteries. *J Thorac Cardiovasc Surg* 1986;91:17.
54. Svennson LG, Crawford ES, Hess KR. Composite valve graft replacement of the proximal aorta: Comparison of techniques in 348 patients. *Ann Thorac Surg* 1992;54:427.
55. Frist WH, Miller DC. Repair of ascending aortic aneurysms and dissections. *J Card Surg* 1986;1(1):33.
56. Webb TH, Williams GM. Abdominal aortic tailoring for renal, visceral, and lower extremity malperfusion resulting from acute aortic dissection. *J Vasc Surg* 1997;26:474.

57. Oliver HF, Maher TD, Liebler GA. Use of Biomedicus centrifugal pump in traumatic tears of the thoracic aorta. *Ann Thorac Surg* 1984;38:586.
58. Gott VL. Heparinized shunts for thoracic vascular operations [editorial]. *Ann Thorac Surg* 1972;14:219.
59. Carpentier A, Deloche A, Fabiani JN, et al. New surgical approach to aortic dissection: Flow reversal and thromboexclusion. *J Thorac Cardiovasc Surg* 1981; 81:659.
60. Elefteriades JA, Hartleroad J, Gusberg RJ, et al. Long-term experience with descending aortic dissection: The complication specific approach. *Ann Thorac Surg* 1992;53:11.
61. Elefteriades JA, Louvoules CJ, Coady MA. Management of descending aortic dissection. *Ann Thorac Surg* 1999; 67:2002.
62. Fann JI, Smith JA, Miller DC, et al. Surgical management of aortic dissection during a 30-year period. *Circulation* 1995;92:113.

CHAPTER

38 ENDOVASCULAR REPAIR OF THORACIC AORTIC PATHOLOGY

Susanna L. Matsen, James H. Black III

INTRODUCTION

Traditional open surgical repair of thoracic aortic disease continues to be associated with significant morbidity and mortality. Endovascular stent grafts have emerged as an exciting new technology to treat thoracic aortic pathologies. This minimally invasive approach decreases operation risk by minimizing aortic manipulation, avoiding large incisions and surgical hemorrhage, and circumventing the complications associated with cardiopulmonary bypass. This chapter presents the advantages and challenges of thoracic endovascular repair of the following pathologies of the thoracic aorta: aneurysm, dissection, penetrating atheromatous ulcers, intramural hematomas, and traumatic lesions.

RESULTS OF OPEN REPAIR

Before one begins a review of endovascular repair of thoracic aortic pathology, a review of the current state of open thoracic replacement is required. It is important to draw the clinical distinction between thoracic aortic replacement and thoracoabdominal aortic replacement. The current literature is replete with series of studies of thoracoabdominal aortic surgery,[1,2] but series detailing the results of lesser thoracic aortic operations are sparse. In thoracic aortic replacement, the duration of renal-visceral ischemia is minimal as thoracic aortic anastomosis often can be accomplished with less than 30 min of aortic interruption. Indeed, if distal perfusion techniques are employed, renal-visceral ischemia may be avoided totally. Thus, extrapolat-

KEY CONCEPTS

- Traditional open surgical repair of thoracic aortic disease is associated with significant morbidity and mortality.
- Endovascular stent graft therapies have emerged as a minimally invasive approach to treating thoracic aortic pathologies.
- Stent graft devices consist of membrane material mounted on an expandable metal stented framework.
- Although several imaging modalities have proved useful in planning and executing stent graft deployment, computed tomography has emerged as the dominant imaging modality because of its wide availability, high resolution, and ability to obtain a variety of three-dimensional reconstructions of the thoracic and abdominal aorta.
- Endovascular stent grafts are deployed through sheaths placed in the common femoral or iliac artery. It is often useful to obtain vascular access through an extension conduit anastomosed to the common iliac artery via a retroperitoneal approach.
- There are four types of "endoleaks," or seepage of blood between the walls of the aorta and/or from graft material.
- Endovascular stent grafts have been used to repair aortic aneurysms, Stanford type B aortic dissections, penetrating atherosclerotic ulcers, and aortic transections. The results of these repairs are promising but still are accumulating.
- Complications of endovascular stent graft repairs of the thoracic aorta include spinal cord ischemic injury, retrograde aortic dissection, and iliofemoral arterial injury.

ing the series detailing thoracoabdominal aortic replacement to the arena of thoracic replacement is likely to overestimate the attendant risk of the pathologies now being addressed by endovascular means. Nonetheless, reviewing the literature of thoracic aortic replacement elucidates the risks both avoided (large cavitary incisions and blood loss) and assumed (paraplegia).

The largest series reporting results of thoracic aortic surgery for repair of degenerative aneurysms—not thoracoabdominal aneurysms—was published by Coselli and associates in 2004.[3] That series compared the results of surgical repair employing either a clamp-and-sew technique with the results of distal aortic perfusion via a left heart bypass circuit (LHB). Over a 15-year period, 387 patients underwent surgical repair by clamp and sew (341 patients; 88.1 percent) or distal perfusion (46 patients; 11.9 percent). Patients who underwent repair using profound circulatory arrest because of inability to cross-clamp the aorta (as a result of rupture, large size, or arch involvement) were excluded from the analysis. Cerebrospinal fluid drainage was used in 24 patients (6.2 percent). The preoperative characteristics of the two groups were compared, and the only factor that reached statistical significance was the fact that the presence of acute dissection was associated more often with the use of LHB ($p = 0.02$). All other variables [age, chronic obstructive pulmonary disease (COPD), coronary artery disease (CAD), renal insufficiency, rupture] were not significantly different between the clamp-and-sew and LHB groups. Intraoperative variables in the two groups were statistically similar in regard to the extent of the thoracic aorta replaced, the emergent presentation, and reattachment of intercostal arteries. The LHB patients required a longer cross-clamp time (35.9 ± 10.4 min versus 26.9 ± 9.9 min, $p = 0.0001$). In addition, LHB patients required more packed red blood cells (PRBC) and fresh frozen plasma (FFP) units than did clamp-and-sew patients (5.9 ± 3.3 and 10.3 ± 8.3 units versus 4.1 ± 3.5 and 7.3 ± 8.1 units, $p = 0.002$ and $p < 0.03$, respectively). More patients treated with LHB (76 percent, $p = 0.006$) required proximal clamp placement between the left common carotid and the left subclavian than did those treated with clamp and sew (54 percent). Postoperative complications were encountered at similar rates whether LHB or clamp-and-sew techniques were employed. Thirty-day mortality data revealed 2 percent mortality in the LHB group and 2.9 percent mortality in the clamp-and-sew group ($p = 0.1$). Renal failure was noted in 7 percent of patients in both groups. Paraplegia rates were quite similar: a striking 4 percent in LHB patients and 2.3 percent in the clamp-and-sew group ($p = 0.3$). The authors hypothesized that the risk profile for the patients in the LHB group was higher; thus, the similar rates of paraplegia noted in the series may indicate a subtle protective effect of LHB. However, after further propensity analysis scoring and stratification, the conclusion that LHB prevents paraplegia could not be supported. Thus, the application of LHB in patients undergoing thoracic aortic replacement for thoracic aneurysms may be left to the discretion of an experienced aortic surgeon.

Apart from distal perfusion techniques to prevent the most dreaded complication of paraplegia, strategies have been developed to protect the cord from interruption of spinal blood flow. Epidural cooling using an iced saline infusion into the intrathecal space is done to produce a temperature of 25 to 28°C in the spinal canal, decreasing the neuronal energy requirement.[4] The flow rate into the epidural space may be limited by the measured cerebrospinal fluid (CSF) pressure (CSFP), as the target CSF perfusion pressure [mean arterial pressure(MAP) – CSFP] should be above 40 mmHg.[5] Admirable paraplegia rates (6 percent) were reported from the Massachusetts General Hospital in its series of over 300 thoracoabdominal repairs. That series included a substantial number of ruptures and acute presentations that are associated clearly with elevated risk.[6] As was stated by Cambria and associates,[6] in that series, the application of local hypothermia avoids the need for systemic moderate hypothermia and the associated coagulopathy. Besides cooling, other mechanisms have been explored to lower spinal metabolism. Acher and associates reported the use of naloxone therapy and barbiturate-based anesthetics to decrease energy expenditure during the critical period of interruption of spinal blood flow.[7] As was reported in their series of 110 thoracic aortic repairs, an admirable 1.6 percent paraplegia rate was observed with this strategy, which also included the deliberate oversewing of intercostal arteries in the critical thoracolumbar zone.

Cerebrospinal fluid drainage (CSFD) is perhaps the most studied and widely accepted strategy employed for the prevention of paraplegia in thoracic aortic surgery. Experimental data suggest that CSF pressure may rise with proximal aortic clamping and that reducing that pressure may improve spinal perfusion pressure.[4] Thus, placement of a drainage catheter into the subarachnoid space to allow efflux of fluid during the operation and in the postoperative period may benefit the fragile circulation of the spinal cord. Generally, the fluid is able to drain when the CSF pressure exceeds 10 mmHg as measured at the level of the spine. The beneficial effect of CSFD was demonstrated in a randomized trial comparing repair of type 1 and type 2 thoracoabdominal aneurysms performed with or without CSFD.[8] A total of 145 patients underwent repair, with 76 receiving CSFD and the other 69 undergoing repair without CSFD. Aortic clamp times, LHB use, and the number of intercostal artery reattachments were similar between the groups. Nine patients (13.0 percent) in the control group had paraplegia or paraparesis; in contrast, only two patients in the CSFD group (2.6 percent) had deficits. Overall, CSFD delivered an 80 percent reduction in the risk of postoperative spinal ischemic complications after type 1 and type 2 thoracoabdominal aneurysm repairs. To reiterate, the combined spinal and visceral ischemia encountered in type 2 thoracic-abdominal aortic aneurysm (TAAA) repairs confers a higher spinal cord complication threat as the spinal ischemic injury may be compounded by the concomitant visceral ischemia. However, in this series, 3 of the 11 patients with deficits received only type 1 TAAA repairs, and all underwent CSFD. As CSFD catheter placement is not risk-free, it generally is accepted that CSFD is clearly beneficial in operations in which aortic topography may mandate combined spinal and visceral ischemia: most type 1 TAAAs and all type 2 TAAAs.

Johns Hopkins approach to open thoracic aortic replacement

The authors' approach to type 1 and type 2 TAAAs and thoracic aortic aneurysms (TAAs) has been to employ CSFD, LHB, and moderate hypothermia (32°C) via a heat exchanger on a Bio-Medicus centrifugal pump. Sequential clamping is used, and intercostal reattachment is performed on the basis of clinical inspection of patent intercostals or as dictated by preoperative spinal arteriographic localization of the artery of Adamkiewicz. For thoracic replacement confined to the supradiaphragmatic aorta, a similar strategy is used, without the spinal arteriographic mapping. For suprarenal or type 3 and type 4 TAAAs, LHB and CSFD rarely are employed as no data exist to support their salutary effect in those groups.

DEVICE OVERVIEW

First-generation stent grafts for repair of thoracic aortic pathology were bulky handmade devices that employed pressed Dacron material hand-sewn onto Gianturco stainless steel stents. The packaging of those handmade devices required large-diameter sheaths (26F) and stiff delivery systems, all of which made accurate delivery and deployment difficult. In addition, the large-caliber devices often required that conduits be sewn onto the iliac or abdominal aorta to accommodate the diameter of the delivery system. Newer-generation devices offer improved flexibility with small introducer systems (Fig. 38-1). After these advances, the U.S. Food and Drug Administration (FDA) approved the first endovascular device for the treatment of degenerative thoracic aneurysms in late 2004.

The current FDA-approved device is manufactured by WL Gore (Flagstaff, AZ) and is called the Excluder Thoracic Endoprosthesis. This device consists of a series of self-expanding nitinol stents affixed to a polytetrafluoroethylene (PTFE) membrane. The outer diameter of the sheath for the delivery of the largest-diameter endoprosthesis (40 mm in diameter) is 9.2 mm. The device is available in lengths of 10, 15, and 20 cm, and device diameters range from 26 to 40 mm. The device is constrained in a PTFE membrane that is removed by withdrawing a "rip-cord" to deploy the device from the middle toward the ends.

Currently undergoing investigation are thoracic devices manufactured by Cook, Inc. (Bloomington, IN), called the

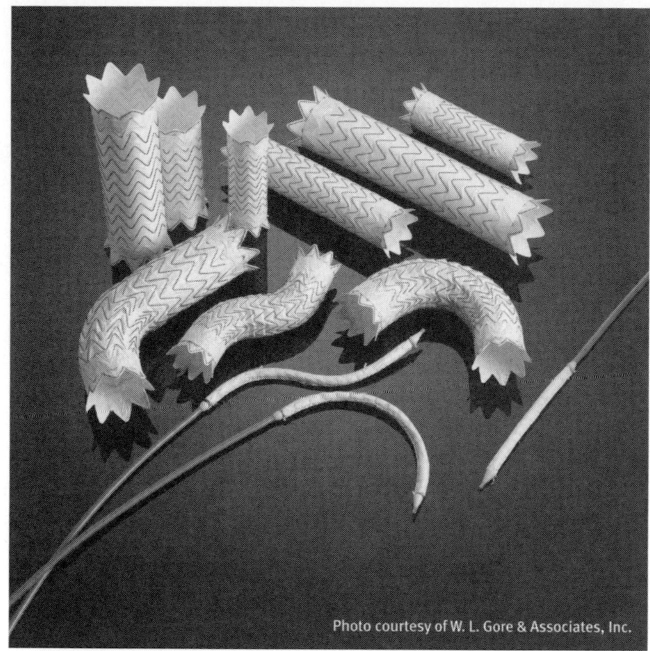
Photo courtesy of W. L. Gore & Associates, Inc.

Figure 38-1 Stent grafts and deployment devices. (Courtesy of W.L. Gore & Associates, Inc.)

Zenith TX2 thoracic endograft and by Medtronic Vascular (Santa Rosa, CA) called the Talent Endoluminal Stent-Graft. The Zenith TX2 device employs woven polyester affixed by sutures to stainless steel Z stents. Barbs are oriented off the ends of the device to promote fixation to the aortic seal zone. Device diameters ranging from 28 to 42 mm are under trial. The Talent graft features an uncovered proximal stent to cross arch vessels and aid fixation. The device is deployed by withdrawing the introduction sheath to allow self-expansion of the endograft into the aorta.

IMAGING FOR DIAGNOSIS

A wide range of imaging modalities are helpful in confirming suspected thoracic aortic pathology: chest radiography, aortography, transthoracic or transesophageal echocardiography, magnetic resonance imaging (MRI), and computed tomography (CT). The benefits and limitations of each of those modalities are reviewed below, along with their applicability to aneurysmal and dissection pathology.

Plain radiography

Classically, widening of the cardiac or aortic silhouette is cited as indicative of aortic disruption, along with pleural effusions and the displacement of aortic calcifications. Specifically, widening of the aortic silhouette was found in 60 to 90 percent of cases of aortic dissection by Spitell and associates and Hagan coworkers in their reviews.[9,10] However, chest radiography has limited specificity and sensitivity.

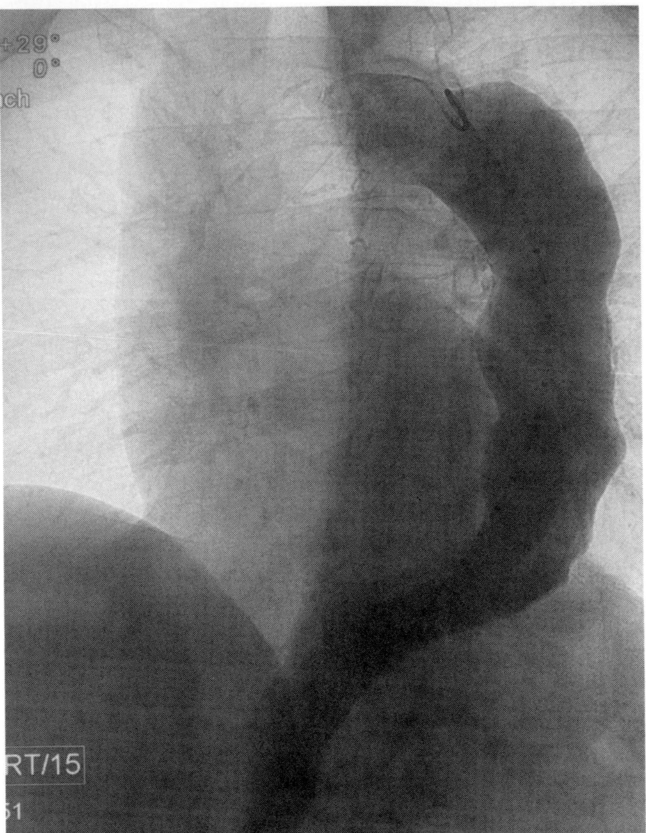

Figure 38-2 Angiography is a vital adjunct to preprocedure planning.

Aortography

This modality has both high sensitivity and high specificity 86 to 88 percent and 75 to 94 percent, respectively, for the diagnosis of aortic dissection.[11–13] Findings suggestive of dissection include distortion of the normal contrast column, flow reversal or stasis into a false channel, failure of major branches to fill, and aortic valvular regurgitation.[13] For the diagnosis of thoracic aortic aneurysm and treatment planning, aortography may improve the accuracy of length measurements of intended aortic seal zones (Fig. 38-2). In addition, aortography may be of benefit in defining aortoiliac occlusive disease, which may require angioplasty or a planned conduit for access for the stent graft delivery. Nonetheless, enthusiasm for this modality is tempered by the potential for diagnostic confusion about malperfusion after pressurized injection, the risk of contrast nephropathy, the time delay to diagnosis, and the expense.

Transthoracic echocardiography and transesophageal echocardiography

Transthoracic echocardiography (TTE) has a sensitivity of 35 to 80 percent and a specificity of 40 to 95 percent for the detection of aortic dissection,[14,15] whereas the sensitivity of transesophageal echocardiography (TEE) is reportedly as high as 98 percent, with 63 to 96 percent specificity.[16–18] TTE may be limited technically by body habitus, emphysema, and narrow intercostal spaces. Although TEE is more invasive, it greatly expands the diagnostic ability of echocardiography. TEE may demonstrate entry tear sites, flow within the false lumen, involvement of the arch or coronary arteries, degrees of aortic valvular regurgitation, and pericardial effusions. Although TEE is especially useful in documenting pathology of the ascending aorta, one must be mindful of its limitations in imaging the anatomic blind spot in the distal ascending aorta and arch secondary to the air-filled trachea and left mainstem bronchus. Additionally, TEE cannot image aortic pathologies past the diaphragm.[19]

Magnetic resonance imaging

MRI has unparalleled sensitivity and specificity for detecting aortic pathology, for instance, 95 to 100 percent for dissection.[20–22] Recent advances in three-dimensional (3-D) reconstruction of gadolinium-enhanced magnetic resonance angiography (MRA) are beneficial in planning thoracic aortic stent graft treatment in patients whose comorbidity profile includes renal insufficiency. However, this enthusiasm must be tempered by the realities of long examination times, inability to monitor critically ill patients,

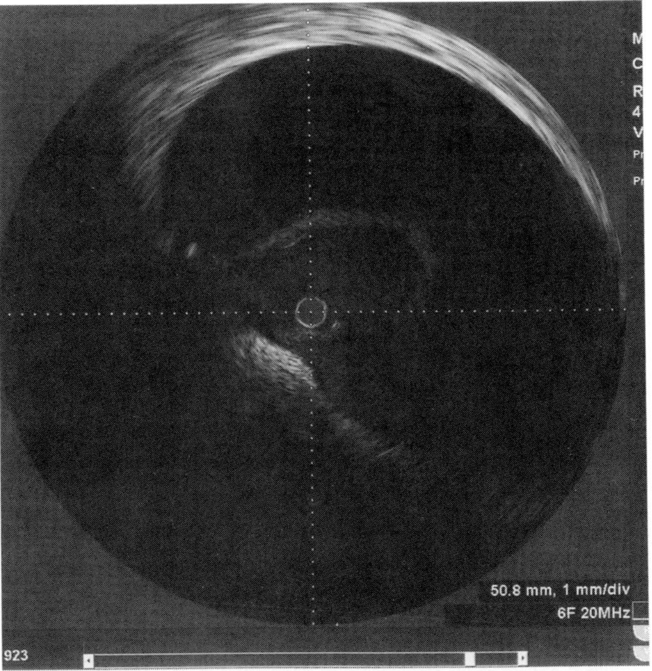

Figure 38-3 Intravascular ultrasound of the aorta. Although not reviewed here, this new imaging modality has had clinical utility in the diagnosis of malperfusion syndromes in aortic dissection. Note collapsed true lumen and surrounding larger, expanded false lumen in this patient with gut and renal ischemia after type B dissection.

expense, and lack of immediate availability. Moreover, MRI is contraindicated for patients with implants or pacemakers.

Computed tomography

CT offers multiple benefits, as reflected by the fact that it is the most commonly used diagnostic test in patients with suspected aortic pathology.[20] Readily available, CT scanning carries a sensitivity of 83 to 95 percent with a specificity of 87 to 100 percent for the detection of acute aortic dissection.[23–25] This modality can be particularly helpful in examination of the true versus the false lumen. A slitlike compressed true lumen should heighten suspicion for branch vessel compromise and malperfusion syndrome substantially (Fig. 38-3). Because of its benefits, CT scanning is a vital adjunct for operative planning. Computed tomography angiography (CTA) has evolved so that multiple reconstructions can be created from the source axial images. Such reconstructions are vital in determining accurate aortic diameters for the prediction of the suitability of stent graft therapies (Fig. 38-4).

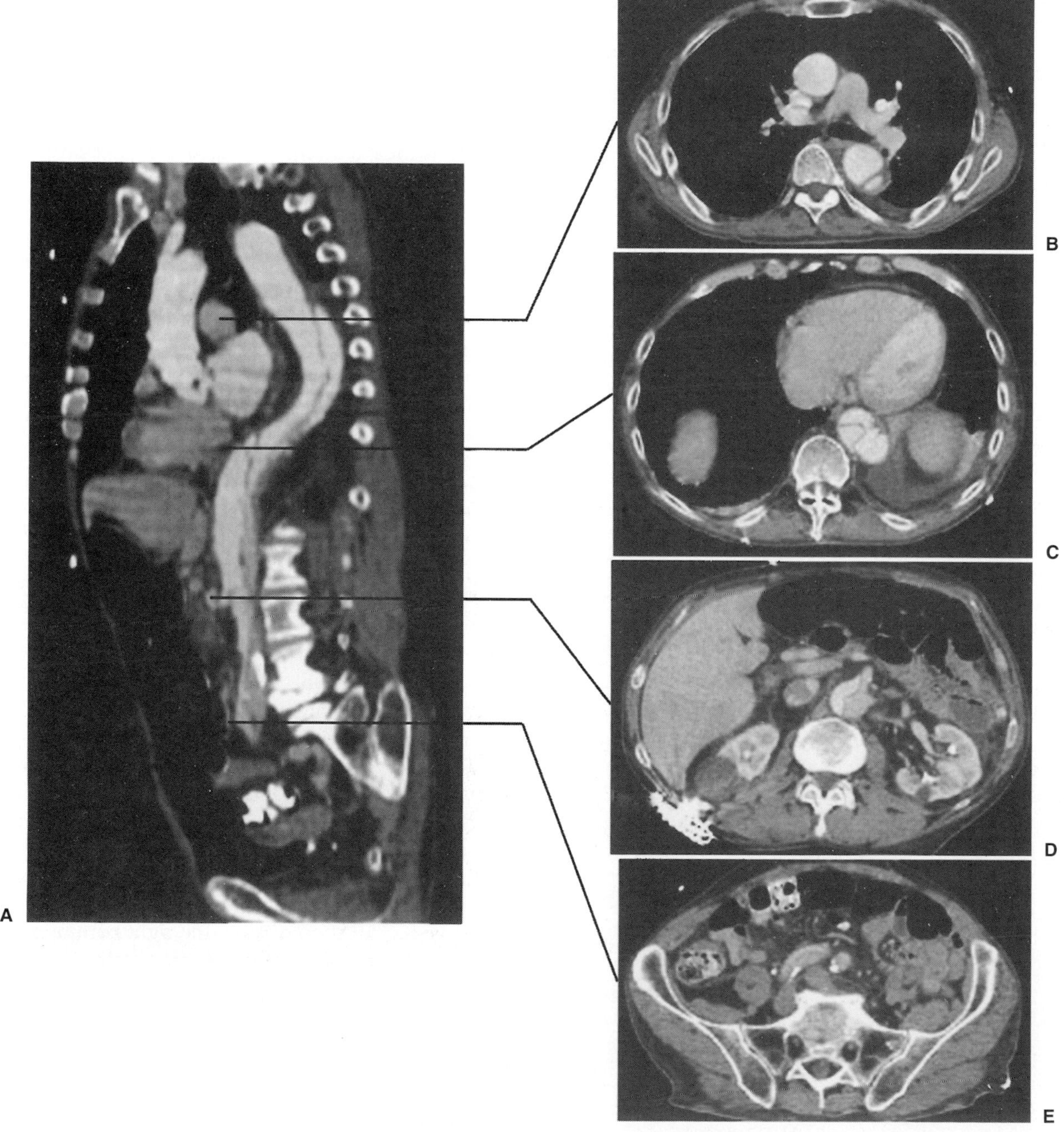

Figure 38-4 Three-dimensional computed tomography has a sensitivity of 83 to 95 percent and a specificity of 87 to 100 percent for the detection of acute aortic dissection.

IMAGING FOR PLANNING THERAPY

Endovascular repair of thoracic aortic pathology requires facility with the interpretation of axial imaging such as CTA and MRA to inspect aortic topography for device insertion and fixation. In addition, planning of thoracic aortic endografting may be aided by conventional diagnostic arteriography, using both subtracted and unsubtracted techniques, especially when 3-D imaging cannot be obtained from available axial data. A key tenet of thoracic aortic endovascular repair is the understanding that device selection and operative planning should be confirmed and verified to the greatest extent possible preoperatively. Furthermore, independent review of available data for device planning should be done by separate physicians as errors in device measurements often translate into immediate treatment failures.

Insertion planning for endovascular devices requires a thorough understanding of the aortic diameters at the proximal and distal sealing sites as measured from outer wall to outer wall. For the FDA-approved Gore device, an aortic diameter of no less than 23 mm to no more than 37 mm allows for implantation using the range devices (26 mm to 40 mm) to yield an oversizing of graft to aorta of 10 to 20 percent (Fig. 38-5).

Oversizing the graft too aggressively may place undue forces on the aortic endograft and result in migration or collapse of the entire graft.[26] The length of proximal fixation should be more than 20 mm with an acceptable aortic diameter throughout this seal zone. If an adequate proximal fixation length is not immediately obtainable, the left subclavian artery can be crossed and excluded with little consequence to the patient (mean left arm pressure decreased, with few symptoms); if the patient has a prior left internal mammary-to-coronary bypass, a left-carotid-to-left-subclavian bypass is required to maintain coronary circulation before coverage. Further encroachment into the arch generally requires salvage of the left common carotid circulation by a prior carotid-carotid bypass. If excessive tortuosity is encountered in either fixation zone, a longer seal length of up to 30 mm may be needed to prevent blood from escaping around the ends of the stent (type 1 endoleak). When multiple devices are required to cover long lengths of aortic pathology, each piece should be made to overlap 3 to 5 cm with the neighboring endograft. The distal aortic seal zone is usually cephalad to the celiac axis.

A common theme in complications of aortic endografting, whether abdominal aortic or thoracic aortic techniques, is the occurrence of damage to access vessels such as the common femoral and iliac arteries. Therefore, if the measured diameter of an intended access vessel is demonstrated to be less than 8 mm, serious consideration should be given to a surgical conduit. The 10-mm Dacron conduits generally are anastomosed to the common iliac or abdominal aorta via a miniflank incision with retroperitoneal exposure of the vessel. In particular, severe calcification of an access vessel may increase the risk of tear, perforation, dissection, or frank rupture. It is not uncommon for such iatrogenic injuries to become obvious when the device sheath is being withdrawn, not at the time of sheath insertion. As the device sheath is removed, the obturation of the injury is relieved and hemorrhage ensues.

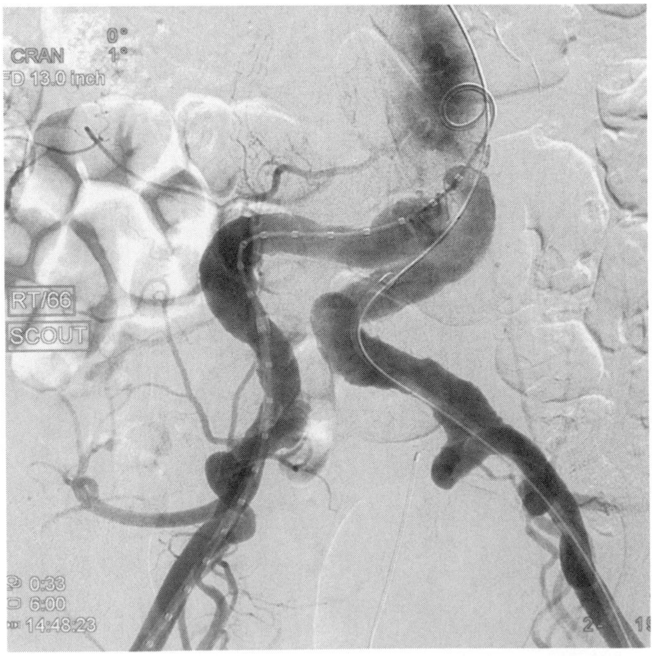

Figure 38-5 Tortuosity and ectasia make stent graft introduction more difficult.

IMPLANTATION TECHNIQUE

The procedure of aortic endografting for thoracic aortic pathologies should be performed in an operating room with a mandatory high-resolution digital imaging system and a radiolucent table. The choice of anesthetic generally is based on preoperative cardiac risk stratification and may include local, epidural, and general anesthesia. The application of CSF drainage should be considered when coverage of the entire thoracic aorta is planned or if a prior abdominal aortic aneurysm (AAA) repair has been performed. Grafts are inserted via cutdown on the intended access vessel, most commonly the right common femoral artery. After this surgical exposure, systemic anticoagulation is achieved, using heparin to maintain an activated clotting time (ACT) greater than 250 s. An angiographic catheter is inserted percutaneously via the opposite common femoral artery or brachial artery to the level of the aortic arch. Using digital subtraction angiography, aortic arch or thoracic aortic angiography is performed to determine the approximate positioning of the endoprosthesis. To view the landing areas in the arch, it often is necessary to view the arch with a 60- to 90-degree left anterior

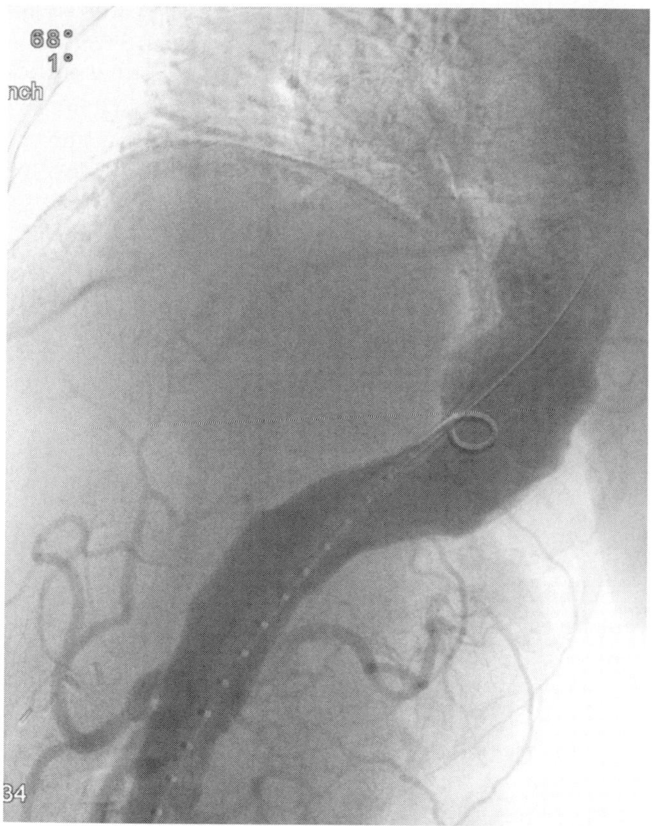

Figure 38-6 Distal aortic projection with a 68-degree left anterior oblique view often is required for proper visualization of the celiac axis for sizing. The figure shows a larger graduated device posterior to the pigtail catheter.

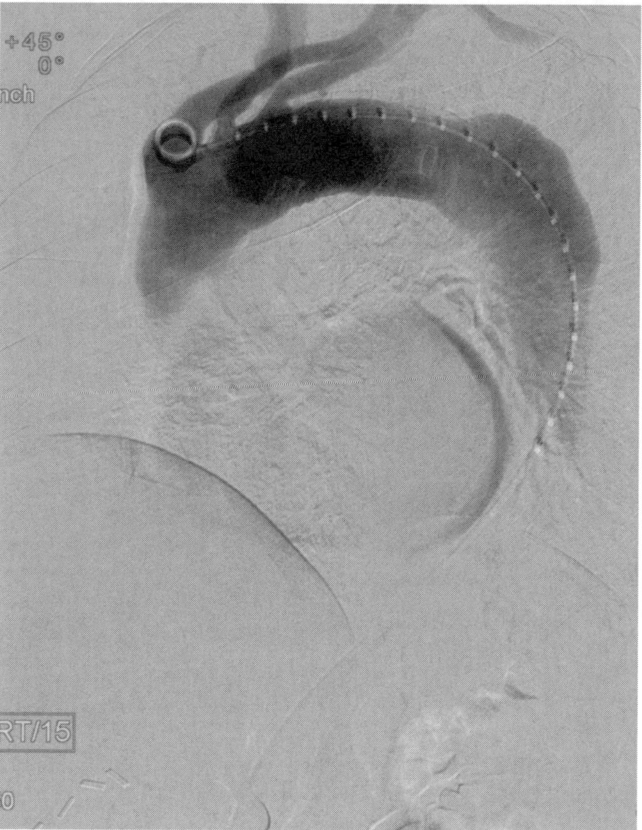

Figure 38-7 A 6-cm seal zone appreciated distal to the left subclavian artery on a left anterior oblique projection.

oblique (LAO) projection. To view the distal seal zone, a similar steep, nearly lateral projection best depicts the level of the celiac axis (Fig. 38-6).

To minimize manipulation, particularly in the arch, the final diagnostic studies before deployment should be performed with the device nearly in place; the stiffness of the wires and delivery systems may alter the course of the aortic arch and affect the landmarks being used to mark the proximal limits of deployment. "Road-mapping" techniques or "fluoro-fade" may improve operator accuracy in proximal fixation. Maneuvers to minimize stroke include flushing of all air from the device sheaths and lumens carefully. Also, manipulation of stiff wires into and from the arch should be done carefully under fluoroscopic guidance (Fig. 38-7). After deployment, fixation should be improved by using a large-diameter compliant occlusion balloon to maximize apposition of the stent graft to the aortic seal zones and regions of device overlap in a distal-to-proximal order (Fig. 38-8). The access sheath is removed carefully, with attention paid to mean arterial pressure as an early indicator of hemorrhage from iatrogenic insertion injury. If a tear in a vessel is suspected, the sheath can be reintroduced to obturate the injury. If the sheath will not pass, an occlusion balloon can be passed proximal to the injury and inflated to achieve vascular control. Frank transections usually require a flank incision and reconstruction, whereas small tears or dissections often are salvaged for endovascular stent placement without conversion.

Johns Hopkins approach to thoracic aortic stent grafting

In light of the preponderance of iatrogenic access injuries, the authors liberally apply retroperitoneal conduits via a flank incision. Most patients undergo general anesthesia both for flexibility of access approach and to avoid patient movement at critical imaging moments. The operations are performed in an endovascular operating room with a ceiling-mounted imaging device.

THORACIC AORTIC ANEURYSM

With an estimated incidence of 6 to 10 cases per 100,000 person-years,[27] a thoracic aortic aneurysm carries a substantial risk of mortality. Coady and associates[28] found a 27.9 percent total incidence of rupture or dissection for descending thoracic aneurysms larger than 6.0 cm. The long-term survival of patients with untreated thoracic aneurysms at 1 and 5 years was 88 percent and 69 percent,

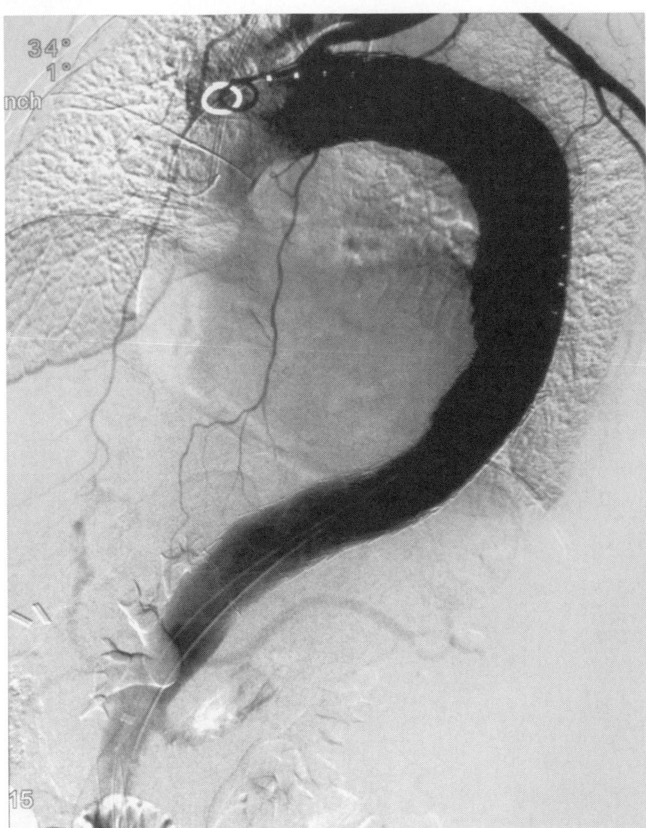

Figure 38-8 Deployed stent graft.

respectively.[28] As with AAAs, the yearly risk of rupture or dissection for thoracic aneurysms has been found to correlate with size: 2 percent for small aneurysms, 3 percent for aneurysms 5.0 to 5.9 cm, and 6 percent for those equal to or larger than 6.0 cm. The risk of death along with rupture and dissection increases markedly at 6.0 cm: 6.5 percent yearly for aneurysms 5.0 to 5.9 cm but 14.1 percent for those equal to or greater than 6.0 cm.[29]

The results of endovascular repair of TAA are summarized in Table 38-1. In the table, endoleak refers to the

Table 38-1 Results of endovascular repair of thoracic aortic aneurysms

	Dake 1994	Cambria 2002	Czerny 2004	Demers 2004
Technical success	100%	100%	94.4%	73%
Mortality	0%	5.6%	3.7%	9 ± 3%
Complication rate	7.7%	NA	1.9%	11%
Paraplegia	0%	0%	0%	NA
Endoleak	30.8%	NA	28.9%	21%
Mean follow-up	11.6 months	17.9 months	38	4.5 ±2.5 years

seepage of blood between the previously sealed walls of the aorta and graft material. Endoleaks are divided into four types: Type I endoleaks occur as a consequence of a poor seal between the aorta and the proximal or distal attachment sites of the graft, type II endoleaks are characterized by back bleeding from branch vessels, type III leaks involve blood excursion between multiple components of grafts, and type IV endoleaks occur when blood transgresses from the lumen through the material of the graft itself.

The use of stent grafts to treat descending thoracic aortic aneurysms was pioneered by Dake and colleagues in 1994.[30] Although endovascular repair previously had been described for AAAs, subclavian artery aneurysms, arteriovenous fistulas, and femoral occlusive disease, this group from Stanford extended the technology to the thoracic aorta. They noted that the potential benefits of an endovascular approach include less invasiveness, lower cost, and lower risk. Their series of 13 patients had 100 percent technical success, 0 percent mortality, and 0 percent paraplegia. The authors reported that two patients had "small patent proximal tracts communicating with the aneurysm" that resolved over the ensuing months and that two more patients required a second procedure to eliminate "residual filling from either a proximal communication or a distal communication," presumably type I endoleaks (30.8 percent). In light of those promising early results, the authors advocated endovascular treatment for highly selected patients.

Cambria and associates[31] from the Massachusetts General Hospital described their initial experience in 2002 with 28 patients, 18 of whom had degenerative aneurysms. All the patients treated for aneurysms had technical success, but one patient died on postoperative day 12. Among their 28 patients (including patients with degenerative aneurysm, chronic dissection, pseudoaneurysm, intramural hematoma, and coarctation), 6 (21 percent) developed endoleaks, 8 (28 percent) had "local complications" that usually (75 percent) were related to access, and 2 (7 percent) had device complications: one dissection and one kinking of the device. Notably, complication rates exclusively for aneurysm patients are not clear from the report. In light of the relatively high occurrence of access complications (including the disruption of the iliofemoral artery that led to the single mortality), those authors urged provider vigilance, including the use of general anesthesia, arterial lines, and a fully equipped operating room with the equipment needed for emergent open conversion. Moreover, they attributed their favorable result profile to their insistence on a minimum 2-cm fixation length and the avoidance of aortic tortuosity for fixation points.

A group from Austria summarized its midterm results for stent grafts in 54 patients with atherosclerotic descending TAAs in 2004.[32] There was 3.7 percent mortality (two patients) from dislocation of the device and multiorgan system failure, giving a device complication rate of 1.9 percent. In that report, the authors focused on endoleak as an outcome, finding 7.7 percent type I endoleaks, 13.5 percent type II, 7.7 percent type III, and no type IV. They attributed most type I endoleaks to technical mistakes. Of note, they found that the majority of endoleaks presented within the first year of intervention. Those authors therefore advocated heightened observation and follow-up in the first year after stent graft placement.

Demers and associates[33] presented their experience with 103 patients who were treated endovascularly for descending thoracic aneurysms in their 2004 midterm report. They reported a perioperative mortality rate of 9 percent (18 percent at 1 year), a primary success rate of 73 percent, and an 11 percent rate of complications (aortic rupture). A primary endoleak was detected in 21 patients, 11 of whom underwent a second successful endovascular repair, yielding a secondary success rate of 84 percent. At 1, 5, and 8 years, actuarial survival estimates were 82 percent, 49 percent, and 27 percent, respectively. Of note, patients deemed to be reasonable open surgical candidates had significantly higher survival rates than did the nonsurgical candidates ($p < 0.001$). Independent risk factors for death in patients receiving endovascular repair were identified as older age harm ratio (HR) 1.1, $p = 0.008$, 95 percent confidence interval (CI) 1.0 to 1.2), previous stroke (HR 2.8, $p = 0.003$), and identification as an inoperable candidate (HR 1.9, $p = 0.04$). That series reported a surprisingly high rate of late aortic rupture in the stented segment: 11 of the 103 patients, with death ensuing in 10 of those patients. Endoleaks had been documented in each of those patients previously. In light of the mixed results of that study, the authors concluded that stent grafting of descending TAAs should not be offered to young patients lacking contraindications to open repair. Like other investigators before them, they emphasized the importance of patient selection, with a keen eye to the identification of favorable anatomic targets.

THORACIC AORTIC DISSECTION (STANFORD TYPE B)

Acute aortic dissection is the most common catastrophe of the aorta, with an annual incidence of 5 to 30 cases per million people per year.[9,10,34,35] Age, hypertension, and structural abnormalities of the aortic wall contribute to the actual incidence within a population.[10,36] A male:female ratio of 5:1 is consistent across many series,[37] the incidence of dissection peaks at 50 to 60 years of age for type A and at 60 to 70 years for type B,[10] and hypertension contributes to 70 to 80 percent of cases.[9,10]

Despite marked treatment advancements since Shekelton's first efforts in the early 1800s, acute aortic dissection remains a lethal affliction. In the International Registry of Acute Aortic Dissection (IRAD) study from 2000, overall mortality stood at 27.4 percent, ranging from 26 percent for patients undergoing graft placement for ascending dissections to 58 percent for those managed medically for ascending dissections. Mortality for patients with descending dissections stood at 10.7 percent for medical treatment for descending dissections, compared with 31.4 percent for surgery.[10] Similarly, Meszaros and colleagues found that 21 percent of patients succumbed before hospital admission. Each hour left untreated increases the risk of death: 22.7 percent within 6 h, 50 percent within 24 h, and 68 percent within the first week (Meszaros and associates 2000[37a]). When the dissection involves the ascending aorta, mortality follows rupture into the pericardium, dissection of the coronary ostia, and acute aortic regurgitation.[38,39] In dissection of the descending aorta, mortality may result from visceral or extremity vessel obstruction or from aortic rupture.[40,41]

Like descending thoracic aneurysms, aortic dissections may result from myriad pathologic processes. For instance, bicuspid aortic valves and the resultant aortic root dilatation are a well-established risk factor that is found in 7 to 14 percent of all aortic dissections.[9,10] Other aortic diseases ranging from the genetic to the congenital contribute to dissection: Marfan's syndrome, Ehlers-Danlos syndrome, Turner's syndrome, Noonan's syndrome, coarctation of the aorta, annuloaortic ectasia, aortic arch hypoplasia, and aortic arteritis.[42] Common to many of those diseases is degeneration of the medial collagen and elastin, leading to diminished structural integrity of the aortic layers.[43–45] Beyond these diseases, medial degeneration seems to arise in dissection patients as a consequence of aging or hypertension; repetitive or excessive dP/dt (change in pressure over change in time) slowly contributes to the breakdown of medial collagen and elastin.[45–47]

The acute versus chronic differentiation occurs at diagnosis 2 weeks after the initial onset of symptoms. Anatomically, two classification schemes prevail: the one proposed by DeBakey and colleagues in 1965 and the Stanford classification, although the former has more widespread use[48]:

- Type I: Dissection originates in the ascending aorta and extends through the aortic arch and into the descending aorta and/or abdominal aorta for a varying distance.
- Type II: Dissection originates in and is confined to the ascending aorta.
- Type III: Dissection originates in the descending aorta and is limited to that structure in type IIIa; type IIIb involves descending and variable extents of the abdominal aorta.

Daily and colleagues developed the Stanford classification scheme in 1970.[49] That system divides dissections into those originating in the ascending aorta (Stanford type A; DeBakey types I and II) and those confined to the descending aorta (Stanford type B; DeBakey types IIIa and IIIb). Here the discussion is limited to Stanford type B.

Over 93 percent of patients with acute aortic dissections present with pain, with 85 percent experiencing an abrupt onset.[10,50] Because dissection may occur anywhere along the course of the aorta, the precise location of the pain varies: anterior or pain radiating to the arm or jaw for type A dissections compared with back or intrascapular region for type B processes.[9,10] Complaints of abdominal pain in this setting raise the specter of mesenteric vascular compromise. True to traditional teachings, patients characterize the pain as "the worst ever" in 90 percent of cases, with a sharp (68 percent), ripping or tearing (50 percent), or migratory character (19 percent).[10] Although syncope presents in less than 3 percent of patients with acute dissection, it is a harbinger of a complex and often fatal course.[10] Patients who present with syncope are more likely to have a type A than a type B dissection (19 percent versus 3 percent, $p < 0.001$), more often have cardiac tamponade (28 percent versus 8 percent, $p < 0.001$), may have suffered a stroke (18 percent versus 4 percent, $p < 0.001$), and are more likely to die in the hospital (34 percent versus 23 percent, $p = 0.01$).[51] Spinal cord ischemia occurs in 2 to 10 percent of type B dissections as a consequence of the interruption of intercostal vessels.[52] Less commonly, patients may experience neuropathies from direct compression of a peripheral nerve: paresthesias from lumbar plexopathy, hoarseness from compression of the recurrent laryngeal nerve, and Horner's syndrome secondary to sympathetic ganglion compression.[53–55]

The natural history of aortic dissection predicts progression to aneurysmal dilatation. In fact, 20 percent of cases of TAAs are attributable to chronic dissection in most series.[1,2,56] Factors that contribute to this evolution to aneurysm include poorly controlled hypertension, a maximal aortic diameter equal to or greater than 4 cm in the acute phase, and continued patency of the false lumen.[57–59] Ten to 20 percent of those with dissection subsequently have late rupture of the aneurysm.[57,60] Moreover, aneurysms that result from chronic dissection tend to be more extensive and occur in younger patients compared with degenerative aneurysms. Open surgical repair of type B dissections rarely is indicated emergently, except in the setting of threatened or actual rupture at the aortic intimal tear. In light of the substantial morbidity and complications associated with extensive aortic replacement in the emergent setting, Lauterbach and associates[40] argued for the abandonment of central aortic repair in the setting of type B dissection. The surgical results of open central aortic repair for dissection have not been overwhelming: Twenty-five to 50 percent of these patients persistently have false lumen flow,[61,62] and surgeons have variable success in relieving distal malperfusion. More important, perioperative mortality ranges from 6 to 67 percent.[63]

Endovascular repair may emerge as the definitive and superior method to treat aortic dissection confidently. An intuitive advantage of endovascular treatment is its ability to obliterate the false lumen by sealing the aortic tear with an aortic endograft. Continued patency of the false lumen has been noted to lead to aneurysmal dilatation.[58,64–69] Certain technical aspects of stent graft placement merit emphasis. First, it is ill advised to place uncovered stents over the site of the entry tear within the proximal true lumen. It is not known whether an acutely dissected intimal flap can tolerate aggressive oversizing of the proximal aorta with a stent. Furthermore, the radial force of a stent may overdistend the true lumen in tortuous portions of the aorta. By these two mechanisms, deployment of such uncovered stents may cause aortic rupture, as has been confirmed in multiple animal studies.[70–72]

A summary of select trials using stent grafts for aortic dissection is provided in Table 38-2. Dake and colleagues

Table 38-2 Results of endovascular repair of type B thoracic aortic dissection

	Dake 1999	Nienaber 1999	Bortone 2002—immediate treatment	Bortone 2002—delayed treatment (>2 weeks)	Eggebrecht 2005	Kusagawa 2005	Nathanson 2005
Technical success	100%	100%	100%	57%	100%	91%	95%
Mortality	20%	0%	0%	7%	3% (20% at 1 year)	6%	2.5% (15% at 1 year)
Complication rate	20%	0%	15%		18.4%	12%	38%
Paraplegia	0%	0%	0%	0%	0%	0%	2.5%
Endoleak	20% (immediate); 7% (1 month)	0%	0%	0%	0%	6%	2.5%
False lumen thrombosis	83% (immediate); 100% (3 months)	83% (immediate); 100% (3 months)	100%	100%	72%	86%	68%
Mean follow-up	10.9 months	1 year	9.7 ± 8.5 months		18 months	3.8 years	NA

reported outcomes of stent graft therapy for type B dissections after their initial experience with homemade devices in 15 patients.[65] Two patients required deployment of a second stent because of residual flow in the false lumen from proximal or distal communication. In that initial series, three patients died (20 percent): two from false lumen rupture hours to days after stent grafting and the third from sepsis 7 days later, apparently as a result of malperfusion syndrome. Their complication rate stood at 20 percent, including gut infarction, leg gangrene, pneumonia, and renal failure. However, stent grafting was successful in achieving complete thrombosis of the false lumen in 12 of the 15 surviving patients. Those authors advocated stent grafts to protect against end-organ ischemia but also emphasized the importance of promptly sealing an intimal tear to preclude progression to aneurysm.

Nienaber and colleagues published their early endovascular experience concurrently with the study mentioned above.[73] Their trial compared 12 consecutive patients with type B dissections treated with stent grafts to matched controls who were treated operatively. Whereas Dake and coinvestigators had used custom-designed stents, Nienaber used commercially available components with uncovered proximal fixation. Although surgical treatment accrued 33 percent morbidity ($p = 0.09$) and 42 percent mortality ($p = 0.04$), those with stent grafts experienced no morbidity or mortality within 12 months. Ten of the 12 patients experienced immediate thrombosis of the false lumen after graft deployment, with the remaining patients demonstrating thrombosis at 3-month follow-up. Compared with surgical therapy, those undergoing endovascular treatment had a shorter stay in the intensive care unit (ICP) ($p < 0.001$), a shorter hospital course ($p < 0.001$), and lower overall mortality ($p = 0.04$). That group concluded that not only may stent graft treatment of thoracic aortic dissections offer substantial cost savings, it is associated with lower morbidity and mortality than open repair.

More recently, Eggebrecht and colleagues[74] summarized stent graft outcomes in 10 patients with acute type B dissections and 28 patients with chronic dissections. They achieved 100 percent technical success with stenting. Predictably, patients undergoing stent graft placement for acute indications experienced higher mortality than did those treated for chronic dissections (40 percent versus 0 percent, $P = 0.001$), as did patients with an American Society of Anesthesiologists (ASA) class higher than 3 ($p = 0.001$). Their complication rate of 18.4 percent was attributable largely to injuries to access vessels, although disruption of the dissecting membrane, subintimal dissection of the aortic arch, hemoptysis, subclavian steal, and aortoesophageal fistula occurred as well. Like previous authors, those investigators determined that endovascular treatment of aortic dissection is both safe and highly successful. However, they did identify pretreatment health status as the most important determinant of a successful outcome.[74]

Kusagawa and colleagues later demonstrated that complete obliteration of the false lumen was more likely in acute-onset than in chronic dissection.[75] That study of 49 consecutive patients included 34 type B dissections (half acute, half chronic), and patients were followed radiographically by CT scan for more than 2 years after endovascular treatment. Those authors concluded that if no endoleaks or intimal tears occur, the false lumen is completely obliterated within 6 months for acute dissections. Although the false lumens in the chronic cases did decrease in size over the initial 6 months, they remained larger than those in the acute group. Moreover, in their 2002 study, Bortone and colleagues could not deploy stent grafts satisfactorily in the setting of delayed treatment (more than 2 weeks) for dissection in 61.5 percent of patients (8 of 13).[63] Two of those patients required deployment of multiple grafts for correction. This was attributed to progression of the false lumen and multiple reentrant intimal tears. Those authors therefore advocated immediate endovascular treatment of aortic dissections.

Nathanson and associates[76] recently summarized their experience treating 40 patients over a 5-year period. Their report listed 95 percent technical success, one perioperative death, one endoleak, one patient with postoperative paraplegia, and 85 percent 1-year survival. The 38 percent of their patients with complications included those with pleural effusions, pneumonia, renal failure, hematoma, pseudoaneurysm, and lymphocele. There were no postoperative thoracic aortic ruptures, and all but one patient experienced regression or stabilization of aortic diameter. Thus, exclusion of the proximal entry point with an endoprosthesis ultimately may decrease the incidence of rupture. Like the authors discussed previously, Nathanson and colleagues advocated early intervention in acute dissection for optimal results.[76]

PENETRATING ATHEROSCLEROTIC ULCERS AND INTRAMURAL HEMATOMAS

First described by Shennan in 1934, penetrating atherosclerotic ulcers (PAUs) were characterized fully by Stanson and colleagues in 1986.[77] Intramural hematomas were described earlier by Krukenberg in 1920.[78] Diagnostically, intramural hematomas are confirmed by a regional aortic wall thickening over 7 mm on CT scan or MRI in the absence of an intimal flap and without enhancement after contrast injection.[79] Each of these entities presents much like aortic dissection, with sharp chest (ascending aorta) or back (descending aorta) pain.[80] In fact, among patients with acute aortic symptoms, 5 to 15 percent of cases are attributable to intramural hematomas.[28,81,82]

Cases of intramural hematoma (IMH) with PAU tend to occur in the descending thoracic aorta (type B), whereas cases of IMH without PAU are grouped in the ascending aorta (type A). Mortality rates follow this delineation: Ascending PAUs led to 57 percent mortality, whereas descending PAUs resulted in 12 percent dissection and death in 5 percent of cases in the study by Ganaha and colleagues.[81] Similarly, 28 percent of cases of type A IMH ended in aortic rupture, compared with only 9 percent of cases of type B IMH in the study by von Kodolitsch and Nienaber.[83] Moreover, 25 percent of cases of IMH without PAU progressed to dissection in the ascending aorta, whereas 13 percent did in the descending aorta. Thus, it has been suggested that type B IMH may be treated conservatively, whereas type A IMH warrants aggressive management.[79,82]

From the pathologic perspective, penetrating atherosclerotic ulcers and intramural hematomas seem to exist on a continuum: When a PAU gains intramural access of sufficient depth, the dissecting process commences, leaving the crescentic ring of blood in the aortic wall characteristic of IMHs. Intramural hematomas originate in severely diseased aortas that have been subject to severe hypertension. Unlike dissection, in which an intimal tear explains this false passage, no such entry is visualized radiographically with IMHs. Nonetheless, a crescentic column of clotted blood fills the space that would be the false lumen in a typical dissection.[80,82,84] Explanations for the origin of this blood have ranged from the spontaneous rupture of the vasa vasorum, to the fracture of an atheromatous plaque, to disruption of a penetrating atherosclerotic ulcer that violates the internal elastic lamina, allowing transit of blood into the layers of the aortic wall.[28,77,85–87]

The natural history of IMHs has been reported to range from progression, to false aneurysm, to spontaneous regression, to dissection, and even to rupture.[79,80,88,89] A recent report correlated initial aortic diameter with progression to a catastrophic result from IMH; patients presenting with an initial aortic diameter greater than 40 mm had a 30-fold increased risk of progression to aneurysm formation or rupture. Furthermore, progression was ninefold more common in patients with an initial aortic wall thickness greater than 1 cm.[88] However, PAUs carry a more severe prognosis than do IMHs: Forty to 50 percent of acutely symptomatic patients progress to acute dissection or aortic rupture during the initial hospital admission.[90,91] Uncontrollable pain, increasing pleural effusion, and larger diameter and depth of PAU all portend progressive disease courses.[81] Therefore, early surgical intervention is recommended for symptomatic penetrating ulcers.[86,90]

Patients with PAU tend to be older and to have multiple comorbidities. Coady and associates[90] found a mean age of 77 years compared with 54 years for type A and 67 years for type B dissections ($p = 0.01$).[90] Associated comorbidities include hypertension,[77,79] COPD, and CAD.[28,81] Fully 40 percent of patients with PAU have been treated previously for AAA, a figure that indicates their extensive degenerative disease. Moreover, these patients carry a more severe prognosis than do those with dissection: 40 percent versus 7.3 percent for type A and 4 percent for type B dissection.

Table 38-3 Results of endovascular repair of penetrating atheromatous ulcer/intramural hematoma

	Schoder 2002	Demers 2004
Technical success	100%	100%
Mortality	0%	12% (15% at 1 year)
Complication rate	12.5%	19%
Paraplegia	12.5%	0%
Endoleak	12.5%	8%
Mean follow-up	14.1 months	51 ± 37 months

Numerous small studies have examined outcomes for stenting grafting of PAUs (Table 38-3). Schoder and associates[92] reported their experience with eight patients with symptomatic PAUs in 2002, including patients with hemoptysis, bloody pleural effusion, and mediastinal bleeding. Six of those patients underwent emergent stent graft repair; all had technical success, although one required an additional stent graft after stent migration (12.5 percent complication rate). There was no periprocedural mortality, but one patient developed fatal hemoptysis 23 months after the procedure. Postmortem examination of that patient raised the question of type I endoleak or a type II endoleak over a patent bronchial artery. Those authors noted that penetrating ulcers can result in pseudoaneurysms, potentially leading to life-threatening aortobronchial fistulas. Thus, the relatively noninvasive approach of endovascular therapy may have a salutary effect on patient safety beyond treatment for the PAU immediately at hand.[92]

In their 2004 paper, Demers and colleagues[93] followed 26 consecutive patients for 8 years after endovascular PAU treatment. They achieved primary success in 92 percent of patients: Two patients had a type I endoleak. One of them was fixed immediately, leading to a 96 percent secondary success rate. Survival at 1 and 5 years was 81 percent and 65 percent, respectively, similar to that seen with open repair. Of note, this series of 26 patient included 14 (54 percent) judged to be unacceptable candidates for thoracotomy. Both larger maximal aortic diameter and female gender were identified as significant independent predictors of treatment failure, pointing to the importance of careful patient selection.[93]

THORACIC AORTIC TRAUMA

Endovascular repair has been explored as a treatment modality for traumatic aortic disruption. Trauma of sufficient severity to cause aortic disruption is often immediately fatal: Sudden death ensues in 75 to 90 percent of those patients, with only 15 to 20 percent able to enter the hospital in a stable condition.[94,95] Those surviving

Table 38-4 Results of endovascular repair of thoracic aortic trauma

	Bartone 2002		Sam 2003	Amabile 2004	Wellons 2004	Demers 2004
Traumatic pathology	Traumatic aortic pseudoaneurysm—immediate	Traumatic aortic pseudoaneurysm—delayed (> 2 weeks)	Blunt traumatic aortic transection	Blunt traumatic aortic rupture	Blunt traumatic aortic disruption	Chronic aneurysm secondary to trauma
Technical success	100%	100%	100%	100%	100%	100%
Mortality	0%	0%	0%	0%	11%	7%
Complication rate	10%		0%	0%	22%	27%
Paraplegia	0%	0%	0%	0%	0%	0%
Endoleak	0%	0%	0%	0%	11%	87%
Mean follow up	14.8 ± 7.8 months		NA	15.1 months	12 months	55 ± 29 months

the immediate injury often have multisystem injuries, making open surgical repair an unattractive option. Mortality rates for open surgical repair in this setting range from 18 to 28 percent, with paraplegia rates of 2.3 to 14 percent.[96,97] Moreover, standard medical therapy carries mortality rates of 20 percent.[35,65,73]

Twenty years of the results of open surgery in 108 patients with traumatic aortic aneurysm were tracked by a group from Duke. Whereas overall mortality was 39 percent, only 26 percent of deaths were directly attributable to aortic trauma, with the rest being the sequelae of multiorgan trauma. The authors concluded that death from intact traumatic aortic aneurysms is attributable mainly to associated injuries and remained relatively constant over the 20-year period of review.[98]

The results of endovascular treatment for traumatic aortic pathology are summarized in Table 38-4. The 2002 study by Bortone and colleagues[63] included a subset of patients with traumatic aortic pseudoaneurysms. Those authors achieved 100 percent technical success with no deaths or paraplegia. There was 1 patient among 10 who required removal of his stent at 2 weeks secondary to compression of the left mainstem bronchus. As with thoracic aortic dissections, those authors advocated immediate endovascular repair rather than waiting more than 2 weeks: Delayed treatment is thought to be associated with the creation of fibrous and calcified connective tissue in the aortic wall, leading to further complications in treatment. In contrast, in the 6 patients (of 10) treated within 2 weeks of traumatic aortic pseudoaneurysm, aortic wall healing was seen in the 1-year follow-up CT scan.[63]

Sam and associates treated three blunt aortic transactions with endovascular cuffs, all successfully.[99] Untreated traumatic thoracic aortic transection has an estimated mortality of 85 percent, whereas standard emergent operative repair is associated with 20 to 30 percent mortality. Each patient was treated with a commercially available device: one with AneuRx aortic cuffs (Medtronic/AVE) and two with Excluder abdominal aortic excluder cuffs (Gore). As these devices are intended for the abdominal aorta, the investigators had to counter their short lengths with the deployment of multiple cuffs. They preferred the Excluder system to that of AneuRx because of its 5 cm of additional length, flexible profile, and smaller delivery sheath.

A group from France retrospectively compared endovascular and surgical treatment of blunt traumatic aortic rupture in 20 patients, 3 of whom had fallen from a great height and the rest of whom sustained their injuries in motor vehicle accidents.[100] Eleven patients were treated surgically, and nine endovascularly. In the surgical group, one patient died, one developed left phrenic paralysis, one had left-sided recurrent nerve injury, and one developed cardiac tamponade. In contrast, the endovascular group had no deaths, no complications (including no endoleaks), and no surgical conversion. However, two patients did require partial coverage of the ostium of the left subclavian with the endostent secondary to insufficient neck length, with no ill effect. Those authors highlighted certain advantages of endovascular treatment for aortic rupture in the post-trauma setting: There is no need for single-lung ventilation in patients who may have lung contusions or rib fractures, systemic heparinization may be avoided in patients with concomitant injuries, and the avoidance of circulatory assistance staves off the systemic inflammatory response in trauma patients.

Wellons and colleagues[101] reviewed their experience with the endovascular treatment of nine hemodynamically stable patients who had sustained severe blunt aortic trauma after motor vehicle accidents. Blood loss ranged from 100 to 200 mL. All the patients underwent successful endovascular repair, although one patient developed a type I endoleak 1 month after repair. There were no procedure-related deaths, no paraplegia, and no renal failure. However, there was a 22 percent complication rate that was ascribable to iliac and femoral artery injuries during access. In light of those admirable results, the authors have adopted two unique strategies. First, they place a superstiff wire into the right axillary artery from the access artery. This allows tracing of the device to the left subclavian artery. Second, they place a percutaneous left brachial artery sheath and diagnostic catheter, allowing continuous aortography during and after device deployment.[101]

Thoracic aortic aneurysms may occur as chronic sequelae of trauma. Demers and colleagues[102] reported their endovascular experience in this setting in 15 patients at an average interval of 18 ± 14 years after the initial injury (motor vehicle accidents in all but one of the patients). This series achieved 100 percent technical success, a 7 percent mortality rate, and a 27 percent rate of complications (left subclavian artery thrombosis and "postimplantation syndrome": fever and leukocytosis). As was discussed previously, in their results for nontraumatic descending TAAs, those authors concluded that endovascular treatment should not be offered to healthy young patients who lack strong contraindications to open repair.[102]

COMPLICATIONS

The emergence of thoracic aortic stent grafting as a primary and often preferred treatment modality for many aortic pathologies has introduced a new spectrum of complications. Because of the rapid evolution of this technology, reports of serious complications and risk analysis are just being appreciated in the literature. Three areas merit mention: spinal ischemic injury, retrograde dissection into the arch, and the consequences of left subclavian coverage.

Spinal cord ischemic injury (SCI) manifesting as paraplegia or paraparesis has been reported in several series, with an incidence of 0 to 12 percent.[103–105] The mechanism of the occurrence of SCI is not completely understood but may involve both primary spinal artery interruption by coverage by stent grafting and hypoperfusion caused by hypotension, which renders the collateral supply ineffective in spinal cord homeostasis. Evidence for such a hypothesis stems from the open surgical literature and the elevated risk appreciated in patients undergoing thoracic endografting in whom prior AAA repair was performed (because lumbar arteries were oversewn).[106]

A recent report by Cheisa and associates[107] examined perioperative risk factors to attempt to predict which patients would be at the highest risk for SCI. Over 5 years, 103 patients underwent endovascular repair of thoracic aortic disease ($N = 88$ TAA, $N = 10$ type B dissection, $N = 5$ PAU). CSF drainage was employed in seven patients on the basis of prior AAA repair or the need to cover T8 to L2 critical intercostals/lumbars. SCI was noted in four patients (4 percent), with all deficits occurring 24 to 96 h after the primary procedure. All deficits resolved with the institution of CSF drainage, steroids, and maintenance of MAP above 90 mmHg. All patients with SCI were noted to have the lowest perioperative MAP below 70 mmHg ($p < 0.001$). No other preoperative demographic or anatomic correlate of the procedure was significant on univariate analysis. Accordingly, vigilance should be maintained in the perioperative period to avoid arrhythmia, anemia, and hypotension as spinal perfusion pressure may be marginal in the immediate perioperative period.[107]

Retrograde dissection (into the arch and ascending aorta) created by the mechanical force of the thoracic stent graft interfacing with the proximal aorta has been described.[108,109] It is important to recognize that this may occur during, immediately after, or weeks after the primary thoracic stent graft implantation. In a report by Neuhauser and coworkers,[108] procedure-related mortality after retrograde type A dissection was 40 percent, with a median time to diagnosis of 21 days postoperatively. Although it may occur more often with stent graft treatment of type B dissection, retrograde dissection has been reported in the treatment of degenerative thoracic aneurysms.[109] The most likely explanation is procedure-related damage to the aortic wall resulting from instrumentation. Violation of the aortic wall creates the nidus that subsequently blossoms into a florid dissection. The variability in presentation, timing, and location underscores the need for regular surveillance of all patients who have been treated with the emerging technology of thoracic aortic endografting.

Coverage of the left subclavian artery for purposes of extending the length of a proximal aortic seal has undergone a significant change in its treatment paradigm. Theoretical concerns about left upper extremity ischemia have not been realized as clinically significant. Such a posture may be clinically predicted from the uncommon presentation of true subclavian steal in patients with subclavian occlusive disease.[110] Recently, a series of 171 patients in whom 22 (12.9 percent) underwent stent graft occlusion of the left subclavian artery was reported.[111] Although a pressure difference was noted between the right (138.4 ± 14.0 mmHg) and left arms (101.8 ± 21 mmHg), no patient manifested a malperfusion syndrome during the primary hospitalization. In follow-up, seven patients reported mild symptoms (mostly exercise-induced weakness), yet none required secondary bypass procedures. In conclusion, it would not appear imperative that subclavian revascularization precede thoracic aortic stent graft coverage of the left subclavian artery; however, if a left internal mammary graft is patent to the coronary circulation, a prophylactic bypass is medically wise.

SUMMARY

Stent graft therapy of the full spectrum of thoracic aortic pathologies is a rapidly developing and emerging technology. On the basis of satisfactory early and middle-term results combined with the obvious avoidance of major cavitary incisions and recovery thereafter, it is very likely that thoracic aortic stent grafting will assume a role as primary therapy for aneurysms, dissections, and traumatic lesions or penetrating ulcers. Not only have endovascular surgeons recognized the advantages of thoracic stent grafts, patients are demanding consideration for such "minimally invasive" options. Open thoracic aortic surgery may become reserved for cases in which anatomy and topography eliminate the viability of graft implantation. Surgeons who want to apply this technology to benefit their patients must do appropriate preoperative planning and imaging, have a solid base of fundamental skill with catheter-based interventions, and recognize the need for regular, lifelong surveillance of all patients treated with thoracic aortic endografts.

References

1. Cambria RP, Davison JK, Zannetti S, et al. Thoracoabdominal aneurysm repair: Perspectives over a decade with the clamp-and-sew technique. *Ann Surg* 1997;226(3):294–303; discussion 303–305.
2. Coselli JS, LeMaire SA, de Figueiredo LP, et al. Paraplegia after thoracoabdominal aortic aneurysm repair: Is dissection a risk factor? *Ann Thorac Surg* 1997;63(1):28–35; discussion 35–36.
3. Coselli JS, LeMaire SA, Conklin LD, et al. Left heart bypass during descending thoracic aortic aneurysm repair does not reduce the incidence of paraplegia. *Ann Thorac Surg* 2004;77:1298–1303.
4. Black JH, Albadawi H, Casey PJ, et al. Acute limb ischemia produces unique systemic and local responses prior to reperfusion. *J Am Coll Surg* 2003; 197(S):98.
5. Levine WC, Lee JJ, Black JH, et al. Thoracoabdominal aneurysm repair: Anesthetic management. *Int Anesthesiol Clin* 2005;43(1):39–60.
6. Cambria RP, Clouse WD, Davison JK, et al. Thoracoabdominal aneurysm repair: Results with 337 operations performed over a 15-year interval. *Ann Surg* 2002;226(4):471–479.
7. Acher CW, Wynn MM, Hoch JR, et al. Combined use of cerebral spinal fluid drainage and naloxone reduces the risk of paraplegia in thoracoabdominal aneurysm repair. *J Vasc Surg* 1994;19(2):236–246.
8. Coselli JS, LeMaire SA, Köksoy C, et al. Cerebrospinal fluid drainage reduces paraplegia after thoracoabdominal aortic aneurysm repair: Results of a randomized clinical trial. *J Vasc Surg* 2002;35:631–639.
9. Spitell PC, Spitell J, Joyce JW. Clinical features and differential diagnosis of aortic dissection: Experience with 236 cases. *Mayo Clin Proc* 1993;68:897–903.
10. Hagan PG, Nienaber CA, Isselbacher EM, et al. The International Registry of Acute Aortic Dissection (IRAD): New insights into an old disease. *JAMA* 2000;283(7): 897–903.
11. Dinsmore RE, Wedeen VJ, Miller SW, et al. MRI of dissection of the aorta: Recognition of the intimal tear and differential flow velocities. *AJR Am J Roentgenol* 1986;146(6):1286–1288.
12. Guthaner DF, Miller DC. Digital subtraction angiography of aortic dissection. *AJR Am J Roentgenol* 1983;141(1):157–161.
13. Petasnick JP. Radiologic evaluation of aortic dissection. *Radiology* 1991;180(2):297–305.
14. Erbel R, Engberding R, Daniel W, et al. Echocardiography in diagnosis of aortic dissection. *Lancet* 1989;1(8636):457–461.
15. Victor MF, Mintz GS, Kotler MN, et al. Two dimensional echocardiographic diagnosis of aortic dissection. *Am J Cardiol* 1981;48(6):1155–1159.
16. Adachi H, Omoto R, Kyo S, et al. [Diagnosis of acute aortic dissection with transesophageal echocardiography and results of surgical treatment.] *Nippon Kyobu Geka Gakkai Zasshi* 1991;39(11):1987–1994.
17. Keren A, Kim CB, Hu BS, et al. Accuracy of biplane and multiplane transesophageal echocardiography in diagnosis of typical acute aortic dissection and intramural hematoma. *J Am Coll Cardiol* 1996;28(3): 627–636.
18. Vignon P, Spencer KT, Rambaud G, et al. Differential transesophageal echocardiographic diagnosis between linear artifacts and intraluminal flap of aortic dissection or disruption. *Chest* 2001;119(6):1778–1790.
19. Erbel R, Bednarczyk I, Pop T, et al. Detection of dissection of the aortic intima and media after angioplasty of coarctation of the aorta: An angiographic, computer tomographic, and echocardiographic comparative study. *Circulation* 1990;81(3):805–814.
20. Moore AG, Eagle KA, Bruckman D, et al. Choice of computed tomography, transesophageal echocardiography, magnetic resonance imaging, and aortography in acute aortic dissection: International Registry of Acute Aortic Dissection (IRAD). *Am J Cardiol* 2002;89(10): 1235–1238.
21. Fruehwald FX, Neuhold A, Fezoulidis J, et al. Cine-MR in dissection of the thoracic aorta. *Eur J Radiol* 1989;9(1):37–41.
22. Tomiguchi S, Morishita S, Nakashima R, et al. Usefulness of turbo-FLASH dynamic MR imaging of dissecting aneurysms of the thoracic aorta. *Cardiovasc Intervent Radiol* 1994;17(1):17–21.
23. Fisher ER, Stern EJ, Godwin JD 2nd, et al. Acute aortic dissection: Typical and atypical imaging features. *Radiographics* 1994;14(6):1263–1271; discussion 1271–1274.
24. Hartnell G, Costello P. The diagnosis of thoracic aortic dissection by noninvasive imaging procedures. *N Engl J Med* 1993;328(22):1637; author reply 1638.
25. Clague J, Magee P, Mills P. Diagnostic techniques in suspected thoracic aortic dissection. *Br Heart J* 1992; 67(6):428–429.
26. Idu MM, Reekers JA, Balm R, et al. Collapse of a stent-graft following treatment of a traumatic thoracic aortic rupture. *J Endovasc Ther* 2005;12(4):503–507.
27. Bickerstaff LK, Pairolero PC, Hollier LH, et al. Thoracic aortic aneuryms: A population-based study. *Surgery* 1982;92:1103–1108.

28. Coady MA, Rizzo JA, Elefteriades JA. Developing surgical intervention criteria for thoracic aortic aneurysms: Penetrating atherosclerotic ulcers and intramural hematomas. *Cardiol Clin North Am* 1999;17:827–839.
29. Davies RR, Goldstein LJ, Coady MA, et al. Yearly rupture or dissection rates for thoracic aortic aneurysms: Simple prediction based on size. *Ann Thorac Surg* 2002;73:17–27.
30. Dake MD, Miller DC, Semba CP, et al. Transluminal placement of endovascular stent-grafts for the treatment of descending thoracic aortic aneurysms. *N Engl J Med* 1994;331(26):1729–1734.
31. Cambria RP, Brewster DC, Lauterbach SR, et al. Evolving experience with thoracic aortic stent graft repair. *J Vasc Surg* 2002;35:1129–1136.
32. Czerny M, Cejna M, Hutschala D, et al. Stent-graft placement in atherosclerotic descending thoracic aortic aneurysms: Midterm results. *J Endovasc Ther* 2004; 11:26–32.
33. Demers P, Miller DC, Mitchell RS, et al. Midterm results of endovascular repair of descending thoracic aortic aneurysms with first-generation stent grafts. *J Thorac Cardiovasc Surg* 2004;127:664–673.
34. Pate JW, Richardson RL, Eastridge CE. Acute aortic dissections. *Am Surg* 1976;42(6):395–404.
35. Kouchoukos NT, Dougenis D. Surgery of the thoracic aorta. *N Engl J Med* 1997;336(26):1876–1888.
36. Khan IA, Nair CK. Clinical, diagnostic, and management perspectives of aortic dissection. *Chest* 2002;122(1): 311–328.
37. Hirst AE, Johns V, Dougenis D. Dissecting aneurysm of the aorta: A review of 505 cases. *Medicine (Baltimore)* 1958;37:217–219.
37a. Meszaros I, Morocz J, Szalvi J, et al. Epidemiology and dinicopathology of aorch dissection. chest 2000;117(5): 1271–1278
38. Cambria RP. Surgical treatment of complicated distal aortic dissection. *Semin Vasc Su*rg 2002;15(2):97–107.
39. Mehta RH, Suzuki T, Hagan PG, et al. Predicting death in patients with acute type A aortic dissection. *Circulation* 2002;105(2):200–206.
40. Lauterbach SR, Cambria RP, Brewster DC, et al. Contemporary management of aortic branch compromise resulting from acute aortic dissection. *J Vasc Surg* 2001;33(6):1185–1192.
41. Cambria RP, Brewster DC, Gertler J, et al. Vascular complications associated with spontaneous aortic dissection. *J Vasc Su*rg 1988;7(2):199–209.
42. Larson EW, Edwards WD. Risk factors for aortic dissection: A necropsy study of 161 cases. *Am J Cardiol* 1984;53(6):849–855.
43. Wheat MW, Jr. Acute dissection of the aorta. *Cardiovasc Clin* 1987;17(3):241–262.
44. O'Gara PT, DeSanctis RW. Acute aortic dissection and its variants: Toward a common diagnostic and therapeutic approach. *Circulation* 1995;92(6):1376–1378.
45. Marsalese DL, Moodie DS, Lytle BW, et al. Cystic medial necrosis of the aorta in patients without Marfan's syndrome: Surgical outcome and long-term follow-up. *J Am Coll Cardiol* 1990;16(1):68–73.
46. Mehta RH, Manfredini R, Hassan F, et al. Chronobiological patterns of acute aortic dissection. *Circulation* 2002;106(9):1110–1115.
47. Reed D, Reed C, Stemmermann G, et al. Are aortic aneurysms caused by atherosclerosis? *Circulation* 1992;85(1):205–211.
48. DeBakey ME, Henly WS, Cooley DA. Surgical management of dissecting aneurysms of the aorta. *Thorac Cardiovasc Surg* 1965;49:130–148.
49. Daily PO, Trueblood HW, Stinson EB, et al. Management of acute aortic dissections. *Ann Thorac Surg* 1970;10: 237–247.
50. Nienaber CA, Eagle KA. Aortic dissection: New frontiers in diagnosis and management. Part II: Therapeutic management and follow-up. *Circulation* 2003;108(6): 772–778.
51. Nallamothu BK, Mehta RH, Saint S, et al. Syncope in acute aortic dissection: Diagnostic, prognostic, and clinical implications. *Am J Med* 2002;113(6):468–471.
52. Syed MA, Fiad TM. Transient paraplegia as a presenting feature of aortic dissection in a young man. *Emerg Med J* 2002;19(2):174–175.
53. Khan I, Wattanasauwan N, Ansari AW. Painless aortic dissection presenting as hoarseness of voice: Cardiovocal syndrome: Ortner's syndrome. *Am J Emerg Med* 1999;17(4):361–363.
54. Greenwood WR, Robinson M. Painless dissection of the thoracic aorta. *Ann Emerg M*ed 1986;4:330–333.
55. Lefebre V, Leduc J, Choteau PH. Painless ischemic lumbosacral plexopathy and aortic dissection. *J Neurol Neurosurg Psychiatry* 1995;58:641.
56. LeMaire SA, Miller CC 3rd, Conklin LD, et al. Estimating group mortality and paraplegia rates after thoracoabdominal aortic aneurysm repair. *Ann Thorac Surg* 2003;75(2):508–513.
57. Juvonen T, Ergin M, Galla JD, et al. Risk factors for rupture of chronic type B dissections. *J Thorac Cardiovasc Surg* 1999;117:776–786.
58. Bernard Y, Zimmermann H, Chocron S, et al. False lumen patency as a predictor of late outcome in aortic dissection. *Am J Cardiol* 2001;87(12):1378–1382.
59. Marui A, Mochizuki T, Mitsui N, et al. Toward the best treatment for uncomplicated patients with type B acute aortic dissection: A consideration for sound surgical indication. *Circulation* 1999;100(Suppl 19):II275–280.
60. Neya K, Omoto R, Kyo S, et al. Outcome of Stanford type B acute aortic dissection. *Circulation* 1992;86(Suppl 5):II1-7.
61. Sasaki S, Yasuda K, Kunihara T, et al. Surgical results of Stanford type B aortic dissection: Comparisons between partial and subtotal replacement of the dissected aorta. *J Cardiovasc Surg (Torino)* 2000;41(2):227–232.
62. Lansman SL, Hagl C, Fink D, et al. Acute type B aortic dissection: Surgical therapy. *Ann Thorac Surg* 2002;74(5):S1833–1835; discussion S1857–1863.
63. Bortone AS, Schena S, D'Agostino D, et al. Immediate versus delayed endovascular treatment of post-traumatic aortic pseudoaneurysms and type B dissections: Retrospective analysis and premises to the upcoming European trial. *Circulation* 2002;106 [12 Suppl 1]: I-234–240.
64. Cambria RP, Brewster DC, Moncure AC, et al. Spontaneous aortic dissection in the presence of coexistent or previously repaired atherosclerotic aortic aneurysm. *Ann Surg* 1988;208(5):619–624.

65. Dake MD, Kato N, Mitchell RS, et al. Endovascular stent-graft placement for the treatment of acute aortic dissection. *N Engl J Med* 1999;340(20):1546–1552.
66. Erbel R, Alfonso F, Boileau C, et al. Diagnosis and management of aortic dissection. *Eur Heart J* 2001;22(18): 1642–1681.
67. Finkbohner R, Johnston D, Crawford ES, et al. Marfan syndrome: Long-term survival and complications after aortic aneurysm repair. *Circulation* 1995;91(3): 728–733.
68. Hausegger KA, Tiesenhausen K, Schedlbauer P, et al. Treatment of acute aortic type B dissection with stent-grafts. *Cardiovasc Intervent Radiol* 2001;24(5):306–312.
69. Ergin MA, Phillips RA, Galla JD, et al. Significance of distal false lumen after type A dissection repair. *Ann Thorac Surg* 1994;57(4):820–824; discussion 825.
70. Kato N, Hirano T, Takeda K, et al. Treatment of aortic dissections with a percutaneous intravascular endoprosthesis: Comparison of covered and bare stents. *J Vasc Interv Radiol* 1994;5(6):805–812.
71. Moon MR, Dake MD, Pelc LR, et al. Intravascular stenting of acute experimental type B dissections. *J Surg Res* 1993;54(4):381–388.
72. Trent MS, Parsonnet V, Shoenfeld R, et al. A balloon-expandable intravascular stent for obliterating experimental aortic dissection. *J Vasc Surg* 1990;11(5): 707–717.
73. Nienaber CA, Fattori R, Lund G, et al. Nonsurgical reconstruction of thoracic aortic dissection by stent-graft placement. *N Engl J M*ed 1999;340(2): 1585–1586.
74. Eggebrecht H, Herold Ulf, Kuhnt O, et al. Endovascular stent-graft treatment of aortic dissection: Determinants of post-interventional outcome. *Eur Heart J* 2005; 26(5):489–497.
75. Kusagawa H, Shimono T, Ishida M. Changes in false lumen after transluminal stent-graft placement in aortic dissections. *Circulation* 2005;111:2951–2957.
76. Nathanson DR, Rodriguez-Lopez JA, Ramaiah VG, et al. Endoluminal stent-graft stabilization for thoracic aortic dissection. *J Endovasc Ther* 2005;12:354–359.
77. Stanson AW, Kazmier FJ, Hollier LH, et al. Penetrating atherosclerotic ulcers of the thoracic aorta: Natural history and clinicopathologic correlations. *Ann Vasc Surg* 1986;1(1):15–23.
78. Krukenberg E. Beiträge zur Frage des Aneuysma dissecans. *Bietr Pathol Anat Allg Pathol* 1920;67:329–351.
79. Muluk SC, Kaufman JA, Torchiana DF, et al. Diagnosis and treatment of thoracic aortic intramural hematoma. *J Vasc Surg* 1996;24(6):1022–1029.
80. Von Kodolitsch Y, Csosz SK, Koschyk DH, et al. Intramural hematoma of the aorta: Predictors of progression to dissection and rupture. *Circulation* 2003;107(8):1158–1163.
81. Ganaha F, Miller DC, Sugimoto K. Prognosis of aortic intramural hematoma with and without penetrating atherosclerotic ulcer: A clinical and radiological analysis. *Circulation* 2002;106:342–348.
82. Nienaber CA, von Kodolitsch Y, Petersen B, et al. Intramural hemorrhage of the thoracic aorta: Diagnostic and therapeutic implications. *Circulation* 1995;92(6): 1465–1472.
83. Von Kodolitsch Y, Nienaber CA. Intramural hemorrhage of the thoracic aorta: Natural history, diagnostic and prognostic profiles of 209 cases with in vivo diagnosis. *Z Kardiol* 1998;87:797–807.
84. Yamada T, Tada S, Harada J. Aortic dissection without intimal rupture: Diagnosis with MR imaging and CT. *Radiology* 1988;168(2):347–352.
85. Mohr-Kahaly S, Erbel R, Kearney P, et al. Aortic intramural hemorrhage visualized by transesophageal echocardiography: Findings and prognostic implications. *J Am Coll Cardiol* 1994;23(3):658–664.
86. Sueyoshi E, Imada T, Sakamoto I, et al. Analysis of predictive factors for progression of type B aortic intramural hematoma with computed tomography. *J Vasc Surg* 2002;35(6):1179–1183.
87. Cambria RP. Regarding "Analysis of predictive factors for progression of type B aortic intramural hematoma with computed tomography." *J Vasc Surg* 2002;35: 1295–1296.
88. Savini C, Casselman F, Ergenoglu MU, et al. Surgical management of progression to type A dissection from an intramural hematoma previously treated with endovascular stent graft placement. *J Thorac Cardiovasc Surg* 2004;128:773–775.
89. Ohmi M, Tabayashi K, Moizumi Y, et al. Extremely rapid regression of aortic intramural hematoma. *J Thorac Cardiovasc Surg* 1999;118(5):968–969.
90. Coady MA, Rizzo JA, Hammond GL, et al. Penetrating ulcer of the thoracic aorta: What is it? How do we recognize it? How do we manage it? *J Vasc Surg* 1998;27(6):1006–1015; discussion 1015–1016.
91. Tittle SL, Lynch RJ, Cole PE et al. Midterm follow-up of penetrating ulcer and intramural hematoma of the aorta. *J Thorac Cardiovasc Surg* 2002;123:1051–1059.
92. Schoder M, Grabenwöger M, Hölzenbein T, et al. Endovascular stent-graft repair of complicated penetrating atherosclerotic ulcers of the descending thoracic aorta. *J Vasc Surg* 2002;36:720–726.
93. Demers P, Miller DC, Mitchell RS, et al. Stent-graft repair of penetrating atherosclerotic ulcers in the descending thoracic aorta: Mid-term results. *Ann Thorac Surg* 2004;77:81–86.
94. Parmley LJ, Mattingly TW, Manion WC, et al. Nonpenetrating traumatic injury of the aorta. *Circulation* 1958;17:1086–1100.
95. Williams JS, Graff JA, Uku JM, et al. Aortic injury in vehicular trauma. *Ann Thorac Surg* 1994;57:726–730.
96. Cowley RA, Turney SZ, Hankins JR, et al. Rupture of thoracic aorta caused by blunt trauma: A fifteen-year experience. *J Thorac Cardiovasc Surg* 1990;100:652–661.
97. Von Oppell UO, Dunne TT, De Groot MK, et al. Traumatic aortic rupture: Twenty-year meta-analysis of mortality and risk for paraplegia. *Ann Thorac Surg* 1994; 58:585–593.
98. Duhaylongsod FG, Glower DD, Wolfe WG. Acute traumatic aortic aneurysm: The Duke experience from 1970 to 1990. *J Vasc Surg* 1992;15:331–343.
99. Sam A, Kibbe M, Matsumura J, et al. Blunt traumatic aortic transection: Endoluminal repair with commercially available aortic cuffs. *J Vasc Surg* 2003;38(5): 1132–1135.
100. Amabile P, Collart F, Gariboldi V, et al. Surgical versus endovascular treatment of traumatic thoracic aortic rupture. *J Vasc Surg* 2004;40:873–879.

101. Wellons ED, Milner R, Solis M, et al. Stent-graft repair of traumatic thoracic aortic disruptions. *J Vasc Surg* 2004;40:1095–1100.
102. Demers P, Miller C, Mitchell RS, et al. Chronic traumatic aneurysms of the descending thoracic aorta: Mid-term results of endovascular repair using first and second-generation stent-grafts. *Eur J Cardiothorac Surg* 2004;25:394–400.
103. Bell RE, Taylor PR, Aukett M, et al. Mid-term results for second-generation thoracic stent grafts. *Br J Surg* 2003;91:811–817.
104. White RA, Donayre CE, Walot I, et al. Endovascular exclusion of descending thoracic aortic aneurysms and chronic dissections: Initial clinical results with the AneuRx device. *J Vasc Surg* 2001;31:927–934.
105. Leurs LJ, Bell R, Degreick Y, et al. Endovascular treatment of thoracic aortic diseases: Combined experience from the EUROSTAR and United Kingdom Thoracic Endograft registries. *J Vasc Surg* 2001;41:670–679.
106. Gravereaux EC, Faries PL, Burks JA, et al. Risk of spinal cord ischemia after endograft repair of thoracic aortic aneurysms. *J Vasc Surg* 2001;34(6):997–1003.
107. Chiesa R, Melissano G, Marrocco-Treischitta MM, et al. Spinal cord ischemia after elective stent-graft repair of the thoracic aorta. *J Vasc Surg* 2003;42:11–17.
108. Neuhauser B, Czermak CV, Fish J, et al. Type A dissection following endovascular thoracic aortic stent-graft repair. *J Endovasc Ther* 2005;12(1):74–81.
109. Pasic M, Bergs P, Knollmann F, et al. Delayed retrograde aortic dissection after endovascular stenting of the descending thoracic aorta. *J Vasc Surg* 2002;36(1):184–186.
110. Hennerici M, Klemm C, Rautenberg W. The subclavian steal phenomenon: A common vascular disorder with rare neurological deficits. *Neurology* 1988;38(5):669–673.
111. Rehders TC, Petzsch M, Ince H, et al. Intentional occlusion of the left subclavian artery during stent-draft implantation in the thoracic aorta: Risks and relevance. *J Endovasc Ther* 2004;11(6):659–666.

CHAPTER

39 PACEMAKER AND DEFIBRILLATOR THERAPY IN CARDIAC SURGERY PATIENTS

Kenneth C. Bilchick, Ronald D. Berger

INTRODUCTION

Permanent pacemakers (PPM) were introduced in the 1950s for use in patients with pathologic conditions of the sinus node, atrioventricular (AV) node, or His-Purkinje system. Since that time they have been refined to allow more complex programming. In addition, periprocedural morbidity has been reduced significantly. As a result, the number of devices implanted has increased steadily, with over 150,000 new pacemakers implanted in the United States each year.[1]

ANATOMY OF THE CONDUCTION SYSTEM

The sinus node is an oval piece of tissue in the roof of the right atrium that is 10 to 20 mm long and 2 to 3 mm wide. It is less than 1 mm from the epicardial surface between the superior and inferior venae cavae.[2,3] Its blood supply is derived from the right coronary artery (RCA) 55 to 60 percent of the time and from the circumflex artery 40 to 45 percent of the time.[2]

The atria are anatomically complex structures and differ significantly from each other. The right atrium is heavily trabeculated over the lateral wall and appendage and is characterized by significant heterogeneity, for example, with abrupt changes in muscle fiber orientation over short distances. In contrast, the left atrium is a more uniform structure. Unlike ventricular myocardium, which contains Purkinje fibers, it now is generally accepted that the atria do not contain specialized conduction tissue. Instead, the spread of the impulse depends on the properties of the atrial muscle bundles. Simultaneous electrical mapping of canine left and right atria demonstrate that the left atrium consistently activates approximately 10 ms later than does the right atrium. Rapid activation of the anterior surface of the left atrium is facilitated by a muscle bundle known as Bachmann's bundle. The wave fronts then converge in the posterior left atrium inferior to the pulmonary veins. Human atria demonstrate similar activation patterns, although the activation times are twice as long because of the larger atrial surface area.[3]

The compact portion of the atrioventricular node (AVN) is just beneath the right atrial endocardium anterior to coronary sinus ostium and directly above the insertion of the septal leaflet of the tricuspid valve (TV). The AVN is located at the apex of the triangle of Koch, which is defined by the TV inferiorly, the tendon of Todaro superiorly, and a line drawn between the coronary sinus and the tricuspid annulus posteriorly. Of note, the node is well removed anteriorly from the coronary sinus. The AVN becomes the penetrating bundle of His at the central fibrous body. In 85 to 90 percent of people, the blood supply to the AVN is via the RCA; in the remainder, blood is supplied via the circumflex artery.[2]

The branching portion of the His bundle begins at the muscular intraventricular septum and becomes the left bundle branch (LBB) and the right bundle branch (RBB). The LBB arises and continues onto the septum beneath the noncoronary cusp of the aortic valve. The LBB may divide into anterior and posterior branches or may have a different branching pattern. The RBB continues as an unbranched extension of the AV node and continues along the right side of interventricular septum to the apex of the right ventricle (RV) and the base of the anterior papillary muscle. Purkinje fibers continue from the bundle branches as networks of conduction fibers on the endocardial surface of both ventricles.[2]

ELECTRICAL PRINCIPLES OF CARDIAC PACING

The conducting tissues of the heart may be divided into fast-response and slow-response tissues. The distribution of ions and their associated electrical voltage gradients are responsible for the cardiac action potential. The baseline of this potential is −90 mV, and the peak is +20 mV for fast-response tissues (Fig. 39-1). The depolarization of fast-response tissues such as the atria, the bundle of His, bundle branches, and Purkinje fibers is due to an inward sodium current, whereas repolarization of those tissues is due primarily to outward potassium currents. In slow-response tissues such as the sinus node and the AVN, the baseline is about −70 mV and depolarization depends primarily on the L-type calcium current.

Cardiac pacing is based on the principle that myocardial cells can be depolarized repeatedly by electrical stimulation. In cardiac pacing, voltage is applied across two electrodes, at least one of which is in contact with myocardium. In bipolar leads, the two electrodes usually are separated from each other on the lead by about 1 cm. In unipolar leads, only one electrode is in contact with the myocardium, and the other electrode is typically the outer can of the pacemaker generator.

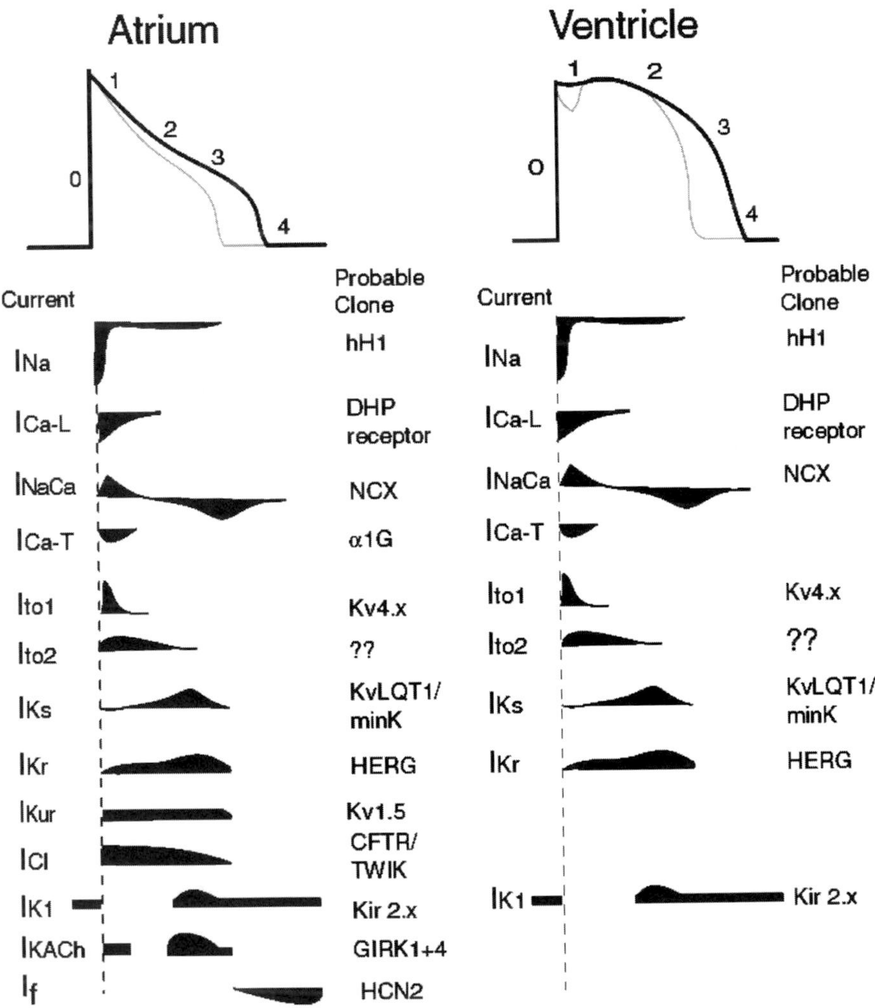

Figure 39-1 Atrial and ventricular action potentials. Schematic of inward and outward ionic currents, pumps, and exchangers that underlie atrial and ventricular action potentials in the mammalian heart. Control and failing (*bold line*) action potential profiles are shown on top. Each phase of the action potential is labeled. Under the action potentials, a schematic of the time course of each current is shown, and the gene product (probable clone) that underlies the current is indicated. (From Akar FG, Tomaselli GF. Genetic basis of cardiac arrhythmias. In: Fuster V, Alexander A, O'Rourke RA (eds). *Hurst's the Heart*, 11th ed. New York: McGraw-Hill; 2004.)

The voltage, current, resistance, and energy of a pacing system are related to one another according to the following equations:

$$V = I \times R$$

where V = voltage (volts), I = current (milliamperes), and R = resistance (kilohms).

$$E = V \times I \times t \text{ (time the current is applied) or } E = (V^2/R) \times t$$

Electrical sensing is based on the detection of the intrinsic current between the two electrodes on bipolar leads or between the lead tip and the pacemaker generator in a unipolar system, with a filter system in place. Unipolar systems are subject to much more noise and/or cross talk than are bipolar leads because the distance between the two electrodes is greater.

CLINICAL INDICATIONS FOR PACING

Indications for permanent pacing

Current indications for permanent pacing are based on the 1998 practice guidelines and the 2002 update to those guidelines devised by the American College of Cardiology (ACC), the American Heart Association (AHA), and the North American Society of Pacing and Electrophysiology (NASPE).[4] The indications follow the standard evidence-based tiered system. A class I indication means that a procedure generally is agreed to be beneficial; class IIa indications are those for which there is conflicting evidence or a divergence of opinion but the weight of evidence is in favor of a procedure. Class IIb is similar to class IIa except that the efficacy of a procedure is less well established.

Permanent pacing should be considered for all patients with irreversible symptomatic bradycardia and selected patients with asymptomatic bradycardia. In addition, the use of biventricular permanent pacing (see below) is increasing in patients with dilated cardiomyopathies accompanied by conduction delay and medically refractory symptoms, whereas right ventricular pacing may be considered in selected patients with hypertrophic cardiomyopathies. Pacing needs in specific cardiac surgeries are considered individually later in this section but are based on the general indications given below.

Common causes of symptomatic bradycardia include sinus node dysfunction (SND), AV block (second or third degree), and carotid sinus hypersensitivity (CSH). The following is a summary of the recommendations for permanent pacemaker implantation in each of these conditions[4]:

SND: Class I with symptomatic bradycardia
Atrioventricular block (AVB), third degree:
  Class I with symptomatic bradycardia
  Class I if ventricular rate less than 40 beats per minute (bpm) or asystole more than 3 s
  Class IIa without symptoms, rate greater than 40 bpm, no asystole more than 3 s
AVB-Mob.2:
  Class I with symptomatic bradycardia
  Class I if wide QRS is present
  Class IIa without symptoms and narrow QRS
AVB-Mob.1:
  Class I with symptomatic bradycardia not recommended without symptoms
CSH: Class I with sinus pause more than 3 s or hypotension

In addition to these indications, the current guidelines give specific indications for permanent pacing in patients with bifascicular block (right bundle branch block accompanied by left hemiblock or left bundle branch block alone):

Class I: Intermittent or persistent Mobitz 2 AV block
  Third-degree AV block
  Alternating bundle branch block
Class IIa: Syncopal episode as long as other causes (specifically ventricular tachycardia) have been excluded[4]

Permanent pacing after coronary artery bypass grafting

After coronary artery bypass grafting (CABG) or valve surgery, patients may develop a number of conduction disturbances, including a left hemiblock, right bundle branch block (RBBB), left bundle branch block (LBBB), bifascicular block, and AV block. The significance of the various fascicular blocks after CABG has been controversial. In contrast to some early studies from the 1970s and 1980s, more recent studies of patients after CABG have not demonstrated any association between bundle branch block or intraventricular conduction defects and cardiac mortality over 3 to 5 years[5–7] even though these conduction disturbances probably indicate some degree of intraoperative myocardial damage.

The natural history of AV block in patients after CABG is that it may resolve within hours after the surgery; last for days, weeks, or months and then resolve; or persist.[8,9] In a series of 348 consecutive patients undergoing CABG, 56 of whom developed AV block postoperatively, the AV block lasted for less than 6 h in 32 (57 percent) and for more than 6 h in 24 (43 percent).[10] In another series of 93 consecutive patients undergoing CABG, all four patients who developed third-degree AV block after the surgery were no longer in AV block after 2 months (AV block resolved in one patient on the second postoperative day; the other three patients had permanent pacemakers implanted before discharge).[8] Another study evaluated 26 patients who had a PPM implanted for AV block and 10 patients with a PPM implanted for SND after CABG. The pacemaker dependency rate (defined as the need for pacing with mode set to VVI 50) after 3 years was 65 percent for the AV block group and 30 percent for the SND group.[9] If the AV block resolves, permanent pacing is unnecessary. Although it may be reasoned that selected patients may not need a generator change at the time of battery end of life because of potential recovery of the conduction system, the authors generally maintain the PPM in most patients because it is difficult to establish with certainty that these patients will not require pacing at some point in the future. Furthermore, it should be noted that a generator change is a very low-risk procedure.

It has been estimated that overall 0.4 to 1.1 percent of patients who undergo CABG will require permanent pacing.[11] Risk factors for AV block and other conduction disturbances include advanced age, the number of vessels bypassed, left main coronary artery stenosis accompanied by total occlusion of a dominant right coronary artery, the presence of an ungraftable right coronary artery, proximal left anterior descending artery (LAD) stenosis involving the first septal perforator, aortic cross-clamp time, and prolonged hypothermic cardioplegia.[8–10,12,13] Of note, the use of normothermic cardioplegia for shorter periods may be responsible for the decreased incidence of AV block after CABG in some series.[14]

Permanent pacing after valvular surgery

Compared with the approximately 1 percent of patients undergoing CABG who have a need for permanent pacing, 3 to 6 percent of patients undergoing valve surgery require permanent pacing.[11,15] The most likely reason for the increased need for permanent pacing after valve surgery is the risk of trauma to the conduction system with this procedure. An estimation of the likelihood of the need for permanent pacing at the time of the surgery informs the choice of the temporary epicardial pacing configuration. Since temporary leads may be associated with bleeding, tamponade, bypass graft injury, and infection, only the necessary number of leads should be implanted. For example, whereas a single ventricular epicardial lead may be appropriate for a low-risk patient, a dual-lead configuration with an additional ventricular lead (in case one lead fails) may be appropriate for higher-risk patients.

A recently published series of 4694 patients undergoing valve surgery between 1992 and 2002 at the Brigham and Women's Hospital established in a multivariate analysis the following as risk factors for conduction disturbances requiring permanent pacemaker implantation: RBBB [odds ratio (OR) 3.6], LBBB (OR 2.0) and PR interval more than 200 ms (OR 1.9) on the preoperative electrocardiogram, multivalve surgery involving the tricuspid valve (OR 3.7) or not involving it (OR 2.1), advanced age (OR 1.4), and a history of prior valve surgery (OR 1.8).[15] For surgery involving only one

Table 39-1 Risk score to predict permanent pacing after valve surgery

Variable	Points
Preoperative electrocardiogram	
Right bundle branch block	2
Left bundle branch block	1
PR interval > 200 ms	1
Multivalve surgery	
Tricuspid valve included	2
Tricuspid valve not included	1
Other	
Age 70 years or above	1
Prior valve surgery	1

Source: Koplan BA, Stevenson WG, Epstein LM, et al. Development and validation of a simple risk score to predict the need for permanent pacing after cardiac valve surgery. *J Am Coll Cardiol* 2003;41: 795–801.

valve, the risk was lowest for mitral valve surgery (3.5 percent), somewhat higher for aortic valve surgery (5.1 percent), and highest for tricuspid valve surgery (12 percent). On the basis of the preoperative electrocardiogram, the need for permanent pacing was greatest in those with a preexisting isolated RBBB (18 percent) or an RBBB accompanied by a left hemiblock (bifascicular block; 16 percent) and somewhat lower in those with a preexisting LBBB (10 percent). A prediction rule for the need for permanent pacing was developed according to the point system shown in Table 39-1. The need for permanent pacing for total point scores of 0, 1, 2, 3, 4, 5, and 6 was 1.9 percent, 5.2 percent, 8.7 percent, 12 percent, 21 percent, 36 percent, and 50 percent, respectively.[15]

Prophylaxis for postoperative atrial fibrillation

Postoperative atrial fibrillation occurs in 10 to 40 percent of all patients undergoing open heart surgery.[16–19] The issue of prophylactic pacing after cardiac surgery as prophylaxis for atrial fibrillation was addressed in a metanalysis of eight trials that enrolled a total of 776 patients and compared control patients with patients randomized to right atrial, left atrial, or biatrial pacing.[20] The patients could be paced at a fixed high rate (fixed high-rate pacing) or at a rate just fast enough to overcome the intrinsic rate (overdrive pacing). Risk reductions for postoperative atrial fibrillation of 2.6-fold and 1.8-fold were found for overdrive biatrial and right atrial pacing, respectively, and a there was a 2.5-fold reduction for fixed high-rate biatrial pacing. Whether biatrial pacing confers an advantage over right atrial pacing is controversial.[21,22] Ongoing studies should help clarify these issues. Although temporary atrial pacing to decrease atrial fibrillation after cardiac surgery has gained general acceptance, the data supporting permanent pacing are less strong.

Although medical therapy with prophylactic beta blockers, amiodarone, and sotalol has been shown to reduce postoperative atrial fibrillation, pacing therapy offers several advantages, including minimal expense; no association with ventricular proarrhythmia, bradycardia, or hypotension; and no need for the initiation of therapy before surgery. In summary, the approximately 2.5-fold risk reduction associated with biatrial pacing (either overdrive or fixed high rate) and overdrive right atrial pacing makes pacing an attractive nonpharmacologic method for preventing atrial fibrillation after cardiac surgery, particularly since atrial epicardial wires are in place.

Pacing in cardiac transplantation

Bradycardia after cardiac transplantation is common, usually temporary, and often due to SND. Although the most common cause for this SND is probably surgical trauma at the time of transplantation,[23] several other causes have been implicated, including disruption of the blood supply to the sinus node,[24] ischemic time,[25] rejection,[26] donor age,[27] and pretransplant amiodarone use.[28]

Until the early 1990s, the standard anastomosis between the recipient and donor hearts was a biatrial anastomosis, as originally described by Lower and Shumway in the canine heart in 1960.[29] As the biatrial anastomosis requires opening the recipient right atrium from the inferior vena caval orifice with transection and oversewing of the recipient superior vena cava, the suture line may result in direct damage to the donor sinus node as well as the blood supply to the sinus node.[30] In the bicaval anastomosis, which came into widespread use in the 1990s, there are direct donor-recipient anastomoses of the inferior and superior vena cava, although the left-sided anastomosis may occur at the level of the pulmonary vein or left atrium, depending on the technique used.[31,32] As might be expected, several studies have documented a decreased need for pacing with the use of the bicaval anastomosis compared with the standard biatrial anastomosis.[30,33–35] In the two randomized studies that compared the need for permanent pacing on the basis of the type of anastomosis used, permanent pacing was required in 5 (6.5 percent) of 75 patients with the biatrial anastomosis but was not required in any of the 81 patients with the bicaval anastomosis. According to a compilation of six studies, permanent pacing was required in 60 (9.2 percent) of 651 patients with biatrial anastomoses compared with only 1 (0.3 percent) of 340 patients with bicaval anastomoses.

The initial approach to a cardiac transplant patient with postoperative bradycardia resulting from SND is medical therapy with chronotropic agents and the use of operatively placed temporary epicardial leads if necessary. Theophylline has been shown to improve prolonged chronotropic dysfunction in transplant recipients and is the drug of choice.[36] Isoproterenol and terbutaline also may be used. Published commentaries generally have recommended permanent pacing if bradycardia caused by SND persists for 2 to 3 weeks.[30,37] Ambulatory Holter monitoring may aid in the decision whether to implant a permanent pacemaker. The reason to wait as long as possible to implant a permanent system is that SND after transplantation is usually manifest by the first week and resolves over 1 to 3 months. Serial electrophysiologic studies in 40 posttransplant patients demonstrated that the sinus node recovery time (SNRT) became abnormal by the first week in 6 (15 percent) patients and by 3 months in 1 other patient. In all six patients with early sinus node dysfunction, the SNRT returned to normal by 6 weeks, although sinoatrial conduction abnormalities persisted in two patients.[38] Because maintaining AV synchrony will maximize cardiac output, a dual-chamber pacemaker system usually is used and programmed to DDDR, although permanent atrial pacing without a ventricular lead is an option (albeit one rarely used in the United States) if AV conduction is intact. One advantage of using an atrial lead only is the decreased likelihood of dislodgment with biopsy, although this is uncommon with experienced operators. If a biatrial anastomosis is present, the pacemaker lead should be implanted in the anteroseptal right atrium rather than the lateral right atrium near the anastomosis.

Cardiac resynchronization therapy (biventricular pacing)

Cardiac resynchronization therapy (CRT) is intended for patients with dilated cardiomyopathy, intraventricular conduction delay, and heart failure. The objective is to correct dyssynchrony by pacing the left ventricle alone or both ventricles (biventricular). Since the left ventricle usually is paced via the coronary sinus, transvenous left ventricular pacing is more technically difficult than is endocardial right ventricular pacing. These transvenous leads can be placed successfully about 90 percent of the time. For the remaining cases, an epicardial approach may be used, as discussed below.

The Multisite Stimulation in Cardiomyopathy (MUSTIC) study has shown statistically significant improvements in the 6-min walk and quality of life (but not mortality) with biventricular pacing,[39] and the Multisite InSync Randomized Clinical Evaluation (MIRACLE) study has shown improvements in functional class, quality of life, and left ventricular dimensions.[40] Results from the recent COMPANION study in dilated cardiomyopathy patients with intraventricular conduction delay demonstrated a 43 percent reduction in mortality with a combination device capable of both CRT and defibrillation (CRT-D) and a 24 percent reduction in mortality for CRT only (borderline, $p = 0.059$).[41] On the basis of the 2002 guideline update, there is now a class IIa indication for biventricular pacing in patients with idiopathic dilated or ischemic cardiomyopathy who meet the following criteria: class III or IV heart failure symptoms refractory to medical therapy, QRS width greater than or equal to 130 ms, left ventricular ejection fraction (LVEF) less than or equal to 35 percent, and LV end-diastolic diameter greater than 55 mm.[4] In light of recent SCD-HeFT trial data showing a survival benefit with defibrillators in patients with class II or III heart failure and an ejection fraction greater than or equal to 35 percent regardless of etiology (nonischemic or ischemic),[42,43] most patients who receive CRT will get a combination biventricular pacemaker-defibrillator.

Hypertrophic obstructive cardiomyopathy

The objective of permanent pacing in patients with hypertrophic obstructive cardiomyopathy is to improve outflow obstruction with early stimulation of the right ventricular apex. The pacemaker is programmed to DDD mode with leads in the right atrium and right ventricle. In randomized clinical studies such as the Pacemaker in Cardiomyopathy study[44] and the M-PATHY study,[45] DDD pacing resulted in statistically significant reductions in the left ventricular outflow tract pressure gradient but only mild improvement in functional status. Myomectomy and ethanol septal ablation are probably more effective treatment options for patients with hypertrophic obstructive cardiomyopathy. The decision whether to implant a pacemaker alone or a pacemaker-defibrillator is based on clinical judgment but may be guided by several factors that, if present, favor a pacemaker-defibrillator. These factors are a personal history of syncope or sudden cardiac death, a family history of sudden cardiac death, nonsustained ventricular tachycardia, massive hypertrophy (wall thickness of 30 mm or more), a pathologic drop in blood pressure with exercise, and hypertrophic cardiomyopathy mutations associated with an increased risk for sudden cardiac death.

Pacing after a myocardial infarction

In patients who have had a myocardial infarction, temporary pacing is indicated for the following conditions:

1. Asystole (class I)
2. Symptomatic bradycardia (class I)
3. Bilateral BBB [alternating BBB or RBBB with alternating left anterior/posterior fascicular block (LAFB/LPFB)] (class I)
4. Asymptomatic Mobitz 2 AV block (class I)
5. New bifascicular block (LBBB or RBBB with left hemiblock) (class I with a prolonged PR interval or class IIa with a normal PR interval)
6. Recurring sinus pauses not responsive to atropine (class IIa)

Permanent pacing is indicated for the following conditions:

1. Symptomatic and persistent second- or third-degree AV block (class I)
2. Transient Mobitz second- or third-degree infranodal AV block (suggested by wide QRS but may require electrophysiologic study) (class I)[4]

Permanent pacing usually is not indicated after a myocardial infarction for transient second- or third-degree AV block in the absence of a wide QRS (e.g., with an isolated LAFB).

PACEMAKER LEADS AND TECHNIQUES FOR IMPLANTATION

Temporary endocardial leads

Temporary endocardial leads usually are introduced via a sheath system in a jugular or subclavian vein. The right internal jugular vein is generally the vein of choice, as it allows for easy passage of the pacing lead through the right atrium and into the right ventricle. As these leads usually are placed in the intensive care unit, often without the aid of fluoroscopy, the position of the lead initially is gauged by viewing the intracardiac electrogram (the distal end of the pacing lead is attached to a cardiac monitoring system). Premature ventricular beats and injury current indicate that the lead is in contact with the right ventricular myocardium. A common pitfall is pacing the tricuspid annulus. Because this is an unstable position, the lead should be advanced amply into the right ventricle. After the introduction of the lead and verification of appropriate pacing thresholds, the lead should be locked into place in the sheath and its position should be verified with chest radiography.

Permanent endocardial leads

Endocardial leads may be fixated actively or passively. The technique for the introduction of permanent endocardial leads is discussed in detail below. In active fixation, a screw mechanism attaches the lead to the endocardium. Passive fixation leads have polyurethane or silicon tines that facilitate attachment to trabeculae. Pacing thresholds may be slightly higher with active fixation, although this is rarely of any consequence. Pacing thresholds may increase after active fixation as a result of inflammation and fibrosis at the site of injury. In general, active fixation leads are more likely to perforate but easier to extract. The two leads have similar sensing characteristics.

Atrial pacemaker leads are designed for placement in the right atrial appendage with trabeculae that stabilize the lead tip. Passive ventricular leads are designed for placement in the apex of the right ventricle with its trabeculations. Placement of leads in other areas of the atrium and ventricle generally requires active fixation for stabilization.

Technique for implantation of permanent endocardial leads

The subclavian approach is currently the standard approach for the placement of endocardial leads and is used for the placement of over 75 percent of those leads.[1] This approach has evolved since Furman and Schwedel[46] reported successful transvenous endocardial pacing via the brachial vein in 1959. Because of a high rate of lead dislodgement, this approach was replaced briefly by the external jugular vein approach.[47] The cephalic cut-down approach became the standard in the late 1960s[48] and remained the standard for over a decade. As a result of the introduction of the peel-away sheath for the percutaneous introduction of leads, the subclavian approach emerged and remains the standard.[49] In a series of 200 consecutive patients randomized to endocardial lead insertion via a subclavian approach or a cephalic approach, successful lead placement was achieved in 99 percent randomized to the subclavian approach and 64 percent of cases with the cephalic approach.[50] The total procedure time was 86 +/−22 min with the subclavian approach and 98 +/− 35 min with the cephalic approach ($p < 0.01$). Blood loss was also less with the subclavian approach (55+/−13 mL versus 115 +/−107mL; $p < 0.01$).

The following approach is the one described by Calkins and coworkers and is used at the authors' institution[50]:

1. The patient is positioned supine on the table with fluoroscopy available.
2. Local anesthesia is given (this may be sufficient, but light sedation often is needed).
3. A sterile field is created.
4. A subcutaneous generator pocket is created by an incision 2 cm below and parallel to the clavicle. The pocket is created along the pectoralis fascia (Fig. 39-2).
5. Subclavian venipuncture is accomplished using a 5F micropuncture introducer needle attached to extension tubing and a 10-mL syringe (Figs. 39-3 and 39-4). Approximately 10 to 20 mL of 1:1 contrast dye and normal saline solution is injected via an intravenous (IV) line placed distally in an ipsilateral vein and then flushed with 25 to 50 mL of saline.
6. Once the axillary and subclavian veins have been opacified, the micropuncture needle is positioned at a 60-degree angle to the plane of the skin and parallel to the axillary vein. Adjustment of the site of needle entry may be necessary to ensure that the needle enters the vein as it crosses over the first rib.

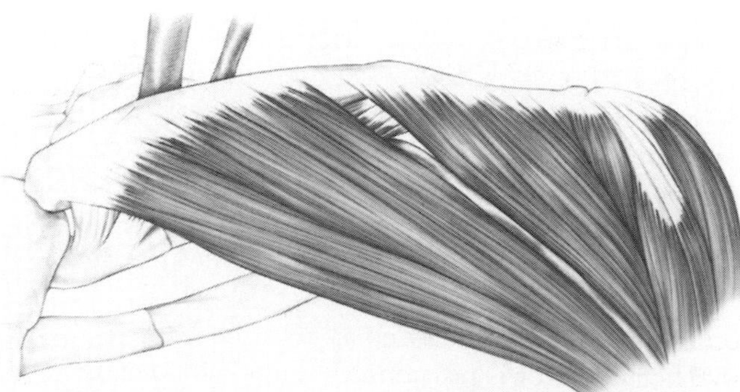

Figure 39-2 Superficial clavicular anatomy. (From Calkins H, Ramza BM, Brinker J, et al. Prospective randomized comparison of the safety and effectiveness of placement of endocardial pacemaker and defibrillator leads using the extrathoracic subclavian vein guided by contrast venography versus the cephalic approach. *Pacing Clin Electrophysiol* 2001;24:456–464.)

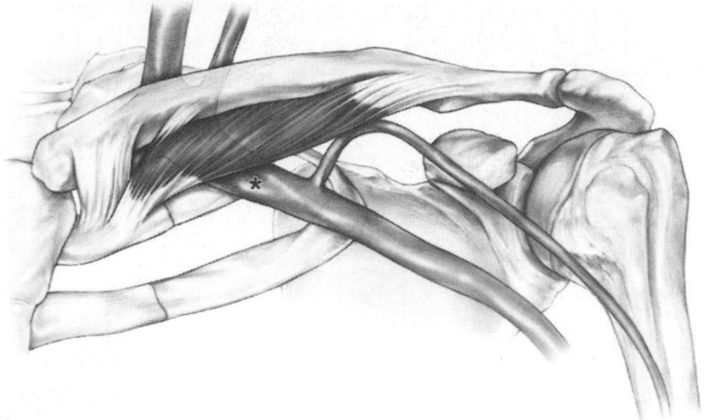

Figure 39-3 Left subclavian vein and associated anatomic structures. (From Calkins H, Ramza BM, Brinker J, et al. Prospective randomized comparison of the safety and effectiveness of placement of endocardial pacemaker and defibrillator leads using the extrathoracic subclavian vein guided by contrast venography versus the cephalic approach. *Pacing Clin Electrophysiol* 2001;24:456–464.)

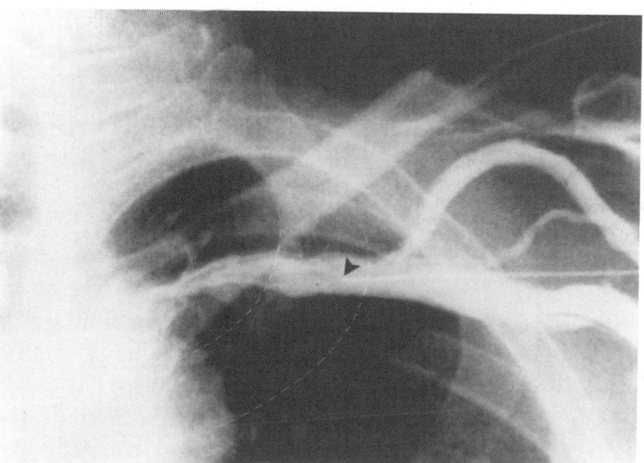

Figure 39-4 Subclavian venography. (From Calkins H, Ramza BM, Brinker J, et al. Prospective randomized comparison of the safety and effectiveness of placement of endocardial pacemaker and defibrillator leads using the extrathoracic subclavian vein guided by contrast venography versus the cephalic approach. *Pacing Clin Electrophysiol* 2001; 24:456–464.)

7. A micropuncture guidewire is advanced through the needle to the superior vena cava and is replaced by a 5F micropuncture sheath that allows the introduction of a 50-cm, 0.035-in. J-tipped guidewire. A 9F peel-away sheath is advanced over the 0.035-in. guidewire.
8. The ventricular lead is advanced through this sheath, and the sheath then is peeled and removed. The ventricular lead is advanced into the right ventricular apex under fluoroscopy.
9. If an atrial lead is planned as well, a second subclavian venipuncture is made, and the atrial lead is placed with the use of the same technique.
10. The leads are connected to the generator, and then pacing and sensing measurements are obtained.
11. If measurements are satisfactory, the lead is screwed in (active fixation) or securely placed among trabeculae (passive fixation). The leads are secured by suture sleeves within the device pocket.
12. The pocket is irrigated with antibiotic solution.
13. The excess lead is coiled and placed into pocket along with the generator.[50]

In general, if the leads are placed too far laterally, there is a greater risk of arterial puncture, whereas if the placement is too medial, there is increased risk of entrapment by the costoclavicular ligament and/or the subclavius muscle.[51]

If the cephalic approach is used, an oblique incision is made just lateral to the deltopectoral groove at the level of the coracoid process of the scapula. A pocket is created, using standard techniques. After dissection down to the pectoralis fascia and identification of the fat pad, the cephalic vein is dissected free, with proximal and distal control of the vein obtained by using permanent silk sutures. A small venotomy is made in the cephalic vein, which is held open with a vein pick. A standard 50-cm 0.035-in. J-tipped guidewire is introduced, and one or two endocardial leads are placed, using standard peel-away sheaths.[50]

Antibiotic prophylaxis for endocardial leads

Antibiotics are given empirically before and after the procedure. Before the procedure, 1 g cefazolin (or 1 g clindamycin for patients with penicillin allergy) should be given. After the procedure, 1 g cefazolin should be given three times daily during the first day. For the second and third days, 500 mg cephalexin three or four times daily should be given. The periprocedural IV antibiotic doses are more important than the postprocedural oral doses. Of note, the choice of the duration of postprocedural antibiotics is somewhat arbitrary.

Temporary epicardial leads

Temporary atrial and ventricular epicardial pacing wires are passed superficially through the epicardial surface, with the atrial wires secured superficially with fine Prolene sutures. The duration of capture with these wires varies, but most start to fail after a week or two. Once they no longer are needed, they generally are extracted, with traction applied to the leads as they emerge from the thorax; this usually causes the suture to break or the lead to pull out from underneath it. This usually does not result in any bleeding.

Permanent epicardial leads

Permanent epicardial leads either screw into the myocardium or are fixed actively in contact with the epicardial surface with deeper Prolene sutures. As is discussed below, placement of permanent epicardial leads requires a small thoracotomy. Any lead can be placed through such a thoracotomy, using standard open surgical techniques. Despite the small size of the thoracotomy, placement of these leads may result in significant postoperative pain, probably because significant force must be applied to spread the ribs during the procedure. There has been increasing experience with placement of epicardial leads using a robotic arm, particularly when a left ventricular lead has to be placed for a biventricular pacing system, as is discussed below. One advantage of this technique is a significant reduction in postoperative pain as a result of the need for only a few small incisions for the arm, camera, and so on.

Technique for standard surgical placement of epicardial leads

Epicardial leads may be placed with the subxiphoid approach or an anterior thoracotomy approach. The subxiphoid approach is preferred in patients without prior cardiac surgery and is performed as follows:

1. With local anesthesia, a vertical midline incision is made below the xiphoid process.
2. The rectus sheath and anterior diaphragm are exposed.
3. The xiphoid process is retracted superiorly or removed, and the subcutaneous fat is dissected.
4. The diaphragmatic portion of the pericardial surface is exposed and opened.
5. Epicardial screw-in leads are attached to the right ventricular free wall.
6. The pericardium is closed around the leads.
7. The generator is placed in the subcutaneous tissue.

The anterior thoracotomy approach often is reserved for patients with prior cardiac surgery and is performed as follows:

1. Access is via the fifth intercostal space.
2. The anterolateral left ventricle is exposed.
3. The leads are fixed and then tunneled subcutaneously to the pulse generator, which usually is placed in the left upper quadrant of the abdomen.

Robotic arm placement of the left ventricular lead for biventricular pacing systems

In approximately 10 percent of patients referred for a biventricular pacing system, placement of the coronary sinus is unsuccessful. In these situations, a surgical left ventricular (LV) epicardial lead may be considered. There has been increasing experience with minimally invasive LV epicardial lead placement, using a robotic surgical system such as the da Vinci Robotic Surgical System (Intuitive Surgical, Sunnyvale, CA). In a series of 10 patients[52] in which 19 epicardial leads were placed (1 patient received only one lead), mean robotic operative time for all cases was 83 ± 53 min (range 30 to 80 min) and was significantly lower in the last 5 cases (50 ± 16 min) compared with the first 5 cases (108 ± 54 min). All the patients were alive and well 25 ± 10 weeks after follow-up with significant improvement in New York Heart Association (NYHA) class and LVEF observed. Reported complications included one inadvertent injury to the LV free wall (corrected with robotically placed pledgeted sutures) early in the series. This was attributed to mediastinal shift associated with mechanical ventilation that allowed the LV to move toward the chest well; in subsequent cases, mechanical ventilation was held during lead placement. One patient developed left lower lobe pneumonia 3 days after the procedure. No blood transfusions or reoperations for bleeding were required.

According to the authors, their surgical approach is as follows. In the seventh intercostal space at the posterior axillary line, a camera port was placed, and the left and right arms of the robot were positioned in the ninth and fifth intercostal spaces, respectively. The left chest was insufflated to a pressure of 8 to 10 mmHg, and a 10-mm working port (for the introduction of the lead and sutures) was inserted posterior to the camera port. The pericardium was opened and retracted posterior to the phrenic nerve. The first and second obtuse marginal (OM) vessels were identified. The pacing lead was introduced through the working port and then secured in place with the robotic arms. (More commonly, a screw-in lead was used, but epicardial steroid-eluting sew-on leads were used in two patients.) In most cases, the lead was placed between the second and third OM vessels, which corresponded to the time of latest ventricular activation as measured by a temporary pacing lead. The pericardium was closed over the permanent leads, which were tunneled to a counterincision in the axilla. After chest tube placement for evacuation of air, the port sites were closed and the patient was reprepared and redraped. The leads then were connected to a preexisting device in the pocket or to a new device.[52]

PROGRAMMING PACEMAKERS

Nomenclature

Pacing modes usually are described with codes consisting of three or four letters. The first letter refers to the chambers paced: A for atrium, V for ventricle, D for both, and O for neither (pacing is turned off). The second letter refers to the chambers sensed, using the same abbreviations employed for pacing (O denotes that sensing is turned off and asynchronous pacing will occur). The third letter refers to the action taken by the pacemaker in response to a sensed signal and may be one of the following: I (inhibit), T (trigger), or D (dual response of inhibiting or triggering for dual-chamber devices). If a fourth letter is used, it is usually R, which refers to rate-responsive pacing. Rate-responsive devices contain a sensor that can adjust the rate in response to temperature, minute ventilation, oxygen saturation, vibration, and other variables. This facilitates appropriate adjustment in heart rate that is based on an individual's physical activity. Dual-chamber pacing often is referred to as physiologic pacing.

DDD mode

In the DDD(R) mode, the pacemaker paces and senses both chambers, with the ability to inhibit or trigger a cardiac depolarization in response to a sensed signal. For example, if an intrinsic atrial beat is sensed within a time interval that corresponds to a programmed heart rate threshold (typically 60 bpm), the pacer will not trigger an artificial atrial beat (atrial pacing is inhibited). If the intrinsic atrial rate is slower than the programmed rate, the atrial lead will trigger an artificial atrial depolarization. As the atrial beat travels through the AV conduction system, the ventricular lead will sense whether the impulse has propagated into the ventricle within a preprogrammed time interval (e.g., 200 ms). If the ventricular lead senses intrinsic depolarization, it will not trigger an artificial ventricular beat (i.e., ventricular pacing is inhibited). If after the set time interval the ventricular lead does not sense intrinsic depolarization, it will trigger an artificial ventricular beat. This mode is especially useful for patients with AV block, a need for AV synchrony to maximize cardiac output, or a history of pacemaker syndrome (see "Pacemaker Complications," below).

DDI mode

In the DDI(R) mode, the pacemaker is programmed to pace and sense in both the atrium and the ventricle. In response to a sensed signal, the pacemaker will inhibit the output of an artificial depolarization. For example, if the intrinsic atrial rate is slower than the programmed rate, the atrial lead will trigger an artificial atrial depolarization. Unlike the DDD mode, DDI will not trigger a ventricular artificial depolarization on the basis of atrial activity. The only scenario in which the ventricular lead will trigger an artificial depolarization occurs when the intrinsic ventricular rate is below a programmed threshold.

VVI mode

In the VVI(R) mode, the pacemaker paces and senses only the ventricle. If an intrinsic ventricular signal is detected, the ventricular lead will not trigger an artificial ventricular depolarization. This mode is particularly useful for patients with persistent atrial arrhythmias such as atrial fibrillation. Unlike the DDI(R) mode, the VVI(R) mode does not pace the atrium if an intrinsic atrial signal is absent. The disadvantage of this mode compared with DDI(R) is AV dyssynchrony with possible compromise of cardiac output as a result of impaired diastolic filling of the left ventricle if there is a native organized atrial rhythm.

Mode switching

Mode switching refers to switching to a mode that is not capable of tracking atrial beats. This is useful in patients with intermittent atrial tachyarrhythmias. Examples are switching from DDDR to DDIR and from DDD to VVI. Although patients with AV nodal ablation for atrial fibrillation may receive greater symptomatic benefit with DDDR and mode switching compared with VVIR,[53] the MOST trial suggested that among patients with SND and paroxysmal atrial fibrillation, DDDR and mode switching do not have any symptomatic benefit.[54]

Other modes

In the AAI(R) mode, the pacemaker paces and senses only the atrium. If an intrinsic atrial signal is sensed, the pacemaker will not trigger an atrial depolarization. This mode may be appropriate for patients with SND and intact AV conduction. The disadvantage of this mode is the lack of ventricular pacing if AV block occurs. In a selected group of patients who were screened to find out if they had intact AV node function, the occurrence of clinically significant AV nodal disease was less than 2 percent per year. This mode is used rarely in the United States.

In the DOO mode, both chambers are paced but not sensed. This mode may be used as a temporary mode during surgery to prevent an interaction between the electrocautery and pacemaker sensing. Such an interaction could result in bradycardia or asystole as a result of inappropriate inhibition of ventricular pacing or rapid ventricular pacing resulting from inappropriate electrocautery sensing by the atrial lead with triggered pacing of the ventricle. In the VOO mode, the ventricle is paced but not sensed. The indication is the same as for DOO. Pacemaker-dependent patients who are undergoing cardiac surgery should be switched to one of these modes before surgery.

PACEMAKER COMPLICATIONS

Complications related to implantation

Pacemaker complications can be divided into complications associated with implantation, pacemaker infections, subsequent loss of capture, pacemaker syndrome, and pacemaker-mediated tachycardia.

Implantation complications may be related to venous access, the endocardial lead, or the pocket. Complications related to venous access are (1) pneumothorax and hemothorax, (2) incidental arterial puncture, and (3) brachial plexus injury. The incidence of pneumothorax or hemothorax with the subclavian endocardial approach has been estimated to be 1 to 3 percent.[55,56] Complications associated with the endocardial lead are (1)atrial or ventricular perforation, tamponade, and complete heart block, (2) chest wall or diaphragmatic stimulation, and (3) venous thrombosis or endocarditis. Complications associated with the pocket are (1) hematoma (appropriate electrocautery use helps avoid this complication), (2) infection, (3) skin compromise, and (4) generator migration. A complete discussion of pacemaker lead and generator infections follows.

Pacemaker lead infections

Patients may present with systemic infection and pacemaker lead endocarditis or local infection. According to a series involving 52 patients, patients with pacemaker lead endocarditis may present early after pacemaker implantation or late with chronically infected leads. In this series, there was fever in 87 percent, pulmonary involvement in 38 percent, positive blood cultures in 88 percent (most frequently *Staphylococcus* in 94 percent of positive cultures), and abnormalities on the lead by transesophageal echocardiography in 94 percent, often not seen with transthoracic echocardiography.[57]

In patients with local infection, conservative therapy may be considered for very low grade infections or minor skin erosions. In patients who present with a pocket abscess or significant skin erosions, conservative treatment (antibiotics, limited debridement, and irrigation) probably will result in failure.[58,59] Generator removal only and/or partial lead extraction are also likely to result in persistent infection.[58–60]

The decision whether to perform percutaneous or surgical lead extraction for vegetations larger than 1 to 2 cm is controversial. In the series mentioned above, the 10 patients with vegetations larger than 10 mm were referred for surgical lead removal, and 2 of them died of septic complications.[57] Although the authors documented a significant rate of septic pulmonary embolism of 30 percent in the entire cohort,[57] most of those cases were without significant clinical sequelae, and so there is still no strong evidence that surgical extraction is preferable to percutaneous extraction for large vegetations.

Loss of capture

Loss of capture may be due to (1) lead dislodgment, (2) lead fracture, (3) a break in lead insulation, and (4) fibrosis at the lead-myocardial interface (increased pacing threshold). Pacemaker interrogation and echocardiography are useful in determining the cause of the loss of capture. For example, lead fracture is associated with high impedance, whereas loss of lead insulation is associated with low impedance.

Other complications

Pacemaker syndrome is caused by the absence of AV synchrony during ventricular pacing, usually resulting in atrial contraction against closed AV valves. Since the atrial contraction may result from retrograde conduction of a ventricular pacing impulse, this syndrome may be more common in patients with SND and intact AV conduction than it is in those with AV block. Symptoms of pacemaker syndrome include light-headedness, weakness, flushing, exercise intolerance, and palpitations. The syndrome may be treated by restoration of AV synchrony with DDD pacing.

In pacemaker-mediated tachycardia, the ventricular impulse is conducted retrograde through the AVN to the atria, where it is sensed by the atrial lead in a dual-lead system, with the resulting ventricular-paced beat triggered by the atrial-sensed beat. The acute remedy is to place a magnet over the pacemaker. The long-term remedy is to reprogram the pacemaker to increase the postventricular atrial refractory period (PVARP) or change the mode from DDD to DDI.

EXTRACTION OF PACING AND DEFIBRILLATING LEADS

Indications

After the initial implantation of a pacing lead, some degree of thrombosis develops and, on areas that are in contact with the endothelium or endocardium, organizes into fibrosis that may propagate along the lead and over time become increasingly dense and calcified (calcification is more common in very old leads). This fibrotic tissue makes lead removal difficult, necessitating extraction with more sophisticated tools. The most common sites for fibrosis are the venous entry site, the curve into the superior vena cava, and the region from the anode ring to the lead tip.[61]

According to a recent North American Society of Pacing and Electrophysiology (NASPE) statement, the term *extraction* should be reserved for pacemaker leads implanted for at least 1 year and leads requiring more than stylets and simple traction for removal.[62] The most common indication for lead extraction is infection, sometimes involving only the pocket but often resulting in vegetations on the pacemaker leads. The most recent class I and class II indications for extraction of chronically implanted leads are listed in Table 39-2.

Procedural strategies

Although infected epicardial leads must be removed surgically, infected endocardial leads usually can be removed

Table 39-2 Indications for extraction of chronically implanted transvenous pacing and defibrillator leads[a]

Class I Indications

- Sepsis (including endocarditis) as a result of documented infection of any intravascular part of the pacing system or as a result of a pacemaker pocket infection when the intravascular portion of the lead system cannot be separated aseptically from the pocket
- Life-threatening arrhythmias secondary to a retained lead fragment
- A retained lead, a lead fragment, or extraction hardware that poses an immediate or imminent physical threat to the patient
- Clinically significant thromboembolic events caused by a retained lead or a lead fragment
- Obliteration or occlusion of all usable veins, with the need to implant a new transvenous pacing system
- A lead that interferes with the operation of another implanted device (e.g., pacemaker or defibrillator)

Class II Indications

- Localized pocket infection, erosion, or chronic draining sinus that does not involve the transvenous portion of the lead system when the lead can be cut through a clean incision that is totally separate from the infected area
- An occult infection for which no source can be found and for which the pacing system is suspected
- Chronic pain at the pocket or lead insertion site that causes significant discomfort for the patient, is not manageable by medical or surgical technique without lead removal, and for which there is no acceptable alternative
- A lead that because of its design or failure may pose a threat to the patient, though the threat is not immediate or imminent if the lead is left in place
- A lead that interferes with the treatment of a malignancy
- A traumatic injury to the entry site of the lead where the lead may interfere with reconstruction of the site
- Leads preventing access to the venous circulation for newly required implantable devices
- Nonfunctional leads in a young patient

[a]Class I indications are those for which there is general agreement that leads should be removed. Class II indications are those for which leads often are removed but there is some divergence of opinion with respect to the benefit versus risk of removal.

Source: Love CJ, Wilkoff BL, Byrd CL, et al. Recommendations for extraction of chronically implanted transvenous pacing and defibrillator leads: Indications, facilities, training: North American Society of Pacing and Electrophysiology Lead Extraction Conference Faculty. *Pacing Clin Electrophysiol* 2000;23:544–551.

percutaneously. As the following discussion primarily refers to endocardial leads, subsequent use of the term *lead(s)* will refer to endocardial leads unless otherwise stated.

Early strategies for lead removal made use of simple traction (later modified to prolong the period of traction with a weight and pulley system) or open chest surgery with cardiopulmonary bypass. As earlier generations of leads were thicker and had greater resistance to loss of integrity during simple traction, this method was often successful. Excessive force, however, created the risk of avulsion of myocardium with resulting tamponade. Experience with surgical extraction of pacemaker leads has been described.[63,64] Generally, surgery is reserved for patients who fail percutaneous extraction and those with large pacemaker lead vegetations, as discussed below.[57] There is no evidence that surgery is associated with lessened mortality compared with the percutaneous technique when used as an initial approach.

The need for a safer, faster, and more consistent technique was satisfied by the development of the countertraction technique that was developed in the late 1980s and evolved during the 1990s.[65,66] This technique employs stylets that are attached to the lead to apply traction while the operator uses a sheath surrounding the lead to free the lead from the fibrotic myocardium and apply countertraction, as shown in Table 39-2.

The extraction procedure is as follows. The generator is removed from the pocket, and the fibrous tissue is separated from the leads down to the subclavian vein, using electrocautery and/or sharp dissection. If a brief trial of gentle, simple traction fails, the countertraction tools are employed. A special locking stylet is chosen according to the size of the lead and advanced as far as possible along the lead and then fixed to the inner coil. A suture is placed tightly around the lead in an attempt to maintain the integrity of the lead during the extraction process. While traction is applied to the lead, the sheath is advanced along the lead to lyse fibrous attachments. The sheath is advanced to within 1 to 2 cm of the electrode tip. As shown in Fig. 39-5, the lead and myocardium are pulled up to the sheath for countertraction, and then continued traction results in release of the lead tip.

The overall complete extraction success rate for conventional countertraction in recent series has been reported to be between 87 and 93 percent, with a major complication rate between 1.4 and 2.5 percent.[67,68] Conversion to a femoral approach sometimes is required because of failure with the subclavian approach. The femoral approach allows the operator to grasp the lead and pull it down from the subclavian implant site and then retrieve it by using countertraction from below with a specially designed sheath. The need for a femoral approach occurs about 5 to 10 percent of the time and increases the overall success rate.

The risk of failed extraction increases significantly with increasing age of the lead.[68] Potential major complications of the procedure include death, cardiac tamponade, pneumothorax, hemothorax, pulmonary embolism, arteriovenous fistulas, and stroke.

Recently, there has been the development of an excimer laser sheath composed of thin inner and outer polymer walls between which a single layer of optical fibers is embedded. Proximally, the optical fibers are attached to an excimer laser generator. Distally, pulses of light with wavelengths of 308 nm are delivered to the tissue. Since the penetration of this wavelength of light in vascular tissue is approximately 100 μm, only the fibrous tissue immediately surrounding the sheath tip is destroyed, facilitating lead extraction. The PLEXES

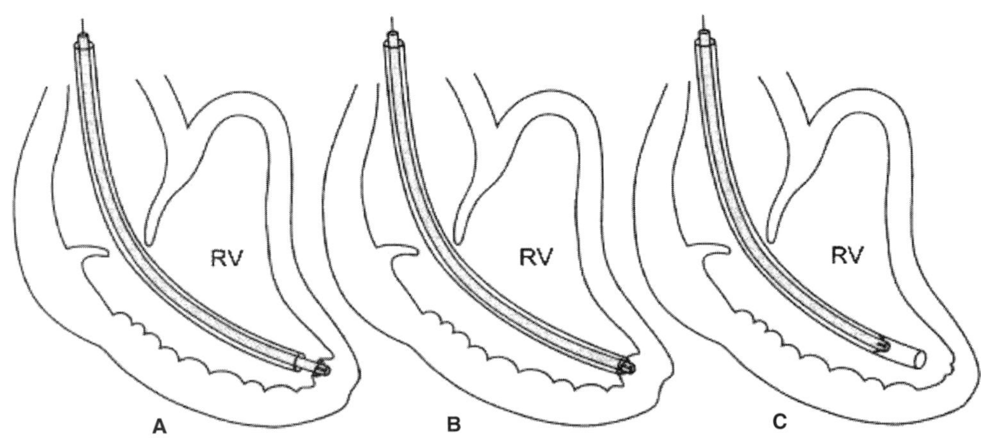

Figure 39-5 Countertraction sequence. A. The sheath is advanced to within 2 cm of the lead tip. B. The lead and myocardium are pulled up to the sheath to apply countertraction. C. The tip releases, and the myocardium falls away. (From Love CJ. Current concepts in extraction of transvenous pacing and ICD leads. *Cardiol Clin* 2000;18:193–217.)

(Pacing Lead Extraction with the Excimer Sheath) trial randomized 301 patients with 465 chronic leads to extraction via a subclavian approach with a conventional sheath or the excimer sheath. Complete removal was achieved in 94 percent of the laser group but in only 64 percent of the conventional group. Rather than converting to a femoral approach, leads that failed with the conventional approach were removed with the laser sheath, with a success rate of 88 percent. Significant complications were encountered in less than 2 percent of the patients, but none was attributed directly to the use of the laser.[69]

Even though the laser sheath has brought new technology to lead extraction, it should be noted that complication rates including death are generally similar to those observed with the conventional approach. The U.S. laser experience encompassing almost 1700 patients was associated with a 1.9 percent major complication rate and an 0.8 percent death rate, compared with a 2.5 percent major complication rate and an 0.6 percent death rate in a registry involving the conventional approach.[70] Furthermore, although the overall success rate is higher using the laser technique compared with traditional countertraction methods from the cephalic approach, this difference is negligible if the femoral route is used when necessary. Published guidelines for training requirements for lead extraction should be followed regardless of the technique used.[71]

Other considerations

Nonfunctional leads do not require routine extraction. In most cases, the leads may be abandoned and new leads can be inserted ipsilaterally. A special case is that of Accufix (Telectronics) and Encor™ (Telectronics) atrial leads, which have been implicated as a cause of death in 6 of over 30,000 patients as a result of fracture of the small retention wire used to form the J shape. This family of leads was withdrawn from the market in 1994; however, some 8000 patients still have these leads implanted. Fracture of this retention wire may work its way through the insulation and perforate the heart. Although some physicians initially elected to remove the leads, the incidence of death (about 0.5 percent) from this procedure was found to be higher than that resulting from the lead itself. On the basis of those findings, physicians were advised to manage patients more conservatively by following them with serial fluoroscopy, with consideration of extraction only for certain indications that were based on patient age, duration of implant, and fracture class of the retention wire.[72] In cases of perforation of the insulation by retention wire (class 3 fracture), it may be possible to snare and selectively retrieve the fractured wire fragment by using percutaneous techniques.

For occlusion of the subclavian vein, conservative management, including short-term anticoagulation, is often adequate, as these patients generally develop venous collaterals. For patients with superior vena cava syndrome in whom dilatation and stenting is planned, extraction of the lead should be considered.[73,74] The occurrence of pulmonary emboli generally does not mandate lead extraction unless the emboli are recurrent despite appropriate anticoagulation.[72]

Pacing leads implanted inadvertently in the left ventricle should be removed immediately. Chronic left ventricular leads can be treated with anticoagulation, with surgical extraction reserved for recurrent cardioembolic stroke despite anticoagulation. Percutaneous extraction is less desirable because of the potential embolization associated with passing the sheaths over the leads and rarely is performed. In regard to tricuspid regurgitation, lead extraction rarely has been of any benefit and can worsen the condition by damaging the valve.

Defibrillator leads can be extracted with the same percutaneous techniques described for pacing leads, with similar success. There has been some concern about the safety of extracting chronically implanted coronary venous leads used for biventricular pacing. Thus far, however, those leads have been removed with remarkably little difficulty, although their implant duration has been relatively short. Determining whether this remains the case years after implantation requires further study.

DEFIBRILLATORS

General considerations

Implantable cardioverter defibrillators (ICDs) were introduced in the 1980s as a means of rescuing patients from life-threatening ventricular tachyarrhythmias. When the rate exceeds a programmed threshold, the device delivers a shock to restore the normal rhythm. The detection of ventricular tachycardia is based primarily on the ventricular rate rather than the width of the QRS complex on the surface electrocardiogram (ECG). Current ICD systems may consist of either one or two leads, with the second configuration designed to allow dual-chamber pacing if necessary. The procedure for implanting an ICD system is similar to that for implanting a pacemaker. With the patient under conscious sedation and local anesthesia, a cardiologist or surgeon inserts a pulse generator subcutaneously and inferior to the left clavicle. The pulse generator is connected to the lead(s) in the right ventricle (and the right atrium with two-lead systems). When the ICD fires, the circuit consists of a ventricular coil as one pole and the pulse generator and/or another coil in the superior vena cava (SVC)/right atrium as the other pole. The pulse generator typically is positioned on the patient's left side, allowing the maximum amount of current to traverse the heart. Of note, ICD leads, like pacemaker leads, may be extracted, but the extraction procedure is more complex because of the ingrowth of tissue into the shock coils. This may be mitigated by the introduction of Gore-Tex-coated coils.

Modes of ICD therapy

The ICD classifies a rhythm on the basis of the ventricular rate. For example, most ICDs are programmed to have one to three zones of tachytherapy plus bradycardia pacing. The device delivers the programmed therapy on the basis of the heart rate it detects. Available therapies include bradycardia pacing, antitachycardia pacing (ATP), and shock delivery. In ATP, the device initiates a short burst of rapid ventricular pacing in an effort to interrupt the reentrant tachycardia by creating a critical zone of conduction within the reentrant circuit that is refractory to additional ventricular activation. The shock may be delivered in the form of low-energy cardioversion or defibrillation. Most ICDs are capable of delivering 30 J or more to terminate unstable ventricular tachycardia and ventricular fibrillation.

Interpreting an ICD interrogation

All ICDs can be interrogated noninvasively to obtain the program that describes what the device will do for a given abnormal heart rate and/or to verify that a reported shock was indeed a shock and was delivered appropriately for a ventricular tachycardia or fibrillation. An ICD interrogation slip is shown in Fig. 39-6. Intracardiac electrograms are depicted. From top to bottom, these are the near-field atrial electrogram, the near-field ventricular electrogram, and the far-field electrogram, which represents a closer approximation to the surface ECG. Inspection of this episode shows initial atrial and ventricular depolarizations in a sequence consistent with sinus rhythm. A premature ventricular depolarization follows and initiates ventricular fibrillation at a cycle length less than 200 ms. During the episode of ventricular fibrillation, the activity depicted in the near-field atrial electrogram is unrelated to that in the near-field ventricular electrogram, consistent with ventricular fibrillation. The ventricular fibrillation is treated successfully with a 21-J biphasic shock. After the shock, the ensuing bradycardia prompts the device to initiate postshock atrioventricular pacing, which is manifested as a wide-complex ventricular rhythm on the far-field electrogram. Interrogation of the device after a shock is

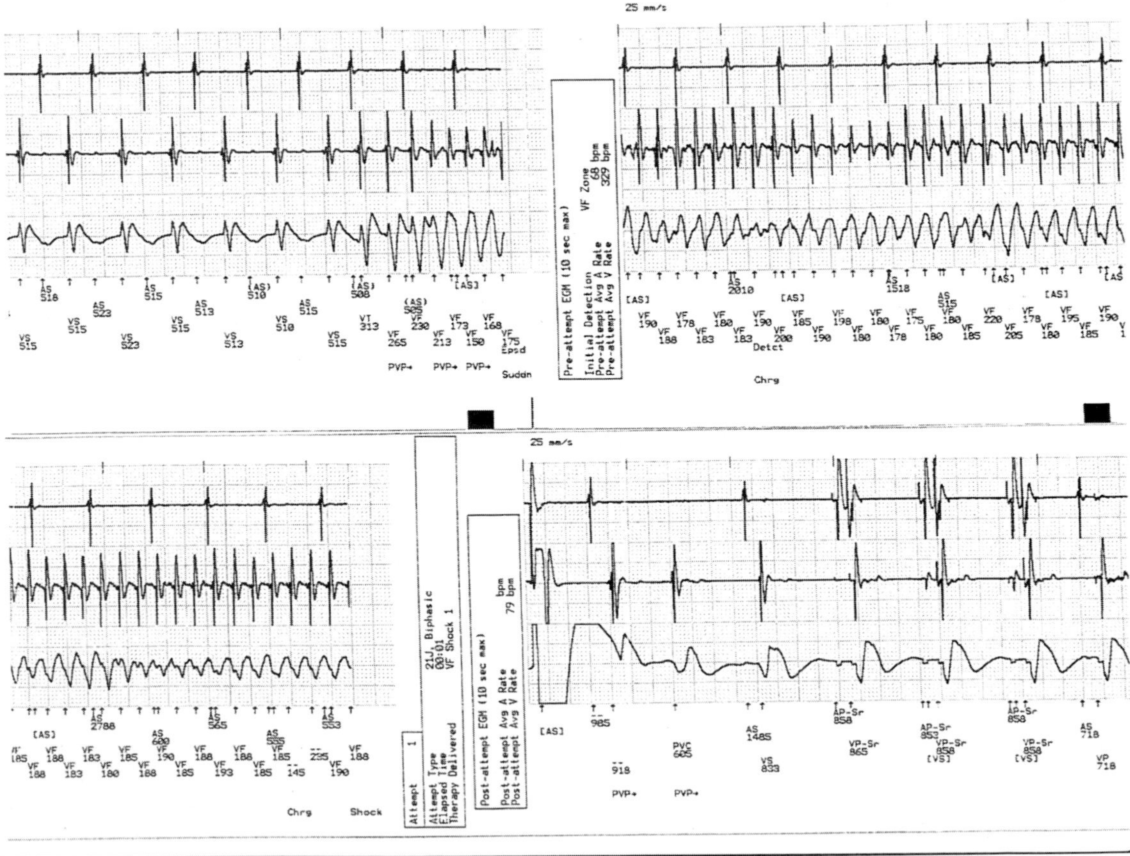

Figure 39-6 ICD interrogation slip. In order from top to bottom, atrial near-field electrogram, ventricular near-field electrogram, and far-field electrogram are shown. Sinus rhythm is followed by a premature ventricular contraction initiating ventricular fibrillation (cycle length < 200 ms), which resolves with a 21-J biphasic shock and is followed by postshock ventricular pacing. Note that during ventricular fibrillation, AV dissociation is present.

important to document appropriate sensing and treatment of the ventricular arrhythmia.

Major indications for ICD implantation

Four important indications for ICDs based on the 1998 and 2002 ACC-AHA-NASPE guidelines follow. (The significance of class I, IIa, and IIb indications is described above.)

1. Cardiac arrest caused by ventricular tachycardia (VT) or ventricular fibrillation (VF) that has an irreversible cause (class I): A mortality benefit has been demonstrated in the Antiarrhythmics versus Implantable Defibrillator (AVID) trial.[75]
2. Sustained VT in the presence of structural heart disease (class I): A mortality benefit for this indication also has been demonstrated in the AVID trial.[75]
3. Nonsustained VT with coronary disease, prior myocardial infarction, left ventricular dysfunction, and inducible VF or sustained VT on electrophysiologic study (EPS) that is not suppressible by class I antiarrhythmic drugs (class I). A mortality benefit has been demonstrated in the Multicenter Automatic Defibrillator Implantation Trial (MADIT-I).[76]
4. Ischemic cardiomyopathy with an ejection fraction (EF) less than or equal to 0.30 at least 1 month after a myocardial infarction and 3 months after coronary artery revascularization surgery (class IIa): This indication is based on the Multicenter Automatic Defibrillator Implantation Trial II (MADIT-II), in which patients with a prior myocardial infarction and an EF less than or equal to 0.30 who received an ICD had 31 percent lower mortality after 20 months of follow-up than did those given conventional therapy.[77] An important task that lies ahead is to find more specific ways to risk stratify this large population as the economic burden of having all patients in this group receive ICDs would be quite large.

There are now trial data to support implantation of defibrillators in patients with ischemic or nonischemic cardiomyopathy and an EF less than or equal to 0.35. Of note, the SCD-HeFT trial showed a similar magnitude of survival benefit whether the cardiomyopathy was of ischemic or nonischemic etiology.[42,43]

Defibrillators in Cardiac Surgery Patients

When considering therapy with an ICD for patients referred for cardiac surgery or with recent cardiac surgery, the following points should be considered. First, revascularization constitutes excellent antiarrhythmic therapy. The CABG-Patch trial[78] randomized 900 patients scheduled for CABG, EF equal to or less than 0.35, and an abnormal signal-averaged ECG (SAECG) indicates an increased arrhythmia risk. Even with an overall 42-month mortality rate of 24 percent as would be expected for higher-risk patients, there was no significant decrease in mortality associated with ICDs after 32 ± 6 months of follow-up. Many trials showing benefit for ICDs, such as the AVID,[75] MADIT-I,[76] and MADIT-II[77] trials, excluded patients referred for CABG and those with recent CABG. For example, MADIT-II excluded patients who had undergone CABG within 3 months.[77] As a result, patients with EF equal to or less than 0.30 shortly after CABG do not meet the criteria for an ICD on the basis of the MADIT-II study. Of note, a post hoc analysis of 281 patients excluded from the AVID trial because they were referred for CABG showed a trend for ICD benefit compared with antiarrhythmic drugs.[75] However, these results are difficult to interpret in light of the post hoc analysis, nonrandomized patients, and lack of statistical significance.

In regard to ICDs in early postsurgical patients, it is important to note that an ICD does not constitute acute therapy for sustained ventricular arrhythmias. On the contrary, ICDs are meant to be a mode of chronic primary or secondary prevention of sudden death associated with ventricular arrhythmias. If a postsurgical patient is having frequent sustained ventricular arrhythmias, that patient should be rendered arrhythmia-free with medical therapy first. The drug of choice in patients with recent CABG is usually amiodarone if there are no contraindications, although other antiarrhythmic drugs may be considered. If amiodarone is chosen and the patient has breakthrough ventricular arrhythmias, additional IV loading doses of amiodarone are frequently effective. In a postsurgical patient who already has an ICD, there still may be a need for external defibrillation. Since most devices assess the need for therapy on the basis of heart rate, a patient may have symptomatic ventricular tachycardia at a rate that is below the threshold for initiating automated therapy (particularly if the patient has been on an antiarrhythmic drug such as amiodarone). In patients referred for both cardiac surgery and an ICD, the ICD should be implanted after the surgery because of the chance for lead displacement during surgery.

Finally, patients with a history of cardiac surgery may be referred at some point for cardiac resynchronization therapy (discussed earlier) for class III or IV heart failure associated with a dilated cardiomyopathy (EF less than 0.35) and intraventricular conduction delay. Results from the COMPANION trial demonstrated a 43 percent reduction in mortality compared with optimal medical therapy in patients who met all the criteria and received a combined defibrillator and biventricular pacemaker.[41] As a result, such patients should be considered for an ICD in addition to CRT. Patients who meet the implant criteria for a CRT device and are referred for cardiac surgery may be considered for LV lead implantation to obviate the later potential need for transvenous placement via the coronary sinus.

References

1. Bernstein AD, Parsonnet V. Survey of cardiac pacing and implanted defibrillator practice patterns in the United States in 1997. *Pacing Clin Electrophysiol* 2001;24: 842–855.
2. Braunwald EJ, ed. *Heart Disease*, 5th ed. Philadelphia: Saunders; 1997.
3. Zipes DP, Jalife J. *Cardiac Electrophysiology: From Cell to Bedside*, 2d ed. Philadelphia: Saunders; 1995.
4. Gregoratos G, Abrams J, Epstein AE, et al. ACC/AHA/NASPE 2002 guideline update for implantation of cardiac pacemakers and antiarrhythmia devices: Summary article: A report of the American College of Cardiology/American Heart Association Task Force on Practice Guidelines (ACC/AHA/NASPE Committee to Update the 1998 Pacemaker Guidelines). *Circulation* 2002;106: 2145–2161.
5. Mustonen P, Hippelainen M, Vanninen E, et al. Significance of coronary artery bypass grafting-associated conduction defects. *Am J Cardiol* 1998;81:558–563.
6. Tuzcu EM, Emre A, Goormastic M, et al. Incidence and prognostic significance of intraventricular conduction abnormalities after coronary bypass surgery. *J Am Coll Cardiol* 1990;16:607–610.
7. Caspi Y, Safadi T, Ammar R, et al. The significance of bundle branch block in the immediate postoperative electrocardiograms of patients undergoing coronary artery bypass. *J Thorac Cardiovasc Surg* 1987;93:442–446.
8. Baerman JM, Kirsh MM, de Buitleir M, et al. Natural history and determinants of conduction defects following coronary artery bypass surgery. *Ann Thorac Surg* 1987; 44:150–153.
9. Feldman S, Glikson M, Kaplinsky E. Pacemaker dependency after coronary artery bypass. *Pacing Clin Electrophysiol* 1992;15:2037–2040.
10. Caspi J, Amar R, Elami A, et al. Frequency and significance of complete atrioventricular block after coronary artery bypass grafting. *Am J Cardiol* 1989;63:526–529.
11. Gordon RS, Ivanov J, Cohen G, Ralph-Edwards AL. Permanent cardiac pacing after a cardiac operation: Predicting the use of permanent pacemakers. *Ann Thorac Surg* 1998;66:1698–1704.
12. Flack JE III, Hafer J, Engelman RM, et al. Effect of normothermic blood cardioplegia on postoperative conduction abnormalities and supraventricular arrhythmias. *Circulation* 1992;86:II385–II392.
13. Mosseri M, Meir G, Lotan C, et al. Coronary pathology predicts conduction disturbances after coronary artery bypass grafting. *Ann Thorac Surg* 1991;51:248–252.
14. Mustonen P, Poyhonen M, Rehnberg S, et al. Conduction defects after coronary artery bypass grafting—A disappearing problem? *Ann Chir Gynaecol Suppl* 2000;89:33–39.
15. Koplan BA, Stevenson WG, Epstein LM, et al. Development and validation of a simple risk score to predict the need for permanent pacing after cardiac valve surgery. *J Am Coll Cardiol* 2003;41:795–801.
16. Ormerod OJ, McGregor CG, Stone DL, et al. Arrhythmias after coronary bypass surgery. *Br Heart J* 1984;51: 618–621.
17. White HD, Antman EM, Glynn MA, et al. Efficacy and safety of timolol for prevention of supraventricular tachyarrhythmias after coronary artery bypass surgery. *Circulation* 1984;70:479–484.
18. Gomes JA, Ip J, Santoni-Rugiu F, et al. Oral d,l sotalol reduces the incidence of postoperative atrial fibrillation in coronary artery bypass surgery patients: A randomized, double-blind, placebo-controlled study. *J Am Coll Cardiol* 1999;34:334–339.
19. Daoud EG, Strickberger SA, Man KC, et al. Preoperative amiodarone as prophylaxis against atrial fibrillation after heart surgery. *N Engl J Med* 1997;337:1785–1791.
20. Daoud EG, Snow R, Hummel JD, et al. Temporary atrial epicardial pacing as prophylaxis against atrial fibrillation after heart surgery: A meta-analysis. *J Cardiovasc Electrophysiol* 2003;14:127–132.
21. Saksena S, Prakash A, Hill M, et al. Prevention of recurrent atrial fibrillation with chronic dual-site right atrial pacing. *J Am Coll Cardiol* 1996;28:687–694.
22. Levy T, Walker S, Rochelle J, Paul V. Evaluation of biatrial pacing, right atrial pacing, and no pacing in patients with drug refractory atrial fibrillation. *Am J Cardiol* 1999; 84:426–429.
23. Heinz G, Kratochwill C, Schmid S, et al. Sinus node dysfunction after orthotopic heart transplantation: The Vienna experience 1987–1993. *Pacing Clin Electrophysiol* 1994;17:2057–2063.
24. DiBiase A, Tse TM, Schnittger I, et al. Frequency and mechanism of bradycardia in cardiac transplant recipients and need for pacemakers. *Am J Cardiol* 1991;67: 1385–1389.
25. Miyamoto Y, Curtiss EI, Kormos RL, et al. Bradyarrhythmia after heart transplantation: Incidence, time course, and outcome. *Circulation* 1990;82: IV313–IV317.
26. Blanche C, Czer LS, Fishbein MC, et al. Permanent pacemaker for rejection episodes after heart transplantation: A poor prognostic sign. *Ann Thorac Surg* 1995;60: 1263–1266.
27. Chau EM, McGregor CG, Rodeheffer RJ, et al. Increased incidence of chronotropic incompetence in older donor hearts. *J Heart Lung Transplant* 1995;14:743–748.
28. Bacal F, Bocchi EA, Vieira ML, et al. Permanent and temporary pacemaker implantation after orthotopic heart transplantation. *Arq Bras Cardiol* 2000;74:5–12.
29. Lower R, Shumway N. Study on orthotopic homotransplantation of the canine heart. *Surg Forum* 1960;11: 18–19.
30. Herre JM, Barnhart GR, Llano A. Cardiac pacemakers in the transplanted heart: Short term with the biatrial anastomosis and unnecessary with the bicaval anastomosis. *Curr Opin Cardiol* 2000;15:115–120.
31. Yacoub M, Mankad P, Ledingham S. Donor procurement and surgical techniques for cardiac transplantation. *Semin Thorac Cardiovasc Surg* 1990;2:153–161.
32. Sarsam MA, Campbell CS, Yonan NA, et al. An alternative surgical technique in orthotopic cardiac transplantation. *J Card Surg* 1993;8:344–349.
33. Parry G, Holt ND, Dark JH, McComb JM. Declining need for pacemaker implantation after cardiac transplantation. *Pacing Clin Electrophysiol* 1998;21: 2350–2352.

34. El Gamel A, Yonan NA, Grant S, et al. Orthotopic cardiac transplantation: A comparison of standard and bicaval Wythenshawe techniques. *J Thorac Cardiovasc Surg* 1995; 109:721–729.
35. Deleuze PH, Benvenuti C, Mazzucotelli JP, et al. Orthotopic cardiac transplantation with direct caval anastomosis: Is it the optimal procedure? *J Thorac Cardiovasc Surg* 1995;109:731–737.
36. Ellenbogen KA, Szentpetery S, Katz MR. Reversibility of prolonged chronotropic dysfunction with theophylline following orthotopic cardiac transplantation. *Am Heart J* 1988;116:202–206.
37. Melton IC, Gilligan DM, Wood MA, Ellenbogen KA. Optimal cardiac pacing after heart transplantation. *Pacing Clin Electrophysiol* 1999;22:1510–1527.
38. Scott CD, Dark JH, McComb JM. Sinus node function after cardiac transplantation. *J Am Coll Cardiol* 1994;24: 1334–1341.
39. Cazeau S, Leclercq C, Lavergne T, et al. Effects of multisite biventricular pacing in patients with heart failure and intraventricular conduction delay. *N Engl J Med* 2001; 344:873–880.
40. Abraham WT, Fisher WG, Smith AL, et al. Cardiac resynchronization in chronic heart failure. *N Engl J Med* 2002; 346:1845–1853.
41. Bristow MR, Saxon LA, Boehmer J, et al. Cardiac-resynchronization therapy with or without an implantable defibrillator in advanced chronic heart failure. *N Engl J Med* 2004;350:2140–2150.
42. Kadish A, Dyer A, Daubert JP, et al. Prophylactic defibrillator implantation in patients with nonischemic dilated cardiomyopathy. *N Engl J Med* 2004;350: 2151–2158.
43. Bardy GH, Lee KL, Mark DB, et al. Amiodarone or an implantable cardioverter-defibrillator for congestive heart failure. *N Engl J Med* 2005;352:225–237.
44. Kappenberger L, Linde C, Daubert C, et al. Pacing in hypertrophic obstructive cardiomyopathy: A randomized crossover study: PIC Study Group. *Eur Heart J* 1997; 18:1249–1256.
45. Maron BJ, Nishimura RA, McKenna WJ, et al. Assessment of permanent dual-chamber pacing as a treatment for drug-refractory symptomatic patients with obstructive hypertrophic cardiomyopathy: A randomized, double-blind, crossover study (M-PATHY). *Circulation* 1999; 99:2927–2933.
46. Furman S, Schwedel J. An intracardiac pacemaker for Stokes-Adams seizures. *N Engl J Med* 1959;261: 943–948.
47. Chardack WM, Gage AA, Federico AJ, et al. The long-term treatment of heart block. *Prog Cardiovasc Dis* 1966;9:105–135.
48. King SM, Arrington JO, Dalton ML. Permanent transvenous cardiac pacing via the left cephalic vein. *Ann Thorac Surg* 1968;5:469–473.
49. Littleford PO, Parsonnet V, Spector SD. Method for the rapid and atraumatic insertion of permanent endocardial pacemaker electrodes through the subclavian vein. *Am J Cardiol* 1979;43:980–982.
50. Calkins H, Ramza BM, Brinker J, et al. Prospective randomized comparison of the safety and effectiveness of placement of endocardial pacemaker and defibrillator leads using the extrathoracic subclavian vein guided by contrast venography versus the cephalic approach. *Pacing Clin Electrophysiol* 2001;24:456–464.
51. Magney JE, Flynn DM, Parsons JA, et al. Anatomical mechanisms explaining damage to pacemaker leads, defibrillator leads, and failure of central venous catheters adjacent to the sternoclavicular joint. *Pacing Clin Electrophysiol* 1993;16:445–457.
52. DeRose JJ, Ashton RC, Belsley S, et al. Robotically assisted left ventricular epicardial lead implantation for biventricular pacing. *J Am Coll Cardiol* 2003;41: 1414–1419.
53. Marshall HJ, Harris ZI, Griffith MJ, et al. Prospective randomized study of ablation and pacing versus medical therapy for paroxysmal atrial fibrillation: Effects of pacing mode and mode-switch algorithm. *Circulation* 1999;99: 1587–1592.
54. Sweeney MO, Hellkamp AS, Ellenbogen KA, et al. Prospective randomized study of mode switching in a clinical trial of pacemaker therapy for sinus node dysfunction. *J Cardiovasc Electrophysiol* 2004;15:153–160.
55. Chauhan A, Grace AA, Newell SA, et al. Early complications after dual chamber versus single chamber pacemaker implantation. *Pacing Clin Electrophysiol* 1994;17: 2012–2015.
56. Aggarwal RK, Connelly DT, Ray SG, et al. Early complications of permanent pacemaker implantation: No difference between dual and single chamber systems. *Br Heart J* 1995; 73:571–575.
57. Klug D, Lacroix D, Savoye C, et al. Systemic infection related to endocarditis on pacemaker leads: Clinical presentation and management. *Circulation* 1997;95: 2098–2107.
58. Lewis AB, Hayes DL, Holmes DR Jr, et al. Update on infections involving permanent pacemakers: Characterization and management. *J Thorac Cardiovasc Surg* 1985; 89:758–763.
59. Molina JE. Undertreatment and overtreatment of patients with infected antiarrhythmic implantable devices. *Ann Thorac Surg* 1997;63:504–509.
60. Parry G, Goudevenos J, Jameson S, et al. Complications associated with retained pacemaker leads. *Pacing Clin Electrophysiol* 1991;14:1251–1257.
61. Love CJ. Current concepts in extraction of transvenous pacing and ICD leads. *Cardiol Clin* 2000;18: 193–217.
62. Love CJ, Wilkoff BL, Byrd CL, et al. Recommendations for extraction of chronically implanted transvenous pacing and defibrillator leads: Indications, facilities, training: North American Society of Pacing and Electrophysiology Lead Extraction Conference Faculty. *Pacing Clin Electrophysiol* 2000;23:544–551.
63. Brodman R, Frame R, Andrews C, Furman S. Removal of infected transvenous leads requiring cardiopulmonary bypass or inflow occlusion. *J Thorac Cardiovasc Surg* 1992;103:649–654.
64. Frame R, Brodman RF, Furman S, et al. Surgical removal of infected transvenous pacemaker leads. *Pacing Clin Electrophysiol* 1993;16:2343–2348.
65. Byrd CL, Schwartz SJ, Hedin NB, et al. Intravascular lead extraction using locking stylets and sheaths. *Pacing Clin Electrophysiol* 1990;13:1871–1875.

66. Fearnot NE, Smith HJ, Goode LB, et al. Intravascular lead extraction using locking stylets, sheaths, and other techniques. *Pacing Clin Electrophysiol* 1990;13:1864–1870.
67. Smith HJ, Fearnot NE, Byrd CL, et al. Five-years experience with intravascular lead extraction: U.S. Lead Extraction Database. *Pacing Clin Electrophysiol* 1994; 17:2016–2020.
68. Byrd CL, Wilkoff BL, Love CJ, et al. Intravascular extraction of problematic or infected permanent pacemaker leads: 1994–1996: U.S. Extraction Database, MED Institute. *Pacing Clin Electrophysiol* 1999;22:1348–1357.
69. Wilkoff BL, Byrd CL, Love CJ, et al. Pacemaker lead extraction with the laser sheath: Results of the pacing lead extraction with the excimer sheath (PLEXES) trial. *J Am Coll Cardiol* 1999;33:1671–1676.
70. Byrd CL, Wilkoff BL, Love CJ, et al. Clinical study of the laser sheath for lead extraction: The total experience in the United States. *Pacing Clin Electrophysiol* 2002;25: 804–808.
71. Hayes DL, Naccarelli GV, Furman S, et al. NASPE training requirements for cardiac implantable electronic devices: Selection, implantation, and follow-up. *Pacing Clin Electrophysiol* 2003;26:1556–1562.
72. Bracke FA, Meijer A, van Gelder LM. Pacemaker lead complications: When is extraction appropriate and what can we learn from published data? *Heart* 2001;85: 254–259.
73. Porath A, Avnun L, Hirsch M, Ovsyshcher I. Right atrial thrombus and recurrent pulmonary emboli secondary to permanent cardiac pacing—A case report and short review of literature. *Angiology* 1987;38:627–630.
74. Mazzetti H, Dussaut A, Tentori C, et al. Superior vena cava occlusion and/or syndrome related to pacemaker leads. *Am Heart J* 1993;125:831–837.
75. A comparison of antiarrhythmic-drug therapy with implantable defibrillators in patients resuscitated from near-fatal ventricular arrhythmias: The Antiarrhythmics versus Implantable Defibrillators (AVID) Investigators. *N Engl J Med* 1997;337:1576–1583.
76. Moss AJ, Hall WJ, Cannom DS, et al. Improved survival with an implanted defibrillator in patients with coronary disease at high risk for ventricular arrhythmia: Multicenter Automatic Defibrillator Implantation Trial Investigators. *N Engl J Med* 1996;335:1933–1940.
77. Moss AJ, Zareba W, Hall WJ, et al. Prophylactic implantation of a defibrillator in patients with myocardial infarction and reduced ejection fraction. *N Engl J Med* 2002;346: 877–883.
78. Bigger JT Jr. Prophylactic use of implanted cardiac defibrillators in patients at high risk for ventricular arrhythmias after coronary-artery bypass graft surgery: Coronary Artery Bypass Graft (CABG) Patch Trial Investigators. *N Engl J Med* 1997;337:1569–1575.

CHAPTER

40 SURGICAL TREATMENT OF CHRONIC PULMONARY THROMBOEMBOLIC DISEASE

Michael M. Madani, Stuart W. Jamieson

INTRODUCTION

Chronic thromboembolic pulmonary hypertension is a common condition that is underdiagnosed significantly. The disease is caused by chronic obstruction of the pulmonary vasculature that results from long-standing pulmonary thromboembolism. Once it is diagnosed, there is only one curative option: surgical removal. Medical therapy is palliative at best, and lung transplantation for this condition is outdated. Pulmonary thromboendarterectomy (PTE) for the treatment of CTEPH is an uncommon procedure but offers a surgical cure with excellent short- and long-term results.

Although pulmonary embolism is one of the more common cardiovascular diseases that affect Americans and despite clinical and statistical evidence of progression of the disease in survivors, the majority of these patients continue to be misdiagnosed. Perhaps a contributing factor is the fact that no specific signs and symptoms are associated with this condition. Furthermore, most patients do not have a definitive history of DVT or PE. The vague nature of the symptoms, including dyspnea on exertion and occasional angina-like chest pains, coupled with lack of awareness among common practitioners, makes the diagnosis quite difficult; unfortunately, these patients often progress to severe degrees of pulmonary

KEY CONCEPTS

- Epidemiology
  - The precise incidence of pulmonary embolism (PE) is unknown, although acute PE is the third most common cause of death. Approximately 75 percent of autopsy-proven PEs are not detected clinically. PE is particularly common in hospitalized elderly patients.
- Pathophysiology
  - PE is usually an embolic manifestation of deep venous thrombosis (DVT), which is caused by venous stasis, vein wall injury, and hypercoagulopathy. Other etiologies include malignancy, chronic indwelling central venous catheters, and spontaneous thrombosis. Emboli become lodged in the pulmonary artery bed and lead to pulmonary vascular hypertension by several proposed processes: redirected pulmonary blood flow, neurovascular perturbation, and hormonal changes.
- Clinical features
  - Chronic thromboembolic pulmonary hypertension (CTEPH) presents insidiously with vague symptomatology. Suspicion should be raised when predisposing factors for DVT (e.g., leg swelling, lower extremity venous stasis changes, chest pain, hemoptysis) are encountered. The most common symptoms associated with pulmonary hypertension are exertional dyspnea, presyncope/syncope, and nonspecific chest pain or pressure. The physical signs of CTEPH are related to right heart failure, including a large A wave progressing to a predominant V wave component in the jugular venous pulse. The S_2 sound often is narrowly split, and P_2 is accentuated; a sharp systolic

ejection click may be heard over the pulmonary artery in the second intercostal space. A right ventricular heave and hypoxia/cyanosis are observed with advanced disease.

- Diagnostics
  - Characteristic findings on plain chest radiography are central pulmonary vascular enlargement, vascular pruning, and right ventricular enlargement. Electrocardiography may demonstrate criteria for right ventricular hypertrophy, including right axis deviation and a dominant R wave in V_1. Pulmonary function tests usually reveal minimal changes in lung volume and ventilation with normal or slightly restricted mechanics; the diffusing capacity of the lung for carbon monoxide (DLCO) often is reduced and is the only abnormality on this test. The ventilation-perfusion lung scan is essential for diagnosis. An entirely normal scan excludes the diagnosis, whereas most patients with CTEPH demonstrate one or more segmental or larger perfusion defects in otherwise normal lung regions. The magnitude of perfusion defects in chronic thromboembolic disease often underestimates the actual degree of vascular obstruction. A positive scan should prompt right heart catheterization and pulmonary angiography. Pulmonary angioscopy may be helpful in cases of equivocal angiographic studies. High-resolution helical computed tomography is being used more frequently in the diagnosis of pulmonary thromboembolic disease.
- Treatment
  - Medical therapy for CTEPH is limited and is generally palliative; chronic anticoagulation is the mainstay. Surgical removal of chronic thromboembolic material is the only curative option for patients with CTEPH.
- Outcomes and prognosis
  - A complication specific to pulmonary thromboendarterectomy is a "reperfusion response" that appears to be related to reperfusion injury. A 30-year experience at the University of California–San Diego (UCSD) Medical Center indicated an overall operative mortality of 9 percent, which has declined to a current rate of about 4.4 percent. In most treated patients, a significant reduction in pulmonary pressures, pulmonary vascular resistance, pulmonary blood flow, and cardiac output is observed immediately and sustained. One year postoperatively, 95 percent of treated patients have improved from New York Hospital Association functional class III or IV to functional class I or II.

hypertension and right heart failure before a diagnosis is established and a treatment strategy is sought.

The precise incidence of PE is unknown, but there are some legitimate estimates. Acute PE is the third most common cause of death (after heart disease and cancer). Approximately 75 percent of autopsy-proven PEs are not detected clinically.[1] Dalen[2] calculated that pulmonary embolism results in 630,000 symptomatic episodes in the United States yearly, making it about half as common as acute myocardial infarction and three times as common as cerebrovascular accidents. This is, however, a low estimate, since in 70 to 80 percent of patients in whom the primary cause of death was PE, The diagnosis was unsuspected before death.[3,4] The disease is particularly common in hospitalized elderly patients. Among hospitalized patients who develop PE, 12 to 21 percent die in the hospital and another 24 to 39 percent die within 12 months.[5–7] Thus, approximately 36 to 60 percent of patients who survive the initial episode live beyond 12 months and may present later in life with a wide variety of symptoms.

The mainstay of treatment of patients with DVT and acute PE is medical management. There are few indications for surgical intervention in the acute setting, and they are specific to hospitalized patients who have had a massive embolus that causes life-threatening acute right heart failure and severe hemodynamic compromise. The presence of a large amount of embolic material in the right atrium or right ventricle, as evidenced by echocardiography, in the setting of severe right heart failure and hemodynamic compromise is another instance in which surgery would be indicated. These indications are, however, few and far between. In contrast, in the chronic form of the disease, the only treatment is surgical removal of the thromboembolic material by means of pulmonary thromboendarterectomy. Medical management in these patients is only palliative and does not address the obstructive nature of the disease. The only other potential surgical cure is transplantation. However, lung or heart-lung transplantation as a surgical cure for this condition is an outdated form of therapy and should be considered an inappropriate use of resources that yields less than satisfactory results.

The prognosis for patients with pulmonary hypertension is poor, and it is worse for those who do not have intracardiac shunts. Thus, patients with primary pulmonary hypertension and those with pulmonary hypertension secondary to PEs fall into a higher-risk category than do those with Eisenmenger's syndrome and have a higher mortality rate. In fact, once the mean pulmonary pressure in patients with thromboembolic disease reaches 50 mmHg or more, 3-year mortality approaches 90 percent.

Regardless of the exact incidence or the circumstances, it is clear that acute embolism and its chronic form, fixed chronic thromboembolic occlusive disease, are both much more common than generally appreciated and are significantly underdiagnosed. Calculations extrapolated from mortality rates and the random incidence of major thrombotic occlusion found at autopsy support the postulate that more than 100,000 people in the United States currently have pulmonary hypertension that could be relieved by an operation. The procedure appears to be permanently curative, but fewer than 3000 of these procedures have been performed; most of them (over 2000 cases) have been done at the authors' center, the University of California–San Diego. This chapter provides an overview of the pathophysiology of this disease and outline the surgical management as it is performed at UCSD.

PATHOPHYSIOLOGY

In 1856, Rudolf Virchow made the association between DVT and PE and suggested that the causes of DVT are related to venous stasis, vein wall injury, and hypercoagulopathy. This triad of etiologic factors remains relevant today and is supported by an ever-growing body of evidence. Although a majority of individuals with chronic pulmonary thromboembolic disease are unaware of a preceding thromboembolic event and do not give a history of DVT, the foundation of most cases of unresolved PEs is acute embolic episodes. Why some patients have unresolved emboli is not certain, but a variety of factors must play a role alone or in combination.

In some cases, the volume of acute embolic material may overwhelm the lytic mechanisms. In other cases, total occlusion of a major arterial branch may prevent lytic material from reaching, and therefore dissolving, the embolus completely. Recurring emboli may not be able to be resolved. The embolic material may be made of substances that cannot be resolved by normal mechanisms (already well-organized fibrous thrombus, fat, or tumor). In some patients, the lytic mechanisms may be abnormal, and other patients may have a propensity for thrombus or a hypercoagulable state.

Synchronized preservation of the fluidity of blood and the integrity of the vascular system entails a balance between blood pro- and anticoagulants. Some patients have deficiencies in natural anticoagulants. Three uncommon familial deficiencies associated with venous thrombosis are deficiencies in antithrombin, protein C, and protein S. Antithrombin is a natural plasma protease that inhibits thrombin after it is formed and, to a lesser extent, before it is formed. Antithrombin is also the cofactor that is accelerated 1000-fold by heparin. Protein C is a potent inhibitor of factor V and platelet-bound factor VII and requires protein S as a cofactor for anticoagulant activity. Both protein C and protein S are vitamin K–dependent zymogens that are activated by thrombin and accelerated by thrombomodulin produced by endothelial cells.

A much more common coagulation deficiency that results from a mutation of factor V (factor V Leiden) that prevents its degradation by protein C has been described and is present in approximately 6 to 7 percent of study populations of Swedes and North American males.[8–11] Both homozygous and heterozygous mutants are associated strongly with venous thrombosis and PE but are not associated with stroke, myocardial infarction, and other manifestations of arterial thrombosis.[11,12]

The presence of the lupus anticoagulant, which is an acquired immunoglobulin G (IgG) or IgM antibody against prothrombinase, increases the likelihood of venous thrombosis by poorly understood mechanisms.[12] The disease may be associated with lupus-like syndromes, immunosuppression, or the intake of specific drugs such as procainamide.

In most cases, regardless of the etiology of the embolus, after the clot becomes wedged in the pulmonary artery, one of two processes occurs[13]: organization of the clot proceeding to canalization, producing multiple small endothelialized channels separated by fibrous septa (i.e., bands and webs), or complete fibrous organization of the fibrin clot without canalization, leading to a solid mass of dense fibrous connective tissue that totally obstructs the arterial lumen.

In addition to the usual pattern of venous thrombosis and subsequent embolization, usually from the legs or pelvis, there are special circumstances that may lead to PEs. Chronic indwelling central venous catheters and pacemaker leads sometimes are associated with PEs. Rarer causes include tumor emboli, and tumor fragments from stomach, breast, and kidney malignancies have been demonstrated to cause chronic pulmonary arterial occlusion. Right atrial myxomas may fragment and embolize.

In addition to the embolic material, a propensity for thrombosis or a hypercoagulable state may result in spontaneous thrombosis in the pulmonary vascular bed or encourage proximal propagation of thrombus after an embolus. However, regardless of the predisposing factors to residual thrombus in the vessels, the final genesis of the resultant pulmonary vascular hypertension may be complex. With the passage of time, the increased pressure and flow that result from redirected pulmonary blood flow in the previously normal pulmonary vascular bed can create a vasculopathy in the small precapillary blood vessels similar to what occurs in Eisenmenger's syndrome.

Factors other than the simple hemodynamic consequences of redirected blood flow probably also are involved in this process. For example, after a pneumonectomy, 100 percent of the right ventricular output flows to one lung, yet there is little increase in pulmonary pressure even with follow-up to 11 years.[14] In patients with thromboembolic disease, however, one frequently detects pulmonary hypertension even when less than 50 percent of the vascular bed is occluded by thrombus. It thus appears that sympathetic neural connections, hormonal changes, or both may initiate pulmonary hypertension in the initially unaffected pulmonary vascular bed. This process can occur when the initial occlusion is in the same lung or the contralateral lung.

Regardless of the etiology, the advancement of pulmonary hypertension as a consequence of changes in the previously unobstructed bed is serious, since this process may lead to an inoperable condition. Thus, with accumulating experience in patients with thromboembolic pulmonary hypertension, surgeons increasingly have been inclined toward early operation to avoid those changes.

CLINICAL FEATURES

Chronic thromboembolic pulmonary hypertension is underdiagnosed severely because there are no specific clinical features. Although the majority of pulmonary thromboembolic material originates form a DVT, more than half of patients with CTEPH do not have a history of DVT or PE. The clinical history therefore may not be helpful, making a diagnosis even more difficult. Nevertheless, during clinical evaluation, predisposing factors for DVT should be sought, as should a history of leg swelling, chest pain, hemoptysis, or any symptom that indicates episodes of PE.

The diagnosis in most patients may be quite difficult since the onset of the disease is insidious. The most common symptom coupled with thromboembolic pulmonary hypertension, as with all other sources of pulmonary hypertension, is exertional dyspnea. This dyspnea is out of proportion to any anomalies found on clinical examination. Similar to complaints of easy fatigability, dyspnea that initially occurs only with exertion often is attributed to anxiety or being "out of shape." Syncope or presyncope (light-headedness during exertion) is another common symptom in patients with pulmonary hypertension. Generally, it occurs in patients with more advanced disease and higher pulmonary arterial pressures.

Another relatively common complaint with CTEPH is nonspecific chest pains or chest pressure. These symptoms occur in approximately 50 percent of patients with more severe pulmonary hypertension. Hemoptysis can occur in all forms of pulmonary hypertension, including CTEPH. It probably results from abnormally dilated vessels that are distended by increased intravascular pressures. Peripheral edema, early satiety, and epigastric or right upper quadrant fullness or discomfort may develop as the right heart fails (cor pulmonale). Some patients with CTEPH present after a small acute pulmonary embolus that may produce acute symptoms of right heart failure. A careful history brings out symptoms of dyspnea on minimal exertion, easy fatigability, diminishing activities, and episodes of angina-like pain or light-headedness. Further examination may reveal signs of pulmonary hypertension.

As is the case with the symptoms, the physical signs of CTEPH are far from uniform. The physical examination may be surprisingly unrewarding if right heart failure has not occurred, even if the patient complains of severe dyspnea. Another important point is that the physical signs of pulmonary hypertension are the same regardless of the underlying pathophysiology.

In the early stages, the jugular venous pulse is characterized by a large A wave. As the right heart fails, the V wave becomes predominant. The right ventricle is usually palpable near the lower left sternal border, and pulmonary valve closure may be audible in the second intercostal space. Occasional patients with advanced disease are hypoxic and slightly cyanotic. Cyanosis, if it is present at all, is usually peripheral and is related to low cardiac output. Central cyanosis may be present from a persistent foramen ovale or atrial septal defect with right-to-left shunting. Clubbing is an uncommon finding.

Examination of the chest may be normal initially. Later, jugular venous distention with prominent A and V waves, as described above, may become evident. Auscultation of the chest may reveal some specific and nonspecific anomalies. The second heart sound is often narrowly split and varies normally with respiration; P_2 is accentuated. A sharp systolic ejection click may be heard over the pulmonary artery. As the right heart fails, a right atrial gallop usually is present, and tricuspid insufficiency develops. Because of the large pressure gradient across the tricuspid valve in patients with pulmonary hypertension, the murmur is high-pitched and may not exhibit respiratory variation. These findings are quite different from those usually observed in patients with tricuspid valvular disease. A murmur of pulmonary regurgitation also may be detected.

A specific sign is flow murmurs, which are heard especially over the back beneath the scapula. Moser and colleagues[15] pointed out that these murmurs often are heard in patients with CTEPH. The murmur is portrayed as maximal over the lung fields, increasing in intensity with inspiration, and frequently spilling beyond the second sound.[15] These murmurs probably result from turbulent flow past a segmental tapering; it is also conceivable that they correspond to aggressive bronchial flow. An important observation is that these flow murmurs have not been described in patients with primary pulmonary hypertension, the major differential diagnosis for this condition.

Signs of chronic venous stasis may be present in the legs, with skin discoloration and perhaps with healed varicosities or varicose ulcers. Peripheral edema is variable among these patients and, if present, may be especially difficult to detect if a patient has chronic lower extremity venous stasis with or without ulceration.

Thus, the clinical signs and symptoms of CTEPH are not by any means specific and are far from uniform. A suspicion for the diagnosis should be raised once the degree of symptomatology is out of proportion to the patient's general condition. Once the suspicion arises, the clinician should pursue key points in the patient's past history and physical findings that may relate to this condition. The diagnosis, however, is confirmed only and finally with the aid of a broad variety of diagnostic modalities.

DIAGNOSTIC MODALITIES

To ensure the diagnosis in patients with CTEPH, a consistent evaluation is recommended for all patients who

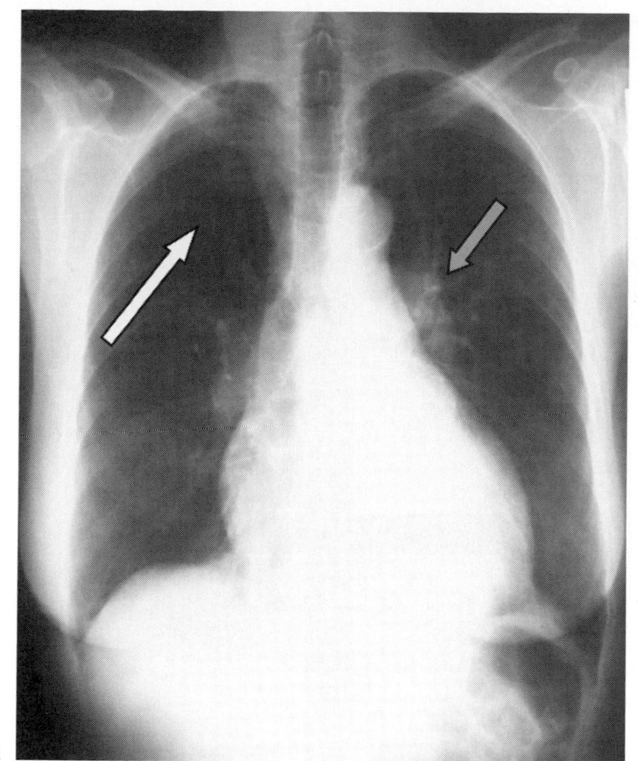

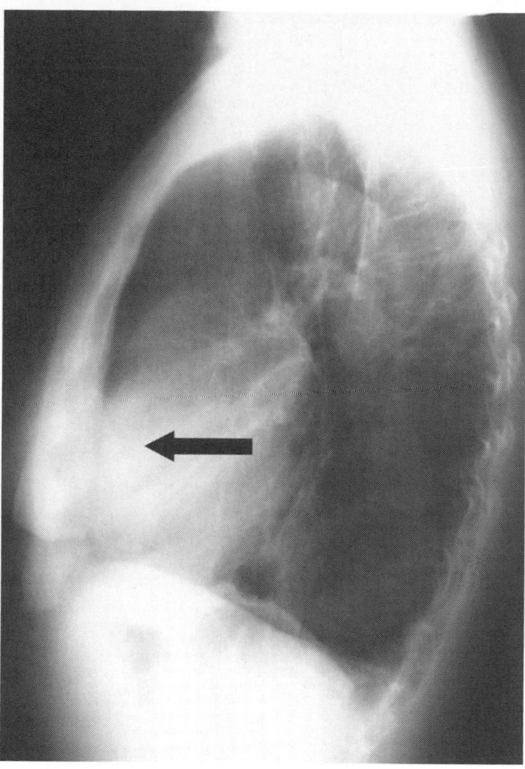

Figure 40-1 Typical anteroposterior and lateral chest radiograph of a patient with chronic thromboembolic pulmonary hypertension. Note an enlarged right atrium and right ventricle (*black arrow on the lateral view*), disparity of size between the left and right pulmonary arteries, and hypoperfusion in several areas of the lung (*white arrow*).

present with unexplained pulmonary hypertension. The nonspecificity of the clinical presentation and symptoms contributes to the diagnostic delay that most patients with CTEPH experience. In the authors' center, it is common to see patients who have gone undiagnosed for several years, typically 2 to 3 years.

The workup generally starts with a chest radiograph. Chest radiography may be deceptively normal in the early stages of CTEPH. However, with the development of significant pulmonary hypertension and right heart enlargement, some characteristic findings may point the examiner toward the diagnosis. Central pulmonary arteries may be enlarged, and the right ventricle may be enlarged without enlargement of the left atrium or ventricle, unlike the case in mitral stenosis (Fig. 40-1). The chest radiograph also may show either apparent vessel cutoffs of the lobar or segmental pulmonary arteries or regions of oligemia that suggest vascular occlusion. However, one should keep in mind that despite these classic findings, a large number of patients may present with a relatively normal chest radiograph even in the setting of high degrees of pulmonary hypertension. The electrocardiogram demonstrates findings of right ventricular hypertrophy (right axis deviation, dominant R wave in V_1).

Pulmonary function tests are necessary to exclude obstructive or restrictive intrinsic pulmonary parenchymal disease as the cause or the hypertension but generally are not helpful. They reveal minimal changes in lung volume and ventilation; these patients by and large have normal or slightly restricted pulmonary mechanics. DLCO often is reduced and may be the only abnormality on pulmonary function testing.

Most of these patients are hypoxic; room air arterial oxygen tension ranges between 50 and 83 torr, with the average being 65 torr.[16] CO_2 tension is slightly reduced and is compensated by reduced bicarbonate. Dead space ventilation is increased. Ventilation-perfusion studies show a moderate mismatch with some heterogeneity among various respirator units within the lung and correlate poorly with the degree of pulmonary obstruction.[17]

The ventilation-perfusion lung scan is the essential test for establishing the diagnosis of unresolved pulmonary thromboembolism. An entirely normal lung scan excludes the diagnosis of both acute and chronic unresolved thromboembolism. Patients with CTEPH invariably demonstrate one or more segmental or larger perfusion defects in lung regions that typically have normal ventilation (Fig. 40-2). The usual lung scan pattern in most patients with pulmonary hypertension is relatively normal or shows diffuse nonuniform perfusion.[18–20] The magnitude of perfusion defects in chronic thromboembolic disease often underestimates the actual degree of vascular obstruction. When subsegmental or larger perfusion defects are noted on the scan, even when they are matched with ventilatory

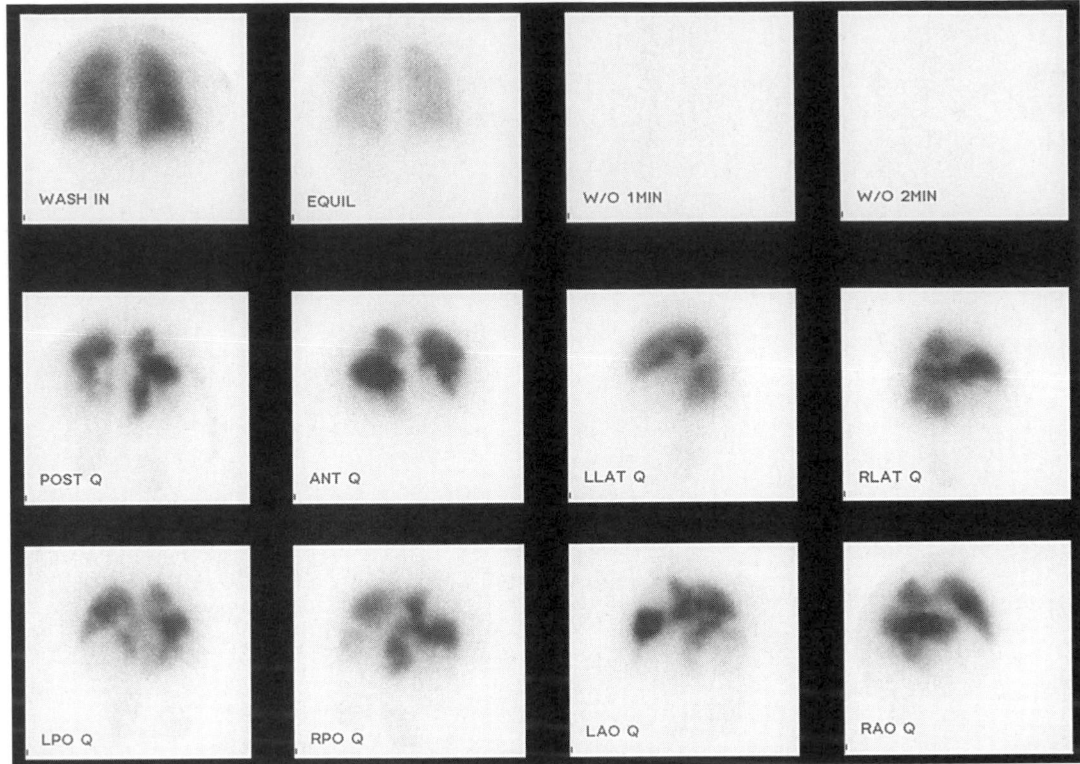

Figure 40-2 Lung ventilation and perfusion study (V/Q scan) in a patient with chronic thromboembolic pulmonary hypertension. Note that the ventilation portion of the study is normal.

defects, pulmonary angiography is appropriate to confirm or rule out thromboembolic disease.

Right heart catheterization and pulmonary angiography should be pursued in any patient with suspected chronic thromboembolic disease. Despite advances in computed tomography and increasing reliance on it in the evaluation of the pulmonary vascular bed, its role in this population remains somewhat undefined, and pulmonary angiography still should be considered the gold standard in establishing the diagnosis of CTEPH. Organized thromboembolic lesions do not have the appearance of the intravascular filling defects seen with acute pulmonary emboli, and experience is essential for the proper interpretation of pulmonary angiograms in patients with unresolved chronic embolic disease. Organized thrombi appear as unusual filling defects, webs, or bands or as completely thrombosed vessels that may resemble congenital absence of the vessel[20] (Fig. 40-3). Organized material along a vascular wall of a recanalized vessel produces a scalloped or serrated luminal edge. Because of both vessel wall thickening and dilatation of proximal vessels, the contrast-filled lumen may appear relatively normal in diameter. Distal vessels demonstrate the rapid tapering and pruning characteristic of pulmonary hypertension (Fig. 40-3).

Historically, angiography in persons with pulmonary hypertension was thought to carry a disproportionate risk. The authors have found that not to be the case, and at the authors' institution, pulmonary angiographies are performed daily in these patients with minimal associated risks. Several thousand angiograms in pulmonary hypertensive patients have been performed at the authors' institution without mortality. Although some risk remains, the benefit of establishing the presence of a treatable cause of the hypertension far outweighs the small risk, and pulmonary angiography should be performed whenever there is a possibility that chronic thromboembolism is the etiology of pulmonary hypertension.

In addition to pulmonary angiography, patients over age 45 undergo coronary arteriography and other cardiac investigations as necessary. If significant disease is found, additional cardiac surgery is performed at the time of pulmonary thromboendarterectomy.

Despite the accuracy and value of pulmonary angiography, in approximately 15 to 20 percent of cases, the differential diagnosis between primary pulmonary hypertension and distal and small vessel pulmonary thromboembolic disease is unclear and hard to establish. Pulmonary angioscopy may be helpful in these patients. The pulmonary angioscope is a fiber-optic telescope that is placed through a central line into the pulmonary artery. The tip contains a balloon that is filled with saline and pushed against the vessel wall. A bloodless field thus can be obtained to view the pulmonary artery wall. The classic appearance of chronic pulmonary thromboembolic disease by angioscopy consists of intimal thickening with intimal

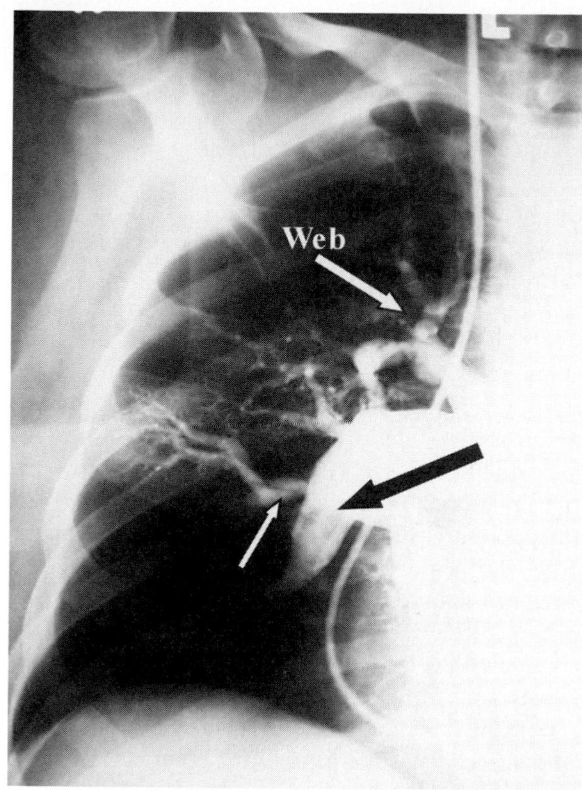

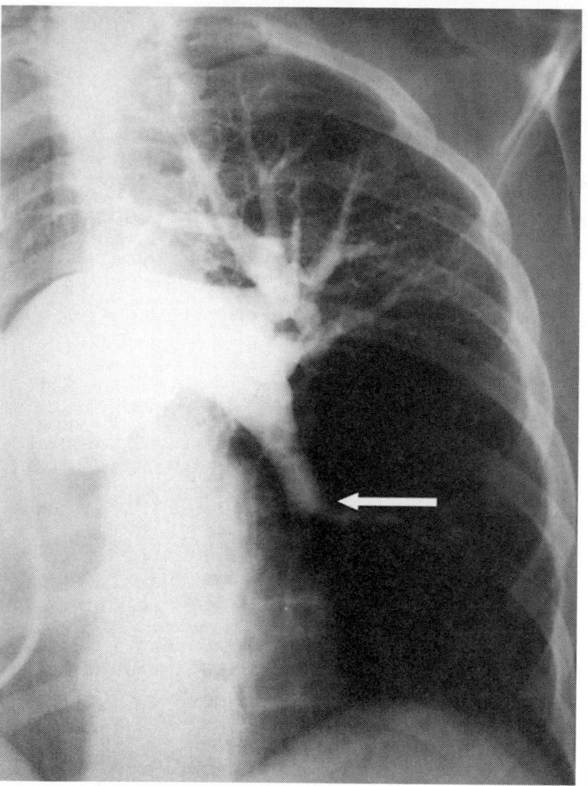

Figure 40-3 Pulmonary angiogram in a patient with chronic thromboembolic pulmonary hypertension. Note the extensive areas of hypoperfusion as a result of complete occlusion, as well as luminal irregularities, webs, bands, and pouches, as shown by the arrows.

irregularity and scarring and webs across small vessels. Those webs are thought to be the residue of resolved occluding thrombi of small vessels but are important diagnostic findings. The presence of embolic disease, occlusion of vessels, or thrombotic material is diagnostic.

In recent years, higher-resolution helical computed tomography (CT) scans of the chest have been used more frequently in the diagnosis of pulmonary thromboembolic disease. The presence of large clots in lobar or segmental vessels generally confirms the diagnosis. CT features of CTEPH include evidence of organized thrombus lining the pulmonary vessels in an eccentric fashion, enlargement of the right ventricle and the central arteries, variation in the size of segmental arteries, and parenchymal changes characteristic of pulmonary infarction. In addition, in rare situations in which there are concerns about external compression or occlusion of main pulmonary arteries is present, CT scans can be helpful in differentiating thromboembolic disease from other causes, such as mediastinal fibrosis, lymph nodes, and tumors.

MEDICAL THERAPY

Medical therapy for CTEPH is of limited value and is palliative at best. In light of the occlusive nature of this disease, there is no curative medical regimen that can alleviate the degree of pulmonary hypertension present in these patients. Right ventricular failure generally is treated with diuretics and vasodilators. A wide variety of pharmacologic agents are in current use for the treatment of primary pulmonary hypertension. They include calcium channel blockers such as diltiazem and nifedipine, prostacyclins such as epoprostenol (Flolan, Remodulin), prostacyclin analogues, endothelin receptor antagonists (Tracleer), and nitric oxide. However, these agents are practically useless in the setting of CTEPH because of the fixed mechanical obstructive nature of the disease. Rarely, patients with CTEPH may have temporary relief with medical management; however, this is not curative, and the symptoms do recur. In general, medical therapy should be regarded as only supportive. Similarly, the prognosis is not affected by medical therapy.

Chronic anticoagulation is the mainstay of the medical regimen. Anticoagulation is used primarily to prevent future embolic episodes, but it also serves to limit the development of thrombus in regions of low flow within the pulmonary vasculature. Inferior vena caval filters also are used routinely to prevent recurrent embolization. If caval filtration and anticoagulation fail to prevent recurrent emboli, immediate thrombolysis may be beneficial, but lytic agents cannot alter the chronic component of the disease.

SURGICAL THERAPY

Surgical removal of the chronic thromboembolic material is the only curative option for patients with CTEPH. In an experienced center, the procedure can be performed with low operative morbidity and mortality and can produce a tremendous hemodynamic benefit with an excellent prognosis. The only other surgical alternative for these patients is transplantation. However, as was mentioned earlier, the authors consider transplantation inappropriate for the treatment of this disease and believe it to be obsolete in the management of patients with CTEPH. In light of the mortality and morbidity rates of patients on the waiting list, the higher risk of the operation, and the less desirable or inferior survival rates (i.e., approximately 80 percent at 1 year at centers experienced in transplantation versus 95 percent for pulmonary endarterectomy), pulmonary thromboendarterectomy is still the superior choice. Furthermore, pulmonary endarterectomy appears to be permanently curative, and the issues of a continuing risk of rejection and immunosuppression are not present.

Allison and coworkers performed the first successful pulmonary "thromboendarterectomy" through a sternotomy, using surface hypothermia, in 1960, but only fresh clots were removed.[21] That operation took place 12 days after a thigh injury that led to PE, and an endarterectomy was not performed. Since that time, there have been occasional reports of the surgical treatment of chronic pulmonary thromboembolism, but most of the surgical experience in pulmonary endarterectomy has been reported from the UCSD Medical Center. Braunwald began the UCSD experience with this operation in 1970, which now totals over 2000 cases. The operation described below, using deep hypothermia and circulatory arrest, is now the authors' standard procedure.

Guiding principles of the operation

Once the diagnosis of thromboembolic pulmonary hypertension has been established firmly, the decision to do an operation is based on the severity of symptoms and the general condition of the patient. In general, suitable candidates with CTEPH have excellent hemodynamic results, with an outstanding long-term prognosis. Early in the pulmonary endarterectomy experience, Moser[19] pointed out that there were three major reasons for considering thromboendarterectomy: hemodynamic, alveolorespiratory, and prophylactic.

The hemodynamic goal is to prevent or ameliorate right ventricular compromise caused by pulmonary hypertension. The respiratory objective is to improve respiratory function by removing a large ventilated but unperfused physiologic dead space. The prophylactic goal is to prevent progressive right ventricular dysfunction or retrograde extension of the obstruction, which might result in further cardiorespiratory deterioration or death. The authors' subsequent experience has added another prophylactic goal: the prevention of secondary arteriopathic changes in the remaining patent vessels.

Although the essential techniques of pulmonary thromboendarterectomy are quite similar to those for other open heart operations, several guiding principles are specific to this procedure. For pulmonary hypertension to be a major factor, both pulmonary arteries must be involved substantially. The surgery is therefore always bilateral, although the volume of chronic thromboembolic material may vary significantly between the two lungs. The only reasonable approach to both pulmonary arteries is through a median sternotomy incision. Historically, there were many reports of unilateral operations, and occasionally this still is done in inexperienced centers through a thoracotomy. However, the unilateral approach ignores the disease on the contralateral side, subjects the patient to hemodynamic jeopardy during the clamping of the pulmonary artery, and does not allow good visibility because of the continued presence of bronchial blood flow. In addition, collateral channels develop in patients with chronic thrombotic hypertension not only through the bronchial arteries but also from diaphragmatic, intercostal, and pleural vessels. The dissection of the lung in the pleural space via a thoracotomy incision therefore can be extremely bloody. The median sternotomy incision, apart from providing bilateral access, avoids entry into the pleural cavities and allows the institution of cardiopulmonary bypass.

A thorough and successful endarterectomy of the pulmonary arteries can be performed only in a bloodless field and under circulatory arrest. Cardiopulmonary bypass is therefore essential not only to ensure cardiovascular stability when the operation is performed but also to allow cooling of the patient for periods of circulatory arrest. Exceptional visibility of the pulmonary vasculature is required, and a bloodless field is an absolute requirement to define an adequate endarterectomy plane and then follow the pulmonary endarterectomy specimen deep into the subsegmental vessels. Because of the copious bronchial blood flow usually present in these cases, periods of circulatory arrest are necessary to ensure perfect visibility. Again, there have been sporadic reports of the performance of this operation without circulatory arrest. However, it should be emphasized that although endarterectomy is possible without circulatory arrest, a complete and full endarterectomy is not. Without a complete endarterectomy all the way to the distal tail end of each branch, successful hemodynamic improvement is not achievable, leaving the patients with residual pulmonary hypertension and a subsequent poor prognosis in the short term and the long term.

The authors always initiate the procedure without circulatory arrest; depending on the collateral flow, a variable amount of dissection is possible before the circulation is stopped, but never complete dissection. The circulatory arrest periods are limited to 20 min, with restoration of flow after each arrest. With experience, the endarterectomy generally is performed with a single period of circulatory arrest on each side.

A true endarterectomy in the plane of the media must be accomplished. It is essential to appreciate that the removal of visible thrombus is largely incidental to this operation. Indeed, in most patients, no free thrombus is present, and on initial direct examination, the pulmonary vascular bed may appear normal to an inexperienced eye. The early literature on this procedure is filled with reports of thrombectomy performed without a complete endarterectomy, and in those cases the pulmonary artery pressures did not improve, often with the resultant death of the patient.

Surgical techniques

After a median sternotomy is performed, the pericardium is incised longitudinally and attached to the wound edges. Typically, the right heart is enlarged, with a tense right atrium and a variable degree of tricuspid regurgitation. There is usually severe right ventricular hypertrophy. These patients are generally quite sensitive to any manipulation of the heart, and with critical degrees of obstruction, the patient's condition may become quite unstable.

Anticoagulation is achieved with the use of beef-lung heparin sodium (400 units/kg intravenously) administered to prolong the activated clotting time beyond 400 s. Full cardiopulmonary bypass is instituted with high ascending aortic cannulation and two caval cannulas. The cannulas must be inserted into the superior and inferior venae cavae sufficiently to enable subsequent opening of the right atrium. The heart is emptied on bypass, and a temporary pulmonary artery vent is placed in the midline of the main pulmonary artery 1 cm distal to the pulmonary valve. This marks the beginning of the left pulmonary arteriotomy.

When cardiopulmonary bypass is initiated, surface cooling with both a head jacket and a cooling blanket is begun. Cooling generally takes 45 min to an hour. When ventricular fibrillation occurs, an additional vent is placed in the left atrium through the right superior pulmonary vein. This prevents atrial and ventricular distention from the large amount of bronchial arterial blood flow that is common in these patients.

The primary surgeon starts the operation on the patient's left side. During the cooling period, some preliminary dissection can be performed, with full mobilization of the right pulmonary artery from the ascending aorta. The superior vena cava also is mobilized fully. The approach to the right pulmonary artery is made medial, not lateral, to the superior vena cava. All dissection of the pulmonary arteries takes place intrapericardially, and neither pleural cavity should be entered. An incision is made in the right pulmonary artery from beneath the ascending aorta out under the superior vena cava and entering the lower lobe branch of the pulmonary artery just after the take-off of the middle lobe artery (Fig. 40-4). It is

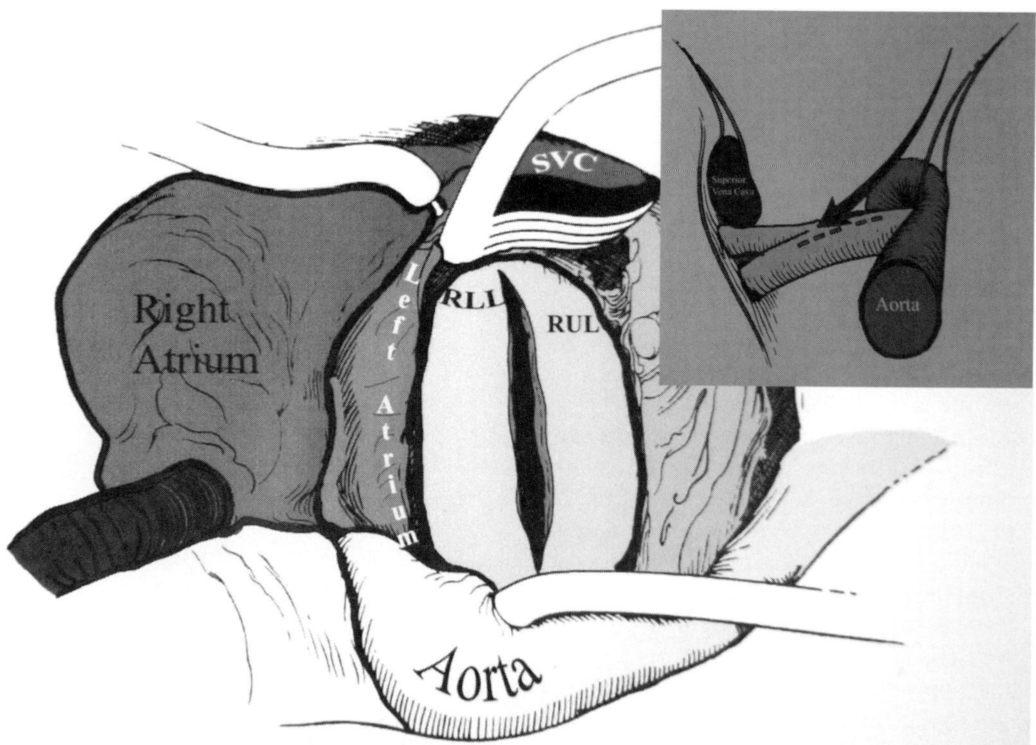

Figure 40-4 Exposure of the right pulmonary artery. The incision is placed between the superior vena cava (SVC) and the aorta, not lateral to the SVC (as shown in the insert). It is imperative that the incision toward the right lower lobe artery be made in the middle of the vessel.

important that the incision stay in the center of the vessel and continue into the lower rather than the middle lobe artery.

A modified cerebellar retractor is placed between the aorta and the superior vena cava. When the pulmonary artery is opened, a varying degree of loose thrombus may be present. This material is removed to ensure good visualization of the vascular bed. It is most important to recognize, however, that an embolectomy without a subsequent endarterectomy is ineffective regardless of the size of thromboembolic material and that in most patients with CTEPH, direct examination of the pulmonary vascular bed at operation generally shows no obvious embolic material. Therefore, to the inexperienced or cursory glance, the pulmonary vascular bed may appear normal even in patients with severe chronic embolic pulmonary hypertension.

When the patient's temperature reaches 20°C, the aorta is cross-clamped and a single dose of cold cardioplegic solution (1 L) is administered. Additional myocardial protection is obtained with the use of a cooling jacket. The entire procedure now is performed with a single aortic cross-clamp period with no further administration of cardioplegic solution.

If the bronchial circulation is not excessive, the endarterectomy plane can be found during this early dissection. However, although a small amount of dissection can be performed before the initiation of circulatory arrest, it is unwise to proceed unless perfect visibility is obtained because the development of a correct plane is essential. Recognizing the plane is perhaps the most crucial and technically challenging part of the operation.

When blood obscures direct vision of the pulmonary vascular bed, thiopental is administered (500 mg to 1 g) until the electroencephalogram (EEG) becomes isoelectric. In most cases, the EEG is isoelectric once the core temperature reaches 20°C. Circulatory arrest is initiated, and the patient is exsanguinated. All monitoring lines to the patient are turned off to prevent aspiration of air. Snares are tightened around the cannulas in the superior and inferior venae cavae.

A microtome knife is used to develop the endarterectomy plane posteriorly because any inadvertent egress in this site can be repaired readily or simply left alone. Dissection in the correct plane is critical because if the plane is too deep, the pulmonary artery may perforate, with fatal results, and if the plane is not deep enough, inadequate amounts of the chronic thromboembolic material will be removed, leaving the patient with residual pulmonary hypertension.

Once the plane is developed correctly, a full-thickness layer is left in the region of the incision to ease subsequent repair. The endarterectomy is performed with an eversion technique. Because the vessel is everted and subsegmental branches are being worked on, a perforation in this area will be inaccessible later. This is why the absolute visualization in a completely bloodless field provided by circulatory arrest is essential. It is important that each subsegmental branch be followed and freed individually until it ends in a "tail," beyond which there is no further obstruction. Residual material never should be cut free; the entire specimen should "tail off" and come free spontaneously. Although retrograde cerebral perfusion has been advocated for total circulatory arrest in other procedures, it is not helpful in this operation because it does not allow a completely bloodless field; also, with the short arrest times that can be achieved with experience, it is not necessary.

Once the right-sided endarterectomy is completed, circulation is restarted, and the arteriotomy is repaired with a continuous 6-0 polypropylene suture. The hemostatic nature of this closure is aided by the nature of the initial dissection, with the full thickness of the pulmonary artery being preserved immediately adjacent to the incision.

After the completion of the repair of the right arteriotomy, the surgeon moves to the patient's right side. The pulmonary vent catheter is withdrawn, and an arteriotomy is made from the site of the pulmonary vent hole laterally to the pericardial reflection, avoiding entry into the left pleural space. Additional lateral dissection does not enhance intraluminal visibility, may endanger the left phrenic nerve, and makes subsequent repair of the left pulmonary artery more difficult (Fig. 40-5). The left-sided dissection is virtually analogous in all respects to that accomplished on the right. The duration of circulatory arrest intervals during the performance of the left-sided dissection is subject to the same restriction that applies to the right.

After completion of the endarterectomy, cardiopulmonary bypass is reinstituted and warming is commenced.

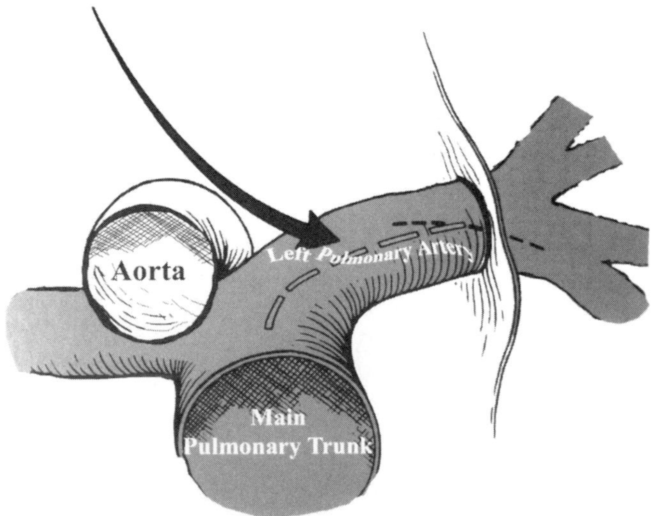

Figure 40-5 Exposure of the left pulmonary artery with its corresponding incision. Note that the incision begins in the midportion of the main pulmonary artery at the site of the insertion of the pulmonary artery vent.

The rewarming period generally lasts approximately 90 min but varies with the body mass of the patient.

The pulmonary artery is closed, and the pulmonary vent is replaced. The right atrium then is opened and examined. Any intraatrial communication is closed. Although tricuspid valve regurgitation is invariable in these patients and is often severe, tricuspid valve repair is not performed. Right ventricular remodeling occurs within a few days, with the return of tricuspid competence. If other cardiac procedures are required, such as coronary artery or mitral or aortic valve surgery, those procedures are performed conveniently during the systemic rewarming period. Myocardial cooling is discontinued once all cardiac procedures have been concluded. The left atrial vent is removed, and the vent site is repaired. All air is removed from the heart, and the aortic cross-clamp is removed.

When the patient has rewarmed, cardiopulmonary bypass is discontinued. Dopamine hydrochloride is administered routinely at renal doses, and other inotropic agents and vasodilators are titrated as necessary to sustain acceptable hemodynamics. The cardiac output is generally high, with low systemic vascular resistance. Temporary atrial and ventricular epicardial pacing wires are placed.

Despite the duration of extracorporeal circulation, hemostasis is achieved readily, and the administration of platelets or coagulation factors is generally unnecessary. Wound closure is routine. A vigorous diuresis is the usual procedure for the next few hours, also a result of the previous systemic hypothermia.

OUTCOMES AND PROGNOSIS

The ages of the patients in the authors' series have ranged from 8 to 86 years. A typical patient will have a severely elevated pulmonary vascular resistance (PVR) level at rest, the absence of significant comorbid disease unrelated to right heart failure, and the appearance of chronic thrombi on angiography that appears to be in balance with the measured PVR level. Exceptions to this general rule, of course, occur.

Although most patients have a PVR level in the range of 800 dyne·s/cm^5 and pulmonary artery pressures that are lower than systemic pressures, the hypertrophy of the right ventricle that occurs over time makes pulmonary hypertension to suprasystemic levels possible. Therefore, many patients (perhaps 20 percent in the authors' practice) have a level of PVR well in excess of 1000 dyne·s/cm^5 and suprasystemic pulmonary artery pressures. There is no upper limit of PVR level, pulmonary artery pressure, or degree of right ventricular dysfunction that excludes patients from the operation.

As was mentioned above, surgeons have become increasingly aware of the changes that can occur in the remaining patent (unaffected by clot) pulmonary vascular bed subjected to the higher pressures and flow that result from obstruction in other areas. Therefore, with the increasing experience and safety of the operation, the authors tend to offer surgery to symptomatic patients whenever an angiogram demonstrates thromboembolic disease. A rare patient may have a PVR level that is normal at rest but elevated with minimal exercise. This is usually a young patient with total unilateral pulmonary artery occlusion and unacceptable exertional dyspnea caused by an elevation in dead space ventilation. In this circumstance, and operation is performed to reperfuse lung tissue, reestablish a more normal ventilation-perfusion relationship (thereby reducing minute ventilatory requirements during rest and exercise), and preserve the integrity of the contralateral circulation.

Thromboembolic classification and surgical outcome

There are four broad types of pulmonary occlusive disease related to thrombus that can be appreciated. These types are based on the anatomic location of the thromboembolic material as well as vessel wall pathology. This classification allows one to estimate the patient's outcome and prognosis after an endarterectomy.[20,22,23] Type I disease (approximately 20 percent of cases of thromboembolic pulmonary hypertension) (Fig. 40-6) refers to the situation in which a major vessel clot is present and readily visible on the opening of the pulmonary arteries. As was mentioned earlier, all central thrombotic material has to be removed completely before the endarterectomy.

In type II disease (approximately 70 percent of cases) (Fig. 40-7), no major vessel thrombus can be appreciated. In these cases, only thickened intima can be seen, occasionally with webs, and the endarterectomy plane is raised in the main, lobar, or segmental vessels. Type III disease (approximately 10 percent of cases) (Fig. 40-8) presents the most challenging surgical situation. The disease is very distal and is confined to the segmental and subsegmental branches. No occlusion of vessels can be seen initially. The endarterectomy plane must be raised carefully and painstakingly in each segmental and subsegmental branch. Type III disease is associated most often with presumed repetitive thrombi from indwelling catheters (such as pacemaker wires) or ventriculoatrial shunts.

Type IV disease (Fig. 40-9) does not represent primary thromboembolic pulmonary hypertension and is inoperable. It represents microscopic distal arteriolar vasculopathy without visible thromboembolic disease. In this entity, there is intrinsic small vessel disease, although secondary thrombus may occur as a result of stasis. Small vessel disease may be unrelated to thromboembolic events ("primary" pulmonary hypertension) or may occur in relation to thromboembolic hypertension as a result of a high-flow or high-pressure state in previously unaffected vessels, similar to the generation of Eisenmenger's syndrome. The authors believe that there also may be sympathetic "cross-talk" from an affected contralateral side or stenotic areas in the same lung.

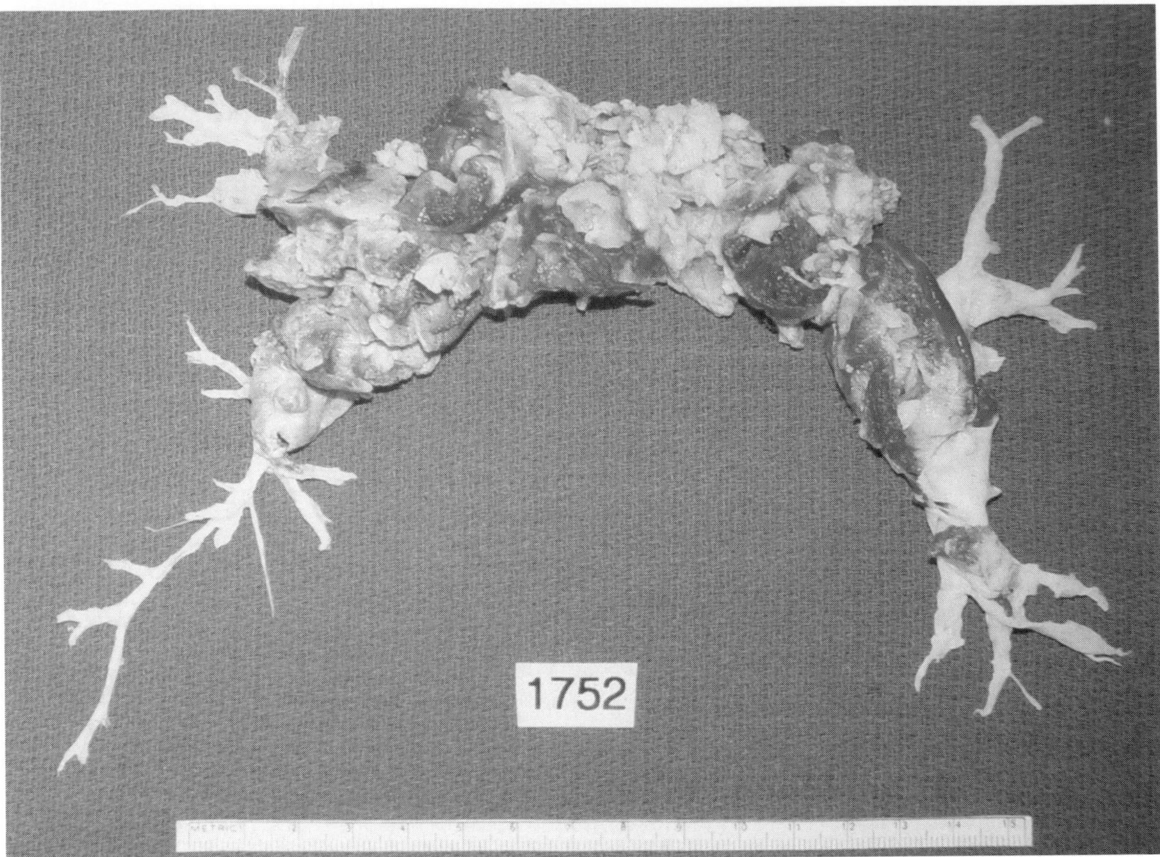

Figure 40-6 Surgical specimen removed from the right and left pulmonary arteries. Fresh thrombus in major arteries indicates type I disease on both sides. Note that removal of only the fresh material leaves a large amount of disease behind. The ruler measures 15 cm.

In general, patients with type III disease have some degree of residual pulmonary hypertension, with higher levels of postoperative PVR and more postoperative tricuspid regurgitation than do those with type I and type II disease. Type IV patients always do. These patients generally require longer inotropic support and ventilatory support and have longer intensive care unit (ICU) and hospital stays. They also have higher incidences of postoperative complications and in fact account for the vast majority of the authors' cases of perioperative morbidity and mortality.

Complications of pulmonary thromboendarterectomy

Patients with CTEPH are subject to all the complications associated with open heart and major lung surgery (arrhythmias, atelectasis, wound infection, pneumonia, mediastinal bleeding, etc.) but also may develop complications specific to this operation. One complication is the development of the "reperfusion response." This is a specific complication that is related to localized pulmonary edema. Reperfusion injury is defined as a radiologic opacity seen in the lungs within 72 h of a pulmonary endarterectomy. This loose definition therefore may encompass many causes, such as fluid overload and infection.

True reperfusion injury that has a direct adverse impact on the clinical course of the patient now occurs in approximately 8 to 10 percent of patients. In its most dramatic form, it occurs soon after operation (within a few hours) and is associated with profound desaturation. Edema-like fluid, sometimes with a bloody tinge, is suctioned from the endotracheal tube. Frank blood from the endotracheal tube, however, signifies a mechanical violation of the blood-airway barrier that has occurred at operation and stems from a technical error. This complication should be managed, if possible, by identification of the affected area by bronchoscopy and balloon occlusion of the affected lobe until coagulation can be normalized.

A common cause of reperfusion pulmonary edema (PE) is persistent high pulmonary artery pressures after operation when a thorough endarterectomy has been performed in certain areas but a large part of the pulmonary vascular bed still is affected by type IV change. However, the reperfusion phenomenon also occasionally

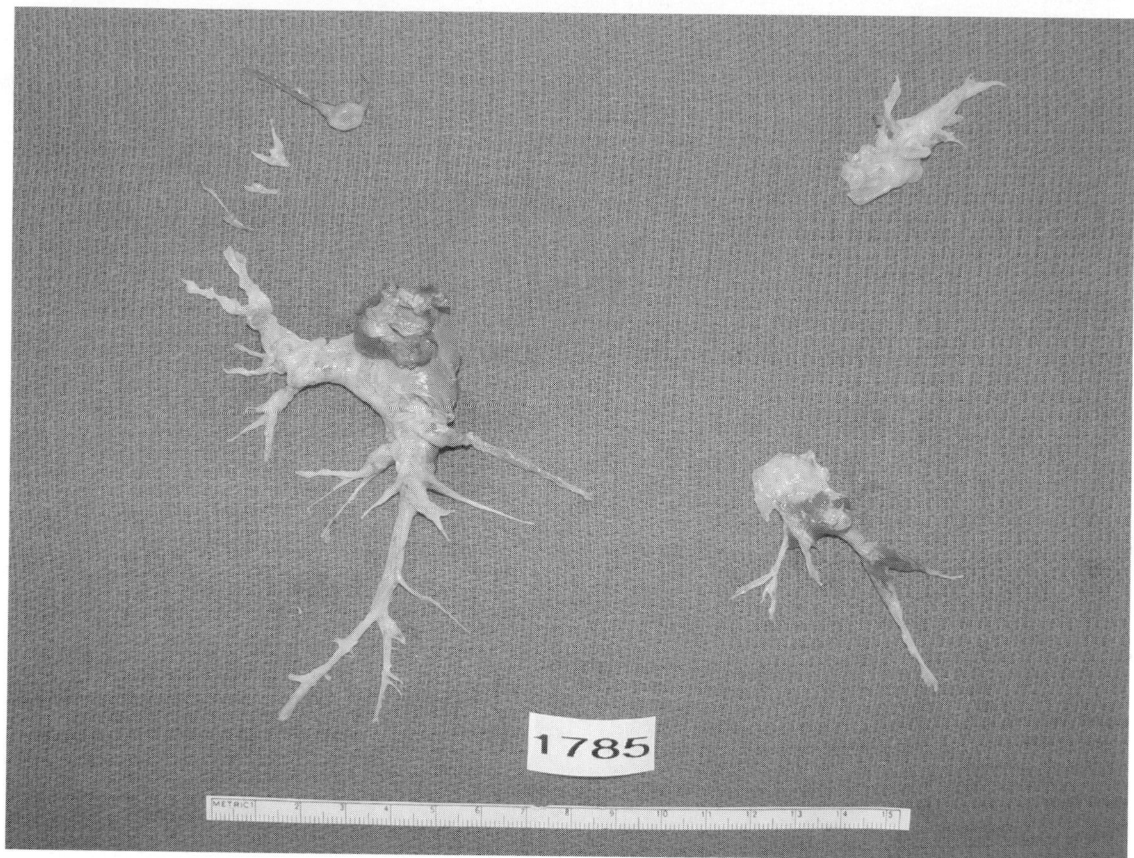

Figure 40-7 Surgical specimen removed from the right and left pulmonary arteries indicating evidence of type II disease. Note the extent of dissection down to the tail end of each one of the branches. The ruler measures 15 cm.

is encountered in patients after a seemingly technically perfect operation with complete resolution of high pulmonary artery pressures. In these cases, the response may be one of reactive hyperemia after the revascularization of segments of the pulmonary arterial bed that have long experienced no flow. Other contributing factors may include perioperative pulmonary ischemia and conditions associated with high-permeability lung injury in the area of the now-denuded endothelium. Fortunately, the incidence of this complication is very much lower now in the authors' series, probably as a result of the more complete and expeditious removal of the endarterectomy specimen that has come with experience over the last decade.

Management of the reperfusion response

Early measures should be taken to minimize the development of PE with diuresis, maintenance of the hematocrit levels, and the early use of peak end-expiratory pressure. Once the capillary leak has been established, treatment is supportive because reperfusion PE eventually will resolve if satisfactory hemodynamics and oxygenation can be maintained. Careful management of ventilation and fluid balance is required. The hematocrit is kept high (32 to 36 percent), and the patient should undergo aggressive diuresis even if this requires ultrafiltration. The patient's ventilatory status may be dramatically position-sensitive. The FiO_2 level is kept as low as is compatible with an oxygen saturation of 90 percent. A careful titration of positive end-expiratory pressure is carried out, with a progressive transition from a volume-limited to a pressure-limited inverse ratio of ventilation and the acceptance of moderate hypercapnia. The use of steroids is discouraged because they are generally ineffective and may lead to infection. Infrequently, inhaled nitric oxide at 20 to 40 parts per million can improve gas exchange. On rare occasions, the authors have used extracorporeal perfusion support (extracorporeal membrane oxygenator or extracorporeal carbon dioxide removal) until ventilation can be resumed satisfactorily, usually after 7 to 10 days.

Results of pulmonary thromboendarterectomy

Pulmonary endarterectomy is performed at several major cardiovascular centers around the world; however, the greatest experience with this operation has been at the UCSD Medical Center, where the technique was pioneered and has been refined to its current state over the

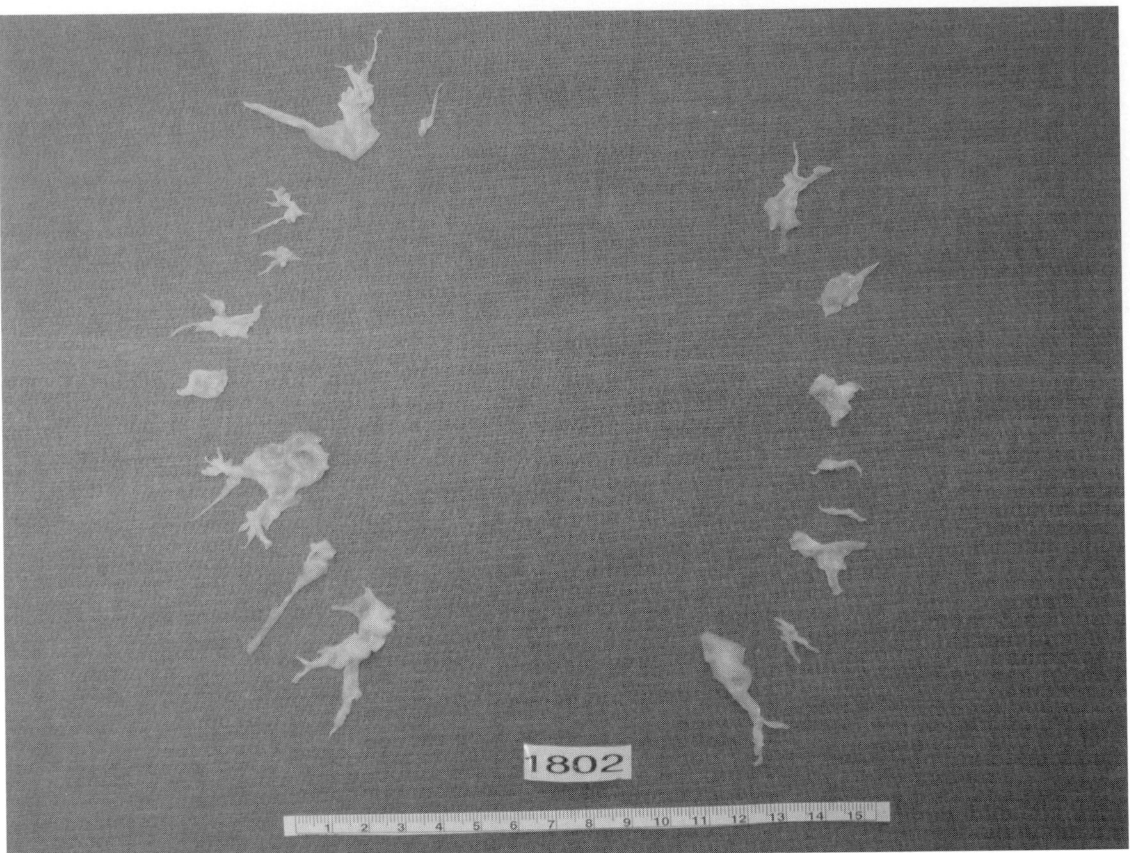

Figure 40-8 Surgical specimen removed from the right and left pulmonary arteries in a patient with type III disease. Note that in this patient the dissection plane has to be developed and raised at each segmental level. The ruler measures 15 cm.

last decade and half. Over 2000 pulmonary endarterectomies have been performed.

The mean age for the authors' patients is 52, with a range of 8 to 86, with a slight male predominance. In nearly a third of the patients, at least one additional cardiac procedure generally is performed at the time of operation. Most commonly, the concurrent procedure is closure of a patent foramen ovale or an atrial septal defect (26 percent) or coronary artery bypass grafting (8 percent).

An immediate reduction of pulmonary pressures and vascular resistance down to normal levels generally is achieved. These hemodynamic accomplishments are usually permanent. The right heart failure resolves rapidly, as does the tricuspid regurgitation. These changes are usually evident immediately postoperatively or as late as a few days postoperatively on follow-up transthoracic echocardiograms. Patients experience a dramatic improvement in their symptoms and have a very low risk of recurrence so long as they are anticoagulated and have received a preoperative inferior caval filter.

An analysis of the authors' data encompassing a time span of 30 years indicates an operative mortality of about 9 percent. However, most recently the authors published[22] an overall mortality of 4.4 percent in their last 500 patients. This reflects the learning curve for performing this operation safely and the refinements in surgical technique that have occurred.

With growing experience, the authors now are able to offer this procedure to some very high-risk patients, with an overall mortality rate of about 4.5 percent. The majority of patients experience dramatic hemodynamic improvement postoperatively. A reduction in pulmonary pressures and resistance to normal levels and a corresponding improvement in pulmonary blood flow and cardiac output are generally immediate and sustained. Echocardiographic studies have demonstrated that with the elimination of chronic pressure overload, right ventricular geometry rapidly reverts toward normal. Right atrial and right ventricular enlargement regresses. Tricuspid valve function returns to normal within a few days as a result of restoration of tricuspid annular geometry after the remodeling of the right ventricle, and tricuspid repair therefore is not part of the operation. In general, these changes can be assumed to be permanent. Whereas before the operation more than 95 percent of the patients are in NYHA functional class III or IV, at 1 year after the operation 95 percent of patients remain in New York Heart Association (NYHA) functional class I or II.[20,22–25]

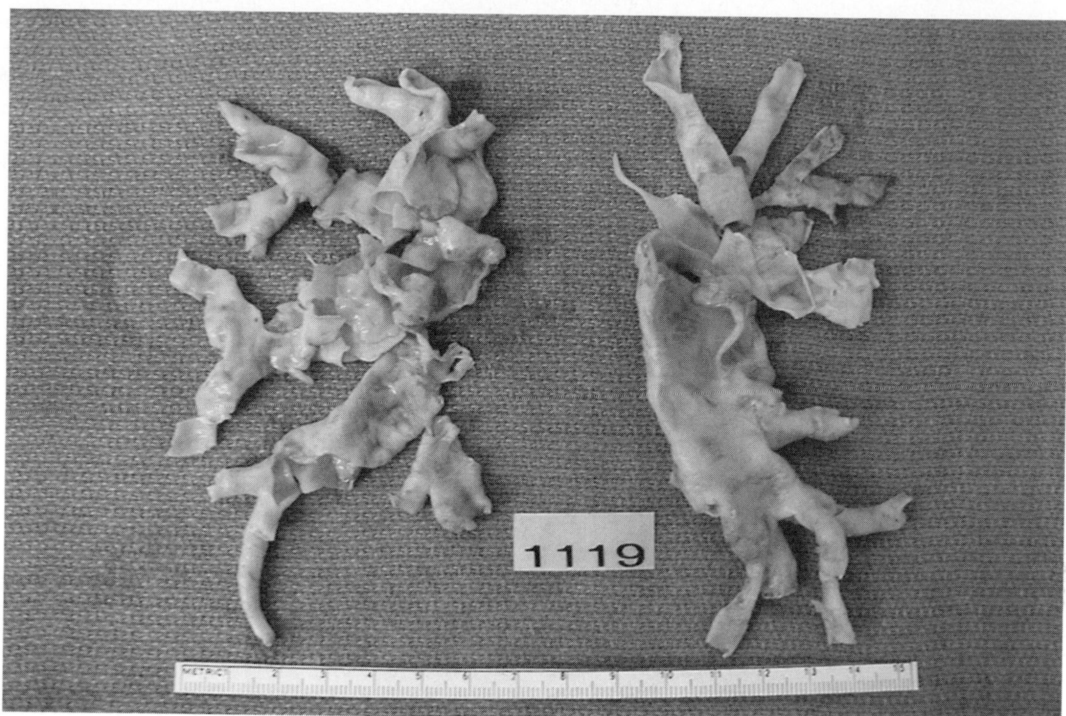

Figure 40-9 Surgical specimen removed from a patient with type IV disease. Note that despite the impressive appearance of the endarterectomy specimen, there are no distal tails. This patient had primary pulmonary hypertension and had no change in pulmonary hemodynamics.

SUMMARY

It is increasingly apparent that pulmonary hypertension caused by chronic pulmonary embolism is a relatively common condition that is underrecognized and carries a poor prognosis. Medical therapy is ineffective in prolonging life and improves the symptoms only transiently. The only therapeutic alternative to pulmonary thromboendarterectomy is lung transplantation. The advantages of thromboendarterectomy include lower operative morbidity and mortality and excellent long-term results without the risks associated with chronic immunosuppression and chronic allograft rejection. The mortality for thromboendarterectomy at the authors' institution is now in the range of 4.5 percent, with sustained benefit. These results are clearly superior to those for transplantation in both the short term and the long term.

Although pulmonary thromboendarterectomy is technically demanding for the surgeon, requiring careful dissection of the pulmonary artery planes and the use of circulatory arrest, excellent short- and long-term results can be achieved. Pulmonary endarterectomy now can be offered to patients with an acceptable mortality rate and anticipation of excellent clinical improvement. With this growing experience, it has become clear that a unilateral operation is obsolete and that circulatory arrest is essential.

Despite an increase in awareness over the last few years and continuous efforts in education through publications and presentations, the principal difficulty is that this still is an underrecognized condition. Increased understanding of both the prevalence of this condition and the possibility of a surgical cure should give more patients an opportunity for relief from this debilitating and ultimately fatal disease.

References

1. Landefeld CS, Chren MM, Myers A, et al. Diagnostic yield of the autopsy in a university hospital and a community hospital. *N Engl J Med* 1988;318:1249
2. Dalen JE, Alpert JS. Natural history of pulmonary embolism. *Prog Cardiovasc Dis* 1975:17:259–270
3. Goldhaber SZ, Hennekens CH, Evens DA, et al. Factors associated with correct antemortem diagnosis of major pulmonary embolism. *Am J Med* 1982;73: 822–826.
4. Rubinstein L, Murray D, Hoffstein V. Fatal pulmonary emboli in hospitalized patients: An autopsy study. *Arch Intern Med* 1988;148:1425–1426.
5. Kniffin WD Jr, Baron JA, Barrett J, et al. The epidemiology of diagnosed pulmonary embolism and deep venous thrombosis in the elderly. *Arch Intern Med* 1994;154:861.
6. Martin M. PHLECO: A multicenter study of the fate of 1647 hospital patients treated conservatively without fibrinolysis and surgery. *Clin Investig* 1993:71:471.

7. Carson JL, Kelley MA, Duff A, et al. The clinical course of pulmonary embolism. *N Engl J Med* 1992;326:1240.
8. Weiss HJ, Turitto VT, Baumgartner HR, et al. Evidence for the presence of tissue factor activity on subendothelium. *Blood* 1989;73;968.
9. Bertina RM, Koeleman BPC, Koster T, et al. Mutation in blood coagulation factor V associated with resistance to activated protein C. *Nature* 1994;369:64.
10. Svensson PJ, Dahlback B. Resistance to activated protein C as a basis for venous thrombosis. *N Engl J Med* 1994;330:517.
11. Ridker PM, Hennekens CH, Lindpaintner K, et al. Mutation in the gene coding for coagulation factor V and the risk of myocardial infarction, stroke, and venous thrombosis in apparently healthy men. *N Engl J Med* 1995;332:912.
12. Feinstein DI. Immune coagulation disorders. In: Colman RW, Hirsh J, Marder VJ, Salzman EW (eds). *Hemostasis and Thrombosis: Basic Principal and Clinical Practice,* 3d ed. Philadelphia: Lippincott; 1994:881.
13. Dibble JH. Organization and canalization in arterial thrombosis. *J Pathol Bacteriol* 1958;75:1–4.
14. Cournad A, Rilev RL, Himmelstein A, Austrian R. Pulmonary circulation in the alveolar ventilation perfusion relationship after pneumonectomy. *J Thorac Surg* 1950;19:80–116.
15. Moser KM, Houk VN, et al. Chronic, massive thrombotic obstruction of the pulmonary arteries: Analysis of four operated cases. *Circulation* 1965; 32:377–385.
16. Benotti JR, Ockene IS, Alpert JS, Dalen JE. The clinical profile of unresolved pulmonary embolism. *Chest* 1983;84:669–678.
17. Moser KM, Auger WF, Fedullo PF. Chronic major-vessel thromboembolic pulmonary hypertension. *Circulation* 1990;81:1735–1743.
18. Moser KM, Daily PO, Peterson K, et al. Thromboendarterectomy for chronic, major vessel thromboembolic pulmonary hypertension: Immediate and longterm results in 42 patients. *Ann Intern Med* 1987;107:560.
19. Moser KM. Pulmonary vascular obstruction due to embolism and thrombosis. In: Moser KM (ed). *Pulmonary Vascular Disease.* New York: Marcel Dekker; 1979:341.
20. Jamieson SW, Kapalanski DP: Pulmonary endarterectomy. *Curr Probl Surg* 2000;37(3):165–252.
21. Allison PR, Dunnill MS, Marshall R. Pulmonary embolism. *Thorax* 1960;15:273–283.
22. Jamieson SW, Sakakibara N, Manecke G, et al. Pulmonary endarterectomy—experience and lessons learned in 1500 cases. *Ann Thorac Surg* 2003;76:1457–1464.
23. Thistlethwaite PA, Mo M, Madani MM, et al. Operative classification of thromboembolic disease determines outcome after pulmonary thromboendarterectomy. *J Thorac Cardiovasc Surg* 2002;124:1203–1211.
24. Mayer E, Dahm M, Hake U, et al. Mid-term results of pulmonary thromboendarterectomy for chronic pulmonary hypertension. *Ann Thorac Surg* 1996;61: 1788–1792.
25. Kramm T, Mayer E, Dahm M, et al. Long-term results after thromboendarterectomy for chronic pulmonary embolism. *Eur J Cardiothorac Surg* 1999;15: 579–584.

CHAPTER

41 SURGICAL MANAGEMENT OF HYPERTROPHIC OBSTRUCTIVE CARDIOMYOPATHY

Pramod Bonde, Akhil Seth, David D. Yuh

INTRODUCTION

Hypertrophic cardiomyopathy is an autosomal dominant cardiac disorder in which there is muscular hypertrophy of the left ventricle. Massive, usually asymmetric, left ventricular hypertrophy (LVH) occurs most often at the level of the basal septum. This results in encroachment on the ventricular chamber, reducing chamber area and volume and leading to increased systolic function and impaired diastolic function. In obstructive forms of the disease, there is an associated obstruction to left ventricular outflow (HOCM). The majority of these patients are asymptomatic throughout life, although some present with severe activity-limiting symptoms. Surgical treatment remains the gold standard for alleviating symptoms. Although other interventional strategies have been proposed, including alcohol septal ablation and dual-chamber pacing, these treatments have not proved to have the same benefit as surgery.[1]

HISTORICAL PERSPECTIVE

The underlying pathology of HOCM first was described by two pathologists, Hallopeau[2] and Liouiville,[3] in the late nineteenth century and later was described by Schmincke[4] in the early twentieth century. Further reports by Davies[5] in 1952 and Brock[6] in 1957 described

KEY CONCEPTS

- Epidemiology
  - The prevalence of hypertrophic cardiomyopathy (HCM) is about 0.2 percent in the general adult population, with autosomal dominant inheritance. Mortality among patients with HCM is less than 1 percent per year, although the stratified risk for sudden death may be higher within some HCM subgroups.
- Pathophysiology
  - HCM is characterized by massive asymmetric idiopathic left ventricular muscular hypertrophy, most often at the level of the basal interventricular septum. The hypertrophy encroaches on the left ventricular chamber, reducing chamber area and volume, and leads to increased systolic function and impaired diastolic function. Hypertrophic obstructive cardiomyopathy (HOCM) represents obstructive forms of this disease. HOCM often is associated with systolic anterior motion (SAM) of the mitral valve, resulting in dynamic obstruction of the left ventricular outflow tract (LVOT).
- Clinical features
  - The most common presenting symptoms include dyspnea, syncope, and angina, resulting from a complex interaction of diastolic dysfunction, arrhythmias, myocardial ischemia, and outflow gradients.
- Diagnostics
  - Suspicion of HCM often is prompted by a systolic ejection murmur that is worsened by preload reduction maneuvers and left ventricular hypertrophic

criteria on 12-lead electrocardiography. Echocardiography confirms the diagnosis, demonstrating asymmetric hypertrophy of the heart, among other characteristics of HCM.

- Treatment
  - Treatment is based on symptomatology. Medical management is based on reducing cardiac contractility to relieve LVOT obstruction partially and reducing the heart rate to enhance diastolic filling (beta blockers and calcium channel blockers). Surgical treatment is considered when medical therapies fail or when obstruction occurs at rest or with provocation. Operations focus on relieving LVOT obstruction with a septal myectomy, sometimes in conjunction with mitral valve replacement.
- Outcomes
  - Surgical complications include heart block requiring pacemaker placement, the need for a reoperation, ventricular septal defect, aortic insufficiency, and mitral regurgitation. Overall, large reductions in LVOT gradients and symptomatic improvement are observed in most clinical series. Early mortality ranges from 0 to 6 percent, with late mortality less than 10 percent. Ten-, 15-, and 20-year survival rates of 80 percent, 72 percent, and 53 percent, respectively, have been observed.

diffuse forms of muscular subaortic stenosis. In 1958, Teare[7] reported a group of young people who had died suddenly and whose postmortem examinations demonstrated myocardial fiber disarray and disproportionate thickening of the ventricular septum. Considerable confusion about this single disease entity stemmed from the fact that each author or group described the disorder by using different nomenclature. The clinical features associated with the previously seen pathology were categorized by Braunwald and coworkers,[8] who called the disease idiopathic hypertrophic subaortic stenosis (IHSS). Goodwin and Fix and associates[9,10] coined the term hypertrophic obstructive cardiomyopathy because they felt that left ventricular outflow obstruction is the distinctive feature of the disease. The involvement of the anterior mitral leaflet first was documented in 1964,[10] when that leaflet was shown to display abnormal SAM. The fact that both obstructive and nonobstructive forms exist became evident after the introduction of echocardiography.[11] This allowed the detection of asymmetric septal hypertrophy (ASH) and SAM.[12]

The first myotomy was reported by Fix and coworkers.[10] A simple myotomy via an aortic approach was a popular alternative introduced by the Toronto group[13] and has been modified since that time by Morrow and coworkers to include the myectomy.[14] The addition of mitral valve replacement was proposed by Cooley and colleagues.[15] The use of a left ventricular–aortic valve conduit to bypass the obstruction is essentially of historical significance only.[16]

EPIDEMIOLOGY

A comprehensive review by Maron and associates reported that the prevalence of HCM was 0.2 percent (1 in 500) in the general adult population.[17–19,21] Therefore, approximately 500,000 persons in the United States may have HCM, with similar trends being reported in other parts of the world.[20,21] General cardiology practices encounter only about 1 percent of these patients.[22] Mortality among patients with HCM is less than 1 percent per year.[23] However, the stratified risk for sudden death within the HCM disease spectrum may be higher.[21]

ETIOLOGY

The inheritance of the familial form of HCM occurs through a Mendelian autosomal dominant trait. Most of the mutations occur in the genes that encode the myocardial sarcomere.[24,25] The most commonly reported mutations occur in the beta-myosin heavy chain, the myosin-binding protein C, and cardiac troponin-T.[26]

PATHOPHYSIOLOGY

Morphologically, the idiopathic muscular hypertrophy of the interventricular septum in HOCM primarily affects the left ventricle and varies in terms of site and severity. In the classic form of HOCM, which often is associated with SAM, hypertrophy occurs maximally in the basal ventricular septum just below the free edge of the anterior mitral leaflet in its open position.[27] Occasionally, hypertrophy may be maximal adjacent to the papillary muscles, a so-called midcavity obstruction.[28] It also may occur within the cardiac apex, as is seen most commonly in the Japanese.[29] Neither of these variants involves SAM. Both free-wall hypertrophy and ASH occur in obstructive forms of the disease.[30] The left ventricular cavity has a sigmoid shape on echocardiography.[31] Other structural abnormalities include a dilated, thickened left atrial wall; elongated, thickened mitral valve leaflets positioned close to the ventricular septum; a distorted right ventricular chamber caused by the hypertrophied interventricular septum; and abnormal wall thickening and luminal narrowing of coronary arterioles within the ventricular septum.[32–36]

Histologically, HOCM can be seen in the ventricular septum as a disorganized myocardial architecture composed of hypertrophied (wider and shorter) cardiac muscle cells with bizarre shapes and multiple intercellular connections.[37] An increase in the number of cell layers and the amount of fibrous tissue also contributes to increased wall thickness.[37] Other histologic features include intramural coronary arteries with luminal narrowing, thickened walls, and increased intimal and medial collagen deposition. This represents a form of small vessel coronary disease that is responsible for the ischemia and myocardial scarring seen in HOCM patients.[37]

Improvements in echocardiography and other forms of real-time cardiac imaging have improved the mechanistic understanding of SAM.[38] The role of the anterior mitral leaflet in dynamic obstruction of the LVOT[39] and SAM was demonstrated by ventriculography and echocardiography. This subsequently was confirmed on autopsy examination.[40] The obstruction is due to a combination of factors, including a hypertrophied interventricular septum, an elongated mitral valve, and papillary muscles that are displaced inward and anterior toward the center of the ventricle (Figs. 41-1 and 41-2). Mitral valve SAM with mitral-septal contact is due primarily to the subaortic septal bulge that narrows the LVOT and causes a Venturi effect. Another proposed mechanism is drag on the anterior mitral leaflet that aggravates this septal-to-mitral contact.[38,41,42]

NATURAL HISTORY

Left ventricular hypertrophy associated with HOCM may not always be present at birth. It may change markedly in early life, but progression of hypertrophy is rare once adulthood is reached.[43,44] These patients commonly present in the second or third decade of life, although clinical courses vary. Older patients tend to be more symptomatic.[45] Infants and young children, however, show severe LVH with congestive heart failure and a higher incidence of sudden death.[46] Sudden death may be much more common in patients with a family history.[47] The mortality of the disease without surgery has been demonstrated to be 15 percent at 5 years and 25 percent at 10 years in symptomatic patients.[48] The most common cause of death is ventricular arrhythmia or cerebral embolism caused by atrial fibrillation.[49]

CLINICAL FEATURES

The clinical manifestations of HOCM correlate well with the underlying pathophysiology regardless of the patient's age at presentation. The most common presenting symptoms include dyspnea, syncope, and angina. These symptoms result from a complex interaction of diastolic dysfunction, arrhythmias, myocardial ischemia, and outflow gradients.[50] Generally, the hypertrophy of

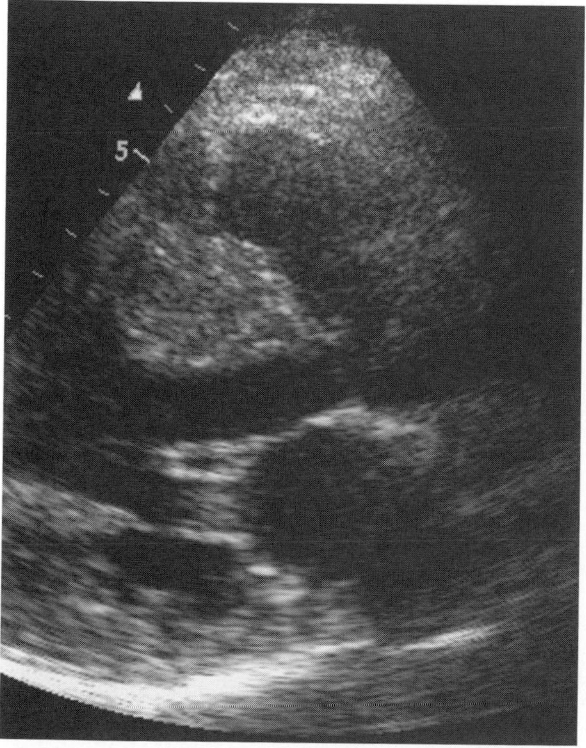

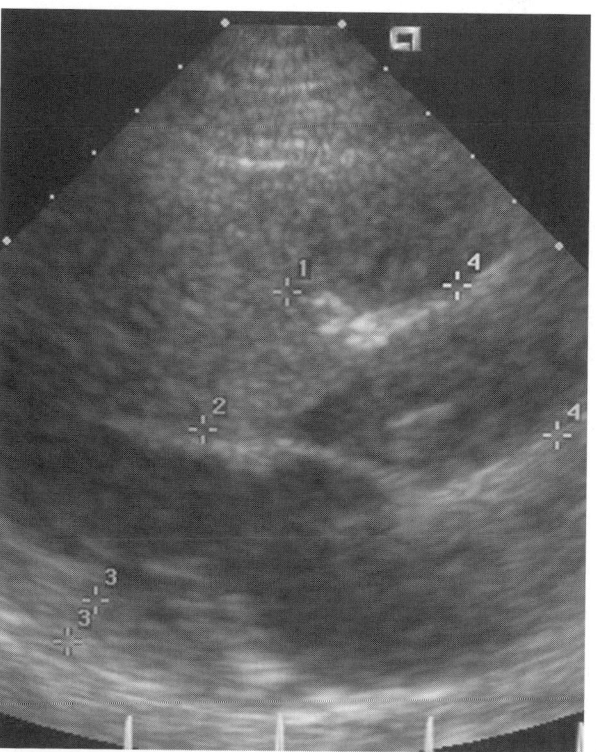

Figure 41-1. Echocardiographic images showing septal hypertrophy (A) and systolic anterior motion (B). (Courtesy of Dr. Raveen Bazaz, MD, and Dr. Angel Lopez-Candales, MD, Echocardiography Laboratory, University of Pittsburgh.)

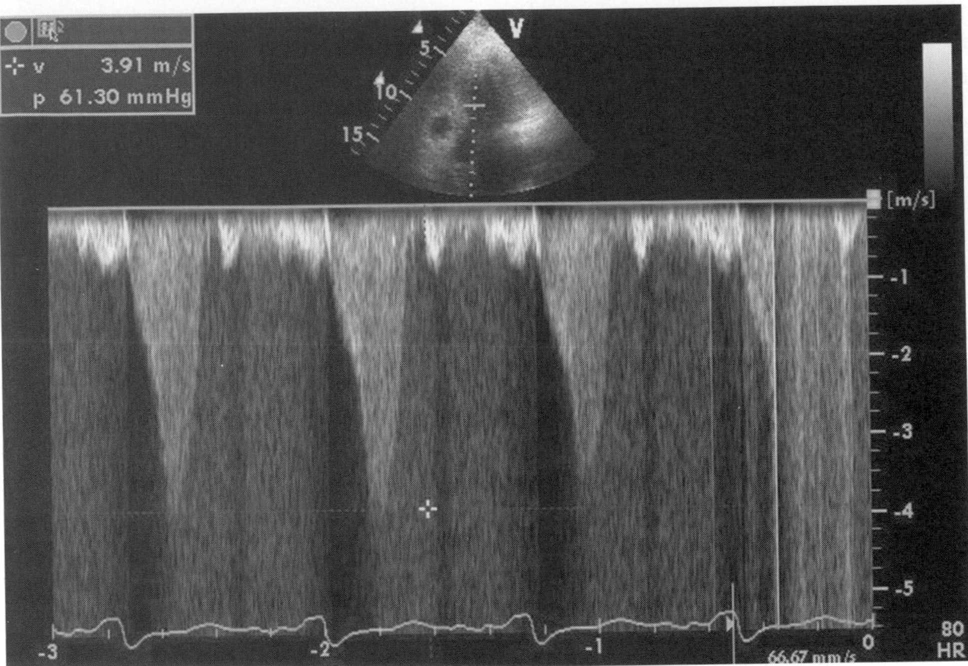

Figure 41-2 Characteristics of late peaking on M-mode echocardiography. (Courtesy of Dr. Raveen Bazaz, MD and Dr. Angel Lopez-Candales, MD, Echocardiography Laboratory, University of Pittsburgh.)

the left ventricle leads to abnormal increases in left ventricular filling pressures that lead to increased back pressure in the lungs, causing subsequent dyspnea on exertion. The narrowing of the LVOT impedes blood flow to the aorta and the periphery, aggravating the symptoms. At the same time, LVH continues to progress as the heart attempts to maintain cardiac output.

The anteriorly placed mitral valve that leads to SAM also impairs left ventricular filling as a result of an elevated transvalvular pressure gradient. The resultant pulmonary vascular congestion manifests as dyspnea.[51] Palpitations usually result from atrial fibrillation and can be permanent in approximately 10 percent of patients.[52]

DIAGNOSIS

A diagnosis of hypertrophic cardiomyopathy first may be suspected on a routine physical examination when a heart murmur or an abnormal electrocardiogram (ECG) is detected. A systolic ejection murmur results from subaortic obstruction, and the hypertrophied ventricle becomes evident on a 12-lead ECG. However, these signs may be absent in patients who do not have significant obstruction.[41] The murmur becomes louder during maneuvers that decrease preload, such as having the patient change position from squatting to standing.[53] The ECG, which is abnormal in 75 to 95 percent of HCM patients, generally shows a left ventricular strain pattern, although Q waves still may be present. Giant negative T waves sometimes are seen in leads V_4 to V_6.[54]

An echocardiogram confirms the diagnosis. This diagnostic modality computes muscle thickness, determines the presence and degree of obstruction, evaluates valve motion, delineates the direction of blood flow, and demonstrates the asymmetric hypertrophy of the heart.[41] Continuous-wave Doppler flow echocardiography is used to diagnose the resting obstruction, which is seen as a high-velocity, late-peaking jet across the LVOT (Fig. 41-2).

Cardiac catheterization and ventriculography are indicated for patients in whom surgery is an option.[55] LVOT obstruction increases with any maneuver that increases left ventricular contractility or decreases left ventricular preload or afterload. Increasing the obstruction through the administration of isoproterenol, exercise, or the Valsalva maneuver decreases pulse pressure and increases the total left ventricular ejection time. However, although obstruction can be exacerbated during exercise, the problem becomes most apparent immediately after exercise is completed as opposed to during exercise.[56] Catheterization reveals that a prominent septal bulge forms the anterior boundary of the LVOT and the anterior mitral leaflet forms its posterior boundary. Catheterization demonstrates SAM in patients with obstruction.[57]

INDICATIONS FOR TREATMENT

Treatment of hypertrophic obstructive cardiomyopathy is based on the symptomatology. Patients with a genetic predisposition who do not have symptoms should be followed regularly.[1,43] Symptoms in nonobstructive patients are caused by left ventricular (LV) diastolic dysfunction and myocardial ischemia caused by narrowing of intramural coronary arteries. Pharmacologic therapy helps control symptoms and is individualized on the basis of their severity. Most patients with an obstruction are controlled with medical therapy, although a minority require intervention for refractory obstruction.[41,43]

Patients who present with risk factors for sudden arrhythmic death, such as those with a family history of premature HCM-related death, prior cardiac arrest, or spontaneous sustained ventricular tachycardia, require the prophylactic placement of an implantable cardioverter-defibrillator. Patients with atrial fibrillation require pharmacologic rate control and anticoagulation.[41]

Patients should be considered for surgery when medical management fails or when obstruction occurs at rest or with provocation.[49] These patients generally have large outflow gradients (equal to or greater than 50 mmHg) and severe symptoms of heart failure.[58,59] Relative contraindications to surgical intervention include concomitant medical conditions, advanced age, and prior cardiac surgery.[43] Therapeutic options for patients with nonobstructive HCM who do not respond to medical management are limited. Those with end-stage heart failure may be candidates for heart transplantation.[60]

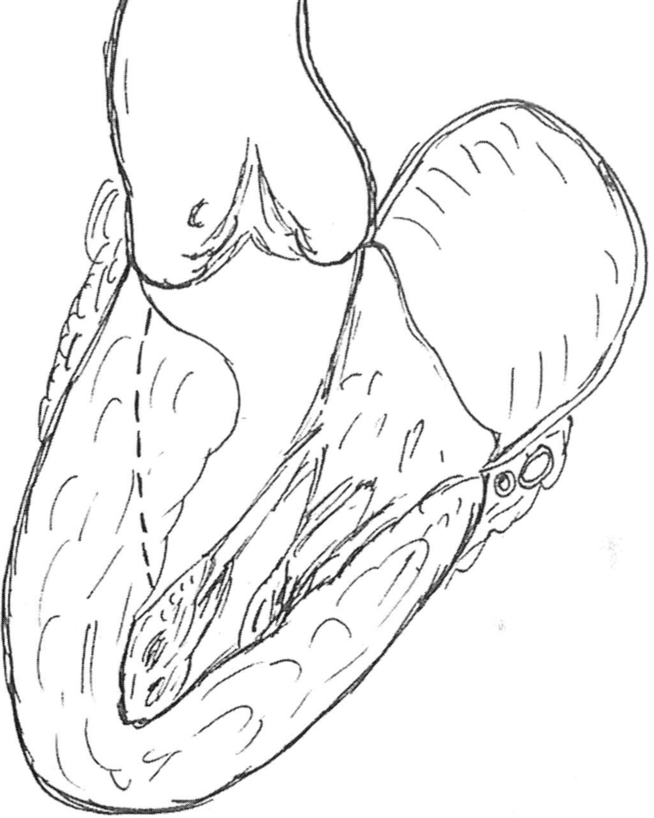

Figure 41-3 The extent of surgical resection of the hypertrophied septum in a patient with hypertrophic obstructive cardiomyopathy.

SURGICAL MANAGEMENT

Morrow initially described the surgical approach to relieving LVOT obstruction, and its modification remains the mainstay of surgical treatment today (Fig. 41-3).[32] Other surgical approaches include transaortic myectomy, extended myectomy, repair of the mitral apparatus, and plication of the anterior mitral leaflet.

Morrow myectomy via aortic approach

Under cardiopulmonary bypass and cardioplegic arrest, an oblique hockey stick incision is made on the anterior ascending aortic wall, extending inferiorly to the noncoronary sinus. Starting beneath the right coronary cusp and up to the junction of the left and right coronary cusps, a deep U-shaped incision is made in the septum (Fig. 41-4). Care is taken not to extend too far to the right side to avoid left bundle branch block. The excision continues toward the ventricular apex as far as possible. Visibility of the septum is improved by depressing the anterior wall of the right ventricle with a swab on a stick. An extension toward the left side can be done if there is significant hypertrophy of the anterior wall of the left

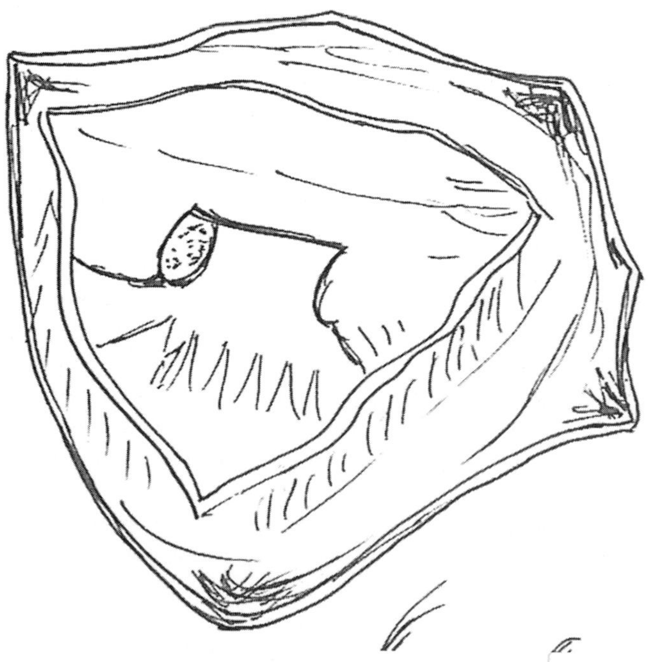

Figure 41-4 Transaortic view of the resected septum in a patient with hypertrophic obstructive cardiomyopathy.

ventricle. In such instances, the incision extends downward toward the base of the anterior papillary muscle and then joins the trough that was created previously.

Morrow myectomy via combined aortic and ventricular approach

The initial steps in this procedure are similar to the ones described above. Once the septal resection is completed via the aortic incision, a left ventriculotomy is performed through a 4-cm oblique incision in the lower anterior wall. This incision should be inferior and parallel to the diagonal vessels as it enters the lumen of the left ventricle below the origin of anterior papillary muscle. The excision then is continued from below into the outflow tract to meet the incision from above. Upon completion of the excision, a thorough inspection is performed to ensure adequate excision of the obstructing muscle.

Extended septal myectomy via aortic approach

This approach concentrates on the resection of the midseptal bulge to abolish SAM. In an extended myectomy, the septal bulge is resected to the base of the papillary muscles.[61] This leaves a more even distribution of the septal thickness and spares 3 to 5 mm below the aortic valve.[62,63] Resection of the midseptal bulge allows flow to track anteriorly and medially away from the mitral valve, minimizing the drag on the mitral leaflets.

The septal bulge is defined by using a trefoil hook retractor, as described by Messmer[62] and by Schoendube and colleagues.[63] The trefoil hook is embedded into the farthest portion of the septal bulge with an orientation between the right coronary ostium and the right and left coronary commissures. It stabilizes the muscle mass during resection. Two parallel incisions, one below the right coronary ostium and the second below the left coronary commissure, are created and are connected 3 mm below the aortic annulus. The trough is extended into the ventricular cavity to the base of the anterior papillary muscle. Digital palpation of the septum often helps the surgeon judge the extent of resection. The papillary muscles are partially excised and mobilized from any abnormal connections to the anterior wall of the left ventricle, allowing the mitral valve to assume a more posterior position.[41] Similar mobilization is performed on the posterior papillary muscle.

Plication of the anterior mitral leaflet

The mitral valve often is enlarged in both area and length with regard to a small left ventricular cavity in patients with HOCM. On the basis of these findings, certain authors advocate plication of the anterior mitral leaflet to reduce the size of the leaflet and chordal length, thus reducing SAM.[64,65] Once the degree of redundancy is assessed, three to four mattress sutures are placed horizontally to plicate the anterior mitral leaflet.

Mitral valve replacement

Mitral valve repair or replacement is indicated clearly when valve abnormalities such as prolapse and calcification are likely to lead to regurgitation. Cooley and coinvestigators[66] and others[67–69] have proposed mitral valve replacement as a therapeutic option for abolishing SAM. However, significant prosthesis-related morbidity has been reported by those investigators that raises concerns about this therapeutic option. In the absence of structural mitral regurgitation, septal myectomy is usually sufficient to abolish SAM.[70]

SURGICAL COMPLICATIONS

Postoperative complications after surgical myectomy for relief of HOCM are shown in Table 41-1. Implantation of a pacemaker was needed in up to 10 percent of patients, and up to 7.2 percent of patients required a reoperation after the myectomy procedure. Relatively few patients experienced the less common complications of postoperative ventricular septal defect, aortic insufficiency, and mitral regurgitation (a maximum of 2.9 percent, 2.6 percent, and 3.4 percent, respectively).

Table 41-1 Postoperative complications after surgical myectomy for hypertrophic obstructive cardiomyopathy

Study	Patient, *n*	Follow-up, years	PM,%	VSD,%	AI,%	MR,%	Reop,%
Van der Lee et al[76]	29	3.4±2.1	0	0	0	3.4	3.4
Schonbeck et al[77]	110	11.7±7.5	4.5	1.8	1.0	1.8	7.2
Minakata et al[78]	56	2.8±2.6	5.4	0	0	0	1.8
Merrill et al[79]	22	6.6	0	0	0	0	4.5
Heric et al[80]	178	3.7±0.33	10.0	1.0	1.0	1.1	2.8
McCully et al[81]	65	2.4±1.7	1.5	0	1.5	1.5	6.2
Minami et al[82]	75	6.7±4.1	8	1.3	0	1.3	1.3
Ten Berg et al[83]	38	6.8	2.6	2.6	2.6	0	0
Gol et Al[84]	69	3.7±2.4	0	2.9	0	0	0

PM = pacemaker implantation; VSD = ventricular septal defect; AI = aortic insufficiency; MR = mitral regurgitation; Reop = reoperation.

Table 41-2 Postoperative outcomes after surgical correction of hypertrophic obstructive cardiomyopathy

Study	Patient, *n*	Follow-up, years	ΔLVOTG, mm Hg	NYHA class I/II %	Early mortality %	Late mortality, %
Van der Lee et al[76]	29	3.4±2.1	100→17	100	0	0
Schoubeek et al[77]	110	11.7±7.5	81→13	91	3.6	27.2
Minakata et al[78]	56	2.8±2.6	97→11	98	0	5.4
Merriff et al[79]	22	6.6	80→12	NA	0	9.1
Heric et al[80]	178	3.7±0.33	93→21	93	6.0	10.7
McCully et al[81]	65	2.4±1.7	73→87	89	4.6	2.0
Minami et al[82]	75	6.7±4.1	125→22	NA	1.3	6.7
Ten Berg et al[83]	38	6.8	72→6	95	0	2.6
Gol et al[84]	69	3.7±2.4	78→18	97	4.3	0

ΔLVOTG = change in left ventricular outflow tract gradient (reduction); NYHA = New York Heart Association status; NA = not available.

OUTCOMES AND PROGNOSIS

Overall, large reductions in LVOT gradients were seen across all the studies surveyed (Table 41-2)[76–84], with a maximum reduction of 103 mmHg. The majority of studies demonstrated that the percentage of patients in New York Heart Association (NYHA) class I or II was 89 percent and above postoperatively. Early mortality ranged from 0 to 6 percent, and late mortality was generally less than 10 percent. Survival data from numerous longitudinal studies demonstrate the long-term efficacy of surgical relief of the obstruction (Table 41-3). The average yearly mortality rate was 1.3 percent, with 5-year expected survival being 84 percent or above in all the studies surveyed. Schonbeck and colleagues[-77] demonstrated 10-, 15-, and 20-year survival rates of 80 percent, 72 percent, and 53 percent, respectively.

MEDICAL MANAGEMENT

The majority of the medications used for symptomatic control in patients with HCM decrease cardiac contractility, partially relieving the obstruction, and slow the heart rate to enhance diastolic filling.[1,41,43] Medications commonly employed include beta blockers and calcium channel blockers (e.g., verapamil) and disopyramide.

Beta blockers have been shown to be effective in 60 to 80 percent of these patients, relieving symptoms of angina and dyspnea while improving their NYHA class. Verapamil similarly suppresses myocardial contractility and has a better effect than do beta blockers. For patients who do not respond to other medications, disopyramide can be administered for its negative inotropic effect, which decreases the outflow gradient and further improves symptoms.[1]

THE ROLE OF CARDIAC TRANSPLANTATION

Heart transplantation should be reserved for HCM patients in end-stage heart failure who are refractory to medical management and in whom surgical correction is not an option. It also is indicated for symptomatic HCM patients without obstruction who have developed end-stage heart failure. Coutu and colleagues[71] reviewed 14 patients who underwent heart transplantation for HCM from 1984 to 2001. Short-term survival (30-day) was 100 percent, and 5-, 10-, and 15-year survival was shown to be 100 percent, 85 percent, and 64 percent, respectively. Ninety-two percent of the long-term survivors maintained NYHA functional class I.

Table 41-3 Postoperative expected survival after surgical correction of hypertrophic obstructive cardiomyopathy

Study	Patient, *n*	HOCM yearly mortality,%	Survival, %		
			5 years	10 Years	15 Years
Cohn et al,1992[85]	31	1.0	100	86	N/A
Heric et al, 1995[80]	178	0.6	86	70	N/A
McCully et al, 1996[81]	65	NA	92	N/A	N/A
Mohr et al, 1989[86]	115	1.0	84	73	N/A
Robbins et al, 1996[87]	158	1.7	85	72	46
Schulte et al, 1993[88]	364	0.6	92	88	84
Ten Berg et al, 1994[83]	38	0.0	100	N/A	N/A
Williams et al, 1987[89]	61	1.1	93	93	N/A
Schonbeck et al, 1998[77]	110	1.5	93	80	72

N/A = not available.

INTERVENTIONAL TECHNIQUES

Dual-chamber pacemaker

The role of dual-chamber pacemaker placement for HOCM is controversial, with initial studies reporting subjective improvement. Unfortunately, prospective randomized trials did not demonstrate any advantage.[72,73] The principle behind pacemaker use is based on the theory that the initiation of the electrical impulse in the apex of the right ventricle alters the systolic contraction sequence of the basal septum, theoretically reducing the outflow gradient. However, there is little evidence to support the continued use of this method of treatment.[1]

Alcohol septal ablation

Balloon occlusion of a perforating artery can lead to dysfunction of the myocardium. This observation forms the basis for septal ablation using absolute alcohol. Alcohol is injected in the septal perforator that supplies the hypertrophic septum, and this induces infarction and remodeling.[74] The results are not comparable with those of surgery in abolishing SAM, probably because of the anatomic variations that exist in the septal perforators.[75]

Complications reported after alcohol ablation include coronary dissection, ethanol leakage into the left anterior descending coronary artery, ventricular arrhythmias, complete heart block, pericardial effusion and/or tamponade, other conduction disturbances, and death.[1] Considerable concerns remain over the potential for infarct progression, iatrogenic ventricular septal rupture, and the creation of permanent scarring that can lead to a long-term arrhythmogenic focus. Currently, the follow-up data are limited for interventional strategies, and surgical correction remains the gold standard against which those therapies will be scrutinized.

References

1. Maron BJ, McKenna WJ, Danielson GK, et al. American College of Cardiology/European Society of Cardiology clinical expert consensus document on hypertrophic cardiomyopathy: A report of the American College of Cardiology Foundation Task Force on Clinical Expert Consensus Documents and the European Society of Cardiology Committee for Practice Guidelines. *J Am Coll Cardiol* 2003;42(9):1687–1713
2. Hallopeau L. Retrecissement ventriculo-aortique. *Gaz Med Paris* 1869;24:683.
3. Liouiville H. Retrecissement cardiaque sous mortique. 1869;24:161.
4. Schmincke A. Ueber linksseitige muskulose conusstenosen. *Dtsch Med Wochenschr* 1907;2:2082.
5. Davies LG. A familial heart disease. *Br Heart J* 1952; 14:206.
6. Brock RC. Functional obstruction of the left ventricle. *Guys Hosp Rep* 1957;106:221.
7. Teare RD. Asymmetrical hypertrophy of the heart in young adults. *Br Heart J* 1958;20:1.
8. Braunwald E, Lambrew CT, Rockoff SD, et al. Idiopathic hypertrophic subaortic stenosis: I. A description of the disease based upon analysis of 64 patients. *Circulation* 1964;29/30(Suppl IV):IV-1.
9. Goodwin JF. Cardiac function in primary myocardial disorders. Part 1. *Br Med J* 1964;1:1527.
10. Fix P, Moberg A, Soderberg H, Karnell J. Muscular subvalvular aortic stenosis: Abnormal anterior mitral leaflet possibly the primary factor. *Acta Radiol (Diagn) (Stockh)* 1964;2:177.
11. Abasi AS, MacAlpin RN, Eber LM, Pearce ML. Echocardiographic diagnosis of idiopathic without outflow obstruction. *Circulation* 1972;46:897.
12. Henry WI, Clark CE, Epstein SE. Asymmetric septal hypertrophy: Echocardiographic identification of the pathognomonic anatomic abnormality of IHSS. *Circulation* 1973;47:225.
13. Trimble AS, Bigelow WG, Wigle ED, Chrysohon A. Simple and effective surgical approach to muscular subaortic stenosis. *Circulation* 1964;29(Suppl):125.
14. Morrow AG, Reitz BA, Epstein SE, et al. Operative treatment in hypertrophic subaortic stenosis: Techniques and the results of pre- and post-operative assessments in 83 patients. *Circulation* 1975;52:88–102.
15. Cooley DA, Wukasch DC, Leachman RD. Mitral valve replacement for idiopathic hypertrophic subaortic stenosis: Results for 27 patients. *J Cardiovasc Surg (Torino)* 1976; 17:380.
16. Dembitsky WP, Weldon CS. Clinical experience with the use of a valve-bearing conduit to constrict a second left ventricular outflow tract in cases of unresectable intraventricular obstruction. *Ann Surg* 1976;184:317.
17. Maron BJ, Gardin JM, Glack JM, et al. Assessment of the prevalence of hypertrophic cardiomyopathy in a general population of young adults: Echocardiographic analysis of 4111 subjects in the CARDIA Study. *Circulation* 1995; 92:785–789.
18. Maron BJ, Mathenge R, Casey SA, Poliac LC, Longe TF. Clinical profile of hypertrophic cardiomyopathy identified de novo in rural communities. *J Am Coll Cardiol.* 1999;33: 1590–1595.
19. Maron BJ, Spirito P, Roman MJ, et al. Prevalence of hypertrophic cardiomyopathy in a population-based sample of American Indians aged 51 to 77 years (the Strong Heart Study). *Am J Cardiol* 2004;93;12:1510–1514.
20. Maron BJ, Estes NAM III, Maron MS, et al. Primary prevention of sudden death as a novel treatment strategy in hypertrophic cardiomyopathy. *Circulation* 2003;107:2872–2875.
21. Maron BJ. Hypertrophic cardiomyopathy: A systematic review. *JAMA* 2002;287:1308–1320.
22. Maron BJ, Peterson EE, Maron MS, Peterson JE. Prevalence of hypertrophic cardiomyopathy in outpatient population referred for echocardiographic study. *Am J Cardiol* 1994;73:577–580.

23. Spirito P, Seidman CE, McKenna WJ, Maron BJ. The management of hypertrophic cardiomyopathy. *N Engl J Med* 1997;336:775–785.
24. Marian AJ, Roberts R. Recent advances in the molecular genetics of hypertrophic cardiomyopathy. *Circulation* 1995;92:1336–1347.
25. Maron BJ, Niimura H, Casey SA, et al. Development of left ventricular hypertrophy in adults in hypertrophic cardiomyopathy caused by cardiac myosin-binding protein C gene mutations. *J Am Coll Cardiol* 2001;38:315–321.
26. Seidman JG, Seidman CE. The genetic basis for cardiomyopathy: From mutation identification to mechanistic paradigms. *Cell* 2001;104:557–567.
27. Epstein SE, Henry WL, Clark CE, et al. NIH Conference: Asymmetric septal hypertrophy. *Ann Intern Med* 1974; 81:650.
28. Falicov RE, Resnekov L. Mid-ventricular obstruction in hypertrophic obstructive cardiomyopathy: New diagnostic and therapeutic challenge. *Br Heart J* 1977;39:701.
29. Yamaguchi H, Ishimura T, Nishiyama S, et al. Hypertrophic unobstructive cardiomyopathy with giant negative T waves (apical hypertrophy): Ventriculographic and echocardiographic features in 30 patients. *Am J Cardiol* 1979;44:401.
30. Maron BJ. Asymmetry in hypertrophic cardiomyopathy: The septal to free wall thickness ratio revisited [editorial]. *Am J Cardiol* 1985;55:835.
31. Lever HM, Karam RF, Currie PJ, Healy BP. Hypertrophic cardiomyopathy in the elderly: Distinctions from the young based on cardiac shape. *Circulation* 1989;79:580.
32. Maron BJ, Gottdiener JS, Roberts WC, et al. Left ventricular outflow tract obstruction due to systolic anterior motion of the anterior mitral leaflet in patients with concentric left ventricular hypertrophy. *Circulation* 1978; 57:527.
33. Corday SR, Virmani R, Waller B, Shah PM. Necropsy evaluation of anterior mitral leaflet elongation in cardiomyopathies: Possible role in hypertrophic cardiomyopathy. *Circulation* 1979;60(Suppl):243.
34. Unverferth DV, Baker PB, Pearce LI, et al. Regional myocyte hypertrophy and increased interstitial myocardial fibrosis in hypertrophic cardiomyopathy. *Am J Cardiol* 1987;59:932.
35. Maron BJ, Wolfson JK, Epstein SE, Roberts WC. Intramural ("small vessel") coronary artery disease in hypertrophic cardiomyopathy. *J Am Coll Cardiol* 1986; 8:545.
36. Spray TL, Maron BJ, Morrow AG, et al. Clinical pathologic conference: A discussion on hypertrophic cardiomyopathy. *Am Heart J* 1978;95:511.
37. Maron BJ, Anan TJ, Roberts WC. Quantitative analysis of the distribution of cardiac muscle cell disorganization in the left ventricular wall of patients with hypertrophic cardiomyopathy. *Circulation* 1981;63:882–894.
38. Sherrid MV, Chaudhry FA, Swistel DG. Obstructive hypertrophic cardiomyopathy: Echocardiography, pathophysiology, and the continuing evolution of surgery for obstruction. *Ann Thorac Surg* 2003;75:620–632.
39. Fix P, Moberg A, Soderberg H, Karnell J. Muscular subvalvular aortic stenosis: Abnormal anterior mitral leaflet possibly the primary factor. *Acta Radiol Diagn* 1964; 2:177–193.
40. Shah PM, Graniak R, Kramer DH. Ultrasound localization of left ventricular outflow tract obstruction in hypertrophic cardiomyopathy. *Circulation* 1969;40:3–11.
41. Sherrid MV, Gunsburg DZ, Moldenhauer S, Pearle G. Systolic anterior motion begins at low left ventricular outflow tract velocity in obstructive hypertrophic cardiomyopathy. *J Am Coll Cardiol* 2000;36:1344–1354.
42. Roberts CS, McIntosh CL, Brown PS, et al. Reoperation for persistent outflow obstruction in hypertrophic cardiomyopathy. *Ann Thorac Surg* 1991;51:455–460.
43. Maron BJ, Spirito P, Wesley Y, Arce J. Development and progression of left ventricular hypertrophy in children with hypertrophic cardiomyopathy. *N Engl J Med* 1986; 314:610.
44. Spirito P, Maron BJ. Absence of progression of LVH in adult patients with hypertrophic cardiomyopathy. *J Am Coll Cardiol* 1987;9:1013.
45. Adelman AG, Wigle ED, Ranganathan N, et al. The clinical course in muscular subaortic stenosis: A retrospective and prospective study of 60 hemodynamically proved cases. *Ann Intern Med* 1972;77:515.
46. Deanfield J, McKenna WJ. Recognition and management in children. In: ten Cate JF (ed). *Hypertrophic Cardiomyopathy: Clinical Recognition and Management.* New York: Dekker; 1985:143.
47. Cecchi F, Maron BJ, Epstein SE. Long-term outcome of patients with hypertrophic cardiomyopathy successfully resuscitated after cardiac arrest. *J Am Coll Cardiol* 1989; 13:1283.
48. Swan DA, Bell B, Oakley CM, Goodwin J. Analysis of symptomatic course and prognosis and treatment of hypertrophic obstructive cardiomyopathy. *Br Heart J* 1971;33:671.
49. Shah PM, Adelman AG, Wigle ED, et al. The natural (and unnatural) history of hypertrophic obstructive cardiomyopathy: A multicenter study. *Circ Res* 1974; 34/35(Suppl II):179.
50. Maron BJ. New observations on the interrelation of dynamic sub-aortic obstruction and exercise in hypertrophic cardiomyopathy [editorial comment]. *J Am Coll Cardiol* 1992;19:534.
51. Nishimura RA, Ommen SR, Tajik AJ. Hypertrophic cardiomyopathy: A patient perspective. *Circulation* 2003;108:e133–e155.
52. Glancy DL, O'Brien KP, Gold HK, Epstein SE. Atrial fibrillation in patients with idiopathic hypertrophic subaortic stenosis. *Br Heart J* 1970;32:652.
53. Nishimura RA, Holmes DR Jr. Hypertrophic obstructive cardiomyopathy. *N Engl J Med* 2004;350:1320–1327.
54. Maron BJ, Wolfson JK, Cirjo E, Spirito P. Relation of electrocardiographic abnormalities and patterns of left ventricular hypertrophy identified by 2-dimensional echocardiography in patients with hypertrophic cardiomyopathy. *Am J Cardiol* 1983;51:189.
55. Goodwin JF. The frontiers of cardiomyopathy. *Br Heart J* 1982;48:1.
56. Klues HG, Leuner C, Kuhn H. Left ventricular outflow tract obstruction in patients with hypertrophic cardiomyopathy: Increase in gradient after exercise. *J Am Coll Cardiol* 1992;19:527.
57. Desilets DT, Kadell BM, Buttenberg HD, et al. Angiographic demonstration of the ventricular septum: A new technique. *Radiology* 1968;91:329.

58. Maron BJ. Hypertrophic cardiomyopathy. *Lancet* 1997;350: 127–133.
59. Wigle ED, Rakowski H, Kimball BP, Williams WG. Hypertrophic cardiomyopathy: Clinical spectrum and treatment. *Circulation* 1995;92:1680–1692.
60. Shirani J, Maron BJ, Cannon RO III, et al. Clinicopathologic features of hypertrophic cardiomyopathy managed by cardiac transplantation. *Am J Cardiol* 1993;72: 434–440.
61. Nakatani S, Schwammenthal E, Level HM, et al. New insights into the reduction of mitral valve systolic anterior motion after ventricular septal myectomy in hypertrophic obstructive cardiomyopathy. *Am Heart J* 1996;131: 294–300.
62. Messmer BJ. Extended myectomy for hypertrophic obstructive cardiomyopathy. *Ann Thorac Surg* 1994;58: 575–577.
63. Schoendube FA, Klues HG, Reith S, et al. Long-term clinical and echocardiographic follow-up after surgical correction of hypertrophic obstructive cardiomyopathy with extended myectomy and reconstruction of the subvalvular mitral apparatus. *Circulation* 1995;92:122–127.
64. McIntosh CL, Maron BJ, Cannon RO, Klues H. Initial results of combined anterior mitral valve plication and ventricular septal myotomy-myectomy for relief of left ventricular outflow obstruction in patients with hypertrophic cardiomyopathy. *Circulation* 1992;86:60–67.
65. Cooley DA. Surgical techniques for hypertrophic left ventricular obstructive myopathy including mitral valve plication. *J Cardiac Surg* 1991;6:29–33.
66. Cooley DA, Leachman RD, Wukasch DC. Mitral valve replacement for idiopathic hypertrophic cardiomyopathy. *J Cardiovasc Surg* 1976;17:380–387.
67. Krajcer Z, Leachman RD, Cooley DA, et al. Mitral valve replacement and septal myomectomy in hypertrophic cardiomyopathy: Ten-year follow-up in 80 patients. *Circulation* 1988;78:I35–43.
68. Walker WS, Reid KG, Cameron EW, et al. Comparison of ventricular septal surgery and mitral valve replacement for hypertrophic obstructive cardiomyopathy. *Ann Thorac Surg* 1989;48:528–535.
69. McIntosh CL, Greenberg GJ, Maron BJ, et al. Clinical and hemodynamic results following mitral valve placement in patients with obstructive hypertrophic cardiomyopathy. *Ann Thorac S*urg 1989;47:236–246.
70. McIntosh C, Maron B. Current operative treatment of obstructive hypertrophic cardiomyopathy. *Circulation* 1988;78:487–495.
71. Coutu, MC, Perrault LP, White M, et al. Cardiac transplantation for hypertrophic cardiomyopathy: A valid therapeutic option. *J Heart Lung Transplant* 2004;23:413–417.
72. Fananapazir L, Epstein ND, Curiel RV, et al. Long-term results of dual-chamber (DDD) pacing in obstructive hypertrophic cardiomyopathy: Evidence for progressive symptomatic and hemodynamic improvement and reduction of left ventricular hypertrophy. *Circulation* 1994;90:2731–2742.
73. Maron BJ, Nishimura RA, McKenna WJ, et al. Assessment of permanent dual-chamber pacing as a treatment for drug-refractory symptomatic patients with obstructive hypertrophic cardiomyopathy: A randomized, double-blind, crossover study. (M-PATHY). *Circulation* 1999; 99:2927–2933.
74. Sigwart U. Non-surgical myocardial reduction for hypertrophic obstructive cardiomyopathy. *Lancet* 1995;346: 211–214.
75. Singh M, Edwards WD, Holmes DR Jr, et al. Anatomy of the first septal perforating artery: A study with implications for ablation therapy for hypertrophic cardiomyopathy. *Mayo Clin Proc* 2001;76:799–802.
76. Van der Lee C, Kofflard MJM, van Herwerden LA, et al. Sustained improvement after combined anterior leaflet extension and myectomy in hypertrophic obstructive cardiomyopathy. *Circulation* 2003;108:2088–2092.
77. Schonbeck MH, Brunner-La Rocca, HP, Vogt PR, et al. Long-term follow-up in hypertrophic obstructive cardiomyopathy after septal myectomy. *Ann Thorac Surg* 1998;65:1207–1214.
78. Minakata K, Dearani JA, Nishimura RA, et al. Extended septal myectomy for hypertrophic obstructive cardiomyopathy with anomalous mitral papillary muscles or chordae. *J Thorac Cardiovasc Surg* 2004;127:481–489.
79. Merrill WH, Friesinger GC, Graham TP Jr, et al. Long-lasting improvement after septal myectomy for hypertrophic obstructive cardiomyopathy. *Ann Thorac Surg* 2000;69:1732–1736.
80. Heric B, Lytle BW, Miller DP, et al. Surgical management of hypertrophic obstructive cardiomyopathy: Early and late results. *J Thorac Cardiovasc Surg* 1995;110: 195–208.
81. McCully RB, Nishimura RA, Tajik AJ, et al. Extent of clinical improvement after surgical treatment of hypertrophic obstructive cardiomyopathy. *Circulation* 1996;94: 467–471.
82. Minami K, Boethig D, Woltersdorf H, et al. Long term follow-up of surgical treatment of hypertrophic obstructive cardiomyopathy (HOCM): The role of concomitant cardiac procedures. *Eur J Cardiothorac Surg* 2002;22: 206–210.
83. Ten Berg JM, Suttorp MJ, Knaepen PJ, et al. Hypertrophic obstructive cardiomyopathy: Initial results and long-term follow-up after Morrow septal myectomy. *Circulation* 1994;90:1781–1785.
84. Gol MK, Emir M, Keles T, et al. Septal myectomy in hypertrophic obstructive cardiomyopathy: Late results with stress echocardiography. *Ann Thorac Surg* 1997; 64(3):739–745.
85. Cohn LH, Trehan H, Collins JJ. Long-term follow-up of patients undergoing myotomy/myectomy for obstructive hypertrophic cardiomyopathy. *Am J Cardiol* 1992;70: 657–660.
86. Mohr R, Schaff HV, Danielson GK, et al. The outcome of surgical treatment of hypertrophic obstructive cardiomyopathy. *J Thorac Cardiovasc Surg* 1989;97:666–674.
87. Robbins RC, Stinson EB. Long-term results of left ventricular myotomy and myectomy for obstructive hypertrophic cardiomyopathy. *J Thorac Cardiovasc Surg* 1996; 111:586–594.
88. Schulte HD, Bircks WH, Loesse B, et al. Prognosis of patients with hypertrophic obstructive cardiomyopathy after transaortic myectomy. *J Thorac Cardiovasc Surg* 1993;106:709–717.
89. Williams WG, Wigle ED, Rakowski H, et al. Results of surgery for hypertrophic obstructive cardiomyopathy. *Circulation* 1987;76(Suppl 5):104–108.

CHAPTER

42 PERICARDIAL DISEASE

Eric A. Okum, Abe DeAnda, Jr.

INTRODUCTION

Historical highlights

Galen was the first to describe pericardial disease in animals (circa 160 A.D.) and subsequently described the surgical drainage of purulent pericardial effusions in two patients.[1] This long predated Lower's 1669 description of pericarditis in humans.[2] There are apocryphal references to penetrating heart wounds being treated, usually by the removal of the offending object, without much information about how subsequent drainage of the pericardial space was handled. Francisco Romero, a Catalonian physician, was probably the first heart surgeon, earning that title when he performed open drainage of a pericardial effusion in 1801. He presented his work 15 years later, but it was suppressed for being too aggressive.[3] This predates the "birth of heart surgery" by almost 100 years; Rehn first successfully sutured a heart wound in 1896.[4]

In 1929, Beck showed experimentally that constrictive pericarditis could be produced and treated surgically in laboratory animals[5,6] using Dakin's solution. His observations of the extent of the adhesions formed (and the concomitant neovascular supply) probably contributed to the development of his later procedures for ischemic heart disease.[7] Pericardiectomy then was

KEY CONCEPTS

- Epidemiology
  - Pericarditis and pericardial effusions have many etiologies, including inflammation, infection, immunologic disorders, malignancy, myxedema, uremia, pregnancy, aortic dissection, cardiac rupture, trauma, myocardial infarction, cirrhosis, and heart failure. The three most common etiologies are neoplasia, uremia, and idiopathic causes. Cardiac tamponade usually is caused by bleeding, followed by other sources of chronic effusions.
- Pathophysiology
  - The pathophysiology of pericardial inflammation relates to the underlying causes of pericardial effusions and pericarditis. Effusions generally arise when pericardial fluid production exceeds reabsorption. With pericardial tamponade, there is a rapid increase in intrapericardial pressure and diminished diastolic compliance, ultimately resulting in equalization of right and left atrial, right and left ventricular, pulmonary artery wedge, and intrapericardial pressures. Pericarditis arises from inflammation of the pericardial sac. In constrictive pericarditis, there is a limitation in cardiac filling that is reflected in a "square root" sign seen in ventricular pressure tracings during cardiac catheterization.
- Clinical features
  - The symptoms of pericardial effusions include dyspnea, fever, and chest pain, although many effusions are asymptomatic. The signs include a pericardial friction rub, global electroencephalographic (ECG) changes, and pulsus paradoxus. Cardiac tamponade presents as hypotension and decreased cardiac output; Beck's triad includes muffled heart sounds, elevated venous pressure, and decreased systemic arterial pressure. Significant constrictive pericarditis manifests with symptoms of right-sided heart failure, including jugular venous distention, worsening peripheral edema, and pleural effusions.
- Diagnostics
  - Echocardiography is the gold standard for the diagnosis of pericardial effusions. Cardiac tamponade is a clinical diagnosis but can be confirmed or

substantiated with echocardiography. Computed tomography is useful in identifying the thickened pericardial sac in patients with pericarditis, although magnetic resonance imaging is more sensitive and specific in diagnosing constrictive pericarditis. Right and left cardiac catheterization is the gold standard for diagnosing constrictive pericarditis.

- Treatment
  - Pericardial effusions are treated most readily with drainage, pericardiocentesis, or a pericardial window. Adjunctive medical therapy can be successful, depending on the etiology of the effusion. Depending on the etiology, tamponade can be treated with pericardiocentesis, a pericardial window, or surgical (re)exploration. Medical treatment of constrictive pericarditis is predicated on treating the underlying cause; however, the mainstay of therapy is pericardiectomy.
- Outcomes and prognosis
  - The outcomes and prognoses for pericardial effusions and tamponade depend on the etiology. Early mortality for pericardiectomy ranges from 5 to 10 percent, with 5-year survival ranging from 65 to 90 percent. Predictors of poor outcome are prior radiation, renal insufficiency, poor ventricular function, pulmonary hypertension, New York Heart Association functional class IV, hyponatremia, ascites, and hyperbilirubinemia.

translated into clinical practice. By 1941, Blalock[8] reported a series of 28 patients who had undergone this procedure.

This chapter focuses on many aspects of pericardial disease, including cardiac tamponade, pericardial effusion, and pericarditis, with an emphasis on the surgical aspects of the disease.

Anatomy

The pericardium is a conical sac that encloses the heart and the great vessels. It is situated posterior to the body of the sternum, bounded by the second and sixth costal cartilages anteriorly and thoracic vertebrae 5 through 8 posteriorly. The ascending aorta, pulmonary artery, and superior vena cava exit from the cephalad opening of the pericardium. The base is fused with the central tendon of the diaphragm. Loose connective tissue called the sternopericardial ligaments attaches the anterior surface of the pericardium to the posterior table of the sternum.

The pericardium is composed of an outer membrane and an inner membrane. A thick layer termed the fibrous pericardium is external, and a thin transparent membrane called the serous pericardium is internal. The serous pericardium is divided further into parietal and visceral layers. The parietal layer is fused to the fibrous portion, and the visceral layer is reflected onto the epicardium. The visceral layer of the serous pericardium is in fact the epicardium of the heart and thus is also in continuity with the adventitia of the coronary vessels. The thin layer of fluid between the two layers allows the heart to move in a nearly frictionless environment.

By virtue of the anatomic reflection of the pericardium, two sinuses exist: the transverse and oblique pericardial sinuses (Fig. 42-1). The transverse sinus is behind the ascending aorta and the pulmonary trunk. If the pericardium is opened anteriorly, one can place a finger easily into this space and go from right lateral to left lateral pericardium. The larger sinus is the oblique sinus, which cradles the heart. One can see this space when the heart is lifted toward the right shoulder. This is a cul-de-sac that is bordered to the right by the inferior vena cava (IVC). It therefore prevents passage around the IVC without sharp dissection. The two sinuses are in near continuity, with only a thin layer of serous pericardium separating them.

The arterial supply of the pericardium comes mainly from the internal thoracic arteries. Smaller branches of the bronchial, esophageal, and superior phrenic arteries also contribute to the blood supply. The visceral layer of the serous pericardium is supplied by the coronary arteries. Venous drainage flows into the internal thoracic veins and the azygous system. The nerve supply comes from the vagus, phrenic, and sympathetic trunks.[9]

Embryology

The pericardium is derived, beginning in the third week of gestation, from the progressive invagination of the intraembryonic coelomic cavity. This results in the creation of the visceral and parietal layers of the serous membrane, which later become the serous pericardium. By the fourth week, with growth of the lung buds, pleuropericardial membranes develop on each side. With continued growth and eventual fusion of the pleuropericardial membranes, the thoracic cavity becomes divided into the pericardial cavity and two pleural cavities. This membrane will become the fibrous pericardium. The failure of these membranes to fuse results in congenital defects of the pericardium.[10]

PERICARDIAL EFFUSION

Epidemiology

The finding of a pericardial effusion is common in modern cardiology and cardiothoracic surgical practice. The evolution and prevalence of noninvasive technology (i.e., echocardiography) have made the diagnosis of

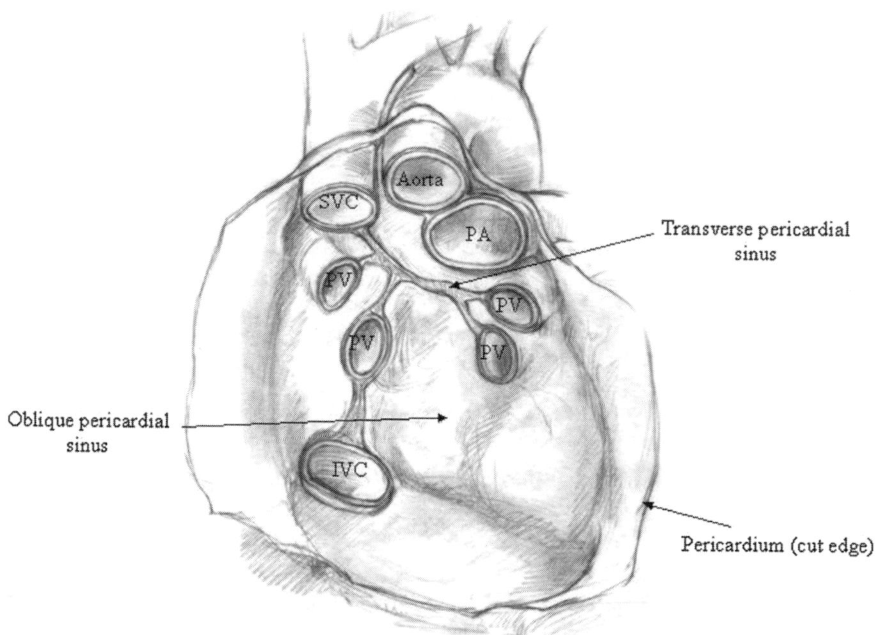

Figure 42-1 Pericardial attachments and reflections. PA = pulmonary artery; PV = pulmonary vein; IVC = inferior vena cava; SVC = superior vena cava. (Reproduced with permission from Mangi AA, Torchiana DF. Pericardial disease. In: Cohn LH, Edmunds LH Jr (eds). *Cardiac Surgery in the Adult.* New York: McGraw-Hill; 2003:1359–1372.)

pericardial effusion easier and apparently more common. Such incidental effusions often are discovered while patients are being evaluated for cardiac valvular disease. However, many systemic processes other than cardiac processes can contribute to the development of pericardial effusions. All types of pericarditis (discussed later in this chapter) can lead to the development of effusions. The etiologies of pericarditis include infection, inflammation, immunologic disorders, malignancy, myxedema, uremia, pregnancy, aortic dissection, cardiac rupture, trauma, chylopericardium, myocardial infarction, cirrhosis, heart failure, and idiopathic causes.[11] Tuberculosis now is an uncommon cause of pericardial effusion but once was one of the more common etiologies of infective pericarditis. The clinical constellation of hemodynamic compromise, cardiomegaly, pleural effusion, and large pericardial effusion was more common in those with tuberculosis than were malignancy and idiopathic causes.[12]

Multiple studies have shown that the three most common etiologies for pericardial effusion are neoplasia, uremia, and idiopathic causes.[13–15] Approximately 40 percent of these patients present with cardiac tamponade.

Pathophysiology

The pathophysiology of pericardial effusion relates to the underlying cause. As was described above, fluid naturally exists between the two layers of the serous pericardium. When that fluid accumulates in the pericardial space, the pericardial effusion can become pathologic. The production of fluid is balanced by the corresponding absorption of fluid by lymphatic channels. The parietal pericardium is drained by the anterior and posterior mediastinal lymph nodes; visceral pericardium is drained via the tracheal and bronchial lymph nodes.[16] Pericardial mesothelial cells contain dense microvilli that facilitate ion and fluid exchange.[17] Effusions arise when production exceeds reabsorption. Thus, effusions can arise from either overproduction or underabsorption.

Clinical features

There is a wide spectrum of clinical presentations for pericardial effusions. Many are asymptomatic and are found incidentally on echocardiography (ECHO), especially in elderly women.[18] On the other end of the spectrum are patients who present in cardiac tamponade.

The symptoms of pericardial effusions may include dyspnea, fever, chest pain, and hemodynamic instability. The signs include a pericardial friction rub, ECG abnormalities, and pulsus paradoxus (described in the section on cardiac tamponade, below).

Posner and associates[19] found that the initial presentation of cardiac tamponade was suggestive of malignancy, especially with very large effusions. Fever, pericardial friction rub, and improvement after the administration of nonsteroidal anti-inflammatory drugs are suggestive of idiopathic pericardial effusion.[19] In 60 percent of these patients, a known previous condition that could cause a pericardial effusion was present. The underlying condition was the cause in more than 90 percent of these patients. The presence of inflammatory signs (chest pain, pericardial friction rub, fever, or ECG changes) was predictive for acute idiopathic pericarditis. Furthermore, a large effusion without tamponade or inflammatory signs was predictive of chronic idiopathic effusion. Tamponade without inflammatory signs was predictive of malignancy.[20]

Diagnostic modalities

Before the advent of ECHO, the diagnosis of a hemodynamically significant pericardial effusion was difficult and had to be confirmed by physical examination. ECHO now is considered the gold standard for the diagnosis of effusions (Fig. 42-2) and can help confirm the diagnosis of a hemodynamically significant effusion (i.e., tamponade). Importantly, a "negative" ECHO does not eliminate the possibility of tamponade. Cardiac catheterization can aid in the diagnosis of tamponade or pericardial constrictive disease but does not affect the diagnosis of effusion.

Attention must be paid to specific ECHO findings. Some patients with evidence of right atrial and ventricular collapse have no clinical evidence of tamponade. Levine and associates[21] performed right-sided heart catheterization and pericardiocentesis on a group of patients with ECHO evidence of tamponade. Many of those patients had no hemodynamic evidence of tamponade. Systolic blood pressure was higher than 100 mmHg in 94 percent of those patients. Pulsus paradoxus was present in only one-third. Right atrial collapse had a positive predictive value of only 50 percent.

Treatment

Medical therapy

The success of medical therapy for pericardial effusions depends on the underlying disease processes that cause the effusion to occur. If systemic signs of inflammation are present, a course of nonsteroidal anti-inflammatory agents or steroids should be started unless hemodynamic compromise is suspected. Any underlying infection should be treated if known.

Medical therapy is most useful with malignant effusions. Chemotherapy or radiotherapy may be useful in preventing recurrence after aspiration of the fluid. Vaitkus and associates[22] reported a success rate of 78 percent in preventing recurrence after systemic chemotherapy was given. Radiation therapy also had good results, especially with radiosensitive tumors such as lymphoma, with success rates greater than 90 percent. Instillation of a sclerosing agent (e.g., tetracycline or bleomycin) through an indwelling catheter also reduced recurrence in some small series.[22]

Surgical therapy

Surgical therapy for pericardial effusion consists of pericardiocentesis with or without catheter placement, a pericardial window, and pericardiectomy. The indications and techniques are described below.

Pericardiocentesis and other modes of surgical drainage are indicated for patients with clinical aspects of cardiac tamponade, suspicion of infection, and a large idiopathic

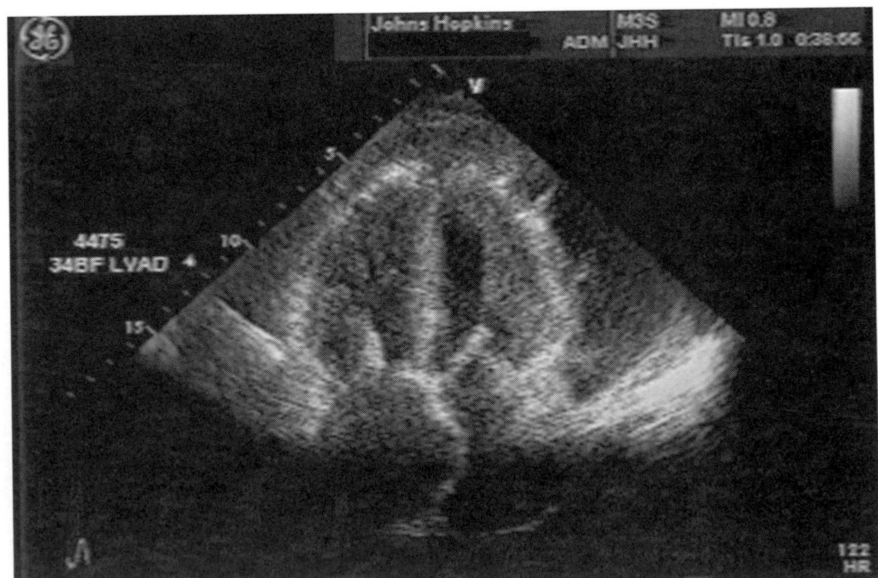

Figure 42-2 Large pericardial effusion detected on echocardiogram. Note the large non-echogenic (*dark*) fluid-filled space around the entire heart.

chronic pleural effusion. Pericardiocentesis or drainage is not warranted in the initial management of asymptomatic patients with a large effusion. However, when large asymptomatic effusions persist for more than 3 months, the risk of tamponade without a specific inciting event approaches 30 percent.[23]

Pericardiocentesis can be performed in the catheterization laboratory (under fluoroscopic guidance) or at the bedside. It should be the initial therapy for those in overt tamponade when such a procedure can be performed easily and safely and for patients who are not in the immediate postoperative period. Once it has been decided to proceed with pericardiocentesis, the decision is made to perform either simple aspiration or percutaneous catheter drainage. The authors favor the latter approach. With this approach, the subxiphoid area is infiltrated with 1% lidocaine for local anesthesia. An 18-gauge spinal needle is inserted to the left of the xiphoid process at a 45-degree angle toward the left shoulder. A "pop" is felt when the needle enters the pericardial sac. This can be aided with fluoroscopic or ECHO guidance. An 8F pigtail catheter then is placed, using the Seldinger technique. The fluid should be aspirated and then sent for culture and cytology. If blood is withdrawn, it is placed in a small basin and observed. Clotted blood suggests that a cardiac chamber was entered. If ECHO is used for guidance, a simple bubble study can be done to verify extracardiac positioning of the catheter needle. A follow-up chest x-ray (CXR) evaluates catheter placement and any evidence of pneumothorax. Techniques have been described in which an alligator clip is attached to the needle and one lead of the ECG. When the myocardium is violated with the needle, a deflection is noted on the ECG.

Pericardial drainage also can be achieved with a pericardial window. Surgical approaches include subxiphoid, left anterior thoracotomy, and thoracoscopy [video-assisted thorascopic surgery (VATS)]. General anesthesia is preferred for all these approaches. Especially when tamponade is the presumptive diagnosis, the patient should be prepped and draped before the induction of anesthesia since hypotension and hemodynamic instability may ensue and rapid thoracotomy may be necessary.

The subxiphoid approach consists of a 6- to 8-cm incision that starts at the junction of the sternum and the xiphoid. The xiphoid process is either resected or split. An Army-Navy retractor is placed under the sternum. Dissection is continued under the sternum until the pericardium is identified and incised. The fluid is drained and sent for culture and cytology. The largest possible piece of pericardium is resected, and any loculations should be broken with finger dissection. A 28F right-angle chest tube is placed into the pericardial space through a separate stab incision. The surgical pericardial incision can be closed, left open, or drained into the peritoneal space.

Pericardial drainage can be approached by a left anterior thoracotomy. A double-lumen tube is not necessary for this approach. A small roll should be placed under the patient's left shoulder so that the patient is at a 30-degree angle from the table. A 6- to 8-cm incision is made in the inframammary crease, with the nipple as its most medial portion. Subcutaneous dissection is continued superiorly for one rib space. The fourth intercostal space is entered; the intercostal muscles are taken off the fifth rib medially and laterally. A sponge stick is used to push the lung away. The pericardium is identified and incised. The fluid is drained and sent for culture and cytology. The pericardium is resected anterior to the phrenic nerve, with the largest section possible being taken. The incision is closed after a 28F chest tube is placed through a separate stab incision. The pericardial space can be drained directly with the chest tube, or the tube can be left in the pleural space under the assumption that any reaccumulation of pericardial fluid will drain into the pleural space.

Thoracoscopy can be used for the pericardial window. However, this approach requires the placement of a dual-lumen endotracheal tube and subsequent single-lung ventilation. Patients with clinical tamponade often will not tolerate this approach. A port for the camera and two working ports are placed. The chest cavity is inspected, including identification of the phrenic nerve. The pericardium then is incised anterior to the nerve, and a large piece of pericardium is resected. Care is taken not to leave a defect so large that cardiac herniation may occur. A single 28F chest tube is left in the pleural space.

Outcomes and prognosis

The outcomes and prognoses for pericardial effusions relate to the underlying disease process. Patients with malignant effusions have a median survival of 2 to 3 months.[24] A study by McDonald and associates[25] compared the subxiphoid pericardial window to percutaneous catheter placement. No direct procedural mortality occurred in either group. However, in-hospital mortality and recurrence rates were significantly higher in the percutaneous group. Allen and coworkers[26] reviewed combined results in the literature, and similar results were noted. Surgical drainage had mortality, complication, and recurrence rates of 0.6 percent, 1.5 percent, and 3.2 percent, respectively. Catheter drainage had rates of 1.9 percent, 10.6 percent, and 13.8 percent, respectively. Thus, despite the relatively short-term benefit of any procedure, compared with percutaneous approaches, surgical drainage may allow patients to be discharged from the hospital.

CARDIAC TAMPONADE

Epidemiology

Cardiac tamponade occurs when the increase in pericardial fluid leads to a significant rise in pericardial pressure, subsequently causing hemodynamic consequences. Etiologies include bleeding (spontaneous, traumatic, postoperative) and other sources of chronic effusions.

Cardiac surgeons are most familiar with cardiac tamponade in the immediate postoperative period. In series, there have been reports that the overall incidence is 0 to 8 percent[27,28] after cardiac surgery. Tamponade in the postoperative period can be difficult to diagnose since typical signs and symptoms may be related to expected (or assumed) cardiac dysfunction (e.g., low-output syndrome). Because of this, tamponade is a diagnosis of exclusion but one that must be entertained early in the postoperative period for unstable patients.

Pathophysiology

In normal circumstances, interpericardial pressure is similar to pleural pressure, with both being subatmospheric. As left ventricular volume increases as a result of rapid infusion of blood during early diastole, interpericardial pressure increases. Understandably, during this time the right ventricle also is filling. However, because it is thin-walled, increases in interpericardial pressure (or extrinsic compression from a clot) can have a deleterious effect on the right ventricle. With tamponade, accumulation of fluid in the pericardial space causes the interpericardial pressure to increase rapidly. The tough fibrous pericardium stretches minimally, preventing the ventricles from filling. Additional increases in fluid result in lost diastolic compliance and reduced heart function.

As the consequences of tamponade progress, higher pressures are required for the ventricles to fill. Compensatory mechanisms include higher systemic and pulmonary artery pressures by vasoconstriction,[29] tachycardia, time-dependent pericardial stretch, and blood volume expansion.[30] The last mechanism aids only in compensating for slow-growing pericardial effusions.

Interpericardial pressure rises initially to levels higher than left and right atrial pressures with the previously mentioned compensatory mechanisms occurring. When right and left atrial, right and left ventricular, pulmonary artery wedge, and interpericardial pressures equalize, cardiovascular collapse ensues.

Clinical features

Cardiac tamponade presents as hypotension and/or decreased cardiac output. Venous pressures are elevated, and jugular venous distention may be present. The classic Beck's triad[31] of muffled heart sounds, elevated venous pressure, and decreased systemic arterial pressure may or may not be present.

Cardiac surgeons encounter cardiac tamponade most often in the immediate postoperative period. Although the classic signs of tamponade (equalization of right and left heart pressures, decreased cardiac output, and hypotension) may be present, the clinical diagnosis is often more subtle. Other features can include decreased urine output, worsening acidosis, increased inotrope or pressor dependence, and new hemodynamic instability. The authors advocate prompt surgical reexploration if any of these criteria are met.

Diagnostic modalities

Physical examination may aid in making the diagnosis of cardiac tamponade. Beck's triad, as described above, may be present. Jugular venous distention and pulsus paradoxus also may be present. Pulsus paradoxus is characterized by a decrease in systolic blood pressure by 10 mmHg during quiet inspiration.[32] The mechanism results from increased caval blood flow during inspiration in a nonintubated patient. With increased venous return, right ventricular volume increases. Because of the increased pressure in the pericardium, the septum is shifted and left ventricular volume is decreased. This translates into decreased cardiac output and arterial hypotension.

Echocardiography confirms the diagnosis and can confirm the size and extent of effusions. ECHO can confirm pulsus paradoxus when inspiration increases right ventricular size and decreases left ventricular size in the presence of a large pericardial effusion. Compression of the right ventricular free wall during late diastole–early systole lasting more than one-third of the cardiac cycle is a sensitive sign. Right ventricular indentation during early diastole is more specific.[33] One must remember that tamponade is not an all-or-none phenomenon. The use of echocardiography in the immediate postoperative period can be problematic. Transthoracic views can be limited by chest tubes or dressings. In the immediate postoperative period, some degree of effusion always exists. Although ECHO may give the diagnosis of tamponade, it does not rule out tamponade. The authors abide by the dictum that postoperative cardiac tamponade is a clinical, not an echocardiographic, diagnosis.

Treatment

Medical therapy

Very little medical therapy exists for cardiac tamponade. The mainstay is volume expansion to optimize preload while operative intervention is planned.

Surgical therapy

Surgical therapy for cardiac tamponade depends on the circumstances in which tamponade arises. The goal of surgical therapy is twofold: relieve extrinsic cardiac compression and reverse the inciting event. Surgical therapy for pericardial effusions with tamponade physiology was discussed in the previous section.

In the postoperative period, sternal reentry is the approach of choice. Careful attention should be paid to the specific location of the clot. For example, thrombus around the aorta should lead the surgeon to the aortic cannulation site or proximal anastomoses as a source of bleeding. Nevertheless, complete exploration and verification of all surgical sites is paramount. Aggressive correction of any coagulopathy also should be done; this includes ensuring that the patient is warm. All too often surgeons forget that a cause of coagulopathy is hypothermia. Rapid infusion of cold volume can exacerbate the problem.

Cardiac tamponade from trauma poses a more difficult problem. In this setting, the surgical approach is dictated by the mode of injury. Penetrating injuries should be explored in accordance with the direction of the trajectory. Pericardiocentesis may alleviate tamponade in the emergency room until the operating room is available. When the authors have planned an exploration via the left chest, they occasionally have started with a subxiphoid window to eliminate blood in the pericardium before placing the patient in the lateral decubitus position. Left thoracotomy, median sternotomy, and clamshell incisions all provide access to the pericardium and drainage of blood. The presence of other suspected injuries should dictate which approach is taken.

PERICARDITIS

Epidemiology

Over the last half century, etiologies for pericarditis have changed. Historically, tuberculosis (TB) was the major cause of infective pericarditis. Infectious diseases cause fewer cases of pericarditis since the emergence of other etiologies, such as previous cardiac surgery, malignancy, radiation, and trauma.[34]

Infection remains a common cause of pericarditis. Sources include the heart, the surrounding tissues, septicemia, and the incision in postoperative patients. Sources can be both bacterial and viral. As expected, infections are much more serious in immunosuppressed patients such as transplant patients and AIDS patients. Viral pericarditis is usually mild and self-limiting and in fact may be subclinical. In contrast, acute bacterial pericarditis can be life-threatening. The most common agents of bacterial pericarditis are streptococci, pneumococci, and staphylococci.[35] Although now less common now, TB remains an etiology, especially in immunocompromised patients. The pathologic stages seen in tubercular pericarditis are characterized by fibrinous exudation followed by serosanguineous effusions. These effusions absorb and organize into caseating granulomas, pericardial thickening, fibrosis, and constriction.[36]

Pericarditis can be seen in renal failure patients because of infection (from dialysis access, for example) as a result of their relative immunosuppressed state or as a result of uremia. Although the exact etiology of uremic pericarditis is unknown, nitrogen retention is required for its development. This condition first was described by Bright in 1836.[37]

A few drugs classically are associated with pericarditis. They are procainamide, hydralazine, methylsergide, emetine, and minoxidil.

Other metabolic causes of pericarditis include systemic lupus erythematosus (SLE), hypothyroidism, and rheumatoid arthritis (RA). Approximately half of patients with RA have pericardial effusions or pericardial adhesions. Patients with more severe RA tend to have worse pericardial issues; this is thought to be related to the deposition of immune complexes in the pericardium.[39]

Radiation is the most common cause of constrictive pericarditis in the United States[39] and was dominant in an era when mediastinal irradiation was a common form of treatment for lymphoma. Postmastectomy irradiation and treatment of some lung cancers also contribute. The degree of inflammation and subsequent constriction relates to the total dose of radiation. One series reported that over 20 percent of patents with radiation-induced pericarditis ultimately required pericardiectomy.[40]

Trauma, cardiac surgery, and myocardial infarction account for additional cases of pericarditis. Both blunt and penetrating trauma can result in pericarditis as a sequela to even a small bloody pericardial effusion. Approximately 50 percent of patients who have had a transmural myocardial infarction develop a form of pericarditis known as Dressler's syndrome. Constrictive pericarditis can be a result of cardiac surgery, but this occurs in less than 5 percent of these patients.[41]

Pathophysiology

Pericarditis by definition is an inflammation of the pericardial sac. The degree and extent of inflammation vary from patient to patient, as do the events that follow this inflammation. For pathologic pericarditis (i.e., resulting in constrictive pericarditis), the basic premise is that inflammation leads to scarring and fibrosis (Fig. 42-3). This in turn leads to constriction and the pathophysiologic processes described below.

The sine qua non of constrictive pericarditis is limitation in cardiac filling. The atria serve three functions: a conduit, a reservoir, and a pump. The primary function is that of a conduit, and this contributes to the rapid early filling of the ventricles during diastole. The majority of diastolic filling occurs in early diastole. This process of filling becomes abnormal when the distention of the ventricles is limited by the fibrous pericardium. Pressures within the heart chambers are relatively normal until the distention of the ventricles becomes limited. End-diastolic pressures suddenly increase, manifested by the "square root" sign seen on ventricular pressure tracings during cardiac catheterization.

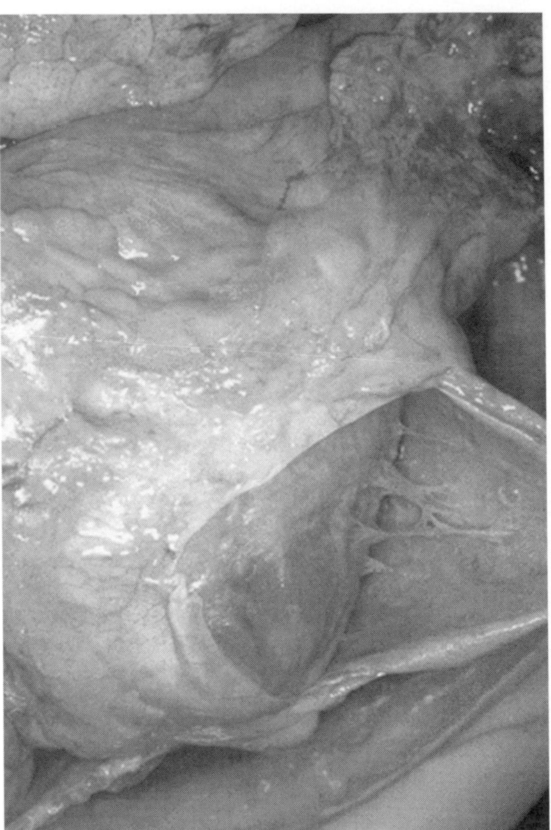

Figure 42-3 Fibrinous pericarditis. Note the characteristically thickened walls of the opened pericardial sac and the intrapericardial adhesions. (Reproduced with permission from WEBPATH, courtesy of Edward C. Klatt, MD.)

Clinical features

Clinical findings depend on the severity of constriction. Patients with mild constriction may be asymptomatic. As constriction becomes more severe, signs and symptoms of heart failure become more pronounced; the heart failure may be limited to one side or may be biventricular. Venous pressures become higher, and symptoms of right-sided heart failure become more prominent. Early symptoms include jugular venous distention, hepatomegaly, and peripheral edema. As the symptoms progress, ascites, worsening peripheral edema, and pleural effusions may develop.

Diagnostic modalities

A few signs may be present with constrictive pericarditis. During inspiration, jugular venous distention may worsen; this is the so-called Kussmaul's sign. Pulsus paradoxus (described earlier) also may be present. A prominent S_3 heart sound may be heard. This pericardial knock is secondary to the rapid ventricular filling during diastole. Murmurs are often absent.

Basic studies such as CXR and ECG may be useful in directing the clinician to the diagnosis. Nonspecific ST elevation or T-wave abnormalities are present in more than 90 percent of these patients. On CXR, pericardial calcification is seen in 40 percent[42] of these patients. Computed tomography (CT) can demonstrate a thickened pericardium (Fig. 42-4). Isolated findings must be supported by physiologic criteria. A newer modality is magnetic resonance imaging (MRI), which is more sensitive and specific than CT in the diagnosis of constrictive pericarditis. MRI can show right atrial dilatation and right ventricular compression. The sensitivity and specificity of MRI are higher than 90 percent.[43]

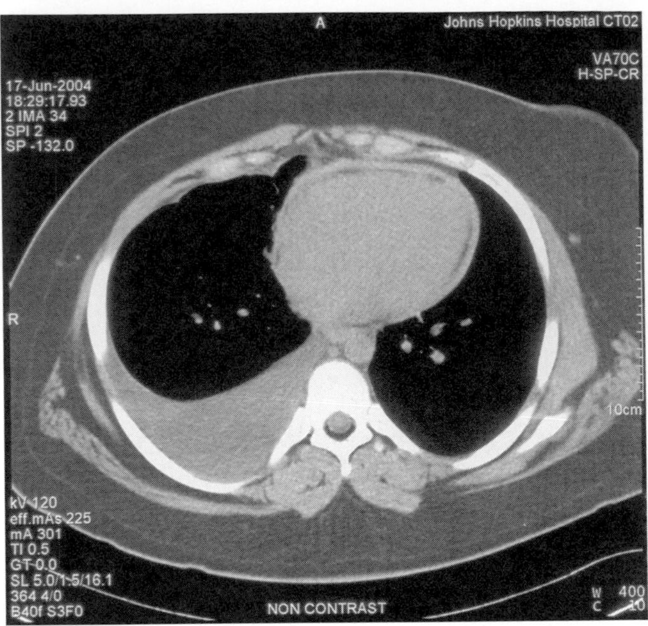

Figure 42-4 Computed tomogram revealing thickened pericardium consistent with constrictive pericarditis.

Although echocardiography is very useful in diagnosing cardiac tamponade and pericardial effusions, it has far less utility with constrictive pericarditis. Thickened pericardium rarely is seen, but pericardial calcification can be evident. ECHO visualization of the pathophysiologic processes can lead to the diagnosis. Specifically, inspection of right ventricular (RV) filling during inspiration may show the interventricular septum bowing to the left.

Right and left heart cardiac catheterization remains the gold standard in the diagnosis of constrictive pericarditis. Hallmark features include equalization of end-diastolic pressures in the right atrium, left atrium, and pulmonary artery. Right ventricular and left ventricular pressures are also equal.[44] Mean atrial pressures should be above 10 mmHg on the right and left sides of the heart. The "square root" sign described earlier is seen on ventricular tracing during catheterization (Fig. 42-5). The right atrial tracing demonstrates a prominent Y descent. The left ventricular ejection fraction should be greater than 40 percent. Right ventricular end-diastolic pressure (RVEDP) is elevated and should be greater than one-third of RV systolic pressure. This finding has

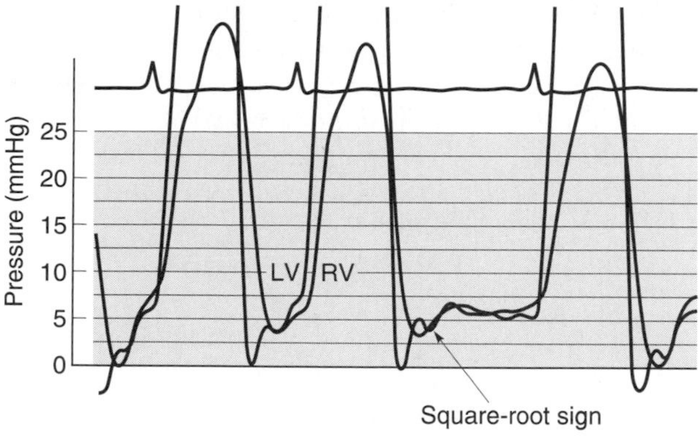

Figure 42-5 Square root sign in a right ventricular pressure tracing in a patient with constrictive pericarditis. (Modified with permission from Spodick DH. *The Pericardium: A Comprehensive Textbook.* New York: Marcel Dekker; 1997:4.)

95 percent sensitivity for the diagnosis of constrictive pericarditis.[45]

The clinician often has difficulty differentiating restrictive cardiomyopathy from constrictive pericarditis. Making the diagnosis is critical, because constrictive pericarditis can be cured surgically. Transplantation is the only surgical treatment for restrictive cardiomyopathy. The criteria mentioned above are neither very sensitive nor very specific in making this distinction. Criteria suggestive of restrictive cardiomyopathy include a small or normal-size heart, reduced left ventricular function, pulmonary and hepatic congestion, and prominent X and Y descents on atrial tracing. However, none of them is pathognomonic.

Ventricular interdependence is the most sensitive and specific test for constrictive pericarditis. This is observed during cardiac catheterization. During the respiratory cycle, concordant increases in right and left ventricular pressure are expected with inspiration. With constrictive pericarditis, a discordance is seen. This observation has a sensitivity of 100 percent and a specificity of 95 percent.[46]

When the diagnosis is unclear after cardiac catheterization, more invasive means can be used to aid in making the diagnosis. Endomyocardial biopsy may be useful. If it is normal or if there are mild inflammatory changes, the biopsy does not help in distinguishing restrictive from constrictive pericarditis. The results of amyloid are diagnostic for restrictive cardiomyopathy. Schoenfeld and associates[47] found that the diagnosis of restrictive cardiomyopathy was made in 39 percent of patients when the diagnosis was unclear after less invasive testing.

When all other modes of testing fail, the diagnosis can be made by miniexploratory thoracotomy. If no pericardial pathology is present, the patient is closed. If constrictive pericarditis is found, a formal pericardectomy is done.

Treatment

Medical therapy

Treatment of the underlying cause of pericarditis is the only medical therapy. However, most often the etiology is unknown. Surgical therapy remains the mainstay of treatment.

Surgical therapy

Once the diagnosis of constrictive pericarditis is confirmed, operative intervention is employed. Many patients present with advanced heart failure. An arterial line and a pulmonary artery catheter should be placed. Surgical approaches are median sternotomy, left anterior thoracotomy, and bilateral anterior thoracotomy and vary with surgeon preference and patient history.

The approach from median sternotomy starts in the usual manner. The sternum is divided, and hemostasis is obtained with electrocautery and bone wax. The pump should be set up and be ready for cardiopulmonary bypass. The thymic fat pad is dissected to the innominate vein. The anterior aspect of the pericardium is palpated and inspected. A scalpel is used to incise the pericardium in the midline, starting anterior to the aorta. Care must be taken during this step, as the pericardium often is densely adherent to the heart. Pericardial flaps are lifted inferiorly and laterally. The dissection over the left side of the heart may have to be done on cardiopulmonary bypass. The pericardium has to be stripped from phrenic nerve to phrenic nerve laterally, off the diaphragm inferiorly, and off the atrioventricular groove superiorly. Bands between the right ventricle and the pulmonary artery must be excised. Failure to do this may lead to pulmonary hypertension.[48] One may need to leave islands of unstripped pericardium over the coronaries, remembering that the serous visceral pericardium is in continuity with the adventitia of the coronary arteries. The pericardium over the right atrium and the cavoatrial junction does not need to be stripped; there is no hemodynamic advantage to this, and the risk of bleeding is substantial.[49]

The authors prefer starting with a left anterior thoracotomy for a pericardiectomy. The patient is intubated with a dual-lumen endotracheal tube. An arterial line and a pulmonary artery catheter are placed. The groins should be prepped in case of a need for bypass. A small roll is placed under the left shoulder. The lung is deflated, and the fourth intercostal space is entered through a left inframammary incision. The phrenic nerve is identified, and the pericardium is incised anteriorly. Dissection is continued anteriorly to the right atrium, inferiorly to the diaphragm, and superiorly to the pulmonary artery.

Sometimes the dissection of the right ventricle is very difficult through this incision. The left anterior thoracotomy can be extended across the sternum to a right anterior thoracotomy (clamshell incision). This exposure is outstanding. Only rarely is cardiopulmonary bypass needed with this approach. All surgical approaches offer equal results and should be dictated by surgeon preference.

Outcomes and prognosis

Early mortality for patients with pericardiectomy ranges from 5 to 10 percent, with 5-year survival ranging between 65 and 90 percent. Patients with idiopathic cardiomyopathy have had the best survival (88 percent 7-year survival). Predictors of a poor outcome were prior radiation, renal insufficiency, poor ventricular function, higher pulmonary artery pressures, New York Heart Association (NYHA) class IV, low serum sodium, ascites, and hyperbilirubinemia.[36,50,51]

References

1. Siegel RE. Galen on surgery of the pericardium: An early record of the therapy based on anatomic and experimental studies. *Am J Cardiol* 1970;26(5):524–527.
2. Lower R. *Tractatus de Corde item de motu, et colore sanguinis et chyli in eum transitu*. London: J. Allestry; 1669:104.
3. Aris A. Francisco Romero, the first heart surgeon. *Ann Thorac Surg* 1997;64:870–871.
4. Aris A. One hundred years of cardiac surgery. *Ann Thorac Surg* 1996;62:636–637
5. Beck CS. The effect of surgical solution of chlorinated soda (Dakin's solution) in the pericardial cavity. *Arch Surg* 1929;18:1659
6. Beck CS, Griswold RA. Pericardiectomy in the treatment of the Pick syndrome: Experimental and clinical observations. *Arch Surg* 1930;21:1064
7. Beck CS. Development of a new blood supply to the heart by operation. *Ann Surg* 1935;102:801–813.
8. Blalock A, Burwell CS. Chronic pericardial disease. *Surg Gynecol Obstet* 1941;73:433.
9. Moore KL. *Clinically Oriented Anatomy*, 3d ed. Philadelphia: Lippincott Williams & Wilkins, 1992: 80–87.
10. Moore KL. *The Developing Human, Clinically Oriented Embryology*, 4th ed. 1988:160–167.
11. Soler-Soler J, Sarista-Sauleda J, Permanyer-Miralda G. Management of pericardial effusion. *Heart* 2001;86(2): 235–240.
12. Agner RC, Gallis HA. Pericarditis: Differential diagnosis and considerations. *Arch Intern Med* 1979;139:407–412.
13. Colombo A, Olsen HG, Egan J, et al. Etiology and prognostic implications of a large pericardial effusion in men. *Clin Cardiol* 1988;11:389–394.
14. Corey GR, Campbell PT, Van Tright P, et al. Etiology of large pericardial effusions. *Am J Med* 2000;109:95–101.
15. Guberman BA, Fowler NO, Engel PJ, et al. Cardiac tamponade in medical patients. *Circulation* 1981;64:633–640.
16. Miller AJ, Pick R, Johnson PJ. The production or acute pericardial effusion: The effects of various degrees of interference with venous return and lymph drainage from heart muscle in the dog. *Am J Cardiol* 1971;28:463.
17. Spodick DH. The normal and diseased pericardium: Current concepts of pericardial physiology, diseases and treatment. *J Am Coll Cardiol* 1983;1:240.
18. Savage DD, Garrison RJ, Brand F, et al. Prevalence and correlates of posterior extra echocardiographic spaces in a free-living population based sample (The Framingham Study). *Am J Cardiol* 1983;51:1207–1212.
19. Posner MR, Cohen GI, Sarkin AT. Pericardial disease in patients with cancer: The differentiation of malignant from radiation-induced pericarditis. *Am J Med* 1981;7:407–413.
20. Sagrista-Sauleda J, Merce J, Permanyer-Miralda G, et al. Clinical clues to the causes of large pericardial effusion. *Am J Med* 2000;109:95–101.
21. Levine MJ, Lorell BH, Divier DJ, et al. Implications of echocardiographically assisted diagnosis of pericardial tamponade in contemporary medical patients: Detection before hemodynamic embarrassment. *J Am Coll Cardiol* 1991:17:58–65.
22. Vaitkus PT, Herrmann HC, LeWinter MM. Treatment of malignant pericardial effusion. *JAMA* 1994;272(1):59–64.
23. Sagrista-Sauleda J, Angel J, Parmanyer-Miralda G, et al. Long-tem follow-up of idiopathic chronic pericardial effusion. *N Engl J Med* 1999;341:2054–2059.
24. Girardi LN, Ginsburg RJ, Burt ME. Pericardiocentesis and intrapericardial sclerosis: Effective therapy for malignant pericardial effusions. *Ann Thorac Surg* 1999;67:437–440.
25. McDonald JM, Meyers BF, Guthrie TJ, et al. Comparison of open subxiphoid pericardial drainage with percutaneous catheter drainage for symptomatic pericardial effusion. *Ann Thorac Surg* 2003;76:811–816.
26. Allen KB, Faber LP, Warren WH, et al. Pericardial effusion: Subxiphoid pericardiostomy versus percutaneous catheter drainage. *Ann Thorac Surg* 1999;67:427–440.
27. Malouf JF, Alam S, Gharzeddine W, Stefadouros MA. The role of anticoagulation in the development of pericardial effusion and late tamponade after cardiac surgery. *Eur Heart J* 1993;14:1451–1457.
28. Shabetai R. The effects of pericardial effusion on respiratory variations in hemodynamic and ventricular function. *J Am Coll Cardiol* 1991;17:249–250.
29. Spodick DH. Pathophysiology of cardiac tamponade. *Chest* 1998;113:1372.
30. Reddy PS, Curtis EI, Uretsky BF. Spectrum of hemodynamic changes in cardiac tamponade. *Am J Cardiol* 1990;66:1487
31. Beck CS. Two cardiac compressor triads. *JAMA* 1935;104:714.
32. Savitt MA, Tyson GS, Elbeery JR, et al. Physiology of cardiac tamponade and paradoxical pulse in conscious dogs. *Am J Physiol* 1992;265:H1996.
33. Schiller NB, Botvinick EH. Right ventricular compression as a sign of cardiac tamponade: An analysis of ventricular dimensions and their clinical implications. *Circulation* 1983;56:774.
34. Ling LH, Oh JK, Schaff HV. Constrictive pericarditis in the modern era: Evolving clinical spectrum and impact on outcome after pericardectomy. *Circulation* 1999;100:1380.
35. Spodick DH. Infectious pericarditis. In: Spodick DH (ed). *The Pericardium: A Comprehensive Textbook*. New York: Marcel Dekker, 1997:260.
36. Tirilomis T, Univerdoben S, von der Emde J. Pericardiectomy for chronic constrictive pericarditis: Risks and outcome. *Eur J Thorac Cardiovasc Surg* 1994;8:487.
37. Bright R. Tabular view of the morbid appearance in 100 cases connected with albuminous urine: With observations. *Guys Hosp Rep* 1836;1:380.

38. Turesson C, Lacobsson L, Bergstrom U. Extra-articular rheumatoid arthritis: Prevalence and mortality. *Rheumatology* 1999;38:668.
39. Schiavone WA: The changing etiology of constrictive pericarditis in a large referral center. *Am J Cardiol* 1986;58:373.
40. Fajardo LF, Stewart JR. Radiation induced heart disease: Human and experimental observations. In: Bristow MR (ed). *Drug Induced Heart Disease.* New York: Elsevier, 1980:241.
41. Kutcher MA, King SB, Alimurung, et al. Constrictive pericarditis as a complication of cardiac surgery: Recognition of an entity. *Am J Cardiol* 1982;50:742.
42. McCaughan BC, Schaff HV, Piehler JM, et al. Early and late results of pericardiectomy for constrictive pericarditis. *J Thorac Cardiovasc Surg* 1985;89:340.
43. Masui T, Finck S, Higgins CB. Constrictive pericarditis and restrictive cardiomyopathy: Evaluation with MR imaging. *Radiology* 1992;182:369.
44. Shabeti R, Fowler NO, Guntheroth WG. The hemodynamics of cardiac tamponade and constrictive pericarditis. *Am J Cardiol* 1970;26:480.
45. Aroney CN, Ruddy TD, Dighero H, et al. Differentiation of restrictive cardiomyopathy from pericardial constriction: Assessment of diastolic function by radionuclide angiography. *J Am Coll Cardiol* 1989;13:1007.
46. Hurrell DG, Nishimura RA, Higano ST, et al. Value of dynamic respiratory changes in left and right ventricular pressures for the diagnosis of constrictive pericarditis. *Circulation* 1996;93:2007.
47. Schoenfeld MH, Supple EW, Dec GW et al. Restrictive cardiomyopathy versus constrictive pericarditis: Role of endomyocardial biopsy in avoiding unnecessary thoracotomy. *Circulation* 1987;75:1012–1017.
48. Portal RW, Besterman EM, Chambers RJ, et al. Prognosis after operation for constrictive pericarditis. *Br Med J* 1966;5487:563.
49. Kloster FE, Crislip RL, Bristow JD, et al. Hemodynamic studies following pericardiectomy for constrictive pericarditis. *Circulation* 1965;32:415.
50. Bertog SC, Thanbidorai SK, Parakh K, et al. Constrictive pericarditis: Etiology and cause-specific survival after pericardiectomy. *J Am Coll Cardiol* 2004;43(8):1450.
51. Arsan S, Mercan S, Sarigul A, et al. Long-term experience with pericardiectomy: Analysis of 105 consecutive patients. *J Thorac Cardiovasc Surg* 1994;42(6):344.

CHAPTER

43 PRIMARY CARDIAC TUMORS

Prashanth Vallabhajosyula, David D. Yuh

BACKGROUND

Definition

Primary cardiac tumors are neoplasms that originate in the heart, including the myocardium, the heart valves, the conduction fibers, and the nerve and lymph tissue in the heart. Primary cardiac tumors often infiltrate into the pericardium and are not discussed here as pericardial tumors. Conditions of the pericardium are discussed in Chapter 42.

Historical highlights

The first description of a primary cardiac tumor was a report of an atrial myxoma in 1845.[1] The first antemortem diagnosis of a primary cardiac tumor was made in 1951 through the use of angiocardiography.[2] The first successful surgical excision of a primary cardiac tumor was a left atrial myxoma performed in 1954. Cardiac papillary fibroelastoma first was described by Yater in 1931.[3] In 1975, the term *papillary fibroelastoma* first was used, and in the same year, its microscopic properties

KEY CONCEPTS

- Epidemiology
  - Primary cardiac tumors are quite rare, with incidences ranging from 0.0017 to 0.2 percent in autopsy series. About 75 percent of primary tumors are benign, and about half of those tumors are myxomas. Papillary fibroelastoma is the second most common benign tumor. Most of the malignant tumors are sarcomas.
- Pathophysiology
  - Myxomas originate from multipotential mesenchymal cells in the heart. They are considered embryonal remnants during septation and differentiation of cardiac tissues, possibly generated from clonal structural aberrations in certain chromosomes (i.e., chromosomes 2, 12, and 17). Papillary fibroelastomas are avascular masses covered by a single layer of endocardial cells, with the matrix containing variable amounts of elastic fibrils. They predominantly originate from the cardiac valves; are typically solitary, although they can be multiple; and originate from the same location or different locations. Sarcomas are mesenchyme-derived sessile, infiltrative, or polypoid masses of various morphologic types.
- Clinical features
  - The clinical manifestations of cardiac tumors are based on the location, size, and mobility of a tumor rather than its histology. Such tumors can cause valvular dysfunction, embolic sequelae, conduction disturbances, outflow tract obstruction, and systemic manifestations (e.g., weight loss, fever, arthralgias, rash). Malignant cardiac tumors can metastasize and irreversibly damage the heart.
- Diagnostics
  - Plain chest radiography findings can be suggestive of a primary cardiac tumor but usually are not diagnostic. Echocardiography is the most important diagnostic technique, although magnetic resonance imaging and computed tomography can provide detailed characteristics.
- Treatment
  - Treatment for primary cardiac tumors is dependent on the benign versus malignant nature of a tumor. Surgical

resection is the primary curative modality for benign tumors, with much documented success (e.g., myxomas). Cardiac sarcomas and lymphomas have dismal prognoses that usually are not altered by surgical resection; there may be a potential role for chemotherapy and/or radiation therapy for some of these malignancies. Surgical resection is usually palliative.

- Outcomes and prognosis
  - Most benign primary cardiac tumors can be resected to achieve a cure. Malignant primary cardiac tumors generally have a poor prognosis (less than 25 percent 1-year survival) despite surgical resection and adjuvant chemotherapy and radiotherapy.

were reported.[4,5] By 1980, the importance of echocardiography in the antemortem diagnosis of primary cardiac tumors was evident.[6]

Overview

Primary cardiac tumors are quite rare, with an incidence ranging from 0.0017 to 0.2 percent in autopsy series.[7–12] Metastatic tumors to the heart are far more common[12] and can occur 100- to 500-fold more commonly than primary tumors. About three-quarters of primary tumors are benign, and about half of the benign tumors are myxomas. The second most common benign tumor is the papillary fibroelastoma. Other benign tumors include lipomas, rhabdomyomas, fibromas, angiomas, teratomas, cystic tumors, mesotheliomas of the atrioventricular node, hamartoma, and endocrine tumors of the heart. The pathophysiology of a cardiac tumor is more dependent on its size and location than on its histology, although malignant tumors behave differently than do primary cardiac tumors. Most of the malignant tumors are sarcomas. Primary malignant tumors of the heart include angiosarcomas, rhabdomyosarcomas, mesotheliomas, fibrosarcomas, lymphomas, liposarcomas, leiomyosarcomas, and malignant teratomas. The mobility of these tumors in the intraatrial-intraventricular spaces also can affect their presenting features.

The primary process underlying the symptoms from benign cardiac tumors is based on their location, size, and mobility. Malignant tumors can be far more infiltrative and thus cause symptoms of contractility dysfunction, pericardial tamponade, and arrhythmias secondary to invasion into the conduction apparatus. The prognosis for benign tumors is significantly better than that for malignant tumors, especially with surgical intervention.

In contrast to the important role for surgical intervention in treating benign primary cardiac tumors, the prognosis for malignant tumors is dismal. Many malignant tumors are metastatic at the time of diagnosis, and the survival benefit of surgical intervention is minimal to nonexistent. This chapter concentrates primarily on benign primary cardiac tumors. Because the clinical presentation of these tumors is more dependent on their location and size than on their histology, it is appropriate to discuss this aspect on the basis of the location of a tumor rather than its type.

BENIGN PRIMARY CARDIAC TUMORS

Myxomas

Nearly 50 percent of benign tumors of the heart are myxomas, making this the most common primary cardiac tumor. Myxomas typically develop in the atria, with over 75 percent originating in the left atrium and 15 to 20 percent originating in the right atrium. Most tumors arise from the interatrial septum, near the border of the fossa ovalis. This is not surprising because the origin of cells that develop into myxomas is believed to be mesenchymal cells. Myxomas also originate from the posterior atrial wall, the anterior wall, and the atrial appendage.[13,14] The occurrence of myxomas in the ventricles is only approximately 8 percent, with equal distribution on the right and left sides.[15] Myxomas of the heart valves are rare.[16,17] There have been reported cases of multifocal, multilocular, and biatrial myxomas.[16,18,19] In these cases, it is not unusual for a myxoma to extend through the foramen ovale into the contralateral atrium. It is important to note that multifocality of myxomas is seen more frequently in patients with familial myxoma.

Epidemiology

The mean age of patients with nonfamilial myxomas is 56 years, and 60 to 70 percent of these patients are female.[13,20,21] These myxomas occur most frequently between the third and sixth decades of life, although the range extends from a stillborn infant to a 95-year-old woman with myxoma.[22] With the advent of improved noninvasive techniques, more myxomas are being diagnosed in the elderly with cardiac symptoms and signs that are attributed to factors besides tumors. Most myxomas occur sporadically, but familial myxomas do occur. Patients with familial myxomas present with symptoms at an earlier age. Studies in these families suggest an autosomal dominant pattern of inheritance with a variable phenotype.[23,24]

Some patients present with cardiac myxoma as part of a syndrome called syndrome myxoma or Carney's syndrome. It is characterized by myxomas in other locations, spotty pigmentation, and endocrine overactivity.[25–27] In addition to cardiac myxomas, these patients typically have myxomas of the breast or skin, lentigines and pigmented nevi of the skin, and endocrine overactivity secondary to pituitary adenomas, adrenocortical disease, or testicular tumors. Cardiac myxomas in patients with Carney's syndrome have a greater tendency to originate outside the left atrium, are at time bilateral, and recur more frequently. It is proposed that syndrome myxoma is a result of hyperproliferation of certain mesenchymal cells that overproduce glycosaminoglycans.[28]

Patients with a family history of cardiac myxomas should be evaluated carefully for multifocality and other symptoms associated with familial syndromes. It is reasonable for first-degree relatives of these patients to undergo echocardiographic evaluation. Postoperatively, these patients should be followed carefully for recurrence and new tumors. Recurrence rates in these patients are reported to be 12 to 22 percent.[29]

Pathology

Because of improvements in the ability to achieve antemortem diagnosis of primary cardiac tumors, most myxomas are examined after surgical resection (Fig. 43-1). Myxomas are well described, and their gross pathology and histology are not changed by their location (Fig. 43-2).[30,31] Most myxomas are grossly round or oval in shape with polypoid features, and others are gelatinous; many are prone to fragment spontaneously. The rate of growth of myxomas is unknown, but they generally are believed to grow quite quickly.[32,33] They are essentially nonmalignant, although there are reports of myxomatous growth after embolization of these tumors.[34–37]

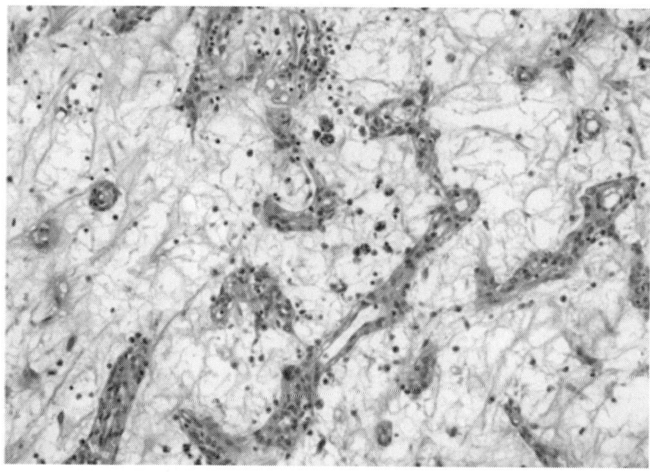

Figure 43-2 Atrial myxoma. Typical microscopic appearance of atrial myxoma with nests of small stellate cells and blood vessels immersed in abundant acellular matrix that is rich in proteoglycans. These tumors often contain smooth muscle, areas of hemorrhage and calcification, hemosiderin-laden macrophages, and chronic inflammatory cells. Hematoxylin-eosin ×200. (Reproduced, with permission, from Reardon MJ, Smythe WR. Cardiac neoplasms. In: Cohn LH, Edmunds LH Jr (eds). *Cardiac Surgery in the Adult.* New York: McGraw-Hill; 2003:1373–1400.)

Histogenesis

Myxomas are primarily of endocardial origin. The cells of origin are multipotential mesenchymal cells in the heart. They are considered to be resident cells that persist as embryonal residues during septation of the heart and its differentiation into myoblasts, smooth muscle cells, angioblasts, and endothelial cells.[38] There is evidence suggesting that the underlying mechanism is clonal structural aberrations in certain chromosomes.[39–44] Both sporadic and familial myxomas have been shown to have clonal telomeric rearrangements and other aberrations at several foci that involve chromosomes 2, 12, and 17. Other reported chromosomal aberrations include rearrangement in 1q32, loss of chromosome Y, and telomeric association between chromosome 13 and chromosome15.[39–43] A study conducted on 11 kindreds with Carney's syndrome reported aberrations in the short arm of chromosome 2.[39] Another report noted a gene defect on chromosome 17q in four unrelated families with Carney's syndrome.[41] Refined linkage analysis in Carney's complex families showed mutations in the chromosome 17q24 gene *PRKAR1-alpha*, which encodes the R1 alpha-regulatory subunit of protein kinase (PKA).[45–47] It is believed that this gene may be involved in tumor suppressor activity; thus, haplotype deficiency of the gene may result in Carney's complex. A recent report noted mutations in the perinatal myosin heavy chain gene involved in the cause of a Carney's complex variant known as trismus–pseudocamptodactyly syndrome.[48] One study conducted on a cardiac myxoma from a patient reported a complex rearrangement at chromosome 12p12 at the site of the *ki-ras* oncogene.[44] Together, these studies support chromosomal aberrations as one of the underlying causes of myxoma formation.

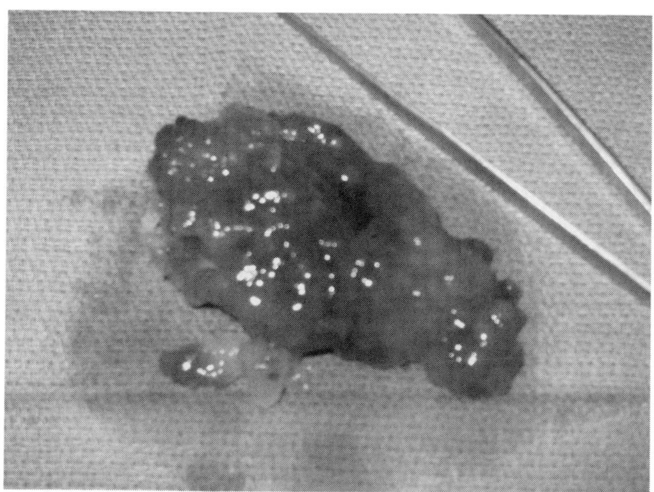

Figure 43-1 Left atrial myxoma. Note the polypoid gelatinous features of this tumor, predisposing it to spontaneous embolization.

Histology

On gross pathology, myxomas are typically gelatinous, polypoid, often pedunculated, smooth, and round. They are rarely sessile, and at times they display a gently lobulated surface. In 90 percent of cases, the tumors originate in the atria, and the pedunculated masses typically have a base of attachment in the atrial septa. This is not surprising in light of the origin of the cells that develop into myxomas. Myxomas analyzed in surgical series typically average 4 to 8 cm in diameter, but the range varies from 1 to 15 cm in the literature. One study reported the weight of resected myxomas ranging from 8 to 175 g.[49]

Polypoid myxomas can be quite mobile, depending on their consistency and collagen content and the length of the stalk. They show little tendency toward spontaneous fragmentation. Villous myxomas are typically not smooth and show fine villous extensions that are fragile. Therefore, they have a higher tendency for spontaneous fragmentation. The surface of myxomas often is covered with thrombi, and it is common to see areas of thrombi inside these tumors.[13]

A diagnosis of myxoma requires the presence of myxoma cells. On microscopy, myxoma characteristically shows patterns of lipidic cells embedded in a myxoid stroma. The stroma is classically rich in glycosaminoglycans.[30,31] The tumor cells have a round, elliptical, or polyhedral shape and may be multinuclear; there is pink cytoplasm; and the nuclei typically have an open chromatin pattern. Myxoma cells are typically present in cords or small clusters and at times may occur as layers of cells surrounding vascular structures. Ten to 20 percent of myxoma specimens contain calcifications, and it is not uncommon to find areas of hemorrhage, lymphocytes, and macrophage infiltration. Small areas of cellular atypia may be present, but mitoses are not seen; these feature may simulate malignancy.[50] Foci of extramedullary hematopoiesis also may be present. The surface of a myxoma usually is covered by polygonal cells and partially covered by endothelial cells.[51] At the base of myxoma there are abundant blood vessels that originate from the subendocardium. Emboli from myxomas may not be sufficient to make the diagnosis as they have less definitive histologic features than does the primary tumor. Analyses of emboli do not show any malignant features in them. There is no invasion of myxoma cells into adjacent structures in the embolized specimen.

On immunohistochemical studies, myxoma cells show positivity on staining for vimentin, supporting their mesenchymal origin.[38] They also show variable positivity to endothelial cell markers such as factor VIII–related antigen and some neuroendocrine and smooth muscle cell markers. On ultrastructural analysis, myxoma cells display cytoplasmic filaments that look like smooth muscle cells.[31] They closely resemble embryonic mesenchymal cells and embryonic endocardial cushion tissue.[31,38] It is important to note that immunohistochemical and ultrastructural findings are sufficient for a definitive diagnosis of myxoma.

Papillary fibroelastoma

Papillary fibroelastomas were described by Yater in 1931.[3] They are benign endocardial papillomas that originate primarily in the cardiac valves. They are the second most common benign primary cardiac tumors and account for 75 percent of all cardiac valvular tumors. The majority of patients with papillary fibroelastomas are asymptomatic, but fibroelastomas can cause life-threatening complications such as stroke, embolism, valve dysfunction, and death. They may be single or multiple and can occur on any valvular surface, papillary muscle, chordae tendineae, or endocardium. Typically, they occur on mitral and aortic valves in adults and in the tricuspid valve in children.

Epidemiology

Papillary fibroelastomas occur primarily occur in the fourth to eighth decades of life, with a predominance for the eighth decade. About 2 percent of reported cases are in the pediatric population. The mean age of detection is 60 years, with a slight male sex predominance (55 percent). There are no familial syndromes with papillary fibroelastomas, and most of these lesions appear to be acquired.[52,53] They occur sporadically, and few congenital cases have been reported. The etiology of these tumors is not known, and there are no long-term follow-up studies that indicate their growth rate. Reports in the literature note the development of fibroelastomas ranging from 6 months to 15 years.[54–56] They are typically slow-growing tumors but can function as a platform for the formation of large thrombi in a short period.[55] There are no clear risk factors for the development of the tumor.

Pathology

Grossly, papillary fibroelastomas have a frondlike appearance, with papillary fronds attaching to the endocardium via a short pedicle.[57] The fronds are narrow and branching and can merge into the valve substance. They are described classically as appearing like a sea anemone, and this is the hallmark of this tumor on gross examination. Cystic fibroelastomas have been reported but are very rare.[58] It is not uncommon for these tumors to be hidden in large thrombi; therefore, the thrombi should be examined carefully. Typically, the size of these tumors in surgical series is around 1 cm in diameter, but the reported range varies from 2 to 70 mm.[59] Fibroelastomas are typically avascular.

The distribution of papillary fibroelastomas is marked by their predominant origin from the cardiac valves. Three-fourths of these tumors originate from the valves, with other sites, in decreasing order of frequency, being the aortic valve, mitral valve, tricuspid valve, and pulmonary valve. Valvular tumors primarily arise from the middle of the valve rather than the edge. Tumors originating from the semilunar valves more commonly project into the arterial lumen. Those from the atrioventricular valves tend to project into the atria. One-fourth of these tumors occur on the endocardial, nonvalvular surface. Papillary fibroelastomas have been reported to originate from the left ventricle,[60] atrial septum,[61,62] ostia of the left and right coronary arteries,[60,63] left and right atrial appendages,[59,64,65] and both the left and the right ventricular outflow tracts.[53,66] Ninety-five percent of these tumors arise in the left heart. Fibroelastomas are typically solitary but can be multiple and may originate from the same location or different locations.[54,67]

The pathogenesis of these tumors is very poorly understood, and there is a lack of understanding of the genetic aberrations that underlie their development. It is evident that these lesions are benign, and they are morphologically distinct from other primary cardiac tumors.

Histology

Papillary fibroelastomas are avascular masses that are covered by a single layer of endocardial cells, with the matrix containing variable amounts of elastic fibrils. Ultrastructurally, the endocardial cells resemble endothelial cells.[68] These cells are hyperplastic and contain many organelles and pinocytic vesicles. The matrix is typically rich in proteoglycans and elastic fibers. Spindle cells similar to smooth muscle cells or fibroblasts also may be seen in the matrix, along with primitive mesenchymal-type cells. The elastic fibers in the matrix are highly variable and therefore may not be seen in certain processed sections. However, the layers of elastic fibers are the hallmark of papillary fibroelastomas. Calcifications are not as common as they are in myxomas. The connective tissue is characteristically marked by mature collagen and irregular elastic fibers that are arranged longitudinally.[4]

Immunohistochemical analysis is not sufficient for a definitive diagnosis of papillary fibroelastoma. Similar to myxomas, the surface cells of fibroelastomas can be positive for vimentin, factor VIII–related antigen, CD34, and S-100 protein.[68] Staining for collagen IV showed a pattern resembling that of elastic tissue. Unlike cardiac myxomas, fibroelastomas lack muscle-specific actin in the stellate cells of the stroma.[68] Other studies demonstrated the presence of dendritic cells and cytomegalovirus proteins in the intermediate layers of fibroelastomas. This suggested the possibility of a chronic viral endocarditis as the possible underlying cause of papillary fibroelastoma development. Evidence strongly supporting a hamartomatous, neoplastic, infective, or reparative process as the cause of fibroelastoma is lacking.

Lipomas

Lipomas are relatively common benign tumors of the heart. They occur in equal frequency in both sexes and are typically sessile or polypoid. The majority of lipomas occur in the subendocardium or subpericardium, and one-fourth are intramuscular. Depending on their location and size, lipomas may manifest clinical symptoms. Many of these tumors are clinically silent and typically are found incidentally or during autopsy. Subendocardial lesions may cause intracavitary extension and produce symptoms that are based on their location. Subpericardial lesions may produce symptoms of pericardial tamponade or effusion. Intramuscular tumors can cause mechanical interference, arrhythmias, and intraventricular or interventricular conduction abnormalities. The majority of lipomas occur in the left ventricle, followed by the right atrium and the interatrial septum.

The size range of reported lipomas is from 1 to 15 cm, with a weight up to 2000 g. These lesions are well encapsulated and contain mature fat cells with occasional fibrous connective tissue or muscular tissue (fibrolipoma and myolipoma). The molecular and genetic basis of cardiac lipomas is poorly understood. Unlike cutaneous lipomas that frequently are associated with rearrangement of chromosome band 12q15, resulting in disruption of the high-mobility group protein gene *HMG1C*, this aberration is not noted in cardiac lipomas. One study noted abnormalities involving a translocation between chromosomes 2 and 19.[69] On diagnosis, it may be difficult to distinguish a lipoma from a myxoma, as at times a lipoma may present as an intraatrial filling defect on diagnostic workup. In these situations, the definitive diagnosis can be made only after surgical resection of the mass.

Cardiac neurilemomas

Cardiac neurilemomas are extremely rare, with 10 reported cases in the literature.[70] These benign tumors are believed to originate from the cardiac branches of the vagus nerve and the cardiac plexus. They occur primarily in the adult population and by location are predominantly present on the right side of the heart. Grossly, the tumor is a solid mass, and on histology, fascicular proliferation of spindle-shaped cells can be noted. Immunohistochemistry is consistent with a neural origin, and staining is typically positive for S-100 and negative for actin.

Angiomas

Hemangiomas and lymphangiomas are extremely rare lesions.[71] They are composed of benign proliferations of endothelial cells that occur as collections of small and large vascular spaces. On histopathology, angiomas are red, hemorrhagic subendocardial nodules that range in size from 2 to 4 cm. They are marked by endothelium-lined spaces filled with blood, lymph, or thrombi. Based on the type of tissue with the higher proliferation, they are classified as hemangiomas or lymphangiomas. Microscopically, the two most common variants are capillary and cavernous hemangiomas. They are typically intramural, usually in the interventricular septum or the atrioventricular node, but may show a preference for the epicardium. Depending on their location, they may cause sudden death or complete heart block. Hemopericardium causing tamponade physiology also may be a presenting symptom. Hemangiomas can be confused with thrombosed, subendocardial blood vessels on gross examination.

Cardiac lymphangiomas are rarer than hemangiomas. They occur primarily in the pediatric population, but adult cases have been reported.[72] There have been fewer than 10 reported cases of primary cardiac lymphangioma.[73] The tumor is often multicystic, with collections of lymphatic vessels noted on histology.

Mesothelioma of the atrioventricular node

Even though the name indicates a specific histogenesis for these benign lesions, their origin is controversial. On histology, these tumors resemble adenomatoid tumors of the ovary and testis, and they are believed to originate from mesothelial rests. They are marked by tubules and cysts that are lined by flat or cuboidal cells. However, other studies suggest an endodermal origin.[74,75] Mesotheliomas of the atrioventricular (AV) node are typically small tumors (less than 1.5 cm) and often cause death by precipitating complete heart block, ventricular arrhythmias, or cardiac tamponade.[76] They do not have a specific age or sex distribution and occur as multicystic nodules that are unencapsulated, located in the atrial septum in the region of the AV node.

Purkinje cell tumors

These lesions have been described only in young infants, associated with tachyarrhythmias.[77] They are best described as cardiac hamartomas, but other popular names include foamy myocardial transformation of infancy, infantile cardiomyopathy with histiocytoid change, and infantile xanthomatous cardiomyopathy.[78] These lesions have a close association with infantile cardiac arrhythmias. They can occur as discrete or diffusely dispersed lesions in both ventricles.[77A] On pathology, they are usually subendocardial lesions and show clusters of myocardial cells with cytoplasmic changes consistent with increased vacuolations and increased eosinophilic staining.

Teratomas

Teratomas are rare tumors with an even lower occurrence rate in the heart than in the anterior mediastinum.[79] They classically contain elements of all three germ layers on histology. Grossly, these tumors contain multiloculated cysts intermingled with solid areas. They are seen more frequently in children and occur predominantly in the right atrium, right ventricle, and interventricular septum.

Endocrine tumors of the heart

These tumors are extremely rare. Most of them are paragangliomas, but pheochromocytomas and benign thyroid tumors also have been reported.[78A] Most intrathoracic paragangliomas occur in the posterior mediastinum. Some may originate in the epicardium of the left atrium or ventricle and, more rarely, in the interatrial septum. Paragangliomas of the heart are thought to originate from the sympathetic fibers to the heart. Similar to pheochromocytomas, paragangliomas may secrete catecholamines.

Very rarely, benign thyroid tumors arise in the heart after originating from ectopic thyroid tissue. They commonly present from the interventricular septum and can cause symptoms of right ventricular outflow obstruction.

Fibromas

As the name indicates, fibromas arise from fibroblasts in the connective tissue of the heart. They occur primarily in children and are the second most common primary cardiac tumor in the pediatric population. About 40 percent of the diagnosed tumors occur in infants, with equal distribution between the sexes. The biologic behavior of fibromas is similar to that of fibromas in other sites in the body. In some cases, cardiac fibromas may be associated with Gorlin's syndrome, which is characterized by multiple basal cell carcinomas, cysts of the jaw, and skeletal deformities.[80]

On gross pathology, fibromas appear as gray, firm, well-circumscribed, but unencapsulated masses (Fig. 43-3). They range in size from 3 to 10 cm. Focal calcifications and cystic degeneration are not uncommon findings. The majority of fibromas arise from the ventricular myocardium, predominantly in the anterior left ventricle and the interventricular septum. On histology, fibromas display elongated fibroblasts amid connective tissue rich in collagen, similar to fibromatoses (Fig. 43-4). Mitotic figures rarely are seen, and the distribution of the fibroblasts is variable. At times, elastin fibers may be seen, and the diagnosis of fibroelastic hamartoma may be made. In light of the association between cardiac fibromas and Gorlin's syndrome, the genetic causes of the latter may be involved in the former[80A]. Gorlin's syndrome results from mutations in the *PTC* gene, a tumor suppressor gene that is believed to be involved in controlling cell fate, growth, and development.[81,82] However, the role of the *PTC* gene in cardiac development is unclear.

Almost three-fourths of cardiac fibromas cause clinical manifestations that are determined by their size and location. These manifestations include mechanical interference with left-sided blood flow, contraction problems, and conduction abnormalities. The most common symptom is cardiomegaly. These tumors can lead to murmurs, congestive heart failure, right ventricular hypertrophy, arrhythmias, and sudden death. The mainstay of treatment is

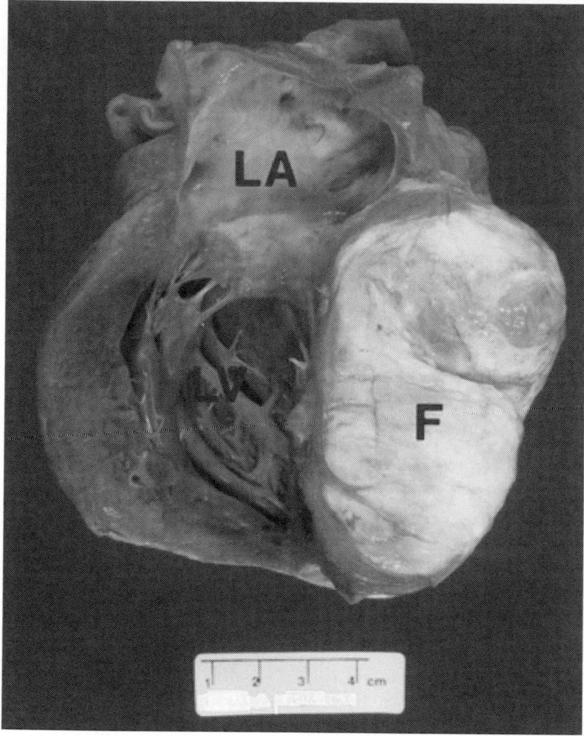

Figure 43-3 Cardiac fibroma. Gross pathologic specimen demonstrates a 7 × 4 × 4-cm pale, tan, firm, well-demarcated intramural mass in the posterior free wall of the left ventricle. LA = left atrium; F = fibroma. (Reproduced, with permission, from Wong JA, Fishbein MC. Cardiac fibroma resulting in fatal ventricular arrhythmia. *Circulation* 2000; 101(16):168.)

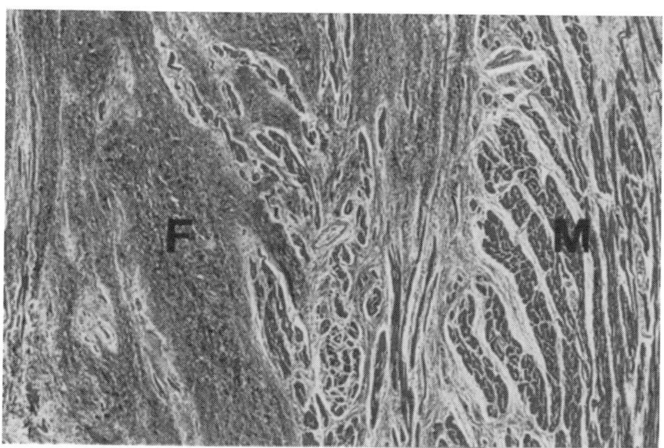

Figure 43-4 Cardiac fibroma. Light microscopy demonstrates infiltrating border of fibroma (F) and normal myocardium (M) (trichrome stain, magnification × 25). (Reproduced, with permission, from Wong JA, Fishbein MC. Cardiac fibroma resulting in fatal ventricular arrhythmia. *Circulation* 2000;101(16):168.)

surgical resection, and successful surgical excision of fibromas has been reported.[83,84]

Rhabdomyomas

Rhabdomyomas are benign tumors that are seen primarily in the pediatric population, with three-fourths occurring in children less than 1 year old.[223] The majority of rhabdomyomas are multiple, and over two-thirds of them occur with equal frequency in the left and right ventricles and the ventricular septum (Fig. 43-5).[85] One-third involve the atria. In children who present with symptoms, at least one of the tumors causes intracavitary obstruction. They also can cause right- and left-sided heart failure, murmurs, and symptoms resembling aortic, pulmonary, and mitral stenosis. Tumors that cause significant cavitary obstruction can lead to death in the first 24 h of life. Otherwise, these children may remain asymptomatic or have progressive symptoms. These tumors are typically multiple and lobulated. Spontaneous regression of rhabdomyomas has been reported.[87,197] Approximately 50 to 75 percent of rhabdomyomas are operable. Because these tumors may regress, observation with careful follow-up is recommended when possible.

There is a strong association between rhabdomyomas and tuberous sclerosis, with a 50 to 85 percent case association.[87,88] Tuberous sclerosis is characterized by hamartomas, seizures, mental deficiency, and adenoma sebaceum.[89,90] About 80 percent of children with

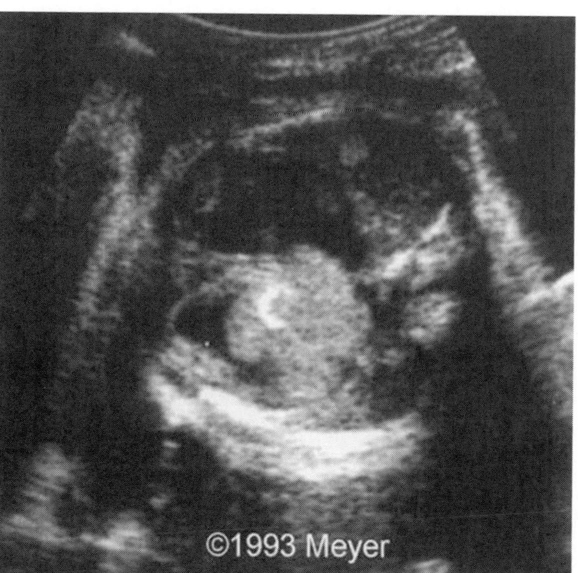

Figure 43-5 Cardiac rhabdomyoma. Echocardiographic four-chamber view of fetal thorax illustrating cardiac rhabdomyoma, which is represented by a bright, shaped lesion in the area of the mitral valve. (Reproduced, with permission, from William J. Meyer, MD, www.TheFetus.net, Department of Obstetrics and Gynecology, Division of Maternal-Fetal Medicine, University of Illinois at Chicago.)

rhabdomyomas may have tuberous sclerosis, and 60 percent of patients with tuberous sclerosis have rhabdomyomas.[90] Tumors that occur in association with tuberous sclerosis are usually multiple and smaller than are sporadic lesions.

On gross pathology, these tumors are smooth, well circumscribed, unencapsulated, and grayish in color. They range in size from 1 mm to 2 to 3 cm in diameter. On histology, they are characterized by "spider cells" that are up to 80 μm and have a cytoplasmic mass in the center with radiating fibrils extending to the periphery (thus the name *spider cells*). These tumors can be distinguished from normal myocardium as clusters with spider cells in them.[91] Ultrastructural studies show tumor cells containing myofibrils, glycogen, and intercellular junctions similar to intercalated discs. On immunohistochemistry, they are similar to muscle tissue, staining positive for myoglobin, actin, desmin, and vimentin. There is some controversy about the origin of rhabdomyomas. It is possible that these lesions are actually hamartomas of the heart. This idea is supported by the close association between rhabdomyomas and tuberous sclerosis and the predominance of hamartomas in patients with tuberous sclerosis. Molecular genetic studies in tuberous sclerosis patients have revealed two disease genes: *TSC1* and *TSC2*. Both seem to function as tumor suppressor genes, and loss of heterozygosity is associated with tumor development.[92,93] Quite possibly, these genes play a role in rhabdomyoma formation.

MALIGNANT PRIMARY CARDIAC TUMORS

Approximately 25 percent of all primary cardiac tumors are malignant.[7] Almost all malignant cardiac neoplasms are sarcomas, and of those sarcomas, rhabdomyosarcomas and angiosarcomas are the most common. Therefore, sarcomas are the second most common primary tumors of the heart after myxomas. Other sarcoma subtypes of the heart include fibrosarcomas, osteosarcoma, neurogenic sarcoma, leiomyosarcomas, liposarcomas, and synovial sarcomas.[94,95] Other malignant tumors of the heart are very rare and include malignant lymphomas, mesotheliomas, and thymomas. In general, malignant cardiac tumors display a rapid downhill course and have a high mortality rate.

Often it may be difficult to distinguish a cardiac mass from a malignant or benign lesion before operation, but it is important to look for signs and symptoms that suggest malignant disease preoperatively. Findings suggestive of a malignant cardiac lesion include gross evidence of distant metastatic disease, local invasion of the tumor into adjacent mediastinal or pleural structures, tumor originating from the right side of the heart or from free atrial wall, echocardiography showing intramural and intracavitary extension of the tumor, chest pain, and a hemorrhagic pericardial effusion. If a patient's cardiac tumor is being followed, a rapid growth rate of the tumor is more suggestive of a malignant process. It is important to note that benign cardiac tumors can mimic a malignant process. Fragments of benign tumor and/or thrombi can embolize to distant sites and mimic metastases. At times, an angioma can cause a hemorrhagic pericardial effusion. In patients with peripheral tumor emboli, it may be possible to attain the correct diagnosis by biopsying the emboli.[11,96–98] Making the right diagnosis can alter the treatment algorithm significantly, especially the decision to do surgery. It is equally important to know that surgeons can offer the only chance for a complete cure. Especially in cases in which benign disease mimics malignancy, it is imperative that surgical intervention be pursued if it is indicated. Even though benign primary cardiac tumors are nonmalignant, they can cause significant morbidity and mortality.

Sarcomas

As was mentioned earlier, sarcomas are the second most common primary cardiac tumors. The morphologic types of sarcomas were mentioned above. These patients frequently have rapid rates of clinical deterioration. These tumors proliferate and invade the myocardium and the adjacent structures rapidly. They generally cause death by infiltration into the myocardium, causing severe contractility problems, obstruction of flow, or distant metastases. Seventy-five percent of patients who present with cardiac sarcomas have metastatic disease at presentation; therefore, the mortality rates for these patients, even with surgical intervention, are high. The most common sites of metastases are the lungs, mediastinal nodes, and vertebral column, followed by intraabdominal organs such as the liver, kidneys, and adrenals.

The presenting symptoms of these patients depend on the location and the size of the tumor and the extent of metastasis. Patients usually present with worsening congestive heart failure, especially on the right side; chest pain; pericardial effusion; conduction abnormalities; obstruction of the venae cavae; weight loss; elevated inflammatory markers; visceral congestion; superior vena cava (SVC) syndrome; and sudden death. Because of the rapid growth of sarcomas, they typically extend into the pericardial space and the cardiac chambers. Of note, sarcomas are more common on the right side of the heart; therefore, symptoms of right-sided obstruction leading to congestion can be an important indicator of malignancy. Obstruction of the right atrium, tricuspid valve, right ventricle, or pulmonary valve may occur. Pulmonary artery sarcomas may present as tumor emboli to the lungs or as right ventricular outflow obstruction. SVC syndrome may result from extension of the tumor outside the heart, leading to obstruction of the superior vena cava.

Epidemiology

Sarcomas can occur at any age but are most common during the third to fifth decades of life. They are distributed equally between the sexes and are predominantly a disease of adults. The exceptions are angiosarcomas, which have a 2:1 male:female ratio,[99–102] and pulmonary artery sarcomas, which have a 2:1 female predominance. Unlike benign tumors of the heart, sarcomas are primarily a disease of the right side of the heart. The sites involved include the right atrium, left atrium, right ventricle, left ventricle, and interventricular septum, in decreasing order of frequency. Angiosarcoma and Kaposi's sarcoma of the heart show an especially strong predilection to originate in the right atrium.[99]

Pathology

Sarcomas may be sessile, infiltrative, or polypoid. All sarcomas derive from the mesenchyme and therefore can be of various morphologic types. Angiosarcomas are typically infiltrative or polypoid in nature (Fig. 43-6) and on histology are characterized by variable anastomotic vascular channels with poorly defined endothelial lining. The endothelial cell layers are irregular and clustered.[100A] Ultrastructural studies show endothelial cells, primitive pericytes, and undifferentiated mesenchymal cells.

Rhabdomyosarcomas often show an infiltrative pattern but also may have polypoid extensions into the cardiac chambers.[101A] They grow rapidly and thus diffusely infiltrate into the myocardium. They are characterized by distinct rhabdomyoblasts seen on microscopy. These cells display cross-striations and on ultrastructural studies display thick and thin filaments and Z bands. It is not uncommon to find mitoses and clusters or heaps of rhabdomyoblasts.

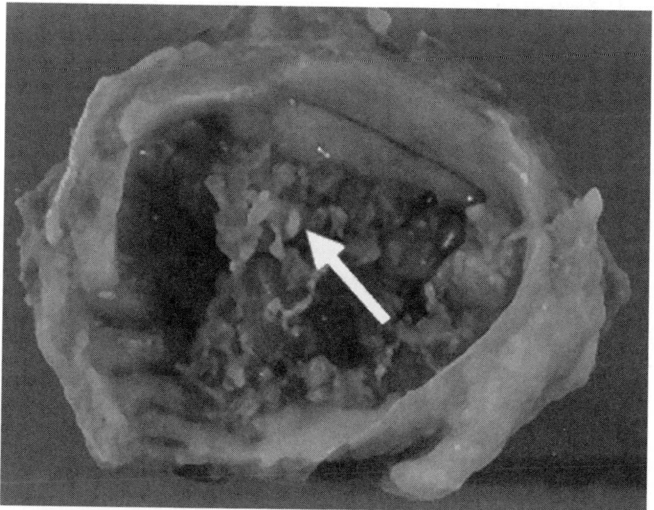

Figure 43-6 Cardiac angiosarcoma. Photograph of the resected specimen shows a portion of the right atrium and intraatrial tumor. Arising from the free wall of the right atrium, the angiosarcoma shows frondlike papillary projections (*arrow*). (Reproduced, with permission, from Best AK, Dobson RL, Ahmad AR. Cardiac angiosarcoma. *Radiographics* 2003;23:S141–145.)

Fibrosarcomas appear whitish and have a soft consistency on gross examination. These tumors tend to infiltrate the heart extensively and often contain areas of hemorrhage and necrosis. On histology, multiple clusters of spindle-shaped cells with elongated nuclei are seen.[102A] Mitoses are seen frequently.

Pulmonary artery sarcomas are very rare and potentially originate from the bulbus cordis. Most reported cases are diagnosed at autopsy. If an early diagnosis is made, surgical resection and chemotherapy are possible treatment options.

Primary lymphoma of the heart

Primary lymphoma of the heart is a very rare and often fatal neoplasm. These lymphomas constitute about 1 to 2 percent of all primary cardiac tumors and less than 0.5 percent of all extranodal lymphomas in immunocompetent patients.[86,103–105] They occur with a slight male predominance (1.5:1 male:female), and approximately 25 percent are diagnosed postmortem. In two-thirds of cases, primary cardiac lymphoma was noted in a single focus, with its size ranging from 3 to 12 cm.[106] A majority of these tumors are diffuse, large B-cell lymphomas that account for almost 70 percent of the cases.

On histology, cardiac lymphoma appears as a dense proliferation of large and intermediate-size cells that invade the myocardium (Fig. 43-7). The cells have a large basophilic cytoplasm with round nuclei.

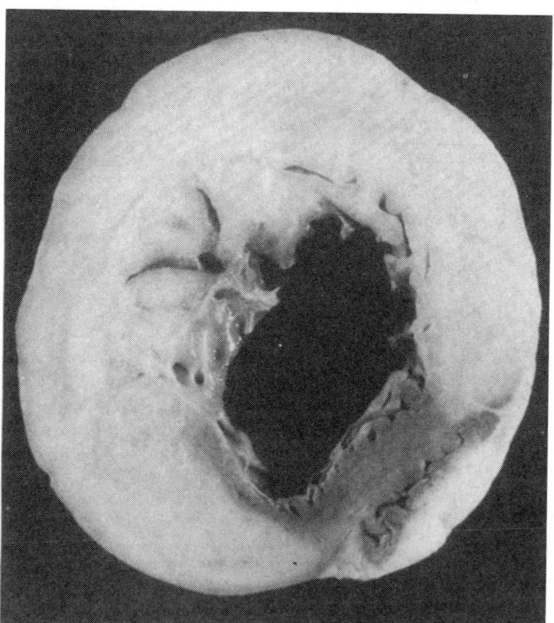

Figure 43-7 Primary cardiac lymphoma. Cross-sectional view of the heart shows replacement of myocardium with lymphoma. (Reproduced, with permission, from Yuh DD, Kubo SH, Francis GS, et al. Primary cardiac lymphoma treated with orthotopic heart transplantation: A case report. *J Heart Lung Transplant* 1994;13(3):538–542.)

CLINICAL PRESENTATION OF CARDIAC TUMORS

Some tumors cause systemic manifestations and cardiac manifestations, whereas other benign tumors may cause only cardiac manifestations.

Cardiac manifestations

The clinical manifestation of cardiac tumors is based on the location and size and the mobility of the tumor rather than its histology.[107] Though malignant tumors may present with other symptoms of local invasion and metastatic disease, the cardiac manifestations of these tumors also usually are based on their location and size. It is important to note that primary cardiac tumors can affect the pericardium through direct infiltration or by causing pericardial effusion. Although pericardial diseases and symptoms are discussed elsewhere, primary cardiac tumors should be included in the differential diagnosis of pericardial disease. Below, there is a discussion of clinical manifestations based on tumor location.

Left atrium

The most common primary cardiac tumor that presents in the left atrium is the benign myxoma. These tumors can be mobile and pedunculated and thus cause symptoms of mitral valve disease.[7,11,108] Left atrial tumors can prolapse into the mitral valve orifice and result in obstruction of AV blood flow. The symptoms can mimic those of mitral regurgitation or mitral stenosis, including dyspnea, orthopnea, paroxysmal nocturnal dyspnea, edema, pulmonary congestion, and fatigue. Symptoms that are not common to mitral valve disease also may occur, such as weight loss, pallor, syncope, and even sudden death.[11,109] Symptoms that are sudden and intermittent in nature are more suggestive of an atrial tumor than of mitral valve disease.[11,109] The most common initial symptoms of left atrial myxoma are dizziness, palpitations, dyspnea, cough, pulmonary edema, and congestive heart failure, followed by embolic manifestations and constitutional symptoms.[110] The classic triad of clinical symptoms seen with left atrial myxomas is obstructive cardiac signs, embolic phenomena, and systemic manifestations.

On examination, signs of pulmonary congestion may be evident, along with mitral valve disease. An audible S_4 and a loud and widely split S_1 suggest pulmonary congestion.[111] A holosystolic murmur that is heard best at the apex may indicate mitral regurgitation. A diastolic murmur suggestive of mitral stenosis may occur secondary to obstruction of the mitral valve orifice by the tumor. In several cases, an early diastolic sound called a tumor plop may be noted.[111] Probably it is secondary to sudden halting of the pedunculated and mobile tumor or results from the tumor hitting the endocardial wall.

Right atrium

Sarcomas are the most common tumor of the right atrium, followed by myxomas. The classic symptoms secondary to these tumors are right heart failure, fatigue, edema, and visceral congestion.[109,112–115] On examination, prominent *a* waves may be noted on the jugular venous pulse. These symptoms can be misdiagnosed as Ebstein's anomaly of the tricuspid valve, constrictive pericarditis, tricuspid valve disease, and SVC syndrome. Because sarcomas are the most common right atrial tumors, these patients often present with other systemic symptoms and metastases. The onset and progression of right-sided heart failure may be acute and rapid and frequently is associated with new systolic or diastolic murmurs.[116] Patients may develop pulmonary embolism and pulmonary hypertension, similar to the presentation of venous thromboembolic disease.[113] Murmurs are typically secondary to tricuspid stenosis from tumor obstruction of the valve or tricuspid regurgitation from failure of the valve to close as a result of tumor interference. In patients with right atrial tumors and a patent foramen ovale, right atrial hypertension can result in right-to-left shunting, leading to systemic hypoxia, cyanosis, and polycythemia.

On examination, these patients may have signs of SVC obstruction, signs of visceral congestion (hepatomegaly and ascites), peripheral edema, and jugular venous distention with a prominent *a* wave.[117] A holosystolic murmur may occur secondary to tricuspid regurgitation, or an early diastolic murmur may be heard as a result of valve stenosis. A diastolic tumor plop has been reported for right atrial tumors, similar to that with left atrial myxomas.[117]

Left ventricle

Tumors with extension into the cardiac chamber can cause obstructive symptoms, including syncope, and symptoms of left heart failure. Tumors with a significant intramural component can cause contractility problems and conduction abnormalities or arrhythmias. At times, these patients may complain of chest pain. On examination, there may be a systolic murmur, and blood pressure variations may occur that are caused by the position of the patient. Examination findings may mimic those seen with aortic stenosis or subaortic stenosis.

Right ventricle

Tumors of the right ventricle can cause symptoms of right heart failure. This may be secondary to obstruction of the right ventricle outflow tract or its filling. Right-sided heart failure may manifest in jugular venous distention, prominent *a* waves on jugular venous pulse, hepatomegaly, and ascites secondary to visceral congestion. Sudden nonfilling of the right side may cause syncope and death.[109,118] Tumor emboli to the pulmonary arteries may cause pulmonary hypertension and sudden shortness of breath. These patients may develop a presystolic murmur and a diastolic rumble.[109] A systolic murmur may result from tricuspid regurgitation. The onset and progression of right sided cardiac manifestations are typically rapid in patients with right ventricular tumors. Similar symptoms can develop secondary to pulmonary stenosis or tricuspid regurgitation, but these symptoms are quite slow in their progression.

Myocardium

Depending on their location and size, myocardial tumors can cause conduction abnormalities or rhythm disturbances.[76,119] Tumors such as angiomas and mesotheliomas can occur predominantly in the area of the AV node and thus cause AV conduction abnormalities, including complete heart block, asystole, and sudden death. Other arrhythmias of the heart can occur with tumors in other locations, including atrial fibrillation, premature ventricular beats, ventricular tachycardia, and ventricular fibrillation.[109] Tumor size and infiltration into the myocardium can cause contraction problems as well, leading to heart failure.

Valves

The most common tumors of the valves are papillary fibroelastomas. Patients with these tumors are typically asymptomatic but may present with a wide range of clinical manifestations. The most common findings include embolic phenomena to the brain, heart, lungs, and periphery. In light of the fact that a majority of fibroelastomas are in the left heart, most embolic phenomena are systemic. There have been several reports of emboli to the cerebral circulation; the emboli present as transient ischemic attacks, stroke, sudden visual loss, and sudden death.[120–125] Embolic phenomena to the visceral organs that cause mesenteric ischemia, renal infarcts, and limb ischemia also have been reported.[126,127] These patients also may develop heart failure and at times have sudden death.[128,129]

Larger tumors of the AV valves may cause symptoms of obstruction of the left or right ventricle, leading to heart failure. Tumors that cause significant and acute obstruction can lead to sudden death.[59,63] At times, the mechanism of sudden death may be an aortic valve tumor causing obstruction of the ostia of the right or left coronary arteries.[130] Valvular tumors may cause incomplete closure of the AV valves, leading to tricuspid or mitral insufficiency.[131,132] This may lead to the new onset of systolic murmurs on physical examination. Narrowing of other aortic outflow tract by a valvular tumor also may cause systolic murmurs. Diastolic murmurs may result from obstructed filling of the ventricles.

Systemic findings

Primary malignant tumors of the heart may cause several systemic manifestations, including fevers, embolic phenomena to the pulmonary vasculature and the systemic circulation, fever, and weight loss. The presence of these symptoms in patients with cardiac manifestations should alert the physician to the possibility of a malignant process. In addition, cardiac myxoma may cause systemic manifestations that can cloud the differentiation of a benign from a malignant underlying process. A wide variety of systemic manifestations of cardiac myxoma have been reported, including weight loss, fevers, arthralgias, rash, clubbing, anorexia, and embolic phenomena.[107,133,134] Abnormalities in laboratory values also have been reported, such as an elevated erythrocyte sedimentation rate, polycythemia, thrombocytosis, and leukocytosis.

Several reports support a role for interleukin-6 (IL-6) in the spectrum of systemic findings seen in patients with myxoma.[135–138] Myxomas constitutively synthesize and secrete IL-6, a proinflammatory cytokine associated with leukocytosis, acute-phase response, pyrexia, and activation of complement and clotting cascades. Elevation in several of the laboratory values mentioned above also may be secondary to IL-6 upregulation. IL-6 levels have shown to decrease after the removal of a cardiac myxoma, along with normalization of several laboratory values. Because of these systemic findings, the diagnosis of myxomas often is delayed, and these patients frequently are misdiagnosed with collagen vascular diseases, vasculitis syndromes, and other autoimmune conditions.[139–141]

Emboli

Embolic phenomena from tumor fragmentation or dislodged superimposed thrombi are well documented.[96,142–144] Most embolic phenomena are secondary to myxomas, but their occurrence also is reported secondary to other primary cardiac tumors. Myxomas are intracavitary lesions and are friable in consistency; therefore, they have a higher rate of tumor embolization. The clinical manifestations depend on the tumor location and the regions of embolization. Right-sided tumors frequently cause pulmonary emboli, leading to symptoms of shortness of breath, oxygenation problems, tachypnea, and tachycardia. They can be confused easily with thromboembolic disease. These patients may develop pulmonary hypertension and cor pulmonale.[145]

Embolization to the systemic circulation results from left-sided tumors, although with a patent foramen ovale, a right-sided atrial tumor may cause systemic embolization. This can result in mesenteric ischemia and infarction of visceral organs, cerebral embolization leading to transient ischemic attacks or stroke, syncope, seizures, peripheral limb ischemia, and infarctions of the heart secondary to coronary embolization. At times, patients with primary cardiac tumors may present only with neurologic sequelae. Biopsies of peripheral embolic material have been documented to aid in the diagnosis of primary cardiac tumors and therefore should be pursued actively.[94,95]

Systemic embolization can be widespread and thus mimic systemic vasculitis syndromes such as polyarteritis nodosa.[139] This is especially true when numerous vascular aneurysms are noted secondary to tumor emboli in conjunction with an elevated erythrocyte sedimentation rate, weight loss, fever, and arthralgias.

DIAGNOSIS

Dramatic improvements in noninvasive techniques to assess cardiac anatomy and function have helped tremendously in the management of cardiac tumors. With techniques such as computed tomography (CT), magnetic resonance imaging (MRI), and echocardiography becoming fixtures in algorithms of cardiac workup, the natural history of cardiac tumors has been altered dramatically. Benign tumors of the heart frequently are discovered incidentally, and the ability to do antemortem diagnosis is significantly better today.

Though physical findings in patients are helpful in the diagnosis of cardiac tumors, they are in no way pathognomonic. Most cardiac tumors, if symptomatic, produce symptoms and signs that are common to many other heart conditions. It is not uncommon for primary cardiac tumors to be diagnosed incidentally, primarily through echocardiography but also by MRI and CT.[146] Cardiac catheterization and angiography continue to play important roles in diagnosis, but it is important to note that this technique should not be pursued before other noninvasive modalities, preferably echocardiography and MRI, are used.

Clinical findings

Common physical findings for tumors in different locations of the heart were discussed in detail earlier in this chapter. These signs and symptoms are also common to other cardiac conditions. A few atypical physical findings may trigger a closer workup for cardiac tumors. For left atrial myxomas, there can be changes in the level of intensity of a systolic or diastolic murmur that are dependent on the position of the patient. This is not the case with valvular heart disease. These patients often have a loud S_1 that typically is split widely. A tumor plop heard after S_2 can be very helpful in strengthening the suspicion for a cardiac tumor. Right atrial tumors can produce a widely split and loud S_1. There may be a paradoxically split S_2 as a result of early closure of the pulmonary valve.

Plain chest radiography

The findings on plain films of the chest are suggestive but not pathognomonic of cardiac tumors. Suggestive findings include overall enlargement of the heart, pulmonary congestion, specific chamber enlargement, a widened mediastinum, and cardiac calcifications. In patients with malignant tumors, mediastinal adenopathy, pleural effusions, and pericardial effusions may be evident. If follow-up films show rapid progression of cardiac enlargement or the new onset of cardiac irregularity or cardiac calcifications, they may suggest a malignant process such as a primary sarcoma. Specific chamber enlargement may suggest cavitary obstruction secondary to a myxoma. Calcifications of the heart may be secondary to many cardiac tumors. Those seen in children should raise the suspicion of a tumor immediately.

Computed tomography

The role of CT in the diagnosis and management of primary cardiac tumors is not clear, but it may be important, especially as advances in CT technology continue to be made. CT can be very helpful in providing a high degree of tissue discrimination, evaluating extracardiac and pericardial structures, and evaluating the degree of intramural tumor extension.[147] Gating the CT image acquisition to the cardiac cycle improves image quality. Moreover, ultrafast CT technology allows for a short scanning acquisition time that reduces motion artifact and thus significantly improves the assessment of intracardiac masses.[147]

Magnetic resonance imaging

The ability of MRI to diagnose and delineate intracardiac masses is proven.[148] MRI may be more helpful in understanding tumor size, shape, and surface than is two-dimensional echocardiography. Contrast enhancement with gadolinium and multiple axial and sagittal views of the cardiac chambers and the tumor may provide precise information about the tumor and aid in surgical planning.[149] In addition, MRI may aid in depicting the tissue composition of cardiac lesions and/or masses, helping differentiate thrombi from tumors and benign from malignant tumors.

Echocardiography

Echocardiography is the most important diagnostic technique for diagnosing primary cardiac tumors. Tumors diagnosed by echocardiography can provide enough information to allow appropriate operative intervention without the need for preoperative angiography.[11] Compared with M-mode echocardiography, two-dimensional echocardiography is better for the diagnosis and classification of primary cardiac tumors.[11] It can provide information about tumor size, mobility, attachment, and location; all these findings are valuable in preoperative planning for potential surgery.

Two-dimensional echocardiography is especially helpful in the diagnosis of left ventricular tumors and tumors that do not prolapse through the mitral and tricuspid valves. It also aids in the detection of small tumors. Left atrial masses and/or lesions can be differentiated with this technique. On echocardiography, atrial thrombus is seen as a layered mass, typically in the posterior atrium, whereas atrial myxomas often appear as mottled masses with areas of echolucency. They are usually not in the posterior atrium. The areas of echolucency in the tumor correspond to regions of hemorrhage in the tumor. Echocardiography also can aid in understanding the hemodynamic changes caused by the tumor. The consequences of valvular disturbances and changes in cardiac contractility may be seen on echocardiography.

Left atrial myxomas can be classified on the basis of their appearance on echocardiography:[150] class I, small tumors prolapsing through the mitral valve; class II, small tumors that do not prolapse; class III, large tumors prolapsing through the mitral valve; class IV, large tumors that do not prolapse.

Transesophageal echocardiography

Transesophageal echocardiography (TEE) is more effective than transthoracic echocardiography in delineating tumor attachment and resolution and especially in detecting right atrial tumors.[151] It provides great visualization of both atria and the atrial septum. TEE even has been used to perform percutaneous biopsy of a right atrial tumor.[152] This method may be especially helpful when the transthoracic modality fails to diagnose the tumor. Studies also suggest that TEE has lower false-positive and false-negative rates than does transthoracic echocardiography.[151]

Angiography

Not all patients with a suspicion or known diagnosis of a primary cardiac tumor need to undergo cardiac catheterization and angiography. In fact, echocardiography, CT, or MRI may provide adequate information for proper diagnosis and treatment planning. The risks and costs of cardiac catheterization often outweigh the benefits of the supplemental information that it may provide. Conditions in which angiography may be helpful include the following situations: Noninvasive techniques are not sufficient in delineating a cardiac lesion, noninvasive techniques fail to provide necessary information about cardiac function and anatomy, and studies suggest the possibility of a malignant tumor. If supplemental information from angiography may alter a surgical approach and treatment planning, it can be beneficial.[153]

On coronary angiography, primary cardiac tumors may show deformity of cardiac chambers, filling defects in the cardiac chambers, compression of the cardiac chambers, wall motion abnormalities, and pericardial effusion. The most common finding is an intracavitary filling defect. Mobile filling defects reflect the possibility of pedunculated tumors, especially myxomas. Irregularities in the myocardial wall also may be observed and suggest an infiltrating tumor of the myocardium, raising the possibility of a malignant tumor. At times, angiography may show the vascular supply of a tumor and its source of blood supply.[153] This can help in surgical planning for an operable tumor.

It is imperative that noninvasive evaluation of a tumor be performed before cardiac catheterization. The performance of catheterization risks dislodging a fragment of a tumor, leading to embolic phenomena. The transseptal approach also may cause dislodgement of a tumor that is present in the region of the fossa ovalis.

TREATMENT

The treatment algorithm for primary cardiac tumors is primarily dependent on the nature of the tumor: benign versus malignant. Surgical resection is the only curative modality among the treatment options for primary cardiac tumors. Though malignant tumors may be candidates for potential tumor resection, operative resection is the treatment of choice for most benign cardiac tumors.[11,154,155] In fact, reports show complete cure of benign cardiac tumors, especially myxomas.[154,155] It is important to note that even benign tumors of the heart can cause severe complications, including embolic phenomena to the pulmonary and systemic circulation, heart failure, and sudden death. Therefore, it is imperative that treatment of all primary cardiac tumors be prompt, especially in patients with clinical manifestations. It is not rare for patients to die or have major complications while waiting for a complete diagnostic workup or surgical resection.[14,21,156]

Benign tumors

There are multiple reports of complete curative resection of benign cardiac tumors, mostly for cardiac myxomas.[154,155,186] The standard approach for resection of benign tumors is through a median sternotomy. Some epicardial tumors can be removed without placing the patient under extracorporeal circulation, but most benign cardiac tumors require that resection be performed under hypothermia, cardioplegic cardiac arrest, and cardiopulmonary bypass.[157,158] It is highly recommended that the tumor be removed under direct visualization rather than with closed approaches. It is critical that during resection tumor fragments not be dislodged and that excision be complete. It is also important to check the other chambers and valves for alternative tumor foci and tumor fragments.[21,159] If possible, the tumor should be removed en bloc. There are reports of large cardiac resections resulting from large benign tumors.[160] In one report, adequate resection of a large left atrial myxoma originating from the posterior wall required complete removal of the heart, followed by autotransplantation.[160] Some reports recommend laser photocoagulation around an attachment site of a myxoma stalk to prevent pretumorous cells from causing recurrence.[161] This also may help reduce the size of the atrial septal defect, facilitating post-excision repair of the defect.

The most common cardiac tumor reported in surgical series is atrial myxoma. Several reports document cure of atrial myxomas after surgical resection.[162,163] Some studies include postoperative follow-up to 10 to 15 years. A complete resection of an atrial myoma is advocated, including the root of the pedicle and the full thickness of the adjacent interatrial septum.[16,157–159] This often leaves an atrial septal defect that can be closed primarily, using a pericardial patch or a Dacron patch. If the tumor attaches to or lies in the vicinity of a heart valve, it may mandate a valve repair by annuloplasty or valve replacement with a prosthetic valve.[17,159,164] The reported long-term outcomes for atrial myxoma resection are excellent, with postoperative mortality ranging from 0 to 3 percent.[159,165] Because of the location of most atrial myxomas, resection of these tumors may precipitate supraventricular arrhythmias and AV conduction disturbances.[166,167]

In 1 to 3 percent of operative cases of sporadic atrial myxoma, there have been reports of recurrences.[34,157,168,169] The time of recurrence after resection has been reported to be as long as 14 years.[169] Possible causes of recurrence include incomplete resection, dislodging of tumor fragments preoperatively or intraoperatively, metasynchronous tumor, tumor embolization, malignant transformation, and the multifocal genesis of a myxoma. Many studies suggest the multifocality of atrial myxomas as the reason for the relatively high recurrence rates in patients with familial myxomas.[166,169,170] In cases of familial cardiac myxomas, it is not uncommon to see multilocular recurrences.[35] Recurrence rates are much higher in patients with familial myxomas, ranging from 12 to 22 percent.[171] The primary cause of recurrence in sporadic myxomas is proposed to be incomplete resection upon initial operation.[169,172] It is highly recommended that all patients undergoing surgical intervention for cardiac tumors get adequate follow-up through serial echocardiographic studies.[171]

As with myxomas, successful curative resections of other benign tumors of the heart are well documented in the literature.[173,174] These tumors include papillary fibroelastomas, rhabdomyomas in children, hemangiomas, lipomas, and fibromas. The intraoperative and postoperative concerns with these lesions are similar to those for myxomas. Depending on the location of the tumors, complete resection of the lesions is recommended. Patients with valvular tumors may undergo local excision with annuloplasty or a prosthetic valve replacement. For intramural tumors and those in the AV conduction pathway, it is critical to have a thorough understanding of the consequences of resection of myocardium or components of the AV conduction system. Preservation of adequate myocardium, preservation of the AV conduction system, and good AV valve function are high priorities. Still, the most important criterion is a complete resection. Therefore, it is not uncommon to sacrifice the papillary muscles, the AV conduction system, one of the AV valves, or the chordae tendineae to attain a complete resection. Of course, this necessitates the replacement of an AV valve, the placement of a permanent pacemaker, or both.

Similar to atrial myxomas, papillary fibroelastomas, which constitute 75 percent of all valvular tumors, have a high rate of curative surgical resection.[175–177] Therefore, surgical resection is the primary treatment modality for a majority of symptomatic and some asymptomatic papillary fibroelastomas. At diagnosis, it is recommended that anticoagulation be initiated immediately. Resection should include the root of the pedicle and the full thickness of the involved endocardium. After excision, repair may involve primary closure or the use of a pericardial or Dacron patch. If there is extensive valve involvement, it may warrant valve repair or replacement. For patients with unresectable tumors, some reports suggest long-term anticoagulation.[178,179] In one report reviewing mitral valve papillary fibroelastomas, 20 patients had simple tumor excision, 7 required mitral valve replacement, and 9 required mitral valve repair.[180] For asymptomatic patients, the decision to do surgical resection typically is based on the mobility of the tumor. Asymptomatic, nonmobile tumors can be followed closely, but mobile tumors should undergo prompt surgical resection. It is important to note that there are no randomized, controlled data to support these recommendations. There are some reports suggesting the use of video-assisted surgery for the resection of papillary fibroelastomas.[181–183] Procedures for resection include methods to avoid ventriculotomy. Left aortic valve tumors can be approached by a transaortic route, and mitral valve tumors can be approached through a left atriotomy.

Since a majority of cardiac myxomas arise in the left atrial septum, three generalized approaches can be conceived:[186] (1) biatriotomy, (2) left atriotomy, and (3) right atriotomy. There is no consensus on the ideal approach. Some argue that a biatriotomy is the best approach as it enables the surgeon to examine all four chambers and thus decreases the risk of recurrence.[185,194] Others report success with a right atrial approach.[184,187] Although biatrial and right atrial approaches are reported most commonly, a selective left atriotomy may be required for myxomas arising from the left atrial posterior wall.

For nonmyxomatous benign tumors, the surgical approach can be variable and has to be based on the location and size of the tumor. Several reports discuss variable approaches to resecting these tumors.[16,154,188–196] Importantly, though various cardiotomy procedures have been discussed, it is crucial that complete excision of all the tumor be performed, using negative margins. Complete excision of malignant tumors may not be possible because of the extensive infiltrative nature of these tumors.

In the pediatric population, rhabdomyomas are the most common benign tumors. In fact, intracavitary masses in this age group (especially under 1 year age) should be considered rhabdomyomas until proved otherwise. The diagnosis of a rhabdomyoma changes the treatment, as it is well known that these tumors can regress spontaneously.[197–199] Regression rates as high as 50 percent have been reported in the literature.[200]

Surgical intervention is indicated only if there are clinical manifestations from the tumor.

It is unclear whether a complete resection of a fibroma is always required.[201,202] There have been reports of partial resection of cardiac fibromas with no further growth on follow-up. Therefore, the recommendation is that in symptomatic patients, if surgical intervention is indicated, there is no need to do a complete resection if it endangers postoperative cardiac function. For symptomatic cardiac angiomas, it is recommended that a complete resection be undertaken as these tumors tend to persist unless excised. Similarly, resection of cardiac teratomas has had good results.[203] For cardiac fibromas in children and infants, the tumor often is unresectable; if this is the case, cardiac transplantation is an option.[200] Reports of surgical intervention for Purkinje cell tumors of the heart show a dismal prognosis.[204,205]

Malignant tumors

The primary algorithm in the treatment of malignant primary cardiac tumors is not surgical resection. As was mentioned earlier in this chapter, a majority of these tumors are sarcomas, and 75 percent of cardiac sarcomas have known metastases at presentation and/or diagnosis. Also, unlike benign tumors, malignant cardiac tumors tend to infiltrate extensively into the ventricular myocardium. Therefore, surgical resection is frequently not a viable option as a result of overt metastases or extensive myocardial infiltration.

There are reports that support a limited role for surgical intervention in the care of patients with malignant tumors. Surgery may aid in the palliation of hemodynamics and the alleviation of the cardiac and systemic manifestations of a malignant tumor. Some reports cite extension of life achieved by pursuing aggressive and combined modalities of treatment, including surgical resection with chemotherapy, radiation therapy, or orthotopic heart transplantation.[206–209] There may be a potential role for chemotherapy and/or radiation therapy in the treatment of cardiac sarcomas, especially lymphosarcomas.[206–209] Otherwise, most of the literature reports a dismal outcome for patients with cardiac sarcomas that is not altered by surgical resection, chemotherapy, radiation therapy, or a combination of any of these treatments.

In patients with primary cardiac lymphoma, surgical resection does not appear to improve patient survival.[210–213] However, some studies report remission of the tumor after treatment with chemotherapy, especially with anthracyclines.[210,214–216] Radiotherapy alone or combined with chemotherapy may confer a further survival benefit.[217,218] Overall, primary cardiac lymphoma has a dismal prognosis, and late diagnosis seems to be a major factor in the poor outcome in these patients. Reports show that about 60 percent of these patients die within 2 months of the diagnosis of the tumor.[106]

In the pediatric population, the occurrence of primary malignant cardiac tumors is exceedingly rare. Outside individual case reports, there is no consensus on the treatment and prognosis of these tumors. Treatment often is based on the information available from similar malignancies originating in other parts of the body.

Overall, unlike benign primary cardiac tumors, the prognosis for malignant primary cardiac tumors is very poor.[16,186,188–195] Most of these patients undergo surgical resection for palliative reasons (often incomplete) and then courses of chemotherapy and radiation therapy and still have poor outcomes (less than 25 percent 1-year survival).[83] Very few series report survival beyond 3 years in a few patients.[186,189,193,219,220] There is some evidence that complete resection, if possible, with adjuvant therapy can double the survival rate.[94] One alternative for these patients may be orthotopic heart transplantation.[221] Goldstein and associates reported that in six patients, if a complete resection was obtained with cardiectomy, orthotopic heart transplantation enabled long-term survival.[221] In an analysis of 21 patients with malignant primary cardiac tumors who underwent cardiectomy plus heart transplant, mean survival was only 12 months.[222] Among those 21 patients, 15 had sarcomas, 3 had malignant fibrohistiocytomas, and 3 had lymphomas. Seven patients in that group had a mean survival of 27 months after transplantation. In contrast, patients with benign tumors who received orthotopic heart transplantation had a mean survival of 46 months. Among the causes of death in the malignant tumor group, over 70 percent of the patients died of recurrent disease or metastases. In the seven patients with improved survival, only one had evidence of recurrent disease. Therefore, it seems that orthotopic heart transplantation may be an option for patients with malignant cardiac tumors only if complete resection of the tumor is possible.

References

1. King TW. 1845. On simple vascular growths in the left auricle of the heart. *Lancet* 2:428.
2. Goldberg HP, Glenn F, Dotter CT, et al. Myxoma of the left atrium: Diagnosis made during life with operative and postmortem findings. *Circulation* 1952;6:762.
3. Yater WM. Tumors of the heart and the pericardium: Pathology, symptomatology and report of nine cases. *Arch Intern Med* 1931;48:627.
4. Fishbein MC, Ferrans VJ, Roberts WC. Endocardial papillary elastofibromas. *Arch Pathol* 1975;99:335.
5. Cheitlin MD, McAllister HA, De Castro CM. Myocardial infarction without atherosclerosis. *JAMA* 1975;231:951.
6. Flotte T, Pinar H, Feiner H. Papillary elastofibroma of the left ventricular septum. *Am J Surg Pathol* 1980;4:585.

7. Allard MF, Taylor GP, Wilson JE, McManus BM. Primary cardiac tumors. In: Goldhaber SZ, Braunwald E (eds). *Cardiopulmonary Diseases and Cardiac Tumors: Atlas of Heart Diseases*, vol. 3. Philadelphia: Current Medicine; 1995:15.1–15.22.
8. Reynan K. Frequency of primary tumors of the heart. *Am J Cardiol* 1996;77:107.
9. Lam KYL, Dickens P, Chan ACL. Tumors of the heart. *Arch Pathol Lab Med* 1993;117:1027.
10. Tazelaar HD, Locke TJ, McGregir CGA. Pathology of surgically excised primary cardiac tumors. *Mayo Clin Proc* 1992;67:957.
11. Salcedo EE, Cohen GL, White RD, Davison MB. Cardiac tumors: Diagnosis and treatment. *Curr Probl Cardiol* 1992;17:73.
12. Pollia JA, Gogol LJ. Some notes on malignancies of the heart. *Am J Cancer* 21996;7:329.
13. Prichard RW. Tumors of the heart: Review of the subject and report of one hundred and fifty cases. *Arch Pathol* 1951;51:98.
14. Livi U, Bortolotti U, Milano A, et al. Cardiac myxomas: Results of 14 years experience. *Thorac Cardiovasc Surg* 1984;32:143.
15. Meller J, Teichholz LE, Pichard AD, et al. Left ventricular myxoma: Echocardiographic diagnosis and review of the literature. *Am J Med* 1977;63:816.
16. Blondeau P. Primary cardiac tumors—French study of 533 cases. *Thorac Cardiovasc Surg* 1990;38:192.
17. Sandrasagra FA, Oliver WA, English TAH. Myxoma of the mitral valve. *Br Heart J* 1979;42:221.
18. Balk AHM, Wagenaar SS, Bruschke AVG. Bilateral cardiac myxomas and peripheral myxomas in a patient with recent myocardial infarction. *Am J Cardiol* 1979; 44:767.
19. Dittmann H, Voelker W, Karsch KR, et al. Bilateral atrial myxomas detected by transesophageal two dimensional echocardiography. *Am Heart J* 1989;118:172.
20. Heath D. Pathology of cardiac tumors. *Am J Cardiol* 1968;21:315.
21. Peters MN, Hall RJ, Cooley DA, et al. The clinical syndrome of atrial myxoma. *JAMA* 1974;230:695.
22. Reddy DJ, Rao TS, Venkaiah KR, et al. Congenital myxoma of the heart. *Indian J Pediatr* 1956;23:210.
23. Carney JA, Hruska LS, Beauchamp GD, et al. Dominant inheritance of the complex of myxomas, spotty pigmentation and endocrine overactivity. *Mayo Clin Proc* 1986;61:165.
24. Van Galder HM, O'Brien DJ, Staples ED, et al. Familial cardiac myxoma. *Ann Thorac Surg* 1992;53:419.
25. Carney JA, Gordon J, Carpenter PC, et al. The complex of myxomas, spotty pigmentation and endocrine overactivity. *Medicine (Baltimore)* 1985;64:270.
26. Vidaillet HJ, Seward JB, Fyke FE, et al. Syndrome myxoma: A subset of patients with cardiac myxoma associated with pigmented skin lesions and peripheral and endocrine neoplasms. *Br Heart J* 1987;57:247.
27. Bennett WS, Skelton TN, Lehan PH. The complex of myxomas, pigmentation and endocrine activity. *Am J Cardiol* 1990;65:399.
28. Carney JA, Behnaz CT. Myxoid fibroadenoma and allied conditions (myxomatosis) of the breast. *Am J Surg Pathol* 1991;15:713.
29. McCarthy PM, Peihler JM, Schaff HV, et al. The significance of multiple, recurrent, and complex cardiac myxomas. *Thorac Cardiovasc Surg* 1986;91:389.
30. Burke AP, Virmani R. Cardiac myxoma: A clinicopathologic study. *Am J Clin Pathol* 1993;100:671.
31. Ferrans VJ, Roberts WL. Structural features of cardiac myxomas: Histology, histochemistry and electron microscopy. *Hum Pathol* 1973;4:111.
32. Malekzadeh S, Roberts WC. Growth rate of left atrial myxoma. *Am J Cardiol* 1989;64:1075.
33. Roudaut R, Gosse P, Dallocchio M. Rapid growth of a left atrial myxoma shown by echocardiography. *Br Heart J* 1987;58:413.
34. Desousa AL, Muller J, Campbell RL, et al. Atrial mycomas: A review of the neurological complications, metastases, and recurrences. *J Neurol Neurosurg Psychiatry* 1978;41:1119.
35. Markel ML, Armstrong WF, Waller BF, et al. Left atrial myxoma with multicentric recurrence and evidence of metastases. *Am Heart J* 1986;111:409.
36. DeMorias CF, Falzoni R, Alves VAF. Myocardial infarct due to a unique atrial myxoma with epithelial-like cells and systemic metastases. *Arch Pathol Lab Med* 1988;112:185.
37. Diflo T, Cantelmo NL, Haudenschild CC, et al. Atrial myxoma with remote metastasis: Case report and review of the literature. *Surgery* 1992;111:352.
38. Lie JT. The identity and histogenesis of cardiac myxomas: A controversy put to rest. *Arch Pathol Lab Med* 1989;113:724.
39. Stratakis CA, Carney JA, Lin JP, et al. Carney complex, a familial multiple neoplasia and lentiginosis syndrome: Analysis of 11 kindreds and linkage to the short arm of chromosome 2. *J Clin Invest* 1996;97:699.
40. Basson CT, MacRae CA, Korf B, Merliss A. Genetic heterogeneity of familial atrial myxoma syndromes. *Am J Cardiol* 1997;79:994.
41. Casey M, Mah C, Merliss AD, et al. Identification of a novel genetic locus for familial cardiac myxomas and Carney complex. *Circulation* 1998;98:2560.
42. Dobin S, Speights VO, Donner LR. Addition [1] [q32] as the sole clonal chromosomal abnormality in a case of cardiac myxoma. *Cancer Genet Cytogenet* 1007;96:181.
43. Miluncky J, Huang XL, Baldwin CT, et al. Evidence for genetic heterogeneity of the Carney complex. *Cancer Genet Cytogenet* 1998;106:173.
44. Dijkhuizen T, van den Berg E, Molenaar WM. Cytogenetics of a case of cardiac myxoma. *Cancer Genet Cytogenet* 1992;73:73.
45. Casey M, Vaughan CJ, He J, et al. Mutations in the protein kinase R1alpha regulatory subunit cause familial cardiac myxomas and Carney complex. *J Clin Invest* 1996;106:31.
46. Kirschner LS, Carney JA, Pack SD, et al. Mutations of the gene encoding the protein kinase A type 1-alpha regulatory subunit in patients with the Carney complex. *Nat Genet* 2000;26:89.
47. Kirschner LS, Sandrini F, Monbo J, et al. Genetic heterogeneity and spectrum of mutations of PRKAR1 alpha gene in patients with the Carney complex. *Hum Mol Genet* 2000;9:3037.
48. Veugelers M, Bressan M, McDermott DA, et al. Mutation of the perinatal myosin heavy chain associated

with a Carney complex variant. *N Engl J Med* 2004; 351:460.
49. Wold LE, Lie JT. Cardiac myxomas: A clinicopathologic profile. *Am J Pathol* 1980;101:219.
50. Goldman BI, Frydman C, Harpaz N, et al. Glandular cardiac myxomas. *Cancer* 1987;59:1767.
51. Kirkler DM, Rode J, Davies MJ, et al. Atrial myxoma: A tumor in search of its origins. *Br Heart J* 1992;67:89.
52. Prichard RW. Tumors of the heart: Review of the subject and report of one hundred and fifty cases. *Arch Pathol* 1951;151:98.
53. Anderson KR, Fiddler GI, Lie JT. Congenital papillary tumor of the tricuspid valve. *Mayo Clin Proc* 1977; 52:665.
54. Levinsky L, Srinivasan V, Gingell RL, et al. Papillary fibroelastoma of aortic and mitral valves following myectomy for idiopathic hypertrophic sub-aortic stenosis. *Thorac Cardiovasc Surg* 1981;29:187.
55. Jaffe II, Jacobs LE, Owen AN, et al. Rapid development of papillary fibroelastoma with associated thrombus: The role of transthoracic and transesophageal echocardiography. *Echocardiography* 1997;14:287.
56. Cesena FH, Pereira AN, Dallan LA, et al. Papillary fibroelastoma of the mitral valve 12 years after mitral valve commissurotomy. *South Med J* 1999;92:1023.
57. Burn CG, Bishop MB, Davies JNP. A stalked papillary tumor of the mural endocardium. *Am J Clin Pathol* 1969;51:344.
58. Braile DM, Rossi MA, Jacob JL, et al. 1993. Cystic fibroelastoma of the mitral valve: Report of a case. *J Thorac Cardiovasc Surg* 1993 ;106:1228.
59. Tsukube T, Ataka K, Taniguchi T, et al. Papillary fibroelastoma of the left atrial appendage: Echocardiographic findings. *Ann Thorac Surg* 2000;70:1416.
60. Rona G, Feeney N, Kahn D. Fibroelastic hamartoma of the aortic valve producing ischemic heart disease: Associated pulmonary glomus bodies. *Am J Cardiol* 1963;12:869.
61. Nakao T, Hollinger I, Attai L, et al.. Incidental finding of papillary fibroelastoma on the atrial septum. *Cardiovasc Surg* 1994;2:423.
62. Watchell M, Heritage DW, Pastore L, et al. Cytogenetic study of cardiac papillary fibroelastoma. *Cancer Genet Cytogenet* 2000;120:174.
63. Bossert T, Diegeler A, Spyrantis N, et al. Papillary fibroelastoma of the aortic valve with temporary occlusion of the left coronary ostium. *J Heart Valve Dis* 2000;9:842.
64. Howard RA, Aldea GS, Shapira OM, et al. Papillary fibroelastoma: Increasing recognition of a surgical disease. *Ann Thorac Surg* 1999;68:1881.
65. Schwinger ME, Katz E, Rotterdam H, et al. Right atrial papillary fibroelastoma: Diagnosis by transthoracic and transesophageal echocardiography and percutaneous transvenous biopsy. *Am Heart J* 1989;118:1047.
66. Uchida S, Obayashi N, Yamanari H, et al. Papillary fibroelastoma in the left ventricular outflow tract. *Heart Vessels* 1992;7:164.
67. Li Mandri G, Homma S, Di Tullio MR, et al. Detection of multiple papillary fibroelastomas of the tricuspid valve by transesophageal echocardiography. *J Am Soc Echocardiogr* 1994;7:315.
68. Rubin MA, Snell JA, Tazelaar HD, et al. Cardiac papillary fibroelastoma: An immunohistochemical investigation and unusual clinical manifestations. *Mod Pathol* 1995;8:402.
69. Vaughan CJ, Weremowicz S, Goldstein MM, et al. A t(2;19)(p13;p13.2) in a giant invasive lipoma from a patient with multiple lipomatosis. *Genes Chromosomes Cancer* 2000;28:133.
70. Nakamura K, Onitsuka T, Yano M, et al. Surgical resection of right atrial neurilemoma extending to pulmonary vein. *Eur J Thor Surg* 2003;24:840.
71. Chao JC, Reyes CV, Hwang MH. Cardiac hemangioma. *South Med J* 1990;83:44.
72. Anbe DT, Fine G. Cardiac lymphangioma and lipoma: Report of a case of simultaneous occurrence in association with lipomatous infiltration of the myocardium and cardiac arrhythmia. *Am J Heart* 1973;86:227.
73. Kaji T, Takamatsu H, Noguchi H, et al. Cardiac lymphangioma: Case report and review of the literature. *J Pediatr Surg* 2002;37:1.
74. Monma N, Satodate R, Tashiro A, et al. Origin of so-called mesothelioma of the atriventricular node. *Arch Pathol Lab Med* 1991;115:1026.
75. Burke MAP, Anderson PG, Virmani R, et al. Tumor of the atrioventricular nodal region. *Arch Pathol Lab Med* 1990;114:1057.
76. Balasundaram S, Halees SA, Duran C. Mesothelioma of the atrioventricular node: First successful follow-up after excision. *Eur Heart J* 1992;13:718.
77. Meysman M, Noppen M, Demeyer G, Vincken W. Malignant epithelial mesothelioma presenting as cardiac tamponade. *Eur Heart J* 1993;14:1576.
77A. Garson A Jr, Smith RT Jr, Moak JP, et al. Incessant ventricular tachycardia in infants: Myocardial hamartomas and surgical cure. *J Am Coll Cardiol* 1987; 38:241.
78. Kearney DL, Titus JL, Hawkins EP, et al. Pathologic features of myocardial hamartomas causing childhood tachyarrhythmias. *Circulation* 1987;75:705.
78A. David TE, Lenkei SC, Marquez-Julio A, et al. Pheochromocytoma of the heart. *Ann Thorac Surg* 1986;41:98.
79. Becker AE. Primary heart tumors in the pediatric age group: A review of salient pathologic features relevant for clinicians. *Pediatr Cardiol* 2000;21:317.
79. Cox JN, Friedli B, Mechmeche M, et al. Teratoma of the heart. *Virchows Arch* 1983;402:163.
80. Feldman PS, Meyer MW. Fibroblastic hamartoma of the heart. *Cancer* 1976;38:314.
80A. Jones KI, Wolf PL, Jensen P, et al. The Gorlin syndrome: A genetically determined disorder associated with cardiac tumor. *Am Heart J* 1986;111:1013.
81. Cotton JL, Kavey RW, Palmier CE, et al. Cardiac tumors and the nevoid basal cell carcinoma syndrome. *Pediatrics* 1991;87:725.
82. Hahn H, Wicking C, Zaphiropoulos PG, et al. Mutations of the human homolog of Drosophila patched in the nevoid basal cell carcinoma syndrome. *Cell* 1996;85:841.
83. Miralles A, Bracamonte L, Soncul H, et al. Cardiac tumors: Clinical experience and surgical results in 74 patients. *Ann Thorac Surg* 1991;52:886.

84. Tazelaar HD, Locke TJ, McGregor CGA. Pathology of surgically excised primary cardiac tumors. *Mayo Clin Proc* 1992;67:957.
85. Elderkin RA, Radford DJ. Primary cardiac tumors in a pediatric population. *J Pediatr Child Health* 2002; 38:173.
86. Rolla G, Bertero MT, Pastena G, et al. Primary lymphoma of the heart: A case report and review of the literature. *Leuk Res* 2002;26:117.
87. Alkalay AL, Ferry DA, Lin B, et al. Spontaneous regression of cardiac rhabdomyoma in tuberous sclerosis. *Clin Pediatr* 1987;26:532.
88. Harding CO, Pagon RA. Incidence of tuberous sclerosis in patients with cardiac rhabdomyoma. *Am J Med Genet* 1990;37:443.
89. Gibbs JL. The heart and tuberous sclerosis: An echocardiographic and electrocardiographic study. *Br Heart J* 1985;54:596.
90. Webb DW, Thomas RD, Osborne JP. Cardiac rhabdomyomas and their association with tuberous sclerosis. *Arch Dis Child* 1993;68:367.
91. Moriarty AT, Nelson WA, McGahey B. Fine needle aspiration of rhabdomyosarcoma of the heart. *Acta Cytol* 1990;34:74.
92. Green AJ, Johnson PH, Yates JR. 1994. The tuberous sclerosis gene on chromosome 9q34 acts as a growth suppressor. *Hum Mol Genet* 1994;31:1833.
93. Green AJ, Smith, Yates JR. Loss of heterozygosity of chromosome 16p13.3 in hamartomas from tuberous sclerosis patients. *Nat Genet* 1994;6:193.
94. Putnam JB, Sweeney MS, Colon R, et al. Primary cardiac sarcomas. *Ann Thorac Surg* 1991;51:906.
95. Burke AP, Cowan D, Virmani R. Primary sarcoma of the heart. *Cancer* 1992;69:387.
96. Eriksen UH, Baandrup U, Jensen BS. Total disruption of left atrial myxoma causing a cerebral attack and a saddle embolus in the iliac bifurcation. *Int J Cardiol* 1992;35:127.
97. Weerasena NA, Groome D, Pollock JG, et al. Atrial myxoma as the cause of acute lower limb ischemia in a teenager. *Scott Med J* 1989;34:440.
98. Reed RJ, Utz MP, Terezakis N. Embolic and metastatic cardiac myxoma. *Am J Dermatopathol* 1989;11:157.
99. Klima U, Wimmer-Greinecker G, Harringer W, et al. Cardiac angiosarcoma—a diagnostic dilemma. *Cardiovasc Surg* 1993;1:674.
100. Hermann MA, Shankerman RA, Edwards WD, et al. Primary cardiac angiosarcoma: A clinicopathologic study of six cases. *J Thorac Cardiovasc Surg* 1992; 103:655.
100A. Keohane ME, Lazzam C, Halperin JL, et al. Angiosarcoma of the left atrium mimicking myxoma. *Hum Pathol* 1989;20:599.
101. Dennig K, Lehmann G, Richter T. 2000. An angiosarcoma in the left atrium. *N Engl J Med* 2000;342:443.
101A. Proctor MS, Tacy GP, Von Koch L. Primary cardiac B cell lymphoma. *Am Heart J* 118:179.
102. Butany J, Yu W. Cardiac angiosarcoma: Two cases and a review of the literature. *Can J Cardiol* 2000;16:197.
102A. Basso C, Stefani A, Calabrese F, et al. Primary right atrial fibrosarcoma diagnosed by endocardial biopsy. *Am Heart J* 1996;131:399.
103. Cairns P, Butany J, Fulop J, et al. Cardiac presentation of non-Hodgkin's lymphoma. *Arch Pathol Lab Med* 1987;111:80.
104. Holladay AO, Siegel RJ, Schwartz DA. Cardiac malignant lymphoma in acquired immune deficiency syndrome. *Cancer* 1992;70:2203.
105. Burke A, Virmani R. Tumors of the heart and great vessels. In: Rosai J (ed). *Atlas of Tumor Pathology*, fascicle 16, third series. Washington, DC: Armed Forces Institute of Pathology; 1995;231–235.
106. Chalabreysse L, Berger F, Loire R, et al. Primary cardiac lymphoma in immunocompetent patients: A report of three cases and review of the literature. *Virchows Arch* 2002;441:456.
107. St. John Sutton MG, Mercier L, Guliani ER, Lie JT. Atrial myxomas: A review of clinical experience in 40 patients. *Mayo Clin Proc* 1980;55:371.
108. Lantz DA, Dougherty TH, Lucca MJ. Primary angiosarcoma of the heart causing cardiac rupture. *Am Heart J* 1989;118:186.
109. Harvey WP. Clinical aspects of cardiac tumors. *Am J Cardiol* 1968;21:328.
110. Pinede L, Duhaut P, Loire R. Clinical presentation of left atrial cardiac myxoma: A series of 112 consecutive cases. *Medicine (Baltimore)* 2001;80:159.
111. Gershlick AH, Leech G, Mills PG, et al. The loud first heart sound in left atrial myxoma. *Br Heart J* 1984; 52:403.
112. Teoh KH, Mulji A, Tomlinson CW, et al. Right atrial myxoma originating from the Eustachian tube. *Can J Cardiol* 1993;9: 41.
113. Heck HA, Gross CM, Houghton JL. Longterm severe pulmonary hypertension associated with right atrial myxoma. *Chest* 1992;102:301.
114. Pessotto R, Santini F, Piccin C, et al. Cardiac myxoma of the tricuspid valve: Description of a case and review of the literature. *J Heart Valve Dis* 3:344.
115. Savino JS, Weiss SJ. Right atrial tumor. *N Engl J Med* 1995;333:1608.
116. Waxler EB, Kawai N, Kasparian H. Right atrial myxoma: Echocardiographic, phonocardiographic and hemodynamic signs. *Am Heart J* 1972;82:251.
117. Keren A, Chenzbruna A, Schuger L, et al. The etiology of tumor plop in a patient with huge right atrial myxoma. *Chest* 1989;95:1147.
118. Hada Y, Wolfe C, Murry CF, et al. Right ventricular myxoma: Case report and review of phonocardiographic auscultatory manifestations. *Am Heart J* 1980;100:871.
119. Kawano H, Okada R, Kawano Y, et al. Mesothelioma in the atrioventricular node: Case report. *Jpn Heart J* 1994;35:255.
120. Fowles RE, Miller C, Ebgert BM, et al. Systemic embolization from a mitral valve papillary endocardial fibroma detected by two dimensional echocardiography. *Am Heart J* 1981;102:128.
121. Ong S, Nanda NC, Barold SS. Two dimensional echocardiographic detection and diagnostic features of left ventricular papillary fibroelastoma. *Am Heart J* 1982;103:916.
122. Topol EJ, Biern RO, Reitz BA. Cardiac papillary fibroelastoma and stroke. *Am J Med* 1986;80:129.

123. McFadden PM, Lacy JR. Intracardiac papillary fibroelastoma: An occult cause of embolic neurologic deficit. *Ann Thorac Surg* 1987;43:667.
124. Giannesini c, Kubis N, N'Guyen A, et al.. Cardiac papillary fibroelastoma: A rare cause of ischemic stroke in the young. *Cerebrovasc Dis* 1999;9:45.
125. Lopez-Sanchez E, Munoz EF, Avino Martinez JA, et al. Central retinal artery occlusion as the initial sign of aortic valve papillary fibroelastoma. *Am J Opthalmol* 2001; 131:667.
126. Harris LS, Adelson L. Fatal coronary embolism from a myxomatous polyp of the aortic valve: An unusual cause of death. *Am J Clin Pathol* 1965;43:61.
127. Pasteuning WH, Zijnen P, van der Aa MA, et al. Papillary fibroelastoma of the aortic valve in a patient with an acute myocardial infarction. *J Am Soc Echocardiogr* 1996;9:897.
128. Fitzgerald D, Gaffney P, Dervan P, et al. Giant Lambl's excrescence presenting as a peripheral embolus. *Chest* 1982;81:516.
129. Klarich KW, Enriquez-Sarano M, Gura GM, et al. Papillary fibroelastoma: Echocardiographic characteristics for diagnosis and pathologic correlation. *J Am Coll Cardiol* 1997;30:784.
130. Bussani R, Silvestri F. Sudden death in a woman with fibroelastoma of the aortic valve chronically occluding the right coronary ostium. *Circulation* 1999;100:2204.
131. Bedi HS, Sharma VK, Mishra M, et al. Papillary fibroelastoma of the mitral valve associated with rheumatic mitral stenosis. *Eur J Cardiothorac Surg* 1995;9:54.
132. Di Mattia DG, Assaghi A, Mangini A, et al. Mitral valve repair for anterior leaflet papillary fibroelastoma: Two case descriptions and a literature review. *Eur J Cardiothorac Surg* 1999;15:103.
133. Goodwin JF. Symposium on cardiac tumors: The spectrum of cardiac tumors. *Am J Cardiol* 1968;21:307.
134. Idir M, Oysel N, Guibaud JP, et al. Fragmentation of a right atrial myxoma presenting as a pulmonary embolism. *J Am Soc Echocardiogr* 2000;13:61.
135. Wada A, Kanda T, Hayashi R, et al. Cardiac myxoma metastasized to the brain: Potential role of endogenous interleukin-6. *Cardiology* 1993;83:208.
136. Seino Y, Ikeda U, Shimada K. Increased expression of interleukin-6 mRNA in cardiac myxomas. *Br Heart J* 1993;69:565.
137. Seguin JR, Beigbeder JY, Hvass U, et al. Interleukin-6 production by cardiac myxomas may explain constitutional symptoms. *J Thorac Cardiovasc Surg* 1992; 103:599.
138. Jourdan M, Bataille R, Sequin J, et al. Constitutive production of interleukin-6 and immunologic features in cardiac myxomas. *Arthritis Rheum* 1990;33:398.
139. Leonhardt ETG, Kullenberg KPG. Bilateral atrial myxomas with multiple arterial aneurysms: A syndrome mimicking polyarteritis nodosa. *Am J Med* 1977;62:792.
140. Byrd WE, Matthews OP, Hunt RE. Left atrial myxoma presenting as a systemic vasculitis. *Arthritis Rheum* 1980;23:240.
141. Feldman AR, Keeling JH. Cutaneous manifestation of atrial myxoma. *J Am Acad Dermatol* 1989;21:1080.
142. De Carli S, Sechi LA, Ciani R, et al. Right atrial myxoma with pulmonary embolism. *Cardiology* 1994; 84:368.
143. Miyauchi Y, Endo T, Kuroki S, et al. Right atrial myxoma presenting with recurrent episodes of pulmonary embolism. *Cardiology* 1992;81:178.
144. Boussen K, Moalla M, Blondeau P, et al. Embolization of cardiac myxomas masquerading as polyarteritis nodosa. *J Rheumatol* 1991;18:283.
145. Heath D, Mackinnon J. Pulmonary hypertension due to myxoma of the right atrium: With special reference to the behavior of emboli of myxoma in the lung. *Am Heart J* 1964;68:227.
146. Lane GE, Kapples EJ, Thompson RC, et al. Quiescent left atrial myxoma. *Am Heart J* 1994;127:1629.
147. Bleiweis MS, Georgiou D, Brundage BH. Detection of intracardiac masses by ultrafast computed tomography. *Am J Card Imaging* 1994;8:69.
148. Fujita N, Caupto GR, Higgins CB. Diagnosis and characterization of intracardiac masses by magnetic imaging. *Am J Card Imaging* 1994;8:69.
149. Reddy DB, Jena Col A, Venugopal P. Magnetic resonance imaging (MRI) in evaluation of left atrial masses: An in vitro and in vivo study. *J Cardiovasc Surg* 1994; 35:289.
150. Charuzi Y, Bolger A, Beeder C, Lew AS. A new echocardiographic classification of left atrial myxoma. *Am J Cardiol* 1985;55:614.
151. Edwards LC, Louie EK. Transthoracic and transesophageal echocardiography for the evaluation of cardiac tumors, thrombi, and valvular vegetations. *Am J Card Imaging* 1994;8:45.
152. Azuma T, Ohira A, Akagi H, et al. Transvenous biopsy of a right atrial tumor under transesophageal echocardiographic guidance. *Am Heart J* 1996;131:402.
153. Fueredi GA, Knetchtges TE, Czarnecki DJ. Coronary angiography in atrial myxoma: Findings in 9 cases. *AJR Am J Roentgenol* 1989;152:737.
154. Wiatrowska BA, Walley VM, Masters RG, et al. Surgery for cardiac tumors: The University of Ottawa Heart Institute experience (1980-1991). *Can J Cardiol* 1993;9:65.
155. Aru GM, Falchi S, Cardu G, et al. The role of transesophageal echocardiography in the monitoring of cardiac mass removal: A review of 17 cases. *J Card Surg* 1993;8:554.
156. Thomas KE, Winchel CP, Varco RL. Diagnostic and surgical aspects of left atrial tumors. *J Thorac Cardiovasc Surg* 1967;53:535.
157. Gerbode F, Kerth WJ, Hill JD. Surgical management of the tumors of the heart. *Surgery* 1967;61:94.
158. Dein JR, Frist WH, Stinson EB, et al. Primary cardiac neoplasms: Early and late results of surgical treatment in 42 patients. *J Thorac Cardiovasc Surg* 1987;93:502.
159. Hanson EC, Gill CC, Razavi M, et al. The surgical treatment of atrial myxomas: Clinical experience and late results in 33 patients. *J Thorac Cardiovasc Surg* 1985;89:298.
160. Scheld HH, Nestle HW, Kling D, et al. Resection of a heart tumor using autotransplantation. *Thorac Cardiovasc Surg* 1988;36:40.
161. Mesnildrey P, Bloch G, Cachera JP, Piwicna A. Atrial myxoma: A new surgical approach using neodymium: yttrium-aluminum-garnet laser photocoagulation. *J Thorac Cardiovasc Surg* 1989;98:313.

162. Larson S, Lepore V, Kennergren C. Atrial myxomas: Results of 25 years experience and review of the literature. *Surgery* 1989;105:695.
163. Bortolotii U, Maraglino G, Rubino M, et al. Surgical excision of intracardiac myxomas: A 20 year followup. *Ann Thorac Surg* 1990;49:449.
164. Sharma SC, Kulkarni A, Bhargava V, et al. Myxoma of the tricuspid valve. *J Thorac Cardiovasc Surg* 1991;101:938.
165. Fang BR, Chiang CW, Hung JS, et al. Cardiac myxoma— clinical experience in 24 patients. *Int J Cardiol* 1990;29:335.
166. Martin LW, Wasserman AG, Goldstein H, et al. Multiple cardiac myxomas with multiple recurrences: Unusual presentation of a benign tumor. *Ann Thorac Surg* 1987; 44:77.
167. Bateman TM, Gray RJ, Raymond MJ, et al. Arrhythmias and conduction disturbances following cardiac operation for the removal of left atrial myxomas. *J Thorac Cardiovasc Surg* 1983;86:601.
168. Read RC, White HJ, Murphy ML, et al. The malignant potentiality of left atrial myxoma. *J Thorac Cardiovasc Surg* 1974;68:857.
169. Gray IR, Williams WG. Recurring cardiac myxoma. *Br Heart J* 1985;53:645.
170. Liebler GA, Margovern GJ, Park SB, et al. Familial myxomas in four siblings. *Thorac Cardiovasc Surg* 1976;71:605.
171. McCarthy PM, Piehler JM, Schaff HV, et al. The significance of multiple, recurrent, and complex cardiac myxomas. *Thorac Cardiovasc Surg* 1986;91:389.
172. Waller DA, Ettles DF, Saunders NR, et al. Recurrent cardiac myxoma: The surgical implications of two distinct groups of patients. *Thorac Cardiovasc Surg* 1989;37:226.
173. Corno A, deSimone G, Catena G, Marcelletti C. Cardiac rhabdomyoma: Surgical treatment in the neonate. *Thorac Cardiovasc Surg* 1984;37:725.
174. Orringer MB, Sisson JC, Glazer G, et al. Surgical treatment of cardiac pheochromocytomas. *J Thorac Cardiovasc Surg* 1985;89:753.
175. Ragni T, Grande M, Cappuccio G, et al. Embolizing fibroelastoma of the aortic valve. *Cardiovasc Surg* 1994;2:639.
176. Shahian DM, Labib SB, Chang G. Cardiac papillary fibroelastoma. *Ann Thorac Surg* 1995;59:538.
177. Grinda JM, Couetil JP, Chauvaud S, et al. Cardiac valve papillary fibroelastoma: Surgical excision for revealed or potential embolization. *J Thorac Cardiovasc Surg* 1999;117:106.
178. Pinelli G, Carteaux JP, Mertes PM, et al. Mitral valve tumor revealed by stroke. *J Heart Valve Dis* 1995;4:199.
179. Sastre-Garriga J, Molina C, Montaner J, et al. Mitral papillary fibroelastoma as a cause of cardiogenic embolic stroke: Report of two cases and a review of the literature. *Eur J Neurol* 2000;7:449.
180. DiMattia DG, Assaghi A, Mangini A, et al. Mitral valve repair of anterior leaflet papillary fibroelastoma: Two case descriptions and a literature review. *Eur J Thor Surg* 1999;15:103.
181. Allen KB, Goldin M, Mitra R. Transaortic video-assisted excision of a left ventricular papillary fibroelastoma. *J Thorac Cardiovasc Surg* 1996;112:199.
182. Espada R, Talwalker NG, Wilcox G, et al. Visualization of ventricular fibroelastoma with a video-assisted thoracoscope. *Ann Thorac Surg* 1997;63:221.
183. Reuthebuch O, Roth M, Skwara W, et al. Cardioscopy: Potential applications and benefit in cardiac surgery. *Eur J Cardiothorac Surg* 199;15:824.
184. Centofanti P, Rosa ED, Deorsola L, et al. Primary cardiac tumors: Early and late results of surgical treatment in 91 patients. *Ann Thorac Surg* 1999;68:1236.
185. Jones DR, Warden HE, Murray GF, et al. Biatrial approach to cardiac myxomas: A 30 year clinical experience. *Ann Thorac Surg* 1995;59:851.
186. Kamiya H, Yasuda T, Nagamine H, et al. Surgical treatment of primary cardiac tumors: 28 years experience in Kanazawa University Hospital. *Jpn Circ J* 2001;65:315.
187. Bjessmo S, Ivert T. Cardiac myxoma: 40 years experience in 63 patients. *Ann Thorac Surg* 1997;63:697.
188. Molina JE, Edwards JE, Ward HB. Primary cardiac tumors: Experience at the University of Minnesota. *Thorac Cardiovasc Surg* 1990;38:183.
189. Murphy MC, Sweeney MS, Putnam JB, et al. Surgical treatment of cardiac tumors: A 25 year experience. *Ann Thorac Surg* 1990;49:612.
190. Basso C, Valente M, Poletti A, et al. Surgical pathology of primary cardiac and pericardial tumors. *Eur J Cardiothorac Surg* 1997;12:730.
191. Perchinsky MJ, Lichtenstein SV, Tyers GF, et al. Primary cardiac tumors: Forty years experience with 71 patients. *Cancer* 1997;79:1809.
192. Tschirkov A, Michev B, Topalov V, et al. Incidences and surgical aspects of cardiac myxomas in Bulgaria. *Thorac Cardiovasc Surg* 1990;38:196.
193. Moosdorf R, Scheld H, Hehrlein FW. Tumors of the heart: Experiences at the Gissen University Clinic. *Thorac Cardiovasc Surg* 1990;38:208.
194. Dein JR, Frist WH, Stinson EB, et al. Primary cardiac neoplasms: Early and late results of surgical treatment in 42 patients. *J Thorac Cardiovasc Surg* 1987;93:502.
195. Grande AM, Ragni TR, Vigano M. Primary cardiac tumors: A clinical experience of 12 years. *Tex Heart Inst J* 1993;20:223.
196. Kotsuka Y, Furuse A, Yagyu K, et al. Long term results of surgical treatment of intracardiac tumors: Effectiveness and limitation of surgical treatment. *Jpn Heart J* 1995;36:213.
197. Farooki ZQ, Ross RD, Paridon SM, et al. Spontaneous regression of cardiac rhabdomyoma. *Am J Cardiol* 1991;67:897.
198. Matsuoka Y, Nakati T, Kawaguchi K, et al. Disappearance of a cardiac rhabdomyoma complicating congenital mitral regurgitation as observed by serial two dimensional echocardiography. *Pediatr Cardiol* 1990;11:98.
199. Nir A, Tajik AJ, Freeman WK, et al. Tuberous sclerosis and cardiac rhabdomyoma. *Am J Cardiol* 1995p76:419.
200. Freedom RM, Lee KJ, MacDonald C, Taylor G. Selected aspects of cardiac tumors in infancy and childhood. *Pediatr Cardiol* 2000;21:299.
201. Smythe JF, Dyck MD, Smallhorn JF, et al. Natural history of cardiac rhabdomyoma in infancy and childhood. *Am J Cardiol* 1990;66:1247.
202. Konkol RJ, Walsh EP, Power T, et al. Cerebral embolism resulting from an intracardiac tumor in tuberous sclerosis. *Pediatr Neurol* 1986;2:108.

203. Molina JE, Edwards JE, Ward HB. Primary cardiac tumors: Experience at the University of Minnesota. *Thorac Cardiovasc Surg* 1990;38:183.
204. Garson A, Gillette PC, Titus JL, et al. Surgical treatment of ventricular tachycardia in an infant. *N Engl J Med* 1984;310:1443.
205. McGregor W, Deanfield J, Farugui A, et al. Infantile cardiomyopathy with histiocytoid change in cardiac muscle cells: Successful intervention with prolonged survival. *Am J Cardiol* 1984;53:982.
206. Auflero TX, Pae WE Jr, Clemson BS, et al. Heart transplantation for tumor. *Ann Thorac Surg* 1993;56:1174.
207. Yuh DD, Kubo SH, Francis GS, et al. Primary cardiac lymphoma treated with orthotopic heart transplantation: A case report. *J Heart Lung Transplant* 1994; 13:536.
208. Baay P, Karawande SV, Kushner JP, et al. Successful treatment of a cardiac angiosarcoma with combined modality therapy. J *Heart Lung Transplant* 1994; 13:923.
209. Crespo MG, Pulpon LA, Pradas G, et al. Heart transplantation for cardiac angiosarcoma: Should its indication be questioned? *J Heart Lung Transplant* 1993; 82:527.
210. Bishop WT, Chan NHL, McDonald IL, et al. Malignant primary cardiac tumor presenting as superior vena cava obstruction syndrome. *Can J Cardiol* 1990;6:259.
211. Castelli MJ, Mihalov ML, Posniak HV, et al. Primary cardiac lymphoma initially diagnosed by routine cytology: Case report and literature review. *Acta Cytol* 1989;33:355.
212. Margolin DA, Fabian V, Mintz U, et al. Primary cardiac lymphoma. *Ann Thorac Surg* 1996;61:1000.
213. Serrano A, Iglesias A, Bellas C, et al. Left atrial ball thrombus with histologic features of extranodal B cell lymphoma: Prolonged survival after surgery. *Acta Oncol* 1994;33:575.
214. Begueret H, Labouyrie E, Dubus P, et al. Primary cardiac lymphoma in an immunocompetent woman. *Leuk Lymphoma* 1998;31:423.
215. Ceresoli GL, Ferreri AJ, Bucci E, et al. Primary cardiac lymphoma in immunocompetent patients: Diagnostic and therapeutic management. *Cancer* 1997;80:1497.
216. Chao TY, Han SC, Nieh S, et al. Diagnosis of primary cardiac lymphoma: Report of a case with cytologic examination of pericardial fluid and imprints of transvenously biopsied intracardiac tissue. *Acta Cytol* 1995; 39:955.
217. Roller M, Manoharan A, Lvoff R. Primary cardiac lymphoma. *Acta Haematol* 1991;85:47.
218. Sommers KE, Edmundowicz D, Katz WE, et al. Primary cardiac lymphoma: Echocardiographic characterization and successful resection. *Ann Thorac Surg* 1996;61:1001.
219. Rossi NP, Kioschos JM, Aschenbrener CA, et al. Primary angiosarcoma of the heart. *Cancer* 1976; 37:891.
220. Sorlie D, Myhre ESP, Stalsberg H. Angiosarcoma of the heart: Unusual presentation and survival after treatment. *Br Heart J* 1984;51:94.
221. Goldstein DJ, Oz MC, Rose EA, et al. Experience with heart transplantation for cardiac tumors. *J Heart Lung Transplant* 1995;14:382.
222. Gowdamarajan A, Michler RE. Therapy for primary cardiac tumors: Is there a role for heart transplantation? *Curr Opin Cardiol* 2000;15:121.
223. Black MD, Kadletz M, Smallhorn JF, et al. Cardiac rhabdomyomas and obstructive left heart disease: histologically but not functionally benign. *Ann Thorac Surg* 1998;65:1388–1390.

CHAPTER

44 CARDIAC TRANSPLANTATION

Jason A. Williams, Brian T. Bethea, David D. Yuh

INTRODUCTION

Over the last two decades, advances in the pharmacologic treatment of end-stage heart failure have improved the quality of life of these patients; however, cardiac transplantation remains the only definitive therapy. Although it once was considered merely an experimental solution, advances in immunology, microbiology, and surgical techniques have allowed cardiac transplantation to blossom into a dynamic and evolving treatment modality with excellent clinical results. Patients who receive transplants attain both long-term survival and an excellent quality of life as a result of this therapy.

HISTORY OF CARDIAC TRANSPLANTATION

Well before Barnard and colleagues performed the first successful human cardiac transplant, the field of cardiac transplantation was developing in basic science laboratories around the world.[1] Alexis Carrel and Charles Guthrie[2] reported the first heterotopic canine heart transplant in 1905. As a result of that breakthrough, pioneers such as Frank Mann at the Mayo Clinic were able to investigate the etiologies of rejection and bioincompatibility between donor and recipient.

Advances in the laboratory were accompanied by technical progress in the field of cardiac surgery. The

KEY CONCEPTS

- Epidemiology
  - Over 2200 cardiac transplants are performed in the United States each year.
- Pathophysiology
  - Cardiac transplantation is indicated for patients who have end-stage New York Heart Association (NYHA) class III or IV heart failure that is refractory to medical management and for whom 1-year survival is estimated to be less than 50 percent without transplantation. Leading diagnoses include idiopathic and ischemic cardiomyopathy, followed by intractable angina or ventricular arrhythmias and end-stage failure from valvular or congenital heart disease.
- Clinical features
  - Most candidates for cardiac transplantation are in end-stage NYHA class III or IV heart failure, with a left ventricular ejection fraction less than 20 percent, pulmonary capillary wedge pressure greater than 25 mmHg, and maximal oxygen consumption less than 10 to 15 mL/kg/min. Status I candidates require strict intensive care unit monitoring and/or intravenous inotropic or mechanical support to maintain adequate hemodynamics. Status II candidates account for all other potential recipients.
- Diagnostics
  - Initial evaluation for cardiac transplant candidacy includes a comprehensive history and physical examination; serum chemistries; serologic assays for hepatitis, human immunodeficiency virus, herpes, and cytomegalovirus; human leukocyte antigen (HLA) tissue typing; maximal oxygen consumption (Vo_2); echocardiography; electrocardiography; Holter monitoring; and pulmonary function testing. Cardiac catheterization is performed to evaluate pulmonary hypertension and coronary anatomy. Other studies are directed toward ruling out malignancy, severe peripheral vascular disease, and psychiatric illness.

- Treatment
  - The donor cardiac allograft is arrested with cardioplegic solution and excised from the donor. With orthotopic cardiac transplantation, after the recipient's native heart has been excised, anastomoses are constructed between the donor's and recipient's left atria, venae cavae (or right atria), and great vessels. Issues specific to cardiac transplant recipients include the early maintenance of adequate allograft function; surveillance and treatment of acute and chronic allograft rejection; aggressive prophylaxis and treatment of bacterial, viral, and fungal infections; and maintenance of a satisfactory immunosuppressive regimen that strikes a balance between pharmacologic side effects and inadequate immunosuppression that can lead to allograft rejection.
- Outcomes and prognosis
  - Orthotopic cardiac transplantation is associated with a 5 to 10 percent mortality rate in the first 30 postoperative days, usually resulting from early graft failure, and 1-, 5-, and 10-year survival rates of approximately 80 percent, 65 percent, and 50 percent, respectively. The majority of deaths in the late posttransplantation period result from accelerated allograft coronary artery disease. Retransplantation for accelerated allograft coronary artery or refractory rejection is associated with a 55 percent 1-year survival rate if it is performed within 2 years of the initial transplant.

development of hypothermic cardiopulmonary bypass eventually led to Richard Lower and Norman Shumway performing the first orthotopic cardiac transplantation in a canine model; that set the stage for the future of cardiac transplantation.[3] Using the technique described by Lower and Shumway, the South African Christiaan Barnard successfully accomplished the first human cardiac transplant on December 3, 1967.[1] Unfortunately, poor clinical outcomes over the ensuing years all but halted the progression of this emerging field within cardiac surgery.

However, the persistent efforts of Shumway and his colleagues at Stanford led to the resurgence of cardiac transplantation as a viable and effective treatment modality in the late 1970s. Further improvements in surveillance of rejection by using endomyocardial biopsy techniques, the emergence of cyclosporine, and advances in cardiac surgical techniques have resulted in today's excellent clinical results.[4,5] The United Network for Organ Sharing (UNOS) reported an annual cardiac transplant rate of over 2200 in the United States alone.[6,7] Only donor organ availability limits this number from growing further, and that limitation is the next large barrier that pioneers in the field of cardiac transplantation will have to surmount.

THE CARDIAC TRANSPLANT RECIPIENT

Indications for transplantation

Because of the severe shortage of available donors and the inherent morbidity associated with cardiac transplantation, strict selection criteria and indications for transplantation are necessary for the judicious allocation of organs (Table 44-1).[8] Most of the patients referred for evaluation are NYHA class III or IV as a result of ischemic heart disease or idiopathic cardiomyopathy.[8] Other common indications include dilated cardiomyopathy as a result of viral, inflammatory, toxic, metabolic, and familial etiologies. Less common indications include intractable angina, refractory malignant ventricular arrhythmias, allograft coronary artery disease from a previous transplant, and cardiac failure caused by valvular and congenital heart disease. Selected candidates are deemed appropriate only if the cause of their end-stage heart failure is irreversible by other means of medical or interventional therapy (revascularization, angioplasty, etc.).[9]

Regardless of the specific etiology, patients become listed candidates on the basis of a variety of clinical parameters determined by each individual institution and selection committee. The prognosis at listing should be less than 50 percent survival at 1 year without transplantation. Prognostication, however, requires considerable clinical judgment and is subjective. Certain parameters have been shown to predict a poor outcome and often are used to aid clinicians in this process. They include a left ventricular ejection fraction less than 20 percent, serum sodium less than 135 meq/dL, pulmonary capillary wedge pressure greater than 25 mmHg, plasma norepinephrine greater than 600 pg/mL, increased

Table 44-1 Indications for cardiac transplantation
Systolic heart failure (ejection fraction < 35%)
• Ischemic cardiomyopathy
• Dilated cardiomyopathy
• Valvular cardiomyopathy
• Hypertensive cardiomyopathy
Ischemic heart disease with intractable angina not amenable to revascularization and not responsive to maximal medical therapy
Intractable arrhythmia not amenable to ablative therapy and not responsive to maximal medical therapy
Hypertrophic cardiomyopathy that has failed maximal medical and surgical therapy

Source: Reproduced, with permission, from Steinman TI, Becker BN, Frost AE, et al. Guidelines for the referral and management of patients eligible for solid organ transplantation. *Transplantation* 2001;71:1189.

cardiothoracic ratio on chest roentgenography, and maximal oxygen consumption (Vo_2) less than 10 to 15 mL/kg/min.[10–17] Among these criteria, the most important independent risk factors for poor survival are reduced left ventricular ejection fraction and reduced Vo_2.[18]

Contraindications for transplantation

A list of absolute and relative contraindications is given in Table 44-2. Although there are few absolute medical contraindications, experts generally agree that fixed pulmonary hypertension with a transpulmonary gradient greater than 15 mmHg and a pulmonary vascular resistance greater than 6 Woods units is an absolute contraindication to heart transplantation.[18–21] Fixed pulmonary hypertension is defined as failure to reduce pulmonary vascular resistance (PVR) by 50 percent after 72 h of vasodilator and parenteral inotropic therapy. Orthotopic heart allografts experience acute right heart failure in the immediate postoperative period in this scenario.[22,23] In this clinical setting, these patients may be evaluated for heterotopic heart or heart-lung transplantation.[24,25]

Recipient age remains the most controversial relative contraindication to transplantation. A number of leading transplant centers report excellent results in patients over age 50 as well as fewer episodes of rejection than in younger patient populations.[26,27] However, older patient populations have more comorbidities and occult systemic illnesses that frequently hinder their postoperative recovery.[26] Thus, most centers focus on physiologic rather than chronologic age, with age being used as an exclusion criterion when there are significant comorbidities.[27]

Systemic illness often excludes patients from transplantation. Diabetes mellitus, if accompanied by evidence of end-organ damage, is a relative contraindication.[28,29] In addition, irreversible renal, hepatic, pulmonary, and noncardiac atherosclerotic vascular disease portends poor outcomes in transplant recipients.[17] The restrictions on transplanting patients infected with human immunodeficiency virus (HIV) are evolving, but this remains a relative contraindication to transplantation. Finally, patients with known systemic malignancy are usually not candidates for transplantation unless there has been a sufficient period of remission and the patient has been deemed cancer-free.[17]

Psychosocial factors also require strict attention during the evaluation process.[30] Patients without the capacity to adhere to rigorous medical regimens and doctors' visits cannot be expected to have acceptable posttransplant outcomes. Psychiatric illness, substance abuse, and a history of noncompliance negatively affect the chances of listing a patient for transplantation.[30,31] Because of the limited resources available, these issues must be addressed in the preoperative assessment to ensure optimal use of available donor hearts.

Table 44-2 Contraindications for cardiac transplantation

Age >70
Fixed pulmonary hypertension
Life-threatening/life-limiting systemic illness, including but not limited to
- Presence of uncured malignancy other than skin neoplasms
- Diabetes mellitus with end-organ damage
- Irreversible renal, hepatic, or pulmonary dysfunction
- End-stage peripheral vascular disease or cerebrovascular disease
- HIV/AIDS
- Sepsis or other systemic infections
- Active multisystem systemic lupus erythematosus or sarcoid
- Any systemic process likely to recur in the transplanted cardiac allograft

Active alcohol or drug abuse
Inability to adhere to strict medical compliance and follow-up
Severe, intractable psychiatric illness
Limited or absent psychosocial support

Recipient evaluation, selection, and prioritization

The process of listing a patient for heart transplantation begins with the initial determination of NYHA end-stage heart disease functional class. Patients generally are referred for transplant evaluation once their class reaches III or IV, although some class II patients with evidence of rapid disease progression are referred.[17] Each transplant center has a multidisciplinary committee of surgeons, cardiologists, psychologists, and nurses that ensures optimal allocation of resources. These committees generally establish institution-specific guidelines, since there is no national or international governing body for heart transplantation. The selection process is used to identify patients who have failed optimal medical alternatives but have the postoperative potential for resumption of a normal active lifestyle and the ability for compliance with a rigorous medical regimen.

These patients undergo an initial evaluation with a comprehensive history, physical examination, and chest x-ray. Routine blood sampling is performed for hepatitis, HIV, and cytomegalovirus (CMV) serologies; thyroid function and glucose tolerance; electrolyte panels and creatinine clearance; lipid panels; fungal serologies; and panel reactive antibody and HLA typing. Routine exercise test measuring Vo_2 consumption is performed along with electrocardiography, echocardiography, Holter monitoring, and pulmonary function testing. Cardiac catheterization is performed to rule out irreversible pulmonary hypertension and reevaluate coronary anatomy. Other frequently indicated studies include malignancy screening, abdominal ultrasonography, carotid and lower extremity Doppler studies, and esophagogastroduodenoscopy. Finally, these patients undergo rigorous psychiatric and social support evaluations.

Once a patient becomes medically eligible for transplantation, he or she is placed on the UNOS regional transplant list. Three hundred patients are added each month to the 2500 patients currently on the waiting list, but only half those patients will receive transplants.[17] Heart transplant candidates are listed as status I if their condition requires strict intensive care unit monitoring and/or the use of intravenous inotropes or mechanical support to maintain hemodynamics. All other patients are listed as status II. Although only 5 to 10 percent of patients listed for transplantation are status I, they account for nearly 60 percent of patients receiving transplants.[17,26]

Preoperative management

In recent years, the use of beta blockers, angiotensin-converting enzyme (ACE) inhibitors, and diuretics has been shown to improve survival in patients with congestive heart failure.[32–34] In decompensated patients who are awaiting heart transplantation, intravenous inotropic support using milrinone, dobutamine, and dopamine has become the standard of care.[35,36] When these measures fail, patients often require the use of intraaortic balloon pumps (IABPs) to maintain hemodynamic stability. For patients who decompensate despite maximal medical intervention, long-term improvements in clinical symptoms have been demonstrated with the use of mechanical assist devices.[37,38] Placement of a ventricular assist device (VAD) or a total artificial heart (TAH) is indicated in patients who do not stabilize after 1 to 2 days of maximal medical therapy.[39,40] Mechanical support acts as an effective bridge, with 70 percent of patients surviving to transplantation in one series.[41] In addition, assist devices are emerging as an acceptable long-term treatment modality for end-stage heart failure in patients who are not amenable to transplantation. The REMATCH trial was the first randomized control trial to demonstrate a distinct survival advantage in patients treated with a left ventricular assist device (LVAD) as destination therapy as opposed to those managed with optimal medical therapy for end-stage heart failure.[42] Approximately 23 percent of the LVAD cohort survived to 2 years in that trial, whereas mortality in the medical group approached 100 percent over the same period. In addition, there was improved quality of life in patients who underwent placement of mechanical assist devices compared with those maintained on medical therapy alone.

Sudden cardiac death continues to be the most common cause of death in patients with end-stage heart failure who are awaiting a transplant.[43] For patients with a known history of life-threatening arrhythmias, the placement of an automatic implantable cardioverter-defibrillator (AICD) and/or treatment with long-term amiodarone often are warranted. These measures can lead to improved survival and thus higher transplant rates in this patient population.[44]

THE CARDIAC DONOR

Donor evaluation and selection

In 1981, an independent council was established to determine standardized universal criteria for brain death that were intended to prevent many of the difficulties in harvesting donor organs during the previous two decades. Brain death was defined as loss of cortical function, apnea, and the absence of brainstem function not caused by reversible processes such as metabolic derangements, drugs, and hypothermia.[45,46] A consensus on brain death within the medical community resulted in numerous laws passed by Congress allowing individuals to donate some or all of their organs for transplantation and requiring medical workers to discuss these options with patients' families.[47–51]

Most organ donors are victims of a cerebrovascular accident or an isolated blunt or penetrating head trauma. Once potential donors have been identified, a three-phase evaluation process is initiated.[45] In the initial phase, transplant representatives collect background information on the potential donor, including age, height, weight, blood type, gender, history of illness leading to brain death, routine blood chemistries, and standard viral [i.e., CMV, hepatitis B virus (HBV), hepatitis C virus (HCV), and HIV] serologies. The next phase requires a more detailed clinical investigation of the cardiac health of the donor. This includes establishment of the amount of hemodynamic support necessary to sustain the patient; review of the electrocardiogram (ECG), plain chest film, and echocardiogram; blood gas parameters; and coronary angiography in the presence of advanced donor age or other risk factors for coronary artery disease. Once the patient passes these initial evaluations and a suitable recipient is found, the final evaluation occurs at the time of organ procurement. Surgeons inspect the heart for the presence of coronary calcification, valvular dysfunction, infarction, or contusion. Once the donor heart passes final inspection, the procurement begins and the recipient center prepares to accept the organ.

Table 44-3 outlines both the relative and the absolute contraindications for cardiac donation.[45] Because of the shortage of donor organs, researchers continue to push the envelope of donor criteria to expand the donor pool. Many centers now accept donors over age 50 or 60 who otherwise are in good health and have shown similar clinical outcomes to the outcomes with younger donor organs.[52,53] One study demonstrated effective clinical outcomes with the use of organs with some evidence of myocardial dysfunction, undersized donors with a donor-to-recipient weight ratio below 0.45, extended ischemic times, positive blood cultures, positive HCV titers, and/or conduction abnormalities.[54] However, despite these efforts, organ donation remains limited, with only 2000 to 2500 hearts becoming available each year.

Table 44-3 Contraindications for cardiac donation

Absolute contraindications
- HIV
- Death from carbon monoxide poisoning (carboxyhemoglobin levels >20%)
- Intractable ventricular arrhythmia
- Sao2 <80% on maximal ventilatory support
- Previous myocardial infarction or documented severe coronary artery disease
- Clinically significant structural heart disease or ejection fraction <10% by echo

Relative contraindications
- Age >60
- Hepatitis B surface antigen positivity
- Sepsis
- Hepatitis C positivity
- Presence of metastatic cancer
- Cardiac contusion as a result of chest wall trauma
- Prolonged hypotension (systolic blood pressure <60 mmHg for more than 6 h)
- Recurrent supraventricular tachycardia
- Prolonged (>24 h) need for high-dose inotropic support (dopamine >20 μg/kg/min)
- Need for cardiopulmonary resuscitation (CPR) >30 min within 24 h of harvest
- Multiple episodes of CPR
- Severe left ventricular hypertrophy
- Moderate hypokinesia seen on echo
- History of intravenous drug abuse

Source: Reproduced, with permission, from Baldwin JC, Anderson JL, Boucek MM, et al. Bethesda conference: Cardiac transplantation: Task Force 2: Donor guidelines. *J Am Coll Cardiol* 1993;22:15.

Donor management

In the interval between evaluation as a potential donor and organ harvesting, the heart donor must be monitored intensely for variations in hemodynamics, fluids, electrolytes, hormonal fluctuations, and ventilatory and acid-base alterations. Because of the complex physiology encountered in patients who have been declared brain-dead, these measures are vital to the successful harvesting and survival of the allograft. This becomes especially important as centers begin to use more donors who meet extended donor criteria.

Optimization of the donor includes maintaining a mean arterial pressure of 80 to 89 mmHg by using intravenous vasopressors, inotropes, or afterload reducers as the situation dictates. Fluid requirements of 100 mL/h, in addition to replacement of the previous hour's urine output, are essential. A goal urine output of 100 mL/h is adequate. For patients with diabetes insipidus, volume replacement and the use of vasopressin are warranted, whereas patients with oliguria may require either fluid boluses or diuretics as clinically indicated.[55,56]

Donors with devastating cerebral incidents such as trauma and spontaneous hemorrhage often have electrolyte imbalances such as hypernatremia, hypokalemia, hypophosphatemia, and hypomagnesemia.[57] These electrolyte abnormalities should be corrected adequately in the preharvest period, and donors should be monitored strictly for the prevention and correction of accompanying acid-base disorders. The goals for optimal ventilator management need to be addressed, with close attention paid to frequent tracheal suctioning.[58] Hypothermia should be prevented by using warming blankets and warm intravenous fluids as necessary. In cardiac donors, hemoglobin should be maintained above 10 g/dL to maximize myocardial oxygen delivery before harvesting. Finally, studies have shown the benefits of pretreatment with hormone replacement therapies such as free triiodothyronine (T_3), cortisol, and insulin, since a variety of hormones become depleted in brain death.[59–61]

Organ preservation

Decades of research on optimal organ storage and preservation have failed to increase the acceptable ischemic time of cardiac allografts past 4 to 6 h. Current preservation techniques continue to use a combination of cardioplegia, organ preservation solution, and hypothermic storage. A variety of storage solutions exist, the studies of which demonstrate little benefit of one particular solution over another.[62] Solutions vary in their composition, with each containing ions in concentrations that resemble those of either intracellular or extracellular fluids. Theoretically, storage solutions with intracellular compositions (high-potassium, low-sodium concentrations), such as University of Wisconsin (UW) and Euro-Collins solutions, prevent intracellular edema by minimizing fluid shifts into the myocardial cells.[63] Conversely, extracellular storage solutions (low-potassium, high-sodium concentrations), such as Stanford and Hopkins solutions, purportedly avoid the cellular damage and increased vascular resistance imposed by high potassium concentrations. The optimal storage temperature during transportation also remains a matter of controversy, although most investigators agree on temperatures between 4 and 10°C.[64]

Approximately 20 percent of perioperative transplant deaths are related to myocardial dysfunction, indicating the need for more research in the field of cardiac allograft preservation. Current promising strategies revolve around the use of impermeants, substrates, and antioxidants in storage solutions. Impermeants such as mannitol and lactobionate, among others, decrease intracellular edema by reducing the intracellular osmotic gradient. Adenosine, L-pyruvate, and L-glutamate, the three substrates most widely studied, have theoretical application in the preservation of high-energy phosphates during storage and the rapid regeneration of those phosphates upon reperfusion.[65] Ischemia-reperfusion injury is the target of antioxidants currently under investigation in many transplant laboratories. In addition, the successes of continuous perfusion seen in renal transplantation have inspired investigators to apply this strategy to heart allografts. Although promising, this technology is limited by the development of extracellular myocardial edema and by the technical limitations of the complex perfusion apparatus.[66]

OPERATIVE TECHNIQUES

Cardiac allograft procurement

Donor organ procurement begins with a median sternotomy and a longitudinal pericardiotomy. The procurement team visually and manually inspects the donor heart for any evidence of cardiac disease or injury. The major vessels are dissected, mobilized, and circumferentially isolated with suture ligatures or vessel loops. The cardiac team then defers to the liver, kidney, pancreas, and pulmonary procurement teams for their harvest preparations.

The anesthesia team administers 30,000 units of intravenous heparin, and the superior vena cava is ligated proximal to the ligated azygous vein (Fig. 44-1). Division of the inferior vena cava at the level of the diaphragm permits efflux of cardioplegia once it is administered. Retrograde administration of a 500 mL flush of cardioplegic solution just proximal to the aortic cross-clamp is followed by rapid cooling of the heart and division of the pulmonary veins, with care taken to leave enough of the left atrial cuff for the implantation. The surgeon divides the aorta just proximal to the innominate artery and then divides the pulmonary artery just proximal to the bifurcation, taking care to spare as much length on those vessels as possible so that later modification can occur in the recipient. This is especially important in recipients with congenital anomalies. Final inspection of the valves and the atrial septum (for patent foramen ovale) is conducted before the allograft is stored in an ice cooler and the graft is transported to the recipient center.

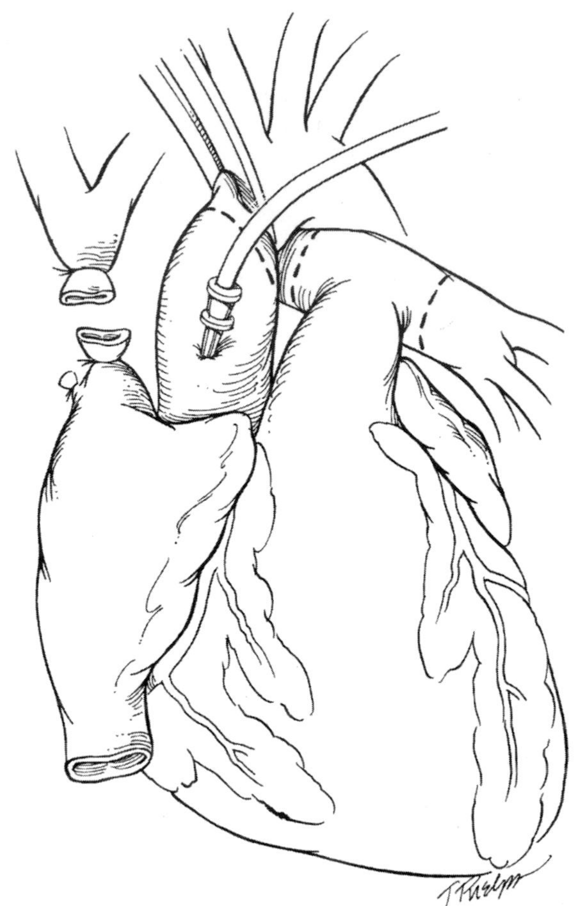

Figure 44-1 Donor pericardiectomy. Lines of transaction of both venae cavae, aorta, and pulmonary arteries. (Reproduced, with permission, from Bethea BT, Yuh DD, Conte JV, Baumgartner WA. Heart transplantation. In: Cohn LH, Edmunds LH Jr (eds). *Cardiac Surgery in the Adult.* New York: McGraw-Hill; 2003:1427–1460.)

Recipient preparation and cardiectomy

Once the procurement team notifies the recipient center that the allograft is acceptable, the recipient undergoes general anesthesia with high-dose intravenous narcotics and avoidance of inhaled agents because of their cardiac depressive effects.[67,68] Vasopressors and inotropes are titrated as necessary to counteract the effects of anesthesia-induced hypotension. In some settings, the administration of aprotinin or aminocaproic acid helps minimize perioperative bleeding.[69]

Either the bicaval or the biatrial anastomosis (originally described by Lower and Shumway) is the surgical technique used for allograft implantation, although most centers prefer the bicaval technique.[3] The recipient is prepared for cardiopulmonary bypass in the standard fashion and cooled to 28°C. The great vessels are transected above the semilunar commissures, and the atria are excised along the atrioventricular grooves (Fig. 44-2). Atrial cuffs are left for allograft implantation unless the bicaval anastomosis technique is used. In that case, the entire right atrium is excised, leaving the superior and inferior vena cava on the right and a small left atrial cuff for anastomosis to the pulmonary veins on the left.[70] Excision of the atrial appendages is performed to reduce the risk of thrombus formation.[71] The proximal 1 to 2 cm of aorta and pulmonary artery are dissected free from each other as the final step in recipient preparation. The timing of donor and recipient cardiectomies is optimally arranged so that completion of the recipient cardiectomy occurs just before the arrival of the allograft.[72]

Cardiac allograft implantation

Final preparation of the cardiac allograft is performed after arrival at the transplant center. The great vessels are dissected and isolated, and the left atrium is

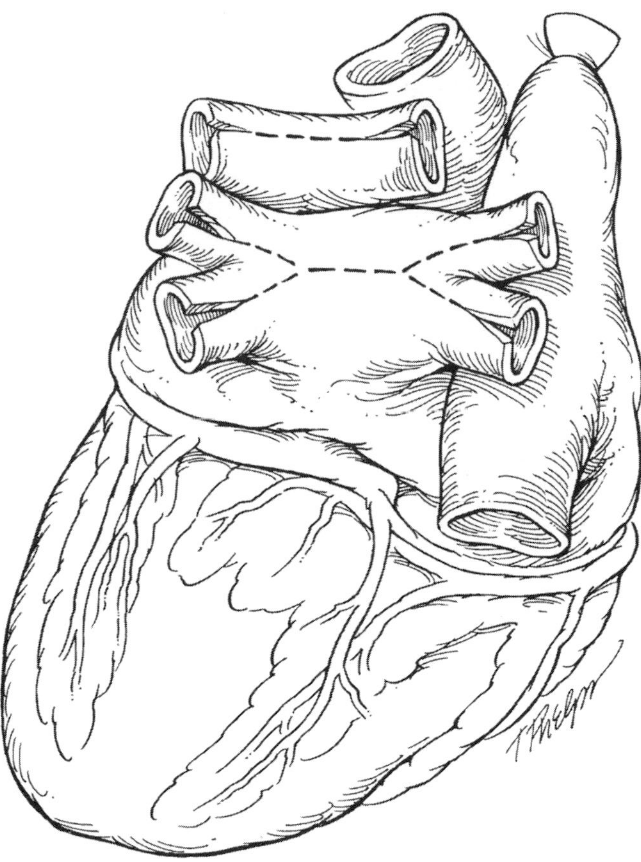

Figure 44-2 Donor allograft preparation for orthotopic cardiac transplantation. The pulmonary vein orifices are joined to form the graft left atrial cuff. (Reproduced, with permission, from Bethea BT, Yuh DD, Conte JV, Baumgartner WA. Heart transplantation. In: Cohn LH, Edmunds LH Jr (eds). *Cardiac Surgery in the Adult.* New York: McGraw-Hill; 2003:1427–1460.)

trimmed to the size appropriate for the recipient atrial cuff that was developed during the recipient's cardiectomy (Fig. 44-2). The right atrium is prepared in a similar fashion for the biatrial anastomotic technique, but this step is omitted when the bicaval technique is used. The transplant team begins implantation with a running 3-0 polypropylene suture for the left atrial anastomosis (Fig. 44-3A). The heart is lowered into the pericardial space and is irrigated continuously with ice-cold saline, and the posterior suture line is completed. The patient then is positioned in a left side down–head up position to keep continuous irrigation in contact with the heart while avoiding interference with the anastomosis. The anterior limb of the anastomosis is carried around the remainder of the atrium and is completed at the interatrial septum (Fig. 44-3B). To prepare the right atrium for anastomosis, the atrium is incised from the inferior vena cava to the right atrial appendage. The atrium is inspected, and care is taken to close any atrial septal defect or patent foramen ovale. Once the surgeon is confident about the integrity of the atrium, the anastomosis on the right is performed in a similar fashion to that on the left (Fig. 44-4).

Next, the pulmonary artery from the allograft is sewn end to end with running 4-0 polypropylene sutures, taking care to trim redundant tissue to prevent kinking of the vessel. The aortic anastomosis completes the procedure, performed in a fashion similar to that for the pulmonary anastomosis (Fig. 44-5). Just before the aortic anastomosis is begun, rewarming of the patient to 37°C is initiated. This allows the cardioplegic infusion to be stopped as soon as the aortic anastomosis is completed. Once the aortic cross-clamp is removed and the heart begins contracting, a final inspection of the suture lines is performed. Epicardial pacing wires and mediastinal tubes are placed in the standard fashion, and the sternum is closed. Intravenous inotropic and vasopressor support helps maintain optimal blood pressure and cardiac output in the immediate postoperative period.

Instead of using the technique described above for a right atrial anastomosis, many institutions now routinely use the bicaval technique.[70] With this technique, the donor allograft is harvested with the superior and inferior vena cava intact, and these vessels are anastomosed individually with the corresponding recipient vessels. This technique circumvents some of the technical shortfalls of the biatrial technique. Studies have shown an improvement in the incidence of atrial fibrillation and flutter and mitral and tricuspid regurgitation when the bicaval technique is employed.[73,74] In addition, improvements in right and left atrial emptying have been demonstrated with this newer technique, with one study reporting improved survival in these patients.[75,76]

Heterotopic cardiac transplantation

A small subset of patients does not qualify for orthotopic heart transplantation. Heterotopic heart transplantation is an option in patients with severe, irreversible pulmonary hypertension and patients with a significant donor-to-recipient size mismatch.[77] In rare pediatric patients, heterotopic heart transplantation has been used to permit recovery of native cardiac function.[78] This technique involves placing the donor heart in parallel with the recipient's diseased heart. There is free communication between the donor and recipient hearts at the atrial level, and the donor pulmonary artery and aorta are anastomosed in an end-to-side fashion to their respective recipient vessels (Fig. 44-6). The donor heart acts in a physiologic manner similar to a biventricular assist device. Since the native heart remains in place and continues to have depressed function, risks include those which are inherent in any

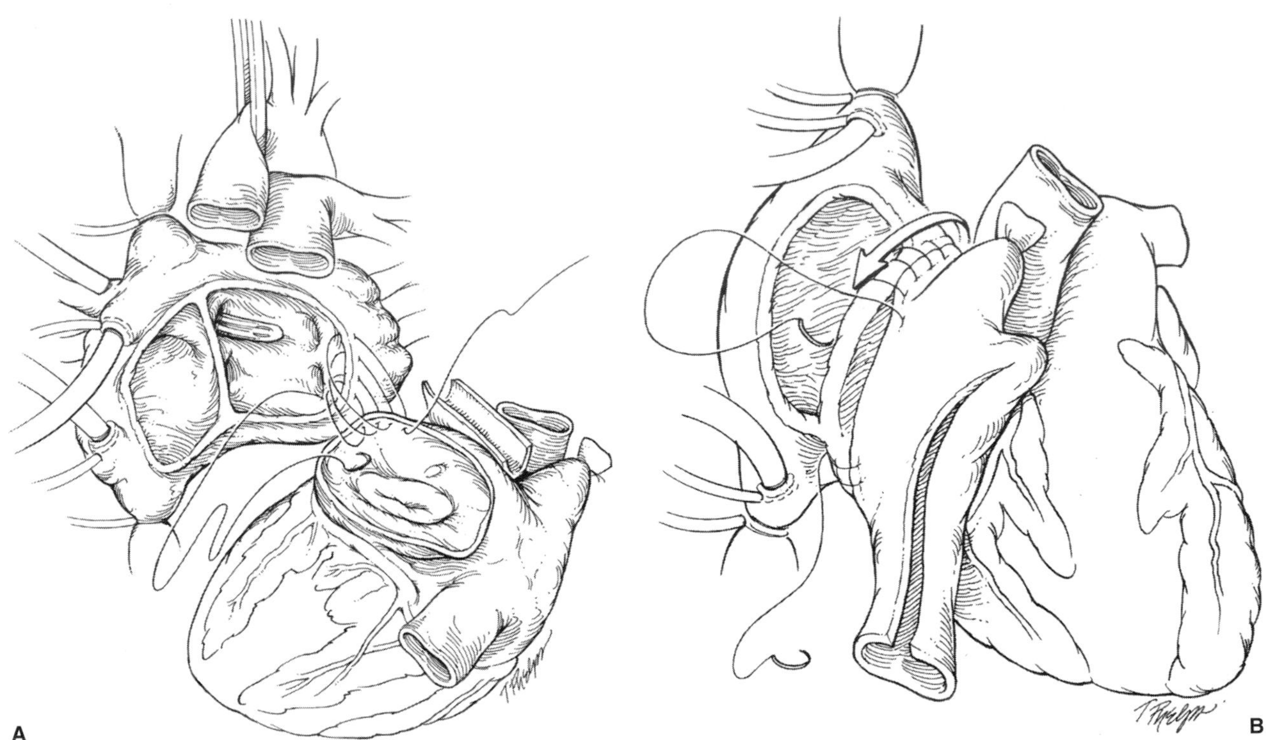

Figure 44-3 **A.** Implantation of a cardiac allograft. The left atrial anastomosis is shown commencing at the left superior pulmonary vein. (Reproduced, with permission, from Bethea BT, Yuh DD, Conte JV, Baumgartner WA. Heart transplantation. In: Cohn LH, Edmunds LH Jr (eds). *Cardiac Surgery in the Adult.* New York: McGraw-Hill; 2003:1427–1460.) **B.** Implantation of cardiac allograft. The left atrial anastomosis is completed. (Reproduced, with permission, from Bethea BT, Yuh DD, Conte JV, Baumgartner WA. Heart transplantation. In: Cohn LH, Edmunds LH Jr (eds). *Cardiac Surgery in the Adult.* New York: McGraw-Hill; 2003:1427–1460.)

patient with end-stage heart failure, including arrhythmias, thromboembolism, angina, and valvular heart disease.

POSTOPERATIVE MANAGEMENT

Hyperacute allograft rejection

The presence of preformed donor-specific antibodies in the transplant recipient leads to the clinical syndrome of hyperacute rejection.[79] This form of early allograft failure occurs within minutes to hours of implantation and is often apparent before the patient leaves the operating room. Histologic evaluation of these failed allografts reveals diffuse interstitial hemorrhage and the absence of a lymphocytic infiltrate. Immunoglobin and complement are seen along the vascular endothelium on immunofluorescent staining. Patients who have this fatal complication can be offered no effective treatment except retransplantation. It should be noted that outcomes remain poor in this patient population even in the rare instances when a new donor heart becomes available. Preoperative testing of ABO blood type matching and panel reactive antibody (PRA) can help predict this devastating complication. Patients with a PRA greater than 10 to 15 percent undergo mandatory T-lymphocyte cross-matching before surgery.[80,81]

Early postoperative period

Because of hypothermia and extended ischemic periods during allograft preservation, recipient hemodynamics fluctuates in the immediate postoperative period as a result of decreased ventricular compliance and contractility.[82–84] This physiologic state often requires 2 to 4 days of parenteral inotropic support, after which most patients regain hemodynamic stability.[85] Unfortunately, some patients are unable to regain adequate cardiac performance quickly because of early allograft failure. This causes approximately 25 percent of early postoperative deaths and is usually secondary to pulmonary hypertension, prolonged allograft ischemia, or acute rejection.[85,86] In the case of right heart failure, the transplant team employs medical measures such as inhaled or intravenous nitrates or prostaglandin E_1 to combat excessive pulmonary pressures. If improvements in right heart function are not seen after these therapies, an IABP or

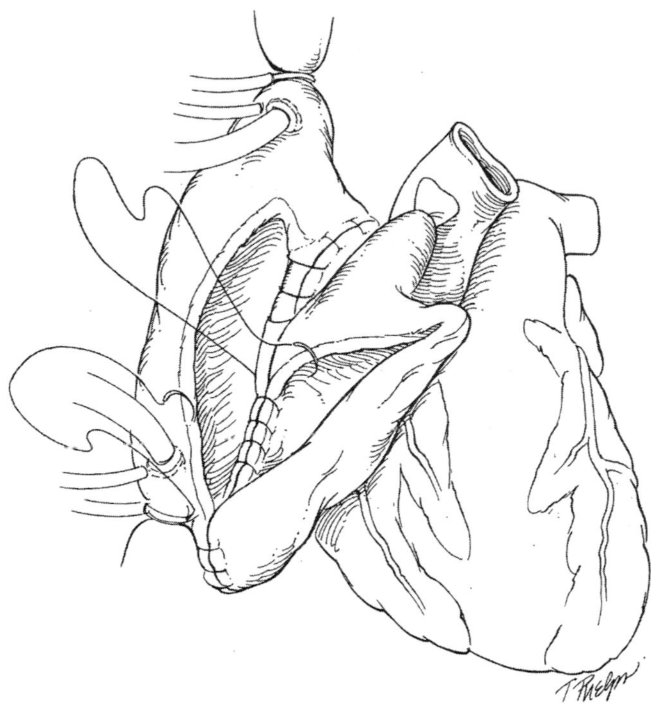

Figure 44-4 Implantation of cardiac allograft. The right atrial anastomosis is shown. (Reproduced, with permission, from Bethea BT, Yuh DD, Conte JV, Baumgartner WA. Heart transplantation. In: Cohn LH, Edmunds LH Jr (eds). *Cardiac Surgery in the Adult.* New York: McGraw-Hill; 2003: 1427–1460.)

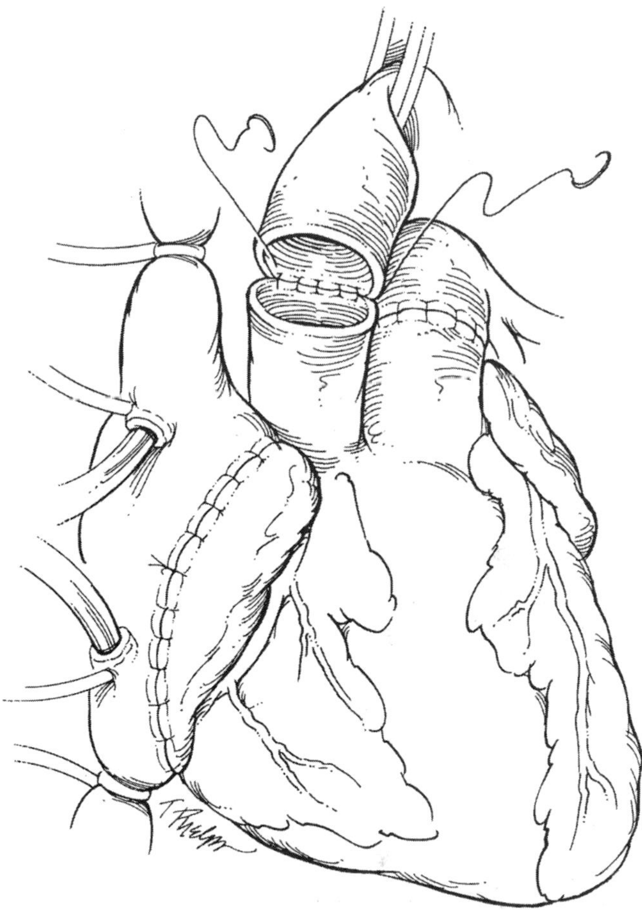

Figure 44-5 Implantation of cardiac allograft. The main pulmonary artery and aorta are anastomosed end to end. (Reproduced, with permission, from Bethea BT, Yuh DD, Conte JV, Baumgartner WA. Heart transplantation. In: Cohn LH, Edmunds LH Jr (eds). *Cardiac Surgery in the Adult.* New York: McGraw-Hill; 2003:1427–1460.)

right ventricular assist device permits the maintenance of hemodynamics until a suitable new donor can be found.[87–89] High-dose immunosuppression combats the effects of early severe allograft rejection, although failure of this therapy may result in the need for mechanical hemodynamic assistance. Myocardial dysfunction resulting from allograft ischemia has few therapeutic options and often requires inotropic or mechanical assistance as a bridge to retransplantation. Unfortunately, regardless of the cause, retransplantation in the early postoperative period is a scenario fraught with poor outcomes and high mortality rates.[90,91]

Normal cardiac allograft physiology is unique in several key respects. First, the allograft myocardium is denervated so that sympathetic responses require hormonal action from distant sites rather than nervous stimulation of the myocardial fibers. Similarly, vagal tone plays no part in cardiac physiology after transplantation, leading to higher resting heart rates and inability to respond to maneuvers such as carotid massage, Valsalva, and atropine injection.[92] These differences lead to a blunted, slower response to alterations in stress and physiology in the transplant recipient.[93–95]

The lack of nervous system input and altered response to circulating catecholamines also can lead to dysrhythmias in the transplant recipient. Bradyarrhythmias occur in more than half of heart transplant recipients, with prolonged allograft ischemia representing the primary risk factor for these arrhythmias.[96] Theophylline, inotropic infusion, and epicardial pacing all effectively treat this problem, with most bradyarrhythmias resolving 1 to 2 weeks after transplantation.[97] Patients who do not respond to these therapies require permanent pacemakers. Atrial fibrillation and/or flutter also affects many transplant recipients and is treated effectively with digoxin.[98] Ventricular dysrhythmias such as premature ventricular contractions and nonsustained ventricular tachycardia are seen in up to 60 percent of transplant recipients but rarely signify an ominous process.[99–101] However, new-onset arrhythmias may herald acute rejection and may warrant further investigation in the proper clinical setting.

Other considerations in the postoperative intensive care setting are similar to those in standard cardiac intensive

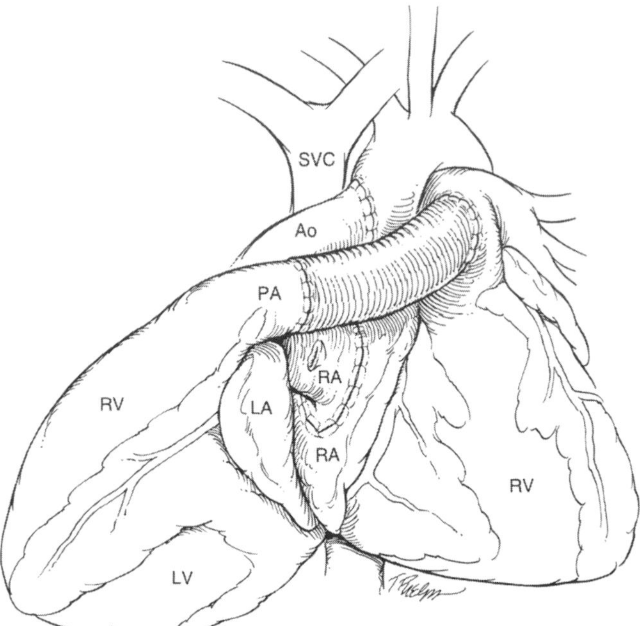

Figure 44-6 Heterotopic cardiac transplantation. The donor heart is placed in parallel with the recipient's native failing heart. There is free communication between the donor and recipient hearts at the atrial level, and the donor's pulmonary artery and aorta are anastomosed in an end-to-side fashion to their respective recipient vessels. Ao = aorta; SVC = superior vena cava; PA = pulmonary artery; RV = right ventricle; LV = left ventricle; LA = left atrium; RA = right atrium. (Reproduced, with permission, from Bethea BT, Yuh DD, Conte JV, Baumgartner WA. Heart transplantation. In: Cohn LH, Edmunds LH Jr (eds). *Cardiac Surgery in the Adult.* New York: McGraw-Hill; 2003: 1427–1460.)

care units. Mean arterial pressures ideally remain below 80 mmHg to reduce afterload on the allograft myocardium. Pulmonary function and ventilator weaning occur in accordance with intensive care unit protocols. Renal function often worsens in transplant patients as a result of preoperative renal insufficiency coupled with the addition of nephrotoxic immunosuppressants. Early use of cytolytic agents instead of tacrolimus or cyclosporine can help prevent this complication, and the addition of mannitol can have a nephroprotective effect. Most patients resume a diet within the first few posttransplant days, and so nutritional and gastrointestinal issues are often not a concern. However, patients who require prolonged intubation or hemodynamic support often benefit from some form of enteral or parenteral nutritional supplementation.

Step-down care and outpatient follow-up

After the early postoperative period, treatment goals focus on early hospital discharge and patient education. To prevent nosocomial infections, patients should be scheduled to leave the hospital within 1 to 2 weeks after surgery.[102] During the recipient's convalescence, the multidisciplinary transplant team focuses on educating patients about their medications, follow-up goals, exercise strategies, diet, and clinical signs of infection or rejection. Routine follow-up allows these patients to maintain active, productive lifestyles within the bounds of a difficult medical regimen. The transplant team performs routine surveillance for rejection, titrates immunosuppressive medications, and cares for the general and cardiac health of the transplant recipient. Close clinical follow-up in the outpatient setting allows patients and clinicians to recognize problems early, permitting adequate treatment while avoiding prolonged hospital stays. The goal of this phase of recipient management is to allow the patient to become an active, healthy, and productive member of society while minimizing the burden of his or her treatment regimen.

IMMUNOSUPPRESSIVE MANAGEMENT

Pharmacologic Strategies

Apart from infectious complications, the most important risk to both patient and graft survival is rejection of the donor allograft as a result of the host's immune response. Immunosuppressive regimens are directed toward attenuating the host's response to foreign allograft tissue while maintaining adequate native immune function to prevent the detrimental effects of infection and malignancy. To accomplish this task, transplant centers initially treat cardiac transplant recipients with high doses of induction immunosuppression. This usually consists of triple-drug regimens in addition to a preoperative induction agent such as muromonab-CD3 (OKT3) or antithymocyte globulin (ATG).

During the early period of clinical cardiac transplantation, corticosteroids were the mainstay of immunosuppression. Treatment began with the administration of intravenous methylprednisolone during an early induction phase, followed by a transition to an oral steroid regimen. Steroids act in a nonselective manner at the nuclear level by inhibiting cytokine synthesis. The transcription of factors such as interleukin-1 (IL-1), IL-2, IL-3, IL-6, tumor necrosis factor-alpha (TNF-α), IF-γ, and granulocyte macrophage colony-stimulating factor (GM-CSF) is inhibited, leading to a diminished immune response.[103] Unfortunately, the nonspecific actions of steroids also lead to numerous unwanted side effects, such as weight gain, glucose intolerance, gastrointestinal distress, hypercholesterolemia, and hyperlipidemia, among many others. Thus, reduction or elimination of steroids from long-term immunosuppression regimens is warranted.[104]

The development of cyclosporine A (cyclosporine) in the 1980s is considered by many to be the single most important advancement in cardiac transplantation. Cyclosporine A inhibits the transcription of IL-2 by helper T lymphocytes, thereby diminishing the effects of cytotoxic T lymphocytes that target the cardiac allograft.[105] These actions are more specific than those of corticosteroids and allow other arms of the immune response to function adequately. This minimizes side effects while maximizing target therapy in the host. Because of this increased specificity in immunosuppression, host defenses maintain the ability to fight infection and certain types of malignancy without compromising the integrity of the allograft. Furthermore, cyclosporine A permits the reduction or in some cases the withdrawal of corticosteroids from immunosuppression regimens. Although these patients still require induction therapy with corticosteroids, these medications can be withdrawn slowly over several weeks to months after the transplantation, leading to steroid-free maintenance regimens in many patients.[106–108] Unfortunately, cyclosporine A therapy is not without complications. Numerous drug interactions and variable interpatient pharmacokinetics mandate close monitoring to maintain systemic drug levels in the therapeutic range.[109–111] The major side effects of this medication are nephrotoxicity and hypertension, the first of which can be dose-limiting or inhibit the use of cyclosporine A altogether.[112]

FK-506 (tacrolimus) also inhibits IL-2 transcription and was developed with the aim of minimizing the unwanted nephrotoxicity of cyclosporin A while maintaining the same therapeutic effects.[113] Clinical trials have proved the efficacy of tacrolimus both in cardiac transplant maintenance regimens and in treating acute cardiac allograft rejection.[114,115] However, certain patients still experience difficulty with glucose intolerance and nephrotoxicity while taking this medication. Therefore, transplant centers tailor their use of IL-2 inhibitors on the basis of individual patient tolerance and often use FK-506 as "rescue" therapy in cases of recalcitrant rejection.

Sirolimus (Rapamycin) blocks the IL-2 pathway at the level of the IL-2 receptor.[103,116] Helper T lymphocytes produce IL-2 that never reaches its target on the cytotoxic T lymphocytes, thus inhibiting the proliferation of this cell type. Rapamycin is still an investigational drug, and studies of its effectiveness are ongoing. Preliminary studies have demonstrated its promise as a treatment for refractory rejection.[117]

The third major class of maintenance therapy inhibits purine synthesis, thus preventing the proliferation of T lymphocytes.[118,119] The first agent in this class, azathioprine, largely has been replaced by mycophenolate mofetil (MMF, CellCept). Rejection rates are similar between the two drugs, but MMF has a better side effect profile, causing less bone marrow suppression and decreased mortality compared with azathioprine.

Polyclonal and monoclonal antibodies play a large role both in immunosuppressive induction and in the treatment of rejection refractory to corticosteroids. Mice or other animals are injected with human T lymphocytes, stimulating the animal's immune system to create antibodies to those cells. Those antibodies, in the form of antithymocyte serum (ATS) or antilymphocyte globulin (ALG), are infused into the transplant recipient. The antibodies bind to the recipient's circulating T lymphocytes, causing opsonization and destruction of those cells. For patients with clinical rejection refractory to steroids, this treatment reduces circulating levels of T lymphocytes to less than 10 percent of normal, assisting in the treatment of T lymphocyte–mediated rejection.[120,121] In addition, infusion of these antibodies is an effective induction strategy for minimizing the amount of corticosteroids and cyclosporine A needed in the immediate postoperative period, thus decreasing some of their unwanted side effects.[122,123]

OKT3 is a similar treatment strategy, using mouse monoclonal antibodies to the CD3 receptor on cytotoxic T lymphocytes.[124,125] OKT3 eliminates the volume of circulating T lymphocytes in a more specific manner by targeting only those cells with CD3 receptors, thus preventing some of the nonspecific effects seen with ATS/ALG.[126] OKT3 has been used both as an induction agent and as a treatment for refractory rejection, showing its greatest benefit as a rescue therapy.[127–130] As with other antibody treatments, side effects include high fevers, malaise, nausea, vomiting, respiratory distress, increased risk of viral infection, and increased risk of malignancy.

Nonpharmacologic strategies

There are other treatments beyond the standard pharmacotherapies discussed above for the treatment of rejection and the reduction of circulating immune cell volumes. Total lymphoid irradiation is intended to reduce lymphocyte volume by irradiating the lymphatic tissues that are known to produce those cell types. Photopheresis uses ultraviolet light to activate mononuclear cells that suppress the effector arm of the T-lymphocyte pathway. Apheresis uses plasma exchange to remove circulating antibodies and activated lymphocytes to suppress the host immune response. These therapies are in the early phases of development, and much research will be required to determine their exact mechanism of action. However, initial studies show promise with all three of these strategies in treating refractory rejection.[131–135]

ACUTE CARDIAC ALLOGRAFT REJECTION

Diagnosis of acute allograft rejection

Most cardiac transplant recipients experience at least one episode of acute rejection mediated by the cellular limb of the immune response early in the recovery period. Eighty percent of rejection episodes occur during the first 3 months after a transplant, and most are treated adequately with pulse doses corticosteroids.[136,137] However, unrecognized or refractory rejection can be a significant complication in the patient's recovery, and rejection continues to account for some of the major morbidities in transplant recipients.

The introduction of cyclosporine A into the immunosuppression regimens of transplant recipients has suppressed the clinical manifestations of rejection dramatically. Currently, cardiac allograft biopsy is the only means of diagnosing a rejection episode. Caves, Stinson, Billingham, and colleagues developed the technique of endomyocardial biopsy that still is used for surveillance and diagnosis of rejection.[138] Their technique involves cannulation of the right internal jugular vein. Subsequently, right interventricular septal specimens are taken for pathologic evaluation. The complications with this procedure are rare and include complications associated with central venous cannulation as well as right ventricular perforation. The histopathologic classification of rejection is shown in Table 44-4.[139]

Table 44-4 Grades of rejection

Grade	Definition
0	No rejection
1A[a]	Focal (perivascular or interstitial) infiltrate without necrosis
1B	Diffuse but sparse infiltrate without necrosis
2	One focus only with aggressive infiltration and/or focal myocyte damage
3A	Multifocal aggressive infiltrates and/or myocyte damage
3B	Diffuse inflammatory process with necrosis
4	Diffuse, aggressive polymorphous ± infiltrate ± edema ± hemorrhage ± vasculitis, with necrosis

[a]Some recent authors and clinicians now combine grades 1A and 1B into a single grade and eliminate grade 2 as a category.
Source: Reproduced, with permission, from Billingham ME, Cary NB, Hammond ME, et al. A working formulation for the standardization of nomenclature in the diagnosis of heart and lung rejection: Heart rejection study group. *J Heart Lung Transplant* 1990;9(6):587.

Investigators continue to seek less invasive modalities for surveillance of rejection. Studies of voltage changes on ECG, computerized heart allograft monitoring, echocardiography, magnetic resonance imaging (MRI), and immunosurveillance have shown promise but lack the sensitivity needed to rule out rejection.[140–147] Because of the lethal consequences associated with unrecognized and untreated rejection, endomyocardial biopsy remains the gold standard for the diagnosis of allograft rejection.

Treatment of acute allograft rejection

During the first three postoperative months, the treatment of choice for episodes of acute rejection is intravenous high-dose pulsed corticosteroids for approximately 3 days. Episodes that occur at a longer interval after transplantation often are treated initially with increased oral steroid doses, followed by a steroid taper and follow-up endomyocardial biopsy to document adequate treatment.[148] Repeat courses of high-dose steroids are attempted if the follow-up biopsy shows inadequate treatment or progression of rejection. However, failure of this second course of steroids or progression to hemodynamic instability warrants rescue therapy with additional agents.

Many of the therapies currently used as rescue protocols were discussed above. They include agents such as OKT3, polyclonal antibodies such as ATS and ALG, FK506, Rapamycin, and MMF.[149–151] In addition, nonpharmacologic treatments using apheresis, photopheresis, and total lymphoid irradiation have shown promising results in some series. Retransplantation formerly was performed for severe rejection that was not amenable to conventional therapies, but the results were so poor that this indication for retransplantation no longer exists.

Treatment of low-grade (I and II) rejection remains controversial, since most episodes of this type of rejection do not progress to higher-grade rejections.[152,153] Pathology demonstrating higher-grade lesions with myocyte necrosis and large lymphocytic infiltrates is accepted universally as an indication for treatment because of the ominous progression of this type of rejection. In addition, any patient experiencing hemodynamic instability and allograft dysfunction will receive treatment regardless of the rejection grade.

Acute vascular (antibody-mediated) rejection

Although most episodes of rejection are a consequence of cell-mediated rejection, the humoral limb of the immune response can cause devastating damage to a cardiac allograft.[154–156] Most patients with antibody-mediated rejection demonstrate hemodynamic instability, endothelial swelling, and antibody-complement deposits within the allograft vasculature.[157,158] Treatment consists of high-dose corticosteroids, plasmapheresis, immunoglobulin G (IgG), and cyclophosphamide, but even maximal treatment often fails in patients with this complication. Mortality from acute antibody-mediated rejection is high, and the development of allograft coronary artery disease is thought to be a direct response to multiple or chronic episodes of humoral rejection.[159–162]

COMPLICATIONS OF CARDIAC TRANSPLANTATION

Bacterial infection

Although allograft rejection significantly complicates the course of a transplant recipient's recovery, infection remains the leading cause of both morbidity and mortality in heart transplant patients.[163,164] The risk of life-threatening infection is greatest within the first 3 postoperative months, and the timing of infections varies with the causative organism. Nosocomial bacterial infections account for the greatest number of infections during the first posttransplant month.[165] Within the first 6 months, opportunistic infections account for the greatest morbidity, with the incidence equilibrating between community-acquired organisms and opportunistic infections after the first year.[166–168]

The primary organisms that cause bacterial infection in transplant recipients are gram-negative bacilli, with *Escherichia coli* and *Pseudomonas aeruginosa* being the most common.[169] In addition, as with surgical patients who are not immunocompromised, infections with *Staphylococcus* species account for the majority of gram-positive infections.

Prevention of infections is centered on two different strategies. The first is meticulous hand washing and isolation of recipients in private rooms to prevent the spread of nosocomial organisms from patient to patient. This has been shown to be as effective as the elaborate isolation procedures used during the first years of cardiac transplantation.[170,171] The second revolves around antibiotic prophylaxis. Recipients receive 48 h of gram-positive antibiotic coverage in the perioperative period to prevent early nosocomial infections from skin flora. In addition, antibiotic prophylaxis is given before any procedure known to cause large bacteremic loads to prevent endocarditis. Patients are treated routinely with trimethoprim-sulfamethoxazole (TMP-SMX) for *Pneumocystis carinii* prophylaxis. Patients with a positive purified protein derivative (PPD) skin test often receive standard *Mycobacterium tuberculosis* prophylactic therapy.[172–174]

Viral infection

Infection with viral pathogens can result from reactivation of latent virus in the recipient or primary infection from donor-to-recipient transmission. All potential donors and recipients are screened for HIV, HBV, HCV, and CMV. Positive titers for HIV, HBV, or HCV generally preclude transplantation, and efforts are made to transplant CMV-negative recipients with CMV-negative organs.[175–178] However, the development of intravenous ganciclovir has conferred such effective prophylaxis and treatment of CMV infections that these standards have become more relaxed. In addition, a few centers are using HCV-positive allografts in HCV-positive recipients.

Patients with CMV are treated with intravenous ganciclovir initially and then are transitioned to oral medication once the infection is under control. CMV remains the most common viral pathogen in transplant recipients and can lead to superinfection with bacterial or fungal pathogens because of its immunosuppressive actions if it is not treated appropriately. Standard treatment of herpes simplex (HSV) and varicella-zoster viral (VZV) infections usually reduces the severity of these infections.[179]

Common prophylaxis for viral pathogens remains controversial, although CMV-negative patients who receive CMV-positive organs usually are given a postoperative course of prophylactic therapy. Patients who are known to have negative titers for VZV, HBV, or measles and are exposed to these pathogens require treatment with specific immune globulins to prevent life-threatening complications. Vaccinations with the live attenuated viruses normally used to prevent some of these infections should be avoided in immunocompromised patients.

Other infections

Fungal infections often manifest as mucocutaneous candidiasis and can be treated easily with topical agents. Esophageal fungal infections that are not responsive to topical agents generally respond to fluconazole. Fungal sepsis in an immunocompromised host warrants aggressive treatment with fluconazole or amphotericin B as indicated by the culture results. *Aspergillus* can cause life-threatening pneumonia in a small subset of the transplant population, necessitating extended treatment with amphotericin B or itraconazole. Fungal infections that disseminate into the central nervous system are usually fatal.[180]

Protozoal infection with *Toxoplasma gondii* can result from donor-to-recipient transmission or acquired infection. This life-threatening complication can be treated effectively with appropriate antiprotozoal medications.[181] As was discussed above, TMP-SMX effectively prevents and treats infections with *P. carinii*, which are the most common cause of late pneumonia in transplant recipients.[172,173,182]

Allograft coronary artery disease

After the first posttransplant year, the leading cause of graft failure and patient death is allograft coronary artery disease (ACAD).[183,184] This poorly understood entity results from multiple inciting factors that lead to concentric coronary intimal hyperplasia and diffuse narrowing of vessels throughout the myocardium.[185,186] Risk factors include but are not limited to immunologic factors such as humoral rejection and nonimmunologic factors such as hypertension, hypercholesterolemia, increased donor age, and infection with CMV.[187–190] Because the cardiac allograft has been denervated, this disease process leads to episodes of silent myocardial ischemia that ultimately lead to allograft demise.

The diagnosis of ACAD generally requires invasive studies, including annual coronary angiography and/or intravascular ultrasound. Less invasive methods such as thallium stress testing have proved insensitive for the detection of these lesions. Once ACAD has been discovered, the only management options currently available are risk reduction practices such as smoking cessation, diet modification, and the use of agents such as antilipid medications and calcium channel blockers.[187–200] As the disease progresses, retransplantation remains the only treatment option since revascularization procedures are ineffective because of the pathophysiology of the disease.

Other chronic complications

Renal dysfunction generally results from immunosuppressive toxicity, as is seen most often with the IL-2 inhibitors cyclosporine A and FK506.[201,202] Frequent monitoring of drug levels and the substitution of one drug for another offer these patients the best chance to avoid long-term serious renal impairment if early renal dysfunction occurs.[203] The kidneys remain the organ system most often affected during the first few months after transplantation. However, they usually recover once the highest doses of these nephrotoxic drugs are reduced.[204]

Refractory hypertension resulting from nephrotoxicity, peripheral vasoconstriction, and fluid retention continues to be a significant complication in cardiac transplant recipients.[205–207] Management of this complication is difficult, and most clinicians treat patients on an individual basis. No single antihypertensive medication or combination of medications has proved effective for most patients.

Transplant recipients are at high risk for the development of certain types of malignancies. The unopposed proliferation of Epstein-Barr virus (EBV) in lymphocytic cells leads to a high rate of posttransplant lymphoproliferative disorder.[208–212] This is best treated with reduction of immunotherapy and antiviral medications such as acyclovir that directly attack the replication of this virus.[213] In addition, carcinomas frequently develop in transplant recipients because of the decreased surveillance of the immune system for those cancers.[214] Skin cancers are the malignancies most commonly seen in transplant recipients.[215] Carcinomas are best treated with conventional chemotherapy, radiation therapy, and surgical excision.

CURRENT RESULTS AND FUTURE DIRECTIONS

The last two decades have witnessed a vast improvement in the survival of cardiac transplant recipients and a significant decrease in morbidity. Current 1-year survival data demonstrate 5 to 10 percent mortality within the first 30 postoperative days, with 1- and 5-, and 10-year survival rates of approximately 80 percent, 65 percent, and 50 percent, respectively.[216,217] Studies show that initial postoperative mortality generally results from early graft failure; most of the remaining deaths in the first 6 months are caused by infection or uncontrollable rejection. Once patients survive this early posttransplantation period, accelerated allograft coronary artery disease is responsible for the majority of the remaining deaths, with an annual death rate of 4 percent per year in the initial transplant population.

Retransplantation for either accelerated ACAD or acute refractory rejection accounts for approximately 3 percent of transplants annually. Cyclosporine A has improved survival dramatically in this population, although the mortality rate in the retransplantation group far exceeds that in primary allograft recipients. Current 1-year survival is only 55 percent if retransplantation occurs within 2 years of the initial transplant.[89] However, if the primary allograft lasts longer than this 2-year interval, survival in the retransplant population can approach that in primary allograft recipients.[7]

These results demonstrate marked improvement in survival among cardiac transplant recipients since the early days, but significant obstacles remain. Limited availability of donor organs has remained constant for decades, and this has led to investigations of alternative sources of donor hearts. Xenotransplantation is one option with innumerable resources, but multiple challenges currently preclude its use. The technologic advances in VADs now allow clinicians to use these devices as "destination therapy" for some patients who otherwise would not qualify for cardiac transplantation.

Another limitation continues to be donor organ preservation, which is currently effective for only 4 to 6 h. This necessitates transplantation within a small regional area that often precludes transplantation into more ideal recipients. Researchers continue to seek better storage methods that will enable clinicians to match and disseminate donor organs to the most ideal recipients. Rejection surveillance continues to require invasive monitoring that can occur only at selected intervals, leading to extended periods of subclinical rejection that cause irreversible long-term damage to allografts. Improvements in monitoring for rejection using noninvasive equipment are needed to permit clinicians to detect rejection earlier and perhaps extend the viability of a donor allograft. Finally, continued improvements in immunosuppression may eliminate the damaging side effects of current immunosuppressive regimens. Since many investigators feel that current medications often perpetuate or accelerate allograft coronary artery disease, the ability to improve on these medications may extend the lives of allografts and their recipients dramatically.

SUMMARY

Since Barnard and colleagues performed the first cardiac transplantation in 1967, advances in the field have led to tremendous improvements in patient outcomes. Patients now undergo transplantation for a variety of etiologies of heart failure, and identification of the ideal recipients for heart transplantation has become key to the success of the procedure. More important, recipient prioritization has become a dominant focus of organ procurement agencies across the country, as the list of eligible recipients continues to grow.

Donor selection and management have as much to do with the success of transplantation as does recipient management. The use of donors who meet extended criteria has the potential to expand the number of cardiac transplants performed each year. Other advances in the field of organ preservation, such as the use of additives in storage solutions and the use of perfusion devices, will increase the safe storage period of cardiac allografts, potentially improving donor-recipient matching and increasing the number of transplants performed annually.

Operative techniques and postoperative care have been refined over the last two decades, improving early outcomes after transplantation. The introduction of cyclosporine was one of the most important advances in the field of heart transplantation, leading to significantly improved middle-term and long-term outcomes. However, infectious complications and chronic allograft rejection in the form of allograft coronary artery disease continue to have a negative effect on patients who receive cardiac allografts.

Cardiac transplantation has progressed from an experimental and often fatal endeavor to the definitive treatment option for congestive heart failure, with excellent medium-term and long-term results in this patient population. However, the field of cardiac transplantation must overcome many obstacles before this treatment option can achieve extended survival results comparable to those of other forms of cardiac and medical interventions. The advances being developed today will bring more questions tomorrow. However, the goal of patient survival and improved cardiac health in today's population will come closer to being reached as research in this field continues.

References

1. Barnard CN. A human cardiac transplant: An interim report of a successful operation performed at the Groote Schuur Hospital, Cape Town. *S Afr Med J* 1967; 41:1271.
2. Carrel A, Guthrie CC. The transplantation of veins and organs. *Am Med* 1905;10:1101.
3. Lower RR, Shumway NE. Studies on the orthotopic homotransplantation of the canine heart. *Surg Forum* 1960;11:18.
4. Caves PK, Stinson EB, Billingham ME, et al. Percutaneous endomyocardial biopsy in human heart recipients: Experience with a new technique. *Ann Thorac Surg* 1973; 16:325.
5. Oyer PE, Stinson EB, Jameison SA, et al. Cyclosporine A in cardiac allografting: A preliminary experience. *Transplant Proc* 1983;15:1247.
6. Go to http://www.unos.org, the website of this organization.
7. Steinman TI, Becker BN, Frost AE, et al. Guidelines for the referral and management of patients eligible for solid organ transplantation. *Transplantation* 2001;71:1189.
8. Hosenpud JD, Leah BE, Keck BM, et al. The registry of the International Society for Heart and Lung Transplantation: Eighteenth official report—2001. *J Heart Lung Transplant* 2001;20:805.
9. Ad Hoc Committee for Cardiothoracic Surgical Practice Guidelines. Transplantation (heart, lung, heart-lung) and heart assist devices: I. *Ann Thorac Surg* 1994;58:903.
10. Stevenson LW, Tillisch JH, Hamilton M, et al. Importance of hemodynamic response to therapy in predicting survival with ejection fraction <20 percent secondary to ischemic or non-ischemic dilated cardiomyopathy. *Am J Cardiol* 1990;66:1348.
11. Lee WH, Packer M. Prognostic importance of serum sodium concentration and its modification by converting enzyme inhibition in patients with severe heart failure. *Circulation* 1986;73:257.
12. Mancini DM, Eisen H, Kussmaul W, et al. Value of peak exercise oxygen consumption for optimal timing of cardiac transplantation in ambulatory patients with heart failure. *Circulation* 1991;83:778.
13. Unverferth DV, Magorien RD, Moeschberger ML, et al. Factors influencing the one year mortality of dilated cardiomyopathy. *Am J Cardiol* 1984;54:147.
14. Cohn JN, Levine TB, Olivari MT, et al. Plasma norepinephrine as a guide to prognosis in patients with chronic congestive heart failure. *N Engl J Med* 1984;311:819.
15. Keogh AM, Baron DW, Hickie JB. Prognostic guides in patients with idiopathic or ischemic dilated cardiomyopathy assessed for cardiac transplantation. *Am J Cardiol* 1990;65:903.
16. Cohn JN, Johnson GR, Shabetai R, et al. Ejection fraction, peak exercise oxygen consumption, cardiothoracic ratio, ventricular arrhythmias, and plasma norepinephrine as determinants of prognosis in heart failure. *Circulation* 1993;87(Suppl):VI-5.
17. Mudge GH, Goldstein S, Addonizio LZ, et al. Twenty fourth Bethesda conference on cardiac transplantation: Task Force 3: Recipient guidelines. *J Am Coll Cardiol* 1993;22:21.
18. Myers J, Gullestad L, Vagelos R, et al. Clinical, hemodynamic, and cardiopulmonary exercise test determinants

of survival in patients referred for evaluation of heart failure. *Ann Intern Med* 1998;129:286.
19. Erickson KW, Costanzo-Nordin MR, O'Sullivan EJ, et al. Influence of preoperative transpulmonary gradient on late mortality after orthotopic heart transplantation. *J Heart Transplant* 1990;9:526.
20. Kormos RL, Thompson M, Hardesty RL, et al: Utility of pre-operative right heart catheterization data as a predictor of survival after heart transplantation. *J Heart Transplant* 1986;5:391.
21. Kirklin JK, Naftel DC, Kirklin JW, et al. Pulmonary vascular resistance and the risk of heart transplantation. *J Heart Transplant* 1988;7:331.
22. Addonizio LJ, Gersony WM, Robbins RC, et al. Elevated pulmonary vascular resistance and cardiac transplantation. *Circulation* 1987;76(Suppl V):52.
23. Stinson EB, Griepp RB, Schroeder JS, et al. Hemodynamic observation two years after cardiac transplantation in man. *Circulation* 1972;45:1183.
24. Griepp RB, Stinson EB, Dong EJ, et al. Determinants of operative risk in human heart transplantation. *Am J Surg* 1971;122:192.
25. Losman JG, Barnard CN. Heterotopic heart transplantation: A valid alternative to orthotopic transplantation: Results, advantages, and disadvantages. *J Surg Res* 1982; 32:297.
26. Miller LW. Listing criteria for cardiac transplantation. *Transplantation* 1998;66:947.
27. Miller LW, Pennington DG, Kanter K, et al. Heart transplantation in patients over 55 years of age. *J Heart Transplant* 1986;5:367.
28. Munoz E, Lonquist J, Radovancevic B, et al. Long-term results in diabetic patients undergoing cardiac transplantation. *J Heart Transplant* 1991;10:189.
29. Rhenman MJ, Rhenman B, Icenogle T, et al. Diabetes and heart transplantation. *J Heart Transplant* 1988; 7:356.
30. Mai FM, McKenzie FN, Kotsuk WJ, et al. Psychiatric aspects of heart transplantation: Preoperative evaluation and postoperative sequelae. *Br Med J* 1986;292:311.
31. Holland C, Hagan M, Volkman K, et al. Substance abuse: Does this warrant exclusion for transplant [abstract]. *J Heart Transplant* 1988;7:70.
32. Bristow MR, O'Connell JB, Gilbert EM, et al. Dose response of chronic beta-blocker treatment in heart failure from either idiopathic dilated or ischemic cardiomyopathy. *Circulation* 1994;89:1632.
33. The SOLVD Investigators. Effect of enalapril on survival in patients with reduced left ventricular ejection fractions and congestive heart failure. *N Engl J Med* 1991;325:293.
34. Pitt B, Zannad F, Remme WJ, et al. The effect of spironolactone on morbidity and mortality in patients with severe heart failure. *N Engl J Med* 1999;341:709.
35. Leier CV, Binkley PF. Parenteral inotropic support for advanced congestive heart failure. *Prog Cardiovasc Dis* 1998; 41:207.
36. Canver CC, Chanda J. Milrinone for long-term pharmacologic support of status 1 heart transplant candidates. *Ann Thorac Surg* 2000;69:1823.
37. Bank AJ, Mir SH, Nguyen DQ, et al. Effects of left ventricular assist devices on outcomes in patients undergoing heart transplantation. *Ann Thor Surg* 2000;69:1369.
38. Morales DLS, Catanese KA, Helman DN, et al. Six year experience of caring for forty-four patients with left ventricular assist device at home: Safe, economical, necessary. *J Thorac Cardiovasc Surg* 2000;119:251.
39. Pennington DG, McBride LR, Kanter KR, et al. Bridging to heart transplantation with circulatory support devices. *J Heart Trans* 1989;8:116.
40. Miller LW. Mechanical assist devices in intensive cardiac care. *Am Heart J* 1991;121:1887.
41. Birovlejv S, Radovancevic B, Burnell BL, et al. Heart transplantation after mechanical circulatory support: Four years experience. *J Heart Lung Trans* 1992; 11:240.
42. Rose EA, Gelijns AC, Moskowitz AJ, et al. Long-term use of a left ventricular assist device for end-stage heart failure. *New Engl J Med* 2001;345:1435.
43. Stevenson WG, Stevenson LW, Weiss J, et al. Programmed ventricular stimulation in severe heart failure: High, short-term risk of sudden death despite non-inducibility. *Am Heart J* 1988;116:1447.
44. Moss AJ, Hall WJ, Cannon DS, et al. Improved survival with an implanted defibrillator in patients with coronary disease at high risk for ventricular arrhythmia. *N Engl J Med* 1996;335:1933.
45. Baldwin JC, Anderson JL, Boucek MM, et al. Bethesda conference: Cardiac transplantation: Task Force 2: Donor guidelines. *J Am Coll Cardiol* 1993;22:15.
46. Guidelines for determination of death: Report of the medical consultants on the diagnosis of death to the President's Commission for the Study of Ethical Problems in Medicine and Biomedical and Behavioral Research. *JAMA* 1981;246:2184.
47. National Task Force on Organ Transplantation. Final report. Rockville, MD: Office of Organ Transplantation, Health Resources, and Services Administration; 1986.
48. Report of Ad Hoc Committee of the Harvard Medical School to Examine the Definition of Brain Death. A definition of irreversible coma. *JAMA* 1968;205:337.
49. Mohandas A, Chou SN. Brain death: A clinical and pathological study. *J Neurosurg* 1976;35:211.
50. Walker AE. The neurosurgeon's responsibility for organ procurement. *J Neurosurg* 1976;44:1.
51. Uniform Brain Death Act, approved at Annual Conference of National Conference of Commissioners on Uniform State Laws, Washington, DC, July 28–August 4, 1978.
52. Tenderich G, Koerner MM, Stuettgen B, et al. Extended donor criteria: Hemodynamic follow-up of heart transplant recipients receiving a cardiac allograft from donors ≥ 60 years of age. *Transplantation* 1998;668:1109.
53. Young JB, Naftel DC, Bourge RC, et al. Matching the heart donor and heart transplant recipient: Clues for successful expansion of the donor pool: A multivariable, multi-institutional report: The Cardiac Transplant Research Database Group. *J Heart Lung Transplant* 1994;13:353.
54. Jeevanandam V, Furukawa S, Pendergast TW, et al. Standard criteria for an acceptable donor heart are restricting heart transplantation. *Ann Thorac Surg* 1996;62:1268.
55. Harms J, Isemer FE, Kolenda H. Hormonal alteration and pituitary function during course of brain stem death

in potential organ donors. *Transplant Proc* 1991; 23:2614.
56. Davis FD. Coordination of cardiac transplantation: Patient processing and donor organ procurement. *Circulation* 1987;75:29.
57. Lentz RD, Brown DM, Kjellstrand CM. Treatment of severe hypophosphatemia. *Ann Intern Med* 1978; 89:941.
58. Salter DR, Dyke CM, Fabian JA (eds). *Anesthesia for Organ Transplantation*. Philadelphia: Lippincott; 1992:81.
59. Gifford RPM, Weaver AS, Burg JE, et al. Thyroid hormone levels in heart and kidney cadaver donors. *J Heart Transplant* 1986;5:249.
60. Novitzky D, Wicomb WN, Cooper DKC, et al. Improved cardiac function following hormonal therapy in brain dead pigs: Relevance to organ donation. *Cryobiology* 1987; 24:1.
61. Novitzky D, Cooper DKC, Zuhdi N. The physiological management of cardiac transplant donors and recipients using triiodothyronine. *Transplant Proc* 1988; 20:803.
62. Demmy TL, Biddle JS, Bennett LE, et al. Organ preservation solutions in heart transplantation: Patterns of usage and related survival. *Transplantation* 1997; 63:262.
63. Stringham JC, Love RB, Welter D, et al. Impact of University of Wisconsin solution on clinical heart transplantation: A comparison with Stanford solution for extended preservation. *Circulation* 1998;98(Suppl 19): II157.
64. Keon KJ, Hendry PJ, Taichman GC, et al. Cardiac transplantation: The ideal myocardial temperature for graft transport. *Ann Thorac Surg* 1988;46:337.
65. Segel LD, Follette DM, Contino JP, et al. Importance of substrate enhancement for long-term heart preservation. *J Heart Lung Transplant* 1993;12:613.
66. Wicomb WN, Cooper DKC, Barnard CN. Twenty four hour preservation of the pig heart by a portable hypothermic perfusion system. *Transplantation* 1982; 34:246.
67. Wynands JE, Wong P, Whalley DG, et al. Oxygen-fentanyl anesthesia in patients with poor left ventricular function. *Anesth Analg* 1983;62:476.
68. Hensley FA, Martin DE, Larach DR, et al. Anesthetic management for cardiac transplantation in North America—1986 survey. *J Cardiothorac Anesth* 1987; 1:429.
69. Royston D. Aprotinin therapy in heart and heart-lung transplantation. *J Heart Lung Transplant* 1993;12:19.
70. Blanche C, Czer LS, Valenza M, et al. Alternative technique for orthotopic heart transplantation. *Ann Thorac Surg* 1994;57:765.
71. Ross D. Report of a heart transplant operation. *Am J Cardiol* 1968;22:838.
72. Yacoub M, Mankad P, Ledingham S. Donor procurement and surgical techniques for cardiac transplantation. *Semin Thorac Cardiovasc Surg* 1990;2:153.
73. Brandt M, Harringer W, Hirt SW, et al. Influence of bicaval anastomosis on late occurrence of atrial arrhythmia after heart transplantation. *Ann Thorac Surg* 1997;64:70.
74. Traversi E, Pozzoli M, Grande A, et al. The bicaval anastomosis technique for orthotopic heart transplantation yields better atrial function than the standard technique: An echocardiographic automatic boundary detection study. *J Heart Lung Transplant* 1998;17:1065.
75. Grande AM, Rinalde M, D'Armini AM, et al. Orthotopic heart transplantation: Standard versus bicaval technique. *Am J Cardiol* 2000;85:1329.
76. Aziz T, Burgess M, Khafagy R, et al. Bicaval and standard techniques in orthotopic heart transplantation: Medium term experience in cardiac performance and survival. *J Thorac Cardiovasc Surg* 1999;118:115.
77. Tagusari O, Kormos RL, Kawai A, et al. Native heart complications after heterotopic heart transplantation: Insight into the potential risk of left ventricular assist device. *J Heart Lung Transplant* 1999;18:1111.
78. Khaghani A, Santini F, Dyke CM, et al. Heterotopic cardiac transplantation in infants and children. *J Thorac Cardiovasc Surg* 1997;113:1042.
79. Trento A, Hardesty RL, Griffith BP, et al. Role of the antibody to vascular endothelial cells in hyperacute rejection in patients undergoing cardiac transplantation. *J Cardiovasc Surg* 1988;95:37.
80. Braun WE. Laboratory and clinical management of the highly sensitized organ transplant recipient. *Hum Immunol* 1989;26:245.
81. Loh E, Bergin JD, Couper GS, et al. Role of panel-reactive antibody cross-reactivity in predicting survival after orthotopic heart transplantation. *J Heart Lung Transplant* 1994;13:194.
82. Tischler MD, Lee RT, Plappert T, et al. Serial assessment of left ventricular function and mass after orthotopic heart transplantation: A four-year longitudinal study. *J Am Coll Cardiol* 1992;19:60.
83. Stinson EB, Griepp RB, Bieber CP, et al. Hemodynamic observations after orthotopic transplantation of the canine heart. *J Thorac Cardiovasc Surg* 1972;63:344.
84. Stinson EB, Caves PK, Griepp RB, et al. The transplanted heart in the postoperative period. *Surg Forum* 1983;24:189.
85. Bourge RC, Naftel DC, Costanzo-Nordin MR, et al. Pretransplantation risk factors for death after heart transplantation: A multi-institutional study. *J Heart Lung Transplant* 1993;12:549.
86. Costanzo-Nordin MR, Heroux AL, Radcany R, et al. Role of humoral immunity in acute cardiac allograft dysfunction. *J Heart Lung Transplant* 1993;12:S143.
87. Reemtsma K, Hardy MA, Drusin RE, et al. Cardiac transplantation: Changing patterns in evaluation and treatment. *Ann Surg* 1985;202:418.
88. Kanter KR, Pennington DG, McBride LR, et al. Mechanical circulatory assistance after heart transplantation. *J Heart Transplant* 1987;6:150.
89. Odom NJ, Richens D, Glenville BE, et al. Successful use of mechanical assist device for right ventricular failure after orthotopic heart transplantation. *J Heart Transplant* 1990;9:652.
90. Srivastava R, Keck BM, Bennett LE, et al. The results of cardiac retransplantation: An analysis of the Joint International Society for Heart and Lung Transplantation/United Network for Organ Sharing Thoracic Registry. *Transplantation* 2000;70:606.

91. Karwande SV, Ensley RD, Renlund DG, et al. Cardiac retransplantation: A viable option? *Ann Thorac Surg* 1992;54:840.
92. Stinson EB, Schroeder JS, Griepp RB, et al. Observations on the behavior of recipient atria after cardiac transplantation in man. *Am J Cardiol* 1972;30:615.
93. Fowles RE, Reitz BA, Ream AK, Kaplant J (eds). *Cardiac Anesthesia II: Cardiovascular Pharmacology.* New York: Grune & Stratton; 1983.
94. Griepp RB, Stinson EB, Dong E Jr., et al. Hemodynamic performance of the transplanted human heart. *Surgery* 1971;70:88.
95. Pope SE, Stinson EB, Daughters GT II, et al. Exercise response of the denervated heart in long-term cardiac transplant recipients. *Am J Cardiol* 1980;46:213.
96. Jacquet L, Ziady G, Stein K, et al. Cardiac rhythm disturbances early after orthotopic heart transplantation. *J Am Coll Cardiol* 1990;16:832.
97. Cameron DE, Augustine SM, Gardner TJ, et al. Preoperative amiodarone therapy causes graft bradycardia following orthotopic heart transplantation. *J Heart Transplant* 1988;7:67.
98. Goodman DJ, Rossen RM, Cannon DS, et al. Effect of digoxin on atrioventricular conduction: Studies in patients with and without cardiac autonomic innervation. *Circulation* 1975;51:251.
99. Corcos T, Tamburino C, Leger P, et al. Early and late hemodynamic evaluation after cardiac transplantation. *J Am Coll Cardiol* 1988;1:264.
100. Romhilt DW, Doyle M, Sagar KB, et al. Prevalence and significance of arrhythmias in long term survivors of cardiac transplantation. *Circulation* 1982;66(Suppl 1):219.
101. Little RE, Kay GN, Epstein AE, et al. Arrhythmias after orthotopic cardiac transplantation: Prevalence and determinants during initial hospitalization and late follow-up. *Circulation* 1989;80:111.
102. Holt C, Fandrich R, Leonard L, et al. Nursing strategy to allow early discharge after cardiac transplantation: Is it safe? *J Heart Transplant* 1990;9:84.
103. Hardman JG, Lee LE (eds). *The Pharmacological Basis of Therapeutics.* New York: McGraw-Hill; 1996:1291–1308.
104. Livi U, Luciani GB, Boff GM, et al. Clinical results of steroid-free induction immunosuppression after heart transplantation. *Ann Thorac Surg* 1993;55:1160.
105. Hess AD, Tutschka PJ. Effect of cyclosporin A on human lymphocytic responses in vivo. *J Immunol* 1980;124:2601.
106. Miller LW, Wolford T, McBride LR, et al. Successful withdrawal of corticosteroids in heart transplantation. *J Heart Lung Transplant* 1992;11:431.
107. Kobashigawa JA, Stevenson LW, Brownfield ED, et al. Initial success of steroid weaning late after heart transplantation. *J Heart Lung Transplant* 1992;11:428.
108. Olivari MT, Jessen ME, Baldwin BJ, et al. Triple-drug immunosuppression with steroid discontinuation by six months after heart transplantation. *J Heart Lung Transplant* 1995;14:127.
109. Kahan BD, Ried M, Newberger J, Pharmacokinetics of cyclosporine in human renal transplantation. *Transplant Proc* 1983;15:446.
110. Keown PA, Stiller CR, Sinclair NR, et al. The clinical relevance of cyclosporine in blood vessels as measured by radioimmunoassay. *Transplant Proc* 1983;15(Suppl I):I-2438.
111. Lemaire M, Fahr A, Maurer G: Pharmacokinetics of cyclosporine: Inter and intra-individual variations and metabolic pathways. *Transplant Proc* 1990;22:1110.
112. Myers BD, Ross J, Newton L, et al. Cyclosporine-associated chronic nephropathy. *N Engl J Med* 1984;311:699.
113. Cotts WG, Johnson MR. The challenge of rejection and cardiac allograft vasculopathy. *Heart Fail Rev* 2001;6:227.
114. Yamani MH, Starling RC, Pelegrin D, et al. Efficacy of tacrolimus in patients with steroid-resistant cardiac allograft cellular rejection. *J Heart Lung Transplant* 2000; 19:337.
115. Taylor DO, Barr ML, Radovancevic B, et al. A randomized, multicenter comparison of tacrolimus and cyclosporine immunosuppressive regimens in cardiac transplantation: Decreased hyperlipidemia and hypertension with tacrolimus. *J Heart Lung Transplant* 1999;18:336.
116. Jain A, Khanna A, Molmenti E, et al. Immunosuppressive therapy. *Surg Clin North Am* 1999;79:1.
117. Haddad H, MacNeil DM, Howlett J, et al. Sirolimus, a new potent immunosuppressant agent for refractory cardiac transplantation rejection: Two case reports. *Can J Cardiol* 2000;16:221.
118. Koegh A, Bourge R, Costanzo M, et al. Three year results of the double-blinded randomized multicenter trial of mycophenolate_luconaz in heart transplant patients. *J Heart Lung Transplant* 1999;18:53.
119. Elion GB. Pharmacologic and physical agents: Immunosuppressive agents. *Transplant Proc* 1978;9:975.
120. Griepp RB, Stinson EB, Dong EJ, et al. The use of antithymocyte globulin in human heart transplantation. *Circulation* 1972;45(Suppl 2):147.
121. Szenpetery S, Mohanakumar T, Barnhart G, et al. Beneficial effects of prophylactic use of rabbit antihuman thymocyte globulin in heart transplant recipients immunosuppressed with cyclosporine. *J Heart Transplant* 1986;5:365.
122. Carey JA, Frist WH. Use of polyclonal antilymphocyte preparations for prophylaxis in heart transplantation. *J Heart Transplant* 1990;9:297.
123. Kawaguchi A, Szenpetery S, Mohanakumar T, et al. Effects of prophylactic rabbit antithymocyte globulin in cardiac allograft recipients treated with cyclosporine. *J Heart Transplant* 1987;6:214.
124. Kung PC, Goldstein G, Reinhertz EL, et al. Monoclonal antibodies defining distinctive human T cell surface antigens. *Science* 1979;206:347.
125. Reinhertz EL, Neuer S, Fitzgerald KA, et al. Antigen recognition by human T lymphocytes is linked to surface expression of the T3 molecular complex. *Cell* 1982;30:735.
126. Chatenoud L, Jonker M, Villemain F, et al. The human immune response to murine OKT3 monoclonal antibody is oligoclonal. *Science* 1986;232(4756):1406–1408.
127. Haverty TP, Sanders M, Sheahan M. OKT3 treatment of cardiac allograft rejection. *J Heart Lung Transplant* 1993;12:591.
128. Frist WH, Gerhardt EB, Merrill WH, et al. Therapy of refractory, recurrent heart rejection with multiple courses of OKT3. *J Heart Transplant* 1990;9:724.

129. Gilbert EM, Dewitt CW, Eiswirth CC, et al. Treatment of refractory cardiac allograft rejection with OKT3 monoclonal antibody. *Am J Med* 1987;82:202.
130. Normann DJ. The clinical role of OKT3. *Cardiol Clin* 1990;8:97.
131. Rubin RH. Prevention and treatment of cytomegalovirus disease in heart transplant patients. *J Heart Lung Transplant* 2000;19(8):731.
132. Frist WH, Winterland AW, Gerhardt EB, et al. Total lymphoid irradiation in heart transplantation: Adjunctive treatment for recurrent rejection. *Ann Thorac Surg* 1989;48:863.
133. Salter MM, Kirklin JK, Bourge RC, et al. Total lymphoid irradiation in the treatment of early or recurrent heart rejection. *J Heart Lung Transplant* 1992;11:902.
134. Wieland M, Randels MJ, Strauss RG, et al. Photopheresis: A promising therapy for intractable cardiac allograft rejection. *J Clin Apheresis* 1992;7:42.
135. Barr ML, Mesiner BM, Eise HJ, et al. Photopheresis for the prevention of rejection in cardiac transplantation. *N Engl J Med* 1998;339:1744.
136. Hunt SA, Stinson EB. Cardiac transplantation. *Annu Rev Med* 1981;32:213.
137. Miller LW. Treatment of cardiac allograft rejection with intravenous corticosteroids. *J Heart Transplant* 1990; 9:283.
138. Caves PK, Stinson EB, Billingham ME, et al. Percutaneous endomyocardial biopsy in human heart recipients: Experience with a new technique. *Ann Thorac Surg* 1973; 16:325.
139. Billingham ME, Cary NB, Hammond ME, et al. A working formulation for the standardization of nomenclature in the diagnosis of heart and lung rejection: Heart rejection study group. *J Heart Lung Transplant* 1990;9(6):587.
140. Warnecke H, Schuler S, Goetze HJ, et al. Non-invasive monitoring of cardiac allograft rejection by intramyocardial electrogram recordings. *Circulation* 1986;75 (Suppl III):72.
141. Keren A, Gillis AM, Freedman RA, et al. Heart transplant rejection monitored by signal average electrocardiography in patients receiving cyclosporine. *Circulation* 1984;70(Suppl I):124.
142. Hsu DT, Spotritz HM. Echocardiographic diagnosis of cardiac allograft rejection. *Prog Cardiovasc Dis* 1990;33:149.
143. Desruennes M, Corocos T, Cabrol A, et al. Doppler echocardiography for the diagnosis of acute allograft rejection. *J Am Coll Cardiol* 1988;12:63.
144. Revel D, Chapelon C, Mathieu D, et al. Magnetic resonance imaging of human orthotopic heart transplantation correlation with endomyocardial biopsy. *J Heart Transplant* 1989;8:139.
145. Schaffellner S, Grasser B, Kniepeiss D, et al. Noninvasive heart monitoring after heart transplantation with CHARM (computerized heart allograft recipient monitoring): Clinical experience. *Transplant Proc* 2000;32:642.
146. Ballester M, Bordes R, Tazelaar HD, et al. Evaluation of biopsy classification for rejection: Relation to detection of myocardial damage by monoclonal antimyosin antibody imaging. *J Amer Coll Cardiol* 1998;31:1357.
147. Abdallah AN, Billes MA, Attia Y, et al. Evaluation of plasma levels of tumour necrosis factor alpha and interleukin-6 as rejection markers in a cohort of 142 heart-grafted patients followed by endomyocardial biopsy. *Eur Heart J* 1997;18:1024.
148. Michler RE, Smith CR, Drusin RE, et al. Reversal of cardiac transplant rejection without massive immunosuppression. *Circulation* 1986;74(Suppl III):68.
149. Carrier M, Jenicek M, Pelletier LC. Value of monoclonal antibody OKT3 in solid organ transplantation: A meta-analysis. *Transplant Proc* 1992;24:2586.
150. Olsen SL, O'Connell JB, Bristow MR, et al. Methotrexate as an adjunct in the treatment of persistent mild cardiac allograft rejection. *Transplantation* 1990;50:773.
151. Bourge RC, Kirklin JK, Williams CW, et al. Methotrexate pulse therapy in the treatment of recurrent acute heart rejection. *J Heart Lung Transplant* 1992;11:1116.
152. Laufer G, Lackovics A, Wollenek G, et al. The progression of mild acute cardiac rejection evaluated by risk factor analysis. *Transplantation* 1991;51:184.
153. Lloveras JJ, Escourrou G, Delisle MG, et al. Evolution of untreated mild rejection in heart transplant recipients. *J Heart Lung Transplant* 1992;11:751.
154. Yowell RL, Hammond EH, Bristow MR, et al. Acute vascular rejection involving the major coronary arteries of a cardiac allograft. *J Heart Lung Transplant* 1988;7:191.
155. Miller LW, Wesp A, Jennison SH, et al. Vascular rejection in heart transplant recipients. *J Heart Lung Transplant* 1993;12:S147.
156. Jambroes G, Borleffs JC, Slootweg PJ, et al. Acute humoral rejection afte5 heart transplantation. *Transplantation* 1988;46:603.
157. Herskowitz A, Soule LM, Ueda K, et al. Arteriolar vasculitis on endomyocardial biopsy: A histological predictor of poor outcome in cyclosporine-treated heart transplant recipients. *J Heart Transplant* 1987;6:127.
158. Hammond EH, Yowell RL, Nunoda S, et al. Vascular (humoral) rejection in heart transplantation: Pathologic observations and clinical implications. *J Heart Transplant* 1989;8:430.
159. Olsen SL, Wagoner LE, Hammond EH, et al. Vascular rejection in heart transplantation: Clinical correlation, treatment options, and future considerations. *J Heart Lung Transplant* 1993;12:S135.
160. Hammond EH, Yowell RL, Price GD, et al. Vascular rejection and its relationship to allograft coronary artery disease. *J Heart Lung Transplant* 1992;11:S111.
161. Hammond EH, Ensley RD, Yowell RL, et al. Vascular rejection of human cardiac allografts and the role of humoral immunity in chronic allograft rejection. *Transplant Proc* 1991;23:26.
162. Rose AG, Pepino P, Barr ML, et al. Relation of HLA antibodies and graft atherosclerosis in human cardiac allograft recipients. *J Heart Lung Transplant* 1992;11:S120.
163. Miller LW, Naftel DC, Bourge RC, et al. Infection after heart transplantation: A multi-institutional study. *J Heart Lung Transplant* 1994;13:381.
164. Petri WA Jr. Infections in heart transplant recipients. *Clin Infect Dis* 1994;18:141.
165. Gentry LO, Zeluff BJ. Diagnosis and treatment of infection in cardiac transplant patients. *Surg Clin North Am* 1986;66(3):459.

166. Hosenpud JD, Herschberger RE, Pantely GA, et al. Late infection in cardiac allograft recipients: Profiles, incidence, and outcome. *J Heart Transplant* 1987;10:80.
167. Dummer SJ. Infectious complications of transplantation. *Cardiovasc Clin* 1990;20:163.
168. Garibaldi R. Infections in organ transplant recipients. *Infect Control* 1983;4:460.
169. Montoya JG, Giraldo LF, Efron B, et al. Infectious complications among 620 consecutive heart transplant patients at Stanford University medical center. *Clin Infect Dis* 2001;33:629.
170. Walsh TR, Gyttendorf J, Dummer S, et al. The value of protective isolation procedures in cardiac allograft recipients. *Ann Thorac Surg* 1989;47:539.
171. Wade JC, Schimpf SC, Rubin RH, Young LS (eds). Epidemiology and prevention of infection in the compromised host. In: *Clinical Approach to Infection in the Compromised Host,* 2d ed. New York: Plenum; 1988:5.
172. Hughes WT, Rivera GK, Schell MJ, et al. Successful intermittent chemoprophylaxis for *Pneumocystis carinii* pneumonitis. *N Engl J Med* 1987;316:1627.
173. Jules-Elysee KM, Stover DE, Zaman MB, et al. Aerosolized pentamidine: Effect on diagnosis and presentation of *Pneumocystis carinii* pneumonia. *Ann Intern Med* 1990; 112: 750.
174. The use of preventive therapy for tuberculous infection in the United States: Recommendations of the Advisory Committee for Elimination of Tuberculosis. *MMWR Morb Mortal Wkly Rpt* 1990;39:9.
175. Love KR, Emery RW, Pritker MR (eds). Nonbacterial infections in thoracic transplantation. In: *State of the Art Reviews: Cardiac Surgery.* Philadelphia: Hanley & Belfus; 1988:647.
176. Lake K, Milfred T, Reutzel J, et al. Practices of cardiothoracic transplant center regarding hepatitis C positive candidates and donors—A follow-up survey [abstract]. *J Heart Lung Transplant* 1995;14(1):S70.
177. Pereira BG, Milford EL, Kirkman RL. Transmission of hepatitis C virus organ transplantation. *N Engl J Med* 1991;325:454.
178. Snydman DR, Werner BG, Heinze-Lacey B, et al. Use of cytomegalovirus immune globulin to prevent cytomegalovirus disease in renal transplant recipients. *N Engl J Med* 1987;317:1049.
179. Seale L, Jones CJ, Kathpalia S, et al. Prevention of herpes virus infection in renal allograft recipients by low-dose oral acyclovir. *JAMA* 1985;254:3435.
180. Hummel M, Thalmann U, Jautzke G, et al. Fungal infections following heart transplantation. *Mycoses* 1992; 35:23.
181. Carey RM, Kimball AC, Armstrong D, et al. Toxoplasma: Clinical experiences in a cancer hospital. *Am J Med* 1973; 54:30.
182. Montgomery JR, Barett FF, Williams TW Jr. Infectious complications in cardiac transplant patients. *Transplant Proc* 1973;5:1239.
183. Urelsky BR, Murali S, Reddy PS, et al. Development of coronary artery disease in cardiac transplant patients receiving immunosuppressive therapy with cyclosporine and prednisone. *Circulation* 1987;76:827.
184. Bieber CP, Hunt SA, Schwinn DA, et al. Complications in long-term survivors of cardiac transplantation. *Transplant Proc* 1981;8:2073.
185. Johnson DE, Gao SZ, Schroeder JS, et al. The spectrum of coronary artery pathologic findings in human cardiac allografts. *J Heart Transplant* 1989;8:349.
186. Billingham ME. Cardiac transplant atherosclerosis. *Transplant Proc* 1987;19(Suppl 5):19.
187. Fields BL, Hoffman RM, Berkoff HA. Assessment of the impact of recipient age and organ ischemic time on heart transplant mortality. *Transplant Proc* 1988;20:1035.
188. Johnson MR. Transplant coronary artery disease: Non-immunologic risk factors. *J Heart Lung Transplant* 1992;11:S124.
189. Winters GL, Kendall TJ, Radio SJ, et al. Post-transplant obesity and hyperlipidemia: Major predictors of severity of coronary arteriopathy in failed human allografts. *J Heart Lung Transplant* 1990;9:364.
190. Grattan MT, Moreno-Cabral CE, Starnes VA, et al. Cytomegalovirus infection is associated with cardiac allograft rejection and atherosclerosis. *JAMA* 1989;261:3561.
191. Rose EA, Pepino P, Barr ML, et al. Relation of HLA antibodies and graft atherosclerosis in human cardiac allograft recipients. *J Heart Lung Transplant* 1992;11:S120.
192. Johnson DE, Gao SZ, Schroeder JS, at al. The spectrum of coronary artery pathologic findings in human cardiac allografts. *J Heart Transplant* 1989;8:349.
193. Billingham ME. Cardiac transplant atherosclerosis. *Transplant Proc* 1987;19(Suppl 5):19.
194. St. Goar FG, Pinto FJ, Alderman EL, et al. Detection of coronary atherosclerosis in young adult hearts using intravascular ultrasound. *Circulation* 1992;86:756.
195. Smart FW, Ballantyne CM, Farmer JA, et al. Insensitivity of noninvasive tests to detect coronary artery vasculopathy after heart transplant. *Am J Cardiol* 1991;67:243.
196. Johnson DE, Alderman EL, Schroeder JS, et al. Transplant coronary artery disease: Histopathologic correlations with angiographic morphology. *J Am Coll Cardiol* 1991;17:449.
197. St. Goar FG, Pinto FJ, Alderman EL, et al. Intravascular ultrasound imaging of angiographically normal coronary arteries: An in vivo comparison with quantitative angiography. *J Am Coll Cardiol* 1991;18:952.
198. Anderson TJ, Meredith IT, Uehata A, et al. Functional significance of intimal thickening as detected by intravascular ultrasound early and late after cardiac transplantation. *Circulation* 1993;88:1093.
199. Mehra MR, Ventura HO, Stapleton DD, et al. The prognostic significance of intimal proliferation in cardiac allograft vasculopathy: A paradigm shift. *J Heart Lung Transplant* 1995;14(6 Pt 2):S207.
200. Wenke K, Meiser B, Thiery J, et al. Simvastatin reduces graft vessel disease and mortality after heart transplantation: A 4 year randomized trial. *Circulation* 1997;96(5):1398.
201. Myers BD, Sibley R, Newton L, et al. The long-term course of cyclosporine-associated chronic nephropathy. *Kidney Int* 1988;33:590.
202. Myers BD. Cyclosporine nephrotoxicity. *N Engl J Med* 1986;30:964.
203. Moyer TP, Post GR, Sterioff S, et al. Cyclosporine nephrotoxicity is minimized by adjusting dosage on the basis of drug concentration in blood. *Mayo Clin Proc* 1988;63:241.
204. Miller LW, Pennington DG, McBride LR. Long-term effects of cyclosporine in cardiac transplantation. *Transplant Proc* 1990;22(Suppl 1):15.
205. Schacter M. Cyclosporine A and hypertension. *J Hypertens* 1988;6:511.

206. Starling RC, Cody RJ. Cardiac transplant hypertension. *Am J Cardiol* 1990;65:106.
207. Mark AL. Cyclosporine, sympathetic activity, and hypertension. *N Engl J Med* 1990;323:748.
208. Armitage JM, Kormos RL, Stuart RS, et al. Post-transplant lymphoproliferative disease in thoracic organ transplant patients: Ten years of cyclosporine-based immunosuppression. *J Heart Lung Transplant* 1991;10:877.
209. Randhawa PS, Yousem SA, Paradis IL, et al. The clinical spectrum, pathology, and clonal analysis of Epstein-Barr virus-associated lymphoproliferative disorders in heart-lung transplant recipients. *Am J Clin Pathol* 1989;92:177.
210. Nalesnik MA, Makowka L, Starzl TE. The diagnosis and treatment of post-transplant lymphoproliferative disorders. *Curr Probl Surg* 1988;25:371.
211. Hanto DW, Sakamoto K, Purtilo DT, et al. The Epstein-Barr virus in the pathogenesis of post-transplant lymphoproliferative disorders. *Surgery* 1981;90:204.
212. Klein G, Purtilo DT. Summary: Symposium on Epstein-Barr virus induced lymphoproliferative diseases in immunodeficient patients. *Cancer Res* 1981;41:4302.
213. Sullivan JL, Medveczky P, Forman SJ, at al: Epstein-Barr virus induced lymphoproliferation: Implications for antiviral chemotherapy. *N Engl J Med* 1984; 311:1163.
214. Penn I. Cancers following cyclosporine therapy. *Transplantation* 1987;43:32.
215. Krikorian JG, Anderson JL, Bieber CP, et al. Malignant neoplasms following cardiac transplantation. *JAMA* 1978;240:639.
216. Sarris GE, Moore KA, Schroeder JS, et al. Cardiac transplantation: The Stanford experience in the cyclosporine era. *J Thorac Cardiovasc Surg* 1994;108:240.
217. Suvarna S, Kennedy A, Ciulli F, Locke T. Revision of the 1990 working formulation for cardiac allograft rejection: The Sheffield experience. *Heart* 1998;79:432.

CHAPTER

45 LUNG AND HEART-LUNG TRANSPLANTATION

Susan D. Moffatt-Bruce, Bruce A. Reitz

INTRODUCTION

Lung and heart-lung transplantation has evolved over several decades to become an accepted modality for patients with end-stage lung and heart disease. To date, more than 8000 lung and 1000 heart-lung transplants have been reported in the United States.[1] Lung transplants have been divided relatively equally between unilateral and bilateral procedures, with about 67 percent of all lung transplant procedures being performed in U.S. centers (Fig. 45-1). Heart-lung transplantation has specific indications that have been redefined since its inception in 1981. More recently, a constant decline in heart-lung activity has paralleled a continuous increase in

KEY CONCEPTS

- Epidemiology
  - To date, more than 8000 lung and 1000 heart-lung transplantations have been reported in the United States. Single-lung and bilateral lung transplants are performed equally often, with about 67 percent of all lung transplants being performed in the United States.
- Pathophysiology
  - Lung and heart-lung transplantation is performed for patients who have end-stage cardiopulmonary disease with no contraindications and have the potential to be rehabilitated completely. Most lung transplants are done for chronic obstructive pulmonary disease, cystic fibrosis, idiopathic pulmonary fibrosis, and pulmonary hypertension. Primary pulmonary hypertension and Eisenmenger's syndrome are the most common indications for heart-lung transplantation.
- Clinical features
  - Candidates typically experience severe dyspnea, cyanosis, hemoptysis, and syncope and have New York Heart Association functional class III and IV status. Lung transplant candidates typically have a life expectancy of 24 to 36 months and are less than 60 (bilateral) to 65 (single) years of age. Patients with chronic obstructive pulmonary disease generally have a forced expiratory volume in 1 second (FEV_1) of less than 20 percent predicted, whereas patients with cystic fibrosis usually have an FEV_1 of less than 30 percent predicted, an increasing oxygen requirement, nutritional decline, and an increasing requirement for hospitalization. Candidates for heart-lung transplant have a life expectancy between 12 and 18 months and are less than 55 years of age.
- Diagnostics
  - Candidates for lung and heart-lung transplants undergo an extensive workup to evaluate underlying cardiopulmonary function and exclude malignancy, active infection, end-organ dysfunction, and vascular disease. Diagnostic modalities include pulmonary function tests, endoscopy (especially bronchoscopy), echocardiography, cardiac catheterization, duplex ultrasonography, computed tomography and/or magnetic resonance imaging, serologic screens, and metabolic panels.
- Treatment
  - *Lung transplantation:* chronic obstructive pulmonary disease, cystic fibrosis, idiopathic pulmonary fibrosis, and pulmonary hypertension. *Heart-lung transplantation:* primary pulmonary hypertension, Eisenmenger's syndrome, and cystic fibrosis.

- Outcomes
  - Lung transplant survival rates are 73 percent, 57 percent, 45 percent, and 23 percent at 1, 3, 5, and 10 years, respectively; these are the best survival rates among patients with chronic obstructive pulmonary disease. Significant functional improvement is immediate and durable beyond the first 3 years of follow-up. For heart-lung transplantation, survival rates are 61 percent, 40 percent, and 25 percent at 1, 5, and 10 years, respectively. Early morbidity and mortality stem from technical complications, noncytomegalovirus (CMV) infections, and graft failure. Late complications are usually manifestations of bronchiolitis obliterans.

isolated lung transplantation, and fewer centers now perform this highly specialized transplantation procedure (Fig. 45-2).[2]

Donor availability continues to limit both lung and heart-lung transplantation. Ways in which to broaden donor criteria are being sought to reduce the clear numeric discrepancy between donors and recipients. Improving donor, awaiting patient and recipient management is paramount to optimizing a limited resource.

Tailoring immunosuppression and pre- and postoperative care has resulted in improved survival and quality of life for recipients of lung and heart-lung transplants. Transplant recipients now can experience good early transplant outcomes with fewer infectious and neoplastic complications. However, chronic rejection in the form of obliterans bronchiolitis remains a seemingly insurmountable obstacle that limits the long-term outcomes of transplant recipients. Surveillance and aggressive attempts at preventing obliterans bronchiolitis are the only currently available treatment modalities.

HISTORICAL BACKGROUND

Thoracic transplantation has developed in conjunction with vascular anastomotic techniques, cardiopulmonary bypass support, and an understanding of immunologic barriers. Alexis Carrel is credited with the earliest work in developing experimental vascular surgery, with a description in 1905 of transplanting a puppy's heart into the neck of an adult dog (Table 45-1).[3] Frank Mann at the Mayo Clinic, prompted by Carrel's experiments, recognized that although transplants were technically feasible, a "biological incompatibility" between donor and recipient limited their success.[4] The earliest reports of experimental lung transplantation are those of Demikhov, who in 1947 performed individual canine lung lobe transplantation. He also demonstrated the technical feasibility of intrathoracic heterotopic heart transplants and is credited with the first successful canine heart-lung transplant, with a total of 8 of 67 dogs surviving more than 48 h.[5] In the western world, Marcus and associates from the Chicago

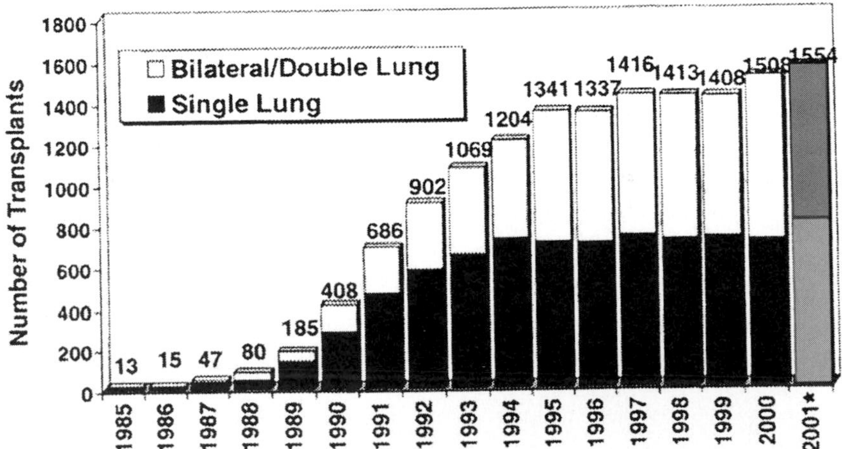

Figure 45-1 Number of lung transplants reported by year and procedure type in the International Society for Heart and Lung Transplantation Registry. (Reprinted from the *Journal of Heart and Lung Transplantation*, Volume 21(9), Hertz MI, Taylor DO, Trulock EP, et al. The Registry of the International Society of Heart and Lung Transplantation: Nineteenth Official Report-2002, 957-962, 2002, with permission from the International Society for Heart and Lung Transplantation.)

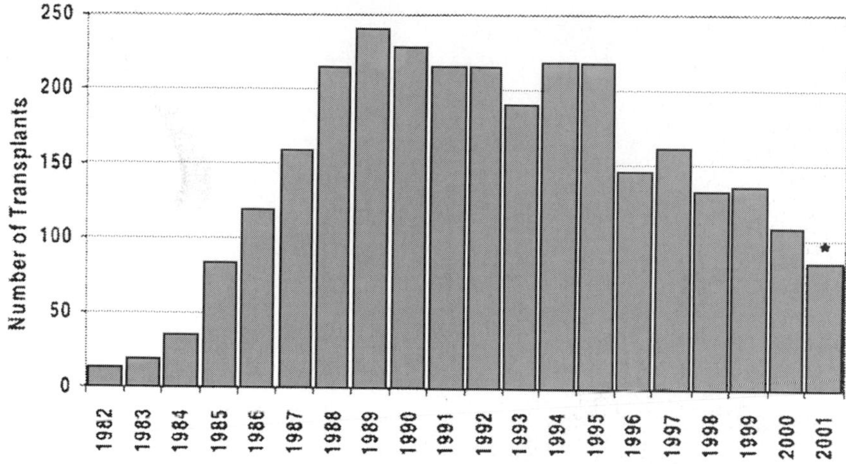

Figure 45-2 Number of heart-lung transplants reported by year of transplant in the International Society of Heart and Lung Transplantation Registry. (Reprinted from the *Journal of Heart and Lung Transplantation*, Volume 21(9), Hertz MI, Taylor DO, Trulock EP, et al. The Registry of the International Society of Heart and Lung Transplantation: Nineteenth Official Report-2002, 957-962, 2002, with permission from the International Society for Heart and Lung Transplantation.)

Medical School described their experiments in heterotopic heart-lung transplantation to the intraabdominal aortas and venae cavae of recipient animals.[6] In 1957, Webb and Howard first reported the use of a pump oxygenator to perform heart-lung transplantation in dogs.[7]

The clinical application of heart and heart-lung transplantation developed concurrently in the late 1960s. Lower and Shumway[8] described the currently used, although somewhat modified, technique of orthotopic heart transplantation in 1960. Human heart transplantation became a clinical reality in 1967, when Christiaan Barnard did a transplant in a 24-year-old woman in South Africa.[9] Three days later, an infant heart transplant was performed but was not successful. Shumway went on to perform the first adult American heart transplant in 1968, initiating the Stanford transplant program, which continues to be active and innovative.

Cooley and associates were the first to attempt heart-lung transplantation in 1968, when they did a transplant in a 2½-year-old girl with an atrioventricular canal defect and pulmonary hypertension; the patient died 14 h postoperatively.[10] Lillehei and colleagues[11] transplanted a heart and lungs into a 43-year-old man in 1969; the patient lived 8 days. Canine studies were ongoing during those years in an attempt to optimize the results of heart-lung transplantation, but it was not until the late 1970s, when Reitz and colleagues at Stanford, using cyclosporin, achieved clinically acceptable results in primates.[12] In 1981, the first successful heart-lung transplant was performed at Stanford in a 45-year-old woman who went on to do well for more than 5 years after the procedure.[13]

Dr. James Hardy at the University of Mississippi performed the first human lung transplant and also is credited with early investigation of immunosuppressive therapy to prolong lung allograft survival in dogs.[14] The first human lung transplant procedure was performed in a prisoner with severe emphysema and an obstructing carcinoma of the left mainstem bronchus. The recipient lived only 18 days and died of multiorgan failure. That disappointing result was followed by several other attempts over a 20-year period until the first successful single lung transplant was reported by Joel Cooper at the University of Toronto.[15] The success of that procedure was attributed to both the introduction of cyclosporin and the use of omental pedicle grafts to supply blood to the tracheal anastomosis. In 1988, Alexander Patterson and coworkers described the technique of en bloc double-lung transplantation.[16] That technique was associated with tracheal anastomotic complications as a result of poor vascularity. As a result, bilateral sequential single-lung transplantation has become the standard of care for patients who require bilateral lung replacement.

INDICATIONS FOR LUNG AND HEART-LUNG TRANSPLANTATION

Most lung transplants are performed for four major disease processes: chronic obstructive pulmonary disease (COPD), cystic fibrosis (CF), idiopathic pulmonary fibrosis (IPF), and pulmonary hypertension (PH). A wide variety of rare conditions contribute fewer than 10 percent of lung transplant recipients, as is shown in Table 45-2.[17]

Table 45-1 Landmark dates in thoracic transplantation

Year	Event
1905	Alexis Carrel transplants a puppy heart into the neck of an adult dog
1933	Frank Mann recognizes rejection as a biologic factor that limits transplantation
1947	Demikhov performs individual canine lung lobe transplants
1953	Marcus and associates describe heterotopic heart-lung transplantation
1956	Demikhov reports technical feasibility of intrathoracic heterotopic heart transplantation
1956	Webb and Howard use the pump oxygenator for heart-lung transplantation in dogs
1960	Lower and Shumway at Stanford report orthotopic heart transplantation in dogs
1963	James Hardy at the University of Mississippi performs the first human lung transplant
1964	James Hardy implants a chimpanzee heart into a 68-year-old man
1967	Christiaan Barnard performs the first human-to-human heart transplant in South Africa
1967	Kantrowitz at Maimonides Hospital performs the first American baby heart transplant
1968	Cooley performs the first heart-lung transplant in a 2-year-old girl
1968	Shumway at Stanford performs the first American adult heart transplant
1969	Lillehei and colleagues transplant heart and lungs into a 50-year-old woman
1978	Reitz and colleagues at Stanford perform heart-lung autotransplants in primates
1981	Reitz and colleagues transplant a heart-lung block into a 45-year-old woman
1986	Joel Cooper performs the first successful single-lung transplant
1987	Alexander Patterson describes the technique of en bloc double-lung transplantation

Table 45-2 Indications for lung and heart-lung transplantation

- Lung transplantation
  - Chronic obstructive pulmonary disease
  - Idiopathic pulmonary fibrosis
  - Cystic fibrosis
  - Alpha$_1$-antitrypsin disease
  - Primary pulmonary hypertension
  - Bronchogenic carcinoma
  - Lymphangioleiomyomatosis
  - Septic lung disease
- Heart-lung transplantation
  - Primary pulmonary hypertension
  - Eisenmenger's syndrome
  - Cystic fibrosis
  - End-stage lung disease and cardiac dysfunction
  - Septic lung disease
  - Cardiac neoplasm

According to the International Society for Heart and Lung Transplantation (ISHLT) database, 39 percent of lungs transplants were performed for COPD, 17 percent for IPF, 16 percent for CF, 9 percent for alpha$_1$-antitrypsin deficiency, and 5 percent for PH.[2] The majority of single-lung transplants were performed for COPD (54 percent) or IPF (24 percent), and most bilateral transplants were performed for CF (33 percent) or COPD (23 percent). Interestingly, the indication of PH for lung transplantation decreased from 13 percent in 1990 to only 4 percent in 2001, whereas the indication of emphysema increased from 21 percent to 42 percent over the last decade.[2]

Severe pulmonary vascular disease in the form of primary pulmonary hypertension (PPH) and Eisenmenger's syndrome secondary to congenital heart disease were the initial disease processes for which heart-lung transplantation was intended. PPH and Eisenmenger's syndrome remain the most common indications for heart-lung transplantation in adults. In addition, the ISHLT database recorded that CF accounted for 19 percent of the heart-lung transplants performed between 1996 and 2001, probably reflecting the role of the domino procedure, in which a CF heart-lung recipient's healthy heart is donated to a cardiac recipient. Less often, heart-lung transplantation is performed for patients with end-stage lung disease and cardiac dysfunction as well as septic lung disease (Table 45-2).[18]

The use of both single- and double-lung transplantation for patients with end-stage COPD has been shown to result in good outcomes.[19] The paucity of donors, however, makes single-lung transplantation more practical. Several groups have reported that bilateral lung transplantation for COPD patients is associated with superior lung function, exercise tolerance, and a trend toward enhanced survival with an excellent quality of life compared with single-lung transplantation.[20] Therefore, in younger candidates with COPD, double-lung transplantation may be more appropriate although not always feasible.

Cystic fibrosis is an indication for both double-lung and heart-lung transplantation. Transplantation often is performed in the setting of chronic pulmonary colonization and infection and additional organ system dysfunction. These are typically young patients, and survival on the transplant waiting list is very limited. It is perceived that patients with CF stand to benefit more from transplantation than does any other transplant candidate group.[21] The decision to perform double-lung or heart-lung transplantation in these patients has evolved as surgical acceptance of these techniques has changed.[22] In a review of Stanford's experience with transplantation in CF patients, the use of heart-lung transplantation predominated between 1988 and 1992, when confidence in the procedure peaked. As the use of double-lung transplantation became more widespread and the shortage of organ donors persisted, bilateral lung transplantation became the preferred method.[23] Nonetheless, the Stanford experience has not revealed any difference between the techniques in terms of actuarial survival, and heart-lung transplantation continues to have a role in small pediatric CF patients.

Congenital heart lesions that have been reported to result in the irreversible pulmonary hypertension known as Eisenmenger's disease include atrial and ventricular septal defects, patent ductus arteriosus, and truncus arteriosis.[24] Patients who undergo thoracic transplantation for congenital heart disease have survival rates comparable to those of adults with noncongenital heart disease.[24] Heart-lung transplantation has provided good results in patients with Eisenmenger's disease and remains the preferred transplant technique among many groups.[25,26] However, because of a donor shortage, lung transplantation with or without intracardiac repair has become an alternative transplant strategy.[27] It has been shown that bilateral single-lung transplantation can be performed as an alternative without an increase in mortality or morbidity. Drug therapy has improved the quality of life for patients with PPH. However, this condition remains lethal, necessitating the use of lung and heart-lung transplantation as a treatment modality. Primary pulmonary hypertension can be approached with single-lung, double-lung, or heart-lung transplantation. The Stanford and Washington University groups both found that lung and heart-lung transplantations provide similar survival benefits and are associated with dramatic improvements in quality of life.[28–30]

Suppurative or septic lung disease poses several problems in regard to transplantation. Bilateral sepsis caused by underlying CF or bronchiectasis mandates excision of both lungs. In addition, extensive pleural adhesions make operative time and the risk of bleeding high. Both heart-lung and bilateral lung transplantations have been advocated for this form of lung disease, and the Stanford and Newcastle groups have reported similar results with either technique.[31–33]

Transplantation for patients with bronchogenic or cardiac malignancy is highly controversial.[34–37] Talbot and coworkers at Columbia have had experience with unresectable cardiac sarcoma and subsequent heart-lung transplantation.[34] All their patients received chemotherapy before transplantation, and median survival after transplantation was 31 months. All those patients had tumor recurrence, and it therefore was concluded that a high incidence of metastatic disease severely limited the role of transplantation for cardiac sarcoma patients. Single- and double-lung transplantation for bronchogenic carcinoma also has been investigated.[35–37] Although transplantation has been found to palliate cancer patients, in particular those with advanced bronchioloalveolar carcinoma, the recurrence rate is high.

Lymphangioleiomyomatosis (LAM) is a rare disease found primarily in white women of childbearing age.[38] Unfortunately, recurrence in the lung allograft has been reported.[39] However, in a single institution review, early outcome and late survival were found to be equivalent to or better than those of lung transplantation for other diagnoses.[40]

RECIPIENT SELECTION CRITERIA

The decision to perform lung or heart-lung transplantation requires the selection of appropriate patients with end-stage cardiopulmonary disease who have no contraindications and the potential to be rehabilitated completely. Symptoms that prompt evaluation for lung or heart-lung transplantation include dyspnea, cyanosis, hemoptysis, and syncope, with patients normally in New York Heart Association functional class III and class IV.[41] This decision process requires a multidisciplinary team that includes thoracic transplant surgeons, cardiologists, pulmonologists, social workers, and psychologists.

Lung transplantation

The criteria for listing a candidate for lung transplantation have changed little since the first transplants were performed. One characteristic that has changed, however, is the life expectancy of the intended recipient at the time of listing. During the early years, 12 to 24 months of life expectancy was deemed sufficiently poor. Current recommendations now propose that a recipient's life expectancy should be 24 to 36 months.[41] Age criteria for bilateral lung transplantation are usually less than 60 years of age compared with 65 years for single-lung transplantation. Patients with COPD generally have an FEV_1 of less than 20 percent predicted, whereas patients with CF usually have an FEV_1 of less than 30 percent predicted, an increasing oxygen requirement, nutritional decline, and an increasing requirement for hospitalization.[17] Absolute contraindications to lung transplantation include other organ end-stage dysfunction; substance abuse, including tobacco; active malignancy; and HIV infection (Table 45-3). The investigation of organ system damage is particularly necessary in patients with CF, in which pancreatic insufficiency is prevalent, as well as periodic sinus inspection for underlying infection. Patients who have a history significant for smoking should undergo a vascular workup to ensure that the carotids and peripheral vasculature are free of disease.

Relative contraindications have changed as the medical management of transplant patients has improved. Neither the use of corticosteroids nor the presence of treatable coronary artery disease with good ventricular function is a contraindication to lung transplantation.[41,42] Reports suggest that patients can have coronary disease stented preoperatively or be revascularized at the time of transplantation without increased morbidity.[42] Clinically significant osteoporosis is a concern, but aggressive preoperative management has improved posttransplant disease progression in those patients.[43] A well-debated

Table 45-3 Lung and heart-lung transplantation: Recipient criteria and contraindications

Recipient criteria
Severe disease with optimal medical management
New York Heart Association class III or IV symptoms
Limited life expectancy (2–3 years)
Stable nutritional status
Patient motivated for rehabilitation
Stable support system
Absolute contraindications
Irreversible dysfunction of other organs (e.g., renal, hepatic)
Current smoking, alcohol, or drug abuse
Active malignancy
HIV infection
Relative contraindications
Mechanical ventilation
Coronary artery disease without left ventricular dysfunction
Significant peripheral vascular disease
Severe osteoporosis
Active pulmonary infection
Hepatitis B or C infection
Sputum with panresistant bacteria, fungi, or atypical mycobacterium
Psychosocial instability
Weight <70% or >130% of ideal body weight
Recent acute steroid use
Chest wall deformity

issue concerning transplanting patients with CF is the presence of multiple or panresistant bacterial organisms. International guidelines suggest that the presence of panresistant bacteria is not an absolute contraindication, but many centers limit transplantation in patients with *Burkholderia cepacia* colonization.[44] Mechanical ventilation, which once was considered an absolute contraindication to lung transplantation because of perceived decreased survival, is no longer a contraindication. Recent reports indicate that although patients intubated before lung transplant have significantly longer intubation times postoperatively, lung function and overall survival are not affected.[45,46]

Heart-lung transplantation

The generally accepted recipient age criterion for heart-lung transplantation is less than 55 years, and the projected recipient life span should be 12 to 18 months despite optimal medical management of the underlying disease. The absolute contraindications to lung transplantation pertain to heart-lung transplantation as well (Table 45-3). Similarly, the relative contraindications listed in Table 45-3 are evaluated on an individual basis for each potential heart-lung transplant candidate. During the early years of heart-lung transplantation, previous cardiothoracic surgery and pleurodesis were deemed absolute contraindications to transplantation because of bleeding from chest wall adhesions and difficulty preserving the vagus, recurrent laryngeal, and phrenic nerves. However, with improved surgical hemostatic devices, the use of antifibrinolytic agents, and greater experience, these patients are now eligible for transplantation.

MANAGEMENT OF PATIENTS AWAITING TRANSPLANTATION

Once they are listed for transplantation, patients ideally should be seen by the transplant team every 3 to 6 months to ensure that they remain in good pretransplant condition. Medications should be reviewed, and signs of infection must be sought aggressively. Renal and hepatic function should be monitored closely with creatinine clearance and liver function tests. Patients awaiting heart-lung transplantation are in some degree of heart failure, and medical management must be aggressive. The use of oxygen and pulmonary vasodilators may improve a patient's comfort and physiologic well-being before transplantation. In patients with primary or secondary PH, the use of continuous epoprostenol therapy should be monitored closely because these patients can develop worsening disease or tachyphylaxis related to drug therapy.[30] Long-term vascular access in all transplant candidates must be monitored closely because of the risk of infection and thrombosis. In patients with CF, pulmonary hygiene is of principal importance because of the danger of chronic bacterial colonization. Various airway clearance techniques, including chest physiotherapy, postural drainage, airway oscillation with flutter valves, and cough techniques, are used.[47] Patients with dilated cardiomyopathy, congestive heart failure, and PPH are predisposed to pulmonary and systemic thrombosis and embolization; therefore, prophylactic anticoagulation often is used before a transplant is performed.

Lung transplant candidates with emphysema and pulmonary fibrosis have been found to have the highest chance of being transplanted. Those with pulmonary fibrosis have the highest risk of dying while awaiting lung transplantation, whereas patients with pulmonary hypertension have the second highest risk of dying on the lung and heart-lung transplant list.[48] The clearest survival benefit from lung transplantation is in the CF group.[17] Independent factors that have been found to be crucial for the highest chance of transplantation include recipient size and ABO blood group. A higher chance of transplantation has been reported for patients whose height is between 176 and 185 cm and for ABO-AB blood group patients. Conversely, lower chances exist for patients whose height is below 156 cm and who are in the ABO-O blood group.[48]

Donor evaluation and graft preservation

The United Network for Organ Sharing (UNOS) reported 201 heart-lung and 3877 lung potential recipients awaiting transplantation as of early 2003, with fewer than 1000 donors having been identified in 2002. Among the 300 patients awaiting heart-lung transplants in 2001, 40 died on the waiting list, resulting in a risk of dying rate of 191.0 per 1000 patient years. Among the 5447 patients awaiting lung transplants in 2001, 488 died on the waiting list, resulting in a risk of dying rate of 133.8 per 1000 patient years. UNOS further reported that the median waiting time for lung transplantation has ranged between 600 and 1000 days over the last 5 years, with waiting times for heart-lung transplant being even longer. There obviously is a discrepancy between demand and donor availability that has a significant clinical impact.

Donor selection and management

The shortage of available organs for donation makes it essential to maximize the utilization of potential donor lungs and heart-lung blocks. Optimal lung function is notoriously difficult to preserve in a multiple-organ donor.[17] Chest trauma, aspiration, infection, and neurogenic pulmonary edema are common causes for poor donor lung and heart-lung quality. In general, patients with a history of malignancy, with the exception of diagnosed brain and nonmelanoma skin cancer; positive serologies for hepatitis B or C; or HIV are not considered suitable donor candidates.[18]

Evaluation of the donor history with respect to preexisting lung disease, smoking, aspiration, and intubation dates provides valuable information about the suitability of the lungs. Donors ideally should be younger than age 55 years, and the chest x-ray should be clear of infiltrates and parenchymal disease. Ventilatory settings should be optimized at a tidal volume of around 10 ml/kg and a positive end-expiratory pressure of 5 cmH_2O, and the fluids administered should be limited so that central venous pressures do not exceed 8 mmHg. Donor lungs are matched to recipients on the basis of ABO blood group compatibility and height and weight for similarity in thoracic size, ideally with less than a 25 percent difference. Early bronchoscopy and lavage may help in clearing secretions, determining the degree of lung injury that may exist, and diagnosing significant lung infection. Lung function can be estimated by measuring a "challenge gas," which is the partial pressure of oxygen (Pao_2) while the donor is on 100% oxygen. Ideally, the challenge gas Pao_2 is 300 mmHg or higher. The patient should be bronchoscoped by the retrieving surgeon before a decision is made to retrieve the lung. Massive purulent secretions and evidence of fungus or gram-negative rods on Gram stain normally preclude retrieval and use of lungs by most transplant teams.

Currently, heart-lung donors are ideally younger than age 50 years. Coronary artery angiograms are performed in patents over 40 years of age and those with multiple risk factors. Cardiac function normally is assessed by echocardiography. Chest trauma, resuscitation, long-term pressure support, or brain death may cause cardiac dysfunction. Sequential cardiac assessment may be necessary to determine the appropriateness of the heart in a heart-lung transplant donor. It has been shown that the administration of triiodothyronine may improve cardiac function in donor patients.[49,50] In general, potential donors with elevated troponin I and T levels and significant left ventricular hypertrophy are not considered suitable for heart donation[51,52] (Table 45-4).

Table 45-4 Lung and heart-lung donor criteria

Conventional donors
ABO compatibility
Thoracic size match
Age less than 50 years (heart-lung)
Age less than 55 years (lung)
Normal troponin levels (heart-lung)
Lack of ventricular hypertrophy (heart-lung)
No history of respiratory disease
No significant smoking history
No active pulmonary infection
No significant chest trauma or history of aspiration or cardiopulmonary resuscitation
No prior cardiac or pulmonary surgery
Short intubation time
Lack of purulent secretions; no gram-negative bacteria or fungi on Gram stain
Clear chest x-ray without infiltrates
Challenge gas greater than 300 mmHg on 100% oxygen
Marginal donors
Age over 55 years (lung)
Age over 50 years (heart-lung)
Tobacco history longer than 20 pack-years
Presence of infiltrate on chest x-ray
Donor ventilation time longer than 5 days
Donor use of inhaled drugs

In an effort to increase successful retrieval of donor lungs, donor criteria have been scrutinized carefully.[53–56] Liberalization of donor criteria has created what is referred to as a marginal donor lung. These marginal lungs are defined as having one of the following criteria: donor age over 55 years, tobacco history longer than 20 years, presence of infiltrate on chest x-ray, donor ventilation time greater than 5 days, and donor use of inhaled drugs. Compared with conventional donor lungs, early mortality was increased, but at 1 year, morbidity and mortality were not found to be affected.[55,56] Marginal lungs are paired to recipients, with relative contraindications to transplantation including older age, hepatitis-positive serology, and high-risk behavior rendering these candidates ineligible for optimal allografts.[55]

Lung and heart-lung preservation and procurement

Thoracic organs normally are retrieved as part of a multi-organ procurement that requires coordinated activity with other thoracic and abdominal retrieval surgeons. Although on-site donor lung procurement was considered necessary in the early 1980s because of poor lung preservation, remote donor procurement is now the standard. Throughout the procedure, hemodynamic stability is maintained by monitoring volume status and minimizing blood loss during the dissection. A median sternotomy is performed, and the pericardium and pleura are opened widely. The heart and lungs are inspected closely and palpated to rule out coronary artery disease in the case of heart–lung procurement and lung lesions in the case of both lung and heart-lung procurement. The aorta is separated from the pulmonary artery and encircled with an umbilical tape. The superior and inferior venae cavae are dissected, and a snare is placed around the superior vena cava after the azygous vein has been ligated and divided. The trachea can be isolated posterior to the left atrium or in the superior mediastinum. Care is taken not to enter the membranous portion of the trachea while an umbilical tape is used to encircle it. The aorta and the pulmonary artery are cannulated with low-profile cannulas for the administration of preservation fluid. Once the abdominal team has completed its dissection, 30,000 units of heparin is administered to the donor. Just before cross-clamping, 500 μg of prostacyclin is administered directly into the pulmonary artery. The superior vena cava is ligated, and the inferior vena cava and left atrial appendage are incised to allow good drainage from both ventricles. The aortic cross clamp is placed, and the heart and lungs are perfused with ice-cold cardioplegia and lung preservation fluid, respectively. The Stanford formulation is a commonly used cardioplegic formulation that consists of potassium chloride (30 meq/L), sodium bicarbonate (44.6 meq/L), and mannitol (12.5g/L) in 5% dextrose water. Gentle ventilation is continued during the perfusion time, and ice-cold balanced solution is poured over the heart and lungs. The heart-lung block is mobilized after resection of the pericardium, and the lungs are inflated completely before the trachea is stapled across and the inflated lungs and heart are removed en bloc. If the heart and lungs are to be taken separately, the heart usually is removed in situ, leaving the lungs in the thorax. Great care must be taken in separating the heart from the lungs in that a large enough left atrial cuff must remain around the pulmonary veins and a sufficient length of pulmonary artery is needed for implantation. The organs then are triple-bagged in cold physiologic solution and transported on ice. Ischemic times of 5 to 6 h for the heart and 4 to 6 h for the lungs are usually permissible. Coordination and constant communication with the recipient surgical team are very important in minimizing ischemic times.

Lung preservation solution is used to minimize reperfusion injury after allograft implantation. The ideal preservation solution should meet the energy requirement of the organ as well as have increased intravascular osmolality to counteract cell swelling. Although Euro-Collins (EC) was used for many years as the gold standard, the use of University of Wisconsin (UW) solution and more recently low-potassium dextran (LPD) has shown clinically favorable results.[57] In animal models, the advantages of an extracellular LPD solution compared with EC or UW were demonstrated in terms of better graft function.[58] In clinical studies, a decrease in reperfusion injury was demonstrated in lungs and heart-lungs perfused with LPD, as well as better long-term survival.[58,59] It has been suggested that these improved results are due to the fact that EC has a high potassium content that impairs pulmonary arterial endothelial cell function and increases the production of reactive oxygen species. Conversely, LPD has been shown to preserve type II pneumocytes, improve cellular metabolic activity, and possibly limit the production of reactive oxygen species.[59] Consequently, many groups, including the Toronto and Stanford lung transplant programs, now use LPD routinely for lung and heart-lung procurements, although many groups continue to use EC with satisfactory results.[60–62] Active research continues to find the best preservation fluid to improve clinical outcomes.[63]

OPERATIVE TECHNIQUES

Carrel's early work with vascular anastomoses coupled with Lower and Shumway's landmark paper paved the way to technically successful thoracic transplantation.[3,8] Today, there are standard recipient operations that permit timely placement of the thoracic organs. Recipients are monitored with an arterial line, a central venous pressure monitor, pulse oximetry, a continuous electrocardiogram, a urinary bladder catheter, and a pulmonary artery catheter on rare occasions. A double-lumen endotracheal tube is often helpful for the dissection of the lung recipient during explantation. Ventilation often is maintained with a fraction of inspired oxygen concentration (FiO_2) of 1.0, and pulmonary hypertension is controlled by using systemic vasodilators as well as inhaled nitric oxide. Care must be taken to suction the trachea carefully during and at the completion of the procedure to facilitate ventilation in the recovery phase.

The use of cardiopulmonary bypass is required in heart-lung transplantation but not for every single- and double-lung transplant. Patients with pulmonary fibrosis and poor functional capacity preoperatively and patients with right heart failure and pulmonary hypertension are likely to require bypass. On bypass, the surgeon is able to clamp the pulmonary artery without causing right heart failure and subsequent cardiovascular collapse. This benefit outweighs the potential negative effects of cardiopulmonary bypass, including fluid retention and activation of inflammatory mediators.

Single-lung transplantation

The recipient is placed in a lateral decubitus position so that the organ recipient side faces up. A posterior lateral thoracotomy is used, entering at the fourth or fifth intercostal space. Good retraction and deflation of the affected lung are essential. The recipient's superior and inferior pulmonary veins, pulmonary artery, and bronchus are identified and dissected out with good hemostasis. The requirement for cardiopulmonary bypass has to be determined at this point. For right lung transplantation, the ascending aorta and the right atrium are used as cannulation sites. For left lung transplantation, the femoral vessels can be used, and the descending thoracic aorta can be used for arterial cannulation. If the venous drainage from the femoral vein is insufficient, a venous cannula can be placed in the pulmonary artery proximal to the clamp. Using vascular staplers, the pulmonary veins and artery are dissected and divided. The bronchus also is dissected carefully, maintaining good vascularity, and then stapled.

The donor lung is brought to the operative field. The donor bronchus is opened, resulting in deflation of the lung, and secretion samples are sent for culture. The donor atrial cuff, pulmonary artery, and bronchus are trimmed, with remaining pericardium and lymphatic tissue being removed. The lung then is placed into the chest and covered with ice-cold laparotomy pads. The sequence of the anastomosis is a matter of institutional preference.[64] The Stanford technique is to start with the bronchus, followed by the pulmonary vein and finally the pulmonary artery, using polypropylene sutures for all anastomoses (Fig. 45-3A). The bronchial anastomosis can be performed a number of ways, including telescoped and end to end[65,66] (Fig. 45-3B). The telescoping technique uses a running suture for the membranous portion and multiple interrupted U stitches for the cartilaginous portion, intussuscepting one airway (usually the donor's) inside the other. This technique leaves a shelf of bronchial tissue protruding into the bronchial lumen that may necrose or serve as a nidus for retention of secretions or invasive airway infection.[65] The end-to-end anastomosis technique involves using a continuous suture but may be associated with delayed bronchial healing such as malacia or subcritical stenosis that manifests months after transplantation.[66] The reported incidence of airway complications is around 5 percent and can be minimized with good surgical technique for donor procurement, good organ preservation, and early postoperative extubation.[67] Bronchial artery revascularization to improve tracheal anastomotic healing has been reported in which direct revascularization of the bronchial artery with the internal mammary artery is performed.[68,69] This technique requires procurement of the donor descending thoracic aorta with preservation of the bronchial arteries, significantly complicating both the donor and recipient operations, with uncertain benefit.

To complete the atrial-to-pulmonary-vein anastomosis, the atrium is clamped with a side-biting Satinsky clamp (Fig. 45-4). A 4.0 polypropylene running suture is used, and the suture is not tied until the lung allograft is perfused to ensure that the anastomosis is not stenosed. The pulmonary artery anastomosis normally is done last and is completed with a 5.0 polypropylene running suture. Great care must be taken in completing the vascular anastomoses because although rare, vascular complications have a high mortality rate.[70] Once the anastomoses are completed (Fig. 45-5), steroids are administered to help reduce reperfusion injury and the pulmonary artery anastomosis is de-aired. The lung is inflated, and the atrial anastomosis is completed. The superior pulmonary vein is aspirated with a 21-gauge needle to aspirate any additional air, and the pulmonary artery clamp must be taken off slowly to prevent overperfusion of the allograft. Although great care is taken to match the size of the donor and recipient lungs, a size discrepancy may result and require downsizing of the recipient lung. Wedge resections with stapling devices can be used as well as formal lobectomies so that the lung can fit comfortably in the recipient's thoracic cavity.[71]

Double-lung transplantation

The original technique of en bloc double-lung transplantation was described by Patterson and coworkers in 1988.[16] This technique was not successful because of poor vascularity of the tracheal anastomosis and therefore was abandoned in favor of bilateral sequential lung transplantation. Since that time, several groups have shown that bronchial artery revascularization improves tracheal perfusion and may allow en bloc implantation.[72–74] The anastomotic techniques are the same as those for single-lung transplantation with cardiopulmonary bypass.

For bilateral single-lung transplantation, the patient is positioned supine. A bilateral anterior thoracosternotomy incision that is referred to as a clamshell is made, extending from the midaxillary line across the sternum through the fourth intercostal space. Cardiopulmonary bypass can be used after the ascending aorta and the right atrium have been cannulated. Alternatively, in an attempt to decrease the perceived morbidity of the clamshell incision, bilateral anterior thoracotomies can be used.[75] This approach, however, does not seem to provide the same exposure of the thoracic apices and mediastinum as the clamshell approach.

A unique form of double-lung transplantation involves lobar transplantation.[76,77] This technique originally was devised for patients who required bilateral lung transplants but could not wait for a double-lung donor block.[78] Two lobes from a living donor, right and left lower lobes, or a single lung divided into two separate lobes from a cadaveric donor are used. A continuous infusion of prostaglandin is administered to the donor

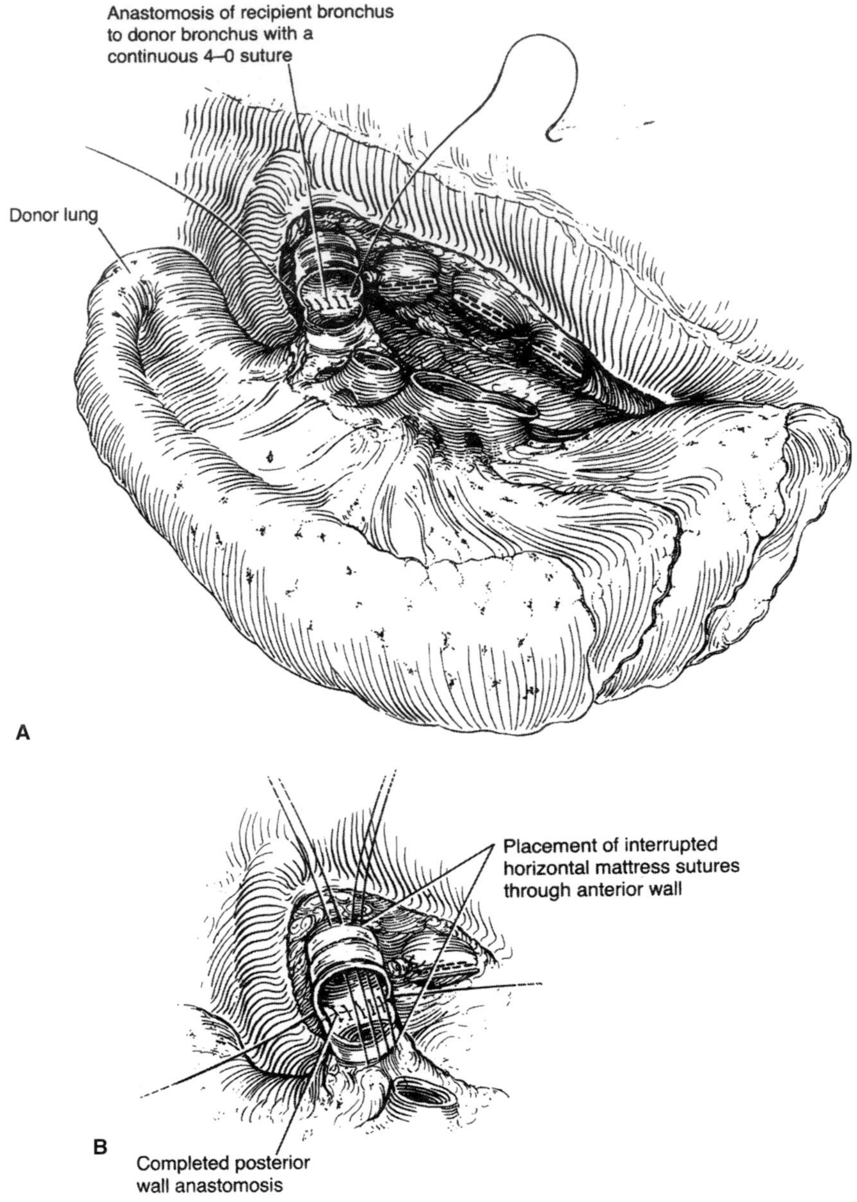

Figure 45-3 Single-lung transplantation. The donor lung is anastomosed to the recipient hilum, starting with the bronchus (A). The bronchial anastomosis can be performed by using a continuous (A) or an interrupted suture technique (B). (Reprinted, with permission, from Van Trigt P. Right lung transplantation. In: Sabiston DC Jr. *Atlas of Cardiothoracic Surgery.* Philadelphia: Saunders; 1995:516.)

during explantation with ex vivo flushing of the lobe with preservation fluid. Using a recipient clamshell incision, the right and left lobes are anastomosed as previously described into the right and left thorax after donor pneumonectomies.[77] Alternatively, the donor left lung is divided and the left upper lobe is rotated 180 degrees and implanted into the right thorax, and the left lower lobe is transplanted in the left thorax. The actuarial survival rates have been reported as being similar to those for conventional double-lung transplantation, but the numbers are small.[76,77] This innovative technique may alleviate the shortage of donor organs.

Heart-lung transplantation

The operation for heart-lung transplantation initially described by Reitz and colleagues was done through a median sternotomy approach.[13] The clamshell incision,

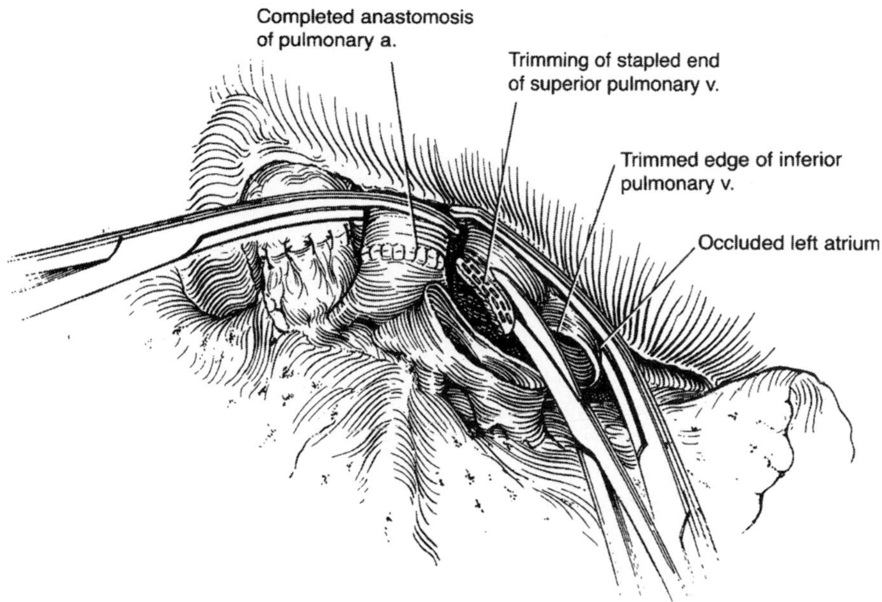

Figure 45-4 Single-lung transplantation. To complete the atrial-to-pulmonary-vein anastomosis, the atrium is clamped with a side-biting Satinsky clamp after the bronchus and pulmonary artery anastomoses have been completed successfully. (Reprinted, with permission, from Van Trigt P. Right lung transplantation. In: Sabiston DC Jr. *Atlas of Cardiothoracic Surgery.* Philadelphia: Saunders; 1995:518.)

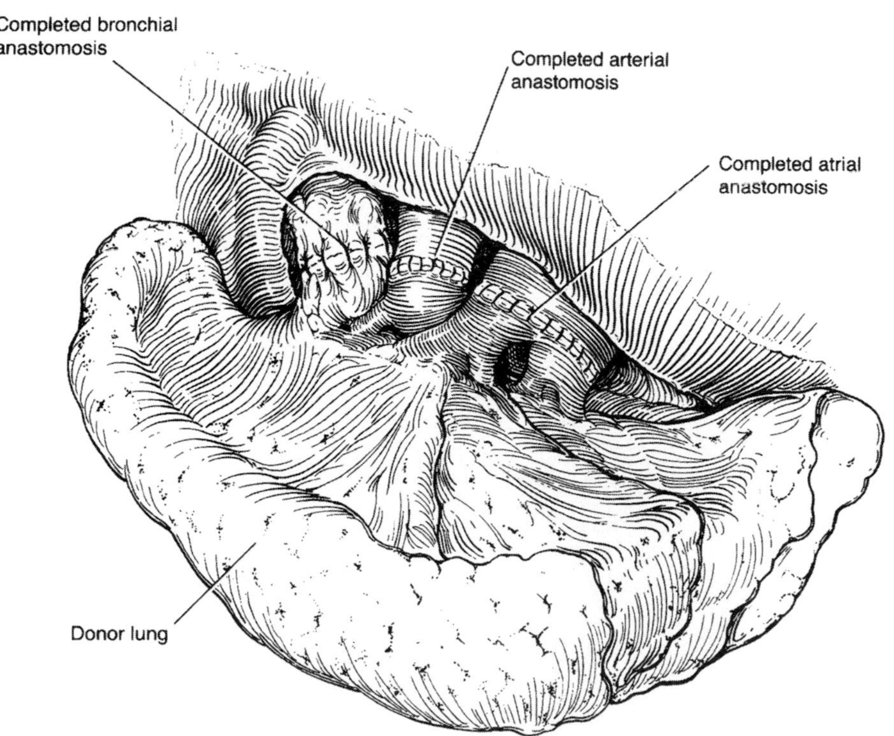

Figure 45-5 Single-lung transplantation. Successful completion of donor-to-recipient bronchus, pulmonary artery, and pulmonary vein anastomoses. (Reprinted, with permission, from Van Trigt P. Right lung transplantation. In: Sabiston DC Jr. *Atlas of Cardiothoracic Surgery.* Philadelphia: Saunders; 1995:520.)

however, has become a popular approach, particularly in patients with congenital heart disease who have multiple adhesions and distorted anatomy. Cardiopulmonary bypass is required for heart-lung transplantation. After the pleura and the pericardium are opened, the aorta and both cavae are cannulated. Once on bypass, the patient is cooled to 28°C. The aorta and the pulmonary artery are divided above their valves. The right atrium is divided so that there is sufficient tissue to perform the atrial anastomosis. The atrial septum is incised, and the dissection is carried around the dome of the left atrium, joining the ostium of the coronary sinus. The heart then is removed. An extrapericardial pneumonectomy is performed bilaterally, taking care to preserve the phrenic nerves. The left pneumonectomy is technically easier and usually is performed first, using staplers to divide the pulmonary vein and artery and mainstem bronchi (Fig. 45-6). The left lung then is removed, and the right pneumonectomy is performed. The trachea is mobilized and divided above the carina. The pulmonary artery and veins are dissected as they exit the pericardium and are excised. The right pulmonary artery is removed completely, whereas a small button of pulmonary artery is left on the left side at the site of the ductus arteriosis to prevent injury to the recurrent laryngeal nerve. At this point, hemostasis must be secured in the posterior mediastinum by using electrocautery, suture ligature, hemoclips, or an argon-beam coagulator.

The heart-lung block is lowered into the chest, and the right lung must pass posterior to the right atrium. The graft is kept cold with topical iced saline. The tracheal end-to-end anastomosis is performed first, using a continuous 4-0 polypropylene suture. Wrapping of the trachea with autologous tissue is not necessary. The atrial anastomosis is performed next, typically with a continuous 3-0 polypropylene suture. Some may opt for a bicaval anastomosis in which the superior and inferior venae cavae are anastomosed individually with 4-0 polypropylene sutures. The aortic anastomosis is the last one and is performed with a 4-0 polypropylene continuous suture. The intraoperative steroids are administered, a vent is placed, and the aortic cross clamp is removed.

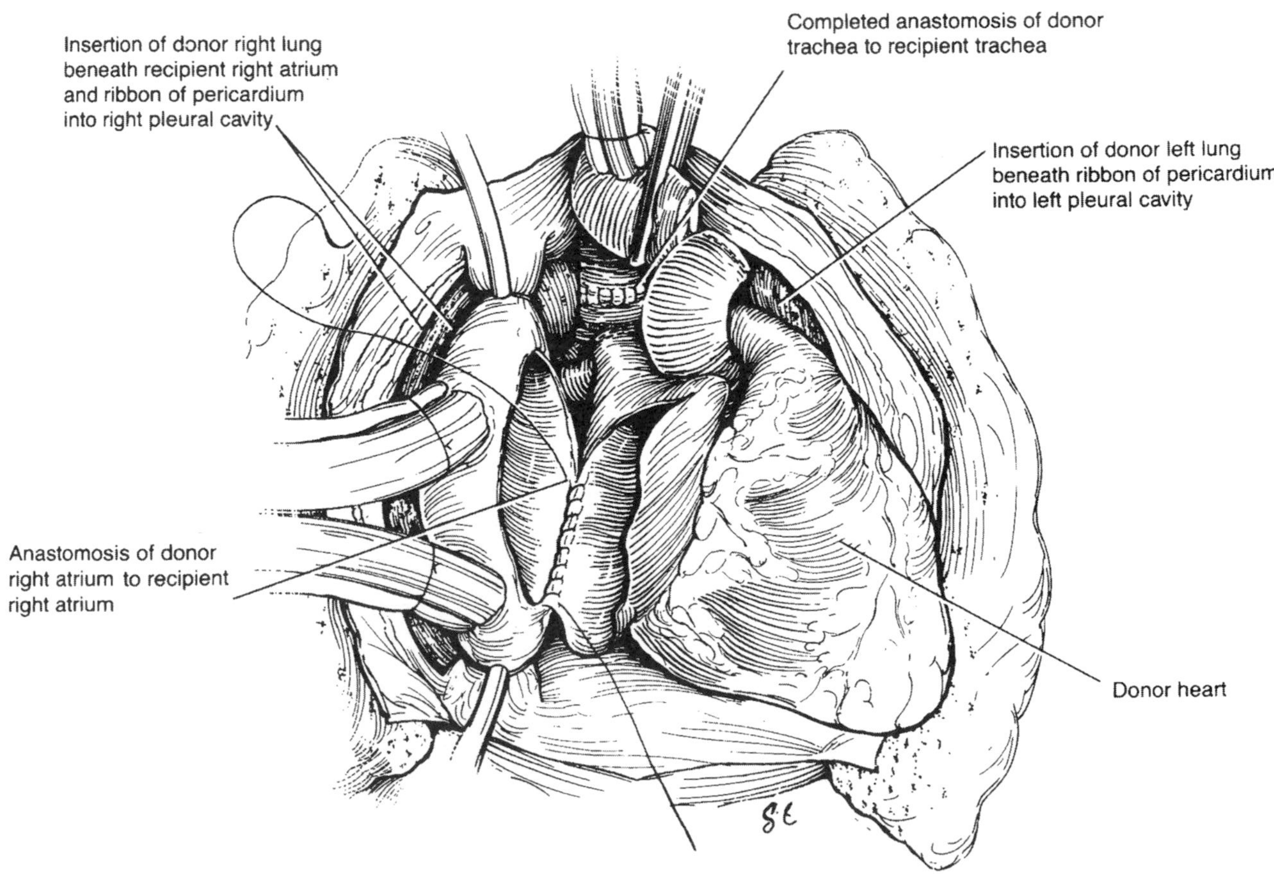

Figure 45-6 Heart-lung transplantation. The donor right lung is passed beneath the right atrium and venae cavae, and the left lung is passed beneath the left phrenic nerve and its pedicle. The tracheal anastomosis is preformed first, followed by the right atrial anastomosis. (Reprinted, with permission, from Van Trigt P. Right lung transplantation. In: Sabiston DC Jr. *Atlas of Cardiothoracic Surgery.* Philadelphia: Saunders; 1995:524.)

An alternative to heart and double-lung transplantation is heart and single-lung transplantation.[79,80] In the reported case of a patient with end-stage congenital heart disease and a protected right lung as a result of a right Glenn and a left Potts shunt, the patient needed only the heart and the left hypertensive lung to be transplanted.[79] Conte and colleagues similarly described the use of this procedure and in a review of the literature found other case reports in which patients with Eisenmenger's syndrome with one unapproachable single pleural space were found to be optimal candidates.[80] This form of heart-lung transplantation reduces the use of donor organs and may mitigate the clinical effect of obliterans bronchiolitis in the transplanted lung.

The "Domino" procedure

In 1989 the first "domino-donor" operation performed in the United States was reported by Baumgartner and associates.[81] A heart-lung block was transplanted into a patient with end-stage CF, and the recipient's heart was transplanted into a second recipient with end-stage cardiomyopathy. The main advantages of this procedure include technical simplicity compared with double-lung transplantation and the preservation of coronary-bronchial collaterals, resulting in improved airway vascularization and the ability to transplant a donor heart with a right ventricle that had been conditioned to chronically elevated pulmonary artery pressures.[82–85] Although various groups have reported using this procedure worldwide and it has been found to account for 7 percent of heart transplants in the United Kingdom, it is now virtually nonexistent in the United States.[85] Yacoub's group at Harefield Hospital, London, has performed 131 domino procedures over the last 10 years. The overall survival is similar to that of recipients of cadaveric hearts, but recipients of hearts from donors with cystic fibrosis were found to survive longer, supporting the theory that the domino heart is better conditioned.[86]

POSTOPERATIVE CARE

Early postoperative period

At the completion of the transplant implantation, the patient is transported to the cardiac intensive care unit. With the assistance of continuous blood pressure, oxygen saturation, urine output, and heart rate monitoring, these patients can be managed carefully. Swan-Ganz catheters are not placed routinely at the time of operation, but if hemodynamic stability cannot be achieved with less invasive monitoring, one can be placed in the intensive care or cardiac catheterization laboratory.

Central filling pressures should be kept low, and if a mean arterial pressure of 50 mmHg and above cannot be maintained, low-dose vasopressors should be instituted. Urine output, acid-base status, and skin perfusion aid in assessing the adequacy of systemic circulation while a patient is on vasopressors.

The ventilatory settings in the intensive care are similar to those after any patient has received cardiopulmonary bypass. FiO_2 should be weaned from 1.0 to a level such that PaO_2 is maintained above 80 mmHg. A partial end-expiratory pressure (PEEP) of 5 to 8 cmH_2O may help prevent atelectasis and should be used if hemodynamically permissible. Early experience with lung transplantation revealed that although ventilatory capacity is restored in patients with new lung allografts, carbon dioxide levels do not return to normal for up to a month after the transplant.[87] Therefore, these patients should be extubated when clinically indicated despite somewhat elevated carbon dioxide levels.

Chest physiotherapy and incentive spirometry should be initiated immediately after extubation. Bronchodilators may have to be prescribed in patients who have bronchospasm. If pain control becomes an issue, an epidural can be placed at the bedside to facilitate deep breathing and coughing. While the patient is in bed, antiembolic stockings and sequential compression devices help reduce the incidence of deep vein thrombosis; low-dose heparin can be administered after the epidural catheter has been removed.

Immunosuppression

Immunosuppression is started upon reperfusion of the allografts, with methylprednisolone being administered to the patient (10 mg/kg) intravenously. Immunosuppression consists of induction and maintenance therapy that is cyclosporin-based. The immunosuppressive regimen used at Stanford is outlined in Table 45-5.

Induction immunosuppression consists of immunosuppressive agents used before the institution of regular maintenance immunosuppression in an attempt to induce allograft tolerance. Advocates for induction therapy believe that it reduces the incidence of early acute rejection as well as the development of chronic rejection in the form of obliterans bronchiolitis.[88,89] Induction therapy also permits late introduction of cyclosporin if there is renal dysfunction.[90] Those opposed to induction therapy believe that it increases the risk of infection and lymphoproliferative disorders.[91] Currently available induction agents include OKT3 (Orthobiothec Corp., Raritan, NJ), antithymocyte globulin (ATG), and Daclizumab (Zenpax, Roch Pharmaceuticals, Nutley, NJ). OKT3 is a murine monoclonal that targets the CD3 antigen on T lymphocytes, ATG is an antithymocyte preparation that reduces the number of effector T lymphocytes, and Daclizumab is a humanized monoclonal antibody that targets the interleukin-2 (IL-2) receptor on activated T lymphocytes. OKT3 has been associated with hemodynamic instability during administration and has had questionable outcomes; it no longer is used routinely at the authors' institution.[92] Instead, either ATG

Table 45-5 Lung and heart-lung immunosuppression regimen

Induction therapy		
Corticosteroids		
	Methylprednisolone 500 mg IV coming off bypass	
RATG	1.5 mg/kg IV postoperative days 1, 2, 3, 5, and 7	
or		
Daclizumab	First dose in operating room 1mg/kg IV: dose every other week for a total of 5 doses	
Maintenance immunosuppression		
Azathioprine	2mg/kg PO daily	
Corticosteroids	Methylprednisolone 125 mg IV q8h for 3 doses postoperatively Prednisone 1.0 mg/kg PO days 1–7 Prednisone 0.60 mg/kg PO divided into two doses days 8–12 Prednisone tapered over 2 months	
Cyclosporin	100 mg PO BID, postoperative day 2 or 3	
	Drug levels:	325 ng/mL 1–6 weeks
		275 ng/mL 6 weeks–3 months
		225 ng/mL 3–6 months
		200 ng/mL beyond 6 months

BID = twice daily; IV = intravenous; PO = orally; RATG = rabbit antithymocyte globulin.

at a dose of 1.5 mg/kg intravenously (IV) on postoperative days 1, 2, 3, 5, and 7 or, more recently, Daclizumab 1 mg/kg in the operating room and then every other week for five doses is used in the induction phase. Earlier studies revealed that ATG is superior to OKT3 in terms of the incidence of acute rejection and overall survival.[92,93] However, more recently, when OKT3, ATG, and Daclizumab were compared in the long-term, no difference in overall survival or development of obliterans bronchiolitis was demonstrated.[94]

Maintenance immunosuppression used in lung and heart-lung transplantation consists of corticosteroids, azathioprine, and cyclosporin. Corticosteroids are used, with the initial dose administered in the operating room upon graft reperfusion. Methylprednisolone 125 mg IV is given every 8 h for three doses, and prednisone 0.25 mg/kg divided twice daily is given orally between days 1 and 5. On day 6, prednisone 1.0 mg/kg divided twice daily is started until day 14, when it is weaned slowly.

Cyclosporin is a T-cell inhibitor that works by inhibiting the intracellular protein calcineurin, which regulates T-cell proliferation. Cyclosporin is given in an oral formulation 2 to 3 days after transplantation, when renal function has stabilized. The usual dose is 5 to 10 mg/kg divided twice daily. The whole blood cyclosporin target level is 325 ng/mL for 1 to 6 weeks, 275 ng/mL from 6 weeks to 3 months, 225 ng/mL from 3 to 6 months, and 200 ng/mL thereafter. Unfortunately, cyclosporin is associated with renal dysfunction, neurotoxicity, and hypertension.

Traditionally, if cyclosporin is not well tolerated by the patient or steroid-resistant rejection occurs, tacrolimus is used.[95,96] Tacrolimus is a macrolide antibiotic isolated from *Streptomyces tsukubaensis* that has a mode of action similar to that of cyclosporin. It is given in an oral dose of 0.05 to 0.075 mg/kg twice daily, and the target trough levels are maintained at 10 to 20 ng/mL for the first month, 10 to 15 ng/mL in the first to third months, and 5 to 10 ng/mL after 3 months. Furthermore, the use of tacrolimus has been associated with attenuation of the progression of obliterans bronchiolitis in lung transplant recipients.[97,98] The use of tacrolimus in lung transplantation has been shown to be associated with a lower incidence of early acute rejection and similar overall survival compared with cyclosporin-based therapy.[99]

Azathioprine is a purine analogue that inhibits DNA and RNA synthesis by blocking the de novo and salvage pathways for purine biosynthesis. It is given in an oral dose of 2 mg/kg daily starting on postoperative day 1. It is associated with bone marrow suppression and hepatotoxicity. When it is not well tolerated, mycophenolate mofetil (MMF) is used in its place at an oral dose of 1000 mg twice daily. This is a newer agent that is an antimetabolite that specifically inhibits inosine monophosphate dehydrogenase, thus affecting only the de novo purine biosynthetic pathway. MMF is not associated with bone marrow suppression or hepatotoxicity but has gastrointestinal side effects that are self-limiting. Recent literature suggests that MMF may prove to be more beneficial in lung transplantation than is azathioprine, especially in combination with tacrolimus.[100,101]

Sirolimus is a macrolide antibiotic that is structurally similar to tacrolimus. Sirolimus binds to the same cytoplasmic protein, FK-binding protein, as tacrolimus but does not inhibit calcineurin. Instead, it appears to inhibit T-cell proliferation later in the intracellular activation pathway. The renal toxicity and neurotoxicity of both cyclosporin and tacrolimus have been attributed to their blockade of calcineurin and therefore are potentially avoidable with the use of sirolimus.[102,103] A dose of 2 mg orally per day is given, and a level of 10 to 13 ng/mL is desirable. Early experience using sirolimus in patients with declining lung function secondary to obliterans bronchiolitis has been favorable, but case reports of sirolimus-induced pneumonitis may limit its use in lung and heart-lung transplantation patients.[104,105] Table 45-6 outlines currently used immunosuppressants and their mechanisms of action and associated toxicities.

Monitoring of lung and heart-lung allograft rejection

Surveillance of allograft function is key for successful transplant outcomes. In the case of single- or double-lung transplantation, bronchoscopy with endobronchial

Table 45-6 Currently used immunosuppressive drugs: Mode of action and toxicities

	Mechanism of Action	Toxicities
Induction immunosuppression drugs		
Antilymphocyte/ antithymocyte immunoglobulin	Deplete activated lymphocytes Deplete activated thymocytes	Antibody response Allergic reaction
OKT3	Sequestration of CD3+ T cells	Cytokine release syndrome Antibody response
Interleukin-2 receptor blocker (Dacliximab)	Inhibits T-cell activation	None known
Maintenance immunosuppression drugs		
Corticosteroids	Anti-inflammatory	Cushingoid habitus Glucose intolerance Osteoporosis Cataracts Hypertension Hyperlipidemia Poor wound healing
Cyclosporin	Calcineurin inhibitor: inhibits T-cell proliferation	Nephrotoxicity Neurotoxicity Hypertension Gingival hyperplasia Hyperlipidemia
Tacrolimus	Calcineurin inhibitor: inhibits T cell proliferation	Nephrotoxicity Neurotoxicity Hypertension Gingival hyperplasia Diabetes Alopecia
Azathioprine	Purine analogue: Inhibits de novo and salvage purine synthesis pathways	Marrow toxicity Hepatotoxicity
Mycophenolate Mofetil	Inhibits inosine monophosphate dehydrogenase; inhibits de novo purine synthesis	Hepatotoxicity Gastrointestinal disturbance
Sirolimus	Inhibits T-cell activation	Hyperlipidemia Myelosuppression

biopsies and clinical parameters, including FEV_1 and forced expiratory flow (FEF_{25-75}) and arterial blood gases, are followed on a routine basis. At Stanford, bronchoscopy and endobronchial biopsies are initiated at 2, 4, 8, and 12 weeks after a transplant and then at 6 months and 1 year. Yearly bronchoscopy is performed with spirometry, blood gases, and chest x-ray at every clinic visit or when clinically indicated.

The monitoring of heart-lung allografts differs somewhat from that of lung allografts alone. Early in the experience of heart-lung transplantation, endomyocardial biopsies were done weekly, and once it was recognized that the cardiac and pulmonary allografts might not be rejected at the same time, surveillance bronchoscopy and endobronchial biopsies and lavage were started. Thereafter, with the realization that cardiac rejection was uncommon in heart-lung allograft recipients, the number of cardiac biopsies was decreased dramatically.[106] Currently, patients undergo surveillance bronchoscopy at 2, 4, 8, and 12 weeks and then at 6 months and 1 year. Yearly bronchoscopic surveillance occurs after the first year or when clinically indicated. Pulmonary function tests, chest x-ray, and arterial blood gases are done at each clinic visit. Endomyocardial biopsies are performed roughly twice in the first 6 months after a transplant and then annually. Coronary angiography is performed at odd-numbered annual anniversaries after a transplant or when clinically indicated.

The Stanford cardiothoracic transplant group described the association between a decrease in FEV_1 and FEF_{25-75} and ongoing acute rejection.[107] Similar findings have been reported for heart-lung allograft recipients in the determination of acute rejection.[108] A 10 percent decrease in spirometry parameters has been associated with a 35 to 50 percent chance of an associated abnormal transbronchoscopic biopsy.[109]

Studies of lung and heart-lung transplant recipients have described bronchial hyperreactivity of the airways to increasing concentrations of methacholine and ultrasonic nebulized distilled water.[110–112] The interpretation of this hyperactivity and its association with inflammation and rejection has been difficult. In a retrospective review of bronchodilator spirometric responses of either FEF_{50} or FEF_{75}, the Toronto group noted a predisposition to the development of obliterans bronchiolitis in cases in which bronchodilation was observed.[108] In that early study, the sensitivity of bronchial responsiveness to inhaled albuterol in predicting obliterans bronchiolitis was 51 percent. More recently, other groups have found that positive methacholine challenges are an early marker of chronic rejection.[110,111]

Chest x-rays of patients with acute allograft rejection may show perihilar or lower lung zone interstitial infiltrates, septal lines, or pleural effusions. These changes have been associated with acute rejection in heart-lung recipients in up to 75 percent of episodes.[113] Radiographic changes are nonspecific, however, and can be associated with lung injury secondary to allograft reperfusion or infectious pneumonitis. Computed tomography (CT) has been used to characterize and diagnose postoperative complications of lung transplantation with varying success.[114–116] CT has been shown to be useful in diagnosing acute and chronic rejection, infection, lymphoproliferative disorders, and recurrence of the initial disease. However, processes demonstrated by CT may be attributed to one of several causes, and therefore treatment is difficult to determine. Sequential CT scans after a transplant are probably the most informative when changes in the lung parenchyma are seen over a defined period. Because of the diagnostic shortcomings of CT scans, the use of magnetic resonance imaging (MRI) has been investigated. A novel approach to the detection of acute lung allograft rejection using MRI coupled with injection of ultrasmall superparamagnetic iron oxide particles has been described, with anticipated success.[117]

Surveillance bronchoscopy with transbronchial biopsy and lavage is currently the best-accepted way to follow lung and heart-lung transplant patients, but controversy exists.[118–122] In performing surveillance bronchoscopy and taking 10 to 12 transbronchial specimens, a high diagnostic yield and low complication rates have been reported.[118] The most common complications include pneumothorax and minor endobronchial bleeding. In reviewing the use of transbronchial biopsies in heart-lung transplants, it has been observed that surveillance biopsies rarely yield findings 2 or more years after a transplant and that surveillance biopsies rarely alter the management of patients with clinically stable lung function.[120] Other large groups have confirmed success in lung transplantation without surveillance bronchoscopy, which they have found poses greater risk to the patient and does not alter the natural course of the development of obliterans bronchiolitis.[121,122]

Endomyocardial biopsies have been the cornerstone of diagnosing cardiac rejection.[123] Although this type of biopsy is used much more routinely in heart transplantation, its role in heart-lung transplantation is important. Animal and clinical evidence suggests that the heart allograft is protected by the lung allograft.[106,124,125] Acute and chronic allograft vasculopathy is monitored by using angiographic evidence of coronary artery vasculopathy in combination with echocardiographic evidence of decreased ventricular dysfunction.[126,127] More recently, Doppler tissue imaging of heart allograft rejection has been described in which patients undergo Doppler tissue imaging at the time of their endomyocardial biopsies.[128] It is suggested that the lymphocytic extracellular infiltration and edema of acute rejection result in increased myocardial stiffness that can be seen as depressed myocardial relaxation velocities on Doppler.[129] This hypothesis has been verified clinically, although it has not replaced routine endomyocardial biopsy protocols clinically.

Prevention of postoperative infectious complications

Immunosuppression places the transplant recipient at increased risk of infectious complications. Therefore, prophylactic measures are instituted early in an attempt to reduce subsequent morbidity. The prophylaxis regimen used at Stanford is outlined in Table 45-7. This regimen provides prophylaxis against CMV, *Pneumocystis carinii* pneumonia (PCP), and *Aspergillus* infections. In

Table 45-7 Antimicrobial prophylaxis regimen for lung and heart-lung transplantation

Cytomegalovirus prophylaxis	
DHPG (ganciclovir IV)	
34-day Regimen:	5 mg/kg IV BID for 14 days 6 mg/kg IV BID for 20 days
Valcyte (ganciclovir oral)	900 mg PO daily for 6 weeks
CytoGam (IgG gamma globulin)	
Within 72 h posttransplant:	150 mg/kg IV
Weeks 2, 4, 6, and 8 posttransplant:	100 mg/kg IV
Weeks 12 and 16 posttransplant:	50 mg/kg IV
Pneumocystis carinii pneumonia prophylaxis	
Trimethoprim-sulfamethoxazole (Bactrim SS) 1 tablet every day for life	
If Bactrim-allergic: Pentamidine 300 mg nebulized once per month	
Aspergillus prophylaxis	
Amphotericin B aerosolized: 20 mg BID while hospitalized	
Itraconazole oral suspension 200 mg every morning, 100 mg every afternoon; start POD 3 for 90 days	

BID = twice a day; IV = intravenous; PO = orally; POD = Post operative day.

addition, these patients receive nystatin oral rinse to protect them from oral candidiasis, and if the donor is positive for toxoplasmosis, the recipient receives pyrimethamine 25 mg and folinic acid daily for 6 weeks.

CMV prophylaxis currently consists of a 34-day course of intravenous ganciclovir followed by oral ganciclovir (Valcyte) for 6 weeks and concurrent hyperimmune globulin therapy (CytoGam). CMV infection can occur as a primary or secondary infection or a reactivation or superinfection.[129] A number of randomized, prospective clinical trials have demonstrated that prophylactic anti-CMV therapy during the first 3 months after transplantation can reduce the incidence of any form of CMV infection.[129–132] Furthermore, ganciclovir prophylaxis has been found to improve survival in lung and heart-lung transplant recipients by reducing the incidence of CMV pneumonitis and delaying the onset of obliterans bronchiolitis.[133] The introduction of CMV hyperimmune globulin to the prophylaxis protocol also has proved to decrease the incidence of CMV infection.[134]

Early fungal infections are related to surgical complications and involve *Aspergillus* species, *Candida*, *Pneumocystis*, and *Cryptococcus*.[135] While the transplant recipient is in the hospital, Amphotericin B aerosolized solution is administered, and itraconazole oral suspension 200 mg qAM and 100 mg qPM starts on postoperative day 3 and is continued until day 90. Trimethoprim-sulfamethoxazole also is started immediately postoperatively, and one tablet daily is given for life for PCP prophylaxis.

POSTOPERATIVE COMPLICATIONS

Early acute respiratory distress ("reperfusion injury")

Early acute respiratory distress ("reperfusion injury") is characterized as nonspecific alveolar damage, lung edema, and hypoxia that occurs within 72 h after lung or heart-lung transplantation.[136] The donor lungs that are retrieved are flushed with preservation fluid and hypothermically preserved to decrease the metabolic rate and cellular energy requirement. Although it is required for organ storage, hypothermia is associated with oxidative stress and apoptosis that may induce upregulation and release of proinflammatory mediators that are probably responsible for allograft reperfusion injury.[136] The incidence of reperfusion injury is reportedly as high as 15 percent and, in addition to hypothermia, has been attributed to preservation solutions, brain death physiology, donor pneumonia or aspiration, chest trauma, and surgical technical difficulties.[136–140] Reperfusion injury has not been found to be dependent on the duration of donor organ ischemia but has been reported to increase in the presence of recipient preoperative pulmonary hypertension.[140]

The clinical spectrum of reperfusion injury can range from mild hypoxia associated with chest x-ray infiltrates to full-blown acute respiratory distress syndrome that requires prolonged intubation, pharmacologic therapy, extracorporeal membrane oxygenation, or retransplantation.[136,149] The most severe form leading to primary graft failure is a major cause of mortality, lengthy hospitalization, and protracted recovery time among survivors.[137]

Pulmonary allograft perfusion fluids have changed over the decade, with a decrease in reperfusion injury demonstrated in lungs and heart-lungs perfused with LPD.[58,59] It has been suggested that improved results are due to the fact that EC has a high potassium content that impairs arterial endothelial cell function, whereas LPD has been shown to preserve type II pneumocytes and improve cellular metabolic activity.[59] Furthermore, controlling the rate of allograft reperfusion has been shown to decrease the incidence of reperfusion injury significantly.[141] Other strategies to reduce reperfusion injury are being investigated actively in animal models and include the administration of melatonin, which is a radical scavenger and antioxidant;[142] blockade of adhesion molecules with monoclonal antibodies at the time of reperfusion;[143] and endobronchial gene transfer using adenovirus that encodes human interleukin-10.[144] At Stanford, leukocyte filtering is used on cardiopulmonary bypass to deplete cells before reperfusion; this has been shown to reduce the incidence of allograft reperfusion injury.[145]

Once reperfusion injury is clinically evident, treatment is dependent on the extent and duration of the injury. Treatment using nitric oxide has been suggested because of its potent vasoregulatory and immunomodulatory properties.[136,146] Nitric oxide has been shown to improve ventilation-perfusion mismatch and decrease pulmonary artery pressures.[147] The use of nitric oxide to prevent reperfusion injury, however, is controversial.[148] Prostaglandin E_1 has been shown to be beneficial when added to preservation fluids because of its vasodilator properties, reduction of endothelial permeability, neutrophil adhesion, and platelet aggregation.[149] The continuous intravenous infusion of prostaglandin E_1 during the early phase of reperfusion has been shown to reduce the incidence of lung reperfusion injury in animal models; however, clinical application is lacking.[150] The combination of inhaled nitric oxide and surfactant replacement also has been used with success in patients with severe reperfusion injury.[146]

Acute rejection

Monitoring and diagnosis

Acute allograft rejection is a major source of morbidity after lung and heart-lung transplantation. As was outlined above, immunosuppressive therapy is administered immediately after transplantation to prevent acute allograft rejection, which is a T-cell-mediated process. Acute rejection has the highest incidence during the first year

Table 45-8 Grading system for acute lung rejection diagnosed by transbronchial biopsy

Grade	Histologic Appearance
0	No significant inflammation; normal specimen
1	Small, infrequent perivascular infiltrates with or without bronchiolar lymphocytic infiltrates
2	Larger, more frequent perivascular lymphocytic infiltrates with or without moderate bronchiolar lymphocytic inflammation; occasional neutrophils and eosinophils
3	Extension of infiltrates into alveolar septa and alveolar spaces with or without bronchiolar mucosal ulceration

after a transplant, particularly during the first 6 months. In heart-lung transplant recipients, cardiac rejection is rare, and therefore surveillance of pulmonary rejection predominates.[106,107] Routine transbronchial biopsies are part of postoperative care at Stanford for both lung and heart-lung transplant recipients. Acute pulmonary rejection is based on perivascular and interstitial mononuclear infiltrates, and each grade of acute rejection specifies the presence of coexistent airway inflammation, the intensity of which also is graded, as outlined in Table 45-8.[151]

Treatment of rejection

Unless clinical deterioration is evident, only grade 2 and greater rejection is treated, as outlined in Table 45-9. Corticosteroids are the cornerstone for treating acute rejection, but in addition, the patient's maintenance immunosuppressive regimen should be reviewed and optimized. Bronchoscopy and biopsy should be repeated 2 to 3 weeks after the initial treatment to ensure that the rejection episode has resolved.

Refractory acute rejection is more clinically challenging to treat. Changing from cyclosporin to tacrolimus has been successful in treating steroid-refractory rejection in both lung and heart transplantation patients.[95,99] Further therapy includes the use of antilymphocyte globulins and OKT3, with varying success.[152,153] Azathioprine is normally part of the maintenance regimen, and conversion to MMF has been attempted in the treatment of refractory rejection. MMF has been shown to both reduce the incidence of rejection and improve pulmonary function after treatment.[154] There is limited experience using total lymphoid irradiation for refractory acute rejection, but at Stanford, a total of 800 cGy of total lymphoid irradiation has been used, resulting in attenuation of rejection but reduced 3-year survival.[155] Photophoresis is an immunomodulatory treatment in which the patient's mononuclear cells are separated and irradiated with ultraviolet light in the presence of 8-methoxypsoralen and then are returned to the patient. Studies in both cardiac and lung transplant recipients with severe refractory rejection have shown this to be a well-tolerated and effective therapy.[156]

Table 45-9 Treatment of lung and heart-lung rejection

Cellular acute grade 2 rejection or greater
Methylprednisolone 1000 mg IV QD for 3 days
Prednisone 0.6 mg/kg PO tapering to 0.2 mg/kg over 3 weeks
Cellular recurrent rejection grade 2 or greater
Methylprednisolone 500–1000 mg IV QD for 3 days
Prednisone 0.6 mg/kg PO with 3-week taper
Optimize azathioprine and cyclosporin
Change cyclosporin to tacrolimus
Change azathioprine to CellCept
Consider addition of sirolimus
Cellular intractable rejection
Total lymphoid irradiation 800 cGy total dose twice weekly (Mantel and inverted Y distribution)

IV = intravenous; QD = every day; PO = orally.

Chronic rejection

Monitoring and diagnosis

Chronic rejection in lung transplantation is known as obliterans bronchiolitis (OB), and in heart transplantation it is referred to as allograft coronary artery vasculopathy. In lung and heart-lung transplantation, the majority of episodes of chronic rejection involve the process of OB since the heart seems to be protected by the lung allografts.[106,107] As seen in Fig. 45-7, the incidence of allograft coronary artery vasculopathy is overshadowed by that of OB, and by 5 years, 42 percent of heart-lung recipients develop OB. The diagnosis of OB is based on histologic confirmation,[151] but because this process can be difficult to diagnose, a proposed clinical description of OB termed bronchiolitis obliterans syndrome (BOS) was established by the ISHLT.[157] Therefore, lung and heart-lung transplant centers have adopted a descriptor of lung allograft dysfunction that is clinically diagnosed with or without histologic confirmation.[151,157] BOS is defined by a greater than 20 percent decrease from baseline in FEV_1 and/or a greater than 25 percent decline in FEF_{25-75} in the absence of acute rejection or infection.[157,158] This decline should be determined by the average of two measurements made at least 3 weeks apart. In addition to clinical criteria and/or histologic biopsies to diagnose BOS, spirometrically gated CT can be used to predict the onset of BOS after lung transplantation.[159,160]

Clinically, progressive airflow limitation of BOS develops because of small airway obstruction caused by fibrous scarring of the terminal bronchioles. Some patients experience rapid loss of lung function, whereas others have a slow but progressive course. Prediction of the clinical course for each transplant recipient is difficult, and BOS remains a major source of morbidity and mortality among all lung transplant recipients.

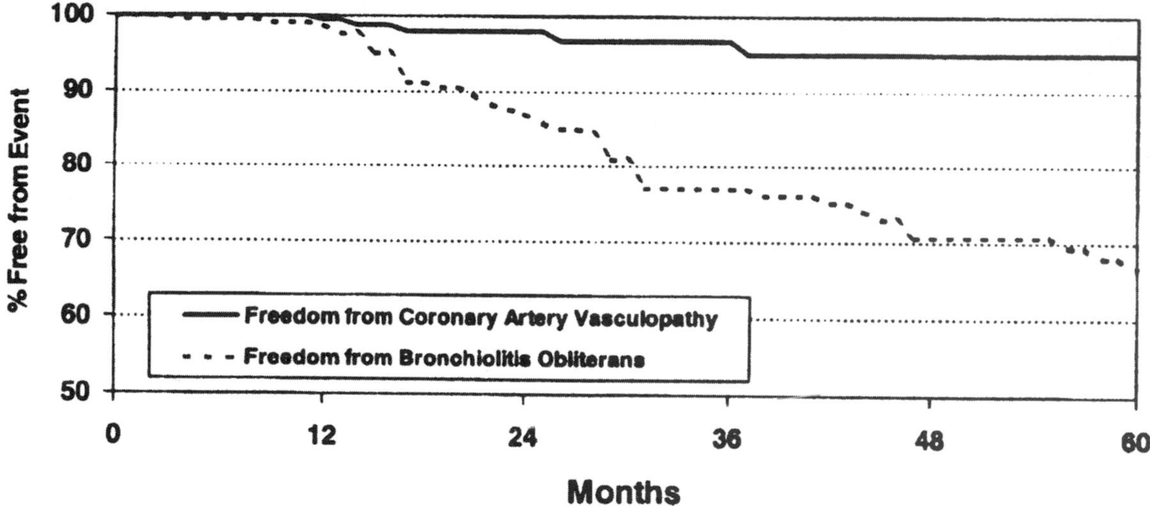

Figure 45-7 Freedom from coronary artery vasculopathy and freedom from bronchiolitis obliterans for heart-lung transplant recipients (April 1994–December 2000). (Reprinted from the *Journal of Heart and Lung Transplantation*, Volume 21(9), Hertz MI, Taylor DO, Trulock EP, et al. The Registry of the International Society of Heart and Lung Transplantation: Nineteenth Official Report-2002, 957-962, 2002, with permission from the International Society for Heart and Lung Transplantation.)

Causes and prevention

BOS is the major factor limiting long-term survival in lung and heart-lung transplant recipients.[161] Donor and recipient characteristics such as sex, age, underlying disease, type of transplant, and graft ischemic time do not appear to affect the onset of BOS.[161–163] Lymphocytic bronchiolitis, early and frequent acute rejection episodes, CMV and bacterial infection, reperfusion injury, gastroesophageal reflux, and anti-human leukocyte antigen (HLA) antibodies have all been implicated in the pathogenesis of BOS, as shown in Table 45-10.[164–168] Increased expression of transforming growth factor–beta (TGF-β) is also a risk factor, suggesting that the inflammatory response that may be instigated by immunologic and nonimmunologic causes can be made worse by an aberrant repair process caused by excessive TGF-β production.[169]

Table 45-10 Risk factors for the development of bronchiolitis obliterans syndrome
Acute rejection episodes
Lymphocytic bronchiolitis
Cytomegalovirus pneumonitis
Medication noncompliance
Reperfusion injury
Bacterial pneumonia
Donor antigen–specific reactivity
Gastroesophageal reflux
Elevated transforming growth factor–beta expression

Treatment of bronchiolitis obliterans syndrome

After the onset of BOS, the average survival at 3 years is only 50 percent because of the progressive and incurable nature of this entity.[170] The main complication of BOS is superimposed infections that can cause rapid deterioration in the patient's condition.[161] Aggressive treatment with suitable antibiotics is key to improving patient well-being. At present the only treatment available is optimization of immunosuppressive regimens and surveillance. When BOS is diagnosed, changing immunosuppressive agents has been shown to slow the progress of the clinical course. Tacrolimus has been successful in slowing the course in patients treated with cyclosporin, and MMF substituted for azathioprine has been promising.[97,101] The use of catalytic therapy in the form of ATG and OKT3 has been investigated, and although the effect can be rapid, BOS ultimately progresses in most of these patients.[171,172] In the future, the use of newer immunosuppressive agents, including sirolimus and Daclizumab, may help prevent and treat this unrelenting process.

Infection

Although prophylaxis against CMV, PCP, toxoplasmosis, and *Aspergillus* infection is prescribed, infectious complications after transplantation remain a problem. Global cellular dysfunction as a result of immunosuppression predisposes transplant recipients to infections with opportunistic as well as nonopportunistic pathogens. Usually, infections unique to transplant recipients are not seen until 1 month after transplantation. In the first month

Table 45-11 Opportunistic infections after lung and heart-lung transplantation

Bacterial
Nocardia asteroides
Listeria monocytogenes
Mycobacterium tuberculosis
Legionella pneumophila
Legionella micdadei
Fungi
Candida albicans
Candida glabrata
Candida krusei
Candida tropicalis
Candida parapsilosis
Aspergillus niger
Cryptococcus neoformans
Histoplasma capsulatum
Blastomyces dermatitidis
Coccidioides immitis
Pseudallescheria boydii
Viruses
Cytomegalovirus
Herpes simplex virus
Varicella-zoster virus
Epstein-Barr virus
Human herpesvirus-6 and -8

after transplantation, infection is attributed to a preexisting infectious condition, transmission from the donor graft, iatrogenic infectious exposure, or early reactivation of viruses. After 6 months, immunosuppression usually is reduced, and the recipients are normally most at risk for disease similar to the risk among nonimmunocompromised hosts. A comprehensive list of opportunistic infections in transplant recipients is given in Table 45-11.

Bacterial opportunistic infections include *Nocardia asteroides, Listeria monocytogenes, Mycobacterium tuberculosis,* and *Legionella pneumophila* and *Legionella micdadei.* Pulmonary bacterial infection is most common, but disseminated infection accompanied by systemic sepsis is not uncommon.[174,175] Respiratory failure and sepsis are the predominant causes of intensive care unit (ICU) admission after a transplant and have an associated mortality rate as high as 37 percent.[174]

Many types of fungi can cause opportunistic infections in transplant recipients, ranging from the common *Candida albicans* to the rare *Pseudallescheria boydii,* with infections ranging from mild to life-threatening. Risk factors for the development of fungal infection include high-dose immunosuppression, diabetes mellitus, prolonged use of indwelling catheters, and administration of broad-spectrum antibiotics.[173] In a review of the prevalence and outcomes of invasive fungal infections in nearly 2000 thoracic organ transplant recipients, *Aspergillus* was the organism found most frequently. Although the incidence of invasive fungal infections was low, the associated mortality rate was found to be as high as 52 percent.[175,176]

Viruses cause the majority of opportunistic infections among transplant recipients. CMV is the most common opportunistic viral infection, with three types of infection possible: (1) primary, (2) secondary or reactivation, and (3) superinfection.[173] The diagnosis of CMV can be made with great accuracy by using antibody-based tests or quantitative polymerase chain reaction assays. Prophylaxis and newer antiviral agents have exhibited considerable efficacy against CMV, although the emergence of ganciclovir-resistant infection needs to be dealt with actively.[177,178]

Posttransplant malignancy

Allograft function depends on maintaining an immunosuppressive state that leaves transplant recipients with a threefold to fourfold increased risk of developing neoplasms.[179] Apart from skin malignancies, common malignancies seen in the general population are not increased in lung and heart-lung recipients; instead, rare tumors, including posttransplant lymphoproliferative disorders (PTLDs) and various sarcomas, occur. The Epstein-Barr virus (EBV) has been associated with PTLD, which is characterized by abnormal monoclonal B-cell proliferation and is frequently extranodal, having a predilection for brain and allograft involvement.[179–181] Treatment of PTLD involves antiviral therapy, chemotherapy, local therapy that includes photodynamic therapy, reduction of immunosuppression, and anti-CD20 monoclonal antibodies.[179,182] The incidence of nonmelanoma skin cancers after transplantation outweighs the incidence of PTLD.[179] Transplant recipients tend to have a greater tendency toward developing squamous cell carcinoma compared with basal cell carcinoma; this is opposite to the pattern in the general population. Most therapy follows standard dermatologic approaches and varies with the histology and clinical stage of the disease.

RESULTS OF LUNG AND HEART-LUNG TRANSPLANTATION

The ISHLT reports survival outcomes for lung transplantation of 73 percent, 57 percent, and 45 percent at 1, 3, and 5 years, respectively.[2] At 10 years, however, long-term survival is only 23 percent. Improvement in 1-year lung transplant survival is indicated by a rise from 47 percent in 1988 to 74.8 percent in 1999.[1] The functional results of lung transplantation have been shown to be immediate and durable beyond the initial 3 years of follow-up.[17] Early results for bilateral lung transplantation have demonstrated an improvement of FEV_1 from 16 percent predicted preoperatively to 84 percent predicted 12 weeks postoperatively. A comparison of survival with and without transplantation in patients with

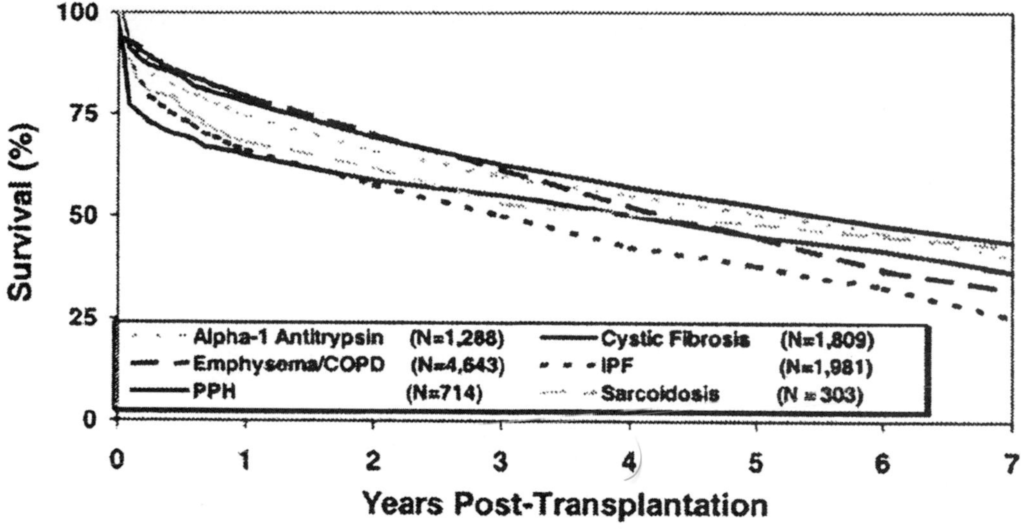

Figure 45-8 Actuarial survival after adult lung transplantation performed between 1990 and 2000 according to the underlying diagnosis. (Reprinted from the *Journal of Heart and Lung Transplantation*, Volume 21(9), Hertz MI, Taylor DO, Trulock EP, et al. The Registry of the International Society of Heart and Lung Transplantation: Nineteenth Official Report-2002, 957-962, 2002, with permission from the International Society for Heart and Lung Transplantation.)

end-stage lung disease has shown that there is a statistically significant improved effect.[183] The best results have been obtained in patients with COPD, who have been reported to experience a 94 percent 1-year and 2-year survival rate.[184] There is controversy about whether double- or single-lung transplantation is best for these patients. Currently, there is evidence that double-lung transplantation results in better long-term survival for COPD patients.[19,185] The worst results have been in patients with idiopathic pulmonary fibrosis, with 1- and 2-year survival of 73 percent. Patients with emphysema and pulmonary fibrosis have the highest chance of receiving a transplant despite the fact that pulmonary fibrosis patients have the highest probability of dying while waiting for a transplant.[46,186,187] Postoperatively, the risk of death has been shown to fall below preoperative risk levels for all patient diagnoses; this also indicates a survival advantage.[188] The survival rates according to diagnosis are given in Fig. 45-8. In general, the results of single right or left and double-lung transplantation are equal in terms of overall survival and improvement in quality of life, although there has been an increased risk of airway complications with left lung transplantation.[189–191] The causes of death in lung transplant patients vary with the time after a transplant. During the first 30 days, graft failure and non-CMV infections are the principal fatal complications. After the first year, obliterans bronchiolitis is the primary cause of death.[2]

Survival analysis of heart-lung transplant recipients reveals high early postoperative mortality, with only 70 percent survival at 3 months (Fig. 45-9).[2] The survival rates at 1, 5 and 10 years have been reported by ISHLT as 61 percent, 40 percent, and 25 percent, respectively. However, Stanford has presented data that reveal that outcomes may be even better than what had been reported previously.[192] Among the heart-lung transplants performed between 1991 and 2000 at Stanford, actuarial survival at 1, 5, and 10 years was 77 percent, 53 percent, and 49 percent, respectively. During the first 30 days, fatalities are dominated by technical complications, infections, and graft failure. For the remainder of the first year, non-CMV infections are the leading cause of death. Beyond the first year after transplantation, obliterans bronchiolitis is the main source of mortality.[1,2,193–195]

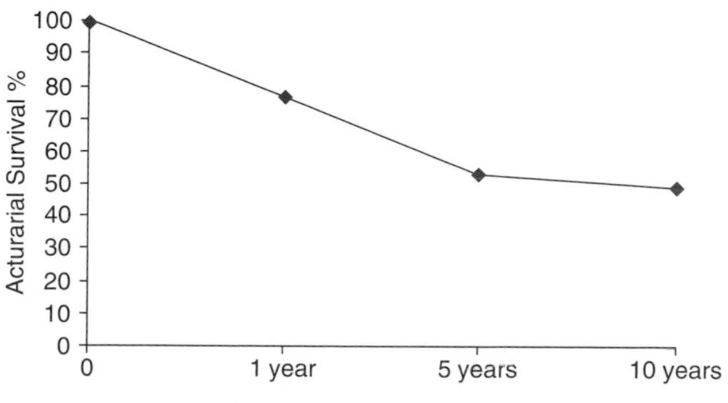

Figure 45-9 Actuarial survival of heart-lung transplant recipients who were transplanted between 1991 and 2000 at Stanford University.

The types of end-stage lung disease found to affect the chance of dying before heart-lung transplantation are CF and PF predominantly, followed by pulmonary hypertension.[187] However, overall survival rates and rates of obliterans bronchiolitis have been affected positively by improved immunosuppressive regimens over the years.[194,195] Functional status and quality of life have been reported to be very good in survivors, and up to 50 percent of these patients return to work.[2,191] In addition, pregnancy after heart-lung transplantation has been reported to be associated with good outcomes for both the mother and the child.[196]

The outcomes of patients who receive cardiac transplants from live donors in the form of the domino procedure have been encouraging.[197,198] The United Kingdom experience has revealed that although there is a higher rate of early mortality after the domino procedure compared with cadaveric heart transplantation, long-term survival is the same. This further emphasizes the usefulness of this procedure for patients with high pulmonary vascular resistance.

Risk factors for poor outcomes among lung and heart-lung transplant recipients have been investigated extensively. The role of cause of donor death in outcomes has not been found to be significant, but there is some evidence that traumatic brain injury may predispose transplanted lungs to severe early rejection episodes and early onset of obliterans bronchiolitis.[199] In fact, freedom from obliterans bronchiolitis at 5 years was only 34 percent for recipients of traumatic head injury donor lungs compared with 50 percent for recipients from donors without head injury.

The role of graft ischemia in outcomes has long been debated.[200–202] Currently, there is little evidence that prolonged ischemic times up to 8 h affect outcomes, and these data may help cautiously extend the normally accepted ischemic time of 6 h and thus geographically expand the donor pool.

The role of human leukocyte antigens and ABO blood groups has been investigated not only to determine the effect on the development of obliterans bronchiolitis and survival but also to expand the donor pool.[202,203] It has been found that although the number of HLA mismatches at the HLA-A and HLA-DR loci predict 1-year mortality and the total number of mismatches predicts 3- and 5-year mortality after lung transplantation, the overall effect is small.[202] Comparing ABO-identical and ABO-compatible recipients, outcomes did not differ in terms of survival or incidence of rejection or lung function.[203] Again, this could be a means to expand the donor pool without compromising outcomes.

The role of CMV and the development of obliterans bronchiolitis ultimately affecting overall survival constitute another variable that is debated actively.[161–164] The exact effect of CMV on the development of bronchiolitis obliterans is controversial, but routine prophylaxis against developing postoperative infections is thought to be paramount.

The understanding and successful treatment of obliterans bronchiolitis will prove to be a major factor in the success of lung transplantation. Currently, obliterans bronchiolitis or BOS is the limiting factor; it is relentless, and once it is diagnosed, the median survival is 1084 days, resulting in a 10-year survival rate of only 27 percent.[204]

RETRANSPLANTATION

Retransplantation is the only option available for irreversible allograft dysfunction and accounts for approximately 4 percent of all lung transplants performed yearly. Retransplantation may be required acutely or later in the course of a transplant recipient. Acute retransplantation occurs days to weeks after transplantation and can be due to acute reperfusion injury, irreversible acute rejection, and vascular and bronchial technical difficulties. Chronically, obliterans bronchiolitis or BOS is the cause for retransplantation in lung and heart-lung recipients. With improvements in the early results of lung transplantation, increasing numbers of recipients are being retransplanted. The pulmonary retransplant registry was founded in 1991 to determine the predictors of outcomes in this patient population.[205–207] This international registry collects data from 47 centers, and the most recent update included 203 patients. The most common indications for retransplantation were obliterans bronchiolitis and acute graft failure. Among these patients, 20 percent underwent ipsilateral single-lung retransplantation, 24 percent contralateral single-lung retransplantation, 19 percent repeat double-lung transplantation, 13 percent double-lung transplantation after a single-lung transplantation, and 24 percent single-lung transplantation after a previous double-lung or heart-lung transplant.[205] Factors that were associated with survival after retransplantation included being ambulatory before retransplantation, being non-ventilator-dependent, more than 2 years after the original transplant, ABO blood group match, CMV-negative donor, and extensive center experience. Factors found not to affect survival included the original diagnosis requiring transplantation, the type of transplant, and the recipient's CMV status.[205] These patients had a 1-year retransplantation survival rate of 64 percent compared with only 33 percent for nonambulatory ventilated recipients. Eighty-one percent and 56 percent of survivors were free of obliterans bronchiolitis 1 and 3 years after retransplantation, respectively. Other centers have reported that the best survival is among patients retransplanted for chronic graft dysfunction. However, when favorable circumstances are not present upon retransplantation, survival rates as low as 22 percent at 1 month have been reported, with sepsis and multiorgan failure being the most common causes of death.[207,208]

The largest series of heart-lung recipients undergoing retransplantation was published in 1994 by the Harefield Hospital transplant team. Only chronic rather than acute graft dysfunction, led to retransplantation in these heart-lung recipients. One- and 2-year survival rates of 25 percent were reported when the entire heart-lung block was retransplanted, with bleeding being a significant contributor to death. These results led transplant centers to perform single-lung retransplantation in heart-lung transplant recipients who develop obliterans bronchiolitis, with a resultant 1-year survival of 67 percent.[209]

Patients undergoing pulmonary retransplantation do not achieve functional status comparable to that of the first transplant. Also, obliterans bronchiolitis occurs after repeat lung transplantation at rates similar to those seen in first-time lung transplantation. Therefore, economic factors, inferior functional status, decreased survival, and an ever-increasing number of patients on the waiting list contribute to arguments against retransplantation. Ethical concerns and financial considerations have to be addressed because the supply of donors does not meet the demand for first-time transplantation. It has been suggested that a yearly cap be enforced for the number of lung retransplantations performed; 2 to 5 percent has been suggested to match the current yearly percentage of heart retransplantation.[210]

SUMMARY

Lung and heart-lung transplantations have come to be accepted modalities for end-stage pulmonary and cardiac disease. The results have improved over more than a decade of experience. Gains in survival and quality of life have been a result of better donor selection, improved operative and perioperative care, and tailored immunosuppression. Nonetheless, lung and heart-lung transplantation remains expensive in terms of monetary and personal costs because of substantial mortality and morbidity. Much progress must be made in lung and heart-lung transplantation if graft loss, immunosuppressive toxicity, and insufficient donor numbers are to be improved on. Perseverance and ongoing research coupled with continuous institutional review of clinical results will help improve outcomes in lung and heart-lung transplantation.

References

1. Bennett LE, Keck BM, Daily OP, et al. Worldwide thoracic organ transplantation: A report from the UNOS/ISHLT International Registry for Thoracic Organ Transplantation. *Clin Transpl* 2000:31–44.
2. Trulock EP, Edwards LB, Taylor DO, et al. The Registry of the International Society for Heart and Lung Transplantation: Twentieth official adult lung and heart-lung transplant report—2003. *J Heart Lung Transplant* 2003;22:625.
3. Carrel A, Guthrie CC. The transplantation of veins and organs. *Am J Med* 1905;10:1101.
4. Mann FC, Priestly JT, Markowitz J, et al. Transplantation of the intact mammalian heart. *Arch Surg* 1933; 26:219.
5. Demikhov VP. *Experimental Transplantation of Vital Organs.* New York: Consultants Bureau; 1962.
6. Marcus E, Wong SNT, Luisada AA. Homologous heart grafts. *Arch Surg* 1953;66:179.
7. Webb WR, Howard HS. Cardiopulmonary transplantation. *Surg Forum* 1957;8:313.
8. Lower RR, Shumway NE. Studies on the orthotopic homotransplantations of the canine heart. *Surg Forum* 1960;11:18.
9. Barnard CN. A human cardiac transplant: An interim report of a successful operation performed at Groote Schuur Hospital, Capetown. *S Afr Med J* 1967;41:1271.
10. Cooley DA, Bloodwell RD, Hallman GL, et al. Organ transplantation for advanced cardiopulmonary disease. *Ann Thorac Surg* 1969;8:300.
11. Lillehei CW. Discussion of Wildevuur CRH, Benfield JR: A review of 23 human lung transplantations by 20 surgeons. *Ann Thorac Surg* 1970;9:489.
12. Reitz BA, Burton NA, Jamieson SW, et al. Heart and lung transplantation, autotransplantation and allotransplantation in primates with extended survival. *J Thorac Cardiovasc Surg* 1980;80:360.
13. Reitz BA, Wallwork JL, Hunt SA, et al. Heart-lung transplantation: Successful therapy for patients with pulmonary vascular disease. *N Engl J Med* 1982;306:557.
14. Hardy JD, Erasian S, Dalton ML. Autotransplantation and homotransplantation of the lung: Further studied. *J Thorac Cardiovasc Surg* 1953;46:606.
15. The Toronto Lung Transplant Group. Unilateral lung transplantation for pulmonary fibrosis. *N Engl J Med* 1986;314:1140.
16. Patterson G, Cooper J, Goldman B, et al. Techniques of successful clinical double-lung transplantation. *Ann Thorac Surg* 1988;45:626.
17. Meyers BF, Patterson GA. Lung transplantation: Current status and future prospects. *World J Surg* 1999;23:1156.
18. Harringer W, Haverich A. Heart and heart-lung transplantation: Standards and improvements. *World J Surg* 2002;26:218.
19. Bavaria JE, Kotloff R, Palevsky H, et al. Bilateral versus single lung transplantation for chronic obstructive pulmonary disease. *J Thorac Cardiovasc Surg* 1996; 112:520.
20. Pochettino A, Kotloff RM, Rosengard BR, et al. Bilateral versus single lung transplantation for chronic obstructive pulmonary disease: Intermediate-term results. *Ann Thorac Surg* 2000;70:1813.
21. Hosenpud JD, Bennett LE, Keck BM, et al. Effect of diagnosis on survival benefit of lung transplantation for end-stage lung disease. *Lancet* 1998;351:24.

22. Yacoub M, Gyi K, Khaghani A, et al. Analysis of 10-year experience with heart-lung transplantation for cystic fibrosis. *Transplant Proc* 1997;29:632.
23. Vricella LA, Karamichalis JM, Ahmad S, et al. Lung and heart-lung transplantation in patients with end-stage cystic fibrosis: The Stanford experience. *Ann Thorac Surg* 2002;74:13.
24. Pigula FA, Gandhi SK, Ristich J, et al. Cardiopulmonary transplantation for congenital heart disease in the adult. *J Heart Lung Transplant* 2001;20:297.
25. Stoica SC, McNeil KD, Perreas K, et al. Heart-lung transplantation for Eisenmenger syndrome: Early and long-term results. *Ann Thorac Surg* 2001;72:1887.
26. Waddell TK, Bennett L, Kennedy R, et al. Heart-lung or lung transplantation for Eisenmenger syndrome. *J Heart Lung Transplant* 2002;21:731.
27. Ueno T, Smith JA, Snell GI, et al. Bilateral sequential single lung transplantation for pulmonary hypertension and Eisenmenger's syndrome. *Ann Thorac Surg* 2000; 69:381.
28. Whyte RI, Robbins RC, Altinger J, et al. Heart-lung transplantation for primary pulmonary hypertension. *Ann Thorac Surg* 1999;67:937.
29. Mendeloff EN, Meyers BF, Sundt TM, et al. Lung transplantation for pulmonary vascular disease. *Ann Thorac Surg* 2002;73:209.
30. Pielsticker EJ, Martinez FJ, Rubenfire M. Lung and heart-lung transplant practice patterns in pulmonary hypertension centers. *J Heart Lung Transplant* 2001; 20:1297.
31. Hasan A, Corris PA, Healy M, et al. Bilateral sequential lung transplantation for end-stage septic lung disease. *Thorax* 1995;50:565.
32. Egan TM, Frank CD, Mill MM, et al. Improved results of lung transplantation for patients with cystic fibrosis. *J Thorac Cardiovasc Surg* 1995;109:224.
33. Barlow CW, Robbins RC, Moon MR, et al. Heart-lung versus double-lung transplantation for suppurative lung disease. *J Thorac Cardiovasc Surg* 2000;119:466.
34. Talbot SM, Taub RN, Keohan ML, et al. Combined heart and lung transplantation for unresectable primary cardiac sarcoma. *J Thorac Cardiovasc Surg* 2002; 124:1145.
35. Zorn GL, McGiffin DC, Young KR, et al. Pulmonary transplantation for advanced bronchioalveolar carcinoma. *J Thorac Cardiovasc Surg* 2003;125:45.
36. Egan TM, Detterbeck FC. The ABCs of LTX for BAC. *J Thorac Cardiovasc Surg* 2003;125:20.
37. De Perrot M, Fischer S, Waddell TK, et al. Management of lung transplant recipients with bronchogenic carcinoma in the native lung. *J Heart Lung Transplant* 2003;22:87.
38. Taylor JR, Ryu J, Colby TV, et al. Lymphangioleiomyomatosis: Clinical course in 32 patients. *N Engl J Med* 1990;323:1254.
39. Bittmann I, Rolf B, Amann G, et al. Recurrence of lymphangioleiomyomatosis after single lung transplantation: New insights into pathogenesis. *Hum Pathol* 2003; 34:95.
40. Pechet TT, Singhal AK, Meyers BF, et al. Lung transplantation for lymphangioleiomyomatosis. *J Heart Lung Transplant* 2001;20:174.
41. DeMeo DL, Ginns LC. Clinical status of lung transplantation. *Transplantation* 20001;72:1713.
42. Patel VS, Palmer SM, Messier RH, et al. Clinical outcome after coronary artery revascularization and lung transplantation. *Ann Thorac Surg* 2003;75:372.
43. Shane E, Papadopoulos A, Staron RB, et al. Bone loss and fracture after lung transplantation. *Transplantation* 1999;68:220.
44. Aris RM, Gilligan PH, Neuringer IP, et al. The effects of pan-resistant bacteria in cystic fibrosis patients on lung transplant outcome. *Am J Respir Crit Care Med* 1998; 19:473.
45. Bartz RR, Love RB, Leverson GE, et al. Pre-transplant mechanical ventilation and outcome in patients with cystic fibrosis. *J Heart Lung Transplant* 2003;22:433.
46. Algar FJ, Alvarez A, Santos LF, et al. Lung transplantation in patients under mechanical ventilation. *Transplant Proc* 2003;35:737.
47. Ramsey BW. Management of pulmonary disease in patients with cystic fibrosis. *N Engl J Med* 1996;335:179.
48. De Meester J, Smits JMA, Persijn GG, et al. Lung transplant waiting list: Differential outcome of type of end-stage lung disease, one year after registration. *J Heart Lung Transplant* 1999;18:563.
49. Timek T, Bonz A, Dillmann R, et al. The effect of triiodothyronine on myocardial contractile performance after epinephrine exposure: Implications for donor heart management. *J Heart Lung Transplant* 1998;17:931.
50. Bouda C, Lalot JM, Perrier JF, et al. Evaluation of donor cardiac function for heart transplantation: Experience of a French academic hospital. *Ann Transplant* 2000;5:51.
51. Potapov EV, Ivanitskaia EA, Loebe M, et al. Value of cardiac troponin I and T for selection of heart donors and as predictors of early graft failure. *Transplantation* 2001;71:1394.
52. Marelli D, Laks H, Fazio D, et al. The use of donor hearts with left ventricular hypertrophy. *J Heart Lung Transplant* 2000;19:496.
53. Chen JM, Sinha P, Rajasinghe HA, et al. Do donor characteristics really matter? Short- and long-term impact of donor characteristics on recipient survival, 1995-1999. *J Heart Lung Transplant* 2002;21:608.
54. Potapov EV, Matthias H, Hubler M, et al. Medium-term results of heart transplantation using donors over 63 years of age. *Transplantation* 1999;68:1834.
55. Bhorade SM, Vigneswaran W, McCabe MA, et al. Liberalization of donor criteria may expand the donor pool without adverse consequence in lung transplantation. *J Heart Lung Transplant* 2000;19:1200.
56. Pierre AF, Sekine Y, Hutcheon MA, et al. Marginal donor lungs: A reassessment. *J Thorac Cardiovasc Surg* 123:421.
57. Hausen B, Beuke Maike, Schroeder F, et al. In vivo measurement of lung preservation solution efficacy: Comparison of LPD, UW, EC and low K^+-EC following short and extended ischemia. *Eur J Cardiothorac Surg* 1997;12:771.
58. Muller C, Furst H, Reichenspurner H, et al. Lung procurement by low-potassium dextran and the effect on preservation injury. *Transplantation* 1999;68:1139.
59. Struber M, Wilhelmi M, Harringer W, et al. Flush perfusion with low potassium dextran solution improves early

graft function in clinical lung transplantation. *Eur J Cardiothorac Surg* 2001;19:190.
60. Fischer S, Matte-Martyn A, de Perrot M, et al. Low-potassium dextran preservation solution improves lung function after human lung transplantation. *J Thorac Cardiovasc Surg* 2001;120:594.
61. Aziz TM, Pillay TM, Corris PA, et al. Perfadex for clinical lung procurement: Is it an advance? *Ann Thorac Surg* 2003;75:990.
62. Hopkinson DN, Bhabra MS, Hooper TL. Pulmonary graft preservation: A worldwide survey of current clinical practice. *J Heart Lung Transplant* 1998;17:525.
63. Vaida AM, Tang DG, Allen C, et al. Novel protection strategy for pulmonary transplantation. *J Surg Res* 2003;109:8.
64. Gaissert HA, Patterson GA. Surgical techniques of single and bilateral lung transplantation. In: Cooper DKC (ed). *Transplantation of Thoracic Organs.* Boston: Kluwer; 1990:457.
65. Garfein ES, McGregor CC, Galantowicz ME, Schulman LL. Deleterious effects of telescoped bronchial anastomosis in single and bilateral lung transplantation. *Ann Transplant* 2000;5:5.
66. Aigner C, Jaksch P, Seebacher G, et al. Single running suture—the new standard technique for bronchial anastomoses in lung transplantation. *Eur J Cardiothorac Surg* 2003;23:488.
67. Alvarez A, Algar J, Santos F, et al. Airway complications after lung transplantation: A review of 151 anastomoses. *Eur J Cardiothorac Surg* 2001;19:381.
68. Yacoub M, Al-Kattan KM, Tadjkarimi S, et al. Medium term results of direct bronchial arterial revascularisation using IMA for single lung transplantation (SLT with direct revascularisation). *Eur J Cardiothoracic Surg* 1997;11:1030.
69. Norgaard MA, Efsen F, Arendrup H, et al. Surgical and arteriographic results of bronchial artery revascularization in lung and heart lung transplantation. *J Heart Lung Transplant* 1997;16:302.
70. Clark SC, Levine AJ, Hasan A, et al. Vascular complications of lung transplantation. *Ann Thorac Surg* 1996; 61:1079.
71. Wissner W, Klepetko W, Wekerle TT, et al. Tailoring of the lung to overcome size disparities in lung transplantation. *J Heart Lung Transplant* 1996;15:239.
72. Sundset A, Tadjkarimi S, Khaghani A, et al. Human en bloc double-lung transplantation: Bronchial artery revascularization improves airway perfusion. *Ann Thorac Surg* 1997;63:790.
73. Pettersson G, Norgaard MA, Arendrup H, et al. Direct bronchial artery revascularization and en bloc double lung transplantation—surgical techniques and early outcome. *J Heart Lung Transplant* 1997;16:320.
74. Hyytinen TA, Heikkila LJ, Verkkala KA, et al. Bronchial artery revascularization improves tracheal anastomotic healing after lung transplantation. *Scand Cardiovasc J* 2000;34:213.
75. Macchiarini P, Ladurie F, Cerrina J, et al. Clamshell or sternotomy for double lung or heart-lung transplantation. *Eur J Cardiothorac Surg* 1999;15:333.
76. Cohen RG, Starnes VA. Living donor lung transplantation. *World J Surg* 2001;25:244.
77. Barr ML, Baker CJ, Schenkel FA, et al. Living donor lung transplantation: Selection, technique, and outcome. *Transplant Proc* 2001;33:3527.
78. Couteil JP, Tolan MJ, Loulmet DF, et al. Pulmonary bipartitioning and lobar transplantation: A new approach to donor organ shortage. *J Thorac Cardiovasc Surg* 1997;113:529.
79. Fann JI, Wilson MK, Theodore J, et al. Combined heart and single-lung transplantation in complex congenital heart disease. *Ann Thorac Surg* 1998;65:823.
80. Conte JV, Jhaveri R, Borja MC, et al. Combined heart-single-lung transplantation: A unique operation for unique indications. *J Heart Lung Transplant* 2002; 21:1250.
81. Baumgartner WA, Traill TA, Cameron DE, et al. Unique aspects of heart and lung transplantation exhibited in the "domino-donor" operation. *JAMA* 1989; 261:3121.
82. Klepetko W, Wollenek G, Laczkovics A, et al. Domino transplantation of heart-lung and heart: An approach to overcome the scarcity of donor organs. *J Heart Lung Transplant* 1991;10:129.
83. Smith JA, Cochrane AD, Esmore DS. Technique and results of cardiac transplantation using "domino-donor" hearts. *J Card Surg* 6:381.
84. Oaks TE, Aravot D, Dennis C, et al. Domino heart transplantation: The Papworth experience. *J Heart Lung Transplant* 1994;13:433.
85. Anyanwu AC, Rogers CA, Murday AJ. Variations in cardiac transplantation: Comparisons between the United Kingdom and the United States. *J Heart Lung Transplant* 1999;18:297.
86. Anyanwu AC, Banner NR, Radley-Smith R, et al. Long-term results of cardiac transplantation from live donors: The domino heart transplant. *J Heart Lung Transplant* 2002;21:971.
87. Trachiotis GD, Knight SR, Hann M, et al. Respiratory responses to CO_2 rebreathing in lung transplant recipients. *Ann Thorac Surg* 1994;58:1709.
88. Girgis RE, Tu I, Berry GJ, et al. Risk factors for the development of obliterative bronchiolitis after lung transplantation. *J Heart Lung Transplant* 1995;15:1200.
89. Reichenspurner H, Girgis RE, Robbins RC, et al. Obliterative bronchiolitis after lung and heart lung transplantation. *Ann Thorac Surg* 1995;60:1845.
90. Wain JC, Wright CD, Ryan DP, et al. Induction immunosuppression for lung transplantation with OKT3. *Ann Thorac Surg* 1999;67:187.
91. Weibe K, Harringer W, Wahlers T, et al. ATG induction therapy and the incidence of bronchiolitis obliterans after lung transplantation: Does it make a difference? *Transplant Proc* 1998;30:1517.
92. Barlow CW, Moon MR, Green GR, et al. Rabbit antithymocyte globulin versus OKT3 induction therapy after heart-lung and lung transplantation: Effect on survival, rejection, infection and obliterative bronchiolitis. *Transpl Int* 2001;14:234.
93. Palmer SM, Miralles AP, Lawrence CM, et al. Rabbit antithymocyte globulin decreases acute rejection after lung transplantation. *Chest* 1999;116:127.
94. Brock MV, Borja Marvin C, Ferber L, et al. Induction therapy in lung transplantation: A prospective, controlled

clinical trial comparing OKT3, anti-thymocyte globulin, and Daclizumab. *J Heart Lung Transplant* 2001; 20:1282.
95. Yamani MH, Starling RC, Pelegrin D, et al. Efficacy of tacrolimus in patients with steroid-resistant cardiac allograft cellular rejection. *J Heart Lung Transplant* 2000;19: 337–342.
96. DeBonis M, Reynolds L, Barros J, Madden BP. Tacrolimus as a rescue immunosuppressant after heart transplantation. *Eur J Cardiothorac Surg* 2001;19: 690–695.
97. Kesten S, Chaparro C, Scavuzzo M, et al. Tacrolimus as rescue therapy for bronchiolitis obliterans syndrome. *J Heart Lung Transplant* 1997;16:905.
98. Revell MP, Lewis ME, Llewellyn-Jones CG, et al. Conservation of small-airway function by tacrolimus/ cyclosporine conversion in the management of bronchiolitis obliterans following lung transplantation. *J Heart Lung Transplant* 2000;19:1219.
99. Treede H, Klepetko W, Reichenspurner H, et al. Tacrolimus versus cyclosporine after lung transplantation: A prospective, open, randomized two-center trial comparing two different immunosuppressive protocols. *J Heart Lung Transplant* 2001;20:511.
100. Zuckermann A, Reichenspurner H, Birsan T, et al. Cyclosporine A versus tacrolimus in combination with mycophenolate mofetil and steroids as primary immunosuppression after lung transplantation: One-year results of a 2-center prospective randomized trial. *J Thorac Cardiovasc Surg* 2003;125:891.
101. Izbicki G, Shitrit D, Aravot D, et al. Improved survival after lung transplantation in patients treated with tacrolimus/mycophenolate mofetil as compared with cyclosporine/azathioprine. *Transplant Proc* 2002; 34:3258.
102. Snell GI, Levvey BJ, Chin W, et al. Rescue therapy: A role for sirolimus in lung and heart transplant recipients. *Transplant Proc* 2001;33:1084–1085.
103. Snell GI, Levvey BJ, Chin W, et al. Sirolimus allows renal recovery in lung and heart transplant recipients with chronic renal impairment. *J Heart Lung Transplant* 2002; 21:540–546.
104. Cahill BC, Somerville KT, Crompton JA, et al. Early experience with sirolimus in lung transplant recipients with chronic allograft rejection. *J Heart Lung Transplant* 2003;22:169.
105. McWilliams TJ, Levvey BJ, Russell PA, et al. Interstitial pneumonitis associated with sirolimus: A dilemma for lung transplantation. *J Heart Lung Transplant* 2003; 22:210.
106. Lim TT, Botas J, Ross H, et al. Are heart-lung transplant recipients protected from developing transplant coronary artery disease? *Circulation* 1996;94:1573.
107. Starnes VA, Theodore J, Oyer PE, et al. Evaluation of heart-lung transplant recipients with prospective, serial transbronchial biopsies and pulmonary function studies. *J Thorac Cardiovasc Surg* 1989;98:683.
108. Otulana BA, Higenbottam T, Scott J, et al. Lung function associated with histologically diagnosed acute lung rejection and pulmonary infection in heart-lung transplant patients. *Am Rev Respir Dis* 1990; 142:329.
109. Becker FS, Martinez, Brunsting LA, et al. Limitations of spirometry in detecting rejection after single-lung transplantation. *Am J Respir Crit Care Med* 1994;150:159.
110. Van Muylem A, Paiva M, Estenne M. Involvement of peripheral airways during methacholine-induced bronchoconstriction after lung transplantation. *Am J Respir Crit Care Med* 2001;164:1200.
111. Stanbrook MB, Kesten S. Bronchial hyperreactivity after lung transplantation predicts early bronchiolitis obliterans. *Am J Respir Crit Care Med* 1999;160:2034.
112. Liakakos P, Snell GI, Ward C, et al. Bronchial hyperresponsiveness in lung transplant recipients: Lack of correlation with airway inflammation. *Thorax* 1997; 52:551.
113. Millet B, Higenbottam TW, Flower CDR. The radiographic appearances of infection and acute rejection of the lung after heart-lung transplantation. *Am Rev Respir Dis* 1989;140:62.
114. Soyer P, Devine N, Frachon I, et al. Computed tomography of complications of lung transplantation. *Eur Radiol* 1997;7:847.
115. Ikonen T, Kivisaari L, Taskinen E, et al. High-resolution CT in long-term follow-up after lung transplantation. *Chest* 1997;111:370.
116. Gotway MB, Dawn SK, Sellami D, et al. Acute rejection following lung transplantation: Limitations in accuracy of thin-section CT for diagnosis. *Radiology* 2001; 221:207.
117. Kanno S, Lee PC, Dodd SJ, et al. A novel approach with magnetic resonance imaging used for the detection of lung allograft rejection. *J Thorac Cardiovasc Surg* 2000; 120:923.
118. Hopkins PM, Aboyoun CI, Chhajed PN, et al. Prospective analysis of 1,235 transbronchial lung biopsies in lung transplant recipients. *J Heart Lung Transplant* 2002;21:1062.
119. Swanson SJ, Mentzer SJ, Reilly JJ, et al. Surveillance transbronchial lung biopsies: Implications for survival after lung transplantation. *J Thorac Cardiovasc Surg* 2000;119:27.
120. Girgis RE, Reichenspurner H, Robbins RC, et al. The utility of annual surveillance bronchoscopy in heart-lung transplant recipients. *Transplantation* 1995;60:1458.
121. Valentine VG, Taylor DE, Dhillon GS, et al. Success of lung transplantation without surveillance bronchoscopy. *J Heart Lung Transplant* 2002;21:319.
122. Tamm M, Sharples LD, Higenbottam TW, et al. Bronchiolitis obliterans syndrome in heart-lung transplantation surveillance biopsies. *Am J Respir Crit Care Med* 1997;155:1705.
123. Billingham ME, Carry NRB, Hammond ME, et al. A working formulation for the standardization of nomenclature in the diagnosis of heart and lung rejection: Heart Rejection Study Group. *J Heart Lung Transplant* 1990;9:587.
124. Kutlu HM, Sadeghi AM, Norton JE, et al. Effect of simultaneous lung transplantation on heart transplant survival in rats. *J Heart Transplant* 1987;6:29.
125. Westra AL, Petersen AH, Prop J, et al. The combi-effect—reduced rejection of the heart by combined transplantation with the lung or spleen. *Transplantation* 1996;52:952.

126. Fauchier L, Sirinelli A, Aupart M, et al. Performances of Doppler echocardiography for diagnosis of acute, mild or moderate cardiac allograft rejection. *Transplant Proc* 1993;12:411.
127. Dodd DA, Brady LD, Carden KA, et al. Pattern of echocardiographic abnormalities with acute cardiac allograft rejection in adults: Correlation with endomyocardial biopsy. *J Heart Lung Transplant* 1993;12:1009.
128. Puleo JA, Aranda JM, Weston MW, et al. Noninvasive detection of allograft rejection in heart transplant recipients by use of Doppler tissue imaging. *J Heart Lung Transplant* 1998;17:176.
129. Dunn DL. Hazardous crossing: Immunosuppression and nosocomial infections in solid organ transplant recipients. *Surg Infect (Larchmt)* 2001;2:102.
130. Uknis ME, Dunn DL. Cytomegalovirus infection and disease after solid organ transplantation: Epidemiology, prevention and therapy. *Transplant Rev* 2000;14:199.
131. Gerbase MW, Dubois D, Rothmeier C, et al. Costs and outcomes of prolonged cytomegalovirus prophylaxis to cover the enhanced immunosuppression phase following lung transplantation. *Chest* 1999;116:1265.
132. Brumble LM, Milstone AP, Loyd JE, et al. Prevention of cytomegalovirus infection and disease after lung transplantation. *Chest* 2002;121:407.
133. Soghikian MV, Valentine VG, Berry GJ, et al. Impact of ganciclovir prophylaxis on heart-lung and lung transplant recipients. *J Heart Lung Transplant* 1996;15:881.
134. Valentine HA, Luikart H, Doyle R, et al. Impact of cytomegalovirus hyperimmune globulin on outcome after cardiothoracic transplantation: A comparative study of combined prophylaxis with CMV hyperimmune globulin plus ganciclovir versus ganciclovir alone. *Transplantation* 2001;72:1647.
135. Kubak BM. Fungal infection in lung transplantation. *Transpl Infect Dis* 2002;4:24.
136. De Perrot M, Liu M, Waddel TK, et al. Ischemic-reperfusion-induced lung injury. *Am J Respir Crit Care Med* 2003;167:490.
137. Christie JD, Bavaria JE, Palevsky HI, et al. Primary graft failure following lung transplantation. *Chest* 1998; 114:51.
138. Chatila WM, Furukawa S, Gaughan JP, et al. Respiratory failure after lung transplantation. *Chest* 2003;123:165.
139. Thabut G, Vinatier I, Stern JB, et al. Primary graft failure following lung transplantation. *Chest* 2003; 121:1876.
140. King RC, Binns OAR, Rodriguez F, et al. Reperfusion injury significantly impacts clinical outcome after pulmonary transplantation. *Ann Thorac Surg* 2000; 69:1681.
141. Fiser SM, Kron IL, Long SM, et al. Controlled perfusion decreases reperfusion injury after high-flow reperfusion. *J Heart Lung Transplant* 2002;21:687.
142. Inci I, Inci D, Dutly A, et al. Melatonin attenuates post-transplant lung ischemia-reperfusion injury. *Ann Thorac Surg* 2002;73:220.
143. Levine AJ, Parkes K, Rooney SJ, et al. The effect of adhesion molecule blockade on pulmonary reperfusion injury. *Ann Thorac Surg* 2002;73:1101.
144. Tagawa T, Suda T, Daddi N, et al. Low-dose endobronchial gene transfer to ameliorate lung graft ischemia-reperfusion injury. *J Thorac Cardiovasc Surg* 2001;123:795.
145. Levine AJ, Parkes K, Rooney S, Bonser RS. Reduction of endothelial injury after hypothermic lung preservation by initial leukocyte-depleted reperfusion. *J Thorac Cardiovasc Surg* 2000;120:47–54.
146. Rocca GC, Pierconti F, Costa MG, et al. Severe reperfusion lung injury after double lung transplantation. *Crit Care* 2002;6:240.
147. Kemming GI, Merkel MJ, Schallerer A, et al. Inhales nitric oxide (NO) for the treatment of early allograft failure after lung transplantation: Munich Lung Transplant Group. *Intensive Care Med* 1998;24:1173.
148. Meade M, Granton JT, Matte-Martyn A, et al. A randomized trial of inhaled nitric oxide to prevent reperfusion injury following lung transplantation. *J Heart Lung Transplant* 2001;20:254.
149. De Perrot M, Fischer S, Liu M, et al. Prostaglandin E1 protects lung transplants from ischemia-reperfusion injury: A shift from pro- to anti-inflammatory cytokines. *Transplantation* 2001;72:655.
150. DeCampos KN, Keshavjee S, Liu M, et al. Prevention of rapid reperfusion-induced injury with prostaglandin E1 during the initial period of reperfusion. *J Heart Lung Transplant* 1998;17:1121.
151. Yousem SA, Berry GJ, Cagle PT, et al. Revision of the 1990 working formulation for the classification of pulmonary allograft rejection: Lung Rejection Study Group. *J Heart Lung Transplant* 1996;15:1.
152. Shennib H, Massard G, Reynaud M, et al. Efficacy of OKT3 therapy for acute rejection in isolated lung transplantation. *J Heart Lung Transplant* 1994;13:514.
153. Bonnefoy-Berard N, Revillard J-P. Mechanisms of immunosuppression induced by antithymocyte globulins and OKT3. *J Heart Lung Transplant* 1996;15:435.
154. Ross DJ, Waters PF, Levin M, et al. Mycophenolate mofetil versus azathioprine immunosuppressive regimens after lung transplantation: Preliminary experience. *J Heart Lung Transplant* 1998;17:768.
155. Ross HJ, Gullestad L, Pak J, et al. Methotrexate or total lymphoid radiation for treatment of persistent or recurrent allograft cellular rejection: A comparative study. *J Heart Lung Transplant* 1996;16:179.
156. Salerno CT, Park SJ, Kreykes NS, et al. Adjuvant treatment of refractory lung transplant rejection with extracorporeal photophoresis. *J Thorac Cardiovasc Surg* 1999; 117:1063.
157. Estenne M, Maurer JR, Boehler A, et al. Bronchiolitis obliterans syndrome 2001: An update of the diagnostic criteria. *J Heart Lung Transplant* 2001;21:297.
158. Nathan SD, Barnett SD, Wohlrab J, et al. Bronchiolitis obliterans syndrome: Utility of the new guidelines in single lung transplant recipients. *J Heart Lung Transplant* 2003;22:427.
159. Knollmann FD, Ewert R, Wundrich T, et al. Bronchiolitis obliterans syndrome in lung transplant recipients: Use of spirometrically gated CT. *Radiology* 2002;225:665.
160. Bankier AA, Van Muylem A, Knoop C, et al. Bronchiolitis obliterans syndrome in heart-lung transplant recipients: Diagnosis with expiratory CT. *Radiology* 2001; 218:533.
161. Heng D, Sharples LD, McNeil K, et al. Bronchiolitis obliterans syndrome: Incidence, natural history, prognosis

and risk factors. *J Heart Lung Transplant* 1998; 17:1255.
162. Estenne M, Hertz MI. Bronchiolitis obliterans after human lung transplantation. *Am J Crit Care Med* 2000;166:440.
163. Brugiere O, Pessione F, Thabut G, et al. Bronchiolitis obliterans syndrome after single-lung transplantation: Impact of time of onset on functional pattern and survival. *Chest* 2002;121:1883.
164. Sharples LD, McNeil K, Stewart S, et al. Risk factors for bronchiolitis obliterans: A systematic review of recent publications. *J Heart Lung Transplant* 2002;21: 271.
165. Sundaresan S, Mohanakumar T, Smith MA, et al. HLA-A locus mismatches and development of antibodies to HLA after lung transplantation correlate with the development of bronchiolitis obliterans syndrome. *Transplantation* 1998;65:648.
166. Husain AN, Siddiqui MT, Holmes EW, et al. Analysis of risk factors for the development of bronchiolitis obliterans syndrome. *Am J Respir Crit Care Med* 1999; 159:829.
167. Fisher AJ, Wardle J, Dark JH, et al. Non-immune acute graft injury after lung transplantation and the risk of subsequent bronchiolitis obliterans syndrome (BOS). *J Heart Lung Transplant* 2002;21:1206.
168. Fiser SM, Tribble CG, Long SM, et al. Ischemia-reperfusion injury after lung transplantation increases risk of late bronchiolitis obliterans syndrome. *Ann Thorac Surg* 2002;73:1041.
169. El-Gamel A, Sim E, Hasleton P, et al. Transforming growth factor beta (TGF-β) and obliterative bronchiolitis following pulmonary transplantation. *J Heart Lung Transplant* 1999;18:828.
170. Reichenspurner H, Girgis RE, Robbins RC, et al. Stanford experience with obliterative bronchiolitis after lung and heart-lung transplantation. *Ann Thorac Surg* 1996;62:1467.
171. Snell GI, Esmore DS, Williams TJ. Cytolytic therapy for the bronchiolitis obliterans syndrome complicating lung transplantation. *Chest* 1996;109:874.
172. Date H, Lynch JP, Sundaresan S, et al. The impact of cytolytic therapy on bronchiolitis obliterans syndrome. *J Heart Lung Transplant* 1998;17:869.
173. Dunn DL. Hazardous crossing: Immunosuppression and nosocomial infections in solid organ transplant recipients. *Surg Infect (Lrchmt)* 2001;2:103.
174. Pietrantoni C, Minai OA, Yu NC, et al. Respiratory failure and sepsis are the major causes of ICU admissions and mortality in survivors of lung transplants. *Chest* 2003;123:504.
175. Grossi P, Farina C, Fiocchi R, et al. Prevalence and outcome of invasive fungal infections in 1,963 thoracic organ transplant recipients: A multicenter retrospective study. *Transplantation* 2000;70:112.
176. Singh N, Husain S. *Aspergillus* infections after lung transplantation: Clinical differences in type of transplant and implications for management. *J Heart Lung Transplant* 2004;22:258.
177. Milstone AP, Brumble LM, Loyd JE, et al. Active CMV infection before lung transplantation: Risk factors and clinical implications. *J Heart Lung Transplant* 2000; 19:744.
178. Bhorade SM, Lurain NS, Jordan A, et al. Emergence of ganciclovir-resistant cytomegalovirus in lung transplant recipients. *J Heart Lung Transplant* 2002;21:1274.
179. Penn I. Post-transplant malignancy: The role of immunosuppression. *Drug Saf* 2000;23:101.
180. Levine SM, Angel L, Anzueto A, et al. A low incidence of posttransplant lymphoproliferative disorder in 109 lung transplant recipients. *Chest* 1999;116:1273.
181. Legere BM, Saad CP, Mehta AC, et al. Endobronchial post-transplant lymphoproliferative disorder and its management with photodynamic therapy: A case report. *J Heart Lung Transplant* 2003;22:474.
182. Swinnen LJ. Treatment of organ transplant-related lymphoma. *Hematol Oncol Clin North Am* 1997;11:963.
183. Geertsma A, Ten Vergert EM, Bonsel GJ, et al. Does lung transplantation prolong life? A comparison of survival with and without transplantation. *J Heart Lung Transplant* 1998;17:511.
184. Cassivi SD, Meyers BF, Battafarano RJ, et al. Thirteen-year experience in lung transplantation for emphysema. *Ann Thorac Surg* 2002;74:1663.
185. Sundaresan RS, Shiraishi Y, Trulock EP, et al. Single or bilateral lung transplantation for emphysema? *J Thorac Cardiovasc Surg* 1996;112:1485.
186. Charman SC, Sharples LD, McNeil KD, et al. Assessment of survival benefit after lung transplantation by patient diagnosis. *J Heart Lung Transplant* 2002; 21:226.
187. De Meester J, Smits JM, Persijn GG, et al. Listing for lung transplantation: Life expectancy and transplant effect, stratified by type of end-stage lung disease, the Eurotransplant experience. *J Heart Lung Transplant* 2001;20:518.
188. De Meester J, Smits JM, Persijn GG, et al. Lung transplant waiting list: Differential outcome of type of end-stage lung disease, one year after registration. *J Heart Lung Transplant* 1999;18:563.
189. Snell GI, Shiraishi T, Griffiths A, et al. Outcomes from paired single-lung transplants from the same donor. *J Heart Lung Transplant* 2000;19:1056.
190. Lanuza DM, Lefaiver C, McCabe M, et al. Prospective study of functional status and quality of life before and after lung transplantation. *Chest* 2000;118:115.
191. Fink G, Lebzelter J, Blau C, et al. The sky is the limit: Exercise capacity 10 years post-heart-lung transplantation. *Transplant Proc* 2000;32:733.
192. Demers P, Robbins RC, Doyle R, et al. Twenty years of combined heart-lung transplantation at Stanford University. *J Heart Lung Transplant* 2002;21:77.
193. Hummel M, Michauk I, Hetzer R, et al. Quality of life after heart and heart-lung transplantation. *Transplant Proc* 2001;33:3546.
194. Reichart B, Gulbins H, Meiser BM, et al. Improved results after heart-lung transplantation: A 17-year experience. *Transplantation* 2003;75:127.
195. Sarris GE, Smith JA, Shumway NE, et al. Long-term results of combined heart-lung transplantation: The Stanford experience. *J Heart Lung Transplant* 1994; 13:940.
196. Baron O, Hubaut JJ, Galetta D, et al. Pregnancy and heart-lung transplantation. *J Heart Lung Transplant* 2002;21:914.

197. Anyanwu AC, Banner NR, Radley-Smith R, et al. Long-term results of cardiac transplantation from live donors: The domino heart transplant. *J Heart Lung Transplant* 2002;21:971.
198. Oaks TE, Aravot D, Dennis C, et al. Domino heart transplantation: The Papworth experience. *J Heart Lung Transplant* 1994;13:433.
199. Ciccone AM, Stewart KC, Meyers BF, et al. Does donor cause of death affect the outcome of lung transplantation? *J Thorac Cardiovasc Surg* 2002;123:429.
200. Fiser SM, Kron IL, Long SM, et al. Influence of graft ischemia time on outcomes following lung transplantation. *J Heart Lung Transplant* 2001;20:1291.
201. Ueno T, Snell GI, Williams TJ, et al. Impact of graft ischemic time on outcomes after bilateral sequential single-lung transplantation. *Ann Thorac Surg* 1999;67:1577.
202. Quantz MA, Bennett LE, Meyer DM, et al. Does human leukocyte antigen matching influence the outcome of lung transplantation? An analysis of 3,549 lung transplantations. *J Heart Lung Transplant* 2000;19:473.
203. Yu NC, Haug MT, Khan SU, et al. Does the donor-recipient ABO blood group compatibility status predict subsequent lung transplantation outcomes? *J Heart Lung Transplant* 1999;18:764.
204. Valentine VG, Robbins RC, Berry GJ, et al. Actuarial survival of heart-lung and bilateral sequential lung transplant recipients with obliterative bronchiolitis. *J Heart Lung Transplant* 1996;15:371.
205. Novick RJ, Stitt LW, Al-Kattan K, et al. Pulmonary retransplantation: Predictors of graft function and survival in 230 patients. *Ann Thorac Surg* 1998;65:227.
206. Novick RJ, Stitt L, Schafers H-J, et al. Pulmonary retransplantation: Does the indication for operation influence postoperative lung function? *J Thorac Cardiovasc Surg* 1986;112:1504.
207. Novick RJ, Schafers H-J, Stitt L, et al. Seventy-two pulmonary retransplantations for obliterative bronchiolitis: Predictors of survival. *Ann Thorac Surg* 1995;60:111.
208. Wekerle T, Klepetko W, Wisser W, et al. Lung retransplantation: Institutional report on a series of twenty patients. *J Heart Lung Transplant* 1996;15:182.
209. Adams DH, Cochrane AD, Khaghani A, et al. Retransplantation in heart-lung recipients with obliterative bronchiolitis. *J Thorac Cardiovasc Surg* 1994;107:450.
210. Novick RJ. Heart and lung retransplantation: Should it be done? *J Heart Lung Transplant* 1998;17:635.

CHAPTER

46 MECHANICAL SUPPORT OF THE HEART

Pramod Bonde, John V. Conte

INTRODUCTION

The history of mechanical circulatory assistance parallels that of cardiac surgery and begins with the introduction of the Gibbon bubble oxygenator.[1] That revolutionary device opened up the field of cardiac surgery and was one of the major medical advances of the last century. Soon after the widespread use of cardiopulmonary bypass (CPB) became commonplace, failure to wean from CPB became recognized as a problem whose solution required temporary cardiac support to enable postcardiotomy cardiac recovery. Spencer and coworkers utilized postoperative femoral CPB in three patients, one of whom survived and ushered in the modern era of temporary mechanical circulatory support.[2] This was soon followed by the use of the first extracorporeal mechanical assist device by DeBakey et al. in 1964[3] and the subsequent development of the intraaortic balloon counterpulsation device, variations of which are still in use today. Kantrovitz,[4] Cooley,[5] Oyer,[6] Devries,[7] and others were responsible for other notable firsts including the first successful bridge to transplant and first successful total artificial heart (TAF) implant. Notable clinical landmarks in the history of mechanical circulatory support are shown in Table 46-1. In this chapter, we review the major indications for mechanical circulatory support as well as the various options available.

CLASSIFICATION OF DEVICE THERAPY

Mechanical circulatory support can be viewed from a variety of different perspectives. One of the most useful is to look at the devices from the perspective of the intention of the treating team. Devices can be broken down into short- and long-term devices. Short-term devices can be considered devices intended to support the circulation for hours to weeks. Indications for short-term support can include "bridge to recovery," where there is hope for cardiac recovery, weaning, and removal of the device (Table 46-2). Such bridge-to-recovery indications include postcardiotomy support following cardiac surgery, acute viral cardiomyopathic syndromes, percutaneous coronary intervention, and myocardial infarction. Another short-term scenario can be labeled a "bridge to a bridge." This would apply to those patients in extremis whose neurologic status is unknown, whose candidacy for cardiac transplant or longer-term support is unknown, or who do not recover their cardiac function and need longer-term support. In these situations, short-term devices, whose cost is generally lower and implantation easier than that of longer-term devices, are often used.

Longer-term support devices are intended for treatment periods of weeks to months or longer. Indications include "bridge to transplant" use, which is the most common application for the long-term left ventricular assist devices (LVADs) (Table 46-2). Less common indications include "bridge to recovery" with or without experimental treatments such as clenbuterol or, more recently, alternative to transplant indications.[8] "Destination therapy" (DT) is the phrase coined to describe the use of left ventricular assist devices as a final therapy to support patients until their death. The landmark Randomized Evaluation of Mechanical Assistance for the Treatment of Congestive Heart Failure (REMATCH) trial[9] was the first to compare survival with mechanical circulatory support to that of optimal medical management. It demonstrated improved survival in patients supported with LVADs compared to medical management and validated the use of these devices for long-term support in patients who were not candidates for transplantation (Fig. 46-1).

Table 46-1 Clinical milestones in the development of mechanical circulatory assistance

Year	Investigator	Type of Device	Comments
1953[1]	Gibbon	Heart-lung machine	Closure of ASD in human
1959[2]	Spencer	Femoral bypass	First case of successful recovery postcardiotomy
1963[3]	DeBakey	Pneumatic paracorporeal VAD	Postcardiotomy failure; 4 days survival
1968[4]	Kantrovitz	IABP	Clinical application of IABP
1969[5]	Cooley	Liotta TAH	Successful bridge to transplant but patient died posttransplant
1984[6]	Oyer	Novacor	Successful bridge to transplant, patient survived
1980[7]	DeVries	Jarvik TAH	First human implant

IABP = intraaortic balloon pump; TAH = total artificial heart; VAD = ventricular assist device.

SPECIFIC DEVICES

Devices can be classified according to their mode of action. The pulsatile versus nonpulsatile distinction is commonly used. The former are usually pneumatically or pusher plate–activated devices, while the latter are centrifugal or axial flow pumps (Table 46-3). Some FDA-approved devices are listed in Table 46-4.

Nonpulsatile devices

Centrifugal/rotodynamic/radial flow pumps

These are the cheapest and most easily available assist devices available for short-term support lasting hours to days. They are mostly employed after postcardiotomy failure, but some newer experimental devices are being developed for long-term use. Blood flow is generated by rotating blades or impellers.[10] These devices do not have valves or multiple moving or occluding parts (Fig. 46-2), theoretically reducing the potential for hemolysis. Priming volumes (52 to 87 mL) differ from pump to pump. Devices of this class are capable of providing high flow rates with low rises in pressure. Several commercial devices are available, including the Carmeda Bio-Pump and the BIO-PUMP (Medtronic Inc, Minneapolis, MN), the Sarns pump (3M Healthcare Inc., Ann Arbor, MI), the St. Jude pump (Bard Cardiopulmonary Division, Haverhill, MA), and the Nikkiso pump (Nikkiso Pumps America Inc., Plumsteadville, PA). These devices are not designed for long-term use. Indications include left heart bypass for thoracic aortic surgery, postcardiotomy ventricular failure, extracorporeal membrane oxygenation (ECMO), and bridge to transplantation or to another VAD. Cannulation sites commonly used for left heart

Table 46-2 Classification of ventricular assist devices by use

Short term (days to weeks)
Bridge to recovery
Bridge to a bridge
Bridge to transplant
Long term (weeks or longer)
Bridge to recovery
Bridge to transplant
Destination therapy

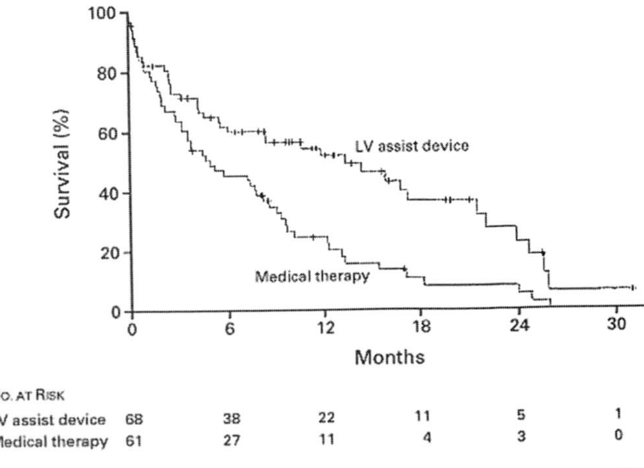

Figure 46-1 Survival benefit in patients receiving mechanical circulatory support. (From REMATCH trial.)

Table 46-3 Types of assist devices classified by mechanisms

Extracorporeal support
Centrifugal pumps (radial flow/rotodynamic)
Sarns 3M
St. Jude
Nikkiso
Medtronic Biopump
Newer centrifugal pumps
HeartQuest System
VentrAssist
HeartMate III
Terumo Dura Heart
Kriton VAD
Paracorporeal support
ABIOMED BVS 5000
Thoratec device
Berlin Heart Excor
Tandem Heart
Intracorporeal support
Aortic compression/counterpulsation
IABP
Kantrovitz CardioVad Systems
Ventricular assist devices
HeartMate LVAD
Novacor LVAD
Next Generation LVAS (Heart Saver VAD)
Arrow Lion heart LVAD (Penn State LVAS)
Model-7 Abdominal Left Ventricular Assist Device (ALVAD)
Total artificial heart (TAH)
Liotta TAH
Jarvik 7 TAH
Aktsu III TAH
AbioCor TAH
Cardiowest TAH (Jarvik 7, Symbion)
Penn State/3M TAH (ABIOMED Inc., acquired from BeneCor)
Axial flow pumps
Jarvik 2000
Heartmate II
MicroMed-DeBakey VAD
Pittsburgh Streamliner mixed flow pump
CorAid LVAS (Arrow Inc.)
Berlin Heart INCOR
Epicardial compression devices
Anastedt cup
CardioSupport Systems
Heart Booster (ABIOMED)
CorCap (Acorn)
Myosplint (Myocor)
Skeletal Muscle Systems
Extracorporeal membrane oxygenation (ECMO)

bypass include the left superior pulmonary vein or left atrium (inflow) and the ascending aorta or femoral artery (outflow). For right heart bypass, inflow is obtained via right atrial cannulation with outflow directed into the pulmonary artery. Cannula fixation is important with these and other devices, since most hemorrhagic complications are due to cannula dislodgement. Anticoagulation is required after device insertion and must be monitored closely.

There are no firm criteria for device weaning and removal, but the achievement of hemodynamic stability and a nominal cardiac output in conjunction with the original indication for instituting support dictate the removal strategy. When a device of this class fails, it is often due to breakdown of the pump head seal, leading to the entry of fluid into the magnetic chamber.[11] Clinical experience has shown that these pumps are especially well suited for left heart bypass and for short-term postcardiotomy left ventricular failure. In one study, 62 patients were supported using the centrifugal pump for postcardiotomy failure; 22 patients required left ventricular support, 9 required right ventricular support, and 31 required biventricular support. Support was extended for up to 19 days, with 42 patients weaned successfully, 27 patients discharged home, and 18 patients surviving more than 1 year.[12] Other studies have reported similar results for-short term support.[13,14]

Paracorporeal pulsatile devices

ABIOMED BVS 5000

This device was approved by the FDA in 1992 for use in all types of recoverable heart failure. It is an external pulsatile VAD capable of supporting the right and/or left ventricles for days to weeks. This device is a pneumatically driven, asynchronous, pulsatile, automated, self-regulating, polycarbonate-housed dual-chamber pump system (Fig. 46-3). The atrial chamber of this two-chamber pump fills passively by gravity drainage; the volume is usually about 100 mL, and the internal chamber is made of flexible polyurethane. The atrial chamber drains into the ventricular chamber through a trileaflet valve made of proprietary material. During systole, compressed air is delivered into the ventricular chamber; it compresses the polyurethane bladder and ejects its contents toward the patient. The pumping unit and console are located outside the body; the inflow and outflow cannulas are tunneled subcutaneously into the mediastinum. Each pump is capable of delivering a maximal output of 6 L/min at a constant stroke volume of 80 mL.

The implantation technique for the BVS 5000 varies from center to center. For right ventricular support, the inflow cannula is placed into the mid-right atrium and secured firmly with pledgeted purse-string sutures. Another alternative is to insert this cannula directly into the right ventricle through its diaphragmatic surface, particularly if there are adhesions from previous surgery. The outflow cannula is anastomosed to the main pulmonary artery. For left ventricular support, the inflow cannula is placed into the left atrium via the right superior pulmonary vein or dome or directly into the left

Table 46-4 Mechanical assist devices used in the United States

Device	FDA-Approved	Ventricle Supported	Duration of Support	Home Discharge
ABIOMED BVS 500	1992	L, R, B	S	No
Thoratec	1996	L, R, B	S, LG	Yes
HeartMate IP	1994	L	LG	No
HeartMate VE	1996	L	LG	Yes
Novacor	1993	L	LG	Yes
	Year Trial Began			
Jarvik	2002	L	LG	Yes
Micromed	2002	L	LG	Yes
HeartMate II	2003	L	LG	Yes
LionHeart	2001	L	LG	Yes
AbioCor	2002	L	LG	Yes
Thoratec	2002	L	LG	Yes

L = left ventricular support; R = right ventricular support; B = biventricular support; S = short-term support; LG = long-term support.

ventricle via the apex. Left ventricular apical cannulation permits complete ventricular decompression, optimizing its chance for recovery. Left ventricular apical cannulation is also advantageous if a mechanical mitral prosthesis is in place, since it permits opening and closing of the leaflets and may reduce thrombotic complications. The outflow cannula is anastomosed to the ascending aorta.

Heparin anticoagulation is required during BVS 5000 support and must be closely monitored; an activated clotting time (ACT) of 180 to 200 s is the goal. The pump is easy to manage and operated based on the principles of preload and afterload management. Limitations of this device include limited patient mobility, restricted flow capacity, and heparinization requirements.

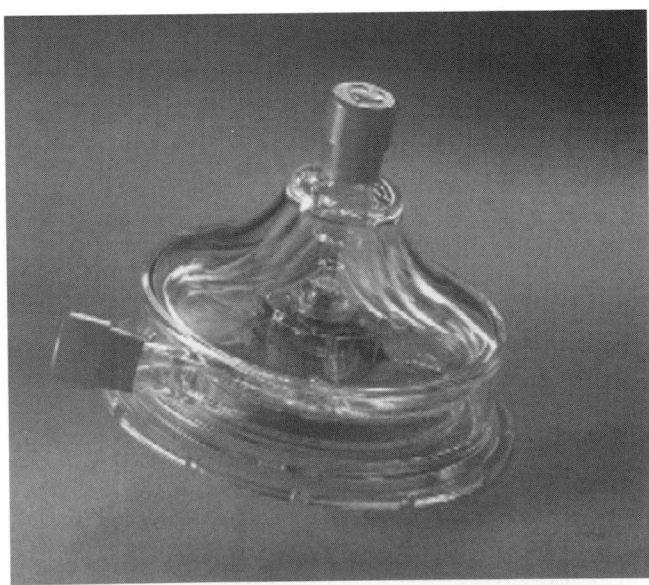

Figure 46-2 BioMedicus (Medtronic Inc.) Centrifugal pump. (With permission from Medtronic Inc.)

A prospective multicenter trial evaluated the safety and efficacy of the BVS 5000 in 31 patients with hemodynamic instability despite maximal pharmacologic and IABP support. There was an improvement in mean arterial pressure from 50.1 ± 15.3 mmHg prior to support to 77.1 ± 8.0 mmHg after support was initiated ($p < 0.01$). The cardiac index increased from 1.6 ± 0.6 L/min/m^2 before support to 2.3 ± 0.3 L/min/m^2 after support was initiated ($p < 0.01$) a total of 76 percent of the cohort (42 patients) experienced bleeding; 17 (55 percent) were successfully weaned from support, and 9 (29 percent) were discharged.[15]

In a retrospective review, the BVS 5000 was implanted in 47 patients exhibiting postcardiotomy acute heart failure. There were 38 patients in the bridge-to-recovery group and 9 in the bridge-to-transplantation group. A total of 25 patients (66 percent) in the bridge-to-recovery group were weaned, and 16 patients (42 percent) went on to discharge. In the bridge-to-transplantation group, 1 patient recovered myocardial function and 1 died while awaiting transplantation, while 7 patients (77 percent) underwent successful cardiac transplantation with a posttransplant survival rate of 66 percent. Patients were supported in the isolated left ventricular (28 percent), biventricular (45 percent), and right ventricular modes (28 percent).[16] In a more recent study involving 202 patients, survival at 3 days, 30 days, and 5 years was 76, 38, and 24 percent, respectively. Patients surviving 30 days experienced a 63 percent 5-year survival. A total of 48 patients (21 percent) were bridged to transplantation, and 71 patients (35.5 percent) were weaned with intent for survival.[17] Similar results are reported from other centers.[18] The wean and

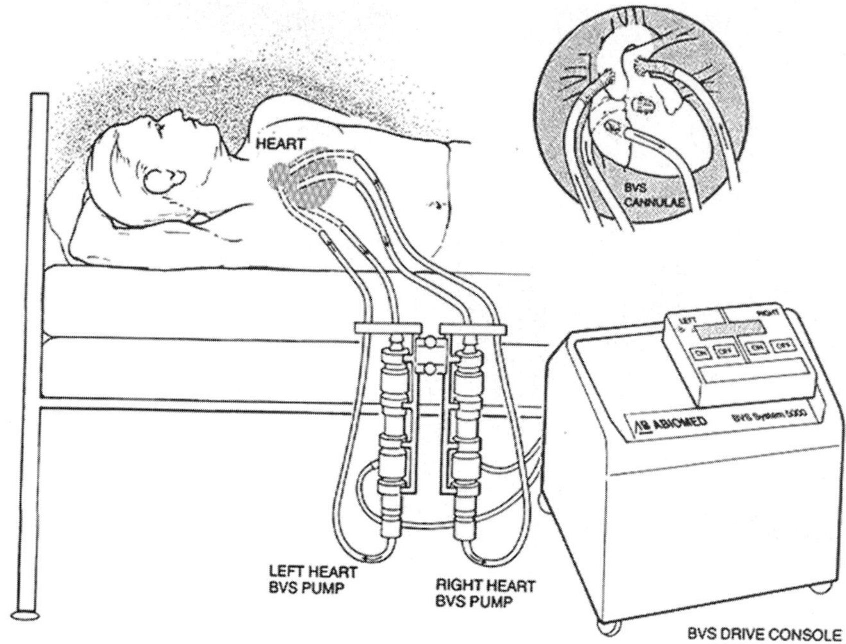

Figure 46-3 ABIOMED BVS 5000. (With permission from ABIOMED Inc.)

discharge rates is generally around 60 and 40 percent, respectively, and this approach has been shown to be cost-effective as well.[19]

Thoratec VAD

Approved by the FDA in 1996 for use as a bridge to cardiac transplantation and subsequently as a bridge to recovery, the Thoratec VAD is the only approved dual-use device on the market. It was first used clinically in 1982 for postcardiotomy failure. This device is flexible and can be employed for short- or long-term use in both large and small patients because of its paracorporeal design. It is a pneumatically driven paracorporeal pump. It uses Delirin tilting monostrut mechanical disk valves for maintaining unidirectional blood flow (Fig. 46-4). There is a flexible blood sac housed in a rigid outer casing; this sac is compressed by air to achieve ejection. Separate pumps are needed for each side of the heart. Three modes of operation are available: fill-to-empty, fixed-rate, and electrocardiogram (ECG)-synchronous modes. The most commonly used mode is the fill-to-empty mode, which pumps at a rate determined by VAD filling. The inflow and outflow cannulas being the only internal components, this pump can be used for small patients, including children. It is approved for bridge-to-transplantation and bridge-to-recovery applications and is the most flexible device available. The cannulas are made of polyurethane except for the distal part, which is made of polyester Dacron. Usually CPB is needed for implantation of the cannulas. For left ventricular support, inflow can be achieved via the left ventricular apex or the left atrium; outflow is usually to the ascending aorta. For right heart support, inflow is via the right atrium and outflow is directed into the main pulmonary artery. Proper positioning of the cannulas is essential for reducing undue kinking of the cannulas and optimal device positioning on the abdominal wall. Anticoagulation with heparin followed by warfarin is required. The main limitations of this device include

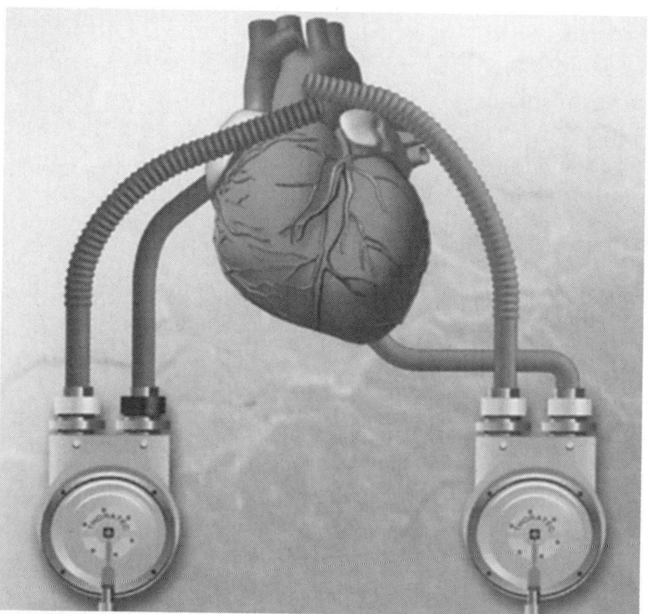

Figure 46-4 Thoratec Paracorporeal VAD. (With permission from Thoratec Corporation.)

Table 46-5 Clinical results of Thoratec VAD

Number of patients	2517
Mean age (range)	46 (6–77)
Gender	
Males (%)	1812 (72)
Females (%)	705 (28)
VAD implant (*n* = 1711)	
LVAD	605
RVAD	111
Bi-VAD	988
Unknown	7
Etiology (*n* = 1589)	
Ischemic cardiomyopathy (%)	566 (36)
Idiopathic cardiomyopathy (%)	521 (33)
Myocardial infarction (%)	113 (7)
Posttransplant failure or rejection (%)	40 (3)
Other diagnosis (%)	349 (22)
Mean bridge to transplant (days) (*n* = 1446)	50
Total implant duration (years)	254

From Thoratec registry, with permission from Thoratec Corporation.

rather bulky paracorporeal pumping chambers and restricted patient mobility due to a large drive console.

To date, more than 2500 patients have undergone Thoratec device implantation for left, right, and biventricular support (Table 46-5). This device has been particularly useful for short-term bridging to transplant in patients suffering from biventricular failure.[20] In an analysis of 828 bridge-to-transplant patients,[20] this system was used for biventricular support in 472 cases, left ventricular support in 326 cases, and right ventricular support in 30 cases for up to 515 days. During the support periods, cardiac indices increased significantly from 1.4 ± 0.8 to 3.0 ± 0.5 L/min/m^2 (with biventricular assistance and left ventricular cannulation). Of the 828 patients, 60 percent underwent transplantation, and the posttransplant survival rate was 86 percent. In the 195 patients who needed postcardiotomy support, the device was used for up to 80 days for cardiac recovery. Thirty-eight percent of the patients were weaned from the device, with 59 percent of these patients discharged. Of 49 postcardiotomy patients considered for transplantation, 32 underwent transplantation and 23 were discharged. Other series reflect similar results.[21,22]

Intracorporeal pulsatile devices

HeartMate LVAD

The Heartmate LVAD (Thoratec Corp., Pleasanton, CA) was designed in 1975 as an implantable, pulsatile, pneumatically actuated (HeartMate IP), intracorporeal left ventricular assist system.[23] The pneumatically driven unit is made of sintered titanium and houses a flexible, textured polyurethane diaphragm. It is driven by a pusher-plate mechanism that, in turn, is driven by compressed air and controlled by a console (Fig. 46-5). The design was modified to a vented electrical system (HeartMate VE) in 1991,[24] with a much smaller console, which confers greater patient mobility. The inflow and outflow conduits utilize porcine xenograft valves (Medtronic-Hancock, Minneapolis, MN). The maximum stroke volume generated is about 85 mL and maximum output can reach up to 11 L/min. The blood-contacting surfaces, unlike those of other devices, are made up of textured polyurethane, which facilitates deposition of a fibrin-collagen matrix, forming a pseudointimal layer. This feature reduces the anticoagulation requirement, calling for aspirin only. To accommodate the device, the patient's body surface area (BSA) must to be at least 1.5 m^2. The pump is inserted either pre- or intraperitoneally in the left upper quadrant of the abdomen. There are two modes of operation: fixed mode (20 to 140 bpm for IP and 50 to 120 bpm for VE) and automatic mode. In the latter mode, the pump senses when its chamber is full and activates the pusher-plate mechanism (fill-to-empty). The battery life usually ranges from 4 to 6 h, with a portable hand pump backup available for device malfunction or power failure. In 2002, the enhanced version of the HeartMate SNAP-VE, the HeartMate XVE LVAS, was approved by the FDA for destination therapy. The notable modification was the inflow valve conduit, which was designed to be six times more durable than in previous versions. To date, more than 1300 patients have undergone HeartMate IP LVAS implantation, while close to 2500 patients have received the HeartMate VE LVAS, with cumulative patient-years of 330 and 964 years, respectively (Table 46-6).

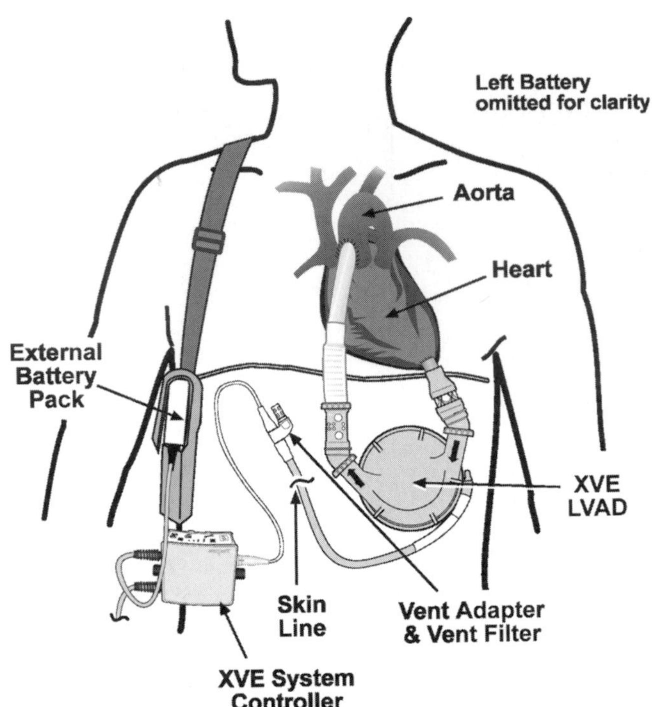

Figure 46-5 Schematic representation of HeartMate XVE LVAS in situ. (With permission from Thoratec Corporation.)

Table 46-6 **Clinical results of HeartMate LVAS**

	IP LVAS	VE LVAS
Number of patients	1322	2476
Mean age (range)	49 (8–74)	51 (11–80)
Gender		
Males (%)	1103 (84)	2076 (85)
Females (%)	216 (16)	368 (15)
Ischemic cardiomyopathy (%)	527 (41)	992 (46)
Idiopathic cardiomyopathy (%)	664 (52)	1036 (48)
Myocardial infarction (%)	48 (4)	44 (2)
Other diagnosis (%)	41 (3)	81 (4)
Mean implant duration (days)	95	147
Maximum support for patients with outcomes (days)	805	1071
Patient-years of experience	331	964

From Thoratec registry, with permission from Thoratec Corporation.

Experience from Columbia University of 243 patients undergoing implantation of HeartMate devices included 52 pneumatic, 17 dual-lead vented electrical, and 174 single-lead vented electrical devices. Overall actuarial survival rates at 1, 3, 5, and 10 years posttransplant were 90.5, 85.1, 69.6, and 39.6 percent, respectively. The overall incidence of infection was 17.7 percent ($n = 43$). Device malfunctions occurred in 32 patients.[25,26] A pivotal prospective multicenter clinical trial was conducted at 24 centers in the United States. There were 280 transplant candidates (232 men, 48 women; median age 55 years) unresponsive to inotropic drugs, intraaortic balloon counterpulsation, or both who received the device. These patients were compared with a control group of 48 patients who were not supported with a device. HeartMate VE support lasted an average of 112 days, with 54 patients supported for more than 180 days. Device-related adverse events included bleeding in 31 (11 percent), infection in 113 (40 percent), neurologic dysfunction in 14 (5 percent), and thromboembolic events in 17 (6 percent) of patients. Successful bridge to transplant was observed in 35.3 percent of HeartMate patients, compared with 67 percent of the control group ($p < 0.001$). A total of 198 patients survived, with 188 patients undergoing cardiac transplantation. One-year posttransplant survival was significantly better in device-supported patients compared with the control population [84 percent (158 of 188) vs. 63 percent (10 of 16); log rank analysis $p = 0.0197$)]. These results are similar to those of the REMATCH trial.[9,27]

Novacor LVAS

The Novacor LVAS (World Heart Corp., Ottawa, Canada) was developed in collaboration with Stanford University and was originally planned as a totally implantable system. It was the first device to bridge a patient successfully to transplant in 1984. Over the years it has evolved into a console-based VAD. The pump drive unit incorporates a dual pusher-plate sac-type pump with a smooth blood-contacting surface. The stroke volume is about 70 mL. It has two porcine-valved polyester inflow and outflow conduits. The system has a high-efficiency linear motor using a pulsed solenoid energy converter with a two-armature assembly. Thus it requires no gears, cams, or intermediate hydraulic conversion, reducing the potential for mechanical failure. There are three modes of operation: single-stroke, fixed-rate, and automatic or synchronus (fill-to-empty) modes. The pump fills passively, aided by the large circular dual-pusher-plate surface area (Fig. 46-6). The power packs usually have 6 h of work life and can be worn on a belt, vest, shoulder bag, or backpack. Anticoagulation with warfarin is necessary and must be closely monitored. The primary cause of mechanical failure is wearing out of the energy converter, although this usually can be detected at least 3 months prior to its ultimate failure.[28]

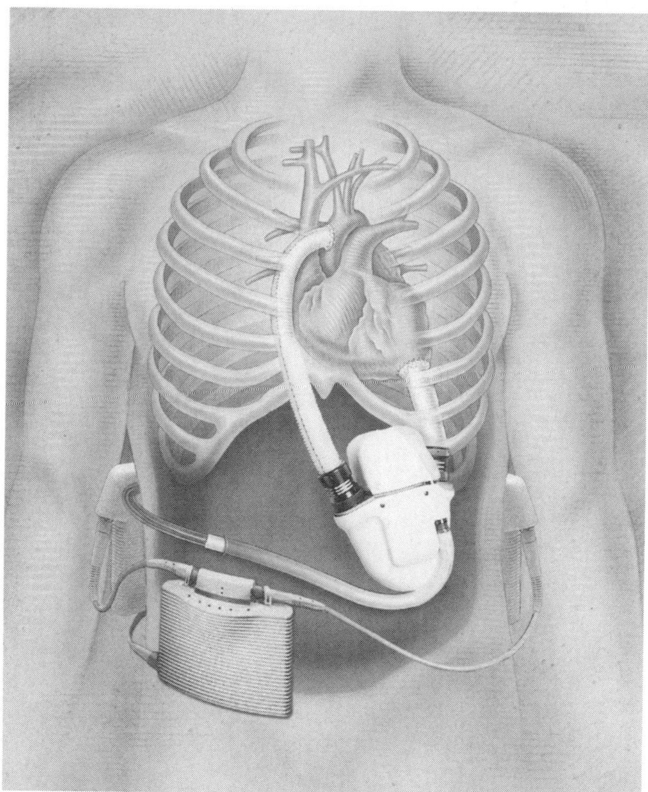

Figure 46-6 Novacor VAD. (With permission from WorldHeart Corporation, Ottawa, Canada.)

The Novacor LVAS has been successfully used for the past two decades as a bridge to cardiac transplantation in patients with end-stage congestive heart failure. Stanford University reported a series of 53 Novacor patients (48 male, 5 female) with a mean age of 44 years (range of 16 to 62 years) and a mean support time of 56 days (range of 1 to 374). Complications consisted of bleeding (43 percent), infection (30 percent), and embolic cerebrovascular events (24.5 percent). Sixty-six percent of the supported patients were successfully bridged to cardiac transplantation.[29] A recent study suggested that, in terms of durability, the Novacor device exceeded the HeartMate VE at 2 months (93.5 percent). Novacor's durability at 3 years was 85.9 percent, with 78 percent of supported patients surviving to transplantation.[30] Another study has reported improvement in cardiac output, wedge pressure, pulmonary vascular resistance, and mean pulmonary pressure after Novacor implantation. Most of the complications observed were related to thromboembolism and occurred in the first 3 months after implantation.[31]

LionHeart LVAS

Developed at Penn State University, the LionHeart LVAS (Arrow International, Reading, PA) was specifically designed for destination therapy in patients with end-stage chronic heart failure.[32] The system is fully implantable without any external conduits for power. It utilizes a brushless motor that actuates a pusher plate using a roller-and-screw mechanism and Delirin disk monostrut valves. The blood-contact surfaces consist of polyurethane sacs, which fill passively. The stroke volume is approximately 65 mL and the maximum achievable flow rate is 8 L/min. The LionHeart requires a gas-filled compliance chamber implanted in the left pleural space to accommodate pump volume displacement (Fig. 46-7). In addition, there is a subcutaneous infusion port that must replaced every 2 to 4 weeks. The battery and system controller are all implanted in the right lower quadrant of the abdomen. The LionHeart's pumping characteristics, based on end-diastolic volumes, are automatically adjusted by a software algorithm, which attempts to provide maximal filling of the pump with each stroke by altering pump speed. The unique feature of this LVAS system is the transcutaneous energy transmission system (TETS), in which electrical energy is supplied to the pump's drive unit by radiofrequency induction. Warfarin anticoagulation is required with this device.

The first clinical implantation of the LionHeart was performed in 1999[33]; the first implantation in the United States was performed in 2001. The Clinical Utility Baseline Study (CUBS) was designed to determine the safety and performance of the LionHeart LVAS to serve as a permanent mode of circulatory support for patients with end-stage heart failure who were ineligible for heart transplantation. As a part of this trial, 26 male patients underwent implantation at seven European Centers; actuarial survival rates were 86 percent at 1 month, 45 percent at 6 months, 41 percent at 1 year, and 34 percent at 2 years.

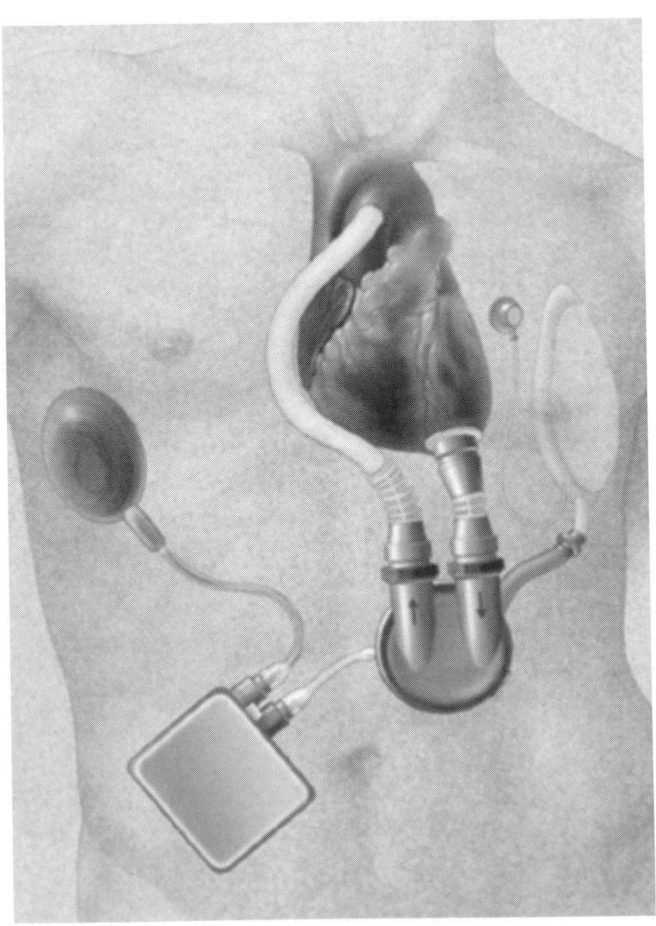

Figure 46-7 Arrow LionHeart. (With permission from Arrow International.)

Total artificial heart

AbioCor total artificial heart

The AbioCor TAF (ABIOMED Inc., Denver, MA) is inserted orthotopically after excising the native ventricles. The energy converter is situated between the two ventricles and consists of a high-efficiency miniature centrifugal pump.[34] A two-position switching valve is used to alternate the direction of the hydraulic flow between the right and left pumping chambers, thus alternating systole between the two chambers. The stroke volume of each chamber is 70 mL (Fig. 46-8). Pumping rates can be adjusted between 75 to 150 bpm with a resultant flow rates of 4 to 8 L/min. All blood-contacting surfaces of the AbioCor TAH, including the trileaflet valves, are made of polyether urethane, resulting in a smooth, continuous blood-contacting surface. An atrial balance chamber permits adjustment of stroke volumes and maintains balance between right and left chambers. This unique feature obviates the need for a compliance chamber. The energy transfer is achieved by a transcutaneous energy transmission and telemetry system (TETTS). The controller and the battery modules (Ni-Cad) are implanted preperitoneally. Externally worn components include the TETTS primary and Ni-Ion battery modules. Anticoagulation with warfarin is required.

Initial clinical trials of the AbioCor TAH are underway. Inclusion criteria include patient age of 18 years or more, ineligibility for cardiac transplantation, a high likelihood of dying within 30 days while on optimized medical management, an acceptable device-fitting evaluation,

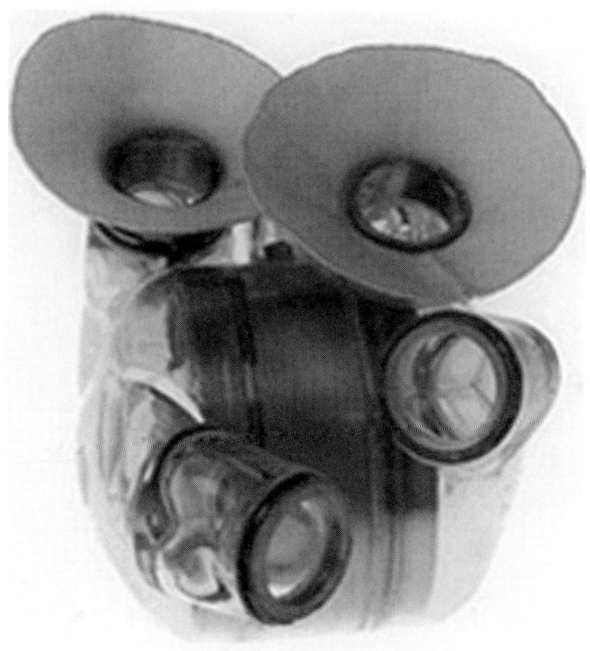

Figure 46-8 Abiocor TAH. (With permission from ABIOMED Inc.)

and biventricular failure with inability to be weaned from temporary mechanical circulatory support. Exclusion criteria include heart failure with significant potential for reversibility, patients on chronic dialysis, irreversible liver failure, blood dyscrasias, suspected or active systemic infection, a positive serum pregnancy test result, severe peripheral vascular disease, transient ischemic attack or stroke secondary to atherosclerosis, psychiatric illness (including drug or alcohol abuse), and lack of an adequate social support system. All patients who are candidates have a 30-day predicted mortality of more than 70 percent based on the AbioScore prognostic model or acute myocardial infarction shock scores. The AbioScore mortality prediction model was developed based on previous prognostic models, including measurements that had the highest prognostic value for mortality in patients with end-stage heart failure. These factors include age, serum sodium, renal function, need for inotropic or intraaortic balloon pump support, body-mass index, left ventricular end-diastolic diameter, peak exercise oxygen consumption, and New York Heart Association (NYHA) functional class. Eligible candidates are screened for device fitting using a proprietary software program (AbioFit, ABIOMED).[35] The primary end point of these first trials is the AbioCor's impact on all-cause mortality in patients with severe heart failure and a predicted life expectancy of less than 30 days despite optimized medical management. Secondary end points include a determination of adverse events, device malfunction, complications related to the device, and quality of life. Thus far 14 implants have been performed in the United States,[34] with most of the patients completing 60 days successfully.[35] The preliminary results revealed two intraoperative deaths (due to intraoperative bleeding or aprotinin reaction) and four late deaths (one from multisystem organ failure and three related to cerebrovascular accidents). Six patients recovered to the point of being able to take multiple trips outside of the hospital, with two patients reaching hospital discharge.[35]

CardioWest TAH

This TAF (CardioWest Technologies Inc., Tucson, AZ) was developed at the University of Utah by Robert Jarvik. Its precursor, the Jarvik 7, was implanted by DeVries in 1980.[7] This is a pneumatically driven biventricular pulsatile device, which is implanted orthotopically.[36] It consists of two ventricular chambers connected to the native atria and incorporates a 27-mm Medtronic-Hall mechanical tilting-disk valve (inflow). The blood-contacting surface consists of an air-compressed polyurethane sac (Fig. 46-9). The pneumatic hose and drive line exit transcutaneously to a console that controls the pump and delivers the compressed air. The pump delivers a stroke volume of 70 mL and is capable of achieving a maximum flow rate of 8 L/min. Warfarin anticoagulation is required. A strict size criterion is observed in selecting patients for this device (Table 46-7). Limitations

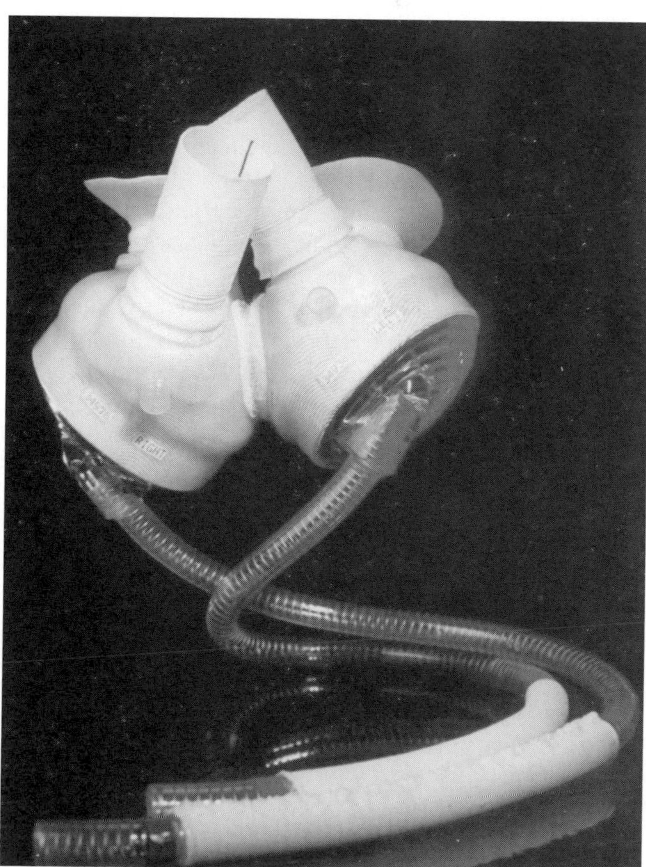

Figure 46-9 Cardiowest TAH. (With permission from SynCardia Inc.)

Table 46-7 CardioWest total artificial heart: criteria for implantation

Body surface area ≥ 1.7 m^2
Cardiothoracic ratio > 0.5
Left ventricular diastolic dimension > 66 mm
Anteroposterior distance (sternum to T10, by computed tomography) > 10 cm
Combined ventricular volume (measured by computed tomography) > 1500 mL

of this device include the large, cumbersome console and frequent maintenance of the pneumatic inlets and outlets.

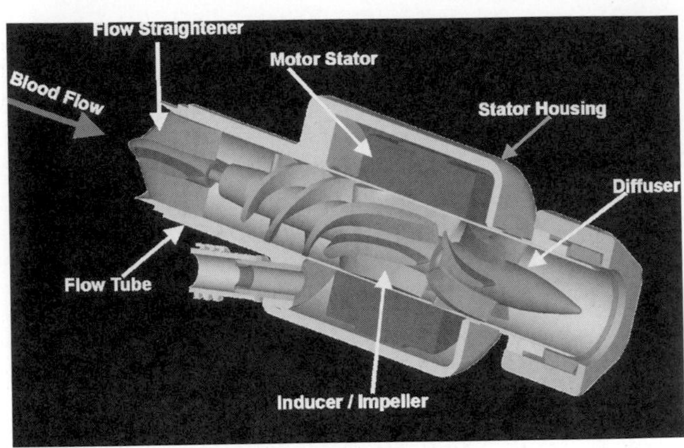

Figure 46-10 DeBakey MicroMed pump. (With permission from MicroMed Inc.)

Rotary axial pumps

Existing pulsatile LVADs are hampered by percutaneous drive lines and bulky consoles and support systems. Additionally, these assist devices are generally not suitable for patients with body surface areas of less than 1.5 m^2 or in pediatric patients with the exception of the paracorporeal Thoratec VAD. Other characteristics of these devices include bleeding complications and difficulty in explantation. These limitations prompted the development of axial flow pumps. Technically, nonpulsatile flow pumps are more attractive than pulsatile systems because they have one moving part, permitting compactness in design, ease of insertion, and lower energy consumption. These devices are inserted into the ventricular apex (inflow) and anastomosed to the thoracic ascending or descending aorta (outflow). They do not require valves and compliance chambers, affording additional simplicity. Despite these advantages, several potential drawbacks exist. Device failure can result in significant backflow of 1.5 to 2.0 L/min from the aorta into the left ventricle. Also, blood-washed bearings have not been studied adequately with respect to thrombogenic complications. Furthermore, earlier concerns about the nonphysiologic nature of nonpulsatile blood flow persists, although initial results from rotary axial flow pumps have been encouraging. Several systems in preclinical and clinical stages of development are showing promise.

DeBakey VAD

The DeBakey VAD (MicroMed Technology Inc., Houston, TX) resulted from a collaboration between the Baylor College of Medicine and NASA[39]; it is undergoing clinical trials in U.S. and European centers.[40] A small (30 mm diameter, 76 mm length, 95 g weight) titanium axial flow pump, the DeBakey VAD is based on an axial impeller-inducer supported by an inflow straightener and outflow diffuser housing ceramic blood-lubricated bearings. The pump produces a flow of 5 to 6 L/min and generates a pressure of 100 Torr at 10,000 rpm (Fig. 46-10). An ultrasonic flow probe continuously measures the pump output. The inflow cannula is placed in the left ventricular apex and the outflow cannula can be anastomosed to the ascending or descending aorta. The pump is placed in a small preperitoneal pocket. A percutaneous drive line connects the power supply and control to the pump from an external console. Pump flow is nonpulsatile and requires warfarin anticoagulation. Laboratory indices reveal no significant hemolysis or changes in plasma free hemoglobin.

Worldwide experience with the DeBakey VAD includes 150 patients who underwent placement of the device as a bridge to transplantation. In this series, 82 patients (55 percent) were bridged to transplantation/recovery or are currently supported and 68 patients (45 percent) died with the device.[41] Reoperation for bleeding was the most common adverse event in 48 patients (32 percent), followed by hemolysis (12 percent) and device infection (3.3 percent). Device failure occurred in 4 cases. Seventeen pumps (11 percent) were noted to have detectable thrombus; of these, 11 cases (64 percent) were successfully resolved with transplantation, pump exchange, or thrombolysis. Thromboembolic events occurred in 10.7 percent of patients. The FDA has recently approved a destination therapy trial (DELTA: Destination Evaluation Long-Term Assist) using the DeBakey VAD and Thoratec HeartMate XVE.

Flowmaker (Jarvik 2000)

The Flowmaker (Jarvik Heart Inc., New York, NY) is a titanium pump (25 mm diameter, 51 mm length, 90 g weight) that is implanted in the left ventricular cavity via the apex; an outflow graft is anstomosed to the descending thoracic aorta (Fig. 46-11).[42] The pump can be implanted through a left thoracotomy. The pump mechanism is similar to that of the DeBakey VAD.[43]

Three different options are available for energy transmission: a percutaneous lead, a skull-mounted titanium pedestal, and TETTS.[42] The Flowmaker is capable of producing flows of 7 L/min at 8000 to 12,000 rpm and requires warfarin anticoagulation. Pump flow rates can be adjusted manually in times of increased activity or can

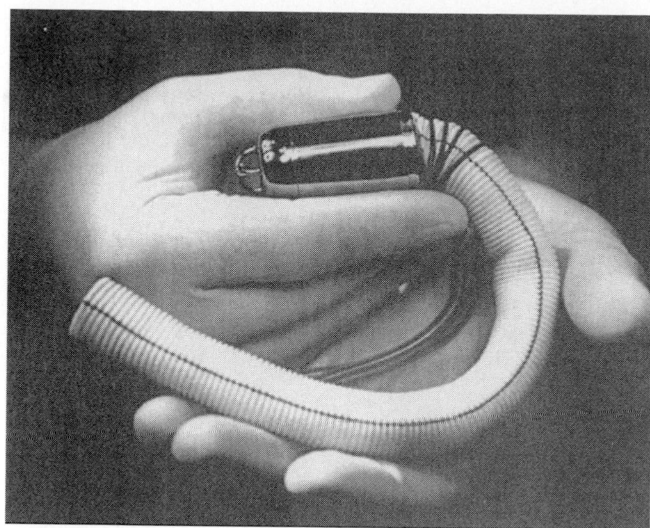

Figure 46-11 The Flowmaker. (Jarvik 2000, with permission from Jarvik Inc.)

be set at a fixed rate. In 35 patients who received the device, the average and cumulative support periods were 67 days and 2348 days, respectively. Eighteen patients underwent successful transplantation and 12 died during the support period.[44]

HeartMate II

The HeartMate II (Thoratec Corp., Pleasanton, CA) was born out of research conducted at the University of Pittsburgh in collaboration with Nimbus. It has a 40-mm diameter, 70-mm length, 176-g weight.[45] The pump mechanism is similar to that of the DeBakey VAD and Jarvik 2000. It is capable of achieving flow rates of 10 L/min and can generate 120 Torr of aortic pressure, operating at 6000 to 13,000 rpm (Fig. 46-12). The pump receives its inflow via the left ventricular apex and delivers outflow to the ascending aorta; it is placed in a small preperitoneal pocket. The current system uses a percutaneous drive line to supply power and control from an external console. Currently, clinical trials are underway in Europe and the United States. The first human implant was performed in 2000.[46]

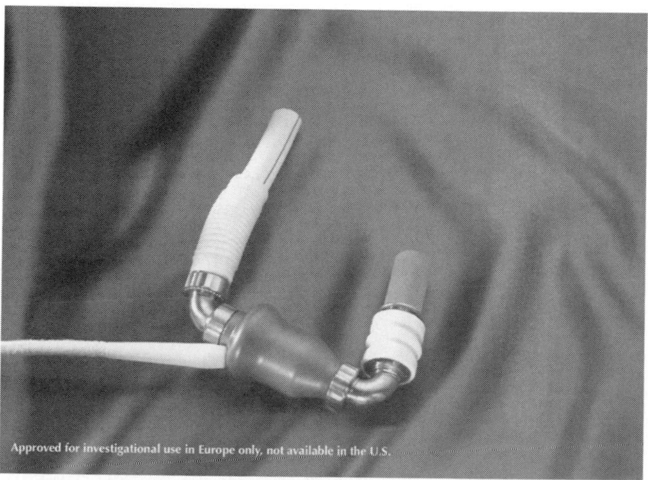

Approved for investigational use in Europe only, not available in the U.S.

Figure 46-12 HeartMate II. (With permission from Thoratec Corporation.)

PATIENT SELECTION

Currently, mechanical circulatory support can be considered for bridge-to-transplantation, bridge-to-bridge, bridge-to-recovery, and destination therapy. Consideration is based on the indication for support and the operative risk involved for the patient. Profound heart failure due to chronic congestive heart failure or acute postcardiotomy pump failure are the most common indications for the institution of mechanical circulatory support. Candidates for support typically display clinical indices of chronic heart failure, with PCWPs in excess of 20 mmHg, cardiac indices less than 2.0 L/min/m^2, and systolic blood pressures less than 80 mmHg despite inotropic support.

For bridge-to-recovery indications, including postcardiotomy failure, short-term support with a centrifugal pump or a pulsatile paracorporeal device is appropriate, since these devices are relatively easy to implant and maintain. If necessary, these devices can be exchanged for longer-term pulsatile or axial flow devices. The option of implanting a TAF for destination therapy is still impeded by the limited experience with these devices, but as the experience grows, TAH and the smaller axial flow devices with portable consoles may be suitable devices for these patients.

The REMATCH trial was designed to compare the results of mechanical assistance versus optimal medical management for patients suffering from end-stage heart failure.[9,47] The efficacy, safety, and cost-effectiveness of "wearable" LVADs versus optimal medical therapy and the impact of LVAD support on all-cause mortality were evaluated. Secondary objectives included analysis of cardiovascular-related mortality, worsening of heart failure, functional status, health-related quality of life, and quality-adjusted survival. The inclusion criteria are listed in Table 46-8.

The lessons from REMATCH indicate that there is a cohort of patients who benefit from LVAD support over medical therapies. These include inotrope-intolerant patients (e.g., ventricular arrythmias), patients requiring complex and/or multistage operations, patients with life threatening coronary lesions not amenable for coronary revascularization, and patients with severe end-stage heart failure. Patients who received an LVAD were more than twice as likely to experience a serious adverse event, including device infections (28 percent at 3 months), bleeding (42 percent at 6 months), device malfunction (35 percent at 24 months), and device failure (10 patients).[48]

Table 46-8 Inclusion criteria for the REMATCH trial

Initial Criteria:

1. Contraindication for heart transplantation
   - Age > 60 years
   - Insulin-dependent diabetes mellitus with end-organ damage
   - Chronic renal failure with serum creatinine > 2.5 mg/dL for 90 days
   - Major comorbidity (physical or psychiatric)
2. End-stage heart failure
3. NYHA class IV for at least 90 days despite ACE inhibitors, diuretics, and digoxin therapy
4. Left ventricular ejection fraction ≤ 25%
5. Peak oxygen consumption ≤ 12 mL/kg body weight/min
6. Inotropic dependence
   - Due to: Symptomatic hypotension
   - Decreasing renal function
   - Worsening pulmonary function

Revised criteria:

1. NYHA class IV status for 60 days
2. Peak oxygen consumption < 12 mL/kg/min

These risks must be balanced with the survival benefit provided by mechanical support. Hence, it is important to identify high-risk candidates who might be optimized prior to device implantation to avoid associated morbidity and mortality.[9]

PREOPERATIVE RISK FACTORS FOR VAD THERAPY

One of the first studies to identify risk factors predictive of postoperative outcomes in VAD patients[49] used a weighted assessment of 24 individual variables in a series of 26 patients. Different types of devices were used, with 70 percent of the subjects receiving biventricular support. The risk factors most strongly associated with adverse outcomes included age greater than 50 years, preoperative cardiopulmonary resuscitation, mechanical ventilation or FiO_2 greater than 70 percent, ECMO, and blood urea nitrogen greater than 60 or a serum creatinine greater than 2.2 mg/dL.[49] Similarly, a review of 56 patients from the Cleveland Clinics and Columbia Presbyterian Hospital between 1990 and 1994 identified oliguria, central venous pressure greater than 16, mechanical ventilation, coagulopathy, and repeat sternotomy as risk factors.[50,51] Survival associated with VAD implantation also correlated well with APACHE II scores, which were significantly improved in patients supported by LVADs. Survival times determined by Kaplan-Meier analysis and Cox proportional analysis after adjustment for APACHE II scores were better for mechanical circulatory support ($p < 0.02$).[52]

In a multivariate analysis of 464 VAD patients obtained from the Novacor European Registry revealed that independent risk factors for death after device

Table 46-9 Columbia University and Cleveland Clinics scoring system for predicting mortality after LVAD implantation

Variable	Score
Revised system	
Ventilation	4
Redo surgery	2
Previous LVAD insertion	2
Central venous pressure > 16 mmHg	1
Prothrombin time > 16 s	1
Original system	
Urine output < 30 mL/h	3
Ventilation	2
Central venous pressure > 16 mmHg	2
Prothrombin time > 16 s	2
Redo surgery	1

implantation included respiratory failure associated with septicemia, right heart failure, age greater than 65 years, acute postcardiotomy failure, and acute myocardial infarction. In the absence of any risk factors, the 1-year survival rate was 60 percent, including posttransplant survival. Any risk factors reduced survival rates to 24 percent.[53] In a prospective multicenter clinical trial conducted at 24 centers in the United States with 280 transplant candidates treated with the HeartMate XVE LVAD, increasing age, prior heart surgery, and hepatic/renal dysfunction were the major predictors of adverse outcomes following device implantation.[27] In a retrospective analysis of 97 LVAD patients, including 64 pneumatic devices and 36 electric devices, significant risk factors for death included a preoperative need for ventilator support or ECMO, elevated blood urea nitrogen, elevated serum creatinine, hyperbilirubinemia, and low pulmonary artery pressures. Postoperative risk factors included reoperation for bleeding, RVAD support requirement, dialysis, and device failure.[54]

In 1995, Columbia University and the Cleveland Clinics proposed a scoring system to predict successful outcomes after LVAD implantation[50]; it was further expanded with evolving technology[55] (Table 46-9). The scoring system is based upon 130 patients who received the vented electrical HeartMate device from 1996 to 2001 (Table 46-10). A score higher than 5 corresponds with a 47 percent mortality, compared with a 9 percent mortality for a score less than 5 (79 percent positive predictive value vs. 70 percent negative predictive value).[55]

CARDIAC CONSIDERATIONS

Valvular heart disease

Valvular stenosis and regurgitation often have significant implications for assist device function. Mitral stenosis can lead to impaired LVAD filling and flow rates. A competent aortic valve is necessary for proper LVAD function;

Table 46-10 Factors important in selecting a mechanical assist device

Factor	Device
Duration of support	
Short term	Centrifugal pumps Paracorporeal devices (e.g., Thoratec VAD, ABIOMED BVS 5000)
Short to medium term	Ventricular assist devices (Novacor, HeartMate, LionHeart)
Long term	Ventricular assist devices (e.g., Novacor, HeartMate, LionHeart) Total artificial heart (e.g., AbioCor TAH, CardioWest TAH)
Aim of support	
Bridge to transplant	Centrifugal pumps Paracorporeal devices (e.g., Thoratec VAD, ABIOMED BVS 5000) Ventricular assist devices (e.g., Novacor, HeartMate, LionHeart)
Bridge to recovery	Ventricular assist devices (e.g., Novacor, HeartMate, LionHeart) Axial flow pumps (e.g., DeBakey, HeartMate II, Jarvik 2000)
Destination therapy	Ventricular assist devices (e.g., Novacor, HeartMate, LionHeart) Axial flow pumps (e.g., DeBakey, HeartMate II, Jarvik 2000) Total Artificial Heart (e.g., AbioCor, CardioWest)
Type of support	
Univentricular	All devices
Biventricular	Paracorporeal devices (Thoratec VAD, ABIOMED BVS 5000) Total Artificial Heart (e.g., AbioCor, CardioWest)
Technical factors	
Small body size	Axial flow devices (e.g., DeBakey, Jarvik
Size of device	2000, HeartMate II)
Anticoagulation	Extracorporeal pumps

severe aortic regurgitation should be corrected with device implantation. Mild to moderate aortic regurgitation can worsen once left ventricular support is initiated because of a reduction in left ventricular pressure and an increase in aortic root pressure. VADs do not completely unload the left ventricle, leading to some flow across the aortic valve. This low, intermittent flow is inadequate to wash an existing mechanical aortic prosthesis. Therefore such valves should be replaced by bioprosthetic valves to prevent thrombus formation and subsequent embolism.

Right ventricular function

When significant right ventricular dysfunction exists, biventricular support should be considered. If right ventricular failure is not recognized prior to the implantation of left ventricular support, unique problems can arise that may necessitate a device change and possibly lead to significant morbidity and mortality.[56] Unfortunately, current biventricular support devices are cumbersome, with large consoles limiting patient mobility. Preoperative risk factors for right ventricular failure after LVAD insertion include hyperbilirubinemia, elevated creatinine, and mechanical ventilatory support.[57] Ochiai and colleagues found that several factors had an 80 percent predictive value in determining the need for right ventricular assistance: right ventricular end-diastolic dimension of 8.5 cm, right ventricular end-diastolic volume of 200 mL, a mean pulmonary artery pressure of 60 mmHg, and a mean right atrial pressure of 70 mmHg.[58]

Atrial and ventricular arrhythmias

Atrial fibrillation and atrial flutter can lead to inadequate right ventricular filling and thrombus formation. Both cardioversion and anticoagulation are essential, even if the device does not otherwise require anticoagulation. Ventricular arrythmias can be considered as a relative contraindication for mechanical support, although it has been shown that device flow can be maintained adequately during ventricular fibrillation in the setting of low pulmonary vascular resistance. In conclusion, arrhythmias should be treated prior to VAD implantation.

Intracardiac shunts

Because of the significant right-to-left shunting that can result after unloading the left ventricle, it is important to close any patent foramen ovale or atrial septal defects with assist device implantation.

OTHER CONSIDERATIONS

Noncardiac organ function plays an important role in clinical outcomes with mechanical device support. Also important is the timing of device insertion, but this is largely influenced by the referral pattern, institutional preferences, and surgeon-specific factors. Some poor outcomes following device therapy are due to delay in instituting device implantation. Ideally, device implantation should be considered prior to the onset of organ failure.

Pulmonary function

Although there are no consensus criteria for pulmonary function testing prior assist device implantation, a FEV_1 greater than 50 percent predicted, FVC of 50 percent predicted, and DL_{CO} of 50 percent predicted are usually baseline requirements in selecting candidates for a mechanical support. Although LVAD therapy has been shown to reduce pulmonary vascular resistance, this is not always observed. When pulmonary vascular resistance is fixed, unloading of the left ventricle by the device does not lead to a significant reduction of right ventricular afterload and increased pulmonary blood flow. In patients with severe pulmonary disease, preoperative computed tomography of the chest is warranted.

Renal function

Many studies have identified renal dysfunction as a significant predictor of poor outcome following assist device implantation. A thorough preoperative evaluation of renal dysfunction is important to determine reversibility. A candidate's baseline renal function prior to the onset of cardiac failure or cardiogenic shock and the potential for recovery should be considered. Many centers now employ aggressive renal support via hemodialysis and hemofiltration, which to some extent has made many patients suitable for mechanical device therapy who would otherwise have been denied. An elevated creatinine has been shown to be a negative risk factor for LVAD insertion.[59] Similarly, elevated blood urea nitrogen greater than 40 mg/dL has been shown to be a risk factor for bridge-to-transplant survival. Severe right ventricular dysfunction and volume overload with a right atrial pressure above 20 mmHg can lead to changes in glomerular filtration, with a resultant decrease in urine output and resistance to diuretic therapy.

Hepatic function

Significant hepatic dysfunction or failure can be detrimental in assist device patients. Prolongation of the international normalized ratio (INR) is one of the most significant risk factors for complications in mechanical assist patients, associated with significant perioperative bleeding and transfusion requirements, worsening coagulopathy, right ventricular dysfunction, and multi-organ-system failure.[60] A total bilirubin greater than 3.6 mg/dL or a direct bilirubin greater than 1.2 mg/dL (e.g., cardiac congestion, drug toxicity, hepatitis, alcohol abuse) is an independent risk factor for an adverse outcomes.[61] If these markers are found to be elevated in a candidate's evaluation, a thorough investigation to assess the degree and severity of hepatic dysfunction is warranted. Patients with right heart failure with resultant hepatic congestion may need right ventricular support in addition to left ventricular support. These and other considerations are particularly important when destination therapy is being considered.

CNS function

The potential for postoperative long-term rehabilitation after device insertion is based on an understanding of the workings of the device, consoles, various alarms, and device maintenance. Hence a major irreversible neurologic deficit or cognitive impairment, which would render patients incapable of managing their devices, is generally a contraindication for device implantation. However, limited motor deficits are not singular contraindications to mechanical device support; in such cases, determinations should be made in consultation with neurologists and support staff.

DEVICE SELECTION

The selection of a mechanical support device is largely dependent on the candidate's clinical situation. Selection is first and foremost dependent on the duration of support needed (e.g., short, medium, or long term); the aim of support (i.e., bridge to transplant, bridge to recovery, or destination therapy); whether univentricular or biventricular support is needed; patient size (many devices are limited to a BSA > 1.5 m^2); and the size of the device itself, particularly when pediatric support is being considered. Anticoagulation requirements and the degree of support represent important secondary issues. Patients requiring total left ventricular support are best supported by a pulsatile device (e.g., HeartMate or Novacor), while lesser degrees of support can be provided by the newer axial-flow devices. Long-term durability and mechanical robustness are important factors when destination therapy is considered. How some of the factors determine device selection is outlined in Table 46-10. A decision-making flowchart for device selection is offered in Fig. 46-13.

SURGICAL MANAGEMENT

Preoperative preparation

As outlined earlier, every attempt should be made to optimize distal organ function. Common interventions include IABP, forced diuresis, pulmonary vasodilators

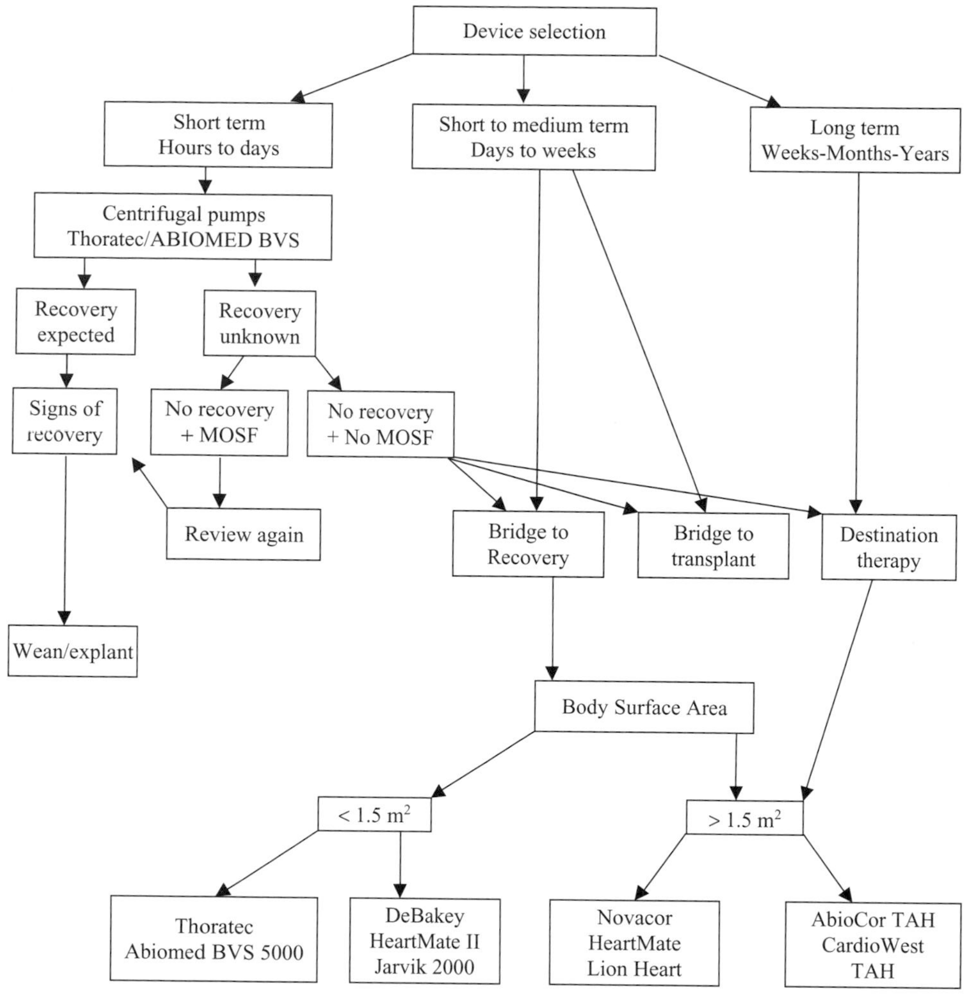

Figure 46-13 Decision-making flowchart: device selection.

(e.g., prostaglandin E_1), hemodialysis/hemofiltration, and the replacement of coagulation factors. A right atrial pressure below 12 mmHg, PCWP less than 20 mmHg, and cardiac index greater than 2.0 are target indices prior to insertion of the device. Pre- or intraoperative echocardiographic studies can help identify a patent foramen ovale or small atrial septal defect and assess valvular and ventricular function.

Operative technique

Most VADs are implanted through a median sternotomy on CPB. The devices can be placed within intra- or preperitoneal pockets. A preperitoneal pump pocket is created by extending the median sternotomy incision. The size of the device affects its location in many patients. Early attempts at placing the device intraperitoneally resulted in colonic perforations, intestinal obstruction, and diaphragmatic hernias; this has led most surgeons to place these devices extraperitoneally. Care is taken to achieve meticulous hemostasis during pocket construction, since hemorrhage and the formation of pocket hematomas are among the most common complications. After the pocket is created, the device is primed and the drive line tunneled from the pocket to exit the right upper abdominal quadrant. The patient is then heparinized and the heart cannulated for CPB.

An off-pump end-to-side anastomosis between the aorta and the outflow conduit can be performed in some patients using a partially occluding clamp. Left ventricular apical inflow cannulation is performed on CPB, creating a circular apical ventriculotomy, placing circumferential mattress sutures to anchor the apical sleeve connector, and connecting the LVAD inflow cannula to this connector. Some surgeons feel that apical inflow cannulation should be performed first to permit more accurate sizing of the outflow graft.

Once the inflow and outflow connections have been made, the LVAD chamber is passively filled, followed by pump de-airing maneuvers. CPB is then weaned concomitantly with initiation of VAD function.

Postoperative care

After LVAD implantation, early postoperative care focuses on optimizing and monitoring native right ventricular function in addition to the usual ICU procedures following cardiac surgery. Adequate right heart function can be fostered with pulmonary vasodilators (e.g., milrinone, nitric oxide). Patients can be weaned to extubation once hemodynamics have been stabilized and hemostasis has been assured. Following this, early patient mobilization and nutritional repletion are undertaken. Postoperative anticoagulation regimens usually include aspirin in addition to warfarin.

VAD explantation

In bridge-to-transplant patients, VAD explantation at the time of transplantation can be complicated by dense adhesions around the device conduits. This situation can be somewhat ameliorated by wrapping the conduits with Gore-Tex. Regardless, upon reentry through the sternum, care must be taken to avoid damage to underlying cardiac and device structures.

COMPLICATIONS

Bleeding

Hemorrhage is the most common complication after assist device implantation.[22,62] Technical factors that can lead to increased bleeding include the creation of large pockets for device placement and loose device connectors and conduits as well as insufficient hemostasis (e.g., cannulation sites, sternal edges). Bleeding can be caused by coagulopathy due to liver failure, prior antiplatelet and antithrombotic medications, and CPB-related platelet consumption.[51] The incidence of significant bleeding is reported to be as high as 50 percent in some series.[22,62,63] Consequently, meticulous hemostasis, a low threshold for reexploration, and judicious use of blood products and clotting factors are mandatory in device implantation.

Infection

The reported incidence of device-related infections varies,[63] but remains one of the most frequent complications after bleeding. Infection rates ranges from 49 to 66 percent, and around 48 percent for the HeartMate device, and is around 48 percent for the Novacor and Thoratec devices.[63] The lack of standardized definitions and criteria for device-related infections have rendered reported infection rates rather inexact.[64]

Thromboembolism

Thromboembolism is associated with all devices. The HeartMate device, which only requires aspirin and dipyridamole has a reported incidence of thromboembolic rate of 7.4 percent. All other devices require warfarin anticoagulation with reported thromboembolic rates ranging between 7 and 47 percent. Better conduits that promote neointimal growth have reduced thromboembolic complications. The newer-generation devices, including axial flow and TAF devices, also suffer from thromboembolic complications.

Multisystem organ failure

Multisystem organ failure after VAD implantation often results from preexisting unrecognized organ dysfunction. On the other hand, infection leading to sepsis, excessive hemorrhage and blood product transfusions, and prolonged ventilation can also contribute to postoperative multisystem organ failure. The incidence of postimplantation organ failure is reported to be between 10 and 30 percent. Careful preoperative assessment and proper timing for device insertion should serve to reduce this incidence.

Right ventricular failure

Early right ventricular failure after LVAD implantation can lead to poor filling of the LVAD and low pump outputs. Occasionally, severe right ventricular failure necessitates placement of a right VAD (RVAD) to sustain LVAD output. Significant primary right ventricular failure has been defined as a right atrial pressure greater than 20 mmHg on maximal drug support or a right atrial pressure greater than the PCWP. Implantable LVADs with portable drivers, permitting patients to be sent home, have led to the increasing use of these devices in preference to biventricular support systems. Nevertheless, 20 to 30 percent of patients experience some degree of right ventricular failure at the time of LVAD implantation. These patients may require prolonged inotropic and ventilatory support and experience hepatic dysfunction and limited mobility.[58] A study from the Cleveland Clinics identified risk factors for RVAD support after LVAD implantation in a retrospective review of 245 patients. In this series, RVADs were required after LVAD insertion for 23 patients: 13 percent of HeartMate IP patients, 4 percent of Novacor patients, and 10 percent of HeartMate VE patients. Eighteen of 23 patients required RVAD support in the first 4 h after LVAD implantation. The strongest predictors for RVAD requirements after LVAD implantation were the need for preoperative circulatory support, female gender, and nonischemic etiology. When survival to transplantation was investigated, it was greater in patients not requiring RVAD support than in those who did not require such support.[58] In another study from the Cleveland Clinics, an elevated right ventricular end-diastolic volume, increased right atrial pressure, elevated transpulmonary gradient, and pulmonary vascular resistance greater than 3.8 were found to be risk factors for right ventricular failure after LVAD implantation.[65,66] Early recognition of right ventricular failure after LVAD insertion and the prompt institution of support are important in reducing morbidity and mortality.

NEWER DEVICES

HeartQuest VAD

The HeartQuest VAD (MedQuest Products Inc.) is an implantable, centrifugal pump housed in a titanium casing. It uses magnetic levitation to suspend and drive a self-centering impeller. The inflow cannula is placed in the left ventricular apex with the outflow cannula anastomosed to the ascending aorta. This device can provide 1.5 to 9 L/min of blood flow. It has a bench durability of 5 years, with low anticoagulation requirements.[67]

VentrAssist LVAS

The VentrAssist (VentraCor Limited) is a small implantable centrifugal pump designed for destination therapy and as a bridge to transplant. It uses a hydrodynamic rotor suspension, which avoids areas of slow and turbulent blood flow. The absence of bearings reduces rotor wear, enhancing the device's durability. It uses large rare-earth magnets with small gaps and a harmonic drive system. Weighing 298 g, it is 6 cm in diameter and 6.5 cm in length. The externally worn battery and controller provide power and control; the battery holds sufficient charge for up to 8 h. The small size of the device should permit its use in smaller adults as well as in children. The short inflow cannula connects to the left ventricular apex and the outflow cannula is anastomosed to the ascending aorta. It has a low potential for thrombosis due to a reduction of stasis. Preclinical tests have been satisfactory and the device is currently undergoing pilot studies.[68]

HeartMate III

The HeartMate III (Thoratec Corp.) is a fully implantable, magnetically suspended centrifugal pump. It incorporates the textured blood surface used in previous Thoratec devices. It measures 6.9 cm by 3.5 cm, has a displacement volume of 195 mL, and weighs 500 g (Fig. 46-14). This device produces a mean blood flow of 4.3 L/min (± 1.5 L/min) and is powered by TETS (Transcutaneous Energy Transfer System).[69]

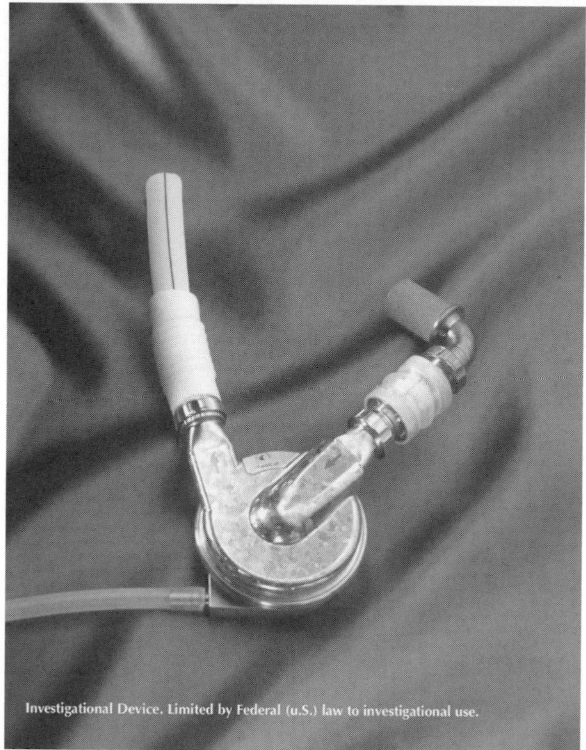

Investigational Device. Limited by Federal (u.S.) law to investigational use.

Figure 46-14 HeartMate III. (With permission from Thoratec Corporation.)

TandemHeart pVAD

The TandemHeart pVAD (CardiacAssist Technologies, Inc., Pittsburgh, PA) is a centrifugal pump that can be rapidly deployed by cardiologists in the cardiac catheterization laboratory by femoral arterial access. It is light in weight (280 g) and requires only 7 mL of priming fluid to accommodate both small and large patients. It is intended for reversible causes of cardiac failure following percutaneous revascularization.[70] The pump is powered by a stationary electromagnetic motor, which drives a rotor and impeller. Rotating at 2700 to 4700 rpm, it is capable of generating flows up to 6 L/min and pressures up to 90 mmHg.[71]

AB-180 iVAD

The AB-180 iVAD (CardiacAssist Technologies, Inc., Pittsburgh, PA) is a surgically implantable version of the TandemHeart pVAD (described above). A 10-mm polytetrafluoroethylene (PTFE) graft conducts outflow to the aorta. A percutaneous cable connects to an integrated infusion pump delivering lubrication and anticoagulation fluid, a flow estimator, and a power line to the VAD. This device can be deployed for postcardiotomy syndrome, acute myocarditis, and acute postinfarction myocardial failure and shock.[71,72]

Kriton VAD

The Kriton VAD (Kriton Medical, Miramar, FL) is a small centrifugal pulsatile device that is fully implantable. The impeller of the pump is supported by a passive radial magnetic bearing that acts in synergy with hydrodynamic bearings. Torque is transmitted to the impeller by electromagnetic coupling via an integrated axial flux gap motor. It can displace 48 mL and generate an output up to 15 L/min. Weighing only 195 g with an extracardiac volume of 28 mL, this device is intended for long-term use and has undergone extensive preclinical testing.[73]

DuraHeart LVAS

The DuraHeart LVAS (Terumo Corporation) is a magnetically suspended centrifugal pump. The impeller is suspended between permanent magnets and electromagnets. It weighs 400 g, displaces about 196 mL, and can generate flows up to 10 L/min.[74] The heparin-bonded inflow and outflow cannulas comprise the blood contact surfaces.

Next Generation LVAS

Formerly known as the HeartSaver VAD, the Next Generation LVAS (WorldHeart Corp.) is a fully implantable pulsatile device (Fig. 46-15). Unlike the Novacor LVAS, it does not require a volume compensator and is smaller in size. Energy transfer is via a transcutaneous energy and information transfer coil. It combines the blood sac, volume displacement chamber, electrohydraulic axial flow pump, and internal control electronics in a single implantable unit. Unlike other VADs, it is intended to be placed in the thorax.[72–74] The device can be implanted via a median sternotomy, eliminating the need for more extensive dissection in the abdomen. The VAD unit incorporates an axial flow, bidirectional brushless DC motor that pumps hydraulic fluid during systole from the volume displacement chamber into the pumping chamber. The hydraulic fluid actuates a flexible diaphragm by exerting external pressure on the flexible polyurethane blood sac. During diastole, the blood sac fills passively, displacing the hydraulic fluid from the pumping chamber back to the volume displacement chamber through a one-way valve mounted on the bulkhead. This device is intended both for left and right ventricular support.[75]

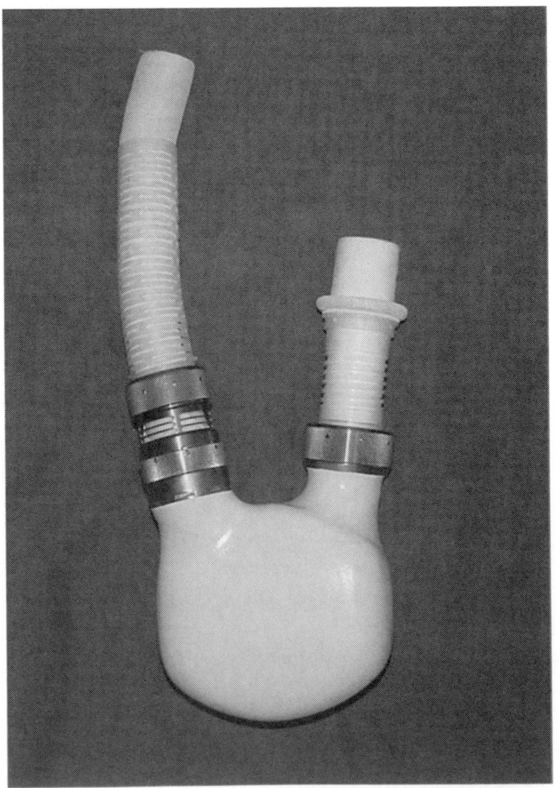

Figure 46-15 Next Generation LVAS. (With permission from WorldHeart Corporation, Ottawa, Canada.)

CorAide LVAS

Developed at Cleveland Clinics, the CorAide LVAS (Arrow Int.) is a small continuous-flow centrifugal pump. It has a magnetically suspended rotor, weighs 293 g, and capable of generating blood flows up to 6 L/min. In preclinical trials. it has shown promise without requiring anticoagulation.[76]

Kantrovitz CardioVad

The Kantrovitz CardioVad (LVAD Technologies Inc., Detroit, MI) has three main parts: a blood pump that is implanted on the lateral aspect of the descending thoracic aorta, a connector for an external power source, and a drive unit to power the pump. The pump, an inflatable avalvular polyurethane bladder, is sutured in place after excising a lateral portion of the aorta. It is about 6.5 cm in length and capable of displacing 60 mL of blood when inflated. The blood-contacting surface is textured so that pseudointima may form on it.[77] No anticoagulation is needed and an external air pump mounted in the external drive unit inflates and deflates the blood pump synchronously but out of the phase with heart contractions. The diastolic augmentation reduces left ventricular afterload, increases cardiac output, and improves coronary perfusion.

Pittsburgh Streamliner mixed flow pump

The Streamliner, the first magnetic-bearing LVAD, is named for the way it provides minimal disturbance to blood flow. Developed at the McGowan Center for Artificial Organ Development, a subdivision of the Department of Surgery at the University of Pittsburgh School of Medicine, the Streamliner operates at approximately 7500 rpm, supplementing the action of a weak or damaged heart.[72]

Penn State TAH

The Penn State TAH (ABIOMED Inc., Danvers, MA) was developed at Penn State University with funding from the National Heart, Lung, and Blood Institute (NHLBI). It is a fully implantable, orthotopically placed biventricular electromechanical total replacement system. The pump consists of a rigid titanium casing enclosing polyurethane blood sacs and an energy converter. This device utilizes Delrin monostrut valves to provide unidirectional flow. [78] The energy converter is composed of a brushless DC electric motor, which actuates a roller screw with pusher plates. Mechanical compression of the blood sacs by the pusher plates against the rigid housing results in alternate emptying of the blood. It has low associated vibrations and minimal noise. It has a stroke volume of about 64 mL and can reach a maximum output of about 8 L/min. Physiologic sensing is through the end-diastolic volume estimated from the motor speed and voltage; this provides the balance between the left- and right-sided pump outputs (akin to the LionHeart). The energy source is comprises TETTS and quick-charging Ni-Cad batteries. A compliance chamber is connected to the motor housing and implanted internally. This device is currently in preclinical testing and is undergoing feasibility and durability studies.[78]

EXCOR

The EXCOR (Berlin Heart Inc.) is a pneumatically actuated paracorporeal pump that can support both ventricles. The EXCOR stroke volume ranges from 10 to 80 mL, permitting its use in adults and children. It is available with two alternative types of valve systems: a mechanical tilting disk and a polyurethane velum valve. The cannulas are made of silicone and are designed to reduce the incidence of thromboembolism and entry/exit site infections. There are two systems available for pneumatic support. One is a stationary drive and the other is a mobile unit. The stationary unit (called Ikus) is capable of supporting both ventricles and can run in synchronous and asynchronous modes; each ventricle can be operated independently. The mobile unit (called Excor) weighs 8.7 kg with two power packs and features a physiologically adaptive synchronous operation.[75]

INCOR

The INCOR (Berlin Heart Inc.) is a magnetically levitated, fully implantable axial flow pump. The impeller is capable of rotating at a speed of 12,000 rpm and can generate flows of 7 L/min at pressures up to 150 mmHg. It is currently undergoing clinical trials in China and Europe.[75] The INCOR requires about 8.5 W of power, weighs 200 g, and is 30 mm in diameter. The pump is titanium-based with silicone conduits. The battery and power pack weigh about 1.5 kg and can be carried on one's person, with a TETTS energy transfer system.

Other devices in development and preclinical testing are the MiTi Heart VAD (MiTi Heart Corporation), MagScrew for VAD and TAH (Foster Miller Technologies), an external cardiac support device called ParaCor (Paracor Surgical Inc.), and a magnetic levitation-based axial flow pump called CentrMag pump (Levitronix Inc.). Other heart failure support devices that alter the geometry of the left ventricle are the CorCap Cardiac Support Device (Acorn Cardiovascular Inc.)[79] and the Myosplint System (Myocor Inc., Maple Grove, MN).[80]

References

1. Gibbon J. Application of a mechanical heart and lung apparatus to cardiac surgery. *Minn Med* 1954;37:171.
2. Spencer FC, BE, Trinkle JK, et al. Assisted circulation for cardiac failure following intracardiac surgery with cardiorespiratory bypass. *J Thorac Cardiovasc Surg* 1959; 49:56.
3. DeBakey ME. Left ventricular bypass pump for cardiac assistance: 1. Clinical experience. *Am J Cardiol* 1971;27 (1):3–11.
4. Kantrowitz A, Tjonneland S, Freed PS, et al. Initial clinical experience with intraaortic balloon pumping in cardiogenic shock. *JAMA* 1968;203(2):113–118.
5. Cooley DA, Liotta D, Hallman GL, et al. Orthotopic cardiac prosthesis for two-staged cardiac replacement. *Am J Cardiol* 1969;24(5):723–730.
6. Pierce WS. Permanent heart substitution: Better solutions lie ahead. *JAMA* 1988;259(6):891.
7. DeVries W, Anderson J, Joyce L, et al. Clinical use of the total artificial heart. *N Engl J Med* 1984;310(5): 273–278.
8. Hon JK, Yacoub MH. Bridge to recovery with the use of left ventricular assist device and clenbuterol. *Ann Thorac Surg* 2003;75(6 Suppl):S36–S41.
9. Rose EA, Gelijns AC, Moskowitz AJ, et al. Long-term use of a left ventricular assist device for end-stage heart failure. *N Engl J Med* 2001;345(20):1435–1443.
10. Curtis JJ, Walls JT, Wagner-Mann CC, et al. Centrifugal pumps: Description of devices and surgical techniques. *Ann Thorac Surg* 1999;68(2):666–671.
11. Curtis JJ, Boley TM, Walls JT, et al. Frequency of seal disruption with the sarns centrifugal pump in postcardiotomy circulatory assist. *Artif Organs* 1994;18(3): 235–237.
12. Hoy FBY, Mueller DK, Geiss DM, et al. Bridge to recovery for postcardiotomy failure: Is there still a role for centrifugal pumps? *Ann Thorac Surg* 2000;70 (4):1259–1263.
13. Magovern GJ Jr. The biopump and postoperative circulatory support. *Ann Thorac Surg* 1993;55(1): 245–249.
14. Noon GP, Ball JW Jr, Papaconstantinou HT. Clinical experience with BioMedicus centrifugal ventricular support in 172 patients. *Artif Organs* 1995;19(7):756–760.
15. Guyton R, Schonberger J, Everts P, et al. Postcardiotomy shock: Clinical evaluation of the BVS 5000 biventricular support system. *Ann Thorac Surg* 1993;56(2):346–356.

16. Dekkers RJ, FitzGerald DJ, Couper GS. Five-year clinical experience with Abiomed BVS 5000 as a ventricular assist device for cardiac failure. *Perfusion* 2001;16(1): 13–18.
17. Smedira NG, Moazami N, Golding CM, et al. Clinical experience with 202 adults receiving extracorporeal membrane oxygenation for cardiac failure: Survival at five years. *J Thorac Cardiovasc Surg* 2001;122(1):92–102.
18. Samuels LE, Holmes EC, Thomas MP, et al. Management of acute cardiac failure with mechanical assist: experience with the Abiomed BVS 5000. *Ann Thorac Surg* 2001;71(3 Suppl):S67–S72; discussion S82–S85.
19. Couper GS, Dekkers RJ, Adams DH. The logistics and cost-effectiveness of circulatory support: Advantages of the Abiomed BVS 5000. *Ann Thorac Surg* 1999;68(2): 646–649.
20. Farrar DJ. The Thoratec ventricular assist device: A paracorporeal pump for treating acute and chronic heart failure. *Semin Thorac Cardiovasc Surg* 2000;12(3):243–250.
21. El-Banayosy A, Korfer R, Arusoglu L, et al. Bridging to cardiac transplantation with the Thoratec ventricular assist device. *Thorac Cardiovasc Surg* 1999;47(Suppl 2): 307–310.
22. Minami K, El-Banayosy A, Sezai A, et al. Morbidity and outcome after mechanical ventricular support using Thoratec, Novacor, and HeartMate for bridging to heart transplantation. Artif Organs 2000;24(6):421–426.
23. DeRose JJ Jr, Umana JP, Argenziano M, et al. Implantable left ventricular assist devices provide an excellent outpatient bridge to transplantation and recovery. *J Am Coll Cardiol* 1997;30(7):1773–1777.
24. Frazier O. First use of an untethered, vented electric left ventricular assist device for long-term support [published erratum appears in *Circulation* 1995 Jun 15;91(12): 3026]. *Circulation* 1994;89(6):2908–2914.
25. Morgan JA, John R, Rao V, et al. Bridging to transplant with the HeartMate left ventricular assist device: The Columbia Presbyterian 12-year experience. *J Thorac Cardiovasc Surg* 2004;127(5):1309–1316.
26. Sun BC, Catanese KA, Spanier TB, et al. 100 long-term implantable left ventricular assist devices: The Columbia Presbyterian interim experience. *Ann Thorac Surg* 1999; 68(2):688–694.
27. Frazier OH, Rose EA, Oz MC, et al. Multicenter clinical evaluation of the HeartMate vented electric left ventricular assist system in patients awaiting heart transplantation. *J Thorac Cardiovasc Surg* 2001;122(6):1186–1195.
28. Wheeldon DR, LaForge DH, Lee J, et al. Novacor left ventricular assist system long-term performance: Comparison of clinical experience with demonstrated in vitro reliability. *ASAIO J* 2002;48(5):546–551.
29. Robbins RC, Kown MH, Portner PM, Oyer PE. The totally implantable Novacor left ventricular assist system. *Ann Thorac Surg* 2001;71(90030):162S–165S.
30. Pasque MK, Rogers JG. Adverse events in the use of HeartMate vented electric and Novacor left ventricular assist devices: Comparing apples and oranges. *J Thorac Cardiovasc Surg* 2002;124(6):1063–1067.
31. Di Bella I, Pagani F, Banfi C, et al. Results with the Novacor assist system and evaluation of long-term assistance. *Eur J Cardiothorac Surg* 2000;18(1):112–116.
32. Mehta SM, Pae WE Jr, Rosenberg G, et al. The LionHeart LVD-2000: A completely implanted left ventricular assist device for chronic circulatory support. *Ann Thorac Surg* 2001;71(90030):156S–161S.
33. El-Banayosy A, Arusoglu L, Kizner L, et al. Preliminary experience with the LionHeart left ventricular assist device in patients with end-stage heart failure. *Ann Thorac Surg* 2003;75(5):1469–1475.
34. Dowling RD, Etoch SW, Stevens KA, et al. Current status of the AbioCor implantable replacement heart. *Ann Thorac Surg* 2001;71(90030):147S–149S.
35. Dowling RD, Gray LA Jr, Etoch SW, et al. The AbioCor implantable replacement heart. *Ann Thorac Surg* 2003; 75(6 Suppl):S93–S99.
36. Copeland JG. Mechanical assist device–my choice: The CardioWest total artificial heart. *Transplant Proc* 2000;32(7):1523–1524.
37. Leprince P, Bonnet N, Rama A, et al. Bridge to transplantation with the Jarvik-7 (CardioWest) total artificial heart: A single-center 15-year experience. *J Heart Lung Transplant* 2003;22(12):1296–1303.
38. Copeland JG III, Smith RG, Arabia FA, et al. Comparison of the CardioWest total artificial heart, the Novacor left ventricular assist system, and the Thoratec ventricular assist system in bridge to transplantation. *Ann Thorac Surg* 2001;71(90030):92S–97s.
39. Wieselthaler GM, Schima H, Hiesmayr M, et al. First clinical experience with the DeBakey VAD continuous-axial-flow pump for bridge to transplantation. *Circulation* 2000;101(4):356–359.
40. Noon GP, Morley DL, Irwin S, et al. Clinical experience with the MicroMed DeBakey ventricular assist device. *Ann Thorac Surg* 2001;71(90030):133S–138S.
41. Goldstein DJ. Worldwide experience with the MicroMed DeBakey ventricular assist device as a bridge to transplantation. *Circulation* 2003;108(90101):272II–277II.
42. Frazier OH, Myers TJ, Jarvik RK, et al. Research and development of an implantable, axial-flow left ventricular assist device: The Jarvik 2000 heart. *Ann Thorac Surg* 2001;71(90030):125S–132S.
43. Kaplon RJ, Oz MC, Kwiatkowski PA, et al. Miniature axial flow pump for ventricular assistance in children and small adults. *J Thorac Cardiovasc Surg* 1996;111(1):13–18.
44. Frazier OH, Shah NA, Myers TJ, et al. Use of the Flowmaker (Jarvik 2000) left ventricular assist device for destination therapy and bridging to transplantation. *Cardiology* 2004;101(1–3):111–116.
45. Burke DJ, Burke E, Parsaie F, et al. The Heartmate II: Design and development of a fully sealed axial flow left ventricular assist system. *Artif Organs* 2001;25(5): 380–385.
46. Griffith BP, Kormos RL, Borovetz HS, et al. HeartMate II left ventricular assist system: From concept to first clinical use. *Ann Thorac Surg* 2001;71(90030):116S–120S.
47. Rose EA, Moskowitz AJ, Packer M, et al. The REMATCH trial: Rationale, design, and end points. Randomized evaluation of mechanical assistance for the treatment of congestive heart failure. *Ann Thorac Surg* 1999;67(3):723–730.
48. Lazar RM, Shapiro PA, Jaski BE, et al. Neurological events during long-term mechanical circulatory support for heart failure. The Randomized Evaluation of Mechanical

Assistance for the Treatment of Congestive Heart Failure (REMATCH) experience. *Circulation* 2004.
49. Pennington DG, McBride LR, Kanter KR, et al. Bridging to heart transplantation with circulatory support devices. *J Heart Transplant* 1989;8(2):116–123.
50. Oz MC, Rose EA, Levin HR. Selection criteria for placement of left ventricular assist devices. *Am Heart J* 1995; 129(1):173–177.
51. Oz MC, Goldstein DJ, Pepino P, et al. Screening scale predicts patients successfully receiving long-term implantable left ventricular assist devices. *Circulation* 1995;92(9 Suppl):II169–II173.
52. Gracin N, Johnson MR, Spokas D, et al. The use of APACHE II scores to select candidates for left ventricular assist device placement. Acute physiology and chronic health evaluation. *J Heart Lung Transplant* 1998;17 (10):1017–1023.
53. Deng MC, Weyand M, Hammel D, et al. Selection and management of ventricular assist device patients: The Muenster experience. *J Heart Lung Transplant* 2000;19 (8 Suppl):S77–S82.
54. McCarthy PM, Smedira NO, Vargo RL, et al. One hundred patients with the HeartMate left ventricular assist device: Evolving concepts and technology. *J Thorac Cardiovasc Surg* 1998;115(4):904–912.
55. Williams MR, Oz MC. Indications and patient selection for mechanical ventricular assistance. *Ann Thorac Surg* 2001;71(90030):86S–91S.
56. Kavarana MN, Pessin-Minsley MS, Urtecho J, et al. Right ventricular dysfunction and organ failure in left ventricular assist device recipients: A continuing problem. *Ann Thorac Surg* 2002;73(3):745–750.
57. Farrar DJ, Hill JD, Pennington DG, et al. Preoperative and postoperative comparison of patients with univentricular and biventricular support with the thoratec ventricular assist device as a bridge to cardiac transplantation. *J Thorac Cardiovasc Surg* 1997;113(1):202–209.
58. Ochiai Y, McCarthy PM, Smedira NG, et al. Predictors of severe right ventricular failure after implantable left ventricular assist device insertion: Analysis of 245 patients. *Circulation* 2002;106(90121):198I–202I.
59. Farrar DJ, Hill JD. Recovery of major organ function in patients awaiting heart transplantation with Thoratec ventricular assist devices. Thoratec Ventricular Assist Device Principal Investigators. *J Heart Lung Transplant* 1994;13(6):1125–1132.
60. Miller LW. Patient selection for the use of ventricular assist devices as a bridge to transplantation. *Ann Thorac Surg* 2003;75(6 Suppl):S66–S71.
61. Reinhartz O, Farrar DJ, Hershon JH, et al. Importance of preoperative liver function as a predictor of survival in patients supported with Thoratec ventricular assist devices as a bridge to transplantation. *J Thorac Cardiovasc Surg* 1998;116(4):633–640.
62. El-Banayosy A, Korfer R, Arusoglu L, et al. Device and patient management in a bridge-to-transplant setting. *Ann Thorac Surg* 2001;71(90030):98S–102S.
63. Minami K, El-Banayosy A, Sezai A, et al. Morbidity and outcome after mechanical ventricular support using Thoratec, Novacor, and HeartMate for bridging to Heart Transplantation. *Artif Organs* 2000;24 (6):421–426.
64. Bentz B, Hupcey JE, Polomano RC, Boehmer JP. A retrospective study of left ventricular assist device–related infections. *J Cardiovasc Mgt* 2004;15(1):9–16.
65. Morgan JA, John R, Lee BJ, et al. Is severe right ventricular failure in left ventricular assist device recipients a risk factor for unsuccessful bridging to transplant and post-transplant mortality. *Ann Thorac Surg* 2004;77(3): 859–863.
66. Nakatani S, Thomas JD, Savage RM, et al. Prediction of right ventricular dysfunction after left ventricular assist device implantation. Circulation 1996;94(9 Suppl): II216–II221.
67. Chen C, Paden B, Antaki J, et al. A magnetic suspension theory and its application to the HeartQuest ventricular assist device. *Artif Organs* 2002;26(11): 947–951.
68. James NL, van der Meer AL, Edwards GA, et al. Implantation of the VentrAssist implantable rotary blood pump in sheep. *ASAIO J* 2003;49(4):454–458.
69. Loree HM, Bourque K, Gernes DB, et al. The Heartmate III: Design and in vivo studies of a Maglev centrifugal left ventricular assist device. *Artif Organs* 2001;25(5):386–391.
70. Kar B, Butkevich A, Civitello AB, et al. Hemodynamic support with a percutaneous left ventricular assist device during stenting of an unprotected left main coronary artery. *Texas Heart Inst J* 2004;31(1):84–86.
71. Pitsis AA, Dardas P, Mezilis N, et al. Temporary assist device for postcardiotomy cardiac failure. *Ann Thorac Surg* 2004;77(4):1431–1433.
72. Song X, Throckmorton AL, Untaroiu A, et al. Axial flow blood pumps. *ASAIO J* 2003;49(4):355–364.
73. Wampler R, Lancisi D, Indravudh V, et al. A sealless centrifugal blood pump with passive magnetic and hydrodynamic bearings. *Artif Organs* 1999;23(8): 780–784.
74. Nojiri C. [Left ventricular assist system with a magnetically levitated impeller technology]. *Nippon Geka Gakkai Zasshi* 2002;103(9):607–610.
75. Portner PM. Permanent mechanical circulatory assistance. In: Baumgartner WARB, Kasper E, Theodore J (eds). *Heart and Lung Transplantation*, 2d ed. Philadelphia: Saunders, 2001.
76. Doi K, Golding LA, Massiello AL, et al. Preclinical readiness testing of the Arrow International CorAide left ventricular assist system. *Ann Thorac Surg* 2004;77(6): 2103–2110.
77. Jeevanandam V, Jayakar D, Anderson AS, et al. Circulatory assistance with a permanent implantable IABP: Initial human experience. *Circulation* 2002;106 (12 Suppl 1):I183–I188.
78. Weiss WJ, Rosenberg G, Snyder AJ, et al. Steady state hemodynamic and energetic characterization of the Penn State/3M Health Care total artificial heart. *ASAIO J* 1999;45(3):189–193.
79. Magliato K. Surgical intervention with the CorCap device: Implications of early results. *Congest Heart Fail* 2004;10(2):105.
80. Fukamachi K, Inoue M, Doi K, et al. Device-based left ventricular geometry change for heart failure treatment: Developmental work and current status. *J Card Surg* 2003;18(Suppl)2:S43–S437.

CHAPTER

47 SURGICAL VENTRICULAR REMODELING

John V. Conte

INTRODUCTION

Congestive heart failure (CHF) is the leading medical problem in Western society. It is the leading cause of death in the United States and is expected to become even more significant in the years ahead. Ischemic cardiomyopathy (ICM) is the leading cause of CHF, affecting some 75 percent of patients with CHF.[1,2]

The etiology of ICM is a full-thickness myocardial infarction. Following infarction, the left ventricle (LV) undergoes a well-described process of ventricular remodeling. Left unchecked, this process can lead to a progressive

KEY CONCEPTS

- Epidemiology
  - Congestive heart failure (CHF) is the most prevalent medical problem in Western society, as the leading cause of death in the United States. Ischemic cardiomyopathy is the leading cause of CHF, affecting 75 percent of patients with CHF.
- Pathophysiology
  - Ischemic cardiomyopathy is generally caused by a full-thickness myocardial infarction, followed by ventricular remodeling. This remodeling process can result in progressive dilation of the ventricle, leading to an increase in the end-diastolic diameter and volume, an increase in left ventricular wall stress and oxygen demand, a loss of the left ventricle's natural elliptical shape with the development of a more rounded form, the development of mitral insufficiency, and, ultimately, a worsening of global systolic function.
- Clinical features
  - Progressive CHF due to ischemic cardiomyopathy results in debilitating congestive symptoms, including dyspnea, fatigue, peripheral edema, and, in its end stages, acute and/or chronic multisystem organ failure. Classically, patients are candidates for surgical ventricular remodeling (SVR) if they have had an anterior myocardial infarction, have a large area of akinesis or dyskinesis, and have clinical evidence of CHF.
- Diagnostics
  - Preoperative diagnostics include cardiac catheterization with coronary angiography. Other potentially useful diagnostics include myocardial viability and magnetic resonance imaging studies.
- Treatment
  - The surgical goals of SVR includes complete revascularization of all viable territories, exclusion of akinetic and dyskinetic segments with a concomitant reduction in the size of the nonfunctioning anteroseptal portion of the heart, recreation of the elliptical shape of the heart, and repair of any valvular incompetence by valve repair or replacement.
- Outcomes/prognosis
  - SVR has been shown to improve ventricular size, morphology, left ventricular ejection fraction, stroke volume index, endocrine markers of CHF, ventricular energetics, ventricular synchrony, and mechanical efficiency. Clinically, it results in improved functional capacity (New York Heart Association class) and an excellent 5-year survival in very sick patients. Further study and experience are needed to optimize patient selection and timing for surgical intervention as well as to better define the mechanistic basis behind the beneficial effects of SVR.

dilation of the ventricle, resulting in an increase in the end-diastolic diameter and volume, an increase in LV wall stress and oxygen demand, a loss of the ventricle's natural elliptical shape with the development of a more rounded contour, the development of mitral insufficiency, and ultimately a worsening of global systolic function.[3,4] The development of mitral regurgitation is due to factors specific to ventricular remodeling as well as unrelated leaflet issues. The first factor related to the remodeling process is annular dilation due to global ventricular enlargement. The second is restricted leaflet motion and reduced coaptation due to the global LV dilation or involvement of the papillary muscles with the infarction itself. These factors combine to prevent leaflet coaptation or limit it in the proper plane, resulting in central regurgitation. Superimposed leaflet pathology can worsen the functional regurgitation.

Postinfarction dysfunction is further affected by both the electrical and mechanical dysynchrony that develops following infarction.[5] The concept of electrical dysynchrony is simply that abnormalities in the conduction system following infarction result in differential timing of left and right ventricular contraction. This dysynchronous contraction results in diminished overall LV function, a condition treated, in appropriate circumstances, with biventricular pacing. Mechanical dysynchrony is a phenomenon of impaired LV function caused by nonuniform contraction, relaxation, and filling of the ventricle due to juxtaposed areas of akinesis, dyskinesis, and hypokinesis alongside normal areas. This has been associated with reduced survival.[5,6]

The prognosis of patients with ischemic cardiomyopathy is related to the size of the LV and the impact that remodeling has had on the function of the remote noninfarcted zones.[4] Progressive thinning and dilation of the remote areas leads to the development of a spherical rather than the normal elliptical shape of the heart. Clinically, the ongoing remodeling generates a progressive reduction in contractile force, thus worsening congestive heart failure and ultimately leading to death.[5,6]

Coronary artery revascularization, details of which are presented elsewhere in this book, has been shown to improve survival in both normal and abnormal ventricles. Improved blood flow cannot improve the function of the scarred, noncontractile areas of the heart. Furthermore, it does not change the evident dyssynchrony. Surgical techniques have been developed to arrest the progression and reverse the morphologic changes induced by the pathologic process of postinfarction ventricular remodeling. Such techniques are commonly referred to as surgical ventricular remodeling (SVR). The goal of SVR is to reduce the size and restore a more normal elliptical shape to these enlarged spherical hearts so as to improve cardiac function. SVR is often performed in conjunction with coronary artery revascularization and mitral valve repair/replacement. In this chapter, these techniques are presented and the clinical outcomes discussed.

HISTORY

The history of the surgical approach to postinfarction remodeling begins with the approach to postinfarction LV aneurysms. Denton Cooley was the first to attempt to change the shape of the ventricle when he performed the first linear LV aneurysmectomy on cardiopulmonary bypass to treat a calcified LV aneurysm in 1958.[7]

Many other techniques and approaches were developed over the years to treat postinfarction ventricular aneurysms.[8] Jatene developed a technique of septoplasty and modified linear closure in the early 1980s.[9] At the same time, Vincent Dor and colleagues introduced the technique of endoventricular circular patch plasty, which later, in 1985, came to bear his name.[10] His approach was unique in that it approached akinetic areas and dyskinetic aneurysms equally. He later began to apply this technique to treat congestive heart failure and altered the way in which changes in ventricular morphology are approached. Cooley and colleagues later utilized a similar technique for aneurysmal resection by patching the anterior wall from within the ventricle but without the encircling purse-string suture to reduce the volume of the anterior wall of the LV.[11]

The concept of reconstructing the ventricle to a prescribed size based on the patient's body size was introduced by Dor and popularized by Menicanti.[12] The best methodology to determine the appropriate size of the reconstructed ventricle has yet to be determined. Some surgeons base it on the enlarged end-diastolic dimensions and others by indexed body surface area.[12] Additional technical approaches that merit mention include a linear closure and septoplasty approach described by Mickleborough and a concentric purse-string or "cerclage" technique followed by linear closure utilized by McCarthy.[17,18] The end result of two decades of surgical innovation is four techniques used for ventricular remodeling procedures today.

INDICATIONS FOR SURGERY

Classically, patients are candidates for SVR if they have had an anterior myocardial infarction, have a large area of akinesis or dyskinesis, and have clinical evidence of CHF. Specific characteristics of patients who have successfully undergone SVR are shown in Table 47-1. Ideal candidates have akinesis/dyskinesis in the anteroseptal area, have retained function of the basilar and lateral portions of the heart, and have good right ventricular function. They should also be candidates for revascularization and mitral valve repair if needed. Included in many clinical series of SVR are patients who have had anterior infarctions with areas of akinesis or dyskinesis who do not have heart failure. The indication for surgery in such patients is angina and the need for coronary artery revascularization. In such patients, the goal of therapy is to prevent dilation and the clinical development of CHF, which is an inevitable part of postinfarction remodeling.

Table 47-1	Indications for surgical ventricular restoration
Anteroseptal myocardial infarction	
NYHA Class 3 or 4 congestive heart failure	
Retained basilar heart function	
Depressed ejection fraction %	
Large area of akinesis/dyskinesis	
Asynergy of > 35% of left ventricle	
Enlarged ventricle	
End-diastolic volume index > 120 mL/m^2	
End-systolic volume index > 60 mL/m^2	
Candidate for valve repair/replacement	
Candidate for revascularization	
Good right ventricular function	

Relative contraindications are shown in Table 47-2. Many patients have additional cardiac conditions that will necessitate repair or replacement, and they should be candidates for surgical repair of any lesion that exists.

SURGICAL APPROACHES

The surgical goals of SVR include complete revascularization of all viable territories, exclusion of akinetic and dyskinetic segments with a concomitant reduction in the size of the nonfunctioning anteroseptal portion of the heart, recreation of the elliptical shape of the heart, and a repair of any valvular incompetence by valve repair or replacement.

Several different surgical approaches are used to achieve the goals stated above. Common among each of the approaches is the median sternotomy incision, which is standard in cardiac surgery. The surgical procedure begins with standard arterial and venous cannulation for cardiopulmonary bypass (CPB). If mitral valve repair or replacement is a strong possibility, cannulation of both the inferior and superior venae cavae is recommended. The LV can be vented directly through its apex, through the left atrium via the right superior pulmonary vein, or through the aortic root. Prior to systemic heparinization, femoral arterial access is obtained to make the later placement of an intraaortic balloon pump easier if necessary. Since concomitant coronary artery bypass grafting (CABG) is usually performed, the standard approach for CABG at that institution is utilized, including myocardial protection.

Once the patient is on CPB, the sequence of procedures performed is a matter of personal preference. Most commonly, CABG is performed first. Once this is accomplished, the SVR or mitral valve replacement (MVR) can be performed next. The author performs the MVR to avoid potential disruption of the ventricular reconstruction with retraction to expose the mitral valve.

Table 47-2	Relative contraindications to surgical ventricular restoration
Multiple areas of infarction	
Loss of basilar myocardial function	
Pulmonary hypertension and right ventricular dysfunction	
Unreconstructable coronary artery disease	

If necessary, the mitral repair can be done at any time utilizing any technique preferred. An intraventricular repair as described by Menicanti is done through the ventriculotomy prior to performing the SVR.[12] Our standard approach is to perform a reduction posterior annuloplasty through a standard interatrial groove incision prior to performing the SVR to avoid the remote possibility of disrupting our ventricular closure.

With the heart vented, the LV will often collapse, demonstrating the area of thinned out scar. If this does not happen, it may be due to a partial-thickness infarction. The absence of collapse does not contraindicate SVR; it simply means that revascularization occurred early enough to prevent full-thickness infarction.

The technique employed at Hopkins is a variation of the endoventricular circular patch plasty popularized by Vincent Dor. It is depicted in Figs. 47-1 to 47-7. The morphology of a normal ventricle and that of a ventricle with an abnormal anterior wall following an anterior infarction is shown in Figs. 47-1 and 47-2. An incision is made into the anterior wall of the LV through the area of scar (Fig. 47-3). In a typical anterior infarction, the incision is extended distally to the apex and proximally parallel to the course of the left anterior descending coronary artery until normal muscle is encountered. Retention sutures are placed into scar to aid in achieving and maintaining exposure (Fig. 47-4).

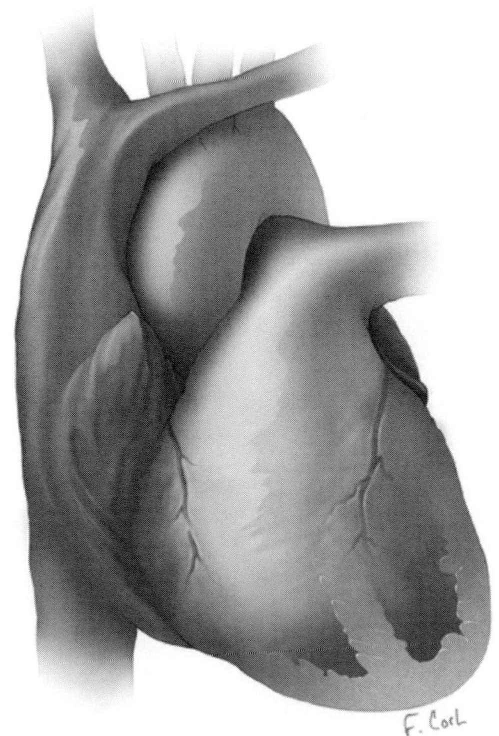

Figure 47-1 Normal heart.

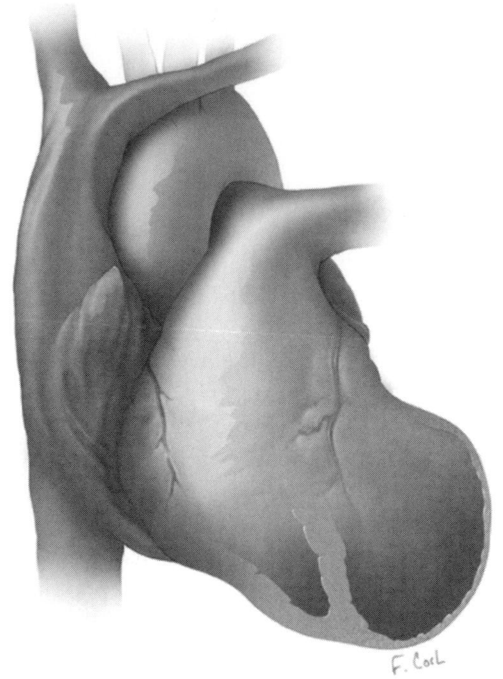

Figure 47-2 Heart with thinned akinetic ventricle following anterior wall myocardial infarction.

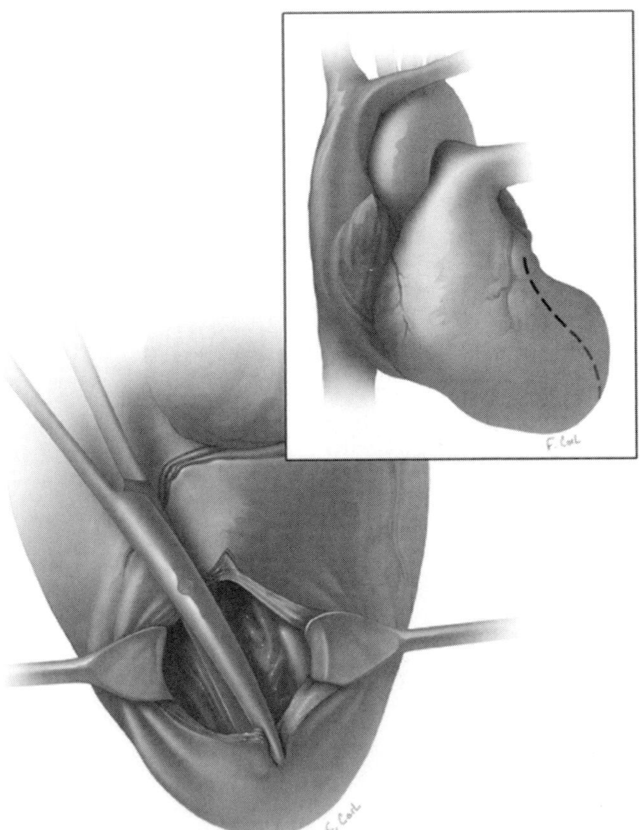

Figure 47-3 Anterior ventriculotomy parallel to the course of the left anterior descending coronary artery.

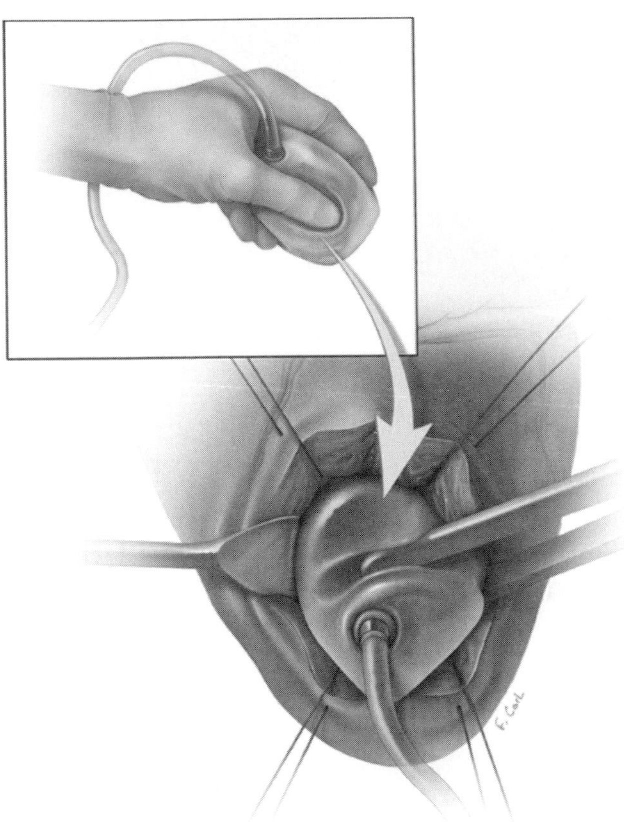

Figure 47-4 Insertion of ventricular sizing device following placement of retention sutures for exposure. The volume of the sizing device is selected on the basis of body surface area (50 to 60 mL/m^2).

The ventricle is inspected. Any thrombus is removed. During inspection of the ventricle, the extent as well as the transmurality of the scar are noted. A transition zone between infarcted and noninfarcted muscle is often palpable. This is particularly so with full-thickness infarctions but is notably absent in some patients who have received thrombolytics or percutaneous revascularization prior to widespread cell death. These patients demonstrate a mosaic pattern of ventricular scarring. Such ventricles often show akinesis rather than dyskinesis. The presence or absence of a transition zone is not known to be of clinical significance. The differences in the various operations are apparent from this point forward in the operation.

A sizing device is inserted into the ventricle to aid in ventricular sizing (Fig. 47-4). Our device is selected based on a volume of 50 to 70 mL/m^2 body surface area, with 55 to 60 mL/m^2 being chosen for most patients. Obese patients will have the volume titrated down to 50 mL/m^2 and cachectic patients will have it titrated up to 70 mL/m^2. At this point in the procedure, an encircling a purse string of 2-0 polypropylene suture is placed along the anterior border of the sizing device. Placement of the purse string is one of the key steps in the operation. It chooses the new apex of the heart and defines the outline of the new anterior wall. Selecting the location of the

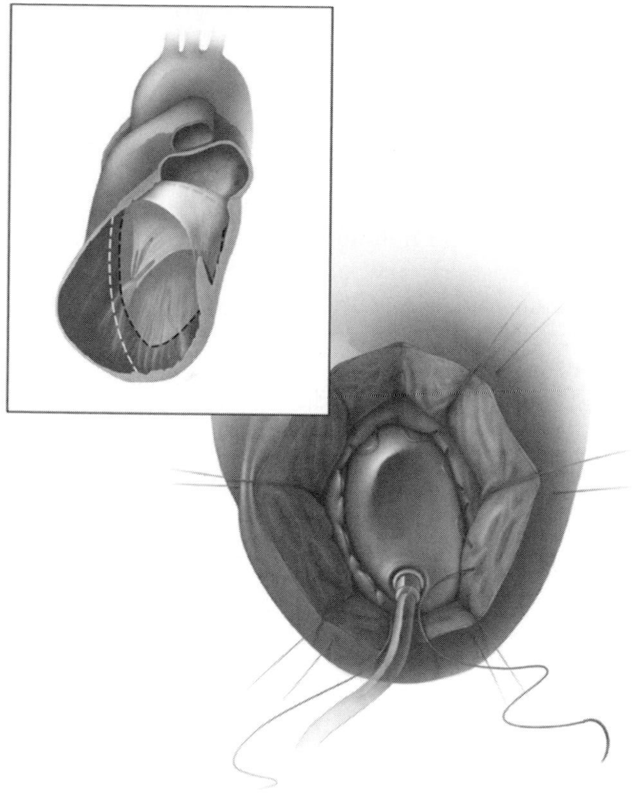

Figure 47-5 Placement of purse-string suture to define margins of reconstruction of anterior wall.

purse strings is usually done by personal preference. It can be done in a measured fashion, using one of several commercially available sizing devices, by selecting a site based on experience or proximity to a landmark such as the papillary muscles, or at the border of infarcted and noninfarcted tissue. Use of the "border zone" was most commonly recommended before the development of commercially available devices. If a sizing device is used, a variety of methods of determining the size of the device to be used have been recommended (Fig. 47-4).

Once the anterior wall is encircled with the purse-string suture, it is reconstructed utilizing a variety of techniques. It is important to place the purse string in such a fashion as to create an elliptical ventricle (Fig. 47-5). A patch of Dacron is used if the remaining defect is greater than 2 to 3 cm long. An oval patch is cut to the appropriate size and sutured in place, closing the defect. Care is taken to place the patch sutures around the anterior purse string. The patch may be sutured using a continuous or interrupted technique. Prior to completing the patch, the left ventricular vent is shut off, allowing the ventricle to fill with blood and forcing air to escape the ventricle through the partially completed closure (Fig. 47-6). After the patch is sutured into place, a linear closure is performed superficial to the patch or purse string. Horizontal mattress sutures, buttressed with bovine pericardium, are used as a first layer of closure. The second layer is a continuous running stitch of 2-0 polypropylene (Fig. 47-7).

If the defect is moderate in size but not large enough for patching, a series of anterior purse-string sutures can be placed to narrow the ventricular defect prior to placement of the mattress sutures.

A word should be mentioned about performing the SVR with the heart beating. One advantage is that poorly functioning, often ischemic ventricles are not further injured during the period of cardiac arrest. Another is that the degree of mitral regurgitation and the result of mitral repair can be assessed in a beating heart, which is felt by some to be advantageous. A final advantage is that it allows the border between contracting and noncontracting segments of the heart to be seen more clearly from within the ventricle, which may aid in performing the SVR. The disadvantage is that it is much more difficult to place the sizing device on the mitral annulus and keep it there to allow accurate placement of sutures. This disadvantage can be partially compensated for by tracing the outline of the margins of the sizer on the endocardium and then deflating the sizer. No good evidence supports any approach; however, the novice may be aided with cardiac arrest until experience is gained.

An alternative technique advocated by Linda Mickleborough employs a primary or patch septoplasty in conjunction with a linear closure to accomplish the same SVR surgical goals. This technique uses the same

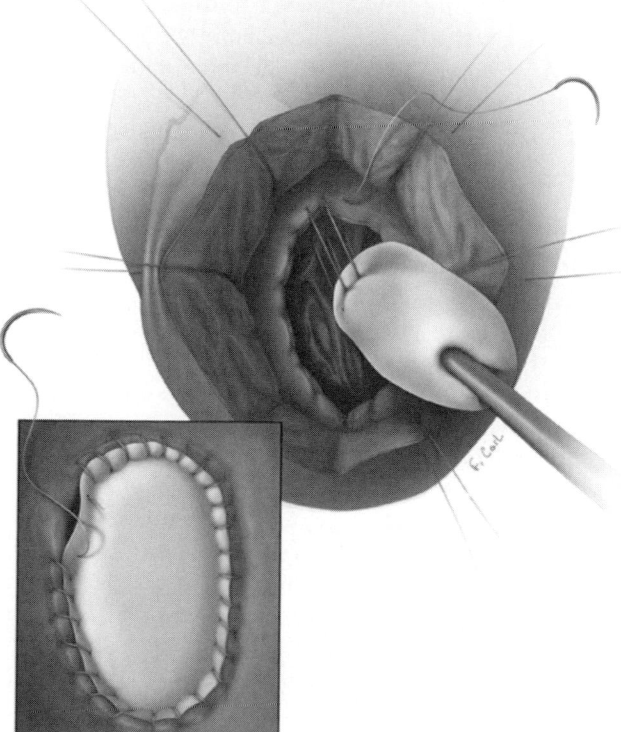

Figure 47-6 Patch closure reconstruction of anterior wall for residual ventriculotomy openings of greater than 3 cm. Smaller residual defects are closed primarily.

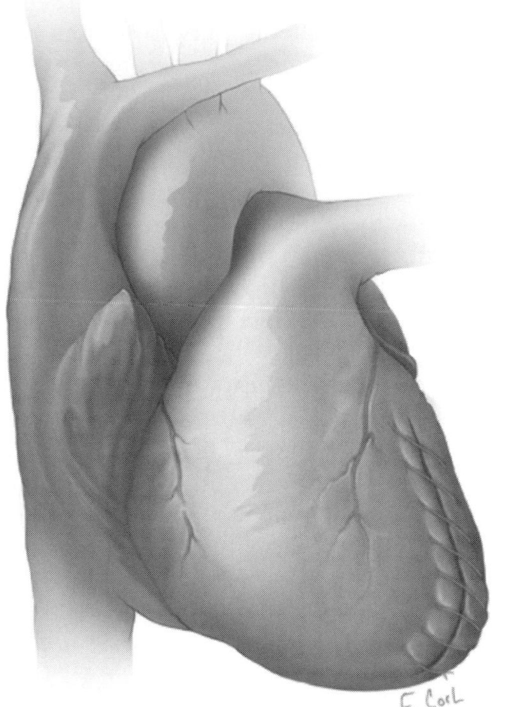

Figure 47-7 Two-layer closure of ventriculotomy. Horizontal mattress sutures are used for the first layer, followed by continuous running suture for the second layer.

anterior ventriculotomy approach to expose the septum and anterior wall. This technique employs a more traditional linear closure to exclude the akinetic or dyskinetic areas of the anterior wall. Additionally, the dilated, fibrotic areas of the infarcted septum are addressed by either including the septum in the linear closure of the anterior wall or patching the septum and including the patch in the linear closure.[13]

A technique of multiple purse strings is employed by Pat McCarthy. Also called the cerclage technique, it begins as do the previous two techniques. Once the anterior wall purse string is placed and tied, additional purse strings are placed a few millimeters superficial to the previous purse string. This continues anteriorly until the final remaining defect is small and is closed with a standard linear closure.[14]

A modified septoplasty technique, employed by Jatene, aimed to reduce the volume of the infarcted septum in conjunction with a patch or primary closure. This technique also begins in the same way as other SVR procedures. An anterior encircling purse string is placed to define the borders of the anterior wall, as is done in some of the other SVR techniques. The distinguishing characteristic of this technique is the placement of mattress sutures in the septum to reduce the horizontal length of the septum. Once the septal reduction is performed, the anterior encircling purse string is tied and the anterior wall closed primarily or with a patch.[9]

OUTCOMES

There is no consensus as to the optimal treatment of ischemic cardiomyopathy. Part of the reason for that is that there are no contemporary prospective randomized trials comparing similar groups of patients between medical therapy, CABG, and SVR with or without revascularization. There is an unlimited number of characteristics that any one study may not specify to ensure that the populations studied are the same as those of other studies. The presence or absence of viability, the presence of targets for revascularization, the location of infarction, and the presence of valvular disease or pulmonary hypertension are but a few making the point.

Much of the data on SVR often involve large, heterogeneous historical groups of patients whose diagnostic studies and evaluation, indications for surgery, surgical procedure, surgeon, follow-up, and many other factors may or may not have been the same, and the papers themselves may not spell them out very clearly.[18] Although most of the published data on outcomes from SVR procedures comes from single-center studies from centers with a great deal of experience, some published data come from a limited number of multicenter studies. Both types provide useful clinical information.[12,16–19]

The effectiveness of SVR can be assessed from a variety of different perspectives. Survival, morbidity, and functional outcomes are the most commonly utilized benchmarks. In a procedure whose functional outcomes are in part based on changing the size and shape of the heart, morphologic assessments are important considerations.

Menicanti and colleagues from Milan have a large experience of over 1000 patients. Their overall experience reflects many of the complicating issues noted above. The overall operative mortality was 7.2 percent for their group. It was lower (4.8 percent) in patients who underwent concomitant CABG, higher in patients with a preoperative EF below 30 percent (12.3 percent), with concomitant mitral valve procedures (15 percent), and in patients with NYHA class 4 symptoms (15.2 percent).[16] What is not easy to discern in this or any other single-institutional experience is exactly what the interplay of two or three of these factors is. It is logical that the risk would be higher. These investigators have identified that factors associated with adverse outcomes include worse NYHA functional class, EF below 20 percent, age above 70 years, urgent intervention, mitral valve procedure, pulmonary hypertension (Pulmonary $\text{Artery}_{\text{systolic pressure}} > 60$ mmHg), larger ventricles (End Diastolic Volume Index > 180 mL/m^2), the number and sites of previous myocardial infarctions, and right ventricular dysfunction.[12]

The optimal technique for performing SVR has not been determined. The personal beliefs of authors have been either implicitly suggested by the surgical technique utilized or studied by direct comparison, usually with a single institutional retrospective study.[16,17] Mickleborough and colleagues reported on 285 patients over a 20-year period utilizing a linear closure technique with (25 percent) or without septoplasty (75 percent). The excellent 5- and 10-year survival was 82 and 62 percent, respectively. As mentioned above, it is unclear whether the patient populations are the same. The study group included posterior infarcts and the data are presented together. In the anterior infarct group (appropriate for SVR), only 62 percent had CHF of an unknown severity despite having a low EF percent (mean 24 + 11 percent). Patients had to have a palpably thinned area in the anterior wall, and severe mitral regurgitation was an exclusion (only 1 percent had a valve intervention); moreover, the presence of calcified aneurysms excluded some patients. Despite these differences, the risk factors for poor outcomes were EF below 20 percent, CHF, ventricular tachycardias and hypertension—in all, not too dissimilar from the conclusions of other investigators.[19–21]

The returning RESTORE group (Reconstructive Endorventricular Surgery Torsion Original Radius Elliptical) is a collection of international centers performing SVR that have combined data to study the outcomes of the SVR procedure. The combined number of patients followed up by this group is 1198, operated on between 1998 and 2003. Most patients were in NYHA class 3 (40 percent) and class 4 (29 percent). Concomitant procedures included CABG in 95 percent, mitral valve repair in 22 percent, and replacement in 1 percent. This study represents what is probably the best large study to date in performing SVR in a heart failure population.

The RESTORE investigators found that global systolic function increased postoperatively and ventricular size decreased as measured by ventriculography, magnetic resonance imaging, or echocardiography. The ejection fraction increased from 29.6 + 11 to 39.5 + 12.3 percent. The LV end-systolic volume index (LVESVI) decreased from 80.4 + 51.4 mL/m^2 to 56.6 + 34.3 mL/m^2.

Survival was excellent in this group. Thirty-day mortality was 5.3 percent and the overall 5-year survival was 68.6 + 2.8 percent (Fig. 47-8). Logistic regression analysis was performed to identify risk factors for death at any time following surgery. These included preoperative EF below 30 percent, LVESVI above 80 mL/m^2, advanced NYHA functional class, and age above 75 years. Patients with an EF above 30 percent had a survival of 63.8 + 3.9 percent compared to 76.7 + 3.2 percent 76.7 + 3.2 percent for those with an EF above 30 percent and 83.0 + 4.0 percent with an EF of greater than 40 percent. The fact that many of these risk factors are the same or similar to those identified by both Menicanti and Mickleborough suggests the ability of single institutions to discover the same findings as seen in multicenter studies.[12,19,20]

Our group at Johns Hopkins has looked at the outcomes of groups of patients with severe advanced CHF. In one study, 100 percent of the patients had class 3 (34 percent) or class 4 (66 percent) CHF and

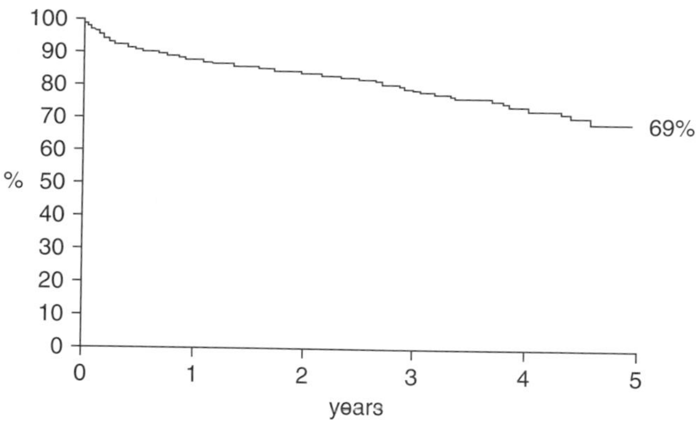

Figure 47-8 Overall 5-year survival curve from the RESTORE group. (Adapted from Athanasuleas et al.[19] with permission.)

an EF by magnetic resonance imaging below 20 percent, with 65 percent having an EF below 15 percent. Despite how sick these patients were, 69 percent improved to NYHA class 1 or 2, with a 1-year survival of 81 percent. Cox regression analysis demonstrated that preoperative diabetes, the use of an intraaortic balloon pump during surgery, incomplete revascularization, and a preoperative LV end-systolic volume index greater than 130 mL/m^2 were significant predictors of overall mortality.[21]

The Hopkins group also looked at the outcomes of SVR in patients who had multi-territory infarctions that had been contraindications in all previously published series. The finding that standard treatment of the anterior wall infarction, along with suture plication of the inferior wall for infarctions in the territory of the right coronary artery and the lateral wall for infarctions in the lateral wall opens the door to a potentially new patient population for this procedure.[22]

The group at the Cleveland Clinic investigated the impact of ventricular remodeling on the neuroendocrine axis following SVR. Several markers of the neurohormonal axis are elevated in congestive heart failure. This group investigated the plasma levels of norepinephrine, renin, and angiotensin II before and 1 year following SVR as well as brain natriuretic peptide before and 3 months following SVR. They found that SVR reduced norepinephrine by 56 percent, angiotensin II by 60 percent, renin activity by 56 percent, and brain natriuretic peptide by 36 percent.[23]

One of the most interesting studies of the effect of SVR on cardiac function was performed by DiDonato and colleagues at the Center Cardiothoracique do Monaco. They looked at 30 patients undergoing SVR who did not have electrical dysynchrony by QRS definition but did have mechanical dysynchrony. Pressure/volume (P/V) loops were obtained with intraventricular micromanometer-tipped catheters and

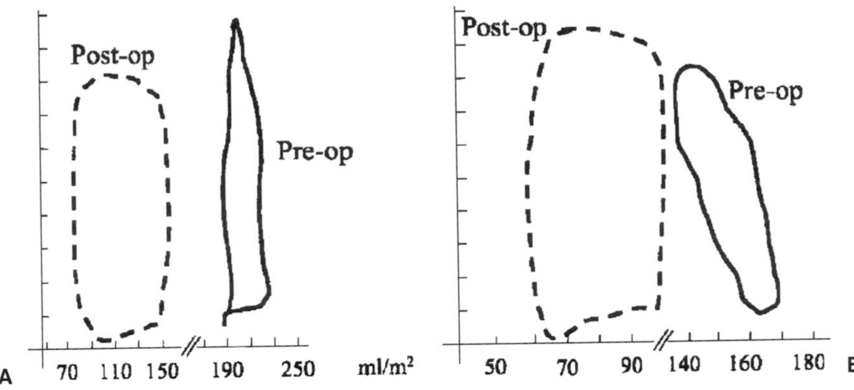

Figure 47-9 Pre- and post-operative pressure volume loops. (Adapted from DiDonato et al.[18] with permission.)

pressure/length (P/L) loops were created by analysis of ventriculograms utilizing the centerline method at 45 discrete intervals. The P/V loops of these patients were very abnormal in size, shape, and orientation, with impaired isometric phases and a rightward shift. Endocardial time motion was either early or late, yielding P/L loops that were abnormal in size, shape, and orientation. Postoperatively, SVR resulted in a leftward shift of the P/V loops, with their near normalization, as well as normalization of endocardial motion and P/L loops (Fig. 47-9). These physiologic results of SVR occurred in concert with improved EF (30 + 13 to 45 + 12 percent), reduced end-diastolic and systolic volume indices (202 + 76 to 122 + 48 mL/m^2 and 144 + 69 to 69 + 40 mL/m^2, respectively), a more rapid peak filling rate (1.75 + 0.7 to 2.32 + 0.7 EDV/s), peak ejection rate (1.7 + 0.07 to 2.6 + 0.09Sv/s), and calculated measurements of mechanical efficiency.[18]

CONCLUSIONS

In summary, SVR is a procedure that has evolved from a treatment for ventricular aneurysms and has become a treatment of CHF. It has been shown to improve ventricular size, morphology, LV ejection fraction, stroke-volume index, endocrine markers of CHF, ventricular energetics, ventricular synchrony, and mechanical efficiency. Clinically, it results in improved functional capacity (NYHA class) and an excellent 5-year survival in very sick patients. It is an excellent treatment option in appropriately selected patients with ischemic cardiomyopathy. Where SVR will fit in the armamentarium of a heart failure team will be institution-dependent based on their expertise and experience. Further studies are needed to better define the appropriate patients, the basis of the beneficial response (ventricular physiology versus relief of ischemia), the optimal technique, and the appropriate time to perform the procedure. Much remains to be worked out.

References

1. Gheorghiade M, Bonow R. Chronic heart failure in the United States: A manifestation of coronary artery disease. *Circulation* 1998;97:282–289.
2. Levy D, Kenchaiah S, Larson MG, et al. Long-term trends in the incidence of and survival with heart failure. *N Engl J Med* 2002;347:18.
3. Ghaudron P, Eilles CI, Kugler I, Ertl G. Progressive left ventricular dysfunction and remodeling after myocardial infarction: Potential mechanisms and early predictors. *Circulation* 1993;87:755–763.
4. DiDonato M, Sabatier M, Toso A, et al. Regional myocardial performance of non-ischemic zones remote from anterior wall left ventricular aneurysm. *Eur Heart J* 1995; 16:1285–1292.
5. Fauchier L, Marie O, Cassett D, et al. Intraventricular and interventricular dyssynchrony in idiopathic dilated cardiomyopathy: A prognostic study with Fournier phase analysis of radionucleotide angioscintigraphy. *J Am Coll Cardiol* 2002;40:2022–2030.
6. White HD, Norris RM, Brown PW, et al. Left ventricular end systolic volume as the major determinant of survival after recovery from myocardial infarction. *Circulation* 1987;76:44–51.
7. Cooley DA, Collins HA, Hall GA, et al. Ventricular aneurysm after myocardial infarction: Surgical excision with use of temporary cardiopulmonary bypass. *JAMA* 1958;167:557.
8. Mills NL, Everson CT, Hockmuth D, et al. Technical advances in the treatment of left ventricular aneurysm. *Ann Thorac Surg* 1993:55:972–800.
9. Jatene AD. Left ventricular aneurysmectomy: Resection or reconstruction? *J Thorac Cardiovasc Surg* 1985;89: 321–331.
10. Dor V, Kreitmann P, Jourdan J. Interest of "physiological" closure of left ventricle after resection and endocardiectomy for aneurysm or akinetic zone comparison with classical technique about a series of 209 left ventricular resections (abstr). *J Cardiovasc Surg* 1985;26:73.

11. Cooley D. Ventricular endoaneurysmorrhaphy: A simplified repair for extensive postinfarction aneurysm. *J Cardiac Surg* 1989;4:200–205.
12. Menicanti L, DiDonato M. The Dor procedure: What has changed after fifteen years of clinical practice? *J Thorac Cardiovasc Surg* 2002;124:886–890.
13. Mickelborough LL. Left ventricular reconstruction for ischemic cardiopathy. *Semin Thorac Cardiovasc Surg* 2002; 14:144–149.
14. Caldiera C, McCarthy PM. A simple method of left ventricular reconstruction without patch for ischemic cardiomyopathy. *Ann Thorac Surg* 2001;72:2148–2149.
15. Doenst T, Velazquez EJ, Beyersdorf B, et al. To STITCH or not to STITCH: We know the answer, but do we know the question? *J Thorac Cardiovasc Surg* 2004;129: 246–249.
16. Tavakoli R, Bettex, Webber A, et al. Repair of postinfarction dyskinetic LV aneurysm with either linear or patch technique. *Eur J Cardiothorac Surg* 2002;22:129–134.
17. Lunblad R, Abdelnoor M, Svenning JL. Surgery for left ventricular aneurysm: Early and late survival after simple linear repair and endoventricular patch plasty. *J Thorac Cardiovasc Surg* 2004;128:449–456.
18. DiDonato M, Toso A, Dor V, et al. Surgical ventricular restoration improves mechanical ventricular dyssynchrony in ischemic cardiomyopathy. *Circulation* 2004;109: 2536–2543.
19. Athanasuleas CL, Buckberg GD, Stanley AW, et al. Surgical ventricular restoration in the treatment of congestive heart failure due to post–infarction ventricular dilation. *J Am Coll Cardiol* 2004;44:1439–1445.
20. Mickleborough LL, Merchant N, Ivanov I, et al. Left ventricular reconstruction: Early and late results. *J Thorac Cardiovasc Surg* 2004;128:127–137.
21. Patel ND, Williams JA, Barreiro CD, et al. Surgical ventricular remodeling for multi territory myocardial infarction: Defining a new patient population. *J Thorac Cardiovasc Surg* 2005,130:1698–1706.
22. Patel ND, Williams JA, Barreiro CD, et al. Surgical ventricular remodeling for patients with clinically advanced congestive heart failure and severe left ventricular dysfunction (EF < 20%). *J Heart Lung Transplant* 2005;29: 2202–2210.
23. Schenk S, McCarthy PM, Starling RC, et al. Neurohormonal response to left ventricular reduction surgery in ischemic cardiomyopathy. *J Thorac Cardiovasc Surg* 2003;128:38–43.

CHAPTER

48 MINIMALLY INVASIVE CARDIAC SURGERY

François Dagenais, Pierre Voisine, Patrick Mathieu

INTRODUCTION

The midline sternotomy incision offers excellent access to all cardiac structures and has been the traditional route for the performance of most cardiac operations. Improvements in myocardial protection techniques and intensive care unit management, coupled with refinements in perfusion techniques, have reduced perioperative mortality and morbidity linked to cardiac surgery. Results of conventional coronary artery bypass grafting (CABG) have been overtly studied and demonstrate exceptional outcomes, as evidenced by graft patency rates of over 90 percent at 15 years for the anastomosis of left internal mammary artery (LIMA) to the left anterior descending artery (LAD).[1] On the other hand, with the growth and advancement of percutaneous interventional techniques (e.g., coronary angioplasty and stenting), patients have demonstrated a willingness to undergo procedures with less favorable mid- and long-term outcomes compared to CABG largely to enjoy lower periprocedural risks and less invasiveness. In response to this, cardiac surgeons have, over the past decade, progressively developed less invasive operations to provide the benefits of standard cardiac procedures with less morbidity. Through the use of innovative surgical approaches combined with new technology, cardiac surgeons introduced a new spectrum of minimally invasive operations. The avoidance of cardiopulmonary bypass (CPB) and/or the full median sternotomy incision is the main feature common to this new generation of procedures. This chapter describes and discusses the evolution and results of minimally invasive CABG, mitral and aortic valve replacement and repair, and other cardiac operations.

MINIMALLY INVASIVE CORONARY ARTERY BYPASS GRAFTING

Although the first attempts to revascularize ischemic myocardium were accomplished on a beating heart, the advent of CPB with cardioplegic arrest offered a reliable and highly reproducible means to perform CABG.

KEY CONCEPTS

- Innovations in alternative methods for cannulation and cardiopulmonary bypass, new visualization systems, retractors and stabilizers, and robotic platforms have facilitated the development of minimally invasive cardiac surgery.
- Compared to conventional surgical approaches, early experiences with minimally invasive valve surgery have produced acceptable, reproducible results in experienced centers with measurable benefits in the form of reduced perioperative morbidity and enhanced patient satisfaction.
- Totally endoscopic coronary bypass grafting remains hindered by the inherent technical complexities of the operation.
- Early experiences with robot-assisted mitral valve repair have proved promising.
- Minimally invasive robot-assisted approaches are being successfully applied to other cardiac operations, including the closure of atrial septal defects, resection of cardiac tumors, and laser transmyocardial revascularization.
- High-quality training programs in minimally invasive approaches will be required to ensure safe outcomes.

During the mid 1990s, in an attempt to circumvent the need for sternotomy, surgeons developed a procedure to create a LIMA-to-LAD anastomosis through a small left anterior thoracotomy. In this procedure, termed minimally invasive direct coronary artery bypass (MIDCAB), the LIMA is harvested through a left anterior thoracotomy or limited sternal split incision with the assistance of a variety of chest retractors. A stabilizer is subsequently applied on the beating heart, thus facilitating performance of the coronary anastomoses (Fig. 48-1). Coronary occlusion is obtained proximally by snaring the coronary artery with a Silastic tape. Early experiences reported good graft patency rates.[2,3] In a literature review, Baer and colleagues[4] reported early mortality rates of 0 to 4.9 percent, conversion rates of 0 to 6.2 percent, and a peak reintervention rate (i.e., graft failure) of 8.9 percent. Furthermore, the incidence of postoperative pulmonary dysfunction, pain management, and atrial fibrillation appeared to be reduced with MIDCAB procedures compared to single-vessel bypasses performed under CPB through a midline sternotomy.[5–7] MIDCAB procedures have also been applied with success to coronary reoperations.[8] Comparisons of MIDCAB to LAD angioplasty and stenting demonstrate significantly higher rates of repeat revascularization with angioplasty, particularly in diabetic patients.[9] Other surgical approaches (e.g., subxiphoid) were developed to revascularize other coronary arteries.[10] Despite the purported advantages of MIDCAB, these minimally invasive procedures remain technically more challenging and require longer operative times with a higher rate of anastomotic revision compared to LIMA-to-LAD anastomoses performed through a standard sternotomy.[11,12]

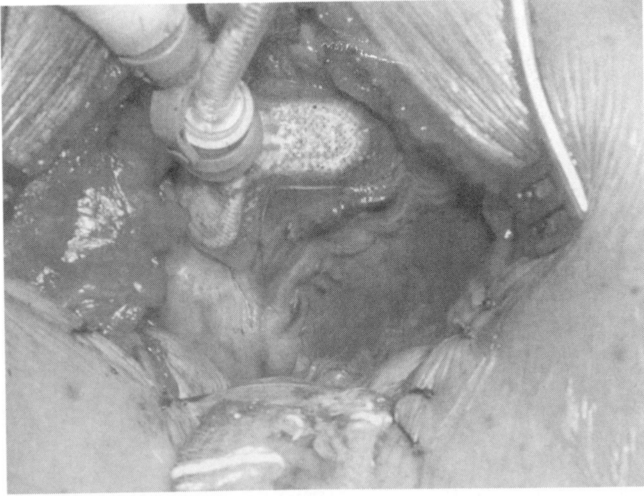

Figure 48-1 Exposure and stabilization of right coronary artery (RCA) and posterior descending artery (PDA) using EndoStarfish via a transabdominal approach. [From Subramanian VA, Patel NU, Patel NC, et al. Robotic assisted multivessel minimally invasive direct coronary artery bypass with port-access stabilization and cardiac positioning: Paving the way for outpatient coronary surgery? *Ann Thorac Surg* 2005;79(5):1590–1596. With permission.]

Parallel to the development of MIDCAB procedures, a Port-Access thoracoscopic system was designed to permit the use of cardiopulmonary bypass and cardioplegic arrest via peripheral cannulation. Through a similar left anterior thoracotomy used with MIDCAB, surgeons have performed multivessel coronary bypass on the arrested heart using this thoracoscopic approach. However, this approach did not gain widespread acceptance owing to its technical complexity and high procedural costs. Furthermore, as for MIDCAB procedures, wound complications—including incisional hernia, wound dehiscence or infection, and chronic pain—have been reported in up to 9.1 percent of patients[13] undergoing thoracoscopic coronary revascularization. Such wound complications, which are often a source of significant morbidity, are mainly linked to the excessive rib spreading required to harvest the LIMA through a limited thoracotomy. To minimize wound complications, surgeons developed a procedure to harvest the LIMA with a standard thoracoscope, thus minimizing such rib spreading.[14] Although reports demonstrate the feasibility of this procedure, long operative times and technical pitfalls limited the use of this approach.

More recently, with the advent of surgical robotics, robot-assisted LIMA harvest has been developed. The enhanced stereoscopic vision and dextrous instrumentation afforded by robotics greatly facilitate the LIMA harvest; robot-assisted LIMA harvest can be performed in as little as 30 to 40 min in most experienced centers. The LIMA is harvested as a pedicle or may also be skeletonized. The right IMA may also be mobilized by opening the right pleural space.[15] Once the LIMA is harvested, the pericardium is opened, the LAD is identified, and the anterior thoracotomy is tailored accordingly. The anastomosis is performed on a stabilized beating heart. A randomized trial comparing pain scores after manual and robot-assisted endoscopic LIMA takedown showed a significant decrease in postoperative pain with the endoscopic technique.[16]

TOTALLY ENDOSCOPIC CORONARY ARTERY BYPASS (TECAB)

Several dedicated centers have actively pursued the development of robot-assisted totally endoscopic coronary artery bypass (TECAB) grafting on the beating and arrested heart. The first successful TECAB performed on a human arrested heart was performed by Loulmet and colleagues in 1998.[17] With this approach, the LIMA is harvested, femorofemoral cardiopulmonary bypass is initiated, and the heart is arrested by occluding the ascending aorta with an endovascular balloon (e.g., Endoclamp) and infusing cardioplegic solution into the aortic root. The coronary anastomosis is performed in a running fashion using robotic instrumentation passed into the chest via modified thoracoscopic ports.

Despite the initial successes, significant technical limitations are associated with TECAB. First, aortic cross-clamp and cardiopulmonary bypass times are usually much greater than with standard techniques. Second, the procedure is generally limited to a single bypass to the LAD, although successful double-vessel TECAB operations have also been reported.[18] In experienced hands, conversion rates to sternotomy are less than 10 percent. Graft patency rates range from 95 to 100 percent at discharge and 96 percent at 3 months postoperatively.[19] The added cost of the Port-Access system and the prolonged cardiopulmonary bypass times have currently limited widespread adoption of this procedure. In an attempt to eliminate the use of cardiopulmonary bypass, TECAB procedures have also been performed on the beating heart. Significant technical challenges had to be surmounted, including the determination of optimal robotic thoracoscopic port placement, the limited working space, vessel stabilization, anastomotic construction, and the lack of tactile feedback. Continuous CO_2 insufflation of the thoracic cage augments working space, although pressures exceeding 10 mmHg have been demonstrated to induce significant hemodynamic changes.[20] Development of an endoscopic stabilizer (Fig. 48-2) coupled to an irrigation port facilitates the performance of a continuous anastomosis. Successful clinical cases have been described using either the da Vinci (Fig. 48-3) (Intuitive Surgical, Sunnyvale, CA) or the Zeus (Computer Motion, Goleta, CA) telemanipulation systems.[21,22] However, as expected, operative and LAD occlusion times are long and the conversion rates remain high. To ensure a safer and more reliable operation, further technological refinements are needed. Improvements in imaging technologies, telemanipulation systems, and endoscopic stabilizers will optimize surgical exposure and anastomotic construction. Direct suturing of the coronary anastomosis remains difficult and time-consuming. Development of distal anastomotic devices may facilitate the performance of TECAB anastomoses on the beating heart. However, variations in patient anatomy, such as intramyocardial LAD or excessive epicardial fat, significantly limit the applicability of these techniques. In such circumstances, the use of endoscopic ultrasound or other imaging modalities may prove useful for the accurate identification of coronary vessels. Although the current literature supports the feasibility of TECAB on the beating heart using computer-assisted surgical robotic systems, cost issues, limited clinical indications, and a steep learning curve currently limit the widespread use of this technology. Robot-assisted minimally invasive coronary artery bypass surgery remains in its evolutionary stage. Its success will be predicated on a methodical approach, combining improvements in both technology and in surgical techniques.

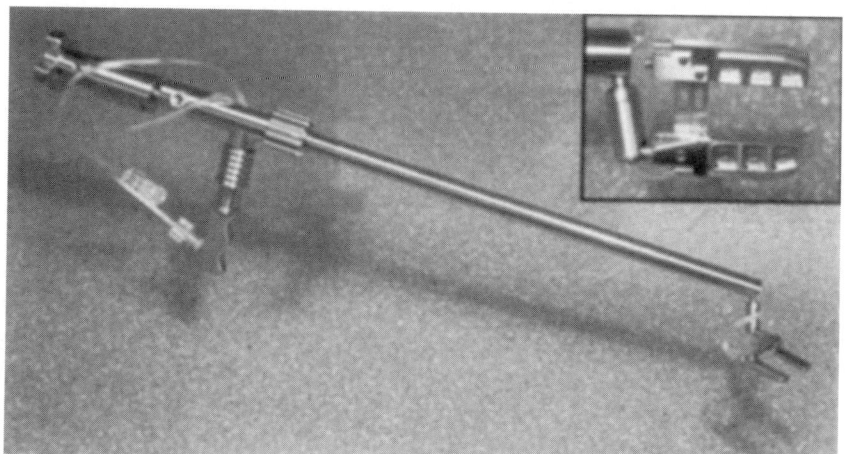

Figure 48-2 A novel, deployable EndoOctopus tissue stabilizer, also fixed to the operating table rail like the original Octopus,[8] was introduced through the right upper trocar for local cardiac wall immobilization. Insert: enlargement of endoscopic suction stabilizer pods viewed from below. [Photograph from Grundeman PF, Budde R, Beck HM, et al. Endoscopic exposure and stabilization of posterior and inferior branches using the EndoStarfish cardiac positioner and the EndoOctopus stabilizer for closed-chest beating heart multivessel CABG: Hemodynamic changes in the pig. *Circulation* 2003;108(Suppl 1):II34–II38. With permission.]

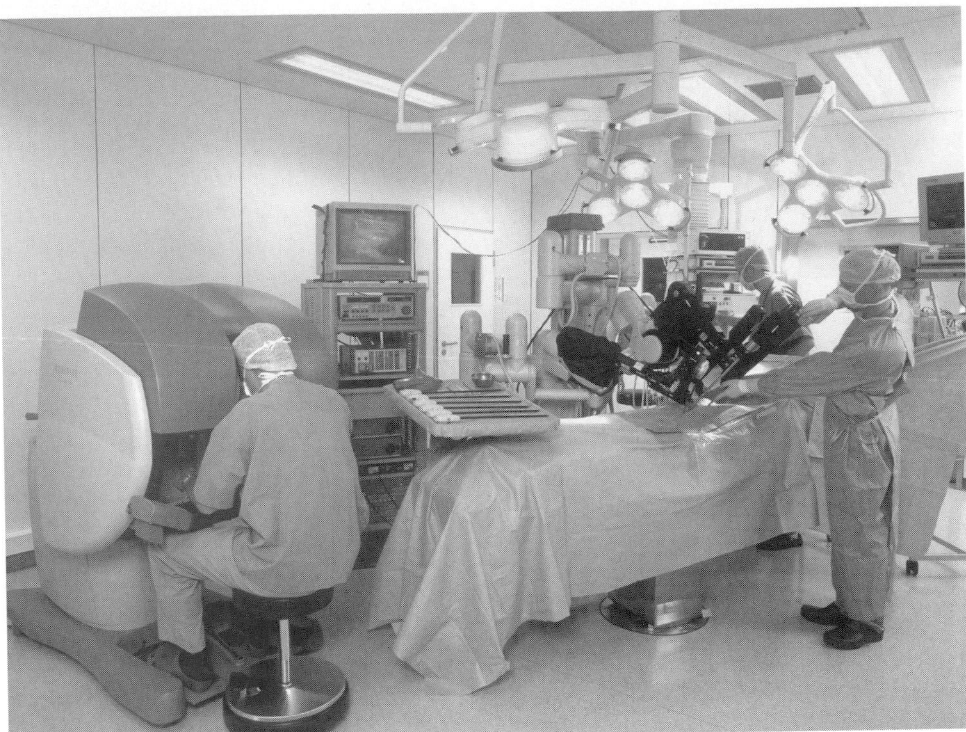

Figure 48-3 The da Vinci surgical robotic system. This system consists of a "slave" robotic platform controlled by the surgeon, who sits at a "master" console equipped with manual actuators and a dual-camera stereoscopic optical system. (Photograph courtesy of Intuitive Surgical, Sunnyvale, CA.)

MINIMALLY INVASIVE VALVE SURGERY

Although mitral valve operations have been performed through thoracotomy incisions during the modern era of cardiac surgery, the midline sternotomy remains the standard approach for mitral and aortic valve operations. Since the 1980s, mitral valve repair techniques have evolved to a high art. Experiences gained with mitral valve repair operations have proved them safe, reproducible, and durable procedures. Recent advancements in surgical techniques and myocardial protection for mitral and aortic valve surgery performed via midline sternotomy are reflected in lower rates of mortality and morbidity. During the mid-1990s, surgeons designed new minimally invasive approaches to the mitral and aortic valves to decrease morbidity while maintaining the excellent outcome standards previously set with mitral and aortic valve operations.

Minimally invasive mitral valve operations

In efforts to avoid a complete midline sternotomy, surgeons found that the mitral valve could be exposed adequately through different incisional approaches. The Cleveland Clinic group initially advocated a parasternal route but subsequently shifted to an upper partial sternotomy. Reporting their experience in a large cohort of patients using an upper partial sternotomy, Cosgrove and colleagues showed similar perioperative results as obtained through a standard complete sternotomy.[23] Other partial sternotomy approaches have also been described, such as the subxiphoid approach, consisting of a transverse skin incision overlying the xiphoid process with an inverted J-type ministernotomy carried out after skin undermining.[24] These techniques have the advantage of allowing central cannulation for CPB and good valve exposure. On the other hand, sternal splitting is still required.

During the same time frame, experimental work conducted at Stanford University led to the development of the Port-Access Endo-CPB system[25] (Fig. 48-4). As described previously, this technology utilizes peripheral CPB perfusion and an endovascular balloon catheter for aortic occlusion. Initial reports by groups in Leipzig and at New York University demonstrated the feasibility of mitral valve repair through a limited right thoracotomy incision and CPB conducted with the Port-Access platform.[26,27] The operation requires meticulous planning. Physical examination and peripheral Doppler studies may be required to exclude significant peripheral vascular disease. The procedure is carried out with a double-lumen endotracheal tube to permit selective single-lung ventilation. The right chest is elevated at approximately

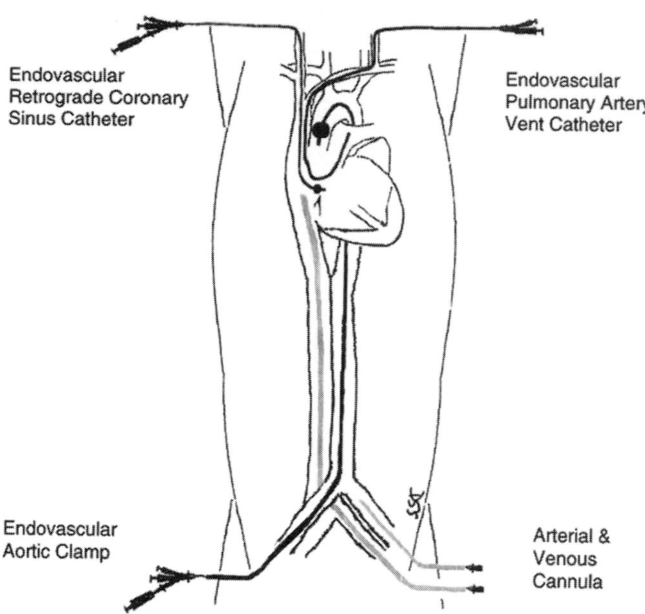

Figure 48-4 Schematic diagram outlining the Port-Access EndoCPB system. The venous and arterial cannulas are connected to the bypass pump. The endovascular aortic clamp is inserted through the femoral artery. The pulmonary artery vent is inserted through the left jugular vein, and the percutaneous venting catheter is inserted through the right jugular vein. [From Schwartz DS, Ribakove GH, Grossi EA, et al. Minimally invasive mitral valve replacement: Port-Access technique, feasibility, and myocardial functional preservation. J Thorac Cardiovasc Surg 1997;113(6):1022–1030. With permission.]

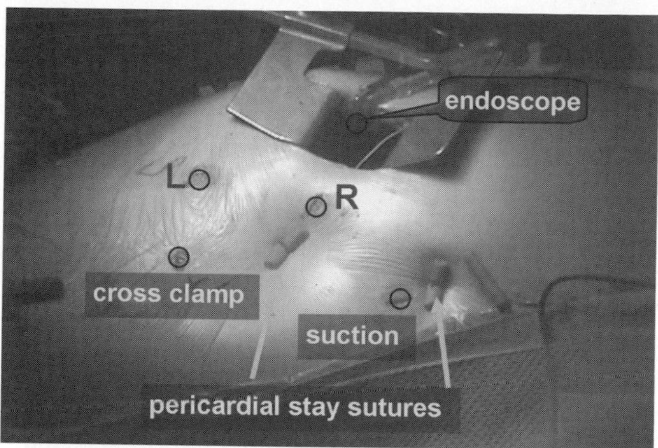

Figure 48-5 Right minithoracotomy approach to the mitral valve using the Port-Access EndoCPB platform. The thoracotomy extends from a point just lateral to the right nipple's areola along a 4- to 8-cm course laterally along the fourth intercostal space. (Photo courtesy of Intuitive Surgical, Sunnyvale, CA.)

30 degrees from the plane of the operating table. The anesthesiologist inserts a percutaneous retrograde coronary sinus catheter and pulmonary vent under transesophageal echocardiographic guidance and confirms their position by fluoroscopy. A 5- to 7-cm incision in the right inframammary fold is created and the thorax is entered at the level of the fourth intercostal space (Fig. 48-5). A soft-tissue retractor is inserted within the wound. Femoral vessel cannulation for CPB is performed through a transverse groin skin incision. A 21F or 23F dual-limb arterial cannula is inserted into the common femoral artery using the Seldinger technique. A 21F venous cannula is subsequently inserted into the femoral vein and directed into the superior vena cava under echocardiographic guidance. Venous drainage is augmented by vacuum assist once CPB has been initiated. In patients with significant peripheral vascular disease, central aortic cannulation may be initiated through a third intercostal incisional approach. The ascending aorta is either clamped with an external cross clamp or by inflating an intraaortic Endoclamp. After selecting the Endoclamp, a 10.5F triple-lumen catheter is inserted through the side arm of the arterial cannula. The catheter tip is positioned 1 to 2 cm above the sinotubular junction and the balloon is inflated. Position is verified throughout the operation by echocardiography; pressure damping in the right radial pressure may suggest balloon migration. Cardioplegia is delivered either through the proximal port of the Endoclamp or through the coronary sinus catheter in cases of external aortic clamping. The intracardiac procedure is conducted according to standard techniques using specifically designed long-shafted instruments. Such a procedure requires a dedicated team experienced with the operative technique and knowing the procedure pitfalls. Anaesthesiologists must be skilled echocardiographers, particularly for catheter positioning and identifying balloon migration. Perfusionists must be accustomed to the peripheral CPB platform and Endoclamp technology. A new "comfort zone" must be established among the surgical team members, since cardiac structures are not as easily accessible as through a standard sternotomy. Early experience demonstrated similar outcomes compared to a standard sternotomy in terms of valvuloplasty success and operative mortality.[28] Compared to the standard sternotomy, perioperative morbidity in terms of blood loss, ventilator time, analgesic requirement, and hospital stay appears to be reduced with the right thoracotomy approach.[29] Patient satisfaction is high and hospital costs are reduced.[30] Moreover, sternal wound complications are avoided and patients usually return to work within a month after the operation. The right minithoracotomy approach is particularly useful in reoperative mitral valve surgery in the setting of patent coronary artery bypass grafts.[31] In cases where a right thoracotomy approach is contraindicated (e.g., previous right thoracotomy, prior right chest irradiation), a left posterior minithoracotomy approach using endoCPB support has been shown to be feasible with acceptable perioperative morbidity and mortality.[32] Complications reported with

this approach include femoral or iliac artery perforations and aortic dissection, thus reemphasizing the necessity of training and expertise with this new technology.

The encouraging results obtained with the right minithoracotomy Port-Access procedure stimulated surgeons to pursue experimentation to further develop the field of minimally invasive mitral surgery. With the advent of videoscopic technology in most surgical specialities, cardiac surgeons investigated the possibility of adding videoscopic assistance to minimally invasive mitral surgery. Carpentier was the first to perform a video-assisted mitral repair via a minithoracotomy in 1996.[33] With videoscopic assistance, the length of the minithoracotomy may be shortened to 4 to 6 cm with minimal rib spreading. Initially, simple valve repair or mitral valve replacement procedures were performed with this approach. With experience, complex valve repairs were successfully performed. In an attempt to ensure camera stability and image quality, the AESOP 3000 (Computer Motion, Santa Barbara, CA), a voice-activated robotic camera, was evaluated in minimally invasive videoscopic mitral surgery. With this device, the operating surgeon verbally commands the camera movements, providing direct eye-brain coordination. Camera motion is predictable, image stability is reliable, and the need for lens cleaning is minimized. The AESOP 3000 enables the surgeon to perform most of the mitral procedure under videoscopic guidance. Similar clinical outcomes were realized in comparisons of the direct vision and the AESOP 3000 videoscopic approaches, although significantly shorter CPB and cross-clamp durations were observed with the AESOP videoscopic procedures, thus validating the advantages of augmented imaging modalities.[34]

With the development of telemanipulation systems came the advent of fully endoscopic mitral surgery. The da Vinci surgical robotic system utilizes stereoscopic optics, articulated tip instruments with seven degrees of freedom similar to the human wrist, and computer-mediated motion scaling and tremor filtering. In May 1998, using the da Vinci system, Carpentier and colleagues performed the first complete robot-assisted mitral valve repair.[35] Further reports by Mohr and Chitwood documented the feasibility of the technique.[36,37] Within a recent phase II FDA trial involving 10 institutions, 112 patients underwent complete robotic mitral repair (Fig. 48-6).[38] Although the perioperative morbidity and mortality as well as early mitral valve competence were acceptable, the 2.1 ± 0.1 h of cross-clamp time and 2.8 ± 0.1 h of cardiopulmonary bypass duration reflected the complexity of this approach. Although operative times appear to decrease with experience, the annuloplasty band placement remains rate-limiting owing to the difficulties in knot tying during robotic procedures. New innovations such as nitinol "U clips" (Coalescent Surgical Inc., Sunnyvale, CA) have replaced manual knot tying and significantly reduced the time required for annuloplasty band placement. In summary, minimally invasive mitral valve surgery has proven to be a safe, reliable, and durable operation in competent hands. Reported benefits have taken the form of less blood product requirements, fewer short-term complications, shorter recovery times, and enhanced patient satisfaction. The introduction of robotics to cardiac surgery has ushered in a new era in the development of fully endoscopic cardiac operations. Widespread use of this expensive technology within the cardiac surgical community will require new innovations to simplify the procedure and the establishment of comprehensive training programs.

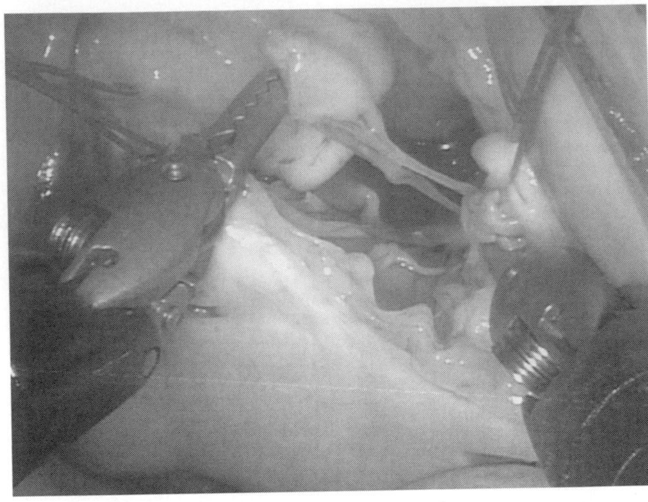

Figure 48-6 Visualization of the mitral valve using the da Vinci surgical robotic system. (Photo courtesy of Intuitive Surgical, Sunnyvale, CA.)

Minimally invasive aortic valve surgery

During the last decade, the quest to reduce patient morbidity from cardiac operations led surgeons to develop approaches to avoid a complete sternotomy in performing aortic valve surgery. Various surgical techniques have been proposed. The inverted "T" partial upper sternotomy was reported initially (Fig. 48-7).[39] Variations were subsequently proposed, such as a "J" upper partial sternotomy, an "I" sternotomy performed between the second and fifth intercostal spaces, a "T"-shaped lower sternotomy, and a "C" ministernotomy, leaving the upper and lower ends of the sternum intact.[40–42] Other authors advocated a right parasternal incision. Cosgrove and colleagues initially advocated a right parasternal incision, with excision of the third and fourth costal cartilages.[43] They abandoned this approach in favor of a partial upper ministernotomy due to occasional anterior chest wall instability after costal resection. Other authors proposed the same parasternal approach without rib resection, thus maintaining the integrity of the chest wall.[44] All of these approaches permit central cannulation and good exposure of the left ventricular outflow track, aortic valve, and ascending aorta.

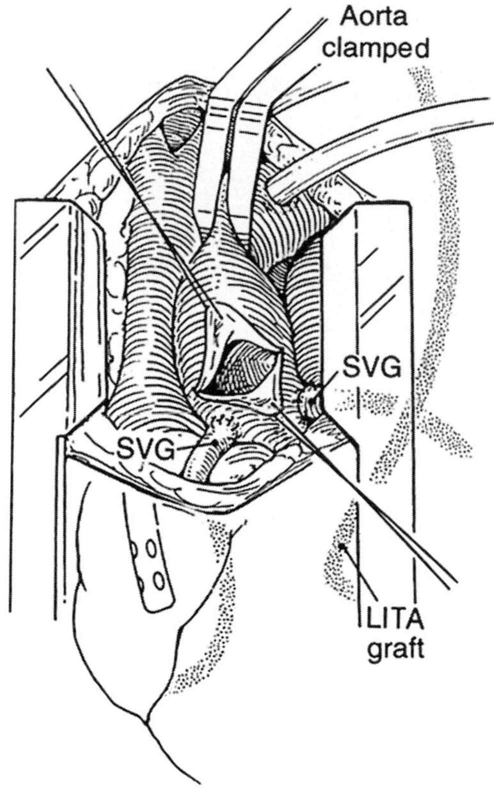

Figure 48-7 Inverted "T" upper partial sternotomy approach to the aortic valve after prior coronary bypass. The previous sternotomy incision is exposed to the third (or fourth) intercostal space and extended laterally to the right or bilaterally, as needed, for exposure. After dissection of the ascending aorta, with particular attention to the position of patent CABG conduits and their proximal anastomoses, cannulation is performed. (In this example, the ascending aorta and innominate vein, but frequently other cannulation sites, are required because of space limitations.) The ascending aorta is cross-clamped and aortic valve replacement is conducted in standard fashion. LITA = left internal thoracic artery; SVG = saphenous vein graft. [From Byrne JG, Aranki SF, Couper GS, et al. Reoperative aortic valve replacement: Partial upper hemisternotomy versus conventional full sternotomy. *J Thorac Cardiovasc Surg* 1999;118(6):991–997.]

Cardioplegia is usually administered in an antegrade fashion. A retrograde coronary sinus catheter may be inserted through the right atrium or percutaneously through the jugular vein. Continuous carbon dioxide is infused within the mediastinum to minimize the risk of liberated air emboli after aortic unclamping. Following the initiation of cardiopulmonary bypass, the aortic valve operation is conducted using standard techniques.

Reports assessing outcomes of minimally invasive aortic valve procedures show early mortality comparative to procedures performed with the conventional median sternotomy approach.[45,46] Reported benefits took the form of reduced blood product requirements, mechanical ventilation times, postoperative pain, and incidence of postoperative supraventricular arrhythmias.[47,48] Candaele and colleagues, comparing outcomes of a partial upper sternotomy to a standard full sternotomy, showed improved postoperative pulmonary function linked to a reduction in pain.[49] Conversely, Szwerc and colleagues were unable to demonstrate any advantage among patients undergoing a minimally invasive aortic valve approach,[50] and Riess cautioned that incomplete opening of the pericardium in minimally invasive aortic valve procedures may lead to earlier tamponade.[51] Consequently adequate chest tube drainage should be used and instruments for emergent sternotomy should be available in the intensive care unit.

OTHER MINIMALLY INVASIVE CARDIAC OPERATIONS

The acceleration of new technologies supporting minimally invasive cardiac surgery has encouraged surgeons to design new approaches to treat different cardiac diseases. Robotic surgery has been applied to correct some congenital defects, including coarctation of the aorta, atrial septal defects, and congenital mitral abnormalities.[52,53] Measurable benefits in terms of quality of life have been documented in patients undergoing robotic closure of atrial septal defects (Fig. 48-8).[54]

With the combined development of new devices and innovative surgical techniques, the surgical treatment of atrial fibrillation ablation has seen a spectacular transformation from the classic time-consuming cut-and-sew Maze operations to fully robotic procedures for epicardial isolation of the pulmonary vein (Fig. 48-9).[55]

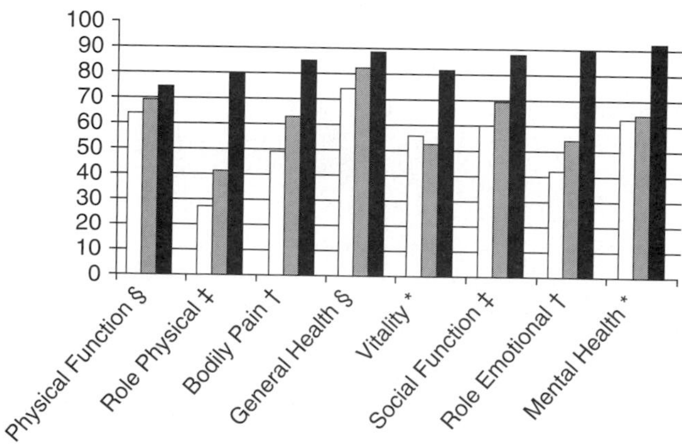

Figure 48-8 Results of SF-36 for robotic (black bars), minithoracotomy (striped bars), and sternotomy (white bars) patients on postoperative day 30. * = $p < 0.001$; † = $p < 0.01$; ‡ = $p < 0.05$; § = $p < 0.05$. (From Morgan et al.[54] With permission.)

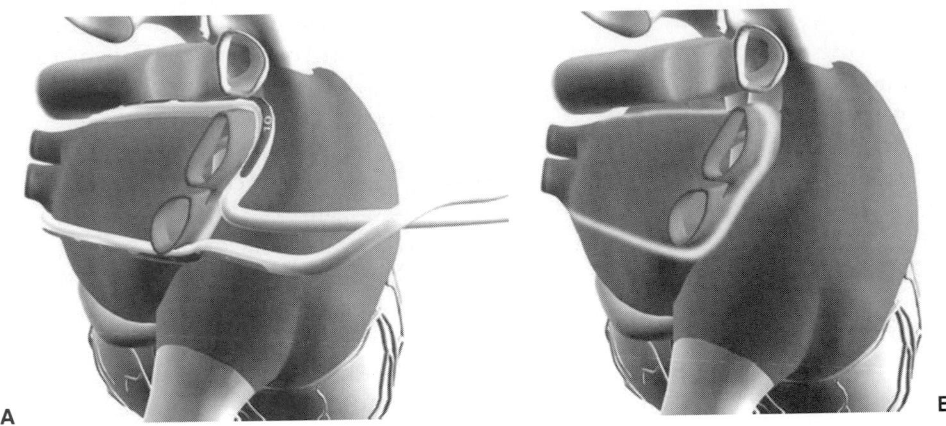

Figure 48-9 Minimally invasive pulmonary vein isolation for atrial fibrillation. A flexible radiofrequency antenna is deployed around all four pulmonary veins via a minimally invasive technique (e.g., robotic right minithoracotomy). An isolating lesion is then created, thus ablating aberrant conduction pathways. (Reproduced with permission from Guidant Corp., Indianapolis, IN.)

Minimally invasive procedures have also been applied to epicardial biventricular lead placement (Fig. 48-10), pericardial window, tricuspid valve surgery, the excision of cardiac tumors[56,57] as well as laser transmyocardial revascularization (Fig. 48-11).[58] Further research will be required to optimize patient selection for these types of procedures and determine the full benefits of these new operations.

CONCLUSIONS

During the past decade, innovations in alternative methods for cannulation and cardiopulmonary bypass, new visualization systems, retractors and stabilizers, and robotic platforms have paved the way for new and exciting developments in minimally invasive cardiac surgery. Compared to conventional surgical approaches, early experiences

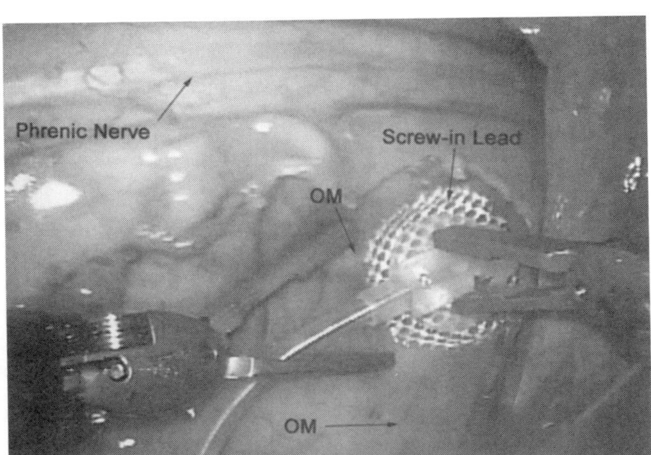

Figure 48-10 Robot-assisted biventricular epicardial lead placement using the da Vinci system. [From Derose JJ Jr, Belsley S, Swistel DG, et al. Robotically assisted left ventricular epicardial lead implantation for biventricular pacing: The posterior approach. *Ann Thorac Surg* 2004;77(4): 1472–1474.]

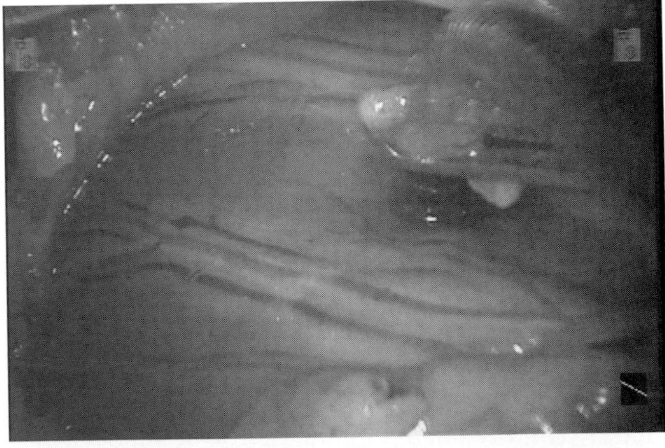

Figure 48-11 Robot-assisted transmyocardial revascularization. A flexible transmyocardial laser probe is manipulated by the da Vinci instrumentation and precisely placed over the segment of the left ventricular wall to be treated. (From Yuh DD, Simon BA, Fernandez A, et al. Totally endoscopic robot-assisted transmyocardial revascularization. *J Thorac Cardiovasc Surg* 2005;130(1):120–124. In press. With permission.)

with minimally invasive valve surgery have produced excellent reproducible results in experienced centers with measurable benefits in the form of reduced perioperative morbidity and enhanced patient satisfaction. TECAB procedures remain hindered by the inherent technical complexities of the operation. Through further technological advancements and the development of new surgical strategies, TECAB procedures may be performed with more ease, safety, and reproducibility. Cardiac surgeons will apply these new technologies to other cardiac applications. Although this expensive technology is currently restricted to centers dedicated to minimally invasive approaches, technical refinements and evidence-based data confirming the benefits of these approaches should contribute to the widespread adoption of these techniques. To ensure the maintenance of the high standards set by conventional cardiac surgery, high-quality training programs in minimally invasive approaches will be required and will definitely constitute a challenge in the upcoming years.

References

1. Camcron A, Davis KB, Green G, et al. Coronary bypass surgery with internal-thoracic-artery grafts: Effects on survival over a 15–year period. *N Engl J Med* 1996;334:216–219.
2. Mack MJ, Magovern JA, Acuff TA, et al. Results of graft patency by immediate angiography in minimal invasive coronary artery surgery. *Ann Thorac Surg* 1999;68: 383–389.
3. Diegler A, Spyrantis N, Matin M, et al. The revival of surgical treatment for isolated proximal high grade LAD lesions by minimally invasive coronary artery bypass grafting. *Eur J Cardiothorac Surg* 2000;17:501–504.
4. Kettering K, Dapunt O, Baer FM. Minimally invasive direct coronary artery bypass grafting: A systematic review. *J Cardiovasc Surg (Torino)* 2004;45:255–264.
5. D'Amato TA, Savage EB, Wiechmann RJ, et al. Reduced incidence of atrial fibrillation with minimally invasive direct coronary artery bypass. *Ann Thorac Surg* 2000;70: 2013–2016.
6. Lichtenberg A, Hagl C, Harringer W, et al. Effects of minimal invasive coronary artery bypass on pulmonary function and postoperative pain. *Ann Thorac Surg* 2000;70: 461–465.
7. Wray J, Al-Ruzzeh S, Mazrani W, et al. Quality of life and coping following minimally invasive direct coronary artery bypass (MIDCAB) surgery. *Qual Life Res* 2004;13: 915–924.
8. Miyaji K, Wolf RK, Flege JB Jr. Minimally invasive direct coronary artery bypass for redo patients. *Ann Thorac Surg* 1999;67:1677–1681.
9. Shirai K, Lansky AJ, Mehran R, et al. Minimally invasive coronary artery bypass grafting versus sternotomy for patients with proximal left anterior descending coronary artery disease. *Am J Cardiol* 2004;93:959–962.
10. Benetti F, Dullum MK, Stamou SC, et al. A xiphoid approach for minimally invasive coronary artery bypass surgery. *J Card Surg* 2000;15:244–250.
11. Detter C, Reichenspurner H, Boehm DH, et al. Single vessel revascularization with beating heart techniques: Minithoracotomy or sternotomy? *Eur J Cardiothorac Surg* 2001;19:464–470.
12. Vicol C, Nollert G, Mair H, et al. Midterm results of beating heart surgery in 1-vessel disease: Minimally invasive direct coronary artery bypass versus off-pump coronary artery bypass with full sternotomy. *Heart Surg Forum* 2003;6:341–344.
13. Ng PC, Chua AN, Swanson MS, et al. Anterior thoracotomy wound complications in minimally invasive direct coronary artery bypass. *Ann Thorac Surg* 2000;69: 1338–1340.
14. Nataf P, Al-Attar N, Ramadan R, et al. Thoracoscopic IMA takedown. *J Card Surg* 2000;15:278–282.
15. Cichon R, Kappert U, Schneider J, et al. Robotically enhanced "Dresden technique" with bilateral internal mammary artery grafting. *Thorac Cardiovasc Surg* 2000; 48:189–192.
16. Bucerius J, Metz S, Walther T, et al. Pain is significantly reduced by cryoablation therapy in patients with lateral minithoracotomy. *Ann Thorac Surg* 2000;70:1100–1104.
17. Loulmet D, Carpentier A, d'Attellis N, et al. First endoscopic coronary artery bypass grafting using computer assisted instruments. *J Thorac Cardiovasc Surg* 1999; 118:4–10.
18. Aybeck T, Dogan S, Andreben E, et al. Robotically enhanced totally endoscopic right internal thoracic coronary artery bypass to the right coronary artery. *Heart Surg Forum* 2000;3:322–324.
19. Dogan S, Aybeck T, Anderson E, et al. Totally endoscopic coronary artery bypass grafting on cardiopulmonary bypass with robotically enhanced telemanipulation: Report of forty-five cases. *J Thorac Cardiovasc Surg* 2002;123: 1125–1131.
20. Falk V, Jacobs S,Gummert JF, et al. Computer-enhanced endoscopic coronary artery bypass grafting: The da Vinci experience. *Semin Thorac Cardiovasc Surg* 2003;15: 104–111.
21. Falk V, Diegler A, Walther, et al. Total endoscopic off-pump coronary artery bypass grafting. *Heart Surg Forum* 2000;3:29–31.
22. Boyd WD, Kodera K, Stahl KD, et al. Current status and future directions in computer-enhanced video- and robotic-assisted coronary bypass surgery. *Semin Thorac Cardiovasc Surg* 2002;14:101–109.
23. Cosgrove DM III, Sabik JF, Navia JL. Minimally invasive valve operations. *Ann Thorac Surg* 1998;65:1535–1538.
24. Karagoz HY, Bayazit K, Battaloglu B, et al. Minimally invasive mitral valve surgery: The subxiphoid approach. *Ann Thorac Surg* 1999;67:1328–1332.
25. Stevens JH, Burdon TA, Peters WS, et al. Port-access coronary artery bypass grafting: A proposed surgical method. *J Thorac Cardiovasc Surg* 1996;111:567–573.
26. Falk V, Walther T, Diegler A, et al. Echocardiographic monitoring of minimally invasive mitral valve surgery using an endoaortic clamp. *J Heart Valve Dis* 1996;5:630–637.
27. Colvin SB, Galloway AC, Ribakove G, et al. Port-access mitral valve surgery: Summary of results. *J Card Surg* 1998;13:286–289.

28. Galloway AC, Grossi EA, Applebaum RM, et al. Minimally invasive port-access valvular surgery: Initial clinical experience. *Circulation* 1997;96 (suppl 1):508.
29. Felger JE, Chitwood WR Jr, Nifong LW, et al. Evolution of mitral valve surgery: Toward a totally endoscopic approach. *Ann Thorac Surg* 2001;72:1203–1208.
30. Grossi EA, LaPietra A, Ribakove GH, et al. Minimally invasive versus sternotomy approaches for mitral reconstruction: Comparison of intermediate-term results. *J Thorac Cardiovasc Surg* 2001;121: 708–713.
31. Onnasch JF, Schneider F, Falk V, et al. Minimally invasive approach for redo mitral valve surgery: A true benefit for the patient. *J Card Surg* 2002;17:14–19.
32. Saunders PC, Grossi EA, Sharony R, et al. Minimally invasive technology for mitral valve surgery via left thoracotomy: Experience with forty cases. *J Thorac Cardiovasc Surg* 2004;127:1026–1032.
33. Carpentier A, Loulmet D, LeBret E, et al. Chirurgie à Coeur ouvert par video-chirurgie et mini-thoracotomie: Premier cas (valvuloplastie mitrale) opéré avec succès. *Comptes Rendus de L`Académie des Sciences: Sciences de la vie* 1996;319:219–223.
34. Chitwood WR. Robot-assisted mitral valve surgery. In: *Advanced Therapy of Cardiac Surgery.* Hamilton, Ontario, Canada: Decker, 2003:220–229.
35. Carpentier A, Loulmet D, Aupecle B, et al. Computer assisted open-heart surgery. First case operated on with success. *CR Acad Sci II* 1998;321:437–442.
36. Chitwood WR Jr, Nifong LW, Elbeery JE, et al. Robotic mitral valve repair: Trapezoidal resection and prosthetic annuloplasty with the da Vinci surgical system. *J Thorac Cardiovasc Surg* 2000;120:1171–1172.
37. Falk V, Walter T, Autschbach R, et al. Robot-assisted minimally invasive solo mitral valve operation. *J Thorac Cardiovasc Surg* 1998;115:470–471.
38. Kypson AP, Nifong W, Chitwood WR Jr. Robotic mitral valve surgery. *Semin Thorac Cardiovasc Surg* 2003; 15:121–129.
39. Navia JL, Cosgrove DM III. Minimally invasive mitral valve operations. *Ann Thorac Surg* 1996;62:1542–1544.
40. Svensson LG. Minimal-access ¨J¨ or ¨j¨ sternotomy for valvular, aortic, and coronary operations or reoperations. *Ann Thorac Surg* 1997;64;1501–1503.
41. Aris A. Reversed ¨C¨ ministernotomy for aortic valve replacement. *Ann Thorac Surg* 1999;67:1806–1807.
42. Doty DB, DiRusso GB, Doty JR. Full-spectrum cardiac surgery through a minimal incision: Ministernotomy (lower half) technique. *Ann Thorac Surg* 1998;65: 573–577.
43. Arom KV, Emery RW. Minimally invasive mitral operations. *Ann Thorac Surg* 1997;63:1219–1220.
44. Sharony R, Grossi EA, Ribakove GH, et al. Minimally invasive cardiac valve surgery. In: *Advanced Therapy of Cardiac Surgery.* Hamilton, Ontario, Canada: Decker, 2003:147–155.
45. Mihaljevic T, Cohn LH, Unic D, et al. One thousand minimally invasive valve operations: Early and late results. *Ann Surg* 2004;240:529–534.
46. Gillinov AM, Banbury MK, Cosgrove DM. Hemisternotomy approach for aortic and mitral valve surgery. *J Card Surg* 2000;15:15–20.
47. Liu J, Sidiropoulos A, Konertz W. Minimally invasive aortic valve replacement (AVR) compared to standard AVR. *Eur J Cardiothorac Surg* 1999;16:S80–S83.
48. Lee JW, Lee SK, Choo SJ, et al. Routine minimally invasive aortic valve procedures. *Cardiovasc Surg* 2000;8: 484–490.
49. Candaele S, Herijgers P, Demeyere R, et al. Chest pain after partial upper versus complete sternotomy for valve surgery. *Acta Cardiol* 2003;58:17–21.
50. Szwerc MF, Benckart DH, Wiechmann RJ, et al. Partial versus full sternotomy for aortic valve replacement. *Ann Thorac Surg* 1999;68:2209–2213.
51. Riess FC, Löwer C, Bleese N. Prevention of potential complications after minimal access aortic valve replacement. *Ann Thorac Surg* 1998;66:1866.
52. Cannon JW, Howe RD, Dupont PE, et al. Application of robotics in congenital cardiac surgery. *Semin Thorac Cardiovasc Surg Pediatr Surg Annu* 2003;6:72–83.
53. Torracca L, Ismeno G, Quarti A, et al. Totally endoscopic atrial septal defect closure with a robotic system: Experience with seven cases. *Heart Surg Forum* 2002;5: 125–127.
54. Morgan JA, Peacock JC, Kohmoto T, et al. Robotic techniques improve quality of life in patients undergoing atrial septal defect repair. *Ann Thorac Surg* 2004;77: 1328–1333.
55. Gerosa G, Bianco R, Buja G, et al. Totally endoscopic robotic-guided pulmonary veins ablation: An alternative method for treatment of atrial fibrillation. *Eur J Cardiothorac Surg* 2004;26:450–452.
56. DeRose JJ, Ashton RC, Belsley S, et al. Robotically assisted left ventricular epicardial lead implantation for biventricular pacing. *J Am Coll Cardiol* 2003;41: 1414–1419.
57. Kypson AP, Glower DD. Minimally invasive tricuspid operation using port access. *Ann Thorac Surg* 2002;74: 43–45.
58. Yuh DD, Simon BA, Fernandez A, et al. Totally endoscopic robot-assisted transmyocardial revascularization. *J Thorac Cardiovasc Surg* 2005;130:120–124.

CHAPTER

49 ECHOCARDIOGRAPHY IN CARDIAC SURGERY

Samia Mora, Katherine C. Wu

PRINCIPLES OF ECHOCARDIOGRAPHY

Since 1976, echocardiography (echo) has been used to evaluate cardiac structure and function. Echo uses sound in the high-frequency range (2 to 10 MHz). Frequency ranges between 2 and 5 MHz are typically used for imaging adults, while frequencies of 7.5 to 10 MHz are used for children and specialized adult applications. The transducer contains a piezoelectric crystal that converts electrical to sound energy, producing sound waves that are transmitted in the form of a beam. A complete transthoracic echocardiogram (TTE) consists of a group of interrelated applications including two-dimensional (2D) anatomic imaging, M-mode, and three Doppler techniques: pulsed-wave (PW), continuous-wave (CW), and color-flow (CF) imaging.[1–7] In addition, the quantification of cardiac chamber dimensions, areas, and volumes is an important aspect of a complete examination. Using a combination of these ultrasound techniques, one can assess the anatomy and function of the cardiac valves, myocardium, and pericardium.

TWO-DIMENSIONAL ECHOCARDIOGRAPHY

Standard views are obtained along three orthogonal planes of the left ventricle (LV): long-axis, short-axis, and the 4-chamber plane (Fig. 49-1A to C). The long axis is parallel to the long axis of the LV. The short axis cuts the LV cross-sectionally, similar to slices of bread in a loaf, and is orthogonal to the long axis. Four standard transducer locations are used to obtain complete visualization of the entire heart: parasternal, apical, subcostal, and suprasternal.

M-MODE ECHOCARDIOGRAPHY

M mode is a one-dimensional "ice pick" view of the heart (Fig. 49-1D) and is often used for measuring LV systolic and diastolic chamber dimensions and wall thickness.

DOPPLER ECHOCARDIOGRAPHY

The Doppler effect is the phenomenon whereby the frequency of sound waves increases or decreases as the sound source moves toward or away from the observer. The resultant Doppler frequency shift can be detected and translated into blood-flow velocity. The velocity of blood can then be used to calculate valvular gradients and areas, intracardiac pressures, and volumetric flow.

Pulsed-wave doppler

Pulsed-wave (PW) Doppler is obtained when a pulse of ultrasound is transmitted intermittently, allowing for estimation of blood-flow velocity at a specific region of interest. It is thus "site-specific." Its disadvantage is aliasing (or wraparound) of the signal at velocities that are one-half of the pulse repetition frequency (Nyquist limit). This property limits the maximal velocity that can be accurately measured with PW.

Continuous-wave doppler

Continuous-wave (CW) Doppler records all the velocities along the path of the ultrasound beam. Using CW, the magnitude of the blood-flow velocity and its direction can be accurately recorded. Its disadvantage is that it does not allow localization of the specific site of the velocity obtained along the beam path. CW is used to measure high-velocity jets associated with valvular dysfunction or intracardiac pressure gradients. The simplified Bernoulli equation can then be used to convert velocities into pressure gradients ($\Delta P = 4V^2$).

Color-flow doppler

Color-flow (CF) Doppler transforms Doppler velocity information into a color-coded scheme. Red denotes

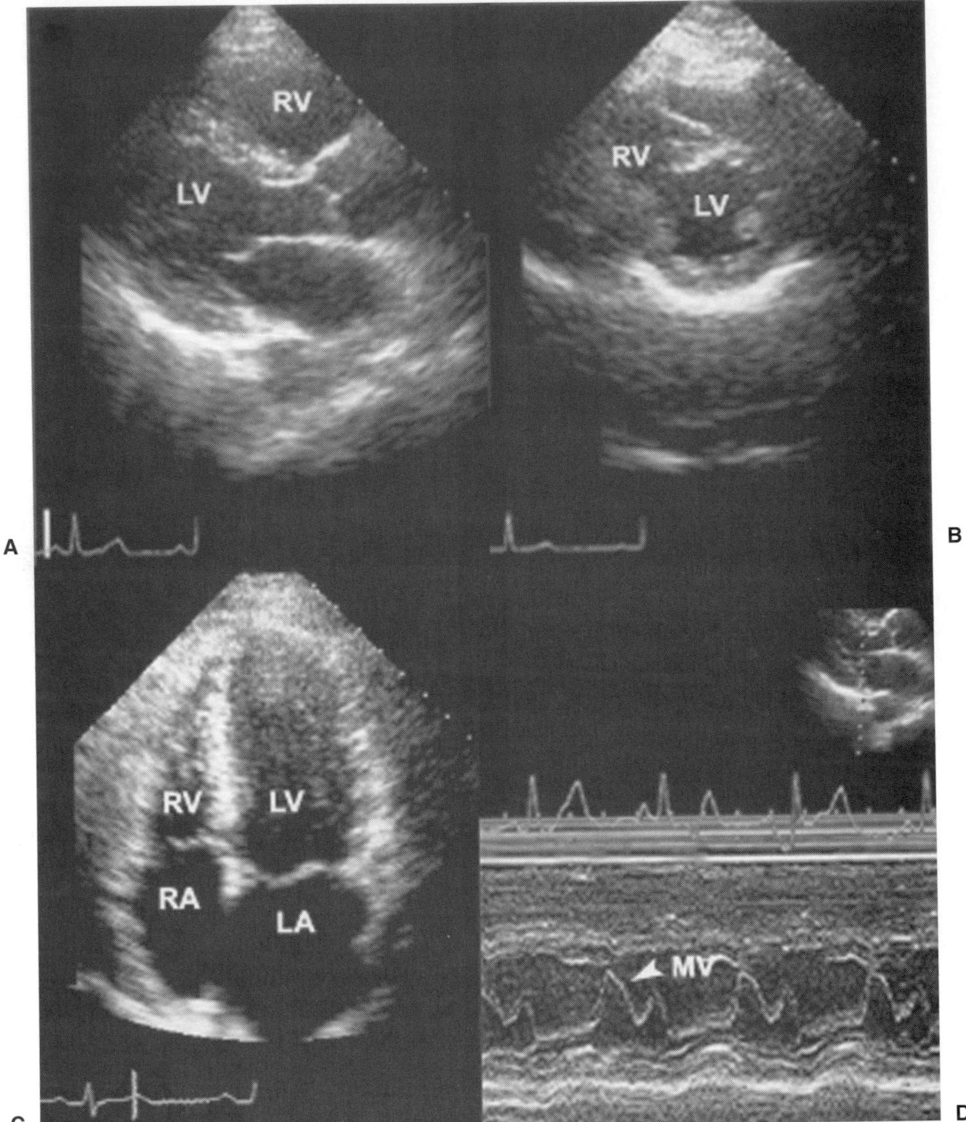

Figure 49-1 Standard 2D TTE (A to C) and M-mode (panel D) views in a normal individual. A. Parasternal long-axis view of the right ventricle (RV), interventricular septum, left ventricle (LV) cavity and posterior wall, and both mitral and aortic valves. Since the RV is the most anterior structure, it will be located closest to the transducer beam and is seen at the top of the image display, while the LV and LA (both posterior structures) are farther away from the transducer and are seen at the bottom of the image. B. Parasternal short-axis view of the ventricles at the papillary muscle midventricular level obtained by rotating the transducer 90 degrees. C. Apical four-chamber view, important for evaluation of ventricular function, apical thrombus, mitral and tricuspid valve function. D. M-mode view through the RV and mitral leaflets. This view is useful for detecting RV diastolic collapse in tamponade.

flow toward the transducer, while blue represents flow away from the transducer. The relative velocity of blood flow is also depicted, with brighter shades of blue or red representing higher velocities. Turbulent flow is seen as multicolored jets (e.g., due to valvular disease or intracardiac shunts).

TRANSESOPHAGEAL ECHOCARDIOGRAPHY

TEE was first introduced clinically in the United States in the 1980s. By placing an echocardiographic probe in the esophagus, which is in close proximity to cardiac structures, TEE obtains significantly enhanced images with excellent resolution. The development of transducer crystals that rotate from 0 to 180 degrees also allows for examination of each cardiac structure from different planes and angles. Acquisition of images is from two basic locations: midesophageal (30 to 35 cm from the incisors) and midgastric (40 to 45 cm from the incisors).

Indications

TEE is useful for the evaluation of patients with limiting body habitus, such as obesity or emphysema, who are not optimally imaged by the transthoracic approach. In addition, certain structures that are not well visualized by transtracheal echo (TTE) [such as the left atrial (LA) appendage, thoracic aorta, and prosthetic valves] can be assessed by the transesophageal approach. A third common indication is to guide intraoperative management during cardiac surgery. Class I indications for perioperative TEE (conditions for which there is evidence and/or general agreement that TEE is useful and effective) are listed in Table 49-1.[8] There are other situations in which TEE may also be useful but is not required (i.e., class II indications: conditions in which there is a divergence of opinion about the usefulness/efficacy of a procedure but in which the weight of opinion is in favor of usefulness/efficacy). These include ongoing surgical procedures in patients at increased risk of myocardial ischemia or hemodynamic instability, during minimally invasive surgery or the Cox-Maze procedure cardiac tumor resection or aneurysm repair, intracardiac thrombectomy or pulmonary embolectomy, for detection of intracardiac air or aortic atheromatous disease, and for selecting anastomotic sites during heart/lung transplantation.[8] Antibiotic prophylaxis for infective endocarditis is usually unnecessary but is optional in the high-risk patient (e.g., complex congenital heart disease, prosthetic valve, poor dentition, or prior history of endocarditis).[9]

Contraindications and complications

Relative contraindications for TEE include significant esophageal pathology (e.g., strictures, varices), history of radiation therapy to the mediastinum, and recent esophageal or gastric surgery. Serious complications of TEE are uncommon (< 1 percent) but may include aspiration and other problems related to oversedation, mucosal trauma, laryngospasm, esophageal or pharyngeal laceration or perforation, methemoglobinemia, and rarely death. TEE probe passage is "blind" and is done without direct visualization. The more severe complications of esophageal or pharyngeal trauma are signaled by patient complaints of severe pain and inability to swallow, which usually occur after the procedure has ended and sedation has worn off. Esophageal perforation during intraoperative TEE can go undetected for a period of time because of the anesthetized state of the patient and the lack of patient feedback regarding pain during probe passage.

Table 49-1 Class I indications for perioperative transesophageal echocardiography

Acute and life-threatening hemodynamic instability
Valve repair or complex valve replacements
Hypertrophic obstructive cardiomyopathy
Aortic dissection with possible aortic valve involvement
Endocarditis (perivalvular involvement)
Congenital heart surgery
Pericardial windows (posterior or loculated effusions)
Placement of intracardiac devices

Source: Data modified from Cheitlin MD, Armstrong WF, Aurigemma GP, et al. ACC/AHA/ASE 2003 guideline update for the clinical application of echocardiography: summary article: a report of the American College of Cardiology/American Heart Association Task Force on Practice Guidelines (ACC/AHA/ASE Committee to Update the 1997 Guidelines for the Clinical Application of Echocardiography). *Circulation* 2003;108:1146–1162.

ASSESSMENT OF VENTRICULAR FUNCTION

Routinely, a qualitative "eyeball" estimate of global LV systolic function is obtained visually by examining LV wall thickening and motion. In addition, quantitative measures of LV systolic function can also be obtained. LV segmental wall function can be analyzed using a semiquantitative grading scale (wall motion score).

LEFT VENTRICULAR EJECTION FRACTION

Ejection fraction (EF) is often reported qualitatively as increased (hyperdynamic), normal, mildly, moderately, or severely reduced.[8] In addition, the reader often assigns an estimated value to the qualitative assessment. Normal LV EF is 61 ± 10 percent.[10]

Visual estimation of EF by experienced readers is generally reliable but is limited by reader variability and depends on optimal echocardiographic delineation of the endocardium.

EF can also be quantified from the equation below after determining end-diastolic volume (EDV) and end-systolic volume (ESV):

$$EF = SV/EDV = (EDV - ESV)/EDV$$

Where SV = stroke volume, EDV = end-diastolic volume, and ESV = end-systolic volume.

Volumes can be obtained by the modified Simpson's method, which divides the LV cavity into a series of stacked cylinders of equal height that are summed to estimate the entire ventricular volume at end-diastole and end-systole. Further details of the technique can be found in several of the references.[1,2,11]

LEFT VENTRICULAR FRACTIONAL SHORTENING (PERCENT FRACTIONAL SHORTENING)

Percent FS is another method for estimating LV systolic function and reflects a percent change in LV dimension with systolic contraction. It is calculated from LV end-diastolic and end-systolic dimensions measured by M mode. For ventricles that are roughly symmetrical without regional wall motion abnormalities, EF is approximately 2 (percent FS).

$$\text{Percent FS} = (\text{EDD} - \text{ESD}) / \text{EDD} \times 100$$

Where EDD = end-diastolic dimension and ESD = end-systolic dimension.

LEFT VENTRICULAR REGIONAL WALL MOTION

For the assessment of LV regional wall motion, the LV is divided into 16 segments (Fig. 49-2), each of which is given a score from 1 to 5 (1, normal or hyperkinetic; 2, hypokinetic; 3, akinetic; 4, dyskinetic; 5, aneurysmal or

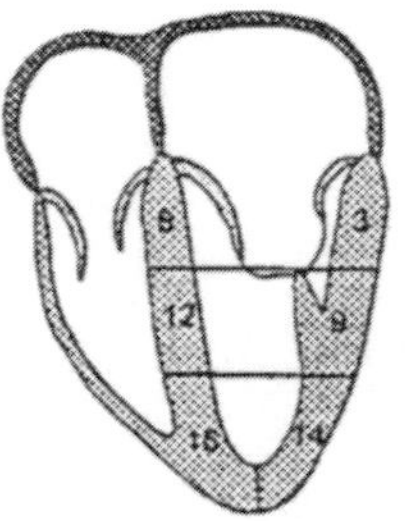

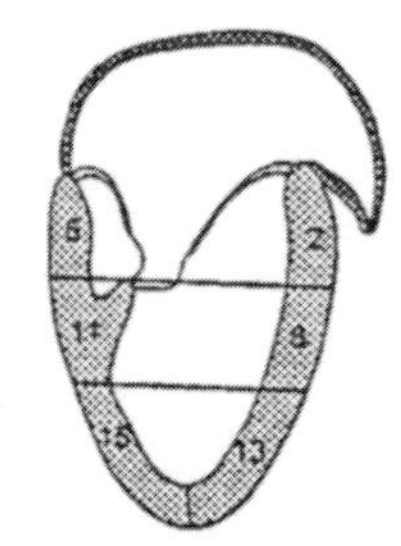

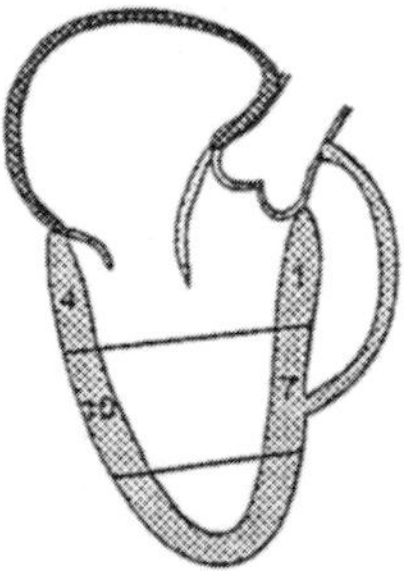

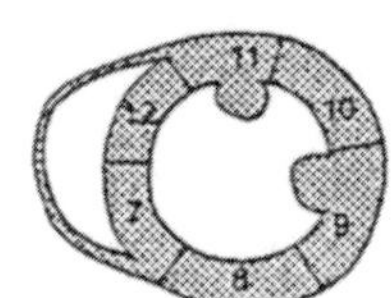

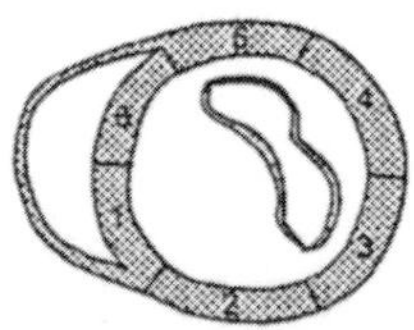

Figure 49-2 Sixteen-segment model of the left ventricle. According to guidelines of the American Society of Echocardiography and the Society of Cardiac Anesthesia, the left ventricle is divided into 16 segments (6 basal, 6 mid ventricular, and four apical segments) for evaluation of wall motion and calculation of the wall motion score. (From Shanewise et al.[12] With permission.)

diastolically deformed). This grading system differs from the 1-to-5 grading system of TEE often used by cardiac anesthesiologists[12] [1, normal (> 30 percent thickening); 2, mildly hypokinetic (10 to 30 percent thickening); 3, severely hypokinetic (< 10 percent thickening); 4, akinetic (no thickening); 5, dyskinetic (paradoxical systolic motion)]. The wall motion score index is calculated as the sum of segmental wall motion scores divided by the number of segments seen. A score of 1 is normal and higher wall motion scores indicate more extensive ventricular dysfunction. However, this grading system is more useful for research databases than for clinical use.

LEFT VENTRICULAR FILLING

LV preload is the LV volume at end-diastole. Normal LV end-diastolic size is 3.5 to 5.7 cm in the parasternal long-axis view. The size of the ventricles and atria may be used for the qualitative evaluation of filling pressures and assessment of hyper- or hypovolemia, particularly intraoperatively with TEE.[13] Small LA size and near cavity obliteration of the LV can indicate hypovolemia.[14] Conversely, ventricular and atrial enlargement may indicate hypervolemia. Doming of the interatrial septum toward the right suggests elevated LA pressure and increased LV preload (the septum bulges toward the side with lower pressure). One limitation to using TEE for indirect measurement of volume status is that the LV may be foreshortened; it is therefore recommended that the LV be imaged from several different planes to get a more accurate estimate of LV volume.[14]

LEFT VENTRICULAR DIASTOLIC FUNCTION

Doppler echo is the most common diagnostic tool for assessing diastolic function. Indices of transmitral and pulmonary venous Doppler flows are commonly used to identify patterns of diastolic dysfunction.[11]

Mitral valve inflow

When sinus rhythm is present, PW Doppler at the level of the mitral valve (MV) leaflets records two velocities separated by a period of diastasis (no flow), as shown in Fig. 49-3. After the MV opens, early rapid (E wave) diastolic filling of the LV occurs, followed by a period of diastasis, after which late filling occurs due to atrial contraction (A wave). Normally, in individuals less than 60 years old, the peak E:A wave velocity ratio is greater than 1. When there is impaired relaxation without elevated filling pressures, the peak E decreases, hence the E:A ratio becomes less than 1. In contrast, a "restrictive" filling pattern is seen when both impaired relaxation and elevated filling pressures are present, resulting in a smaller contribution of atrial contraction and an increased E:A ratio (> 1.5 to 2).

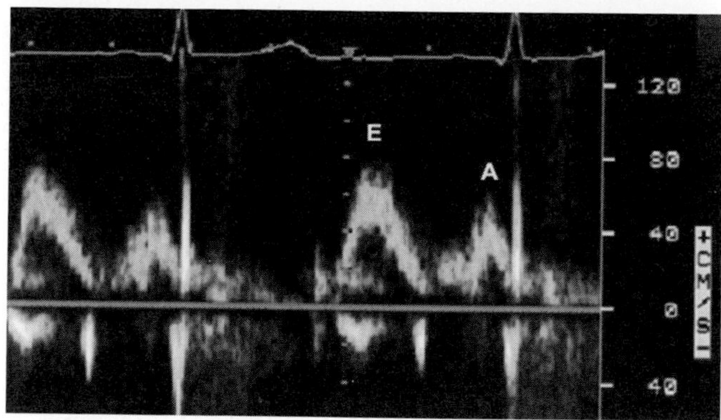

Figure 49-3 Pulsed-wave (PW) Doppler of the mitral valve inflow. This figure shows a normal pattern of blood flow through the mitral valve in diastole. The two peaks indicate early (E wave) and late (A wave) diastolic filling separated by a brief period of diastasis (no flow). In individuals less than 65 years old, a normal E:A ratio is 2:1. Deceleration time is the time interval from peak E velocity to baseline.

Pulmonary vein flow

Four velocities are seen in PW Doppler of the pulmonary veins (Fig. 49-4). Occurring in early systole, the first systolic forward flow velocity (PV_{S1}) is due to the relaxation of the LA, which promotes pulmonary venous flow into the LA. In mid- to late systole, a second systolic forward flow (PV_{S2}) occurs that is produced by the increase in pulmonary venous pressure occurring after right ventricular (RV) systole. In diastole, a third pulmonary vein velocity is seen (PV_D). This is related to the decrease in LA pressure seen after MV opening. The fourth velocity is the atrial flow reversal velocity (PV_a) that is related to LA contraction. A pulmonary vein systolic velocity peak less than the diastolic velocity peak is suggestive of elevated LA pressures. Restrictive filling indicative of very high filling pressures is seen when PV_{S2} is much less than PV_D. When higher filling pressures are present, both the duration and peak velocity of PV_a are increased. Another sign of elevated LA pressure is when the duration of PV_a is longer than the duration of the mitral inflow A wave (by > 0.03 s).

RIGHT VENTRICULAR FUNCTION AND FILLING PRESSURES

Qualitative evaluation of RV wall thickening and motion is done visually, as in the evaluation of LV function, although it is more difficult to estimate RV function. Normal RV size is less than two-thirds of LV size (see Fig. 49-1). Septal wall flattening (resulting in a D-shaped LV in the short-axis view) or septal deviation into the LV can be see in both pressure- and volume-overload conditions of the RV.[12]

When tricuspid regurgitation is present, the RV systolic pressure (RVSP) can be estimated (see also "Pulmonary Hypertension," below), although TTE is preferred to TEE for measuring RVSP because of better alignment of the transducer beam with the direction of the regurgitant jet.

Examination of the size and respiratory changes of the venae cavae and hepatic veins can give helpful clues to the patient's volume status and is also used in the evaluation of pericardial disease. Although TTE is preferred for examination of respirophasic collapse of the inferior vena

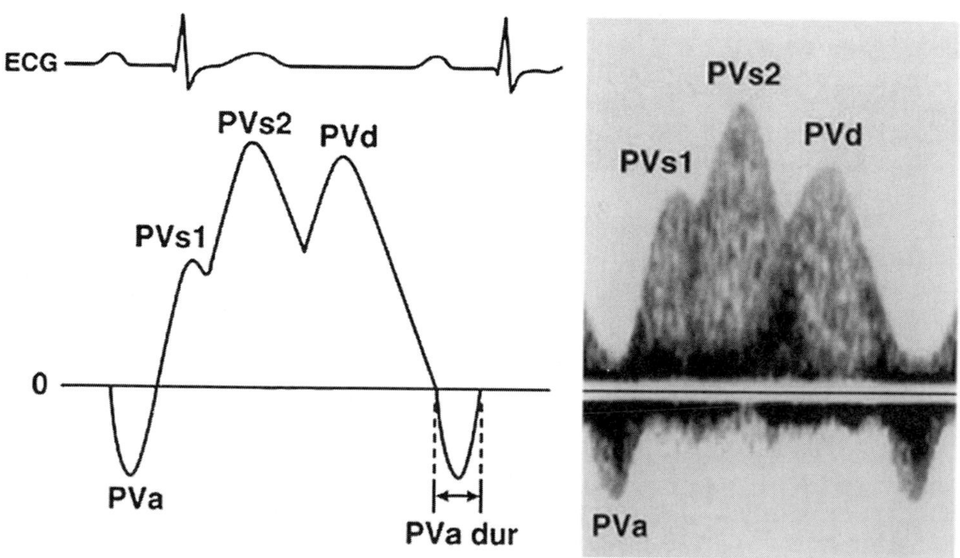

Figure 49-4 Pulsed-wave (PW) Doppler of the pulmonary vein. This figure shows a normal pattern of blood flow through the pulmonary veins with four velocities seen (PV_{S1}, PV_{S2}, PV_D, PV_a). Duration of peak reverse flow velocity during atrial contraction (PV_a dur) is also measured. (From Oh et al.[11] With permission.)

cava, TEE provides better visualization of the superior vena cava. Dilatation of the superior vena cava (greater than one-half the aortic dimension in the short-axis view) is suggestive of hypervolemia.[14]

VALVULAR DISEASE

MITRAL VALVE

Mitral valve morphology

Normal MV function depends on the normal function of all its component parts, including the mitral leaflets, annulus, chordae tendineae, papillary muscles, and LV. The rectangular posterior leaflet is composed of three scallops (P1, P2, P3), while the semicircular anterior leaflet is divided into thirds for descriptive purposes (Fig. 49-5). Normal MV area is 4 to 6 cm^2.

Mitral stenosis

Rheumatic heart disease is the most common cause of mitral stenotic lesions (Fig. 49-6), with leaflet thickening and fusion of the commissures (characteristic fish-mouth valve in the short-axis view and hockey-stick appearance in the long-axis view).

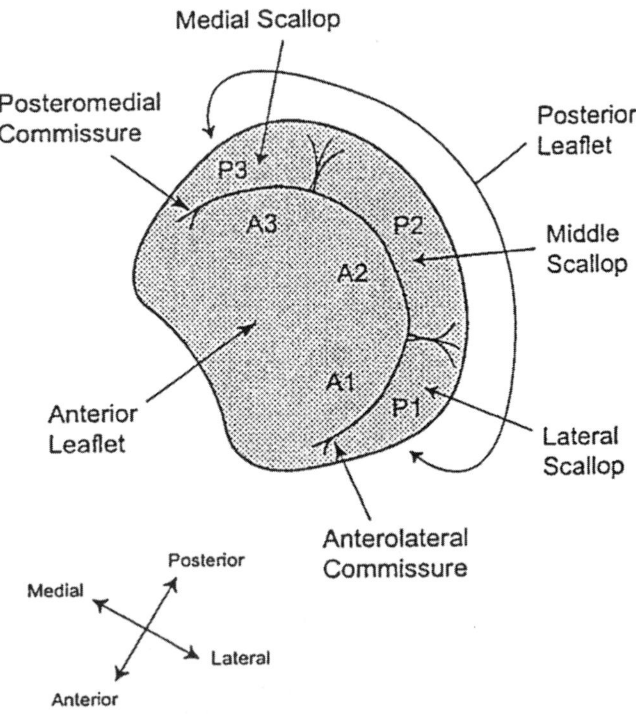

Figure 49-5 Mitral valve structure. The mitral valve consists of two leaflets, the anterior and posterior leaflets, which are separated at the annulus by the posteromedial and anterolateral commissures. The posterior leaflet is rectangular and composed of three scallops (P1, P2, P3). The anterior leaflet is semicircular and is divided into three segments for descriptive purposes (A1, A2, A3). (From Shanewise et al.[12] With permission.)

Two-dimensional (2D) echo is the "gold standard" for evaluating mitral stenosis (MS) and allows assessment of the structure and function of the mitral annulus, leaflets, chordae, papillary muscles, LV size and function, LA size, and pulmonary hypertension (RVSP). The Wilkins echo score[15] for rheumatic MS is based on four variables (leaflet mobility, leaflet thickening, subvalvular thickening, and calcifications). Each variable receives a score of 1 to 4 and the individual scores are summed up. A total score equal to or greater than 8 is associated with better outcomes for mitral balloon valvuloplasty. For valves with less favorable scores (> 8), cardiac surgery with valve replacement may be the preferred treatment modality.

Mitral valve area

Calculation of MV area is usually obtained using the pressure half-time (PHT) method. PHT is the time (milliseconds) for the maximal pressure gradient to decrease by half and is usually equal to the deceleration time multiplied by 0.29.

$$\text{MV area (cm}^2\text{)} = 220 / \text{PHT (ms)}$$

The PHT method has several important shortcomings. It is affected by concomitant aortic regurgitation or decreased LV compliance.[4] The rapid increase in LV diastolic pressure associated with either of these conditions may shorten the PHT and underestimate the extent of stenosis. Other techniques to estimate valve area include planimetry and the continuity equation.[1,4] The latter approach is also less reliable in the presence of significant aortic and mitral regurgitation. Details of this approach are outlined in the references 1 through 11.

Mitral valve pressure gradients

As the degree of obstruction to blood flow caused by a stenotic valve increases, the velocity of the blood flow also increases in order to maintain constant flow (conservation of mass or flow). Velocities can then be transformed into pressures with the simplified Bernoulli equation:

$$\Delta P = 4V^2$$

Where ΔP = MV pressure gradient (mmHg) and V = velocity of blood flow across the MV (ms).

Severity of mitral stenosis

The mean MV pressure gradient and MV area are used to estimate the severity of mitral stenosis and the need for intervention (Table 49-2).

Mitral regurgitation

There are three basic mechanisms of mitral regurgitation (MR): primary abnormalities of the mitral leaflets, commissures, or annulus; malfunctioning of the subvalvular

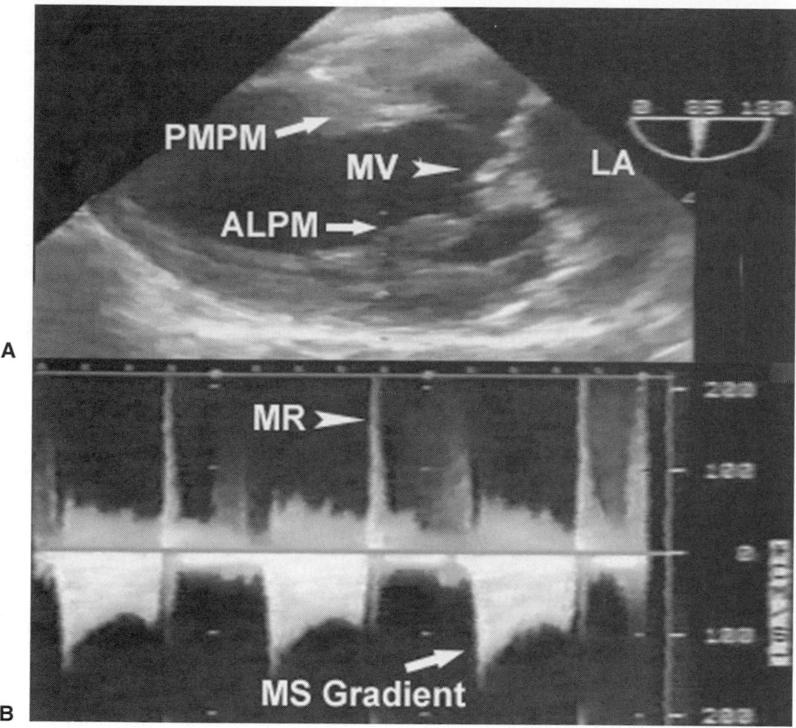

Figure 49-6 Rheumatic mitral stenosis. A. Transesophageal transgastric long-axis view of the left ventricle, the anterolateral papillary muscle (ALPM), the posteromedial papillary muscle (PMPM), mitral valve (MV) leaflets, and left atrium (LA). Note the thickened and partially calcified subvalvular and valvular structures (short arrow). The patient had severe three-vessel coronary artery disease in addition to rheumatic aortic stenosis and atrial fibrillation and underwent successful mitral and aortic valve replacements and coronary artery bypass grafting. B. Continuous-wave (CW) Doppler of the mitral valve intraoperatively. MR = mitral regurgitation; MS = mitral stenosis.

structures (chordae tendineae and papillary muscles); and alterations in LV and LA dimensions and function.

The most common cause of isolated severe MR is myxomatous degeneration (Fig. 49-7). The valve itself can also be deformed from rheumatic fever, mitral annular calcification, infective endocarditis, and congenital lesions (cleft MV). Other less common causes of leaflet abnormalities include endomyocardial fibrosis, carcinoid disease, drugs (e.g., fenfluramine hydrochloride and phentermine, or Fen-Phen), radiation therapy, trauma, and collagen vascular disease.

Table 49-2 Severity of mitral stenosis

Severity	Mitral valve area (cm^2)	Mean gradient[a] (mmHg)
None	4–6	—
Mild	1.6–2.0	<5
Moderate	1.1–1.5	5–10
Severe	≤1	>10

[a]Assumes normal cardiac output.
Source: ACC/AHA Guidelines for the Management of Patients with Valvular Heart Disease.[9] With permission.

Abnormalities in the subvalvular structures include dysfunctional and/or ruptured chordae tendineae and papillary muscles. Ruptured chordae tendineae account for a large proportion of MR lesions. Etiologies include idiopathic causes, MV prolapse, infective endocarditis, and thoracic trauma. Papillary muscle dysfunction (with or without frank rupture) is most often seen in the setting of myocardial ischemia or infarction. The posteromedial head of the papillary muscle is most vulnerable to ischemia because of its end-artery vascular supply. Other causes of dysfunction include dilated cardiomyopathy, myocarditis, hypertension, and chest trauma.

Global or regional LV enlargement may dilate the mitral annulus and change the position and axis of contraction of the papillary muscles, leading to dysfunction. Progressive LA and LV enlargement associated with chronic MR further exacerbate the extent of MR because of continued changes in chamber geometry.

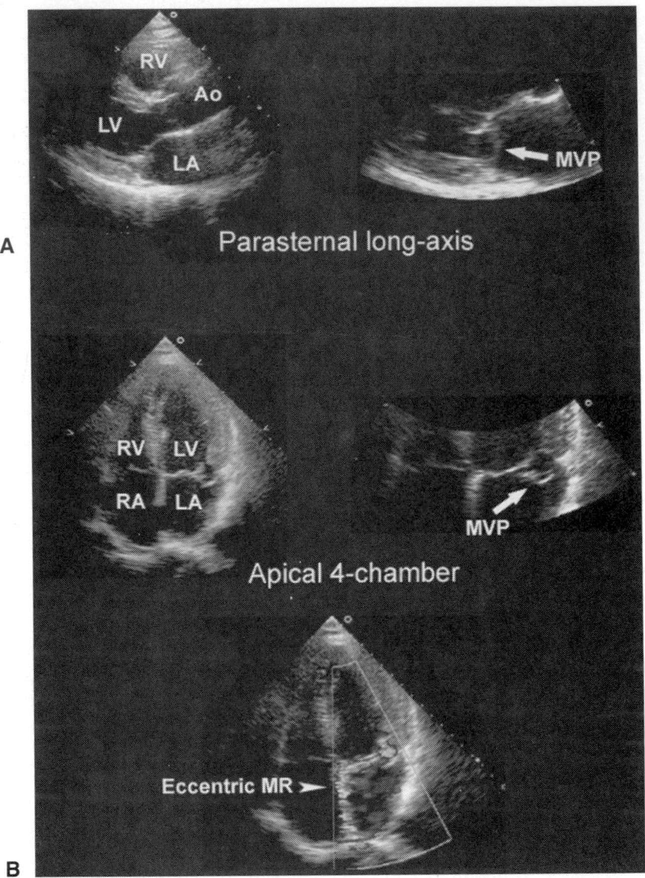

Figure 49-7 Myxomatous mitral valve prolapse and mitral regurgitation. A. Transthoracic parasternal long-axis view of the mitral valve with a greater than 2-mm prolapse of the posterior leaflet (MVP) beyond the plane of the annulus. B. Apical four-chamber view shows biatrial enlargement. C. Color-flow Doppler shows severe mitral regurgitation (MR) with an eccentric jet that is "wall hugging" and anteriorly directed (opposite the side of leaflet prolapse).

Two-dimensional echocardiography

Unlike the case in MS, where echo is the accepted gold standard for diagnosis, there is no gold standard for the assessment of MR; therefore multiple parameters are used in estimating the severity of MR.[16] The purpose of echo in MR is to determine the etiology, mechanism, and severity of regurgitation; determine the need for surgery and the type of surgery that is necessary; and evaluate other valves, RV and LV function, and the presence of pulmonary hypertension. The most important aspect is to determine the hemodynamic significance of the regurgitation based on LV size (particularly end-systolic dimension), LV systolic function (EF), and the presence and degree of LA enlargement and pulmonary hypertension (RVSP). Regurgitant jet size and area may contribute to the assessment of MR but often correlate poorly with MR severity.[16] The degree of MR intraoperatively may appear less or more severe compared to the degree preoperatively, particularly for ischemic MR, because of different hemodynamic and ischemic conditions (e.g., lower blood pressure or relief of ischemia will reduce the amount of regurgitation).[17]

Severity of mitral regurgitation

Echo findings in severe MR[4,16] include:

- Large regurgitant jet: > 40 percent of LA area.
- Wide vena contracta (the narrowest part of the regurgitant color jet at its origin): ≥ 7 mm.
- Eccentric wall-impinging regurgitant jet (Fig. 49-7B).
- Dilated LV: end-systolic dimension ≥ 45 mm or end-diastolic dimension ≥ 70 mm.
- LV EF < 55 to 60 percent.
- Dilated LA (≥ 5.5 cm), although the LA may not be dilated in acute MR.
- Pulmonary hypertension: resting RVSP > 50 mmHg.
- Restrictive mitral filling pattern: high peak early transmitral velocity (E wave) > 1.5 ms.
- Pulmonary vein systolic flow reversal: A normal pulmonary vein Doppler pattern has a systolic (S) wave larger than the diastolic (D) wave. As the MR progresses, the S wave decreases until it may become reversed. While a reduced S wave is a nonspecific finding,[18] the presence of a reversed S wave has high specificity for significant MR. The absence of a reversed S wave does not exclude significant MR.
- Effective orifice area (ERO) ≥ 0.4 cm^2.

Table 49-3 summarizes the important echo features of MV stenosis and regurgitation.

Mitral valve prolapse

Mitral valve prolapse (MVP) is the most common cause of MR in patients undergoing cardiac surgery in the United States.[19] MVP is the systolic billowing or displacement of at least 2 mm of either mitral leaflet into

Table 49-3	Echocardiographic assessment of the mitral valve
Morphology	Mitral annulus, leaflets, chordae, papillary muscles, LV size and function, LA size, pulmonary hypertension (RVSP)
Stenosis	Often rheumatic Echo score: leaflet mobility, thickening, subvalvular thickening, calcifications, < 8 favors valvuloplasty Severe MS: area ≤ 1 cm^2 or mean gradient > 10 mmHg
Regurgitation	Regurgitant jet size does not correlate well with severity Severe MR: dilated LV (ESD > 45 mm), ↓ LV systolic function (EF < 55–60%), dilated LA, pulmonary hypertension (RVSP > 50)

LV = left ventricle; RVSP = right ventricular systolic pressure; MS = mitral stenosis; MR = mitral regurgitation; ESD = end-systolic dimension; LA = left atrium; EF = ejection fraction.

the LA beyond the plane of the mitral annulus in the parasternal or apical long-axis views (see Fig. 49-7). Recent criteria for echo diagnosis of MVP[20] have become more stringent, leading to increased specificity of the criteria for MVP while at the same time preserving sensitivity for the detection of MVP complications. Classic MVP is defined as equal to or greater than 5 mm of leaflet thickening (myxomatous changes) of the prolapsing leaflet, while nonclassic prolapse is leaflet thickening less than 5 mm. Compared to nonclassic MVP, classic MVP has a worse prognosis, with most complications of MVP (significant MR and congestive heart failure, MV surgery, infectious endocarditis) arising in patients with classic MVP.[19] Asymmetrical prolapse of the leaflets is associated with progression to more significant disease (flail leaflet and severe MR).

Determining which segment of the mitral leaflet tissue is prolapsing is essential for proper MV repair. MR associated with MVP often has an eccentric jet directed opposite to the prolapsing leaflet (e.g., anteriorly directed jet if posterior leaflet prolapse is present). In contrast, in MR associated with rheumatic mitral stenosis, the regurgitant jet is directed toward the affected leaflet due to restricted leaflet motion (e.g., anteriorly directed jet if the anterior leaflet is calcified). MR associated with MVP may be due to flail leaflet or chordal rupture resulting from myxomatous involvement of the chordae or leaflet. Chordal rupture is diagnosed when the chords are seen as mobile echodensities attached to a flail or partially flail leaflet (Fig. 49-8).[21] These may be confused with or may be difficult to distinguish from vegetations of infective endocarditis. Mitral annulus calcification (MAC) may also be seen in patients who have MVP.

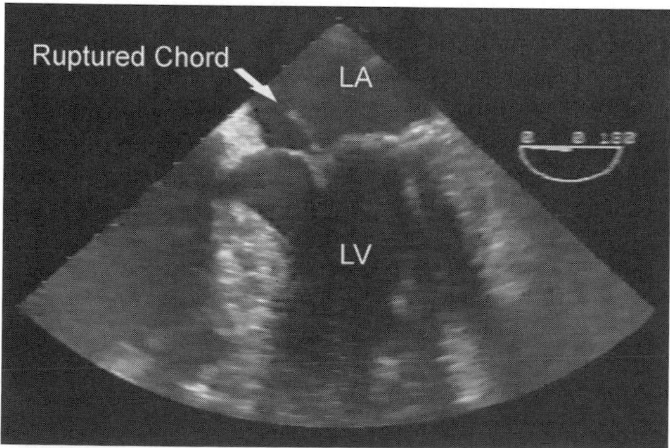

Figure 49-8 Ruptured chord attached to a flail segment of the posterior mitral leaflet due to myxomatous disease. Intraoperative transesophageal echocardiogram showing the ruptured chord as an echodense linear filament attached to the flail leaflet, prolapsing into the left atrium during systole.

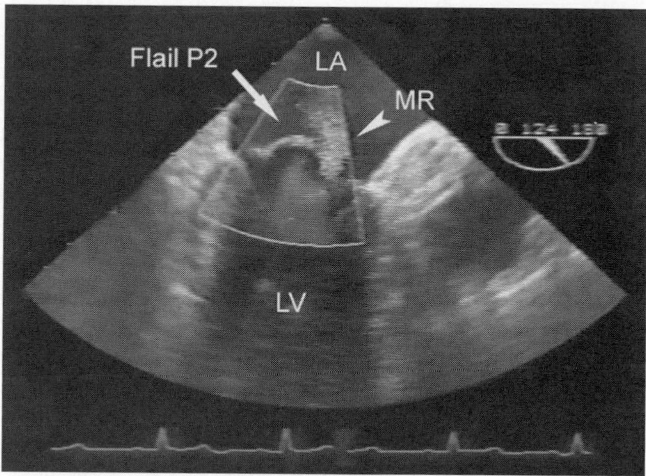

Figure 49-9 Flail mitral leaflet with severe mitral regurgitation. Intraoperative transesophageal echocardiogram with color-flow Doppler consistent with severe mitral regurgitation. This patient underwent successful mitral valve repair with posterior leaflet quadrangular resection and an annuloplasty band.

Flail leaflet

Flail leaflet encompasses a spectrum of disease severity from partially to completely flail leaflets, resulting in excessive motion of the mitral leaflets and various degrees of MR (Fig. 49-9). Flail mitral leaflet is diagnosed when the leaflet tip is "upturned" toward the LA during MV closure (due to loss of coaptation). Most commonly, it is caused by MVP or endocarditis resulting in chordal rupture, but it may also be caused by ischemia or infarction of the papillary muscle (usually affecting the posteromedial papillary muscle). A partially flail leaflet (due to chordal rupture) is usually associated with moderate to severe MR, while a completely flail mitral leaflet is almost always associated with severe MR necessitating surgery.[21]

Ruptured papillary muscle

Dysfunction of the papillary muscle results in severe MR and is most often due to acute myocardial infarction. Papillary muscle dysfunction should be differentiated from acute chordal rupture. Papillary muscle rupture is diagnosed in the appropriate clinical context when a triangular mass (the head of the papillary muscle), seen attached to the flail leaflet, prolapses into the LA during systole, accompanied by severe MR.[17]

Leaflet perforation

This is most commonly caused by valvular endocarditis, while less common etiologies include congenital (cleft MV) or iatrogenic causes. With leaflet perforation, the regurgitant jet is often eccentric and originates at the site of perforation.

Mitral valve repair

TEE is essential in determining the suitability of a valve for repair. It can assess the mechanism and severity of

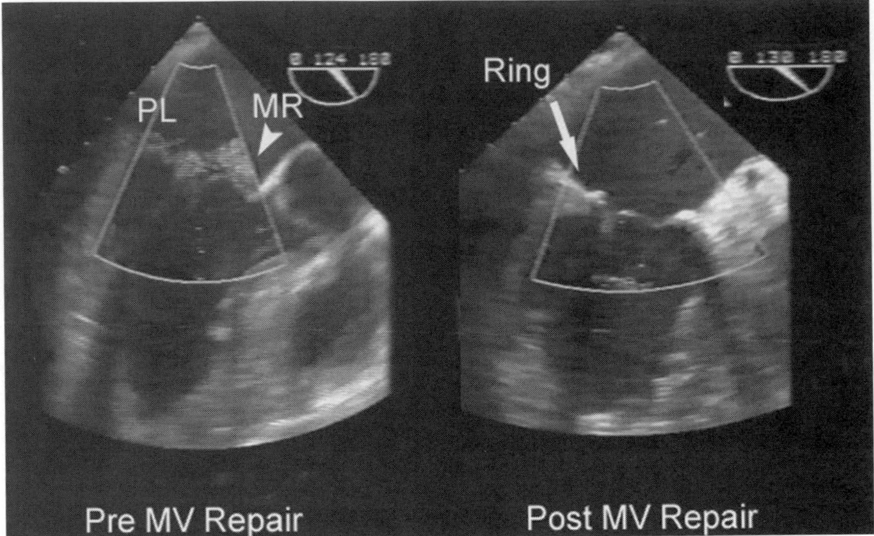

Figure 49-10 Posterior leaflet prolapse and dilated mitral annulus. Note the anteriorly directed eccentric jet of mitral regurgitation seen on transesophageal echocardiography. Following the repair (posterior leaflet quadrangular resection and annuloplasty ring), the patient had good ventricular function and no residual mitral regurgitation.

MR, identify the affected leaflets, determine the presence of coexisting valvular lesions, and estimate RV and LV function. The prognosis of MV repair differs based on the mechanism of MR (organic/primary vs. functional/secondary) and is strongly influenced by the preoperative EF. The most common indication for MV repair is myxomatous disease. Determining which leaflet or segment is involved is important in deciding on the suitability of the repair, the likelihood of successful repair (better with posterior leaflet prolapse), and the method of repair. This is done by analyzing the motion of the leaflets and the direction of the regurgitant jet.

TEE is also helpful intraoperatively to assess the success of the repair. Immediately postrepair (Fig. 49-10), the competency of the valve can be assessed for residual MR (1+, mild; 2+, moderate; 3+, moderate to severe; 4+, severe). Phenylephrine and volume may be administered in order to assess the effect of increased afterload and preload on the degree of residual MR. If there is MR postrepair equal to or greater than 2+, further surgery is indicated. Repeat imaging is also done after the patient is off cardiopulmonary bypass. Other findings that may be detected on TEE include residual mitral stenosis, global or regional LV systolic dysfunction, suture dehiscence or leaflet perforation, and MV systolic anterior motion (SAM) with outflow obstruction. Limitations to intraoperative TEE include the effect of changing hemodynamics, which may significantly affect the appearance and severity of valvular lesions, since the evaluation depends on preload and afterload conditions as well as ventricular function. Hence, it is important that loading conditions be similar in comparing the severity of MR.

AORTIC VALVE

Aortic valve morphology

Normally, the aortic valve (AV) is composed of three semilunar leaflets (cusps) that open and close passively due to pressure differences between the LV and the aorta. Small strands may be seen on the cusps (Lambl's excrescences), particularly on TEE, and represent a normal variant. Bicuspid and rarely unicuspid or quadricuspid valves may be seen on echo (Fig. 49-11). The normal valve area is 3 to 4 cm^2 with a 2-cm leaflet separation during systole.

A bicuspid AV is the most common congenital heart defect and occurs in about 1 to 2 percent of the U.S. population. The morphologic features of a bicuspid AV are somewhat variable. In some patients, there are two equal-sized cusps with a single central commissure. In many others, the cusps may be unequal in size with an eccentric commissure, with the larger of the two cusps containing a raphe.[1,22] In the parasternal long-axis views, bicuspid valves are characterized by systolic doming. In the short-axis views, the hallmark is an elliptical "football"-shaped systolic orifice. The valve leaflets themselves may be thickened and fibrotic, particularly with increasing patient age. A bicuspid valve may be functionally normal with no significant stenosis or regurgitation, particularly in adolescents and young adults, among whom up to one-third have no significant valvular dysfunction.[23] However, over time, progressive "wear and tear" with resulting fibrosis and valve calcification leads to functional abnormalities. By the age of 60 years, over 50 percent of bicuspid valves are significantly stenotic. Valve regurgitation is frequently present

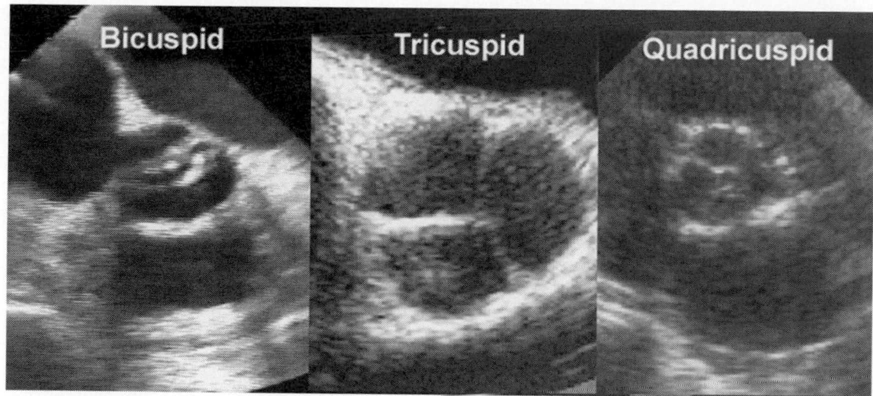

Figure 49-11 Bicuspid, tricuspid, and quadricuspid aortic valves. The normal aortic valve is trileaflet (central panel). Bicuspid valve is the most common congenital anomaly of the aortic valve (left panel), with quadricuspid (right panel) aortic valves being much less common.

as well and may be the predominant functional abnormality in younger patients. Etiology of the regurgitation may be retraction and fibrosis of the commissures or leaflets, cusp prolapse, dilatation of the aortic root or valve annulus, or damage from infective endocarditis.

It is important to recognize that bicuspid AVs are often associated with abnormalities of the aorta. Concomitant aortic coarctation occurs in a minority. Aortic dissection is another known association, with 5 to 9 percent of patients with dissecting aortic aneurysms having bicuspid valves. Aortic root dilatation may be due to a common developmental defect that affects both the aorta and the valve.[24] Poststenotic dilatation of the ascending aorta can also occur.

Aortic stenosis

Rheumatic aortic stenosis (AS) (Fig. 49-12A) is usually associated with MV disease. Calcium deposits are present on both sides of the aortic cusps, resulting in commissural fusion and aortic regurgitation. Degenerative calcific disease is the most common cause of AS in the United States. It is often associated with MAC and coronary artery disease. Nodular calcification is often present on the aortic aspect of the valve along the bases of the cusps and may protrude into the sinuses of Valsalva (Fig. 49-12B and C). In contrast to rheumatic AS, there is no commissural fusion in degenerative AS, hence aortic regurgitation is rare.

Two-dimensional echocardiography

A thorough echo evaluation includes assessing the thickness and calcification of the leaflets, their mobility, looking for the etiology of stenosis (e.g., bicuspid, rheumatic, degenerative calcific) and its extent, the presence of other valvular lesions, and assessing LV size and function. TTE is often superior to TEE in assessing the severity of AS because obtaining maximal velocity jets (i.e., absolutely parallel to flow) is often difficult with TEE.

Aortic valve area

In aortic stenotic lesions, the AV area decreases by approximately 0.1 cm^2 per year, although large variations from patient to patient exist.[25] The AV area is usually determined using the continuity equation. Direct planimetry (visualization of the orifice area) is less reliable for patients with heavily calcified valves (due to shadowing of the valve) and for critical ("pinhole") stenoses.[22] The continuity equation is based on the principle of conservation of flow (or mass), whereby flow before the valve must equal flow across the valve. Since the area of the LV outflow tract (LVOT) can be directly measured, as can velocities in the LVOT and across the valve, the AV area can then be calculated:

$$A_1V_1 = A_2V_2$$

Where A = area or πr^2; V = velocity; A_1V_1 = flow proximal to the valve (LVOT); A_2V_2 = flow across the valve.

The major limitation to the continuity equation is that small errors in the LVOT diameter become magnified in estimating the AV area (since the radius is squared in the equation). As a general rule, one may assume that the LVOT diameter is 2 cm (r_1 = 1 cm) with generally good estimates of the AV area. Another limitation is in obtaining the maximal aortic jet velocity, which requires that the echocardiographic Doppler beam be exactly parallel to the direction of blood flow.

Aortic valve pressure gradients

Like pressure gradients obtained for mitral stenosis, the simplified Bernoulli equation is used for estimating AV pressure gradients:

$$\Delta P = 4V^2$$

Where ΔP = AV pressure gradient (mmHg) and V = velocity of blood flow across the AV (ms).

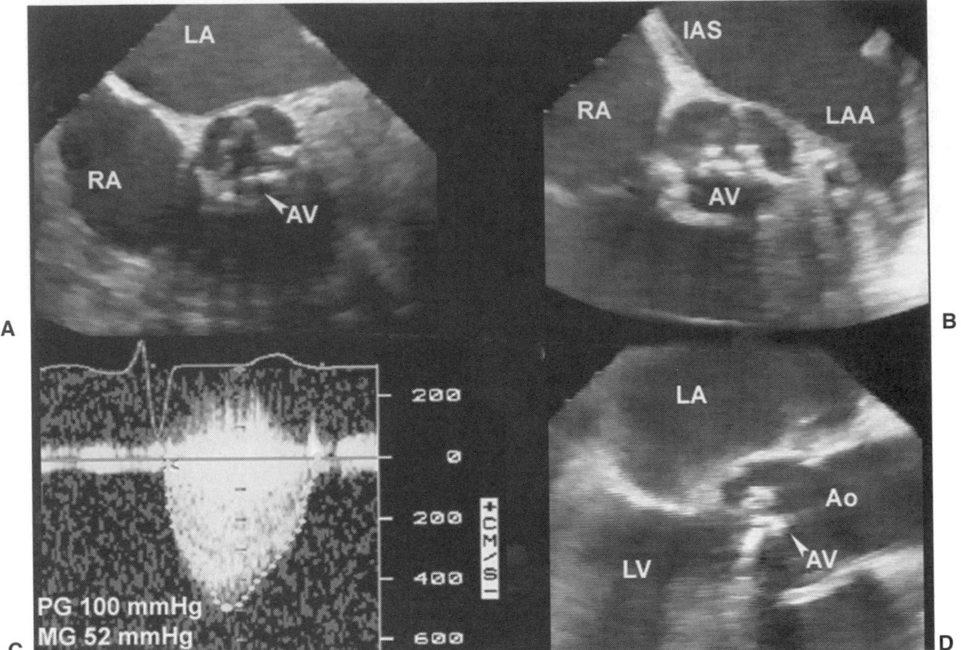

Figure 49-12 Rheumatic and calcific aortic stenosis. A. Rheumatic aortic stenosis with calcium deposits in the commissures resulting in commissural fusion. B and D. Short and long-axis views: Calcific aortic stenosis, with calcium deposits on the aortic aspect of the valve on the bases of the cusps and no commissural fusion. C. Continuous-wave (CW) Doppler of the aortic valve (shown in B and C) is consistent with severe aortic stenosis (aortic velocity > 4 ms, mean gradient > 50 mmHg). RA = right atrium; LA = left atrium; AV = aortic valve; LAA = left atrial appendage; IAS = interatrial septum; Ao = aorta; PG = peak gradient; MG = mean gradient.

AV pressure gradients may be significantly underestimated because of inadequate envelopes (because the Doppler beam is not parallel to the blood flow) or an inadequate number of measurements from different locations. Maximal velocities may be present or obtainable from only certain locations in an individual patient. Hence complete assessment from all locations is needed. In addition, the velocity of flow is highly dependent on overall LV function. Pressure gradients may significantly underestimate the severity of AS in the presence of severe LV dysfunction ("low-gradient AS"). The opposite is also true, whereby increased flow velocity across the valve is seen in situations of increased cardiac output (i.e., anemia, aortic regurgitation, hyperthyroidism) and may not reflect true aortic stenosis. In such situations, valve area calculations may be more accurate, and correlation with valve morphology and visual assessment of leaflet mobility is important.

Severity of aortic stenosis

The mean AV pressure gradient and the AV area are used to estimate severity of AS and the need for surgical intervention (Table 49-4). If there is a significant discrepancy between the pre- and intraoperative grading of the severity of AS, the following should be considered:

1. Change in hemodynamic conditions: changes in heart rate or rhythm, contractility, and hemodynamics influence the gradients across the AV. The AV area is usually less affected by loading conditions.
2. Measurement variability in data recording: measurement errors in the LVOT diameter greatly influence the AV area, since the LVOT radius is squared in the continuity equation.

Table 49-4 Severity of aortic stenosis

Severity	Velocity (ms)	Area (cm^2)	Mean gradient[a] (mmHg)
None	1	3–4	—
Mild	2.5–2.9	> 1.5	< 25
Moderate	3–4	1–1.5	25–50
Severe	> 4	< 1	> 50

[a]Assumes normal cardiac output.
Source: ACC/AHA Guidelines for the Management of Patients with Valvular Heart Disease.[9] With permission.

Aortic regurgitation

Echo assessment of aortic regurgitation (AR) includes a comprehensive examination of AV morphology, aortic root dilatation, and LV size and function.[16] TTE is generally the initial diagnostic test used for evaluating the severity of AR. However, TEE is also helpful particularly for patients with poor transthoracic windows, if prosthetic valves are present, and intraoperatively to guide surgical repair. TEE is particularly useful for determining the mechanism of regurgitation by distinguishing valvular from nonvalvular causes of AR. Common etiologies for AR include congenital malformations (bicuspid valves); degenerative calcific, rheumatic, and infective endocarditis; aortic aneurysm (Fig. 49-13) or dissection, Marfan's syndrome, drug-induced (e.g., Fen-Phen) AR, and prosthetic valve dysfunction.[9] Acute and chronic AR differ in both pathophysiology and echo findings. Many of the echo findings in chronic AR (e.g., LV dilatation and systolic dysfunction) may not be present in acute AR. Chronic AR is a state of both pressure and volume overload of the LV, resulting in LV hypertrophy and dilatation.

Two-dimensional echocardiography

This is helpful for evaluating LV size and function, AV structure and leaflet mobility, aortic root dilatation, aortic dissection, associated vegetations, diastolic fluttering motion of MV leaflets, and premature MV closure (indicative of significant AR).

Severity of aortic regurgitation

In assessing the severity of chronic AR, it is essential to combine data on LV size and function with Doppler data and not to rely solely on color Doppler, since it is often misleading. No study has yet demonstrated that quantification of the severity of AR by Doppler criteria alone is predictive of outcome. Instead, LV size and function are used for risk stratification of asymptomatic patients with chronic AR. Echo findings in severe AR include:

- Dilated LV: minor-axis dimension > 50 to 55 mm in systole or > 70 to 75 mm in diastole
- LV ejection fraction < 55 percent
- Pressure half-time < 200 ms
- Proximal regurgitant color jet width/LVOT diameter ≥ 65 percent
- Vena contracta > 6 mm
- Holodiastolic flow reversal in the descending thoracic aorta
- Restrictive filling pattern to the MV inflow

In comparison to men, women with AR should be considered for surgery before severe symptoms have developed

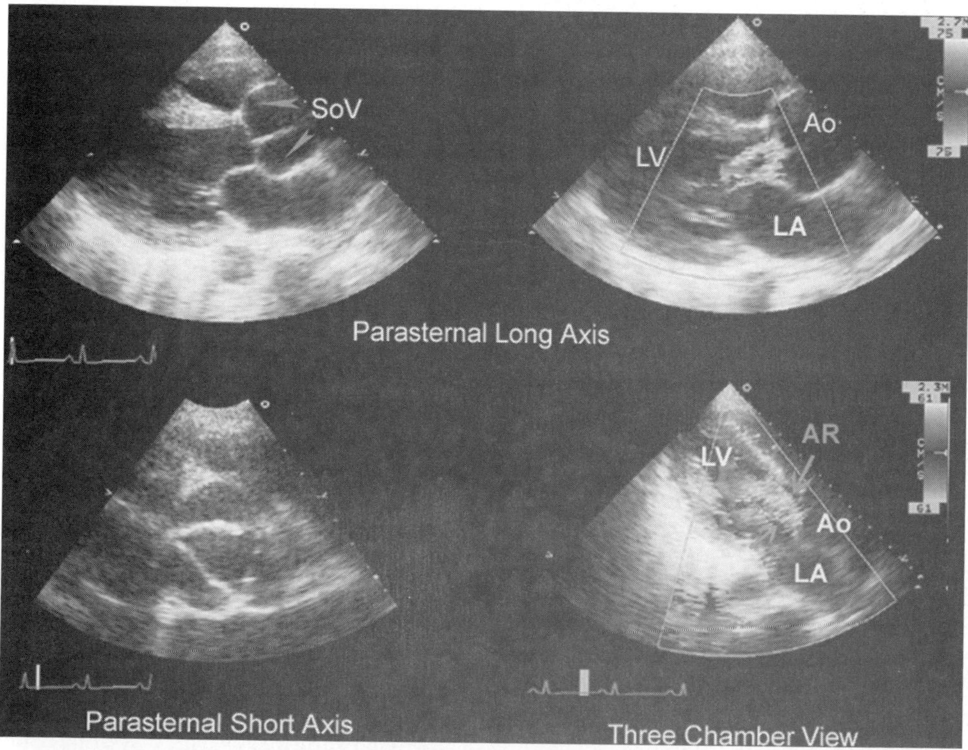

Figure 49-13 Aortic aneurysm of the sinuses of Valsalva and secondary aortic regurgitation. The aortic wall is thin at the sinuses of Valsalva and aneurysmal dilatation results in aortic regurgitation. Note the wide base of the regurgitant jet (vena contracta) consistent with severe aortic regurgitation (arrow). SoV = sinuses of Valsalva; LV = left ventricle; Ao = aorta; LA = left atrium; AR = aortic regurgitation.

Table 49-5 Echocardiographic assessment of the aortic valve

Morphology	Three semilunar leaflets/cusps, LV size and function
Stenosis	Often degenerative/calcific Severe AS: area < 1 cm^2 or mean gradient > 50 mmHg
Regurgitation	Regurgitant jet size does not correlate well with severity Severe AR: dilated LV (ESD > 50–55 mm), LVH, ↓ LV systolic function (EF < 55%) Acute AR: LV dilatation/systolic dysfunction may be absent

LV = left ventricle; AS = aortic stenosis; AR = aortic regurgitation; ESD = end-systolic dimension; LVH = left ventricular hypertrophy; EF = ejection fraction.

and for smaller LV dimensions. In a recent study, intraoperative mortality was similar for men and women, but 10-year survival was significantly worse for women than for men (39 vs. 72 percent, respectively).[26]

In acute AR, many of the features of chronic volume overload will not be present. The severity will be need to be assessed by evaluation of color-flow Doppler jet width, presence of significant pulmonary hypertension, and evidence by Doppler of rapid equilibration of aortic and LV diastolic pressure (short diastolic half-time <200 ms, short mitral deceleration time <150 ms, or premature closure of the MV). Echo assessment of the AV is summarized in Table 49-5.

TRICUSPID VALVE

Tricuspid valve morphology

Normal function of the TV depends on the normal function of its components: annulus, leaflets, chordae, papillary muscles, right atrium, and ventricle.

Tricuspid stenosis

The most common cause of tricuspid stenosis (TS) is rheumatic, which results in both stenosis and regurgitation of the TV and is often associated with concomitant mitral or AV disease. Echo assessment of TS is similar to that of MS. The mean gradient across the TV is normally < 2 mmHg. Tricuspid stenosis is considered severe when the mean gradient is ≥ 7 mmHg and the pressure half-time (PHT) is ≥ 190 ms.

Tricuspid regurgitation

As in the case of the AV and MV, TTE or TEE evaluation of tricuspid regurgitation (TR) focuses on the identification of the etiology or mechanism of TR as well as its hemodynamic severity. TR is the most common abnormality of the TV. Mild TR is a normal finding in 70 percent of individuals.[16] Pathologic TR is often secondary to RV dysfunction, RV dilatation, or significant systolic pulmonary hypertension (systolic pulmonary artery pressures > 55 mmHg). Primary causes of TR are less common (Ebstein's anomaly, endocarditis, trauma, anorectic drugs, carcinoid, myxomatous or rheumatic valvular disease, radiation). Patients with severe TR of any cause have poor long-term outcomes because of RV dysfunction and/or systemic venous congestion. TV reconstruction, annuloplasty, or valve replacement is indicated in some cases of severe TR.

TEE is useful intraoperatively to assess the need for TV surgery when TR is secondary to annular dilatation and/or elevated pulmonary artery pressures, particularly during MV surgery. After correction of MV disease, TV surgery may be required if persistent severe TR or annular dilatation (≥ 30 mm) is still present (Fig. 49-14).[27]

Severity of tricuspid regurgitation

Echo findings in severe TR include[16]:

- A large regurgitant (color) jet (> 10 cm^2), vena contracta > 7 mm, or eccentric jet
- Annular dilatation (≥ 30 mm), leaflet coaptation, anatomic clues (e.g., vegetations, myxomatous disease)
- Dilated right atrial (RA)
- Dilated RV and paradoxical interventricular septal wall motion
- Pulmonary hypertension
- Dilated venae cavae and hepatic veins with minimal respiratory flow variation and systolic flow reversal

Pulmonary hypertension

In the absence of pulmonary stenosis, pulmonary artery systolic pressure is equal to RV systolic pressure (RVSP). RVSP is estimated using the simplified Bernoulli equation ($\Delta P = 4V^2$) from the peak TR velocity (V). ΔP is then the pressure gradient across the TV, or the pressure difference between the RA and RV ($\Delta P = P_{RV} - P_{RA}$). In the absence of elevated RA pressures, the right atrial pressure (P_{RA}) is estimated at 10 mmHg. Therefore,

$$\boxed{RVSP = P_{RA} + \Delta P = 10 + 4V^2}$$

Where RVSP = RV systolic pressure and V = peak TR velocity (ms).

Severity of pulmonary hypertension

Normal pulmonary artery systolic values are 18 to 25 mmHg with a mean of 12 to 16 mmHg.[2] Pulmonary hypertension is defined as systolic pulmonary artery pressure greater than 30 mmHg or mean pulmonary artery pressure less than 20 mmHg at rest.[2] Commonly used values using RVSP to estimate the severity of pulmonary hypertension are shown in Table 49-6.

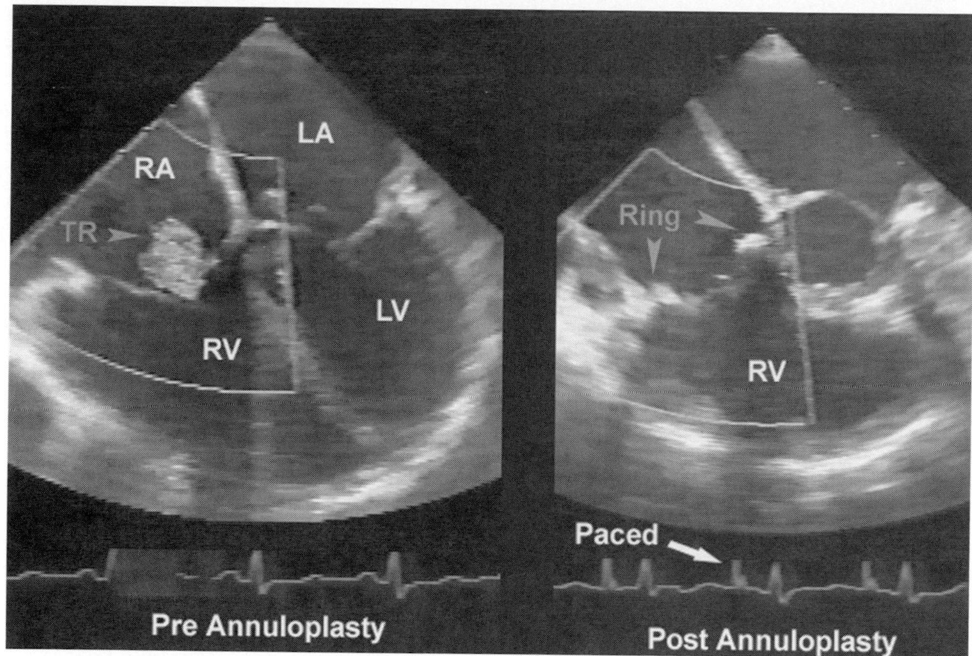

Figure 49-14 Tricuspid valve annuloplasty. This patient had infective endocarditis resulting in flail posterior mitral valve leaflet and tricuspid regurgitation. He underwent mitral valve repair and tricuspid valve annuloplasty. Note the dilated atria and tricuspid annulus preprocedure and the pacer spikes on the rhythm strip postprocedure. RA = right atrium; TR = tricuspid regurgitation; RV = right ventricle.

PROSTHETIC VALVES

Any evaluation of prosthetic valve function should include an assessment of transvalvular pressure gradients and valve area, similar to the evaluation of native valve function. TTE is helpful in the initial assessment of prosthetic valve dysfunction. However, its sensitivity is impaired by difficulty in visualizing structures around and behind the prosthesis, particularly for mechanical valves. Prosthetic material attenuates the ultrasound beam and causes multiple reverberations, hampering interpretation. TEE is often required for the complete evaluation of prosthetic valve structure and function. Cinefluoroscopy may also be a relatively quick and useful method for determining leaflet mobility in mechanical valves and is indicated when mechanical valve thrombosis is suspected. When valve dysfunction is suspected, 2D echo with Doppler and color flow in addition to TEE may be necessary for a comprehensive evaluation of valve function. Such an evaluation of valve function is summarized in Table 49-7.[28] TEE findings in common complications of prosthetic valves are shown in Table 49-8.[28]

Table 49-6 Severity of pulmonary hypertension

	RVSP (mmHg)
Normal	18–25
Mild	30–40
Moderate	40–70
Severe	>70

RVSP = right ventricular systolic pressure.

Prosthetic valve pressure gradients

Like native valve gradients, prosthetic valve pressure gradients can be obtained using the simplified Bernoulli

Table 49-7 Evaluation of prosthetic valves

Pressure gradients	$\Delta P = 4V^2$
Valve area	MV prostheses: area = 220/PHT AV or MV prostheses: $A_1V_1 = A_2V_2$
Regurgitation/leaks	Size, symmetry, velocity, eccentricity
Leaflet mobility/restriction	Degree of leaflet excursion
LV size/function	LV dimensions, EF
Pulmonary hypertension	RVSP = $4V^2 + 10$
Compare with prior echo	Change in gradients, area, leaks

ΔP = pressure gradient; V = velocity; MV = mitral valve; PHT = pressure half-time; AV = aortic valve; A_1V_1 = flow (area$_1$ × velocity$_1$) proximal to the valve prosthesis; A_2V_2 = flow (area$_2$ × velocity$_2$) across the valve prosthesis; LV = left ventricle; EF = ejection fraction; RVSP = right ventricular systolic pressure.
Source: From Zabalgoitia.[28] With permission.

Table 49-8 TEE Findings in prosthetic valve complications

Paravalvular leak	Large, wide, eccentric jet with high-velocity turbulent flow
	Dehiscence, regurgitation, stenosis
	Calcific degeneration (bioprostheses)
	Often due to inappropriate sizing, stenosis, or regurgitation
	Decreased range of motion or maximum excursion
	Stenosis (± regurgitation)
	Distinguish from fibrin strands, which are small filaments on the atrial aspect of mitral or ventricular aspect of aortic valves
Pannus formation	Stenosis
Structural deterioration	Irregular echogenic mobile mass or masses on valve
	Regurgitation (± stenosis)
	Leaflet destruction (bioprostheses)
	Perivalvular abscess (valve rocking, periaortic root thickening, echolucency)
	Perivalvular dehiscence, fistular tract
Nonstructural dysfunction	
Thrombosis	

Source: From Zabalgoitia.[28] With permission.

equation ($\Delta P = 4V^2$). Compared to normal native valves, homografts and the newer nonstented bioprostheses have similar velocities and pressure gradients, while mechanical valves have higher flow velocities. Prosthetic valves except ball-cage valves normally have pressure gradients since they are by design obstructive, with gradients increasing as valve size decreases. High gradients are often seen with 19-mm AV prostheses. High gradients in prosthetic valves may be seen for other reasons as well, such as high cardiac output, valve obstruction, or significant valvular regurgitation (due to increased flow).

Prosthetic valve area

As in the case of native valves, prosthetic valve area can be calculated using the continuity equation or pressure half-time method. For AV prostheses, the continuity equation ($A_1V_1 = A_2V_2$) is usually used. The LV outflow tract (LVOT) diameter or outer diameter of the sewing ring (not its internal diameter) should be measured for accurate estimation of A_1. For MV prostheses, use of the continuity equation is preferred, since the pressure half-time equation may overestimate the true prosthetic MV area. The continuity equation should not be used if there is significant aortic regurgitation or MR. The same equations may be used for the calculation of prosthetic TV areas.

Paravalvular leaks

Normal amounts of regurgitation are expected with prosthetic valves owing to the built-in transvalvular regurgitation ("closing volume"). The amount of regurgitation increases with valve size, the size of the gap between the occluder and the rim, and lower heart rates. Echo findings[4] of normal prosthetic valve regurgitation include:

1. AV: regurgitant area < 1 cm^2 and length of jet < 1.5 cm
2. MV: regurgitant area < 2 cm^2 and length of jet < 2.5 cm
3. Characteristic flow patterns (Medtronic-Hall, one central jet; Star-Edwards, two curved side jets; Bjork-Shiley, two unequal side jets; St. Jude Medical, two side jets and one central jet)

Larger leaks in other locations (Fig. 49-15) are abnormal and may be associated with significant hemodynamic compromise, hemolysis, or valve dehiscence.[28] TEE is often required to fully assess prosthetic valve regurgitation because of the limited sensitivity of TTE. Echo characteristics that differentiate physiologic from nonphysiologic regurgitation are summarized in Table 49-9.[28]

INFECTIVE ENDOCARDITIS

TEE is the procedure of choice for the detection of vegetations in infective endocarditis, with better sensitivity (50 percent for TTE vs. 90 percent for TEE) and specificity (95 percent for TTE vs. >95 percent for TEE) for native valve endocarditis compared to TTE.[29,30] Characteristics of valvular vegetations are listed in Table 49-10.[29] However, early in the course of infective endocarditis, vegetations may not have these typical characteristics and TEE should be repeated if the clinical suspicion is high. Compared with native valve endocarditis, it is more difficult to identify vegetations on prosthetic valves because of artifact from the prosthetic materials. Often both TTE and TEE are useful to detect vegetations, although TTE has lower sensitivity compared with TEE for prosthetic valve endocarditis.[8] TEE is particularly sensitive for identifying ring abscesses. Complications of infective endocarditis (Fig. 49-16) include:

1. Paravalvular abscesses
2. Valve destruction or perforation, leaflet rupture, or dehiscence of prosthetic valves
3. Fistulas
4. Pseudoaneurysms
5. Emboli

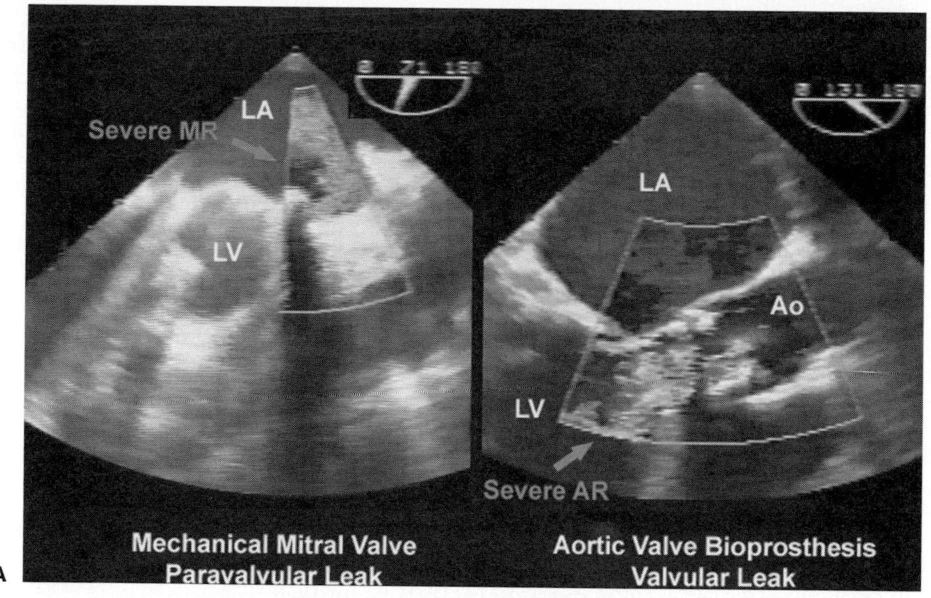

Figure 49-15 Paravalvular and valvular leaks. A. Bileaflet mechanical mitral prosthesis with severe paravalvular regurgitation secondary to endocarditis and partial valve dehiscence, requiring valve replacement. B. Aortic bioprosthesis with severe aortic regurgitation due to calcific degeneration and a torn leaflet. LA = left atrium; LV = left ventricle; MR = mitral regurgitation; Ao = aorta.

EVALUATION OF SPECIFIC DISORDERS

CORONARY ARTERY DISEASE

Myocardial ischemia/infarction

The echo manifestation of myocardial ischemia is a decrease in contractility or systolic wall thickening of the ischemic territory that is manifest within seconds of the onset of ischemia, prior to evidence of electrocardiographic ischemia.[4] Abnormal wall thickening is a better indicator of ischemia than wall motion, since infarcted myocardium may be passively pulled or tethered by adjacent normal myocardium, resulting in apparent wall motion without active contraction. Ancillary signs of ischemia include an increase in end-systolic LV volume and a decrease in global contractility or EF.[4] Hypokinesis is decreased contractility (<30 percent wall thickening); akinesis is the absence of contractility (<10 percent wall thickening); and dyskinesis is outward motion during systole. Echo is accurate at localizing the site of coronary obstruction (Fig. 49-17). However, it usually overestimates infarct size due to myocardial stunning, which has resulted in a lack of correlation between wall motion abnormalities detected on echo in the setting of an acute myocardial infarction and infarct extent.[31]

Table 49-9 Physiologic and nonphysiologic valvular regurgitation

Regurgitant Jet	Physiologic	Nonphysiologic
Size	Small, narrow	Large, wide
Symmetrical	Yes	No
Velocity	Low	High
Eccentric	No	Yes

Source: Modified from Zabalgoitia.[28] With permission.

Ischemic, infarcted, stunned, or hibernating myocardium?

Myocardial segments may be dysfunctional secondary to ischemia, infarction/scar, or stunned or hibernating myocardium. Stunned myocardium is postischemic ventricular dysfunction that occurs when reperfusion of the occluded artery has been achieved but the wall motion and thickening of the corresponding myocardial segment remain abnormal—a condition that may last for days to weeks. Hibernating myocardium results from chronic ischemic dysfunction when the myocardial tissue is chronically hypoperfused owing to inadequate blood flow, resulting in abnormal wall motion and thickening, but it usually recovers after successful revascularization. Resting echo may help differentiate viable (stunned or hibernating) myocardium from nonviable (infarcted or scarred) myocardium based on wall thickness. Thicker myocardium is more likely to be viable, while thinned and fibrotic myocardium most likely represents scar.[4] The specificity of these criteria is quite low, however. Viability assessment

Table 49-10 Echocardiographic characteristics of vegetative and nonvegetative valvular masses

Characteristic	Vegetation	Nonvegetation
Echogenicity	Similar to myocardium Low echogenicity/gray	Similar to pericardium High echogenicity/white
Location	Upstream surface of valve near the regurgitant jet	Downstream surface of valve
Motion	Mobile, prolapses	Less mobile
Shape	Amorphous, lobulated Wide base of attachment	Filamentous, strand-like narrow base of attachment
Regurgitation	Severe regurgitant jet Vegetation located near jet	Mild or no regurgitant jet
Other	Paravalvular abscess/leak Fistula Valve dehiscence	None

Source: Modified from Schiller.[29] With permission.

can be significantly improved with dobutamine or stress echocardiography.[8] A biphasic response on dobutamine echo is the most sensitive parameter for viable myocardium and is associated with improved survival after revascularization. This is evidenced by an improvement in wall motion and thickening or recruitment at low-dose dobutamine (10 to 20 μg/kg/min) followed by worsening of wall motion and thickening at higher doses (30 to 40 μg/kg/min) when the ischemic threshold is reached.

Left ventricular aneurysm and mural thrombus

A true ventricular aneurysm consists of a thin wall (< 7 mm) that is echogenic (and sometimes calcified) and has

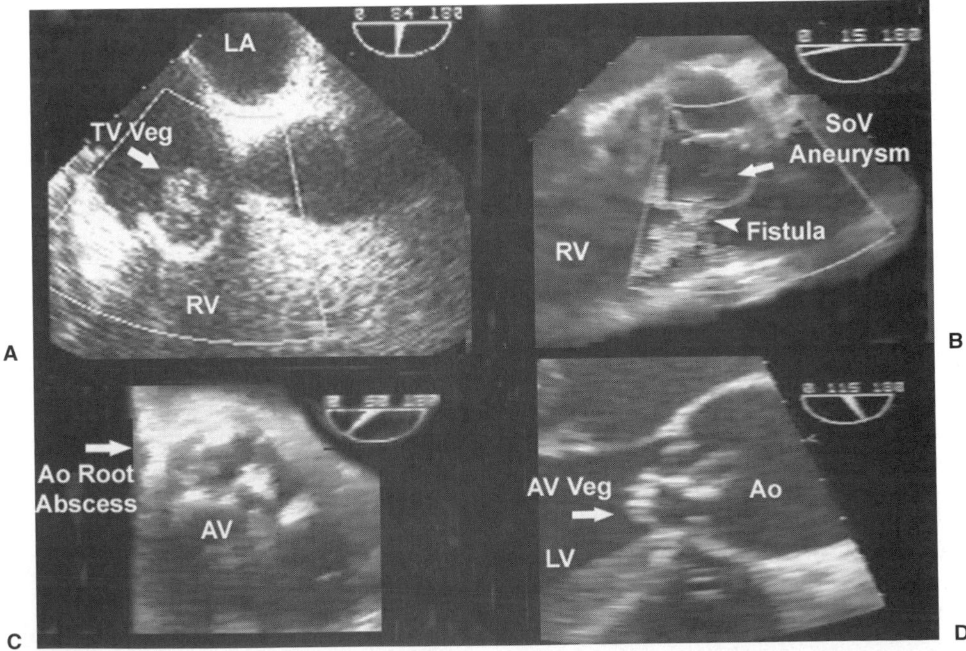

Figure 49-16 Complications of infective endocarditis. A. Large vegetation on bioprosthetic tricuspid valve seen on transesophageal echocardiogram. B. Sinus of Valsalva aneurysm and aortic–right ventricular fistula. C. Bicuspid aortic valve with bacterial endocarditis complicated by large aortic root (annular) abscess (note the thickened perivalvular tissue) and complete heart block requiring emergent surgery. D. Large aortic valve vegetation prolapsing into the left ventricular outflow tract during systole. LA = left atrium; TV = tricuspid valve; RV = right ventricle; SoV = sinus of Valsalva; Ao = aorta; AV = aortic valve; LV = left ventricle.

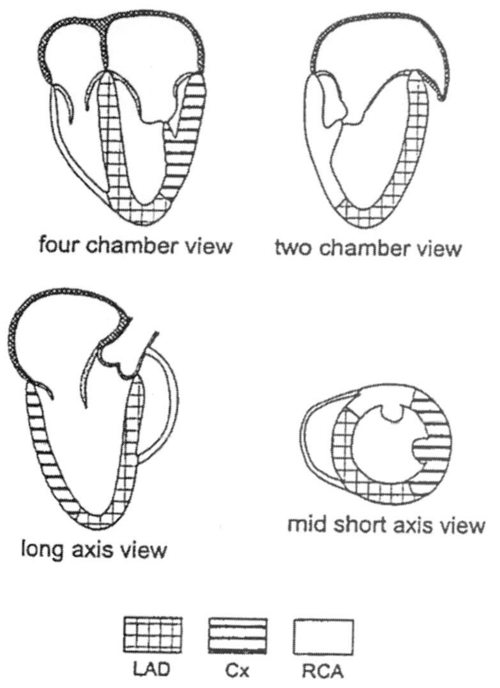

Figure 49-17 Common myocardial perfusion patterns by each of the three major coronary arteries. LAD = left anterior descending; Cx = left circumflex; RCA = right coronary artery. (From Shanewise et al.[12] With permission.)

outward motion in both systole and diastole.[31] Most aneurysms occur apically, with inferobasal aneurysms being the second most common. Aneurysms are complications of adverse remodeling following transmural myocardial infarcts. Spontaneous echo contrast (SEC) or mural thrombus may be present within an LV aneurysm and is associated with an increased risk of embolic events. The appearance of an acute mural thrombus (same echogenicity as myocardium) generally differs from that of a chronic thrombus, which tends to be layered with areas of calcification.[31] Compared to TTE, TEE may be limited in detecting apical thrombi because of the often suboptimal visualization of the true LV apex with TEE.

Pseudoaneurysms can also be complications of acute myocardial infarction and are characterized by the lack of a true myocardial wall. They result from contained free wall myocardial rupture in which a portion of the pericardial space limits frank rupture. Pseudoaneurysms can generally be differentiated from true aneurysms by the presence of a narrow neck (less than half of the maximum diameter) compared to the wider base of a true aneurysm.[31]

Postinfarct ventricular septal defect

Life-threatening mechanical complications after acute myocardial infarction include free wall rupture, papillary muscle dysfunction/rupture, and ventricular septal defect (VSD) (Fig. 49-18). TTE is usually sufficient for the diagnosis of mechanical complications, although TEE may be used as an adjunct. Postinfarct VSD is uncommon (less than 1 percent of total infarcts), although it is associated with the worst outcome of mechanical complications in patients with cardiogenic shock. Unlike postinfarct papillary muscle rupture, VSD occurs with approximately equal frequency after anterior and inferior infarcts. The posteroapical septum is the most common site of postinfarct

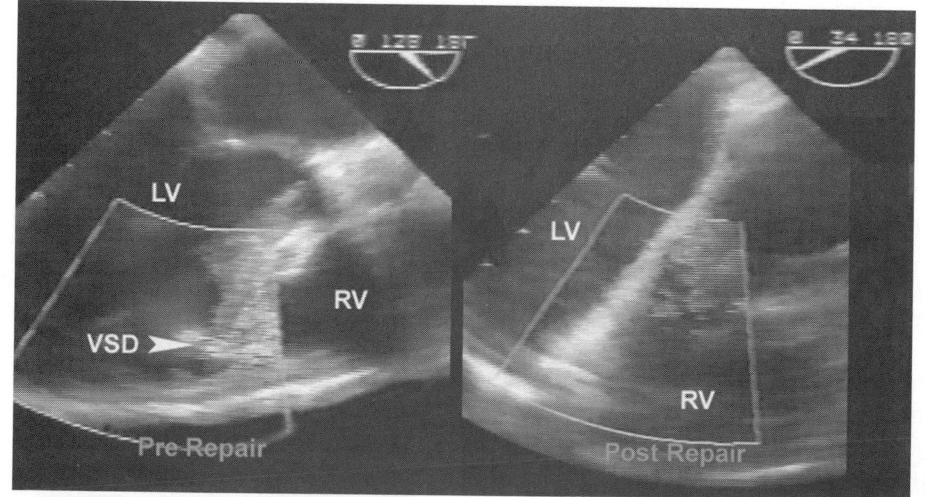

Figure 49-18 Postinfarct ventricular septal defect (VSD). This patient had suffered an acute anterior myocardial infarction that was treated with thrombolytics but subsequently developed a high septal VSD. A. Intraoperative transesophageal echocardiogram with color-flow Doppler diagnostic of VSD with high-velocity turbulent flow across the septum. B. Surgical repair with a pericardial patch and coronary artery bypass grafting to the ostial left anterior descending artery was successful. Color-flow Doppler shows no flow across the septum. LV = left ventricle; RV = right ventricle.

Table 49-11 Diagnostic tests for acute aortic dissection

Test	Sensitivity (%)	Specificity (%)	Pluses and minuses
TEE	99–100	> 89	*Pluses*: Quick, semi-invasive, assesses AR, coronaries, pericardial effusion, may assess IH *Minuses*: Limited assessment of IH, "blind spot" of distal ascending aorta and anterior aortic arch, reverberation artifact
CT	> 90	> 85	*Pluses*: Quick, noninvasive *Minuses*: Cannot assess branch vessels or IH, dye load/allergy
MRI	98–100	100	*Pluses*: Noninvasive, assesses branch vessels, IH *Minuses*: Slow, may not be available, pacemakers/device, breath-hold necessary
Angiography	88–91	> 95	*Pluses*: Assesses coronaries, AR, branch vessels *Minuses*: Slow, invasive, dye load, may miss dissection if lumen is completely thrombosed, does not detect IH

IH = intramural hematoma; AR = aortic regurgitation.
Sources: From Erbel et al.,[32] Sabatine,[33] and Nienaber et al.[34] With permission.

VSD. Echo is the gold standard for diagnosing ventricular septal rupture complicating myocardial infarction. TTE using color-flow Doppler has a sensitivity of 85 to 95 percent, while TEE has a sensitivity and specificity of 100 percent.[31] Echo characteristics of postinfarct VSD, in addition to the septal defect, include the presence of a small pericardial effusion with possible intrapericardial thrombus (echogenic mobile mass in the pericardial space) and echo evidence of tamponade.[31]

THORACIC AORTIC ANEURYSM AND DISSECTION

TTE may diagnose aortic dissection by detecting an intimal flap in the aorta (specificity 95 percent), but it has low sensitivity (80 percent) for ascending aortic dissection and even lower sensitivity for distal thoracic aortic dissection (70 percent).[32] TEE is one of three imaging modalities used for the diagnosis of acute aortic dissection—TEE, computed tomography (CT), and magnetic resonance imaging (MRI)[33,34]—and for the diagnosis of perioperative aortic dissections (Table 49-11). The choice of imaging modality depends primarily on the availability of the imaging procedure and patient characteristics (e.g., hemodynamic instability, presence of a pacemaker, or contrast allergy), since the overall diagnostic accuracy for TEE, CT, and MRI is comparable.[32] TEE is the imaging procedure of choice for patients who are hemodynamically unstable. Compared to CT or MRI, one limitation of TEE is that it cannot image the aortic segment located between the distal ascending aorta and the proximal arch, which may decrease its sensitivity for detection of aortic dissection, hematoma, or atheroma in this region.

The main criterion for TEE diagnosis of suspected acute aortic dissection is the presence of two lumina (false and true) separated by an intimal flap (Table 49-12 and Fig. 49-19). Other findings for diagnosing aortic dissection by TEE[32] include:

1. Tear or disruption of the flap continuity or jets seen with color Doppler across the flap
2. Complete obstruction of the false lumen; presence of thrombus
3. Central displacement of intimal calcification or separation of intimal layers from thrombus
4. Periaortic hematoma (echo-free spaces around the aorta)
5. Intramural hematoma (crescent-shaped echodensity with vacuolization within it on the aortic short-axis view)
6. Pericardial or pleural effusion
7. AR

It is important to define the anatomic site and extension of the dissection, the degree of AR, involvement of the coronary arteries, LV dysfunction, and the presence of pericardial effusion or tamponade.

Intraoperatively, TEE is used during reconstructive surgery for hemodynamic status, entry/exit sites, evaluation of decompression of the false lumen, and assessment of concomitant valve surgery.[13] Postoperatively, TEE is used for the detection of residual regurgitation and LV dysfunction. TEE is also indicated for defining the anatomic site and size of aortic aneurysms.

Table 49-12 True versus false lumen in aortic dissection

	True lumen	False lumen
Systole	Expansion	Collapse
Diastole	Collapse	Expansion
SEC/thrombus	Absent or minimal	Present
Blood flow	Systolic forward flow	Reversed or absent flow

SEC = spontaneous echo contrast.
Source: Erbel et al.[32] With permission.

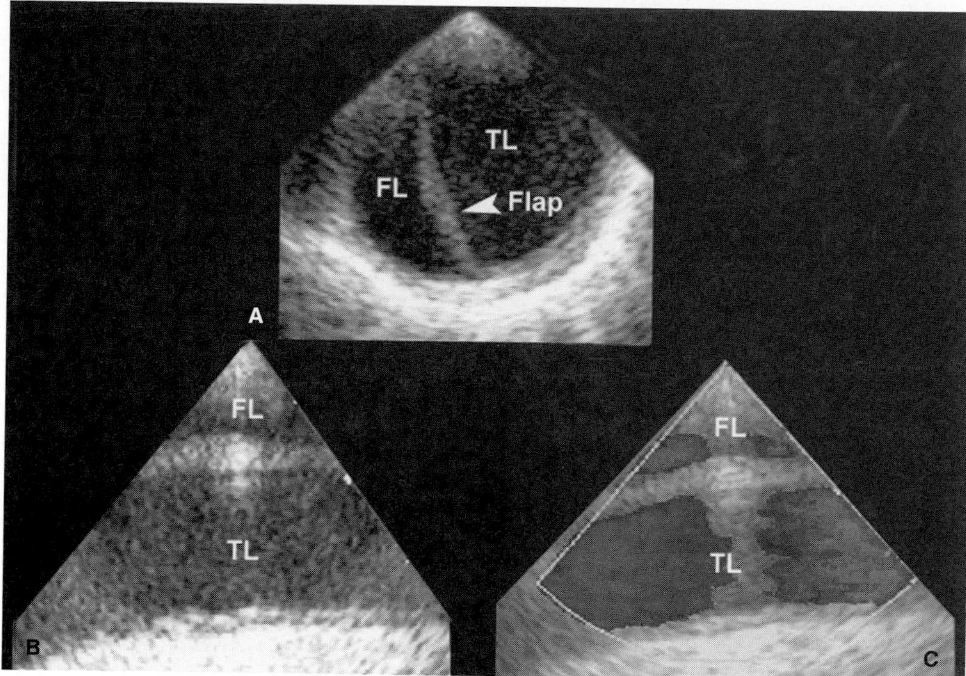

Figure 49-19 Dissection of the descending thoracic aorta. Transesophageal echocardiogram showing a large aortic dissection with the diagnostic flap separating the true (TL) and false lumen (FL). A. Short-axis view. B. Long-axis view. C. Long-axis with color-flow Doppler shows flow in both the true and false lumens.

PERICARDIAL DISEASE

Pericardial effusion and tamponade

Echo is the diagnostic test of choice for detection of pericardial effusion (PE) and assessing its hemodynamic significance. TEE is usually superior to TTE for evaluating pericardial thickness and adjacent structures, although CT and/or MRI are preferred for evaluating the pericardium. Normally, the pericardial space contains 10 to 50 mL of fluid and the pericardium measures 1 to 3 mm in thickness. An increase in the volume of the pericardial fluid results in elevated pericardial pressures, leading to reduced RV filling, followed by reduced LV filling (Fig. 49-20). PE usually appears as an echo-free space surrounding the myocardium, although as protein or cellular debris increases in the fluid, it becomes increasingly echogenic.[35] PE is differentiated from pleural effusion by the anterior location of PE relative to the proximal descending thoracic aorta, while pleural effusion is located posteriorly to the aorta. Epicardial fat may be confused with PE, since it is also echolucent, although epicardial fat is usually more echogenic than pericardial fluid and is usually located anteriorly.[35] TEE is useful in the postoperative patient with tamponade and a small loculated PE that may be difficult to visualize on TTE. Loculated PE in postoperative cardiac surgery patients may cause tamponade in the absence of typical

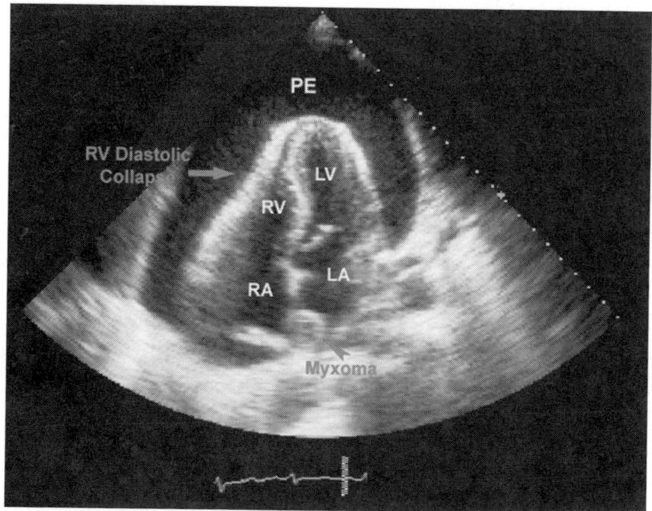

Figure 49-20 Large pericardial effusion and cardiac tamponade. Transthoracic echocardiogram of the apical four-chamber view reveals an atrial myxoma attached to the interatrial septal with a large echolucent circumferential pericardial effusion (PE) and evidence of elevated intrapericardial pressure. Classic features of tamponade are shown with right ventricular (RV) diastolic collapse and abnormal interventricular septal motion (shifted toward the left during inspiration). RA = right atrium; LA = left atrium; LV = left ventricle.

Table 49-13	Echocardiographic signs of cardiac tamponade
RA collapse	Sensitive but not specific.
RV diastolic collapse	Ranges from inward dip to complete collapse of RV free wall in diastole; specific sign but may be absent if elevated RV pressures or adhesions tether RV.
LA, LV collapse	May be the only sign of tamponade in postoperative cardiac surgery patients.
Abnormal interventricular septal motion	Inspiration: septum shifts to the left.
Respiratory variation in ventricular size	Inspiration: LV becomes smaller, RV larger.
Respiratory variation in transvalvular inflow velocities	Inspiration: mitral inflow E velocity decreases, tricuspid inflow velocity increases.
Respiratory variation in PV and HV velocities	Inspiration: PV velocities decrease and HV velocities increase.
Dilated IVC and blunted respiratory changes	Not very specific.

RA = right atrium; RV = right ventricle; LA = left atrium; LV = left ventricle; PV = pulmonary vein; HV = hepatic vein; IVC = inferior vena cava.
Sources: From Oh[4] and Munt et al.[35] With permission.

Table 49-14	Echocardiographic signs of constriction
Pericardial thickening and calcification	TEE better than TTE, but additional imaging with CT or MRI may be necessary
Dilated RA, LA, IVC	Nonspecific findings
Diastolic flattening of the LV posterior wall	Secondary to reduced filling in mid- to late diastole, sensitive but not specific
Abnormal interventricular septal motion	Inspiration: septum shifts to the left
Premature pulmonary valve opening	RV diastolic pressure > PA diastolic pressure in middiastole
Respiratory variation in ventricular size	Inspiration: LV becomes smaller, RV larger
Respiratory variation in transvalvular and venous (pulmonary/hepatic) flow velocities	As in tamponade, respiratory variation may be more prominent in constriction

RA = right atrium; LA = left atrium; IVC = inferior vena cava; LV = left ventricle; RV = right ventricle; PA = pulmonary artery.
Sources: From Oh,[4] Munt et al.,[35] and Hoit.[36] With permission.

echo signs (Table 49-13). In these patients, any evidence of LA or LV collapse or other localized chamber compression may be indicative of hemodynamically significant elevated intrapericardial pressures.

Constrictive pericardial disease

In constrictive pericardial disease, the pericardium is thickened (>3 mm) and often calcified, which reduces ventricular filling in diastole and causes diastolic heart failure. However, the absence of pericardial calcification does not rule out the diagnosis of constriction. Although echo signs of constriction (Table 49-14) are not very sensitive or specific, a completely normal echo study usually rules out constriction.[36] Other imaging modalities, such as CT or MRI, may be necessary to further evaluate the pericardium and distinguish constriction from restriction.

CARDIAC SOURCES OF EMBOLI

One of the most common indications for TEE is for the evaluation for cardiac sources of emboli, since TTE does not visualize well the potential sources of emboli (LA appendage thrombus, aortic atheroma, patent foramen ovale or atrial septal defect, LV thrombus, valvular lesions, intracardiac tumors). Small thrombi in the LA or LA appendage can be detected using TEE. In addition, factors that may contribute to or accompany atrial thrombi are often seen in the absence of an obvious thrombus: LA or LA appendage enlargement, SEC consistent with blood stasis, and decreased LA appendage contraction with low PW Doppler velocities (< 20 mm/s). Aortic atheromas are evaluated for mobile components, plaque rupture, and ulceration and are graded as mild (< 1 mm), moderate (1 to 3.9 mm), and severe (≥ 4 mm).

ATRIAL SEPTAL DEFECTS

TEE is superior to TTE for visualizing atrial septal defects (ASDs). The anatomic defect is visualized using two-dimensional echo and confirmed with Doppler and contrast (bubble study) using maneuvers that increase RA pressure, such as Valsalva or cough. The hemodynamic significance of the shunt is assessed using Doppler by quantifying the shunt size and determining the presence of pulmonary hypertension. Shunt quantification is obtained as the ratio of pulmonary to systemic flow (Q_p:Q_s) using Doppler cardiac outputs across the pulmonary valve and AV.[4] All four pulmonary veins should be visualized and the presence of associated anomalies excluded. TEE plays an important role in determining the suitability of ASDs for device closure versus cardiac surgery based on the size of the ASD and the rim of tissue surrounding it as well as the degree of septal tissue redundancy.[23] TEE has become essential for guiding placement of catheter-deployed closure devices and in assessing residual shunts (Fig. 49-21).

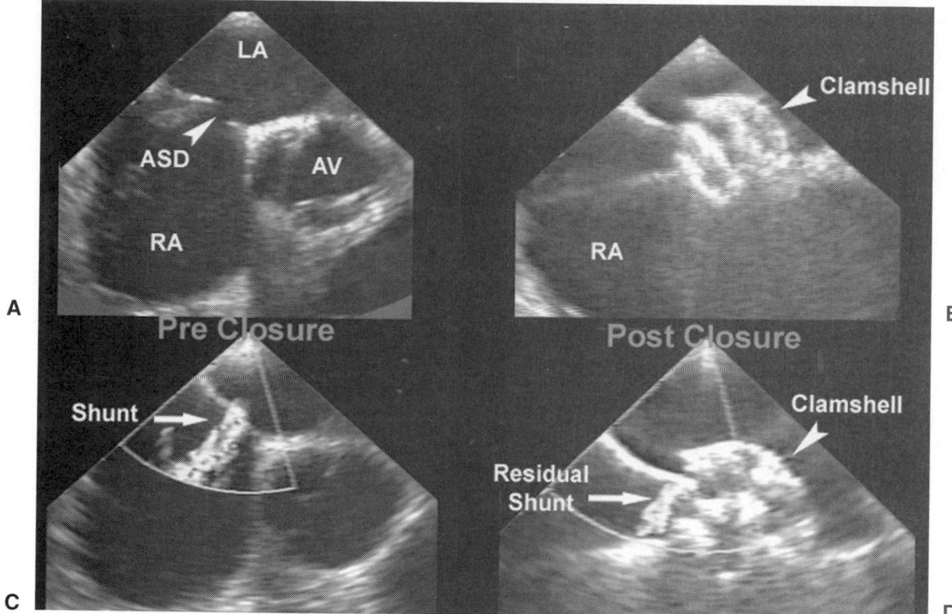

Figure 49-21 Secundum atrial septal defect (ASD) and clamshell closure. A. Secundum ASD seen as a defect in the mid-interatrial septum along with a dilated right atrium (RA) on transesophageal echocardiography. The size of the rim of tissue between the ASD and the aortic valve is critical in determining likelihood of success with device closure. C. Color-flow Doppler of the ASD shows a high-turbulence jet consistent with shunt (arrow). B. The clamshell has been deployed across the ASD. D. Postprocedure color-flow Doppler with small residual shunt that usually resolves spontaneously after a period of several weeks to months. AV = aortic valve.

CARDIAC TUMORS

TEE, because of its high sensitivity, is the imaging modality of choice and is superior to TTE, CT, MRI, and angiography for detecting cardiac tumors.[1,4] Although MRI may not detect small cardiac tumors, it is usually performed after TEE for further differentiation of thrombus (presence of methemoglobin or hemosiderin) from neoplasm, since it is superior to TEE for tissue characterization. MRI examinations are multiplanar and typically include fast T1- and T2-weighted techniques with administration of gadolinium (a paramagnetic contrast agent) and a technique for imaging moving structures with single-slice breath-hold, such as fast gradient-echo sequences (e.g., FLASH). Primary tumors are more likely to affect the myocardium, while secondary tumors usually involve the pericardium with secondary intramyocardial infiltation.[37] Atrial myxomas are the most common (up to 25 percent) primary cardiac tumors. Atrial myxomas as seen on TEE or TTE show several typical features[37] (Fig. 49-22A):

- Ninety percent originate in the interatrial septum, near the fossa ovalis.
- A spherical mass with a speckled appearance is often seen in RA myxomas, while a villous amorphous mass may be seen in LA myxomas.
- Ninety percent attach to the wall of the atrium via a stalk, which may allow prolapse through the MV.
- Intramural hemorrhage (cysts) and necrosis result in a heterogeneous appearance of echodensity; calcifications are uncommon but may be seen.
- They may be highly mobile and a cardiac source of embolus.

Metastatic tumors to the heart most commonly arise from the breast or lung but may include leiomyosarcoma (Fig. 49-22B). Metastatic tumors usually affect the pericardium and result in pericardial effusion. In addition, some tumors metastasize through the inferior vena cava (renal cell, hepatoma), affecting the right heart more than the left; TEE allows for visualization of the route of extension.[37] Tumors involving the cardiac valves are rare (often fibroelastomas) and may affect valve competence and global LV function. MRI and ultrafast CT may be a useful adjunct in delineating tumors of the cardiac valves.[38]

LEFT VENTRICULAR OUTFLOW TRACT OBSTRUCTION

TEE is used intraoperatively for septal myectomy for treatment of obstruction of the LV outflow tract (LVOT) due

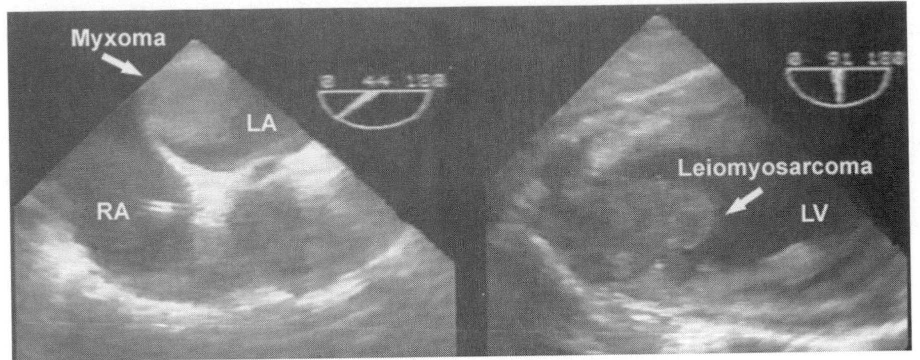

Figure 49-22 Cardiac tumors. A. Large atrial myxoma attached to the interatrial septum, seen as a spherical mass with a speckled appearance. B. Metastatic leiomyosarcoma of genitourinary tract origin with myocardial invasion of the left ventricular (LV) apex.

to hypertrophic cardiomyopathy. Systolic anterior motion (SAM) of the MV may cause LVOT obstruction; TEE is used to define the structures involved in the SAM (e.g., chordae, anterior leaflet). As in aortic stenosis, LVOT gradients may differ intraoperatively versus preoperatively owing to different hemodynamics. Color-flow Doppler typically demonstrates turbulent blood flow (mosaic pattern) at the site of LVOT obstruction. An eccentric jet of MR may also be seen if there is abnormal coaptation of the mitral leaflets (usually a posteriorly directed jet owing to abnormal coaptation of the anterior mitral leaflet).

TEE is also helpful during resection of lesions causing subaortic stenosis. It can determine the location and severity of obstruction. It is also useful for evaluating the success of the surgery in relieving the obstruction and in detecting MR that may result from the surgery.[22]

References

1. Otto CM. *The Practice of Clinical Echocardiography.* Philadelphia: Saunders, 2002:977.
2. Braunwald EB. *Heart Disease.* Philadelphia: Saunders, 2001:2297.
3. Maurer G, Mohl W. *Echocardiography and Doppler in Cardiac Surgery.* New York: Igaku-Shoin, 1989:355.
4. Oh JK. *The Echo Manual.* Philadelphia: Lippincott Williams & Wilkins, 1999:278.
5. Murphy JG. *Mayo Clinic Cardiology Review.* Philadelphia: Lippincott Williams & Wilkins, 2000:1381.
6. Quinones MA, Otto CM, Stoddard M, et al. *American Society of Echocardiography: Recommendations for Quantification of Doppler Echocardiography.* Raleigh, NC: American Society of Echocardiography, 2001.
7. Hagan AD, DeMaria AN. *Clinical Applications of Two-Dimensional Echocardiography and Cardiac Doppler.* Boston/Toronto: Little, Brown, 1989:1556.
8. Cheitlin MD, Armstrong WF, Aurigemma GP, et al. ACC/AHA/ASE 2003 guideline update for the clinical application of echocardiography: Summary article: A report of the American College of Cardiology/American Heart Association Task Force on Practice Guidelines (ACC/AHA/ASE Committee to Update the 1997 Guidelines for the Clinical Application of Echocardiography). *Circulation* 2003;108:1146–1162.
9. ACC/AHA Guidelines for the Management of Patients with Valvular Heart Disease. A report of the American College of Cardiology/American Heart Association. Task Force on Practice Guidelines (Committee on Management of Patients with Valvular Heart Disease). *J Am Coll Cardiol* 1998; 32:1486–1588.
10. Goldstein SA, Harry M. *American Society of Echocardiography Core Curriculum for Physicians.* Raleigh, NC: American Society of Echocardiography, Vol. 2003.
11. Oh JK, Appleton CP, Hatle LK, et al. The noninvasive assessment of left ventricular diastolic function with two-dimensional and Doppler echocardiography. *J Am Soc Echocardiogr* 1997;10:246–270.
12. Shanewise JS, Cheung AT, Aronson S, et al. ASE/SCA guidelines for performing a comprehensive intraoperative multiplane transesophageal echocardiography examination: Recommendations of the American Society of Echocardiography Council for Intraoperative Echocardiography and the Society of Cardiovascular Anesthesiologists Task Force for Certification in Perioperative Transesophageal Echocardiography. *J Am Soc Echocardiogr* 1999;12:884–900.
13. Practice guidelines for perioperative transesophageal echocardiography. A report by the American Society of Anesthesiologists and the Society of Cardiovascular Anesthesiologists Task Force on Transesophageal Echocardiography. *Anesthesiology* 1996;84:986–1006.
14. Schiller NB. Hemodynamics derived from transesophageal echocardiography (TEE). *Cardiol Clin* 2000;18:699–709.
15. Wilkins GT, Weyman AE, Abascal VM, et al. Percutaneous balloon dilatation of the mitral valve: An analysis of echocardiographic variables related to outcome and the mechanism of dilatation. *Br Heart J* 1988; 60:299–308.
16. Zoghbi WA, Enriquez-Sarano M, Foster E, et al. Recommendations for evaluation of the severity of native valvular regurgitation with two-dimensional and Doppler echocardiography. *J Am Soc Echocardiogr* 2003;16:777–802.

17. Griffin BP, Stewart WJ. Echocardiography in patient selection, operative planning, and intraoperative evaluation of mitral valve repair. In: Otto CM (ed). *The Practice of Clinical Echocardiography.* Philadelphia: Saunders, 2002:417–434.
18. Thomas JD. Doppler echocardiographic assessment of valvular regurgitation. *Heart* 2002;88:651–657.
19. Playford D, Weyman AE. Mitral valve prolapse: Time for a fresh look. *Rev Cardiovasc Med* 2001;2:73–81.
20. Freed LA, Levy D, Levine RA, et al. Prevalence and clinical outcome of mitral-valve prolapse. *N Engl J Med* 1999;341:1–7.
21. Zaroff JG, Picard MH. Transesophageal echocardiographic (TEE) evaluation of the mitral and tricuspid valves. *Cardiol Clin* 2000;18:731–750.
22. Shively BK. Transesophageal echocardiographic (TEE) evaluation of the aortic valve, left ventricular outflow tract, and pulmonic valve. *Cardiol Clin* 2000;18:711–729.
23. King MEE. Echocardiographic evaluation of the adult with unoperated congenital heart disease. In: Otto CM (ed). *The Practice of Clinical Echocardiography.* Philadelphia: Saunders, 2002:868–899.
24. Hahn RT, Roman MJ, Mogtader AH, Devereux RB. Association of aortic dilation with regurgitant, stenotic and functionally normal bicuspid aortic valves. *J Am Coll Cardiol* 1992;19:283–288.
25. Otto CM, Burwash IG, Legget ME, et al. Prospective study of asymptomatic valvular aortic stenosis. Clinical, echocardiographic, and exercise predictors of outcome. *Circulation* 1997;95:2262–2270.
26. Klodas E, Enriquez-Sarano M, Tajik AJ, et al. Surgery for aortic regurgitation in women. Contrasting indications and outcomes compared with men. *Circulation* 1996;94:2472–2478.
27. Raman SV, Wooley CF. Tricuspid valvular regurgitation. *Curr Treat Options Cardiovasc Med* 2001;3:37–43.
28. Zabalgoitia M. Echocardiographic recognition and quantitation of prosthetic valve dysfunction. In: Otto CM (ed). The Practice of Clinical Echocardiography. Philadelphia: Saunders, 2002:525–550.
29. Schiller NB. Clinical decision making in endocarditis. In: Otto CM (ed). *The Practice of Clinical Echocardiography.* Philadelphia: Saunders, 2002:451–468.
30. Ryan EW, Bolger AF. Transesophageal echocardiography in the evaluation of infective endocarditis. *Cardiol Clin* 2000;18:773–787.
31. Foster E, Tseng ZH. Echocardiography in the coronary care unit. In: Otto CM (ed). *The Practice of Clinical Echocardiography.* Philadelphia: Saunders, 2002:251–274.
32. Erbel R, Alfonso F, Boileau C, et al. Diagnosis and management of aortic dissection. *Eur Heart J* 2001;22:1642–1681.
33. Sabatine MS. *Pocket Medicine.* Philadelphia: Lippincott Williams and Wilkins, 2000:31.
34. Nienaber CA, von Kodolitsch Y, Nicolas V, et al. The diagnosis of thoracic aortic dissection by noninvasive imaging procedures. *N Engl J Med* 1993;328:1–9.
35. Munt BI, Kinnaird T, Thompson CR. Pericardial disease. In: Otto CM (ed). *The Practice of Clinical Echocardiography.* Philadelphia: Saunders, 2002:639–657.
36. Hoit BD. Management of effusive and constrictive pericardial heart disease. *Circulation* 2002;105:2939–2942.
37. Goldman JH, Foster E. Transesophageal echocardiographic (TEE) evaluation of intracardiac and pericardial masses. *Cardiol Clin* 2000;18:849–860.
38. Wintersperger BJ, Becker CR, Gulbins H, et al. Tumors of the cardiac valves: Imaging findings in magnetic resonance imaging, electron beam computed tomography, and echocardiography. *Eur Radiol* 2000;10:443–449.

CHAPTER

50 CARDIAC MAGNETIC RESONANCE IMAGING

Jens Vogel-Claussen, David A. Bluemke

INTRODUCTION

The availability of high-field-strength magnets, high-performance-gradient hardware, and ultrafast sequence technology in recent years has transformed cardiac magnetic resonance imaging (MRI) into a multifunctional tool. Cardiac MRI can provide three-dimensional analysis of cardiac anatomy, viability, motion, and function with high accuracy and reproducibility.[1,2] Because of the complex cardiac anatomy and motion, cardiac MRI can be challenging and previously had been performed primarily at specialized centers. More recently, a comprehensive cardiac MRI exam has become a reliable clinical tool in a wide range of healthcare centers. In this article we briefly outline imaging techniques and illustrate the various applications of cardiac MRI.

GENERAL PRINCIPLES

Communication between the surgeon and the MRI center is essential for efficient and accurate diagnosis. The examination will then be tailored to the specific clinical question. Instructing patients as to the nature of the examination will likely significantly improve the quality of the test. During the MRI examination, patients will need to perform multiple breath-holds of about 10 to 20 s duration. Patients with severe shortness of breath or who cannot lie flat on the MRI table are often poor candidates for cardiac MRI. Such patients should be discussed with the MRI center prior to referral. Overall, a directed examination requires about 20 to 30 min, whereas a comprehensive examination will require 45 to 60 min. There are no restrictions on eating or drinking before the MRI examination except if stress examinations are performed (see below).

CONTRAINDICATIONS

Compatibility of a patient's devices with the MRI scanner is a frequent issue and changes frequently with technology development. In general, all prosthetic cardiac valves are MRI-compatible. Pacemakers and implantable cardioverters/defibrillators (ICDs) are generally considered to be incompatible with MRI. However, there have been recent reports at our institution and others of patients who have safely undergone MRI at 1.5 T with certain types of these devices in place.[3,4] Currently, MRI scanning with pacemakers or ICDs in place is considered experimental, but there is rapid development in this area. Older devices manufactured before the year 2000 and certain manufacturers' devices are less likely to be MRI-compatible. Thus, consultation with the MRI center should be performed when an MRI examination is deemed essential to patient care.

Coronary and other vascular stents are increasingly common. Most stents have not been explicitly tested by the manufacturer for MRI compatibility. Package labels from the manufacturer may indicate that MRI may be performed 6 weeks after implantation, with the rationale that the stent is endothelialized at that time and less likely to move in the magnetic field. Our approach is to evaluate these devices on a case-by-case basis. In many instances, the risk of performing the MRI examination with such a device may be outweighed by the benefit of performing the examination. Lists of devices that have been tested for MRI compatibility have been published in the literature as well as listed on websites, such as www.MRIsafety.com.

There is no known adverse effect of MRI on the fetus; MRI examination is frequently preferred compared to imaging examinations using x-rays. The decision to scan during pregnancy should be made on an individual basis. The contrast agents used for MRI cross the placenta, so deferring the examination to a later trimester would also reduce any potential risk.[5]

If cardiac stress imaging is performed with dobutamine, adenosine, or dipyridamole, the patient should be questioned about relative contraindications to these agents and specifically counseled to avoid theophylline-containing drugs or foods for at least 24 h prior to the exam. A gadolinium-based contrast agent is frequently used in association with cardiac MRI. Unlike iodine-based contrast agents for computed tomography or angiography, the MRI contrast agents have no significant effect on renal function. Patients with renal insufficiency are frequently referred to MRI for this reason. Reactions to the MRI contrast agent are very rare, but a prior severe reaction would constitute a contraindication to the contrast injection.

CARDIAC GATING

Cardiac MRI makes use of electrocardiographic (ECG) gating to suppress cardiac motion artifacts and arterial pulsation. The objective of cardiac gating is to acquire an R wave that is taller than the S or T wave. Even after obtaining a strong ECG signal initially, the signal may become obscured by additional noise from the magnetic field or regurgitant fraction (RF) pulses. Therefore optimal electrode-to-skin contact is necessary and skin shaving and cleansing is often necessary at the electrode placement sites. Nevertheless, imaging with an impaired ECG signal (i.e., pericardial effusion) or cardiac arrhythmias can be challenging.[6] For patients with arrhythmia who can tolerate a beta blocker, a short-acting agent (e.g., metoprolol) may be administered 30 min before the MRI examination.

UNDERSTANDING CARDIAC MAGNETIC RESONANCE IMAGES

Terminology in MRI can be quite confusing to both the cardiovascular imager and the cardiovascular surgeon. The method of creating the images is termed the "pulse sequence," and pulse sequence names often change in order to give a manufacturer a perceived marketing advantage over competitors. Therefore a brief review of some principles underlying the terminology is worthwhile.

Images may be rather simply classified by the relative brightness of blood in the vessels or in the ventricular chambers. The blood can be made to be dark ("black-blood images") when the ventricular or arterial walls are the primary focus of the examination (Fig. 50-1). For example, to visualize a myocardial infarction, it is useful to make the blood in the ventricle very dark so as not to obscure the ventricular wall. Although it is entirely acceptable to refer to such images as "black-blood images," more specific terminology can be used to indicate how the image was generated. Thus, the term *black-blood image* is a very generic way of describing more specific terminology such as fast spin-echo or turbo spin-echo images.

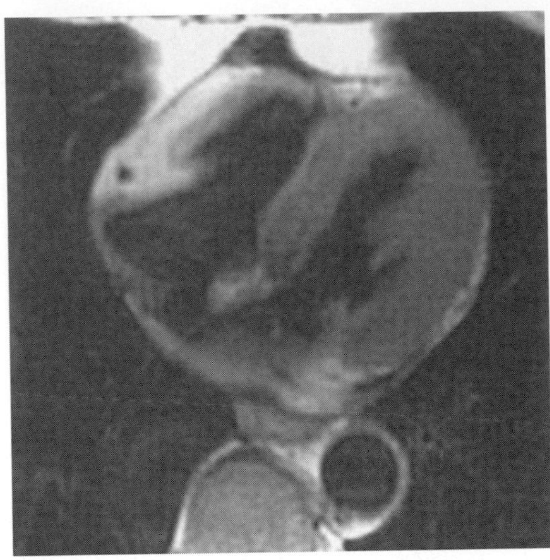

Figure 50-1 Transverse black-blood MRI of the heart and descending thoracic aorta. Because of the double-inversion technique, the blood in the cardiac chambers and descending aorta appears black.

The most important type of black-blood image generation for the cardiovascular system is termed a double-inversion recovery fast spin-echo sequence. These images are acquired in a breath-hold and are used to image myocardial edema, tumors, or complex anatomic regions. The method involves a specific pulse ("inversion pulse") that is used to make the blood dark relative to the myocardium. Advantages of the method are very high soft tissue contrast, similar to that seen in brain or musculoskeletal imaging. Spatial resolution is usually quite good, between 0.5 and 2 mm. The disadvantage is a relatively long imaging time. In addition, the images are static rather than cine images.[7]

Black-blood MR images can be further categorized. "T1-weighted" MR images display myocardium and fluid as intermediate signal and fat as bright signal. T1-weighted MR images are also used to show enhancement of abnormal tissues after intravenous administration of a gadolinium-based MR contrast agent (discussed further below). "T2-weighted" MR images show fluid and edema as bright signal. These are most commonly used to depict inflammation, tumor edema, or edema from myocardial infarction.

Besides black-blood images, the most commonly used MR images are "bright-blood images" (Fig. 50-2). Typically, these are viewed as cine images of the ventricle or valve planes. These methods have the advantage of taking less time to acquire than the black-blood images; thus visualization of motion is possible. The temporal resolution of these images is 25 to 50 ms or less if needed.

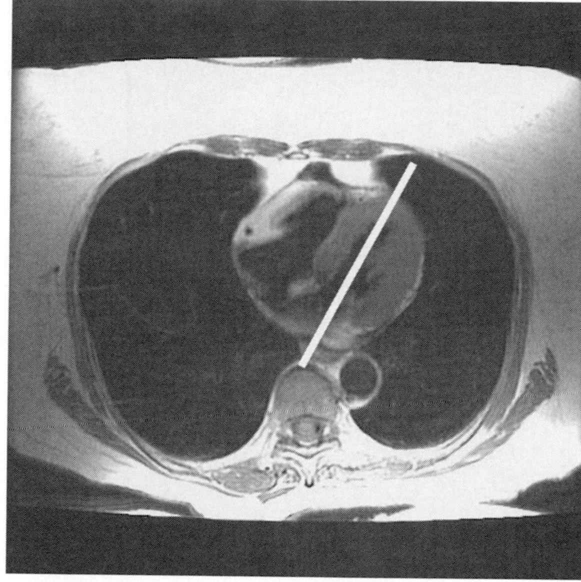

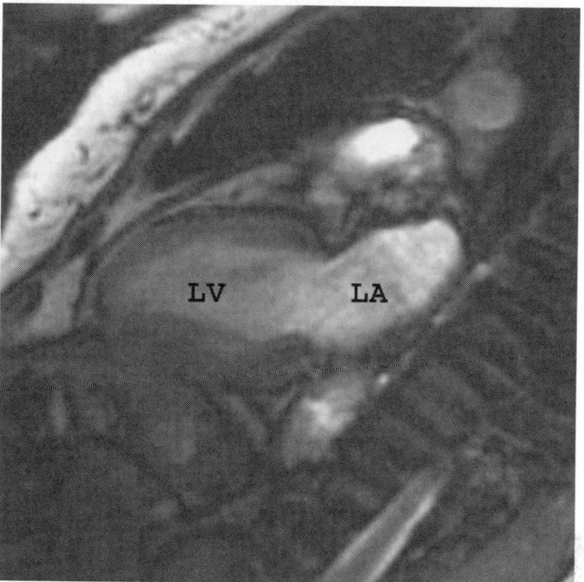

Figure 50-2 By imaging in the plane through the left ventricle and left atrium prescribed by the white bar on the transverse view (A), an oblique vertical long-axis two-chamber view of the left ventricle and left atrium is obtained (B). The long-axis view is acquired with the bright-blood (FIESTA) MRI technique (B). LA = left atrium; LV = left ventricle.

The bright-blood cine images are generated using a method generally known as gradient echo (GRE) imaging. The newest GRE methods have trade names such as balanced fast-field echo, FIESTA, or TrueFISP, depending on the vendor of the MR scanner. These sequences are of specific advantage for cardiac MR and represent substantial improvement in image quality compared to older methods of cardiac cine imaging.[8] The spatial resolution of the images is about 2 mm, which is substantially greater than the resolution possible with nuclear techniques (6 mm). The blood pool in the ventricle has very bright signal, so that the border between the ventricle and blood pool is easily distinguished. Turbulent jets at sites of stenosis or regurgitation are dark and readily distinguished using the newest sequences. Gradient-echo images are also used for imaging myocardial infarction.

Disadvantages of bright-blood gradient-echo images include large amounts of image distortion around metal, including sternal wire implants, stents, and embolization coils. The most frequent problem we have observed arose in patients with congenital heart disease who had embolization coils placed and required later evaluation with MRI. These coils distort large areas of anatomy, with the area of distortion centered on the device.

Other techniques—such as flow-sensitive MRI, myocardial viability techniques, and vascular imaging—are discussed later in this chapter.

CARDIAC IMAGING PLANES

Since the cardiac axes differ significantly from the axial, sagittal, and coronal planes of the body, specific imaging planes are necessary for adequate cardiac visualization and evaluation. Recently three-dimensional acquisitions have been developed, so that the heart can be sliced and viewed from any desirable angle at postprocessing. This further shortens the acquisition time. A brief illustration of key imaging planes and how these images are derived is provided below.

Axial, sagittal, and coronal planes

The first imaging plane is usually a transverse image of the chest with black-blood techniques (Fig. 50-1). Radiologists and surgeons are most familiar with this plane; it can not only permit evaluation of the anatomic position of the cardiac chambers, coronary artery origins, and great vessels but also detect extracardial intrathoracic pathology. Further sagittal and coronal planes can be obtained. The coronal plane is useful in evaluating the left ventricular outflow tract, aortic valve anatomy, diaphragmatic portion of the left ventricular wall, and the extension of the pericardium over the proximal portion of the great vessels. The plane parallel to the aortic arch on axial images is called the double-oblique or oblique sagittal plane. This plane is used to evaluate the aortic arch and aortic dissection.

Vertical long-axis view

The vertical long-axis plane, sometimes referred to as a two-chamber view, is named based on visualization of the left ventricle and left atrium (Fig. 50-2A and B). The mitral valve is readily depicted in this plane.

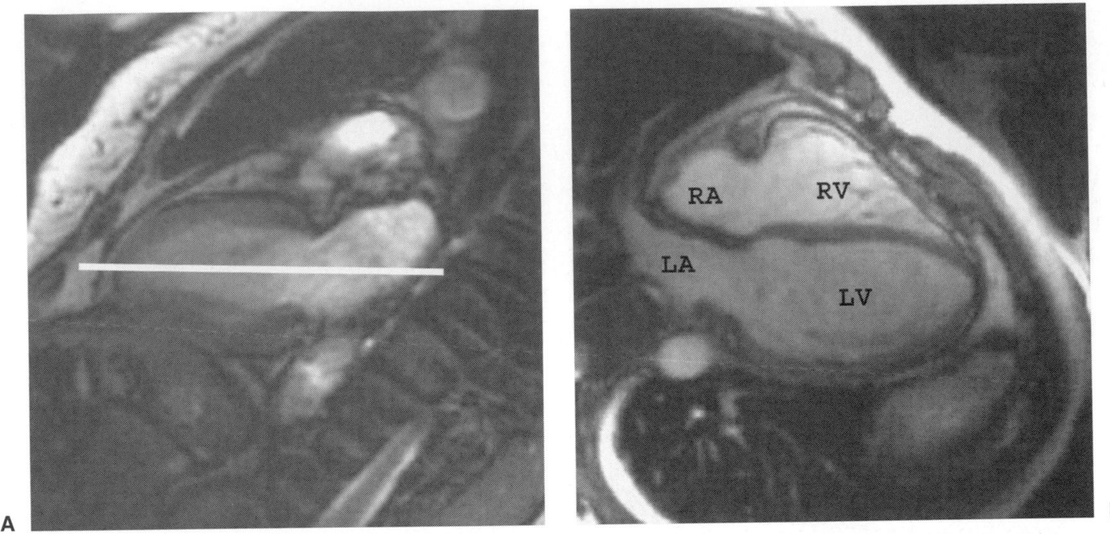

Figure 50-3 By imaging along the axis prescribed by the white bar on the long-axis view (A), the horizontal long-axis view is obtained (B). The horizontal long-axis view is acquired with the FIESTA MRI technique. RA = right atrium; RV = right ventricle; LA = left atrium; LV = left ventricle.

Horizontal long-axis view

The horizontal long-axis plane, sometimes referred to as a four-chamber view, is oriented 90 degrees to the vertical long-axis view. This view is obtained from a line through the posterior wall of the left atrium, the middle of the mitral valve, and the left apex on the two-chamber view (Fig. 50-3A and B). The horizontal long-axis view depicts the right and left atria and both ventricles as well as the mitral and tricuspid valves and displays the relationship of the four chambers on a single image. Cine GRE images in this plane can evaluate mitral and tricuspid valve function, atrial or ventricular septal defects (VSDs), and bilateral ventricular contraction.

Short-axis view

Images in the short-axis plane can be obtained by obtaining images perpendicular to the left ventricular long axis seen on the horizontal or vertical long-axis views (Fig. 50-4A and B). The short-axis images show the cross-sectional anatomy of the right and left ventricle. Short-axis cine images are ideal to evaluate left and

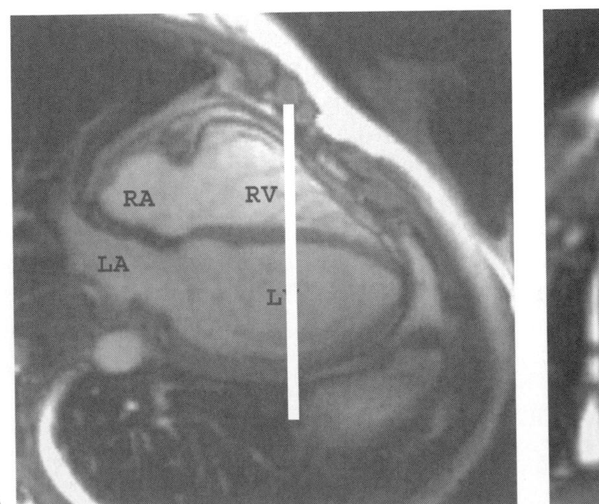

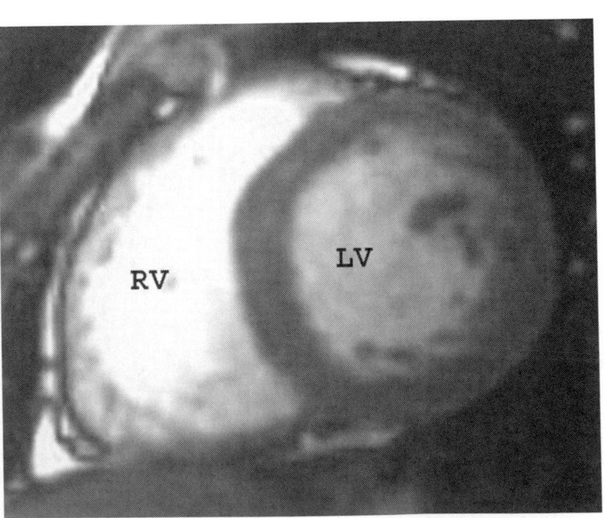

Figure 50-4 By imaging along the axis prescribed by the white bar on the long-axis image (A), the short-axis view is obtained (B). The short-axis view is acquired with the bright-blood FIESTA MRI technique (B). RV = right ventricle; LV = left ventricle.

right ventricular mass, volumes, and function in order to obtain end-diastolic volume (EDV), end-systolic volume (ESV), and ejection fraction (EF). Differences in stroke volume from the left heart compared to the right heart quantify shunt volumes or valvular regurgitation. Furthermore, this plane is suitable for identifying focal wall motion abnormalities.

CLINICAL APPLICATIONS OF CARDIAC MAGNETIC RESONANCE IMAGING

CARDIAC MASS AND FUNCTION

Left ventricular mass is a strong independent predictor of fatal and nonfatal cardiovascular events.[9,10] Cardiac MRI is currently the most accurate and reproducible method for the assessment of cardiac volumes, mass, and function.[11] To evaluate the left ventricular mass, short axis cine MR images are used. The endocardial and epicardial contours of the left myocardial wall are automatically or semiautomatically traced on each slice using special software. The contours of the cardiac chambers are then summed and multiplied by the slice thickness and slice gap (Simpson method) to obtain the contour volumes (Fig. 50-5). Finally, left ventricular wall mass is calculated from the volumes based on a myocardial density of 1.05 g/cm^3. By tracing end-systolic and end-diastolic volumes, cardiac function parameters like end-diastolic volume, end-systolic volume, and ejection fraction can be calculated according to the same principle.

Cardiac MRI using bright-blood cine imaging is used to assess cardiac wall motion. Most centers grade wall motion visually, as either normal, hypokinetic, akinetic,

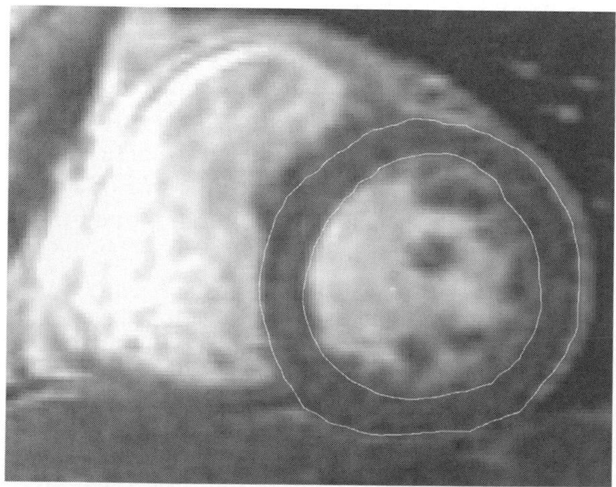

Figure 50-5 Short-axis fast-gradient echo MRI demonstrates automatic outline of endo- and epicardial borders of the left ventricle for left ventricular mass evaluation with dedicated software.

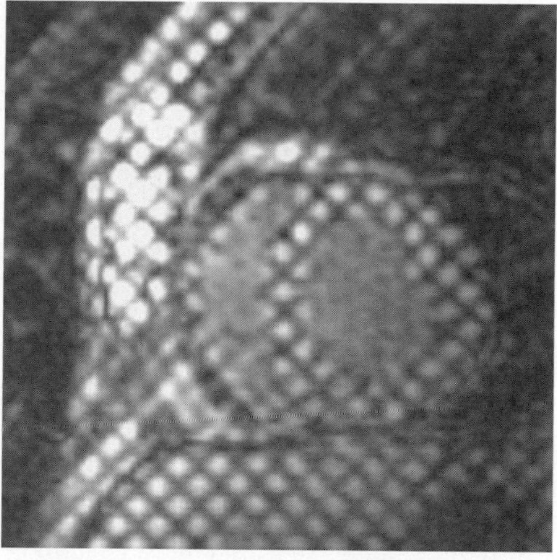

Figure 50-6 To assess for focal wall motion abnormalities, MR tagging can be used, as demonstrated on this short-axis view of the heart. During myocardial contraction, the distance between magnetically placed tag lines decreases, directly measuring regional shortening.

or dyskinetic at the base, middle, and apex of the left ventricle. Qualitative assessment of wall motion by MRI, like that of echocardiography, depends on the use of experienced readers for greatest reproducibility.

A limited number of centers have experience using "tagged MRI" to quantitatively measure regional cardiac wall motion. These methods, developed by Zerhouni and colleagues,[12] represent the most precise way for measuring both systolic and diastolic function. The method involves placing a magnetic strip on the myocardium at end diastole. As the heart contracts, the magnetic strip moves and bends along with the motion and contraction of the myocardium. Measuring the distances between the magnetic strips on each image assesses regional contractility. By using these methods, the contraction of the heart in any direction (circumferential, radial, and longitudinal) may be accurately measured (Fig. 50-6). Currently the primary use of quantitative methods to measure regional cardiac contraction has been in specific research protocols. Given the nature of cardiovascular imaging, however, it is likely that these methods will gain further importance in the future. Tagged MRI has other specialized uses, such as the detection of pericardial to myocardial adhesions in constrictive pericarditis.

ASSESSMENT OF VALVULAR HEART DISEASE

Conventional and transesophageal echocardiography are still the most widely applied methods to evaluate valvular cardiac anatomy, such as leaflet number, valvular thickness, vegetations, and valvular function. Recent developments in cardiac MRI techniques demonstrate that valve

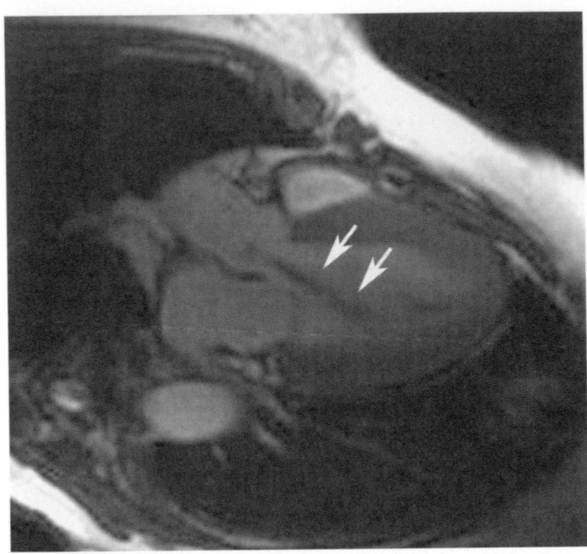

Figure 50-7 Bright-blood (FIESTA) image of the heart demonstrates moderate aortic valve regurgitation (arrows).

evaluation by MRI can be an attractive alternative or complementary to echocardiography. MRI evaluation is noninvasive and provides three-dimensional anatomic and functional data, which are potentially more accurate and reproducible than those of echocardiography.[13,14]

Black-blood sequences are used to analyze valvular anatomy (e.g., valve thickening or bicuspid valves). Cine MRI bright-blood techniques are used to evaluate abnormal flow patterns such as valvular stenosis or regurgitation, which cause loss of signal and appear as a dark signal void (Fig. 50-7). This signal void is caused by turbulent flow and the acceleration of flow within the normal bright-blood pool, similar to aliasing in Doppler ultrasonography. This signal void also depends on technical factors, which may vary in appearance depending on the MRI scanner. Thus, this signal void is usually evaluated only qualitatively. The degree of valvular regurgitation is measured by the area of volume of signal void and maximum length of the signal void in the receiving chamber.

A method to quantitate valvular regurgitation is to calculate the RF with ventricular volumetric measurements. As described above, end-systolic and end-diastolic volumetric measurements of the blood pool are first performed. In the normal heart, the right and left ventricular stroke volumes (end-diastolic volume minus end-systolic volume) are equal. If there is unilateral valvular regurgitation, the end-diastolic volume is higher on the affected side than on the unaffected side of the heart; therefore the stroke volume on the affected side is also higher. The difference in stroke volume between a regurgitant and a normal ventricle is the regurgitant volume.

The RF can be calculated by dividing the regurgitant volume by the stroke volume of the regurgitant ventricle. An RF of 15 to 20 percent corresponds to mild valvular regurgitation; an RF of 20 to 40 percent to moderate regurgitation; and an RF of more than 40 percent to marked regurgitation. In the presence of unilateral combined valvular insufficiency (e.g., mitral and aortic regurgitation), this technique can calculate only the combined volume of regurgitation. In cases of bilateral valvular regurgitation (e.g., pulmonary and aortic valves), this technique will not provide accurate results. The method, however, may be used to assess the functional consequences of a VSD.

Flow-sensitive or velocity-encoded MRI (VEC-MRI) is the best way to quantify valvular regurgitation. In this method, the velocity of blood flow is linearly related to the brightness of the MR image. Stationary tissue appears gray, whereas antegrade or retrograde flow along the phase-encoding axis appears as black or bright pixels. VEC-MRI makes it possible to quantify of blood-velocity profiles at different time points of the cardiac cycle. Blood velocity can be encoded for imaging planes perpendicular to the blood flow (through plane velocity measurement) or parallel to the direction of flow (in-plane velocity measurement). Flow-volume curves can map the absolute stroke volume and regurgitant volume in different phases of the cardiac cycle.

ISCHEMIC HEART DISEASE

Compared to nuclear medicine techniques such as single photon emission computed tomography (SPECT) or positron emission tomography (PET), cardiac MRI is capable of visualizing subendocardial or even papillary muscle infarctions owing to its superior spatial resolution.[15] Furthermore, cardiac MRI is more cost-effective than PET imaging. Recently, three-dimensional single-breath-hold and myocardial suppression techniques have improved the depiction of myocardial infarction and shortened imaging time. These methods are increasingly important for surgical planning prior to coronary artery bypass surgery in patients with prior myocardial infarction. The accuracy and ease of use of these methods suggest that they may also be applied to clinical trials of therapeutic agents that may reduce the size of a myocardial infarct or assess the morphologic and functional consequences of surgery (Fig. 50-8).

MYOCARDIAL VIABILITY

Viable myocardium is myocardium that may recover function following coronary revascularization. Hibernating myocardium (with reduced blood flow) will recover function, but scar/fibrosis in an area of infarction will not. After myocardial infarction, accurate assessment of myocardial viability is crucial for optimal clinical decision making. Cardiac MRI is capable of accurately delineating nonviable or infracted myocardium from potentially

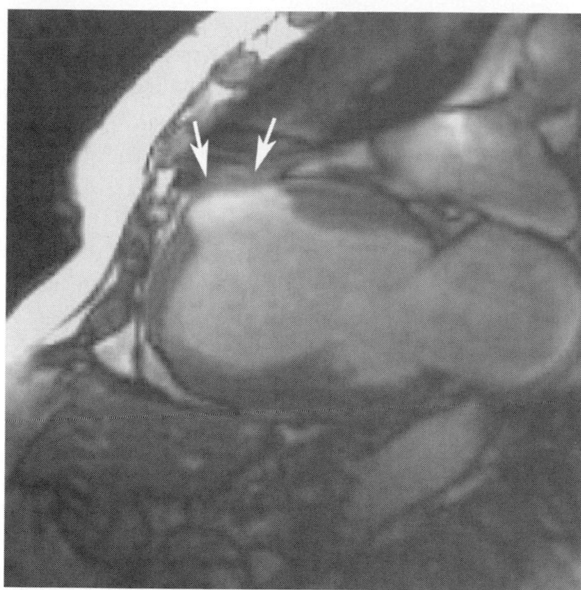

Figure 50-8 Bright-blood (FIESTA) long-axis view demonstrates focal thinning and outpouching of the anterior left ventricular wall (arrows), compatible with aneurysm formation after myocardial infarction.

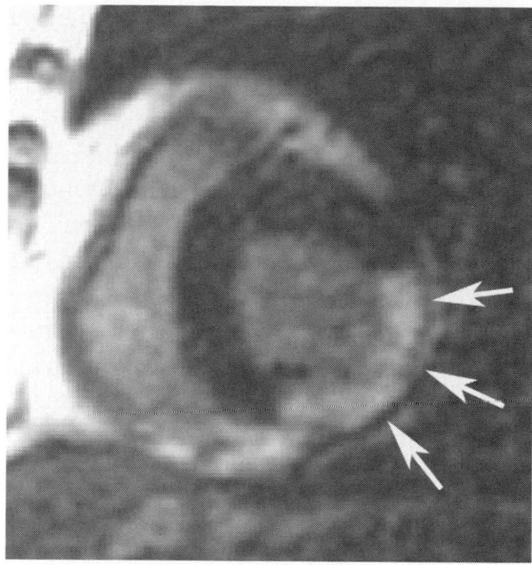

Figure 50-9 Short-axis gadolinium-enhanced delayed MRI demonstrates transmural delayed enhancement of the myocardium in the distribution of the left circumflex coronary artery due to myocardial infarction (arrows).

salvageable myocardium. The advantages of cardiac MRI as compared with nuclear, echocardiographic, or PET methods include (1) high spatial resolution, (2) lack of need for pharmacologic stress agents, and (3) short examination time. Disadvantages include (1) reduced image quality in patients with arrhythmias and (2) patient safety exclusions, as discussed under "Contraindications," above.

For identifying viable versus nonviable myocardium, an intravenous injection of a gadolinium-based contrast agent is used. On delayed images, obtained 10 to 20 min after contrast injection, myocardial scar ("nonviable") retains the gadolinium contrast agent, while washout of the contrast agent occurs in viable myocardium (Fig. 50-9). MR images are optimized so that normal myocardium is "suppressed" on gradient-echo images. Another commonly used term for MRI of this type is *myocardial delayed enhancement* (MDE), or "viability" imaging. This terminology refers to the characteristic 10- to 20-min delay during which the contrast agent in scar/fibrosis distributes differently to normal, viable myocardium.

In viability imaging, scar/fibrosis is depicted as an area of high signal intensity that is typically subendocardial or transmural in a coronary artery distribution. Images are readily interpreted at the base, middle, and apex of the heart on short- and long-axis views. The concept that "bright is dead" is that myocardium with high signal on these MR images corresponds to noncontracting scar/fibrosis. The basis for this relates to both animal models following myocardial infarction and human studies that show lack of contraction of the enhanced myocardium following coronary revascularization.[16,17]

Because of the high spatial resolution of MRI, subendocardial and transmural infarction can be readily identified. In chronic myocardial infarction, myocardial scar may also show thinning of the ventricular wall, particularly in transmural infarction. In addition, thrombus in regions of aneurysm formation may be identified. In general, myocardial scar/fibrosis involving more than 50 percent of myocardial wall thickness by cardiac MRI is unlikely to recover contractile function following coronary revascularization.[17]

ACUTE MYOCARDIAL INFARCTION/MYOCARDIAL NECROSIS

With acute myocardial infarction, there is loss of integrity of myocyte cellular membranes. In addition, large myocardial infarction may be associated with capillary occlusion and plugging with cellular debris, termed microvascular obstruction. This is more commonly observed in large Q-wave myocardial infarction. Cardiac MRI may be used to image both infarction resulting in myocardial necrosis and microvascular obstruction. The MRI methods are similar as those described above for assessing myocardial scar/necrosis. In addition, MRI perfusion imaging is performed in order to assess microvascular obstruction.

After acute myocardial infarction, first-pass perfusion images obtained immediately after bolus administration of the gadolinium contrast agent demonstrate lack of enhancement at the region of microvascular obstruction. This is typically at the "core" of the area of myocardial necrosis. Lack of enhancement of this infarct core, or microvascular obstruction, is related to poor patient prognosis, as documented by Wu and coworkers, with increased incidence of congestive heart failure, recurrent infarction, and chest pain.[18]

The delayed-enhancement MR images in this setting typically show diffuse enhancement of the entire infarct area, or the zone of myocardial necrosis, which may be either subendocardial or transmural. The mechanism of enhancement is likely related to increased volume of distribution of the gadolinium contrast agent due to disruption of cell membranes in the area of myocardial infarction. Areas of stunned myocardium, which have decreased function but intact cell membranes, do not show delayed enhancement on MRI. Cine MR images are obtained in conjunction with the delayed enhancement MR images and show akinesis in areas of myocardial stunning.

Note that areas of acute or chronic infarction may be difficult to distinguish using these methods. Both acute and chronic infarctions show bright areas on delayed enhancement MRI. If the infarction is transmural and chronic, the myocardium will show thinning. However, enhancement of the myocardium on MRI is very nonspecific and requires interpretation with respect to the correct clinical setting. Knowledge of the coronary catheterization results may aid in interpretation of the MRI results. For example, patients with large acute myocardial infarctions often have microvascular obstruction with delayed first-pass enhancement on MRI. However, a patient with chronic infarction and total occlusion of a coronary territory may also show delayed first-pass enhancement in that coronary distribution. Both types of patients will have delayed enhancement on MR images obtained 10 to 20 min after injection of the gadolinium contrast agent.

If the clinical setting is ambiguous, T2-weighted images may be applied for increased specificity for acute versus chronic infarction. T2-weighted MR images depict the distribution of edema in acute myocardial infarction, which is not present in scar/fibrosis.

MYOCARDIAL ISCHEMIA

Myocardial ischemia induced by exercise or pharmacologic stress may be evaluated using MRI.[19] The principles of these stress tests are identical to those used in nuclear medicine techniques except that exercise-induced ischemia is difficult to achieve in the magnetic MRI environment. MRI stress testing is currently done at relatively few institutions, although the results have rivaled those of nuclear pharmacologic stress testing. Advantages of MRI in this setting include a higher spatial resolution than can be obtained with nuclear methods (2 mm versus 6 mm, respectively); lack of the false positives due to breast or soft tissue attenuation, as seen with nuclear methods; and direct identification of myocardial scar/fibrosis with MRI. Compared to dobutamine stress echocardiography, MRI may be an alternative in patients with poor acoustic windows and indeterminate echocardiography results. Disadvantages of MRI include nonstandardized methodology, inability to accurately monitor 12-lead ECG changes in the magnetic environment, and limited access to the patient during the stress examination.

MRI stress testing has been performed with either dobutamine, dipyridamole, or adenosine as a pharmacologic stress agent. Dobutamine causes increased contractility of the myocardium. Ischemia-induced wall motion abnormality at peak stress is readily visualized on cine MR images. In addition, chronic ischemic or hibernating myocardium will demonstrate increased contractility with dobutamine, resulting in improved wall motion in the affected areas compared to rest imaging. Dobutamine MRI is performed by performing MR cine imaging at increasing levels of dobutamine infusion, typically from 5 to 50 μg/kg/min. MRI must be done rapidly in near real time and the examining physician must detect wall motion abnormalities, at which time the test is terminated.

Dipyridamole and adenosine are direct vasodilators. These agents result in augmented blood flow in normal coronary arteries, while stenotic vessels will show lack of increased blood flow. At peak vasodilatation, the gadolinium-based contrast agent is rapidly injected intravenously; as a result, myocardial territories with vascular stenosis show less enhancement than nonstenotic territories on MR perfusion images. Perfusion stress MRI is usually combined with cine MRI to assess ventricular function. In addition, delayed MRI is performed to assess for areas of scar/fibrosis, as discussed above for viability imaging.

CORONARY ARTERY IMAGING

Direct visualization of the coronary artery wall and lumen is crucial for the diagnosis of coronary artery arteriosclerosis. It is also necessary to determine the degree of lumenal stenosis in evaluating a patient and planning treatment by coronary artery angioplasty, stenting, or bypass surgery. Conventional coronary digital subtraction angiography (DSA) remains the "gold standard" to visualize the coronary artery lumen and the degree of stenosis. However, this procedure is not risk-free, owing to its invasive nature. Furthermore, the cost of conventional angiography exceeds by far the cost of coronary artery MRI.

In the last decade, MRI coronary angiography has made significant advances and demonstrated its feasibility.[20,21] At present, pilot studies with healthy volunteers can depict nearly the full length of the left circumflex, left anterior descending, and right coronary arterial lumen and wall (Figs. 50-10 and 50-11). The current spatial resolution ranges between 0.7×0.7 and 0.9×0.9 mm^2. However, in vivo coronary artery imaging can be

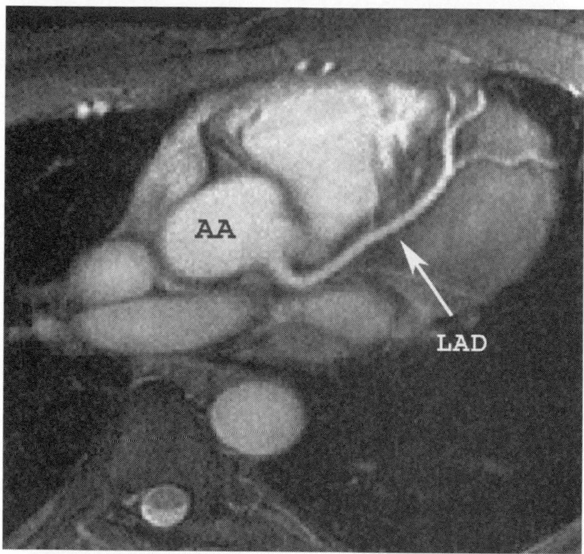

Figure 50-10 Navigator free-breathing (3-tesla) MRI of the left anterior descending (LAD) coronary artery in a healthy volunteer. AA = ascending aorta. (Courtesy M. Stuber, Johns Hopkins University, Baltimore, MD.)

challenging because of artifacts caused by complex cardiac, respiratory, and patient movement. For patients with normal sinus rhythm, cardiac motion can be reliably suppressed by electrographic gating. Respiratory gating can be challenging owing to more unpredictable diaphragmatic motion.

Several strategies have been pursued to minimize these factors. At present three-dimensional gradient-echo coronary MR angiography (MRA) techniques are state of the art. Most recently, stronger field magnets (up to 3 tesla compared to most of the current 1.5-tesla MRI scanners) have become available commercially. These are likely to be applied to the challenging area of coronary MRI because they offer an improved tissue signal.[22]

Coronary artery calcifications may cause signal void and can mimic stenosis, although these effects appear to be less severe than with coronary CT angiography. Coronary artery bypass grafts and stents are difficult to evaluate because of artifacts from surgical clips, sternal wires, and stent material. Tantalum stents have more favorable MRI characteristics than stents made of stainless steel.

At present, the most common clinical indication for coronary MRA is the evaluation of aberrant coronary arteries. Knowledge of coronary anomalies is useful in planning cardiac surgery and in the prevention of sudden cardiac death (Fig. 50-12A and B). Coronary MRA has been proven to be equal or even superior to DSA in the analysis of congenital vascular anomalies and has become the gold standard for their evaluation. There may be additional application in patients with Kawasaki's disease in order to avoid repeat catheterization. Coronary MRA can reliably detect coronary aneurysms and is the preferred method for noninvasive follow-up of such patients (Fig. 50-13).[23]

MAGNETIC RESONANCE IMAGING OF CARDIAC MASSES

MRI is the examination of choice to confidently exclude cardiac masses in cases where echocardiography is equivocal. MRI has superior tissue characterization capabilities to better define cardiac masses compared to cardiac CT imaging and does not require irradiation.

The most common cardiac mass is a ventricular or atrial thrombus. Acute thrombi may appear mass-like, whereas chronic thrombi conform to the contour of the cardiac cavity and may be more difficult to detect. The vascular supply of most thrombi is poor, so that the majority do not enhance after the administration of gadolinium contrast (Fig. 50-14).

Metastases to the heart and pericardium are 20 to 40 times more common than primary tumors and are generally associated with a poor prognosis.[24] Noncardiac tumors may spread to the heart or myocardium via hematogenous dissemination, lymphatic spread, direct local invasion, or via the transvenous route (Fig. 50-15). Tumors that most likely metastasize to the heart are malignancies of the lung and breast, melanoma, and lymphoma. Melanoma is the most common tumor metastasizing hematogenously to the heart. Melanoma metastasis to the myocardium may show the characteristic MRI appearance of bright lesions on T1 and T2 images, which enhance with intravenous contrast. The brightness is attributed to paramagnetic metals bound to melanin.

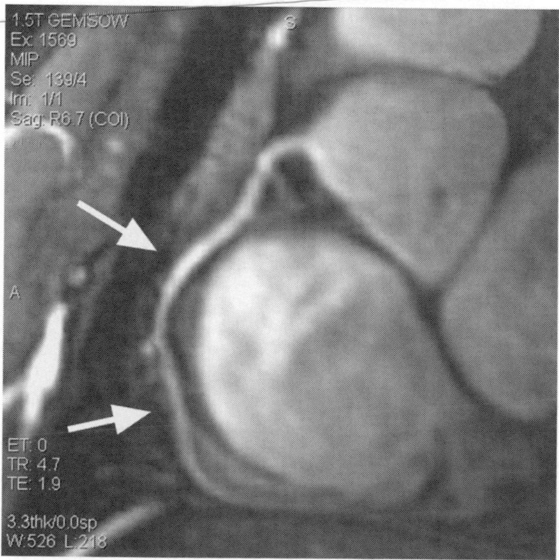

Figure 50-11 A high-resolution MRI of the right coronary artery with intravenous contrast (arrows). (Courtesy M. Stuber, Johns Hopkins University, Baltimore, MD.)

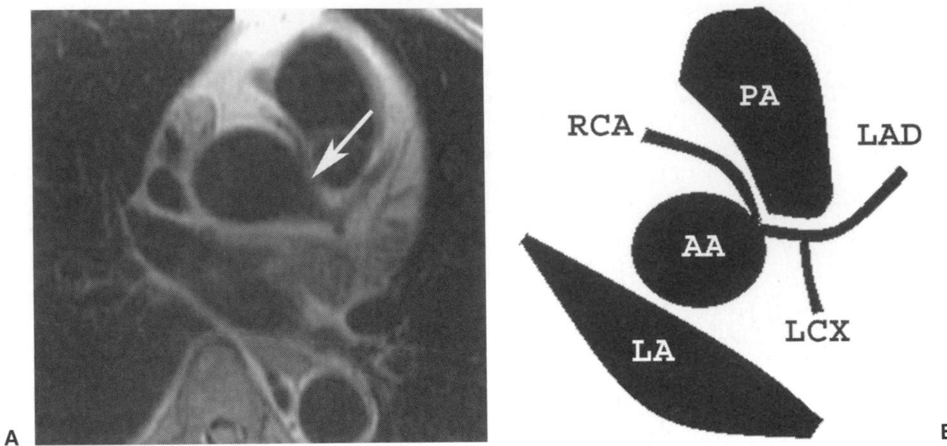

Figure 50-12 A black-blood axial MRI demonstrating anomalous origin of the right coronary artery (arrow). The anomalous RCA travels between the pulmonary artery and the aortic root. This anomaly is potentially lethal and requires surgical reimplantation of the RCA (A). The anatomy is illustrated in the diagram (B). RCA = right coronary artery; LAD = left anterior descending coronary artery; AA = aortic artery; LCX = left circumflex coronary artery; PA = pulmonary artery; LA = left atrium.

MRI can depict direct invasion of the heart by bronchogenic or esophageal carcinomas, lymphoma, invasive thymoma, or mesothelioma. Obliteration of the pericardial fat plane by the tumor on MR images is a sign of involvement of the myocardium.

Hepatocellular carcinoma, renal cell carcinoma, and adrenal tumors are the most likely to spread via direct extension into the inferior vena cava and the heart. Coronal and sagittal MRI is useful to depict this process. Gadolinium-enhanced MRI can further distinguish between tumor extension versus thrombus in the inferior vena cava and right atrium. In contrast to echocardiography, MRI can detect not only intracardial but also extracardial masses, as in the lungs.

Primary tumors of the heart are rare and most often benign. In general most benign tumors are intralumenal and are attached by a narrow stalk. Most malignant primary and secondary malignancies are broad-based or

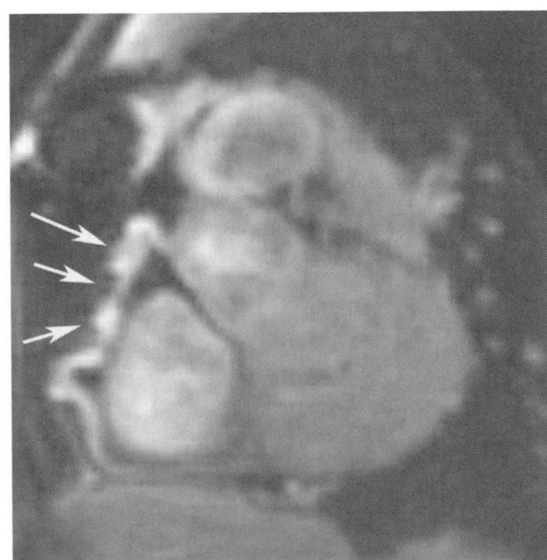

Figure 50-13 This 16-year-old male presented with acute chest pain. Coronary MR angiography demonstrates aneurysmal dilatation and intermittent narrowing of the proximal right coronary artery (arrows) compatible with Kawasaki's disease.

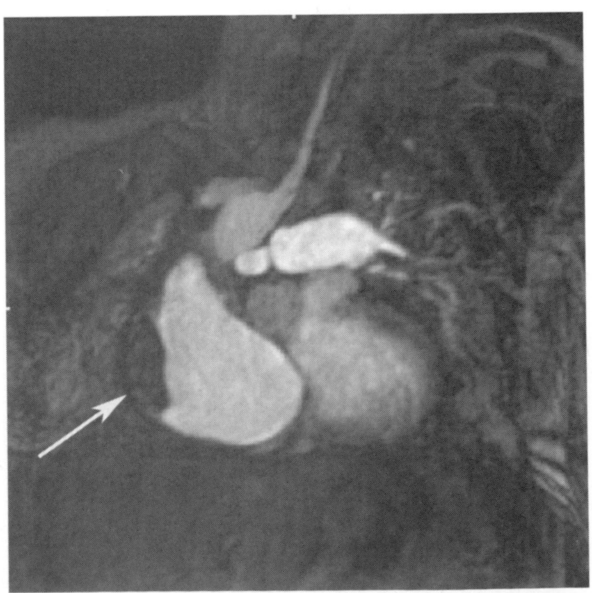

Figure 50-14 This gadolinium-enhanced coronal oblique image demonstrates a nonenhancing mass in a patulous right atrium compatible with thrombus (arrow).

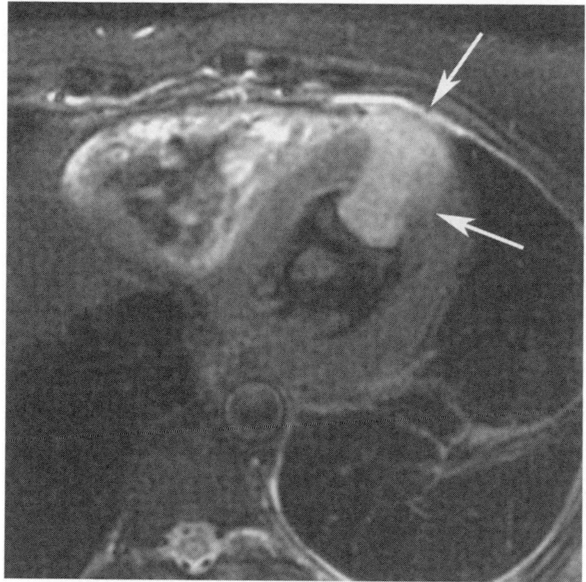

Figure 50-15 Metastatic leiomyosarcoma involving the left ventricle. This axial cardiac black-blood MRI with fat suppression demonstrates a high-signal-intensity mass in the apex of the left ventricle (arrows). The tumor was resected surgically.

invade the myocardium. Most tumors enhance with intravenous contrast.

The benign cardiac myxoma is the most common primary cardiac tumor, representing 50 percent of all primary cardiac neoplasms.[25] It is usually located in the left atrium in the region of the fossa ovalis of the intraatrial septum (Fig. 50-16A and B). The MRI appearance of cardiac myxoma varies depending of the amount of myxomatous and fibrous tissue. In general, myxomas will show increased T2 signal because of the myxomatous components of the tumor.

The second most common benign tumor is cardiac fibroma. It commonly arises from the interventricular septum, right ventricle, or atria and can be quite large. Because of their homogeneous fibrous nature these tumors are hypointense on T2-weighted images and isointense on T1-weighted images, usually showing little or no contrast enhancement. Calcifications may occur; these are not well appreciated with MRI and better evaluated by CT.

Cardiac lipomas usually occur in the pericardial space and less frequently in a cardiac chamber. Owing to their fat content, they have a homogeneous, bright T1 signal and usually do not enhance with intravenous gadolinium-based contrast agents. MRI can specifically identify fat because of the chains of fatty acid present; it is the method of choice to diagnose this tumor (Fig. 50-17A and B, Fig. 50-18A and B). Paragangliomas are commonly located in the left atrium, coronary arteries, or aortic root. Characteristically, they show marked enhancement with gadolinium. Nuclear medicine imaging with iodine 123 or iodine-131 metaiodobenzylguanidine (MIBG) is also widely used to localize and diagnose extraadrenal paragangliomas.[26]

Primary malignant cardiac tumors are extremely rare.[27] Angiosarcoma is the most common neoplasm of this kind, usually presenting as a bulky, infiltrative, right-sided cardiac mass, the right atrium being the most frequent site of origin (Fig. 50-19). Pericardial involvement is common, and patients may present with a hemorrhagic pericardial effusion. Metastatic disease to bone, liver, adrenal gland, and spleen is often present at the time of diagnosis. Owing to their high vascularity, angiosarcomas enhance with gadolinium. Depending on the degree of tumor necrosis, MRI will show high signal in these areas on T2-weighted

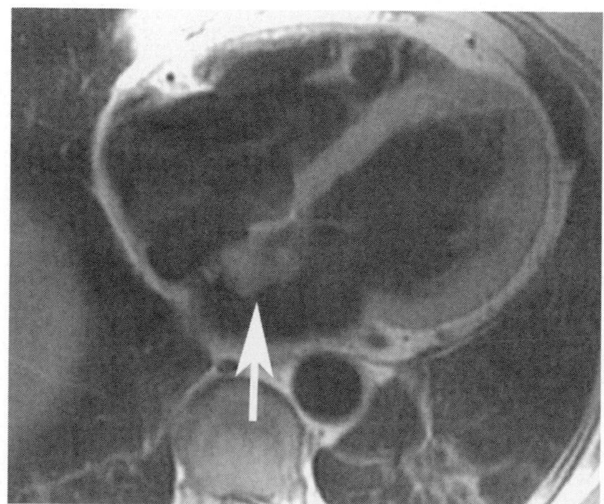

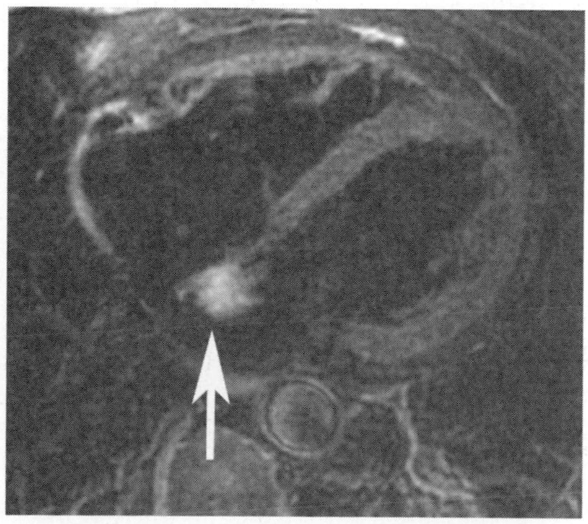

Figure 50-16 Cardiac myxoma. This T1-weighted axial black-blood MRI of the heart shows a lobulated mass (arrow) in the left atrium arising from the atrial septum (A); it has high signal intensity on the fat-suppressed T2-weighted axial black-blood MRI due to the myxomatous component in this tumor (B).

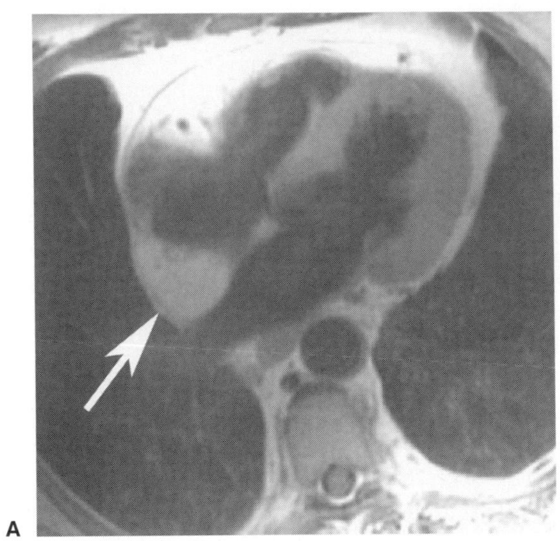
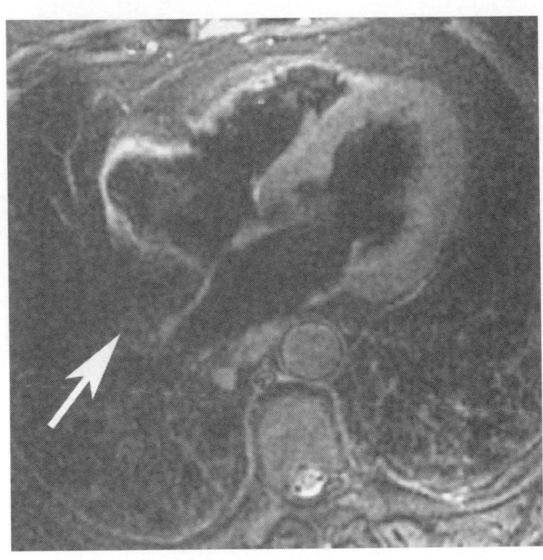

Figure 50-17 This T1-weighted axial black-blood image without (A) and with (B) fat suppression demonstrates a paracardial lipoma (arrows). In (B), the fat signal was selectively suppressed in a manner that is chemically specific for lipid.

images. Rhabdomyosarcomas arise from cardiac striated muscle; their signal characteristics are similar to the myocardial signal and they enhance after gadolinium administration. Leiomyosarcomas and fibrosarcomas are exceedingly rare cardiac malignancies with variable signal characteristics and contrast enhancement.

PERICARDIAL DISEASE

The pericardium is a double-walled sac, of which the outer wall is fibrous. Beneath this is an internal sac called the serous pericardium, which consists of outer (parietal) and inner (visceral) layers separated by a potential space, the pericardial cavity. Echocardiography is usually the initial examination of choice to evaluate pericardial disease. MRI is complementary and more definitive in the evaluation of constrictive pericarditis, pericardial thickening, or loculated pericardial effusion, for example.

The normal pericardium appears as a low-signal band around the heart usually measuring 1 to 2 mm in thickness; it is outlined by the high signal intensity of mediastinal and epicardial fat. The actual pericardium is thinner and measures about 0.4 to 1.0 mm. This discrepancy between MRI

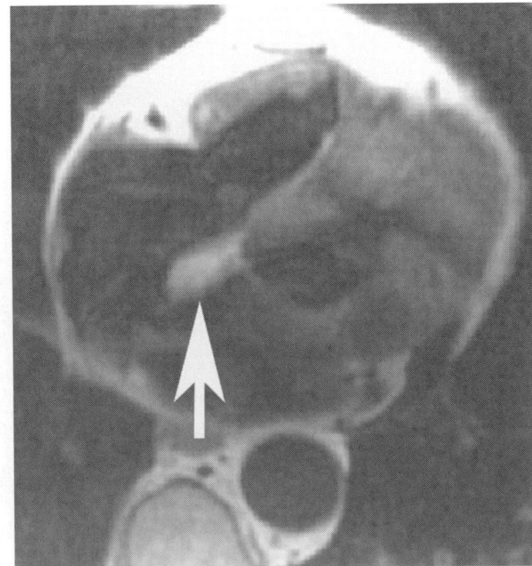
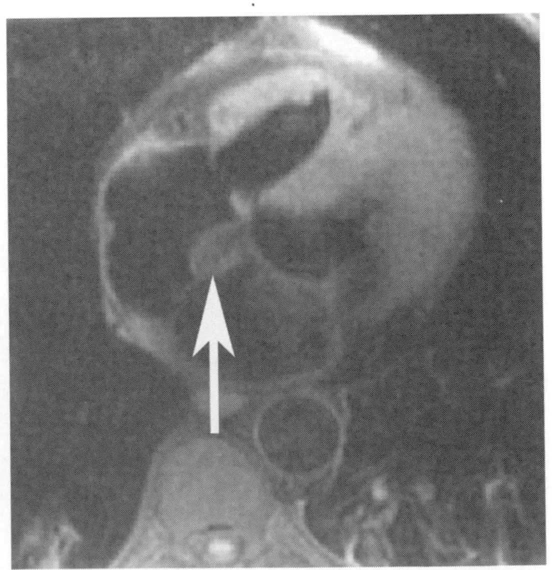

Figure 50-18 Lipomatous hypertrophy of the atrial septum. This axial T1-weighted black-blood MRI demonstrates bright signal within a prominent atrial septum (A), which drops in signal with fat suppression (B).

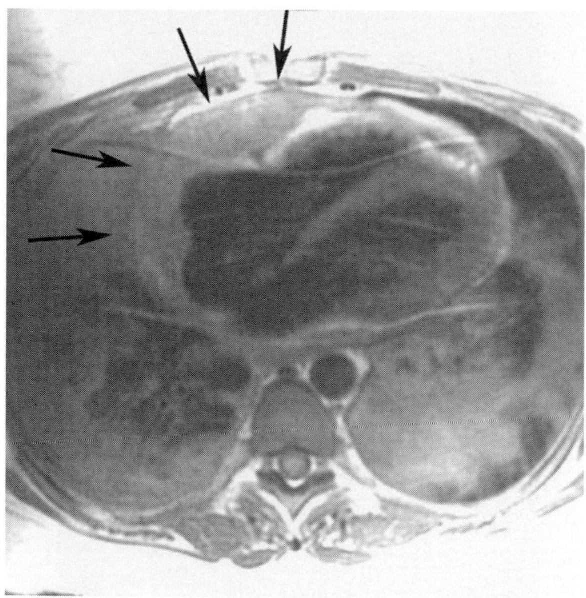

Figure 50-19 Cardiac angiosarcoma. This T1-weighted axial black-blood MRI demonstrates an ill-defined mass (arrows) involving the right atrial and right ventricular wall (A), which avidly enhances with intravenous gadolinium. Note the pulmonary edema in both lower lungs.

and pathologic measurements is likely due to a combination of chemical shift artifact (caused at fat-fluid interfaces), motion artifact, volume averaging, and the inclusion of small amounts of pericardial fluid in MRI measurements.[28] Small amounts of pericardial fluid also accumulate in the superior pericardial recess, a normal structure between the aortic root and main pulmonary artery, which should not be confused with a mass or focal aortic dissection.

Multiple pathologies can cause pericardial effusion. Pericardial fluid in excess of 50 mL is considered abnormal. Pericardial effusions are usually easily detected with ultrasound; however, loculated pericardial fluid or a limited acoustic window (e.g., in patients with chronic obstructive pulmonary disease) can make evaluation with ultrasound difficult. Simple effusions demonstrate low signal intensity on proton density–weighted spin-echo sequences or double-inversion sequences and high signal intensity on T2-weighted spin-echo, fast spin-echo, and steudy state free precession (SSFP) as well as fast cine sequences. However, the movement of pericardial fluid during the cardiac cycle can result in signal void, especially on proton density–weighted and T2-weighted sequences. Hemorrhagic, proteinaceous, or exudative pericardial effusions often show increased signal intensity on T1-weighted images. Blood products of varying age within the pericardial space demonstrate variable T1 and T2 signal. Contrast enhancement with gadolinium may be seen in pericarditis or neoplastic effusions.

MRI findings of pericarditis include pericardial thickening of 4 mm or more and an associated simple or complex effusion. MRI is particularly helpful in diagnosing constrictive pericarditis; this is a common indication for MRI of the pericardium at our institution. The diagnostic hallmark of constrictive pericarditis in the correct clinical setting is pericardial thickening with or without calcifications (Fig. 50-20). Before antibiotic treatment was available, tuberculosis was the most common cause of constrictive pericarditis, often associated with large, extensive calcifications. Today the most common cause of constrictive pericarditis is idiopathic (49 percent), followed by iatrogenic causes such as previous pericardiotomy (30 percent) and irradiation (11 percent).[29] Less common etiologies include viral pericarditis, connective tissue disease, neoplasm, and uremia. Gross calcifications are present in only 28 percent of cases of constriction. CT is more sensitive than MRI in detecting calcifications; however, owing to superior soft tissue contrast, MRI is superior in the distinction of pericardial thickening from pericardial effusion. In a series of 29 patients with clinical symptoms, pericardial thickening determined by MRI was associated with constrictive pericarditis with a sensitivity of 93 percent.[30] However, constrictive pericarditis can be seen without evidence of pericardial thickening; therefore clinical history and additional findings (e.g., tubular ventricles, enlarged atria, focal contour deformities of the ventricles, enlarged inferior vena cava, ascites, and pleural effusions) are helpful.[31] Also, postoperative pericardial adhesions can be seen in the setting of constrictive pericarditis.

Pericardial cysts derive from embryonic pericardium, which is pinched off during development. The most common location is the right anterior costophrenic angle. Pericardial cysts have a thin, nonenhancing rim and are indistinguishable from bronchogenic cysts by MRI. If pericardial cysts contain simple fluid, they are dark on T1-weighted sequences and bright on T2-weighted images. If they contain proteinaceous fluid or

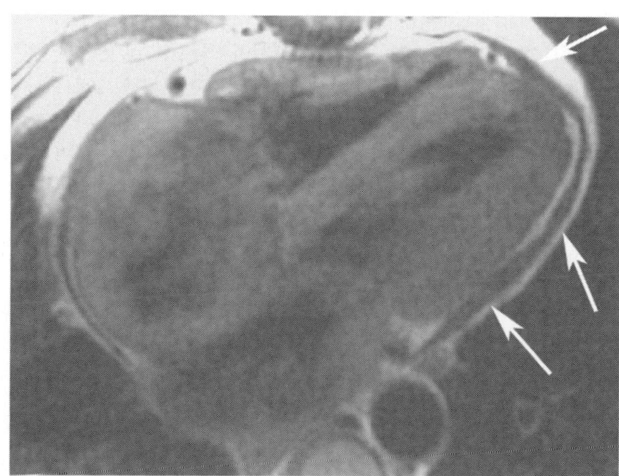

Figure 50-20 Constrictive pericarditis. A T1-weighted axial black-blood MRI of the heart shows moderate thickening of the pericardium (arrows).

blood products, they may have a bright signal on T1-weighted images.

Rarely, complete or partial absence of the pericardium occurs, and these conditions can be diagnosed by MRI. However, portions of the pericardium overlying the left lateral ventricle and right atrium may not normally be visualized. Partial absence of the pericardium can be challenging in these cases.

Metastatic pericardial involvement is far more common than primary pericardial malignancies. Imaging of primary and secondary malignancies does occur and is described in the chapter on the MR imaging of cardiac masses.

MAGNETIC RESONANCE IMAGING OF CONGENITAL HEART DISEASE

Cardiac MRI complements echocardiography in the evaluation of congenital heart disease and provides explicit depiction of the morphology of the chambers and great vessels. Often MRI makes invasive angiocardiography in pediatric and adult patients unnecessary and decreases the morbidity in diagnostic workup in these patients.

Dedicated imaging coils for infants for higher signal-to-noise acquisitions allow thinner slice selection and smaller fields of view for higher resolution. This improves image quality and the confidence in diagnosis of congenital heart disease. Single-breath-hold MRI is obtained in ventilated patients by suspending respiration for short periods.

For the evaluation of aortic coarctation, the oblique sagittal plane is most useful in defining the location and anatomy of the isthmus in relation to the aortic arch arteries (Fig. 50-21). Most frequently, gadolinium-enhanced three-dimensional MRA techniques are used to depict collateral circulation and vascular variants, such as a right aberrant subclavian artery. After surgical treatment, MRI is routinely used for postoperative follow-up. Other great vessel variants, such as double aortic arch, pulmonary sling, or transposition, are easily depicted with MRI (Fig. 50-22).

MRI of a patent ductus arteriosus can be challenging due to the generally small size, length, and orientation of the duct and limited MRI resolution (Fig. 50-23). Therefore optimized coils, software, and patient sedation, which is especially vital in newborns and infants, is necessary. On coronal imaging, communication between the underside of the distal aortic arch and the superior aspect of the origin of the left pulmonary artery is often demonstrated. Finally, flow-sensitive imaging (VEC-MRI) can further quantify the amount of shunting.

As in the evaluation of cardiac valves, the anatomy and severity of intracardiac shunts with depiction of changes in secondary chamber morphology (e.g., hypertrophy or dilatation) can also be performed with MRI. Axial or left anterior oblique projections are useful for evaluating the

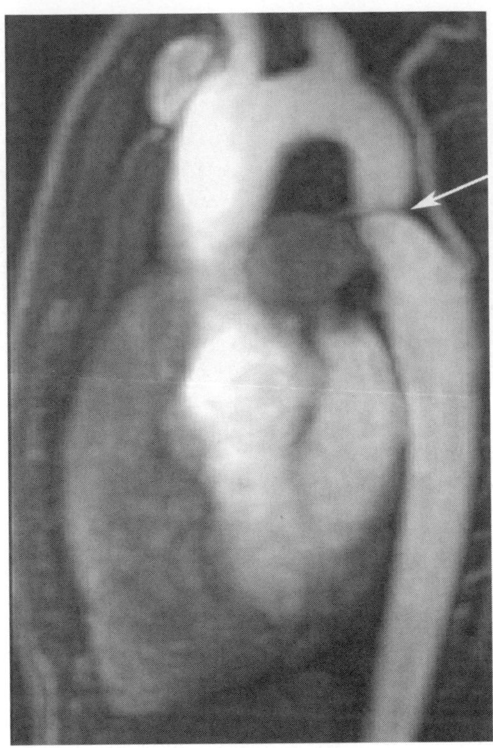

Figure 50-21 A double-oblique MR angiogram of the aortic arch with intravenous gadolinium shows an aortic coarctation of the distal arch (arrow) with mild poststenotic dilatation of the descending thoracic aorta.

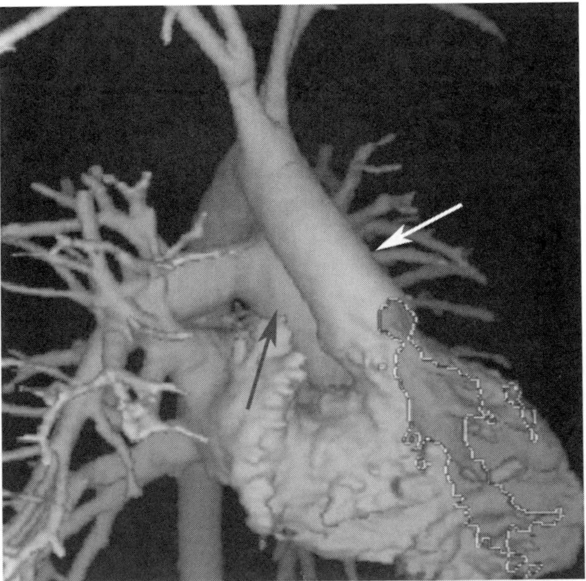

Figure 50-22 Transposition of the great arteries. A multiplanar reconstructed gadolinium-enhanced MRI of the heart shows an anomalous pulmonary artery arising from the left ventricle (black arrow) and an anomalous ascending aorta arising from the right ventricle (white arrow).

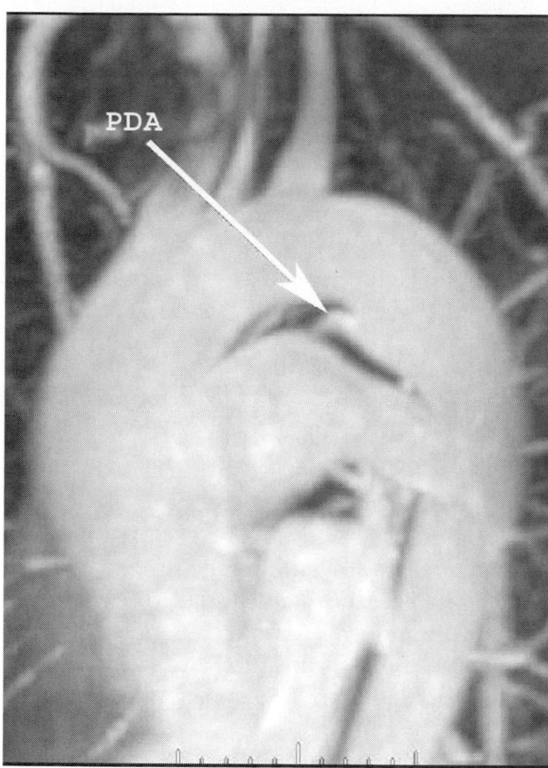

Figure 50-23 Patent ductus arteriosus (PDA). A double-oblique MRI of the aortic arch with intravenous gadolinium shows a patent vascular connection (arrow) between the main pulmonary artery and distal aortic arch.

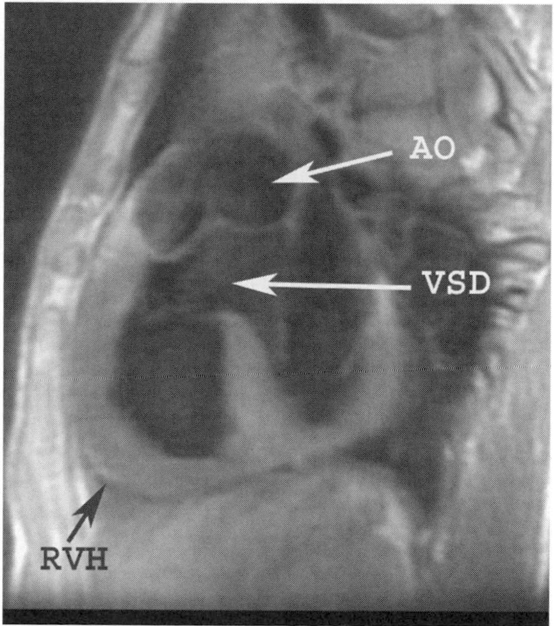

Figure 50-24 Tetralogy of Fallot. A black-blood MRI of the heart demonstrates the key features of tetralogy of Fallot: a large ventricular septal defect (VSD), high-riding aorta (AO), and right ventricular hypertrophy (RVH) due to pulmonary artery stenosis.

intraatrial septum. Axial MRI has 97 percent sensitivity and 90 percent specificity for detection of atrial septal defects.[32] Often the atrial septum is infiltrated with fat, which produces good contrast in evaluating the signal void due to turbulent flow and the direction of shunt flow with bright-blood cine GRE or FIESTA MRI. Flow-sensitive imaging (VEC-MRI) can further quantify the amount of shunting. Accordingly, membranous and muscular defects of the ventricular septal wall can be depicted with MRI. Muscular VSDs may be difficult to detect with black-blood imaging and may be diagnosed indirectly by signal-void jets of the shunted blood. Careful evaluation of cine images allows distinction between left-to-right, right-to-left, and bidirectional shunts.

MRI is capable of confidently diagnosing the tetralogy of Fallot anomaly (Fig. 50-24). MRI evaluation in these patients includes characterization of the VSD, degree of pulmonary stenosis and aortic insufficiency, as well as depiction of the right ventricular morphology. The usually large subaortic VSD is well demonstrated in axial, long-axis, or sagittal views. MRI evaluation of flow dynamics across the VSD is very important to assess for Eisenmenger physiology (right-to-left shunting). Coronal imaging is useful in evaluating the extent of systemic-to–pulmonary artery collaterals and degree of pulmonary artery stenosis. Sagittal views are helpful in examining the overriding aortic root and degree of aortic regurgitation. Furthermore, MRI is vital for the preoperative planning and postoperative evaluation of surgical shunts. For example, Blalock-Taussig shunts are best evaluated along the long axis of the graft.

In infants with Ebstein's anomaly, imaging is necessary to diagnose the anatomic displacement and malfunction of the tricuspid valve and degree of right-sided cardiac dilatation due to tricuspid valve insufficiency. Postoperative MRI is helpful in evaluating the artificial tricuspid valve as well as chamber morphology. Sometimes MRI of artificial valves in postoperative hearts can be challenging owing to artifacts caused by artificial valves and surgical clips.

MAGNETIC RESONANCE IMAGING OF ARRHYTHMOGENIC RIGHT VENTRICULAR DYSPLASIA

Arrhythmogenic right ventricular dysplasia (ARVD) is a rare disease in which tachyarrhythmias are associated with predominantly right-sided cardiomyopathy. These tachyarrhythmias are associated with sudden cardiac death. MRI is the preferred noninvasive imaging test for this condition.

The diagnosis of ARVD is challenging because clinical signs may be absent or ECG changes inconclusive. MRI findings in ARVD include an abnormal right ventricular myocardium with fatty infiltration and regional right

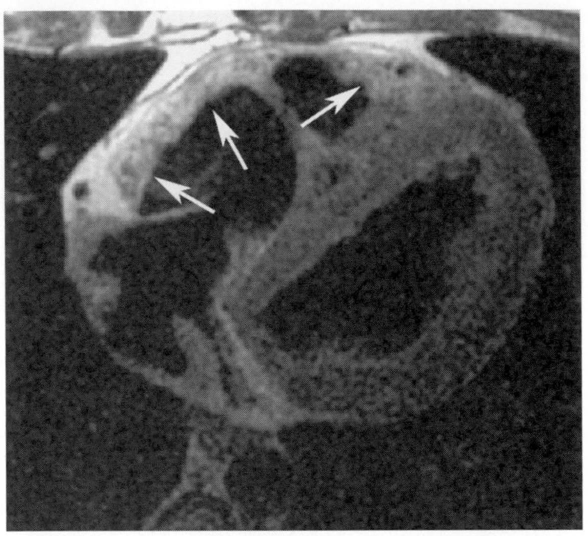

Figure 50-25 Arrhythmogenic right ventricular dysplasia (ARVD). An axial black-blood cardiac MRI demonstrates fat infiltration and focal thinning of the right ventricular wall (arrows), key features of ARVD.

ventricular akinesia or dyskinesia (Fig. 50-25).[33] Increased end-diastolic volume and decreased right ventricular ejection fraction are also be observed. The high resolution of spin-echo and double-inversion recovery images permits confident differentiation between epicardial fat, myocardium with trabeculations, and blood pool of the right ventricle. In addition, the high temporal resolution of cine gradient-echo and SSFP images provides adequate temporal resolution of right ventricular wall motion abnormalities and permits calculations of EF and EDV.

SUMMARY

Because of the high prevalence of cardiovascular disease and its socioeconomic impact, there is a need for improved means of noninvasive diagnosis. Cardiac MRI is a noninvasive technique that allows comprehensive examination of cardiac anatomy, function, and vasculature. With rapidly emerging and improving MRI techniques and the more widespread availability of this modality, cardiac MRI continues to play an important role in patient management.

References

1. Wagner S, Auffermann W, Buser P, et al. Functional description of the left ventricle in patients with volume overload, pressure overload, and myocardial disease using cine magnetic resonance imaging. *Am J Card Imaging* 1991;5(2):87–97.
2. Kim RJ, Fieno DS, Parrish TB, et al. Relationship of MRI delayed contrast enhancement to irreversible injury, infarct age, and contractile function. *Circulation* 1999;100(19): 1992–2002.
3. Martin ET, Coman JA, Shellock FG, et al. Magnetic resonance imaging and cardiac pacemaker safety at 1.5-Tesla. *J Am Coll Cardiol* 2004;43(7):1315–1324.
4. Roguin A, Zviman MM, Meininger GR, et al. Modern pacemaker and implantable cardioverter/defibrillator systems can be magnetic resonance imaging safe: In vitro and in vivo assessment of safety and function at 1.5 T. *Circulation* 20043;110(5):475–482.
5. Ahmed S, Shellock FG. Magnetic resonance imaging safety: Implications for cardiovascular patients. *J Cardiovasc Magn Reson* 2001;3(3):171–182.
6. Gaba RC, Carlos RC, Weadock WJ, et al. Cardiovascular MR Imaging: Technique optimization and detection of disease in clinical practice. *Radiographics* 2002;22(6):e6.
7. Greenman RL, Shirosky JE, Mulkern RV, Rofsky NM. Double inversion black-blood fast spin-echo imaging of the human heart: A comparison between 1.5T and 3.0T. *J Magn Reson Imaging* 2003;17(6):648–655.
8. Carr JC, Simonetti O, Bundy J, et al. Cine MR angiography of the heart with segmented true fast imaging with steady-state precession. *Radiology* 2001;219(3):828–834.
9. Levy D, Garrison R, Savage D, et al. Prognostic implications of echocardiographically determined left ventricular mass in the Framingham Heart Study. *N Engl J Med* 1990;322:1561–1566.
10. Koren MJ, Devereux RB, Casale PN, et al. Relation of left ventricular mass and geometry to morbidity and mortality in uncomplicated essential hypertension. *Ann Intern Med* 1991;114:345–352.
11. Francois CJ, Fieno DS, Shors SM, Finn JP. Left ventricular mass: Manual and automatic segmentation of true FISP and FLASH cine MR images in dogs and pigs. *Radiology* 2004;230(2):389–395.
12. Zerhouni EA, Parish DM, Rogers WJ, et al. Human heart: Tagging with MR imaging—A method for noninvasive assessment of myocardial motion. *Radiology* 1988;169(1): 59–63.
13. Sondergaard L, Stahlberg F, Thomsen C. Magnetic resonance imaging of valvular heart disease. *J Magn Reson Imaging* 1999;10(5):627–638.
14. Didier D. Assessment of valve disease: Qualitative and quantitative. *Magn Reson Imaging Clin N Am* 2003;11(1):115–134, vii.
15. Klein C, Nekolla SG, Bengel FM, et al. Assessment of myocardial viability with contrast-enhanced magnetic resonance imaging: Comparison with positron emission tomography. *Circulation* 2002;105(2):162–167.
16. Fieno DS, Kim RJ, Chen EL, et al. Contrast-enhanced magnetic resonance imaging of myocardium at risk: Distinction between reversible and irreversible injury throughout infarct healing. *J Am Coll Cardiol* 2000;36(6):1985–1991.
17. Kim RJ, Wu E, Rafael A, et al. The use of contrast-enhanced magnetic resonance imaging to identify reversible myocardial dysfunction. *N Engl J Med* 2000;343(20):1445–1453.
18. Wu KC, Kim RJ, Bluemke DA, et al. Quantification and time course of microvascular obstruction by contrast-enhanced echocardiography and magnetic resonance imaging following acute myocardial infarction and reperfusion. *J Am Coll Cardiol* 1998;32(6):1756–1764.
19. Wagner A, Mahrholdt H, Sechtem U, et al. MR imaging of myocardial perfusion and viability. *Magn Reson Imaging Clin N Am* 2003;11(1):49–66.

20. Danias PG, Stuber M, Botnar RM, et al. Coronary MR angiography: Clinical applications and potential for imaging coronary artery disease. *Magn Reson Imaging Clin N Am* 2003;11(1):81–99.
21. Kim WY, Danias PG, Stuber M, et al. Coronary magnetic resonance angiography for the detection of coronary stenoses. *N Engl J Med* 2001;345(26): 1863–1869.
22. Botnar RM, Stuber M, Lamerichs R, et al. Initial experiences with in vivo right coronary artery human MR vessel wall imaging at 3 tesla. *J Cardiovasc Magn Reson* 2003;5(4):589–594.
23. Greil GF, Stuber M, Botnar RM, et al. Coronary magnetic resonance angiography in adolescents and young adults with Kawasaki disease. *Circulation* 2002;105(8): 908–911.
24. Gilkeson RC, Chiles C. MR evaluation of cardiac and pericardial malignancy. *Magn Reson Imaging Clin N Am* 2003;11(1):173–186, viii.
25. Araoz PA, Mulvagh SL, Tazelaar HD, et al. CT and MR imaging of benign primary cardiac neoplasms with echocardiographic correlation. *Radiographics* 2000;20(5):1303–1319.
26. Maurea S, Cuocolo A, Reynolds JC, et al. Iodine-131 metaiodobenzylguanidine scintigraphy in preoperative and postoperative evaluation of paragangliomas: Comparison with CT and MRI. *J Nucl Med* 1993;34(2):173–179.
27. Gilkeson RC, Chiles C. MR evaluation of cardiac and pericardial malignancy. *Magn Reson Imaging Clin North Am* 2003;11(1):173–186, viii.
28. Glockner JF. Imaging of pericardial disease. *Magn Reson Imaging Clin N Am* 2003;11(1):149–162, vii.
29. Oh KY, Shimizu M, Edwards WD, et al. Surgical pathology of the parietal pericardium: A study of 344 cases. *Cardiovasc Pathol* 2001;10(4):157–168.
30. Sechtem U, Tscholakoff D, Higgins CB. MRI of the abnormal pericardium. *AJR* 1986;147(2):245–252.
31. Glockner JF. Imaging of pericardial disease. *Magn Reson Imaging Clin N Am* 2003;11(1):149–162, vii.
32. Boxt LM, Rozenshtein A. MR imaging of congenital heart disease. *Magn Reson Imaging Clin N Am* 2003;11(1): 27–48.
33. Castillo E, Tandri H, Rodriguez ER, et al. Arrhythmogenic right ventricular dysplasia: Ex vivo and in vivo fat detection with black-blood MR imaging. *Radiology* 2004;232(1): 38–48.

PART

III

CONGENITAL CARDIAC SURGERY

CHAPTER

51 MILESTONES IN CONGENITAL CARDIAC SURGERY

Luca A. Vricella, Vincent L. Gott, Duke E. Cameron

"There is nothing more difficult to take in hand, more perilous to conduct, nor uncertain in its success, than to take the lead in the introduction of a new order of things. For the innovator has for enemies all of those who have done well under the old, and lukewarm defenders in all of those who may do well under the new."

—Niccoló Macchiavelli (1469–1527)

Few other medical disciplines have required for their development the degree of daring courage, tenacity, and drive that characterized the efforts of the early pioneers in the field of congenital cardiac surgery. Only a century ago, Theodore Billroth publicly condemned the dream of cardiac surgical intervention by stating that "Any surgeon who wishes to preserve the respect of his colleagues would never attempt to operate on the heart."[1] Over the last six decades, the specialty of pediatric cardiac surgery has evolved from a heroic effort with occasional success into a consolidated, sophisticated specialty with excellent outcomes and, essentially, few limits imposed by pathology or age of the patient.

The history of pediatric heart surgery initially coincided with that of cardiac surgery itself. By far the majority of early extra- and intracardiac procedures were in fact performed to address various forms of congenital (rather than acquired) heart disease. The adventure of intracardiac repair of congenital malformations, in turn, paved the way for technical advancements that pushed forward the field of adult cardiac surgery.

Each of the chapters in Part III of this book touches briefly on the historical highlights that pertain to specific malformations. In this chapter, the reader is offered a broad overview and key historical references that pertain to the initial evolution of this challenging field (Table 51-1), identifying four successive eras: (1) that of closed extracardiac operations, (2) the era of early closed or semiclosed intracardiac operations, (3) the initial phase of complete intracardiac repair, and (4) a subsequent period marked by the refinement of techniques and the expansion of the field to the correction or palliation of virtually any type of congenital heart disease.

THE INITIAL PHASE: EARLY EXTRACARDIAC OPERATIONS

At a time when transpleural surgery was at its dawn,[2–4] the repair of simple cardiovascular malformations was a natural initial surgical goal. Although these conditions were anatomically simple, the too often advanced disease state of the patients and the threat of infection in the preantibiotic era often made these initial daring attempts unsuccessful.

John Strider of Boston first performed surgical ligation of a patent ductus arteriosus on March 6, 1937, immediately noticing that the palpable thrill had disappeared after duct interruption.[5] The 22-year-old patient was correctly diagnosed preoperatively with subacute bacterial endocarditis of the ductus arteriosus and succumbed to overwhelming sepsis on the fourth postoperative day. Necropsy disclosed a large endocarditic vegetation, extending from the arterial duct to the level of the pulmonary valve.

Robert Gross (Fig. 51-1) ushered in the field of congenital heart surgery by successfully interrupting a patent ductus arteriosus at Boston Children's Hospital on August 26, 1938.[6] Although he was the chief resident at the time, Gross performed the procedure in a very ill 7-year-old child, apparently against the advice of his chairman William Ladd.[7,8] The procedure took place while the latter was in Europe; the patient was uneventfully discharged in 10 days and survived for many years. Even though primacy of this milestone in cardiothoracic surgery has been debated,[9] this landmark operation demonstrates that intervention on the great vessels within the depth of the chest was possible, with curative outcome.

Table 51-1 The Evolution of Cardiac Surgery: Time Line[a]

Year	Event
1938	Ligation of patent ductus arteriosus (Gross)
1944	Coarctation repair (Crafoord)
1944	Blalock-Taussig shunt
1946	Potts' shunt
1946	Closed pulmonary valvotomy (Sellors)
1948	Blalock-Hanlon atrial septectomy
1952	Pulmonary artery band (Muller and Dammann)
1952	Atrial well for ASD closure (Gross)
1952	ASD closure with inflow occlusion and hypothermia (Lewis)
1954	Controlled cross-circulation (Lillehei)
1957	Pacemaker for complete heart block (Lillehei, Bakken, and Gott)
1958	Superior cavopulmonary anastomosis (Glenn)
1962	Waterston's shunt
1966	Balloon atrial septostomy (Rashkind)
1968	Atriopulmonary connection (Fontan and Baudet)
1971	Complex repair in neonates and infants with PHCA (Barratt-Boyes)
1975	Arterial switch operation (Jatene)
1976	Introduction of PGE_1 (Elliott)
1981	First-stage palliation of hypoplastic left heart syndrome (Norwood)
1984	Neonatal heart transplantation (Bailey)

PGE_1 = Prostaglandin E_1; PHCA = profound hypothermic circulatory arrest.
[a]Chronological sequence of major contributions to the development of the field of congenital heart surgery.

Following this initial procedure, coarctation of the aorta was addressed. Alfred Blalock was the first to attempt correction of this problem in a canine model, by turning down the distally transected left subclavian artery and anastomosing the vessel to the proximal descending aorta (Blalock-Park procedure).[10] A discouragingly high rate of paraplegia was noted—likely the consequence of relatively long clamp times, which limited flow through a normal-caliber subclavian artery and poor collateral circulation. Clarence Crafoord (Fig. 51-2) routinely clamped the aorta during ligation of the arterial duct, and first reported coarctation repair with end-to-end anastomosis in two patients operated at the Karolinska Institute in 1944.[11] Robert Gross described a case of successful coarctation repair shortly thereafter[12] and was first in addressing this malformation with an interposition homograft in 1949.[13]

These initial interventions were indeed curative, but the long-term outlook of children with complex cyanotic congenital heart disease remained dismal until the mid-1940s. Although somewhat approximative, preoperative diagnosis was possible and solely relied on clinical examination, chest radiographs, and electrocardiography; at Johns Hopkins, Helen Taussig was able, with such a rudimentary diagnostic armamentarium, to place children with congenital heart disease into broad diagnostic categories, underscoring the urgency of developing a method for stable palliation of cyanotic patients. The

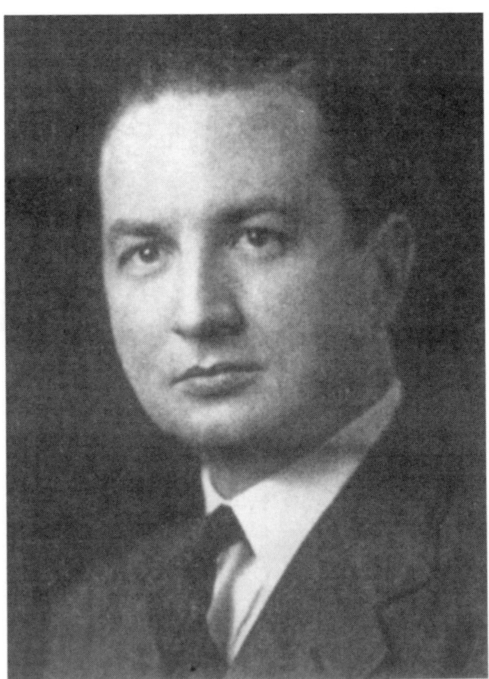

Figure 51-1 Robert E. Gross (1905–1988). (From Westaby,[1] p. 110. With permission.)

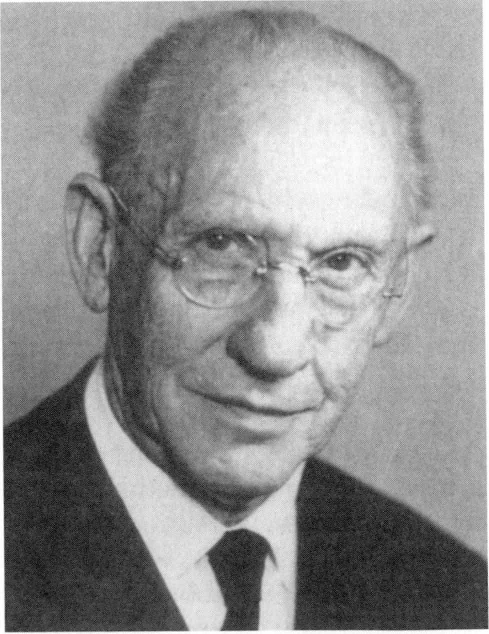

Figure 51-2 Clarence Crafoord (1899–1984). (From Shumaker HB Jr. The Evolution of Cardiac Surgery. Indianapolis: Indiana University Press, 1992:56. With permission.)

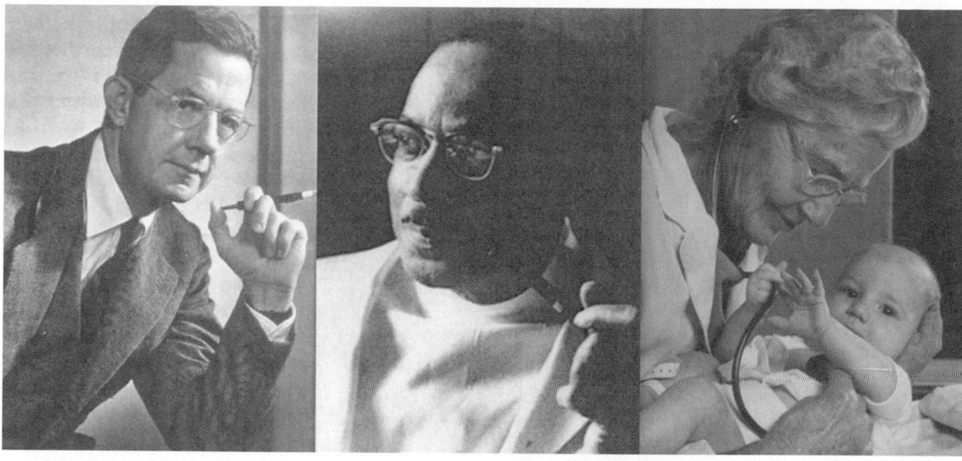

Figure 51-3 Protagonists of the first systemic-to-pulmonary shunt on November 29, 1944, at the Johns Hopkins Hospital. Left to right: Alfred Blalock (1890–1964), Vivien Thomas (1910–1985), and Helen Taussig (1898–1986). (Courtesy of the Johns Hopkins University photographic archives.)

creation of an "artificial ductus arteriosus" was deemed unfeasible by Robert Gross; Taussig then turned to Alfred Blalock, the newly appointed chief of surgery at the Johns Hopkins Hospital (Fig. 51-3). While in Nashville, Dr. Blalock and Vivien Thomas (his laboratory technician) had established an experimental model of pulmonary hypertension that entailed ligation of the pulmonary artery and anastomosis between the subclavian and left branch pulmonary arteries.[14] Although they were unable to increase pulmonary pressure because of the low impedance of the pulmonary vascular bed, the technique provided the increase in pulmonary blood flow that cyanotic children so desperately needed. This concept was introduced in the clinical arena on November 29, 1944, when Blalock successfully performed the first systemic-to-pulmonary shunt, thus opening the doors to the long-term palliation of cyanotic patients (Fig. 51-4).[15,16] Eileen Saxon, then a 16-month-old infant with pulmonary stenosis (Fig. 51-5), had barely reached the operative weight of 4 kg from a nearly prohibitive birth weight of 1.1 kg.

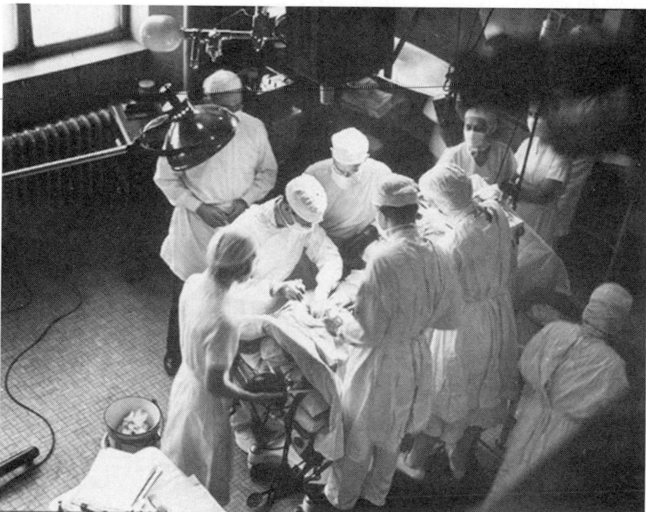

Figure 51-4 One of the first "blue baby" operations at the Johns Hopkins Hospital, circa 1945. In the center of the photograph, to the left of the operating table, Dr. Alfred Blalock. Behind him, Vivien Thomas, and, to his left, the then chief resident Dr. William Longmire. Standing as first assistant, opposite to Dr. Blalock, is the assistant resident, Dr. Denton Cooley. (Courtesy of the Johns Hopkins University photographic archives.)

Several modifications of this initial concept have followed and were all eventually rendered obsolete by the introduction of the "modified" Blalock-Taussig shunt.[17] Among these, anastomosis of the descending aorta to the left pulmonary artery (Potts shunt)[18] and of the ascending aorta to the right pulmonary artery (Waterston shunt)[19] were reported in 1946 and 1962, respectively. These approaches often proved to be unreliable in grading pulmonary blood flow, and were extraordinarily difficult to control at the time of late complete intracardiac repair.

Over the ensuing decades, systemic-to-pulmonary shunts—rather than the initial approach to staged repair of biventricular hearts—became the mainstay of palliation for univentricular heart disease (Fig. 51-6). Extracardiac palliative procedures are now more typically performed as the initial step toward achievement of complete right heart bypass, the so-called Fontan circulation (Fig. 51-7).[20–26]

For children with malformations characterized by left-to-right shunting and pulmonary overcirculation, initial treatment of pulmonary hypertension by pulmonary

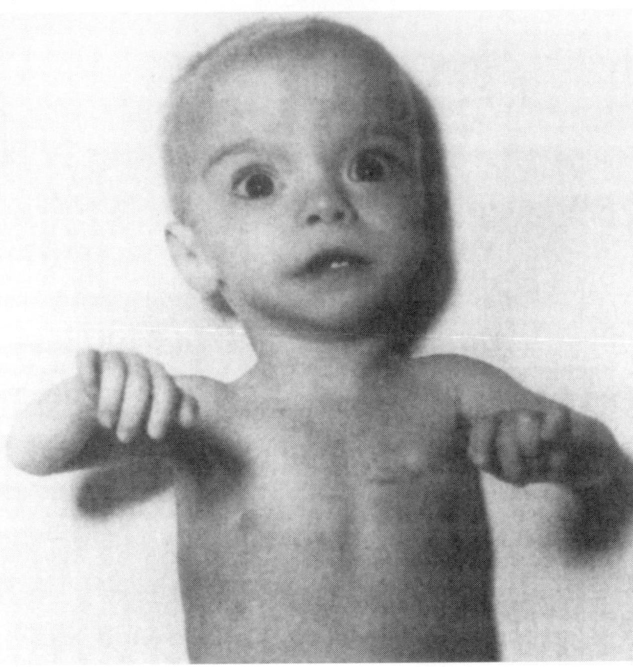

Figure 51-5 Eileen Saxon, the first infant to undergo a systemic-to-pulmonary shunt for palliation of cyanotic heart disease. Note the left-sided thoracotomy scar. In the first few patients undergoing the procedure, the thoracotomy was performed on the side ipsilateral to the aortic arch. The technique very rapidly evolved to a turndown of the subclavian artery contralateral to the side of the aortic arch, as technically more straightforward. (Courtesy of Or. WP Longmire. *Alfred Blalock. His Life and Times.* Privately published by the author, 1991, p. 99. With permission.).

arterial banding was first introduced by Muller and Dammann in 1952.[27] Although rarely utilized in biventricular hearts, pulmonary arterial banding still finds a role in the initial staging of cardiac malformations characterized by univentricular morphology and pulmonary hyperperfusion (Chap. 69).

EARLY CLOSED OR SEMICLOSED INTRACARDIAC OPERATIONS

The first attempts at closed intracardiac intervention were made to address pulmonic stenosis in cyanotic infants. T. Holmes Sellors of London reported the first successful transventricular pulmonary valvotomy in December 1946.[28] He had originally intended to perform a systemic-to-pulmonary shunt, but the chronic sequelae of tuberculosis made this initial plan unfeasible in his patient with Fallot's tetralogy. This approach was subsequently popularized by Lord Brock at Guy's Hospital and became the standard of care for pulmonic stenosis for much of the following decade. This approach was later to be largely supplanted by open valvotomy on cardiopulmonary bypass and, eventually, by the much more often utilized percutaneous balloon valvotomy, first introduced in 1982 by Jean Kan at the Johns Hopkins Hospital.[29]

The initial growing success of palliative and closed procedures in prolonging the lives of patients affected by pathologies that would then, without intervention, have been unsurvivable[30] led to the development of several semiclosed procedures to address simple malformations (such as atrial septation defects) or to achieve initial palliation for more complex congenital anomalies.

Although an initial partially successful attempt at closure of an atrial septal defect (ASD) with the external suturing technique was described by Murray in 1948,[31] Robert Gross in 1952 reported the ingenious use of an "atrial well" to close ASDs.[32] The well was constructed by suturing a rubber funnel to the right atrial wall (Fig. 51-8), which made it possible to prevent exsanguination and air embolization. Through the well and under the stable and contained column of blood, the surgeon identified the defect by palpation and repaired it primarily without any direct visualization. Although the technique was of necessity quite rudimentary and imperfect, John Kirklin in 1956 reported a series of 29 patients undergoing successful ASD closure with the atrial well technique and without operative mortality.[33]

The atrial well could also be utilized to create an interatrial communication in patients with cyanotic lesions characterized by poor mixing. Atrial septectomy was nevertheless mainly performed in the era of semiclosed techniques with the method introduced by Blalock and Hanlon in 1948.[34] In this method, right lung isolation was performed by temporarily occluding the right pulmonary artery and veins and by applying an appositely designed clamp (Fig. 51-9) to the groove of Sondergaard. The dorsal and right-lateral portion of the interatrial septum could then be excised and the interatrial groove closed primarily. These difficult operations[35,36] were eventually rendered obsolete by Rashkind's introduction of balloon septostomy in 1966.[37]

INITIAL PHASE OF COMPLETE INTRACARDIAC REPAIRS

Closed- or semiclosed operations failed to successfully address more complex morphologic problems, for which a true correction under direct vision was considered utopic until the early 1950s. The parallel investigation of hypothermia by the pioneering work of Wilfred Bigelow[38] and the introduction and development of extracorporeal circulation by John Gibbon (Fig. 51-10), and the groups at the University of Minnesota and the Mayo Clinic made true intracardiac surgery a reality.

On September 2, 1952, John Lewis (Fig. 51-11) first achieved closure of an atrial septal defect under direct vision in a 5-year-old child at the University of Minnesota.[39,40] The procedure lasted 58 min and was

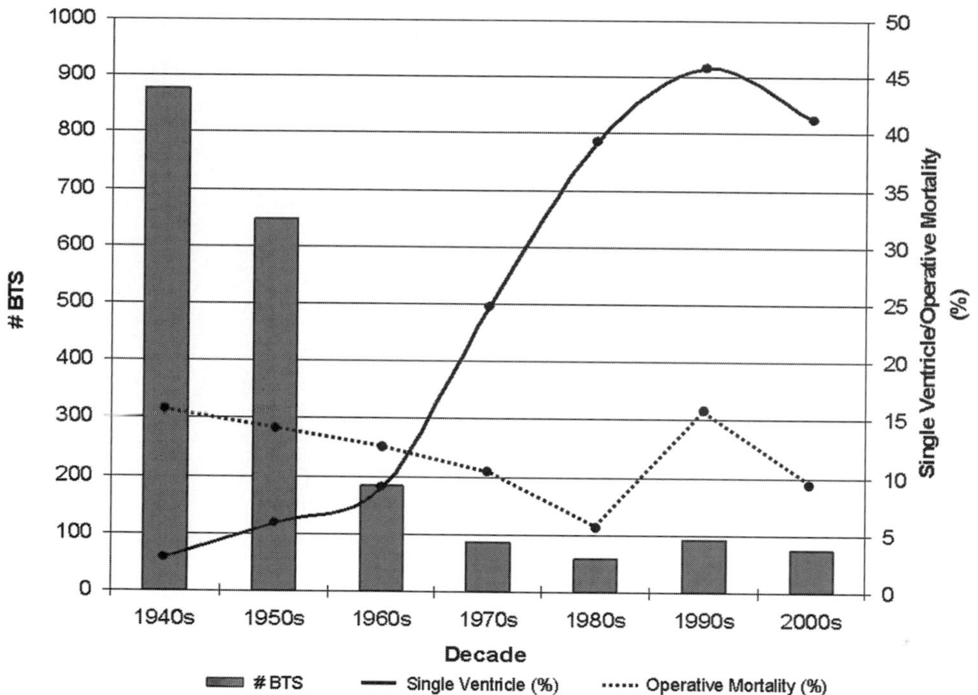

Figure 51-6 Trends in systemic-to-pulmonary shunts: the Johns Hopkins experience with 2029 shunts over six decades (1944–2006). A decrease in the total number of procedures is paralleled by a rise of the percentage of shunts performed as palliation for univentricular heart disease. A reduction in mortality and the subsequent peak in the late 1980s and early 1990s is possibly related to shunts being mainly utilized as part of the initial treatment of hypoplastic left heart syndrome. (From Williams JA et al. Two thousand Blalock-Taussig shunts: A six decade experience. Unpublished data.)

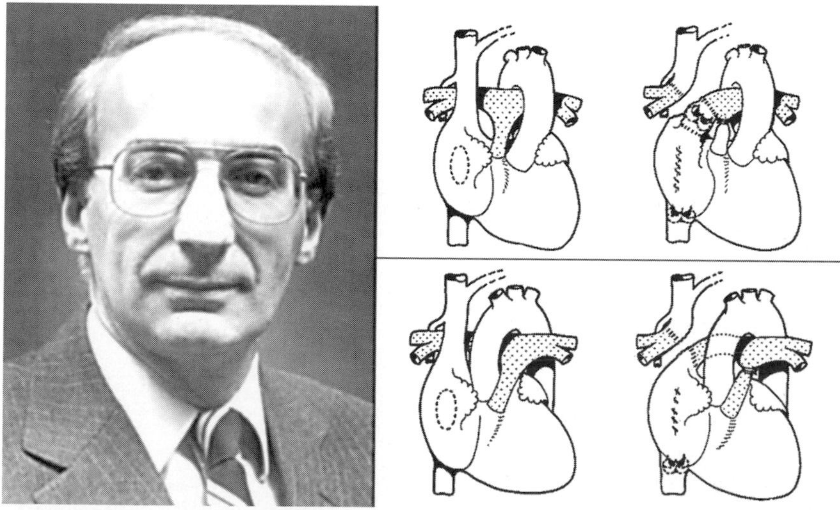

Figure 51-7 Francois Maurice Fontan (left).[1] Right: Illustration from the original 1971 article detailing a novel surgical approach to tricuspid atresia and univentricular heart disease.[21] Atriopulmonary connection with (upper panel) and without (lower panel) interposition of a valved homograft.

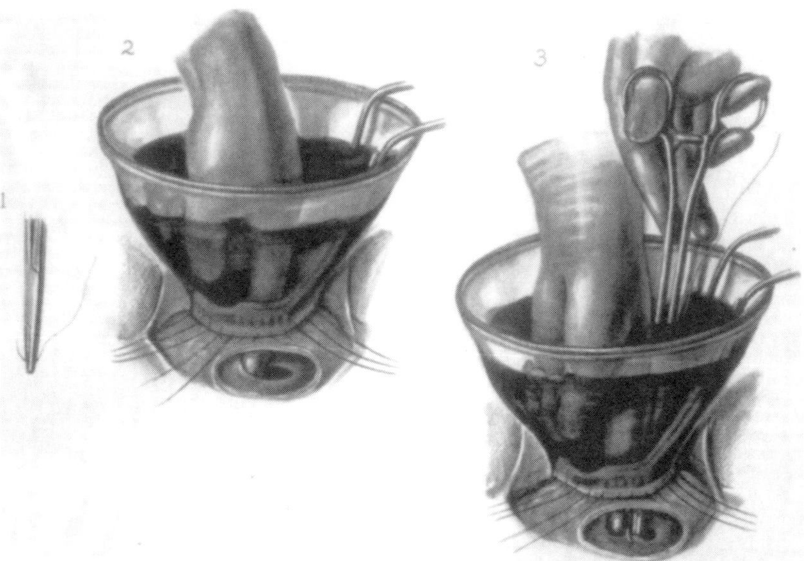

Figure 51-8 The "atrial well" technique for closure of atrial septal defects, introduced by Robert E. Gross in 1952. A rubber cone is anastomosed to the convexity of the right atrium and the defect is palpated by the index finger of the operator under the column of blood (2). An appropriately loaded suture (1) is then utilized to close the defect (3). (From Westaby,[1] p. 400. With permission.)

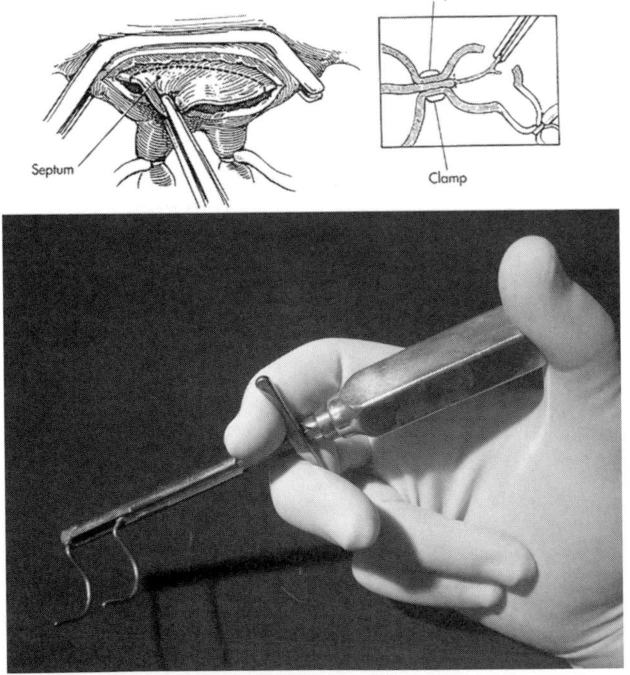

Figure 51-9 Blalock-Hanlon atrial septectomy. Upper panel: following isolation of the right pulmonary artery and veins, an incision is made in Sondergaard's groove (left) and the dorsal and leftward portion of the interatrial septum excised (right). (From Waldhausen JA. The early history of congenital heart surgery: Closed heart operations. *Ann Thorac Surg* 1997;64:1533. With permission.) Lower panel: appositely designed clamp, utilized by Alfred Blalock to perform closed atrial septectomy. (Courtesy of Vivien Thomas, given to the Division of Cardiac Surgery, The Johns Hopkins Hospital.)

preceded by a period of systemic surface cooling of 2 h and 10 min. At a core temperature of 28°C, a right thoracotomy was performed and, during 5 min of inflow occlusion, the 2-cm ASD was primarily closed. In merely a decade, the mortality for ASD closure was lowered from 30.2 percent (Gross's original series on ASD closure using the atrial well) to 12.1 percent (Lewis's inflow occlusion series).[41]

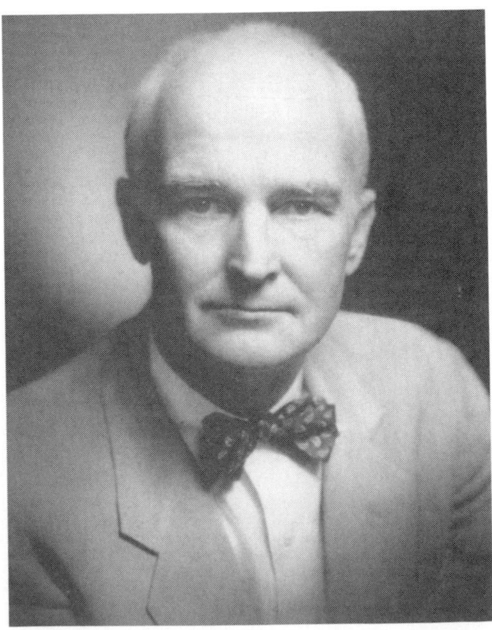

Figure 51-10 John Gibbon Jr. (1903–1973). (From Shumaker HB Jr. The evolution of cardiac surgery. Indianapolis: Indiana University Press, 1992: ii. With permission.)

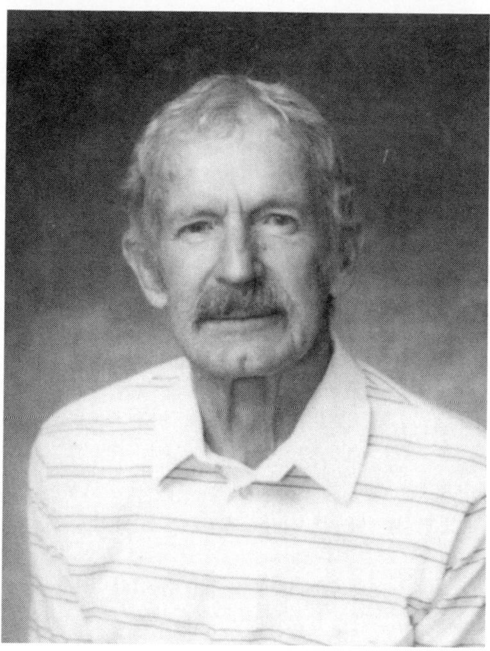

Figure 51-11 Floyd John Lewis (1916–1993). (From Westaby,[1] p. 75. With permission.)

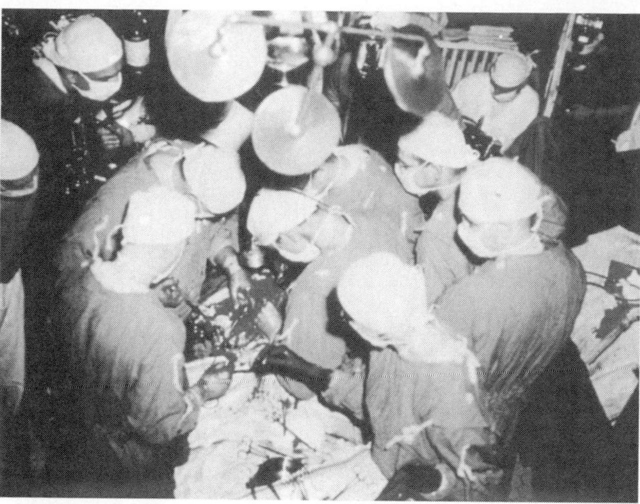

Figure 51-13 University of Minnesota, Operating Room B, March 26, 1954: the first case of controlled cross-circulation. Dr. C. Walton Lillehei, to the right of the scrub nurse, is seen wearing a head light. Opposite to Dr. Lillehei is Richard Varco. The patient's father is in the right background, and visible is the femoral donor cannulation site. Morley Cohen and Herbert Warden are seen behind Dr. Lillehei. Vincent Gott, the surgical intern on the cardiac service, is seen at the left upper corner of the picture, while assistant resident Norman Shumway is to his right. (Image courtesy of the University of Minnesota photographic archives.)

With the inflow occlusion technique, the time allowed for repair was below 10 min; to allow some degree of safety, the next natural evolution of intracardiac repair techniques was the introduction of extracorporeal circulation. John Gibbon was first to report successful direct closure of an ASD with the assistance of extracorporeal circulation in an 18-year-old patient at the University of Pennsylvania in 1953.[42]

Success and failure rapidly alternated in the early history of extracorporeal circuits. Two main techniques rapidly emerged: controlled cross-circulation and mechanical extracorporeal perfusion, championed by the University of Minnesota and the Mayo Clinic, respectively.

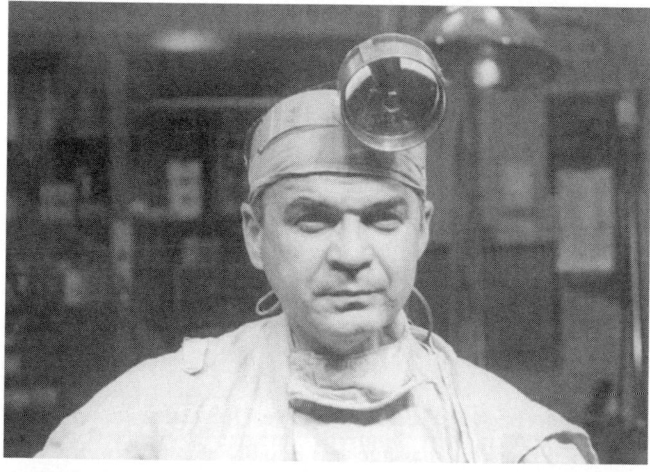

Figure 51-12 Clarence Walton Lillehei (1918–1999). (From Westaby,[1] p. 45. With permission.)

C. Walton Lillehei (Fig. 51-12) spearheaded the efforts to achieve intracardiac repair of complex cardiac lesions with the clinical introduction of controlled cross-circulation on March 26, 1954.[43] Lillehei, Varco, Cohen, and Warden pioneered this technique after extensive laboratory investigation in canines.[44,45] The first patient, a 1-year-old boy with an operative weight of 6.9 kg, was supported by his father (Figs. 51-13 and 51-14) for 19 min while the ventricular septal defect was closed primarily. The patient succumbed to pneumonia after 11 days, but this partial success did not undermine the morale of the surgeons at the University of Minnesota. Against institutional bias but with the support of Owen Wangensteen (Fig. 51-15), Lillehei, 2 weeks later, closed the ventricular septal defect of a 4-year-old girl, achieving long-term survival. Lillehei and coworkers performed a total of 45 operations with controlled cross-circulation. Among these was the first successful repair of tetralogy of Fallot, ventricular septal defect, and atrioventricular canal.[46–48] In this extraordinary series, operative mortality was 38 percent, and 79 percent of hospital survivors were alive at 30-year follow-up.[49] No operative deaths was directly attributable to extracorporeal perfusion, and postoperative heart block most certainly was implicated in several of the early failures. Because of this early, apparently insurmountable

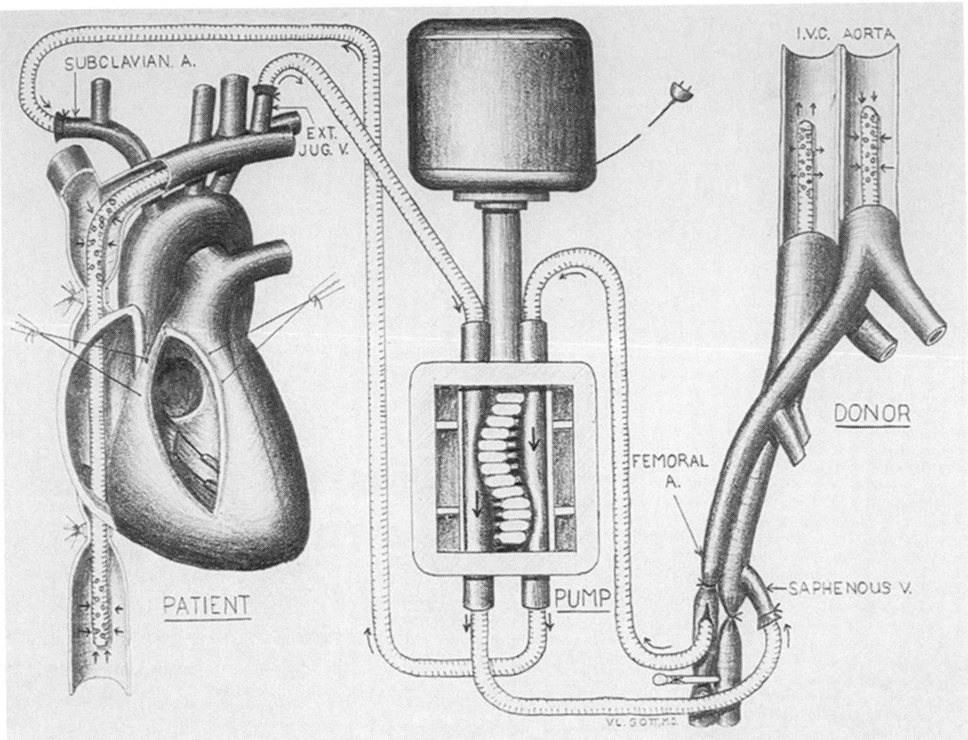

Figure 51-14 Schematic illustration of the first case of controlled cross circulation, 1954. Original drawing by the intern on C. Walton Lillehei's service, Vincent L. Gott. Reproduced with permission from Lillehei CW. Section III: Cardiopulmonary bypass and myocardial protection. In: Stephenson LW, Ruggero R, eds. *Heart surgery classics*. Boston, Adams Publishing Group, Ltd, 1994:130.

complication, Lillehei, Bakken, and coworkers also developed, from pressing necessity, the first temporary and, eventually, permanent implantable pacemakers.[50,51] By the 1950s, the University of Minnesota turned to circulatory support with the DeWall-Lillehei oxygenator[52] and abandoned controlled cross-circulation.

John Kirklin (Fig. 51-16) at the Mayo Clinic concentrated all his efforts on cardiopulmonary bypass, developing the Mayo-Gibbon apparatus and its modifications.[53]

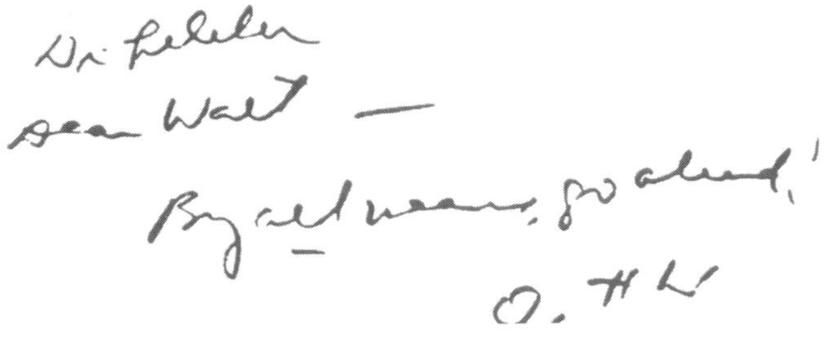

Figure 51-15 Note from Owen H. Wangensteen written to C. Walton Lillehei on March 25th 1954, the eve of the first parental cross-circulation.
Dr. Lillehei
Dear Walt –
By all means, go ahead!
OHW
[From Lillehei,[49] p. 126. With permission.)

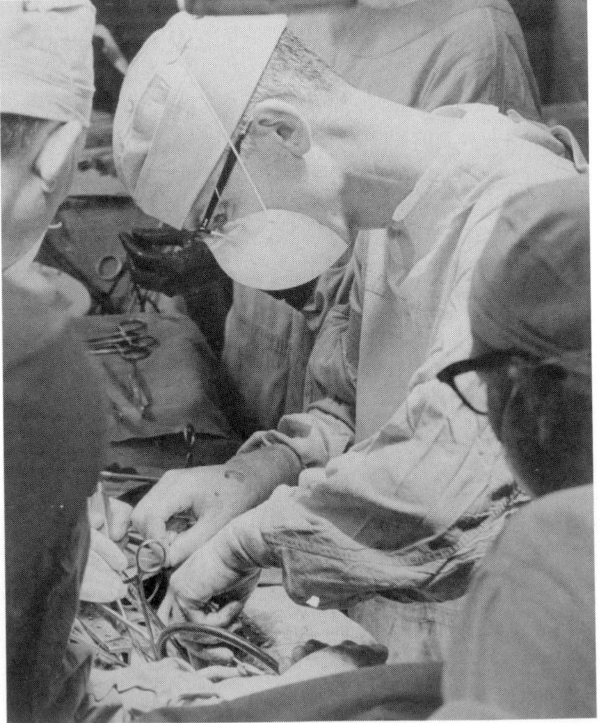

Figure 51-16 John Kirklin (1917–2004). (Courtesy of Dr. Joseph Dearani, Division of Cardiac Surgery, The Mayo Clinic. With permission.)

In 1955, Kirklin reported a cohort of 38 patients with ventricular and other septation defects corrected with the aid of mechanical cardiopulmonary support.[54] This initial work established the relative safety of mechanical extracorporeal circulation and served as a platform for the development of the field of pediatric cardiac surgery. Utilizing the techniques developed in Minnesota, more complex anomalies could be successfully approached in the early 1960s without excessive mortality.[55–61]

In spite of this initial success, intracardiac repair remained as a daring undertaking in neonates and infants, largely because of the deleterious effects of cardiopulmonary bypass in children.[62] The size of the bypass circuits, the crudeness of the materials, and the underdevelopment of pediatric critical care made correction of cardiac anomalies in early infancy prohibitive. Between 1955 and the mid-1960s, smaller patients underwent correction almost exclusively following initial palliation by closed cardiac techniques.

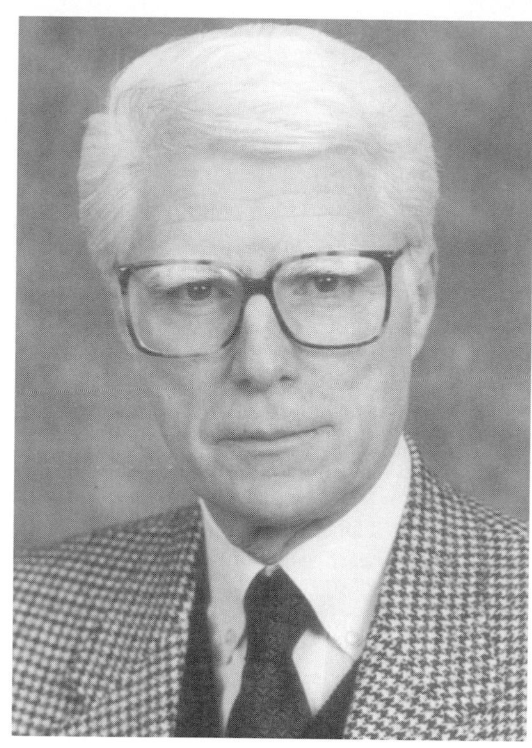

Figure 51-18 Aldo Castaneda (1930 –). (From Westaby S. The foundation of cardiac surgery. In: *Landmarks in Cardiac Surgery*. Oxford, UK: Isis Medical Media, 1997:135. With permission.)

EXPANSION OF THE FIELD OF CONGENITAL CARDIAC SURGERY

Brian Barratt-Boyes (Fig. 51-17) was without doubt one of the most influential figures in the further advancement of congenital cardiac surgery. He returned to Green Lane Hospital (Auckland, New Zealand) after 2 seminal years at the Mayo Clinic (1953–1955). Sir Brian pioneered the concept of profound hypothermia and hypothermic circulatory arrest. This approach aggressively minimized the duration of exposure to extracorporeal surfaces and the subsequent inflammatory response, limiting it mainly to that needed for cooling and rewarming. The actual intracardiac repair could then be carried out expeditiously with no cannulae crowding an asanguinous field, thus greatly facilitating exposure in neonates and small infants. Furthermore, systemic cooling permitted relatively reliable myocardial protection before the routine introduction of cardioplegia[63–65] in surgery involving congenital cardiac surgical procedures. This radical innovation made possible the intracardiac repair of complex anomalies in neonates and infants, with excellent outcomes.[66,67] Of the 37 infants reported in his original 1971 article,[68] 33 had operative weights below 10 kg, and 25 patients were between 8 days and 12 months of age at the time of surgical correction. A gradual but steady shift toward early, complete one-stage intracardiac repair rather than initial palliation followed.[69–73] Complex anomalies such as total anomalous pulmonary venous connection, transposition of the great arteries,[72,73] complete atrioventricular canal,[74–76] and aortic arch anomalies[77] could be repaired in the neonatal period or in early infancy with much more acceptable morbidity and mortality as compared with the results of earlier corrective attempts.

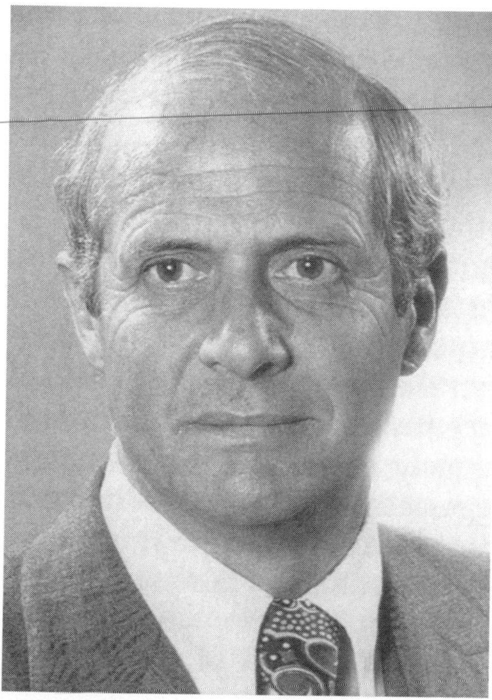

Figure 51-17 Sir Brian Barratt-Boyes (1924–2006). (From Shumaker HB Jr. The evolution of cardiac surgery. Indianapolis: Indiana University Press, 1992:283. With permission.)

This pioneering work was further developed by Castaneda (Fig. 51-18),[70–71] Jatene,[79,80] Norwood,[81,82] Bailey[83,84] and others.[85–88] Thanks to the vision and determination of these contributors and to the exponential progress of perioperative care (Chap. 53),[37,89] the field had evolved over a mere 25-year period from treacherous attempts at palliation in older children to routine complete correction in neonates and infants.

References

1. Westaby S. The foundation of cardiac surgery. In: *Landmarks in Cardiac Surgery.* Oxford, UK: Isis Medical Media Ltd, 1997:15.
2. Brewer LA III. Historical notes on lung cancer before and after Graham's successful pneumonectomy in 1933. *Am J Surg* 1980;143:650.
3. Naef AP. Forgotten pioneers in thoracic surgery. *Thorac Cardiovasc Surg* 1992;40:1.
4. Waldhausen JA. The early history of congenital heart surgery: Closed heart operations. *Ann Thorac Surg* 1997;64:1533.
5. Graybiel A, Strieder JW, Boyer NH. An attempt to obliterate the patent ductus arteriosus in a patient with subacute bacterial endocarditis. *Am Heart J* 1938;15:621.
6. Gross RE, Hubbard JP. Surgical ligation of a patent ductus arteriosus. Report of first successful case. *JAMA* 1939;112:729.
7. Xydas S, Widmann WD, Hardy MA, William E. Ladd: Father of pediatric surgery. *Curr Surg* 2003;60:47.
8. Moore FD, Folkman J. Robert Edward Gross. *Biogr Mem Natl Acad Sci* 1995;66:130.
9. Kaemmer H, Meisner H, Hess J, et al. Surgical treatment of patent ductus arteriosus: A new historical perspective. *Am J Cardiol* 2004;94:1153.
10. Blalock A, Park EA. The surgical treatment of experimental coarctation (atresia) of the aorta. *Ann Surg* 1944;119:445.
11. Crafoord C, Nylin G. Congenital coarctation of the aorta and its surgical treatment. *J Thorac Surg* 1945;14:347.
12. Gross RE, Hufnagel CA. Coarctation of the aorta. Experimental studies regarding its surgical correction. *N Engl J Med* 1945;223:287.
13. Gross RE, Bill AH Jr, Pierce EC II. Methods for preservation and transplantation of arterial grafts. Observations on arterial grafts in dogs. Report of transplantation of preserved arterial grafts in 9 human cases. *Surg Gynecol Obstet* 1949;88:689.
14. Levy SE, Blalock A. Experimental observations on the effects of connecting by suture the left main pulmonary artery to the systemic circulation. *J Thorac Surg* 1939;8:525.
15. Blalock A, Taussig HB. The surgical treatment of malformations of the heart in which there is pulmonary stenosis or atresia. *JAMA* 1945;132:189.
16. Taussig HB, Bauersfeld R. Congenital malformations of the heart: Follow-up studies on the first 1000 patients operated on for pulmonic stenosis or atresia. *Ann Intern Med* 1953;38:1.
17. De Leval MR, McKAy R, Jones M, et al. Modified Blalock-Taussig shunt. Use of subclavian artery orifice as flow regulator in systemic–pulmonary artery shunts. *J Thorac Cardiaovasc Surg* 1981;81:112.
18. Potts WJ, Smith S, Gibson S. Anastomosis of the aorta to a pulmonary artery. *JAMA* 1946;132:627.
19. Waterston DJ. Treatment of Fallot's tetralogy in children under one year of age. *Rozhl Chir* 1962;41:181.
20. Glenn WWL. Circulatory bypass of the right side of the heart. *N Engl J Med* 1958;259:117.
21. Fontan F, Baudet E. Surgical repair of tricuspid atresia. *Thorax* 1971;26:240.
22. Galankin NK. Proposition and technique of cavopulmonary anastomosis. *Exp Surg* 1957;5:33.
23. Carlon CA, Mondini PG, de Marchi R. Surgical treatment of some cardiovascular diseases. *J Int Coll Surg* 1951;16:1.
24. Haller JA, Adkins JC, Worthington M, et al. Experimental studies on permanent bypass of the right heart. *Surgery* 1966;59:1128.
25. Kreutzer G, Bono H, Galindez E, et al. Una operacion para la correction de la atresia tricuspidea. Proceedings from the 9th Argentinean Congress of Cardiology, Buenos Aires, Argentina, Oct 31–Nov 6, 1971.
26. DeLeval MR, Kilner P, Gewillig M, et al. Total cavopulmonary connection: A logical alternative to atriopulmonary connection for complex Fontan operations. *J Thorac Cardiovasc Surg* 1988;96:682.
27. Muller WH Jr, Dammann JF Jr. The treatment of certain congenital malformations of the heart by the creation of pulmonic stenosis to reduce pulmonary hypertension and excessive pulmonary blood flow. A preliminary report. *Surg Gynecol Obstet* 1952;95:213.
28. Sellors TH. Surgery for pulmonary stenosis: A case in which the pulmonary valve was successfully divided. *Lancet* 1948;1:988.
29. Kan SJ, White RI Jr, Mitchell SE, et al. Percutaneous balloon valvuloplasty: A new method for treating congenital pulmonary valve stenosis. *N Engl J Med* 1982;307:540.
30. Gross RE. Surgical closure of an aortic septal defect. *Circulation* 1952;5:858.
31. Murray G. Closure of defects in cardiac septa. *Ann Surg* 1948;128:843.
32. Gross RE, Pomerantz AA, Watkins E Jr, et al. Surgical closure of defects of the interauricular septum by use of an atrial well. *N Engl J Med* 1952;247:455.
33. Barratt-Boyes BG, Ellis FH, Kirklin JW. Technique for repair of atrial septal defect using the atrial well. *Surg Gynecol Obstet* 1956;103:646.
34. Blalock A, Hanlon CR. The surgical treatment of complete transposition of the aorta and pulmonary artery. *Surg Gynecol Obstet* 1950;90:1.
35. Results of the Blalock-Hanlon operation in 90 patients with transposition of the great vessels. *J Thorac Cardiovasc Surg* 1966;52:525.
36. Zamora R, Moller JH, Lucas RV Jr, et al. Complete transposition of the great vessels: Surgical results of emergency Blalock-Hanlon operation in infants. *Surgery* 1970:67:706.

37. Rashkind WJ, Miller WW. Creation of an atrial septal defect without thoracotomy. A palliative approach to complete transposition of the great arteries. *JAMA* 1966;196:991.
38. Bigelow WG, Lindsay WK, Greenwood WF. Hypothermia. Its possible role in cardiac surgery: An investigation of factors governing survival in dogs at low body temperatures. *Ann Surg* 1950;132:849.
39. Lewis FJ, Taufic M. Closure of atrial septal defects with the aid of hypothermia: Experimental accomplishments and the report of one successful case. *Surgery* 1953; 33:52.
40. Shumway NE. F John Lewis, MD: 1916–1993. *Ann Thorac Surg* 1996;61:250.
41. Lewis FJ. Discussion of Bigelow WG, Mustard WT, Evans JG. Some physiologic concepts of hypothermia and their applications to cardiac surgery. *J Thorac Cardiovasc Surg* 1954;28:463.
42. Gibbon JH Jr. Application of a mechanical heart and lung apparatus to cardiac surgery. *Minn Med* 1954;37:171.
43. Lillehei CW, Cohen M, Warden HE, et al. The results of direct vision closure of ventricular septal defects in eight patients by means of controlled cross-circulation. *Surg Gynecol Obstet* 1955;101:446.
44. Warden HE, Cohen MC, Read RC, et al. Controlled cross circulation for open intracardiac surgery. *J Thorac Cardiovasc Surg* 1954;28:331.
45. Cohen M, Lillehei CW. A quantitative study of the "azygos factor" during vena caval occlusion in the dog. *Surg Gynecol Obstet* 1954;98:225.
46. Lillehei CW. Controlled cross circulation for direct-vision intracardiac surgery. Correction of ventricular septal defects, atrioventricularis communis, and tetralogy of Fallot. *Postgrad Med* 1955;17:388.
47. Lillehei CW, Cohen M, Warden HE, et al. Direct vision intracardiac surgical correction of the tetralogy of Fallot, pentalogy of Fallot, and pulmonary atresia defects. Report of first 10 cases. *Ann Surg* 1955;142:418.
48. Lillehei CW, Cohen M, Warden HE, et al. Complete anatomical correction of the tetralogy of Fallot defects. Report of a successful surgical case. *Arch Surg* 1956;73: 1956.
49. Lillehei CW. Section III: Cardiopulmonary bypass and myocardial protection. In: Stephenson LW, Ruggero R, eds. *Heart Surgery Classics.* Boston: Adams Publishing Group, 1994:126–128.
50. Wierich WL, Paneth M, Gott VL. Control of complete heart block by the use of an artificial pacemaker and a myocardial electrode. *Circ Res* 1958;6:410.
51. Lillehei CW, Gott VL, Hodges PC, et al. Transistor pacemaker for treatment of complete atrioventricular dissociation. *JAMA* 1960;76:2006.
52. DeWall RA, Warden HE, Read RC, et al. A simple, expendable, artificial oxygenator for open heart surgery. *Surg Clin North Am* 1956;36:1025.
53. Kirklin JW, DuShane JW, Patrick RT, et al. Intracardiac surgery with the aid of a mechanical pump oxygenator system (Gibbon-type): Report of eight cases. *Proc Staff Mayo Clin* 1955;30:201.
54. DuShane JW, Kirklin JW, Patrick RT, et al. Ventricular septal defects with pulmonary hypertension. Surgical treatment by means of a mechanical pump-oxygenator. *JAMA* 1956;160:950.
55. Rastelli GS, Ongley PA, Kirklin JW, et al. Surgical repair of the complete form of persistent common atrioventricular canal. *J Thorac Cardiovasc Surg* 1968;55:299.
56. McGoon DC, Rastelli GC, Ongley PA. An operation for the correction of truncus arteriosus. *JAMA* 1968: 205:59.
57. Rastelli GC. A new approach to "anatomic" repair of transposition of the great arteries. *Mayo Clin Proc* 1969;44:1.
58. Kirklin JW, Harp RA, McGoon DC. Surgical treatment of origin of both vessels from right ventricle, including cases of pulmonary stenosis. *J Thorac Cardiovasc Surg* 1964;48:1026.
59. Hardy KL, May IA, Webster CA, et al. Ebstein's anomaly: A functional concept and successful definitive repair. *J Thorac Cardiovasc Surg* 1964;48:927.
60. Senning A. Surgical correction of transposition of the great arteries. *Surgery* 1959;45:966.
61. Mustard WT. Successful two-stage correction of transposition of the great vessels. *Surgery* 196;55:469.
62. Kirklin JK, Westaby S, Blackstone EH, et al. Complement and the damaging effects of cardiopulmonary bypass. *J Thorac Cardiovasc Surg* 1983;86:845.
63. Melrose DG, Dreyer B, Bentall HH. Elective cardiac arrest. *Lancet* 1955;269:21.
64. Hearse DJ, Stewart DA, Brainbridge MV. Cellular protection during myocardial ischemia: The development and characterization of a procedure for the induction of reversible ischemic arrest. *Circulation* 1976;54:193.
65. Laks H, Barner HB, Kaiser G. Cold blood cardioplegia. *J Thorac Cardiovasc Surg* 1979;77:319.
66. Barratt-Boyes BG. Cardiac surgery in neonates and infants. *Circulation* 1971;44:924.
67. Seelye ER, Harris EA, Squire AW, et al. Metabolic effects of deep hypothermia and circulatory arrest in infants during cardiac surgery. *Br J Anaesth* 1971;43:449.
68. Barratt-Boyes BG, Simpson M, Neutze JM. Intracardiac surgery in neonates and infants using deep hypothermia with surface cooling and limited cardiopulmonary bypass. *Circulation* 1971;43(5 Suppl):I25.
69. Kirklin JW, Blackstone EH, Pacifico AD, et al. Routine primary repair vs two-stage repair of tetralogy of Fallot. *Circulation* 1979;60:373.
70. Kirklin JW. The movement of cardiac surgery to the very young. In: Crupi G, Parenzan L, Anderson RH, eds: *Perspectives in Pediatric Cardiology*. Armonk, NY: Futura, 1989:3–22.
71. Bacha EA, Scheule AM, Zurakowski D, et al. Long-term results after early primary repair of tetralogy of Fallot. *J Thorac Cardiovasc Surg* 2001;122:154.
72. Castaneda AR, Lamberti J, Sade RM, et al. Open-heart surgery in the first three months of life. *J Thorac Cardiovasc Surg* 1974;68:719.
73. Castaneda AR, Norwood WI, Jonas RS, et al. Transposition of the great arteries and intact ventricular septum: Anatomical repair in the neonate. *Ann Thorac Surg* 1984;5:438.
74. Norwood WI, Dobell AR, Freed MD, et al. Intermediate results of the arterial switch operation. A 20-institution study. *J Thorac Cardiovasc Surg* 1988;96:854.
75. Castaneda AR, Mayer JE, Jonas RA, et al. Repair of complete atrioventricular canal in infancy. *World J Surg* 1985; 9:590.

76. Hanley FL, Fenton KN, Jonas RA, et al. Surgical repair of complete atrioventricular canal defects in infancy. Twenty-year trends. *J Thorac Cardiovasc Surg* 1993;106:387.
77. Ilbawi M, Cua C, Deleon SY, et al. repair of complete atrioventricular septal defect and tetralogy of Fallot. *Ann Thorac Surg* 1990;50:407.
78. Sell JE, Jonas RA, Mayer JE, et al. The results of a surgical program for interrupted aortic arch. *J Thorac Cardiovasc Surg* 1988;96:871.
79. Jatene AD, Fontes VF, Paulista PP, et al. Successful anatomic correction of transposition of the great vessels: A preliminary report. *Arq Brasil Cardiol* 1975;28:461.
80. Jatene AD, Fontes VF, Paulista PP, et al. Anatomic correction of transposition of the great vessels. *J Thorac Cardiovasc Surg* 1976;72:364.
81. Norwood WI, Lang P, Hansen DD. Physiologic repair of aortic atresia-hypoplastic left heart syndrome. *N Engl J Med* 1983;308:22.
82. Norwood WI, Lang P, Castaneda AR, et al. Experience with operations for hypoplastic left heart syndrome. *J Thorac Cardiovasc Surg* 1981;82:511.
83. Bailey LL, Nehlsen-Cannarella SL, Concepcion W, et al. Baboon-to-human cardiac xenotransplantation in a neonate. *JAMA* 1985;254:3321.
84. Bailey LL, Nehlsen-Cannarella SL, Doroshow RW, et al. Cardiac allotransplantation in newborns as therapy for hypoplastic left heart syndrome. *N Engl J Med* 1986;315:949.
85. Konno S, Imai Y, Lida Y, et al. A new method for prosthetic valve replacement in congenital aortic stenosis associated with hypoplasia of the aortic valve ring. *J Thorac Cardiovasc Surg* 1975;70:909.
86. Ross DN, Somerville J. Correction of pulmonary atresia with a homograft aortic valve. *Lancet* 1966;2:1446.
87. Ross DN. Replacement of aortic and mitral valves with a pulmonary autograft. *Lancet* 1967;2:956.
88. Yacoub MH, Radley-Smith R, Hilton CJ. Anatomical correction of complete transposition of the great arteries and ventricular septal defect in infancy. *Br Med J* 1976; 1:1112.
89. Elliott RB, Starling MB, Neutze JM. Medical manipulation of the ductus arteriosus. *Lancet* 1975;1:140.

CHAPTER

52 THE ANATOMY OF CONGENITAL CARDIAC MALFORMATIONS

Robert H. Anderson, Andrew C. Cook

INTRODUCTION

The results of the surgical treatment of congenital cardiac malformations have been transformed within the last half-century. Prior to the development of cardiopulmonary bypass, it was impossible even to contemplate the repair of major malformations, even though ingenious surgeons had successfully closed simple intracardiac lesions such as holes between the atrial chambers. Even when it proved possible for the surgeon to work within the heart in the setting of a bloodless operative field, the results of operative repair were far from perfect, and many patients died subsequent to the operative procedure. Nowadays, it is unusual for any patient with a relatively simple defect to die, and even those with "complex" lesions are now expected to survive. There have been many reasons for these truly remarkable advances, but without question one has been the knowledge of detailed intracardiac anatomy accrued within recent decades. In the past, it was often thought that, in the setting of so-called complex malformations, this anatomy was difficult to understand. It is now recognized that, although the combination of given lesions can truly be complex, the anatomy itself is relatively straightforward provided that it is approached in straightforward fashion and using a system of analysis that is simple and logical. To achieve success, therefore, the budding pediatric cardiac surgeon must hone not only the surgical skills but also the intellectual rigor needed to analyze the structure of the congenitally malformed heart. It would be foolish to suggest that problems do not still exist in obtaining the necessary morphologic understanding, but these problems can be minimized by using a simple philosophy combined with use of words in their vernacular sense. Too many of the problems of the past have reflected linguistic rather than scientific disagreements. It remains appropriate to remember the aphorism attributed to Rudolf Virchow, namely that "those who fail to learn from the mistakes of the past are condemned to repeat them." In this chapter, therefore, we describe the basics of cardiac anatomy that permit the surgeon to diagnose and recognize the arrangement of the cardiac chambers during surgical procedures and at the same time appreciate the likely position of the vital conduction tissues. The concomitant advances made over recent years in diagnostic techniques are now such that the basic layout of the heart will have almost certainly been established prior to commencement of intracardiac procedures. Nonetheless, even in the most complex cases, preliminary diagnosis demands little more, in terms of morphology, than the distinction of a right atrium from a left atrium, a right ventricle from a left ventricle, and an aorta from a pulmonary trunk. It is such distinctions that provide the basis for simple sequential segmental analysis.[1] For the surgeon, the anatomy of holes and blockages within the heart and great vessels are of equal or even greater significance. This morphology is addressed elsewhere in the appropriate chapters of this book; therefore we confine ourselves to showing how the anatomy of some important defects differs markedly from the normal arrangement. Our primary concern, however, is to establish the requirements for a systematic and simple approach to cardiac anatomy.

APPROACHES TO THE HEART

The heart lies in the mediastinum. In most instances, it is found with its apex pointing to the left, and with about two-thirds of its bulk to the left of the midline. If not thus located, the surgeon should immediately consider the possibility that complex malformations lurk within the heart. When the heart is abnormally located, it is our preference to describe the arrangement in simple terms, such as "heart mostly in the right chest with the apex pointing to the left" or as appropriate. In this way, we avoid the need to define arcane terms, such as "pivotal dextrocardia" and comparable locutions. The surgeon usually approaches the heart through the midline anteriorly or via the thoracic cavities. Nowadays, a median sternotomy or a variation on this approach is used most frequently. It is fortunate for the surgeon that the area of the mediastinum immediately behind the sternum is devoid of vital structures. Separate incisions can be made in the suprasternal notch and beneath the xiphoid process, the two being joined by blunt dissection. Splitting of the sternum exposes the pericardial sac lying between the pleural cavities. An important structure in this area is the thymus gland, particularly well developed in infants, which wraps itself over the pericardium in the area of the arterial pole. In dividing or excising the gland, the surgeon must take care of both the arterial supply, from the internal thoracic and inferior thyroid arteries, and the venous drainage through the thymic veins. The latter structures are fragile and often empty via a common trunk to the left brachiocephalic vein, which may be inadvertently damaged by undue traction.

Having exposed the pericardium, the surgeon should then remember that the vagus and phrenic nerves traverse its length, albeit well clear of the operative field (Fig. 52-1). The phrenic nerves, nonetheless, can be damaged should the pericardium be harvested for use as an intracardiac patch or baffle. Excessive traction on the pericardial cavity should be avoided, since it is easy to avulse the origin of the pericardiophrenic arteries, which accompany the phrenic nerves.

Lateral thoracotomies are made most frequently in the fourth intercostal space, using the posterior bloodless triangle between the edges of the latissimus dorsi, trapezius, and teres major muscles. An incision midway between the ribs avoids the intercostal neurovascular bundle, protected beneath the lower margin of the fourth rib. Such an incision takes the surgeon into the pleural space.

On the left side, posterior retraction of the lung exposes the middle mediastinum, revealing the left lobe of the thymus overlying the pericardium and the aortic arch, with its associated nerves and vessels. The aortic isthmus and descending aorta are readily approached in this fashion, dividing the parietal pleura posterior to the vagus nerve. Care must be taken to avoid the left recurrent laryngeal nerve, which takes its origin from the vagus and curves around the inferior border of the arterial ligament or, if this structure is still patent, the arterial duct (Fig. 52-2). The thoracic duct should also be avoided; this vessel drains at the junction of the left subclavian and internal jugular veins.

A right thoracotomy provides access to the right pulmonary artery and adjacent structures. On the right side, the right recurrent laryngeal nerve passes around the subclavian artery as it runs superiorly from the vagus toward the larynx. The stellate ganglion from the sympathetic trunk is also at potential danger in this region, inappropriate damage to this structure resulting in Horner's syndrome.

SURFACE ANATOMY OF THE HEART

The nature of the cardiac chambers is readily determined by external inspection. The morphology of the appendages best distinguishes the right from the left atrium. These out-

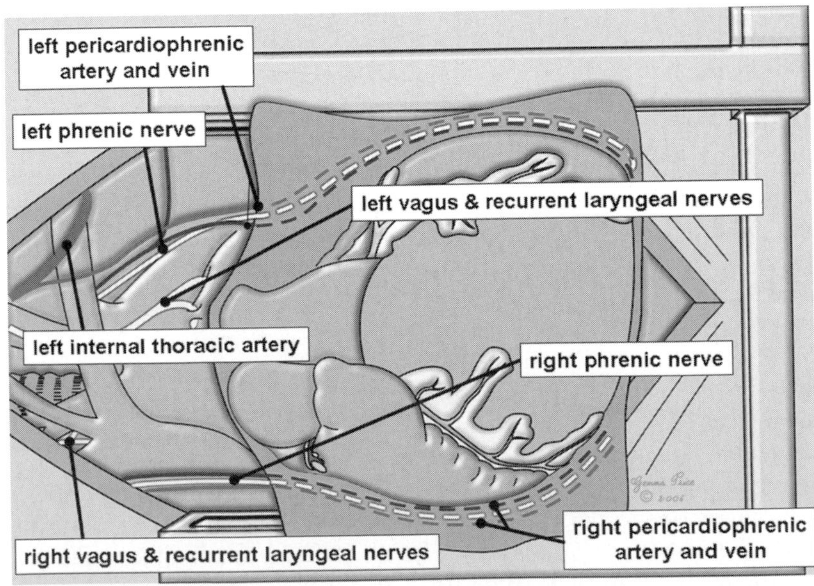

Figure 52-1 The diagram shows the relationships between the vagus and phrenic nerves and the heart contained within its pericardial sac as seen by the surgeon approaching the heart through a median sternotomy.

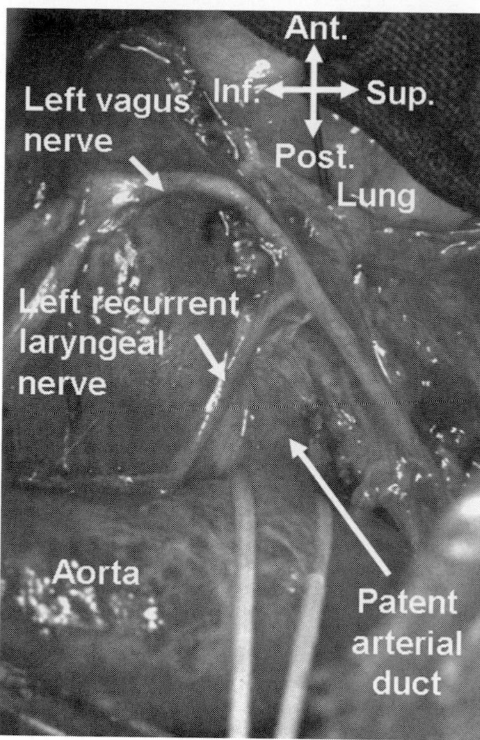

Figure 52-2 This operative view through a left thoracotomy shows the relationships of the recurrent laryngeal nerve relative to the arterial duct. (Courtesy of Benson Wilcox, MD, with permission.)

pouchings usually clasp the arterial pedicle, with one appendage to each side (Fig. 52-3). The arrangement in which both appendages are on the same side of the pedicle is called juxtaposition of the atrial appendages. Should the two appendages both be left-sided, then the cardiac chambers and arterial trunks are almost always abnormally joined together. If both appendages are to the right, however, this being a much rarer finding, the heart is again likely to be malformed, but in much simpler fashion, sometimes with no more that an atrial septal defect. Juxtaposition of the appendages also distorts the internal atrial architecture, particularly the atrial septum—a situation that can produce problems unless properly recognized.

In this chapter, we use the terms "right" and "left" to indicate morphology rather than position, this being one of the basic rules of congenital cardiac morphology. If position is also abnormal, this should be described separately. The appendages are the best structures with which to distinguish the morphologically right and left atriums. The right appendage has an obviously triangular shape, in contrast to the tubular left appendage. Shape, however, can be modified by abnormal hemodynamics. In situations of uncertainty therefore, the surgeon should examine carefully the junctions between the appendages and the remainder of the atrial chambers.[2] The essential feature of the right atrium is that the pectinate muscles extend all around the atrioventricular junction to the back of the heart. In the left atrium, in contrast, the posterior wall is entirely smooth, the pectinate muscles being confined within the tubular appendage. When the triangular appendage is right-sided and the tubular appendage left-sided, this usual arrangement is frequently called "situs solitus." Our preference, as already stated, is to use words which have currency in normal language, so we prefer simply to describe it as "the usual arrangement." On rare occasion, the tubular appendage will be right-sided, with the triangular one on the left side. This is best described as "the mirror-imaged arrangement." Although often called "situs inversus," the appendages in this setting are truly mirror-imaged rather than being turned upside down. Mirror-imagery is rare. In

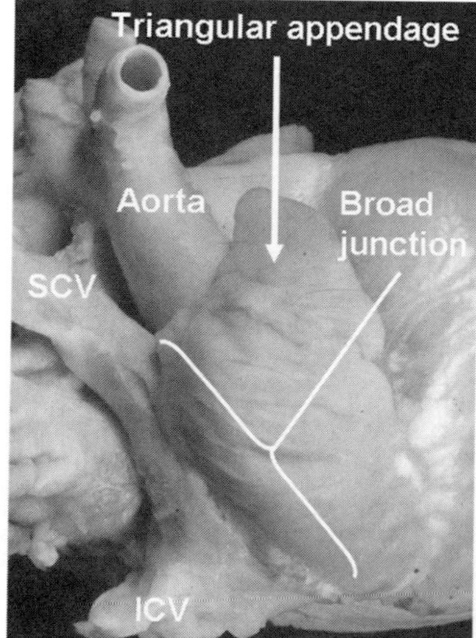

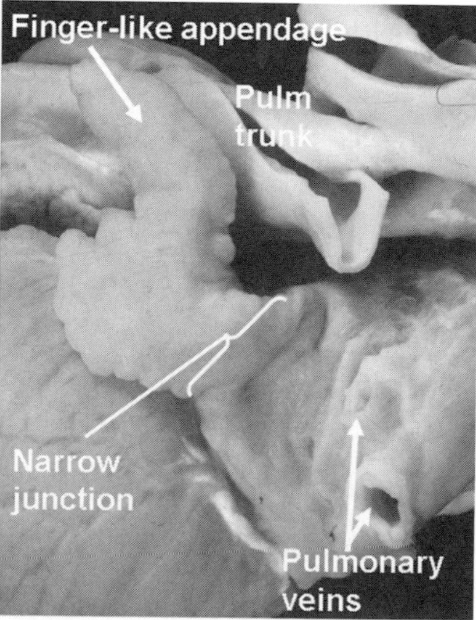

Figure 52-3 These lateral views of the heart, taken in anatomic position, show the different shapes of the right and left atrial appendages.

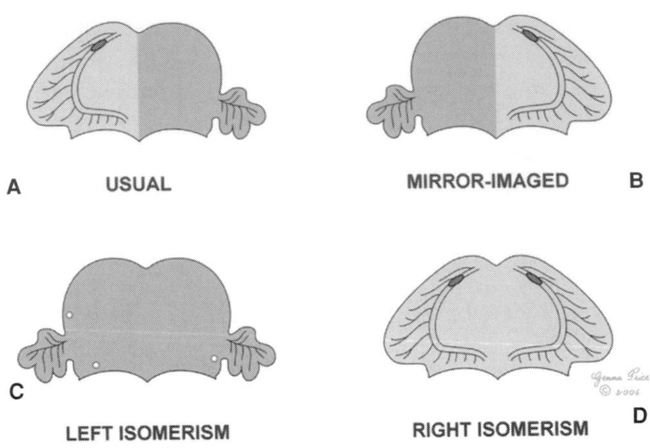

Figure 52-4 The potential arrangement of the atrial appendages. Note the location of the sinus node (hatched commas or dots; see text for further discussion).

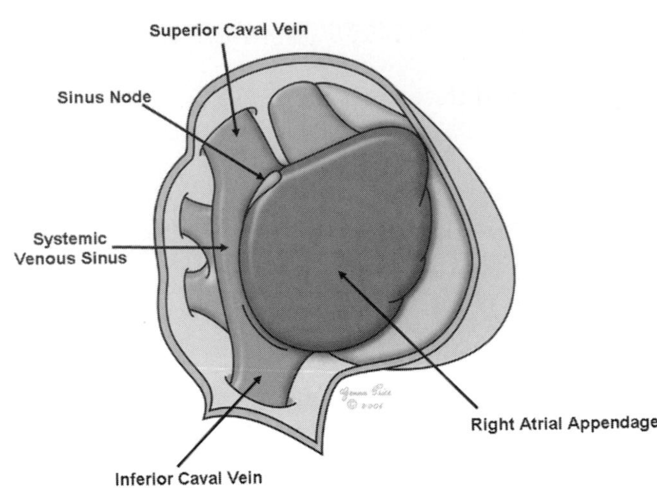

Figure 52-5 The drawing shows how the terminal groove interposes between the right atrial appendage and the systemic venous component. The heart is shown in anatomic orientation, with the subepicardial position of the sinus node marked.

the setting of complex malformations, it is more frequent to find the arrangements in which both the appendages have comparable morphology. Both appendages can then either be broad and triangular, with pectinate muscles extending all around the atrioventricular vestibules, or else both can be tubular and narrow, with smooth posterior atrial walls on both sides (Fig. 52-4). These arrangements are accurately described as isomerism of the right or left atrial appendages, respectively. Patients with such arrangements of the appendages also typically have jumbled-up abdominal organs, along with an isomeric arrangement of the lungs and bronchial tree.[1,2] The overall arrangement is called visceral heterotaxy and, in the past, was often categorized on the basis of splenic morphology. These syndromes are the harbingers of the most complex combinations of intracardiac lesions, but it is now unusual for such patients to be denied attempted surgical correction. By the simple expedient of inspecting the appendages, the surgeon now has the means of diagnosing these entities directly in the operating room, should the conditions not have been recognized during the diagnostic workup. Indeed, recognition of the appendages is the more important to the surgeon, since sometimes there is discordance between splenic anatomy and the arrangement of the appendages.[3] It is accurate recognition of the appendages that guides the surgeon to an appreciation of the likely location of the sinus node.[4]

Thus, the surgeon should examine carefully the junctions between the appendages and the atrial venous components. If the junction is morphologically right, there will be an extensive terminal groove, marking the site of the terminal crest internally (Fig. 52-5). The sinus node is always located in the immediately subendocardial position within this groove, positioned lateral to the crest of the atrial appendage (Fig. 52-6). The morphologically left junction is never marked by any such prominent groove and similarly lacks a sinus node. Should both junctions be morphologically right, the sinus node will be duplicated and the surgeon should respect both junctions. In the setting of isomeric left appendages, in contrast, the sinus node will be hypoplastic or even absent, and the surgeon should be aware that the nodal remnant can be positioned in the smooth atrial wall close to the atrioventricular junctions.[4]

Having inspected the appendages, the surgeon should turn attention to the venoatrial connections, ensuring that all the pulmonary veins, along with the caval veins and the coronary sinus, are in their appropriate positions.

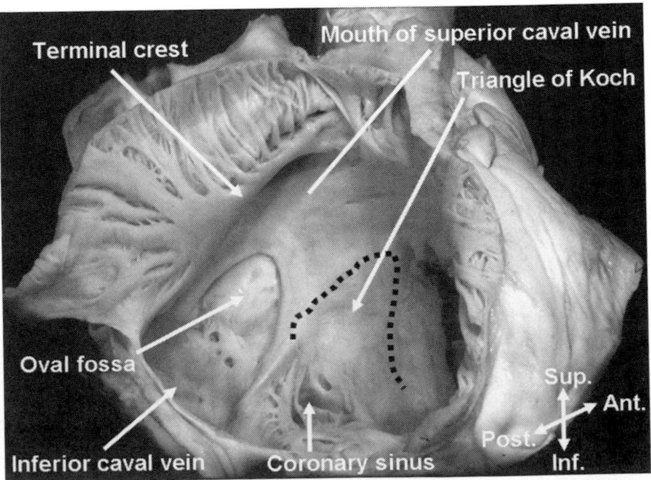

Figure 52-6 The right atrium has been opened with the heart in anatomic position to show the terminal crest and the location of the triangle of Koch. Note the apparent extensive area occupied by the septal surface.

Search should always be made for a persistent left superior caval vein. This will be found between the left appendage and the left pulmonary veins. If the surgeon has already established that there is isomerism of the left atrial appendages, then attention should be directed to the inferior caval vein, which is often interrupted in this setting, venous flow from the abdomen being returned through the azygos venous system, which will be correspondingly enlarged. External inspection also provides significant information concerning the structure of the ventricular mass. It is the positions of the interventricular branches of the coronary arteries that are the guide.[5] In the usual situation, the anterior interventricular coronary artery is a branch of the main stem of the left coronary artery, descending close to the obtuse margin of the ventricular mass. Should this artery take its origin from a coronary artery arising in right-sided position from the aortic root, the aorta itself being anterior to the pulmonary trunk, then almost always the ventricles themselves will be arranged in mirror-imaged fashion (so-called left-hand ventricular topology) with the morphologically left ventricle then positioned on the right. Identification of such a coronary arterial pattern should alert the surgeon to the likely presence of congenitally corrected transposition, the combination of discordant atrioventricular and ventriculoarterial connections (see below). Equally obvious should be the arrangement in which two arteries of comparable size take origin from an anteriorly positioned aorta, delimiting the position of a small ventricle on the anterior surface of the ventricular mass. Such a finding is indicative of disproportion between the sizes of the ventricles. The most frequent disproportion is seen when the left ventricle is dominant and the right ventricle is small, as in double-inlet left ventricle or tricuspid atresia. Should prominent interventricular arteries not be evident on the anterior ventricular surface, suspicion should be raised that there is a solitary ventricle of indeterminate morphology. This pattern, however, is exceedingly rare. Much more frequently in this setting, the right ventricle will be dominant, with the small left ventricle hidden on the diaphragmatic surface of the ventricular mass. This is the typical pattern seen in hypoplasia of the left heart.

In examining the ventricular mass, note should also be taken of the relationship of the arterial trunks, confirming first that there are separate aortic and pulmonary trunks as opposed to a common or solitary trunk. There will usually be separate trunks, and typically the aortic trunk is then posterior and right-sided, with the pulmonary trunk spiraling around the aorta as it divides into right and left pulmonary arteries. This is the "normal relationship."

Abnormal relationships of the great arterial trunks are indicative of intracardiac malformations, albeit that the positions and connections of the cardiac chambers themselves cannot be inferred from such knowledge. Abnormal arterial positions, nonetheless, give important clues to the presence of particular lesions, which nowadays will almost certainly have been diagnosed with consummate accuracy before the patient reaches the operating room. An anterior and right-sided aorta is the typical feature of discordant ventriculoarterial connections, usually known as "transposition," but is also seen when both arterial trunks arise from the right ventricle. When the aorta is anterior and left-sided, most frequently the transposition will be congenitally corrected as discussed above, but this pattern can also be seen with double outlet from the right ventricle. The aorta can also be anterior and left-sided when the connections are concordant across both the atrioventricular and ventriculoarterial junctions, a rare situation sometimes called "anatomically corrected malposition."[6] A left-sided and anterior aorta can also be found with regular transposition. All this variation serves to emphasize that relationships of the arterial trunks are at best a guide to the specific connections of the cardiac segments.

ANATOMY OF THE CARDIAC CHAMBERS

The perceptive reader will have ascertained from our descriptions thus far that one of the major features of the congenitally malformed heart is that the cardiac chambers are not always in their usual position, nor are they joined as expected to their neighbors. The most important rule of congenital cardiac anatomy, nonetheless, is that each chamber has a relatively constant anatomy irrespective of its position or its connections, albeit that a subtle change in morphology is found when the chambers are connected in abnormal fashion or when the junctions between the cardiac segments are themselves malformed. In this section, therefore, we concentrate our attention on the expected normal morphology, emphasizing when the surgeon should expect to find abnormal arrangements.

THE RIGHT ATRIUM

As already discussed, the most distinctive feature of the right atrium is its extensive triangular appendage, which is separated from the venous component of the atrium by the terminal groove (Fig. 52-5). When viewed by the surgeon, the superior caval vein enters the left-hand side of the venous component, with the inferior caval vein to the right-hand side. The venous component itself is then seen by the surgeon as a sleeve, being separated inferiorly from the right pulmonary veins by the extensive interatrial groove. This groove, also known as Waterston's or Sondergaard's groove, is a deep infolding between the right and left atrial walls.

Opening of the right atrium reveals the extensive terminal crest (Fig. 52-6). This muscular bundle underlies the terminal groove, encasing the orifices of both the superior and inferior caval veins, and extending anteriorly toward the atrial septum. In the region of the septum, it becomes a muscular ridge, the eustachian ridge, which separates the orifice of the inferior caval vein from the mouth of the coronary sinus. The mouths of these venous structures are often guarded by sickle-shaped fibrous folds of varying dimensions, the eustachian and thebesian valves. The fibrous commissure of these two valves buries itself in the musculature between the coronary sinus and the oval fossa; as viewed by the surgeon, it runs toward the left-hand margin of the tricuspid vestibule. This important structure, the tendon of Todaro, forms one boundary of the crucial triangle of Koch (Fig. 52-6). When seen in the operating room, the tendon forms the most distant border of the triangle, while the site of annular attachment of the septal leaflet of the tricuspid valve is closer to the surgeon. The atrioventricular node is found at the apex of this triangle, with the atrioventricular bundle penetrating from the apex to pass into the left ventricular outflow tract.

When the right atrium is viewed as shown in Fig. 52-6, the impression is gained of an extensive septal surface between the right and left atriums. Sectioning shows that this is not the case (Fig. 52-7). The atrial septum, defined as the tissue that can be removed without encroaching on the pericardial cavity,[7] is confined to the floor of the oval fossa and its anteroinferior margins.[7,8] The left-hand side of the fossa, as viewed by the surgeon, is the atrial wall overlying the aortic root. The septum secundum, between the fossa and the orifice of the superior caval vein, positioned superiorly with the heart in anatomic location but seen as an inferior structure by the surgeon, is no more than the deeply infolded walls of the interatrial groove.

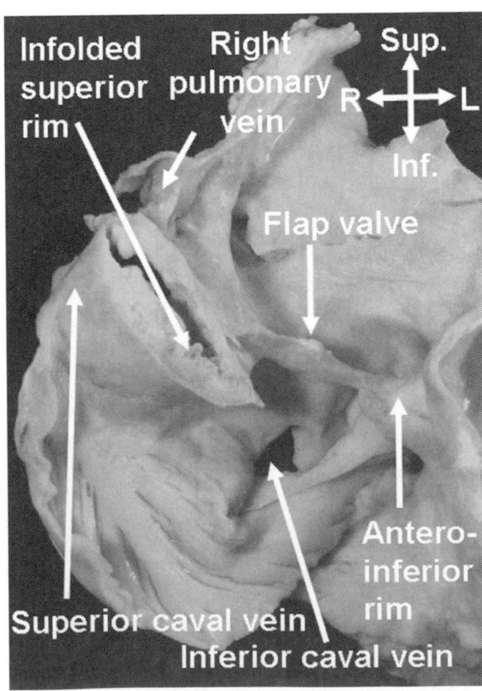

Figure 52-7 Sectioning of the heart reveals that only the oval fossa and its inferoanterior rim are true septal structures. The other borders are infoldings of the atrial walls.

THE LEFT ATRIUM

Overall, the left atrium (Fig. 52-8) has a much simpler structure than the right atrium but also possesses an extensive body, which is lacking in the right atrium. The appendage accounts for less of the chamber than on the right side. The venous component, located posteriorly and superiorly, receives the four pulmonary veins, one at each corner. When seen by the surgeon entering through the atrial roof, the narrow opening of the tubular appendage is to the left hand, while the septal surface is to the right. The smooth inferior and posterior margin of the mitral vestibule overlies the coronary sinus as it runs round from the obtuse margin of the ventricular mass. The septal surface of the left atrium is much simpler than that of the right, being formed by the flap valve of the oval fossa (Fig. 52-8).

THE ATRIOVENTRICULAR AND VENTRICULOARTERIAL JUNCTIONS

Knowledge of the structure of the junctions between the cardiac components is fundamental to the proper understanding of several congenital anomalies, particularly atrioventricular septal defects in the setting of common atrioventricular junctions.[9] The salient anatomy of both these junctions, and the relationship between the valves

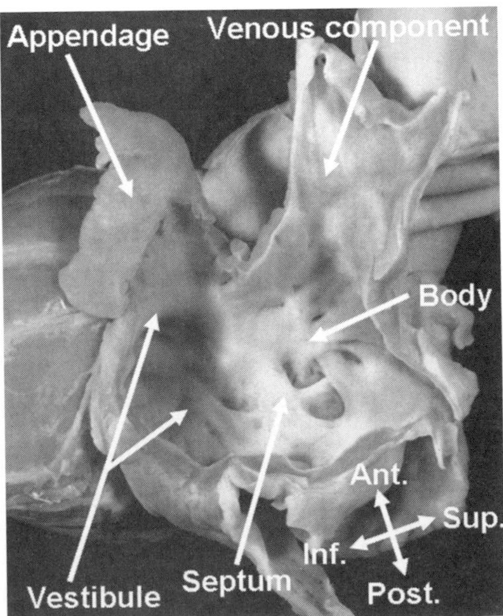

Figure 52-8 The components of the left atrium are shown in anatomic orientation as seen in left lateral position.

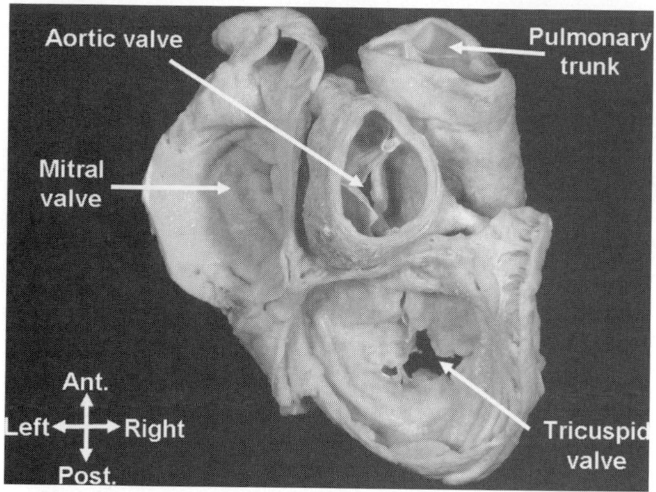

Figure 52-9 The atrial myocardium has been removed from the base of the heart, which is photographed from above and from the right to show the arrangement of the atrioventricular junctions relative to the ventriculoarterial junctions.

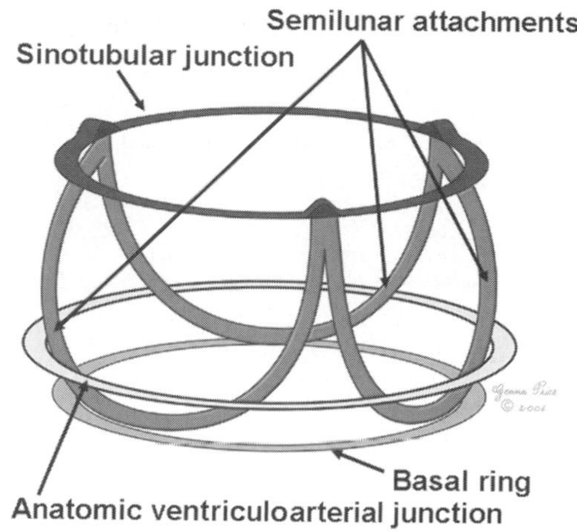

Figure 52-10 The drawing shows how the arterial roots are formed in the style of a coronet, with the semilunar attachments of the valvar leaflets crossing the anatomic ventriculoarterial junction. The basal ring is a virtual ring, made by joining together the basal attachments of the leaflets. The sinotubular junction, in contrast, is a true annular structure and marks the distal boundary of the arterial root.

guarding them, is well seen when the musculature of the atrial chambers and the arterial trunks is dissected away from the ventricular base, which can then be viewed from its superior aspect (Fig. 52-9). Although each of the four cardiac valves is usually described as possessing an annulus, in reality none has a true and complete fibrous ring supporting its leaflets. It is the mitral annulus that approximates most closely to the concept of a ring, albeit that it is more akin to an oval saddle, and parietally there is often very little collagenous tissue supporting the mural leaflet of the valve. In the tricuspid orifice, it is very rare to find a collagenous annulus. Instead, it is the fibro fatty tissues of the atrioventricular groove that separate the atrial muscle from the ventricular mass. In the case of the arterial valves, the concept of a "ring" is totally deficient. For both the aortic and pulmonary valves, each of the three leaflets is attached to the underlying ventricular structures in semilunar fashion. Although encased in a circular tube, the attachments of the arterial valvar leaflets, when considered as a whole, take the form of a coronet, with the hinge lines of the leaflets tenting up to reach the sinotubular junction and sweeping down to the nadir of the attachments at the ventricular bases (Fig. 52-10). In the right ventricle, these basal attachments are exclusively supported by ventricular muscle, specifically by the free-standing subpulmonary infundibulum. For the aortic valve, in contrast, a good half of the valvar circumference is supported by fibrous and collagenous tissues. This is because the leaflets of the aortic valve usually have extensive fibrous continuity with those of the mitral valve and, via the membranous septum, also with the leaflets of the tricuspid valve (Fig. 52-11). The two ends of the region of aortic-mitral valvar continuity are thickened to form the right and left fibrous trigones, with the right trigone itself forming an integral part of the fibrous mass where the aortic root is continuous with the leaflets of the tricuspid valve (Fig. 52-12). This whole area is called the central fibrous body, incorporating the so-called membranous septum, which forms the medial wall of the subaortic outflow tract beneath the zone of apposition

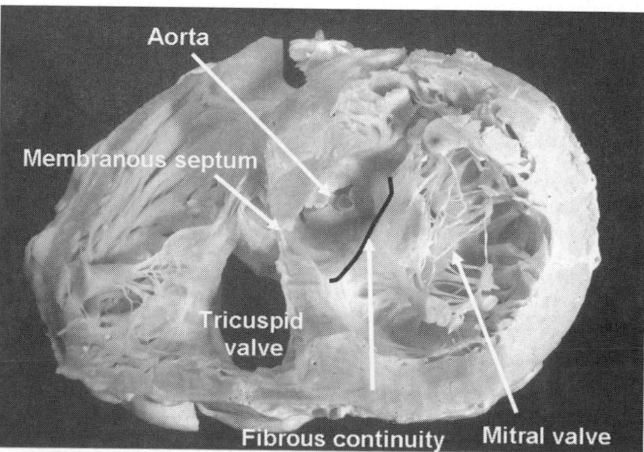

Figure 52-11 The short axis of the ventricular mass is photographed from beneath in left anterior oblique orientation, showing the relationship between the leaflets of the aortic and mitral valves. Note also the fibrous continuity with the tricuspid valve through the substance of the membranous septum.

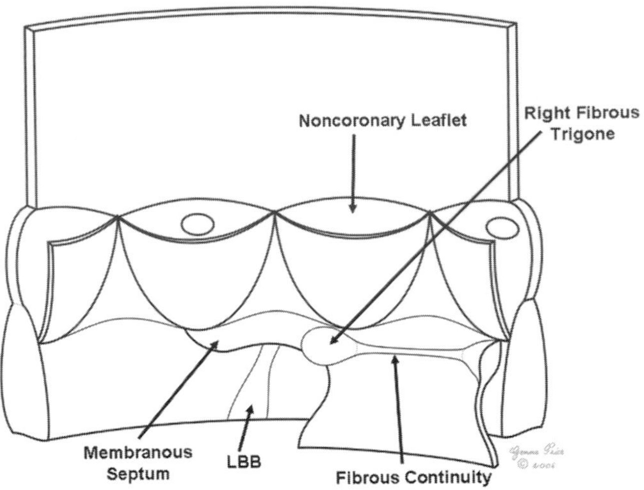

Figure 52-12 The drawing shows how the right trigone and the membranous septum form the so-called central fibrous body.

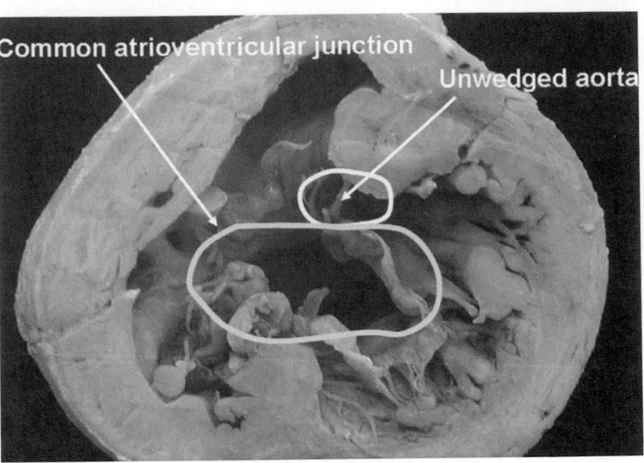

Figure 52-13 An atrioventricular septal defect with the common atrioventricular junction has been sectioned in the short axis of the ventricular mass and photographed from beneath (compare with Fig. 52-11). The essence of the lesion is the common atrioventricular junction.

between the right coronary and noncoronary leaflets of the aortic valve. The attachment of the septal leaflet of the tricuspid valve divides this membranous septum into its atrioventricular and interventricular components.

Viewing the atrioventricular junctions from their ventricular aspect (Fig. 52-11) shows how the subaortic outflow tract "lifts" the aortic leaflet of the mitral valve away from the muscular ventricular septum. Because of this, the two atrioventricular valves are attached to opposite sides of the septum over a remarkably short distance. In this short area, the tricuspid valve is attached to the septum more toward the ventricular apex than is the mitral valve, producing the well-recognized echocardiographic feature of valvar off setting. In times gone by, we considered this area to be the "atrioventricular muscular septum."[9] We now know that, in this area, an extension of the inferior atrioventricular groove interposes between the atrial and ventricular musculatures. The area is better likened to a sandwich rather than a septum.[10] It is into the atrial aspect of the sandwich that the coronary sinus opens to the right atrium, having traversed the posterior and inferior aspect of the left atrioventricular junction. The atrial components of the "atrioventricular muscular sandwich" contain the atrioventricular node, which lies on the sloping atrial aspect of the junction. From this position, the atrioventricular bundle is able to penetrate the central fibrous body and reach the crest of the muscular ventricular septum in the left ventricular outflow tract. The surgical landmark to this point of penetration is the zone of apposition between the right and noncoronary aortic valvar leaflets. As seen from the right atrium, it is the landmarks of the triangle of Koch that delineate the site of the specialized atrioventricular conduction tissues. Seen from the left atrium, the septal end of the zone of apposition between the leaflets of the mitral valve demarcates the area of danger. In approaching from the right ventricle, so as to protect the conduction tissue, the surgeon must avoid the area immediately adjacent to the medial papillary muscle and the zone of apposition between the septal and anterosuperior leaflets of the tricuspid valve.

It is the atrioventricular muscular sandwich together with the atrioventricular component of the membranous septum that are lacking in the group of lesions known as atrioventricular canal malformations, or more recently as atrioventricular septal defects.[9] Attention to the junctional morphology of these lesions shows that the phenotypic feature is a common atrioventricular junction (Fig. 52-13). The valve guarding the common junction closes in the fashion of a pentafoliate structure, irrespective of whether there is a common valvar orifice, or separate orifices for the right and left ventricles, the latter morphology being the phenotypic feature of the so-called ostium primum defect.[9] Attention to the pattern of closure of the left ventricular component of this common valve shows that it possesses three leaflets, one being exclusive to the left ventricle and the other two being the left ventricular components of leaflets that bridge the ventricular septum (Fig. 52-14). Analysis in this fashion shows that the "cleft" in the left atrioventricular valve, a source of appreciable confusion over the years, is no more than the zone of apposition between the left ventricular components of these two leaflets bridging the ventricular septum.

THE RIGHT VENTRICLE

Traditionally, it has been customary to divide ventricles into sinus and conus. This convention is adequate for the

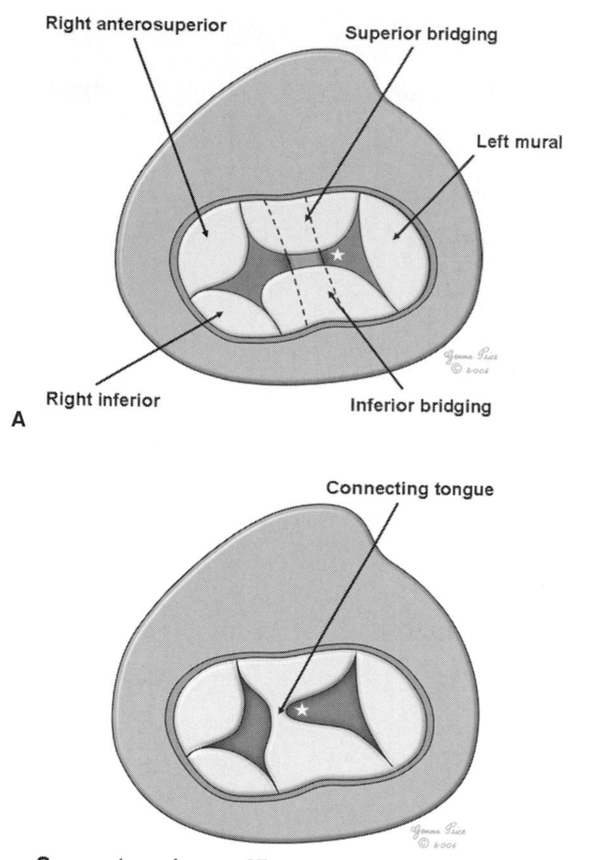

Figure 52-14 The drawing shows the arrangement of the leaflets of the common valve that guards the common atrioventricular junction, as shown in Fig. 52-13, when (A) there is a common atrioventricular junction and (B) there are separate valvar orifices for the right and left ventricles. Note that the left atrioventricular valve possesses three leaflets and that the so-called cleft (asterisk) is the zone of apposition between the left ventricular components of the leaflets, which bridge the ventricular septum.

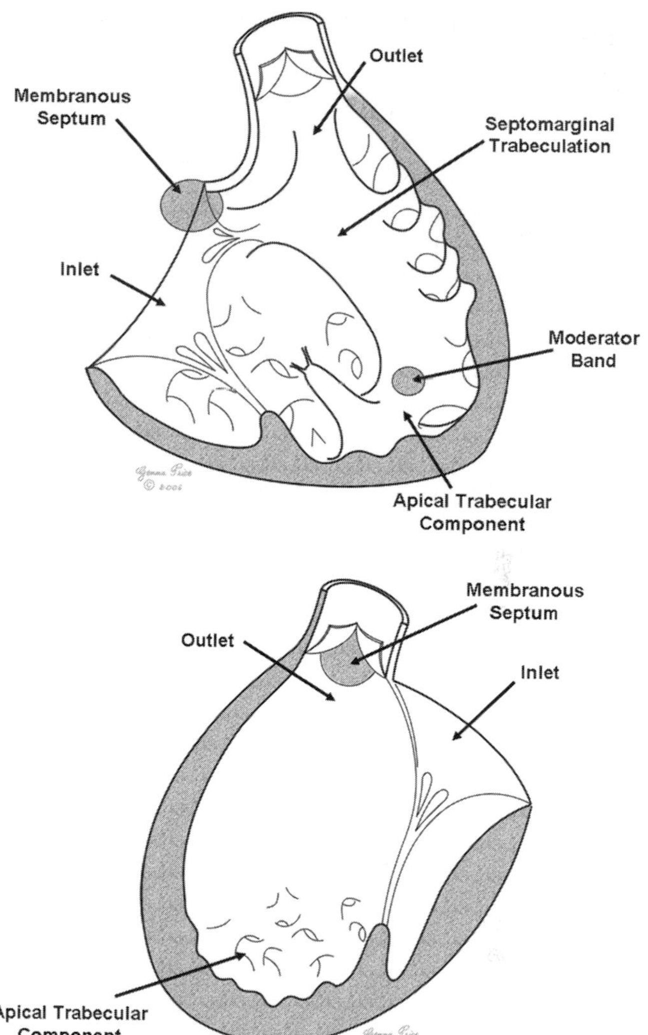

Figure 52-15 The drawing shows how both right and left ventricles can be described as possessing inlet, apical trabecular, and outlet components.

normal heart, although less than ideal. In our opinion, it is better to consider ventricles as possessing three rather than two components, namely the inlet, apical trabecular, and outlet portions (Fig. 52-15). All ventricles, no matter how deformed, are readily described using this tripartite convention. For instance, the small ventricles in functionally univentricular hearts with a dominant left ventricle, whether produced by double-inlet or tricuspid atresia, possess apical trabecular and outlet components. As such they are logically described as ventricles, and the hole between them and the dominant left ventricle appropriately described as the ventricular septal defect.[11]

In describing the atrioventricular valves, integral components of most ventricles, we must be able to distinguish their leaflets. This is best done by viewing the valves in their closed rather than open positions. It is then an easy matter to recognize the number of zones of apposition within the components of the skirt of leaflet tissue. Such an approach is much better than taking the “commissural cords” as the criterion of division between leaflets. In using the criterion of commissural cords, it is difficult to determine whether the mitral valve has two or four leaflets.[12] When viewed from the stance of the closed valve, there is no question but that the mitral valve possesses two leaflets with a solitary zone of apposition between them.[13] In similar fashion, viewing the closed tricuspid valve shows that it truly possesses three leaflets.[14] And, when seen in attitudinally appropriate orientation, these leaflets are located septally, anterosuperiorly, and inferiorly within the valvar orifice.

The right ventricle, when normally constituted, possesses the tricuspid valve in its inlet portion. The zone of apposition between its septal and anterosuperior leaflets, supported by the medial papillary muscle, is intimately

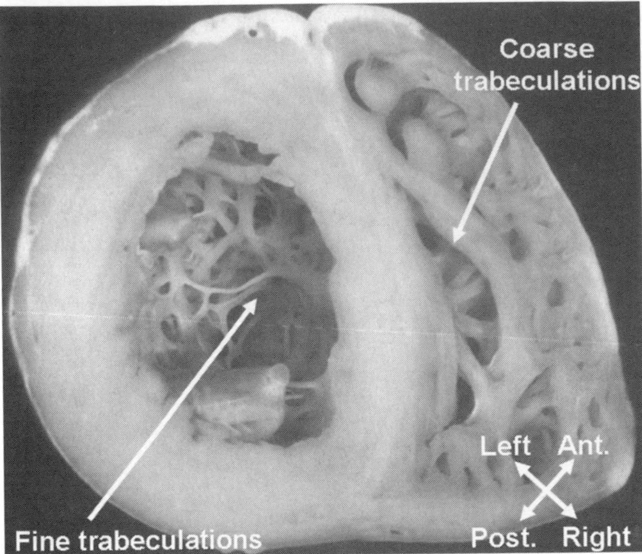

Figure 52-16 The view of the apical part of the ventricular mass, seen from above, shows the difference in apical trabeculations between the right and left ventricles.

related to the site of penetration of the atrioventricular bundle. The feature of the apical trabecular component is its typically coarse trabeculations. Indeed, it is on this basis that the ventricle is most reliably differentiated from the finely trabeculated left ventricle (Fig. 52-16).

In the normal right ventricle, the outlet component is a free-standing muscular sleeve, the infundibulum (Fig. 52-17). The apparently "septal" aspect of this infundibulum is part of the supraventricular crest, which interposes between the attachments of the leaflets of the tricuspid and pulmonary valves. Dissection shows that this structure is no more than the parietal wall of the heart, its removal emphasizing the important relationship to the right coronary artery (Fig. 52-18). The crest inserts between the limbs of the extensive septal muscle bundle, which runs down into the apical trabecular component, splitting into various trabeculations including the moderator band, the anterior papillary muscle, and various septoparietal trabeculations (Fig. 52-18). In the past, this extensive bundle was often viewed as part of the supraventricular crest, and it still retains the designation of "septal band." Logic dictates that this structure cannot, at the same time, be both septal and supraventricular. It is better to distinguish this important structure as the septomarginal trabeculation, separating it in this way from both the ventriculoinfundibular fold, which forms the supraventricular crest, and the outlet component of the ventricular septum.[15] In the normal heart, however, it is not possible to distinguish with certainty that small part of the muscular septum between the subaortic and subpulmonary outlets. This part of the septum is better seen when the ventricular septum itself is deficient and is most obvious when both arterial trunks take their origin predominantly or completely from the right ventricle, as

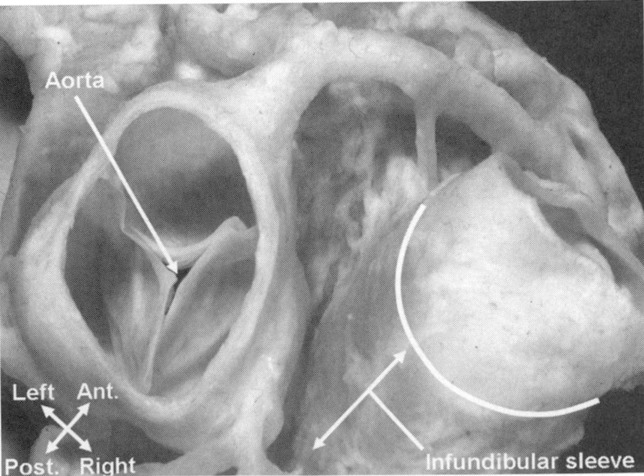

Figure 52-17 The free-standing muscular infundibulum of the right ventricle has been swung away from the aortic root, showing the deep tissue plane that separates the two arterial roots. The white line shows the circular junction between the infundibular musculature of the right ventricle and the wall of the pulmonary trunk.

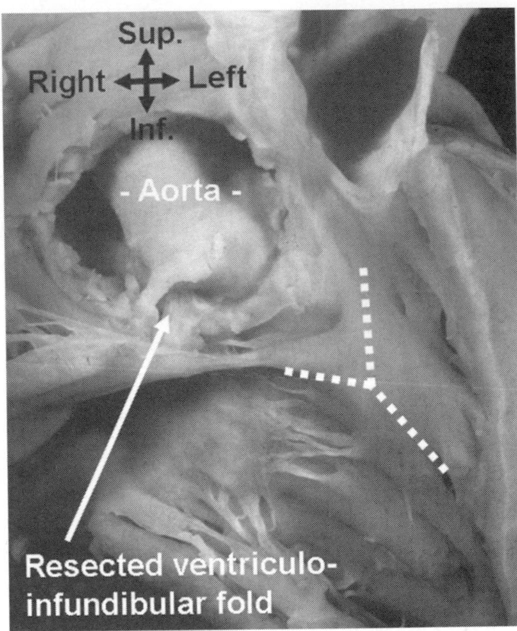

Figure 52-18 The larger part of the supraventricular crest has been cut away, showing that it is no more than a fold in the parietal ventricular wall. Note the aorta giving rise to the right coronary artery. The dissection also shows how the crest inserts between the limbs of the septomarginal trabeculation (Y-dotted lines). This extensive trabeculation extends to the apex of the right ventricle, with multiple septoparietal trabeculations taking origin from its anterior aspect.

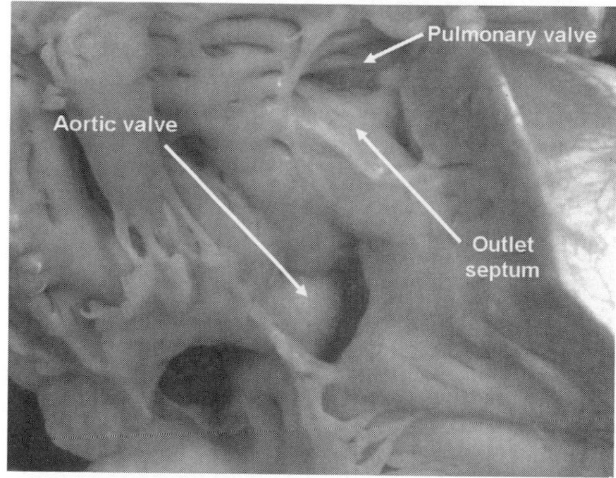

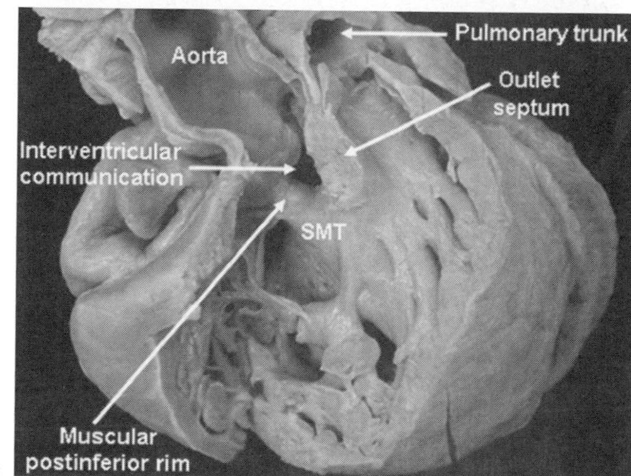

Figure 52-19 These illustrations show the extensive outlet septum, seen in the setting (A) of tetralogy of Fallot and (B) double-outlet right ventricle.

in tetralogy of Fallot (Fig. 52-19A) or double-outlet right ventricle (Fig. 52-19B).

THE LEFT VENTRICLE

As with the right ventricle, we find it best to analyze the left ventricle as possessing inlet, apical trabecular, and outlet components (Fig. 52-13). The inlet component contains the mitral valve, which has a solitary zone of apposition between its aortic and mural leaflets (Fig. 52-20). The aortic leaflet is relatively short, guarding only about one-third of the valvar circumference, albeit that it has considerable depth.[13] The mural leaflet, although having a much more extensive annular attachment, has much less depth. In most hearts, this leaflet is divided into a series of "scallops," usually three, but five or even six may be seen on occasion. Although guarding different lengths of the junction, the two leaflets have more or less equal surface area. The left ventricle is characterized by its particularly fine trabeculations. Unlike the right ventricle, however, the trabecular

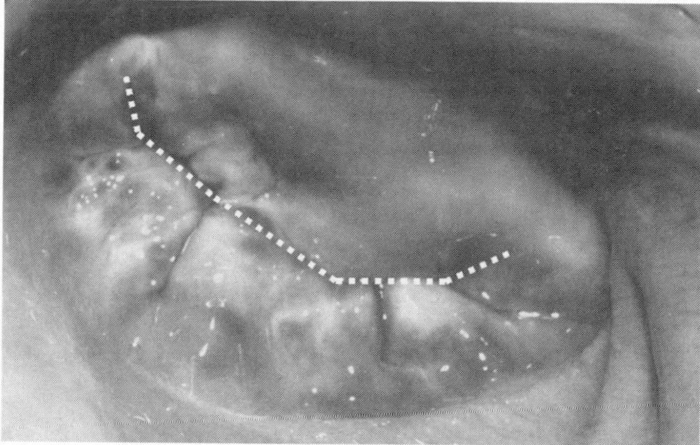

Figure 52-20 The mitral valve is photographed from above with the leaflets in their closed position. Note the solitary zone of apposition of the leaflets (dotted line), which guard markedly dissimilar proportions of the atrioventricular junction. The anterior leaflet is also known as the aortic leaflet of the valve.

component of the left ventricle has a smooth septal surface, down which cascades the fan-like left bundle branch of the ventricular conduction tissues. The outlet portion is well formed in the left ventricle but does not have completely muscular walls because of the fibrous continuity between the leaflets of the aortic and mitral valves. As we have already emphasized, because of the coronet-like attachment of the valvar leaflets (Fig. 52-10), it is inappropriate to describe either arterial valve as possessing an "annulus." It is the semilunar attachments of the valvar leaflets that constitute the surgical "annulus," and it is these structures that the surgeon typically uses as an anchorage for sutures in replacing the aortic valve. We should emphasize again, therefore, that the leaflets are attached within the arterial root in crown-like rather than circular fashion.

SEQUENTIAL SEGMENTAL ANALYSIS OF CONGENITAL HEART DISEASE

In the preceding paragraphs, we have discussed the basic morphology of the cardiac chambers and emphasized the features of surgical note. Thus far, this has been considered mostly in the setting of the normal heart, albeit with emphasis being placed on the differences seen in the setting of a common atrioventricular junction (Figs. 52-14 and 52-15) or when the ventricular septum itself is deficient (Fig. 52-19). The majority of patients undergoing surgery will have their intracardiac lesions in the setting of the normal heart. Persistent patency of the arterial duct, for example, or a simple aortic coarctation, does not alter the basic cardiac morphology. Similarly, the presence of a simple atrial septal defect does not distort the basic arrangement to such an extent that the heart is not readily recognized as being normal. In a few cases, nonetheless, the anatomy can be exceedingly bizarre, often with the heart itself abnormally positioned. Even in these complex cases, description is straightforward if the surgeon follows the logical approach we have tried to establish in the previous paragraphs. This is because, as we have already discussed, the atrial appendages, the markers of atrial identity, can be arranged in only one of four patterns (Fig. 52-4). Irrespective of these patterns, the ways in which the atrial chambers can connect to the ventricles are also strictly limited, as are the possibilities for the ventricles to make connection with the arterial trunks. We conclude our discussion of cardiac morphology, therefore, with a brief account of the principles and philosophy of sequential segmental analysis.[1,17]

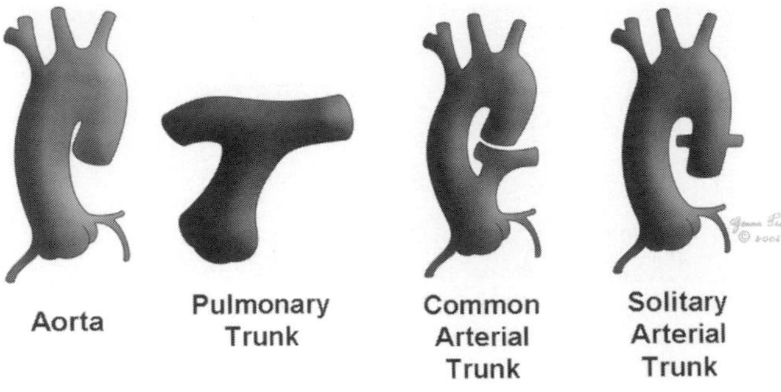

Figure 52-21 The features permitting distinction of an aorta from a pulmonary trunk and a common from a solitary arterial trunk.

PHILOSOPHY OF SEQUENTIAL SEGMENTAL ANALYSIS

To provide an unambiguous account of any abnormally formed heart, it is necessary to separate, for the purposes of description, the morphology of the individual cardiac segments, the way that the segments are joined one to the other, and the interrelationships of the components within each segment.[17] Provided that each of these features is described using mutually exclusive terms, the specific words themselves are less important, although it surely makes sense to use words in the fashion that they are also employed in day-to-day activities. We have used a multiplicity of terms during the evolution of our own approach. It is these experiences that have convinced us of the value of using simple everyday words in description rather than retaining a lexicon deeply rooted in classic etymology. One of our rules, therefore, is to eschew Latin and Greek words, since American English has now become the scientific "lingua franca." Another of our rules is to follow the "morphologic method." This requires that cardiac components, however deformed or abnormal, should always be identifiable in terms of their own intrinsic characteristics.[18,19] Venous connections, therefore, cannot be used to identify an atrium, since the veins themselves may connect anomalously. In similar fashion, the structure of an atrioventricular valve cannot always be used as the final arbiter of the morphology of a ventricle, simply because some ventricles do not possess atrioventricular valves. Thus, as we have already discussed, it is the morphology of the atrial appendages that provides the most reliable feature for atrial recognition, and it is the nature of the apical trabeculations that is most useful for distinguishing between the ventricles. Although the arterial trunks have no intrinsic distinguishing features, almost always their pattern of branching is sufficiently discrete to permit distinction of an aorta from a pulmonary trunk and both of these from a common or solitary trunk (Fig. 52-21). On the basis of the philosophy outlined above, it also follows that we always account separately for the way that the cardiac chambers are joined as opposed to their relationships in space. It could be argued that each of these features should then have equal weight in description. There is little doubt, however, that the surgeon is most concerned with the way that the cardiac components are joined or not joined. In our system, therefore, we delegate primary importance to the connections between the cardiac components, relegating relationships to a secondary role.

ATRIAL ARRANGEMENT

Recognition of the arrangement of the appendages is the starting point of diagnosis. We depicted the four possible arrangements for the appendages in Fig. 52-4. When both morphologically right and left appendages are present, as in the usual and mirror-imaged patterns, the arrangements can be said to be lateralized. The other two patterns are isomeric. As we discussed, it is the morphology of the atrial appendages that dictates the disposition of the sinus node, hence the importance to the surgeon of recognizing the position of the morphologically right appendage.

VARIATIONS AT ATRIOVENTRICULAR JUNCTIONS

Once the atrial arrangement is known, the other information needed to analyze the structure of the atrioventricular junctions is the morphology of the ventricular chambers. Separate attention should then be paid to the fashion in which the atria are joined to the ventricles and the morphology of the atrioventricular valve or valves, which guard the junctions. The commonest patterns are found when each atrium is joined to its own separate ventricle. Such biventricular atrioventricular connections can be found either with lateralized or isomeric atrial appendages. With lateralized appendages, there are two possible patterns of connection across the atrioventricular junctions (Fig. 52-22). The first gives the concordant pattern and is seen when the right atrium is joined to the

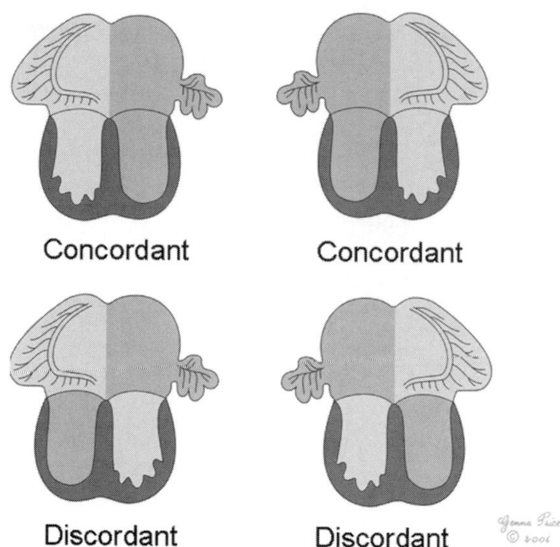

Figure 52-22 The diagram shows the essence of concordant and discordant atrioventricular connections, which can both exist in either usually arranged or mirror-imaged variants.

right ventricle and the left atrium to the left ventricle. In the second pattern, producing discordant connections, the right atrium is connected to the left ventricle and the left atrium to the right ventricle. Should the appendages be isomeric, then irrespective of the arrangement of the ventricles, the atrioventricular connections are biventricular but ambiguous (Fig. 52-23). It is also important in this situation, therefore, to take note of the topologic arrangement of the ventricular mass. There are two basic patterns (Fig. 52-24). In the usual pattern, as seen in the normal heart with usual atrial arrangement and concordant atrioventricular connections, the right ventricle is related to the left ventricle, so that, figuratively speaking, it is the palmar surface of the right hand of the observer that can be placed on the septal surface of the ventricle, with the thumb in the inlet, the wrist in the apex, and the fingers in the outlet. It is appropriate, therefore, to describe this as right-hand topology (Fig. 52-24, left panel). In the mirror-imaged variant, as seen typically in the patient with congenitally corrected transposition, it is the left hand that can be placed on the septal surface of the morphologically right ventricle; hence its designation as left-hand topology (Fig. 52-24, right panel). Either of these two arrangements can be found when hearts with isomeric atrial appendages have biventricular atrioventricular connections (Fig. 52-23). It follows, therefore, that complete description requires an account of atrial arrangement and ventricular topology. The topologic arrangement is also important to the surgeon, since this feature dictates the disposition of the conduction tissues.[4]

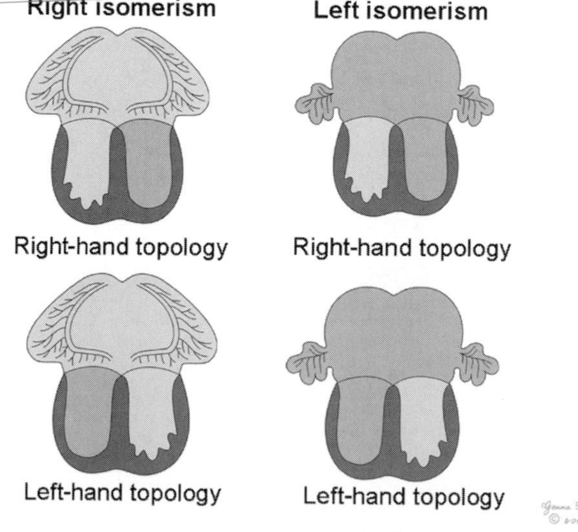

Figure 52-23 When the atrial appendages are isomeric, the atrioventricular connections are perforce ambiguous. Description of ventricular topology is then essential so as fully to characterize the anatomic arrangement.

There is then a much smaller second group of hearts that do not exhibit biventricular atrioventricular connections, having as their unifying feature the fact that the atria are joined to only one ventricle. Thus, the hearts have univentricular atrioventricular connections.[20] In this group, all variants can exist irrespective of whether the atrial appendages are lateralized or isomeric. The junctional morphologies making up the group are double-inlet ventricle and absence of either the right or the left atrioventricular connection (Fig. 52-25). With any of these patterns,[21] the atria can be connected to a dominant left ventricle, a dominant right ventricle, or a solitary and indeterminate ventricle. When the atria are connected to either a dominant left or a right ventricle, the complementary ventricle is incomplete and hypoplastic, since of necessity it will lack at least the greater part of its inlet portion. Incomplete right ventricles, as found with the atria, are connected to a dominant left ventricle and are always positioned anterosuperiorly relative to the ventricular mass, although they may be either right- or left-sided (Fig. 52-26, right). Incomplete left ventricles, as seen in the presence of univentricular connection to a dominant right ventricle, are always positioned posteroinferiorly, but again may be either right- or left-sided (Fig. 52-26, left). The feature of solitary and indeterminate ventricles is that they do not possess second ventricles.

The arrangement of the atrioventricular valves depends on the number of atrioventricular junctions. In the setting of concordant, discordant, ambiguous, and double-inlet connections, the atria are joined across two atrioventricular junctions to the ventricular mass. The dual atrioventricular junctions, however, can be guarded by two separate valves (Fig. 52-11) or by a common

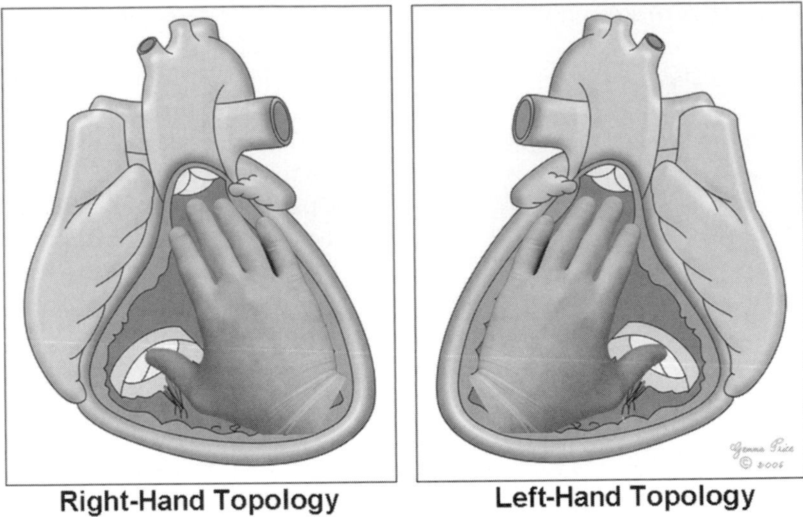

Figure 52-24 The two patterns of ventricular topology, which can be likened to the palms of the hands placed on the septal surfaces of the right ventricles.

atrioventricular valve (Fig. 52-14). One of two valves, or rarely both, may straddle the ventricular septum when the tension apparatus is attached on both sides of the septum. When a valve straddles, then usually its junction also overrides the septum. The degree of this override determines the commitment of the valve to the two ventricles. For the purposes of categorization of the precise connection present in such hearts, the overriding valve is assigned to the ventricle connected to its greater part. Common valves usually straddle, but not always. A common valve, nonetheless, always guards two atrioventricular junctions (Fig. 52-13), so note must be taken of this feature in assessing the degree of override. When there are two valves, it is also possible for one of the valves to

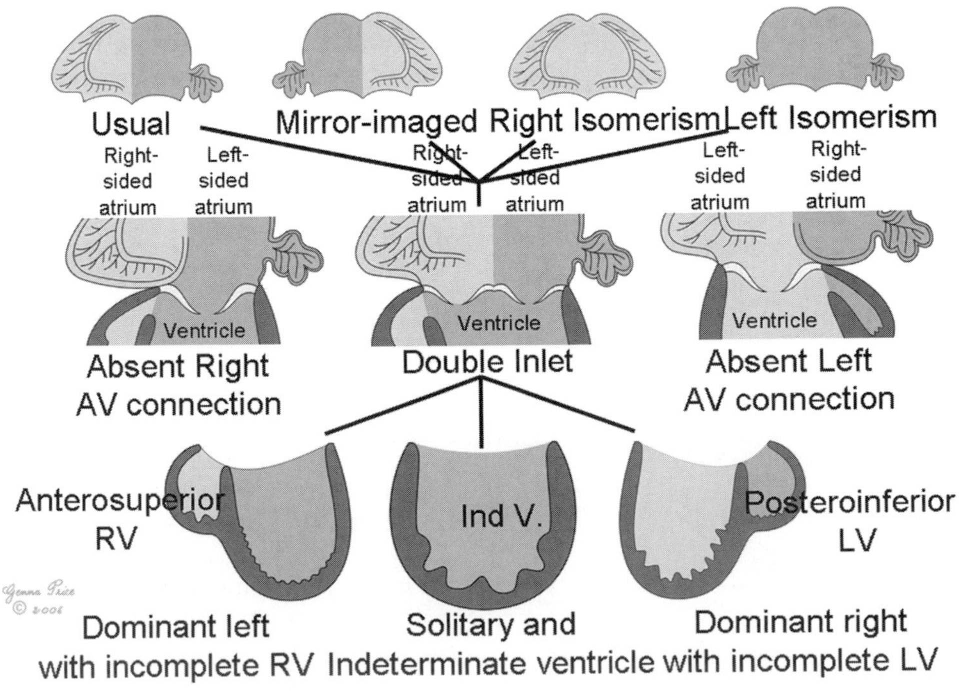

Figure 52-25 The arrangements that produce univentricular atrioventricular connections.

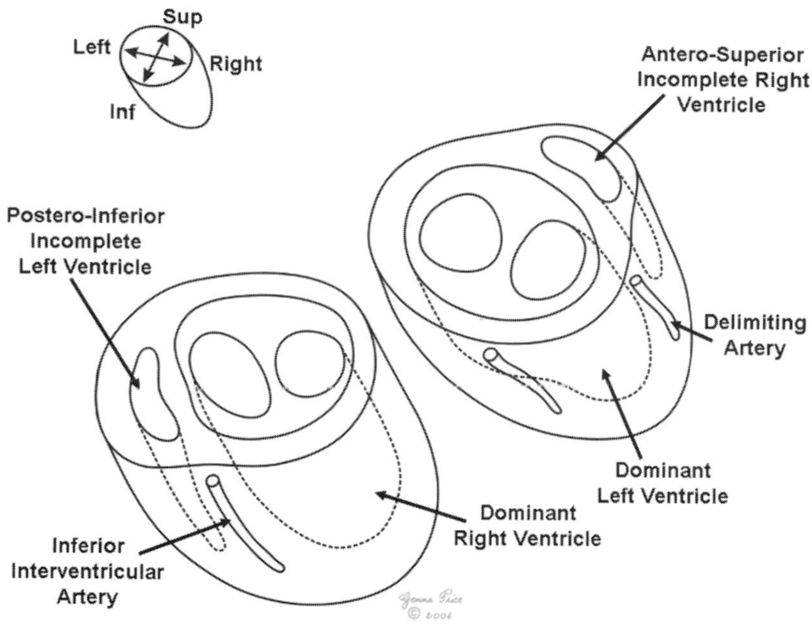

Figure 52-26 The drawing shows how incomplete right ventricles are always found anterosuperiorly relative to a dominant left ventricle, albeit in right-sided or left-sided position (upper panels), whereas incomplete left ventricles are positioned inferoposteriorly relative to dominant right ventricles, but again can be left-sided or right-sided (lower panels).

be imperforate. This morphology must be distinguished from absence of an atrioventricular connection, since both patterns produce atrioventricular valve atresia.[22] When one atrioventricular connection is absent, the modes of connection of the persisting junction are strictly limited. The atrioventricular valve may either be exclusively connected to one ventricle or alternatively may straddle or override.[23] The latter arrangement gives a connection that is uniatrial but biventricular (Fig. 52-27).

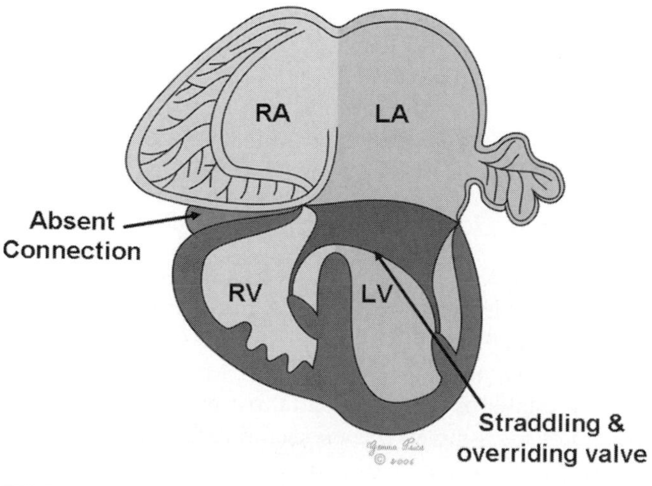

Figure 52-27 The drawing illustrates the uniatrial but biventricular atrioventricular connection.

VARIATIONS AT THE VENTRICULOARTERIAL JUNCTIONS

In analyzing the ventriculoarterial junctions, it is again necessary to distinguish between the specific junctional morphology and the structure of the arterial valve or valves guarding the junctions. At this level, attention should also be paid to arterial relationships as well as the morphology of the ventricular outflow tracts—so-called infundibular or conal anatomy.

The ventriculoarterial connections are concordant when the aorta takes origin from the left ventricle and the pulmonary trunk from the right ventricle. When the aorta arises from the right ventricle and the pulmonary trunk from the left ventricle, the ventriculoarterial connections are discordant. These descriptions hold good irrespective of whether the ventricles themselves are complete or incomplete. Double outlet exists when the larger parts of both ventriculoarterial junctions take origin from the same ventricle, which can be of right, left, or solitary and indeterminate morphology. Single outlet from the heart describes the situation in which only one patent arterial trunk can be traced from the ventricular mass. The trunk may be common or solitary (Fig. 52-21) or, alternatively, it may be an aortic trunk with pulmonary atresia or a pulmonary trunk with aortic atresia. Because arterial valves lack tension apparatus, they cannot straddle. Thus, variations in valvar morphology are more limited than for the atrioventricular valves. Furthermore, a common arterial valve exists only when there is a common arterial trunk. When there are two arterial valves, however, one of them may be imperforate. One or both may also override the septum. As with overriding atrioventricular valves, the precise connection of an overriding arterial valve is determined by using the "50 percent" law.

Arterial interrelationships are of no significance in determining the fashion in which the trunks take their origin from the ventricular mass. Indeed, it is impossible to infer the ventricular connection of the intrapericardial arterial trunks from their relationships. Relationships can be of help in predicting connections. For example, a right-sided and anterior aorta is seen most frequently with concordant atrioventricular and discordant ventriculoarterial connections. At best, however, such associations are no more than a guide to the possibility of abnormal connections. In describing the abnormal relationships, it is also necessary to account for both the positions of the arterial valves and for the orientation of the ascending portions of the arterial trunks. Relationships can be described by accounting for the position of the aortic valve relative to the pulmonary valve, taking note of right/left and anterior/posterior coordinates. For the arterial trunks, the possibilities are for the pulmonary trunk to spiral around the aorta toward its bifurcation, or else for the trunks to ascend in parallel fashion. Combining these two variables makes it an easy matter to describe all anticipated patterns of arterial interrelationships.

In the past, great emphasis was placed on the role of the bilateral conus, or bilateral infundibulum, in diagnosis. Again, however, there is no specificity in these findings. Each arterial valve can potentially be supported by a complete muscular infundibulum irrespective of the ventriculoarterial connection. It is more important, therefore, to analyze the infundibular components. There are three parts of significance.[15] The first separates the arterial valves and their subvalvar outflow tracts from each other. This structure is the muscular outlet—the infundibular or conal septum. The second part is the free parietal component of the ventricular wall. The third part is the inner heart curvature of the ventricles between the atrium and the great arterial trunks. This muscular fold separates the arterial valves from the atrioventricular valves and is well described as the ventriculoinfundibular fold. The most frequent variability in infundibular morphology depends on the integrity of this fold. When it is intact, then there is discontinuity between the atrioventricular and arterial valvar leaflets; in other words there is usually a complete muscular infundibulum or indeed bilateral infundibula (Fig. 52-19B). When the fold is deficient, there is continuity between the leaflets of the atrioventricular and arterial valves, and part of the infundibulum is deficient (Fig. 52-19B). We purposely use the term "usually," since it is rarely possible for the ventriculoinfundibular fold to be intact, producing arterial-atrioventricular discontinuity, and yet for the outlet septum to be deficient, permitting valvar continuity between the leaflets of the aortic and pulmonary valves. In this setting, the muscular infundibula would be incomplete. The integrity of the ventricular outflow tracts, therefore, depends on the morphology of both the ventriculoinfundibular fold and the outlet septum. The interrelationship between these structures is well demonstrated in the "supracristal ventricular septal defect." In the past, such defects were held to be "supracristal" because they were positioned superiorly relative to the so-called septal band (Fig. 52-28A). But the allegedly infracristal defects (Fig. 52-28A) are also positioned superiorly relative to this "band." It is because of such difficulties than we believe it is better to describe the septal band as the septomarginal trabeculation, this being an integral component of the muscular ventricular septum. Nowadays, fortunately, ventricular septal defects are more usually described as being perimembranous, muscular, or doubly committed and subarterial.[24] It is failure of muscularization of the outlet septum, combined with failure of formation of the subpulmonary infundibulum, which is the phenotypic feature of the doubly committed, or supracristal, defect (Fig. 52-28B). There is a common ventriculoarterial junction, albeit guarded by separate aortic and pulmonary valves. The lesion is closely related, therefore, to a common arterial trunk (Fig. 52-29), albeit that the doubly committed defect can be found when both arterial trunks arise from the right ventricle or even when they take their origin predominantly from the left ventricle. Because of this variation, it has been suggested that the lesion would best be described as "double outlet both ventricles."[25]

SUBSEQUENT STEPS IN SEQUENTIAL ANALYSIS

The analysis described thus far accounts only for the segmental combination of the heart. In most instances, this will be normal. But it will have cost the surgeon nothing to prove this normality. Indeed, it is essential to do so. Having established the segmental pattern, analysis is concluded by assessing all the associated defects present. This is also best done in segmental fashion, commencing by confirming the normality of the venoatrial connections. Attention can then be directed to the atrial segment, the ventricular segment, and the arterial segment in turn, at the same time looking for any junctional malformations

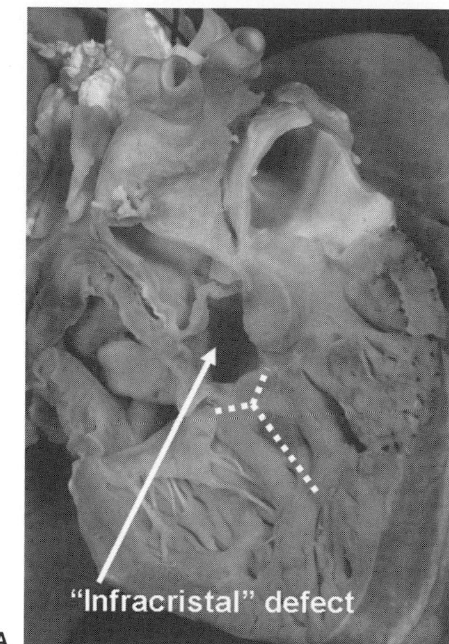

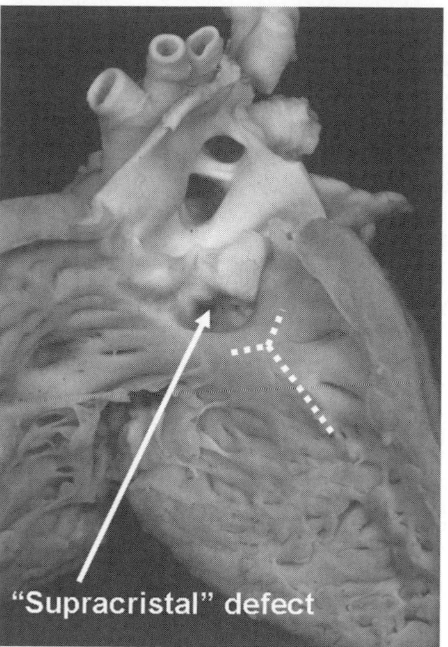

Figure 52-28 The "supracristal" defect (B) is compared with the allegedly "infracristal" variant (A); in reality both defects are located within the limbs of the "septal band" or septomarginal trabeculation (dotted Y). The phenotypic feature of the supracristal defect, which is doubly committed and juxtaarterial, is failure of muscularization of the outlet septum and failure to form the subpulmonary infundibulum. Because of this, there is a common ventriculoarterial junction.

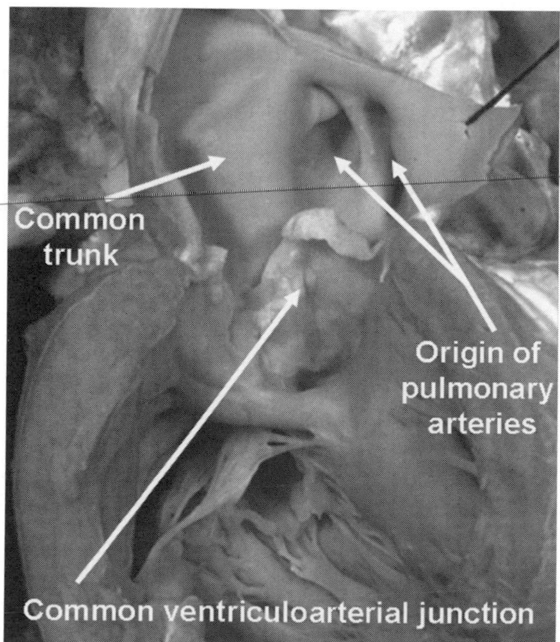

Figure 52-29 The picture shows the doubly committed ventricular septal defect seen in the setting of a common arterial trunk. Note the similarity to the defect shown in Fig. 52-28B. The phenotypic feature of both hearts is the common ventriculoarterial junction, albeit guarded by separate aortic and tricuspid valves in the heart shown in Fig. 52-28B.

that may not have been accounted for during the analysis of the connections. Then the anatomy of the aortic and pulmonary pathways is assessed. In this way, any congenital cardiac lesion or combination of lesions, however simple or complex, is accounted for and understood in the segmental setting of the heart itself. Separate description is then provided for the location of the heart, the direction of its apex, and the arrangement of the thoracic and abdominal organs, taking care to describe each system separately when discrepancies from the anticipated patterns are encountered. To the best of our knowledge, it has proved possible to describe and categorize in unambiguous fashion all lesions thus far known and encountered.

ACKNOWLEDGMENT

The research on which our account is based has been supported over a period of 30 years by the British Heart Foundation together with the Joseph Levy Foundation. Research at the Institute of Child Health and Great Ormond Street Hospital for Children NHS Trust benefits from R&D funding received from the NHS Executive. The text of this chapter is based upon a comparable account written for the textbook edited by Gardner and Spray.[26] The illustrations are adapted from the third edition of *Surgical Anatomy of the Heart*.[27]

References

1. Anderson RH, Ho SY. Sequential segmental analysis: Description and categorisation for the millennium. *Cardiol Young* 1997;7:98.
2. Uemura H, Ho SY, Devine WA, et al. Atrial appendages and venoatrial connections in hearts with patients with visceral heterotaxy. *Ann Thorac Surg* 1995;60:561.
3. Uemura H, Ho SY, Devine WA, et al. Analysis of visceral hetertotaxy according to splenic status, appendage morphology, or both. *Am J Cardiol* 1995;76:846.
4. Smith A, Yen Ho S, Anderson RH, et al. The diverse cardiac morphology seen in hearts with isomerism of the atrial appendages with reference to the disposition of the specialized conduction system. *Cardiol Young* 2006;16:437–454.
5. Anderson RH, Becker AE. Coronary arterial patterns: A guide to identification of congenital heart disease. In: Becker AE, Losekoot TG, Marcelletti C, Anderson RH (eds). *Paediatric Cardiology*, vol 3. Edinburgh: Churchill Livingstone, 1981:251.
6. Van Praagh R. The story of anatomically corrected malposition of the great arteries. *Chest* 1976;69:2.
7. Anderson RH, Webb S, Brown NA. Clinical anatomy of the atrial septum with reference to its developmental components. *Clin Anat* 1999;12:362.
8. Sweeney LJ, Rosenquist GC. The normal anatomy of the atrial septum in the human heart. *Am Heart J* 1979;98:94.
9. Becker AE, Anderson RH. Atrioventricular septal defects. What's in a name? *J Thorac Cardiovasc Surg* 1982;83:461.
10. Anderson RH, Ho SY, Becker AE. Anatomy of the human atrioventricular junctions revisited. *Anat Rec* 2000;260:81.
11. Jacobs ML, Anderson RH. Nomenclature of the functionally univentricular heart. *Cardiol Young* 2006;16:3.
12. Yacoub M. Anatomy of the mitral valve chordae and cusps. In: Kalmanson D (ed). *The Mitral Valve. A Pluridisciplinary Approach.* London: Edward Arnold, 1976:15–20.
13. Kanani M, Anderson RH. Editorial: The anatomy of the mitral valve: A retrospective analysis of yesterday's future. *J Heart Valve Dis* 2003;12:543.
14. Sutton JP III, Ho SY, Vogel M, et al. Is the morphologically right atrioventricular valve tricuspid? *J Heart Valve Dis* 1995;4:571.
15. Anderson RH, Becker AE, Van Mierop LHS. What should we call the "crista"? *Br Heart J* 1977;39:856.
16. Anderson RH. Clinical anatomy of the aortic root. *Heart* 2000;84:670.
17. Anderson RH. How should we optimally describe complex congenitally malformed hearts? *Ann Thorac Surg* 1996;62:710.
18. Lev M. Pathologic diagnosis of positional variations in cardiac chambers in congenital heart disease. *Lab Invest* 1954;3:71.
19. Van Praagh R, David I, Wright GB, et al. Large RV plus small LV is not single RV. *Circulation* 1980;61:1057.
20. Anderson RH, Quero-Jimenez M, Rigby ML, et al. Univentricular atrioventricular connection: The single ventricle trap unsprung. *Pediatr Cardiol* 1983;4:273.
21. Cook AC, Anderson RH. The functionally univentricular circulation: Anatomic substrates as related to function. *Cardiol Young* 2005;15(Suppl 3):7.
22. Orie JD, Anderson C, Ettedgui J, et al. Echocardiographic-morphologic correlations in tricuspid atresia. *J Am Coll Cardiol* 1995;26:750.
23. Anderson RH, Rigby ML. The morphological heterogeneity of "tricuspid atresia" (editorial note). *Int J Cardiol* 1987;16:67.
24. Soto B, Becker AE, Moulaert AJ, et al. Classification of ventricular septal defects. *Br Heart J* 1980;43:332.
25. Brandt PWT, Calder AL, Barratt-Boyes BG, et al. Double outlet left ventricle. Morphology, cineangiography, diagnosis and surgical treatment. *Am J Cardiol* 1976;38:897.
26. Anderson RH. The anatomy of congenital cardiac malformations. In: Gardner TJ, Spray TL (eds). *Operative Cardiac Surgery*, 5th ed. London: Edward Arnold, 2004:535–558.
27. Wilcox BR, Cook AC, Anderson RH. *Surgical Anatomy of the Heart*, 3[d] ed. Cambridge, UK: Cambridge University Press, 2004.

CHAPTER

53 MANAGEMENT OF THE PEDIATRIC CARDIAC SURGICAL PATIENT

Cho Ng, Allan Goldman

INTRODUCTION

In recent years, as the operative mortality in pediatric cardiac surgery has fallen, attention has been directed toward the reduction of perioperative morbidity. The aim of this chapter is to focus on postoperative care and, in particular, on understanding the underlying pathophysiology and effects of cardiopulmonary bypass. The special circumstances of the postoperative neonate are also discussed. The emphasis is on an anticipatory (rather than reactive) approach. Last, we present a review of complications specific to the pediatric cardiac surgical patient.

CARDIORESPIRATORY INTERACTIONS

There are important interactions among the components of the functional unit comprising the heart and lungs. If untreated, cardiac failure will lead to respiratory failure. Conversely, respiratory failure will exacerbate preexisting cardiac failure. It is also important to appreciate the effects of positive-pressure ventilation on the cardiovascular system. Appropriate tidal volumes should be used to ensure adequate gas exchange while minimizing lung trauma and other morbidities. In our practice, we utilize tidal volumes of 5 to 7 mL/kg with the specific goal of avoiding barotrauma. Carbon dioxide clearance is determined by minute ventilation (i.e., tidal volume times respiratory rate) and oxygenation by inspired oxygen levels and mean airway pressure. Neonates with congenital heart disease may have parenchymal lung disease as well, and may therefore require higher levels of ventilatory support. Inspired oxygen levels are set according to the underlying pathology. For example, patients with lesions characterized by duct-dependent systemic perfusion or balanced circulation will usually need low inspired oxygen (i.e., preferably room air) to prevent pulmonary overcirculation. Advantages and disadvantages of mechanical ventilation must be weighed during the pre- and postoperative periods. Positive-pressure ventilation has been demonstrated to have negative effects on cardiac output[1,2] by elevating intrathoracic pressure, impeding venous return, and lowering preload and cardiac output. It is also associated with increased right ventricular afterload and decreased systemic vascular resistance. In the patient who has undergone cardiopulmonary bypass, this phenomenon is exacerbated by the need for higher inflation pressures to overcome the fall in lung compliance that accompanies bypass.

In describing cardiopulmonary interactions, two categories deserve particular mention: patients undergoing Glenn and Fontan-type repairs (see Chap. 69) and those undergoing repair of tetralogy of Fallot. In infants and children with univentricular heart disease palliated by a Glenn or Fontan-type repair, pulmonary blood flow is dependent on systemic venous pressure, pulmonary vascular resistance, and the end-diastolic pressure of the systemic ventricle. In this setting, there is no ventricular impulse to overcome any rise in pulmonary vascular resistance, and positive-pressure ventilation may lower cardiac output by increasing pulmonary vascular resistance.[3] Patients who have undergone repair of various forms of tetralogy of Fallot with pulmonary atresia or stenosis disclose preoperative right ventricular hypertrophy, which, coupled with a right ventriculotomy, may result in right ventricular dysfunction. In particular, the right ventricle may show diastolic dysfunction with impaired diastolic filling following correction, resulting in a fall in cardiac output. Pulmonary blood flow then becomes more dependent on right atrial contraction and central venous pressure (i.e., preload); in such instances, it is often useful to minimize ventilatory pressures as much as possible.

In the clinical scenarios described, there have been favorable experiences with "negative-pressure" ventilation, which is thought to be more physiologic and is associated with improved hemodynamics.[1] Negative-pressure ventilation involves placing a fitted "jacket" around the chest. Suction is intermittently applied to the device, effectively displacing the anterior chest wall up and outward and resulting in lung inflation, improved venous return and cardiac output.

MONITORING MODALITIES IN THE INTENSIVE CARE UNIT

Routine monitoring modalities

The patient who has undergone cardiac surgery is subject to a number of insults due to direct myocardial injury and the systemic inflammatory response related to cardiopulmonary bypass. The first 24 h after surgery is the period of maximum instability; therefore close monitoring and timely interventions are essential. Monitoring techniques may be divided into noninvasive and invasive techniques (Table 53-1).

Table 53-1 Postoperative monitoring techniques

Noninvasive	Invasive
Pulse and blood pressure:	Systemic arterial blood pressure
ECG monitoring	Central venous pressure
Cuff blood pressure	Left atrial pressure
Respiration:	Pulmonary arterial pressure
Pulse oximetry, end-tidal CO_2	Cardiac output (thermodilution and similar techniques)
Temperature:	
Core and peripheral	
Cardiac output monitoring:	
Doppler flow measurements	
Neuromuscular junction monitoring:	
Single-twitch, tetanic, and train-of-four stimulation	
Depth of sedation:	
Bispectral index monitoring	
Cerebral function analysis monitor (CFAM)	

Paramount to monitoring is the ability to interpret the resultant data and make appropriate, timely interventions. Clinical observations such as palpation of pulse and observation of respiratory rate and pattern are critical in the assessment. Monitoring techniques have different levels of *accuracy* (i.e., difference between the measurement utilized and the "gold standard" measurement) and *precision* (i.e., reproducibility of the measurement), but all are prone to some form of error; therefore it is important to take the overall clinical picture into account in making therapeutic decisions (e.g., saturation monitor reads 100 percent but patient appears cyanotic).

Electrocardiography

The electrical activity of the heart was first noted in 1856.[5] It was not until the 1890s that devices were developed to record surface potentials. Over the next 20 years, normal and abnormal patterns were recognized. Most modern ECG monitors use three monitoring leads and display three standard "leads" (i.e., leads I, II, and III). Surface electrodes detect changes in electrical potential, which are amplified and filtered to remove interference from electrical devices (e.g., AC current) and from noncardiac sources in the patient (e.g., shivering).

The main purpose of the ECG (Fig. 53-1) is to help identify changes in heart rate and rhythm that may accompany significant changes in physiology; sinus tachycardia is still considered an important sign that "something is not right."

Sources of error

1. Surface contact. Most ECG leads have gel pads to improve contact with the skin. Problems may arise if the pads are dry or there is skin contamination (e.g., oil-based ointments). Changing the lead for a new one and cleaning the skin with an alcohol wipe can often correct the problem.
2. Interference. Interference from the patient (e.g., shivering) or other electrical equipment can make interpretation of the ECG pattern difficult. Ensure that the appropriate electronic filters on the ECG monitor are active.
3. Lead placement error. Misplaced leads may lead to abnormal or altered ECG patterns (e.g., ST-segment elevation) that may be misinterpreted.

Noninvasive measurement of blood pressure

There are a number of different noninvasive methods to measure blood pressure (NIBP), all of which rely on the principle of occluding a limb with a cuff and then lowering the cuff pressure until the return of blood flow is detected. The following methods have been employed:

Palpation
Auscultation
Oscillotonometry
Oscillometry (e.g., Dynamap)

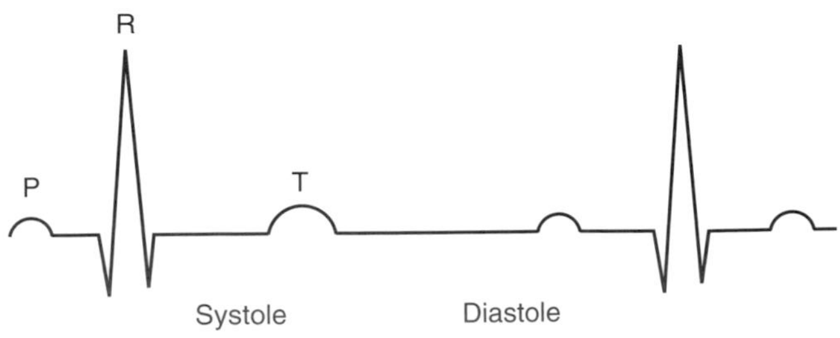

Figure 53-1 Normal electrocardiogram.

NIBP tends to *overestimate* low blood pressures and *underestimate* high blood pressures. Its downside in critically ill patients is that it gives only intermittent readings, which have a high interobserver variability. However, NIBP does permit blood pressure measurements without employing invasive catheters and is useful in following trends.

Pulse oximetry

This technique uses the differential absorption of infrared light by oxygenated and deoxygenated hemoglobin to determine oxygen saturations. Since its introduction in the 1970s by Hewlett-Packard, the technology has evolved to become a standard bedside monitoring technique. In the intensive care unit (ICU) environment, it is invaluable in allowing continuous monitoring of the patient's oxygen saturation (SpO_2) and pulse rate. It is particularly useful for the rapid detection of falls in saturation (e.g., ventilation problems) or undesirably rapid rises in saturation in univentricular circulations (i.e., trying to balance pulmonary and systemic circulations).

However, there are important limitations to the use of pulse oximetry (Fig. 53-2):

The technique requires detection of pulsatile blood flow; therefore, if perfusion is poor (e.g., with vasoconstriction), it can give erroneous readings.

Movement and outside interference (e.g., fluorescent lights, diathermy) can disrupt the readings. The SpO_2 readings are reliable only if a regular pulsatile trace is visible.

The oxygen saturation is derived from standard curves obtained from healthy volunteers. It is accurate at 90 percent and above but loses accuracy below 70 percent and is inaccurate below 50 percent.

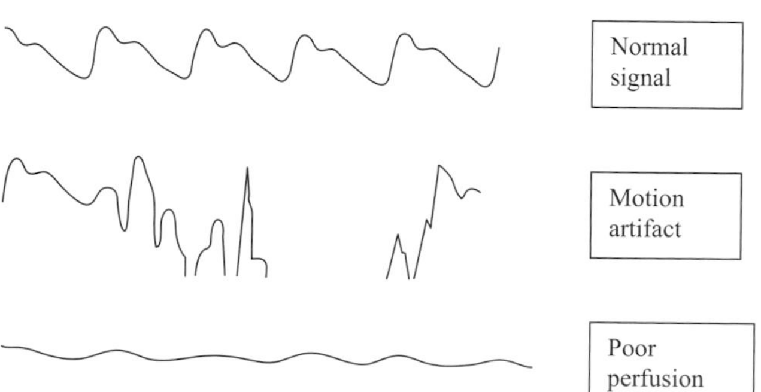

Figure 53-2 Pulse oximetry. There are important limitations to the use of this modality: (1) It requires detection of pulsatile blood flow, so that, where there is poor perfusion (e.g., vasoconstriction) it can give erroneous readings, and (2) movement and outside interference (e.g., fluorescent lights, diathermy) can disrupt the readings. The SpO_2 readings are reliable only if a regular pulsatile trace is visible.

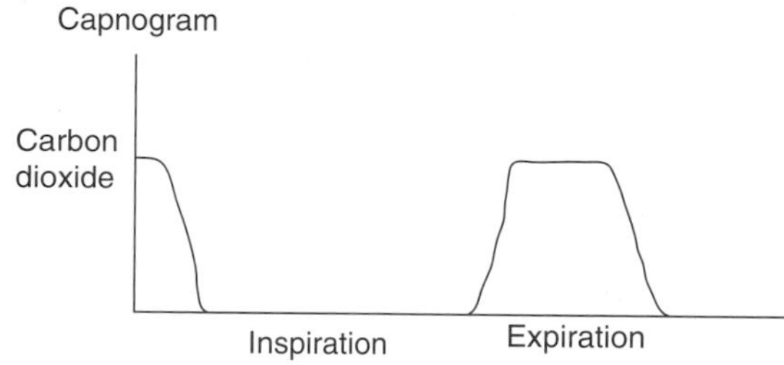

Figure 53-3 Sample capnogram.

The absorption characteristics of carboxyhemoglobin and methemoglobin will lead to erroneously high saturation values.

Capnography

End-tidal expired carbon dioxide (CO_2) tensions (Fig. 53-3) closely approximate actual arterial CO_2 tensions. Thus, the technique of measuring end tidal CO_2 ($ETCO_2$) permits reasonable estimations of arterial CO_2 levels. $ETCO_2$ monitoring is standard practice in anesthesia and increasingly common in the ICU. It is used to confirm correct endotracheal tube placement, monitor adequacy of ventilation, and identify ventilatory problems early (Tables 53-2 and 53-3). The usual technique uses infrared light absorption to detect CO_2. This is either measured "inline" (i.e., with light shone through a clear cuvette that sits between the endotracheal tube and ventilator), or "sidestream" (i.e., a sampling line draws off gas from the ventilator tubing for analysis at the machine).

Sedation monitoring

Electroencephalographic (EEG) waveforms become attenuated when patients are sedated or anesthetized and can be used as a means to monitor the level of sedation. In practice, full continuous EEG monitoring is impractical on the ICU due to the need for many electrodes and skilled personnel for interpretation. An adapted form of EEG monitoring, bispectral index monitoring (BIS), gives a single score that can be used as a measure of the level of

Table 53-2 Causes of elevated end-tidal CO_2

Inadequate ventilation	Obstructed endotracheal tube Inadequate ventilation (e.g., respiratory depression, inadequate tidal volume)
Excess production	Fever Hypercatabolic state
High inspired CO_2	Rebreathing of expired gases CO_2 entrained into ventilation circuit (e.g., management of hypoplastic left heart)

Table 53-3 Causes of reduced end-tidal CO_2	
Excessive alveolar minute ventilation	High tidal volume High respiratory rate Improvement in lung compliance without appropriate weaning of ventilator
Increased alveolar dead space	Pulmonary embolus Low cardiac output
Low CO_2 production	Hypothermia Hypocatabolic state
Equipment problem	Sampling error (e.g., water in sampling tubing) Leak around endotracheal tube

sedation and shows some promise for use in the ICU.[6,7] There is also new interest in the use of continuous cerebral function monitoring (CFAM) in the ICU or in the operating room (OR) for the early identification of seizures.

Cardiac output monitoring

Invasive techniques have been available to measure cardiac output for many years. All involve the Fick principle, originally described in 1870, and are based on oxygen consumption:

Oxygen consumption = cardiac output × (arterial oxygen content – venous oxygen content)

By reworking the formula and measuring oxygen consumption and blood gas values, a cardiac output can be derived. Different "indicators" in blood (e.g., temperature in thermodilution, lithium in the lithium dilution catheters) can also be measured. These techniques require an intact circulation with no intracardiac shunt. Any shunting [e.g., due to a ventricular septal defect (VSD)] will lead to erroneous results. This makes the technique invalid for many pediatric patients. Until recently, the only form of reliable cardiac output monitoring required invasive techniques such as pulmonary artery (PA) flotation catheters (i.e., thermodilution catheters). Their use in children has been limited because of the technical difficulties in catheter placement in small patients. The development of Doppler ultrasound techniques has permitted noninvasive monitoring of cardiac output. In simple terms, by using the Doppler principle, blood velocity in a vessel can be calculated from the frequency shift of the reflected ultrasound wave. This is most commonly measured in the aorta. By integrating the velocity together with the cross-sectional area of the aorta (i.e., measured using echocardiography or estimated based on weight), flow and hence cardiac output can be estimated. The development of small esophageal probes has permitted continuous monitoring. The technique is still evolving in the pediatric ICU, requiring placement of a relatively invasive esophageal probe, which is prone to error from misplacement or rotation. However, it can give useful data on trends in cardiac output.[8,9]

Invasive blood pressure monitoring

Invasive blood pressure monitoring is now a standard technique in the ICU. It permits continuous blood pressure monitoring. A combination of systemic arterial, central venous, and left atrial pressures can give much information about a patent's circulatory status, leading to sensible interventions to treat low cardiac output.

Invasive arterial pressure

This monitoring is now routine in the postoperative cardiac patient to permit real-time monitoring of blood pressure and easy blood gas sampling. Postoperative cardiac patients are likely to be hemodynamically unstable and on vasoactive agents, so it is imperative that their hemodynamics be closely monitored. The common monitoring sites are:

Radial artery
Femoral artery
Dorsalis pedis artery
Umbilical artery (in neonates)
Axillary artery

The brachial artery may also used, but because of less collateralization at the elbow, distal ischemia is a significant risk (Table 53-4).

Central venous pressure monitoring

Central venous pressure (CVP) can be measured from one of the lumens of a multilumen central venous line. CVP can be used to ascertain intravascular filling status and as a marker of right heart function. Potential CVP line sites include:

Internal jugular vein (use with caution if considering a univentricular route as it will form part of Glenn and Fontan circulations)
Subclavian vein
Femoral vein
Umbilical vein (neonates)

Left atrial lines

Direct left atrial (LA) lines are used in some patients to help assess left heart filling and left heart failure in the immediate postoperative period. Once the patient is stable hemodynamically, they should be removed. There is a small risk of bleeding and cardiac tamponade during removal of these lines. Usually pleural drains are left in place until the LA line has been removed. Prior to removal, the platelet count and clotting parameters should be checked and surgical backup should be available in case of excessive bleeding or tamponade.

Table 53-4 Problems with invasive arterial monitors

Problem	Causes/Solutions
Distal ischemia	Arterial line sites should always be regularly monitored for ischemia, which varies in appearance from local skin blanching to obvious distal ischemia with pallor of the affected area. Anything other than momentary skin blanching should prompt siting of a new catheter and removal of the old one.
Reading errors	Check "zero calibration" on system regularly (e.g., transducer at level of tricuspid valve). Damped traces may result from air or clots in the line or use of soft tubing in the transducer line.
Infection	Both local and systemic infection is a risk due to regular sampling from the line. Concern about infection should prompt removal of the line. There is no optimal time to remove a line, but lines should be removed as soon as possible, and certainly there should be good reason to keep one beyond 7 to 10 days.
Drug error	Arterial lines must not be used for drug administration, as there is a risk of vasospasm and distal necrosis. They should be well labeled (e.g., with red stickers) to avoid confusion with venous lines.

Pulmonary artery catheters

There are two main types of PA catheters. In the operative patient where pulmonary hypertension is thought to be a risk (e.g., truncus arteriosus repair, obstructed anomalous pulmonary veins), a catheter is placed directly at the time of surgery. It permits monitoring of PA pressures and the response to interventions such as administration of inhaled nitric oxide. There are potential problems of overreacting to changes in PA pressures and cardiac tamponade upon line removal. Postoperative pulmonary hypertension is also now less common (e.g., earlier surgery, modified ultrafiltration), so that PA lines are less commonly used in current practice. PA line removal procedures are the same as those for LA lines.

The second type of PA catheter is the PA flotation catheter, which is placed via the internal jugular vein and "floated" through the right atrium, right ventricle, and PA. It provides data on pulmonary arterial and left-sided filling pressures (i.e., wedge pressure). It can also be used to measure cardiac output via thermodilution. A relatively high rate of complications is associated with these catheters in pediatric patients, so they are rarely used.

THE ICU "HANDOFF"

The transfer of a sick child from the operating team to the cardiac ICU team is one of the most critical interfaces affecting patient outcome. This should therefore follow a fixed protocol, which includes:

1. Setting up stable ventilatory and cardiac support and establishing appropriate monitoring
2. Providing comprehensive hand-over of information

The postoperative cardiac surgical patient has often undergone prolonged surgery and cardiopulmonary bypass; therefore he or she is also likely to have a significantly altered physiology. The keys to anticipating and dealing with postoperative problems are understanding what interventions occurred in the operating room, how the native physiology was altered, and the patient's hemodynamic status (Table 53-5). Particularly important is how the patient responded to separation from bypass and to therapeutic interventions (e.g., fluid boluses, inotropes).

EFFECTS OF CARDIOPULMONARY BYPASS

Cardiopulmonary bypass (CPB) is usually used to support the circulation and respiration of the patient during complex heart surgery. Although it has many side effects, it is a "necessary evil" that allows the surgeon to achieve repair or palliation. There are three main areas where CPB has significant detrimental effects:

Table 53-5 Essential areas to cover in transfers from OR to ICU

Anesthetist	Surgeon
Details of any preoperative concerns (infection, hemodynamic status)	Preoperative diagnosis, hemodynamic status
Details of anesthetic induction and problems encountered	Previous surgical procedures
Airway problems	Details of bypass times, cross-clamp times and whether hypothermia was used
Vascular access and any problems encountered	Details of the surgical procedure, including prostheses used (e.g., homografts, Gore-Tex tubes) and areas of concern (e.g., coronary artery patterns or implantation problems)
Fluids and drugs administered, antibiotics used	Any postoperative concerns or instructions to be aware of (e.g., anticoagulation)
Rhythm and hemodynamic parameters at the start and on coming off bypass	
Vasoactive drugs in use	
Clinical responses to fluid boluses (i.e., ventricular compliance, especially in neonates)	
Information from intraoperative echocardiography	
Analgesics and sedatives used	

1. CPB has a major effect on the immune system. Its impact on the balance of pro- and anti-inflammatory responses is still poorly understood. In some cases, CPB is thought to elicit a pathologic systemic inflammatory response syndrome (SIRS).
2. CPB causes dysfunction of the coagulation cascade at all levels.
3. Low cardiac output is often noted in the first 24 h after CPB.

The body's stress response to CPB involves the activation of an inflammatory cascade with the production of multiple proinflammatory cytokines (e.g., interleukins 1, 6, and 8 and tumor necrosis factor) and the activation of the complement cascade. This response helps the host deal with the additional stress of bypass and surgery and is also thought to aid in the process of healing and recovering from surgery. The cascade is augmented from contact activation of blood with artificial surfaces (i.e., the bypass circuit) and the consequences of ischemia and reperfusion.[10] It is now becoming apparent that the inflammatory response is also modulated by anti-inflammatory mediators (e.g., IL-10). It is likely that this imbalance affects patient outcomes. An early fall of monocyte HLA-DR activity (i.e., immune paresis) has been associated with increased morbidity after congenital heart surgery.[11]

Coagulopathy

Coagulopathy is common after cardiac surgery for a number of reasons:

1. Dilution of blood clotting factors during bypass. The bypass circuit volume is several hundred milliliters, equivalent to the circulating volume of a 3-kg neonate. In particular, low fibrinogen levels will prevent clot formation.
2. Activation of the clotting cascade by contact with artificial surfaces leads to the consumption of clotting factors and platelets.
3. Platelet consumption and dysfunction. This occurs because platelets exposed to the artificial surfaces of the bypass circuit and surfaces of damaged tissues become activated and degranulate, contributing to the inflammatory cascade. Bypass and the resulting cytokine cascades also appear to cause impairment of platelet function (e.g., change in shape, resulting in lower surface area for adhesion). Platelet transfusions may be used to treat bleeding (platelet count $< 100 \times 10^9/L$); however, prophylactic transfusions are not necessary unless there is marked thrombocytopenia ($< 20 \times 10^9/L^9$).
4. Hypothermia. Our metabolic systems evolved to function best at 37°C. The clotting cascade, like other enzyme systems, is less efficient during hypothermic conditions. Cooling to 33°C leads to a 50 percent reduction in enzymatic activity.[14]
5. Fibrinolysis. CPB activates not only the coagulation cascade but also its counterpart, the fibrinolytic pathways. Generally this does not cause clinically significant bleeding. Aprotinin may help reduce bleeding by reducing fibrinolysis and preserving platelet function.
6. Disseminated intravascular coagulation (DIC) is characterized by widespread microvascular thromboses and ongoing fibrinolysis, causing consumption of platelets and clotting factors. This results in widespread bleeding (e.g., skin puncture sites, mucous membranes, widespread petechiae). Bypass and cardiac surgery may lead to DIC in a number of circumstances.
7. Heparin. Heparin is used to prevent thrombosis during CPB. Inadequate heparinization may lead to a consumptive coagulopathy. At the conclusion of bypass, heparin is usually reversed with protamine, which forms a stable neutralizing complex with heparin. Underdosing of protamine will lead to residual heparin anticoagulation, potentially causing postoperative bleeding. Under dosing can lead in fact to a "heparin rebound" effect, where initially there is an apparent normalization of clotting factors and cessation of bleeding, followed by rebleeding and an abnormal clotting profile within the ensuing hours. This is usually not problematic since, with reasonable renal function, heparin is cleared in the first few hours after its discontinuation.

Coagulation tests and bleeding

Bleeding in the postoperative period is relatively common. This may result from tissue and vessel trauma from surgery, residual effects of anticoagulants used during bypass, or from clotting factor deficiencies. Clearly significant surgical bleeding (> 4mL/kg/h in the first hour) often requires surgical intervention. It is necessary to exclude or treat coagulation defects or residual anticoagulant effects before embarking on surgical exploration.

Routine coagulation screen

This panel includes the activated partial thromboplastin time (APTT), prothrombin time (PT), and fibrinogen. A normal screen implies no clotting defects; excessive residual bleeding is frequently "surgical." An elevated APTT suggests a heparin effect or clotting factor deficiency. An elevated PT may indicate factor deficiencies or a residual heparin effect. Low fibrinogen levels will impair clot formation and should be treated.

The thromboelastogram (TEG)

This test is a whole-blood bedside test that has been in use for many years and is gaining acceptance as a rapid test to assess the entirety of the coagulation cascade. In its simplest form, two samples are run simultaneously, one with heparinase to remove the effects of heparin. If both samples are normal, then excessive bleeding is often considered surgical. If the plain sample is abnormal but the heparinase sample is normal, then the coagulation defect is due to residual heparin. If both samples are abnormal, there may be a deficit in either clotting factors or platelet activity (i.e., number or function). The TEG can also help differentiate between platelet and clotting factor deficiencies. A prolonged R time is suggestive of a factor deficiency, whereas low maximum amplitude suggests a platelet deficiency.

Most coagulopathies are mild and self-correcting, with minimal clinical effects. Clotting factors and platelet counts usually return to normal levels after 24 h. In some cases, particularly after prolonged bypass times, coagulopathies may be severe and require blood product support (Table 53-6). Our practice in case of significant hemorrhage is the early use of cryoprecipitate or platelets (or both as necessary) and aprotinin. When bleeding persists despite repletion of clotting factors and normalization of coagulation tests, surgical exploration is undertaken.

Factor VIIa

Activated factor VII was developed for use in hemophiliacs and essentially bypasses part of the coagulation cascade. In the presence of tissue factor (exposed in traumatized tissues), activated factor VII will convert prothrombin to thrombin, generating a "thrombin burst" that will allow a fibrin clot to form rapidly at the site of trauma. In theory, it should target sites of tissue damage and bleeding. In practice, it has been used successfully to help control bleeding after cardiac surgery and ECMO.[12,13]

Cardiac tamponade

Cardiac tamponade can complicate any cardiac operation and should always be excluded in the setting of sustained hypotension or low cardiac output. Classic signs include systemic hypotension, low pulse pressure, thready pulse, high atrial pressures, and decreased urine output. The diagnosis may be confirmed by echocardiography. Treatment generally requires reopening of the chest and relieving the tamponade to restore hemodynamic stability. If the patient is in a severe state of low cardiac output, there should be no delay in chest reopening. One should be cautious when chest drainage suddenly ceases, as this may reflect chest tube occlusion with ongoing bleeding into the pleural spaces. If clinical suspicion is high, chest reopening should occur without delay, even before a confirmatory diagnostic echocardiogram is performed. While preparing to reexplore the chest, resuscitation includes fluid boluses, increasing or starting inotropes, and stopping vasodilators and diuretics.

Table 53-6 Summary of therapies for coagulopathy

Abnormal coagulation parameter	Therapy
Platelet count < 100,000 × 10^9/L	Platelets 10–15 mL/ kg
PT > 24 s	Fresh frozen plasma 10–15 mL/kg
Fibrinogen < 1 g/L	Cryoprecipitate 5 mL/kg
APTT > 60 s and normal PT	Protamine 0.5–1.0 mg/kg
APTT and PT equally prolonged	Fresh frozen plasma 10–15 mL/kg

PT = prothrombin time; APTT = activated partial thromboplastin time.

Ameliorating the effects of CPB

For open heart surgery, CPB cannot be avoided. However, there are a number of ways in which its effects may be blunted. Several techniques are used to attenuate these effects:

1. Steroids. Endogenous steroids are produced in response to stress. They help maintain vascular integrity and mobilize energy sources (e.g., lipolysis, protein breakdown). Steroids are potent anti-inflammatory agents that work by suppressing leukocyte activity. Leukocyte migration and the release of cytokines are all suppressed.[16] Steroids have been proposed as a therapy to ameliorate the effects of cardiopulmonary bypass. Although there are many studies on the use of steroids for CPB, the evidence is still inconclusive.[17–19] There is some evidence that high-dose steroids given pre- and intraoperatively reduce morbidity.[20] The most commonly used steroids are methylprednisolone, dexamethasone, and hydrocortisone. Although there are potential side effects (e.g., hyperglycemia, hypertension, increased susceptibility to infection), these are mild compared to the problems related to SIRS.
2. Modified ultrafiltration (MUF) is a technique of performing hemofiltration toward the end of bypass with the aim of removing fluid and cytokines. The immediate benefits include an increase in hematocrit, reduction in total body water, and reduction in cytokine load. These effects may help minimize postoperative capillary leak and tissue edema.[21–23]
3. Mild therapeutic hypothermia can be protective in a number of circumstances. This has been studied in cardiac arrest[24,25] and traumatic head injury,[26] with some evidence suggesting a possible reduction in metabolic turnover and inflammatory damage.
4. Surfaces with which blood comes into contact during bypass stimulate an inflammatory response. The use of new "biocompatible" surfaces such as heparin-coated circuits may reduce the degree of inflammatory activation.
5. There is emerging interest in the concept of "remote preconditioning" to reduce reperfusion injury. This concept is based on a brief period of limb ischemia induced by a blood pressure cuff to protect against cardiac reperfusion injury in cardiac surgery.

LOW CARDIAC OUTPUT

A low cardiac output state may complicate any cardiac procedure but is to be expected if the repair has been difficult, necessitating prolonged CPB, aortic cross-clamping, and/or circulatory arrest. Moreover, neonates and smaller infants have more bypass-related morbidity. Ideally, low cardiac output should be diagnosed using cardiac output monitoring; however, as discussed previously, current techniques have a number of drawbacks, such that cardiac output monitoring at the bedside is rarely performed in the postoperative period. Low cardiac output is manifest by indicators of inadequate tissue perfusion:

- Low pulse volume, prolonged capillary refill time, and low blood pressure
- Metabolic acidosis
- Oliguria or anuria
- Low mixed venous saturation, which will be due to excessive oxygen extraction (i.e., < 75 percent of the systemic saturation).

The nadir for cardiac output occurs between 8 and 12 h after CPB. The typical clinical course reflects this pattern of an initially adequate output followed by a slow decline over the ensuing 12 to 24 h after bypass. Thus, the patient may be hemodynamically stable immediately postoperatively but then deteriorates overnight in the ICU, with escalating inotropic and fluid requirements and falling urine output.[27] In many cases, this nadir is followed by steady improvement by the following postoperative day.

There are a number of key steps in the assessment and treatment of low cardiac output:

1. The repair. Data from the surgeons performing the repair, hemodynamic monitoring data, and echocardiography are vital to assessing the repair and whether residual or undiagnosed lesions are present, causing hemodynamic compromise. Such data are useful in excluding pericardial effusion and tamponade, and can help to assess cardiac function. Although esophageal or epicardial echocardiography may have been performed in the operating room, it is still useful to perform a repeat study in the ICU for any unexplained deterioration in the patient's hemodynamics.
2. Assess filling pressures and ventricular physiology to guide the need for preload (i.e., fluid boluses).
3. Measure PA pressures. Pulmonary hypertension may impair cardiac output by affecting left-sided preload.
4. Inotropic support. A number of inotropes are available, each with different pharmacokinetics (Table 53-7). Each institution will have its individual preference, but there is little evidence to favor any one of the agents other than the routine use of high-dose milrinone infusion (0.7 μg/kg/min) after cardiopulmonary bypass for congenital heart surgery.
5. Vasodilators. In the postoperative patient, there may be increased afterload secondary to a number of things including pain, hypothermia, and endogenous/

Table 53-7 Inotropic pharmacology

Drug	Action	Pharmacology	Drawbacks
Dopamine	Increases contractility, vasodilates coronary arteries, chronotrope, increases cardiac index, peripheral vasodilator	Agonist at adrenergic beta receptors (and alpha receptors at higher doses) and dopaminergic receptors; half-life: 2 min; renal, liver, and monoamine oxidase metabolism	Tachycardia, vasoconstriction at higher doses (> 10 μg/kg/min)
Dobutamine	Inotrope and peripheral vasodilator	Predominantly a $beta_1$ agonist; synthetic sympathomimetic amine; half-life 2 min; liver metabolism	Tachycardia at higher doses
Epinephrine/adrenaline	Inotrope, chronotrope	Agonist at alpha and beta receptors; liver metabolism, but also uptake by neurons and metabolized by monoamine oxidase and catechol-O-methyl transferase	Marked vasoconstrictive effect at higher doses, leading to peripheral ischemia
Isoproterenol	Chronotropy, some inotropy, peripheral vasodilator; used predominantly as a chronotrope (e.g., after cardiac transplantation)	Synthetic sympathomimetic amine; $beta_1$ agonist; half-life 2 min; conjugated mainly in liver and lungs	Contraindicated in hypertrophic cardiomyopathy (may exacerbate)

exogenous catecholamines. Increased afterload will increase myocardial work and oxygen consumption and can impair cardiac output by elevating end-diastolic volume, thus effectively reducing stroke volume. Judicious use of systemic vasodilators can improve cardiac output. Calcium channel blockers (e.g., nifedipine) causes vasodilatation by inhibiting calcium influx in smooth muscle cells, thereby causing muscle relaxation. Phosphodiesterase inhibitors (e.g., enoximone, milrinone) are known to reduce the degradation of cyclic nucleotides and therefore increase tissue concentrations of cAMP and cGMP. The heart possesses a specific subtype of phosphodiesterase III, the inhibition of which results in an elevation of cAMP only. As cAMP is the second messenger for $beta_1$ adrenergic receptors in the heart, elevation of its concentrations by use of selective phosphospodiesterase III inhibitors such as milrinone or enoximone mimics the effects of $beta_1$-adrenoceptor stimulation. These drugs are therefore useful for increasing contractility in cardiac failure. Additionally, this class of drugs affects the sarcoplasmic reticulum and increases the rate of Ca^{2+} reabsorption, which allows for better diastolic relaxation (lusitropic action) and acts as a potent vasodilator. There is good evidence that milrinone can reduce the incidence and severity of low cardiac output after congenital heart surgery and bypass and that it also decreases the length of stay.[28]

6. Antiplatelet agents (e.g., aspirin, clopidogrel) are used to reduce the risk of intracardiac thrombosis in chronic states of low cardiac output.
7. Angiotensin converting enzyme inhibitors. These drugs block conversion of angiotensin I to angiotensin II, thereby causing peripheral arteriolar vasodilatation and reducing systemic afterload. They have a reasonably long half-life and are used orally, so are of use in the recovery phase or in chronic heart failure; they are less useful acutely.
8. Systemic cooling may be useful in low-cardiac-output states:
   a. Pyrexia increases metabolic rate, causes tachycardia, and increases myocardial metabolism as well as myocardial oxygen demand; therefore avoidance of pyrexia minimizes additional stress on the heart.
   b. Therapeutic cooling to 33 to 35°C may reduce metabolic rate and myocardial oxygen consumption, and thus help to control tachycardia.[29]
10. Mechanical circulatory support. For low-cardiac-output states refractory to the conventional therapies outlined above, mechanical support should be considered provided that there is no residual anatomic lesion as well as a reversible etiology. The modes employed currently include:
   a. Extracorporeal membrane oxygenation (ECMO). Cannulas are placed either via the neck through the right internal jugular vein (i.e., cannula tip in the right atrium) and common carotid artery (i.e., cannula tip at the junction of the innominate artery and aortic arch) or via direct chest cannulation (i.e., direct right atrial and aortic cannulas). ECMO has the advantage of providing both heart and lung support. The need to anticoagulate means that bleeding can be a major issue in the immediate postoperative period, requiring significant blood and blood product support. Cannulation via the neck can reduce bleeding complications but may be technically difficult owing to the need to reposition the patient while on bypass. Most patients will also require LA decompression to allow full decompression of the left heart. This can be achieved using atrial septostomy or by placing a direct LA "vent."
   b. Ventricular assist devices (VADs). These devices are generally classified into pulsatile and nonpulsatile types. The most common pulsatile devices used in children are paracorporeal devices that can be used to support either the left heart (LVAD) or the right heart (RVAD) or both (BiVAD). The advantages of these devices are that they are smaller, can achieve full cardiac decompression and rest (not always achievable on ECMO), and are more suitable for longer-term support. As these devices are implantable, patients may be extubated and even mobile on VAD support. The main limitations are that they require median sternotomy for direct cannulation of the atria or ventricles and do not possess an oxygenator, so adequate lung function is necessary.
   c. Centrifugal pumps are useful in providing short-term support for isolated left or right ventricular failure in the postoperative period.
11. Intraaortic balloon pump (IABP). Intraaortic balloon counterpulsation is synchronized with the ECG or arterial pressure tracing such that inflation occurs in diastole and deflation just before ventricular systole. The balloon reduces afterload during ejection while deflating. During diastole, the balloon is inflated, augmenting the diastolic pressure and improving coronary filling. Thus, myocardial oxygen consumption is reduced while myocardial perfusion is enhanced. There is extensive experience with IABP counterpulsation in adults; until recently, however, there has been a limitation to its use in children owing to the size of the balloons.[32] IABP can support only the left ventricle, and its role is probably in bigger children with predominant left ventricular failure in whom it may obviate the need for ECMO.
12. Thyroid hormone replacement. There is some evidence that thyroid function is depressed in the postoperative period and that thyroid hormone replacement (i.e., intravenous T_3) therapy reverses this and may shorten ICU stays.[30,31]

13. Replacement steroids. Adrenal dysfunction may occur after bypass and surgery. Low plasma cortisol levels may result in hypotension, which can be relatively resistant to inotropic therapy until steroid replacement is effected.

SPECIAL CONSIDERATIONS IN NEONATAL PATIENTS UNDERGOING CARDIAC SURGERY

Most newborn infants admitted to the cardiac ICU are "term" babies (i.e., 37 to 42 weeks' gestation) and are referred with proven or suspected cardiac pathology. The following notes highlight areas in which the care of neonates differs substantially from that of older infants and children. Congenital heart disease should be considered in any term neonate that presents soon after birth or to the emergency department. It should also be suspected in babies who are cyanotic but hemodynamically stable. The neonatal heart is also different from that in other age groups in that there is less muscle and hence a limited ability to increase stroke volume; any increase in cardiac output is therefore rate-dependent. In cases where myocardial function is borderline (e.g., late switch for transposition of the great arteries), tachycardia is observed to maintain cardiac output (up to 180 beats per minute).

Intracranial bleeding

Neurologic injury can occur as a result of cardiovascular collapse. This is particularly true in those patients with systemic duct-dependent lesions. Few diagnostic tools are available to help assess the degree of neurologic damage, and prognostication may not be possible at this early stage. Newborn infants and, in particular, preterm neonates have an increased susceptibility to intracranial bleeding, which may occur at the germinal matrix (i.e., periventricular matter near the lateral ventricles) or choroid plexus. In severe cases, it may extend into the brain parenchyma. Risk factors include prematurity, difficult delivery with perinatal asphyxia (Apgar score < 4 at 1 min), male gender, and coagulopathy or anticoagulation. The following grading system is based on cranial ultrasound appearance:

Grade 1: periventricular only
Grade 2: blood visible in ventricles but no ventriculomegaly
Grade 3: Blood in ventricles plus ventricular dilatation
Grade 4: Hemorrhage extending into brain parenchyma

Grades 1 and 2 are not associated with increased morbidity. Grades 3 and 4 imply increased risk of neurologic damage. Treatment of any coagulopathy is essential. In addition, cranial ultrasound should be performed routinely to exclude bleeding in any baby that has been unwell. If there has been bleeding, regular follow-up by a neurosurgeon is essential. Marked ventricular dilatation may require fluid drainage or ventricular shunting.

Cranial ultrasound

Applicable to neonates and infants up to approximately 10 months of age, cranial ultrasound provides a view of the brain parenchyma. Visualization requires an open anterior fontanelle. Items that can be assessed include bleeding, infarction, ventricular dilatation, and the presence of cerebral edema (Fig. 53-4).

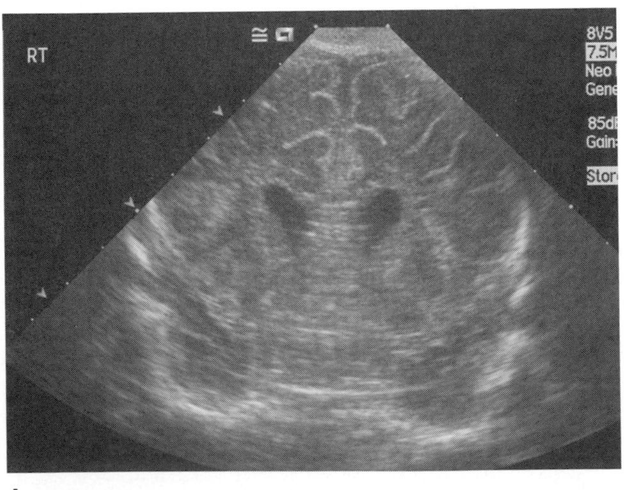

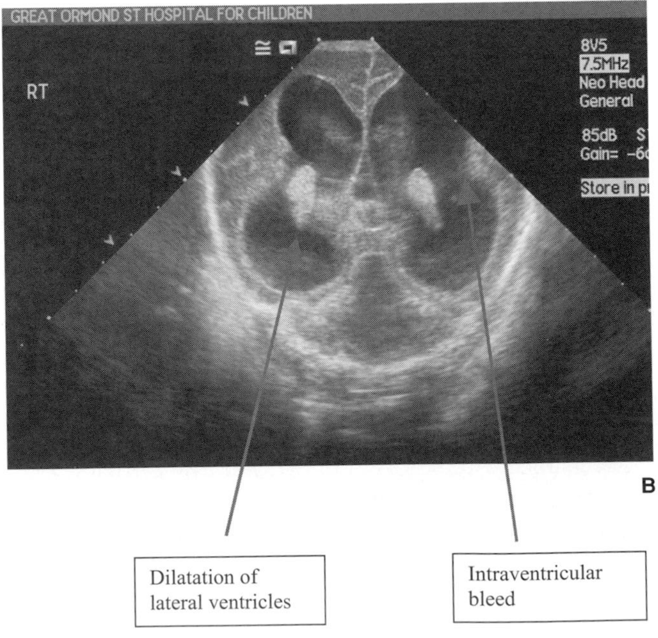

Figure 53-4 Cranial ultrasound images in neonates. Panel **A** shows a normal exam. Panel **B** shows ventricular dilatation and intraventricular bleeding.

Temperature control

Hypothermia

Neonates have a large ratio of surface area to body mass, and therefore lose heat more readily. They also have a limited ability to control their temperature because they cannot sweat or shiver. Neonates have a reduced capacity to generate heat using "nonshivering thermogenesis." Measures to prevent excessive cooling should be taken, including the following:

1. Maintaining the neonate in a radiant heater or incubator
2. Checking core temperatures regularly
3. Avoiding exposure or excessive handling, particularly in areas where the environmental temperature is low

Hyperthermia

Neonates can overheat easily; therefore care should be taken when overhead radiant heaters or phototherapy lights (to treat hyperbilirubinemia) are used. This is particularly important in the postbypass period when hyperthermia is associated with SIRS. In fact, one may choose to cool these patients to 34 or 35°C as a means of treating low cardiac output or dysrhythmias.

FLUID MANAGEMENT

Healthy term infants will consume as much fluid as they require from breast or bottle feeding. Recommended feeding schedules for *healthy infants* are as follows:

Age (days)	1	2	3	4	5	6	7+
Term infants (oral/NG)	60	90	120	120	140	140	160

Fluid intake is frequently restricted in sick infants of all gestational ages. Requirements must therefore be based on the following clinical and laboratory assessments:

Weight:	Regular weighing can help gauge fluid balance
Clinical assessment:	Skin turgor Condition of anterior fontanelle Mucous membranes Urine output
Measured fluid balance:	Accurate if measured correctly, but it does not take account of insensible losses
Laboratory:	Plasma sodium Osmolality Creatinine Hematocrit

Fever, radiant heaters, and phototherapy increase insensible losses substantially. Fluid therapies for the premature infant are listed in Table 53-8.

Table 53-8 Fluid therapy for the premature infant (day 1)

Birth weight	Fluid volume (mL/kg/day)	Glucose	Sodium
> 1.5kg	50–60	10%	None
1.0–1.5	60–70	10%	None
0.75–1.0	80–100	10%	None

Body weight may be allowed to decrease 5 to 15 percent over the first 10 days.
Prescribe fluid on basis of:
Weight loss/gain
Plasma sodium concentration
Factors increasing insensible fluid losses
Edema or overt fluid losses
Fluid balance
Underlying pathophysiology

Insensible losses are increased by phototherapy and the use of radiant heaters, pyrexia, and skin breakdown. Fluid retention and tissue edema are common after surgery and bypass. For this reason, fluid intake is generally restricted after surgery (Table 53-9).

FEEDING AND NUTRITION

Nutrition is a vital component of the treatment plan for sick children in the ICU, particularly for patients who have also undergone surgery. When caloric and protein intake is inadequate, catabolic processes start to occur, with consequent loss of body mass and tissue integrity. Adequate nutrition, particularly when given enterally, reduces morbidity and mortality and can shorten ICU stay. Well babies can be fed soon after birth. Sick infants of whatever birth weight should not be fed enterally until:

The baby's general condition is improving
There are normal bowel sounds and no abdominal distention
Meconium has been passed

Fluid restriction may limit caloric intake (Table 53-10), but enteral nutrition should be commenced as soon as possible unless there are concerns about bowel function. Where enteral nutrition is not possible, total

Table 53-9 Fluid management in the immediate postoperative period

	Nonbypass	Postbypass
Day 1	70% of normal maintenance	50% of normal maintenance
Day 2 onward	Increase gradually to 100%, based on clinical and biochemical indicators of fluid status	

Table 53-10 Recommended daily caloric intake

Age	Recommended daily caloric intake
Less than 1 year	100 kcal/kg
1–6 years	90–75 kcal/kg
7–16 years	75–45 kcal/kg

parenteral nutrition (TPN) should be commenced without delay (see "Total Parenteral Nutrition," below).

Stresses, such as infection or surgery, increase caloric requirements. In practice, it is difficult to achieve adequate caloric intake with TPN; this is really only achievable with enteral feeding.

Enteral feeding has many advantages over TPN. First, administration of enteral feeds is less invasive, with a correspondingly lower risk of infection, since TPN requires the use of an indwelling central line to deliver sufficient calories. Second, enteral feeding stimulates gut function and appears to reduce "translocation" of bacteria—the phenomenon whereby gut organisms enter the bloodstream, leading to bacteremia and sepsis.

Routes for feeding

When they are sufficiently well, patients should ideally be taking their usual oral diet. During recovery in the ICU, possible routes for feeding include nasogastric, gastrostomy and jejunal (transpyloric) feeding.

- Nasogastric tubes are relatively easy to place and are easily replaceable. They should be positioned such that the tip is in the stomach; this can be confirmed radiographically. Some children have relative gut immobility, particularly if they are unwell or on large doses of sedatives. Prokinetic agents, such as metoclopramide, may be useful. Small doses of erythromycin have also been useful in this context, with relatively few side effects.
- Transpyloric feeding. In some patients with gastroparesis, a transpyloric tube can be placed once a mechanical obstruction has been ruled out. This can be done at the bedside or under fluoroscopic guidance.
- Caloric demands may require supplementation with carbohydrate complexes. Large amounts of carbohydrate may be difficult to absorb (e.g., mucosal dysfunction following surgery or trauma), resulting in diarrhea. By reducing the amount of caloric supplementation or changing to a hydrolyzed formula, the diarrhea may be reduced or eliminated.

An umbilical arterial catheter (UAC) is not per se a contraindication to enteral feeding. Particular caution must be exercised where there has been or is continuing concern over bowel perfusion (e.g., after cardiac arrest or hypoplastic left heart syndrome). Our practice is to delay enteral feeds in this group for 3 to 5 days depending on the clinical situation. Babies should generally not be fed:

- If the gastric aspirate over 3 to 4 h is consistently greater than the volume of feedings.
- If there are signs of intestinal obstruction or suspicion of necrotizing enterocolitis.
- For 4 to 6 h before extubation. There should be no concern about the need for reintubation before feeds are restarted after extubating the patient.
- If you suspect an inborn error of metabolism.

Total parenteral nutrition

When enteral nutrition is not possible (e.g., in patients with enterocolitis or bowel ischemia), TPN should be commenced as soon as possible in order to maintain nutrition. The essential components of a balanced solution include:

1. Carbohydrate, usually provided in the form of a glucose solution.
2. Lipids, provided in the form of a lipid emulsion. This is generally started at a low dose, aiming to build up to 1 g/kg/day. Lipids are usually given as a separate infusion.
3. Protein is provided in the form of an amino acid solution, aiming for 2 to 4 g/kg/day of nitrogen.
4. Electrolytes. Sodium, potassium, calcium, phosphorus, and magnesium are all supplemented and guided by laboratory values.
5. Vitamins. Essential vitamins are given in the form of a vitamin solution added to the main TPN solution.
6. Trace elements such as zinc, copper, and selenium may be added in individual amounts. Patients on long-term TPN should have these levels monitored to ensure adequate replacement.

TPN can be associated with complications. Central line infection is a risk, particularly in the case of nontunneled lines. TPN solutions are hypertonic, and venous thrombosis may occur as a result. Cholestasis may occur with TPN and sometimes results in marked jaundice. This is usually reversible and resolves when enteral feeds are reestablished.

Necrotizing enterocolitis

Preterm neonates and sick term neonates are vulnerable to necrotizing enterocolitis (NEC), where extensive areas of bowel become necrotic and occasionally perforate. Predisposing factors include ischemia during either the prenatal and postnatal periods. It is essential to keep a high index of suspicion for this condition, particularly with cardiac lesions associated with left ventricular outflow tract obstruction (e.g., severe coarctation, hypoplastic left heart syndrome). Classic signs include large bilious gastric aspirates, abdominal distention, and gastrointestinal bleeding. Affected babies typically undergo an acute deterioration in their general condition, with hemodynamic instability and the development of a lactic acidosis. Examination of the abdomen reveals distention and tenderness. Abdominal radiography shows distended loops of bowel and free gas if there has been a perforation (Fig. 53-5). There may also be pneumatosis coli (i.e., presence of gas in the bowel wall or "intramural gas").

An urgent general surgical consultation should be sought if this diagnosis is suspected. After the baby is stabilized, an exploratory laparotomy to confirm the diagnosis and resect any affected bowel is frequently recommended for the most severe cases (i.e., perforation). Broad-spectrum antibiotics to cover bowel organisms are also started (e.g., metronidazole, penicillin, gentamicin). Bowel rest is recommended for at least 10 days, during which time nutrition must be maintained parenterally.

Milk feeds

Nutritionally, we aim to achieve at least 100 kcal/kg/day. In babies that have been sick or have residual cardiac lesions, more calories are needed. Various nutritional sources include:

- Mother's breast milk
  - 70 kcal/100 mL.
  - Suitable for all infants.
  - Can be supplemented with additives or additional formula feeds.
- Standard infant formula
  - 65 kcal/100 mL.
  - Term infants.
  - Adequate caloric intake only if the infant is not fluid-restricted; otherwise caloric supplements will be needed.
- Preterm formula
  - Typically 80 kcal/100 mL.
  - Higher protein and mineral content than "term" formulas.

Most well term infants tolerate feedings every 3 to 4 h. Otherwise healthy low-birth-weight infants may need bolus feeding every 2 h. Sicker infants of all ages may better tolerate frequent small-volume feeds or continuous nasogastric feeds.

OTHER MANAGEMENT ISSUES

Blood transfusion

Neonates should always receive cytomegalovirus-negative blood. Babies with proved or suspected Di George syndrome (i.e., truncus arteriosus, aortic interruption) should receive irradiated blood products to prevent graft-versus-host disease stemming from transfused white cells. Prior to transfusing any baby, the question of whether additional tests are required should be answered (e.g., chromosomal analysis). Although babies receive blood that is usually leukocyte-depleted and are transfused through a white cell filter, there is a small chance that some leukocytes may get through and contaminate any testing.

Drug dosing

Liver and renal functions are inefficient at birth. All drug doses must be checked against an authoritative reference.

Ranges for pathology tests

Normal ranges for many tests differ in the neonatal period. Check carefully with your local laboratory for relevant reference values.

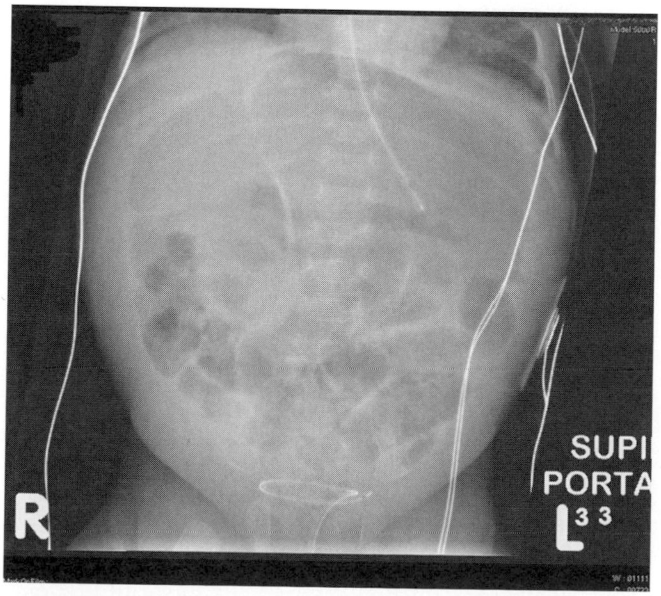

Figure 53-5 Abdominal roentgenogram showing free peritoneal gas with gas outlining the falciform ligament.

Apneic episodes

Apneic episodes are respiratory pauses that extend beyond the normal interval (i.e., up to 20 s). They are common in babies born before 34 weeks but uncommon in well term babies. They are of significance if their duration is in excess of 15 to 20 s and accompanied by a fall in heart rate or oxygen saturation. Apneic episodes are frequently a nonspecific sign of an underlying problem. Potential problems include:

Sepsis
Lung disease (respiratory distress syndrome, pulmonary edema, pneumonia)
Hypoxia
High ambient temperature
Hypocalcemia
Hypoglycemia
Heart failure (pulmonary edema)
Intracranial bleeding
Fits
Aspiration/gastroesophageal reflux
Sedative/analgesia drugs

Rare metabolic disorders (e.g., "Ondine's curse," Leigh disease)

Apneic episodes should be treated with stimulation and, if necessary, gentle bag-and-mask ventilation. These patients should be monitored with an apnea alarm and pulse oximetry. Underlying causes should be excluded with the following:

Septic workup
Chest x-ray
CBC, glucose, calcium
Cranial ultrasound
Cardiac ultrasound

Theophylline may be useful in preterm infants if episodes persist and there is no obvious cause. If this fails, nasal continuous positive airway pressure (CPAP) will usually prevent further recurrences.

MANAGEMENT OF UNIVENTRICULAR CIRCULATIONS

A number of congenital malformations lead to functionally univentricular circulations [e.g., hypoplastic left heart syndrome (HLHS), tricuspid atresia]. Adequate circulation depends on adequate mixing of oxygenated and deoxygenated blood at the atrial level, adequate cardiac output generated by the ventricle, and adequate distribution of blood flow between the pulmonary and systemic circulations. Neonatally, ductal patency must be maintained to allow the single ventricle to supply the pulmonary (tricuspid atresia) or systemic circulation (HLHS). The usual surgical strategy is to secure adequate mixing, secure systemic blood supply, and add a conduit or shunt to supply the lungs (e.g., stage 1 Norwood procedure).

The most important consideration both pre- and postoperatively is to maintain adequate cardiac output (i.e., fluids, inotropes). The division of blood between the pulmonary (Qp) and systemic (Qs) circulations will also need balancing, and the ideal balance is where there is equal flow (i.e., Qp:Qs ratio at 1:1). Excessive systemic flow may lead to inadequate pulmonary blood flow and hypoxia. Excessive pulmonary blood flow may result in inadequate systemic flow, leading to a low-cardiac-output state. More importantly, excessive pulmonary runoff can result in a low diastolic pressure, causing myocardial ischemia. A 1:1 balance will result in arterial oxygen saturations around 75 percent. However, in the setting of adequate cardiac output, achieving a 1:1 ratio is not as crucial as was previously believed. The usual measures of adequate systemic oxygen delivery (e.g., lactate, urine output, blood pressure) should also be looked at before aggressive interventions to alter Qp:Qs are instituted. There are many strategies to alter Qp:Qs; they all essentially work on the principle of altering the relative resistances (Table 53-11).

Table 53-11 Strategies for altering Qp:Qs

Problem	Strategies
Excessive Qp (high oxygen saturations, systemic hypotension, wide pulse pressure, low diastolic pressure, lactic acidosis)	In the unoperated hypoplastic left heart, ensure ductal patency with prostaglandin E_1 infusion and verify with echocardiography. Manage in air (oxygen is a pulmonary vasodilator) unless systemic saturations are low (e.g., < 60%). If ventilated, use relative hypoventilation or entrain carbon dioxide into breathing mixture to raise blood carbon dioxide tensions (pulmonary vasoconstriction), with low normal pH. Maintain Hb at 14–16 g/dL to increase viscosity Some centers use hypoxic respiratory mixture (inspired oxygen 18%). This technique requires using nitrogen to dilute the oxygen content of air. It has the major disadvantage of causing pulmonary venous desaturation, so that total delivered oxygen will fall; it should be reserved for extreme circumstances.
Low Qp (low systemic oxygen saturations)	Newborn: pulmonary vascular resistance may still be high soon after birth, but it will fall over a few days. Poor lung compliance (e.g., infection, fluid overload). Positive-pressure ventilation will lower work of breathing. Noninvasive support (e.g., nasal CPAP) may be beneficial. In tricuspid atresia, ensure ductal patency with prostaglandin E_1 infusion and check with echocardiography.

It is vital to appreciate that emphasis is placed on increasing cardiac output by reducing systemic afterload rather than by attempting to increase pulmonary vascular resistance (Table 53-12).

GENERAL COMPLICATIONS AFTER CARDIAC SURGERY

Arrhythmias

Sinus tachycardia

Baseline heart rates vary with age, but heart rates above 180/min are of concern. An ECG should be performed to assess the rhythm. If the rhythm is unclear (i.e., atrial fibrillation/flutter), an atrial ECG should be performed (with one of the ECG leads connected to the atrial pacing wires instead of the skin) to aid diagnosis. Sinus tachycardia is a nonspecific but important sign of

Table 53-12	Postoperative management principles for norwood patients
Sedation and paralysis	In the initial postoperative period, we want to minimize metabolic demands. Sedation and paralysis can improve stability by minimizing demands on cardiac output. Patients may also return from the operating room with the chest open.
Hemodynamics	Optimize cardiac output **1.** Afterload reduction (e.g., milrinone) **2.** Judicious use of inotropes **3.** Ventilatory strategies to balance the circulation
Fluids	Fluid restrict postbypass as usual. Use small aliquots of fluid when giving fluid boluses for filling (5mL / kg). Initially avoid enteral feeding (for possible gut ischemia); use TPN to maintain caloric intake.
Lines	Norwood patients should routinely return with arterial, CVP, and central lines for infusions. It is important to remove any neck jugular venous lines as soon as possible to minimize chances of clots forming and jeopardizing future operations (e.g., Glenn, Fontan).

abnormal physiology. Additionally, the tachycardia itself increases myocardial oxygen demand and stress. It is vital to differentiate and treat (Table 53-13) the underlying causes, which include:

Central: pain, anxiety, fever, seizures
Drugs: catecholamines (dobutamine, dopamine, epinephrine, isoproterenol)
Cardiac: hypovolemia, low cardiac output state (bypass, residual lesion)
Miscellaneous: hypercarbia, hypoxia, pulmonary hypertension

In the normal heart, atrial contraction improves ventricular filling and may contribute up to 20 percent of the cardiac output. In relatively well patients, the loss of atrioventricular synchrony may not have a severe effect on hemodynamic status. However, in the postoperative cardiac patient, the effects of bypass and surgery may lead to a state low cardiac output where a loss of atrioventricular synchrony can be significant. This is particularly true with restrictive physiology (e.g., repair of tetralogy of Fallot, Fontan procedure) when the atrial contribution to cardiac output is significant.

Pulmonary hypertension

Pulmonary hypertension may be preexisting or may occur in cases where a predisposition exists (e.g., high pulmonary blood flow, obstructed pulmonary venous drainage). There appears to be a trend toward less severe pulmonary hypertension in congenital cardiac patients which may be related to earlier repair of lesions and the use of modified ultrafiltration.[22] Conditions in which pulmonary hypertension may complicate the postoperative course include:

- Truncus arteriosus
- Late repair of ventricular septal defects or atrioventricular septal defects
- Late repair of transposition of the great arteries
- Obstructed anomalous pulmonary venous drainage
- Obstruction to pulmonary venous drainage (e.g., pulmonary venous stenosis, mitral valve stenosis)
- Chromosomal anomalies (e.g., trisomy 21)

Table 53-13 Arrhythmia management		
Junctional/ectopic tachycardia	Rhythm arising from AV junction or His bundle. More common with procedures on right ventricular outflow tract. May be more common with more sympathetic drive or sympathomimetics. Loss of AV synchrony. Tachycardia increases myocardial oxygen consumption and impairs diastolic filling. This is a malignant rhythm that requires aggressive treatment.	Treat pain, sedate. Minimize inotrope doses. Prevent pyrexia; consider therapeutic cooling (to 33–34° C). Correct electrolyte disturbances. Consider magnesium supplements (≥ 2 mmol/L). Antiarrhythmics: Amiodarone will usually achieve chemical cardioversion or can slow the rate sufficiently to permit the use of AV sequential pacing.
Complete heart block	May be related to localized edema of the conduction system; will usually recover in 1–2 weeks.	Even if the escape rate is adequate, AV sequential pacing should be instituted to prevent patient compromise if bradycardia develops. If pacing wires are not functional, chronotropic agents such as isoproterenol can raise the rate of the escape rhythm sufficiently to temporize while a pacing system is being placed.

Treatment

When there is an expectation that pulmonary hypertension will complicate the postoperative course, a PA catheter to monitor pressures may be helpful. The PA pressure (PAP) may be elevated at baseline, with additional episodic sharp rises in PAP to systemic or suprasystemic levels. These episodes may be associated with hypoxemia and hypotension (i.e., lack of pulmonary blood flow leading to impaired left heart filling). PA pressure lines also allow continuous pressure monitoring and can help identify when hypertensive crises begin, allowing prompt intervention:

Treatment strategies for pulmonary hypertension

1. Prevention. Pulmonary vasodilators can lower PAP, but there is no evidence that prophylactic use will prevent postoperative problems. However, when there is established pulmonary hypertension with hemodynamic compromise, we can prevent further crises by minimizing patient agitation and stressful procedures and using adequate sedation (e.g., opioid boluses, benzodiazepines) in performing procedures likely to be agitating (e.g., airway suctioning).
2. Ventilation strategies. Ventilating to normal or mildly alkalotic pH and maintaining high inspired oxygen can reduce both pulmonary vascular resistance and lability.[35]
3. Pulmonary vasodilators. There are an increasing number of pharmacologic agents (Table 53-14) that act as pulmonary vasodilators.[35–38]

Table 53-14 Commonly used medications for postoperative pulmonary hypertension

Inhaled nitric oxide	Works via cGMP, causing pulmonary vasodilatation. As it is inhaled, it is truly selective for the pulmonary vascular bed and should improve ventilation/perfusion match in the lungs. It is still considered the treatment of choice for severe pulmonary hypertension.
Milrinone	This phosphodiesterase III inhibitor elevates intracellular cGMP levels. It has beneficial effects on hemodynamics postbypass but also acts as a pulmonary vasodilator.
Sildenafil	A phosphodiesterase V inhibitor that also elevates intracellular cGMP levels but is more specific to the pulmonary circulation than milrinone. Risk of worsening ventilation/perfusion matching and systemic hypotension. Has been used as a means to wean off inhaled nitric oxide.
Epoprostenol (prostaglandin I)	An inhibitor of cAMP breakdown that causes vasodilatation (pulmonary and systemic). It also has antiplatelet effects, which may reduce microvascular thrombosis. Limitations to its use are similar to those of sildenafil.

Infection

Preoperative infections

Children with congenital heart lesions are more vulnerable to respiratory tract infections and are ideally cleared of infection preoperatively. There are occasional risk-benefit decisions to be made; waiting for the infection to clear versus the likelihood that the unrepaired lesion will leave the patient prone to greater morbidity (e.g., heart failure, more infections). In cases of recent respiratory tract infections (i.e., within about 6 weeks) the postoperative course may be complicated by prolonged ventilatory support.

Early infections (within 1 week) Patients receive perioperative prophylaxis, with the choice of drug and its duration depending on the institution. These drugs will generally cover common skin organisms, so that nosocomial infections will dominate. Nosocomial infections affect up to 10 percent of ICU patients. Common sites include:

- The bloodstream (central lines, bowel "translocation")
- The respiratory tract (preoperative infection, endotracheal intubation)
- The urinary tract (urinary catheterization)
- Wounds

Late infections (after 1 week) Mediastinitis is a deep-seated infection involving structures and tissues deep in the sternum. Mediastinitis may present a few days to a few weeks postoperatively, with symptoms and signs varying widely from patient to patient. Classically, body temperature and hematologic markers of infection are elevated (e.g., white cell count, C-reactive protein). Physical examination may reveal evidence of sternal wound infection with purulent discharge. Sternal instability is almost pathognomonic of mediastinitis. Patients may also present with general malaise or, in the case of infants, "irritability," which may or may not be accompanied by fever. Therefore, if there is a delayed recovery from surgery but no obvious residual surgical lesion or other obvious cause, mediastinitis should be considered. The most common infecting organism is *Staphylococcus aureus*, which is often grown from both wound and blood cultures. These patients require surgical exploration followed by mediastinal irrigation. Our practice is to use a povidone-iodine-based

(Betadine) irrigant for 48 h followed by saline irrigation until the effluent fluid is free of organisms on culture. Appropriate antibiotics are given for 3 to 6 weeks.

Failure to wean from mechanical ventilatory support

Failure to separate from ventilatory support may have several etiologies:

1. Residual cardiac lesion. Failure to wean from ventilatory or inotropic support should raise the suspicion of a residual or undiagnosed cardiac lesion. This may range from a residual shunt (e.g., VSD or ASD) to valvular stenosis. Clinical examination may reveal an obvious cause, but frequent imaging with plain chest radiographs to exclude pulmonary causes and echocardiography to look for residual cardiac lesions are usually necessary. If there is doubt about the hemodynamic significance of a lesion, further imaging such as cardiac catheterization, computed tomography (CT), or magnetic resonance imaging (MRI) should be considered to aid in decision making. Patients who have significant residual lesions will suffer significant morbidity (e.g., prolonged mechanical ventilation, prolonged inotropic support, more infections) if these are left untreated.
2. Lung disease. Pulmonary disease may delay ventilator weaning and extubation. The etiologies of lung disease in the cardiac patient are manifold, and there may be preexisting disease to complicate an operation. Common lesions include:
   a. Segmental consolidation or collapse. This may be secondary to infection or retained secretions. The likelihood of this complication rises with prolonged mechanical ventilation.[29] Treatment involves physiotherapy and appropriate antibiotics.
   b. Interstitial lung fluid may accumulate as a result of cardiopulmonary bypass or where fluid balance becomes excessively positive. This will lead to reduced lung compliance, increased work of breathing, and failure to successfully separate from ventilatory support. Treatment generally consists of diuretics and bronchodilators. Failure to respond to medical treatment should prompt a search for a residual cardiac lesion.
   c. Pleural effusions will also reduce overall chest compliance. Likely causes include:
      i. High central venous pressures (e.g., restrictive right ventricular physiology, Fontan circulation, superior vena caval thrombosis).
      ii. Residual cardiac lesions causing cardiac failure (e.g., residual VSD).

      Treatment should include drainage of the effusion and treatment of the underlying problem.

Table 53-15 Strategies for reducing lymphatic leaks

Medium-chain triglyceride (MCT) feeds	These are absorbed directly into the portal circulation, avoiding stimulation of lymphatic flow by absorption of triglycerides into the intestinal lymphatics.
Somatostatin	Elicits gut paracrine effects, reducing lymphatic flow.

3. Chylothorax. Accumulation of lymphatic fluid in the chest has multiple consequences, including reduced chest compliance and the loss of lymphatic components (i.e., white cells, proteins, fluids). Lymphatic leaks may occur due to damage to the thoracic duct or other lymphatic vessels at the time of surgery or when there is a prolonged elevation of central venous pressure. Diagnosis is confirmed by examination of the fluid (e.g., high triglyceride content, predominance of lymphocytes on microscopy). Chylous effusions should be drained and any underlying cause treated. Further lymphatic leaks can be minimized using a number of strategies (Table 53-15). Usually, minimizing lymphatic flow will allow lymphatic leaks to seal. Medium-chain triglycerides (MCT) feeds are usually continued for 6 to 8 weeks. If a lymphatic leak is prolonged or large in volume, protein losses may be significant. Albumin and immunoglobulin levels should be assessed and replacement considered. In refractory cases, there may need to be surgical intervention (e.g., thoracic duct repair or ligation, pleurodesis).
4. Phrenic nerve palsy. The course of the phrenic nerves in the mediastinum makes them prone to injury during cardiac surgery. This is usually reversible, resulting in a neuropraxia that may recover over a number of weeks. In infants, most quiet breathing is diaphragmatic, so that loss of diaphragmatic function causes significant respiratory distress. Clinically, there is "paradoxical breathing" whereby, on inspiration, there is indrawing of the abdomen on the affected side instead of outward movement; this is due to diaphragmatic flattening. The diagnosis should be confirmed with ultrasound or fluoroscopy. It is important that the patient be breathing spontaneously or only on CPAP during any diagnostic test, as positive-pressure ventilation will abolish any paradoxical movements. In larger patients (i.e., older than 1 year), a longer interval of support (e.g., CPAP) may permit adequate recovery. In neonates and smaller infants, surgical plication of the affected diaphragm will usually be necessary.
5. Tracheobronchomalacia. Relative weakness of the main airways will result in partial or complete collapse during inspiration (i.e., intrathoracic pressures lower than atmospheric). The severity may vary from mild symptoms present only during deep breaths or crying

Table 53-16 Categories of renal failure in the pediatric cardiac patient

Prerenal causes	Heart failure, hypotension, dehydration (e.g., excessive diuresis)
Renal parenchymal causes	Preexisting renal disease (e.g., reflux nephropathy, glomerulonephritis)
Postrenal causes	Obstruction in the renal tract (e.g., calculi, urinary tract infection)

to severe stridor and recession at rest. Tracheobronchomalacia is more common in preterm infants. It may occur in association with cardiac disease where there has been vascular compression of the main airways (e.g., PA sling). A definitive diagnosis can be made using dynamic bronchography or bronchoscopy. Management includes CPAP, airway stenting, or even tracheostomy and long-term positive-pressure ventilation to "stent" the airways. In many cases, growth and strengthening of the airway with time permits weaning from support.

Renal failure and fluid imbalance

Renal failure is generally classified into three broad categories (Table 53-16).

Preoperative considerations

While awaiting surgery for congenital heart disease, children may require diuretics to control heart failure. Prolonged and high-dose diuretic therapy may lead to a degree of renal impairment. This may be exacerbated by impaired renal perfusion related to the heart failure itself. Postoperatively, continued diuretic therapy will be needed to help control fluid balance.

Postoperative considerations

The kidneys are highly vascular structures with a large endothelial surface area. Consequently, the inflammatory cascade related to bypass adversely affects renal function. Perioperative hypotension will also contribute to this. Risk factors for postoperative renal failure are listed in Table 53-17.

Treatment

Treatment is generally predicated on addressing the underlying problem. Any potentially nephrotoxic drugs should be avoided if possible. Careful attention to fluid balance and fluid restriction may be necessary. Electrolyte balance requires close monitoring, avoiding hyperkalemia or hypocalcemia in particular. If nitrogen clearance is impaired, special low-protein feeds containing essential amino acids will be necessary.

The point at which to start renal support can be difficult to determine. Clear indications include:

Table 53-17 Risk factors for postoperative renal failure

Preoperative renal failure	Improved hemodynamics should result in gradual improvement in renal function.
Preoperative cardiac arrest or low cardiac output	Impaired renal perfusion, resulting in acute tubular necrosis (ATN). Often reversible if adequate perfusion is restored. ATN may take several weeks to resolve.
Prolonged cardiopulmonary bypass	
Nephrotoxic drugs	Many drugs in regular use—including aminoglycosides, furosemide, and nonsteroidal agents—have a potential for nephrotoxicity.
	Immunosuppressants, such as tacrolimus and cyclosporine, adversely affect renal function and can cause postoperative renal failure in heart or lung transplant recipients.

- Fluid overload
- Hyperkalemia (potassium > 6.0 or rising rapidly)
- Uncontrollable metabolic acidosis

Relative indications include acutely rising urea and creatinine levels. There are no clear cutoff values; a rapidly rising trend should prompt consideration of renal support. Additionally, with symptoms of uremia and urea levels above 40 mmol/L, renal support should be considered.

Oliguria or anuria will clearly result in fluid accumulation and overload if not promptly treated. Early intervention to correct hypotension and low cardiac output will prevent progression to anuric renal failure (Table 53-18).

As mentioned previously, potassium homeostasis is a central issue in renal failure. Potassium levels above 6.0 mmol/L or rapidly rising levels will require prompt treatment. These measures include:

1. Immediately stopping any intravenous fluids containing potassium.
2. Correcting pH with bicarbonate.
3. Consider specific measures to lower potassium:
   a. Salbutamol bolus or infusion drives potassium intracellularly.
   b. Glucose and insulin bolus drives potassium intracellularly.
   c. Calcium resonium is a potassium chelating agent.

Many drugs are cleared by renal mechanisms, so alterations in medication dose and frequency are often necessary in renal failure (Table 53-19).

Table 53-18 Treatment algorithm for oliguria or anuria

Action	Rationale
"Fluid challenge" and diuretics.	Hypovolemia may cause oliguria.
Administer 10–20 mL/kg of crystalloid or colloid.	Urine output may be restored by diuretics in some cases where renal insult has resulted in oligo-/anuria.
Administer furosemide bolus or infusion (0.1–1.0 mg/k/h)	Requires fluid restriction to maintain fluid balance.
Administer aminophylline bolus and Infusions; particularly useful with tacrolimus induced failure	If patient is anuric set limit at 300mL/m²/day.
Peritoneal dialysis (PD)	Relatively easy to institute and maintain and minimally invasive, but much less effective as a form of acute renal support in patients > 1 year old. Diaphragmatic splinting from PD fluid may require increased ventilatory support.
Hemofiltration (continuous veno-venous hemofiltration; CVVH)	Indications for CVVH include fluid overload.

Table 53-19 Medications requiring special consideration in renal failure

Medication	Considerations
Morphine	Effects prolonged.
Penicillins, cephalosporins, aminoglycosides	Reduced renal clearance, so dose and frequency requires alteration.
Neuromuscular blockers	Avoid pancuronium and vecuronium, as they accumulate. Atracurium is safe due to Hoffman degradation (i.e., hydrolyses spontaneously at body temperature).
Digoxin, amiodarone	Will need lower doses to avoid accumulation.
Angiotensin converting enzyme inhibitors	Avoid, as they can worsen renal function due to effects on renal perfusion.
Heparin	Unfractionated heparin may be used in usual doses. Low-molecular-weight heparin has a prolonged half-life, so lower doses and monitoring of anti-Xa activity are necessary.

Neurologic protection and seizures

Cardiac surgery and CPB may be complicated by neurologic injury. Risk factors include:

1. Perioperative cardiac arrest and severe low cardiac output
2. Air or particulate emboli
3. Use of hypothermic circulatory arrest during bypass

If an intraoperative event occurs that has placed the patient at significant risk of brain injury, a number of measures may be useful in limiting potential neurologic injury:

1. Maintain cerebral perfusion and oxygenation.
   a. Maintain good arterial oxygenation ($PaO_2 > 90$ mmHg if possible) for biventricular repairs.
   b. Aim for normocapnia and normal pH to prevent vasoconstriction related to low PCO_2 or vasodilatation related to high CO_2.
   c. Aim for supranormal arterial blood pressure.
   d. Maintain the patient in a slight head-up tilt (reverse Trendelenburg around 15 degrees) and head in a midline position. This should encourage venous return and minimize venous congestion. Neck vessel cannulation should also be avoided if possible to minimize venous obstruction.
2. Therapeutic hypothermia. There is some evidence that moderate cooling to 34°C for 24 to 48 h may confer benefits following cardiac arrest.[24,25] Cooling to moderate temperatures has relatively few side effects and is easy to institute using a water-filled cooling mattress. Most experience has been in adults, with limited neurologic follow up. Patients who have had prolonged cardiac arrests (e.g., 10 min or longer) or where significant low cardiac output has been a concern may be cooled for 24 h with minimal risk of side effects. There are also preliminary data suggesting benefit in cooling babies with moderate birth asphyxia for 48 h to 34°C.[43]

CONCLUSION

The care of critically ill children after heart surgery is challenging and best performed in dedicated pediatric ICUs with staff trained in cardiac critical care.

Particular attention must be paid to appropriate ventilation, inotropic support, nutrition, and multiorgan protection. It is important to understand the differences in treatment of the neonate, particularly differences in myocardial function and response to drugs. Similarly, it is vital to understand the management of univentricular physiology in both parallel and series circulations. The management of the infant or child in a state of low cardiac output is particularly challenging; it is crucial to exclude anatomic defects to understand the pathophysiology of the underlying lesion and operation. Cardiorespiratory interactions are also important in this context. Last, as mortality falls, more attention will focus on morbidity, the length of ICU stay, and neurologic injury and its long-term effects.

References

1. Pinsky MR. Determinants of pulmonary arterial flow variation during respiration. *J Appl Physiol* 1984;56:1237–1245.
2. Henning RJ. Effects of positive end-expiratory pressure on the right ventricle. *J Appl Physiol* 1986;61:819–826.
3. Pecora DV, Hohenberger M. Reflex pulmonary vascular response to distention of lung vessels and left heart. *J Appl Physiol* 1970;29(3):318–322.
4. Shekerdemian LS, Schulze-Neick I, Redington AN, et al. Negative pressure ventilation as haemodynamic rescue following surgery for congenital heart disease. *Intens Care Med* 2000;26(1):93–96.
5. von Koelliker A, Muller H. Nachweis der negativen Schwankung des Muskelstroms am naturlich sich kontrahierenden Herzen. *Verhandlungen Physikalisch-Medizinischen Gesellschaft Wurzberg* 1856;6:528–533.
6. Courtman SP, Wardurgh A, Petros AJ. Comparison of the bispectral index monitor with the Comfort score in assessing level of sedation in critically ill children. *Intens Care Med* 2003;29: 2239–2246.
7. Triltsch AE, Nestmann G, Orawa H, et al. Bispectral index versus COMFORT score to determine the level of sedation in paediatric intensive care unit patients: A prospective study. *Crit Care* 2005;9:R9–R17.
8. Tibby SM, Hatherill M, Murdoch IA. Use of transesophageal Doppler ultrasonography in ventilated pediatric patients: Derivation of cardiac output. *Crit Care Med* 2000;28:2045–2050.
9. Tibby Sm, Murdoch IA. Monitoring cardiac function in intensive care. *Arch Dis Child* 2003;88:46–52.
10. Paparella D, Yau TM, Young E. Cardiopulmonary bypass induced inflammation: Pathophysiology and treatment. An update. *Eur J Cardiothorac Surg* 2002;21:232–244.
11. Allen ML, Peters MJ, Goldman A, et al. Early postoperative monocyte deactivation predicts systemic inflammation and prolonged stay in pediatric cardiac intensive care. *Crit Care Med* 2002;30(5):1140–1145.
12. Tobias JD, Simsic JM, Weinstein S, et al. Recombinant factor VIIa to control excessive bleeding following surgery for congenital heart disease in pediatric patients. *J Intens Care Med* 2004;19(5):270–273.
13. Wittenstein B, Ng C, Ravn H, Goldman A. Recombinant factor VII for severe bleeding during extracorporeal membrane oxygenation following open heart surgery. *Pediatr Crit Care Med* 2005;6(4):473–476.
14. Johnston TD, Chen Y, Reed RL II. Functional equivalence of hypothermia to specific clotting factor deficiencies. *J Trauma-Injury Infect Crit Care* 1994;37(3):413–417.
15. Slichter SJ. Relationship between platelet count and bleeding risk in thrombocytopenic patients [review]. *Transf Med Rev* 2004;18(3):153–167.
16. Riad M, Mogos M. Thangathurai D, Lumb PD. Steroids. *Curr Opin Crit Care* 2002;8(4):281–284.
17. Kilger E, Weis F, Briegel J, et al. Stress doses of hydrocortisone reduce severe systemic inflammatory response syndrome and improve early outcome in a risk group of patients after cardiac surgery. *Crit Care Med* 2003;31(4): 1068–1074.
18. Rubens FD, Mesana T. The inflammatory response to cardiopulmonary bypass: A therapeutic overview [review]. *Perfusion* 2004;19(Suppl 1):S5–S12.
19. Bourbon A, Vionnet M, Leprince P, et al. The effect of methylprednisolone treatment on the cardiopulmonary bypass–induced systemic inflammatory response. *Eur J Cardiothorac Surg* 2004;26(5):932–938.
20. Schroeder VA, Pearl JM, Schwartz SM, et al. Combined steroid treatment for congenital heart surgery improves oxygen delivery and reduces postbypass inflammatory mediator expression. *Circulation* 2003;107(22): 2823–2828.
21. Dittrich S, Aktuerk D, Seitz S, et al. Effects of ultrafiltration and peritoneal dialysis on proinflammatory cytokines during cardiopulmonary bypass surgery in newborns and infants. *Eur J Cardiothorac Surg* 2004;25(6):935–940.
22. Berdat PA, Eichenberger E, Ebell J, et al. Elimination of proinflammatory cytokines in pediatric cardiac surgery: Analysis of ultrafiltration method and filter type. *J Thorac Cardiovasc Surg* 2004;127(6):1688–1696.
23. Elliott MJ. Ultrafiltration and modified ultrafiltration in pediatric open heart operations. *Ann Thorac Surg* 1993;56: 1518–1522.
24. Journois D, Israel-Biet D, Pouard P, et al. High-volume, zero-balanced hemofiltration to reduce delayed inflammatory response to cardiopulmonary bypass in children. *Anesthesiology* 1996;85:965–976.
25. Bernard SA, Gray TW, Buist MD, et al, Treatment of comatose survivors of out-of-hospital cardiac arrest with induced hypothermia. *N Engl J Med* 2002;346:557–563.
26. Hypothermia after Cardiac Arrest Study Group. Mild therapeutic hypothermia to improve the neurologic outcome after cardiac arrest. *N Engl J Med* 2002;346:549–556.
27. Zhi D, Zhang S, Lin X. Study on therapeutic mechanism and clinical effect of mild hypothermia in patients with severe head injury. *Surg Neurol* 2003;59:381–385.
28. Wernovsky G, Wypij D, Jonas RA, et al. Postoperative course and hemodynamic profile after the arterial switch operation in neonates and infants. A comparison of low-flow cardiopulmonary bypass and circulatory arrest. *Circulation* 1995;92(8):2226–2235.
29. Hoffman TM, Wernovsky G, Atz AM, et al. Efficacy and safety of milrinone in preventing low cardiac output syndrome in infants and children after corrective surgery for congenital heart disease. *Circulation.* 2003;107(7):996–1002.
30. Dalrymple-Hay MJ, Deakin CD, Knight H, et al. Induced hypothermia as salvage treatment for refractory cardiac failure following paediatric cardiac surgery. *Eur J Cardiothorac Surg* 1999;15(4):515–518.
31. Chowdhury D, Ojamaa K, Parnell VA, et al. A prospective randomised clinical study after thyroid treatment after operations for complex CHD. *J Thorac Cardiovasc Surg* 2001;122(5):1023–1025.
32. Mainwaring N. Supplementation of thyroid hormone in children undergoing cardiac surgery. *Cardiol Young* 2002;12(3):211–217.
33. Akomea-Agyin C, Kejriwal NK, Franks R, et al. Intraaortic balloon pumping in children. *Ann Thorac Surg* 1999:67: 1415–1420.
34. Hyllner M, Houltz E, Jeppsson A. Recombinant activated factor VII in the management of life-threatening bleeding in cardiac surgery. *Eur J Cardiothorac Surg* 2005;28(2): 254–258.

35. Dominguez TE, Mitchell M, Friess SH, et al. Use of recombinant factor VIIa for refractory hemorrhage during extracorporeal membrane oxygenation. *Pediatr Crit Care Med* 2005;6(3):348–351.
36. Schulze-Neick I, Li J, Penny DJ, Redington AN. Pulmonary vascular resistance after cardiopulmonary bypass in infants: Effect on postoperative recovery. *J Thorac Cardiovasc Surg* 2001;121(6):1033–1039.
37. Lamarche Y, Gagnon J, Malo O, et al. Ventilation prevents pulmonary endothelial dysfunction and improves oxygenation after cardiopulmonary bypass without aortic cross-clamping. *Eur J Cardiothorac Surg* 2004;26(3):554–563.
38. Gothberg S, Edberg KE. Inhaled nitric oxide to newborns and infants after congenital heart surgery on cardiopulmonary bypass. A dose-response study. *Scand Cardiovasc J* 2000;34(2):154–158.
39. Lyons JM, Duffy JY, Wagner CJ, Pearl JM. Sildenafil citrate alleviates pulmonary hypertension after hypoxia and reoxygenation with cardiopulmonary bypass. *J Am Coll Surg* 2004;199(4):607–614.
40. Fortier S, DeMaria RG, Lamarche Y, et al. Inhaled prostacyclin reduces cardiopulmonary bypass-induced pulmonary endothelial dysfunction via increased cyclic adenosine monophosphate levels. *J Thorac Cardiovasc Surg* 2004;128(1):109–116.
41. Elward AM, Warren DK, Fraser VJ. Ventilator-associated pneumonia in pediatric intensive care unit patients: Risk factors and outcomes. *Pediatrics* 2002;109(5):758–764.
42. Gurgueira GL, Leite HP, Taddei JA, de Carvalho WB. Outcomes in a pediatric intensive care unit before and after the implementation of a nutrition support team. *J Parenter Enteral Nutr* 2005;29(3):176–185.
43. Gluckman PD, Wyatt JS, Azzopardi D, et al. Selective head cooling with mild systemic hypothermia after neonatal encephalopathy: Multicentre randomised trial. *Lancet* 2005;365(9460):663–670.

CHAPTER

54 PALLIATIVE OPERATIONS FOR CONGENITAL HEART DISEASE

Christopher T. Salerno, Brian L. Reemsten, Gordon A. Cohen

INTRODUCTION

Alfred Blalock and Helen Taussig ushered in the surgical treatment of congenital heart disease with the introduction in clinical practice of a systemic artery-to-pulmonary artery shunt in 1944 (Fig. 54-1). In the current era of early complete correction of congenital heart disease, the Blalock-Taussig shunt still plays an important role in the surgical management of newborns and infants with malformed hearts.[1–3] Although this trend toward repair is founded in part on recognition of the complications associated with palliative procedures and the realization that infants can tolerate fully corrective procedures, some malformations have demonstrated improved results with a staged approach. A staged repair is often favored when there are extenuating technical issues that stem from morphologic complexity or severe extracardiac pathology that would make one-stage correction prohibitive. The functionally single ventricle (Chap. 69) is an example of this strategy, by which a staged palliative approach eventually achieves the goal of separating pulmonary and systemic circulations.

For any one anomaly amenable to early biventricular repair [for example, tetralogy of Fallot, pulmonary atresia, and ventricular septal defect (VSD) plus aortic coarctation and double-outlet right ventricle), there are very few randomized studies comparing staged repair to early complete repair, and those that do exist suffer from limited study power. In most centers palliation is furthermore usually reserved for sicker or smaller patients, making all comparisons subject to surgical bias.

Palliative procedures are primarily designed to alter pulmonary blood flow, enhance intracardiac mixing, or train a ventricle prior to definitive surgery. For example, aortopulmonary shunts will increase pulmonary blood flow, while a pulmonary artery band (PAB) will limit pulmonary perfusion. Despite often being considered lower-risk procedures, palliative operations often pose challenging issues of technique and patient management and are subject to nonnegligible operative complications and interoperative attrition rates.

SYSTEMIC-TO-PULMONARY SHUNTS

As early complete repair has become increasingly more common, indications for systemic-to-pulmonary artery shunts are in some respects controversial. However, there are some lesions with well-balanced ventricles and some duct-dependent single-ventricle lesions for which, in most centers, a shunt still remains as the initial procedure. In those instances, a systemic-to-pulmonary artery shunt may be an absolute necessity for early survival, at the expense of further procedures.

A systemic-to-pulmonary artery shunt could be indicated in any anomaly that presents with obstruction of blood flow either entering or exiting the right heart (in tricuspid or pulmonary stenosis or atresia, for example). Other indications include anomalies with unbalanced pulmonary blood flow where a systemic-to-pulmonary artery shunt (alone or, rarely, with a PAB) can also be used to reliably regulate pulmonary blood flow.

CLASSIC BLALOCK-TAUSSIG SHUNT

The development of palliative procedures began at the Johns Hopkins Hospital with the goal of providing improved blood flow to the pulmonary vascular bed in cyanotic children; the right subclavian-to-right pulmonary artery shunt was introduced clinically in 1944.[3] This method of systemic-to-pulmonary artery (PA) shunt followed the pioneering experimental work by Alfred Blalock and Vivien Thomas, who created a canine

THE SURGICAL TREATMENT OF MALFORMATIONS OF THE HEART

IN WHICH THERE IS PULMONARY STENOSIS OR PULMONARY ATRESIA

ALFRED BLALOCK, M.D.
AND
HELEN B. TAUSSIG, M.D.
BALTIMORE

Heretofore there has been no satisfactory treatment for pulmonary stenosis and pulmonary atresia. A "blue" baby with a malformed heart was considered beyond the reach of surgical aid. During the past three months we have operated on 3 children with severe degrees of pulmonary stenosis and each of the patients appears to be greatly benefited.

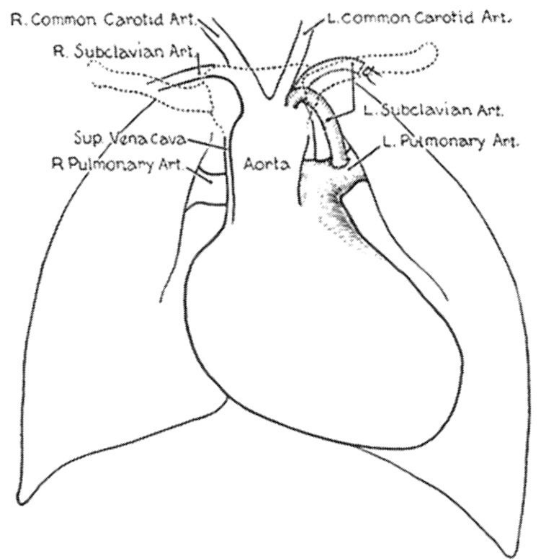

Fig. 3 (case 1).—Procedure used. The end of the left subclavian artery was anastomosed to the side of the left pulmonary artery.

Figure 54-1 Title page and Figure 3 from the original manuscript by Blalock and Taussig describing the first "Blue baby operation", performed at the Johns Hopkins Hospital on November 29th, 1944. (Reprinted with permission from: Blalock A, Taussig HB. The surgical treatment of malformations of the heart in which there is pulmonary stenosis or atresia. *JAMA* 1945;132:189.)

model of pulmonary artery hypertension by anastomosing the subclavian artery to the transected end of the PA; this concept was adopted as a palliative attempt to augment pulmonary blood flow in patients with tetralogy of Fallot. In the 2 years following the first successful case, hundreds of cyanotic children traveled to Baltimore to undergo a classic Blalock-Taussig shunt. The reported early mortality was 16 percent, and only 6 percent of the patients were refused surgery.

The shunt is classically performed on the side opposite the aortic arch by anastomosing the subclavian artery to the ipsilateral pulmonary artery in an end-to-side fashion. There is usually an innominate artery on the side opposite the aortic arch, and it provides adequate length and orientation to allow for the subclavian to form a gentle curve inferiorly toward the PA. Access to the subclavian artery is typically described via a thoracotomy (Fig. 54-

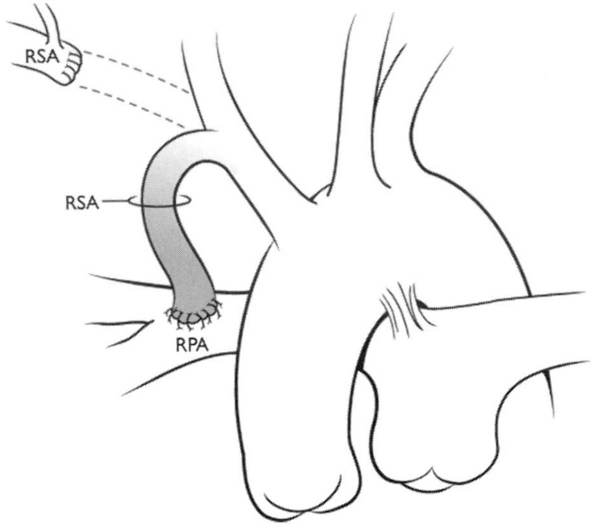

Figure 54-2 Classic Blalock-Taussig shunt. RPA = right pulmonary artery, RSA = right subclavian artery.

2). The branches of the subclavian artery are also ligated. Additional mobilization can be obtained by dissecting the proximal carotid artery. The subclavian artery is then brought through the loop of the recurrent laryngeal nerve and oriented down toward the pulmonary artery. The artery is spatulated and sewn to the main pulmonary artery. Division of the inferior pulmonary ligament will often help in facilitating this anastomosis.

The classic Blalock-Taussig shunt has the advantages of avoiding prosthetic materials, having a limited amount of flow, and growing with the child. However, in some this procedure may lead to arm or hand ischemia. At the time of corrective surgery, the shunt may be taken down via median sternotomy by entering the plane posterior to the superior vena cava (SVC).

MODIFIED BLALOCK-TAUSSIG SHUNT

A significant modification of the classic Blalock-Taussig shunt, first performed by Redo and Ecker in 1963, involved the interposition of a prosthetic graft to connect the systemic circulation to the PA (Fig. 54-3).[4–6] This procedure was later reported by Gazzaniga in 1976 and termed the "modified" Blalock-Taussig shunt by deLeval in 1975.[7] This modification provides several advantages over the standard Blalock-Taussig shunt: less tendency to deform hypoplastic pulmonary arteries, less need for mediastinal dissection, preservation of upper extremity blood flow, consistent shunt flow (regulated by the internal diameter of the ostia of the innominate or subclavian arteries), and adequate length. Disadvantages include a 10 to 15 percent incidence of seroma formation and the rare possibility of endocarditis or thrombosis (3 to 5 percent). Because of the significant advantages, the modified Blalock-Taussig shunt remains the most widely used systemic-to-

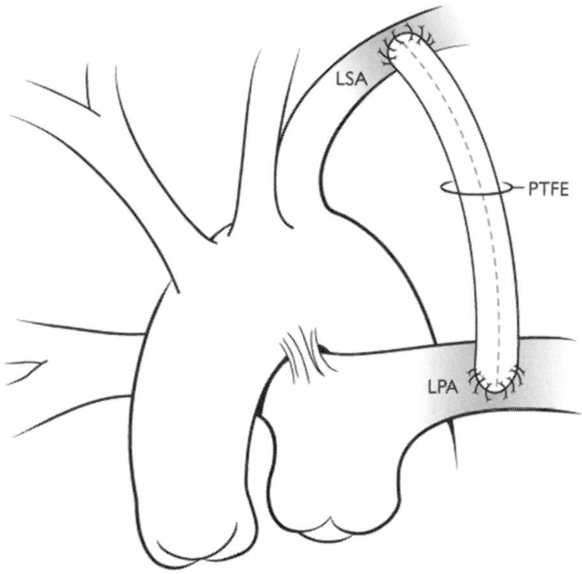

Figure 54-3 Modified Blalock-Taussig shunt. LPA = left pulmonary artery, LSA = left subclavian artery. PTFE = polytetrafluoreethylene shunt.

pulmonary shunt today. Initial concerns that there may be a risk of impaired growth of the contralateral PA have been discredited by current literature, which demonstrates that equivalent growth without distortion can be accomplished with the modified shunt.[5] Compared to the classic Blalock-Taussig shunt, the modified Blalock-Taussig shunt has a more predictable life span, which is limited by the lack of growth potential. These shunts are destined for short-interval use and generally require some other surgical intervention to provide a reliable source of pulmonary blood flow as the child grows.

The modified Blalock-Taussig shunt can be performed through either right or left thoracotomy, or via a median sternotomy. In reality, the decision to perform a sternotomy versus a thoracotomy is usually dictated by surgeon preference. However, in some circumstances the approach is dependent on the vascular anatomy and the location of the ductus arteriosus. The three different approaches have subtle advantages and disadvantages. Some authors have suggested that a right-sided shunt is easier to take down, while others suggest that a thoracotomy is preferred because, at the time of the next operation, the pericardium will be relatively free of adhesions. A median sternotomy allows for duct ligation, a shorter and more centrally located shunt with less distortion and eventual loss of the upper lobe pulmonary artery branch, and affords the ability to initiate cardiopulmonary bypass in case of hemodynamic instability or intolerable levels of hypoxemia.

In performing the procedure via thoracotomy, the chest is usually entered through the fourth intercostal space. The lung is retracted inferiorly and medially and the mediastinal pleura opened posterior to the SVC. The innominate and/or subclavian arteries are dissected free from the surrounding tissues and controlled with vessel loops. During this portion of the dissection, great care is taken to avoid the recurrent laryngeal nerve, which, on the right side, passes around the distal innominate artery at its bifurcation into subclavian and common carotid arteries. Next, the PA is mobilized, first proximally toward the pericardial reflection and then distally to the first bifurcation. The vessels are controlled with vascular tapes. An expanded polytetrafluoroethylene (ePTFE, Gore-Tex) graft is then beveled with scissors to conform to the natural curve of the systemic artery. A Cooley or Castaneda vascular clamp is applied to the subclavian artery, and an arteriotomy is made on the inferior aspect of the artery. The anastomosis is performed with 7-0 nonabsorbable monofilament suture in a running fashion. Some authors prefer systemic heparinization prior to systemic vessel clamping; we prefer to heparinize the patient after the first anastomosis is complete. The clamp is then repositioned on the graft to minimize systemic arterial trauma. If at this point the azygos vein lies in the direct path of the shunt, it is ligated and divided. The distal anastomosis is performed by first placing a stay suture in the direct center of the superior margin of the unmanipulated PA to make sure that there will be no torsion or kinking during occlusion. Prior to initiating the anastomosis, vascular tapes are used for a test occlusion of the PA. Once the surgeon is assured that the patient will tolerate single-lung perfusion, the pulmonary arteriotomy is made by excising a circular portion of the PA. The excised portion should be larger than the diameter of the graft so as to avoid distal stenosis. The graft is then cut to length, attempting to avoid any redundancy. The anastomosis is again performed with 7-0 monofilament nonabsorbable suture in a running fashion. Clamps and tapes are then released, hemostasis is assured, and the chest closed with an indwelling drain. There should be a nearly instantaneous increase in the patient's oxygen saturation and a drop in the diastolic blood pressure, with a palpable thrill in both shunt and pulmonary artery.

If a sternotomy is chosen, the sequence remains the same. Following sternotomy and thymectomy, the pericardium is left undisturbed and the innominate artery is mobilized to the bifurcation. A small pericardial incision is then made in order to mobilize the PA between the aorta and SVC. The anastomosis is performed as described above.

The size of the shunt is left to the surgeon's discretion. Most infants of normal birth weight require a 3.5-mm shunt. Infants weighing less than 3.5 kg should be treated with a shunt of no less than 3 mm. Larger infants may receive shunts as large as 4 or 5 mm, especially if it is performed through a thoracotomy. The decision is based upon the size of the patient and the alternate sources of pulmonary blood flow that exist.

Although originally described via thoracotomy (actually from the left), the sternotomy approach tends to be favored by most units. In addition to the benefits outlined above, it provides superior vascular exposure and likely reduces the potential for injuries to either recurrent nerve or phrenic nerve during both creation and takedown of the shunt. There is a substantial body of literature comparing the various techniques used to create a classic or modified Blalock-Taussig shunt. To date no randomized study has identified the best method to maximize advantages and minimize disadvantages. Regardless of the approach used to create the shunt, it is usually relatively straightforward to take down a modified Blalock-Taussig shunt through a median sternotomy at the time of the next procedure. A right-sided shunt can be found by dissecting the plane between the aorta and SVC. A left-sided shunt presents more difficulty at the time of takedown and is usually identified by dissecting along the left PA, the inferior aspect of the aorta, or by entering the pleural space. The ePTFE graft can be interrupted with hemoclips and simply divided. The distal end of the graft does not need to be removed unless access to the PA is required as part of the procedure (e.g., in case of a superior cavopulmonary anastomosis or a pulmonary arterioplasty).

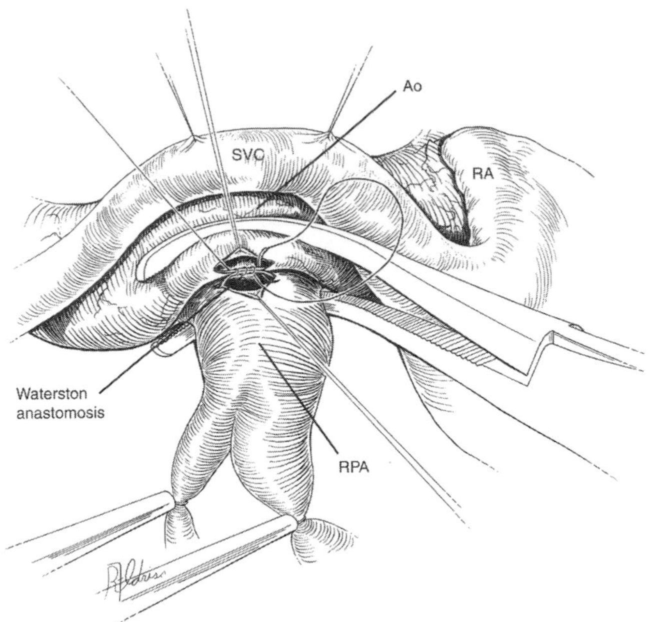

Figure 54-4 Waterston shunt. Side-to-side anastomosis between the ascending aorta and right branch pulmonary artery. Ao = ascending aorta, RA = right atrium, RPA = right pulmonary artery, SVC = superior vena cava. (From Kaiser LR, Kron IL, Spray TL (eds). *Mastery of Cardiothoracic Surgery*. Philadelphia: Lippincott-Raven, 1998:641. With permission.)

WATERSTON AND POTTS SHUNTS

The success of Blalock-Taussig procedure spawned a number of other systemic shunts. In 1946, Potts described an aortopulmonary shunt.[8] This shunt was performed by creating an anastomosis from the descending aorta to the left PA through a left thoracotomy in patients with a right-sided aortic arch. To facilitate this procedure, a special partial occluding clamp was devised to minimize the risk of paraplegia. The Potts shunt was used throughout the 1940s and 1950s in patients thought to be too small for a classic Blalock-Taussig shunt. The Potts shunt was also associated with several serious complications, including PA aneurysms and sizing difficulties, which often led to persistent cyanosis or chronic pulmonary hypertensive changes. In time, the Potts shunt was abandoned owing to its unnecessary difficulty and the risk associated with shunt takedown. Simple ligation of the shunt often leads to uncontrollable hemorrhage, requiring peripheral bypass and circulatory arrest to achieve control and repair.

In 1955 Davidson and colleagues first described a shunt from the ascending aorta to the PA. In 1962, Waterston reported a similar intrapericardial anastomosis between the posterior ascending aorta and the right PA (Fig. 54-4).[9] The procedure was performed through a right thoracotomy; the right PA and ascending aorta are both partially occluded with the same clamp. After making two opposing arteriotomies, the PA and ascending aorta were sewn side to side. This shunt was very effective in infants but was prone to PA kinking, with resultant unequal pulmonary blood flow and subsequent hypoplasia of the underperfused PA. The Waterston shunt is taken down intrapericardially at the time of definitive repair, the aorta is primarily closed, and the PA is patched.

In performing both the Waterston and Potts shunts, notorious difficulty was found in estimating the correct size that would prevent pulmonary hypertension or cyanosis. These shunts have been replaced by the central shunt (Fig. 54-5).

The central shunt is a modification of the Potts and Waterston shunts, created with an interpositioned ePTFE graft. These shunts are most often used when

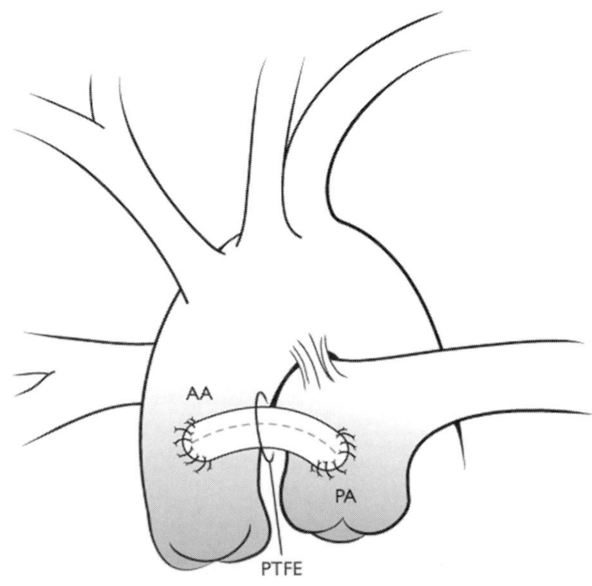

Figure 54-5 Central shunt. AA = ascending aorta, PA = pulmonary artery, PTFE = polytetrafluoroethylene shunt.

branch pulmonary arteries are small, in the hope of encouraging pulmonary arterial growth. In creating a central shunt, a small-caliber graft is preferable so as to avoid the potential for pulmonary overcirculation.

All systemic-to-PA shunts are designed to enhance pulmonary blood flow, but they also result in greater pulmonary venous return with subsequent left ventricular volume overload and an increase in left ventricular end–diastolic dimension. In general, it is necessary to replace the systemic inflow with a venous source at around 6 months of age in patients with single ventricle and by 2 years in patients with well-balanced ventricular chambers.

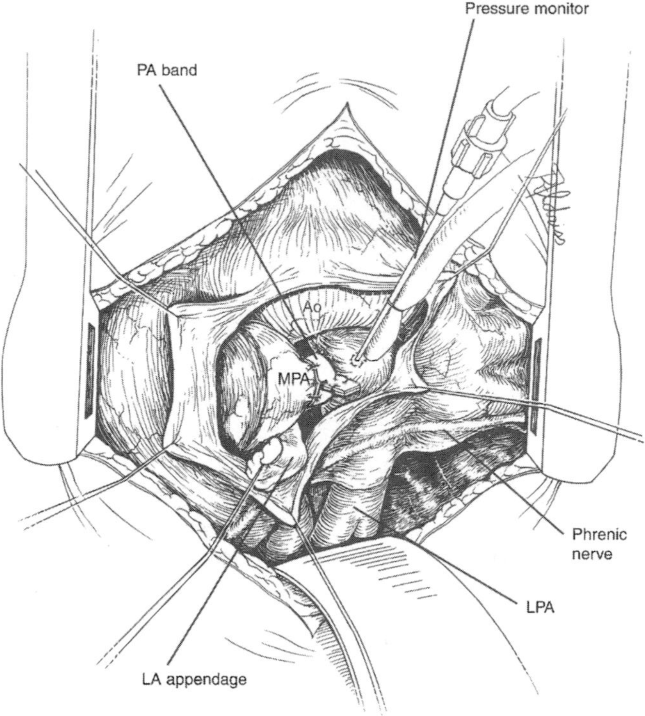

Figure 54-6 Pulmonary artery band. Seen through a left thoracotomy, with a pressure monitoring line inserted in the distal main pulmonary artery. Ao = aorta, LA = left atrial artery, LPA = left pulmonary artery, MPA = main pulmonary artery, PA = pulmonary artery. (From Kaiser LR, Kron IL, Spray TL (eds). *Mastery of Cardiothoracic Surgery*. Philadelphia: Lippincott-Raven, 1998:641. With permission.)

PULMONARY ARTERY BANDING

First conceived by Muller and Dammann in 1952, PA banding (Fig. 54-6) was the only treatment for complex congenital heart disease with unrestricted pulmonary blood flow (large left-to-right shunt or single ventricle with unrestrictive pulmonary blood flow).[10] For many years, the PA band (PAB) was the procedure of choice for large VSDs, atrioventricular canal, or truncus arteriosus. This form of palliation was initially effective, but it has fallen out of favor because of the increasing safety associated with primary repair of most lesions and also owing to some of the known complications associated with PA banding.

A few congenital lesions still lend themselves to primary palliation with PAB.[11,12] Current indications for PA banding include "swiss cheese" VSDs, multiple VSDs with coarctation, unbalanced atrioventricular septal defects in small patients, single-ventricle lesions, and to prepare the systemic ventricle for the arterial switch operation in cases with intact septum and late presentation. In most cases, the goal of PAB is to protect the pulmonary vascular bed from systemic or near systemic pressures associated with these lesions and to facilitate future venoarterial shunts or delayed complete repair.

The presence of a concurrent illness in a patient with an otherwise correctable lesion would be an acceptable reason for PAB placement. Patients with pulmonary overcirculation are more prone to respiratory illness and have less reserve to cope with viral illnesses such as pneumonia due to the respiratory syncytial virus (RSV). This disease state can last for weeks, often with the need for prolonged mechanical ventilation as the lungs recover; PAB in the short term may allow the child to improve and have the lesion corrected in a better clinical condition.

SURGICAL TECHNIQUE

Except in cases of aortic coarctation associated with a VSD not suitable for simultaneous repair, PAB is usually approached by most surgeons via a median sternotomy. After partial thymectomy, the pericardium is opened from the base of the innominate artery to the level of the pulmonary annulus. Pericardial stay sutures are placed to enhance exposure. The aorta and PA are carefully separated with cautery, and the PA is then encircled with careful blunt dissection. It is crucial to do as little vertical dissection between the aorta and PA as possible so as to minimize band migration. Although some authors recommend Teflon-impregnated Dacron, we use a 3.0-mm ePTFE conduit to create the band. We prefer this technique because the PTFE band causes less of an inflammatory response and can usually be removed off bypass without any further intervention on the debanded PA if the PAB has been in place for less than 6 months. In addition, we have found that where a VSD closes spontaneously during the period that the band is applied, the band can be removed in the cardiac catheterization laboratory by balloon dilatation, thus avoiding resternotomy. Bands constructed of either Teflon, silk or Dacron will often require a period of cardiopulmonary bypass with PA reconstruction in order to remove the band.

The banding material is advanced around the PA. The band is sequentially tightened using small Weck clips until the band is fixed to the desired circumference. In 1972, Mustard and Trusler introduced a formula to estimate the size of the band needed in patients with VSDs.[13] This formula suggested that the circumference of the band in millimeters should be equal to the child's weight in kilograms plus 20. This formula may be helpful as a guideline; however, intraoperative pressure measurements should be used to individualize the band size for each patient. The distal pulmonary arterial pressure should be reduced to somewhere between one-third and one-half of systemic, and systemic arterial saturations should remain between 75 and 85% on 50 percent inspired oxygen. The systemic pressure will usually increase by 10 to 15 mmHg after proper banding.

Several complications are specific to PA banding. Improper band sizing can produce pulmonary under- or overcirculation, with resulting congestive heart failure or cyanosis from excessive right-to-left shunting. However, this is an unusual problem if intraoperative pressures are taken correctly. Another possible complication is band migration. This problem may lead to impingement on the PA bifurcation, causing stenosis of one or both branch pulmonary arteries. It is most common for the right PA to be compromised during banding, producing left PA hypertension and right PA ostial stenosis. Banding of the PA has been also associated with injury to the left phrenic nerve at the time of PAB placement or reentry. This is, of course, particularly detrimental in patients with functionally single ventricles staged toward Fontan-type physiology. Last, in palliating single-ventricle lesions with a posteriorly displaced conal septum, banding is thought to contribute to obstruction of left ventricular outflow.

VENOARTERIAL SHUNTS

The goal of a venoarterial shunt is to improve oxygenation by channeling the systemic venous return in part or in whole to the pulmonary vasculature. These procedures are commonly used in patients with a cyanotic defect who are tracking to a Fontan-type procedure or total cavopulmonary connection (see Chap. 69). Glenn first introduced the principle of systemic venous-to-PA connections, effectively bypassing the ventricle.[14] The connection is an end-to-end SVC-to-right PA anastomosis. The Glenn shunt provides reliable pulmonary blood flow and relieves the volume overload on the left ventricle imposed by left-to-right and systemic-to-pulmonary shunts. Furthermore, it unloads the right ventricle in cases of right ventricular hypoplasia and Ebstein's malformation of the tricuspid valve (see Chaps. 62 and 76). This palliative procedure is particularly useful in young infants thought not to be candidates for a single-stage procedure. The classic Glenn procedure (Fig. 54-7) was later followed by the bidirectional Glenn (Fig. 54-8), a modification in which an end-to-side PA anastomosis is created.[15] The major limitation to early palliation with a Glenn-type anastomosis is the need for low pressures in the pulmonary bed, which are usually not present until 3 or 4 months of age.

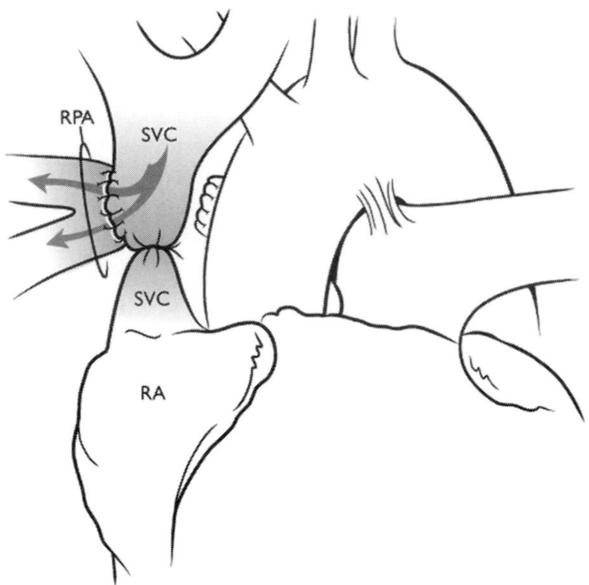

Figure 54-7 Classic Glenn superior cavopulmonary connection. RA = right atrium, RPA = right pulmonary artery, SVC = superior vena cava.

Although initially successful, the classic Glenn procedure fell out of favor as a definitive procedure when the Fontan total caval pulmonary connection was popularized for patients with single-ventricle physiology. Although a trend toward early completion of a total cavopulmonary connection (at less than 2 years of age) has been established, not all children are ideal candidates for immediate bicaval connection to the PA. In these patients, a superior cavopulmonary anastomosis became an intermediate step in management of the single ventricle. The usual palliative sequence is the creation of a systemic-to-pulmonary shunt for palliation in the neonatal period, followed by a Glenn or hemi-Fontan (see Chap. 70) connection at around 6 months of age and, last, by completion of the Fontan operation when the child reached about 15 kg in size.

SURGICAL TECHNIQUE, BIDIRECTIONAL GLENN

The approach is typically through a sternotomy. Following reoperative sternotomy, sharp dissection is undertaken to gain control of the systemic-to-pulmonary shunt. Next, the right PA and SVC (including division of the azygos vein) are fully mobilized. Stay sutures are placed in the lateral extent of the SVC and the exact midpoint of the

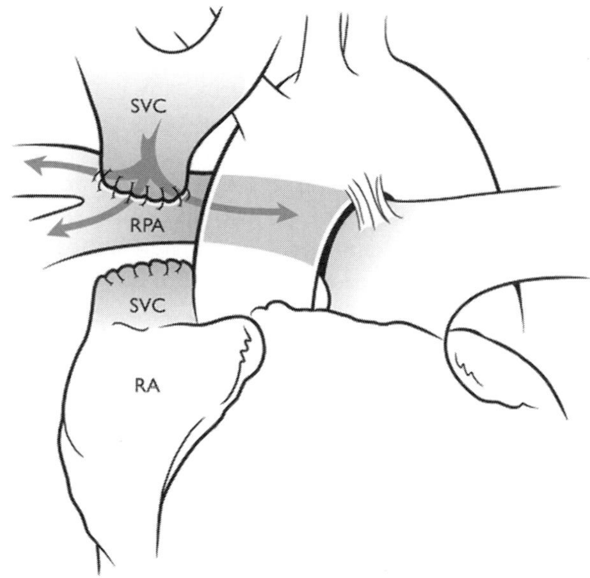

Figure 54-8 Bidirectional Glenn cavopulmonary anastomosis. RA = right atrium, RPA = right pulmonary artery, SVC = superior vena cava.

superior portion of the PA to avoid distraction during clamping. The patient is then systemically heparinized. Cardiopulmonary bypass is routinely initiated with aortic and venous cannulas. Of the two venous cannulas, one is placed in the very proximal SVC or innominate vein while another is either placed at the inferior atriocaval junction (if a concomitant transatrial procedure is required) or through the right atrial appendage. Alternatively, a shunt can be utilized between SVC and right atrium, while in rare instances (when redundant blood flow to the pulmonary vasculature exists) the procedure can be performed by avoiding shunting or cardiopulmonary bypass altogether.

As bypass is instituted and the systemic-to-pulmonary shunt is ligated, the cardiac portion of the SVC is cross-clamped, divided, and oversewn with great care not to injure the sinus node. In the case of a previous Blalock-Taussig shunt, the graft-to-PA anastomosis is taken down and the arteriotomy widened so that the caliber is larger than that of the SVC. The anastomosis is performed in a running fashion, taking care to avoid purse stringing the suture line. In cases were purse stringing appears likely, intermittent locking sutures or interrupted sutures may prove useful. This portion of the procedure is usually performed at normothermia with the heart beating. Cardioplegic arrest may be necessary if an atrial septectomy or tricuspid valve repair is required. At the conclusion of bypass, it is important to monitor both SVC pressure and arterial saturation. In cases where the arterial saturation is intolerably low or the SVC pressure is significantly elevated, a technical problem should be considered. If no technical error can be identified and the arterial saturation is unresponsive to ventilatory or pharmacologic manipulation, placement of a small additional systemic-to-pulmonary shunt may be considered. The need for postoperative anticoagulation is a controversial subject, but most authors usually recommend at least the use of antiaggregant therapy.

The Glenn shunt has a reported operative mortality of 4 to 5 percent and can sustain palliation for 5 to 7 years.[16] Patients normally maintain saturations in the low to mid 80s, which generally persist to the fourth year of life, when cyanosis becomes symptomatic. A well-known complication of the superior cavopulmonary connection is the development of venovenous collaterals (superior to inferior vena cava) which result in shunting of the upper body venous return away from the PA to the right atrium and hence accelerated cyanosis. Once this condition becomes evident, the patient should undergo evaluation for completion of the total cavopulmonary connection.

ATRIAL SEPTECTOMY AND SEPTOSTOMY

For some lesions, palliation can be provided by increasing the intracardiac mixing of venous and arterial blood. This can be accomplished either through a surgical atrial septectomy or a percutaneous balloon or blade septostomy. There are various ways of performing a surgical septectomy without cardiopulmonary bypass. The Blalock-Hanlon septectomy was first performed in 1950 through a right thoracotomy.[17] The right and left atrium are occluded with a single clamp. The atria are opened within the clamp with two parallel incisions (on either side of the septum); a portion of the atrial septum is then grasped and excised. The clamp is repositioned to allow the septum to fall back into the atria, and the resulting common atriotomy is then closed. With few exceptions, this difficult and often high-risk procedure is no longer performed. Another technique for performing a surgical septectomy is that of inflow occlusion. This is usually performed through a median sternotomy. To perform this operation, the SVC and the inferior vena cava are both encircled with a heavy tie, which can be snared. A large purse-string suture is placed in the right atrial appendage and the patient is placed in the head-down position. Both cavae are then snared and the heart beats for about 5 to 10 s, at which time the aorta is cross-clamped. The right atrium is opened within the boundary of the large purse-string suture. The tissue in the fossa ovalis is then excised. With the purse-string suture still open, the cavae are unsnared and the right atrium fills with blood and de-airs the heart. The purse-string suture in the atrium is closed and the aorta is unclamped. The whole procedure should take less than 60 s of cross clamping.

Most patients who now require correction of an atrial septal defect (e.g., transposition of the great arteries without VSD) undergo a Rashkind balloon septostomy. The procedure is usually performed under either fluoroscopic or echocardiographic guidance.[18] The septostomy itself is accomplished by passing a balloon-tipped catheter via the femoral vein across the foramen ovale. The balloon is inflated and rapidly pulled back. Because the procedure is performed with an imaging study, the effectiveness of the shunt can be assessed immediately, and the septostomy can be repeated if the result is suboptimal. In patients with a thick atrial septum recalcitrant to balloon septostomy, an atrial septectomy can be performed alternatively.[19–21]

SUMMARY

Despite the current trend to perform early correction of most cardiac lesions, palliative procedures remain an indispensable tool in the armamentarium of the surgeon treating congenital heart disease. These operations are designed to alter pulmonary blood flow, augment intracardiac mixing, or train a downregulated ventricle. In some cases, several procedures are performed in sequence as part of a multistage palliation strategy or with the aim of delaying complete intracardiac repair. Each of these procedures is associated with drawbacks and specific complications, making complete repair of malformed hearts with well-balanced ventricles ideal.

References

1. Najm HK, Van Arsdell GS, Watzka S, et al. Primary repair is superior to initial palliation in children with atrioventricular septal defect and tetralogy of Fallot. *J Thorac Cardiovasc Surg* 1998;116:905–913.
2. Cardiac surgery of the neonate and infant. In: Castaneda AR, Jonas RA, Mayer JE, Hanley FL (eds). Philadelphia: Saunders, 1994:270–271.
3. Blalock A, Taussig HB. The surgical treatment of malformations of the heart in which there is pulmonary artery stenosis or pulmonary atresia. *JAMA* 1945;128:189.
4. Gladman G, McCrindle BW, Williams WG, et al. The modified Blalock-Taussig shunt: Clinical impact and morbidity in Fallot's tetralogy in the current era. *J Thorac Cardiovasc Surg* 1997;114:25–30.
5. Jahangiri M, Lincoln C, Shinebourne EA. Does the modified Blalock-Taussig shunt cause growth of the contralateral pulmonary artery? *Ann Thorac Surg* 1999;67:1397–1399.
6. Bove EL, Kohman L, Sereika S, et al. The modified Blalock-Taussig shunt: Analysis of adequacy and duration of palliation. *Circulation* 1987;76(Suppl):III1923.
7. DeLeval MR, Mckay R, Jones M, et al. Modified Blalock-Taussig shunt. *J Thorac Cardiovasc Surg* 1981;81:112.
8. Potts WJ, Smith S, Gibson S. Anastomosis of aorta to pulmonary artery: Certain types in congenital heart disease. *JAMA* 1945;132:627.
9. Waterston DJ. Treatment of Fallot's tetralogy in infants under the age of 1 year. *Rozhl Chir* 1962;41:181.
10. Muller WH Jr, Danimann JF Jr. The treatment of certain congenital malformations of the heart by creation of pulmonic stenosis to reduce pulmonary hypertension and excessive pulmonary blood flow: A preliminary report. *Surg Gyencol Obstet* 1952;95:213–219.
11. Amin Z, Backer CL, Duffy CE. Does banding of the pulmonary artery affect pulmonary valve function after the Damus-Kaye-Stansel operation? *Ann Thorac Surg* 1998;66:836–841.
12. Takayama H, Sekiguchi A, Chikada M, et al. Mortality of pulmonary artery banding in the current era: Recent artery mortality of PA banding. *Ann Thorac Surg* 2002;74:1219–1223.
13. Albus RA, Trusler GA, Izukawa T, et al. Pulmonary artery banding. *J Thorac Cardiovasc Surg* 1984;88: 645–653.
14. Glenn WW, Patino JF. Circulatory bypass of the right heart. IV. Shunt between superior vena cava and distal right pulmonary artery: Report of clinical applications. *N Engl J Med* 1958;259:117–123.
15. Pizarro C, DeLeval MR. Surgical variations and flow dynamics in cavopulmonary connections: A historical review. *Semin Thorac Cardiovasc Surg Pediatr Cardiac Surg Annu* 1998;1:53–60.
16. Kouchoukos NT, Blackstone EH, Doty DB, et al (eds). *Kirklin/Barratt-Boyes Cardiac Surgery*, 3d ed. Philadelphia: Churchill Livingstone, 2003:1140.
17. Blalock A, Hanlon CR. Surgical treatment of complete transposition of the aorta and pulmonary artery. *Surg Gynecol Obstet* 1950;90:1–15.
18. Rashkind WJ, Miller WW. Creation of an atrial septal defect without thoracotomy: A palliative approach to complete transposition of the great vessels. *JAMA* 1966;196: 991–992.
19. Kaiser LR, Kron IL, Spray TL (eds). *Mastery of Cardiothoracic Surgery.* Philadelphia: Lippincott-Raven, 1998:635.
20. del Nido PJ, Wilian WG, Coles JG, et al. Closed heart surgery for congenital heart disease in infancy. *Clin Perinatol* 1988;15:681–697.
21. Perry SB, Lang P, Keane JF, et al. Creation and maintenance of an adequate interatrial communication in left atrioventricular valve atresia or stenosis. *Am J Cardiol* 1986;15:622–626.

CHAPTER

55 PATENT DUCTUS ARTERIOSUS

Tain-Yen Hsia, Jeffrey J. Wu, Richard Ringel

INTRODUCTION

The ductus arteriosus is a normal vascular connection between the pulmonary arterial trunk and the proximal descending thoracic aorta, and an essential component of the fetal circulation. During fetal life, it allows right-to-left shunting of maternally derived oxygenated placental blood to the systemic circulation, bypassing the high-resistance pulmonary bed. Following birth, increases in oxygen tension and a drop in pulmonary vascular resistance trigger spontaneous closure (contraction and subsequent fibrosis) of the ductus. Patent ductus arteriosus (PDA) is the persistence of the ductus as a vascular structure (rather than a ligamentous connection) beyond the early neonatal period, leading to unabated left-to-right shunting between the aorta and pulmonary artery with subsequent pulmonary overcirculation.

With an incidence of between 1 in 2500 to 5000 births, PDA is the second most common congenital cardiac malformation.[1] While recognition of the presence of the ductus arteriosus during fetal circulation dates to Galen, it was not until 1907 that John Monro first suggested surgical ligation of PDA in an address to the Philadelphia Academy of Surgery.[2] Thirty-one years later, in 1938, the first operation was attempted by Graybiel and Stieder in a 22-year-old woman with

KEY CONCEPTS

- **Epidemiology**
  - The ductus arteriosus is a normal fetal structure, arising from the left sixth aortic arch, connecting the left main pulmonary artery to the upper descending thoracic aorta. Persistent patency beyond the neonatal period occurs in approximately 1 in 2500 term live births, with a male-to-female ratio of 2:1. Patent ductus arteriosus (PDA) accounts for 5 to 10 percent of all congenital heart defects, with up to 30 percent of cases observed in preterm infants.
- **Pathophysiology**
  - The presence of a large, nonrestrictive PDA leads to left-to-right shunting with pulmonary overcirculation, subsequent left atrial dilatation, left ventricular volume overload, and congestive heart failure; if left untreated, irreversible pulmonary hypertension and Eisenmenger's physiology with right-to-left shunting and cyanosis ultimately ensue.
- **Clinical features**
  - Presentation may range from absence of symptoms to the presence of a "machinery-like" murmur with poor feeding, failure to thrive, tachypnea, and recurrent respiratory infections.
- **Diagnosis**
  - Chest x-ray typically discloses increased pulmonary vascular markings, pulmonary edema, and cardiomegaly. Transthoracic echocardiography demonstrates the ductal anatomy and any coexisting defects.
- **Treatment**
  - Treatment strategies include pharmacologic closure with indomethacin in premature infants, catheter-based closure with coil occlusion in older children and adults, video-assisted thoracoscopic closure, and conventional thoracotomy and ligation. Whereas operative outcomes in premature newborns are heavily dependent on associated comorbidities, morbidity and mortality from surgical or percutaneous closure in infants and children are almost negligible.

bacterial endocarditis involving the arterial duct.[3] Although the PDA was successfully ligated, the patient succumbed to infection and gastrointestinal complications a week later. Robert Gross reported, later in that same year, the first surgical cure for a congenital cardiac defect by ligating a duct in a 7-year-old child with severe heart failure.[4] This heralded an amazing era of innovation and discovery in the surgical treatment of congenital heart disease. Although a PDA can today be interrupted through interventional or minimally invasive techniques, operative ligation remains a model of finest surgical practice: predictable anatomy, minimal morbidity, and excellent outcomes.

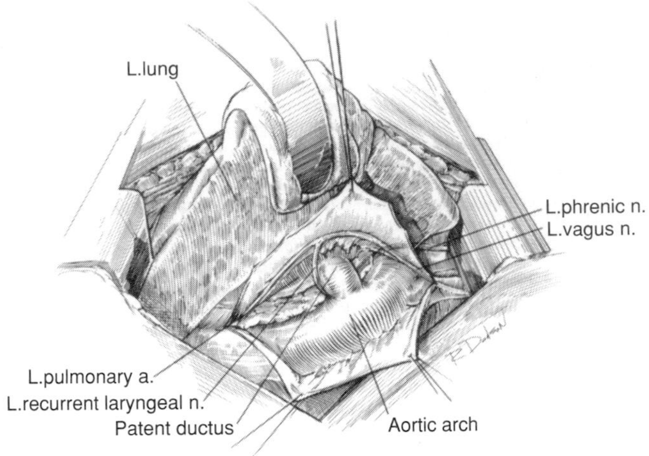

Figure 55-1 Patent ductus arteriosus and contiguous structures through a left thoracotomy (surgeon's perspective). [From Castaneda AR, Jonas RA, Mayer JE, Hanley FL (eds). *Cardiac Surgery of the Neonate and Infant.* Philadelphia: Saunders, 1994:208. With permission.]

ANATOMY AND EMBRYOLOGY

Early in fetal development, the aortic sac is connected to paired dorsal aortae through six arterial arches (see Chap. 75).[5,6] The normal ductus arteriosus develops from the dorsal portion of the left sixth arch. However, because of the bilateral symmetry of the arterial system, arterial ducts can be bilateral or absent, right- or left-sided (the latter being by far the most common variant). The sixth arches develop from the plexus of capillaries that supply the developing buds. These capillaries initially arise from the aortic sac but later join the dorsal aorta. When the arterial segments separate to form the aorta and pulmonary trunk, the sixth arches remain connected to the pulmonary trunk. On the right, the dorsal sixth arch regresses and the ventral portion becomes the proximal right pulmonary artery. On the left, the ventral sixth arch is incorporated into the main pulmonary trunk, while the dorsal portion remains to become the ductus arteriosus.

The fetal ductus arteriosus normally originates from the pulmonary trunk as a continuation of the lesser curve of the aortic arch, a few millimeters distal and opposite to the origin of the left subclavian artery. It is a short, wide vessel of variable length, lying posteriorly to the left main bronchus with the vagus nerve coursing anterior to it. When there is a right-sided aortic arch, the ductus usually arises from the proximal descending aorta in conjunction with the left subclavian artery. The pulmonary end of the ductus is narrower than the aortic end and is invested by the pericardial reflection, while the aortic end is invested by the parietal pleura. The length of the ductus in infancy varies between 2 and 8 mm, with the diameter ranging from 4 to 12 mm. The left recurrent laryngeal nerve branches off the vagus and encircles the inferomedial wall of the duct before ascending behind the aortic arch into the tracheoesophageal groove (Fig. 55-1).

The wall of the ductus arteriosus differs histologically from that of the adjoining aorta and pulmonary artery. Instead of the circumferential layers of elastic fibers, the media of the ductus is made up of smooth muscle cells arranged into a poorly organized spiral outer layer and a longitudinal inner layer that protrudes centrally to join the intima at "cushion" points. Large gaps between intimal cushions are filled with mucinous substance and called "mucoid lakes." The internal elastic intima is thicker than that of other vascular structures, forming wavy layers adjacent to the intimal cushions. The medial smooth muscle is particularly sensitive to PGE_1 and PGI_2, which cause relaxation and dilatation as well as increased oxygen tension, which promotes ductal constriction.[7,8]

The first stage of ductal closure occurs within 15 to 20 h of birth. This is triggered by a rapid decrease of prostaglandins (due to loss of maternal supply) and accelerated metabolism (by increased pulmonary blood flow). In addition, increased PaO_2 inhibits prostaglandin synthetase, further blunting the level of circulating prostaglandins. The physiologic consequence of these changes is contraction of the smooth muscle in the ductal wall media, with subsequent thrombosis. The second stage of ductal closure is completed within 2 to 3 weeks of birth. This occurs by fibrous proliferation in the intima with necrosis of the inner layer of the media and hemorrhage into the wall. Development of neointimal mounds is stimulated by vascular endothelial growth factor. The result is the permanent sealing of the lumen and the development of a fibrous ligamentum arteriosum. The ductus is closed by 8 weeks of age in 88 percent of infants with a normal cardiovascular system. Failure of this process results in persistent patency of the ductus arteriosus. Because of the immaturity of the ductal tissue, preterm infants respond poorly to increases in oxygen tension and therefore become the patient population at highest risk of developing PDA persistence. Inability of the immature lungs to clear circulating vasodilators may also contribute to ductal persistence. The incidence of PDA increases from 7 percent in very low birth weight infants to as high as 42 percent in extremely low birth weight neonates.

CLINICAL PRESENTATION

As pulmonary vascular resistance falls shortly after birth, increased left-to-right shunting across the PDA results in decreased systemic perfusion and a high left ventricular volume load, with decreased pulmonary compliance. The magnitude of the shunt (Qp:Qs) depends on the size of the ductus as well as on the balance between systemic and pulmonary vascular resistance. In the absence of fixed pulmonary hypertension, when Qp:Qs is low, the hemodynamic effect of the PDA is insignificant, and physiologic derangements are minimal. With a hemodynamically significant PDA, Qp:Qs is high, and increased pulmonary runoff in systole and diastole becomes detrimental to systemic pressure, leading to end-organ malperfusion. Furthermore, high pulmonary blood flow increases pulmonary artery pressure and, if left uncorrected, can lead to permanent pulmonary vascular disease. The clinical features of a hemodynamically significant PDA are similar to those of left-sided heart failure, with tachypnea, frequent respiratory infections, pulmonary edema, and failure to thrive. Premature infants with a PDA may present with substantial metabolic acidosis, oliguria, respiratory decompensation, and necrotizing enterocolitis.

A hemodynamically insignificant PDA may present subtly later in life. In this setting, left ventricular failure does not develop and symptoms are absent in infancy and childhood. A murmur is usually detected on routine physical examination, leading to the echocardiographic diagnosis of PDA.

A rare late mode of presentation of a PDA is infective endocarditis. The presence of a PDA may alter the local vascular immune response mechanisms or cause endothelial damage, providing a nidus for bacterial colonization. In the preantibiotics era, the average age of death in patients with a PDA surviving beyond infancy was 36 years, and infective endocarditis accounted for 45 percent of such deaths.[9]

DIAGNOSIS

Physical examination and echocardiography represent the cornerstones for the diagnosis of PDA. The patient will present with a widened pulse pressure, a hyperactive precordium, and an occasional systolic thrill. A continuous "machinery-like" murmur radiating from the pulmonic area to the midclavicle is characteristic. Electrocardiography may demonstrate left ventricular

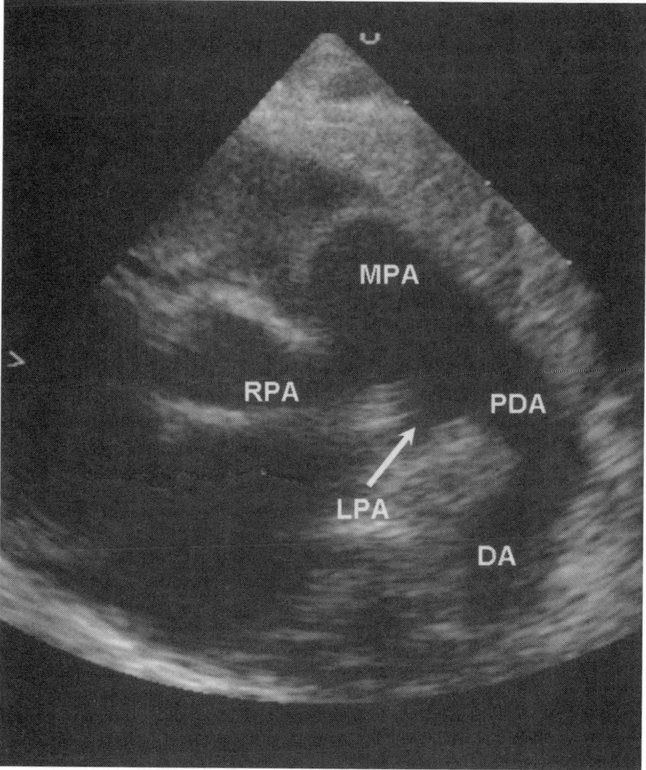

Figure 55-2 Echocardiographic image of a patent ductus arteriosus from a high parasternal view. DAO = descending aorta, AI = aortic isthmus, PDA = patent ductus arteriosus. (Courtesy of William Ravekes, MD, Division of Pediatric Cardiology, the Johns Hopkins Hospital.)

hypertrophy and left atrial enlargement. Chest radiography may show cardiomegaly with increased pulmonary markings and enlarged pulmonary trunk. Transthoracic Doppler echocardiography is diagnostic, showing the accelerated, narrow jet flow originating from the proximal descending aorta into the left pulmonary artery (Fig. 55-2). Cardiac catheterization is currently reserved for interventional device closure after echocardiographic diagnosis. Catheterization is also indicated in the older child with a large ductus and cyanosis due to right-to-left shunting at the ductal level, in order to define the reversibility of pulmonary hypertension. If pulmonary resistance is over 75 percent of systemic and is unresponsive to nitric oxide and oxygen administration, PDA closure is contraindicated.

SURGICAL TREATMENT

Traditionally, the presence of a PDA is an indication for closure. With the improved sensitivity of diagnostic modalities, the very small and hemodynamically insignificant ductus can be detected. While likely not warranting early intervention, small PDAs can still be a potential site for bacterial endarteritis and will require monitoring.

Treatment strategies include pharmacologic closure, percutaneous closure in the catheterization laboratory, video-assisted thoracoscopic (VATS) hemoclip occlusion, and conventional open posterolateral thoracotomy with ligation. Percutaneous closure is effective in the treatment of children and adults with PDA. Primary surgical closure is reserved for premature newborns, small infants, and patients who have failed device closure. A randomized trial has demonstrated that early surgical ligation of PDA in neonates reduces the need for mechanical ventilation and oxygen supplementation, shortens hospital stay, and decreases the incidence of retrolental fibroplasia and necrotizing enterocolitis when compared to pharmacologic closure.[10] However, initial attempt at pharmacologic PDA closure remains the initial therapeutic modality at most institutions.

Pharmacologic treatment is successful in achieving PDA closure in up to 60 percent of premature infants.[5] A combined strategy of fluid restriction, diuretics, and indomethacin is used. Indomethacin has been utilized clinically since 1976 to facilitate ductal closure in premature infants[11] but is rarely successful in full-term neonates. Contraindications to indomethacin use in preterm infants include hyperbilirubinemia, sepsis, coagulopathy, gastrointestinal bleeding, and renal insufficiency. If indomethacin use is contraindicated or fails, surgical closure is undertaken. Preterm infants typically undergo two to three courses of indomethacin (12 to 24 h apart) before being considered for surgical closure.

Early operative PDA closure carries low operative morbidity and mortality. Ductal ligation is now frequently performed at the bedside in the neonatal intensive care unit in order to minimize the risks of hypothermia and transport of the critically ill neonate. Several series have in fact reported results of bedside PDA closure to be comparable to those of procedures performed in the operating room.[12] Surgical intervention in the premature infant requires close attention to maintenance of body temperature, precise ventilatory management, and fluid administration. The size and shape of the ductus can be variable. A wide, short ductus can be difficult to ligate, whereas a long, tortuous ductus is easier to interrupt. The ductal tissue in neonates tends to be extremely fragile and therefore must be handled with great caution. Care should be taken to avoid scissoring through the ductus with overaggressive ligation. A short, wide ductus may be better divided between clamps if tissue integrity is a concern. As described previously, the left recurrent laryngeal nerve makes its loop around the ductus. Care must be taken to identify and protect this nerve during surgical closure.

In the setting of a left-sided aortic arch, the patient should be positioned in the right lateral decubitus position with the left arm supported over the head to elevate the scapula. The chest is entered through a left posterolateral thoracotomy, with division of the muscle layers and entrance into the third or fourth intercostal space. The left lung is retracted anteriorly with a narrow malleable retractor, and the mediastinal pleura is incised over the descending aorta. The left recurrent laryngeal nerve should be identified and preserved. Extensive dissection of the ductus itself should be avoided owing to the friable nature of the tissue. The left pulmonary artery, arch of the aorta, and subclavian artery should all be carefully identified (Fig. 55-2). The ductus is frequently larger than the aortic arch and isthmus. The most common technical error is the inadvertent ligation of the left pulmonary artery, which is mistaken for the ductus. The pleura is incised just above and below the ductus using fine scissors. We prefer to apply a hemoclip to close the PDA (Fig. 55-3); however, if the duct is unusually large or the patient is an older infant or child, it may be encircled with silk ties, doubly ligated, and divided. Prior to ductal ligation, test occlusion of the ductus with DeBakey forceps should be performed. A rise in diastolic pressure should be noted, as well as maintained pulsatility in the descending aorta and unaltered oximetric signal in the lower extremities. A medium-sized hemoclip is applied, with the tip of the clip visible posteriorly beyond the inferior margin of the ductus. The mediastinal pleura is typically left open. A chest tube may be placed if there is concern for pulmonary parenchymal injury. Several specific considerations should be made for adults presenting with a PDA. Historical series from the 1960s suggest that 40 percent of patients with untreated PDA would die by age 45 because of chronic pulmonary vascular disease or Eisenmenger's syndrome. When patients present in

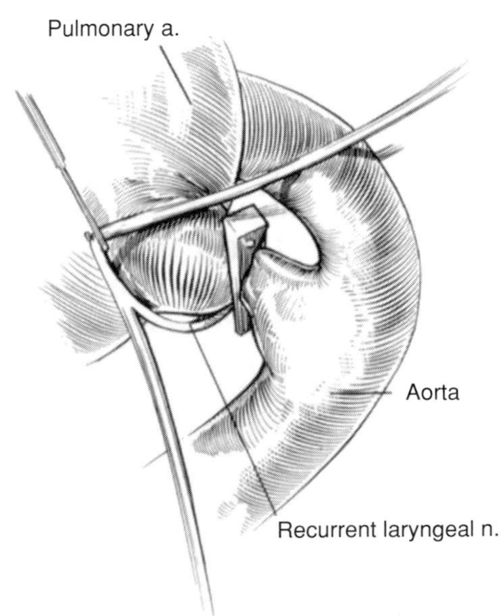

Figure 55-3 A hemoclip is utilized to interrupt the patent ductus arteriosus in premature infants. [From Castaneda AR, Jonas RA, Mayer JE, Hanley FL (eds). *Cardiac Surgery of the Neonate and Infant.* Philadelphia: Saunders, 1994:209. With permission.]

adulthood, diagnostic catheterization should be performed to determine operability by assessing the degree of pulmonary hypertension and responsiveness to nitric oxide and oxygen. Since adult patients may have significant calcification of the ductus, the PDA should be approached through a median sternotomy with cardiopulmonary bypass. A median sternotomy may also be useful in patients with a wide, short PDA. The transpulmonary artery approach described by Goncalves-Estella[13] with support of cardiopulmonary bypass can be used in these cases, with temporary occlusion of the branch pulmonary arteries. The aorta and the main pulmonary arterial trunk are dissected apart. Cardiopulmonary bypass is established with a single venous cannula and aortic return line, cooling is begun, and the patient is placed in the Trendelenburg position. The opening of the ductus is controlled by digital compression on the pulmonary arterial confluence, avoiding excessive pulmonary arterial runoff on institution of corporeal circulation. When adequate systemic cooling is achieved, low-flow cardiopulmonary bypass is instituted. The pulmonary artery is opened and the incision extended onto the left pulmonary artery opposite the orifice of the PDA. The ductal opening is next closed with pledgeted mattress sutures if no calcification is present. If significant calcification of the pulmonary arterial end of the ductus is noted, the orifice should be closed using a bovine pericardial or Dacron patch. Alternatively, the duct can be controlled with a balloon-tipped catheter inserted though the pulmonary artery into the descending aorta at low-flow perfusion. In a variation of this technique, a patch can be slid over the catheter and secured in place.[14]

Aneurysmal dilatation of the arterial duct has been described, with potential risks of rupture, erosion, infection, and thromboembolism. Neonatal ductal aneurysms usually resolve spontaneously by thrombosis. Any patients above 2 months of age with a ductal aneurysm should undergo prompt surgical repair. These patients may present with hoarseness from recurrent laryngeal nerve traction, vocal cord paralysis, or obstruction of the left mainstem bronchus. Surgical treatment is performed on cardiopulmonary bypass, with aneurysmal excision and patch aortoplasty under circulatory arrest.

The first VATS PDA closure was performed in 1991 by Laborde.[15] Video-assisted closure can be performed with three to four small incisions for instrumentation. Port incisions are placed in a line to facilitate posterolateral thoracotomy extension should conversion to a conventional approach be required. This innovative approach minimizes chest wall trauma, division of muscular planes, and rib retraction. The ductus is dissected free of surrounding tissues, the recurrent laryngeal nerve is identified, and the duct is interrupted with clips. Good results from VATS closure have been obtained in low-birth-weight infants. Purported advantages are reduced patient discomfort and hospital length of stay. This technique has been used in neonates, children, and adults. In Laborde's series of 332 consecutive pediatric patients, mortality was zero, with minimal morbidity.

Closure with robotic assistance has also been performed. The limitations, however, are due to the physically large size of the instruments, requiring 7-mm ports. Current robotic systems use widely spaced operating arms, thus limiting their use to adults. No tactile feedback is available to indicate to the surgeon the degree of force applied.

Results of surgery with a traditional posterolateral thoracotomy approach have a long-standing record of providing a durable repair with minimal morbidity and mortality. In 1994, Mavroudis and coworkers reported the results of the traditional surgical approach at their institution between 1947 and 1993.[16] This series included 1108 patients who underwent ligation and division of a PDA. There were no mortalities and no recurrences. The authors concluded that these results represent the standard of care to which video-assisted and catheter-based closure should be compared. Recent series describing results with the VATS approach have shown comparable results with minimal residual shunts and no important complications.[14] Only three patients in a series of 300 endoscopic cases required conversion to a standard posterolateral thoracotomy, and only two experienced transient functional impairment of the recurrent laryngeal nerve.

TRANSCATHETER OCCLUSION OF A PATENT DUCTUS ARTERIOSUS

The first nonsurgical PDA closure was reported by Porstmann in 1967.[18] Closure was accomplished by implantation of an expandable plug within the arterial duct. Although the required delivery system was much too large to be of practical use in small children, this report pointed to the possibility that repair of congenital heart defects could be accomplished by transcatheter techniques. Twelve years later, Rashkind developed a double umbrella device to close the ductus arteriosus of a 3.5-kg infant.[19] Clinical trials met with some success, but rates of residual leakage and technical difficulties precluded wide acceptance or FDA approval of the device. In 1992, Gianturco embolization coils (Cook Inc., Bloomington, IN) were first used to produce embolization of the ductus arteriosus by modification of the technique used in the preceding decade to embolize fistulae, arteriovenous malformations, and other vascular abnormalities. Cambier and colleagues reported the first case of successful transcatheter PDA coil embolization in 1992.[20] This technique immediately gained wide popularity for its low cost, excellent safety, efficacy, and for its adaptability to a wide spectrum of patients ranging from infancy to adulthood. Coil embolization is still used to close small PDAs, but the technique can be cumbersome and the

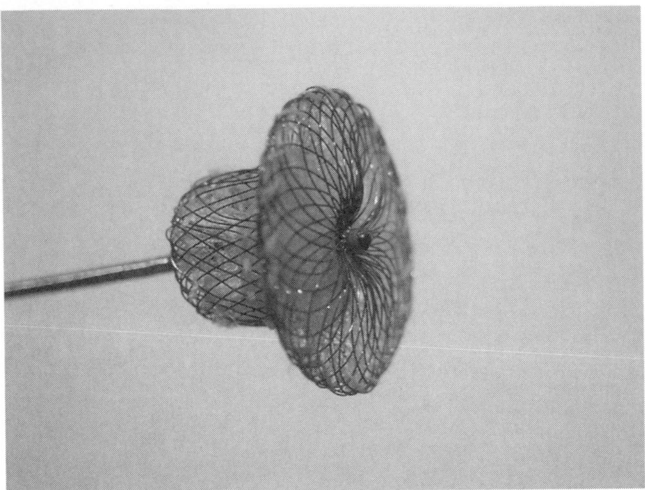

Figure 55-4 Amplatzer ductal occluder (ADO) device. (Courtesy of Richard Ringel, MD, Division of Pediatric Cardiology, The Johns Hopkins University Hospital.)

residual leak rate is higher when larger PDAs are encountered, particularly in small infants. Thus a number of investigators have continued to work on the challenge of developing a device specifically designed to close the ductus arteriosus. In 2002 the first such device to obtain FDA approval was the Amplatzer ductal occluder (ADO); it remains to date the only device specifically approved for nonsurgical closure of the ductus arteriosus in the United States.[21] The device consists of 72 strands of nitinol wire woven into a mushroom-shaped plug with a core of polyester fiber (Fig. 55-4). It is particularly helpful for closure of moderate-to-large PDAs in patients above 6 months of age. For infants younger than 6 months, the right-angle orientation of the flat aortic retention disk to the plug portion of the device that fits within the ductus itself does not truly conform to aortic anatomy, and may protrude excessively into the aortic lumen of a smaller infant. However, a newly modified version of the device with the aortic retention disk angled back 32 degrees and with its concavity toward the aorta is showing great promise for use in younger infants.[22] Device closure of the PDA offers the obvious advantage of avoiding a surgical incision. The procedure at most centers is performed on an outpatient basis under moderate sedation, with use of percutaneous femoral venous and arterial access (Fig. 55-5). Contraindications to the use of nonsurgical techniques currently include a large (≥ 4 mm diameter) PDA in infants weighing 6 kg or less, active endocarditis, or pulmonary hypertension with right-to-left shunting through the ductus arteriosus.

Several treatment algorithms have emerged, wherein smaller PDAs (minimum diameter ≤ 2.5 mm) are closed by coil embolization[20,21] and larger PDAs are closed with an ADO; with this strategy, successful implantation with complete closure will approach 98 percent or greater.[22]

Complications of coil embolization are uncommon. Femoral artery thrombosis is rare and essentially seen only in smaller infants. Almost all of these problems are

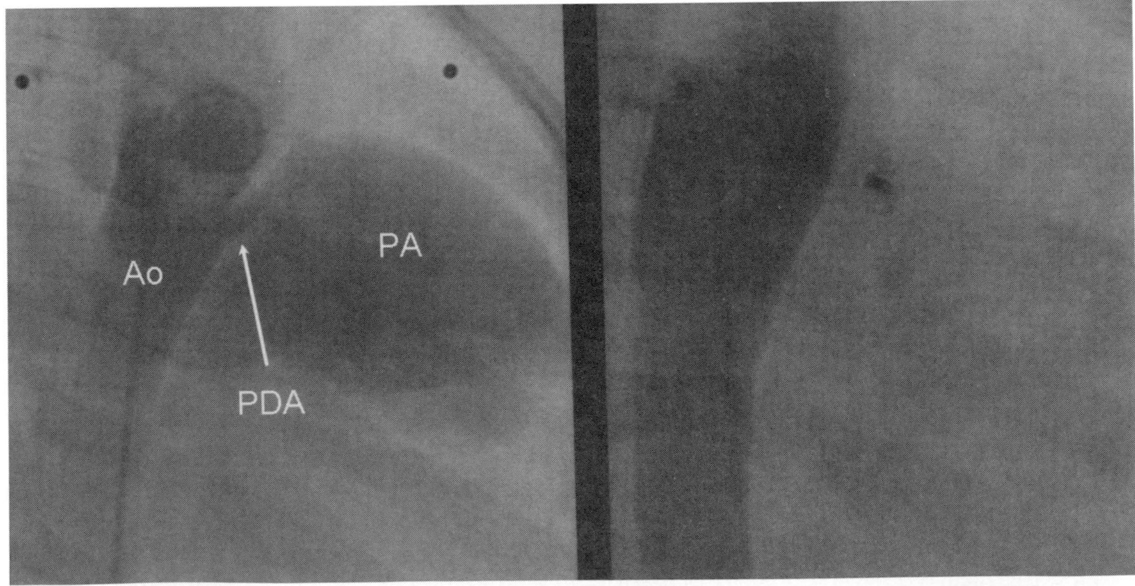

Figure 55-5 Interruption of patent ductus arteriosus with Amplatzer ductal occluder (ADO) device. Left: Contrast is seen within the ductus arteriosus with injection in the thoracic aorta. Right: successful closure of the arterial duct. (Courtesy of Richard Ringel, MD, Division of Pediatric Cardiology, The Johns Hopkins University Hospital.

transient, responding to anticoagulant or thrombolytic therapy. Embolization of the coil into the pulmonary arteries is the most frequently described complication, occurring in up to 16 percent of procedures;[23] but virtually all of these embolized coils can be removed immediately during catheterization without sequelae. Embolization into a systemic artery is very unusual, occurring in 0 to 3 percent of cases. Hemolysis following coil embolization is very rare and can be avoided by implanting additional coils[24,25] to eliminate any residual shunting identified on the postimplant aortic contrast study. Creation of left pulmonary artery stenosis or aortic obstruction has been described infrequently, but is almost exclusively seen in the small infant with a PDA that requires three or more coils to achieve adequate closure. Complications associated with the Amplatzer device are likewise uncommon, and usually minor when use of the device is restricted to patients over 6 months of age. Major adverse events (i.e., device embolization, partial pulmonary artery obstruction, loss of femoral pulse, bleeding requiring transfusion) occurred in 10 of 439 (2.3 percent) patients during phase III FDA trials, with most of these occurring in smaller infants.[21]

SUMMARY

Treatment of PDA can be performed with low mortality and morbidity. Multiple options are now available, ranging from medical to surgical to interventional catheter-based treatment. Nonsurgical device closure of the ductus arteriosus can be performed with a success rate of about 98 percent and a complication rate below 3 percent with the use of an interventional strategy that employs embolization coils for small PDAs and ADOs for moderate to large PDAs. Operative closure is recommended for infants with congestive heart failure who weigh 6 kg or less; such patients should not wait until they are of more appropriate size for a nonsurgical approach.

References

1. Anderson RC. Causative factors underlying congenital heart malformations. Patent ductus arteriosus. *Pediatrics* 1954;14:143.
2. Monro JC. Ligation of the ductus arteriosus. *Ann Surg* 1907;46:335.
3. Graybiel A, Strieder JW, Boyer NH. An attempt to obliterate the patent ductus arteriosus in a patient with bacterial endocarditis. *Am Heart J* 1938;15:621.
4. Gross RE, Hubbard JP. Surgical ligation of a patent ductus arteriosus. A report of first successful case. *JAMA* 1939; 112:729.
5. Pierone AR, Benson LN. The patent arterial duct. In: Freedom RM, Yoo SJ, Mikailian H, et al (eds). *The Natural and Modified History of Congenital Heart Disease.* Boston: Blackwell, 2004:72–82.
6. Jonas RA. Patent ductus arteriosus, aortopulmonary window, sinus of Valsalva fistula, aortoventricular tunnel. In: Jonas RA (ed). *Comprehensive Surgical Management of Congenital Heart Disease.* New York: Arnold, 2004:187–206.
7. Silver MM, Freedom RM, Silver MD, et al. The morphology of the human newborn ductus arteriosus: A reappraisal of its structure and function with special reference to prostaglandin E_1 therapy. *Hum Pathol* 1981;12:1123.
8. Coceani F, Olley PM. Role of prostaglandin, prostacyclin, and thromboxane in the control of prenatal patency and postnatal closure of the ductus arteriosus. *Semin Perinatol* 1980;4:109.
9. Balzer DT, Spray TL, McMullin D, et al. Endarteritis associated with a clinically silent patent ductus arteriosus. *Am Heart J* 1993;125:1192.
10. Hawkins JA, Minich LL, Tani LY, et al. Cost and efficacy of surgical ligation versus transcatheter coil occlusion of patent ductus arteriosus. *J Thorac Cardiovasc Surg* 1996; 112:1635.
11. Heymann MA, Rudolph AM, Silverman NH. Closure of the ductus arteriosus in premature infants by inhibition of prostaglandin synthesis. *N Engl J Med* 1976;295:530.
12. Gould DS, Montenegro LM, Gaynor JW, et al. A comparison of on site and off site patent ductus arteriosus ligation in premature infants. *Pediatrics* 2003;112:1298.
13. Goncalves-Estella A, Perez-Villoria J, Gonzales-Reoyo F, et al. Closure of a complicated ductus arteriosus through the transpulmonary route using hypothermia. Surgical considerations in one case. *J Thorac Cardiovasc Surg* 1975;69:698.
14. Omari BO, Shapiro S, Ginzton L, et al. Closure of short, wide patent ductus arteriosus with cardiopulmonary bypass and balloon occlusion. *Ann Thorac Surg* 1998; 66:277.
15. Laborde F, Noirhomee P, Karam J, et al. A new video-assisted thoracoscopic surgical technique for interruption of patent ductus arteriosus in infants and children. *J Thorac Cardiovasc Surg* 1993;105:278.
16. Mavroudis C, Backer CL. Forty-six years of patient ductus arteriosus division at Children's Memorial Hospital of Chicago. Standards for comparison. *Ann Surg* 1994; 220:402.
17. Nezafati MH, Mahmoodi E, Hashemian SH, et al. Video-assisted thoracoscopic surgical (VATS) closure of patent ductus arteriosus: Report of three-hundred cases. *Heart Surg Forum* 2002;5:57.
18. Porstmann W, Wierny L, Warnke H. Der Verschluss des Ductus Arteriosus Persistens ohne Thorakotomie. *Thoraxchirurgie* 1967;15:199.
19. Rashkind WJ, Cuaso CC. Transcatheter closure of patent ductus arteriosus: Successful use in a 3.5 kg infant. *Pediatr Cardiol* 1979;1:3.
20. Cambier PA, Kirby WC, Wortham DC, et al. Percutaneous closure of the small (< 2.5 mm) patent ductus arteriosus using coil embolization. *Am J Cardiol* 1992;69:815.
21. Pass RH, Hijazi Z, Hsu D, et al. Multicenter USA Amplatzer patent ductus arteriosus occlusion device trial: Initial and one-year results. *J Am Coll Cardiol* 2004; 44:513.

22. Masura J, Gavora P, Podnar T. Transcatheter occlusion of patent ductus arteriosus using a new angled Amplatzer duct occluder: Initial clinical experience. *Cardiovasc Intervent* 2003;58:261.
23. Galal MO. Advantages and disadvantages of coils for transcatheter closure of patent ductus arteriosus. *J Intervent Cardiol* 2003;16:157.
24. El Sisi A, Tofeig M, Arnold R, et al. Mechanical occlusion of the patent ductus arteriosus with Jackson coils. *Pediatr Cardiol* 2001;22:29.
25. Podnar T, Gavora P, Masura J. Percutaneous closure of patent ductus arteriosus: Complementary use of detachable Cook patent ductus arteriosus coils and Amplatzer duct occluders. *Eur J Pediatr* 2000;159:293.

CHAPTER

56 ATRIAL SEPTAL DEFECTS AND PARTIAL ANOMALOUS PULMONARY VENOUS CONNECTION

Dario Troise, Richard E. Ringel, Luca A. Vricella, Paolo Arciprete

DEFINITION

We define an atrial septal defect (ASD) as a deficiency of any size in the atrial septum (Fig. 56-1). We do not consider as a true ASD (even though it is briefly mentioned in this chapter) the patent foramen ovale (PFO), namely an open flap-valve bordered superiorly by the upper limbic tissue and inferiorly by the valve of the fossa ovalis, which opens only in specific circumstances, as during coughing or the Valsalva maneuver. The ostium primum (OP) defect is part of the spectrum of atrioventricular septal defects and is discussed in detail in Chap. 58.

A partial anomalous pulmonary venous connection (PAPVC) is a condition presenting with variable anatomic patterns where some but not all pulmonary venous flow lacks drainage into the left atrium. This condition, characterized therefore by one or more pulmonary veins functionally draining into the right atrium, may or may not be associated with an ASD. Similar considerations apply to scimitar syndrome (SS).

This chapter covers clinical and surgical aspects that pertain to these malformations (ASD, PAPVC, and SS) and eventually focuses briefly on current nonsurgical alternatives for ASD closure.

KEY CONCEPTS

- **Epidemiology**
  - Atrial septal defects and partial anomalous pulmonary venous connection (PAPVC) are among the most common congenital heart defects, with a prevalence (including persistence of a patent foramen ovale, or PFO) greater than 15 percent for the general population and, when other cardiac anomalies are present, as high as 35 to 50 percent; there is a slight female predominance.
- **Morphology**
  - Atrial septal defects (ASDs) can be categorized according to the area of deficient interatrial septum: Secundum-type/PFO (most common), superior/inferior sinus venosus, primum defects, and coronary sinus ASDs. PAPVC and scimitar syndrome often occur in the setting of an ASD. Defects are variable in size: from restrictive to unrestrictive to virtual absence of any septal rim.
- **Pathophysiology**
  - The magnitude of the left-to-right shunt depends on the respective compliance of the right and left ventricles and on the diameter of the defect. Because of streaming of systemic venous return toward the left atrium, superior and inferior sinus venosus defects can present with mild cyanosis. A minority of patients with very large defects will develop PVOD over several decades and, eventually, fixed PHTn and right-to-left shunting.
- **Clinical features**
  - In the absence of other malformations, ASDs are rarely symptomatic in early infancy. Features of pulmonary overcirculation (dyspnea, failure to thrive, recurrent respiratory infections) are rare in infancy and early childhood. Arrhythmias or paradoxical emboli can be initial modes of presentation.

- **Diagnosis**
  - Physical exam (split and fixed second heart sound) and chest x-ray (cardiomegaly, anomalous vascular markings in PAPVC) suggest the diagnosis, confirmed by transthoracic echocardiography. In equivocal cases and for PAPVC/scimitar syndrome, transthoracic echocardiography, magnetic resonance imaging, and computed tomography might be utilized. Cardiac catheterization has almost no role in the diagnostic workup except for patients with evidence of PHTn considered for surgical closure.
- **Treatment**
  - Surgical closure is rarely indicated in infancy but should be performed for unrestrictive defects in pre-school-age children and for symptomatic adults and cases of paradoxical embolization. When the anatomy is permissive, percutaneous device closure can be considered. Conventional primary or patch closure of the defect can be accomplished via a right thoracotomy or limited/full sternotomy and, in the current era, should be associated with virtually no mortality or significant morbidity.

HISTORICAL HIGHLIGHTS

Following the successes of surgical closed heart procedures in the 1940s, surgeons focused their attention, mainly because of its relative simplicity, on the correction of ASDs.

This pathologic condition was described as a "perforating channel in the atrial septum" by Leonardo da Vinci in 1513,[1] but it was only in the mid-1930s that the first antemortem diagnosis was made by Rossler, in his report on 62 cases of ASD found at autopsy.[2] It was only between the late 1940s and early 1950s that, with the introduction of cardiac catheterization, a definite diagnosis became possible.

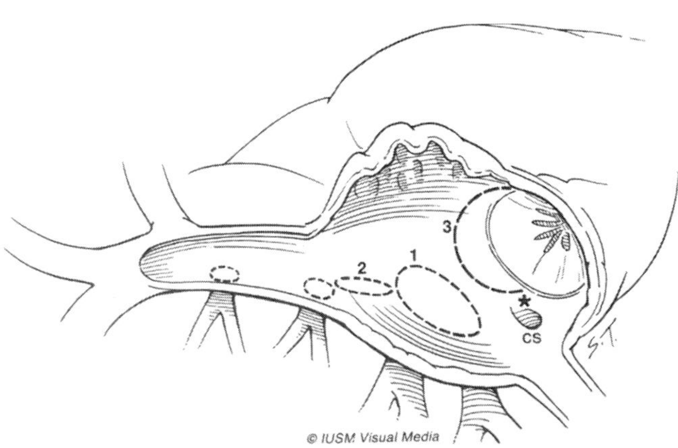

Figure 56-1 Different locations of atrial septal defects as schematically seen through a right atriotomy. Along the superior vena cava, an anomalous pulmonary vein enters the systemic atrium just cephalad to the superior sinus venosus ASD (2). 1 = ostium secundum ASD; 3 = ostium primum ASD; CS = coronary sinus; * = location of the atrioventricular conduction system. [From Turrentine MW. Atrial septal defects. In: Yang SC, Cameron DE (eds). *Current Therapy in Thoracic and Cardiovascular Surgery.* Philadelphia: Mosby, 2004:731. With permission.]

On account of the brief temporal mismatch between the possibility of safely diagnosing the condition during life and the feasibility of treating it surgically, three eras in the surgical treatment of the ASD can be identified: the closed-heart era, the semiclosed era, and the open-heart era.

Murray was the first surgeon to report, in 1948, the closure of an ASD in a 12 year-old boy, using the external suturing technique.[3] The patient survived, but success was subtotal owing to a residual shunt, later discovered on cardiac catheterization. In the early 1950s, various closed methods were investigated, including the intussusception technique of Santy,[4] the invagination technique of Swan,[5] the digital palpation closed technique proposed by Bailey,[6] and the Sondergaard circumclusion technique.[7] All these attempts led to unacceptable mortality and a high incidence of morbidity, such as atrial distortion, coronary sinus stenosis, and the persistence of significant residual defects.

In 1953, Robert Gross utilized a semiopen technique that entailed the introduction of a cone within the atrium, allowing for closure of the defect without direct vision in the depth of a blood-filled well.[8] John Kirklin reported a series of 29 patients corrected with this technique at Mayo Clinic without operative mortality.[9]

The experiments of a short period of inflow occlusion under surface hypothermia gave way to the era of open-heart correction. Inspired by the laboratory work of Wilfred Bigelow, John Lewis at the University of Minnesota first reported successful closure of an ASD under direct vision in a 5-year-old girl.[10] Shortly thereafter, closure was accomplished with cross-circulation by C. Walton Lillehei.

With the construction of the first heart-lung machine, John Gibbon opened the current era of open-heart surgery in the treatment of ASDs.[11]

In 1858, Peacock described for the first time the anatomic findings of a sinus venosus defect (SVD) in a 6 year-old girl who died of scarlet fever.[12] After initial approaches to PAPVC with palliative and closed techniques, Kirklin and colleagues first reported successful outcomes with open correction of various types of PAPVC.[13]

EMBRYOLOGY

The cardiac tube is formed by an inner layer of endocardium separated from the external myocardium by an extracellular matrix, known as cardiac jelly.[14] At the fifth week of embryonic life, the primary septum (septum primum) appears as a partition, of mesenchymal origin, in the dome of the common atrium. With further development, it occupies more space and, at the same time, incorporates two segments of mesenchymal origin that are also concomitantly forming: the endocardial cushions of the atrioventricular canal and the vestibular spine (spina vestibuli), which originate from the dorsal mesocardium and are situated between the endocardial cushions and the anteriorly and inferiorly located septum primum. In this early phase, the space between the septum primum and the endocardial cushions is called ostium primum. It has not yet been established whether the development of the septum primum consists in growth from the roof of the common atrium toward the inferiorly displaced endocardial cushions[15] or, as stated by Van Praagh[16] and apparently in contrast to mainstream embryology, in an upward growth, starting from the inferior vena cava (IVC), the left wall of which is in direct continuity with the septum primum) toward the roof of the common atrium.

Before complete fusion of all mesenchymal segments of the interatrial septum, the superior part of the primary septum is reabsorbed, forming multiple fenestrations that converge into a single defect known as the ostium secundum.

From the dorsal aspect of the common atrium emerges to follow an infolding of the atrial wall (septum secundum), which will be directed toward (but on the right side of) the septum primum. The plane of growth of the two septa is not identical and may thus overlap for a variable extent (Fig. 56-2). The conformation of the septum resembles a flap valve in which a superoinferior plane as well as a lateral plane of growth may be identified. The development of this structure allows for half of the oxygenated placental blood to cross the interatrial communication. The septum primum becomes involved in this process, leaving vestigial remnants in the segments located in proximity of the endocardial cushions. This vestigial part, which is not overlapped by the more superior septum secundum, is the floor of the fossa ovalis. The upper edge of the flap valve does not fuse with it but simply overlaps it. With postnatal changes in heart chamber pressures, the superior edge of the fossa ovalis fuses completely (in approximately 60 percent of cases) with the lower edge of the septum secundum. In the remaining part, the fusion is incomplete and a communication between the atria persists as a patent foramen ovale.

Development of the muscular septum primum and of the ventral proliferation of extracardiac mesenchyme from the dorsal mesocardium aligns the common pulmonary vein (CPV), which, once incorporated into the posterior aspect of the left-sided atrium, eventually differentiates into the left and right pulmonary veins. The sinus venosus segment is that part of the atrium which, in postnatal life, will be responsible for draining systemic and coronary return as well as for the development of the smooth venous tissue between the venous ostia. The connection of the sinus with the atrial segment after the primary tube is formed is represented by the sinoatrial orifice, which, forced by the predominant development of the right-sided sinus, migrates from its midline position toward the right. The sinoatrial orifice is surrounded by venous valves on the right and left sides. Once incorporated into the dorsal aspect of the right-sided atrium, the development of the sinus segment pushes the right side of the venous valve toward a ventral line and crosses two bands developing perpendicular to it: the superior and the inferior limbic bands. These bands develop underneath the endocardium at the periphery of the fossa ovalis. The superior band, from the upper edge of the fossa ovalis (superior limbus of the

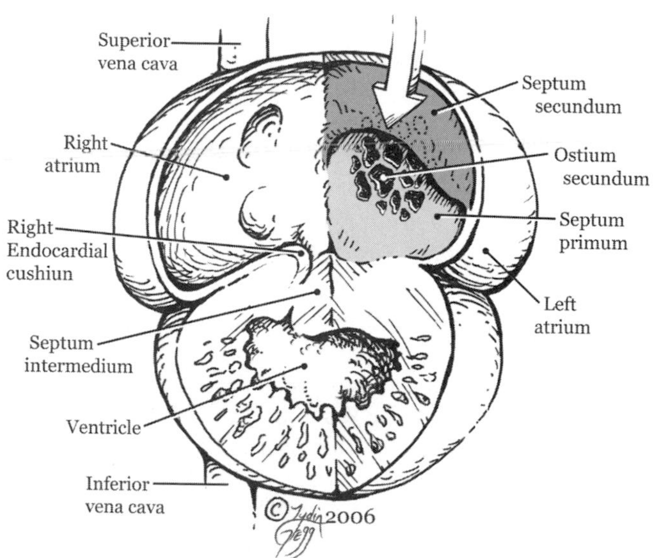

Figure 56-2 Development of the interatrial septum (6 weeks' gestation). The atria are partitioned by the developing septum. On the left of the midline, the septum primum has obliterated the ostium primum and is in the process of partial reabsorption in its cephalad portion (ostium secundum). The septum secundum originates to the right of the septum primum and covers the ostium secundum for a variable length. [Image by Lydia Gregg, with permission]

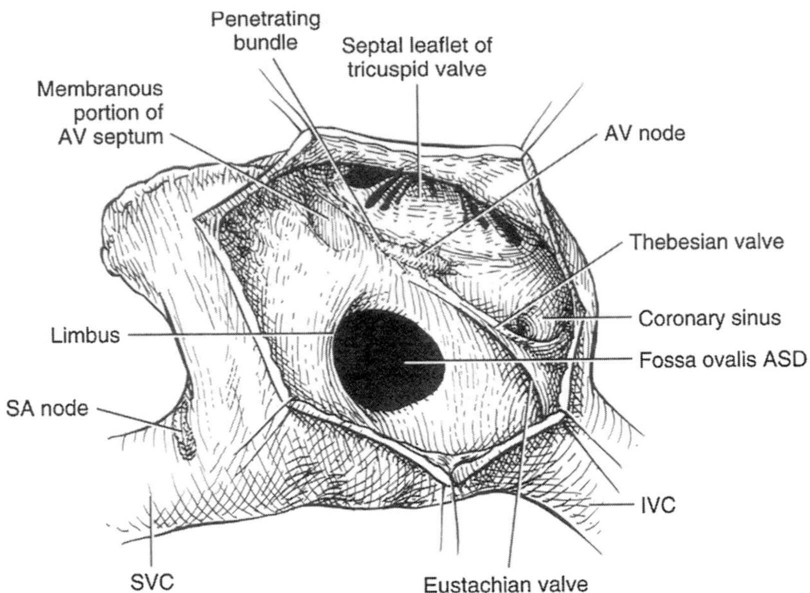

Figure 56-3 Secundum-type atrial septal defect (fossa ovalis ASD). Schematic view as seen through a right atriotomy. AV = atrioventricular; IVC = inferior vena cava; SA = sinoatrial; SVC = superior vena cava. [From Atrial septal defect and partial anomalous pulmonary venous connection. In: Kouchoukos NT, Blackstone EH, Doty DB, et al (eds). *Kirklin/Barratt-Boyes Cardiac Surgery.* 3d ed. Philadelphia: Churchill-Livingstone, 2003:730. With permission.]

fossa ovalis) crosses the venous valve between superior and inferior caval orifices; the inferior band (inferior limbus of the fossa ovalis), crosses the venous valve between the IVC and the coronary sinus (CoS) orifices and, eventually, forms the base of the sinus septum.

The incomplete development of the septum primum results in a defect within the fossa ovalis (Fig. 56-3). This process may be related to different mechanisms, such as incomplete overlapping of the superior limbus of the fossa ovalis (patent foramen ovale); redundancy of the foraminal valve (aneurysm of the atrial septum); partial or total breakdown of the septum primum, resulting in a single perforation of the septum primum (ostium secundum defect); or in multiple fenestrations.

As previously pointed out, after maturation of the septum primum, the infolding of the dorsal common atrial cavity positions the CPV in its definitive location behind the left atrium. Hence, various theories have been advanced to explain the development of PAPVC. Hartley[17] suggested that the incomplete migration of the sinoatrial orifice, from the midline, was the main cause of the development of a superior vena cava (SVC) medially, with displacement of the septum primum toward the septum secundum and subsequent underdevelopment of the latter. This theory would indeed account for the overriding of the SVC typically observed in the superior caval ASD but not for the high prevalence of PAPVC associated with it. An elegant echocardiographic study on sinus venosus defects (SVD) from the Children's Hospital in Boston has shown that the deficiency in the wall that normally separates the right pulmonary veins or SVC and the right atrium (RA) is the leading cause of this particular defect.[18] Depending on the structures involved in this anomalous process, different subsets of ASDs, with one or more right pulmonary veins overriding the septum secundum, will occur.

Finally, a CoS defect may be due to a deficiency in the remnant of the left horn of the sinus venosus, which extends along the entire length of the coronary sinus to reach its orifice. This defect is generally found in association with the persistence of a left SVC.

Advances in genetic analysis and molecular biology have striven to investigate the embryonic mechanisms of cardiac looping, chamber development, myocardial cell growth, and cardiac valve formation. At present, the origin of most of the complex genetic traits of congenital heart disease remains to be completely defined. Studies focused on chromosomal abnormalities, autosomal dominant syndromes, and genetic linkage analysis of relatives of patients presenting with minor degrees of congenital heart disease have led to the detection of only a handful of the genes responsible for the development of congenital heart malformations.

Specifically (with regard to atrial septation defects), it is known that the Holt-Oram syndrome (association of ventricular septal defect and ASD with limb abnormalities) is the product of mutation of gene TBX5 in locus 12q24. Several investigations have revealed a heterozygous mutation in gene NKX2.5 in locus 5q34 in families with ASDs and conduction abnormalities.[14]

ANATOMIC CONSIDERATIONS

The five more commonly occurring variants[19] of defects of the interatrial septum are (1) ostium secundum (OS) defect and PFO, (2) ostium primum (OP) defect, (3) coronary sinus (CoS) defect, (4) sinus venosus (SV) ASD and its association in the superior position with PAPVC, and (5) scimitar syndrome (SS).

The OS defect is the most common of all types of interatrial communications (80 percent). This defect is confined within the borders of the fossa ovalis (see Fig. 56-3), and its name is in fact almost a misnomer, since the OS defect is actually the final result of deficiency in the development of the septum primum. Ostium secundum defects may differ in size and morphology, depending on the degree of reabsorption of the septum primum and the deficiency of the flap valve of the fossa ovalis. The degree of its absence varies from partial deficiency to complete absence, when the inferior border of the septum primum becomes continuous with the posterior wall of the IVC. Surgeons must bear this anatomic peculiarity in mind in order to distinguish the inferior edge of the defect from the eustachian valve: this misperception may result in a surgical disaster following inadvertent baffling of the IVC to the left atrium (LA). A patent foramen ovale (PFO) is found in approximately 30 percent of normal hearts. In the absence of left-to-right shunt (and with LA pressure > RA pressure), the lack of closure of the natural flap valve may be considered not a true interatrial communication. Intermittent shunting across the PFO may occur spontaneously or during provoking maneuvers that increase RA pressure, such as coughing or the Valsalva maneuver.

Because of the direct continuity between the leftward aspect of the IVC wall and the septum primum, when the floor of the fossa ovalis is absent and an ASD extends toward the IVC, the inferior caval ostium overrides the defect onto the left atrium. This anatomic pattern, or inferior SV ASD, may occasionally promote right-to-left shunt with cyanosis. Moreover, the proximity of right pulmonary veins to the deficient posteroinferior rim of the ASD favors a functional hemianomalous pulmonary venous connection.

At the extreme of septal maldevelopment is the common atrium, which may be described as an association of several defects involving structures of different embryonic origin. The association of a complete lack of the septum primum and of the superior and inferior limbi has been classified by some authors as the common atrium. This lesion is generally found in atrial isomerism in association with a persistent left SVC draining into an unroofed coronary sinus.

Defects located beneath the inferior limb of the primary septum (10 percent of all ASDs) are associated with morphologic abnormalities of the atrioventricular valves and are described in Chap. 58. Even if these are to be invariably classified as atrioventricular septal (AVSD) or endocardial cushion defects, the OP defect has been reported in hearts with no evidence of AVSD morphology.[20]

The CoS defect (Fig. 56-4) results from variable fenestrations along the common wall between the CoS and the posterior aspect of the LA. It represents an infrequent type of ASD, accounting for only 1 to 2 percent of all defects of the interatrial septum. The ostium of the CoS is invariably present in its expected position along the posteroinferior margin of the triangle of Koch (see Chap. 52). This defect is generally found in association with a number of lesions, most frequently the persistence of the left SVC: these associated lesions (with the extreme form being the total absence of the CoS wall) determine the spectrum of the "unroofed coronary sinus syndrome." A surgical classification has been proposed that categorizes CoS defects into proximal, medial, and distal according to the site of the deficiency of the CoS wall along its length.[21–23]

The superior sinus venosus defect (SV ASD) is associated with PAPVC in 5 to 10 percent of cases. This malformation, also known as superior caval ASD, is located in the posterosuperior atrial septum, cranial to the superior limbic band. The most common position for the site of drainage of the anomalous pulmonary veins is at the superior atriocaval junction (Fig. 56-5). In 95 percent of cases with PAPVC, two right pulmonary veins (upper and middle lobes) are involved, but there may be three or even four pulmonary veins connected to the proximal SVC or SVC–right atrial junction. The SVC typically overrides the atrial septum and may result in right-to-left shunting across the ASD. When this defect is associated with the lack of the posterior limbus (posterior ASD), pulmonary venous drainage is somewhat anatomically unclear, although it flows functionally into the right atrium (RA). When anomalous drainage of the right pulmonary veins is found with an intact posterior limbus or OS ASD, the anatomy is clear and a true PAPVC is present.

In scimitar syndrome (Fig. 56-6), an anomalous right pulmonary venous trunk (generally draining the entirety of the right lung) descends in a craniocaudal direction to connect to the IVC, generally above the IVC-RA junction.[24] This anomalous trunk usually descends along the right border of the pericardium. It has a crescent-like morphology (scimitar shape) and, at the level of the right hemidiaphragm, passes transversely and anteriorly to the hilum of the right lung to connect to the IVC. The radiologic appearance of this pathology is characteristic (Fig. 56-7). The interatrial septum may be intact or an OS/ PFO defect may be associated to SS. Scimitar syndrome generally occurs in association with several extracardiac malformations,

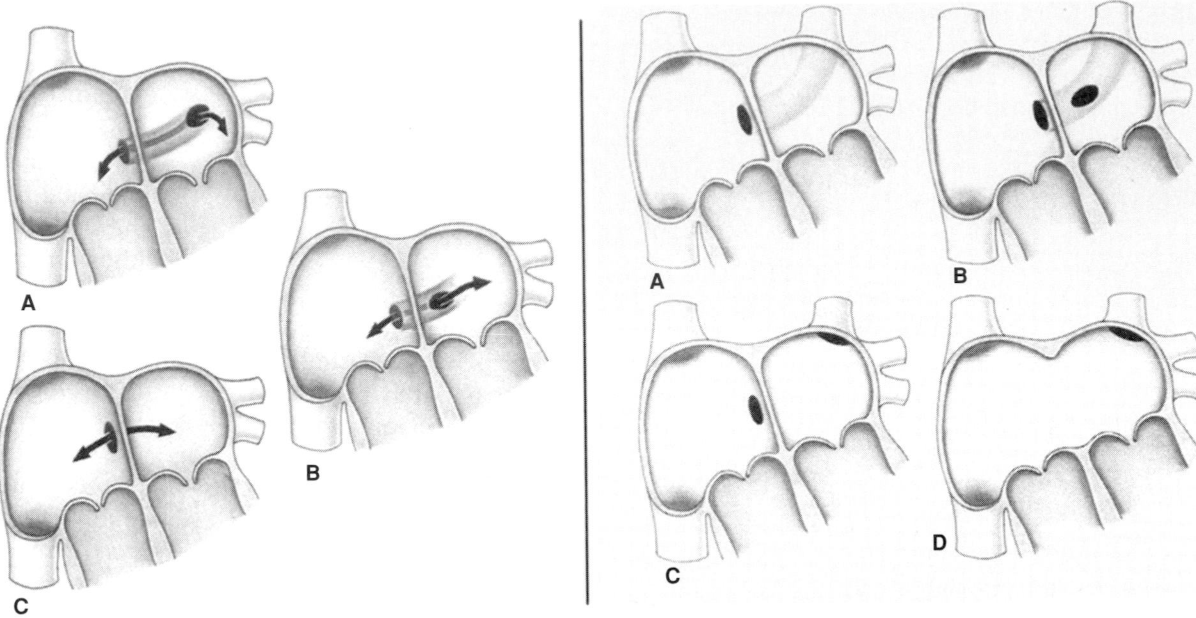

Figure 56-4 Coronary sinus (CoS) defect with and without left superior vena cava (LSVC). Left panel: proximal (a) and midportion unroofing of the coronary sinus, resulting in interatrial communication. (c) Complete absence of the roof. Right panel: (a) Persistent LSVC with intact CoS roof. The roof of CoS draining the LSVC can be fenestrated (b) or absent (c) and can be associated with absence of the interatrial septum (d). [From deLeval M. Anomalies of the systemic venous return. In: Stark J, deLeval M (eds). *Surgery for Congenital Heart Defects,* 2d ed. Philadelphia: Saunders, 1994:320,323. With permission.]

such as right lung hypoplasia (invariably associated with a marked right mediastinal shift with dextrocardia), right pulmonary artery stenosis and/or hypoplasia and right lower lobe (RLL), or bronchopulmonary sequestration. Diaphragmatic anomalies occur in approximately 20 percent of cases, and consist of right lung herniation through the foramen of Bochdalek or of abnormal attachment of the hemidiaphragm. Very occasionally, a common pulmonary vein trunk drains the entire right lung and descends in a craniocaudal direction to connect with the posterior LA. This peculiar arrangement shares similar radiologic findings with SS but has no clinical significance.

Two or more of the above-mentioned types may be associated within the same heart, and are referred to as confluent ASDs.

PATHOPHYSIOLOGY

The magnitude of left-to-right shunting is determined by the size of the communication and relative compliance of the ventricles. As for ventricular septal defects (VSDs), the location of the ASD has very limited influence on the magnitude of the pulmonary-to-systemic flow ratio (Qp:Qs). If a relatively small subtricuspidal shunt (because of the high pressure gradient between the ventricles) can give rise to a large left-to-right shunt, only a large ASD leads on the contrary to a large shunt. In the presence of a large ASD with an area similar to that of the mitral valve (MV), pulmonary venous return will be equally distributed between the ASD and the MV. If the ASD is restrictive, blood flow will be diverted preferentially toward the MV, and the Qp:Qs will rarely exceed 2:1.[19] Only in cases of associated acquired and/or congenital heart defects that increase LA pressure (as in systemic hypertension, MV stenosis, coarctation of the aorta, patent ductus arteriosus, and VSD) will flow across the atrial septum be increased independently of ASD area. If a large defect is present, atrial pressures will equalize. In this circumstance, the respective flows across mitral and tricuspid valves will vary according to the relative compliance of the ventricles. In the early months of life, the thickness of the right ventricle (RV) exceeds the thickness of the left (LV), resulting in right-to-left shunting. After the neonatal period, the LV exceeds in thickness the RV, yielding a net left-to-right shunt. The effect of atrial-level shunting results in enlargement of the RA, RV, and pulmonary arteries (PAs). The overload is usually well tolerated by the RV, and heart failure seldom develops in childhood. Occasionally, heart failure occurs in infancy, but it is very rare and is generally related to various extracardiac conditions. In cases of

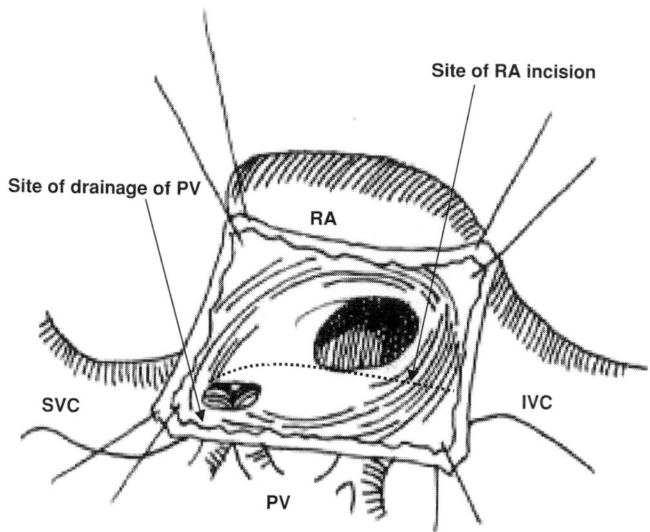

Figure 56-5 Superior sinus venosus ASD, as seen through a right atriotomy. Ao = aorta; MPA = main pulmonary artery; SA = sinoatrial; SVC = superior vena cava. (From Jonas RA. *Comprehensive Surgical Management of Congenital Heart Disease.* London: Arnold, 2004:228. With permission.)

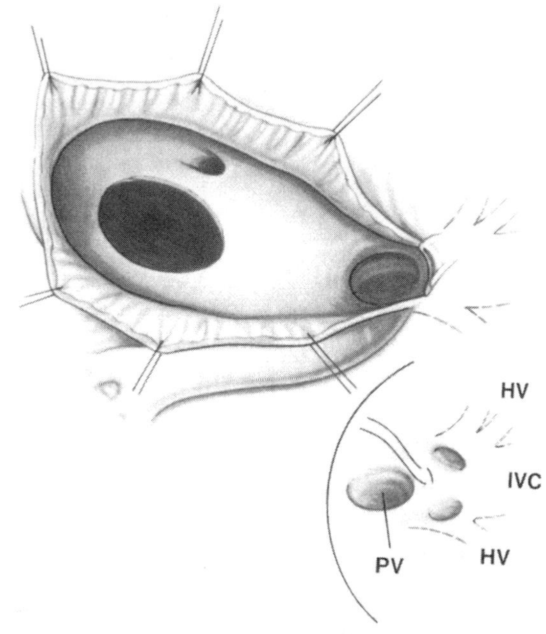

Figure 56-6 Schematic representation of scimitar syndrome as seen through the right atrium. In the figure, a large fossa ovalis ASD is also represented. The anomalous draining vein enters the IVC right above the hepatic veins (insert). IVC = inferior vena cava; HV = hepatic vein; PV = pulmonary vein. [From Stark J. Secundum atrial septal defect and partial anomalous pulmonary venous return. In: deLeval M, Stark J (eds). *Surgery for Congenital Heart Defects,* 2d ed. Philadelphia: Saunders, 1994:350. With permission.]

ASD with pulmonary hypertension (PHT)–as in rare pediatric cases and in some adult patients–RV thickness will increase and compliance of the RV may be similar and/or higher than that of the LV. In these cases, a right-to-left shunt will appear with a marked degree of cyanosis and hypoxia, with clinically evident heart failure.

The increase in pulmonary blood flow, over several years, may promote the development of PHT in adulthood. The onset of PHT is variable and, at present, it is not possible to establish which patient will develop PHT and at what age. This variability may depend on the multiple factors involved in the pathogenesis of PHT: recurrent pulmonary infections with microatelectasis, progressive increase in left-to-right shunt with enlargement of the ASD, individual endothelial vascular hyperreactivity, thrombotic and thromboembolic lesions of lung arteries, failure of the pulmonary vascular resistance to drop, and association with acquired heart diseases, promoting LV dysfunction such as MV prolapse, coronary artery disease, and systemic hypertension.[25]

In the presence of an interatrial communication, a potential reverse shunt at atrial level may account for paradoxical embolization in the cerebral circulation. This condition may depend on instantaneous trans-ASD gradient modifications, as well as the size, morphology, and position of the defect along the atrial septum. A large metaanalysis has indicated the presence of interatrial septal abnormalities as significantly associated to paradoxical embolism.[26] Furthermore, the incidence of PFO among adults suffering from cerebrovascular accidents was found to be higher than in the unaffected population. Coagulation disorders or thrombocytosis may play a role in the pathogenesis of paradoxical embolization.

CLINICAL FEATURES

The reported incidence of isolated ASD ranges from 7 to 14 percent, with a slight female predominance. This fairly broad range is due to the inclusion criteria used in the reports over the last few decades that considered ASDs and PFOs referred to surgery as identical pathologic entities. In the setting of other congenital heart defects, their incidence ranges from 33 to 50 percent.[27] The wide use of echocardiography has led to the detection of ASDs of any size and at any age. Several investigators have reported the results from populations of children bearing an ASD at long-term follow-up.[28–29]

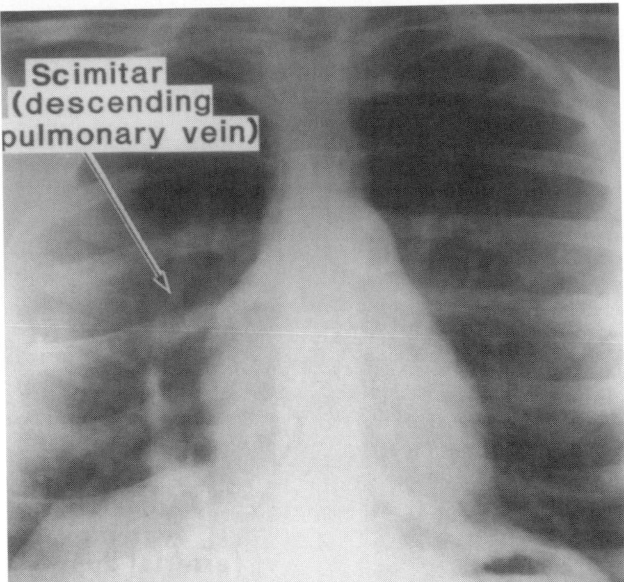

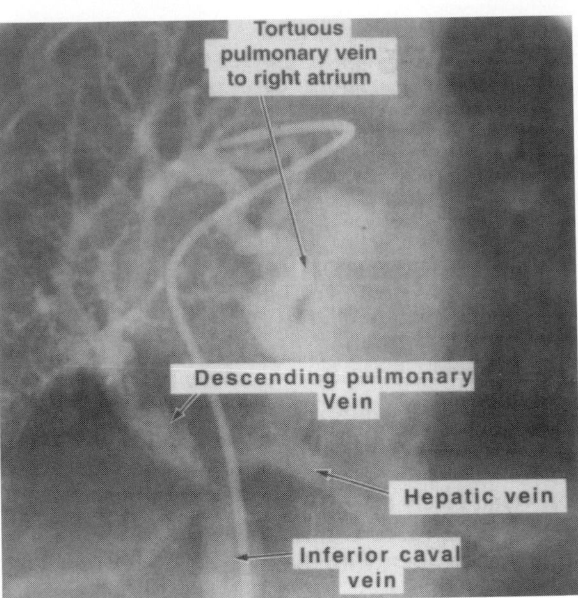

Figure 56-7 Characteristic radiologic appearance of scimitar syndrome. On Chest x-ray, a right-lower-lung-field crescentic vascular marking is visible (left). Cardiac catheterization discloses the anomalous right inferior pulmonary vein draining into the inferior vena cava (right). Tortuous anomalous venous return from the upper and middle lobes to the right atrium is also seen. [From Anderson RH, Baker EJ, Mccartney FJ, Rigby ML (eds). *Paediatric Cardiology*, 2d ed. Philadelphia: Churchill Livingstone, 2000. With permission.]

The conclusions emerging from these studies may be summarized as follows:

- ASDs less than 6 mm in diameter, detected in infancy, almost always restrict spontaneously.
- ASDs 6 to 8 mm in diameter, classified as hemodynamically insignificant, may restrict even after 5 years of age and not necessarily below 18 months of age, as once held.
- ASDs greater than 8 mm in diameter may increase in size during childhood, although a restrictive physiology is still a more common possibility.

Among all diagnosed ASDs, the reported incidence of sinus venosus defects varies between 2 and 10 percent.[30] This relatively high incidence may be due to diagnostic bias, the incidence of SVD being higher in studies focusing on cohorts with more "complex" ASDs.

The signs and symptoms of ASD and PAPVC are strictly related to the direction and magnitude of the shunt and with the age of the patient at detection. Qp:Qs is greater than 1 in predominant left-to-right shunt. When Qp:Qs is below 1.5 to 1.8:1,[31] clinical signs and symptoms are typically mild or absent in both pediatric and adult patients. When Qp:Qs exceeds 2:1, signs and symptoms become clinically evident. In this subset of patients the classic "fixed split second heart sound" and systolic pulmonary flow murmur are typically audible. Reduced exercise capacity and a history of recurrent respiratory infections may be present in childhood as well as in adolescence. Several other conditions must be taken into consideration in the differential diagnosis, such as innocent murmur associated with a normal cardiovascular state and pulmonary valve stenosis; this is usually audible in the higher upper left sternal border, presents with an early systolic ejection sound, and, in cases of stenosis of the pulmonary artery branches, is transmitted toward the back. In these conditions, however, splitting of the second heart sound is absent.

In cases of PAPVC, the amount of shunt through the abnormally connected veins will often result in heart failure, pulmonary infections, growth retardation, and poor effort tolerance even in infancy.

In adult patients, an episode of paroxysmal atrial fibrillation may represent the first clinical event.

The development of PHT and poor exercise capacity with cyanosis, dyspnea, and migraine often represents the pathophysiologic evolution of an ASD toward irreversible changes within the pulmonary vasculature (Eisenmenger's syndrome).

Lastly, PFO with or without associated aneurysm of the atrial septum may promote paradoxical embolism and should be clinically ruled out in the context of an acute cerebrovascular event.[31,32]

Scimitar syndrome is a rare cardiac malformation diagnosed in approximately 2 of 100,000 live-births and is often associated with other congenital heart lesions, variable hypoplasia of the right lung, and PHT.[33] As mentioned in the morphologic considerations, the constant feature is a single trunk draining venous return from the entire right lung into the IVC. There are often accessory systemic-to-pulmonary collaterals from the abdominal aorta to the RLL. When symptoms emerge during infancy, other anomalies (such as septation defects or left ventricular outflow tract obstruction) are often associated. The presence of aortopulmonary collaterals does not generally have a critical impact on the development of heart failure, since the hypoplastic lung is typically underperfused. Furthermore, pulmonary sequestration of the right lung (in the absence of hypoplasia) usually involves a maximum of two pulmonary segments. When SS is discovered in late childhood or in adulthood, the patient may be asymptomatic or, more often, refer to a history of recurrent respiratory tract infections, cough, and dyspnea. Heart failure, if present, is of mild degree. Intracardiac lesions are generally absent, and extralobar sequestration of a RLL is observed in approximately 50 percent of cases. Qp:Qs usually ranges from 1.5 to 3.1.[33]

As mentioned above, physical examination in early childhood is often less than revealing unless the shunt is substantial or there are associated lesions.[34] In large ASDs, a left parasternal lift can be detected, while a fixed, split second heart sound is typically audible, together with a soft "crescendo-decrescendo" systolic flow murmur over the pulmonary valve's auscultation focus. The second heart sound can be prominent in case of PHT. Clinical evidence of overcirculation is rare, as is cyanosis in cases without severe PHT. Cyanosis with streaming can be observed in superior or inferior defects where the SVC or IVC "straddles" the interatrial septum at the site of the defect, resulting in a functional right-to-left shunt of variable magnitude. This is, from a clinical standpoint, often underdetected. In a recent review of infants and children with ASDs without associated lesions treated at our institution, only 1 of 255 patients was cyanotic on presentation.

Even though symptoms might not present until the fifth decade of life, approximately 50 percent of adults will manifest exertional dyspnea by the age of 20; among adults with sizable defects, almost all will be symptomatic by the sixth decade of life.[24] If untreated, adults with large ASDs show a 75 percent mortality rate within the fifth decade, rising to nearly 90 percent in the sixth decade of life.[36]

Symptomatic supraventricular arrhythmias often complicate the natural history of ASDs diagnosed in adulthood, the most common among them being atrial fibrillation, followed by atrial flutter. In the elderly, sick sinus syndrome might be the initial rhythm abnormality upon presentation; given the risk of paradoxical embolization, insertion of a transvenous pacing system without percutaneous or surgical ASD closure is contraindicated.

Paradoxical embolization should be strongly suspected as the pathophysiologic entity underlying cryptogenic strokes, although the very low prevalence of venous thrombosis and procoagulant conditions make this a rare entity in infants and children. The presence of an atrial septal aneurysm (in the absence of interatrial communication) was considered a predisposing factor for paradoxical embolism; data from the SPARC study[37] and the Patent Foramen Ovale and Atrial Septal Aneurysm Study Group[38] did not find this morphologic variant of septal morphology to be an independent risk factor for embolism in the absence of a PFO or ASD.

DIAGNOSTIC STUDIES

In children, electrocardiographic examination almost always discloses normal sinus rhythm and incomplete right bundle branch block, with a right axis deviation on the frontal plane between 90 and 120 degrees. In adulthood, atrial flutter and fibrillation are more frequent after the fourth decade of life, and they increase in incidence with advanced age. In this subset of patients, the counterclockwise loop on the frontal plane shows less rightward shift and complete right bundle branch block, with a prominent R' wave (> 15 mm) on the right precordial leads in almost 50 percent of patients with PHT.

Radiologic findings are dependent on the magnitude of Qp:Qs, with plethoric lung fields typically seen in the presence of larger defects. Cardiomegaly also reflects the amount of blood flow across the ASD, with heart diameter increasing with a higher degree of left-to-right shunt, usually associated with a prominent radiologic projection of the pulmonary artery trunk. Once obstructive pulmonary vascular changes and structural PHT worsen (leading to Eisenmenger's syndrome and right-to-left shunting) cardiac size decreases, the central pulmonary arteries become prominent and their branches appear truncated, with oligemic peripheral lung fields (Fig. 56-8).

Sinus venosus ASDs may be associated with additional pathognomonic findings, such as a significant prominence of the upper right vascular pedicle, in cases of superior caval ASD with right PAPVC or the right inferior crescentic shadow of the anomalous pulmonary vein on the frontal plane in SS.

Transthoracic echocardiography (TTE) is the diagnostic modality of choice for ASD. M-mode echocardiography provides indirect evidence of ASD, revealing right ventricular (RV) overload with increased RV diameter and, in most cases, flattened or paradoxical ventricular septal motion. Even though these ultrasonographic findings clearly support the evidence of increased right chamber preload, they are not specific; similar findings are in fact observed with several other cardiac diseases, such as, for example, tricuspid and pulmonary regurgitation and total or partial anomalous pulmonary venous connection, among others. Two-dimensional echocardiography is much more specific for the diagnosis of an ASD. The reported detection rate ranges from 89 to 99

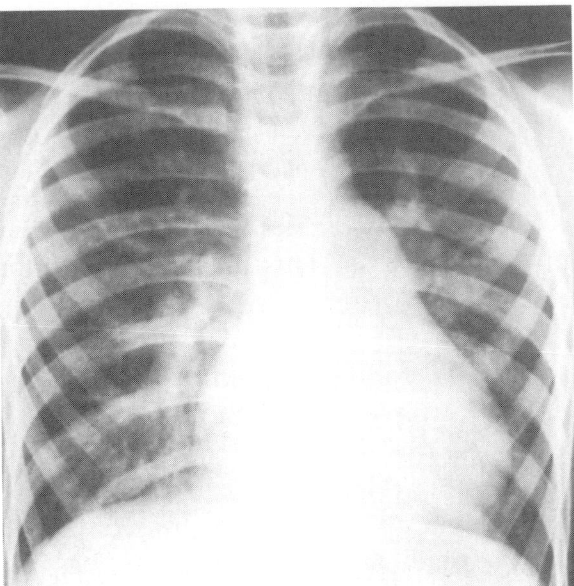
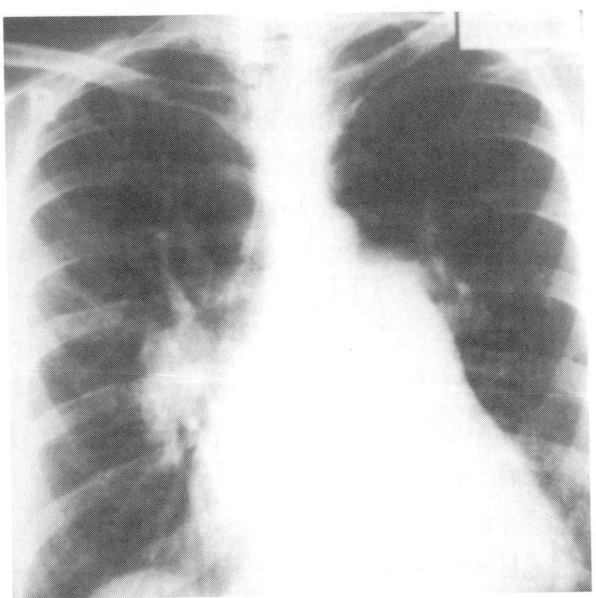

Figure 56-8 Radiologic findings in atrial septal defect. Left: pulmonary overcirculation with increased interstitial vascular markings and cardiomegaly. Right: patient with advanced pulmonary vascular obstructive disease in the setting of an untreated atrial septal defect. Cardiomegaly, prominent central pulmonary arteries, and oligemic peripheral lung fields. [From Anderson RH, Baker EJ, Mccartney FJ, Rigby ML (eds). *Paediatric Cardiology,* 2d ed. Philadelphia: Churchill Livingstone, 2000. With permission.]

percent for OS defects[39] with the use of subcostal and modified longitudinal scans (Fig. 56-9). Color Doppler-flow mapping techniques can be performed to confirm the presence of an ASD and to visualize the direction of the shunt, with good correlation with findings at cardiac catheterization.[40]

Coronary sinus ASDs may be suspected in patients with echocardiographic evidence of a dilated CoS. Besides the common findings of dilated RV, more posterior scanning views (subcostal and apical four-chamber) can directly reveal the communication between the CoS and LA.

Contrast echocardiographic evaluation may better reveal the suspected ASD. In cases of unidirectional left-to-right shunt, the observation of a negative washout into the RA may confirm the suspicion of a shunt at the atrial level, whereas in cases of right-to-left shunting, the detection of contrast bubbles of agitated saline in the LA provides direct evidence of an inverted shunt.

Trans-thoracic echocardiography is much less reliable in patients with uncommon defects at the atrial level, such as SV ASDs and PAPVCs, with a sensitivity of approximately 70 percent.[41] Because of the shorter distance between probe and defect, transesophageal echocardiography (TEE) overcomes inadequate visualization, especially in older children and adults, in whom diagnostic sensitivity and specificity for SV ASDs/PAPVC approach 100 percent.[42] Longitudinal scans are particularly useful in the delineation of the upper atrial septum, while short-axis views may be fundamental for assessment of the pulmonary-systemic venous connection.

Three-dimensional TEE currently represents the most sophisticated tool for the morphologic evaluation of ASDs that are potential candidates for percutaneous closure (Fig. 56-10). Three-dimensional reconstruction allows for precise localization of the defect. delineation of its proximity to valvular structures, visualization of the venous ostia and adequacy of margins, as well as provision of an immediate assessment of defect's obliteration following device deployment (Fig. 56-11).[43] Similar advantages have been reported with the recent introduction of intravascular ultrasound (IVUS) techniques for diagnosis and treatment of ASDs.[44,45]

Although the vast majority of ASDs are diagnosed accurately with conventional ultrasonography, imaging techniques (magnetic resonance imaging and computed tomography) have gained wide acceptance in defining anomalous venous connections in patients with complex ASDs.[46]

Cardiac catheterization is not indicated in the preoperative diagnostic workup of ASDs in children, adolescents, and young adults. Given the reliability of TTE and TEE, cardiac cathterization is currently indicated only in those cases with inadequate imaging or for complete assessment of complicated ASDs. Such conditions may include severe heart failure in infants, cases of suspected PAPVC not clearly defined by ultrasound, SS, and, in the adult population, associated acquired heart lesions (such as valvular pathology and/or coronary obstructive disease).

A full invasive diagnostic study with hemodynamic evaluation is indicated in patients with secondary PHT

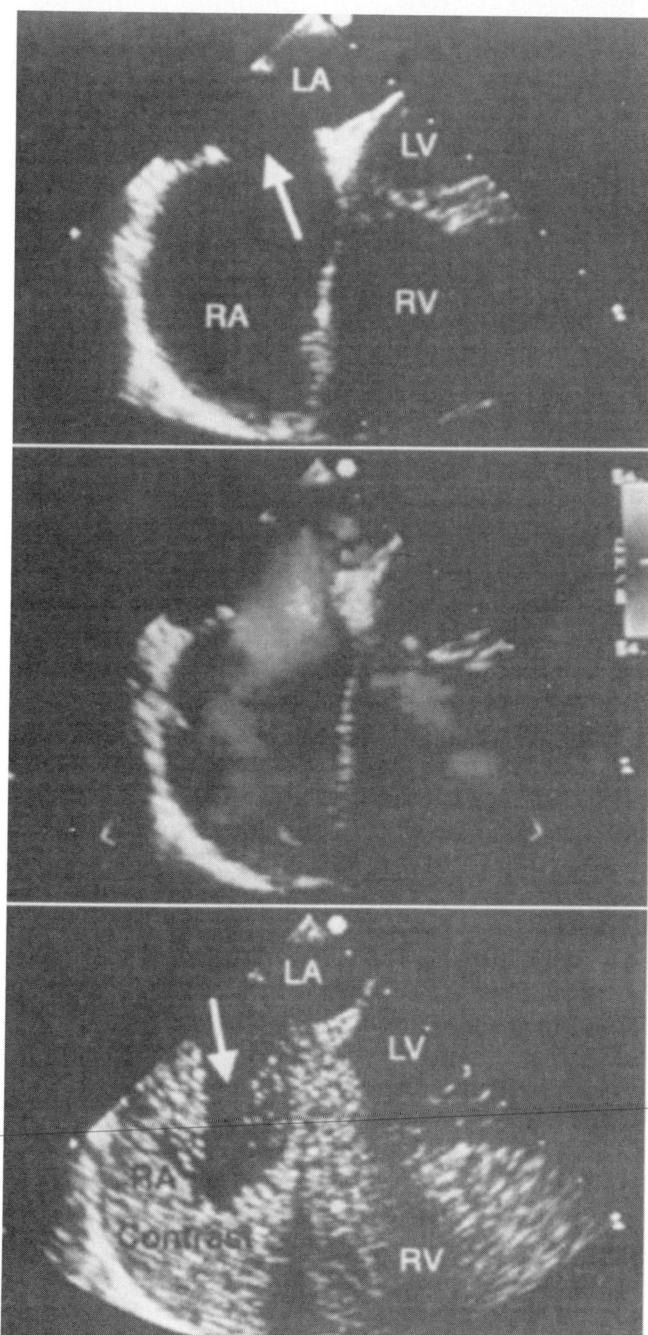

Figure 56-9 Transesophageal echocardiography in a patient with a large secundum-type ASD. A large defect (arrow, top panel) is visible between the right and left atria. Color-flow Doppler interrogation reveals unrestricted left-to-right shunting (middle). Systemic venous injection of agitated saline reveals a "negative washout" of saline bubbles secondary to the left-to-right shunt, with paucity of contrast seen in the left atrium. [From Atrial septal defect and partial anomalous pulmonary venous connection. In: Kouchoukos NT, Blackstone EH, Doty DB, et al (eds). *Kirklin/Barratt-Boyes Cardiac Surgery,* 3d ed. Philadelphia: Churchill-Livingstone 2003:735. With permission.]

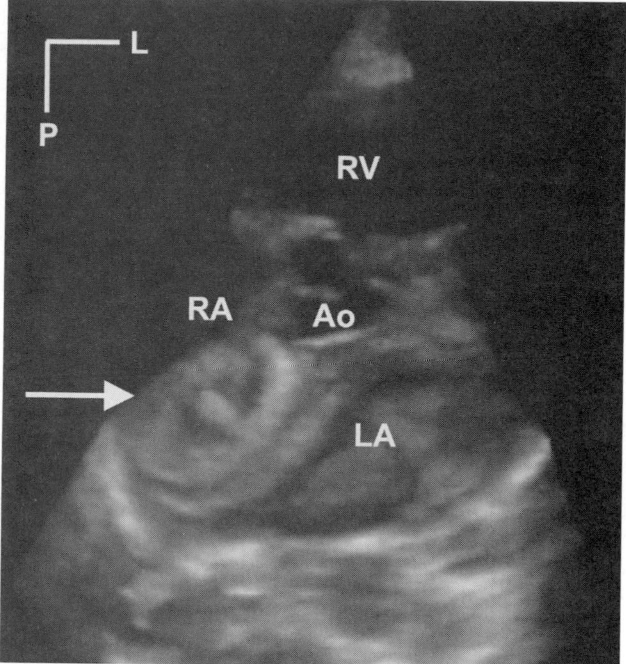

Figure 56-10 Three-dimensional transesophageal echocardiogram. (Courtesy of Dr. William Ravekes, Division of Pediatric Cardiology, Johns Hopkins Hospital.

and an ASD. Feasibility of surgery is judged upon calculation of pulmonary vascular resistance and its eventual decrease according to the administration of oxygen, inhaled nitric oxide (iNO), and infusion of prostacyclin analogues. With a significant decrease in pulmonary arterial pressure and resistance, the patient should be considered a surgical candidate. Lack of response to the abovementioned pulmonary vasodilators contraindicates surgical intervention. In intermediate cases, fenestrated ASD closure can be considered.

NONOPERATIVE MANAGEMENT

As already mentioned, indications for surgical intervention are rarely met in children younger than 2 years of age. Failure to thrive and need for medical therapy or correction is, however, more frequent in infants and children with a common atrium or chromosomal abnormalities.[35,46] There are also other conditions in which early crossover from medical to surgical management might be indicated, such as otherwise unexplained PHT in infancy[47] and concomitant association of an enlarged coronary sinus (atypical left cor triatriatum), functionally similar to totally anomalous pulmonary venous connection.[48] If the child presents symptoms and/or evidence of RA/RV enlargement at echocardiography, continuing medical management until 5 years of age could be justified. Several investigators have in fact reported spontaneous restriction, even in those cases with heart failure in

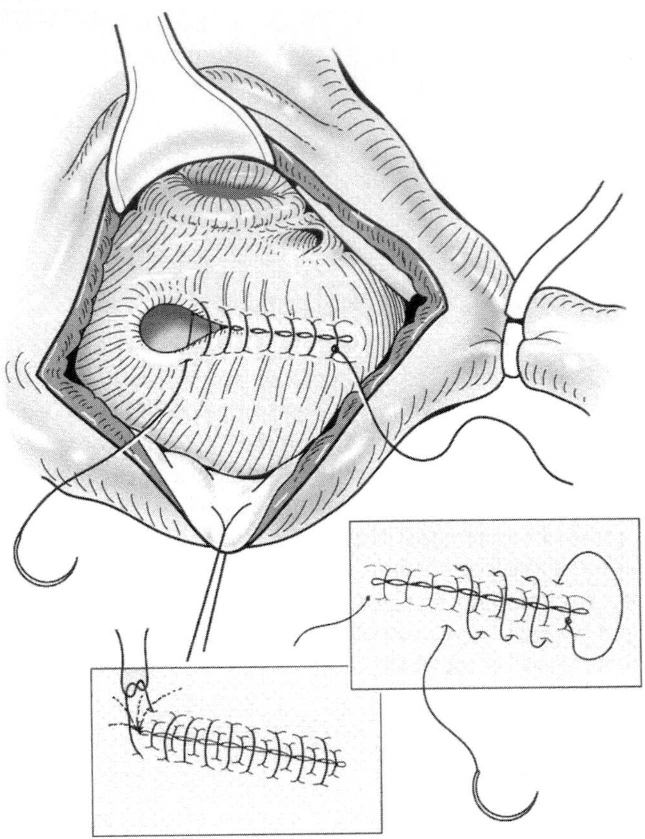

Figure 56-11 Direct closure of ASD. A two-layer closure with nonreabsorbable suture is started at the inferior aspect of the oval-shaped defect and run in a cephalad direction (left side of the figure). [From Manning PB. Atrial septal defect. In: Gardner TJ, Spray TL (eds). *Operative Cardiac Surgery,* 5th ed. London: Arnold 2004:595. With permission.]

infancy.[29] In the interim (even though rarely needed), diuretics and angiotensin antagonists can be used to control symptoms and progression of heart failure while cardiac status is monitored echocardiographically on a yearly basis. In cases not amenable to a conservative approach and not showing a tendency toward restriction, intervention can usually be postponed until 1 to 2 years of age, at a time when morbidity and mortality from ASD closure are usually negligible.[49]

The advantage of surgical intervention in ASD and/or PAPVC in adult and elderly patients has been debated.[50] The Canadian consensus conference on adult congenital heart disease[51] clearly underscored that any "significant ASD warrants intervention," implying that any ASD with RV volume overload, atrial arrhythmias, and/or late heart failure should be treated, given the low risk of surgical and percutaneous intervention.

Closure of the defect is not recommended in patients presenting with advanced pulmonary vascular obstructive disease. Medical treatment is indicated and should be individually tailored according to symptoms, comorbidities, and cardiovascular complications.

SURGICAL TREATMENT

Closure of ASDs is typically approached through a median sternotomy, although a right thoracotomy with central or peripheral cannulation can be considered in postpuberal patients and young adults. We advocate a low median sternotomy or inferior hemisternotomy in prepuberal females, given the possibility of distortion and permanent cosmetic damage to the developing breast with an anterolateral thoracotomy.

Below is outlined the surgical approach to closure of ASDs, along with a brief description of specific considerations that apply to more complex variants of ASD, namely CoS, SV ASD/PAPVC, and SS. A description of the techniques utilized for more complex subtypes of anomalous systemic venous connections and atrial septation is beyond the scope of this chapter.[52,53]

A median sternotomy is performed with conventional cannulation including bicaval drainage. Cardiopulmonary bypass with moderate hypothermia (30° to 32°C) is instituted and the repair accomplished either with fibrillatory or cardioplegic arrest. Following cardiac arrest, caval snares are tightened and an oblique atriotomy is

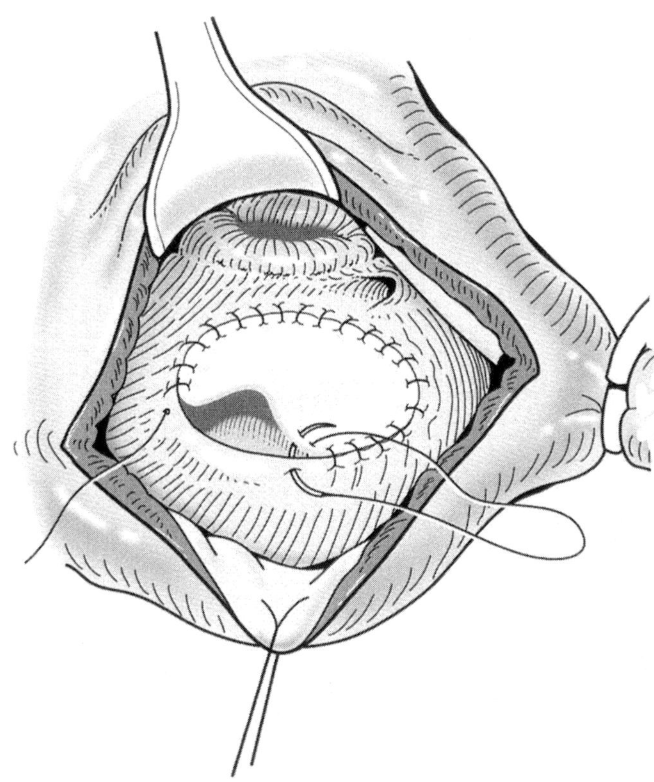

Figure 56-12 Patch ASD closure. A patch of autologous pericardium is secured around the circumference of the defect with a running polypropylene suture. [From Manning PB. Atrial septal defect. In: Gardner TJ, Spray TL (eds). *Operative Cardiac Surgery,* 5th ed. London: Arnold 2004:596. With permission.]

performed. Depending on preoperative localization of the defect, cephalad or caudad extension of the atriotomy is considered. The left atrium is usually vented directly across the defect and the anatomic situation evaluated, including the morphology of the mitral and tricuspid valves. The RV outflow tract is also assessed, and all pulmonary and systemic venous ostia are accounted for.

The technique chosen (primary or patch closure) to repair the defect is determined by the size, location, and shape of the ASD. In our opinion, the majority of ASDs (within the fossa ovalis, with the exception of the single atrium) can be closed with a continuous double-layer nonabsorbable suture (see Fig. 56-11), catching strong bits of the posterior and anterior limbic tissue of the atrial septum and starting from the caudal edge of the defect. It is obviously recommended that the right pulmonary veins not be restricted, the mitral valve not distorted and the nodes not injured. Patch closure can be easily performed with a portion of autologous pericardium, harvested at the beginning of the procedure and tanned in 0.6 percent glutaraldehyde for 30 min (Fig. 56-12). Alternatively, polytetrafluoroethylene, bovine pericardium, or Dacron patches can be utilized. The latter should, however, be avoided in the presence of known mitral regurgitation, as persistent regurgitant jets on the Dacron fabric have been associated with hemolysis. Given the known thrombogenicity of the aneurysmal fossa ovalis ASD, we routinely resect the aneurysmal tissue and then perform patch closure rather than plicating or patching the redundant tissue. For the defects outlined above, several minimally invasive approaches have been devised to accomplish direct or patch closure of "simple" septation defects.[54]

In inferiorly located ASDs, when there is deficiency of an inferoposterior rim, it is best to start patch closure in this area, proceeding from the IVC toward the more developed ASD rim. Modified ultrafiltration is carried out in our practice in all children with operative weight below 20 kg. Blood-conservation strategies (i.e., minimal priming of the circuit with autologous blood after cannulation and utilization of a "cell saver" system to scavenge and reinfuse shed blood) are considered for children with operative weight above 20 kg.

For closure of an isolated CoS defect, it is sufficient to simply close off the coronary sinus (Fig. 56-13), bearing in mind that the cephalad margin is very close to the atrioventricular node. Since the tissue on that side is fairly soft, surgical closure with a patch secured with a continuous nonabsorbable suture is advisable. To avoid the atrioventricular node, the suture line should remain (anteriorly and superiorly) very deep within the coronary sinus, taking small bites of tissue. Simple closure of the coronary sinus will allow for a small obligatory right-to-left shunt from the coronary sinus to the left atrium.

As mentioned in the morphology section, superior SV defects are located high in the septum secundum and are generally associated with anomalous connections of the right pulmonary veins in proximity of the superior cavoatrial junction. Direct cannulation of the SVC (as opposed to transatrial indirect cannulation) is optional and depends on SVC diameter and site of drainage of the anomalous pulmonary veins. A vertical incision (posterior to the sulcus terminalis and sinoatrial node and anterior to the pulmonary veins) is the approach we have utilized in nearly all patients (n = 49) with superior SV ASD

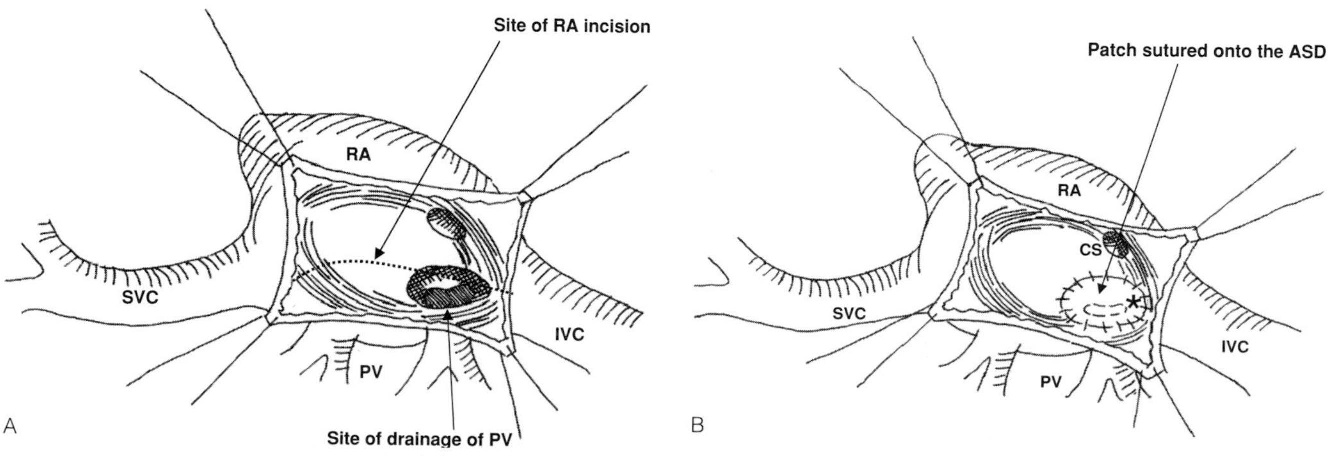

Figure 56-13 Closure of unroofed coronary sinus ASD with otherwise intact interatrial septum and no left superior vena cava. Left: unroofed sinus with intact septum and large coronary sinus. Right: patch closure of the coronary sinus with atologous pericardium, with deep suture line along the superior edge to avoid damage to the atrioventricular conducton system. Ao = aorta; IVC = inferior vena cava; LA = left atrium; RPA = right pulmonary artery; SVC = superior vena cava. (From Jonas RA. *Comprehensive Surgical Management of Congenital Heart Disease*. London: Arnold, 2004:230. With permission.]

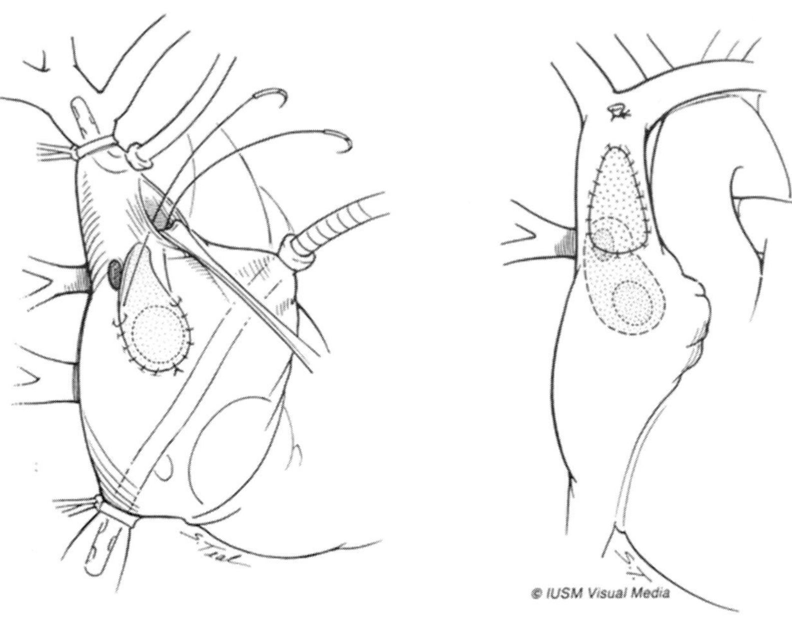

Figure 56-14 Closure of superior sinus venosus atrial defect with partial anomalous pulmonary venous connection. Left: through a superior right atriotomy, the defect is closed with a patch of autologous pericardium, rerouting the right superior pulmonary vein to the left atrium. Right: an additional pericardial patch is used to close the atriotomy extended across the superior atriocaval junction. [From Turrentine MW. Atrial septal defects. In: Yang SC, Cameron DE (eds). *Current Therapy in Thoracic and Cardiovascular Surgery.* Philadelphia: Mosby, 2004:735. With permission.]

undergoing correction at our institution. The right atriotomy is extended across the superior atriocaval junction, well above the superior margin of the anomalously connected pulmonary vein. The left atrium is usually vented via the atrial septal defect. The defect is closed with a patch of autologous pericardium, baffling the right-sided pulmonary veins toward the left atrium (Fig. 56-14). To prevent undue stenosis of the SVC, the atriotomy is closed with a generous patch of autologous pericardium or, when the SVC is large, by direct running closure.

In those uncommon cases in which the SVC lumen appear to be extremely small or the anomalously connected veins drain very high above the RA-SVC junction, a fairly radical procedure should be considered (Warden procedure, Fig. 56-15). Through the right atriotomy, the anomalous return is rerouted to the LA. The atriocaval junction is transected and the distal aspect of the SVC is oversewn. The SVC is then anastomosed directly to the right atrial appendage. In older children, a polytetrafluoroethylene interposition graft can be used. In cases of PAPVC not associated with an ASD, the floor of the fossa ovalis can be excised, and the resulting unrestrictive communication utilized to baffle the anomalous return to the left atrium.

The surgical correction of SS is based on pre- and intraoperative localization of the anomalous pulmonary venous return. The anomaly is often amenable to rerouting toward the left atrium from within the IVC-RA junction (Fig. 56-16). If the anomalous pulmonary vein ostium is too low, the vein can be alternatively ligated at the diaphragm and either transected and anastomosed to the left or right atrium or connected to the left atrium in a side-to-side fashion (Fig. 56-17). Variable depth of hypothermia is usually needed to aid in exposure.

SURGICAL OUTCOMES

The postoperative course that follows correction of ASD and PAPVC is generally uneventful, and the majority of patients can be separated from mechanical ventilation in the operating room and discharged home within 3 to 4 days.[55]

Aside from morbidity that can be observed in any cardiac operation, specific minor early complications are represented by postpericardiotomy syndrome (typically 7 to 14 days after the operation) and arrhythmias, particularly following SV ASD/PAPVC repair.[53–55]

Excellent long-term outcomes for patients of all ages have been reported[56–60] and, in the current era, morbidity and mortality for surgical closure of any type of ASD should approach zero.[31] Between 1993 and 2004, 255

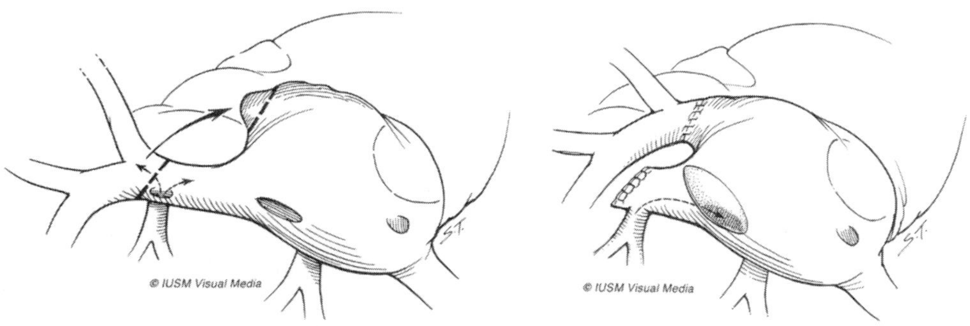

Figure 56-15 Warden procedure. When the partial anomalous return to the superior vena cava is remote from the superior atriocaval junction, the superior vena cava (SVC) is transected (left). Pulmonary venous return is rerouted to the left atrium via an existing or surgically performed atrial septal defect and the SVC is anastomosed to the right atrial appendage (right). [From Turrentine MW. Atrial septal defects. In: Yang SC, Cameron DE (eds). *Current Therapy in Thoracic and Cardiovascular Surgery.* Philadelphia: Mosby, 2004:735. With permission.]

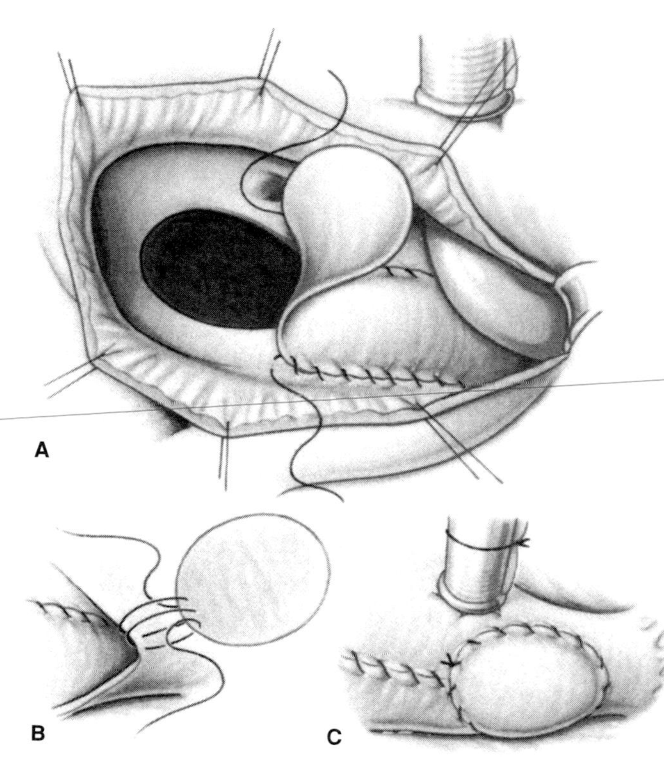

Figure 56-16 Surgical correction of scimitar syndrome. An intracardiac baffle of autologous pericardium (a) is used to rerout pulmonary venous return to the left atrium via an ASD. The lower portion of the atriotomy is enlarged with a second patch to avoid stenosis of the inferior vena cava (b,c).[From Stark J. Secundum atrial septal defect and partial anomalous pulmonary venous return. In: deLeval M, Stark J (eds). *Surgery for Congenital Heart Defects,* 2d ed. Philadelphia: Saunders, 1994:351. With permission.]

children (age < 18 years) underwent surgical ASD closure at our institution. Most patients had isolated secundum-type defects, 49 patients had SVD ± PAPVC, one infant had a CoS ASD, and two had scimitar syndrome; there were no operative mortalities and no cerebrovascular accidents, while the incidence of delayed pericardial effusions was 5 percent.

When surgery is indicated in smaller infants, mortality is similar (but not quite as low) as in older children, while reported morbidity ranges between 2.5 and 11 percent.[49,58,61]

PERCUTANEOUS CLOSURE OF ATRIAL SEPTAL DEFECTS

Transcatheter ASD closure was first described in 1976 by King and coworkers.[62] In the subsequent two decades, multiple ingenious devices were developed to effectively close secundum ASDs. The goal has been to design a device that could be delivered through a small vascular sheath, produce complete closure in 98 percent or more of patients, be technically easy to insert, and remain removable until the point of final deployment. Most of the devices invented to date have failed to accomplish these goals for one reason or another. The Amplatzer Septal Occluder (ASO) was introduced in 1995 and subsequently proven to be safe and effective in producing closure of OS ASDs, gaining FDA approval in November 2001 (Fig. 56-18). By the end of 2005, the manufacturer estimated that 80,000 implants had been performed worldwide. The ASO remains to date the only FDA-approved ASD closure device in the United States.

As part of the FDA approval process, a study of 596 patients was performed, with 442 undergoing ASO device closure of their ASDs and 154 having surgical

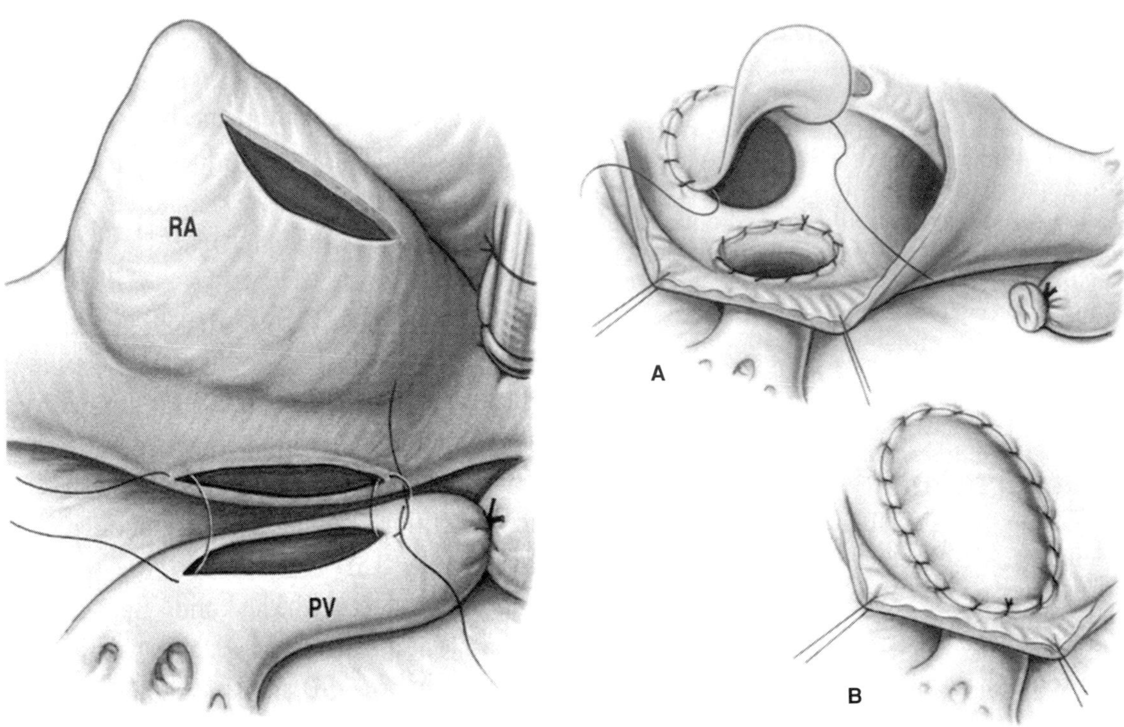

Figure 56-17 Surgical correction of scimitar syndrome. When return of the anomalous pulmonary vein is very low, a side-to-side anastomosis can be constructed between the vein and the left atrium (left). Alternatively, the vein can be transected distally and anastomosed in an end-to-side fashion, with pericardial baffle rerouting to the left atrium (right). PV = pulmonary vein; RA = right atrium. [From Stark J. Secundum atrial septal defect and partial anomalous pulmonary venous return. In: deLeval M, Stark J (eds). *Surgery for Congenital Heart Defects,* 2d ed. Philadelphia: Saunders, 1994:351. With permission.]

repair of their defects.[63] Successful ASO implantation rate was 96 percent, with a successful closure (≤ 2-mm residual shunt) rate of 99 percent at 12 months. Patients undergoing catheterization remained in the hospital for 1 day on average (versus 3.4 days for surgical patients), and outcomes compared favorably with those of the surgical cohort.

Device closure of secundum-type ASDs can be safely performed even on small children (under 5 years of age). Butera and coworkers reported a complete closure rate of 100 percent at 1 year in 48 children under the age of 5 (mean age and weight 3.6 years and 15 kg)[64] with no device-related complications. However, it is important to note that in this study of 99 children, 51 patients had defects considered too large for safe implantation of a device and were referred for surgical repair. Eligibility rates for device closure are much higher for older children and adults, with only 3.7 percent of all subjects enrolled in the initial FDA trial[63] having ASDs that were judged inappropriate for device closure.

Although closure of very large ASDs (greater than 30 mm) can be challenging, most defects are readily occluded using standard technique. Simultaneous use of fluoroscopy and transesophageal or intracardiac echocardiography is now standard practice and makes it possible to exclude from device implantation those defects with diminutive rims or locations that would jeopardize valvular function or inflow. The procedure typically requires 60 to 90 min, with 10 to 20 min of fluoroscopy time. Overnight observation is strongly advised, with

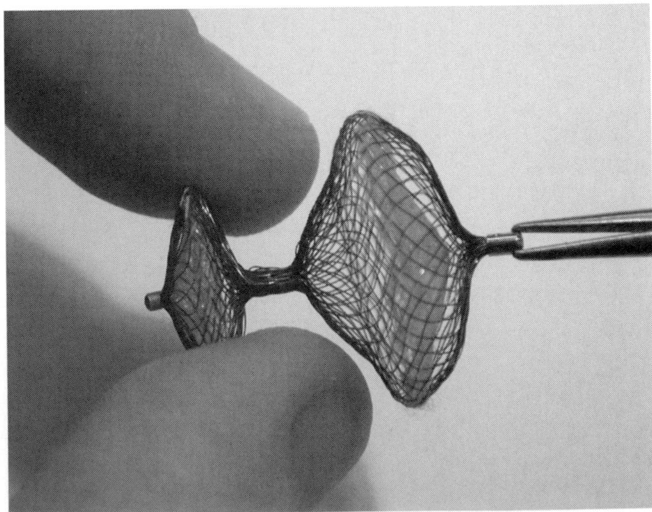

Figure 56-18 Amplatzer atrial septal occluder.

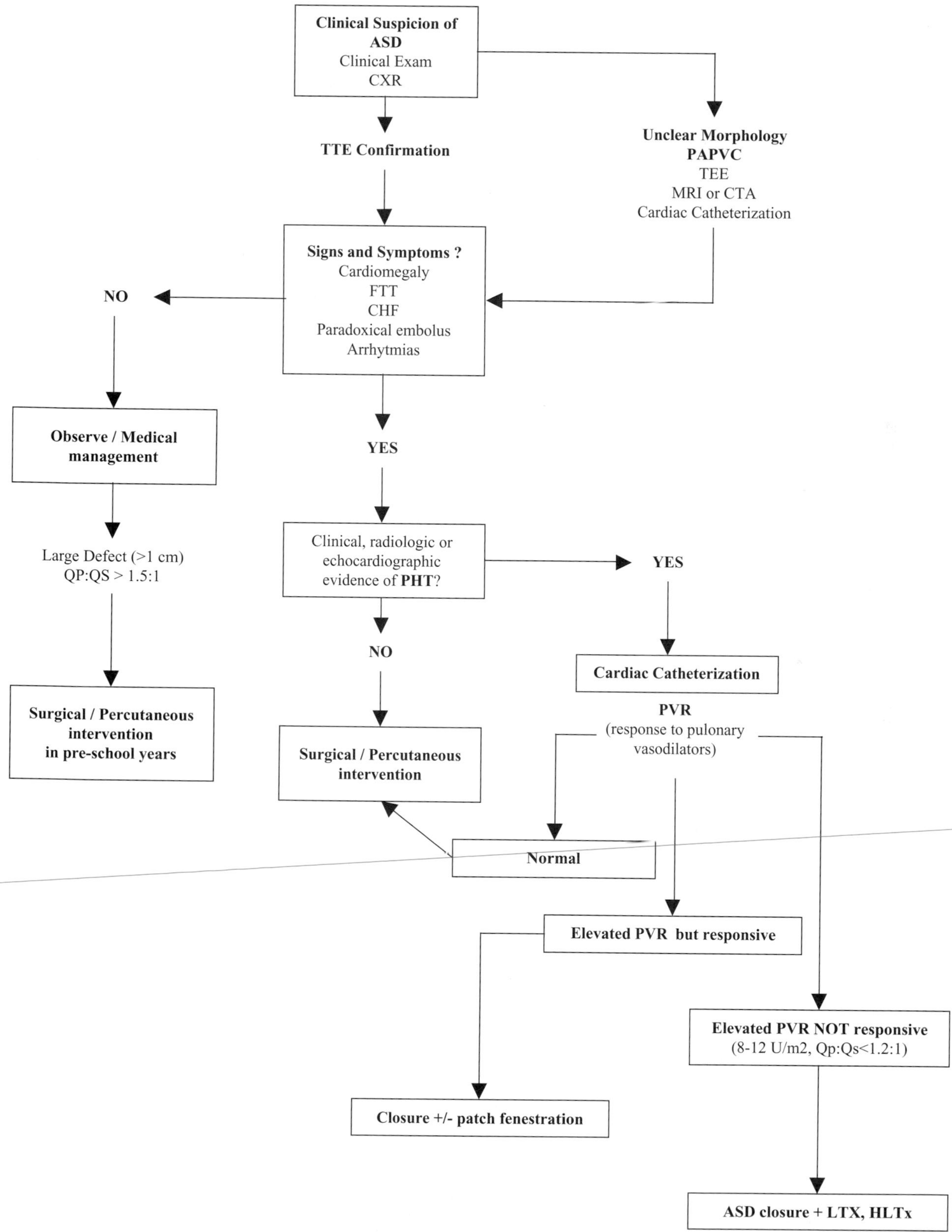

Figure 56-19 Clinical decision-making algorithm for management of isolated atrial septal defects and partial anomalous venous connection. ASD = atrial septal defect; CHF = congestive heart failure; CTA = CT angiography; CXR = chest x-ray; FTT = failure to thrive; HLTx = heart-lung transplantation; LTX = lung transplantation; MRI = magnetic resonance imaging; PAPVC = partial anomalous pulmonary venous connection; PHT = pulmonary hypertension; PVR = pulmonary vascular resistance; TEE = transesophageal echocardiography; TTE = transthoracic echocardiography.

next-day discharge after echocardiographic confirmation of stable device position, minimal or no residual shunting, absence of pericardial effusion or interference with atrioventricular valve function or venous drainage.

Postmarketing surveillance has identified 37 instances of device erosion through the atrial wall into either the pericardial space or the ascending aorta, leading to hemopericardium and, in some cases, cardiac tamponade. Three deaths have been attributed to this phenomenon. A detailed review of all reported cases identified device oversizing to be the greatest risk factor for device erosion.[65,66]

References

1. Rashkind WJ. Historical aspects of congenital heart disease. *Birth Defects* 1982;8:2.
2. Roesler H. Interatrial septal defect. *Arch Intern Med* 1954; 54:339.
3. Murray G. Closure of defects in cardiac septa. *Ann Surg* 1948;128:843.
4. Santy P, Bret J, Marion P. Communication interauricolaire traitee par invagination transseptale de l'auricule droit. *Lyon Chir* 1950;45:359.
5. Swan H, Maresh G, Johnson ME, et al. The experimental creation and closure of auricular septal defect. *J Thorac Surg* 1950;20:542.
6. Bailey CP, Bolton HE, Jamison WL, et al. Atrio-septopexy for interatrial septal defects. *J Thorac Surg* 1953;26:184.
7. Soondergaard T, Gotsche H, Ottoson P, et al. Surgical closure of interatrial septal defects by circumclusion. *Acta Chir Scand* 1955;109:188.
8. Gross RE. Surgical closure of defects of the interauricular septum by use of an atrial well. *N Engl J Med* 1952;247: 455.
9. Kirklin JW, Swan HJ, Wood EH, et al. Anatomic, physiologic, and surgical consideration in repair of interatrial communications in man. *J Thorac Surg* 1955;29:37.
10. Lewis FJ, Taufic M. Closure of atrial septal defects with the aid of hypothermia: Experimental accomplishments and the report of the one successful case. *Surgery* 1953; 33:53.
11. Gibbon JH. Application of a mechanical heart-lung apparatus to cardiac surgery. *Minn Med* 1954;37:171.
12. Peacock TB: Malformations dependent on arrest of development at an early period of fetal life. In: Peacock TB (ed). *Malformations of the Human Heart.* London: John Churchill, 1858:24.
13. Kirklin JW. Surgical treatment of anomalous pulmonary venous connection (partial anomalous pulmonary venous drainage). *Mayo Clin Proc* 1953;28:476.
14. Molecular and morphogenetic cardiac embryology: Implications for congenital heart disease. In: Artman M, Mahony L, Teitel DF (eds). Neonatal Cardiology. New York: McGraw-Hill, 2002:1.
15. McCarthy KP, Ho SE, Anderson RHA. Defining the morphological phenotypes of atrial septal defects and interatrial comunication. *Images Pediatr Cardiol* 2003;15:1.
16. Van Praagh R. Congenital heart disease: Embryology, anatomy and approach to diagnosis. 1997;27:25a.
17. Hartley HRS. The sinus venous type of the atrial septal defect. *Thorax* 1958;13:12.
18. Van Praagh S, Carrera ME, Sanders SP, et al. Sinus venous defect: Unroofing of the right pulmonary veins–anatomic and echocardiographic findings and surgical treatment. *Am Heart J* 1994;128:365.
19. Jacobs JP, Burke RP, Quintessenza JA, et al. Atrial septal defect. *Ann Thorac Surg* 2000;69(suppl):S18.
20. Keith A. The anatomy of valvular mechanisms around the various orifices of the right and left auricles with some observations on the morphology of the heart. *J Anat* 1903;2:37.
21. Mantini F, Grondin CF, Lillehei CW, et al. Congenital anomalies involving the coronary sinus. *Circulation* 1966;33:317.
22. De Leval MR, Ritter DG, McGoon DC, et al. Anomalous systemic venous connection. Surgical considerations. *Mayo Clin Proc* 1975;50:599.
23. Anomalies of the systemic venous return. In: Stark J, de Leval MR (eds). *Surgery of the Congenital Heart Defects.* Philadelphia: Saunders, 1994:320.
24. Gudjohnson U, Brown JW. Scimitar syndrome. *Semin Thorac Cardiothorac Surg Pediatr Card Surg Annu* 2006;25-62.
25. Tozzini S, Anichini C, Nesi G, et al. Secundum atrial septal defect and pulmonary hypertension in an 86-year-old woman: A case report and a review of the literature. *Ital Heart J* 2002;3:682.
26. Overell JR, Bone I, Leeks KR. Interatrial septal abnormalities and stroke: A meta-analysis of case-control studies. *Neurology* 2000;55:1172.
27. Atrial septal defect. In: Corno AF (ed). Congenital heart defects. Darmstadt, Germany: Springer Steinkopff Verlag, 2003:13.
28. Mc Mahon CJ, Feltes TF, Fraley JK, et al. Natural history of growth of secundum atrial septal defects and implications for transcatheter closure. *Heart* 2002;87:256.
29. Brassard M, Fouron JC, van Daesburg NH, et al. Outcome of children with atrial septal defect considered too small for surgical closure. *Am J Cardiol* 1999;83: 1552.
30. Oliver JM, Gallego P, Gonzalez A, et al. Sinus venosus syndrome: Atrial septal defect or anomalous venous connection? A multiplane transoesophageal approach. *Heart* 2002;88:634.
31. Atrial septal defect and partial anomalous pulmonary venous connection. In: Kirklin JW, Barrat-Boyes BG (eds). *Cardiac Surgery.* Philadelphia: Churchill Livingstone, 2003:715.
32. Schrader R. Indications and techniques of transcatheter closure of patent foramen ovale. *J Intervent Cardiol* 2003;16:543.
33. Brown JW, Ruzmetov M, Minnich DJ, et al. Surgical management of scimitar syndrome: An alternative approach. *J Thorac Cardiovasc Surg* 2003;125:238.
34. Huddleston CB, Vernat E, Canter CE, et al. Scimitar syndrome presenting in infancy. *Ann Thorac Surg* 1999;67:154.

35. Mainwaring RD, Mirali-Akbar H, Lamberti JJ, et al. Secundum-type atrial septal defects with failure to thrive in the first year of life. *J Card Surg* 1996;11:116.
36. Campbell M. Natural History of atrial septal defect. *Br Heart J* 1970;32:820.
37. Meissner I, Whisnant JP, Kandheria BK, et al. Prevalence of potential risk factors for stroke assessed by transoesophageal echocardiography and carotid ultrasonography: The SPARC study. Stroke and Prevention: Assessment of Risk in a Community. *Mayo Clin Proc* 1999;74:862.
38. Mas JL, Arquizan C, Lamy C, et al. Recurrent cerebrovascular events associated with patent foramen ovale, atrial septal aneurysm or both. *N Engl J Med* 2001;345:1740.
39. Pascoe RD, Oh JK, Warnes CA, et al. Diagnosis of sinus venosus atrial septal defect with trans-esophageal echocardiography. *Circulation* 1996;94:1049.
40. Defects in cardiac septations. In: Snider RA, Serwer GA, Ritter SB (eds). *Echocardiography in Pediatric Heart Disease.* St Louis: Mosby-Year Book, 1997:237.
41. Congenital heart disease. In: Oh JK, Seward JB, Tajik AJ (eds). *Echo Manual.* Philadelphia: Lippincott Williams & Wilkins, 1999:223.
42. Nanda NC, Pinhero L, Sanyal RS, et al. Transesophageal biplane echocardiography imaging: Technique, planes and clinical usefulness. *Echocardiography* 1990;7:771.
43. Magni G, Hijazi ZM, Pandian NG, et al. Two- and three-dimensional transesophageal echocardiography in patient selection and assessment of atrial septal defect closure by the new DAS-Angel Wings device: Initial clinical experience. *Circulation* 1997;96:1722.
44. Zanchetta M, Pedon L, Rigatelli G, et al. Intracardiac echocardiography: Evaluation in secundum atrial septal defect transcatheter closure. *Cardiovasc Intervent Radiol* 2003;26:52.
45. Ungerleider RM, Greeley WJ, Sheikh KH, et al. Routine use of intraoperative epicardial echocardiography and Doppler color flow imaging to guide and evaluate repair of congenital heart lesions. A prospective study. *J Thorac Cardiovasc Surg* 1990;100:297.
46. Congenital heart disease assessed with magnetic resonance techniques. In: Skorton DJ, Schelbert HR, Wolf GL, Brundage BH (eds). *Cardiac Imaging.* Philadelphia: Saunders, 1996:672.
47. Bull C, Deanfield J, de Leval M, et al. Correction of isolated secundum atrial septal defect in infancy. *Arch Dis Child* 1981;56:784.
48. Cochrane AD, Marath A, Mee RB. Can a dilated coronary sinus produce left ventricular inflow obstruction? An unrecognized entity. *Ann Thorac Surg* 1994;58:1114.
49. Galal MO, Wobst A, Halees Z, et al. Peri-operative complications following surgical closure of atrial septal defect type II in 232 patients: A baseline study. *Eur Heart J* 1984;15:1381.
50. Shah D, Azhar M, Oakley CM, et al. Natural history of secundum atrial septal defect in adults after medical or surgical treatment: A historical prospective study. *Br Heart J* 1994;71:224.
51. Connelly MS, Webb GD, Somerville J. Canadian consensus conference on adult congenital heart disease. *Can J Cardiol* 1996;14:395.
52. Stark J, deLeval M. *Surgery for Congenital Heart Defects.* Philadelphia: Saunders, 1994.
53. Atrial septal defect, partial anomalous pulmonary venous connection and scimitar syndrome. In: Mavroudis K, Backer C (eds). *Pediatric Cardiac Surgery,* 3d ed. St Louis: Mosby, 2003:283.
54. Del Nido PJ, Bichell DP. Minimal accass surgery for congenital heart defects. *Semin Thorac Cardiovasc Surg Pediatr Card Surg Annu* 1998;1:75.
55. Vricella LA, Dearani JA, Gundry SR, et al. Ultra fast track in congenital heart surgery. *Ann Thorac Surg* 2000; 69:86.
56. Nieminen HP, Eero VJ, Heikki S. Late results of pediatric cardiac surgery in Finland: A population-based study with 96% follow-up. *Circulation* 2001;104:570.
57. Murphy GJ, Gersh BJ, Mc Goon MD, et al. Long-term outcome after surgical repair of isolated atrial septal defect: Follow-up at 27–32 years. *N Engl J Med* 1990;323: 1644.
58. Iyer RS, Hoschtitzky A, Jacobs J, et al. Closure of isolated secundum atrial septal defect in infancy. *Asian Cardiovasc Thorac Ann* 2000;8:38.
59. St John Sutton MG, Tajik AJ, Mc Goon DC. Atrial septal defect in patients ages 60 years or older: Operative results and long-term postoperative follow-up. *Circulation* 1981;64:402.
60. Konstantinides S, Geibel A, Olschewski M, et al. A comparison of surgical and medical therapy for atrial septal defects in adults. *N Engl J Med* 1995;333:469.
61. Kalmar P, Irrgang E. Cardiac surgery in the Federal Republic of Germany during 1990: A report by the German Society of Thoracic and Cardiovascular Surgery. *Thorac Cardiovasc Surg* 1001;39:167.
62. King TD, Mill NL. Secundum atrial septal defects: Nonoperative closure during cardiac catheterization. *JAMA* 1976;235:2506.
63. Du Z, Hijazi Z, Kleinman CS, et al. Comparison between transcatheter and surgical closure of secundum atrial septal defect in children and adults. *J Am Coll Cardiol* 2002;39: 1836.
64. Butera G, De Rosa G, Chessa M, et al. Transcatheter closure of atrial septal defect in young children. *J Am Coll Cardiol* 2003;42:2410.
65. Amin Z, Hijazi ZM, Bass JL, et al. Erosion of Amplatzer septal occluder device after closure of secundum atrial septal defects: Review of registry of complications and recommendations to minimize future risk. *Cathet Cardiovasc Intervent* 2004;63:496.
66. Gougeon F. *Hemodynamic Compromise with the Amplatzer Septal Occluder: Importance of Proper Balloon Sizing Techniques.* AGA Medical Corporation, January 2, 2006.

CHAPTER

57 VENTRICULAR SEPTAL DEFECTS

David L. S. Morales , Charles D. Fraser, Jr.

DEFINITION AND EPIDEMIOLOGY

A ventricular septal defect (VSD) is a deficiency in the ventricular septum that can vary in size, number, or location on the septum. All three determine its physiology, while the location alone determines its nomenclature. VSD is the most commonly recognized congenital heart defect excluding bicuspid aortic valve. Approximately 20 percent of patients with congenital defects have isolated VSDs and, if one includes VSDs in combination with other defects, VSDs are diagnosed in 50 percent of all patients with congenital heart disease.[1] VSDs occur at a rate of 0.5 per 1000 live births and in 4.5 to 7 of 1000 premature infants,[1,2] with a slightly higher prevalence in females (56 percent).[3] About 5 percent of VSDs are related to chromosomal syndromes (such as 22q11 deletion and trisomy 21), in which VSD is the most common cardiac defect identified.[4]

HISTORICAL NOTE

In 1891, Dupren coined the term *Maladie de Roger* in honor of Henry-Louis Roger, who first described the

KEY CONCEPTS

- Epidemiology
  - Ventricular septal defect (VSD) is the most common noncyanotic cardiac anomaly (20 percent of all malformations); it is present in over 50 percent of children with complex congenital heart disease. VSDs occur in 0.5 of 1000 live births, and 5 percent are related to chromosomal syndromes.
- Morphology
  - VSDs vary in size, number, and location along septum. They are classified as (1) perimembranous (most common), (2) inlet type, (3) nonmuscular outlet, and (4) muscular. The conduction system and aortic valve leaflets are in anatomic proximity and are at risk during repair.
- Pathophysiology
  - Degree and direction of shunting between the right and left ventricles depend on size (restrictive or nonrestrictive) and balance between the systemic vascular resistance (SVR) and pulmonary vascular resistance (PVR). Aortic regurgitation can ensue as a consequence of leaflet prolapse through the defect.
- Clinical features
  - Small, restrictive defects are often asymptomatic. Symptoms of overcirculation are present in unrestrictive VSDs; with development of irreversible pulmonary vascular changes in untreated large shunts, fixed pulmonary hypertension and cyanosis develop (Eisenmenger's syndrome).
- Diagnosis
  - Echocardiography accurately defines the anatomy of VSD and associated lesions. Cardiac catheterization is rarely required.
- Treatment
  - Timing of closure is indicated by the degree of shunting and aortic valve involvement and is most typically performed in infancy. Transatrial or transventricular approaches are most commonly utilized, with minimal morbidity and mortality. Percutaneous or periventricular device closure is still experimental, while a staged approach (with pulmonary arterial banding and delayed complete repair) is now considered only in selected cases .

clinical and pathologic findings of a VSD in 1879.[5] Eisenmenger then chronicled the natural history of an unrestrictive VSD by his account of the postmortem findings in a cyanotic patient who died at age 32 with a large VSD, a severely hypertrophied right ventricle (RV), pulmonary and tricuspid valve insufficiency, and thickened pulmonary arteries.[6] However, the term *Eisenmenger's syndrome* was not introduced until Abbott delineated the pathophysiology of a VSD in the 1930s.[7]

Muller first surgically addressed a VSD in 1952 by placement of a pulmonary artery band (PAB).[8] Lillehei, using controlled cross circulation, was the first to perform a VSD repair in 1954.[9] DuShane reported transventricular repair in 1956, while a transatrial approach was introduced the following year by Stirling.[10,11] Truex's description in 1958 of the atrioventricular node (AVN) and the conduction pathway in patients with VSDs is an integral part of all modern surgical techniques of VSD closure.[12] Kirklin and associates established in 1961 the ability to repair VSDs in small infants, therefore avoiding the two-staged approach of banding of the pulmonary artery (PA) followed by VSD closure.[13]

ANATOMY

In order to comprehend the different nomenclatures that are used for VSDs and the approaches and techniques for repairing this anomaly, one must understand the anatomy of the RV, the conduction system, and the tricuspid valve (TV).

The TV has three leaflets: septal, anterior, and posterior (Fig. 57-1). The posterior papillary muscle, which is located on the inferior wall of the RV near the septum, gives rise to the chordae of the septal and posterior leaflets. The anterior papillary muscle gives rise to the chordae of the anterior and posterior leaflets. It is anchored at the acute margin of the RV and fuses with the RV muscle to become the moderator band, which travels inferiorly and becomes the septal band (alternatively termed trabeculum septomarginalis or septomarginal trabeculation), which travels toward the RV outflow tract. The septal band then divides into its posterior and anterior arms. Between these two arms is the infundibular septum, also known as the conal, outlet, or supracristal septum. The medial papillary muscle (the muscle of Lancisi), which gives chordae to the anterior and septal leaflets of the TV, is most prominent and identifiable during infancy and attaches to the septal band or its posterior arm. The parietal band is the continuation of the septal band's posterior arm anteriorly onto the RV free wall. The parietal band and both arms of the septal band join to form the supraventricular crest (crista supraventricularis), the C-shaped nonobstructive entrance into the outlet region (subpulmonary conus) of the RV. This muscle shelf between the tricuspid and pulmonary valve (PV) creates pulmonary–tricuspid valve discontinuity.

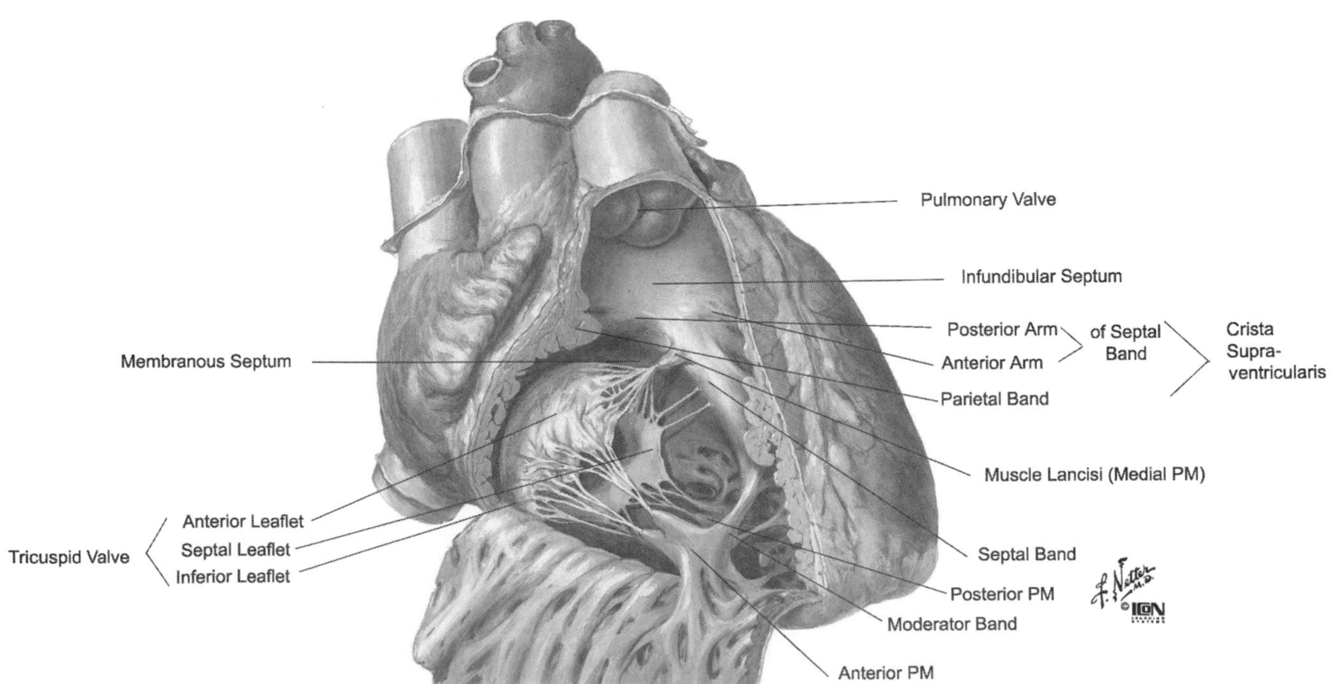

Figure 57-1 Anatomy of the right ventricle. (From Netter F. *The Netter Collection*, vol 5, sec 1. Illustrations. Icon Learning Systems, MediaMedia USA, Inc. All rights reserved. With permission. The drawing has not been modified; however the labeling is that of the authors.)

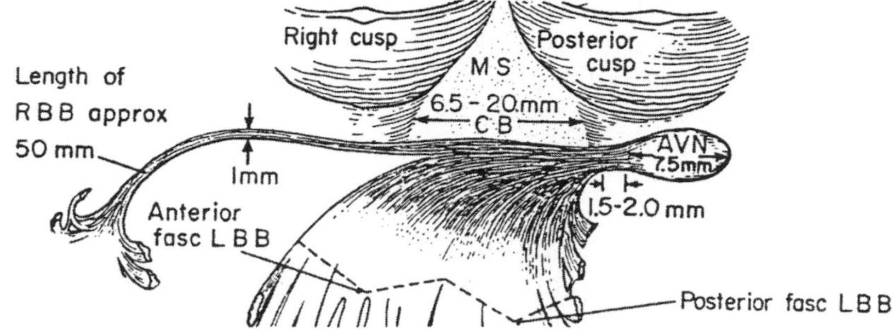

Figure 57-2 A view of the atrioventricular conduction system from the left ventricle and its relationship to the membranous septum and the aortic valve. AVN = atrioventricular node, MS = membranous septum, fasc = fasciculus, RBB = right bundle branch, LBB = left bundle branch. (From Titus JL. Normal anatomy of the human cardiac conduction system. *Mayo Clin Proc* 1973;48:24–30. With permission.)

It is essential to know the location of the AVN and the bundle of His in order to perform safe closure of a VSD. The AVN is located in the triangle of Koch (formed by the tendon of Todaro, the coronary sinus os, and the septal leaflet of the TV). More precisely, it is in the muscular region right below the triangle's apex and directly on the right atrial side of the central fibrous body. From another perspective, the AVN is under the nadir of the noncoronary (posterior) cusp of the aortic valve (Fig. 57-2). The AV bundle (Bundle of His) arises from the AVN and exits at the apex of the triangle of Koch, passing to the ventricular side through the right aspect of the central fibrous body. At this point, the bundle is on the posteroinferior margin of the membranous septum, which lies just posterior to the commissure of the septal and anterior leaflets of the TV (Fig. 57-3). The bundle penetrates the ventricular septum and continues on the left ventricular (LV) side in 75 percent of patients.

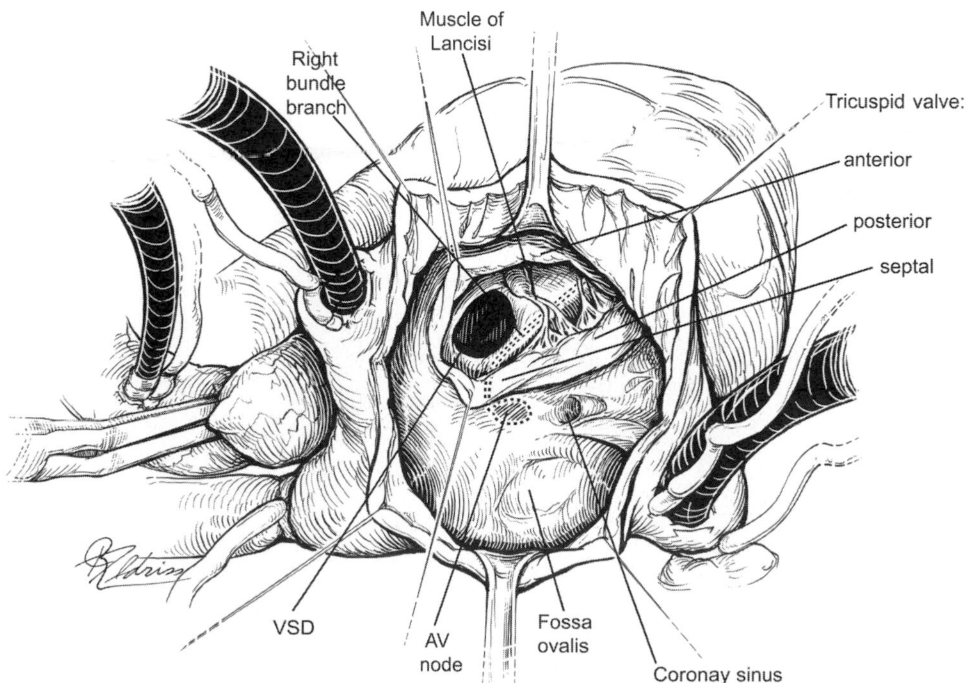

Figure 57-3 Depiction of the atrioventricular node and its course on the inferior border of a perimembranous VSD; viewed from a right atrial surgical approach. (Drawing by Rachid Idriss. Used with the artist's permission, who reserves all rights. The drawing has not been modified, however the labeling is that of the authors.)

Whether on the right or left, it courses along the inferior border of the membranous septum and begins to give off fibers to the left bundle branch over a distance of 1 to 2 cm. When the membranous septum is intact, this area is just below and to the left of the commissure between noncoronary and right coronary cusps of the aortic valve. In considering the bundle from the aortic valve perspective, one should perceive its path as coursing a few millimeters below the area between the right noncoronary (posterior in Fig. 57-2) commissure and the nadir of the right coronary sinus. The remaining fibers of the bundle, which now surface to the anteroinferior border of the membranous septum, become the right bundle branch. The left bundle branch fans out over the septum while the right bundle branch courses as a single radiation (Fig. 57-3). From the anteroinferior border of the membranous septum, the right bundle passes below the muscle of Lancisi and then to the inferior borders of the septal and moderator bands until it reaches the anterior papillary muscle, where it disperses to innervate the RV. Therefore the bundle of His is most often in harm's way during operations on a perimembranous (PM) VSD. The bundle of His runs along a PM VSD's inferior border from where it penetrates the TV annulus to the most inferior papillary muscle on the VSD's muscular rim (the muscle of Lancisi) (Fig. 57-4). The fact that the AVN and bundle of His are specialized myocytes and thus exist only in muscular tissue and not in fibrous tissue is an important fact to consider in placing sutures for VSD repair. The conduction system can also be at risk at the superior edge of a muscular inlet VSD, where the conduction system runs in the muscle between the VSD and the membranous septum.

NOMENCLATURE AND PATHOLOGIC ANATOMY

There are many classifications of VSDs that have been proposed and used; our preference is a modification of the classic Anderson classification. However, to make our classification useful to the reader, we will compare other terms and classification to this terminology.

The ventricular septum can be sectioned into four regions: (1) the *inlet septum*, which is the area of the septum bounded by the attachments of the TV; (2) the *muscular septum*, which is the area from apex to the crista supraventricularis outside these attachments; (3) the *outlet septum*, which is the area from the crista supraventricularis to the PV, and (4) the *perimembranous septum*, which is quite small and lies under the commissure of the anterior and septal leaflets of the TV. The muscular region is further subdivided into anterior, posterior, apical, and midmuscular regions. The Anderson classification names

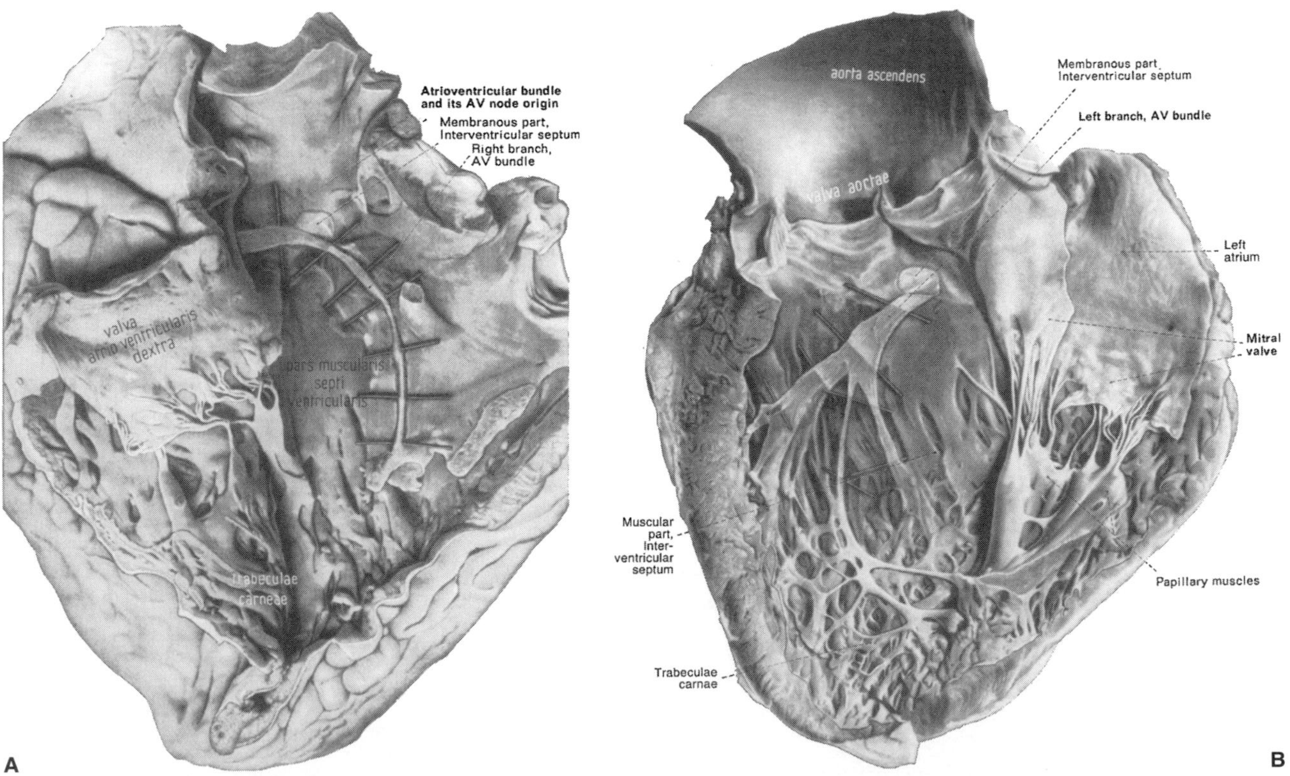

Figure 57-4 Anatomy of the atrioventricular conduction system. A. The atrioventricular bundle and its right branch dissected in the right ventricle. B. The atrioventricular bundle and its left branch dissected in the left ventricle. (From Sobotta. *Atlas der Anatomie des Menschen*, 16th ed. Munich: Urban & Schwarzenberg, 1963. With permission.)

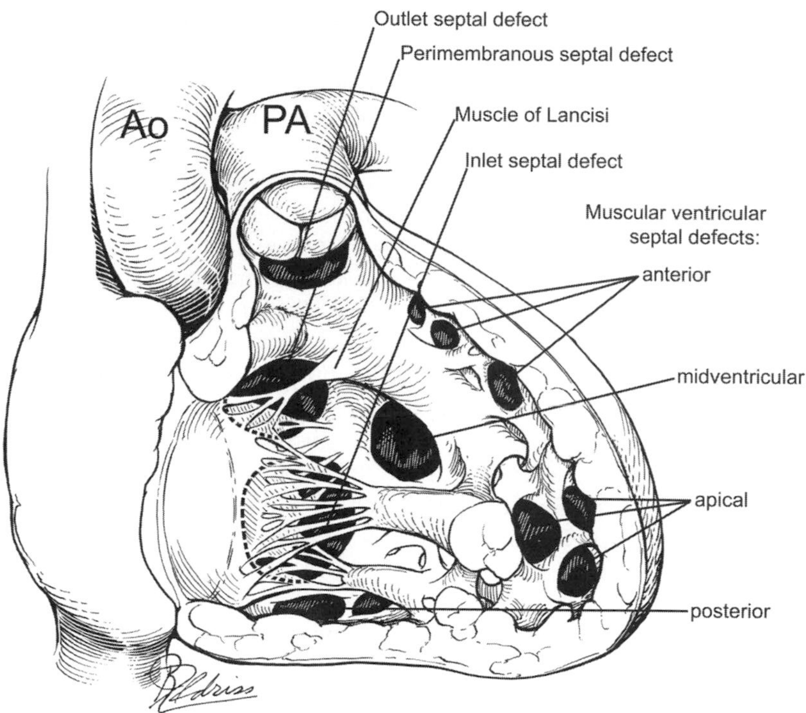

Figure 57-5 The different types of VSDs as viewed via the right ventricle. (Drawing by Rachid Idriss. Used with the artist's permission, who reserves all rights. The drawing has not been modified, however the labeling is that of the authors.)

VSDs according to the region in which they are located. However, from a surgical perspective, one wants to know not only the location of the defect but also its relation to the conduction system. The latter can be transmitted to the surgeon by first defining whether the defect is PM (an absence of the membranous septum) or not (all other types of defects). This automatically tells the surgeon whether or not the conduction system is remote, and if not remote, where it is (inferior to a PM defect for a d-looped heart and superior to a PM defect for a l-looped heart). The exception to this rule is an inlet VSD, which is discussed further on. One can also describe the type of PM VSDs by the areas defined by Anderson. Therefore a PM VSD can be one with muscular extension, outlet extension, inlet extension, or any combination. Non-PM VSDs can be muscular in type (outlet, inlet, anterior, posterior, apical, midmuscular) or outlet or inlet types bound by valve tissue (Fig. 57-5). The synonyms in other classifications for all the terms used above can be found in Table 57-1. The table lists all the different names by which a VSD within a certain region can be designated. The different names listed under a certain region are sometimes used imprecisely to denote any VSD in the area, but most of the terms are not interchangeable and refer to a very specific type of VSD. For example, some might use the

Table 57-1 Nomenclature utilized for ventricular septal defects

Preferred terminology	Synonyms
Perimembranous VSD	
PM VSD with inlet extension	Membranous, infracristal, paramembranous
PM VSD with outlet extension	Membranous, conoventricular, subaortic
PM VSD with muscular extension	Membranous, infracristal, paramembranous
Non-muscular-outlet VSD	Conal, supracristal, subarterial, subaortic, subpulmonary, infundibular, intracristal, doubly committed, conal septal, juxtaarterial
Inlet VSD	Canal type, atrioventricular
Muscular	
Inlet	Canal type
Outlet	Conal, supracristal, subarterial, infundibular, conal septal
Midmuscular VSD	Central
Apical muscular VSD	
Anterior muscular VSD	Marginal
Posterior muscular VSD	Inferior

terms *subaortic* and *supracristal* to refer to the same VSD; however, the former is a general term that refers to any VSD abutting the aortic valve, whereas the latter specifically refers to an outlet VSD abutting a semilunar valve.

The PM VSD represents approximately 80 percent of all VSDs; the remaining 20 percent are evenly distributed among inlet, outlet, and muscular VSDs. A notable exception to this distribution is the almost 30 percent overall prevalence of outlet-type VSDs in the Asian population with VSDs.[14] Small asymptomatic muscular VSDs, which are probably the most common heart defect (present in about 5 percent of all neonates), are grossly underestimated in these statistics, since the vast majority close in the first months of life without recognition.[15]

Perimembranous VSDs are intimately related to the tricuspid and aortic valves. In fact, the absence of the PM septum often creates tricuspid–aortic valve fibrous continuity. “Spontaneous closure” of PM VSDs usually occurs from partial or complete occlusion of the VSD by aneurysmal TV tissue. This aneurysmal tissue is formed from the sheer force of the left-to-right (L-R) shunt resulting in creation of fibrotic tissue, “accessory valve tissue,” and/or, perhaps, remnants of endocardial cushion tissue. Some have described a defect of just the atrioventricular septum causing a shunt from the left ventricle to the right atrium, known as a “Gerbode defect.”[16] When seen on echocardiography, this almost always represents a PM VSD with a jet directed through a cleft in the TV or the septal-anterior commissure, giving the echocardiographic appearance of a Gerbode defect. A consequence of this physiologic shunting from the LV to the right atrium can be extensive right atrial enlargement; if an atrial septal defect exists, streaming of the blood can possibly cause right to left atrial (LA) shunting with resulting cyanosis.

Malalignment of the infundibular septum is also associated with PM VSDs, usually with outlet extension. If one considers the infundibular septum as being in the coronal plane with the RV outflow tract above and the LV outflow tract below, then comprehension of the malaligned VSDs is more straightforward. In an anteriorly malaligned VSD, the infundibular septum is deviated anteriorly into the RV outflow tract, causing obstruction. The aortic valve also moves anteriorly, so that it overrides the ventricular septum. In a posteriorly malaligned VSD, the infundibular septum deviates posteriorly into the LV outflow tract, causing obstruction.

Outlet defects are often differentiated between defects that are completely bound by muscle and those that are bounded on one side by aortic valve tissue (subaortic, juxtaarterial VSDs), by pulmonary valve tissue (subpulmonary VSDs), or both (doubly committed, subarterial VSDs). This differentiation is useful in terms of the pathophysiology. The nonmuscular outlet defects along with PM VSDs with outlet extension can both be associated with aortic valve insufficiency, characterized by lengthening and eventual prolapsing of the right coronary leaflet (outlet defect) or noncoronary leaflet (PM VSD). This valve tissue can partially or completely close the defect. The conduction system is remote to outlet defects.

Inlet defects are beneath the septal leaflet of the TV, just inferior and posterior to the membranous septum. These defects can be an atrioventricular septal defect or a muscular inlet defect. The former is an endocardial cushion defect, characterized by absence of the PM septum, atrioventricular valve abnormalities, and a conduction system traveling along the inferior aspect of the defect. A muscular inlet defect is a VSD that can be remote to the conduction system or have the conduction system border the defect superiorly.

Muscular VSDs can be multiple or appear to be so because of the overlying trabeculae in the RV. This topography and multiplicity may cause difficulty in closure of these defects. When these impediments become prohibitive to conventional surgery, the term “Swiss cheese septum” is usually used to describe them. However, it should be noted that some believe that a Swiss cheese septum is actually an entity distinct from multiple VSDs. The morphology of the Swiss cheese septum is believed to originate from septal noncompaction during embryologic development; thus, unlike a group of muscular VSDs, Swiss cheese defects cannot close spontaneously.[17,18]

PATHOPHYSIOLOGY

The pathophysiology of a VSD is determined by the size of the defect and its location. If the defect is smaller than the aortic annulus (a restrictive VSD), then the shunt’s direction and volume is determined by the difference in systolic pressures of the ventricles. If the defect is larger than the aortic valve, then the defect is nonrestrictive and the pressure in the ventricles should equalize. The direction and volume of this shunt is determined by the difference in pulmonary and systemic vascular resistance.

Restrictive VSDs can be further categorized as small or moderate in size. A small VSD has a large resistance to flow, resulting in a small L–R shunt, and the pulmonary vasculature is well protected. The small shunt volume does not increase ventricular work or volume, so the LA and LV tend not to dilate. The large pressure gradient across the small VSD favors L-R flow throughout the cardiac cycle, which can produce a continuous murmur. Moderate-sized defects remain restrictive but allow a large enough L-R shunt to cause left-sided volume overload, characterized by LA and LV dilation. The pulmonary vasculature remains protected; however, some pulmonary hypertension can exist, which will cause RV pressure and work to increase. This results in mild RV hypertrophy.

Nonrestrictive VSDs allow the RV and LV to have equal pressures, with the determination of flow across the defect resulting from outflow resistance. In the LV, this is determined by systemic vascular resistance or by LV outflow tract anomalies (subaortic stenosis, aortic stenosis, coarctation, etc.). In the RV, this is determined by PVR or by RV outflow tract anomalies (PV stenosis, tetralogy of Fallot, etc.). PVR is high at birth and decreases the L-R shunt; however, the PVR naturally decreases as the pulmonary vascular bed matures. The decline in PVR occurs mostly over the first few days, but the process is not completed until 2 to 6 weeks after birth.[19,20] The thinning of the vascular media, the enlargement and proliferation of the peripheral PAs, and the regression of the PA's perinatal muscularity mark the normal maturation of the pulmonary vessels. However, a large L-R shunt disturbs the growth and remodeling of the pulmonary vasculature, so that medial hypertrophy develops, muscularization of PAs persists, and the size and number of peripheral PAs is reduced. These structural changes are the basis of pulmonary vascular disease.[21,22] Any patient with a nonrestrictive VSD and no RV outflow tract obstruction has pulmonary hypertension, but this does not necessarily indicate that the patient has pulmonary vascular disease. The latter is a disease state of the pulmonary vasculature correlating to specific pathologic changes in the PAs, while pulmonary hypertension is simply a hemodynamic state of the PAs at any given time. A nonrestrictive VSD is characterized by a large L-R shunt, which will cause volume overload of the LA and LV, resulting in significant dilation of these chambers. This shunt will also result in pulmonary hypertension, which in time will cause RV hypertrophy and increasing PVR. As the PVR increases, the L-R shunt decreases. When end-stage pulmonary vascular disease ensues, the shunt can even reverse direction to a right-to-left shunt (i.e. Eisenmenger's syndrome). Reversal of shunting and cyanosis rarely present in children below age 5 with isolated VSDs and is usually seen in adolescents and adults.

CLINICAL FEATURES

The presentation of a patient with a VSD varies according to the size of the defect, the amount of L-R shunting, and PVR (Fig. 57-6). The majority of VSDs are small; these patients are asymptomatic and are diagnosed because of a loud systolic murmur, prompting an echocardiogram. The murmur is often not heard until the first postnatal visit, after PVR has dropped. Many of these defects will close spontaneously by muscle hypertrophy, fibrosis of the defect's margins, or leaflet adherence

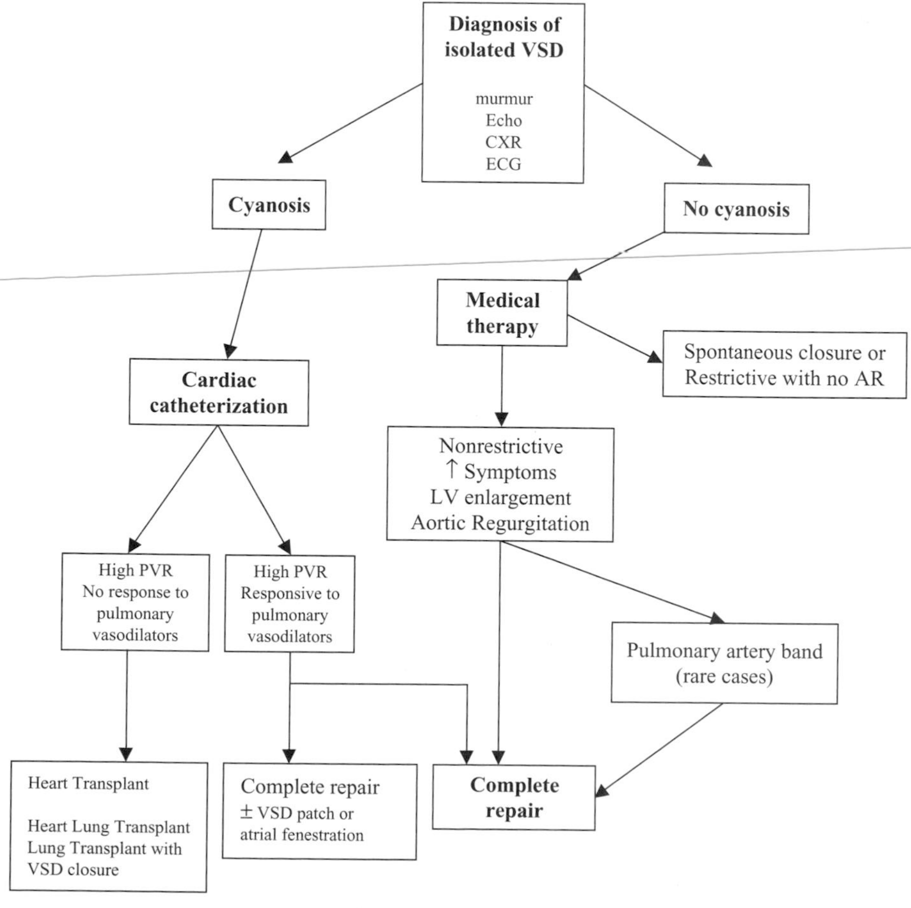

Figure 57-6 Decision-making flowchart for isolated ventricular septal defect.

to the defect. In a study by Turner and colleagues, 290 children with isolated VSDs of all sizes were followed for a mean of 65 months.[23] The study revealed that 68 percent of VSDs with complete muscular borders closed spontaneously, and 29 percent of PM VSDs closed. There were no cases of endocarditis in this nonoperative series. The aortic valve can also contribute to the narrowing of defects that have an outlet component, which can cause aortic insufficiency; this is a situation that demands prompt surgical treatment. Despite therapy, the natural history of the damaged aortic valve may no longer be normal. Thus waiting for spontaneous closure of PM VSDs or outlet VSDs, even with close follow-up, is not without risk.

Patients with large VSDs present with varying degrees of pulmonary overcirculation. The amount of overcirculation usually determines their age at presentation. Patients with larger defects and significant overcirculation can present in the first months of life, as PVR falls. These patients present with tachypnea, poor feeding, slow weight gain, and diaphoresis with activity. They are at risk for repeated upper respiratory infections, "cardiac asthma," and failure to thrive. Shunt size and the length of exposure to the resulting pulmonary hypertension will determine the time frame for the development of the varying degrees of pulmonary vascular disease. Patients with trisomy 21 have a shorter time course to reach significant pulmonary vascular disease than most children.[24] The end stage of pulmonary vascular disease is termed Eisenmenger's syndrome: PVR greater than systemic vascular resistance, reversal of shunt flow from L-R to R-L, cyanosis, and eventually RV failure.[25]

DIAGNOSIS

Physical examination

Small defects usually have minimal physical findings and a normal chest x-ray (CXR) and electrocardiogram (ECG). Precordial activity is typically normal, but a thrill may be palpable on the lower left sternal border. The murmur is a loud, high-frequency holosystolic murmur that includes and sometimes goes beyond the second heart sound and is heard best over the left lower sternal border. The murmur's continuous nature in systole provides evidence of a large pressure gradient between the RV and LV. Small muscular defects can sometimes have short murmurs that cut off at midsystole because of septal contraction.[26] Heart sounds are usually normal.

Moderate to large defects with minimal elevation of PVR present with similar exams that vary according to the amount of shunting. Precordial activity is accentuated and can span from the left apical area at first, indicating increased LV volume, to the right parasternal area eventually, indicating pulmonary hypertension and RV hypertrophy. As LV volume increases, the left thorax may begin to bulge, especially in younger infants. As the shunt increases, the third heart sound becomes more prominent, as does a middiastolic rumble, which indicates increased pulmonary blood flow at least double systemic blood flow. The holosystolic nature and the loudness of the murmur begin to dissipate as defects become larger and the pressure gradient between the RV and LV decreases. As pulmonary hypertension increases, the second heart sound has a narrower split and the pulmonary component becomes louder. There are no specific ECG patterns that are pathognomonic for VSDs and most patients' ECGs are normal. There can be ECG evidence of increased left heart volume (left atrial enlargement), but these findings are not specific to VSDs. On CXR, as the LV volume increases, there is a downward and leftward elongation of the cardiac silhouette on the anteroposterior (AP) film, whereas left atrial enlargement is seen on the lateral film or, when severe, by carinal widening on the AP film (Fig. 57-7). The increase in vascular markings denotes the amount of overcirculation.

Large VSDs coupled with high PVR allow for minimal shunting. Therefore the LV work is close to normal, resulting in little precordial activity. There will, however, be a notable RV lift. A short or absent VSD murmur is usually heard. Murmurs that may be heard are a result of tricuspid regurgitation (harsh holosystolic murmur) or pulmonary insufficiency (early diastolic murmur). There is usually no third heart sound or diastolic rumble. The pulmonary component of the second heart sound is quite prominent; however, more than 50 percent of the time, the second heart sound is single. ECG may show RV hypertrophy. The CXR on these patients can demonstrate

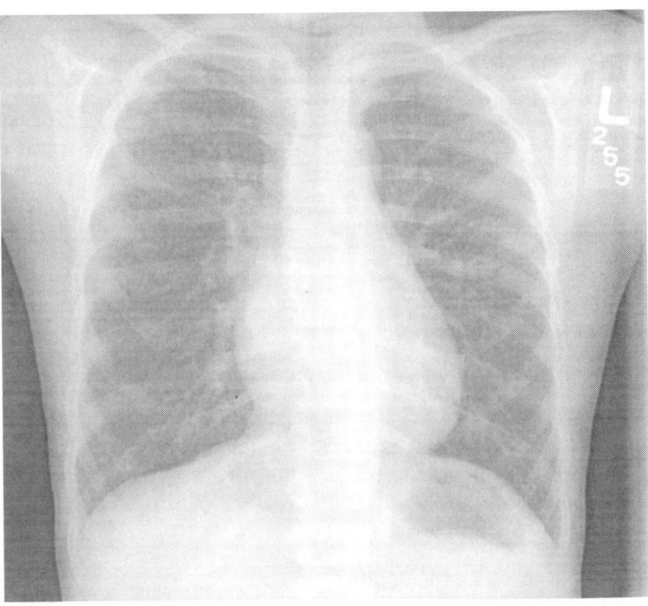

Figure 57-7 Anteroposterior chest x-ray of a patient with a VSD. Note the leftward elongation of the cardiac silhouette, representing an increase in left ventricular volume, and the plethoric lung fields.

a normal-size heart or RV hypertrophy, both accompanied by marked prominence of the main PA and its immediate branches. There is a paucity of vascular markings on the outer third of the lung fields.

Diagnostic Imaging

Two-dimensional echocardiography with color Doppler flow evaluation is the most widely used imaging to diagnose and characterize a VSD. To assess a VSD completely, one must not only localize it but also define its shape and dimensions, which is accomplished by viewing the defect from multiple imaging planes. Color Doppler allows for small VSDs not seen on two-dimensional echocardiography (usually < 2mm) to be identified and, more importantly, provides physiologic information about the VSD. One can measure the peak velocity across the VSD, which, if placed in the modified Bernoulli formula [4 x (peak velocity)^2], can yield the interventricular pressure gradient.[27] If this velocity is high, one has a restrictive VSD. If this velocity is low, one usually has a nonrestrictive VSD with near equalization of RV and LV pressures. However, at times a low velocity can be seen with a restrictive VSD if there is high RV pressure secondary to RV outflow obstruction or elevated perinatal PVR that has not yet fallen. Therefore a low intraventricular pressure gradient does not necessarily correlate with pulmonary vascular disease, even in the presence of a nonrestrictive VSD. RV pressure may be estimated by measuring the velocity of the tricuspid regurgitant jet [4 (TR jet velocity)^2 + (central venous pressure ≈ RV pressure)]. If a pulmonary insufficiency jet exists, then an estimation of the diastolic PA pressure can be calculated by measuring its velocity [4(PI jet velocity)^2 + (RV diastolic pressure)]. One can also get a sense of where the patient is in the spectrum of VSD pathophysiology by assessing the amount of LV and LA dilation as well as RV hypertrophy. The echocardiogram should obviously assess for other cardiac anomalies in particular patent ductus arteriosus, aortic coarctations, and RV or LV outflow tract obstruction.

The principal indication for diagnostic cardiac catheterization of a VSD patient is when echocardiography and the clinical assessment indicate the possibility of advanced pulmonary vascular disease. Again, this would be rare for young children. One should keep in mind that the PVR of a child with an isolated VSD would have to be extremely elevated not to attempt a repair in this era of multiple pulmonary vascular bed dilators [inhaled nitric oxide (iNO), prostacyclin, sildenafil milrinone, etc.] Therefore one may question exposure to the risks of catheterization to quantify the echocardiographic findings more precisely when the results will not change the therapeutic decision. Catheterization of a VSD patient is also useful in attempts to define the anatomy of multiple apical VSDs, which magnetic resonance imaging (MRI) and echocardiography sometimes cannot identify. Catheterization of a patient with an isolated VSD should result in (1) a Qp:Qs that can be estimated by (aortic O_2 sat − SVC O_2 sat) / (pulmonary venous O_2 sat − PA O_2 sat); (2) the calculated PVR = (mPAP – LA mean pressure) / pulmonary blood flow (Qp) resulting in Wood units (= mmHg/L/min); (3) the PA pressures; (4) if PVR is high, the determination of the pulmonary vasculature reactivity to vasodilators such as 100 percent FiO_2 and iNO; and (5) the delineation of any unclear anatomy.

MRI has recently been used to provide accurate information about the morphology of VSDs. When surgical referral is being considered, MRI may be recommended in those patients in whom it is difficult to discern ventricular volume overload. The MRI can supply a noninvasive estimate of the Qp:Qs as well as an accurate account of the heart's volumes and of associated anomalies that are sometimes difficult to diagnose by echocardiography (anomalous pulmonary venous return, for example). Also, three-dimensional intracardiac reconstruction MRI may soon be more widely available.

THERAPEUTIC MANAGEMENT

Medical therapy

The medical treatment of VSD patients is oriented toward decreasing L-R shunting and the symptoms of overcirculation. This is usually done with a combination of diuretics (i.e., furosemide), afterload-reducing agents (ACE inhibitors), and digoxin. Patients may also require nutritional support such as nasogastric tube feedings. Close surveillance for and aggressive treatment of upper respiratory infections is an important aspect of these children's care. Most children presenting with VSDs have some degree of pulmonary vascular disease; however, the presentation of an older cyanotic child with end-stage pulmonary vascular disease requires catheterization. The treatment and workup of such cases is outside the scope of this chapter. One should exercise caution when a patient requires intubation or inotropic support for a supposedly isolated VSD. Before embarking on surgical therapy, a careful investigation should be performed to make sure that no other cardiac anomaly (for example, left-sided obstruction or an additional source of L-R shunting) or primary pulmonary disease exists.

Invasive Therapy

Surgical Therapy

Surgical techniques for VSD closure have progressed tremendously over the past three decades and have allowed for neonatal surgical therapy to move from palliation to repair. At most institutions, all patients with isolated VSDs that require surgical correction undergo single-stage closure.

At the authors' institution, all repairs are generally performed with aortic and bicaval cannulation. Once the heart is arrested with cold cardioplegia, the right atrium is opened and the left heart is vented via the atrial septum. This should produce a bloodless and still intracardiac surgical field in which to work. There are several approaches to VSDs at this point, depending on the location.

The majority of VSDs (perimembranous, inlet, and the majority of muscular defects) can be addressed via a right atrial approach (Fig. 57-8). The leaflets of the TV are retracted to visualize the defect. A particular variation in technique to visualize transatrially inlet defects or PM VSDs with outlet extension is the incision of the septal and/or anterior leaflet(s) of the TV via a radial incision or one parallel to the annulus. This will often provide excellent visualization for repair; once this has been completed, the TV is reconstructed. The actual closure of the VSD can be done with a patch secured to the septum with interrupted pledgetted stitches, a running stitch, or a combination of the two. The patch can be made of various materials, including autologous pericardium tanned in glutaraldehyde, Dacron, or Gore-Tex. Primary (no patch) closure is usually reserved for a small muscular VSD. A key to successful VSD closure is the surgeon's awareness of the conduction system and the aortic valve. The TV annulus, which is the structure to which the VSD patch is often anchored posteriorly and superiorly, is just anterior to and sometimes in fibrous continuity with the aortic valve. Therefore the aortic valve leaflets are at risk for injury when these superior sutures are being placed. The conduction system is at risk in stitching the inferior rim of a PM VSD between the muscle of Lancisi (the most inferior papillary muscle bundle on the VSD rim) and the TV annulus (Fig. 57-4). In this area, interrupted sutures can be taken far from the rim or a running suture can be placed very superficially along the rim. It is important to remember that the conduction system exists only in muscular tissue and not in fibrous tissue.

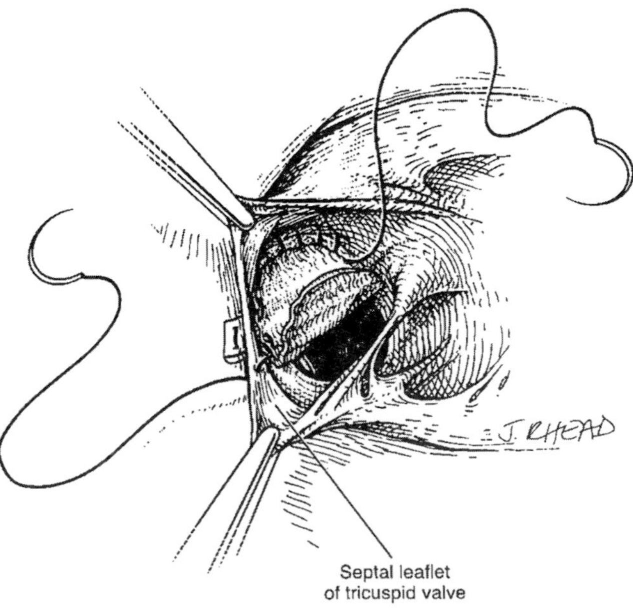

Figure 57-8 Transatrial approach to VSD patch closure. In the illustration, a running suture technique is utilized. (From Kouchoukos NT, Blackstone EH, Doty DB, et al (eds). *Kirklin/Barratt-Boyes Cardiac Surgery,* 3d ed. Philadelphia: Churchill Livingstone, 2003:874. With permission.)

Approach through the pulmonary artery is usually reserved for outlet defects. The pure outlet muscular defects can be closed with a simple primary or patch technique. However, the majority of outlet defects abut the PV annulus. These defects are also closed with a patch, but several unique factors must be considered. These particular VSDs have the highest incidence of significant aortic valve involvement. The aortic valve leaflets (usually the right coronary cusp) can prolapse and/or fill the defect. Therefore it is essential to identify the aortic valve and not to include it in the repair. The patch will not only close the defect but also serve to support the aortic valve and eliminate the Venturi effect, which can be the cause of aortic valve prolapse. Some mild forms of aortic insufficiency will improve with repair of the defect alone, but this is unpredictable. If the aortic insufficiency is moderate or greater and/or the aortic leaflet clearly has a pathologic change, then the aortic valve should be addressed. Perimembranous defects can also be associated with aortic insufficiency and usually involve prolapse of the noncoronary cusp. A discussion of aortic valve repair techniques—which include triangular resection, subcommissural stitches, Trussler-type repair (horizontal plication of the redundant leaflet to the aortic wall), and Yacoub-type repair (primary closure of the VSD with vertical plication of the sinus and leaflet)—are beyond the scope of this chapter. There is no superior rim to outlet defects, so interrupted pledgetted sutures are usually placed through the fibrous base of the pulmonary valve leaflets and then through the patch. Interrupted or running sutures can anchor the remainder of the patch, with little concern for the conduction system, which is remote. However, if the posterior limb of the septal band (part of the crista supraventricularis) is not identified, the VSD may be a PM defect with outlet extension. Thus the conduction system would be on the inferior border of the defect.

A transaortic approach is usually applied in addressing a VSD that is associated with another left-sided lesion such as aortic valve insufficiency or valvular/subvalvular stenosis. Our practice is still to close these defects from the RA approach to avoid left bundle branch block; however many still use this approach, and discussion of it is helpful in contemplating the relationship of VSDs and the conduction system.

An RV approach (Fig. 57-9) for an isolated VSD is unnecessary except in very rare situations in which the VSD is inaccessible from the different approaches; for

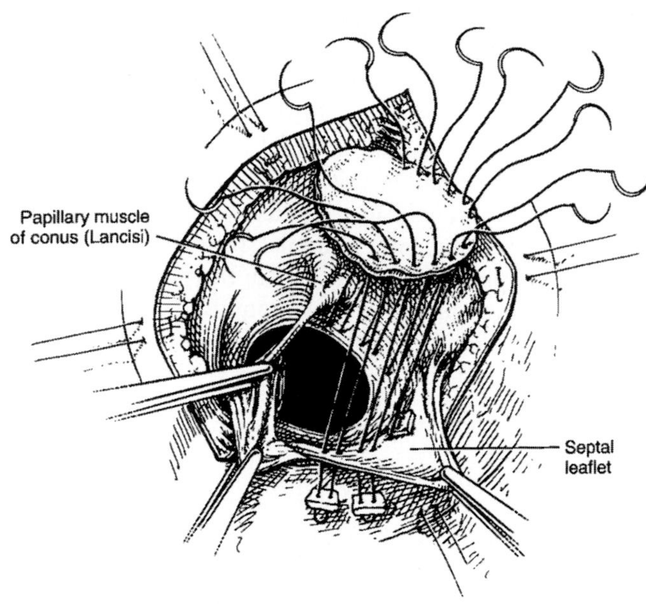

Figure 57-9 Transatrial approach to VSD closure. In the illustration, an interrupted suture technique is utilized. (From Kouchoukos NT, Blackstone EH, Doty DB, et al (eds). *Kirklin/Barratt-Boyes Cardiac Surgery*, 3d ed. Philadelphia: Churchill Livingstone, 2003:876. With permission.).

example: (1) When the posterior limb of the septal band is absent in a large outlet VSD, it is difficult to approach its inferior border from the PA or its superior border from the right atrium; thus neither approach suffices. (2) Visualization of a PM VSD with outlet extension can be hindered by hypertrophied infundibular muscle bundles. Resection of such bundles may at times be difficult from the RA or PA approaches; thus exposure is optimized by a small right ventriculotomy. Mapping out the ventricular incision in relation to the coronary anatomy is essential in avoiding significant ischemic complications, such as disruption of an anomalous anterior descending artery coming from the right coronary artery or of a large conal branch responsible for the proximal septal perforators. Again, we emphasize that right ventriculotomy is rarely needed to close an isolated VSD.

The LV approach is used even more infrequently than the RV approach and is reserved only for addressing those patients with multiple apical defects. Swiss cheese defects are difficult to approach from the right side because the trabeculations make the identification of distinct VSD borders impossible. However, this sieve-like defect on the right is fairly clear cut on the nontrabeculated smooth septum of the LV. After careful mapping of the coronary arteries, an incision parallel and to the left of the anterior descending artery is started at the apex and extended vertically. These incisions are obviously avoided whenever possible because of pseudoaneurysms, ventricular dysfunction, and ventricular arrhythmias arising from scar tissue. These complications are why many authors still attempt closure of these Swiss cheese defects from the right side of the heart.

RESULTS

Surgical outcomes

Complications from surgical VSD closure are infrequent; they include the following:

1. Tricuspid valve insufficiency from chordal shortening, leaflet entrapment by the VSD patch, or leaflet distortion if incised for exposure.
2. Possible aortic valve insufficiency if the sutures in the superior aspect of the patch catch or damage the aortic valve leaflets.
3. Complete heart block if the bundle of His is damaged or transected by sutures. Temporary block can occur secondary to edema in the area or trauma caused by careless suctioning or manipulation around the AVN area with instruments. The decision of when to place a pacemaker depends on the individual situation. Factors in one's decision include preoperative AVN function, the nature of the procedure and cardiac anatomy, and the postoperative course. The frequency of this complication should be approximately 1 percent. Right bundle branch block, on the other hand, is a frequently seen rhythm (about 35 percent) change postoperatively.[28]
4. Residual VSD: Leaving the operating room with a clearly significant residual VSD has been greatly reduced with the use of intraoperative transesophageal echocardiography (TEE). The difficulty arises when one must decide whether a small residual defect is physiologically and clinically significant enough to warrant rearresting the heart and attempting complete closure. A Qp:Qs of less than 1.5:1 is used as a general guideline for a residual VSD shunt that could be observed. However, in practice, the decision to leave a residual VSD is multifactorial and based on such aspects of the case as the difficulty of the VSD closure, one's perception of how the heart will tolerate another arrested period, and the residual shunt that is left.

Operative mortality for isolated VSD closure is quite low ranging from 0 to 3 percent.[29,30] The most common mode of death is acute cardiac failure, which usually is a result of one of the following: poor intraoperative myocardial protection, pulmonary hypertensive crises, a preoperative viral pulmonary process, or any combination of these with a small malnourished infant in heart failure. The risk factors for hospital death have changed significantly over the past decade. Young age, multiple VSDs, location, aortic insufficiency, PAB, and patient size, which all have been predictive of hospital mortality at various times in the past, are no longer risk factors.[28]

In the current era, only major associated cardiac anomalies, especially when associated with multiple VSDs, are risk factors for hospital mortality. Preoperative PA pressures or resistance do not affect hospital mortality but do affect long-term results, which manifest as late deaths secondary to progression of pulmonary vascular disease.[31] Late mortality after repair, when pulmonary pressures are low, is less than 2.5 percent; most of these deaths result from ventricular arrhythmias.[28] The surgical repair of an isolated VSD before complications begin to arise (usually before 2 years of age, depending on the VSD) can return a patient to a normal life expectancy with full functional activity and normal growth.[28]

Device closure

Device closure of VSDs is an emerging field that should be offered as a therapeutic option in selected cases. These devices are usually introduced via percutaneous catheterization techniques but can also be alternatively introduced via a periventricular approach. The periventricular technique, which is performed off bypass and uses TEE guidance, passes an occluding device through the right ventricular free wall and deploys it.[32] This technique can be repeated for multiple muscular VSDs. Experience with percutaneous device closure is greatest with muscular defects. The two devices presently offered in the United States for closure of muscular defects is the Cardio-SEAL (NMT, Boston, MA) device (a modified ASD clamshell occluder, FDA-approved for high-risk surgical VSD patients) and the Amplatzer Muscular VSD occluder, a specifically designed nitinol wire with polyester mesh device, which is currently under FDA review. Clinical experience with percutaneous closure of muscular VSDs has reached a point that it can be considered in the management of VSDs that are challenging to address surgically. On the other hand, closure of perimembranous VSDs using percutaneous device closure is still very much experimental, with only one available device (the Amplatzer Membranous VSD occluder, currently under study for patients weighing more than 8 kg). The largest report in the literature consists of only 25 patients collected from 9 different institutions.[33] This study has less than 1-month follow-up and an average patient age of 14 years and weight of 43 kg. The challenge for this therapeutic approach is that PM VSDs are almost always surgically approachable with negligible mortality and minimal morbidity. Also, the possible complications for devices in this position include not only device embolization, air embolism, perforation, residual shunt, and hemolysis but also are expanded to heart block and aortic insufficiency.

Palliation

The list of clinical and anatomic features that discourage early primary repair of VSDs becomes shorter with every year; thus the frequency of surgical palliation for isolated VSDs using pulmonary artery banding has continued to decline. Size of the patient, which in the past was one of the most frequent reasons for a PAB, is no longer a contraindication for complete repair in major centers, where the expansion of neonatal heart surgery has rendered this consideration almost null. Successful repair in a premature neonate of 700 g has been reported.[34] For patients with isolated VSDs, a "Swiss cheese septum" and multiple VSDs are the most frequent diagnoses to be palliated with a PAB. Pulmonary artery banding is performed off bypass, can be approached either via a median sternotomy or a left thoracotomy, and is described in detail in Chap. 54. Although it may be done palliatively, placement of a PAB may not be a simple or low-morbidity procedure. It is not always straightforward to balance the pulmonary and systemic circulations, especially with a reactive and/or high PVR; PA banding can carry a hospital mortality of 8 percent and even higher in neonates.[37] It may require early reoperation for PAB adjustment; furthermore, 29 percent of PABs can be inadequate (too loose or tight)[37] and after PAB removal, PA reconstruction is often required at the time of complete intracardiac repair.

References

1. Wells WJ, Lindesmith GG. Ventricular septal defect. In: Arciniegas E (ed). *Pediatric Cardiac Surgery.* Chicago: Year Book, 1985.
2. Moe DG, Guntheroth WG. Spontaneous closure of uncomplicated ventricular septal defect. *Am J Cardiol* 1987;60:674–678.
3. Hoffman JLE, Rudolph AM. The natural history of ventricular septal defects in infancy. *Am J Cardiol* 1965; 16:634–653.
4. Nora JJ, Fraser FLC. *Medical Genetics.* Philadelphia: Lea & Febiger, 1974:334.
5. Roger H. Recherches cliniques sur la communication congenitale des duex coeurs, par inocclusion du septum interventriculaire. *Bull Acad Nat Med (Paris)* 1879;8:1074–1075.
6. Wood P. The Eisenmenger syndrome or pulmonary hypertension with reversed central shunt. *Br Med J* 1958;46: 755–762.
7. Abbott ME. Congenital heart disease. In: *Nelson's Loose-Leaf Medicine,* vol 5. New York: Thomas Nelson, 1932:207.
8. Muller WH Jr, Dammann JF. The treatment of certain congenital malformations of the heart by the creation of pulmonic stenosis to reduce pulmonary hypertension and excessive pulmonary blood flow. *Surg Gynecol Obstet* 1952;95:213–219.
9. Lillehei CW, Cohen M, Warden HE, et al. The results of direct vision closure of ventricular septal defects in eight patients by means of controlled cross circulation. *Surg Gynecol Obstet* 1955;101:446–466.

10. DuShane JW, Kirklin JW, Patrick RT, et al. Ventricular septal defects with pulmonary hypertension: Surgical treatment by means of a mechanical pump-oxygenator. *JAMA* 1956;160:950–953.
11. Stirling GR, Stanley PH, Lillehei CW. Effect of cardiac bypass and ventriculotomy upon right ventricular function. *Surg Forum* 1957;8:433–438.
12. Truex RC, Bishof JK. Conduction system in human hearts with interventricular septal defects. *J Thorac Surg* 1958;35: 421–439.
13. Kirklin JW, DuShane JW. Repair of ventricular septal defect in infancy. *Pediatrics* 1961;27:61–66.
14. Tatsuno K, Ando M, Takan A, et al. Diagnostic importance of aortography in conal ventricular-septal defect. *Am Heart J* 1975;89:171–177.
15. Johnson WH Jr, Moller JH. *Pediatric Cardiology*. Philadelphia: Lippincott Williams & Wilkins, 2001:99.
16. Velebit V, Schoneberger A, Ciaroni S, et al. "Acquired" left ventricular-to-right atrial shunt (gerbode defect) after bacterial endocarditis. *Tex Heart Inst J* 1995;22:100–102.
17. Seddio F, Reddy VM, McElhinney DB, et al. Multiple ventricular septal defects: How and when should they be repaired? *J Thorac Cardiovasc Surg* 1999;117:134–139.
18. Agmon Y, Connolly HM, Olson LJ, et al. Noncompaction of the ventricular myocardium. *J Am Soc Echocardiogr* 1999;12:859–863.
19. Krovetz LJ, Goldbloom S. Normal standards for cardiovascular data. II. Pressure and vascular resistance. *John Hopkins Med J* 1972;130:187–195.
20. Rudolph AM, Auld PAM, Golinko RJ, et al. Pulmonary vascular adjustments in the neonatal period. *Pediatrics* 1961;28:28–34.
21. Wennik ACG, Oppenheimer-Dekker A, Moulaert AJ. Muscular ventricular septal defects: A reappraisal of the anatomy. *Am J Cardiol* 1979;43:259–264.
22. Van Praagh R, McNamara JJ. Anatomic types of ventricular septal with aortic insufficiency. *Am Heart J* 1968;75: 604–619.
23. Turner SW, Hornung T, Hunter S. Closure of ventricular septal defects: A study of factors influencing spontaneous and surgical closure. *Cardiol Young* 2002;12:357–363.
24. Hasegawa N, Oshima M, Kawakami H, et al. Changes in pulmonary tissue of patients with congenital heart disease and Down syndrome: A morphological and histochemical study. *Acta Paediatr Jpn* 1990;32:60–66.
25. Lucas RV Jr, Adams P Jr, Anderson RC, et al. The natural history of isolated ventricular septal defect: A serial physiologic study. *Circulation* 1961;24:1372–1387.
26. Moss AJ, Adams FH. In: Emmanouilides GC, Allen HD, Riemenschneider TA, Gutgesell HP (eds). *Heart Disease in Infants, Children, and Adolescents, Including the Fetus and Young Adult,* 5th ed. Baltimore: Williams & Wilkins, 1995:734.
27. Murphy DJ, Ludomirsky A, Huhta JC. Continuous wave Doppler in children with ventricular septal defect: Noninvasive estimation of pressure gradient. *Am J Cardiol* 1986;57:428–432.
28. Kouchoukos NT, Blackstone EH, Doty DB, et al (eds). *Kirklin/Barratt-Boyes Cardiac Surgery,* 3d ed. Philadelphia: Churchill Livingstone, 2003:880.
29. Richardson JV, Schieken RM, Lauer RM, et al. Repair of large ventricular septal defects in infants and small children. *Ann Surg* 1982;195:318–322.
30. Backer CL, Winters RC, Zales VR, et al. The restrictive ventricular septal defect: How small is too small to close? *Ann Thorac Surg* 1993;56:1014–1018.
31 Blackstone EH, Kirklin JW, Bradley EL, et al. Optimal age and results in repair of large ventricular septal defects. *J Thorac Cardiovasc Surg* 1976;72:661–679.
32. Bacha EA, Cao QL, Starr JP, et al. Perventricular device closure of muscular ventricular septal defect. *J Thorac Cardiovasc Surg* 126:1718, 2003.
33. Bass JL, Kalra GS, Arora R, et al. Initial human experience with the Amplatzer perimembranous ventricular septal occluder device. *Cath Cardiovasc Intervent* 2003;58: 238–239.
34. Reddy VM, McElhinney DB, Sagrado T, et al. Results of 102 cases of complete repair of congenital heart defects in patients weighing 700 to 2500 grams. *J Thorac Cardiovasc Surg* 1999;117:324–331.
35. Trusler GA, Mustard WT. A method of banding the pulmonary artery for large isolated ventricular septal defect with and without transposition of the great arteries. *Ann Thorac Surg* 1972;13:351–355.
36. Albus RA, Trusler GA, Izukawa T, et al. Pulmonary artery banding. *J Thorac Cardiovasc Surg* 1984;88: 645–653.
37. Pinho P, Von Oppell UO, Brink J, et al. Pulmonary artery banding: Adequacy and long-term outcome. *Eur J Cardiothorac Surg* 1997;11:105–111.

CHAPTER

58 ATRIOVENTRICULAR SEPTAL DEFECTS

Mazyar Kanani, Martin J. Elliott

INTRODUCTION

Following the first successful repair of atrioventricular septal defects (AVSDs) at the dawn of modern cardiac surgery, significant advances have been made in many aspects of overall patient management. In line with improvements in cardiopulmonary bypass, postoperative care, and refinement of surgical technique together with morphologic understanding,[1] there has been a striking reduction in both postoperative mortality and early morbidity. As a counterpoint to this phenomenon, attention has in the last decade focused away from mortality as the single most important outcome measure and moved onto the long-term outlook.

Reflecting this increased confidence in the operative management in the last quarter century,[2] there has been an evolution in the timing of surgery from a staged approach to an era of complete repair in early infancy (Fig. 58-1).[1,3]

KEY CONCEPTS

- Epidemiology
  - The prevalence of atrioventricular septal defect (AVSD) is 0.19 per 1000 live births, accounting for 2.9 percent of congenital cardiac malformations. In about 60 percent of these cases, shunting is confined to the atrial level. Tetralogy of Fallot (ToF) is associated in 2 to 10 percent of cases of AVSD, while Down's syndrome is seen in 75 percent of infants with complete AVSD.
- Morphology
  - This is variable, according to extent and presence of atrial and ventricular components; however, a common atrioventricular valve and displacement of the AV node are common features. These defects typically fall into three categories: (A) partial (primum component only); (B) complete atrial septal defect (ASD) and ventricular septal defect (VSD), and (C) transitional (restrictive VSD). Complete AVSD is further subdivided according to the degree of bridging of the superior leaflet. Although Rastelli type A is most common (70 percent of all complete AVSDs), type C is the one most frequently associated with ToF.
- Pathophysiology
  - Pathophysiology varies with the degree of shunting, left ventricular atrioventricular valve regurgitation, and pulmonary vascular resistance, as well as with associated anomalies.
- Clinical features
  - Larger left-to-right shunts (complete AVSDs) will present early with congestive heart failure and pulmonary hypertension, while presentation of partial and transitional AVSDs (in the absence of significant left atrioventricular valve regurgitation) will present later and have a similar presentation and natural history as ASDs.
- Diagnosis
  - Chest x-ray (CXR) will disclose an enlarged cardiac silhouette and increased pulmonary markings in large shunts. Echocardiography is diagnostic and defines type of defect, valvar morphology and degree of regurgitation, relative ventricular balance, and associated anomalies. Cardiac catheterization is used in selected cases and shows the characteristic "gooseneck deformity" from subaortic elongation of the left ventricular outflow tract (LVOT).

- Treatment
  - A staged approach [pulmonary artery banding (PAB) followed by complete repair] is relegated to selected cases of complete AVSD. Most such cases should be repaired before 6 months of age, whereas partial defects without valvar regurgitation and defects with a restrictive VSD component can be repaired between 2 and 4 years of age.
- Outcomes
  - Operative mortality for complete AVSDs is currently below 5 percent, and incomplete defects have similar morbidity and mortality as ASDs. Long-term prognosis is defined by long-term valvar patency and associated lesions.

EPIDEMIOLOGY

The prevalence of AVSD has been put at 0.19 per 1000 live births, accounting for 2.9 percent of congenital cardiac malformations. In about 60 percent of these defects, the shunting is confined to the atrial level.

ANATOMIC CONSIDERATIONS

The principal malformation that defines the AVSD lies at the atrioventricular junction. The normal arrangement is considered first.

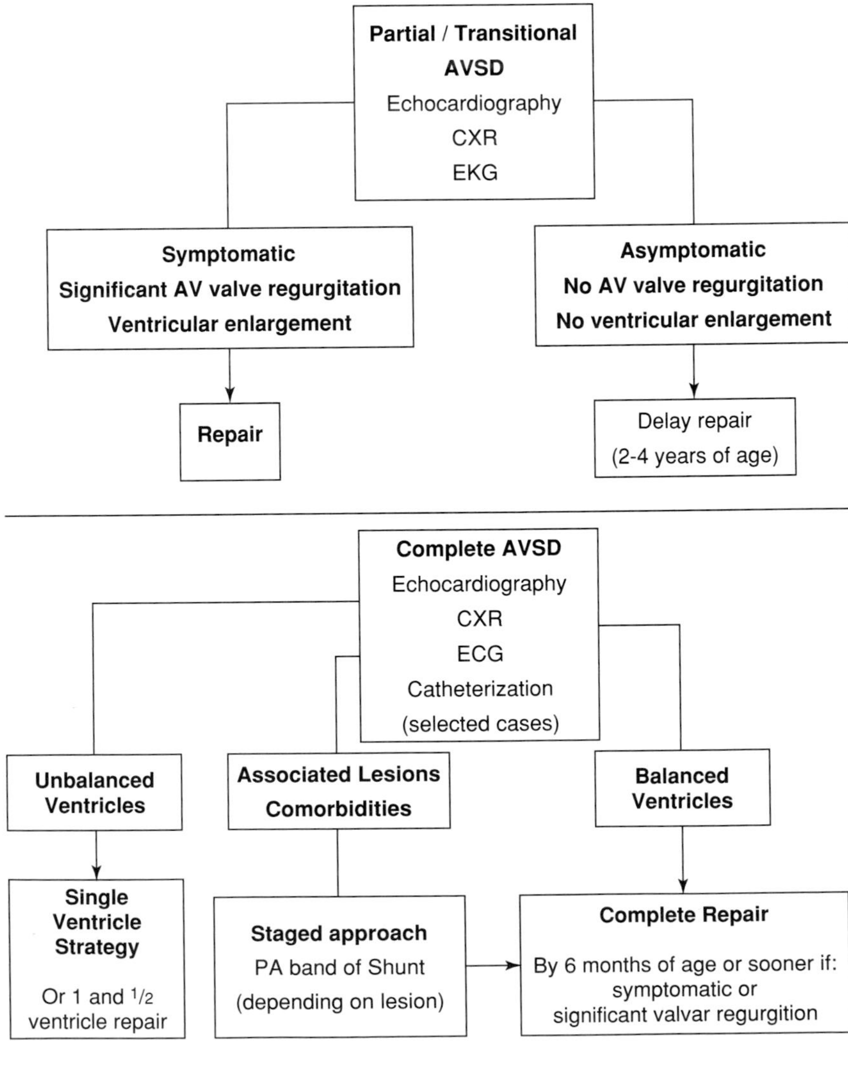

Abbreviations:
AV = atrioventricular;
CXR = chest x-ray;
ECG = electrocardiogram.

Figure 58-1 Decision-making flowchart for atrioventricular septal defects (AVSDs). AV = atrioventricular; CXR = chest x-ray; ECG = electrocardiogram.

The normal atrioventricular junction

The atrioventricular (AV) junction is defined as the muscular area that surrounds the orifices of the AV valves and marks the point at which the distal margins of the atrial musculature meet the ventricular myocardium. Thus, there are two AV junctions in the normal heart, one supporting the tricuspid and the other the mitral orifices. Although the musculature of the two chambers abuts over the circumference of this junction, they are nevertheless separable apart from the area of the muscular axis of AV conduction—the bundle of His. Wedged in between the two junctions is the subaortic outflow tract, incorporating the indwelling aortic valve. Beyond this anteriorly is the subpulmonary outflow tract, mounted on its free-standing infundibulum (Fig. 58-2).

In considering junctional morphology, it is possible to distinguish the points of attachment of the AV valvar hinges from the points of muscular AV contiguity. At the right AV junction, where the hinges of the tricuspid valve are anchored by muscle throughout, these two areas are essentially the same apart from the short length where the septal leaflet of the valve crosses the membranous septum. In doing so, it divides the membranous septum into AV and interventricular components (Fig. 58-3).

This disparity between the muscular AV junction and the valvar annulus is most clearly seen at the mitral valve, where the fibrous tissue of the aortomitral fibrous continuity supports one-third of the annulus (Fig. 58-4).

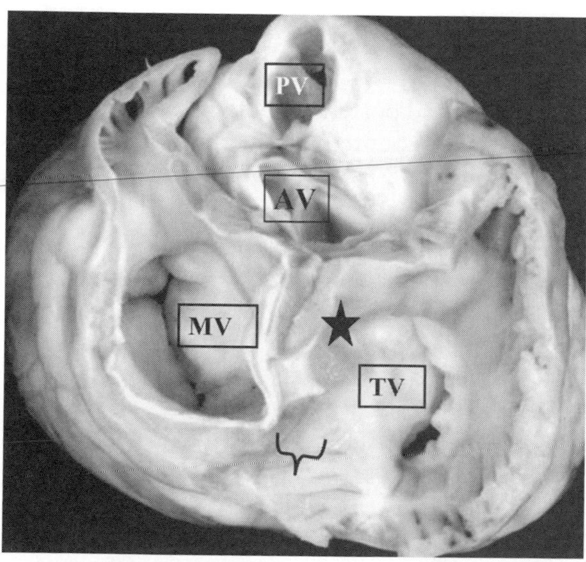

Figure 58-2 The normal heart from above, with the atrial roof removed. There is normal atrioventricular septation, resulting in two separate atrioventricular junctions. The black star indicates the site of the atrioventricular septum that is bisected by the septal leaflet of the tricuspid valve. The black parenthesis is the position of the atrioventricular muscular sandwich. AV = aortic valve; MV = mitral valve; TV = tricuspid valve; PV = pulmonary valve.

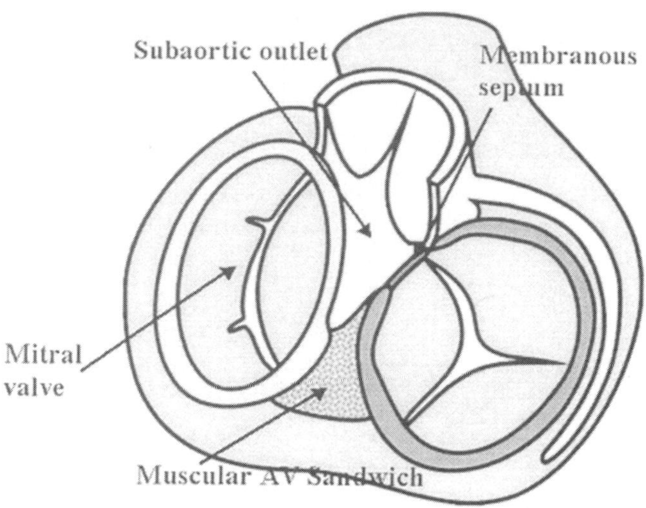

Figure 58-3 A diagrammatic representation of the normally septated heart, showing the relationship between the subaortic outflow tract and the atrioventricular septum and sandwich. Note how the subaortic outflow tract is wedged between the two atrioventricular junctions. AV = atrioventricular.

The atrioventricular septum and sandwich

Observed in the four-chamber view, the tricuspid annulus is seen to lie at a more apical position than its mitral counterpart. Consequently, in the region immediately caudal and posterior to the area where the septal leaflet traverses the membranous septum, the muscular atrial septum overlaps the crest of the ventricular septum. This area between

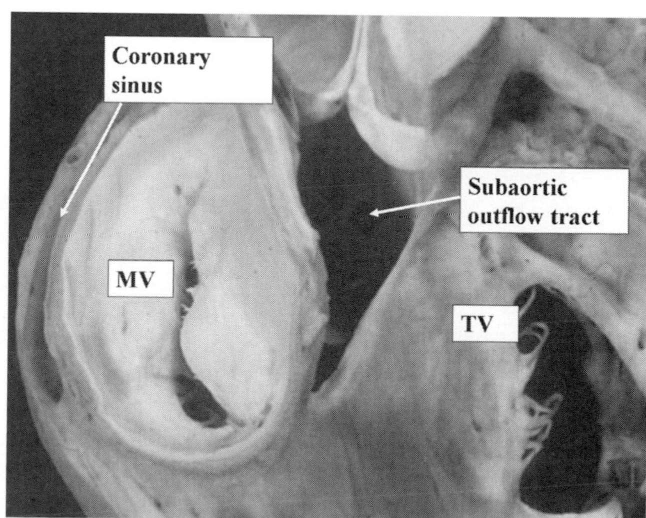

Figure 58-4 A photographic equivalent of Fig. 58-3. The coronary sinus and circumflex branch of the left coronary artery skirt around the parietal left atrioventricular junction.

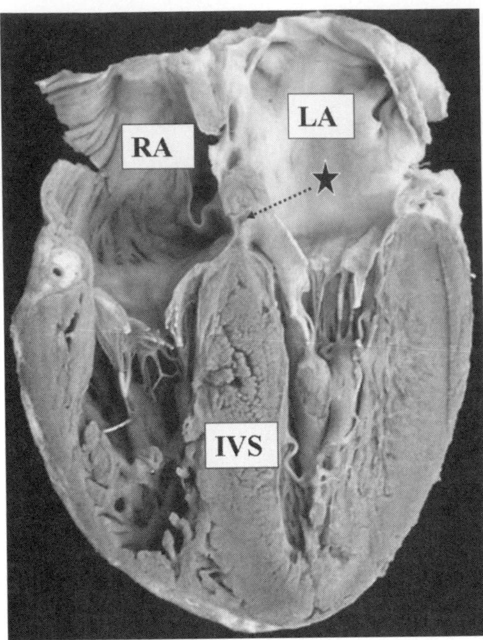

Figure 58-5 A specimen of the normal heart taken in four-chamber section. The normal offsetting of the hinge points of the mitral and tricuspid valves gives rise to the atrioventricular septum (marked by the black star). IVS = interventricular septum; LA = left atrium; RA = right atrium.

the offset hinges of the AV valves has previously been called the muscular AV septum,[4] but it is, in fact, none other than an extension of the fibrofatty tissue of the posteroinferior AV groove (Fig. 58-5). The term *AV septum* should therefore be reserved for the AV component of the fibrous membranous septum. It is the absence of these two components—the fibrous membranous septum and the fibrofatty muscular sandwich—that define hearts with AVSDs more than any other anatomic feature.

THE COMMON ATRIOVENTRICULAR JUNCTION IN ATRIOVENTRICULAR SEPTAL DEFECTS

The common AV junction is the fundamental feature that sets the AVSD apart from the normal heart (Fig. 58-6).

It occurs irrespective of the number of valvar orifices and is seen even in the absence of septal deficiency. All other morphologic features seen in this defect arise as a direct consequence of this singular arrangement of the junctional structures. Other morphologic markers can be considered under the following subheadings:

- Leaflets arrangement
- Septal deficiency
- The ventricular mass
- The subaortic outflow tract
- The conduction axis

Leaflet arrangement and the subvalvar apparatus

The oval-shaped common AV junction in AVSDs surrounds an orifice guarded by a valve that usually possesses five leaflets. There is some variability in this arrangement, depending on the permutation of leaflet fusion. Variable fusion may result in separate right and left orifices or may produce any number of accessory orifices, depending on the location and extent of fusion.

Lying across the crest of the ventricular septum, to a variable extent, are the superior and inferior bridging leaflets (SBLs and IBLs). These were previously known as the anterior and posterior bridging leaflets, respectively, and have no counterparts in the normally septated heart (left in Fig. 58-6).

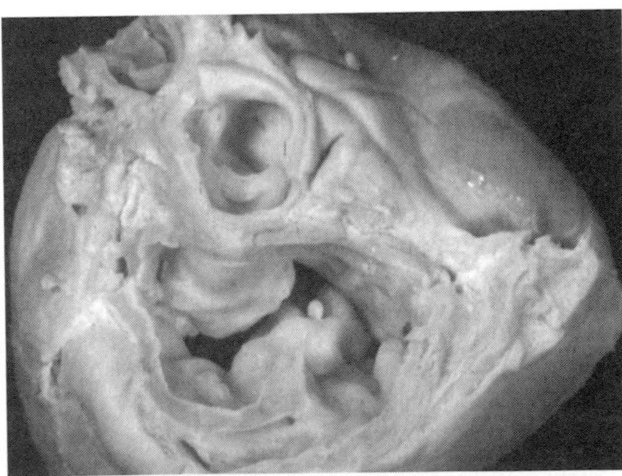

Figure 58-6 Left: schematic representation of a heart with atrioventricular septal defect and common atrioventricular junction, looking from the atrial aspect. The atrial roof has been removed. There is a common annulus that serves both ventricles, being surrounded by a common atrioventricular valve with five leaflets. The rightward black arrow indicates the position of the zone of apposition between the left sides of the superior and inferior bridging leaflets, which has previously been called a "cleft." Right: a photographic equivalent of the left panel. Anderson RH, Becker AE. *Controversies in the description of malformed hearts.* London: Imperial College Press, 1997.

Adjacent to the SBL over the orifice of the right ventricle is the anterosuperior leaflet (ASL), which is analogous to its tricuspid counterpart. Supported by the parietal margins of the common junction on both sides are the right and left mural leaflets. The right mural leaflet lies against the ASL and IBL, the left leaflet lies in apposition with the SBL and IBL.

The subvalvar apparatus is similarly abnormal, most conspicuously in the arrangement of the papillary muscles. The two left-sided papillary muscles normally lie obliquely, assuming anterolateral and posteromedial attitudes. In AVSD, these two muscles are located in the same vertical plane, being positioned superiorly and inferiorly; hence their names (Fig. 58-7).

The superior muscle supports the zone of apposition at the SBL-mural leaflet interface, and the inferior muscle supports the zone of apposition between the IBL and mural leaflets. Unlike the case on the right side, the position of these left-sided muscles is consistent. However, they may be found in clusters, as in the so-called parachute arrangement, where the cords from all leaflets converge onto only one papillary muscle (Fig. 58-8).

Rastelli classification and right ventricular papillary muscles

The papillary muscle arrangement of the right side depends on the degree of bridging of the SBL across the VSD. This forms the basis for the Rastelli classification.[2,5]

When there is minimal bridging of the SBL into the left ventricle, or Rastelli class A, the edge of the leaflet is tethered to the crest of the septum (left in Fig. 58-9). Here, the ventricular septum is analogous to a papillary muscle, supporting the zone of apposition between the SBL and IBL. In this situation, the ASL of the right AV valve is well developed and morphologically similar to its tricuspid counterpart. At operation, this arrangement gives the appearance of the SBL being divided over the septum (Fig. 58-10A). Subsequent anatomic observation determined that this "division" of the SBL over the septum merely represents the zone of apposition between the SBL and well-formed ASL in the class A defect and that the SBL is undivided over the ventricular septum in all classes of the defect.[6–8]

In the class B defect, the SBL extends even more into the right ventricle, with further reduction in the size of the ASL (Fig. 58-10B). It is usually unattached to the ventricular septum but at its right margin is supported solely by an anomalous right ventricular papillary muscle that arises from the septomarginal trabeculation. In the so-called type C defect (Fig. 58-9, right panel), the SBL extends even further into the right ventricle and floats freely above the ventricular septum, extending from the anterior papillary muscle of the right ventricle to the superior papillary muscle of the left ventricle (Fig. 58-10C). The ASL is necessarily smaller, accommodating the greater encroachment of the SBL into the right side.

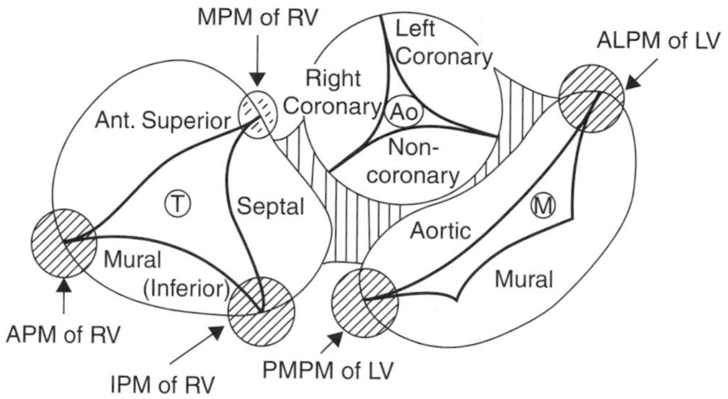

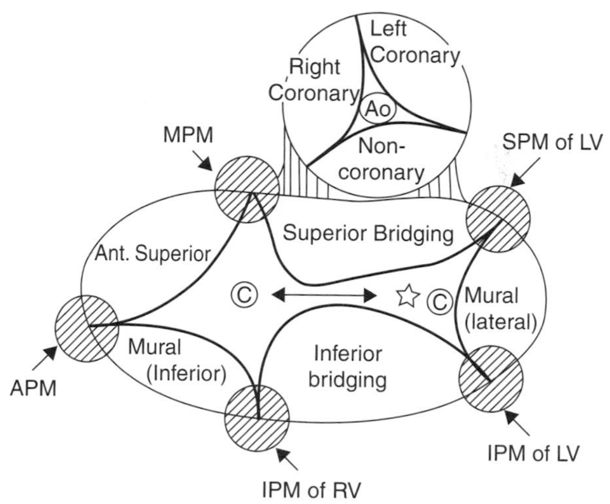

Figure 58-7 Diagrams of the atrioventricular arrangement in the normal heart **(A)** and in the heart with deficient atrioventricular septation **(B)**. View is from the ventricles (below). This shows not only the abnormal atrioventricular arrangement in atrioventricular septal defects but also the abnormal leaflet and papillary muscle positioning. ALPM = anterolateral papillary muscle; Ao = aortic orifice; APM = anterior papillary muscle; C = common orifice; IPM = inferior papillary muscle; LV = left ventricle; M = mitral orifice; MPM = medial papillary muscle; PMPM = posteromedial papillary muscle; RV = right ventricle; SPM = superior papillary muscle; T = tricuspid orifice. (From Frifti E, Bonacchi M, Bernabei M, et al. Repair of complete atrioventricular septal defects in patients weighing less than 5 kg. *Ann Thorac Surg* 2004;77:1717. With permission.)

Lack of cordal attachments to the septum ensures unhindered access to the aortic valve beneath.[9,10] In the type C defect, there is a high association with ToF. The reasons for this are developmental, as rightward displacement of the outlet septum during the development may limit cordal attachment to the septum.[11,12]

Epidemiologically, the type A defect has the greatest prevalence, both in morphologic and clinical series,

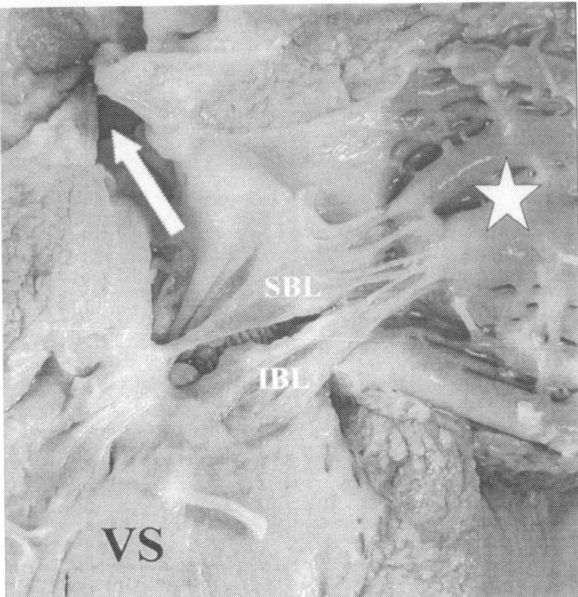

Figure 58-8 A specimen of atrioventricular septal defect looking from the left ventricular aspect. There is a solitary papillary muscle arrangement in which the superior (SBL) and inferior (IBL) bridging leaflets converge to a single papillary muscle (white star). The white arrow indicates the position of the subaortic outflow tract. VS = ventricular septum.

ranging from 50 to 75 percent of cases.[7,13–15] Variability in the degree of bridging of the SBL may also be seen in cases of AVSD with separate orifices, or the "partial defect," where minimal bridging of the SBL is the most common pattern.

The nature of the zone of apposition: "cleft" or "commissure"?

The area between left sides of the bridging leaflets has been the subject of much controversy. The principal question is whether it represents a cleft, as in the so-called isolated cleft of the anterior leaflet of the mitral valve,[16] or whether it is the commissure between the leaflets of a left AV valve. A commissure is the functional division between the leaflets of a valve that is supported by a fan-shaped tendinous cord atop a papillary muscle. A cleft is defined as a space or opening made by splitting the anterior leaflet.[17] Given these definitions, this space between the bridging leaflets may be best thought of as septal commissure in a trifoliate leaflet AV valve.

Morphology of the atrial and ventricular septal defects

Although septal deficiency is almost uniformly seen in hearts with this defect, the pattern of blood flow between the chambers is largely determined by the cordal and leaflet anatomy.

The ventricular septum in AVSD is "scooped," with a gentle curve extending from the crux of the heart to the left ventricular outflow tract (LVOT) (Fig. 58-11). The depth of the scoop and the resulting deficiency are very variable, being more extensive in hearts with common orifices.[7,18,19]

Above the plane of the annulus is the so-called ostium primum defect (Fig. 58-12), which in some instances may be obliterated through attachments of the leaflets to its edge, giving rise to obligatory ventricular shunting. If combined with a secundum atrial septal defect, it may produce a common atrium.

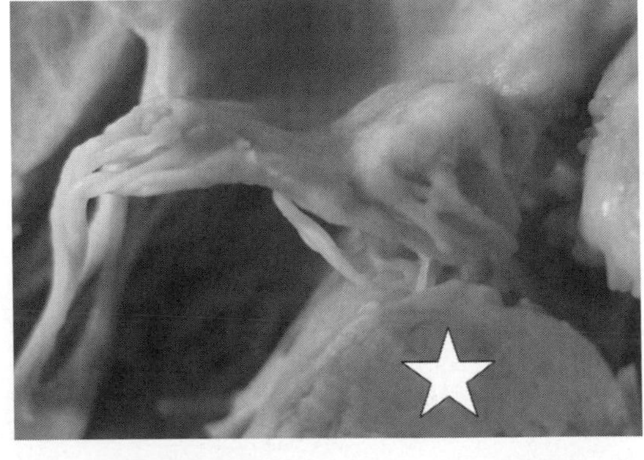

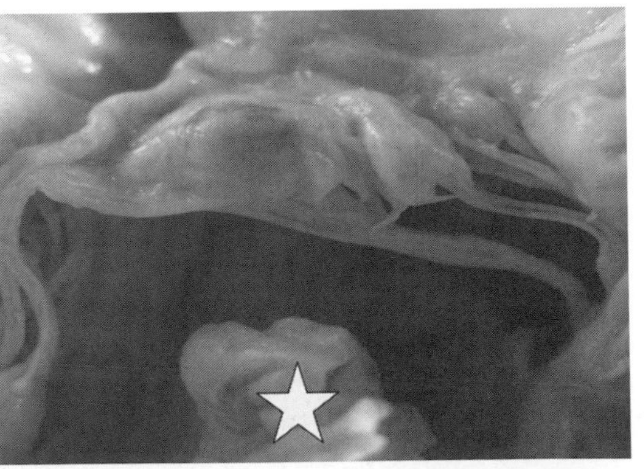

Figure 58-9 Specimens showing variations in the degree of bridging of the superior bridging leaflets, forming the basis of the Rastelli classification. This is a four-chamber orientation; the white stars indicate the position of the ventricular septum. Left panel: Rastelli type A arrangement where the SBL is minimally bridged and bound to the crest of the ventricular septum. Right panel: the type C arrangement where the superior bridging leaflet bridges the septum to the greatest extent and floats freely. Rastelli GC, Ongley PA, Kirklin JW, et al. Surgical repair of the complete form of persistent common atrioventricular canal. *J Thorac Cardiovasc Surg* 1968;55:299–308.

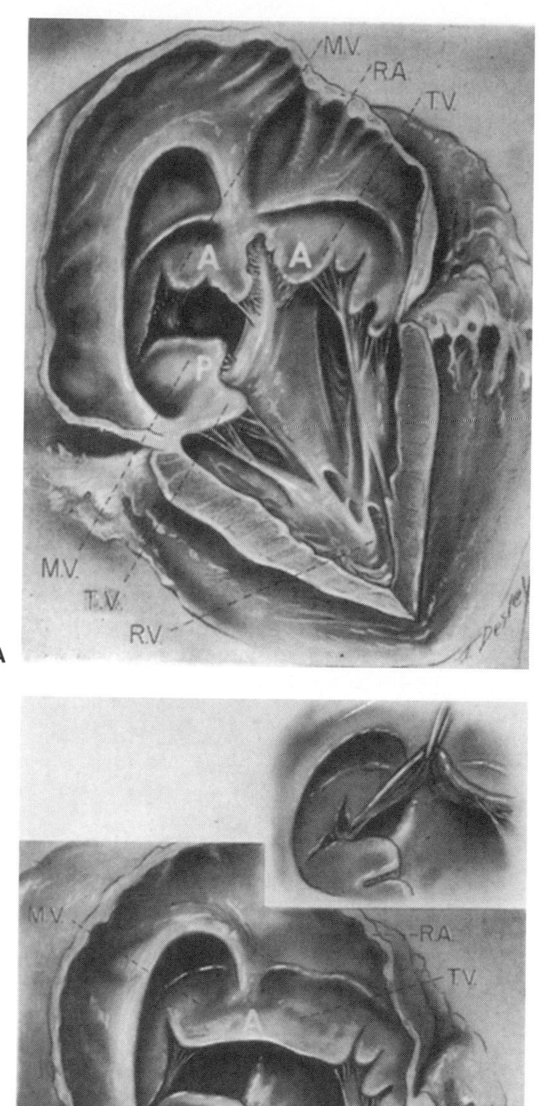

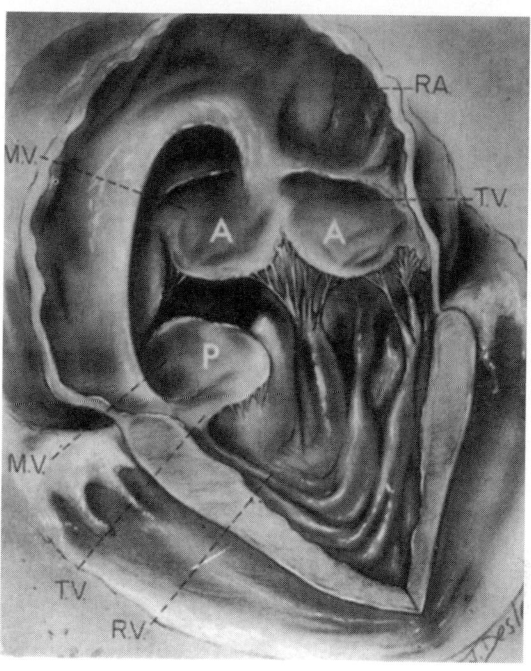

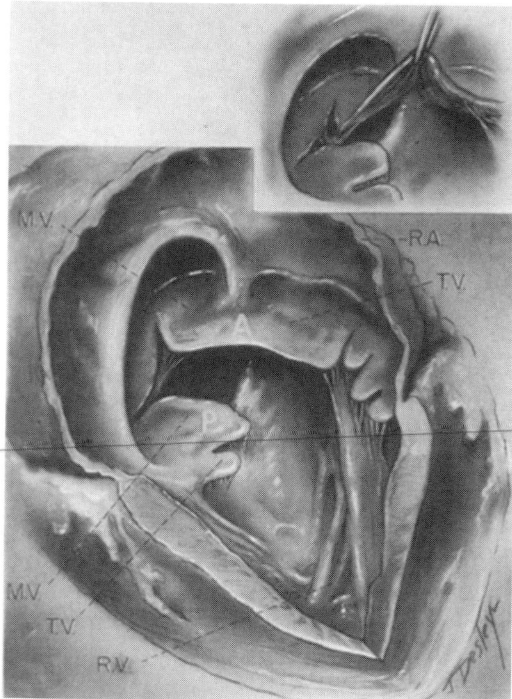

Figure 58-10 Figures taken from Rastelli's original study on the arrangement of the superior bridging leaflet in atrioventricular septal defects (**A** to **C**). In type **A**, the superior bridging leaflet is minimally bridged, with most of the leaflet confined to the left ventricle and tethered to the septum. In Type **B**, the degree of bridging is greater, with its right ventricular attachment being to an anomalous papillary muscle. In type **C**, the leaflet is maximally bridged, being free-floating and attached onto the medial papillary muscle of the right ventricle with the anterosuperior leaflet. (From Rastelli G, Kirklin JW, Titus JL. Anatomic observations on complete form of persistent common atrioventricular canal with special reference to atrioventricular valves. *Mayo Clin Proc* 1966;41:296. With permission.)

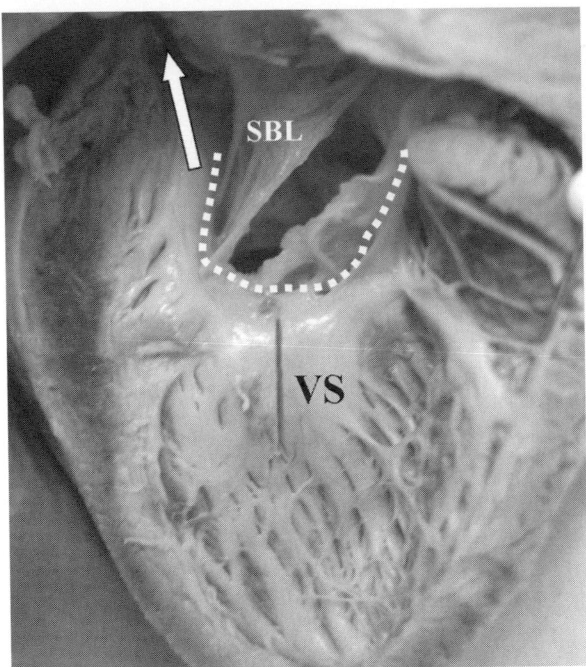

Figure 58-11 A specimen of atrioventricular septal defect looking from the left ventricle in long-axis section. The "scooped out" appearance of the crest of the ventricular septum (VS) has been marked by the white line. The white arrow points to the narrowed subaortic outflow tract. SBL = superior bridging leaflet.

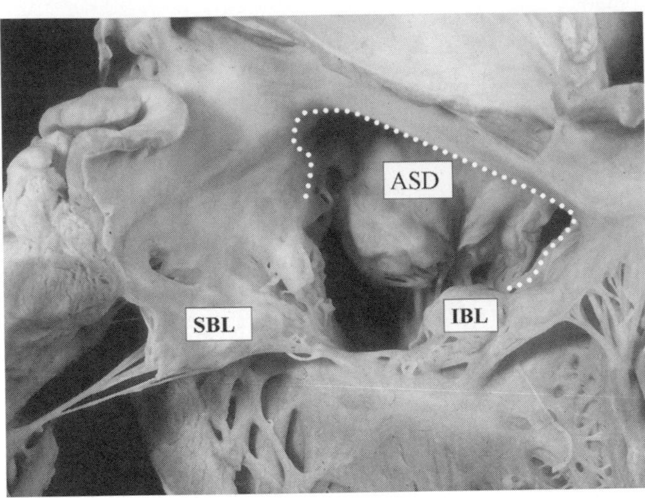

Figure 58-12 Specimen of atrioventricular septal defect looking from the left ventricle, showing the relationships between the atrial septal defect (ASD), ventricular septal defect, and bridging leaflets (SBL and IBL). The white line shows the characteristically crescentic shape to the primum ASD component.

Common versus separate orifices

There are two varieties of AVSD, depending on the level of intracardiac shunting caused by the pattern of leaflet fusion. However, when the leaflets are stripped from both variations, their junctional morphology is identical.[4]

In the defect with separate orifices, also known as the partial AVSD, there is a tongue of leaflet connecting the bridging leaflets over the ventricular septal crest. Therefore, the septal communication beneath the leaflets is obliterated, limiting shunting to the atrial level (Figs. 58-13 and 58-14).

Although this fusion results in separate AV orifices, the connecting tongue is not a continuation of the common annulus across the septum. The morphologic extent of this tongue again shows variability. In some instances, the bridging leaflets are fused with each other, but multiple intercordal spaces beneath the leaflets leave the potential for interventricular shunting (Fig. 58-15).

Hearts exhibiting this latter phenomenon have been termed the "intermediate" or "transitional" AVSD, emphasizing separate orifices in the context of persisting ventricular shunting, as if it were embryologically a transitional form between two extremes. We believe that this term is misleading and loses sight of the fact that the defining feature of hearts with this defect is deficiency of AV septation and not leaflet morphology. As such, septation may be deficient or otherwise, with no intermediate arrangement.[20] Despite the clinically more benign course of the defect with separate orifices, there is a greater prevalence of subaortic obstruction, papillary muscle anomalies, and leaflet dysplasia. Nevertheless, the association with other complex malformations is more common in hearts with a common orifice.

Ventricular morphology and balance

In the normal heart, the inlet/outlet ratio is the same (Fig. 58-16, left panel). This is also seen in hearts with perimembranous VSDs and those with an isolated "cleft" in the anterior leaflet of the mitral valve, which have all been previously described as the "forme fruste" of AV septal defect.[21] In the latter, the outlet length is significantly longer than the inlet and can be appreciated from the "goose-neck" deformity of the subaortic outflow tract (Fig. 58-16, right panel). This has been explained in terms of a shorter inlet[22] or a longer outlet.[23] These ratios are the same in AVSDs with common and separate orifices.

The diameters of the inlets of both ventricles as well as the volumes of the ventricles are the same, or balanced, with the atrial and ventricular septa being in line. In the era of two-staged repair, a reduction in the volume of the right ventricle was occasionally observed after pulmonary trunk banding, owing to hypertrophy of the trabecular layer of the myocardium. Aside from this specific

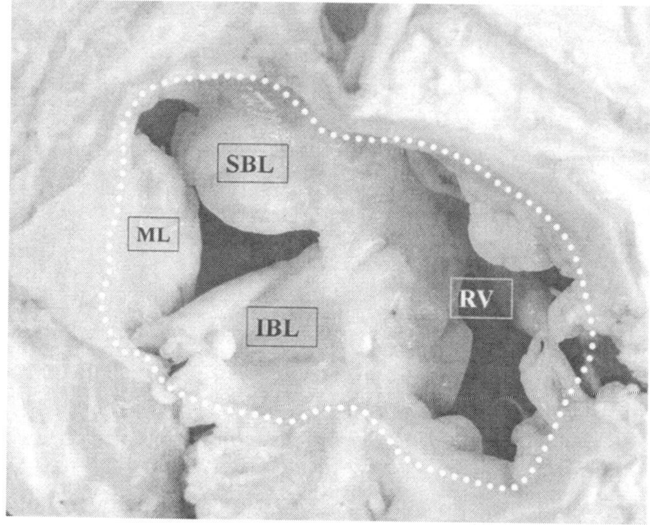

Figure 58-13 A specimen of atrioventricular septal defect with common atrioventricular junction (encircled by the white line) but with separate orifices. The orifices are divided by a connecting tongue of tissue between superior and inferior (SBL and IBL) bridging leaflets, which is also bound to the crest of the ventricular septal defect. This closes off the ventricular communication. ML = mural leaflet of the left atrioventricular valve; RV = right ventricle.

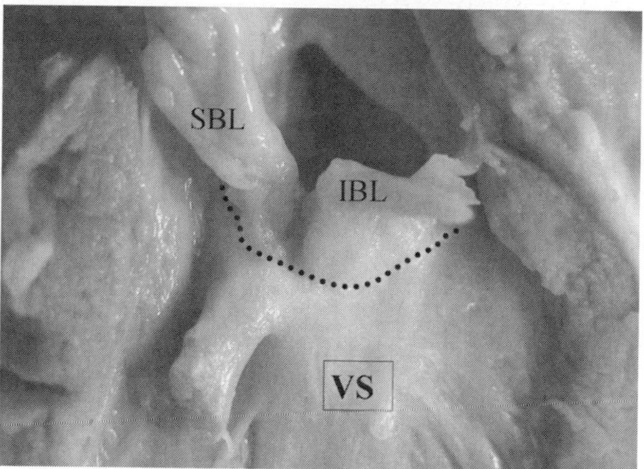

Figure 58-14 Specimen of atrioventricular septal defect with separate orifices, looking from the left ventricle. The dotted line shows the position of the crest of the ventricular septum (VS), which is bound to the bridging leaflets (SBL and IBL), thus closing off any ventricular communication. Note how the zone of apposition has a three-dimensional configuration in that is rises up from the septum before continuing forward.

situation, left dominance may occur with hypoplasia of the right ventricular and pulmonary arterial components, typically in association with malalignment of the atrial and ventricular septa. This leads to the most extreme case of double-inlet left ventricle with common AV valve.[24] In the case of right dominance, there is usually hypoplasia of the left ventricular and aortic structures, with normal alignment of the atrial and ventricular structures.[25]

The subaortic outflow tract and subaortic stenosis

Although the subaortic outflow tract is narrower[26] and longer[10] than normal (as seen on angiography), obstruction is surprisingly uncommon (Fig. 58-16, right panel).[27]

The principal source of obstruction derives from the anterior and unwedged position of the subaortic ouflow tract, which is a direct product of failure of AV septation. This exaggeration of the subaortic outflow tract is also more pronounced in hearts with the Rastelli type A leaflet morphology, where the SBL is tethered to the crest of the ventricular septum, narrowing the outflow tract even further. This also explains why obstruction is more frequent in the setting of separate orifices.

Additionally, the superior papillary muscle or an anomalous portion of it may extend into the subaortic outflow tract, or there may be a prominent anterolateral trabecular muscle bundle. Similarly, there may be accessory tissue tags or cordal attachments from the SBL, further obstructing the path. Such hearts may also become obstructed through mechanisms that affect normally septated hearts, such as fibrous subaortic shelves.

There may also be a further, dynamic component to the potential for obstruction in these hearts. The elongated outflow tract is a muscular tube that constricts during systole, heard as a persisting systolic murmur in the absence of clinically significant left AV valve regurgitation. Obstruction is also well recognized in the postoperative setting, as after left AV valvar replacement, where it accounts in part for the high mortality.

The morphology of the atrioventricular conduction axis

The displacement of the conduction axis is the direct result of deficient septation, with absence of the central fibrous body that normally marks the point at which the AV node continues as the AV bundle. There is some variability among hearts with the AV septal defect, depending on the alignment of the atrial and ventricular septa. Thus, the nodal triangle is displaced posteriorly and inferiorly and lies in the posterior right atrial wall, between the orifice of the coronary sinus and the crux of the heart.

From this position, the bundle of His passes to the crest of the ventricular septum through the crux, which is the first point of contact of the atrial and ventricular musculature. It runs along the crest of the septum under the cover of the IBL, giving off left bundle branches. At

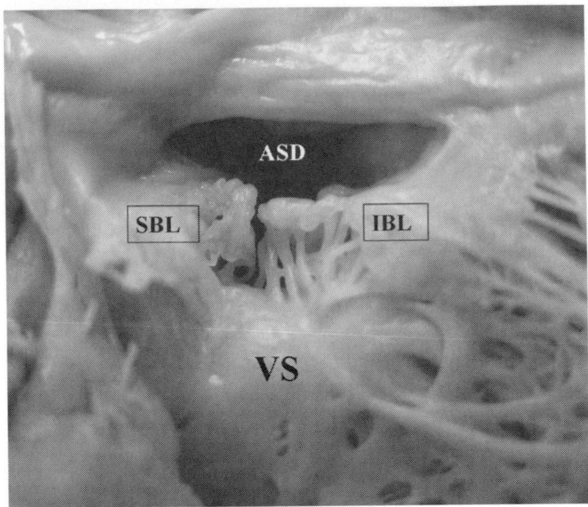

Figure 58-15 Specimen of atrioventricular septal defect, looking from the left ventricle. This is a defect with a common orifice, but there are multiple small intercordal communications between the ventricles. This has previously been called the "intermediate" or "transitional" defect.

about the midpoint of the ventricular septum, it becomes the right bundle branch, which descends to the medial papillary muscle of the right ventricle (Fig. 58-17). Thus, at operation, the greatest danger is at the time of securing the atrial septal patch, when the node is approached at the crux.

CLINICAL FEATURES

Aside from synchronous congenital malformations, the presentation and clinical findings of patients with AVSD are determined by several factors, among which are the level of shunt and the competence of the left AV valve. Both variables may be the cause of acute and severe presentation.

In the presence of isolated atrial shunting and minimal valvar regurgitation, the presentation is often delayed, akin to a defect in the oval fossa. The findings may be made incidentally, or suspicion may be raised by recurrent chest infections or reduced exercise tolerance.

With a common orifice and shunting at both levels, presentation is usually in infancy, with cardiac failure. The child is diaphoretic and short of breath on feeding and fails to thrive. These problems are compounded if there is severe left AV valvar regurgitation. On examination, the child is undernourished, breathless, and tachycardic, with hepatomegaly. There is a hyperactive precordium with a systolic thrill and a pansystolic murmur of variable grade.

DIAGNOSIS

On CXR, there is variable cardiomegaly, reflected in the cardiothoracic ratio. If the valve is severely regurgitant, the heart is enlarged in the absence of significant shunting. The pulmonary trunk is similarly engorged, with prominence of the pulmonary vascular markings. With

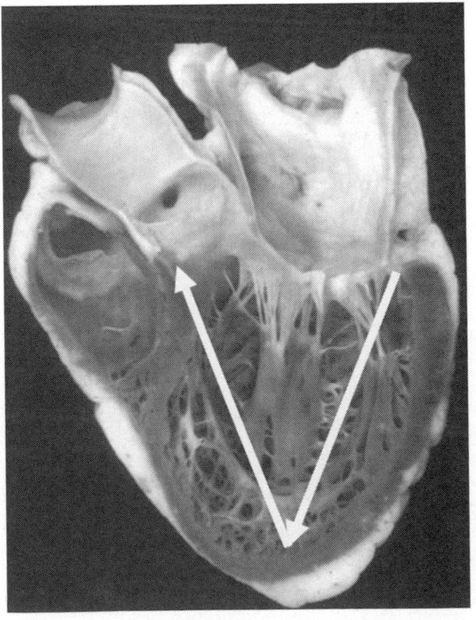
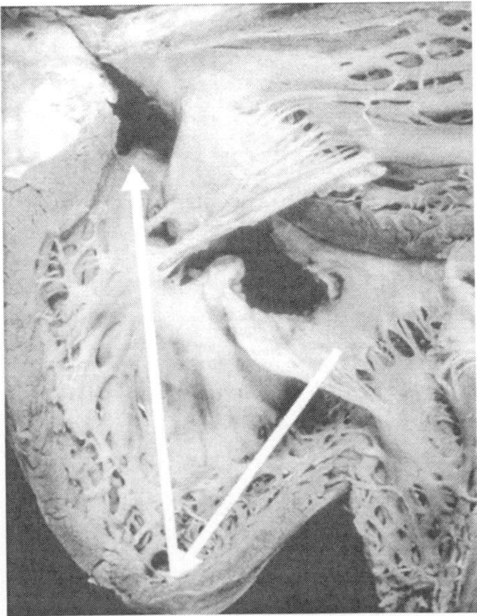

Figure 58-16 Left-hand panel: the comparable inlet and outlet dimensions of the normal heart. Right-hand panel: the inlet dimension of the heart with the atrioventricular septal defect, which is much smaller than the elongated outlet. This accounts for the scooping of the ventricular septum.

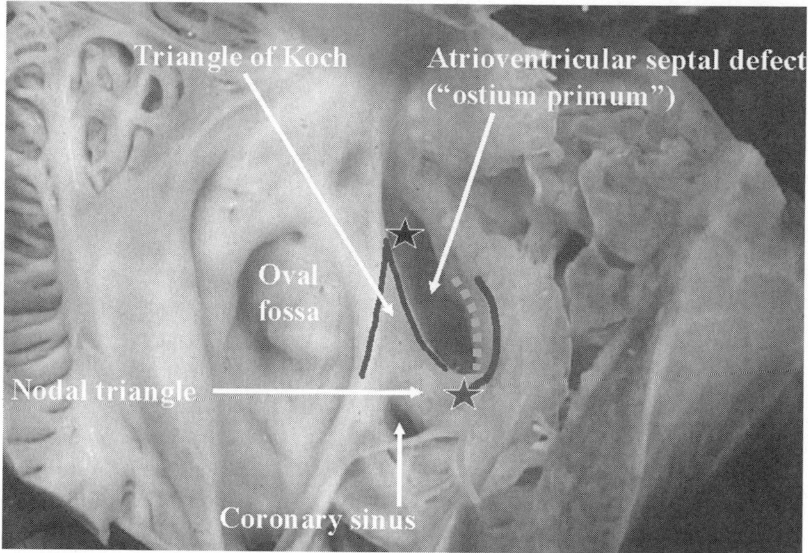

Figure 58-17 The position of the conduction axis in atrioventricular septal defects. The view is from the opened right atrium. The margins of the triangle of Koch are indicated; the superior black star indicates where one would normally expect to find the atrioventricular node (i.e., at the apex of the triangle). However, in this defect, the node has been displaced to the area between the coronary sinus and the crux of the heart (inferior black star). From here, the conduction axis runs along the proximal part of the ventricular crest (dotted line).

persisting pulmonary hypertension, the heart is not as greatly enlarged, but the pulmonary trunk is engorged, with "pruning" of the markings of the vascular tree.

Although superseded by echocardiography,[43] cardiac catheterization is presently reserved for those patients with complex defects where the intracardiac shunt must be calculated and when operability must be determined in the face of raised pulmonary vascular resistance. Information provided includes the anatomy, degree of AV valvar regurgitation, and quantification of the shunt. The diagnostic hallmark is the "gooseneck" appearance of the LVOT in the anteroposterior projection[22] (Fig. 58-18).

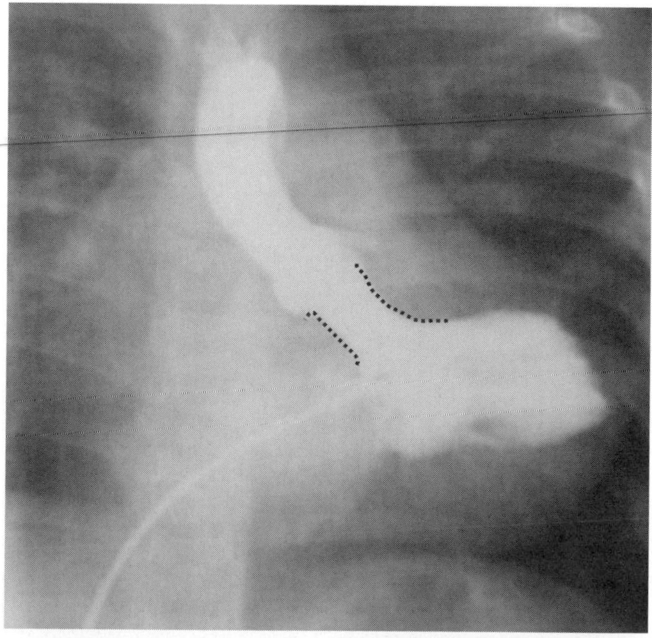

Figure 58-18 An anteroposterior angiocardiographic projection of the heart with an atrioventricular septal defect and common atrioventricular junction. The left ventricular outflow tract is elongated as a "gooseneck" (outlined), since it lies in an unwedged position anterior to the common atrioventricular junction.

ECHOCARDIOGRAPHY

This has superseded all other modalities as the pre-,[44,45] intra-,[46–48] and postoperative[49] investigation of choice. Doppler interrogation reveals intracardiac shunting, AV valve function, and patency of the LVOT while also determining the pulmonary vascular pressures. It has also, in recent years, been applied for prenatal diagnosis.[50]

There are a number of anatomic hallmarks. On the four-chamber view, the common AV junction causes loss of the normal offsetting of the AV valves (Fig. 58-19, left). Furthermore, the relationship of the leaflets to the crest of the ventricular septum can be appreciated on this view (Fig. 58-19, right). On the long-axis section, the

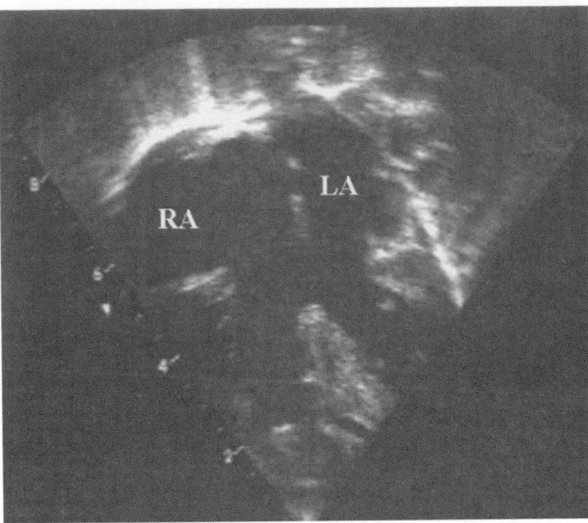

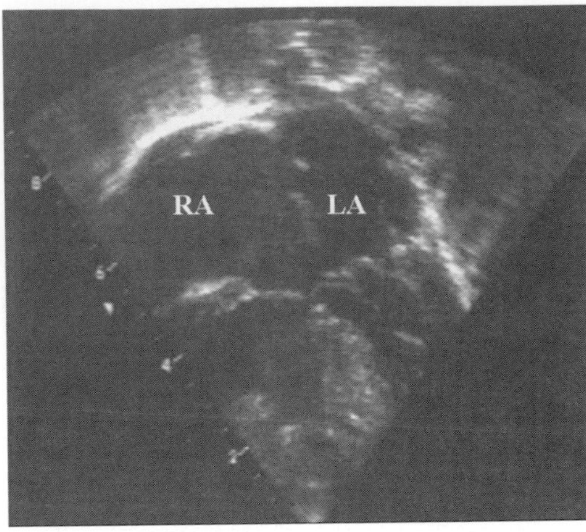

Figure 58-19 Two-dimensional transthoracic echocardiogram of the heart with atrioventricular septal defect in four-chamber view, taken in diastole (left panel) and systole (right panel). Note the tethering of the bridging leaflets to the crest of ventricular septum in systole, as well as the lack of off-setting of the AV valve. LA = left atrium; RA = right atrium.

"gooseneck" deformity of the LVOT is also visible; on the short-axis view, the common AV valve annulus is seen (Fig. 58-20). With separate right and left orifices, the trifoliate left AV valve is seen on short-axis with an exclusive orientation of the leaflets.

The size of the VSD is variable, often being larger beneath the superior bridging leaflet. There will also be variable cordal tethering to its crest. This septal tethering is greatest beneath the inferior bridging leaflet, as seen on the four-chamber section. It is therefore important to look for subtle ventricular shunting in the intercordal spaces with color-flow Doppler interrogation. Thus, because of this cordal obstruction, the degree of interventricular shunting is greatest with a free-floating superior bridging leaflet.

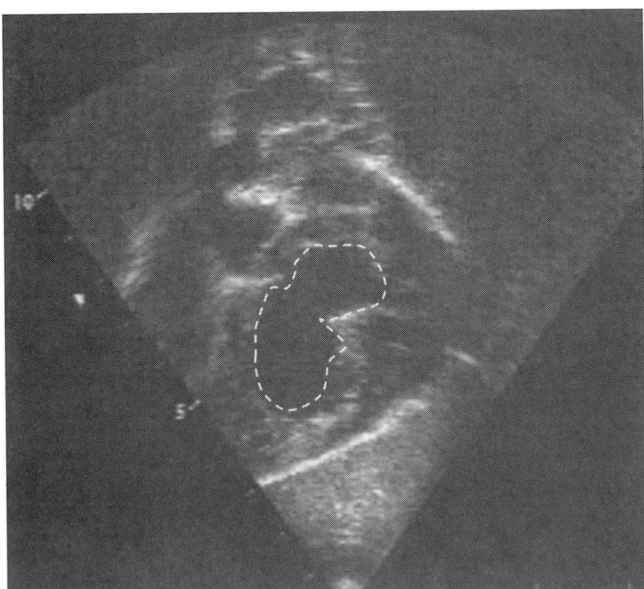

Figure 58-20 The same heart as in Fig. 58-18 in short-axis orientation showing the characteristic shape of the common atrioventricular junction (outlined).

NATURAL HISTORY

Without surgical intervention, the natural course will be determined by a number of factors, principally the level and degree of the intracardiac shunting, the pulmonary vascular resistance, and the competence of the left AV valve. It also follows that these factors will affect the timing of surgical intervention and subsequent outcome.

In the absence of significant left AV valvar regurgitation, the natural history of defects with separate orifices will be similar to that of a defect in the oval fossa. Therefore up to 15 percent of these patients will develop pulmonary hypertension by adulthood, and symptomatic deterioration may coincide with the development of atrial fibrillation.[51]

As predicted, the clinical course of the defect with a common orifice is more pernicious, with early deterioration from pulmonary hypertension, cardiac failure or respiratory infections. It is estimated that up to 80 percent of patients who do not undergo correction die by the age of 2 years.[52]

SURGICAL MANAGEMENT

Two pivotal events have transformed the surgical repair of AVSDs. The first and most conspicuous was the introduction of cardiopulmonary bypass; this could not have been successful without the other crucial event: mapping of the conduction tissue, by Lev.[53] Up to then, repair was hazardous, even in the best of hands. In 1954, Kirklin and associates successfully closed a defect with separate orifices using the atrial well of Gross. By 1955, defects were being closed under cardiopulmonary bypass using the DeBakey roller pump and wire-mesh screen oxygenator.[54]

Lillehei and associates performed the first repair of the so-called complete defect in 1954 by suturing the inferior rim of the atrial septum directly to the crest of the ventricular septum. Unsurprisingly, this often caused complete heart block, thus worsening valvar regurgitation and subaortic stenosis. It led to the introduction, in 1962,[55] of the single-patch technique as a way of overcoming early mortality. Over the last four decades, results have continued to improve, owing to better surgical techniques, more refined bypass circuits, and tailored postoperative care together with the use of permanent pacemaker systems.

One- versus two-stage repair

In the modern era, attention has shifted from a two-stage repair (involving initial pulmonary artery banding) to complete primary repair in infancy. What factors have brought about this change of strategy? There are two. First, there is greater understanding of the morphology, as mentioned. This also advanced the appreciation of the abnormal pathophysiology. Thus it was recognized quickly that banding was often ineffective in alleviating heart failure in the presence of severe left AV valvar incompetence.[56] Overall, the mortality associated with banding approached 50 percent.[56–58] Within face of these concerns, complete repair before the age of 2 years was called for, bringing the timing of intervention into line with that of simple VSDs. By the late 1970s, early primary repair had become the norm.[59,60]

Today, initial banding is reserved for complex defects, such as multiple VSDs, concurrent sepsis, and in some cases of the so-called unbalanced AVSDs, when it is possible to delay biventricular repair to a later date.[61,62]

Timing of repair

Hand in hand with primary repair is a decline in the age at operation. Independent of age, the timing will also be determined by other factors, such as the pulmonary vascular resistance, size of the intracardiac shunt and the degree of left AV valvar regurgitation. Aside from the protective effects on the pulmonary circulation,[28] earlier age at repair may confer benefits to the competence of the left AV valve. Chronic valvar regurgitation and volume overload lead to progressive annular dilatation with poorer leaflet coaptation. This is accompanied by leaflet dysplasia at the zone of apposition, further affecting the coapting mechanism. This cycle of "regurgitation begets regurgitation" is broken early by timely intervention. As a counterargument to early repair is the possibility of tearing of the sutures at the zone of apposition in patients weighing less than 5 kg at operation.[63]

Until 1973, only 6 patients below the age of 6 years had undergone attempts to repair defects with a common orifice, with only 2 survivors. By the late 1990s, the timing had reached the contemporary practice of repair within the first 6 months of life.

With AV septal defect with separate orifices in the absence of symptoms and left AV valvar regurgitation, repair is performed electively at 3 to 4 years of age, in line with defects in the oval fossa. Surgery is suitably earlier in those presenting with symptoms.

Principles of repair

The goals of repair are ventricular septation where there is a common orifice, atrial septation together with repair of the AV valves while avoiding heart block, residual defects, and obstruction of the LVOT. Competence of the left AV valve must be achieved while preventing stenosis of its orifice.

Several techniques have been used to achieve these ends, essentially being variations on the single- or double-patch themes. However, unusual leaflet morphologies add to the complexity.

Approach to the heart, cannulation, and cardioplegic arrest

The technique currently used at Great Ormond Street Hospital is described below. Median sternotomy is used in all cases. After thymectomy, the pericardiotomy is veered slightly to the left of the midline and the pericardium left attached on its right border. The aorta, arterial duct, and caval veins are then mobilized with diathermy. A silk ligature is passed around the arterial duct once this has been identified. In small infants, it may be very delicate, so it is often not ligated until cardiopulmonary bypass is established. This is followed by insertion of 5-0 polypropylene purse-string sutures in the aorta, superior caval vein, and right atrial appendage.

For aortic cannulation, a flexible DLP cannula is used (Medtronic, Grand Rapids, MI). A temporary angled metal Great Ormond Street venous cannula (GU Company, Tricomed, Addiscombe, Surrey, UK) is placed through the right atrial appendage, allowing rapid establishment of cardiopulmonary bypass, followed by ligation of the arterial duct. The superior caval vein is cannulated with a second angled metal cannula appropriate for the caliber of the vessel. Following cannulation of the superior caval vein, the metal cannula is removed from the right atrial appendage and replaced with a vent. The inferior caval vein is then dissected to the first hepatic vein. Once this has been exposed, a 5-0 polypropylene purse-string suture is placed, followed by cannulation. Nylon tape is then used to snare both caval veins.

The patient is cooled to 25°C in the case of the common orifice defect and above 32°C in the defect with separate orifices. The aorta is then cross-clamped and cardioplegia is administered. The right atrium is opened with an incision running parallel to the right AV groove. The left atrium may be vented through either the oval fossa or the right superior pulmonary vein. The latter structure may eventually be used for insertion of a left atrial pressure monitoring line.

The double-patch technique

Irrespective of the patch technique, there are a number of initial stages prior to septation:

1. Inspection: this commences with the position and size of the coronary sinus, proceeding to assessment of the size of the atrial component and patency of the oval fossa. The leaflets of the common AV valve are assessed for accessory orifices. The leaflets are elevated to reveal the ventricular component beneath as well as the state of the subvalvar apparatus. The ventricular septum is also inspected for additional septal defects.
2. Definition of the "kissing point" (Fig. 58-21): Bringing together the bridging leaflets over the left side of the ventricular septum allows their natural line of closure to be determined, forming a vital part of valvar repair. Once determined, the kissing point is marked with a 6-0 polypropylene suture.
3. Closure of the ventricular component (Fig. 58-22). This is closed with a 0.4-mm polytetrafluoroethylene (Gore-Tex) suture, although other materials may be used. The dimensions of the defect are assessed using silk, which is used to fashion out a crescentic patch of Gore-Tex. This is sutured to the right side of the ventricular septum with a continuous 5-0 polypropylene suture. To facilitate this, some small secondary cords may have to be sacrificed. The suture line is commenced close to the annulus through the inferior bridging leaflet, where it is well away from the position of the bundle. The first one or two bites are placed with the patch outside the heart. Once fixed, the prosthetic patch is slid into position beneath the bridging leaflets. The suture line then runs deeply along the right side of the septum toward the superior bridging leaflet, weaving through the cords. Finally, it is brought through the superior bridging leaflet, avoiding the aortic valve. A rubber-shod clamp is placed on the free end of the suture.
4. Atrial septation (Fig. 58-23). The atria are septated while separating the common valve into right and left components. Interrupted 6-0 polypropylene sutures, double-armed, are placed along the horizontal margin of the ventricular patch. The sutures are then

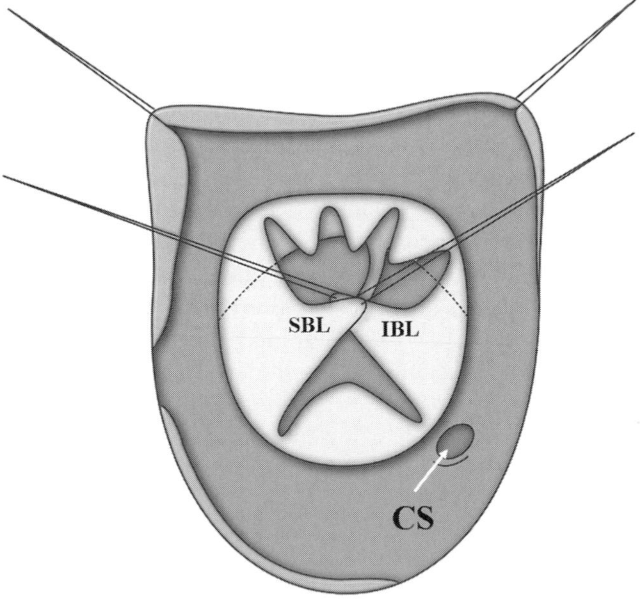

Figure 58-21 Drawing of the surgical repair of the atrioventricular septal defect with a common orifice, using the two-patch technique. The view is in surgical orientation, through the right atrium. The "kissing point" of the superior and bridging leaflets are initially brought together and marked with polypropylene marking sutures. (Modified from Jacobs JP, Elliott MJ. Atrioventricular septal defects. In: Kaiser LR, Kron IL, Spray TL (eds). *Mastery of Cardiothoracic Surgery.* Philadelphia: Lippincott-Raven; 1998. With permission.)

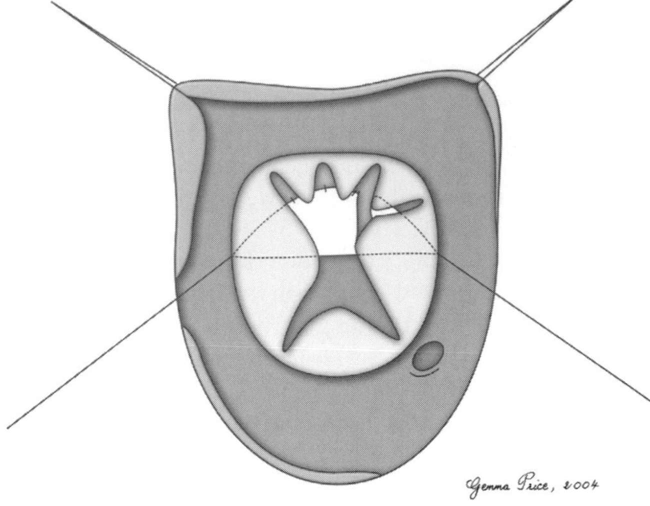

Figure 58-22 The crescentic patch of 0.4-mm Gore-Tex is sutured to the crest of the ventricular septum, keeping the suture line to the right side of the ventricular septum in order to avoid injury to the conduction tissue. (Modified from Jacobs JP, Elliott MJ. Atrioventricular septal defects. In: Kaiser LR, Kron IL, Spray TL (eds). *Mastery of Cardiothoracic Surgery.* Philadelphia: Lippincott-Raven; 1998. With permission.)

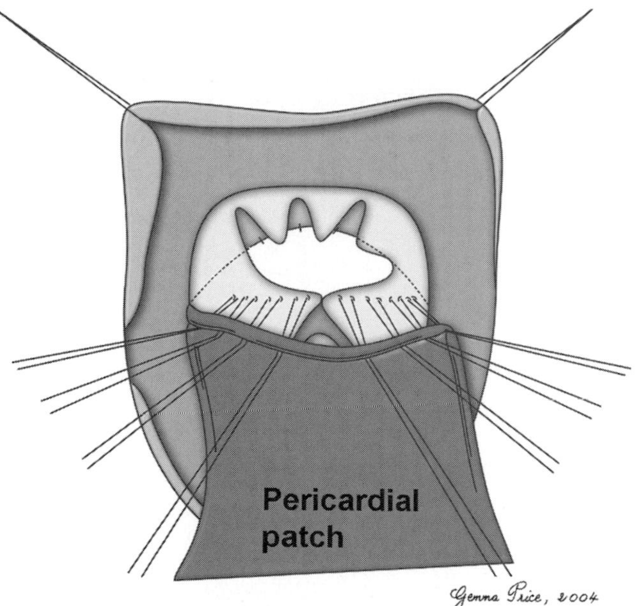

Figure 58-23 Next, the patch of autologous pericardium is secured to the ventricular septal patch and bridging leaflets by a line of double-armed interrupted sutures, released from its pericardial attachment, and slid down into place. (Modified from Jacobs JP, Elliott MJ. Atrioventricular septal defects. In: Kaiser LR, Kron IL, Spray TL (eds). *Mastery of Cardiothoracic Surgery*. Philadelphia: Lippincott-Raven; 1998. With permission.)

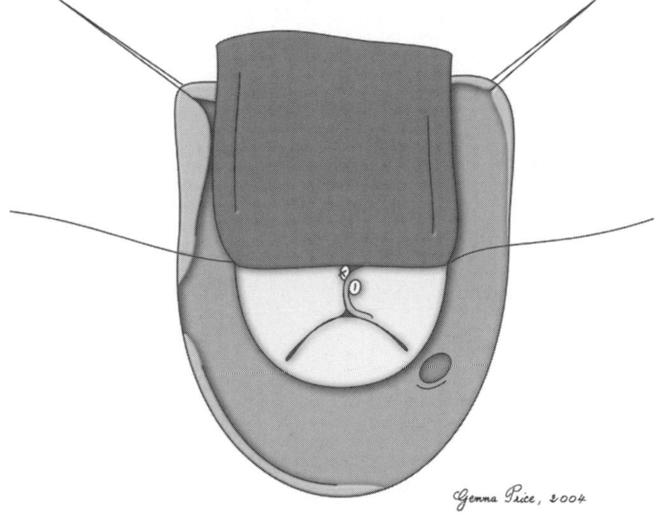

Figure 58-24 Once in place, the pericardial patch is elevated to allow the zone of apposition to be closed with pericardially pledgetted polypropylene sutures. (Modified from Jacobs JP, Elliott MJ. Atrioventricular septal defects. In: Kaiser LR, Kron IL, Spray TL (eds). *Mastery of Cardiothoracic Surgery*. Philadelphia: Lippincott-Raven; 1998. With permission.)

passed through the bridging leaflets and through the edge of the prepared autologous pericardium. This suture line runs from the inferior to the superior margin of the annulus. Thus, the line passes in an axis that bisects the common junction, its axis defined by the kissing points of the bridging leaflets. The sutures are then tied after the right side of the pericardium has been detached.

5. Consequently, the bridging leaflets are sandwiched between the two septal patches. Once this has been performed, the pericardial patch is swung over, exposing the newly created left AV orifice. The zone of apposition between the bridging leaflets is closed with one or two interrupted 6-0 polypropylene sutures supported with a small patch of pericardium (Fig. 58-24). The left atrioventricular valve is tested with a bulb syringe of cold saline. A commisuroplasty or annuloplasty may improve competence if there is persisting central regurgitation. A Hegar dilator ensures that the repaired valve is not stenotic.
6. The atrial patch is sutured in place with continuous 5-0 polypropylene, avoiding the position of the AV node. The coronary sinus may be left on either side of the patch, but it is committed to the right side in the face of a left superior caval vein. The first suture of the atrial patch is the free end of the ventricular patch suture that was held in a rubber-shod clamp. If the coronary sinus is committed to the right side, the suture line passes around the coronary sinus, close to the eustachian valve of the inferior caval vein, well inferior to the bundle. If the sinus is on the left side, the suture line binds the patch to the left AV valve at the annular margin (Fig. 58-25).

Once the heart is septated, the heart is de-aired and the aortic cross clamp is removed. Once warm, cardiopulmonary bypass is weaned.

The single-patch technique

This method has changed little since 1962. In the modern era, a pericardial patch is almost always used to close both ASDs and VSDs. The bridging leaflets are divided in order to accommodate the solitary patch.[64] Given that both bridging leaflets must be anchored to the patch, the suture line is more extensive than with the two-patch technique.

The techniques compared

Extensive comparisons have been made of the benefits of one technique over the other. The single-patch technique has been hailed as simpler (and therefore superior), with greater exposure of the VSD and subvalvar apparatus[65] and even associated with reduced duration of postoperative ventilator support.[34] However, it has also

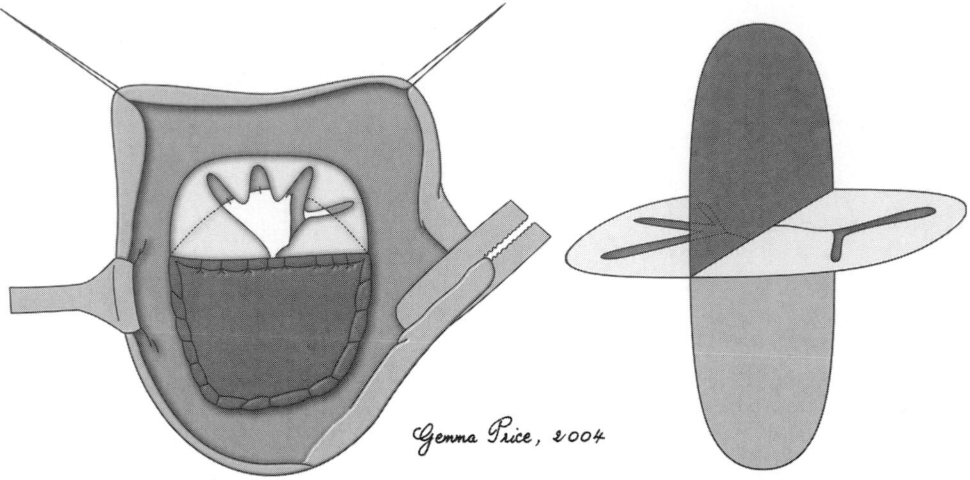

Figure 58-25 The repair is complete when the free edge of the pericardial patch is secured to the leading edge of the atrial septum. In this case, the coronary sinus is committed to the left ventricle. The right-hand panel shows the anterosuperior view of the newly septated heart. (Modified from Jacobs JP, Elliott MJ. Atrioventricular septal defects. In: Kaiser LR, Kron IL, Spray TL (eds). *Mastery of Cardiothoracic Surgery.* Philadelphia: Lippincott-Raven; 1998. With permission.)

been criticized for its theoretical effects on valvar competence,[66] since relatively more of the left AV valve is taken up in the suture line, with the risk of dehiscence.[28,67,68] This has caused some to change their technique over time.[28] Furthermore, it has been argued that closure of the zone of apposition may be inappropriate with this technique, since division of the leaflets and resuspension of the valve results in restricted mobility of the superior bridging leaflet.[69] Nevertheless, results are comparable and depend on operator preference.

The modified single-patch technique

This was initially introduced by Rastelli but refined and expanded by Wilcox[70] and the Australian group.[71] Here, the AV valves are sutured directly to the crest of the ventricular septum, simultaneously incorporating a single patch that is anchored to the leaflets and closing the atrial septal defect. Thus, in essence, the defect with the common orifice is converted to one with separate orifices where the valves are bound to the septal crest.

Several centers have adopted it as their standard, including Boston,[72] where it is defended on anatomic principles. Although it is known that the septal scoop is greatest in the setting of a common orifice, this is not the case in 30 to 40 percent of hearts.[19] It follows, therefore, that direct suturing of the leaflets to the septal crest is entirely feasible without distortion of the left ventricular outflow or disruption of the natural line of valvar closure. Another argument for this simplified technique is that ventricular septal patches have been getting progressively smaller with time, so that discarding them altogether is the next natural step in surgical evolution.

Attaining and maintaining leaflet atrioventricular valvar competence

Attainment of a competent left AV valve involves more than closure of the zone of apposition between the bridging leaflets.

Correct sizing of the ventricular patch is the first method, since it supports the annulus. If the patch is too long, the bridging leaflets will fail to coapt. If it is too short, valvar stenosis will ensue.[73]

Despite the observation that the zone of apposition is the most incompetent part of the left AV valve, its closure has not always been advocated. Carpentier[74] has stated that the trifoliate left AV valve is well adapted to its role. Thus, closure of the zone of apposition would reduce valvar opening during diastole and produce undue tension on the suture line.[69,75] Therefore an integrated trileaflet repair was advocated, based on the native trifoliate appearance.

Nevertheless, others have argued that the zone does not have the characteristic features and support of commisures in the normal AV valves and should therefore be closed.[61]

Some authors have taken the middle ground, repairing only those valves that were incompetent on saline testing[14,76] and not those in the very young because of the risk of tearing the leaflets.[63]

There are certain situations where it is agreed that the zone should be left open to prevent valvar stenosis. One well-recognized situation is that of the solitary left ventricular papillary muscle, or so-called parachute valve. Here, the bridging leaflets have a common papillary muscle insertion, leading to a slit-like valvar orifice.

There is a similar risk of stenosis when one is faced with a small left ventricle or in the presence of an accessory left ventricular orifice.[19,77–79] One way of standardizing the decision as to whether or not close has called for assessing the size of the left mural leaflet, the angular size of which has been found to be inversely related to the size of the inferior bridging leaflet.[19] An angular size of greater than 45 degrees has been used as the determinant of closure.[80]

Commissuroplasty or annuloplasty may also be used to improve competence, either at the commissures or centrally. They have also been used as a "belt and braces" measure in older patients with the defect of separate orifices where there has been chronic annular dilatation.[61,62]

ATRIOVENTRICULAR SEPTAL DEFECT WITH TETRALOGY OF FALLOT

Tetralogy of Fallot (ToF) complicates 2.7 to 10 percent of cases of AVSD. Conversely, AVSD complicates only 1 to 2 percent of cases of ToF.[81] There are a number of issues that must be considered during repair. First is the issue of whether complete primary repair can be carried out at an early stage. Even in the contemporary era, the majority of patients are palliated initially with a systemic-to-pulmonary shunt, the decision being guided by the severity of preoperative cyanosis. However, some have advocated early primary repair, stating that this aggressive strategy negates the risks associated with shunting.[82] However, there is no consensus, so that the age at complete repair varies greatly among different centers, ranging from a few months to several years.

Another issue is the finding that in the combined defect, the superior bridging leaflet is free-floating.[12] This has affected the decision as to whether to use a single- or double-patch strategy.[82,83] Some advocate two-patch repair on the understanding that it reduces the incidence of LVOT obstruction.[84–87] This is because the ventricular septal patch can be easily fashioned into a teardrop shape to accommodate the contour of the deviated outlet septum. Given this and other unresolved issues, such as the impact of both AV and pulmonary valvar dysfunction, mortality is still highly variable, ranging from less than 5 percent[81,84] to 33 percent.[85]

RESULTS OF REPAIR AND COMPLICATIONS

MORTALITY

There has been a striking reduction in the early and late postoperative mortality since the dawn of repair. In the current era, in the situation of a common orifice with no associated defects, balanced ventricles, and in the absence of vascular pulmonary hypertension, the mortality in most reporting centers is less than 5 percent and usually on the order of 1.5 to 3 percent. This is in contrast to three decades ago, when mortality was anywhere from 30 to 60 percent. The analysis of these results has also enabled some risk factors to be identified for mortality, some with more consistency than others (Table 58-1).

Table 58-1 Predictors of postoperative mortality in patients with complete atrioventricular septal defects

Risk factors for operative mortality	References
Preoperative pulmonary hypertension	35, 88, 89
Preoperative LAVV regurgitation, leaflet dysplasia or dysplastic LAVV	31,88, 90–92
Unbalanced ventricles	15, 90, 93
Double-orifice LAVV or solitary papillary muscle	28, 31, 64
Additional ventricular septal defects	31
Early era of operation	34, 64, 92
Postoperative pulmonary hypertensive crisis	28
Postoperative LAVV regurgitation	28, 64
Young age at repair	29 (before 1976), 92 (before 1990), 89
Low body weight	35, 89, 90
Long aortic cross-clamp time	35, 89
Requirement for preoperative inotropic support	88
Requirement for preoperative ventilatory support	94
Nonclosure of the zone of apposition	89, 95
Coarctation of the aorta	92

LAVV = left atrioventricular valve.

POSTOPERATIVE COMPLICATIONS

Aside from the general risks associated with anesthesia and cardiopulmonary bypass, the following complications are observed with this defect.

Pulmonary hypertensive crisis

The incidence of this complication has fallen with the advent of reduced age at primary repair, but the risk is still significant in older patients, those with preoperative pulmonary hypertension, and those with moderate to severe preoperative left AV valvar regurgitation. In these cases, concurrent use of both pulmonary artery and left atrial pressure lines is invaluable in the first 24 to 36 h after surgery. Scenarios that may trigger a crisis—such as acidosis, hypoxia, or agitation—must be avoided. Thus, older patients are intubated and sedated for longer periods in the postoperative phase. Alpha-adrenergic blockers, such as phenoxybenzamine, may be used prophylactically, preoperatively, and during rewarming. During a crisis, the patient is sedated and hyperventilated, so that the $PaCO_2$ falls to below 3.5 kPa. Paralysis may also be instituted, together with intravenous nitroprusside or inhaled nitric oxide.

Heart block

In the modern era, when the position of the conduction bundle has been defined, the prevalence of this complication has fallen to 1 to 2 percent. The key is careful suture placement in the region of the coronary sinus, remembering that the conduction system runs the same course irrespective of the number of orifices. Following operation, in the case of temporary heart block that may occur in the context of regional conduction tissue edema, the patient should leave the operating room with temporary pacing wires.

Left atrioventricular valvar regurgitation

This may be considered as an early or late postoperative complication that might require reoperation. It may be recognized as a persistently elevated left atrial pressure and failure to wean from intubation, being confirmed by echocardiography. Early reoperation for regurgitation has been consistently reported in 5 to 7 percent of patients, with little change over the years.[15,64,96] It may be associated with technical factors, such as closing the zone of apposition; but in some series the use of closure of the zone with annuloplasty did not affect the overall incidence of regurgitation.[64] Some have also suggested that the severity of preoperative regurgitation correlated with the degree of postoperative insufficiency,[28] whereas others have found no relationship between the two.[32]

Late regurgitation, measured as freedom from reoperation, is found with varying degree, ranging from about 80 to 90 percent at 10 years.[89,92,95] The incidence of this complication has similarly shown little change over the years, being more common in such situations as in the setting of a double-orifice valve, nonclosure of the zone of apposition, non-Down's patients,[90,96] and a dysplastic left AV valve. Recently, division of the superior bridging leaflet at operation during patch placement has also been associated with an increased incidence of long-term left AV valve regurgitation.[97] Table 58-2 summarizes the risk factors identified in the literature for early and late AV valvar regurgitation.

Table 58-2 Predictors of postoperative left atrioventricular valve (LAVV) regurgitation in patients with complete atrioventricular septal defects

Risk factors for postoperative left atrioventricular valvar regurgitation	References
Preoperative LAVVR	96–98
Nonclosure of the zone of apposition	61, 90 ,96, 99
Non-Down's AVSD	38, 90
Leaflet dysplasia	100
Double-orifice left atrioventricular valve	96, 97, 99, 100
Solitary papillary muscle arrangement	97
Older age at operation	38
Division of the bridging leaflets at operation	97
Earlier era of operation	95
Unbalanced atrioventricular septal defects	90, 100
Preoperative pulmonary hypertension	100

THE FUTURE

Although, in terms of both mortality and morbidity, surgical repair of this defect has come a very long way, the main issue for the future involves long-term durability of the repair and quality of life. With this in mind, the stagnant incidence of long-term left AV valvar deterioration will be tackled successfully only by thoroughly understanding the form and function of the valve, with all of its morphologic nuances.

References

1. Castaneda AR, Mayer JE Jr, Jonas RA. Repair of complete atrioventricular canal in infancy. *World J Surg* 1985;9:590.
2. Rastelli GC, Ongley PA, Kirklin JW, et al. Surgical repair of the complete form of persistent common atrioventricular canal. *J Thorac Cardiovasc Surg* 1968;55:299.
3. Bender HW Jr, Hammon JW Jr, Hubbard SG, et al. Repair of atrioventricular canal malformation in the first year of life. *J Thorac Cardiovasc Surg* 1982;84:515.
4. Becker AE, Anderson RH. Atrioventricular septal defects: What's in a name? *J Thorac Cardiovasc Surg* 1982;83:461.
5. Rastelli G, Kirklin JW, Titus JL. Anatomic observations on complete form of persistent common atrioventricular canal with special reference to atrioventricular valves. *Mayo Clin Proc* 1966;41:296.
6. Anderson RH, Zuberbuhler JR, Penkoske PA, et al. Of clefts, commissures and things. *J Thorac Cardiovasc Surg* 1985;90:605.
7. Penkoske PA, Neches WH, Anderson RH, et al. Further observations on the morphology of atrioventricular septal defects. *J Thorac Cardiovasc Surg* 1985;90:611.

8. Ugarte M, Enriquez DS, Quero M. Endocardial cushion defects: An anatomical study of 54 specimens. *Br Heart J* 1976;38:674.
9. Gallo P, Formigari R, Hokayem NJ, et al. Left ventricular outflow tract obstruction in atrioventricular septal defects: A pathologic and morphometric evaluation. *Clin Cardiol* 1991;14:513.
10. Ebels T, Ho SY, Anderson RH, et al. The surgical anatomy of the left ventricular outflow tract in atrioventricular septal defect. *Ann Thorac Surg* 1986;41:483.
11. Uretzky G, Puga FJ, Danielson GK, et al. Complete atrioventricular canal associated with tetralogy of Fallot. Morphologic and surgical considerations. *J Thorac Cardiovasc Surg* 1984;87:756.
12. Suzuki K, Ho SY, Anderson RH, et al. Morphometric analysis of atrioventricular septal defect with common valve orifice. *J Am Coll Cardiol* 1998;31:217.
13. Backer CL, Mavroudis C, Alboliras ET, et al. Repair of complete atrioventricular canal defects: Results with the two-patch technique. *Ann Thorac Surg* 1995;60:530.
14. Bove EL, Sondheimer HM, Kavey RE, et al. Results with the two-patch technique for repair of complete atrioventricular septal defect. *Ann Thorac Surg* 1984; 38:157.
15. Redmond JM, Silove ED, De Giovanni JV, et al. Complete atrioventricular septal defects: The influence of associated cardiac anomalies on surgical management and outcome. *Eur J Cardiothorac Surg* 1996;10:991.
16. McGoon DC, Puga FJ. Atrioventricular canal. *Cardiovasc Clin* 1981;11:311.
17. Van Praagh S, Porras D, Oppido G, et al. Cleft mitral valve without ostium primum defect: Anatomic data and surgical considerations based on 41 cases. *Ann Thorac Surg* 2003;75:1752.
18. Gutgesell HP, Huhta JC. Cardiac septation in atrioventricular canal defect. *J Am Coll Cardiol* 1986;8:1421.
19. Ebels T, Anderson RH, Devine WA, et al. Anomalies of the left atrioventricular valve and related ventricular septal morphology in atrioventricular septal defects. *J Thorac Cardiovasc Surg* 1990;99:299.
20. Ebels T, Anderson RH. The concept and definition of an "intermediate form" of atrioventricular septal defect. *J Thorac Cardiovasc Surg* 1991;102:799.
21. Di Segni E, Edwards JE. Cleft anterior leaflet of the mitral valve with intact septa. A study of 20 cases. *Am J Cardiol* 1983;51:919.
22. Blieden LC, Randall PA, Castaneda AR, et al. The "goose neck" of the endocardial cushion defect: Anatomic basis. *Chest* 1974;65:13.
23. Van Groningen JP, Hartel ME, Wenink ACG. Septal deficiency in atrioventricular septal defect. *Ann NY Acad Sci* 1990;588:449.
24. Smallhorn JF, Tommasini G, Macartney FJ. Two-dimensional echocardiographic assessment of common atrioventricular valves in univentricular hearts. *Br Heart J* 1981;46:30.
25. Drinkwater DC Jr, Laks H. Unbalanced atrioventricular septal defects. *Semin Thorac Cardiovasc Surg* 1997;9:21.
26. Chang CI, Becker AE. Surgical anatomy of left ventricular outflow tract obstruction in complete atrioventricular septal defect: A concept for operative repair. *J Thorac Cardiovasc Surg* 1987;94:897.
27. Piccoli GP, Ho SY, Wilkinson JL, et al. Left-sided obstructive lesions in atrioventricular septal defects: An anatomic study. *J Thorac Cardiovasc Surg* 1982;83:453.
28. Bando K, Turrentine MW, Sun K, et al. Surgical management of complete atrioventricular septal defects. A twenty-year experience. *J Thorac Cardiovasc Surg* 1995; 110:1543.
29. Studer M, Blackstone EH, Kirklin JW, et al. Determinants of early and late results of repair of atrioventricular septal (canal) defects. *J Thorac Cardiovasc Surg* 1982;84:523.
30. Abbruzzese PA, Livermore J, Sunderland CO, et al. Mitral repair in complete atrioventricular canal. Ease of correction in early infancy. *J Thorac Cardiovasc Surg* 1983;85:388.
31. Chin AJ, Keane JF, Norwood WI, et al. Repair of complete common atrioventricular canal in infancy. *J Thorac Cardiovasc Surg* 1982;84:437.
32. Weintraub RG, Brawn WJ, Venables AW, et al. Two-patch repair of complete atrioventricular septal defect in the first year of life. Results and sequential assessment of atrioventricular valve function. *J Thorac Cardiovasc Surg* 1990;99:320.
33. Kirklin JW, Blackstone EH, Bargeron LM Jr, et al. The repair of atrioventricular septal defects in infancy. *Int J Cardiol* 1986;13:333.
34. Tweddell JS, Litwin SB, Berger S, et al. Twenty-year experience with repair of complete atrioventricular septal defects. *Ann Thorac Surg* 1996;62:419.
35. McGrath LB, Gonzalez-Lavin L. Actuarial survival, freedom from reoperation, and other events after repair of atrioventricular septal defects. *J Thorac Cardiovasc Surg* 1987;94:582.
36. Baird PA, Sadovnick AD. Life expectancy in Down syndrome. *J Pediatr* 1987;110:849.
37. Marino B. Atrioventricular septal defect: Anatomic characteristics in patients with and without Down's syndrome. *Cardiol Young* 1992;2:308.
38. Michielon G, Stellin G, Rizzoli G. Repair of complete common atrioventricular canal defects in patients younger than four months of age. *Circulation* 1997;96(9 Suppl):II–22.
39. De Biase L, Di Ciommo V, Ballerini L, et al. Prevalence of left-sided obstructive lesions in patients with atrioventricular canal without Down's syndrome. *J Thorac Cardiovasc Surg* 1986;91:467.
40. Chi TL, Krovetz JL. The pulmonary vascular bed in children with Down's syndrome. *J Pediatr* 1975;86:533.
41. Clapp S, Perry BL, Farooki ZQ, et al. Down's syndrome, complete atrioventricular canal, and pulmonary vascular obstructive disease. *J Thorac Cardiovasc Surg* 1990;100:115.
42. Bull C, Rigby ML, Shinebourne EA. Should management of complete atrioventricular canal defect be influenced by coexistent Down syndrome? *Lancet* 1985;1(8438): 1147.
43. Lipshultz SE, Sanders SP, Mayer JE, et al. Are routine preoperative cardiac catheterization and angiography necessary before repair of ostium primum atrial septal defect? *J Am Coll Cardiol* 1988;11:373.
44. Cabrera A, Pastor E, Galdeano JM, et al. Cross-sectional echocardiography in the diagnosis of atrioventricular septal defect. *Int J Cardiol* 1990;28:19.

45. Lange A, Mankad P, Walayat M, et al. Transthoracic three-dimensional echocardiography in the preoperative assessment of atrioventricular septal defect morphology. *Am J Cardiol* 2000;85:630.
46. Zellers TM, Zehr R, Weinstein E, et al. Two-dimensional and Doppler echocardiography alone can adequately define preoperative anatomy and hemodynamic status before repair of complete atrioventricular septal defect in infants < 1 year old. *J Am Coll Cardiol* 1994;24: 1565.
47. Ungerleider RM, Kisslo JA, Greeley WJ, et al. Intraoperative prebypass and postbypass epicardial color flow imaging in the repair of atrioventricular septal defects. *J Thorac Cardiovasc Surg* 1989;98:90.
48. Canter CE, Spray TL, Huddleston CB, et al. As originally published in 1989: Intraoperative evaluation of atrioventricular septal defect repair by color flow mapping echocardiography. Updated in 1997. *Ann Thorac Surg* 1997;63:592.
49. Kececioglu D, Kehl HG, Schmid C, et al. Morphologic characterization and assessment of mitral regurgitation after repair of atrioventricular defects in children. *Thorac Cardiovasc Surg* 1997;45:70.
50. Fesslova V, Villa L, Nava S, et al. Spectrum and outcome of atrioventricular septal defect in fetal life. *Cardiol Young* 2002;12:18.
51. Somerville J.Ostium primum defect: Factors causing deterioration in the natural history. *Br Heart J* 1965; 27:413.
52. Berger TJ, Blackstone EH, Kirklin JW, et al. Survival and probability of cure without and with operation in complete atrioventricular canal. *Ann Thorac Surg 1979*; 27:104.
53. Lev M. The architecture of the conduction system in congenital heart disease. I. Common atrioventricular orifice. *AMA Arch Pathol* 1958;65:174.
54. Kirklin JW, Burchell HB. Repair of the partial form of persistent common atrioventricular canal: So-called ostium primum type of atrial septal defect with interventricular communication. *Ann Surg* 1955;142:858.
55. Maloney JV Jr, Marable SA, Mulder DG. The surgical treatment of common atrioventricular canal. *J Thorac Cardiovasc Surg* 1962;43:84.
56. Hunt CE, Formanek G, Levine MA. Banding of the pulmonary artery: Results in 111 children. *Circulation* 1971;43:395.
57. Stark J, Aberdeen E, Waterston DJ. Pulmonary artery constriction (banding): A report of 146 cases. *Surgery* 1969; 65:808.
58. Newfeld EA, Sher M, Paul MH. Pulmonary vascular disease in atrioventricular canal defect. *Am J Cardiol* 1976; 37:159.
59. Mair DD, McGoon DC. Surgical correction of atrioventricular canal during the first year of life. *Am J Cardiol* 1977;40:66.
60. Kirklin JW, Blackstone EH. Management of the infant with complete atrioventricular canal. *J Thorac Cardiovasc Surg* 1979;78:32.
61. Capouya ER, Laks H, Drinkwater DC, et al. Management of the left atrioventricular valve in the repair of complete atrioventricular septal defects. *J Thorac Cardiovasc Surg* 1992;104:196.
62. Reddy VM, McElhinney DB, Brook MM, et al. Atrioventricular valve function after single patch repair of complete atrioventricular septal defect in infancy: How early should repair be attempted? *J Thorac Cardiovasc Surg* 1998;115:1032.
63. Prifti E, Bonacchi M, Bernabei M, et al. Repair of complete atrioventricular septal defects in patients weighing less than 5 kg. *Ann Thorac Surg* 2004;77:1717.
64. Hanley FL, Fenton KN, Jonas RA, et al. Surgical repair of complete atrioventricular canal defects in infancy. Twenty-year trends. *J Thorac Cardiovasc Surg* 1993; 106(3):387–394.
65. Merrill WH, Hammon JW Jr, Graham TP Jr. Complete repair of atrioventricular septal defect. *Ann Thorac Surg* 1991;52:29.
66. Pacifico AD, Ricchi A, Bargeron LM Jr, et al. Corrective repair of complete atrioventricular canal defects and major associated cardiac anomalies. *Ann Thorac Surg* 1988;46:645.
67. Culpepper W, Kolff J, Lin CY, et al. Complete common atrioventricular canal in infancy–Surgical repair and postoperative hemodynamics. *Circulation* 1978;58:550.
68. Yasui H, Nakamura Y, Kado H, et al. Primary repair for complete atrioventricular canal: Recommendation for early primary repair. *J Cardiovasc Surg (Torino)* 1990; 31:498.
69. Ashraf MH, Amin Z, Sharma R. Atrioventricular canal defect: Two-patch repair and tricuspidization of the mitral valve. *Ann Thorac Surg* 1993;55:347.
70. Wilcox BR, Jones DR, Frantz EG, et al. Anatomically sound, simplified approach to repair of "complete" atrioventricular septal defect. *Ann Thorac Surg* 1997; 64:487.
71. Nicholson IA, Nunn GR, Sholler GF, et al. Simplified single patch technique for the repair of atrioventricular septal defect. *J Thorac Cardiovasc Surg* 1999;118:642.
72. Jonas RA. Complete atrioventricular canal. In: *Comprehensive Surgical Management of Congenital Heart Disease*. London: Hodder Arnold; 2004:386.
73. Lacour-Gayet F, Comas J, Bruniaux J. Management of the left atrioventricular valve in 95 patients with atrioventricular septal defects and a common atrioventricular orifice: A ten-year review. *Cardiol Young* 1991; 1:367.
74. Carpentier A. Surgical anatomy and management of the mitral component of atrioventricular canal defects. In: Anderson RH, Shinebourne EA (eds). *Paediatric Cardiology 1977*. Edinburgh: Churchill Livingstone; 1977:477.
75. Enriquez de Salamanca F, Ugarte M. Anatomy of atrioventricular malformations. In: Anderson RH, Shinebourne EA (eds). *Paediatric Cardiology 1977*. London: Churchill Livingstone; 1977:429.
76. Mavroudis C, Weinstein G, Turley K. Surgical management of complete atrioventricular canal. *J Thorac Cardiovasc Surg* 1982;83:670.
77. Mace L, Dervanian P, Houyel L, et al. Surgically created double-orifice left atrioventricular valve: A valve-sparing repair in selected atrioventricular septal defects. *J Thorac Cardiovasc Surg* 2001;121:352.
78. Abbruzzese PA, Napoleone A, Bini RM, et al. Late left atrioventricular valve insufficiency after repair of partial

atrioventricular septal defects: Anatomical and surgical determinants. *Ann Thorac Surg* 1990;49:111.

79. Meijboom EJ, Ebels T, Anderson RH, et al. Left atrioventricular valve after surgical repair in atrioventricular septal defect with separate valve orifices ("ostium primum atrial septal defect"): An echo-Doppler study. *Am J Cardiol* 1986;57:433.
80. Ebels T, Anderson RH. Atrioventricular septal defects. In: Anderson RH, Baker E, Macartney F, et al (eds). *Paediatric Cardiology*. London: Churchill Livingstone; 2002:939.
81. Karl TR. Atrioventricular septal defect with tetralogy of Fallot or double-outlet right ventricle: Surgical considerations. *Semin Thorac Cardiovasc Surg* 1997;9:26.
82. McElhinney DB, Reddy VM, Silverman NH, et al. Atrioventricular septal defect with common valvar orifice and tetralogy of Fallot revisited: Making a case for primary repair in infancy. *Cardiol Young* 1998;8:455.
83. Ilbawi M, Cua C, DeLeon S, et al. Repair of complete atrioventricular septal defect with tetralogy of Fallot. *Ann Thorac Surg* 1990;50:407.
84. Alonso J, Nunez P, Perez DL, et al. Complete atrioventricular canal and tetralogy of Fallot: Surgical management. *Eur J Cardiothorac Surg* 1990;4:297.
85. Bertolini A, Dalmonte P, Bava GL, et al. Surgical management of complete atrioventricular canal associated with tetralogy of Fallot. *Cardiovasc Surg* 1996;4:299.
86. Chiu IS, Hung CR, Wang JK. Surgical treatment of complete atrioventricular septal defect associated with tetralogy of Fallot. *Int J Cardiol* 1995;48:225.
87. Vouhe PR, Neveux JY. Surgical repair of tetralogy of Fallot with complete atrioventricular canal. *Ann Thorac Surg* 1986;41:342.
88. Alexi-Meskishvili V, Ishino K, Dahnert I, et al. Correction of complete atrioventricular septal defects with the double-patch technique and cleft closure. *Ann Thorac Surg* 1996;62:519.
89. Boening A, Scheewe J, Heine K, et al. Long-term results after surgical correction of atrioventricular septal defects. *Eur J Cardiothorac Surg* 2002;22:167.
90. Ross DA, Nanton M, Gillis DA. Atrioventricular canal defects: Results of repair in the current era. *J Card Surg* 1991;6:367.
91. Tlaskal T, Hucin B, Marek J, et al. Individualized repair of the left atrioventricular valve in spectrum of atrioventricular septal defect. *J Cardiovasc Surg (Torino)* 1997; 38:233.
92. Gunther T, Mazzitelli D, Haehnel CJ. Long-term results after repair of complete atrioventricular septal defects: Analysis of risk factors. *Ann Thorac Surg* 1998;65:754.
93. Schaffer R, Berdat P, Stolle B. Surgery of the complete atrioventricular canal: Relationship between age at operation, mitral regurgitation, size of the ventricular septum defect, additional malformations and early postoperative outcome. *Cardiology* 1999;91:231.
94. Alexi-Meskishvili V, Hetzer R, Dahnert I, et al. Results of left atrioventricular valve reconstruction after previous correction of atrioventricular septal defects. *Eur J Cardiothorac Surg* 1997;12:460.
95. Crawford FA Jr, Stroud MR. Surgical repair of complete atrioventricular septal defect. *Ann Thorac Surg* 2001; 72:1621.
96. Michielon G, Stellin G, Rizzoli G, et al. Left atrioventricular valve incompetence after repair of common atrioventricular canal defects. *Ann Thorac Surg* 1995;60(6 Suppl):S604–S609.
97. Fortuna RS, Ashburn DA, Carias DO, et al. Atrioventricular septal defects: Effect of bridging leaflet division on early valve function. *Ann Thorac Surg* 2004; 77:895.
98. Pozzi M, Remig J, Urban AE. Atrioventricular septal defects. Analysis of short- and medium-term results. *J Thorac Cardiovasc Surg* 1991;101:138.
99. Najm HK, Coles JG, Endo M, et al. Complete atrioventricular septal defects: Results of repair, risk factors, and freedom from reoperation. *Circulation* 1997;96(9 Suppl):II-5.
100. lapp SK, Perry BL, Farooki ZQ, et al. Surgical and medical results of complete atrioventricular canal: A ten year review. *Am J Cardiol* 1987;59:454.

CHAPTER

59 AORTOPULMONARY WINDOW

Anthony Azakie, Michael M. Brook, Tom R. Karl

INTRODUCTION

Aortopulmonary (AP) window or AP septal defect is a rare congenital anomaly that consists of an abnormal communication between the ascending aorta and main or branch pulmonary artery. The lesion has also been called an AP fenestration or AP fistula. It occurs in 0.2 to 0.5 percent of patients with congenital cardiac disease.[1] Embryologically, the lesion results from aplasia, malalignment, or failure of fusion of the AP and truncal septa.

In 1952, Robert Gross reported the first surgical ligation of an AP window.[2] The use of cardiopulmonary bypass to correct the anatomic defect was first described in 1957 by Cooley and associates.[3]

PATHOPHYSIOLOGY

The pathophysiology of AP window depends on the size of the defect and the presence of associated cardiac anomalies. The lesion usually produces a significant left-to-right shunt and resembles, with regard to pathophysiology and natural history, other septation defects such as large ventricular septal defects or patent arterial duct, truncus arteriosus, or anomalous origin of branch pulmonary arteries from the aorta (Fig. 59-1).

The aortic and pulmonary artery (PA) pressures may be equal, and flow to the lungs (QP:QS) is determined by the pulmonary vascular resistance (PVR) and size of the communication. As PVR typically declines in the first few weeks of life, congestive cardiac failure, left ventricular volume

KEY CONCEPTS

- Epidemiology
  - Aortopulmonary (AP) window is a rare congenital anomaly, representing 0.2 to 0.5 percent of all cases of congenital heart disease.
- Pathophysiology
  - An abnormal communication between the ascending aorta and main or branch pulmonary artery results in severe left-to-right shunting. The degree of pulmonary overcirculation, pulmonary hypertensive vascular changes, congestive heart failure, and failure to thrive depend on associated anomalies and the size of the defect, which is often large enough to allow equalization of pulmonary and aortic pressures. Associated malformations are present in 50 to 60 percent of cases and include interrupted aortic arch, tetralogy of Fallot, and anomalous origin of the right pulmonary or coronary artery.
- Diagnosis
  - Two-dimensional echocardiography provides accurate identification and localization of AP window as well as definition of associated lesions.
- Treatment
  - Surgical closure of large defects is indicated at the time of diagnosis in order to avoid early development of fixed pulmonary hypertension. Patch repair using a transaortic, transpulmonary, or "sandwich" approach has excellent outcomes. Small defects can be ligated or approached by percutaneous techniques.
- Outcomes/prognosis
  - Operative mortality is reported at less than 10 percent, with long-term prognosis largely dependent on the development of pulmonary hypertensive changes.

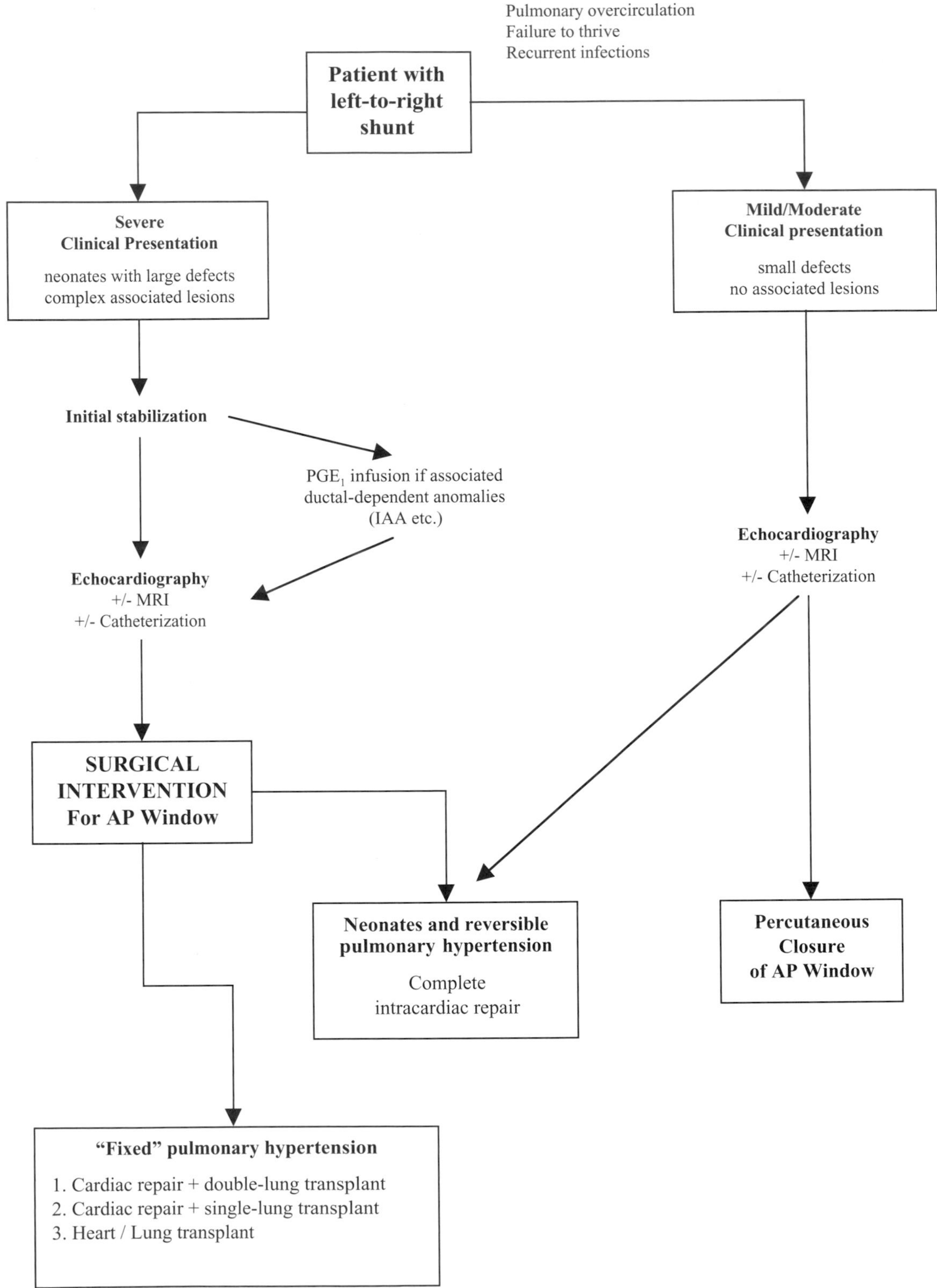

Figure 59-1 Decision-making flowchart.

overload, and pulmonary congestion develop. There is a widened pulse pressure with a relatively lower diastolic blood pressure, and coronary perfusion can be significantly reduced. If PVR does not drop significantly in the early postnatal period, cardiac failure does not ensue. The natural history of the lesion mimics that of a large left-to-right shunt, with failure to thrive and persistent, severe pulmonary overcirculation. If the child survives untreated beyond infancy, progression to severe (and sometimes irreversible) pulmonary vascular disease ensues.

EMBRYOLOGY AND MORPHOLOGY

Embryologically, aortopulmonary septation defects result from aplasia, malalignment, or failure of fusion of the AP and truncal septa. In the avian embryo, both inhibition of bone morphogenetic protein (BMP) function by the inhibitor Noggin as well as impairment of cardiac neural crest migration result in failure of AP septation.[4–6] The defects observed in this model, however, are not limited to the AP septum but also include the common arterial trunk, double-outlet right ventricle, and defects in atrioventricular septation. AP window has been reported to occur also in the context of trisomy 13 and in fetuses with terminal deletions of the long arm of chromosome 2.[7,8]

The pathologic anatomy and morphologic classification most commonly used is that proposed by Mori and colleagues,[9] with three basic subtypes of AP window or AP septal defect (Fig. 59-2A to C). Type I involves a defect in the septum above the sinotubular junction of the great vessels, on the left side of the ascending aorta and proximal to the PA bifurcation (Fig. 59-2A). The lesion or defect is circular and oriented in a sagittal plane. The second type (type II) is a more distal and oblique defect, which extends into the PA bifurcation with involvement of the right PA in the defect (Fig. 59-2B). The proximal right PA is "unroofed," and the defect involves the posterior aspect of the ascending aorta. The third type of AP window is a combination of types I and II (Fig. 59-2C). The defect is usually large and characterized by almost complete absence of the AP septum, such that there is a common vascular origin to the aortic arch, ductus arteriosus, and pulmonary arteries. Associated anomalies are present in 50 to 60 percent of

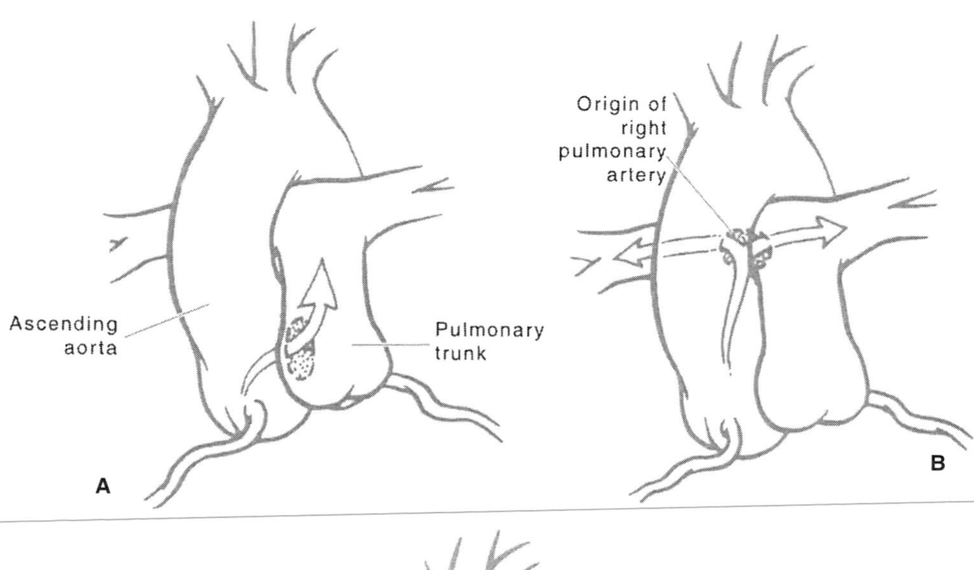

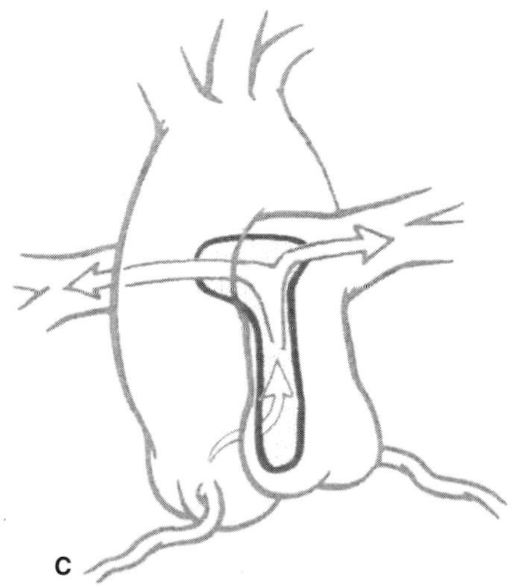

Figure 59-2 Classification of AP window. **A.** Type I involves a defect in the aortopulmonary septum, proximal to the pulmonary artery bifurcation. **B.** Type II is a more distal and oblique defect. **C.** The third type of AP window is a combination of types I and II. (From Kouchoukos NT, Blackstone EH, Doty DB, et al. (eds). *Kirklin/Barratt-Boyes Cardiac Surgery*, 3d ed. Philadelphia: Churchill-Livingstone, 2003. With permission.)

cases of AP window.[10–32] Interrupted aortic arch is one of the most common lesions associated with AP window. In distinction to the type B interruption seen in truncus arteriosus (and typically associated with ventricular septal defect and DiGeorge syndrome), type A arch interruption with intact ventricular septum is more often seen in association with AP window. The "Berry syndrome" describes the association between AP window, right PA origin from the aorta, and arch obstruction or interruption.[22] Anomalous origin of the right, left, or circumflex coronary arteries has been described in association with AP window, stressing the importance of defining the coronary anatomy during preoperative imaging.[14,26,27,32,33] Other associated lesions include tetralogy of Fallot, ventricular and atrioventricular septal defects, transposition of the great arteries, and double aortic arch. Concomitant PA vegetations or endocarditis changes can also be observed.

CLINICAL FEATURES

AP window is a rare lesion with male preponderance (1.8:1 male:female ratio) that is also associated with the VACTERL syndrome (i.e., *v*ertebral anomalies, *a*nal atresia, *c*ardiovascular anomalies, *t*racheoesophageal fistula, *e*sophageal atresia, *r*enal anomalies, and *l*imb anomalies). The timing and mode of presentation depend on associated lesions and the size of the defect. For isolated (and usually large) AP window, presentation usually occurs in the neonatal period or in early infancy. Signs and symptoms at the time of presentation include respiratory distress, failure to thrive, poor weight gain, and recurrent pulmonary infections. Physical examination usually reveals a systolic and middiastolic murmur along the left upper sternal border; in some cases, the murmur is continuous. The heart is enlarged. Small restrictive defects may present as an asymptomatic murmur on routine physical examination.

Electrocardiography may show signs of biventricular hypertrophy due to elevated pulmonary blood flow, increased pulmonary vascular resistance, and left ventricular volume overload. There is prominent left atrial enlargement. Chest x-ray discloses increased pulmonary vasculature and an enlarged heart.

DIAGNOSIS AND IMAGING

Echocardiography

In the current era, the diagnosis can be completely made by two-dimensional echocardiography (Fig. 59-3A to C). Echocardiography provides accurate identification of the AP window and characterization of associated lesions.[17,34–36] Care must be taken to distinguish "dropout" that may be normally seen in the AP septal region from true AP window or AP septal defect.[37] Doppler echocardiography shows abnormal continuous flow in the pulmonary arteries. Forward flow into the distal main PA helps in differentiating AP window from patent ductus arteriosus (PDA). Retrograde diastolic aortic flow can be seen and, if tricuspid regurgitation is present, right ventricular pressure can be estimated. The ventricles may show hypertrophy, while pulmonary and systemic veins and atrioventricular/semilunar valves are usually normal.

Cardiac catheterization and angiography

In the current era, cardiac catheterization is usually not necessary, since echocardiography can usually provide a complete and accurate diagnosis with identification of all associated lesions. However, cardiac catheterization can be useful to further define the anatomy and size of the defect as well as origins of the pulmonary arteries when echocardiography is inconclusive. Aortic root angiography is extremely useful in delineating the anatomy of the pulmonary arteries and the origins of the coronary arteries, essential features in planning the surgical repair. Cardiac catheterization is also important in assessing the arborization of the pulmonary vasculature as well as the presence and reversibility of increased pulmonary vascular resistance.

Magnetic resonance imaging

AP window can be successfully diagnosed by magnetic resonance imaging (MRI).[38-42] Spin-echo T1-weighted axial and coronal magnetic resonance images show a window-like communication between the left side of the ascending aorta and the right wall of the main pulmonary arterial trunk. Associated anomalous origin of the right PA from the ascending aorta can also be identified by MRI.

SURGICAL MANAGEMENT AND OUTCOMES

As stated above, the management and outcome of AP window depends on the size and location of the lesion and its associated cardiovascular defects.[20,21,30,43–49] The surgical repair must be tailored to the specific anatomic and physiologic features of each patient. Isolated AP window is usually repaired through a median sternotomy with the use of cardiopulmonary bypass (Fig. 59-4A to C). Arterial cannulation is performed in the distal ascending aorta or transverse aortic arch. Bicaval cannulation is used for venous return. Upon institution of cardiopulmonary bypass, both pulmonary arteries are dissected and controlled with tourniquets in order to avoid excessive runoff into the pulmonary vascular tree, with consequent hypotension (Fig. 59-4A). The aorta is clamped distally and cold-blood antegrade cardioplegia

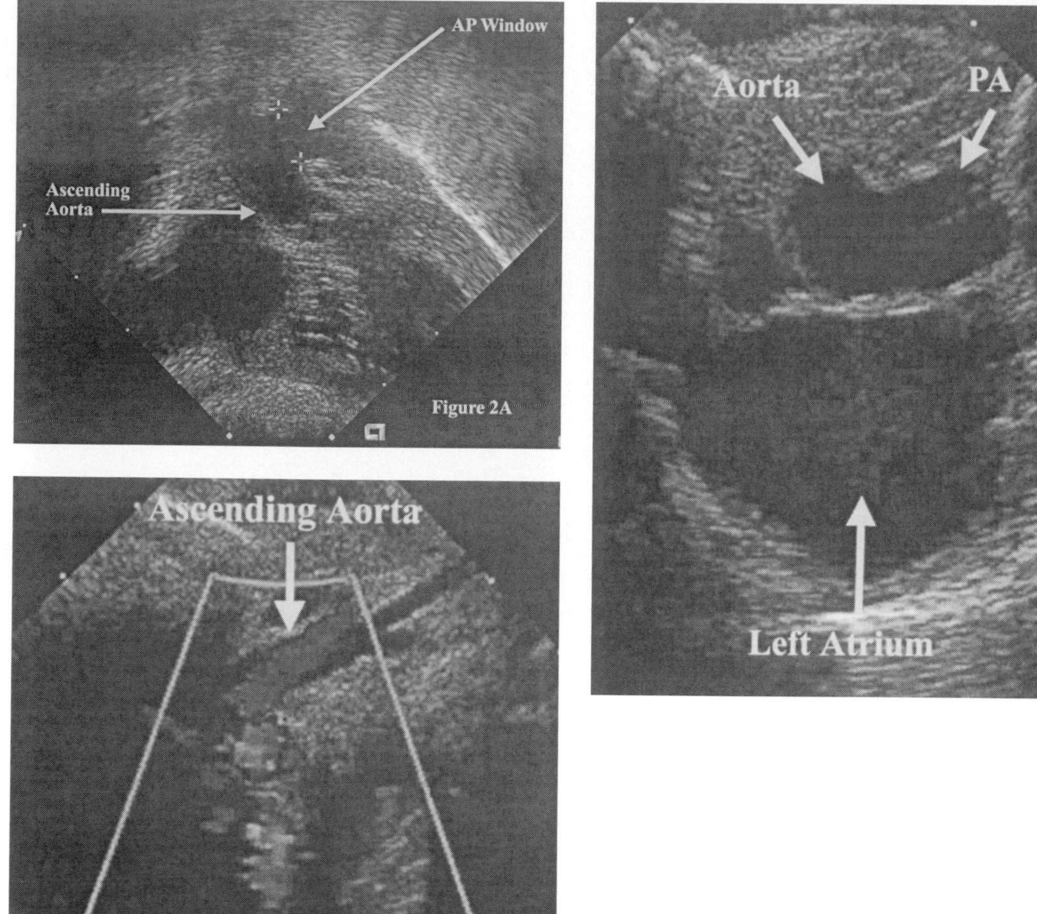

Figure 59-3 Echocardiographic image of AP window with interrupted aortic arch and anomalous origin of the right pulmonary artery. **A.** Longitudinal image of ascending aorta with aortopulmonary septal defect. **B.** Coronal image showing the window between the ascending aorta and pulmonary artery. **C.** Interruption of the aortic arch beyond the innominate artery.

is delivered either into the aortic root or in a retrograde fashion through the coronary sinus. After diastolic arrest has been achieved, the right atrium is opened and the left heart vented through an interatrial communication.

Exposure of the AP defect is accomplished via an incision in the ascending aorta, main PA, or both. Alternatively, a superior and anterior incision can be made through the defect itself (Fig. 59-4B). The transaortic approach utilizes a longitudinal or transverse aortic incision, which allows optimal visualization and inspection of both coronary ostia as well as the origins of both branch pulmonary arteries.[43,50,51] The aortic and pulmonary roots are inspected as well as the semilunar valves, and the location and size of the defect are determined. The defect is usually repaired with a patch. Patch materials include synthetic Dacron, expanded polytetrafluoroethylene, and autologous pericardium fixed in glutaraldehyde. The patch is tailored so as to be extended on the roof of the right PA if the defect extends into its origin. For lesions in which the right coronary artery originates anomalously from the PA, the transaortic incision is extended leftward onto the PA to create a flap that includes the right coronary artery and is large enough to close the AP window.[52,53] The residual defect in the pulmonary arterial wall is repaired with an autologous pericardial patch.

The "sandwich technique"[54–56] utilizes an incision in the superior and anterior portion of the AP window that extends one-third to one-half of the circumference of the defect. The incision exposes both aortic and pulmonary roots while allowing inspection of the pulmonary arteries. A patch is sewn to the posterior ridge of the defect, and the anterior portion of the patch is sandwiched between the aortic and pulmonary arterial walls (Fig. 59-4C). The coronary arteries must be identified using this approach. If a coronary artery originates on the pulmonary arterial

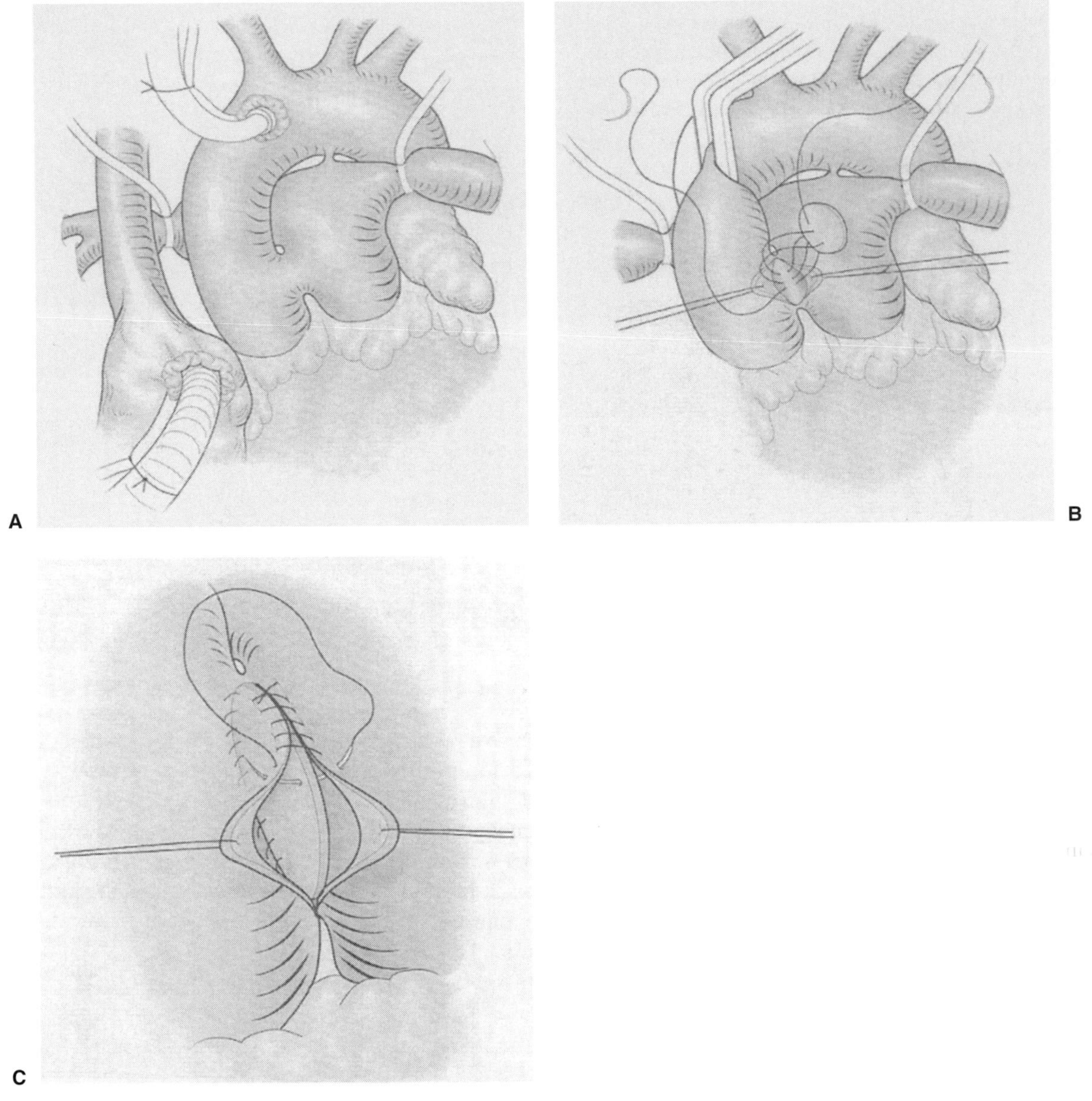

Figure 59-4 Repair of AP window with the "sandwich" technique. A. Upon institution of cardiopulmonary bypass, both pulmonary arteries are dissected and controlled with tourniquets. B. After diastolic cardioplegic arrest, an incision is made in the superior and anterior portion of the AP window extending one-third to one-half of the circumference of the defect. C. A patch is "sandwiched" between the aortic and pulmonary arterial walls and sewn in place to seal the defect. (From Spray TL, Gardner TJ (eds). *Operative Cardiac Surgery*, 5th ed. London: Hodder Arnold, 2004. With permission.)

side of the defect, the incision is made so that the patch is sewn in a way to incorporate the coronary ostium onto the aortic side. Alternatively a coronary button can be dissected, the AP window closed with a patch, and the coronary button reimplanted into to the aortic root.

Small AP windows can be exposed through limited skin incisions and an upper hemisternotomy. This involves dissecting and encircling the diminutive communication and then ligating it. Kawata and coworkers have reported successful repair of an AP window with a clip through a left thoracotomy in an infant with extremely low birth weight (758 g).[57] Cardiac catheterization 7 months after the operation showed no residual shunt and no stenosis of ascending aorta, PA, or coronary arteries.

Several reports have described the percutaneous transcatheter deployment of devices to close relatively small AP septal defects in infants and children. Complete occlusion of the defect can be achieved without complications.[58–62] Significant residual defects after surgical closure of AP windows have traditionally required reoperation. More recently, transcatheter approaches have been used to occlude hemodynamically significant residual defects.

Patients with AP window and fixed/severe pulmonary hypertension (Eisenmenger's syndrome) can be surgically treated by lung transplantation with intracardiac repair for selected patients, reserving heart-lung transplantation for those with unreconstructable heart disease.[63] Selected patients with major intracardiac defects and pulmonary hypertension may have good early results after cardiac repair and single-lung transplantation. However, sequential double-lung transplantation and cardiac repair for AP window may have advantages over single-lung transplantation with intracardiac repair or heart-lung transplantation.[64]

Outcomes for surgical repair of isolated AP windows are excellent, with morbidity and mortality rates approaching zero in the current era. Early outcomes depend on the complexity of associated defects and the metabolic condition of the child on initial presentation. Overall, actuarial survival ranges between 70 and 90 percent at 10 years.[28,43,45,47,49] Freedom from reintervention is 70 to 80 percent at 10 years.[45,49] Patients undergoing repair via a transaortic approach generally show favorable growth of the pulmonary arteries and the aortic root. Some authors have, in fact, advocated against exposure through a pulmonary arteriotomy, since its use is associated with increased need for late reintervention.[45]

ACKNOWLEDGMENTS

The authors would like to thank Mr. Leonard A. Moon and Ms. Kala Garner for assisting with preparation of this chapter and imaging support.

References

1. Kutsche LM, Van Mierop LH. Anatomy and pathogenesis of aorticopulmonary septal defect. *Am J Cardiol* 1987;59: 443–447.
2. Gross RE. Surgical closure of an aortic septal defect. *Circulation* 1952;5:858–863.
3. Cooley DA, McNamara DG, Latson JR. Aorticopulmonary septal defect: Diagnosis and surgical treatment. *Surgery* 1957;42:101–120.
4. Roberts KE, McElroy JJ, Wong WP, et al. BMPR2 mutations in pulmonary arterial hypertension with congenital heart disease. *Eur Respir J* 2004;24:371–374.
5. Allen SP, Bogardi JP, Barlow AJ, et al. Misexpression of noggin leads to septal defects in the outflow tract of the chick heart. *Dev Biol* 2001;235:98–109.
6. Takahashi K, Kido S, Hoshino K, et al. Frequency of a 22q11 deletion in patients with conotruncal cardiac malformations: A prospective study. *Eur J Pediatr* 1995;154: 878–881.
7. Sharma J, Saleh M, Das BB. Berry syndrome with trisomy 13. *Pediatr Cardiol* 2002;23:205–209.
8. Waters BL, Allen EF, Gibson PC, et al. Autopsy findings in a severely affected infant with a 2q terminal deletion. *Am J Med Genet* 1993;47:1099–1103.
9. Mori K, Ando M, Takao A, et al. Distal type of aortopulmonary window. Report of 4 cases. *Br Heart J* 1978;40: 681–689.
10. Somerville J. Aortopulmonary septal defect: Five cases treated by operation. *Guys Hosp Rep* 1959;108:177–193.
11. Morrow AG, Greenfield LJ, Braunwald E. Congenital aortopulmonary septal defect. Clinical and hemodynamic findings, surgical technic, and results of operative correction. *Circulation* 1962;25:463–476.
12. Faulkner SL, Oldham RR, Atwood GF, et al. Aortopulmonary window, ventricular septal defect, and membranous pulmonary atresia with a diagnosis of truncus arteriosus. *Chest* 1974;65:351–353.
13. Rosenquist GC, Taylor JF, Stark J. Aortopulmonary fenestration and aortic atresia. Report of an infant with ventricular septal defect, persistent ductus arteriosus, and interrupted aortic arch. *Br Heart J* 1974;36: 1146–1148.
14. Bourlon F, Kreitmann P, Jourdan J, et al. Anomalous origin of left coronary artery with aortopulmonary window: A case report with surgical correction and delayed control. *Thorac Cardiovasc Surg* 1981;29:91–92.
15. Shore DF, Ho SY, Anderson RH, et al. Aortopulmonary septal defect coexisting with ventricular septal defect and pulmonary atresia. *Ann Thorac Surg* 1983;35: 132–137.
16. Tiraboschi R, Salomone G, Crupi G, et al. Aortopulmonary window in the first year of life: Report on 11 surgical cases. *Ann Thorac Surg* 1988;46:438–441.
17. Carminati M, Borghi A, Valsecchi O, et al. Aortopulmonary window coexisting with tetralogy of Fallot: Echocardiographic diagnosis. *Pediatr Cardiol* 1990;11:41–43.
18. Amato JJ. Complete transposition of the great arteries with aortopulmonary window. *J Thorac Cardiovasc Surg* 1992;104:1490–1491.
19. Boonstra PW, Talsma M, Ebels T. Interruption of the aortic arch, distal aortopulmonary window, arterial duct and aortic origin of the right pulmonary artery in a neonate: Report of a case successfully repaired in a one-stage operation. *Int J Cardiol* 1992;34:108–110.
20. Bertolini A, Dalmonte P, Bava GL, et al. Aortopulmonary septal defects. A review of the literature and report of ten cases. *J Cardiovasc Surg (Torino)* 1994;35: 207–213.
21. Serraf A, Lacour-Gayet F, Robotin M, et al. Repair of interrupted aortic arch: A ten-year experience. *J Thorac Cardiovasc Surg* 1996;112:1150–1160.
22. Abbruzzese PA, Merlo M, Chiappa E, et al. Berry syndrome, a complex aortopulmonary malformation: One-stage repair in a neonate. *Ann Thorac Surg* 1997;64: 1167–1169.
23. Gouri SR, Rao SG, Dandekar C. Aortopulmonary window with atrial septal defect. *J Indian Med Assoc* 1997;95:203–205.
24. Codispoti M, Mankad PS. One-stage repair of interrupted aortic arch, aortopulmonary window, and anomalous origin of right pulmonary artery with autologous tissues. *Ann Thorac Surg* 1998;66:264–267.

25. De Caro E, Pongiglione G, Ribaldone D. Interruption of the aortic arch, ventricular septal defect, aortic atresia and aortopulmonary fistulous communication. *Int J Cardiol* 1998;65:19–21.
26. Morell VO, Feccia M, Cullen S. Anomalous coronary artery with tetralogy of Fallot and aortopulmonary window. *Ann Thorac Surg* 1998;66:1403–1405.
27. Izumoto H, Ishihara K, Fujii Y, et al. AP window and anomalous origin of right coronary artery from the window. *Ann Thorac Surg* 1999;68:557–559.
28. Soares AM, Atik E, Cortez TM, et al. Aortopulmonary window. Clinical and surgical assessment of 18 cases. *Arq Bras Cardiol* 1999;73:59–74.
29. Pauliks LB, Bharati S, Magid MS, et al. A cross between truncus arteriosus communis and aortopulmonary septal defect: A hitherto undescribed entity. *Pediatr Cardiol* 2000;21:477–479.
30. McElhinney DB, Paridon S, Spray TL. Aortopulmonary window associated with complete atrioventricular septal defect. *J Thorac Cardiovasc Surg* 2000;119:1284–1285.
31. Alborino D, Guccione P, Di Donato R. Aortopulmonary window coexisting with tetralogy of Fallot. *J Cardiovasc Surg (Torino)* 2001;42:197–199.
32. Mahadevan C, Kareem S, Jitendra V, et al. Pulmonary origin of circumflex artery in aortopulmonary window. *Asian Cardiovasc Thorac Ann* 2003;11:80–81.
33. Chopra PS, Reed WH, Wilson AD, et al. Delayed presentation of anomalous circumflex coronary artery arising from pulmonary artery following repair of aortopulmonary window in infancy. *Chest* 1994;106:1920–1922.
34. Vargas Barron J, Castro MC, Guadalajara JF, et al. Echocardiographic aspects of the aortopulmonary window. Report of a case with angiocardiographic correlations. *Arch Inst Cardiol Mex* 1980;50:591–597.
35. Reyes de la Cruz L, Vizcaino Alarcon A, et al. Echocardiographic diagnosis of anomalous origin of one pulmonary artery from the ascending aorta. *Arch Cardiol Mex* 2003;73:115–123.
36. Alva-Espinosa C, Jimenez-Arteaga S, Diaz-Diaz E. Diagnosis of Berry syndrome in an infant by two-dimensional and color Doppler echocardiography. *Pediatr Cardiol* 1995;16:42–44.
37. Balaji S, Burch M, Sullivan ID. Accuracy of cross-sectional echocardiography in diagnosis of aortopulmonary window. *Am J Cardiol* 1991;67:650–653.
38. Huggon IC, Baker EJ, Maisey MN, et al. Magnetic resonance imaging of hearts with atrioventricular valve atresia or double inlet ventricle. *Br Heart J* 1992;68:313–319.
39. Incesu L, Baysal K, Kalayci AG, et al. Magnetic resonance imaging of proximal aortopulmonary window. *Clin Imaging* 1998;22:23–25.
40. Kim TK, Choe YH, Kim HS, et al. Anomalous origin of the right pulmonary artery from the ascending aorta: Diagnosis by magnetic resonance imaging. *Cardiovasc Intervent Radiol* 1995;18:118–121.
41. Sieverding L, Klose U, Apitz J. Morphological diagnosis of congenital and acquired heart disease by magnetic resonance imaging. *Pediatr Radiol* 1990;20:311–319.
42. Teo EL, Goldberg CS, Strouse PJ, et al. Aortopulmonary window with interrupted aortic arch and pulmonary artery sling: Diagnosis by echocardiography and magnetic resonance imaging: Case report and literature review. *Echocardiography* 1999;16:147–150.
43. Backer CL, Mavroudis C. Surgical management of aortopulmonary window: A 40-year experience. *Eur J Cardiothorac Surg* 2002;21:773–779.
44. Di Bella I, Gladstone DJ. Surgical management of aortopulmonary window. *Ann Thorac Surg* 1998;65: 768–770.
45. Hew CC, Bacha EA, Zurakowski D, et al. Optimal surgical approach for repair of aortopulmonary window. *Cardiol Young* 2001;11:385–390.
46. Malec E, Brzegowy P, Mroczek T. Surgical treatment of aortopulmonary window with tetralogy of Fallot. *Scand Cardiovasc J* 2001;35:159–160.
47. Tanoue Y, Sese A, Ueno Y, et al. Surgical management of aortopulmonary window. *Jpn J Thorac Cardiovasc Surg* 2000;48:557–561.
48. Sharma R, Saha K, Kothari SS. Neonatal correction of interrupted aortic arch, aortopulmonary window and ascending aortic origin of right pulmonary artery. *Indian Heart J* 1996;48:717–720.
49. Tkebuchava T, von Segesser LK, Vogt PR, et al. Congenital aortopulumonary window: Diagnosis, surgical technique and long-term results. *Eur J Cardiothorac Surg* 1997;11:293–297.
50. Clarke CP, Richardson JP. The management of aortopulmonary window: Advantages of transaortic closure with a Dacron patch. *J Thorac Cardiovasc Surg* 1976;72: 48–51.
51. Doty DB, Richardson JV, Falkovsky GE, et al. Aortopulmonary septal defect: Hemodynamics, angiography, and operation. *Ann Thorac Surg* 1981;32: 244–250.
52. Luisi SV, Ashraf MH, Gula G, et al. Anomalous origin of the right coronary artery with aortopulmonary window: Functional and surgical considerations. *Thorax* 1980;35: 446–448.
53. Gula G, Chew C, Radley-Smith R, et al. Anomalous origin of the right pulmonary artery from the ascending aorta associated with aortopulmonary window. *Thorax* 1978;33: 265–269.
54. Preusse CJ. The surgical management of aortopulmonary window using the anterior sandwich patch closure technique. *J Cardiovasc Surg (Torino)* 1989;30:713.
55. Ravikumar E, Whight CM, Hawker RE, et al. The surgical management of aortopulmonary window using the anterior sandwich patch closure technique. *J Cardiovasc Surg (Torino)* 1988;29:629–632.
56. Johansson L, Michaelsson M, Westerholm CJM, et al. Aortopulmonary window: A new operative approach. *Ann Thorac Surg* 198;25:564–567.
57. Kawata H, Kishimoto H, Ueno T, et al. Repair of aortopulmonary window in an infant with extremely low birth weight. *Ann Thorac Surg* 1996;62:1843–1845.
58. Richens T, Wilson N. Amplatzer device closure of a residual aortopulmonary window. *Catheter Cardiovasc Interv* 2000;50:431–433.
59. Tulloh RM, Rigby ML. Transcatheter umbrella closure of aorto-pulmonary window. *Heart* 1997;77:479–480.

60. Pavcnik D, Wright KC, Wallace S, et al. Device for percutaneous transcatheter closure of cardiac septal defects. *Cardiovasc Intervent Radiol* 1993;16:308–312.
61. Atiq M, Rashid N, Kazmi KA, et al. Closure of aortopulmonary window with Amplatzer duct occluder device. *Pediatr Cardiol* 2003;24:298–299.
62. Stamato T, Benson LN, Smallhorn JF, et al. Transcatheter closure of an aortopulmonary window with a modified double umbrella occluder system. *Cathet Cardiovasc Diagn* 1995;35:165–167.
63. Lupinetti FM, Bolling SF, Bove EL, et al. Selective lung or heart-lung transplantation for pulmonary hypertension associated with congenital cardiac anomalies. *Ann Thorac Surg* 1994;57:1545–1548.
64. Charpentier A, Levy F, Mettauer B, et al. Successful sequential double lung transplantation and cardiac repair for aortopulmonary window: Technical and functional advantages over heart-lung transplantation. *Transplant Proc* 1996;28:2878–2879.

CHAPTER

60 TETRALOGY OF FALLOT

Duccio Di Carlo, Maria Cristina Digilio, Luigi Ballerini

DEFINITION

Although this malformation was first described by Nicolas Steno in 1873,[1] it owes its eponym to a series of papers published by Etienne-Louis Fallot in 1888.[2]

Tetralogy of Fallot (ToF) is a relatively common congenital cardiac anomaly characterized by a large ventricular septal defect (VSD), RV outflow tract obstruction (RVOTO), dextroposition of the aorta, and RV hypertrophy. A precise definition of the anomaly nevertheless presents some difficulty because, as Lev and Eckner stated,[3] no two cases of ToF are the same. It can be argued that ToF is not a discrete entity, forming part of a spectrum of cardiac anomalies that range between tetralogy with mild pulmonary stenosis (PS) on one end and tetralogy with pulmonary atresia and aortopulmonary collaterals on the other. Nonetheless, all hearts having ToF are unified by the anatomic hallmark of subpulmonary infundibular narrowing due to anterior and cephalad deviation of the infundibular septum, associated with aortic dextroposition and thus defining the VSD.[4]

KEY CONCEPTS

- **Epidemiology**
  - Tetralogy of Fallot (ToF) accounts for 5.4 percent of all congenital heart defects and is associated with extracardiac malformations in 32 percent and chromosomal abnormalities in 12 percent.
- **Morphology**
  - This involves dextroposition of the aorta with 50 percent override of a large ventricular septal defect associated with anterosuperior deviation of the outlet septum, resulting in right ventricular outflow tract obstruction (RVOTO) and RV hypertrophy. A right-sided aortic arch and an anomalous left anterior descending coronary artery (LAD) from the right coronary artery (RCA) are observed in 25 and 5 percent of cases, respectively. RVOTO can occur at the subvalvar, valvar, and supravalvar levels; stenosis can be associated with an absent pulmonary valve in rare cases.
- **Pathophysiology**
  - Symptoms are dictated by the degree of right-to-left shunting across the ventricular septal defect (VSD) and the degree of RVOTO, with resulting cyanosis. Anoxic/hypoxic spells are rare in the neonatal period.
- **Clinical features**
  - In patients with mild stenosis, signs and symptoms are similar to those of VSD, while more severe RVOTO is characterized by severe cyanosis.
- **Diagnosis**
  - This is established by electrocardiography (ECG) significant for RV hypertrophy and, in cyanotic children, clear lung fields and diminished pulmonary arterial prominence on chest x-ray (CXR). Echocardiography usually suffices to proceed to correction or palliation, delineating all intra- and extracardiac features. Cardiac catheterization, computed tomography (CT), and magnetic resonance imaging (MRI) are useful in selected cases with unclear anatomy and in patients requiring reoperation.
- **Treatment**
  - Prostaglandin (PGE_1) infusion is administered in patients with severe RVOTO and duct-dependent pulmonary perfusion. Surgical intervention is

indicated in symptomatic newborns and later in infancy for asymptomatic patients. As age is no longer a factor for increased mortality, the choice between complete repair and palliation depends on institutional preferences and associated anomalies.

- **Outcomes**
  - Outcomes are excellent, with operative mortality below 3 percent in contemporary series. One-third of patients require late reintervention for residual RVOTO, VSD, or chronic pulmonary regurgitation.

EPIDEMIOLOGY

Tetralogy of Fallot accounts for 5.4 percent of all congenital heart defects and, excluding transposition of the great arteries, represents for about 60 percent of conotruncal defects.[5] A higher incidence of this anomaly has been observed in males, with a male:female ratio of 3:2. Several factors have been excluded as important in the development of this cardiac anomaly.[5,6] In one-third of patients with ToF with either concomitant chromosomal abnormalities or genetic syndromes, extracardiac malformations are observed.[5,7]

SYNDROMIC TETRALOGY OF FALLOT

According to the epidemiologic results of the Baltimore-Washington Infant Study,[5] ToF is associated with extracardiac anomalies in 32.2 percent of cases and chromosomal abnormalities are involved in 11.9 percent.[5] The most frequently diagnosed chromosomal syndromes are related to trisomy of chromosomes 13 (Patau), 18 (Edwards) and 21 (Down). Recent advances in cytogenetic and molecular genetic techniques have led to the identification of syndromes due to submicroscopic defects, such as the microdeletion of chromosome 22q11.2 (Del22), associated with the DiGeorge/velo-cardio-facial syndrome. Among single-gene defects, Alagille syndrome is known to be frequently associated with ToF. The syndrome is due to mutations in the *JAGGED1* gene and is clinically characterized by paucity of the interlobular bile ducts, coronary artery disease (CAD), skeletal anomalies, ocular abnormalities, and a characteristic facial phenotype.[8]

Several conditions with multiple malformations have ToF as their cardiac component. These include CHARGE (C: coloboma of the eye, H: heart defect, A: atresia choanae, R: retardation in growth and development, G: genital hypoplasia, and E: ear anomalies),[9] VACTERL (V: vertebral defects, A: anal atresia, C: cardiac defect, TE: tracheoesophageal fistula/esophageal atresia, R: renal anomalies, and L: limb malformations)[5] and the facio-auriculo-vertebral spectrum.[10]

Tetralogy in Del22

DiGeorge and velo-cardio-facial syndromes are genetic conditions associated with Del22 and present with overlapping features. Clinical characteristics include palatal anomalies, facial dysmorphisms, neonatal hypocalcemia, immune deficit, and speech/learning disabilities. Congenital heart disease is present in 75 percent of patients, and ToF and ToF–pulmonary atresia each account for 25 percent of cases.[11,12] Microdeletions in chromosome 22 are seen on karyotype analysis in approximately 10 percent of all patients with tetralogy[7,13] and 35 percent of patients with ToF and pulmonary atresia.[14] Additional cardiac defects are found in 59 percent of patients with ToF and del22; these include (1) right or cervical aortic arch with or without aberrant left subclavian artery, (2) hypoplasia or absence of the infundibular septum, (3) absence of the pulmonary valve, and (4) discontinuity and diffuse hypoplasia of the pulmonary arteries.[12,14,15]

Tetralogy in Down's syndrome

ToF is the only conotruncal anomaly described in patients with Down's syndrome, occurring in 8 percent of cases. The VSD in these patients is particularly large; if a common atrioventricular valve is also present, the morphology is almost invariably that of a Rastelli type C atrioventricular septal defect (see Chap. 58). Cardiac defects commonly associated with ToF in nonsyndromic or in Del22 patients (such as pulmonary atresia, absent pulmonary valve, discontinuity of pulmonary arteries and absent infundibular septum) are very rare in Down's syndrome.[16]

NONSYNDROMIC TETRALOGY OF FALLOT

Nonsyndromic ToF is often a sporadic occurrence in families, but multiple affected family members can also occasionally be found. In 1968, Nora introduced the "multifactorial" model of inheritance for the etiology of nonsyndromic congenital heart disease, suggesting that several genetic loci can interact together in association with environmental factors.[6] However, familial recurrence of concordant ToF within affected family members supports monogenic or oligogenic inheritance in selected cases.

In practical genetic counseling, the recurrence risk for congenital heart disease among siblings of patients affected by ToF is quoted at approximately 3 percent.[6,17] The results of a British collaborative study suggested a three-gene model for nonsyndromic ToF as the best-fitting model in familial and sporadic cases.[18] The genetic basis of ToF is therefore complex and heterogeneous.

Chromosomal anomalies, (Del22 in particular), are not detectable in familial cases of nonsyndromic ToF,[17] pointing to the implication of genes located on different chromosomes. The number of genes known to be involved in nonsyndromic ToF is low. Up to now, only low-penetration mutations in *NKX2.5* (4 percent of ToF cases) have been found.[19] A missense mutation of the *JAGGED1* gene[20] and low-penetrance mutations in the *ZFPM2/FOG2* gene (4 percent of patients with tetralogy)[21] have been found.

MORPHOLOGY

The usual segmental anatomy of ToF is levocardia and situs solitus with concordant atrioventricular and ventriculoarterial connection. Situs inversus is uncommon (<5 percent), and isolated dextrocardia and left atrial isomerism are rare. The anterosuperior (or cephalad) deviation of the infundibular septum and its malalignment is considered the essence of ToF. This results in malalignment between the infundibular and trabecular septum, producing a very typical type of infundibular pulmonary stenosis (PS) and VSD (Fig. 60-1). Van Praagh has suggested that ToF is truly a "monology" resulting from this septal displacement and that, in ToF, the outlet septum is "too short, too narrow and too shallow."[22] Not all authors agree that the infundibular septum is constantly hypoplastic. In typical cases, the model of "pulmonary stenosis" nevertheless relates to the deviated infundibular septum; the resulting obstruction is muscular and tends to be progressive. Although the malalignment of infundibular septum and trabecula septomarginalis is primary responsible for RVOTO, other mechanisms may also contribute to it. In many patients, a hypoplastic pulmonary annulus, a stenotic, often bicuspid pulmonary valve with thickened leaflets and commissural fusion (75 percent of cases), as well as variable degrees of hypoplasia of the pulmonary trunk and branches can be observed as well. Abnormal muscle bands are also found in 11 percent of cases.[23]

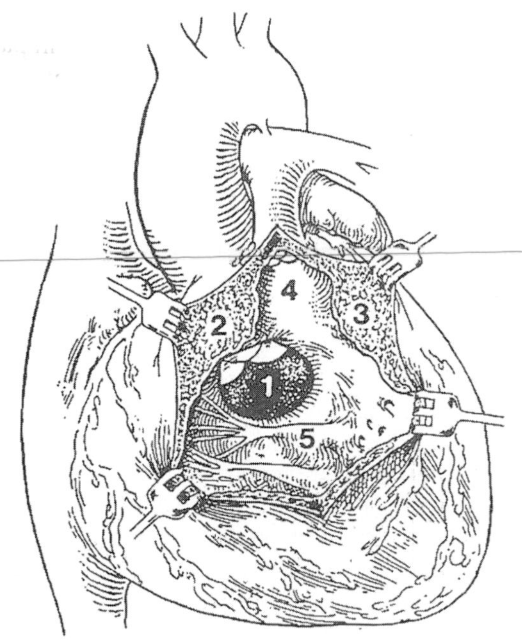

Figure 60-1 Morphologic features of "classic" ToF. Large VSD (1) with overriding aorta and (2) seen behind the ventriculoinfundibular fold. Superior and leftward deviation of the outlet septum and hypertrophic parietal (3) and ventricular muscular bands result in RVOTO (4), with a diminutive infundibulum and pulmonary valve. Papillary muscle of the conus (5). [From Bove EL, Lupinetti FM. Tetralogy of Fallot. In: Mavroudis C, Backer CL (eds). *Pediatric Cardiac Surgery*, 2d ed. St. Louis: Mosby; 1994:277. With permission.]

The degree of aortic override varies from 30 to 90 percent, with usually 50 percent of the aortic origin above the right ventricle.[24] Kirklin and Barratt-Boyes have pointed out that aortic override is associated with a variable degree of clockwise rotation of the aortic root. The aortic valve cusps are abnormally positioned in ToF, with the noncoronary cusp positioned more anteriorly and to the right than in normal hearts. The amount of override and clockwise rotation of the aortic root is related to the degree of hypoplasia of the RVOT and malalignment of the infundibular septum.[24]

The right ventricle is almost invariably normal in size, but cases are described with hypoplasia of the RV cavity and tricuspid valve (1 to 2 percent of patients).[25] In typical tetralogy, the ventricular septal defect is large and subaortic, reflecting in its very nature the deviation of the outlet septum. Some defects are perimembranous; in this case, the roof of the left ventricular margin of the VSD is formed by the area of fibrous continuity between the leaflets of the aortic and tricuspid valves.[26] Inlet or outlet extensions of the VSD are frequently observed. Controversy exists as to whether a subpulmonary or doubly-committed ("subarterial") VSD should be considered part of a variant of tetralogy. In these cases, the infundibular septum is severely hypoplastic or is absent and is not responsible for RVOTO. In some cases, the VSD is restrictive. This is rare in the neonate but has been diagnosed with increasing frequency in older infants and children.[27,28] The most common mechanism of restriction is represented by mobile tricuspid valve accessory tissue.

The pulmonary arterial circulation in patients with ToF has been the subject of much attention because of the important pathophysiologic and surgical implications.

There is a tremendous variability in pulmonary artery size; the smallest confluent pulmonary arteries are seen in patients with tetralogy and pulmonary atresia. Left pulmonary stenosis at the site of ductal insertion has been observed with increasing frequency. One pulmonary artery, usually the left, may originate from the ascending aorta or may have a ductal origin.[29] Multiple aortopulmonary collaterals are uncommon in ToF with confluent pulmonary arteries, but their coexistence is possible in "classic" tetralogy as well as in the variant with an absent pulmonary valve.[29] A pulmonary artery sling (origin of LPA from the RPA; see Chap. 75) has rarely been seen in association with ToF.[30]

The left ventricle is usually normal in size and morphology. Rarely, the left ventricular (LV) end-diastolic volume is truly reduced.[31]

The association of mitral stenosis and supravalvular mitral ring has been observed,[32] while an isolated mitral cleft may rarely be seen.

Bicuspid aortic valve, aortic valve stenosis, and aortic regurgitation have all been reported.[33] Aortic regurgitation is uncommon in early infancy but may develop later in adolescence or adulthood, especially in nonoperated patients.[23] Twenty-five percent of patients with tetralogy have a right-sided aortic arch. Other rare anomalies of the aortic arch have been described.[34–36]

The anatomy of the coronary arteries in ToF is of considerable surgical importance because of the hazard of damage during ventriculotomy. The most common anomaly is origin of the left anterior descending coronary artery (LAD) from the right coronary artery, occurring in about 5 percent of patients.[24] In this situation, the anterior descending coronary artery crosses the RVOT at a variable distance from the pulmonary valve. Less frequently, cases have been recorded of (1) single right or left coronary artery (4 percent), (2) origin of the left coronary artery or anterior descending from the pulmonary trunk,[37] and (3) origin of both coronary arteries from the pulmonary trunk.[38]

A variety of other structural cardiac defects have been found in association with ToF.[23,24,41–50]

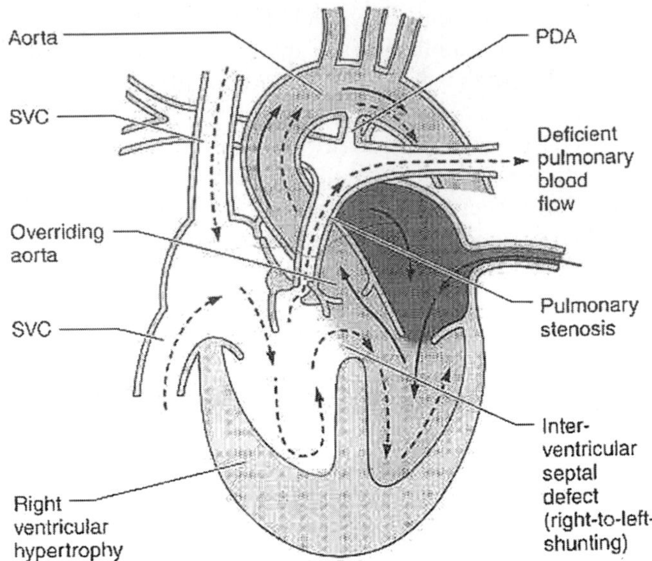

Figure 60-2 Pathophysiology of ToF. [From Reitz BA, Yuh DD (eds). *Congenital Cardiac Surgery.* New York: McGraw-Hill; 2002:134. With permission.]

PATHOPHYSIOLOGY

The pathophysiology of ToF reflects the severity of the RVOT stenosis in the presence of a wide interventricular communication (Fig. 60-2). Pressures in the ventricles and aorta are equal, independently of the degree of RVOTO. The relative pulmonary (Qp) and systemic (Qs) blood flow depends on the respective resistance to flow. When RVOTO is mild, Qp may exceed Qs and there will be a predominantly left-to-right shunt, with a clinical picture similar to that of an isolated VSD ("pink" tetralogy). With increasing degrees of RVOTO, a dominant right-to-left shunt occurs, with variable cyanosis. A fall in systemic resistance with no change in RV afterload will result in increased right-to-left shunt.

CLINICAL PRESENTATION

Signs and symptoms are determined by the degree of RVOTO and are sometimes influenced by associated anomalies.

When the RVOTO is severe, presentation occurs in the neonatal period. Persistent cyanosis becomes apparent within the first days of life and patients may develop metabolic acidosis, partly compensated by an increase in respiratory rate. Nonetheless, the majority of children are acyanotic at birth. A systolic heart murmur is typically present and is associated with a single second heart sound. An aortic ejection click may also be heard at the lower left sternal border. When the RVOTO is moderate, cyanosis will become evident at the end of the first year of life, with a strong systolic murmur audible over the pulmonary valve.

A dramatic feature observed in patients with tetralogy is the "blue spell" (anoxic/hypoxic spell). These episodes, lasting 15 to 60 min, are commonest between 6 months and 2 years of age. They typically occur on awakening and may be precipitated by crying, straining, feeding, heat intolerance, and other forms of physical stress.

These events are extraordinarily frightening to parents and are characterized by an increase in rate and depth of respiration, cyanosis and possibly syncope or seizures. In 1958, Wood first postulated that the spells were due to infundibular "spasm" and also observed that the systolic murmur frequently disappeared during the spelling episode.

DIAGNOSIS

In the newborn, the electrocardiogram (ECG) may be normal for age. Failure of right-sided T waves to invert is

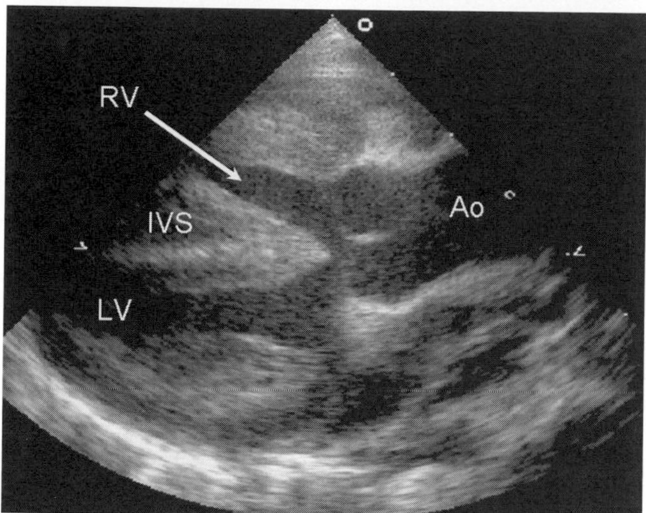

Figure 60-3 Echocardiographic imaging in ToF. Parasternal long-axis window showing the aorta (Ao) overriding the interventricular septum (IVS). RV = right ventricle; LV = left ventricle. (Courtesy of Dr. Craig Sable, Department of Cardiology, Children's National Medical Center, Washington, DC.)

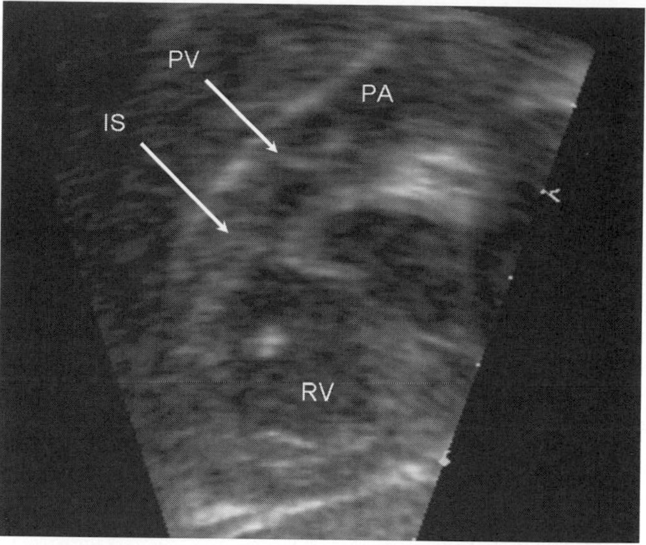

Figure 60-4 Subcostal short-axis echocardiographic window in an infant with ToF and subpulmonary obstruction. IS = infundibular stenosis; PA = pulmonary artery; PV = pulmonary valve; RV = right ventricle. (Courtesy of Dr Craig Sable, Department of Cardiology, Children's National Medical Center, Washington, DC.)

often (but not always) found in the first 2 to 3 months. The mean frontal QRS axis is between 90 and 150 degrees. RV hypertrophy with dominant R waves in V_1 and dominant S in V_6 is usually found in younger patients. A counterclockwise QRS loop in the frontal plane may suggest a coexisting atrioventricular septal defect.

The typical radiographic findings of ToF are those of reduced pulmonary vascular markings with normal heart size and a typical pulmonary concavity seen below the left-sided aortic arch, reflecting a diminutive pulmonary trunk.

Echocardiographic imaging is almost always the only required diagnostic modality prior to proceeding to operative repair or palliation of ToF. This modality provides definition of all anatomic details crucial for surgical intervention. The subxyphoid right oblique window (Fig. 60-3) nicely shows the RVOT and enables quantification of the degree of anterior deviation of the conal septum as well as definition of pulmonary valve morphology, the size of the annulus, and visualization of the main and right branch pulmonary arteries. If the valve is nearing atresia, continuity between the pulmonary trunk and infundibulum is also appropriately shown with this view.[51] The subxyphoid left oblique and parasternal long-axis views allow for visualization of the VSD and the degree of aortic dextroposition (Fig. 60-4). With the four-chamber view, the posterior extension of the VSD (inlet septum) is identified, as well as the presence of additional VSDs. The suprasternal window helps to define the size and morphology of the main pulmonary branches, as well as the side of the aortic arch.[28,52,53]

Finally, the ability to image the coronary arterial pattern by echocardiography often plays a significant role in surgical decision making (Fig. 60-5).[54]

In cases where cardiac catheterization is needed preoperatively, complete angiographic imaging requires biplane RV angiography, biplane left ventricular angiography, imaging of the pulmonary arteries, and assessment of coronary arteries as well as descending aortography (to exclude significant aortopulmonary collaterals). RV angiography, using biplane angiography with caudocranial angulation, can demonstrate the RV anatomy and the size and distribution of pulmonary arteries (Fig. 60-6). Left ventricular angiography, in the long axial oblique view, is useful to demonstrate the size of subaortic and, if present, additional muscular VSDs. Coronary anatomy is defined with angiography and helps in differentiating an anomalous LAD from large conal branches.

MEDICAL MANAGEMENT

Recent advances in surgical treatment have progressively reduced the need for medical therapy. Two situations may still deserve the attention of the pediatric cardiologist before cardiac surgery is undertaken: (1) Duct-dependent ToF with near atresia of the pulmonary artery (PA) in the newborn, in which PGE_1 infusion is required before the surgical treatment pathway of choice of the individual unit is undertaken. (2) Tetralogy of Fallot with major associated extracardiac anomalies, which may

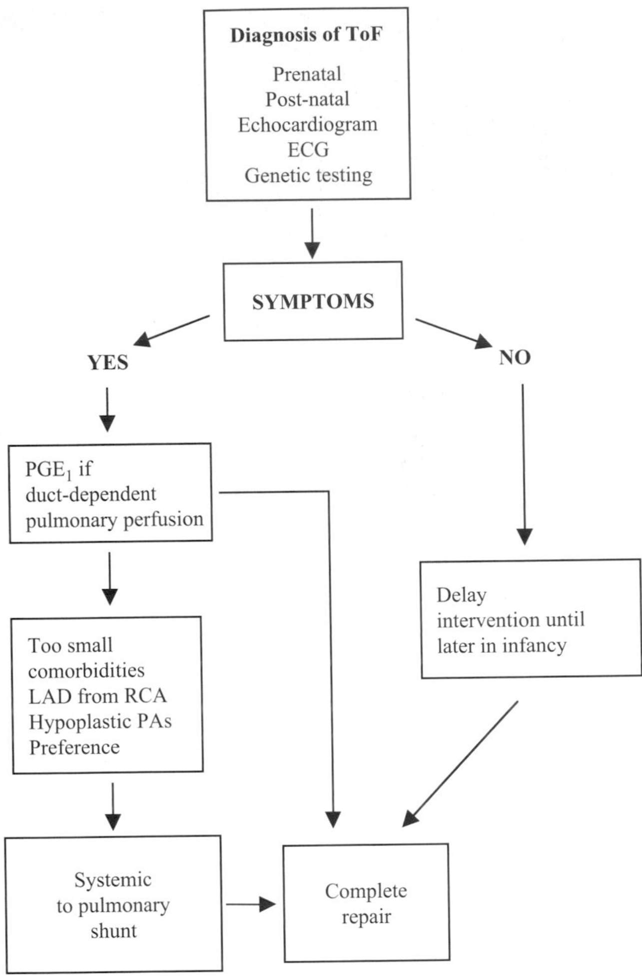

Figure 60-5 Decision-making algorithm for patients with ToF.

need initial management; in these cases, treatment with beta blockers may be instituted to prevent hypoxic spells during other interventions.

PERCUTANEOUS INTERVENTION

Palliative interventional treatment, intended to relieve the RVOTO, was first reported by Lababidi in 1983.[55] Following this pioneering work, this approach has been applied by several groups in order to avoid palliative surgery in exceedingly high-risk and low-weight babies.[56,57] The technique is similar to that used in isolated pulmonary valve stenosis; there is an inherent risk of triggering a hypoxic spell secondary to infundibular spasm.

The results with this technique vary widely according to the morphology of the RVOT and the presence of mainly valvular obstruction. Good results have also been described with balloon dilatation in patients with hypoplastic pulmonary branches; in this approach, "cutting" balloon catheters have proven to be much more effective than the common high-pressure devices.[58]

Congenital absence of the pulmonary valve

This rare malformation was first described by Chevers in 1847.[59] In the majority of cases, this lesion is associated with VSD, obstructive pulmonary annulus, and massive dilation of the main and one or both branch pulmonary arteries; this combination of lesions is known as ToF with absent pulmonary valve syndrome (ToF APVS).[60]

Nonetheless, APVS has been described as an isolated lesion with intact ventricular septum and also in association with atrial septal defect (ASD), patent ductus arteriosus (PDA), double-outlet right ventricle,[61] atrioventricular canal, and transposition of the great arteries.[62, 65] In APVS, the pulmonary valve may be absent or represented by hypoplastic nodules.[60,63] The pulmonary valve

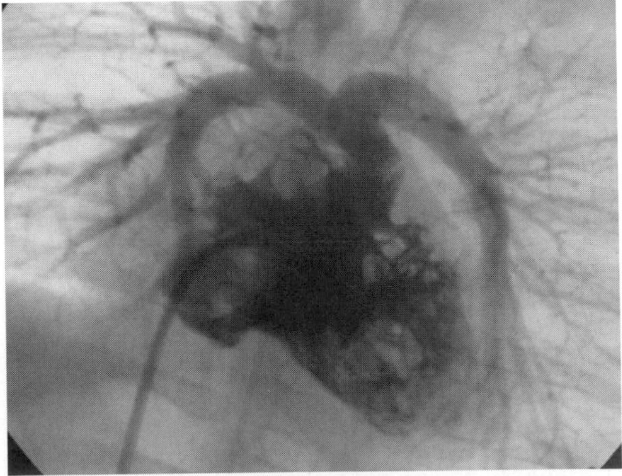
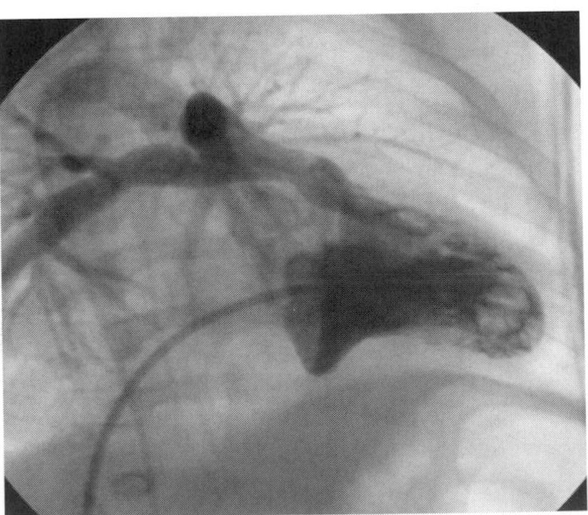

Figure 60-6 Cardiac catheterization in an infant with ToF. Craniocaudal view (left) with delineation of valvar and subvalvar obstruction as well as branching of the pulmonary arteries. Right anterior oblique view (right), demonstrating valvar obstruction and the diminutive RVOT.

annulus is usually obstructive and is often associated with a long, hypoplastic infundibulum that is rarely critically narrowed because of chronic pulmonary regurgitation.

The main and one or both pulmonary arteries are aneurysmal. The aneurysmal dilatation of the pulmonary arteries is mainly responsible for symptoms in neonates and young infants, causing bronchial compression and respiratory distress.[64] Compression involves the anterior aspect of the trachea and major bronchi, most commonly on the right, producing massively hyperinflated lungs and spontaneous pneumothorax. Rabinovitch has suggested that the intrapulmonary proximal bronchial ramifications are subject to compression as well,[65] explaining why some patients do not experience respiratory improvement after surgical repair.

The pulmonary arteries may be nonconfluent, with one pulmonary artery usually the left arising from a left-sided arterial duct.[63]

The laterality of the aortic arch and the abnormalities of the coronary arteries have the same frequency as that in classic ToF.

Data from the New England Regional Infants Cardiac Program suggests a prevalence of about 0.0065 per 1000 live births,[66] with the majority of patients developing varying degrees of respiratory distress in the neonatal period or early infancy. Physical examination reveals a characteristic harsh systolic-diastolic murmur ("to-and-fro"), best auscultated at the upper left sternal border, with a single second heart sound. In those patients who survive the first year of life, respiratory symptoms often improve spontaneously.

Aside from the massively dilated pulmonary arteries, electrocardiography and intracardiac findings on echocardiography are similar to those observed in "classic" tetralogy. Chest X-ray demonstrates air trapping and pronounced central vascular markings, while cardiac catheterization defines the huge pulmonary arteries, with annular obstruction and a well-represented infundibulum (Fig. 60-7).

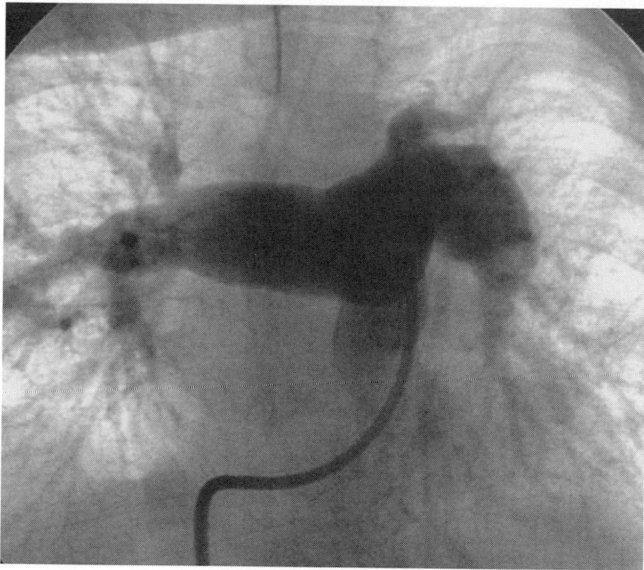

Figure 60-7 Pulmonary arteriogram in a patient with ToF and APVS. There is impressive enlargement of the branch pulmonary arteries.

SURGICAL TREATMENT

The ominous natural history of ToF was changed forever by the efforts of pioneers such as Blalock and Potts, who conceived and first performed palliative procedures to increase pulmonary blood flow.[67] In 1954, Lillehei and colleagues first demonstrated the feasibility of total repair using controlled cross circulation.[68] After these astonishing surgical breakthroughs, Waterston[69] and Cooley[70] developed other palliative procedures and, in the following years, important contributions and refinement of the technique of repair on cardiopulmonary bypass were made by Kirklin,[24,67] Castaneda,[71] and Bove.[72]

As a consequence of this massive effort, age at the time of repair has dropped dramatically, while the need for palliation has become increasingly rare.[73]

Repair of ToF in any age group remains nevertheless challenging; while early mortality approaches zero in many contemporary series, attention is now also focusing on means to prevent or treat long-term postoperative complications that often require late surgical reintervention.

Transventricular repair

Cardiopulmonary bypass is instituted with moderate hypothermia, and any prior aortopulmonary shunts are immediately ligated and divided. Deep hypothermia and circulatory arrest are seldom necessary but are still liberally used in some centers.

Myocardial protection is obtained with cold blood or crystalloid cardioplegia. Following aortic cross clamping, a longitudinal right ventriculotomy is performed (Fig. 60-8). This is extended, when necessary, across the pulmonary valve annulus: the size of the annulus (after pulmonary valvotomy if required) is measured with a Hegar dilator and compared to the classic tables published in 1977 by Pacifico and colleagues (reporting normal annular values by body weight and confidence limits). If a transannular incision is elected, it is usually continued across the origin of the left pulmonary artery. Ideally, the ventriculotomy should be extended proximally 3 to 4 mm beyond the edge of the conal septum.[74] Resection of the displaced conal (infundibular) septum is mostly confined to the parietal insertion. Several muscular bands are surrounded by a right-angle clamp and divided in sequence; fibrous tissue is completely removed as well as other hypertrophic trabeculae. The septal insertion of the malaligned septum is usually left untouched in order to preserve the septal branches of the LAD.[75] The same

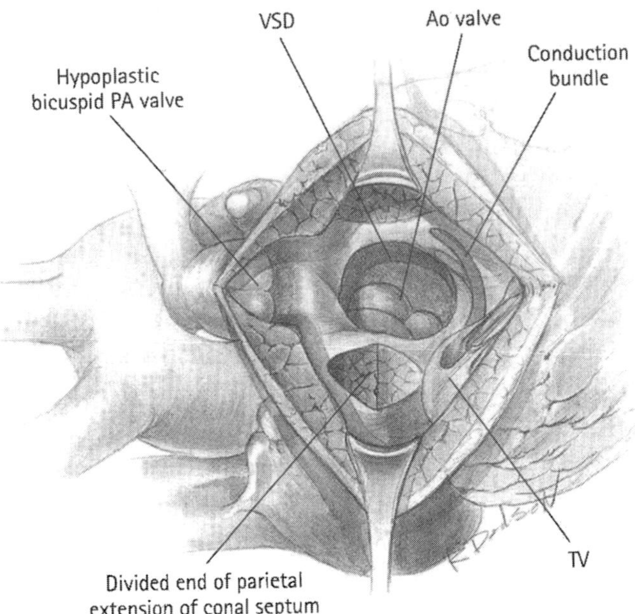

Figure 60-8 Exposure of the VSD through a ventriculotomy (surgeon's perspective). (From Jonas RA. *Comprehensive Surgical Management of Congenital Heart Disease.* London: Arnold; 2004:288. With permission.)

applies to the moderator band, deep in the ventricular cavity, which supports the anterior papillary muscle of the tricuspid valve. A circular patch of Dacron/Gore-Tex/heterologous or autologous pericardium is used to close the VSD with interrupted, pledgeted sutures (Fig. 60-9). This technique is highly recommended for small infants, in whom the myocardium is delicate and friable and may tear on a running suture.

Transatrial closure of a ventricular septal defect

Exposure of a VSD and repair through the tricuspid valve was first described by Pacifico[75] and offers several advantages. Through the same approach, transatrial closure and subpulmonary resection can be accomplished, avoiding or reducing to a minimum the need for a ventriculotomy where valvotomy or transannular patch are required.

Through the generous right atriotomy, the patent foramen ovale can be utilized for venting and is usually only partially closed in neonates and small infants. This will act as a decompressing pathway in the early postoperative phase should dangerous right-sided hypertension develop. The perspective of the VSD through the atriotomy is very different for the surgeon (Fig. 60-10). The tricuspid margin of the VSD comes easily in to view, while its conal and upper margins are remote. With the aid of one or two small right-angle retractors, the lower part of the RVOTO is exposed and resection of the parietal band of the septum performed. This maneuver greatly helps to visualize the upper margin of the VSD. In neonates and infants, bundle division, rather than muscle resection, may be sufficient. Again, the outflow tract is sized with a Hegar dilator and a decision is made as to whether or not the pulmonary annulus is hypoplastic.

When the resection is complete, the VSD is closed, preferably with multiple pledgeted interrupted sutures.

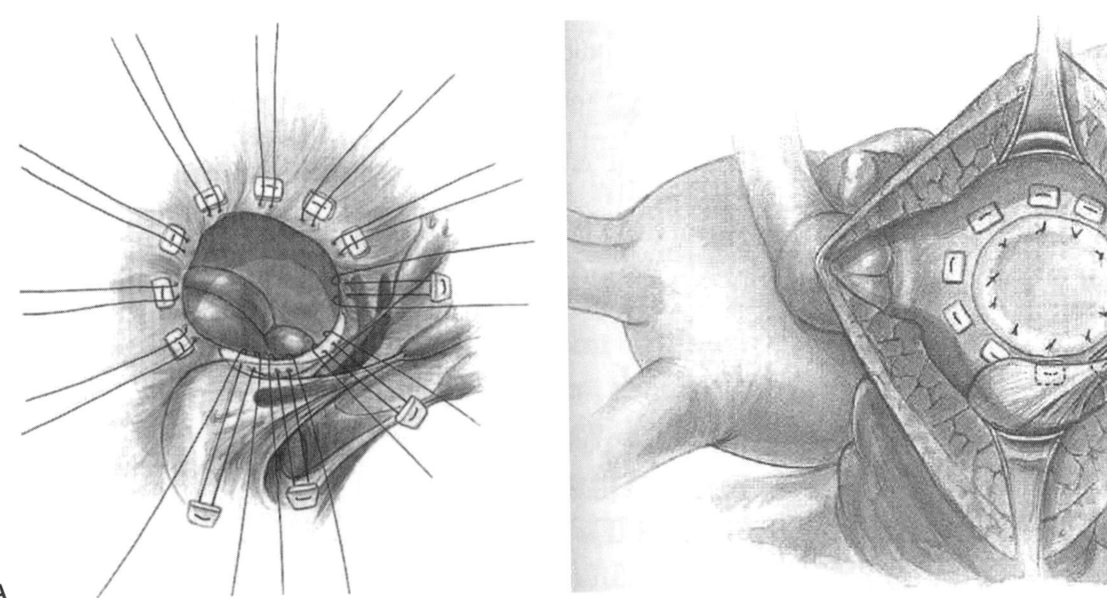

Figure 60-9 Transventricular closure of VSD in ToF. Interrupted pledgeted sutures are placed around the perimeter of the defect (left), with great care not to injure the conduction system (in dark gray). Patch in place (right). (From Jonas RA. *Comprehensive Surgical Management of Congenital Heart Disease.* London: Arnold; 2004:289. With permission.)

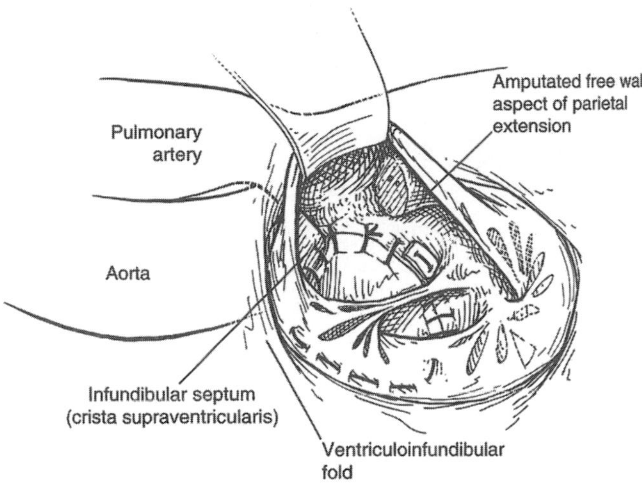

Figure 60-10 Transatrial approach to VSD closure in ToF (surgeon's perspective). [From Kouchoukos NT, Blackstone EH, Doty DB, et al (eds). *Kirklin/Barratt-Boyes Cardiac Surgery,* 3d ed. Philadelphia: Churchill Livingstone/Elsevier; 2003:974. With permission.]

The first sutures, placed just below the insertion of the muscle of Lancisi, are gently pulled downward by the assistant, thereby progressively exposing the upper margin of the VSD. In older infants or children, a continuous running suture may be used, starting at the same point with a pledgeted 5-0 monofilament suture. The position of the main His bundle has been the subject of considerable study and debate.[76] Traditionally, sutures passed through the septal leaflet of the tricuspid valve and through the adjacent muscle, staying away from the apex of the VSD muscle, are believed to be safe. Injury to the right bundle may be more difficult to avoid, as several possible levels of damage have been described.[77]

Surgical management of right ventricular outflow tract obstruction

This is the most controversial aspect of the surgical management of ToF.[80] The surgeon is often faced with a difficult choice between residual obstruction and a severely regurgitant pulmonary valve. Both may lead to RV dysfunction.

In the transventricular approach, a smaller than normal pulmonary annulus is not acceptable, and the ventriculotomy is immediately carried across it. In the transatrial-transpulmonary repair,[79] an extensive pulmonary valvotomy is first performed, followed by further resection of muscular bands through the pulmonary annulus. If the annulus itself is hypoplastic, the incision is carried across it into the infundibulum for a short (5- to 6-mm) length.

In our experience, a full transatrial repair of ToF is rarely possible. An infundibular ventriculotomy, in our hands, is usually insufficient to relieve the obstruction that is most often sited at the lower level of the conal septum. This is particularly true when repair is performed in small infants. That is why we, like others,[74] recommend that the incision be carried downward slightly beyond the level of the malaligned conal septum.

Autologous/heterologous pericardium or Gore-Tex are commonly employed for the infundibular/transannular reconstruction of the RVOT (Fig. 60-11). This part of the procedure can be carried out on the beating heart, after aortic unclamping.

In the contracting heart, the need for further resection of the ventricular incision may become evident. The shape of the patch is usually elliptical, and care must be taken not to enlarge the pulmonary annulus excessively (ideally, 1.5 times the normal pulmonary annular size per body weight). A valve-bearing transannular patch has been recommended in the past by some authors.[80–86] Most favor the use of a Gore-Tex monocusp or an aortic homograft; with the latter, the aortic cusp is utilized as a monocusp valve, while the anterior leaflet of the mitral valve in continuity with the ascending aorta is used to fashion the transannular patch. Although most series of monocusp valves claim competency in the early postoperative phase, there is no convincing evidence that valvar function is preserved at long-term follow-up with these techniques.

At completion of the procedure, RV pressure is measured directly, and the ratio between peak systolic RV and aortic pressures is calculated. Any value below 0.8 is accepted, as a drop in systolic RV pressure does commonly occur in the first 24 h postoperatively. Higher values imply the need for further RVOT enlargement. Bypass is resumed under normothermic condition and the RVOT patch explored: muscle resection and extension of the ventricular incision are both performed and a new patch is inserted.

Specific considerations

Major coronary anomaly

This complicating feature is found in less than 10 percent of cases. The most common type consists of an LAD branching off the right coronary artery and crossing the RV infundibulum. A dual LAD or very prominent conal branch may be also found. Pulmonary origin of the LAD has been reported.[37] If a transannular patch is required for repair, inadvertent transection of the anomalous vessel could be life-threatening.[87]

Proposed solutions include (1) adjustment of the site/orientation of the ventriculotomy alone[88,89]; (2) conduit placement between a low ventriculotomy and the pulmonary artery confluence in a end-to-side or end-to-end fashion; and (3) creation of a double outflow with a native pulmonary artery flap.[90,91] Unless pulmonary atresia or extreme hypoplasia of the pulmonary trunk is present, we favor the last option in order to

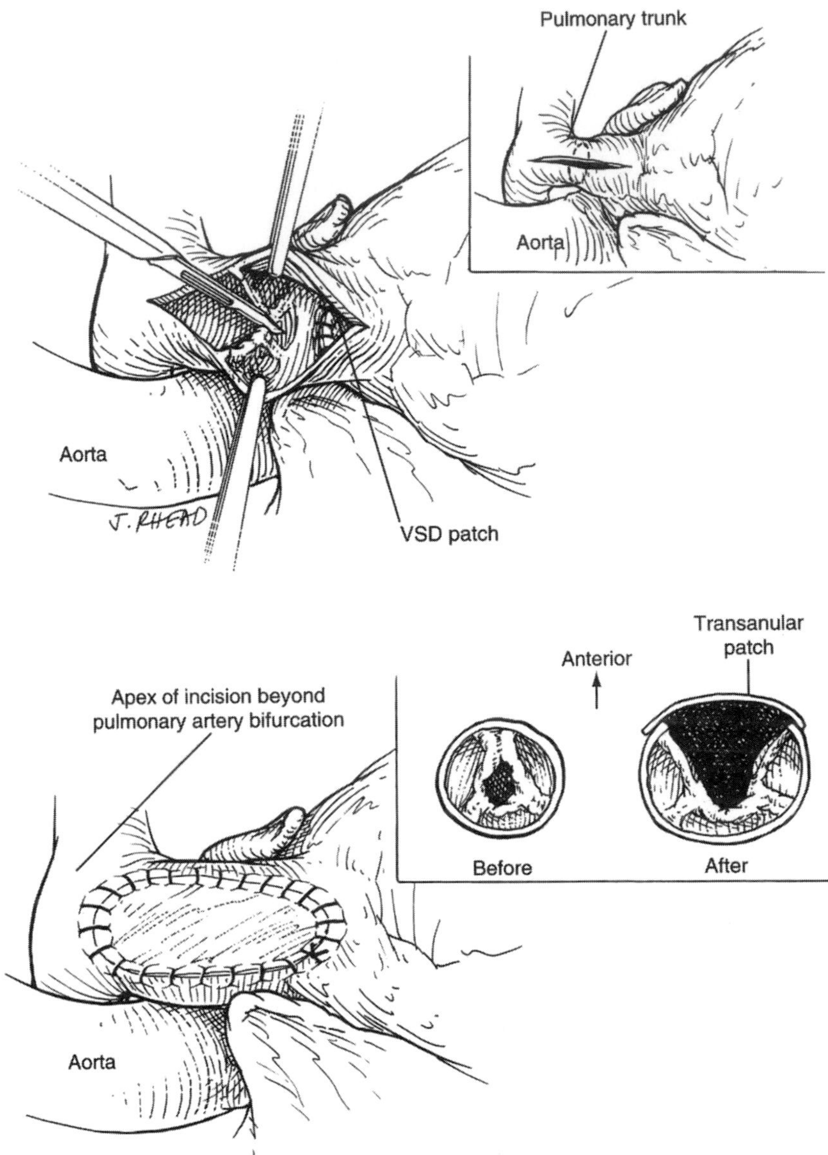

Figure 60-11 Pulmonary valvotomy (top) in a severely stenotic valve and hypoplastic annulus. A transannular patch is secured in place with a running suture (bottom). Should the valve be stenotic and the annulus be of adequate diameter for body weight, a valvotomy is performed and the pulmonary arteriotomy is not carried across the annulus. Two separate patches (pulmonary artery and ventriculotomy) can be used in a subvalvar stenosis that is not amenable to transatrial resection. [From Kouchoukos NT, Blackstone EH, Doty DB, et al (eds). *Kirklin/Barratt-Boyes Cardiac Surgery,* 3d ed. Philadelphia: Churchill Livingstone/Elsevier; :974. With permission.]

avoid the serious long-term implications of conduit placement.

Hypoplastic right ventricle

This variant of ToF is exceedingly rare. Only a few cases have been reported, mainly in papers detailing partial biventricular repair ("one and one-half" ventricle repair).[25,92] The tricuspid valve annulus is significantly smaller than normal for body surface area and the trabecular RV portion is poorly represented. A frequent consequence of RV hypoplasia is inability to close the VSD through the tricuspid valve; ventriculotomy is most often necessary to accomplish closure of the defect. In addition, these patients also require a bidirectional cavopulmonary anastomosis to avoid right-sided failure.

Multiple ventricular septal defects

Multiple VSDs constitute a major surgical challenge in ToF. The peculiar hypertrophy of RV myocardium tends in fact to conceal the position and size of the defects. Fortunately, a single, apically displaced muscular VSD is the most common occurrence. Transatrial repair for the anatomic features mentioned above is most likely to be unsuccessful; the infundibulotomy required to enlarge the RVOT is also remote from the ventricular apex. A small, transverse apical ventriculotomy[93] is usually required, and division of a few muscular bands greatly aids in exposure of the defect and all its margins. Closure may be performed with a patch, with interrupted pledgeted suture, or, more recently, with a percutaneous VSD closure device deployed in the operating room under direct vision. The ventriculotomy is closed directly with a double layer running monofilament suture or with a patch.

RESULTS

Perioperative outcomes

Hospital mortality approaches zero in most series. It was 1.6 percent in a series of symptomatic neonates reported by Hirsch and coworkers[94] and 0.5 percent among older children in a large series from Melbourne.[79] Similar results have been reported by other groups.[74,95–97] In a recent 4-year period, we operated on 116 patients with ToF, with 3 deaths (2.5 percent). In the Toronto experience,[98,99] age at surgery of less than 3 months and previous palliation were not associated with increased mortality, but rather with longer ventilation times and intensive care unit stay, as well as with a higher incidence of multi-organ-system failure.

In many institutions, repair of symptomatic individuals with ToF can be therefore safely accomplished at any age. Nonetheless, repair in neonates may require deep hypothermia and circulatory arrest,[94] the long-term outcome of which remains uncertain at present; this patient population tends to have a longer and more complicated postoperative course and a high incidence of early reoperation, particularly due to RVOTO.[94] For these reasons, repair of asymptomatic neonates with ToF is not considered in our institution; in symptomatic patients, an individualized choice is made between repair and palliation, based on anatomy of the pulmonary arteries, associated defects, and extracardiac anomalies.

Long-term results

The pioneering series from two institutions in Minnesota offer the longest follow-up interval for repair of ToF.[68,100] Late survival (30 to 32 years) was 77 and 86 percent. These series truly established a surgical landmark, demonstrating that a potentially lethal condition can be defeated, and that quality of life and life expectancy for those treated was only slightly inferior to that of the normal population.[101] More recent series, with considerably shorter follow-up, report even better results.[72,102] Transatrial repair with minimal infundibulotomy seems to achieve less RV dilatation in the medium-term follow-up interval.[103] Factors that appeared to be related to reduced early and long-term survival (such as early age at operation or transannular patching) have been almost neutralized. Several long-term issues have been correlated with decreased length of survival.[104–108]

Arrhythmias have been implicated in poor outcomes. In the early postoperative period, junctional ectopic tachycardia[96] may occur, and prompt treatment must be implemented in order to prevent acute cardiac failure. Complete heart block is a rare occurrence, with an incidence in modern series of less than 2 percent. At late follow-up, symptomatic arrhythmias and sudden deaths (commonly attributed to ventricular ectopy) are reported in several series.[68,100,109,110] Older age at repair[100] and long-standing pulmonary regurgitation have also been implicated in the genesis of arrhythmias. The presence of a ventriculotomy scar is an important concomitant factor.

RVOTO is a common cause of reoperation (14 percent of early survivors in Knott-Craig's experience).[102] Patients who are younger at the time of repair (particularly neonates) face a higher risk of reoperation. Conversely, repair in infancy is not believed to pose an increased risk for reoperation. Attempts at preservation of the pulmonary valve[111] have also achieved satisfactory intermediate-term results. Unfortunately, these strenuous efforts to maintain the native pulmonary valve in situ do no consistently achieve postoperative competency (in one series, only 68 percent were competent 12 months postoperatively).[111]

In ToF, the surgeon constantly faces the dilemma of whether a residual systolic gradient with an intact pulmonary valve, small ventriculotomy, and small patch is better that no gradient, a longer ventriculotomy, and wider patch with an absent or incompetent pulmonary valve. The study of Cullen and associates[104] suggests that the right ventricle may show a peculiar postoperative behavior subsequent to new onset of pulmonary regurgitation, termed "restrictive physiology": this, in turn, produces different effects, depending on the elapsed time from surgery. Shortly after the operation, diastolic dysfunction will occur, as indicated by high RV filling pressure and poor response to inotropic support.[104] In the long term, on the contrary, a favorable effect of restrictive physiology is noted, as it tends to minimize pulmonary regurgitation, with better exercise performance.[106] Other studies suggest that "restrictive physiology" is prevented by early age at repair.[107] Pulmonary regurgitation can be avoided or reduced, at least temporarily, in numerous ways. Many would agree that a residual gradient associated to a peak systolic RV/LV ratio between 0.5 and 0.75 is auspicious in terms of a possible late postoperative advantage.

A large number of publications have addressed the problem of long-term pulmonary regurgitation (PR) after repair.[106,112–121] As pulmonary valvotomy or transannular patching is commonly required, PR is the most frequent residual defect after surgery. After having been considered a benign event for a considerable time, there is now concern for its negative effect on RV size and function. Nonetheless, the amount of PR that can be tolerated and the timing of reoperation are still strongly debated. One major difficulty is that patients with PR are asymptomatic for a prolonged period in the postoperative phase. Geva and coworkers found, with MRI imaging, that impaired systolic function of either the left or right ventricle was associated with symptoms in a group of patients with an median time interval of 21 years from repair.[118] Conversely, PR and RV dilatation (increased end-diastolic volume) were not associated with clinical deterioration. There is general consensus that surgery is required in symptomatic patients.[119] In many of these patients, PR is only one of residual defects, with only one-third having isolated PR.[114]

Therrien and colleagues[121] tried to establish, with MRI studies, the degree of RV dilatation and dysfunction that would not improve to normal after pulmonary valve replacement (PVR). In studying 17 adult patients, they found that an RV end-diastolic volume greater that 170 mL/m^2 or an RV end-systolic volume greater than 85 mL/m^2 were not associated with normalization of RV function after PVR. Most authors report low mortality, relief of symptoms, and rapid reduction of RV volumes after appropriately timed PVR.[113,117,120,121] Finally, PVR appears to be associated with hindering of progressive prolongation of the PR interval on ECG and with a reduction in the incidence of atrial and ventricular arrhythmias.

PVR can be performed in association with ablative surgery in patients with preoperative documented arrhythmias. In a multicenter study, PVR was performed on 70 patients with atrial flutter/fibrillation or monomorphic ventricular tachycardia, and cryoablation was carried out in 15 (21 percent). The prevalence of arrhythmias was globally reduced, but complete abolition occurred only in patients who were also treated with cryoablation. Even in these high-risk patients, operative mortality was acceptable (4 percent).[116]

First-time PVR in infancy and early childhood is usually performed with a pulmonary homograft. A number of reoperations, unfortunately, are anticipated after the initial one. Repeat homograft implantation may elicit an immunologic response, possibly detrimental to homograft function; bioprosthetic heterograft conduits, bovine jugular vein, and even mechanical valves have been utilized.[115,122,123]

Percutaneous valve replacement[124] is an ingenious alternative to reoperation. The valve implanted is a bovine venous valved conduit, mounted on a nitinol stent and delivered transvenously in patients without aneurysmal dilation of the RVOT.

Patients with ToF or pulmonary atresia may also develop progressive aortic insufficiency.[125] A dilatation of the ascending aorta with loss of the sinotubular junction is often associated to this condition. In the past, aortic valve replacement was recommended for these patients. With the current strong interest in aortic valve repair, alternative solutions have been used[126,127] in order to avoid the drawbacks of mechanical and bioprosthetic prostheses.

Surgical treatment and results in patients with tetralogy and absent pulmonary valve syndrome

In this complex anomaly, cardiac and respiratory symptoms are closely entwined.[128] As a consequence, the search for the optimal surgical solution has often swung from one side to the other. The ideal candidate for surgery is an infant or child with mild cardiac and respiratory symptoms. In such conditions, several surgical strategies have been employed. On the opposite side of the spectrum, there is the neonate with severe respiratory symptoms or small infant with tracheobronchomalacia. In such patients, aortopulmonary collateral vessels may play a role in exacerbating the symptoms of respiratory and cardiac failure.[129]

The most severe form of the disease typically features absence of segmental pulmonary arteries at the hila, replaced by tufts of vessels compressing the intraparenchymal bronchi. The number of alveoli is also globally reduced.[65] At present, there is no treatment for this extreme form of APVS.

Presentation in neonates and infants has prompted attempts at palliation[130] with pulmonary artery banding, ligation of the pulmonary trunk and placement of a central shunt, or simple sternotomy.[131] Medical measures have consisted of preoperative ventilation in the prone position and prevention of air trapping in the lung parenchyma.[131] In the last two decades, primary surgical repair has been attempted,[130,132,133] following the trend of every earlier repair of classic ToF. In ToF with APVS, this strategy would seem most appropriate, taking into account the severity of symptoms in neonates and infants and the possibility of preventing the development or progression of tracheobronchomalacia.

Surgical treatment should ideally accomplish two goals: VSD repair with RVOT reconstruction and relief of bronchial compression. Most authors agree that after VSD closure, a valved conduit repair is indispensable in the neonatal period.[130,132–135] Presumably some degree of pulmonary hypertension does persist after surgery, and a pulmonary valve is instrumental in counteracting its negative effect on the RV. Pulmonary artery resection (anterior), pulmonary plication (posterior), or a combination of the two[136] as well as total resection of the central pulmonary branches and replacement with a bifurcated homograft[135] have been adopted.

Some authors[136] recommend aortic transection in order to obtain optimal exposure of the pulmonary arteries down to the respective hila. The Lecompte maneuver (bringing the pulmonary bifurcation anterior to the aorta) has been used to maximize the displacement of the pulmonary artery away from the bronchi.[137] Bronchial stents have been utilized only in extreme cases.

Hospital mortality is high among neonates and infants with APVS, ranging from 17 to 33 percent.[130–135] In small, more recent series, more favorable results have been reported.[137] Surgery in older children is considerably less hazardous and outcomes tend to parallel those of ToF. In older children, results seem to be equally good with conduits, transannular patches, or monocusp valved patches.[138] Late survival in ToF with APVS is considerably lower than in "classic" ToF, with survival at 5 and 10 years reported at 80 percent and 70 percent, respectively.[135] In a large series from Boston,[135] the presence of respiratory distress and year of operation before 1990 were predictors of poor early and late outcome.

The need for further surgery frequently arises in this group of patients. Besides residual VSD, RVOTO, and PR, respiratory symptoms secondary to unrelieved compression of the trachea and bronchi are common causes for reoperation, often in the first 24 months after initial correction. Repeat plication of the pulmonary arterial branches and implantation of a valved conduit are the most frequently performed procedures at reintervention.[133]

References

1. Marquis RM. Longevity and early history of tetralogy of Fallot. *Br Med J* 1956;1:819–822.
2. Fallot A. Contribution a l'anatomie pathologique de la maladie bleue (cyanose cardiaque). *Marseille Med* 1888;25:77–403.
3. Lev M, Eckner FA. The pathologic anatomy of tetralogy of Fallot and its variants. *Dis Chest* 1964;45:251–261.
4. Becker A, Connor M, Anderson R. Tetralogy of Fallot: A morphometric and geometric study. *Am J Cardiol* 1975;35:402–412.
5. Ferencz C, Rubin JD, Loffredo C, et al. Epidemiology of congenital heart disease. The Baltimore-Washington Infant Study. 1981–1989. Mount Kisco, NY: Futura; 1993.
6. Nora JJ, Berg K, Nora AH. Cardiovascular diseases: Genetics, epidemiology and prevention. New York: Oxford University Press; 1991;53–80.
7. Marino B, Digilio MC, Grazioli S, et al. Associated cardiac anomalies in isolated and syndromic patients with tetralogy of Fallot. *Am J Cardiol* 1996;77:505–508.
8. Li L, Krantz ID, Deng Y, et al. Alagille syndrome is caused by mutations in human Jagged1, which encodes a ligand for Notch1. *Nat Genet* 1997;16:243–251.
9. Wyse RKH, Al-Mahdawi S, Burn J, et al. Congenital heart disease in CHARGE association. *Pediatr Cardiol* 1993;14:75–81.
10. Kumar A, Friedman JM, Taylor GP, et al. Pattern of cardiac malformation in oculoauriculovertebral spectrum. *Am J Med Genet* 1993;46:423–426.
11. Ryan AK, Goodship JA, Wilson DI, et al. Spectrum of clinical features associated with interstitial chromosome 22q11 deletions: A European collaborative study. *J Med Genet* 1997;34:798–804.
12. Marino B, Digilio MC, Toscano A, et al. Anatomic patterns of conotruncal defects associated with deletion 22q11. *Genet Med* 2001;3:45–48.
13. Goldmuntz E, Clark BJ, Mitchell LE, et al. Frequency of 22q11 deletions in patients with conotruncal defects. *J Am Coll Cardiol* 1998;32:492–498.
14. Digilio MC, Marino B, Grazioli S, et al. Comparison of occurrence of genetic syndromes in ventricular septal defect with pulmonic stenosis (classic tetralogy of Fallot) versus ventricular septal defect with pulmonic atresia. *Am J Cardiol* 1996;77:1375–1376.
15. Anaclerio S, Marino B, Carotti A, et al. Pulmonary atresia with ventricular septal defect: Prevalence of deletion 22q11 in the different anatomic patterns. *Ital Heart J* 2001;2:384–387.
16. Marino B. Patterns of congenital heart disease and associated cardiac anomalies in children with Down syndrome. In: Marino B, Pueschel SM (eds). *Heart Disease in Persons with Down Syndrome.* Brookes; 1996:133–140.
17. Digilio MC, Marino B, Giannotti A, et al. Recurrence risk figures for isolated tetralogy of Fallot after screening for 22q11.2 microdeletion. *J Med Genet* 1997;34: 188–190.
18. Burn J, Brennan P, Little J, et al. Recurrence risks in offspring of adults with major heart defects: Results from first cohort of British collaborative study. *Lancet* 1998; 351:311–316.
19. Goldmuntz E, Geiger E, Benson W. NKX2: Mutations in patients with tetralogy of Fallot. *Circulation* 2001;104:2565–2568.
20. Eldadah ZA, Hamosh A, Biery NJ, et al. Familial tetralogy of Fallot caused by mutation in the Jagged1 gene. *Hum Molec Genet* 2001;10:163–169.
21. Pizzuti A, Sarkozy A, Newton AL, et al. Mutations of ZFPM2/FOG2 gene in sporadic cases of tetralogy of Fallot. *Hum Mutat* 2003;22:372–377.
22. Van Praagh R, Van Praagh S, Nebesor RA. Tetralogy of Fallot: Underdevelopment of the pulmonary infundibulum and its sequelae. *Am J Cardiol* 1970;26:25–33.
23. Zuberbuhler JR. Tetralogy of Fallot. In: Emmanouilides GC, Allen HD, Riemenschneider TA et al (eds). *Moss and Adams' Heart Disease in Infants, Children, and Adolescents, Including the Fetus and Young Adult.* Baltimore: Williams & Wilkins; 1995:998–1018.
24. Kirklin JW, Barratt-Boyes BG. *Cardiac Surgery,* 2d ed. New York: Churchill Livingstone; 1993;861–1012.
25. Muster AJ, Zales VR. Ilbawi MN, et al. Biventricular repair of hypoplastic right ventricle assisted by pulsatile bidirectional cavopulmonary anastomosis. *J Thorac Cardiovasc Surg* 1993;105:112–119.
26. Suzuky A, Ho SY, Anderson RH, et al. Further morphology studies on tetralogy of Fallot, with particular emphasis on the prevalence and structure of the membranous flap. *J Thorac Cardiovasc Surg* 1990;99: 528–535.

27. Hoffman JIE, Rudolph AM, Nadas AS, et al. Pulmonary stenosis, ventricular septal defect and RV pressure above systemic level. *Circulation* 1960;22:405–411.
28. Musewe NN, Smallhorn JF, Moes CAF, et al. Echocardiographic evaluation of obstructive mechanism of tetralogy of Fallot with restrictive ventricular septal defect. *Am J Cardiol* 1988;61:664–668.
29. Burrows PE, Freedom RM, Rabinovitch M, et al. The investigation of abnormal pulmonary arteries in congenital heart disease. *Radiol Clin North Am* 1985;23: 689–717.
30. Gikony BM, Juc KL, Edwards JE. Pulmonary vascular sling: Report of seven cases and review of the literature. *Pediatr Cardiol* 1989;10:81–89.
31. Graham TP Jr, Faulkner S, Bender H Jr. Hypoplasia of the left ventricle: Rare cause of postoperative mortality in tetralogy of Fallot. *Am J Cardiol* 1977;40:454–457.
32. Hohn AR, Jain KK, Tamer DM. Supravalvular mitral stenosis in tetralogy of Fallot. *Am J Cardiol* 1968;22: 733–737.
33. Glancy DI, Morrow AG, Roberts WC. Malformations of the aortic valve in patients with the tetralogy of Fallot. *Am Heart J* 1968;76:755–759.
34. Nakajima Y, Nishibatake M, Ikeda K, et al. Abnormal development of fourth aortic arch derivatives in the pathogenesis of tetralogy of Fallot. *Pediatr Cardiol* 1990;11:69–71.
35. Virdi IS, Keeton BR, Shore DF, et al. Surgical management in tetralogy of Fallot and vascular ring. *Pediatr Cardiol* 1987;8:131–134.
36. Komula RJ, Bais A, Lal N. Interrupted aortic arch with tetralogy of Fallot. *J Cardiovasc Surg* 1991;32:541–543.
37. Yamaguchi M, Tsukube T, Hosokawa Y, et al. Pulmonary origin of left anterior descending coronary artery in tetralogy of Fallot. *Ann Thorac Surg* 1991;52:310–312.
38. Heifetz SA, Rabinovitch M, Mueller KH, et al. Total anomalous origin of the coronary arteries from the pulmonary artery. *Pediatr Cardiol* 1986;7:11–18.
39. Soto B, Pacifico AD. Tetralogy of Fallot. In: *Angiocardiography in Congenital Heart Malformations.* Mount Kisco, NY: Futura; 1990:353–375.
40. Sharma S, Rafani M, Mukhopadhyay S, et al. Collateral arteries arising from the coronary circulation in tetralogy of Fallot. *Int J Cardiol* 1988;19:237–243.
41. Nagao GI, Daoud GI, McAdams AJ, et al. Cardiovascular anomalies associated with tetralogy of Fallot. *Am J Cardiol* 1967;20:206–211.
42. Abdallah HI, Marks LA, Balsara RK, et al. Staged repair of pentalogy of Cantrell with tetralogy of Fallot. *Ann Thorac Surg* 1993;56:979–980.
43. Piot JD, Leriche H, Losay J, et al. Malformations de la valve tricuspide associées a la tetralogie de Fallot operées. *Arch Mal Coeur Vaiss* 1985;78:757–761.
44. Sahai S, Kothari SS, Wasir HS. Tetralogy of Fallot with Ebstein's anomaly of the tricuspid valve. *Indian Heart J* 1994;46:53–54.
45. Redington AN, Raine J, Shinebourne EA, et al. Tetralogy of Fallot with anomalous pulmonary venous connections: A rare but clinically important association. *Br Heart J* 1990;64:325–328.
46. Gerlis LM, Fiddler GI, Pearse RG. Total anomalous pulmonary venous drainage associated with tetralogy of Fallot: Report of a case. *Pediatr Cardiol* 1984;4: 297–300.
47. Vargas FJ, Coto EO, Mayer JE Jr, et al. Complete atrioventricular canal and tetralogy of Fallot: Surgical considerations. *Ann Thorac Surg* 1986;42:258–263.
48. Gatzoulis MA, Shore D, Yacoub M, et al. Complete atrioventricular septal defect with tetralogy of Fallot: Diagnosis and management. *Br Heart J* 1994;71: 579–583.
49. Kothari SS, Rajani M, Shrivastava S. Tetralogy of Fallot with aorto-pulmonary window. *Int J Cardiol* 1988;18: 105–108.
50. Van Praagh R, Corwin RD, Dahlquist E, et al. Tetralogy of Fallot with severe left ventricular outflow tract obstruction due to anomalous attachment of the mitral valve to the ventricular septum. *Am J Cardiol* 1970;26: 95–101.
51. Marino B, Ballerini L, Marcelletti C, et al. Right oblique subxyphoid view for two-dimensional echocardiographic visualization of the right ventricle in congenital heart disease. *Am J Cardiol* 1984;54:1064–1068.
52. Freedom RM, Benson LN, Smallhorn JF. Neonatal heart disease. London: Springer-Verlag; 1992:213–228.
53. Santoro G, Marino B, Di Carlo D. Echocardiographically guided repair of tetralogy of Fallot. *Am J Cardiol* 1994;73:808–811.
54. Jureidini SB , Appleton RS, Nouri S, et al. Detection of coronary abnormalities in tetralogy of Fallot by two-dimensional echocardiography. *J Am Coll Cardiol* 1989;14:960–967.
55. Lababidi Z, Wu JR. Percutaneous balloon pulmonary valvuloplasty. *Am J Cardiol* 1983;52:560–562.
56. Qureshi SA, Kirk CR, Lamb RK, et al. Balloon dilatation of the pulmonary valve in the first year of life in patients with tetralogy of Fallot. *Br Heart J* 1988;60:232–235.
57. Piechaud JF, Delogu AB, Iserin L, et al. Palliative treatment of tetralogy of Fallot by percutaneous dilatation of the right ventricular outflow tract; 40 cases. *Arch Mal Coeur Vaiss* 1994;86:573–579.
58. Bergersen LJ, Perry SB, Lock JE. Effect of cutting balloon angioplasty on resistant pulmonary artery stenosis. *Am J Cardiol* 2003;91:185–189.
59. Chevers N. Rechèrches sur les maladies de l'àrtere pulmonaire. *Arch Gen Med* 1847;15:488–508.
60. Rowe RD, Vlad P, Keith JD. Atypical tetralogy of Fallot. A non-cyanotic form with increased lung vascularity. *Circulation* 1955;12(2):230–238.
61. Baker WP, Kelminson LL, Turner WM. Absence of pulmonic valve associated with double outlet right ventricle. *Circulation* 1967;36(3):452–455.
62. Oppido G, Carotti A, Albanese SB, et al. Transposition with absent pulmonary valve syndrome: Early repair of a rare case. *Ann Thorac Surg* 2001;71(5):1686–1688.
63. Calder AL, Brandt PW, Barratt-Boyes BG. Tetralogy of Fallot with absent pulmonary valve leaflets and origin of one pulmonary artery from the ascending aorta. *Am J Cardiol* 1980;46:106–116.
64. Corno A, Picardo S, Ballerini L, et al. Bronchial compression by dilated pulmonary artery. *J Thorac Cardiovasc Surg* 1985;90:705–710.
65. Rabinovitch M, Grady S, David I, et al. Compression of intrapulmonary bronchi by abnormally branching

pulmonary arteries associated with absent pulmonary valves *Am J Cardiol* 1982;50:804–812.
66. Fyler DC. Report of the New England Regional Infant Cardiac Program. *Pediatrics* 1980;65(suppl 2): 376–461.
67. Kirklin JW, Karp RB. *The Tetralogy of Fallot from a Surgical Viewpoint.* Philadelphia: Saunders; 1970:vii–x.
68. Lillehei CW, Varco RL, Cohen M, et al. The first open heart corrections of tetralogy of Fallot. A 26–31 year follow-up of 106 patients. *Ann Surg* 1986;204(4): 490–502.
69. Waterston DJ. Treatment of Fallot's tetralogy in children under one year of age. *Rozhl Chir* 1962;41:181–183.
70. Cooley DA, Hallman GL. Intrapericardial aortic-right pulmonary arterial anastomosis. *Surg Gynaecol Obstet* 1966;122:184–187.
71. Castaneda AR, Mayer JE Jr, Jonas RA, et al. Repair of tetralogy of Fallot in infancy. Early and late results. *J Thorac Cardiovasc Surg* 1977;74:372–381.
72. Hennein HA, Mosca RS, Urceley G, et al. Intermediate results after complete repair of tetralogy of Fallot in neonates. *J Thorac Cardiovasc Surg* 1995;109: 332–344.
73. Galdman G, McCrindle BW, Williams WG, et al. The modified Blalock-Taussig shunt: Clinical impact and morbidity in Fallot's tetralogy in the current era. *J Thorac Cardiovasc Surg* 1997;114:25–30.
74. Pozzi M, Trivedi DB, Kitchiner D, et al. Tetralogy of Fallot: What operation, at which age. *Eur J Cardiothorac Surg* 2000;17:631–636.
75. Pacifico AD, Sand ME, Bargeron LM Jr, et al. Transatrial-transpulmonary repair of tetralogy of Fallot. *J Thorac Cardiovasc Surg* 1987;93:919–924.
76. Kurosawa H, Imai Y, Becker AE. Surgical anatomy of the atrioventricular conduction bundle in tetralogy of Fallot: New findings relevant to the position of sutures. *J Thorac Cardiovasc Surg* 1988;95:586–591.
77. Horowitz NL, Alexander AJ, Edmunds LH. Postoperative right bundle branch block: Identification of three levels of block. *Circulation* 1980;62:319–328.
78. Hanley FL. Management of the congenitally abnormal right ventricular outflow tract: What is the right approach? *J Thorac Cardiovasc Surg* 2000;119:1–3.
79. Karl TR, Sano S, Pornviliwan S, et al. Tetralogy of Fallot: Favourable outcome of nonneonatal transatrial, transpulmonary repair. *Ann Thorac Surg* 1992;54:903–907.
80. Yamagishi M, Kurosawa H. Outflow reconstruction of tetralogy of Fallot using a Gore-Tex valve. *Ann Thorac Surg* 1993;56:1414–1417.
81. Turrentine MW, McCarthy RP, Vijay P, et al. Polytetrafluoroethylene monocusp valve technique for right ventricular outflow tract reconstruction. *Ann Thorac Surg* 2002;74:2202–2205.
82. Quintessenza JA, Jacobs JP, Morell VO, et al. Initial experience with a bicuspid polytetrafluoroethylene pulmonary valve in 41 children and adults: A new option for right ventricular outflow tract reconstruction. *Ann Thorac Surg* 2005;79:924–931
83. Isomatsu Y, Shin'oka T, Aoki M, et al. Establishing right-ventricle-to-pulmonary artery continuity by autologous tissue: An alternative approach to prosthetic conduit repair. *Ann Thorac Surg* 2004;78:173–180.
84. Kurosawa H, Imai Y, Nakazawa M, et al. Standardized patch infundibuloplasty for tetralogy of Fallot. *J Thorac Cardiovasc Surg* 1986;92:396–401.
85. Kurosawa H, Imai Y, Nakazawa M, et al. Conotruncal repair of tetralogy of Fallot. *Ann Thorac Surg* 1988;45: 661–666.
86. Kurosawa H, Morita K, Yamagishi M, et al. Conotruncal repair of tetralogy of Fallot: Midterm results. *J Thorac Cardiovasc Surg* 1998;115:351–360.
87. Di Carlo D, De Nardo D, Ballerini L, et al. Injury to the left coronary artery during repair of tetralogy of Fallot: Successful aorta-coronary PTFE graft. *J Thorac Cardiovasc Surg* 1987;93:468–470.
88. Kalra S, Sharma R, Choudhary SK, et al. Right ventricular outflow tract after non-conduit repair of tetralogy of Fallot with coronary anomaly. *Ann Thorac Surg* 2000; 70:723–726.
89. Brizard CP, Mas C, Sohn YS, et al. Transatrial-transpulmonary tetralogy of Fallot repair is effective in the presence of anomalous coronary arteries. *J Thorac Cardiovasc Surg* 1998;116:770–779.
90. van Son JAM. Repair of tetralogy of Fallot with anomalous origin of left anterior descending coronary artery. *J Thorac Cardiovasc Surg* 1995;110:561–562.
91. Dandolu BR, Baldwin HS, Norwood WI, et al. Tetralogy of Fallot with anomalous coronary artery: Double outflow technique. *Ann Thorac Surg* 1999;67: 1178–1180.
92. Kreutzer C, Mayorquim RdC, Kreutzer G, et al. Experience with one and a half ventricle repair. *J Thorac Cardiovasc Surg* 1999;117:662–668.
93. Stellin G, Padalino M, Milanesi O, et al. Surgical closure of apical ventricular septal defects through a right ventricular apical infundibulotomy. *Ann Thorac Surg* 2000; 69:597–601.
94. Hirsch JC, Mosca RS, Bove EL. Complete repair of tetralogy of Fallot in the neonate. Results in the modern era. *Ann Surg* 2000;232(4):508–514.
95. Sousa Uva M, Lacour-Gayet F, Komiya T, et al. Surgery for tetralogy of Fallot at less than six months of age. *J Thorac Cardiovasc Surg* 1994;107(5):1291–1300.
96. Parry AJ, McElhinney DB, Kung GC, et al. Elective primary repair of acyanotic tetralogy of Fallot in early infancy: Overall outcome and impact on the pulmonary valve. *J Am Coll Cardiol* 2000;36:2279–2283.
97. Alexiou C, Chen Q, Galogavrou M, et al. Repair of tetralogy of Fallot in infancy with a transventricular or a transatrial approach. *Eur J Cardiothorac Surg* 2002;22: 174–183.
98. Van Arsdell GS, Maharaj GS, Tom J, et al. What is the optimal age for repair of tetralogy of Fallot? *Circulation* 2000;102(suppl III):123–129.
99. Dyamenahalli U, McCrindle BW, Barker GA, et al. Influence of preoperative factors on outcomes in children younger than 18 months after repair of tetralogy of Fallot. *Ann Thorac Surg* 2000;69:1236–1242.
100. Murphy JG, Gersh BJ, Mair DD, et al. Long-term follow-up in patients undergoing surgical repair of tetralogy of Fallot. *N Engl J Med* 1993;329:593–599.
101. Veldtman GR, Connolly HM, Grogan M, et al. Outcomes of pregnancy in women with tetralogy of Fallot. *J Am Coll Cardiol* 2004;44:174–180.

102. Knott-Craig CJ, Elkins RC, Lane MM, et al. A 26-year experience with surgical management of tetralogy of Fallot: Risk analysis for mortality and late reintervention. *Ann Thorac Surg* 1998;66:506–511.
103. Atallah-Yunes NH, Kavey RW, Bove EL, et al. Postoperative assessment of a modified surgical approach to repair of tetralogy of Fallot. Long-term follow-up. *Circulation* 1996;94(suppl II):22–26.
104. Cullen S, Shore DF, Redington A. Characterization of right ventricular diastolic performance after complete repair of tetralogy of Fallot. Restrictive physiology predicts slow postoperative recovery. *Circulation* 1995;91: 1782–1789.
105. Norgard G, Gatzoulis MA, Moraes F, et al. Relationship between type of outflow tract repair and postoperative right ventricular diastolic physiology in tetralogy of Fallot. Implications for long-term outcome. *Circulation* 1996;94:3276–3280.
106. Gatzoulis MA, Clark AL, Cullen S, et al. Right ventricular diastolic function 15 to 35 years after repair of tetralogy of Fallot. Restrictive physiology predicts superior exercise performance. *Circulation* 1995;91: 1775–1781.
107. Munkhammar P, Cullen S, Jögi P, et al. Early age at repair prevents restrictive right ventricular (RV) physiology after surgery for tetralogy of Fallot (TOF). Diastolic RV function after TOF repair in infancy. *J Am Coll Cardiol* 1998;32:1083–1087.
108. Frigiola A, Redington AN, Cullen S, et al. Ventricular contractile dysfunction in patients with surgically repaired tetralogy of Fallot. *Circulation* 2004; 110(Suppl II):II153–II157.
109. Gatzoulis MA, Balani S, Webber SA, et al. Risk factors for arrhythmia and sudden cardiac death after repair of tetralogy of Fallot: A multicentre study. *Lancet* 2000; 356:975–981.
110. Hamada H, Terai M, Jibiki T, et al. Influence of early repair of tetralogy of Fallot without an outflow patch on late arrhythmias and sudden death: A 27-year follow-up study following a uniform surgical approach. *Cardiol Young* 2002;12:345–351.
111. Rao V, Kadletz M, Hornberger LK, et al. Preservation of the pulmonary valve complex in tetralogy of Fallot: How small is too small? *Ann Thorac Surg* 2000;69: 176–180.
112. Rowe SA, Zahka KG, Manolio TA, et al. Lung function and pulmonary regurgitation limit exercise capacity in postoperative tetralogy of Fallot. *J Am Coll Cardiol* 1991;17:461–466.
113. Warner KG, Anderson JE, Fulton DR, et al. Congenital heart disease: Restoration of the pulmonary valve reduces right ventricular volume overload after previous repair of tetralogy of Fallot. *Circulation* 1993;88(Suppl II):II189–II197.
114. Yemets IM, Williams WG, Webb G, et al: Pulmonary valve replacement late after repair of tetralogy of Fallot. *Ann Thorac Surg* 1997;64:526–530.
115. Rosti L, Murzi B, Colli AM, et al. Pulmonary valve replacement: A role for mechanical prostheses? (letter) *Ann Thorac Surg* 1998;65:888.
116. Therrien J, Siu S, Harris LJ, et al. Impact of pulmonary valve replacement on arrhythmia propensity late after repair of tetralogy of Fallot. *Circulation* 2001;103: 2489–2494.
117. Lim C, Lee J, Kim W, et al. Early replacement of pulmonary valve after repair of tetralogy: Is it really beneficial? *Eur J Cardiothorac Surg* 2004;25:728–734.
118. Geva T, Sandweiss BM, Gauvreau K, et al. Factors associated with impaired clinical status in long-term survivors of tetralogy of Fallot repair evaluated by magnetic resonance imaging. *J Am Coll Cardiol* 2004;43: 1068–1074.
119. Davlouros PA, Karatza AA, Gatzoulis MA, et al. Timing and type of repair for severe pulmonary regurgitation after repair of tetralogy of Fallot. *Int J Cardiol* 2004;97: 91–101.
120. Van Straten A, Vliegen HW, Hazekamp MG, et al. Right ventricular function after pulmonary valve replacement in patients with tetralogy of Fallot. *Radiology* 2004; 233(3):824–829.
121. Therrien J, Provost Y, Merchant N, et al. Optimal timing for pulmonary valve replacement in adults after tetralogy of Fallot repair. *Am J Cardiol* 2005;95:779–782.
122. Pearl JM, Cooper DS, Bove KE, et al. Early failure of the Shelhigh pulmonary valve conduit in infants. *Ann Thorac Surg* 2002;74:542–549.
123. Tiete AR, Sachweh JS, Roemer U, et al. Right ventricular outflow tract reconstruction with the Contegra bovine jugular vein conduit: A word of caution. *Ann Thorac Surg* 2004;77:2151–2156.
124. Lutter G, Ardehali R, Cremer J, et al. Percutaneous valve replacement: Current state and future prospects. *Ann Thorac Surg* 2004;78:2199–2206.
125. Niwa K, Siu S, Webb GD, et al. Progressive aortic root dilatation in adults late after repair of tetralogy of Fallot. *Circulation* 2002;106(11):1374–1378.
126. Ishizaka T, Ichikawa H, Sawa Y, et al. Prevalence and optimal management strategy for aortic regurgitation in tetralogy of Fallot. *Eur J Cardiothorac Surg* 2004;26: 1080–1086.
127. Di Carlo D, Santilli A, Amodeo A, et al. Acquired aortic regurgitation after repair of congenital heart defects: Another pitfall of "corrective" surgery? (letter) *Eur J Cardiothorac Surg*. In press.
128. Fouron JC. Tetralogy of Fallot with absent pulmonary valve. Clarification of a complex malformation and of its therapeutic challenge. *Circulation* 1990;82(4): 1525–1527.
129. Knauth AL, Marshall AC, Geva T, et al. Respiratory symptoms secondary to aortopulmonary collateral vessels in tetralogy of Fallot absent pulmonary valve syndrome. *Am J Cardiol* 2004;93:503–505.
130. Snir E, de Leval MR, Elliott MJ, et al. Current surgical technique to repair Fallot's tetralogy with absent pulmonary valve syndrome. *Ann Thorac Surg* 1991;51: 979–982.
131. Heinemann MK, Hanley FL. Preoperative management of neonatal tetralogy of Fallot with absent pulmonary valve syndrome. *Ann Thorac Surg* 1993;55: 172–174.
132. Godart F, Houyel L, Lacour-Gayet F, et al. Absent pulmonary artery valve syndrome: Surgical treatment and considerations. *Ann Thorac Surg* 1996;62: 136–142.

133. McDonnell B, Raff G, Gaynor WJ, et al. Outcome after repair of tetralogy of Fallot with absent pulmonary valve. *Ann Thorac Surg* 1999;67:1391–1395.
134. Kirshbom PM, Jaggers JJ, Ungerleider RM. Tetralogy of Fallot with absent pulmonary valve: Simplified technique for homograft repair. *J Thorac Cardiovasc Surg* 1999;118:1125–1127.
135. Hew CC, Daebritz S, Zurakowski D, et al. Valved homograft replacement of aneurysmal pulmonary arteries for severely symptomatic absent pulmonary valve syndrome. *Ann Thorac Surg* 2002;73:1778–1785.
136. Conte S, Serraf A, Godart F, et al. Technique to repair Tetralogy of Fallot with absent pulmonary valve. *Ann Thorac Surg* 1997;63:1489–1491.
137. Hraska V, Kantorova A, Kunovsky P, et al. Intermediate results with correction of tetralogy of Fallot with absent pulmonary valve using a new approach. *Eur J Cardiothorac Surg* 2004;21:711–715.
138. Kreutzer C, Schlichter A, Kreutzer G. Tetralogy of Fallot with absent pulmonary valve: A surgical technique for complete repair. *J Thorac Cardiovasc Surg* 1999;117: 192–194.

CHAPTER

61 PULMONARY ATRESIA WITH VENTRICULAR SEPTAL DEFECT AND MAJOR AORTOPULMONARY COLLATERALS

Malcolm J. MacDonald, Frank L. Hanley

INTRODUCTION

Pulmonary atresia (Pa) with ventricular septal defect (VSD) and major aortopulmonary collateral arteries (MAPCAs) is a complex lesion with great morphologic variability. It is characterized by atresia of the pulmonary valve, a tetralogy-type of VSD, and pulmonary collateral vessels originating from the aorta. Major variability occurs in the pulmonary vascular circulation. Development of the pulmonary arterial system occurs by fusion of the left and right sixth dorsal aortic arch with the plexus of systemic arteries carried by the lung buds from the

KEY CONCEPTS

- Epidemiology
  - Pulmonary atresia (Pa) with ventricular septal defect (VSD) and major aortopulmonary collateral arteries (MAPCAs) is a complex lesion with great morphologic variability representing approximately 2 percent of congenital heart defects, with a prevalence of 0.07 per 1000 live births.
- Morphology
  - There is an association of atresia of the pulmonary valve, a tetralogy-type VSD, and pulmonary collateral vessels originating usually from the descending thoracic aorta.
- Pathophysiology
  - Pathophysiology and degree of cyanosis depend on the contribution of aortopulmonary collaterals to oxygenation.
- Clinical features
  - Neonates born with Pa, VSD, and MAPCAs may have very unpredictable presentations owing to the anatomic variability of the lesion. Patients may be minimally symptomatic or severely cyanotic or may develop congestive heart failure.
- Diagnosis
  - Diagnostic evaluation includes echocardiography, cardiac catheterization, and, in selected cases, magnetic resonance imaging to elucidate the anatomy of MAPCAs.
- Treatment
  - Definitive therapy is surgical. The ultimate goal of surgical therapy is creation of separated in-series pulmonary and systemic circulations. Achievement of this goal requires "unifocalization" of the vascular systems, VSD closure, and reconstruction of the right ventricular outflow tract (RVOT). "Single stage" unifocalization with or without concurrent VSD closure is favored by the authors.
- Outcomes
  - In over 300 patients managed by the author's protocol, complete unifocalization via median sternotomy was achieved at the initial operation in 85 percent. Intracardiac repair was achieved at initial operation in 56 percent and in 83 percent within 2 years. Recent early mortality was 2 percent. Kaplan-Meier survival was 91 percent at 1 year and 86 percent at 10 years.

foregut. Failure of the normal fusion process results in Pa. Development of the true pulmonary arteries (PAs) is variable and depends on the point in gestation at which connection of the lumen of the true PAs with the right ventricle is lost.[1] True central PAs vary from normal in size to absent. The mean diameter of the central PAs in the author's series of over 300 patients was 1.5 mm. A small central confluence is usually present. When confluent PAs are present, there is typically no ductus arteriosus. When the right and left main PAs are discontinuous, bilateral ducts may exist, the right typically originating from innominate or subclavian artery.

Persistent connections from the aorta (MAPCAs) probably originate from splanchnic vessels. Aortopulmonary collaterals vary widely in origin, course, size, and histologic characteristics. The mean number of collaterals in the author's series was 3.8 ±1.4. Aortopulmonary collaterals originate most commonly from the proximal descending aorta. There is great variation in connection of MAPCAs into the pulmonary circulation. A given lung segment may have its blood supply derived from the true PA system, MAPCAs, or both; collateral vessels may supply anything from a small proportion of the total lung parenchyma to most of the pulmonary vascular bed. Variable degrees of obstruction of the collateral vessels may occur, and obstructions may be inconsistent in their location (proximally or distally) within the vessels. Diffuse collateralization from the systemic circulation (especially the chest wall) is common, particularly after surgical intervention.

The pulmonary microcirculation is healthiest at birth and declines progressively thereafter. The natural history of the MAPCAs is frequently characterized by progressive stenosis, which may result in distal microvascular hypoplasia. In the absence of stenosis, the systemic level pressure may cause pulmonary vascular obstructive disease (PVOD). Surgical interventions requiring use of systemic-to-pulmonary arterial connections (e.g., Blalock-Taussig shunt or aortopulmonary window) may also result in PVOD due to systemic-pressure pulmonary vascular perfusion.

The intracardiac anatomy is typified by an anteriorly malaligned VSD (hence the alternative designation as tetralogy of Fallot with Pa; see Chap. 60 for VSD morphology). The ventricles are typically normally developed, although the infundibulum of the right ventricle (RV) may be small. There are normal atrioventricular and ventriculoarterial connections. Figure 61-1 is a decision-making flowchart to be used in the treatment of this condition.

EPIDEMIOLOGY AND ASSOCIATED ANOMALIES

Pulmonary artery with VSD represents approximately 2 percent of congenital heart defects. In the Baltimore-Washington Infant Study a prevalence of 0.07 per 1000 live births was reported.[2] Pa with VSD accounted for 1.4 percent of all forms of congenital heart disease and 20.3 percent of all forms of tetralogy of Fallot. Infants of diabetic mothers are at an approximately tenfold greater risk of developing Pe with VSD. Genetic factors are considered likely to be etiologically contributory in that there is an increased risk of occurrence in siblings (2.5 to 3 percent) and in the offspring of adults with tetralogy of Fallot (1.2 to 8.3 percent).

Associated cardiac and extracardiac anomalies may occur. Commonly associated cardiac anomalies include secundum atrial septal defect (ASD), coronary anomalies, and multiple VSDs. Other less common cardiac anomalies have also been reported. A significant proportion of patients with Pa and VSD have associated syndromic or extracardiac anomalies. Associated extracardiac anomalies include the VATER syndrome (i.e., vertebral anomalies, anal atresia, tracheoesophageal fistula, esophageal atresia, and renal anomalies), Alagille syndrome, DiGeorge (velocraniofacial) syndrome, and trisomy 21, among others. There may be an unusually high incidence of tracheobronchial anomalies, particularly originating from the right-upper-lobe bronchus of the trachea (bronchus suis), which may result in right-upper-lobe complications postoperatively while the patient is intubated.

CLINICAL FEATURES

Children born with Pa, VSD, and MAPCAs may have very unpredictable presentations owing to the anatomic variability of the lesion. The VSD is typically unrestrictive. Patients with valvar atresia but little collateralization may be severely cyanotic. Patients with severe atresia and/or hypoplastic true pulmonary arteries but extensive collateralization may be minimally symptomatic. Such patients may eventually develop congestive heart failure due to pulmonary overcirculation or may develop progressive cyanosis. In these patients, cyanosis is due to paucity of pulmonary flow because of inadequate collaterals, stenosis of the collaterals, or pulmonary microvascular obstructive disease. Development of these complications may occur at very variable rates, resulting in unpredictably delayed presentation. Cyanotic spells may occur. In patients with Pa, these symptoms occur because of decreases in systemic vascular resistance, resulting in markedly decreased pulmonary blood flow (rather than owing to right ventricular infundibular spasm, as is usual in tetralogy without atresia). Late presentation may occur[3] and may include polycythemia, "clubbing," cerebral embolism, and abscesses.

DIAGNOSTIC EVALUATION

Following presentation with typical symptoms, patients require complete diagnostic investigation. Pulse oximetry is a useful indicator of adequacy of pulmonary blood flow. Patients with oxygen saturation greater

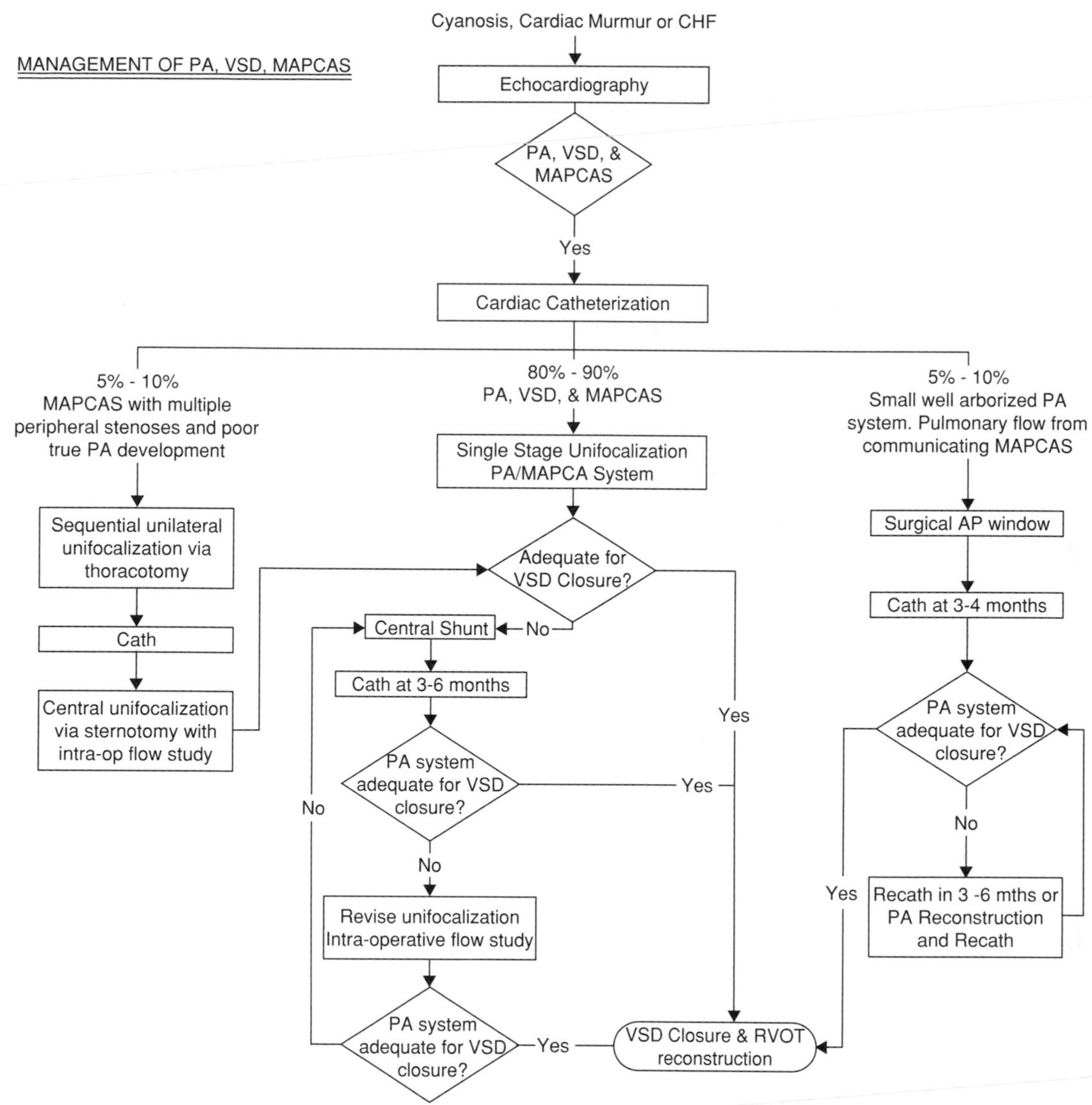

Figure 61-1 Clinical decision-making algorithm in pulmonary atresia with VSD and multiple aortopulmonary collaterals. PA, pulmonary artery; VSD, ventricular septal defect; MAPCA, major aorto-pulmonary collateral arteries.

than 85 to 90 percent typically have well-developed collateral systems and are at risk for pulmonary overcirculation. Patients with oxygen saturations less than 75 to 80 percent may have poorly developed pulmonary vascular and collateral systems.

Chest radiographs may demonstrate pulmonary plethora or hypoperfusion of the lung fields. The electrocardiogram is typically normal at birth but will gradually develop evidence of right ventricular hypertrophy, comparable to tetralogy of Fallot.

Echocardiography is highly reliable in making the diagnosis of Pe, VSD, and MAPCAs but is typically inadequate for complete evaluation. Echocardiography is sensitive for the detection of aortopulmonary collaterals but inadequate for complete delineation, which is essential for surgical management. The intracardiac anatomy is well delineated by echocardiography. Echocardiography may also show other associated cardiac lesions including ASD (in contrast to a patent foramen ovale), multiple VSDs, and coronary anomalies.

Cardiac catheterization is essential in evaluating the true PA and aortopulmonary collateral system (Fig. 61-2). It is particularly important to clarify the complete true PA and aortopulmonary collateral distribution. Evaluation of the true PA system may be difficult unless there is duct-dependent pulmonary circulation or a connection between a collateral and the true PA system. Retrograde venous wedge angiography may be needed to evaluate the true PA system. The true central PA system appears as a "seagull"-like vascular structure and is best visualized in the left lateral or left anterior oblique view. Following surgical and percutaneous interventions, repeated cardiac catheterization is essential to assess their effects and to plan for subsequent procedures when staged repair is necessary. In addition to imaging, hemodynamic data are important. The presence of elevated

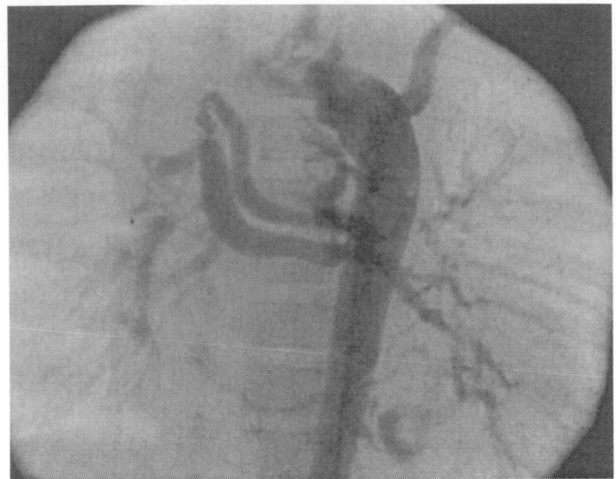

A

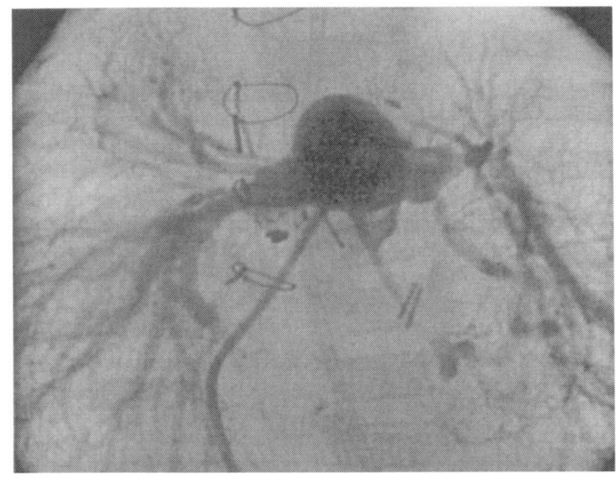

B

Figure 61-2 Aortic arch angiogram before **(A)** and main pulmonary arteriogram after **(B)** one-stage complete unifocalization in a 2-month-old infant with five MAPCAs and 1.5-mm confluent PAs. The VSD was left open. The postoperative angiogram demonstrates complete perfusion of both lungs. (From Reddy et al.[12] With permission.)

distal pressure within collateral vessels (mean pressure greater than 20 to 25 mmHg) suggests significant PVOD within the affected lung segments. Evaluation of right ventricular (RV) pressure may be helpful in assessing for VSD closure in patients who have been managed by complete unifocalization and placement of an RV-PA conduit without VSD closure, as advocated by some authors. RV pressure less than 50 percent systemic (under optimal circumstances) or, at most, up to 75 percent systemic suggests that the VSD can be closed. After unifocalization and RVOT reconstruction without VSD closure, the presence of a left-to-right shunt at the ventricular level indicates adequacy of the pulmonary vasculature to tolerate at least one full cardiac output and suitability for VSD repair.

Magnetic resonance imaging (MRI) is gaining prominence in evaluating the anatomy of complex collaterals. Owing to difficulty in the evaluation of angiograms, three-dimensional MRI reconstructions may be helpful in achieving detailed anatomic assessments and appropriate operative planning.

GOALS AND PRINCIPLES OF THERAPY

The initial management of patients presenting with Pa, VSD, and MAPCAs is based on medical stabilization, such that full evaluation and proper therapeutic planning can be undertaken. Some patients with excessive pulmonary blood flow may require anticongestive management. Interventional cardiac catheterization is important in both short and long-term management. Interventional procedures may include coil occlusion of collaterals providing duplicate flow to individual pulmonary segments and balloon dilatation of stenoses. Pulmonary valve perforation and dilatation may be performed in the very rare instance of Pa with VSD and an adequately developed main PA system.

The ultimate goal of surgical therapy is the creation of separated in-series pulmonary and systemic circulations. The ideal age for repair of this lesion is unknown. If the patient is well balanced physiologically, we prefer to perform the repair when the patient is between 3 and 6 months of age, and to perform single-stage repair. There are many advantages to early one-stage repair. Cardiovascular physiology is normalized and cyanosis is corrected. The patient is protected against pulmonary hypertension related to high flow through either collaterals or systemic shunts. The number of operations is reduced, reducing the complexity and morbidity of reoperative surgery. The major problem in management is the natural and intervened history of the MAPCAs and the complexity of surgical intervention in the pulmonary vascular bed (Fig. 61-3).

Reconstruction must achieve unobstructed flow from the right ventricle to the PA system. Achieving this goal requires "unifocalization" of the vascular systems, recruiting as much of the true PA-supplied and MAPCA-supplied systems as possible and, eventually, closure of the VSD. The most important physiologic factor indicating a favorable ultimate outcome is postrepair RV pressure, which depends on the number of lung segments included in the pulmonary vascular bed and the status of the pulmonary microvasculature. The goal of early intervention is to incorporate as many lung segments in the pulmonary vascular circuit as possible and to close the VSD such that the pulmonary circulation is exposed to normal pulmonary arterial pressures. Surgical approaches have included staged reconstruction via thoracotomies with subsequent pulmonary arterial centralization and ultimate VSD closure via sternotomy, staged reconstructions via sternotomies, and single-stage reconstruction.[4–9]

"Single-stage" unifocalization with or without concurrent repair of the VSD is favored by the authors.[10–12] The operation is achievable via sternotomy in most

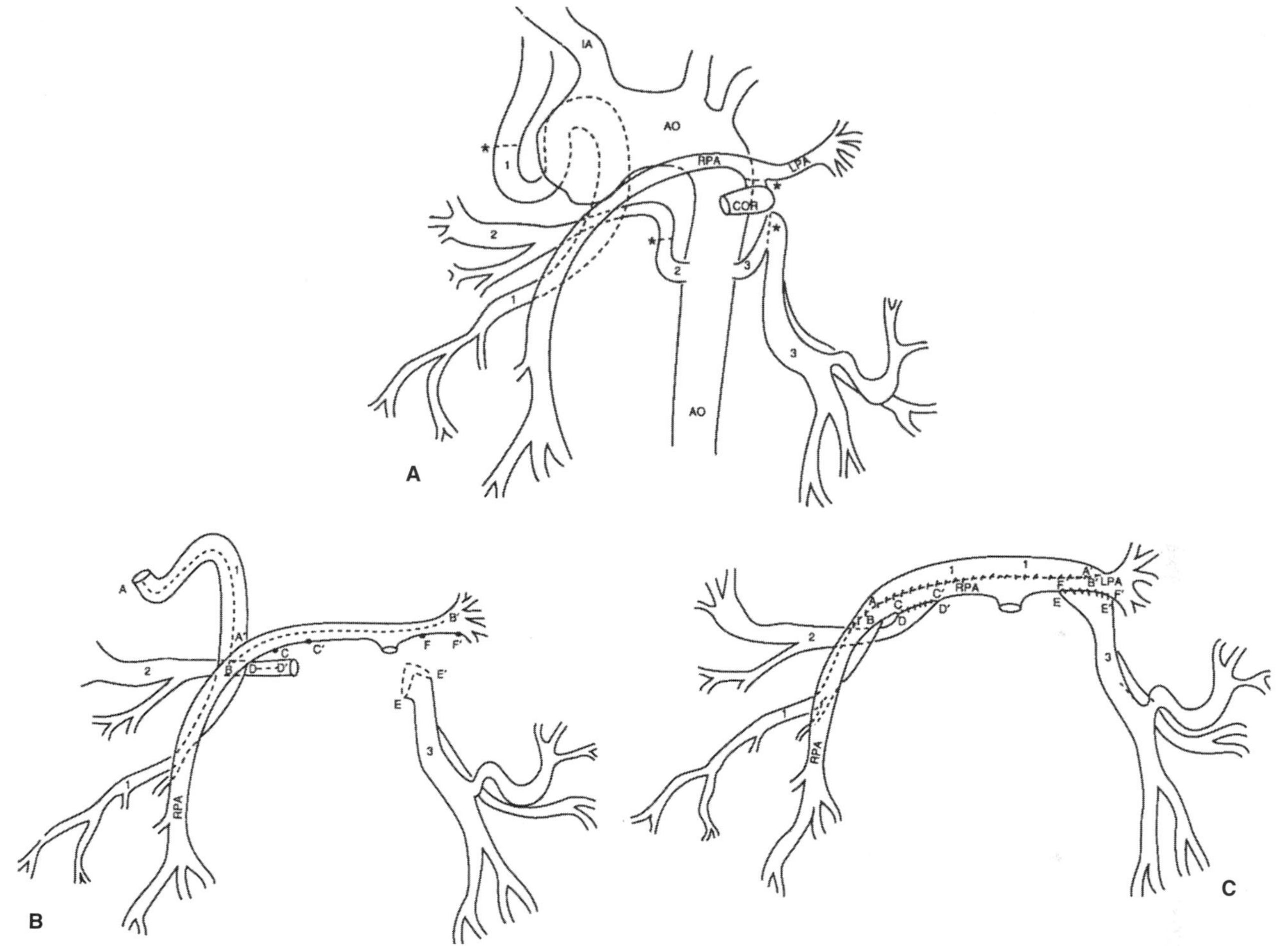

Figure 61-3 Anatomy of pulmonary blood supply and unifocalization in a 3.5-month-old child who underwent one-stage complete unifocalization and repair of tetralogy of Fallot with MAPCAs. **A.** Illustration of pulmonary blood supply with left (LPA) and right (RPA) pulmonary arteries, a coronary collateral (COR) connecting to the true pulmonary artery, and three MAPCAs (1 to 3) from the innominate artery (IA) and descending aorta (AO). **B.** MAPCAs are opened along the dashed lines A-A′, D-D′, and E-E′, whereas the true pulmonary arteries are filleted open from hilum to hilum (B-B′). **C.** Unifocalization and reconstruction of the pulmonary artery is completed with full native tissue continuity. Collateral 1 A-A′ is anastomosed side to side to the incision B-B′ in the true pulmonary artery as a long onlay. Collateral 2 is anastomosed end-to-side to the undersurface of the RPA from D-D′ to C-C′. Collateral 3 is anastomosed end to side to the undersurface of the LPA from E-E′ to F-F′. (From Reddy et al.[10] With permission.)

patients, avoiding the potential long-term complications of thoracotomy. In patients whose PA system is inadequate to support a full cardiac output due to distal stenosis or hypoplasia, unifocalization of the collaterals and creation of a shunt from the ascending aorta to the unifocalized PA system is performed whenever possible. The VSD is left open and early follow-up and reintervention planned.

In a small minority of patients, minute centrally confluent true PAs are present with a relatively complete arborization pattern to most or all lung segments. Pulmonary blood flow is from MAPCAs, which share dual-supply vascular distribution with the true pulmonary arteries. In these patients we construct a neonatal "aortopulmonary window" by transecting the main PA close to the infundibulum and anastomosing the small main PA to the ascending aorta to encourage pulmonary vascular growth (Fig. 61-4).[13] Important MAPCAs are ligated. These patients are evaluated for intracardiac repair at 3 and 6 months of age. In a few patients, the majority of MAPCAs have multiple stenoses at the segmental and subsegmental branches. True PAs may or may not be present. This small subgroup of patients with Pa, VSD, and MAPCAs are managed by sequential staged thoracotomies.

Patients who have severe cyanosis, an inadequate collateralization, or a pulmonary vascular bed not amenable to reconstruction or those who fail unifocalization and complete correction may eventually require pulmonary or heart-lung transplantation. Patients who have had

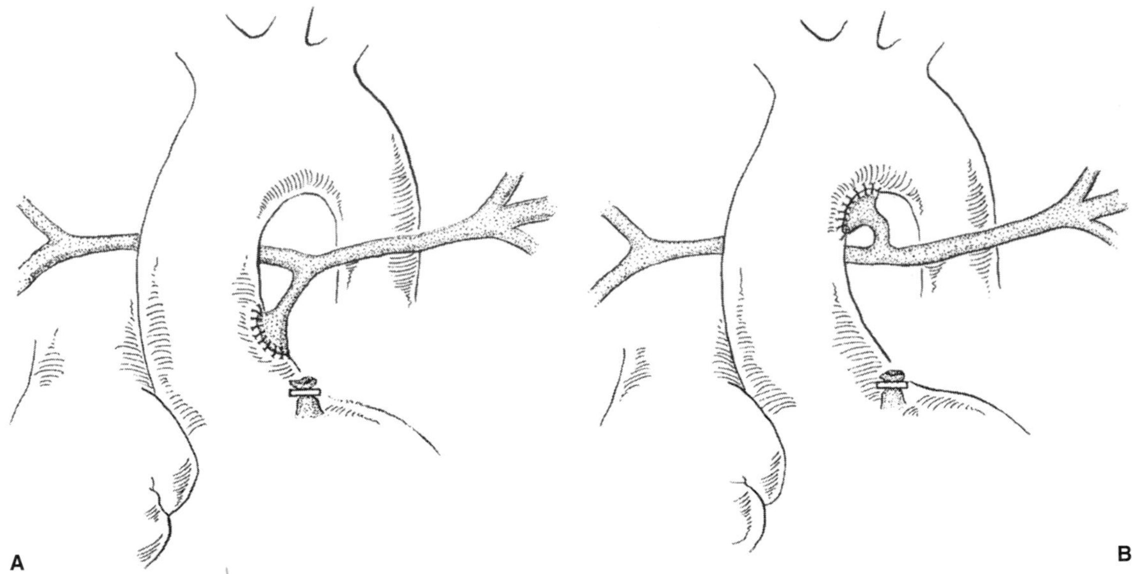

Figure 61-4 Surgical aortopulmonary window. The ideal location for anastomosis varies according to patient-specific anatomic variables and may be dictated not only by pulmonary artery anatomy but also by aortic size and position. **A.** Most common anastomotic position at left posterolateral aspect of ascending aorta, just above the sinotubular junction. **B.** Less common pulmonary artery confluence has better positional lie when located superiorly to the undersurface of the aortic arch. (From Rodefeld et al.[13] With permission.)

bilateral thoracotomies who require pulmonary transplantation due to failure of unifocalization are very difficult subjects for transplant, due to severe cyanosis and the development of extensive collateral vessels from the chest wall. Thoracotomy approaches to pulmonary vascular reconstruction are therefore used only when unavoidable.

SURGICAL THERAPY

The first priority is to completely unifocalize the PA and MAPCA complex. Our current approach is to perform the first intervention at 3 to 6 months of age (the median age of first operation in the authors' series was 8 months). Complete bilateral unifocalization via median sternotomy can usually be achieved (85 percent in the authors' series). Intracardiac repair is achieved as early as possible (56 percent at first operation and 83 percent within 2 years in the authors' series). In patients who are severely cyanotic or overshunted, earlier intervention is feasible and may be necessary. Customizing the therapeutic approach to the individual patient and creative, meticulous surgical technique is essential in achieving good surgical outcomes.

Timing of VSD closure may be a significant challenge.[14] Patients who have previously undergone pulmonary artery reconstruction and unifocalization and who have demonstrated satisfactory pulmonary vascular growth on follow-up angiography typically are amenable to VSD closure and RV-to-PA conduit RVOT reconstruction. When there is a question regarding the adequacy of the pulmonary bed to accommodate a full cardiac output, the authors have used an intraoperative flow study. When the VSD is closed, a patent foramen ovale is left to allow for right-to-left shunt in the event of elevated right ventricular pressure in the postoperative period.

Other authors have advocated using an "adjustable VSD" closure.[15] In this particular technique, the VSD is closed with a patch, leaving a deliberate defect in the superior portion of the patch, which is encircled with a purse-string suture. The RVOT is reconstructed, and a pressure-monitoring cannula is placed in the right ventricle. Occlusion of the deliberate "residual" VSD is then attempted. If the VSD can be occluded with resulting RV pressure half or less of the systemic pressure, the defect is completely closed. Otherwise the defect is maintained patent to allow for right-to-left shunt. The purse-string suture is enclosed in a tourniquet snare and brought to the subcutaneous tissue, where it may be easily located and exposed later.

Operative technique

The surgical approach to the mediastinum favored by the authors is via a wide midline incision and a median sternotomy. Subtotal thymectomy is performed. The right pleura is widely opened anterior to the phrenic nerve, the right lung is lifted out of the pleural cavity, and the right-sided collaterals are identified and dissected. Similarly, the left pleura is opened and the left-sided collaterals are identified and dissected. Collaterals are rerouted by opening the pleura on both sides posterior to the phrenic nerves. The descending aorta is exposed in the posterior mediastinum and all the collaterals from it are identified, dissected, and controlled. The pericardium is then opened, partial anterior pericardiectomy is performed, and the excised portion of pericardium is preserved in 0.6% glutaraldehyde. The native pulmonary arteries, if present, are completely mobilized from hilum to hilum. Any further collaterals from the upper descending aorta are identified and dissected in the subcarinal space between the tracheobronchial angle and the roof of the left atrium by an approach between the right superior vena cava and the aorta. The floor of the pericardial reflection in the transverse sinus is opened and the posterior mediastinal soft tissues are dissected to expose the aortic segment and the collaterals in this region. This is an important maneuver for gaining access to collaterals, which quite often arise from this location (Fig. 61-5). Opening this space also provides the most direct avenue for collateral rerouting for direct tissue-to-tissue anastomosis. In patients in whom collaterals originate from the aortic arch or the neck vessels, the vessels are exposed and mobilized. All collaterals are controlled with snares or neurovascular clips before cardiopulmonary bypass is instituted to avoid excessive PA runoff and systemic overcirculation. As many collaterals as possible are permanently ligated at their origin, mobilized, and unifocalized without cardiopulmonary bypass. When the patient's oxygenation reaches an unacceptably low level, cardiopulmonary bypass is instituted, and the remainder of the collaterals are unifocalized at mild to moderate hypothermia, with the heart beating. A calcium supplemented blood prime is used in the cardiopulmonary bypass pump circuit to maintain normal cardiac function. During unifocalization, emphasis is placed on avoiding synthetic or allograft conduits in the periphery and on achieving unifocalization by native tissue-to-tissue anastomosis. Surgical techniques used to achieve native tissue-to-tissue continuity may include side-to-side anastomosis of collaterals to the central PAs (thus augmenting the hypoplastic true PAs), side-to-side anastomosis of collateral-to-collateral or of collateral-to-peripheral true PAs, end-to-side anastomosis of collateral-to-collateral or of collateral-to–true PA, anastomosis of a button of aorta (giving rise to multiple unobstructed collaterals) to the native PAs, end-to-end or end-to-side anastomosis of collateral to central conduit, allograft patchplasty of stenotic distal segments of the collaterals, or allograft patch augmentation of the reconstructed neocentral PAs. These anastomoses are achieved directly by bringing collaterals either through the transverse sinus, below the hilum of the lung, or above the hilum to achieve the optimal anatomic result and by making use

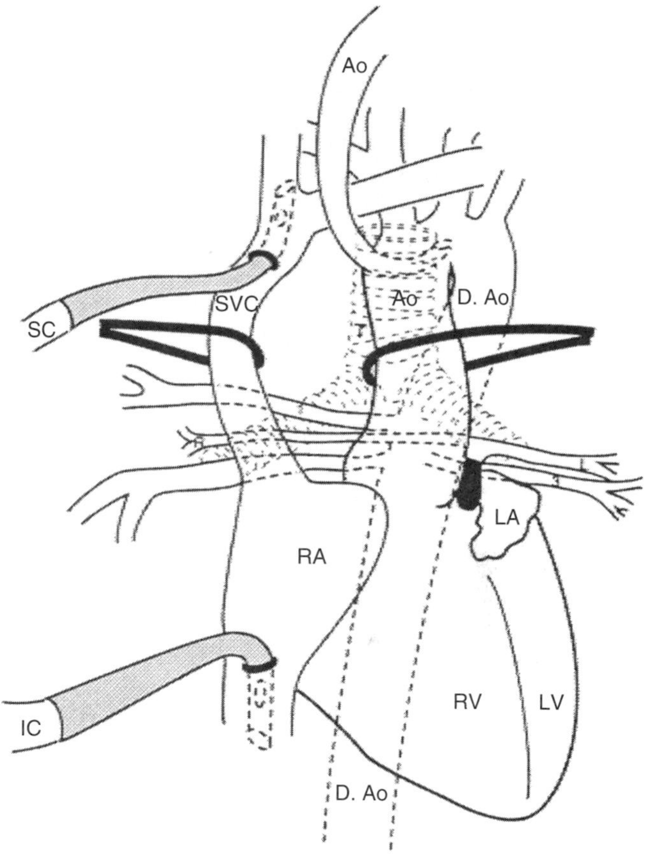

Figure 61-5 The transverse sinus is an important avenue for dissecting, routing, and unifocalizing the collaterals that arise from the descending aorta in the region of the subcarinal space. In this diagram, the MAPCAs are depicted anterior to the tracheobronchial tree. However, collaterals in this region have a variable relation to the extraparenchymal airways and esophagus, and the technique of rerouting and unifocalization must be individualized to optimize the lie of each collateral. Ac = Aortic cannula; Ao = ascending aorta; D.Ao = descending aorta; IC = inferior caval cannula; L = left pulmonary artery; LA = left atrium; LV = left ventricle; PA = atretic main pulmonary artery; R = right pulmonary artery; RA = right atrium; RV = right ventricle; SC = superior caval cannula; SVC = superior vena cava. (From Reddy et al.[10] With permission.)

of as much of the collateral length as possible. Tension-free tissue-to-tissue anastomosis is essential; collateral length is therefore critically important. Collateral length is consequently given the highest priority in order to achieve tissue-to-tissue anastomosis. If a discrete stenosis is present in the midportion of a collateral, the collateral is used and the stenosis is managed by side-to-side reconstruction at the stenotic area or, if that is not possible, by augmentation patching. Collaterals that provide a dual supply to a lung segment in conjunction with the true PA are unifocalized in order to build up the size of the reconstructed PAs. Particularly difficult aspects of unifocalization may occasionally be completed after aortic cross-clamping and cardioplegic arrest is induced, at moderate hypothermia. If use of patch material is unavoidable, we use it noncircumferentially so that the growth potential of the native tissue is preserved. We limit the use of circumferential nonviable conduits to the central mediastinum. Essential concepts necessary to achieve this type of unifocalization are flexibility regarding reconstruction, aggressive mobilization, maximizing the length of the MAPCAs, and creative rerouting.

In a total of more than 1100 unifocalized collaterals, only a small number have been reconstructed with circumferential nonviable conduit (expanded polytetrafluoroethylene). In patients with absent or string-like true PAs, a nonvalved allograft conduit may sometimes be necessary to reconstruct the central left and right PAs. In such patients, in whom growth potential is an issue, the hilar regions are reconstructed with native tissue only (using the techniques described), and the conduit serves as the main left and right PAs with the graft limited to the pericardial cavity.

Following completion of the unifocalization, the VSD is closed when indicated. Suitability for closure of the VSD may be determined by preoperative studies or may require an intraoperative flow study to assess the total resistance of the pulmonary vascular bed. The flow study is performed with the patient on cardiopulmonary bypass. The recreated main PA supplying the entire pulmonary vascular bed is cannulated and perfused using a calibrated pump head from the cardiopulmonary bypass pump. Flow from the pump head is progressively increased up to the equivalent of at least one cardiac output. A pressure catheter is placed in the PA system, and the left atrium is vented. If the mean PA pressure is less than 25 mmHg, the VSD can be closed. If the mean PA pressure is greater than 25 mmHg, a central shunt is created.

If VSD closure is indicated, a longitudinal ventriculotomy is made in the right ventricular infundibulum and hypertrophied muscle bundles are resected. The VSD is closed with a glutaraldehyde-fixed autologous pericardial patch or a polyester (Dacron) patch. The right atrium is opened to inspect the atrial septum. An atrial septal defect or patent foramen ovale, if present, is closed, leaving a small unidirectional interatrial communication as a "pop-off" valve for right to left shunt of venous blood in case of postoperative right ventricular dysfunction. In occasional cases with an intact atrial septum, a small one-way interatrial communication is created. A homograft valved conduit is tailored and used to connect the right ventricle to the reconstructed neopulmonary arterial system. A valved bovine jugular vein conduit (Contegra) may provide a useful alternative.[16] The distal conduit is anastomosed to the reconstructed PAs using a 6-0 or 7-0 monofilament nonabsorbable suture. The distal anastomosis may be performed prior to cardioplegic arrest in order to minimize ischemic time when the decision has been made to close the VSD. If needed, a distal extension of the conduit tissue can be shaped to augment the reconstructed central branch PAs. The proximal right ventricle-to-conduit anastomosis is made with a continuous monofilament nonabsorbable suture by directly anastomosing the conduit around a portion of its circumference and augmenting the anastomosis with a "hood" of either pericardium or homograft tissue to complete the anastomosis. The proximal conduit anastomosis may be constructed after removal of the aortic cross clamp and reperfusion of the heart during the rewarming period. A pressure-monitoring catheter is placed into the PAs across the RVOT. Following adequate rewarming, the patient is weaned from cardiopulmonary bypass with constant monitoring of the systemic arterial, PA, and atrial pressures. After separation from bypass, these pressures are measured continuously and transesophageal echocardiography is performed to ensure that there are no significant residual defects.

Bilateral pleural and mediastinal drains are placed and the sternum is closed. If bleeding or ventilation is a significant concern, we electively leave the sternum open and close the chest incision with a siliconized rubber (Silastic) patch. Secondary sternal closure is performed on the second or third postoperative day once the patient is physiologically stable.

Postoperative management

In the postoperative phase, patients are ventilated, kept well sedated, and, if necessary, pharmacologically paralyzed until they are hemodynamically stable and on minimal ventilatory support. Inotropic support is provided using dopamine, milrinone, calcium chloride, and epinephrine infusions as needed. Important postoperative problems include pulmonary parenchymal reperfusion injury, pulmonary hemorrhage, bronchospasm, and phrenic nerve injury. Reperfusion injury most typically occurs in pulmonary segments that are severely hypoperfused preoperatively. Bronchospasm may occur due to extensive hilar and intraparenchymal dissection. Phrenic nerve injury is uncommon and can be avoided by meticulous attention during dissection. Splanchnic organ dysfunction has previously been described and was a problem in the early experience of the authors. The problem typically presents as acute hepatic dysfunction or, rarely, intestinal necrosis. Visceral organ dysfunction is now not common; maintenance of perfusion pressure above 40 mmHg during cardiopulmonary bypass appears to have been of significant importance in resolving the problem.

Postoperative follow-up and evaluation

After repair, all patients are closely followed clinically. Routine echocardiography and nuclear pulmonary flow scans are performed at least every 3 months. In patients in whom the VSD is left open or a shunt is made to the unifocalized PA system, cardiac catheterization is performed approximately 3 months postoperatively. If the Qp:Qs ratio is over 2:1, the VSD is closed. If less than 2:1, the PA system is assessed for stenotic lesions that may be amenable to percutaneous catheter-based or surgical intervention. Following VSD closure, the status of the conduit from the right ventricle to the PA is closely followed by serial clinical and echocardiographic evaluation in order to look for stenosis or insufficiency. Cardiac catheterization is performed electively approximately 1 year following complete repair.

CURRENT OUTCOMES

Reddy and colleagues reported the outcomes of 85 patients with Pa, VSD, and MAPCAs.[12] Fifty-six underwent complete one-stage unifocalization and intracardiac repair. In 23 patients, the VSD was left open at the time of complete unifocalization. There were 6 early and 7 late deaths. Actuarial 3-year survival was 80 percent.

Rodefeld and colleagues[13] reported on patients with diminutive PAs who required creation of an aortopulmonary window. In the series of 18 patients with confluent diminutive PAs who underwent the procedure, there was 100 percent early survival; the 2 late deaths were unrelated to the procedure. Follow-up angiography demonstrated excellent development of the true PAs.

Hanley and associates have now accumulated data on 307 patients with VSD and MAPCAs who were managed as described.[17] Median age at first surgery was 8 months. Initial operation was complete unifocalization via median sternotomy in 85 percent. Intracardiac repair was achieved at initial operation in 56 percent and in 83 percent within 2 years. Early mortality was 9.7 percent in the first half of the experience and 2 percent in the second half. Late follow-up was 81 percent complete up to 12 years, with 6.3 percent mortality. Kaplan-Meier survival was 91 percent at 1 year, 86 percent at 5 years, and 86 percent at 10 years.

References

1. Rabinovitch M, Herrera-DeLeon V, Casteneda AR, et al. Growth and development of the pulmonary vascular bed in patients with tetralogy of Fallot with or without pulmonary atresia. *Circulation* 1981;64:1234–1249.
2. Perry LW, Neill CA, Ferencz C, et al. Infants with congenital heart disease: The cases. In. Ferencz C, Rubin JD, Loffredo CA et al (eds). *Perspectives in Pediatric Cardiology: Epidemiology of Congenital Heart Disease.* The Baltimore-Washington Infant Study 1981–1989. Armonk, NY: Futura; 1993:33–62.
3. Marelli AJ, Perloff JK, Child JS, et al. Pulmonary atresia with ventricular septal defect in adults. *Circulation* 1994;89:243–251.
4. Puga FJ, Leoni FE, Julsrud PR, et al. Complete repair of pulmonary atresia, ventricular septal defect, and severe peripheral arborization abnormalities of the central pulmonary arteries. *J Thorac Cardiovasc Surg* 1989;98:1018–1028.
5. Sawatari K, Imai Y, Kurosawa H, et al. Staged operation for pulmonary atresia and ventricular septal defect with major aortopulmonary collateral arteries. *J Thorac Cardiovasc Surg* 1989;98:738–750.
6. Iyer KS, Mee RBB. Staged repair of pulmonary atresia with ventricular septal defect and major systemic to pulmonary artery collaterals. *Ann Thorac Surg* 1991;51:65–72.
7. Cho JM, Puga FJ, Danielson GK, et al. Early and long term results of the surgical treatment of tetralogy of Fallot with pulmonary atresia with or without major aortopulmonary collateral arteries. *J Thorac Cardiovasc Surg* 2002;124:70–81.
8. Duncan B, Mee RB, Prieto L, et al. Staged repair of tetralogy of Fallot with pulmonary atresia and major aortopulmonary collateral arteries. *J Thorac Cardiovasc Surg* 2003;126:692–704.
9. Gupta A, Odim J, Levi D, et al. Staged repair of pulmonary atresia with ventricular septal defect and major aortopulmonary collateral arteries: Experience with 104 patients. *J Thorac Cardiovasc Surg* 2003;126:1746–1752.
10. Reddy VM, Liddicoat JR, Hanley FL. Midline one stage complete unifocalization and repair of pulmonary atresia with ventricular septal defect and major aorto-pulmonary collaterals. *J Thorac Cardiovasc Surg* 1995;109:832–845.
11. McElhinney DB, Reddy VM, Hanley FL. Tetralogy of Fallot with major aortopulmonary collaterals: Early total repair. *Pediatric Cardiol* 1998;19:289–296.
12. Reddy VM, McElhinney DB, Amin Z, et al. Early and intermediate outcomes after repair of pulmonary atresia with ventricular septal defect and major aortopulmonary collateral arteries: Experience with 85 patients. *Circulation* 2000;101:1826–1832.
13. Rodefeld MD, Reddy VM, Thompson LD, et al. Surgical creation of aortopulmonary window in selected patients with pulmonary atresia and with poorly developed aortopulmonary collaterals and hypoplastic pulmonary arteries. *J Thorac Cardiovasc Surg* 2002;123:1147–1154.
14. Reddy VM, Petrossian E, McElhinney DB, et al. One stage unifocalization in infants: When should the ventricular septal defect be closed? *J Thorac Cardiovasc Surg* 1997;113:858–866.
15. Hanley FL , Reddy VM. Pulmonary atresia with ventricular septal defect and major Aortopulmonary collaterals (Spray TL, editor's comments). In: *Mastery of Cardiothoracic Surgery.* Philadelphia: Lippincott-Raven; 1998:830.
16. Scavo VA, Turrentine MW, Antifiero TX, et al. Valved bovine jugular venous conduits for right ventricular to pulmonary artery reconstruction. *ASAIO J* 1999;45: 482–487.
17. Hanley FL, Reinhartz O, Suleman S, et al. Management of major aortopulmonary collateral arteries. Abstract submitted to AHA 2005.

CHAPTER

62 PULMONARY STENOSIS AND PULMONARY ATRESIA WITH INTACT VENTRICULAR SEPTUM

Mark D. Plunkett, Fotios Mitropoulos, Hillel Laks

PULMONARY STENOSIS

Pulmonary stenosis accounts for 8 to 10 percent of all congenital heart defects. The pulmonary valve is dome-shaped, with commissural fusion and variable subvalvar right ventricular outflow tract (RVOT) obstruction. The pulmonary annulus may be normal in size or smaller than predicted, and a patent foramen ovale (PFO) or atrial septal defect (ASD) is usually present. Clinical presentation is variable. Although severe pulmonary stenosis may present in the newborn period, most of these lesions do not manifest significant signs and symptoms until later in childhood. Clinical findings are directly related to the severity of the stenosis and degree of shunting across the atrial septum. Timing of intervention is based on severity of clinical findings and an RVOT gradient in excess of 50 mmHg. Both catheterization with balloon valvotomy and surgical valvotomy are associated with low morbidity and mortality and excellent long-term survival.

PULMONARY ATRESIA WITH INTACT INTERVENTRICULAR SEPTUM

Pulmonary atresia (Pa) with intact interventricular septum (IVS) is an uncommon lesion that represents between 1 and 3 percent of all congenital heart lesions. There is no communication between the right ventricle and the pulmonary arteries, and a patent ductus arteriosus (PDA) is essential for early survival. The defect presents with varying degrees of hypoplasia of the right ventricle and tricuspid valve and often involves right ventricle-to-coronary artery fistulas (45 percent) and right ventricle (RV) dependent coronary circulation (10 percent).

In neonates with Pa/IVS, surgical classification of right ventricular hypoplasia into mild (more than two-thirds of normal) moderate (one-third to two-thirds of normal), and severe (less than one-third of normal) is useful in selecting the surgical management, requiring either valvotomy, shunting, and possibly tricuspid valvotomy.

KEY CONCEPTS

- Pulmonary Stenosis
  - Right ventricular outflow tract obstruction at the level of the pulmonary valve.
  - Pulmonary annulus may be stenotic or normal.
  - Treatment is often with balloon valvotomy versus surgical valvotomy.
  - Recurrent stenosis and insufficiency is common with surgical or balloon valvotomy.
- Pulmonary atresia with intact ventricular septum
  - Complex defect with complete absence of communication between right ventricle and pulmonary arteries.
  - Characterized by varying degrees of right ventricle and tricuspid valve hypoplasia.
  - Multiple surgical interventions common in childhood.
  - Surgical treatment strategies based on size and development of right ventricle and tricuspid valve.

A similar classification is used in older children. Patients are stratified into those who will benefit from an attempt to achieve a biventricular repair and those who are best suited for a Fontan palliation scheme.

PULMONARY STENOSIS

DEFINITION

Pulmonary stenosis (PS) with intact ventricular septum (IVS) is characterized by right ventricular outflow tract (RVOT) obstruction at the level of the pulmonary valve. The pulmonary valve is typically dome-shaped, with commissural fusion of the leaflets and a small central orifice. The pulmonary annulus may be either normal in size or smaller than predicted by the patient's weight. The right ventricle is usually of normal size and morphology but may develop right ventricular hypertrophy very early in life and lead to further obstruction at the infundibular level.

HISTORICAL NOTE

The initial pathologic description of PS is credited to Morgagni in 1761. The first attempt at surgical treatment of this lesion is attributed to Doyen in 1913. In his report, Doyen described a transventricular valvotomy using a tenotomy knife, with an unsuccessful outcome.[1] In 1948, Sellors and Brock reported successful blunt valve dilatation using a transventricular approach.[2] Several successful cases of open pulmonary valvotomy using systemic hypothermia and ventricular fibrillation also followed. Open pulmonary valvotomy with the use of cardiopulmonary bypass was successfully introduced in 1955. This remained the primary treatment for patients with pulmonary stenosis until the technique of balloon valvotomy was introduced by Semb and associates in 1979. In 1982, Kan and associates first reported successful percutaneous balloon valvotomy in patients with pulmonary stenosis.[3]

EPIDEMIOLOGY

Obstructive lesions of the RVOT are found in 25 to 30 percent of children with congenital heat disease. Isolated PS at level of the pulmonary valve with an intact IVS accounts for approximately 8 to 10 percent of all congenital heart defects, with a slightly higher incidence in females. Without intervention, the onset of hypoxia and heart failure in neonates carries an extremely high mortality. There is a reported increased incidence of 2 to 4 percent in siblings of patients with this particular defect.

ETIOLOGY AND PATHOGENESIS

As in the case of most congenital heart defects, the etiology of this lesion is unknown. Failure of the pulmonary valve leaflets to form and separate adequately during embryonic development results in limited mobility and stenosis of the valve. The consequent turbulence of blood flow across this region during subsequent growth and development leads to fibrous distortion of the valve leaflets and further increases the degree of stenosis. Right ventricular hypertrophy develops secondarily and is directly related to the severity of the obstruction. Rarely, neonates may present with enlarged right ventricles and cardiomyopathy, which is associated with poor prognosis despite early intervention.

CLINICAL FEATURES

Neonates with critical PS who present in the newborn period develop severe cyanosis and congestive heart failure. The clinical findings are directly related to the severity of the stenosis as well as to the degree of shunting across the interatrial septum. On physical examination, most children with pulmonary stenosis present with a harsh holosystolic ejection murmur, an ejection click, and a palpable thrill over the pulmonic valve region. These neonates often appear irritable, tachypneic, and hypoxic due to right-to-left shunting at the atrial level. Although severe PS may present in the newborn period, most of these lesions do not manifest significant clinical findings until later in childhood. The timing of intervention is usually determined by the severity of clinical findings or a documented gradient of 50 mmHg or greater across the RVOT. The results of treatment are directly related to the size of the right ventricle and the patient's age at presentation.

LABORATORY AND DIAGNOSTIC FEATURES

An electrocardiogram typically reveals right axis deviation, prominent p waves, and right ventricular hypertrophy. On the chest radiograph, prominent pulmonary artery (PA) shadows secondary to poststenotic dilatation can be observed. The cardiac shadow is usually normal except in severe cases with associated congestive heart failure. Transthoracic echocardiographic examination establishes the severity of the stenosis and identifies any associated anomalies. Cardiac catheterization is performed to obtain other additional diagnostic information and possibly to perform therapeutic intervention with a balloon valvotomy.

DIFFERENTIAL DIAGNOSIS

The differential diagnosis includes all congenital heart defects that have RVOT obstruction as an anatomic finding. They include defects such as tetralogy of Fallot, PS with ventricular septal defect (VSD), Pa/IVS, and all morphologic cardiac abnormalities characterized by infundibular obstruction. Echocardiography can easily delineate these defects in most patients, and identify those with isolated PS with an intact ventricular septum.

THERAPY

The medical management of these patients is similar to that for any neonate or child with RVOT obstruction. In the neonate with severe PS and cyanosis, ductal patency must be maintained with prostaglandin infusion and pulmonary vascular resistance reduced to ensure adequate pulmonary blood flow. Systemic hypotension is avoided, as it may result in reduced ductal flow and subsequent hypoxemia. These patients may also have dynamic obstruction in the infundibular region secondary to right ventricular myocardial hypertrophy. Inotropic agents must therefore be used with caution, as increased contractility may, in turn, worsen functional obstruction across the RVOT, further compromising pulmonary perfusion. After initial stabilization (with or without percutaneous intervention), operative valvotomy can be performed as a semielective procedure, as either an open technique using cardiopulmonary bypass or with a transventricular approach without extracorporeal circulation.

Operative procedures

Open pulmonary valvotomy using cardiopulmonary bypass

Open pulmonary valvotomy is performed through a median sternotomy using cardiopulmonary bypass and bicaval cannulation. The patent ductus arteriosus (PDA) is ligated or snared prior to the initiation of cardiopulmonary bypass. An aortic cross clamp is applied and antegrade cardioplegia is administered through the aortic root to achieve myocardial arrest. Cardioplegic arrest may be omitted and the procedure performed on bypass with the heart beating if no septation defect is present. The patent foramen ovale or ASD is closed through a right atriotomy incision, either primarily or with a patch of autologous pericardium. A vertical arteriotomy is then performed on the anterior wall of the main PA and extended down to the level of the pulmonary valve. The stenotic valve is inspected, and the fused commissures are carefully incised with a no. 11 scalpel or fine vascular scissors. The incisions in the valve should extend to the annulus (Fig. 62-1). Any valvular adhesions to the PA wall are sharply incised. A partial valvectomy may be necessary to remove thickened valve tissue or dense fibrous scarring on dysplastic leaflets. The infundibulum is then inspected through the valve for any subvalvular stenosis, and sharp infundibular resection may be performed if necessary. The arteriotomy may be closed primarily or with a patch of autologous or bovine pericardium to reduce any residual obstruction. A transannular patch may be required if the annulus is small.

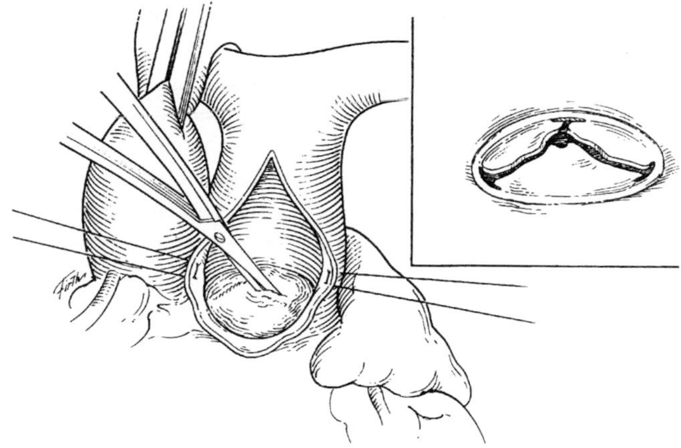

Figure 62-1 Open pulmonary valvotomy using cardiopulmonary bypass. The pulmonary valve is approached through a vertical arteriotomy and the fused commissures are incised with a no. 11 scalpel or fine scissors.

Off-Pump transventricular pulmonary valvotomy

If no ASD is present, a pulmonary valvotomy may be performed through a median sternotomy using an off-pump transventricular technique. A purse-string suture is placed in the anterior wall of the right ventricle. An angiocatheter connected to a pressure transducer is first introduced through the purse-string suture in the right ventricle and into the PA. Using the same technique, progressively larger metal dilators are then introduced across the valve membrane. If the valve tissue does not dilate easily, a long vascular clamp can be used to initially disrupt the valve tissue. After adequate dilation is achieved, the purse string is tied and reinforced. If adequate relief of obstruction is not achieved, then open valvotomy may be performed or a systemic-to-pulmonary shunt may be added to augment pulmonary flow.

Results

Most patients with PS are operated on electively and require routine pre- and postoperative care. In neonates, the management of acidosis, electrolyte derangements, and congestive heart failure should be aggressively pursued prior to surgery. Following operative correction, there is often a residual gradient across the RVOT. Inotropic support should be used cautiously during postoperative care in order to avoid exacerbation of any residual infundibular obstruction. Mild and moderate residual gradients often resolve with age and the patient's growth.

Both balloon valvotomy and surgical valvotomy are associated with low morbidity and mortality rates and excellent long-term survival. Each has a significant incidence of recurrent stenosis, requiring additional early or late interventions. There is also a significant incidence of pulmonary valve insufficiency following both procedures. Mild to moderate pulmonary insufficiency is tolerated remarkably well by most patients, and its long-term clinical importance is a current topic of investigation. Although late mortality is not reportedly changed in patients with significant pulmonary insufficiency, the development of right ventricular enlargement, right ventricular dysrhythmias, and abnormal right ventricular response to exercise may lead to increased morbidity in these patients and a resultant need for late pulmonary valve replacement.

A multi-institutional study by Hanley and associates reported a 30-day survival of 89 percent and a 4-year survival of 81 percent for all modes of intervention in neonates with critical PS.[4] Of note, 26 percent of these patients required reintervention within 2 years for residual stenosis (defined as a gradient greater than or equal to 30 mmHg). Following successful pulmonary valvotomy (after either initial intervention or reintervention), right ventricular size approaches normal in more than 90 percent of these patients. A report by Rao and associates on 80 patients treated initially with balloon valvotomy with follow-up between 3 and 10 years showed a freedom from repeat balloon valvotomy or surgery of 88 and 84 percent at 5 and 10 years, respectively.[5] Furthermore, surgical reintervention in older children is associated with minimal morbidity and mortality and excellent short- and long-term outcomes.

PULMONARY ATRESIA WITH INTACT VENTRICULAR SEPTUM

DEFINITION

By definition there is no communication between the right ventricle (RV) and pulmonary arteries; patency of the ductus arteriosus is essential for early survival. The defect presents with varying degrees of hypoplasia of the RV and tricuspid valve and often involves fistulas from the RV to the coronary artery. Morphologically and functionally, the hypoplastic tricuspid valve usually varies in direct correlation to the size of the RV. Coronary artery fistulas are present in 45 percent of cases and are more common in patients with severely hypoplastic RVs and small but competent tricuspid valves. Additionally, it should be noted that an Ebstein's malformation of the tricuspid valve might be present in some cases. These patients may present with marked cardiomegaly due to right atrial enlargement, severe tricuspid regurgitation, and a relatively normal RV size.

HISTORICAL NOTE

Surgical treatment of this pulmonary atresia/intact ventricular septum (Pa/IVS) was historically associated with very high morbidity and mortality. The low incidence of this defect combined with its extreme morphologic variability delayed the development of a standardized approach to surgical therapy.

The original Greenwold classification[6] of Pa/IVS described this defect by two types of RVs: type I with a hypoplastic RV and type II with a normal or dilated RV. A further refinement of this classification was offered by Goor and Lillihei, who described the tripartite morphology of the RV (a sinus inlet part, a trabecular part, and a conus or outlet portion) and used this as a basis for surgical therapy.[7] Bull and associates introduced as part of the pre- and intraoperative decision-making process the actual annular diameter of the tricuspid valve.[8] More recently, the surgical approach to Pa/IVS has been based primarily on a quantitative Z-score assessment of the tricuspid valve diameter.[9] The Z score is determined by comparing the estimated diameter of the tricuspid valve (as measured by echocardiography) to the expected "normal" size and calculating the difference in standard deviations. In 1989, Billingsley and associates from UCLA introduced a surgically oriented classification of mild, moderate, and severe hypoplasia of the RV, as described below.[10] With a more systematic approach to this defect, increasing surgical experience, and improved diagnostic modalities, outcomes from the surgical treatment of Pa/IVS have steadily improved.

EPIDEMIOLOGY

In contrast to other forms of RVOT obstruction, Pa/IVS is an uncommon congenital cardiac malformation, representing between 1 and 3 percent of all congenital heart defects.[11] Without early surgical intervention, children with Pa/IVS have an extremely high mortality rate. The natural history in untreated patients is a 50 percent mortality rate at 2 weeks of life and approximately 85 percent at 6 months.[12] Death occurs as a consequence of severe hypoxemia and progressive metabolic acidosis secondary to closure of the ductus arteriosus. In general, most children with Pa/IVS will require multiple surgical interventions during childhood.

ETIOLOGY AND PATHOGENESIS

The etiology of this defect remains unknown. A failure of formation of a patent pulmonary valve during embryonic development results in a completely obstructed RVOT.

Since the ventricular septum remains intact, forward blood flow through the RV is precluded. The growth and development of the RV and tricuspid valve (TV) are severely compromised by this lack of forward flow. Both structures tend to follow a similar pattern of hypoplasia, which is reflected by the TV annular size and the reduced size and volume of the RV chamber. RV–to–coronary artery fistulas are present in 45 percent of cases and are more common in those patients with a severely hypoplastic RV and a small competent TV.[13] In 10 percent of patients, the coronary circulation may by dependent on RV pressure for perfusion by way of fistulous communications associated with proximal coronary stenosis. Pulmonary blood flow is dependent almost entirely on a PDA, as aortopulmonary collaterals are uncommon with this defect. Ebstein's malformation of the TV is seen in some patients, adding to the severity of the defect. No specific genetic pattern of inheritance has been identified.

CLINICAL FEATURES

Although prenatal diagnosis is increasing for many congenital heart defects, most neonates with Pa/IVS are diagnosed shortly after birth. The diagnosis is often prompted by varying degrees of hypoxia and cyanosis within the first week of life. Physical examination is often remarkable for prominent venous pulsations. A significant systolic murmur may be indicative of tricuspid regurgitation. This must be differentiated from the continuous murmur of a PDA. Neonates with hypoxia and poor perfusion in spite of medical management should be evaluated for the presence of a restrictive ASD. In this case, balloon septostomy should be performed to relieve the obstruction at the atrial level. Neonates with severely hypoplastic RVs may also require open atrial septostomy. Classification of the defect is determined by echocardiography; cardiac catheterization and an appropriate operative procedure are selected based on assessment of RV morphology, TV size, the RVOT and the coronary circulation.

LABORATORY AND DIAGNOSTIC FEATURES

In neonates with Pa/IVS, an electrocardiogram shows progressive evidence of RA enlargement with prominent P waves. The pattern of RV hypertrophy that is present in most neonates is absent. A chest radiograph is usually unremarkable at birth but may later reveal an increased heart shadow secondary to RA and left ventricular enlargement. The lung fields are usually clear with normal to diminished vascular markings. Echocardiography remains the initial diagnostic study to identify the anatomic abnormalities and assess RV morphology. The size of the ventricular cavity, valve dimensions and function, and the nature of the RVOT obstruction can be evaluated. Because of the complexity and morphologic variability of Pa/IVS, the anomaly must be defined by both echocardiography and right/left heart catheterization. Catheterization should determine the size and competency of the TV, the degree of RV hypoplasia, the size of the pulmonary arteries, the coronary anatomy and presence of coronary sinusoids and fistulas, and ventricular function. Selective coronary injections and an injection into the RV are also required for a complete evaluation. RV–to–coronary artery fistulas are frequently accompanied by the development of fibrous intimal hyperplasia, resulting in stenosis or complete obstruction of the native coronary circulation. The presence of obstructive lesions in the proximal coronaries may produce a "RV-dependent coronary circulation" (RVDCC). Such patients are at high risk for myocardial ischemia, as desaturated blood from the RV perfuses a significant portion of the myocardium. An even greater risk of myocardial ischemia is incurred by the reduction of diastolic aortic pressure resulting from the creation of a systemic-to-PA shunt. In such patients, decompression of the RV by either an outflow tract patch or a pulmonary or tricuspid valvotomy is poorly tolerated and may lead to acute myocardial infarction and intraoperative demise. The presence or absence of a RVDCC must be established in a neonate prior to determining the operative strategy.

DIFFERENTIAL DIAGNOSIS

The differential diagnosis encompasses all congenital heart defects with Pa. This includes such defects as Pa with VSD and single-ventricle defects associated with Pa. Echocardiography can easily delineate these defects in most patients, and correctly identify those with isolated PA/IVS. Cardiac catheterization is furthermore performed in almost all affected neonates to confirm the diagnosis and define the anatomy.

THERAPY

Previous surgical experience has indicated that the surgical management of patients with Pa/IVS should be based primarily on an anatomic classification system that specifically defines the degree of RV hypoplasia. A variety of surgical strategies have been proposed for the treatment of these infants.[14–19] We and others have found classification of the RV hypoplasia more accurate and consistent with surgical outcomes.[20–24] Using this approach, neonates with Pa/IVS are initially separated into three groups of mild, moderate, and severe RV hypoplasia. In patients with mild RV hypoplasia, the TV and RV cavity are approximately two-thirds or greater of the calculated normal size, and the RVOT is well developed. This usually correlates with a Z score for the TV between 0 and –2. In patients with moderate RV hypoplasia, the TV and the RV cavity are approximately one-half of calculated normal size (with a range of one-third to two-thirds of normal) and the pulmonary outflow tract is usually developed enough to perform an effective pulmonary valvotomy. This usually correlates with a Z score for the TV of –2 to –4. In patients with severe RV hypoplasia, the TV and RV cavity are one-third or less of calculated normal size and the pulmonary outflow tract is not amenable to an effective pulmonary valvotomy. This usually correlates with a Z score for the TV of –4 to –6. This approach is not based on any single anatomic component such as the size of the tricuspid annulus but instead assesses the overall RV morphology and the degree of both TV and RV hypoplasia.

During the initial evaluation of patients with Pa/IVS, special attention must be paid to the anatomy of the coronary circulation. Abnormalities of the coronary circulation are often found in the severely hypoplastic group and dictate which surgical management options are indicated.[25] During fetal development, RV hypertension may cause intramyocardial sinusoids to develop. These sinusoids may branch extensively into blind channels or communicate by fistulas with the coronary artery circulation. The morphology of these sinusoids and their specific communications are extremely variable. Proximal coronary artery stenoses or obstructions may develop in a coronary artery supplied by these intramyocardial sinusoids. If the distal coronary artery flow is dependent on these sinusoids for adequate myocardial perfusion, they are termed RV-dependent coronary circulations (RVDCC).[26] Decompression of the RV in these patients is contraindicated and may lead to acute myocardial ischemia and death.

Surgical management of neonates

Almost all neonates with Pa/IVS will require surgical management early in life in order to survive. Treatment with prostaglandin E_1 maintains pulmonary flow through the PDA and allows time for medical stabilization, diagnostic evaluation, and surgical decision making. Once the anatomy and morphology of these lesions have been defined by echocardiography and right/left cardiac catheterization, classification is determined and an appropriate operative strategy initiated. Delay in surgical treatment is hazardous and may reduce early survival.

The surgical approach to most patients is based on the degree of RV hypoplasia (Table 62-1). Initial surgical management of most neonates with Pa/IVS involves the establishment of a reliable and adequate source of pulmonary blood flow while optimizing the potential for growth and development of the RV and TV.

Table 62-1 Surgical management of pulmonary atresia with intact ventricular septum in neonates according to the degree of right ventricular hypoplasia

Classification of RV hypoplasia	Classification	Treatment
Mild	Tricuspid valve and RV cavity more than two-thirds normal size, well-developed RVOT	Pulmonary valvotomy and shunt or valvotomy only
Moderate	Tricuspid valve and RV cavity one-third to two-thirds normal size, moderately hypoplastic RVOT	Pulmonary valvotomy and shunt
Severe	Tricuspid valve and RV cavity less than one-third normal size, severely hypoplastic or absent RVOT	Shunt only or shunt and tricuspid valvotomy

RV = right ventricle; RVOT = right venticular outflow tract.

Neonates with mild right ventricular hypoplasia

Neonates with Pa/IVS and mild RV hypoplasia are best treated with a pulmonary valvotomy, insertion of an aorta-to-PA shunt, and ligation of the ductus arteriosus. Occasionally there are patients in whom a pulmonary valvotomy alone will restore adequate pulmonary blood flow. Experience has shown that initial valvotomy alone often fails to produce effective palliation despite favorable anatomy. In most instances, it is preferable to perform a small shunt to ensure adequate pulmonary blood flow and promote subsequent growth of the branch PAs.

Neonates with moderate right ventricular hypoplasia

Neonates with PA/IVS and moderate RV hypoplasia are best treated with a pulmonary valvotomy, augmentation of the pulmonary outflow tract, insertion of an aorta-to-PA shunt, and ligation of the ductus arteriosus. Pulmonary valvotomy and augmentation of the pulmonary outflow tract relieves RV hypertension, reduces tricuspid regurgitation, and potentiates the growth of both the tricuspid annulus and the RV cavity. This may allow for a subsequent biventricular repair as the definitive procedure. A transannular pericardial patch may be necessary to augment the RVOT. This procedure can be performed off pump without using cardiopulmonary bypass, which is preferred in neonates where a mixed circulation will persist postoperatively.

Neonates with severe right ventricular hypoplasia

Neonates with Pa/IVS and severe RV hypoplasia are more difficult to manage surgically. Balloon atrial septostomy is recommended at the time of cardiac catheterization, and stenting of the ductus arteriosus may be considered as well. Pulmonary valvotomy is usually not effective in relieving RV hypertension. These neonates are best treated with an aorta-to-PA shunt or a subclavian artery-to-PA (modified Blalock-Taussig) shunt. If there are no RV sinusoids or there are tortuous, narrow sinusoids without broad coronary artery fistulas, the RV is decompressed by incising the TV. This can be performed using a closed technique without cardiopulmonary bypass. In most cases, decompression of the RV results in regression of the narrow, tortuous type of sinusoid and does not result in myocardial ischemia (if the native coronary circulation is intact). Frequently, broad fistulas from the coronary arteries to the RV can be identified on the epicardial surface of the heart and directly ligated.

Specific operative procedures for neonates

Below are described some specific techniques utilized in patients with Pa/IVS. Details on systemic-to-pulmonary shunts are presented in Chap. 54, while insertion of a transannular patch is described in Chap 60.

Insertion of a transannular right ventricular outflow tract patch via sternotomy

A transannular patch can be placed with relative ease on cardiopulmonary bypass, with aortic and right atrial cannulation and ligation of the ductus arteriosus. In some cases with moderate RV hypoplasia, the infundibulum is long and narrow but reaches the pulmonary valve membrane. In these cases, a pericardial transannular patch may be inserted without bypass (Fig. 62-2A to C). A median sternotomy incision is used. A pediatric cross clamp is placed immediately beneath the bifurcation of

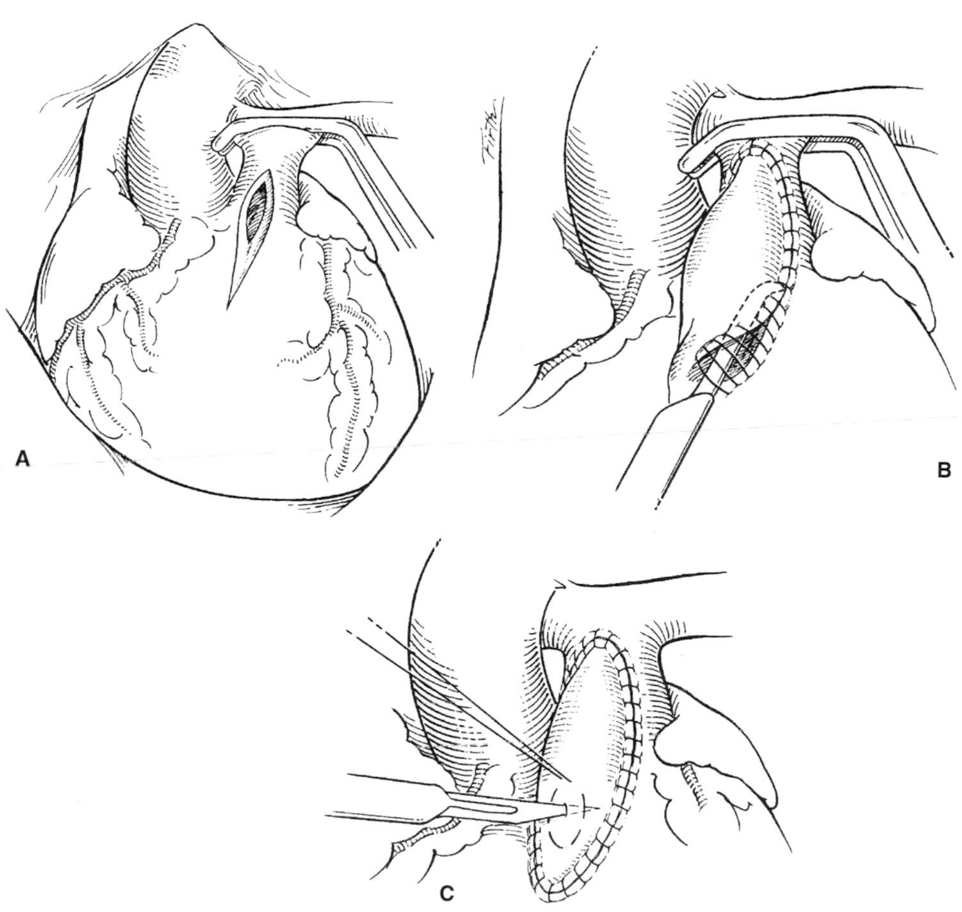

Figure 62-2 Off-pump transannular pulmonary outflow tract pericardial patch. **A.** A cross clamp is placed on the main pulmonary artery as shown. The main pulmonary artery is incised and extended with a partial-thickness incision of the myocardium. **B.** The pericardial patch suture is left loose along the inferior edge until the annulus is divided and the right ventricular myocardium is completely incised into the outflow tract. **C.** Additional opening of the right ventricular outflow tract can be achieved with a no. 11 scalpel through a purse-string suture in the patch.

the PA. The ductus is kept open to provide pulmonary blood flow. A vertical incision is made in the main PA down to the RV junction. A partial thickness incision is made over the RV for a distance to bring the incision over the RV cavity. Part of the muscle is resected to a depth of 2 to 3 mm to thin out the RV. A pericardial patch is then sutured to the pulmonary arteriotomy with a running polypropylene down to the RV junction. The suture line is continued to the edges of the RV incision leaving the sutures loose inferiorly. A no. 12 scalpel is then used to incise the valve membrane and to cut into the RV cavity under the pericardial patch. The sutures are pulled up to control bleeding and the cross clamp is removed. If the RV pressure is not adequately reduced, a rhizotomy knife is introduced through a purse-string suture in the pericardial patch and the RV muscle is further incised until an adequate outflow tract has been created to reduce the RV pressure to an acceptable level.

Off-Pump pulmonary valvotomy via left thoracotomy

A pulmonary valvotomy may be performed using a closed technique through a left thoracotomy. The approach is through the fourth intercostal space, with the lung retracted to expose the hilar region. The overlying pericardium is incised and the left PA identified. The main PA and PDA are then identified and the main PA is dissected from surrounding tissue. Care is taken to avoid dissection of the PDA to maintain its patency during the procedure. The main PA is cross-clamped immediately below the bifurcation, allowing pulmonary perfusion to continue via the ductus arteriosus. The artery is then incised longitudinally and retracted to expose the valve. The fused commissures are identified and incised sharply with a no. 11 scalpel. A thin-bladed vascular C clamp is applied to the incision in the PA and the cross clamp is removed. A Gore-Tex shunt can then be sutured to the main PA and to the subclavian artery using techniques similar to those used for a modified Blalock-Taussig shunt. The ductus arteriosus is ligated prior to releasing flow into the shunt.

Closed tricuspid valvotomy

This technique is used in patients with severe RV hypoplasia where the possibility of a subsequent biventricular repair is reduced. As mentioned above, preoperative catheterization must determine the absence of sinusoids or RVDCC prior to decompression of the RV. The closed tricuspid valvotomy can be performed through a median sternotomy or via a right thoracotomy. The pericardium is incised anterior to the phrenic nerve and a purse-string suture is placed in the right atrial appendage. An instrument is made using a rhizotomy knife with a small curved blade passed through a segment of red rubber tubing as described in previous reports.[22] A pressure-measuring needle is placed into the tubing and connected to a transducing monitor. The tubing is then introduced into the right atrium and passed into the RV while monitoring the pressure. The knife blade is then exposed in the RV and the TV is cut anteriorly. Care is taken to avoid incising the area of the conduction system posteriorly. When the RV pressure has fallen to one-half systemic or less, the knife is retracted into the tubing, which is then removed from the right atrium. The purse-string suture is tied to achieve hemostasis. We have found that decompression of the RV results in regression of the narrow, tortuous type of sinusoid and does not result in myocardial ischemia if the native circulation is intact.

Surgical management of older children

Infants with Pa/IVS are followed closely after their initial palliative procedures. With improving results, an increasing number of patients are presenting for later interventions. A cardiac catheterization is performed at 3 to 6 months of age, depending on the infant's initial morphology and subsequent echocardiographic findings. In patients with severe RV hypoplasia, repeat catheterization at 2 to 3 months is recommended, as there may be a high mortality in this group while awaiting repair. The selection of operative procedures is once again based primarily on RV morphology and an assessment of the TV and RV growth since the previous intervention. Whereas in neonates the size of the TV and the RV usually correlate, in older children there can be a significant discrepancy between these two measurements. Definitive procedures will be determined based on the anatomic findings at catheterization. These patients are again divided into those with mild, moderate, or severe hypoplasia (Table 62-2).

The use of an adjustable snare to close the ASD permits right-to-left shunting at the atrial level in children where RV volume and compliance may limit forward outflow to the pulmonary arteries. The ability to adjust the size of the ASD allows for postoperative control of right-to-left shunting and the adjustment of forward flow through the RV.[27,28] This can be helpful in optimizing cardiac output and avoiding excessive cyanosis.

Biventricular repair for patients with mild right ventricular hypoplasia

In patients with mild RV hypoplasia, later surgical intervention includes closure of the ASD with an adjustable snare, enlargement of the RV cavity and outflow tract by myocardial resection, and patch augmentation of the RVOT. In order to achieve a competent pulmonary valve, either a pericardial monocusp valve or a bioprosthetic tissue valve is inserted in the RVOT. A successful biventricular repair is achieved in the majority of these patients. Some patients with mild hypoplasia treated by valvotomy may not require subsequent surgery unless the obstruction to the outflow tract has recurred.

Biventricular and partial biventricular repair for patients with moderate right ventricular hypoplasia

In the patient with moderate RV hypoplasia, definitive repair is dictated by the previous growth and development

Table 62-2 Approaches for definitive repair of patients with pulmonary atresia with intact ventricular septum

Classification of RV hypoplasia	Treatment options
Mild	Closure of ASD (adjustable snare), enlargement of RV and RVOT, and transannular patch with monocusp valve. Ligation of previous shunt.
	Closure of ASD (adjustable snare), enlargement of RV and RVOT, and valved pulmonary homograft. Ligation of previous shunt.
Moderate	Closure of ASD (adjustable snare), bidirectional Glenn shunt, enlargement of RV and RVOT, and transannular patch with oversized bioprosthetic valve. Ligation of previous shunt.
	Closure of ASD (adjustable snare), bidirectional Glenn shunt, enlargement of RV and RVOT, and valved pulmonary homograft. Ligation of previous shunt.
Severe	Staged bidirectional Glenn shunt for later Fontan procedure.
	Adjustable ASD. Partial ligation of previous shunt.
	Lateral tunnel Fontan with adjustable ASD. Ligation of previous shunt.
	Extracardiac Fontan with adjustable ASD. Ligation of previous shunt.

ASD = atriel septal defect; RV = right ventricle; RVOT = right venticular outflow tract.

of the RV and the TV. If the TV diameter is one-half to two-thirds normal size, then repair consists of partial closure of the ASD with an adjustable snare, enlargement of the RV cavity by myocardial resection, and insertion of a valved conduit between the RV and the PA. A monocusp trans-annular patch from native pericardium may be used in smaller patients. If the TV diameter is one-third to one-half of normal, then repair consists of partial closure of the ASD with an adjustable snare, enlargement of the RV cavity, creation of a bidirectional Glenn shunt, and insertion of a valved conduit between the RV and PA. The Glenn shunt reduces the volume load on the small RV and provides an obligatory source of pulmonary blood flow. This allows the channeling of approximately one-third of the systemic venous return from the superior vena cava directly to the pulmonary arteries while the inferior vena cava (two-thirds of the systemic venous return) continues to pass through the TV and RV. This has been termed the "one-and-one-half ventricle" or "partial biventricular" repair. The ASD is adjustable to create a gradient between right atrium (RA) and left atrium to encourage forward flow through the RV. This will in turn enhance its development (as well as that of the TV) increasing the likelihood of a two-ventricle repair. Based on the subsequent growth of the RV and the TV, either a two-ventricle repair (with take-down of the Glenn shunt) or a completion Fontan reconstruction may follow.

Staged Fontan procedures for patients with severe right ventricular hypoplasia

In patients with Pa/IVS and severe RV hypoplasia (one-third of normal size or less), a biventricular repair is usually not possible. Most of these patients will have undergone placement of a systemic-to-PA shunt in the neonatal period with or without tricuspid valvotomy, depending on the presence or absence of RVDCC. The Glenn bidirectional cavopulmonary shunt is performed in the first 3 to 6 months of life with a plan for a Fontan procedure (total cavopulmonary connection, see also Chap. 69) within the first 3 to 4 years of life. A fenestration of the Fontan is used in our practice as an ASD with an adjustable snare. The Fontan may be performed either as a lateral tunnel or as an extracardiac conduit.

Surgical management of children with Pa/IVS with Ebstein's malformation

Ebstein's malformation of the TV is present in 10 percent of patients with Pa/IVS. This group of neonates should be considered separately. Most of these patients will have severe TV insufficiency and a normal-sized or enlarged RV. There is also massive dilatation of the RA. The left ventricle is often compromised in these infants because of the dilated dysfunctional RV. While an aorta-to-PA shunt may establish adequate pulmonary blood flow, left ventricular output remains compromised by the dilated RV. Surgical intervention in these patients is associated with greater than 50 percent mortality.[29] Orthotopic heart transplantation should be considered as a therapeutic option.

Surgical management of children with right ventricle–dependent coronary circulation

An RVDCC is one in which there are sinusoidal connections between the cavity of the RV and the coronary circulation, either with obstruction in the native coronary circulation or with broad sinusoidal connections that would result in runoff from the coronary circulation into the low-pressure RV. Tortuous sinusoidal connections without coronary stenoses do not usually denote an RVDCC. Decompression of the RV at the time of the bidirectional Glenn anastomosis will usually result in closure of these sinusoids as opposed to the broad-based fistulous connections. In some cases the large fistulous connections can be identified on the surface of the heart and be suture ligated at the time of the bidirectional Glenn shunt, allowing RV decompression at that time.

In infants with RVDCC, systemic RV pressure must be maintained to ensure adequate coronary perfusion to the myocardium.[30] Even in older children, decompression of the RV by augmentation of the outflow tract or tricuspid valvotomy may lead to severe myocardial ischemia and acute cardiac failure. If an RVDCC is identified, a single-ventricle surgical strategy is pursued and a bidirectional Glenn shunt placed at 3 to 6 months of age without RV decompression. Any additional source of pulmonary blood flow, such as a previously placed shunt, is reduced to give a estimated Qp:Qs of 1.3:1 or less from the Glenn shunt and the systemic-to-PA shunt combined.

At 2 to 4 years of age, depending on the state of the patient, the Fontan procedure is completed. In order to bring oxygenated blood to the TV, the septum is excised and the coronary sinus unroofed at the time of Fontan completion.

If there are signs of myocardial ischemia, either preoperatively or intraoperatively, the RVDCC may be improved by creating an aortic-to-RV shunt.[31] This shunt theoretically changes the RV systolic pressure to equal the systemic pressure, elevating the diastolic pressure and maintaining coronary perfusion. Flow through such a shunt appears to be bidirectional and biphasic. If myocardial ischemia results from decompression of an undiagnosed RVDCC, coronary artery bypass grafting using the internal mammary artery may be attempted. The use of coronary artery bypass grafting in these patients is limited by technical difficulties, conduit options, and the limited long-term patency of the grafts.

Finally, in patients with RVDCC and severe RV dysfunction, early shunt placement may be followed by orthotopic heart transplantation.

Specific operative procedures in older children

Enlargement of the right ventricular cavity and right ventricular outflow tract

The RV cavity is enlarged by sharp resection of trabecular muscle and cardiopulmonary bypass with bicaval cannulation and both antegrade and retrograde blood cardioplegic arrest. The RA is opened longitudinally and the TV inspected; the annulus is measured and compared to normal values and its competence tested with cold saline. An incision is made longitudinally from the main PA through the annulus and across the infundibulum to the main RV cavity. The cavity is enlarged by resection of trabecular muscle. Care is taken to work between the papillary muscles, which must not be incised. A glutaraldehyde-treated pericardial outflow patch is then placed on the RV incision. In infants, we generally prefer a pericardial patch with a pericardial monocusp valve. In older children, we have used a homograft or porcine valve within the RV outflow tract.

Adjustable atrial septal defect

If the ASD is large, it is closed with a Gore-Tex vascular patch. If the defect is small with firm edges, it may be closed with the purse-string suture of the "adjustable ASD." The adjustable ASD is created by placing a no. 1 polypropylene suture as a purse string around the tissue edges of the existing septal defect, with a pericardial pledget used as a reinforcement. Both ends of the suture are then brought out through the intertrial groove. An 8F polyethylene tube is cut to length to reach the linea alba and passed over the ends of the polypropylene suture to construct the snare. The tubing is sutured to the atrial wall with a single chromic suture (Fig. 62-3A). The snare is adjusted by tightening or loosening the polypropylene suture at the end of the tubing and securing the length with medium clips. The end of the snare is left under the subxiphoid linea alba, where it can be retrieved under local anesthesia postoperatively for subsequent adjustment. The same technique can be used to create an adjustable defect in a patch repair using Gore-Tex (expanded polytetrafluoroethylene, or ePTFE). The defect in the suture line is left on the right side where it is surrounded by a polypropylene suture as described above (Fig. 62-3B). The ASD is left open until the patient is weaned from bypass. The ASD is then slowly closed, using the snare while monitoring the RA pressure and arterial oxygen saturations. An RA pressure of about 12 to 14 mmHg with an oxygen saturation of 88% or above on 100 percent inspired oxygen is considered ideal.

Bioprosthetic valve insertion with transannular patch

A transannular incision is made vertically across the pulmonary outflow tract and extended onto the left PA and down into the RV. Any residual membrane in the region of the annulus is resected. The distance between the RVOT and the PA bifurcation is assessed. If it is short, use of a homograft may not be possible, as the proximity of the proximal and distal suture lines will result in bulging of the homograft. For this situation, a larger porcine valve can be placed under a pericardial (autologous or bovine) patch within the RVOT. The porcine valve may be implanted at the level of the native valve annulus (Fig. 62-4A) or in the subvalvular region below the level of the true pulmonary annulus (Fig. 62-4B) to accommodate a larger valve and reduce the amount of compression that may result from closure of the sternum. A running polypropylene suture is used to insert the valve, which is also sutured to the patch anteriorly (Fig. 62-4C).

Homograft valve insertion

If the distance between the RVOT and the PA bifurcation is adequate, an appropriate aortic or pulmonary homograft is chosen. A running polypropylene suture is used distally just below the PA bifurcation. Proximally, the homograft is sutured to the RVOT just below the pulmonary valve with a running suture. The proximal anastomosis of the homograft and the RVOT are augmented with a pericardial or synthetic (ePTFE or Dacron) patch.

Transannular patch with pericardial monocusp valve

This technique is used for neonates and infants but can also be used for smaller children. It should be used for

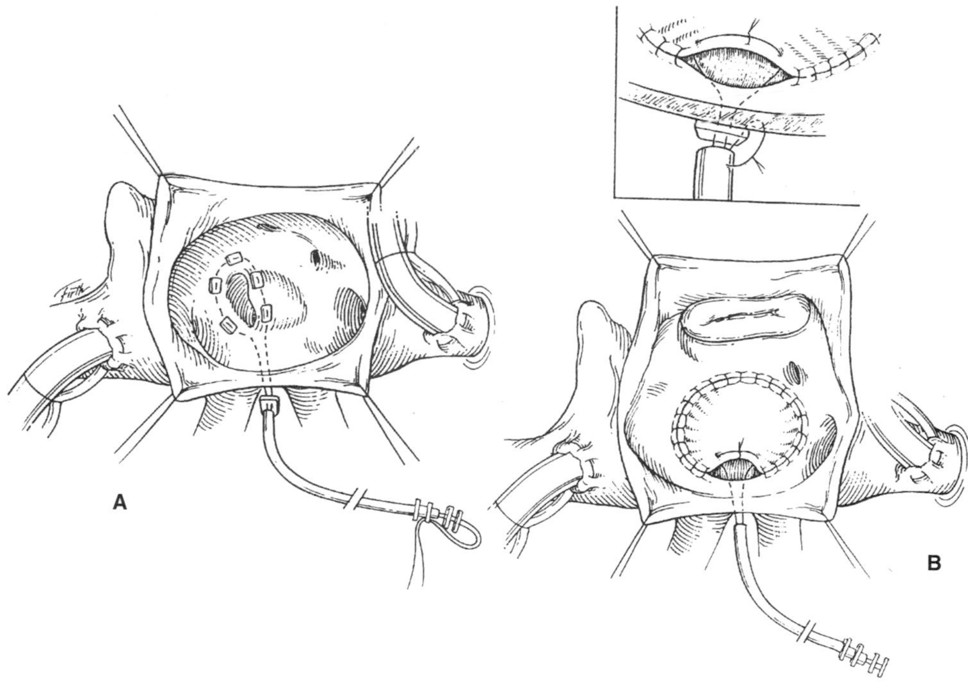

Figure 62-3 Adjustable atrial septal defect with and without patch closure of the native atrial septal defect. **A.** A no. 1 polypropylene purse-string suture is secured around the border of the atrial septal defect using pericardial or felt pledgets. The snare is constructed using 8F polyethylene tubing placed over the no. 1 polypropylene suture and measured to reach the linea alba. **B.** If a large secundum atrial septal defect is present, it is closed with a Gore-Tex or pericardial patch, and a defect is left in the lateral wall. A no. 1 polypropylene suture is brought in through the interatrial groove and placed as a horizontal mattress stitch through the edge of the patch. The no. 1 polypropylene suture is then anchored to the edge of the patch with a 5-0 polypropylene suture.

patients with mild or moderate RV hypoplasia and with acceptable PA size, as the valve will remain competent for a shorter period of time than a complete tissue valve. It has the advantage, however, of rarely causing obstruction even when the valve has become incompetent.

Bidirectional glenn shunt

A median sternotomy incision is used for a Glenn cavopulmonary anastomosis. The right PA and superior vena cava are dissected free from surrounding tissues and the azygos vein is divided between ligatures. Excessive dissection in this region may disrupt lymphatic tissue and result in postoperative chylothorax. The PA pressure is measured on both sides. A left superior vena cava (SVC) may be identified anterior to the left PA. The SVC is clamped just above the RA and the proximal pressure is monitored. If the pressure does not rise above a mean of 30 mmHg, a left SVC should be suspected. If both right and left SVCs are present, cardiopulmonary bypass or a temporary shunt may not be necessary. If the proximal pressure in the clamped SVC is 30 mgHg or greater, a temporary shunt should be used. If possible, the use of cardiopulmonary bypass is avoided in our practice. A vertical purse-string suture is placed on the SVC at its junction with the innominate vein. A second purse-string suture is placed in the right atrial appendage. The patient is heparinized and a temporary bypass shunt is created using two venous cannulas and a Y connector with a chapeau attachment. The SVC is cannulated with the bevel of the cannula placed toward the right internal jugular vein. The second cannula is placed in the right atrial appendage. The circuit is connected after air is completely evacuated from the cannulas and the clamps are removed, with visualization of flow. The SVC is then clamped at its junctions with the RA and the innominate vein. The anterior aspect of the SVC and the superior margin of the right PA are marked to ensure proper alignment of the cavopulmonary anastomosis. The SVC is divided at the atrial junction and the open end of the SVC is enlarged by an incision in the posterior wall of the vessel. The anastomosis is performed with a running 6-0 or 7-0 polypropylene suture (Fig. 62-5).

Any previously placed systemic-to-PA shunt is now reduced in size to give an estimated QP:QS of 1.3:1 or less. The SVC and PA pressures are measured, as well as the arterial oxygen saturations on 100 percent oxygen.

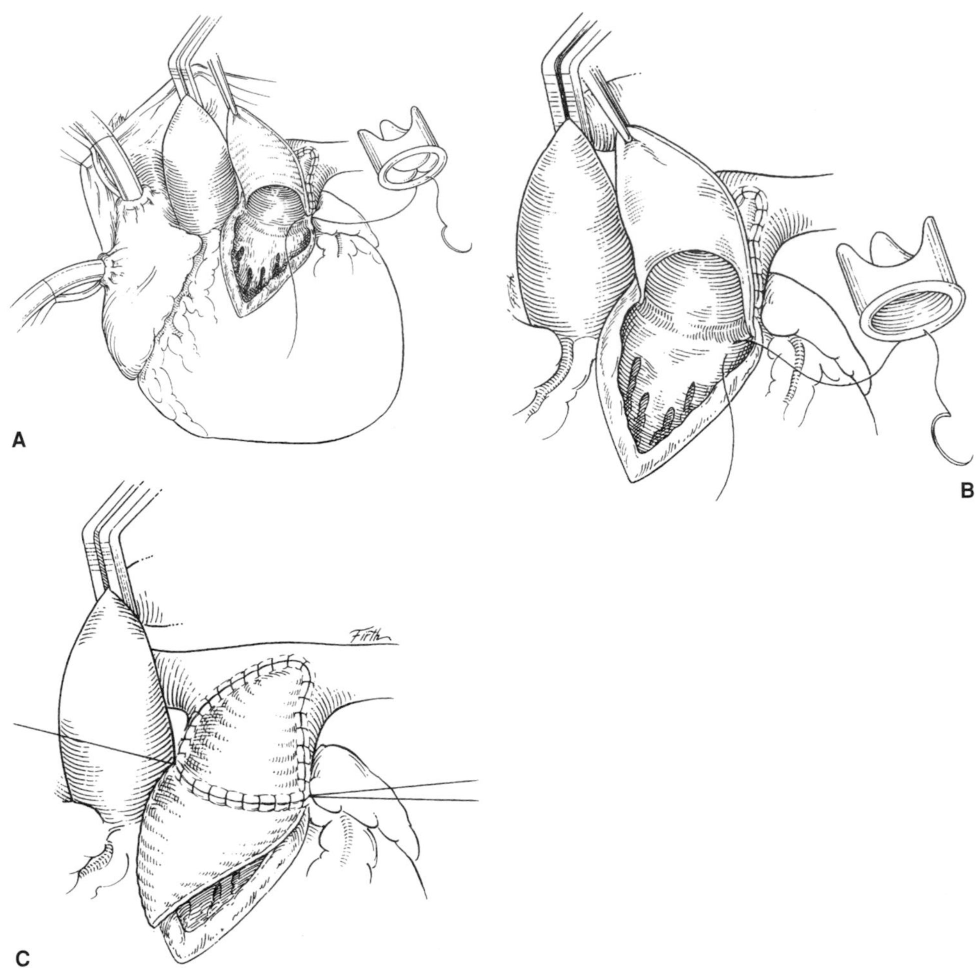

Figure 62-4 Insertion of bioprosthetic valve under a transannular patch. An oversized bioprosthetic valve is chosen and is sutured to the native annulus **(A)**. A patch of native pericardium is treated with glutaraldehyde and used to enlarge the RVOT. An alternate technique is to suture the bioprosthetic valve to the outflow tract wall just below the native annulus **(B)**. The anterior sewing ring of the valve is anchored to the patch at the completion of the reconstruction **(C)**.

An ePTFE membrane is left as a pericardial substitute to facilitate reentry at the time of total cavopulmonary connection.

Lateral tunnel Fontan with adjustable atrial septal defect

A Fontan procedure is usually performed as a second-stage operation following the creation of a Glenn cavopulmonary shunt. Most patients undergo a bidirectional Glenn shunt prior to the Fontan procedure. A median sternotomy is performed and bicaval venous cannulation between the superior and inferior venae cavae is carried out. Systemic hypothermia to 24°C is used in addition to cold blood cardioplegic arrest.

A right atriotomy is performed just anterior to the linea terminalis and the edges are retracted with stay sutures. The coronary sinus is identified and cannulated with a retrograde cardioplegia catheter. Cold blood cardioplegia is delivered intermittently both antegrade and retrograde.

The atrial septum is excised. The SVC orifice is identified from within the RA. It is important that this orifice be widely open and not restrictive. The right PA is incised adjacent to the opening in the SVC stump. The posterior wall of the anastomosis is created by suturing the adjacent PA and RA together with polypropylene suture. Anteriorly, the connection is bridged with a pericardial patch to assure patency without obstruction.

After the RA-to-PA anastomosis has been completed, the lateral tunnel is constructed. A rectangular Gore-Tex patch is cut from 0.8-mm-thick Gore-Tex vascular patch material. The length is carefully measured from the orifice of the inferior vena cava (IVC) to that of the SVC. The width is left about two-thirds

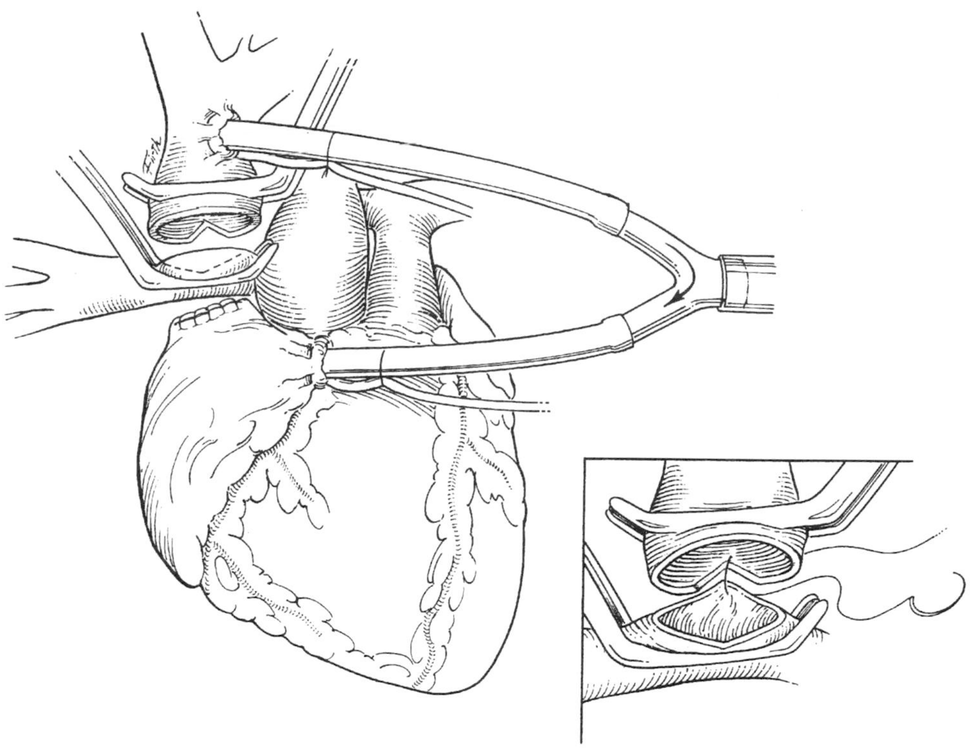

Figure 62-5 Bidirectional Glenn shunt. The Glenn shunt operation is performed using a superior vena cava–to–PA shunt. The cannulas are placed in the superior vena cava and the RA, allowing continuous flow of venous return to the RA during the reconstruction. To avoid stenosis, the anastomosis is tailored as shown in the insert.

of the length to be trimmed after completion of the posterior suture line. A running polypropylene suture is used for the posterior suture line, which is begun at the IVC orifice (Fig. 62-6A). The suture line is carried superiorly to the site of the orifice of the adjustable ASD, where it ends. This site is chosen because it comprises a natural recess close to the right superior pulmonary vein at the superior and lateral end of the fossa ovalis. A second polypropylene suture line is begun at the superior end of the ASD defect and carried superiorly around the SVC orifice. The ASD is sized according to the patient's age and made large in diameter so that it may be reduced in size if necessary after the patient comes off bypass. As a rule of thumb, the defect's size is 4 mm for 2-year-olds, 6 mm for 4-year-olds, and 8 mm for children 6 years old and older. The patch is trimmed appropriately as the suture line advances. Before the anterior suture line is completed, the snare control is placed for the adjustable ASD. A no. 1 polypropylene suture is brought through a pericardial pledget, through the interatrial septum at the lower border of the ASD, and through the edge of the Gore-Tex patch. It is then brought back through the upper edge of the Gore-Tex patch and out through the interatrial septum and through the pericardial pledget. An 8F polyethylene tube is cut to the appropriate length to reach the linea alba and the polypropylene sutures are brought through this snare. The no. 1 polypropylene is sutured to the edge of the Gore-Tex patch with a 5-0 polypropylene suture, the polyethylene tubing is sutured to the lateral wall with 2-0 chromic catgut, and the polypropylene is fixed to the heavy polypropylene with a medium-sized hemaclip. These three points of fixation prevent inadvertent closure of the ASD by tugging on the polypropylene. The patch is now trimmed to create a wide open connection and to reach just anterior to the linea terminalis. The anterior part of the suture line is completed using full thickness sutures to avoid a suture-line leak. The right atrial incision is then closed with a polypropylene suture (Fig. 62-6B).

Transthoracic lines are generally placed in the left and RA. If an internal jugular line is not inserted, the right atrial line can be inserted to measure the pressure in the pulmonary system via the Fontan tunnel or the Glenn shunt. The patient is now weaned from cardiopulmonary bypass and the ASD snare is adjusted to achieve arterial saturations of 80 to 85 percent with an FIO_2 of 50 percent while attempting to maintain pressure in the Fontan circuit at or below 16 mmHg.

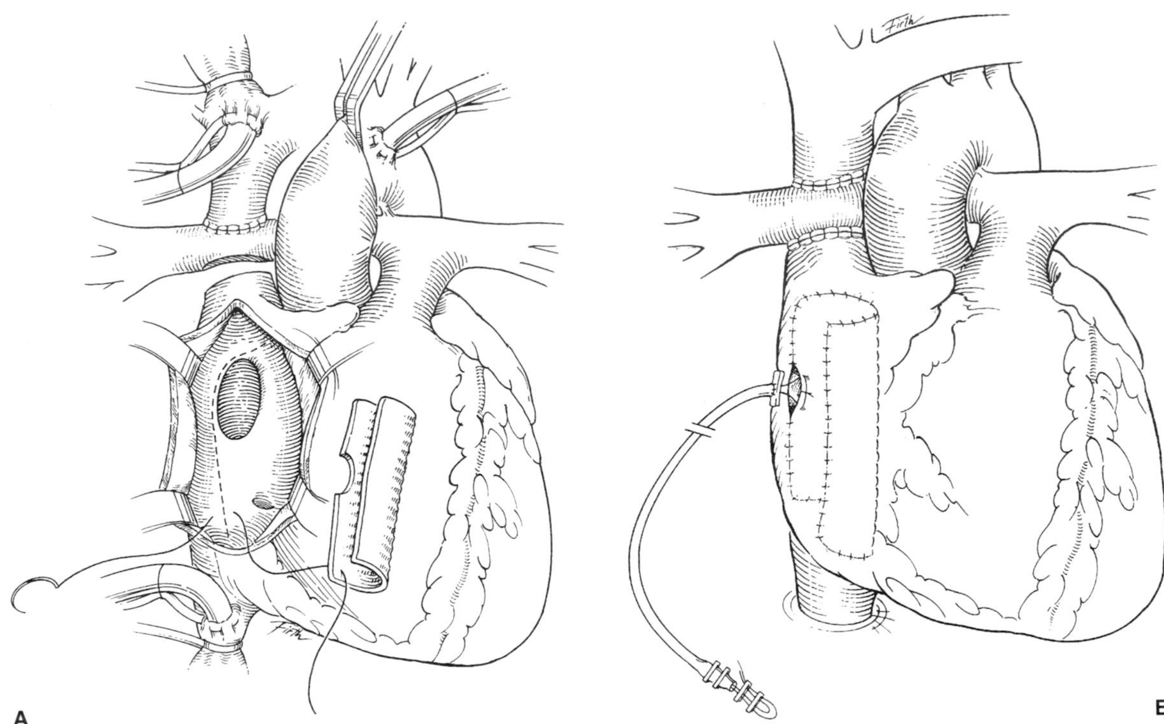

Figure 62-6 Lateral tunnel Fontan with an adjustable atrial septal defect. A tunnel of uniform caliber is constructed by suturing a Gore-Tex vascular patch to the orifice of the inferior vena cava and the superior vena cava and to the lateral atrial wall **(A)**. A defect is left in the tunnel and an adjustable atrial septal defect is achieved by passing a no. 1 polypropylene suture through the lateral portion of the interatrial septum and through the edge of the Gore-Tex tunnel. The no. 1 polypropylene suture is then secured to the edge of the Gore-Tex with a 5-0 polypropylene suture. The suture is brought back out the inter-atrial septum and through a pericardial pledget. The snare is constructed with a #8 Fr polyethylene tubing and anchored to the heart through a pledget as shown **(B)**. The completed lateral tunnel Fontan reconstruction is shown with the adjustable atrial septal defect left open.

Extracardiac Fontan with adjustable atrial septal defect

The extracardiac Fontan is performed through a median sternotomy using cardiopulmonary bypass and bicaval cannulation. The procedure can be completed in most patients without the need for cardioplegic arrest of the heart. A clamp is placed on the inferior vena cava near its junction to the RA. The inferior vena cava is then divided between the snared venous cannula and the clamp. The atrium is repaired and the clamp is removed.

The open end of the inferior vena cava is anastomosed end-to-end to a Gore-Tex conduit (16 to 20 mm in diameter) using a running Gore-Tex suture. The proximal anastomosis is performed end-to-side between the Gore-Tex conduit and the inferior aspect of the right PA. The clamps are released and flow is established between the inferior vena cava and the pulmonary arteries.

To create the adjustable atrial septal defect, a partially occluding vascular C clamp is placed on the Gore-Tex graft. A direct anastomosis is performed between the extra-cardiac conduit and the RA. A snare is inserted to control the opening and closing of this "ASD" (Fig. 62-7A). An alternate method uses a conduit for the defect. With this technique an 8.0-mm Gore-Tex graft is anastomosed end to side to the middle of the larger conduit. A similar technique is used to create an opening in the RA and the other end of the 8.0-mm graft is anastomosed to this site. A snare is inserted around the smaller conduit (Fig. 62-7B). A distinct drawback to the extracardiac Fontan is the need for anticoagulation with warfarin postoperatively for up to a year, with subsequent conversion to aspirin therapy.

Aorta-to–right ventricle shunt

The aorta-to-RV shunt is performed through a median sternotomy using cardiopulmonary bypass and bicaval cannulation. Cardioplegic arrest of the heart may or may not be necessary. The shunt is created using a 5.0-mm ringed Gore-Tex graft. A partially occluding clamp is placed on the anterior wall of the ascending

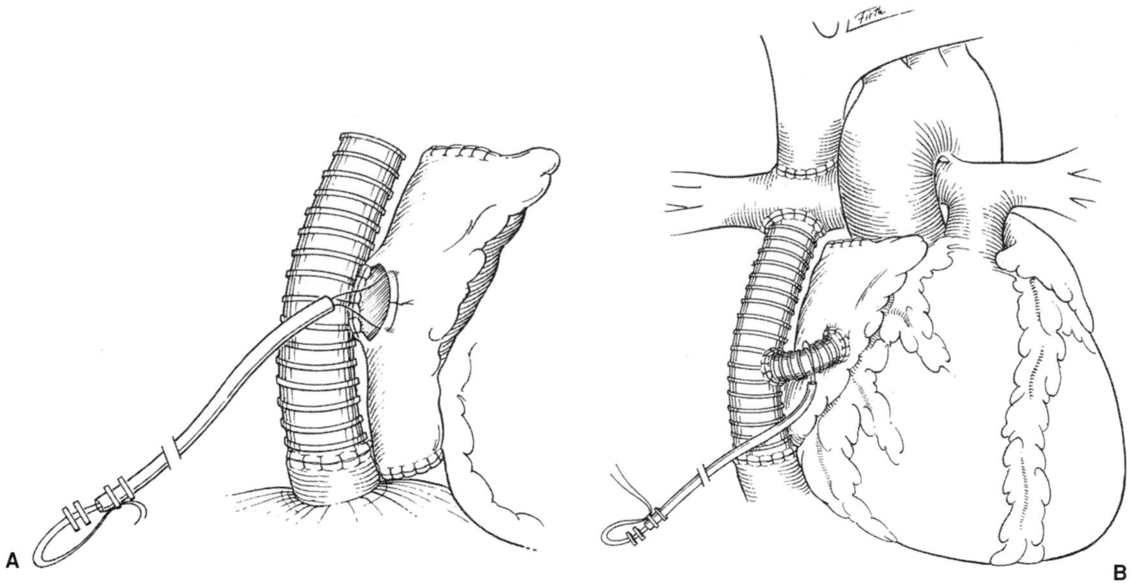

Figure 62-7 Extracardiac Fontan with an adjustable fenestration. The extracardiac conduit is implanted and a direct anastomosis is made between the conduit and the atrial wall. The defect is controlled with an adjustable snare **(A)**. The extracardiac conduit is implanted and a communication is established between the conduit and the atrium using an 8.0-mm Gore-Tex graft. The graft diameter is then controlled by an adjustable snare **(B)**.

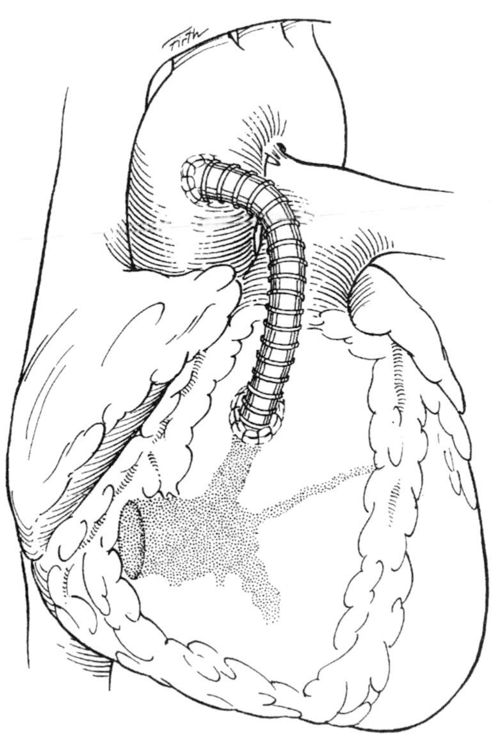

Figure 62-8 Aorta-to-right ventricle ringed Gore-Tex conduit. The shunt is inserted between the ascending aorta and the right ventricular cavity with or without cardiopulmonary bypass.

aorta. An aortotomy is created and an end-to-side anastomosis performed between the graft and the ascending aorta using a running polypropylene suture. A ventriculotomy is made in the infundibular portion of the RV and the distal end of the graft is anastomosed to this site using a running polypropylene suture (Fig. 62-8).

COURSE AND PROGNOSIS

POSTOPERATIVE CARE IN NEONATES

Neonates may be critically ill in the early postoperative period following operative intervention for Pa/IVS. The presence of low cardiac output may require substantial inotropic support. In the presence of a systemic-to-PA shunt, balanced pulmonary and systemic blood flow must be achieved. The management of pulmonary and systemic vascular resistance is critical to maintaining adequate oxygenation and cardiac output. Episodes of pulmonary hypertension must be managed quickly and may require the use of inhaled nitric oxide. An excessively large shunt may lead to pulmonary overcirculation and require adjustment or replacement of the shunt. Postoperative ischemia can develop due to unrecognized RVDCC and may be associated with electrocardiographic changes, ventricular dysrhythmias, and segmental wall dyskinesis on echocardiography. In patients with persistent hypoxemia despite adequate medical management, residual RVOT obstruction or severe tricuspid hypoplasia should be excluded.

POSTOPERATIVE CARE IN OLDER CHILDREN

Early management after the Fontan procedures should focus on optimizing cardiac output and reducing systemic venous pressure. Inotropes are routinely used, starting with dopamine and dobutamine. If additional inotropic support is needed, milrinone may be added. If systemic vascular resistance is low and additional inotropic support is required, the use of epinephrine may be indicated. The adjustable ASD is useful because it allows as much as one-third of the systemic venous return to traverse the defect to the atrium, thus lowering the systemic venous pressure while increasing left ventricular preload and the cardiac output. With a QP:QS ratio of 1.5:1, the arterial oxygen saturation should be approximately 85%. A systemic venous pressure of 12 to 15 mmHg is optimal. It should be noted that the presence of a patent right-to-left shunt increases the risk of paradoxical emboli from thrombus, which may develop in the RA or the hepatic veins. Therefore complete closure of the adjustable ASD should be performed when it is hemodynamically tolerated.

If the pulmonary vascular resistance is elevated postoperatively following a Glenn or Fontan procedure, it is reduced with an infusion of nitroglycerin and prostaglandin (PGE_1). These medications are more effective in lowering pulmonary vascular resistance if delivered directly into a catheter in the Glenn or Fontan tunnel. If these medications are not sufficient, nitric oxide is administered through the ventilator. Unlike intravenous medications, nitric oxide does not result in the lowering of systemic vascular resistance.

Extubation within the first 24 h is generally attempted for both Glenn and Fontan procedures. The development of pleural and pericardial effusions is anticipated and mediastinal and pleural chest tubes are left for several days postoperatively until drainage is minimal.

If a jugular vein line has been inserted, it is used for measuring the PA pressure and for the infusion of pulmonary vasodilators if necessary. The line is removed within 12 h to avoid venous thrombosis.

OUTCOMES

Historically, the surgical treatment of Pa/IVS was associated with very high morbidity and mortality.[4,32] Previous extensive reviews of the clinical and pathologic aspects of this defect have allowed for a greater understanding of the disease and the development of surgical therapy.[35] With increasing surgical experience, a more standardized approach has evolved and outcomes from many institutions have steadily improved.[36–42] The role of catheter-based interventions in these patients, including balloon valvotomy and stenting of the RVOT and the ductus arteriosus, is evolving and remains to be defined.[43] At the UCLA School of Medicine, our surgical approach to patients with Pa/IVS has been based on classification of the degree of RV hypoplasia. Between 1982 and 2001, a total of 111 patients with a diagnosis of Pa/IVS underwent surgical intervention at our institution. Six patients had Ebstein's anomaly of the TV and were excluded from analysis.[21] A total of 63 patients with Pa/IVS underwent palliative procedures at UCLA as neonates. Twenty patients were classified as severe RV hypoplasia and/or demonstrating severe coronary abnormalities with RVDCC. There were three early deaths in this group. Forty-three patients were classified as mild to moderate RV hypoplasia, without significant RV sinusoids or fistulas. These patients all underwent procedures to open the RVOT with or without a shunt. There were three early deaths and two late deaths in this group. Early survival in this total group is 90 percent and late survival is 87 percent. A total of 82 patients surviving palliative procedures from UCLA and referring institutions underwent later interventions at UCLA based on our classification system.

Fifty-seven patients underwent complete or partial biventricular repair. Nineteen of these patients underwent partial biventricular repair with a bidirectional cavopulmonary shunt and an adjustable ASD. There were three deaths in this group. Twenty-three of these patients underwent Fontan operations as a later intervention. Two patients underwent cardiac transplantation following initial palliation. There were two early deaths and one late death following discharge. Actuarial survival in this total group is 96 percent at 1 year, 89 percent at 5 years, and 86.3 percent at 10 years. As evidenced by our experience, the prognosis for children with Pa/IVS continues to improve as a more structured and methodical surgical approach based on RV morphology is taken.

References

1. Dumont J. Chirurgie des malformations congenitales ou acquises du coeur. *Presse Med* 1913;21:860.
2. Sellors TH. The surgery of pulmonary stenosis. *Lancet* 1948;1:988–993.
3. Kan JS, White RI, Mitchell SE, Gardner TJ. Percutaneous balloon valvuloplasty: A new method for treating congenital pulmonary stenosis. *N Engl J Med* 1982;307:540–546.

4. Hanley FL, Sade RM, Freedom RM, et al. Outcomes in critically ill neonates with pulmonary stenosis and intact ventricular septum: A multi-institutional study. *J Am Coll Cardiol* 1993;22:183–192.
5. Rao PS, Galal O, Patnana M, et al. Results of three to ten year follow up of balloon dilatation of the pulmonary valve. *Heart* 1998;80:591–595.
6. Greenwold WE, Dushane JW, Burchell HB, et al. Congenital pulmonary atresia with intact ventricular septum: Two anatomic subtypes. *Circulation* 1956;14: 945–950.
7. Goor DA, Lillehei CW. *Congenital Malformations of the Heart.* New York: Grune & Stratton, 1975.
8. Bull C, De Leval MR, Mercanti C, et al. Pulmonary atresia and intact ventricular septum: A revised classification. *Circulation* 1982;66(2):266–272.
9. Hanley FL, Sade RM, Blackstone, et al. Outcomes in neonatal pulmonary atresia with intact ventricular septum: A multiinstitutional study. *J Thorac Cardiovasc Surg* 1993;105:406–427.
10. Billingsley AM, Laks H, Boyce SW, et al. Definitive repair in patients with pulmonary atresia and intact ventricular septum. *J Thorac Cardiovasc Surg* 1989;97: 745–754.
11. Subramanian S, Wagner H, Teshai G, et al. Pulmonary atresia with intact ventricular septum. *Ann Clin Inf* 1972;13:225–230.
12. Trusler GA, Yamamoto N, Williams WG, et al. Surgical treatment of pulmonary atresia with intact ventricular septum. *Br Heart J* 1976;38:957–965.
13. Daubeney P, Delany D, Anderson R, et al. Pulmonary atresia with intact ventricular septum: Range of morphology in a population-based study. *J Am Coll Cardiology* 2002;39:1670–1679.
14. De Leval M. Bull C, Hopkins R, et al. Decision making in the definitive repair of the heart with a small right ventricle. *Circulation* 1985;72(Suppl II):52–60.
15. De Leval M, Bull C, Stark J, et al. Pulmonary atresia and intact ventricular septum: Surgical management based on a revised classification. *Circulation* 1982;66:272–280.
16. Foker JE, Braunlin EA, Ste Cyr JA, et al. Management of pulmonary atresia with intact ventricular septum. *J Thorac Cardiovasc Surg* 1986;92:706–715.
17. Joshi SV, Brown WJ, Mee RBB. Pulmonary atresia with intact ventricular septum. *J Thorac Cardiovasc Surg* 1986;91:192–199.
18. Cobanoglu A, Metzdroff MT, Pinson CW, et al. Valvotomy for pulmonary atresia with intact ventricular septum and a disciplined approach to achieving a functioning right ventricle. *J Thorac Cardiovasc Surg* 1985;89:482–490.
19. Leung MP, Mok C, Lee J, et al. Management evolution of pulmonary atresia and intact ventricular septum. *Am J Cardiol* 1993;71:1331–1336.
20. Yoshimura N, Yamaguchi M, Ohashi H, et al. Pulmonary atresia with intact ventricular septum: Strategy based on right ventricular morphology. *J Thorac Cardiovasc Surg* 2003;126:1417–1426.
21. Odim JN, Laks H, Plunkett M, et al. Successful management of patients with pulmonary atresia with intact ventricular septum using a three tier grading system for right ventricular hypoplasia. *Ann Thorac Surg.* 2006;81: 678–684.
22. Laks H, Plunkett MD. Pulmonary stenosis and pulmonary atresia with intact septum. In: Kaiser LR, Kron IL, Spray TL (eds). *Mastery of Cardiothoracic Surgery.* Philadelphia: Lippincott-Raven, 1998:805–818.
23. Laks H, Billingsley A. Advances in the treatment of pulmonary atresia with intact ventricular septum. *Cardiol Clin* 1989;7(2):387–392.
24. Mainwaring RD, Lamberti JL. Pulmonary atresia with intact ventricular septum: Surgical approach based on ventricular size and coronary anatomy. *J Thorac Cardiovasc Surg* 1993;106:733–738.
25. Calder AL, Co EE, Sage MD. Coronary arterial abnormalities in pulmonary atresia with intact ventricular septum. *Am J Cardiol* 1987;59:436–442.
26. Gittenberg-deGroot AC, Sauer U, Bindl L, et al. Competition of coronary arteries and ventriculo-coronary arterial communications in pulmonary atresia with intact ventricular septum. *Int Cardiol* 1988;18:243–258.
27. Laks H, Pearl JM, Drinkwater DC, et al. Partial biventricular repair of pulmonary atresia with intact ventricular septum: Use of an adjustable atrial septal defect. Circulation 1992;86(Suppl II):159–166.
28. Laks H, Pearl JM, Haas GS, Drinkwater DC, et al. Partial Fontan: Advantages of an adjustable interatrial communication. *Ann Thorac Surg* 1991;52:1084–1095.
29. Stellin G, Santini F, Thiene G, et al. Pulmonary atresia, intact ventricular septum, and Ebstein's anomaly of the tricuspid valve: Anatomic and surgical considerations. *J Thorac Cardiovasc Surg* 1993;106:255–261.
30. Giglia TM, Mandell VS, Connor AR, et al. Diagnosis and management of right ventricle–dependent coronary circulation in pulmonary atresia with intact septum. *Circulation* 1992;86:1516–1528.
31. Laks H, Gates RN, Grant PW, et al. Aortic to right ventricular shunt for pulmonary atresia and intact ventricular septum. *Ann Thorac Surg* 1995;59:342–347.
32. Cole RB, Muster AJ, Lev M, et al. Pulmonary atresia with intact ventricular septum. *Am J Cardiol* 1968;21: 23–24.
33. Moulton AL, Bowman FO, Edie RN, et al. Pulmonary atresia with intact ventricular septum. *J Thorac Cardiovasc Surg* 1979;78:527–530.
34. Shams A, Fowler RS, Trusler GA, et al. Pulmonary atresia with intact ventricular septum: Report of 50 cases. *Pediatrics* 1971;47:370–377.
35. Freedom RM. The morphologic variations of pulmonary atresia with intact ventricular septum: Guidelines for surgical intervention. *Pediatr Cardiol* 1983;4:183–188.
36. Hawkins JA, Thorne JK, Boucek MM, et al. Early and late results in pulmonary atresia with intact ventricular septum. *J Thorac Cardiovasc Surg* 1990;100:492–497.
37. Coles JG, Freedom RM, Lightfoot NE, et al. Long-term results in neonates with pulmonary atresia with intact ventricular septum. *Ann Thorac Surg* 1989;47: 213–217.
38. Lightfoot NE, Coles JG, Dasmahapatra HK, et al. Analysis of survival in patients with pulmonary atresia and intact ventricular septum treated surgically. *Int J Cardiol* 1989;24:159–164.
39. Rychik J, Levy H, Gaynor JW, et al. Outcome after operations for pulmonary atresia with intact ventricular septum. *Cardiovasc Surg* 1998;116:924–931.

40. Hanley FL, Sade RM, Blackstone EH, et al. Outcomes in neonatal pulmonary atresia with intact ventricular septum: A multiinstitutional study. *J Thorac Cardiovasc Surg* 1993;105:406–427.
41. Milliken JC, Laks H, Hellenbrand W, et al. Early and late results in the treatment of patients with pulmonary atresia and intact ventricular septum. *Circulation* 1985;72(Suppl II),II61–II69.
42. Najm HK, Williams WG, Coles JG, et al. Pulmonary atresia with intact ventricular septum: Results of the Fontan procedure. *Ann Thorac Surg* 1997;63:669–675.
43. Weber H. Initial and late results after catheter intervention for neonatal critical pulmonary valve stenosis and atresia with intact ventricular septum: A technique in continual evolution. *Cath Cardiovasc Intervent* 2002;56: 394–399.

CHAPTER

63 DOUBLE-OUTLET RIGHT VENTRICLE

Umar S. Boston, Joseph A. Dearani

BACKGROUND

HISTORIC HIGHLIGHTS

Double-outlet right ventricle (DORV) is a complex form of congenital heart disease that encompasses a wide spectrum of anatomic variability and associated physiology. The anatomic and physiologic spectrum can range from tetralogy of Fallot (ToF) to transposition of the great arteries with ventricular septal defect (VSD) to true single-ventricle physiology. As a result of this variable anatomy, the terminology and definition of DORV has undergone many modifications.[1–3] Using pathologic specimens, Vierordt in 1898 described DORV as a "partial transposition" (i.e., there was only one overriding great vessel in the form of the aorta over the right

KEY CONCEPTS

- Epidemiology
  - Relatively uncommon (0.09 per 1000 births).
- Pathophysiology
  - Considerable variability in pathophysiology is seen with double-outlet right ventricle (DORV), depending on the location of the ventricular septal defect (VSD), the relationship of great arteries, and presence of outflow-tract stenosis.
- Clinical features
  - Patients usually present by 2 months of age. Presentation is variable and depends on type of DORV and associated cardiac anomalies. Congestive heart failure is seen in patients with unrestricted subaortic, doubly committed or noncommitted VSDs without right ventricular outflow tract obstruction (RVOTO). Cyanosis results from RVOTO, leading to restriction of pulmonary blood flow or from preferential streaming of blood from the left ventricle to the pulmonary artery, as seen in the Taussig-Bing anomaly.
- Diagnosis
  - Echocardiography defines the relationship of the great arteries to the right ventricle and to each other and delineates size and position of the VSD. Magnetic resonance imaging may provide complementary information about intracardiac anatomy as well as the size and status of the aortic arch and pulmonary arteries and the three-dimensional relationship of the cardiac chambers and great arteries. Catheterization can be performed to determine hemodynamics, exclude pulmonary vascular disease, and assess coronary anatomy.
- Treatment
  - Definitive management includes operation, preferably complete repair during infancy. Surgical repair is tailored to address the variable anatomic abnormalities. In patients with subaortic or doubly committed VSDs without RVOTO, the repair is performed as an intraventricular tunnel from VSD to aorta. If RVOTO exists, RVOT augmentation or conduit placement is performed. The Taussig-Bing anomaly is treated with the arterial switch operation and tunneling of the VSD to the pulmonary artery. Patients with a remote VSD, other complex valvar abnormalities, or unbalanced ventricles may require staged palliative single-ventricle surgery.
- Outcomes/prognosis
  - Outcomes are determined by the anatomy and repair performed. Late results may range from tetralogy of Fallot to complex intraventricular

tunnels with potential use of conduit; such patients are at subsequent risk for subaortic obstruction, conduit failure, and need for reoperation. Patients undergoing the arterial switch procedure have excellent late survival but may have a greater incidence of neo-aortic valve regurgitation, requiring subsequent reoperation. Complex biventricular intracardiac repairs are associated with a higher risk of reoperation. Fontan procedures for complex anatomy are associated with less operative mortality and lower rates of reoperation. Functional benefits of complex biventricular repairs compared to single-ventricle palliation have not been defined.

ventricle).[4] In 1950 the "Taussig-Bing heart" was described as a form of partial transposition with a subpulmonic VSD.[2] In 1957, Witham used the term *DORV* as it is used today.

DEFINITION

In order to account for the anatomic variability seen in DORV, it is best to simplify its definition. DORV is best defined as a type of ventriculoarterial connection whereby both great arteries arise entirely or predominantly from the right ventricle.[5] Consequently it is not a specific congenital malformation; rather, it is a term used to define the relationship of the great arteries to the right ventricle. To further delineate DORV, most authors agree that the degree of aortic override of the right ventricle has to be greater than 50 percent. In the past, some authors felt this needed to be greater than 90 percent. More rigid criteria can be seen in the literature to define DORV.[6] Others have advocated that DORV be defined by the lack of aortic-mitral fibrous continuity and the presence of both subaortic and subpulmonic coni. However, the transition from aortic-mitral fibrous continuity to the presence of conus is gradual, making it difficult to clearly demarcate the division between fibrous continuity and discontinuity. As a result, it is recommended that fibrous aortic-mitral discontinuity and bilateral coni not be a prerequisite in the definition of DORV.[7]

EPIDEMIOLOGY

DORV is a rare congenital cardiac anomaly. Its frequency has been reported as approximately 0.09 per 1000 births. There is no racial or gender predominance.[1]

MORPHOLOGY AND CLASSIFICATION

The pathophysiology and type of surgical repair are influenced by three main factors: (1) location of the VSD in relation to the great arteries, (2) the relationship of the great arteries to each other, and (3) commonly occurring associated abnormalities (Fig. 63-1).

VENTRICULAR SEPTAL DEFECT

The classification of DORV is based on the location of the VSD in relation to the semilunar valves.[5] This is not an anatomic definition but a classification system that describes the distance the VSD is located from the semilunar valves. VSDs in close proximity are "committed." Committed VSDs are classified as subaortic, subpulmonic, or doubly committed.[8] Committed VSDs are perimembranous (i.e., conoventricular) and thus are located between the anterior and posterior limbs of the trabecula septomarginalis (TSM). The attachment of the infundibular septum to either the anterior or posterior limb predicts which great artery is related to the VSD. Subaortic VSD is associated with the infundibular septum being attached or aligned with the anterior limb of the TSM. Conversely, posterior limb alignment of the TSM with the infundibular septum results in a subpulmonary VSD (Fig. 63-2A and B). The infundibular septum is absent with the doubly committed VSD (Fig. 63-2C). Noncommitted VSDs are away from the semilunar valve(s). It has been proposed that this distance should be greater than the diameter of the aortic valve.[9] Noncommitted VSDs are located in the inlet septum (atrioventricular canal defects or muscular) or the trabecular ventricular septum (Fig. 63-2D). The majority of VSDs in DORV are unrestrictive, but restrictive VSDs may be seen in approximately 10 percent of patients. Although restrictive VSDs are diagnosed preoperatively in approximately 1.6 percent, an additional 11 percent of patients require VSD enlargement at the time of repair to prevent subaortic obstruction.[10,11] Multiple VSDs can be seen in 13 percent; it is extremely rare for no VSD to be present. In the absence of a VSD, there is an atrial septal defect (ASD), which serves as the left-to-right shunt. In this situation the left ventricle is usually hypoplastic.[7]

Subaortic VSD

This is the most common type of VSD and occurs in approximately 50 to 55 percent of patients undergoing repair of DORV. The VSD is unrestrictive. Bilateral coni are present in 77 percent of patients and a subpulmonary conus is present in 23 percent (Table 63-1).[9] The length of the conus determines the distance of the VSD from

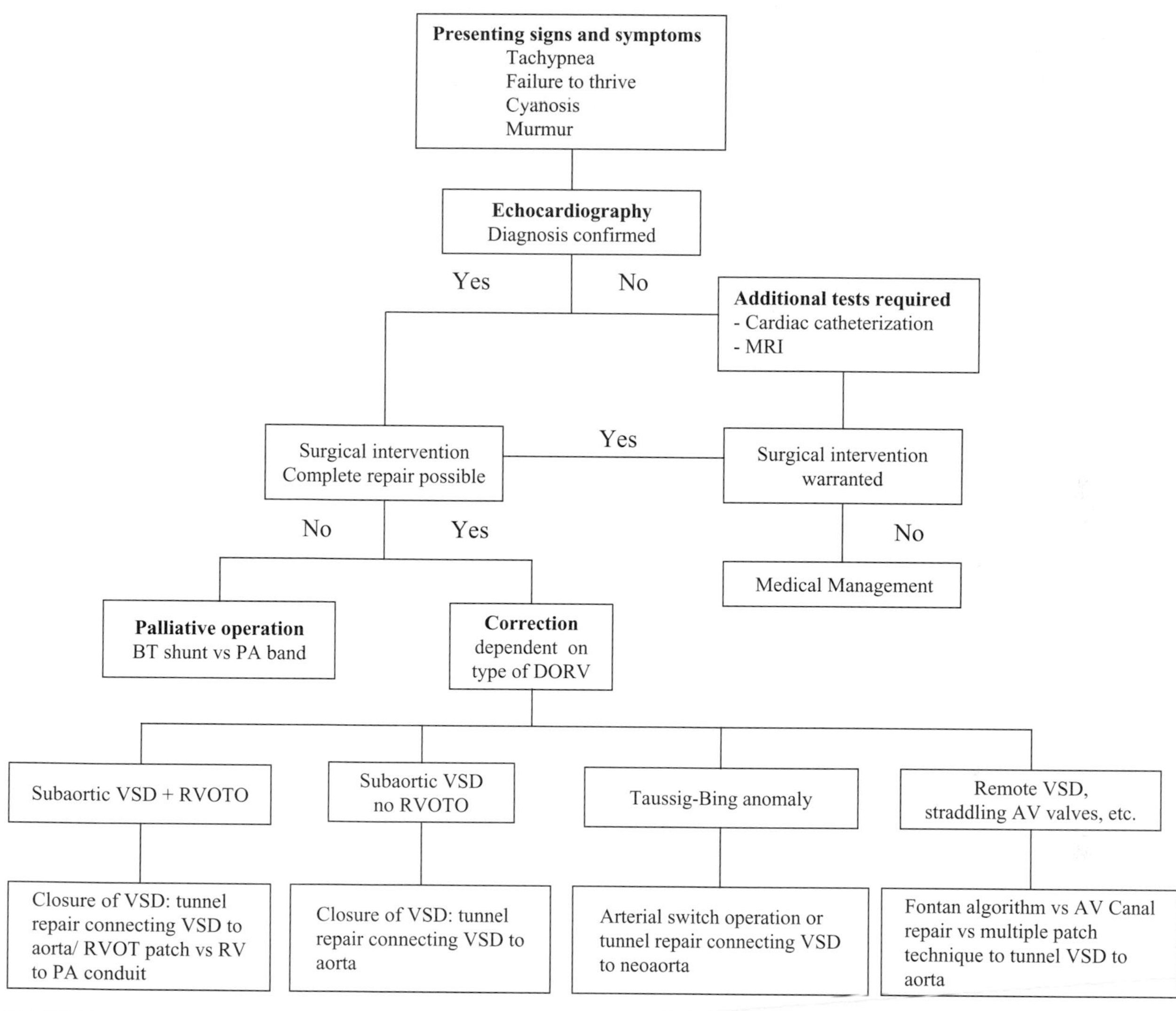

Figure 63-1 Decision-making flowchart

the aortic valve. Because the infundibular septum is aligned with the anterior limb of the TSM, the subaortic VSD is located in a posterior position in the ventricular septum (Fig. 63-2A). In the presence of aortic-mitral fibrous continuity (i.e., absent subaortic conus) the left cusp or the base of the anterior leaflet of the mitral valve forms the posterosuperior margin of the VSD. This morphologic variant is termed juxtaaortic VSD.

Subpulmonic VSD

This type of VSD is often seen in the Taussig-Bing anomaly. It is located in a more anterior position in the ventricular septum, since the posterior limb of the TSM is rotated and aligned with the infundibular septum (Fig. 63-2B). Pulmonary stenosis is usually absent and the VSD is unrestrictive. Subpulmonary VSDs are present in approximately 30 percent of patients with DORV undergoing surgical repair.[10,11] As with the subaortic VSD, the length of the pulmonary conus determines the distance between VSD and the pulmonary valve. In this anatomic variation, the conus forms the anterosuperior margin of the VSD. The absence of subpulmonary conus results in pulmonary-mitral and occasionally pulmonary-tricuspid continuity. This results in the VSD being juxtapulmonary.

Doubly committed VSD

This type of VSD is seen in 3 to 10 percent of surgical series.[12] The VSD is usually large owing to a deficient or absent infundibular septum. The semilunar valves form the superior border, while the limbs of the TSM form the anterior, inferior, and posterior margins (Fig. 63-2C).

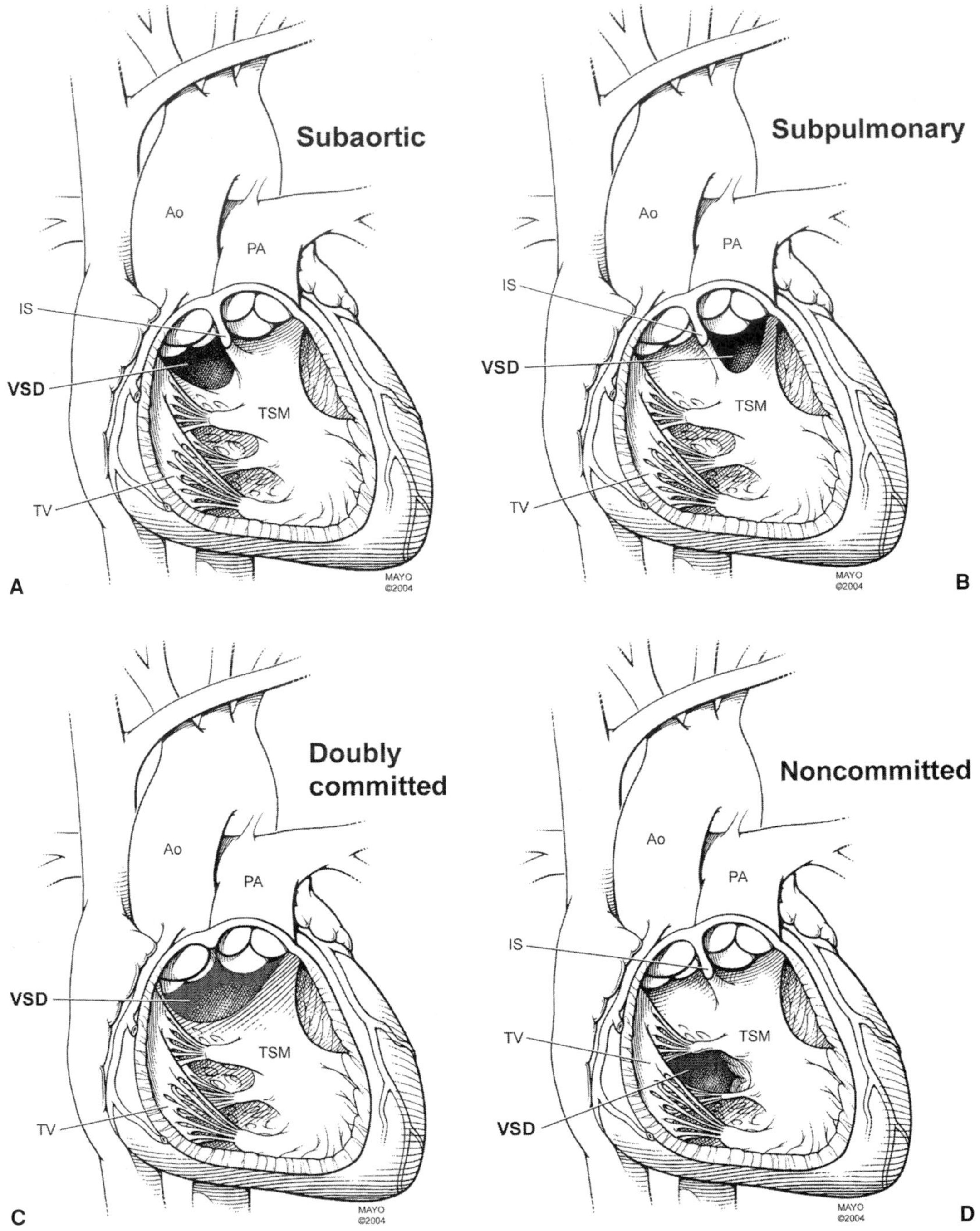

Figure 63-2 A. Diagram illustrating double-outlet right ventricle with subaortic VSD. B. Diagram illustrating double-outlet right ventricle with subpulmonic VSD. C. Diagram illustrating double-outlet right ventricle with doubly committed VSD. D. Diagram illustrating double-outlet right ventricle with noncommitted VSD. Ao = aorta; IS = interventricular septum; PA = pulmonary artery; TSM = trabecula septomarginalis; TV = tricuspid valve.

Noncommitted VSD

This type of VSD is remote from the semilunar valves and is reported in 3 to 20 percent of surgical series.[9] Most are associated with DORV and complete ASDs. Straddling of the atrioventricular valve may be present with this type of VSD (Fig. 63-2D).

RELATIONSHIP OF THE GREAT ARTERIES

The relationship of the great arteries at the level of the semilunar valves in DORV can be grouped into two broad categories: spiraling and parallel. Spiraling great arteries is the normal anatomic relationship with the

Table 63-1 Relationship of ventricular septal defect and conus pattern in double-outlet right ventricle

	Type of conus			
Position of VSD	Bilateral (%)	Subaortic (%)	Subpulmonary (%)	Absent (%)
Subaortic	77	0	23	0
Subpulmonary	45	55	0	0
Doubly committed	67	0	0	33
Noncommitted	50	50	0	0

Source: Data from Green Lane Hospital's report of 42 autopsy specimens; adapted from Kirklin and Barratt-Boyes.[10] With permission.

aortic trunk positioned posterior and to the right of the pulmonary trunk. This is the most common relationship of the great vessels in DORV.[7] When the great arteries are parallel, the aortic trunk is in a more anterior position relative to the pulmonary trunk. There are multiple degrees of variability in the anteroposterior relationship of the aortic trunk to the pulmonary trunk. In general, however, this relationship can be broken down into the following: (1) aorta located to the right and side by side with the pulmonary artery (Taussig-Bing), (2) aorta located to the right and anterior to the pulmonary artery (D-TGA), and (3) aorta located anterior and to the left of the pulmonary artery (similar to that observed in L-TGA or congenitally corrected transposition).

It must be noted that the relationship of the great arteries and the type of VSD present are independent of each other. In general terms, however, spiraling and L-malposition of the great arteries are most commonly associated with subaortic VSDs. Side-by-side (parallel) great arteries are most often associated with subpulmonic VSDs.[7]

OTHER CARDIAC ANOMALIES

Associated cardiac anomalies are common with DORV, and almost any type of congenital cardiac anomaly can be present. At the Mayo Clinic, 179 patients with a diagnosis of DORV were operated on from 1972 to 1992 and 87 (48.6 percent) had concomitant congenital anomalies. Table 63-2 shows the concomitant anomalies present in this series. ASD was the most common associated anomaly, followed by persistent left superior vena cava (SVC) and coronary artery anomalies. Multiple VSDs were seen in approximately 12 percent of patients; these have been shown to be a risk factor for early mortality.[13] Coarctation of the aorta is a commonly associated anomaly and is observed in approximately 50 percent of patients with the Taussig-Bing form of DORV.[14,15]

Overriding and/or straddling of the atrioventricular valve apparatus may be present in DORV, making biventricular repair difficult. Straddling of the right atrioventricular (AV) valve may permit a biventricular repair.[16] Significant overriding of the right AV valve may result in a small inlet portion of the right ventricle after VSD closure and a concomitant bidirectional cavopulmonary shunt may be necessary ("one-and-one-half ventricle" repair). [17] Associated mitral valve anomalies include mitral atresia, parachute valve, straddling, and supravalvular stenosing ring.

Pulmonary stenosis occurs commonly in DORV hearts, particularly in those with subaortic and doubly committed VSDs. The stenosis is most often at the level of the infundibulum, clinically presenting as right-to-left shunting.

The coronary artery anatomy in DORV is predominantly of the normal pattern.[18] However, anomalous coronary patterns can be seen in up to 16 percent of patients undergoing operation. The most common is anomalous origin of the left anterior descending artery from the right coronary artery. This pattern is typically seen in the subgroup of DORV with subaortic VSD and right ventricular outflow tract obstruction (RVOTO).[19] Coronary arterial patterns that are seen with transposition of the great arteries can also be present with DORV.

Table 63-2 Concomitant congenital cardiac anomalies in 179 patients undergoing repair for double-outlet right ventricle (exclusive of pulmonary stenosis) at the Mayo Clinic from 1972 to 1992[a]

	Number	Frequency (%)
ASD	99	55
Persistent left SVC	34	19
Coronary anomalies	28	16
Multiple VSDs	22	12
Nonconfluent PA	21	12
Situs inversus	18	10
PDA	18	10
Right aortic arch	16	9
AV discordance	5	3
Common atrium	5	3
Coarctation	6	3
AV canal	6	3
Mitral stenosis	4	2
TAPVC/PAPVC	3	2
Unroofed coronary sinus	1	1

ASD = atrial septal defect; AV = atrioventricular; PA = pulmonary artery; PDA = patent ductus arteriosus; PAPVC = partial anomalous pulmonary venous connection; SVC = superior vena cava; TAPVC = total anomalous pulmonary venous connection; VSD = ventricular septal defect.

[a]Unpublished data.

With regard to the conduction system, the AV node and the bundle of His follow pathways that are specific for the type of AV connections. In AV concordance, the VSD is usually perimembranous (conoventricular) and the conduction tissue would be along the posteroinferior border of the defect. In the presence of AV discordance, the conduction pathways would be anterior and adjacent to the pulmonary artery.

PATHOPHYSIOLOGY AND CLINICAL MANIFESTATIONS

Clinical presentation is variable and depends on the particular morphology of DORV, type of VSD, and the presence or absence of associated RVOTO.

SUBAORTIC VENTRICULAR SEPTAL DEFECT

The position of the infundibular septum and the presence of RVOTO determine the clinical presentation. Anterior deviation of the infundibular septum producing RVOTO presents with cyanosis, much like ToF. Concomitant pulmonary stenosis may be present. Other symptoms that can be seen as a result of RVOTO include failure to thrive, dyspnea on exertion, squatting, and polycythemia.

Management is similar to that of ToF. In the absence of RVOTO, the clinical presentation is like that of a large VSD, with heart failure and pulmonary overcirculation as typical presenting features.

SUBPULMONARY VENTRICULAR SEPTAL DEFECT

Clinical presentation is usually cyanosis due to unfavorable streaming of deoxygenated blood into the aorta and oxygenated blood into the pulmonary artery via the subpulmonary VSD. This presentation is very similar to that of patients with D-TGA. Subaortic stenosis may be present in up to 35 percent of patients with Taussig-Bing anomaly.[15] Concomitant coarctation or arch hypoplasia may occur in up to 50 percent of infants with DORV and subpulmonary VSD.[15] Patients are seen in the newborn period or in early infancy with cyanosis, heart failure, failure to thrive, and frequent respiratory infections. If surgical correction is not undertaken, high pulmonary blood flow in this subgroup of DORV patients results in pulmonary vascular obstructive disease at an early age.

DOUBLY COMMITTED VSD

This lesion is uncommon, and the mode of clinical presentation depends on the presence of favorable or unfavorable streaming. Pulmonary stenosis may also be present.

REMOTE VENTRICULAR SEPTAL DEFECT

Clinical presentation is similar to that of patients with single ventricle physiology, i.e., oxygen saturations usually reflect complete mixing due to the remoteness of the VSD from the great arteries. Pulmonary blood flow may be balanced, increased, or decreased.

PHYSICAL EXAMINATION

There are no specific findings on physical exam that are pathognomonic of DORV. Patients in heart failure can present with tachypnea and failure to thrive, while cyanosis is seen in patients with inadequate pulmonary blood flow.

A VSD murmur is almost always present in the form of a pansystolic murmur, best heard over the left lower sternal border. If RVOTO is present a systolic ejection murmur is best heard over the second intercostal space on the left.

DIAGNOSIS

ELECTROCARDIOGRAPHY

There are no electrocardiographic (ECG) findings that are pathognomonic for DORV. However, certain ECG abnormalities can be seen in DORV (Fig. 63-3). The most common abnormality seen is right ventricular hypertrophy and right axis deviation. This is a result of systemic pressurization of the right ventricle. Left ventricular hypertrophy can be observed in the presence of a restrictive VSD or from volume overload in the presence of high pulmonary blood flow, as can be seen in DORV with subpulmonic VSD (Taussig-Bing anomaly). Right atrial enlargement is commonly seen with pulmonary stenosis. In contrast, left atrial enlargement is seen in the absence of pulmonary stenosis or when functional mitral stenosis is present. Other ECG abnormalities include first-degree atrioventricular block and left axis deviation due to posterior displacement of the conduction tissue.

CHEST X-RAY

Variable chest x-ray (CXR) findings can be associated with DORV. Patients with pulmonary stenosis will have diminished pulmonary vascular markings. In contrast, patients with high pulmonary blood flow will show plethoric lung fields. Patients presenting late with pulmonary vascular obstructive disease usually have diminished pulmonary vascular markings and prominent central pulmonary arteries. Cardiomegaly can be present. Double-outlet right ventricle with RVOTO (i.e., with ToF-like physiology) may reveal right ventricular hypertrophy, poor prominence of the pulmonary artery, and upward displacement of the cardiac apex (*coeur en*

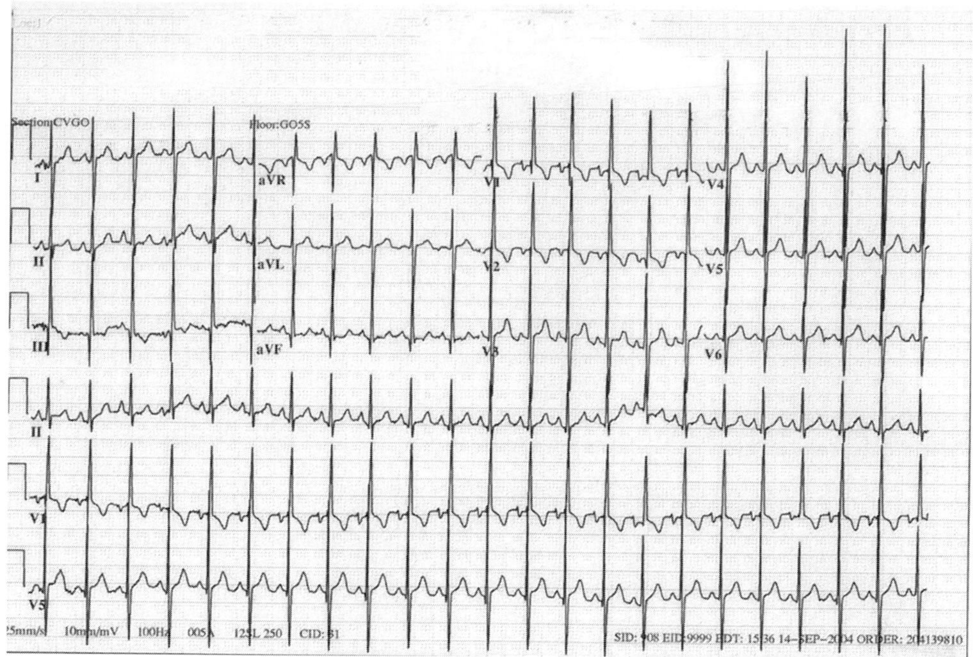

Figure 63-3 ECG of 6-month-old patient with double-outlet right ventricle and subaortic VSD exhibiting some of the features that can be seen with this anomaly: normal sinus rhythm with biatrial enlargement, right ventricular hypertrophy, and right axis deviation.

Sabot). Left ventricular hypertrophy and enlargement, which may be seen in the presence of an unrestrictive VSD, may disclose on CXR an apex that is downwardly turned and displaced below the diaphragm.

ECHOCARDIOGRAPHY

Transthoracic echocardiography is the imaging technique most commonly used for making the diagnosis of DORV. Transesophageal echocardiography is utilized to further define more complex abnormalities of the atrioventricular valves (i.e., overriding and straddling). Diagnosis is established by demonstrating both great arteries predominately arising from the anterior right ventricle and VSD as the sole outlet of the left ventricle. Echocardiography can also delineate aortic-mitral fibrous discontinuity. Concomitant cardiac anomalies (i.e., coronary artery patterns, coarctation, etc.) are usually readily noted on echocardiographic examination. Echocardiography is therefore usually the only diagnostic modality needed for establishing the appropriate plan of management in an infant. Figure 63-4 illustrates some of the characteristic echocardiographic findings that establish the diagnosis of DORV. Additional diagnostic techniques are usually required in older children and adults.

CARDIAC CATHETERIZATION

Cardiac catheterization may be indicated to assess hemodynamic characteristics and suitability of repair, exclude pulmonary vascular obstructive disease, and determine coronary artery anatomy.

MAGNETIC RESONANCE IMAGING

MRI provides complementary information about associated intracardiac defects and the status of the aorta and pulmonary arteries. In addition, MRI can provide data regarding the three-dimensional relationship of the cardiac chambers and arrangement of the great arteries as well as an accurate assessment of left and right ventricular function. MRI may be able to predict the feasibility of biventricular repair in DORV hearts with noncommitted VSDs.[21]

SURGICAL THERAPY

In 1957, Kirklin, at the Mayo Clinic, performed the first repair of DORV in a child. This technique involved an intraventricular tunnel establishing left ventricular-aortic continuity via a subaortic VSD.[11] Since that time, many surgical procedures have been developed to repair some of the more complex anatomic variations seen with DORV.[13,22–26] The optimal surgical approach is tailored to the specific anatomic anomaly present. Complete anatomic repair is the goal when feasible. This includes establishing continuity of the left ventricle with the systemic circulation, of the right ventricle with the pulmonary circulation, and of VSD closure.

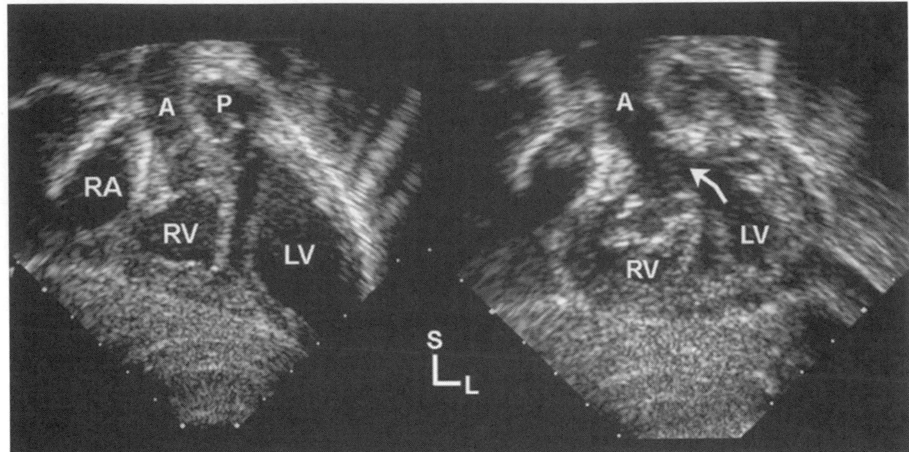

A

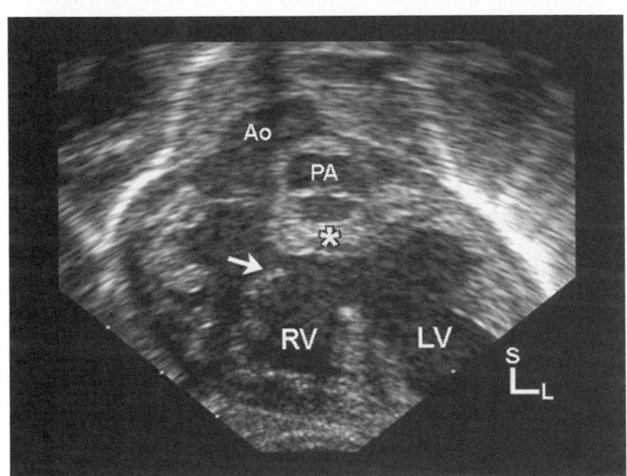

B

Figure 63-4 A. Transthoracic echocardiogram in a patient with double-outlet right ventricle with subaortic VSD. Left image: subcostal four-chamber view with anterior angulation demonstrates both great arteries arising from the RVOT with aorta (A) to the right and pulmonary artery (P) to the left. Right image: slight posterior angulation of the scan plane reveals that the VSD (arrow) is closely related to the aorta. There is infundibular muscle interposed between the VSD and the pulmonary valve. There is no pulmonary or subpulmonary stenosis and no important structures or valve attachments lying between the VSD and the aortic valve. Repair in this situation requires placement of an intraventricular tunnel to direct LV outflow across the VSD toward the aorta, allowing the RV to eject anteriorly to the patch directly into the PA. B. Transthoracic echocardiogram illustrating double-outlet right ventricle with remote VSD. Subcostal four-chamber view with anterior angulation demonstrates both great arteries arising from the RVOT. Note, however, that the semilunar valves are relatively further away as compared to the echocardiogram (A). The pulmonary valve is to the left and is separated from the VSD by a thick wall of malpositioned infundibular septum (asterisk). The tricuspid valve has an outlet attachment that is positioned between the VSD and the aortic valve (arrow). Simple septation in this case is not possible. There are three options for complete repair: (1) To construct a complex intraventricular tunnel (multiple-patch technique) with tricuspid valve replacement. (2) To perform an arterial switch operation with resection of the leftward portion of the malpositioned infundibular septum. (3) To treat this complex anatomic DORV variant as a functionally univentricular heart and direct the patient to a Fontan palliation strategy.

A palliative operation prior to complete repair may be required and occurs in 42 to 75 percent of patients with DORV.[13,22,23] Furthermore, approximately 25 percent will undergo more than one palliative operation, thus illustrating the complexity of this anomaly. Palliative operations (detailed in Chap. 54) have included systemic-to-pulmonary artery shunts, pulmonary artery banding, and repair of other anomalies such as coarctation. Anatomic anomalies precluding complete repair include ventricular hypoplasia, straddling or overriding of the atrioventricular valves, multiple VSDs, pulmonary vascular obstructive disease, and other associated complex cardiac anomalies.

It is helpful to the surgeon to categorize DORV into one of four groups, as this helps in guiding the appropriate surgical management:

1. Subaortic or doubly committed VSD without RVOTO (VSD type)
2. Subaortic or doubly committed VSD and RVOTO (ToF type)
3. Subpulmonary VSD (TGA type, Taussig-Bing)
4. Noncommitted VSD with or without RVOTO

SUBAORTIC OR DOUBLY COMMITTED VSD WITHOUT RVOTO (VSD TYPE)

The VSD is usually exposed through a longitudinal right ventriculotomy with care taken not to injure large conal branches or the left anterior descending artery. A right atrial approach can also be utilized. However, with this approach, it is difficult to assess proper alignment of the intraventricular tunnel from the VSD to the aorta. After the right ventriculotomy is made, the size and location of the VSD is established, particularly noting whether the VSD abuts the tricuspid valve or has a rim of muscle along its posterior border. The diameter of the VSD must be at least equal to the diameter of the aortic annulus to prevent outflow tract obstruction to the aorta. If the VSD is restrictive, it is enlarged by incising or resecting a wedge of muscle in an anterosuperior direction. Obstructing muscle bundles of the right ventricle and a small portion of the infundibular septum are often excised for proper alignment of the patch, which is shaped like a tunnel. RVOTO (from "crowding of the right ventricle") is a potential complication of this procedure. This problem is avoided by establishing that the distance between the tricuspid annulus and the pulmonary annulus is at least equal to the diameter of the aortic annulus. This can be assessed preoperatively by subxiphoid views on echocardiography and by intraoperative assessment. The patch material used is often a Sauvage Dacron patch (USCI Sauvage filamentous Dacron fabric, C.R. Bard, Inc., Bellerica, MA), Gore-Tex (W. L. Gore and Associates, Inc., Flagstaff, AZ), or a tailored Dacron tube graft. The patch is sewn to channel blood flow from the left ventricle across the VSD to the aortic annulus. It is important to note that the patch should not be flat but rather fashioned as an open tube or tunnel, thus providing an unobstructed channel between the VSD and the aorta. Superiorly, the patch is sewn to the aortic annulus. Posteroinferiorly, the suture line is deviated away from the edge of the VSD to avoid injury to the conduction tissue. Posteriorly, the patch is sewn to the base of the septal leaflet of the tricuspid valve. If muscle interposes the tricuspid annulus and VSD, the VSD repair sutures can be placed in this muscle (conus) without damaging the conduction tissue (Fig. 63-5). If a transventricular approach is used, the right ventriculotomy is closed with a patch to avoid RVOTO created by the intraventricular tunnel.

Complete intraventricular tunnel repair is performed within the first 6 months of life because of the increased risk of developing pulmonary vascular obstructive disease. In previous years, initial palliation with a pulmonary artery band followed by an intraventricular tunnel and debanding in early childhood was performed. Doubly committed VSDs (with or without RVOTO) are uncommon. When present, repair is usually accomplished in early infancy. Closure of the superior aspect of the VSD may be challenging because of the absence of the infundibular septum. If needed, enlargement of the VSD is performed. If the VSD is more closely related to the pulmonary artery, the arterial switch operation as described for the Taussig-Bing anomaly is preferred.

SUBAORTIC OR DOUBLY COMMITTED VSD WITH RVOTO (TETRALOGY-TYPE DORV)

The repair of this anomaly is similar to repairs described in the chapter on ToF (Chap. 60). Exposure of the VSD is usually accomplished via a right ventriculotomy or a transatrial approach. The os of the infundibulum is resected to enlarge the RVOT. The VSD is closed using the tunnel technique described above. The right ventriculotomy is closed with a transannular patch to prevent RVOTO. An anomalous coronary artery crossing the right ventricular outflow tract can limit the ventriculotomy, resulting in inadequate relief of RVOTO. In this situation, a valved extracardiac conduit from right ventricle to pulmonary artery can be used. In the current era, most centers would perform complete repair in the first year of life. Alternatively, palliation with a systemic-to-pulmonary shunt can be performed if surgical treatment is required in the first 2 to 3 months of life because of worsening cyanosis.

SUBPULMONARY VENTRICULAR SEPTAL DEFECT (TAUSSIG-BING TYPE)

The operation of choice for DORV with subpulmonary VSD and no RVOTO (i.e., Taussig-Bing anomaly) is the arterial switch operation with patch closure of the VSD, resulting in the rerouting of left ventricular ejection

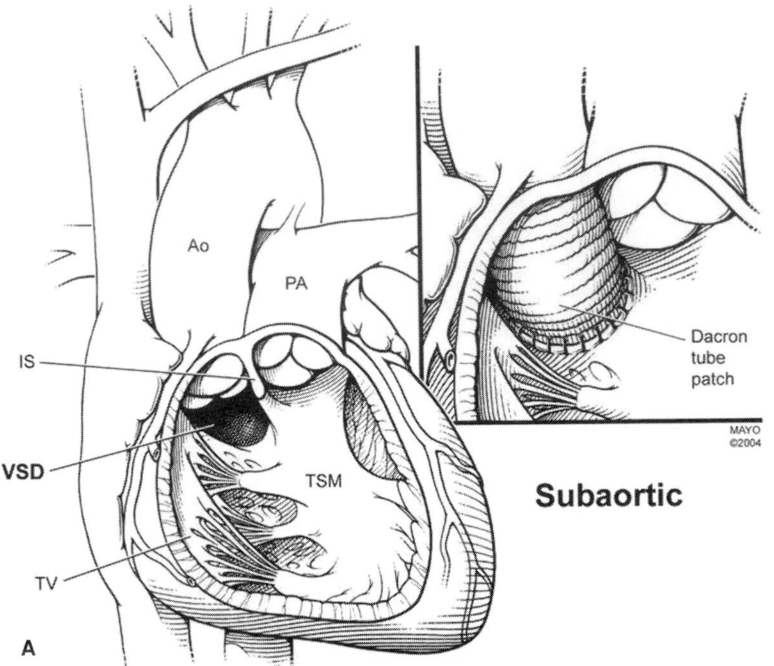

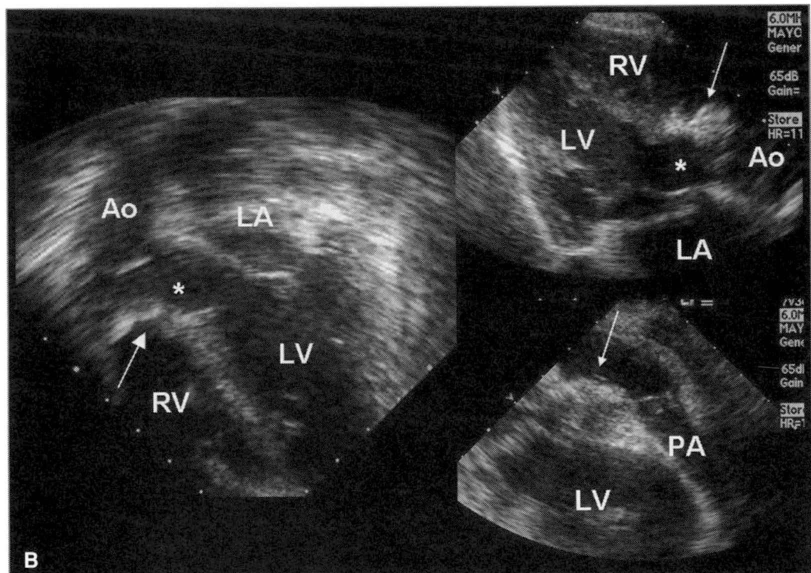

Figure 63-5 A. Diagram illustrating intraventricular tunnel repair of double-outlet right ventricle with subaortic VSD. Left ventricular ejection is directed via the VSD to the aorta. B. Postoperative transthoracic echocardiogram illustrating repair in a patient with DORV and subaortic VSD with no postoperative LVOT or RVOT obstruction. The left panel is an anteriorly angulated apical view illustrating deviation of the VSD patch (subaortic VSD) in order to channel flow from the VSD to the aorta. The arrow points to the RV surface of the VSD patch. The asterisk indicates the pathway from the LV to the aortic valve created by the patch. The upper right panel is a parasternal long-axis image in the same patient. Again, the arrow points to the RV surface of the patch and asterisk indicates the pathway from the LV to the aortic valve created by the patch. The lower right panel is a modified parasternal view focused on the long axis of the main PA. The RV outflow has been deviated anterior to the patch (arrow) but remains widely patent.

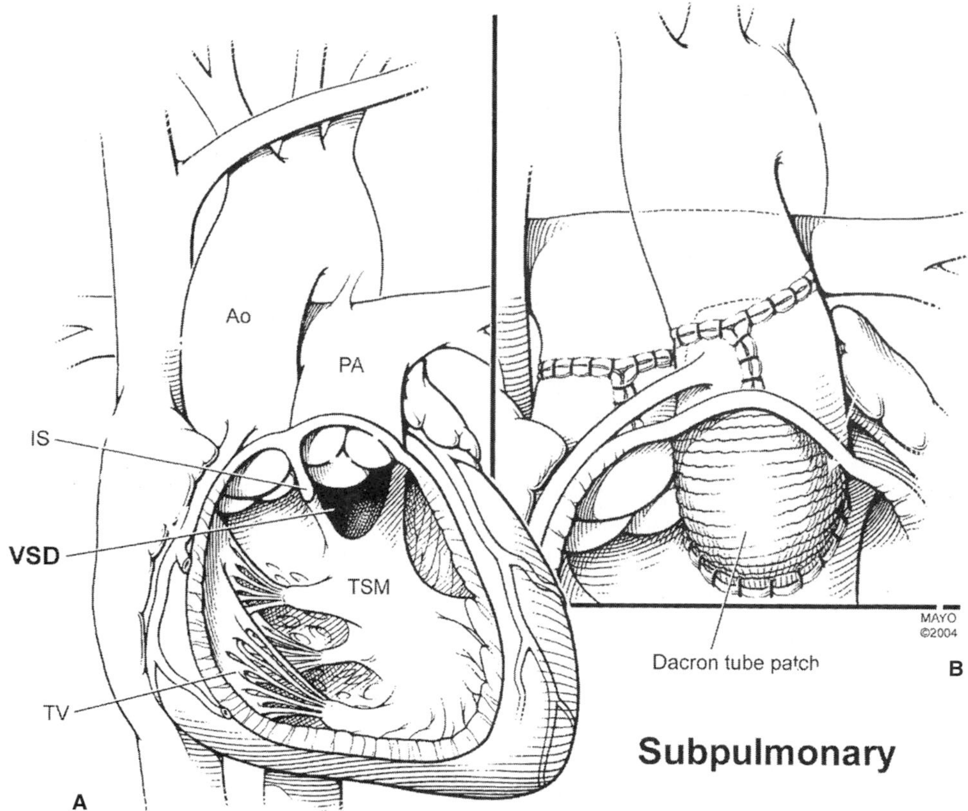

Figure 63-6 Diagram illustrating the arterial switch operation and tunneling of LV flow through the VSD to the neoaorta for a Taussig-Bing anomaly.

blood flow from the left ventricle to the pulmonary (neoaortic) valve (Fig. 63-6). Details of the arterial switch operation are described in the chapter on transposition of the great arteries (Chap. 66). Closure of the VSD can be approached via the right atrium, right ventricle, or aortic root (neopulmonary artery), depending on the location of the VSD.

Results of the arterial switch operation for this anomaly have been excellent, and the operative mortality for this form of DORV has significantly decreased in recent years.[26]

Intraventricular tunnel repair techniques such as the Kawashima operation are performed less commonly for patients with Taussig-Bing anomaly.[27] Increasing expertise with the arterial switch operation has made the Kawashima repair less appealing.

Concomitant aortic arch hypoplasia can be present with Taussig-Bing hearts and can be addressed as a single-stage complete repair. In the presence of arch hypoplasia, there is a high likelihood of hypoplasia of the RVOT, leading to clinically important infundibular obstruction. As such, RVOT obstruction should always be evaluated in the presence of arch hypoplasia.

The REV operation (*réparation à l'etage ventriculaire*) introduced by Lecompte is yet another repair designed for patients in whom an arterial switch and simple intraventricular tunnel repair of the VSD is not feasible. This situation arises when there is coexisting LV outflow tract obstruction (i.e., pulmonary stenosis). In this operation, the LV outflow is directed to the aorta and the pulmonary trunk transected, with its distal segment anastomosed directly to the right ventricle.[28,29]

NONCOMMITTED VENTRICULAR SEPTAL DEFECT WITH OR WITHOUT RVOTO

Surgical repair in this group is complex and challenging. Although a biventricular repair is desirable in this particular subgroup because of the presence of two normally functioning ventricles and atrioventricular valves, the complexity of the intracardiac repair and tunnel can be associated with high early mortality. In selected instances, long complex tunnel repairs can be undertaken. VSD enlargement with some infundibular resection is almost always required. An arterial switch operation may be preferred to bring the aorta closer to the remote VSD and make the intraventricular tunnel less complex. Some have reported the use of a multiple- (two to four) patch technique to create the tunnel between the VSD and aorta.[30]

In the majority of these cases, the best treatment algorithm appears to be a single-ventricle management strategy (see Chap. 69). This usually involves placement of a pulmonary artery band during the neonatal period. A bidirectional cavopulmonary anastomosis is usually performed when the patient is between 4 and 6 months of age. The Fontan procedure is generally performed between 18 months and 4 years of age.

The Fontan procedure has undergone many modifications; at present, medium-term results are quite favorable.[13] This operation has therefore been advocated in order to channel some of the more complicated anatomic variants of DORV toward a single-ventricle physiologic track.[24] In their 20-year experience in treating DORV, Brown and coworkers performed modified Fontan operations in 26.6 percent of their patients. In addition to remote VSD, indications for Fontan-type operations have included complex anomalies such as straddling AV valves, AV septal defects or hypoplastic left ventricle, or a combination of AV septal defects and hypoplastic ventricle, atrial isomerism, multiple VSDs, and major pulmonary artery anomalies including atresia, slings, and discontinuous branch pulmonary arteries. Early mortality when Fontan-type operations are performed has been shown to be 7.9 percent in this complex group of patients.[22]

PALLIATIVE OPERATIONS

Palliative operations are less frequently performed in the current era owing to the lower mortality rates achieved with complete repair in neonates and infants. Furthermore, recent series have shown that patient age and weight do not adversely impact mortality.[22,23] However, these studies were undertaken in centers that perform a large number of operations in neonates and infants. Many reported surgical series continue to show between 42 and 75 percent of patients having had an initial palliative operation mostly in the form of a modified Blalock-Taussig shunt or pulmonary arterial band.[11,23] This may reflect in part the fact that many patients were operated on in an earlier era. This percentage will continue to decrease as results of complete repair during infancy continue to improve.

RESULTS

Results of complete repair for DORV have been reported in several large contemporary series, and early mortality has been shown to range from 2.6 to 9 percent.[11,13,22,23,25,31] In general, late outcome is determined by anatomy and postrepair physiology.

Patients with ToF-type DORV have results similar to those achieved currently with tetralogy. When repair requires the use of a RV-to-PA conduit, repeat operation(s) for conduit replacement are required. The REV procedure (pulmonary artery directly attached to the right ventricle) may lessen the need for reoperation,[32] but this may occur at the expense of RV dilatation and subsequent RV failure from long-standing pulmonary regurgitation.

Patients undergoing arterial switch operations have excellent late survival. In contrast to standard transposition, the incidence of neoaortic valve regurgitation is more common in this group and may require the need for reoperation for valve repair or replacement.[33] Also, the side-by-side relationship of the great vessels can lead to branch pulmonary stenosis following the LeCompte maneuver.

Subaortic obstruction is a complication that can be seen immediately as well in the late postoperative period in patients who have undergone complete repair for DORV. This complication is a result of intracardiac tunneling of

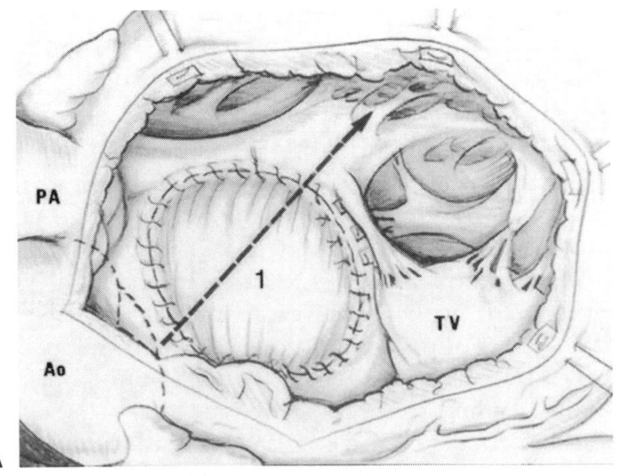

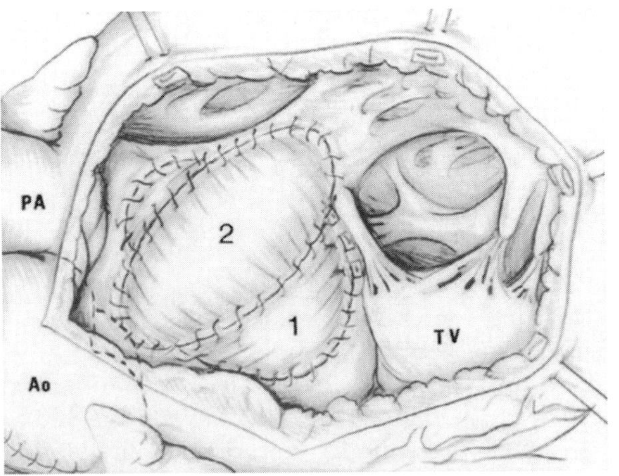

Figure 63-7 Extended septoplasty for management of late subaortic obstruction following complete repair for DORV. A. Right ventriculotomy approach. The arrow illustrates the septal incision made through the patch and toward the apex (leftward). B. Following a septal incision, a second patch is placed, resulting in augmentation of the LVOT. (From Belli et al.[34] With permission.)

the VSD to the aorta. Late development of subaortic obstruction results from protrusion of the inferior rim of the tunnel into the left ventricular outflow tract (LVOT) or from fibrous tissue below the aortic valve.[35] The risk of this complication can range from 5 to 50 percent, depending on the individual anatomy.[23,34] Treatment of subaortic obstruction is surgical and involves an extended septoplasty (Fig. 63-7) and subaortic resection of fibrous tissue.

Brown and colleagues reported a 20-year experience in 124 patients. Survival at 15 years was 96 percent for simple intracardiac repairs, 90 percent for subpulmonary VSD, and 90 percent for straddling AV valves or hypoplastic ventricles. The freedom for reoperation at 15 years was 87 percent for simple intracardiac repairs, 72 percent for subpulmonary VSD, and 100 percent for those with more complex intracardiac anatomy who underwent an arterial switch operation and VSD closure, thus avoiding a complex intracardiac tunnel repair.

Risk factors for early mortality include simultaneous obstruction of the aortic arch, AV septal defects, mitral stenosis or regurgitation, multiple VSDs, and age less than 1 month.[13,22,23]

CONCLUSIONS

DORV is a type of ventriculoarterial connection whereby both great arteries arise from the right ventricle. It is a form of complex congenital heart disease that can be associated with many other cardiac anomalies. The physiology and clinical presentation ranges from VSD-like to tetralogy of Fallot to transposition and to single-ventricle physiology. A full understanding of both the anatomy and physiology of this complex lesion leads to the proper surgical management strategy. The current trend is for complete repair in early infancy when feasible. Late results are favorable for most patients, although the potential need for reoperation remains.

References

1. Abbott ME, McRae T, Funk D (eds). Transposition or reversed torsion of the arterial trunks. In: *Modern Medicine: Its Theory and Practice.* Philadelphia: Lea & Febiger, 1927:716–736.
2. Lev M, Volk BM. The pathologic anatomy of the Taussig-Bing Heart: Riding pulmonary artery. Report of a case. *Bull Int Assoc Med Mus* 1950;31:54–64.
3. Witham AC. Double-outlet right ventricle: A partial transposition complex. *Am Heart J* 1952;43:773–780.
4. Vierordt H. Die Angeborenenherzkrankheiten. *Nothnagel's Speziale Pathologische Therapie* 1898 ;15:244.
5. Lev M, Bharati S, Meng CCL, et al. A concept of double-outlet right ventricle. *J Thorac Cardiovasc Surg* 1972;64: 271–281.
6. Neufeld HN, Lucas RV, Lester RG, et al. Origin of both great vessels from the right ventricle without pulmonary stenosis. *Br Heart J* 1962;24:393–399.
7. Walters HL, Mavroudis C, Tchervenkov CI, et al. Congenital Heart Surgery and Database Project: Double outlet right ventricle. *Ann Thorac Surg* 2000;69:S249–S263.
8. Anderson RH. Double-outlet right ventricle. *Cardiol Young* 2001;II:329–344.
9. Belli, E, Serraf, A, Lacour-Gayet F. Double-outlet right ventricle with non-committed ventricular septal defect. *Eur J Cardiothorac Surg* 1999;15:747–752.
10. Kirklin JW, Barratt-Boyes BG. Double–outlet right ventricle. In: Kirklin JW, Barratt-Boyes BG (eds). *Cardiac Surgery,* 3d ed. New York: Churchill Livingstone, 2003:1509–1539.
11. Kirklin JW, Harp RA, McGoon DC. Surgical treatment of origin of both arteries from right ventricle, including cases of pulmonary stenosis. *J Thorac Cardiovasc Surg* 1964;48: 1026–1036.
12. Musumeci F, Shumway S, Lincoln C, et al. Surgical treatment for double-outlet right ventricle at the Brompton Hospital, 1973 to 1986. *J Thorac Cardiovasc Surg* 1988;96:278–287.
13. Kleinert S, Sano T, Weintraub RG, et al. Anatomic features and surgical strategies in double-outlet right ventricle. *Circulation* 1997;96:1233–1239.
14. Parr GV, Bharati S, Lev M, et al. Fetal coarctation in complete transposition of the great arteries with ventricular septal defect vs Taussig-Bing group of hearts. Surgical significance. *Circulation* 1982;66:II195–II199.
15. Sondheimer HM, Freedom RM, Olley PM. Double-outlet right ventricle: Clinical spectrum and prognosis. *Am J Cardiol* 1977:39:709–715.
16. Serraf A, Piot D, Belli E, et al. Biventricular repair of transposition of the great arteries and unbalanced ventricles. *J Thorac Cardiovasc Surg* 2001;122:1199–1203.
17. Van Arsdell GS, Williams WG, Freedom RM. A practical approach to 1 and 1/2 ventricle repairs. *Ann Thorac Surg* 1998;66:678–680.
18. Hagler J. Double-outlet right ventricle. In: *Moss and Adams' Heart Disease in Infants, Children, and Adolescents,* 5th ed. Baltimore: Williams & Wilkins, 1995:1246.
19. Sridaromont S, Feldt RH, Ritter DG, et al. Double-outlet right ventricle: Hemodynamic and anatomic correlations. *Am J Cardiol* 1976;38:85–89.
20. Mitchell SC, Korones Sb, Berendes HW. Congenital heart disease in 56,109 births: Incidence and natural history. *Circulation* 1971;43:323–329.
21. Beekman RP. Spin echo MRI in the evaluation of hearts with a double outlet right ventricle: Usefulness and limitations. *Magn Res Imaging* 2000;18:245–253.
22. Brown JW, Ruzmetzov M, Okada Y, et al. Surgical results in patients with double outlet right ventricle: A 20-year experience. *Ann Thorac Surg* 2001;72:1630–1635.
23. Belli E, Serraf A, Lacour-Gayet F, et al. Biventricular repair for double-outlet right ventricle: Results and long-term follow-up. *Circulation* 1998;98(Suppl II):360–365.

24. Russo P, Danielson GK, Puga F, et al. Modified Fontan procedure for biventricular hearts with complex forms of double-outlet right ventricle. *Circulation* 1988;78(Suppl III):20–25.
25. Lacour-Gayet F. Biventricular repair of double outlet right ventricle with non-committed ventricular septal defect (VSD) by VSD rerouting to the pulmonary artery and arterial switch. *Eur J Cardiothorac Surg* 2002;21: 1042–1048.
26. Masuda M. Clinical results of arterial switch operation for double-outlet right ventricle with subpulmonary VSD. *Eur J Cardiothorac Surg* 1999;15:283–288.
27. Kawashima Y, Fujita T, Miyamoto T, et al. Intraventricular rerouting of blood for the correction of Taussig-Bing malformation. *J Thorac Cardiovasc Surg* 1971;62:825–829.
28. Borromee L, Lecompte Y, Batisse A, et al. Anatomic repair of anomalies of ventriculoarterial connection associated with ventricular septal defect. Clinical results in 50 patients with pulmonary outflow tract obstruction. *J Thorac Cardiovasc Surg* 1988;95:96–99.
29. Lecompte Y, Neveux JY, Leca F, et al. Reconstruction of the outflow tract without prosthetic conduit. *J Thorac Cardiovasc Surg* 1994;58:1146–1149.
30. Barbero-Marcial M, Tanamati C, Atik E, et al. Intraventricular repair of double-outlet right ventricle with noncommitted ventricular septal defect: Advantages of multiple patches. *J Thorac Cardiovasc Surg* 1999;118: 1056–1067.
31. Takeuchi K, McGowan F, del Nido P, et al. Surgical outcome of double-outlet right ventricle with subpulmonary VSD. *Ann Thorac Surg* 2001;71:49–53.
32. Rubay J, Lecompte Y, Batisse A, et al. Anatomic repair of anomalies of ventriculo-arterial connection. *Eur J Cardiothorac Surg* 1988;2:305–311.
33. Haas F, Wottke M. Long-term survival and functional follow-up in patients after arterial switch operation. *Ann Thorac Surg* 1999;86:1692–1697.
34. Belli E, Serraf A, Lacour-Gayet F, et al. Surgical treatment of subaortic stenosis after biventricular repair of double-outlet right ventricle. *J Thorac Cardiovasc Surg* 1996;112:1570–1578.

CHAPTER

64 TOTAL ANOMALOUS PULMONARY VENOUS CONNECTION

Nicholas Kang, Victor T. Tsang

INTRODUCTION

Total anomalous pulmonary venous connection (TAPVC) can be defined as absence of any direct connection between the pulmonary veins and the left atrium. In this malformation, the pulmonary veins drain into the right heart via the systemic venous circuit, resulting in mixing of oxygenated and deoxygenated blood in the right atrium. An interatrial communication is necessary for postnatal survival. In addition, there may be obstruction to the pulmonary venous pathway, resulting in pulmonary venous hypertension.

Obstructed TAPVC remains one of the few true surgical emergencies in congenital heart disease. The first attempts at surgical repair were made in the 1950s, initially using closed methods[1,2] and, later, with inflow occlusion.[3] Complete intracardiac repair with cardiopulmonary bypass was first reported by Burroughs and Kirklin, who described three cases in 1956.[4]

ANATOMIC CLASSIFICATION

The most commonly used classification system[5] for TAPVC describes four anatomic subtypes: supracardiac (40 to 50 percent of cases), cardiac (20 to 25 percent), infracardiac (25 percent) and mixed (5 percent) (Fig. 64-1). This refers to the direction of the venous pathway from the pulmonary

KEY CONCEPTS

- Epidemiology
  - Total anomalous pulmonary venous connection (TAPVC) is a rare congenital anomaly, found in 1 to 3 percent of all cases of congenital heart disease. It is either found in isolation (most commonly) or associated with complex atrial isomerism.
- Morphology
  - The hallmark is the absence of connection between pulmonary veins and left atrium. Return is routed via the systemic venous system to the right atrium and, via an atrial septal defect (ASD), to the left atrium. These malformations are classified as supracardiac (45 percent), cardiac (25 percent), infracardiac (25 percent) and mixed (5 percent).
- Pathophysiology
  - This depends on the morphology and obstruction to pulmonary venous egress toward the right atrium. The latter often causes severe pulmonary venous hypertension.
- Clinical features
  - The typical presentation, if associated with some degree of venous obstruction somewhere between the pulmonary veins and left atrium, is that of severe respiratory distress and cyanosis in the newborn. Patients with no venous obstruction or with cardiac TAPVC and nonrestrictive ASD will present later with pulmonary overcirculation.
- Diagnosis
  - Echocardiography is diagnostic. Angiography is not indicated. Computed tomography and/or magnetic resonance imaging may be useful in selective and reoperative cases.
- Treatment
  - Obstructed TAPVC represents a true surgical emergency. The operative procedure involves creation of a connection between the pulmonary venous confluence and the left atrium.
- Outcomes
  - Mortality is correlated with preoperative status and the development of pulmonary venoocclusive disease (10 percent of cases). Patients who do not develop this nearly uniformly fatal complication have an excellent long-term outlook.

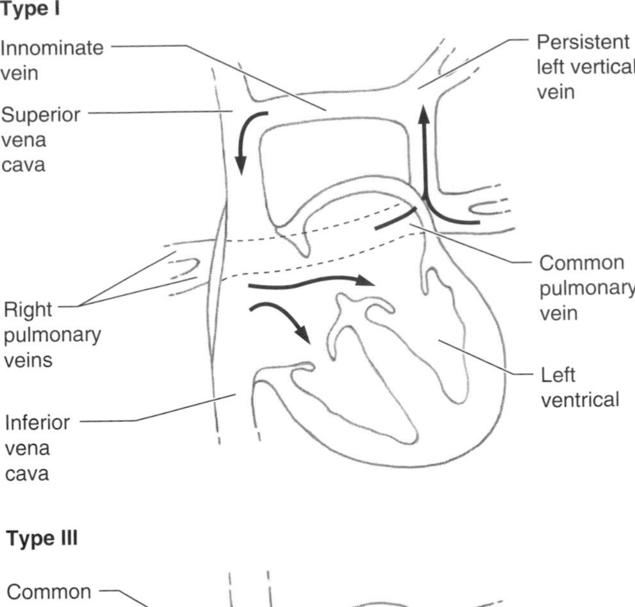

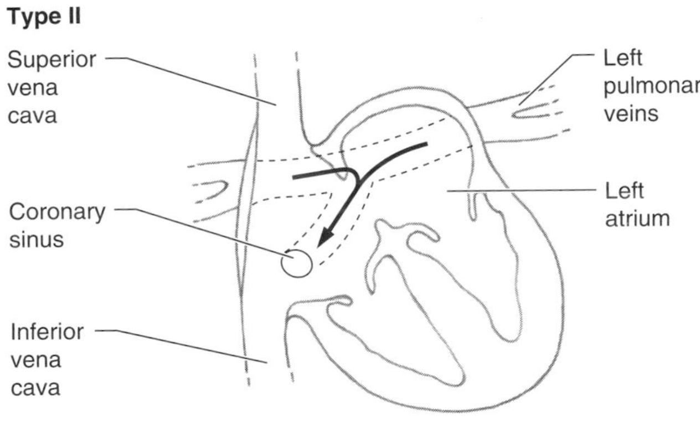

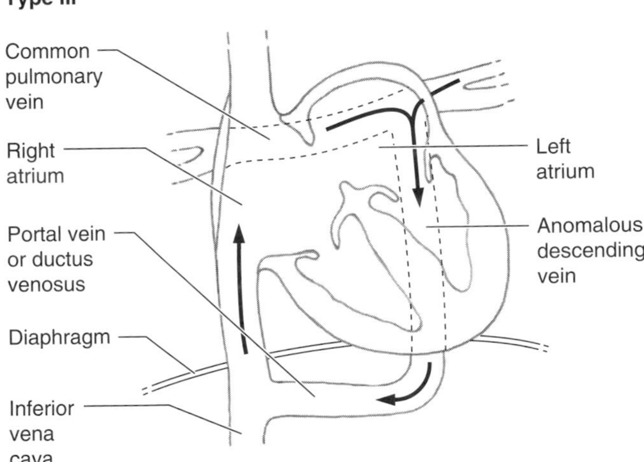

Figure 64-1 Schematic illustration of total anomalous pulmonary venous connection (TAPVC), supracardiac (I), cardiac (II), and infracardiac (III) types. [From Reitz BA, Yuh DD (eds). *Congenital Cardiac Surgery.* New York: McGraw-Hill 2002:148-149. With permission.]

venous confluence, which receives the individual pulmonary veins. The confluence itself is situated behind the heart, typically immediately posterior to the posterior pericardium.

In supracardiac TAPVC, the confluence gives rise to an ascending vertical vein, which usually connects to the left innominate vein. However, it may connect directly with the superior vena cava (SVC)[6] or, rarely, with one of the tributaries to the SVC. In cardiac TAPVC, the confluence typically drains into the coronary sinus, the ostium of which appears enlarged within the right atrium. In infracardiac TAPVC, there is a descending vertical vein, which passes through the diaphragm to join either the portal vein or ductus venosus or rarely some other infradiaphragmatic vein; return to the right atrium is therefore via the inferior vena cava. Mixed-type TAPVC, as the name implies, is a combination of the above, most often with the left-upper-lobe vein connected via an ascending vertical vein to the left innominate vein and the other pulmonary veins draining into the coronary sinus.

Obstruction to the pulmonary venous pathway may be due to a localized stenosis or to an inadequate aggregate caliber of the connecting vein or veins. Obstructed TAPVC occurs most often in the infracardiac variety, followed by supracardiac, mixed, and cardiac types in decreasing order of frequency. The interatrial communication may occasionally be restrictive and therefore also be a possible cause of pulmonary venous obstruction.

TAPVC usually occurs as an isolated lesion (aside from the associated interatrial communication). However, a patent ductus arteriosus may also be present. In right and left atrial isomerism, TAPVC is usually part of the complex of multiple lesions found in these rare conditions and mostly occurs as an infracardiac type.

PATHOPHYSIOLOGY

TAPVC is a mixing lesion in which oxygenated and deoxygenated blood eventually meets at the atrial level, resulting in cyanosis. There may be a degree of streaming, with blood from the inferior vena cava (IVC) preferentially directed through the patent foramen ovale (PFO) into the left atrium, theoretically favoring higher systemic saturation in the infracardiac type of TAPVC. In all variants, the left atrium is typically small and underfilled,[7] which adversely affects its compliance.

The feature that most importantly determines the pathophysiology and clinical presentation is the presence or absence of pulmonary venous obstruction. When present, this is often severe and results in marked pulmonary venous hypertension and edema, leading to severe hypoxemia. Right ventricular pressure may become systemic or even suprasystemic in this situation, and heart failure quickly ensues if the lesion is left uncorrected.

CLINICAL FEATURES

TAPVC is an uncommon lesion, representing about 2 percent of congenital heart defects. The clinical presentation usually occurs in the neonatal period when obstruction is present, with diffuse pulmonary edema and respiratory distress. Neonates may be critically sick and develop marked hypoxemia and acidosis, requiring resuscitation and mechanical ventilation, especially if the diagnosis is delayed and venous obstruction prominent. When obstruction is absent, the presentation is less acute. However, the natural history is still for heart failure to develop, typically within the first few months of life.[8] In patients surviving untreated beyond the first year of life, cyanosis is generally mild and there may be fairly nonspecific failure to thrive or limited exercise tolerance.

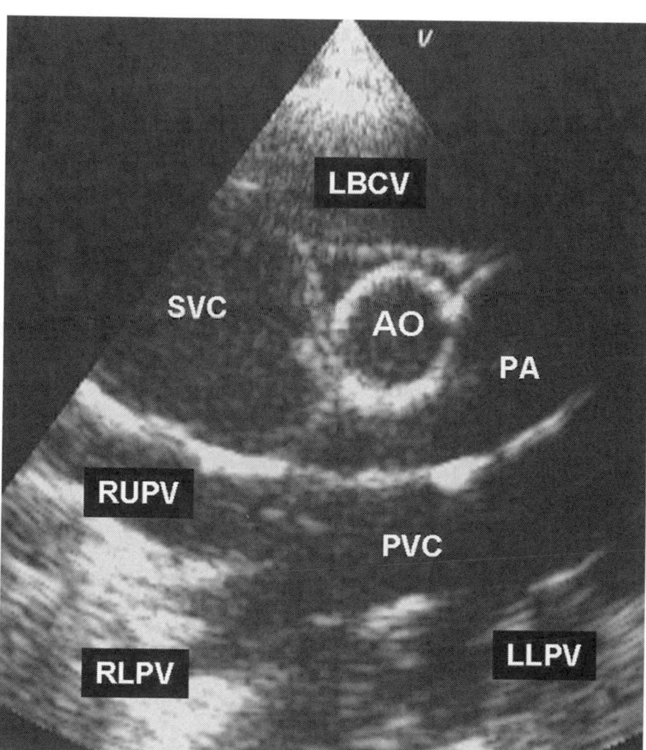

Figure 64-2 Echocardiographic findings in supracardiac TAPVC, suprasternal view. SVC = superior vena cava; LBCV = left brachiocephalic vein; AO = aorta; PA = pulmonary artery; PVC = pulmonary venous confluence; RUPV = right upper pulmonary vein; RLPV = right lower pulmonary vein; LLPV = left lower pulmonary vein.

DIAGNOSTIC MODALITIES

Neonates presenting with obstructed TAPVC typically have normal heart size with diffuse pulmonary interstitial "ground-glass" shadowing due to pulmonary edema. Older infants with increased pulmonary blood flow may have mild cardiomegaly. A prominent superior mediastinal shadow due to the ascending vertical vein and dilated SVC may be seen in older patients with supracardiac TAPVC and has been labeled the "snowman sign."[9]

Echocardiography is usually diagnostic (Figs. 64-2, 64-3, and 64-4) and identifies the absence of pulmonary veins entering the left atrium. The anatomic subtype can usually be reliably defined and the connecting vein(s) to the systemic venous circuit also visualized. Right heart volume overload is an associated feature. Color Doppler imaging also provides information about turbulence in the venous pathway, indicative of obstruction.

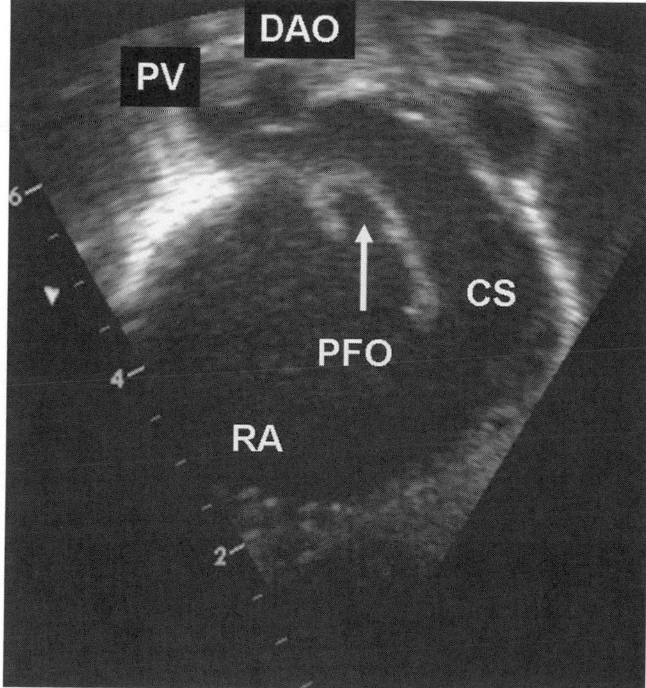

Figure 64-3 Intracardiac TAPVC. CS = coronary sinus; DAO = descending thoracic aorta; PV = pulmonary veins; PFO = patent foramen ovale; RA = right atrium.

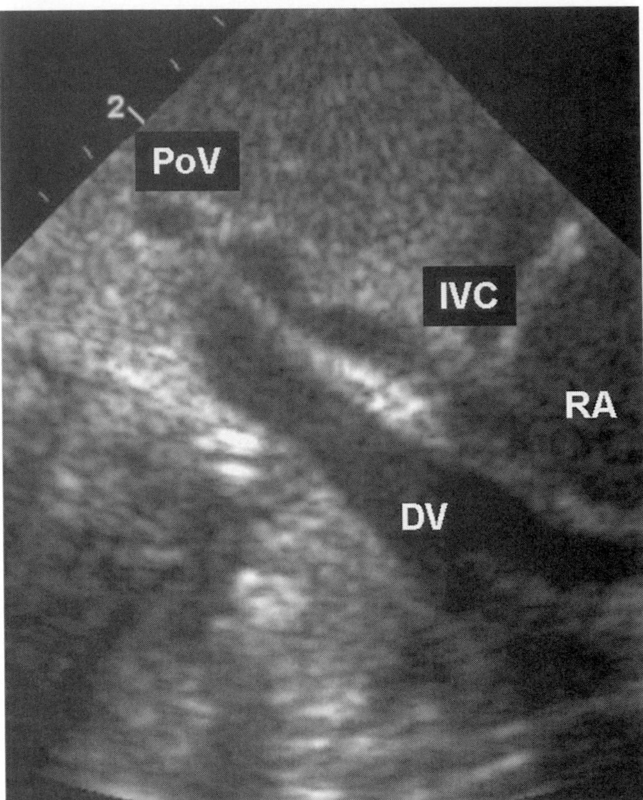

Figure 64-4 Infracardiac TAPVC. The descending vein is seen parallel to the inferior vena cava. DV = descending vein; IVC = inferior vena cava; PoV = portal vein; RA = right atrium.

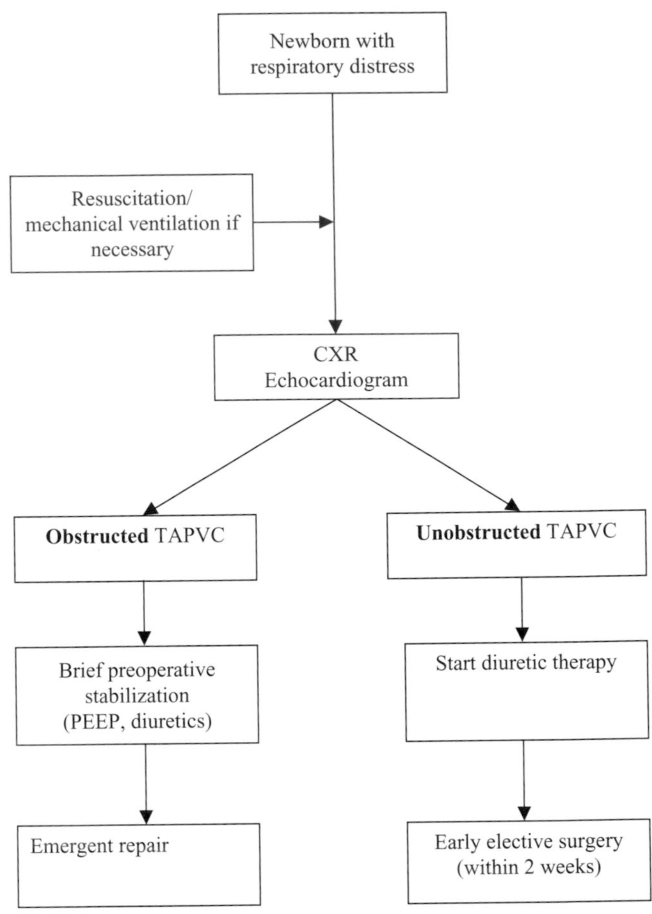

Figure 64-5 Decision-making flowchart.

Cardiac catheterization is no longer used in the current era of echocardiographic diagnosis. The contrast load also exacerbates pulmonary edema and therefore may be hazardous in sick neonates.

Recent advances in image resolution and three-dimensional reconstruction have made computed tomography (CT) and magnetic resonance imaging (MRI) promising modalities for assessment of the pulmonary veins. Although echocardiography is usually sufficient for the initial diagnosis, CT and MRI may be valuable in the postoperative situation where recurrent pulmonary vein stenosis is suspected. At present, CT is probably more accurate in identifying precise pulmonary vein anatomy. However, MRI has the ability to quantify flow and velocity and can potentially provide more information about differential lung perfusion and individual pulmonary vein stenosis (Fig. 64-5).

MEDICAL THERAPY

Preoperative medical therapeutic options are limited. Patients requiring resuscitation should be intubated and ventilated, keeping the inspired oxygen concentration as close to 21 percent as possible in order to minimize pulmonary congestion. Positive end-expiratory pressure helps to maintain alveolar opening and limit pulmonary edema. Diuretics are also helpful, and excessive volume loading must be avoided. Inotropic support may be required. Once the diagnosis of obstructed TAPVC is confirmed by echocardiography, surgery should not be delayed. However, Ward and colleagues have reported success with balloon or blade atrial septostomy in patients without extracardiac obstruction but having a restrictive interatrial communication. Using this strategy, surgery could be postponed for a mean of 12 months in their series.[10] Nowadays, early repair is strongly advocated once the hemodynamic status has been optimized.

Patients without obstruction require less urgent operation but usually still have signs of pulmonary plethora. Treatment with diuretics can be initiated and supplemental oxygen avoided while awaiting early elective surgery. Prostaglandin infusion is contraindicated in patients with TAPVC, as pulmonary vasodilation and left-to-right shunting across the arterial duct will exacerbate pulmonary congestion.

SURGICAL THERAPY

Supracardiac and infracardiac total anomalous pulmonary venous connection

TAPVC requires surgical correction and remains one of the true surgical emergencies in neonates with obstruction. The principles of operation in supracardiac and infracardiac TAPVC are (1) to identify the anatomy precisely, (2) to interrupt the anomalous connection to the systemic venous circuit, (3) to create an anastomosis between the pulmonary venous confluence and left atrium and (4) to close the interatrial communication (although some surgeons may prefer to leave behind an atrial communication as a "blow-out" valve in anticipation of postoperative pulmonary hypertension). Several different techniques exist for performing the anastomosis, some of which also include enlarging the left atrium.[11–17] Whatever method is used, the most important aspect of surgical correction is to create an unobstructed return for pulmonary venous blood into the left atrium. We describe our preferred technique below, followed by a summary of other methods.

Surgery is performed with cardiopulmonary bypass. The duct is routinely ligated, as this may be patent in up to 20 percent of cases. During cooling, pH stat is employed and the hematocrit maintained around 30 percent. At 18°C, the heart is arrested with a single dose of cold-blood cardioplegia, following which the circulation is stopped and the patient exsanguinated into the venous reservoir. Deep hypothermic circulatory arrest has the advantages of single venous cannulation and a bloodless operative field, avoiding any clamping of the pulmonary veins. The head is packed in ice during this period. At this point, the heart is reflected into the right pleural space, which is opened deliberately for this purpose. The pulmonary veins and their connections are then dissected where they lie immediately posterior to the pericardium. Although this dissection can be performed on bypass while the patient is still cooling, we prefer to disturb the heart as little as possible during this period. All the veins must be identified accurately as they enter the confluence. The connecting vein (ascending or descending vertical vein) is then ligated and divided. Care must be taken to avoid injuring the left phrenic nerve in cases of an ascending vertical vein to the left innominate vein. A ligature is placed around the tip of the left atrial appendage and retracted toward the patient's left shoulder in order to help align the anastomosis of the left atrium with the confluence. Corresponding incisions (Fig. 64-6) are made in the pulmonary venous confluence and the body of the left atrium, and a generous anastomosis performed. We use a continuous 7-0 polypropylene suture, locking the suture line intermittently to avoid purse-stringing of the anastomosis. No attempt is made to augment the size of the left atrium. The ASD is then closed by direct suture through the

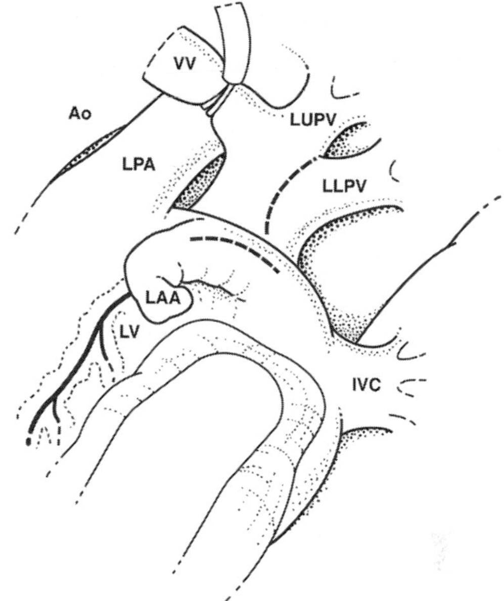

Figure 64-6 Posterior approach to the supracardiac TAPVC. Description in text. Ao = aorta; IVC = inferior vena cava; LAA = left atrial appendage; LLPV = left lower pulmonary vein; LPA = left pulmonary artery; LUPV = left upper pulmonary vein; LV = left ventricle; VV = vertical vein.

right atrium, although it is often wise (given the diminutive size of the left atrium) to close the interatrial communication with a patch. Bypass is reestablished and the heart de-aired prior to unclamping the aorta. Slow rewarming is commenced. A pulmonary artery pressure-monitoring line is inserted and a peritoneal dialysis catheter placed. Weaning from bypass is undertaken at 36°C. Mild hypothermia is preferred to minimize neurologic morbidity and also because of the anticipated low-cardiac-output state postoperatively. In our practice, the repair is checked with intraoperative transesophageal or epicardial echocardiography. Some authors would argue against insertion of a transesophageal probe, as this may be compressive of the newly performed anastomotic site. After modified ultrafiltration, protamine is given and the heart decannulated. Atrial and ventricular pacing wires are attached and drains inserted. The chest is usually closed but can be electively left open in very sick neonates.

The method of exposure described above (retracting the cardiac apex and performing the anastomosis from outside the heart) was described by Williams and coworkers in 1964.[11] A commonly used alternative technique involves approach through the right atrium (Fig. 64-7).[12] The rim of the fossa ovalis that encircles the interatrial communication is excised to gain wide access to the left atrium. The posterior wall of the left atrium is

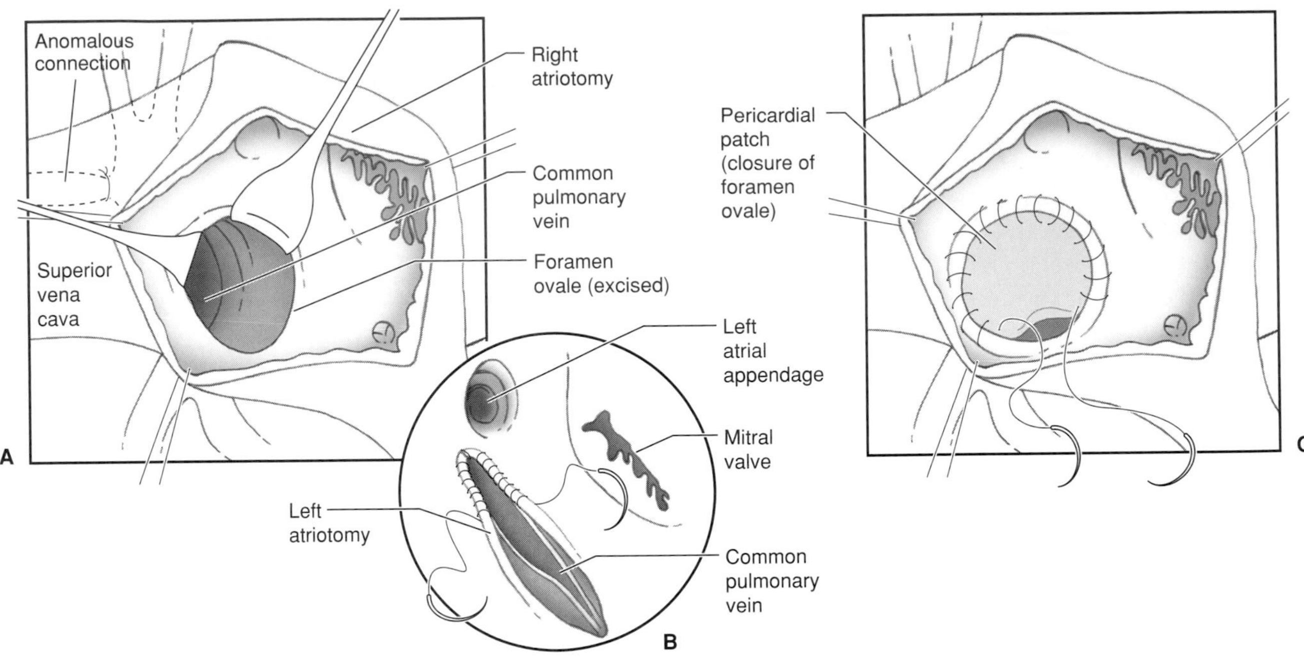

Figure 64-7 Transatrial approach for repair of TAPVC. The venous confluence is exposed through the foramen ovale and the back wall of the left atrium (A). The venotomy made in the venous confluence is anastomosed to the left posterior atriotomy (B). The interatrial communication is closed with autologous pericardium (C). [From Reitz BA, Yuh DD (eds). *Congenital Cardiac Surgery*. New York: McGraw-Hill 2002:151. With permission.]

then opened transversely and anastomosed to a corresponding transverse incision in the common pulmonary vein, which lies immediately behind the left atrium. The PFO is closed with a patch to augment the size of the left atrium. This method has the theoretical advantage of avoiding distortion in creating the anastomosis, which is done without displacing the heart. A modification of this technique involves a transverse right atriotomy, which is extended onto the lateral left atrial wall.[13,14] The anastomosis is then essentially extracardiac, with a pericardial patch used to simultaneously augment the anastomosis and the left atrium. Another approach described involves exposing the common pulmonary vein and left atrium through the transverse sinus between the aorta and superior vena cava.[15]

Cardiac Total anomalous pulmonary venous connection

In this variant (in which the pulmonary venous confluence joins the coronary sinus to drain into the right atrium), the operative strategy differs slightly in principle and is usually somewhat simpler. Total cardiopulmonary bypass with bicaval cannulation is used and only mild hypothermia to 34°C is employed. After the heart has been arrested, the right atrium is opened and the anatomy identified. An incision is made to connect the ostium of the coronary sinus with the ASD. The combined hole is then closed with a patch of autologous pericardium, thus diverting the coronary sinus blood into the left atrium (Fig. 64-8). In this way, the pulmonary venous return is directed back to the left heart. A small and clinically unimportant right-to-left shunt is created as the desaturated myocardial venous blood that drains normally via the coronary sinus is diverted to the left atrium.

An alternative method of repair of cardiac TAPVC has been proposed by van Praagh and associates[18] to avoid late stenosis at the repair site. This technique involves "unroofing" of the coronary sinus into the left atrium, closure of the ostium of the coronary sinus in the right atrium, as well as closing of the interatrial defect. Care must be taken to avoid damage to the AV node with either technique. Jonas and colleagues[19] have reported cases of obstructed cardiac TAPVC that may necessitate anastomosing the back of the left atrium to the junction of the pulmonary veins rather than the simpler unroofing operation.

SURGICAL OUTCOME

Early postoperative mortality

Neonatal repair of obstructed TAPVC still carries a significant mortality in many centers and is generally

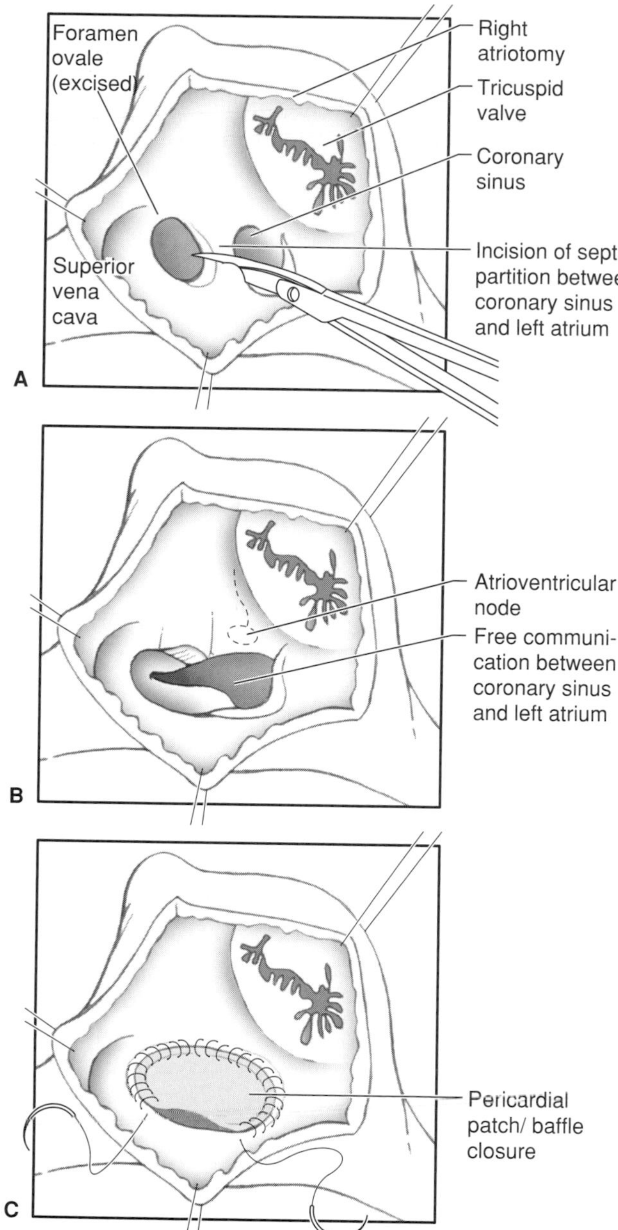

Figure 64-8 Repair of cardiac TAPVC (return to coronary sinus). Through a right atriotomy, the coronary sinus is unroofed (A). This creates a free communication between coronary sinus and left atrium (B). The atria are partitioned with a baffle of autologous pericardium (C). [From Reitz BA, Yuh DD (eds). *Congenital Cardiac Surgery*. New York: McGraw-Hill 2002:152. With permission.]

considered a high-risk operation in modern risk-stratification schemes.[20–22] The patient's preoperative status is an important determinant of outcome and, unlike the case with other neonatal conditions (such as transposition or interrupted aortic arch), these patients have limited potential for preoperative medical stabilization. Cardiopulmonary bypass and ischemic cardioplegic arrest (with or without deep hypothermic circulatory arrest) predictably imposes a major insult on cardiac and other end-organ function in critically sick neonates. Multivariate analysis has previously identified infracardiac subtype, pulmonary venous obstruction, and poor preoperative status as incremental risk factors for death owing to low-cardiac-output syndrome in most cases.[23] However, a large study by Bando and colleagues[24] found that a small pulmonary confluence associated with diffuse pulmonary vein stenosis was the only independent risk factor for mortality and need for reoperation. They also documented (despite the increased frequency of neonatal repair) a decline in pulmonary hypertensive crises and operative mortality over the last 30 years, reflecting the improved management of sick neonates in the perioperative period.

Pulmonary vein stenosis

This formidably challenging complication occurs in approximately 5 to 10 percent of patients operated for TAPVC.[25] It usually develops within the first few months after initial repair, although it rarely may become manifest a year or more later. Patients re-present with tachypnea and pulmonary venous congestion, and echocardiography identifies accelerated turbulent flow in the pulmonary veins, usually at the site of anastomosis. Although anastomotic technical failure may occasionally be implicated, the stenosis is more often related to a poorly understood process of neointimal hyperplasia and has been associated with all surgical techniques used for primary repair. A sclerosing vasculopathy develops, which can be remote from or extend beyond the anastomotic site and progress inexorably into the pulmonary veins despite recurrent attempts at repair.

This dreaded complication has led to a number of innovative reoperative techniques. The "sutureless" technique of repair[26,27] involves enlarging the strictured pulmonary venous openings and anastomosing the atrium to the fibrous or pericardial margins surrounding the veins, rather than to the intima itself. This concept was derived from modifications of the Senning operation,[28] in which the in situ pericardium was used to augment the pulmonary venous pathway. Some surgeons have advocated this repair as the primary operation for TAPVC as a means of avoiding development of this usually fatal complication. Other techniques for reoperation include patching the stenosed veins with pericardium or in situ left atrial appendage[29] or simple incision into the stenosed vein from within the left atrium, allowing the venous drainage to be contained by surrounding adhesions. All methods have been associated with significant failure rates, further supporting the notion that the disease process is intrinsic to the veins themselves rather than the surgical technique.

Attempts have also been made to prevent recurrences using pharmacologic agents. Steroids[30] and cytotoxic drugs have been used to try to suppress the proliferation of fibroblasts that characterizes these lesions. However, there is limited evidence at present to support their use and they therefore remain experimental. A phase II trial of vinblastine and methotrexate has recently been conducted at Boston Children's Hospital, for which results are presently awaited. Interventional catheterization with dilatation and stenting of pulmonary vein stenoses has generally met with very limited success.[31]

Long-term functional outcome

Patients with isolated TAPVC who survive surgery and do not develop early pulmonary vein stenosis can be expected to grow normally and are usually asymptomatic in NYHA functional class 1 at late follow-up.[24] In atrial isomerism, the long-term prognosis is much more guarded and dictated by the associated complex cardiac and extracardiac lesions. Several small series report long-term survival of less than 40 percent in this group of patients, with survival of 5 to 13 percent in the subgroup who require neonatal surgical intervention.[32–34] Whereas operative mortality for "simple" TAPVC has improved over the years, the group of patients with isomerism (or other complex associated lesions) has remained fairly constant. Part of the explanation for this may be the difficulty in regulating pulmonary blood flow in situations where (1) a systemic-to-pulmonary shunt is required for right ventricular outflow tract obstruction or (2) when pulmonary artery banding is required for pulmonary overcirculation.

References

1. Muller WH. The surgical treatment of transposition of the pulmonary veins. *Ann Surg* 1951;134:683–693.
2. Gross RE, Watkins E Jr, Pomeranz AA, et al. A method for surgical closure of interauricular septal defects. *Surg Gynecol Obstet* 1953;96:1–23.
3. Lewis FJ, Varco RL, Taufic M, et al. Direct vision repair of triatrial heart and total anomalous pulmonary venous drainage. *Surg Gynecol Obstet* 1956;102:713–720.
4. Burroughs JT, Kirklin JW. Complete surgical correction of total anomalous pulmonary venous connection: Report of three cases. *Mayo Clin Proc* 1956;31:182–188.
5. Craig JM, Darling RC, Rothney WB. Total pulmonary venous drainage into the right side of the heart: Report of 17 autopsied cases not associated with other major cardiovascular anomalies. *Lab Invest* 1957;6:44–48.
6. Warembourg H, Dubost C, Soyer R, et al. A rare case of total anomalous pulmonary venous return into the base of the superior vena cava. *Ann Chir Thorac Cardiovasc* 1972;11:239–246.
7. Mathew R, Thilenius OG, Replogle RL, Arcilla RA. Cardiac function in total anomalous pulmonary venous return before and after surgery. *Circulation* 1977;55:361–370.
8. Bonham-Carter RE, Capriles M, Noe Y. Total anomalous pulmonary venous drainage. A clinical and anatomical study of 75 children. *Br Heart J* 1969;31:45–51.
9. Golden RL, Bertrand CA. "Snowman" heart. Manifestation of total anomalous pulmonary venous connection. *JAMA* 1960;173:1102–1105.
10. Ward KE, Mullins CE, Huhta JC, et al. Restrictive interatrial communication in total anomalous pulmonary venous connection. *Am J Cardiol* 1986;57:1131–1136.
11. Williams GR, Richardson WR, Campbell GS. Repair of total anomalous pulmonary venous drainage in infancy. *J Thorac Cardiovasc Surg* 1964;47:199–204.
12. Hawkins JA, Clark EB, Doty DB. Total anomalous pulmonary venous connection. *Ann Thorac Surg* 1983;36:548–560.
13. Doty DB. *Cardiac Surgery: Operative Technique*. St Louis: Mosby-Yearbook, 1997.
14. Schumacker HB Jr, King H. A modified procedure for complete repair of total anomalous pulmonary venous drainage. *Surg Gynecol Obstet* 1961;112:763–774.
15. Tucker BL, Lindesmith GG, Stiles QR, et al. The superior approach for correction of the supracardiac type of total anomalous pulmonary venous return. *Ann Thorac Surg* 1976;22:374–377.
16. Goor DA, Yellin A, Frand M, et al. The operative problem of small left atrium in total anomalous pulmonary venous connection: Report of 5 patients. *Ann Thorac Surg* 1976;22:245–248.
17. Corno A, Giamberti A, Carotti, A et al. Total anomalous pulmonary venous connection: Surgical repair with double patch technique. *Ann Thorac Surg* 1990;49:492–494.
18. Van Praagh R, Harken AH, Delisle G, et al. Total anomalous pulmonary venous drainage to the coronary sinus. A revised procedure for its correction. *J Thorac Cardiovasc Surg* 1972;64:132–135.
19. Jonas RA, Smolinsky A, Mayer JE, et al. Obstructed pulmonary venous drainage with total anomalous pulmonary venous connection to the coronary sinus. *Am J Cardiol* 1987;59:431–435.
20. Jenkins KJ, Gauvreau K, Newburger JW, et al. Consensus-based method for risk adjustment for surgery for congenital heart disease. *J Thorac Cardiovasc Surg* 2002;123:110–118.
21. Kang N, Cole T, Tsang V, et al. Risk stratification in paediatric open-heart surgery. *Eur J Cardiothorac Surg* 2004;26:3–11.
22. Lacour-Gayet F, Clarke D, Jacobs J, et al. The Aristotle score: A complexity-adjusted method to evaluate surgical results. *Eur J Cardiothorac Surg* 2004;25:911–924.
23. Kouchoukos NT, Blackstone EH, Doty DB, et al. *Kirklin/Barratt-Boyes Cardiac Surgery*, 3d ed. Philadelphia: Churchill Livingstone, 2004.
24. Bando K, Turrentine MW, Ensing GJ, et al. Surgical management of total anomalous pulmonary venous connection. Thirty-year trends. *Circulation* 1996;94(Suppl II):12–16.
25. Lacour-Gayet F, Zoghbi J, Serraf AE, et al. Surgical management of progressive pulmonary venous obstruction

after repair of total anomalous pulmonary venous connection. *J Thorac Cardiovasc Surg* 1999;117:679–787.
26. Lacour-Gayet F, Rey C, Planche C. Pulmonary vein stenosis. Description of a sutureless surgical procedure using the pericardium in situ. *Arch Mal Coeur Vaiss* 1996;89:633–636.
27. Caldarone CA, Najm HK, Kadletz M, et al. Relentless pulmonary vein stenosis after repair of total anomalous pulmonary venous drainage. *Ann Thorac Surg* 1998;66: 1514–1520.
28. Senning A. Correction of the transposition of the great arteries. *Ann Surg* 1975;182:287–292.
29. Ricci M, Elliott M, Cohen GA, Catalan, et al. Management of pulmonary venous obstruction after correction of TAPVC: Risk factors for adverse outcome. *Eur J Cardiothorac Surg* 2003;24:28–36.
30. Sands A, Craig B, Casey F. A possible role for steroid therapy in preventing postoperative stenosis in totally anomalous pulmonary venous connection. *Cardiol Young* 1998;8:240–246.
31. Hyde JAJ, Stümper O, Barth MJ, et al. Total anomalous pulmonary venous connection: Outcome of surgical correction and management of recurrent venous obstruction. *Eur J Cardiothorac Surg* 1999;15:735–740.
32. Hashmi A, Abu-Sulaiman R, McCrindle BW, et al. Management and outcomes of right atrial isomerism: A 26-year experience. *J Am Coll Cardiol* 1998;31: 1120–1126.
33. Sadiq M, Stumper O, De Giovanni JV, et al. Management and outcome of infants and children with right atrial isomerism. *Heart* 1996;75:314–319.
34. Caldarone CA, Najm HK, Kadletz M, et al. Surgical management of total anomalous pulmonary venous drainage: Impact of coexisting cardiac anomalies. *Ann Thorac Surg* 1998;66:1521–1526.

CHAPTER

65 TRUNCUS ARTERIOSUS

D. Michael McMullan, Gordon A. Cohen

HISTORY AND EPIDEMIOLOGY

Truncus arteriosus (also termed common arterial trunk) is an unusual[1–4] developmental anomaly, characterized by incomplete conotruncal septation, leading to a common aortopulmonary trunk and ventricular septal defect. The disorder was first described by Wilson in 1798.[5] Initial surgical management focused on palliative pulmonary artery banding; however, long-term survival associated with this treatment was poor. The first surgical repair was

KEY CONCEPTS

- Epidemiology
  - Truncus arteriosus is a rare cyanotic cardiac malformation with an incidence of 0.07 per 1000 live births (1.1 percent of all cardiac anomalies), with 40 percent of patients disclosing 22q11 deletion on genetic testing. There is also a variable phenotypic association with DiGeorge syndrome and craniofacial defects.
- Morphology
  - A single truncal valve usually overrides a large ventricular septal defect. The different classification schemes are based on the origin of the pulmonary arteries (from truncus, ductus arteriosus, or descending aorta), the association of aortic arch interruption, and ventricular septal defects.
- Pathophysiology
  - Typically, there is intracardiac mixing (atrial and/or ventricular septal defect) with pulmonary overcirculation and, (if IAA is present), features of duct-dependent distal aortic perfusion. If untreated, chronic pulmonary vascular changes ensue, leading to fixed pulmonary hypertension.
- Clinical features
  - Presentation is in the neonatal period with pulmonary overcirculation and worsening symptoms as pulmonary vascular resistance falls. Hemodynamic collapse, acidosis, and lower body malperfusion are seen in patients with associated IAA and closure of the patent ductus arteriosus.
- Diagnosis
  - Echocardiography is usually all that is needed to proceed to surgical correction. Truncal anatomy, truncal valve morphology and function, location of the ventricular septal defect, and coronary anatomy are usually well defined echocardiographically. Additional diagnostic modalities include cardiac catheterization, computed tomography, and magnetic resonance imaging with three-dimensional reconstruction.
- Treatment
  - Complete repair in the neonatal period is standard treatment, following resuscitation and prostaglandin (PGE_1) infusion in newborns with IAA and ductal closure. Repair entails closure of the ventricular septal defect, truncal septation with reestablishment of continuity from the right ventricle (RV) to the pulmonary artery (PA) with a valved conduit, and, if required, IAA and truncal valve repair. Pulmonary arterial banding is currently very rarely performed in neonates and infants, in whom complete correction is contraindicated.
- Outcomes
  - In contemporary series, operative mortality ranges between 4 and 7 percent and is correlated to the reactivity of the pulmonary vascular bed and operative weight below 3 kg. Long-term prognosis is dependent on need for reintervention for truncal valve repair/replacement and structural failure of the RV-PA conduit.

performed in 1962, when Behrendt and colleagues closed the ventricular septal defect and used a valveless conduit to establish continuity between the right ventricle and the pulmonary artery.[6] Complete repair of truncus arteriosus with a valved conduit was first reported by McGoon in 1967[7] and remains the procedure of choice for these patients.

A recent prospective population-based study estimated the prevalence of truncus arteriosus to be approximately 0.07 per 1000 live births, representing 1.09 percent of all congenital cardiac malformations.[3,8] The incidence may be more than threefold higher in infants of diabetic mothers.[9] Twenty years ago, the 1-year mortality rate for truncus arteriosus was estimated at 2.6 per 100,000 live births, representing 3.7 percent of all deaths due to congenital heart disease during that period.[10] Median 1-month mortality was 23 percent. With contemporary advancements in surgical technique and perioperative management, survival is likely higher. Without surgical correction, approximately 70 percent of infants die within the first 3 months of life,[11] whereas some individuals who are diagnosed later in life may survive for years without surgical intervention.[12–15] This subset likely represents those individuals with relatively balanced pulmonary-systemic circulations during infancy and in whom severe pulmonary vascular obstructive disease inevitably develops.

EMBRYOLOGIC DEVELOPMENT

The heart and great vessels develop from primitive mesoderm and neural crest cells. At approximately 20 days' gestation, blood islands of the cardiogenic plate coalesce to form the left and right endocardial tubes within the intraembryonic coelom (early pericardial cavity). The endocardial tubes fuse to become the bulbus cordis at approximately 23 days. The most cephalad portions of the bulbus cordis become the truncus arteriosus and conus cordis. During this period, the bulboventricular structures begin rotating anteriorly and to the right to form the heart loop. At approximately 29 days, truncoconal swellings begin to develop into truncoconal ridges. As these ridges grow, they fuse to form the truncal septum, which divides the aorta from the pulmonary artery and the conal septum, which becomes the supraventricular crest and the subpulmonic infundibulum. Spiral rotation along an axis similar to the heart loop separates the posterolateral aortic root from the more anteromedial pulmonary arterial root at approximately 37 days. Fusion of the conal septum with the endocardial cushions during this period establishes ventricular separation, with resultant left ventricle–aorta and right ventricle–pulmonary artery concordance.

Persistent truncus arteriosus results from incomplete or altered septation and rotation of components of the bulbus cordis. There is strong evidence that dorsal and ventral neural crest cells migrate into the heart and contribute to conotruncal ridge formation.[16–18] Experimental ablation of these regions of the neural crest is associated with hypoplasia or aplasia of the thymus, thyroid, and parathyroid glands and persistent truncus arteriosus. Although the mechanisms by which neural crest cells regulate conotruncal development have not been clearly elucidated, it is believed that alterations in neural crest cell migration may explain the association between conotruncal malformations and craniofacial defects such as those of DiGeorge syndrome. Recent experimental studies have implicated abnormal bone morphogenetic protein signaling in inappropriate conotruncal septation.[19] These proteins constitute the largest group of the transforming growth factor beta family and appear to mediate several aspects of normal cardiac development.

GENETIC FACTORS

The genetic basis for persistent truncus arteriosus is likely multifactorial. An association between persistent truncus arteriosus and chromosome 22q11 deletion is well established. Chromosome 22q11 deletion affects approximately 700 infants annually in the United States and is present in 1.5 percent of patients with congenital heart defects[20] and in up to 40 percent of patients with truncus arteriosus.[21,22] Moreover, truncus arteriosus is present in approximately 10 percent of patients with chromosome 22q11 deletion.[23] In addition to cardiovascular malformations, chromosome 22q11 deletion has also been clearly linked to aplasia and hypoplasia of the thymus.[20,24,25] It is now recognized that 22q11.2 deletion syndrome encompasses the phenotypes previously described as DiGeorge syndrome and velocardiofacial syndrome. Because of these strong associations, genetic testing for chromosome 22q11 deletion in patients diagnosed with truncus arteriosus or thymic aplasia or hypoplasia is warranted. Additional potential etiologic genetic alterations linked to truncus arteriosus include chromosomal duplication of 8p and 8q[26,27] and mutations in transcription factors NKX2.5[28] and Pitx2.[29] Evidence supporting rare autosomal recessive inheritance of truncus arteriosus in the absence of 22q11.2 deletion has been reported.[30]

MORPHOLOGY

Truncus arteriosus is characterized by a single aortopulmonary trunk arising from the base of the heart, which gives rise to the coronary, systemic, and pulmonary arteries. An obligatory ventricular septal defect is present. The origin of the pulmonary arteries varies considerably and forms the basis of the two major classification systems. Collett and Edwards[14] proposed the first widely accepted classification scheme in 1949. In their system, the spectrum of truncal variations is divided into four general categories based on the origin of the pulmonary arteries. In type I truncus arteriosus, the left and right branch pulmonary arteries arise from a single short main pulmonary trunk. The main pulmonary trunk commonly arises from the posterior aspect of the truncus, just above the truncal valve. In type II truncus arteriosus, the origins of the left and right pulmonary arteries are in close proximity to one another along the posterior aspect of the truncus. In type III truncus arteriosus, the origins of the left and right pulmonary arteries arise more laterally and separate from one another. In type IV truncus arteriosus, the pulmonary arteries arise from the descending aorta rather than the truncus. Although this configuration has historically been referred to as pseudotruncus, it is now generally believed to represent a form of pulmonary atresia with aorticopulmonary collateral vessels and should not be classified as a variation of truncus arteriosus.

An additional classification system was developed by Van Praagh and Van Praagh in 1965.[31] Like the Collett and Edwards classification systems, this system also divides truncus arteriosus into four categories. Type A1 is characterized by a main pulmonary artery segment arising from the truncus due to a partially formed aorticopulmonary septum. Type A2 is characterized by the presence of left and right pulmonary arteries arising independently from the truncus, irrespective of the proximity of their origins. Type A3 is characterized by the presence of a single pulmonary artery arising from the truncus. In this form, often referred to as hemitruncus, the contralateral lung is supplied by a pulmonary collateral vessel arising from either the distal aorta or ductus arteriosus. Type A4 is characterized by a hypoplastic or interrupted aortic arch with pulmonary arteries arising from a large ductus arteriosus. In this classification scheme the designation of type B indicates absence of a ventricular septal defect. However, because the presence of a true truncus arteriosus in these patients is questionable, the Van Praagh B classification is seldom used. These classification schemes share overlapping features and are schematically represented in Fig. 65-1. Collett and Edwards type I and Van Praagh type A1 are essentially the same. Van Praagh type A2 encompasses the Collett and Edwards types II and III.

In 2000, a new classification system was developed by the STS Congenital Heart Surgery Database Committee and representatives of the European Association for Cardiothoracic Surgery.[32] This system, based on the Van Praagh scheme, divides truncus arteriosus into three main categories: truncus arteriosus with confluent or near confluent pulmonary arteries, truncus arteriosus with absence of one pulmonary artery, and truncus arteriosus with interrupted aortic arch or coarctation. In this system, modifiers are used to denote the number of truncal valve leaflets, the presence and degree of truncal valve stenosis or insufficiency, and the presence of ventricular hypoplasia, coronary artery anomaly, overriding

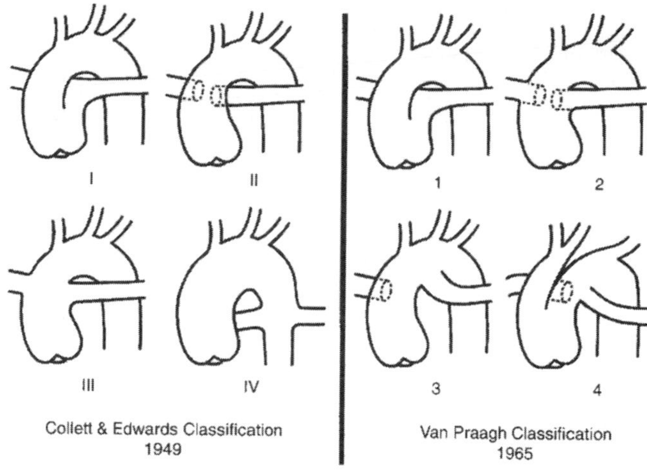

Figure 65-1 Morphologic classifications of truncus arteriosus. The Collet-Edwards classification describes truncus types I to IV according to the origin of the branch pulmonary arteries, whereas Van Praagh's types 1 to 4 are subdivided according to presence (subtype A) or absence (subtype B) of associated ventricular septal defects (details in text). (From Vricella LA, Tsang VT. Truncus arteriosus. In: Yang SC, Cameron DE (eds). *Current Therapy in Thoracic and Cardiovascular Surgery*. Philadelphia: Mosby; 2004:751. With permission.)

truncal valve, transposition, or thymic aplasia. A similar nomenclature scheme to describe various methods of repairing or palliating truncus arteriosus has also been proposed. Although these classification systems may be very useful for risk-stratification analysis, the Van Praagh and Collett and Edwards classification systems continue to be widely used.

The truncal valve is most commonly bicuspid (about 5 percent), tricuspid (about 50 percent), or quadricuspid (about 30 percent). More than four cusps and, rarely, a single cusp may also be seen. Valve leaflets may be thickened and dysplastic, contributing to valvular insufficiency or stenosis. Despite these functional and morphologic variations, fibrous continuity between the truncal valve and the mitral valve is preserved. The tricuspid valve may be in fibrous continuity or may be separated from the truncal valve by a thin muscular band. The truncal valve typically overrides the interventricular septum and the subarterial ventricular septal defect in a balanced manner or more further over the right ventricle. Less frequently, the truncus arises predominantly from the left ventricle. The ventricular septal defect is normally located in the subarterial portion of the infundibular septum. The ventriculoinfundibular fold typically forms the posterior margin of the defect and separates it from the anterior leaflet of the tricuspid valve. Less commonly, the ventricular septal defect may extend posteriorly to the tricuspid valve annulus in the perimembranous outlet portion of the septum. The inferior margin of the ventricular septal defect is made up by the trabecula septomarginalis, and the superior margin typically extends to the truncal valve.

Coronary artery anatomy in truncus arteriosus may exhibit significant variability.[33] Two coronary ostia are generally present. The left coronary artery typically originates from the left portion of the truncus. It may originate high in the sinus of Valsalva or above the sinus near in proximity to the takeoff of the pulmonary artery. The left coronary artery normally supplies the left ventricular myocardium. The right coronary artery typically originates from the right anterior portion of the truncus. The right coronary artery normally supplies the right ventricle. However, an anterior descending coronary artery may originate from the right coronary artery and cross the right ventricle. In up to 18 percent of cases, a single coronary ostium originating from either the left or right is present. Additional coronary anomalies that have been reported include the circumflex artery originating from the right coronary artery, ostial stenosis due to structural deformation related to the adjacent commissure, the right coronary artery originating from the anterior descending coronary artery, and major coronary branches of the right coronary artery crossing the right ventricular outflow tract to supply anterobasal surfaces of both ventricles and the upper portion of the interventricular septum.[34] Abnormal coronary anatomy must be carefully considered in planning surgical correction, because failure to recognize variations in coronary anatomy may cause or contribute to perioperative morbidity or mortality.[35]

Truncus arteriosus is generally associated with a left aortic arch, but a right aortic arch is present in approximately 30 percent of cases. Association with double aortic arch[36] and persistent embryonic fifth aortic arch[37,38] has also been reported. In approximately 10 percent of cases, the aortic arch is either interrupted or severely hypoplastic. The interruption usually occurs distal to the origin of the left common carotid artery (type B aortic arch interruption; see Chap. 68) and is accompanied by ductal continuity with the descending thoracic aorta. In this morphologic variant, the pulmonary arteries arise from the ductus arteriosus. Other associated abnormalities of the great vessels include interrupted aortic arch with postductal origin of all brachiocephalic vessels[39] and the absence of one PA.[40] Absence of one pulmonary artery occurs most frequently on the same side as the aortic arch. Truncus arteriosus is also commonly associated with patent foramen ovale/secundum atrial septal defect or tricuspid insufficiency or stenosis.[41]

PATHOPHYSIOLOGY

The physiologic features of truncus arteriosus are typical of those seen in other forms of cyanotic congenital heart disease with increased pulmonary blood flow. The single aortopulmonary trunk results in parallel pulmonary-systemic circulations, making intracardiac mixing of systemic and pulmonary blood at the level of the ventricular septum obligatory to maintain adequate systemic oxygenation. Additional mixing occurs at the level of the atrial septal defect when present (Fig. 65-2). During fetal development pulmonary blood flow represents less than 10 percent of the cardiac output due to increased pulmonary vascular resistance. At birth, the combined cardiac output traverses the truncal valve and the amount of pulmonary blood flow is determined by the change in pulmonary vascular resistance and the presence of any pulmonary arterial narrowing. Because the pulmonary vascular resistance initially falls below the systemic vascular resistance, severe hypoxia rarely occurs. When it does, proximal or distal pulmonary artery narrowing must be suspected. As the pulmonary vascular resistance continues to fall during early postnatal life, pulmonary blood flow increases. Increased pulmonary venous return leads to volume overload of the right ventricle, cardiopulmonary inefficiency, and congestive heart failure. The large, nonrestrictive ventricular septal defect enables pressure equilibration between the left and right ventricles, which leads to right ventricular hypertrophy. Increased pulmonary blood flow, combined with systemic level arterial pressures within the pulmonary circulation, ultimately brings about pulmonary vascular changes that, in turn, increase pulmonary vascular resistance. Because the pulmonary arteries originate above the truncal valve, the pulmonary circulation is exposed to systemic-level pressures

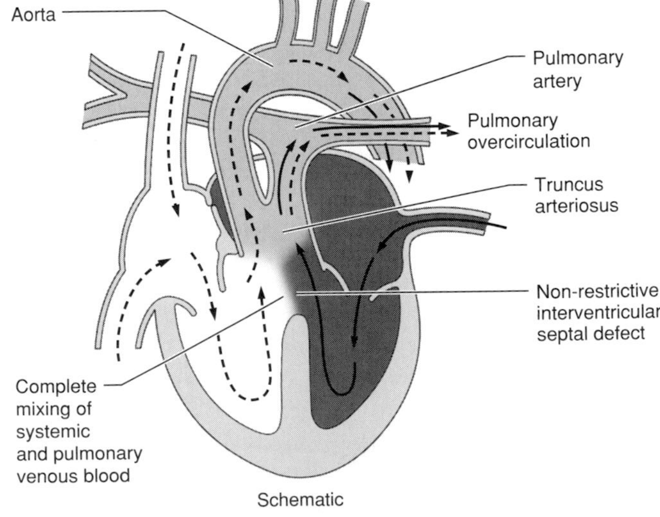

Figure 65-2 Diagram illustrating the pathophysiology of tricuspid atresia. (From Reitz BA, Yuh DD (eds). *Congenital Cardiac Surgery*. New York: McGraw-Hill; 2002:153. With permission.)

during both systole and diastole. It is believed that this accelerates the abnormal pulmonary vascular changes leading to increased pulmonary vascular resistance and pulmonary hypertension. Although increased pulmonary vascular resistance and pressure generally occur several months later in life, there is evidence that early molecular and cellular changes occur within a few weeks in the presence of increased pulmonary blood flow[42] and that observed vascular changes are related to alterations in nitric oxide and endothelin activity.[43] These findings may explain the improved outcomes associated with earlier surgical repair.

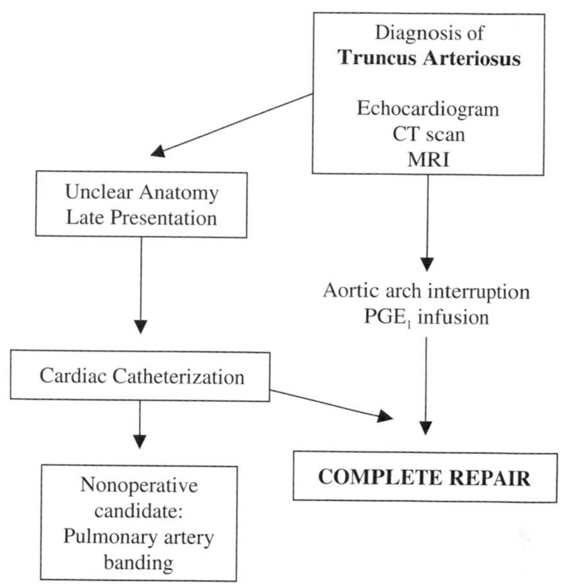

Figure 65-3 Decision-making flowchart. Clinical decision-making algorithm for neonates with truncus arteriosus.

CLINICAL FINDINGS

The clinical findings associated with truncus arteriosus depend on the degree of truncal valve competence, pulmonary vascular resistance, and coexisting cardiac defects. Shortly after birth, infants exhibit generally mild cyanosis, tachycardia, tachypnea, costosternal retractions, and diaphoresis, which may worsen during feeding. The second heart sound is single and a harsh systolic ejection murmur may be audible at the left lower sternal border. A precordial thrill may be present. Pulmonary runoff produces a low diastolic pressure and widened pulse pressure. Truncal valve stenosis and insufficiency may produce a more pronounced ejection murmur or a diastolic decrescendo murmur, respectively. Cyanosis may improve as pulmonary vascular resistance continues to fall over the first few weeks. Increasing pulmonary overcirculation leads to progressive worsening symptoms of congestive heart failure, including pulmonary edema, hepatomegaly, and failure to thrive. These findings may develop at an accelerated rate or may be more pronounced in the setting of truncal valve insufficiency. Those who fail to undergo surgical correction during infancy may exhibit improvement in heart failure symptoms but worsening of cyanosis as maladaptive pulmonary vascular changes progress and pulmonary blood flow decreases. Infants with Van Praagh type A4 truncus arteriosus (interrupted aortic arch, ductal origin of pulmonary arteries) may exhibit symptoms of systemic hypoperfusion and ischemia as well as hypoxia as the ductus arteriosus begins to close shortly after birth. Features such as micrognathia, choanal atresia, and cleft palate may be found in patients with coexisting chromosome 22q11 deletion syndromes (Fig. 64-3).

Diagnostic studies

Truncus arteriosus is most commonly diagnosed shortly after birth; however, prenatal diagnosis is becoming increasingly common as prenatal care becomes more accessible. All cyanotic infants should undergo careful diagnostic testing, including blood gas analysis, pulse oximetry, electrocardiography, chest radiography, and transthoracic or transesophageal echocardiography. Early pulse oximetric screening may detect evidence of truncus arteriosus before symptoms develop.[44] Biventricular hypertrophy is generally evident on the electrocardiogram and may become more pronounced over time. Although initial chest radiographs may appear normal, subsequent studies typically demonstrate cardiomegaly and increased pulmonary vascular markings. Absence of the thymic shadow may be observed in patients with coexisting neural crest disorders such as DiGeorge syndrome. A right-sided aortic arch may be apparent in approximately 30 percent of cases. Two-dimensional and Doppler echocardiography accurately detect truncus arteriosus and characterize important anatomic and hemodynamic features, including type of truncus, truncal valve morphology and function, presence of pulmonary arterial stenosis, size and location of the ventricular septal defect, location of coronary ostia, pulmonary blood flow and resistance, and presence of associated lesions.[45] Although the echocardiographic distinction between different conotruncal abnormalities is challenging in the fetus, truncus arteriosus may be accurately diagnosed by fetal echocardiography.[46] Accurate in utero diagnostic studies are invaluable in counseling parents. Cardiac catheterization and coronary angiography are useful for accurate anatomic and physiologic assessment of the pulmonary arteries and to determine the precise orientation and course of the coronary arteries. This is especially important in older infants, who may exhibit pulmonary vascular hypertrophic changes, and in infants with echocardiographic evidence of coronary artery abnormalities. Computed tomography and resonance magnetic imaging with three-dimensional reconstruction are gaining wide acceptance as additional diagnostic tools.

CLINICAL MANAGEMENT

The initial medical management of these patients should focus on the treatment of congestive heart failure and ensuring adequate oxygen delivery. Initial hypoxia may necessitate endotracheal intubation and mechanical ventilation. As pulmonary vascular resistance falls, decreased diastolic coronary perfusion may lead to worsening of heart failure symptoms, especially during feeding and crying. Diuretics, digoxin, and occasionally more powerful inotropic agents are useful in managing heart failure. Hypocalcemia must be corrected in patients with coexisting syndromes involving the deletion of chromosome 22q11. The findings of progressive tachycardia, hypotension, acidosis, and hypoxemia during early postnatal life suggest Van Praagh type A4 truncus arteriosus. Intravenous prostaglandin therapy must be initiated to arrest closure of the ductus arteriosus. Genetic screening for chromosome 22q11 deletion should be undertaken in all patients with truncus arteriosus. Patients presenting later in life, with evidence of advanced pulmonary vascular obstructive disease and pulmonary hypertension, may benefit from inhaled nitric oxide therapy. However, the prognosis for these children remains poor.

Surgical therapy

Initial surgical management of truncus arteriosus was limited to palliative pulmonary artery banding, which resulted in survival rates similar to those observed in untreated patients. The first reported surgical repair utilizing a nonvalved Teflon conduit was performed in 1962.[6] Following this, McGoon and colleagues performed the first successful repair with a valved conduit in an older child in 1967.[7] Reports of successful repair and improved outcomes in younger infants[47] subsequently led to earlier repair and avoidance of maladaptive pulmonary vascular changes. Currently, banding of the pulmonary arteries should be considered only when coexisting conditions such as sepsis, shock, or intracranial hemorrhage prevent surgical repair.

The timing of surgical intervention in these patients has received considerable attention. Overall, the trend has been toward earlier repair in infants and neonates. Repair of truncus arteriosus during the first few weeks of life may be safely accomplished in the majority of patients[48] and appears to improve survival.[49] Early repair ameliorates congestive heart failure and failure to thrive and prevents irreversible pulmonary vascular disease. However, the overall operative mortality associated with early repair of the truncus arteriosus remains relatively high compared with repair of other forms of complex congenital cardiac disease.[50,51] The reason for this discrepancy is unclear. A review of the strategy for management of truncus arteriosus by Brizard and colleagues[52] found that weight less than 3 kg is an independent risk factor for early perioperative mortality and that deferring surgery until 2 to 3 months of age decreases surgical risks. Although such a policy results in surgical intervention on infants of greater body weight and the use of larger valved conduits with associated longer freedom from reoperation, this may represent policy-driven selection of patients without specific risk factors. It is our policy to operate on patients diagnosed with truncus arteriosus during the neonatal period. Factors such as very low birth weight or the presence of unbalanced systemic-to-pulmonary circulations direct the precise timing of surgery. Because most neonates exhibit some degree of unbalanced circulation and hemodynamic sequelae, earlier surgical correction seems prudent in order to prevent the complications of pulmonary vascular disease associated with increased pulmonary blood flow.

Operative technique

We routinely employ intraoperative transesophageal echocardiography to evaluate valve function, intracardiac shunting, and wall motion before and after repair. Repair of a type 1 truncus is depicted in Fig. 65-4. Following median sternotomy, a generous portion of pericardium is harvested and treated with glutaraldehyde. The origin and course of the coronary arteries are carefully evaluated. The common arterial trunk, complete aortic arch, and great vessels are extensively mobilized. The pulmonary arteries are mobilized well into the hilum and snares are placed. When the ductus arteriosus is present, care must be taken to avoid injuring it. In the presence of an interrupted aortic arch, snares are also placed around the great vessels. Arterial cannulation should be performed in the most distal ascending aorta or the transverse arch. Bicaval cannulas and a left ventricular vent are used to adequately decompress the heart. Snares are tightened to occlude the pulmonary arteries upon initiation of cardiopulmonary bypass. If a ductus arteriosus is present, it is ligated. After distal aortic cross clamping, cold blood cardioplegia is administered via an ascending aortic cannula and readministered intermittently throughout the procedure. In the setting of significant truncal valve insufficiency, retrograde cardioplegia may be delivered via the coronary sinus. Alternatively, the common trunk may be opened just distal to the origin of the pulmonary arteries and cardioplegia given directly into the coronary ostia. Topical iced slush is applied and the patient is cooled to 32°C.

In the presence of a clearly defined common pulmonary artery, it is transected close to the common arterial trunk and the resultant truncal defect is closed with a Dacron patch and a running polypropylene suture. When the pulmonary arteries arise separately, the common arterial trunk should be opened in a transverse fashion just distal to the origin of the pulmonary arteries, which are divided proximally. This approach often enables primary closure of the aorta without distortion of the coronary ostia. When insufficiency is detected by

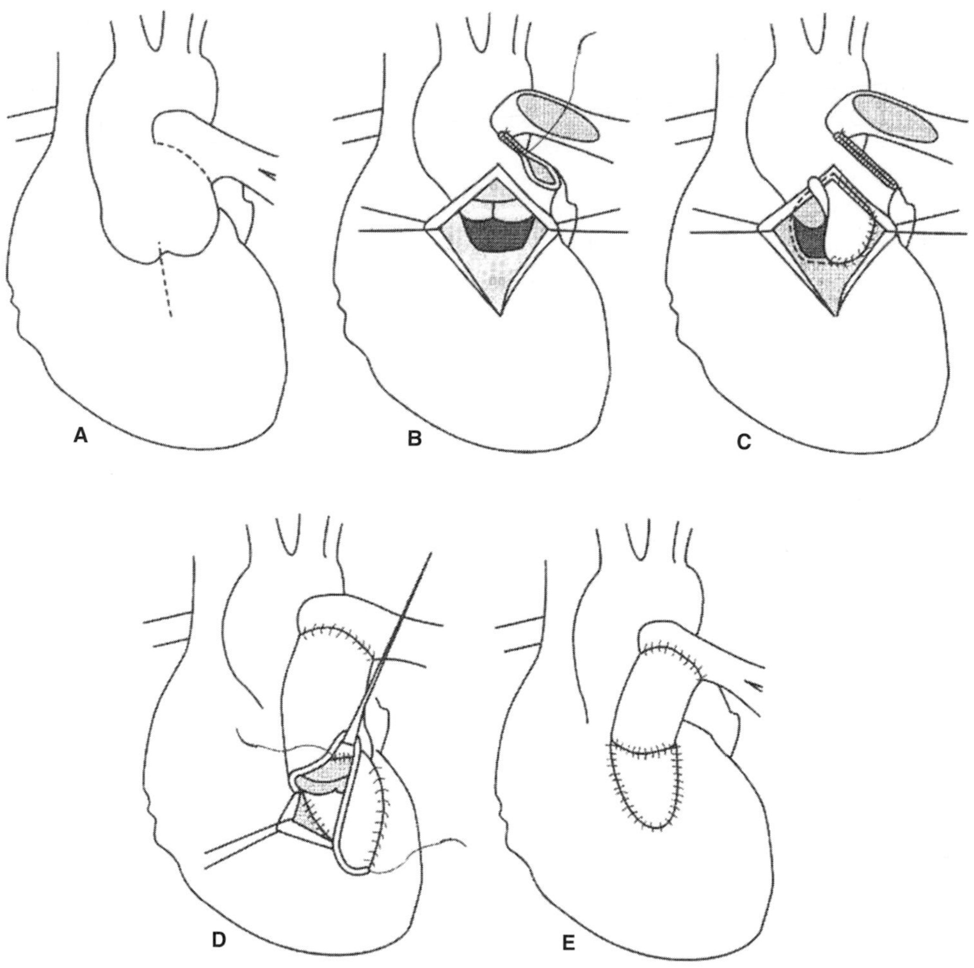

Figure 65-4 Schematic rendition of complete repair of truncus arteriosus, Collet-Edwards, type I. The procedure entails septation of the truncus and a right ventriculotomy to perform VSD closure [dotted lines, (A)]. Following septation of the truncus, the large VSD is exposed through a right ventriculotomy (B). The VSD is closed with a patch (C). Continuity between right ventricle and pulmonary arterial confluence is reestablished with a valved conduit and a proximal hood (D). Completed procedure (E). (From Vricella LA, Tsang VT. Truncus arteriosus. In: Yang SC, Cameron DE (eds). *Current Therapy in Thoracic and Cardiovascular Surgery*. Philadelphia: Mosby; 2004:753. With permission.)

echocardiography, complete transection of the common arterial trunk facilitates thorough evaluation of the truncal valve.

A longitudinal incision, originating at the base of the common arterial trunk, is performed in the anterior surface of the right ventricular outflow tract. This incision must be modified if a significant coronary artery crosses this area.[34,35] The edges of the cardiotomy are trimmed to create a smooth oval opening. When a subarterial ventricular septal defect is present, it is easily visualized and repaired though this incision. The septal defect is closed with a Dacron sauvage patch and either running or interrupted 6-0 polypropylene suture. Subarterial ventricular septal defects are commonly surrounded by a clearly defined circumferential rim of muscle. The superior aspect of the patch is sewn to the subvalvular aspect of the ventriculotomy by passing pledget-supported interrupted sutures through the anterior wall of the right ventricular outflow tract. Injury to the conduction system is unlikely, as the system is separated from the septal defect by the posterior muscle tissue of the ventriculoinfundibular fold. In contrast, the conduction system is at risk in the setting of a perimembranous inlet type of ventricular septal defect, in which the defect extends to the tricuspid annulus. In this setting, we have found that approaching the defect through the right atrium provides the best exposure and facilitates suture placement through the base of the septal leaflet of the tricuspid valve. Sutures should be placed well away from the edge of posteroinferior margin of the defect so as to avoid injury to the conduction system. A patent foramen ovale or secundum atrial septal defect is typically present. Rather than completing closure of the defect, we prefer to leave in place some interatrial communication to allow right-to-left shunting. This may be accomplished by partial closure or by closing the defect with a fenestrated autologous pericardial patch. The 2- to 4-mm fenestration may easily be closed at a later time using percutaneous techniques. With this approach, cardiac output can be safely maintained in the setting of postoperative pulmonary hypertensive crises.

A valved conduit is most commonly used to establish right ventricle-to–pulmonary artery continuity. Several types of conduit have been used successfully for this purpose, including aortic and pulmonary homografts,[53–56] composite bioprosthetic conduits,[57–59] pulmonary xenografts,[60,61] aortic xenografts,[62] autologous pericardial valved conduits,[63,64] and valved venous xenografts.[65–68] Choice of conduit is generally based on availability of homograft tissue and surgeon experience and preference. Generally, homograft tissue is preferred because it offers improved valve longevity and is technically easier to sew than composite (Dacron) valved conduits.[55,69] The reported longevity of homograft conduits varies widely, with reported freedom from homograft replacement ranging from approximately 50 percent at 3 years[54] to approximately 75 percent at 10 years.[53] Conduit stenosis is the most common reason for reintervention (i.e., conduit replacement).[70] In multivariate analysis, small homograft size has been identified as a predictor of conduit failure.[56] Limited availability of small homografts is a significant limitation to the use of homograft conduits. Large adult homografts have been successfully downsized by longitudinal wall excision and conversion to bicuspid conduits.[71] This technique may be useful when an appropriate-size homograft is unavailable.

In general, composite xenograft conduits are more prone to calcification and early failure than homografts. Significant obstruction of the right ventricular outflow tract occurs in up to 77 percent of patients within 12 months of surgery.[72] Actuarial freedom from reintervention following implantation ranges from 48 percent at 18 months[57] to 64 percent at 4 years,[73] depending on the type of conduit used. Small conduit size has also been identified as a risk factor for conduit failure in composite xenograft conduits.[73] Initial reports describing the use of stentless xenograft root conduits in these patients also describe limited conduit durability.[61,62]

The Contegra (Medtronic Inc., Minneapolis, MN) bovine jugular vein graft has recently been approved for use as a right ventricle–to–pulmonary artery conduit. The graft is derived from a segment of bovine jugular vein that contains a naturally integrated tricuspid valve with associated sinuses. This graft offers several advantages, including the availability of several sizes (12 to 22 mm) and the ability to position the valve near the distal anastomosis. Initial reports indicating durability at least equivalent to that of homografts[67] have been tempered by limited cases of aneurysmal dilation,[74] thrombus formation,[75] and fibrotic membrane formation leading to distal conduit stenosis.[76]

Several methods have been devised to establish right ventricle–to–pulmonary artery continuity without the use of homografts or xenografts. Fresh autologous pericardial valved conduits have been constructed and used in patients with truncus arteriosus.[64] Although preliminary follow-up indicates 66 percent freedom from reoperation at approximately 7 years, the mean age of these patients at initial operation was 6 months. Performed in younger patients, this technique has been associated with excellent freedom from reoperation but increased in-hospital mortality.[77] Direct right ventricle–to–pulmonary artery anastomosis has also been employed to reconstruct the right ventricular outflow tract in patients with favorable pulmonary artery anatomy.[78] Following direct posterior approximation, an anterior patch, with or without a pericardial monocusp, is fashioned from pericardium or Dacron. This repair is also associated with increased early mortality but improved freedom from reoperation at 8 to 10 years.[77,79] Although debatable, significant pulmonary insufficiency may be detrimental during the early postoperative period. The potential benefit of conduit growth must be weighed against pulmonary regurgitation in considering each of these repair techniques.

The distal conduit–to–pulmonary artery anastomosis is completed first. In cases where the branch pulmonary arteries arise from a single common pulmonary trunk, the common orifice may have to be enlarged to accommodate an appropriately sized conduit. This is especially true when a pulmonary artery band has been placed previously. Enlargement of the pulmonary artery orifice may be accomplished by incising the common pulmonary trunk laterally along the course of the one or both proximal branch pulmonary arteries. The extent of lateral incision must be modified when there is a significant discrepancy in the size of the branch pulmonary arteries. The incisions may have to be extended into the hilum in cases of severe branch stenosis or hypoplasia. The distal conduit is trimmed accordingly and anastomosed to the common pulmonary orifice using 6-0 polypropylene suture. In the setting of type I truncus with a relatively long common arterial segment, the pulmonary orifice may be sewn directly to the right ventriculotomy. Advantages of this method include capacity for growth and relative freedom from conduit stenosis.

The aortic cross clamp may be removed prior to construction of the proximal ventricle–to-conduit anastomosis. However, we find that the proximal anastomosis may be performed efficiently and most accurately on an arrested heart during a period of active rewarming. When an aortic homograft is used, it should be oriented so that the anterior leaflet of the mitral valve can be used as a hood to close the right ventriculotomy without distorting the homograft valve. Alternatively, a segment of Gore-Tex, Dacron, or homograft tissue may be used as an extension to close the remaining ventriculotomy. The valved portion of the homograft may be advanced toward the distal anastomosis to reduce the possibility of valve distortion caused by sternal compression. In this technique, the homograft is divided and the distal segment utilized for the proximal anastomosis. Irrespective of the technique used, narrowing of the ventriculotomy opening and distortion of the homograft valve must be avoided. After air has been carefully evacuated from the heart via an aortic root vent, the aortic cross clamp is removed. Once cardiac activity has been reestablished, the patient is weaned from cardiopulmonary bypass support. Transesophageal echocardiography provides important information regarding truncal and neopulmonic valve function and the presence of retained intracardiac air. Greater than mild truncal valve insufficiency should be addressed immediately by reinstituting full cardiopulmonary bypass, cooling, cardioplegic arrest, and valve repair. Consideration should be given to temporary left atrial and pulmonary artery catheters. The additional hemodynamic information may be very helpful during the early postoperative period.

Specific technical considerations

Discontinuous pulmonary arteries

In cases where the left and right pulmonary arteries arise from the common trunk in a noncontiguous manner, direct primary anastomosis of a common pulmonary arterial orifice to the right ventriculotomy is not possible. The left pulmonary artery, which generally arises from the ductus arteriosus, is first mobilized and separated from ductal tissue at its origin. The right pulmonary artery is then detached and the common trunk defect closed as described above. An aortic homograft is prepared for use as a conduit by removing the two proximal brachiocephalic vessels at their origin and ligating the left subclavian stump at its origin. The homograft is then anastomosed end-to-end to the shorter of the two pulmonary arteries. The remaining pulmonary artery is anastomosed end-to-side to the homograft at the site of the excised brachiocephalic vessels. The proximal anastomosis is performed as described above. Alternatively, pulmonary homograft may be used if the branches are of sufficient length. A composite bioprosthetic conduit may be used in the absence of an appropriate homograft; however, the conduit's inherent stiffness may lead to distortion of the branch pulmonary arteries.

Truncus arteriosus with interrupted aortic arch

Correction of truncus arteriosus with interrupted aortic arch is generally performed under hypothermic circulatory arrest. The ascending aorta, brachiocephalic vessels, and pulmonary arteries are widely dissected to facilitate extensive mobilization of these structures. The origins of the first two to three intercostal arteries are divided to enable adequate mobilization of the descending aorta and permit a tension-free aortic reconstruction. We prefer to conduct cardiopulmonary bypass using bicaval and aortic/selective right subclavian artery cannulation. This approach provides excellent exposure for aortic reconstruction and permits low-flow antegrade cerebral perfusion during lower-body circulatory arrest. The branch pulmonary arteries are occluded with snares on initiation of cardiopulmonary bypass. A left ventricular vent is used to keep the heart adequately decompressed. The patient is cooled to 18°C and cerebral cooling packs are applied. Snares are used to occlude the innominate, left common carotid, and left subclavian arteries, and a clamp is used to occlude the descending aorta distal to the isthmus. Lower-body circulatory arrest is accompanied by low-flow antegrade cerebral perfusion. Care must be taken to avoid injury to the coronary arteries in separating the proximal main pulmonary artery from the aorta. After carefully inspecting the truncal valve through this defect, the latter is closed using a patch, as described above. When an anomalous right subclavian artery arises from the descending aorta, it may be simply divided and ligated. After all ductal tissue has been resected, the lateral aspect of the aorta is incised at the origin of the left common carotid artery and the descending aorta is anastomosed end-to-side using 6-0 polypropylene suture. After the cannula has been removed from the descending aorta and air from the aorta, the brachiocephalic snares are removed and rewarming is initiated. Right ventricle–to–pulmonary artery continuity is established as above and the patient is weaned from cardiopulmonary bypass.

Critical compression of the left mainstem bronchus may occur following repair of truncus arteriosus with interrupted arch. This can be avoided by adequate mobilization of structures during surgical correction and high vascular anastomosis at the level of the origin of the left common carotid artery to prevent direct airway compression by the reconstructed aorta. Critical bronchial compression must be considered in the setting of postoperative air trapping in the left lung, pneumonia, or failure to wean from ventilator support. Radiographic confirmation of bronchial compression warrants immediate revision of the aortic reconstruction. A 10-mm Gore-Tex interposition graft placed distal to the left subclavian artery may be used to lengthen the aortic arch and relieve tension on the bronchus. Replacement of this segment with a larger Dacron interposition graft can be performed safely through a left thoracotomy later in life.

Truncal valve dysfunction

Morphologic and functional dysfunction of the truncal valve must be carefully evaluated using preoperative and postoperative transesophageal echocardiography and direct inspection during surgical correction. Preoperative insufficiency or stenosis may be caused by structural valve abnormalities, abnormal flow characteristics related to systemic-to-pulmonary runoff, or a combination of the two. Therefore the degree of dysfunction noted during preoperative echocardiography may not accurately predict truncal valve function following surgical partition of the truncus arteriosus. We believe that any truncal valve dysfunction should be addressed during the initial corrective procedure. Every effort should be made to repair a dysfunctional truncal valve rather than replace it. Some degree of truncal valve insufficiency is present in more than one-third of patients.[80,81] Using a mechanistic approach to valve insufficiency, numerous repair techniques have been successfully employed.[81–87] The surgeon should be familiar with several repair methods because of the variability of underlying structural defects. Prolapsing cusps may be resuspended from the annulus using a pledget-reinforced 6-0 polypropylene mattress suture through the adjacent commissure. Careful resection of thickened cusp edges may improve leaflet apposition. Cusp augmentation, using autologous pericardium, has also been used in the setting of scarred and retracted leaflets. Insufficiency associated with four or more leaflets may improve following suture approximation of incomplete commissures in partially fused leaflets to create a functionally bicuspid or tricuspid valve. Alternatively, leaflet excision and reduction annuloplasty with or without coronary reimplantation may be required in the setting of annular enlargement. Irrespective of the technique utilized, the fundamental goal of repair is to correct truncal insufficiency without narrowing the valve orifice.

Truncal valve stenosis is less common.[49] Stenosis due to leaflet abnormalities may also be amenable to valvuloplastic techniques, such as commissurotomy and debulking of myxomatous zones of coaptation. Resection of a subvalvular fibromuscular membrane should be undertaken when it contributes to stenosis. However, stenosis due to a critically small annulus or continued regurgitation following valve repair generally necessitates valve replacement with an aortic valve homograft (Fig. 65-5).[88,89] The truncus is transected just distal to the origin of the pulmonary arteries and a right ventriculotomy is created, extending from the free wall of the right ventricular outflow tract to the annulus of the truncal valve. The truncal root and leaflets are excised and coronary ostia buttons preserved. The aortic homograft is then sewn into place using 6-0 polypropylene suture. The homograft should be oriented so that the anterior leaflet of its mitral valve is used to close the ventricular septal defect. Alternatively, the mitral leaflet may be removed and the defect closed with a Dacron patch. The site for attachment of each coronary button is carefully planned to ensure a tension-free, unobstructed anastomosis. Windows are cut into the homograft and the ostia are sewn into place using 8-0 polypropylene. After completion of the distal aortic anastomosis with 6-0 polypropylene, a second homograft (aortic of pulmonic) is used to construct a right ventricle–to–pulmonary artery conduit as described above.

POSTOPERATIVE MANAGEMENT

During the early postoperative period, the patient must be vigilantly observed for evidence of right ventricular dysfunction. Pulmonary hypertensive crises may occur in these patients, especially if surgical repair is undertaken after the neonatal period. Early extubation and appropriate use of analgesic and anxiolytic agents are recommended to decrease the risk of pulmonary hypertensive episodes. A hemodynamically significant rise in pulmonary arterial pressure should prompt the critical care staff to expeditiously initiate measures to reduce pulmonary vascular resistance, including increasing mechanical minute ventilation and fraction of inspired oxygen, administration of analgesics/anxiolytics, and inhaled nitric oxide. Echocardiographic evidence of acute truncal insufficiency, regional wall motion abnormalities, or right ventricle–to–pulmonary artery conduit obstruction or insufficiency warrants immediate surgical reintervention.

Right ventricular compliance may be poor because of prior exposure to systemic blood pressure. Accordingly, increased filling pressure may be required to optimize ventricular function. Significant right-to-left shunting through the fenestrated atrial septum is not uncommon but generally decreases as right ventricular compliance improves. Significant shunting may lead to cyanosis and suggests critical pulmonary hypertension. Postoperative dysrhythmia can contribute to significant myocardial dysfunction and decreased cardiac output. However, junctional ectopic tachycardia appears to occur less commonly following surgical intervention for truncus arteriosus than for other congenital cardiac anomalies.[90] Because truncus arteriosus is associated with an increased risk of developing necrotizing enterocolitis,[91] postoperative abdominal distention and feeding intolerance should be carefully evaluated.

OUTCOMES

Outcome measures for patients with truncus arteriosus have changed greatly since the introduction of surgical correction in the neonatal period. Increasing numbers of patients undergo nonpalliative, corrective surgery at an earlier age.[92] The trend of improved short- and long-term survival appears to be strongly related to earlier surgical intervention.[49] Surgical repair during the early neonatal period may prevent the development of detrimental pulmonary vascular changes and reduce the risk of postoperative death.[93] Factors associated with increased mortality in these patients include other coexisting cardiac anomalies,[94] truncal valve insufficiency

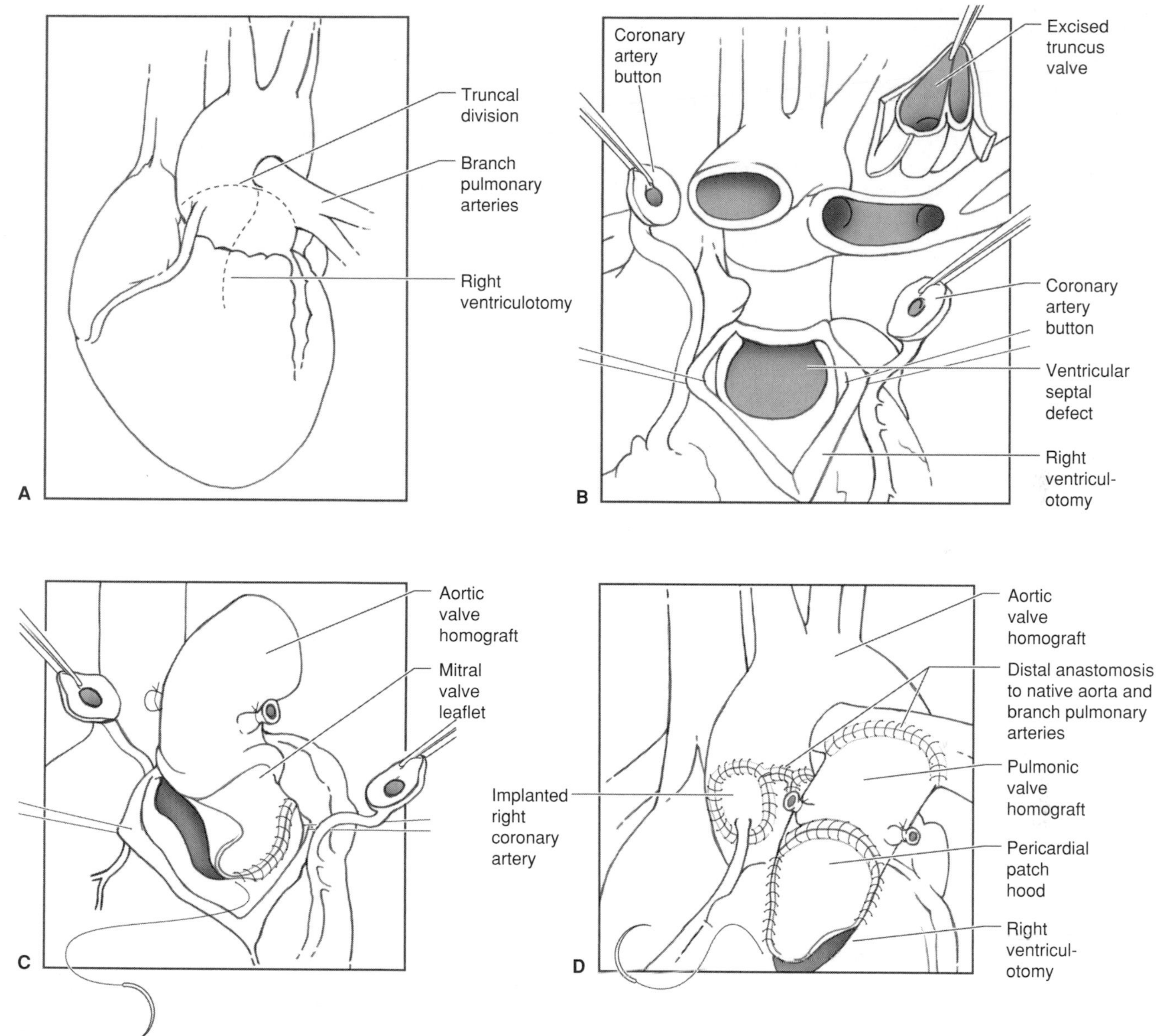

Figure 65-5 Repair of truncus arteriosus, including truncal root replacement. The truncus is septated and the root excised (A and B). The VSD is closed with the anterior mitral valve leaflet attached to an aortic root homograft (C). The coronary buttons are reimplanted and a homograft is utilized to restore RV–PA continuity (D). (From Reitz BA, Yuh DD (eds). *Congenital Cardiac Surgery*. New York: McGraw-Hill; 2002:155. With permission.)

prior to repair,[95] and truncal valve replacement.[96] Early postoperative mortality is approximately 4 to 7 percent at 30 days.[83,96,97] The recent trend toward earlier surgical intervention complicates accurate determination of current long-term survival data; however, recent series have reported long-term survival rates up to 92 percent at 1 year,[96] 90 percent at 5 years,[95] 71 to 85 percent at 10 years,[95,98,99] 83 percent at 15 years,[95] and 60 percent at 20 years.[99] A significant number of late deaths may be related to reoperations.[95,97] Approximately two-thirds of patients require truncal valve replacement within 10 years if truncal insufficiency is present at the time of initial repair, whereas up to 95 percent of patients without truncal insufficiency at time repair do not require truncal valve replacement at 10 years.[95] Freedom from right ventricle–pulmonary artery conduit replacement varies according to several factors, including conduit size, type, and age at operation. Cumulative freedom from conduit failure has been reported as approximately 80 percent at 1 year,[97] 50 percent at 10 years,[98,99] and 33 percent at 15 years.[99] Both surgical and nonsurgical methods may be employed to address the recurring problem of conduit failure in these patients. Conduit stenosis has been successfully managed using a percutaneous self-expanding stent.[100] Such nonsurgical methods may improve long-term outcomes by postponing higher-risk surgical interventions. Trends toward improved short- and long-term survival indicate that increasing numbers of these patients will be cared for by members of the emerging field of adult congenital cardiac surgery.

References

1. Tandon R, Hauck AJ, Nadas AS. Persistent truncus arteriosus. A clinical, hemodynamic, and autopsy study of nineteen cases. *Circulation* 1963;28:1050–1060.
2. Calder L, Van Praagh R, Van Praagh S, et al. Truncus arteriosus communis. Clinical, angiocardiographic, and pathologic findings in 100 patients. *Am Heart J* 1976;92: 23–38.
3. Samanek M, Voriskova M. Congenital heart disease among 815,569 children born between 1980 and 1990 and their 15-year survival: A prospective Bohemia survival study. *Pediatr Cardiol* 1999;20:411–417.
4. Tennstedt C, Chaoui R, Korner H, et al. Spectrum of congenital heart defects and extracardiac malformations associated with chromosomal abnormalities: Results of a seven year necropsy study. *Heart* 1999;82:34–39.
5. Wilson J. A description of a very unusual malformation of the human heart. *Phil Trans R Soc London (Biol)* 1798;18:346.
6. Behrendt DM, Kirsh MM, Stern A, et al. The surgical therapy for pulmonary artery–right ventricular discontinuity. *Ann Thorac Surg* 1974;18:122–137.
7. McGoon DC, Rastelli GC, Ongley PA. An operation for the correction of truncus arteriosus. *JAMA* 1968;205: 69–73.
8. Samanek M. Children with congenital heart disease: Probability of natural survival. *Pediatr Cardiol* 1992;13: 152–158.
9. Wren C, Birrell G, Hawthorne G. Cardiovascular malformations in infants of diabetic mothers. *Heart* 2003;89: 1217–1220.
10. Gillum RF. Epidemiology of congenital heart disease in the United States. *Am Heart J* 1994;127:919–927.
11. Stark J, Gandhi D, de Leval M, et al. Surgical treatment of persistent truncus arteriosus in the first year of life. *Br Heart J* 1978;40:1280–1287.
12. Gutierrez PS, Binotto MA, Aiello VD, et al. Chest pain in an adult with truncus arteriosus communis. *Am J Cardiol* 2004;93:272–273.
13. Niwa K, Perloff JK, Kaplan S, et al. Eisenmenger syndrome in adults: Ventricular septal defect, truncus arteriosus, univentricular heart. *J Am Coll Cardiol* 1999;34: 223–232.
14. Collett RW, Edwards JE. Persistent truncus arteriosus: A classification according to anatomic types. *Surg Clin North Am* 1949;29:1245–1271.
15. Marcelletti C, McGoon DC, Mair DD. The natural history of truncus arteriosus. *Circulation* 1976;54: 108–111.
16. Hutson MR, Kirby ML. Neural crest and cardiovascular development: A 20-year perspective. *Birth Defects Res Part C Embryo Today* 2003;69:2–13.
17. Ali MM, Farooqui FA, Sohal GS. Ventrally emigrating neural tube cells contribute to the normal development of heart and great vessels. *Vascul Pharmacol* 2003;40: 133–140.
18. Webb S, Qayyum SR, Anderson RH, et al. Septation and separation within the outflow tract of the developing heart. *J Anat* 2003;202:327–342.
19. Delot EC, Bahamonde ME, Zhao M, et al. BMP signaling is required for septation of the outflow tract of the mammalian heart. *Development* 2003;130:209–220.
20. Botto LD, May K, Fernhoff PM, et al. A population-based study of the 22q11.2 deletion: Phenotype, incidence, and contribution to major birth defects in the population. *Pediatrics* 2003;112:101–107.
21. Boudjemline Y, Fermont L, Le Bidois J, et al. Prevalence of 22q11 deletion in fetuses with conotruncal cardiac defects: A 6-year prospective study. *J Pediatr* 2001;138: 520–524.
22. McElhinney DB, Driscoll DA, Emanuel BS, et al. Chromosome 22q11 deletion in patients with truncus arteriosus. *Pediatr Cardiol* 2003;24:569–573.
23. Ryan AK, Goodship JA, Wilson DI, et al. Spectrum of clinical features associated with interstitial chromosome 22q11 deletions: A European collaborative study. *J Med Genet* 1997;34:798–804.
24. Chaoui R, Kalache KD, Heling KS, et al. Absent or hypoplastic thymus on ultrasound: A marker for deletion 22q11.2 in fetal cardiac defects. *Ultrasound Obstet Gynecol* 2002;20:546–552.
25. Marino B, Digilio MC, Toscano A, et al. Anatomic patterns of conotruncal defects associated with deletion 22q11. *Genet Med* 2001;3:45–48.
26. Fan YS, Siu VM. Molecular cytogenetic characterization of a derivative chromosome 8 with an inverted duplication of 8p21.3–>p23.3 and a rearranged duplication of 8q24.13–>qter. *Am J Med Genet* 2001;102: 266–271.
27. Digilio MC, Angioni A, Giannotti A, et al. Truncus arteriosus and duplication 8q. *Am J Med Genet* 2003;121A: 79–81.
28. McElhinney DB, Geiger E, Blinder J, et al. NKX2.5 mutations in patients with congenital heart disease. *J Am Coll Cardiol* 2003;42:1650–1655.
29. Franco D, Campione M. The role of Pitx2 during cardiac development. Linking left-right signaling and congenital heart diseases. *Trends Cardiovasc Med* 2003;13:157–163.
30. Abushaban L, Uthaman B, Kumar AR, et al. Familial truncus arteriosus: A possible autosomal-recessive trait. *Pediatr Cardiol* 2003;24:64–66.
31. Van Praagh R, Van Praagh S. The anatomy of common aorticopulmonary trunk (truncus arteriosus communis) and its embryologic implications. A study of 57 necropsy cases. *Am J Cardiol* 1965;16:406–425.
32. Jacobs ML. Congenital Heart Surgery Nomenclature and Database Project: Truncus arteriosus. *Ann Thorac Surg* 2000;69:S50–S55.
33. De la Cruz MV, Cayre R, Angelini P, et al. Coronary arteries in truncus arteriosus. *Am J Cardiol* 1990;66: 1482–1486.

34. Anderson KR, McGoon DC, Lie JT. Surgical significance of the coronary arterial anatomy in truncus arteriosus communis. *Am J Cardiol* 1978;41:76–81.
35. Lenox CC, Debich DE, Zuberbuhler JR. The role of coronary artery abnormalities in the prognosis of truncus arteriosus. *J Thorac Cardiovasc Surg* 1992;104: 1728–1742.
36. Paul JF, Serraf A. Images in cardiovascular medicine. Truncus arteriosus and double aortic arch. *Circulation* 2002;105:170.
37. Lim C, Kim WH, Kim SC, et al. Truncus arteriosus with coarctation of persistent fifth aortic arch. *Ann Thorac Surg* 2002;74:1702–1704.
38. Parmar RC, Pillai S, Kulkarni S, et al. Type I persistent left fifth aortic arch with truncus arteriosus type A3: An unreported association. *Pediatr Cardiol* 2004;25: 432–433.
39. Ishizaka T, Allen SW, Strouse PJ, et al. Postductal origin of the left carotid, left subclavian, and aberrant retroesophageal right innominate arteries in truncus arteriosus with interrupted aortic arch. *Pediatr Cardiol* 2003;24:581–584.
40. Wong MN, Kirk R, Quek SC. Persistent truncus arteriosus with absence of right pulmonary artery. *Heart* 2003; 89:549.
41. Castaneda AR, Jonas RA, Mayer JE, et al. Truncus arteriosus. In: *Cardiac Surgery of the Neonate and Infant.* Philadelphia: Saunders; 1994:281–293.
42. Black SM, Fineman JR, Steinhorn RH, et al. Increased endothelial NOS in lambs with increased pulmonary blood flow and pulmonary hypertension. *Am J Physiol* 1998;275:H1643–H1651.
43. Black SM, Bekker JM, McMullan DM, et al. Alterations in nitric oxide production in 8-week-old lambs with increased pulmonary blood flow. *Pediatr Res* 2002;52:233–244.
44. Koppel RI, Druschel CM, Carter T, et al. Effectiveness of pulse oximetry screening for congenital heart disease in asymptomatic newborns. *Pediatrics* 2003;111:451–455.
45. Silverman NH. Truncus arteriosus. In: *Pediatric Echocardiography.* Baltimore: Williams & Wilkins; 1993: 229–243.
46. Duke C, Sharland GK, Jones AM, et al. Echocardiographic features and outcome of truncus arteriosus diagnosed during fetal life. *Am J Cardiol* 2001;88:1379–1384.
47. Ebert PA, Turley K, Stanger P, et al. Surgical treatment of truncus arteriosus in the first 6 months of life. *Ann Surg* 1984;200:451–456.
48. Bove EL, Beekman RH, Snider AR, et al. Repair of truncus arteriosus in the neonate and young infant. *Ann Thorac Surg* 1989;47:499–505.
49. Hanley FL, Heinemann MK, Jonas RA, et al. Repair of truncus arteriosus in the neonate. *J Thorac Cardiovasc Surg* 1993;105:1047–1056.
50. Stark JF, Gallivan S, Davis K, et al. Assessment of mortality rates for congenital heart defects and surgeons' performance. *Ann Thorac Surg* 2001;72:169–174.
51. Stark J, Gallivan S, Lovegrove J, et al. Mortality rates after surgery for congenital heart defects in children and surgeons' performance. *Lancet* 2000;355:1004–1007.
52. Brizard CP, Cochrane A, Austin C, et al. Management strategy and long-term outcome for truncus arteriosus. *Eur J Cardiothorac Surg* 1997;11:687–695.
53. Alexiou C, Keeton BR, Salmon AP, et al. Repair of truncus arteriosus in early infancy with antibiotic sterilized aortic homografts. *Ann Thorac Surg* 2001;71: S371–S374.
54. Perron J, Moran AM, Gauvreau K, et al. Valved homograft conduit repair of the right heart in early infancy. *Ann Thorac Surg* 1999;68:542–548.
55. Mayer JE Jr. Uses of homograft conduits for right ventricle to pulmonary artery connections in the neonatal period. *Semin Thorac Cardiovasc Surg* 1995;7:130–132.
56. Forbess JM, Shah AS, St Louis JD, et al. Cryopreserved homografts in the pulmonary position: Determinants of durability. *Ann Thorac Surg* 2001;71:54–59.
57. Ishizaka T, Ohye RG, Goldberg CS, et al. Premature failure of small-sized Shelhigh No-React porcine pulmonic valve conduit model NR-4000. *Eur J Cardiothorac Surg* 2003;23:715–718.
58. Imai Y, Takanashi Y, Hoshino S, et al. The equine pericardial valved conduit and current strategies for pulmonary reconstruction. *Semin Thorac Cardiovasc Surg* 1995;7:157–161.
59. Barbero-Marcial M, Baucia JA, Jatene A. Valved conduits of bovine pericardium for right ventricle to pulmonary artery connections. *Semin Thorac Cardiovasc Surg* 1995;7:148–153.
60. Guadalupi P, Spadoni I, Vanini V. Repair of hemitruncus with autologous arterial ring and valved bioconduit. *Ann Thorac Surg* 2000;70:1708–1710.
61. Brawn WJ. The use of a glutaraldehyde-preserved bovine pulmonary valve, as a pulmonary valve substitute in infants. *Semin Thorac Cardiovasc Surg* 1995;7:154–156.
62. Chard RB, Kang N, Andrews DR, et al. Use of the Medtronic Freestyle valve as a right ventricular to pulmonary artery conduit. *Ann Thorac Surg* 2001;71: S361–364.
63. Attanawanich S, Withurawanit W. Correction of truncus arteriosus using a fresh autologous pericardial trileaflet valve conduit. *J Med Assoc Thai* 2002;85:380–384.
64. Schlichter AJ, Kreutzer C, Mayorquim RC, et al. Five- to fifteen-year follow-up of fresh autologous pericardial valved conduits. *J Thorac Cardiovasc Surg* 2000;119: 869–879.
65. Carrel T, Berdat P, Pavlovic M, et al. The bovine jugular vein: A totally integrated valved conduit to repair the right ventricular outflow. *J Heart Valve Dis* 2002;11: 552–556.
66. Corno AF, Hurni M, Griffin H, et al. Bovine jugular vein as right ventricle–to–pulmonary artery valved conduit. *J Heart Valve Dis* 2002;11:242–247.
67. Breymann T, Thies WR, Boethig D, et al. Bovine valved venous xenografts for RVOT reconstruction: Results after 71 implantations. *Eur J Cardiothorac Surg* 2002;21: 703–710.
68. Chatzis AC, Giannopoulos NM, Bobos D, et al. New xenograft valved conduit (Contegra) for right ventricular outflow tract reconstruction. *Heart Surg Forum* 2003;6: 396–398.
69. Reddy VM, Rajasinghe HA, McElhinney DB, et al. Performance of right ventricle to pulmonary artery conduits after repair of truncus arteriosus: A comparison of Dacron-housed porcine valves and cryopreserved allografts. *Semin Thorac Cardiovasc Surg* 1995;7:133–138.

70. Wells WJ, Arroyo H Jr, Bremner RM, et al. Homograft conduit failure in infants is not due to somatic outgrowth. *J Thorac Cardiovasc Surg* 2002;124:88–96.
71. Hiramatsu T, Miura T, Forbess JM, et al. Downsizing of valve allografts for use as right heart conduits. *Ann Thorac Surg* 1994;58:339–342.
72. Levine AJ, Miller PA, Stumper OS, et al. Early results of right ventricular–pulmonary artery conduits in patients under 1 year of age. *Eur J Cardiothorac Surg* 2001;19: 122–126.
73. Aupecle B, Serraf A, Belli E, et al. Intermediate follow-up of a composite stentless porcine valved conduit of bovine pericardium in the pulmonary circulation. *Ann Thorac Surg* 2002;74:127–132.
74. Boudjemline Y, Bonnet D, Agnoletti G, et al. Aneurysm of the right ventricular outflow following bovine valved venous conduit insertion. *Eur J Cardiothorac Surg* 2003;23:122–124.
75. Tiete AR, Sachweh JS, Roemer U, et al. Right ventricular outflow tract reconstruction with the Contegra bovine jugular vein conduit: A word of caution. *Ann Thorac Surg* 2004;77:2151–2156.
76. Kadner A, Dave H, Stallmach T, et al. Formation of a stenotic fibrotic membrane at the distal anastomosis of bovine jugular vein grafts (Contegra) after right ventricular outflow tract reconstruction. *J Thorac Cardiovasc Surg* 2004;127:285–286.
77. Lacour-Gayet F, Serraf A, Komiya T, et al. Truncus arteriosus repair: Influence of techniques of right ventricular outflow tract reconstruction. *J Thorac Cardiovasc Surg* 1996;111:849–856.
78. Lecompte Y, Neveux JY, Leca F, et al. Reconstruction of the pulmonary outflow tract without prosthetic conduit. *J Thorac Cardiovasc Surg* 1982;84:727–733.
79. Danton MH, Barron DJ, Stumper O, et al. Repair of truncus arteriosus: A considered approach to right ventricular outflow tract reconstruction. *Eur J Cardiothorac Surg* 2001;20:95–103.
80. Di Donato RM, Fyfe DA, Puga FJ, et al. Fifteen-year experience with surgical repair of truncus arteriosus. *J Thorac Cardiovasc Surg* 1985;89:414–422.
81. McElhinney DB, Reddy VM, Rajasinghe HA, et al. Trends in the management of truncal valve insufficiency. *Ann Thorac Surg* 1998;65:517–524.
82. Mavroudis C, Backer CL. Surgical management of severe truncal insufficiency: Experience with truncal valve remodeling techniques. *Ann Thorac Surg* 2001;72:396–400.
83. Jahangiri M, Zurakowski D, Mayer JE, et al. Repair of the truncal valve and associated interrupted arch in neonates with truncus arteriosus. *J Thorac Cardiovasc Surg* 2000;119:508–514.
84. Elami A, Laks H, Pearl JM. Truncal valve repair: Initial experience with infants and children. *Ann Thorac Surg* 1994;57:397–401.
85. Imamura M, Drummond-Webb JJ, Sarris GE, et al. Improving early and intermediate results of truncus arteriosus repair: A new technique of truncal valve repair. *Ann Thorac Surg* 1999;67:1142–1146.
86. Pigula FA, Mahnke CB, Anagnostopoulos PV, et al. Closed correction of systemic semilunar valve insufficiency in the neonate. *J Thorac Cardiovasc Surg* 2003;126: 1650–1652.
87. Van Son JA, Reddy VM, Black MD, et al. Morphologic determinants favoring surgical aortic valvuloplasty versus pulmonary autograft aortic valve replacement in children. *J Thorac Cardiovasc Surg* 1996;111:1149–1156.
88. Sierra J, Beghetti M, Kalangos A. Truncus arteriosus repair with double aortic homograft. *J Card Surg* 2004;19: 252–253.
89. Elkins RC, Steinberg JB, Razook JD, et al. Correction of truncus arteriosus with truncal valvar stenosis or insufficiency using two homografts. *Ann Thorac Surg* 1990;50: 728–733.
90. Dodge-Khatami A, Miller OI, Anderson RH, et al. Surgical substrates of postoperative junctional ectopic tachycardia in congenital heart defects. *J Thorac Cardiovasc Surg* 2002;123:624–630.
91. McElhinney DB, Hedrick HL, Bush DM, et al. Necrotizing enterocolitis in neonates with congenital heart disease: Risk factors and outcomes. *Pediatrics* 2000;106:1080–1087.
92. Williams JM, de Leeuw M, Black MD, et al. Factors associated with outcomes of persistent truncus arteriosus. *J Am Coll Cardiol* 1999;34:545–553.
93. Rodefeld MD, Hanley FL. Neonatal truncus arteriosus repair: Surgical techniques and clinical management. *Semin Thorac Cardiovasc Surg Pediatr Card Surg Annu* 2002;5:212–217.
94. Brown JW, Ruzmetov M, Okada Y, et al. Truncus arteriosus repair: Outcomes, risk factors, reoperation and management. *Eur J Cardiothorac Surg* 2001;20: 221–227.
95. Rajasinghe HA, McElhinney DB, Reddy VM, et al. Long-term follow-up of truncus arteriosus repaired in infancy: A twenty-year experience. *J Thorac Cardiovasc Surg* 1997;113:869–878.
96. Thompson LD, McElhinney DB, Reddy M, et al. Neonatal repair of truncus arteriosus: Continuing improvement in outcomes. *Ann Thorac Surg* 2001;72:391–395.
97. Tatebe S, Nagakura S, Boyle EM Jr, et al. Right ventricle to pulmonary artery reconstruction using a valved homograft. *Circ J* 2003;67:906–912.
98. Monro JL, Alexiou C, Salmon AP, et al. Reoperations and survival after primary repair of congenital heart defects in children. *J Thorac Cardiovasc Surg* 2003;126: 511–520.
99. Dearani JA, Danielson GK, Puga FJ, et al. Late follow-up of 1095 patients undergoing operation for complex congenital heart disease utilizing pulmonary ventricle to pulmonary artery conduits. *Ann Thorac Surg* 2003;75: 399–410.
100. Frias PA, Meranze SG, Graham TP Jr, et al. Relief of right ventricular to pulmonary artery conduit stenosis using a self-expanding stent. *Cath Cardiovasc Intervent* 1999;47:52–54.

CHAPTER

66 TRANSPOSITION OF THE GREAT ARTERIES

Richard G. Ohye, Eric J. Devaney, Zuhab A. Qamar, Edward L. Bove

INTRODUCTION AND MORPHOLOGY

Transposition of the great arteries (TGA) is a common congenital cardiovascular malformation characterized by ventriculoarterial discordance. This discordant anatomy is defined by the fact that the aorta arises from the morphologic right ventricle (RV) and the pulmonary artery (PA) from the morphologic left ventricle (LV). The anatomy of TGA is best understood in the context of Van Praagh's segmental anatomy, a three-letter nomenclature

KEY CONCEPTS

- Epidemiology
  - Transposition of the great arteries (TGA) is the most common cyanotic cardiac anomaly, accounting for approximately 10 percent of congenital cardiac malformations.
- Morphology
  - The aorta arises from the right ventricle and the pulmonary artery from the left ventricle. More than 50 percent of patients have an intact ventricular septum, while the remainder are split between a ventricular septal defect (VSD) with and without pulmonary stenosis (PS). The coronary artery pattern is variable; the most common one involves the left circumflex and left atrial descending (LAD) arteries arising from leftward and the right coronary artery (RCA) from the rightward sinus, respectively.
- Pathophysiology
  - Systemic and pulmonary circuits are in parallel, with the degree of cyanosis depending on mixing at the ASD, patent ductus arteriosus (PDA), or VSD level and coexisting PS.
- Clinical features
  - In the absence of PS, pulmonary overcirculation ensues, with variable cyanosis determined by the adequacy of mixing. Cases of TGA with adequate PS and VSD can remain asymptomatic for a prolonged period. Infants with late presentation exhibit left ventricular (LV) deconditioning from prolonged exposure of the LV to low pulmonary pressures.
- Diagnosis
  - Electrocardiography (ECG) and chest x-ray (CXR) suggest the diagnosis in the cyanotic newborn. Echocardiography defines the relationship between the great vessels, associated ASD/VSD and PDA, and coronary patterns and estimates LV pressures. Cardiac catheterization is rarely required in current era.
- Treatment
  - In patients with an intact ventricular septum, severe cyanosis can be improved with percutaneous intervention (balloon or blade atrial septostomy). The arterial switch operation with or without VSD closure is the operation of choice, performed after LV training with PA banding in patients with a deconditioned LV. In patients with significant PS and cyanosis, temporary palliation with a modified Blalock-Taussig shunt can be performed before repair with a Rastelli operation (VSD baffled to aorta) and RV-to-PA conduit.
- Outcomes
  - Excellent outcomes are seen, with an operative mortality of less than 5 percent; long-term complications are represented by supravalvar PS, neoaortic regurgitation or stenosis, and coronary insufficiency.

system in which the atria, the cardiac looping, and the position of the great vessels are used to describe cardiac malformations. The first letter (S, I, or A) describes atrial *situs* (solitus, inversus, or ambiguus). The second letter (D or L) refers to the *dextro* or *levo* looping of the primitive cardiac tube during fetal development, which determines whether atria and ventricles are concordant (d-looping, right atrium attaches to right ventricle and left atrium attaches to left ventricle) or discordant. The third letter describes the relative position of the great vessels. The letter S signifies normally related great vessels and I denotes normally related but inverted great vessels. D or L describes the rightward or leftward position of the aorta relative to the pulmonary artery in the setting of transposition. Hence in a normal heart, there is atrial *situs solitus*, *dextro* looping, and normally related great vessels, or (S, D, S).

In general, TGA is subclassified in *dextro* (or d-TGA) and *levo* (or l-TGA) transposition, referring to the position of the aorta relative to the pulmonary artery (the last letter of the segmental anatomy classification scheme described above). In TGA, there is generally *situs solitus* of the atria. D-transposition of the great arteries is invariably associated with d-looping, resulting in a segmental anatomy of (S, D, D). L-transposition of the great arteries is characterized by atrioventricular and ventriculoarterial discordance (right atrium attaches to left ventricle and left atrium to right ventricle) and is alternatively termed congenitally corrected TGA. This association of l-looping with l-TGA results in an anatomy coded as (S, L, L). Other extremely rare forms of TGA, including (S, D, L), have been described but are beyond the scope of this chapter. However, the treatment options are generally similar. From a strictly morphologic standpoint, there should only be two forms of transposition: d-TGA, properly termed *transposition of the great arteries,* and l-TGA, which should be referred to as *congenitally corrected transposition.*

These are distinct clinical entities, each with several subtypes requiring a number of diverse reconstructive approaches; they are dealt with in separate sections of this textbook. With all forms of d-TGA, there is the need to maintain adequate mixing of oxygenated and deoxygenated blood between the right and left sides of the heart. The circulation in d-TGA is one of two separate circuits, pulmonary and systemic, in parallel (Fig. 66-1). Without communication between the two sides of the heart, deoxygenated blood does not reach the lungs and oxygenated blood does not reach the systemic circulation.

Although TGA was first described by Baillie in 1797,[1] the term *transposition* is credited to Farre, who used "transposition of the aorta and pulmonary artery" to describe the malformation in 1814.[2] The term was further refined by Van Praagh[3] in 1971 to clarify *transposition* as describing ventriculoarterial discordance, while *malposition* referred to positional anomalies of the great arteries observed in other lesions.

Initial surgical therapies for TGA were palliative, aimed at increasing intracardiac mixing and improving systemic oxygen saturation. In 1950, Blalock and Hanlon described a technique for performing an atrial septectomy without cardiopulmonary bypass to improve

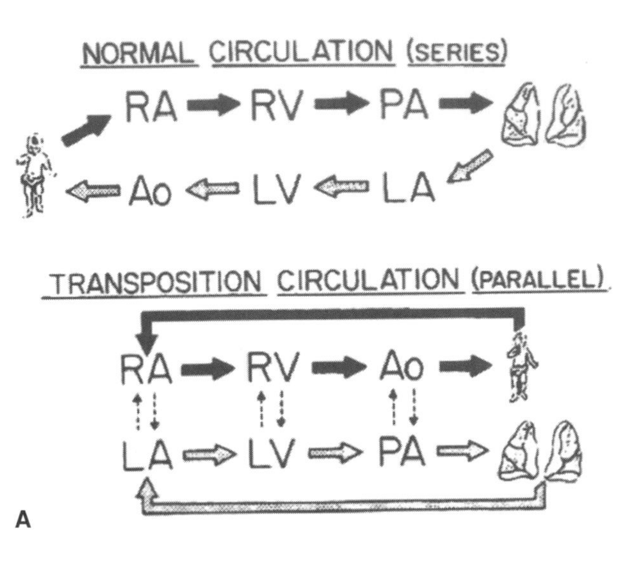

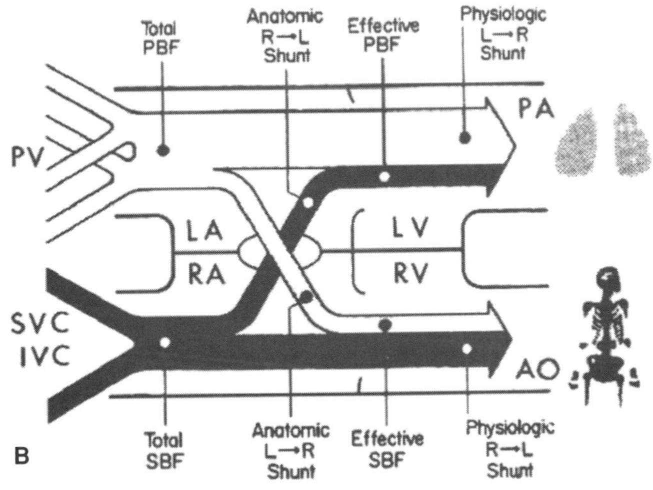

Figure 66-1 Pathophysiology of d-transposition of great arteries (dTGA). A. Systemic and pulmonary circuits in series with normally-related great vessels and in parallel with d-TGA. B. Flows and shunts in d-TGA with intact ventricular septum. Solid arrows = deoxygenated blood; stippled arrows = oxygenated blood; dashed arrows = intercirculatory shunts; Ao = aorta; IVC = inferior vena cava; L = left; LA = left atrium; LV = left ventricle; PA = pulmonary artery; PBF = pulmonary blood flow; PV = pulmonary veins; R = right; RA = right atrium; RV = right ventricle; SBF = systemic blood flow; SVC = superior vena cava. [From Wernovsky G. Transposition of the great arteries. In: Allen HD, Gutgesell HP, Clark EB, Driscoll DJ (eds). *Moss and Adams' Heart Disease in Infants, Children and Adolescents,* 6th ed. Philadelphia: Lippincott, Williams & Wilkins; 2001:1038. With permission.]

mixing at the atrial level.[4] Edwards, Bargeron, and Lyons later reported a modification of the Blalock-Hanlon atrial septectomy in which the atrial septum was repositioned posterior to the right pulmonary veins, baffling them to the right atrium (RA).[5] Other partial atrial-level switch procedures were devised by Lillihei and Varco,[6] who anastomosed the right pulmonary veins to the RA and the inferior vena cava (IVC) to the left atrium (LA), and Baffes, who performed a similar procedure with a homograft conduit from the IVC to LA.[7]

The first attempts at anatomic correction were directed at switching the two great vessels. Throughout the 1950s, a number of techniques for arterial-level switch operations were described, some including the transfer of one or both coronaries, but most leaving them in the pulmonary circuit. Although they were universally unsuccessful, these pioneering procedures laid the groundwork for the understanding of critical concepts for future procedures, including coronary anatomy and the importance of an LV prepared to handle system workloads. The first successful repairs were once again directed at the atrial level. In 1959, Senning accomplished the first successful atrial-level switch with a series of complex intraatrial baffles of native atrial tissue.[8] This technique was simplified in 1963 by Mustard with the use of prosthetic material.[9] The "Mustard procedure" quickly became the treatment of choice for d-TGA and remained such until Jatene reported the first successful arterial switch operation (ASO) in 1975.[10] Jatene and other authors demonstrated the long-term benefits of a true anatomic repair, which could be achieved with acceptable operative mortality. While the Mustard and Senning operations are no longer used as primary therapy for d-TGA, they remain important for the treatment of l-TGA, which is discussed in greater detail in Chap. 67.

Several theories have been put forth regarding the embryology of d-TGA. Some authors support the theory that the normal spiral septation of the conotruncus does not occur and development of a straight septum results in transposition.[11–13] Van Praagh and Van Praagh have postulated that the etiology is persistence of the subaortic conus and reabsorption of the subpulmonary conus, leading to pulmonary-mitral continuity and ultimately transposition of the great arteries.[14] Other theories also propose a similar abnormal development of pulmonary-mitral continuity or of the area below the semilunar valves, or an abnormality of hemodynamics and blood flow as the etiology.[15]

D-TGA can be subdivided into d-TGA with intact ventricular septum (IVS) (55 to 60 percent), and d-TGA with ventricular septal defect (VSD) (40 to 45 percent). In d-TGA/VSD, one-third of the ventricular defects are hemodynamically insignificant. The VSDs are most commonly of the perimembranous or outlet morphologic types. Pulmonic stenosis (PS), causing significant left ventricular outflow tract obstruction (LVOTO), occurs rarely with an IVS. It is not uncommon to measure a preoperative gradient across the LVOT due to shifting of the septum from the high pressure RV outflow tract (RVOT) to the lower-pressure LVOT in d-TGA/IVS. However, the gradient will resolve with anatomic correction and shift of the septum rightward. Hemodynamically significant PS occurs in approximately 10 percent of d-TGA/VSD and may affect operative decision making.[16]

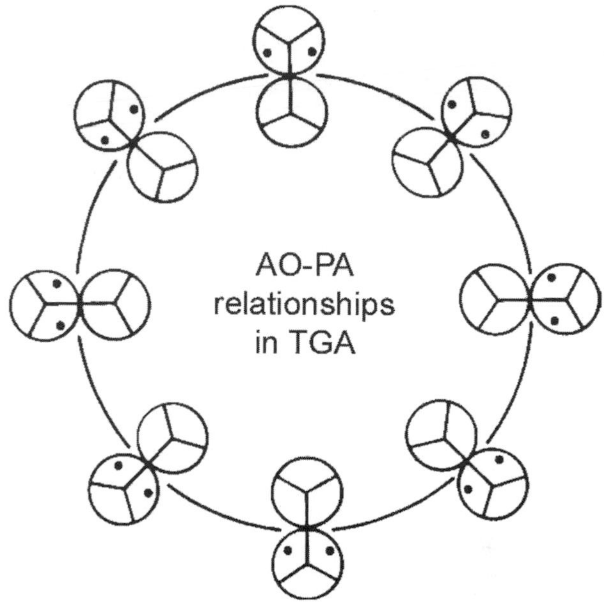

Figure 66-2 The range of the relative positions of the aorta and pulmonary artery in transposition of the great arteries. (AO = aorta; PA = pulmonary artery; TGA = transposition of the great arteries. [From Mavroudis C, Backer CL. Transposition of the great arteries. In: Mavroudis C, Backer CL (eds). *Pediatric Cardiac Surgery,* 3d ed. Philadelphia: Mosby; 2003:442. With permission.]

The relative positions of the aorta and PA are variable in TGA (Fig. 66-2). Fortunately the sinuses of Valsalva of the aorta and PA tend to be in mirror-image alignment. This arrangement facilitates coronary transfer during the ASO. Similarly, the coronary artery arrangement can be variable. In the current era, most of these coronary artery patterns do not represent an obstacle to surgical correction (as discussed below). To standardize the definition of the coronary anatomy, the sinuses are conventionally numbered 1 and 2. If one imagines oneself standing in the nonfacing aortic sinus looking at the pulmonary root (Fig. 66-3), the right-hand sinus is numbered 1 and the left hand sinus 2. Using this convention (also known as the "Leiden" convention), the coronary anatomy is then described based on the sinuses of origin of the various coronary artery branches. For example, in the most common arrangement, the left anterior descending and circumflex coronary arteries arise from sinus 1 and the right coronary artery from sinus 2. This pattern, as seen in Fig. 66-3, is described as 1LCx2R.

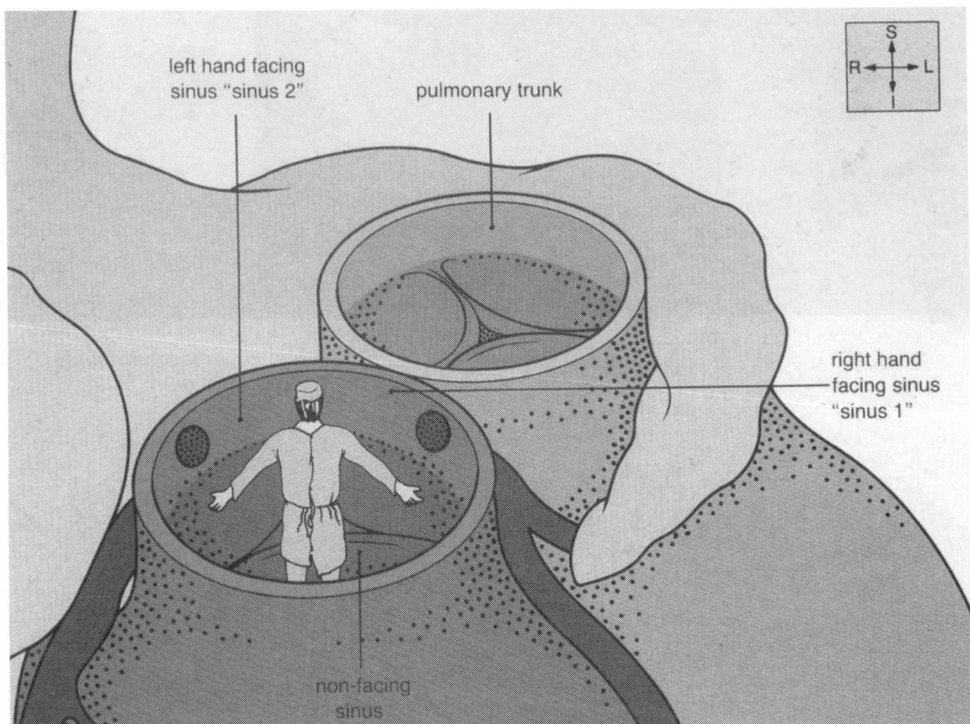

Figure 66-3 Conventional numbering (Leiden convention) of the aortic sinuses for defining the coronary patterns. The illustration shows the typical coronary arrangement in d-TGA. [From Lesions in abnormally connected hearts. In: Wilcox BR, Andreson RH (eds). *Surgical Anatomy of the Heart,* 2d ed. London: Gower, 1992:819. With permission.]

The common coronary arrangements are summarized in Figs. 66-4 and 66-5.

PATHOPHYSIOLOGY

As mentioned above, the circulation in d-TGA consists of two circuits in parallel (Fig. 66-1A). Deoxygenated blood is ejected to the body from the RV into the aorta, returning via the venae cavae to the RA and back to the RV. The oxygenated blood cycles from the LV to the PA and through the lungs to return once again to the LA and LV. Thus, intercirculatory shunting is required for mixing to occur. As reflected in Fig. 66-1B, the *effective* pulmonary blood flow (the amount of deoxygenated blood reaching the lungs) is composed of only the anatomic right-to-left shunted blood. Similarly, the *effective* systemic blood flow (the amount of oxygenated blood reaching the body) is equal to the amount of anatomic left-to-right shunting. There are several potential levels of mixing, including an atrial septal defect (ASD), a VSD, and a patent ductus arteriosus (PDA). In d-TGA/IVS, this is achieved by maintaining a PDA with prostaglandin E_1 (PGE_1) infusion and ensuring an adequate ASD. This may require performance of a blade or balloon atrial septostomy, a cardiac catheterization, or an echocardiographically guided method of opening the atrial septum, as described by Rashkind in 1966.[17] Rarely, an open atrial septectomy will be required to stabilize a patient prior to an ASO. In d-TGA/IVS and d-TGA/VSD with mild or no PS, there may be adequate mixing at the atrial and/or ventricular levels to allow for the discontinuation of PGE_1. In the presence of significant PS, PGE_1 will be necessary to provide sufficient pulmonary blood flow.

For patients escaping early diagnosis, the evolution of the intermediate-term pathophysiology depends on the anatomy. In the majority of patients with d-TGA/IVS, the closure of the PDA with the resultant loss of mixing will lead to severe cyanosis and cardiovascular decompensation. Although they are generally significantly cyanotic, a minority of patients may survive undiagnosed with d-TGA/IVS owing to adequate atrial-level mixing. In these patients, the LV will become deconditioned as it becomes acclimated to ejecting against the low resistance pulmonary circulation. After 4 to 6 weeks, this deconditioning progresses to the point where an ASO would result in LV failure, as the LV would be abruptly required to assume systemic workloads. These ventricles require reconditioning prior to an ASO, as detailed below.

Patients with d-TGA and a nonrestrictive VSD will have pulmonary overcirculation, as in the case of any patient with a large systemic-to-pulmonary shunt. However, unlike the typical patient with a large VSD,

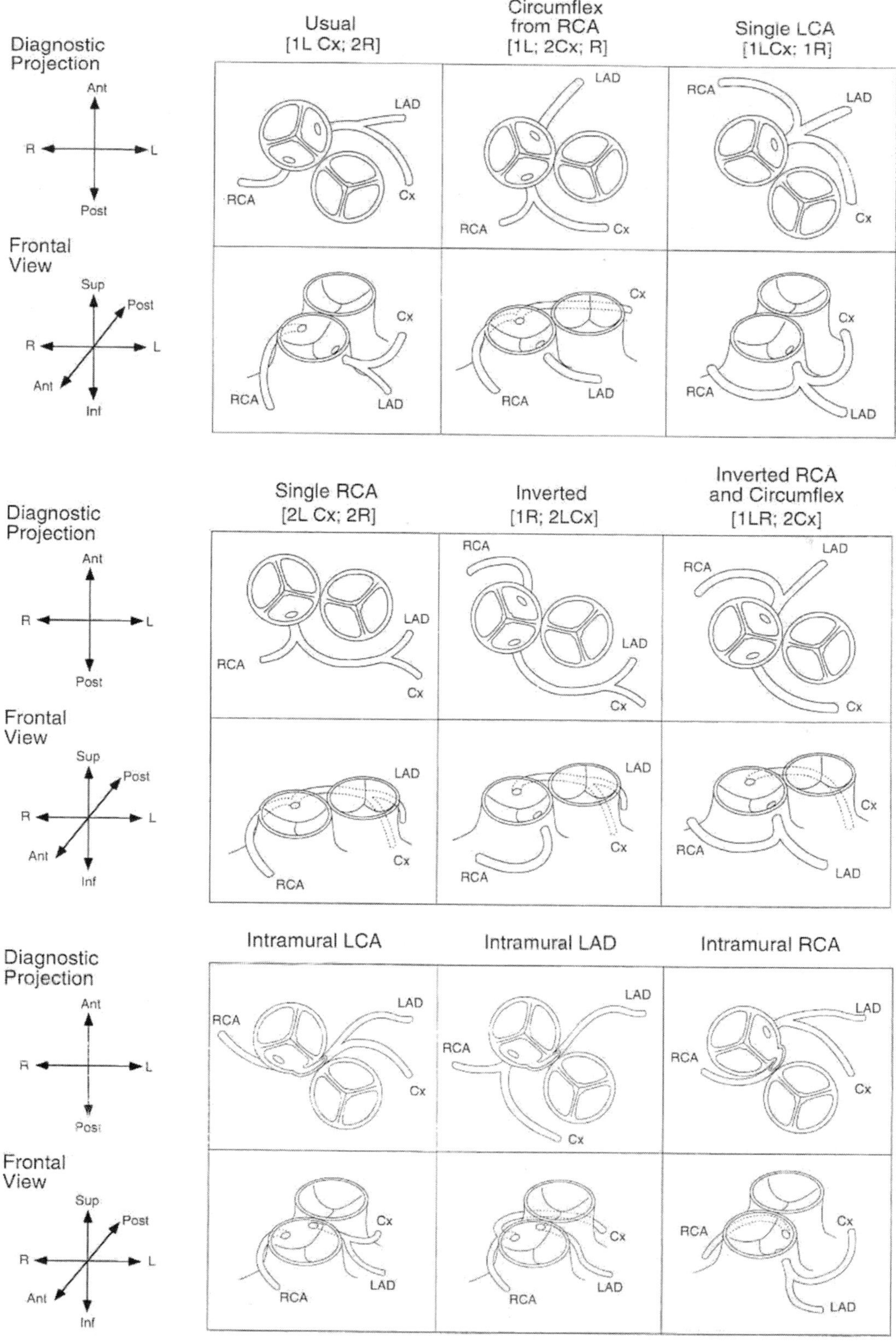

Figure 66-4 Coronary artery patterns in TGA. Upper panel: Two-dimensional echocardiographic view. Lower panel: "surgeon's view." Ant = anterior; Cx = circumflex; Inf = inferior; L = left; R = right; LAD = left anterior descending; Post = posterior; RCA = right coronary artery; Sup = superior. [From Wernovsky G. Transposition of the great arteries. In: Allen HD, Gutgesell HP, Clark EB, Driscoll DJ (eds). *Moss and Adams' Heart Disease in Infants, Children and Adolescents,* 6th ed. Philadelphia: Lippincott, Williams & Wilkins; 2001:1038. With permission.]

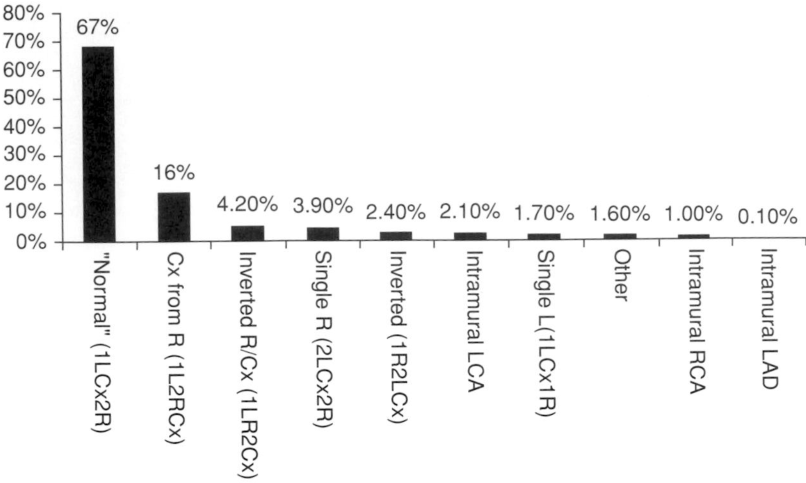

Figure 66-5 Distribution of coronary patterns. [Modified from Wernovsky G. Transposition of the great arteries. In: Allen HD, Gutgesell HP, Clark EB, Driscoll DJ (eds). *Moss and Adams' Heart Disease in Infants, Children and Adolescents,* 6th ed. Philadelphia: Lippincott, Williams & Wilkins; 2001:1033. With permission.]

patients with transposition are at significant risk for the accelerated development of pulmonary vascular obstructive disease (PVOD). As early as 2 months of age, 20 percent of patients with d-TGA and a nonrestrictive VSD will have Heath-Edwards grade 3 or greater histologic pulmonary vascular changes.[18] By 12 months, up to 89 percent will have grade 4 changes.[19] Although the LV remains conditioned due to the pressure load from the nonrestrictive VSD, the development of PVOD may preclude anatomic repair. Patients with d-TGA/VSD/PS can have a more benign natural history, as the appropriate degree of PS leaves them well balanced between adequate effective pulmonary blood flow and protection from PVOD. The LV in patients with d-TGA/VSD/PS remains conditioned due to the pressure load of both the VSD and the PS.

CLINICAL FEATURES

D-TGA is the most common cause of cyanosis in infants and accounts for approximately 10 percent of all congenital cardiovascular malformations.[20] The clinical manifestations of a patient with d-TGA are based upon the amount of intercirculatory shunting of the specific anatomy. In the patient with d-TGA/IVS (or a virtually intact septum), cyanosis is essentially universal. Cyanosis is recognized by nursing or physician staff in 56 percent of neonates within the first hour of life and 92 percent by 1 day.[21] The remainder of the physical exam is often nondiagnostic. Systolic cardiac murmurs are present in approximately half of the patients but are usually of grade 2 or less. In the presence of a large VSD, the cyanosis may be very mild and initially overlooked. Signs of congestive heart failure (CHF), including tachycardia and tachypnea, generally become evident by 2 to 6 weeks as pulmonary vascular resistance falls and pulmonary blood flow increases. Murmurs may increase, and other ausculatory findings typically associated with CHF may become evident. These findings may include a grade 3 to 4/VI pansystolic murmur, a gallop, a mid-diastolic rumble, and a narrowly split second heart sound with a prominent pulmonary component. The addition of significant PS leads to diminished pulmonary blood flow and severe cyanosis.

DIAGNOSTIC MODALITIES

The electrocardiogram (ECG) at birth is generally normal for age. Within the first weeks, abnormal RV hypertrophy with right axis deviation becomes evident with d-TGA/IVS. In the presence of a large VSD, biventricular hypertrophy predominates in the majority of patients, while the axis remains normal in approximately one-third. The chest radiograph (CXR) is often initially normal in d-TGA with IVS or VSD. The classic triad of an egg-shaped heart, mild cardiomegaly, and mildly increased pulmonary vascular markings occurs in only about one-half of patients (Fig. 66-6).[21] With d-TGA/IVS approximately one-half to two-thirds of CXRs demonstrate the classic "egg on a string" sign (globular heart with mild or no cardiomegaly below a narrow mediastinal shadow due to the anteroposterior

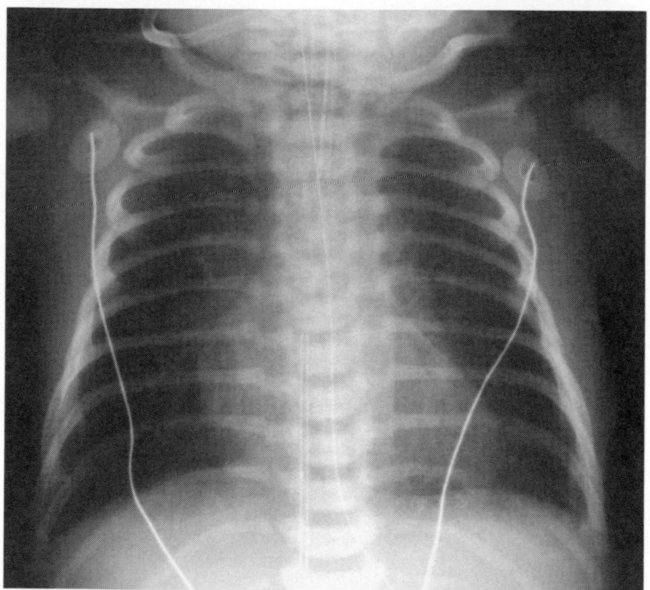

Figure 66-6 Chest radiograph of a patient with d-TGA with intact ventricular septum, demonstrating the classic "egg on a string" radiographic finding.

alignment of the great vessels). The pulmonary vasculature is normal in one-third to one-half of patients and mildly increased in the remainder. Over the first few weeks, cardiomegaly may become more apparent, and the pulmonary vascular markings invariably increase. In the presence of a VSD, the cardiac *silhouette* is generally noticeably larger and the pulmonary vasculature more prominent than in d-TGA/IVS, as pulmonary vascular resistance falls over the first few weeks of life.

Two-dimensional and Doppler echocardiography is the diagnostic modality of choice. Echocardiography can accurately diagnose the origins of the great arteries arising from the incorrect ventricles. Classically, in a long-axis view, the two great vessels can be seen in parallel rather than wrapping around each other in their normally related configuration. In the short-axis view, the two semilunar valves, which normally lie in different planes, can be imaged in the same two-dimensional slice, resulting in the "double-barreled shotgun" appearance. Doppler/echocardiography can also accurately diagnose the common associated lesions, including the number, size, and location of VSDs, the degree and cause of LVOTO, and assess the patency of the atrial septum and ductus arteriosus. In addition, coronary anatomy can usually be effectively defined. Cardiac catheterization is rarely required for diagnostic purposes in d-TGA except to define particularly complex coronary anatomy, occasionally to clarify multiple or complex VSDs, and to assess pulmonary vascular resistance or LV pressures in the patient presenting late.

MEDICAL THERAPY

Medical management strategies are utilized to palliate the patient until definitive surgical correction can be undertaken. For patients identified at the time of birth or presenting soon thereafter with cardiovascular compromise, PGE_1 is instituted to maintain ductal patency. The ASD is examined on Doppler and/or echocardiography. It is essentially always necessary to have a minimally or nonrestrictive ASD to allow adequate mixing. Even in the setting of d-TGA with a large VSD, a significant ASD is usually necessary. This is because mixing at the atrial level tends to be more effective, as it occurs in both systole and diastole, unlike the case with a VSD, where shunting occurs primarily during systole. If a restrictive ASD is present, a balloon atrial septostomy is performed under fluoroscopic or echocardiographic guidance. Occasionally, if the atrial septum is particularly thick, a blade and/or static balloon septostomy may be necessary. Rarely is it necessary to proceed with an urgent ASO or, for the patient in poor clinical condition, an open septostomy for a failed percutaneous intervention. Once a nonrestrictive ASD is identified or created, PGE_1 can occasionally be weaned and the PDA allowed to close in d-TGA with a large VSD while oxygen saturations are closely monitored for adequate intercardiac shunting. This may also be the case for d-TGA/IVS, where atrial-level mixing may be adequate to maintain systemic oxygenation until surgery can be performed.

SURGICAL THERAPY

In the absence of mitigating factors that would preclude major open-heart surgery—such as poor clinical condition, prematurity, or low birth weight—our current policy for the treatment of all forms of d-TGA is complete repair in the neonatal period.

D-Transposition of the great arteries without pulmonic stenosis

The current treatment for d-TGA is an arterial switch operation (ASO), which is performed via a median sternotomy. A portion of autologous pericardium is harvested and placed in dilute glutaraldehyde solution for later use in reconstructing defects created in the proximal aorta where the coronary arteries are removed. Standard techniques of cardiopulmonary bypass (CPB) using bicaval cannulation and moderate hypothermia are employed. The arterial cannula is placed slightly higher on the ascending aorta, near the base of the innominate artery, than for other procedures. For straightforward d-TGA/IVS or VSD, deep hypothermic circulatory arrest or low-flow CPB is not necessary. After the initiation of CPB, a left atrial vent is inserted via the right upper pulmonary vein. The antegrade cardioplegia needle is placed in the ascending aorta at the line of planned division or above for later de-airing. A cross clamp is applied on the distal ascending aorta and the heart is arrested with antegrade cardioplegia. Interval doses of maintenance cardioplegia may be given throughout the case in a retrograde fashion or administered directly within the coronary ostia. The aorta and main PA are divided (Fig. 66-7A). The PA is translocated anterior to the aorta (Lecompte maneuver) and the distal aorta anastomosed to the proximal PA (Fig. 66-7B). In the technique, currently favored at our institution, the neoaorta is reconstructed prior to translocating the coronary arteries. Once the neoaortic anastomosis is completed, the cross clamp can be temporarily removed, allowing the neoaortic root to fill and assume its post-repair three-dimensional shape. We have found that this technique facilitates optimal reimplantion of each coronary artery without tension, kinking or twisting. The coronary arteries are removed from the aorta with buttons of adjacent artery and transferred to the proximal PA (Fig. 66-7C). The proximal aorta is reconstructed using a pantaloon-shaped patch of autologous pericardium (Fig. 66-7D), and anastomosed to the distal PA. It is important to properly align the coronary buttons in the neoaortic root. As illustrated in Fig. 66-7E, the original inferior-most point of the coronary button on the aorta is seldom the same for the new location on the neoaorta. It is imperative to allow the button to sit in the most natural position, which is usually not the same orientation as on the native aorta. The ASD and, if present, the VSD are closed transatrially (Fig. 66-7F).

D-Transposition of the great arteries with vsd and pulmonic stenosis

The management strategy of d-TGA with VSD and *significant* PS is determined by the severity and etiology of the PS. Occasionally, in the case of focal subpulmonic stenosis, it may be possible to resect the area of obstruction through the pulmonary valve and proceed with an ASO. However, this resection is technically difficult through the posteriorly located and often hypoplastic pulmonary valve associated with the PS. More commonly, the subvalvar and associated valvar PS precludes an ASO. Although, as mentioned above, our policy is to generally perform complete neonatal repair, there are other options to delay anatomic repair; these may be employed for the management of this particular subset of patients. These strategies are also useful for the patient presenting in poor clinical condition or with prematurity or low birth weight. It is possible for these patients to have well-balanced circulations, with a degree of PS that is significant enough to protect the pulmonary vasculature from the development of PVOD without causing prohibitive levels of hypoxemia. Although the PS tends to be progressive, owing to the continued increase in LVH, it is possible to delay operation in this subset of patients with d-TGA/VSD/PS. However, careful monitoring for an increase in cyanosis is imperative. In the presence of severe PS and significant cyanosis, a palliative modified Blalock-Taussig shunt can be performed to delay definitive repair.

Whether performed initially or as a staged procedure, d-TGA in the presence of significant PS and a VSD requires a Rastelli procedure to be performed. The Rastelli operation utilizes the VSD to allow the LV to eject into the aorta. The operation is performed via a median sternotomy with standard aortic and bicaval cannulation. After the initiation of CPB, a left atrial vent and antegrade cardioplegia needle are placed. A cross clamp is applied and the heart is arrested. A right infundibulotomy is performed (Fig. 66-8A). Resection of the infundibular septum may facilitate the creation of continuity from the LV to the aorta (Fig. 66-8B). The PA is divided at the level of the pulmonary annulus and the proximal end is oversewn. The VSD patch is constructed to incorporate both the VSD and the aortic valve, creating a tunnel from the LV to the aorta (Fig. 66-8C). RV-to-PA continuity is established using a conduit from the right ventricular infundibulum to the distal PA (Fig. 66-9).

Left ventricular retraining

Because pulmonary vascular resistance falls rapidly during the first days of life, the PA and LV pressures drop. In the absence of a nonrestrictive VSD, significant PS, or large PDA, the LV becomes deconditioned, losing muscle mass and the ability to function at systemic workloads. These left ventricles require retraining prior to an ASO. The point at which an LV becomes unprepared can be difficult to determine; however, patients presenting after 4 to 6 weeks are certainly of concern. Objective data to make this determination are few, although LV posterior wall thickness or an LV muscle mass normal for age suggests that the LV will be able to perform at systemic pressures. For patients with moderate PS or a restrictive VSD, an LV pressure that is 70 percent of the systemic pressure generally indicates a prepared LV. Patients who present with a marginally or clearly unprepared LV require a two-stage approach. The first stage entails the placement of a PA band (PAB) to raise the LV pressure and recondition the ventricle, followed by an ASO. It may also be necessary to add a modified Blalock-Taussig shunt with the PAB to augment pulmonary blood flow. In general, a goal of an LV/RV pressure ratio of 0.7 is desirable. Although this may be achieved in a single banding in patients presenting in the first weeks to months of life, sequential tightening may be necessary in the older patient. Echocardiographic guidance can also be useful during the placement of the PAB to assist in deciding how tight a PAB will be tolerated. One measure of an effective PAB on echocardiogram is rightward shift of the ventricular septum. The echocardiogram can

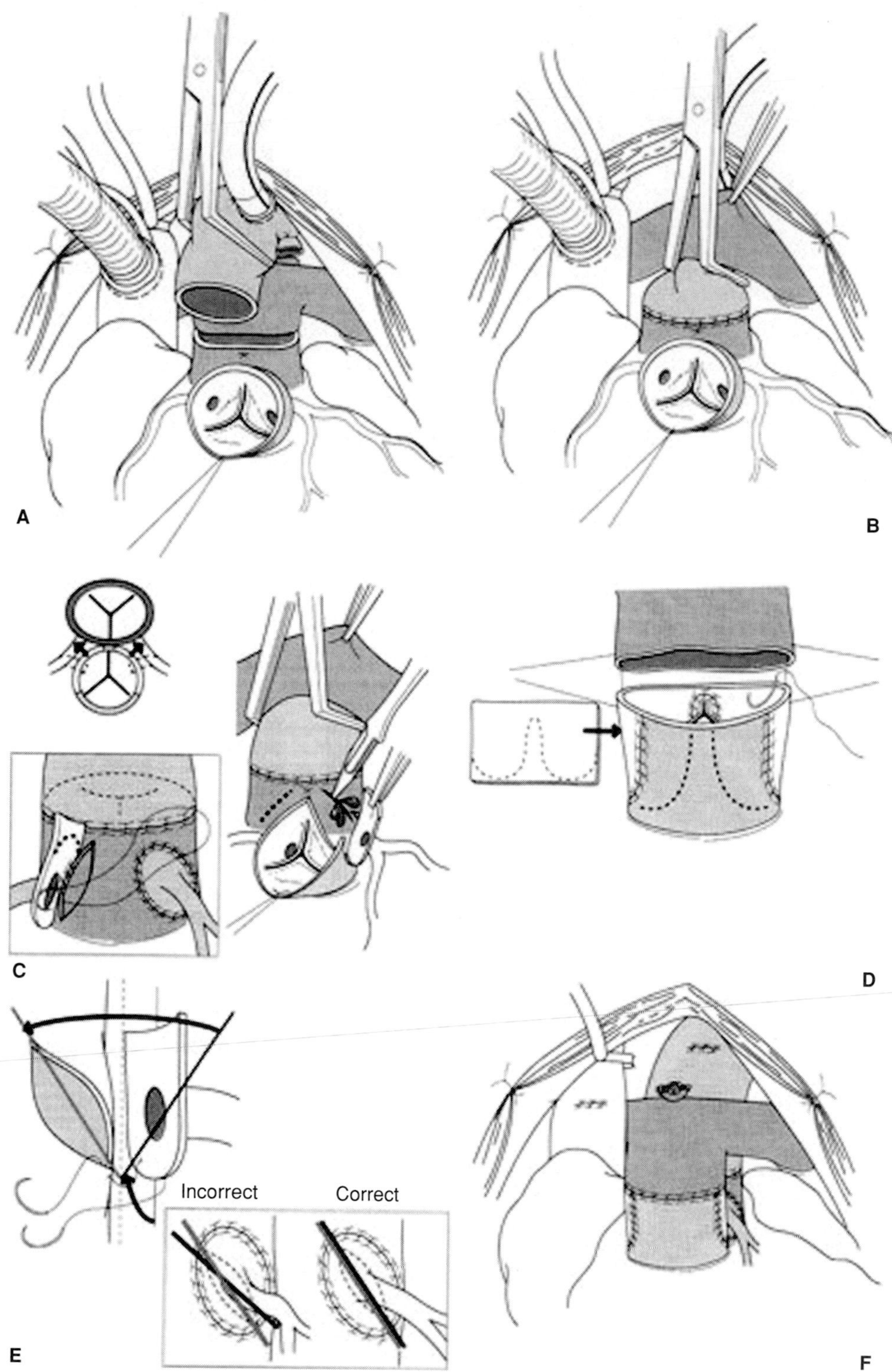

Figure 66-7 The arterial switch operation. A. Division of the aorta and pulmonary artery (PA). B. The "Lecompte maneuver" with the distal aorta anastomosed to the PA. C. Translocation of the coronary arteries. D. Reconstruction of the aorta with a pantaloon-shaped patch of autologous pericardium. E. Proper alignment of the coronary arteries. F. The completed repair. [From Devaney EJ, Ohye RG, Hirsch JC, Bove EL. Congenital heart disease. In: Mulholland MW, Lillemoe KD, Doherty GM, et al (eds). *Greenfield's Surgery: Scientific Principles and Practice*. Philadelphia: Lippincott, Williams & Wilkins; 2006:1442.

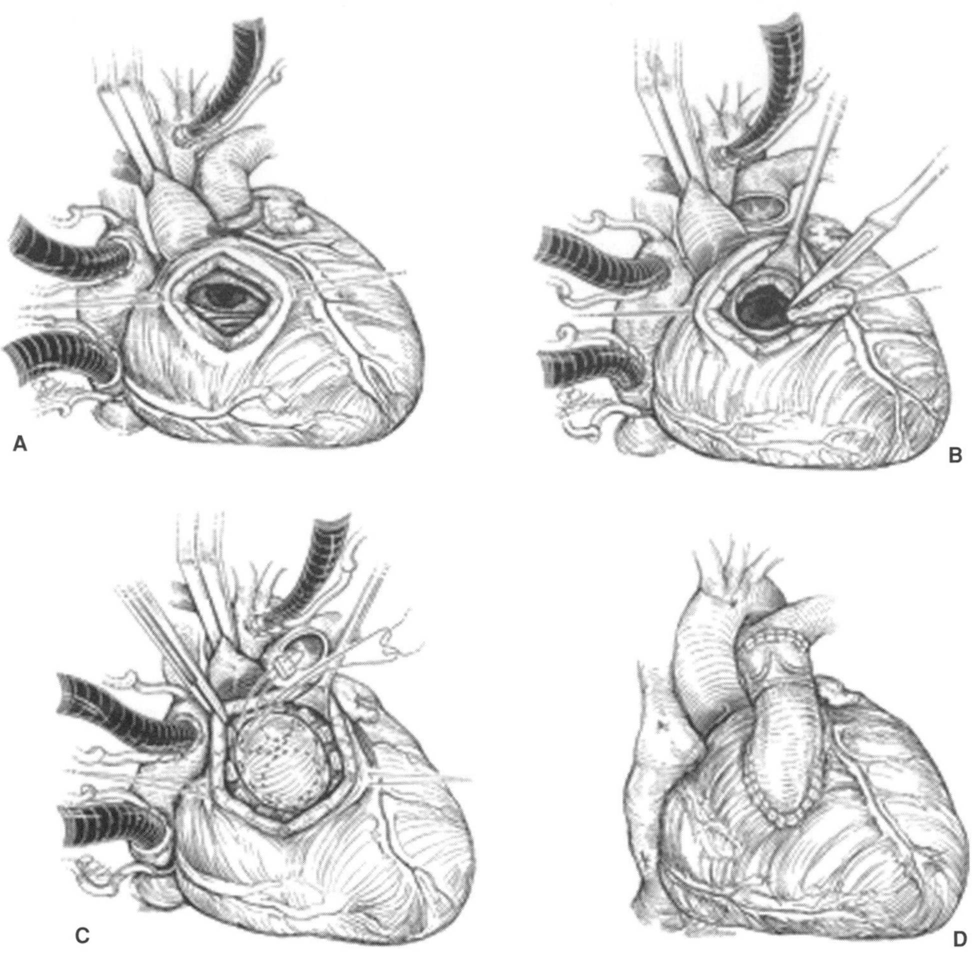

Figure 66-8 The Rastelli procedure. [From Mavroudis C, Backer CL. Transposition of the great arteries. In: Mavroudis C, Backer CL (eds). *Pediatric Cardiac Surgery,* 3d ed. Philadelphia: Mosby; 2003:465. With permission.]

also be employed to guard against ventricular failure from a PAB that is excessively tight. In patients presenting within the first few weeks to months of life, the retraining process can usually be accomplished within a few weeks. Indications that the LV has been properly reconditioned include an LV/RV pressure ratio of greater than 0.7 and an LV wall thickness or muscle mass that are normal for age.

A particularly challenging group of patients for ventricular retraining are those who present very late or, more commonly, those who present with a failed atrial-level switch. These patients present with RV failure generally associated with severe tricuspid regurgitation. Tricuspid valve replacement has often been unrewarding, as the underlying problem is the RV failure. Among this population of patients, a percentage may be amenable to ventricular retraining. This reconditioning may require several weeks to months, with sequential PAB tightening to achieve a prepared LV. Although similar measures of LV preparedness can be utilized, the determination remains difficult. In addition, many patients may not tolerate the banding and develop biventricular failure. Orthotopic cardiac transplantation remains a viable alternative to ventricular retraining and ASO.

Special coronary considerations

Although older series have often identified certain coronary artery patterns, particularly a retropulmonary circumflex or a single left coronary artery from sinus 2 (1L2RCx, 2RLCx), as risk factors for early mortality, most centers are currently able to perform successful coronary transfers for all arterial patterns.[22–25] Of note, Brown and associates[23] found that the coronary artery pattern was neutralized as a risk factor after switching to the technique of completing the neoaortic anastomosis prior to transferring the aortic buttons, as described above. However, despite these advances, the intramural coronary artery still requires special consideration (Fig. 66-10). Most importantly, the intramural course of the

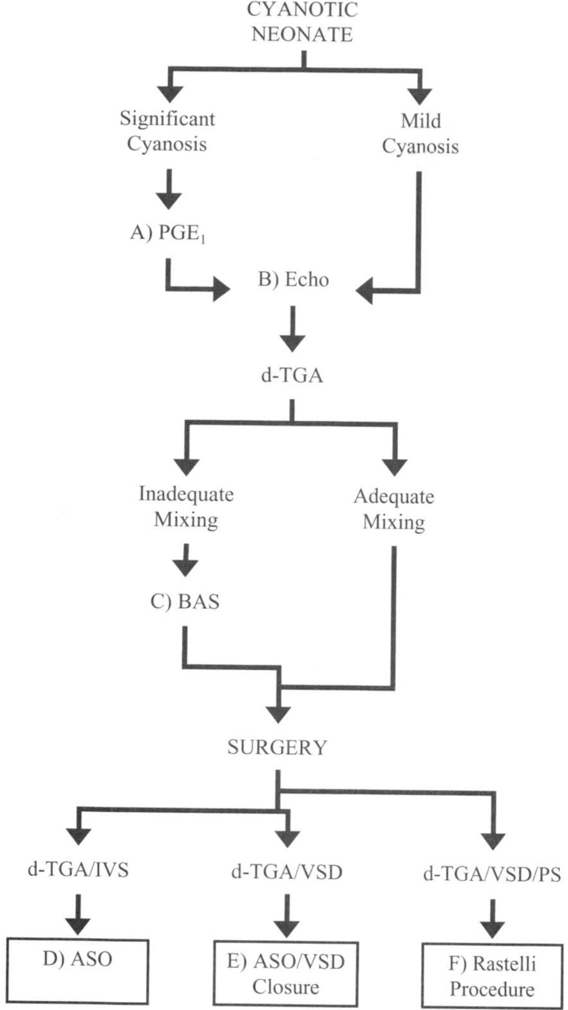

Figure 66-9 Decision-making flowchart.

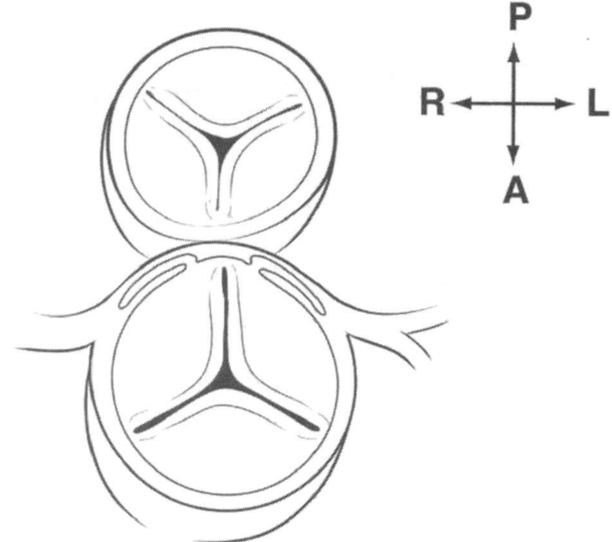

Figure 66-10 An example of double intramural coronary arteries. A = anterior; P = posterior; R = right; L = left. [From Padalino MA, Ohye RG, Devaney EJ, Bove EL. Double intramural coronary arteries in d-transposition of the great arteries. *Ann Thorac Surg* 2004;78:2181–2183. With permission.]

coronary artery must be recognized prior to harvesting the coronary artery button in order to avoid coronary transection. Skilled echocardiographers can often identify suspicious coronary pathways, but careful intraoperative determination of coronary artery entrance and exit points remains crucial. Once the course of the coronary artery is positively identified, the button can generally be successfully and uneventfully harvested, splitting the aortic wall to elevate valve commissures or cusps as necessary (Fig. 66-11). Unroofing of the coronary orifice might be helpful to ensure a widely patent artery. The two arteries can alternatively be left together and transferred to the neoaorta as a single unit.

RESULTS

Currently published hospital survival for the ASO ranges from approximately 90 to 95 percent.[16,23,24,26] D-TGA/IVS generally has a lower mortality than d-TGA/VSD or d-TGA/VSD/PS. Hospital mortality for d-TGA/IVS ranges from 3.5 to 7.6 percent, compared with 9.4 to 13.1 percent for d-TGA/VSD.[23,24] Long-term survivals at 5 to 10 years and at 15 years range between 87.9 and 93 percent and 86 and 88 percent, respectively.[23,24,26] The most common cause for reintervention after ASO is supravalvar pulmonic stenosis, occurring in 3.9 to 16 percent.[24,26] A recent study over a 25-year period of 101 patients undergoing a Rastelli operation revealed a hospital mortality of 7 percent, with no deaths in the last 7 years of the study.[27] Actuarial survival at 5, 10, 15, and 20 years was 82, 80, 68, and 52 percent. At the C.S. Mott Children's Hospital at the University of Michigan, from January 1999 to January 2004, a total of 114 infants with d-TGA underwent operation. Patients with double-outlet right ventricle or other malformations associated with d-malposition of the great arteries were excluded. Of the 114 patients, 60 had d-TGA/IVS (53 percent); the remaining 54 had d-TGA/ VSD (47 percent). Pulmonary stenosis was present in 2 patients among those with d-TGA/IVS (3 percent) and in 13 patients with d-TGA/VSD (24 percent). Coronary patterns were 1LCx2R in 75 patients (66 percent), 1L2RCx in 20 (18 percent), and other patterns in 19 patients (16 percent), including 8 intramural coronaries. D-TGA was corrected via a simple ASO in 71 patients (62 percent), ASO with VSD closure in 31 patients (27 percent), and a Rastelli procedure in 12 patients (11 percent). There were two hospital mortalities, both in patients with

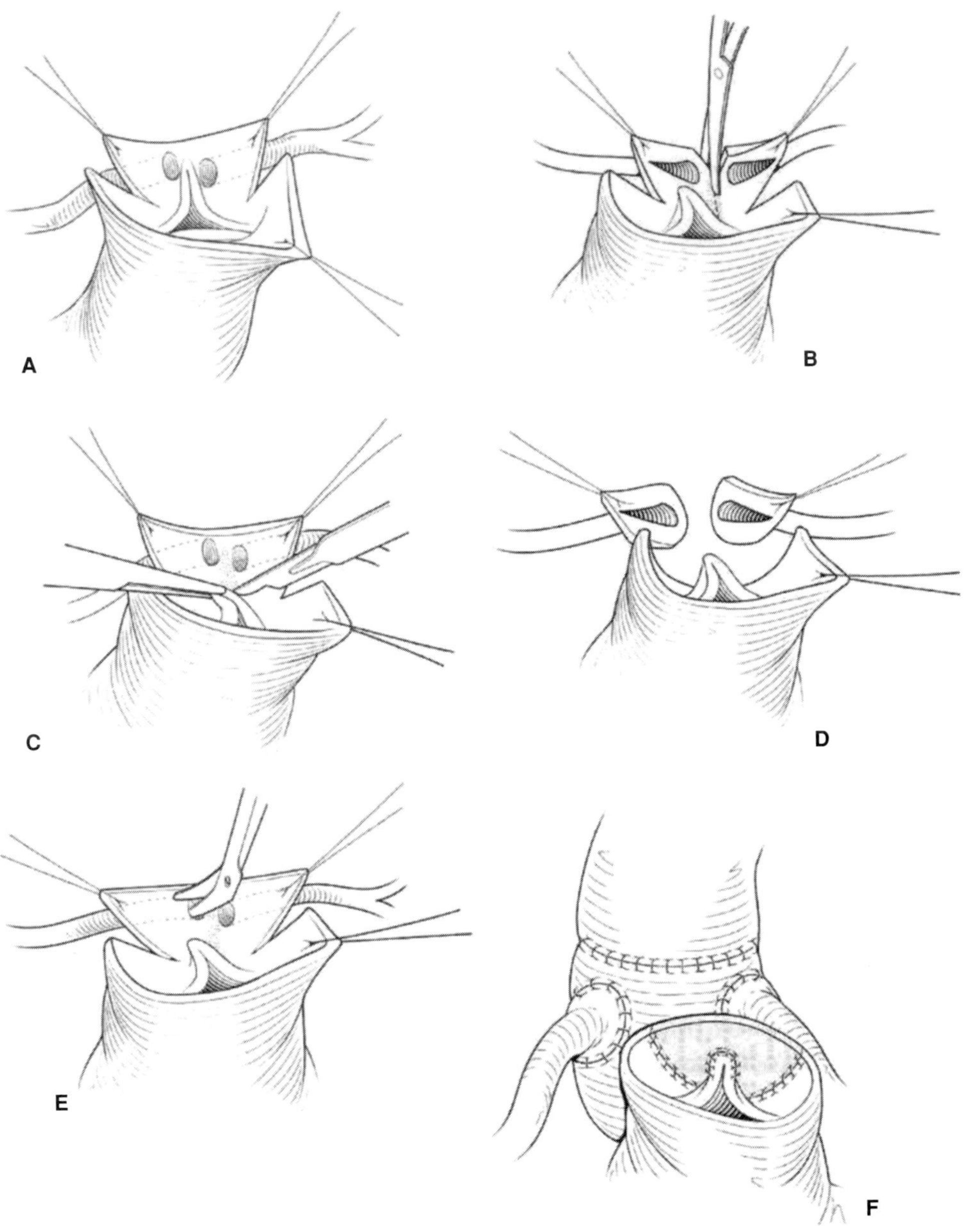

Figure 66-11 The method for coronary transfer of double intramural coronary arteries. A. A single button is mobilized. B. The commissure is elevated from the aortic wall. C. The orifices are unroofed. D and E. The buttons are excised and divided. F. The coronaries are translocated to the neoaorta and the aortic root is reconstructed with autologous pericardium with resuspension of valve commissure. [From Padalino MA, Ohye RG, Devaney EJ, Bove EL. Double intramural coronary arteries in d-transposition of the great arteries. *Ann Thorac Surg* 2004;78:2181–2183. With permission.]

d-TGA/VSD, for an overall mortality of 1.8 percent. One died unexpectedly following an uneventful repair, presumably of cardiac causes, and the second died from necrotizing enterocolitis.

Staged conversion for failed atrial-level switches has been a more challenging problem. In a recent report by Mavroudis and colleagues,[28] 11 patients underwent 15 PA bandings in an attempt at LV retraining; 4 required cardiac transplantation for biventricular failure, 6 have undergone ASO, and 1 awaits conversion. There were no early deaths in the transplanted patients and 1 late death at 7 years from chronic rejection. There were 2 early and no late deaths in the group undergoing ASO, for an overall successful conversion rate of 40 percent (4 of 10). Overall survival was 64 percent (7 of 11), including the patients awaiting ASO.

References

1. Baillie M. The *Morbid Anatomy of Some of the More Important Parts of the Body*. London: Johnson and Nichols; 1797:38.
2. Farre JR. Pathological researches. In: *Malformations of the Human Heart*. London: Longman, 1814:28.
3. Van Praagh R, Perez-Trevino C, Lopez Cuellar M, et al. Transposition of the great arteries with posterior aorta, anterior pulmonary artery, subpulmonary conus and fibrous continuity between aortic and atrioventricular valves. *Am J Cardiol* 1971;28(6):621–631.
4. Blalock A, Hanlon CR. The surgical therapy of complete transposition of the aorta and pulmonary arteries. *Surg Gynecol Obstet* 1950;90(1):1–15.
5. Edwards WS, Bargeron LM, Lyons C. Reposition of right pulmonary veins in transposition of great vessels. *JAMA* 1964;118:522–523.
6. Lillehi CW, Varco RL. Certain physiologic, pathologic, and surgical features of complete transposition of the great vessels. *Surgery* 1953;34(3):376–400.
7. Baffes TG. A new method for surgical correction of transposition of the aorta and pulmonary artery. *Surg Gynecol Obstet* 1956;102(2):227–233.
8. Senning A. Surgical correction of transposition of the great vessels. *Surgery* 1959;45(6):966–980.
9. Mustard WT. Successful two-stage correction of transposition of the great vessels. *Surgery* 1963;55:469–472.
10. Jatene AD, Fontes VF, Paulista PP, et al. Successful anatomic correction of transposition of the great vessels. A preliminary report. *Arq Bras Cardiol* 1975;28(4): 461–464.
11. De La Cruz MV, Da Rocha JP. An ontogenic theory for the explanation of congenital malformations involving the truncus and conus. *Am Heart J* 1956;51(5): 782–805.
12. Peacock T. On malformations etc. of the human heart. London: Churchill; 1958.
13. Shaner RF. Anomalies of the heart bulbus. *J Pediatr* 1949; 61:223–229.
14. Van Praagh R, Van Praagh S. Isolated ventricular inversion: A consideration of morphogenesis, definition and diagnosis of nontransposed and transposed great arteries. *Am J Cardiol* 1966;17(3):395–406.
15. Mavroudis C, Backer CL. Transposition of the great arteries. In: Mavroudis C, Backer CL (eds). *Pediatric Cardiac Surgery*. Philadelphia: Mosby; 2003:442.
16. Kirklin J. Complete transposition of the great arteries. In: Kirklin J (ed). *Cardiac Surgery*. New York: Churchill Livingstone; 1993:1383–1467.
17. Rashkind WJ, Miller WW. Creation of an atrial septal defect without thoracotomy: A palliative approach to complete transposition of the great arteries. *JAMA* 1966;196(11):991–992.
18. Clarkson PM, Neutze JM, Wardill JC, et al. The pulmonary vascular bed in patients with complete transposition of the great arteries. *Circulation* 1976;53 (3): 539–543.
19. Newfeld EA, Paul MH, Munster AJ, et al. Pulmonary vascular disease in transposition of the great vessels and intact ventricular septum. *Circulation* 1979;59(3):525–530.
20. Report of the New England Regional Infant Cardiac Program. *Pediatrics* 1980;65(2 Pt 2):375–461.
21. Levin DL, Paul MH, Munster AJ, et al. d-Transposition of the great vessels in the neonate: A clinical diagnosis. *Arch Intern Med* 1977;137(10):1421–1425.
22. Kirklin JW, Blackstone EH, Tchervenkov CI, et al. Clinical outcomes after the arterial switch operation for transposition: Patient, support, procedural, and institutional risk factors. Congenital Heart Surgeons Society. *Circulation* 1992;86(5):1501–1515.
23. Brown JW, Park HJ, Turrentine MW. Arterial switch operation: Factors impacting survival in the current era. *Ann Thorac Surg* 2001;71(6):1978–1984.
24. Haas F, Wottke M, Poppert H, et al. Long-term survival and functional follow-up in patients after the arterial switch operation. *Ann Thorac Surg* 1999;68(5):1692–1697.
25. Quaegebeur J, Auteri J. Transposition of the great arteries: The arterial switch operation. In: Baue A, Geha AS, Hammond GL, et al (eds). *Glenn's Thoracic and Cardiovascular Surgery*, 6th ed. Stamford, CT: Appleton & Lange; 1996:1393–1407.
26. Losay J, Touchot A, Serraf A, et al. Late outcome after arterial switch operation for transposition of the great arteries. *Circulation* 2001;104(12 Suppl 1):I121–I126.
27. Kreutzer C, De Vive J, Oppido G, et al. Twenty-five-year experience with Rastelli repair for transposition of the great arteries. *J Thorac Cardiovasc Surg* 2000;120 (2): 211–223.
28. Mavroudis C, Backer CL. Arterial switch after failed atrial baffle procedures for transposition of the great arteries. *Ann Thorac Surg* 2000;69(3):851–857.

CHAPTER

67 CONGENITALLY CORRECTED TRANSPOSITION

Nicoletta Salviato, Salvatore Ocello, Carlo F. Marcelletti

INTRODUCTION

Corrected transposition, when first encountered, resembles an unreal apparition....All of the important people were there doing their expert job. The operation began well. The individual cardiac chambers and structures were present and accounted for, and the ventricular septal defect was in the perimembranous location. But something else was fundamentally wrong. Almost everything was out of place in a weird mime of normal, clearly an illusion characteristic of another nightmare. There seemed no choice but to press on even in the face of this confusion, hoping as always that by applying basic principles one could win out. The ventricular septal defect was therefore carefully patched so as to avoid the conduction system, and perfusion was discontinued. Heart block ensued, cardiac output became poor, and tragedy loomed.

Dwight McGoon, 1983[1]

DEFINITION AND SEQUENTIAL ANALYSIS

The classic definition of "congenitally corrected transposition of great arteries" derived from the observation that

KEY CONCEPTS

- Epidemiology
  - Congenitally corrected transposition of the great arteries is a rare condition, comprising less than 1 percent of all congenital heart defects.
- Morphology
  - In the most common variety, there is situs solitus with discordant atrioventricular and ventriculoarterial connection (double discordance). Associated anomalies include Ebstein's malformation of the tricuspid (systemic) valve, ventricular septal defect, obstruction of the right ventricular outflow tract, situs inversus, and anomalous course of the atrioventricular conduction system.
- Pathophysiology and clinical features
  - These are based on the cumulative effects of the associated lesions and the long-term performance of a morphologic right ventricle facing systemic afterload. Cyanosis and pulmonary overcirculation can ensue, with great variability in the timing of presentation.
- Diagnosis
  - Chest x-ray discloses mesocardia. Echocardiography and cardiac catheterization are complementary in determining the necessity and timing of intervention.
- Treatment
  - Some patients may remain asymptomatic, whereas others will require pacemaker insertion for heart block. Early in infancy, shunting or pulmonary artery banding of symptomatic patients is indicated. Eventually, one of three pathways can be chosen: (1) anatomic repair; (2) physiologic repair, with recruitment of the morphologic right ventricle and left ventricle to the pulmonary and systemic circulations; and (3) staged palliation to single-ventricle physiology.
- Outcomes
  - Classic anatomic repair (closure of the ventricular septal defect and relief of the right ventricular outflow tract obstruction) has substantial morbidity and mortality. Physiologic repair is difficult but offers the long-term advantage of biventricular physiology. Fontan palliation is often a valid alternative to repair, with acceptable outcomes (see Chap. 69).

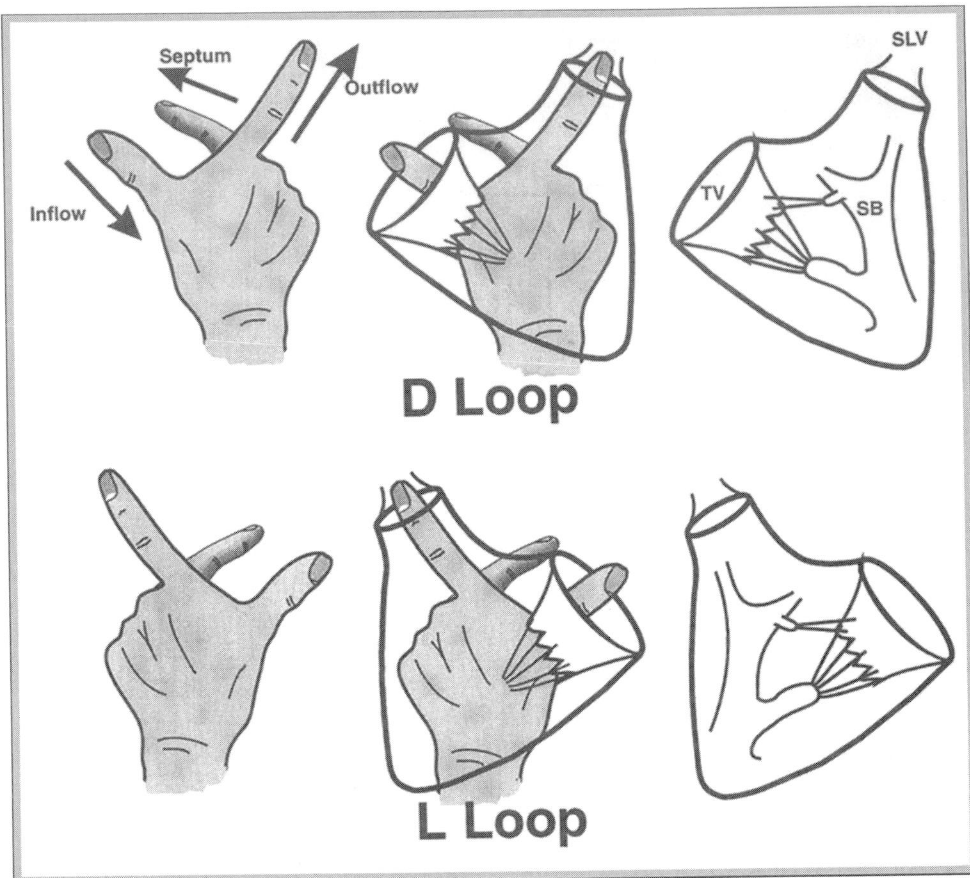

Figure 67-1 Hand topology (loop) in normally connected hearts (D loop, top) and congenitally corrected transposition (L loop, bottom). Explanation in text. (From Kaiser LR, Kron IL, Spray TL (eds). *Mastery of Cardiothoracic Surgery*. Philadelphia: Lippincott-Raven, 1998:591. With permission.)

the effects of such transposition are "corrected" by the congenital inversion of the two ventricles, with the two circulatory pathways "physiologically" in series despite morphologic derangements. Basically the same as "two negative gives a positive," this condition comprises less than 1 percent of all congenital heart defects.

Congenitally corrected transposition of the great arteries (CC-TGA) configures the condition of the "double discordance" where the atrioventricular discordance is associated with ventriculoarterial discordance: the right atrium is connected with a mitral valve to a morphologic left ventricle, from which arises the pulmonary artery; conversely, the left atrium is connected with a tricuspid valve to the anatomic right ventricle, from which arises the aorta. To avoid confusion throughout this chapter, we have set aside the morphologic characteristics that define a right or left ventricle and utilize (unless otherwise indicated) the terms *right* or *left* as they apply to the anatomic and physiologic location of the ventricular chamber. Therefore the "right" ventricle is subpulmonary, whereas the "left" is subaortic.

The atrioventricular and ventriculoarterial sequence is most frequently associated with a visceroatrial "situs solitus," in which the ventricular loop is located on the left side (L loop). The concept of "loop" and "handedness" is simplified in Fig. 67-1 by imagining a hand positioned on the convexity of the septum, with the thumb through the atrioventricular valve and the index finger through the ventriculoarterial connection. The hand that can be placed with the palm following the convexity of the septum defines the loop. In normally connected hearts, the right hand will be positioned on the septum, the index finger through the pulmonary valve, and the thumb through the tricuspid (D loop) (Fig. 67-1). L loop is seen in CC-TGA, where the left hand is positioned on the septum and the thumb goes through the tricuspid valve (morphology of the atrioventricular valve follows and defines that of the underlying ventricle) and the index through the aortic valve.

Rarely, CC-TGA can present with visceroatrial situs inversus, with the right ventricle regularly sited with a normal ventricular "loop" (D loop). The cardiac apex in the most common form of congenitally corrected transposition is related to the peculiar position of the anatomic left ventricle, and it is located in a more central position than normal (Fig. 67-2). This location exists

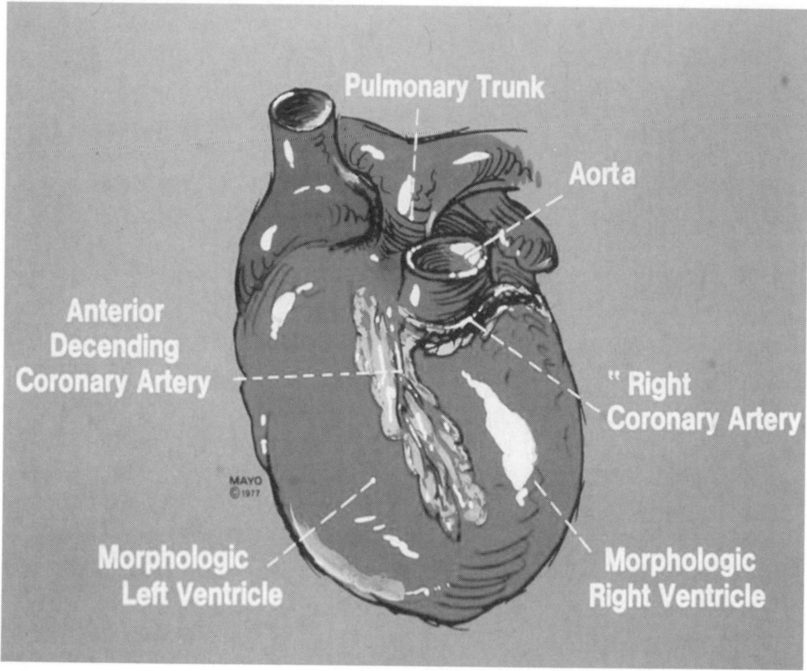

Figure 67-2 Most common external cardiac anatomy in congenitally corrected transposition, with the aorta anterior and to the left, the pulmonary trunk centrally, and mesocardia. (Courtesy of Mayo Clinic photographic archives.)

even in situs inversus, where the cardiac apex is rotated on the right side and more centrally in comparison with the classic "mirror-image" dextrocardia. Heterotaxy is not observed in congenitally corrected transposition.

PATHOPHYSIOLOGY

In isolated CC-TGA, blood from inferior and superior venae cavae and from the coronary sinus drains into the right atrium and through a bicuspid (mitral) atrioventricular orifice into the morphologic left ventricle (physiologic right ventricle). The pulmonary veins drain into the left atrium and blood is transported via the tricuspid atrioventricular orifice into the morphologic right ventricle (physiologic left). This ventricle pumps the blood into the aorta and therefore into the systemic and coronary circulation. Thus, in congenitally corrected transposition, the basic circulation is normal. As a consequence, oxygen saturation within heart chambers and in the great arteries is normal, even if the blood flows through "wrong" atrioventricular valves and ventricles. The pulmonary artery is in the pathway of the unsaturated blood and the aorta in the pathway of oxygenated blood. In these hearts there is another important physiologic aspect that dominates the natural history of CC-TGA: the morphologic right ventricle has to propel blood into the aorta against systemic resistance and high afterload.

ASSOCIATED LESIONS

Patients with congenitally corrected transposition of the great arteries are usually seen because of the additional lesions that are commonly associated. The most relevant associations are tricuspid valve regurgitation (the systemic atrioventricular valve), varying degrees of Ebstein's malformation of the tricuspid valve (TV), ventricular septal defect (VSD), right ventricular outflow tract obstruction (RVOTO, typically pulmonary stenosis or atresia), malposition of the cardiac apex, and conduction defects (more frequently complete heart block). The clinical presentation of CC-TGA is dependent on the cumulative effect of associated lesions on pulmonary blood flow. Indication for surgery is also determined by the nature and severity of the associated cardiac defects.[2–4]

CONDUCTION TISSUE

As mentioned above, the most frequent form of "double discordance" occurs with situs solitus and L loop. The course of the atrioventricular conduction tissue therefore differs from that in the normal heart with ventricular D loop. Although the sinus node is normally located at the superior atriocaval junction, the atrioventricular conduction tissue is grossly abnormal. Because of its malalignment with the ventricular septum, the node fails to give rise to a penetrating bundle.[5–8]

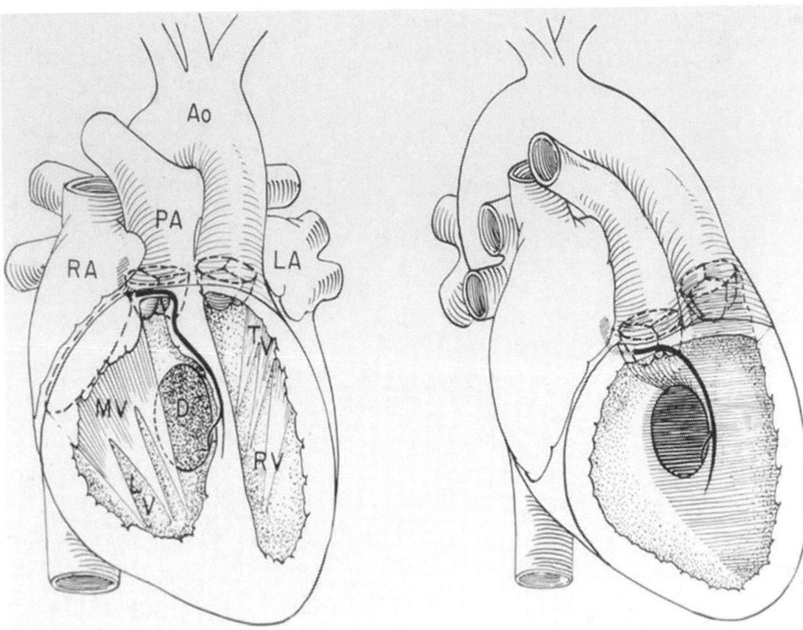

Figure 67-3 Conduction tissue in congenitally corrected transposition with situs solitus. The bundle of His courses in a superoinferior trajectory along the leftward margin of the ventricular septal defect. Ao = aorta; D = ventricular septal defect; LA = left atrium; LV = left ventricle; MV = mitral valve; PA = pulmonary artery; TV = tricuspid valve; conduction system in black.

In the normal heart, the bundle of His runs in an inferoposterior position with respect to the membranous septum; in CC-TGA (with situs solitus), however, the bundle of His is located in a specular fashion in an anterosuperior position and has a much longer course than normal. Such a condition poses the risk that the subject with CC-TGA will go on to develop complete atrioventricular block. On the other hand, when CC-TGA presents with situs inversus, the normal anatomic position of the right ventricle (D loop) allows the bundle of His to follow a normal course.

The surgical history of double discordance revolves around the identification and localization of the conduction system (Fig. 67-3). The studies of Anderson and coworkers in 1973 first clarified the distribution of the conduction tissue.[8–10]

> No wonder that great appreciation was felt by surgeons when the studies of Anderson et al. identified the location of the specialised conduction tissue in corrected transposition. I well remember that my reaction to this news was one of great relief, a sense of returning to reality.
>
> Dwight C. McGoon, 1983[1]

DIAGNOSIS AND CLINICAL PRESENTATION

When congenitally corrected transposition is isolated, without associated cardiac defects, it can remain totally asymptomatic for life, and the diagnosis is often incidental. The electrocardiogram (ECG) is typical for the absence of a QRS transition complex in the precordial leads. The chest x-ray shows a midline cardiac position in the frontal view, with a linear left cardiac border due to the levoposition of the aorta.

The subxiphoid and apical four-chamber echocardiographic views allow identification of the sequential anatomy and visualization of associated ventricular perimembranous defects, valvar and subvalvar pulmonary obstruction, and TV morphology and function.

Cardiac catheterization and angiography complete the functional and structural assessment. The clinical presentation depends on the associated defects and pathophysiologic patterns.

In forms associated with a nonrestrictive VSD, pulmonary overcirculation with left-to-right shunting is observed, with elevated pulmonary blood flow and various degrees of pulmonary hypertension. In such cases, the infant may present with active precordium, tachypnea, failure to thrive, and recurrent pulmonary infections.

When the VSD is associated with valvular and/or subvalvular pulmonary stenosis, progressive cyanosis secondary to right-to-left shunting is seen.

Sometimes (mainly in the presence of dysplastic TV, VSD, and valvular or subvalvular pulmonary stenosis) cyanosis and concomitant right-sided heart failure may develop.

NATURAL HISTORY

In the isolated form, symptoms may be absent until the sixth or seventh decade of life, and the individual may have a near normal life expectancy. Onset of complete atrioventricular block or systemic atrioventricular valve incompetence with congestive heart failure is not rare. However, in atrial situs inversus, because of the considerably higher prevalence of a normally positioned atrioventricular node, there is less likelihood of the spontaneous development complete heart block. When heart block develops, pacemaker implantation is of course necessary.

SURGICAL TREATMENT

The surgical history of patient with double discordance can start either with palliative procedures and continue with intracardiac repair or begin with primary complete surgical correction.

Palliative procedures

Many of these patients undergo anatomic or physiologic intracardiac repair after one or more surgical palliations, which may produce functional and/or anatomic alterations. Chronic volume overload secondary to systemic-to-pulmonary artery shunt and/or atrioventricular valve regurgitation result in an increase in size of the ventricular cavity, followed by a proportional degree of eccentric hypertrophy. Chronic pressure overload secondary to pulmonary artery banding and/or subaortic obstruction, inducing ventricular hypertrophy, alter both systolic and diastolic function. Correct timing of surgery in such patients is another determining factor of early and late outcome, with the goal of preserving biventricular systolic and diastolic function. If any surgical palliations should be needed before repair, it should aim at obtaining a Qp/Qs of approximately 1:1.[11]

In general terms, two major categories can be identified according to the pattern of pulmonary blood flow (PBF): those with restrictive PBF and those with unrestricted PBF. Patients with restrictive PBF, depending on the severity of pulmonary stenosis, might require surgical palliation at different ages. We believe that a systemic-to-pulmonary artery shunt should be preferred in patients younger than 4 to 6 months. In older patients, a bidirectional cavopulmonary anastomosis (Glenn shunt, see Chap. 69) should be the palliation of choice, allowing growth and protection of the pulmonary vascular bed. A bidirectional cavopulmonary anastomosis brings the advantage of dramatically reducing the volume load of the right ventricle to normal values and diverting desaturated blood only to the lungs, thus increasing effective pulmonary blood flow. Patients with unrestricted PBF have a rather usual clinical presentation, with congestive heart failure during the first months of life and failure to thrive: these are babies with a Qp/Qs often greater than 2:1. This represents a significant volume overload, which in the long run may impair ventricular function. All these findings indicate the need for surgical intervention early in life. If the great arteries do not show severe discrepancy in size (aorta not too small compared with pulmonary artery) pulmonary artery banding (PAB) may represent a good surgical option.

Intracardiac repairs

Biventricular repair of CC-TGA is possible, but complete physiologic or anatomic connections are complex and associated with significant long-term problems, such as arrhythmias, subaortic obstruction, valvular dysfunction, obstruction of the ventricular-to-pulmonary artery conduit, and deteriorating ventricular function. Recent advances have supported a variety of surgical strategies.

Physiologic biventricular repair

Intracardiac repair of VSD in CC-TGA has presented technical problems and has been associated with a high operative risk. Progressive definition of the relative merits of the different approaches to the VSD, the use of conduits in establishing unobstructed flow between the pulmonary ventricle and the pulmonary artery, and better knowledge of the anatomic relations of the conduction system to the VSD and pulmonary outflow tract have provided a more favorable basis for physiologic repair of this malformation.

The approach for VSD closure can be through the right-sided mitral valve, through the aorta, or through the left-sided TV. Exposure of the VSD through a right atriotomy can also be enhanced by partially detaching the leaflet of the right atrioventricular (AV) valve. In patients in whom replacement of the right AV valve is required, the valve can be excised before VSD closure. If an initial atriotomy gives inadequate exposure, a ventriculotomy may be necessary to allow closure of the defect. Only under exceptional circumstances are bilateral ventriculotomies required.

As Anderson and colleagues[12] have indicated, in CC-TGA "as a consequence of malalignment of interatrial, interventricular, and conal septal, the pulmonary outflow tract is an obliquely oriented channel which is particularly prone to obstruction." Right ventricular outflow tract obstruction (RVOTO) may be at valvular or subvalvular level.[9–15]

It is also to be recalled that in CC-TGA, the abnormal origin of the pulmonary artery is just posterior to the right coronary artery: the pulmonary outflow tract is wedged deeply into the ventricular chamber between the atrioventricular valves. Pulmonary valvotomy or infundibulectomy (or both) or interposition of an extracardiac

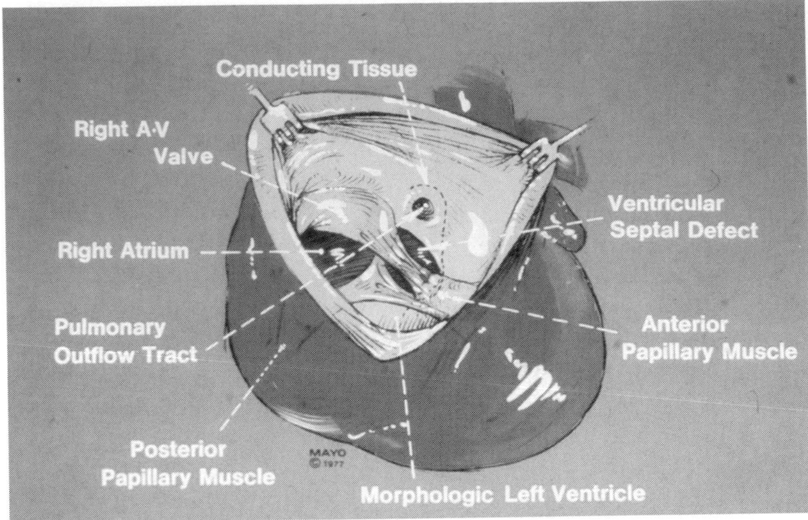

Figure 67-4 Exposure of the ventricular septal defect through a ventriculotomy (oversized for graphic purposes) in the right-sided morphologic left ventricle. (Courtesy of Mayo Clinic photographic archives.)

conduit from the pulmonary ventricle to the pulmonary artery may therefore be particularly difficult.

Pulmonary valvular stenosis in the absence of annular hypoplasia is managed by valvotomy. Relief of subvalvular or annular stenosis by direct resection or patch enlargement is contraindicated because of the presence of specialized conduction tissue in this region. Patch enlargement of the pulmonary outflow tract is further contraindicated because of the overlying coronary artery. Thus an extracardiac conduit extending from the morphologic left ventricle (pulmonary ventricle) to the pulmonary artery seems to provide the most effective means for relief of isolated RVOTO.[16]

A particular technique has been developed in order to reduce the risk of heart block in attempting relief of pulmonary stenosis in CC-TGA by means of a valved conduit. The VSD is closed with a large patch in such a way that both great arteries and the major conduction bundles lie to the left of the patch. This technique requires use of an extracardiac conduit to reconstruct the RVOT. The procedure is completed by dividing the pulmonary trunk and closing its proximal stump or by ligating it (Figs. 67-4, 67-5, and 67-6).

Despite knowledge of the anomalous location of the conduction system[9,13,16] in CC-TGA, the risk of heart

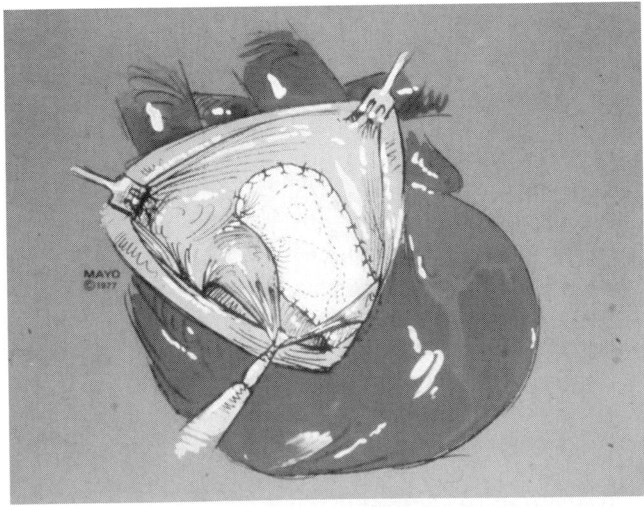

Figure 67-5 The ventricular septal defect is closed with a patch, then secured anteriorly and to the left away from the conduction system. (Courtesy of Mayo Clinic photographic archives.)

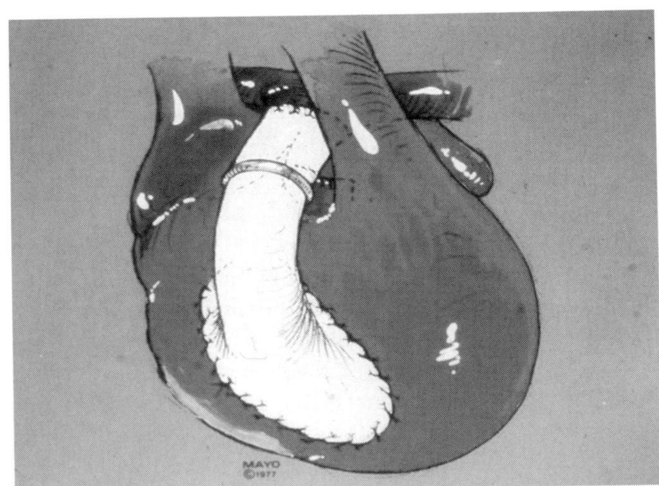

Figure 67-6 A valved conduit is interposed between the subpulmonary ventricle and the pulmonary arterial confluence; the proximal pulmonary artery stump is then oversewn. (Courtesy of Mayo Clinic photographic archives.)

block remains a major concern.[6,17,19,20] Nevertheless, physiologic repair by means of VSD closure and RVOT reconstruction in patients with CC-TGA/VSD/RVOTO can be recommended with greater optimism than earlier experience would justify.

Atrioventricular valve malformation was first reported by Edwards.[21] Becu[2] and Allwork[13] have recently demonstrated the high frequency of associated left atrioventricular valve anomalies resembling Ebstein's malformation (see Chap. 76) and suggest that the morphologic TV is anatomically abnormal in the majority of cases but functionally deficient in only about one-third.[12] Depending on the anatomy encountered, incompetence of one or both AV valves can be managed by valvuloplasty, annuloplasty, or valve replacement.

Anatomic biventricular repair

In patients with atrioventricular and ventriculoarterial discordance and following physiologic repair, the morphologic right ventricle and TV may progressively deteriorate while functioning in the systemic circuit. Therefore the strategy of placing the morphologic left ventricle and mitral valve into the systemic circulation can be achieved only by a double-switch operation, which has been proposed by Ilbawi and associates[22] and Marcelletti and colleagues[23] to limit this functional deterioration. It consists in switching both venous return and arterial outflow. The concept of a double switch was initially suggested for patients with CC-TGA, VSD, and pulmonary stenosis and subsequently applied to CC-TGA without pulmonary stenosis, with or without VSD.

In this setting, a Mustard or Senning intraatrial transposition of venous return is performed as usual for simple TGA. It is not uncommon for CC-TGA of the {SLL} and {IDD} types to have associated cardiac positioning abnormalities, such as mesocardia or apicocaval juxtaposition. In these cases the free wall of the systemic venous atrium is likely to be deficient, making the Mustard preferable to the Senning technique.[24]

For patients with VSD and pulmonary stenosis, a morphologic left ventricle–to–aortic intracardiac baffle is accomplished through a subaortic incision in the infundibulum of the morphologic left-sided right ventricle. Finally, a left ventricle–to–pulmonary trunk conduit is placed (Rastelli operation, Fig. 67-7).[23]

A connection from the superior vena cava to the pulmonary artery (Glenn anastomosis) may be associated with a double-switch procedure, in which the pulmonary ventricle is made anatomically and functionally smaller by the intracardiac baffle and ventriculotomy so as to unload the venous atrium and ventricle. With this approach, the superior limb of the atrial switch is eliminated, the atrial baffle is simplified, the number of atrial suture lines is diminished, and the aortic cross-clamp time is shortened.

For patients without pulmonary stenosis, a classic arterial switch operation is performed (see Chap. 66). If a VSD is present, it is closed as described previously. When these procedures are considered for patients without VSD, in whom the morphologic left ventricle is working at low pressure, preparation of the left ventricle for systemic workload can be done by progressively increasing afterload by means of a pulmonary artery band (ventricular retraining).

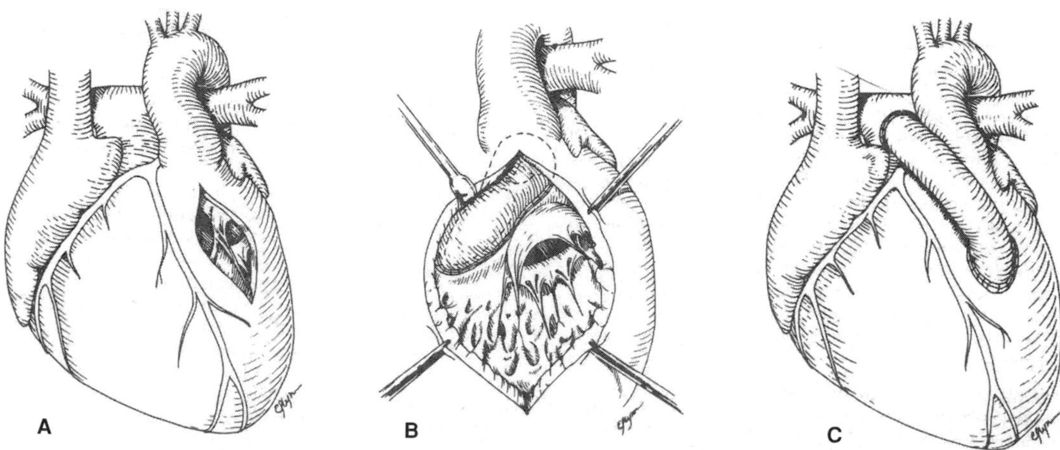

Figure 67-7 Anatomic correction of congenitally corrected transposition with ventricular septal defect. A subaortic ventriculotomy is made in the morphologic right ventricle **(A)**. A baffle is created, channeling blood from the subpulmonary morphologic right ventricle **(B)**. Continuity between morphologic right ventricle and pulmonary artery is established with a valved conduit **(C)**. In cases without situs inversus, a Mustard intraatrial baffle is also placed to redirect venous return (not seen in the illustration). (From Kaiser LR, Kron IL, Spray TL (eds). *Mastery of Cardiothoracic Surgery*. Philadelphia: Lippincott-Raven, 1998:803. With permission.)

When severely unbalanced ventricles exist and a biventricular repair is not reasonable, a single-ventricle repair is indicated. Also, in case of straddling atrioventricular valves or an uncommitted VSD, a single-ventricle approach is preferable to complex biventricular repair.[11] The Fontan principle is, even in the best of circumstances, a palliative one, although most biventricular repairs requiring a valved conduit are palliative as well. A biventricular repair has the advantage of maintaining normal physiology, thus leading to better exercise tolerance and fewer atrial arrhythmias. In physiologic terms, the incorporation of a ventricle in the pulmonary circulation allows lower central venous pressure and better adaptation to exercise. There are situations in which the short- and intermediate-term results after a complex biventricular repair have been suboptimal. In such cases the application of the Fontan principle, even in the presence of two well-balanced ventricles, may improve results.

Physiologic versus anatomic repair: controversies and future guidelines

There is currently a tendency to prefer the anatomic repair (double-switch procedure). Since 1992, when our group described the Mustard and Rastelli operation,[13] this new option has been adopted by most groups.[25,26] We reported on three patients with congenitally corrected transposition of the great arteries and situs inversus who underwent successful anatomic repair of associated anomalies (VSD and pulmonary outflow tract obstruction). We now believe that this option may also be applied in the presence of situs solitus. The principles of the correction are as follows: (1) Patch rerouting of venous flows at the atrial level; (2) patch closure of the VSD through a right ventriculotomy, baffling the left ventricle to the aorta; and (3) valved conduit interposition between the left ventricle and the pulmonary artery in situs inversus.

If the VSD is restrictive, it can be safely enlarged by extensive resection of the anterosuperior border because of the posteroinferior location of the His bundle in the presence of situs inversus. With this technique, the morphologic left ventricle and the native mitral and aortic valves are recruited for systemic work, with intrinsic long-term advantages. It is, however, a complex procedure involving substantial use of prosthetic material. More experience is necessary to establish whether this approach is superior to the physiologic repair.[25,26]

Physiologic repair of CC-TGA (leaving the morphologic right ventricle in support of the systemic circulation) has been accomplished by different techniques of VSD closure combined with relief, or bypass, of associated RVOTO.

Although TV anomalies resembling Ebstein's anomaly are not prevalent in situs inversus, this approach is potentially frustrated by progressive right ventricular failure and ensuing complete heart block.

Pascal Vouhé and coworkers reported the results of 52 patients with CC-TGA and VSD who underwent a physiologic repair between 1974 and 1996,[25] noting a high operative mortality and the incidence of heart block. Anatomic complete repairs in future years, especially for early correction of severe TV regurgitation in CC-TGA without LVOTO, may prove to have better outcomes. We have recently reviewed our last consecutive 108 patients with double discordance and associated anomalies undergoing surgical repair, and these data strongly suggest the need for further comparison between two-ventricle repair and extracardiac Fontan palliation. Total cavopulmonary connection was performed in this study, with no mortality. This particular approach has eliminated, in our series, the surgical risks of heart block and acceleration of progressive tricuspid regurgitation often seen following VSD closure. Another potential advantage results from retaining both ventricles in the systemic circulation. In cases involving complex VSD and tricuspid anatomy or abnormal systemic or pulmonary venous return, this approach also provides excellent intermediate-term results.

The main theoretical advantage of anatomic correction (double switch or Senning-Rastelli) arises from its use of the left ventricle as the systemic pumping chamber and of the mitral valve as the systemic atrioventricular valve. Performance of an anatomic correction should be strongly considered for patients with tricuspid regurgitation before surgical intervention, Ebstein's malformation of the TV, and right ventricular dysfunction. Heart transplantation remains another option for this difficult patient population but is associated with the drawback of immune suppression; moreover, it provides an uncertain long-term outlook.

In our opinion, the long-term outcome of patients with CC-TGA who have been treated by a classic surgical approach is unsatisfactory. Systemic right ventricular and TV dysfunction (especially if requiring valve replacement) predicts a poor prognosis for many of these patients.

CONCLUSION

In conclusion, the management of CC-TGA should proceed as follows:

1. Postponement of surgery until the patient becomes symptomatic.
2. Palliation should be the initial step. Pulmonary artery banding, systemic-to-pulmonary artery shunt, and bidirectional cavopulmonary anastomosis are optimal tools for treating the symptoms and staging the patient toward later complete separation of pulmonary and systemic circulations.
3. Finally, repair should obtain an anatomic arrangement avoiding all intrinsic risks related to "double discordance." When one or more of the mentioned risk factors would make correction prohibitive, single-stage palliation should be considered as a preferred alternative to anatomic repair.

References

1. Losekoot TG, Anderson RH, Becker AE, et al. *Congenitally Corrected Transposition.* New York: Churchill Livingstone, 1983: foreword.
2. Becu LM, Swan HJC, DuShane JW, et al. Cardiac clinics. CXLIV. Ebstein's malformation of the left atrioventricular valve in corrected transposition of the great vessels with ventricular septal defect. *Mayo Clin Proc* 1955;30: 483–490.
3. Friedberg DZ, Nadas AS. Clinical profile of patients with congenital corrected transposition of the great arteries: A study of 60 cases. *N Engl J Med* 1970;282: 1053–1059.
4. Hallman GL, Gill SS, Bloodwell RD, et al. Surgical treatment of cardiac defects associated with corrected transposition of the great vessels. *Circulation* 1967;35(Suppl 1): 133–142.
5. Kinsley RH, McGoon DC, Danielson GK. Corrected transposition of the great arteries: Associated ventricular rotation. *Circulation* 1974;49:574–578.
6. Kupersmith J, Krongrad E, Gersony WM, et al. Electrophysiologic identification of the specialized conduction system in corrected transposition of the great arteries. *Circulation* 1974;50:795–800.
7. Lev M, Licata RH, May RC. The conduction system in mixed levocardia with ventricular inversion (corrected transposition). *Circulation* 1963;28:232–237.
8. Skow JR, Mulder DG. Atrial approach for repair of ventricular septal defect in corrected transposition. *J Thorac Cardiovasc Surg* 1974;67:426–429.
9. Anderson RH, Arnold R, Wilkinson JL. The conducting system in congenitally corrected transposition. *Lancet* 1973;1:1286–1288.
10. Danielson GK, McGoon DC, Wallace RB, et al. Surgery of corrected transposition. In: Anderson RH, Shinebourne EA (eds). Pediatric *Cardiology*. Edinburgh: Churchill Livingstone, 1978:224–230.
11. De Leval MR, Bastos P, Stark J, et al. Surgical technique to reduce the risks of heart block following closure of ventricular septal defect in atrioventricular discordance. *J Thorac Cardiovasc Surg* 1979;78:515–526.
12. Marcelletti C, Maloney JD, Ritter DG, et al. Corrected transposition and ventricular septal defect. Surgical experience. *Ann Surg* 1980;191(6):751–759.
13. Allwork SP, Bentall HH, Becker AE, et al. Congenitally corrected transposition of the great arteries: Morphologic study of 32 cases. *Am J Cardiol* 1976;38:910–923.
14. Anderson RC, Lillehei CW, Lester RG. Corrected transposition of the great vessels of heart: A review of 17 cases. *Pediatrics* 1957;20:626–646.
15. Anderson RH, Becker AE, Arnold R, et al. The conducting tissues in congenitally corrected transposition. *Circulation* 1974;50:911–923.
16. Anderson RH, Becker AE, Gerlis LM. The pulmonary outflow tract in classically corrected transposition. *J Thorac Cardiovasc Surg* 1975;69:747–757.
17. Maloney JD, Ritter DG, McGoon DC, et al. Identification of the conduction system in corrected transposition and common ventricle at operation. *Mayo Clin Proc* 1975;387–394.
18. Van Praagh R, Vlad P, Keith JD. Complete transposition of the great arteries. In: Keith JP, Rowe RD, Vlad P (eds). *Heart Disease in Infancy and Childhood*, 2d ed. New York: Macmillan, 1967:682–744.
19. Waldo AL, Pacifico AD, Bargeron LM Jr, et al. Electrophysiological delineation of the specialized A-V conduction system in patients with corrected transposition of the great vessels and ventricular septal defect. *Circulation* 1975;52:435–441.
20. Fox LS, Kirklin JW, Pacifico AD, et al. Intracardiac repair of cardiac malformations with atrioventricular discordance. *Circulation* 1976;54:123–127.
21. Edwards JE. Differential diagnosis of mitral stenosis: A clinico-pathologic review of simulating conditions. *Lab Invest* 1954;3:89–92.
22. Ilbawi MN, DeLeon SY, Backer CL, et al. An alternative approach to the surgical management of physiologically corrected transposition with ventricular septal defect and pulmonary stenosis or atresia. *J Thorac Cardiovasc Surg* 1990;100:410–415.
23. Marcelletti C, Mair DD, McGoon DC, et al. The Rastelli operation for transposition of the great arteries: Early and late results. *J Thorac Cardiovasc Surg* 1976;72:427–434.
24. Di Donato RM, Troconis CJ, Marino B, et al. Combined mustard and Rastelli operations. An alternative approach for repair of associated anomalies in congenitally corrected transposition in situs inversus [IDD]. *J Thorac Cardiovasc Surg* 1992;104:1246–1248.
25. Termignon J-L, Leca F, Vouhè PR, et al. "Classic" repair of congenitally corrected transposition and ventricular septal defect. *Ann Thorac Surg* 1996;62:199–206.
26. Hraska V, Duncan BW, Mayer JE, et al. Long-term outcome of surgically treated patients with corrected transposition of the great arteries. *J Thorac Cardiovasc Surg* 2005;129:182–191.

CHAPTER

68 HYPOPLASTIC LEFT HEART SYNDROME

Peter J. Gruber, Thomas L. Spray

DEFINITION

Hypoplastic left heart syndrome includes a wide spectrum of anatomic abnormalities with the common feature of left ventricular hypoplasia and hypoplasia of the ascending aorta. At one end of the spectrum there may be some mild left ventricle hypoplasia, mild aortic stenosis, and aortic coarctation. At the other end of the spectrum, however, there is complete absence of the left ventricle, aortic atresia, or an association with an interrupted aortic arch. All these neonates present a serious challenge to congenital heart surgeons, cardiologists, and their families; the condition is uniformly fatal in the absence of intervention. There is now little argument about the utility of staged operative repair in these children as a result of continued improvements in operative techniques and perioperative care.

HISTORICAL HIGHLIGHTS

Therapy for HLHS has been one of the great successes of treatment of congenital heart disease (CHD). Before

KEY CONCEPTS

- Epidemiology
  - Hypoplastic left heart syndrome (HLHS) accounts for 5 percent of all congenital heart anomalies and is responsible for 25 percent of cardiac deaths in the first week of life. Its incidence is 1.8 in 10,000 live births, with 25 percent of cases showing associated noncardiac malformations and 5 percent showing chromosomal abnormalities.
- Morphology
  - HLHS includes a wide spectrum of anatomic abnormalities with the common feature of hypoplasia of the left ventricle (LV) and the ascending aorta. At one end of the spectrum there may be some mild LV hypoplasia, mild aortic stenosis, and aortic coarctation. At the other end there is complete absence of the LV, aortic atresia, and aortic arch interruption.
- Pathophysiology
  - Systemic venous return is channeled via an interatrial communication to the right ventricle (RV) and, through the pulmonary artery and patent ductus arteriosus (PDA), to the systemic and pulmonary circulations. Balanced physiology ensues, with QP:QS varying according to systemic and pulmonary vascular resistance as well as the unrestrictive nature of an atrial septal defect (ASD).
- Clinical features
  - HLHS is uniformly fatal if it is not treated as a result of ductal closure in the postnatal period. Evidence of pulmonary overcirculation is provided by QP:QS on clinical examination.
- Diagnosis
  - Prenatal echocardiography can be used to detect unbalanced ventricles as early as 20 weeks of gestational age. Postnatal echocardiography readily establishes the diagnosis and guides medical and surgical decision making.
- Treatment
  - Prostaglandin E_1 (PGE_1) infusion is the cornerstone of early resuscitation, coupled with balloon atrial septostomy in case of restrictive ASD. A three-stage single-ventricle palliation approach has been adopted by most centers. The first stage involves aortic arch reconstruction and establishment of a reliable source of pulmonary blood flow, and the

second and third stages consist of sequential partitioning of the systemic and pulmonary circulations. Transplantation has been used as the initial approach or, more commonly, for those who fail palliative strategy. In high-risk neonates, initial palliation with a hybrid approach (stenting of coarctation and pulmonary arterial banding) should be considered.

- Outcomes
  - Operative survival of stage I Norwood palliation depends on several variables, including anatomic factors (diameter of ascending aorta, operative weight, restrictive ASD, associated anomalies), and nears 80 percent in several series. Operative mortality between 5 and 10 percent has been observed for second- and third-stage palliation. Long-term complications [ventricular failure, atrioventricular (AV) valve regurgitation, arrhythmias, and protein-loosing enteropathy, among others] dictate a late prognosis and the need for reintervention or transplantation.

the 1980s, HLHS was a uniformly lethal condition. Over the last 25 years, palliation of HLHS has become a standard operation in nearly all institutions. In 1952, Lev[1] first described maldevelopment of the left-sided cardiac structures in combination with a small ascending aorta and transverse arch. By 1958, Noonan and Nadas[2] had defined the syndrome further to describe a variety of cardiac malformations of left heart structures. The first report of any attempt to palliate a patient with mitral atresia was by Redo and associates,[3] who in 1961 performed an atrial septectomy, using inflow occlusion through a right thoracotomy; the patient died soon after the operation. In 1968, Sinha and coworkers[4] outlined management principles that remain in use today that include creation of an unobstructed atrial communication, unrestricted ductal flow, and control of pulmonary blood flow. Cayler and colleagues[5] described an anastomosis between the right pulmonary artery (PA) and the ascending aorta with banding of both right and left pulmonary arteries. Interestingly, 35 years later, PA banding is being employed in certain centers for selected children who present with a medical or anatomic situation that is not suitable for stage 1 Norwood reconstruction; this first-stage hybrid procedure involves stenting the ductus arteriosus and atrial septal defect and bilateral PA bands.[6,7] Litwin, Mohri, and others all performed operations that were variations of these principles that were unsuccessful but contributed to the development of the knowledge of the disease and its palliation.[8,9] In 1977, Doty and Knott[10] described primary reconstruction that included atrial septation and a right atrium (RA) to PA Fontan circuit. Again, though no patients survived, this experience confirmed that one-stage reconstruction would not be successful because of high neonatal pulmonary vascular resistance (PVR).[10] Levitsky, Behrendt, and others described multiple possible surgical procedures; although the procedures demonstrated no long-term success,[11,12] they established the principle of staged reconstruction as first described for tricuspid atresia by Fontan and Kreutzer, with a strategy of initial palliation followed by later separation of the systemic and pulmonary circulations.[13,14] However, it was Norwood who provided the seminal contribution as the first to palliate infants successfully in 1980 and in 1983 with the first report of a successful staged approach.[15,16] The Norwood procedure remains the primary reconstructive approach to this day.

EMBRYOLOGY AND ANATOMIC CONSIDERATIONS

From a molecular standpoint, the developmental mechanisms that underlie HLHS are obscure, as there are no mutations that have been associated robustly with this part of the heart. Despite the existence of rare family clustering of HLHS, linkage analysis has been unproductive.[17–20] However, embryologically, there are clues. The severe hypoplasia of left heart structures is probably a consequence of limited flow during development secondary to a primary abnormality of either left ventricular inflow or left ventricular outflow. Primary defects of myocardial growth are unlikely to be a mechanism for this disease, since the myocardium appears normal.[21,22] Additionally, in approximately 5 percent of patients with aortic atresia, an unrestrictive ventricular septal defect coexists, and in such cases, there is nearly always normal development of the left ventricle and the mitral valve.

Patients can be categorized on the basis of atrioventricular and semilunar valvular morphology into three primary subsets: (1) aortic atresia with mitral atresia (40 percent), (2) aortic stenosis with mitral stenosis (30 percent), and (3) aortic atresia with mitral stenosis (30 percent) (Fig. 68-1). Aortic stenosis with mitral atresia is rare. HLHS variants include a malaligned AV canal, a double-outlet right ventricle with mitral atresia, tricuspid atresia with transposed great arteries, and a univentricular heart with aortic stenosis. There is frequently leftward and posterior deviation of the septal attachment of the septum primum, but this is unlikely to be a common developmental mechanism, since it is seen commonly in other CHD patients. Usually, the superior and inferior venae cavae (SVC and IVC) are connected normally to the right atrium, though in about 15 percent of these patients a left SVC draining to the coronary sinus is present. Other structural abnormalities of the heart are rare, with less than 5 percent of patients demonstrating AV valvular dysplasia. Also rare (less than 5 percent) is an association with abnormalities of pulmonary venous return or aortic arch interruption. Abnormalities in brain

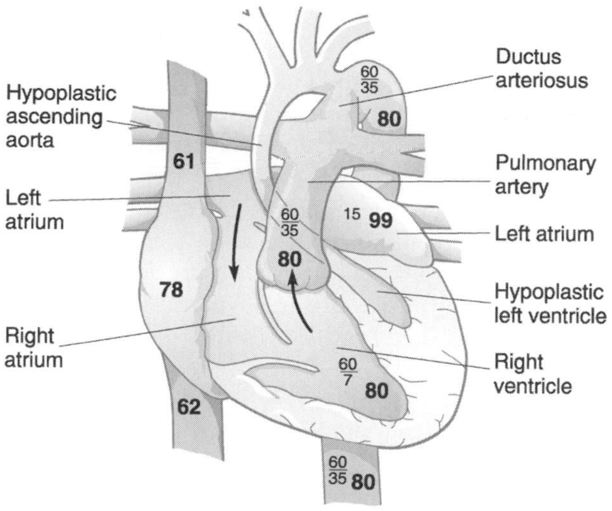

Figure 68-1 Anatomy and physiology of hypoplastic left heart syndrome. Hypoplastic left-sided structures force pulmonary venous blood to flow from the left atrium through the interatrial communication to the right atrium (*downward arrow*). Blood from the right ventricle flows both to the pulmonary circulation via the pulmonary artery (*upward arrow*) and to the systemic circulation via the ductus arteriosus. Maintenance of ductal patency is critical for survival. The surgical principles of repair aim at maintaining this stable physiology. (Reprinted with permission from Gruber P, Spray T, et al. Hypoplastic left heart syndrome. In Kaiser LK, Kron IL (eds.), *Mastery of cardiothoracic surgery*, 2nd ed. Philadelphia: Lippincott Williams & Wilkins, 2006:936.)

development increasingly are being associated with children with severe congenital heart disease and may define a high-risk group for operative repair.[23] The pulmonary vascular tree also harbors abnormalities with an increase in number of vessels as well as muscularity.[24,25]

PATHOPHYSIOLOGY

A normal fetus has a parallel circulation that adequately supports single-ventricle physiology before birth. Three communications (the ductus venosus, foramen ovale, and ductus arteriosus) shunt oxygenated placental blood largely past the hepatic and pulmonary beds to supply the splanchnic circulation. Hypoplastic left heart syndrome is well supported in this situation, and as a result, it is rarely a cause of fetal demise. Hypoplastic left heart syndrome is probably a secondary result of early obstructive lesions of either mitral or aortic valvular development. This has been supported in animal models of mitral or aortic stenosis with resulting left ventricular hypoplasia.[22] However, the primary cause of the obstructive flow lesion that leads secondarily to HLHS is unknown. Interestingly, there are no known genetic animal models that recapitulate HLHS despite the existence of a large number of mutations that affect valvular development. This argues for a complex early multifactorial event or, more likely, a transient early insult.

EPIDEMIOLOGY

Hypoplastic left heart syndrome is a uniformly fatal disease if it is not treated. It represents 5 percent of all cases of CHD and is responsible for nearly 25 percent of cardiac deaths in the first week of life. Among 10,000 live births, approximately 1.8 will be born with HLHS, with a slight male predominance. Of these, 25 percent also will have a noncardiac anomaly, and 5 percent a chromosomal abnormality (most typically trisomy 13, 18, or 21). Syndromic lesions are rare, but among these patients, Turner's syndrome(monosomy X) is the most common. The recurrence risk is 2.2 percent for one affected sibling and 6 percent for two affected siblings, suggesting a genetic predisposition but arguing against a simple effect.

CLINICAL PRESENTATION

The presentation of infants with CHD has changed dramatically over the last 10 years. In most large centers, the majority of patients are identified through prenatal echocardiography; this early identification has not been correlated consistently with a better outcome. Although some tachypnea and mild cyanosis may be present, it is not until the ductus arteriosus begins to close that children with HLHS manifest evidence of impaired systemic perfusion with pallor, lethargy, and diminished femoral pulses. Cardiac examination reveals a dominant right ventricular impulse, a single second heart sound, and often a nonspecific soft systolic murmur. Electrocardiographic examination reveals right atrial enlargement and right ventricular hypertrophy. Chest x-ray occasionally shows mild cardiomegaly and increased pulmonary vascular markings.

DIAGNOSIS

Physical examination of children with HLHS is usually normal. The examination is determined by the underlying anatomy as well as the chronicity of the disease (ductal closure and PVR). Poor perfusion, weak distal pulses that may not be present because of the size of the ductus, acidosis, and a sepsis-like picture may confound the diagnosis. In the absence of risk factors or laboratory findings consistent with sepsis, one should look for left-sided obstructive lesions.

There are no specific laboratory indicators of HLHS. These patients usually exhibit normal values. With ductal closure and malperfusion, end-organ compromise may be reflected by altered hepatic and renal function tests.

At 20 weeks of gestation, a fetal echocardiogram allows reasonable visualization of the cardiac structures. It is neither feasible nor cost-effective to screen all pregnancies; a selective approach therefore is taken currently in which only mothers at high risk are screened. Frequently, a ventricular size discrepancy is the first hint of impending problems. Certainly, the presence of an intact or restrictive atrial septum should prompt term high-risk delivery in an institution where an urgent postdelivery atrial septectomy can be performed safely and rapidly. The use of prenatal screening improves the prenatal condition of the child but may not translate into an improved outcome (at least in cases of transposition of the great arteries or HLHS).[26,27] After delivery, the infant should undergo two-dimensional and Doppler echocardiography to define anatomy to an extent sufficient for medical and surgical decision making. It is important to distinguish HLHS from other diseases that may mimic certain of its features, as their management differs.

Chest radiography often demonstrates mild cardiomegaly and excessive pulmonary blood flow. Head ultrasound should be obtained in all patients to rule out intracranial hemorrhage and minimize the risks of heparinization and circulatory arrest. Patients with medical necrotizing enterocolitis should have a 7-day course of intravenous antibiotics before first-stage palliation.

MEDICAL THERAPY

Regardless of the anatomic subtype, preoperative stabilization is critical to the ultimate outcome of patients with HLHS. Nearly all patients with suspected HLHS are transported to the authors' center on PGE_1 at a dose of 0.01 to 0.025 μg/kg/min. Two clinically important dose-dependent side effects of PGE_1 are hypotension and apnea, though they are infrequently clinically important. Umbilical arterial and umbilical venous lines are used for monitoring and central access in most patients. Most infants can ventilate with a natural airway and indeed often have more favorable hemodynamics while extubated. Supplemental oxygen generally should be avoided as it will act as a pulmonary vasodilator, decreasing PVR, increasing Qp:Qs, and thus decreasing systemic perfusion. Inotropic support is required in patients who have had a perinatal insult but otherwise is rarely necessary. The goal of these maneuvers is to get the patient to the operating room in as stable condition as possible.

SURGICAL THERAPY

There are two primary therapies for HLHS: (1) staged reconstructive surgery leading to a modified Fontan-Kreutzer procedure and (2) heart transplantation. Heart transplantation is discussed in detail in Chapter 80; this chapter focuses on staged reconstructive surgery.

Over the last 20 years, the Norwood procedure has evolved and become the standard approach in nearly all institutions that care for neonates and infants with HLHS. There are three primary goals to first-stage palliation: (1) establishment of unrestricted interatrial communication to provide complete mixing and avoid pulmonary venous hypertension, (2) establishment of a reliable source of pulmonary blood flow, allowing for the development of pulmonary vasculature and minimization of volume load on the single ventricle, and (3) provision of unobstructed outflow from the ventricle to the systemic circulation.

The Children's Hospital of Philadelphia offers surgical palliation to nearly all patients with HLHS, including very low birth weight infants and those with nonlethal genetic syndromes.

Stage I reconstructive procedure

Two perfusion techniques can be used for first-stage palliation: deep hypothermic circulatory arrest (DHCA) and selective antegrade continuous cerebral perfusion. At present, there is no consensus on the superiority of one approach over the other, although DHCA is used more commonly.

The child is brought to the operating room and ventilated on room air, with care taken to avoid hyperventilation. A full midline sternotomy is performed, and the thymus is removed in its entirety, with care being taken to avoid the phrenic nerves. The pericardium is opened, and an obligatory mediastinal inspection is performed to confirm the echocardiographic findings, especially to identify abnormalities of the aortic arch and coronary arteries. The ascending and descending aorta, head vessels, ductus arteriosus, and pulmonary arteries are mobilized extensively, with care taken to preserve the integrity of the recurrent laryngeal nerve. No attempt is made to dissect the systemic veins. Purse-string sutures are placed in the proximal main pulmonary artery and generously around the right atrial appendage, through which heparin is administered. A previously thawed pulmonary homograft hemiartery patch is trimmed in an extended arrowhead shape and set aside. After the activated clotting time reaches 300 s, the patient is cannulated, with the arterial cannula inserted at the base of the main pulmonary artery and a single venous cannula inserted in the right atrium (Fig. 68-2). Cardiopulmonary bypass is initiated, and tapes are brought down around the branch pulmonary arteries. The patient is cooled to 18°C over 15 min, during which time any remaining dissection is performed. A side-biting clamp is placed on the innominate artery, and a Gore-Tex graft (usually 4.0 mm for patients over 3.2 kg) is anastomosed in an end-to-side fashion. The clamp is removed, and flow is assessed. If blood does not flow easily out of the open shunt, the anastomosis should be revised. A large hemoclip is placed gently to occlude the shunt temporarily.

On initiation of circulatory arrest, tapes are brought down around the head vessels and a spoon clamp is

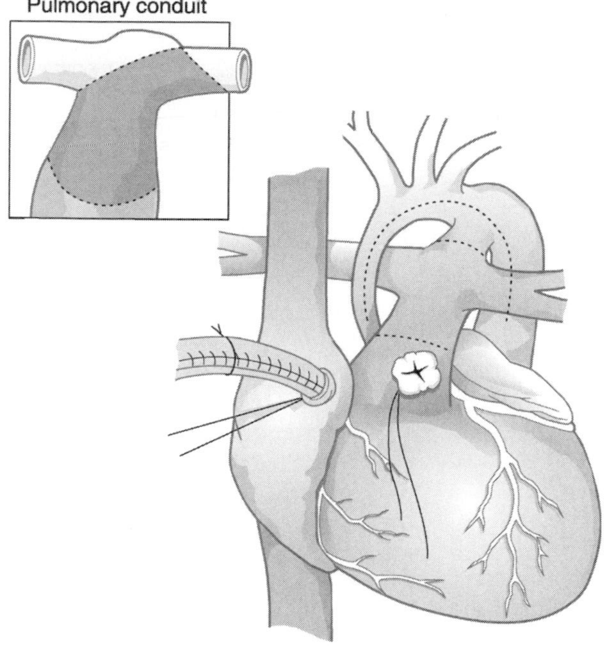

Figure 68-2 Incisions for hypoplastic left heart syndrome first-stage palliation. Cannulation is performed with an arterial cannula in the base of the main pulmonary artery and a single venous cannula through a generous purse string around the right atrial appendage. Subsequent incisions, as described in the text, are indicated by the dotted lines. The patch for aortic augmentation and completion of the aortopulmonary anastomosis is fashioned from a pulmonary homograft (*insert*). (Reprinted with permission from Gruber P, Spray T, et al. Hypoplastic left heart syndrome. In Kaiser LK, Kron IL (eds.), *Mastery of cardiothoracic surgery*, 2nd ed. Philadelphia: Lippincott Williams & Wilkins, 2006:938.)

placed on the descending aorta distal to the ductal insertion site. Cardioplegia is administered retrograde through a side port on the arterial cannula. After the patient's blood volume has been drained into the reservoir, all cannulas and PA tapes are removed. The ductus arteriosus is ligated on the PA side and divided on the aortic side. The atrial septum is excised completely, working through the atrial purse-string sutures. Though this is seldom necessary, visualization can be improved through a right atriotomy. Next, the main PA is divided close to the branch PAs, and the defect in the distal main PA segment is closed with an oval homograft patch or primarily, in a vertical fashion. At a point beginning immediately adjacent to the divided main pulmonary artery (MPA) the diminutive aorta is incised medially and the aortotomy is carried superiorly along the underside of the transverse arch through the ductal insertion site to a point approximately 1 cm distal to it. Importantly, all redundant ductal tissue is excised and the coarctation shelf is debrided (alternatively, the segment is excised and the isthmus and proximal descending aorta are reanastomosed). The proximal-aortic-to-proximal-PA connection is performed using interrupted fine polypropylene sutures to connect the root of the great vessels. Next, the arch is reconstructed using the homograft patch, carrying this suture line down to complete the Damus-Kaye-Stansel (DKS) anastomosis proximally (Fig. 68-3). The distal Blalock-Taussig shunt anastomosis is performed

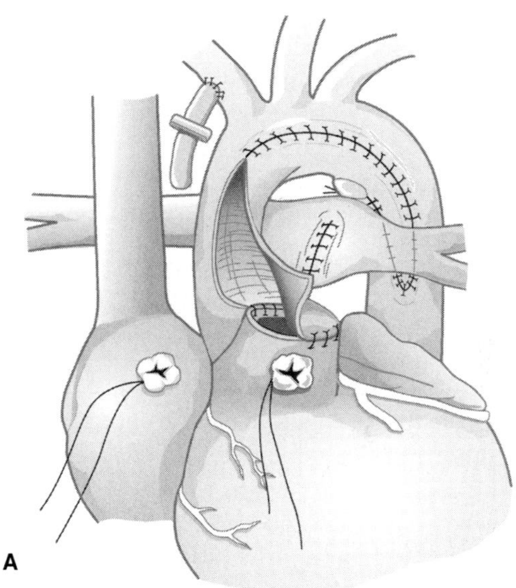

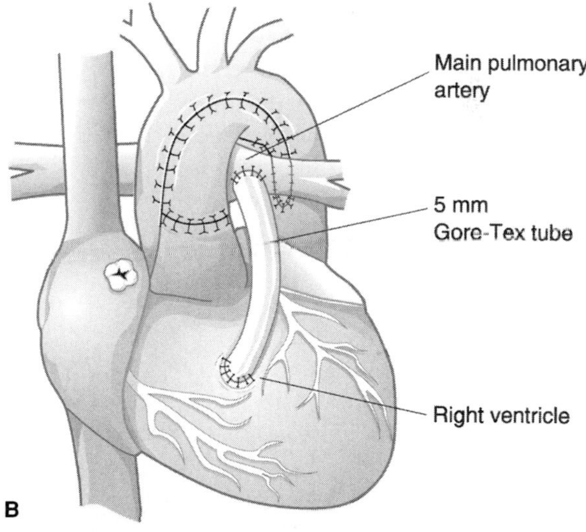

Figure 68-3 Damus-Kaye-Stansel anastomosis (DKS) and aortic arch reconstruction. After complete excision of ductal tissue and an interrupted anastomosis of the medial aspects of the aorta and the main pulmonary artery, the homograft patch is used to augment the hypoplastic aortic arch and complete the DKS. The modified right Blalock-Taussig shunt is completed from the innominate artery to the right pulmonary artery (**A**). An alternative approach (Sano modification, **B**) substitutes a right ventricle–pulmonary artery Gore-Tex conduit for the Blalock-Taussig shunt. (Reprinted with permission from Gruber P, Spray T, et al. Hypoplastic left heart syndrome. In Kaiser LK, Kron IL (eds.), *Mastery of cardiothoracic surgery*, 2nd ed. Philadelphia: Lippincott Williams & Wilkins, 2006:938–939.)

to the origin of the right PA, although some prefer to do this with rewarming after removal of the aortic cross-clamp. The arch is infused with cold saline to assess the geometry and rule out kinking or residual obstruction, the atrium is infused with cold saline to de-air, and the cannulas are replaced. Cardiopulmonary bypass is begun, and the patient is warmed to 37°C over 22 min. It is important at this point to assess prompt and equivalent filling of the coronary distributions, and any perfusion defect should be addressed immediately with revision of the aortopulmonary anastomosis. During warming, obvious bleeding should be controlled. The average duration of hospitalization is 7 to 21 days, with the limiting factor often being the establishment of adequate oral intake of formula.

Stage II procedure

Two important observations by Norwood and colleagues early in the reconstructive experience prompted the institution of an intermediate stage between the initial palliation and the completion of a total cavopulmonary connection. The first observation was that there was time-related interstage mortality; the second was that the chronic volume load of a systemic-to-pulmonary shunt could create diastolic ventricular dysfunction. Thus, an intermediate stage was initiated as either a bidirectional cavopulmonary (Glenn) shunt or a hemi-Fontan procedure (see Chapter 69). A bidirectional cavopulmonary anastomosis sets the patient up for an extracardiac conduit, whereas a hemi-Fontan sets the patient up for a lateral tunnel completion Fontan. No long-term data prove the superiority of one approach over the other. In general, at approximately 4 to 6 months of age, stage I survivors are catheterized to evaluate both pressures throughout the heart and the anatomy of the pulmonary arteries. The use of a cavopulmonary anastomosis before 3 months of age usually is associated with increased hypoxia and upper body venous congestion. The technique for a bidirectional cavopulmonary anastomosis is fairly standard (Fig. 68-4A). The approach is through a reoperative median sternotomy during which care is taken in regard to the dissection of the neoaorta, which is often adherent to the left side of the sternum and somewhat fragile. The patient is cannulated in a standard fashion with an arterial cannula in the neoaorta, a small angled venous cannula in the SVC, and a straight cannula in the body of the RA. Although it is possible to perform this procedure without cardiopulmonary bypass (CPB), the authors find it considerably easier to use CPB and believe that the anatomic result is improved. Extracorporeal circulation is begun, and a tape is brought down around the SVC cannula after ligation and division of the azygous vein. The previous shunt is divided and ligated near the innominate artery. A vascular clamp is placed at the SVC-RA junction, and the SVC is divided. The atrial portion is closed in two layers with fine monofilament sutures. The PA is opened in the superior portion and inspected carefully. If preoperative catheterization revealed pulmonary arterial stenosis, this is addressed with pulmonary homograft patch augmentation. The SVC then is anastomosed to the superior aspect of the right pulmonary artery as medially as possible toward the left PA. The tape is removed from the SVC cannula, and one or two right atrial lines are brought into the mediastinum percutaneously from the right and placed in the body of the right atrium. The patient is weaned from CPB, and the SVC cannula is removed. Modified ultrafiltration is performed, and during that

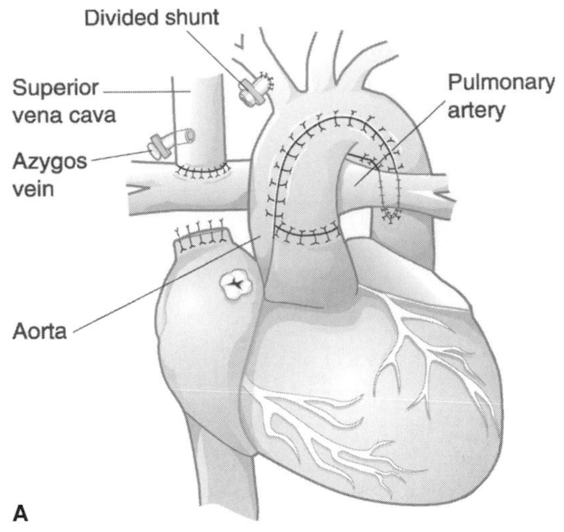

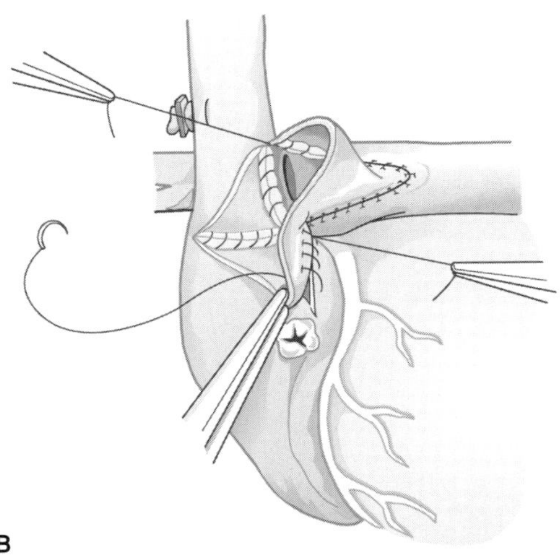

Figure 68-4 Superior cavopulmonary anastomosis. **A.** The bidirectional Glenn replaces the source of obligatory pulmonary blood flow from the Blalock-Taussig shunt to the superior vena cava. **B.** The hemi-Fontan results in precisely the same physiology but uses a single piece of homograft to augment the pulmonary arteries, complete the superior cavopulmonary anastomosis, and create the right atrium–pulmonary artery dam simultaneously. (Reprinted with permission from Gruber P, Spray T, et al. Hypoplastic left heart syndrome. In Kaiser LK, Kron IL (eds.), *Mastery of cardiothoracic surgery*, 2nd ed. Philadelphia: Lippincott Williams & Wilkins, 2006:940–941.)

time, all suture lines are checked for hemostasis. At the completion of modified ultrafiltration, the SVC pressure can be measured directly. The SVC monitoring line is removed, and the cannulation purse string is tied securely. All cannulas are removed, and protamine is administered. The chest is closed in a standard fashion, and the patient is returned to the intensive care unit (ICU). In general, these patients can be extubated soon after their return to the ICU.

An alternative operative approach is the hemi-Fontan, which the authors perform under deep hypothermic circulatory arrest. The details of this procedure are summarized in Fig. 68-4B and are described in Chapter 69. The hemi-Fontan is performed under DHCA, using a piece of folded homograft to augment the pulmonary arteries and create the superior cavopulmonary anastomosis and the RA-PA dam simultaneously. This dam subsequently will be removed for the lateral tunnel completion Fontan operation.

Stage III procedure

Between ages 2 and 5, usually on the basis of a combination of the patient's weight, growth characteristics, and arterial saturations, the patient is reimaged by echocardiography and occasionally with cardiac catheterization. If there are no anatomic issues to be addressed with catheter-based intervention (e.g., distal arch coarctation), the patient is referred for Fontan reconstruction via an extracardiac conduit or a lateral tunnel completion Fontan. For the extracardiac conduit, DHCA or continuous bypass with or without aortic cross-clamping is employed, whereas DHCA is used for the lateral tunnel. The approach is through a reoperative median sternotomy. The following material describes the basic steps of the extracardiac Fontan.

The patient is cannulated bicavally in a standard fashion, and an arterial cannula is placed high in the aortic reconstruction. Cardiopulmonary bypass is begun, and tourniquets are applied around the caval cannulas. A vascular clamp is placed at the IVC-RA junction, and the IVC is divided. The atrial portion is closed partially in two layers with fine monofilament sutures. The conduit (18- to 22-mm Gore-Tex) is trimmed to the appropriate length to avoid compression of the right pulmonary vein (which typically is shorter than one might expect), and a 4-mm fenestration is punched in the medial aspect near the IVC portion. The IVC-conduit anastomosis is completed with monofilament sutures, followed by a side-to-side anastomosis of the remaining cardiac portion of the IVC opening with the exterior conduit, leaving a rim of conduit around the fenestration. Next, the PAs are opened in the inferior portion and inspected directly. If preoperative studies revealed any pulmonary arterial stenosis and the beveled end of the Gore-Tex conduit will not span the area of stenosis, this situation is addressed with pulmonary homograft patch augmentation. The conduit then is anastomosed to the inferior aspect of the pulmonary arteries, angled slightly medially to the SVC. Practically, the angled nature of the superior portion of the conduit augments the pulmonary confluence from the right to the left PA (Fig. 68-5A). The conduit is infused with saline to de-air, and the patient is weaned off CPB. The SVC cannula is removed, and a period of modified ultrafiltration is begun. All suture

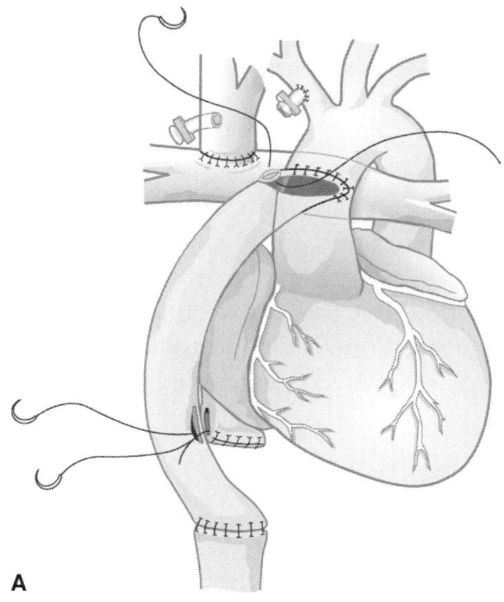

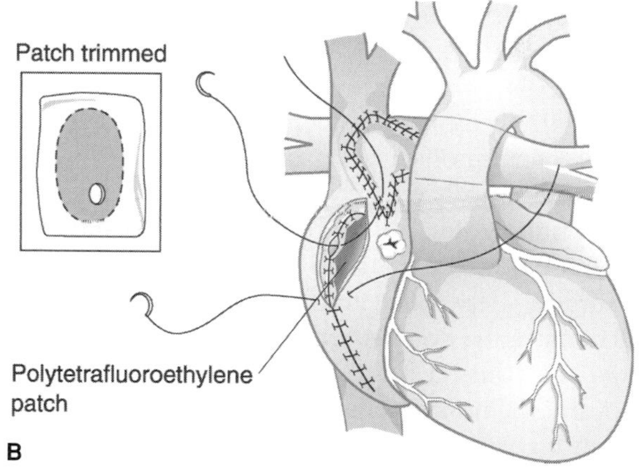

Figure 68-5 Fontan completion. **A.** The extracardiac Fontan uses a Gore-Tex tube graft to channel inferior vena cava (IVC) blood *outside* the heart to the pulmonary circuit. A 4-mm fenestration is fashioned between the remnant cardiac portion of the IVC and the side of the conduit. **B.** The lateral tunnel Fontan baffles blood from the IVC along the lateral aspect of the atrium inside the heart to the pulmonary circuit. The homograft dam created during the hemi-Fontan is excised to create continuity with the pulmonary arteries. Fenestration patency has proved more reliable in this procedure than in the extracardiac Fontan. (Reprinted with permission from Gruber P, Spray T, et al. Hypoplastic left heart syndrome. In Kaiser LK, Kron IL (eds.), *Mastery of cardiothoracic surgery*, 2nd ed. Philadelphia: Lippincott Williams & Wilkins, 2006:943–944.)

lines are checked for hemostasis. At the completion of modified ultrafiltration, the SVC pressure is measured directly with a transthoracic line. An additional monitoring line is placed in the right atrium. All cannulas are removed, and protamine is administered. The chest is closed in a standard fashion, and the patient is returned to the ICU. In general, these patients can be extubated soon after their return to the ICU.

An alternative operative approach is the lateral tunnel Fontan, which the authors perform under deep hypothermic circulatory arrest. The technical details of this procedure are summarized in Fig. 68-5B. The lateral tunnel Fontan is performed under DHCA, using a piece of fenestrated Gore-Tex patch to baffle blood from the IVC to the pulmonary arteries. The previously constructed PA-RA homograft dam is excised. There are no long-term data suggesting the superiority of one technique over the other, but the lack of an atrial suture line with the extracardiac Fontan has led to a preference for its use when extensive PA reconstruction is necessary.

OUTCOMES

Despite continued improvement in outcomes, patients with HLHS continue to present a formidable challenge. The authors' group reported the results of the 15-year Children's Hospital of Philadelphia (CHOP) experience with 840 patients undergoing stage I surgery for HLHS between 1984 and 1999. The 1-, 2-, 5-, 10-, and 15-year survivals for the entire cohort were 51 percent, 43 percent, 40 percent, 39 percent, and 39 percent, respectively. A later era of stage I palliation was associated with significantly improved survival, with 3-year survival for patients undergoing stage I reconstruction from 1995 to 1998 of 66 percent versus 28 percent for those undergoing surgery between 1984 and 1988.[28] More recent studies have shown further improvement and demonstrated that the variability in outcome is influenced by anatomy. One retrospective study of risk factors for operative and 1-year mortality in 158 patients who underwent the Norwood procedure demonstrated that the diagnosis of HLHS is not a predictor of mortality. HLHS was present in 102 patients, and other forms of functional single ventricle with systemic outflow tract obstruction were observed in the remaining 56. Operative survival for the entire cohort was 77 percent (78 percent for patients with HLHS and 75 percent for patients with other diagnoses). Birth weight, associated cardiac anomalies, total support time, and the need for extracorporeal membrane oxygenation (ECMO) or ventricular assist device (VAD) support were predictors of operative mortality. Survival to 1 year was 86 percent after successful first-stage palliation, although the presence of an extracardiac anomaly, a genetic syndrome, or an additional cardiac defect was predictive of worse survival in the first year of life.[29]

Additional perioperative or operative treatment strategies may improve morbidity and mortality rates. A consecutive series of 115 patients who underwent stage I palliation from Milwaukee identified the risk factors for mortality and the impact of new treatment strategies. Between 1996 and 2001, hospital survival was 93 percent compared with 53 percent for the time interval between 1992 and 1996. Survival to stage II palliation also was improved significantly, increasing from 44 percent to 81 percent. Anti-inflammatory treatment strategies, continuous saturated venous oxygen (Svo_2) monitoring, and the use of phenoxybenzamine were factors favoring survival to stage II.[30]

Another approach has been the development of home surveillance programs. One study compared patients discharged before the initiation of home surveillance with those discharged with an infant scale and a pulse oximeter. The parents maintained a daily log of weight and arterial oxygen saturation according to pulse oximetry and were instructed to contact their physicians in case of arterial oxygen saturation less than 70 percent according to pulse oximetry, an acute weight loss of more than 30 g/24 h, or failure to gain at least 20 g during a 3-day period. Interstage mortality was 15.8 percent in the historic group and 0 percent in the monitored group, suggesting that monitoring programs may provide significant benefit in reducing interstage attrition.[31]

Recent reports advocate that an RV-PA conduit (rather than a modified Blalock-Taussig shunt) as reintroduced by Sano and colleagues may improve the outcome after stage I reconstruction.[32–34] However, further studies have indicated the need for caution before broad adoption of the RV-PA conduit. The CHOP group compared the outcomes of all neonates who underwent a stage I reconstruction between 2002 and 2004 with the use of the RV-PA conduit and modified Blalock-Taussig shunt. In all, 149 infants underwent a stage I reconstruction for HLHS or its variants. There was no difference in surgical mortality, time to extubation, or length of hospital stay between the two techniques. Although there was no difference in overall mortality, patients with an RV-PA conduit required more conduit-related reinterventions and returned earlier for stage II reconstruction.[35]

Patients who have completed staged palliation for HLHS frequently require reintervention. A study examining these reinterventions during a 6-year period between 1995 and 2001 found that 123 procedures were performed in 71 patients. The median time from Fontan completion to reoperation was 3.6 years, with indications for reintervention including arrhythmia, cyanosis, exercise intolerance, protein-losing enteropathy (PLE), atrioventricular valve (AVV) regurgitation, and other indications. The procedures included pacemaker insertion or revision (48 percent), reinclusion of previously excluded hepatic veins (13 percent), revision to a lateral tunnel or extracardiac conduit pathway (11 percent), cardiac transplantation (7 percent), enlargement or creation of a baffle fenestration (5 percent), isolated AVV repair or replacement (2 percent), and other procedures (14 percent). There were five early and five late deaths. Hospital mortality was greatest among patients undergoing cardiac transplantation (44 percent), who accounted for 80 percent of the early deaths. Most reinterventions can be performed with minimal morbidity and mortality. However, patients who require cardiac transplantation after a Fontan procedure fare poorly.[36]

For high-risk infants, some have advocated catheter-based hybrid approaches (stage I: ductal stenting and PA banding; stage II: septectomy, arch augmentation, and cavopulmonary anastomosis; stage III: catheter-based Fontan completion). One report of the hybrid stage I procedure in 14 high-risk neonates between 2003 and 2005 demonstrated promising results, with a 78.5 percent hospital survival rate. Eight patients underwent stage II procedures, with two operative deaths. These techniques may be limited in certain anatomic subsets, such as patients with aortic atresia in which preductal retrograde coarctation is a significant problem.[6,37]

The results from stage III palliation with Fontan circulation also continue to improve. The authors' group reviewed the outcomes of 332 patients: 281 with a lateral tunnel and 51 with an extracardiac Fontan procedure. There was a 93.4 percent hospital survival rate, and by questionnaire, 94.6 percent of guardians described their children's overall health as excellent or good and 5.4 percent reported it as fair or poor. School performance was described as above average in 30.2 percent, average in 39.9 percent, and below average in 29.8 percent. With regard to cardiac functional status, 34.2 percent responded that their children had no limitations to physical activity, 52.5 percent reported a slight limitation, 12.1 percent reported a significant limitation, and 1.2 percent reported a severe limitation. Although these data suggest that acceptable survival outcomes have been observed at intermediate follow-up of the Fontan operation, much work remains to be done.[38]

In comparing outcomes of extracardiac conduit and lateral tunnel Fontan connections, the results have been conflicting. The Toronto group reported the results of 60 extracardiac conduit and 47 lateral tunnel total cavopulmonary connections performed between 1994 and 1998. Overall operative mortality was 5.6 percent and did not differ between groups. The lateral tunnel group had a significantly higher incidence of postoperative sinoatrial node dysfunction, supraventricular tachycardia, and need for temporary postoperative pacing. The median duration of ICU stay and the need for ventilatory support were longer in the lateral tunnel group. Holter analysis showed a higher incidence of atrial arrhythmias in the lateral tunnel group.[39]

However, other authors have not found support for one technique over the other. For example, the Charleston group found an incidence of sinus node dysfunction of 21 percent in the lateral tunnel group and 59 percent in the extracardiac group. No permanent pacemaker was placed in the lateral tunnel group, whereas three were placed in the extracardiac group group.[40] Another report from that group demonstrated identical operative mortality and similar mean Fontan pressure, transpulmonary gradient, and common atrial pressure in the first 24 h after the completion of a cavopulmonary connection. Duration of mechanical ventilation, ICU stay, chest tube drainage, and hospital stay did not differ. Again, extracardiac conduit patients had a higher incidence of sinus node dysfunction both in the postoperative period and at hospital discharge.[41] These techniques also appear equivalent in the situation of a failing Fontan, with no hospital deaths and no arrhythmias at hospital discharge or differences in mean duration of intubation, inotropic support, ICU stay, hospital stay, or episodes of acute postoperative arrhythmias.[42]

References

1. Lev M. Pathologic anatomy and interrelationship of hypoplasia of the aortic tract complexes. *Lab Invest* 1952;1:61.
2. Noonan JA, Nadas AS. The hypoplastic left heart syndrome: An analysis of 101 cases. *Pediatr Clin North Am* 1958;5:1029.
3. Redo SF, Farber S, Gross RE. Atresia of the mitral valve. *Arch Surg* 1961;82:696.
4. Sinha SN, Rusnak SL, Sommers HM, et al. Hypoplastic left ventricle syndrome: Analysis of thirty autopsy cases in infants with surgical considerations. *Am J Cardiol* 1968; 21:166.
5. Cayler GG, Smeloff EA, Miller GE Jr. Surgical palliation of hypoplastic left side of the heart. *N Engl J Med* 1970; 282:780.
6. Bacha EA, Daves S, Hardin J, et al. Single-ventricle palliation for high-risk neonates: The emergence of an alternative hybrid stage I strategy. *J Thorac Cardiovasc Surg* 2006;131:163.
7. Pizarro C, Norwood WI. Pulmonary artery banding before Norwood procedure. *Ann Thorac Surg* 2003;75: 1008.
8. Litwin SB, Friedberg DZ. Surgical management of a neonate with interrupted aortic arch, transposition of the great Arteries, and tricuspid atresia. *Cardiovasc Dis* 1975; 2:182.
9. Mohri H, Horiuchi T, Haneda K, et al. Surgical treatment for hypoplastic left heart syndrome: Case reports. J Thorac *Cardiovasc Surg* 1979;78:223.
10. Doty DB, Knott HW. Hypoplastic left heart syndrome: Experience with an operation to establish functionally normal circulation. *J Thorac Cardiovasc Surg* 1977;74:624.
11. Behrendt DM, Rocchini A. An operation for the hypoplastic left heart syndrome: Preliminary report. *Ann Thorac Surg* 1981;32:284.

12. Levitsky S, van der Horst RL, Hasteiter AR, et al. Surgical palliation in aortic atresia. *J Thorac Cardiovasc Surg* 1980;79:456.
13. Fontan F, Baudet E. Surgical repair of tricuspid atresia. *Thorax* 1971;26:240.
14. Kreutzer G, Galindez E, Bono H, et al. An operation for the correction of tricuspid atresia. *J Thorac Cardiovasc Surg* 1973;66:613.
15. Norwood WI, Kirklin JK, Sanders SP. Hypoplastic left heart syndrome: Experience with palliative surgery. *Am J Cardiol* 1980;45:87.
16. Norwood WI, Lang P, Hansen DD. Physiologic repair of aortic atresia-hypoplastic left heart syndrome. *N Engl J Med* 1983;308:23.
17. Gelb BD. Molecular genetics of congenital heart disease. *Curr Opin Cardiol* 1997;12:321.
18. Loffredo CA, Chokkalingam A, Sill AM, et al. Prevalence of congenital cardiovascular malformations among relatives of infants with hypoplastic left heart, coarctation of the aorta, and d-transposition of the great arteries. *Am J Med Genet A* 2004;124:225.
19. McBride KL, Fernbach S, Menesses A, et al. A family-based association study of congenital left-sided heart malformations and 5,10 methylenetetrahydrofolate reductase. *Birth Defects Res A Clin Mol Teratol* 2004;70:825.
20. McElhinney DB, Krantz ID, Bason L, et al. Analysis of cardiovascular phenotype and genotype-phenotype correlation in individuals with a JAG1 mutation and/or Alagille syndrome. *Circulation* 2002;106:2567.
21. Chen B, Bronson RT, Klaman LD, et al. Mice mutant for Egfr and Shp2 have defective cardiac semilunar valvulogenesis. *Nat Genet* 2000;24:296.
22. Sedmera D, Hu N, Weiss KM, et al. Cellular changes in experimental left heart hypoplasia. *Anat Rec* 2002;267:137.
23. Forbess JM, Visconti KJ, Bellinger DC, et al. Neurodevelopmental outcomes in children after the Fontan operation. *Circulation* 2001;104:I127.
24. Macedo A, Pinto E, Ramos S, et al. Structural changes in pulmonary vessels and coronary arteries in hypoplastic left heart syndrome. *Acta Med Port* 1991;4:253.
25. Maeda K, Yamaki S, Kado H, et al. Hypoplasia of the small pulmonary arteries in hypoplastic left heart syndrome with restrictive atrial septal defect. *Circulation* 2004;110:II139.
26. Kumar RK, Newburger JW, Gauvreau K, et al. Comparison of outcome when hypoplastic left heart syndrome and transposition of the great arteries are diagnosed prenatally versus when diagnosis of these two conditions is made only postnatally. *Am J Cardiol* 1999;83:1649.
27. Satomi G, Yasukochi S, Shimizu T, et al. Has fetal echocardiography improved the prognosis of congenital heart disease? Comparison of patients with hypoplastic left heart syndrome with and without prenatal diagnosis. *Pediatr Int* 1999;41:728.
28. Mahle WT, Spray TL, Wernovsky G, et al. Survival after reconstructive surgery for hypoplastic left heart syndrome: A 15-year experience from a single institution. *Circulation* 2000;102:III136.
29. Gaynor JW, Mahle WT, Cohen MI, et al. Risk factors for mortality after the Norwood procedure. *Eur J Cardiothorac Surg* 2002;22:82.
30. Tweddell JS, Hoffman GM, Mussatto KA, et al. Improved survival of patients undergoing palliation of hypoplastic left heart syndrome: Lessons learned from 115 consecutive patients. *Circulation* 2002;106:I82.
31. Ghanayem NS, Hoffman GM, Mussatto KA, et al. Home surveillance program prevents interstage mortality after the Norwood procedure. *J Thorac Cardiovasc Surg* 2003;126:1367.
32. Sano S, Ishino K, Kado H, et al. Outcome of right ventricle-to-pulmonary artery shunt in first-stage palliation of hypoplastic left heart syndrome: A multi-institutional study. *Ann Thorac Surg* 2004;78:1951.
33. Sano S, Ishino K, Kawada M, et al. Right ventricle-pulmonary artery shunt in first-stage palliation of hypoplastic left heart syndrome. *Semin Thorac Cardiovasc Surg Pediatr Card Surg Annu* 2004;7:22.
34. Pizarro C, Malec E, Maher KO, et al. Right ventricle to pulmonary artery conduit improves outcome after stage I Norwood for hypoplastic left heart syndrome. *Circulation* 2003;108(Suppl 1):II155.
35. Tabbutt S, Dominguez TE, Ravishankar C, et al. Outcomes after the stage I reconstruction comparing the right ventricular to pulmonary artery conduit with the modified Blalock Taussig shunt. *Ann Thorac Surg* 2005;80:1582.
36. Petko M, Myung RJ, Wernovsky G, et al. Surgical reinterventions following the Fontan procedure. *Eur J Cardiothorac Surg* 2003;24:255.
37. Galantowicz M, Cheatham JP. Lessons learned from the development of a new hybrid strategy for the management of hypoplastic left heart syndrome. *Pediatr Cardiol* 2005;26:190.
38. Mitchell ME, Ittenbach RF, Gaynor JW, et al. Intermediate outcomes after the Fontan procedure in the current era. *J Thorac Cardiovasc Surg* 2006;131:172.
39. Azakie A, McCrindle BW, Van Arsdell G, et al. Extracardiac conduit versus lateral tunnel cavopulmonary connections at a single institution: Impact on outcomes. *J Thorac Cardiovasc Surg* 2001;122:1219.
40. Dilawar M, Bradley SM, Saul JP, et al. Sinus node dysfunction after intraatrial lateral tunnel and extracardiac conduit Fontan procedures. *Pediatr Cardiol* 2003;24:284.
41. Kumar SP, Rubinstein CS, Simsic JM, et al. Lateral tunnel versus extracardiac conduit Fontan procedure: A concurrent comparison. *Ann Thorac Surg* 2003;76:1389.
42. Morales DL, Dibardino DJ, Braud BE, et al. Salvaging the failing Fontan: Lateral tunnel versus extracardiac conduit. *Ann Thorac Surg* 2005;80:1445.

CHAPTER

69 TRICUSPID ATRESIA AND THE FUNCTIONALLY SINGLE VENTRICLE

Carin A. van Doorn, Marc R. de Leval

INTRODUCTION

A wide variety of congenital cardiac lesions lack two well-developed ventricles; from a functional standpoint, they are characterized by a single ventricular chamber that supports both systemic and pulmonary circulations. It is well established that the definitive palliation for these univentricular hearts is the Fontan circulation, whereby the pulmonary and systemic blood flow are placed in series with the single ventricle connected to the systemic circulation. To achieve the Fontan state, many patients need preliminary procedures, either to reduce or augment pulmonary blood flow.

DEFINITIONS AND ANATOMIC CONSIDERATIONS

A truly morphologic univentricular heart is rare; more often there is an additional rudimentary chamber. The most common type of single ventricle is tricuspid atresia, with an incidence of 1 to 3 percent of all congenital heart lesions. In tricuspid atresia there is no direct communication between the right atrium and the right ventricle, and often a dimple or localized fibrous thickening is found at the expected site of the tricuspid valve. The right atrium is large and an interatrial communication is always present. The right ventricle is hypoplastic and

KEY CONCEPTS

- Epidemiology
  - Tricuspid atresia is the most common type of functionally single ventricle. Associated cardiac abnormalities are always present and may lead to obstruction of pulmonary or systemic outflow.
- Morphology and pathophysiology
  - The pulmonary and systemic circulations are in parallel. The degree of hypoxemia depends on pulmonary blood flow, which is determined by the associated cardiac abnormalities and the pulmonary vascular bed, both of which are subject to change over time.
- Diagnosis
  - Echocardiography provides detailed structural and functional information on the heart, particularly in infants. Cardiac catheterization, magnetic resonance imaging, and computed tomography may be necessary to gather additional information.
- Treatment
  - Without surgical treatment the majority of patients will die in infancy, either from severe cyanosis or, less commonly, congestive heart failure. The Fontan circulation is widely accepted as the definitive surgical palliation for patients with tricuspid atresia and other anomalies with functionally single ventricles. There are strict selection criteria for the Fontan operation. In particular, preserved ventricular function and an adequate pulmonary vascular bed are mandatory. Many patients require preliminary operations in infancy to balance pulmonary and systemic circulations. The surgical technique for the Fontan operation has evolved over time.
- Outcome
  - Operative mortality for suitable Fontan candidates in the current era is approximately 5 percent. Late attrition of the Fontan circulation is a serious clinical problem, and its mechanisms are poorly understood.

lacks an inflow portion, but its trabecular and ouflow portion may be well developed.

Tricuspid atresia is uniformly associated with other cardiac malformations. A ventricular septal defect (VSD) is usually present. The ventriculoarterial connection can be concordant or, less commonly, discordant (transposition of the great arteries); rarely, there is double-outlet right or left ventricle. Infundibular obstruction to pulmonary blood flow is often present, but obstruction can also be observed at the level of the ventricular septal defect (restrictive VSD) or the pulmonary valve, which may be atretic. In patients with transposition of the great arteries, there may be subaortic stenosis or coarctation. The associated cardiac malformations determine the balance between pulmonary and systemic blood flow.

Other forms of univentricular hearts include mitral atresia, double-inlet right and left ventricle, hearts with a common atrioventricular valve and only one well-developed ventricle, hearts with heterotaxy syndrome and only one fully developed ventricle, and pulmonary atresia with an intact ventricular septum and hypoplastic right ventricle. In addition, some complex hearts with two well-formed ventricles cannot be septated and become candidates for a single-ventricle strategy as the only viable surgical option. Examples of the latter morphologic group are hearts with major straddling of the atrioventricular valves, or certain forms of double-outlet right ventricle, or transposition of the great arteries with remote VSD. Hypoplastic left heart syndrome, a common form of univentricular heart, is not discussed in this chapter. Chapter 68 is dedicated to that condition.

HISTORICAL HIGHLIGHTS

With the advent of the Blalock-Taussig shunt in 1944,[1] palliation became possible for patients with single-ventricle physiology and cyanosis. Pulmonary artery banding was introduced in 1952 by Muller to alternatively reduce excessive pulmonary blood flow.[2] Following extensive laboratory work, Glenn showed that partial right heart bypass was possible in a patient with tricuspid atresia by anastomosing the superior vena cava (or azygos vein) to the divided right pulmonary artery.[3] This procedure evolved to the bidirectional cavopulmonary shunt, in which the superior vena cava is anastomosed end to side to the undivided pulmonary artery, thus shunting blood into both lungs.[4] In 1968, Fontan and Baudet performed the first total right heart bypass operation by establishing an atriopulmonary connection in a patient with tricuspid atresia.[5] The operation was based on the concept that the right atrium could replace the right ventricle as the driving force for the pulmonary circulation. In addition, separating the systemic and pulmonary circulations and placing them in series improved arterial oxygen saturation and reduced volume load on the single ventricle. Over the years there have been several modifications of the Fontan procedure. It became apparent that the atrial "kick" was not essential to cardiac output, and the atriopulmonary connection has now been largely replaced by the more energy-efficient total cavopulmonary anastomosis.[6] In this palliative configuration, the superior vena cava drains directly into the pulmonary artery and an intraatrial tunnel—or, more recently, an extracardiac conduit[7]—is used to baffle the inferior vena cava to the pulmonary artery. For patients with subaortic obstruction undergoing the Fontan procedure, Waldman described the concurrent use of a modified Damus-Kaye-Stansel procedure to achieve unobstructed systemic outflow.[8]

Staging of Fontan palliation was introduced in an attempt to reduce the operative risk of the Fontan operation. Initial performance of a superior cavopulmonary shunt was followed at a later stage by completion of the total cavopulmonary connection.[9] Another modification in technique was the creation of a fenestration in the Fontan baffle to allow a right-to-left shunt to maintain systemic ventricular filling. This proved to be particularly important in patients with impaired pulmonary blood flow, albeit at the cost of variable degrees of cyanosis. The fenestration can be closed percutaneously.[10]

Improved understanding of the Fontan physiology and evolution of the surgical techniques have extended the original indication of the Fontan operation from tricuspid atresia to many other forms of complex univentricular hearts.

PATHOPHYSIOLOGY

In tricuspid atresia, the systemic venous return crosses the interatrial communication to the left atrium, where it mixes with pulmonary venous blood. As a result, oxygen saturations in the ventricles, aorta, and pulmonary artery are virtually identical (Fig. 69-1). Systemic arterial hypoxemia is always present but is worse when the pulmonary-to-systemic blood flow ratio is low (in case of associated pulmonary stenosis or restrictive VSD). In case of severe hypoxemia, metabolic acidosis will eventually develop. In tricuspid atresia with normally related great vessels, blood reaches the pulmonary artery indirectly through a VSD and hypoplastic right ventricle. Pulmonary blood flow may be unrestricted initially but usually diminishes over time due to restriction of the VSD or the development of infundibular stenosis. In tricuspid atresia with transposition of the great arteries, the left ventricle is connected directly to the pulmonary artery and, unless pulmonary stenosis is present, pulmonary blood flow is high and pulmonary vascular disease will develop. In this anatomic subgroup, the aorta receives blood indirectly via the VSD and the hypoplastic right ventricle. Progressive restriction of the VSD will produce the effect of developing subaortic stenosis.

In patients with functionally single ventricles with other morphologic features, the pathophysiology will be

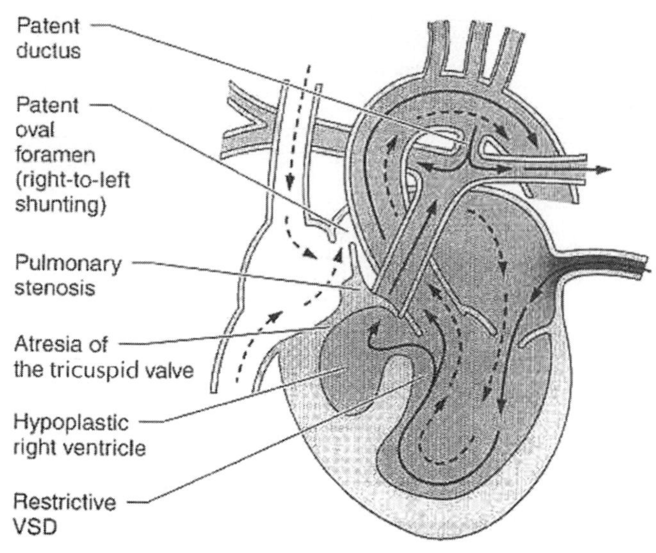

tricuspid atresia. (■)——►, Oxygenated; (□)- - -►, Deoxygenated; (□)- - -⇄, mixed.

Figure 69-1 Diagram illustrating the pathophysiology of tricuspid atresia with restrictive pulmonary blood flow. VSD = ventricular septal defect. [From Reitz BA, Yuh DD (eds). *Congenital Cardiac Surgery.* New York: McGraw-Hill; 2002:144. With permission.]

determined by the balance between pulmonary and systemic blood flow, the effects of intracardiac mixing and streaming, and the presence of other cardiovascular pathology (such as total abnormal pulmonary venous drainage or atrioventricular valve regurgitation). In most single-ventricle circulations, systemic ventricular dysfunction and failure will develop as the result of cyanosis and/or volume overload.

NATURAL HISTORY

The natural history of single-ventricle circulations is predominantly related to the degree of pulmonary blood flow and any associated cardiac lesions. There may also be associated noncardiac abnormalities, which will have an independent impact on outcome. Early onset of cyanosis is a predictor of worst survival, leading to death in 90 percent of untreated cyanotic patients with tricuspid atresia in the first year of life.[11] Patients with unobstructed pulmonary blood flow also fare poorly, often dying in infancy from congestive heart failure or early onset of pulmonary vascular disease. This clinical course may be accelerated in the presence of left-sided obstruction, such a subaortic stenosis or coarctation. A small subset of patients has a balanced circulation with unobstructed systemic blood flow and adequate restriction to prevent pulmonary overcirculation. These patients have a more favorable prognosis, with a mean survival of 8 years.[12] Without surgical intervention, only 10 percent of infants will be alive by the age of 10 years.[13]

CLINICAL PRESENTATION

The clinical features are determined by the degree of pulmonary blood flow and associated cardiac malformations (Fig. 69-2).

Most patients with tricuspid atresia present with cyanosis on the first day of life. Some may have a duct-dependent pulmonary circulation and will become rapidly cyanotic as the ductus arteriosus closes after birth. In the majority of patients, cyanosis is progressive and due to increasing infundibular stenosis and/or restriction of the VSD. Hypoxic spells may occur and are characterized by cyanosis, dyspnea, and occasionally syncope. Clubbing may develop in older children. In a minority of patients, however, there is no obstruction to pulmonary blood flow, and these patients present with congestive heart failure from overcirculation. With falling pulmonary vascular resistance, symptoms will get worse in the first weeks of life. In most univentricular hearts there is mixing of circulations, but streaming may occur, particularly in complex hearts, resulting in differential saturation in the great arteries.

DIAGNOSTIC MODALITIES

Chest x-ray usually shows signs of low pulmonary blood flow, with reduced pulmonary vascular markings and diminutive hilar shadowing. In cases of high pulmonary blood flow (usually tricuspid atresia with discordant ventriculoarterial connection), there is pulmonary plethora and cardiomegaly. Electrocardiography in most patients will demonstrate left axis deviation and, frequently, a tall (> 2.5-mm) notched p-wave consistent with right atrial enlargement.

Echocardiography provides both detailed anatomic diagnosis and functional assessment. The echocardiogram will usually show a hyperechoic shelf at the expected site of the tricuspid valve, in association with reduced right ventricular dimensions. The following information is essential to allow proper surgical planning: size and course of the pulmonary arteries, relationship of the great vessels, degree of right ventricular outflow tract obstruction, size of the interatrial communication, size and position of the VSD, presence of patent ductus arteriosus, aortic coarctation or other structural cardiovascular abnormalities. In addition, ventricular function needs to be assessed. Particularly in infants (who typically have excellent echocardiographic windows), enough information can usually be acquired to proceed directly to operative intervention.

Cardiac catheterization is not routinely performed but remains an important diagnostic adjunct if there is

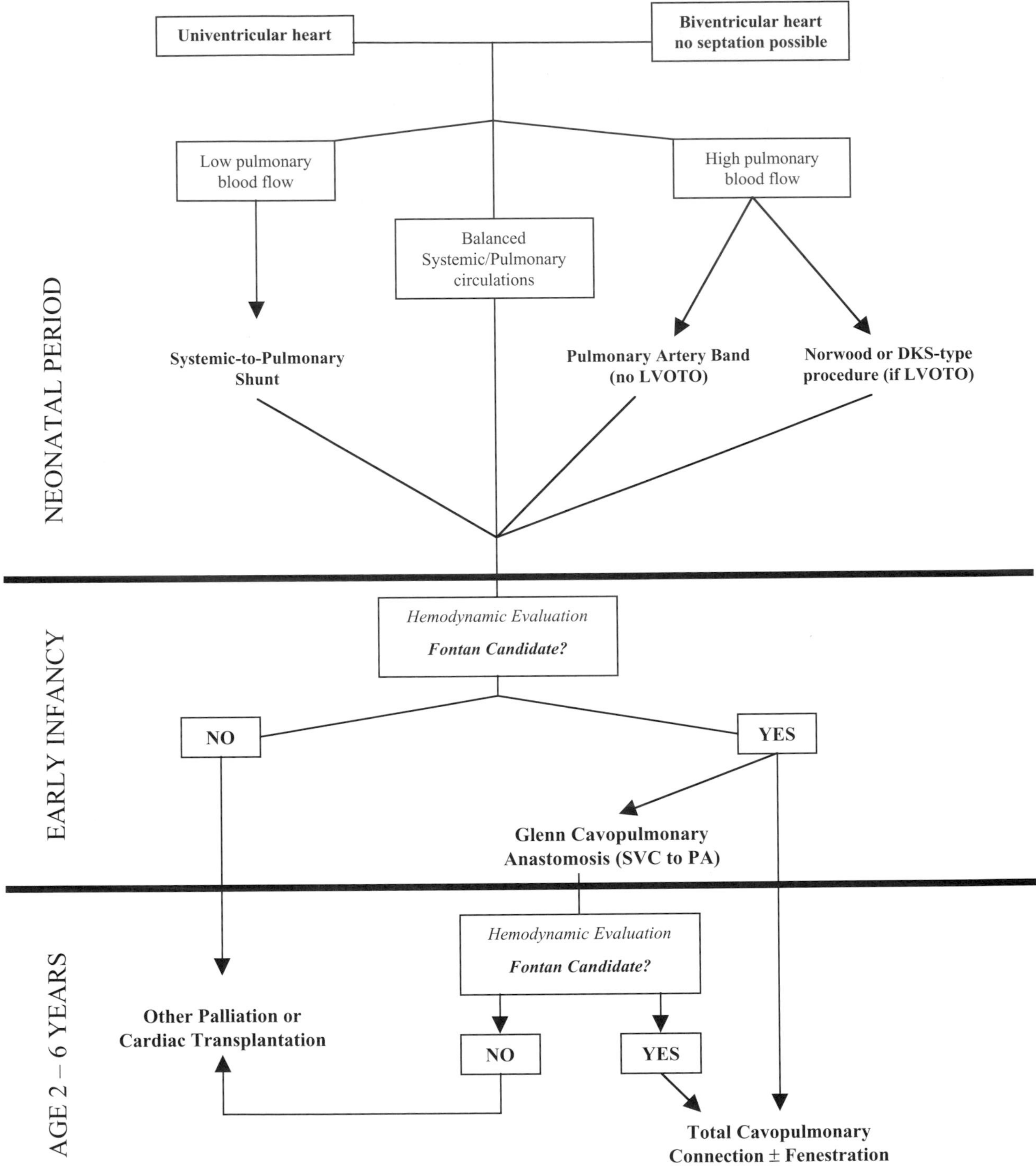

Figure 69-2 Clinical decision-making flowchart for pediatric patients with functionally univentricular hearts.

doubt about the size and distribution of the pulmonary arterial supply and a need for direct pressure measurements. In addition, catheter interventions can be performed to supplement or sometimes avert initial surgical intervention.

Magnetic resonance imaging and computed tomography are being utilized with increasing frequency to investigate patients with congenital heart disease, allowing for three-dimensional reconstruction of the cardiovascular structures and noninvasive assessment of hemodynamic function.

SELECTION CRITERIA FOR THE FONTAN PROCEDURE

The initial selection criteria for the procedure, described by Fontan and colleagues for patients with tricuspid

Table 69-1 The "ten commandments" for selection of patients with tricuspid atresia for the fontan procedure

1. Minimum age 4 years
2. Sinus rhythm
3. Normal caval drainage
4. Right atrium of normal volume
5. Mean pulmonary artery pressure $\leq$ 15 mmHg
6. Pulmonary arterial resistance $<$ 4 U/m^2
7. Ratio of pulmonary artery diameter to aorta diameter $\geq$ 0.75
8. Normal ventricular function (ejection fraction $>$ 0.6)
9. Competent left atrioventricular valve
10. No impairing effects of previous shunts

Source: Choussat A et al.[14] With permission.

atresia, were very strict and known as the "ten commandments" (Table 69-1).[14] With increasing experience, these criteria have been relaxed and, at the same time, the indication for the operation has been extended to many forms of complex single ventricle. However, owing to the unique physiology associated with the Fontan procedure, appropriate patient selection remains of paramount importance.

The minimal age of patients undergoing the Fontan operation has been progressively lowered in an attempt to try to minimize the deleterious effects of long-standing cyanosis and volume overload. The optimal and minimal ages are not known, but successful Fontan operations have been performed in patients as young as 7 months who presented with increasing cyanosis and suitable hemodynamics.[15] It remains to be seen whether a very early Fontan operation has a better long-term outcome, particularly in patients with well-balanced circulations.

Preoperative sinus rhythm, normal caval drainage, and normal right atrial volume are not absolute requirements, but unobstructed pulmonary venous drainage is obligatory.

The pulmonary vasculature remains an important selection criterion for the Fontan procedure. Mean pulmonary arterial pressure ($\leq$ 15 mmHg) and pulmonary arteriolar resistance ($<$ 4 U/m^2) should be low and any pulmonary distortion related to previous shunts should be corrected. Adequate size of the pulmonary arteries is also important. There have been various attempts to standardize pulmonary artery measurements, such as the McGoon ratio[16*] and the Nakata index, [17†] but the usefulness of these indices has been questioned, as they do not account for the compliance of the pulmonary vascular bed.

* The McGoon ratio is obtained from the sum of the diameters of the immediately prebranching portions of the left and right pulmonary arteries divided by the diameter of the descending aorta just above the diaphragm.

† The Nakata index is derived from the sum of the diameters of the left and right pulmonary arteries (measured just before the origin of the upper-lobe branches) divided by the body surface area.

Adequate ventricular function is also crucial for a successful Fontan procedure. Ventricular impairment, however, is not always an absolute contraindication if it can be related to volume overload in the presence of an aortopulmonary shunt that will be taken down at the time of second-stage palliation. The same is true for mild or moderate atrioventricular valve regurgitation in the setting of a volume-loaded heart. More recently, ventricular hypertrophy has also been recognized as an important risk factor for Fontan failure.[18] Predisposing conditions for ventricular hypertrophy, such as subaortic obstruction or coarctation, should be corrected as soon as possible. In the absence of uniform selection criteria, most centers will use a combination of the above criteria and grade patients as being at low, intermediate, or high-risk for the Fontan procedure.

MEDICAL THERAPY

Medical therapy in the management of the functionally single ventricle is limited to supportive measures. Neonates with severe hypoxemia, in whom pulmonary blood flow is dependent on a patent ductus arteriosus, benefit from prostaglandin E_1 infusion until surgical intervention can be undertaken. The same strategy is utilized in patients with associated aortic coarctation and duct-dependent systemic circulation. In those with congestive heart failure, treatment with diuretics is indicated.

SURGICAL THERAPY

Preliminary procedures in preparation for the fontan circulation

The goals of preliminary surgical procedures leading up to the Fontan operation are as follows:

1. Improvement of clinical symptoms
2. Optimization of the pulmonary vascular bed and of ventricular performance
3. Provision of anatomic setup for the Fontan procedure

In the majority of patients with single-ventricle circulation, pulmonary blood flow is restricted; in some it is excessive, and very few have naturally balanced circulations. Within the first year of life, therefore, most patients will require palliative procedures, either to increase pulmonary blood flow or restrict it. The choice of procedure is guided by the underlying anatomy and pulmonary vascular resistance, both of which are subject to change over time. For augmentation of pulmonary blood flow, a systemic-to-pulmonary artery shunt is usually placed. However, in the subset of patients with transposition of the great arteries with aortic coarctation, a Norwood-type procedure is indicated to relieve the obstruction to systemic blood flow at the same time. In those with unrestricted pulmonary blood flow, banding of the main pulmonary artery is used to reduce pulmonary artery flow. Patients with transposition of the great arteries who undergo this procedure need close postoperative monitoring because of the risk for development of subaortic stenosis. Palliative procedures are detailed in Chap. 54. It should always be remembered that improper preliminary procedures can result in the loss of Fontan candidacy.

Bidirectional cavopulmonary shunt

The connection from the superior vena cava to the pulmonary artery (Fig. 69-3) can be performed during the Fontan operation or as the first of two procedures of a staged total cavopulmonary connection. The advantages of a venous-to-pulmonary artery shunt over an arterial shunt are that the venous blood that enters the pulmonary artery is much more desaturated; therefore a higher take up of oxygen per milliliter of blood is possible. In addition, systemic venous blood is diverted to the lungs, thus reducing volume load on the single ventricle.

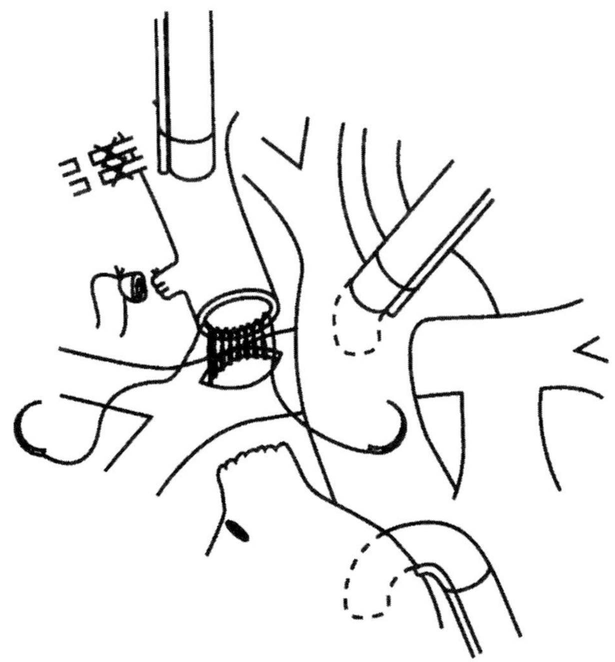

Figure 69-3 Surgical technique for bidirectional cavopulmonary shunt. The superior vena cava (SVC) and branch pulmonary arteries are fully mobilized. The azygos vein and small venous branches near the innominate vein–SVC junction are ligated to prevent runoff into the inferior vena cava (IVC). If there is IVC interruption with azygos continuation, the azygos vein must be preserved. Cardiopulmonary bypass is instituted with two cannulas draining the right atrium and SVC–innominate vein junction and an aortic return line. The aortopulmonary shunt is subsequently taken down (not seen in the diagram). The SVC is divided and the cardiac end oversewn. The SVC is anastomosed end to side to the upper margin of the right pulmonary artery. Additional sources of pulmonary blood supply, such as forward flow over a stenosed pulmonary outflow tract or left-sided arterial pulmonary shunt, are usually left in place.

There is no universal agreement on selection criteria for a cavopulmonary shunt, but it is generally accepted that these are less rigorous than those for the Fontan operation. It remains open to discussion whether any additional source of pulmonary blood flow (such as a patent ductus arteriosus, patent right ventricular outflow tract, or systemic-to-pulmonary artery shunt) should be taken down at the time of the cavopulmonary shunt. Any adverse anatomic features for the Fontan circulation should, if possible, be corrected at the time of operation.

The creation of a cavopulmonary shunt requires complete occlusion of the superior vena cava during the anastomosis. To avoid dangerous levels of upper body venous hypertension, the operation is usually performed on cardiopulmonary bypass. This has the added advantage that the patient's oxygenation will not be compromised if any systemic-to-pulmonary artery shunts are taken down and that, in addition, other cardiac anomalies can be corrected during the operation. An alternative method to achieve decompression of the venous system is the use of a temporary cavoatrial shunt, thus avoiding the deleterious effects of cardiopulmonary bypass. This shunt can be inserted either between the superior vena cava and right atrium or, if pulmonary blood flow is a concern, between the superior vena cava and pulmonary artery.

The hemi-Fontan modification of the cavopulmonary shunt involves patch augmentation of the central pulmonary arteries and an anastomosis between the superior cavoatrial junction and the pulmonary artery. This operation has been particularly popular in patients with hypoplastic left heart syndrome in whom, following first-stage Norwood palliation, pulmonary distortion and hypoplasia are common.[19] The hemi-Fontan operation is described in Chap. 70.

A controversial point in the surgical management plan for the cavopulmonary shunt is whether to leave an additional source of pulmonary blood flow in place (such as an existing aortopulmonary shunt or forward flow over a banded pulmonary artery) with the cavopulmonary shunt. Proponents argue that this adds some pulsatility to pulmonary blood flow, which is more physiologic to the pulmonary vascular bed; those disfavoring this approach are concerned about the increased volume load on the single ventricle.

Complications associated with a cavopulmonary shunt include preferential perfusion of the lower parts of the lung and the formation of arteriovenous pulmonary artery fistulas.[20] Communications between the (higher pressure) superior vena cava territory and lower body veins, left atrium, and pulmonary veins may also be present, promoting left-to-right shunting and increasing cyanosis.[21] Furthermore, aortopulmonary collateral vessels may impose an increased volume load on the heart. With somatic growth of the child, the relative contribution of superior vena cava return to total venous return decreases, and an additional source of pulmonary blood flow is needed. In suitable patients, total cavopulmonary connection should now be completed. If the patient is not a Fontan candidate, another option may be to add a small arterial shunt to increase net pulmonary blood flow.

Completion of total cavopulmonary connection

The original atriopulmonary Fontan operation has now largely been replaced by a total cavopulmonary connection. The inferior vena cava is connected to the pulmonary artery either by means of an intraatrial baffle (Fig. 69-4) or, in the most recently introduced

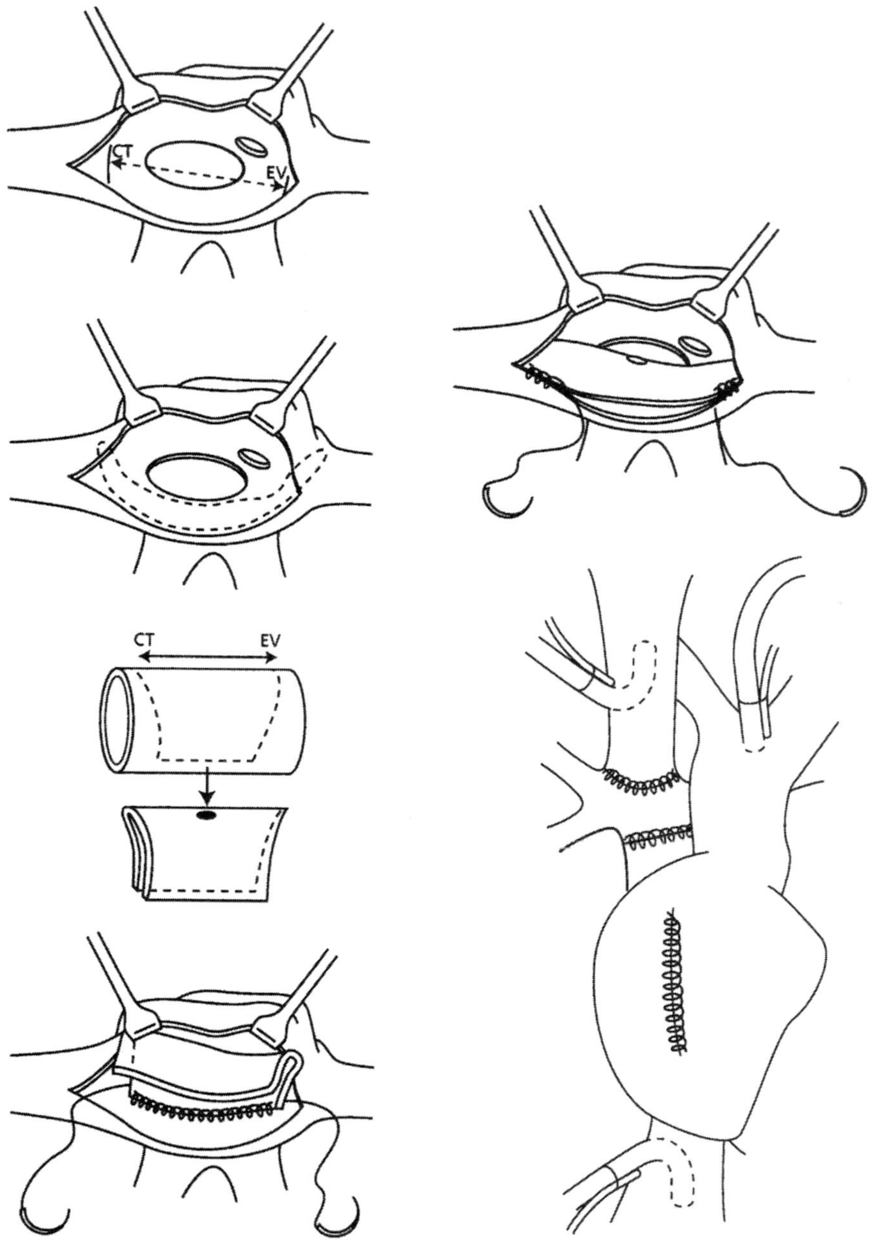

Figure 69-4 Surgical technique for lateral tunnel Fontan. The beginning of the operation may involve performing a bidirectional cavopulmonary anastomosis (see Fig. 69-3), or this may already be in place. Bicaval venous cannulation and aortic return are utilized to institute cardiopulmonary bypass at moderate hypothermia. The right atrium is opened along the crest of the septum (top left) and the size of the intraatrial baffle is measured between the eustachian valve (EV) and the crista terminalis (CT). A polytetrafluoroethylene conduit at least 16 mm in diameter is opened longitudinally and, if required, a 4- to 5-mm fenestration is performed. The prosthetic baffle is sewn halfway around the junction of the inferior vena cava with the right atrium, along the posterior wall of the atrial septum, crista terminalis, and halfway around the junction with the superior vena cava (bottom left and top right). Care is taken to avoid injury to the sinus node. The cardiac end of the transected superior vena cava is anastomosed end to side to the undersurface of the right pulmonary artery (bottom right).

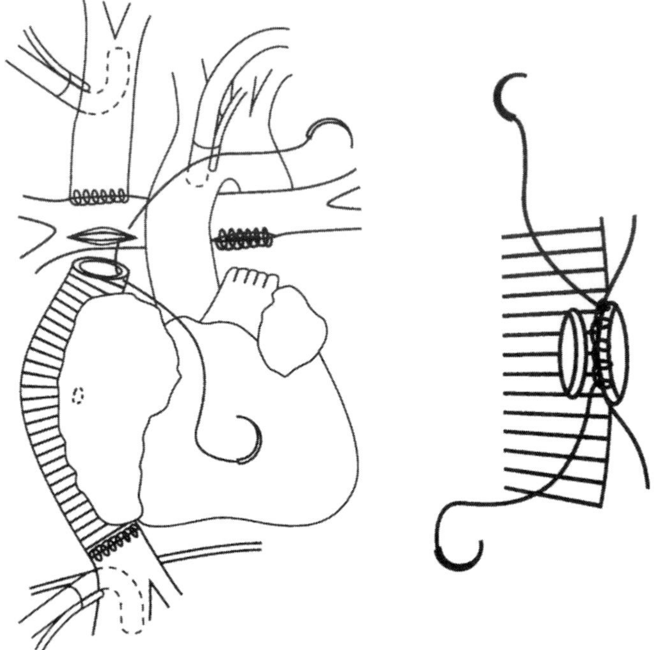

Figure 69-5 Surgical technique for extracardiac Fontan. Cannulation for cardiopulmonary bypass is as described in Fig. 69-4. The cavopulmonary junction is transected and the cardiac end oversewn. A polytetrafluoroethylene conduit at least 16 mm in diameter (22-mm diameter in adults) is anastomosed end to end to the transected inferior vena cava. The conduit is gently curved around the atrium toward the right pulmonary artery, and the top end of the prosthesis is anastomosed end to side to the left pulmonary artery. If a fenestration is required, A 4- to 5-mm hole is cut in the prosthesis and a slightly larger opening is made in the opposite right atrial wall with side-biting clamps. The two orifices are then anastomosed (right).

configuration, with the use of an extracardiac polytetrafluoroethylene conduit. The latter procedure (Fig. 69-5) can be performed without cross-clamping the aorta and, if a temporary shunt between the inferior vena cava and right atrium is used, also without the use of cardiopulmonary bypass.

OUTCOMES

Early mortality and morbidity

Morbidity and mortality from the various preliminary procedures performed for various structural abnormalities with functionally single ventricle are reported elsewhere in this textbook. The operative mortality for the lateral tunnel Fontan and extracardiac Fontan is approximately 5 percent.[22–24] However, in patients with the syndrome of a single ventricle and heterotaxy, syndrome, mortality is two to three times higher owing to the multiple associated cardiovascular abnormalities.[22]

A low cardiac output in the immediate postoperative period can lead to a vicious cycle, resulting in multiple organ failure and death unless early takedown of the connection or fenestration is performed. Such a low-output state can be triggered by various factors, including ventricular dysfunction, raised pulmonary vascular resistance, cardiac arrhythmias, and suboptimal technical procedures. Pleural effusions requiring prolonged chest tube drainage are a common early occurrence after the Fontan operation.

Late results

The Fontan state is associated with a premature decline in functional status and survival compared with the normal population. In 1990, Fontan and colleagues reported that, even if the operation was performed under perfect conditions, predicted long-term survival was 86, 81, and 73 percent at 5, 10, and 15 years respectively.[25] In a recent series of patients who had undergone the lateral tunnel Fontan, long-term survival was 93 percent at 5 years and 91 percent at 10 years. For the more recently introduced extracardiac-conduit Fontan, survival up to 8 years is similar.[24] The reasons for the late attrition after the Fontan operation are poorly understood, but chronic elevation of the systemic venous pressure probably plays a major role.

The distended atrium in the atriopulmonary Fontan is prone to dysrhythmias, especially because of the presence of multiple suture lines. The incidence of this has been much reduced in the lateral tunnel Fontan, with reported freedom from supraventricular tachyarrhythmias of 96 and 91 percent at 5 and 10 years, respectively, and freedom from new bradyarrhythmias of 88 and 79 percent at the same follow-up interval.[23] Risk factors for arrhythmias are related to cardiac morphologic features, such as heterotaxy syndrome and atrioventricular valve abnormalities.[23] Five-year follow-up results for the extracardiac Fontan are similar.[26]

Pulmonary arteriovenous fistulas occur both following the cavopulmonary shunt and the Fontan operation. They can produce significant right-to-left shunting with resultant hypoxemia and cyanosis. Their etiology is unclear, but exclusion of the hepatic effluent from the pulmonary circuit may be a factor; resolution has been reported by redirecting hepatic venous blood to the pulmonary arteries.[27]

Thromboembolism occurs both early and late after the Fontan operation and consists of pathway thrombosis as well as pulmonary and/or cerebral emboli. Although the reported incidence ranges from 3 to 16 percent for venous thrombosis[28,29] and from 3 to 19 percent for stroke,[30,31] many events are probably unrecognized. The etiology is likely to be multifactorial and includes suboptimal flow patterns, arrhythmias, thrombogenicity of vascular conduits, hypercoagulable states, and liver dysfunction. Prophylactic long-term anticoagulation remains a contentious issue but is utilized routinely in many centers.

Protein-losing enteropathy (PLE) is a debilitating, poorly understood complication that involves loss of protein from the gastrointestinal tract. It can occur any time after the Fontan operation, with a reported incidence of up to 15 percent and a mortality of 50 percent at 5 years following initial diagnosis.[32,33] Clinical symptoms are related to the degree of nonselective protein loss and include ascites, effusion, peripheral edema, immunodeficiency, and coagulopathy. An elevated fecal alpha$_1$-antitrypsin level is diagnostic.[33] Medical treatment is often disappointing. High-dose corticosteroids (1 to 2 mg/kg/day for a minimum of 2 to 3 weeks) and unfractionated heparin (5000 U/m^2/day for several weeks)[35] may benefit some patients. Optimization of the hemodynamics through revision of the Fontan pathways, creation of a fenestration, pacing, or cardiac transplantation has been successful in other cases. In refractory cases, takedown of the Fontan circuit or cardiac transplantation have been performed with regression of PLE.

Pathway problems involving baffle leaks and localized stenoses have been increasingly managed by catheter interventions. In the recently introduced extracardiac conduit Fontan, lack of growth of the tube prosthesis is a potential drawback, but this has not been a problem when conduits between 18 and 20 mm in diameter were used.[26] Conversely, oversizing of the conduit has been complicated by poor hemodynamic performance and conduit thrombosis.[37]

Ventricular dysfunction is common and is multifactorial in origin. The Fontan state itself is associated with a reduction in ventricular preload as well as an increase in afterload, but in the absence of the compensatory increase in contractility seen in normal hearts.[38] Other adverse working conditions include volume overload, subaortic stenosis, atrioventricular valve regurgitation, atrial arrhythmias, and coronary sinus hypertension. In addition, the myocardium in some congenitally malformed hearts may be intrinsically abnormal[39] or the anatomic and structural characteristics may be inadequate to support the systemic circulation. Reduced exercise capacity has been demonstrated in Fontan patients with a morphological right ventricle.[40]

MANAGEMENT OF THE FAILING FONTAN CIRCULATION

Hemodynamic failure of the Fontan circulation currently occurs predominantly in patients who received an atriopulmonary connection. In those patients who have structural problems of the Fontan pathways or refractory atrial arrhythmias, Fontan conversion to a total cavopulmonary connection with concomitant arrhythmia surgery has been shown to improve exercise tolerance with low incidence of recurrent arrhythmias.[41] Patients with end-stage ventricular failure or other Fontan-related problems refractory to medical treatment should be considered for transplantation. However, pretransplant evaluation of the pulmonary vascular bed in the Fontan circulation is difficult because of the inability to reliably measure pulmonary blood flow, while low pulmonary arterial pressure and transpulmonary gradient may not be predictive of absence of pulmonary vascular disease. The transplant operation itself can be technically challenging because of multiple previous operations and the need for extensive vascular reconstruction. In small series, operative mortality for transplantation after staged Fontan palliation ranges from 7 to 67 percent,[42,43] with high mortality among potential recipients awaiting a suitable donor allograft.

References

1. Blalock A, Taussig H. The surgical treatment of malformations of the heart in which there is pulmonary atresia. *JAMA* 1945;128:189–193.
2. Muller WH, Dammann JF Jr. The treatment of certain congenital malformations of the heart by the creation of pulmonic stenosis to reduce pulmonary hypertension and excessive pulmonary blood flow. *Surg Gynecol Obstet* 1952;95:213–219.
3. Glenn WW, Patino JF. Circulatory by-pass of the right heart. Preliminary observations on the direct delivery of vena caval blood into the pulmonary arterial circulation. Azygos vein–pulmonary artery shunt. *Yale J Biol Med* 1954;27:147–152.
4. Azzolina G, Eufrate S, Pensa P. Tricuspid atresia: Experience in surgical management with a modified cavopulmonary anastomosis. *Thorax* 1972;17: 111–115.
5. Fontan F, Baudet E. Surgical repair of tricuspid atresia. *Thorax* 1971;26:240–248.
6. de Leval MR, Kilner P, Gewillig M, et al. Total cavopulmonary connection: A logical alternative to atriopulmonary connection for complex Fontan operations. *J Thorac Cardiovasc Surg* 1988;96:682–695.
7. Marcelletti C, Corno A, Giannico S, et al. Inferior vena cavapulmonary artery extracardiac conduit: A new form of right heart bypass. *J Thorac Cardiovasc Surg* 1990; 100:228–232.
8. Waldman JD, Lamberti JJ, George L, et al. Experience with Damus procedure. *Circulation* 1988;78(Suppl III): 32–39.
9. Bridges ND, Jonas RA, Mayer JE, et al. Bidirectional cavopulmonary anastomosis as interim palliation for high risk Fontan candidates. *Circulation* 1990;82(Suppl IV): 170–176.
10. Bridges ND, Lock JE, Castaneda AR. Baffle fenestration with subsequent transcatheter closure: Modification of the Fontan operation for patients at increased risk. *Circulation* 1990;82:1681–1689.

11. Campbell M. Tricuspid atresia and its prognosis with and without surgical treatment. *Br Heart J* 1961;23:699–710.
12. Patel MM, Overy DC, Kozonis MC, et al. Long-term survival in tricuspid atresia. *J Am Coll Cardiol* 1987;9: 338–340.
13. Rao PS. Further observations on the spontaneous closure of physiologically advantageous ventricular septal defects in tricuspid atresia: Surgical implications. *Ann Thorac Surg* 1983;35;121–131.
14. Choussat A, Fontan F, Besse P, et al. Selection criteria for Fontan's procedure. In: Anderson RH, Shinebourne EA (eds). *Paediatric Cardiology*. Edinburgh: Churchill Livingstone; 1978:559–566.
15. Pearl JM, Laks H, Drinkwater DC, et al. Modified Fontan procedure in patients less than 4 years old. *Circulation* 1992;86(Suppl V):100–105.
16. Piehler JM, Danielson GK, McGoon DC, et al. Management of pulmonary atresia with ventricular septal defect and hypoplastic pulmonary arteries by right ventricular outflow construction. *J Thorac Cardiovasc Surg* 1980;80:552–567.
17. Nakata S, Imai Y, Takanashi Y, et al. A new method for the quantitative standardization of cross-sectional areas of the pulmonary arteries in congenital heart diseases with decreased pulmonary blood flow. *J Thorac Cardiovasc Surg* 1984;88:610–619.
18. Kirklin JK, Blackstone EH, Kirklin JW, et al. The Fontan operation. Ventricular hypertrophy, age, and date of operation as risk factors. *J Thorac Cardiovasc Surg* 1986;92: 1049–1064.
19. Douglas WI, Goldberg CS, Mosca RS, et al. Hemi-Fontan procedure for hypoplastic left heart syndrome: Outcome and suitability for Fontan. *Ann Thorac Surg* 1999;68: 1361–1367.
20. Clouter A, Ash JM, Smallhorn JF, et al. Abnormal distribution of pulmonary blood flow after the Glenn shunt or Fontan procedure: Risk of development of arteriovenous fistulae. *Circulation* 1985;72:471–479.
21. Magee AG, McCrindle BW, Benson LN, et al. Systemic venous collaterals after the bidirectional cavopulmonary anastomosis. Prevalence and predictors. *J Am Coll Cardiol* 1998;32:502–508.
22. Azakie A, Merklinge SL, Williams WG, et al. Improving outcomes of the Fontan operation in children with atrial isomerism and heterotaxy syndromes. *Ann Thorac Surg* 2001;72:1636–1640.
23. Stamm C, Friehs I, Mayer JE, et al. Long-term results of the lateral tunnel Fontan operation. *J Thorac Cardiovasc Surg* 2001;121:28–41.
24. Kumar SP, Rubinstein CS, Simsic JM, et al. Lateral tunnel versus extracardiac conduit Fontan procedure: A concurrent comparison. *Ann Thorac Surg* 2003;76:1389–1396.
25. Fontan F, Kirklin JW, Fernandez G, et al. Outcome after a "perfect" Fontan operation. *Circulation* 1990;81: 1520–1536.
26. Alexi-Meskishvili V, Ovroutski S, Ewert P, et al. Mid-term follow-up after extracardiac Fontan operation. *Thorac Cardiovasc Surg* 2004;52:218–224.
27. Pike NA, Vricella LA, Feinstein JA, et al. Regression of severe pulmonary arteriovenous malformations after Fontan revision and "hepatic factor" rerouting. *Ann Thorac Surg* 2004;78:697–699.
28. Dobell ARC, Trusler GA, Smallhorn JF, et al. Atrial thrombi after the Fontan operation. *Ann Thorac Surg* 1986;42:664–667.
29. Rosenthal D, Friedman A, Kleinman S, et al. Thromboembolic complications after Fontan operation. *Circulation* 1995;92(Suppl II):287–293.
30. du Plessis AJ, Chang AC, Wessel DL, et al. Cerebrovascular accidents following the Fontan operation. *Pediatr Neurol* 1995;12:230–236.
31. Matthews K, Bale J, Clark E, et al. Cerebral infarction complicating Fontan surgery for cyanotic congenital heart disease. *Pediatr Cardiol* 1986;7:161–166.
32. Feldt RH, Driscoll DJ, Offord KP, et al. Protein-losing enteropathy after Fontan operation. *J Thorac Cardiovasc Surg* 1996;112:672–680.
33. Mertens L, Hagler DJ, Sauer U, et al. Protein-losing enteropathy after the Fontan operation: An international multicenter study (PLE Study Group). *J Thorac Cardiovasc Surg* 1998;115:1063–1073.
34. Hill RE, Hercz A, Corey ML, et al. Fecal clearance of alpha 1-antitrypsin: A reliable measure of enteric protein loss in children. *J Paediatr* 1981;99:416–418.
35. Rychik J, Piccoli DA, Barber G. Usefulness of corticosteroid therapy for protein loss in late survivors of Fontan surgery and other congenital heart disease. *Am J Cardiol* 1991;68:819–821.
36. Donnelly JP, Rosenthal A, Castle VP, et al. Reversal of protein-losing enteropathy with heparin therapy in three patients with univentricular hearts and Fontan palliation. *J Pediatr* 1997;130:474–478.
37. Alexi-Meskishvili V, Ovroutski S, Ewert P, et al. Optimal conduit size for extracardiac Fontan operation. *Eur J Cardiothorac Surg* 2000;18:690–695.
38. de Leval MR. The Fontan circulation: A challenge to William Harvey? *Nat Clin Pract Cardiovasc Med* 2005;2:202–208.
39. Akiba T, Becker AE. Disease of the left ventricle in pulmonary atresia with intact ventricular septum. The limiting factor for long-lasting successful surgical intervention. *J Thorac Cardiovasc Surg* 1994;108:1–8.
40. Ohuchi H, Yasuda K, Hasegawa S, et al. Influence of ventricular morphology on aerobic exercise capacity in patients after the Fontan operation. *J Am Coll Cardiol* 2001;37:1967–1974.
41. Mavroudis C, Backer SL, Deal BJ, et al. Fontan conversion to cavopulmonary connection and arrhythmia circuit cryoablation. *J Thorac Cardiovasc Surg* 1998;115:547–556.
42. Mitchell MB, Campbell DN, Boucek MM. Heart transplantation for the failing Fontan circulation. *Semin Thorac Cardiovasc Surg Pediatr Cardiac Surg Annu* 2004;7:56–64.
43. Michielon G, Parisi F, Squitieri C, et al. Orthotopic heart transplantation for congenital heart disease: An alternative for high-risk Fontan candidates? *Circulation* 2003;108(Suppl I):140–149.

CHAPTER

70 SURGERY FOR LEFT VENTRICULAR OUTFLOW TRACT OBSTRUCTION IN CHILDREN

Lester C. Permut, Marco Ricci, Gordon A. Cohen

INTRODUCTION

Left ventricular outflow tract obstruction is a relatively common form of congenital heart disease; it occurs in 2.8 per 10,000 births and accounts for 3 to 6 percent of congenital heart defects.[1] The levels of obstruction are classified anatomically as valvar (50 percent), subvalvar (25 percent), and supravalvar (10 percent). Multiple levels of obstruction are present in about 15 percent of cases.[2] Left ventricular outflow tract obstruction may be associated with other congenital heart defects, including atrioventricular canal defect, double-outlet right ventricle, and some forms of functionally single ventricle. This chapter focuses on isolated congenital left ventricular outflow tract obstruction (LVOTO) in functionally biventricular hearts. Aortic arch interruption and coarctation are treated in Chapter 71.

KEY CONCEPTS

- Epidemiology:
  - Left ventricular outflow tract obstruction (LVOTO) occurs in 2.8 of 10,000 live births, accounting for 3 to 6 percent of congenital heart defects.
- Morphology:
  - LVOTO is valvar in 50 percent, subvalvar in 25 percent, and supravalvar in 10 percent of cases. Multilevel obstruction is present in 15 percent of cases.
- Pathophysiology:
  - Obstruction at any level causes increased left ventricular systolic pressure and wall stress and consequent left ventricular hypertrophy. Left ventricular hypertrophy produces subendocardial ischemia and diastolic dysfunction. Eventually, myocardial fibrosis occurs with associated left ventricular systoli dysfunction. Low cardiac output, pulmonary edema, and ventricular arrhythmias occur late and are associated with increased mortality.
- Clinical features:
  - Neonates with critical valvar aortic stenosis (AS) present with low cardiac output and shock, requiring emergency treatment. Other forms of LVOTO are often asymptomatic and are detected by the presence of a heart murmur. Chest pain, dyspnea, and palpitations occur with increased activity as the degree of obstruction worsens. Symptoms at rest occur with long-standing LVOTO.
- Diagnosis:
  - Diagnostic evaluation is performed in children with a characteristic systolic ejection murmur. An ejection click indicates stenosis at the valvar level. Echocardiography allows diagnosis and determines the level(s) of obstruction. The left ventricular outflow tract gradient can be estimated with the use of Doppler flow velocity, and ventricular systolic and diastolic function can be assessed. Diagnostic cardiac catheterization is rarely necessary.
- Treatment:
  - Neonates with critical valvar AS respond well to percutaneous transcatheter balloon valvotomy. Open valvotomy or aortic valve replacement is required in older children. Enlargement of a small annulus may be achieved with the use of Konno aortoventriculoplasty. Options for valve replacement

include a mechanical prosthesis, an allograft, and an autograft (Ross procedure), but all have significant disadvantages in the pediatric population. Discrete subaortic membrane is resected via aortotomy, but diffuse tunnel-like narrowing requires a modified Konno procedure. A variety of aortoplasty techniques are available for patients with supravalvar AS.

- Outcomes:
  - Excellent outcomes, with operative mortality of less than 5 percent, are achieved in most patients. Reoperation to upsize valves is expected in pediatric patients with somatic growth after aortic valve replacement (AVR). Discrete subaortic membrane recurs in approximately 15 to 20 percent of patients despite successful initial repair.

SURGICAL ANATOMY OF THE LEFT VENTRICULAR OUTFLOW TRACT

The left ventricular outflow tract is positioned centrally in the heart in close anatomic relation to other important cardiac structures (Fig. 70-1). Below the level of the aortic valve, the outflow tract is bordered anteriorly and to the left by the infundibular septum. Posteriorly, it is bordered by the anterior leaflet of the mitral valve and the central fibrous body. The membranous septum is positioned anteriorly and to the right, beneath the junction of the right coronary and noncoronary cusps of the aortic valve. This relationship is surgically important, as the bundle of His courses beneath the membranous septum on the left ventricular aspect and may be injured in the course of resection or suture placement, resulting in complete heart block.

The normal aortic valve consists of three thin leaflets of equal size that are attached to the aortic wall in a semilunar fashion. The so-called aortic annulus therefore is not a circular ring but a scalloped coronet.[3] The free edge of each leaflet has an area of central thickening termed the nodulus of Arantius. The leaflet edges coapt in diastole and open freely in systole, creating an unobstructed triangular orifice for the ejection of blood from the left ventricle to the aorta. Leaflets are designated in accordance with the adjacent coronary artery ostia as left, right, and noncoronary cusps.

The proximal ascending aorta constitutes the distal left ventricular outflow tract. Immediately above the ventriculoarterial junction, the aorta enlarges to form the sinuses of Valsalva. These sinuses, like their corresponding valve leaflets, are named for the coronary artery ostia that arise from them. They are important for normal aortic valve function and coronary artery blood flow.[4] The sinotubular junction refers to the normal area of aortic narrowing at the junction between the sinuses of Valsalva and the tubular portion of the ascending aorta. The uppermost point of aortic valve leaflet attachment occurs at the sinotubular junction.

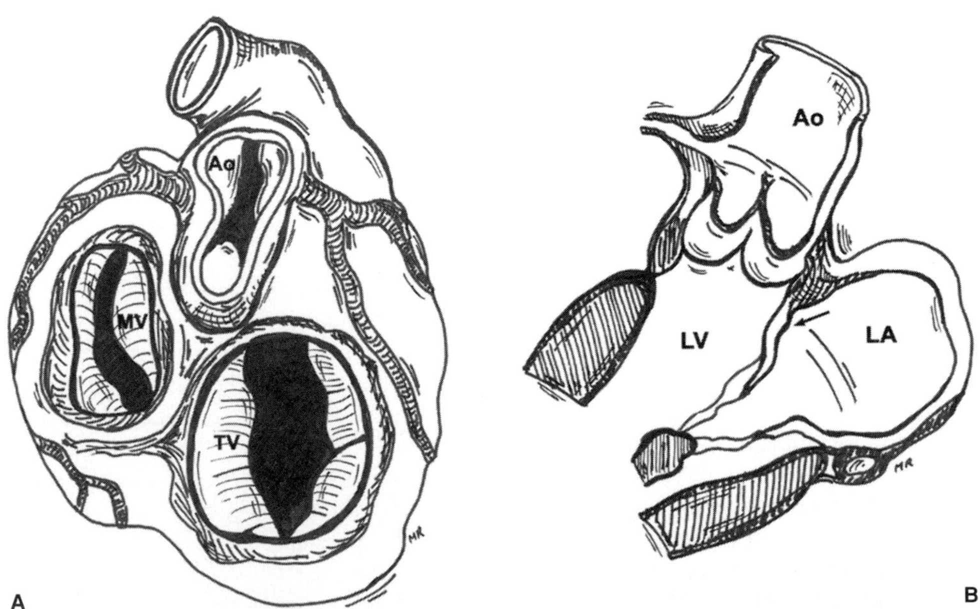

Figure 70-1 Anatomy of the left ventricular outflow tract. A. Cranial view. The aortic valve is centrally positioned between the mitral and tricuspid valves. B. Schematic left-sided view: The noncoronary aortic cusp is in fibrous continuity with the anterior leaflet of the mitral valve. The bundle of His courses below the membranous septum. Ao = aorta; MV = mitral valve; TV = tricuspid valve; LA = left atrium.

PATHOPHYSIOLOGY OF LEFT VENTRICULAR OUTFLOW TRACT OBSTRUCTION

Regardless of the etiology, obstruction to flow through the left ventricular outflow tract results in increased left ventricular systolic pressure and wall stress. Left ventricular hypertrophy develops as a compensatory mechanism that maintains normal wall stress and stroke volume in accordance with Laplace's law. However, increased ventricular wall mass increases myocardial oxygen demand while limiting diastolic coronary blood flow. Oxygen demand eventually exceeds supply, resulting in myocardial ischemia.[5]

Left ventricular systolic function is initially normal or hyperdynamic in the early stages of obstruction. With progressive left ventricular hypertrophy, decreased wall compliance restricts ventricular filling and produces diastolic dysfunction. A decreased preload reduces stroke volume and cardiac output. Left ventricular end-diastolic pressure and left atrial pressure rise, resulting in left atrial hypertrophy. Patients with long-standing obstruction develop myocardial fibrosis, areas of ischemic injury, and decreased ventricular systolic function. Low cardiac output, pulmonary edema, and ventricular arrhythmias ensue, associated with an increasing risk of sudden death.

Relief of LVOTO ideally is achieved before the development of systolic dysfunction. Early relief of obstruction leads to regression of ventricular hypertrophy and normalization of cardiac function. In the later stages, some components of ventricular dysfunction are likely to be irreversible despite relief of obstruction. Surgical repair in these patients is associated with higher risk and poorer outcomes.

VALVAR AORTIC STENOSIS

Pathology

Valvar aortic stenosis in children is most commonly congenital in etiology. The leaflets are thickened and dysplastic, with variable degrees of commissural fusion (Fig. 70-2). The valve is typically bicuspid in morphology but may be tricuspid or even unicuspid. Fusion of the right and left cusps is associated most frequently with stenosis.[6] Obstruction results from decreased leaflet mobility and a reduction in effective orifice size. Small annular size also may be present, further impeding left ventricular ejection.

Clinical presentation

Neonates with critical aortic stenosis develop symptoms soon after birth. After closure of the ductus arteriosus, severe outflow obstruction results in pulmonary congestion and poor peripheral perfusion. Dyspnea, tachypnea, and rales are present on pulmonary examination. A systolic ejection murmur may be present, but it may be difficult to hear when cardiac output is reduced severely. The distal extremities have cold, clammy skin with poor capillary refill and thready, rapid pulses. The differential diagnosis includes other causes of shock, including sepsis and other forms of congenital heart disease. Prompt diagnosis and institution of therapy are necessary to prevent rapid deterioration and death.

Older children present less acutely, often with the finding of an asymptomatic heart murmur on routine physical examination. Difficulty feeding in infants and decreased exercise tolerance in older children may be observed as

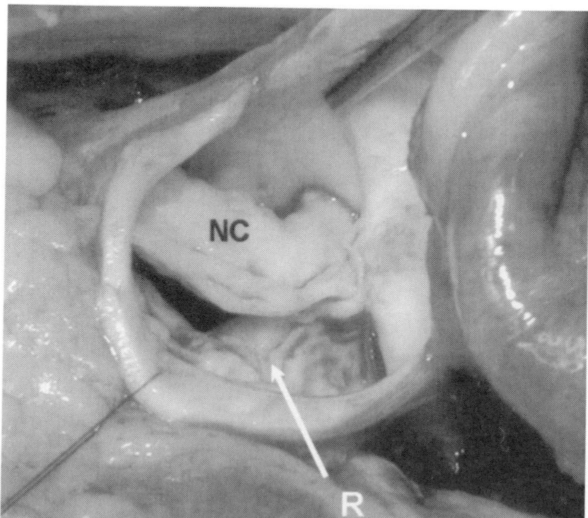

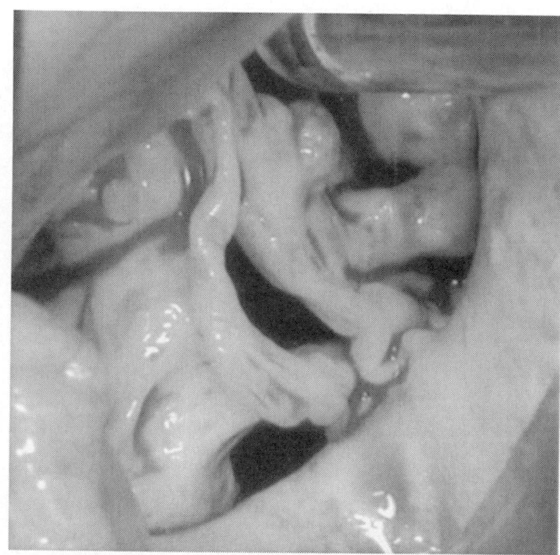

Figure 70-2 Stenotic bicuspid aortic valve. *Left*: The leaflets are asymmetric, with a larger leaflet resulting from the fusion between the left and right coronary cusps at the raphe (R), poorly coapting against the thickened noncoronary leaflet (NC). *Right*: Severe calcific stenosis of the bicuspid aortic valve. (Image courtesy of Dr. Duke Cameron, Division of Cardiac Surgery, Johns Hopkins University Hospital.)

the severity of obstruction increases. Later symptoms include exertional angina, congestive heart failure, and syncope. Physical findings generally are limited to the cardiovascular examination: a harsh systolic ejection murmur at the right upper sternal border radiating to the neck, S_4 gallop, and poor upstroke of the carotid pulse. An ejection click may indicate the presence of a bicuspid valve.

Diagnosis

Chest x-ray is usually nondiagnostic. In neonates with critical stenosis, cardiomegaly and pulmonary congestion are present. Findings in older children generally are limited to moderate left ventricular enlargement, left atrial enlargement, and prominence of the aortic knob.

The electrocardiogram shows left ventricular hypertrophy. Serial findings of increasing QRS voltage and the development of a strain pattern suggest worsening obstruction.

Echocardiography is the principal diagnostic method for the evaluation of LVOTO. Two-dimensional echocardiography allows assessment of aortic valve morphology including leaflet number, degree of thickening, and mobility. Doming of the leaflets is typical (Fig. 70-3). Dimensions of the subvalvar area, annulus, effective valve orifice, and aortic root are measured accurately. Left ventricular cavity size and the presence and severity of left ventricular hypertrophy can be assessed. Indexes of systolic and diastolic function can be calculated. Color Doppler imaging accurately identifies the level of obstruction, allowing a distinction between valvar, subvalvar, and supravalvar stenosis. Doppler measurement of blood flow velocity across the valve provides an estimate of the peak pressure gradient. Progression of disease and timing of intervention therefore can be determined in a noninvasive fashion in most cases.

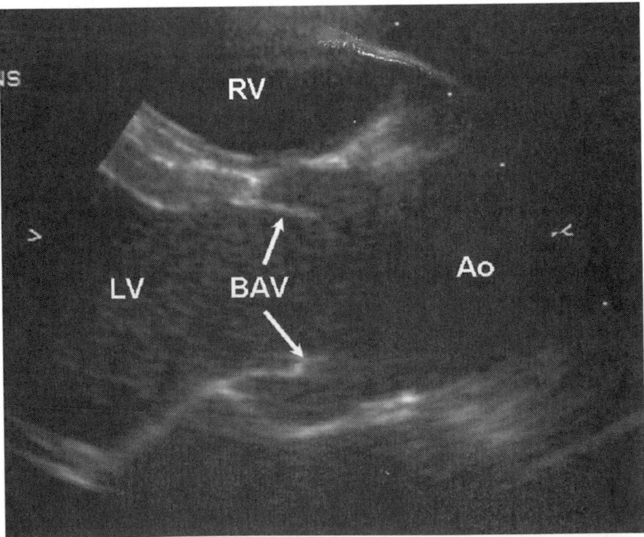

Figure 70-3 Two-dimensional echocardiogram in a patient with congenital aortic stenosis. Long-axis view of bicuspid valve. The leaflets are doming in systole. Ao = aorta; BAV = bicuspid aortic valve; LV = left ventricle; RV = right ventricle. (Image courtesy of Dr. William Ravekes, Division of Pediatric Cardiology, Johns Hopkins Hospital.)

With accurate echocardiographic assessment, cardiac catheterization rarely is required in the diagnostic evaluation of aortic stenosis. It may be indicated to confirm the diagnosis or assess the severity of obstruction when the clinical and echocardiographic findings are equivocal. Direct simultaneous measurement of left ventricular pressure and aortic pressure is the most accurate method for assessing the outflow tract gradient. However, identification of the precise level of obstruction may not be possible. Elevation of left ventricular end-diastolic pressure indicates impaired diastolic function. Left ventriculography allows assessment of ventricular systolic function and may outline the valve leaflets, providing some assessment of morphology.

Treatment

Neonatal critical aortic stenosis

Critical aortic stenosis diagnosed in the newborn period constitutes a medical emergency. A neonatal presentation indicates severe outflow obstruction that requires urgent intervention. Initial stabilization includes endotracheal intubation and inotropic support. Prostaglandin infusion will establish or maintain patency of the ductus arteriosus and improve systemic perfusion. Emergency aortic valvotomy previously was the treatment of choice, performed soon after resuscitation. Recently, however, percutaneous transcatheter balloon aortic valvotomy has supplanted surgical valvotomy in many centers. The procedure is performed in the catheterization laboratory, with the advantages of rapid relief of obstruction and avoidance of cardiopulmonary bypass and aortic cross-clamping. Risk factors for failure include a small aortic annulus, a bicuspid aortic valve, poor left ventricular function, and limited operator experience.[7,8] Outcomes are generally similar to those for open valvotomy. Hospital mortality for either procedure is 0 to 20 percent.[9,10] Mortality is higher in patients with bicuspid valve morphology. Significant aortic regurgitation is more likely after balloon valvotomy, but residual stenosis is more common after surgical valvotomy. The authors' protocol at Children's Hospital and Regional Medical Center in Seattle is to reserve surgical valvotomy for patients in whom balloon valvotomy is unsuccessful. No surgical valvotomy has been required in those patients. Regardless of the technique, neonatal aortic valvotomy is considered a palliative procedure for most patients, with only 48 percent freedom from reoperation after 5 years.[9]

In a small subset of neonates with critical aortic stenosis and small left ventricular size, it may be difficult to determine whether a two-ventricle approach with aortic valvotomy/replacement or a single-ventricle approach with the Norwood procedure is more appropriate.

Rhodes and associates[11] identified criteria, including body surface area, indexed aortic root dimension, ratio of left ventricle to heart length, and indexed mitral valve area, as predictors of successful valvotomy. More recently, a multi-institutional study of 320 patients allowed multiple linear regression analysis of independent factors associated with survival after two-ventricle repair versus Norwood-type palliation.[12] The derived equation requires the following values: age at entry, aortic valve z-score, grade of endocardial fibroelastosis, diameter of ascending aorta, presence of moderate or severe tricuspid regurgitation, and z-score of left ventricular length. A positive result favors the Norwood approach, whereas a negative result favors biventricular repair; the data can be entered and the relative risk of either approach can be estimated by using the website of the Congenital Heart Surgeons Society (www.chssdc.org).

Valvar aortic stenosis in older children

The objectives of surgical treatment of aortic stenosis are relief of symptoms and reduction of the risk of sudden death. Sudden death is related directly to the severity of obstruction and correlates with the peak systolic gradient. Stenosis is considered severe when the gradient is equal to or greater than 75 mmHg, moderate when it is between 50 and 75 mmHg, and mild when it is less than 50 mmHg. Surgery is indicated in any symptomatic patient regardless of severity and in asymptomatic patients with severe stenosis. Surgery is not recommended for asymptomatic patients with mild stenosis. There is controversy about the management of asymptomatic patients with moderate stenosis. Surgical management should be considered on an individual basis. The authors generally recommend surgery in patients who demonstrate a strain pattern on electrocardiography or abnormal exercise testing.

The two options for surgical management of aortic stenosis are valvotomy and aortic valve replacement. Valve replacement in children poses unique challenges that are not seen in the adult population. The smallest mechanical and bioprosthetic valves available (17 to 19 mm) are too large for the annular size of smaller children. Even when replacement is feasible, unless an "adult-sized" valve is used, somatic growth eventually results in recurrent outflow obstruction because the prosthesis size is fixed. Re-replacement with an appropriately sized valve may be limited by restricted annular growth from the original prosthesis.

The choices of prosthetic valves for children are more limited than are those for adults. Bioprostheses do not require anticoagulation, but calcific degeneration occurs at an accelerated rate compared with adults, virtually precluding their use in children.[13] Mechanical prostheses maintain their structural integrity but require anticoagulation with warfarin. Anticoagulation can be achieved safely in children, but issues of compliance, inconsistent diet, and potential for injury increase the risk of bleeding and thromboembolic complications in this patient population.

Allograft replacement of the aortic root became popular in the early 1990s. Small valves with excellent early hemodynamic performance were readily available, and it was hoped that degeneration would not occur. Subsequent reports, however, demonstrated severe accelerated degeneration that required early reoperation in younger children.[14] Severe calcification and inflammatory reaction of surrounding tissues complicate allograft removal and place adjacent structures, including the mitral valve and the bundle of His, at risk during reoperation.

Pulmonary autografting and reconstruction of the right ventricular outflow tract with an allograft (the Ross procedure) is often the best choice for aortic valve replacement in small children. The autograft has growth potential, does not develop calcific degeneration, and does not require anticoagulation. There are, however, a number of important limitations. The aortic and pulmonary annulus sizes must be similar; stretching of the autograft to fit a dilated aortic root will result in neoaortic insufficiency. The operation is technically challenging, requiring longer periods of cardiopulmonary bypass and aortic cross-clamping compared with other techniques for valve replacement. Allograft reconstruction of the right ventricular outflow tract necessitates eventual reoperation for conduit stenosis from somatic growth and calcific degeneration. Finally, it has been recognized that congenitally bicuspid aortic stenosis may be associated with a connective tissue disorder that involves fibrillin-1 production. The pulmonary autograft in these patients may be prone to dilatation and aortic insufficiency, especially when exposed to the higher pressures in the systemic circulation. Further follow-up is necessary, but caution is warranted when one is contemplating pulmonary autograft aortic root replacement in this patient population.[15,16]

In summary, there is no ideal substitute for aortic valve replacement in children. Aortic valvotomy is, whenever feasible, the procedure of choice in this population. Although often not definitive, adequate palliation usually is achieved. Small residual gradients and mild aortic insufficiency are acceptable. Valvotomy can defer the need for valve replacement significantly, allowing insertion of a larger prosthesis at a later time and reducing the total number of re-replacements required over a patient's lifetime.

Aortic valvotomy

Aortic valvotomy is performed via a median sternotomy. A single right atrial cannula provides venous drainage, and the aortic cannula is placed as distally as possible. Some surgeons advocate closed valvotomy that is performed by passing dilators of increasing size through the aortic valve; the dilators are introduced through a purse string in the left ventricular apex. This technique is performed with cardiopulmonary bypass but avoids the need for aortic cross-clamping and cardioplegic arrest. The authors believe that open valvotomy with direct visualization of the aortic valve allows more precise leaflet separation, resulting in better relief of gradient and a decreased risk of significant aortic insufficiency.

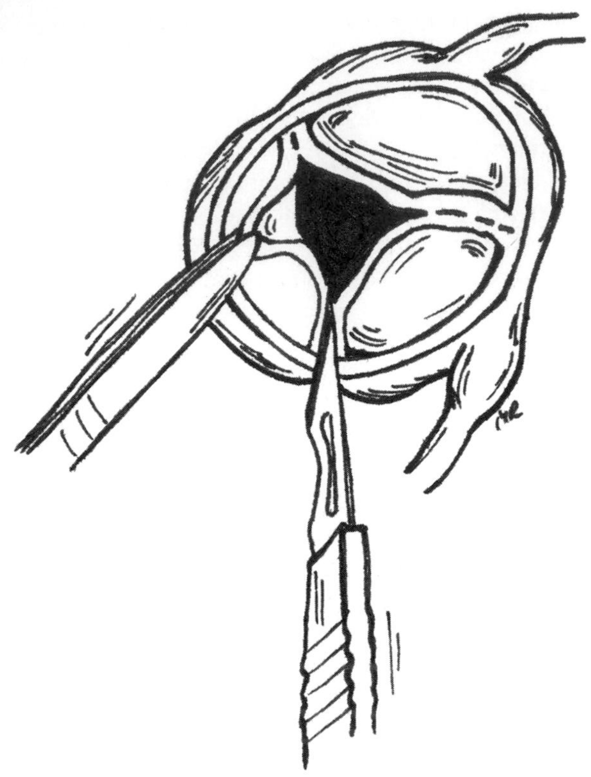

Figure 70-4 Open aortic valvotomy. The incision is performed toward the commissural post of the nonfused leaflets.

The aorta is clamped, and cardioplegia is delivered via the aortic root. A transverse aortotomy is made just above the sinotubular junction, with care taken to avoid injury to the right coronary artery and the aortic valve leaflets. The valve is inspected carefully. Fused commissures are opened precisely with a scalpel (Fig. 70-4). The incisions are not extended to the aortic wall, since this may result in loss of support and aortic insufficiency. Excessive fibrous tissue, if present, is excised from the leaflets. Fibrous attachments between the base of the leaflets and the aortic wall are divided to maximize leaflet mobility. Despite these steps, the effective orifice may be inadequate, particularly in smaller bicuspid valves. Ilbawi and colleagues[17] described a technique of extended valvotomy for these patients. Circumferential incisions are made above the true commissures and raphes (Fig. 70-5). They reported a low incidence of aortic insufficiency and significantly lower gradients compared with standard valvotomy. The aortotomy is closed precisely to avoid supravalvar narrowing, and the cross-clamp is removed. The patient is weaned from cardiopulmonary bypass with mild inotropic support (dopamine 5 μg/kg/min and milrinone 0.5 μg/kg/min). The adequacy of repair is assessed by transesophageal echocardiography and direct measurement of pressure in the left ventricle and ascending aorta. Modified ultrafiltration is performed before decannulation.

Early mortality in older infants and children undergoing aortic valvotomy is reported currently to be less than 2 percent,[2,7] and late mortality is rare. Reintervention for progressive regurgitation or restenosis may be required, but this generally occurs later than in neonates. The reoperation rate in children over 1 year of age at the time of the initial valvotomy is 2 percent at 10 years but then increases 3.3 percent per year.[18]

Aortic valve replacement Aortic valve replacement is required when valvotomy is not sufficient to reduce the transvalvar gradient adequately. In larger children with adequate annular size, simple replacement of the valve is performed as it is in adults. Prosthesis selection should be individualized. The authors generally avoid porcine and bovine bioprostheses as well as allograft implantation because of the rapid degeneration and early failure observed in children. The remaining options therefore are limited to mechanical prosthesis and pulmonary autograft.

Aortic valve replacement with a mechanical prosthesis is performed via a median sternotomy. A single right atrial or two-stage venous cannula provides venous

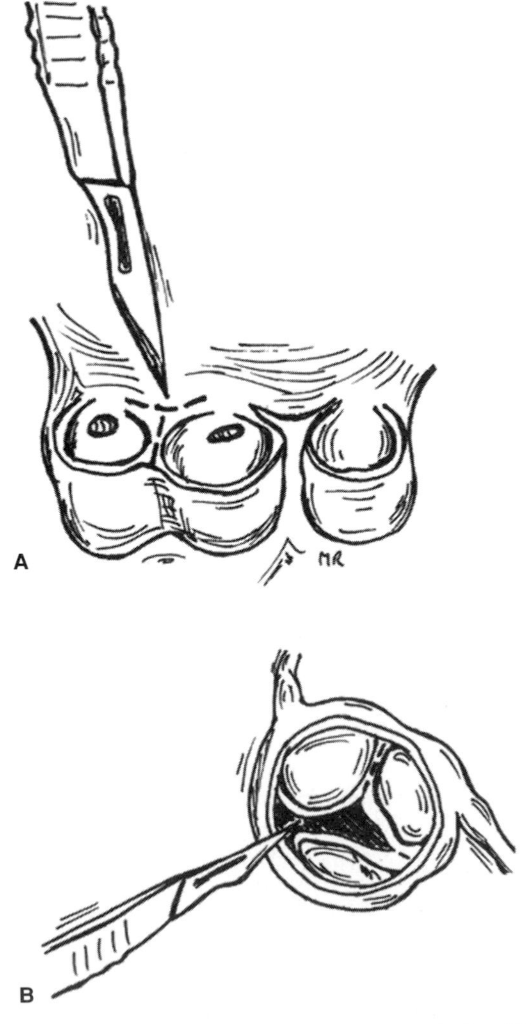

Figure 70-5 Extended aortic valvotomy. A. Lateral view demonstrating incisions at true commissures and raphe. B. Cranial view.

drainage, and the ascending aorta is cannulated distally. The aorta is clamped, and in the absence of significant aortic insufficiency, cardioplegia is infused in the aortic root. After aortotomy, additional cardioplegia is delivered every 30 min through a retrograde coronary sinus catheter or by direct coronary ostial perfusion. A left ventricular vent is placed through the left atrial appendage or the right superior pulmonary vein.

A transverse aortotomy is made and is extended into the noncoronary sinus of Valsalva. The aortic valve leaflets are excised. Interrupted pledgeted mattress sutures are placed circumferentially around the annulus. In smaller patients, intraannular placement may be preferable to avoid coronary ostial obstruction by the sewing ring. The sutures are passed through the sewing ring, and the valve is parachuted into place. After the sutures are tied, the prosthetic leaflets are assessed carefully to ensure unhindered mobility. The aortotomy is closed, and the aortic clamp is removed. The patient is weaned from cardiopulmonary bypass with mild inotropic support. Transesophageal echocardiography is used to assess prosthetic function. Modified ultrafiltration is performed before decannulation.

Hospital mortality after mechanical aortic valve replacement in children is 0 to 5 percent. Early complications include permanent heart block in 3 percent and acute endocarditis in 2 percent of these patients. Late complications relate primarily to anticoagulation. In reports of long-term follow-up, valve thrombosis occurs in 0 to 2 percent of patients. This sometimes can be managed pharmacologically with thrombolytic agents but frequently requires urgent surgical thrombectomy or valve replacement. Embolic events are reported in 2 percent, and significant bleeding episodes occur at a rate of 0.15 percent per patient year.[19,20]

Ross procedure Ross[21] reported aortic valve replacement with a pulmonary autograft and allograft reconstruction of the right ventricular outflow tract in 1967 (Fig. 70-6). In the absence of significant size discrepancy or connective tissue disease, the Ross procedure is the preferred technique for aortic valve replacement in small children. In larger children, it frequently is preferred over mechanical prosthesis to avoid the need for anticoagulation.

The approach is via a median sternotomy. The venae cavae are cannulated individually, and the ascending aorta is cannulated distally. The aorta is clamped, and in the absence of significant aortic insufficiency, cardioplegia is infused in the aortic root. Cardioplegia also may be delivered retrograde through a coronary sinus catheter and by direct coronary ostial perfusion after an aortotomy. Additional cardioplegia is delivered every 30 min during the cross-clamp period. A left ventricular vent is placed through the left atrial appendage or the right superior pulmonary vein.

The aorta and the pulmonary trunk are separated, and the pulmonary trunk is opened transversely just proximal to the bifurcation. The pulmonary valve is inspected to identify any pathology that would preclude its use as an aortic valve replacement. Transection of the pulmonary trunk then is completed. A right-angle clamp is passed carefully through the leaflets into the right ventricular outflow tract, and a site for proximal transection is identified in the infundibular free wall approximately 5 mm below the level of the valve. A transverse infundibular incision is made and carried to the infundibular septum at each end. The infundibular septum is scored with a scalpel blade. A plane can be developed between the subconal muscle and the underlying interventricular septum. Dissection in this plane completes the harvest, and the autograft is stored in normal saline solution before implantation. The resulting posterior raw surface is cauterized. In their practice, the authors also apply a thin layer of biological sealant to ensure hemostasis. In dissecting the autograft, care must be taken at the leftward extent of the septal dissection to avoid injury to the first septal perforating branch of the left anterior descending coronary artery. The pulmonary artery is sized, and an appropriate allograft is thawed and prepared for reconstruction of the right ventricular outflow tract.

The aorta is transected just above the sinotubular junction. The aortic valve leaflets are excised, and the left and right coronary arteries are excised with a generous button of aortic wall. The autograft is oriented by alignment of the commissures. A proximal anastomosis then is constructed. Interrupted simple braided sutures are used for smaller patients, although a continuous technique with polypropylene sutures can be used in larger children and teenagers. The coronary buttons are anastomosed to incisions in the respective autograft sinuses of Valsalva. The distal aortic anastomosis is constructed with a running polypropylene suture. Air is evacuated from the left side of the heart, and the aortic clamp is removed. Continuity between the right ventricle and the pulmonary artery is restored by interposing the previously thawed allograft in the reperfused, beating heart. The patient is weaned from cardiopulmonary bypass with mild inotropic support. Transesophageal echocardiography is used to assess autograft and allograft function as well as left ventricular wall motion. Modified ultrafiltration is performed before decannulation in children with an operative weight below 20 kg.

The results of the Ross procedure are excellent in carefully selected pediatric patients. Early mortality is 0 to 6 percent, occurring primarily in infants under 5 months of age.[22–25] Complications occur infrequently and include bleeding, arrhythmia, heart block, and stroke.[24,25] Actuarial survival at 7 years is over 90 percent,[23,24] and actuarial freedom from reoperation is 93 to 100 percent.[22,23] Aortic root dilatation is common late after the Ross procedure in children and warrants careful echocardiographic follow-up.[26,27]

Konno aortoventriculoplasty Annular enlargement is required in children with small aortic annular size requiring

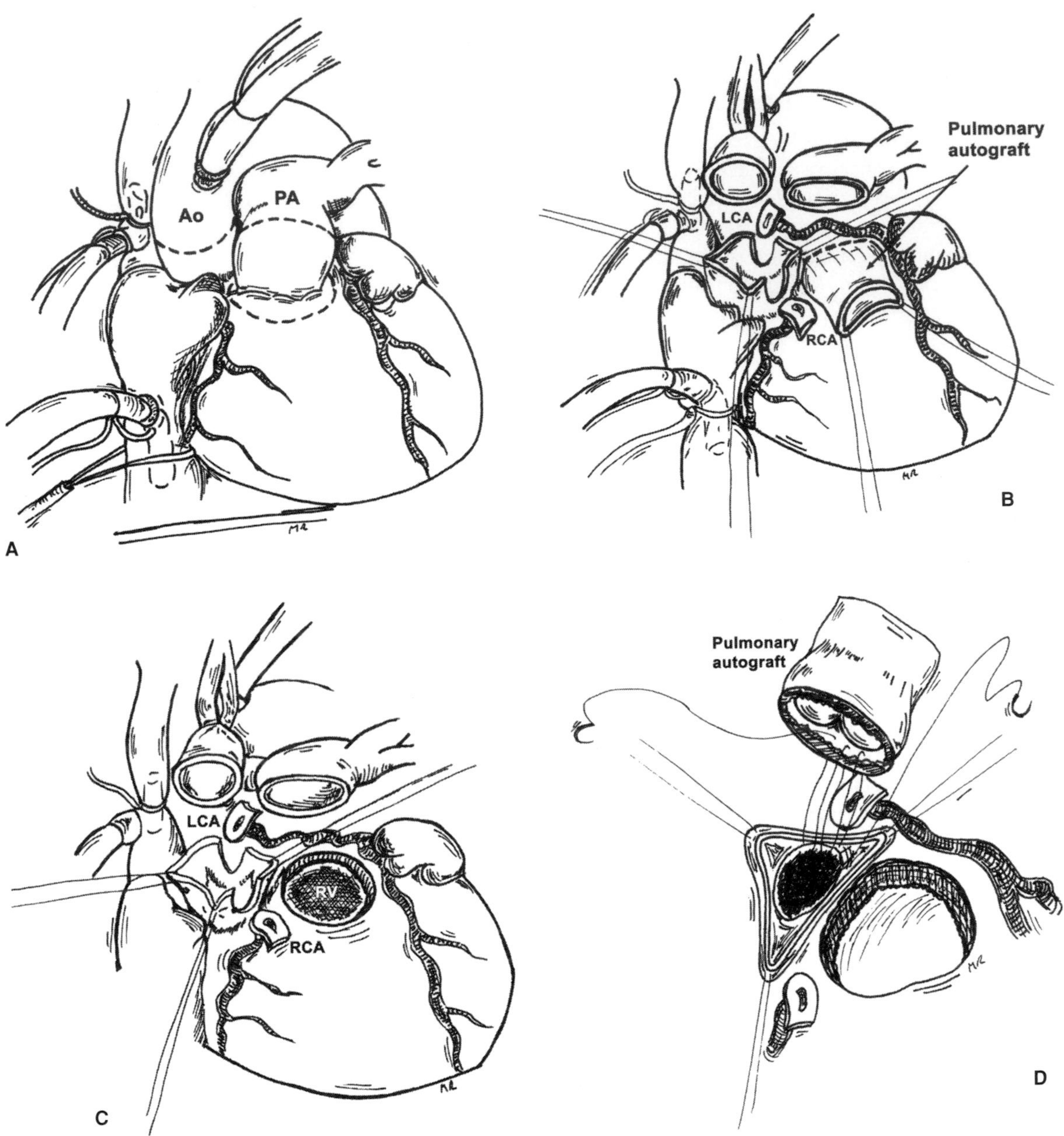

Figure 70-6 Ross procedure. A. Dotted lines indicate incisions in the aorta, pulmonary trunk, and right ventricular infundibulum. B. The aorta and pulmonary artery are transected, and the coronary buttons are excised from the sinuses of Valsalva. C. Removal of the pulmonary autograft. D. The proximal anastomosis of the pulmonary autograft is begun posteriorly.

aortic valve replacement. Nicks and colleagues[28] and Manougian and Seybold-Epting[29] described techniques for posterior annular enlargement that have been used successfully in adults. However, the resulting increase in annular size is generally inadequate to allow insertion of even a small prosthetic valve in small children. Konno and coworkers[30] described a technique of anterior enlargement that more effectively increases annular size and relieves coexistent subvalvar stenosis (Fig. 70-7).

The approach is via a median sternotomy. The venae cavae are cannulated individually, and the ascending aorta is cannulated distally. The aorta is clamped, and in the absence of significant aortic insufficiency, cardioplegia is infused in the aortic root. Additional cardioplegia is delivered every 30 min during the cross-clamp period. A left ventricular vent is placed through the left atrial appendage or the right superior pulmonary vein.

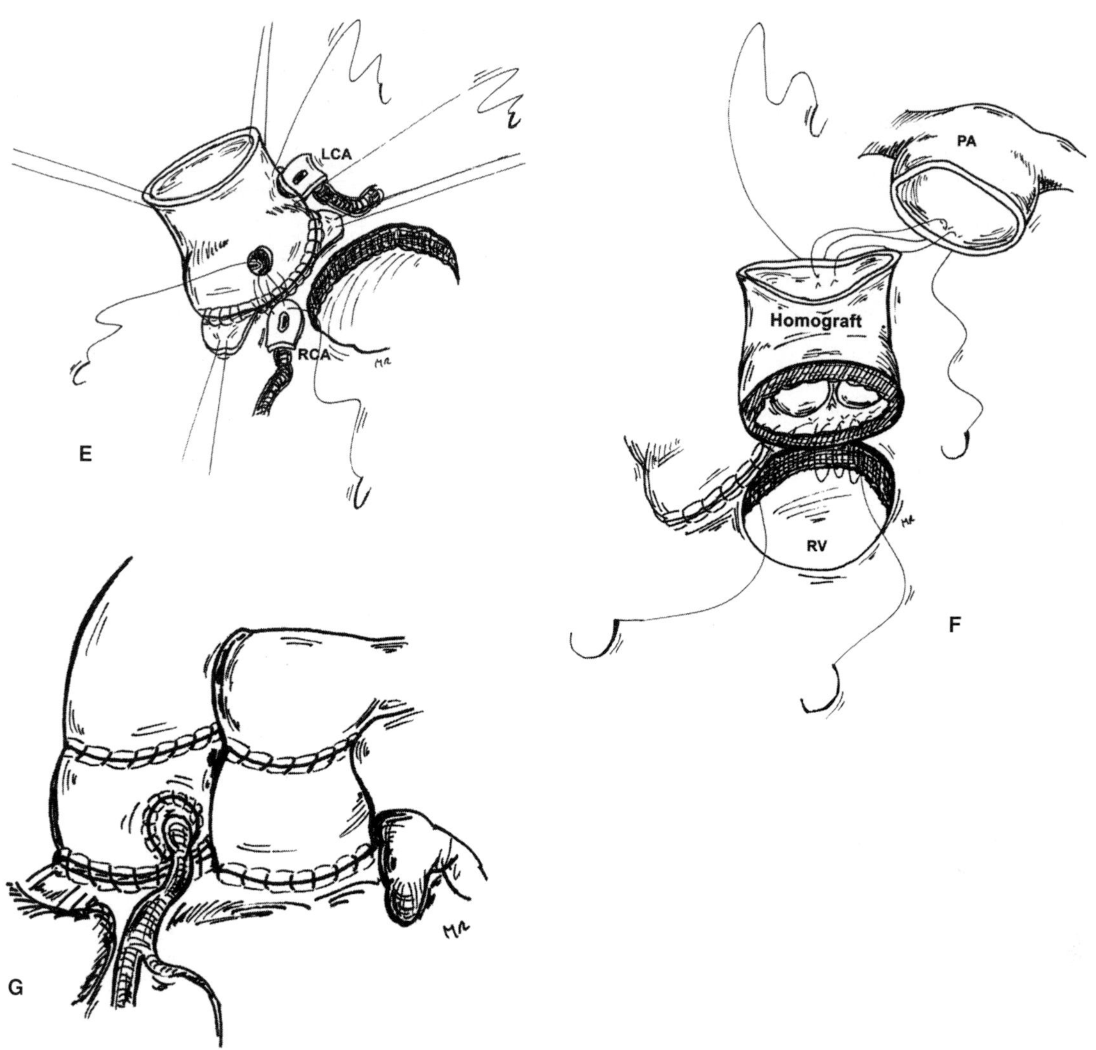

Figure 70-6 (*continued*) E. The proximal autograft anastomosis is completed, and the coronary buttons are sutured to the autograft sinuses of Valsalva. F. A homograft restores continuity of the right ventricular outflow tract. G. The autograft is anastomosed distally to the ascending aorta. Ao = aorta; LAD = left anterior descending coronary artery; LCA = left coronary artery; PA = pulmonary artery; RCA = right coronary artery; RV = right ventricle.

A vertical aortotomy is made and is carried onto the right ventricular outflow tract well to the left of the origin of the right coronary artery. Care is taken to avoid injury to the pulmonary valve. The aortic valve leaflets are excised, allowing visualization of the left and right ventricular aspects of the infundibular septum. An incision is made across the aortic annulus into the infundibular septum. Injury to the conduction tissue is avoided by placing this incision to the left of the papillary muscle of the conus (muscle of Lancisi). A diamond-shaped patch of Dacron is fashioned, and the inferior portion is sutured to the edges of the septal incision with interrupted pledgeted mattress sutures. An appropriately sized prosthetic valve then is inserted as was described for aortic valve replacement. Anteriorly, the valve sutures are passed through the prosthetic patch. The superior portion of the patch is used to close the ascending aorta. The right ventricular free wall is enlarged with a patch of bovine pericardium. Air is evacuated from the left side of the heart, and the aortic clamp is removed. The patient is weaned from cardiopulmonary bypass with mild inotropic support. Transesophageal echocardiography is used to assess prosthetic function, patch leaks, and left ventricular wall motion.

A modification of this technique can be used for annular enlargement in conjunction with the Ross procedure. The pulmonary autograft is harvested with a triangular portion of right ventricular free wall that is used as the septal patch (Fig. 70-8).

In light of the complex form of LVOTO seen in pediatric patients who require the Konno or the Ross-Konno

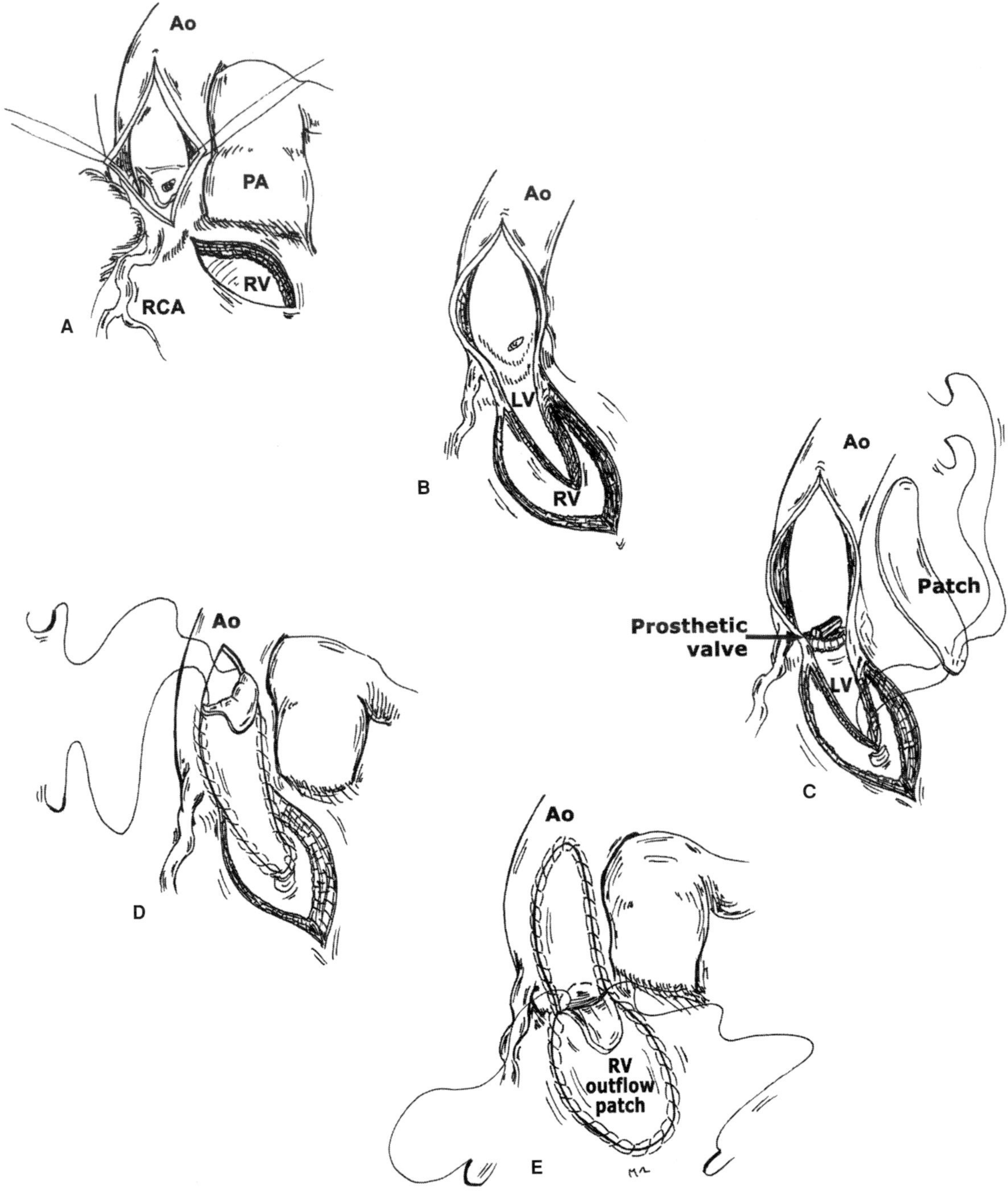

Figure 70-7 Konno aortoventriculoplasty. A. A longitudinal aortotomy is extended to the right ventricular infundibulum. The incision is to the left of the origin of the right coronary artery. B. The aortic leaflets are excised. An incision is made through the annulus and extended into the infundibular septum. C. The aortic valve prosthesis is sutured to the annulus posteriorly. The lower portion of a diamond-shaped patch is sutured to the septum, enlarging the annulus and subvalvar area. D. The prosthetic valve is sutured to the patch anteriorly, and the upper portion of the patch closes the aortotomy. E. The right ventriculotomy is closed with a patch of bovine pericardium. Ao = aorta; PA = pulmonary artery; RCA = right coronary artery; LV = left ventricle; RV = right ventricle.

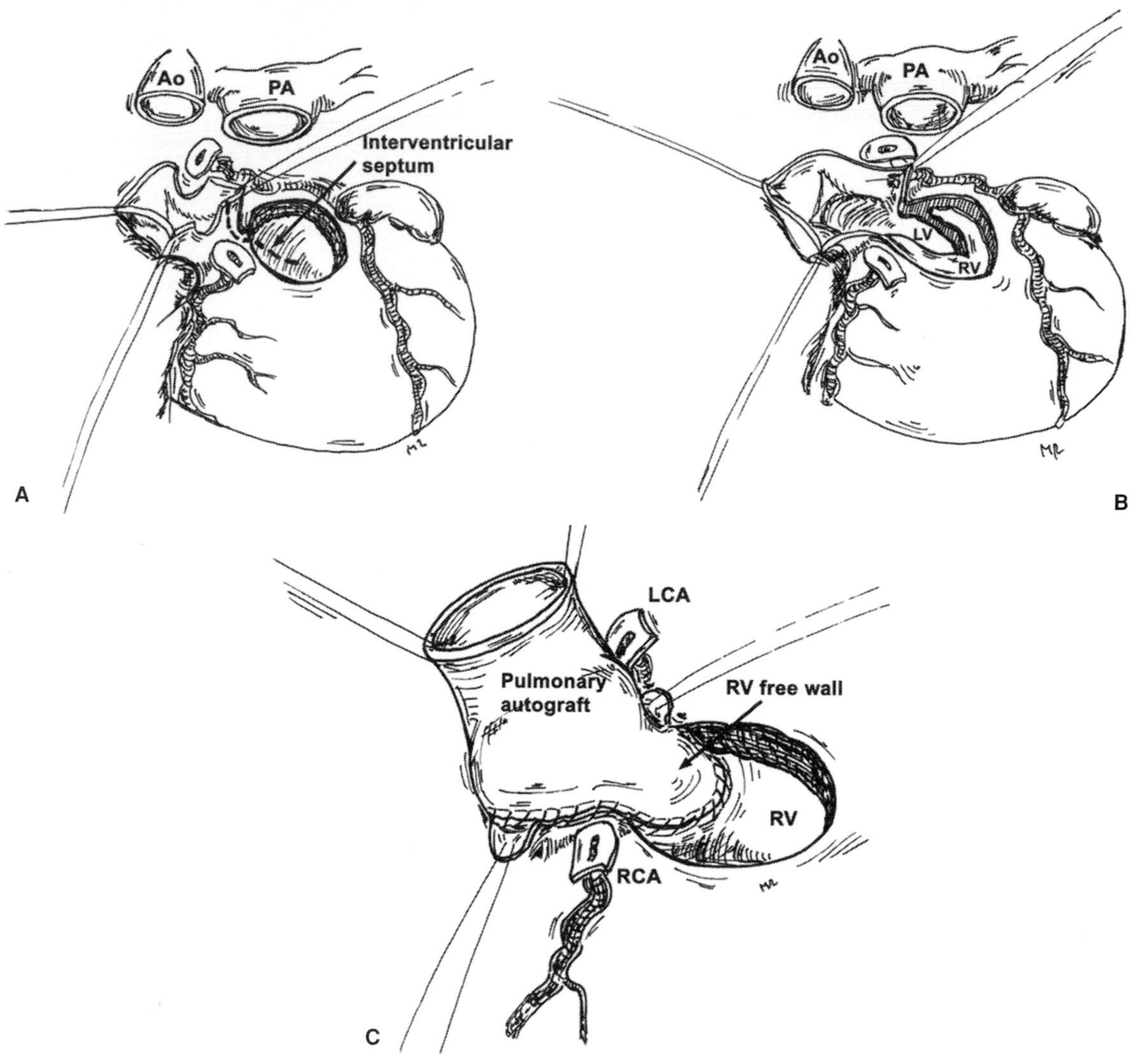

Figure 70-8 Ross-Konno procedure. A. The aorta and autograft are prepared as illustrated in Fig. 70-6A–C. An incision is made across the aortic annulus and extended into the septum. B. The annulus and subvalvar area are enlarged. C. The autograft is harvested with a triangular portion of right ventricular free wall that is used for septal closure. LV = left ventricle; RV = right ventricle.

procedure, early and late results are quite good. On average, the annulus is enlarged to twice the original size.[31] Operative mortality for the Konno procedure with prosthetic valve replacement is 5 to 15 percent. Ten-year actuarial survival is 90 percent. Ten-year freedom from reoperation with a mechanical prosthesis is 80 to 89 percent. At 15 years it falls to 52 percent, largely as a result of valve outgrowth.[31,32] Ten-year freedom from reoperation with a bioprosthesis is 0 percent, primarily because of valve degeneration.[32] Operative mortality for the Ross-Konno procedure is 0 to 7 percent even in children under 1 year of age.[22,32,33] Postoperative complications include bleeding, arrhythmia, heart block, and left ventricular dysfunction. No permanent effects on ventricular function are present at long-term follow-up.[34]

SUBVALVAR AORTIC STENOSIS

Subaortic stenosis in children results from either a discrete fibrous membrane or, less commonly, diffuse, fibromuscular tunnel-like stenosis. The discrete subaortic membrane is probably an acquired lesion that rarely is seen in infants. Turbulence within a small or elongated aortic root causes thickening of the endocardium. A ring of fibrous tissue results that is adherent to the septum anteriorly, extending posteriorly to the right and left fibrous trigones and to the anterior mitral leaflet.[35] Associated subaortic anomalies are present in 31 percent of these patients, including anomalous septal insertion of the mitral valve, accessory mitral valve tissue, anomalous papillary muscles, and anomalous muscular bands.[36] In addition to outflow obstruction, aortic insufficiency develops in more than 50 percent of these patients from turbulence-induced leaflet deformity or direct attachment of the membrane to the aortic leaflets.[37]

Tunnel-like subaortic stenosis is a congenital lesion in which the subaortic region is diffusely hypoplastic. Thickened septal myocardium and endocardial fibrosis contribute to outflow tract obstruction.

Signs and symptoms

Patients with discrete subaortic stenosis usually present after infancy when an asymptomatic murmur is detected on physical examination. Early symptoms include feeding intolerance and easy fatigability. Chest pain, syncope, and congestive heart failure may develop with worsening obstruction. A systolic ejection murmur without an ejection click is heard on auscultation. A diastolic decrescendo murmur may be heard at the left lower sternal border when a discrete subaortic membrane causes aortic insufficiency. Tunnel-like fibromuscular stenosis often presents in infancy but is otherwise indistinguishable from a discrete membrane on the basis of signs and symptoms.

Diagnosis

Chest x-ray is usually nondiagnostic. Findings generally are limited to moderate left ventricular enlargement, left atrial enlargement, and prominence of the aortic knob.

The electrocardiogram shows left ventricular hypertrophy. Serial findings of increasing QRS voltage and the development of a strain pattern suggest worsening obstruction.

Two-dimensional echocardiography is the primary diagnostic method for diagnosing subaortic stenosis and distinguishing a discrete fibrous membrane from the diffuse fibromuscular type of obstruction. A discrete membrane usually is detected below the aortic valve, extending from the anterior mitral leaflet to the septum (Fig. 70-9). Diffuse fibromuscular stenosis is identified as a long hypoplastic outflow tract (Fig. 70-10). A color Doppler flow study reveals the level of obstruction below the aortic valve leaflets and will detect the presence of aortic insufficiency. Doppler measurement of blood flow velocity in the outflow tract provides an estimate of the peak pressure gradient. Progression of disease and timing of intervention therefore can be determined in a noninvasive fashion.

With accurate echocardiographic assessment, cardiac catheterization rarely is required in the diagnostic evaluation of subaortic stenosis. It may be indicated to assess the severity of obstruction when the clinical and echocardiographic findings are equivocal.

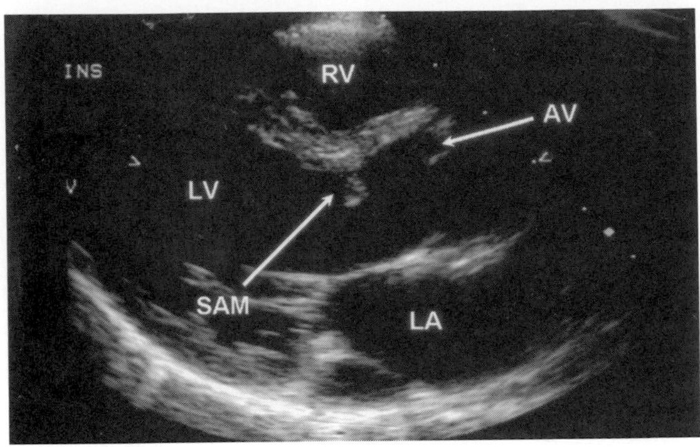

Figure 70-9 Two-dimensional echocardiogram of discrete subaortic membrane. Parasternal long-axis view. AV = aortic valve; LA = left atrium; LV = left ventricle; RV = right ventricle; SAM = subaortic membrane. (Image courtesy of Dr. William Ravekes, Division of Pediatric Cardiology, Johns Hopkins Hospital.)

Treatment

Discrete fibrous subaortic stenosis

Surgical excision of a discrete fibrous subaortic membrane is indicated for relief of symptoms, for severe obstruction (gradient greater than 50 mmHg), and when moderate to severe aortic insufficiency is present. Asymptomatic patients with gradients less than 30 mmHg

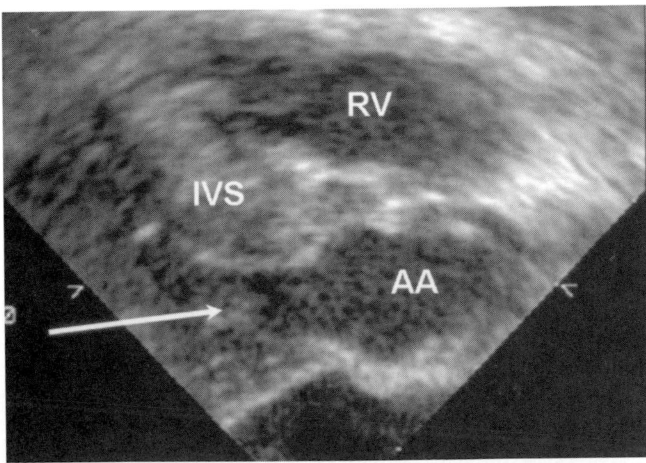

Figure 70-10 Two-dimensional transesophageal echocardiogram of diffuse fibromuscular tunnel-like subaortic stenosis. The arrow points to the subaortic stenotic left ventricular outlet. AA = ascending aorta; IVS = interventricular septum; RV = right ventricle. (Image courtesy of Dr. William Ravekes, Division of Pediatric Cardiology, Johns Hopkins Hospital.)

and without significant aortic insufficiency do not require surgery but should be followed with serial echocardiograms to detect progression. There is controversy about asymptomatic patients with moderate obstruction and mild aortic insufficiency. Some centers advocate prophylactic excision in all cases, citing the low risk of surgery and the benefit of preventing aortic insufficiency.[38] However, natural history studies have demonstrated that many of these patients do not progress beyond mild obstruction or aortic regurgitation over many years.[39] Furthermore, recurrent stenosis and progressive aortic insufficiency may develop despite apparently successful membrane excision.[38–40] Patients with a gradient greater than 30 mmHg, close proximity of the membrane to the aortic valve, and membrane extension to the mitral valve are at higher risk for progressive obstruction and should undergo surgical repair.[41] Older age and a gradient above 50 mmHg are independent risk factors for progressive aortic insufficiency and are indications for repair.[42]

The surgical approach is via a median sternotomy. A single right atrial or a two-stage venous cannula provides venous drainage, and the ascending aorta is cannulated distally. The aorta is clamped, and in the absence of significant aortic insufficiency, cardioplegia is infused in the aortic root. A transverse aortotomy is made and is extended into the noncoronary sinus of Valsalva. The aortic valve leaflets are retracted gently, allowing visualization of the membrane in the left ventricular outflow tract.

The membrane is grasped anteriorly with a skin hook or a traction suture. A radial incision is made into the membrane, extending just into the underlying septal myocardium. The membrane then is excised circumferentially by blunt dissection. Care is taken to avoid injury to the anterior leaflet of the mitral valve and the aortic valve leaflets. Resection of additional septal muscle is performed to ensure complete excision of the membrane. Yacoub and colleagues[35] advocate the additional resection of fibrous tissue in the left and right fibrous trigones.

The aortotomy is closed, and the aortic clamp is removed. The patient is weaned from cardiopulmonary bypass. Transesophageal echocardiography is used to assess relief of obstruction and aortic insufficiency. After resection of discrete subaortic membrane, mortality approaches zero. Permanent heart block and iatrogenic ventricular septal defect occur in fewer than 5 percent of these patients. Reoperation for recurrent obstruction is required in 15 to 20 percent of patients at 5 years.[38,39] Aortic insufficiency progresses in 25 percent of patients at 10-year follow-up but is three times more likely in patients with a preoperative gradient over 40 mmHg.[38]

The indications for excision of recurrent discrete subaortic stenosis are the same as those for the initial operation. Re-resection with more aggressive septal myectomy is the authors' procedure of choice. In the case of a second recurrence, a modified Konno procedure is performed as described below for the treatment of tunnel-like stenosis.

Diffuse fibromuscular subaortic stenosis

Indications for surgery in patients with tunnel-like subaortic stenosis are the same as those for patients with a discrete subaortic membrane, but relief of the obstruction is technically more challenging. Resection of fibromuscular tissue from the septum may be possible, but this is often inadequate because of the long circumferential narrowing of the outflow tract. Conal enlargement with a modified Konno procedure is the preferred approach in these patients (Fig. 70-11).[43]

The modified Konno procedure is performed via a median sternotomy incision. The venae cavae are cannulated individually, and the ascending aorta is cannulated distally. The aorta is clamped, and cardioplegia is infused in the aortic root. A transverse aortotomy is made just above the sinotubular junction. The subaortic area is inspected through the retracted aortic valve leaflets. A transverse incision is made in the right ventricular infundibulum, allowing visualization of the infundibular septum. A right-angle clamp is passed through the aortic annulus, and a safe site for septal incision is identified. A full-thickness longitudinal septal incision is made through the right ventriculotomy, and subaortic fibromuscular tissue is resected. The resulting ventricular septal defect is closed with a Dacron or Gore-Tex patch. The right ventriculotomy is closed with a bovine pericardial patch, and the patient is weaned from cardiopulmonary bypass in the usual fashion. Early mortality was 0 percent in several large series of patients who underwent a modified Konno procedure. Excellent relief of obstruction is obtained, with no permanent heart block and no hemodynamically significant residual ventricular septal defects. More long-term follow-up is required, but freedom from reoperation at 3 years has been found to be 95 to 100 percent.[44,45]

Placement of a left ventricular apicoaortic valved conduit has been described for patients with severe outflow tract obstruction considered not amenable to conventional repair.[46] The authors believe that nearly all patients can be treated more definitively with resection and a modified Konno procedure.

SUPRAVALVAR AORTIC STENOSIS

Supravalvar aortic stenosis is the least common form of LVOTO. The underlying biochemical mechanism is abnormal elastin synthesis that is related to mutations in the chromosome region 7q11.23. This may occur in association with Williams's syndrome, as an autosomal dominant familial trait, or as a sporadic finding.[47]

The pathologic lesion in supravalvar stenosis is a thickening of the aortic wall that results from collagen

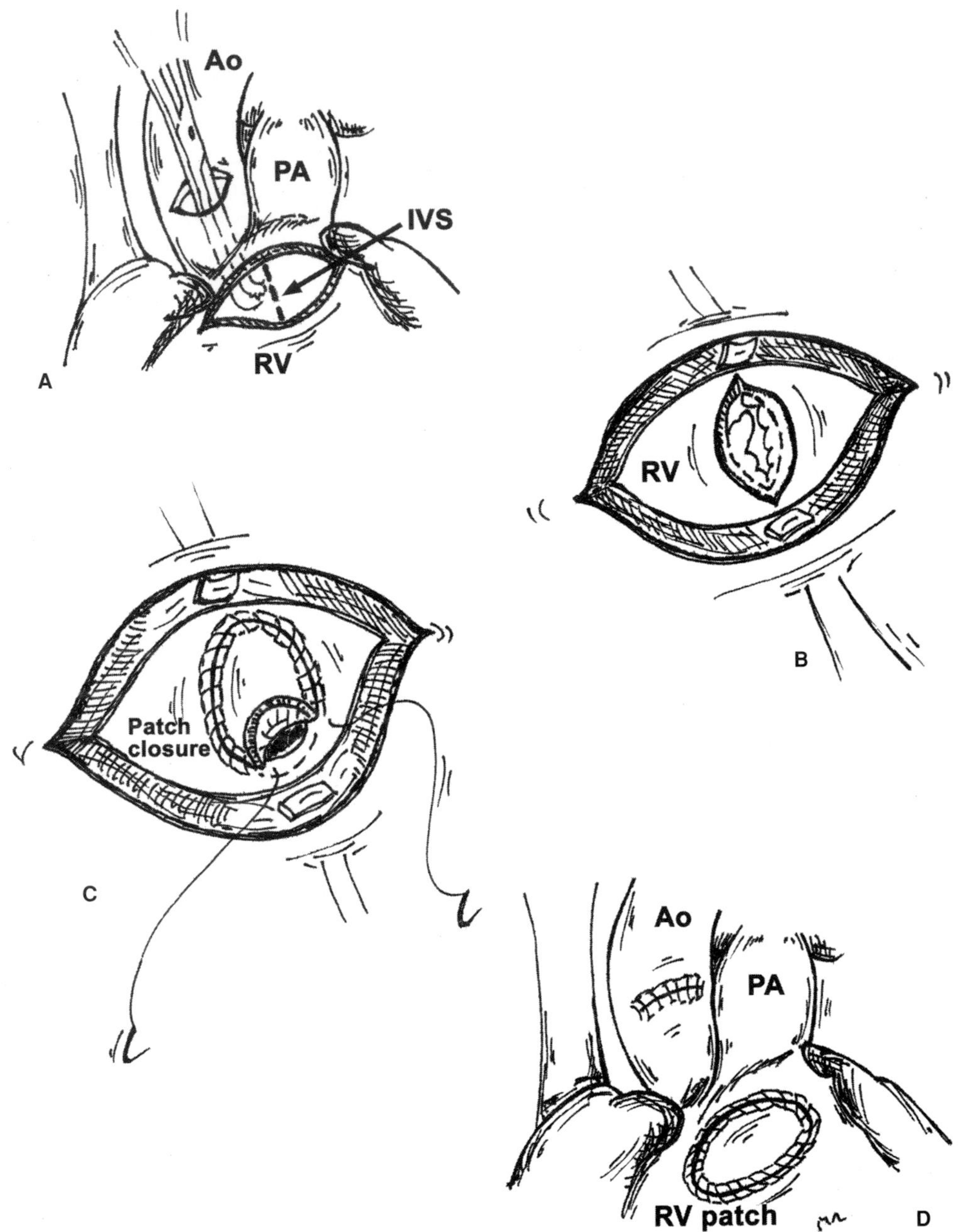

Figure 70-11 Modified Konno procedure. A. Transverse incisions are made in the aorta and right ventricular infundibulum. A right-angle clamp is passed through the aortic valve leaflets to identify the site of septal incision. B. The septum is incised longitudinally, and fibromuscular tissue is resected. C. The ventricular septal defect is closed with a synthetic patch. D. The right ventricular incision is closed with a bovine pericardial patch. Ao = aorta; IVS = interventricular septum; PA = pulmonary artery; RV = right ventricle.

deposition and smooth muscle hypertrophy in the media as well as hyperplasia and fibrosis of the intima.[48] The narrowing is localized to the sinotubular junction in 85 percent of cases, with either an hourglass or a discrete membranous morphology. Diffuse hypoplasia is present in 15 percent of cases and involves the entire ascending aorta, occasionally extending to the transverse arch and the descending aorta.[49]

Although the site of stenosis may be localized, it is important to recognize that the pathologic process involves the entire aortic root.[50,51] Distortion of the aortic valve and sinuses of Valsalva may occur, including leaflet adherence to the stenotic ridge at the sinotubular junction. Concomitant valvar or subvalvar stenosis is present in 20 to 40 percent of these patients.[49,52,53]

Coronary ostial stenosis, most commonly involving the left coronary artery, occurs in 25 percent of these patients.[49] Three mechanisms have been identified: (1) Thickening of the ostial wall may occur as part of the generalized aortopathy, (2) adherence of the aortic valve cusp to the sinotubular junction may isolate the ostium from the lumen of the aorta, and (3) diffuse narrowing of the left main coronary artery may represent a form of premature atherosclerosis that results from the abnormally high sinus of Valsalva pressures.[54] Ischemic lesions are found in 80 percent of autopsy specimens.[55]

Signs and symptoms

Patients with supravalvar aortic stenosis typically present in the first year of life, although cardiovascular findings are present in less than one-third of these newborns.[56] Symptoms include feeding or exercise intolerance, angina, and syncope. About 10 percent of patients are asymptomatic.[53]

Patients with Williams's syndrome may be identified by the presence of dysmorphic "elfin" facies, mental retardation, poor growth, urogenital anomalies, and hypercalcemia. Cardiovascular findings include a systolic ejection murmur with radiation to the neck and poor carotid pulse upstroke.

Diagnosis

As with other causes of LVOTO, chest x-ray findings are nonspecific. Mild to moderate left ventricular and left atrial enlargement may be present.

The electrocardiogram shows left ventricular hypertrophy. ST-segment and T-wave abnormalities consistent with ischemia may be seen in patients with coronary artery involvement. Two-dimensional echocardiography is the usual method of diagnosis in patients with supravalvar aortic stenosis. Decreased aortic caliber, increased wall thickness, and abnormal leaflet mobility are identified. Localized stenosis can be distinguished from the more diffuse pattern, and the extent of distal involvement can be assessed. Coronary ostial involvement as well as concomitant subaortic stenosis also can be detected. In contrast to valvar and subvalvar stenosis, echocardiographic measurement of peak gradients in supravalvar stenosis correlates poorly with catheter-measured gradients. Echocardiography therefore is less helpful in assessing the severity of obstruction and the timing of surgical intervention.[57]

Cardiac catheterization is performed routinely to assess patients with supravalvar stenosis when surgical repair is being considered. It is the only method for accurate measurement of the peak systolic gradient. Aortography distinguishes the localized type from diffuse hypoplasia and accurately defines the distal extent of narrowing (Fig. 70-12). Coronary ostial stenosis can be detected; this is helpful in planning the surgical procedure.

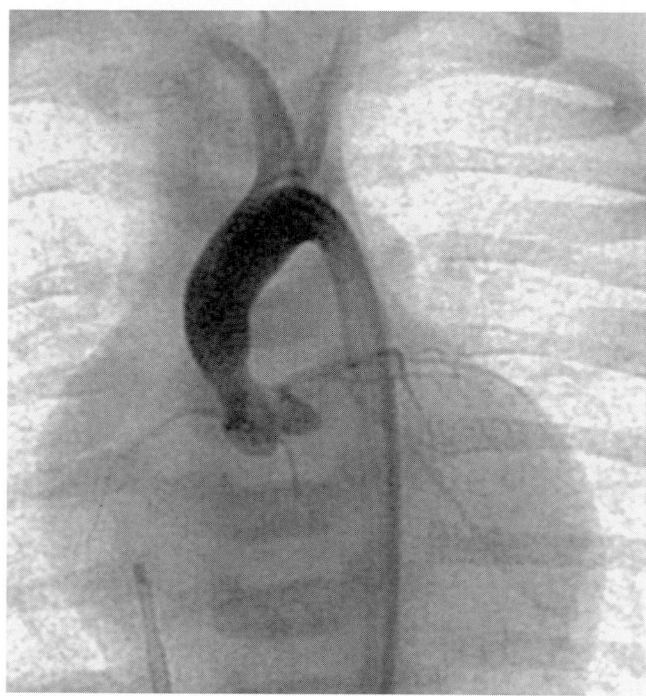

Figure 70-12 Aortogram of supravalvar aortic stenosis. The typical hourglass appearance of the ascending aorta is demonstrated. (Courtesy of Dr. Richard Ringel, Division of Pediatric Cardiology, The Johns Hopkins Hospital.)

Treatment

Surgical repair of supravalvar aortic stenosis is indicated in symptomatic patients as well as in asymptomatic patients with a peak catheter-measured systolic gradient greater than 50 mmHg. The goals of repair are to relieve outflow obstruction and restore normal geometry to the aortic valve and sinuses of Valsalva.

The approach is via a median sternotomy. A single right atrial cannula provides venous drainage, and the aortic cannula is placed as distally as possible. The aorta is clamped, and cardioplegia is delivered via the aortic root. A number of aortoplasty techniques have been described for relief of localized stenosis. McGoon and coinvestigators[58] first performed a longitudinal aortotomy, beginning above the area of narrowing and extending into the noncoronary sinus of Valsalva (Fig. 70-13). The stenotic ridge is excised, and a diamond-shaped patch of bovine pericardium, Dacron, or Gore-Tex is used to augment the ascending aorta. With the recognition that distortion of the aortic valve and

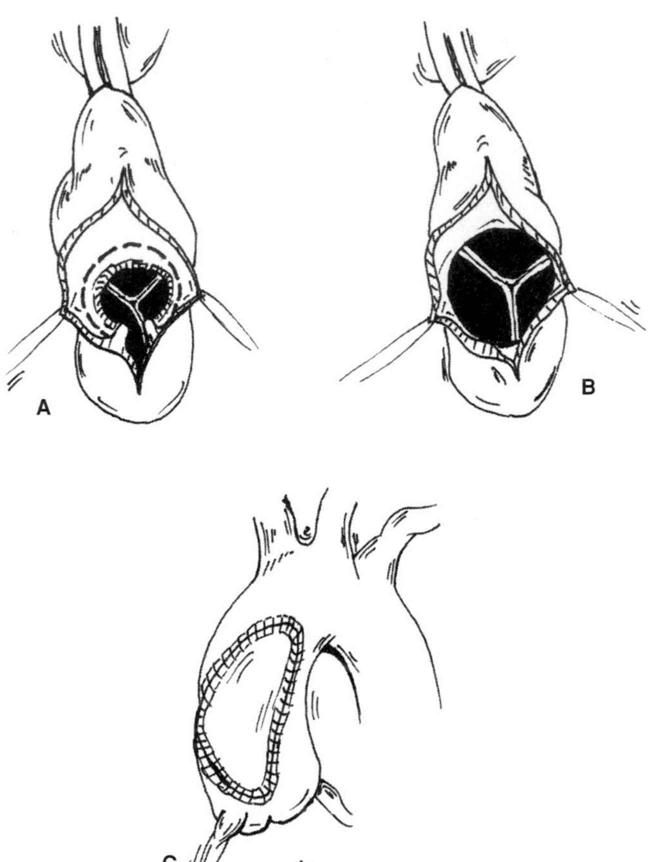

Figure 70-13 McGoon repair of supravalvar aortic stenosis. A. A longitudinal aortotomy is made, extending across the stenotic ridge into the noncoronary sinus of Valsalva. B. The stenotic ridge is resected. C. An elliptical patch of Dacron or bovine pericardium enlarges the ascending aorta.

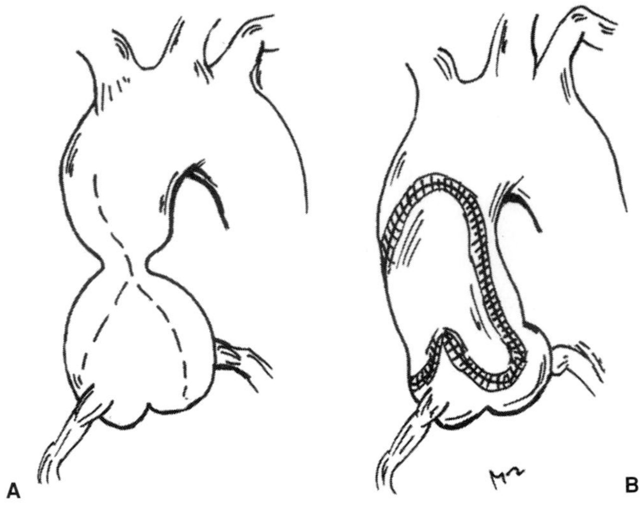

Figure 70-14 Doty repair of supravalvar aortic stenosis. A. An inverted Y-incision is made into the noncoronary and right sinuses of Valsalva. B. The aorta is augmented with a pantaloon-shaped patch.

sinuses of Valsalva may contribute to outflow obstruction, techniques were developed to maintain greater symmetry of the sinuses. Doty and associates[59] described an inverted Y-incision into the noncoronary and right coronary sinuses of Valsalva (Fig. 70-14). The incision in the right sinus is placed well to the left of the origin of the right coronary artery. A pantaloon-shaped patch enlarges both the ascending aorta and the sinuses. Brom[60] advocated augmentation of all three sinuses (Fig. 70-15). The aorta is transected at the area of narrowing. Incisions are made into each sinus of Valsalva. The sinuses are augmented with triangular patches, and the augmented root is reanastomosed to the ascending aorta. Myers and Waldhausen and their associates[61] described an innovative technique to achieve three-sinus augmentation using autologous tissue (Fig. 70-16). The aorta is transected at the area of narrowing, and incisions are made in the sinuses as with Brom's technique. Three incisions are made in the ascending aorta opposite the aortic valve commissures, and the aorta is reapproximated. Variations of this technique include excision of the stenotic segment[62] and the use of an autologous ring of pulmonary artery to enlarge the sinuses.[63]

Regardless of the technique, the coronary ostia should be inspected carefully to identify any obstruction that may be present. Treatment is based on the mechanism of obstruction. When ostial wall thickening is present, a Brom repair is used, with extension of the left coronary sinus incision into the left main coronary artery. Patch repair of the sinus is continued onto the coronary artery, with resultant coronary osteoplasty.[54,64] Coronary obstruction from leaflet adherence to the stenotic ridge is relieved by careful separation of the fused leaflet and resection of residual tissue around the ostium. Diffuse narrowing of the left main coronary artery requires coronary artery bypass. A saphenous vein graft may be preferable since progressive arteriopathy may involve the subclavian artery and limit internal mammary artery flow.[54]

Patients with diffuse hypoplasia pose a greater surgical challenge. A combination of the techniques discussed above must be tailored to the specific findings that are encountered.[65,66] Involvement of the transverse arch and descending aorta requires extensive augmentation using deep hypothermic circulatory arrest or low-flow bypass with continuous cerebral perfusion.[65–67]

It is difficult to assess the results of surgery for supravalvar aortic stenosis because of the variability of pathologic findings, the diversity of the techniques employed, and the relatively small number of patients in

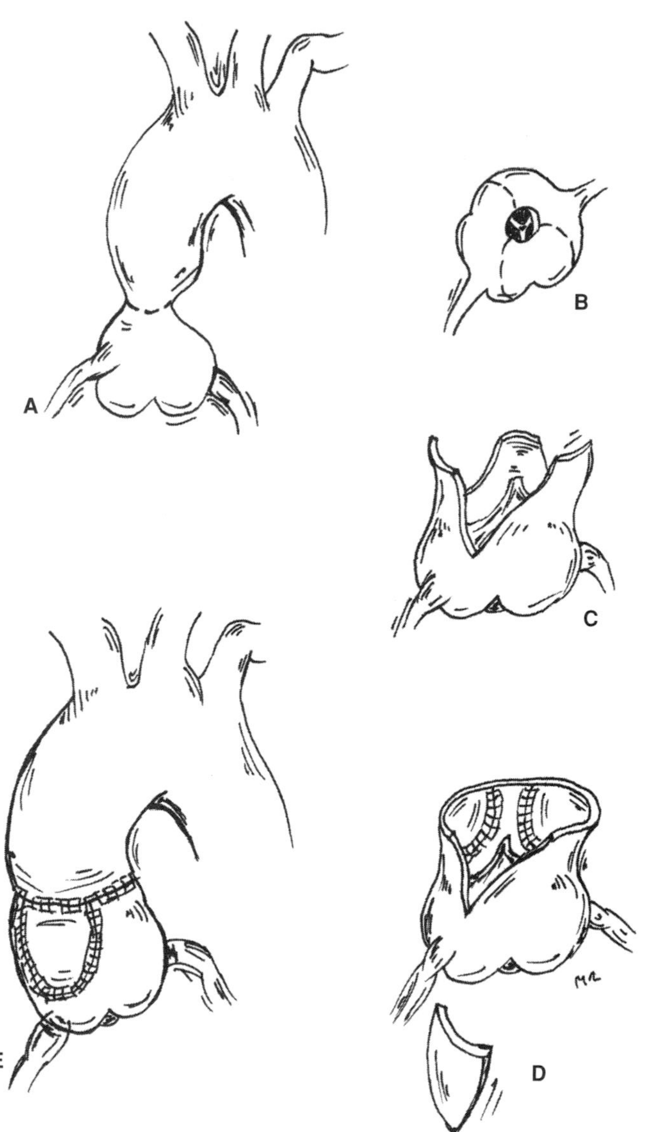

Figure 70-15 Brom repair of supravalvar aortic stenosis. A. The aorta is transected at the area of stenosis. B. Longitudinal incisions are made in each sinus of Valsalva. C. Appearance of the proximal aorta with incisions. D. Triangular patches augment the sinuses of Valsalva. E. The proximal aorta is reanastomosed to the distal aorta.

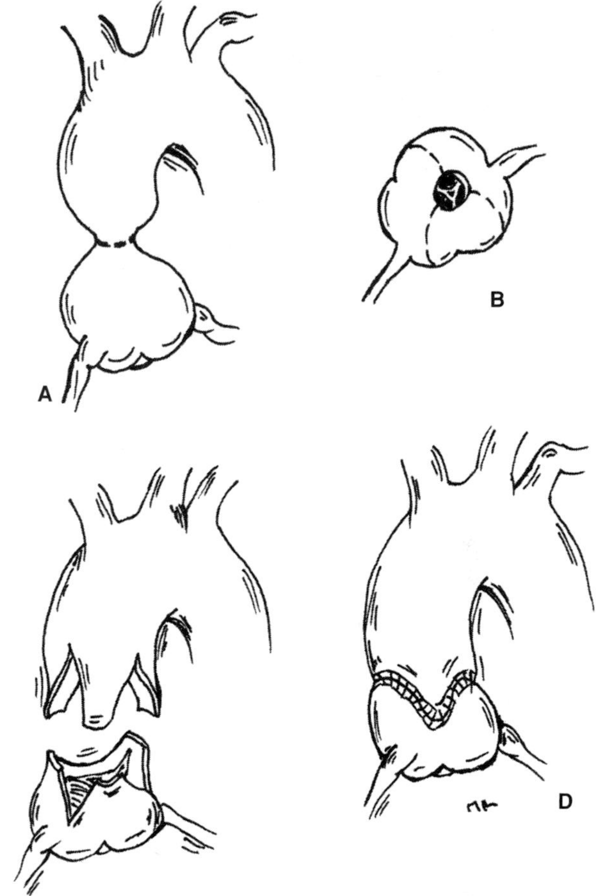

Figure 70-16 Myers-Waldhausen repair of supravalvar aortic stenosis. A. The aorta is transected at the area of stenosis. B. Longitudinal incisions are made in each sinus of Valsalva. C. Longitudinal incisions are made in the ascending aorta opposite the aortic valve commissures. D. The proximal aorta is reanastomosed to the distal aorta.

each reported series. Regardless of the technique, aortoplasty for localized obstruction achieves a long-term reduction of peak gradient from 90 mmHg to 10 to 30 mmHg with an early mortality of 0 to 2 percent.[49,53,68] No differences in short- or long-term outcome were noted between techniques augmenting one, two, or all three sinuses of Valsalva.[49,69] Freedom from reoperation at 10 years is 70 to 85 percent, and 10-year actuarial survival is 90 to 95 percent.[52,53,69] Reoperation and late death most commonly are related to progressive valve dysfunction, not recurrence of supravalvar stenosis.[49,52,53] Surgery for diffuse supravalvar stenosis is less successful. Early mortality is greater than 10 percent, and rates of reoperation and late death also are increased.[70] Poor aortic growth persists in both the localized and the diffuse forms despite successful relief of obstruction, and so long-term serial monitoring is required.[71]

SUMMARY

Left ventricular outflow tract obstruction is a common form of congenital heart disease that affects the aortic valve, the subvalvar region, and the supravalvar region. Severe stenosis results in left ventricular hypertrophy, cardiac failure, and sudden death. Early diagnosis (primarily by two-dimensional echocardiography) allows assessment of the level and severity of obstruction so that an appropriate plan of management can be designed. Surgery is indicated in symptomatic patients and in asymptomatic patients with moderate to severe obstruction or significant aortic regurgitation. Surgical techniques are available to relieve obstruction at all levels. The development of a replacement valve that has growth potential, resists degeneration, and does not require anticoagulation will improve outcomes and quality of life in this group of patients.

References

1. Ferencz C, Neill CA. Cardiovascular malformations: Prevalence at live birth. In Freedom RM, Benson IN, Smallhorn JF (eds). *Neonatal Heart Disease.* New York: Springer-Verlag; 1992:19.
2. Brown JW, Ruzmetov M, Vijay P, et al. Surgery for aortic stenosis in children: A 40-year experience. *Ann Thorac Surg* 2003;76:1398.
3. Anderson RH. Clinical anatomy of the aortic root. *Heart* 2000;84:670.
4. DePaulis R, Tomai F, Ghini AS, et al. Coronary flow characteristics after a Bentall procedure with or without sinuses of Valsalva. *Eur J Cardiothorac Surg* 2004;26:66.
5. Becker AE. Myocardial remodeling and its complications. In Hurst WJ, Anderson RH, Becker AE, Wilcox BR (eds). *Atlas of the Heart.* New York: Lippincott; 1998:2.2.
6. Fernandes SM, Sanders SP, Khairy P, et al. Morphology of bicuspid aortic valve in children and adolescents. *J Am Coll Cardiol* 2004;44:1648.
7. Bhabra MS, Dhillon R, Bhudia S, et al. Surgical aortic valvotomy in infancy: Impact of leaflet morphology on long-term outcomes. *Ann Thorac Surg* 2003;76:1412.
8. Reich O, Marek J, Razek V, et al. Long-term results of percutaneous balloon valvoplasty of congenital aortic stenosis: Independent predictors of outcome. *Heart* 2004;90:70.
9. McCrindle BW, Blackstone EH, Williams WG, et al. Are outcomes of surgical versus transcatheter balloon valvotomy equivalent in neonatal critical aortic stenosis? *Circulation* 2001;104[Suppl I]:I-152.
10. Alexiou C, Chen Q, Langley SM, et al. Is there still a place for surgical valvotomy in the management of aortic stenosis in children? The view from Southampton. *Eur J Cardiothorac Surg* 2001;20:239.
11. Rhodes LA, Colan SD, Perry SB, et al. Predictors of survival in critical aortic stenosis. *Circulation* 1991;84:2325.
12. Lofland GK, McCrindle BW, Williams WG, et al. Critical aortic stenosis in the neonate: A multi-institutional study of management, outcomes, and risk factors. *J Thorac Cardiovasc Surg* 2001;121:10.
13. Kopf GS, Hellenbrand WE, Kleinman CS. Fate of left-sided cardiac bioprosthesis valves in children. *Arch Surg* 1986;121:488.
14. Mitchell MB, Campbell DN, Bishop DA, et al. Surgical options and results of repeated aortic root replacement for failed aortic allografts placed in childhood. *J Thorac Cardiovasc Surg* 2002;124:459.
15. Laudito A, Brook MM, Suleman S, et al. The Ross procedure in children and young adults: A word of caution. *J Thorac Cardiovasc Surg* 2001;122:147.
16. Raja SG. Ross operation for bicuspid aortic valve: The myth, the reality. *Eur J Cardiothorac Surg* 2004;26:660.
17. Ilbawi MN, Wilson WR, Roberson DA, et al. Extended aortic valvuloplasty: A new approach for the management of congenital valvar aortic stenosis. *Ann Thorac Surg* 1991;52:663.
18. DeBoer DA, Robbins RC, Maron BJ, et al. Late results of aortic valvotomy for congenital valvar aortic stenosis. *Ann Thorac Surg* 1990;50:69.
19. Alexiou C, McDonald A, Langley SM, et al. Aortic valve replacement in children: Are mechanical prostheses a good option? *Eur J Cardiothorac Surg* 2000;17:125.
20. Shanmugam G, MacArthur K, Pollock J. Mechanical aortic valve replacement: Long-term outcomes in children. *J Heart Valve Dis* 2005;14:166.
21. Ross DN. Replacement of aortic and mitral valves with a pulmonary autograft. *Lancet* 1967;2:956.
22. Hraska V, Krajci M, Haun C, et al. Ross and Ross-Konno procedure in children and adolescents: Mid-term results. *Eur J Cardiothorac Surg* 2004;25:742.
23. Raja SG, Pozzi M. Ross operation in children and young adults: The Alder-Hey case series. *BMC Cardiovasc Disord* 2004;4:3.
24. Hazekamp MG, Grotenhuis HB, Schoof PH, et al. Results of the Ross operation in a pediatric population. *Eur J Cardiothorac Surg* 2005;27:975.
25. Khwaja S, Nigro JJ, Starnes VA. The Ross procedure is an ideal aortic valve replacement operation for the teen. *Semin Thorac Cardiovasc Surg Pediatr Card Surg Annu* 2005;8:173.
26. Luciani GB, Casali G, Favaro A, et al. Fate of the aortic root late after Ross operation. *Circulation* 2003;108:II-61.
27. Kouchoukos NT, Masetti P, Nickerson NJ, et al. The Ross procedure: Long-term clinical and echocardiographic follow-up. *Ann Thorac Surg* 2004;78:773.
28. Nicks R, Cardmill T, Bernstein L. Hypoplasia of the aortic root: The problem of aortic valve replacement. *Thorax* 1970;25:339.
29. Manougian S, Seybold-Epting W. Patch enlargement of the aortic valve by extending the aortic incision into the anterior mitral leaflet: New operative technique. *J Thorac Cardiovasc Surg* 1979;78:402.
30. Konno S, Imai Y, Nakajima M, et al. A new method for prosthetic valve replacement in congenital aortic stenosis associated with hypoplasia of the aortic valve ring. *J Thorac Cardiovasc Surg* 1975;70:909.
31. Cobanoglu A, Thyagarajan GK, Dobbs J. Konno-aortoventriculoplasty with mechanical prosthesis in dealing with small aortic root: A good surgical option. *Eur J Cardiothorac Surg* 1997;12:766.
32. Erez E, Kanter KR, Tam VKH, et al. Konno aortoventriculoplasty in children and adolescents: From prosthetic valves to the Ross operation. *Ann Thorac Surg* 2002;74:122.
33. Ohye RG, Gomez CA, Ohye BJ, et al. The Ross/Konno procedure in neonates and infants: Intermediate-term survival and autograft function. *Ann Thorac Surg* 2001;72:823.

34. Sharma GK, Wojtalik M, Siwinska A, et al. Aortoventriculoplasty and left ventricular function: Long-term follow-up. *Eur J Cardiothorac Surg* 2004;26:126.
35. Yacoub M, Onuzo O, Riedel B, et al. Mobilization of the left and right fibrous trigones for relief of severe left ventricular outflow obstruction. *J Thorac Cardiovasc Surg* 1999;117:126.
36. Marasini M, Zannini L, Ussia GP, et al. Discrete subaortic stenosis: Incidence, morphology and surgical impact of associated subaortic anomalies. *Ann Thorac Surg* 2003;75:1763.
37. Kitchiner D. Subaortic stenosis: Still more questions than answers. *Heart* 1999;82:647.
38. Brauner R, Laks H, Drinkwater DC, et al. Benefits of early surgical repair in fixed subaortic stenosis. *J Am Coll Cardiol* 1997;30:1843.
39. Rohlicek CV, del Pino SF, Hosking M, et al. Natural history and surgical outcomes for isolated discrete subaortic stenosis in children. *Heart* 1999;82:708
40. Coleman DM, Smallhorn JF, McCrindle BW, et al. Postoperative follow-up of fibromuscular subaortic stenosis. *J Am Coll Cardiol* 1994;24:1558.
41. Bezold LI, Smith EO, Kelly K, et al. Development and validation of an echocardiographic model for predicting progression of discrete subaortic stenosis in children. *Am J Cardiol* 1998;81:314.
42. McMahon CJ, Gauvreau K, Edwards JC, et al. Risk factors for aortic valve dysfunction in children with discrete subvalvar aortic stenosis. *Am J Cardiol* 2004;94:459.
43. DeLeon SY, Ilbawi MN, Roberson DA, et al. Conal enlargement for diffuse subaortic stenosis. *J Thorac Cardiovasc Surg* 1991;102:814.
44. Jahangiri M, Nicholson IA, del Nido PJ, et al. Surgical management of complex and tunnel-like subaortic stenosis. *Eur J Cardiothorac Surg* 2000;17:637.
45. Caldarone CA, Van Natta TL, Frazer JR, et al. The modified Konno procedure for complex left ventricular outflow tract obstruction. *Ann Thorac Surg* 2003;75:147.
46. Khanna SK, Anstadt MP, Bhimji S, et al. Apico-aortic conduits in children with severe left ventricular outflow tract obstruction. *Ann Thorac Surg* 2002;73:81.
47. Keating, MT. Genetic approaches to cardiovascular disease: Supravalvular aortic stenosis, Williams syndrome, and long-QT syndrome. *Circulation* 1995;92:142.
48. O'Connor WN, Davis JB Jr, Geissler R, et al. Supravalvar aortic stenosis. *Arch Pathol Lab Med* 1985;109:179.
49. Van Son JAM, Danielson GK, Puga FJ, et al. Supravalvular aortic stenosis: Long-term results of surgical treatment. *J Thorac Cardiovasc Surg* 1994;107:103.
50. Stamm C, Li J, Ho SY, Redington AN, et al. The aortic root in supravalvular aortic stenosis: The potential surgical relevance of morphologic findings. *J Thorac Cardiovasc Surg* 1997;114:16.
51. Stamm C, Friehs I, Ho SW, et al. Congenital supravalvar aortic stenosis: A simple lesion? *Eur J Cardiothorac Surg* 2001;19:195.
52. Delius RE, Steinberg JB, L'Ecuyer TL, et al. Long-term follow-up of extended aortoplasty for supravalvular aortic stenosis. *J Thorac Cardiovasc Surg* 1995;109:155.
53. Brown JB, Ruzmetov M, Palaniswamy V, et al. Surgical repair of congenital supravalvular aortic stenosis in children. *Eur J Cardiothorac Surg* 2002;21:50.
54. Thistlethwaite PA, Madani MM, Kriett JM, et al. Surgical management of congenital obstruction of the left main coronary artery with supravalvular aortic stenosis. *J Thorac Cardiovasc Surg* 2000;120:1040.
55. Van Son JAM, Edwards WD, Danielson GK. Pathology of coronary arteries, myocardium, and great arteries in supravalvular aortic stenosis: Report of five cases with implications for surgical treatment. *J Thorac Cardiovasc Surg* 1994;108:21.
56. Eronen M, Peippo M, Hiippala A, et al. Cardiovascular manifestations in 75 patients with Williams syndrome. *J Med Genet* 2002;39:554.
57. Tani LY, Minch L, Pagotto LT, et al. Usefulness of Doppler echocardiography to determine the timing of surgery for supravalvar aortic stenosis. *Am J Cardiol* 2000;86:114.
58. McGoon DC, Mankin HT, Vlad P, et al. The surgical treatment of supravalvular aortic stenosis. *J Thorac Cardiovasc Surg* 1961;41:125.
59. Doty DB, Polansky DB, Jenson CB. Supravalvular aortic stenosis. *J Thorac Cardiovasc Surg* 1977;74:362.
60. Brom AG. Obstruction of the left ventricular outflow tract. In: Khonsari S (ed). *Cardiac Surgery: Safeguards and Pitfalls in Operative Technique.* Rockville: Aspen; 1988:276.
61. Myers JL, Waldhausen JA, Cyran SE, et al. Results of surgical repair of congenital aortic stenosis. *J Thorac Cardiovasc Surg* 1993;105:281.
62. Chard RB, Cartmill TB. Localized supravalvar aortic stenosis: A new technique for repair. *Ann Thorac Surg* 1993;55:782.
63. Al-Halees Z, Prabhakar G, Galal O. Reconstruction of suprvalvar aortic stenosis with autologous pulmonary artery. *Ann Thorac Surg* 1998;65:532.
64. Shin H, Katogi T, Yozu R, et al. Surgical angioplasty of left main coronary stenosis complicating supravalvular aortic stenosis. *Ann Thorac Surg* 1999;67:1147.
65. Folliguet TA, Mace L, Dervanian P, et al. Surgical treatment of diffuse supravalvar aortic stenosis. *Ann Thorac Surg* 1996;61:1251.
66. Pretre R, Arbenz U, Vogt PR, et al. Application of successive principles to correct supravalvular aortic stenosis. *Ann Thorac Surg* 1999;67:1167.
67. Yamagishi M, Shuntoh K, Matsushita T, et al. Complete augmentation of diffuse narrowing of the aorta with Williams syndrome by using an overturn approach. *J Thorac Cardiovasc Surg* 2003;125:1556.
68. McElhinney DB, Petrossian E, Tworetzky W, et al. Issues and outcomes in the management of supravalvar aortic stenosis. *Ann Thorac Surg* 2000;69:562.
69. Hazekamp MG, Kappetein AP, Schoof PH, et al. Brom's three-patch technique for repair of supravalvular aortic stenosis. *J Thorac Cardiovasc Surg* 1999;118:252.
70. English RF, Colan SD, Kanani PM, et al. Growth of the aorta in children with Williams syndrome: Does surgery make a difference? *Pediatr Cardiol* 2003;24:566.
71. Sharma BK, Fujiwara H, Hallman GL, et al. Supravalvar aortic stenosis: A 29 year review of surgical experience. *Ann Thorac Surg* 1991;51:1031.

CHAPTER

71 COARCTATION OF THE AORTA AND INTERRUPTED AORTIC ARCH

S. Adil Husain, Nahush A. Mokadam, Lester C. Permut, Mark D. Rodefeld

COARCTATION OF THE AORTA

The etymology of the term *coarctation* derives from the Latin root, *coarctare*, to compress. Coarctation of the aorta (CoA) is defined as a congenital narrowing of the aorta that is hemodynamically significant. CoA occurs in more than 4 in 10,000 live births and accounts for more than 5 percent of anomalies in children born with congenital heart defects.[1] Although isolated coarctation is more common in males, coarctation associated with other cardiac lesions occurs with equal frequency in males and females.

CoA can occur along the entire length of the aorta but is most commonly found just proximal to the junction of the ductus arteriosus and the descending aorta (Fig. 71-1). A posterior protuberance of the media,

KEY CONCEPTS

Coarctation of the Aorta

- Introduction
  - Coarctation of the aorta (CoA) is defined as a hemodynamically significant narrowing of the aorta. It occurs in about 4 in 10,000 births and accounts for more than 5 percent of congenital heart defects.
- Clinical features
  - CoA presents as a spectrum of disease, ranging from neonatal ductal dependence to newly diagnosed, previously unrecognized, long-standing hypertension in an adult. One-third of neonates have an isolated CoA, one-third have a ventricular septal defect, and one-third have complex congenital heart disease. A bicuspid aortic valve is present in 50 percent. Up to 80 percent of neonates with hypoplastic left heart syndrome have a CoA.
- Diagnosis
  - Echocardiography is the diagnostic modality of choice in neonates. In older patients, computed tomography, magnetic resonance imaging, and angiography are employed.
- Treatment
  - Surgical treatment is preferred, with several techniques available. The choice of procedure depends on the anatomy of the aorta and associated anomalies. Native CoA balloon angioplasty is possible but has decreased long-term success in neonates; its use is perhaps of better application in older children and recoarctation. Endovascular stents have emerged as a possible alternative to surgery, but long-term data are not available.
- Results
  - Surgical repair of isolated CoA in the neonatal period can be accomplished with minimal morbidity and mortality, whereas the results of repair of CoA in association with complex coronary heart disease varies according to the dominant cardiac pathology and patient-related variables. Recoarctation occurs in up to 30 percent of patients corrected in the neonatal period, with a similar incidence despite the different techniques utilized. Late hypertension is common in patients operated later in life and is partly responsible for

the slightly decreased long-term survival of this patient population.

Interrupted Aortic Arch

- Morphology
  - In this condition there is anatomic lack of continuity in the aortic arch, classified according to the site of occurrence into type A (distal to left subclavian), type B (between the left common carotid and subclavian), and type C (just distal to the innominate artery). Type B is most common and is associated with thymic agenesis and 22q11 microdeletion. The prevalence is 0.003 per 1000 live births. A ventricular septal defect is nearly always present. Bicuspid aortic valve is found in 50 percent of infants, with left ventricular outflow tract obstruction often seen because of hypoplasia of the aortic root or posterior malalignment of the infundibular septum.
- Clinical features
  - In newborns not prenatally diagnosed, presentation is rapid because of ductal closure and resulting visceral hypoperfusion and shock. Peripheral pulses vary according to the site of interruption and there is variable pulmonary overcirculation. Median time of death if untreated is 4 to 10 days from birth, with 75 percent mortality within 1 year.
- Diagnosis
  - Echocardiography is the diagnostic modality of choice in neonates. In more complex anomalies, computed tomography, magnetic resonance imaging, and angiography are employed.
- Treatment
  - Surgical treatment follows a brief period of stabilization with PGE_1 infusion and restoration of ductal patency. Single-stage repair of aortic arch interruption and coexisting cardiac anomalies is undertaken. Alternatively, a staged approach with initial arch repair and banding of the pulmonary artery followed by delayed correction of intracardiac anomalies can be considered.
- Results
  - In the current era, operative mortality following operative repair of an interrupted aortic arch is less than 10 percent. Five-year survival is reported at greater than 70 percent. Reintervention rates (surgical and percutaneous) for arch obstruction at 3-year follow-up range between 15 and 30 percent.

often augmented by ductal tissue, typically creates a shelf in the aortic lumen. Externally, the aorta is visibly narrowed, but often to a lesser extent than is observed upon entering its lumen. In addition, the aortic isthmus, defined as the segment between the left subclavian artery and the ductus arteriosus, is frequently hypoplastic. In some patients, the hypoplasia involves the entire transverse aortic arch. There are numerous classification systems, all of which are essentially descriptive.

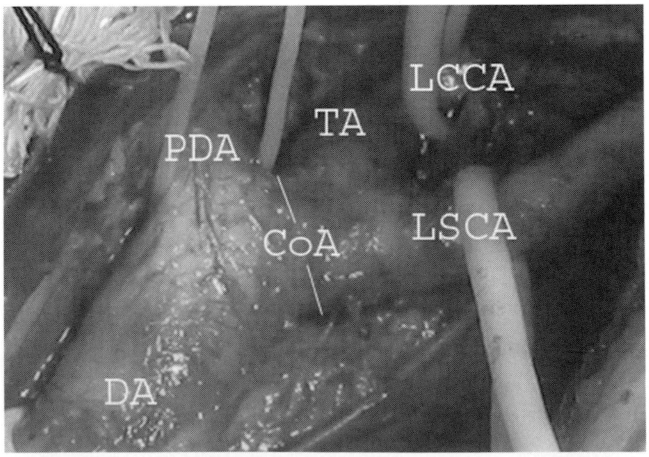

Figure 71-1 Surgical photograph of aortic coarctation in an infant as seen through a left thoracotomy (operating surgeon's view). CoA = coarctation of aorta; DA = descending aorta; LCCA = left common carotid artery; LSCA = left subclavian artery; PDA = patent ductus arteriosus; TA = transverse arch.

The first description of aortic coarctation is credited to Paris in 1791, whereas the first published report of repair by resection and end-to-end anastomosis was by Crafoord in 1944.[2,3] Gross independently described a nearly identical repair in 1945 and was the first to describe the technique of interposition grafting.[4,5] Effective augmentation of the narrowed aortic segment with patch aortoplasty was described by Vossschulte in 1957, while Waldhausen introduced in 1966 the subclavian flap aortoplasty.[6,7]

ETIOLOGY

The etiology of aortic coarctation is unknown. CoA may be associated with genetic anomalies including Turner's syndrome (45 X,O) and Noonan's syndrome; to date, however, no specific or reproducible molecular abnormality has been identified. In the fetal circulation, right-to-left flow through the ductus arteriosus results in decreased flow across the aortic isthmus with respect to either the ascending or descending aorta. Following postnatal ductal closure, the normal aorta presumably expands and grows in response to increased flow and pressure. This concept is corroborated by an increased incidence of CoA in patients with lesions diminishing aortic flow, such as aortic stenosis, ventricular septal defect (VSD), and mitral valve pathology. Furthermore, coarctation is rarely seen in lesions that result in increased aortic flow, such as tetralogy of Fallot.

It has been well recognized that the presence of ductal tissue within the aorta may contribute to this process. The muscular wall of the ductus arteriosus is exquisitely sensitive to changes in neonatal hemodynamics and to pharmacologic agents such as prostaglandin and nonsteroidal anti-inflammatory agents. In some patients, the ductal tissue extends well into the adjacent aortic wall and, during ductal contraction, may contribute to the development of coarctation. These findings have been confirmed in histologic studies.[8] Additional biochemical factors have been identified in patients with CoA. The aortic isthmus and in some the transverse arch exhibit a higher fraction of elastin lamellae and a lower fraction of α actin–positive cells. These findings may account for decreased aortic growth.[9]

CLINICAL FEATURES

Clinical presentation is determined by the location and degree of aortic narrowing as well as the presence of associated intra- or extracardiac anomalies. Although neonates may appear normal at birth, they develop evidence of aortic obstruction with ductal closure. Manifestations include poor feeding, irritability, and tachypnea. A persistent systolic precordial murmur in the setting of weak or absent femoral pulses should raise the suspicion of aortic coarctation. Other presenting signs include differential oxygen saturations between the upper and lower extremities and pulmonary overcirculation from left to right shunting across the patent foramen ovale. In the most severe form, with ductal closure over the first days to weeks of life, the sudden increase in afterload on the nonhypertrophied left ventricle results in a marked decrease in left-sided stroke volume and ejection fraction. Cardiomegaly results from an acute increase in right ventricular end-diastolic volume consequent to increased left-to-right shunting through the patent foramen ovale.[10] Poor perfusion and listlessness may occur. Femoral pulses are not palpable and metabolic acidosis ensues. If CoA is left untreated, end-organ damage (including renal failure and necrotizing enterocolitis) will ultimately result in death.

Infants who undergo more gradual closure of the ductus may develop arterial collaterals, allowing for a less catastrophic presentation. In such cases, the most common finding is usually failure to thrive. These children often have difficulty with feedings and diaphoresis. Physiologically, these infants have compensated for the increase in afterload and present with left ventricular hypertrophy. Older children and adults not diagnosed in infancy (presumably due to a less severe form of disease) commonly present with unexplained hypertension or during the workup of a murmur. Lower extremity pulses are delayed or absent, exercise tolerance may be diminished, and claudication may be a chief complaint. Other symptoms include manifestations of upper body hypertension such as headache, epistaxis, visual field disturbances, and stroke. These patients develop left ventricular hypertrophy to compensate for the persistent hypertension and increased afterload.

ASSOCIATED ANOMALIES

In one report, 82 percent of all coarctations were isolated, 11 percent were associated with a VSD, and complex anatomy was observed in 7 percent.[11] CoA is associated with a bicuspid aortic valve in approximately 50 percent of patients.[12] Since CoA creates a pressure load on the left heart, a patent foramen ovale with a left-to-right shunt is often present. Aortic coarctation occurs in less than 10 percent of patients with transposition of the great vessels and in up to 50 percent of patients with the Taussig-Bing heart (see Chap. 63).[13,14] In these patients, conal malalignment may produce subaortic obstruction with decreased antegrade flow through the transverse arch and isthmus. Hypoplastic left heart syndrome has an 80 percent incidence of CoA.[15] CoA is also associated with other forms of functional single ventricle, including tricuspid atresia with transposition of the great arteries and double-inlet left ventricle. Shone's complex is characterized by a parachute mitral valve, supraannular mitral ring, subaortic stenosis, and CoA. These patients present with a spectrum of disease, some requiring single ventricle palliation.

NATURAL HISTORY

Unrecognized CoA is rare in the current era. Untreated coarctation leads to premature death due to complications of unrelenting hypertension, with its attendant effects on the coronary and cerebral circulation. These effects include coronary artery disease, cerebrovascular accidents (both aneurysmal and atherosclerotic), congestive heart failure, and aortic rupture. In addition (particularly in patients with bicuspid aortic valves) bacterial endocarditis can occur. The survival of untreated patients with isolated CoA is depicted in Fig. 71-2.

DIAGNOSTIC MODALITIES

The principal method of diagnosis early in life is echocardiography. In the neonate and infant, the presence of a large thymus allows for excellent visualization of the arch structures (Fig. 71-3). Surface echocardiography provides specific anatomic information including location,

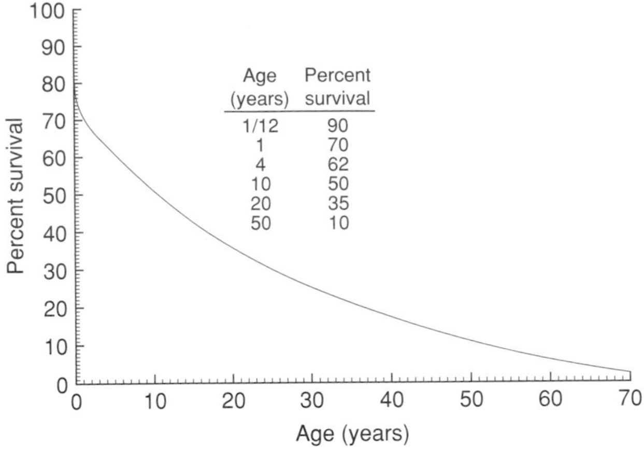

Figure 71-2 Survival of patients with surgically untreated isolated coarctation of the aorta. (From Kouchoukos et al, p. 1328.[11] With permission.)

length (diffuse versus discrete narrowing), and dimension of the coarctation segment. Severity of obstruction can be assessed quantitatively by measurement of Doppler flow velocity and qualitatively by evaluation of abdominal aortic pulsatility and diastolic flow. The presence of left ventricular hypertrophy also suggests increased severity. In addition, echocardiography allows for the detection of associated intracardiac lesions and transverse arch hypoplasia. In the presence of a patent ductus arteriosus, the ability of echocardiography to diagnose a CoA may be limited. As thymic regression ensues, the interposition of lung tissue between the arch and the chest wall obscures echocardiographic details, making echocardiography less useful in older children and adults. In this particular age group, the use of cross-sectional imaging, such as thin-slice computed tomography and magnetic resonance imaging, provides excellent structural detail of the aortic arch and its branches. In addition, as these modalities provide imaging of the entire chest and abdomen, the detection of important collateral arteries is feasible.

Angiography (the traditional "gold standard" for aortic evaluation) is now rarely used for diagnosis, as it is more invasive and exposes the patient to a nephrotoxic contrast load (Fig. 71-4). However, angiography should be performed with the objective of delineating unclear anatomy and when percutaneous intervention is contemplated.

MEDICAL THERAPY

The role of medical therapy in the treatment of hemodynamically significant CoA is limited to temporizing

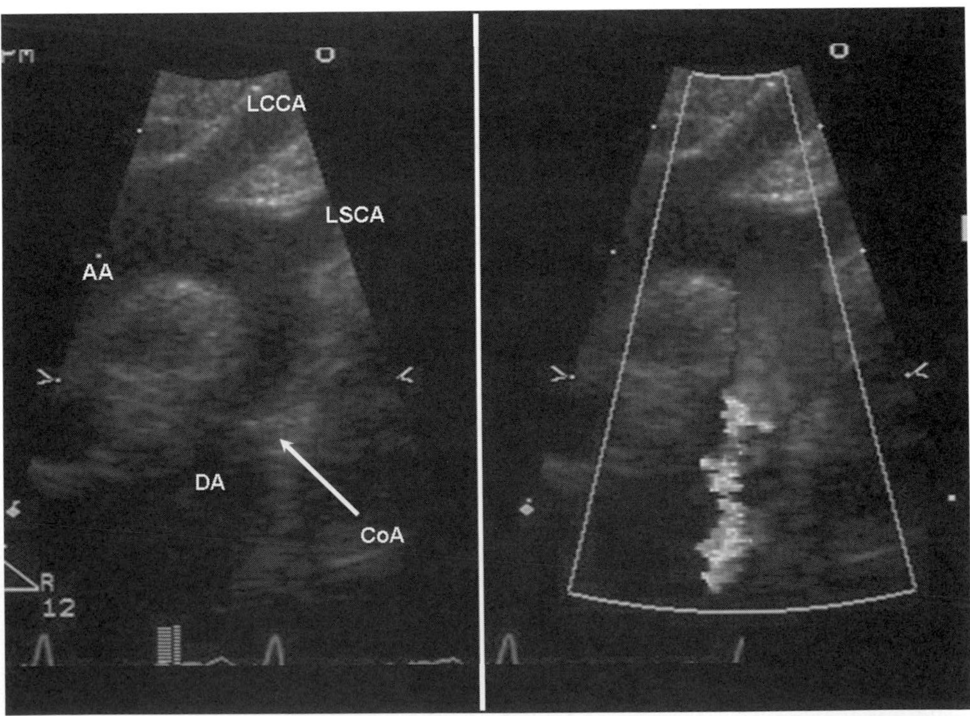

Figure 71-3 Echocardiographic findings in aortic coarctation. AA = ascending aorta; CoA = coarctation of aorta; IA = innominate artery; LCCA = left common carotid artery; LSCA = left subclavian artery; RPA = right pulmonary artery. (Image courtesy of J. Geoffrey Stevenson, MD.)

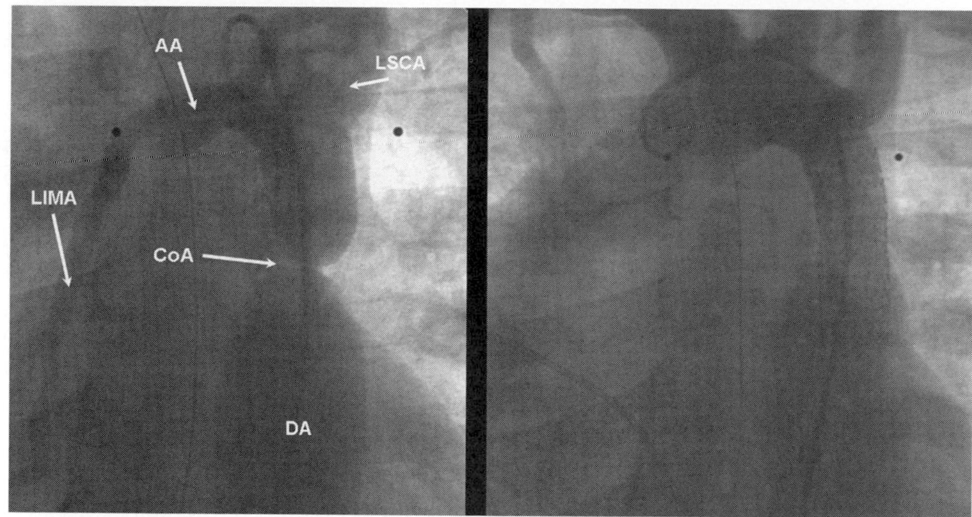

Figure 71-4 Angiographic findings in aortic coarctation. AA = ascending aortic arch; TA = transverse aortic arch; DA = descending aorta; IA = innominate artery; LCCA = left common carotid artery; LSCA = left subclavian artery; CoA = coarctation of aorta. (Image courtesy of Richard Ringel, MD, Division of Pediatric Cardiology, The Johns Hopkins Hospital.)

measures while timing and method of repair are being considered. The mainstay of medical therapy in neonates is prostaglandin (PGE_1) infusion. Intravenous administration maintains patency of the ductus arteriosus, allowing for resuscitation and restoration of end-organ perfusion in compromised infants. Side-effects of PGE_1 include generalized edema and apnea, sometimes requiring preoperative mechanical ventilation.

In patients who have undergone repair and in those in whom the diagnosis is made later in life, the surveillance and treatment of hypertension is paramount. As previously discussed, the limited life span of patients with CoA may be directly related to persistent hypertension despite successful anatomic repair.

CATHETER-BASED INTERVENTION

Successful primary treatment of aortic coarctation by balloon angioplasty has been reported but requires further investigation to define its overall efficacy, safety, and long-term durability. The main limitations of balloon angioplasty, particularly in the neonate, are early recurrence of coarctation, aneurysm formation, and access-related injury to the femoral artery. In a recent retrospective review, nearly 60 percent of neonates undergoing primary balloon angioplasty required subsequent surgical repair, and 13 percent developed saccular aneurysms. In the surgical repair group, 18 percent developed recoarctation responsive to balloon dilatation, and no patients developed aneurysms.[16] Balloon angioplasty appears therefore to be more indicated in critically ill neonates who are poor surgical candidates because of severe left ventricular dysfunction or intercurrent illness, allowing for palliation until surgical correction can be safely undertaken. Balloon angioplasty is nevertheless the treatment of choice for recurrent coarctation following neonatal surgical repair, with a greater than 90 percent success rate at relieving the gradient and a 16 percent incidence of restenosis requiring reintervention.[17]

Endovascular stents provide durable relief of aortic coarctation in older children and adults. Stents have a significant advantage over simple angioplasty in that they prevent elastic recoil of the aortic wall, reducing the likelihood of dissection during the procedure. Stent placement in younger children is generally not preferable. Smaller stents cannot undergo serial dilation to keep pace with somatic growth, resulting in the eventual need for a technically difficult surgical repair. Larger stents may allow serial dilatation, but the size of the femoral artery often precludes stent placement in smaller patients. As with surgical intervention, persistent hypertension despite successful relief of obstruction requires diligent surveillance and treatment. In a recent review of endovascular treatment of CoA in adolescents and adults (1-year follow-up data), all patients had persistent resolution of their aortic gradient, although this group did report a 13 percent incidence of small aneurysms.[18] Although long-term data are not yet available, midterm results appear to compare favorably with surgical repair.

SURGICAL THERAPY

Surgical correction is indicated for all symptomatic neonates and infants or older children and adults who are not candidates for transcatheter therapy. Operation should be considered in asymptomatic patients for an upper-to-lower extremity mean blood pressure gradient in excess of 20 mmHg that is associated with upper extremity hypertension and a greater than 50 percent reduction in luminal diameter in the coarctation segment. A low gradient in the presence of robust collateral development does not exclude severe obstruction and should not be considered a contraindication to surgery.

Following the induction of general anesthesia, a right radial arterial line is inserted and the patient placed in a right lateral decubitus position. A left thoracotomy through the fourth intercostal space provides ideal exposure for most repairs. Alternatively, a muscle-sparing extrapleural approach has been described to provide adequate exposure with comparable results.[19] In cases requiring associated intracardiac repair or complex transverse arch reconstruction, median sternotomy and cardiopulmonary bypass with circulatory arrest may be appropriate; the description of these more complex techniques is beyond the scope of this discussion. Following thoracotomy, the lung is retracted anteroinferiorly and the pleura overlying the aorta incised longitudinally. Any crossing lymphatics are ligated and divided to prevent the occurrence of a chylothorax. Care is taken to preserve the left vagus nerve and the recurrent laryngeal nerve as it passes around the ligamentum arteriosum or patent ductus arteriosus. The pleural edges are suspended by sutures to aid in exposure and retraction of the lung (Fig. 71-5). For all methods of reconstruction, dissection and control of the proximal aortic arch, left common carotid and subclavian arteries, descending aorta, ductus arteriosus, and any enlarged intercostals arteries is essential for a safe repair. Although it is ideal to preserve the intercostal arteries when possible, several pairs may be sacrificed to obtain a tension-free anastomosis.

Resection with end-to-end anastomosis

The ductus arteriosus is ligated and divided. The proximal aorta is clamped obliquely across the left subclavian artery and transverse arch. The distal aorta is clamped well below the planned anastomotic site. The left common carotid artery may be safely occluded by the proximal clamp, but the innominate artery must remain patent to preserve cerebral blood flow via the right common carotid artery. This is confirmed by an adequate waveform on the right radial artery pressure monitor. Care is taken to ensure that the clamps do not distort the area of reconstruction or compress the innominate artery. Intercostal arteries that may backbleed into the field should be controlled by temporary clips or snares. The coarctation is completely resected, including all ductal tissue macroscopically visible within the aorta. The aorta is reapproximated in a running fashion using 7-0 polypropylene suture in neonates and small infants (Fig. 71-6). Interrupted suture placement or the use of absorbable suture material has not been shown to improve results.

The primary advantage of resection and end-to-end anastomosis is the complete excision of all abnormal aortic tissue. However, adequate mobilization is required to create a tension-free anastomosis. Mobilization of the distal aorta risks injury to fragile intercostals collateral vessels in older children and adults. Other techniques may therefore be more appropriate in this age group.

Extended resection with end-to-end anastomosis is necessary in the presence of severe transverse arch hypoplasia. The proximal clamp is placed to the level of the innominate artery and ascending aorta. After coarctation resection, the underside of the aortic arch is

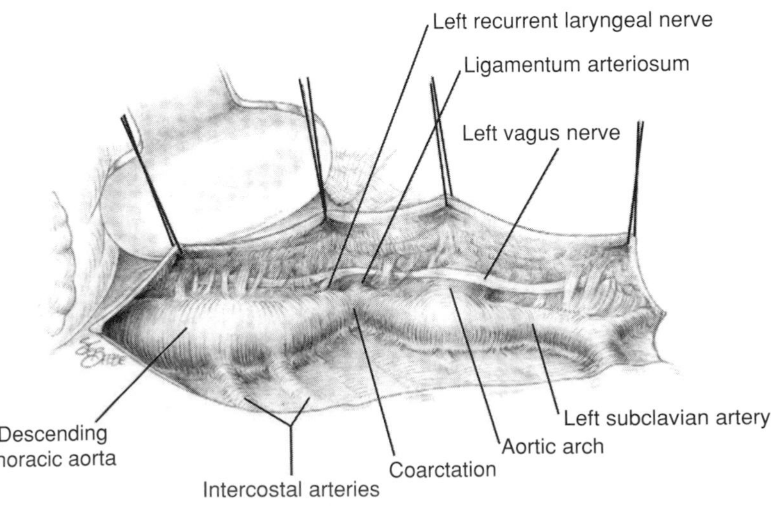

Figure 71-5 Surgical anatomy of a coarctation of the aorta. (From Khonsari and Sintek, p. 188.[52] With permission.)

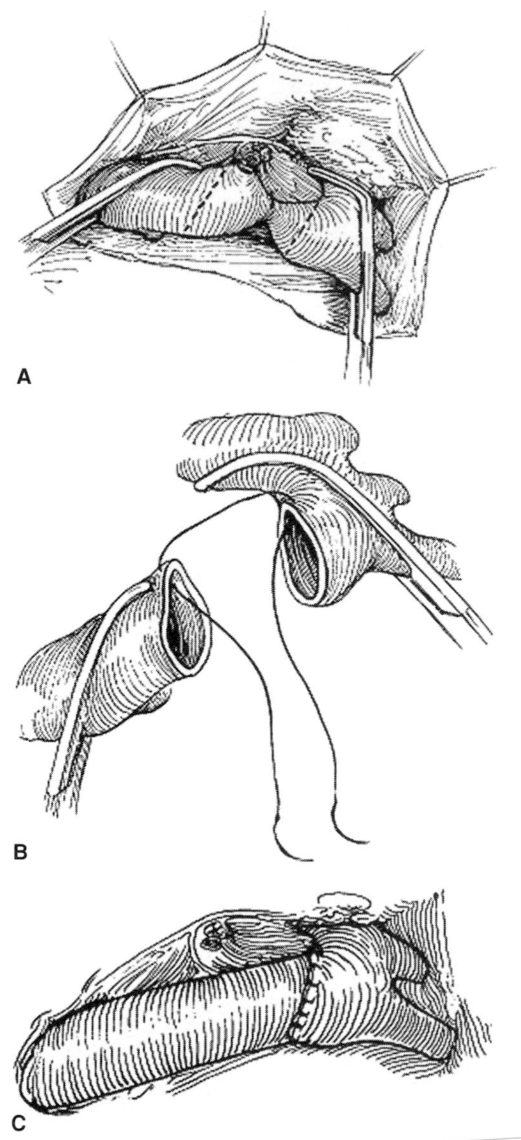

Figure 71-6 Resection of aortic coarctation segment with end-to-end anastomosis. A. Proximal and distal control of the aorta is obtained and the ductus is ligated. B. The coarctation is resected. The aorta is reapproximated using fine polypropylene suture. C. Completed aortic reconstruction. [From Coarctation of the aorta, aortopulmonary shunts, and aortopulmonary collaterals. In: Sellke FW, del Nido PJ, Swanson SJ (eds). *Sabiston and Spencer Surgery of the Chest.* Philadelphia: With permission from *Elsevier,* 2005:1919.]

opened and anastomosed to the appropriately beveled descending aorta (Fig. 71-7). Wide proximal and distal mobilization is necessary to allow tension-free approximation for this repair.

Subclavian flap aortoplasty

Full mobilization of the left subclavian artery is required for this repair. The left subclavian artery is ligated at the level of its first branch, taking care to preserve all distal branches, as they provide the collateral circulation to the left arm. Some surgeons additionally ligate the vertebral artery to prevent late subclavian steal syndrome. The ductus is ligated and a longitudinal aortotomy is begun distal to the area of coarctation. The incision is extended proximally across the coarctation and into the left subclavian artery, ending just proximal to the previously placed ligature. The left subclavian artery is transected and the resulting subclavian flap is turned inferiorly and sutured to the edges of the descending aorta with a running 7-0 polypropylene suture (Fig. 71-8). A "reverse" subclavian flap may be used less commonly for discrete coarctation proximal to the left subclavian artery or distal transverse arch hypoplasia (Fig. 71-9).

The advantages of subclavian flap aortoplasty include ease of repair and the avoidance of extensive mobilization. Adequate length and caliber of the subclavian artery should be ascertained with this technique. Subclavian flap aortoplasty is generally avoided beyond infancy because of concern with arm perfusion.

Patch aortoplasty

Following clamp placement, the aorta is incised longitudinally over the coarctation, from the left subclavian artery origin to the level of the first intercostal artery (Fig. 71-10). The coarctation ridge is typically not excised, and an oval patch of prosthetic material is fashioned and sutured to the aortotomy edge using continuous suture. Care is taken to ensure that the widest portion of the patch overlies the coarctation ridge.

The advantage of this technique is that it is relatively expedient and can be performed with minimal dissection of collaterals, particularly in the older patient in whom mobilization and a tension-free anastomosis might not be easily achieved. Furthermore, the patch can cover a relatively long segment of coarctation and can be made sufficiently redundant to avoid recoarctation. Therefore the recoarctation rate is very low, particularly in children above 1 year of age.

The main disadvantage of patch aortoplasty, as described in early reports, is aneurysmal dilatation in the aortic wall opposite the patch. Rates of aneurysm formation varied widely but in some series occurred in over 50 percent of patients.[20] It is now recognized that this complication was largely related to the use of Dacron as the patch material in earlier series. The noncompliant quality of Dacron generated excessive tension in the aortic wall opposite the patch.[21] This was accentuated in patients in whom the coarctation ridge was excised. Currently, polytetrafluoroethylene is the prosthetic material of choice for patch aortoplasty. A recent series reported no true aneurysm formation in 125 patients between the ages of 4 days and 17 years.[22]

In older children and adults, interposition grafting can be performed with a technique similar to that described for thoracic aortic aneurysms.

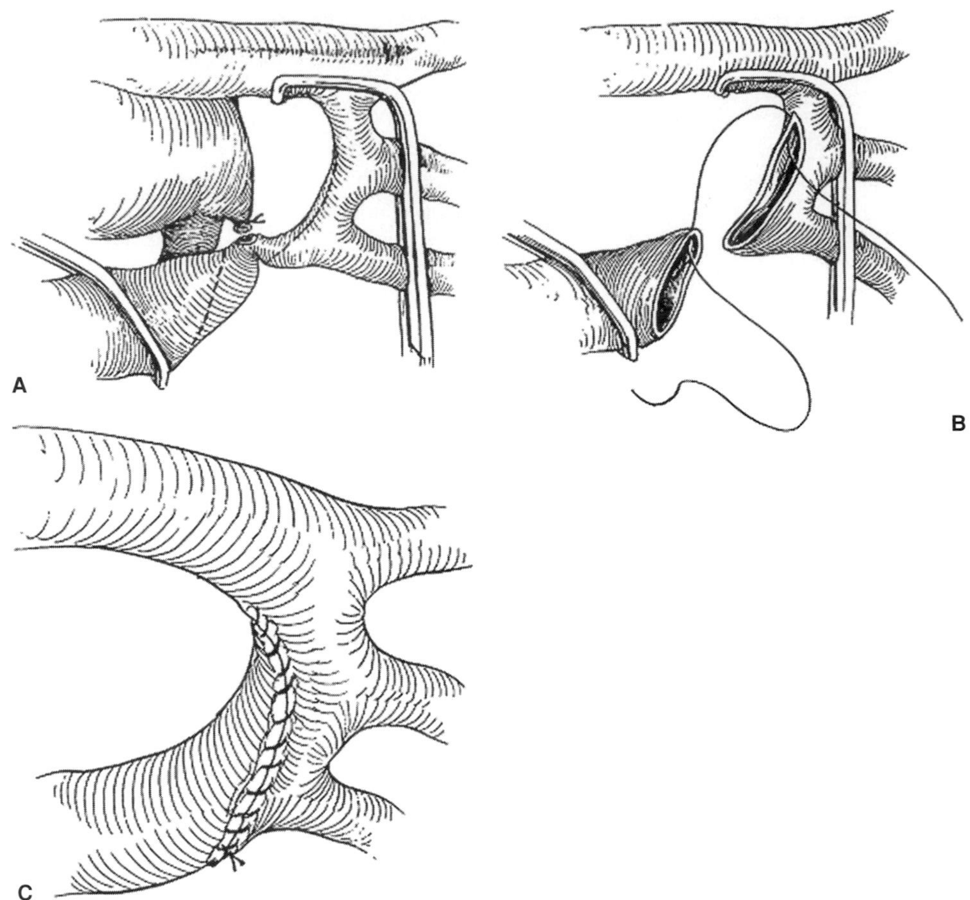

Figure 71-7 Extended resection with end-to-end anastomosis. A. The proximal aortic clamp is placed flush on the innominate artery at the level of the ascending aorta. The ductus is ligated, the coarctation is resected, and the underside of the aortic arch is incised. B. The descending aorta is beveled and enlarged in order to appropriately augment the aortic arch. Reconstruction is carried out using fine polypropylene suture. C. The completed repair. [From Coarctation of the aorta, aortopulmonary shunts, and aortopulmonary collaterals. In: Sellke FW, del Nido PJ, Swanson SJ (eds). *Sabiston and Spencer Surgery of the Chest.* Philadelphia: With permission from Elsevier, 2005:1919. .]

MANAGEMENT OF ASSOCIATED ANOMALIES

In patients with complex associated lesions (e.g., transposition of the great arteries, double-outlet right ventricle), the approach and timing of coarctation repair is usually dictated by the management of the more complex anatomy. This typically entails repair via median sternotomy with hypothermic circulatory arrest or low-flow continuous cerebral perfusion. Coarctation repair is performed by patch aortoplasty or resection and extended end-to-end anastomosis.

The management of CoA associated with a VSD remains controversial. VSDs that are likely to cause congestive heart failure, unlikely to close spontaneously, and have favorable anatomy may benefit from a single-stage repair of both VSD and coarctation via median sternotomy. Gaynor and colleagues advocate simultaneous repair for all infants with aortic coarctation, moderate to large VSDs, and aortic arch hypoplasia.[23] In their retrospective series, median survival at 16 months was 96 percent (actuarial 3-year survival), with actuarial freedom from all reintervention of 71 percent at 1 year and 59 percent at 2 years. Alternatively, some centers advocate pulmonary artery banding at the time of coarctation repair via left thoracotomy. Closure of the VSD and removal of the pulmonary artery band is performed via median sternotomy at 4 to 6 months of age. A multi-institutional study reported a 97 percent 2-year survival in patients undergoing two-stage repair. In this group of 34 patients, 38 percent had undergone subsequent VSD closure and 9 percent had expired,

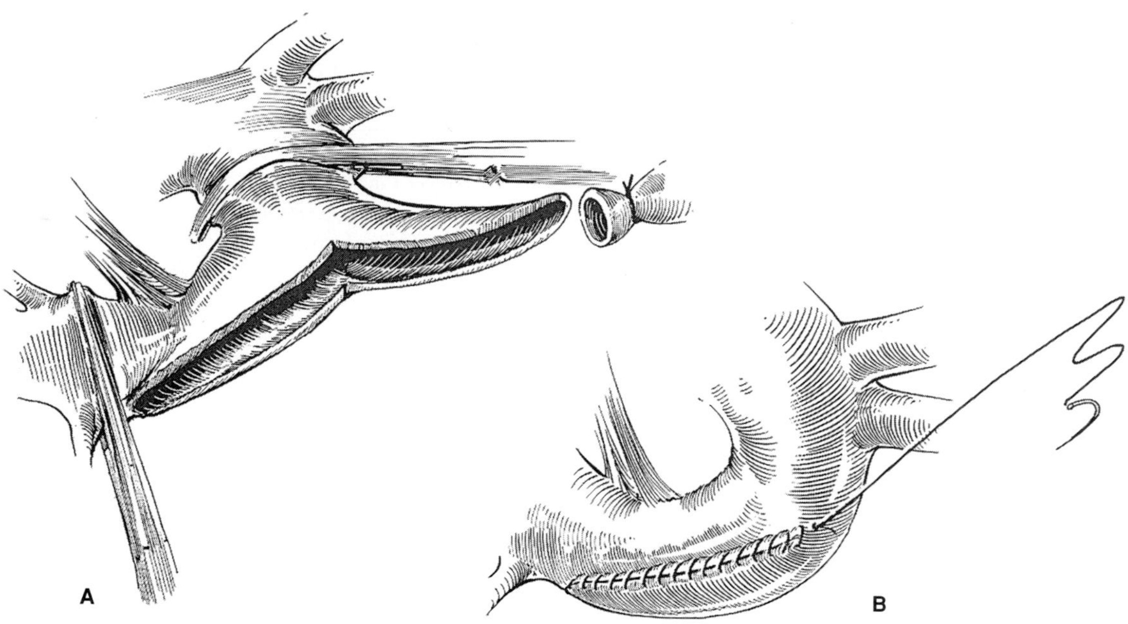

Figure 71-8 Subclavian flap aortoplasty. A. The transverse arch and descending aorta are clamped. An aortotomy extends from the descending aorta across the coarctation into the left subclavian artery. B. The left subclavian artery is sewn over the isthmus of the aorta using a continuous 7-0 polypropylene suture. [From Aortic coarctation. In: Casteneda AR, Jonas RA, Mayer JE, Hanley FL (eds). *Cardiac Surgery of the Neonate and Infant.* Philadelphia: Elsevier, 1994:347. With permission.]

leaving 53 percent free from further surgery at 2-year follow-up.[24] New technology, such as absorbable pulmonary artery bands and catheter-guided septal occluders, may increase the potential benefits of the two-stage approach.

POSTOPERATIVE MANAGEMENT AND EARLY COMPLICATIONS

In the absence of complex congenital heart disease, postoperative management focuses on pain control and

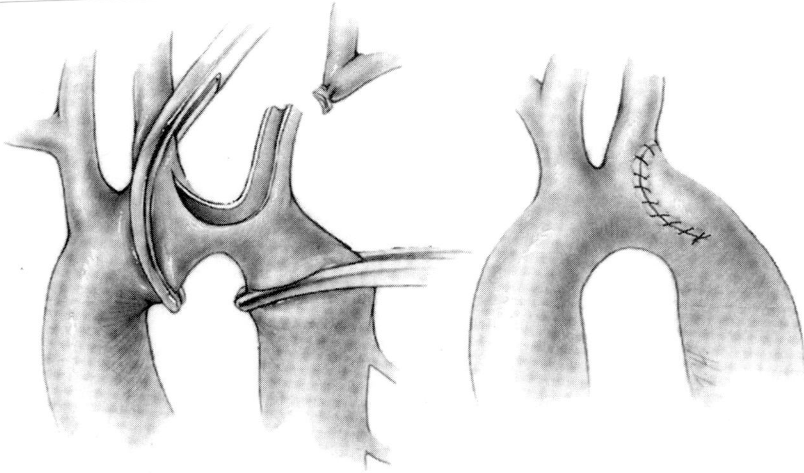

Figure 71-9 Reverse subclavian flap aortoplasty. The left subclavian artery is divided at its first branch (left). An incision is made on the medial aspect of the subclavian artery extending across the superior transverse arch to the origin of the left common carotid artery. The subclavian artery flap is turned medially to augment the transverse aortic arch (right). (From Khonsari and Sintek, p. 188.[52] With permission.)

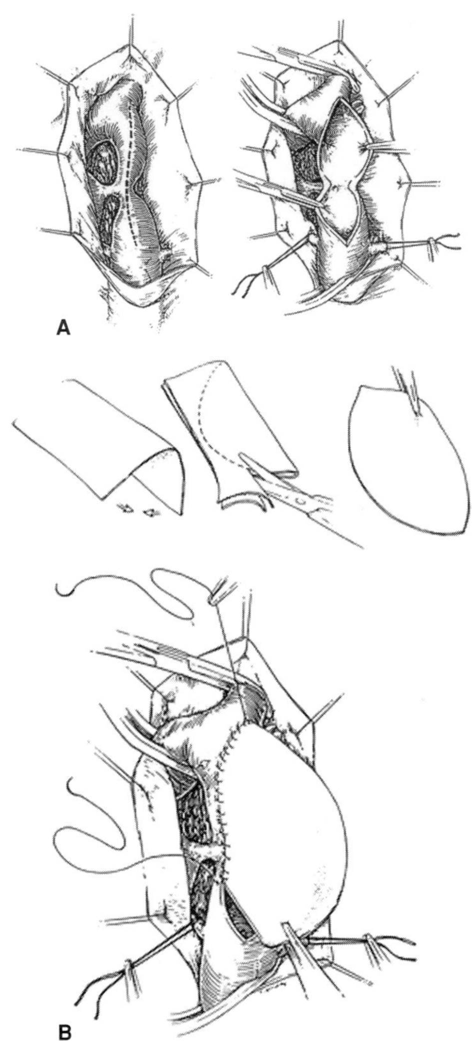

Figure 71-10 Patch aortoplasty. A. The aorta is incised longitudinally (dotted) line after obtaining proximal, distal and branch control. The coarctation ridge is left in situ. B. An oval patch of polytetrafluoroethylene is fashioned and sutured in place using a continuous suture, ensuring substantial redundancy to allow for growth. (From Backer et al, p. 132.[22] With permission.)

pulmonary toilet, as would be expected after any thoracotomy. In neonates, careful monitoring is essential, particularly as this group has a higher incidence of apnea and lobar collapse. Arterial hypertension following repair is common and independent of pain control. So-called paradoxical hypertension can persist for days to weeks following repair and may be related to increased catecholamine levels in a sensitive vascular bed coupled with the overstimulated renin-angiotensin axis. Age-appropriate antihypertensive agents are used carefully in order to avoid hypotension. Some 5 to 10 percent of older patients will report abdominal discomfort for a few days following coarctation repair ("postcoarctectomy syndrome"). This is mild in most cases but in some may require a period of bowel rest and nasogastric decompression. The most malignant form of this process can lead to necrotizing mesenteric arteritis requiring bowel resection. Aggressive management of hypertension appears beneficial. Chylothorax may occur as lymphatics are divided. Tube thoracostomy drainage should be carefully monitored for chylous characteristics, and clinically significant late pleural effusions should be evaluated by thoracentesis. Rarely, reoperation for ligation of lymphatics is required. The most feared complication of coarctation repair is paraplegia, with an incidence of up to 0.5 percent in some series, mostly historical.[25] A number of contributing factors have been identified, including cross-clamp time (greater than 30 min), division of arterial collaterals during dissection, and intraoperative hypotension, among others. The recognition of these factors has resulted in a decreased incidence in the modern era.

OPERATIVE MORTALITY

The development of modern neonatal intensive care has positively impacted the results of surgery for aortic coarctation. Most patients arrive in the operating room in stable condition and are closely monitored in the immediate postoperative period. Although early and late morbidity may occur, perioperative mortality remains rare. Serfontein and Kron reported neonatal mortality of 1.2 percent, which was directly related to preoperative instability.[26] In older patients the operation is even safer unless CoA is accompanied by significant associated anomalies.

LONG-TERM RESULTS

The development of long-term complications is not rare.[27] Table 71-1 summarizes key long-term sequelae, their incidence, and considerations regarding their etiology.

Hypertension

Hypertension is frequently reversed immediately following repair. Unfortunately, there is a significant incidence of late postoperative hypertension independent of recurrent coarctation, which may account for many of the long-term sequelae in these patients. The etiology of hypertension is multifactorial. At least some component is a result of renin overactivity, as renal perfusion is limited by the coarctation. Other contributing factors include deranged baroreceptor and endothelial function and abnormal arterial wall stiffness in the upper extremities.[28] The result is a poorly defined vasculopathic state associated with persistent hypertension throughout life. The roles of prenatal hemodynamics and delayed early treatment are also unknown.

Table 71-1 Risk factors for complications following repair of coarctation of the aorta

Complication	Prevalence (%)	Cause of death (%)	Risk factors
Coronary artery disease	5–23	25–66	Duration of preoperative hypertension Postoperative hypertension
Hypertension	25–75	–	Age at repair Recoarctation Follow-up duration Aortic insufficiency
Cerebrovascular accident	3	0–12	Pre- and postoperative hypertension Berry aneurysm
Heart failure	Unknown	9–35	Hypertension Aortic valve disease Coronary artery disease
Recoarctation	3.1–10.8	–	Repair in infancy Subclavian flap aortoplasty Balloon angioplasty
Aneurysm/rupture	5.4–20	5–35	Patch aortoplasty Balloon angioplasty

Source: Adapted from Jenkins.[27] With permission.

Recurrent coarctation

Recurrence of aortic coarctation is a process largely limited to repairs performed in the neonate. The overall recurrence rate depends on the original morphology, patient's age and weight at repair, associated anomalies, type of repair used, and vigilance of postoperative surveillance. Most centers use the same criteria for recurrence as with initial diagnosis: a pressure gradient across the lesion of greater than 20 mmHg. The recurrence rate in neonates weighing less than 2 kg may be as high as 44 percent,[29] but it is between 15 and 20 percent overall.[16,30] There is a 2 percent recurrence rate following coarctation repair in adults.[31]

Aneurysm formation

As discussed above, the development of aneurysms following patch repair with a polyester prosthetic patch has been well described. In addition, the formation of pseudoaneurysms along suture lines has been reported. These can become further complicated if they are mycotic.

Late mortality

The true incidence of long-term mortality directly related to CoA is difficult to determine. Heterogeneity of patient groups, loss to follow-up, and the underdetection of hypertension-related deaths preclude simple analysis. In the perioperative period, mortality is less than 3 percent, and is more than likely independent of technique of repair.[23,32] More important to the survival of these patients is the presence or absence of complex congenital heart disease. Late mortality appears to be related to the sequelae of uncontrolled hypertension, such as congestive heart failure, cerebrovascular events, and aortic dissection or rupture.[26]

CONCLUSIONS

CoA presents in a diverse population, ranging from critically ill neonates with complex congenital anatomy to adults with newly diagnosed refractory hypertension. The efficacy of surgical therapy has been well established, with several acceptable techniques for resection and repair being available. The presence of associated congenital anomalies is largely responsible for both prognosis and mortality. Catheter-based interventions may be appropriate in some older patients, but surgical repair remains the treatment of choice for the majority of patients with aortic coarctation.

INTERRUPTED AORTIC ARCH

Interrupted aortic arch (IAA) describes a congenital cardiovascular malformation involving an anatomic lack of continuity between the proximal and distal components of this vascular structure. Unlike coarctation, it is a complete disruption of the aorta. It is frequently associated with presence of a VSD and a spectrum of hypoplasia of left-sided heart structures secondary to limited left heart outflow in fetal life. In addition, there is an association with microdeletion of the q11 segment of chromosome 22, which may involve issues of developmental delay and cognitive sequelae.

IAA comprises 1 to 4 percent of autopsy cases of congenital heart disease and represents 1.3 percent of infants presenting with congenital cardiovascular disease. The estimated prevalence is 0.003 per 1000 births.[33] Untreated, this uncommon anomaly has a median age to death of 4 to 10 days, with 75 percent mortality within 1 month.[34] Death occurs with closure of the ductus arteriosus. If the ductus stays open longer, survival is possible; however mortality is then 90 percent by 1 year.[35]

IAA was first described by Steidele in 1778.[36] Surgical intervention was first described by Merrill in 1955, where a direct anastomosis was performed in a patient with short segmented IAA.[37] An associated VSD was not closed at the time of repair. By 1959, Celoria and Patton had collected 28 cases that they classified according to site of obstruction.[38] Villalobos and colleagues as well as Blake and colleagues each reported a successful case during the early 1960s, in which they employed a prosthetic graft for repair.[39,40] Sirak and colleagues were the first to describe the use of "turned down" arch vessels in the reconstruction as well as the first neonate to survive this repair.[41] Barratt-Boyes and coworkers in 1970 performed the first simultaneous repair of aortic arch interruption and VSD closure.[42] This procedure was performed using deep hypothermic circulatory arrest via thoracotomy and median sternotomy. The first simultaneous IAA and VSD repair via the anterior approach and without the use of a prosthetic graft was reported by Trusler in 1975.[43] The treatment of IAA was revolutionized with the introduction of PGE_1 therapy in 1976 by Elliot and colleagues.[44]

EMBRYOLOGY

The aortic arch is described anatomically as having proximal and distal components. In early fetal development, there are six aortic arches. These connect with the right and left dorsal aortas distally (descending aorta) and with the conotruncus proximally (proximal aorta). Arches I to III subsequently regress to become facial and skull vessels.[45]

In normal embryogenesis, the proximal aortic arch originates from the left horn of the aortic sac to develop the portion between the innominate and left carotid arteries. The distal arch (between the left carotid and left subclavian arteries) is derived from the left fourth aortic arch. The aorta between the left subclavian artery and the ductus arteriosus is derived from the confluence of the dorsal aorta and the left sixth arch. The site of interruption is associated morphologically with a specific abnormality in the development of these aortic arches.[45]

MORPHOLOGY AND CLASSIFICATION

Celoria and Patton introduced a classification system (Fig. 71-11) for IAA in 1959.[38] Type A interruption was described as occurring distal to the left subclavian artery. In this scenario, the interruption yields a duct-dependent environment for lower-body perfusion. This form of IAA has been described as "aortic atresia" and classically presents with a fibrous cord across the interruption with no luminal continuity. The length of interruption may vary and may approach up to 3 CM in some cases. Type B interruption occurs between the left common carotid artery and the left subclavian artery. It is the most common type of IAA, with an approximate incidence of 60 to 70 percent.[46] It is important to note that type B IAA can be associated with an aberrant right subclavian artery originating from the distal descending thoracic aorta. This associated anomaly is correlated with the nomenclature of type B_1 versus type B_2 IAA. Type B IAA is also the specific subtype associated with DiGeorge syndrome and 22q11 microdeletion. Type C interruption is found between the innominate artery and left common carotid artery. It is the rarest form, comprising less than 5 percent of IAAs.[47]

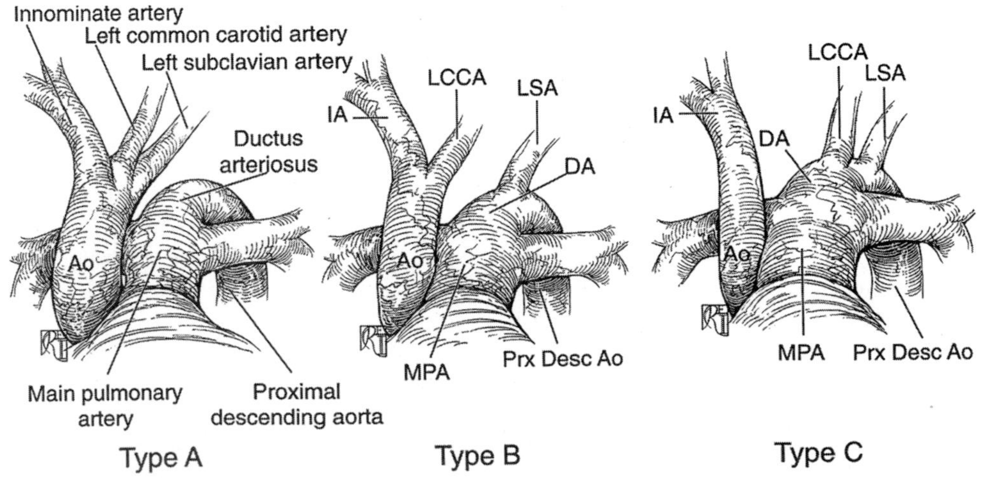

Figure 71-11 Celoria and Patton morphologic classification of aortic arch interruption, according to the site of anatomic discontinuity along the arch. (From Jonas.[50] With permission.)

ASSOCIATED CARDIAC ANOMALIES

Anomalies of the brachiocephalic vessels are relatively common. As mentioned, an aberrant right subclavian artery originating as a fourth brachiocephalic branch from the descending thoracic aorta is common in type B but also may be found in type A. Other abnormal origins of the right subclavian artery include a cervical takeoff from the right common carotid artery or from a right-sided ductus, which itself is originating from the right pulmonary artery.[48]

The aortic valve is bicuspid in approximately 30 to 50 percent of patients with IAA, as is the case with aortic coarctation. Subaortic stenosis may be present or may develop later, especially in cases involving type B IAA and an aberrant origin of the right subclavian artery. This is due to the increased flow via the ductus arteriosus during fetal development and less flow via the left ventricular outflow tract (LVOT).[34]

A coexisting large VSD is nearly always present. Aside from a patent ductus arteriosus, it is the most common associated anomaly, occurring in approximately 75 percent of cases. This anatomic anomaly (with the septum frequently being malaligned and displaced posteriorly) creates a large muscular ridge known as the muscle of Moulaert.[34,49] This structure may protrude into the subaortic region, resulting in left ventricular outflow tract obstruction (LVOTO).

An atrial septal defect can also be seen in association with IAA. It is usually of the patent foramen ovale variety but can at times be large and thus physiologically significant. Other lesions such as truncus arteriosus (common arterial trunk), transposition of the great arteries, or aortopulmonary window may coexist.

CLINICAL PRESENTATION AND DIAGNOSIS

Via ultrasound evaluation, prenatal diagnosis has become more commonplace. In this controlled diagnostic environment, PGE_1 therapy is initiated immediately following birth. In infants in whom a diagnosis has not been made prenatally, clinical sequelae are often not present until ductal closure. Subsequently, generalized tissue malperfusion and profound associated acidosis is typical. End-organ issues such as liver dysfunction with elevated hepatic enzymes, kidney failure with anuria, and ischemic gut injury with necrotizing enterocolitis may occur. Myocardial and cerebral injury may also be present due to prolonged systemic acidosis. In cases where ductal closure does not occur, symptoms of congestive heart failure may result secondary to an increasing left-to-right shunt via the VSD as pulmonary resistance falls.[50]

Clinical examination findings include abnormal pulses, depending on the location of aortic interruption. Differential cyanosis between upper and lower extremities is not often present or conclusive. Cardiac murmurs and electrocardiograms are also nonspecific. Chest radiographs may reveal gross cardiomegaly as well as pulmonary congestion.

Echocardiography, the only specific diagnostic modality, is required prior to operative intervention (Fig. 71-12). Cardiac catheterization, which was challenging in neonates presenting in shock, is no longer considered a requirement for diagnosis unless unusual anatomic features require further definition. Using transthoracic echocardiography, the exact site of aortic arch interruption as well as the presence of an associated VSD can typically be determined. In addition, evaluation of the LVOT as well as any other coexisting intracardiac anomalies can be satisfactorily performed. Additional specific data such as the length of interruption, luminal diameter of the aorta, exact dimensions of the LVOT, anatomy of the aortic valve, and presence or absence of thymic tissue are helpful in designing a therapeutic strategy. Body imaging techniques, such as computed tomography and

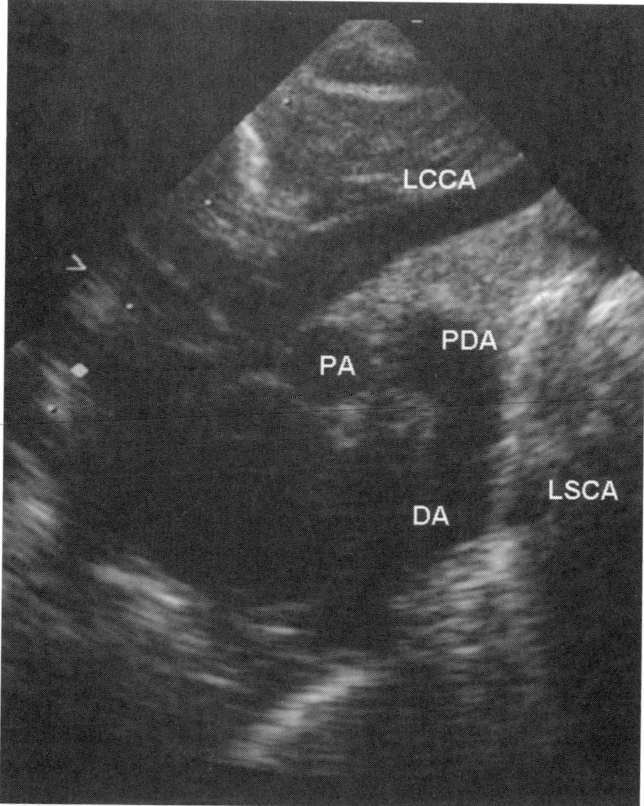

Figure 71-12 Echocardiographic findings in aortic arch interruption type B. No continuity in the arch is noted echocardiographically between the takeoff of the left common carotid and subclavian arteries. AA = ascending aorta; DA = descending aorta; IA = innominate artery; LCCA = left common carotid artery; LSCA = left subclavian artery; PDA = patent ductus arteriosus. (Courtesy of William Ravekes, MD, Division of Pediatric Cardiology, The Johns Hopkins University.)

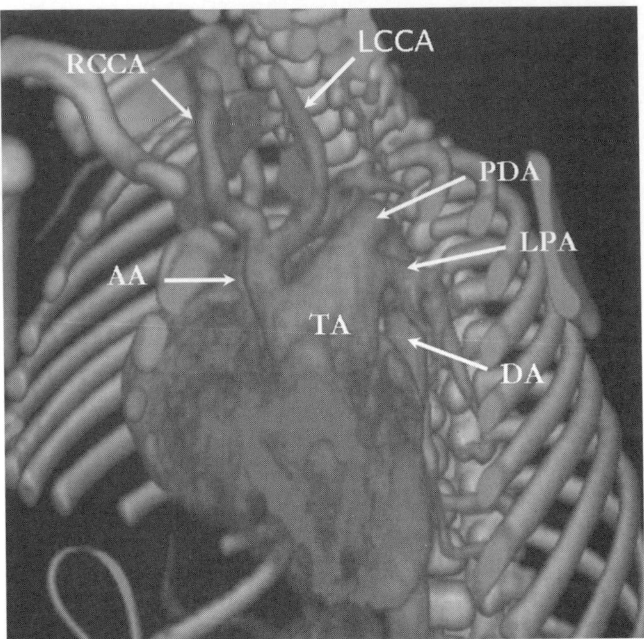

Figure 71-13 Magnetic resonance imaging (MRI) in complex aortic arch interruption. Neonate with truncus arteriosus and interrupted aortic arch (type A). Truncus arteriosus (TA) giving rise to right and left (LPA) pulmonary arteries and in direct continuity with the descending aorta (DA) via a patent ductus arteriosus (PDA). The ascending aorta branched in right (RCCA), left (LCCA) common carotid and left subclavian arteries (LSCA). The right subclavian artery (not visible) originated from the proximal right pulmonary artery and was divided intraoperatively. (Courtesy of Philip J. Spevak, MD, Division of Pediatric Cardiology, the Johns Hopkins University.)

magnetic resonance imaging (Fig. 71-13), can be useful in difficult cases and to aid in surgical planning.

TREATMENT

Medical management

The introduction of PGE_1 in 1976 was revolutionary in the treatment of IAA. The reestablishment of ductal flow is an imperative first step in the initial management of this abnormality. The maximization of pulmonary resistance is also beneficial in regard to increasing systemic blood flow, improving end-organ perfusion, and avoiding associated systemic acidosis. This can be achieved by minimizing administration of oxygen as well as employing a strategy of hypoventilation and permissive hypercapnea via specified ventilatory support. Any evidence of metabolic acidosis should be treated. The achievement of appropriate volume status as well as the use of inotropic agents may also be critical in resuscitation. With appropriate medical management, the neonate may be stabilized and will ultimately be a more appropriate candidate for surgical intervention, with surgical outcomes being markedly improved.

Surgical techniques

Improvements in cardiopulmonary bypass technique as well as the concept of selective antegrade or regional low-flow cerebral perfusion have changed operative strategies for the treatment of this disease entity. Single-stage repair with direct anastomosis with or without the need for circulatory arrest has become a strategy employed at most centers.[51,52] As an alternative, a staged approach with direct repair of the IAA and pulmonary artery banding for palliation of the VSD, followed by subsequent closure of the VSD, may be considered. Using this philosophy, a left thoracotomy is employed not only for cases of IAA without associated VSD but also in a staged approach for neonates with associated VSD. IAA represents a spectrum of entities; thus the surgical approach must take patient-specific factors into consideration.

In the case of type A IAA, the anatomic abnormality can be conceptually classified in the same category as coarctation. An extended end-to-end anastomosis via left thoracotomy and without the need for cardiopulmonary bypass may be the management of choice if no other intracardiac pathology is present. The choice of a single versus a staged approach for treatment of type B IAA with or without associated cardiac anomalies is more complex.

In neonates undergoing one-stage repair, it is very helpful to place invasive arterial monitoring in the right upper extremity. This allows perfusion pressures to be monitored and documented during periods of antegrade cerebral perfusion. Umbilical and/or femoral arterial pressure can also be monitored to document the adequacy of distal perfusion and postrepair gradients. Single or bicaval venous cannulation is employed for venous drainage. An arterial cannula circuit with a Y-connector split is used to perfuse both the aortic arch proximal to the obstruction as well as the descending aorta via cannulation of the pulmonary artery trunk and advancing it toward the patent ductus arteriosus (Fig. 71-14). Cannulation of the ascending aorta should be performed along its right lateral aspect or separately at the base of the innominate artery to keep clear the region of the aorta that will be incised for anastomosis to the distal aortic limb. Also, once cardiopulmonary bypass has been initiated, it is critical to snare tourniquets around the branch pulmonary arteries to limit pulmonary runoff and ensure adequate distal perfusion via the ductus arteriosus into the descending aorta.

Cooling is initiated with a goal of profound hypothermia (16 to 18°C). While cooling occurs, extensive mobilization of the aorta and its branches is undertaken in order to obtain a subsequent tension-free anastomosis.

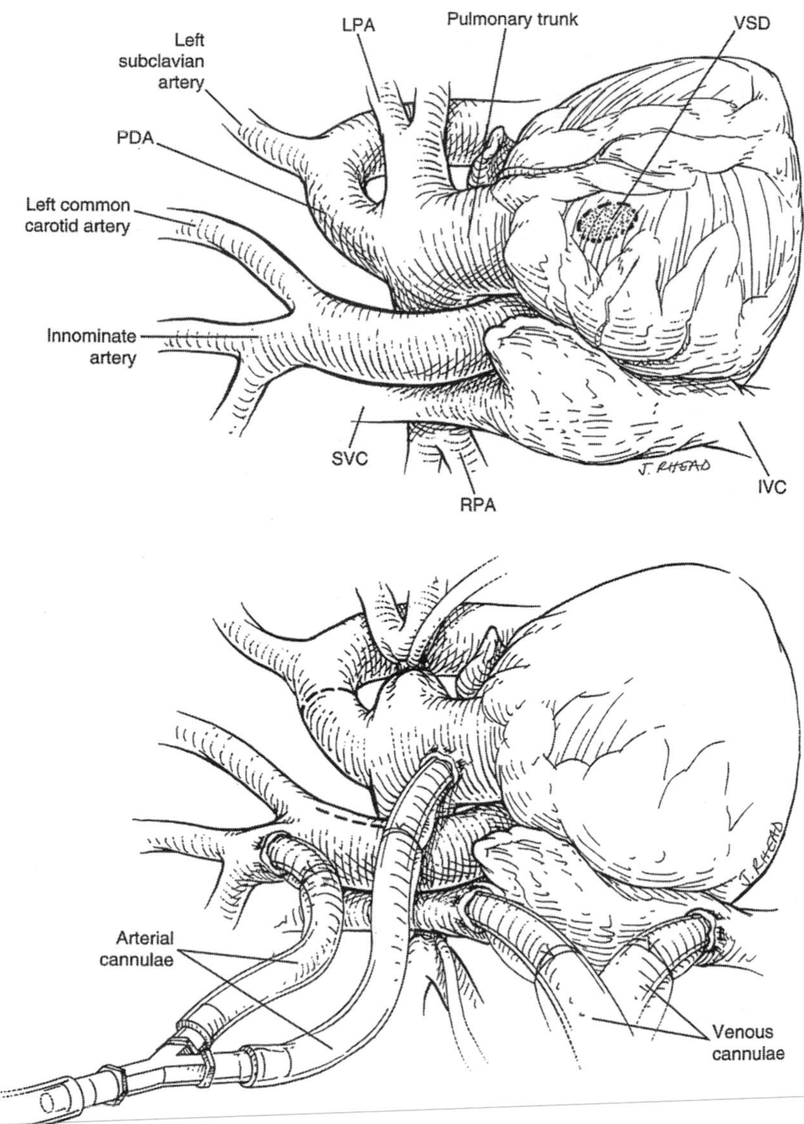

Figure 71-14 Cardiopulmonary bypass (CPB) strategy for repair of type B interrupted aortic arch as schematically represented from the operating surgeon's perspective (top). The arterial return line is bifurcated and introduced into the main pulmonary artery and ascending aorta. The cannulation site for the latter is positioned opposite to the anticipated anastomosis (dotted line, bottom panel). Systemic venous drainage is provided by bicaval or single (in small neonates) venous cannulas. Pulmonary artery snares are tightened on initiation of CPB. IVC = inferior vena cava; LPA = left pulmonary artery; PDA = patent ductus arteriosus; RPA = right pulmonary artery; SVC = superior vena cava; VSD = ventricular septal defect. (From Kouchoukos et al, p. 1358.[11] With permission.)

On achieving the desired cooling, the descending aortic perfusion cannula is removed. The distal aorta is subsequently clamped and all ductal tissue is ligated and excised.

During arch reconstruction, cerebral and cardiac perfusion pressures should be maintained at approximately 50 mL/kg/min at 22°C if selective antegrade cerebral perfusion is utilized.[53] Flows may be further reduced if the patient is cooled more aggressively. Perfusion pressures can be documented via the arterial monitoring line for the right upper extremity. A direct end-to-side aortic anastomosis can then be performed without tension between the distal aorta and an aortotomy in the proximal aortic limb. An incision is made along the left pos-

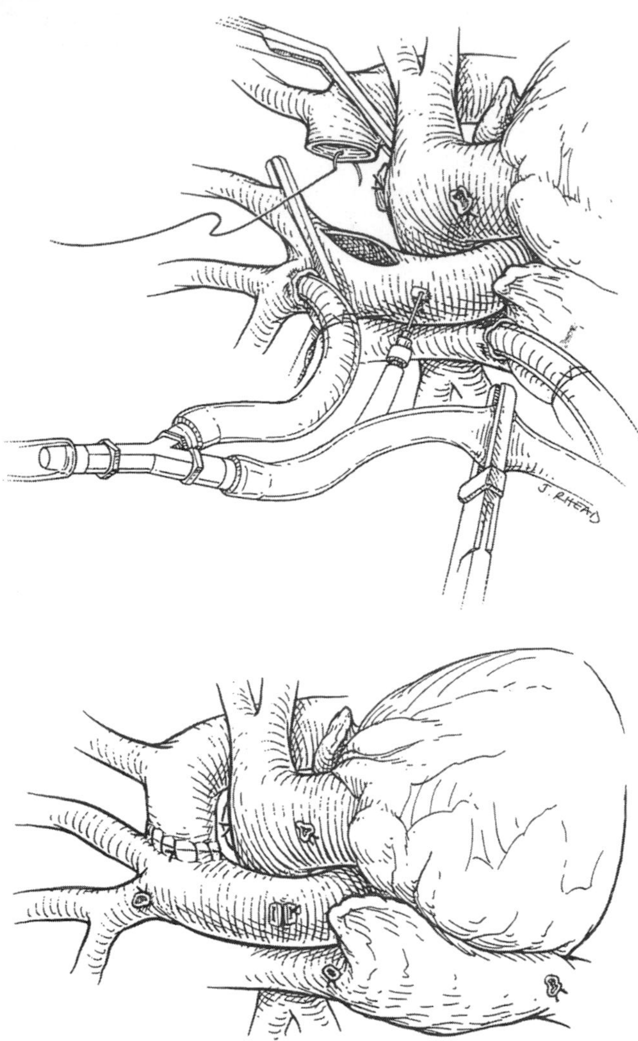

Figure 71-15 End-to-side anastomosis between the ascending and descending aorta in type B aortic arch interruption. The return cannula in the pulmonary artery has been removed and selective antegrade cerebral perfusion is maintained (top). The end-to-side anastomosis is completed with a continuous polypropylene suture (bottom). (From Kouchoukos et al, p. 1358.[11] With permission.)

terolateral aspect of the ascending aorta, and it is enlarged to approximate the lumen of the distal aortic limb. The anastomosis is completed, using continuous suture technique (Fig. 71-15), along the posterior aspect of the vertically oriented ascending aorta. Patch augmentation of any associated regions of hypoplasia may be considered. In case of anomalous right subclavian artery takeoff, division of this structure may aid in the mobilization of the descending thoracic aorta and improve the likelihood of a tension-free anastomosis.

While maintaining distal perfusion and after infusion of cold blood cardioplegia into the aortic root, the ascending aorta can be clamped and the VSD and or other associated anomalies addressed. Issues related to LVOTO may be treated either via subaortic resection or, in extreme cases, via a Damus-Kaye-Stansel (DKS) type of procedure. In this setting, left ventricular outflow may be directed via the VSD toward the pulmonary artery using an intracardiac baffle. The main pulmonary artery is then divided proximal to its bifurcation site and anastomosed to the side of the native aorta. Subsequently, a right ventricular outflow tract reconstruction is undertaken from the right ventricle to the confluence of the main right and left pulmonary arteries.[54,55]

Alternatively, an intracardiac baffle is not performed and ventricular output is directed through both aorta and pulmonary artery (joined with a DKS-type anastomosis) into the aortic arch. A modified Blalock-Taussig shunt is then performed to provide pulmonary blood flow, deferring ventricular baffling and insertion of a right ventricle–pulmonary artery conduit to a later time.

Alternative approaches to the repair of IAA are available and should remain in consideration due to the broad disease spectrum that this entity represents. At the Indiana University School of Medicine–Riley Hospital for Children, a staged approach with the use of a left carotid artery swing-down technique has yielded excellent results. In this technique, via a left fourth interspace thoracotomy, patients underwent division of the left carotid artery with anastomosis of the divided end to the descending aorta (Fig. 71-16). Pulmonary artery banding

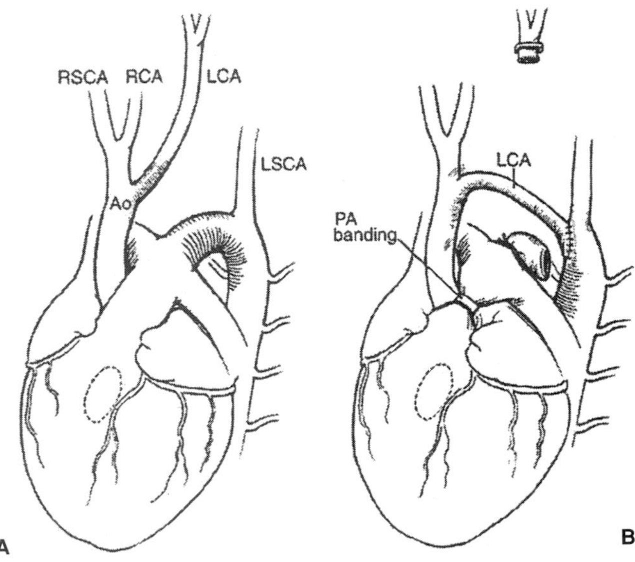

Figure 71-16 Left common carotid (LCA) "turndown" repair of type B (left) aortic arch interruption. The artery is divided distally and anastomosed in an end-to-side fashion to the descending aorta (right). The ventricular septal defect (VSD) is left open and the pulmonary trunk is banded. Ao = aorta; LCA = left carotid artery; LSCA = left subclavian artery; RCA = right carotid artery; RSCA = right subclavian artery. (From Brown et al.[56] With permission.)

was employed in cases with associated VSD. Although this strategy has the disadvantage of being a staged palliative approach, outcome data are quite favorable, especially with respect to early mortality. This strategy may be attractive in cases presenting other complex cardiac anomalies or other significant comorbidities such as very low birth weight.[56]

Postoperative care of patients with complete repair of a simple IAA should be relatively straightforward. Any need for prolonged inotropic support or additional critical care monitoring should prompt a search for additional untreated hemodynamic lesions or other uncorrected pathology. An undiagnosed or residual VSD may be identified by analyzing oxygen saturation data from a pulmonary artery line. Echocardiography may also be utilized. In unusual circumstances, cardiac catheterization may yield important data in regard to residual LVOTO.[48]

OUTCOMES

Hospital mortality for neonatal single-stage repair of IAA in the current era is less than 10 percent.[46] This figure is unchanged by the presence of an associated VSD. Among subtypes of IAA, mortality has been described to be as low as 4 percent for type A interruption and 11 percent for type B. The highest survival is in the subgroup of patients with isolated type A IAA amenable to complete repair via left thoracotomy. Lowest survival data are published for patients with type C IAA. The presence of coexisting anomalies and the location of interruption have been shown to affect mortality risk. Other risk factors for mortality include preoperative clinical status with regard to degree and adequacy of resuscitation in addition to the presence and severity of LVOTO.[51] Following initial complete intracardiac repair, 5-year survival as high as 70 percent has been documented. [57] The most extensive reported long-term follow-up has been to 16 years and has described an overall survival of 59 percent, with a need for arch reintervention of 28 percent.[58] As additional long-term data become available, these figures will likely improve as a reflection of advances in medical and surgical therapy.

In the Indiana University School of Medicine experience using a staged approach and left carotid swing-down for arch reconstruction, operative mortality for patients with IAA and VSD, regardless of interruption subtype, was only 0.3 percent (1 of 44); 27 percent of these patients had associated LVOTO. In patients with more complex associated anomalies, such as Taussig-Bing double-outlet right ventricle or truncus arteriosus, there was no mortality for staged intervention using left carotid swing-down.[56]

Morbidity issues for IAA are somewhat specific to subtype as well as anatomic variations. Left recurrent laryngeal and phrenic nerve injuries may occur owing to the extensive dissection required around the aortic arch and adjacent structures. The left mainstem bronchus passes under the arch of the aorta; as a result, anastomotic tension between the proximal and distal aortic limbs may induce a bowstring effect over the bronchus, yielding airway obstruction and associated pulmonary obstructive issues.

Late morbidity can be divided into two primary categories: persistence of a transaortic gradient or worsening LVOTO. Pressure gradients across the anastomosis are more likely to occur in situations where synthetic patch material has been employed, owing to a lack of growth potential. This should be avoided. Patients with a direct arch anastomosis have as high as a 60 percent incidence of late obstruction (gradient greater than 30 mmHg) within 18 months of surgery.[46] Percutaneous balloon dilatation can relieve residual or recurrent arch obstruction safely in the majority of these patients. In more recent published experiences, however, freedom from reintervention due to gradients across the reconstruction is excellent, at 86 percent at 3 years.[53] A more problematic long-term detrimental outcome is associated with late subaortic obstruction or LVOTO. Freedom from reintervention for such pathology has been reported as high as 77 percent at 3 years.[57]

CONCLUSIONS

IAA represents an extreme, life-threatening form of congenital heart disease; it is a lesion that may be treated by any of several of management strategies. In the current era, surgical options yield excellent outcomes. The presenting clinical picture and effective initiation of medical management is paramount to overall outcome. PGE_1 has revolutionized the ability to temporize these patients, allowing for complete resuscitation and medical stabilization prior to operative intervention. In most centers, single-stage repair is the preferred operative approach. However, a two-stage approach, with initial arch reconstruction using a left carotid artery swing-down and pulmonary artery banding with subsequent intracardiac repair, yields excellent results and may be considered. Early outcomes are dependent on preoperative medical management, subtype of interruption, and extent of associated anomalies. Long-term outcomes are associated with levels of transaortic reconstruction pressure gradients as well as issues of LVOTO. Overall, surgical management of this anatomic abnormality is quite promising.

References

1. Hoffman JIE, Kaplan S. The incidence of congenital heart disease. *J Am Coll Cardiol* 2002;39:1890.
2. Paris M. Rétrècissement considerable de l'aorte pectorale observé à l'Hotel Dieu de Paris. *J Chirurg Desault* 1791; II:107.
3. Crafoord C, Nylin G. Congenital coarctation of the aorta and its surgical treatment. *J Thorac Cardiovasc Surg* 1945; 14:347.
4. Gross RE, Hufnagel CA. Coarctation of the aorta: Experimental studies regarding its surgical corrections. *N Engl J Med* 1945;233:287.
5. Gross RE. Treatment of certain aortic coarctations by homologous grafts. *Ann Surg* 1951;134:753.
6. Vossschulte K. Surgical correction of coarctation of the aorta by an "isthmusplastic" operation. *Thorax* 1961; 16:338.
7. Waldhausen JA, Nahrwold DL. Repair of coarctation of the aorta with a subclavian flap. *J Thorac Cardiovasc Surg* 1966;51:532.
8. Ho SY, Anderson RH. Coarctation, tubular hypoplasia, and the ductus arteriosus. Histological study of 35 specimens. *Br Heart J* 1979;41:268.
9. Machii M, Becker AE. Hypoplastic aortic arch morphology pertinent to growth after correction of aortic coarctation. *Ann Thorac Surg* 1997;64:516.
10. Graham TP, Atwood GF, Boerth RC, et al. Right and left heart size and function in infants with symptomatic coarctation. *Circulation* 1977;56:641.
11. Coarctation of the aorta and interrupted aortic arch. In: Kouchoukos NT, Blackstone EH, Doty DB, et al (eds). *Kirklin/Barratt-Boyes: Cardiac Surgery*, 3d ed. Philadelphia: Churchill-Livingstone, 2003:1315.
12. Becker AE, Becker MJ, Edwards JE. Anomalies associated with coarctation of the aorta: Particular references to infancy. *Circulation* 1970;41:1067.
13. Mohammadi S, Serraf A, Belli E, et al. Left-sided lesions after anatomic repair of transposition of the great arteries, ventricular septal defect, and coarctation: Surgical factors. *J Thorac Cardiovasc Surg* 2004;128:44.
14. Parr GVS, Waldhausen JA, Bharati S, et al. Coarctation in Taussig-Bing malformation of the heart: Surgical significance. *J Thorac Cardiovasc Surg* 1983;86:280.
15. Elzenga NJ, Gittenberger de Groot AC. Coarctation and related aortic arch abnormalities in hypoplastic left heart syndrome. *Int J Cardiol* 1985;8:379.
16. Fiore AC, Fischer LK, Schwartz T, et al. Comparison of angioplasty and surgery for neonatal aortic coarctation. *Ann Thorac Surg* 2005;80:1659.
17. Maheshwari S, Bruckheimer E, Fahey JT, et al. Balloon angioplasty of postsurgical recoarctation in infants. *J Am Coll Cardiol* 2000;35:209.
18. Mahadevan VS, Vondermuhll IF, Mullen MJ. Endovascular aortic coarctation stenting in adolescents and adults. *Cathet Cardiovasc Intervent* 2006;67:268.
19. Dave HH, Buechel ERV, Prêtre R. Muscle-sparing extrapleural approach for the repair of aortic coarctation. *Ann Thorac Surg* 2006;81:243.
20. Parks WJ, Ngo TD, Plauth WH, et al. Incidence of aneurysm formation after Dacron patch aortoplasty repair for coarctation of the aorta: Long–term results and assessment utilizing magnetic resonance angiography with three-dimensional surface rendering. *J Am Coll Cardiol* 1995;26:266.
21. Rheuban KS, Gutgesell HP, Carpenter MA, et al. Aortic aneurysm after patch angioplasty for aortic isthmus coarctation in childhood. *Am J Cardiol* 1986;58:178.
22. Backer CL, Paape K, Zales VR, et al. Coarctation of the aorta: Repair with polytetrafluoroethylene patch aortoplasty. *Circulation* 1995;92:132.
23. Gaynor WJ, Wernovsky G, Rychik J, et al. Outcome following single-stage repair of coarctation with ventricular septal defect. *Eur J Cardiothorac Surg* 2000;18:62.
24. Quaegebeur JM, Jonas RA, Weinberg AD, et al. Outcomes in seriously ill neonates with coarctation of the aorta. *J Thorac Cardiovasc Surg* 1994;108:841.
25. Brewer LA, Fosburg RG, Mulder GA, et al. Spinal cord complications following surgery for coarctation of the aorta. *J Thorac Cardiovasc Surg* 1972;64:368.
26. Serfontein SJ, Kron IL. Complications of coarctation repair. *Pediatr Card Surg Ann Semin Thorac Cardiovasc Surg* 2002;5:206.
27. Jenkins NP, Ward C. Coarctation of the aorta: Natural history and outcome after surgical treatment. *Q J Med* 1999;92:365.
28. de Divitiis M, Pilla C, Kattenhorn M, et al. Vascular dysfunction after repair of coarctation of the aorta: Impact of early surgery. *Circulation* 2001;104:I165.
29. Bacha EA, Almodovar M, Wessel DL, et al. Surgery for coarctation of the aorta in infants weighing less than 2 kg. *Ann Thorac Surg* 2001;71:1260.
30. Cowley CG, Orsmond GS, Feola P, et al. Long-term, randomized comparison of balloon angioplasty and surgery for native coarctation of the aorta in childhood. *Circulation* 2005;111:3453.
31. Carr JA. The results of catheter-based therapy compared with surgical repair of adult aortic coarctation. *J Am Coll Cardiol* 2006;47:1101.
32. Rubay JE, Sluysmans T, Alexandrescu V, et al. Surgical repair of coarctation of the aorta in infants under one year of age: Long-term results in 146 patients comparing subclavian flap aortoplasty and modified end to end anastomosis. *J Cardiovasc Surg* 1992;33:216.
33. Collins-Nakai RL, Dick M, Parisi-Buckley L, et al. Interrupted aortic arch in infancy. *J Pediatr* 1976;88:959.
34. Freedom RM, Bain HH, Esplugas E, et al. Ventricular septal defect in interruption of aortic arch. *Am J Cardiol* 1977;39:572.
35. Dische MR, Tsai M, Baltaxe HA, et al. Solitary interruption of the arch of the aorta. *Am J Cardiol* 1975;35:271.
36. Steidele RJ, *Samml Chir Med Beob* 1778;2:114.
37. Merrill DL, Webster CA, Sampson PC. Congenital absence of the aortic isthmus: Report of a case with successful surgical repair. *J Thorac Cardiovasc Surg* 1957;33:311.
38. Celoria GC, Patton RB. Congenital absence of the aortic arch. *Am Heart J* 1959;58:407.
39. Villalobos MC, Balderrama DP, Lopez JL, et al. Complete interruption of the aorta. *Am J Cardiol* 1961;8:664.
40. Blake HA, Manion WC, Spencer FC. Atresia or absence of the aortic isthmus. *J Urol Nephrol* 1962;43:607.

41. Sirak HD, Ressallat M, Hosier DM, et al. A new operation for repairing aortic arch atresia in infancy: Report of 3 cases. *Circulation* 1968;37:II43.
42. Barratt-Boyes BG, Nicholls TT, Brandt PW, et al. Aortic arch interruption associated with patent ductus arteriosus, ventricular septal defect and total anomalous pulmonary venous connection. *J Thorac Cardiovasc Surg* 1972;63:367.
43. Trusler GA, Izukawa T. Interrupted aortic arch and ventricular septal defect. Direct repair through a median sternotomy incision in a 13-day-old infant. *J Thorac Cardiovasc Surg* 1975;69:126.
44. Elliot RB, Starling MB, Neutze JM. Medical management of the ductus arteriosus. *Lancet* 1975;1:140.
45. Vricella LA, Cameron DE. Aortic arch interruption. In: Yang, Cameron DE (eds). *Current Therapy in Thoracic and Cardiovascular Surgery.* Philadelphia: Mosby, 2004:775–778.
46. Sell JE, Jonas RA, Mayer IE, et al. The results of a surgical program for interrupted aortic arch. *J Thorac Cardiovasc Surg* 1988;96:864.
47. Van Praagh R, Bernhard WF, Rosenthal A, et al. Interrupted aortic arch: Surgical treatment. *Am J Cardiol* 1971;27:200.
48. Kutsche LM, Van Mierop LH. Cervical origin of the right subclavian artery in aortic arch interruption: Pathogenesis and significance. *Am J Cardiol* 1984; 53:892.
49. Fleming WSH, Sarafian LB, Clarke ED, et al. Critical aortic coarctation: Patch aortoplasty in infants less than age 3 months. *Am J Cardiol* 1979;44:687.
50. Jonas RA. Interrupted aortic arch. In: Mavroudis C, Backer CL (eds). *Pediatric Cardiac Surgery,* 3d ed. Philadelphia: Mosby, 2003:345–359.
51. Jonas RA, Quaegebeur JM, Kirklin JW, et al. Outcomes in patients with interrupted aortic arch and ventricular septal defect. A multi-institutional study. *J Thorac Cardiovasc Surg* 1994;107:1099.
52. Khonsari S, Sintek CF. *Cardiac Surgery: Safeguards and Pitfalls in Operative Technique,* 3d ed. Philadelphia: Lippincott, Williams & Wilkins, 2003.
53. Asou T, Kado H, Imoto Y, et al. Selective cerebral perfusion technique during aortic arch repair in neonates. *Ann Thorac Surg* 1996;61:1546.
54. Yasui H, Kado H, Nakano E, et al. Primary repair of interrupted aortic arch and severe aortic stenosis in neonates. *J Thorac Cardiovasc Surg* 1987;93:539.
55. Ilbawi MN, Idriss FS, DeLeon SY, et al. Surgical management of patients with interrupted aortic arch and severe subaortic stenosis. *Ann Thorac Surg* 1988;45:174.
56. Brown JW, Ruzmetov M, Okada Y, et al. Outcomes in patients with interrupted aortic arch and associated anomalies: A 20 year experience. *Eur J Cardiothorac Surg* 2006. In press.
57. Fulton JO, Mas C, Brizard CP, et al. Does left ventricular outflow tract obstruction influence outcome of interrupted aortic arch repair? *Ann Thorac Surg* 1999;67:177.
58. McCrindle BW, Tchervenkov CI, Konstantinov IE, et al. Risk factors associated with mortality and interventions in 472 neonates with interrupted aortic arch: A congenital heart surgeons society study. *J Thorac Cardiovasc Surg* 2005;129:243.

CHAPTER

72 COR TRIATRIATUM

Giancarlo Crupi

DEFINITION

The classic definition of cor triatriatum is based on the recognition that either the left atrium (cor triatriatum sinister) or the right atrium (cor triatriatum dexter) is divided into two chambers by an abnormal fibromuscular membrane. The terms *subdivided left* or *right atrium*[1–4] will be used throughout this chapter, highlighting in a more comprehensible fashion the basic anomaly of this uncommon cardiac malformation.

In the commonest left-sided variant of this lesion, the pulmonary veins enter a proximal common pulmonary venous chamber, which is separated by a fibromuscular membrane from a distal chamber containing the mitral valve and left atrial appendage.

KEY CONCEPTS

- Epidemiology
  - Cor triatriatum is an uncommon congenital cardiac anomaly in which either the left (cor triatriatum sinister) or right (cor triatriatum dexter) atrium is divided into two chambers by a membrane. Subdivided left atrium represents the most frequent anatomic variant of this lesion, which accounts from 0.1 to 0.4 percent of all congenital heart defects.
- Morphology
  - The pulmonary veins enter a proximal chamber (common pulmonary venous chamber) separated by a fibromuscular membrane from a distal chamber where the left atrial appendage and the mitral valve are found. The proximal and distal chambers may communicate through one or more openings within the dividing membrane, and an atrial septal defect (ASD) is usually present.
- Pathophysiology
  - In the absence of associated cardiac lesions, the pathophysiology of subdivided left atrium depends on the resulting obstruction to pulmonary blood flow. Pulmonary overcirculation is present when left-to-right shunting occurs through an ASD between common pulmonary venous chamber and right atrium.
- Clinical features
  - The clinical presentation in infancy is similar to that of total anomalous pulmonary venous connection, with low cardiac output, pallor, tachypnea, poor peripheral pulses and failure to thrive. Death may occur within the first year of life in 75 percent of untreated patients. Children and young adults present with signs of pulmonary venous hypertension of various importance.
- Diagnosis
  - Diagnosis is usually established by transthoracic and transesophageal echocardiography, although magnetic resonance imaging can be used in selected cases. Cardiac catheterization may be indicated in the presence of associated cardiac lesions.
- Treatment
  - Resection of the membrane through a right atrial approach is recommended in infants, whereas a left atrial approach through the common pulmonary venous chamber may be used in older children and adults and in the presence of associated anomalies. Percutaneous catheter disruption of the membrane may represent an alternative to surgery in selected cases of subdivided right atrium. Outcomes are dependent on the preoperative clinical condition.

Subdivided right atrium is a much rarer anomaly in which a membrane, originating from the crista terminalis, divides the trabecular portion of the right atrium from the venae cavae. This entity should be distinguished[5] from the commoner occurrence of prominent eustachian or thebesian valves.

HISTORICAL BACKGROUND

The typical findings of subdivided left atrium were first described in 1868 by Church,[6] although the term *cor triatriatum* was initially applied to this anomaly by Borst in 1905.[7] Subdivided left atrium was first diagnosed angiographically by Miller in 1964[8] and echocardiographically by Ostman-Smith in 1984.[9] Surgical repair was first accomplished in 1956.[10,11] Cor triatriatum dexter was described by Rokitanski in 1875,[12] yet noninvasive diagnosis by means of echocardiography has been increasingly reported only since 1987.[13] Successful surgical repair of subdivided right atrium was reported in 1972.[14,15]

BASIC EMBRYOLOGY

The morphogenesis of subdivided left atrium remains unclear, and the various hypotheses reported thus far[5] fail to explain all the many anatomic variants of this anomaly. The entrapment theory proposed by Van Praagh and Corsini[16] is consistent with the findings observed in most cases of subdivided left atrium and also with the hourglass and the tubular types described by Marin-Garcia and colleagues,[17] where no membrane is seen to divide the common pulmonary venous chamber from the mitral valve and the left atrial appendage. The entrapment theory postulates that subdivided left atrium results from the entrapment of the left atrial ostium of the common pulmonary vein by tissue of the right horn of the sinus venosus, leading to failure in the incorporation of the common pulmonary veins into the left atrium during the fifth week of embryonic development. Consequently, these authors use the term *common pulmonary vein chamber* to describe the proximal chamber, which receives the pulmonary veins. Yet the entrapment theory fails to explain the coexistence of subdivided left atrium with either total or partial anomalous pulmonary venous drainage.[4]

The morphogenesis of subdivided right atrium is less controversial.[3–5] During early cardiac development, the opening of the sinus venosus in the right portion of the common atrium is delineated by two valves, which join superiorly to form the septum spurium. The left valve becomes incorporated in the septum secundum whereas the superior portion of right valve (which regresses at around 12 weeks of gestation) forms the crista terminalis; the remnants of the inferior portion form the eustachian and thebesian valves. According to Gharagozloo,[5] the obstructing membrane in subdivided right atrium originates from the crista terminalis and should be distinguished from the more commonly observed prominent eustachian or thebesian valves. In essence, subdivided right atrium is caused by the persistence of an unusually prominent right valve of the sinus venosus.

MORPHOLOGY

The most comprehensive classification of the anatomic variants of subdivided left atrium was reported by Krabill and Lucas.[18] In its classic form (Fig. 72-1), the right and

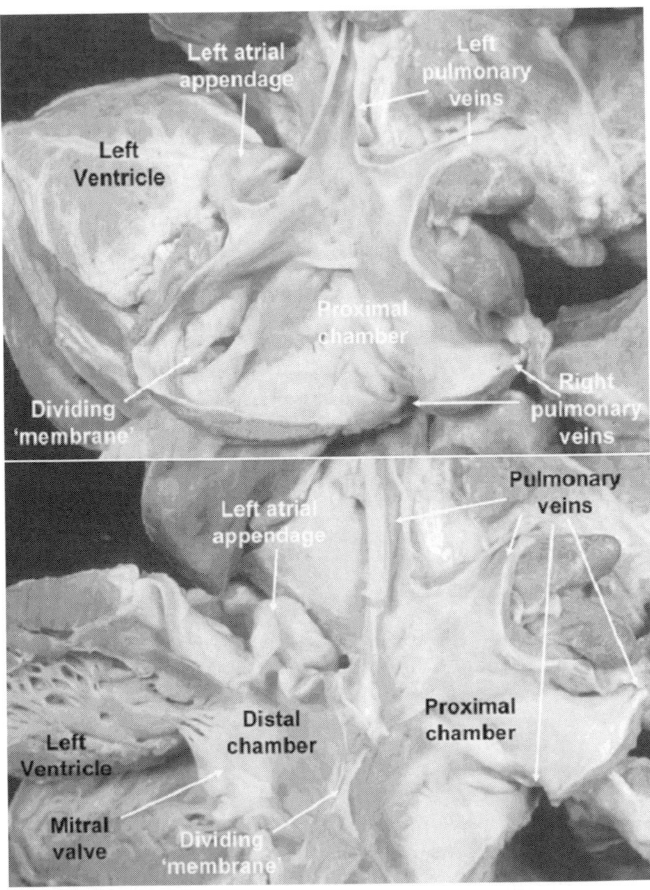

Figure 72-1 Autopsy specimen of subdivided left atrium. Top: The common pulmonary venous chamber (proximal chamber) is opened to show the drainage of the left and right pulmonary veins and the dividing membrane with a fenestration in its center. Bottom: The distal chamber and the left ventricle are opened to show the membrane separating the proximal from the distal chamber, where the mitral valve and the left atrial appendage are seen. (Courtesy of Professor RH Anderson, Institute of Child Health, London.)

left pulmonary veins enter a common pulmonary venous chamber (proximal chamber), which is in most instances separated by a fibromuscular diaphragm from a distal chamber where the mitral valve and the left atrial appendage are found. The dividing membrane may show a single orifice ranging in diameter between less than 3 mm to about 1 cm; occasionally, there may be several small defects. In two unusual variants of subdivided left atrium, the so-called hourglass and tubular types, no membrane is found to divide the left atrium (Fig. 72-2).[16] In these variants, the thicker-walled common pulmonary vein chamber is usually posterior and somewhat superior and medial to the thin-walled proximal chamber. Associated anomalies may be present in more than 50 percent of the patients with this lesion. In addition to the more frequent finding of partial and total anomalous pulmonary venous connection, associated anomalies include ventricular septal defect (VSD), atrioventricular septal defect (AVSD or AV canal), tetralogy of Fallot, and coarctation of the aorta. A left superior vena cava[19] is found more frequently than with other types of congenital heart defects and may be associated with a partially or totally unroofed coronary sinus.[20]

The typical finding of subdivided right atrium is the presence of a membrane separating the right atrial appendage and the tricuspid orifice from the venae cavae and the coronary sinus. According to Gharagozloo,[5] the term *subdivided right atrium* should be reserved for those hearts where the dividing membrane originates from the crista terminalis (Fig. 72-3) and, as mentioned above, this entity should be distinguished from those cases of unusual prominence of either the eustachian or thebesian valves, which do not originate from the crista terminalis.[3] Yet the former lesion has often been described at necropsy, whereas the latter anatomic variant has been increasingly diagnosed clinically by echocardiography. The most commonly observed cardiac malformations associated with subdivided right atrium include pulmonary valve stenosis or atresia, hypoplastic right ventricle, and tricuspid valve stenosis or atresia.[21,22]

PATHOPHYSIOLOGY

Obstruction of pulmonary venous return to the left atrium is the key hemodynamic feature of subdivided left atrium. The severity of obstruction is multifactorial and depends not only on the size of the fenestration in the dividing membrane but also on both the presence and the size of an ASD between the chamber of the common pulmonary veins and the right atrium as well as on associated cardiac lesions. Severe pulmonary venous hypertension, indistinguishable from that observed in obstructed total anomalous pulmonary venous connection, is present when the size of the fenestration is severely restrictive (3 mm or less) and the atrial septum is intact. Conversely, when a large ASD is present between

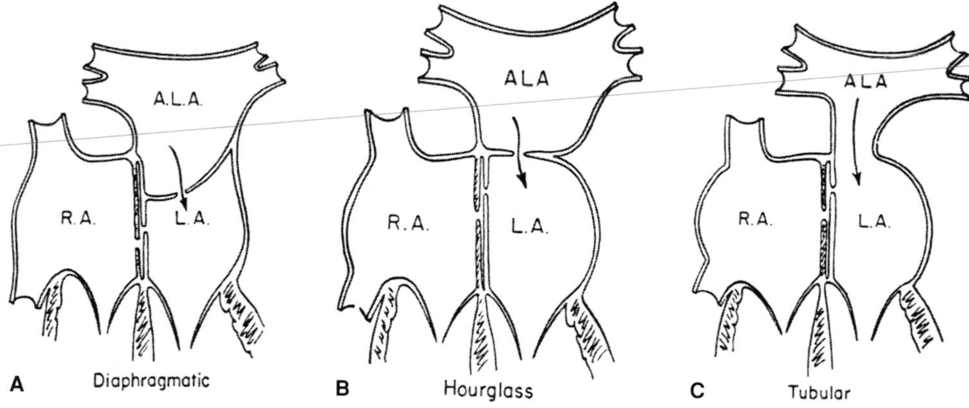

Figure 72-2 Anatomic types of cor triatriatum (subdivided left atrium). Type A is the commonest anatomic variant, where a fibromuscular membrane divides the accessory left atrial chamber (ALA, representing the common pulmonary venous chamber) from the true left atrium (LA, or distal chamber), where the mitral valve and the left atrial appendage are found. In type B, described as the *hourglass type,* a constriction is seen externally at the junction between the common pulmonary venous and distal chambers, where no membrane is found. No dividing membrane can be found also in type C *(tubular type),* where a tubular channel receives all the pulmonary veins (common pulmonary venous chamber) and joins the distal chamber. RA = right atrium. (From Marin-Garcia et al.[17] With permission.)

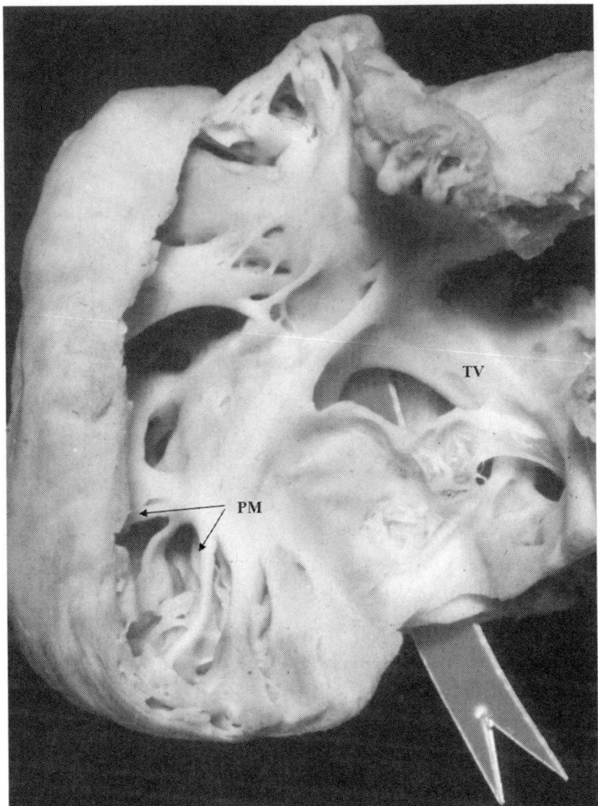

Figure 72-3 Autopsy specimen of subdivided right atrium due to persistence of the right venous valve. The right atrium and the right ventricle are opened to show a large fibrous membrane originating from the crista terminalis and dividing the right atrial appendage and the tricuspid valve from the venae cavae. The membrane deflects blood from the inferior vena cava (through which an arrow is placed) into the left atrium via the fossa ovalis. The opening of the superior vena cava is also behind the venous valve and is not visible. The vestibule of the tricuspid valve is seen to the right lower corner of the figure. PM = pectinates muscles; TV = tricuspid valve. (Courtesy of Professor RH Anderson, Institute of Child Health, London.)

CLINICAL FEATURES

The clinical presentation of patients with subdivided left atrium but without major associated lesions will depend on the degree of obstruction to pulmonary blood flow through the dividing membrane. If the communication between the common pulmonary venous chamber and the mitral valve is small (3 mm or less), the patient may become symptomatic in the first few months of life owing to ongoing low cardiac output with pallor, poor peripheral pulses, tachypnea, and growth failure. In the presence of associated anomalous pulmonary venous return or when an ASD is present between the common pulmonary venous chamber and the right atrium, symptoms due to increased pulmonary blood flow (such as recurrent respiratory infections, congestive heart failure, and failure to thrive) may coexist.[23]

The severity and quality of symptoms in patients with subdivided right atrium also seem to depend largely on two variables: the degree of obstruction produced by the membrane and the state of the interatrial septum. With only a minor degree of obstruction, this lesion is often asymptomatic and may be detected only incidentally at surgery for correction of other cardiac anomalies or during echocardiography. Cyanosis due to shunting of the common pulmonary venous chamber and the right atrium or in presence of either a partial or a total unobstructed pulmonary venous return, left-to-right shunting will be present and pulmonary venous obstruction may not be obvious.

The hemodynamic features of subdivided right atrium are equally based on the severity of obstruction to systemic venous return and to the presence of an ASD. Cyanosis may, in fact, be frequent due to shunting of inferior caval blood into the left atrium through an ASD. Right-sided congestive heart failure with elevated central venous pressure may be present in cases with intact atrial septum and right ventricular inflow or outflow obstruction.

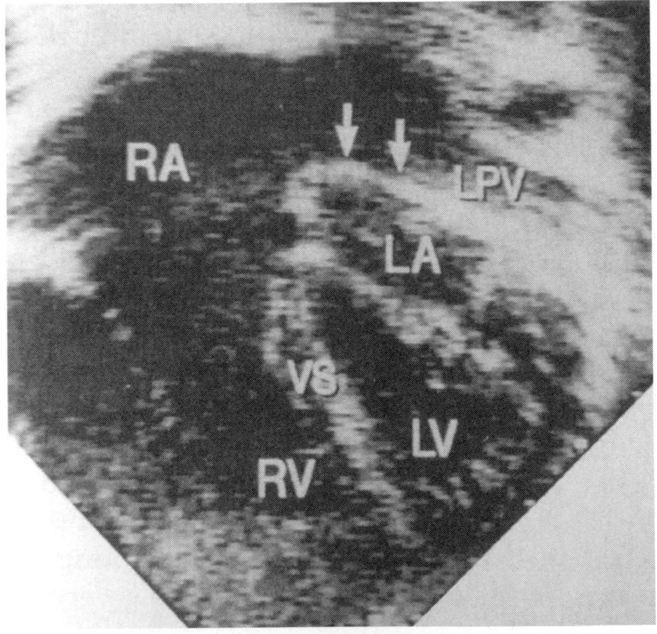

Figure 72-4 Transthoracic echocardiographic imaging (apical four-chamber view) of subdivided left atrium. The common pulmonary venous chamber communicates via a large atrial septal defect with the right atrium and is separated by a membrane (arrow) from the left atrium (distal chamber). LA = left atrium; LV = left ventricle; RA = right atrium; RN = right ventricle; VS = ventricular septum. (From Van Son et al.[20] With permission.)

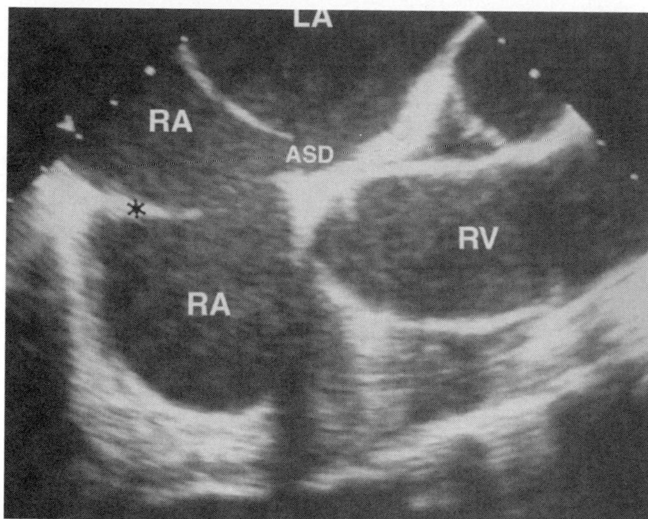

Figure 72-5 Transesophageal echocardiographic imaging of subdivided right atrium. Long axis view demonstrates the dividing membrane (*) in the right atrium. ASD = atrial septal defect; LA = left atrium; RA = right atrium; RV = right ventricle. (From Joe BN, Poustchi-Amin M, Wooddard PK. Cor triatriatum dexter. *Radiology* 2003;226:702. With permission.)

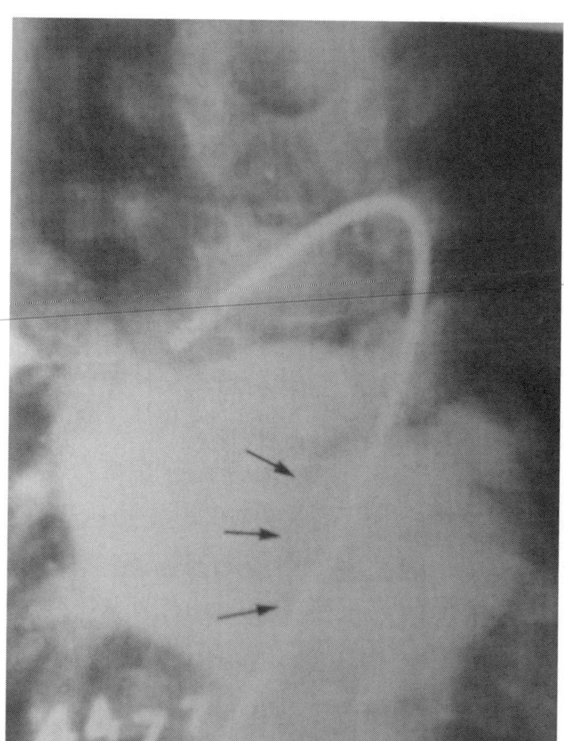

Figure 72-6 Angiographic imaging of subdivided left atrium. Pulmonary artery injection of contrast medium delineates the dividing membrane (arrowed) between the common pulmonary venous chamber and the distal chamber, where the left atrial appendage is seen. The atrial septum was intact. (From Arciniegas et al.[37] With permission.)

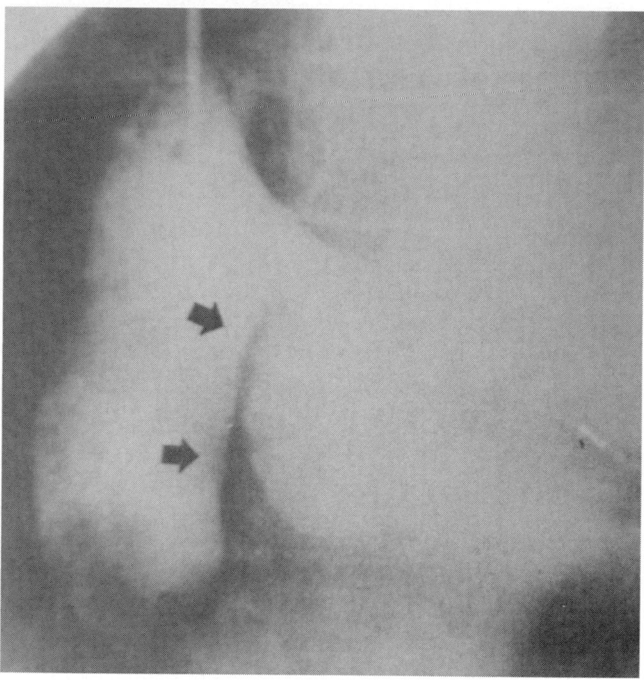

Figure 72-7 Angiographic imaging of subdivided right atrium. Superior vena cava injection of contrast medium demonstrates the division of the right atrium by an abnormal remnant (arrowed) of the right valve of the sinus venosus. (From Ott et al.[40] With permission.)

inferior caval blood in the left atrium through an ASD is the dominant clinical feature when the membrane is severely obstructive. This situation is often well tolerated into adult life and only occasionally may result in severe hypoxemia in infancy. Right-sided heart failure with elevated central venous pressure due to obstruction of the tricuspid valve or the right ventricular outflow tract may occur when the atrial septum is intact.[24]

DIAGNOSTIC MODALITIES

Echocardiography is the method of choice for identification of both subdivided left and right atrium.[25,26] Transthoracic two-dimensional echocardiography (Fig. 72-4) may be supplemented by transesophageal imaging (Fig. 72-5) for further evaluation.[27] The use of magnetic resonance imaging (MRI) has been increasingly reported in recent literature for diagnosis and preoperative planning. MRI is thought to have a higher sensitivity than echocardiography and angiography.[28] In general, MRI provides better spatial resolution and superior tissue contrast compared with echocardiography. Cardiac catheterization and angiography (Figs. 72-6 and 72-7) are no longer indicated for the diagnosis of subdivided atria unless major associated cardiac lesions are suspected.

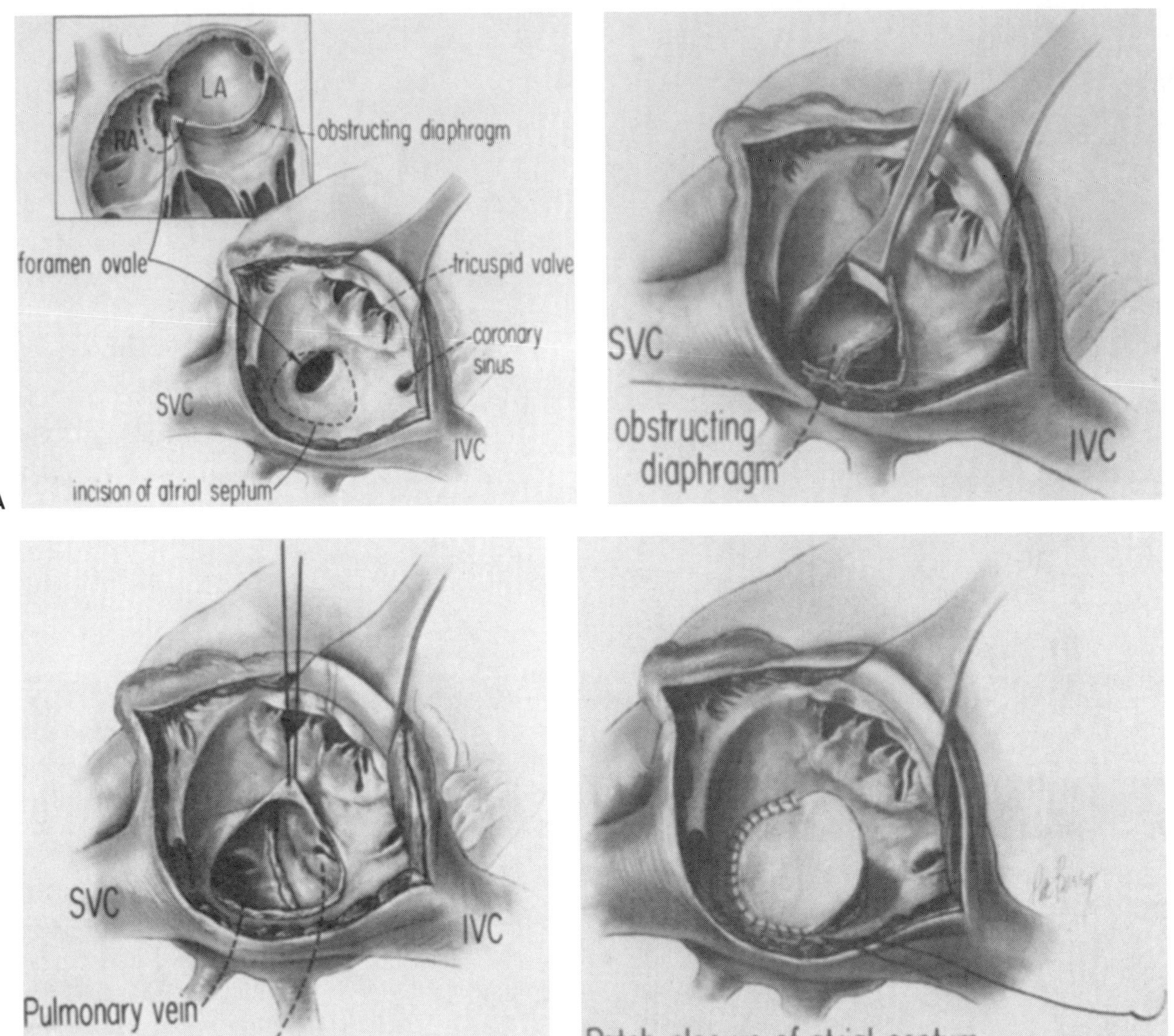

Figure 72-8 Right atrial approach for repair of subdivided left atrium. A. Right atrial incision through the superior and inferior margins of the foramen ovale. B. These incisions are carried to the right atrial wall, providing simultaneous exposure of both the common pulmonary venous chamber and the distal chamber. This allows careful evaluation of the relationship between the dividing membrane and the mitral valve. C. Complete excision of the membrane brings the pulmonary veins and the mitral valve in continuity. D. Reconstruction of the septal incision with a pericardial patch. IVC = inferior vena cava; SVC = superior vena cava. (From Richardson et al.[2] With permission.)

SURGICAL MANAGEMENT

Surgery is the only mode of treatment for symptomatic patients with subdivided left atrium. Timing of operation is based primarily on the clinical status, and prompt surgery is indicated for those infants who present with symptoms of severely obstructed pulmonary blood flow. Without surgical treatment, 75 percent of patients born with such malformations die in infancy.[29] Urgent repair is also indicated in older patients presenting with chronic symptoms. Planning of the operation is based on the coexistence and the complexity of associated lesions. Before operation, the drainage of all pulmonary and systemic veins should be ascertained. In the presence of a left superior vena cava (frequently associated with subdivided left atrium), the possibility that the coronary sinus may be partially or totally unroofed should be ruled out.

Moderately hypothermic or normothermic cardiopulmonary bypass with bicaval cannulation and antegrade cold blood cardioplegia may be routinely used in straightforward cases. The strategy of normothermic versus hypothermic cardiopulmonary bypass remains controversial[30–32]; hypothermic circulatory arrest should be used only in the presence of complex associated lesions.[33]

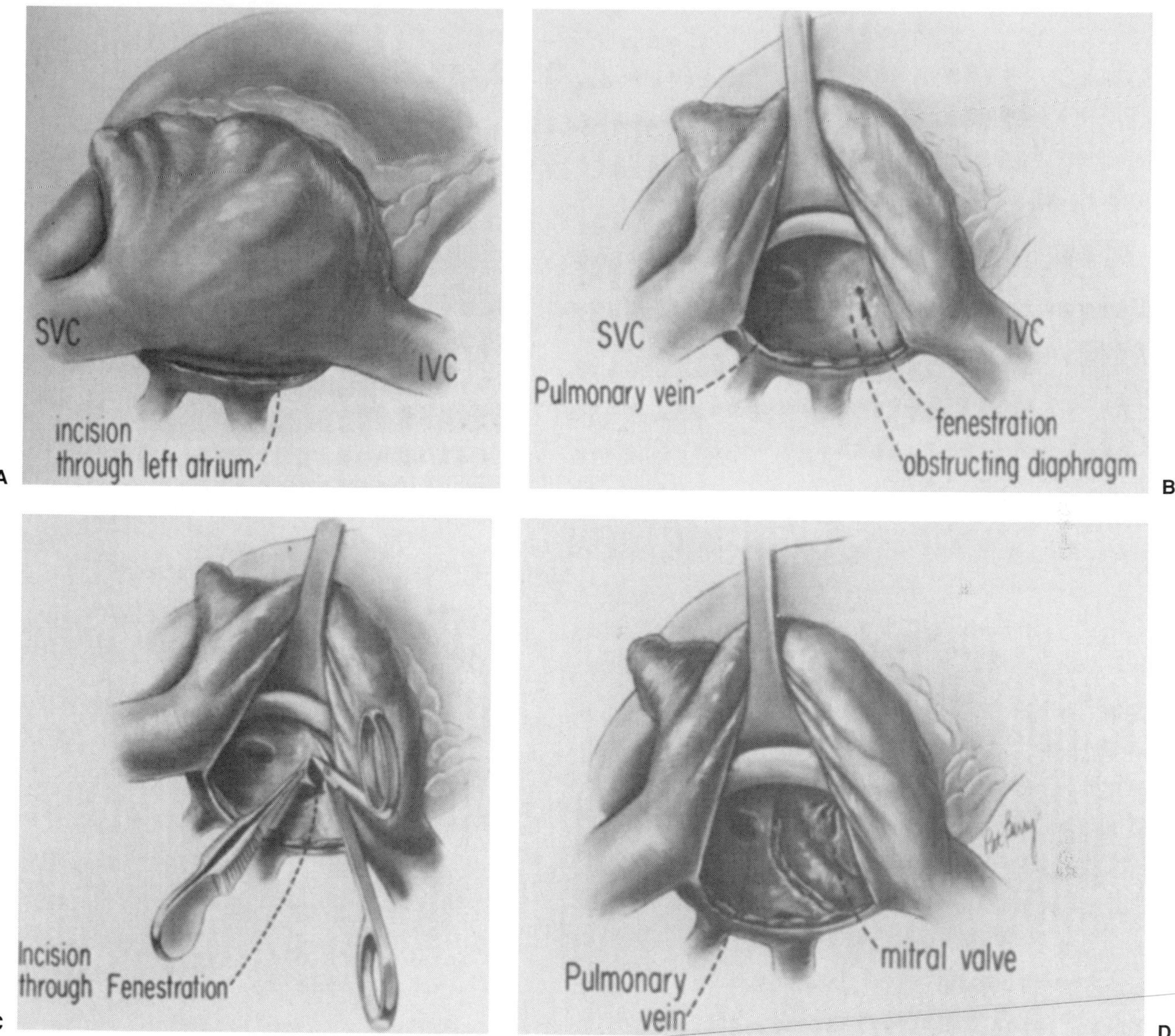

Figure 72-9 Left atrial approach for repair of subdivided left atrium. A. A longitudinal incision is made in the left atrium (common pulmonary venous chamber) posterior to the interatrial groove. B. The atrial septum is retracted superiorly, exposing the dividing membrane with central fenestration. C. Excision of the dividing membrane is commenced by opening the fenestration and continued leftward after visualization of the left inferior pulmonary vein and of the mitral valve. D. The pulmonary veins are seen in continuity with the mitral valve. LA = left atrium (common pulmonary venous chamber); RA = right atrium; SVC = superior vena cava; IVC = inferior vena cava. (From Richardson et al.[2] With permission.)

A right atrial approach (Fig. 72-8) is recommended for infants and small children, especially in the presence of an enlarged common pulmonary venous chamber. After aortic cross-clamping, the right atrium is opened through a longitudinal incision parallel to the atrioventricular groove. A longitudinal septal incision is carried out through the fossa ovalis, obtaining optimal exposure of the fibromuscular membrane and of the mitral valve below it. The membrane can be excised completely while preserving the integrity of the mitral valve. The atrial septum is reconstructed with a pericardial patch.

A longitudinal incision in the common pulmonary vein chamber just posterior to the interatrial groove (Fig. 72-9) can be satisfactorily used in older children and adults. Anterior retraction of the atrial septum allows adequate exposure of the membrane for subsequent resection. A potential pitfall of this approach is the initial difficulty of assessing the relationship between the membrane and the mitral valve below it. Closure of the fossa ovalis or patch reconstruction of the atrial septum may be more technically demanding with this approach. Modified ultrafiltration and the use of nitric oxide in infants with severe pulmonary hypertension can be a very useful therapeutic adjunct in the early postoperative phase.

Resection of the obstructing membrane is the treatment of choice in patients with subdivided right atrium, although percutaneous catheter disruption of the membrane[34] may represent an alternative to surgery in selected cases without associated lesions. Transesophageal echocardiography may be useful for a better definition of the relationship of the membrane with the surroundings structures. Normothermic cardiopulmonary bypass on a beating heart with bicaval cannulation may be used in simple cases of subdivided right atrium without septal defects. The surgical approach in the presence of associated anomalies should be tailored to the individual case.

OUTCOMES

Aside from occasional case reports,[20,35] there are only a few reports of relatively large cohorts of patients with cor triatriatum.[23,36] Most of the literature regarding this topic was published in earlier decades,[2,19,37,38] making any comparison with modern practice in the surgical management of infants and small children not entirely meaningful. Regardless to the timing of publication, it is not surprising that most reported deaths occurred within the first year of life in infants who where severely symptomatic or in the presence of complex associated lesions. In high-risk cases, hospital mortality has been reported between 33 and 60 percent.[23,37] These results underscore the importance of an early and detailed preoperative diagnosis, particularly when complex lesions are associated. In contrast, hospital mortality is uncommon after repair of this lesion in older patients.

Unfavorable late events leading to restenosis—such as pulmonary vein stenosis[2] and incomplete resection of the dividing membrane between the common pulmonary venous and the distal chamber—are exceedingly rare.[39]

The life expectancy of patients with subdivided left atrium without major associated cardiac lesions approaches that of the general population, particularly if repair is performed in infancy.

With the exception of the papers by Hansing and coworkers[14] and Trento and associates,[3] most descriptions of the surgical management of patients with subdivided right atrium have been single case reports.[15,40] This lesion may represent the primary lesion, and successful surgical treatment has been reported even in the first few months of life.[3,15] On the other hand, an obstructing membrane within the right atrium may be found at operation associated with other lesions causing obstruction to pulmonary blood flow, and treatment and prognosis depends on that of the dominant lesion.

References

1. Thilenius OG, Bharati S, Lev M. Subdivided left atrium: An expanded concept of cor triatriatum. *Am J Cardiol* 1976;37:743.
2. Richardson JV, Doty DB, Siewers RD, et al. Cor triatriatum (subdivided left atrium). *J Thorac Cardiovasc Surg* 1981;81:232.
3. Trento A, Zuberbuhler JR, Anderson RH, et al. Divided right atrium (prominence of the eustachian and thebesian valves). *J Thorac Cardiovasc Surg* 1988;96:457.
4. Anderson RH. Understanding the nature of congenital division of the atrial chambers. *Br Heart J* 1992; 68:1.
5. Gharagozloo F, Bulkley BH, Hutchins GM. A proposed pathogenesis of cor triatriatum: Impingement of the left superior vena cava on the developing left atrium. *Am Heart J* 1977;94:618.
6. Church WS. Congenital malformation of the heart: Abnormal septum in the left auricle. *Trans Pathol Soc Lond* 1868;19:188.
7. Borst H. Ein Cor triatriatum. *Zentralbl Allg Pathol* 1905;16:812.
8. Miller GA, Ongley PA, Anderson MW, et al. Cor triatriatum: Hemodynamic and angiographic diagnosis. *Am Heart J* 1964;68:298.
9. Ostman-Smith I, Silverman IM, Oldershaw P, et al. Cor triatriatum sinistrum: Diagnostic on cross sectional echocardiography. *Br Heart J* 1984;51:211.
10. Vineberg A, Gialloreto O. Report of a successful operation for stenosis of common pulmonary vein (cor triatriatum). *J Can Med Assoc* 1956;74:719.
11. Lewis FJ, Varco RL, Taufic M, et al. Direct vision repair of triatrial heart and total anomalous pulmonary venous drainage. *Surg Gynecol Obstet* 1956;713:102.
12. Von Rokitansky C. Die defecte der Scheidewande des Herzens: Pathologish-anatomische Abhandlung. Vienna: Braumuller, 1875.
13. Alboliras ET, Edwards WD, Driscoll DJ, et al. Cor triatriatum dexter: Two-dimensional echocardiographic diagnosis. *J Am Coll Cardiol* 1987;9:334.
14. Hansing CE, Young WP, Rowe GG. Cor triatriatum dexter: Persistent right sinus venosus valve. *Am J Cardiol* 1972;30:559.
15. Mazzucco A, Bortolotti U, Gallucci V, et al. Successful repair of symptomatic cor triatriatum dexter in infancy. *J Thorac Cardiovasc Surg* 1983;85:140.
16. Van Praagh R, Corsini I. Cor triatriatum: Pathologic anatomy and a consideration on morphogenesis based on 13 postmortem cases and a study of normal development of the pulmonary vein and atrial septum in 83 human embryos. *Am Heart J* 1969;78:379.
17. Marin-Garcia J, Tandon R, Lucas RV Jr, et al. Cor triatriatum: Study of 20 cases. *Am J Cardiol* 1975;35:59.
18. Krabill KA, Lucas RV Jr. Abnormal pulmonary venous connection. In: Emmanouilides GC, Allen HA,

Riemenschneider TA, Gutgesell HP (eds). *Moss and Adams' Heart Disease in Infants, Children, and Adolescents Including the Fetus and Young Adult.* Baltimore: William & Wilkins, 1995:863.

19. Oglietti J, Cooley DA, Izquierdo JP, et al. Cor triatriatum: Operative results in 25 patients. *Ann Thorac Surg* 1983;35:415.
20. Van Son JA, Autschback R, Mohr FW. Repair of cor triatriatum with partially unroofed coronary sinus. *Ann Thorac Surg* 1999;68:1414.
21. Yater WM. Variations and anomalies of the venous valves of the right atrium of the human heart. *Arch Pathol* 1929;7:418.
22. Doucoette J, Knoblich R. Persistent right valve of the sinus venosus: So-called cor triatriatum dextrum: Review of the literature and report of a case. *Arch Pathol* 1963;75:105.
23. Rodefeld MD, Brown JW, Heimansohn DA, et al. Cor triatriatum: Clinical presentation and surgical results in 12 patients. *Ann Thorac Surg* 1990;50:562.
24. Embrey RP. Cor triatriatum, pulmonary vein stenosis, atresia of the common pulmonary vein. In: Mavroudis C, Backer CL (eds). *Pediatric Cardiac Surgery,* 2d ed. St. Louis: Mosby–Year Book, 1994:503.
25. Shuler CO, Fyfe DA, Sade R, et al. Transesophageal echocardiographic evaluation of cor triatriatum in children. *Am Heart J* 1995;129:507.
26. Muhiudeen-Russel IA, Silverman NH. Images in cardiovascular medicine. Cor triatriatum in an infant. *Circulation* 1997;95:2700.
27. Fiorilli R, Argento G, Tomasco B, et al. Cor triatriatum dexter diagnosed by transesophageal echocardiography. *J Clin Ultrasound* 1995;23:502.
28. Masui T, Seelos KC, Kersting-Sommerhoff BA, et al. Abnormalities of the pulmonary veins: Evaluation with MR imaging and comparison with cardiac angiography and echocardiography. *Radiology* 1991;181:645.
29. Cor triatriatum. In: Kirklin JW, Barratt-Boyes BG. *Cardiac Surgery,* 2d ed. New York: Churchill Livingstone, 1993: 675.
30. Corno AF. A lost opportunity (letter). *J Thorac Cardiovasc Surg* 2004;127:1857.
31. Jonas RA, Newburger JW, Bellinger DC (reply to letter). *J Thorac Cardiovasc Surg* 2004;127:1858.
32. Carpena C, Colokathis B, Subramanian S. Cor triatriatum. Successful correction in 4 patients including 2 less than 1 year of age. *Ann Thorac Surg* 1974;17:325.
33. Vouhè PR, Baillot-Vernant F, Fermont L, et al. Cor triatriatum and total anomalous pulmonary venous connection: A rare, surgically correctable anomaly. *J Thorac Cardiovasc Surg* 1985;90:443.
34. Savas V, Samyn J, Schreiber TL, et al. Cor triatriatum dexter: Recognition and percutaneous transluminal correction. *Cathet Cardiovasc Diagn* 1991;23:183.
35. Varma PK, Warrier G, Ramachandran P, et al. Partial atrioventricular canal defect with cor triatriatum sinister. Report of three cases. *J Thorac Cardiovasc Surg* 2004;127:572.
36. Salomone G, Tiraboschi R, Crippa M, et al. Cor triatriatum. Clinical presentation and operative results. *J Thorac Cardiovasc Surg* 1991;101:1088.
37. Arciniegas E, Farooki ZQ, Hakimi M, et al. Surgical treatment of cor triatriatum. *Ann Thorac Surg* 1981;32:571.
38. Miller GA, Ongley PA, Anderson MW. Cor triatriatum: Hemodynamic and angiocardiographic diagnosis. *Am Heart J* 1964;68:298.
39. Jorgensen CR, Ferlic RM, Varco RL, et al. Cor triatriatum: Review of the surgical aspects with a follow-up report on the first patient successfully treated with surgery. *Circulation* 1967;36:101.
40. Ott DA, Cooley DA, Angelini P, et al. Successful surgical correction of symptomatic cor triatriatum dexter. *J Thorac Cardiovasc Surg* 1979;78:573.

CHAPTER

73 VALVAR DISEASE IN CHILDREN

Christian P. Brizard, Yves d'Udekem d'Acoz, Nelson Alphonso

This chapter focuses on the pathology and treatment of the mitral and aortic valves, since congenital anomalies of the tricuspid and pulmonary valves are detailed elsewhere in this textbook.

MITRAL VALVE DISEASE IN CHILDREN

This section attempts to cover the vast spectrum of mitral valve disease in children, both congenital and acquired, to the exclusion of mitral valve pathology in atrioventricular discordance, univentricular hearts, and hypoplastic left heart syndrome.

ANATOMY AND EMBRYOLOGY

Precise knowledge of the normal anatomy of the mitral valve and the interpretation of echocardiographic studies is essential to understanding the mechanism of mitral valve regurgitation or stenosis (functional classification), elucidate the location of leaflet dysfunction (segmental valve analysis), and plan and achieve successful surgical repair. The normal anatomy of the mitral valve in the child does not differ from that in the adult.[1]

The embryology of the mitral valve is complex. Our understanding of the formation of the leaflets and suspension apparatus has evolved, so that the current

KEY CONCEPTS

MITRAL VALVE

- Pathophysiology
  - Severe mitral stenosis or regurgitation causes low cardiac output.
- Clinical Features
  - In neonates and infants, signs of cardiac failure, predominantly right. In older children, mitral auscultation signs plus signs of pulmonary hypertension in mitral stenosis.
- Diagnostic
  - 2D echocardiography.

Treatment

- Medical
  - Mitral regurgitation: Unless very aggressive in severely symptomatic children, medical treatment has little impact. ACE inhibitors are commonly prescribed.
  - Mitral stenosis: Diuretics are indicated while afterload reduction is strictly contraindicated.
- Surgical
  - In patients with mitral annulus smaller than 18 mm (smallest mechanical prosthesis), maximal medical therapy is indicated to achieve weight gain. If the surgery cannot be avoided, repair even at the expense of imperfect result. In patients with mitral annulus larger than 18 mm, liberal surgical indication if good repair can be predicted. More conservative approach if repair is unlikely.
  - Mechanical valve in anatomical position has a good prognostic with current anticoagulation protocol.

AORTIC VALVE

- Pathophysiology
  - In neonates and infants, predominantly stenosis (fusion of the zone of apposition of leaflets leads to tricuspid, bicuspid, of unicuspid valve). In adolescents, predominantly regurgitation.

- Clinical Features
  - In critical neonatal aortic stenosis, cardiovascular collapse at the closure of the ductus. Later often asymptomatic.
- Diagnostic
  - Echocardiography (assessment of the suitability of biventricular repair, severity of stenosis-regurgitation, mechanism of valvar dysfunction).

Treatment
- Medical
  - So far, equivalent results for balloon valvuloplasty and aortic commissurotomy.

  Surgical
  - Aortic valve repair is the preferred option. Ross procedure is the best alternative.

approach is mainly based on immunohistochemistry, in vivo labeling of cushion tissue, and scanning electron micrography of human and avian embryos.[2,3] In humans, the mitral valve develops between the 5th and 15th weeks of embryonic life. It is established that leaflets and chordae derive from the endocardial cushion tissue lying on the inner surface of the atrioventricular junction. The separation between atrial and ventricular myocardium is dependent on the sulcus tissue located on the epicardial side of the junction. As the cushion tissue elongates and grows toward the ventricular cavity, it is gradually delaminated from the underlying myocardium and the leaflet becomes progressively shaped as a funnel-like structure totally attached to the myocardium. Perforations then appear into the valve leaflet and grow to form the chordae tendineae. The atrial aspect of the cushion will generate the spongy atrial layer and the ventricular layer will generate the fibrous part of the mitral valve and chordal apparatus. The development of the papillary muscles takes place simultaneously, originating from the myocardium. A horseshoe-shaped ridge lies within the left ventricle. The anterior and posterior parts of this ridge lose contact with the ventricular wall, forming the papillary muscles and increasing in size while maintaining structural continuity with the cushion tissue at the tip of the papillary muscle. The midportion of the muscular ridge will be incorporated into the apical trabeculations of the left ventricle.[4]

Several atrioventricular cushions participate in the embryogenesis of the mitral valve, the most important being the superior and inferior cushions. However, in comparing the respective contribution of these two cushions, there is no true symmetry. The superior cushion tissue will contribute to the development of the majority of the anterior leaflet of the mitral valve, whereas the inferior cushion will generate most of the septal leaflet of the tricuspid valve. Smaller cushions are involved in the formation of the mural leaflet of the mitral valve. The wedging of the aortic root into the superior bridging leaflet (mostly originating from the superior cushion) will separate the developing mitral valve from its septal attachments.

PATHOLOGY

Congenital anomalies of the mitral valve

Congenital stenosis and insufficiency of the mitral valve are presented together, as their pathology and associated lesions are similar. Moreover, they frequently coexist in the same patient.

The supravalvar mitral ring

A common cause of congenital mitral valve stenosis, the supravalvar mitral ring is an acquired fibrous structure attached to the posterior annulus of the mitral valve, running from both commissures to the midheight of the anterior leaflet. The lesion is stenotic and often more significant than the extent of the ring would suggest. This is mostly due to the consequent limitation in the opening mechanism of the anterior leaflet rather than to the actual diaphragm-like effect of the ring. Strictly attached to the mitral valve annulus, it is to be differentiated from cor triatriatum (Chap. 72). The supravalvar mitral ring is secondary to turbulent flow through the mitral orifice. The primary lesion of the mitral valve responsible for this turbulent flow can be stenotic or regurgitant or can be very discrete and difficult to identify (Fig. 73-1). It can be related to a prominent coronary sinus, as found in hearts with persistence of the left superior vena cava

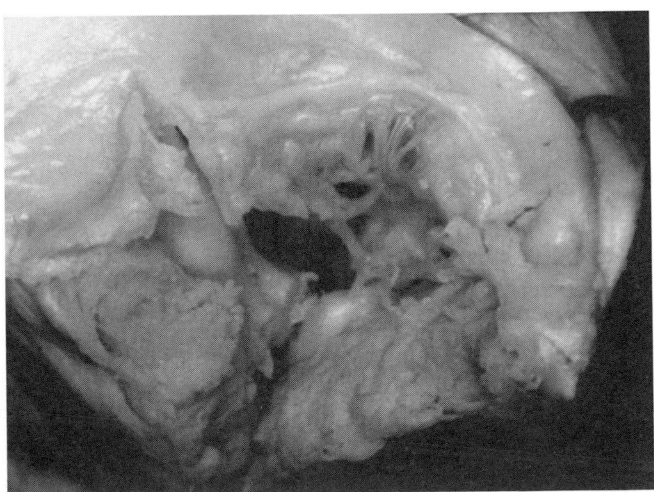

Figure 73-1 Supravalvar-ring and hammock valve (postmortem specimen). Note the high implantation of the supravalvar ring, close to the annulus at the level of the posterior leaflet (right side of picture) and at the midlevel of the anterior leaflet (left side of picture). The free edge of the posterior leaflet is tethered to the posterior wall of the left ventricle, characteristic of the hammock valve.

draining into the coronary sinus.[5] For these reasons, the supravalvar mitral ring is probably prone to recur after surgical resection unless (or even when) the underlying anatomic anomaly has been identified and corrected. The supravalvar ring can be encountered very early in life, in the neonate or young infant. It should be suspected when a transvalvar gradient appears to increase at follow-up or when the Doppler gradient is greater than that defined by Doppler echocardiography.

Cleft mitral valve

Very often isolated, the cleft mitral valve can be easily differentiated from a left atrioventricular valve in a partial atrioventricular septal defect.[6,7] It is an actual cleft with no suspension apparatus on the edges of the defect. The cleft is centered on the aortic commissure between the noncoronary and left coronary cusps.[7] Each half of the anterior leaflet at midportion bears the attachment of the strut chordae. Both papillary muscles are normal. Rarely, the cleft mitral valve is associated with a leaflet tissue defect, which is an acquired defect secondary to chronic regurgitation through the cleft. The defect is never stenotic and may generate only little regurgitation for a long time.

Accessory valve tissue and valvar tags

In this specific anomaly, the interchordal spaces are filled with a dense network of valve tissue. When there is continuity between the anterior and posterior leaflets, the accessory valvar tissue may be generating a gradient inversely correlated with the size of the perforations in the accessory tissue (Fig. 73-2). When the accessory valve tissue is entrapped in the left ventricular outflow tract, the mitral valve may become regurgitant due to the traction exerted by the accessory valvar tissue on the anterior leaflet, making the valve incompetent in midsystole.[8] Left ventricular outflow tract obstruction is nevertheless the predominant hemodynamic lesion observed with this pathology.[9,10]

Lesions associated with lack of valvar tissue

Three major anatomic types of lesions are associated with lack of valvar tissue. The functional endpoint of the lesion can be either normal, predominantly regurgitant or stenotic, or both.

Parachute mitral valve The parachute mitral valve (PMV) can be found in isolation and is also observed in association with Shone's complex.[11,12] The most common finding is that of a predominant single papillary muscle with the orifice of the mitral valve overriding its tip. With this particular pathology, there is a spectrum of abnormality of the suspension apparatus, ranging from complete fusion of the tip of the papillary muscle to the free edge of the valve[4] and relatively normal-looking chordae with good mobility of the leaflet. Accessory papillary muscles are usually very small and connected to only a short segment of the free edge or even to the undersurface of the leaflet tissue (as would be the case in a larger-than-normal secondary chorda). The functional anatomy of the PMV depends on the interaction between the amount of tissue and the mobility of the leaflet; the presence and size of the fenestrations; and the presence, length, and quality of the chordae.[13] The parachute mitral valve almost always has a stenotic component.

Double-orifice mitral valve is an exceedingly rare variant of PMV, with the lesser papillary muscle supporting a complete orifice. This lesion should be differentiated from the left atrioventricular valve, in which an accessory orifice is often found in the case of diminutive or absent

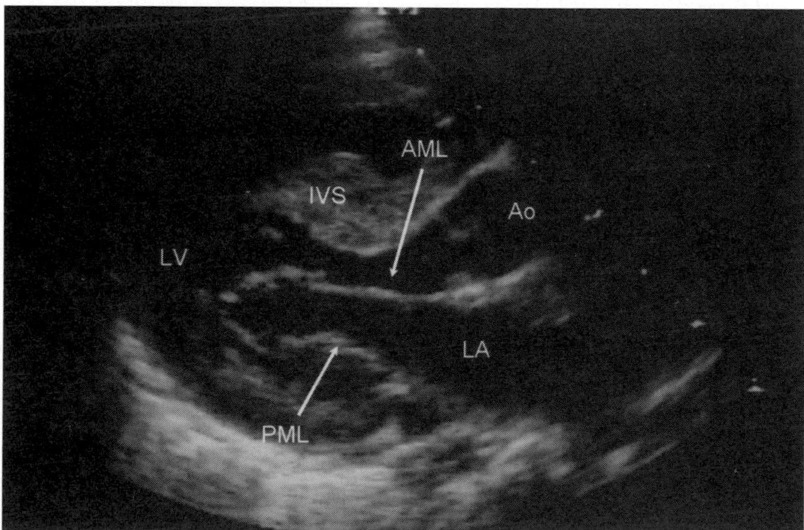

Figure 73-2 Accessory mitral valve tissue in diastole; parasternal long-axis view. AML = anterior mitral leaflet; Ao = aorta; IVS = interventricular septum; LA = left atrium; LV = left ventricle; PML = posterior mitral leaflet.

left lateral leaflet (mural leaflet). The second orifice is almost always competent and should not be closed at the time of the repair.

Papillary muscle–commissure fusion[14] This anomaly, which can be limited to only one papillary muscle, ranges from cases with short chordae to those in which the tip of the papillary muscle is actually directly attached or fused to the commissural area of the free edge. The valve is generally more regurgitant than restrictive; this is due to the lack of valvar tissue and the consequent restriction of leaflet motion. When the papillary muscles are hypertrophied, the bulk of their mass is generally responsible for a predominantly restrictive physiology.

Hammock valve (arcade mitral valve)[13] Here the suspension apparatus may have lost all resemblance to the normal anatomy. No papillary muscle may be identifiable or there may be multiple very small ones behind the posterior leaflet. The leaflets are suspended by a network of chordae directly attached to the posterior wall of the ventricle. This attachment is generally displaced toward the base of the heart, with an excess of tension on the anterior leaflet and extreme limitation in the motion of the posterior leaflet (see Fig. 73-1). The valve is most often predominantly regurgitant.

Regurgitant mitral valves with normal anatomy associated with congenital cardiac lesions

It is difficult to ascertain the congenital origin of these lesions, since the anatomy of the mitral valve is otherwise normal. Although most publications on congenital anomalies of the mitral valve include them,[15] there is no evidence of their congenital origin. Unlike the previously mentioned anomalies, they are in fact not found at birth. They are usually associated with conditions characterized by significant volume loading of the left ventricle (i.e., large ventricular septal defect or large patent ductus arteriosus). The pathophysiology is that of initial dilation of the posterior annulus due to the effect of the increase in volume overload. Secondarily, the marginal chordae elongate and create prolapse of the free edge of the anterior leaflet. These lesions are not rare, as they account for 15 to 40 percent of the patients reported in the literature concerning congenital mitral valve regurgitation. Functional mitral regurgitation secondary to cardiomyopathies is not included in this chapter.

ALCAPA Mitral valve regurgitation found in an anomalous left coronary artery from the left pulmonary artery (ALCAPA) is of ischemic origin and is described in detail in Chap. 74. In this particular anomaly, mitral regurgitation is a constant finding and is quantitatively almost always moderate to severe. The typical patient is between 2 and 4 months of age at diagnosis. Correction of the ALCAPA reduces the grade of regurgitation but rarely suppresses entirely. Structural modification of the suspension apparatus with infarction of the anterolateral papillary muscle and elongation of the chordae originating from the latter prevent complete regression of the regurgitation without concomitant mitral valve repair.[16]

Mitral valve disease with excess leaflet tissue: mitral valve prolapse and connective tissue disorder

Whether to include the mitral valve prolapse syndrome (limited in its more common form to the middle scallop of the posterior leaflet) in the congenital group is debatable. Using strict criteria, the incidence of mild bulging of the anterior leaflet was negligible and no prolapses were detected when a large population of neonates was reviewed, arguing against the congenital nature of this entity.[17] The histologic anomalies are limited in adults to the middle scallop of the posterior leaflet, with predominant alteration of the elastic fibers and proliferation of myxomatous tissue; these anomalies, in all likelihood, have a genetic etiology.[18] In the more extensive form of mitral valve prolapse (Barlow's disease, with excess of tissue distributed to both the anterior and posterior leaflets), histology demonstrates extensive infiltration of the spongiosa with myxomatous tissue. This more extensive form can also be seen in neonates and infants. It is encountered in sporadic cases or in familial forms and has been associated with at least one locus mutation on chromosome 16.[19] The histologic anomalies are identical to those found in Marfan's[20–22] and Elher-Danlos[23] syndromes. Similar valvar alterations are found in Hurler's syndrome (mucopolysaccharidosis type I).

Acquired mitral valve disease

Rheumatic heart disease

Acute rheumatic fever (ARF) is an autoimmune disorder in which the immune response to group A streptococcal (GAS) M protein generates T cells and antibodies that cross-react with cardiac antigens.[24,25] Although ARF does not generate long-term sequelae to brain, joints, or skin, the heart (specifically the mitral and/or aortic valves) may be permanently affected. The acute damage to the valves may cause chronic and evolving lesions secondary to the scarring process and/or to modifications in hemodynamics. This chronic picture is known as rheumatic heart disease (RHD), which is the most common pediatric heart disease in developing countries. Not all individuals are equally susceptible to ARF. Only 3 to 5 percent have an inherited susceptibility, although the basis of this is unknown. Also, only a limited number of GAS strains can initiate ARF in the susceptible host.[26]

Acute lesions Acute lesions are exclusively regurgitant. On inspection, the valvar tissue and chordae are swollen but supple. Prolapse of either leaflet can be seen, but the anterior leaflet is predominantly affected.[27] This prolapse is usually related to elongation of limited groups of chordae, while chordal rupture is rare. Multiple small nodules (2 to 3 mm in diameter) can be seen on the free edge of either of the mitral leaflets. Mitral regurgitation is a

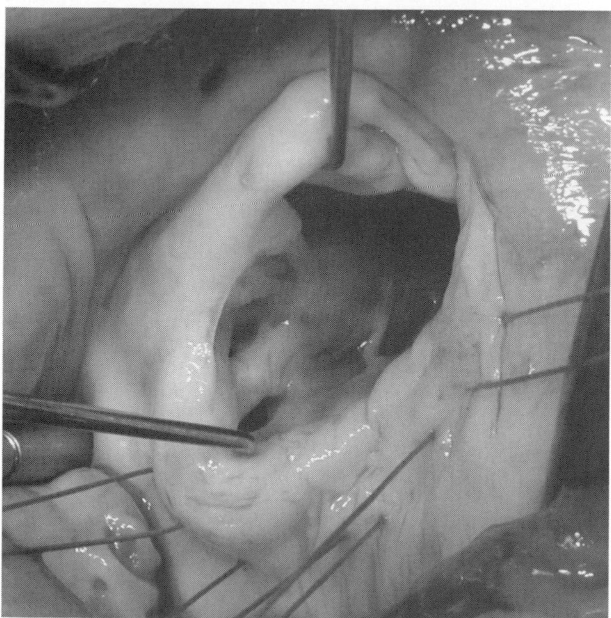

Figure 73-3 Chronic evolution of rheumatic mitral insufficiency. The anterior and posterior leaflets are severely retracted. There is limitation of posterior leaflet motion, prolapse of the anterior leaflet, commissural fusion, and paucity of chordae, which are thickened and fused.

combination of annular dilation (secondary to rheumatic pancarditis) and various degrees of prolapse.

Chronic lesions The scarring process generates retraction of the valvar tissue and, to a lesser degree, of the chordae. This process is sometimes sufficient to correct the prolapse of the acute phase. The healing of the spongiosa induces fusion of chordae, as demonstrated by the dramatic reduction in the number of chordae together with the large increase in their size. The physiology of the regurgitation is a combination of prolapse of the anterior leaflet, retraction of the posterior leaflet, and annular dilation (Fig. 73-3). In the pediatric age group, the mitral valve is exclusively or predominantly regurgitant, while stenosis typically appears later in the chronic phase of the disease with continuation of the retraction process. Calcifications are rare in the pediatric population with RHD.

Infective endocarditis

Bacterial endocarditis (BE) of the mitral valve is rare and, excluding patients with RHD, represents less than 2 percent of all BE in children. At the Royal Children's Hospital, Melbourne, a history of mitral valve anomaly before the diagnosis of BE was uncommon. The resulting physiology is always that of a regurgitant lesion. Intraoperatively, a vegetation is the most common finding and typically grows on the atrial side of the mitral valve; however, vegetations are not always present at the time of surgery. Rarely the vegetation will have embolized, more commonly it has regressed with medical therapy or has never been there. Other findings are perforation of the leaflet (Fig. 73-4), abscess formation within the mitral annulus, or extension toward the aortic valve. Histologic examination of vegetations discloses microorganism-infiltrated fibrin thrombi. Findings in the affected valvar tissue at the vegetation implantation site suggest a strong inflammatory reaction with neovascularization and infiltration of lymphocytes, giant cells, and fibroblasts. At the time of surgical repair, it is very important to differentiate intact valvar tissue (supple, thin, and resistant) from infected tissue (thickened, edematous, and friable).

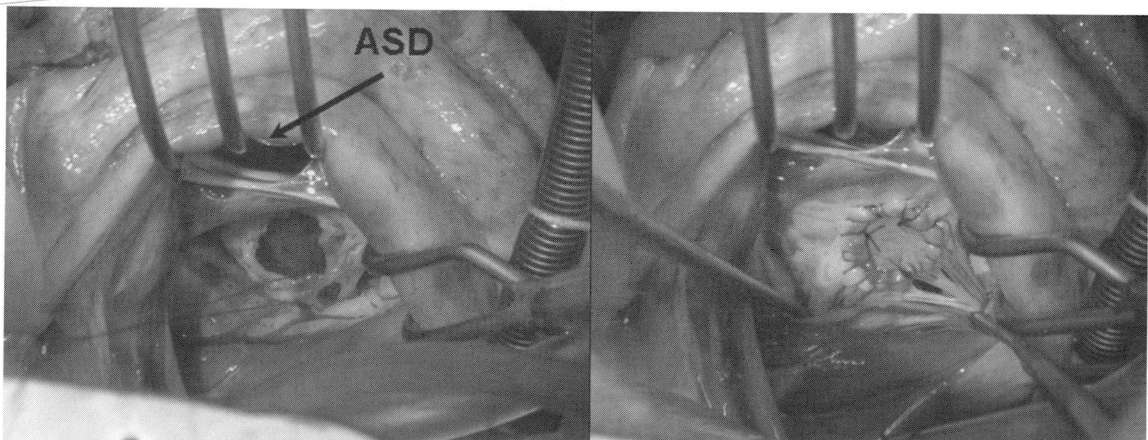

Figure 73-4 Acute endocarditis of the mitral valve. Large endocarditic perforation of the anterior mitral leaflet of a 6 year-old child (left). Result following repair with autologous pericardial patch (right). ASD = atrial septal defect. (Image courtesy of Luca Vricella, MD, Division of Cardiac Surgery, the Johns Hopkins University.)

CLINICAL FEATURES AND PRESENTATION

Neonates and young infants

For both stenosis and regurgitation, the clinical presentation in this age group includes cardiac failure, with dyspnea on exertion (feeding) and tachypnea at rest. Severe failure to thrive is usually present. Clinical examination shows hepatomegaly and cool extremities. Auscultation is difficult, but a strong apical systolic murmur should indicate significant mitral regurgitation, whereas a diastolic murmur in the case of mitral stenosis can be difficult to auscultate or may even be absent in the context of low cardiac output or associated atrial-level left-to-right shunting.

Older infants and toddlers

Beyond the neonatal period, failure to thrive, dyspnea on exertion, and a history of repeated chest infections are predominant in mitral stenosis. Pallor and cold extremities, tachycardia, and dyspnea suggest low cardiac output. Signs of pulmonary hypertension, with an exacerbated second heart sound, prominent right ventricular impulse, and hepatomegaly are frequent. A diminished first sound with a low-intensity middiastolic murmur suggests thickened leaflets with limited excursion and can be absent in a low-output state. Older infants and toddlers with mitral regurgitation present with various degrees of failure to thrive and dyspnea with feeds or on exertion. An enlarged left ventricular impulse—with a high-frequency, high-intensity holosystolic murmur heard at the apex and extending into the axillae—is easily auscultated, with signs of right heart failure rarely being seen.

There is no laboratory test for the diagnosis of ARF; hence the diagnosis remains clinical. The diagnosis requires the evidence of a preceding group A streptococcal infection (elevated or rising antistreptolysin O titers, a positive throat culture or positive rapid antigen test for group A streptococci); although this is necessary, it is not sufficient. The probability of a diagnosis of ARF varies according to geographic location (according to ARF incidence) and ethnicity. For diagnostic purposes, clinicians follow Jones's criteria, updated in 1992.[28]

DIAGNOSTIC MODALITIES IN MITRAL VALVE DISEASE

Electrocardiography

There is left atrial enlargement in both mitral stenosis and regurgitation and left ventricular enlargement in mitral regurgitation; right atrial and right ventricular enlargement is seen when pulmonary hypertension is present. In the pediatric population, the rhythm is almost always sinus.

Chest X-ray

Chest x-ray will typically demonstrate the "double density" seen in left atrial enlargement; this is more often the case in regurgitation than in stenosis; other findings are those of variable pulmonary plethora and enlarged contour of the main pulmonary artery. In the presence of mitral valve regurgitation, left ventricular enlargement is responsible for most of the prominence of the cardiac silhouette.

Echocardiography

The echocardiographic study is obligatory and essential. Systematically conducted, it provides all the information necessary to diagnose the mitral anomaly, assess its severity,[29] and assist the surgeon with the repair.[30]

The transthoracic four-chamber view is best for obtaining an accurate transvalvar gradient and defining the precise amplitude of any prolapse or restriction; in general, it is much more accurate than other views in grading the degree of regurgitation. The short-axis view of the mitral valve (en face view) provides direct imaging of the area of the mitral orifice as well as the location and origin of the regurgitation jet. It allows a precise analysis of the papillary muscles (presence, size, location, and symmetry). Transesophageal echocardiography is superior in defining the anatomic details of the suspension apparatus and in evaluating the functional classification. By moving the probe within the esophagus, the operator can obtain precise localization of the area of prolapse along the free edge of the anterior leaflet, using the anterior commissure (probe up) and the posterior commissure (probe down) as anatomic landmarks.

For mitral stenosis, the peak instantaneous and mean gradients across the valve must be interpreted according to the quality of diastolic function and of any associated lesions. The overall impact of the gradient on the surgical indication must be weighed against pulmonary artery pressure and clinical context.

Functional classification

Transthoracic echocardiography (TTE) and transesophageal echocardiography (TEE) make it possible to classify mitral valve pathology, according to the motion of the leaflets, into one of the three following types (Carpentier's functional classification). This classification is irrespective of anatomy and etiology but can add significant clues to what will eventually be found during surgery.[31]

Type I: normal leaflet motion Mitral regurgitation results from a lack of coaptation between the leaflets.

Type II: leaflet prolapse The free edge of one or both leaflets overrides the plane of the orifice during systole.

Type III: Restricted leaflet motion The motion of one or both leaflets is limited. This can be secondary to short or stiff leaflet tissue or suspension apparatus (type IIIa or diastolic) or because the leaflet is pulled away from the coaptation area by a paradoxical motion of the ventricular wall (type IIIb or systolic).

Three-dimensional echocardiography

Three-dimensional echocardiography has made very important progress in the past few years; however, the spatial definition currently obtained does not warrant a change in the way patients are now being investigated. In those weighing more than 12 kg, very good information on the origin of the regurgitant jet can be obtained, and this seems to be superior to the information generated by the en face view in two-dimensional echocardiography.[32,33]

Magnetic resonance imaging and electron-beam computed tomography

Computed tomography (CT) allows precise calculation of the mitral valve regurgitant fraction with flow measurement; so does magnetic resonance imaging (MRI) when correction for the modification of the plane of the valve with three-directional velocity-encoded MRI is used.[34] The mitral valve area is calculated with MRI, and correlations with echocardiographic findings are very strong.[35] Whatever the imaging technique employed, there are limitations in small patients, in whom resolution is critical. Neither MRI nor CT has enough spatial resolution to visualize the valvar tissue or suspension apparatus in small children.

Diagnostic cardiac catheterization

In the current era, there is very limited indication for an invasive diagnostic and hemodynamic study in the assessment of mitral valve disease. Associated lesion or consideration for balloon valvuloplasty may warrant cardiac catheterization.

TREATMENT

Medical therapy

Medical treatment must be vigorous when the annulus is too small to allow implantation of a mechanical prosthesis in the anatomic position. In the setting of predominant mitral regurgitation, the treatment should include angiotensin-converting enzyme inhibitors, diuretics, and, if necessary, blood transfusion.[36,37] In mitral stenosis, any vasodilator or afterload-reducing agent is obviously contraindicated.

Surgical treatment

Indications

The indications for surgical intervention differ somewhat in pediatric patients as compared with adults. Within the pediatric age group, the cutoff point is more related to the size of the mitral valve annulus than to the age of the patient.

Large mitral valve annulus "Large" implies an annulus greater than 30 mm in female patients and greater than 32 mm in males. Using a wide range of mitral valve repair techniques, the probability of a successful repair of the valve with a large annulus is very high. A mitral annuloplasty or even a remodeling annuloplasty will not be outgrown and will not generate stenosis with the growth of the patient. The repair of virtually all valves is an accessible goal.

The patients should be operated on as soon as the regurgitation is severe, irrespective of the severity of symptoms. The probability of repair is directly related to the experience of the surgical team.

Small mitral valve annulus In neonates (< 28 days), infants (> 28 days and less than 1 year), and generally every pediatric patient with a mitral valve annulus less than 18 to 19 mm in size, the repair is technically very challenging, while replacement is possible only with the use of surgical artifacts associated with significantly increased mortality.[38,39] In these patients, surgical intervention should be deferred as long as the patient can be managed with intense medical therapy, including transfusion and continuous positive airway pressure (CPAP). Aggressive medical therapy allows, in some cases, postponement of surgical intervention for several months, often generating significantly more favorable operating conditions.

Intermediate mitral valve annulus In these patients, with a mitral valve annulus greater than 19 mm but smaller than adult size, mitral valve replacement can be safely performed in the anatomic position. Therefore the timing of the mitral valve repair does not have to be delayed for fear of replacement in an unfavorable position. In this age group, this anatomic situation is found in patients between the ages of 1 to 12 years; it is generally safe to wait for quite a long time (up to several years) in cases of severe regurgitation provided that adequate monitoring of pulmonary artery pressure and ventricular function is achieved.[40,41]

Mitral valve repair

At our institution, cardiopulmonary bypass is conducted with moderate hypothermia (32°C), hemoglobin of 10 to 12 g/dL, pump flow of 150 to 200 mL/min/kg or 2.4 L/min/m^2. Myocardial protection is achieved with cold blood cardioplegia administered every 20 to 30 min. The time for preparation for bypass is used for mandatory intraoperative TEE. Venous cannulation should allow as

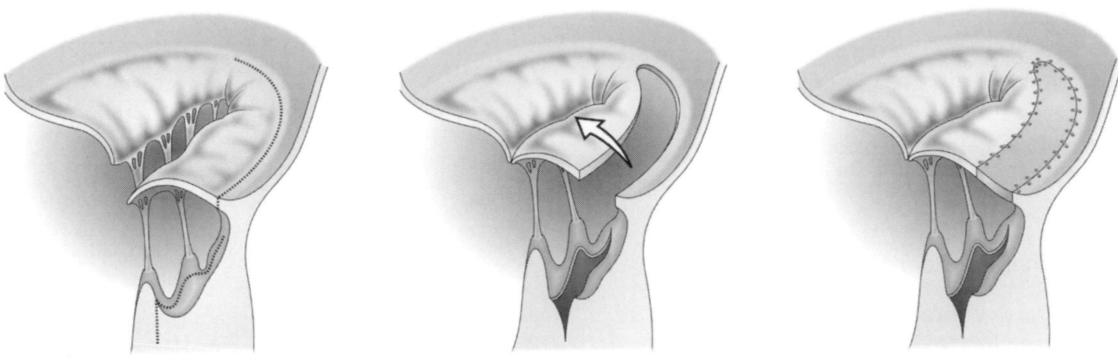

Figure 73-5 Detachment of the posterior leaflet allows access to the suspension apparatus for mobilization (here in a hammock valve). Patch enlargement of the posterior leaflet treats the type III leaflet motion abnormality and allows for a larger annuloplasty.

much access as possible to the atrioventricular groove. Direct cannulation of the superior vena cava and at a distance from the cavoatrial junction and of the inferior vena cava immediately at its origin allows for precise application of the retractor blades. Limited dissection of the groove is performed and, after cross-clamping, the left atrium is entered in the interatrial groove. Exposure is enhanced with mattress sutures inserted into the posterior annulus, pulling the valve upward and toward the operator. The tourniquet on the inferior vena cava is pulled upward and to the left. A self-retaining retractor for mitral surgery adapted to the size of the patient is used in our practice. Approach through the interatrial septum provides a lesser edge for anchoring of the retractor blades and exposes the conduction tissue to more pressure. Approach through the roof of the left atrium does not expose the posterior commissure and the posterior papillary muscle well.

Once satisfactory exposure of the mitral valve is achieved, the valve is systematically analyzed and the observation compared with the preoperative information. The functional classification is confirmed but the extension or restriction of mitral valve prolapse is based on echocardiographic studies of the beating heart. Then analysis of the anatomy follows: a supravalvar ring is confirmed or eliminated; the diameter of the annulus is carefully assessed; texture, aspect, and size of the mitral valve leaflets are noted; the presence and location of any jet lesion is determined as well as the number, aspect, and distribution of the chordae; finally, the presence of commissural tissue and dedicated suspension apparatus as well as the size, location, and morphology of the papillary muscles are assessed. The examination ends with a careful check for accessory mitral valve tissue in the interchordal spaces. The diameter of the annulus and of the opening of the mitral valve is compared to the normal values reported for the patient's body surface area. We use a modification of the sizes provided by Kirklin.[42]

The treatment is adapted to the predominant functional class.

Correction of type I functional abnormalities With the exception of some isolated type I abnormalities without annular dilation (mostly the cleft mitral valve), an annuloplasty is mandatory in all cases of mitral valve insufficiency. In most other cases, attempts to perform mitral valve repair without annuloplasty have resulted in

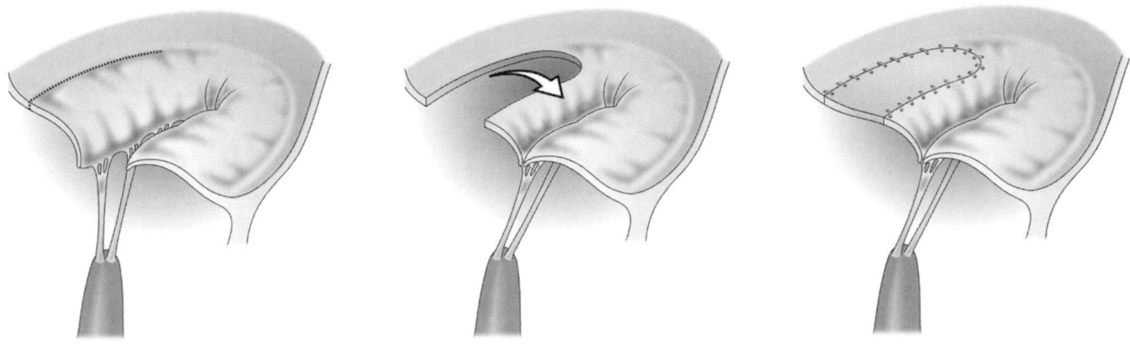

Figure 73-6 Patch enlargement of the anterior leaflet to treat the lack of tissue in a congenital mitral valve or the retraction of the rheumatic leaflet.

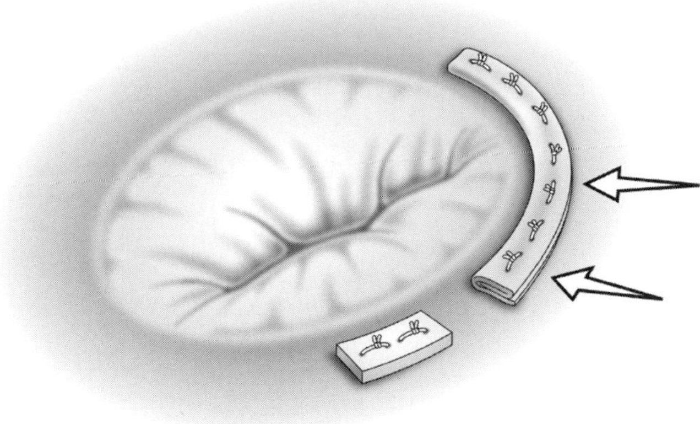

Figure 73-7 Annuloplasty limited to the posterior annulus in patients with less than an adult-sized annulus. A band or short strips of polytetrafluoroethylene or pericardium divided into two or three segments can be used to allow for growth.

recurrence.[14,43] In order to accommodate an adult-size device or a larger-size annulus than what would be indicated from the area of the anterior leaflet, leaflet enlargement with glutaraldehyde-treated pericardium of the posterior leaflet (Fig. 73-5), the anterior leaflet (Fig. 73-6), or both is used.[43–45] When no device is available for the size of the patient or the device is thought to be too small, an annuloplasty limited to the posterior annulus is indicated. The annuloplasty must incorporate both fibrous trigones and can be interrupted in the middle to allow for further growth. Several materials can be used for that purpose, mainly Dacron or polytetrafluoroethylene (PTFE). Mattress sutures should not be tied too tightly (Fig. 73-7). Too thick an annuloplasty may be linked to increased inflow velocity during follow-up.

Correction of type II functional abnormalities Multiple techniques are available to correct the enhanced leaflet motion seen in this functional class. Whether these techniques are to be used in isolation or in combination depends on the extension in width of the prolapse (localized or extended to the whole width of the free edge). It is the height of the prolapse (based on the findings of TEE) and the quality of the chordae that will dictate the choice of technique.

As long as the anatomic correction is adequate (restoring a large surface of apposition between the anterior and posterior leaflets), all techniques are effective and reliable. Overcorrection will generate stress directly on the repaired area and deprive the valve of the relief of stress provided by the surface of apposition. All overcorrections eventually fail, most often in the first few days postoperatively.

Chordal shortening requires thin and flexible chordae.[31] The correction generates important shortening of the chordae and is only adopted when the prolapse is wide (Fig. 73-8). It is a time-consuming procedure and is to be considered if multiple chordae are to be shortened, requiring also access to the midheight of the papillary muscles.

Chordal transfer between secondary chordae and the free edge (more than chordal transfer from the posterior leaflet to the anterior leaflet) allows for correction of localized prolapse. The chorda should be detached from the body of the anterior leaflet with a minimal amount of valvar tissue. It is then attached to the free edge directly at the required length with a small running suture (Fig. 73-9).

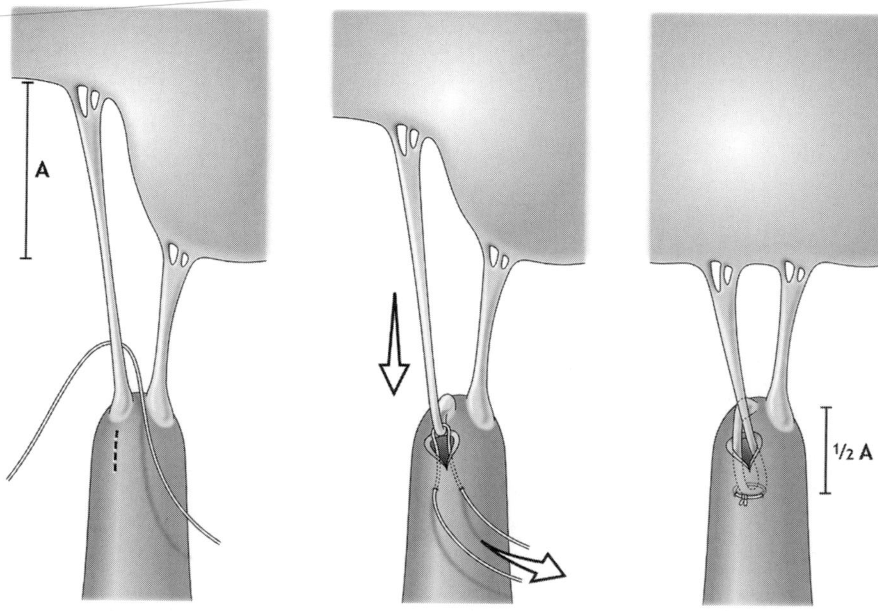

Figure 73-8 Chordal shortening. Note the extent of the shortening achieved.

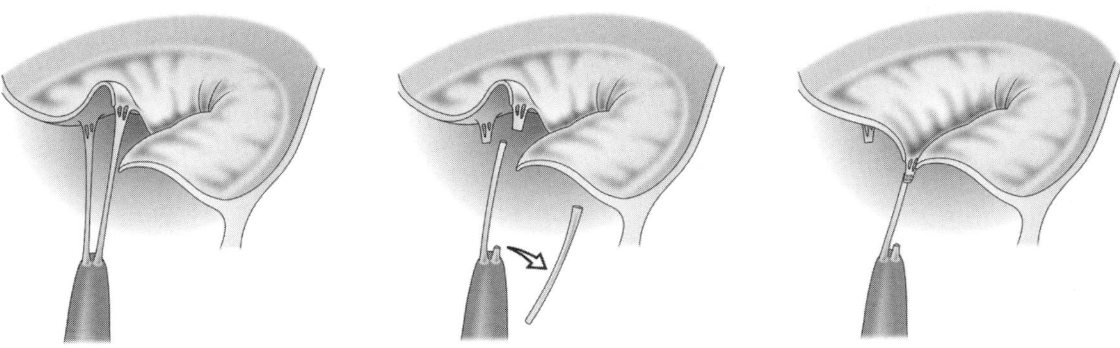

Figure 73-9 Chordal transfer. Only secondary chordae should be used and not the basal chordae.

Wedge resection of the papillary muscle (Fig. 73-10) and sliding plasty generate different degrees of correction of prolapse of multiple chordae (Fig. 73-11). These techniques are very well adapted to prolapse involving a large segment of the anterior leaflet.

Artificial chordae Artificial chordae should be used only in the absence of available chordae of appropriate strength and quality in the area of prolapse. The insertion requires rigorous technique to avoid overcorrection and large knots at the free edge (Fig. 73-12).

Correction of type III functional abnormalities Successful correction of restricted leaflet motion and insufficient leaflet tissue is the essence of working with congenital mitral anomalies, especially in the first year of life. It falls into three general categories:

1. *Posterior leaflet mobilization and enlargement associated with mobilization of the papillary muscles.* Access to the suspension apparatus is the key to adequate mobilization of the latter. It can be done through the mitral valve orifice when it is sufficiently large. Most often, it is very small and does not allow for good access to the suspension apparatus. In these situations, detachment of the posterior leaflet generates a good view of the papillary muscles. Adequate thinning, mobilization from the posterior wall, and splitting and fenestration of the papillary muscles can then be performed safely with good exposure. After full mobilization, the posterior leaflet is reconstructed with enlargement of the valvar tissue (see Fig. 73-5).[15]
2. *Enlargement of valvar tissue using autologous pericardium treated with glutaraldehyde.* Augmentation of the valvar leaflet tissue is the only way to treat a lack of valvar tissue. It can be limited to the anterior leaflet (see Fig. 73-6) or the posterior leaflet or be used for both. Extension of the posterior leaflet

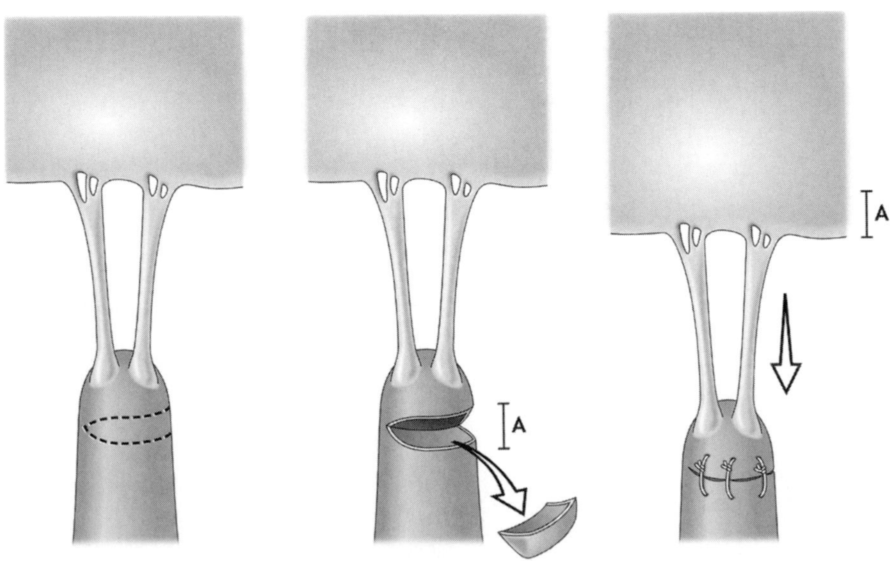

Figure 73-10 Papillary wedge resection. This achieves limited shortening distributed to several chordae.

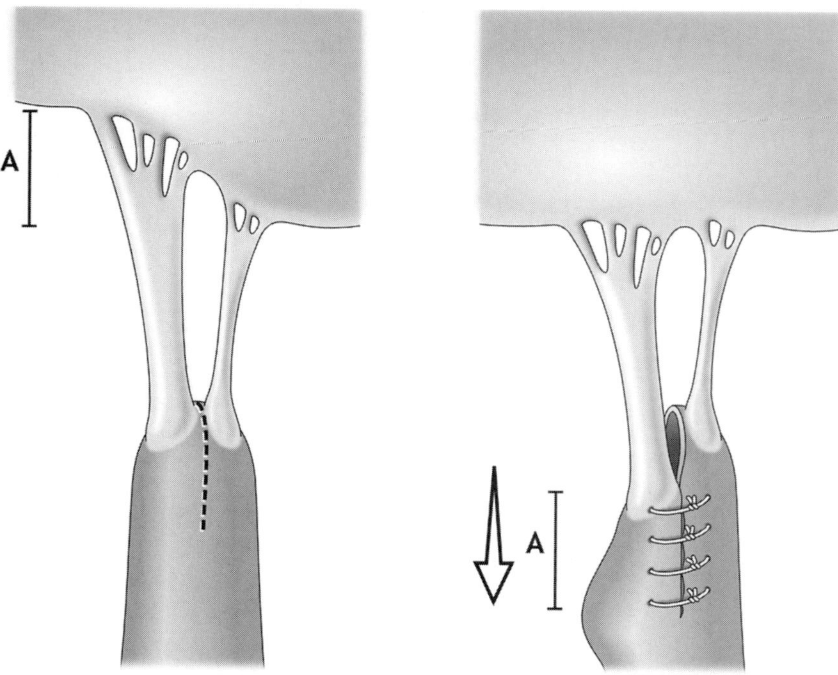

Figure 73-11 Sliding plasty. This technique achieves controlled shortening for thickened chordae.

should be limited to less than half of the height of the leaflet. It can be limited to the area of the middle scallop; alternatively, when the detachment extends from one commissure to another, the extension should reproduce a shape with three scallops and two commissures to allow for a large opening in diastole.

Extension of the anterior leaflet should be done in the body of the leaflet (leaving a strip of valvar tissue close to the hinge point) in order to avoid mechanical stress at this level. The height of the extension should not be greater than two-fifths of the height of the leaflet, leaving the area close to the free edge intact to

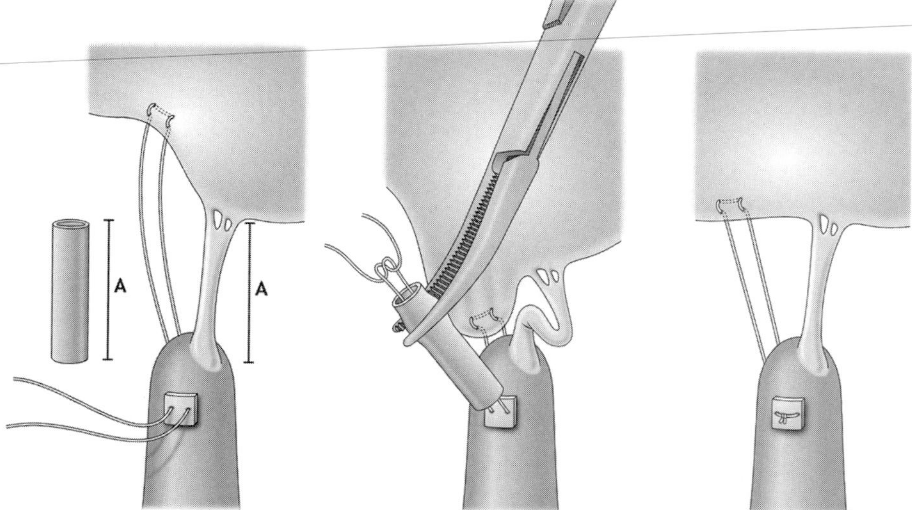

Figure 73-12 Technique for insertion of polytetrafluoroethylene chordae: (1) a template is made from a short plastic tube cut at the required length and slid over the distal part of the stitch. (2) The free edge of the leaflet is lowered to the contact of the papillary muscle. The artificial chorda is tied while the template is clamped. (3) The template is removed and the mattress suture is pulled to bring the knot into contact with the papillary muscle.

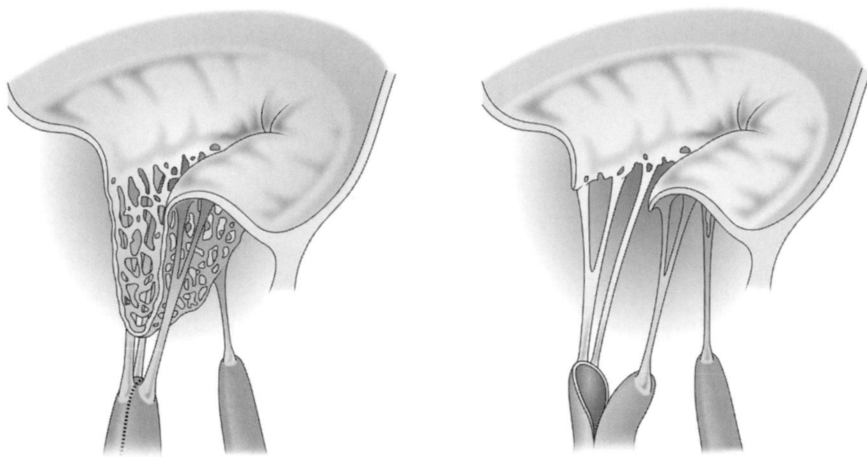

Figure 73-13 Excision of extravalvular tissue, here within a parachute mitral valve. Great care must be taken to preserve the suspension apparatus.

allow for a supple and efficient surface of coaptation. If possible, the enlargement should be symmetrical from trigone to trigone.

3. *Resection of supravalvar rings and accessory mitral valve tissue.* Resection of supravalvar tissue requires excellent exposure of the leaflets. The supravalvar tissue can sometimes be peeled off the valvar tissue. More often, there will be the need for a careful cleavage plane with blunt dissection. Perforation of the anterior leaflet may occur; this should be closed with a figure-of-eight suture. The resection of accessory mitral valve tissue requires a similarly rigorous surgical technique, and very good exposure of the subvalvar apparatus is needed to perfectly differentiate the mitral valve chordae from what can be resected without compromising the integrity of the suspension apparatus. Various approaches to the suspension apparatus may have to be combined: through the mitral valve orifice and the aortic valve or by detachment of the posterior leaflet (Fig. 73-13).

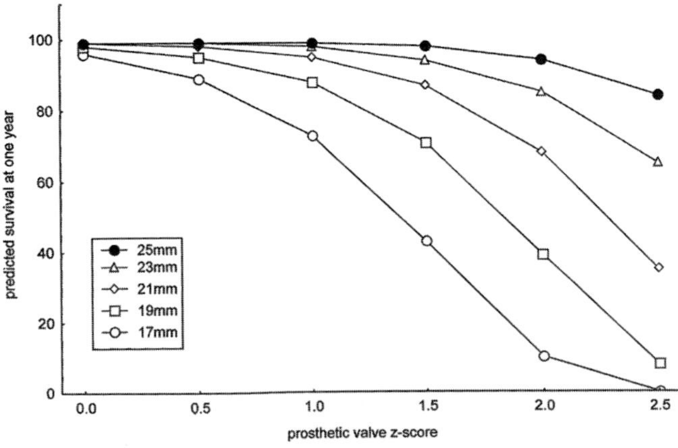

Figure 73-14 Predicted survival at 1 year is plotted against the prosthetic valve z-score. Note that as disparity between the size of the prosthetic valve and the normal mitral annulus increases (increasing z-score), 1-year survival falls precipitously. This effect is greatest at smaller valve sizes. (From Caldarone CA, Raghuveer G, Hills CB, et al. Long-term survival after mitral valve replacement in children aged < 5 years: A multi-institutional study. *Circulation* 2001;104(12 Suppl 1):I143. With permission.)

Valve replacement

Mitral valve replacement should be avoided at all costs in pediatric patients; however, it may be the only option when the valve cannot be repaired. The risk of death in pediatric mitral valve replacement with a mechanical prosthesis increases with the prosthetic size/body-weight ratio, with higher mortality in patients with smaller annular diameters (Fig. 73-14).[46]

Mitral valve replacement in the supraannular position in infants This procedure should be avoided as much as possible because it is responsible for the majority (or totality) of perioperative and late deaths in units with experience with mitral valve replacement in children. Mitral valve repair is often a palliation or a short-term palliation, but allows for annular growth and eventually replacement in with the patient in a satisfactory technical condition.

Mitral valve replacement with a larger annulus This is now possible with excellent long-term results, and only mechanical valves should be implanted in pediatric patients. The introduction of low-profile aortic valves has proven to be very useful in the management of pediatric mitral valve replacement (MVR), since in patients with smaller annular diameters (< 17 mm), an aortic prosthesis can be implanted in an "upside-down" position.

Bioprostheses have been associated with early degeneration and the need for reoperation in younger patients,[47] and mitral valve homografts have not produced satisfactory results in children.[48]

Replacement of mechanical prostheses

This procedure has become not uncommon in most pediatric units. The need for prosthesis replacement is dictated by the size of the first prosthesis implanted and the age at first implantation.[49] The indication is usually the development of a transmitral gradient with pulmonary hypertension, at rest or during exertion. A larger-size prosthesis can usually be implanted, but it is in rare instances more than two sizes larger than the one previously implanted. For a 17-mm mechanical prosthesis implanted in infancy, two further valve replacements will typically be required until a 25-mm mechanical valve can be implanted. On the other hand, a palliative repair should allow for a larger prosthesis to be implanted at the time of the first MVR. Technically, the replacement of a pediatric mechanical prosthesis differs significantly from the same procedure in the adult. Great care must be taken to remove of all cuff tissue and pledgets; everting mattress sutures (especially with pledgets) should be avoided, as they may reduce the size of the annulus. Preference is given in our practice to simple interrupted sutures.

Special considerations

Rheumatic heart disease in children Appropriate timing for mitral valve repair in children with RHD is essential but unfortunately rarely achieved. Surgery should be delayed from the acute rheumatic episode to allow for spontaneous regression of regurgitation with attenuation of the carditis under appropriate treatment. Early surgery is more difficult, as tissues are swollen and fragile. Mitral valve repair during the acute phase of RHD carries high recurrence rates.

At the Royal Children's Hospital, Melbourne, we favor a short period of follow-up (6 to 12 months) when severe mitral regurgitation has become chronic. At that time, morphologic conditions are usually better than those encountered at an earlier intervention or beyond 12 months. The leaflets should still be thin and pliable and the suspension apparatus moderately elongated but not thickened. Under such operating conditions, excellent results can be achieved with a low residual inflow gradient.

Operation on long-standing chronic mitral valve regurgitation will, on the contrary, generate difficult operating conditions: severe retraction of both leaflets, intense thickening of the suspension apparatus, and commissural fusion with calcifications.

Bacterial endocarditis We advocate very aggressive and early intervention for infective BE in children. When mitral regurgitation is greater than moderate, and as soon as the antibiotic therapy is initiated, we believe that surgery is indicated to prevent further damage of the valve or extension of the endocarditic process to the aortic valve.

OUTCOMES

Neonates and infants

Between 1996 and 2004 at the Royal Children's Hospital in Melbourne, 9 patients less than 1 year of age underwent 12 mitral valve procedures for mitral valve regurgitation. All infants underwent initial valve repair, with three reinterventions. Among the latter, one patient received a 21-mm bileaflet prosthesis 7 months after initial repair. The second patient, with Shone complex, underwent homograft MVR (12 mm) after initial repair and a Ross procedure in the neonatal period; eventually, this patient succumbed to bilateral bronchomalacia. The third reoperation was undertaken to make a repair indicated by a previous error in technique. There was one early death in a neonate with severe Marfan's syndrome, which was unrelated to an otherwise successful mitral valve repair.

During the same time interval, 6 patients with a median age of 5 months (range 1 week to 10 months) were operated for congenital mitral stenosis. All had severe failure to thrive and severe pulmonary hypertension. The mean preoperative gradient was 13 ± 2.3 mmHg. The underlying malformations included papillary muscle–commissure fusion (n = 3), parachute mitral valve (n = 2) and supravalvar ring (n = 1). Two patients underwent reoperation. The first patient had three reoperations, leading ultimately to MVR with a mechanical valve (diameter 23 mm). The second patient (neonatal Shone's complex and interrupted aortic arch) underwent reoperation (resection of supravalvar membrane) 2 years following initial intervention.

Outcomes beyond infancy

From the most recent available literature,[15,50–52] repair should be suitable for more than 90 percent of patients in this age group with mitral regurgitation, with operative mortality below 10 percent and expected reoperation rates lower than 15 percent at 15 years. Between 1996 and 2005, 34 patients were operated on for congenital mitral regurgitation at our institution. Their median age was 3 years (range 2 weeks to 15 years). All patients underwent initial repair, with 3 hospital deaths and 2 patients requiring late MVR. At follow-up, 6 patients had moderate residual/recurrent regurgitation (Fig. 73-15). Hospital mortality should be low when mitral stenosis is isolated.[53] Mitral stenosis with associated cardiac lesions generates high mortality and reoperation rates, but such associations are rare beyond infancy. After mitral valve repair for mitral stenosis, residual gradients are frequent but are often well tolerated, with the

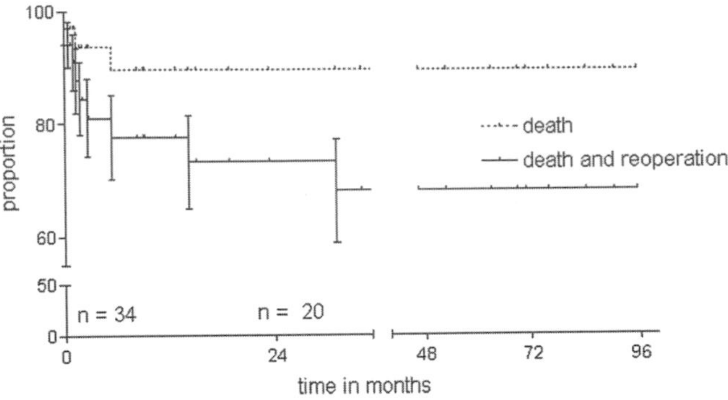

Figure 73-15 Actuarial freedom from reoperation and death or reoperation for repair of congenital mitral valve regurgitation at the Royal Children's Hospital, Melbourne, between 1996 and 2005.

need for reintervention indicated by the level of pulmonary hypertension.

Rheumatic mitral valves

In centers with large surgical volumes, successful mitral valve repair can be accomplished in greater than 90 percent of pediatric patients with RHD, with operative mortality often below 2 percent.[54] Large variations in reoperation rates are reported (from less than 10 to 45 percent at 5 years).[55–57] This variability could be attributed to the quality of the follow-up, but, most importantly, to compliance with secondary antibiotic prophylaxis. In analyzing the success of surgical mitral valve repair, the age of the patient at the time of the first rheumatic episode and the interval to surgical intervention is also to be considered as a potential factor. At our institution, 88 patients 6 to 24 years of age had surgery for rheumatic mitral valve insufficiency between 1996 and 2005. All patients underwent initial mitral valve repair. Freedom from reoperation at 70 months (32 patients at risk) is 78 percent. There were 15 reoperations in 13 patients, of which 7 were replacements and 8 were further repairs. There was one early and one late death.

Mitral valve replacement

Current warfarin therapy in children is safe, with recent advances in INR monitoring that more often allow for a stable value in the range of 3 to 3.5.[58]

Recent series of mechanical MVR in the pediatric age group (including small patients)[59–62] suggest that MVR is performed with low operative mortality provided that the native annulus is large enough to accommodate the prosthesis in the anatomic position. Small series of supraannular implantations have reported elevated early and late mortality.[46] Freedom from second valve replacement is directly related to the age at initial MVR and to the size of the prosthesis implanted.[49]

AORTIC VALVE DISEASE IN CHILDREN

The study of aortic valve disease in children has usually been limited to those born with aortic valve anomalies. But in the present era, an increasing number of children are reaching adulthood with anomalies of the aortic root related to a birth defect or secondary to a surgical procedure. The following discussion also focuses on this developing field. Subaortic membrane stenosis, supravalvar aortic stenosis, Shone's complex, bacterial endocarditis, and rheumatic valve disease, which are treated separately in other chapters, are mentioned here only briefly.

HISTORY

Aortic valvotomy under direct vision was among the first congenital cardiac procedures to be reported as early as 1956.[63,64] Cabrol and Senning later paved the way for the development of modern aortic valve repair.[65,66] The introduction of autograft aortic valve replacement by Ross in 1967 opened an era of alternative replacement for those small children for whom prosthetic valves (excluding root homografts) are unavailable.[67]

EMBRYOLOGY

The mechanisms leading to the formation of the semilunar leaflets are not yet fully elucidated.[68] It is believed that the aortic valve arises from three endocardial cushions appearing on the inner surface of the septated distal primitive outflow tract and that most of the malformations observed result from variable degrees of fusion of the zone of apposition of these primitive leaflets.[69] The fact that most valves (even unicuspid ones) present three interleaflet triangles seems to substantiate this theory.[70] The only exceptions to this rule are aortic valve aplasia, some cases of bicuspid valves, and quadricuspid valves.[71–73] Intrauterine flow restriction through the aortic valve will accordingly model the size of the left ventricle. This seems to be a late phenomenon, because similar midtrimester aortic lesions can result in either a normal-sized or a hypoplastic left ventricle.[74] The modeling of left ventricular size by flow through the aortic valve opens the possibility of fetal aortic valve balloon dilatation to prevent the occurrence of hypoplasia of the left ventricle.[75]

PATHOPHYSIOLOGY

Congenital lesions

Stenosis is the predominant feature of symptomatic congenital aortic valve disease in neonates and infants. With the fusion of the zone of apposition between leaflets, the commissural area supporting the leaflets disappears, leading to a dome-like appearance of the valve. According to the number of such zones between leaflets remaining open, the valve can be tricuspid, bicuspid, or unicuspid.[76] These valves often present a considerable degree of fibrous dysplasia and nodular thickening. Because of the modeling of the heart's components by flow during fetal life, the more severe the obstruction, the smaller the ascending aorta.[77]

Patients who present as teenagers have predominantly regurgitant valves. Bicuspid valve disease is then the most common morphologic abnormality.[78]

Acquired lesions

A variety of congenital cardiac lesions are responsible for the deformity of one or more components of the aortic root.

Tetralogy of fallot and pulmonary atresia

Patients with right-to-left shunts such as tetralogy of Fallot or pulmonary atresia have dilated aortic roots, because their aortas have been subjected to high blood flow over time. Aortic root dilatation may cause central regurgitation by lack of coaptation of the leaflets, related to dilatation of the sinotubular junction. This dilatation can progress even after surgical repair. Patients with pulmonary atresia are more susceptible to aortic root dilatation than those with tetralogy of Fallot, and the later the repair, the higher the risk of dilatation.[79,80] The noninflammatory loss of smooth muscle cells, with mucoid degeneration and fragmentation of the elastic fibers of the media similar to that encountered in bicuspid valve disease or Marfan's syndrome, has been observed in the aortic walls of these patients.[81] It is yet unclear whether these abnormalities of the media are genetically inherited and related to the associated disorder or whether they correspond to apoptosis of the media induced by high flow within the aorta.

Regurgitation related to a ventricular septal defect

Classically, the Venturi effect associated with the high-velocity jet of a restrictive ventricular septal defect (VSD) is responsible for the attraction of aortic leaflets to the VSD orifice, with involvement of the right, the noncoronary, or both leaflets.[82,83] In doubly-committed subarterial VSDs (frequently encountered in the Asian population), the valve is immediately adjacent to the defect and leaflet attraction is much more common in this instance than in perimembranous VSDs.[83,84] Over time, the leaflet elongates and prolapses. At a later stage, the sinus dilates. Finally, the prolapsed leaflet may occlude the opening of the VSD. We believe that the lack of support to the right coronary cusp in doubly-committed VSD is at least as important as the Venturi effect. This would explain why the regurgitation is much less frequent in perimembranous VSD.

Iatrogenic lesions: the arterial switch

All procedures involving the aortic root are likely to alter its geometry. The congenital heart repair that has attracted the most attention is the arterial switch operation (ASO; see Chap. 66). The insertion of the coronary buttons in the neoaortic root at the level of the sinotubular junction may be responsible for late regurgitation. It is disputed whether punch techniques, which insert the buttons in holes created in the sinuses, cause less distortion of the aortic root.[85,86] There is a significant body of evidence that the neoaortic valve is structurally a pulmonary valve and therefore prone to dilation when exposed to systemic pressure. The pathophysiology of the regurgitation is therefore not solely related to the disruption of the sinotubular junction.

Subaortic membrane

Valvar lesions observed in association with the subaortic membrane (see Chap. 70) are thought to be due to the systolic jet and vary from minimal damage to extensive fibrous proliferation extending to the ventricular surfaces of the leaflets, sometimes completely obstructing the interleaflet triangles.[87] Half of the patients present with aortic regurgitation, even when the stenosis is responsible for only mild gradients. The progressive incorporation of the valve in the fibrous proliferation of the membrane may ultimately lead to severe valvar stenosis. In infants and children, valvar lesions are progressive and surgery is recommended when regurgitation appears. This evolution might be slower during adulthood.[88,89]

Supravalvar aortic stenosis

Williams syndrome is found in half of the patients presenting with supravalvar aortic stenosis. It is characterized by an "elfin" facies and outgoing personality, loquacity, deficient cognitive and physical development; it is also associated with renal, skeletal, and vascular anomalies. The most frequent lesions are peripheral stenoses that do not respond to interventional balloon dilatation and supravalvar stenosis. In most instances, supravalvar narrowing is accompanied by considerable abnormalities of the aortic root and the left ventricular outflow tract.[90] The valve is bicuspid or stenotic in up to 50 percent of patients. Thickening and retraction of the sinuses, along with fusion of the commissures to the sinotubular ridge, is frequently responsible for variable coronary ostial stenosis. Left ventricular outflow tract obstruction is identified in as many as one-fourth of patients.[91,92] After operation, regurgitation due to distortion of the aortic root is not uncommon; we therefore advocate repair with Brown's "three-patch technique," described in Chap. 70.[93,94]

CLINICAL FEATURES

Epidemiology

The exact incidence of aortic valve disease in children is difficult to elucidate, as most of the minor deformities of the valve will not become symptomatic for several decades. There seems to be a male predominance of the disease.[95] A bicuspid aortic valve is found in approximately 1 to 2 percent of the general population, with males being affected four times more commonly than females.[78]

Almost 75 percent of the repaired tetralogy patients present with aortic root dilatation once they reach adulthood, accompanied by some degree of regurgitation; however, relatively few become symptomatic.[96] Only 1 percent of tetralogy patients need surgery in the 20 years following their initial repair.[80,96–98]

Aortic valve prolapse is far more frequently encountered in doubly-committed than in perimembranous VSDs. Eleven percent of the patients with perimembranous VSDs will have some degree of aortic valve prolapse, and one-third of the prolapsing valves will cause more than trivial regurgitation. Up to two-thirds of the patients with doubly-committed VSD will show valve prolapse, with 40 percent of those having significant regurgitation. This incidence is even higher in males.[84,99,100] The severity of the regurgitation invariably increases with time. Aortic regurgitation may appear after VSD closure even if the valve was not prolapsing before surgery. When present at the time of surgery, its progression seems to be halted by closure of the VSD.[100,101]

After the ASO, neoaortic regurgitation is very frequent but rarely significant. In 35 percent of the neonates, regurgitation will appear, but only 2 percent of the total will need reoperation for aortic insufficiency in the 10 years following the procedure. Nonetheless, careful examination has revealed that 25 percent of those having aortic regurgitation might have slow progression of their regurgitation.[85,86]

In early infancy, mitral lesions are responsible for most of the mortality of patients affected by Marfan's syndrome. In childhood and adolescence, mitral valve prolapse and aortic dilatation have a similar cumulative incidence. Four out of five Marfan's patients reaching adulthood present aortic root dilatation, and one in five present aortic regurgitation necessitating surgery.[102] Aortic dissection has been only exceptionally reported in pediatric patients with Marfan's syndrome.[103]

Among children and adolescents with RHD, aortic and mitral valves are, respectively, involved in 54 and 85 percent of the cases.[104]

The incidence of active infective BE in children has increased over the last decade, mainly as a result of the improved survival of patients at risk (such as hospitalized neonates and infants with indwelling catheters). Before 1970, the most important factor predisposing to BE was RHD. Today, the predominant predisposing factor has become the presence of congenital heart disease. The incidence is highest among those with cyanotic heart disease, especially if they had operations for restricted pulmonary blood flow or aortic valve replacement.[105]

Clinical features

Neonates and infants below 3 months of age with aortic stenosis and reduced left ventricular function or duct-dependent systemic circulation are described as having critical neonatal aortic stenosis. At the time of ductal closure (if the aortic obstruction is severe), the neonate may be found in cardiovascular collapse with profound desaturation. Later in infancy, the first symptoms may be tachypnea, poor feeding, and failure to thrive.

Most patients presenting after the age of 1 year with aortic stenosis or regurgitation will be asymptomatic. Poor growth, angina, and syncope are found in less than 10 percent of patients with aortic stenosis. Their most frequently encountered symptom is the subjective feeling of fatigability. Awareness of increased neck pulsation comes only in an advanced stages of aortic valve regurgitation.[106,107]

In neonates presenting with critical aortic stenosis, poor pulses, hyperactive precordium, peripheral edema, and hepatomegaly may be noticed. Although a murmur can usually be depicted, the typical murmur at the left sternal edge radiating to the neck is present in only 20 percent of patients.[108] In older children with aortic stenosis, the heave of the apical impulse can be detected on inspection and palpation. Visible bounding arterial pulses accompanying aortic valve regurgitation will become more obvious with increasing severity of the disease.[106,107]

DIAGNOSTIC MODALITIES

The electrocardiogram (ECG) is usually not contributory to the diagnosis of neonatal aortic stenosis and can display signs of left or right ventricular hypertrophy. Below the age of 1 month, the predominant pattern is right ventricular hypertrophy. Older patients with severe aortic stenosis or regurgitation will show signs of left ventricular hypertrophy.[106,107]

The chest x-ray of symptomatic neonates will invariably display cardiomegaly and, in 50 percent of patients, signs of pulmonary congestion. Older patients have a normal-sized heart silhouette. The presence of cardiomegaly with aortic stenosis is associated with a poor prognosis.[109]

Two-dimensional echocardiography provides invaluable information about the morphology of the valve and the severity of the disease. Echocardiography should determine the morphology of the valve leaflets: their quality, mobility, and the presence of calcifications, fibrous nodes, or raphe. The aortic root dimensions should always be evaluated. Diameter at the level of the hinge points of the leaflets, the sinuses, the sinotubular junction and the ascending aorta should be carefully measured. During the evaluation of children with aortic regurgitation, the source of the jet, its orientation, and, if possible, the mechanism of regurgitation should be identified. Dilatation of the aortic root, leaflet prolapse, and restrictive motion of the leaflets can all be responsible for aortic regurgitation. The short-axis view will better determine the opening of the valve and the source of the regurgitation, while the long-axis projection will give details on the direction of the regurgitant jet, the coaptation area, and any eventual prolapse. In the latter view, the leaflet morphology should be carefully examined. Bulging of the core of the leaflet should be distinguished from true prolapse, where the free edge falls below the level of the free edge of the facing leaflets. The coaptation area between the leaflets should be carefully assessed, as should whether coaptation occurs adequately above the hinge points of the valve. Pulsed Doppler echocardiography allows the detection of even mild degrees of obstruction. Continuous-wave Doppler echocardiography provides a way to estimate the instantaneous pressure gradient through the valve by the simplified Bernoulli equation: pressure gradient $= 4 \times$ (peak velocity)^2. This calculated gradient slightly overestimates the peak-to-peak gradient measured invasively.[110] Interpretation of the pressure gradient in the presence of an open duct is difficult and can be misleading. Evaluation of the transaortic flow is essential but necessarily subjective. In that context, left ventricular function, especially shortening fraction and size of the left-to-right shunt at the atrial level, are key factors to consider as well. Eventually, the severity of the obstruction is based on clinical judgment. The severity of aortic regurgitation is best assessed with pulsed Doppler echocardiography. The cross-sectional area of the regurgitant jet in the left ventricular outflow tract and the holodiastolic abdominal aortic flow reversal seem to be better predictors of the degree of regurgitation than the length of the jet or the slope of the aortic regurgitation.[111,112] In the neonate, the dimensions of the left-sided chambers are evaluated, indexed to body surface area, and a z-score is determined. These measurements will help to determine the likelihood that the left heart will sustain the systemic circulation and consequently the patient's suitability for a biventricular repair. In particular, length of left ventricular cavity, mitral valve area, and presence of endocardial fibroelastosis should be recorded.[113,114] Echocardiography is sufficient to elaborate the diagnosis of aortic valve disease in children. A thorough screening of associated anomalies is nonetheless mandatory.

In the neonate, cardiac catheterization should be reserved for the evaluation of associated lesions. Beyond this age, catheterization will be of great help in the decision-making process in cases with borderline indications for surgery or valvuloplasty or when there is a discrepancy between symptoms and echocardiographic findings.

Exercise testing is sometimes performed to assess patients with peak gradients inferior to 60 mmHg in order to demonstrate ST-segment changes or arrhythmias or to obtain a precise evaluation of the exercise capacity of adolescents with vague complaints of fatigability. Its usefulness in determining the indication for an invasive procedure remains to be established.[115]

MEDICAL MANAGEMENT

The lifesaving resuscitative measure in a neonate arriving in cardiovascular collapse is the administration of prostaglandin E_1 (PGE_1). Inotropic support and mechanical ventilation may be required to treat heart failure. The evaluation of the child should thereafter enable the clinician to decide between a biventricular repair or a Norwood-type procedure. The largest study to date examining outcomes for critical aortic stenosis has identified the following parameters, allowing prediction of survival with either of the two options: age, z-score of the aortic valve at the sinuses, grade of endocardial fibroelastosis, diameter of the ascending aorta, presence of moderate or severe tricuspid regurgitation and z-score of ventricular length.[113]

Urgent intervention is mandated for the infant presenting in shock or showing clinical or echocardiographic evidence of poor left ventricular function. Patients presenting with high peak gradients should be offered an early procedure, but there is increasing evidence that, in asymptomatic patients, intervention can be delayed if they are submitted to a close follow-up.[116,117] The cutoff gradient for intervention has usually been set at 50 to 60 mmHg, but this level has been decided arbitrarily. In children and adolescents, surgery or interventional catheterization will be recommended for symptomatic disease, ECG repolarization or ischemic changes at rest or on exercise, and when the transvalvar gradient is greater than 75 mmHg. In aortic regurgitation, the presence of symptoms, left ventricular dysfunction (ejection fraction < 50 percent) and an increase in left end-systolic and end-diastolic diameters are indications for surgery.[118] In RHD, an operation is more frequently indicated for the mitral component of the disease while there is concomitant moderate aortic regurgitation. Valve repair in these circumstances seems rewarding, with freedom from aortic valve dysfunction of 68 percent at 8 years.[119] There has been recent evidence that treatment with angiotensin-converting enzyme inhibitors in growing children with aortic regurgitation limits excessive increases in left ventricular mass and volume.[120]

SURGICAL THERAPY

Many authors have indicated a transverse aortotomy as the preferred approach for aortic valve repair. This statement may not necessarily be true with regard to the pediatric population because the main feature of aortic valve disease in the young is valvar stenosis with its corollary, a small ascending aorta. Therefore the surgeon should not hesitate to perform an oblique aortotomy, extending the incision in the noncoronary sinus almost down to the level of the annulus in order to gain optimal exposure of the aortic valve.

Aortic valve repair

Once stay sutures are placed on the commissures (or at 120 degrees from each other, where commissures should normally be positioned), one can appreciate the valve and the mechanism responsible for regurgitation. In our experience, only lack of mobility of the leaflets at their hinge points will preclude repair. Thereafter, the fused commissures are opened up to the aortic wall. The calcifications and fibrous nodes are resected. Local thickenings are shaved with caution. It has been our policy to remove thickening when it impairs the mobility of the leaflet or it is obstructive in and of itself but to avoid cosmetic shaving of the cusps because this may promote further fibrosis and retraction. Tears from a previous balloon dilatation are then closed directly or, if the regurgitation at this level caused a retraction of the cusps, by the addition of a glutaraldehyde-preserved autologous pericardial patch.

Congenital aortic stenosis often results from the partial or complete fusion of the zone of apposition of adjoining leaflets, followed by the involution of the apposed area. Therefore the valve takes on the appearance of a dome. Classical commissurotomy consists of opening the roof of this dome-like structure, leaving the severed elements unsupported, and thereby causing regurgitation. A typical bicuspid valve would be opened largely between its two main components, leaving the area of the raphe untouched. It has now been shown that valve repair of congenital lesions provides the best chance for long-term success.[121,122] Because the aorta is naturally small in these patients, it has been our policy to transform unicuspid valves into bicuspid valves and bicuspid valves into tricuspid ones by creating new commissures.[123] The surgical instrumentation to achieve good valvotomy and commissuroplasty is very important. We use ophthalmic microblades and specially modified ophthalmic tooth forceps (with 0.2-mm teeth). The area of the potential commissure is identified, and the leaflets are opened in their direction up to the aortic root wall. Calcifications and fibrous thickenings present in the raphe are resected. Stay sutures are placed at the highest point of the planned neocommissures, at the level of the planned sinotubular junction. Two separate patches of glutaraldehyde-preserved autologous pericardium are cut into triangular shapes. Each patch is then sutured with a continuous suture to the severed leaflet, whether it corresponds to an opened doming valve or a previous raphe. The two patches are then secured together at the level where they join on the aortic wall. Both patches are trimmed, if necessary, in order to achieve the appropriate height and leave adequate tension on the free edge of the new leaflets. A continuous suture secures both patches to the aortic wall up to the previously positioned stay suture, marking the superior aspect of the neocommissure (Fig. 73-16).

Some authors have recommended the resection of all thickened leaflet tissue before patch reconstruction by resecting almost the entirety of the body of the valve leaflets and then reconstructing the three leaflets made of pericardial patches. We prefer to leave the native tissue in place as long as mobility along the hinge points is preserved. As patch material, we favor autologous pericardium incubated for 8 min in 0.625% glutaraldehyde and rinsed thoroughly. When used for leaflet reconstruction, bovine pericardium patches undergo rapid fibrocalcific degeneration.[124] Some have postulated that the use of fresh autologous untreated pericardium may allow for patch growth.[125] Three rectangular strips of pericardium patches are tailored as follows: The length of each patch is cut slightly longer than the free edge of the leaflet. The height of the patch should be calculated, so that even with unequal leaflets, the newly created free edges are all at the same level. The patch extensions should not be redundant, to avoid prolapsing, but should be high enough to achieve 4 to 5 mm of apposition in order to reduce stress on the valve. The strips of

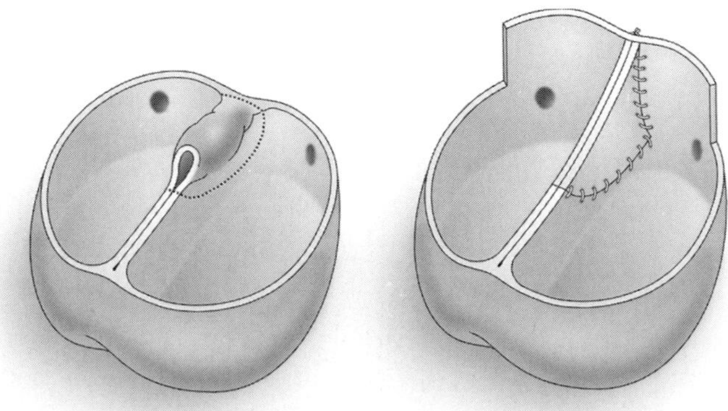

Figure 73-16 Critical aortic stenosis. Commissurotomy of a unicuspid valve and construction of a neocommissure, converting the valve to a bicuspid morphology (details in text).

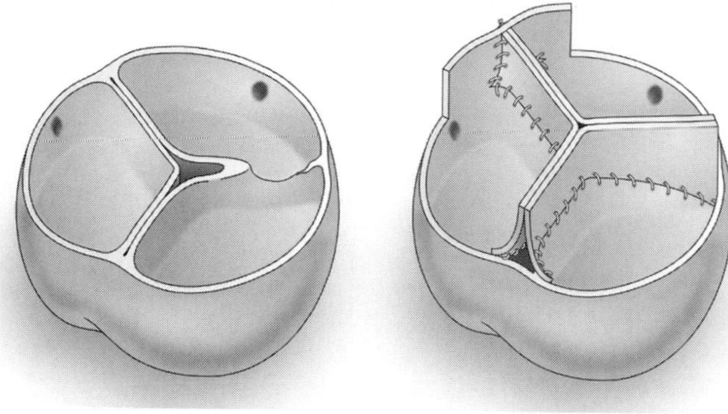

Figure 73-17 Stenotic and regurgitant bicuspid valve. Creation of a tricuspid morphology and cusp extension with glutaraldehyde-related autologous pericardium (details in text).

pericardium are then sutured with a continuous suture to their respective leaflets, with the mesothelial face on the ventricular side and taking great care to avoid any gathering unless there is significant elongation of the free edge (as compared with the adjacent one). Stay sutures are positioned a few millimeters above the apices of the commissures. It is at this stage that the length of the newly created free edge is set by cutting the redundant extremities of each patch. Theoretically, all three patches should have the same length, equal to the diameter of the sinotubular junction. In practice, this is done by bringing the three patches into a closed position with a temporary stitch at the center of the valve, as would be done with a Frater apposition stitch. Then each adjacent half free edge is apposed to give it the appropriate length and minimal tension while maintaining the new commissures in their expected natural position. Each commissure is then recreated by suturing the two adjacent strips of pericardium to the aortic wall, progressing cephalad from the natural commissure. Great care should be taken to achieve perfect alignment with the axis of the natural commissure. The suture is then passed outside of the aorta. A separate suture secures the top of the neocommissure and buries the two joined strips of pericardium (Figs. 73-17 and 73-18).

Specific considerations

Bicuspid valve

Beyond infancy, the dominant feature of the bicuspid aortic valve will guide the surgical strategy. Bicuspid valve patients almost always have some degree of stenosis; however, when the valve is predominantly regurgitant, it is most likely amenable to repair. The type of repair is guided by the size of the aortic root and the quality of the leaflet. If the root is of normal size and the leaflet thickened, we would perform a tricuspidization of the valve by opening the raphe associated with cusp extension. Exceptionally, in pediatric patients we would find a very large aortic root with thin leaflets. The repair would be similar to the one performed in adults (Fig. 73-19) who present late (in the second to fourth decades) with a purely regurgitant bicuspid valve. According to the anatomic finding, triangular resection of the raphe, free-edge reinforcement with a PTFE suture, and subcommissural annuloplasty can be performed.[126,127]

Ventricular septal defect and aortic regurgitation

Many techniques have been reported, but their application depends on the severity of the disease and the extent of prolapse. The primary lesion involves the displacement of the hinge point of the prolapsing leaflet through the VSD orifice, thereby limiting the height of the apposition surface of the right coronary cusp and increasing the stress on its free edge. Then the free edge elongates, the regurgitation increases in volume, and secondary lesions appear on the adjacent cusps. Elongation of the free edge can be corrected by free-edge resuspension.[128]

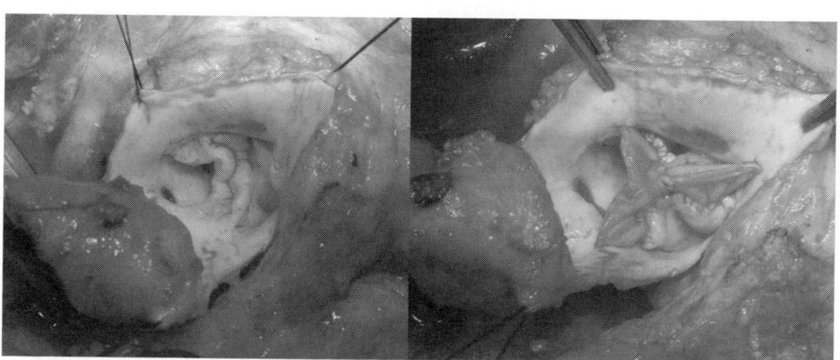

Figure 73-18 Triangular resection at the free edge and pericardial cusp extension (right) of a purely regurgitant bicuspid valve (left).

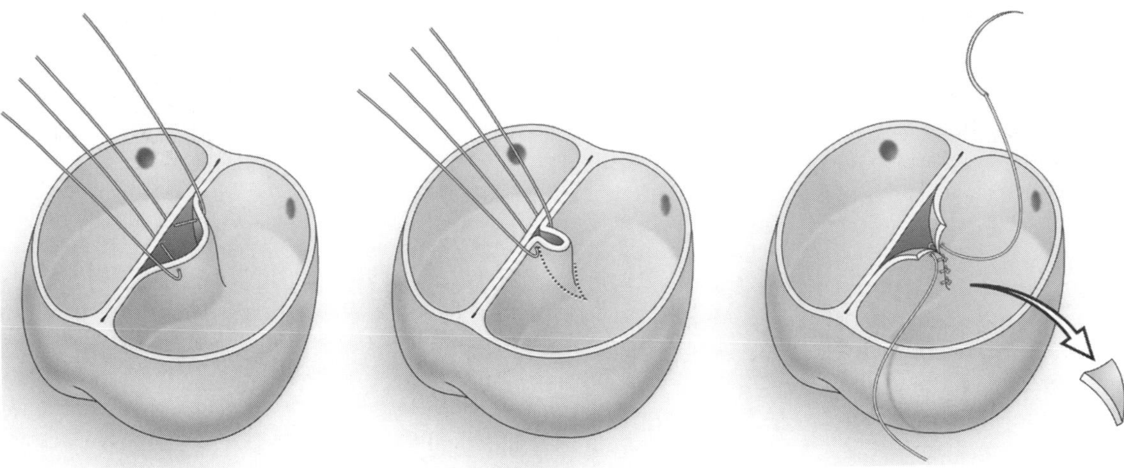

Figure 73-19 Method used to calculate the width of the triangular resection at the free edge in a bicuspid valve, resulting in shortening of the free margin and correction of aortic regurgitation.

To preserve the growth potential together with the fine mechanical properties and stress-relief ability of the commissure, we favor a triangular resection of the mid-portion of the free edge (Fig. 73-20) (or where the valve is most thickened if this allows keeping the relationship with the other noduli of Arantius). Yacoub has described a technique that can be basically applied to all lesions. Through the aortotomy, pledgeted sutures are secured on the edge of the VSD, passed through the leaflet hinge point, and then used to plicate the sinus.[129] Others have described a two-patch technique, using one patch for the VSD and one for the dilated sinus.[130] For this particular lesion, we favor a technique with no patch, where the emphasis is on the repositioning of the hinge point toward the aortic lumen and the restoration of the normal height of the right coronary cusp, together with triangular resection at the free edge whenever indicated.

Subaortic membrane

Extensive resection of all extensions of the membrane is necessary. In the most severe cases, this necessitates resculpting the inferior surface of the interleaflet triangle and thinning the aortic leaflets. The most severe cases are the most prone to recurrence.

Marfan's syndrome

Aortic regurgitation associated with mild aortic root dilatation is best treated with plication of the sinotubular junction and subcommissural annuloplasty, especially if performed in association with mitral valve repair. More severe dilatation of the aortic root may require valve-sparing procedures, as performed in adult patients.[131]

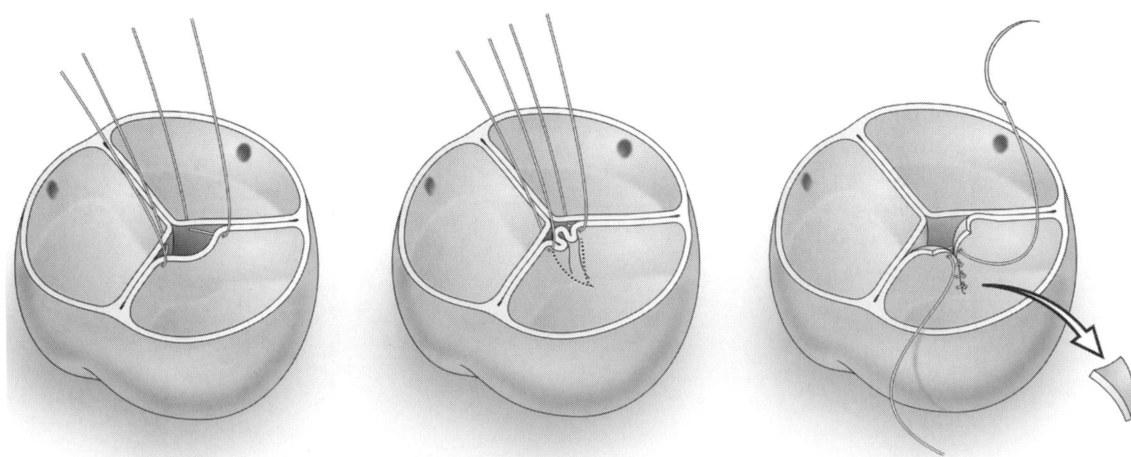

Figure 73-20 Method for correcting cusp prolapse in a tricommissural aortic valve by shortening the free margin (triangular resection) of the prolapsing cusp.

Aortic valve replacement

The techniques of prosthetic valve replacement, Bentall and Ross procedures, are essentially performed much as in adults. The main difference is the limited size of the aortic root. For that reason, we never use pledgeted sutures or horizontal mattress sutures to secure the valve in children. In order to reduce the need for reoperation, at the very least a 19-mm prosthesis should be inserted. Techniques of annular enlargement are often necessary, either by incision and patching of the annulus onto the mitral valve leaflet as described by Manouguian,[132,133] with a Konno procedure, or with both (see Chap. 70).

In performing a Ross procedure (Chap. 70), it is essential to match the diameter of the aortic orifice with that of the pulmonary autograft. In the presence of a small aortic orifice or a subaortic tunnel, a Konno-type aortoventriculoplasty must be performed and is simple after the autograft excision. When the pulmonary autograft is smaller than the aortic annulus, this has to be corrected by subcommissural annuloplasty or even a small triangular resection (reverse Konno or Manouguian procedure). Correction of the mismatch with a larger autograft cuff is strictly prohibited[134,135]; generally, the pulmonary autograft tissue below the nadir of the pulmonary cusps must be kept to a minimum. Funnel obstruction of the left ventricular outflow tract and fibrous remodeling related to subaortic stenosis are substrates for recurrent stenosis and failure of the autograft. Inclusion technique has been recommended as the procedure of choice in performing a Ross in the adults, but it is only exceptionally feasible in children because of the diminutive size of the aortic root.

OUTCOMES

Balloon valvuloplasty versus surgical valvotomy

Since outcomes in infants less than 3 months of age with critical aortic stenosis are significantly worse, the issue of congenital aortic stenosis in the neonatal period should be considered separately from that in older infants and children.[136] In this age group, the mortality seems independent of the type of procedure used and ranges between 0 and 20 percent.[136–139] The cause of death in this group is mostly related to the inability of the left-sided heart structures to sustain the systemic circulation.[140]

Catheter-based procedures and surgical interventions relieve stenosis with fundamentally different modes of action, as reflected by the differences in the clinical consequences of these procedures. Inflation of a balloon angioplasty catheter will tear the valve in the plane of least resistance—in the supple, mobile component of the valve—while classic surgical commissurotomy will open the fibrotic fused zones of apposition, leaving thickened leaflets with reduced mobility. Therefore balloon valvuloplasty will typically decrease the transvalvar gradient by 40 percent, while the surgical procedure will decrease it by 20 percent, but it will also be responsible for more aortic regurgitation.[140,141] Avulsion of the valve with severe aortic regurgitation occurs in 5 percent of balloon dilatations of the aortic valve.[141] Despite these differences, an extensive comparative clinical study performed in neonates failed to demonstrate a significant difference between these procedures in their respective rates of early mortality or long-term reoperation. Thirty percent of patients need a reoperation after 6 months and 50 percent after 5 years (Fig. 73-21). The preprocedural need for inotropic support, lower weight at valvotomy, and moderate to severe aortic valve regurgitation immediately after valvotomy are predictive factors for early reoperation.[140]

In the older age group, the mortality is extremely low and again the results are remarkably comparable to those of surgical valvotomy. The decrease in peak-to-peak gradient is around 50 percent, and freedom from reoperation in this age group is again similar for both techniques. After both types of procedures, the transvalvar gradient and the severity of aortic regurgitation usually increase over time.[141]

Because of the similarity in results offered by interventional catheterization and surgery, the choice between the two procedures should depend on individual center preference and relative experience with both procedures. However, all studies to date have compared balloon valvuloplasty with classic techniques of surgical

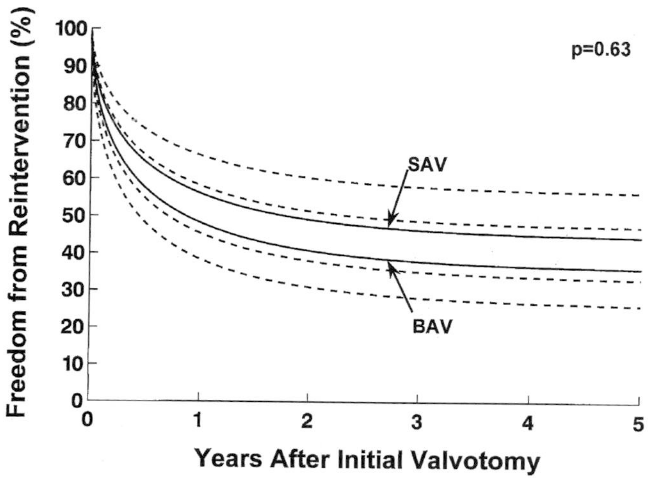

Figure 73-21 Time-related freedom from aortic valve–related reintervention stratified by type of initial aortic valvotomy, adjusted for differences in group characteristics. BAV = balloon valvotomy; SAV = surgical valvotomy. Solid lines represent parametric determination of continuous point estimates, and dashed lines enclose 70 percent CI. (From McCrindle BW, Blackstone EH, Williams WG, et al. Are outcomes of surgical versus transcatheter balloon valvotomy equivalent in neonatal critical aortic stenosis? *Circulation* 2001;104(12 Suppl 1):I152–I158. With permission.)

commissurotomy; we believe that with the more recently developed techniques of repair, improved results with surgery will soon emerge.[123] Interventional procedures preclude a later repair of quality in many patients. It has been clearly demonstrated that the best results after balloon dilatation are achieved in patients with structurally tricuspid valves with fusion at the commissural level.[142] On the other hand, patients with truly bicuspid aortic valves will not have a relief of their stenosis if the raphe is kept intact, and in this setting it is reasonable to think that surgery will achieve superior and more durable results. Therefore, irrespective of the age of the patients, we limit the indication for balloon dilatation to only tricuspid valves with commissural fusion, and prefer surgical correction for all remaining patients.

Aortic valve repair

Modern techniques of valve repair such as neocommissural reconstruction have only recently been introduced in the pediatric population, and long-term results of valve repair in children can only be extrapolated from the adult experience and from the cusp extension techniques applied to rheumatic valves. Some groups have reported a freedom from structural valve deterioration for cusp extension or cusp replacement with autologous pericardium greater than 90 percent at 9 years after repair, without any need for anticoagulation.[124,125] The freedom from reoperation for adults with bicuspid valve repair without cusp extension is 84% at 7 years.[127]

A particular concern for repair is the association of a bicuspid valve with supra- or subvalvar aortic stenosis. Outcomes are influenced by the severity of the outflow tract obstruction. These patients are very likely to necessitate further surgery, with a reported 5-year freedom from reoperation of only 43 percent.[93] In this setting, a Ross or a Ross-Konno procedure should be considered.

Valve-sparing procedures can successfully be performed in children, but only intermediate-term results of these procedures are available for the pediatric population.[131]

We have followed 21 patients with tricuspidization and leaflet extension with a cumulative follow-up of 530 patient-months (1999–2005). Two patients required immediate revision of the repair and retained their valves. There was one late reoperation (pulmonary autograft) at 50-month follow-up. After the same interval, 4 patients had moderate aortic insufficiency and 4 had a gradient less than 30 but greater than 20 mmHg.

Recurrence of regurgitation is rare after valve repair for VSD-related aortic regurgitation; a 15-year freedom from reoperation as high as 81 percent has been reported.[82] In the adult population, results seem much less promising.[143]

The aortic regurgitation associated with subaortic membrane regresses in the majority of operated cases, especially when aggressive resection of all the proliferative tissue is undertaken.[87]

Aortic valve replacement

Bioprostheses

Owing to the unacceptable rate of calcification and degeneration (leading to reoperation in up to 75 percent of patients at 5 years),[144] the use of bioprostheses in children has largely been abandoned. They should be used only as a last resort in patients in whom anticoagulation is strictly contraindicated and who are not candidates for a Ross procedure, such as female patients of childbearing age.[145]

Mechanical valves

The operative mortality of children undergoing a mechanical valve replacement is higher than that for adult patients (between 5 and 13 percent) mainly owing to concomitant risk factors such as previous surgery, associated conditions necessitating repair, and poor ventricular function.[132,146,147] In this age group, major bleeding and thromboembolic events are remarkably rare, with an estimated linearized rate of 0.3 percent per patient-year for each of these complications. When complications of anticoagulation occur, they are usually due to the lack of compliance in the adolescent age group.[132,147,148] Ten-year freedom from reoperation is as high as 92 percent in this age group.[132,146] The 10-year survival is around 75 percent.[146,149] Some authors have pointed out that patients with congenital heart disease may be prone to late pannus formation in the subvalvar area and that they might be more susceptible to late valve failure than their adult counterparts.[150,151]

Homografts

The 10-year freedom from tissue failure for aortic valve replacement with homografts is reported at 62 ± 3 percent in large series of adult patients. The incidence of homograft valve deterioration is higher in the adolescent and young adult and highest in infants; these data clearly preclude the liberal use of such grafts in this age group.[152] The risk of reoperation after allograft valve replacement of the aortic valve is greater than 50 percent in the 3 years following implantation performed in children below the age of 3 years.[153]

Ross procedure

Reported mortality for the Ross procedure in children usually ranges between 0 and 6 percent.[135,154–158] The advantages of the Ross procedure in children are obvious. It allows the best anatomic restoration of the left ventricular outflow tract with no residual gradient and no need for anticoagulation, and it can be performed easily in all age groups. It has also been demonstrated that the growth of the autograft parallels somatic growth.[155,159] Comparative retrospective studies seem to underline the superiority of the pulmonary autograft with regard to both survival and valve-related complications.[151,160] The rate of autograft failure in adults is 4 percent and, in half of the cases, the autograft can be repaired at reoperation. The 25-year freedom from reoperation on the right ventricular outflow tract is greater than 83 percent.[161]

The Ross procedure can also be performed for aortic RHD, but one should be aware that the risk of rheumatic valvulitis of the autograft ranges between 3 and 17 percent and that this risk is higher when the mitral valve is involved.[158,162,163]

Despite its apparent excellent results, the Ross procedure may not be the panacea for all children. Geometric mismatch between the aortic and pulmonary roots seems to be responsible for a high rate of autograft failure, especially when the procedure is performed for aortic valve regurgitation.[134] There is an increasing concern that all autografts implanted as roots (especially bicuspid aortic valves) are subjected to progressive dilatation, and it is not yet known how many will eventually require reoperation for neoaortic regurgitation.[164,165] Several studies have reported that, at 5 years, greater than mild regurgitation occurred in 25 percent of autografts.[157]

We therefore believe that aortic valve repair should be attempted in all circumstances where it seems feasible, especially in infants and children. It is likely that a number of these repairs will fail with time, especially those involving the most extensive reconstruction with pericardium. In addition, because geometric mismatch between the pulmonary root and the aortic root predisposes to the autograft failure after a Ross procedure, we offer primary valve repair for all infants in the hope that it might allow them to have near-normal growth of the aortic root; thus the Ross procedure can be performed at a later age with more favorable long-term results. When the primary concern is aortic regurgitation, the rate of autograft failure is substantial. These lesions seem the best suited for repair, and we strongly recommend repair in these situations. When the lesion is predominantly stenotic and the annulus is small, a Ross procedure is indicated.

Also, in the acute phase of the rheumatic process, we try to avoid operating. The Ross procedure is contraindicated when the valve is still thin and pliable, with an elongated free edge. We perform a triple-cusp extension repair systematically when the valve must be addressed and offer a Ross procedure only when the leaflets are severely retracted and/or calcified.

References

1. Fann JI, Ingels NB Jr, Miller DC. Pathophysiology of mitral valve disease. In: Cohn LH, Edmunds LH Jr (eds). *Cardiac Surgery in the Adult*. New York: McGraw-Hill; 2003:901–931.
2. Oosthoek PW, Wenink AC, Vrolijk BC, et al. Development of the atrioventricular valve tension apparatus in the human heart. *Anat Embryol (Berl)* 1998; 198:317.
3. Wessels A, Markman MW, Vermeulen JL, et al. The development of the atrioventricular junction in the human heart. *Circ Res* 1996;78:110.
4. Oosthoek PW, Wenink AC, Wisse LJ, et al. Development of the papillary muscles of the mitral valve: Morphogenetic background of parachute-like asymmetric mitral valves and other mitral valve anomalies. *J Thorac Cardiovasc Surg* 1998;116:36.
5. Cochrane AD, Marath A, Mee RB. Can a dilated coronary sinus produce left ventricular inflow obstruction? An unrecognized entity. *Ann Thorac Surg* 1994;58:1114.
6. Tamura M, Menahem S, Brizard C. Clinical features and management of isolated cleft mitral valve in childhood. *J Am Coll Cardiol* 2000;35:764.
7. Kohl T, Silverman NH. Comparison of cleft and papillary muscle position in cleft mitral valve and atrioventricular septal defect. *Am J Cardiol* 1996;77:164.
8. Prifti E, Frati G, Bonacchi M, et al. Accessory mitral valve tissue causing left ventricular outflow tract obstruction: Case reports and literature review. *J Heart Valve Dis* 2001;10:774.
9. Schmid AC, Zund G, Vogt P, et al. Congenital subaortic stenosis by accessory mitral valve tissue, recognition and management. *Eur J Cardiothorac Surg* 1999;15:542.
10. Calabro R, Santoro G, Pisacane C, et al. Critical left ventricular outflow tract obstruction due to accessory mitral valve tissue. *Echocardiography* 2000;7:177.
11. Shone JD, Sellers RD, Anderson RC, et al. The developmental complex of "parachute mitral valve," supravalvular ring of left atrium, subaortic stenosis, and coarctation of aorta. *Am J Cardiol* 1963;11:714.
12. Brauner RA, Laks H, Drinkwater DC, et al. Multiple left heart obstructions (Shone's anomaly) with mitral valve involvement: Long-term surgical outcome. *Ann Thorac Surg* 1997;64:721.
13. Carpentier A. Congenital malformations of the mitral valve. In: Stark J, de Leval M (eds). *Surgery for Congenital Heart Defects,* 2d ed. Philadelphia: Saunders; 1994:599–614.
14. Carpentier A, Branchini B, Cour JC, et al. Congenital malformations of the mitral valve in children. Pathology and surgical treatment. *J Thorac Cardiovasc Surg* 1976;72:854.
15. Chauvaud S, Fuzellier JF, Houel R, et al. Reconstructive surgery in congenital mitral valve insufficiency (Carpentier's techniques): Long-term results. *J Thorac Cardiovasc Surg* 1998;115:84.
16. Guerrero RR, Wilkinson JL, Brizard CP. Reconstruction of left main coronary artery with subclavian artery free graft in an infant. *Eur J Cardiothorac Surg* 2005;27:927.
17. Nascimento R, Freitas A, Teixeira F, et al. Is mitral valve prolapse a congenital or acquired disease? *Am J Cardiol* 1997;79:226.
18. Fornes P, Heudes D, Fuzellier JF, et al. Correlation between clinical and histologic patterns of degenerative mitral valve insufficiency: A histomorphometric

study of 130 excised segments. *Cardiovasc Pathol* 1999;8:81.
19. Disse S, Abergel E, Berrebi A, et al. Mapping of a first locus for autosomal dominant myxomatous mitral-valve prolapse to chromosome 16p11.2-p12.1. *Am J Hum Genet* 1999;65:1242.
20. van Karnebeek CD, Naeff MS, Mulder BJ, et al. Natural history of cardiovascular manifestations in Marfan syndrome. *Arch Dis Child* 2001;84:129.
21. Fuzellier JF, Chauvaud SM, Fornes P, et al. Surgical management of mitral regurgitation associated with Marfan's syndrome. *Ann Thorac Surg* 1998;66:68.
22. Boileau C, Jondeau G, Mizuguchi T, et al. Molecular genetics of Marfan syndrome. *Curr Opin Cardiol* 2005;25:194.
23. Pope FM, Burrows NP. Ehlers-Danlos syndrome has varied molecular mechanisms. *J Med Genet* 1997;34:400.
24. Guilherme L, Dulphy N, Douay C, et al. Molecular evidence for antigen-driven immune responses in cardiac lesions of rheumatic heart disease patients. *Int Immunol* 2000;12:1063.
25. Lymbury RS, Olive C, Powell KA, et al. Induction of autoimmune valvulitis in Lewis rats following immunization with peptides from the conserved region of group A streptococcal M protein. *J Autoimmun* 2003;20:211.
26. Bisno AL. Group A streptococcal infections and acute rheumatic fever. *N Engl J Med* 1991;325:783.
27. Marcus RH, Sareli P, Pocock WA, et al. Functional anatomy of severe mitral regurgitation in active rheumatic carditis. *Am J Cardiol* 1989;63:577.
28. Guidelines for the diagnosis of rheumatic fever. Jones Criteria, 1992 update. Special Writing Group of the Committee on Rheumatic Fever, Endocarditis, and Kawasaki Disease of the Council on Cardiovascular Disease in the Young of the American Heart Association. *JAMA* 1992;268:2069.
29. Banerjee A, Kohl T, Silverman NH. Echocardiographic evaluation of congenital mitral valve anomalies in children. *Am J Cardiol* 1995;76:1284.
30. Chauvaud S, Fuzellier JF, Houel R, et al. Reconstructive surgery in congenital mitral valve insufficiency (Carpentier's techniques): Long-term results. *J Thorac Cardivasc Surg* 1998;115:84; discussion, 92.
31. Carpentier A. Cardiac valve surgery: The "French correction." *J Thorac Cardiovasc Surg* 1983;86:323.
32. Acar P, Laskari C, Rhodes J, et al. Three-dimensional echocardiographic analysis of valve anatomy as a determinant of mitral regurgitation after surgery for atrioventricular septal defects. *Am J Cardiol* 1999;83:745.
33. Barrea C, Levasseur S, Roman K, et al. Three-dimensional echocardiography improves the understanding of left atrioventricular valve morphology and function in atrioventricular septal defects undergoing patch augmentation. *J Thorac Cardiovasc Surg* 2005;129:746.
34. Didier D, Ratib O, Lerch R, et al. Detection and quantification of valvular heart disease with dynamic cardiac MR imaging. *Radiographics* 2000;20:1279.
35. Lembcke A, Borges AC, Dushe S, et al. Assessment of mitral valve regurgitation at electron-beam CT: Comparison with Doppler echocardiography. *Radiology* 2005;236:47.
36. Nihill MR, McNamara DG, Vick RL. The effects of increased blood viscosity on pulmonary vascular resistance. *Am Heart J* 1976;92:65.
37. Lister G, Hellenbrand WE, Kleinman CS, et al. Physiologic effects of increasing hemoglobin concentration in left-to-right shunting in infants with ventricular septal defects. *N Engl J Med* 1982;306:502.
38. Gunther T, Mazzitelli D, Schreiber C, et al. Mitral-valve replacement in children under 6 years of age. *Eur J Cardiothorac Surg* 2000;17:426.
39. van Doorn C, Yates R, Tsang V, et al. Mitral valve replacement in children: Mortality, morbidity, and haemodynamic status up to medium-term follow up. *Heart* 2000;84:636.
40. Krishnan US, Gersony WM, Berman-Rosenzweig E, et al. Late left ventricular function after surgery for children with chronic symptomatic mitral regurgitation. *Circulation* 1997;96:4280.
41. Murakami T, Nakazawa M, Nakanishi T, et al. Prediction of postoperative left ventricular pump function in congenital mitral regurgitation. *Pediatr Cardiol* 1999;20:418.
42. Kirklin JW, Barrat-Boyes BG. Anatomy, dimension and terminology. In: Kirklin JW, Barrat-Boyes BG (eds). *Cardiac Surgery*, 2d ed. London: Churchill Livingstone; 1993:3–60.
43. Chauvaud S, Jebara V, Chachques JC, et al. Valve extension with glutaraldehyde-preserved autologous pericardium. Results in mitral valve repair. *J Thorac Cardiovasc Surg* 1991;102:171.
44. Vincentelli A, Zegdi R, Prat A, et al. Mechanical modifications to human pericardium after a brief immersion in 0.625% glutaraldehyde. *J Heart Valve Dis* 1998;7:24.
45. Acar C, de Ibarra JS, Lansac E. Anterior leaflet augmentation with autologous pericardium for mitral repair in rheumatic valve insufficiency. *J Heart Valve Dis* 2004;13:741.
46. Caldarone CA, Raghuveer G, Hills CB, et al. Long-term survival after mitral valve replacement in children aged < 5 years: A multi-institutional study. *Circulation* 2001;104(12 Suppl 1):I143.
47. Antunes MJ, Santos LP. Performance of glutaraldehyde-preserved porcine bioprosthesis as a mitral valve substitute in a young population group. *Ann Thorac Surg* 1984;37:387.
48. Chauvaud S, Waldmann T, d'Attellis N, et al. Homograft replacement of the mitral valve in young recipients: Mid-term results. *Eur J Cardiothorac Surg* 2003;23:560.
49. Raghuveer G, Caldarone CA, Hills CB, et al. Predictors of prosthesis survival, growth, and functional status following mechanical mitral valve replacement in children aged < 5 years, a multi-institutional study. *Circulation* 2003;108(Suppl I):I174.
50. Wood AE, Healy DG, Nolke L, et al. Mitral valve reconstruction in a pediatric population: Late clinical results and predictors of long-term outcome. *J Thorac Cardiovasc Surg* 2005;130:66.
51. McCarthy JF, Neligan MC, Wood AE. Ten years' experience of an aggressive reparative approach to congenital mitral valve anomalies. *Eur J Cardiothorac Surg* 1996;10:534.
52. Okita Y, Miki S, Kusuhara K, et al. Early and late results of reconstructive operation for congenital mitral regurgitation

in pediatric age group. *J Thorac Cardiovasc Surg* 1988; 96:294.

53. Chauvaud S, Mihaileanu S, Gaer J, et al. Surgical treatment of congenital mitral stenosis: "The Hôpital Broussais" experience. *Cardiol Young* 1997;7:15.
54. Deloche A, Jebara VA, Relland JY, et al. Valve repair with Carpentier techniques. The second decade. *J Thorac Cardiovasc Surg* 1990;99:990; discussion, 1001.
55. Antunes MJ, Magalhaes MP, Colsen PR, et al. Valvuloplasty for rheumatic mitral valve disease. A surgical challenge. *J Thorac Cardiovasc Surg* 1987;94:44.
56. Pomerantzeff PM, Brandao CM, Faber CM, et al. Mitral valve repair in rheumatic patients. *Heart Surg Forum* 2000;3:273.
57. Skoularigis J, Sinovich V, Joubert G, et al. Evaluation of the long-term results of mitral valve repair in 254 young patients with rheumatic mitral regurgitation. *Circulation* 1994;90(5 Pt II):II167.
58. Streif W, Andrew M, Marzinotto V, et al. Analysis of warfarin therapy in pediatric patients: A prospective cohort study of 319 patients. *Blood* 1999;94:3007.
59. van Doorn C, Yates R, Tsang V, et al. Mitral valve replacement in children: Mortality, morbidity, and haemodynamic status up to medium term follow up. *Heart* 2000; 84:636.
60. Masuda M, Kado H, Matsumoto T, et al. Mitral valve replacement using bileaflet mechanical prosthetic valve in the first year of life. *Jpn J Thorac Cardiovasc Surg* 2000; 48:643.
61. Ninet J, Sassolas F, Robin J, et al. Mitral valve replacement in infants using the "Saint-Jude Medical" prosthesis. *Arch Mal Coeur Vaiss* 1994;87:643.
62. Daou L, Sidi D, Mauriat P, et al. Mitral valve replacement with mechanical valves in children under two years of age. *J Thorac Cardiovasc Surg* 2001;121:994.
63. Kortz AB, Swan H. Direct vision trans-aortic approach to the aortic valve during hypothermia: Experimental observations and report of successful clinical case. *Ann Surg* 1956;144:205.
64. Benjamin RB, Lewis FJ, Niazi SA, et al. Aortic valvulotomy under direct vision during hypothermia. *J Thorac Surg* 1956;32:81.
65. Cabrol C, Cabrol A, Guiraudon G, et al. Treatment of aortic insufficiency by means of aortic annuloplasty. *Arch Mal Coeur Vaiss* 1966;59:1305.
66. Senning A. Fascia lata replacement of aortic valves. *J Thorac Cardiovasc Surg* 1967;54:465.
67. Ross DN. Replacement of aortic and mitral valves with a pulmonary autograft. *Lancet* 1967;523:956.
68. Rothenberg F, Fisher SA, Watanabe M. Sculpting the cardiac outflow tract. Birth Defects Res Part C *Embryol Today* 2003;69:38.
69. Sans-Coma V, Fernandez B, Duran AC, et al. Fusion of valve cushions as a key factor in the formation of congenital bicuspid aortic valves in Syrian hamsters. *Anat Rec* 1996;244:490.
70. Anderson RH. Understanding the structure of the unicuspid and unicommissural aortic valve. *J Heart Valve Dis* 2003;12:670.
71. Hartwig NG, Vermeij-Keers C, De Vries HE, et al. Aplasia of semilunar valve leaflets: Two case reports and developmental aspects. *Pediatr Cardiol* 1991;12:114.
72. Angelini A, Ho SY, Anderson RH, et al. The morphology of the normal aortic valve as compared with the aortic valve having two leaflets. *J Thorac Cardiovasc Surg* 1989;98:362.
73. Timperley J, Milner R, Marshall AJ, et al. Quadricuspid aortic valves. *Clin Cardiol* 2002;25:548.
74. Hornberger LK, Sanders SP, Rein AJ, et al. Left heart obstructive lesions and left ventricular growth in the midtrimester fetus. A longitudinal study. *Circulation* 1995;92:1531.
75. Tworetzky W, Wilkins-Haug L, Jennings RW, et al. Balloon dilation of severe aortic stenosis in the fetus: Potential for prevention of hypoplastic left heart syndrome: Candidate selection, technique, and results of successful intervention. *Circulation* 2004;110:2125.
76. McKay R, Smith A, Leung MP, et al. Morphology of the ventriculoaortic junction in critical aortic stenosis. Implications for hemodynamic function and clinical management. *J Thorac Cardiovasc Surg* 1992;104(2): 434.
77. Hove JR, Koster RW, Forouhar AS, et al. Intracardiac fluid forces are an essential epigenetic factor for embryonic cardiogenesis. *Nature* 2003;421:172.
78. Ward C. Clinical significance of the bicuspid aortic valve. *Heart* 2000;83:81.
79. Dodds GA III, Warnes CA, Danielson GK. Aortic valve replacement after repair of pulmonary atresia and ventricular septal defect or tetralogy of Fallot. *J Thorac Cardiovasc Surg* 1997;113:736.
80. Niwa K, Siu SC, Webb GD, et al. Progressive aortic root dilatation in adults late after repair of tetralogy of Fallot. *Circulation* 2002;106:1374.
81. Niwa K, Perloff JK, Bhuta SM, et al. Structural abnormalities of great arterial walls in congenital heart disease: Light and electron microscopic analyses. *Circulation* 2001;103:393.
82. Elgamal MA, Hakimi M, Lyons JM, et al. Risk factors for failure of aortic valvuloplasty in aortic insufficiency with ventricular septal defect. *Ann Thorac Surg* 1999; 68:1350.
83. Ishikawa S, Morishita Y, Sato Y, et al. Frequency and operative correction of aortic insufficiency associated with ventricular septal defect. *Ann Thorac Surg* 1994;57:996.
84. Tohyama K, Satomi G, Momma K. Aortic valve prolapse and aortic regurgitation associated with subpulmonic ventricular septal defect. *Am J Cardiol* 1997;79:1285.
85. Formigari R, Toscano A, Giardini A, et al. Prevalence and predictors of neoaortic regurgitation after arterial switch operation for transposition of the great arteries. *J Thorac Cardiovasc Surg* 2003;126:1753.
86. McMahon CJ, Ravekes WJ, Smith EO, et al. Risk factors for neo-aortic root enlargement and aortic regurgitation following arterial switch operation. *Pediatr Cardiol* 2004;25:329.
87. Parry AJ, Kovalchin JP, Suda K, et al. Resection of subaortic stenosis: Can a more aggressive approach be justified? *Eur J Cardiothorac Surg* 1999;15:631.
88. Oliver JM, Gonzalez A, Gallego P, et al. Discrete subaortic stenosis in adults: Increased prevalence and slow rate of progression of the obstruction and aortic regurgitation. *J Am Coll Cardiol* 2001;38:835.

89. Vogt J, Dische R, Rupprath G, et al. Fixed subaortic stenosis: An acquired secondary obstruction? A twenty-seven year experience with 168 patients. *Thorac Cardiovasc Surg* 1989;37:199.
90. Stamm C, Li J, Ho SY, et al. The aortic root in supravalvular aortic stenosis: The potential surgical relevance of morphologic findings. *J Thorac Cardiovasc Surg* 1997; 114:16.
91. McElhinney DB, Petrossian E, Tworetzky W, et al. Issues and outcomes in the management of supravalvar aortic stenosis. *Ann Thorac Surg* 2000;69:562.
92. Sharma BK, Fujiwara H, Hallman GL, et al. Supravalvar aortic stenosis: A 29-year review of surgical experience. *Ann Thorac Surg* 1991;51:1031.
93. Delius RE, Steinberg JB, L'Ecuyer T, et al. Long-term follow-up of extended aortoplasty for supravalvular aortic stenosis. *J Thorac Cardiovasc Surg* 1995;109:155.
94. Hazekamp MG, Kappetein AP, Schoof PH, et al. Brom's three-patch technique for repair of supravalvular aortic stenosis. *J Thorac Cardiovasc Surg* 1999;118:252.
95. Mody MR, Mody GT. Serial hemodynamic observations in congenital valvular and subvalvular aortic stenosis. *Am Heart J* 1975;89:137.
96. Chugh R, Child JS, Perloff JK, et al. Echocardiographic characterization of the aortic root in adults with tetralogy of Fallot. *Circulation* 2001;104:558.
97. d'Udekem Y, Ovaert C, Grandjean F, et al. Tetralogy of Fallot: Transannular and right ventricular patching equally affect late functional status. *Circulation* 2000;102 (19 Suppl 3):III116.
98. Ishizaka T, Ichikawa H, Sawa Y, et al. Prevalence and optimal management strategy for aortic regurgitation in tetralogy of Fallot. *Eur J Cardiothorac Surg* 2004; 26:1080.
99. Eroglu AG, Oztunc F, Saltik L, et al. Evolution of ventricular septal defect with special reference to spontaneous closure rate, subaortic ridge and aortic valve prolapse. *Pediatr Cardiol* 2003;24:31.
100. Sim EK, Grignani RT, Wong ML, et al. Influence of surgery on aortic valve prolapse and aortic regurgitation in doubly committed subarterial ventricular septal defect. *Am J Cardiol* 1999;84:1445.
101. Tomita H, Arakaki Y, Ono Y, et al. Evolution of aortic regurgitation following simple patch closure of doubly committed subarterial ventricular septal defect. *Am J Cardiol* 2000;86:540.
102. van Karnebeek CD, Naeff MS, Mulder BJ, et al. Natural history of cardiovascular manifestations in Marfan syndrome. *Arch Dis Child* 2001;84:129.
103. Zalzstein E, Hamilton R, Zucker N, et al. Aortic dissection in children and young adults: Diagnosis, patients at risk, and outcomes. *Cardiol Young* 2003;13:341.
104. El-said GM, El-Refaee MM, Sorour KA, et al. Rheumatic fever and rheumatic heart disease. In: Garson A, Bricker JT, Fisher DJ, Neish SR (eds). *The Science and Practice of Pediatric Cardiology,* 2d ed. Philadelphia: Williams & Wilkins; 1998:1720.
105. Ferrieri P, Gewitz MH, Gerber MA, et al. Unique features of infective endocarditis in childhood. *Circulation* 2002;105:2115.
106. Perloff JK. Congenital aortic stenosis. Congenital aortic regurgitation. In: Perloff JK (ed). *Clinical Recognition of Congenital Heart Disease,* 5th ed. Philadelphia: Saunders; 2003:81–112.
107. Latson LA. Aortic stenosis: Valvar, supravalvar, and fibromuscular subvalvar. In: Garson A, Bricker JT, Fisher DJ, Neish SR (eds). *The Science and Practice of Pediatric Cardiology,* 2d ed. Philadelphia: Williams & Wilkins; 1998:1257–1276.
108. Moller JH, Nakib A, Eliot RS, et al. Symptomatic congenital aortic stenosis in the first year of life. *J Pediatr* 1966;69:728.
109. Marquis RM, Logan A. Congenital aortic stenosis and its surgical treatment. *Br Heart J* 1955;17:373.
110. Peller OG, Wallerson DC, Devereux RB. Role of Doppler and imaging echocardiography in selection of patients for cardiac valvular surgery. *Am Heart J* 1987;114:1445.
111. Perry GJ, Helmcke F, Nanda NC, et al. Evaluation of aortic insufficiency by Doppler color flow mapping. *J Am Coll Cardiol* 1987;9:952.
112. Tani LY, Minich LL, Day RW, et al. Doppler evaluation of aortic regurgitation in children. *Am J Cardiol* 1997;80:927.
113. Lofland GK, McCrindle BW, Williams WG, et al. Critical aortic stenosis in the neonate: A multi-institutional study of management, outcomes, and risk factors. Congenital Heart Surgeons Society. *J Thorac Cardiovasc Surg* 2001;121:10.
114. Rhodes LA, Colan SD, Perry SB, et al. Predictors of survival in neonates with critical aortic stenosis. *Circulation* 1991;84:2325.
115. Mitchell BM, Strasburger JF, Hubbard JE, et al. Serial exercise performance in children with surgically corrected congenital aortic stenosis. *Pediatr Cardiol* 2003; 24:319.
116. Nishimura RA, Pieroni DR, Bierman FZ, et al. Second natural history study of congenital heart defects. Aortic stenosis: Echocardiography. *Circulation* 1993;87 (2 Suppl):II66.
117. Baram S, McCrindle BW, Han RK, et al. Outcomes of uncomplicated aortic valve stenosis presenting in infants. *Am Heart J* 2003;145:1063.
118. Bonow RO, Carabello B, Edmunds LH Jr, et al. Guidelines for the management of patients with valvular heart disease: Executive summary. A report of the American College of Cardiology/American Heart Association Task Force on Practice Guidelines (Committee on Management of Patients with Valvular Heart Disease). *Circulation* 1998;98:1949.
119. Al Halees Z, Gometza B, Al Sanei A, et al. Repair of moderate aortic valve lesions associated with other pathology: An 11-year follow-up. *Eur J Cardiothorac Surg* 2001;20:247.
120. Mori Y, Nakazawa M, Tomimatsu H, et al. Long-term effect of angiotensin-converting enzyme inhibitor in volume overloaded heart during growth: A controlled pilot study. *J Am Coll Cardiol* 2000;36:270.
121. Bhabra MS, Dhillon R, Bhudia S, et al. Surgical aortic valvotomy in infancy: Impact of leaflet morphology on long-term outcomes. *Ann Thorac Surg* 2003;76:1412.
122. van Son JA, Reddy VM, Black MD, et al. Morphologic determinants favoring surgical aortic valvuloplasty versus pulmonary autograft aortic valve replacement in children. *J Thorac Cardiovasc Surg* 1996;111:1149.

123. Tolan MJ, Daubeney PE, Slavik Z, et al. Aortic valve repair of congenital stenosis with bovine pericardium. *Ann Thorac Surg* 1997;63:465.
124. Duran CM, Gometza B, Shahid M, et al. Treated bovine and autologous pericardium for aortic valve reconstruction. *Ann Thorac Surg* 1998;66(Suppl):S166.
125. Kalangos A, Beghetti M, Baldovinos A, et al. Aortic valve repair by cusp extension with the use of fresh autologous pericardium in children with rheumatic aortic insufficiency. *J Thorac Cardiovasc Surg* 1999;118:225.
126. Carpentier A. Cardiac valve surgery: The "French correction." *J Thorac Cardiovasc Surg* 1983;86:323.
127. Casselman FP, Gillinov AM, Akhrass R, et al. Intermediate-term durability of bicuspid aortic valve repair for prolapsing leaflet. *Eur J Cardiothorac Surg* 1999;15:302.
128. Kalangos A, Beghetti M, Murith N, et al. Leaflet's free edge suspension for correction of aortic insufficiency associated with ventricular septal defect. *Ann Thorac Surg* 1998;65:566.
129. Yacoub MH, Khan H, Stavri G, et al. Anatomic correction of the syndrome of prolapsing right coronary aortic cusp, dilatation of the sinus of Valsalva, and ventricular septal defect. *J Thorac Cardiovasc Surg* 1997;113:253.
130. Bonhoeffer P, Fabbrocini M, Lecompte Y, et al. Infundibular septal defect with severe aortic regurgitation: A new surgical approach. *Ann Thorac Surg* 1992; 53:851.
131. Vricella LA, Williams JA, Ravekes WJ, et al. Early experience with valve-sparing aortic root replacement in children. *Ann Thorac Surg* 2005;80:1622.
132. Alexiou C, McDonald A, Langley SM, et al. Aortic valve replacement in children: Are mechanical prostheses a good option? *Eur J Cardiothorac Surg* 2000;17:125.
133. Manouguian S, Seybold-Epting W. Patch enlargement of the aortic valve ring by extending the aortic incision into the anterior mitral leaflet. New operative technique. *J Thorac Cardiovasc Surg* 1979;78:402.
134. Laudito A, Brook MM, Suleman S, et al. The Ross procedure in children and young adults: A word of caution. *J Thorac Cardiovasc Surg* 2001;122:147.
135. Reddy VM, McElhinney DB, Phoon CK, et al. Geometric mismatch of pulmonary and aortic anuli in children undergoing the Ross procedure: Implications for surgical management and autograft valve function. *J Thorac Cardiovasc Surg* 1998;115:1255.
136. McCrindle BW. Independent predictors of immediate results of percutaneous balloon aortic valvotomy in children. Valvuloplasty and Angioplasty of Congenital Anomalies (VACA) registry investigators. *Am J Cardiol* 1996;77:286.
137. Alexiou C, Langley SM, Dalrymple-Hay MJ, et al. Open commissurotomy for critical isolated aortic stenosis in neonates. *Ann Thorac Surg* 2001;71:489.
138. Gildein HP, Kleinert S, Weintraub RG, et al. Surgical commissurotomy of the aortic valve: Outcome of open valvotomy in neonates with critical aortic stenosis. *Am Heart J* 1996;131:754.
139. Hawkins JA, Minich LL, Tani LY, et al. Late results and reintervention after aortic valvotomy for critical aortic stenosis in neonates and infants. *Ann Thorac Surg* 1998;65:1758.
140. McCrindle BW, Blackstone EH, Williams WG, et al. Are outcomes of surgical versus transcatheter balloon valvotomy equivalent in neonatal critical aortic stenosis? *Circulation* 2001;104(12 Suppl 1):I152.
141. Justo RN, McCrindle BW, Benson LN, et al. Aortic valve regurgitation after surgical versus percutaneous balloon valvotomy for congenital aortic valve stenosis. *Am J Cardiol* 1996;77:1332.
142. Reich O, Tax P, Marek J, et al. Long term results of percutaneous balloon valvoplasty of congenital aortic stenosis: Independent predictors of outcome. *Heart* 2004;90:70.
143. Rao V, Van Arsdell GS, David TE, et al. Aortic valve repair for adult congenital heart disease: A 22-year experience. *Circulation* 2000;102(19 Suppl 3):III40.
144. Schenk MH, Vaugn WK, Reul GJ, O'Lauglin MP. Long-term follow-up in children and adolescents with left-sided artificial valves. *J Am Coll Cardiol* 1993;21(2):81A.
145. Avila WS, Rossi EG, Grinberg M, et al. Influence of pregnancy after bioprosthetic valve replacement in young women: A prospective five-year study. *J Heart Valve Dis* 2002;11:864.
146. Champsaur G, Robin J, Tronc F, et al. Mechanical valve in aortic position is a valid option in children and adolescents. *Eur J Cardiothorac Surg* 1997;11:117.
147. Vosa C, Renzulli A, Lombardi PF, et al. Mechanical valve replacement under 12 years of age: 15 years of experience. *J Heart Valve Dis* 1995;4:279.
148. Tait RC, Ladusans EJ, El Metaal M, et al. Oral anticoagulation in paediatric patients: Dose requirements and complications. *Arch Dis Child* 1996;74:228.
149. Fiane AE, Lindberg HL, Saatvedt K, et al. Mechanical valve replacement in congenital heart disease. *J Heart Valve Dis* 1996;5:337.
150. Cabalka AK, Emery RW, Petersen RJ, et al. Long-term follow-up of the St. Jude Medical prosthesis in pediatric patients. *Ann Thorac Surg* 1995;60:(Suppl):S618-S623.
151. Lupinetti FM, Duncan BW, Scifres AM, et al. Intermediate-term results in pediatric aortic valve replacement. *Ann Thorac Surg* 1999;68:521.
152. Lund O, Chandrasekaran V, Grocott-Mason R, et al. Primary aortic valve replacement with allografts over twenty-five years: Valve-related and procedure-related determinants of outcome. *J Thorac Cardiovasc Surg* 1999;117:77.
153. Clarke DR, Campbell DN, Hayward AR, et al. Degeneration of aortic valve allografts in young recipients. *J Thorac Cardiovasc Surg* 1993;105:934.
154. Al Halees Z, Pieters F, Qadoura F, et al. The Ross procedure is the procedure of choice for congenital aortic valve disease. *J Thorac Cardiovasc Surg* 2002;123:437.
155. Elkins RC, Knott-Craig CJ, Ward KE. Pulmonary autograft in children: Realized growth potential. *Ann Thorac Surg* 1994;57:1387.
156. Elkins RC, Knott-Craig CJ, Ward KE, et al. The Ross operation in children: 10-year experience. *Ann Thorac Surg* 1998;65:496.
157. Hraska V, Krajci M, Haun C, et al. Ross and Ross-Konno procedure in children and adolescents: Mid-term results. *Eur J Cardiothorac Surg* 2004;25:742.
158. Pieters FA, Al Halees Z, Hatle L, et al. Results of the Ross operation in rheumatic versus non-rheumatic aortic valve disease. *J Heart Valve Dis* 2000;9:38.

159. Schoof PH, Gittenberger-De Groot AC, et al. Remodeling of the porcine pulmonary autograft wall in the aortic position. *J Thorac Cardiovasc Surg* 2000;120:55.
160. Turrentine MW, Ruzmetov M, Vijay P, et al. Biological versus mechanical aortic valve replacement in children. *Ann Thorac Surg* 2001;71(5 Suppl):S356.
161. Oury JH, Hiro SP, Maxwell JM, et al. The Ross procedure: Current registry results. *Ann Thorac Surg* 1998;66(6 Suppl):S162.
162. Al Halees Z, Kumar N, Gallo R, et al. Pulmonary autograft for aortic valve replacement in rheumatic disease: A caveat. *Ann Thorac Surg* 1995;60(2 Suppl):S172.
163. Choudhary SK, Mathur A, Sharma R, et al.. Pulmonary autograft: Should it be used in young patients with rheumatic disease? *J Thorac Cardiovasc Surg* 1999;118:483.
164. Kouchoukos NT, Masetti P, Nickerson NJ, et al. The Ross procedure: Long-term clinical and echocardiographic follow-up. *Ann Thorac Surg* 2004;78:773.
165. Solowiejczyk DE, Bourlon F, Apfel HD, et al. Serial echocardiographic measurements of the pulmonary autograft in the aortic valve position after the Ross operation in a pediatric population using normal pulmonary artery dimensions as the reference standard. *Am J Cardiol* 2000;85:1119.

CHAPTER

74 CONGENITAL ANOMALIES OF THE CORONARY ARTERIES

Farzaneh Banki, Christopher T. Salerno, Gordon A. Cohen

Congenital coronary anomalies are defined as any coronary pattern with a feature (origin, course, or termination) rarely encountered in the general population. According to the literature, coronary anomalies are observed in 1 percent of the general population; these prevalence data are derived from cineangiograms performed for suspected obstructive coronary artery disease.[1] Autopsy series have revealed even a lower incidence of 0.3 percent.[2]

Coronary arterial anomalies vary widely in clinical relevance, from those that limit survival to those that are of concern only because of potential injury during cardiac surgery. Coronary anomalies have been implicated in chest pain, sudden death, cardiomyopathy, syncope, dyspnea, ventricular fibrillation, and myocardial infarction.[3] Sudden death can unfortunately often be the initial mode of presentation of a coronary artery anomaly. Van Camp and coworkers reported that coronary anomalies are found in association with 11.8 percent of sudden deaths in U.S. high school and college athletes.[4] According to the Sudden Death Committee of the American Heart Association,[5] coronary anomalies cause 19 percent of deaths in athletes. These anomalies are not all life-threatening. Rigatelli[6] has described a classification of coronary artery anomalies based on their clinical significance. Class I (benign coronary artery anomalies) includes those abnormal patterns that are clinically silent and not related to myocardial ischemia or sudden death (anomalous origin of a coronary artery from the aorta or anomalous origin of the left circumflex coronary from the right coronary artery). Class II comprises anomalies that are associated with myocardial ischemia, such as left coronary artery from the pulmonary artery and coronary artery fistula draining to the right heart, resulting in right heart volume overload. Class III includes those anomalies of the coronary circulation associated with sudden death, such as a true single coronary artery that supports the entire coronary circulation, originates from a normal left coronary artery, and usually courses between the pulmonary artery and aorta. Class IV includes coronary anomalies associated with superimposed coronary artery disease.

In this chapter we describe these anomalies according to (1) origin, (2) course, and (3) termination.

ANOMALOUS ORIGIN OF THE CORONARY ARTERIES

Coronary arteries of anomalous origin arise most commonly from the pulmonary artery or the aorta. In rare instances, coronary arteries can originate from aortic branches such as the carotid and brachiocephalic arteries.[7]

Origin from the pulmonary artery

The right, left main, circumflex, or both coronary arteries may arise from the pulmonary artery; the origin of the left coronary artery from the pulmonary artery is the most common anomaly in this subgroup and was first described by Brooks in 1885.[8]

The different origins of the coronary arteries from the pulmonary artery are described in Table 74-1.

Anomalous origin of the coronary artery from the pulmonary artery (ALCAPA) is compatible with life in utero owing to high prenatal pulmonary pressure and consequent forward flow in the anomalous left coronary artery. As pulmonary vascular resistance decreases in the first 3 months after birth, flow reversal in the anomalous coronary artery resulting in ischemia and the development of collateralization will ensue. This change in pulmonary vascular resistance results, in "coronary steal" of blood toward the low-pressure pulmonary artery.[9] This pathophysiologic sequence may result in ischemia,

Table 74-1 Anomalous coronary arterial pattern: origin from the pulmonary artery

LCA arising from the posterior–facing sinus (ALCAPA)
CX arising from the posterior–facing sinus
LAD arising from the posterior–facing sinusRCA arising from the anterior right–facing sinus (ARCAPA)
Ectopic location (outside–facing sinuses) of any coronary artery from the pulmonary artery
From the anterior left sinus
From the pulmonary trunk
From the pulmonary branch

ALCAPA = anomalous left coronary artery from pulmonary artery; CX = circumflex; LAD = left anterior descending; LCA = left coronary artery; RCA = right coronary artery.

infarction, or mitral insufficiency. The infant may present with dyspnea, profuse sweating, pallor, and fatigue induced by feeding and crying; between these acute events, the physical exam may be normal.[10] This anomaly can be diagnosed by echocardiography or cardiac catheterization. Visualization of the anomalous left coronary artery arising from the pulmonary artery and the demonstration of retrograde flow through collaterals from the dilated coronary artery into the pulmonary trunk is characteristic.[11,12] The right coronary artery (RCA) originating from the aorta is enlarged, and the left coronary artery fills in a retrograde fashion. The ventriculogram characteristically discloses hypokinesis of the anterior wall.

If untreated, the mortality due to this condition is reported to be as high as 80 percent in the first year of life[13]; prompt operation after diagnosis is therefore recommended. Establishment of a dual coronary system is the goal of surgical intervention. Reimplantation of the anomalous left coronary artery into the aorta has been described by Laks and coworkers.[14] During this procedure, the aorta and pulmonary artery are both incised and the left coronary artery and a surrounding cuff of pulmonary arterial wall are excised as a button and transferred to the aorta (Fig. 74-1). The defect in the pulmonary artery is reconstructed with a pericardial patch, and the coronary artery anastomosis is performed with a technique similar to that described for the arterial switch operation in neonates with transposition of the great arteries (Chap. 66). If the coronary artery is too short to reach the aorta, the pulmonary artery can be divided and an intrapulmonary baffle (Takeuchi procedure) or elongation with an autologous pericardial tube can be performed.[15]

The origin of the right coronary from the pulmonary artery is rare[16] and is better tolerated due to the lower right ventricular pressure, which allows easier flow from the pulmonary artery to the myocardium. This condition nevertheless requires prompt surgical repair because of the inherent risk of cardiac arrest and sudden death. The operation of choice is direct implantation of the RCA into the aorta with a technique similar to that described for the ALCAPA.

Separate anomalous origin of the circumflex coronary artery from the pulmonary artery most often occurs in association with other cardiac defects and is therefore usually repaired with a reimplantation technique when the dominant malformation is corrected or palliated.[17]

Origin from the aorta

Origin of a coronary artery from an abnormal site within the aortic root accounts for about one-third of all coronary arterial anomalies (Table 74-2). Each of the three coronary arteries may arise from the wrong aortic sinus of Valsalva or from an excessively high or low position on the appropriate sinus, with resultant anatomic distortion of the arterial ostium. The most common anomalous origin of a coronary artery from the aorta involves the circumflex coronary artery originating from the right sinus of Valsalva or the proximal portion of the RCA; the circumflex coronary artery then courses posterior to the aorta to reach its normal location.[18] This anomaly is of no clinical significance, although the abnormal coronary artery may be at risk for extrinsic compression during aortic or mitral valve replacement.[19]

The next most common anomaly involving abnormal origin from the aorta is that in which the RCA originates from the left sinus of Valsalva, a variant of the single coronary artery. In this situation, the anomalous RCA usually runs between the aorta and the pulmonary artery (Fig. 74-2).[20] Although coronary filling occurs during diastole, compression between the great vessels with or without an associated "slit-like" appearance of the coronary ostium has been postulated as potential mechanism for ischemia.

A true single coronary artery is very rare, with an incidence of 0.04 percent. There is usually a single aortic ostium and, although there has been a single report of sudden death in an infant,[21] its clinical relevance in adults is unknown. This particular anomaly tends to be associated with complex congenital heart disease and is therefore typically detected long before adulthood.[22] Smith and coworkers[23] classified cases of single coronary artery

Table 74-2 Anomalous coronary arterial pattern: origin from the aorta

1. Anomalous left circumflex coronary artery
2. Single coronary artery
a. One artery supplies the entire heart
b. A single coronary divides into two branches
3. Left main coronary artery from the right sinus of Valsalva
4. Right coronary artery originating from left sinus of Valsalva
5. Anomalous left anterior descending artery
6. Fusion of aortic cusp to aortic wall
7. Congenital atresia of the left coronary ostium

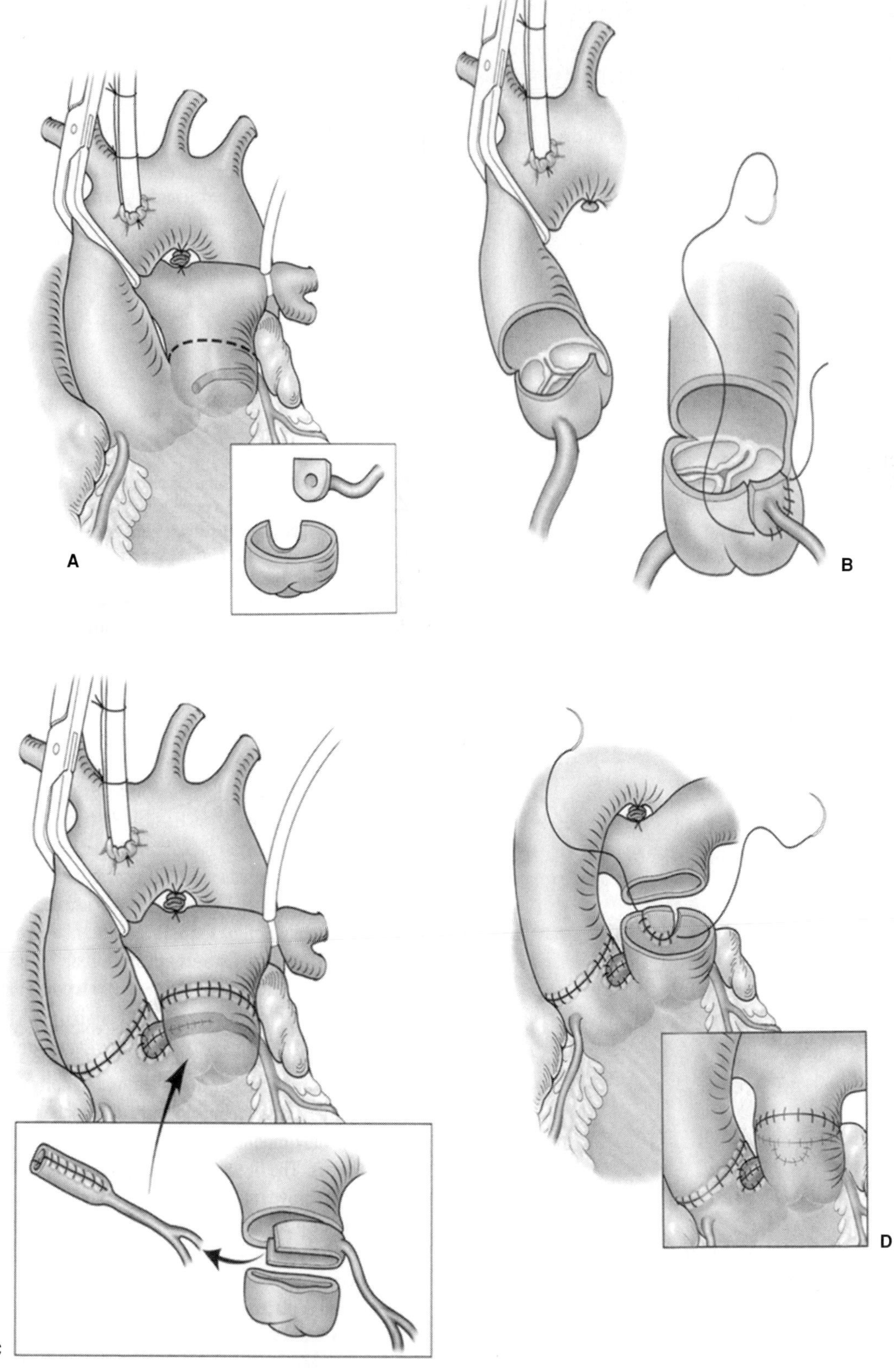

Figure 74-1 Surgical correction of anomalous left coronary artery originating from pulmonary artery (ALCAPA). The coronary button is excised from its origin in the pulmonary artery and transferred as a button to the aortic root. (From Gaynor JW. Coronary anomalies. In: Gardner TJ, Spray TL (eds.). *Operative cardiac surgery,* 5th ed. New York: Arnold, 2004.

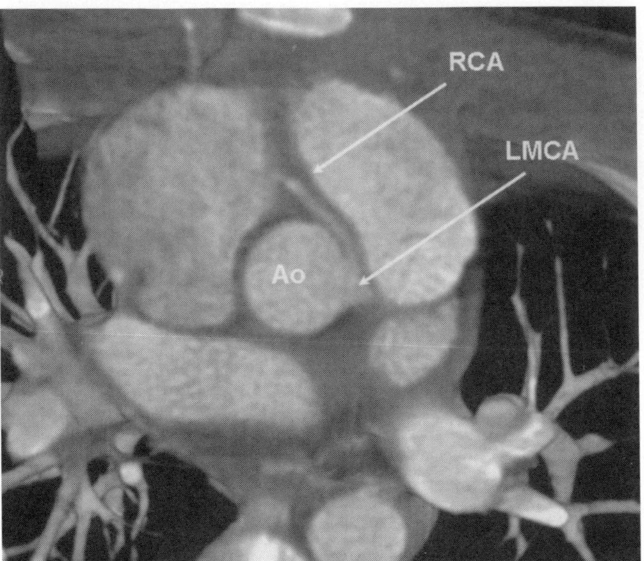

Figure 74-2 Computed tomography of the chest illustrating the anomalous origin of the right coronary artery (RCA) from the left coronary sinus. Note the length of the intramural course of the abnormally originating vessel. Ao = aorta; LMCA = left main coronary artery. The intraoperative findings are shown in Fig. 74-4. (Courtesy of Duke Cameron, MD, Division of Cardiac Surgery, the Johns Hopkins Hospital.)

into those in which there is only one artery supplying the entire heart (type I), those in which the single coronary artery divides into two branches with normal distribution (type II), and those in which the criteria that define type I and II are not met.

Of all possible anomalous origins of a coronary artery from the aorta, the one that is most clearly associated with the risk of sudden death is the origin of the left main coronary artery from the right sinus of Valsalva. Once the left main coronary artery arises from this location, it may course to its normal area of distribution[18] posterior to the aorta,[24] anterior to the right ventricular outflow tract,[10] within the interventricular septum beneath the right ventricular infundibulum, or between the aorta and right ventricular outflow tract.[25] The coursing of the anomalous left coronary artery between the great vessels is associated with sudden cardiac death, which often occurs during or immediately after strenuous physical activity.[26] Diagnostic evaluation includes echocardiography, electrocardiography, and stress testing. Although coronary arteriography is usually indicated prior to surgical intervention, high-resolution computed tomography has a high yield in identifying the course of the aberrant coronary as well as the extent of the intramural course of the vessel and its ostial anatomy (see Fig. 74-2).

For the two above-mentioned coronary anomalies (left main coronary artery from the right sinus and RCA from the left sinus of Valsalva), surgical treatment is recommended.[27] Although intervention is advised by most authors, the optimal technique largely depends on the individual patient's anatomy (extent of the intramural course, morphology of the coronary ostium, age of the patient, and concomitant coronary artery disease, among others). Successful coronary reimplantation has been reported for the treatment of anomalous origin of the RCA from the left sinus of Valsalva.[28] Unroofing of the intramural course of the coronary artery into the appropriate sinus has also been described (Figs. 74-3 and 74-4).[29] The addition of a coronary artery bypass graft has been utilized in older patients, but such an optional safety measure carries the unresolved question of long-term patency of the graft in the setting of unobstructed competitive flow from the unroofed or relocated native coronary.

An anomalous left anterior descending artery from the RCA or sinus of Valsalva is relatively rare and, in the absence of congenital heart disease (most often conotruncal anomalies), is of no clinical significance.[30]

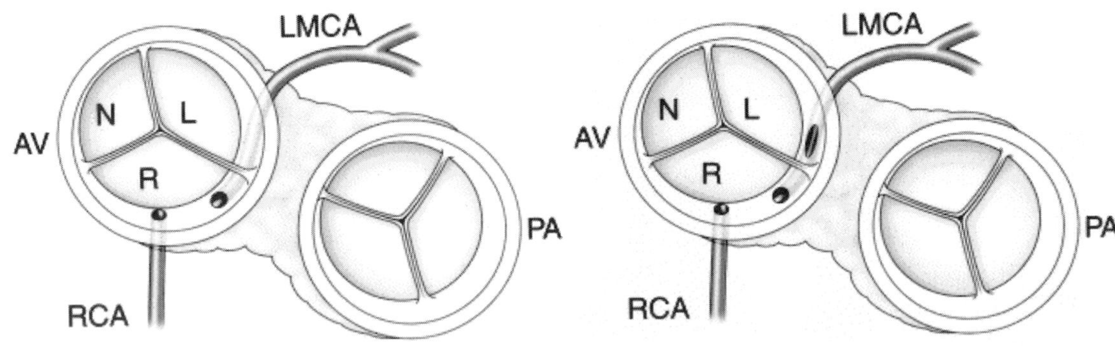

Figure 74-3 Simplified technique for correction of anomalous origin of the left coronary artery from the right coronary sinus (left). The intramural course is unroofed in the left coronary sinus, effectively creating a double-inlet coronary system (right). (From Karamichalis et al.[29] With permission.)

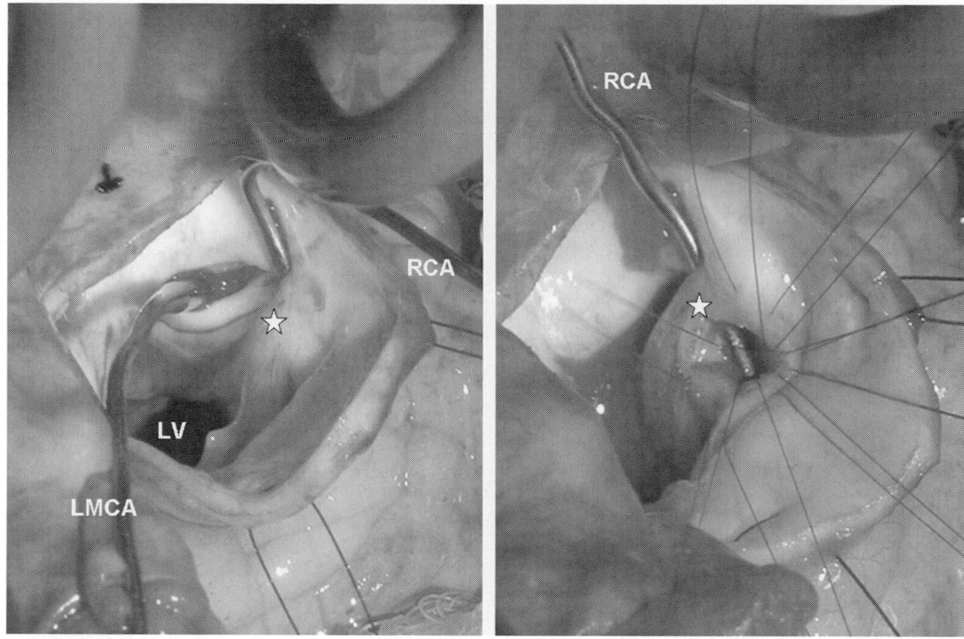

Figure 74-4 Intraoperative photograph of coronary artery unroofing. Left: two coronary probes are utilized to assess ostial anatomy and the proximal course of the coronary arteries. The commissural post between the left and right coronary sinuses is marked with an asterisk. The ostium of the left main coronary artery (LMCA) is separate from that of the right coronary artery (RCA). The RCA courses intramurally between aortic and pulmonary roots. Right: The intramural course of the right coronary originating from the left coronary sinus is unroofed, creating a wide accessory ostium into the right coronary sinus. LV = left ventricle. (Courtesy of Duke Cameron, M.D., Division of Cardiac Surgery, the Johns Hopkins Hospital.)

Ostial obstruction of the left main coronary artery can also be secondary to anomalous left aortic cusp, fusion of the left aortic cusp with the aortic wall,[31] or congenital atresia of the left coronary ostium.[32] Coronary stenosis or atresia may occur as an isolated anomaly; more commonly, however, it occurs in the setting of other congenital lesions, including supravalvular aortic stenosis and pulmonary atresia with intact ventricular septum.[27]

ANOMALOUS COURSE OF THE CORONARY ARTERIES

As mentioned above, these anomalies are commonly associated with an aberrant origin of the coronary arteries, which can be categorized according to the anatomic relationship of the vessel to the aorta and the pulmonary trunk during its course. The aberrant origin of the left main coronary artery or the anterior descending coronary artery from the right sinus of Valsalva can be classified into four different subtypes based on their course: posterior, interarterial, anterior, and septal. In the posterior or retroaortic subtype, the main coronary artery is placed posterior and inferior to the aortic root. In the interarterial or preaortic course, the left main coronary artery courses between the ascending aorta and the pulmonary trunk. In the anterior or prepulmonic course, the left anterior descending artery is anterior to the right ventricular outflow tract. In the septal or subpulmonic variant, the left anterior coronary artery takes an intramyocardial course through the interventricular septum beneath the right ventricular infundibulum.[33]

One of the most common variants of the anomalous course of coronary arteries is the "mural" coronary.[34] In this anatomic variant, a coronary vessel is covered by a bridge of myocardium and is often difficult to visualize. The mural coronary may be constricted by the myocardial bridge during systole; in rare cases, this has been hypothesized as the underlying structural abnormality in cases of ischemia and sudden death.[35]

Last, anomalous course of the RCA in the right atrial wall encountered during coronary artery bypass surgery has been reported.[35]

ANOMALOUS TERMINATION OF THE CORONARY ARTERIES

With regard to anomalous coronary artery termination, coronary arteries may communicate with venae cavae, cardiac chambers, the pulmonary artery and veins, and the coronary sinus.

Patients will typically present with exertional angina, palpitations, and congestive heart failure. These symptoms have been reported in up to 73 percent of patients with anomalies of coronary termination.[37] As a consequence of right-to-left shunting in more severe cases, up to 50 percent of patients disclose cardiomegaly or increased pulmonary vasculature on chest x-ray.[38] Diagnosis is made with echocardiography and cardiac catheterization. A left-to-right shunt (Qp:Qs) of as high 1.6:1 has been reported, with no correlation between shunt magnitude and clinical signs or symptoms.[39]

A coronary arteriovenous fistula is the commonest clinically significant congenital coronary termination abnormality, accounting for approximately 50 percent of all coronary anomalies.[40] Arteriovenous coronary fistulas are present in 1 of 50,000 live births (0.002 percent of the general population) and are found incidentally in approximately 0.2 to 0.25 percent of patients undergoing cardiac catheterization.[37,41] Fistulas are isolated in 55 to 80 percent of patients and associated with other congenital heart defects in 20 to 40 percent of cases.[42]

It is generally recommended that all diagnosed major coronary arteriovenous fistulas be treated as soon as the diagnosis is made owing to increase mortality and morbidity with age.[37,39] Direct ligation has been the most common technique (Fig. 74-5).[38] Recently, endovascular therapy with percutaneous fistulous obliteration has been successfully employed (Fig. 74-6).[43]

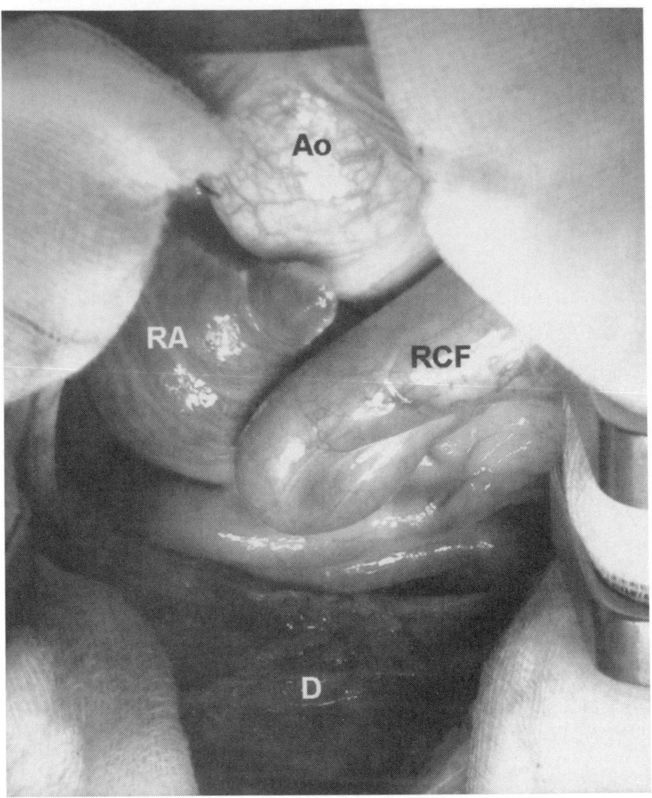

Figure 74-5 Intraoperative photograph of giant right coronary artery arteriovenous fistula. The fistulous tract was ligated distally before entrance in the right atrium. Ao = aorta; D = diaphragm; RA = right atrium; RCF = right coronary fistula. (Courtesy of Mr. Victor Tsang and Sir Magdi Yacoub, Cardiac Unit, Great Ormond Street Hospital for Children NHS Trust, London.)

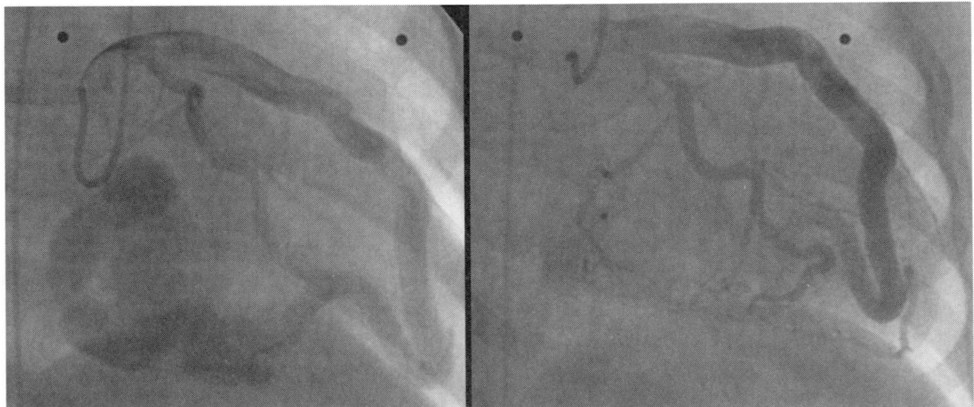

Figure 74-6 Endovascular approach to large right coronary artery arteriovenous fistula (left). The fistulous tract was occluded percutaneously (right). (Courtesy of Richard Ringel, M.D., Division of Pediatric Cardiology, the Johns Hopkins Hospital.)

References

1. Baltaxe HA, Wixon D. The incidence of congenital anomalies of coronary arteries in adult population. *Radiology* 1977;122:47.
2. Click RL, Holmes DR, Vliestra RE, et al. Anomalous coronary arteries: Location, degree of atherosclerosis and effect on survival: Report from the Coronary Artery Surgery Study. *J Am Coll Cardiol* 1989;13:531.
3. Angelini P. Normal and anomalous coronary arteries in humans. In: *Coronary Artery Anomalies: A Comprehensive Approach*. Philadelphia: Lippincott Williams & Wilkins, 1999:27-150.
4. Van Camp SP, Bloor CM, Mueller FO, et al. Nontraumatic sports death in high school and college athletes. *Med Sci Sports Excerc* 1995;27:641.
5. Maron BJ, Thompson PD, Puffer JC, et al. Cardiovascular preparticipation screening of competitive athletes. A statement for health professionals from the Sudden Death Committee (clinical cardiology) and Congenital Cardiac Defects Committee (cardiovascular disease in the young), American Heart Association. *Circulation* 1998;94:850.
6. Rigatelli G. Coronary artery anomalies: What we know and what we have to learn. A proposal for a new clinical classification. *Ital Heart J* 2003;4:305.
7. Davis JS, Lie JT. Anomalous origin of a single coronary artery from the innominate artery. *Angiology* 1977;28:775.
8. Brooks H. Two cases of an abnormal coronary artery of the heart arising from the pulmonary artery. *J Anat Physiol* 1985;20:26.
9. Wright NL, Baue AE, Baum S, et al. Coronary artery steal due to an anomalous left coronary artery originating from the pulmonary artery. *J Thorac Cardiovas Surg* 1970;59:461.
10. Bland EF, Garland J. Congenital anomalies of the coronary arteries: Report of an unusual case associated with cardiac hypertrophy. *Am Heart J* 1933;8:787.
11. Chu E, Cheitlin MD. Diagnostic considerations in patients with suspected coronary artery anomalies. *Am Heart J* 1933;126:1427.
12. Jureidini SB, Nouri S. Reliability of echocardiography in the diagnosis of anomalous origin of the left coronary artery from the pulmonary trunk. *Am Heart J* 1991; 22:61.
13. Wesselhoeft H, Fawcett JS, Johnson AL. Anomalous origin of the left coronary artery from the pulmonary trunk. Its clinical spectrum, pathology, and pathophysiology, based on reviews on 140 cases with seven further cases. *Circulation* 1968;38:403.
14. Laks H, Ardehali A, Grant P, et al. Aortic implantation of anomalous left coronary artery. An improved surgical approach. *J Thorac Cardiovasc Surg* 1995;109: 519.
15. Sese A, Imoto Y. New technique in the transfer of an anomalously originated left coronary artery to the aorta. *Ann Thorac Surg* 1992;53(3):527.
16. Vairo U, Marino B, De Simone G, et al. Early congestive heart failure due to origin of the right coronary artery from the pulmonary artery. *Chest* 1992;102:1610.
17. Alexi-Meskishvili VV, Potapov EV, Hetzer R, et al. Origin of the circumflex coronary artery from the pulmonary artery in infants. *Ann Thorac Surg* 1998; 66:1406.
18. Liberthson RR, Dinsmore RE, Bhatri S, et al. Aberrant coronary artery origin from the aorta: Diagnosis and clinical significance. *Circulation* 1974;50:774.
19. Roberts WC, Morrow AG. Compression of anomalous left circumflex coronary arteries by prosthetic valve fixation rings. *J Thorac Cardiovasc Surg* 1969;57:834.
20. Danias PG, Stuber M, McConnell MV, et al. The diagnosis of congenital coronary anomalies with magnetic resonance imaging. *Coron Artery Dis* 2001;12:621.
21. Moore L, Byard RW. Sudden and unexpected death in infancy associated with a single coronary artery. *Pediatr Pathol* 1992;12:231.
22. Sharbaugh AH, White S. Single coronary artery. Analysis of the anatomic variation, clinical importance, and report of five cases. *JAMA* 1974;230:243.
23. Smith JC. Review of single coronary artery with report of 2 cases. *Circulation* 1950;1:1168.
24. Kardos A, Babai L, Rudas L, et al. Epidemiology of congenital coronary artery anomalies: A coronary arteriography study on a central European population. *Cathet Cardiovasc Diagn* 1997;42:270.
25. Sabiston DC, Floyd WL, McIntosh HD. Anomalous origin of the left coronary artery from the pulmonary artery in adults. Surgical management. *Arch Surg* 1968;97:963.
26. Frescura C, Basso C, Thiene G, et al. Anomalous origin of coronary arteries and risk of sudden death: A study based on an autopsy population of congenital heart disease. *Hum Pathol* 1998;29:689.
27. Walker F, Webb G. Congenital coronary artery anomalies: The adult perspective. *Coron Artery Dis* 2001;12:599.
28. Di Lello F, Mnuck JF, Flemma RJ, et al. Successful coronary reimplantation for anomalous origin of the right coronary artery from the left sinus of Valsalva. *J Thorac Cardiovasc Surg* 1991;102:455.
29. Karamichalis JM, Vricella LA, Murphy DJ, et al. Simplified technique for correction of anomalous origin of left coronary artery from the anterior aortic sinus. *Ann Thorac Surg* 2003;76:266.
30. Kimbiris D, Iskandrian AS, Segal BL, et al. Anomalous aortic origin of coronary arteries. *Circulation* 1978; 58:606.
31. Line DE, Babb JD, Pierce WS. Congenital aortic valve anomaly. Aortic regurgitation with left coronary artery isolation. *J Thorac Cardiovasc Surg* 1979;77:533.
32. Mullins CE, el-Said G, McNamara DG, et al. Atresia of the left coronary artery ostium. Repair by saphenous vein graft. *Circulation* 1972;46:989.
33. Ropers D, Gehling G, Pohle K, et al. Images in cardiovascular medicine. Anomalous course of the left main or left anterior descending coronary artery originating from the right sinus of Valsalva: Identification of four common variations by electron beam tomography. *Circulation* 2002; 105:42.
34. Geiringer E. The mural coronary. *Am Heart J* 1951;41: 359.
35. Cheitlin MD. The intramural coronary artery: Another cause for sudden death with exercise? *Circulation* 1980; 62:238.
36. Jalal A, Shackcloth M, Dihmis WC. Anomalous course of the right coronary artery in the right atrial wall: A word of caution. *Heart Surg Forum* 2002;5:300.

37. Fernandes ED, Kadivar H, Hallman GL, et al. Congenital malformations of the coronary arteries: The Texas Heart Institute experience. *Ann Thorac Surg* 1992;54: 732.
38. Rittenhouse EA, Doty DB, Ehrenhaft JL. Congenital coronary artery–Cardiac chamber fistula. Review of operative management. *Ann Thorac Surg* 1975;20:468.
39. Liberthson RR, Sagar K, Berkoben JP, et al. Congenital coronary arteriovenous fistula. Report of 13 patients, review of the literature and delineation of management. *Circulation* 1979;59:849.
40. Mavroudis C, Backer CL, Rocchini AP, et al. Coronary artery fistulas in infants and children: A surgical review and discussion of coil embolization. *Ann Thorac Surg* 1997; 63:1235.
41. Urrutia-S CO, Falaschi G, Ott DA, et al. Surgical management of 56 patients with congenital coronary artery fistulas. *Ann Thorac Surg* 1983;35:300.
42. Tkebuchava T, Von Segesser LK, Vogt P, et al. Congenital coronary fistulas in children and adults: Diagnosis, surgical technique and results. *J Cardiovasc Surg (Torino)* 1996; 37:29.
43. McElhinney DB, Burch GH, Kung GC, et al. Echocardiographic guidance for transcatheter coil embolization of congenital coronary arterial fistulas in children. *Pediatr Cardiol* 2000;21:253.

CHAPTER

75 VASCULAR RINGS AND PULMONARY ARTERY SLING

Ronald K. Woods, Dale G. Hall

DEFINITION AND HISTORY

The defining feature of the anomalies discussed in this chapter is an abnormality of the ascending aorta, arch, great vessels, descending aorta, or pulmonary artery that causes, to varying degrees, compression of the trachea, esophagus, or both. A complete ring of vascular tissue may or may not be present; nonetheless, the term *ring* is the accepted generic term for these anomalies. The term *sling*, however, is used to refer specifically to a particular anomaly of the pulmonary artery. The Society of Thoracic Surgeons Nomenclature and Data Base Committee has recommended categorization as complete vascular rings (double aortic arch, right arch with

KEY CONCEPTS

- Epidemiology
  - Vascular rings and pulmonary artery sling represent 1 to 3 percent of all congenital cardiac malformations. The most frequent type of vascular ring is aberrant left subclavian artery, whereas the most rare condition is the pulmonary artery sling.
- Morphology
  - Of the over 100 variations in morphology that have been described, 6 are most commonly observed: (1) anomalous left subclavian artery with left aortic arch, (2) double aortic arch, (3) right aortic arch with left ligamentum, (4) right aortic arch with aberrant left subclavian artery, (5) tracheal compression by the innominate artery, and (6) pulmonary artery sling. Cardiac malformations (tetralogy of Fallot, ventricular septal defect, atrial septal defect, and aortic coarctation) are seen in 15 to 20 percent of cases.
- Pathophysiology
  - Structural obstruction of the aerodigestive tract.
- Clinical features
  - Most vascular rings are symptomatic. Compression by the complete or partial ring of the esophagus, trachea, or both dictates the mode of presentation. Patients with an aberrant left subclavian artery are often asymptomatic, whereas pulmonary slings and complete rings are almost uniformly clinically significant.
- Diagnosis
  - Chest x-ray is rarely diagnostic. Barium esophagography is usually able to point to the presence of a vascular ring with reasonable specificity. Computed tomography and magnetic resonance imaging are useful in defining the anatomy and are currently more routinely utilized. Bronchoscopy is important in the diagnosis of both innominate artery compression and pulmonary artery sling and in assessing the degree of tracheobronchomalacia.
- Treatment
  - Treatment is indicated in all symptomatic patients. With the exception of double aortic arch with dominant left component, almost all cases (left aortic arch with right ligamentum, pulmonary artery sling, and innominate artery compression) are approached through a left thoracotomy with division of the vascular ring.
- Outcomes
  - For the vast majority of vascular rings, morbidity and mortality are the same as seen in any simple thoracic procedure involving a thoracotomy. Mortality is much higher for patients with pulmonary artery sling. The degree of tracheobronchomalacia has a significant impact on long-term prognosis.

left ligamentum) and partial vascular rings (pulmonary artery sling, innominate artery compression, aberrant subclavian artery).[1] Although over 100 unique vascular morphologies have been described, only 6 specific anomalies are discussed in this chapter, as they comprise the vast majority of clinically relevant cases. These include aberrant right subclavian artery (ARSA), double aortic arch (DAA), right arch with left ligamentum and/or aberrant left subclavian artery, and Kommerell's diverticulum (RA, ALSA, RALL), innominate artery compression (IAC) of the trachea, and pulmonary artery sling (PAS).

The first description of a vascular ring is probably that of an aberrant right subclavian artery by Hunauld in 1735, reporting an autopsy finding.[2] The term *dysphagia lusoria,* meaning "sport of nature" and referring to the swallowing symptoms, was coined by Bayford in 1794.[3] Hommel provided the first description of double aortic arch in 1737.[4] The first description of pulmonary artery sling was reported much later, in 1897, by Glaevecke.[5] Gross performed the first repairs of vascular rings: double arch in 1945[6] and aberrant right subclavian artery in 1946.[7] In 1954, Potts reported the first repair of pulmonary artery sling.[8]

EPIDEMIOLOGY

Because not all vascular rings are symptomatic, the true prevalence of this group of anomalies is not accurately known. Various estimates include 0.04 to 0.5 percent of live births and approximately 1 to 3 percent of surgical congenital cardiovascular malformations.[9] The most common anomaly is ARSA, with a prevalence estimated at 0.5 percent. Of the types discussed in this chapter, PAS is the least common. For example, two large centers have reported surgical series of 16 patients in 13 years[10] and 18 patients in 23 years.[11] There is no known ethnic, sexual, or geographic disposition.

EMBRYOLOGY AND PATHOGENESIS

The *anlage* consists of an aortic sac and paired ventral and dorsal aortas connected at various stages of development by branchial arch vessels (Fig. 75-1). Formation and selective regression of these components at various stages of embryologic development lead to what is considered a normal arrangement (see Chap. 51). For example, branchial arches 1 and 2 typically regress (do contribute to arteries of the face and stapedial artery). Arch 3 gives rise to the internal carotid arteries. Arch 4 on the right becomes the right subclavian artery up to the takeoff of the internal thoracic artery. On the left, arch 4 contributes to the aortic arch from the left common carotid to the isthmus (region near the ductus arteriosus). Arch 5 regresses bilaterally. It is believed that arch 6 regresses on the right and contributes to the ductus on the left. A more recent contention is that the dorsal aorta contributes most to formation of the main pulmonary artery, not arch 6, as previously believed.[12] The seventh intersegmental arteries contribute to formation of the subclavian arteries bilaterally. The impact of

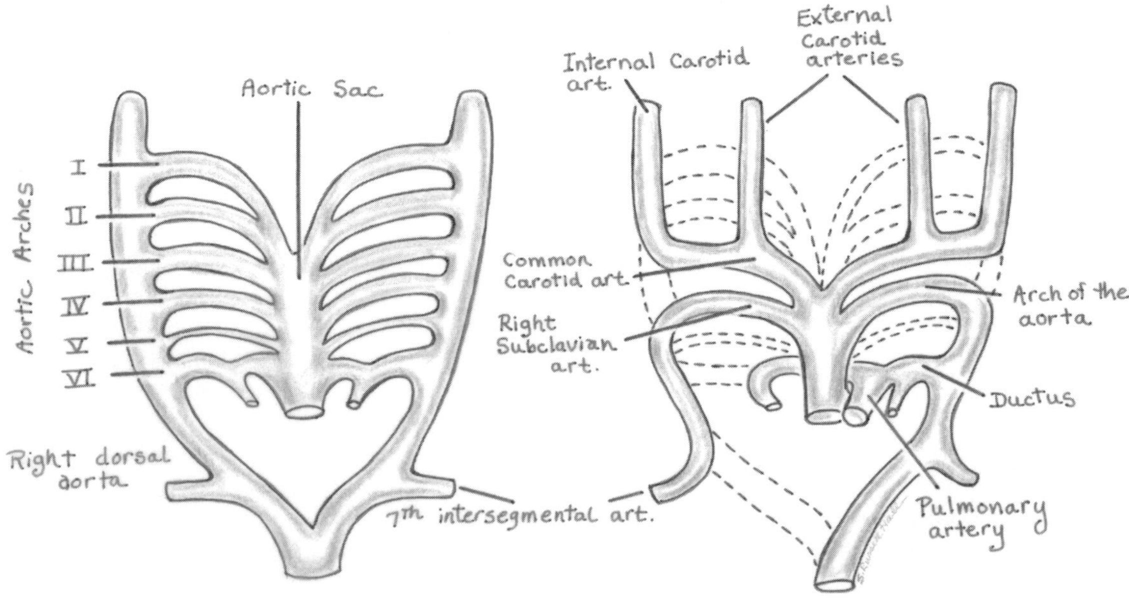

Figure 75-1 Embryologic *anlage* depicting aortic sac and paired aortic arches connected by branchial arches.

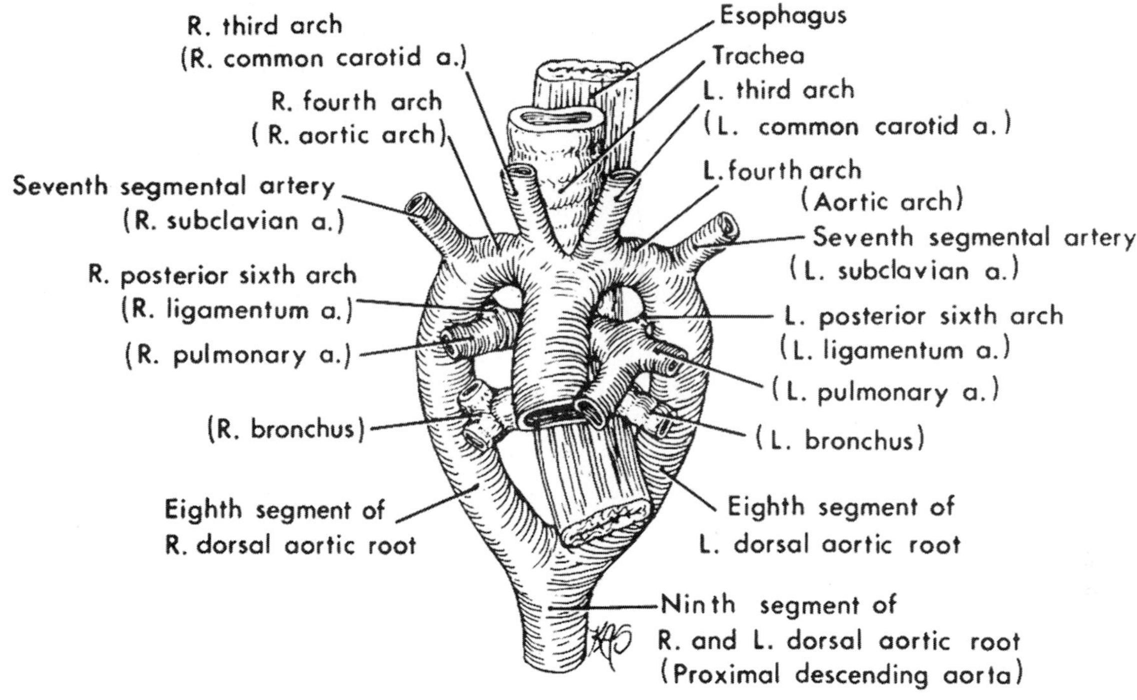

Figure 75-2 Hypothetical double arch system of Edwards.

molecular biology and genetics on embryology continues to evolve. It is acknowledged that such understanding will enhance and may well change the above-described paradigm of arch development.

Failure of certain components to form and/or regress according to the usual program gives rise to vascular rings. The classic hypothetical double arch system of Edwards[13] offers a useful model to aid visualization of the various types of anomalies (Fig. 75-2).

With the exception of confirmed general notions, such as involvement of neural crest migration and association of arch anomalies with 22q11 deletion,[14] the exact cause(s) of vascular rings is not known.

SPECIFIC ANOMALIES DEFINED

Before describing the specific anatomy of these anomalies, it is appropriate to clarify certain terms. *Right* or *left* aortic arch is defined as the side of the trachea by which the arch passes to connect to the descending aorta. A normal arch is left-sided. The descending aorta is described as being right, left, or midline with reference to the center of the vertebral bodies. A normal descending aorta is left-sided.

Aberrant right subclavian artery (ARSA)

The arch and descending aorta are left-sided. Believed due to abnormal regression of the right fourth branchial arch, the ARSA originates from the descending aorta and traverses the mediastinum posterior to the esophagus to reach the apex of the right chest (Fig. 75-3). The degree of posterior esophageal compression varies in severity.

Double aortic arch (DAA)

Due to persistence of both right and left fourth arches, right and left aortic arches connect the ascending aorta to the descending aorta, thereby forming a true ring that encircles both trachea and esophagus. In theory, the ductus could be right, left, or bilateral, and the descending aorta could be right, left, or midline; however, the common arrangement is a left-sided ductus or ligamentum and descending aorta (Fig. 75-4). The right or posterior arch is dominant in 80 percent of cases, whereas codominance occurs in 10 to 20 percent of cases. The compression of the esophagus and trachea is usually prominent.

Right arch anomalies

In this general category of anomalies due to regression of the left fourth arch, both the branching pattern of the great vessels and the location of the descending aorta can vary. The more common branching patterns are a retroesophageal ALSA and, less frequently, mirror-image branching; the sequence is innominate (giving left common carotid and left

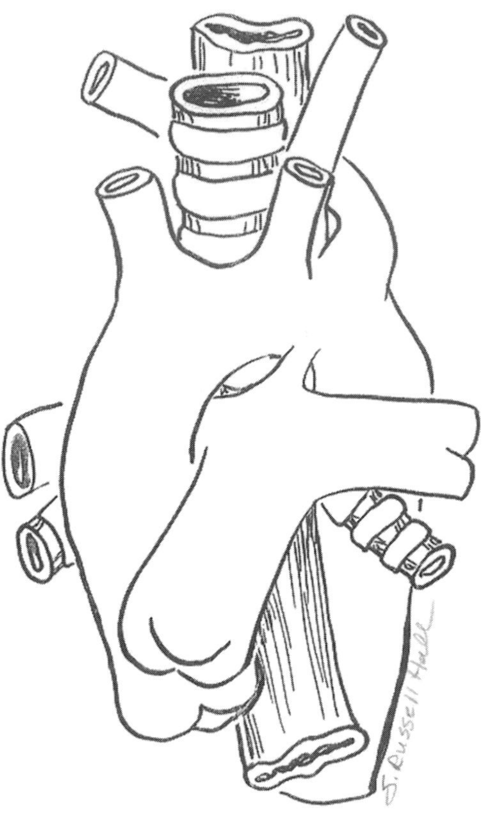

Figure 75-3 Anatomy of aberrant right subclavian artery.

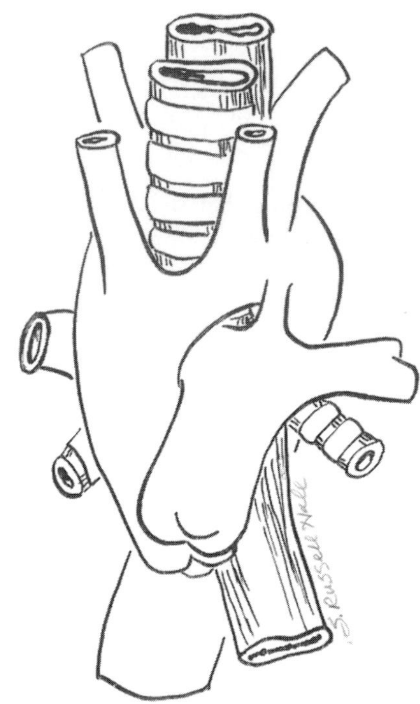

Figure 75-4 Anatomy of double aortic arch.

subclavian), right common carotid, and right subclavian artery (Fig. 75-5).

With right arch and ALSA, there are two other potential contributions to tracheoesophageal compression: left ligamentum or ductus and a Kommerell's diverticulum.[15] The diverticulum is the regressed fourth arch, giving rise to the left subclavian artery. This component may persist to varying degree as a diverticulum that can independently cause symptoms. Depending on the location of the descending aorta (if left-sided), the subclavian artery itself may not directly compress the posterior esophagus; however, a tethering effect and/or the effect of a ligamentum (which may connect to the descending aorta, left subclavian, or diverticulum) or diverticulum usually contributes to posterior esophageal compression and often tracheal compression as well.

With mirror-image branching, a left-sided ligamentum to the descending aorta can lead to compression of the esophagus or the trachea as well. If the ligamentum connects to the innominate or nonretroesophageal left subclavian, compression is less likely.

Innominate artery compression (IAC)

The exact embryologic basis of this anomaly is not known. The arch morphology is typically normal. Compared to the usual arrangement, the innominate artery often originates from a site somewhat more distal and posterior. In coursing cephalad and rightward, it leads to compression of the anterior trachea. There is no esophageal compression (Fig. 75-6).

Pulmonary artery sling (PAS)

In this anomaly, due to abnormal progression of the aortic sac and/or sixth arch development, the left pulmonary artery originates extrapericardially from the posterosuperior aspect of the right pulmonary artery. It courses over the right mainstem bronchus and posterior to the lower trachea/carina and anterior to the esophagus (Fig. 75-7). The duct or ligamentum usually originates at the site of the right pulmonary artery and courses superior to the left main bronchus and anomalous left pulmonary artery to reach the aorta. This arrangement leads to compression of the right main bronchus, distal trachea/carina, and effacement of the anterior esophagus (symptoms from the latter are usually not noted). It does not constitute a complete ring, but the sling imposes an impressive compressive effect. Associated findings include (1) complete tracheal rings in over 50 percent of cases (usually lower trachea), (2) infrequent absence of or unilobar lung, and (3) intracardiac defects.[16]

ASSOCIATED ANOMALIES

Probably the most important associated finding for the group as a whole is congenital heart anomalies, occurring in

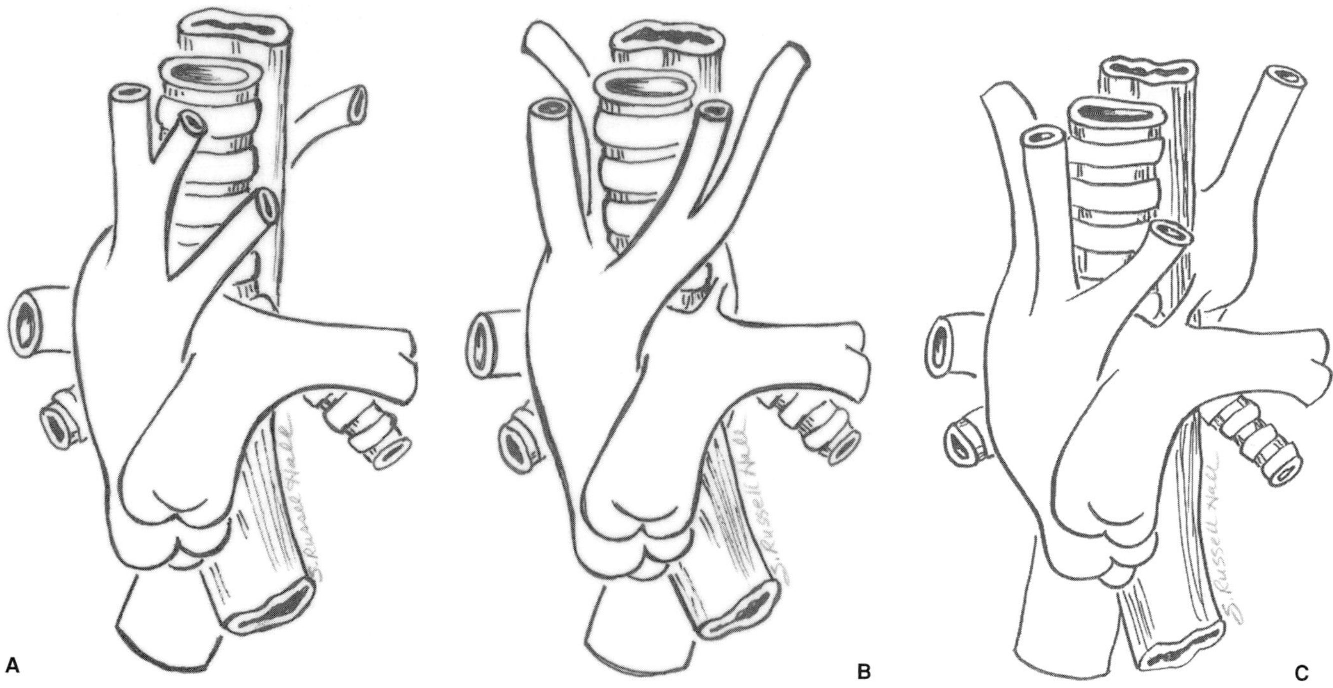

Figure 75-5 Right arch anomalies: **(A)** right arch with aberrant left subclavian artery; **(B)** right arch with mirror-image branching and left ligamentum; and **(C)** right arch with Kommerell's diverticulum, aberrant left subclavian artery, and left ligamentum.

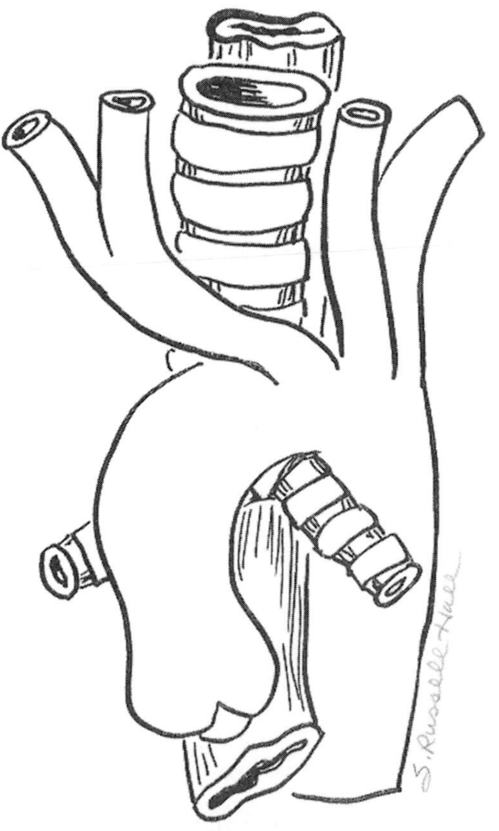

Figure 75-6 Anatomy of innominate artery compression of the trachea.

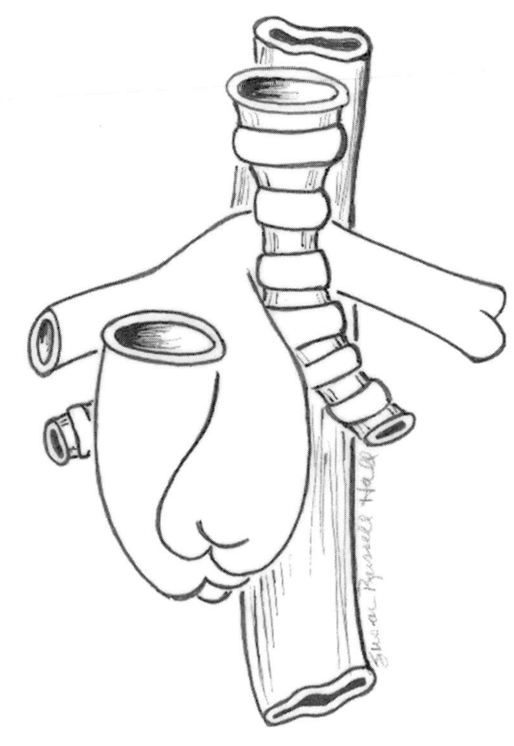

Figure 75-7 Anatomy of pulmonary artery sling.

approximately 15 to 20 percent of patients[17] (the incidence is much lower for IAC). Ventricular septal defect and tetralogy of Fallot each account for approximately one-third of cases, with aortic coarctation and atrial septal defect comprising the majority of the remainder. The presence of congenital heart disease impacts both the treatment strategy and prognosis and cannot be overemphasized. The most common chromosomal abnormality is 22q.11 deletion, occurring in approximately 15 to 20 percent of cases.[14] Depending on the degree of phenotypic expression, this finding has modest implications for short-term prognosis as well as other long-term health and behavioral issues. Complete tracheal rings, noted in over 50 percent of patients with PAS, merit special attention due to their impact on the need for concomitant tracheal reconstruction. Although not an intrinsic abnormality per se, airway malacia is a common secondary finding in patients with symptoms of airway compression. Although not usually requiring specific surgical treatment, airway malacia can have a significant impact on postoperative recovery.

CLINICAL FEATURES

Since the true denominator is not known, the true likelihood of developing symptoms is unknown as well. However, clinical experience clearly supports the variable propensity for symptoms among these anomalies. In general, an ARSA is infrequently symptomatic,[16] whereas a PAS is almost always symptomatic. Symptoms are probably more likely with right arch and ALSA compared to ARSA. Double aortic arch and RALL, with rare exception, produce symptoms.

The mode of presentation includes stridor, feeding difficulty, recurrent pulmonary or upper airway infection, acute life-threatening events, and/or a history of "asthma." Aberrant right subclavian artery and right arch with ALSA (if not tethered by a ligamentum or compressed by a Kommerell's diverticulum) exclusively cause swallowing-related difficulties. Right arch with left ligamentum can present with both airway and swallowing symptoms. With DAA, PAS, and IAC, airway symptoms usually predominate. In general, anomalies causing notable airway compression present in infancy, whereas anomalies causing only esophageal compression may present much later.

DIAGNOSIS

The history and physical examination provide a suggestion of the diagnosis based on the predominance of

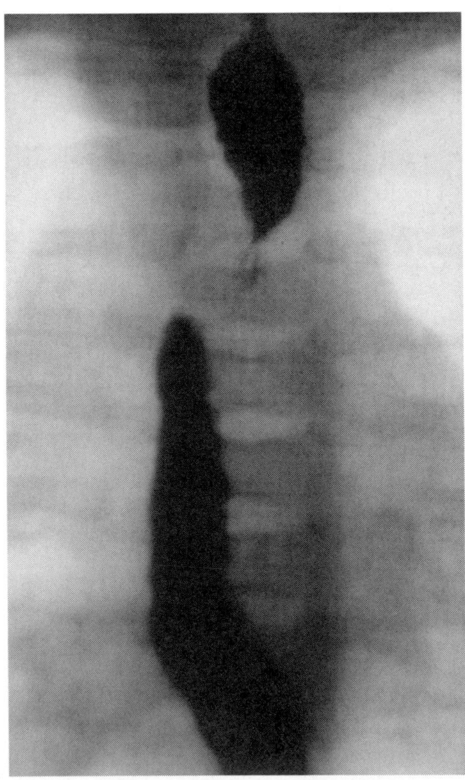

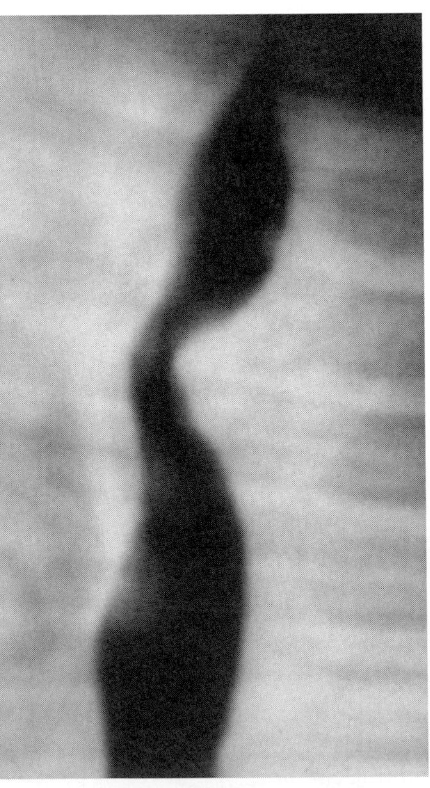

Figure 75-8 Barium swallow depicting double aortic arch. **A.** Posteroanterior view; note the parallel offset of dye columns. **B.** Lateral view; note the more significant posterior rightward effacement from the larger right arch.

airway or esophageal symptoms. Gastroesophageal reflux, asthma, and foreign body are certainly more common than vascular rings and should be regarded accordingly in the workup. Likewise, compression from a mediastinal mass must be excluded. Nonetheless, an index of suspicion for vascular rings is an important first step in making the diagnosis. Before discussing various optimal strategies, it is appropriate to briefly review the various diagnostic modalities and their relative strengths and weaknesses.

Barium swallow

Hallmark findings of vascular rings on plain film and barium swallow have been known since the 1940s.[18] The advent of newer modalities has perhaps diminished the enthusiasm for this diagnostic tool. This is nevertheless a relatively reliable, simple, safe, and cost-effective modality.[17,19–21] Although certain anomalies have characteristic findings, barium swallow detects the presence of an anomaly more reliably than the specific morphology. Nonetheless, it usually provides enough information to plan the operative strategy. It should not be considered a test to detect IAC. Patterns of dye effacement include bilateral effacement (right often more than left); significant posterior effacement; and, often, parallel separation of dye columns for DAA (Fig. 75-8); posterior effacement for aberrant subclavian artery, with perhaps lateral effacement depending on the side of the arch and origin of the subclavian; rightward and posterior effacement for RALL; and anterior effacement of the midesophagus for PAS.

Magnetic resonance imaging and computed tomography

Since the initial reports using CT and MRI to diagnose vascular rings (1960s for CT, 1980s for MRI), the use of these modalities has become commonplace.[22–26] Both provide clear delineations of anatomy and are usually very accurate in specifying the type of anomaly. They also provide good delineation of the airway (they can usually detect IAC but are not considered the "gold standard") and are usually adequate to determine whether airway reconstruction will be necessary. However, bronchoscopy may still be necessary to confirm radiographic findings or to plan the extent of resection. MRI and CT cannot reliably detect ligamentous structure or non-patent vascular lumens; however, this information can usually be inferred based on the clinical context. Figures 75-9 and 75-10A illustrate imaging of a double aortic arch and PAS.

The one disadvantage of both these modalities is the need for sedation and, depending on the availability of breath-hold sequences or sufficiently rapid acquisition, possibly intubation and mechanical ventilation. Such interventions on an infant with a compromised airway may be unsafe and imprudent.

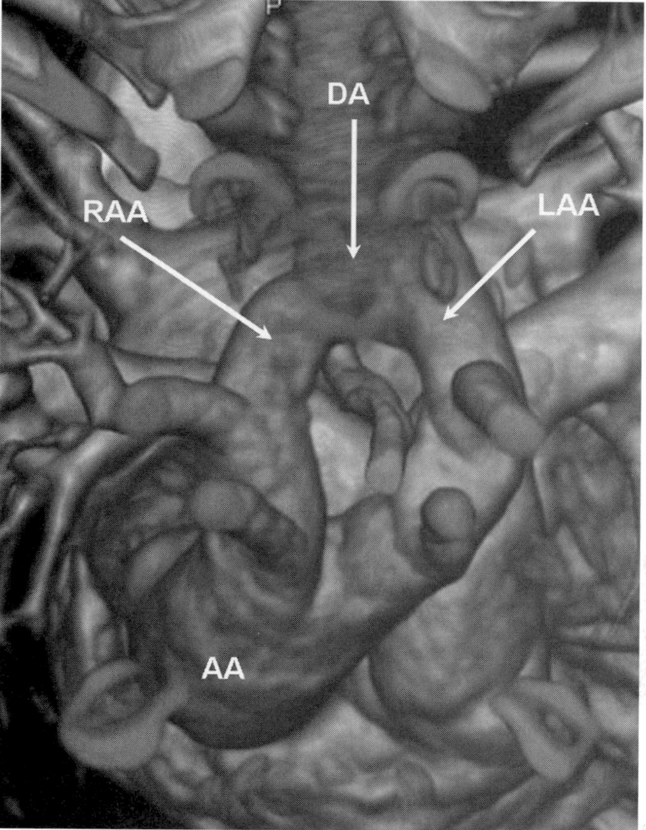

Figure 75-9 Three-dimensional computed tomography imaging in patient with double aortic arch. Right (RAA) and left (LAA) aortic arches give rise to ipsilateral subclavian and carotid arteries. Craniocaudal view. AA = ascending aorta; DA = descending aorta. (Image courtesy of Philip Spevak, MD, Division of Pediatric Cardiology, the Johns Hopkins University Hospital.)

Bronchoscopy

Bronchoscopy represents the gold standard for the diagnosis of IAC, revealing anterior pulsatile compression of the airway.[27] It is extremely relevant to the accurate assessment of the need for, and planning the extent of, airway reconstruction in PAS. Since tracheobronchomalacia is not uncommon after surgery, bronchoscopy is useful to confirm the presence of malacia and help rule out (along with CT or MRI) inadequate surgical therapy as a cause of persistent symptoms.

Echocardiography

Although an experienced echocardiographer can detect many vascular rings,[24,28,29] echocardiography should not be used in most practices as the sole diagnostic method. Of course a major advantage is portability and minimal morbidity. Its real utility in the workup is the reliable detection of concomitant cardiac anomalies. The importance of this

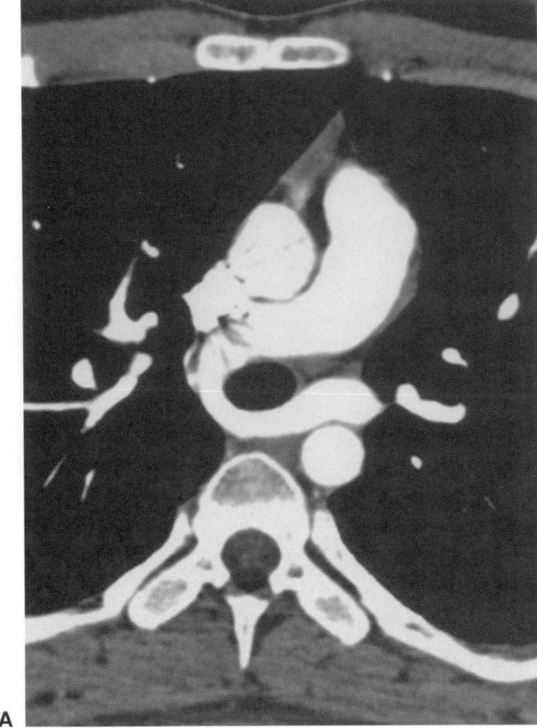

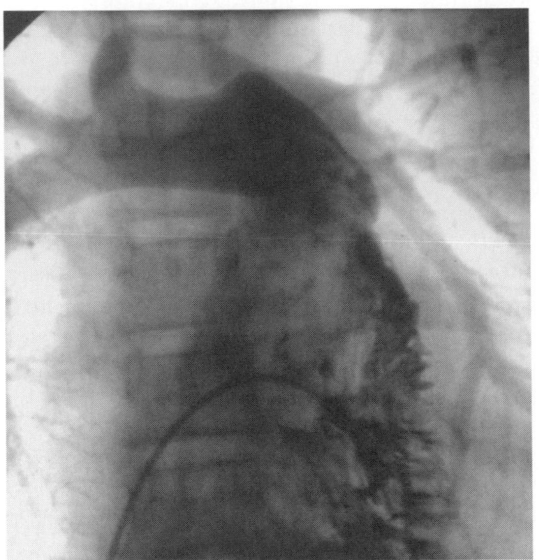

Figure 75-10 Pulmonary artery sling depicted by **(A)** contrast-enhanced CT and **(B)** pulmonary angiography.

knowledge in planning the appropriate management strategy cannot be overemphasized.

Angiography

Angiography can certainly be used to delineate vascular anatomy accurately (see Fig. 10B).[28] Most would agree that this degree of invasiveness is not necessary unless it is mandated by the workup for an intracardiac anomaly.

FORMULATING A STRATEGY

Three questions are relevant to formulating an optimal approach: (1) Does the patient have a symptomatic anomaly? (2) Is there an associated anomaly relevant to the management and outcome? and (3) Would additional tests, not already performed to answer questions 1 and 2, influence the operative strategy? If these three questions are answered correctly, the patient experiences minimal morbidity in the workup, and if an equally effective but less costly alternative is not available, the workup has been optimal. There is no single best test for all cases, nor is there a single optimal strategy or sequence of tests. There is a tendency to rely more on MRI and CT in recent years; however, barium swallow remains a valid option in many cases. Also, bronchoscopy is considered the gold standard for IAC and is very useful in planning reconstruction of the airway in PAS.

Since all tests are imperfect, intraoperative delineation of anatomy is important. For the vast majority of cases, left thoracotomy or thoracoscopy will be appropriate or sufficient.[17,19,30–36] In other words, although it may be preferable to fully delineate the specific anomaly preoperatively, this degree of information rarely alters the surgical approach and the need to delineate anatomy intraoperatively. In fact, in the author's review of over 918 cases, over 99 percent of cases other than PAS or IAC would have been readily repaired via a posterior or lateral left chest approach.[17]

There are important exceptions. The important associated anomaly that probably will change the approach is an intracardiac defect. Although therapy could be sequenced, in many cases it is appropriate to perform both repairs via a median sternotomy under the same anesthesia.[32] The second exception, IAC, is typically repaired via a limited anterior right or left minithoracotomy (it can also be done thoracoscopically). A third exception is PAS, which most surgeons prefer to repair via a median sternotomy with cardiopulmonary bypass. Finally there are infrequent exceptions, such as left arch with right ligamentum or double arch with atretic proximal right arch, for which a right-sided approach or median sternotomy would be appropriate.

Excluding IAC, there are three general approaches that provide enough information to treat the patient correctly: (1) CT or MRI plus echocardiography—bronchoscopy on-table if further information is needed about the airway (e.g., PAS); (2) barium swallow plus echocardiography—bronchoscopy on-table as in 1; (3) in the case of detection of the vascular ring by echocardiography, confirmation with CT (MRI) or barium swallow and bronchoscopy as in 1. Of course, angiography, if otherwise necessary, will obviate the need for other modalities (IAC an exception). For IAC, if a vascular ring is suspected and the CT (MRI) or barium swallow is nondiagnostic, bronchoscopy is warranted.

The best choice may depend on whether the patient is stable in the outpatient setting or being mechanically ventilated in the intensive care unit.

TREATMENT: ARCH AND GREAT VESSELS

General principles

Monitoring is for the most part routine; however, it is a good idea to have blood pressure monitoring capability in the right arm (left, depending on subclavian anatomy) and one leg (noninvasive is often adequate). In some cases, it might be useful to add monitoring of blood pressure or pulse oximetry waveform in the other arm. With test occlusion, such monitoring minimizes the risk of dividing the ring at an incorrect site. Good communication with the anesthesiologist is also important, as many of these children can have compromised airways, and subtle manipulation can lead to loss of ventilation.

For most cases, a left posterolateral thoracotomy in the third or fourth interspace is adequate (see exceptions below).[17,19,30–36] After retraction of the lung from the apex, the mediastinal pleura is opened. The superior intercostal vein and/or lymphatics can be divided between ties or thoroughly cauterized. The vagus and recurrent nerves are identified and carefully preserved throughout the dissection. The arch(es) and great vessels should be mobilized to an extent that allows confident confirmation of the anatomy. For many anomalies, the anatomy and site for division is obvious; however, test occlusion with pressure monitoring ensures a correct location. Depending on the size and patency of the lumen being divided, division can be accomplished between ties (or suture ligatures) or by application of vascular clamps and oversewing of the divided ends. Permanent suture material should be used. Once the ring is divided, it is important to lyse adhesions or fibrous bands that have formed under the site of compression around the esophagus and/or airway. A chest drain is optional, depending on the concern for air leak, bleeding, or lymphatic leak. Refer to Figs. 75-11 to 75-15 for illustrations of the repair techniques.

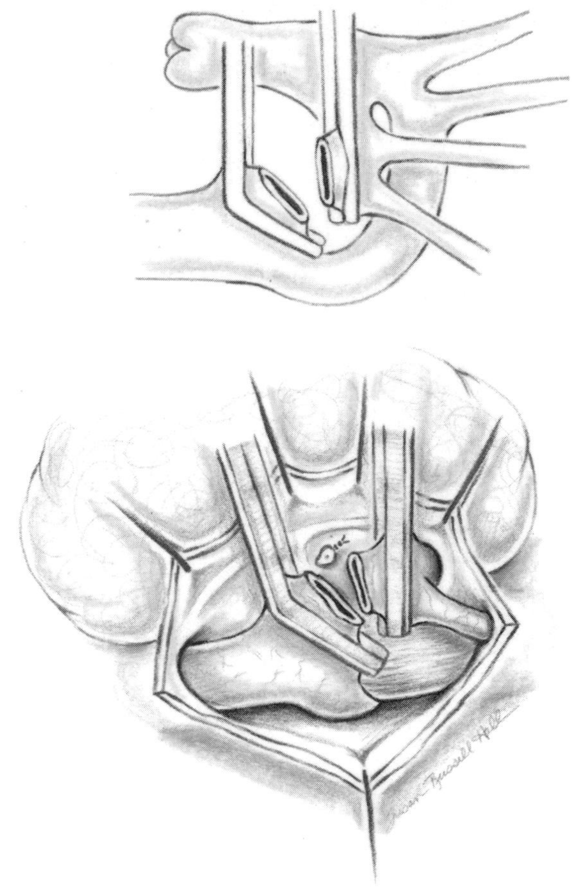

Figure 75-11 Illustration of repair of vascular rings: double aortic arch. The diminutive arch (at the left in this schematic view) and the ligamentum arteriosus are divided. (Schematic drawing, left thoracotomy.)

We regard prophylactic aortopexy as reasonable in selected cases. For example, if a child has significant airway symptoms preoperatively and the access for repair of the ring is permissible, then the minimal additional time and effort to elevate either the distal ascending aorta or the airway toward the sternum may well obviate the need for a second operation to treat tracheomalacia.

Video-assisted thoracoscopic surgery (VATS)

Many of the more straightforward rings can also be repaired using minimally invasive techniques.[37,38] With the exception of one access site that typically is 5 mm wide (a working port), the remainder of the sites can be simple stab incisions or small trocars for 3-mm instrumentation. Optimal placement of ports or access sites is variable among surgeons; however, it is generally more functional to place the camera under the tip of scapula with the left- and right-hand working sites placed anteriorly and posteriorly, respectively (these can be interchanged as needed).

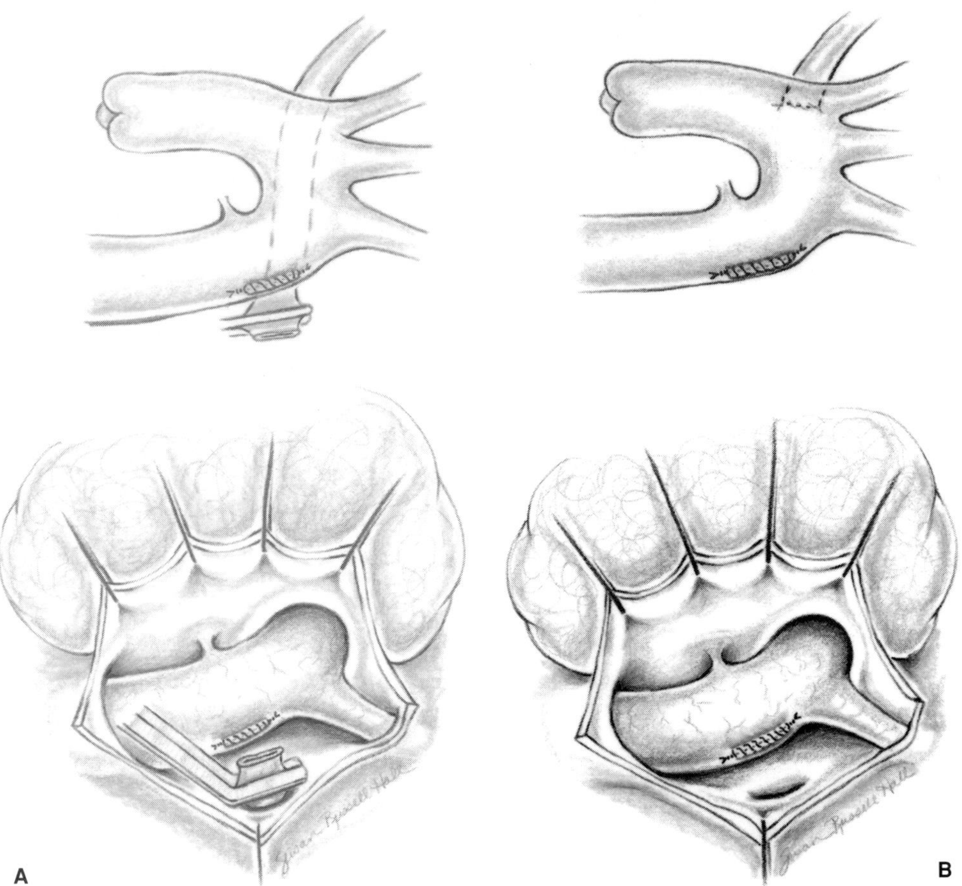

Figure 75-12 Illustration of repair of vascular rings. Aberrant right subclavian artery. The aberrant artery is divided from its takeoff from the descending aorta **(A)** and is allowed to retract behind the esophagus **(B)**. (Schematic drawing, left thoracotomy.)

In small children, the distance from the chest wall (fulcrum point) to the dissection field is quite short; therefore, to achieve a given radius of motion of the instrument tip, considerably more relative motion of the instrument handle is needed when the patient is a child rather than an adult. Placing access sites close together can make the procedure unnecessarily difficult. For left-sided VATS, the endotracheal tube can be advanced to the right mainstem bronchus to provide single-lung ventilation. Still, it may be necessary to add a fourth port to facilitate lung retraction.

The remainder of the operation proceeds as in the open scenario. Division can be accomplished with intra- or extracorporeal tying, or with intracorporeal suturing as needed. For large, patent lumens, the merit and safety of dividing between surgical clips is left to the cautious discretion of the individual surgeon. Enlargement of an access site, if necessary to ensure safe division, can be performed but detracts somewhat from the benefit of the minimally invasive approach. It should be appreciated that the criteria for selecting appropriate candidates are not fully refined.

SPECIFIC ANOMALIES AND SURGICAL CONSIDERATIONS

Innominate artery compression

The repair can be approached via either a right or left anterior minithoracotomy.[16,27,39] Although uncommonly reported, this can also be done via a low transverse cervical incision. The second costal cartilage can be sacrificed if necessary. The internal thoracic vessels are preserved. The thymus is mobilized with preservation of the phrenic nerve, and the pericardial reflection at the distal ascending aorta and proximal arch are identified. The pericardium and outer aorta at the site of origin of the innominate artery is then pexed with two or three pledgetted permanent sutures to the undersurface of the sternum. Additional sutures can be placed if needed to minimize severe angulation of the artery. Intraoperative bronchoscopy can be useful to guide the degree of pexy needed. Although the incision with the open technique is typically very small, VATS can likewise be used to perform the repair.

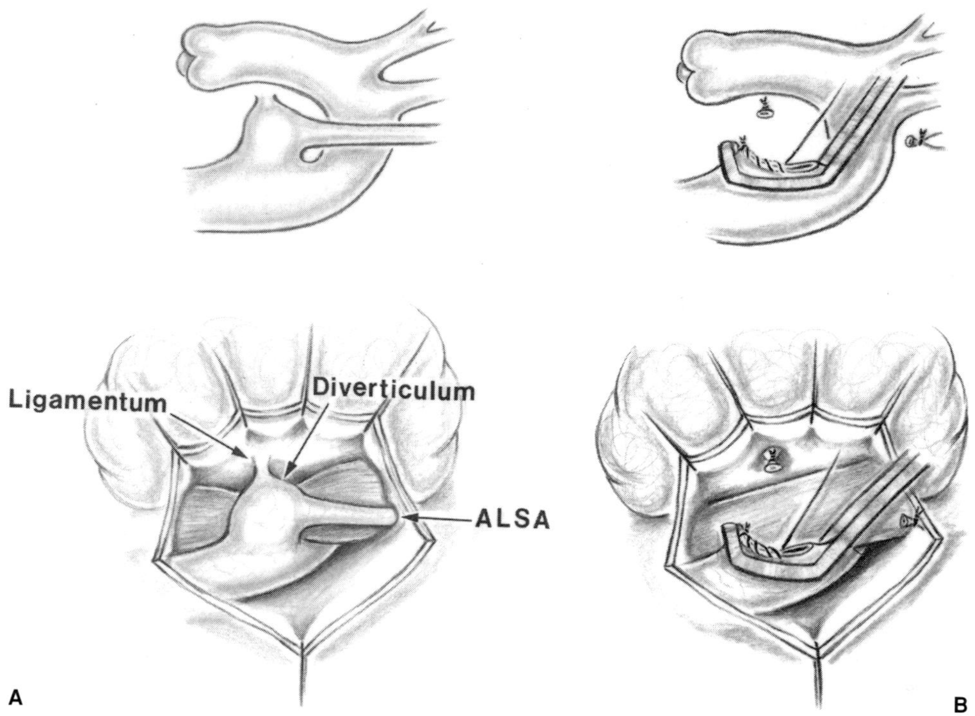

Figure 75-13 Illustration of repair of vascular rings. Kommerell's diverticulum, aberrant left subclavian artery, and left ligamentum **(A)**. Care should be taken when placing the clamp at the base of the diverticulum to avoid narrowing the aorta. The ligamentum is divided **(B)**. (Schematic drawing, left thoracotomy.)

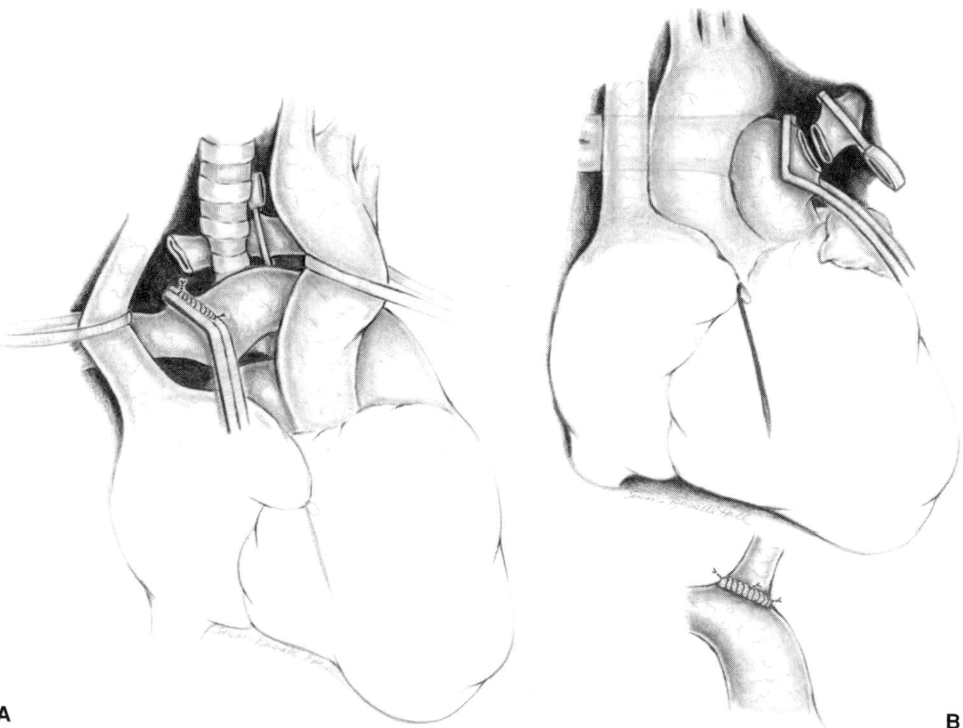

Figure 75-14 Illustration of repair of vascular rings. Left pulmonary artery sling. The left pulmonary artery is mobilized behind the trachea and detached from its origin on the posterior aspect of the right pulmonary artery **(A)**. It is then brought anteriorly and anastomosed to the leftward aspect of the main pulmonary trunk **(B)**. (Schematic drawing, median sternotomy.)

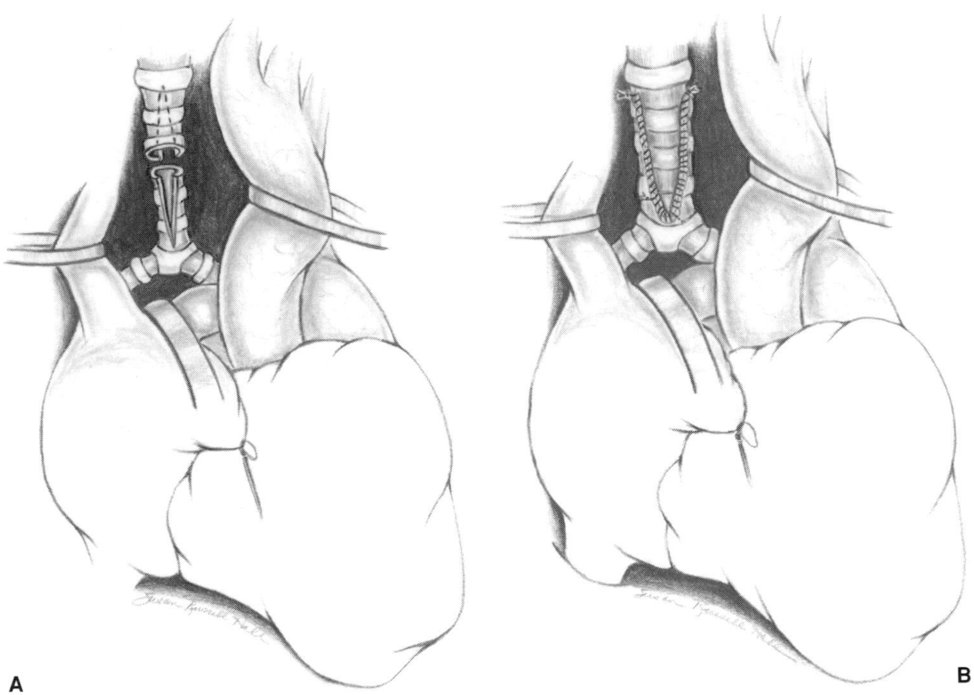

Figure 75-15 Illustration of repair of vascular rings. Tracheal reconstruction (sliding tracheoplasty) after repair of left pulmonary artery sling (Fig. 75-20). On cardiopulmonary bypass, the trachea is divided and longitudinal incisions are made in the anterior portion of the distal segment and on the posterior portion of the proximal segment **(A)**. With the sliding technique, the two ends are anastomosed **(B)**. (Schematic drawing, median sternotomy.)

Kommerell's diverticulum

For the majority of right arch anomalies, with or without an ALSA or Kommerell's diverticulum, the repair can be performed via the left chest (Fig. 75-12).[16,40–42] If a diverticulum is present and the descending aorta is rightward or midline, some surgeons may prefer the right chest. In this case, it is important to ensure that treatment of the diverticulum will also release any tethering effect of a left ligamentum, as direct division of a left ligamentum from the right chest may not be straightforward. We recommend repairing a diverticulum, not simply ligating the subclavian artery. To minimize the risk of inadequate treatment, the diverticulum should be resected and oversewn flush with the aorta (Fig. 75-13). Consideration should be given to resection of any enlarged lymphatic nodes in the immediate vicinity.

Aberrant subclavian artery

With the exception of an ALSA, as noted above, repair can be performed via the left chest.[16,17,19,30–36] With an ALSA or ARSA, after division, the vessel should be mobilized well behind the esophagus and allowed to retract to the opposite side after division.

One factor that can impact the approach is reimplantation of the divided artery. There is no one uniform perspective among surgeons regarding the necessity or appropriateness of reimplantation.[16] The risk of ischemic complications in young children is quite low. Also, estimates of longer-term morbidity, such as limb discrepancy, are low but variable and imprecise. For adults without atherosclerotic disease, the risk of ischemic complication is approximated at 5 to 10 percent. Also relevant is the lack of extensive documentation of long-term patency of reimplantation in infants. Currently, we do not routinely reimplant vessels in infants and small children but do so in older children and adults. If reimplantation is anticipated, the approach can be individualized to the patient's anatomy and the site of reimplantation. For example, we have reimplanted an ARSA via the lateral chest (using the carotid or innominate arteries) or via a limited upper ministernotomy.

Associated cardiac anomalies

For most combinations of ring or sling morphology and intracardiac anomaly, single-stage repair is appropriate.

In certain cases, such as a neonate with tetralogy of Fallot deemed not to be a candidate for complete neonatal repair, the vascular ring can be repaired at the time of the shunt procedure or final repair, depending on the particular circumstance. Essentially every ring or sling morphology can be repaired via a median sternotomy.

Repair of the vascular ring can be performed prior to or during bypass, depending on the amount of retraction needed for exposure for a particular ring.

Pulmonary artery sling

Although various approaches can be used, most surgeons recommend repair via a median sternotomy on cardiopulmonary bypass.[10,11,43,44] The need for and extent of airway reconstruction should be thoroughly assessed prior to incision (by bronchoscopy, MRI, or CT). With the patient supported on bypass, ventilation is discontinued and the endotracheal tube withdrawn proximally from the anticipated field of work. Both the airway and left pulmonary artery are approached between the superior vena cava and the aorta (Fig. 75-14). If airway reconstruction is needed, the airway can be divided first (usually at the narrowest site) to facilitate mobilization of the pulmonary artery. The left pulmonary artery is then reimplanted onto the main pulmonary artery. Patch closure at the site of detachment minimizes risk of narrowing. The airway is then reconstructed using either resection and direct reimplantation for short-segment disease, resection with autograft,[16] or slide tracheoplasty for more extensive disease (Fig. 75-15).[45,46] Standard principles of airway surgery apply: adequate mobilization with release techniques if needed (often not necessary), preservation of lateral blood supply, preservation of vagus nerves, and tension-free, airtight anastomosis. After reconstruction, the endotracheal tube is advanced to an appropriate position. We believe that simply leaving the left pulmonary artery in place and reanastomosing the airway behind the artery should be avoided.[44] Barring particular concerns, the patient can be extubated early to minimize trauma to the airway.

If airway reconstruction is not needed, the left pulmonary artery is simply mobilized, detached, brought anterior to the airway, and reimplanted onto the main pulmonary artery.

COURSE AND PROGNOSIS

For most children without intracardiac anomalies, the clinical course is straightforward. Esophageal compressive symptoms improve promptly. Airway symptoms improve as well, but often less rapidly, typically requiring days to weeks for complete resolution.[17,21,47,48] Most children can be sent home 2 to 3 days postoperatively. Airway issues should dictate follow-up strategy. For a child without any initial airway symptoms, a single wound check is sufficient. For a child with airway symptoms, more thorough and frequent follow-up is appropriate, depending on severity (perhaps every 2 to 5 days in the first 2 to 3 weeks), to ensure progressive resolution and allow prompt intervention when indicated.

Excluding PAS and rings associated with intracardiac anomalies, mortality is very low, typically less than 1 percent.[16,17,19,30–36] Bleeding and sepsis account for most deaths. For PAS, reported mortalities are quite variable, ranging from 6 to 50 percent .[10,11,43,44] Airway complications (leak, dehiscence) are the most common cause of death.

Morbidity is typical of any thoracic vascular procedure ranging from bleeding and infection to recurrent laryngeal nerve palsy, chylothorax, and chest wall deformity. A reasonable estimate for overall morbidity is 10 percent.

Tracheobronchomalacia

One associated morbidity particular to vascular rings with airway compression is tracheobronchomalacia, defined as dynamic collapse of the airway secondary to inadequate structural support. It occurs in approximately 5 to 10 percent of patients,[17,49] most often at the site of compression from the vascular ring. Many children will initially have residual noisy breathing that progressively improves over the first 2 weeks. The diagnosis of malacia is suspected based on initially more severe obstructive symptoms, failure to improve, or progressive worsening. The diagnosis is confirmed by bronchoscopy. There is no uniform agreement on the duration of persistent but improving obstructive symptoms needed to warrant bronchoscopy or a clinical diagnosis of malacia. Certainly many children will demonstrate evidence of malacia if evaluated early by bronchoscopy. In our opinion, it is prudent to continue observation according to the following guidelines: (1) initial postoperative obstructive symptoms are not severe—the child can maintain ventilation without excessive work of breathing and can maintain adequate nutritional intake; (2) there is progressive resolution of symptoms; and (3) by 2 to 3 weeks postoperatively the symptoms are markedly diminished. If any of these criteria are not met, bronchoscopy is indicated. If bronchoscopy does not reveal findings of malacia, CT or MRI is warranted to exclude inadequate surgical treatment or external compression from enlarged reactive lymph nodes. Reoperation is appropriate in such circumstances.

Management of confirmed tracheobronchomalacia is not straightforward. The best guideline is to persist with conservative therapy to the extent possible. If not feasible, options for intervention include aortopexy, intraluminal stenting (thin-walled silicon or wire mesh stents), and extraluminal stenting.[49–55] There is no uniform agreement on the best initial therapy. We favor aortopexy as initial therapy, recognizing there is a role for intraluminal stenting in very select patients. Intraluminal stenting has the advantage of being less invasive and the disadvantage of usually requiring several follow-up bronchoscopies to evacuate mucous plugs or reposition the stent. Pending the availability of newer-generation, thinner-walled silicon stents, the presently available self- or balloon-expandable metallic stents, although not ideal, are probably the best option in infants.[51,52] With larger airways in older children, silicon stents become more appropriate. It is important to recognize that the ease of removal of a metallic stent decreases with time due to ingrowth. Stents should be removed at the earliest possible time. Stents of any kind can also erode into adjacent vascular structures with catastrophic consequences. We strongly recommend against stenting vascular compression of the airway. The final option when all else fails is tracheostomy with supplemental positive-pressure ventilation. Fortunately, very few children require this type of treatment.

ACKNOWLEDGEMENTS

The authors would like to acknowledge the following colleagues for their outstanding contributions for completion of this chapter: Randolf Otto, MD; John P. McCloskey, MD; Chris B. Stefanelli, MD; and Roberta S. Stephenson, MD. We would also like to express sincere appreciation to Susan Russell Hall and Marlene Kennedy for the medical artwork and technical support with manuscript preparation, respectively.

References

1. Backer CL, Mavroudis C. Congenital Heart Surgery Nomenclature and Database Project: Vascular rings, tracheal stenosis, pectus excavatum. *Ann Thorac Surg* 2000;69:3085.
2. Hunauld. Examen de quelques parties d'un singe. *Hist Acad R Sci* 1735:2;516. Cited in Stewart JR, Kincaid OW, Edwards JE. *An Atlas of Vascular Rings and Related Malformations of the Aortic Arch System*. Springfield, IL: Charles C Thomas, 1964.
3. Bayford D. *An Account of a Singular Case of Obstructed Deglutition*. London: Memorial Medical Society, 1794; 2:275.
4. Hommell L. Observationes anatomicae de arcu aortae bifido du dueto thoracico duplica, et de carstidum atque subclaviarum. *Holdomas* 1737;21:161.
5. Glaevecke H, Doehle H. Uber eine seltene angeborene Anomalie der Pulmonalarterie. *Munch Med Wochenschr* 1897;44:950.
6. Gross RE. Surgical relief for tracheal obstruction from a vascular ring. *N Engl J Med* 1945;233:586.
7. Gross RE, Ware PF. The surgical significance of aortic arch anomalies. *Surg Gynecol Obstet* 1946;83:435.
8. Potts WJ, Holinger PM, Rosenblum AH. Anomalous left pulmonary artery causing obstruction to right main stem bronchus. *JAMA* 1954;155:1409.
9. Nikaidoh H, Berendis HW, Mitchel SC, et al. Congenital heart disease in 56,109 births. Incidence and natural history. *Circulation* 1971;43:323.
10. Backer CL, Mavroudis C, Dunham ME, et al. Pulmonary artery sling: Results with median sternotomy, cardiopulmonary bypass, and reimplantation. *Ann Thorac Surg* 1999;67:1738.
11. Pawade A, de Leval MR, Elliott MJ, et al. Pulmonary artery sling. *Ann Thorac Surg* 1992;54:967.
12. Haworth SG. The pulmonary circulation. In: Anderson RH, Baker EJ, Macartney FJ, et al (eds). *Pediatric Cardiology,* 2d ed. London: Harcourt, 2002:57.
13. Stewart JR, Kincaid OW, Edwards JE. *An Atlas for Vascular Rings and Related Malformations of the Aortic Arch System*. Springfield, IL: Charles C. Thomas, 1964.
14. Momma K, Matsuoka R, Takao A. Aortic arch anomalies associated with 22q11 deletion (CATCH 22). *Pediatr Cardiol* 1999;20:97.
15. Kommerell B. Verlagerung des Oesophagus durch eine abnormale verlaufende Arteria subclavia dextra (arteria lusoria). *Fortschr Geb Rontgenstr* 1936;54:590.
16. Mavroudis C, Backer CL. Vascular rings and pulmonary artery sling. In: Mavroudis C, Backer CL (eds). *Pediatric Cardiac Surgery*. Philadelphia: Mosby, 2003:234.
17. Woods RK, Sharp RJ, Holcomb GW, et al. Vascular anomalies and tracheoesophageal compression: A single institution's 25-year experience. *Ann Thorac Surg* 2001;272: 434.
18. Neuhauser EBD. The roentgen diagnosis of double aortic arch and other anomalies of the great vessels. *Am J Radiol* 1946;56:1.
19. Bertolini A, Pelizza A, Panizzon G, et al. Vascular rings and slings. *J Cardiovasc Surg* 1987; 28:301.
20. Chun K, Colombani PM, Dudgeon D, et al. Diagnosis and management of congenital vascular rings: A 22-year experience. *Ann Thorac Surg* 1992;53:597.
21. Bonnard A, Auber F, Fourcade L, et al. Vascular ring abnormalities: A retrospective study of 62 cases. *J Pediatr Surg* 2003;38:539.
22. Julsrud PR, Ehman RL. Magnetic resonance imaging of vascular rings. *Mayo Clin Proc* 1986;61:181.
23. Beekman RP, Beek FJA, Hazekamp MG, et al. The value of MRI in diagnosing vascular abnormalities causing stridor. *Eur J Pediatr* 1997;156:516.
24. Van Son JAM, Julsrud PR, Hagler DJ, et al. Imaging strategies for vascular rings. *Ann Thorac Surg* 1994;57: 604.
25. McLoughlin MJ, Weisbrod G, Wise DJ, et al. Computed tomography in congenital anomalies of the aortic arch and great vessels. *Radiology* 1981;138:399.
26. Lowe GM, Donaldson JS, Backer CL. Vascular rings: 10-year review of imaging. *Radiographics* 1991;11:673.
27. Moes CF, Izukawa T, Trusler GA. Innominate artery compression of the trachea. *Arch Otoloaryngol* 1975; 101:733.
28. Sahn DJ, Valdez-Cruz LM, Ovitt TW, et al. Two-dimensional echocardiography and intravenous digital video subtraction angiography for diagnosis and evaluation of double aortic arch. *Am J Cardiol* 1982;50:342.
29. Lillihei CW, Colan S. Echocardiography in the preoperative evaluation of vascular rings. *J Pediatr Surg* 1992;27:1118.
30. Backer CL, Ilbawi MN, Idriss FS, et al. Vascular anomalies causing tracheoesophageal compression. *J Thorac Cardiovasc Surg* 1989;97:725.
31. Hartyanszky IL, Lozsadi K, Marcsek P, et al. Congenital vascular rings: Surgical management of 111 cases. *Eur J Cardiothorac Surg* 1989;3:250.

32. Kocis KC, Midgley FM, Ruckman RN. Aortic arch complex anomalies: 20-year experience with symptoms, diagnosis, associated cardiac defects, and surgical repair. *Pediatr Cardiol* 1987;18:127.
33. Spiridonov AA, Podzolkov VP, Ivanitskii AV, et al. Vascular ring: Classification, clinical aspects, diagnosis, and principles of surgical treatment. *Grud Serdechnsososudistaia Khir* 1990;11:3.
34. Horvath P, Hucin B, Hruda J, et al. Surgical treatment of congenital vascular anomalies causing tracheoesophageal compression. *Rozhl Chir* 1980;69:504.
35. Van Son JAM, Julsrud PR, Hagler DJ, et al. Surgical treatment of vascular rings: The Mayo Clinic experience. *Mayo Clin Proc* 1993;68:1056.
36. Sharma S, Dobbs JL, Cobanoglu A. Surgical correction of vascular ring anomalies. *Asian Cardiovasc Thorac Ann* 2000;8:344.
37. Burke RP, Rosenfeld HM, Wernovsky G, et al. Video-assisted thoracoscopic vascular ring division in infants and children. *J Am Coll Cardiol* 1995;25:943.
38. Tomislav M, Cannon JW, del Nido PJ. Robotically assisted division of a vascular ring in children. *J Thorac Cardiovasc Surg* 2003;125:1163.
39. Gross RE, Neuhauser EBD. Compression of the trachea by an anomalous innominate artery: An operation for its relief. *Am J Dis Child* 1948;75:570.
40. Backer CL, Hillman N, Mavroudis C, et al. Resection of Kommerell's diverticulum and left subclavian artery transfer for recurrent symptoms after vascular ring division. *Eur J Cardiothorac Surg* 2002;22:64.
41. Malas MB, Barr ML, Starnes VA, et al. Dyspnea lusoria: Compression of the pulmonary artery by a Kommerell's diverticulum. *Ann Thorac Surg* 2002;73:312.
42. Verkroost MW, Hamerlijnck RP, Vermeulen FE. Surgical management of aneurysms at the origin of an aberrant right subclavian artery. *J Thorac Cardiovasc Surg* 1994;107:1469.
43. Jonas RA, Spevak PJ, McGill T, et al. Pulmonary artery sling: Primary repair by tracheal resection in infancy. *J Thorac Cardiovasc Surg* 1989;97:548.
44. van Son JAM, Hambsch J, Haas GS, et al. Pulmonary artery sling: Reimplantation versus antetracheal translocation. *Ann Thorac Surg* 1999;68:989.
45. Tsang V, Murday A, Gillbe C, et al. Slide tracheoplasty for congenital funnel-shaped tracheal stenosis. *Ann Thorac Surg* 1989;48:632.
46. Grillo HC, Wright CD, Vlahakes GJ, et al. Management of congenital tracheal stenosis by means of slide tracheoplasty or resection and reconstruction, with long-term follow-up of growth after slide tracheoplasty. *J Thorac Cardiovasc Surg* 2002;123:145.
47. Anand R, Dooley KJ, Williams WH, et al. Follow-up of surgical correction of vascular anomalies causing tracheobronchial compression. *Pediatr Cardiol* 1994; 15:58.
48. Bertrand JM, Chartrand C, Lamarre A, et al. Vascular ring. Clinical and physiological assessment of pulmonary function following surgical correction. *Pediatr Pulmonol* 1986;2:378.
49. Conti VR, Lobe TE. Vascular sling with tracheomalacia: Surgical management. *Ann Thorac Surg* 1989;47: 310.
50. Greenholz SK, Karrer FM, Lilly JR. Contemporary surgery of tracheomalacia. *J Pediatr Surg* 1986;21: 511.
51. Filler RM, Carolos Frag VFJ, Matute J. The use of expandable metallic airway stents for tracheobronchial obstruction in children. *J Pediatr Surg* 1995;30:1050.
52. Marr EA, Parsons DS, Lally KP. Treatment of severe bronchomalacia with expanding endobronchial stents. *Arch Otolaryngol Head Neck Surg* 1990;116:1087.
53. Kiely EM, Spitz L, Bereton R. Management of tracheomalacia by aortopexy. *Pediatr Surg Int* 1987;2:13.
54. Weber TR, Keller MS, Fiore A. Aortic suspension (aortopexy) for severe tracheomalacia in infants and children. *Am J Surg* 2002;184:573.
55. Abdel-Rahman U, Ahrens P, Fiesuth HG, et al. Surgical treatment of tracheomalacia by bronchoscopic monitored aortopexy in infants and children. *Ann Thorac Surg* 2002;74:315.

CHAPTER

76 EBSTEIN'S ANOMALY

Antonio F. Corno, Christian Schreiber, Norbert Augustin

INTRODUCTION

Ebstein's anomaly is a rare but complex and fascinating congenital heart defect. Since its original description in 1866, dramatic advances have been made in its diagnosis and treatment. The surgical treatment, including tricuspid valve repair and closure of any interatrial communication (with or without appropriate antiarrhythmia procedures), provides improvement in oxygenation, exercise tolerance, and reduction in the incidence of supraventricular arrhythmias. Quality of life and longevity are improved.

KEY CONCEPTS

- Epidemiology
  - Ebstein's anomaly represents 1 percent of all heart defects and 0.3 to 0.8 percent of all cardiac malformations diagnosed in the first year of life.
- Morphology
  - The hallmark of the lesion is apical displacement of the septal and posterior leaflets of the tricuspid valve, with "atrialization" of a variable portion of the right ventricle and various degrees of RVOTO. The right atrium is frequently dilated as a consequence of tricuspid valve insufficiency, rarely because of stenosis. An interatrial communication is almost always present. Ebstein's anomaly is also found in patients with congenitally corrected transposition of the great arteries (CC-TGA).
- Pathophysiology
  - Given the wide morphologic spectrum of this condition, pathophysiology is dependent on the degree of valvular regurgitation, shunting, and RVOTO, with duct-dependent pulmonary circulation in extreme cases. The right ventricle is dilated and the interventricular septum bulges leftward; this may result in impaired left ventricular function. Supraventricular tachycardia, Wolf-Parkinson-White syndrome (WPW), and ventricular arrhythmias are seen in as many as 20 to 25 percent of cases, leading to sudden death in 3 to 10 percent.
- Diagnosis
  - Two-dimensional echocardiography provides complete information regarding cardiac morphology and functional status as well as the presence of associated lesions. Cardiac catheterization is utilized selectively.
- Indication for treatment
  - Surgical intervention is indicated in symptomatic neonates with Ebstein'anomaly, either because of severe tricuspid regurgitation or RVOTO. In older patients, surgery is indicated because of cyanosis, heart failure, or recurrent arrhythmias.
- Treatment
  - Complete repair entails closure of the atrial septal defect, plication of the atrialized portion of the right ventricle, and repair of the tricuspid valve. Tricuspid valve replacement is very rarely required, and it should possibly be avoided. In selected cases, "one and one-half" ventricular repair (intracardiac repair and Glenn cavopulmonary anastomosis) has been performed with success.
- Outcome/prognosis
  - Improvements in surgical techniques, adapted to the morphology and function specific for each individual patient, has allowed for a significant reduction in mortality and rate of reoperation, together with a substantial improvement in quality of life.

INCIDENCE

Representing 1 percent of all congenital heart defects, Ebstein's anomaly is the 18th most common congenital cardiac malformation and is the underlying structural abnormality observed in 0.3 to 0.8 percent of all patients presenting with cardiac disease in the first year of life; the prevalence of this rare condition is 1 in 20,000 to 50,000 live births, with equal male:female occurrence.[1–8]

MORPHOLOGY

With relevance to the surgical management of the condition, five anatomic features[3,9–11] of Ebstein's anomaly have been described:

1. Displacement of the septal and posterior leaflets of the tricuspid valve toward the apex of the right ventricle, with adherence to the myocardium (Fig. 76-1).
2. The anterior leaflet is attached to the appropriate level of the tricuspid valve annulus but is redundant, larger than normal, and with multiple fenestrations and chordal attachments to the ventricular wall.
3. The segment of right ventricle between the level of the true tricuspid annulus and the attachment of the septal and posterior leaflets is unusually thin and dysplastic and described as "atrialized"; the tricuspid annulus and right atrium are extremely dilated.
4. The cavity of the right ventricle (beyond the atrialized portion) is reduced in size, usually with lack of an inlet chamber and with a small trabecular component.
5. The infundibulum is often obstructed by the redundant tissue of the anterior leaflet as well as by the chordal attachments of the anterior leaflet to the infundibulum.

In addition, Carpentier[12–13] described four clinical variants of progressively increasing severity:

1. Type A: the volume of the true right ventricle is adequate.
2. Type B: the volume of the right ventricle is small and there is a large atrialized portion of the right ventricle.
3. Type C: the volume of the right ventricle is small, with right ventricular outflow tract obstruction (RVOTO).
4. Type D: there is almost complete atrialization of the right ventricle with the exception of an extremely diminutive infundibular component; the only communication between atrialized ventricle and infundibulum is through the commissure between the anterior and septal tricuspid valve leaflets.

ASSOCIATED ANOMALIES

The most common associated anomaly[1–8,14–16] is an atrial septal defect, present in about 50 percent of cases. Variable degrees of right ventricular outflow tract obstruction may be present. A Wolff-Parkinson-White type of accessory pathway, often with associated preexcitation, is present in 4 to 26 percent of cases. In symptomatic neonates with severe obstruction to pulmonary blood flow, survival is dependent on the presence of a

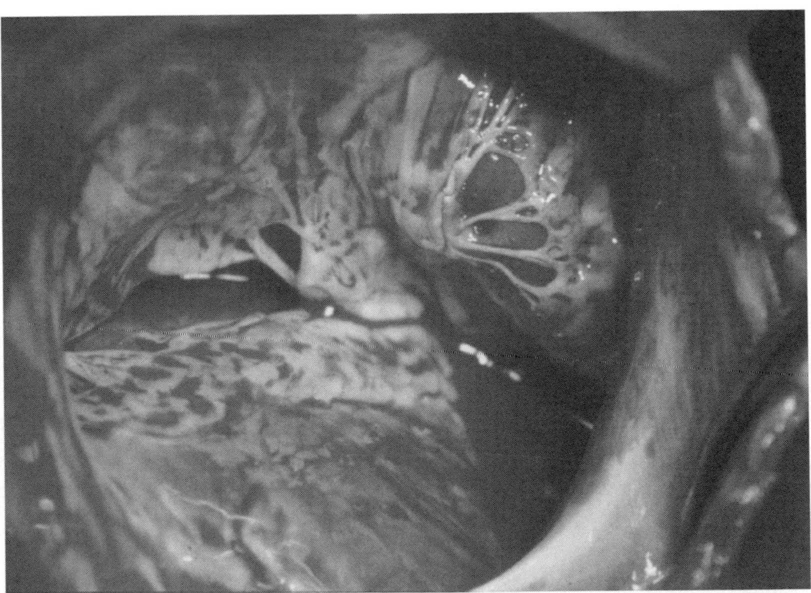

Figure 76-1 Ebstein's anomaly: morphology. Intraoperative photograph from a right atriotomy. (From Corno.[3] With permission. Courtesy of Dr. Sylvain Chauvaud, Hôpital Européen Georges Pompidou, Paris.)

concomitant patent ductus arteriosus. Rarely, there is association with an abnormality of ventriculoarterial connection or double discordance (atrioventricular and ventriculoarterial; see Chap. 67) or with partial anomalous pulmonary venous connection, cor triatriatum, atrioventricular septal defect, ventricular septal defect, tetralogy of Fallot, or aortic coarctation. Ebstein's anomaly can be seen in patients with Down's syndrome, Marfan's syndrome, Ulrich-Noonan syndrome, and Cornelia de Lange syndrome.

PATHOPHYSIOLOGY

The right atrium is usually dilated as a consequence of the abnormal valvular morphology, which most frequently leads tricuspid valve insufficiency. The anterior tricuspid valve leaflet forms a large sail-like structure with or without fenestrations and RVOTO; when there is no fenestration of the tricuspid valve leaflet, tricuspid stenosis can be the dominant valvular lesion. In severe cases, the inferior right ventricular wall is thin and void of muscle cells, thus forming an aneurysmal structure. The right ventricle is dilated and the interventricular septum bulges leftward: this may impair left ventricular function. The foramen ovale is almost always patent, sometimes associated with an ostium secundum atrial septal defect. The shunt at the atrial level can be left-to-right, right-to-left, or bidirectional, according to the presence and degree of right atrial hypertension due to right heart failure, tricuspid valve regurgitation, stenosis, or RVOTO.[3,4,14,15]

Patients with Ebstein's malformation are prone to arrhythmias as a consequence of several anatomic findings: (1) the right atrium is severely dilated, resulting in stretching and fibrosis; (2) in as many as 20 to 25 percent of patients, the poor fibrous development of the atrioventricular annulus results in the presence of bypass tracts from the atria to the ventricles, akin to Wolf-Parkinson-White syndrome; (3) the poor fibrous encasement of the atrioventricular node and bundle of His causes atrioventricular reentry tachycardia; and (4) ventricular arrhythmias result from the stretched, fibrotic, and dysplastic right ventricular myocardium.

Sudden death is encountered in 3 to 10 percent of patients, secondary to supraventricular tachycardia or rapid conduction of atrial fibrillation or flutter, leading to ventricular tachycardia.[1,3,4,6–8,17–18]

DIAGNOSIS

When patients with Ebstein's malformation present with profound cyanosis in the newborn period, this lesion is typically associated with severe tricuspid valve regurgitation and massive right atrial dilatation; in these patients, the presentation is similar to that of newborns with pulmonary atresia/intact ventricular septum or with tricuspid atresia.[1,3–8,19–23]

On the other hand, if the malformation is mild and the right atrium does not dilate significantly soon after birth owing to a drop in the pulmonary vascular resistance, the clinical situation may improve. In older patients, signs and symptoms are due to progressively increasing cyanosis, heart failure, reduced effort tolerance, and arrhythmias.[24,25] Although patients can also present with sudden death or paradoxical embolization,[1,3,4,7,8] the severity of the clinical picture does not necessarily correlate with the extent of the pathologic changes of the tricuspid valve.

On physical examination, cyanosis and clubbing are common, and chest wall deformity secondary to cardiomegaly is often seen. Even though the precordium can be quiet, diastolic or systolic murmurs can be auscultated in the presence of inflow/outflow tract obstruction or tricuspid valve regurgitation. The most striking finding on physical examination is that of a gallop rhythm, with a split S_1 (due to the delay in tricuspid valve closure) and a persistently split S_2 secondary to right bundle branch block and delayed right ventricular semilunar valve closure; also, ventricular filling sounds are present. With a very compliant right atrium, jugular venous distention and hepatosplenomegaly can be minimal.

Electrocardiographic examination discloses prolongation of the PR interval in 16 to 42 percent of cases; right axis deviation, right atrial enlargement and right bundle branch block are also observed, often with a decrease in the R wave amplitude in leads V_1 through V_4. An absent Q wave in V_6 due to ventricular displacement secondary to a dilated right atrium can be seen, while complete or incomplete right bundle branch block is present in 77 to 94 percent of cases; 4 to 26 percent of patients also manifest electrocardiographic evidence of Wolf-Parkinson-White syndrome.

Variable degrees of cardiomegaly are noted on chest x-ray, mainly secondary to right atrial enlargement with posterior apical displacement. The lung fields appear normal or hypoperfused according to the degree of RVOTO.

Echocardiography is diagnostic and allows definition of the following features:

- Presence and degree of right-to-left shunt at the atrial level
- Degree of tricuspid regurgitation (width of jet at origin and retrograde extension toward the hepatic veins (Fig. 76-2)
- Right atrial and ventricular size (Fig. 76-3) and function
- Left ventricular function

In addition, echocardiography can assess the potential response to surgery by assessing the following anatomic variables: displacement of septal leaflet, degree of tethering, dysplasia and fenestration of the anterior leaflet of the tricuspid valve, and right ventricular enlargement.

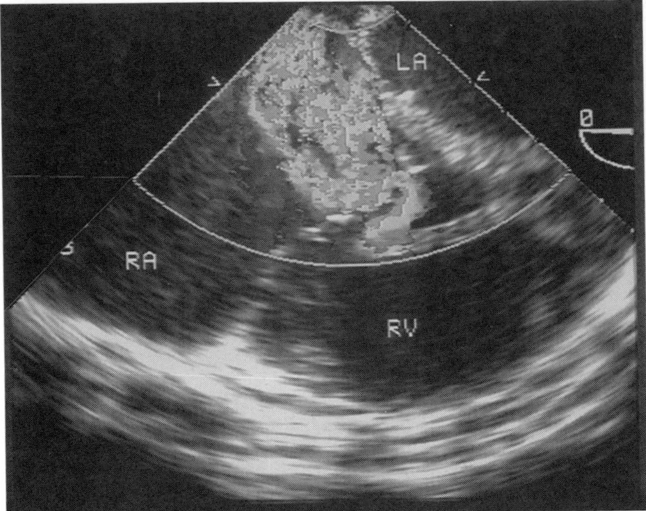

Figure 76-2 Ebstein's anomaly: echocardiographic findings. Transesophageal color Doppler echocardiogram showing severe tricuspid valve regurgitation. LA = left atrium, RA = right atrium, RV = right ventricle. (From Corno.[3] With permission. Courtesy of Dr. Pierre-Guy Chassot.)

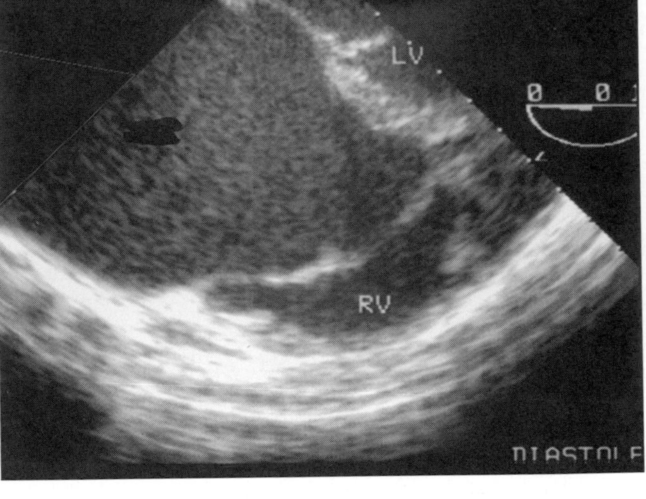

Figure 76-3 Ebstein's anomaly: echocardiographic findings. Transesophageal echocardiogram showing the size of the right atrium and ventricle and the displacement of the anterior leaflet of the tricuspid valve. LV = left ventricle, RV = right ventricle. (From Corno.[3] With permission. Courtesy of Dr. Pierre-Guy Chassot.)

Cardiac catheterization should be performed with great caution, as it may lead to life-threatening arrhythmias; it is indicated only to rule out increased pulmonary vascular resistance or the presence of associated complex cardiac malformations during preoperative investigation.

NATURAL HISTORY

Mortality in untreated children presenting in the neonatal period is 30 to 50 percent and, considering all ages, ranges between 12.5 and 21.0 percent.[1,3–8,19] Mortality is higher in the presence of severe right atrial enlargement, a large atrialized right ventricular portion, and a distally tethered tricuspid valve leaflet with right ventricular dysplasia.

Mortality rates are higher in patients with other associated congenital heart diseases and when presentation is in infancy with severe cyanosis and/or congestive heart failure.

INDICATIONS FOR SURGICAL TREATMENT

Surgery is indicated in symptomatic neonates with Ebstein's anomaly because of severe tricuspid valve regurgitation and often a massively dilated right atrium, right-to-left shunting at the atrial level, and reduced pulmonary blood flow, a clinical picture similar to that of pulmonary atresia with intact ventricular septum (see Chap. 62). In older children and adults, surgery is usually indicated because of cyanosis, heart failure, and arrhythmias.

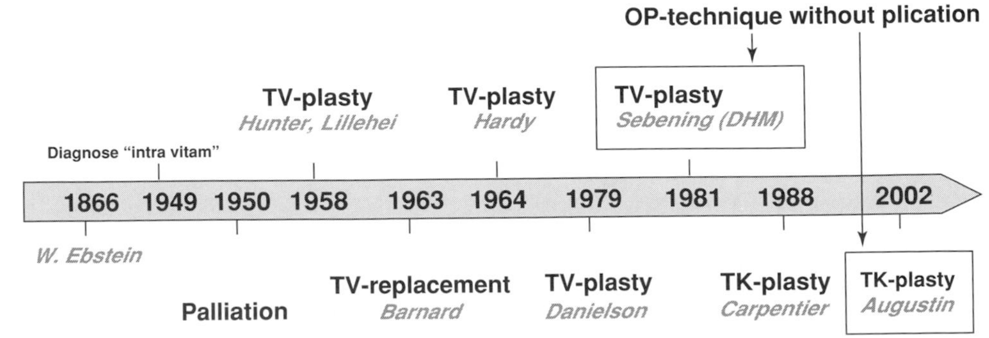

Figure 76-4 Historical evolution of the surgical approach to Ebstein's anomaly.

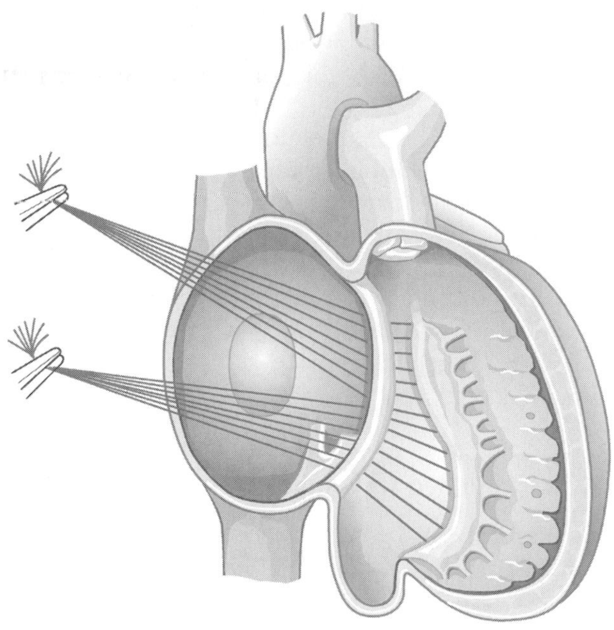

Figure 76-5 Exclusion of the "atrialized" right ventricle with transverse plication. (From Hardy et al.[35] With permission.)

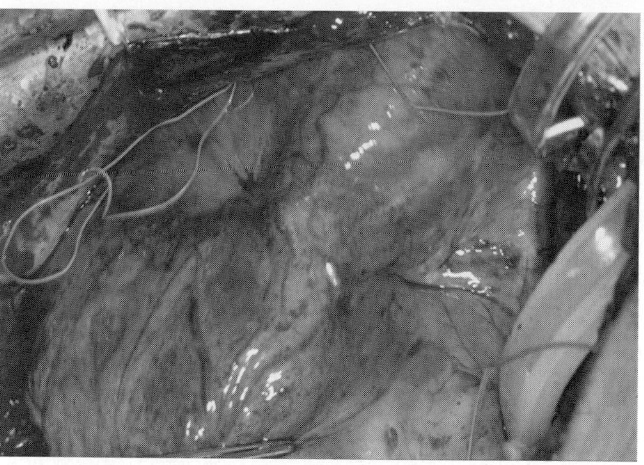

Figure 76-6 Intraoperative photograph showing the external cardiac appearance following plication of the atrialized portion of the right ventricle. (From Corno.[3] With permission.)

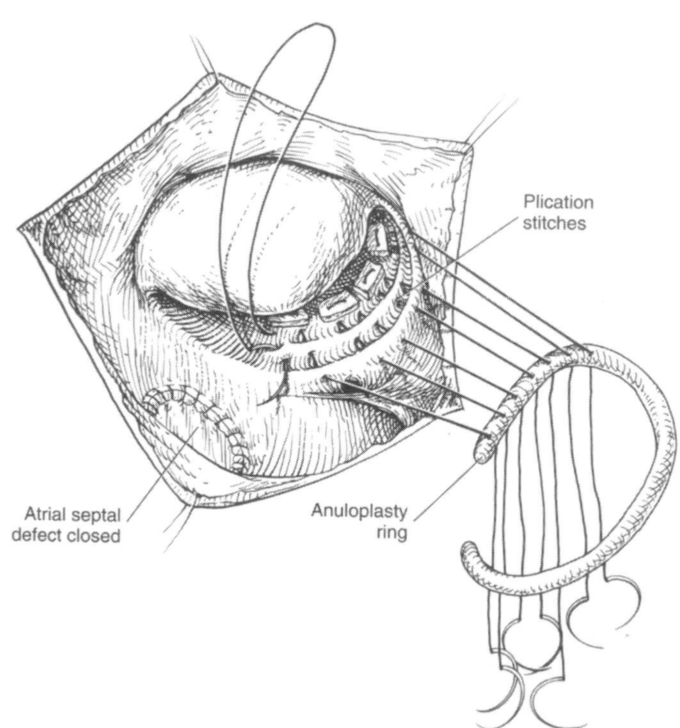

Figure 76-7 Danielson technique for repair of Ebstein's anomaly. Pledgeted sutures are utilized to plicate the atrialized portion of the right ventricle are then used to secure an annuloplasty ring in place. (From *Kirklin/Barratt-Boyes cardiac surgery* 3rd edition. Kouchoukos et al. (eds). Philadelphia: Churchill Livingstone: 2003, 1190. With permission.)

SURGICAL TREATMENT

The surgical approach to Ebstein's anomaly has seen a substantial evolution over the last four decades (Fig. 76-4). First surgical attempts aimed at closing only the interatrial communication or at increasing the pulmonary blood flow with palliative procedures such as aortopulmonary shunts or cavopulmonary connections. The operative results were usually far from satisfactory.[10,23,26,27]

The focus then shifted on tricuspid valve replacement, with Christian Barnard, in 1968, first implanting a mechanical prosthesis in a patient with Ebstein's anomaly.[28] However, initial attempts at treating this malformation with tricuspid valve replacement resulted in an early mortality of up to 54 percent.[8,25,29–33]

Hunter and Lillehei were the first to perform a tricuspid valvuloplasty for Ebstein's anomaly, although with a fatal outcome. They first reported plication of the atrialized right ventricle, thus trying to reposition the valvular plane.[34] A modification of this concept was later brought to clinical practice (Fig. 76-5), but this approach did not initially provide consistent results.[35,36]

The Fontan operation was then reported in a patient with Ebstein's anomaly,[37] opening the way toward a univentricular type of repair in selected cases.[38] Various technical modifications have also been reported, with improving short- and long-term results.[39] However, due to the rare occurrence of this congenital heart defect, most of these techniques were applied in rather small series and in case reports.

Currently adopted techniques

Here we focus on the surgical techniques that are currently most widely utilized, with consistent reports in an

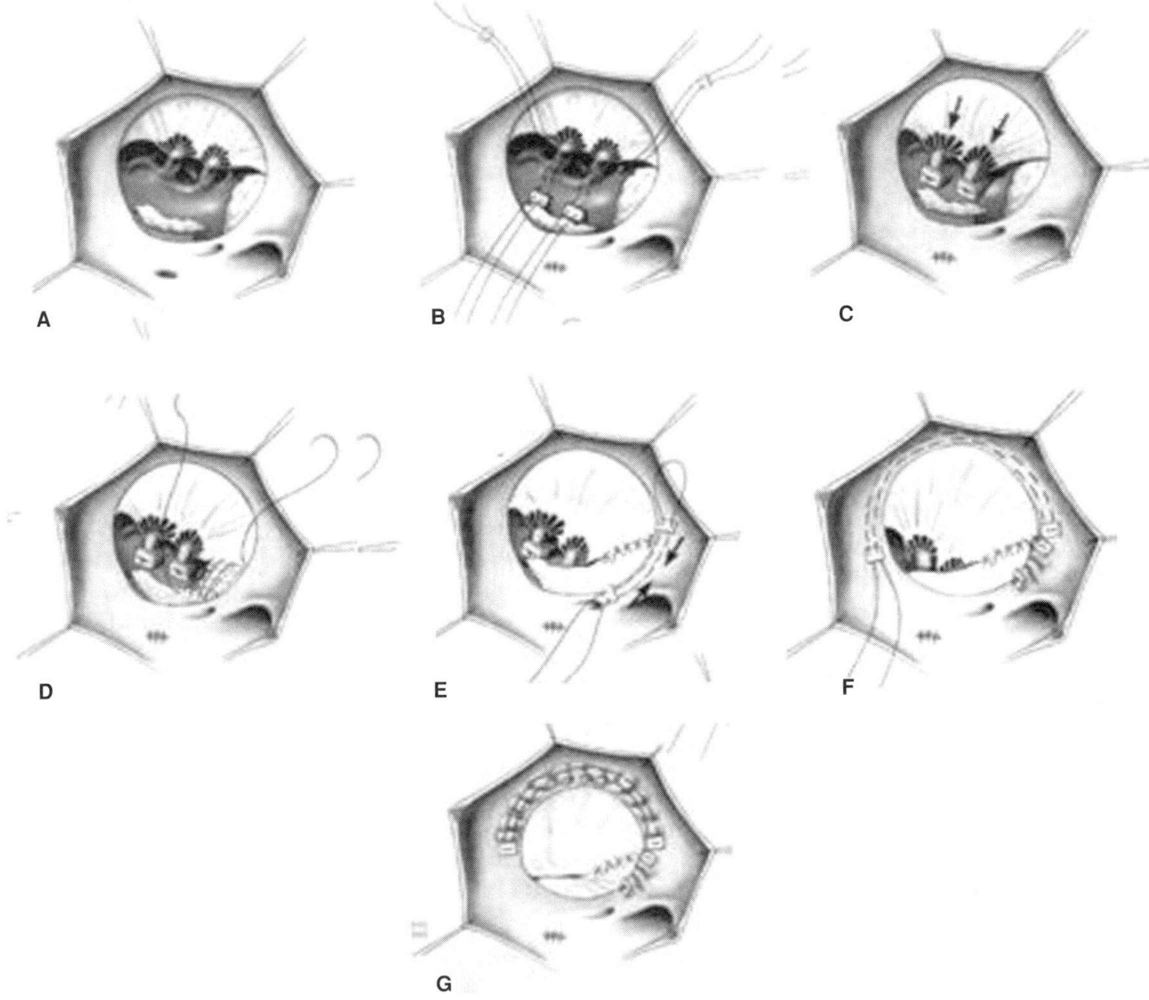

Figure 76-8 Dearani/Danielson technique. Ebstein's morphology (A). The base of the papillary muscle(s) is moved toward the ventricular septum (B and C). The posterior angle of the tricuspid orifice is closed by plication (D). Posterior annuloplasty (E). Anterior purse-string annuloplasty to complete the repair (F and G). (From Dearani and Danielson.[24] With permission.)

adequate number of patients and with particular emphasis on the techniques adopted by the authors.

As a general consideration in repairing Ebstein's anomaly, intraoperative transesophageal echocardiography is an invaluable tool, as it can provide morphologic and functional information to better plan and immediately assess the result of surgical intervention.

Surgical repair typically includes the following steps:

1. Closure of the atrial septal defect
2. Plication of the atrialized portion of the right ventricle (Figs. 76-5 and 76-6) or no plication at all (see Deutsches Herzzentrum München experience)[40–47]
3. Repair of the tricuspid valve[40–50]

Tricuspid valve replacement[51] may be required in cases of unsatisfactory repair or unfavorable anatomy of the valvular tissue (i.e., size of anterior leaflet, grade of tethering, grade of displacement of the valvular plane).

Danielson technique (monocusp-plasty with transverse plication)

Danielson at the Mayo Clinic developed a repair consisting of plication of the free wall of the atrialized portion of the right ventricle, posterior tricuspid annuloplasty, and excision of redundant right atrial wall.[6,30,31,43] The repair was based on the construction of a monocusp valve with the use of the anterior tricuspid leaflet, which is usually enlarged in this anomaly (Fig. 76-7).

Dearani/Danielson technique (monocusp-plasty with anterolateral shifting of the valvular plane, with or without plication)

This most recent modification involves bringing the anterior papillary muscle(s) toward the ventricular septum with one or more pledgeted sutures to facilitate closure of the anterior leaflet against the septum, as well as the addition of an anterior purse-string annuloplasty to repair those hearts that have extensive dilatation of the RVOT and of the anterior portion of the tricuspid annulus (Fig. 76-8).[24] This technique shows similarities to the Augustin/Sebening technique.

Carpentier technique (remodeling with longitudinal plication)

Carpentier developed a complex but efficient method for valve repair (Fig. 76-9). The four systematic surgical steps were as follows: (1) mobilization of the anterosuperior leaflet, (2) longitudinal plication of the atrialized right ventricle, (3) plication of the tricuspid valve annulus with rotation, and (4) reattachment of the anterosuperior leaflet on the right atrioventricular groove. Reinforcement of the tricuspid annulus with a prosthetic ring was used only in adult patients. The interatrial communication was always closed.[12,13,42] Recently, Chauvaud added a bidirectional cavopulmonary shunt in selected patients in order to decrease preload of the compromised right ventricle.[52]

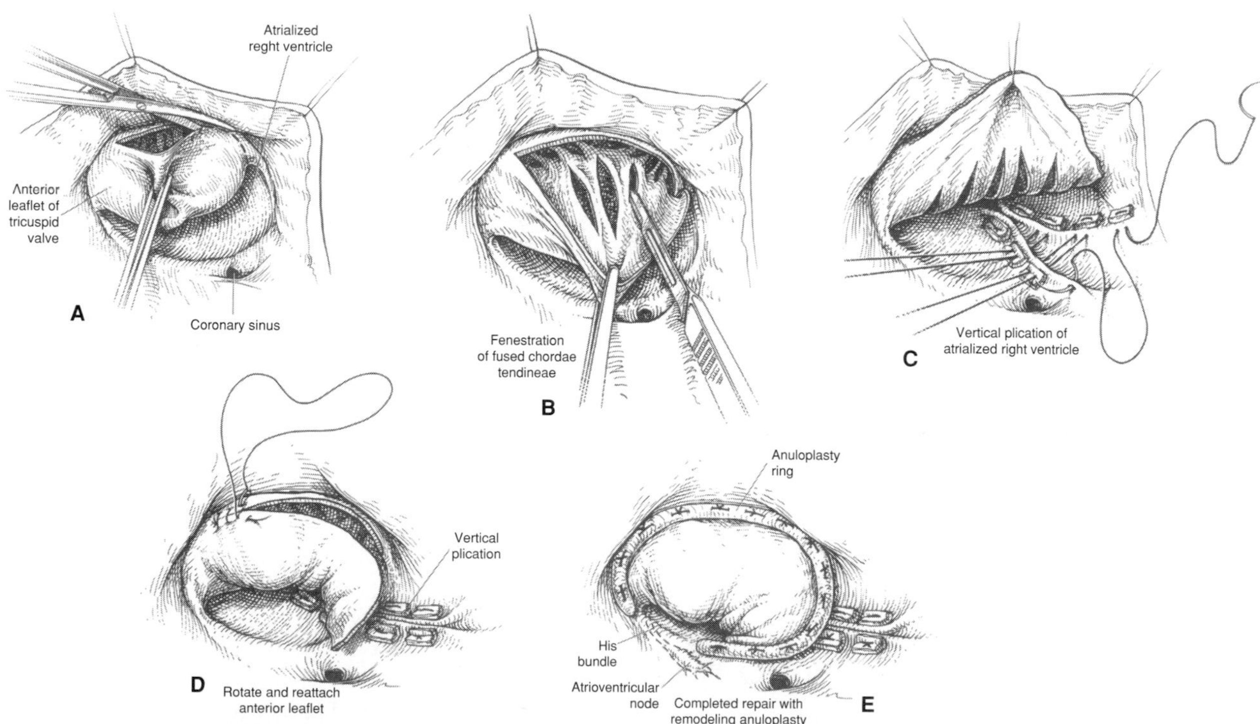

Figure 76-9 Carpentier technique. Initial morphology (A). Mobilization of the anterior leaflet and longitudinal plication of the atrialized portion of the right ventricle (B and C), with clockwise rotation of the anterior leaflet and suture on the atrioventricular junction (D). Final appearance (E). (From Danielson et al.[30] With permission.)

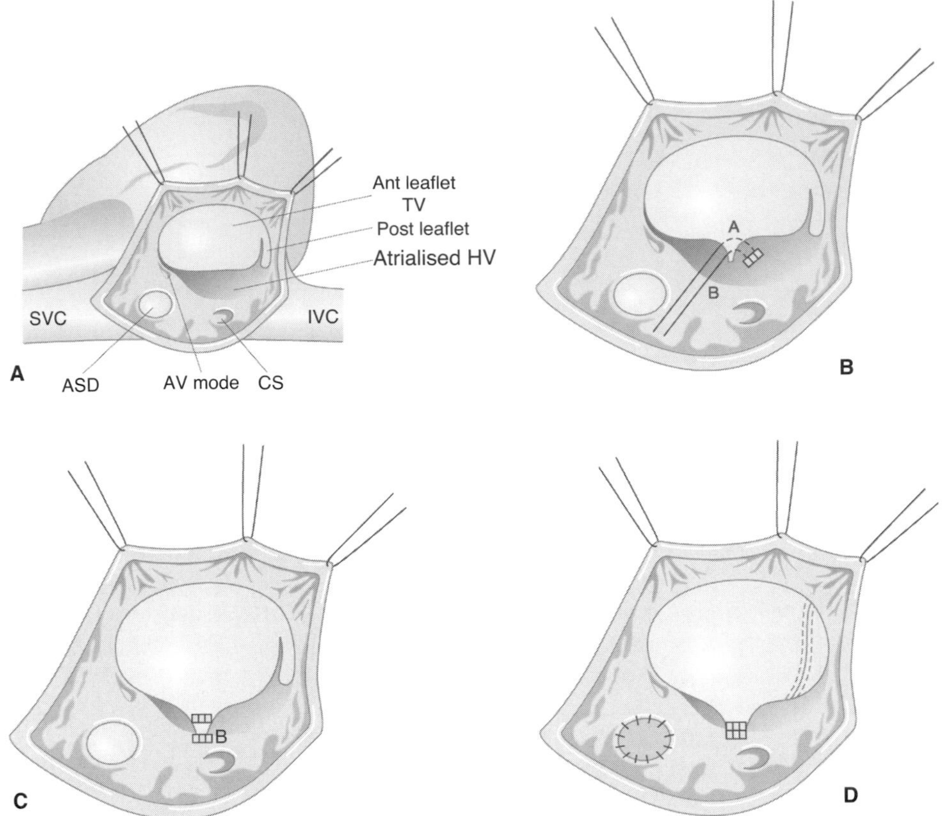

Figure 76-10 Sebening technique. After identification of the papillary muscles (A), placement of a pledgeted stitch (B) and anterolateral relocation (B and C) is accomplished. C. Closure of the "commissure" between the anterior and posterior leaflets (or free wall). A plication of the atrialized portion is not performed. (From Augustin et al.[40] With permission.)

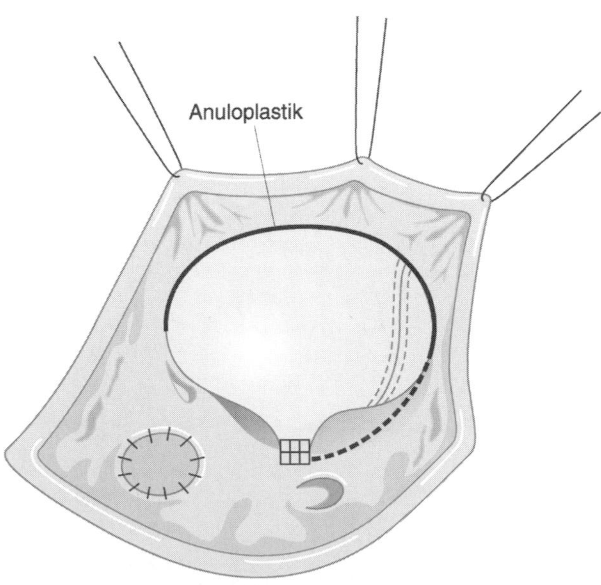

Figure 76-11 Augustin/Sebening technique. Additional stabilization of the valvular plane. Arrows indicate placement of additional stitches at the rightlateral aspect of the anterior leaflet toward the septal leaflet.

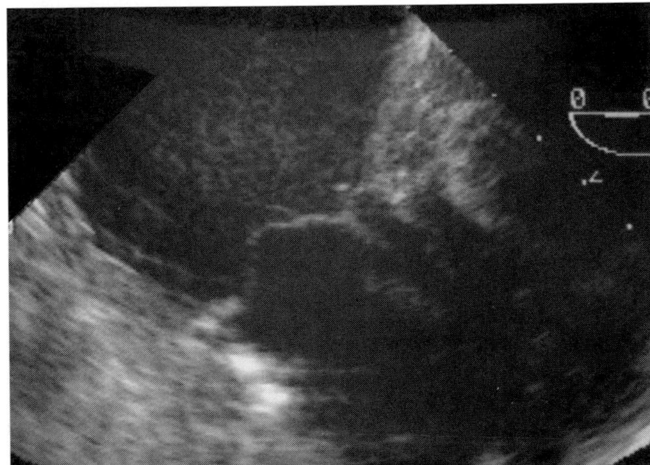

Figure 76-12 Postoperative transesophageal echocardiogram after reconstruction of the tricuspid valve, plication of the atrialized portion of the right ventricle, and end-to-side anastomosis of the superior vena cava to the right pulmonary artery (see Fig. 76-2 for the preoperative echocardiogram of the same patient). (From Corno.[3] With permission. Courtesy of Dr. Pierre-Guy Chassot.)

	Pat n	30-day-mortality %	Plasty %	Re-OP %	OP-technique
Watson (Int. study) 1974	57	54.5	0	0	various
Danielson et al. 1997	323	6.5	42.7	16.7	transverse plication
Renfu et al. 2001	139	8.6	80.0	9.0	various plications
Chauvaud et al. 2003	210	9.0	98.0	9.0	longitudinal plication
Multi-Center study (ECHSA) 2005	152 (28 re-op)	13.0	47.4	9.0	various
DHM 2005	110	1.8	89.1	17.3	no plication

Figure 76-13 Metanalysis of six large clinical series of patients with Ebstein's anomaly undergoing surgical intervention.

Sebening technique (monocusp-plasty with anterolateral shifting of the valvular plane by "relocating" the anterior leaflet without plication)

The "single-stitch technique" was developed at the Deutsches Herzzentrum München. This modification includes a monocusp-plasty with anterolateral shifting of the valvular plane by "relocating" the anterior leaflet. The latter is achieved by stitching the papillary muscle(s) to the septum in the direction of the "true" valvular annulus (Fig. 76-10).

Augustin/Sebening technique (monocusp-plasty with anterolateral shifting of the valvular plane by "relocating" the anterior leaflet, with additional stitches between the anterior leaflet and the septum and annuloplasty techniques)

Another essential modification was introduced by Augustin since, with previous techniques, the rate of reoperation was as high as 17 percent after excellent early results and tricuspid valve function. The main component of this modification (Fig. 76-11) was the additional stabilization of the

n	110
Follow-up	95.5%
Interval	2 m – 28.5 y (Median 8.2 y, mean 10.3 y)

OP-procedure	%	n
Plasty	89.1	98
Replacement	8.2	9
Palliation	2.7	3

Figure 76-14 Clinical data on 110 patients with Ebstein's anomaly who underwent surgery between 1974 to 2004 at the Deutsches Herzzentrum München, Munich, Germany. Follow-up is complete for 105 patients (95.5 percent).

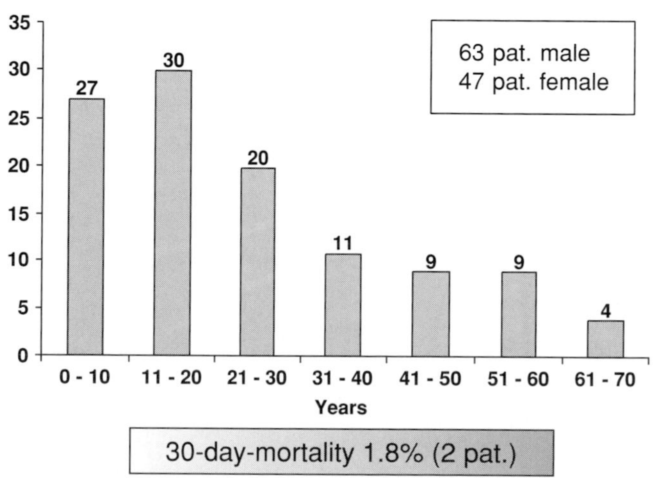

Figure 76-15 Age distribution for 110 patients with Ebstein's anomaly who underwent surgery at the authors' institution.

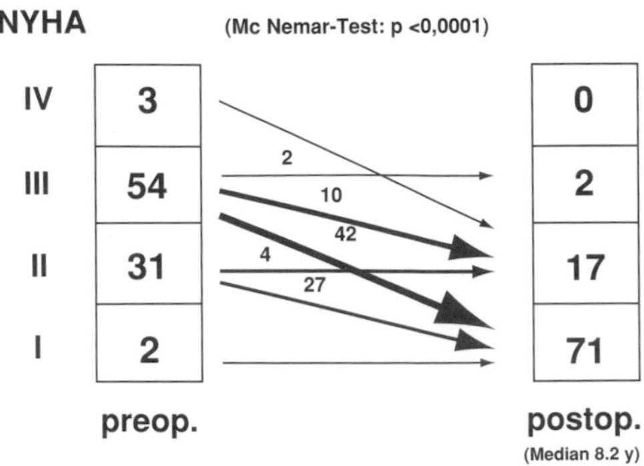

Figure 76-16 Improvement in New York Heart Association (NYHA) functional class after surgery in the authors' series.

annulus, either by placement of stitches at the right-lateral aspect of the anterior leaflet toward the septal leaflet or with reinforcement of the tricuspid annulus with a Teflon-felt strip or a tricuspid ring.[41]

"One–and one-half" ventricular repair

In patients with reduced size or function of the right ventricle, a one–and one-half ventricular repair is performed, with end-to-side anastomosis of the superior vena cava to the right pulmonary artery (in addition to the intracardiac repair) in order to reduce the volume overload imposed on the small, malfunctioning right ventricle following repair.[52–60] In a group of patients with Ebstein's anomaly, cyanosis, severe tricuspid valve regurgitation, and compromised left ventricular function (mean ejection fraction 58 percent, mean shortening fraction 25 percent), the one–and one-half ventricular repair provided complete regression of cyanosis and signs of heart failure,[56] reduced the degree of tricuspid valve regurgitation (Fig. 76-12), and improved left ventricular function (postoperative mean ejection fraction and shortening fraction of 77 and 40 percent, respectively).

Antiarrhythmia procedures

Preoperative electrophysiologic assessment for bypass pathways is necessary in order to perform intraoperative ablation. Concomitant intraoperative procedures for arrhythmias can be performed at the time of intracardiac repair without an increase in early mortality. These procedures should be performed in addition to repair in all patients with Ebstein's anomaly and supraventricular tachyarrhythmias documented preoperatively. Surgical procedures for accessory pathway–mediated tachycardia and atrioventricular nodal reentrant tachycardia provide excellent (up to 100 percent) freedom from recurrence, while recurrence following surgical treatment of atrial flutter/fibrillation is approximately 25 percent.[17,18]

When ventricular pacing is required, it should be done with epicardial rather than transvenous leads, since tricuspid valve function is already compromised.

SURGICAL OUTCOMES

Specific complications can be observed following repair of this complex malformation: residual or recurrent atrial septal defect; residual, recurrent, or surgically induced tricuspid valve stenosis or insufficiency; complete atrioventricular block; right coronary artery obstruction during the process of plication; and right and/or left ventricular dysfunction.

Several groups have gained a vast experience in the treatment of this rare malformation over the years (Fig. 76-13).

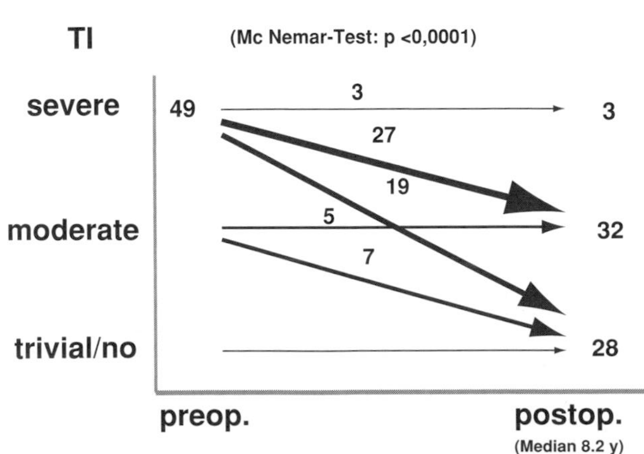

Figure 76-17 Tricuspid valve function following surgery. TI = tricuspid insufficiency.

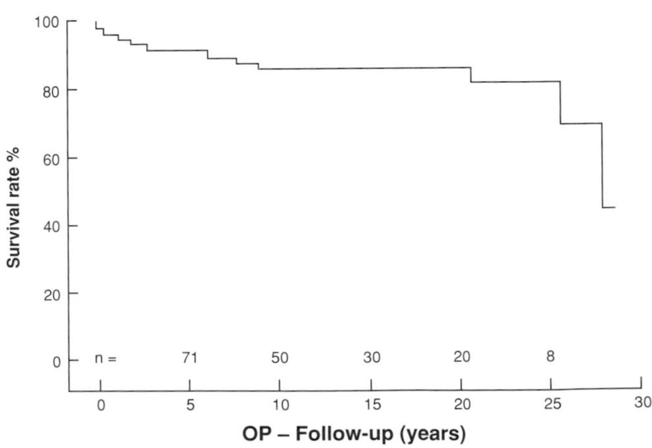

Figure 76-18 Actuarial survival curve for 110 patients with Ebstein's anomaly who underwent surgery at the authors' institution.

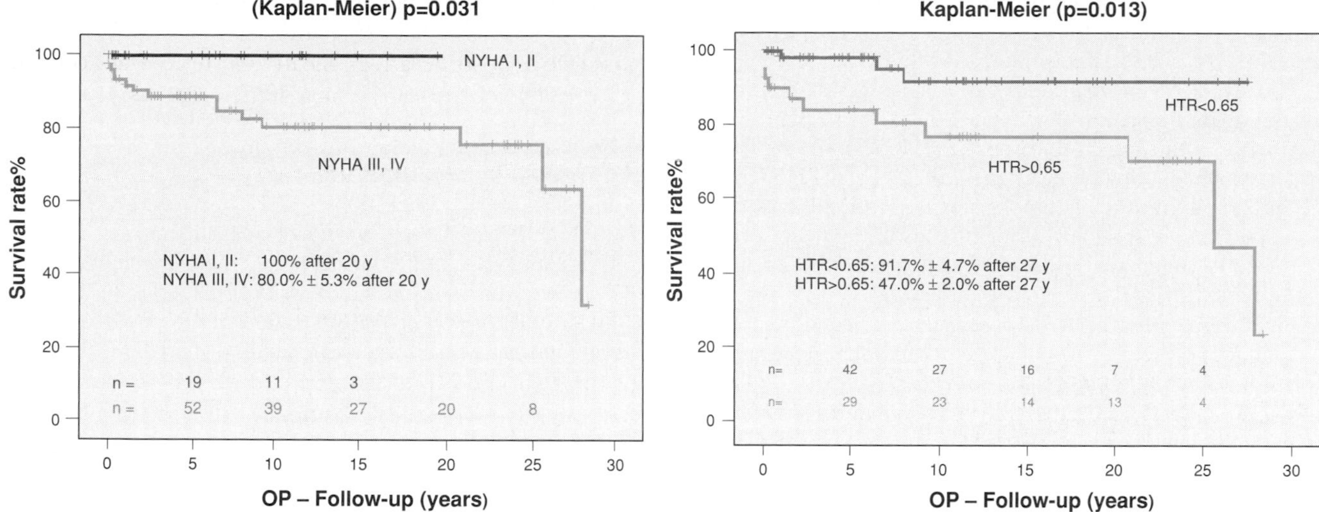

Figure 76-19 Influence of preoperative NYHA functional class (left panel) and preoperative cardiomegaly (as indicated by cardiothoracic ratio, HTR, right panel) on long-term survival in the authors' series.

However, for the purpose of this chapter, focus is solely on the surgical results from the Deutsches Herzzentrum München, as reported in Figs. 76-14 to 76-19).

As evidenced by our outcome data, the reduction of tricuspid valve insufficiency must be seen as the key to surgical repair and successful long-term outcomes. Timely intervention is therefore indicated, even when patients are still in functional New York Heart Association (NYHA) class II, and in the presence of a cardiac/thoracic ratio greater than 0.65.

Despite effective loss of the inlet component, the "functional" right ventricle often remains of moderate or good size in comparison with the size of the left ventricle. Plication of the atrialized right ventricle or mobilization of the valvular apparatus does not seem to be essential from a morphologic standpoint. Other complex repair techniques may even put the right coronary artery at risk.

If none of the tricuspid valve repair techniques mentioned above lead to a reduction of the degree of tricuspid insufficiency to less than moderate (without inducing any stenosis), we strongly advocate primary valve replacement. Valve replacement, with either a mechanical or biological prosthesis, yields satisfactory results in the current era. In this respect, every effort should be made to limit the duration of cardiac ischemia. In the absence of an interatrial communication, valvular repair (especially annuloplasty techniques and even valve replacement) may be performed on the beating heart, therefore avoiding any period of cardioplegic cardiac arrest.

References

1. Attenhofer Jost CH, Connolly HM, Edwards WD, et al. Ebstein's anomaly. Review of a multifaceted congenital cardiac condition. *Swiss Med Wkly* 2005;135:269.
2. Becker AE, Becker MJ, Edwards JE. Pathologic spectrum of dysplasia of the tricuspid valve. Features in common with Ebstein's malformation. *Arch Pathol* 1971;91:167.
3. Corno AF. Congenital heart defects. In: *Decision Making for Surgery.* Vol 1. *Common Defects.* Darmstadt, Germany: Steinkopff Verlag, 2003.
4. Flores Arizmendi A, Fernandez Pineda L, Quero Jimenez C, et al. The clinical profile of Ebstein's malformation as seen from the fetus to the adult in 52 patients. *Cardiol Young* 2004;14:55.
5. Fyler DC, Buckley LP, Hellenbrand WE. Report of the New England Regional Infant Care Program. *Pediatrics* 1980;65(Suppl):375.
6. Mair DD. Ebstein's anomaly: Natural history and management. *J Am Coll Cardiol* 1992;19:1047.
7. Szydlowski L, Rudzinski A, Kordon Z, et al. Clinical picture and treatment in various presentations of Ebstein's anomaly in children. *Acta Cardiol* 2004;59:240.
8. Watson H. Natural history of Ebstein's anomaly of the tricuspid valve in childhood and adolescence: An international cooperative study of 505 cases. *Br Heart J* 1974;36:417.
9. Schreiber C, Cook A, Ho SY, et al. Morphologic spectrum of Ebstein's malformation: Revisitation relative to surgical repair. *J Thorac Cardiovasc Surg* 1999;117:148.
10. Wright JL, Burchell HB, Kirklin JW, et al. Congenital displacement of the tricuspid valve (Ebstein's malformation): Report of a case with closure of an associated foramen ovale for correction of the right-to-left shunt. *Mayo Clin Proc* 1954;29:278.
11. Zuberbuhler JR, Allwork SP, Anderson RH. The spectrum of Ebstein's anomaly of the tricuspid valve. *J Thorac Cardiovasc Surg* 1979;77:202.

12. Carpentier A, Chauvaud S, Macé L, et al. A new reconstructive operation for Ebstein's anomaly of the tricuspid valve. *J Thorac Cardiovasc Surg* 1988;96:92.
13. Chauvaud SM, Mihaileanu SA, Gaer JAR, et al. Surgical treatment of Ebstein's malformation. The Hôspital Broussais experience. *Cardiol Young* 1996;6:4.
14. Haworth SG, Shinebourne EA, Miller GAH. Right-to-left interatrial shunting with normal right ventricular pressure. A puzzling haemodynamic picture associated with some rare congenital malformations of the tricuspid valve and right ventricle. *Br Heart J* 1975;37:386.
15. Schire V, Sutin GL, Barnard CN. Organic and functional pulmonary atresia with intact ventricular septum. *Am J Cardiol* 1961;8:100.
16. Wang RX, Li XR, Qian DJ. Ebstein's malformation with atrial septal defect, right cor triatriatum, and right overt accessory atrioventricular pathway. *Heart* 2005;91:25
17. Bockeria L, Golukhova E, Dadasheva M, et al. Advantages and disadvantages of one-stage and two-stage surgery for arrhythmias and Ebstein's anomaly. *Eur J Cardiothorac Surg* 2005;28:536.
18. Khositeth A, Danielson GK, Dearani JA, et al. Supraventricular tachyarrhytmias in Ebstein anomaly: Management and outcome. *J Thorac Cardiovasc Surg* 2004;128:826.
19. Di Russo GB, Gaynor JW. Ebstein's anomaly: Indications for repair and surgical technique. *Semin Thorac Cardiovasc Surg* 1999;2:35.
20. Knott-Craig CJ, Overholt ED, Ward KE, et al. Repair of Ebstein's anomaly in the symptomatic neonate: An evolution of technique with 7-year follow-up. *Ann Thorac Surg* 2002;73:1786.
21. McElhinney DB, Salvin JW, Colan SD, et al. Improving outcomes in fetuses and neonates with congenital displacement (Ebstein's malformation) or dysplasia of the tricuspid valve. *Am J Cardiol* 2005;15:582.
22. Pfaumer A, Eicken A, Augustin N, et al. Symptomatic neonates with Ebstein anomaly. *J Thorac Cardiovasc Surg* 2004;127:1208.
23. Starnes VA, Pitlick PT, Bernstein D, et al. Ebstein's anomaly appearing in the neonate. A new surgical approach. *J Thorac Cardiovasc Surg* 1991;101:1082.
24. Dearani JA, Danielson GK. Surgical management of Ebstein's anomaly in the adult. *Semin Thorac Cardiovasc Surg* 2005;17:148.
25. McFaul RC, Davis Z, Giuliani ER, et al. Ebstein's malformation: Surgical experience at the Mayo Clinic. *J Thorac Cardiovasc Surg* 1976;72:910.
26. Glenn WWL. Circulatory bypass of the right side of the heart. Shunt between superior vena cava and distal right pulmonary artery. Report of clinical application. *N Eng J Med* 1958;259:117.
27. Timmis HH, Hardy JD, Watson DG. The surgical management of Ebstein's anomaly: The combined use of tricuspid valve replacement, atrioventricular plication, and atrioplasty. *J Thorac Cardiovasc Surg* 1967;53:385.
28. Barnard CN, Schrire V. Surgical correction of Ebstein's malformation with a prosthetic tricuspid valve. *Surgery* 1963;54:302.
29. Cartwright RS, Smeloff EA, Cayler GG, et al. Total correction of Ebstein's anomaly by means of tricuspid replacement. *J Thoracic Cardiovas Surg* 1964;47: 755.
30. Danielson GK, Maloney JD, Devloo RAE. Surgical repair of Ebstein's anomaly. *Mayo Clin Proc* 1979;54:185.
31. Danielson GK, Fuster V. Surgical repair of Ebstein's anomaly. *Ann Surg* 1982;196:499.
32. Pasqué M, Williams WG, Coles JG, et al. Tricuspid valve replacement in children. *Ann Thorac Surg* 1987;44:164.
33. Westaby S, Karp RB, Kirklin JW, et al. Surgical treatment in Ebstein's malformation. *Ann Thorac Surg* 1982;34:388.
34. Hunter SW, Lillehei CW. Ebstein's malformation of the tricuspid valve. Study of a case together with suggestion of a new form of surgical therapy. *Chest* 1958;33:297.
35. Hardy KL, May IA, Webster CA, et al. Ebstein's anomaly: A functional concept and successful definitive repair. *J Thorac Cardiovasc Surg* 1964;48:927.
36. Hardy KL, Roe BB. Ebstein's anomaly: Further experience with definitive repair. *J Thorac Cardiovasc Surg* 1969;58:553.
37. Marcelletti C, Duren DR, Schuilenburg RM, et al. Fontan's operation for Ebstein's anomaly. *J Thorac Cardiovasc Surg* 1980;79:63.
38. Sano S, Ishino K, Kawada M, Kasahara S, et al. Total right ventricular exclusion procedure: An operation for isolated congestive right ventricular failure. *J Thorac Cardiovasc Surg* 2002;123:640.
39. Chen JM, Mosca RS, Altmann K, et al. Early and medium-term results for repair of Ebstein anomaly. *J Thorac Cardiovasc Surg* 2004;127:990.
40. Augustin N, Schmidt-Habelmann P, Wottke M, et al. Results after surgical repair of Ebstein's anomaly. *Ann Thorac Surg* 1997;63:1650.
41. Augustin N, Schreiber C, Badiu C, et al. Ebstein´s anomaly: 30 year Munich experience of surgical treatment. Presented at the fourth WCPCCS, Buenos Aires, September 2005.
42. Chauvaud S, Berrebi A, d'Attellis N, et al. Ebstein's anomaly: Repair based on functional analysis. *Eur J Cardiothorac Surg* 2003;23:525.
43. Danielson GK, Driscoll DJ, Mair DD, et al. Operative treatment of Ebstein's anomaly. *J Thorac Cardiovasc Surg* 1992;104:1195.
44. Hancock Friesen CL, Chen R, Howlett JG, et al. Posterior annular plication: Tricuspid valve repair in Ebstein's anomaly. *Ann Thorac Surg* 2004;77:2167.
45. Ullmann MV, Born S, Sebening C, et al. Ventricularization of the atrialized chamber: A concept of Ebstein's anomaly repair. *Ann Thorac Surg* 2004;78:918.
46. Wu Q, Huang Z. Anatomic correction of Ebstein anomaly. *J Thorac Cardiovasc Surg* 2001;122:1237.
47. Wu Q, Huang Z. A new procedure for Ebstein's anomaly. *Ann Thorac Surg* 2004;77:470.
48. Cherian SM, Varghese R, Sankar NM, et al. De Vega's tricuspid annuloplasty for Ebstein's anomaly. *J Cardiovasc Surg* 2003;44:231.
49. De Vega NG. La annuloplastia selectiva, regulable y permanente. Una technica original para el tratamiento de la insuficiencia tricuspide. *Rev Esp Cardiol* 1972;25:555.
50. Schmidt-Habelmann P, Meisner H, Struck E, et al. Results of valvuloplasty for Ebstein's anomaly. *Thorac Cardiovasc Surg* 1981;29:155.
51. Davtyan HG, Corno AF, Drinkwater DC, et al. Valve replacement for congenital heart disease. *Circulation* 1986;74:II-250.

52. Chauvaud S, Fuzzelier J, Berrebi A, et al. Bi-directional cavopulmonary shunt associated with valvuloplasty in Ebstein's anomaly: Benefits in high risk patients. *Eur J Cardiothorac Surg* 1998;13:514.
53. Chowdhury UK, Airan B, Talwar S, et al. One and one-half ventricle repair: Results and concerns. *Ann Thorac Surg* 2005;80:2293.
54. Corno AF, Mazzera E, Marino B, et al. Bidirectional cavopulmonary anastomosis. *J Am Coll Cardiol* 1989;13:74.
55. Corno AF. Surgery for congenital heart disease. *Curr Opin* Cardiol 2000;15:238.
56. Corno AF, Chassot PG, Payot M, et al. Ebstein's anomaly: One and half ventricular repair. *Swiss Med Weekly* 2002; 132;485.
57. Corno AF. Surgical treatment of complex cardiac anomalies: the "one and half ventricle repair." *Eur J Cardiothorac Surg* (editorial comment) 2002;22:436.
58. Gasul BM, Weinberg M, Luan LL, et al. Superior vena cava–right main pulmonary artery anastomosis. Surgical correction for patients with Ebstein's anomaly and for congenital hypoplastic right ventricle. *JAMA* 1959;171: 1797.
59. Mazzera E, Corno AF, Picardo S, et al. Bidirectional cavopulmonary shunts: Clinical applications as staged or definitive palliation. *Ann Thorac Surg* 1989;47:415.
60. Reddy VM, McElhinney DB, Silverman NH, et al. Partial biventricular repair for complex congenital heart defects: An intermediate option for complicated anatomy or functionally borderline right complex heart. *J Thorac Cardiovasc Surg* 1998;116:21.

CHAPTER

77 EXTRACORPOREAL MEMBRANE OXYGENATION IN PEDIATRIC CARDIAC CARE

Harris Baden, Howard Jeffries, Gordon A. Cohen

INTRODUCTION

From the earliest days, advances in extracorporeal membrane oxygenation (ECMO) have been linked to advances in cardiopulmonary bypass (CPB) and repair of congenital cardiac malformations. Since C. Walton Lillihei[1] first employed the technique of controlled cross-circulation using the patient's parent, efforts to perfect cardiopulmonary support have transitioned from the operating suite to the intensive care bedside. In the intervening years, every facet of cardiopulmonary bypass has been studied and refined. Improvements in these techniques have afforded the surgeon the opportunity to tackle even the most complex anatomic anomalies in even the smallest babies. Likewise, advances in extracorporeal support methods have led clinicians to expand clinical indications and implementation in the ICU. However, despite the fact that these practices usually originated in the cardiac surgical suite, heart disease was, until the last decade or so, usually a contraindication for ECMO. Early experience in adults was discouraging,[2] with better success reported in the care of newborns with respiratory failure.[3] Extension to include older infants and children with respiratory failure followed.[4]

Cardiac ECMO, as it has come to be known, was almost unheard of until the late 1980s. As preoperative, anesthetic, CPB, and surgical techniques evolved and improved, ECMO use for isolated cardiac or combined cardiorespiratory failure expanded, usually as a last-ditch effort for the dying infant or child. With experience, refinement, and successes, cardiac ECMO has begun to make the transition from "rescue" therapy, to "therapeutic" or even "preventive" management. Coincident with advances in pharmacologic and mechanical ventilatory support strategies for respiratory failure, the number of ECMO runs for the cardiac population has steadily increased as a proportion of the Extracorporeal Life Support Organization (ELSO) Registry (Fig. 77-1). Specifically, in 1985 there were only 32 cardiac ECMO cases versus 385 neonatal (noncardiac) cases, increasing to 548 cardiac cases versus 751 neonatal cases in 2003.[5] In this chapter, we take a comprehensive look at cardiac ECMO, with attention to the different types (venoarterial or venovenous), their relative indications, and their respective advantages, disadvantages, and outcomes. In addition, we discuss the myriad equipment options and also review the physiology of ECMO and principles of clinical application. Last, we consider new opportunities and indications for circulatory support.

VENOARTERIAL ECMO

In simplest terms, venoarterial ECMO (VA-ECMO) consists of taking deoxygenated blood from the venous circulation, oxygenating it, and then pumping it back into the arterial circulation. How this is accomplished depends on individual and institutional experience and preference. The obvious benefit is that the patient's entire cardiorespiratory system is bypassed, thereby ensuring adequate end-organ oxygenation even in the settings of respiratory and circulatory collapse. Ideally, the brain, kidneys, and other organs thereby maintain their essential functions in a circumstance that would otherwise almost surely lead to multiorgan failure and possibly death. Importantly, this support system likely creates an environment that is more conducive to functional improvement. There are ample data to support this assertion with regard to the lungs, and advances in the understanding of the pathogenesis of cardiac failure suggest that the same is likely true for the heart.[6]

Indications and experience

In neonates with congenital cardiac malformations, indications for VA-ECMO can arise soon after birth. The infant with obstructed total anomalous pulmonary venous drainage is the classic example of a newborn that can present in extremis and require emergent institution of VA-ECMO. Ideally, with VA-ECMO support, the baby's clinical condition can be optimized prior to surgical correction. Similarly, some neonates with congenital cardiomyopathy (i.e., dysrhythmias) will benefit from support while diagnostic studies and therapeutic interventions are pursued. Without ECMO, these babies might die before a diagnosis is established and therapies implemented.

Postoperative instability is the most common indication for VA-ECMO in the cardiac setting. Whether due to prolonged CPB or circulatory arrest times, complex surgical repair and manipulation of the heart, exaggerated inflammatory response to CPB, or inadequate

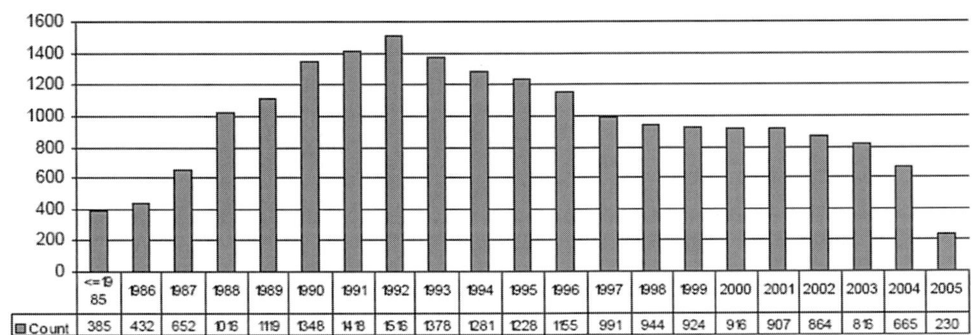

	<=1985	1986	1987	1988	1989	1990	1991	1992	1993	1994	1995	1996	1997	1998	1999	2000	2001	2002	2003	2004	2005
Count	385	432	652	1016	1119	1348	1418	1516	1378	1281	1228	1155	991	944	924	916	907	864	816	665	230

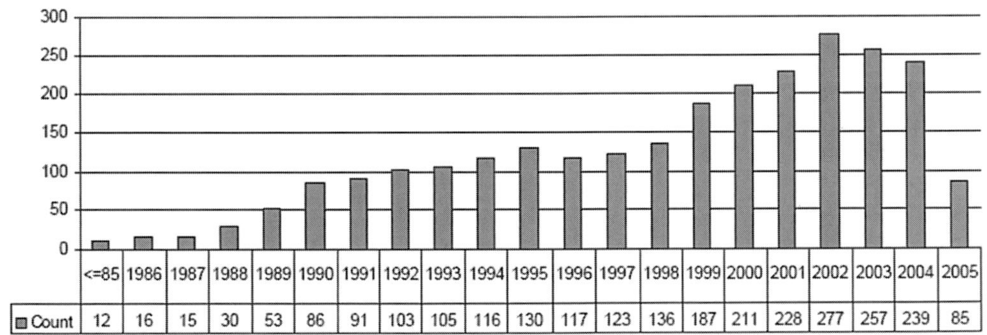

	<=85	1986	1987	1988	1989	1990	1991	1992	1993	1994	1995	1996	1997	1998	1999	2000	2001	2002	2003	2004	2005
Count	12	16	15	30	53	86	91	103	105	116	130	117	123	136	187	211	228	277	257	239	85

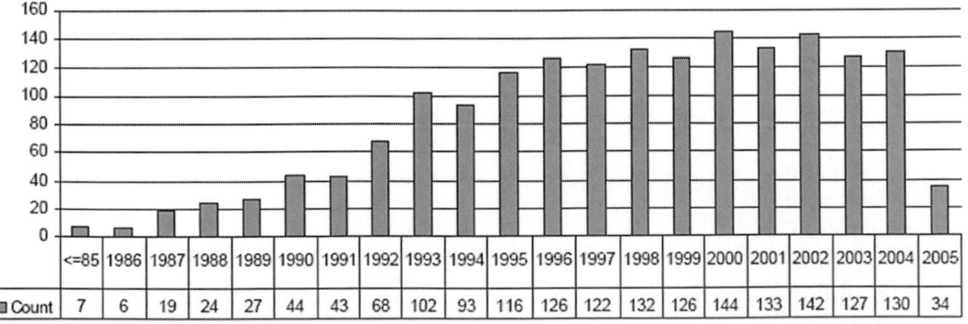

	<=85	1986	1987	1988	1989	1990	1991	1992	1993	1994	1995	1996	1997	1998	1999	2000	2001	2002	2003	2004	2005
Count	7	6	19	24	27	44	43	68	102	93	116	126	122	132	126	144	133	142	127	130	34

Figure 77-1 Annual ECMO neonatal respiratory and neonatal and infant cardiac runs. Note that 2005 entries represent only January through June.

myocardial protection, the availability of VA-ECMO is often lifesaving as a bridge to recovery. Of course it is critical that residual structural lesions be ruled out as the cause for compromise; thus a thorough assessment (i.e. transesophageal echocardiogram) is imperative before initiating VA-ECMO.

In 1987, Kanter and colleagues were the first to report some success with ECMO in patients who had undergone cardiotomy, with 6 of 13 surviving to discharge.[7] Since then, the literature is replete with institutional reports of ECMO use in patients with structural cardiac anomalies. Most recently, Morris and coworkers at the Children's Hospital of Philadelphia (CHOP) reported their experience with 137 patients on cardiac ECMO[8] between 1995 and 2001. Diagnoses encompassed the spectrum of congenital cardiac malformations, including single ventricle with intracardiac mixing and single ventricle with separate circulations, as well as children with structurally normal hearts. Overall survival to discharge was 39 percent. Two-thirds of the patients had undergone cardiac surgery prior to ECMO, with 40 percent of those surviving to discharge. In that subset, risk factors for mortality included age less than 1 month, male gender, duration of mechanical ventilation before initiation of ECMO, and the development of renal or hepatic dysfunction on ECMO. Failure to separate from CPB was not found to be a predictor of death, which means that in those cases ECMO was literally lifesaving. In addition, despite historical bias against placing patients with single ventricle physiology on ECMO, this factor did not prove to be significantly associated with death in this series. No factor analyzed was predictive of mortality in the subset of patients who had not undergone surgery and in whom survival to discharge was 35 percent. Overall, considering the fact that many of the survivors likely would have died without mechanical support, the authors concluded that, "it is imprudent to impose strict indications or contraindications to ECMO support."

Another high-volume pediatric cardiac surgical center, the University of Michigan (UM), described its experience in 74 patients supported with cardiac ECMO between 1995 and 2001.[9] Overall hospital survival was 50 percent. Patients with two ventricles were more likely to survive than those with single-ventricle physiology (58 vs. 34 percent), and patients with renal insufficiency (35 percent needed hemofiltration) were less likely to survive.

Chaturvedi and colleagues at the Great Ormond Street Hospital in London have reported on 81 cardiac patients managed with ECMO between 1992 and 2000.[10] More than half of these patients were placed on ECMO in the OR following multiple unsuccessful attempts at separation from CPB. Overall survival to discharge was 49 percent. Their report includes only patients with two-ventricle anatomy. Patients placed on ECMO in the surgical suite had a 64 percent survival to discharge, as compared to 29 percent in those patients cannulated in the ICU. Like the CHOP and UM groups, they found that renal failure was a significant risk factor for mortality. Also, as with virtually all other reports of pediatric cardiac ECMO, their data support the contention that a residual cardiac lesion bodes poorly for outcome and is a contraindication for initiation of support. In our experience, however, there are situations where a patient can be supported for a period of hours or even days, subsequently return to the OR or the interventional cardiology suite for correction of residual lesions, and then be weaned from ECMO; so even this contraindication is a relative one.

Defining which patients are appropriate candidates for cardiac ECMO support is complicated. Based on univariate and multiple logistic regression analysis of retrospectively collected data in 218 patients, Trittenwein and colleagues proposed inclusion criteria related to lactate and central venous oxygen saturations.[11] We believe that such criteria are too narrow and not universally applicable. Trying to impose strict inclusion and/or exclusion criteria is difficult and imprecise; rather, each case requires thoughtful consideration on an individual and institutional basis.

Timing of initiation of ECMO is probably critically important. Low-cardiac-output syndrome (LCOS)[12,13] is common to most scenarios in which cardiac ECMO is considered. Clinically, LCOS manifests as poor peripheral perfusion, oliguria, and lactic acidosis despite adequate intravascular volume and often elevated filling pressures. Mixed venous oxygen saturations are low, secondary to decreased oxygen delivery. After correcting for anemia, hypoxia, or obstructive cardiac disease, traditional therapy for this type of cardiogenic shock focuses on maximizing pharmacologic support. Usual agents act through a variety of mechanisms, but most cause an increase in biventricular afterload and heart rate. The net effect is to increase myocardial work and oxygen demand in a setting where myocardial oxygen supply is already compromised. This can exacerbate injury and delay or even prevent myocardial recovery. With ECMO, unloading the heart and decreasing its work creates an environment that is more favorable for repair and recovery.[14] In effect, earlier institution of mechanical support helps to ensure adequate perfusion of the heart, brain, kidneys, and other vital organs while minimizing ongoing myocardial insult and enhancing recovery. Most recent reports have documented better outcomes in those patients placed on ECMO in the OR as compared to those cannulated in the ICU.[9,10,15] One could reasonably theorize that this disparity was due to the fact that those patients supported from the OR avoided prolonged periods of LCOS that may have predisposed those cannulated later (in the ICU) to worse outcomes.

Experience with mechanical support of nonsurgical heart failure also merits consideration. In their series, Morris and associates report 35 percent survival in the nonsurgical population, which included patients with cardiomyopathy and myocarditis. Marx and coworkers have reported 67 percent survival in patients supported with ECMO for acute myocarditis and 62 percent survival in patients with cardiomyopathy. Duncan and colleagues report 83 percent survival in 12 pediatric patients with myocarditis who were placed on ECMO.[16] Of their overall population (12 ECMO, 3 VAD), 47 percent recovered with return of native ventricular function, and 33 percent survived following successful ECMO bridge to cardiac transplantation.

Several other series also describe the successful use of ECMO as a bridge to transplantation.[17–21] Kirshbom and colleagues at CHOP described 31 patients supported with ECMO as a bridge to cardiac transplantation.[22] They found no difference in long-term survival between heart transplant recipients who were supported with ECMO prior to transplant versus those who were not. Of the 31 patients, 6 had sufficient recovery of function to be weaned from ECMO and discharged home ("bridged to recovery"), while 12 of the original 31 ultimately underwent cardiac transplantation. Overall survival to discharge was 48 percent (15 of 31).

Interestingly, only 18 percent of patients who were postsurgical survived to transplant, as compared to 64 percent of the nonsurgical patients.

The CHOP experience does not support the enforcement of an arbitrary cutoff for duration of support, as they have had several patients survive after more than 250 h on ECMO, including four who were successfully transplanted after 500 h of support and one who survived 1126 h before transplant. Furthermore, as others have reported, pre-ECMO cardiac arrest was not associated with poorer outcome.[9,19,23]

For patients requiring ECMO after cardiac transplantation, Kirshbom and coworkers report 22 percent survival to discharge in those patients requiring support soon after transplantation as compared to the three patients who required support in the late period; two of the latter survived to discharge. They concluded that ECMO can be an effective tool for management of the peritransplant patient.

Of course survival is not the only marker of a successful ECMO run. Long-term sequelae can be considerable and devastating and should bear considerable weight in any discussion of indications and outcomes. Assessment of neurologic insult directly related to cardiac ECMO is difficult due to the many confounding variables. Cyanotic heart disease alone is, as an example, associated with neurodevelopmental abnormalities.[24–27] Similarly, behavioral and cognitive impairment is well-documented in both adults and children following cardiopulmonary bypass, as are gross and fine motor deficits.[28–30] Additionally, follow-up in neonatal respiratory ECMO survivors has revealed neurobehavioral and functional deficiencies.[31–39] Trying to ascribe neurodevelopmental irregularities to ECMO in a population with each of these known risks is difficult. Acute abnormalities have been described in cardiac ECMO patients at UM, as 14 percent had seizures and 7 percent had radiographic evidence of injury to the central nervous system (CNS).[9] Hamrick and colleagues report significant long-term impairment in their 11-year experience with infants supported by ECMO following cardiac surgery.[40] Of their 53 patients, 7 of the 14 survivors available for long-term follow-up (13 percent overall) were neurologically completely intact.

Golej and Trittenwein have looked critically at the issue of neurologic impairment associated with cardiac ECMO.[41] They advocate for early recognition and rehabilitation in this at-risk population. As with most advances in CPB and operating room management, monitoring devices and strategies are crossing over into the ICU (bispectral index monitoring and near infrared spectroscopy). However, pre-ECMO intracranial imaging is not as universally possible in cardiac patients as it is in neonates with respiratory failure. In that population, evidence of preexisting intracranial hemorrhage is a contraindication for ECMO. In cardiac ECMO patients, serial cranial ultrasounds are routinely obtained after return to the ICU, but even these studies lack adequate capability to detect anything less than gross hemorrhage or infarct.[40] Refinements in the ECMO circuit and devices have allowed for relative minimization of anticoagulation needs (discussed further on), but the risks of hemorrhage and embolic events remain real and may be even more significant on a microvascular level than is currently appreciated.

Implementation

Placing a patient on ECMO for cardiac support requires a cohesive team of surgeons, perfusionists, ECMO specialists, nurses, and cardiac intensivists. ECMO is fraught with potential technical complications, often with disastrous outcomes. Experience and vigilance are critical to ensuring optimal outcomes.

Cannulation

The quality of the cannulation is essential to the success of ECMO support. A poorly cannulated patient will not have a successful ECMO run. Hence, it is of the utmost importance that this procedure not be taken lightly. Proper positioning of the cannulas is mandatory. Venting of the heart is also necessary to achieve appropriate cardiac rest.

It is critically important to decompress the left ventricle in patients with impaired left ventricular function placed on ECMO; failure to do so can be catastrophic. With cervical cannulation, return flow from the arterial cannula is directed at the aortic valve. Particularly in the setting of poor ventricular function, this increased afterload may lead to left ventricular distention. The subsequent increase in wall tension and myocardial oxygen demand will ultimately impede myocardial recovery. The presence of any degree of aortic insufficiency exacerbates this process.

Effective left ventricular venting can be achieved by one of several techniques. In a closed chest setting, the LV can be decompressed by creating or augmenting an interatrial communication. If present, a patent foramen ovale (PFO) can be enlarged at the bedside by balloon septostomy under echocardiographic guidance. If no PFO exists, blade septostomy can be performed in the catheterization laboratory. Cheung and coworkers have described a percutaneous technique for placing a left-sided vent that can be connected to the venous return of the ECMO circuit as an alternate method of decompressing the left heart.[42]

When the chest is open, a cannula can be placed through the left atrial appendage or in the space between the two right-sided pulmonary veins and connected to the venous return of the ECMO circuit (Fig. 77-2). Alternatively, a surgical atrial septectomy can be performed, thus avoiding the need for additional cannulas. Regardless of how, in patients with severely depressed left ventricular function it is essential that left ventricular decompression be achieved soon after initiating support. If this is neglected, severe left ventricular dysfunction may preclude any ejection through an aortic valve that is essentially held shut by the flow from the arterial cannula. Acute left ventricular distention with fulminant pulmonary edema may rapidly ensue. Furthermore, with the standard cervical cannulation for VA-ECMO, the source of coronary artery perfusion depends on the presence or absence of left ventricular ejection.[43] Blood ejected from the left ventricle perfuses the coronary circulation preferentially, even with the high flow emanating from the arterial cannula. Effective left-sided decompression, therefore, will ensure that the highly oxygenated blood coming from the ECMO circuit will preferentially perfuse the coronaries rather than the often desaturated blood coming from the sick left ventricle. Moreover, if the heart continues to eject due to incomplete decompression, moderate levels of ventilation must be continued during ECMO support. Left heart unloading, coupled with moderate respiratory ventilation, should result in decreased myocardial oxygen demand and increased myocardial oxygenation.

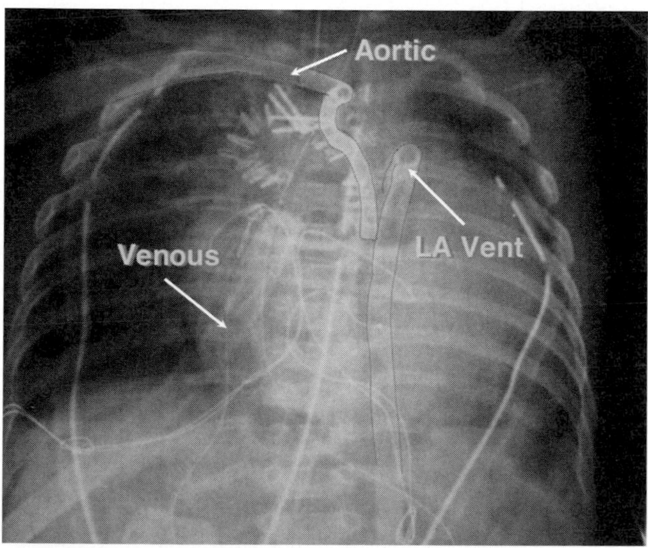

Figure 77-2 Technique for left ventricular decompression.

Management

Unlike the neonate with isolated respiratory failure, in whom ECMO flows and sweep gases are adjusted to maintain adequate oxygenation and ventilation, the infant or child on cardiac ECMO has cardiac insufficiency, often coupled with respiratory insufficiency. The degree to which gas exchange is dependent on ECMO will obviously affect the management strategy. For the patient with isolated cardiac failure, ECMO flows are adjusted to ensure adequate end-organ blood flow. Clinical parameters, such as urine output and toe temperature, should be regularly scrutinized and ECMO flows adjusted to maintain adequate perfusion. Laboratory values, including arterial lactate and mixed venous oxygen saturations, are also important and should be followed serially. In general, flows of 100 to 150 mL/kg/min should be adequate to maintain homeostasis. Some circumstances, as in the case of an infant in whom the pulmonary and systemic circulations are in parallel (single ventricle with aortopulmonary shunt), may require considerably higher flows. It has been and continues to be our practice to keep aortopulmonary shunts open and utilize higher flows. Because of the nonpulsatile nature of generally available circuits, arterial waveform tracings may provide an indication of the degree of native cardiac contribution to systemic output. Lack of discernible pulse pressure indicates that the ECMO circuit is responsible for all the effective systemic blood flow. This circumstance can occur when the heart is completely bypassed, when there is "cardiac stun," or in the setting of cardiac failure. It is important to remember that coronary perfusion results from antegrade ejection of blood out the aortic valve, and it is only in the setting of nearly complete lack of cardiac output that coronary blood flow becomes dependent on the oxygen-rich blood returning via the arterial ECMO cannula. Bearing that in mind, it is important to ensure that whatever blood is being ejected out the left ventricle is well saturated, so that the heart does not suffer ongoing ischemia. Ventilator FiO_2 should thus be maintained around 40 percent.

Serial echocardiograms can be helpful in gauging improvement in cardiac function, particularly in the setting of right ventricular failure where ventricular geometry and pressures can be assessed. It is often necessary to reduce ECMO flows to allow cardiac filling in order to make a determination. Levels of brain natriuretic peptide (BNP) and cardiac troponin I can be followed serially as well. In general, however, assessing improvement and adequacy of cardiac function requires weaning of ECMO flows monitoring systemic blood pressure and perfusion are monitored using the clinical parameters described above. Increases in arterial pulse pressure and perfusion indicate improving cardiac function and should encourage the weaning of ECMO flows. When flows have been sufficiently weaned, echocardiography is favorable, and perfusion is maintained on reasonable levels of inotropes, a trial off ECMO is warranted.

For the patient with combined cardiorespiratory failure, estimation of support needs and weaning preparedness is more complicated. In addition to ECMO flow rate, the sweep gas FIO_2 and flow rate are important determinants of respiratory gas exchange. In many instances, restoration of adequate circulation with initiation of ECMO leads to rapid improvement in respiratory mechanics and gas exchange as interstitial and alveolar lung water is cleared. Likewise, restoration of normal arterial oxygen tensions and pH can precipitate significant improvement in cardiac function. In addition to the clinical and laboratory parameters previously discussed, regular monitoring of arterial blood gases is vital. Weaning involves gradual decreases in FIO_2, sweep flow rate, and ECMO flow rate coupled with corresponding increases in mechanical ventilatory support. Once the patient can maintain physiologic values on reasonable ventilator settings and inotropes, a trial off ECMO is justified.

Other considerations

One consideration for cardiac ECMO is how to handle systemic-to-pulmonary artery shunts. This can be the case in single-ventricle patients or in patients with inadequate pulmonary blood flow. In our practice, we have chosen to leave all shunts open. In fact, most of our cannulations are done via a neck approach; therefore opening or closing of the shunt would require reentering the mediastinum. There are some qualifications to this statement. Our indications for placing a patient with a modified Blalock-Taussig shunt onto ECMO would be low oxygen saturations or a hyperactive pulmonary vascular bed. In both cases, we would employ venovenous ECMO (VV-ECMO) support with a single cannula placed in the internal jugular vein. In this case, the shunt is not affected by the presence of the ECMO cannula. In the case of a palliated HLHS patient, we again would favor VV-ECMO for low saturations. If a patient were in a state of low cardiac output after Norwood repair and required mechanical cardiac assist, we would use VA-ECMO via neck cannulation. However, in our patient population, we use the "Sano shunt" or a conduit from the right ventricle to the pulmonary artery, which would not be affected by an arterial neck cannulation. To date, we have used VV-ECMO only in the Norwood population.

VENOVENOUS ECMO

At first blush, indications for VV-ECMO in the cardiac population may seem limited. In fact, as experience grows, more clinical applications become apparent. VV-ECMO has several potential advantages over VA-ECMO. First, in many instances only a single venous cannula is required and, obviously, no large-caliber arterial vessels are disrupted and potentially sacrificed. Second, physiologic pulsatile flow is maintained. Third, the pulmonary vascular bed is perfused with oxygen-rich blood. And last, the myocardium is perfused with oxygen-rich blood. The last two features deserve particular consideration as they apply to the cardiac population.

Pulmonary hypertension is a common comorbidity in the pediatric cardiac population.[44] In many instances, elevated pulmonary vascular resistance (PVR) and right ventricular dysfunction lead to significant morbidity and even mortality in the perioperative period. In addition, infants with unrepaired cyanotic heart disease are at particular risk when they acquire common viral respiratory illnesses.[44–47] In these settings, we have found VV-ECMO to be the ideal mechanical support mode to affect improvement in oxygenation, correction of respiratory acidosis, and reduction in PVR. Clinically, the result is increased pulmonary blood flow, decreased right ventricular strain, better left-sided filling, enhanced myocardial oxygenation, and improved cardiac output. We consistently note rapid decreases in inotropic requirements following the institution of VV-ECMO.

Imamura and associates at Arkansas Children's Hospital report a similar experience in 10 patients placed on VV-ECMO for support in the setting of acute viral pneumonia and another 8 patients with inadequate pulmonary blood flow.[44] In each of these two groups, VV-ECMO served as a bridge to recovery or surgical intervention. Survival to discharge was 95 percent.

Implementation

Placing a patient on VV-ECMO is much less complicated than placing one on VA-ECMO. Several techniques are available: a purely open technique, a percutaneous technique, or the "semi-Seldinger" technique. We employ all three techniques but believe that there are situation-specific indications for each. Our primary technique is the semi-Seldinger technique because it allows for consistent and accurate cannulation, the internal jugular vein is not ligated, and at the conclusion of ECMO, the cannula can be easily removed at the bedside by nonsurgical staff. Moreover, placing the child on VV-ECMO using this technique can be done with a minimum of help; usually a single surgeon and a single OR nurse are adequate.

Management

The management of VV-ECMO differs from that of VA-ECMO in many ways. Cardiac output is not supported in any way other than the improvement in native function discussed above. As such, adjustments in ECMO flow rates do not directly affect blood pressure and perfusion. Mechanical ventilation is usually maintained using a lung-protective strategy to minimize airway trauma and optimize lung repair. In addition, adequate lung inflation is necessary to avoid elevations in PVR related to interalveolar capillary collapse (Fig. 77-3). In those patients supported due to inadequate pulmonary blood flow, surgical creation of a palliative shunt or full repair can be accomplished when the patient's physiologic parameters have normalized, making him or her a better candidate for anesthesia and/or cardiopulmonary bypass.

Functionally, pump flow rate, sweep gas flow, and FIO_2 are adjusted to achieve the desired oxygen saturations and arterial blood gas parameters. Weaning is attempted when chest x-ray findings and pulmonary mechanics indicate improvement in respiratory function or when indications are that PVR has reduced and right ventricular function has improved. Sweep flow and FIO_2 are weaned and mechanical ventilator settings increased accordingly. When sweep gas settings are minimized and ventilator settings are reasonable, removal of the patient from VV-ECMO can be tried by capping the gas source. In the cases of pulmonary hypertension, initiation of a pulmonary vasodilator (iNO, phosphodiesterase inhibitor V) may facilitate this transition.

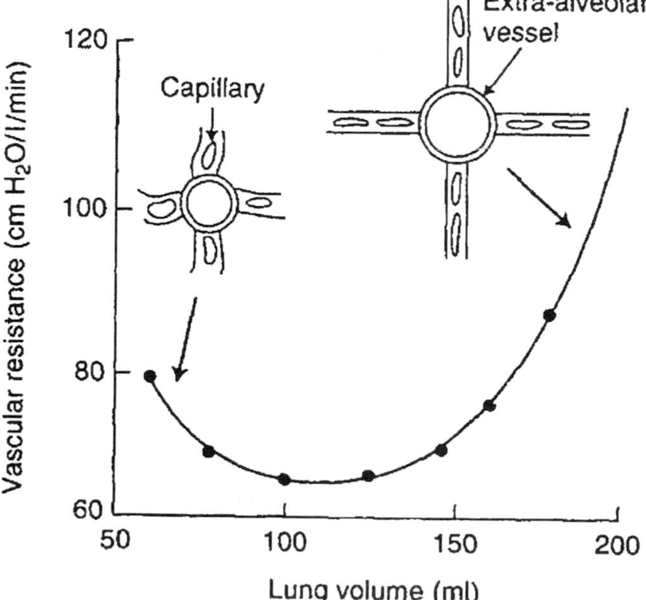

Figure 77-3 Pulmonary vascular resistance in relation to lung volume. Pulmonary vascular resistance is at its nadir when the lung is at functional residual capacity (FRC). In settings of either atelectasis or overdistention, pulmonary vascular resistance increases.

Other considerations

Feeding

Critically ill patients on ECMO typically have significant nutritional requirements. Postoperative cardiac surgical patients have the added burden of wound healing, which further increases their nutritional needs. Parenteral nutrition has traditionally been the primary source of calories for patients on cardiac ECMO because suboptimal splanchnic perfusion is associated with LCOS. However, enteral feedings have been shown to be beneficial by maintaining gut mucosal integrity, improving gastrointestinal immunologic function, and reducing septic morbidity.[48–50] Although there are no studies focusing exclusively on cardiac ECMO patients, a recent large retrospective study in neonates on ECMO demonstrated tolerance of enteral feeding without serious adverse events.[48] In that study, 67 of 77 VA-ECMO patients received enteral feedings. Dopamine infusion was administered to 80 percent of these patients, with a median dose of 7 µg/kg/min and a maximum dose of 20 µg/kg/min. Three patients were on both dopamine and dobutamine, and four patients received both dopamine and epinephrine. The patients on inotropic support did not have an increase in the rate of retained feedings or adverse outcomes. Additional studies have demonstrated success in the enteral feeding of adults on VV-ECMO.[51]

Administration of intravenous lipids in association with parenteral hyperalimentation for patients on ECMO raises particular concerns related to their effect on the extracorporeal circuit. In an in vitro analysis, a fat emulsion was infused into ECMO circuits at a rate of 3 mL/h.[52] All circuits showed layering (separation of fat emulsion from blood) and agglutination at 24 h. Adhesion of the emulsion to the circuit was evident in all samples. This study, along with anecdotal experience at many other ECMO centers, suggests that fat emulsions should be infused through separate intravenous sites whenever possible.

Immune prophylaxis

Some centers routinely utilize immunosuppressive agents prior to initiation of ECMO and during subsequent circuit changes. This practice has intuitive appeal due to the inflammatory cascade that is triggered upon exposure of the patient's blood components to the foreign surfaces of the ECMO circuit. Griffin and colleagues recently published a randomized, double-masked, controlled trial of dexamethasone versus placebo in infants placed on ECMO for respiratory failure.[53] They randomized 59 infants to either group and noted significant improvement in lung injury scores in the dexamethasone arm versus the placebo arm on day 3 of ECMO. However, they did not find a significant difference in outcome between the two groups, as the mean ECMO duration was 143.5 h in the dexamethasone group and 160 h in the placebo group. Therefore, although steroids may ameliorate some of the inflammatory response, their effect on long-term outcome is less certain.

Hypothermia is routinely utilized in cardiopulmonary bypass and appears to play a role in modulation of the immune response to the CPB circuit. Recent laboratory investigations have noted the role of hypothermia in altering the activities of neutrophils, which have been shown to be associated with decreased endothelial adherence and decreased release of L-selectin from the bone marrow in the setting of hypothermia.[54–56] These data are intriguing and suggest a new area of focus as investigators pursue ways to minimize the immunologic response to ECMO.

EQUIPMENT

The typical ECMO circuit comprises three main parts: a pump, an oxygenator, and a heat exchanger. Additional components include the tubing to transport the blood and other pieces of equipment that serve as monitoring devices and ensure safe operation of the ECMO circuit. Regardless of the type of ECMO utilized, the basic principles of the circuit remain the same (Fig. 77-4). Deoxygenated blood is removed from the patient, accelerated in a pump, oxygenated, heated, and then returned to the patient. Tubing size, oxygenator volume, and requisite flow rates will differ based on patient size; these variables have hematologic and immunologic implications for the patient. Platelet consumption will increase in proportion to the surface area of the membrane lung (within the oxygenator), activating the immune response.[57] Neonatal circuits may require the equivalent of twice the patient's circulating blood volume to prime, while in an adult the circuit priming volume may represent only half the circulating blood volume.[58,59] The following sections discuss details related to pumps, oxygenators, heat exchangers, tubing, and safety and monitoring devices.

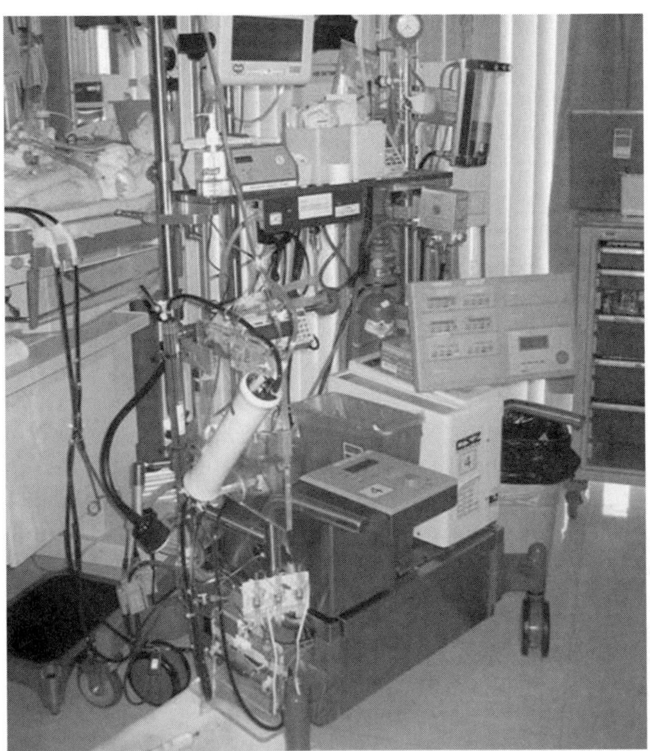

Figure 77-4 ECMO circuit.

Pumps

First developed by Gibbon, the standard roller pump (Fig. 77-5) has been the device most widely used for ECMO over the past 30 years. Its popularity is based on the fact that it is a relatively inexpensive, predictable device with a simple design that responds well to servocontrol. Blood flow is generated by the compression of the tubing that forces blood forward ahead of the moving roller. As one end of the roller completes its compressive phase, the other end is just beginning. Compression is carefully adjusted to be just nonocclusive in order to generate forward flow and minimize hemolysis and tubing wear.[60] However, this device does have the following significant limitations:

1. It requires continuous servoregulation and pressure monitoring to prevent the development of high levels of negative pressure or positive pressure.
   a. High negative pressures may result in hemolysis, damage to the venous and/or atrial structures from which the cannula arises. This may result in cavitation, causing air to be drawn out of solution.[57] The bladder (see below) is utilized to aid in monitoring and servoregulation in the setting of negative pressure.

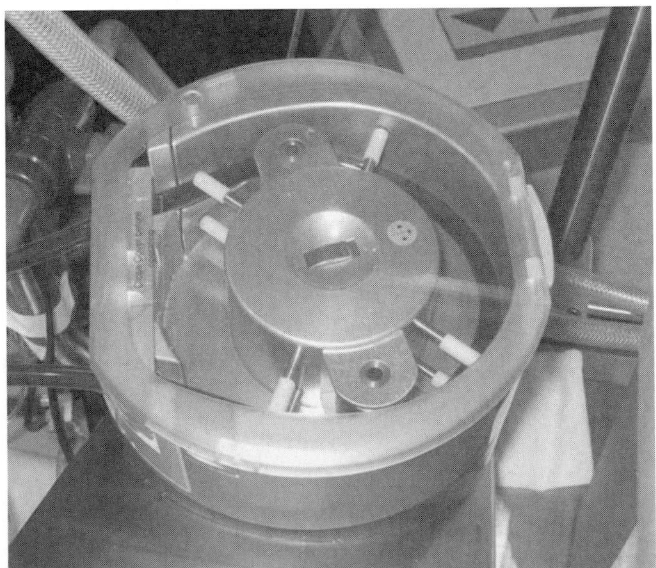

Figure 77-5 Roller pump.

b. High positive pressure may result in circuit rupture.
2. It can pump large quantities of air.
3. It causes spallation of the tubing, which can result in the embolization of particulate matter.
4. It can eventually cause circuit rupture due to repetitive occlusion.
5. It is dependent on gravity drainage from the venous system for inflow pressure.

Owing to the concerns with roller pumps, investigators have experimented with the use of centrifugal pumps. These (Fig. 77-6) use rotating cones activated by a forced vortex pumping action. These pumps cause less trauma to blood elements, although fibrin deposits in the pumping chamber can limit their useful life to 5 to 7 days.[61] Unlike the case with roller pumps, inflow here is gravity-independent, allowing the pumps to be placed at any height. The pump is sensitive to preload and afterload, either of which will affect pump flow. Unlike roller pumps, centrifugal pumps will come to a stop when they have entrained a large amount of air. Centrifugal pumps, however, can generate large negative pressures, which may lead to cavitation and hemolysis. Centrifugal pumps have not been widely adopted at ECMO centers; because of the high resistance in this form of oxygenator, which leads to hemolysis, it is not readily compatible with membrane oxygenators (see below). However, there is now renewed interest in centrifugal pumps owing to the development of next-generation hollow-fiber oxygenators (see below), which have less resistance and appear to interface much better with centrifugal pumps.

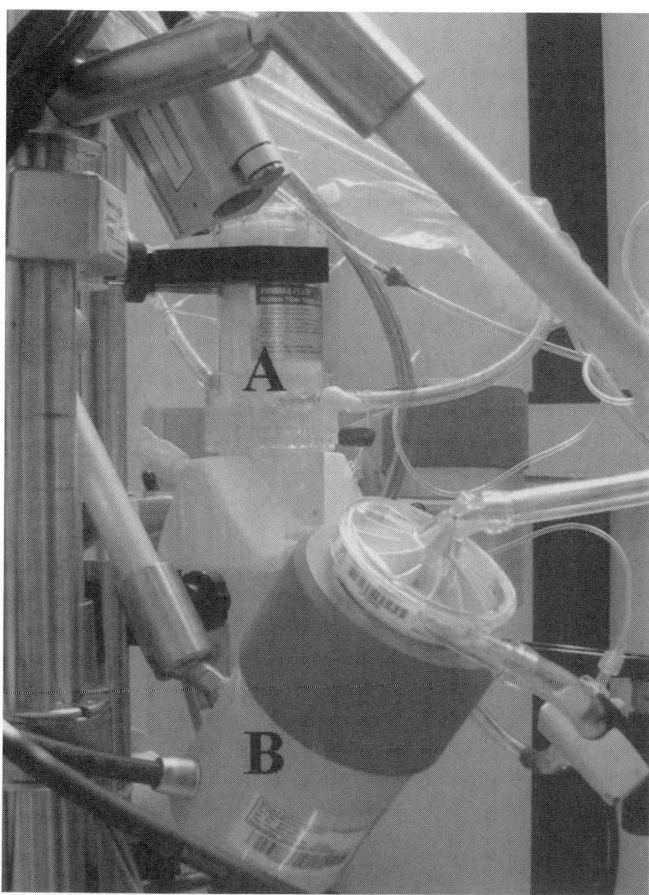

Figure 77-6 A. Hollow-fiber oxygenator. B. Centrifugal pump.

Despite the theoretical advantages and disadvantage of the pumps described above, there has been no definitive proof that either pump is superior.[62]

Oxygenators

The artificial oxygenator functions like a lung, adding oxygen to the circulating blood and removing carbon dioxide. An ideal extracorporeal lung should be noncompliant, so that blood volume remains constant, thus minimizing the risk of thrombosis and hemolysis.[57] In modern oxygenators, blood flows into a manifold region, from which it disperses to either a membrane lung in the case of a *membrane oxygenator* or to the microporous fibers of a *hollow-fiber oxygenator*. Oxygenated gas flows through the device in countercurrent to the flow of blood. Oxygen diffuses across the membrane into the blood and carbon dioxide is eliminated. Because of the high carbon dioxide diffusing capacity of these devices, in some instances carbon dioxide may actually need to be added to the gas mixture in order to normalize the patient's arterial blood gas. Oxygen does not diffuse as readily and is limited by the time period that the hemoglobin molecule is in transit through the oxygenator. As a result, oxygenators are limited in their oxygenating capacity based on the pump flow rate and are differentiated by the threshold rate above which the oxygenator is no longer able to increase the saturation of venous blood from 70 to 95 percent.[63]

Like their natural counterparts, oxygenators are susceptible to clot formation, collapse, edema, hemorrhage, and thrombosis.[63,64] Ventilation/perfusion mismatching can ensue. Water, plasma, and blood may collect in the gas phase of the oxygenator and decrease the rate of carbon dioxide exchange. Accordingly, P_{CO_2} can be a sensitive indicator of edema accumulation, which results in a decrease in the functional gas-exchange surface.[57] Likewise, thrombotic complications within the oxygenator are not an uncommon source of oxygenator failure. Unusually high preoxygenator pressures (> 400 mmHg), a fall in postoxygenator PO_2, or deteriorating patient blood gases should alert the ECMO specialist to such an occurrence.[57]

Currently, two types of oxygenators are most widely used in the United States: *membrane oxygenators* and *hollow-fiber oxygenators*. The membrane oxygenator (Fig. 77-7) is the most widely used for ECMO[65] and is a descendant of the spiral-wound silicone membrane lung

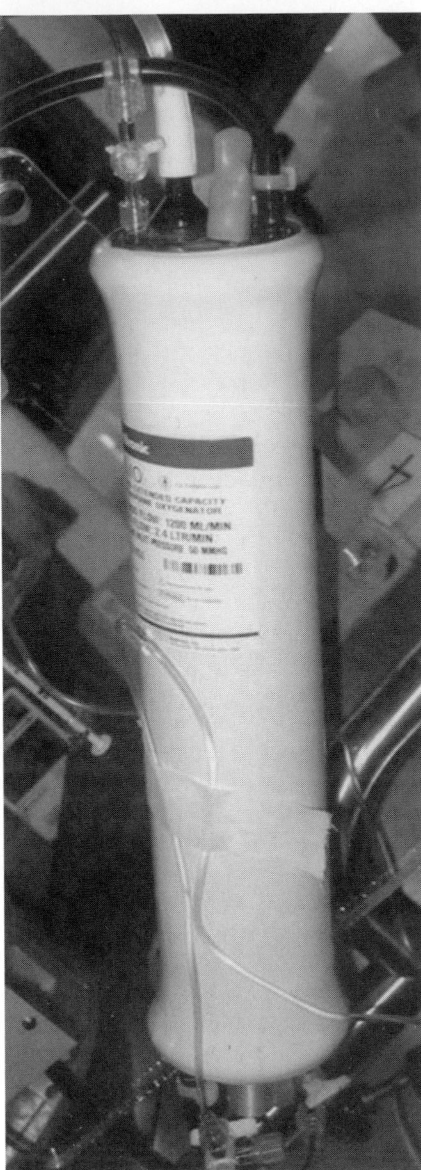

Figure 77-7 Membrane oxygenator.

developed by Kolobow in 1963.[66] This oxygenator is a long, spirally wound envelope of silicone rubber. Gas circulates within the winding spirals of the envelope, which has a high resistance and thereby limits the rate of blood transit and improves the oxygenating capability. Currently available devices provide a wide range of surface areas, from 0.4 to 4.5 m^2. They require a relatively small priming volume, are quite reliable, have excellent long-term gas exchange characteristics, are relatively nonthrombogenic, and are FDA-approved.[57] However, they require high perfusion pressures to overcome the high resistance described above, are difficult to prime, and offer limited capability to modulate oxygen exchange capacity.

Hollow-fiber oxygenators have enjoyed a recent surge of interest due to their low internal resistance, which allows them to be coupled with centrifugal pumps. These devices utilize microporous capillaries, around which blood flows and contacts the ventilatory gas. Advantages include low resistance and low priming volumes. Disadvantages include a propensity for plasma leakage (exacerbated by intralipid use) and undesired ultrafiltration.[57] New-generation hollow-fiber oxygenators appear to be less susceptible to these shortcomings.[67–73] Motomura and colleagues have achieved stable gas performance with minimal plasma leakage over a 2-week period of use.[73] With continued improvements in technology, hollow-fiber oxygenators may increasingly be used with ECMO and will potentially encourage a shift toward centrifugal pumps.

Heat exchangers

The *heat exchanger* is the last part of the circuit through which the blood passes en route back to the patient. In a survey conducted in 2002, Lawson found that 82 percent of ECMO centers used the Medtronic ECMOtherm heat exchanger, 15 percent used a Gish heat exchanger, and 3 percent used the Dideco D720 heat exchanger.[65] Structurally, heat exchangers are composed of silicone-coated stainless steel tubes that allow warm water to flow outside the ECMO circuit in a countercurrent fashion. Blood is heated as it flows vertically from the upper to lower portion, permitting air bubbles to be trapped in the upper section.[64] Heat exchangers are particularly important in the management of neonatal patients due to their propensity for temperature instability. Device failure occurs in some 1 to 2 percent of ECMO cases.[74] Most commonly, failure is due to the leakage of water from the connectors at the top and bottom of the device. Leakage of blood is uncommon and, because of the higher pressure in the ECMO circuit, leakage of water into the blood phase is even less common.[64]

Tubing

Circuit tubing has improved significantly since the advent of ECMO 30 years ago. Most of the circuit consists of polyvinyl chloride tubing, a readily available and relatively inexpensive product. One potential disadvantage with polyvinyl chloride tubing has been the release of the plasticizer di(2-ethylhexyl)phthalate (DEHP), which animal studies show may result in decreased fertility, reduced sperm production in males, and ovarian dysfunction.[75–77] However, a 2004 study by Khodayar, and associates found that adolescents exposed to DEHP as neonates on ECMO showed no adverse effects on their physical growth, maturation, or liver, thyroid, renal, and gonadal function.[78]

Polyvinyl chloride tubing, however, is not durable enough for the "raceway"—the portion of the circuit passing through the roller pump. Instead, most ECMO centers currently utilize Super Tygon tubing, S-65 HL, in the raceway, as it is more resistant to rupture and has been shown to minimize spallation (fragmentation and release of microparticles from plastic). Heparin-bonded circuits have been developed in an effort to reduce thrombotic complications (see the discussion of anticoagulation, below). The Carmeda Bioactive Surface (CBAS; Carmeda, Stockholm, Sweden) is a covalent endpoint bonding coating that attaches the heparin molecule to the plastic while the antithrombin-binding site remains exposed.[79] Systemic heparin requirements are significantly reduced in heparin-bonded circuits versus non-heparin-bonded circuits.[80,81] In addition, the Carmeda coating has been shown to reduce DEHP leakage from polyvinyl chloride tubing.[82]

Safety and monitoring devices

The bladder

A recent survey by Lawson and coworkers found that 92 percent of American ECMO centers utilize a *bladder* (Fig. 77-8) in the ECMO circuit.[65] The bladder is situated just proximal to the pump and serves a variety of functions. Aspiration ports associated with the bladder allow for the removal of any air that may have inadvertently been introduced into the circuit. Likewise, the bladder provides access to the circuit whereby medications, infusions, blood products, and volume may be administered. Last, prebladder pressures are routinely measured via a transducer and provide a quantifiable estimate of the venous return pressure. Servoregulated pumps will decrease and even shut off flow as the bladder pressure approaches or falls below a critical value.

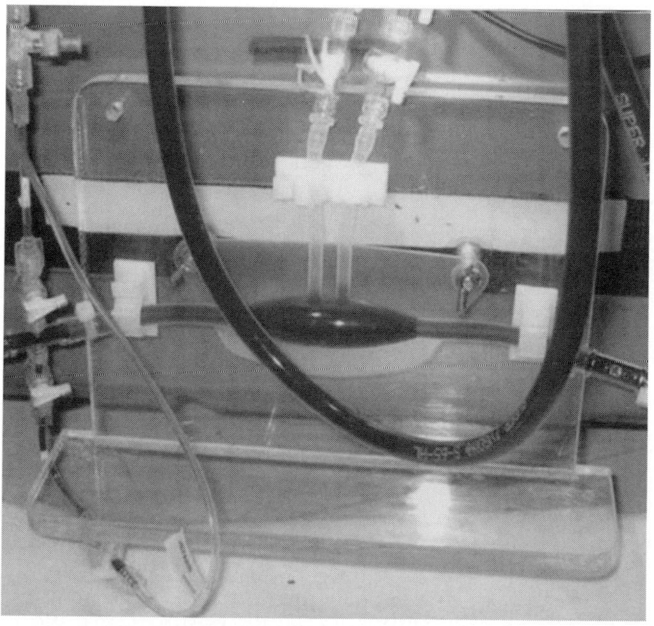

Figure 77-8 Bladder reservoir.

In older children and adults, a bridge may be added under the bladder to allow blood to be diverted directly into the pump. Small bladders may not easily handle the larger volumes in older patients, and this bypass helps to prevent overdistention. In this situation, the pressures are transduced directly from the bladder.

Pressure transducers

In addition to the prebladder pressures, most ECMO centers monitor circuit pressures between pump and patient.[83] In particular, pre- and postoxygenator pressures are usually monitored, so that a pressure increase as a result of distal circuit thrombosis and/or kinking can be detected.[57] Isolated increases in preoxygenator pressure in the setting of a normal postoxygenator pressure alerts the technician to possible thrombosis within the oxygenator. Generally speaking, a rising pressure gradient across an oxygenator predicts oxygenator failure. There is a greater risk of circuit disruption when preoxygenator pressures are above 400 mmHg, probable when they are above 500 mmHg, and imminent when the pressure exceeds 600 mmHg.[57]

Bubble detectors

Bubble detectors are an added safety precaution.[65] Although the bladder, oxygenator, and heat exchanger all scavenge large bubbles, making air-embolism unlikely, bubble detectors typically have automatic shutoff switches and serve as a last check before blood returns to the patient.[84] Once the circuit shut downs, the air bubbles rise to the top of the heat exchanger, where they can be removed through distal circuit aspiration ports.

The bridge

PVC tubing, referred to as "the bridge," usually connects the arterial and venous limbs of the ECMO circuit. Its main function is to allow the patient to be temporarily removed from the ECMO circuit during a trial off support or during an emergency. In such an instance, the bridge is unclamped and the proximal arterial and venous lines are clamped. The patient is thereby excluded from the circuit and blood can continue to circulate within the ECMO circuit. During normal ECMO operation, the bridge remains clamped but must be "flashed" every 20 to 30 min to prevent stagnation and possible thrombosis within that segment. Flashing of the bridge has been associated with an initial decrease and then a secondary increase in mean arterial pressure and mean left carotid artery blood flow.[85] Cerebral oxygen delivery is decreased because of this arteriovenous shunt, which may lead to an increase in cerebral oxygen extraction and vasodilatation and eventually an increase in cerebral blood volume and excess cerebral oxygen delivery.[86] Reperfusion injury, with free-radical formation, could occur in this setting and potentiate or cause cerebral injury. Totapally and colleagues studied an open-bridge ECMO circuit and showed a reduction in systemic arterial pressure fluctuations caused by changes in SVR associated with flashing of the bridge.[87]

Coagulation system

During open cardiac surgical procedures, the patient's entire blood volume is exposed to both the bypass circuit and the surgical wound, both of which stimulate activation of all blood elements involved in the inflammatory cascade.[88] Patients placed on ECMO following cardiac surgery continue to be exposed to a large biomaterial surface and the wound. Over time, equilibrium can eventually be established between the activation and neutralization of blood elements and is required for successful continuation of extracorporeal support. Most of our understanding of the activation of blood components comes from experience with short-term cardiopulmonary bypass, although there is a growing body of literature specific to ECMO.

Once blood contacts the ECMO circuit, plasma proteins are instantly adsorbed onto all nonendothelial surfaces.[89–91] These proteins are tightly packed, irreversibly bound, and stationary.[91] Fibrinogen is adsorbed by the hydrophobic surface of these biomaterials.[89] This surface will eventually stimulate clot formation and activate blood elements, including five plasma protein systems (contact system, intrinsic coagulation pathway, extrinsic coagulation pathway, fibrinolysis, and complement) and five blood cell types (platelets, endothelial cells, neutrophils, monocytes, and lymphocytes).

Platelets adhere to the ECMO circuit and become activated, causing them to degranulate and release substances that in turn activate even more platelets.[92] Thrombin is generated by the coordination of the plasma protein systems and further activates platelets. Platelets change shape by extending pseudopods and begin to express GPIIb/IIIA receptors, which bind platelets, using fibrinogen as a bridge.[93] Adherent platelets will detach and fragment, leading to a decrease in the number of normal platelets in the circulating pool.[94] The activation of the coagulation system is not limited to activity within the ECMO circuit, as patients may develop systemic disseminated intravascular coagulation (DIC).

In addition to the impact of the circuit, the exposure of circulating monocytes to the surgical wound will potentiate the activation of the coagulation system. Monocytes will elaborate tissue factor and continue the activation of the intrinsic and extrinsic coagulation pathways.[93] While this is usually of a self-limited nature in open cardiac procedures, it can have a protracted effect in patients who require transthoracic cannulation for ECMO.

Anticoagulation

The activation of the coagulation system from exposure to the ECMO circuit and the surgical wound makes anticoagulation a necessity. However, it can be exceedingly difficult to achieve the delicate balance between appropriate anticoagulation and hemorrhage control in postoperative cardiac surgical patients. The ideal anticoagulant would inhibit platelet activation and aggregation as well as activation of the coagulation cascade but would maintain enough procoagulant properties to allow for coagulation at the surgical site. Traditionally, heparin has been the most commonly used anticoagulant for all forms of ECLS, although it is far from an ideal agent.

Heparin inhibits thrombin and factor Xa generation, requiring normal levels of circulating thrombin and accelerating its action approximately 1000 times. Heparin's effects can be blocked with protamine, enhancing its attractiveness. However, heparin does not have any effect on platelet activation and does not inhibit the generation of thrombin—merely its activity. Large doses of heparin are routinely required during ECMO, mainly due to inactivation of the heparin molecule by mechanisms in both blood and the circuit that eliminate more than half of the administered heparin.[95] Of additional growing concern is the recent increase in awareness of allergic reactions to heparin, manifesting as heparin-induced thrombocytopenia (HIT).

The majority of ECMO centers continue to follow *activated clotting times* (ACT) to titrate heparin therapy. ACT is a crude measure of the effect of heparin on whole blood, but its ease of use in point-of-care testing makes it the preferred method. Prior to cannulation, patients not already anticoagulated require an initial heparin bolus (usually 75 to 100 U/kg), which is followed by a continuous infusion to maintain the ACT between 180 to 220 s. Postoperative patients will usually require the lower end of the range and may not receive much heparin at all in the first 24 to 48 h in order to promote hemostasis at the surgical site. Other agents and techniques may be on the horizon, including a reduction in circuit thrombogenicity and the development of alternative selective anticoagulants.

Argatroban is a potent, reversible, direct thrombin inhibitor that has been suggested as an alternative therapy in patients who develop heparin sensitivity. In laboratory experiments, Argatroban is associated with absence of clot initiation and a decrease in thrombin generation, raising its potential as a heparin alternative.[96] Its use has been reported to facilitate cardiopulmonary bypass in a heparin-sensitized infant undergoing tricuspid valve removal secondary to bacterial endocarditis.[97] Recent reports from the Oregon Health Sciences University have noted the successful use of argatroban in ECMO patients with probable HIT.[98]

Nafamostat mesylate is a broad-spectrum protease inhibitor that suppresses activation of contact proteins during ECMO.[99] It has been shown to reduce heparin requirements and resulted in a shorter ACT in the patient than the ECMO circuit.[100] Use of this agent during CPB has been shown to reduce postoperative blood loss.[101] A 1997 study by Nagaya and colleagues used nafamostat in 12 newborns that had hemorrhagic complications before or during ECMO.[100] The ACT of the blood delivered to the patient was reduced by 27 s compared to the circuit ACT and was associated with control of bleeding in 66 percent of the patients.

As previously discussed, heparin-bonded circuit have been developed using covalent (Cardmeda systems, described above) and ionic bonding (Duraflo II, Baxter) techniques. Heparin bound to the surface exerts an antithrombin-mediated inhibition of thrombin and factor Xa. The thrombin-antithrombin complexes bind to the surface without functionally blocking the activity of the immobilized heparin and serve to decrease exogenous heparin requirements.[92] A laboratory investigation of heparin-coated and uncoated systems was performed by Urlesberger and coworkers.[102] They found that coagulation system activation and D-dimer formation were significantly delayed in the heparin-coated group. After 6 h, no differences between the groups were detected, and after 24 h, markers had returned to near baseline values. The authors concluded that these circuits may provide only limited advantages in long-term ECMO use. However, they do offer benefits to those patients with a high bleeding risk, as they allow for less systemic heparinization.

Protease inhibitors, such as aprotinin or aminocaproic acid (Amicar), function primarily through inhibition of the fibrinolytic system and to a smaller extent by inhibition of the coagulation system. They have been shown to significantly reduce the requirements for blood products during cardiopulmonary bypass. A 1993 study reported a decrease in the incidence of intracranial hemorrhage and other hemorrhagic complications in patients on ECMO treated with Amicar.[103] In addition, Amicar's use is widely reported in the cardiac ECMO literature as an adjunct for postoperative patients with significant postoperative bleeding.[104] The caveat, however, is that Amicar will likely shorten the life expectancy of the ECMO circuit. Finally, although there seems to be less experience with aprotinin, a recent case report details its successful use in the setting of life-threatening bleeding on ECMO.[105]

There is great potential for more clinically important technologic advances in the near future. As an example, a 2002 article in *Artificial Organs* described a new ECMO system developed in Japan.[106] That circuit utilizes a hollow-fiber oxygenator with an ultrathin, dense layer in contact with blood that is able to prevent plasma leak. A centrifugal pump is utilized and the entire blood-contacting surface of the tubing is coated with a newly developed heparin material (Toyobo-NCVC coating). Venoarterial ECMO was successfully performed for 34 days in a goat without systemic anticoagulation. Plasma leakage was not detected and sufficient gas exchange was maintained throughout, with minimal thrombus formation.

Rapid cardiopulmonary support

Rapid cardiopulmonary support (CPS) refers to the application of ECMO as an immediate life-sustaining therapy in the setting of cardiopulmonary arrest. John Gibbon, the pioneer of CPB, speculated in 1939 on the ability of a heart-lung machine to temporarily take over the function of the heart and lungs during a period of deterioration and provide a time interval for the recovery of organ function, leading to potential survival.[107] CPS has evolved from early reports of use following myocardial infarction, pulmonary embolism, and other emergency conditions.[108–111] Its current form is the result of a slow iterative approach in the design and development of both the equipment and management principles over the last 20 years.

There are several early accounts of the use of the standard ECMO circuit for the resuscitation of patients with cardiac arrest following cardiac surgery.[112,113] A 1998 study by Duncan and associates from Boston Children's Hospital describes a modified rapid-deployment circuit for use in patients undergoing cardiopulmonary resuscitation.[114] The circuit was designed to allow for the provision of cardiopulmonary support within 15 min of notification and is maintained in the ICU; it is completely portable for use throughout the hospital. The circuit is maintained with a vacuum and carbon dioxide–primed 0.8-m^2 membrane oxygenator. This oxygenator is able to support children up to 10 kg; for bigger children, a 1.5-m^2 oxygenator is spliced in. The circuit contains Normosol solution (Abbott Laboratories, Abbott Park, IL) and is primed with 5 percent albumin. If blood is available at the time of cannulation, it is added to the circuit; if not, it is added later. If added later, crystalloid is either removed 1:1 during the infusion of the blood or removed via ultrafiltration. The policy at Boston Children's Hospital is to mobilize the rapid-resuscitation ECMO team after 10 min of cardiopulmonary resuscitation (CPR) in a patient with heart disease. Duncan and colleagues describe 11 patients in this retrospective review. Of these, 10 patients (91 percent) were able to wean from ECMO and 7 (64 percent) survived to discharge; 6 (55 percent) are long-term survivors. One of these children has mild neurologic impairment and one has moderate neurologic impairment.

In 57 of the 137 patients from the CHOP report previously cited, ECMO was initiated during active CPR. The median duration of chest compressions was 45 min (range, 5 to 105 min) in the survivors and 50 min (range, 15 to 90 min) in the nonsurvivors.[8] Fifty-one percent of patients were weaned from ECMO, and 37 percent survived to hospital discharge. Forty-four percent (7 patients) of those with CPR longer than 60 min survived to discharge; 2 patients had new-onset seizure activity prior to discharge. Of note, all patients had ice applied to their heads during resuscitation.

Clearly, rapid-deployment CPS can potentially improve outcome following cardiopulmonary arrest. Long-term neurologic outcome in these patients remains to be determined. The significant resource allocation required to institute and support a rapid-deployment CPS program may limit its widespread implementation and will need to be carefully considered on a hospital-by-hospital basis.

CONCLUSIONS

Exciting advances in extracorporeal membrane support equipment, techniques, and experience have led to a blossoming of its use in the pediatric cardiac population. Consideration of earlier initiation of support is warranted based on outcomes reported in the literature as well as the theoretical advantage of avoiding multiorgan dysfunction associated with LCOS. Furthermore, improved myocardial repair and recovery is possible when demands on the ailing heart are decreased. Nevertheless, thoughtful, realistic consideration of the myriad clinical and programmatic issues associated with cardiac ECMO must be pursued on a case-by-case basis to ensure its judicious use and to avoid offering false hope to families.

References

1. Lillehei CW. Controlled cross circulation for direct vision intracardiac surgery correction of ventricular septal defects, atroventricularis communis, and tetralogy of Fallot. *Postgrad Med* 1955;17:388.
2. Gille JP. Respiratory support by extracorporeal circulation with an artificial lung. *Bull Physiopathol Respir* 1974;10:373.
3. Bartlett RH et al. Extracorporeal membrane oxygenation (ECMO) cardiopulmonary support in infancy. *Trans Am Soc Artif Intern Organs* 1976;22:80.
4. Moler FW et al. Extracorporeal life support for severe pediatric respiratory failure: An updated experience 1991–1993. *J Pediatr* 1994;124:875.
5. July 2004 ELSO Registry Data, International Summary.
6. Deng MC et al. Mechanical circulatory support for advanced heart failure. Effect of patient selection or outcome. *Circulation* 2001;103:231.
7. Kanter RR et al. Extracorporeal membrane oxygenation for postoperative cardiac support in children. *J Thorac Cardiovasc Surg* 1987;93:27.
8. Morris MC et al. Risk factors for mortality in 137 pediatric cardiac intensive care unit patients managed with extracorporeal membrane oxygenation. *Crit Care Med* 2004;32(4):1061.
9. Kovolos NS et al. Outcome of pediatric patients treated with extracorporeal life support after cardiac surgery. *Ann Thorac Surg* 2003;76:1435.
10. Chaturvedi RR et al. Cardiac ECMO for biventricular hearts after paediatric open heart surgery. *Heart* 2004;90:545.
11. Trittenwein G et al. Proposed entry criteria for postoperative cardiac extracorporeal membrane oxygenation after pediatric open heart surgery. *Artif Organs* 1999;23(11): 1010.
12. Black MD et al. Determinants of success in pediatric cardiac patients undergoing extracorporeal membrane oxygenation. *Ann Thorac Surg* 1995;60:133.
13. Marx M et al. Extracorporeal life support in pediatric patients with heart failure. *Artif Organs* 1999;23: 1001.
14. Levin GR et al. Reversal of chronic ventricular dilation in patients with end-stage cardiomyopathy by prolonged mechanical unloading. *Circulation* 1995;91: 2715.
15. Ferrazzi P et al. Assisted circulation for myocardial recovery after repair of congenital heart disease. *Eur J Cardiothorac Surg* 1991;5:419.
16. Duncan BW et al. Mechanical circulatory support for the treatment of children with acute fulminant myocarditis. *J Thorac Cardiovasc Surg* 2001;122(3):440.
17. Dalton HJ et al. Extracorporeal membrane oxygenation for cardiac rescue in children with severe myocardial dysfunction. *Crit Care Med* 1993;21:1020.
18. Delius RE. Prolonged extra corporeal life support of pediatric and adolescent cardiac transplant patients: Updated. *Ann Thorac Surg* 1990;50:791.
19. Del Nido PJ et al. Extracorporeal membrane oxygenation support as a bridge to pediatric heart transplantation. *Circulation* 1994;90:1166.
20. Di Russo GB et al. Prolonged extracorporeal membrane oxygenation as a bridge to cardiac transplantation. *Ann Thorac Surg* 2000;69:925.
21. Frazier EA et al. Prolonged extracorporeal life support for bridging to transplant: Technical and mechanical consideration. *Perfusion* 1997;12(2):93.
22. Kirshbom PM et al. Use of extracorporeal membrane oxygenation in pediatric thoracic organ transplantation. *J Thorac Cardiovasc Surg* 2002;123:130.
23. Mehta U et al. Extracorporeal membrane oxygenation for cardiac support in pediatric patients. *Am Surg* 2000;66:879.
24. Kumar K. Neurological complications of congenital heart disease. *Indian J Pediatr* 2000;67:S15.
25. Mahle WT. Neurologic and cognitive outcomes in children with congenital heart disease. *Curr Opin Pediatr* 2001;13:482.
26. Samango-Sprouse C, Suddaby EC. Developmental concerns in children with congenital heart disease. *Curr Opin Cardiol* 1997;12.
27. Umperopoulos C et al. Neurologic status of newborns with congenital heart defects before open heart surgery. *Pediatrics* 1999;103:402.
28. Bellinger DC et al. Developmental and neurologic status of children after heart surgery with hypothermic circulatory arrest or low-flow cardiopulmonary bypass. *N Engl J Med* 1995;332:549.
29. Fallon P et al. Incidence of neurological complications of surgery for congenital heart disease. *Arch Dis Child* 1995;72:418.
30. Sharma R et al. Neurological evaluation and intelligence testing in the child with operated congenital heart disease. *Ann Thorac Surg* 2000;70:575.
31. Bulas DI et al. Neonates treated with ECMO: Predictive value of early CT and US neuroimaging findings on

short-term neurodevelopmental outcome. *Radiology* 1995;195:407.
32. Glass P et al. Severity of brain injury following neonatal extracorporeal membrane oxygenation and outcome at age 5 years. *Dev Med Child Neurol* 1997;39:441.
33. Glass P et al. Morbidity for survivors of extracorporeal membrane oxygenation: Neurodevelopmental outcome at 1 year of age. *Pediatrics* 1989;83:72.
34. Glass P et al. Neurodevelopmental status at age five years of neonates treated with extracorporeal membrane oxygenation. *J Pediatr* 1995;127:447.
35. Rais-Bahrami K et al. Neurodevelopmental outcome in ECMI) vs near-miss ECMO patients at 5 years of age. *Clin Pediatr (Phila)* 2000;39:145.
36. Andrews AF et al. One- to three-year outcome for 14 neonatal survivors of extracorporeal membrane oxygenation. *Pediatrics* 1986;78:692.
37. Flusser H et al. Neurodevelopmental outcome and respiratory morbidity for extracorporeal membrane oxygenation survivors at 1 year of age. *J Perinatol* 1993;13:266.
38. Schumacher RE et al. Follow-up of infants treated with extracorporeal membrane oxygenation for newborn respiratory failure. *Pediatrics* 1991;87:451.
39. Towne BH et al. Long-term follow-up of infants and children treated with extracorporeal membrane oxygenation (ECMO): A preliminary report. *J Pediatr Surg* 1985;20:410.
40. Hamrick SEG et al. Neurodevelopmental outcome of infants supported with extracorporeal membrane oxygenation after cardiac surgery. *Pediatrics* 2003; 111:544.
41. Golej J, Trittenwein G. Early detection of neurologic injury and issues of rehabilitation after pediatric cardiac extracorporeal membrane oxygenation. *Artif Organs* 1999;23:1020.
42. Cheung MM et al. Percutaneous left ventricular "vent" insertion for left heart decompression during extracorporeal membrane oxygenation. *Pediatr Crit Care Med* 2003;4:447.
43. Shen I et al. Left ventricular dysfunction during extracorporeal membrane oxygenation in a hypoxemic swine model. *Ann Thorac Surg* 2001;71:868.
44. Imamura M et al. Venovenous extracorporeal membrane oxygenation for cyanotic congenital heart disease. *Ann Thorac Surg* 2004;778:1723.
45. Dickson ME et al. Stunned myocardium during extracorporeal membrane oxygenation. *Am J Surg* 1990; 160:644.
46. Khongphatthanayothin A et al. Impact of respiratory syncytial virus infection on surgery for congenital heart disease: Postoperative course and outcome. *Crit Care Med* 1999;27:1974.
47. Boyce TG et al. Rates of hospitalization for respiratory syncytial virus infection among children in Medicaid. *J Pediatr* 2000;137:865.
48. Nanekamp MN, Spoel M, Sharman-Koendjbiharie I, et al. Routine enteral nutrition in neonates on extracorporeal membrane oxygenation. *Pediatr Crit Care Med* 2005;6:275.
49. Heyland DK, Cook DJ, Guyatt GH. Enteral nutrition in the critically ill patient: A critical review of the evidence. *Intens Care Med* 1992;19:435.
50. Moore FA, Moore FA, Feliciano DV, et al. Early enteral feeding, compared with parenteral, reduces postoperative septic complications. The results of a meta-analysis. *Ann Surg* 1992;216:172.
51. Scott LK, Boudreaux K, Thaljeh F, et al. Early enteral feedings in adults receiving venovenous extracorporeal membrane oxygenation. *J Parenter Enter Nutr* 2004;28:295.
52. Buck ML, Ksenich RA, Wooldridge P. Effect of infusing fat emulsion into extracorporeal membrane oxygenation circuits. *Pharmacotherapy* 1997;17:1292.
53. Griffin MP, Woolridge P, Alford BA, et al. Dexamethasone therapy in neonates treated with extracorporeal membrane oxygenation. *J Pediat* 2004;144:296.
54. Le Deist F, Menasche P, Kucharski C, et al. Hypothermia during cardiopulmonary bypass delays but does not prevent neutrophil-endothelial cell adhesion. *Circulation* 1995;92:354.
55. Menasche P, Peynet J, Haeffner-Cavaillon N, et al. Influence of temperature on neutrophil trafficking during clinical cardiopulmonary bypass. *Circulation* 1995;92:334.
56. Cox CS, Lally KP. Extracorporeal life support and the systemic inflammatory response. In: Zwischenberger JB, Steinhorn RB, Bartlett RH (eds). *ECMO Extracorporeal Cardiopulmonary Support in Critical Care*, 2d ed. Extracorporeal Life Support Organization, 2000: 161.
57. Hirschl RB. Devices. In: Zwischenberger JB, Steinhorn RB, Bartlett RH, eds. *ECMO Extracorporeal Cardiopulmonary Support in Critical Care*, 2d ed. Extracorporeal Life Support Organization, 2000:199–236.
58. Hirschl RB, Bartlett RH. Extracorporeal membrane oxygenation (ECMO) in cardiorespiratory failure. Chicago: Yearbook Medical Publishers, 1987. Referenced in Hirschl RB. Devices. In: Zwischenberger JB, Steinhorn RB, Bartlett RH (eds). *ECMO Extracorporeal Cardiopulmonary Support in Critical Care*, 2d ed. Extracorporeal Life Support Organization, 2000: 199–236.
59. Chapman R, Bartlett RH. Extracorporeal life support manual for adult and pediatric patients. Ann Arbor: University of Michigan Medical Center, 1991. Referenced in Hirschl RB. Devices. In: Zwischenberger JB, Steinhorn RB, Bartlett RH (eds). *ECMO Extracorporeal Cardiopulmonary Support in Critical Care*, 2d ed. Extracorporeal Life Support Organization, 2000:199–236.
60. Brabant C. Mechanical pumps for extracorporeal circulation. Children's Hospital Wisconsin Website: Heart Matters—October 2001.
61. Moon YS, Ohtsubo S, Gomez MR, et al. Comparison of centrifugal and roller pump hemolysis rates at low flow. *Artif Organs* 1996;20:579.
62. Yamagishi T, Kunimoto F, Isa Y, et al. Clinical results of extracorporeal membrane oxygenation (ECMO) support for acute respiratory failure: A comparison of centrifugal pump ECMO with roller pump ECMO. *Surg Today* 2004;34:209.
63. Galletti PM, Richardson PD, Snider MT. A standardized method for defining the overall gas transfer performance of artificial lungs. *ASAIO Trans* 1972;18:359.

64. Singh AR. Neonatal and pediatric extracorporeal membrane oxygenation. *Heart Dis* 2002;4:40.
65. Lawson DS, Walczak R, Lawson AF, et al. North American neonatal extracorporeal membrane oxygenation (ECMO) devices: 2002 survey results. *J Extra Corpor Technol* 2004;36:16.
66. Kolobow T, Boman RL. Construction and evaluation of an alveolar membrane artificial heart lung. *Trans ASAIO* 1963;9:238.
67. Kahawito S, Maeda T, Takano T, et al. Gas transfer performance of a hollow fiber silicone membrane oxygenator: Ex vivo study. *Artif Organs* 2001;25:498.
68. Kawahito S, Maeda T, Motomura T, et al. Development of a new hollow fiber silicone membrane oxygenator: In vitro study. *Artif Organs* 2001;25:494.
69. Kawahito S, Maedo T, Motomura T, et al. Feasibility of a new hollow fiber silicone membrane oxygenator for long-term ECMO application. *J Med Invest* 2002;49:156.
70. Kawahito S, Motomura T, Glueck J, Nose Y. *Ann Thor Cardiovasc Surg* 2002;8:268.
71. Kawahito S, Haraguchi S, Maeda T, et al. Preclinical evaluation of a new hollow fiber silicone membrane oxygenator for pediatric cardiopulmonary bypass: Ex-vivo study. *Ann Thorac Cardiovasc Surg* 2002; 8:7.
72. Motomura T, Maeda T, Kawahito S, et al. Extracorporeal membrane oxygenator compatible with centrifugal pumps. *Artif Organs* 2002;36:952.
73. Motomura T, Maeda T, Kawahito S, et al. Development of silicone rubber hollow fiber membrane oxygenator for ECMO. *Artif Organs* 2003;27:1050.
74. Extracorporeal Life Support Organization Registry 2000.
75. Foster PM, Mylchreest E, Gaido KW, Sar M. Effects of phthalate esters on the developing reproductive tract of male rats. *Hum Reprod Update* 2001;7:231.
76. Park JD, Habeebu SS, Klaasen CD. Testicular toxicity of di-(2-ethylhexyl)phthalate in young Sprague-Dawley rats. *Toxicology* 2002;171:105.
77. Poon R, Lecavaliert P, Meueller R, et al. Subchronic oral toxicity of do-n-octyl phthalate and di-(2-ethylhexyl) phthalate in the rat. *Food Chem Toxicol* 1997;35:225.
78. Khodayar RB, Nunez S, Revenis ME, et al. Follow-up study of adolescents exposed to di-(2-ethylhexyl) phthalate (DEHP) as neonates on extracorporeal membrane oxygenation (ECMO) support. *Environ Health Perspect* 2004;112:1339.
79. Larsson R, Olsson P. A new thrombogenic surfaced prepared by selective covalent binding of heparin via a modified reducing terminal residue. *Biomat Med Devices Artif Organs* 1992;2:161.
80. Camel JE, de Csepel J, Atkinson JB. Extracorporeal membrane oxygenation using a Carmeda heparin coated circuit in neonates. Presented at the Extracorporeal Life Support Organization Meeting. Dearborn, Michigan, 1992. Referenced in Hirschl RB. Devices. In: Zwischenberger JB, Steinhorn RB, Bartlett RH (eds). *ECMO Extracorporeal Cardiopulmonary Support in Critical Care,* 2d ed. Extracorporeal Life Support Organization, 2000:199–236.
81. Muehrcke DD, McCarthy PM, Stewart RW, et al. Complications of extracorporeal life support systems using heparin-bound surfaces. The risk of intracardiac clot formation. *J Thorac Cardiovasc Surg* 1995;10:843.
82. Haishima Y. Matsude R, Hayashi Y, et al. Risk assessment of di(2-ethylhexyl)phthalate release from PVC blood circuits during hemodialysis and pump-oxygenation therapy. *Int J Pharm* 2004;274:119.
83. Allison PL, Kurusz M, Graves DF, Zwischenberger JB. Devices and monitoring during neonatal ECMO: Survey results. *Perfusion* 1990;5:193.
84. Faulkner S. ELSO techniques survey. Presented at the Extracorporeal Life Support Organization Meeting. 1995. Referenced in Hirschl RB. Devices. In: Zwischenberger JB, Steinhorn RB, Bartlett RH, eds. *ECMO Extracorporeal Cardiopulmonary Support in Critical Care,* 2d ed. Extracorporeal Life Support Organization, 2000:199–236.
85. Van Heijst A, Liem D, van der Staak F, et al. Hemodynamic changes during opening of the bridge in venoarterial extracorporeal membrane oxygenation. *Pediatr Crit Care Med* 2001;2:265.
86. Leim KD, Kollee LA, Klaessens JH, et al. Disturbance of cerebral oxygenation and hemodynamics related to the opening of the bypass bridge during veno-arterial extracorporeal membrane oxygenation. *Pediatr Res* 1995;38:124.
87. Totapally BR, Sussmane JB, Hultquist K, et al. Variability in systemic arterial pressure during closed and open bridge extracorporeal life support: An in vitro evaluation. *Crit Care Med* 2000;28:2076.
88. Blackstone EH, Kirklin JW, Stewart RW, Chenoweth DE. The damaging effects of cardiopulmonary bypass. In: Wu KK, Roxy ED (eds). *Prostaglandins in Clinical Medicine: Cardiovascular and Thrombotic Disorders.* Chicago: Yearbook, 1982:355.
89. Uniyal S, Brash JL. Patterns of adsorption of proteins from human plasma onto foreign surfaces. *Thromb Haemost* 1982;47:285.
90. Ziats NP, Pankowsky DA, Tierney BP, et al. Adsorption of Hagemann factor (factor XII) and other plasma proteins to biomedical polymers. *J Lab Clin Med* 1990;116:687.
91. Horbett TA. Principles underlying the role of adsorbed plasma proteins in blood interactions with foreign materials. *Cardiovasc Pathol* 1993;2:137S.
92. Muntean W. Coagulation and anticoagulation in extracorporeal membrane oxygenation. *Artif Organs* 1999;23:979.
93. Bowen FW, Edmunds LH. Coagulation, anticoagulation and the interaction of blood and artificial surfaces. In: Zwischenberger JB, Steinhorn RB, Bartlett RH (eds). *ECMO Extracorporeal Cardiopulmonary Support in Critical Care,* 2d ed. Extracorporeal Life Support Organization, 2000:67.
94. Zilla P, Fasol R, Groscurth P, et al. Blood platelets in cardiopulmonary bypass operations. Recovery occurs after initial stimulation, rather than continual activation. *J Thorac Cardiovasc Surg* 1989;97:379.
95. Green TP, Isham-Schopf B, Irmiter RJ, et al. Inactivation of heparin during extracorporeal circulation in infants. *Clin Pharmacol Ther* 1990;48:148.

96. Young G, Yonekawa KE, Nakagawa P, Nugent DJ. Argatroban as an alternative to heparin in extracorporeal membrane oxygenation circuits. *Perfusion* 2004;19:283.
97. Dyke PC, Russo P, Mureebe L, et al. Argatroban for anticoagulation during cardiopulmonary bypass in an infant. *Paediatr Anaesth* 2005;15:328.
98. Mejak B, Giacomuzzi C, Heller E,. Argatroban usage for anticoagulation for ECMO on a post-cardiac patient with heparin-induced thrombocytopenia. *J Extra Corpor Technol* 2004;36:178.
99. Mellegren K, Skogby M, Friberg LG, et al. The influence of a serine protease inhibitor, nafamostat mesilate, on plasma coagulation, and platelet activation during experimental ECLS. *Thromb Haemost* 1998;79:342.
100. Nagaya M, Futamura M, Kato J, et al. Application of a new anticoagulant (nafamostat mesylate) to control hemorrhagic complications during extracorporeal membrane oxygenation: A preliminary report. *J Pediatr Surg* 1997;32:531.
101. Sato T, Tanaka K, Kondo C, et al. Nafamostat mesylate administration during cardiopulmonary bypass decreases postoperative bleeding after cardiac surgery. *ASAIO Trans* 1991;37:194.
102. Urlesberger G, Zobel G, Rodl S, et al. Activation of the clotting system: Heparin-coated versus non-coated systems for extracorporeal circulation. *Int J Artif Organs* 1997;20:708.
103. Wilson JM, Bower LK, Fackler JC, et al. Aminocaproic acid decreases the incidence of intracranial hemorrhage and other hemorrhagic complications or ECMO. *J Pediatr Surg* 1993;28:436.
104. Wessel DL, Almodovar MC, Laussen PC. Intensive care management of cardiac patients on extracorporeal membrane oxygenation. In: Duncan BW (ed). *Mechanical Support for Cardiac and Respiratory Failure in Pediatric Patients.* New York: Marcel Decker, 2001:75–112.
105. Biswas AK, Lewis L, Sommerauer JF. Aprotinin in the management of life-threatening bleeding during extracorporeal support. *Perfusion* 2000;15:211.
106. Nishinaka T, Tasumi E, Taenaka Y, et al. At least thirty-four days of animal continuous perfusion by a newly developed extracorporeal membrane oxygenation system without systemic anticoagulants. *Artif Organs* 2002;26:548.
107. Gibbon JH Jr. Artificial maintenance of circulation during experimental occlusion of pulmonary artery. *Arch Surg* 1927;34:1105.
108. Prichard PA, Kurusz M, Zwischenberger JB. Venoarterial perfusion for resuscitation and cardiac procedures: Cardiopulmonary support. In: Zwischenberger JB, Steinhorn RB, Bartlett RH (eds). *ECMO Extracorporeal Cardiopulmonary Support in Critical Care,* 2d ed. Extracorporeal Life Support Organization, 2000:619–632.
109. Stuckey JH, Newman MM, Dennis C, et al. The use of the heart-lung machine in selected cases of acute myocardial infarction. *Surg Forum* 1957;8:342.
110. Cooley DA, Beall AD. A technique of pulmonary embolectomy using temporary cardiopulmonary bypass: Experimental and clinical considerations. *J Cardiovasc Surg* 1961;2:469.
111. Kennedy JH. The role of assisted circulation in cardiac resuscitation. *JAMA* 1965;197:97.
112. Del Nido PJ, Dalton HJ, Thompson AE, Siewers RD. Extracorporeal membrane oxygenator rescue in children during cardiac arrest after cardiac surgery. *Circulation* 1992;86(5S):300.
113. Dalton HJ, Siewers RD, Fuhrman BP, et al. Extracorporeal membrane oxygenation for cardiac rescue in children with severe myocardial dysfunction. *Crit Care Med* 1993;21:1020.
114. Duncan BW, Ibrahim AE, Hraska V, et al. Use of rapid-deployment extracorporeal membrane oxygenation for the resuscitation on pediatric patients with heart disease after cardiac arrest. *J Thorac Cardiovasc Surg* 1998;116:305.
115. Peek GJ, Firmin RK, Moore HM, Sosnowski AW. Cannulation of neonates for venovenous extracorporeal life support. *Ann Thorac Surg* 1996:61:1851.

CHAPTER

78 VENTRICULAR ASSIST DEVICES IN CHILDREN

Gan Dunnington, Jr., Marc Pelletier, Bruce Reitz

INTRODUCTION

Ventricular assist devices (VADs) can be invaluable tools for the management of refractory heart failure. As pediatric cardiac surgery becomes more prevalent, the use of these devices will also become more commonplace in managing both acute and chronic pediatric heart failure. Pediatric indications for circulatory support are often different from those of the adult population; however, the same goal of bridging the failing heart to recovery or transplant can be accomplished. Since the 1960s, attempts have been made to support failing pediatric hearts. Successful recovery has been reported with extracorporeal membrane oxygenation (ECMO) support as well as with VAD support after initial failure to wean from bypass. Moreover, numerous cases of successful bridging to transplantation have been reported.[1–3] The results of these series indicate a definite benefit in this patient population, although associated with significant morbidity and mortality.

Mechanical support for failing pediatric hearts must be customized to the individual's need, size, and physiology. Certainly, in children from neonatal age to adolescence, one size does not fit all. Unfortunately, many of the promising VADs specifically engineered for pediatric patients are currently being utilized only overseas and have not yet been approved for unrestricted clinical use in the United States. In the United States, the initial reports of mechanical pediatric cardiac support have entailed utilization of devices initially intended for the adult patient population. Therefore many of these devices were too large to accommodate the specific requirements of the small child. For this reason, many of the smallest patients have not had VAD support available and have been rescued or bridged to transplantation or recovery with ECMO as the mainstay of circulatory assist in this particular group.

Pediatric patients in acute need of ventricular assistance often differ from those who present with more chronic heart failure. Indeed, the decision as to which device to use should be based on the indication and prognosis (Fig. 78-1). A patient who cannot be weaned from cardiopulmonary bypass might only need ventricular support for a few days, while the myocardium recovers, while another patient with end-stage heart failure might require a VAD designed for longer use that is both portable and durable in anticipation of a lengthy wait on a heart transplant list.

KEY CONCEPTS

- The parallel growth of pediatric cardiac surgery and ventricular assist device (VAD) technology has led to the development of mechanical support specifically tailored to the management of pediatric heart failure. Pediatric VADs are used for heart failure refractory to conventional medical therapy and act as bridges to either recovery or transplantation. Each one of the numerous devices currently available has specific advantages, but device selection must be individualized to the patient's particular clinical circumstances. Ongoing development of new devices has resulted in promising results in supporting pediatric heart failure. Anticoagulation and infection prophylaxis remain major concerns in the management of pediatric patients undergoing VAD placement.

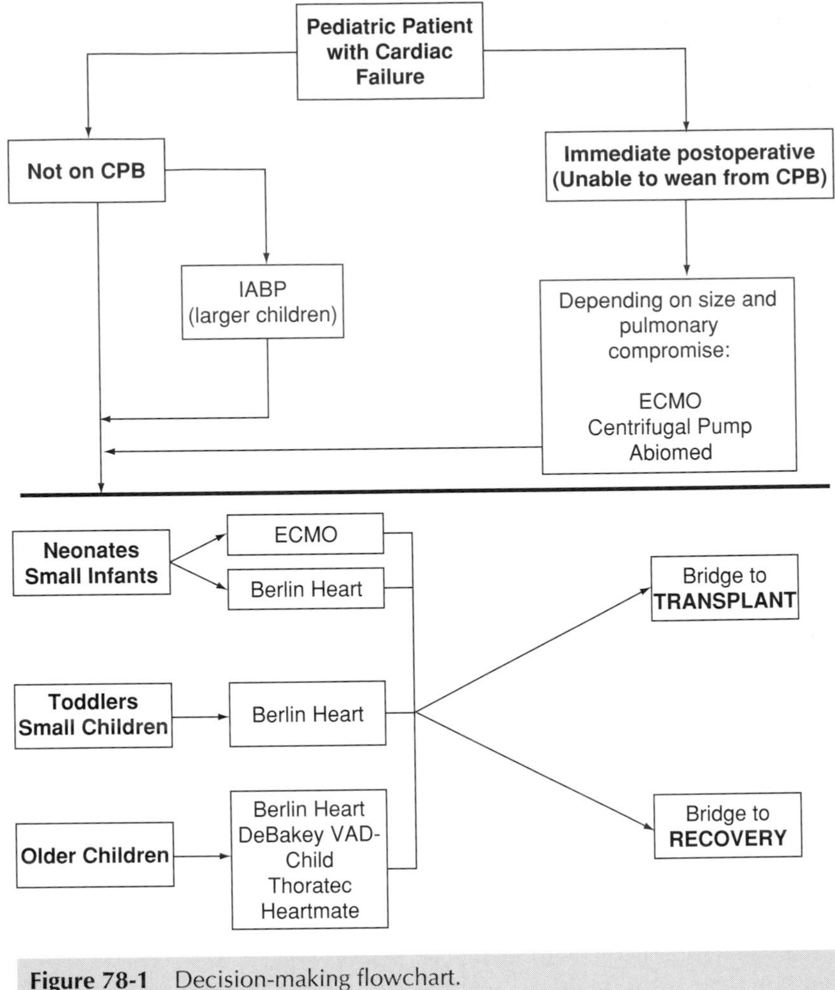

Figure 78-1 Decision-making flowchart.

New devices are constantly being developed, and adult VADs will continue to be adapted to the pediatric patient population. As the technology evolves and becomes more readily available, VADs will likely become a mainstay of the management of pediatric heart failure in both the acute and chronic settings.

PATHOPHYSIOLOGY

Pediatric heart failure severe enough to necessitate a VAD often differs from adult heart failure (Table 78-1). For children, the most common etiologies of myocardial failure include postoperative failure to wean from cardiopulmonary bypass, congenital heart disease, cardiomyopathies, and acute myocarditis.[4] Children usually do not suffer from the typical adult problems of hypertension and ischemic heart disease. Congenital heart disease often entails elements of right/left ventricular and pulmonary dysfunction, which necessitate biventricular support. Much less commonly, isolated right or left heart failure without pulmonary dysfunction exists, necessitating unilateral VAD support alone.

By assuming much of the responsibility for cardiac output, VADs may allow for the failing myocardium to recover. Decompression of the cardiac chambers through mechanical assistance can lower wall stress, reduce myocardial oxygen consumption, and allow for recovery of the myocardium. Other advantages of VAD support include potentially lower requirements for inotropic and vasoactive agents that have, as some of

Table 78-1 Common causes of pediatric cardiac failure

Post-cardiotomy
Congenital heart disease (with or without surgical intervention)
Acute myocarditis
Cardiomyopathy
Toxins
Genetic dystrophy
Infection (viral/HIV)
Nutritional
Ischemic (Kawasaki's disease)
Idiopathic
Hypertrophic
Cardiac arrest (postarrest ventricular dysfunction)

their side effects, arrhythmias, peripheral vasoconstriction, and hyper-/hypotension. For those patients with reasonable pulmonary function, VADs offer isolated ventricular support without the need for oxygenation. In these patients (as opposed to patients on ECMO, for example), the benefits of not requiring an oxygenator in the circuit include lower anticoagulation requirements, less platelet destruction, fewer bleeding complications, and the possibility of mobilization.

CLINICAL FEATURES

Congestive heart failure in children is primarily attributable to congenital heart defects, cardiomyopathies, and myocardial dysfunction following cardiac surgical repair. The yearly incidence of heart failure from structural defects is 0.1 to 0.2 percent of live births, while the yearly incidence of cardiomyopathy in infants and children has been estimated to be 0.6 in 100,000. Repaired or palliated structural defects leave an unknown prevalence of heart failure in this patient population. About 10 to 20 percent of those who have undergone complex repairs of congenital cardiac defects will develop heart failure by young adulthood.[5]

Aside from failure to wean from cardiopulmonary bypass, typical symptoms of heart failure in infants include tachypnea, tachycardia, failure to thrive, and poor feeding. Patients may develop signs of congestion, including an enlarged cardiac silhouette on chest radiographs, pulmonary edema, and hepatic enlargement. In toddlers and older children, jugular venous distention and edema might be findings observed in association with growth failure and fatigue. As children become adolescents, the severity of heart failure can be classified as it is in adults, typically with the New York Heart Association (NYHA) functional classification.

If untreated, heart failure ultimately compromises end-organ perfusion, thus leading to the downward spiral of multi-organ-system failure. Altered mentation, decreased urine output, rising creatinine, increasing liver function indices, and elevated lactic acid levels all point to inadequate perfusion. If cardiac output or perfusion pressures do not meet the metabolic demands of the body, persistent decline and circulatory collapse will ensue.

INDICATIONS FOR VENTRICULAR ASSIST DEVICE IMPLANTATION

Initial therapy for pediatric heart failure will usually include diuretics, digoxin, and beta blockers as well as angiotensin-converting enzyme inhibitors. As heart failure progresses, patients will require admission to the intensive care unit, along with inotropic and vasodilator support to maintain adequate cardiac output. We have preferred the use of milrinone, epinephrine, and dopamine as our customary inotropic agents in these circumstances. With worsening failure, patients will often require intubation and ventilatory support, hemodynamic monitoring with a Swan-Ganz catheter, close monitoring of renal function and placement of an indwelling urinary catheter. Adequate enteral nutrition must also be provided, usually by means of an feeding tube.

The indications for VAD remain the same in larger children as in adults, even though the disease process may differ (Table 78-2). For smaller children, such as infants and toddlers, indications for VAD support are much more vague and often rely on clinical judgment. Signs such as recurrent ventricular arrhythmias, inability to feed, and recurrent pulmonary edema are particularly ominous in this patient population. Catastrophic collapse can occur with great rapidity and without the usual clinical warning signs often seen in adults. Near-death and resuscitation events, even when patients are stabilized, should not be given another chance to occur. In a medically optimized patient, elevated cardiac filling pressures along with persistent acidosis and hypotension indicate poor perfusion, often secondary to poor ventricular function. These are the types of "gray-zone signs" that should lead one to contemplate institution of VAD support. In essence, if clinical deterioration secondary to heart failure continues despite maximal inotropic support, strong consideration should be given to insertion of a VAD.

Pediatric VADs are always "bridging" devices to either recovery or transplantation.[2,3,6] The concept of destination therapy, which is gaining acceptance in the adult population, is not accepted for pediatric patients at this time. Ethical considerations (including futility and hopelessness) must be addressed before placing a VAD, particularly in cases of cardiac arrest.

The indications for VAD placement can be divided into acute and chronic heart failure. This distinction may

Table 78-2 Indications for a Ventricular Assist Device
Inability to wean from cardiopulmonary bypass
Persistent heart failure after maximal treatment with inotropic and IABP support
$BP_{sys} < 90$ mmHg
SVR > 2000 dynes/s/cm^2
PCWP > 20 mmHg
CI < 1.8-2.0 L/min/m^2
End-organ dysfunction:
Altered mental status
Elevated BUN and creatinine levels
Elevated liver enzymes

BPsys = systemic blood pressure; BUN = blood urea nitrogen; CI = confidence interval; IABP = intraaortic balloon pump; PCWP = pulmonary capillary wedge pressure; SVR = systemic vascular resistance.

affect the decision of which device to place once the decision for VAD implantation has been made. For example, postcardiotomy patients can initially be maintained on VADs designed for short-term use. Options like ECMO or placement of an intraaortic balloon pump (IABP) may be equivalent if not better in this setting. Patients with chronic heart failure might benefit more from a pulsatile VAD or a device that allows for earlier mobility and less lifestyle restrictions. There is a rising population of patients who will fail to wean successfully from "acute" devices and will need conversion to more "chronic" support.[6] This will increasingly become the case, as more pediatric VADs become available in the United States.

As pediatric VADs become more commonplace in clinical practice, new indications may arise for their utilization. Rather than merely representing a salvage procedure, VADs may become a standard adjunct for some complex congenital heart operations. One group of investigators has suggested routine ventricular assist after complex congenital reconstructions like the Norwood procedure, citing greater ease of postoperative management as an advantage.[7] With greater use and long-term follow-up, the indications for VAD placement will change and might be further broadened.

SURGICAL THERAPY

At present, only a limited number of pediatric VADs are available in the United States. This should change in the near future, as promising results from European studies are being reported. The range of mechanical assist devices for the pediatric heart includes IABPs and ECMO circuits as well as pulsatile and nonpulsatile VADs. Although ECMO for cardiac support has been directly compared to nonpulsatile VADs in a few series,[8] there are few data directly comparing one VAD to another.

Intraaortic balloon counterpulsation

Although use of the IABP has greatly facilitated the management of adult patients with heart failure, translation to the pediatric population has not been as fruitful. The IABP is a biocompatible balloon that is introduced into the descending thoracic aorta and intermittently inflated/deflated (triggered by the electrocardiogram) to augment diastolic pressure. By deflating prior to the initiation of systole, the device decreases afterload and thus ventricular work. Pediatric anatomy and physiology have posed many obstacles for the use of this technology through the years. Difficulty with insertion remains a challenge even with smaller designs, while higher pediatric heart rates make timing a significant challenge, particularly in a 1:1 setting. Moreover, some feel that the pediatric aorta is considerably more elastic and compliant than that of the adult, which limits the counterpulsation effect; this assertion has nevertheless recently been challenged.[9] Furthermore, most pediatric patients have unobstructed coronaries, rendering the increased coronary perfusion afforded by the IABP less relevant than it is in adults. Patients with IABP suffer from problems with thrombosis and emboli, as well as the destruction and consumption of cellular blood components, therefore requiring transfusion. For these reasons, the IABP has a limited role in the pediatric population.[10] Although they may be reasonable for short-term support in larger children, IABPs have a very limited role in long-term mechanical support or bridging to transplantation.

Extracorporeal membrane oxygenation

ECMO consists of a centrifugal or roller pump combined with an oxygenator, which is used for venoarterial or venovenous bypass (Fig. 78-2). Introduced in 1957, this modality has proven to be most useful for neonates with respiratory failure. However, it has also been widely utilized with some success in pediatric cardiac failure. At this time, it is the most widely used method of pediatric ventricular support in the United States, mostly secondary to its availability and ease of placement. Unlike most other VADs, ECMO can be used for children of all sizes, from premature neonates to adults. It can be placed centrally (through the chest) or peripherally with either carotid artery and jugular vein or femoral artery and vein cannulation. Physiologically, ECMO does result in a decrease in cardiac preload as well as a small decrease in afterload; however, without venting the left heart, it can result in increased ventricular wall stress because of the inability to decompress the left-sided cardiac chambers. Left atrial and ventricular distention occurs to a degree proportional to the number of aortopulmonary collaterals; it may be managed by venting the left atrium either directly or transseptally via the right atrium.[11] ECMO by design improves arterial oxygenation and, if cannulated in a venoarterial fashion, acts to support both ventricles. For those patients with mainly pulmonary dysfunction (meconium aspiration, for example), ECMO can be instituted in a venovenous configuration, thereby improving venous blood oxygenation and myocardial oxygen delivery. Pulmonary hypertension resulting from low venous blood saturations may also be improved, allowing for some off-loading of the right heart. For the most part, venovenous bypass, as opposed to a venoarterial configuration, is uncommonly utilized in the pediatric population.

Since the ECMO circuit involves both a pump and an oxygenator, it is reasonable that the pump alone may suffice for those patients without pulmonary insufficiency. By eliminating the oxygenator, it is possible to decrease the amount of foreign surface contact in the circuit, thus decreasing the inflammatory response. Moreover, if the venous cannula is placed in the left atrium or ventricle, the same pump may be used as a left VAD. For this

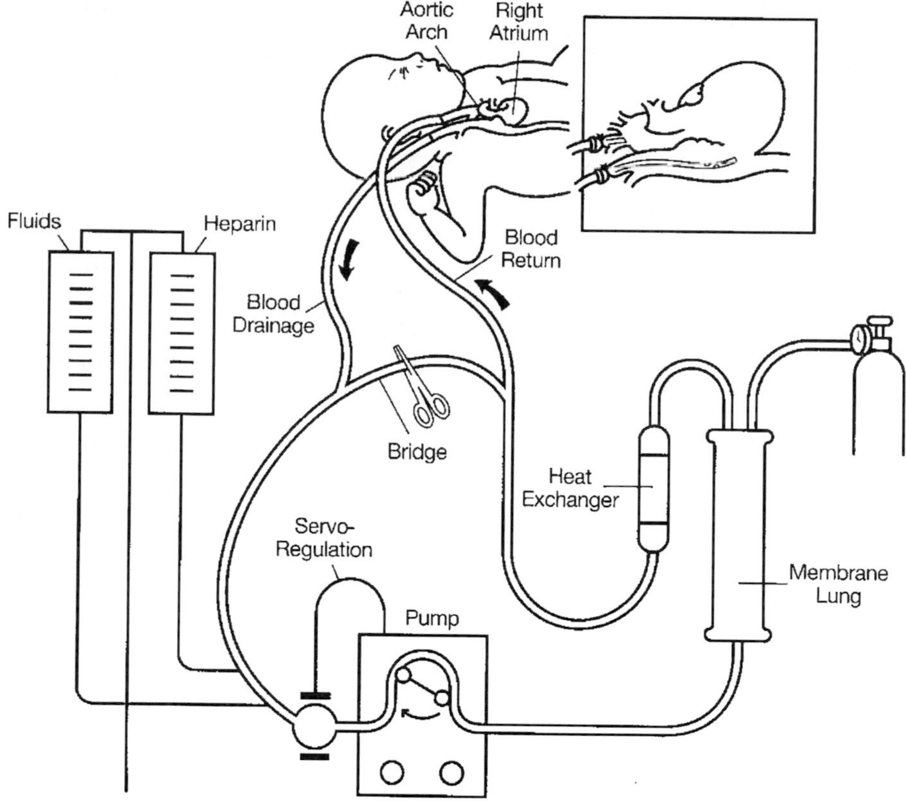

Figure 78-2 Typical extracorporeal membrane oxygenation (ECMO) circuit with right common carotid/internal jugular cannulation.

reason, the most commonly used true VAD in the United States has been the centrifugal pump. Extracorporeal membrane oxygenation is discussed in further detail in Chap. 77. For the purpose of this chapter, we categorize VADs into nonpulsatile and pulsatile types.

Nonpulsatile ventricular assist devices

Centrifugal pump

The centrifugal pump has been the most widely used VAD in pediatric cardiac surgery. These VADs consist of inflow and outflow cannulas connected by a centrifugal pump for blood propulsion. Often, the same cannulas utilized during cardiopulmonary bypass may be used for the institution of postoperative ventricular support. Additional cannulation of a pulmonary vein, left atrial appendage, or the pulmonary artery will allow for univentricular or biventricular support. Centrifugal pumps do not generate pulsatile flow and are considered to cause less hemolysis than roller heads. Roller pumps are less portable and also pose a risk of raceway rupture with resultant gas embolism.[11]

Successful results using centrifugal VADs have been reported in children of all sizes, including one series of 35 neonates weighing less than 6 kg with postcardiotomy failure.[12] Sixty-three percent of these patients were successfully weaned from centrifugal pumps in this series. Intraaortic balloon counterpulsation may also be utilized to add pulsatility to this form of support.

Patients may be weaned from these VADs by progressively decreasing the flow rate while observing the ventricular and hemodynamic response under echocardiographic guidance. Cardiac chamber dilation indicates inability of the native heart to maintain adequate cardiac output, thus necessitating continued support. If the patient fails to wean from the centrifugal pump within a few days, a decision to convert to a longer-term bridging device or withdrawal of care must be considered. In a series from Boston studying pediatric patients who required VAD or ECMO placement, patients who were unable to wean from the VAD or ECMO within 72 h either died or required cardiac transplantation. Lack of ejection (identified by pulsatility of the arterial line waveform) is also regarded as an adverse prognostic indicator for ventricular recovery.[13]

Centrifugal pump VADs are not designed for mobile patients; most remain intubated, sedated, and often pharmacologically paralyzed while recovering. In summary, the centrifugal pump is essentially an ECMO circuit deprived of an oxygenator. The advantage to this type of VAD is avoidance of blood trauma known to be caused by the oxygenator; however, if a patient has

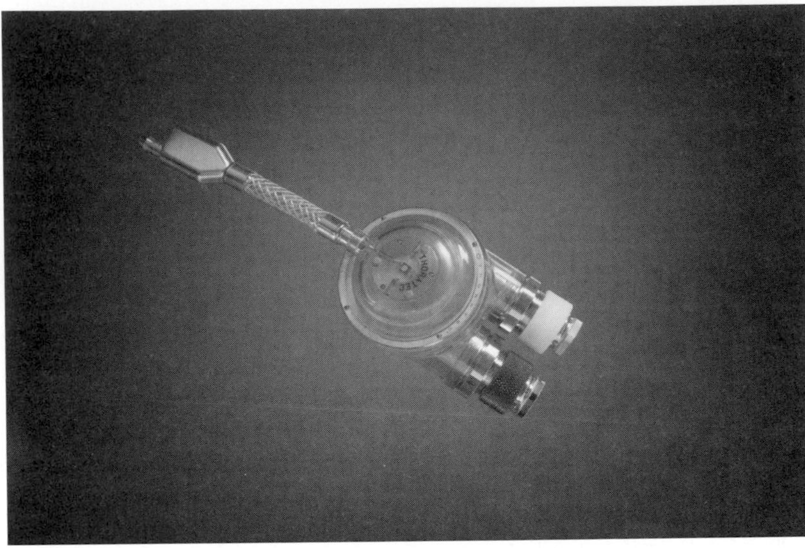

Figure 78-3 Thoratec VAD.

pulmonary compromise or intracardiac shunts, ECMO is probably the better choice for short-term supportive care.

Axial flow pumps

Axial flow pumps (Hemopump, MicroMed DeBakey VAD-Child, Jarvik 2000, Heartmate II, Streamliner, Impella system, Valvo pump, the IVAP VAD, and Berlin INCOR) are the latest devices in an emerging technology that aims at incorporating nonpulsatile flow into miniaturized devices that might someday help support pediatric heart failure patients.[14] They are typically small, tubular, implantable rotary pumps connected either directly to the ventricle or to inflow and outflow cannulas. They operate at higher rotational speeds than centrifugal pumps and generate higher flow with lower increases in pressure. They operate at slightly less power, which might, in turn, facilitate the development of lighter and more portable power supplies in the future. Limited experience with axial flow pumps in larger pediatric patients has been reported.[15] Considering their smaller size and the possibility of implantation via a left thoracotomy, these pumps may become a viable option for VAD support in children awaiting transplant.

Pulsatile ventricular assist devices

In the United States, there is still no pulsatile VAD specifically designed for children. There have nevertheless been reports of adult models (Thoratec, Novacor, Abiomed) adapted in larger children with some success.[16,17] Although there are various different designs, most of these devices involve inflow and outflow cannulas, a pneumatically driven pump with air and blood chambers separated by a biocompatible membrane, and valves assuring unidirectional flow. They are mostly paracorporeal and require central cannulation of the heart and great vessels.

Patients with pulsatile VADs have been shown to have fewer bleeding complications,[18] fewer severe infectious complications, and increased mobility; they can often be weaned from mechanical ventilation. To date, pulsatile VADs have been more effective in treating myocarditis and cardiomyopathy patients than postcardiotomy patients. Furthermore, preliminary data have shown that pulsatile VAD support is less effective for neonates and infants than for older children.[16]

The Thoratec VAD is a pneumatically driven paracorporeal pump with mechanical valves and a maximum stroke volume of 65 mL (Fig. 78-3). In a recent review, a total of 101 children (under 18 years of age) received a Thoratec VAD.[16] Anticoagulation was achieved initially in the postoperative period with heparin, with a goal aPTT of 60 to 80 s. This medication was changed to warfarin, with a target international normalized ratio (INR) of 2.5 to 3.5, which is similar to protocols designed for adults. Overall, 66 patients survived to transplant while 10 were bridged to recovery and VAD explantation. Preoperative weight was greater than 20 kg in all but one patient, with the majority of children weighing more than 50 kg. Pediatric patients supported by Thoratec fared better if treated for myocarditis or cardiomyopathy than for postcardiotomy rescue or congenital heart disease. Patients who had left ventricular cannulation had fewer neurologic events than those who were cannulated via the left atrium.[16]

The Abiomed BVS 5000 is a pneumatically driven pump with an electromagnetic console, a gravity-filled chamber, and an air-actuated ventricular chamber to induce pulsatile contractions (Fig. 78-4). It has been used successfully though only sporadically in a few pediatric

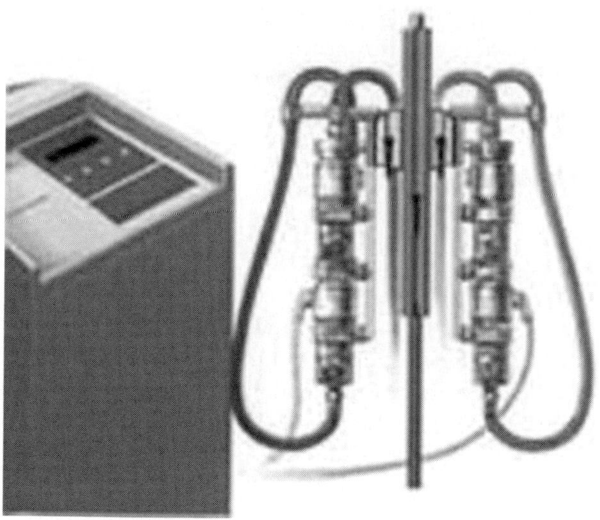

Figure 78-4 Abiomed BVS 5000.

patients, all of whom were adolescents.[10] No series have been reported with this device in smaller children.

The Berlin Heart assist device is the European counterpart of the Thoratec VAD; however, it has been successfully modified to fit smaller patients. Although it is not yet FDA-approved for use in the United States, it has been used very sparingly in cases of compassionate care (Fig. 78-5). The Berlin Heart is also a pneumatically driven paracorporeal pump with either tilting-disk or trileaflet polyurethane valves. The pump is available in numerous stroke-volume sizes down to 10 mL, and there are a variety of different sized cannulas. By 2002, over 85 patients had been supported by a Berlin Heart.[16] Anticoagulation is initially maintained with heparin infusion to maintain aPTT between 60 and 80 s. Forty-five patients were treated at one institution (Deutsches Herzzentrum, Berlin).[19] Patient weight ranged from 2.2 to 81 kg (mean 25 kg), with a mean duration of support of 19 days. Of the 45 patients, 17 survived to transplant and 5 to recovery for a survival of 48.9 percent. In a recently presented subset analysis from the same institution (unpublished data), infant survival at 1 year from implantation was reported as high as 75 percent. Patients of smaller size and those with congenital lesions or postcardiotomy patients fared worse than larger patients with either cardiomyopathy or myocarditis. There was an 11 percent rate of neurologic complications, with equal numbers of intracerebral hemorrhages and thromboembolic events.

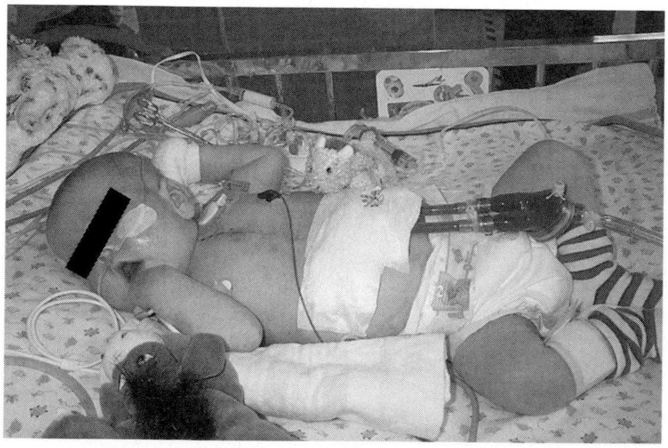

Figure 78-5 Infant with Berlin Heart VAD implanted at Stanford University Medical Center, successfully bridged to cardiac transplantation. (Reproduced with family permission.)

The Medos assist device is another European pneumatically driven paracorporeal pump designed to accommodate pediatric patients, with pump stroke volumes as low as 10 mL as well as several different sized cannulas (Fig. 78-6). Anticoagulation is achieved with intravenous heparin and oral antiaggregant therapy with aspirin. Of 56 patients with known outcome supported by the Medos device, 11 survived to transplantation and 10 were weaned to recovery, for an overall survival rate of 37.5 percent.[16] Again, there was a trend toward a greater survival advantage in patients treated for cardiomyopathy than for postcardiotomy patients.

The Toyobo VAD is a Japanese model with 20-mL stroke volumes and a maximal output of 2.4 L/min; it was reportedly implanted in 8 patients.[20] Three of the patients were weaned and none ultimately survived this small series. Nevertheless, with further refinement and development, this VAD might have pediatric applications in the future.

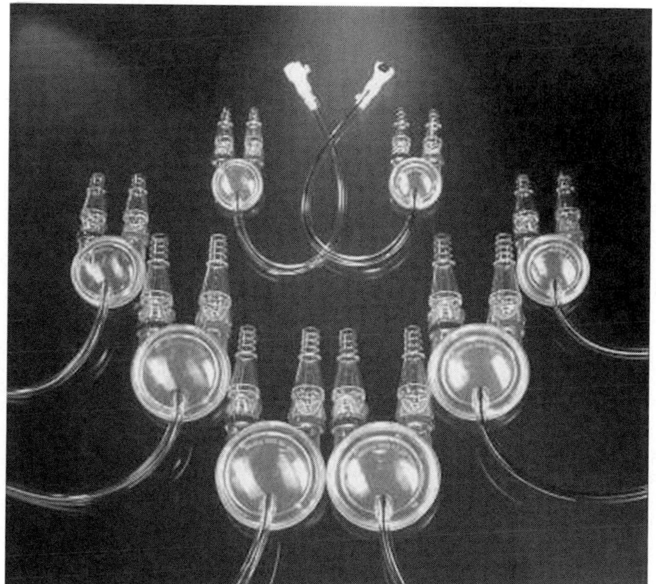

Figure 78-6 Medos VAD.

SURGICAL CONSIDERATIONS

Peripheral cannulation

The most common technique involves a cutdown of the right carotid artery and jugular vein. Alternatively, the femoral artery and vein may be used. An appropriately sized cannula is placed in each vessel and securely fixed. Meticulous de-airing is performed during all connections. The carotid artery must be either ligated or reconstructed after successful weaning from peripheral support such as ECMO.

Central cannulation

Numerous techniques and sites have been used for both inflow and outflow cannulas. Initiation of VAD support in a patient already on cardiopulmonary bypass is usually accomplished with standard bypass cannulas inserted through the superior pulmonary vein into either the left atrium or across the mitral valve into the left ventricle. We place the inflow cannula through a purse-string suture (4-0 polypropylene) in the right superior pulmonary vein. Alternatively, the left ventricular apex can be cannulated using pledgeted 2-0 braided sutures. This may minimize neurologic complications[15] and improve pump inflow, leading to superior flow rates. When possible, cannulas should be brought securely through the skin in the subcostal region and fixed to the skin. Placement of long-term VADs (typically pulsatile devices) usually involves direct apical cannulation with interrupted braided pledgeted mattress sutures fixed to a sewing ring on the VAD cannula. Appropriate de-airing protocols are essential to avoid neurologic complications of air emboli.

CLINICAL ISSUES

Anticoagulation

Anticoagulation is used for all pediatric VADs. One of the major technical difficulties with developing pediatric VADs involves the thrombogenicity of smaller devices.[21] Although there may be slight variations in company recommendations, full anticoagulation is recommended for all devices to keep the aPTT between 60 and 90 s. If the patient is converted to an oral anticoagulation strategy (warfarin), an INR of 2.5 to 3.5 is usually recommended. This regimen does contribute significantly to the bleeding episodes associated with VADs. The risk of thrombosis with resultant embolic phenomena must therefore be weighed against the severity of bleeding as measured by transfusion requirements and hemodynamic instability.

In an effort to reduce anticoagulation requirements and improve safety margin, antithrombotic medications are routinely utilized as well. Recent reports in adults have highlighted the use of heparin-coated lines and more biocompatible bypass circuits that reduce complement activation and fibrinolysis. This might be extrapolated to pediatric VAD circuits.[22,23] Further development of circuit coating might reduce the anticoagulation requirements and therefore the bleeding complications that often accompany the use of VADs.

Antibiotic prophylaxis

Routine antibiotic prophylaxis is mandatory in the perioperative phase. Prophylaxis against gram-positive flora is usually all that is indicated in an otherwise uninfected patient. First-generation cephalosporins are our first choice; these should be given 30 min prior to incision and are routinely administered for 24 h postoperatively. Any signs of infection must be addressed aggressively.

Infection

Despite the use of strict aseptic techniques during both the insertion and maintenance of VADs, infections continue to be a major cause of morbidity and mortality. Because many pediatric VADs are placed at the end of somewhat lengthy operations for the correction of congenital defects, there is already an elevated risk of infection. In these cases, perioperative antimicrobial prophylaxis should be extended for 48 to 72 h, and any suspicion of infection should be aggressively managed with immediate cultures and the administration of broad-spectrum antibiotics, followed by change to a more targeted regimen as soon as culture results and sensitivities are available. Very little has been published regarding pediatric VAD infections; some have advocated antifungal prophylaxis in adults at least for the early perioperative period.[24] Adult studies have shown device-related infections to be very serious and often fatal. Treatment must include timely antimicrobial therapy, surgical drainage or debridement, and, sometimes, device removal.

Bleeding

Owing to the need for anticoagulation, bleeding is an inherent risk that can lead to devastating complications. Intracerebral bleeds occur in 5 to 15 percent of patients supported with pulsatile VADs,[16] with the majority of these proving to be fatal. One study specifically compared the blood transfusion requirements of patients on ECMO versus those supported with a Berlin Heart. They found that patients with the Berlin Heart required significantly less blood, platelet, and plasma replacement than those on ECMO.[18]

Neurologic complications

Poor neurologic outcomes following institution of cardiac support are often multifactorial in etiology, including underlying disease, duration and severity of low-cardiac-output state as well as complications of bleeding and thromboembolism due to the assist device. In long-term follow up of children with cardiac disease who required mechanical support, it has been shown that poor neurologic outcomes were more common in ECMO survivors (60 percent) than nonpulsatile VAD survivors (20 percent).[14] Other data have suggested lower neurologic complications with pulsatile VADs.[12] Finally, left ventricular cannulation might lower the risk of neurologic events in patients with pulsatile VADs.[16]

CONCLUSIONS

In comparison to the adult population, development of pediatric VADs is still in its relative infancy. However, as technology continues to improve, VADs are likely to become invaluable tools in the treatment and management of both acute and chronic heart failure. The decision of which device to use must be tailored to the individual patient. As pediatric patients survive the initial insult of acute cardiac failure with the assistance of short-term VAD support, they must be weaned, changed to more suitable long-term VAD support, or transplanted. Decisions must be made quickly, before refractory infections or end-organ failure occurs. As transplantation is limited by organ availability, there is a need for long-term VADs in small children. As further research and development advances in the field of cardiac support, pediatric patients will soon have more treatment options for their complex medical problems.

References

1. Helman DN, Addonizio LJ, Morales DL, et al. Implantable left ventricular assist devices can successfully bridge adolescent patients to transplant. *J Heart Lung Transplant* 2000; 19(2):121–126.
2. Levi D, Marelli D, Plunkett M, et al. Use of assist devices and ECMO to bridge pediatric patients with cardiomyopathy to transplantation. *J Heart Lung Transplant* 2002;21 (7):760–770.
3. Stiller B, Hetzer R, Weng Y, et al. Heart transplantation in children after mechanical circulatory support with pulsatile pneumatic assist device. *J Heart Lung Transplant* 2003;22 (11):1201–1208.
4. Dadlani GH, Harmon WG, Simbre VC II, et al. Cardiomyocyte injury to transplant: Pediatric management. *Curr Opin Cardiol* 2003;18(2):91–97.
5. Kay J, Colan S, Graham T Jr. Congestive heart failure in pediatric patients. Am Heart J 2001;142(5): 923–928.
6. Dembitsky WP. Bridging from acute to chronic devices. *Ann Thorac Surg* 1999;68(2):724–728.
7. Ungerleider RM, Shen I, Yeh T ,et al. Routine mechanical ventricular assist following the Norwood procedure: Improved neurologic outcome and excellent hospital survival. *Ann Thorac Surg* 2004;77(1):18–22.
8. Duncan BW. Mechanical circulatory support for infants and children with cardiac disease. *Ann Thorac Surg* 2002;73(6):1670–1677.
9. Akomea-Agyin C, Kejriwal NK, Franks R, et al. Intraaortic balloon pumping in children. *Ann Thorac Surg* 1999; 67(3):1415–1420.
10. Throckmorton AL, Allaire PE, Gutgesell HP, et al. Pediatric circulatory support system. *ASAIO J* 2002;48(2): 216–221.
11. Trittenwein G, Goleg J, Burda G, et al. Neonatal and pediatric extracorporeal membrane oxygenation using nonocclusive blood pumps: The Vienna experience. *Artif Organs* 2001;25(12):994–999.
12. Thuys CA, Mullaly RJ, Horton SB, et al. Centrifugal ventricular assist in children under 6 kg. *Eur J Cardiothor Surg* 1998;13(2):130–134.
13. Duncan BW, Hraska V, Jonas RA, et al. Mechanical circulatory support in children with cardiac disease. *J Thorac Cardiovasc Surg* 1999;117(3):529–541.
14. Song X, Throckmorton AL, Untaroiu A, et al. Axial flow blood pumps. *ASAIO J* 2003;49(4):355–356.
15. Morales DL, DiBardino DJ, McKenzie ED, et al. Lessons learned from first application of the De Bakey VAD child: An intra corporeal ventricular assist device for children. *J Heart Lung Transpl* 2005;24(3):331–337.
16. Reinhartz O, Stiller B, Eilers R, et al. Current clinical status of pulsatile pediatric circulatory support. *ASAIO J* 2002;48(5):455–459.
17. Hotz H, Linneweber J, Dohmen PM, et al. Bridge-to-recovery from acute myocarditis in a 12-year-old child. *Artif Organs* 2004;28(6):587–599.
18. Stiller B, Lemmer J, Merkle F, et al. Consumption of blood products during mechanical circulatory support in children: Comparison between ECMO and a pulsatile ventricular assist device. *Intens Care Med* 2004;30(9):1814–1820.
19. Merkle F, Boettcher W, Stiller B. Pulsatile mechanical cardiac assistance in pediatric patients with the Berlin heart ventricular assist device. *J Extra Corpor Technol* 2003; 35(2):115–120.
20. Takano H, Nakatani T. Ventricular assist systems: Experience in Japan with Toyobo pump and Zeon pump. *Ann Thorac Surg* 1996;61(1):317–322.
21. Bachmann C, Hugo G, Rosenberg G, et al. Fluid dynamics of a pediatric ventricular assist device. *Artif Organs* 2000;24(5):362–372.
22. Jensen E, Andreasson S, Bengtsson A, et al. Changes in hemostasis during pediatric heart surgery: Impact of a biocompatible heparin-coated perfusion system. *Ann Thorac Surg* 2004;77(3):962–967.
23. Jensen E, Andreasson S, Bengtsson A, et al. Influence of two different perfusion systems on inflammatory response in pediatric heart surgery. *Ann Thorac Surg* 2003;75(3): 919–925.
24. Holman WL, Skinner JL, Waites KB, et al. Infection during circulatory support with ventricular assist devices. *Ann Thorac Surg* 1999;68(2):711–716.

CHAPTER

79 CONGENITAL ANOMALIES OF THE SINUSES OF VALSALVA AND AORTICO–LEFT VENTRICULAR TUNNEL

Torin P. Fitton, Achintya Moulick, Luca A. Vricella

CONGENITAL ANOMALIES OF THE SINUSES OF VALSALVA

Initially described in 1839,[1] sinus of Valsalva (SoV) aneurysm is a rare condition incidentally found in 0.15 to 1 percent of patients undergoing cardiopulmonary bypass (CPB)[2,3] and five times more frequently in Asians.[4] In 1956, Morrow and Lillehei, using inflow inclusion and a membrane oxygenator, separately reported successful SoV aneurysm repair.[5,6] Since then, surgical repair has been established as the accepted standard of care.

Although acquired SoV aneurysms can occur in the setting of infection or trauma, they are most commonly congenital and are associated with many different connective tissue disorders, including rheumatoid arthritis, Ehlers-Danhlos syndrome, Marfan's syndrome, Klippel-Feil syndrome, Turner's syndrome, trisomies 13 and 15, Loeys-Dietz syndrome, arachnodactyly, and osteogenesis imperfecta. SoV aneurysms are frequently associated with other cardiac abnormalities, including ventricular septal defect (VSD) and aortic valve regurgitation.

SoV aneurysms most commonly originate from the right coronary sinus (RCS), followed by the noncoronary sinus,[7] reflecting the embryologic origin of the RCS and noncoronary (NCS) sinus from fusion of the bulbar septum and truncal ridges. Incomplete fusion of the bulbar septum can in fact result in aneurysm formation when the septum is subjected to long-standing systemic arterial pressure.[8] Aneurysms of the left coronary sinus are exceedingly rare and are usually an acquired phenomenon, as the left coronary cusp does not arise from the bulbar septum.

MORPHOLOGY

On histopathology, SoV aneurysms are characterized by separation of the sinus aortic media adjacent to the hinge point of the aortic valve cusp.[8] Normally the sinuses are thinner than the tubular portion of the aorta and are limited inferiorly by the semicircular hinge point of the corresponding aortic valve cusp. In patients with SoV aneurysms, this otherwise normal characteristic is accentuated, and thinning of the aortic wall with disconnection of the media increases over time, resulting in aneurysm formation.[9]

The anatomic relationship between aortic root and adjacent cardiac structures predicts the clinical findings associated with gradual dilation and rupture of SoV aneurysms (Fig. 79-1). Aneurysms arising from the RCS most commonly involve the right atrium (RA) or right ventricular outflow tract (RVOT), while NCS aneurysms decompress either into the right or left atrium. Rare aneurysmal dilation of the left aortic sinus can eventually rupture into the left atrium. Although aortic root involvement is usually limited to a single sinus, enlargement of two sinuses or the entire aortic root occurs in rare cases. A concomitant VSD is found in up to 50 percent of congenital cases.[10,11]

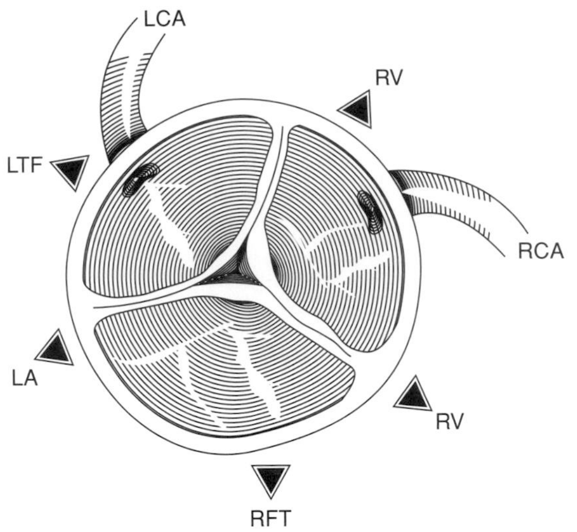

Figure 79-1 Anatomic relationship between aortic root and adjacent cardiac structures as schematically viewed from the operating surgeon's perspective. LA = left atrium; LCA = left coronary artery; LFT = left fibrous trigone; RA = right atrium; RCA = right coronary artery; RV = right ventricle. [From Vricella LA, Cameron DE. Anomalies of the sinuses of Valsalva and aortico–left ventricular tunnel. In: Kaiser LR, Kron IL, Spray TL (eds). *Mastery of Cardiothoracic Surgery,* 2d ed. Philadelphia: Lippincott Williams & Wilkins, 2006 (in press). With permission.]

CLINICAL FEATURES

SoV aneurysms produce symptoms by compression or direct rupture into an adjacent chamber and are often found incidentally. Onset of symptoms is gradual in 50 to 70 percent of patients and occurs most commonly between 20 and 30 years of age but ranges in reported series from infancy to the seventh decade.[12–15] Aortic root rupture into either a neighboring cardiac chamber or within the pericardial cavity is rare in the first two decades of life.[16–18] Although clinical presentation is most commonly indolent, it can be acute depending on aneurysmal size, site of rupture (adjacent chamber versus pericardial sac), and the concomitant presence of a VSD or aortic insufficiency. In case of intracardiac rupture or fistulization, the most common presenting symptom is dyspnea, with nearly all patients exhibiting a continuous systolic-diastolic "machinery-like" murmur.[19] Numerous electrocardiographic findings have been described, including ST-segment depression, onset of Q waves, atrioventricular block, atrial fibrillation, and sudden death. Intrapericardial rupture typically presents with acute hemodynamic collapse and cardiac tamponade. A minority of patients (less than 20 percent) will present with evidence of sepsis associated with bacterial endocarditis.[20]

SURGICAL THERAPY

Urgent operative intervention is clearly indicated for symptomatic patients with rupture or compressive fistulas. SoV aneurysms that are asymptomatic but discovered at the time of CPB should be repaired because of the high likelihood of progressive increase in size, possibility of rupture, or symptom progression. Smaller, asymptomatic SoV aneurysms discovered incidentally during routine echocardiography can be safely followed over time unless progressive enlargement is noted or the patient develops symptoms. Surgical repair may be indicated earlier in patients with significant connective tissue disorder or family history of dissection or rupture.

After induction of general anesthesia, transesophageal echocardiography is routinely performed to confirm the preoperative findings, assess valvular competence, and rule out associated septation defects and endocarditic vegetations. Transesophageal echocardiography is also crucial in defining the course of the fistulous tract in case of intracardiac rupture. The surgical treatment of three-sinus enlargement of the aortic root is detailed elsewhere in this volume and entails either valve-sparing replacement[21,22] of the root or replacement with mechanical or biological prostheses.

Aortotomy is performed to assess the aortic root anatomy and an additional right atriotomy is performed to expose the distal site of rupture or protrusion, especially the "windsock" aneurysmal sac that projects toward the right-sided chambers. A transventricular approach can be utilized alternatively to expose a concomitant VSD. The aortic aspect of the defect is repaired with prosthetic material (Fig. 79-2) to prevent the high risk of aortic valve distortion and recurrence of primary closure. In case of diverticular extension into the RA or right ventricle (RV) (via a VSD), the distal aspect of the SoV aneurysm is corrected with similar technique.

In spite of several well-described repair techniques, the incidence of aortic regurgitation (AR) has been reported between 30 and 50 percent and is severe enough to warrant aortic valve replacement (AVR) in as many as 50 to 80 percent of affected patients.[23] Aortic regurgitation commonly results from prolapse of the affected sinus cusp, which occurs secondary to involvement of the annulus, loss of infundibular support with a conal VSD, or a Venturi effect on the involved cusp.[18] The Ross procedure is to be considered as a viable alternative to root replacement in selected cases.

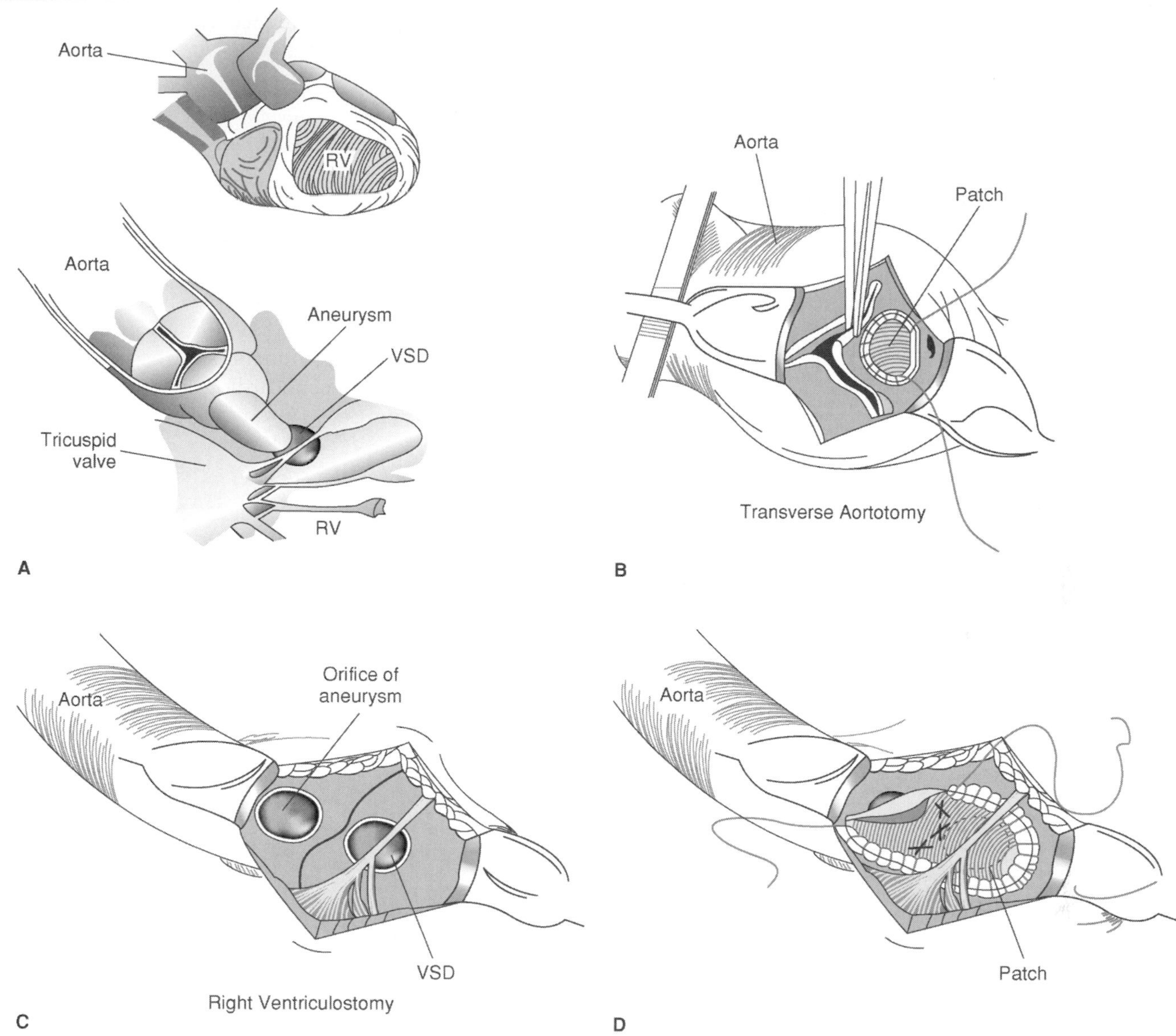

Figure 79-2 Surgical repair of aneurysm of the sinus of Valsalva, originating from the right coronary sinus. (A) schematic view with aneurysm protruding through ventricular septal defect. (B) The inlet to the aneurysm is closed with a patch of bovine or autologous pericardium. C and D. Transventricular repair of the inferior portion of the sinus of Valsalva aneurysm. The defect and the orifice of the aneurysm are closed with a single polyester patch. RV = right ventricle; VSD = ventricular septal defect. [From Vricella LA, Cameron DE. Anomalies of the sinuses of Valsalva and aortico–left ventricular tunnel. In: Kaiser LR, Kron IL, Spray TL (eds). *Mastery of Cardiothoracic Surgery*, 2d ed. Philadelphia: Lippincott Williams & Wilkins, 2006 (in press). With permission.]

RESULTS

Au and coworkers presented the long-term results of 53 patients treated for SoV aneurysms, reporting no operative mortality and a 15-year survival of 83 percent.[14] A retrospective review of 22 patients presenting with intracardiac rupture at the Johns Hopkins Hospital demonstrated an operative mortality of 5 percent, with late survival of 85 and 60 percent at 5 and 10 years, respectively.[19] This decrease in late survival likely reflects the noncongenital etiology of SoV aneurysm more frequently observed in western countries. Although factors such as bacterial endocarditis, need for AVR, and VSD closure do not appear to worsen survival, preoperative aortic regurgitation and VSD have been reported to decrease aortic valve–related freedom from reintervention, with a reported need for AVR of up to 25 percent in the decade following diagnosis and initial intervention.[13,14,24]

AORTICO–LEFT VENTRICULAR TUNNEL

Aortico–left ventricular tunnel (ALVT) is an extremely rare developmental condition consisting of a paravalvular communication between the aortic root and left ventricular cavity. It represents only 0.001 percent of all congenital cardiac anomalies.

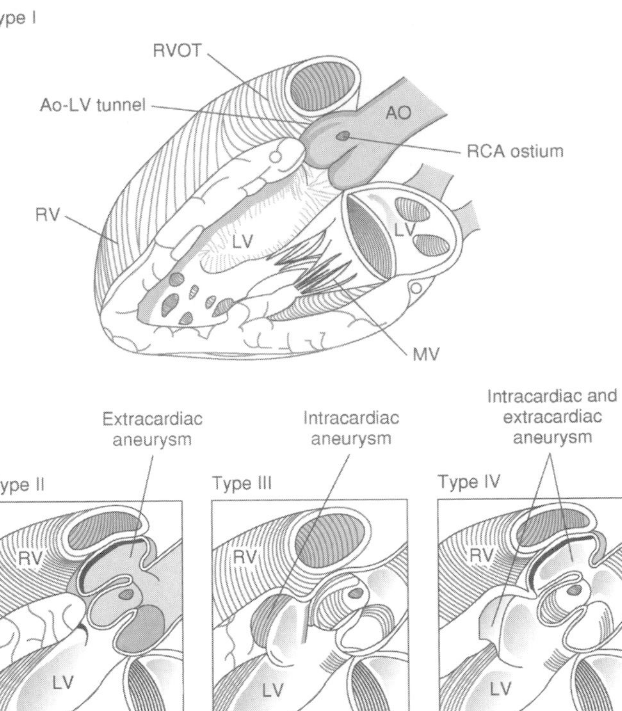

Figure 79-3 Proposed morphologic classification of aortico–left ventricular (Ao-LV) tunnel. Type I: Simple tunnel with slit-like opening at aortic end, no aortic valve distortion. Type II: Large tunnel with oval aortic opening with or without aortic valve distortion. Type III: Intracardiac aneurysm of the ventricular portion of the tunnel with or without right ventricular outflow tract obstruction. Type IV: Combination of types II and III. [From Shum-Tim D, Tchervenkov CI. Aortic–left ventricular tunnel. In: Mavroudis C, Backer CL (eds). *Pediatric Cardiac Surgery,* 3d ed. Philadelphia: Mosby, 2003:576. With permission.]

MORPHOLOGY

The lesion typically originates from the RCS around the coronary ostium and can be appreciated grossly as a palpable, pulsatile mass between aortic and pulmonary artery roots. The course of the aneurysm can be variable, but it usually terminates in the ventricular cavity below the right coronary leaflet. The ventricular opening can be appreciated with retraction of the aortic valve cusps. The most frequently occurring anatomic variants are categorized in the Hovaguimian classification (Fig. 79-3).[25] Almost half of all patients will disclose associated defects (VSD, bicuspid aortic valve) on echocardiographic examination, although the aortic valve is usually competent. Coronary anomalies have been reported in up to one-third of patients.[6]

CLINICAL FEATURES

The clinical presentation is dependent on the size of the fistulous tract and the degree of associated aortic regurgitation. Although an ALVT is an uncommon cause of neonatal congestive heart failure, ALVT should be suspected in neonates with plethoric lung fields, cardiomegaly, a diastolic murmur, and widened pulse pressure. Like SoV aneurysms, large fistulous tracts can also lead to progressive RVOTO and cyanosis.

The diagnostic modality of choice is transthoracic echocardiography, which readily demonstrates the classic "dropout" of the interventricular septum inferior to the RCS. Cardiac catheterization and magnetic resonance imaging are rarely required.

THERAPY

The degree of valvular insufficiency and severity of congestive heart failure often mandate immediate operative intervention, but serial observation with echocardiography is acceptable, as spontaneous closure of small ALVT defects has been reported.

Intraoperatively, bicaval cannulation is employed only if a concomitant septal defect requires surgical correction. Cardiopulmonary bypass with moderate hypothermia and the direct infusion of coronary ostial cardioplegia are employed. We favor closure of both inlet and outlet orifices of the tunnel in a manner similar as that described for SoV aneurysm (Fig. 79-4). Patch closure of both openings of the ALVT provides additional protection from late valvular regurgitation and recurrence of the fistulous tract. As an alternative approach, both orifices of the ALVT can be approached from within the ALVT (Fig. 79-5).

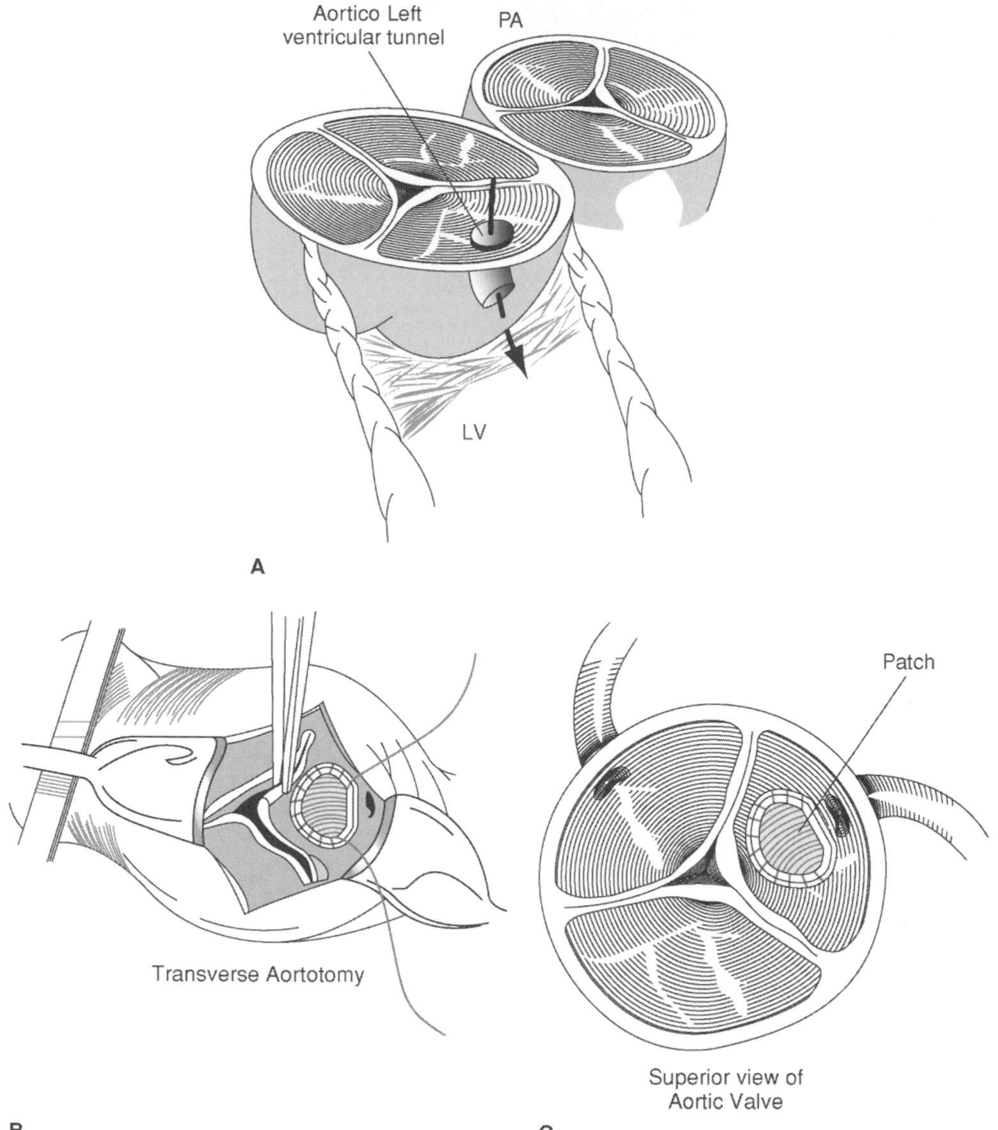

Figure 79-4 Aortico–left ventricular tunnel with the inlet originating (A) in the right coronary sinus (most typical location). Through an aortotomy (B and C), the inlet orifice to the tunnel is closed with an autologous pericardial patch. The ventricular opening of the tunnel is closed through the aorta separately, either primarily or with an additional patch. [From Vricella LA, Cameron DE. Anomalies of the sinuses of Valsalva and aortico–left ventricular tunnel. In: Kaiser LR, Kron IL, Spray TL (eds). *Mastery of Cardiothoracic Surgery,* 2d ed. Philadelphia: Lippincott Williams & Wilkins, 2006 (in press). With permission.]

RESULTS

In contemporary series, operative mortality has been reported to be less than 10 percent, with need for reoperative intervention being the most significant determinant of late outcome. The most common early complications include atrioventricular heart block and aortic valve regurgitation. Aortic regurgitation secondary to postrepair deformity or root dilation due to lack of annular support around the ALVT may result in need for late aortic valve or root replacement in up to 50 percent of patients, particularly if initial correction is delayed beyond infancy.[26,27]

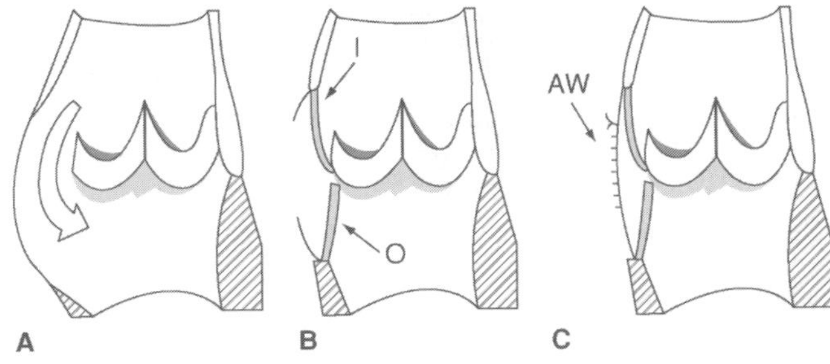

Figure 79-5 Schematic representation of alternative approach for repair of aortico–left ventricular tunnel. A. cross section of the aortic root with the tunnel indicated by the downward-pointing arrow. B. The tunnel is exposed *directly* through an aortotomy, and the inlet (I) an outlet (O) orifices are closed with separate patches. C. The aortic wall (AW) is closed primarily.

References

1. Hope J. *A Treatise on Diseases of the Heart and Great Vessels.* London: Churchill & Sons, 1839.
2. Mayer ED, Ruffman K, Saggau W, et al. Ruptured aneurysms of the sinus of Valsava. *Ann Thorac Surg* 1986;42:81.
3. Verghese M, Jairaj PS, Babuthaman C, et al. Surgical treatment of ruptured aneurysms of the sinus of Valsalva. *Ann Thorac Surg* 1986;41:284.
4. Chu SH, Hung CR. Ruptured aneurysms of the sinus of Valsalva in Oriental patients. *J Thorac Cardiovasc Surg* 1990;99:288.
5. Lillehei CW, Stanley P, Varco RL. Surgical treatment of ruptured aneurysm of the sinus of Valsalva. *Ann Surg* 1957;146:459.
6. Morrow AG, Baker RR, Hansen HE, et al. Successful repair of the aneurysm of the sinus of Valsalva. *Circulation* 1957;16:533.
7. Baek WK, Kim JT, Yoon YH, et al. Huge sinus of Valsalva aneurysm causing mitral valve incompetence. *Ann Thorac Surg* 2002;73:1975.
8. Edwards JE, Burchell HB. The pathological anatomy of deficiencies between the aortic root and the heart, including aortic sinus aneurysms. *Thorax* 1957;12:125.
9. Abbott ME. Clinical and developmental study of a case of ruptured aneurysm of the right anterior aortic sinus of Valsalva, leading to communication between the aorta and base of the right ventricle. Contributions to medical and biological research. New York: Hoeber, 1919:899–914.
10. Gerbode F, Osborn JJ, Johnston JB, et al. Ruptured aneurysms of the aortic sinus of Valsalva. *Am J Surg* 1961;102:268.
11. Takach TJ, Reul GJ, Duncan JM, et al. Sinus of Valsalva aneurysm or fistula: Management and outcome. *Ann Thorac Surg* 1999;68:1573.
12. Pan C, Tsao CH, Chen C, et al. Surgical treatment of the ruptured aneurysm of the aortic sinuses. *Ann Thorac Surg* 1981;32:162.
13. Murashita T, Kubota T, Kamikubo Y, et al. Long-term results of aortic valve regurgitation after repair of ruptured sinus of Valsalva aneurysm. *Ann Thorac Surg* 2002;73:1466.
14. Au WK, Chiu SW, Mok CK, et al. Repair of ruptured sinus of Valsalva aneurysm: Determinants of long-term survival. *Ann Thorac Surg* 1998;66:1604.
15. Azakie A, David TE, Peniston CM, et al. Ruptured sinus of Valsalva aneurysm: Early recurrence and fate of the aortic valve. *Ann Thorac Surg* 2000;70:1466.
16. Shah RP, Ding ZP, Ng A, et al. A ten-year review of ruptured sinus of Valsalva: Clinico-pathological and echo-Doppler features. *Singapore Med J* 2001;42:473.
17. Abe T, Komatsu S. Surgical repair and long-term results in ruptured sinus of Valsalva aneurysm. *Ann Thorac Surg* 1988;46:520.
18. Dong C, Wu QY, Tang Y. Sinus of Valsalva aneurysm: A Beijing experience. *Ann Thorac Surg* 2002;74:1621.
19. Harkness JR, Fitton TP, Barreiro CJ, et al. A 32-year experience with surgical repair of sinus of Valsalva aneurysm. *J Card Surg* 2005;20:198.
20. Choudhary SK, Bhan A, Sharma R, et al. Sinus of Valsalva aneurysms: 20 years' experience. *J Card Surg* 1997;12:300.
21. Cameron DE, Vricella LA. Valve-sparing aortic root replacement in Marfan syndrome. *Semin Thorac Cardiovasc Pediatr Card Surg Ann* 2005;8:103.
22. Vricella LA, Williams JA, Ravekes WJ, et al. Early experience with valve-sparing aortic root replacement in children. *Ann Thorac Surg* 2005;80:1622.
23. Naka Y, Kadoba K, Ohtake S, et al. The long-term outcome of a surgical repair of sinus of Valsalva aneurysm. *Ann Thorac Surg* 2000;70:727.
24. Van Son JAM, Danielson GK, Shaff HV, et al. Long-term outcome of surgical repair of ruptured sinus of Valsalva aneurysm. *Circulation* 1994;90:20.
25. Hovaguimian H, Cobanoglu A, Starr A. Aortico-left ventricular tunnel: A clinical review and a new surgical classification. *Ann Thorac Surg* 1988;45:106.
26. Levy MJ, Schachner A, Blieden LC. Aortico-left ventricular tunnel: Late follow up. *Ann Thorac Surg* 1986;42:304.
27. Martins JD, Sherwood MC, Mayer JE, et al. Aortico-left ventricular tunnel: 35-year experience. *J Am Coll Cardiol* 2004;44:446.

CHAPTER

80 PEDIATRIC CARDIAC TRANSPLANTATION

Nahidh W. Hasaniya, Anees J. Razzouk, Richard E. Chinnock, Leonard L. Bailey

BACKGROUND

Clinical cardiac transplantation (CT) began when Christiaan Barnard performed the first human heart allotransplant on December 3, 1967.[1] After that time, numerous centers began programs of CT. Initially, the recipients in most centers appeared to have a satisfactory operation, but they soon experienced fatal allograft rejection, systemic infection, or both. Enthusiasm waned, and clinical CT was limited to the efforts of Norman Shumway and associates at Stanford University and Richard Lower and associates at Stanford University and later at the Medical College of Virginia in the United States and Christian Cabrol and associates in France.

Cardiac transplantation regained global popularity with the introduction of the immunoregulative drug cyclosporine in the early 1980s.[2] Improved control of the host immune response translated into better survival and fewer infectious complications. Heart transplantation outcomes continued to be enhanced by the application of improved operative techniques and immunosuppression, the use of endomyocardial biopsy for the diagnosis of graft rejection, and the use of viral prophylaxis. Infants and young children, however, largely were excluded from CT during the 1970s and early 1980s. Successful CT in a newborn baby first was accomplished on November 20, 1985, at Loma Linda University (LLU) in southern California.[3] That experience ushered

KEY CONCEPTS

- Epidemiology
  - Since 1982, over 5000 pediatric heart transplants have been recorded in the Registry of the International Society of Heart and Lung Transplantation. The current number of reported pediatric heart transplants is about 350 per year.
- Indications
  - Heart transplantation is the most effective and often the only treatment for end-stage heart disease. Complex congenital heart disease is the main indication for heart transplantation in infants, whereas end-stage cardiomyopathy is the main indication after the first year of life.
- Contraindications
  - The main contraindication is elevated pulmonary vascular resistance that is unresponsive to oxygen and vasodilators.
- Techniques
  - Heart transplantation is performed using either biatrial or bicaval techniques, depending on the size of the recipient child. Graft procurement and implantation are modified to accommodate the specific anatomic variations present in recipients with congenital heart disease.
- Outcomes
  - Mortality while waiting for a donor is 12 to 40 percent. The overall actuarial survival at 10 years ranges between 50 and 66 percent and is 74 percent for newborn recipients. Causes of mortality include graft rejection and failure, infection, posttransplant coronary artery disease (16 percent), and malignancy (8 percent).

in a new era of infant and pediatric CT, representing the major growth area in CT during the 1990s.

Since 1982, over 5000 pediatric CT procedures have been recorded by the Registry of the International Society for Heart and Lung Transplantation (ISHLT). The incidence of pediatric CT has plateaued, with about 350 infant and childhood recipients reported annually to the ISHLT Registry. The United States contributes about half the annual total, with 181 pediatric recipients 0 to 10 years of age reported to the ISHLT Registry in 2003. Today, infants and children (0 to 18 years old) constitute 10 percent of all recipients of CT.[4]

This chapter reviews indications for and contraindications to pediatric CT, timing for surgery, surgical techniques, immunosuppression regimens, rejection surveillance, complications, outcomes (highlighting the LLU experience), and future trends.

INDICATIONS

Cardiac transplantation provides the most effective treatment for end-stage heart disease, whether myopathic or structural (congenital). Data from the ISHLT Registry's annual report suggest that complex congenital heart disease is the primary indication for transplantation among patients in the first year of life, accounting for more than 75 percent of cases.[5,6] End-stage cardiomyopathy (including "burned-out" congenital heart disease) is the predominant indication for transplantation among recipients who are beyond the first year of life. Retransplantation accounts for 1 to 5 percent of all indications (Table 80-1).[4] Cardiac diagnoses that may be considered for orthotropic transplantation in early infancy are shown in Table 80-2.

Table 80-2 Cardiac malformations presenting in early infancy that may be an indication for orthotopic cardiac transplantation

1. Hypoplastic left heart syndrome (hypoplastic aortic tract complex)
2. Hypoplastic left heart equivalent:
   a. D-TGA with hypoplastic right ventricle and aortic tract
   b. Single ventricle with hypoplastic aortic tract
   c. L-TGA with single ventricle and heart block
   d. Shone's complex: severe mitral valve stenosis (atresia), left ventricular outflow obstruction, coarctation of the aorta
3. Symptomatic severe Ebstein's anomaly with normal pulmonary arteries
4. Multiple obstructive rhabdomyomas or fibromas
5. Pulmonary atresia/intact ventricular septum (large sinusoids[a])
6. A-V septal defect with hypoplastic left ventricle and mitral component (frequently associated with coarctation)
7. Single ventricle with subaortic obstruction (bulboventricular foramen)
8. Severe intrauterine A-V valve insufficiency and ventricular dysfunction
9. Straddling A-V valve and tensor apparatus
10. Complex truncus arteriosus
11. Severe congenital or acquired cardiomyopathy at end stage with maximal medical management

[a]Diminutive right heart malformations *must* have adequate-size right and left pulmonary arteries. Neonates unresponsive to PGE_1 may require placement of a systemic-pulmonary shunt while waiting for a donor).
A-V = atrioventricular; D-TGA = D-loop transposition of the great arteries; L-TGA = L-loop transposition of the great arteries.

CONTRAINDICATIONS

The main contraindication to CT is elevated pulmonary vascular resistance (more than 5 to 6 Woods units) that is unresponsive to oxygen and vasodilators. Children with a transpulmonary gradient greater than 15 mmHg are largely unsuitable for isolated CT.[7] Pulmonary vascular resistance is seldom an issue during early infancy but becomes an important contraindication in older children and adolescents. Other contraindications are listed in Table 80-3, and include unstable metabolic

Table 80-1 Indications for and survival after pediatric cardiac transplantation based on age

Age	< 1 Year, %	1–10 Years, %	11–17 Years, %
Indication			
Congenital	76	37	25
Myopathy	20	53	66
Other	3	5	6
Retransplant	1	5	3
Survival			
30-day	87	90	91
1-year	80	85	88
3-year	74	78	80
5-year	63	70	67

Adapted from the International Society of Heart and Lung Transplantation Registry and the United Network for Organ Sharing Registry, published as a bar graph in the *Journal of Heart and Lung Transplantation*, vol. 20, August 2001, from Fig. 5, p. 806.

Table 80-3 Clinical conditions that may contraindicate orthotopic cardiac transplantation

1. Marked prematurity (< 34–36 weeks)
2. Excessively low birth weight
3. Active malignancy
4. Multisystem organ failure
5. Persistent acidosis with pH below 7.0
6. Abnormal neurologic status, suggesting a poor long-term prognosis
7. Active, untreated infection
8. Genetic anomalies or syndromes that significantly limit survival
9. Socioeconomic factors leading to noncompliance
10. Hypoplastic obstructive pulmonary veins

and hemodynamic status, inadequate psychosocial support, profound neurologic and renal dysfunction, untreated clinical infection, and chromosomal abnormalities that limit survival.

TIMING

The decision to proceed with CT is multifactorial, and depends on the transplant facility, the physician, the recipient, and the recipient's family. Pretransplant evaluation of potential recipients nevertheless should be expeditious, leading to early registration with the national organ procurement and distribution center. Delay leads to unnecessary morbidity and mortality. Even when a patient is registered, the waiting time is entirely unpredictable. A waiting recipient may encounter major morbidities such as overwhelming sepsis, cerebral hemorrhage, necrotizing enterocolitis, cardiac arrest, and hepatorenal failure, among others; these morbidities become contraindications to CT. As indications for CT have expanded and organ supply has remained constant, recipient waiting time and the resulting morbidity have increased. Mortality while waiting for a donor heart graft has ranged between 12 and 40 percent.

Experience with mechanical circulatory support as a bridge to pediatric transplantation remains limited. Extracorporeal membrane oxygenation (ECMO; see Chapter 77) is useful for only a relatively short period.[8] Utilization on with infant-sized ventricular assist devices (VADs; see Chapter 78) is just being reported. Outcomes remain indeterminate but promising. In older children and adolescents, the use of VADs has improved waiting time survival without negatively affecting CT outcome. Early listing for CT optimizes recipient survival and reduces the need for intermediate mechanical circulatory support.

GRAFT PROCUREMENT

Donor heart procurement is tailored to the individual anatomic demands of the recipient. En bloc excision of the heart, the pulmonary arterial tree, the superior vena cava (SVC) in continuity with the brachiocephalic vein and the origin of the internal jugular veins, and some or all of the aortic arch may be required to simplify recipient reconstruction. Concomitant lung donation may not be suitable when replacement of the central pulmonary artery is anticipated in a heart recipient or when a cardiac recipient has situs inversus or anomalous pulmonary venous connections, which may require the use of the entire donor left atrium. A general rule of thumb is to procure more rather than less of what the recipient will require. Aggressive trimming of the donor heart should be postponed until its implantation into the recipient.

Heart procurement usually is accomplished in concert with the procurement of additional organs (by other teams) through a long midline incision. The donor is given 25 mg/kg of cephalosporin antibiotic and 25 mg/kg of methylprednisolone. Fifty percent dextrose (0.5 to 1 mL/kg) is administered intravenously to the donor every 15 min until the organ is excised. The aorta is separated from the pulmonary artery, and the aortic arch vessels are doubly ligated and divided. The SVC and the innominate vein (as needed) are isolated. The azygos vein is ligated and divided. Its posterior location becomes a landmark for the future SVC anastomosis, or it can be used to enlarge the donor SVC if there is a size discrepancy. When each team has completed the dissection, the donor receives intravenous heparin in a dose of 500 units per kilogram, and the heart is decompressed by transecting the inferior vena cava (IVC) and one of the left pulmonary veins. The aorta is cross-clamped, and 250 to 500 mL of antegrade cold crystalloid cardioplegia is administered. In their practice, the authors utilize Roe's solution for myocardial protection in a dose of 75 mL/kg in neonates and smaller children. Both pleural spaces are opened to accommodate drainage. If the lungs are being procured, the left heart is vented by amputating the left atrial appendage before the infusion of lung preservation solution. Cardiectomy is accomplished by first transecting the IVC, as was mentioned above, and then the pulmonary veins at the pericardial reflection. If the lungs are being harvested, the pulmonary veins are not divided at the pericardial reflection. Instead, the left atrium is opened and carefully transected to preserve an adequate cuff around the pulmonary veins. The branch pulmonary arteries are transected at the pericardial reflection if the lungs are not being procured, whereas if the lungs are being retrieved, the main pulmonary artery is divided before the bifurcation. The heart is lifted upward, and posterior attachments are divided. The SVC and the aorta are divided on the basis of the amount of tissue needed. The heart is then removed from the field to a back table, where it is examined while being immersed in cold saline solution. If present, a patent foramen ovale is closed, and the graft is packaged in a self-sealing plastic bag placed in a sterile, sealed container and immersed in an ice chest for transportation. Portions of donor thymus, spleen, and hilar or mesenteric lymph nodes are harvested and stored for immunologic testing. Communication between the procurement team and the team at the recipient hospital is essential to minimize graft cold ischemia time. It has been recommended that graft ischemia time be kept to less than 4 h to reduce perioperative mortality.[4] However, longer ischemia times of up to 9.5 h without increased mortality have been reported by investigators at LLU.[9]

GRAFT IMPLANTATION

The original biatrial technique (Fig. 80-1A) of CT was described by Lower and Shumway in 1967.[10] This

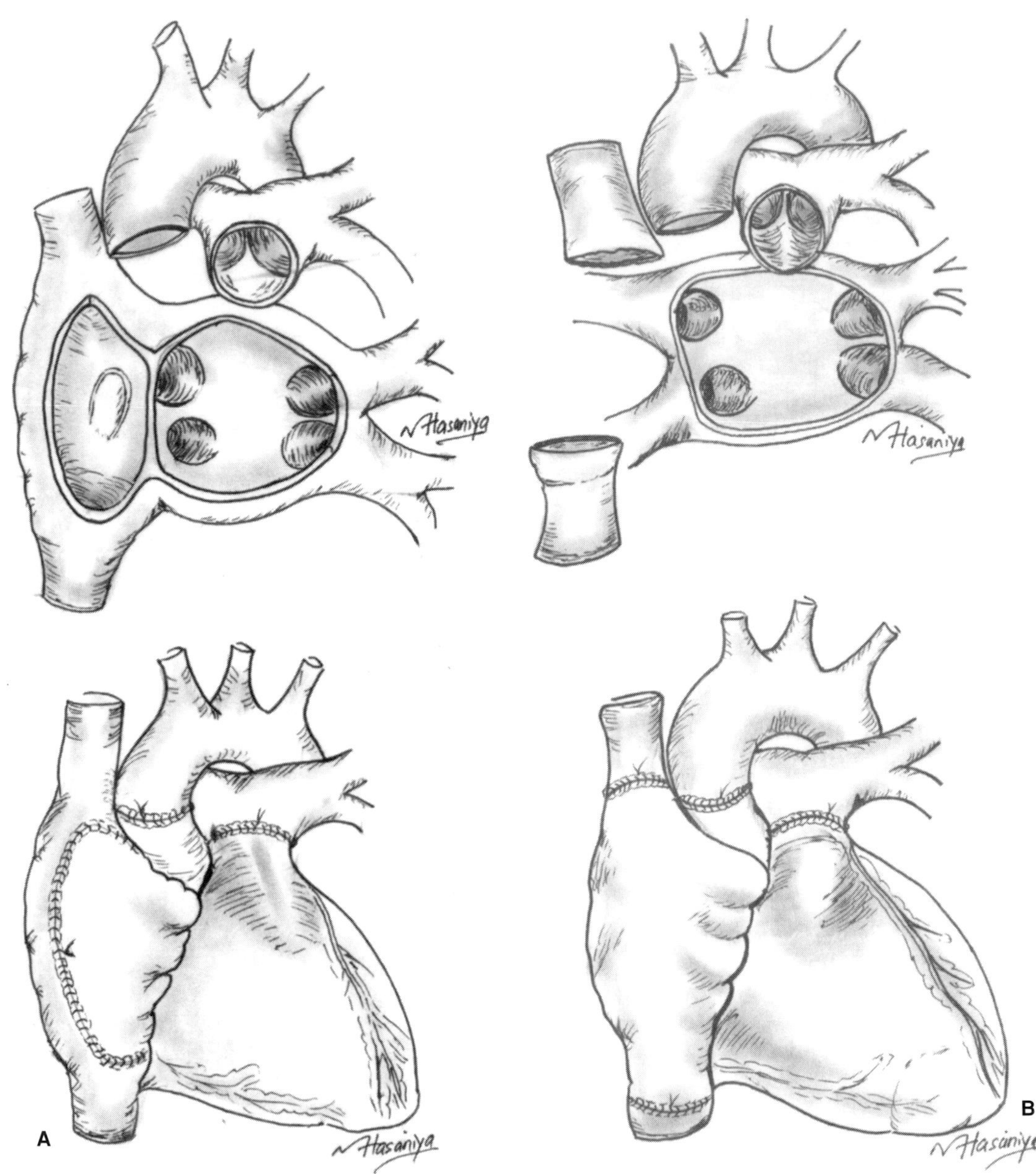

Figure 80-1 Technique of biatrial **(A)** and bicaval **(B)** cardiac transplantation.

technique frequently creates oversized atria and thus may distort right atrial geometry and lead to atrioventricular valve insufficiency and/or arrhythmias. Bicaval anastomosis, which originally was described by Dreyfus and colleagues,[11] is now the technique that is employed most commonly (Fig. 80-1B). Bicaval CT preserves right atrial morphology and is applicable at any age. It is particularly useful during reoperative CT or when space is an issue. The recipient procedure is accomplished with a median sternotomy. The thymus is excised. The recipient is placed on cardiopulmonary bypass, using aortic and right atrial cannulation. At LLU, systemic cooling to a core temperature of 18 to 20°C is achieved routinely. The aorta is cross-clamped, bypass flow is reduced, and the passive venous cannula is replaced by flexible pump suckers. Both the aorta and the pulmonary trunks are divided just above the semilunar valves. Both the SVC and the IVC are divided, preserving a small atrial cuff on each one to facilitate later anastomoses. A left atriectomy is performed, leaving a posterior atrial cuff that contains the pulmonary veins, and the native heart is removed from the chest. The donor heart is evaluated, and the left atrium is trimmed to match the recipient left atrial cuff. The left atrioatrial anastomosis is performed, using the left atrial appendage as a landmark to match donor and recipient atrial cuffs. A small area of the anastomosis is kept incomplete so that cold saline can be flushed intermittently through the left-sided structures. The IVC anastomosis then is completed, followed by an end-to-end anastomosis of the SVC. The aortic anastomosis is completed, and intracavitary air is displaced by flushing of the left heart with cold saline. The aortic clamp is removed, ending graft ischemia, and the pulmonary arterial anastomosis is completed during reperfusion of the allograft. All anastomoses are performed with continuous polypropylene sutures. The graft and the patient are rewarmed and reperfused for at least an hour to allow the heart to fully recover. As the recipient rewarms, inotropic and vasodilating drugs such as dopamine, milrinone, and nitroglycerin are infused intravenously, and the recipient is separated from extracorporeal circulation.

A biatrial anastomosis usually is employed in small babies. The interatrial septum is anastomosed first, followed by the right atrium and then the left atrium. The procurement and trimming of the donor heart and the technique of CT are modified to cope with various anatomic situations, examples of which are discussed below.

Infants with hypoplastic left heart syndrome

The technique of orthotopic CT and aortic arch reconstruction in infants with hypoplastic left heart syndrome (HLHS) (Fig. 80-2) first was described in 1986.[12] The technique later was modified to reduce the duration of circulatory arrest.[13] The chest is opened through a midsternal incision, and thymectomy is accomplished. Cardiopulmonary bypass is initiated, using a single venous drainage cannula in the right atrium, and an arterial perfusion cannula is placed in the pulmonary trunk but directed into the arterial duct and snared to prevent flow into the lungs. Systemic cooling to a core temperature of 18 to 20°C is achieved within 12 to 15 min. During this period, branches of the aortic arch are dissected and surrounded individually with loose tourniquets. Low-flow perfusion is initiated. The passive atrial drainage cannula is replaced with an active pump sucker. The diminutive ascending aorta is ligated and divided just proximal to the brachiocephalic artery. Traction on this ligature facilitates exposure of the proximal descending aorta. The main pulmonary artery is transected at the level of the valve. The hypoplastic heart is excised, leaving in place posterior atrial wall cuffs and a rim of atrial septum.

After inspection of the recipient pulmonary veins, implantation of the donor heart begins with the atrial septum at its inferior aspect, using a continuous monofilament suture that is carried up the septum and around the right atrium first. A flexible suction catheter is repositioned in the right atrial appendage while the graft is retracted toward the operating surgeon and the left atrial anastomosis is completed. With the infant in the Trendelenburg position, the aortic arch vessels are snared, the circulation is arrested, and the arterial perfusion cannula is withdrawn. The arterial duct is ligated and divided, and all ductal tissue is excised. The undersurface of the aortic arch is incised from the level of the brachiocephalic

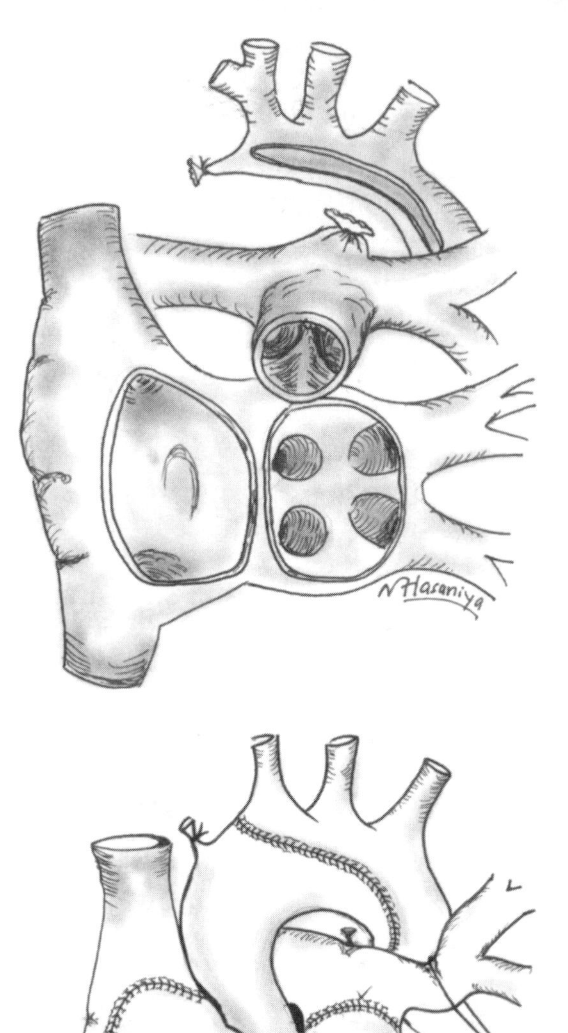

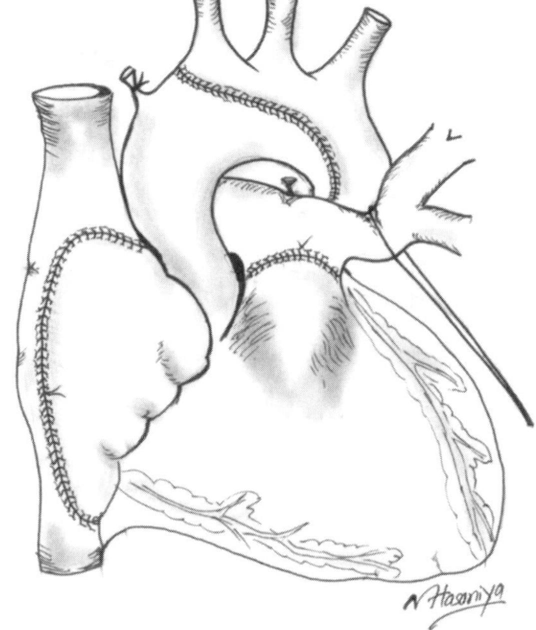

Figure 80-2 Cardiac transplantation of infants with hypoplastic left heart syndrome (note the technique for aortic arch reconstruction).

trunk to several millimeters beyond the ductus arteriosus onto the descending aorta. The neoaortic arch is reconstructed with the opened long segment of the donor arch, starting beyond the amputated duct. A period 20 to 25 min of circulatory arrest provides a bloodless field for this part of the procedure. Special care is exercised to identify and avoid injury of the recurrent laryngeal nerve. The aorta is filled with cold saline via the stump of the donor brachiocephalic artery, which also is used for reinsertion of the arterial cannula. The passive venous cannula is placed back into the donor right atrium through the appendage. Perfusion is resumed, and air is evacuated through a vent site in the donor ascending aorta. The occluders around the arch vessels are removed, and the pulmonary arterial anastomosis is completed during the early warming phase of recirculation. The patient is rewarmed to 37°C, using a minimum of 60 min of extracorporeal reperfusion. In some instances, when cold ischemic time is prolonged, reperfusion is extended to 80 or 90 min to achieve complete functional recovery of the heart.[14]

Infants with HLHS after a failed Norwood procedure

In this special situation, the donor heart procurement includes the central pulmonary arteries and the complete aortic arch. Recipient dissection exposes the aortic arch, the aortopulmonary shunt, and both branch pulmonary arteries. The shunt is closed and divided, the native pulmonary arterial bifurcation is replaced by the donor pulmonary arteries, and the donor aorta is connected end to end to the previously reconstructed aortic arch if the distal arch is unobstructed. Otherwise, the aortic arch is reconstructed completely with donor aorta. Circulatory arrest is unnecessary in the first instance but may be employed to enable arch reconstruction if necessary. The rest of the implantation is similar to the procedure for HLHS described above.[15]

Recipients with situs inversus

Donor cardiectomy is performed with en bloc removal of the SVC and the innominate vein, which together are used to reconstitute cephalic venous drainage in the recipient. The donor left pulmonary vein orifices are oversewn, and the left atrium is opened vertically and, to some extent, horizontally between the right pulmonary veins. This approach helps align the donor graft for anastomosis with the recipient right-sided pulmonary atrium. The procedure is performed with low-flow hypothermic perfusion, as was described above. The left pericardium is excised widely. The recipient heart is removed, leaving behind a small pulmonary atrial cuff and abundant systemic atrial tissue in continuity with the left-positioned IVC. The recipient systemic venous atrial remnant is fashioned into a short conduit, directing IVC drainage toward the right side of the recipient. Graft implantation is started with the left atrial anastomosis. The IVC of the recipient, which is lengthened toward the right, is anastomosed to that of the donor heart. The conduit formed by the donor's SVC and innominate vein is anastomosed to the left-sided SVC of the recipient and positioned in the transverse sinus behind the aorta and pulmonary artery. The donor SVC–innominate vein may also be anastomosed to a large recipient transverse brachiocephalic (innominate) vein anterior to the great arteries. The aortic anastomosis is performed next, the cross-clamp is removed, and the patient is rewarmed. During the warming phase, the recipient's pulmonary artery is opened longitudinally into the left pulmonary artery. The short stump of native main pulmonary artery is closed right to left with a running suture, leaving a left-sided recipient pulmonary arterial orifice for anastomosis with the donor main pulmonary artery. In infants who require aortic arch reconstruction, the aortic anastomosis is performed before the SVC connection, using a short period of circulatory arrest. This is done to facilitate earlier graft reperfusion. In this instance, the donor SVC–innominate vein conduit is positioned anterior to the great arteries.[16] The procedure is illustrated in Fig. 80-3.

Cardiac transplantation after a failed Fontan operation

Multipalliated children may end up with cavopulmonary shunts, destroyed or absent central pulmonary arteries, and failed attempts at achieving satisfactory Fontan physiology. These children may have atrial situs solitus and occasionally situs ambiguus or inversus. The donor heart is harvested with adequate systemic veins and pulmonary arteries for reimplantation, using a cavocaval strategy. Profound hypothermic CPB is achieved with single aortic and venous cannulas, and a low-flow state is established. Using active "sucker" venous drainage, cardiectomy is performed. Graft implantation is started with attachment of the left atria. This is followed by anastomosis of the IVC, the main pulmonary artery (or separate right and left pulmonary arteries), one or both superior cavae or internal jugular veins, and, finally, the aorta.[15] These features are illustrated in Fig. 80-4.

SURVEILLANCE

At LLU, transplant recipients are followed and evaluated by a specialized team that consists of pediatricians, coordinators, pharmacists, and cardiologists. Initially, office surveillance occurs twice weekly, then weekly, and then monthly for the first year. Follow-up visits are less frequent after that time. This is a lifetime commitment that provides mutual benefit to both the recipient and the transplant parents. The outpatient follow-up visits include history and physical examination, electrocardiography, echocardiography, yearly chest roentgenograms, complete blood count, immunosuppression drug levels, and measurement of electrolytes and viral titers. Cardiac biopsy, coronary angiography, and intravascular ultrasound are accomplished annually beyond the first posttransplant year. Testing throughout the patient's life is based on specific protocols.

IMMUNOSUPPRESSION

In the earliest days of CT, therapeutic options for the prevention of allograft rejection were limited.[17] Initial

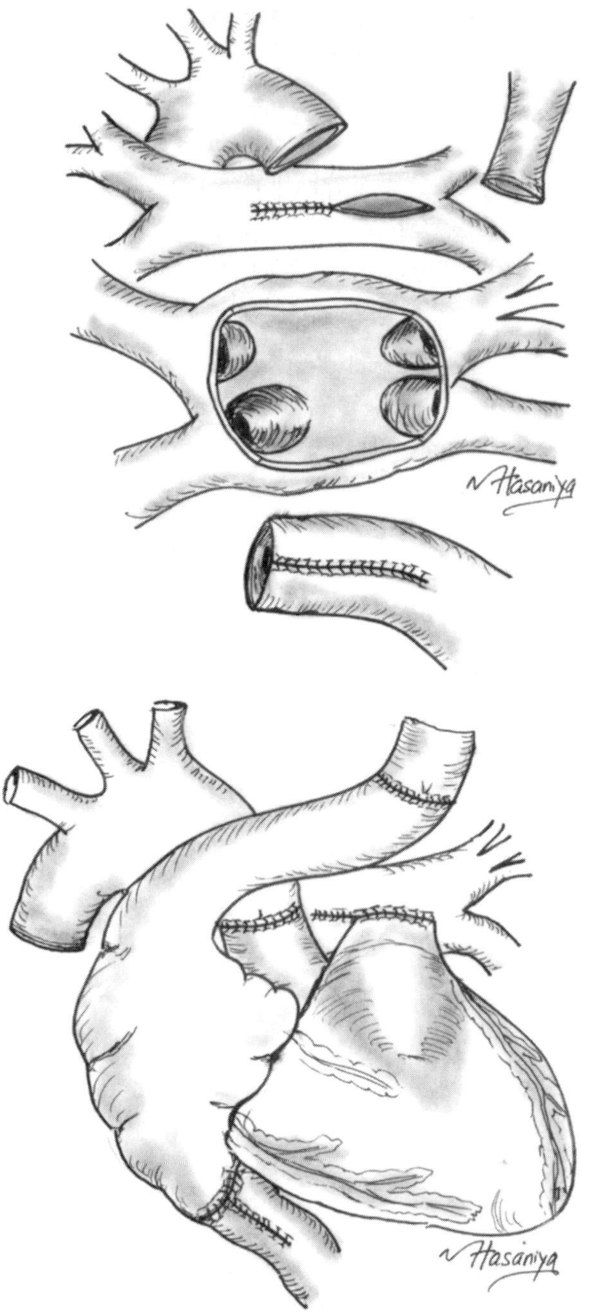

Figure 80-3 Cardiac transplantation in children with situs inversus. Cardiectomy is performed, the pulmonary anastomotic site is relocated to the left, and the inferior vena cava is rerouted to the right of the midline (*top*). Graft implantation is performed in the usual fashion, with the donor's left brachiocephalic vein anastomosed to the left superior vena cava (*bottom*). The superior caval connection can be positioned anterior or posterior to the aorta.

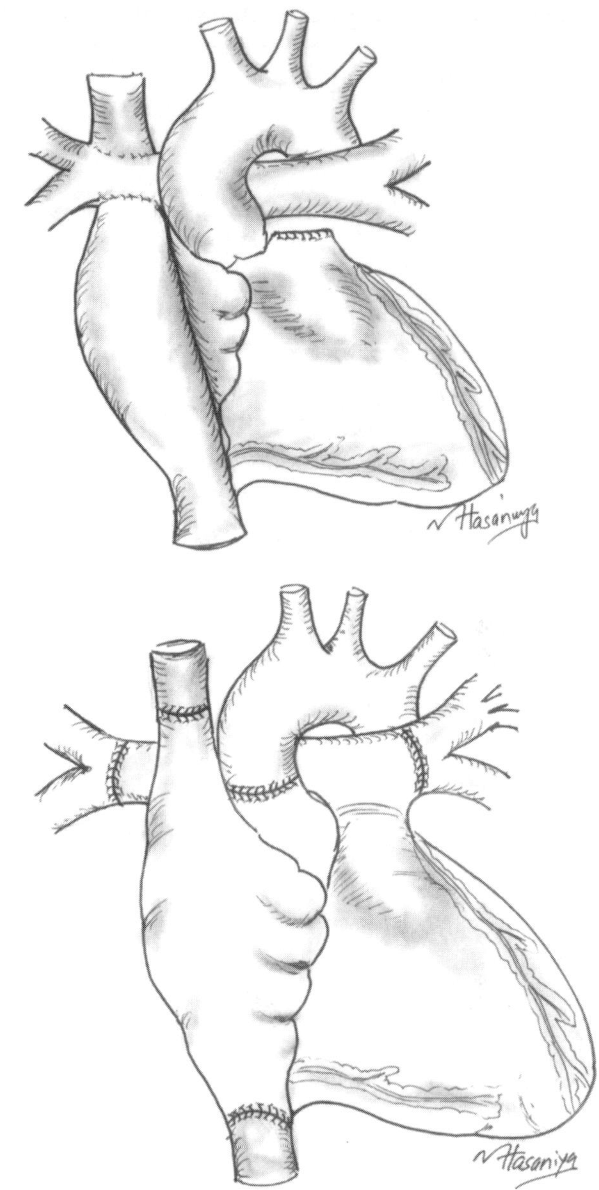

Figure 80-4 Cardiac transplantation after a failed Fontan procedure (top). A cavocaval strategy is employed (bottom). On occasion, the central pulmonary arterial tree may require replacement with en bloc donor pulmonary arteries, as illustrated here.

protocols utilized total body irradiation. This was followed by the use of azathioprine, 6-mercaptopurine, and other myelotoxic agents. Steroids were used systematically beginning in the early 1960s. Consistently successful immunosuppression was not established, however, until the introduction of cyclosporine in the early 1980s. Several other immunoregulative agents have become available and are in use today. The most important immunosuppressive agents that are in current clinical use and their basic mechanisms of action are summarized in Table 80-4.[18]

IMMUNOSUPPRESSION STRATEGIES

Immunosuppression strategies in pediatric CT are built around induction versus no induction and double- versus triple-drug regimens. None of these strategies,

Table 80-4 Immunosuppressive agents: current clinical use and basic mechanism of action

	Corticosteroids	Cyclosporine	Tacrolimus	Azathioprine	Mycophenolate mofetil	Sirolimus	ATG/ATS	OKT3	Basiliximab, Daclizumab	Plasmapheresis	Photophoresis	TLI
Inhibition of T-cell activation												
Decreased APC effectiveness	X											
Inhibition of TCR/antigen binding	X						X	X				
Inhibition of accessory molecules	X						X					
Inhibition of IL-2 production	X	X	X						X			
Inhibition of T-cell production												
Inhibition of IL-2/IL-2R interaction									X			
Inhibition of proliferative response to cytokine	X					X						
Inhibition of DNA synthesis				X	X							X
T-cell depletion							X	X				X
Inhibition of B-cell proliferation	X	X	X	X	X	X	X	X	X			X
B-cell/antibody depletion							X			X		X
Inhibition of smooth muscle proliferation					X	X						
Promotion of suppressor cells											X	X

APC = antigen-presenting cell; TCR = T-cell receptor; IL-2 = interleukin-2; IL-2R = interleukin-2 receptor; ATG/ATS = polyclonal anti-thymocyte preparations; OKT-3 = anti-CD3 monoclonal antibody; TLI = total lymphoid irradiation.

however, have been evaluated in large-scale, randomized, controlled studies. Their use in pediatric CT has been adopted from adult thoracic and pediatric noncardiac solid organ trials. An algorithm for the management of immunosuppression is shown in Fig. 80-5.

Induction

Induction therapy (the use of monoclonal or polyclonal antibody T-cell-depleting agents) has been a controversial subject for a number of years. Induction was employed very early in transplantation and then fell out of favor because of concerns about overimmunosuppression with resultant infections and posttransplant lymphoproliferative disease (PTLD). There has been renewed interest, however, in the use of induction antibody preparations as a means to reduce or eliminate the need for corticosteroids. Several studies have demonstrated the efficacy of this approach.[19–21] In the most recent report from the registry of the ISHLT,[22] 45 percent of pediatric CT patients were treated with induction strategies. With the exception of neonates, rabbit-derived polyclonal antibody is employed in all LLU-managed pediatric recipients in a steroid-avoidance regimen.[23]

Dual-versus triple-drug regimens

Essentially all regimens start with the foundation of a calcineurin inhibitor: either cyclosporine or tacrolimus. There has been only one small-scale trial comparing cyclosporine and tacrolimus in pediatric CT,[24] and it demonstrated essentially equivalent efficacy. In the ISHLT registry report, the use of tacrolimus 1 year after transplantation surpassed the use of cyclosporine. The main advantage of tacrolimus is its reduced cosmetic (hirsutism and gingival hyperplasia) side effects. It has greater potency than cyclosporine and is used successfully in patients with recurrent rejection. There are, however, concerns about an increased incidence of PTLD and posttransplant diabetes among recipients managed with tacrolimus. Newer strategies that use lower target blood levels of tacrolimus have helped ameliorate both of these concerns.

Cyclosporine has been the preferred calcineurin inhibitor at LLU. Target trough levels (whole blood monoclonal assay) are 250 to 300 ng/mL for the first 6 months, 200 to 250 ng/mL for the next 6 months, and 125 to 150 ng/mL thereafter if the rejection history is acceptable. Tacrolimus is used primarily in selected situations such as high-risk candidates (multiple prior cardiac surgeries), high recipient panel-reactive antibody, and/or

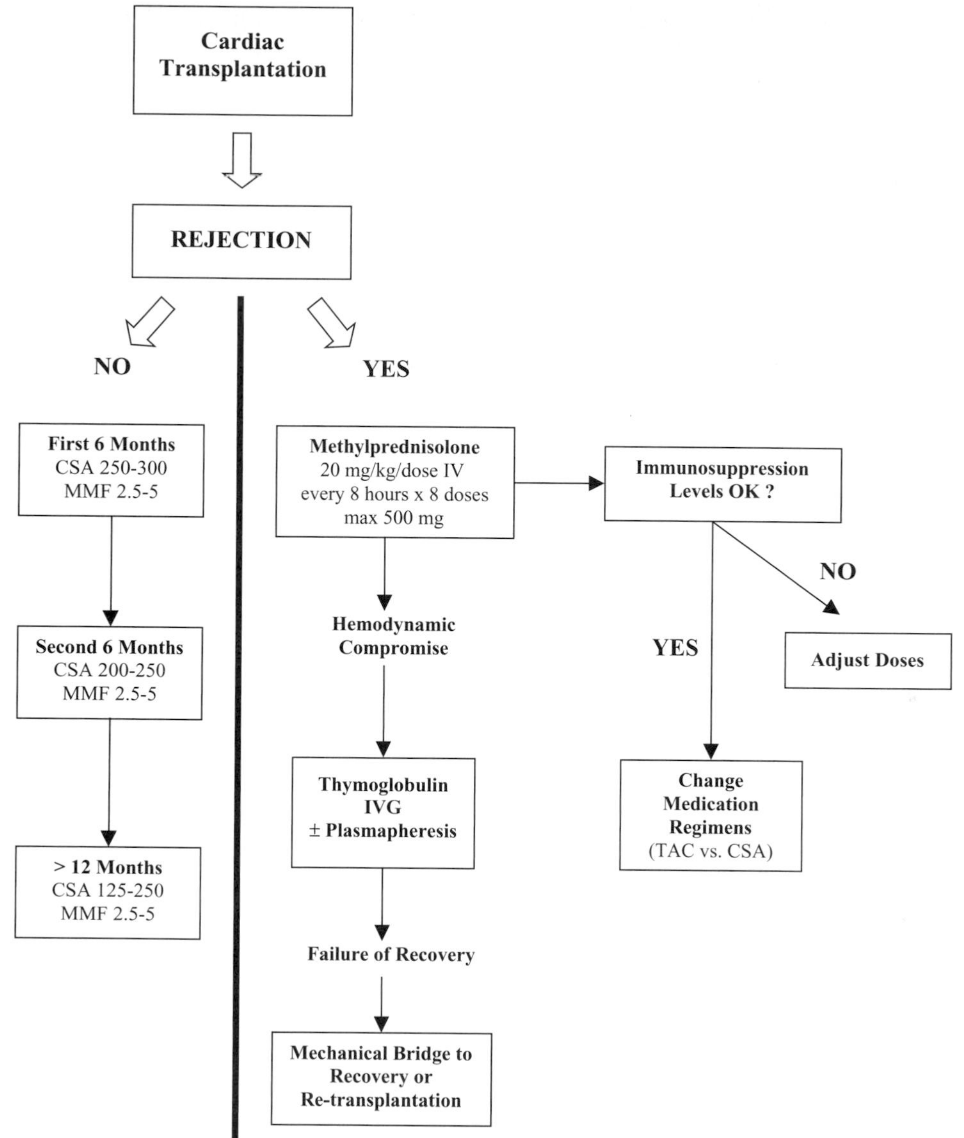

Figure 80-5 Decision-making flowchart for immunosuppression management after pediatric cardiac transplantation (Loma Linda University protocol). CSA = cyclosporine (ng/mL); IVG = intravenous gamma globulin; MMF = mycophenolate mofetil (μg/mL), TAC = tacrolimus, TX = transplant.

African-American recipients. Tacrolimus also is used in patients with recurrent rejection, after retransplantation, and among children for whom cosmetic side effects are problematic.

Antiproliferative agents

Azathioprine (AZA) has been the historic mainstay drug in this class of immunosuppressants. However, ISHLT registry data suggest that mycophenolate mofetil (MMF) is used in 60 percent of pediatric CT patients in place of AZA. Two retrospective studies in children have indicated that potential benefits can result from the use of MMF.[25,26] In adult cardiac transplant trials, MMF has been shown to decrease the progression of coronary intimal thickening.[27] Mycophenolate mofetil, however, like AZA, can induce bone marrow suppression. Significant gastrointestinal side effects may occur with the use of MMF, affecting patient tolerability. The primary immunoregulation regimen at LLU utilizes MMF in a dose of 600 mg/m^2 per day divided twice daily, advancing the dose as tolerated to maintain a blood level of 2.5 to 5 μg/mL (measuring mycophenolic acid levels).

Corticosteroids

Oral prednisone historically has been the mainstay of rejection prophylaxis. Nevertheless, several reports indicate that effective rejection prophylaxis in pediatric CT patients can be achieved without the use of maintenance prednisone therapy.[23] Some believe that steroid avoidance requires antibody induction therapy; however, the use of newer immunosuppressive agents has paved the way for prednisone reduction or elimination regardless of the use of an induction antibody. Programs that use corticosteroids typically start at a dose of 2 mg/kg per day of prednisone, weaning over the first 3 months to a maintenance dose of 0.1 to 0.3 mg/kg per day once daily or every other day.

Steroid avoidance has been practiced at LLU from the inception of the program. Oral prednisone may be used temporarily in the treatment of rejection or chronically in the very few children in whom no other combination of agents is effective or tolerated.

mTOR inhibitors

The mammalian target of Rapamycin (mTOR) inhibitor sirolimus is a newer agent that functions synergistically with calcineurin inhibitors. Pediatric CT data seem to indicate the usefulness of this agent in the management of rejection, and in the reduction of renal dysfunction and side effects of calcineurin inhibitors.[28]

Sirolimus has been employed at LLU for recurrent rejection, in children with renal insufficiency in conjunction with MMF (to decrease or eliminate the calcineurin use), as solo therapy after treatment for PTLD, and in children who have evidence of moderate to severe cardiac allograft vasculopathy.[29,30]

Nonpharmacologic measures

Three other therapies may play a role in pediatric CT. Total lymphoid irradiation (TLI) has been used in the treatment of recalcitrant rejection.[31] It has become less important with the availability of newer immunosuppressive agents. Plasmapheresis has been used[32] either before CT (in highly sensitized patients) or in posttransplant recipients who experience acute antibody-mediated rejection (AMR) or in whom AMR is anticipated. Photophoresis involves the extraction of lymphocytes from recipients. The lymphocytes are pretreated with psoralen, exposed to ultraviolet A light, and reinfused into the recipient. Photophoresis has been helpful in the prevention[33] and treatment of recurrent rejection. There have been no published reports of its use in children.

TREATMENT OF ACUTE REJECTION

Treatment of a first-time acute graft rejection episode involves high-dose intravenous or oral administration of corticosteroids. Intravenous treatment often is followed by the use of oral prednisone, which is tapered gradually to discontinuation over several weeks. Acute rejection in LLU infants and children is treated with intravenous methylprednisolone in a dose of 20 mg/kg per dose to a maximum of 500 mg per dose twice per day for eight doses. Uncomplicated rejection that is diagnosed by biopsy alone may be treated with oral prednisone 2 mg/kg per day for 3 days, with a taper to zero over 3 weeks. Patients with recurrent rejection or with acute rejection manifested by hemodynamic compromise are managed with the use of anti-T-cell antibody in addition to corticosteroids. At LLU, Thymoglobulin in a dose of 1.5 mg/kg per day is administered intravenously over 6 h. The dose is repeated daily for 7 to 10 days. A lymphocyte profile should be obtained on day 3, targeting an absolute CD3 count of less than 200 cells per milliliter. Intravenous immunoglobulin administered in relatively high doses also may be useful in the management of acute rejection.[34]

An acute graft rejection episode, particularly one that occurs late (more than 3 months) after CT, requires investigation of the etiology of the episode. If immunosuppressive doses have been administered faithfully and if the desired therapeutic levels have been maintained, the desired level must be increased or the agent must be changed. Noncompliance must be suspected in any late rejection episode, especially among recipients with low drug levels and among adolescent recipients.

OUTCOMES AND THE LOMA LINDA UNIVERSITY EXPERIENCE

Data from the Pediatric Heart Transplant Study (PHTS) Registry suggest that actuarial survival exceeds 50 percent at 10 years in all pediatric age groups reported since 1982 (Fig. 80-6). Excluding operative and first-year mortality, overall survival at 10 years is 70 percent, with late attrition for adolescent recipients being twice that for infants (4 percent/year versus 2 percent/year). Recent trends suggest generally improved operative and first-year survival. Allograft rejection has been the primary cause of death during the first 3 posttransplant years. Allograft posttransplant coronary artery disease (PTCAD) is the major cause of late mortality. Pediatric recipients who do not require chronic prednisone therapy have a 10 percent increase in late survival.

Since 1985, 420 infants and children under age 18 years have been recipients of CT at LLU. The majority (n = 286) of the recipients have been under 12 months of age. Overall actuarial survival, including operative mortality, at 10 years is 66 percent, whereas three-quarters of newborn recipients are expected to be alive at 10 years. The incidence of documented PTCAD among all recipients is 16 percent. The incidence of posttransplant malignancy is 7.7 percent. A quarter (24.8 percent) of the recipients require treatment for systemic hypertension. Four recipients of isolated CT also have required late kidney transplantation. No recipients are currently on chronic dialysis. One hundred sixty-five recipients (40 percent) have survived 10 or more years with their transplanted hearts.

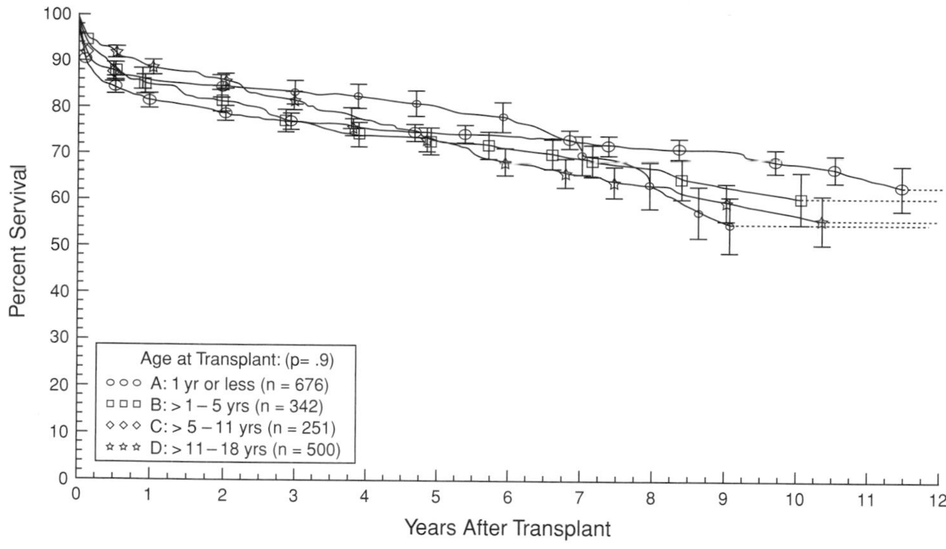

Figure 80-6 Actuarial survival for pediatric age groups from all institutions reported to the Pediatric Heart Transplant Study for the period 1993–2004.

Forty-two (10 percent) have lived 15 or more years since the primary transplantation. The first survivor of neonatal transplantation celebrated his twentieth birthday with his original allograft in November 2005.

The availability of donor organs remains a challenge, particularly for recipients in very early life. Hence, biological replacement of the heart will continue to be reserved only for infants and children who have no other option. Today, for example, just a few young infants with HLHS are ever considered for CT. They fall into two categories: (1) those for whom palliative intervention is judged unlikely to succeed and (2) those who fail to respond favorably to initial palliative reconstruction. Outcomes probably will reflect the nature of this strategy in managing infants with HLHS compared with the results when elective primary transplantation is utilized. Only 17 infants with a diagnosis of HLHS or its equivalent have had primary transplantation at LLU (using the current indications described above) during the last 5 years. Among this small cohort, operative mortality has been 12 percent (2 of 17) and 12-month actuarial survival has been 76 percent.

COMPLICATIONS

The most important untoward consequences of CT are rejection and infection. Others include hypertension, seizure, renal dysfunction, hematologic abnormality, and hepatic dysfunction. Late complications include chronic rejection, neurodevelopmental delay, PTCAD, chronic renal failure, and PTLD. Leading causes of late mortality include PTCAD, chronic graft dysfunction, and malignancies.

Posttransplant coronary artery disease

Posttransplant coronary artery disease is a major issue, resulting in increased morbidity and mortality. The reported prevalence ranges between 10 and 20 percent. Thus far, the prevalence of this dreaded phenomenon appears to be lower among pediatric recipients than it is in the adult population. The most important risk factor associated with increased PTCAD is increased frequency and severity of graft rejection.[35] Prevention of PTCAD includes the use of increased immunosuppression, calcium channel blockers, and lipid-lowering strategies. Treatment of severe established disease consists of elective retransplantation.[36,37]

Retransplantation

Retransplantation is preformed in 1 to 5 percent of patients and certainly will increase in use over time. Indications for retransplantation include primary graft failure, irreversible acute rejection, chronic graft dysfunction, and PTCAD. Thirty-six (8.6 percent) of the 420 LLU recipients have had either urgent ($n = 3$) or elective ($n = 33$) retransplantation for acute allograft failure (including early rejection) or evidence of severe PTCAD, respectively. Five- and 10-year actuarial survival for children after elective retransplantation is 76 percent and 62 percent, respectively.

FUTURE TRENDS

The relatively fixed number of donors for pediatric recipients requires that their distribution and utilization be maximized. Hence, distribution policies have been developed to ensure that adolescent organs reach pediatric recipients preferentially. In addition, a protocol has been devised for the use of ABO-mismatched hearts in young infant recipients.[38] The outcomes of this approach have been excellent, mortality among infants waiting for transplantation has been reduced, and fewer donor hearts have been wasted in this age group. The ABO-mismatched project is being expanded.

As the requirement for CT among young infants with HLHS and its equivalent has diminished, there has been an increasing number of children and adolescents with end-stage congenital heart disease for whom transplantation is the only route to survival. In addition, the demand for retransplantation is on the rise. Devices of one sort or another and perhaps innovative ventricular remodeling procedures will play a more prominent role in bridging these children to transplantation in the future. As CTs become technically more demanding, the relative morbidity and mortality risks will increase.

Finally, the future ability to induce graft-specific tolerance will make organ transplantation an exceedingly attractive therapy. Indications for pediatric CT will expand, as will the demand for donor organs, including organs from other species. Some of today's most promising research in xenotransplantation is focused on a tolerance model.[39,40] Together, tolerance induction and xenografting may become the future of pediatric CT.

References

1. Barnard CN. A human cardiac transplant: An interim report of a successful operation performed at Groote Schuur Hospital, Cape Town. *S Afr Med J* 1967;41:1271.
2. Oyer PE, Stinson EB, Jamieson SW, et al. Cyclosporin-A in cardiac allografting: A preliminary experience. *Transplant Proc* 1983;15:1247.
3. Bailey LL, Nehlsen-Cannarella SU Doroshow RW, et al. Cardiac allotranplantation in newborns as therapy for hypoplastic left heart syndrome. *N Engl J Med* 1986; 315:949.
4. The Registry of the International Society for Heart and Lung Transplantation. Eighteenth official report—2001. *J Heart Lung Transpl*ant 2001;20:805.
5. Boucek MM, Edwards LB, Berkeley JK, et al. The Registry of the International Society for Heart and Lung Transplantation: Fifth official pediatric report—2001 to 2002. *J Heart Lung Transplant* 2002; 21:827.
6. Boucek MM, Edwards LB, Keck BM, et al. Registry of the International Society for Heart and Lung Transplantation: Seventh official pediatric report—2004. *J Heart Lung Transplant* 2004;23:933.
7. Zales VR, Muster AJ, Backer C, et al. Pharmacologic reduction of pretransplantation pulmonary vascular resistance predicts outcome after pediatric cardiac transplantation. *J Heart Lung Transplant* 1993;12:965.
8. Kirshbom PM, Bridges ND, Myung RJ, et al. Use of extracorporeal membrane oxygenation in pediatric thoracic organ transplantation. *J Thorac Cardiovasc Surg* 2002;123:130.
9. Scheule AM, Zimmerman GJ, Johnston JK, et al. Duration of graft cold ischemia does not affect outcomes in pediatric heart transplant recipients. *Circulation* 2002;106[Suppl I]:163-I
10. Stinson EP, Dong E Jr, Iben AB, el al. Cardiac transplantation in man: III. Surgical aspects. *Am J Surg* 1969; 118:l82.
11. Dreyfus G, Jebara V, Mihaileanv S, et al. Total orthotopic heart transplantation: An alternative to the standard technique. *Ann Thorac Surg* 1991;52:1181.
12. Bailey LL, Concepcion W, shattuck H, et al. Method of heart transplantation for treatment of hypoplastic left heart syndrome. *J Thorac Cardiovasc Surg* 1986;92:1.
13. Vricella LA, Razzouk AJ, del Rio M, et al. Heart transplantation for hypoplastic left heart syndrome: Modified technique for reducing circulatory arrest time. *J Heart Lung Transplant* 1998;17:1167.
14. Razzouk AJ, Chinnock R, Gundry SR, et al. Infant heart transplantation in the management of hypoplastic left heart syndrome. In Anderson RH, Pozzi M (eds). *Hypoplastic Left Heart Syndrome.* London: Springer-Verlag; 2005.
15. Bailey LL. Heart transplantation techniques in complex congenital heart disease. *J Heart Lung Transplant* 1993; 12:S168.
16. Vricella LA, Razzouk AJ, Gundry SR, et al. Heart transplantation in infants and children with situs inversus. *J Thorac Cardiovasc Surg* 1998;116:82.
17. Allison AC. Immunosuppressive drugs: The first 50 years and a glance forward. *Immunopharmacology* 2000;47:63.
18. Kirklin JK, George JF. Immuosuppressive modalities. In Kirklin JK, Young JB, McGiffin DC (eds). *Heart Transplantation.* New York: Churchill Livingstone; 2002:390.
19. Boucek RJ, Naftel D, Boucek MM, et al. Induction immunotherapy in pediatric heart transplantation recipients: A multicenter study. *J Heart Lung Transplant* 1999;18(5):460.
20. Parisi F, Danesi H, Squitieri C, et al. Thymoglobulin use in pediatric heart transplantation. *J Heart Lung Transplant* 2003;22(5):591.
21. Di Filippo S, Boissonnat P, Sassolas F, et al. Rabbit antithymocyte globulin as induction immunotherapy in pediatric heart transplantation. *Transplantation* 2003;75(3):354.
22. Boucek MM, Edwards LB, Keck BM, et al. Registry of the International Society for Heart and Lung Transplantation: Eighth official pediatric report—2005. *J Heart Lung Transplant* 2005;24(8):968.
23. Chinnock R, Baum M, Larsen R, et al. Rejection management and long-term surveillance of the pediatric heart

transplantation recipient: The Loma Linda experience. *J Heart Lung Transplant* 1993;12:S255.

24. Pollock-Barziv SM, Dipchand AI, McCrindle BW, et al. Randomized clinical trial of tacrolimus- vs. cyclosporine-based immunosuppression in pediatric heart transplantation: Preliminary results at 15-month follow-up. *J Heart Lung Transplant* 2005;24(2):190.
25. Dipchand AI, Benson L, McCrindle, et al. Mycophenolate mofetil in pediatric heart transplantation recipients: A single-center experience. *Pediatr Transplant* 2001;5(2):112.
26. Morrow WR, Parker JG, Naftel DC, et al. Adjunctive mycophenolate vs. azathioprine for prevention of rejection in pediatric CT recipients. *J Heart Lung Transplant* 2005; 24(2S):S113.
27. Kobashigawa J, Tobis J, Mentzer RM, et al. Ruther analysis of the intravascular ultrasound data from the randomized mycophenolate mofetil (MMF) trial in heart transplantation recipients. *J Heart Lung Transplant* 2004;23(Suppl):S42.
28. Lobach NE, Pollock-Barziv SM, West LJ, et al. Sirolimus immunosuppression in pediatric heart transplantation recipients: A single center experience. *J Heart Lung Transplant* 2005;24(2):184.
29. Shankel TM, Cutler D, Johnston J, et al. Experience with sirolimus in pediatric heart transplantation recipients. *J Heart Lung Transplant* 2004;23(2S):S77.
30. Mancini D, Pinney S, Burkhoff D, et al. Use of rapamycin slows progression of cardiac transplantation vasculopathy. *Circulation* 2003;108(1):48.
31. Asano M, Gundry SR, Razzouk AJ, et al. Total lymphoid irradiation for refractory rejection in pediatric heart transplantation. *Ann Thorac Surg* 2002; 74(6):979.
32. Jacobs JP, Quintessenza JA, Boucek RJ, et al. Pediatric cardiac transplantation in children with high panel reactive antibody. *Ann Thorac Surg* 2004; 78:1703.
33. Barr ML, Meiser BM, Eisen HJ, et al. Photopheresis for the prevention of rejection in cardiac transplantation: Photopheresis Transplantation Study Group. *N Engl J Med* 1998;339(24):1744.
34. Jordan SC, Quartel AW, Czer LS, et al. Posttransplant therapy using high-dose human immunoglobulin (intravenous gamma globulin) to control acute humoral rejection in renal and cardiac allograft recipients and potential mechanism of action. *Transplantation* 1998;66(6):800.
35. Mulla NF, Johnston JK, Dussen LV, et al. Late rejection is a predictor of transplant coronary artery disease in children. *J Am Coll Cardiol* 2001;37:243.
36. Kaiznelson S, Wang XM, Chia D, et al. The inhibitory effects of pravastatin on natural killer cell activity in vivo and on cytotoxic T-lymphocyte activity in vitro. *J Heart. Lung Transplant* 1998;17:335.
37. Dearani JA, Razzouk AJ, Gundry SR, et al. Pediatric heart transplantation: Intermediate-term results. *Ann Thorac Surg* 2001;71:66.
38. West LJ, Pollock-Barziv SM, Dipchand AI, et al. ABO-incompatible heart transplantation in infants. *N Engl J Med* 2001;344(11):793.
39. Fuchimoto Y, Huang CA, Yamada K, et al. Mixed chimerism and tolerance without whole body irradiation in a large animal model. *J Clin Invest* 2000;105:1779.
40. Yamada K, Shimizu A, Utsugi R, et al. Thymic transplantation in miniature swine: II. Induction of tolerance by transplantation of composite thymokidneys to thymectomized recipients. *J Immunol* 2000;164(6):3079.

INDEX

Note: Page numbers followed by f indicate figures; those followed by t indicate tables.